# EMERGENCY MEDICINE

## Clinical Essentials

# EMERGENCY MEDICINE
## Clinical Essentials

### SECOND EDITION


Editor

**James G. Adams, MD**
Professor and Chair, Department of Emergency Medicine, Northwestern University Feinberg School of Medicine, Northwestern Memorial Hospital, Chicago, Illinois

Associate Editors

**Erik D. Barton, MD, MBA**
Chief of Emergency Medicine, Division of Emergency Medicine, University of Utah Health Care; Associate Professor, University of Utah School of Medicine, Salt Lake City, Utah

**Jamie L. Collings, MD**
Associate Professor, Executive Director, Innovative Education, Department of Emergency Medicine, Northwestern University Feinberg School of Medicine, Chicago, Illinois

**Peter M.C. DeBlieux, MD**
Professor of Clinical Medicine, Louisiana State University Health Sciences Center; Professor of Clinical Surgery, Tulane University School of Medicine, New Orleans, Louisiana

**Michael A. Gisondi, MD, FACEP**
Associate Professor, Residency Program Director, Department of Emergency Medicine, Northwestern University Feinberg School of Medicine, Chicago, Illinois

**Eric S. Nadel, MD**
Associate Professor, Harvard Medical School; Program Director, Harvard Affiliated Emergency Medicine Residency, Brigham and Women's Hospital/Massachusetts General Hospital, Boston, Massachusetts



ELSEVIER
SAUNDERS

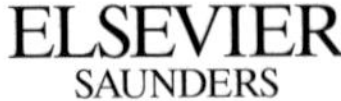

SAUNDERS

1600 John F. Kennedy Blvd.
Ste 1800
Philadelphia, PA 19103-2899

EMERGENCY MEDICINE: CLINICAL ESSENTIALS ISBN: 978-1-4377-3548-2
**Copyright © 2013, 2008 by Saunders, an imprint of Elsevier Inc.**

No part of this publication may be reproduced or transmitted in any form or by any means, electronic or mechanical, including photocopying, recording, or any information storage and retrieval system, without permission in writing from the publisher. Details on how to seek permission, further information about the Publisher's permissions policies, and our arrangements with organizations such as the Copyright Clearance Center and the Copyright Licensing Agency can be found at our website: www.elsevier.com/permissions.

This book and the individual contributions contained in it are protected under copyright by the Publisher (other than as may be noted herein).

**Notices**

Knowledge and best practice in this field are constantly changing. As new research and experience broaden our understanding, changes in research methods, professional practices, or medical treatment may become necessary.

Practitioners and researchers must always rely on their own experience and knowledge in evaluating and using any information, methods, compounds, or experiments described herein. In using such information or methods, they should be mindful of their own safety and the safety of others, including parties for whom they have a professional responsibility.

With respect to any drug or pharmaceutical products identified, readers are advised to check the most current information provided (i) on procedures featured or (ii) by the manufacturer of each product to be administered to verify the recommended dose or formula, the method and duration of administration, and contraindications. It is the responsibility of practitioners, relying on their own experience and knowledge of their patients, to make diagnoses, to determine dosages and the best treatment for each individual patient, and to take all appropriate safety precautions.

To the fullest extent of the law, neither the Publisher nor the authors, contributors, or editors assume any liability for any injury and/or damage to persons or property as a matter of products liability, negligence or otherwise, or from any use or operation of any methods, products, instructions, or ideas contained in the material herein.

Chapter 45, "Emergency Biliary Ultrasonography": Beatrice Hoffman retains copyright to her original images. Chapter 139, "Venomous Snakebites in North America": Robert L. Norris retains copyright to his original images.

**Library of Congress Cataloging-in-Publication Data**

Emergency medicine : clinical essentials / editor, James G. Adams ; associate editors, Erik D. Barton … [et al.].—2nd ed.
p. ; cm.
Includes bibliographical references.
ISBN 978-1-4377-3548-2 (hardcover : alk. paper)
I. Adams, James, 1962 May 8-
[DNLM: 1. Emergency Medicine—methods. 2. Emergencies. WB 105]
616.02′5—dc23

2012023682

*Senior Content Strategist:* Stefanie Jewell-Thomas
*Senior Content Development Specialist:* Dee Simpson
*Publishing Services Manager:* Anne Altepeter
*Senior Project Manager:* Doug Turner
*Designer:* Steve Stave

Printed in the People's Republic of China
Last digit is the print number: 9 8 7 6 5 4 3 2 1

Working together to grow libraries in developing countries

www.elsevier.com | www.bookaid.org | www.sabre.org

ELSEVIER BOOK AID International Sabre Foundation

*To my immediate and extended family, for their love, support, patience, and encouragement. To my friends, mentors, and colleagues, from whom I continue to learn so much. To the faculty and residents, whose great talent and dedication invigorate me. To the authors and editors of this text, in recognition of their knowledge, skill, wisdom, and generosity.*

JGA

*To my family, friends, and faculty, who better understand the virtues of patience and without whose support I could never achieve anything great! I am very blessed to be surrounded by such amazing souls. Thanks for being part of this success!*

EDB

*To Mark, Keaton, and Kameron, you are what is most important in my life. Thanks for supporting me in everything I do. To my students and residents, you give me inspiration and motivation, and you never fail to make "work" fun!*

JLC

*To Karen, Joshua, and Zachary for your love and undying patience with my educational pursuits and being a constant reminder that you are my main thing. To my patients at Charity Hospital, who inspire me to help others. You have taught me best what it means to be a physician. To my students, residents, peer faculty, and especially Keith Van Meter. Thanks for the opportunity to work and learn with all of you.*

PMCD

*To Derek and Abby, with all my love. Thank you for your support, encouragement, love, and advice—here's to many, many years of continued adventures.*

MAG

*To the HAEMR residents and dedicated faculty, who keep me motivated and humble as we perpetuate the cycle of teaching and learning. To my colleagues, who have shared their experience and wisdom to expand the foundation of our field with this text. To my family and friends, who have supported me along the way. To my mother, Harriet, who was always proud and would continue to be so. To my wife, Marianne, and our children, Josh, Emily, and Henry, for their love, patience, and laughter.*

ESN

# Preface

We hope that this edition of *Emergency Medicine: Clinical Essentials* will cover the core content of the specialty of emergency medicine in a practical and useful way. The style and format are constructed with emergency medicine residents in mind. The table of contents specifically mirrors the key topic areas of emergency medicine. The chapters are written by physicians who provide lucid explanations and make the information clinically relevant. The authors are experts, leading educators on the topic, and particularly talented academicians. The chapter format favors short segments, highly readable prose, and many subheadings. Maximal use of pedagogic tools such as boxes, tables, figures, and algorithms helps summarize and synthesize key themes. This facilitates initial learning and later enables quick references and resetting of the learning, especially when used in the electronic version. This text is constructed to be easy to use on electronic reading devices, recognizing that books have quickly evolved from static print to dynamic, interactive electronic tools.

This book is designed so that it can be part of a curriculum and embedded into a training program. There is probably no way to master this specialty's huge amount of content other than continuous, deliberate, concentrated study, so this book hopes to make the study easier through straightforward writing and clear tables and figures. It is never easy to learn large amounts of material and stay current with latest treatment guidelines. This text brings both the latest recommendations and succinct explanations. Eventually, throughout the course of a residency, the core information can be covered in its entirety, at least once but usually twice. The residency program's clinical experiences, case conferences, simulation exercises, and other parts of the curriculum will reinforce themes, teach additional knowledge, assess judgment, and evaluate practical skills. Faculty members can refer to the text to refresh their own knowledge or to use the tables and algorithms for clinical teaching in the emergency department.

This textbook is also intended to be relevant to the practicing physician, from whom society expects the highest level of clinical practice. The next era of clinical physician evaluation will be to assess whether we are practicing according to evidence-based or consensus-based standards. This text emphasizes these areas of practical, applied decision making. It offers explicit, current, and practical recommendations that will be useful for practicing physicians.

Our clinical practice is rapidly changing as diagnostic tools are increasingly incorporated, new therapies applied, and entirely new disorders emerge. Some types of emergencies were unknown a decade ago, such as those related to novel implanted devices, complications of new surgical procedures such as organ transplantation or bariatric surgery, and even fertility treatment. The use of diagnostic testing, whether magnetic resonance imaging, computed tomography, or bedside ultrasound, is changing. Time-dependent therapeutic interventions for resuscitation and even standards of treatment for serious infectious disease have evolved. All these areas and more are covered in the text as core information for the emergency medicine specialist.

In summary, this textbook is well suited as a stand-alone text or a reference tool but also can be used as a component of an emergency medicine residency curriculum. The link to the specialty core content, the readable design, and the content selection is meant to be useful, accessible, and functional, in addition to forward looking as technology transforms our methods of teaching, learning, and evaluation. We are preparing for the electronic future, where this text fits neatly into a world in which reading is done online, a quick retrieval of information is desired, and a screen-friendly format is appreciated. The world will continue to change quickly, and so will this text.

**James G. Adams**
**Erik D. Barton**
**Jamie L. Collings**
**Peter M.C. DeBlieux**
**Michael A. Gisondi**
**Eric S. Nadel**

# Contributors

**Michael K. Abraham, MD**
Clinical Assistant Professor, Department of Emergency Medicine, University of Maryland School of Medicine, Baltimore, Maryland; Attending Physician, Department of Emergency Medicine, Upper Chesapeake Health System, Bel Air, Maryland
*Lung Transplant Complications*

**Fredrick M. Abrahamian, DO, FACEP**
Clinical Professor of Medicine, David Geffen School of Medicine at University of California, Los Angeles, Los Angeles, California; Director of Education, Department of Emergency Medicine, Olive View–UCLA Medical Center, Sylmar, California
*Infections in the Immunocompromised Host*

**Mohammed A. Abu Aish, MD, MEd, FRCPC**
Pediatric Emergency Medicine Physician, Division of Pediatric Emergency Medicine, British Columbia Children's Hospital, Vancouver, British Columbia, Canada
*Submersion Injuries*

**Bruce D. Adams, MD, FACEP**
Professor of Surgery, Chief, The Center for Emergency Medicine, University of Texas Health Science Center at San Antonio, San Antonio, Texas
*Rhabdomyolysis*

**James G. Adams, MD**
Professor and Chair, Department of Emergency Medicine, Northwestern University Feinberg School of Medicine, Northwestern Memorial Hospital, Chicago, Illinois
*Preface*
*Systemic Lupus Erythematosus*

**Nima Afshar, MD**
Assistant Professor of Medicine, University of California, San Francisco, San Francisco, California
*Aortic Dissection*

**James Ahn, MD**
Clinical Instructor, Department of Medicine, University of Chicago, Chicago, Illinois
*Inflammatory Bowel Disease*

**Amer Z. Aldeen, MD, FACEP**
Assistant Professor, Associate Residency Director, Department of Emergency Medicine, Northwestern University Feinberg School of Medicine, Northwestern Memorial Hospital, Chicago, Illinois
*Epidemic Infections in Bioterrorism*

**Paul J. Allegretti, DO, FACOEP, FACOI**
Professor and Program Director, Department of Emergency Medicine, Midwestern University, Downers Grove, Illinois; Professor and Program Director, Department of Emergency Medicine, Provident Hospital of Cook County, Chicago, Illinois
*Vasculitis Syndromes*

**Jennifer F. Anders, MD**
Assistant Professor, Department of Pediatrics, Johns Hopkins University School of Medicine; Fellowship Program Director, Division of Pediatric Emergency Medicine, Johns Hopkins Children's Center, Baltimore, Maryland
*Pediatric Gynecologic Disorders*

**Jana L. Anderson, MD**
Instructor in Emergency Medicine and Pediatrics, Departments of Emergency Medicine and Pediatrics, Mayo Clinic, Rochester, Minnesota
*Child with a Fever*

**Phillip Andrus, MD, FACEP, RDMS**
Assistant Professor of Emergency Medicine, Mount Sinai School of Medicine, New York, New York
*Peripheral Nerve Disorders*

**Christian Arbelaez, MD, MPH**
Assistant Residency Director, Harvard Affiliated Emergency Medicine Residency, Department of Emergency Medicine, Brigham and Women's Hospital; Assistant Professor of Medicine, Harvard Medical School, Boston, Massachusetts
*Health Care Disparities and Diversity in Emergency Medicine*

**Charles B. Arbogast, DO**
Chief of Nephrology, William Beaumont Army Medical Center, El Paso, Texas
*Rhabdomyolysis*

**Chandra D. Aubin, MD, RDMS**
Assistant Professor, Assistant Residency Director, Department of Emergency Medicine, Washington University School of Medicine, St. Louis, Missouri
*Hernias*

**Jennifer Avegno, MD**
Clinical Assistant Professor, Department of Medicine, Section of Emergency Medicine, Louisiana State University Health Sciences Center, New Orleans, Louisiana
*Emergency Medical Services and Disaster Medicine*

**John Bailitz, MD**
Emergency Ultrasound Director, Department of Emergency Medicine, John H. Stroger Hospital of Cook County; Assistant Professor, Department of Emergency Medicine, Rush University Medical Center, Chicago, Illinois
*Thoracic Trauma*

**Patricia Baines, MD**
Assistant Professor, Medical Director of Forensic Program, Department of Emergency Medicine, Emory University, Atlanta, Georgia
*Gastrointestinal Bleeding*

**Aaron E. Bair, MD**
Associate Professor, Department of Emergency Medicine, UC Davis Medical Center, Sacramento, California
*Advanced Airway Techniques*

**Katherine Bakes, MD**
Director, Denver Emergency Center for Children, Associate Director, Emergency Department, Denver Health Medical Center, Denver, Colorado; Associate Professor, Department of Emergency Medicine, University of Colorado School of Medicine, Aurora, Colorado
*Neonatal Cardiopulmonary Resuscitation*
*Pediatric Resuscitation*
*Pediatric Trauma*

**Aaron N. Barksdale, MD**
Assistant Professor, Department of Emergency Medicine, Truman Medical Center/University of Missouri, Kansas City, School of Medicine; Clinical Instructor, Department of Emergency Medicine, Children's Mercy Hospital/University of Missouri, Kansas City, School of Medicine, Kansas City, Missouri
*Allergic Disorders*

**William G. Barsan, MD**
Professor, Department of Emergency Medicine, University of Michigan, Ann Arbor, Michigan
*Altered Mental Status and Coma*

**Erik D. Barton, MD, MBA**
Chief of Emergency Medicine, Division of Emergency Medicine, University of Utah Health Care; Associate Professor, University of Utah School of Medicine, Salt Lake City, Utah
*Preface*

**Benjamin S. Bassin, MD**
Clinical Instructor, Department of Emergency Medicine, University of Michigan, Ann Arbor, Michigan
*Altered Mental Status and Coma*

## CONTRIBUTORS

**Craig G. Bates**, MD, FACEP
Attending Emergency Physician, Metrohealth Medical Center; Clinical Assistant Professor of Emergency Medicine, Case Western University School of Medicine, Cleveland, Ohio
*Asthma*
*Chronic Obstructive Pulmonary Disease*

**Jamil D. Bayram**, MD, MPH, EMDM, MEd
Assistant Professor, Department of Emergency Medicine, Rush University Medical Center, Chicago, Illinois
*Gynecologic Infections*

**Tomer Begaz**, MD
Associate Professor, Department of Emergency Medicine, Medical College of Wisconsin, Milwaukee, Wisconsin
*Traumatic Brain Injury (Adult)*
*Emergency Contraception*

**Kip Benko**, MD
Associate Clinical Professor, Department of Emergency Medicine, University of Pittsburgh School of Medicine, Pittsburgh, Pennsylvania
*Dental Emergencies*

**Kavita Bhanot**, MD
Attending Physician, Department of Emergency Medicine, St. Joseph Mercy Health System, Ann Arbor, Michigan
*Evidence-Based Medicine*

**Kriti Bhatia**, MD
Associate Residency Director, Attending Physician, Department of Emergency Medicine, Brigham and Women's Hospital, Boston, Massachusetts
*Eye Emergencies*

**Paul D. Biddinger**, MD
Director of Operations, Department of Emergency Medicine, Massachusetts General Hospital; Director, Emergency Preparedness and Response Exercise Program, Harvard School of Public Health, Boston, Massachusetts
*Regulatory and Legal Issues in the Emergency Department*

**Andra L. Blomkalns**, MD
Associate Professor and Vice Chair, Department of Emergency Medicine, University of Cincinnati College of Medicine, Cincinnati, Ohio
*Cardiac Imaging and Stress Testing*

**John M. Boe**, MD,
Assistant Clinical Professor, Department of Emergency Medicine, Indiana University School of Medicine, Indianapolis, Indiana
*Anorectal Disorders*

**J. Stephen Bohan**, MD
Executive Vice Chairman, Department of Emergency Medicine, Brigham and Women's Hospital; Assistant Professor, Department of Emergency Medicine, Harvard Medical School, Boston, Massachusetts
*Leadership and Emergency Medicine*

**Keith Boniface**, MD, RDMS
Associate Professor, Department of Emergency Medicine, George Washington University Medical Center, Washington, District of Columbia
*Bowel Obstructions*

**Laura J. Bontempo**, MD
Assistant Professor, Department of Emergency Medicine, Yale University, New Haven, Connecticut
*Maxillofacial Disorders*

**Pierre Borczuk**, MD
Associate in Emergency Medicine, Division of Emergency Medicine, Massachusetts General Hospital; Assistant Professor in Medicine, Harvard Medical School, Boston, Massachusetts
*Cardiac Valvular Disorders*

**Keith Borg**, MD, PhD
Assistant Professor, Department of Medicine, Division of Emergency Medicine, Medical University of South Carolina, Charleston, South Carolina
*Self-Harm and Danger to Others*

**Nicholas A. Borm**, MD
Resident Physician, Department of Emergency Medicine, Northwestern University Feinberg School of Medicine, Chicago, Illinois
*Gynecologic Pain and Vaginal Bleeding*

**Philip Bossart**, MD
Professor, Division of Emergency Medicine, University of Utah School of Medicine, Salt Lake City, Utah
*Hip and Femur Injuries*

**Megan Boysen Osborn**, MD
Assistant Professor, Department of Emergency Medicine, UC Irvine Healthcare, University of California, Irvine, Orange, California
*Potassium*

**William J. Brady**, MD
Professor of Emergency Medicine and Internal Medicine, Chair, Resuscitation Committee, Medical Director, Emergency Preparedness and Response, University of Virginia Health System; Operational Medical Director, Charlottesville—Albemarle Rescue Squad and Albemarle County Fire Rescue; Medical Director, Allianz Global Assistance, Charlottesville, Virginia
*Management of Cardiac Arrest and the Post–Cardiac Arrest Syndrome*
*Renal Failure*

**Jeremy B. Branzetti**, MD
Acting Instructor, Division of Emergency Medicine, University of Washington, Seattle, Washington
*Emergency Delivery and Peripartum Emergencies*

**Bart S. Brown**, MD
Attending Emergency Physician, St. Vincent Emergency Physicians, Indianapolis, Indiana
*Emergency Biliary Ultrasonography*

**David F.M. Brown**, MD
Vice Chairman, Department of Emergency Medicine, Massachusetts General Hospital; Associate Professor, Division of Emergency Medicine, Harvard Medical School, Boston, Massachusetts
*Acute Coronary Syndrome*

**Sean M. Bryant**, MD
Associate Professor, Department of Emergency Medicine, Rush Medical College/John H. Stroger Hospital of Cook County; Assistant Fellowship Director, Toxikon Consortium; Associate Medical Director, Illinois Poison Center, Chicago, Illinois
*Antidepressants and Antipsychotics*

**John H. Burton**, MD
Chair and Professor of Emergency Medicine, Department of Emergency Medicine, Carilion Clinic, Roanoke, Virginia
*Facial Trauma*

**Christine Butts**, MD
Clinical Assistant Professor, Department of Emergency Medicine, Director of Division of Emergency Ultrasound, Louisiana State University Health Sciences Center, New Orleans, Louisiana
*Emergency Cardiac Ultrasound: Evaluation for Pericardial Effusion and Cardiac Activity*
*Ultrasound-Guided Vascular Access*
*Sonography for Trauma*
*Aortic Ultrasound*
*Basic Emergency Ultrasound*

**Mark W. Byrne**, MD
Emergency Ultrasound Fellow, Department of Emergency Medicine, Brigham and Women's Hospital, Boston, Massachusetts
*Emergency Renal Ultrasonography*

**Daniel Cabrera**, MD
Assistant Professor, Department of Emergency Medicine, Mayo Clinic, Rochester, Minnesota
*Management of Emergencies Related to Implanted Cardiac Devices*

**Robert D. Cannon**, DO
Assistant Professor, Department of Medicine, University of South Florida College of Medicine; Assistant Residency Director, Department of Emergency Medicine, Lehigh Valley Health Network, Allentown, Pennsylvania
*Insecticides, Herbicides, and Rodenticides*

**David A. Caro, MD**
Associate Professor, Department of Emergency Medicine, University of Florida College of Medicine—Jacksonville, Jacksonville, Florida
*Basic Airway Management*

**Christopher R. Carpenter, MD**
Assistant Professor, Department of Emergency Medicine, Washington University School of Medicine, St. Louis, Missouri
*Alcoholic Ketoacidosis*

**Wallace A. Carter, MD**
Director, Emergency Medicine Residency, NewYork-Presbyterian Hospital; Associate Professor of Emergency Medicine, Weill Medical College of Cornell University; Associate Professor of Clinical Medicine, College of Physicians and Surgeons of Columbia University, New York, New York
*Endocarditis*

**Cindy W. Chan, MD**
Attending Physician, Department of Emergency Medicine, Advocate Christ Medical Center, Oak Lawn, Illinois
*First Trimester Ultrasonography*

**Gar Ming Chan, MD**
Specialist in Emergency Medicine, Consultant, Launceston General Hospital, Launceston, Tasmania, Australia
*Sympathomimetics*

**Andrew K. Chang, MD**
Associate Professor, Department of Emergency Medicine, Albert Einstein College of Medicine; Attending Physician, Department of Emergency Medicine, Montefiore Medical Center, Bronx, New York
*Vertigo*

**Douglas M. Char, MD**
Associate Professor and Residency Program Director, Division of Emergency Medicine, Washington University School of Medicine, St. Louis, Missouri
*The Emergency Psychiatric Assessment*

**Navneet Cheema, MD**
Resident Physician, Department of Emergency Medicine, Northwestern University Feinberg School of Medicine, Chicago, Illinois
*Soft Tissue Injury*

**Yi-Mei Chng, MD, MPH**
Affiliated Clinical Instructor, Division of Emergency Medicine, Stanford University School of Medicine, Stanford, California; Senior Physician, Department of Emergency Medicine, Kaiser Permanente Santa Clara Medical Center, Santa Clara, California
*Dialysis-Related Emergencies*

**Michael R. Christian, MD**
Assistant Professor of Emergency Medicine and Pediatrics, Department of Emergency Medicine, Truman Medical Center/University of Missouri, Kansas City, School of Medicine; Medical Toxicologist, Division of Clinical Pharmacology and Medical Toxicology, Children's Mercy Hospital, Kansas City, Missouri
*Antidepressants and Antipsychotics*

**Richard F. Clark, MD**
Professor, Department of Emergency Medicine, Director, Division of Medical Toxicology, University of California, San Diego, Medical Center; Medical Director, San Diego Division, California Poison Control System, San Diego, California
*Arthropod Bites and Stings*
*Marine Food-Borne Poisoning, Envenomation, and Traumatic Injuries*

**Kathleen J. Clem, MD**
Professor and Chair, Department of Emergency Medicine, Loma Linda University School of Medicine, Loma Linda, California
*Helminths, Bedbugs, Scabies, and Lice Infections*

**James E. Colletti, MD**
Assistant Professor of Emergency Medicine, Emergency Medicine Residency Program Director, Department of Emergency Medicine, Mayo Clinic, Rochester, Minnesota
*Child with a Fever*

**Jamie L. Collings, MD**
Associate Professor, Executive Director, Innovative Education, Department of Emergency Medicine, Northwestern University Feinberg School of Medicine, Chicago, Illinois
*Preface*
*Gynecologic Pain and Vaginal Bleeding*
*Breast Disorders*

**Christopher B. Colwell, MD, FACEP**
Director of Service, Department of Emergency Medicine, Denver Health Medical Center; Professor and Vice Chair, Department of Emergency Medicine, University of Colorado School of Medicine, Denver, Colorado
*Lightning and Electrical Injuries*

**Justin Cook, MD, FACEP**
Attending Emergency Physician, Legacy Emanuel Medical Center, Portland, Oregon; Clinical Faculty, Department of Emergency Medicine, Alameda County Medical Center—Highland Hospital, Oakland, California
*Ultrasound-Guided Vascular Access*
*Sonography for Trauma*
*Aortic Ultrasound*
*Basic Emergency Ultrasound*

**Jeremy L. Cooke, MD**
Staff Physician, Department of Emergency Medicine, South Sacramento Kaiser Hospital, Sacramento, California
*Altered Mental Status and Coma*

**Julie J. Cooper, MD**
Physician, Doctors for Emergency Services, Christiana Care, Health System, Newark, Delaware
*Biliary Tract Disorders*

**D. Mark Courtney, MD, MSCI**
Assistant Professor, Department of Emergency Medicine, Northwestern University Feinberg School of Medicine, Chicago, Illinois
*Pulmonary Embolism*
*Venous Thrombosis*

**Kirk L. Cumpston, DO**
Assistant Professor, Department of Emergency Medicine, Virginia Commonwealth University, Richmond, Virginia
*Cardiovascular Drugs*

**Rita K. Cydulka, MD, MS**
Professor and Vice Chair, Department of Emergency Medicine, MetroHealth Medical Center/Case Western Reserve University, Cleveland, Ohio
*Asthma*
*Chronic Obstructive Pulmonary Disease*

**Lynda Daniel-Underwood, MD**
Associate Professor, Department of Emergency Medicine, Loma Linda University School of Medicine, Loma Linda, California
*Psychosis and Psychotropic Medication*

**Elizabeth M. Datner, MD**
Vice Chair, Clinical Operations, Department of Emergency Medicine, Hospital of the University of Pennsylvania; Associate Professor, Perelman School of Medicine, University of Pennsylvania, Philadelphia, Pennsylvania
*Resuscitation in Pregnancy*

**Jonathan E. Davis, MD**
Associate Professor, Department of Emergency Medicine, Georgetown University School of Medicine; Program Director, Emergency Medicine Residency Program, Georgetown University/Washington Hospital Center, Washington, District of Columbia
*Male Genitourinary Emergencies*

**Virgil Davis, MD**
Assistant Professor, Division of Emergency Medicine, University of Utah School of Medicine, Salt Lake City, Utah
*Heat-Related Emergencies*

**Mae F. De La Calzada-Jeanlouie, DO**
Medical Toxicology Fellow, Department of Emergency Medicine, North Shore University Hospital, Manhasset, New York
*Sympathomimetics*

**Sarah Steward de Ramirez**
Resident Housestaff, Department of Emergency Medicine, Johns Hopkins Hospital, Baltimore, Maryland
*Thyroid Disorders*

## CONTRIBUTORS


**Peter M.C. DeBlieux, MD**
Professor of Clinical Medicine, Louisiana State University Health Sciences Center; Professor of Clinical Surgery, Tulane University School of Medicine, New Orleans, Louisiana
*Preface*

**Wyatt W. Decker, MD**
Professor of Emergency Medicine, Mayo Clinic, Scottsdale, Arizona
*Management of Emergencies Related to Implanted Cardiac Devices*

**Jorge del Castillo, MD, MBA**
Clinical Associate Professor, Department of Emergency Medicine, University of Chicago, Pritzker School of Medicine, Chicago, Illinois; Associate Head, Division of Emergency Medicine, NorthShore University Healthsystem, Evanston, Illinois
*Foot and Ankle Injuries*

**John Deledda, MD**
Assistant Professor, Department of Emergency Medicine; Chief of Staff, University Hospital, University of Cincinnati, Cincinnati, Ohio
*Cardiac Imaging and Stress Testing*

**Eva M. Delgado, MD**
Pediatric Emergency Medicine Fellow, Pediatric Emergency Department, Children's Hospital & Research Center Oakland, Oakland, California
*Hematuria*

**M. Kit Delgado, MD, MS**
Clinical Instructor, Division of Emergency Medicine, Stanford University School of Medicine; Health Care Research and Policy Fellow, Center for Primary Care and Outcomes Research, Stanford University School of Medicine, Stanford, California
*Hematuria*

**Margaret M. DiGeronimo, MD**
Physician, Emergency Physicians at Porter Hospital, Denver, Colorado
*Arterial and Venous Trauma and Great Vessel Injuries*

**Gail D'Onofrio, MD**
Professor and Chair, Department of Emergency Medicine, Yale University School of Medicine, New Haven, Connecticut
*Seizures*

**Gerard S. Doyle, MD, MPH**
Clinical Assistant Professor, Division of Emergency Medicine, University of Utah School of Medicine, Salt Lake City, Utah
*Low Back Pain*

**Bradley A. Dreifuss, MD**
Assistant Professor, Director of Rural and International Emergency Medicine, Department of Emergency Medicine, University of Arizona, Tucson, Arizona
*Acute Radiation Emergencies*

**Jeffrey Druck, MD**
Associate Professor, Department of Emergency Medicine, University of Colorado School of Medicine, Denver, Colorado
*Thermal Burns*
*Chemical Burns*

**Jonathan A. Edlow, MD, FACEP**
Professor of Medicine, Harvard Medical School; Vice-Chairman and Director of Quality, Department of Emergency Medicine, Beth Israel Deaconess Medical Center, Boston, Massachusetts
*Headache*
*Tick-Borne Diseases*

**Jeffrey M. Elder, MD**
Clinical Instructor, Department of Medicine, Section of Emergency Medicine, Louisiana State University Health Sciences Center; Director of Emergency Medical Services, City of New Orleans, New Orleans, Louisiana
*Emergency Medical Services and Disaster Medicine*

**Kirsten G. Engel, MD**
Research Assistant Professor, Department of Emergency Medicine, Northwestern University Feinberg School of Medicine, Chicago, Illinois
*Patient-Centered Care*

**Ugo A. Ezenkwele, MD, MPH**
Vice Chairman of Emergency Medicine, Woodhull Medical and Mental Health Center; Assistant Professor, Department of Emergency Medicine, New York University School of Medicine, New York, New York
*Emergency Management of Red Blood Cell Disorders*

**Jessica A. Fulton, DO**
Attending Physician, Department of Emergency Medicine, Grand View Hospital, Sellersville, Pennsylvania
*Anticholinergics*

**Fiona E. Gallahue, MD**
Assistant Professor, Division of Emergency Medicine, Department of Medicine, University of Washington, Seattle, Washington
*Postpartum Emergencies*

**Manish Garg, MD, FAAEM**
Associate Professor of Clinical Emergency Medicine, Associate Residency Program Director, Department of Emergency Medicine, Temple University Hospital; Site Primary Investigator of the EMERGEncy ID NET Research Surveillance Group, National Institutes of Health/Centers for Disease Control and Prevention; Director of Global Health Education, Temple University School of Medicine, Philadelphia, Pennsylvania
*Cardiovascular and Neurologic Oncologic Emergencies*

**Gus M. Garmel, MD, FACEP, FAAEM**
Clinical Professor (Affiliated) of Surgery (Emergency Medicine), Stanford University School of Medicine; Co-Program Director, Stanford/Kaiser Emergency Medicine Residency Program; Medical Student Clerkship Director, Surgery 313D (EM), Stanford University School of Medicine, Stanford, California; Senior Emergency Physician, The Permanente Medical Group, Kaiser Permanente Santa Clara Medical Center, Santa Clara, California
*Conflict Resolution in Emergency Medicine*

**Ryan T. Geers, MD, MSW**
Department of Emergency Medicine, University of Cincinnati, Cincinnati, Ohio
*Cardiac Imaging and Stress Testing*

**Carl A. Germann, MD**
Assistant Professor, Tufts University School of Medicine; Director, Maine Medical Center-Tufts Medical School Program; Attending Physician, Maine Medical Center, Portland, Maine
*Imaging of the Central Nervous System*

**Chris A. Ghaemmaghami, MD**
Associate Professor and Vice Chair for Academic Affairs, Medical Director, Emergency Department, University of Virginia; Director, Fellowship in Cardiovascular Emergencies, Department of Emergency Medicine, University of Virginia Health System, Charlottesville, Virginia
*Intracranial Hemorrhages*

**Michael A. Gibbs, MD**
Chief, Department of Emergency Medicine, Maine Medical Center, Portland, Maine; Professor, Department of Emergency Medicine, Tufts University School of Medicine, Boston, Massachusetts
*Genitourinary Trauma*
*Hand and Wrist Injuries*

**Gregory H. Gilbert, MD**
Assistant Clinical Professor, Clerkship Director, Principles of Medicine Associate Director, Stanford University School of Medicine, Stanford, California; Attending Physician and Life Flight Medical Director, Stanford University Hospital, Stanford, California
*Dialysis-Related Emergencies*

**Michael A. Gisondi, MD, FACEP**
Associate Professor, Residency Program Director, Department of Emergency Medicine, Northwestern University Feinberg School of Medicine, Chicago, Illinois
*Preface*

**Steven A. Godwin, MD, FACEP**
Associate Professor, Chair and Chief, Department of Emergency Medicine; Assistant Dean, Simulation Education, University of Florida College of Medicine—Jacksonville, Jacksonville, Florida
*Procedural Sedation*
*Smoke Inhalation*

**Joshua N. Goldstein, MD, PhD**
Assistant Professor, Department of Emergency Medicine, Harvard Medical School and Massachusetts General Hospital, Boston, Massachusetts
*Headache*
*Bleeding Disorders*

**Eric Goralnick, MD**
Assistant Clinical Director, Department of Emergency Medicine, Brigham and Women's Hospital; Instructor, Harvard Medical School, Boston, Massachusetts
*White Blood Cell Disorders*

**Deepi G. Goyal, MD**
Associate Professor, Department of Emergency Medicine, Mayo Clinic, Rochester, Minnesota
*Viral Infections*

**Matthew N. Graber, MD, PhD**
Institutional Research Director, Attending Physician, Department of Emergency Medicine, Kaweah Delta Medical Center, Visalia, California
*Diabetes and Hyperglycemia*

**David D. Gummin, MD, FACEP, FAACT, FACMT**
Departments of Pediatrics and Emergency Medicine, Medical College of Wisconsin; Medical Director, Wisconsin Poison Center, Milwaukee, Wisconsin
*Hydrocarbons*

**Geetika Gupta, MD**
Clinical Instructor, Department of Emergency Medicine, University of Michigan, St. Joseph Mercy Hospital Emergency Medicine Residency Program, Ann Arbor, Michigan
*Medical-Legal Issues in Emergency Medicine*

**Todd A. Guth, MD**
Medical Education Fellow, Department of Emergency Medicine, University of Colorado, Aurora, Colorado
*Esophageal Disorders*

**Azita G. Hamedani, MD, MPH**
Division Chief, Department of Emergency Medicine, University of Wisconsin School of Medicine and Public Health, Madison, Wisconsin
*Quality and Patient Safety in Emergency Medicine*

**Abigail D. Hankin, MD, MPH**
Assistant Professor, Department of Emergency Medicine, Emory University School of Medicine; Assistant Professor, Behavioral Health and Health Education, Rollins School of Public Health, Atlanta, Georgia
*Intimate Partner Violence*

**Benjamin P. Harrison, MD**
Program Director, Madigan Army Emergency Medicine Residency, Tacoma, Washington
*Anxiety and Panic Disorders*

**Stephen C. Hartsell, MD**
Professor of Surgery, Director of Education and Global Health Programs, Division of Emergency Medicine, University of Utah School of Medicine, Salt Lake City, Utah
*Non-Snake Reptile Bites*

**Tarlan Hedayati, MD, FACEP, FAAEM**
Assistant Professor, Assistant Program Director, Department of Emergency Medicine, John H. Stroger Hospital of Cook County; Assistant Professor, Department of Emergency Medicine, Rush Medical College, Chicago, Illinois
*Thoracic Trauma*

**Alan C. Heffner, MD**
Director, Medical Intensive Care Unit, Division of Critical Care, Departments of Internal Medicine and Emergency Medicine, Carolinas Medical Center; Assistant Clinical Professor, University of North Carolina—Charlotte Campus, Charlotte, North Carolina
*Fluid Management*
*Acid-Base Disorders*

**Diane B. Heller, MD, JD**
Assistant Clinical Professor, Department of Emergency Medicine, Mount Sinai School of Medicine, New York, New York; Attending Physician, Department of Emergency Medicine, Morristown Medical Center, Morristown, New Jersey
*Informed Consent and Assessing Decision-Making Capacity in the Emergency Department*

**Robin R. Hemphill, MD, MPH**
Directory of Quality and Safety, Associate Professor, Department of Emergency Medicine, Emory University School of Medicine, Atlanta, Georgia
*Third Trimester Pregnancy Emergencies*

**Gregory L. Henry, MD**
Risk Consultant, The Emergency Physician Medical Group; Clinical Professor, Department of Emergency Medicine, University of Michigan, Ann Arbor, Michigan; Past President, The American College of Emergency Physicians; Past President, Savannah Assurance, Ltd.
*Medical-Legal Issues in Emergency Medicine*

**H. Gene Hern, Jr., MD**
Residency Director, Department of Emergency Medicine, Alameda County Medical Center—Highland Hospital, Oakland, California; Associate Clinical Professor, Department of Emergency Medicine, University of California, San Francisco, San Francisco, California
*Pharynx and Throat Emergencies*

**Sheryl L. Heron, MD, MPH**
Associate Professor, Associate Residency Director, Department of Emergency Medicine, Assistant Dean, Clinical Education, Associate Director for Education and Training, Center for Injury Control, Emory University School of Medicine, Atlanta, Georgia
*Gastrointestinal Bleeding*

**Cherri D. Hobgood, MD, FACEP**
Rolly McGrath Professor and Chair, Department of Emergency Medicine, Indiana University School of Medicine, Indianapolis, Indiana
*Quality and Patient Safety in Emergency Care*

**Beatrice Hoffmann, MD, PhD**
Assistant Professor, Department of Emergency Medicine, Johns Hopkins University, Bayview Medical Center, Baltimore, Maryland
*Emergency Biliary Ultrasonography*

**Lance H. Hoffman, MD**
Associate Professor, Department of Emergency Medicine, University of Nebraska Medical Center, Omaha, Nebraska
*Sodium and Water Balance*

**Christy Hopkins, MD, MPH**
Associate Professor, Division of Emergency Medicine, University of Utah School of Medicine, Salt Lake City, Utah
*Knee and Lower Leg Injuries*

**Russ Horowitz, MD, RDMS**
Director, Emergency Ultrasound, Children's Memorial Hospital; Assistant Professor, Department of Pediatrics, Northwestern University Feinberg School of Medicine, Chicago, Illinois
*Pediatric Abdominal Disorders*
*Pediatric Orthopedic Emergencies*

**Debra E. Houry, MD, MPH**
Vice Chair for Research, Department of Emergency Medicine, Emory University School of Medicine; Director, Center for Injury Control, Emory University, Atlanta, Georgia
*Intimate Partner Violence*

**David S. Howes, MD, FACEP, FAAEM**
Professor of Medicine and Pediatrics, Residency Program Director Emeritus, Section of Emergency Medicine, University of Chicago, Chicago, Illinois
*Lung Infections*

**J. Stephen Huff, MD**
Associate Professor, Department of Emergency Medicine and Neurology, University of Virginia, Charlottesville, Virginia
*Intracranial Hemorrhages*
*Conversion Disorder, Psychosomatic Illness, and Malingering*

**James Q. Hwang, MD, RDMS, RDCS**
Attending Physician, Director of Emergency Ultrasound, Department of Emergency Medicine, Scripps Memorial Hospital La Jolla, La Jolla, California
*Lower Extremity Venous Ultrasonography*

## CONTRIBUTORS

**Eric Isaacs, MD**
Professor, Department of Emergency Medicine, University of California, San Francisco; Attending Physician, Department of Emergency Services, San Francisco General Hospital, San Francisco, California
*The Violent Patient*

**Benjamin F. Jackson, MD**
Assistant Professor, Department of Pediatrics, Division of Emergency Medicine, Medical University of South Carolina, Charleston, South Carolina
*Self-Harm and Danger to Others*

**Andy Jagoda, MD, FACEP**
Professor and Chair, Department of Emergency Medicine, Mount Sinai School of Medicine, New York, New York
*Delirium and Dementia*

**Edward C. Jauch, MD**
Professor and Interim Chief, Division of Emergency Medicine; Professor, Department of Neurosciences; Associate Vice Chair, Research, Department of Medicine, Medical University of South Carolina, Charleston, South Carolina
*Neurologic Procedures*

**Kerin A. Jones, MD,**
Assistant Professor, Department of Emergency Medicine, Detroit Receiving Hospital/Wayne State University, Detroit, Michigan
*Gastrointestinal Devices, Procedures, and Imaging*

**Randall S. Jotte, MD**
Associate Professor, Division of Emergency Medicine, Washington University School of Medicine, St. Louis, Missouri
*Addiction*

**Christopher S. Kang, MD, FACEP, FAWM**
Research Director, Attending Physician, Department of Emergency Medicine, Madigan Army Medical Center, Tacoma, Washington; Assistant Clinical Professor, Division of Emergency Medicine, University of Washington, Seattle, Washington; Assistant Clinical Professor, Department of Emergency and Military Medicine, Uniformed Services University of the Health Sciences, Bethesda, Maryland
*Chemical and Nuclear Agents*
*Anxiety and Panic Disorders*

**Jacqueline Khorasanee, MD**
Resident Physician, Department of Emergency Medicine, Northwestern University Feinberg School of Medicine, Chicago, Illinois
*The Healthy Pregnancy*

**Christopher S. Kiefer, MD**
Assistant Professor of Clinical Emergency Medicine, Department of Emergency Medicine, Indiana University School of Medicine, Indianapolis, Indiana
*Child with a Fever*

**Tae Eung Kim, MD**
Assistant Professor, Department of Emergency Medicine, Loma Linda University Medical Center, Loma Linda, California
*Psychosis and Psychotropic Medication*

**Heidi H. Kimberly, MD, RDMS**
Director of Ultrasound Education, Emergency Department, Brigham and Women's Hospital; Instructor, Emergency Medicine, Harvard Medical School, Boston, Massachusetts
*Emergency Renal Ultrasonography*

**Matthew Kippenhan, MD**
Assistant Professor, Department of Emergency Medicine, Northwestern University Feinberg School of Medicine, Chicago, Illinois
*The Healthy Pregnancy*
*Disorders of Early Pregnancy*

**Niranjan Kissoon, MD, FRCP(C), FAAP, FCCM, FACPE**
Vice President, Medical Affairs, British Columbia's Children's Hospital and Sunny Hill Health Centre for Children, University of British Columbia and British Columbia's Children's Hospital; Professor in Acute and Critical Care—Global Child Health; Professor, Department of Pediatrics and Emergency Surgery, University of British Columbia; Senior Scientist, Child and Family Research Institute, Vancouver, British Columbia, Canada; President, World Federation of Paediatric Intensive and Critical Care Societies
*Submersion Injuries*

**Kevin Klauer, DO, EJD, FACEP**
Chief Medical Officer, Emergency Medicine Physicians, Ltd., Canton, Ohio; Editor in Chief, Emergency Physicians Monthly; Assistant Clinical Professor, Department of Emergency Medicine, Michigan State University College of Osteopathic Medicine, East Lansing, Michigan
*Patient-Centered Care*

**Frederick Korley, MD, FACEP**
Assistant Professor, Department of Emergency Medicine, Johns Hopkins University, Baltimore, Maryland
*Thyroid Disorders*

**Joshua M. Kosowsky, MD**
Clinical Director, Department of Emergency Medicine, Brigham and Women's Hospital; Assistant Professor, Department of Emergency Medicine, Harvard Medical School, Boston, Massachusetts
*Congestive Heart Failure*

**Karen Nolan Kuehl, MD, FACEP**
Clinical Instructor, Department of Emergency Medicine, Carilion Clinic, Roanoke, Virginia
*Facial Trauma*

**Thomas Kunisaki, MD, FACEP, FACMT**
Clinical Associate Professor, Department of Emergency Medicine, Shands-Jacksonville University of Florida Academic Health Center; Medical Director, Florida Poison Information Center—Jacksonville, Shands-Jacksonville, Jacksonville, Florida
*Smoke Inhalation*

**Shana Kusin, MD**
Clinical Instructor, Department of Emergency Medicine, Toxicology Fellow, Oregon Poison Center, Oregon Health and Science University, Portland, Oregon
*Ethanol and Opioid Intoxication and Withdrawal*
*Pediatric Overdoses*

**Michael Lambert, MD, RDMS, FAAEM**
Fellowship Director, Emergency Ultrasound, Department of Emergency Medicine, Advocate Christ Medical Center, Oak Lawn, Illinois
*First Trimester Ultrasonography*

**Patrick M. Lank, MD**
Attending Physician, Department of Emergency Medicine, Northwestern University Feinberg School of Medicine; Toxicology Fellow, Toxikon Consortium, John H. Stroger Hospital of Cook County, Chicago, Illinois
*Ethanol and Opioid Intoxication and Withdrawal*
*Pediatric Overdoses*

**Erin M. Lareau, MD**
Clinical Instructor, Department of Emergency Medicine, Northwestern University Feinberg School of Medicine, Chicago, Illinois
*Tendinitis and Bursitis*

**Sara Lary, DO, DTM&H**
Assistant Professor, International Emergency Medicine Fellow, Department of Emergency Medicine, Loma Linda University Medical Center, Loma Linda, California
*Helminths, Bedbugs, Scabies, and Lice Infections*

**Erik G. Laurin, MD**
Associate Professor, Director of Medical Student Education, Department of Emergency Medicine, University of California, Davis, Sacramento, California
*Advanced Airway Techniques*

**Holly K. Ledyard, MD**
Assistant Professor, Division of Emergency Medicine and Neurology, University of Utah School of Medicine, Salt Lake City, Utah
*Transient Ischemic Attack and Acute Ischemic Stroke*

**Eric L. Legome, MD**
Chief of Service, Department of Emergency Medicine, Kings County Hospital; Visiting Associate Professor, Department of Emergency Medicine, SUNY Downstate College of Medicine, Brooklyn, New York; Associate Professor, Department of Emergency Medicine, New York Medical College, Valhalla, New York
*Blunt Abdominal Trauma*
*Penetrating Abdominal Trauma*

**Tracy Leigh LeGros, MD, PhD**
Associate Professor—Clinical, Department of Medicine, Section of Emergency Medicine, Louisiana State University Health Sciences Center; Program Director, Undersea and Hyperbaric Medicine Fellowship, New Orleans, Louisiana
*Approach to the Pediatric Patient with a Rash*
*Dysbarism, Dive Injuries, and Decompression Illness*
*Local and Regional Anesthesia*
*Approach to the Adult Rash*
*Rash in the Severely Ill Patient*

**Katrina A. Leone, MD**
Education Fellow and Adjunct Instructor, Department of Emergency Medicine, Oregon Health and Science University, Portland, Oregon
*Calcium, Magnesium, and Phosphorus*

**Matthew R. Levine, MD**
Assistant Professor, Director of Trauma Services, Department of Emergency Medicine, Northwestern University Feinberg School of Medicine, Chicago, Illinois
*Soft Tissue Injury*

**Michael Levine, MD**
Department of Emergency Medicine, Section of Medical Toxicology, University of Southern California, Los Angeles, California
*Bleeding Disorders*

**Jason E. Liebzeit, MD**
Assistant Professor, Department of Emergency Medicine, Emory University School of Medicine, Atlanta, Georgia
*Anorexia Nervosa and Bulemia Nervosa*

**Michelle Lin, MD**
Associate Professor, Department of Emergency Medicine, University of California, San Francisco, San Francisco General Hospital, San Francisco, California
*Spine Trauma and Spinal Cord Injury*

**M. Scott Linscott, MD**
Adjunct Professor of Surgery (Clinical), Division of Emergency Medicine, University of Utah School of Medicine, Salt Lake City, Utah
*Injuries to the Shoulder Girdle and Humerus*

**Suzanne Lippert, MD**
Clinical Instructor, Division of Emergency Medicine, Stanford University School of Medicine, Stanford, California
*Pediatric Genitourinary and Renal Disorders*

**John B. Lissoway, MD**
Fellow in Wilderness Medicine, Stanford University School of Medicine, Stanford, California
*Ear Emergencies*

**Robert Lockwood, MD, AM**
Resident Physician, Department of Emergency Medicine, Northwestern University Feinberg School of Medicine, Chicago, Illinois
*Breast Disorders*
*Wound Repair*

**Heather Long, MD**
Director, Medical Toxicology; Associate Professor, Department of Emergency Medicine, Albany Medical Center, Albany, New York
*Acetaminophen, Aspirin, and NSAIDs*

**Dave W. Lu, MD, MBE**
Acting Instructor, Department of Medicine, Division of Emergency Medicine, University of Washington School of Medicine, Seattle, Washington
*Ethics of Resuscitation*

**Binh T. Ly, MD, FACMT, FACEP**
Professor of Emergency Medicine and Medicine, Department of Emergency Medicine; Director, Medical Toxicology Fellowship, Division of Medical Toxicology; Director, Emergency Medicine Residency, Department of Emergency Medicine, University of California, San Diego; Staff Medical Toxicologist, California Poison Control System, San Diego Division, San Diego, California
*Over-the-Counter Medications*

**Catherine A. Lynch, MD**
Clinical Instructor, Department of Emergency Medicine, Emory University School of Medicine, Atlanta, Georgia
*Hypertensive Crisis*

**Troy E. Madsen, MD**
Assistant Professor, Division of Emergency Medicine, University of Utah School of Medicine, Salt Lake City, Utah
*Non-Snake Reptile Bites*

**Swaminatha V. Mahadevan, MD, FACEP, FAAEM**
Associate Professor of Surgery/Emergency Medicine, Associate Chief, Division of Emergency Medicine, Stanford University School of Medicine; Emergency Department Medical Director, Stanford University Medical Center, Stanford, California
*Spine Trauma and Spinal Cord Injury*

**Mamta Malik, MD**
Clinical Instructor, Department of Emergency Medicine, Rush Medical College; Associate Director, International Emergency Medicine Fellowship, Attending Physician, Department of Emergency Medicine, Rush University Medical Center, Chicago, Illinois
*Gynecologic Infections*

**Haney A. Mallemat, MD**
Assistant Professor, Department of Emergency Medicine, University of Maryland School of Medicine, Baltimore, Maryland
*Shock*

**Michael P. Mallin, MD, RDCS**
Assistant Professor, Division of Emergency Medicine, University of Utah School of Medicine, Salt Lake City, Utah
*Emergency Cardiac Ultrasound: Evaluation for Pericardial Effusion and Cardiac Activity*

**Gerald Maloney, DO**
Attending Physician, Department of Emergency Medicine, MetroHealth Medical Center; Assistant Professor, Department of Emergency Medicine, Case Western Reserve University, Cleveland, Ohio
*Renal Transplant Complications*

**Nicole Malouf, MD**
Chief Resident, Department of Medicine, Division of Emergency Medicine, Medical University of South Carolina, Charleston, South Carolina
*Self-Harm and Danger to Others*

**Rita A. Manfredi, MD**
Associate Clinical Professor, Department of Emergency Medicine, George Washington University, Washington, District of Columbia
*Appendicitis*

**David E. Manthey, MD**
Professor and Vice Chair of Education, Department of Emergency Medicine, Wake Forest University School of Medicine, Winston-Salem, North Carolina
*Pneumothorax*
*Pleural Effusion*

**Keith A. Marill, MD**
Attending Physician, Department of Emergency Medicine, Massachusetts General Hospital; Assistant Professor, Division of Emergency Medicine, Harvard Medical School, Boston, Massachusetts
*Tachydysrhythmias*

**Melissa Marinelli, MD**
Resident Physician, Department of Emergency Medicine, Northwestern University Feinberg School of Medicine, Chicago, Illinois
*Abdominal Aortic Aneurysm*

## CONTRIBUTORS

**Joseph P. Martinez, MD**
Assistant Professor, Department of Emergency Medicine, University of Maryland School of Medicine, Baltimore, Maryland
*Pericarditis, Pericardial Tamponade, and Myocarditis*

**Amal Mattu, MD**
Professor and Vice Chair, Department of Emergency Medicine, University of Maryland School of Medicine, Baltimore, Maryland
*Pericarditis, Pericardial Tamponade, and Myocarditis*

**Anna K. McFarlin, MD**
Section of Emergency Medicine, Louisiana State University Health Sciences Center, New Orleans, Louisiana
*Approach to the Pediatric Patient with a Rash*

**Mark McIntosh, MD, MPH**
Associate Professor, Department of Emergency Medicine, University of Florida, Jacksonville, Florida
*Emergencies in Infants and Toddlers*

**Candace D. McNaughton, MD, MPH**
Assistant Professor, Department of Emergency Medicine, Vanderbilt University, Nashville, Tennessee
*Hypoglycemia*

**Ron Medzon, MD**
Associate Professor, Department of Emergency Medicine, Boston Medical Center, Boston University School of Medicine, Boston, Massachusetts
*Penetrating Neck Trauma*

**Carl R. Menckhoff, MD, FACEP**
Medical Director and Chair, Department of Emergency Medicine, Medical Center of Lewisville, Lewisville, Texas; Ultrasound Director, Director of Education, Questcare Partners, Dallas, Texas; Associate Professor, Department of Emergency Medicine, Georgia Health Sciences University, Augusta, Georgia
*Nephrolithiasis*

**Glen E. Michael, MD**
Assistant Professor, Department of Emergency Medicine, University of Virginia, Charlottesville, Virginia
*Conversion Disorder, Psychosomatic Illness, and Malingering*

**Nathan W. Mick, MD**
Director, Clinical Operations, Director, Pediatric Emergency Medicine, Department of Emergency Medicine, Maine Medical Center, Portland, Maine; Assistant Professor, Tufts University School of Medicine, Boston, Massachusetts
*Pediatric Cardiac Disorders*

**Lisa D. Mills, MD**
Associate Professor, Department of Emergency Medicine, University of California, Davis, Sacramento, California
*Tetanus*
*Rabies*

**Trevor J. Mills, MD, MPH**
Professor, Department of Medicine, Section of Emergency Medicine, Louisiana State University Health Sciences Center, New Orleans, Louisiana; Chief of Emergency Medicine Services, VA Northern California Health Care System, Rancho Cordova, California
*Trauma Resuscitation*
*Forearm Fractures*

**Peter P. Monteleone, MD**
Cardiovascular Medicine Fellow, Department of Cardiovascular Medicine, Cleveland Clinic, Cleveland, Ohio
*Management of Cardiac Arrest and the Post–Cardiac Arrest Syndrome*

**Raveendra S. Morchi, MD**
Assistant Professor, Department of Emergency Medicine, Harbor University of California, Los Angeles Medical Center, Torrance, California
*Connective Tissue and Inflammatory Disorders*

**Lisa Moreno-Walton, MD, MSCR**
Associate Professor—Clinical, Department of Medicine, Section of Emergency Medicine; Assistant Professor—Research, Department of Genetics, Louisiana State University Health Sciences Center; Associate Residency Program Director and Research Director, Section of Emergency Medicine, Louisiana State University Health Sciences Center; Associate Professor, Department of Surgery, Tulane University School of Medicine, New Orleans, Louisiana
*Health Care Disparities and Diversity in Emergency Medicine*

**Elizabeth A. Mort, MD**
Instructor in Medicine, Associate Chief Medical Officer, Vice President of Quality and Safety, Massachusetts General Hospital; Instructor of Health Care Policy, Harvard Medical School, Boston, Massachusetts
*Quality and Patient Safety in Emergency Medicine*

**Thomas Morrissey, MD, PhD**
Associate Professor, Department of Emergency Medicine, University of Florida College of Medicine—Jacksonville, Jacksonville, Florida
*Ear Emergencies*

**Heather Murphy-Lavoie, MD**
Associate Professor, Assistant Residency Director, Emergency Medicine Residency; Associate Program Director, Undersea and Hyperbaric Medicine Fellowship, Louisiana State University School of Medicine/Medical Center of Louisiana in New Orleans, New Orleans, Louisiana
*Approach to the Pediatric Patient with a Rash*
*Dysbarism, Dive Injuries, and Decompression Illness*
*Local and Regional Anesthesia*
*Approach to the Adult Rash*
*Rash in the Severely Ill Patient*

**Mark B. Mycyk, MD**
Associate Professor, Department of Emergency Medicine, Rush Medical College; Attending Physician, Department of Emergency Medicine, Cook County Hospital; Research Director, Toxikon Consortium, Chicago, Illinois
*Hallucinogens and Drugs of Abuse*
*Toxic Alcohols*

**Eric S. Nadel, MD**
Associate Professor, Harvard Medical School; Program Director, Harvard Affiliated Emergency Medicine Residency, Brigham and Women's Hospital/Massachusetts General Hospital, Boston, Massachusetts
*Preface*

**Swathi Nadindla, MD**
Senior Resident, Department of Emergency Medicine, Mount Sinai School of Medicine, New York, New York
*Peripheral Nerve Disorders*

**Brian K. Nelson, MD**
Professor and Chair, Department of Emergency Medicine, Paul L. Foster School of Medicine, El Paso, Texas
*Adrenal Crisis*
*Pituitary Apoplexy*

**Lewis S. Nelson, MD**
Professor, Department of Emergency Medicine, New York University School of Medicine; Director, Fellowship in Medical Toxicology, New York City Poison Control Center, New York, New York
*Anticholinergics*

**Sara W. Nelson, MD**
Assistant Professor, Tufts University School of Medicine, Department of Emergency Medicine, Maine Medical Center, Portland, Maine
*Hand and Wrist Injuries*

**David H. Newman, MD**
Director of Clinical Research, Associate Professor of Emergency Medicine, Department of Emergency Medicine, Mount Sinai School of Medicine, New York, New York
*Evidence-Based Medicine*

**Bret A. Nicks,** MD, MHA
Associate Professor, Medical Director of Clinical Operations, Department of Emergency Medicine, Wake Forest University School of Medicine, Winston-Salem, North Carolina
*Pneumothorax*
*Pleural Effusion*

**Vicki E. Noble,** MD, RDMS
Director, Division of Emergency Ultrasound, Department of Emergency Medicine, Massachusetts General Hospital; Associate Professor, Harvard Medical School, Boston, Massachusetts
*Emergency Biliary Ultrasonography*
*Lower Extremity Venous Ultrasonography*
*Emergency Renal Ultrasonography*
*First Trimester Ultrasonography*

**Joshua N. Nogar,** MD
Department of Toxicology and Emergency Medicine, University of California, San Diego, San Diego, California
*Arthropod Bites and Stings*

**Robert L. Norris,** MD
Professor and Chief, Division of Emergency Medicine, Stanford University School of Medicine, Stanford, California
*Venomous Snakebites in North America*

**Ashley Booth Norse,** MD, FACEP
Associate Program Director, Department of Emergency Medicine; Director of Governmental Affairs, Emergency Medicine; University of Florida College of Medicine—Jacksonville, Jacksonville, Florida
*Mammalian Bites*

**Robert E. O'Connor,** MD, MPH
Professor and Chair, Department of Emergency Medicine, University of Virginia, Charlottesville, Virginia
*Management of Cardiac Arrest and the Post–Cardiac Arrest Syndrome*

**Kelly P. O'Keefe,** MD
Program Director, Department of Emergency Medicine, University of South Florida/Tampa General Hospital, Tampa, Florida
*Mesenteric Ischemia*
*Diverticulitis*

**Haru Okuda,** MD
National Medical Director, SimLEARN, Veterans Health Administration; Associate Professor of Emergency Medicine, University of Central Florida College of Medicine, Orlando, Florida
*Delirium and Dementia*

**Brian W. Patterson,** MD, MPH
Resident Physician, Department of Emergency Medicine, Northwestern University Feinberg School of Medicine, Chicago, Illinois
*Introduction to Cost-Effectiveness Analysis*

**Leigh A. Patterson,** MD
Assistant Professor, Residency Director, Department of Emergency Medicine, East Carolina University Brody School of Medicine, Greenville, North Carolina
*Pelvic Fractures*

**Richard Paula,** MD
Chief Medical Informatics Officer, Department of Emergency Medicine, Tampa General Hospital, Tampa, Florida
*Liver Disorders*
*Fungal Infections*

**Joseph F. Peabody,** MD
Attending Physician, Department of Emergency Medicine, Lutheran General Hospital, Park Ridge, Illinois; Clinical Assistant Professor, Department of Emergency Medicine, University of Illinois at Chicago College of Medicine, Chicago, Illinois
*Lung Infections*

**David A. Peak,** MD
Assistant Residency Director, Harvard Affiliated Emergency Medicine Residency, Department of Emergency Medicine, Massachusetts General Hospital; Assistant Professor, Department of Emergency Medicine (Surgery), Harvard Medical School, Boston, Massachusetts
*Acute Compartment Syndromes*

**John Nelson Perret,** MD
Clinical Assistant Professor, Department of Family Medicine, Louisiana State University Health Sciences Center, New Orleans, Louisiana
*Emergencies in the First Weeks of Life*

**Andrew D. Perron,** MD
Professor and Residency Program Director, Department of Emergency Medicine, Maine Medical Center, Portland, Maine
*Imaging of the Central Nervous System*

**Vanessa Maria Piazza,** MD
Clinical and Academic Emergency Medicine Staff and Emergency Ultrasound Staff, Department of Medicine, Section of Emergency Medicine, Carity Interim Hospital, New Orleans, Louisiana
*Aortic Ultrasound*

**Robert F. Poirier,** MD, FACEP
Assistant Professor, Chief of Clinical Operations, Department of Emergency Medicine, Washington University School of Medicine/Barnes-Jewish Hospital, St. Louis, Missouri
*Complications of Bariatric Surgery*

**Emilie S. Powell,** MD, MBA
Assistant Professor, Department of Emergency Medicine, Northwestern University Feinberg School of Medicine, Chicago, Illinois,
*Introduction to Cost-Effectiveness Analysis*

**Susan B. Promes,** MD
Professor and Vice Chair for Education, Department of Emergency Medicine, University of California, San Francisco, San Francisco, California
*Resuscitation in Pregnancy*
*Meningitis, Encephalitis, and Brain Abscess*

**Tammie E. Quest,** MD
Chief of Palliative Medicine, Department of Veterans Affairs, Atlanta VA Medical Center; Associate Professor, Department of Emergency Medicine, Emory University School of Medicine, Atlanta, Georgia
*Ethics of Resuscitation*

**James Quinn,** MD, MS
Professor of Surgery/Emergency Medicine, Division of Emergency Medicine, Stanford University School of Medicine, Stanford, California
*Syncope*

**Claudia Ranniger,** MD, PhD
Assistant Professor, Department of Emergency Medicine; Medical Director, Simulation Center, Office of Interdisciplinary Medical Education, George Washington University, Washington, District of Columbia
*Appendicitis*

**Niels K. Rathlev,** MD
Chair, Department of Emergency Medicine, Baystate Medical Center, Springfield, Massachusetts; Professor and Chair, Department of Emergency Medicine, Tufts University School of Medicine, Boston, Massachusetts
*Penetrating Neck Trauma*

**James W. Rhee,** MD
Director of Medical Toxicology, Department of Emergency Medicine, Loma Linda University School of Medicine; Assistant Program Director, Emergency Medicine Residency, Loma Linda University Medical Center, Loma Linda, California
*Sedative-Hypnotic Agents*

**Keri Robertson,** DO, FACOEP
Assoicate Program Director and Clinical Associate Professor, Department of Emergency Medicine, Midwestern University, Downers Grove, Illinois; Department of Emergency Medicine, Swedish Covenant Hospital, Chicago, Illinois
*Vasculitis Syndromes*

**Matthew T. Robinson,** MD
Assistant Professor of Clinical Emergency Medicine, Division Chief of Medical Quality and Safety, Department of Emergency Medicine, University of Missouri Hospitals and Clinics, Columbia, Missouri
*Fluid Management*
*Acid-Base Disorders*

## CONTRIBUTORS

**Robert L. Rogers,** MD
Associate Professor of Emergency Medicine and Medicine, Director, Medical Education and Teaching Fellowship, Department of Emergency Medicine, University of Maryland School of Medicine, Baltimore, Maryland
*Lung Transplant Complications*

**Carlo L. Rosen,** MD
Program Director and Vice Chair for Education, Department of Emergency Medicine, Beth Israel Deaconess Medical Center, Boston, Massachusetts
*Blunt Abdominal Trauma*
*Penetrating Abdominal Trauma*

**Christopher Ross,** MD, FACEP, FAAEM, FRCPC
Assistant Professor, Rush Medical College; Associate Chair of Planning, Education and Research, Assistant Program Director, Department of Emergency Medicine, John H. Stroger Hospital of Cook County, Chicago, Illinois
*Peripheral Arterial Disease*

**Scott E. Rudkin,** MD, MBA, RDMS, FAAEM, FACEP
Vice Chief, Department of Emergency Medicine, University of California, Irvine, Orange, California
*Demyelinating Disorders*

**Anne-Michelle Ruha,** MD
Fellowship Director, Department of Medical Toxicology, Banner Good Samaritan Medical Center, Phoenix, Arizona
*Insecticides, Herbicides, and Rodenticides*

**Michael S. Runyon,** MD
Director of Global Emergency Medicine, Assistant Program Director, Department of Emergency Medicine, Carolinas Medical Center, Charlotte, North Carolina
*Genitourinary Trauma*

**Annie T. Sadosty,** MD
Assistant Professor, Department of Emergency Medicine, Mayo Clinic, Rochester, Minnesota
*Viral Infections*

**Tracy G. Sanson,** MD
Education Director, Emergency Medicine Residency; Associate Professor, Department of Emergency Medicine, University of South Florida/Tampa General Hospital, Tampa, Florida
*Mesenteric Ischemia*
*Diverticulitis*

**Jairo I. Santanilla,** MD
Clinical Assistant Professor, Department of Medicine, Section of Emergency Medicine, Section of Pulmonary/Critical Care Medicine, Louisiana State University Health Sciences Center; Department of Pulmonary/Critical Care Medicine, Ochsner Medical Center, New Orleans, Louisiana
*Mechanical Ventilation*

**Sally A. Santen,** MD, PhD
Assistant Dean, Educational Research and Quality Improvement; Associate Chair, Education, Department of Emergency Medicine, University of Michigan, Ann Arbor, Michigan
*Third Trimester Pregnancy Emergencies*

**Osman R. Sayan,** MD
Assistant Director, Emergency Medicine Residency, NewYork-Presbyterian Hospital; Assistant Clinical Professor of Medicine, College of Physicians and Surgeons of Columbia University, New York, New York
*Endocarditis*

**Michael J. Schmidt,** MD
Medical Director, Director of Emergency Department Informatics; Assistant Professor, Department of Emergency Medicine, Northwestern University Feinberg School of Medicine, Chicago, Illinois
*Sepsis*

**Kathleen S. Schrank,** MD
Professor of Medicine, Division Chief for Emergency Medicine, Department of Medicine, University of Miami Miller School of Medicine; Emergency Medical Services Medical Director, City of Miami Fire Rescue, Miami, Florida
*Constipation*
*Joint Disorders*

**Jeremiah D. Schuur,** MD, MHS
Director of Quality and Patient Safety, Director of Performance Improvement, Department of Emergency Medicine, Brigham and Women's Hospital; Assistant Professor, Harvard Medical School, Boston, Massachusetts
*Quality and Patient Safety in Emergency Medicine*

**Theresa Schwab,** MD, FRCPC
Attending Physician, Department of Emergency Medicine, Advocate Christ Medical Center, Oak Lawn, Illinois; Assistant Professor, Department of Emergency Medicine, University of Illinois at Chicago College of Medicine, Chicago, Illinois
*Peripheral Arterial Disease*

**Wesley H. Self,** MD, MPH
Assistant Professor, Department of Emergency Medicine, Vanderbilt University School of Medicine, Nashville, Tennessee
*Hypoglycemia*

**Monique I. Sellas,** MD
Attending Physician, Department of Emergency Medicine, Massachusetts General Hospital; Instructor, Department of Surgery, Division of Emergency Medicine, Harvard Medical School, Boston, Massachusetts
*Sexual Assault*

**Andrew W. Shannon,** MD, MPH
Clinical Instructor, Department of Emergency Medicine, Louisiana State University Health Sciences Center, New Orleans, Louisiana
*Ultrasound-Guided Vascular Access*

**Ghazala Q. Sharieff,** MD, MBA
Director of Pediatric Emergency Medicine, Palomar-Pomerado Health System/California Emergency Physicians; Clinical Professor, University of California, San Diego, San Diego, California
*Neonatal Cardiopulmonary Resuscitation*
*Pediatric Resuscitation*
*General Approach to the Pediatric Patient*
*Pediatric Trauma*

**Rahul Sharma,** MD, MBA, CPE, FACEP
Medical Director and Associate Chief of Service, Emergency Department, New York University Langone Medical Center—Tisch Hospital; Assistant Professor of Emergency Medicine, New York University School of Medicine, New York, New York
*Eye Emergencies*

**Philip Shayne,** MD
Associate Professor, Department of Emergency Medicine, Emory University School of Medicine, Atlanta, Georgia
*Hypertensive Crisis*

**Ashley Shreves,** MD
Assistant Professor, Departments of Emergency Medicine and Geriatrics and Palliative Medicine, Mount Sinai School of Medicine, New York, New York
*Evidence-Based Medicine*

**Amandeep Singh,** MD
Physician, Department of Emergency Medicine, Alameda County Medical Center—Highland Hospital, Oakland, California
*Meningitis, Encephalitis, and Brain Abscess*

**Ellen M. Slaven,** MD
Clinical Associate Professor of Medicine, Section of Emergency Medicine, Louisiana State University Health Sciences Center, New Orleans, Louisiana
*Human Immunodeficiency Virus Infection*
*Skin and Soft Tissue Infections*
*Antibiotic Recommendations*

**Mark Sochor,** MD, FACEP
Associate Professor, Department of Emergency Medicine, University of Virginia, Charlottesville, Virginia
*Management of Cardiac Arrest and the Post–Cardiac Arrest Syndrome*

**Mitchell C. Sokolosky,** MD
Associate Professor, Residency Program Director, Department of Emergency Medicine, Wake Forest University School of Medicine, Winston-Salem, North Carolina
*Pancreatic Disorders*

**Jeremy D. Sperling, MD**
Assistant Director, Emergency Medicine Residency Program, NewYork-Presbyterian Hospital; Assistant Professor of Clinical Medicine, Weill Cornell Medical College, New York, New York
*Introduction to Oncologic Emergencies*

**Sarah A. Stahmer, MD**
Associate Professor, Program Training Director, Department of Surgery, Division of Emergency Medicine, Duke University Hospital, Durham, North Carolina
*Bradyarrhythmias*

**Robert L. Stephen, MD**
Associate Professor, Division of Emergency Medicine, University of Utah Health Sciences Center, Salt Lake City, Utah
*Hypothermia and Frostbite*

**Brian A. Stettler, MD**
Residency Program Director, Department of Emergency Medicine, University of Cincinnati Medical Center, Cincinnati, Ohio
*Neurologic Procedures*

**Matthew Strehlow, MD**
Clinical Associate Professor, Director, Clinical Decision Unit, Division of Emergency Medicine, Stanford University School of Medicine, Stanford, California
*Chest Pain*

**Mark Su, MD**
Assistant Professor of Emergency Medicine, Hofstra North Shore–LIJ School of Medicine at Hofstra University; Director, Fellowship in Medical Toxicology, Department of Emergency Medicine, North Shore University Hospital, Manhasset, New York
*Hypoglycemic Agent Overdose*

**Amita Sudhir, MD**
Assistant Professor of Emergency Medicine, University of Virginia Health System, Charlottesville, Virginia
*Renal Failure*

**D. Matthew Sullivan, MD**
Associate Professor, Associate Director of Operations, Department of Emergency Medicine, Carolinas Medical Center, Charlotte, North Carolina
*Tuberculosis*

**Jeffrey Tabas, MD**
Associate Professor of Clinical Emergency Medicine, Department of Emergency Medicine, University of California, San Francisco, San Francisco, California
*Chest Pain*

**Taku Taira, MD**
Clinical Assistant Professor, Assistant Residency Director, Department of Medicine, Division of Emergency Medicine, Olive View–UCLA Medical Center, Sylmar, California
*Platelet Disorders*

**James K. Takayesu, MD,**
Associate Residency Director, Harvard-Affiliated Emergency Medicine Residency, Brigham and Women's Hospital/Massachusetts General Hospital; Attending Physician, Department of Emergency, Massachusetts General Hospital, Boston, Massachusetts
*Documentation*

**Asim F. Tarabar, MD**
Director, Medical Toxicology, Assistant Professor, Department of Emergency Medicine, Yale University School of Medicine; Quality Improvement Director, Emergency Department, Yale New Haven Hospital, New Haven, Connecticut
*Seizures*

**Danny G. Thomas, MD, MPH**
Assistant Professor of Pediatrics, Section of Emergency Medicine, Medical College of Wisconsin, Milwaukee, Wisconsin
*Pediatric Traumatic Brain Injury*

**Kristine M. Thompson, MD**
Assistant Professor, Department of Emergency Medicine, Mayo Clinic, Jacksonville, Florida
*Viral Infections*

**Trevonne M. Thompson, MD**
Assistant Professor, Associate Director of Medical Toxicology, Department of Emergency Medicine, University of Illinois at Chicago College of Medicine, Chicago, Illinois
*Inhaled Toxins*

**Stephen Thornton, MD**
Toxicology Fellow, Division of Medical Toxicology; Clinical Instructor, Department of Emergency Medicine, University of California, San Diego, San Diego, California
*Marine Food-Borne Poisoning, Envenomaton, and Traumatic Injuries*
*Over-the-Counter Medications*

**T. Paul Tran, MD, MS, FACEP**
Associate Professor, Department of Emergency Medicine, University of Nebraska College of Medicine, Omaha, Nebraska
*Allergic Disorders*

**Jacob Ufberg, MD**
Associate Professor and Residency Director, Department of Emergency Medicine, Temple University School of Medicine, Philadelphia, Pennsylvania
*Cardiovascular and Neurologic Emergencies*

**Andrew S. Ulrich, MD**
Associate Professor, Executive Vice-Chair, Department of Emergency Medicine, Boston Medical Center, Boston University School of Medicine, Boston, Massachusetts
*Seizures*

**Michael C. Wadman, MD**
Associate Professor, Department of Emergency Medicine, University of Nebraska College of Medicine, Omaha, Nebraska
*Sodium and Water Balance*

**Ernest E. Wang, MD, FACEP**
Clinical Associate Professor, Assistant Dean for Medical Education, University of Chicago Pritzker School of Medicine; Medical Director, NorthShore Center for Simulation and Innovation, Division of Emergency Medicine, NorthShore University HealthSystem, Evanston, Illinois
*Cranial Nerve Disorders*

**N. Ewen Wang, MD**
Associate Professor, Division of Emergency Medicine, Stanford University School of Medicine, Stanford, California
*Pediatric Genitourinary and Renal Disorders*

**Danielle M. Ware-McGee, MD**
Clinical Instructor, Department of Emergency Medicine, Northwestern University Feinberg School of Medicine, Chicago, Illinois
*Diseases of the Stomach*
*Abdominal Aortic Aneurysm*

**Ian S. Wedmore, MD, FACEP, FAWM, DiMM**
Program Director, Austere and Wilderness Medicine, Department of Emergency Medicine, Madigan Army Medical Center, Tacoma, Washington
*Chemical and Nuclear Agents*

**Natasha Wheaton, MD**
Resident Physician, Department of Emergency Medicine, Northwestern University Feinberg School of Medicine, Chicago, Illinois
*Diseases of the Stomach*

**Beranton Whisenant, MD**
Assistant Professor and Director of Research, Department of Emergency Medicine, University of Florida College of Medicine—Jacksonville, Jacksonville, Florida
*Procedural Sedation*

**Max Wintermark, MD**
Associate Professor of Radiology, Neurology, Neurological Surgery, and Biomedical Engineering, Chief of Neuroradiology, Department of Radiology, University of Virginia, Charlottesville, Virginia
*Intracranial Hemorrhages*

## CONTRIBUTORS

Michael E. Winters, MD, FACEP, FAAEM
Associate Professor of Emergency Medicine and Medicine, University of Maryland School of Medicine; Co-Director, Combined EM/IM/Critical Care Program; Medical Director, Adult Emergency Department, University of Maryland Medical Center, Baltimore, Maryland
*Shock*

Stephen J. Wolf, MD
Senior Associate Program Director, Residency in Emergency Medicine, Department of Emergency Medicine, Denver Health Medical Center, Denver, Colorado; Associate Professor and Director of Medical Education, Department of Emergency Medicine, Assistant Dean for Advanced Studies, Office of Undergraduate Medical Education, University of Colorado School of Medicine, Aurora, Colorado
*Arterial and Venous Trauma and Great Vessel Injuries*

Richard E. Wolfe, MD
Chief of Emergency Medicine, Department of Emergency Medicine, Beth Israel Deaconess Medical Center; Associate Professor of Medicine, Department of Medicine, Harvard Medical School, Boston, Massachusetts
*Blunt Abdominal Trauma*

Todd Wylie, MD, MPH
Program Director, Pediatric Emergency Medicine Fellowship, Assistant Professor, Department of Emergency Medicine, University of Florida College of Medicine—Jacksonville, Jacksonville, Florida
*Emergencies in Infants and Toddlers*

Christine Yang-Kauh, MD
Assistant Program Director, Department of Emergency Medicine, New York Methodist Hospital, Brooklyn, New York
*Complications of Gynecologic Procedures, Abortion, and Assisted Reproductive Technology*

Timothy P. Young, MD
Assistant Professor of Pediatrics and Emergency Medicine, Department of Emergency Medicine, Loma Linda University Medical Center and Children's Hospital, Loma Linda, California
*Sedative-Hypnotic Agents*

Steven M. Zahn, MD
Assistant Medical Director, Department of Emergency Medicine, Sherman Hospital, Elgin, Illinois
*Intracranial and Other Central Nervous System Lesions*

Cristina M. Zeretzke, MD, FAAP
Section Chief, Pediatric Emergency Medicine, Our Lady of the Lake Regional Medical Center, Pediatric Residency Program, Baton Rouge, Louisiana
*Emergencies in the First Weeks of Life*

David K. Zich, MD
Assistant Professor of Medicine, Department of Emergency Medicine, Northwestern University Feinberg School of Medicine, Chicago, Illinois
*Food- and Water-Borne Infections*

Amy E. Zosel, MD, MSCS
Assistant Professor, Department of Emergency Medicine, Medical College of Wisconsin, Milwaukee, Wisconsin
*General Approach to the Poisoned Patient*

# Contents

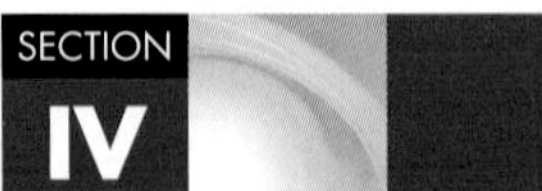

## GASTROINTESTINAL DISEASES



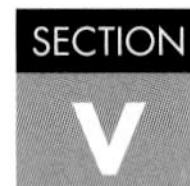

## THORACIC AND RESPIRATORY DISORDERS



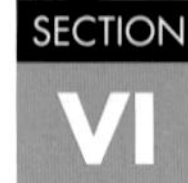

## CARDIAC DISORDERS

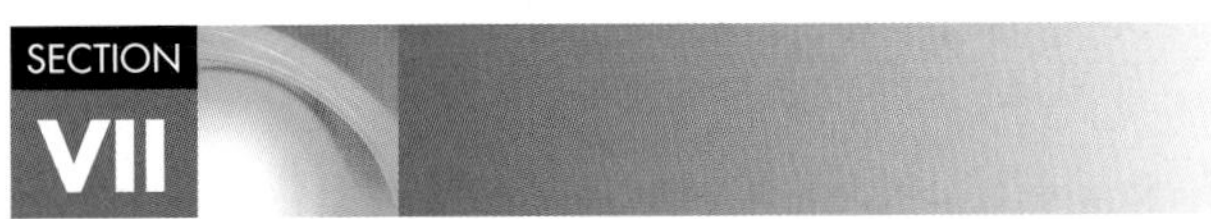

SECTION VII

## VASCULAR DISEASES



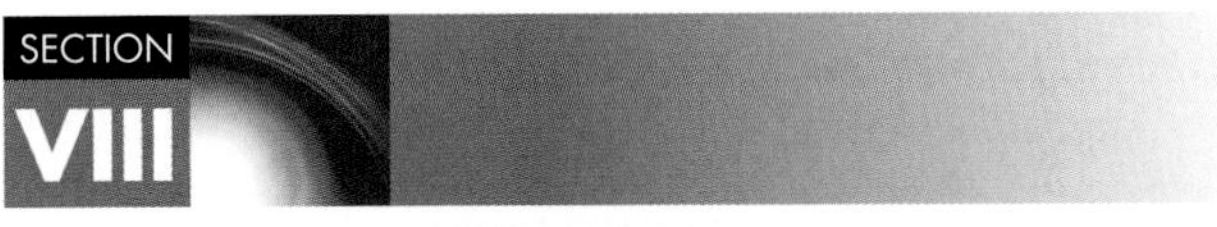

SECTION VIII

## TRAUMATIC DISORDERS

SECTION IX

## NERVOUS SYSTEMS DISORDERS

SECTION X

## IMMUNE SYSTEM DISORDERS

SECTION XI

## GENITOURINARY AND RENAL DISEASES

SECTION XII

## WOMEN'S HEALTH AND GYNECOLOGIC DISEASES

## ENVIRONMENTAL DISORDERS

## BITES, STINGS, AND INJURIES FROM ANIMALS



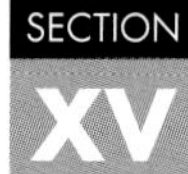


## TOXICOLOGIC EMERGENCIES

## METABOLIC AND ENDOCRINE DISORDERS

## INFECTIONS

## CUTANEOUS DISORDERS

## EMERGENCY PSYCHIATRIC DISORDERS

SECTION XX

## HEMATOLOGY AND ONCOLOGY MANAGEMENT

SECTION XXI

## LEADERSHIP, COMMUNICATION, AND ADMINISTRATION



## ONLINE CONTENT

Available at www.expertconsult.com. To register your account, please follow the activation instructions on the inside front cover of this book.

# Ultrasound Video Contents

Available at www.expertconsult.com. To register your account, please follow the activation instructions on the inside front cover of this book.

# Basic Airway Management 1

David A. Caro

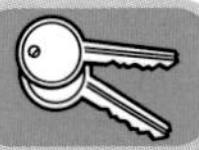

**KEY POINTS**

- Establishment of a patent airway is the cornerstone of successful resuscitation and a defining proficiency of emergency medicine.
- Basic airway management includes the initial airway evaluation and identification and use of interventions to maintain oxygenation and ventilation. These interventions might be simple, such as the application of supplemental oxygen, or complex, such as noninvasive ventilation or emergency tracheal intubation.
- The goal of emergency intubation is safe, successful intubation of the trachea with an endotracheal tube that allows oxygenation and ventilation while protecting the airway from aspiration.
- Patients in the emergency department are always considered high risk because they have not been evaluated beforehand, may have eaten recently, may have anatomic obstacles that are not readily apparent, or may have unstable hemodynamic parameters.

Rapid-sequence intubation (RSI) is the technique of combining sedation and paralysis to create optimal intubating conditions to facilitate emergency intubation. RSI has become the standard in emergency airway management, with intubation success rates greater than 99%.[1] The emergency airway operator should fully understand the risks and benefits and also know when to deviate from its standard algorithm.

## AIRWAY ASSESSMENT

Initial assessment of the patient's airway may identify key features that will help guide airway management. This assessment may have to proceed simultaneously with supportive airway maneuvers.

Anatomically, one should assess the patient by looking for facial distortion and the position in which the airway is held. Drooling or inability to tolerate secretions may be apparent and are ominous signs that suggests significant supraglottic irritation. Patients should be asked to open their mouth, or if they are obtunded, a jaw-thrust and mouth-opening maneuver should be performed carefully to determine how far it can be opened. Palpation of facial structures includes determination of nasal, maxillary, and mandibular stability. Maxillary instability, in particular, should alert the practitioner to be cautious with any nasal intubation, whether by nasal trumpet, nasogastric tube, or blind nasotracheal intubation, because intracranial misplacement of nasal trumpets and nasogastric and nasotracheal tubes has been reported.[2-6] Once past the facial structures, the tongue should be viewed. Similarly, the hard and soft palate, as well as the tonsils, should be evaluated.

Functional assessment is performed to determine whether the patient can move air and phonate. Specific airway noises should be noted, especially stridor.[7] Such assessment leads the clinician to evaluate for specific indications for intubation (**Box 1.1**).[8,9]

Oxygenation failure can be defined as an inability to maintain oxygen saturation greater than 90% despite optimal oxygen supplementation (the exception is a patient with chronic obstructive pulmonary failure, who typically maintains a saturation of 85% to 90%).[8,10] Ventilatory failure is usually measured by clinical features, including respiratory rate, abnormal depth or work of breathing, abnormal breathing patterns, accessory muscle use, inability to speak in complete sentences, presence of abnormal airway sounds (stridor or severe wheezing), or altered mental status. Studies also point to end-tidal carbon dioxide measurement as an aid in procedural sedation,[10] but it is potentially unable to accurately predict $Pa{CO_2}$ in patients with dyspnea.[11]

Acute obtundation diminishes a patient's ability to sense irritant stimuli and therefore spontaneously protect the airway.[9,12] This is part of the rationale for using a Glasgow Coma Scale score of 8 or lower as a cue to intubate trauma patients.[12] Traditionally, the gag reflex has been used to determine whether a patient's airway reflexes are intact. Stimulation of a gag reflex in an obtunded or trauma patient may result in unwanted patient reactions, however, such as bucking, gagging, coughing, or actual vomiting; additionally, up to 37% of healthy volunteers fail to demonstrate a gag reflex.[12,13] Alternatively, a patient who swallows spontaneously while recumbent has sensory and motor paths capable of protecting the airway.[12,14,15] In addition, recent articles have questioned use of the Glasgow Coma Scale score in nontrauma patients and instead emphasize clinical judgment in making the decision to intubate.[16,17]

Finally, the patient's anticipated course will serve as an intubation criterion if loss of airway patency or protection is predicted within the near future.

## CRITICAL AIRWAY PHYSIOLOGY

### OXYGENATION TECHNIQUES

The binding of oxygen to hemoglobin is not linear. Hemoglobin tends to bind oxygen well until the partial pressure of oxygen decreases to 60 mm Hg, and then it rapidly dissociates to allow diffusion of oxygen into blood and surrounding tissue. An oxygen partial pressure of 60 mm Hg correlates with an oxygen saturation of approximately 90%[18] (**Fig. 1.1**). This is an important correlation that should be kept in mind throughout resuscitation (**Table 1.1**).

Patients who require intubation should be preoxygenated with a nonrebreather mask. The goal is to wash as much nitrogen out of the lungs as possible and replace it with oxygen.[19-21]

When the patient is paralyzed during RSI, this reservoir will permit continued delivery of oxygen to the alveoli for some time, thereby allowing the patient to maintain oxygen saturation while apneic. Five or more minutes of preoxygenation allows this reservoir to develop. Alternatively, if pressed for time, the patient can be asked to take eight vital capacity breaths through the nonrebreather in an attempt to build as great a reservoir as possible.[22] Not surprisingly, critically ill patients have decreased oxygen reserve and tolerate apnea less well than do relatively healthy subjects.[19,20,23,24]

Positive pressure will occasionally be required to oxygenate a patient before intubation. A critical feature of RSI is avoidance of active bag-mask ventilation unless it is absolutely necessary.[22] Active bag-mask ventilation with oxygenation is reserved for patients whose oxygen saturation is below 90%.[8] Any positive pressure ventilation will not only ventilate the lungs but also insufflate the stomach. This fact is critical to

**BOX 1.1 Indications for Emergency Intubation**

Failure to oxygenate or ventilate
Failure to protect the airway
Anticipated course that will require intubation

**Table 1.1 Oxygenation Adjuncts**

| DEVICE | RATE | $FIO_2$ (%) |
|---|---|---|
| Nasal cannula | 2 L | 24 |
| Nasal cannula | 4 L | 27 |
| Nasal cannula | 6 L | 30 |
| Venturi mask | — | 40 |
| Nonrebreather mask | 15 L + | 65-70 |
| Bag-mask (one-way inhalation valve + one-way exhalation port, seal maintained without bagging) | 15 L + | 90 |

From Barker TD, Schneider RE. Supplemental oxygenation and bag-mask ventilation. In: Walls RM, Murphy MF, editors. Manual of emergency airway management. 3rd ed. Philadelphia: Lippincott Williams & Wilkins; 2008. pp. 47-61. Available at http://www.loc.gov.lp.hscl.ufl.edu/catdir/enhancements/fy0807/2007050100-d.html; http://www.loc.gov.lp.hscl.ufl.edu/catdir/enhancements/fy0811/2007050100-t.html.

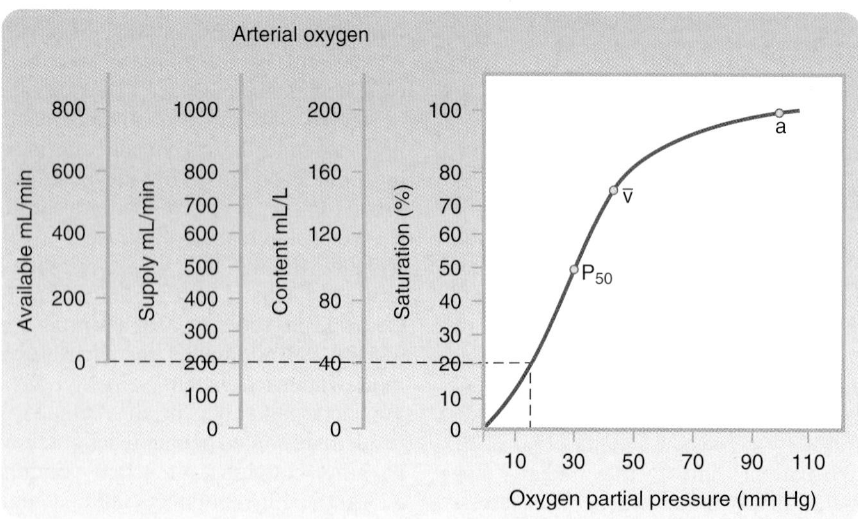


**Fig. 1.1 Oxygen-hemoglobin dissociation curve.** Four different ordinates are shown as a function of oxygen partial pressure (the abscissa). In order from right to left, they are saturation (%), $O_2$ content (mL of $O_2$/0.1 L of blood), $O_2$ supply to peripheral tissues (mL/min), and $O_2$ available to peripheral tissues (mL/min), which is calculated as $O_2$ supply minus the approximately 200 mL/min that cannot be extracted below a partial pressure of 20 mm Hg. Three points are shown on the curve: *a*, normal arterial pressure; $\bar{v}$, normal mixed venous pressure; and $P_{50}$, the partial pressure (27 mm Hg) at which hemoglobin is 50% saturated. (From Miller RD, editor. Miller's anesthesia. 6th ed. Philadelphia: Churchill Livingstone, 2005.)

the performance of RSI because a paralyzed patient is at risk for aspiration as a result of relaxed esophageal sphincter tone, especially if the stomach is distended with air.[22] Active bag ventilation and oxygenation may need to be performed in patients who are experiencing acute oxygenation failure. Most adult bag-mask devices have reservoirs greater than 1 L and can deliver high-flow oxygen if a good mask seal is maintained.[24-26] Alternatively, continuous positive airway pressure or bilevel positive airway pressure can provide a constant level of positive pressure support or two levels of pressure support, respectively, through a tightly fitted mask that fits over the nose or the mouth and nose[27,28]; if applied in a timely manner in the correct patient, the need for intubation might be averted.

### *Bag-Mask Technique*

Bag-mask oxygenation plus ventilation is a critical skill that all airway managers must master before learning to perform RSI (**Boxes 1.2** and **1.3**).[19] Application of the bag and mask requires proper patient positioning and correct application of a mask seal. The ideal position for mask ventilation is with the patient supine and the head and neck in the sniffing position.[19] A proper mask seal is obtained by opposing the mask to the facial skin to create a good air seal. Additionally, new extraglottic devices are available that allow bag ventilation with an inflated balloon surrounding the glottis.[29] These devices can also be used to ventilate and oxygenate patients who do not have contraindications (**Box 1.4**).[7,30-37]

## EMERGENCY AIRWAY ALGORITHM

A patient who merits intubation and is dead or nearly so (a crash airway) requires immediate orotracheal intubation or cricothyrotomy without sedation or paralysis. A patient who is alive and requires intubation will force the airway manager to determine the method of intubation and what medications to use to facilitate it (**Fig. 1.2**).[8]

If the patient is not a crash airway candidate, one should plan to use medications to facilitate intubation. This step requires a determination of expected airway difficulty. Failure to evaluate and anticipate airway difficulty is one of the major causes of failure of intubation.[38,39] The use of paralytics in emergency intubation requires preparation for an alternative airway in the event that a patient cannot be intubated by standard means. A difficult airway may preclude the use of paralytics altogether until the clinician can ensure glottic visualization, which is usually obtained with procedural sedation and topical anesthesia. The approach to a difficult airway is discussed in greater detail in Chapter 2.

Unfortunately, there is no universal definition of a difficult airway. Some patients give the clinician an immediate gestalt that their airway will be difficult. Clinicians tend to be correct when their initial reaction is that an airway will be difficult.[38,39] The converse is not true. Some otherwise normal-appearing patients will have subtle anatomic differences that may make intubation difficult and are not immediately recognizable by a clinician who is not specifically evaluating for such difficulty.

A number of studies have demonstrated various clinical cues that can be used in an attempt to predict a difficult airway (see Box 1.4). No clinical sign, either alone or in combination with other signs, is 100% sensitive in ruling out a difficult airway.[31-35,38,40] However, by using a combination of signs, the vast majority can be identified to make the practitioner aware of potential hazards.

Identification of airway difficulty will require the clinician to give serious thought to performing a sedated examination of the airway with topical anesthesia before proceeding to RSI with neuromuscular blockade (see Chapter 2.)

**BOX 1.2 Failed Airway Fallback**

Mask ventilation is the initial airway management modality of choice for any patient who fails to maintain adequate oxygenation with a nonrebreather mask or begins to desaturate below 90% while apneic during an attempt at rapid-sequence intubation.[8]

**BOX 1.3 Requirements for Adequate Bag-Mask Oxygenation and Ventilation Technique**

Proper positioning
- Sniffing position if possible
- Airway adjuncts such as nasal trumpets or oral airways in appropriate patients

Proper mask seal
- Two-person technique, with one solely responsible for the mask seal, is best
- Jaw-thrust maneuver: pull the mandible up to the mask

**BOX 1.4 Causes of Airway Difficulty**

Problems with bag ventilation: **MOANS** (**M**ask seal, **O**besity, **A**ge [>50 years old], **N**eck mobility, **S**nores)[7,30]

Problems with laryngoscopy: **LEMON** (**L**ook for airway distortion, **E**valuate mouth opening and thyromental distance, **M**allampati score, **O**bstruction, **N**eck mobility)[31-37]

Problems with cricothyrotomy: **SHORT** (previous neck **S**urgery, expanding neck **H**ematomas, **O**besity, previous **R**adiation therapy, and **T**umors and abscesses that might distort the anatomy)[7]

Problems with the use of extraglottic devices: **RODS** (**R**estricted mouth opening, **O**bstruction, **D**isrupted or distorted airway, **S**tiff lungs or cervical spine)[36]

From Murphy MF, Walls RM. Identification of the difficult and failed airway. In: Walls RW, Murphy WF, editors. Manual of emergency airway management. 3rd ed. Philadelphia: Lippincott, Williams & Wilkins; 2008. pp. 81-93. Available at http://www.loc.gov.lp.hscl.ufl.edu/catdir/enhancements/fy0807/2007050100-d.html; http://www.loc.gov.lp.hscl.ufl.edu/catdir/enhancements/fy0811/2007050100-t.html.

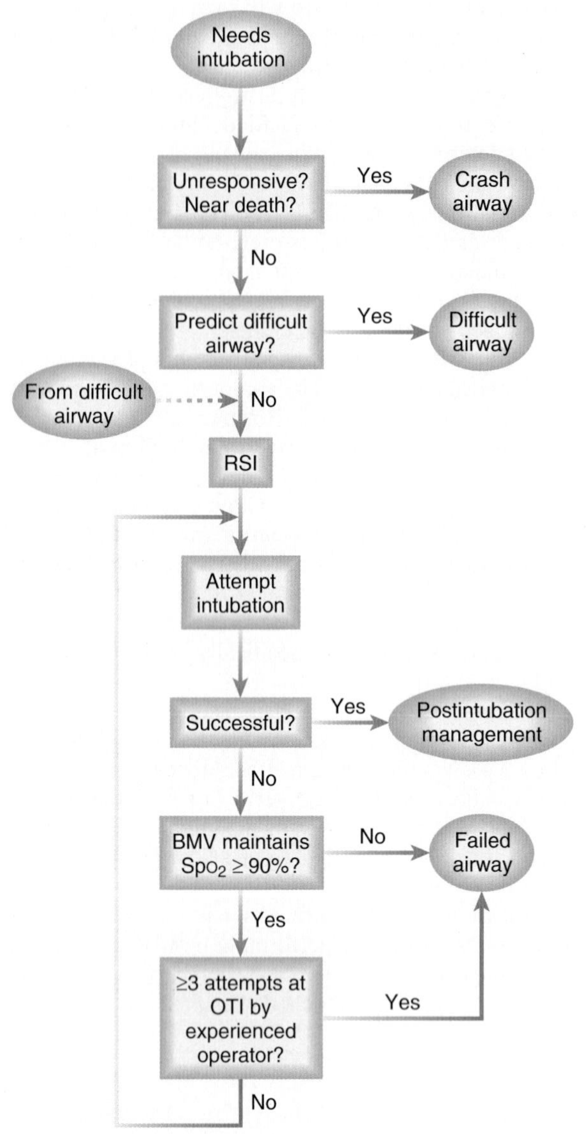


**Fig. 1.2 Main emergency airway management algorithm.** *BMV*, Bag-mask ventilation; *OTI*, orotracheal intubation; *RSI*, rapid-sequence intubation; *$Spo_2$*, pulse oximetry. (Adapted from Walls RM: The emergency airway algorithms. In Walls RM, Luten RC, Murphy MF, et al, editors. Manual of emergency airway management. 2nd ed. Philadelphia: Lippincott Williams & Wilkins, 2004. Copyright 2004: The Airway Course and Lippincott Williams & Wilkins.)

## INTUBATION

Orotracheal intubation is now the preferred method of emergency intubation, either by direct laryngoscopy or by video laryngoscopy.[44-46] The process of intubation includes proper patient positioning, clinician positioning, tool choice and assembly, and technique of laryngoscopy. In performing standard oral intubation, the patient lies flat and supine while positioning of the patient's head is addressed.[44] Patients with immobile cervical spines, whether secondary to trauma, arthritis, or other causes, should not have their heads or necks manipulated, and the head should be maintained in a neutral position with in-line stabilization by a person designated for this task.[45,46] If mobility is not an issue, the age of the patient and size of the occiput determine the need for elevation of the patient's shoulders or head. Infants have a relatively large occiput with respect to their bodies and will therefore passively flex their head forward when lying flat.[47] This makes a more acute angle that the laryngoscopist has to navigate. The airway axes will align better if the infant's shoulders are elevated. An adult's head is relatively smaller and tends to extend at the cervicothoracic junction instead of flexing. This counterintuitively moves the laryngeal and pharyngeal axes into an alignment that is less parallel and can be overcome by placing a roll under the adult's head.[47] A key anatomic relationship to keep in mind is that the head is ideally aligned when an imaginary line drawn between the tragus of the ear and the anterior axillary line is parallel to the floor.

Standard orotracheal intubation is performed with the practitioner at the head of the bed looking down at the patient's face. The clinician gently grasps the laryngoscope with the fingertips of the left hand. Using the right hand, the clinician opens the patient's mouth in either a scissoring technique with the thumb and index finger or by grasping the mentum and moving it caudally to expose the mouth. The blade of the laryngoscope is then gently inserted into the right side of the mouth and advanced into the pharynx.

The direct laryngoscope blades most commonly used for emergency intubation are the curved Macintosh blade and the straight Miller blade. Traditional intubation with the Macintosh blade begins with insertion of the blade at the right corner of the mouth. The blade is advanced under direct visualization, is swept to the midline, and concomitantly sweeps the tongue to the patient's left. The tip of the blade is directed into the vallecula, and the laryngoscope is then pushed up as a unit. The epiglottis is lifted up because of its connection to the hyoepiglottic ligament, which attaches to the posterior surface of the mucosa behind the hyoid and the base of the epiglottis. Lifting of the epiglottis exposes the vocal cords and glottis.

Traditional intubation with the Miller blade is similarly performed by inserting the blade in the right side of the mouth and maintaining the position of the blade on the right side of the tongue while the blade is inserted to the epiglottis, again under direct visualization. Tongue control is a major issue, with the blade pushing the tongue upward and to the left. The laryngoscope is then pushed upward to physically lift the epiglottis and expose the vocal cords.

Video laryngoscopic intubation is the newest method of orotracheal intubation and has developed into a valid option for primary intubation in the majority of patients. Multiple options exist, and each has its own method of how it is used.[48] The benefit of these devices is that they routinely provide a laryngoscopic view superior to that possible with direct laryngoscopy in the vast majority of patients in whom they are used.[42,43,49,50] The angles required for passage of the tube may sometimes present the key challenge, so this is an additional focal point of training. As with any video-based system, the principal downside is the potential for obstruction of the operator's view if blood, vomitus, or excessive secretions are present in the oropharynx.

Finally, nasotracheal intubation is another option for intubation, although its use is decreasing in favor of directly visualized oral intubation. Nasotracheal intubation requires a breathing patient because the patient's breath sounds will guide the intubator in placing the tube. Nasotracheal intubation should not be considered a primary mode of intubation because its success rate has clearly been shown to be lower than that of orotracheal intubation with RSI.[51]

## MEDICATIONS, PHARMACOLOGY, AND PHYSIOLOGIC RESPONSES TO MEDICATION CLASSES

### SEDATIVE AGENTS

Multiple sedatives can be used for RSI. Use of a sedative humanely allows amnesia and sedation, thereby potentially improving laryngoscopy and intubation.[41] The choice of sedative agent for a given clinical scenario differs according to the pathophysiologic parameters that the clinician observes or anticipates to occur during the attempt at RSI. Hemodynamic instability, elevated intracranial pressure, and bronchospasm are some of the most common complicating factors that the clinician must consider during preparation for sedation. A list of sedative agents used for RSI and their side effect profiles can be found in **Table 1.2**.

The most commonly used sedatives in current emergency practice include midazolam (Versed) and etomidate (Amidate). Doses of midazolam recommended in the anesthesia literature are 0.1 to 0.3 mg/kg intravenously. The danger of using midazolam in these doses is the hypotension that it generates, especially in critically ill patients. Most practitioners will intentionally underdose midazolam in the setting of RSI for this specific reason.[52]

Etomidate is administered at a dose of 0.3 mg/kg intravenously and does not cause the hypotension seen with midazolam.[52-54] Etomidate does cause reversible cortisol suppression, however, and is no longer used as a drip for long-term sedation. The effect on cortisol after a single dose has been demonstrated to resolve spontaneously and has not been shown to have an effect on patient outcome.[55] Controversy has recently developed regarding the use of etomidate in patients with sepsis. One major study reportedly identified etomidate as a causal agent in increasing mortality in this patient population.[56,57] However, this study was underpowered and not designed to look for this concern, and its findings were based on post hoc analysis of the study results.[58] At least one small-scale study has demonstrated no increase in mortality between etomidate and midazolam in this setting.[59] No large-scale study exists at the time of this writing to specifically answer this question, but with the overwhelming success of single-dose etomidate in emergency intubations, definitive studies would be necessary to change practice.

### NEUROMUSCULAR BLOCKING AGENTS (PARALYTICS)

The paralytics commonly used for RSI include depolarizing agents (succinylcholine) and nondepolarizing agents (vecuronium, rocuronium). Succinylcholine has been studied extensively and is the classic agent used for RSI. It has a short time of onset (approximately 45 seconds), a short duration of action (approximately 5 to 10 minutes), and a wide dosing margin (the typical dose for RSI is 1.5 mg/kg, but doses up to 6 mg/kg do not change its pharmacokinetics).[60] Succinylcholine also has some significant side effects, including occasionally significant hyperkalemia, fasciculations, and malignant hyperthermia. Any airway manager who plans to use succinylcholine should be well versed in its mechanism of action, as well as its potentially significant and life-threatening side effects[61,62] (**Box 1.5**).

Rocuronium has recently come into favor as a nondepolarizing agent that can provide succinylcholine-like intubating conditions in 45 to 60 seconds, provided that the correct dose (1.0 to 1.2 mg/kg intravenously) is used.[63-66] The benefits of using a nondepolarizing agent include the absence of fasciculations and hyperkalemia. The duration of action of nondepolarizing agents is much longer than that of succinylcholine, however, with rocuronium being the shortest acting at 45 to 60 minutes. See **Table 1.3** for a list of commonly used nondepolarizing paralytic agents.

### PRETREATMENT AGENTS

Some medications have the potential to aid in promoting physiologic responses to intubation if given as pretreatment agents. The typical laryngoscopy in an adult will result in sympathetic stimulation that could be detrimental in certain

**Table 1.2** Sedative Agents

| AGENT | RECOMMENDED DOSE | TIME TO ONSET | DURATION OF ACTION | USEFUL ATTRIBUTES |
|---|---|---|---|---|
| Etomidate | 0.3 mg/kg IV | 15-45 sec | 3-12 min | Hemodynamic stability |
| Midazolam (benzodiazepine) | 0.1-0.3 mg/kg IV | 30-60 sec | 15-30 min | Commonly used, familiarity |
| Ketamine | 1.5 mg/kg IV | 45-60 sec | 10-20 min | Sympathetic "kick," bronchodilation |
| Propofol | 1.5-3 mg/kg IV | 15-45 sec | 5-10 min | Bronchodilation |
| Thiopental (barbiturate) | 1-6 mg/kg IV | <30 sec | 5-10 min | Standard agent before the advent of other classes |

**BOX 1.5 Succinylcholine—Critical Points**

Dose: 1.5 mg/kg intravenously (range, 1-3 mg/kg)
Mechanism of action: depolarizing neuromuscular blockade. Succinylcholine binds to acetylcholine receptors and stimulates continual depolarization, which results in paralysis
Side effects:
- Hyperkalemia (sometimes fatal in patients with preexisting hyperkalemia)
- Fasciculations
- Increased intraocular pressure
- Increased intragastric pressure
- Bradycardia in children
- Malignant hyperthermia
- Masseter spasm in children (requires a nondepolarizing agent [rocuronium, vecuronium] to overcome)

**Table 1.3 Nondepolarizing Agents**

| AGENT | RECOMMENDED DOSE | TIME TO ONSET | DURATION OF ACTION |
|---|---|---|---|
| Rocuronium | 1 mg/kg IV | 45-60 sec | 30-60 min |
| Vercuronium | 0.1 mg/kg IV | 90-120 sec | 60-75 min |

**Table 1.4 Pretreatment Agents**

| AGENT | RECOMMENDED DOSE | PROPOSED ACTION |
|---|---|---|
| Lidocaine | 1.5 mg/kg IV | Blunt bronchospasm, blunt the reflexive response to laryngoscopy |
| Opioid (fentanyl) | 1.5 mcg/kg IV | Blunt the reflexive response to laryngoscopy |
| Atropine | 0.01 mg/kg IV | Avoid bradycardia in children receiving succinylcholine |

cases. Patients with asthma, elevated intracranial pressure, aortic dissection, hypertensive emergencies, and acute myocardial infarction have pathophysiology that could be worsened by an increase in sympathetic stimulation.[67] Intravenous lidocaine, 1.5 mg/kg, has potential benefit in attenuating bronchospasm[68,69] and increases in intracranial pressure[70,71] when given as a premedication 2 to 3 minutes before RSI. Opioids (e.g., fentanyl, 1 to 5 mcg/kg intravenously 2 to 3 minutes before RSI) may have benefit in attenuating increases in intracranial pressure[72] and reflexive, sympathetic hemodynamic responses to intubation.[73,74] A body of literature indirectly supports the select use of these medications in critical airway management (**Table 1.4**). Laryngoscopy or the succinylcholine dosage in pediatric patients can result in

**BOX 1.6 Assumptions for Emergency Rapid-Sequence Intubation**

The airway has to be secured.
The patient's stomach is full.
The patient has unstable hemodynamics or has the potential to become hemodynamically unstable.
The patient's condition is critical and time is of the essence.

**BOX 1.7 The Seven P's of Rapid Sequence Intubation**

1. Preparation (airway assessment, tool assembly, positioning)
2. Preoxygenation
3. Premedications (if indicated)
4. Paralysis with sedation
5. Protection of the airway with the Sellick maneuver
6. Passage of the tube and confirmation
7. Postintubation management

parasympathetic stimulation and resultant bradycardia, which has led some experts to advocate a pretreatment dose of atropine before attempts at pediatric intubation. Current recommendations are to use atropine for all intubations in children younger than 1 year and to have the drug available for those older than 1 year.[47]

## PUTTING IT TOGETHER: RAPID-SEQUENCE INTUBATION

RSI is the technique of combining sedation and paralysis to create the most optimal intubating conditions during emergency intubation (**Box 1.6**).[1,9,22,41,75] Seven checklist points have been identified to help clinicians prepare for emergency RSI (**Box 1.7**).[22] Also known as the 7 P's, this or a similar checklist can be used during each intubation in which airway managers participate.[22] This tool should be viewed as a patient safety device and an error minimization instrument. As with any high-stakes activity, the use of memory aids and algorithms can reduce the cognitive load associated with decision making and allow the practitioner to focus on the specific task at hand.[76]

Protection of the airway refers to the use of cricoid ring pressure (Sellick maneuver) during the process of paralysis, intubation, and confirmation of endotracheal placement. The cricoid ring is compressed with an assistant's index finger and thumb in an attempt to compress the underlying esophagus and prevent passive regurgitation of stomach contents into the trachea.[77,78] The amount of force recommended is equivalent to the amount required to create discomfort when pressing with the same fingers on the bridge of the nose.[19] Some studies have identified improper Sellick maneuver technique as a potential obstruction to laryngoscopy and placement of the endotracheal tube (ETT), but it might help prevent gastric insufflation during attempts at bag-mask ventilation and is currently recommended if resources permit.[19]

The sixth step is passage of the tube. Laryngoscopy is performed at approximately 1 minute after the paralytic agent has been administered. The ETT is placed under direct vision (either line of sight or with video monitoring) through the cords and into the trachea. An adult man should typically have the tube placed orally to a depth of 24 cm, and an adult woman should typically have the tube inserted to 21 cm. A general rule of thumb is that the ETT should be inserted to three times its size.[79] Placement of the ETT is considered complete once objective verification of placement has occurred, typically by end-tidal carbon dioxide detection.[80,81]

## SUMMARY

Emergency airway management involves a combination of techniques and strategies designed to ensure success of intubation in critically ill patients. The approach to an emergency airway is necessarily different from that taken for an elective or urgent case. The airway manager must have a solid foundation in ventilation techniques (bag-mask, extraglottic devices), which will be the first rescue device. Assessment of the airway is a critical skill that mandates a methodic approach to ensure that a difficult airway is recognized and appropriately planned for. The use of RSI has revolutionized emergency intubation, and a set of strategies is required to deal with routine intubations and difficult airways. Management of difficult airways is discussed in Chapter 2.

## SUGGESTED READINGS

Hung OR, Murphy MF. Management of the difficult and failed airway. New York: McGraw Hill; 2008.

Walls RM, Murphy MF. Manual of emergency airway management. 3rd ed. Philadelphia: Lippincott Williams & Wilkins; 2008.

## REFERENCES

***References can be found on Expert Consult @ www.expertconsult.com.***

# 2 Advanced Airway Techniques

*Aaron E. Bair and Erik G. Laurin*

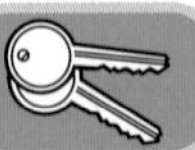

**KEY POINTS**

- Advanced airway management is predicated on selecting the right technical approach for a given patient.
- Anticipated difficult airway management often relies on a sedated (or "awake") technique.
- An organized approach (and backup plan) is essential for success with an unanticipated difficult airway.

## PERSPECTIVE

The cognitive skills to determine when a patient requires airway support are as important as the manual skills to accomplish the task. Currently, rapid-sequence intubation (RSI) is the most frequently used and successful means of intubating the trachea in emergency medical practice.[1-4] It is clear that combining the use of a paralytic agent with a sedative agent has resulted in more successful laryngoscopy.[5,6] This has led to fewer failed airways. Because every attempt at intubation may be difficult, a prepared and practiced backup or contingency plan is vital. The discussion of the various techniques and adjunctive measures that follows in this chapter reflects their application within an overall strategy.

In some cases the use of paralytics (i.e., RSI) is inappropriate because of a relatively high likelihood of intubation failure and subsequent worsening of the clinical condition linked to intubation attempts and the probability of failed ventilation. Accordingly, it is important to distinguish patients who are likely to be difficult to intubate, ventilate, and rescue (which often means performing a cricothyrotomy). These concepts are emphasized by the LEMON, MOANS, and SHORT mnemonics[7] covered in Chapter 1. What follows is an overview of a strategic approach to advanced emergency airway management.

### EPIDEMIOLOGY

A difficult airway (a case in which intubation is difficult to achieve) in the emergency department (ED) is far less studied but is probably experienced more frequently than in the more controlled environment of the operating suite. Patient extremis and lack of patient preparation make encountering both anticipated and unanticipated difficult airways more likely, with some estimates as high as 20%.[8] Fortunately, however, the frequency of intubation failure in the ED is much lower and approximates 1%.[3,9,10] The prevalence of airways requiring rescue from previous failed attempts in the ED is difficult to determine. What is apparent is that rescue devices are not used routinely, although they are commonly available.[11,12]

### ANTICIPATED DIFFICULTY

Multiple predictors related to airway anatomy have been reported in the anesthesia literature, but none have been shown to be useful in isolation for predicting intubation difficulty.[13-18] However, some evidence suggests the use of a limited set of assessments in patients undergoing airway management in the ED. The LEMON mnemonic has been proposed for this purpose[19,20] (**Box 2.1**) (see Chapter 1). If difficulty is predictable and the patient is not a suitable candidate for RSI, the optimal approach depends on the previous training of the intubator and the availability of advanced airway tools.

### UNANTICIPATED DIFFICULTY

Every patient in any environment has the potential for unexpectedly being difficult to intubate. Unexpectedly encountering blood, emesis, a mass, an anatomic variant, or evolving traumatic injury can all result in a challenging airway. In this chapter we attempt to organize and briefly define some of the many rescue techniques that might be used in emergency practice.

## ANTICIPATED DIFFICULT AIRWAY

Only a small fraction of patients undergoing ED intubation are actually deemed poor candidates for RSI, even though many patients are expected to be difficult to intubate. No discreet threshold at which RSI is deemed to be safe and when it is contraindicated has ever been determined, partly because of the lack of sensitivity of the various difficult airway prediction tools. Importantly, many ED patients are in extremis and unable to cooperate with a preprocedural examination.[21,22] Much of what is discussed in the current literature is based on the anesthesia experience, which generally reflects the "elective" intubation of cooperative patients. Nevertheless, it is often useful to perform a preprocedural assessment, as allowed by time constraints and the patient's condition. Some

**BOX 2.1 LEMON Mnemonic for Possible Difficult Intubation**

**L**ook to see whether an obvious abnormality is present
**E**valuate the 3-3-2 rule
**M**allampati assessment
**O**bstruction of the upper airway
**N**eck immobility

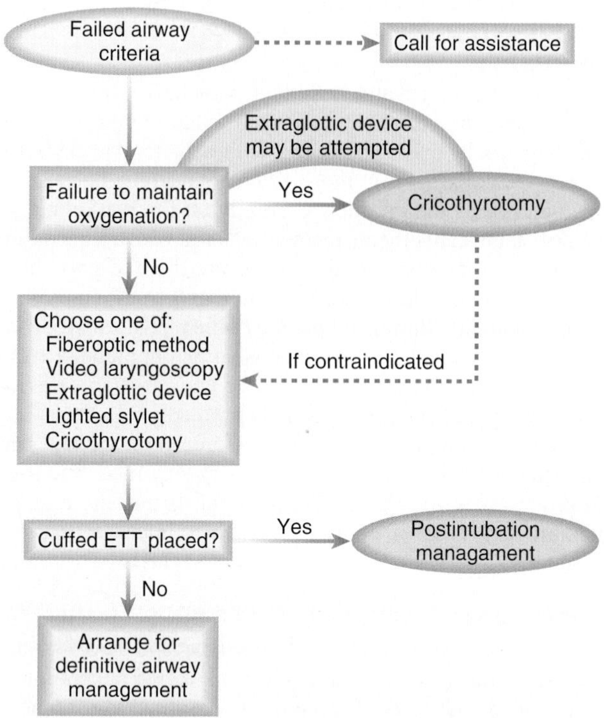


**Fig. 2.1 Difficult airway algorithm.** *ETT*, Endotracheal tube. (Adapted from Walls BM. The emergency airway algorithms. In: Walls RM, Murphy MF, editors. Manual of emergency airway management. 3rd ed. Philadelphia: Lippincott Williams & Wilkins; 2008.)

evaluation is necessary to be able to accurately estimate the potential for encountering a difficult airway.

The algorithm presented in **Figure 2.1** represents a clinical approach to a difficult airway.[7] Application of such an approach is predicated on the answers to several key questions:

- Is there enough time to plan a methodic approach?
- Despite the identified presence of difficult airway predictors, can RSI still be used safely?
- Is the patient's oxygenation adequate?

Understanding these issues in context to a given clinical scenario will help in the decision-making process regarding alternative approaches.

## RAPID-SEQUENCE INTUBATION FOR A DIFFICULT AIRWAY

RSI is preferred for the vast majority of intubations performed in the ED. It is important to realize that provider familiarity will probably be the major determinant regarding device and technique selection beyond the use of RSI. For this reason it is prudent to focus on techniques that are likely to remain familiar through frequent use. Accordingly, the use of optimized and augmented laryngoscopy merits discussion because these concepts are simply extensions of "routine" RSI.

## OPTIMIZED LARYNGOSCOPY

Routine direct laryngoscopy relies on manipulation of the soft tissues of the hypopharynx and the base of the tongue into the relatively fixed proportions of the mandible. The goal of such manipulation is to allow a direct line of sight to the larynx and vocal cords. This, however, can be difficult given certain unalterable variables of patient anatomy. The process of optimizing the view is probably the simplest and often the least appreciated of the skills of an expert airway manager. The features of optimization are discussed in the following sections.

### Head and Neck Positioning

In the absence of cervical spine immobilization, active range of neck flexion and extension can frequently provide markedly improved visualization.[23]

### External Laryngeal Manipulation

External manipulation of the larynx is distinct from the familiar cricoid pressure concept (e.g., the Sellick maneuver). It is, however, related to BURP (**b**ackward, **u**pward, **r**ightward **p**ressure). The process of laryngeal manipulation is active. It requires that the intubator actively move the larynx to maximize visualization of the laryngeal structures. Generally, once the view is optimized, an assistant will be required to maintain the preferred positioning.[24-26]

### Facility with Various Blade Types

Laryngoscope blade types come in various sizes and shapes and therefore have various advantages and disadvantages. In general, two formats are used with regularity: curved (e.g., Macintosh) and straight (e.g., Miller). Curved blades are often best for sweeping the tongue laterally. Some patients may be difficult to intubate because of an elongated or anteriorly oriented vallecula and epiglottis. In such cases, a straight blade may prove to be useful. Although most practitioners will have a preferred blade, it is important to maintain facility with both general blade types because they often have offsetting advantages. Additionally, a multitude of variably profiled laryngoscopes with adjunctive prisms and mirrors are available. These devices are not frequently used in emergency practice.

## AUGMENTED LARYNGOSCOPY

This concept refers to using an assistive device to either extend the view of the intubator (i.e., fiberoptic stylet) or assist in tube placement with use of a narrow-diameter introducer. Such introducers have been used for decades and come in various formats (i.e., Eschmann, Frova). The leading tip of these introducers is angled anteriorly to provide tactile feedback regarding location of the introducer. These devices can be valuable when visualization is limited.

## ALTERNATIVE TECHNIQUES FOR THE ANTICIPATED DIFFICULT AIRWAY

### *Fiberoptics*

As a class, directable and flexible scopes have been available for decades. They have recently been made more portable by replacing the heavy light source with a battery pack. These devices are consequently more convenient in the harried ED. The majority of the products currently on the market consist of a directable cable mechanism associated with a light source and fiberoptic bundle. Notable issues are that the glass fibers that constitute the optics are breakable and small amounts of debris can greatly diminish viewing quality. Historically, these devices were considered too expensive or impractical. In the future, however, these type of flexible and directable devices will probably become more available. To date, relatively little research relevant to emergency medicine practice has been conducted.[2,27-29] A recent query of emergency medicine training programs in the United States suggests that the majority maintain this type of equipment,[11] but clinical expertise is variable.

FLEXIBLE AND DIRECTABLE FIBEROPTICS Flexible and directable fiberoptic models are portable and have variable diameters and lengths. This equipment varies depending on its intended purpose. The shorter nasopharyngoscope is approximately 35 cm in length, in contrast to the 60-cm bronchoscope. The goal is to directly visualize the glottis via the nares or mouth. Once the cords are visualized, the tip of the fiberoptic scope is advanced into the airway to the level of the carina. The preloaded endotracheal tube is then advanced over the scope and into the airway. Efficacy of this technique in an awake patient requires adequate patient and equipment preparation (**Box 2.2**).

FLEXIBLE AND NONDIRECTABLE FIBEROPTICS Flexible and nondirectable fiberoptics have been designed to be used from within the lumen of an endotracheal tube. They all share in common the issues related to obscuration of view with debris. Additionally, any attempt to direct the tip of the device relies on manipulation of the associated endotracheal tube with visual feedback through either an eyepiece or video monitor. Despite these shortcomings, these devices are attractive because the nondirectable group is generally regarded as more durable and tends to be less expensive. An example of this type of device is the Trach View (Parker Medical, Englewood, CO).

SEMIRIGID FIBEROPTICS The semirigid fiberoptic scope is, conceptually, a semimalleable stylet with internal fiberoptic bundles.[34] These devices are similar to the nondirectable class

**BOX 2.2 Patient Preparation**

If using a nasal approach, adequate topical anesthesia and vasoconstriction can be achieved with various agents via an atomizer.

If using an oral approach, various spray anesthetic agents can be used in addition to a nebulized agents (e.g., lidocaine). Additionally, gargled lidocaine (4%) can be effective, patient cooperation permitting.

An antisialagogue (e.g., glycopyrrolate) can be useful to allow better tissue absorption of topical anesthetic agents. However, at least 20 minutes is needed for efficacy as a drying agent.

Sedation is used, as necessary, to achieve reasonable anxiolysis to improve patient cooperation.

Preoxygenation, as always, is fundamental to procedural sedation and airway management.

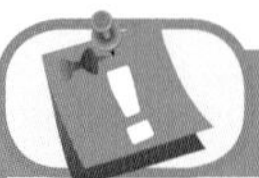

**TIPS AND TRICKS**

Even though a complete tutorial of the technical details of using flexible fiberoptics is beyond the scope of this review, several technique pearls are worth highlighting:

1. Recognize that the procedure will take at least 15 to 20 minutes to accomplish. If the patient cannot tolerate such a wait, use of this technique may be misguided.
2. Stay in the anatomic midline at all times during the procedure. Straying laterally will often result in poor visualization and inability to pass the vocal cords.
3. Keep the slack out of the scope. If slack is present along the length of the scope, rotation of the body of the scope will not translate into rotation of the tip.
4. The size of the working channel in many scopes is often too small for suction to be effective.
5. If the tube is resistant to passage of the scope into the airway, it is likely that the tip of the tube, or Murphy's eye, is caught at the level of the arytenoids. Rotation of the *entire* tube-scope apparatus 45 to 90 degrees will probably overcome the obstruction.
6. Further considerations:
   - Nasal approach. This route may be better tolerated by the patient and will not subject the equipment to damage from biting by the patient. However, it is prone to cause bleeding with passage of the tube. Adequate vasoconstriction is key. Partially intubating the chosen naris with the endotracheal tube can often simplify the procedure by avoiding the obscuring materials in the nasopharynx. Beware, however, that placing the tip of the tube too deep into the posterior pharynx will make subsequent scope manipulation challenging because of the acute angle that will be required for the tip of the scope to reach the glottis. Optimally, the tip of the endotracheal tube should be placed at the level of the uvula before attempting to advance the scope to the vocal cords.
   - Oral approach. This may be advantageous if a larger endotracheal tube is needed. However, a bite block or a device that provides an oropharyngeal conduit may be necessary if there is a possibility of the patient biting the equipment. Additionally, a fiberoptic technique can be used in conjunction with a second provider using a laryngoscope to manipulate the soft tissues of the oropharynx.
   - Adjunctive use. Use of flexible fiberoptics through a laryngeal mask airway or similar device has been described.[30-33]

of fiberoptics with respect to image quality and durability. An example of this type of device is the Shikani optical stylet (Clarus Medical, LLC, Minneapolis, MN).

RIGID FIBEROPTICS Rigid fiberoptic scopes consist of an imaging bundle enclosed within a rigid L- or J-shaped assembly. This shape is designed for placement into the hypopharynx with subsequent indirect visualization of the glottis. One of the chief advantages of these devices is that limited head, neck, and jaw mobility is less of a concern because of the ability to "look around the corner" of the hypopharynx. Examples in this class are the Bullard (Circon Corporation, Stanford, CT),[35-37] WuScope Tubular Fiberoptic Laryngoscope (Achi Corporation, San Jose, CA),[38-41] and UpsherScope (Mercury Medical, Inc., Clearwater, FL).[42,43] These scopes are relatively expensive and their availability in the ED has been limited.[11]

### Optical Laryngoscopy

Optical laryngoscopes use a series of lenses to provide a view of the anterior aspect of the glottis that is often not possible with direct laryngoscopy. Although image quality is inferior to that of video laryngoscopes, optical laryngoscopes are inexpensive, durable, and portable tools for difficult airway management. An example is the Airtraq, a disposable optical laryngoscope with a J-shaped blade that allows visualization of the glottis with the head and neck in a neutral position. In small randomized and nonrandomized studies, the Airtraq improved glottic exposure, reduced intubation difficulty scores, decreased cervical spine motion, and caused less change in the heart rate than did direct laryngoscopy with a Macintosh laryngoscope.[44-46]

### Video Laryngoscopy

Video laryngoscopes use either a micro video camera or more traditional fiberoptic bundles encased in a laryngoscope handle design. Placement of the camera is meant to provide a wide-angle view of the glottis but is somewhat more removed from the various debris issues often encountered with the optics-in-the-tube format. The GlideScope (Verathon, Inc., Bothell, WA) is an example of the micro video camera design. This device is relatively new with limited ED experience.[47] The literature that exists suggests that it can be used with very little motion of the cervical spine and that glottic visualization is generally excellent.[48-51] However, actual intubation may be a bit more of a challenge because it requires an extreme "hockey stick" angulation of the styletted endotracheal tube to reach the glottis. Currently, laryngoscope sizes available correspond roughly to Macintosh No. 4 and No. 2, as well as pediatric sizes.

Additionally, video has been adapted to the more familiar Macintosh blade format in the current C-MAC (Karl Storz, Tuttlingen, Germany). The video element has been shown to improve the grade of view in ED patients[52] and in simulated patients with difficult airways.[53]

### Awake Techniques

In the context of a difficult airway the role of an awake technique may be (1) to determine the status of airway landmarks (with the intention of performing RSI if the landmarks are recognizable) or (2) to perform the intubation given the need for the patient to maintain spontaneous respirations. Either may be accomplished with direct laryngoscopy. A confirmatory look may also be done with a flexible fiberoptic scope.

The term "awake" is a misnomer. It is important to realize that a better descriptor of this concept would be "sedated." In a patient who is currently maintaining some airway tone and respiratory drive, this approach may be indicated when difficult intubation and ventilation are both anticipated. This approach may be somewhat time consuming because adequate sedation and topical anesthesia of the airway are required (**Box 2.3**). However, its advantage is that patients will be able to breathe on their own during attempts at definitively controlling the airway. It is important to understand the underlying pathologic process with respect to its dynamic impact on the airway. For instance, a quick look to determine the risks associated with RSI may be misleading if rapid swelling from burns or angioedema are evolving during the process. This

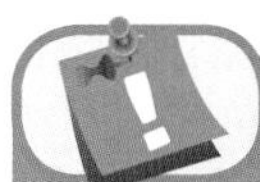

**TIPS AND TRICKS**

**GlideScope Use**

- The GlideScope handle stays in the midline—no tongue sweep.
- The handle is *not* used to lift, unlike a more familiar laryngoscope.
- To accommodate the approach to the glottis, the endotracheal tube with stylet will need an acute angle (approximately 90 degrees).
- To accommodate advancement of the tube off the stylet, it may help to partially withdraw the stylet during tube advancement. Generally, this last step will require coordination with an assistant.

**BOX 2.3 Patient Sedation and Topical Anesthesia: A Recipe**

**Nasal (Anesthesia and Vasoconstriction)**

- Only needed if the nasal route is anticipated
- Oxymetazoline (0.05%)/lidocaine (1%), 1:1 in a mucosal atomizer, 10 mL total
- Use preservative-free (cardiac) lidocaine to avoid the rare allergic reaction to preservatives
- Provides effective anesthesia and vasoconstriction
- Time: 2 to 3 minutes

**Oral**

- Lidocaine (4%), 30 mL gargle and spit
- Time: 1 to 2 minutes

**Glottis**

- Lidocaine (1% to 4%, preservative free), 10 mL in a nebulizer
- Time: 10 minutes

**Sedation**

- The goal is only light sedation
- Deep procedural sedation defeats the purpose and may lead to airway obstruction

concept should be kept in mind inasmuch as an initial look may be reassuring but subsequent attempts may be profoundly disappointing because of a dynamic clinical process.

### Blind Nasotracheal Intubation

The overall success rate of blind nasotracheal intubation is lower than that of RSI.[54,55] Additionally, such intubation can be complicated by nasal hemorrhage and induction of vomiting (with its associated risk of aspiration). However, it is often an expedient option in patients who still have fairly vigorous spontaneous respirations.

### Light Wand

In general, light wand intubation does not rely on visualization of any internal structure. Instead, it relies on a transmitted glow of light through the soft tissues of the neck. The skill required for its application depends largely on recognizing midline (i.e., tracheal) versus lateral soft tissue placement. The Trachlight has been shown to be useful in the operating suite,[56-60] but ED experience has been limited. Its design and the necessity for a pronounced L-shaped curve in the stylet and endotracheal tube make it rather forgiving of difficult anatomy that might otherwise inhibit direct laryngoscopy. It is important to note that proper tube placement and preparation of the device do take a few minutes. To make it more useful as a rescue device and more amenable to quick grab deployment, it should be prepared and stored in a ready-to-use condition.

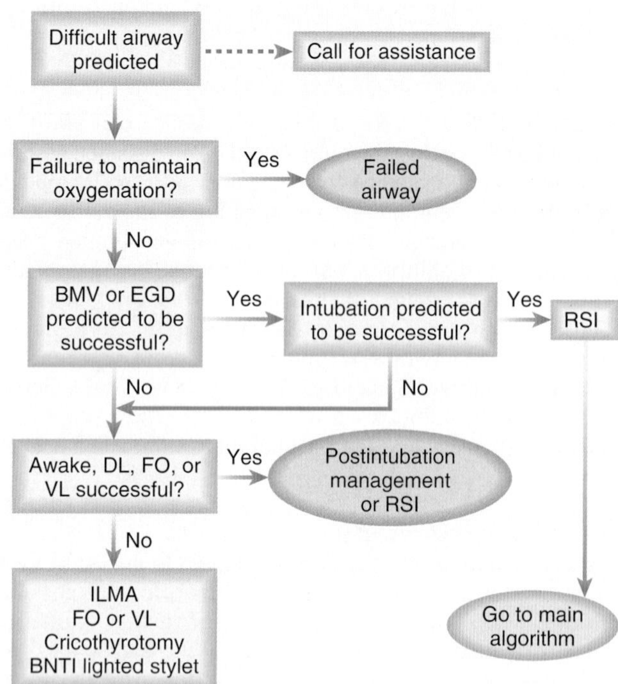


**Fig. 2.2 Failed airway algorithm.** *BMV*, Bag-mask ventilation; *BNTI*, blind nasotracheal intubation; *DL*, direct laryngoscopy; *EGD*, extraglottic device; *FO*, fiberoptic; *ILMA*, intubating laryngeal mask airway; *RSI*, rapid-sequence intubation; *VL*, video laryngoscopy. (Adapted from Walls RM. The emergency airway alorithm. In: Walls RM, Murphy MF, editors. Manual of emergency airway management. 3rd ed. Philadelphia: Lippincott Williams & Wilkins; 2008.)

## THE UNANTICIPATED DIFFICULT AIRWAY

The concept of an unanticipated difficult airway generally presupposes that an attempt at intubation has already been made. It is often a situation that necessitates a change from the original strategy used and requires a fresh perspective. Even though failed intubation attempts are infrequent, they do occur and a rational backup or rescue plan must be in place. Ultimately, the choice of rescue devices is limited by simple availability or experience with use. We will attempt to highlight the various classes of devices that appear promising for use in emergency practice.

The difficult airway and failed airway are related but distinct concepts. A difficult airway becomes a failed airway after three attempts at intubation by a skilled operator. From this point, subsequent maneuvers are in large part directed by operator familiarity and skill. However, the key branch point in the decision-making process depends on the adequacy of ventilation. The "can't intubate, can ventilate" scenario is managed differently from the "can't intubate, can't ventilate" scenario. Each of these situations will be approached within the concept of the failed airway algorithm (**Fig. 2.2**).

### CAN'T INTUBATE, CAN VENTILATE

Successful ventilation is defined as being able to maintain oxygen saturation above 90% with bag-mask ventilation. In this situation the provider has some time to direct further efforts and take advantage of any opportunity for success as identified on previous attempts. A directed response might include optimizing or augmenting a previously failed RSI with maneuvers discussed previously. Additionally, it may include the use of alternative intubation devices.

### Tracheal Introducer

The tracheal introducer has been in use since the 1940s, and several products are currently available on the market. The Eschmann introducer is also known as the gum elastic bougie. Incidentally, this term is a misnomer because it is not a bougie (e.g., dilator), nor is it made from gum. Instead, it is a woven Dacron rod 30 cm long that is coated with resin for durability and added stiffness. Newer products have also recently arrived on the market (e.g., Frova, Cook Medical, Bloomington, IN). These introducers are used in conjunction with direct laryngoscopy, especially when the vocal cords cannot be visualized. Their design helps access an extremely anterior trachea and confirm proper placement. One of these design features is an angulated tip that allows directable manipulation and tactile feedback. The tip clicks as it bumps along the anterior tracheal rings. The absence of clicks may suggest esophageal placement. Additionally, if the introducer is in the airway, a hard stop will be felt as the introducer gently passes from the trachea into a small-diameter airway. In contrast, if the introducer is mistakenly placed in the esophagus, the operator will be able to advance the introducer without a firm end point as the introducer enters the stomach.[61-65] Once these tactile indicators suggest tracheal placement, a standard endotracheal tube can then be advanced over the introducer and into the trachea.

### The Laryngeal Mask Airway

The laryngeal mask airway (LMA) currently has several variations in format, one of which, the intubating LMA (ILMA, e.g., Fastrach), is shown in **Figure 2.3**. This device has been

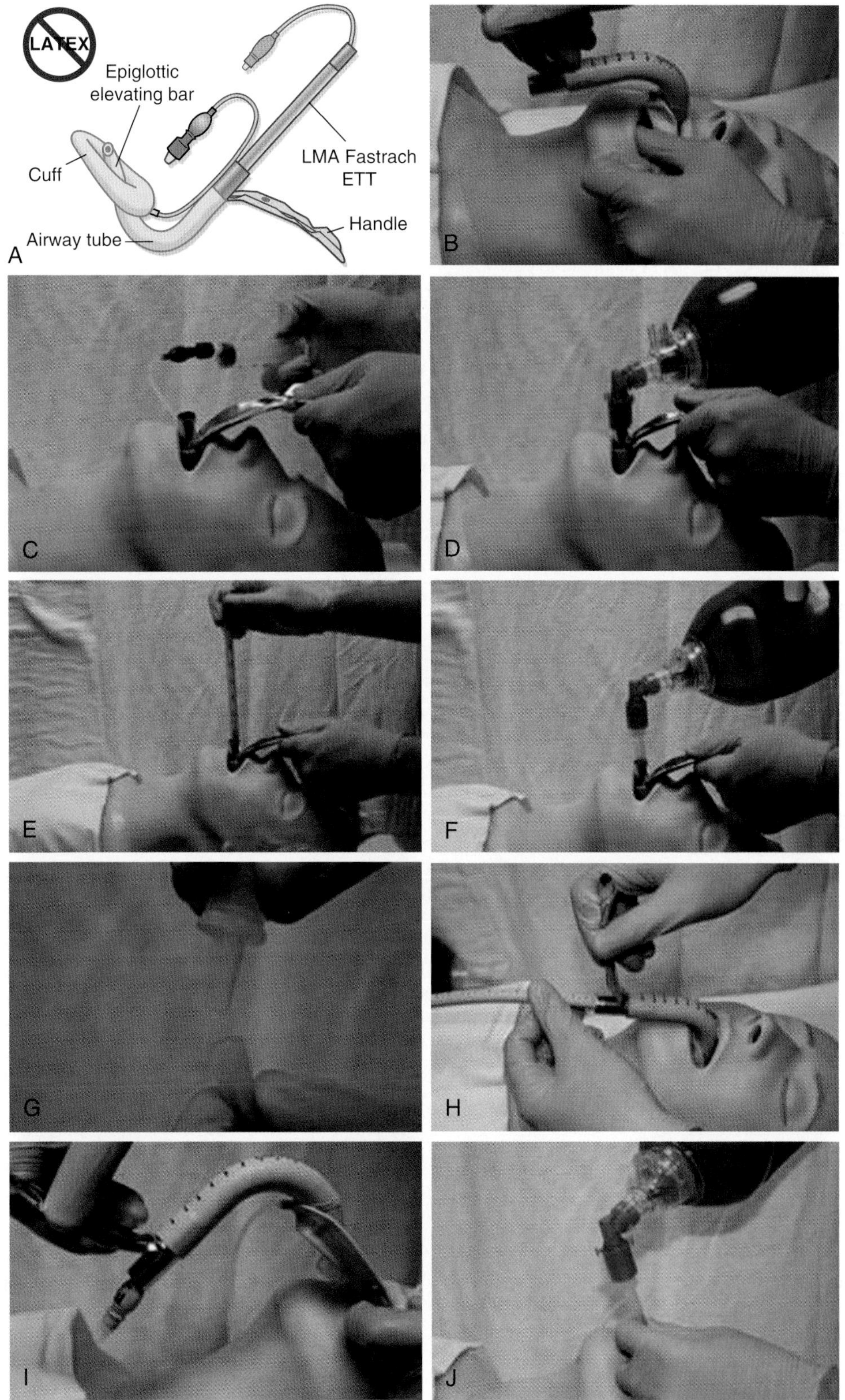


**Fig. 2.3 Intubating laryngeal mask airway (ILMA) (Fastrach). A,** The ILMA. **B,** Place in the oropharynx. **C,** Position and inflate the ILMA cuff. **D,** Ventilate the patient with the ILMA. **E,** Place the ETT into the ILMA. **F,** Ventilate the patient with the ETT. **G,** Remove the adaptor. **H,** Use the stabilizer to remove the ILMA. **I,** Allow the balloon to pass through. **J,** Confirm tube placement and ventilate. *ETT*, Endotracheal tube.

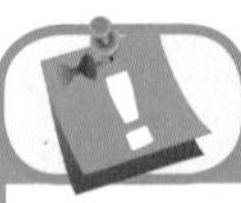

TIPS AND TRICKS

**Success with a Tracheal Introducer**

Ideal use is when the vocal cords are too anterior to visualize them well with direct laryngoscopy.

Have a helper ready to assist in advancing the tube over the introducer.

Once the introducer is in trachea, keep the laryngoscope in place and continue lifting. This will straighten the path for the endotracheal tube to slide over the introducer into the trachea.

If resistance is met as the endotracheal tube is advanced to the level of the glottis, the tube should be withdrawn slightly, rotated 45 to 90 degrees, and then advanced with gentle pressure.

demonstrated to provide adequate ventilation and a good opportunity for success with blind intubation through the LMA.[66-73] Placement of the ILMA is nearly identical to that for a standard LMA, with one notable difference: the rigid handle of the ILMA allows easier manipulation of the device and does not require the operator to place fingers inside the patient's mouth to guide placement. Once the ILMA is placed in the hypopharynx and the cuff is inflated, bag ventilation can begin. If ventilation is adequate (which is the case in the majority of patients and implies good ILMA positioning), the proprietary nonkinking endotracheal tube can be advanced through the lumen of the ILMA. In anesthesia reports such intubation has a high rate of success. The ILMA cuff is then deflated, the ILMA is removed over the endotracheal tube, and the tube is left in place as a definitive airway. The success rate in emergency patients in whom prior intubation attempts have failed and who often have full stomachs is thus far unpublished and unknown.

## CAN'T INTUBATE, CAN'T VENTILATE

In this dire situation the vast majority of patients will require an invasive airway unless the expeditious use of an extraglottic rescue device can convert the situation to "can't intubate, *can* ventilate."

### *Rescue Airway Devices*

Rescue devices establish an airway for oxygenation and ventilation and sit in an extraglottic position instead of passing through the vocal cords. They are critical tools for the management of difficult and failed airways. The most commonly used extraglottic devices are laryngeal masks (LMA [La Jolla, CA], intubating laryngeal airway [ILA]) and laryngeal tubes (King LT, King Systems, Noblesville, IN; Combitube, Nellcor, Boulder, CO). In emergency airway management, an extraglottic device can be used to provide ventilation until a definitive airway is established, thereby converting a "can't intubate, can't ventilate" situation to a "can't intubate, can ventilate" one. Placement of the extraglottic device and verification of successful ventilation must be done rapidly because failure of the device and worsening hypoxemia would necessitate emergency cricothyrotomy.

The LMA and ILA are two devices designed to create a mask seal over the laryngeal inlet to ventilate and oxygenate patients for short to intermediate periods during elective anesthesia or emergency airway management. The mask portions of each of these devices are similar in shape, but the ILA mask is slightly stiffer to prevent folding of the leading edge during insertion. Many clinicians have familiarity with laryngeal masks, thus making them useful rescue devices. Anesthesia studies report that the ILMA is effective in managing difficult and failed airways, but its performance in ED airway management has not been adequately studied.[69,72,74,75] Several models are commercially available, but only two allow placement of a cuffed endotracheal tube in the trachea through the device (ILMA and ILA) and may therefore be more appropriate as rescue devices in the ED.

An additional type of extraglottic device is a laryngeal tube such as the Combitube and the King LT. These devices have a pharyngeal cuff and an esophageal cuff with a port between the cuffs at the level of the laryngeal inlet for ventilation. The King LT is shorter and simpler than the Combitube, has one large lumen instead of two smaller ones, and uses only one inflation valve to fill both cuffs. Few studies comparing extraglottic rescue airway devices have been performed, and data regarding superiority of one over another as rescue devices are lacking.[76,77]

### *Invasive Intubation*

Studies done since the common acceptance of RSI in the ED show that approximately 1% of patients at large trauma centers still require cricothyrotomy.[1,3,10] These procedures have generally been performed via an open surgical technique. However, newer developments have provided a percutaneous option. The advantage of this technique may lie in its familiarity of use because it relies on the routinely used Seldinger technique.

Several key considerations need to be taken into account with respect to cricothyrotomy. First, it should be recognized that providers are often hesitant to perform what may be perceived as a highly problematic and complicated procedure. In current practice it is not uncommon for the person performing the intubation to be the same individual who needs to recognize failure. Additionally, it is this same provider who will need to change course and provide an invasive airway. In this circumstance, overcoming cognitive inertia can be difficult and contribute to a disastrous delay. Many practitioners say that the most difficult portion of performing a cricothyrotomy is simply making the decision to do so. Such a decision is mandated in a "can't intubate, can't ventilate" scenario unless a bridging device can be used successfully. The presence of certain features may influence the actual approach chosen. It should be kept in mind that certain clinical circumstance may make an invasive airway particularly challenging. The mnemonic SHORT (**Box 2.4**) has been proposed for use when considering an invasive airway. Several technical variants of cricothyrotomy are in common use.

OPEN SURGICAL TECHNIQUE Among the techniques described in the literature, two are commonly referenced.

*Standard Technique* The standard technique generally involves the surgeon being positioned over the right shoulder of the patient. The incision is midline and vertical, and a tracheal hook is placed into the thyroid cartilage. Cephalad traction is applied and a horizontal incision of the cricothyroid membrane is created. Dilation of the incision is followed by intubation (**Fig. 2.4**).[78,79]

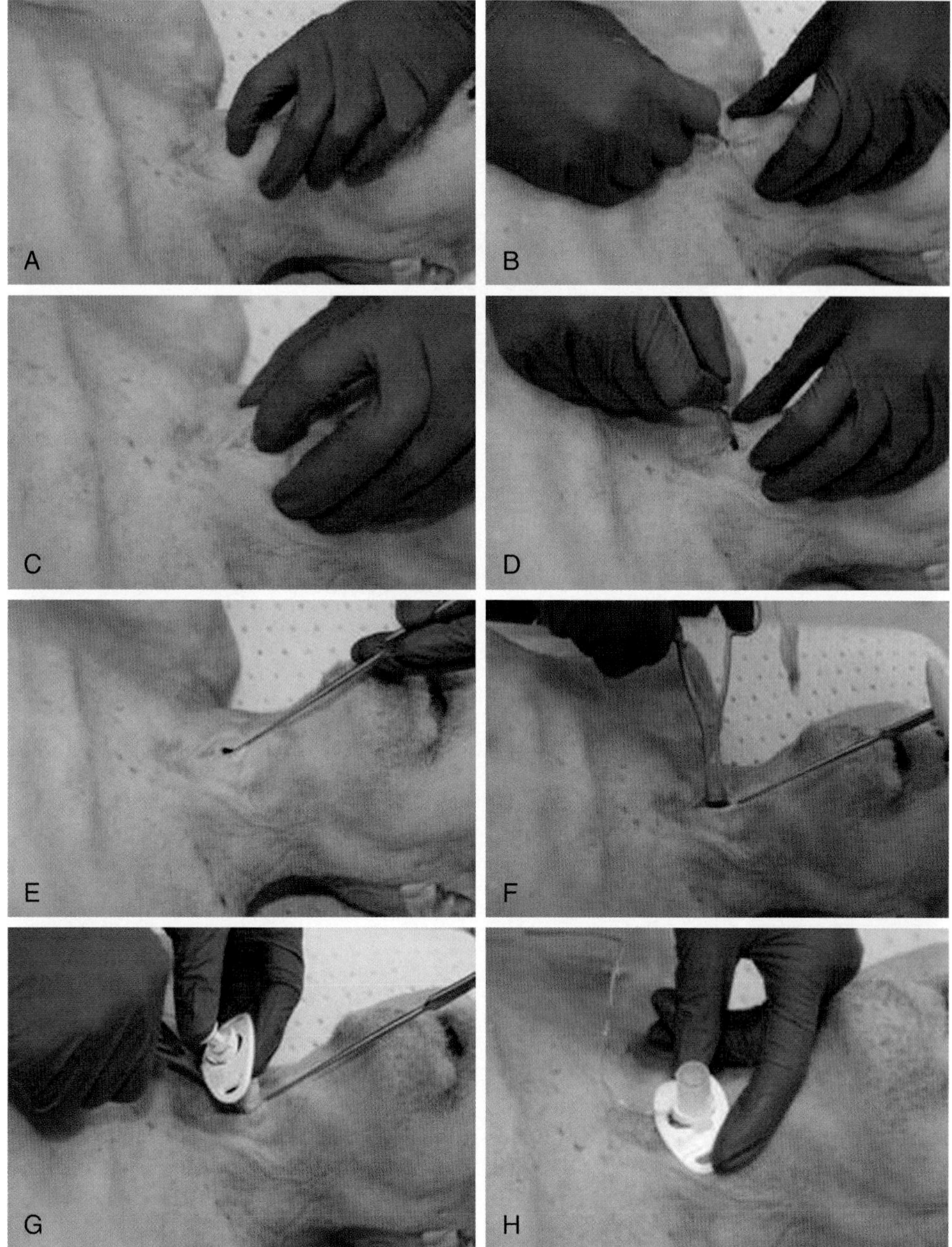


**Fig. 2.4 Standard surgical cricothyrotomy. A,** Palpate the cricothyroid membrane. **B,** Incise the skin vertically and in the midline. **C,** Identify the cricothyroid membrane. **D,** Incise the membrane horizontally. **E,** Use a hook to provide cephalad traction. **F,** Dilate the stoma vertically. **G,** Place the tube and rotate it into position. **H,** Replace the obturator with the inner cannula.

**BOX 2.4 Difficult Cricothyrotomy Mnemonic: SHORT**

**S**urgery (i.e., neck scar)
**H**ematoma
**O**besity
**R**adiation therapy involving the neck with a subsequent scar
**T**rauma with disrupted landmarks

*Rapid Four-Step Technique* This technique has evolved from the standard technique for sake of expediency. The procedure is initiated from the head of the gurney, where the intubator is most likely to be positioned. If the pertinent anatomy is clearly palpable (step 1), the skin and cricothyroid membrane are incised simultaneously with a No. 20 scalpel in a horizontal orientation (step 2). A blunt hook is then applied along the caudal side of the scalpel. The hook is used to apply traction to the cricoid ring (step 3). The incision is thus stabilized and widened for subsequent intubation

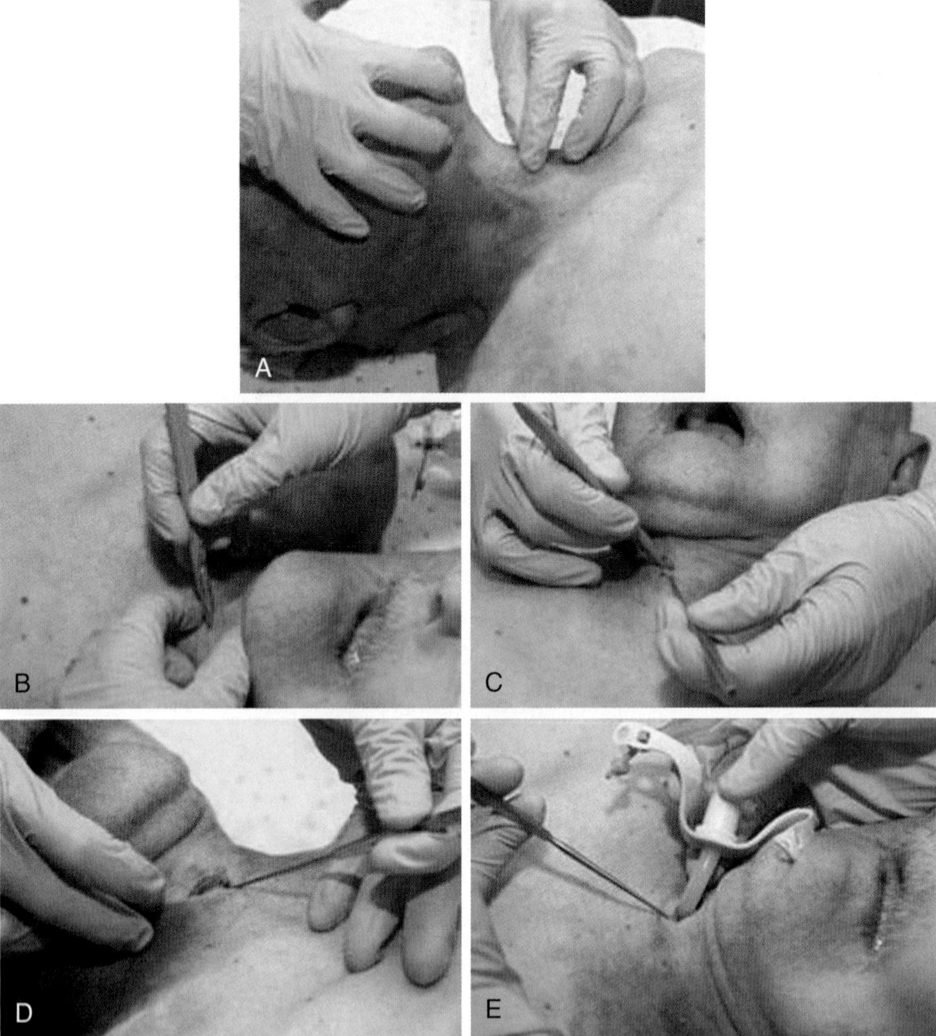

**Fig. 2.5 Rapid four-step technique for cricothyrotomy. A,** Step 1—palpation. **B,** Step 2—incision. **C,** Step 3—hook (placement and pull). **D,** Step 4—intubation.

(step 4) (**Fig. 2.5**). This technique may be a favorable alternative to the standard technique for several reasons. First, the operator performs the procedure from the head of the bed instead of having to step around to the side of the bed. Second, the traction applied to the cricoid ring obliterates the pretracheal potential space, which may inadvertently be intubated when using the standard technique. Third, hand positioning when applying cricoid traction is somewhat similar to that with laryngoscopy. This familiarity can be beneficial in view of the infrequency of performing the procedure and the associated potential for atrophy of skills.[80-84]

PERCUTANEOUS TECHNIQUE In contrast to the open techniques just described, this technique relies on a wire-through-needle (e.g., Seldinger) method for accessing the airway. Recent technologic advances have resulted in the production of cuffed endotracheal tubes that can be placed within the airway by using a dilator over a wire (**Fig. 2.6**).[85,86]

## PEDIATRIC CONSIDERATIONS

Most of the adjunctive devices discussed in this chapter have limited or no application to young children. There is probably overlap among older children and teens as size allows; however, very little research in this area has been performed. What follows is a brief summary of products that have some applicability to infants and children.

### RESCUE DEVICES

#### *Classic Laryngeal Mask Airway*

No intubating form of the LMA is available for pediatric patients. Although the small adult size might accommodate a larger teen, these devices are scaled to fit on the basis of height considerations. The classic (nonintubating) LMA is available in all sizes appropriate for teens to neonates.

#### *King LT*

This device in available in sizes appropriate for children, as well as infants.

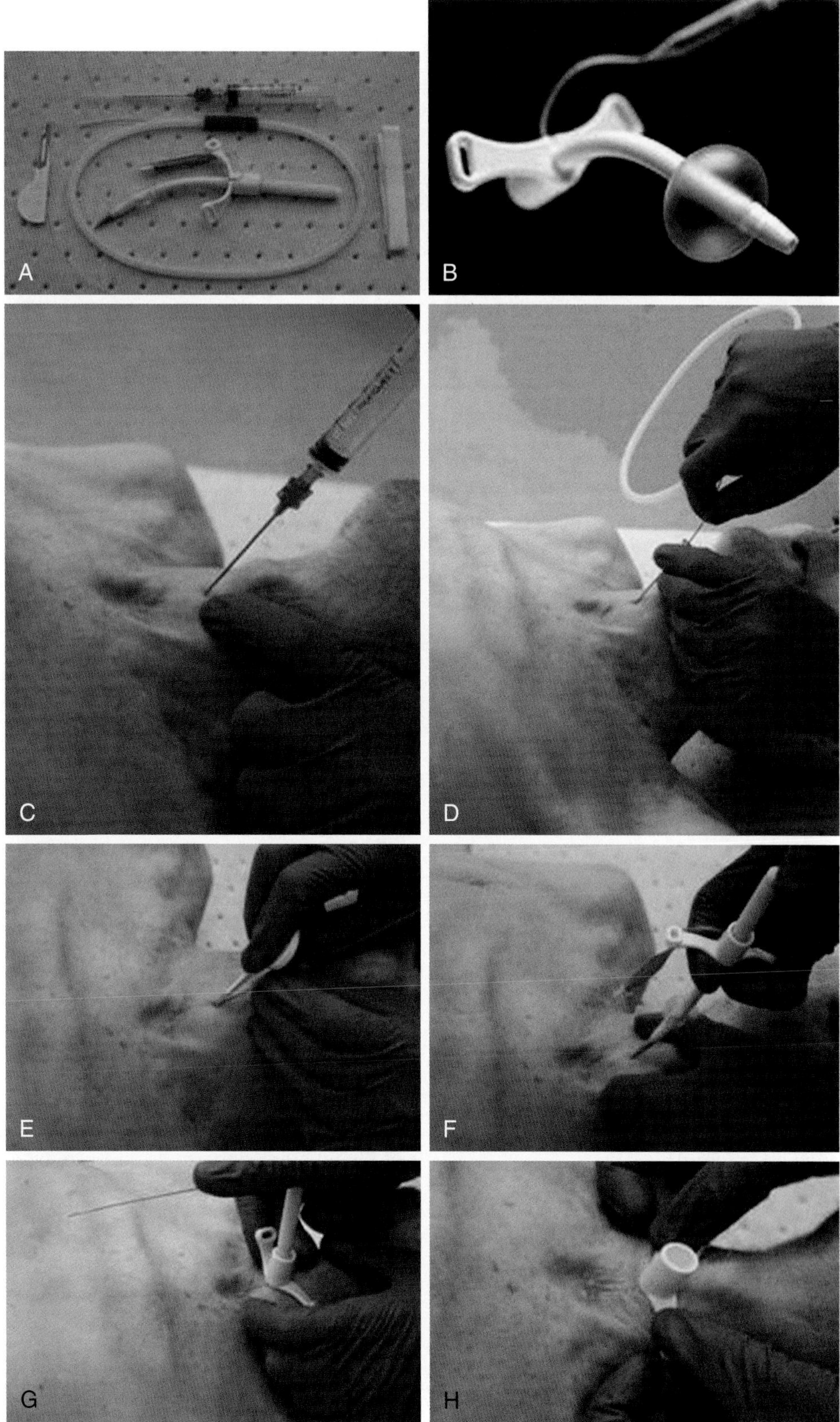

**Fig. 2.6 Percutaneous cricothyrotomy with the Cook (Melker) kit. A,** Kit contents. **B,** Cuffed tube. **C,** Place the needle through the cricothyroid membrane. **D,** Place the wire through the needle. **E,** Incise the skin. **F,** Thread the dilator/tube over the wire. **G,** Advance the tube into the airway. **H,** Remove the dilator and wire.

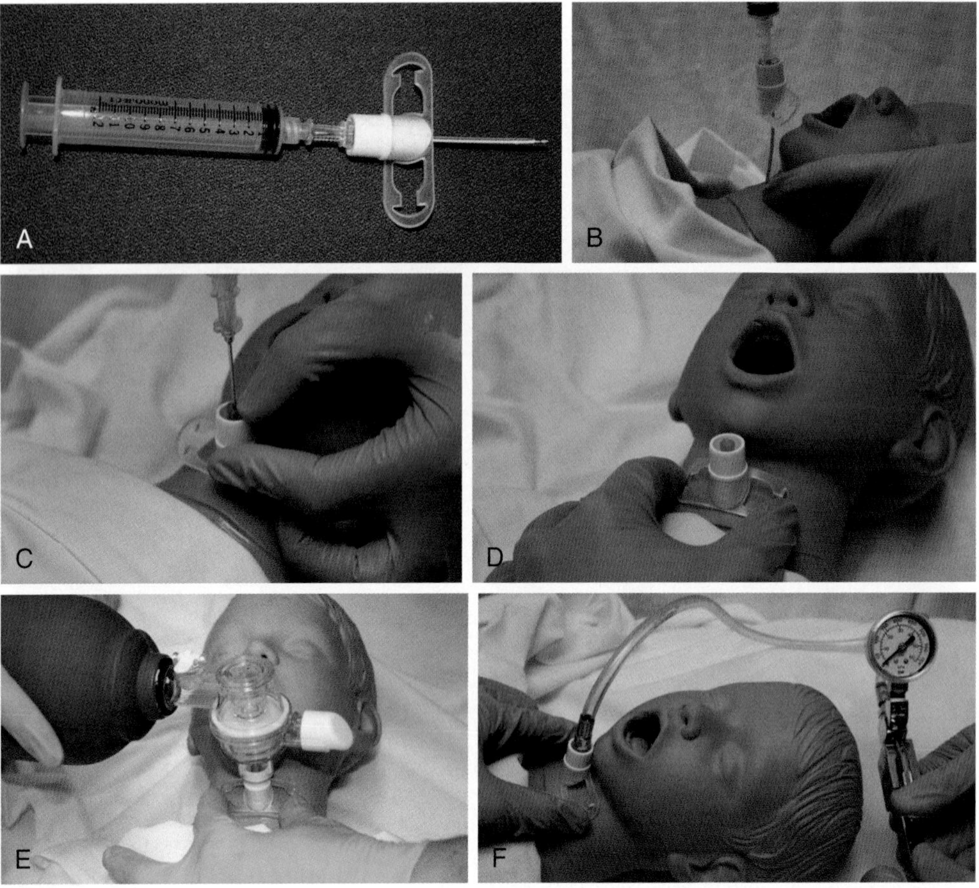

**Fig. 2.7 Needle cricothyrotomy. A,** Transtracheal catheter device. **B,** Palpate and puncture the cricothyroid membrane. **C,** Withdraw the needle. **D,** Hold the catheter in place. **E,** Use the outer adapter for bag ventilation. **F,** Use the inner Luer-Lok for jet ventilation.

### *GlideScope for Children*

Currently, a small GlideScope is available for children as small as 2 kg.

### *Fiberoptics*

Flexible fiberoptic scopes have been developed for very small airways. However, the diameter of these scopes is generally too small to allow easy passage of the endotracheal tube off the scope into the airway. This "railroading" method in thinner scopes is more likely to kink the scope. This risks breaking the scopes and is prone to failure.

## INVASIVE CONSIDERATIONS

In children younger than 10 years, open cricothyrotomy is contraindicated because of airway size. Currently, the only invasive method that is available for use in young children and infants is needle cricothyrotomy, which is commonly discussed in the context of jet insufflation. Such high-pressure oxygen has been shown to provide adequate short-term oxygenation with somewhat less successful ventilation. This technique does nothing to protect the airway because a cuffed tube is not present in the airway. Various adapted combinations have been described to allow the use of a ventilation bag (plus adaptor) with a cricothyrotomy needle. The pressure generated with such a bag is generally inadequate for all except small infants. In general, jet ventilation catheters such as the VBM catheter (Medizintechnik GmbH, Sulz am Neckar, Germany) are used with high-pressure jet ventilation systems (**Fig. 2.7**). Barotrauma is often a concern, and kinking or egress of the catheter from its original placement as a result of the high pressure can be an issue. In such a case, manual stabilization of the catheter assembly is prudent until a definitive airway can be established.

## REFERENCES

*References can be found on Expert Consult @ www.expertconsult.com.*

# Mechanical Ventilation 3

*Jairo I. Santanilla*

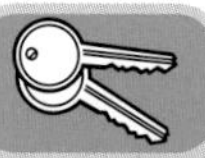

**KEY POINTS**

- Noninvasive positive pressure ventilation reduces the need for endotracheal intubation.
- Rapid titration and adjustment of the noninvasive ventilator to reduce the work of breathing are essential for the success of noninvasive positive pressure ventilation.
- Monitoring of airway pressure and use of a low–tidal volume strategy minimize the risk for ventilator-induced lung injury.
- Appropriate selection of ventilator mode, tidal volume, positive end-expiratory pressure, fraction of inspired oxygen, and inspiratory flow rate is essential to minimize the work of breathing and enhance correction of hypoxemia.
- Correction of hypoxemia is critical, but correction of hypercapnia is not.

## EPIDEMIOLOGY

Patients with severe respiratory complaints account for about 12% of emergency department (ED) visits.[1] Almost 800,000 hospitalizations per year involve mechanical ventilation, which costs nearly $27 billion and represents 12% of all hospital costs. Although the overall number of patients requiring mechanical ventilation is small (2.8%), the relative mortality is as high as 34%.[2] Twenty-six percent of asthmatic patients who required intubation reported the ED as their primary source of health care.[3] Thorough knowledge of noninvasive and invasive mechanical ventilation, lung-protective ventilation strategies, and methods to enhance patient-ventilator synchrony is essential in the practice of emergency medicine.

## PATHOPHYSIOLOGY

A wide variety of conditions can lead to respiratory failure. Generally, respiratory failure is characterized as hypoxic (inability to adequately oxygenate), hypercapnic (inability to adequately ventilate), or both hypoxic and hypercapnic. In addition, respiratory failure can be caused by an inability to protect the airway.

Alterations in the normal physiology and anatomy of the respiratory system can lead to respiratory failure requiring mechanical ventilation. Anatomic alterations causing airway obstruction, such as tumors, edema, direct or indirect trauma, burns, or other such pathology, may result in respiratory failure. Central nervous system alterations caused by traumatic brain injury, intoxicants, and hemorrhagic or ischemic stroke can cause overt respiratory failure or loss of protective reflexes. Diseases of the peripheral nervous system may result in hypoventilation. Primary pulmonary diseases such as pneumonia can be manifested as ventilation-perfusion mismatch. Asthma and chronic obstructive pulmonary disease (COPD) can lead to hypercapnic respiratory failure. Cardiovascular disease may be accompanied by respiratory failure secondary to acute cardiogenic pulmonary edema, cardiac arrest, myocardial infarction, acute valvular insufficiency, cardiomyopathy, or arrhythmias. Finally, global states such as shock from any cause can lead to respiratory failure.

## PRESENTING SIGNS AND SYMPTOMS

Patients requiring mechanical ventilation will typically be seen in extremis. Vital signs are paramount in the initial management. A rapid history and physical examination are also important. Patients may have a wide range of heart rate, respiratory rate (RR), and blood pressure. Pulse oximetry may be difficult to perform. Patients may complain of dyspnea, chest pain, anxiety, or generalized malaise. They may have altered mental status, tachypnea, hypopnea or apnea, diaphoresis, tachycardia, or bradycardia and occasionally arrive in full cardiac arrest. The history and physical examination should be focused on determining the need for mechanical ventilation and the cause of the respiratory failure.

## DIFFERENTIAL DIAGNOSIS AND MEDICAL DECISION MAKING

The decision to place someone on mechanical ventilation should be a clinical one performed at the bedside. Five basic questions can assist in determining the need for mechanical ventilation. First, is the patient failing to maintain an adequate airway or protect the airway? Second, is adequate oxygenation being maintained? Third, is adequate ventilation being maintained? Fourth, is the patient's expected clinical course such that intubation is indicated? "Yes" answers to any of these questions should prompt consideration for intubation. Finally, is the patient a candidate for noninvasive positive pressure ventilation (NPPV)? Selected patients may be given a trial of NPPV instead of intubation.

$SI = \frac{SV}{BSA}$ **FACTS AND FORMULAS**

Ideal body weight (IBW, kg)

- Males: IBW = 50 kg + 2.3 kg for each inch over 5 feet
- Females: IBW = 45.5 kg + 2.3 kg for each inch over 5 feet

## TREATMENT

### PREHOSPITAL SETTING

Mechanical ventilation in the prehospital setting is typically limited to continuous positive airway pressure (CPAP) or NPPV and critical care transport ventilators. The presence of CPAP/NPPV machines is becoming more commonplace in emergency medical system (EMS) vehicles. Patients who require intubation typically need bag-valve ventilation during transport. Critical care transport ambulances are fewer in number but carry transport ventilators, which have become increasingly smaller and more complex. An important step in transporting a patient on a transport ventilator is to test the patient on the transport ventilator before leaving the facility, preferably before moving the patient to the stretcher. This allows paramedics and EMS nurses to coordinate ventilator settings with respiratory therapists at the transferring facility. Critically, it allows early determination of intolerance to the transport ventilator.

### HOSPITAL SETTING

The typical setting for initiation of mechanical ventilation will be the prehospital or hospital setting. Occasionally, patients with chronic respiratory failure managed with home ventilators will arrive at the ED in acute respiratory failure; such patients should be placed on critical care ventilators while the work-up is in progress, and their home ventilator should accompany them to the ED. This functions in two ways: first, it addresses any possible complications caused by the home ventilator, and second, it allows ease of familiarity with the ventilator.

### CONSULTATION

Patients suffering from respiratory failure requiring mechanical ventilation will need to be admitted to a critical care unit or be transferred to a facility able to take care of mechanically ventilated patients. Consultation with a critical care medicine provider is preferable, though not always available.

## TECHNIQUES AND METHODS OF MECHANICAL VENTILATION

Mechanical ventilatory support may be provided through a noninvasive or invasive approach. Furthermore, each technique may be applied with a variety of ventilator modes. The key differences in ventilatory support are determined by the trigger, the limit, and the cycle. The trigger is the event that starts inspiration: either patient-initiated or machine-initiated respiratory effort. Limit refers to the airflow parameter that is regulated during inspiration: either airflow rate or airway pressure. The cycle terminates inspiration: either a set volume is delivered (volume-cycled ventilation [VCV]), a pressure is delivered for a set period (pressure-cycled ventilation [PCV]), or the patient ceases inspiratory effort (pressure support ventilation [PSV]).

The plethora of terms associated with mechanical ventilation can cause confusion and misunderstanding, especially because some terms are used interchangeably. Knowing a few simple terms can improve understanding and aid management. The ventilator can be set to reach either a target volume or a target pressure. Other terms used for this target are cycle and limit. Volume cycled, volume limited, and volume targeted all refer to the same thing. Similarly, pressure cycled, pressure limited, and pressure targeted also refer to the same mode. "Control" breaths are ventilator-initiated breaths. "Assist" breaths are patient-initiated breaths. Therefore, a ventilator that is set on volume-targeted (cycled, limited) assist/control (AC) mode has breaths that are initiated by the patient (assist breaths) and the ventilator (control breaths) and reaches a set volume target (cycle, limit).

## MODES OF INVASIVE MECHANICAL VENTILATION

### CONTROL MODE

Control mode ventilation (CMV) is used almost exclusively in anesthesia, but knowledge of this mode's limitations aids in comprehension of other modes' features (**Fig. 3.1**). In CMV, all breaths are triggered, limited, and cycled by the ventilator.

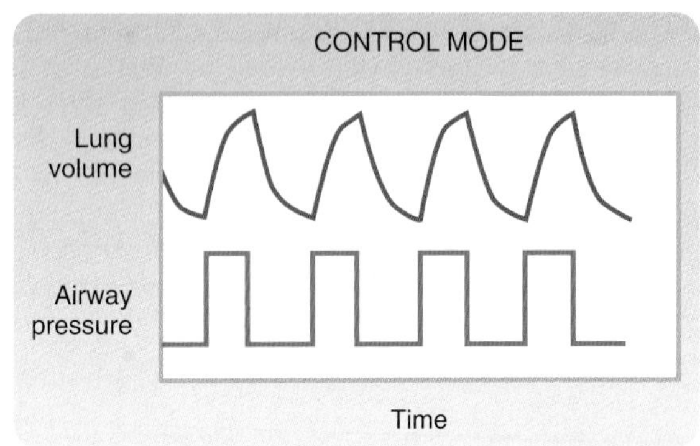


**Fig. 3.1 Control mode.** Tidal volume, respiratory rate, inspiratory flow rate, $FIO_2$, and positive end-expiratory pressure are controlled. In this mode there is no synchronization with the patient's respiratory effort.

In volume-targeted mode, the physician selects a tidal volume (VT), RR, inspiratory flow rate (IFR), fraction of inspired oxygen ($FIO_2$), and positive end-expiratory pressure (PEEP). The machine then delivers positive pressure and applies as much pressure as required to deliver the set VT at the set IFR. (In pressure-targeted mode the physician sets the pressure high, RR, $FIO_2$ and pressure low or PEEP.) Note that patients can set their own flow rate in pressure-targeted modes. The machine then delivers positive pressure and applies as much pressure as required to reach the set pressure high. The VT values generated are a function of respiratory system compliance. The patient is not able to initiate or terminate a breath. If inspiratory effort is initiated before the machine is triggered to deliver a breath, airflow would not occur regardless of the patient's inspiratory effort. If exhalation is incomplete and the time for the machine to deliver a breath has occurred, the ventilator would provide as much pressure as necessary to cause inhalation. Imagine forcibly exhaling, or coughing, when the ventilator begins to deliver a breath. This lack of synchrony would cause distress and risk structural lung or airway injury. For these reasons, CMV is never used except for apneic, paralyzed, or anesthetized patients.

## ASSIST/CONTROL MODE

AC mode usually provides the greatest level of ventilatory assistance (**Fig. 3.2**). In volume-targeted ventilation, the physician sets VT, RR, IFR, $FIO_2$, and PEEP. (In pressure-targeted mode, the physician sets the pressure high, RR, $FIO_2$ and pressure low or PEEP.) In contrast to all other modes, the trigger that initiates inspiration can be either an elapsed time interval (determined by the set RR) or the patient's spontaneous inspiratory effort. When either occurs, the machine delivers the set VT (in volume-targeted mode) or pressure high (in pressure-targeted mode). The machine follows a time algorithm that synchronizes the machine with patient-initiated breaths. If the patient is breathing at or above the set RR, all breaths are initiated by the patient. If the patient breathes below the set RR, machine-initiated breaths are interspersed among the patient's breaths. Work of breathing (WOB) is primarily the effort that the patient exerts to cause airway pressure to drop to the threshold that triggers onset of the ventilator. (Manipulating the sensitivity of the ventilator sets this threshold.) Furthermore, WOB may be performed to a variable degree during inspiration, depending on how much the respiratory muscles are activated. WOB with the volume-targeted AC mode may be extreme in two situations: when the VT drawn by the patient is greater than the set VT and when the patient inspires at a rate that exceeds the set IFR (see later).

In the majority of situations, AC mode is used as described earlier and is termed *volume-targeted* or *volume-cycled ventilation*. As an alternative, some ventilators allow pressure-targeted (cycled) ventilation (PCV, not to be confused with PSV, described later) (**Fig. 3.3**). Instead of IFR, the limit during PCV is a set airway pressure. Instead of VT, the cycle during PCV is a set inspiratory time (TI). On some ventilator models, RR and the inspiratory-to-expiratory (I:E) ratio are set, and TI is calculated from these settings. On other models, TI is available as a setting. Because VT is not set, the VT delivered varies slightly from breath to breath, depending on lung compliance, airway resistance, and patient effort. PCV may offer a slight advantage over VCV in clinical scenarios that require control of the I:E ratio, but a body of literature investigating this concept does not exist. Historically, PCV was commonly used in neonates and infants, although modern ventilators that precisely measure small VT are currently favored. PCV may be the only mode available on some portable and transport ventilators.

## SYNCHRONIZED INTERMITTENT MANDATORY VENTILATION AND PRESSURE SUPPORT

Synchronized intermittent mandatory ventilation (SIMV) is probably the most commonly misunderstood mode of mechanical ventilation (**Fig. 3.4**). The physician sets VT, RR, IFR, $FIO_2$, and PEEP, as in AC mode. In contrast to AC mode, however, the trigger that initiates inspiration depends on the

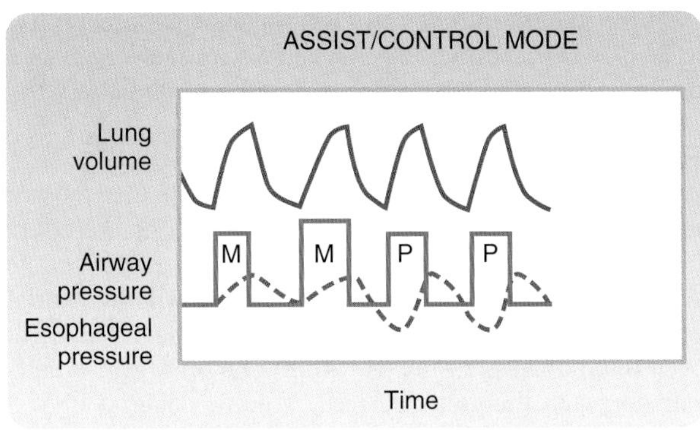


**Fig. 3.2 Volume-targeted, assist/control mode.** Tidal volume is controlled. A minimum mandatory respiratory rate is set and synchronized with patient effort. If the patient breathes at a rate higher than the set rate, all breaths are assisted. The *dashed line* represents esophageal/intrathoracic pressure dynamics. The first two breaths represent machine-initiated (M) breaths; the second two breaths represent patient-initiated (P) breaths.

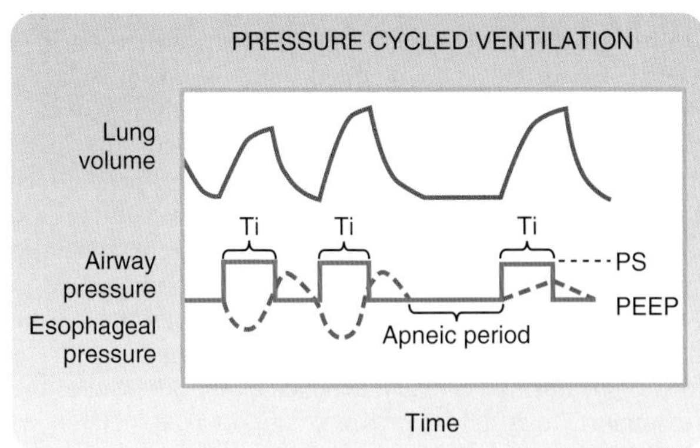


**Fig. 3.3 Pressure-targeted, assist/control mode.** Inspiratory pressure support (PS) and inspiratory time (TI) are controlled. Tidal volume may vary from breath to breath. The minimum mandatory respiratory rate is set and synchronizes with patient effort. The *dashed line* represents esophageal/intrathoracic pressure dynamics. The first two breaths represent patient-initiated breaths; the third breath is a machine-initiated (mandatory) breath. *PEEP*, Positive end-expiratory pressure.

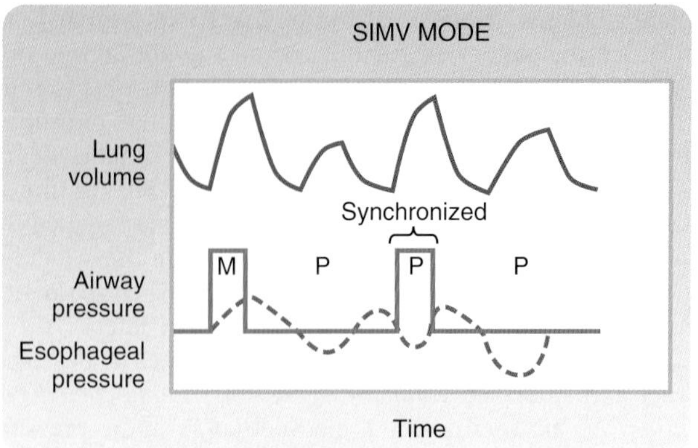


**Fig. 3.4 Volume-targeted, synchronized intermittent mandatory ventilation (SIMV).** Tidal volume is controlled only during machine-assisted breaths. Tidal volume may vary during nonassisted (patient-initiated) breaths. The minimum mandatory respiratory rate is set. If the patient breathes more slowly than the set rate, the machine synchronizes with patient effort (third breath). If the patient breathes faster than the set rate, breaths in excess of the set rate are not assisted (second and fourth breaths). *M*, Machine-initiated breath; *P*, patient-initiated breath. The *dashed line* represents esophageal/intrathoracic pressure dynamics.

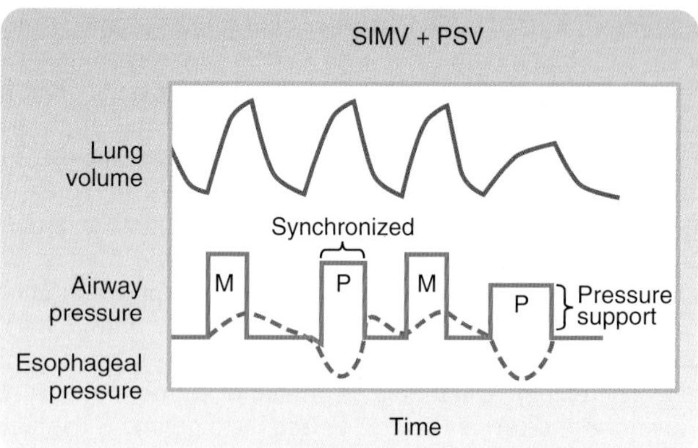


**Fig. 3.5 Volume-targeted, synchronized intermittent mandatory ventilation (SIMV) with pressure support ventilation (PSV).** Tidal volume is controlled during machine-initiated (M) breaths (first and third breaths) and synchronized patient-initiated (P) breaths (second breath). Pressure support is provided whenever the patient initiates a breath over the set rate (fourth breath). Tidal volume may vary during pressure-supported breaths. The dashed line represents esophageal/intrathoracic pressure dynamics.

patient's RR relative to the set RR. When the patient breathes at or below the set RR, the trigger can be either elapsed time or the patient's respiratory effort. In this case, WOB is equivalent to AC. When the patient breathes above the set RR, the ventilator is not triggered to assist in making spontaneous breaths in excess of the set RR. The work associated with such breaths may be quite high because the patient must generate enough negative force to pull air through the ventilator and overcome the resistance to airflow caused by the ventilator circuit tubing and the endotracheal tube (ETT), in addition to the WOB required as a result of the underlying disease process.

This limitation of SIMV can be diminished by the addition of PSV (**Fig. 3.5**). PSV causes inspiratory positive pressure to be applied during patient-initiated breaths that exceed the set RR. The patient initiates and terminates inspiration, thereby determining VT. Once the patient triggers pressure support, it is maintained until the machine detects cessation of patient effort, as indicated by a fall in inspiratory airflow. VT, IFR, and TI are not controlled but instead are determined by patient effort. The WOB performed during PSV involves triggering the ventilator to deliver the pressure and maintaining inspiratory effort throughout inhalation. Contrast this with machine-assisted ventilation in AC or SIMV, where WOB involves triggering the ventilator but lung inflation continues regardless of the patient's inspiratory effort. WOB during PSV also depends on the set level of pressure support. Insufficient pressure support is associated with high WOB, which leads to a small VT and a high RR. Adequate pressure support reduces WOB and improves VT and RR. Many experts view RR as the best index of the adequacy of the level of pressure support. It should be adjusted to maintain an acceptable RR of less than 30 but preferably less than 24 breaths per minute.

SIMV can be used in pressure-targeted ventilation. Essentially, the ventilator is set to reach a target pressure for each of the ventilator-initiated breaths and potentially a different target for patient-initiated breaths. Another way to consider pressure-targeted SIMV is as PSV with a set rate.

## CONTINUOUS POSITIVE AIRWAY PRESSURE

CPAP alone is not a true form of assisted mechanical ventilation because inspiration is not assisted by increasing airway pressure. Pressure greater than ambient atmospheric pressure is supplied, but it is held constant throughout the respiratory cycle. During inhalation, the gradient between the airway and intrathoracic pressure is higher than it would be if breathing ambient air. Conversely, the gradient is lower during exhalation. As a result, inhalation requires slightly less effort than normal breathing does, and the airways are held open during exhalation to allow better expiratory airflow. As in SIMV, PSV may be added to CPAP. CPAP with PSV is a form of assisted ventilation because inspiratory pressure is augmented, and this is more appropriately referred to as simply PSV. As discussed earlier, the patient initiates and terminates each breath; therefore, WOB is performed as the patient initiates each breath and maintains inspiratory effort throughout inhalation.

## OTHER MODES

The most recent innovations in ventilator modes are those that combine volume and pressure targets, which are referred to as dual modes. Pressure-regulated volume control, autoflow, volume ventilation plus, adaptive support ventilation, variable pressure control, and variable pressure support are all dual modes that adjust pressure or volume targets from breath to breath to reach the goals desired. Volume-ensured PSV and pressure augmentation alter parameters within the breath to reach goals. Unfortunately, few studies have compared these latest modes with one another or with conventional modes.

Finally, modes that have rarely been used in the ED setting and are beyond the scope of this chapter include high-frequency ventilation, airway pressure release ventilation, bilevel ventilation, proportional assist ventilation plus, and proportional pressure support.

## MONITORING DYNAMIC PRESSURE DURING INVASIVE VENTILATION

Mechanical ventilation can cause damage to the lungs on a macroscopic and microscopic level. The direct cause of lung injury is believed to be a combination of overdistention of the alveoli and repetitive alveolar opening and closing with shear of the alveolar wall. The concept of ventilator-induced lung injury (VILI) has evolved to encompass all forms of injury at the organ and alveolar level, including pneumothorax, pneumomediastinum, bronchial rupture, diffuse alveolar damage, and acute respiratory distress syndrome (ARDS). Pressure is measured at the ventilator end of the circuit (the proximal part of the airway), and this measurement is used as an index of the pressure within the lung.

### PEAK INSPIRATORY AIRWAY PRESSURE

Peak inspiratory airway pressure ($P_{peak}$) is the highest pressure that is generated during inflation of the lung. Because pressure decreases incrementally along the path at each point of resistance, the pressure delivered at the alveolar level may be significantly less than the measured $P_{peak}$, particularly when resistance to airflow is high. Therefore, $P_{peak}$ is not an ideal surrogate measurement for alveolar pressure and does not correlate with VILI.

### PLATEAU PRESSURE

Plateau pressure ($P_{plat}$) is the end-inspiratory airway pressure and is measured just after airflow has ceased. Because this is a static measurement (absence of airflow), resistance of the circuit and airways does not play a role. Therefore, $P_{plat}$ is a logical surrogate measurement for mean alveolar pressure. Its primary limitation is that compliance is not equal in all regions of the lung. The degree of alveolar distention in healthy regions of the lung may be significantly greater than that in heavily diseased lung regions at the same $P_{plat}$. In a healthy adult undergoing mechanical ventilation with normal lung compliance, $P_{plat}$ is low, usually in the range of 5 to 15 cm $H_2O$. Patients with alveolar disease (pneumonia, cardiogenic pulmonary edema, acute lung injury [ALI], and ARDS) have poor lung compliance, and $P_{plat}$ is typically much higher in these states. Measures to maintain $P_{plat}$ below the currently recommended limit of 30 cm $H_2O$ are discussed later.

### INTRINSIC POSITIVE END-EXPIRATORY PRESSURE

PEEP indicates that the airway pressure measured at the end of exhalation is above ambient air pressure. When PEEP is set by the clinician and applied by the ventilator, it is termed extrinsic PEEP ($PEEP_e$). In contrast, intrinsic PEEP ($PEEP_i$) arises when exhalation is incomplete because of either intrathoracic airway obstruction, early airway closure during exhalation, or inadequate exhalation time. The common end point is trapping of air in the lung at the end of exhalation, which ultimately leads to increased intrathoracic pressure. $PEEP_i$ can cause problems through several mechanisms. First, because exhalation is incomplete, air is progressively being trapped in the lungs, thereby leading to early airway closure and dynamic hyperinflation with an associated risk for VILI. Second, $PEEP_i$ leads to difficulty triggering the ventilator and increased WOB, as discussed previously. Third, $PEEP_i$ can cause patient-ventilator dyssynchrony when the patient continues active contraction of the respiratory muscles at end exhalation as the ventilator is triggered. Lung inflation may begin while the patient is attempting to complete exhalation. Finally, increased intrathoracic pressure can impede venous return to the heart and consequently lead to hemodynamic instability. Simultaneously, impaired venous return may compromise pulmonary blood flow, increase physiologic dead space, and result in worsening hypercapnia. Control of $PEEP_i$ is discussed later.

## MODES OF NONINVASIVE MECHANICAL VENTILATION

The cause of the respiratory failure is the best predictor of whether a patient will respond to noninvasive techniques. The literature supports the application of NPPV for certain conditions—COPD,[4,5] asthma,[6] congestive heart failure (CHF),[7,8] pneumonia, trauma, cancer, and neuromuscular disease—as well as for pediatric patients.

Noninvasive ventilators are more portable because of the use of a smaller air compressor/blower, but they cannot develop pressures as high as larger critical care ventilators can. A noninvasive ventilator can provide up to 20 to 40 cm $H_2O$ of air pressure, as compared with critical care ventilators capable of delivering greater than 100 cm $H_2O$ of air pressure. Newer noninvasive ventilators can be set for volume- or pressure-targeted mode, AC or SIMV, and even proportional assist.

### SPONTANEOUS AND SPONTANEOUS/TIMED MODES

In spontaneous mode, airway pressure cycles between inspiratory positive airway pressure (IPAP) and expiratory positive airway pressure (EPAP). This mode is commonly referred to as biphasic (or bilevel) positive airway pressure, but other proprietary names refer to the same mode. The trigger to switch from EPAP to IPAP is the patient's inspiratory effort. A variety of ventilator models use one or several of the following to indicate patient effort: a drop in airway pressure, measured inspired volume (usually 5 to 6 mL), or an increase in airflow rate. The limit during inspiration is the set level of IPAP. The inspiratory phase cycles off when the machine senses cessation of patient effort, as indicated by a decrease in inspiratory flow below a set threshold (typically 60% of the peak IFR) or attainment of maximum inspiratory time (usually 3 seconds). The latter is a safety mechanism to prevent lung hyperinflation as a result of ventilator "runaway," but it was not available on early generations of noninvasive ventilators. VT may vary from breath to breath, dependent primarily on the magnitude and duration of patient effort, but also on lung compliance. WOB is predominantly related to initiating and maintaining airflow throughout the inspiratory phase. Additional WOB may occur if the patient actively contracts the expiratory muscles.

Spontaneous mode is dependent on the patient's effort to trigger inhalation. Respiratory acidosis will develop in a patient breathing at a slow, inadequate rate. To prevent this adverse consequence, spontaneous/timed mode allows the machine to be triggered either by patient effort or after an elapsed time interval that is calculated from a set minimum

RR. If the patient does not initiate inspiration during the set interval, IPAP is triggered. For machine-initiated breaths, the machine cycles back to EPAP based on a set inspiratory time. For patient-initiated breaths, the ventilator cycles as it would in spontaneous mode.

Pragmatically, NPPV (noninvasive) and PSV (invasive) are similar but have a few noteworthy differences. First, the trigger for PSV is a drop in airway pressure sensed by the ventilator. Some ventilators monitor airflow in the inspiratory and expiratory limbs of the ventilator circuit and will be triggered if airflow in the inspiratory limb is greater than airflow in the expiratory limb. The sensitivity of the trigger can be adjusted on a conventional ventilator by setting the magnitude of the change in pressure required for triggering. This is contrasted with NPPV, in which sensitivity is continuously and automatically adjusted by the noninvasive ventilator based on the amount of air leak and is not able to be adjusted by the physician. Second, because PSV is supplied by a critical care ventilator, leaks are not tolerated or compensated. Because airflow through a leak may be misinterpreted in this mode as patient inspiratory effort, a leak may lead to early triggering before exhalation is complete. Leaks may also cause failure to cycle off in synchrony with cessation of patient effort. These phenomena are less likely to occur when using a noninvasive ventilator. Finally, the nomenclature used for airway pressure is different. Pressure during the expiratory phase is termed PEEP, analogous to the EPAP of NPPV. Pressure during the inspiratory phase is termed peak inspiratory pressure, analogous to the IPAP of spontaneous mode. The distinction is that in PSV the numerical value for pressure support is the equivalent of the difference between IPAP and EPAP.

### INITIATION OF NONINVASIVE POSITIVE PRESSURE VENTILATION

The process of initiating a trial of noninvasive ventilatory support consists of four basic steps. First, the patient must be willing to accept face mask ventilation. Because the patient should remain awake and cooperative during ventilation, the process should be explained before the mask is applied. Initially, an $FIO_2$ of 100% with 3 to 5 cm $H_2O$ of CPAP is provided. Acceptance may improve if the patient holds the mask against the face. The mask is secured with straps once the patient demonstrates acceptance.

Next, after explaining that the pressure will change, ventilation is switched to NPPV with an EPAP of 3 to 5 cm $H_2O$ and an IPAP of 8 to 10 cm $H_2O$. IPAP is titrated in 2- to 3-cm $H_2O$ increments until exhaled VT (measured by the ventilator) is in the range of 6 to 9 mL/kg IBW. Further adjustment of IPAP should be directed toward obtaining an RR of less than 30. Another option is to start with high IPAP (20 to 25 cm $H_2O$) and titrate down based on patient comfort. Of note, no studies have compared a low-to-high IPAP versus a high-to-low IPAP approach.

EPAP is then adjusted to the lowest level that allows synchrony between the patient and ventilator. Understanding this process requires review of the components of WOB related to triggering the ventilator. The patient activates the inspiratory muscles to decrease intrathoracic pressure. As intrathoracic pressure falls below airway pressure, transpulmonary pressure becomes positive, airflow begins, and the ventilator is triggered. In a normal patient, the inspiratory muscle force required to lower intrathoracic pressure to a level that triggers the ventilator is not great. In a patient with high $PEEP_i$ (also known as auto-PEEP), intrathoracic pressure is high at end exhalation. The inspiratory muscle force required to lower intrathoracic pressure below airway pressure is significantly greater. Thus the WOB that is performed to trigger the ventilator is proportional to the amount of $PEEP_i$ that is present.

While delivering NPPV, it is impossible to measure $PEEP_i$ without invasive means. Instead, to detect $PEEP_i$, signs of difficulty triggering the ventilator or signs of expiratory airflow obstruction should be sought. On physical examination, recruitment of the accessory muscles of inspiration suggests that $PEEP_i$ is a problem. A useful technique is palpation of the sternocleidomastoid muscle while simultaneously watching the ventilator flow graphs or listening for the ventilator to trigger. When the muscle is felt to contract before the ventilator triggers, $PEEP_i$ may be the culprit. Observation of active abdominal muscle recruitment during exhalation indicates airflow obstruction as a cause of elevated $PEEP_i$. When elevated $PEEP_i$ is suspected, EPAP should be increased in increments of 2 to 3 cm $H_2O$ until the problem is controlled. The maximum safe level of EPAP that should be used during NPPV has not been determined in an evidence-based manner. Typical initial settings range from 0 to 5 cm $H_2O$; maximum settings described in the methods sections of various trials range from 12.5 to 15 cm $H_2O$. It is prudent to measure the heart rate and blood pressure and perform pulse oximetry after each increase in EPAP because high levels may compromise cardiac output. As EPAP is increased, corresponding increasing increments in IPAP are required to maintain a differential between EPAP and IPAP that ensures adequate VT.

Finally, $FIO_2$ is adjusted to maintain adequate $O_2$ saturation. In many clinical situations, continuous pulse oximetry alone is adequate for this purpose. Arterial blood gas determinations are not routinely required but may be helpful in select patients to assess improvement in respiratory acidosis.

## SPECIFIC DISEASE PROCESSES

### CONTROLLING AIRWAY PRESSURE—LUNG-PROTECTIVE VENTILATOR STRATEGIES

Causes of difficulty with mechanical ventilation fall into four general categories:

- High airway pressure during lung inflation
- High $PEEP_i$ because of obstructive airways disease
- Patient-ventilator dyssynchrony
- Equipment failure

#### *Acute Respiratory Distress, Acute Lung Injury, and Pulmonary Edema*

Elevated plateau pressure is encountered in patients with poor lung compliance as a result of parenchymal lung disease (e.g., pulmonary edema, either cardiogenic or noncardiogenic) or obstructive airways disease with air trapping. The goal is to support the respiratory system while avoiding iatrogenic injury.

Initial studies compared a conventional ventilation strategy (VT of 10 to 15 mL/kg IBW with a goal of obtaining normal $PaO_2$ and $PaCO_2$) with a lung-protective ventilation strategy

(VT of 6 to 8 mL/kg IBW with correction of hypoxia, but allowing hypercapnia in favor of avoiding high airway pressure). The results were conflicting.[9-13] A landmark study, the ARDS Network Trial,[14] prospectively compared a conventional strategy (VT of 12 mL/kg and a $P_{plat}$ limit of 50 cm $H_2O$) with a protective strategy (VT of 6 mL/kg IBW and a $P_{plat}$ limit of 30 cm $H_2O$). After enrollment of 861 patients with ARDS and an interim analysis, the trial was stopped early because of a 22% reduction in mortality, 20% fewer days requiring mechanical ventilation, and fewer cases of organ system failure in the group receiving the lung-protective strategy.

The mechanical ventilation strategy in patients with other disease processes has not been studied as extensively. Extrapolation of these findings to patients with CHF, ALI, pneumonia, pulmonary fibrosis, pulmonary contusion, lung cancer, and other lung pathology is not based on experimental evidence.

In summary, based on the available literature, a lung-protective strategy should be used that involves low VT, limitation of $P_{plat}$ to 30 cm $H_2O$, and permissive hypercapnia in a patient with ARDS or pulmonary edema to avoid iatrogenic lung injury. This ARDSnet strategy should also be considered in patients with the diffuse infiltrative lung diseases mentioned earlier.

### *Obstructive Airways Disease*

Exacerbation of obstructive airways disease requiring mechanical ventilation is often associated with air trapping and dynamic hyperinflation of the lungs. High $P_{peak}$ arises as a result of inspiratory airflow resistance, a phenomenon more common in patients with severe asthma than in those with COPD. High $P_{plat}$ is caused by lung overdistention and consequent diminished compliance. Patients with both high $P_{peak}$ and $P_{plat}$ comprise a group of high-risk patients with both obstruction and overdistention who are at high risk for complications, including pneumothorax, tension pneumothorax, pneumomediastinum, dysrhythmias, and hemodynamic collapse. No prospective trials comparing ventilation strategies in such patients have been conducted. It is common practice to use a strategy of permissive hypercapnia to eliminate $PEEP_i$ and avoid high $P_{plat}$. This strategy makes use of low VT, low RR, and high IFR to shorten the inspiratory time and prolong the expiratory time. Although this strategy often leads to hypercapnia, it is considered safer to allow respiratory acidosis to develop than to ventilate at excessive airway pressure. A lower limit of acceptable pH has not been established, but general recommendations have been to allow pH values as low as 7.15 to 7.2. Permissive hypercapnia is required more often in the management of status asthmaticus than in the management of COPD. Evidence in support comes from retrospective studies. Current recommendations include VT less than 8 mL/kg IBW, an initial RR of 8 to 10 cycles/min, and $FIO_2$ adjusted to obtain a $PaO_2$ of approximately 60 mm Hg or a $PaO_2$ of 85% to 88%. The concept of permissive hypercapnia and controlled hypoventilation in the management of acute asthma exacerbation has been widely accepted.[15] Some reports suggest that $P_{peak}$ and $P_{plat}$ are not adequate indicators of pulmonary hyperinflation[16] and recommend that expiratory volumes be measured in these patients.[17] This latter technique has not gained widespread acceptance, however.

## FOLLOW-UP, NEXT STEPS IN CARE, AND PATIENT EDUCATION

- Admissions (inpatient and outpatient)
- Indication for admission

Patients placed on mechanical ventilation (either invasive or noninvasive) require admission to the hospital. Some centers are able to manage NPPV outside the intensive care unit, but this should be considered only in patients who have demonstrated marked improvement and are on minimal settings. Patients admitted to the floor with NPPV should still be monitored carefully.

Patients who required NPPV during their ED course and subsequently improve to the point where they no longer needed mechanical ventilation should be considered for admission or observation. Asthmatic patients who have improved may be considered for discharge, but only after a period of observation.

Occasionally, patients with chronic respiratory failure will be seen in the ED. Evaluation of such patients should be based on their chief complaint. Determination for admission is essentially the same as for other patients. If admission is required for simple issues, these patients will need to be admitted to the intensive care unit because it is the only location with personnel trained to manage the ventilator.

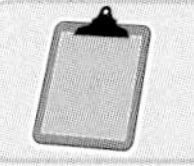

**DOCUMENTATION**

One should strive to document the following:

- Indications for mechanical ventilation
  - Why did the patient require intubation/noninvasive positive pressure ventilation?
- Interventions performed
- Details of intubation
  - What agents were used?
  - How difficult was management of the airway?
- Complications while on the ventilator
- Time spent with the patient

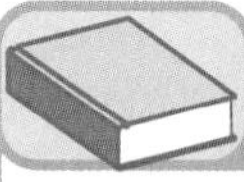

**PATIENT TEACHING TIPS**

Explain what is going on with the patient.
Exude confidence.
Motivate and reassure the patient.
Assume that an intubated patient can hear you.

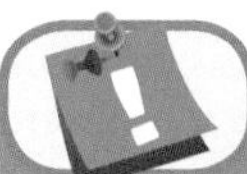

**TIPS AND TRICKS**

When starting noninvasive positive pressure ventilation, have patients hold the mask to their face.

**BOX 3.1 Complications of Mechanical Ventilation**

Pneumothorax
Auto-PEEP, dynamic hyperinflation, breath stacking
Decreased cardiac output and blood pressure
Vocal cord damage
Tracheal stenosis
Unplanned extubations
Ventilator-associated pneumonia

*PEEP,* Positive end-expiratory pressure.

## COMPLICATIONS

### INVASIVE MECHANICAL VENTILATION

In the ED, complications of mechanical ventilation (**Box 3.1**) can begin during the preintubation period. Induction agents may cause or worsen hypotension. Overly aggressive bag-valve-mask ventilation may lead to decreased venous return and hypotension. Airway trauma and mechanical complications may be caused by the act of intubation. Initiating mechanical ventilation and transitioning from negative pressure ventilation to positive pressure ventilation may lead to hypotension. Positive pressure ventilation may worsen an existing pneumothorax or give rise to pneumothorax. Auto-PEEP (also known as $PEEP_i$, dynamic hyperinflation, breath stacking) can lead to hypotension and circulatory collapse. Ventilator-associated lung injury can be caused by barotrauma, volutrauma, or trauma related to atelectasis. Long-term complications can include inability to be liberated from the ventilator, ventilator-associated pneumonia, tracheal stenosis, and vocal cord injury.

Some of the commonly underrecognized problems that arise in the support of critically ill patients fall into the category of patient-ventilator dyssynchrony. These situations can markedly increase WOB and lead to increased $CO_2$ and lactic acid production with both respiratory and metabolic acidosis.

### INTRINSIC POSITIVE END-EXPIRATORY PRESSURE

Maneuvers directed at elimination of $PEEP_i$ have in common the effect of decreasing inspiratory time and therefore providing more expiratory time. Decreasing RR and VT and increasing IFR effectively accomplish this goal. Frequently, this cannot be achieved without sedation, sometimes requiring the addition of pharmacologic paralysis.

#### *Difficulty Triggering the Ventilator*

To trigger a ventilator, a patient must cause either a drop in pressure or an increase in airflow at the proximal part of the airway, depending on the type of ventilator in use. The magnitude of change required to trigger the ventilator is adjusted by setting the sensitivity, usually in the range of −1 to −2 cm $H_2O$ below the level of $PEEP_e$. Difficulty triggering the ventilator is often not easy to detect. When it becomes obvious by physical examination that the patient is using the accessory muscles of respiration to trigger the ventilator, the problem may be severe. The condition can be detected earlier by inspecting the pressure-volume time curve on the ventilator display. A large negative deflection at the beginning of inhalation suggests that ventilator sensitivity needs to be increased.

More commonly, high $PEEP_i$ is the cause. The patient must first lower intrathoracic pressure enough to overcome $PEEP_i$ before airway pressure can drop to the threshold sensitivity. The solution to this problem is to raise $PEEP_e$ to a level one half to three fourths of $PEEP_i$ and allow the patient to perform less work to trigger inhalation. This process mandates frequent reassessment of $PEEP_i$ and manipulation of the ventilator during this dynamic period.

#### *Autocycling*

Autocycling refers to a phenomenon in which the ventilator set in AC mode begins to rapidly trigger without the patient initiating respiration. The cause is usually vacillations in airway pressure that the ventilator interprets as patient effort. Tremors, shivering, voluntary motion, convulsions, and oscillating water in the ventilator circuit are all examples of potential causes. Autocycling should prompt immediate disconnection from the ventilator circuit and ventilation with a bag-valve device until the problem has resolved.

#### *Rapid Breathing*

When attempting to ventilate a patient with an obstructive process, the goal is to eliminate $PEEP_i$. Permissive hypercapnia is best achieved at low RRs, but at the same time hypercapnia is a powerful stimulus to breath. This can typically be quelled by using a combination of sedatives such as benzodiazepines in combination with opiates. Neuromuscular blockade should be considered a last resort undertaken only after careful consideration of the risks associated with prolonged paralysis and the potential development of neuropathy in patients with critical illness. If undertaken, it should be done only to weaken the patient sufficiently to inhibit dyssynchrony with the ventilator. Other common causes of rapid breathing include sepsis, pulmonary emboli, pregnancy, hepatic encephalopathy, intracranial hypertension, stroke or hemorrhage, and posthypercapnic status. Some of these conditions are appropriate physiologic responses, whereas others, though pathologic, are difficult to control and occasionally tolerated.

#### *Outstripping the Ventilator and Double Cycling*

In patients undergoing low-VT ventilation for ARDS or for an obstructive process, hypercapnia and an increased respiratory drive will develop. Outstripping the ventilator refers to the patient's effort to draw a higher VT than is set while in a volume-targeted mode. This can be detected by observing the exhaled VT or by finding a negative deflection at the end of inhalation on the pressure-volume time plot. Double cycling occurs when the patient desires a larger VT than is set and continues to inspire despite the delivery of a breath. The ventilator will then provide a second breath almost immediately after the first. This is especially problematic because the actual VT delivered is twice the set volume. As with controlling rapid breathing, the solution is sedation and analgesia, particularly with opiates. In addition, switching to a pressure-targeted mode or increasing the set VT may alleviate this issue.

### *Straining over the Ventilator*

Straining over the ventilator indicates that the patient is attempting to inhale at a flow rate in excess of the set IFR on a volume-targeted mode. When it is obvious by examination that the patient is actively inhaling, the problem may be severe. On the pressure-volume time plot the rise in pressure during inhalation will be concave rather than convex. Potential solutions are to raise the IFR, switch to pressure-targeted mode or PSV, or use sedation and analgesia.

### *Coughing*

Coughing is a common problem that can arise from increased secretions, a foreign body in the airway (ETT), or the underlying pulmonary disease process. Coughing can lead to autocycling, poor patient comfort, ETT dislodgment, and rarely airway injury. Placement of the ETT above the carina should be confirmed. Suctioning plus provision of warmed, humidified air is often helpful. If these simple measures fail to provide relief, aerosolized lidocaine or suppression with opiates may increase patient comfort.

### EQUIPMENT FAILURE

Whenever a patient decompensates while receiving mechanical ventilation, consideration should be given to equipment failure as the cause. Interruption of the oxygen supply, accidentally rotated knobs, disconnected ventilator circuitry, and obstructed tubes are all potential culprits. Immediate action should include disconnection from the ventilator and bag ventilation with 100% $O_2$. The mnemonic made popular by the American Heart Association's Pediatric Advanced Life Support Course is useful to recall the causes of unexpected decompensation: DOPE (**d**islodgment of the ETT, **o**bstruction of the tube, **p**neumothorax, and **e**quipment failure). Confirmation of ETT placement, suctioning via an endotracheal catheter, auscultation, chest radiography, and equipment troubleshooting are necessary actions.

### NONINVASIVE MECHANICAL VENTILATION

The main complication of NPPV is an inability to tolerate the mask or the pressure. Long-term complications can include an inability to eat or drink, nasal and oral dryness, and pressure necrosis on the bridge of the nose, the cheeks, or the chin or above the ears.

## PROGNOSIS

Because of the wide range of causes of respiratory failure, the prognosis is highly variable and dependent on the cause and severity. The prognosis of patients with respiratory failure caused simply by oversedation from intoxicants can be quite good. Conversely, patients with ARDS as their sole organ dysfunction have a mortality of 20% to 25%. Respiratory failure with multiorgan system failure carries much higher mortality that is based on the severity of the illness. Overall, a requirement for invasive mechanical ventilation carries an approximate 34.5% in-hospital mortality.[2]

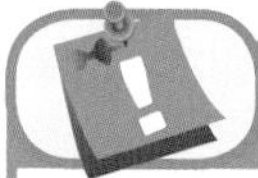

**TIPS AND TRICKS**

**Pitfalls and Pearls for Mechanical Ventilation**

**Pitfalls**

Not considering NPPV
Not using NPPV early enough
Not having the personnel or time to adequately monitor and make adjustments
Not adjusting pressures quickly enough

**Pearls**

Early use of NPPV should be considered in a wide variety of patients.
Proper patient selection is paramount.
Selection of the interface and adjustment of parameters are crucial for success.
A team approach with close observation of the patient is vital.

*NPPV*, Noninvasive positive pressure ventilation.

## SUGGESTED READINGS

Santanilla JI, Daniel B, Yeow ME. Mechanical ventilation. Emerg Med Clin North Am 2008;26:849–62.

Yeow ME, Santanilla JI. Noninvasive positive pressure ventilation in the emergency department. Emerg Med Clin North Am 2008;26:835-47.

## REFERENCES

***References can be found on Expert Consult @ www.expertconsult.com.***

# 4 Shock

*Haney A. Mallemat and Michael E. Winters*

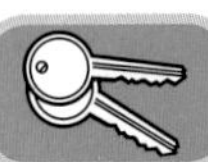

**KEY POINTS**

- Circulatory dysfunction can occur at three levels—the central circulation, the peripheral circulation, and the microcirculation—sometimes with subtle clinical findings.
- The initial history and physical examination should focus on identifying signs of hypoperfusion and detecting any immediately life-threatening circulatory disorders.
- Bedside ultrasonography can be helpful in assessing intravascular volume status and cardiac function and in detecting vascular catastrophes.
- Circulatory support is aimed at restoring adequate oxygen delivery.
- End points of circulatory resuscitation include clinical signs, mean arterial blood pressure, serum lactate level, and central venous oxygenation.

## PERSPECTIVE

The circulatory system is a complex vascular network that stretches more than 60,000 miles and circulates an average of 8000 L of blood each day. When circulatory dysfunction occurs, oxygen delivery is impaired, which leads to progressive cellular dysfunction. If not identified and treated, organ failure and death can ensue rapidly. This chapter discusses important elements of the history and physical examination along with invasive and noninvasive monitoring modalities used by the emergency physician (EP) to assess and support the circulatory system.

## ANATOMY

**Figure 4.1** illustrates the anatomy of the circulatory system.

## PATHOPHYSIOLOGY OF CIRCULATORY DYSFUNCTION

Normal organ function requires adequate perfusion and delivery of oxygen. Oxygen delivery is determined by arterial oxygen content and cardiac output. Arterial oxygen content is a function of hemoglobin concentration and arterial oxygen saturation. Cardiac output is governed by heart rate, contractility, and loading conditions. Any process that adversely affects cardiac output or arterial oxygen saturation can decrease oxygen delivery and result in circulatory dysfunction.

Cardiac output can be affected by the heart rate, arrhythmias, and alterations in ventricular loading. Preload, afterload, and contractility each affect ventricular loading. The Frank-Starling law (**Fig. 4.2**) states that the principal force governing the strength of ventricular contraction is the length of muscle fibers.[1] In a normal heart, muscle fiber length is determined by intravascular volume, often termed preload. As preload increases, myocardial fibers increase in length, which results in increased force of contraction. Increased force of ventricular contraction increases stroke volume and cardiac output. In contrast, depletion of intravascular volume results in muscle fiber shortening, less forceful cardiac contractions, lower stroke volume, and decreased cardiac output.

Increasing ventricular preload improves myocardial contractility only to a point, beyond which myocardial fibers become overstretched. Overstretched fibers can lead to worsening myocardial contractility and, eventually, increased hydrostatic pressure and interstitial edema (e.g., pulmonary edema).

Changes in afterload can also affect ventricular function. For example, severe hypertension impedes ventricular function by reducing cardiac emptying and flow while increasing myocardial workload. Similarly, reducing afterload increases cardiac emptying and flow while decreasing myocardial workload.

Contractility, a measure of ventricular function, is altered by a variety of factors. Medications such as dobutamine can increase the force of contraction for a given preload. In contrast, diseases such as congestive heart failure can reduce contractility and worsen stroke volume and cardiac output.

Circulatory dysfunction can also occur with alterations in regional or microcirculatory blood flow. Disorders that affect arteriolar tone, such as sepsis, cause maldistribution of blood flow between organs and a mismatch of oxygen delivery with demand. Capillary obstruction and endothelial impairment interrupt intraorgan oxygen delivery, thereby potentially resulting in organ failure.

Circulatory dysfunction exists as a spectrum ranging from mild impairment to shock with overt circulatory collapse. Shock is defined as the inability of the circulatory system to

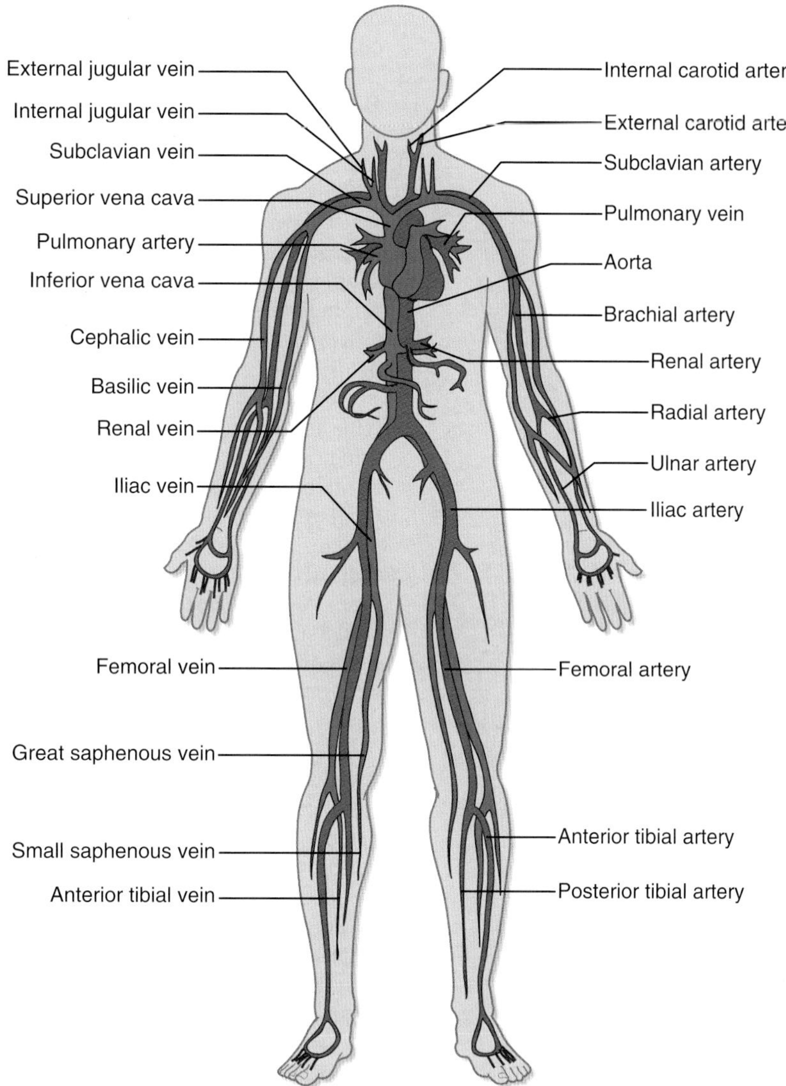


**Fig. 4.1 Anatomy of the circulatory system.**

provide adequate tissue perfusion, which potentially leads to cellular dysfunction.[1] Four categories of shock have been differentiated and defined by the underlying pathophysiology of the circulatory dysfunction: hypovolemic, cardiogenic, distributive, and obstructive **(Box 4.1)**.[2] Because each category requires specialized management, every attempt must be made to determine the exact cause of the shock.

## PRESENTING SIGNS AND SYMPTOMS

Circulatory insufficiency can be accompanied by myriad clinical findings. The signs and symptoms primarily reflect organ dysfunction secondary to hypoperfusion and decreased oxygen delivery. Classic signs of circulatory dysfunction include reduced blood pressure, abnormal heart rate, tachypnea, hypoxemia, mottled extremities, and decreased urine output. The most dramatic manifestation is cardiac arrest with complete circulatory failure. Unfortunately, many emergency department (ED) patients with circulatory dysfunction have vague, nonspecific symptoms. Common nonspecific symptoms of circulatory insufficiency include fatigue, malaise, weakness, lightheadedness, dizziness, altered mental status, diaphoresis, dyspnea, and syncope. Circulatory dysfunction should be considered in every patient with vague, undifferentiated symptoms.

## INITIAL ASSESSMENT

An initial circulatory assessment should be performed for every ED patient within the first minutes after arrival. This assessment consists of a review of triage vital signs, a focused history, physical examination, and possibly bedside ultrasonography. The goal of the initial circulatory assessment is to detect signs of organ hypoperfusion and identify any immediately life-threatening disorders. Life-threatening disorders requiring rapid diagnosis and treatment include pulmonary embolism, acute myocardial infarction, cardiac tamponade,

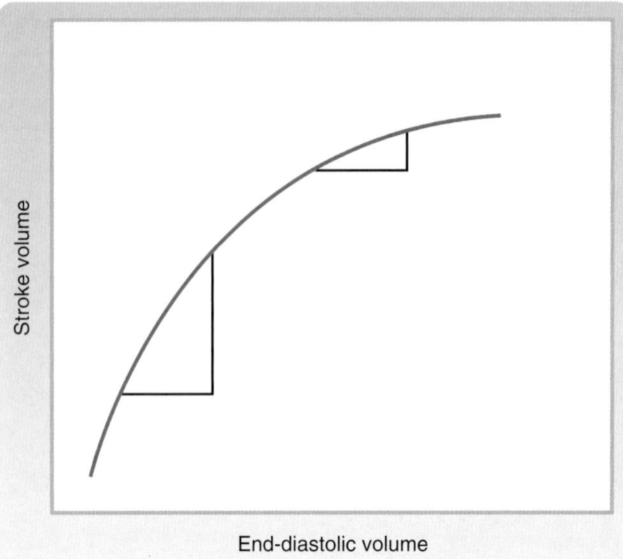


**Fig. 4.2** Frank-Starling curve demonstrating the relationship between end-diastolic pressure (preload) and systolic performance (stroke volume).

**BOX 4.1 Hinshaw and Cox Classification of Circulatory Shock**

**Hypovolemic**
Hemorrhage
Third spacing of fluids
- Ileus
- Burns
- Pancreatitis

**Cardiogenic**
Myocardial infarction
Valvular insufficiency
Arrhythmia

**Obstructive**
Massive pulmonary embolism
Tension pneumothorax
Pericardial tamponade
Aortic stenosis

**Distributive**
Septic shock
Anaphylactic shock
Neurogenic shock

tension pneumothorax, aortic dissection, and ruptured abdominal aortic aneurysm.

## VITAL SIGNS

For nearly all ED patients, circulatory assessment begins with the noninvasive measurement of vital signs. Although blood pressure and heart rate are central to the initial assessment, it is important to note the respiratory rate and oxygen saturation. Any abnormality in the respiratory rate or oxygen saturation may affect arterial oxygen content and impair oxygen delivery. Noninvasive measurement of vital signs correlates poorly with organ perfusion in critically ill patients but serves as an important component of the initial ED assessment of the circulatory system.[3]

### Blood Pressure

Blood pressure, the driving force for organ perfusion, is determined by cardiac output and arterial tone.[1] It is important to understand that no blood pressure value is considered normal for every patient. Normal blood pressure values do not always indicate sufficient oxygen delivery. Blood pressure values should be interpreted in the context of the patient's clinical findings, medical history, and treatment received.

Blood pressure is one of the most common measurements in all of clinical medicine, yet it is often measured incorrectly.[4] In the ED, blood pressure is initially obtained during triage with automated blood pressure devices that apply the oscillometric method. These devices can be adversely affected by ambient noise and cuff position. In addition, automated devices typically overestimate true arterial blood pressure in patients with low-flow states. These limitations, combined with activity in the triage environment and patient anxiety, often result in inaccurate measurements of blood pressure. Understandably, triage values can be an unreliable indicator of true blood pressure. Blood pressure measurements should be repeated serially at the bedside in patients demonstrating any evidence of circulatory insufficiency.

The auscultatory method has long been considered the "gold standard" for noninvasive blood pressure measurement. It determines systolic and diastolic pressure on the basis of detection of Korotkoff sounds. The ideal location is the upper part of the arm. The procedure is performed as follows:

1. Remove all clothing from the arm and place the blood pressure cuff so that the middle of the cuff is approximately at the level of the right atrium. The lower edge of the cuff should be 2 to 3 cm above the antecubital fossa to allow easy palpation and auscultation of the brachial artery.
2. Locate the radial artery and inflate the blood pressure cuff to approximately 30 mm Hg above the point at which the radial arterial pulse disappears.
3. Place the bell of the stethoscope over the brachial artery and deflate the cuff at a rate of 2 to 3 mm Hg per second. The appearance of faint, repetitive sounds for at least two consecutive beats is phase I of the Korotkoff sounds. Phase I is systolic blood pressure. The point at which all sounds disappear is phase V, or diastolic blood pressure.

Measure blood pressure bilaterally during the initial circulatory examination. A difference of more than 10 mm Hg is significant and may indicate an aortic emergency. Unfortunately, up to 20% of individuals have significant blood pressure differences between their arms.[5] Nevertheless, an aortic emergency must be ruled out in any patient with evidence of circulatory insufficiency and blood pressure discrepancies.

Though considered the gold standard, the auscultatory method has several pitfalls. **Box 4.2** lists errors commonly made during measurement of blood pressure with the auscultatory method.

### Heart Rate

The heart rate is an integral component of cardiac output. Tachycardia or bradycardia can impair circulatory function. As with blood pressure, triage measurements of the heart rate

**BOX 4.2 Pitfalls in Blood Pressure Measurement Using the Auscultatory Method**

Failure to use an appropriately sized blood pressure cuff:
- Blood pressure is falsely elevated if the cuff is too small.
- The bladder should measure at least 80% of the length and be 40% of the width of the upper part of the arm.
- Use a thigh cuff if necessary.

Failure to recognize the auscultatory gap:
- Occurs in elderly hypertensive patients with wide pulse pressure.
- Results in overestimation of diastolic pressure.
- Auscultation should be continued until the cuff is fully deflated.

Hypotensive states:
- The auscultatory method overestimates blood pressure in low-flow states.
- Do not use the auscultatory method to monitor unstable patients.

can be inaccurate and unreliable. Therefore, heart rate measurement should be repeated in every patient on initial examination. In addition to the rate, irregularities in rhythm should be noted. Arrhythmias can severely compromise circulatory function and organ perfusion. Furthermore, heart rate variability may be an early indication of circulatory dysfunction.[6] Methods to determine heart rate variability remain investigational and require additional research before clinical application.

### Orthostatic Blood Pressure

Depletion of intravascular volume can impair oxygen delivery by decreasing venous return and cardiac output. Symptoms of volume depletion are attributable to reduced cerebral blood flow and include weakness, lightheadedness, unsteadiness, impaired cognition, tremulousness, and syncope. Orthostatic blood pressure measurements can occasionally aid the EP in detecting otherwise unsuspected intravascular volume depletion, but they must be integrated with specific clinical findings. They are not obtained routinely because they have significant limitations.

A positive orthostatic blood pressure response is defined as a reduction in systolic blood pressure of at least 20 mm Hg or a reduction in diastolic blood pressure of at least 10 mm Hg within 3 minutes after standing in a patient with symptoms of volume depletion.[7] Orthostatic blood pressure should be measured with the patient in the supine and standing positions. For patients who are unable to stand or who are markedly unsteady, a sitting position may be used. Wait at least 2 minutes before obtaining a standing blood pressure measurement because nearly all patients have a brief orthostatic response immediately on standing. Always measure the heart rate with orthostatic blood pressure. In normal patients, the heart rate increases from 5 to 12 beats/min with standing. Increases greater than 30 beats/min are abnormal and indicate significant volume depletion.

Orthostatic blood pressure measurements have several limitations. Numerous conditions in addition to volume depletion impair the postural hemodynamic response and result in orthostatic hypotension. Most notable are the effects of aging and medications. Up to 30% of elderly patients demonstrate an orthostatic response in the absence of volume depletion.[8] Many elderly patients take medications that alter the postural response to changes in position; such medications include antiadrenergics, antidepressants, antihypertensives, neuroleptics, anticholinergics, and antiparkinsonian drugs. In addition, any disorder causing primary or secondary autonomic dysfunction can lead to orthostatic hypotension.

### Pulse Pressure

Increasing evidence demonstrates that abnormal pulse pressure—the difference between systolic and diastolic blood pressure—is an independent risk factor for cardiovascular morbidity and mortality. To date, studies have focused on outpatients with established hypertension. Nevertheless, it is important to determine pulse pressure in the initial circulatory assessment of an ED patient. Acute disorders that alter circulatory function are often manifested as abnormalities in pulse pressure. A narrow pulse pressure (<40 mm Hg) indicates reduced stroke volume and thus reduced cardiac output. Life-threatening conditions resulting in a narrow pulse pressure include tension pneumothorax, cardiac tamponade, pulmonary embolism, acute myocardial infarction with cardiogenic shock, and severe volume depletion. A widened pulse pressure (>40 mm Hg) results from processes that lower systemic vascular resistance. Diseases that can be accompanied by widened pulse pressure include sepsis, anaphylaxis, acute aortic insufficiency, adrenal insufficiency, and neurogenic shock.

## HISTORY

A focused history is essential during the initial circulatory assessment. Key elements are a history of the present illness, previous medical history, medication history, family history, and social history. With respect to the history of the present illness, determine the onset and duration of symptoms, the context in which the symptoms developed, any associated symptoms, and any aggravating or alleviating factors. Important associated symptoms include chest pain, dyspnea, palpitations, syncope, and altered mental status. Review the patient's medical history and direct attention to disorders that may impair cardiac output or arterial oxygen content.

Medications can result in circulatory abnormalities through direct effects or side effects. Two important classes of medications are antiarrhythmic agents and antihypertensive agents. It is crucial to note whether the patient is taking a beta-blocker or calcium channel blocker because both agents can alter the compensatory response to circulatory insufficiency. Always interpret vital signs in the context of the medical history and medication regimen.

Additional key components of the history are the family and social histories. Directly question patients about their family history of sudden death, premature coronary artery disease, venous thromboembolism, and connective tissue disorders (e.g., Marfan syndrome). Similarly, question patients about their use of illicit substances known to have circulatory effects, namely, cocaine.

## PHYSICAL EXAMINATION

Physical examination of the circulatory system begins with the general appearance of the patient. Observe the patient's positioning, mental status, skin color, and respiratory pattern.

Suspect circulatory abnormalities in restless, diaphoretic, delirious, pale, mottled, or tachypneic patients. In addition, note any distinct clinical features implying an underlying medical condition. **Table 4.1** lists the characteristic features of disorders that can affect the circulatory system.

Examine the head and neck for abnormalities suggesting circulatory disease. Facial edema implies impaired venous return resulting from conditions such as superior vena cava thrombosis and constrictive pericarditis. Examination of the jugular venous pulse provides important information about central venous pressure (CVP) and the dynamics of the right side of the heart.[9] Place the patient in a 45-degree recumbent position and shine a light tangentially across the neck. The right side is preferred because of its anatomic alignment with the superior vena cava and right atrium. Beginning at the sternal notch, measure the height (in centimeters) of the internal jugular vein pulsations. Pulsations more than 4 cm above the sternal notch are abnormal and a sign of elevated CVP.[9] **Figure 4.3** illustrates jugular venous distention in a young woman with pericardial effusion.

The cardiopulmonary examination is a quintessential component of circulatory assessment. Observe the rate, depth, and effort of respirations. Tachypnea accompanied by shallow respirations or the use of accessory muscles indicates impending respiratory failure. Auscultate the lungs for asymmetric breath sounds, rhonchi, rales, and wheezing. Recall that any pulmonary process can adversely affect arterial oxygen content and thereby impair oxygen delivery. Auscultate the heart over the right and left upper sternal edges, the lower left sternal edge, and the cardiac apex. Determine the rate and listen for rhythm irregularities, the intensity of heart sounds, murmurs, gallop rhythms, and pericardial rubs. Though difficult with the ambient noise in the ED, attempt to determine whether cardiac murmurs are systolic or diastolic, which can potentially provide valuable information in patients with acute cardiopulmonary dysfunction. Gallop rhythms are low-frequency heart sounds that are heard best with the bell of the stethoscope.

The extremities must be examined as part of the initial circulatory assessment. It is important to observe their color

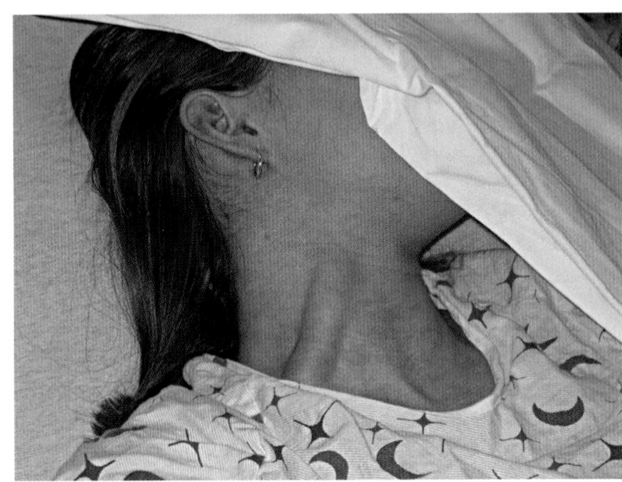

**Fig. 4.3** Jugular venous distention in a young woman with pericardial effusion.

**Table 4.1 Characteristics of Conditions That Affect the Circulatory System**

| CONDITION | CLINICAL APPEARANCE | POTENTIAL CIRCULATORY IMPLICATIONS |
|---|---|---|
| Marfan syndrome | Arachnodactyly<br>Arm span greater than height<br>Longer pubis-to-foot length than pubis-to-head length | Aortic dissection |
| Osteogenesis imperfecta | Blue sclera | Aortic dissection<br>Aortic aneurysm<br>Aortic valve insufficiency<br>Mitral valve prolapse |
| Hyperthyroidism | Exophthalmos | Congestive heart failure |
| Hypothyroidism | Expressionless face<br>Periorbital edema<br>Loss of lateral third of the eyebrows<br>Dry, sparse hair | Congestive heart failure<br>Pericardial effusion |
| Hemochromatosis | Bronze pigmentation of skin<br>Loss of axillary and pubic hair | Cardiomyopathy |
| Turner syndrome | Short stature<br>Webbed neck<br>"Shield" chest<br>Medial deviation of the extended forearm | Aortic coarctation |
| Aortic insufficiency | Bobbing of the head with heartbeat<br>Systolic flushing of the nail beds | — |

and temperature. Signs of poor perfusion include cold, pale, clammy, mottled skin associated with delayed capillary refill (normal capillary refill is less than 2 seconds). Inspect for symmetric or asymmetric edema and clubbing of the fingers and toes. Finally, palpate the carotid, radial, femoral, dorsalis pedis, and posterior tibial pulses for rate, amplitude, and regularity.

## EMERGENCY ULTRASONOGRAPHY

Even after the most careful evaluation of the history, vital signs, and physical examination, the pathophysiology of the circulatory dysfunction may not be completely clear. In this situation, further diagnostic testing is needed to confirm a diagnosis or initiate treatment. Unfortunately, diagnostic testing may require transfer of the patient from the ED to areas in the hospital with significantly less monitoring (e.g., the radiology suite).

Over the past 3 decades, ultrasonography has become essential in the initial assessment of patients with circulatory dysfunction. Ultrasonography is easily performed at the bedside and provides a noninvasive, real-time assessment of causes of circulatory dysfunction. Because ultrasonography may identify the cause of circulatory dysfunction faster than traditional diagnostic testing can, definitive interventions can be initiated rapidly, thereby potentially minimizing end-organ damage.[10]

Many ultrasonography algorithms and approaches for assessing circulatory dysfunction have been published. For the purposes of this discussion, we will use the RUSH (Rapid Ultrasound in SHock) protocol to illustrate the utility of ultrasonography in evaluating circulatory dysfunction.[11] In three systematic steps, the RUSH protocol evaluates circulatory dysfunction as follows:

Step 1: Evaluate the heart (the "pump").
Step 2: Assess intravascular volume status (the "tank").
Step 3: Evaluate the major vascular structures (the "pipes").

### *Step 1: Evaluate the Pump*

Evaluation of the heart with the RUSH protocol is different from a formal echocardiogram obtained by cardiologists. Formal echocardiography examines the heart from multiple views, comments on segmental wall motion abnormalities, and evaluates valvular function and structure. The cardiac component of the RUSH protocol is limited to the following: (1) global left ventricular function, (2) relative size of the left ventricle (LV) to the right ventricle (RV), and (3) evaluation of the pericardial sac for tamponade (**Fig. 4.4**). To perform the assessment, a 3.5-MHz probe is placed on the left anterior aspect of the chest (i.e., parasternal view) (**Fig. 4.5, *A***) or below the costal margin (i.e., subcostal view) (**Fig. 4.5, *B***). Once an adequate view is obtained, global left ventricular function can be described as normal, hyperkinetic, reduced, or severely reduced.

The next cardiac assessment is left and right ventricular size. In normal patients, the RV is 60% the size of the LV. Any increase in the ratio of RV to LV size is considered abnormal and suggests the possibility of pulmonary embolism or right ventricular infarction as the cause of the circulatory dysfunction. In these situations, the thin-walled RV can fail under acutely increased pressure or volume loads. If right ventricular failure occurs, the amount of blood delivered to the left

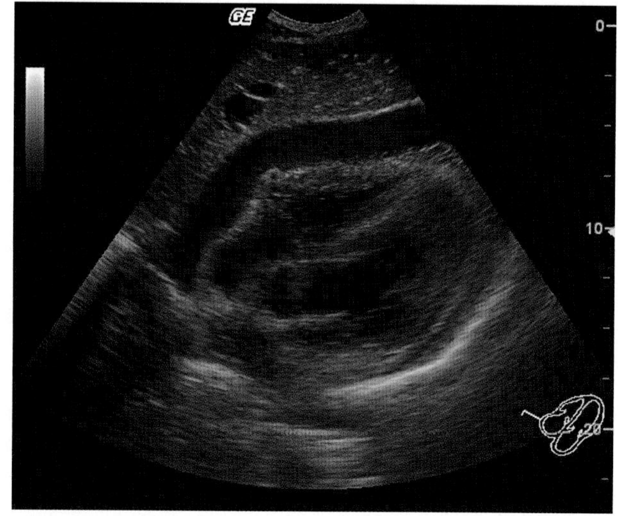


**Fig. 4.4** Subcostal view of the heart demonstrating pericardial effusion.

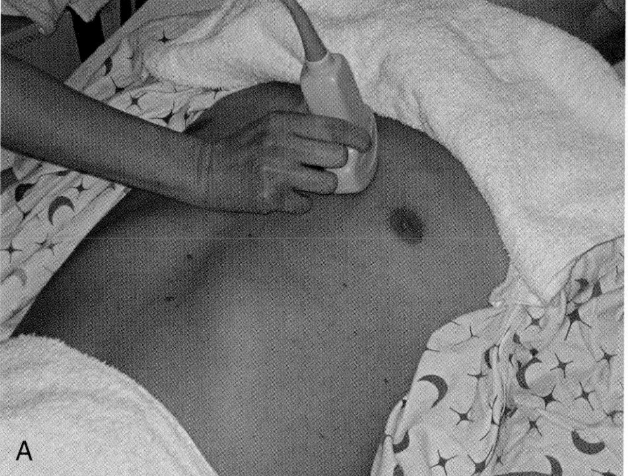


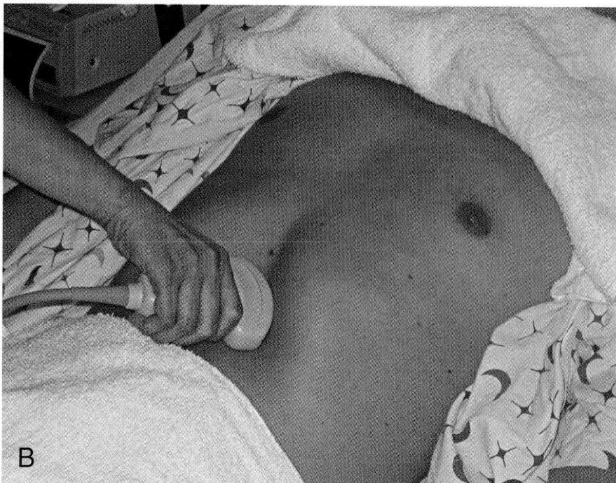


**Fig. 4.5** Proper positioning of the ultrasound probe for parasternal (A) and subxiphoid (B) views of the heart.

side of the heart may not be sufficient for adequate cardiac output.

The final portion of the cardiac examination is evaluation of the pericardial space. Pericardial tamponade can cause obstructive shock and should be diagnosed promptly. The classic echocardiographic images show a large anechoic space (i.e., fluid) around the pericardium that is compressing the RV and can lead to a hyperdynamic and underfilled LV.

### *Step 2: Evaluate the Tank*

The second step in the RUSH protocol is evaluation of intravascular volume status, or "the tank." As stated previously, depletion of intravascular volume reduces preload and decreases left ventricular filling, thereby decreasing cardiac output. Examination of the inferior vena cava (IVC) from a subcostal approach allows evaluation of the tank. For example, a patient with hypovolemic shock may have a small IVC that changes significantly in diameter with respiration. Such a patient probably has low CVP with an empty tank, thus indicating that volume should be administered as part of the resuscitation. Contrast this example with a patient with a full tank; that is, a large and dilated IVC. This condition may occur in cardiogenic or obstructive shock, where volume may assist in resuscitation, but would probably not be the main cause of the underlying pathophysiology.

Following determination of intravascular volume, assess the "leakiness" of the tank; that is, examine major body compartments where fluid may have "leaked." Examination of the abdominal compartment and the thoracic space for free fluid may reveal the source of leakiness (**Fig. 4.6**). Finally, evaluation for the presence of pneumothorax is critical in assessment of the tank because tension pneumothorax can cause obstructive shock secondary to compression of the major vessels and relative hypovolemia and shock.

### *Step 3: Evaluate the Pipes*

The final step in the RUSH protocol is evaluation of the "pipes"; that is, examination of the major arteries and veins for rupture or obstruction. Inspect the thoracic and abdominal portions of the aorta for dissection or aneurysm. Then focus on the venous system and look for deep vein thrombosis (DVT) by compressing the veins of the lower extremity. Hypotensive patients with evidence of DVT may have a hemodynamically significant pulmonary embolus.

All three steps of the RUSH protocol should be completed sequentially and thoroughly. If an abnormality is found, the temptation to terminate the study early should be avoided because of the potential for additional findings. Once the examination has been completed, positive and negative findings should be clinically integrated and interpreted to determine the cause of the shock. Combined findings from the RUSH evaluation and their indication of the type of shock are listed in **Table 4.2**.

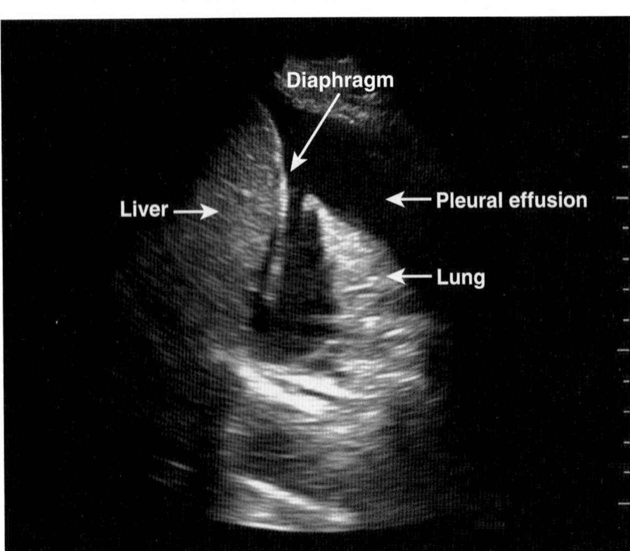


**Fig. 4.6** Free fluid in the thoracic space as demonstrated by bedside ultrasound.

### *Additional Uses of Emergency Ultrasonography*

Ultrasonography can be used for emergency procedures such as establishment of intravenous access, pericardiocentesis, and transvenous cardiac pacing.[12] It can also be used for hemodynamic monitoring (e.g., volume responsiveness, CVP, pulmonary artery occlusion pressure [PAOP], cardiac output).[13,14]

## PROCEDURES AND CIRCULATORY MONITORING

Procedures pertinent to circulatory assessment and support center on obtaining vascular access and placing invasive circulatory monitors. Rapid attainment of intravenous access is required for patients exhibiting signs and symptoms of hypoperfusion. Invasive circulatory monitoring is used to ensure adequate tissue perfusion and oxygen delivery. Invasive monitoring is indicated for patients who continue to exhibit signs of hypoperfusion despite initial resuscitative measures. Common invasive modalities include arterial blood pressure monitoring, CVP monitoring, and pulmonary artery catheterization. A number of new monitoring modalities have been developed to evaluate the adequacy of circulation. These new modalities include esophageal Doppler analysis, pulse contour analysis, thoracic bioreactance, near-infrared retinal spectroscopy, transcutaneous tissue oxygen monitors, central venous oxygen saturation monitoring, and sublingual capnometry.

### INTRAVENOUS ACCESS

Despite the physician's desire to perform central venous catheterization during initial resuscitation, peripheral venous cannulation is preferred. As stated by Poiseuille's law, the rate at which intravenous fluids can be infused depends on the radius and length of the catheter. Greater volume can be infused over a shorter time with short peripheral catheters than with a central venous line. Peripheral catheters should be 18 gauge or larger. The external jugular veins and the veins of the antecubital fossa provide rapid and safe access for peripheral venous cannulation.

Central venous catheterization has become a common bedside procedure in emergency medicine. In the United States, more than 5 million central venous catheters are placed each year. **Table 4.3** lists several indications for and contraindications to establishing central venous access. The procedure presents a risk for a number of complications (see the

**Table 4.2** Differential Diagnosis Based on RUSH Examination Findings

| RUSH EVALUATION | HYPOVOLEMIC SHOCK | CARDIOGENIC SHOCK | OBSTRUCTIVE SHOCK | DISTRIBUTIVE SHOCK |
|---|---|---|---|---|
| Pump | Hypercontractile heart<br>Small chamber size | Hypocontractile heart<br>Dilated heart | Hypercontractile heart<br>Pericardial effusion<br>Cardiac tamponade<br>RV strain<br>Cardiac thrombus | Hypercontractile heart (early sepsis)<br>Hypocontractile heart (late sepsis) |
| Tank | Flat IVC<br>Flat jugular veins<br>Peritoneal fluid (fluid loss)<br>Pleural fluid (fluid loss) | Distended IVC<br>Distended jugular veins<br>Lung rockets (pulmonary edema)<br>Pleural fluid<br>Peritoneal fluid (edema) | Distended IVC<br>Distended jugular veins<br>Absent lung sliding (pneumothorax) | Normal or small IVC (early sepsis)<br>Peritoneal fluid (sepsis source)<br>Pleural fluid (sepsis source) |
| Pipes | Abdominal aneurysm<br>Aortic dissection | Normal | DVT | Normal |

*DVT*, Deep vein thrombosis; *IVC*, inferior vena cava; *RUSH*, Rapid Ultrasound in SHock; *RV*, right ventricular.
From Perera P, Mailhot T, Riley D, et al. The RUSH exam: Rapid Ultrasound in SHock in the evaluation of the critically ill. Emerg Med Clin North Am 2010;28:29-56.

**Table 4.3** Central Line Placement: Indications and Contraindications

| | |
|---|---|
| Indications | Failed peripheral venous access<br>Cardiopulmonary arrest<br>Central venous pressure monitoring<br>Transvenous pacemaker insertion<br>Emergency hemodialysis<br>Administration of medications known to irritate the peripheral veins |
| Contraindications | |
| Absolute | None |
| Relative | Cutaneous infection at the site of puncture<br>Existing venous thrombosis<br>Existing arteriovenous fistula<br>Coagulopathy—subclavian and internal jugular sites<br>Thrombocytopenia—subclavian and internal jugular sites |

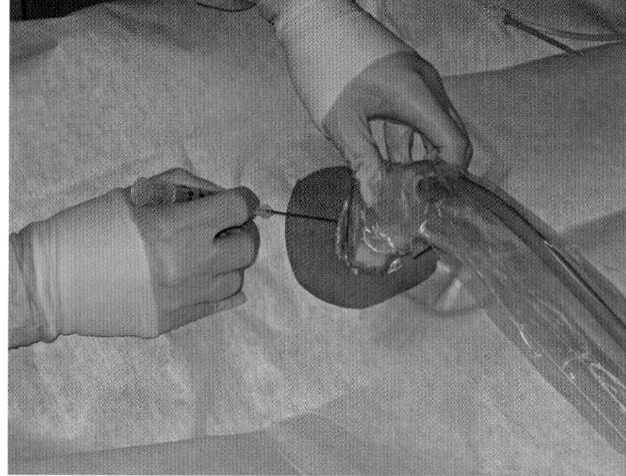

**Fig. 4.7** Proper positioning of the ultrasonography probe for catheterization of the internal jugular vein.

Red Flags box), but their occurrence can be minimized by following the basic rules of good practice (see the Tips and Tricks box). For catheterization of the internal jugular vein, the ultrasonography probe should be positioned on the anterior aspect of the neck, as demonstrated in **Figure 4.7**. Identification of the vein can be facilitated by asking the patient to perform the Valsalva maneuver, which causes engorgement of the neck veins (**Fig. 4.8**, ***A* and *B***).

## ARTERIAL BLOOD PRESSURE MONITORING

Invasive arterial blood pressure monitoring is required for patients with persistent circulatory dysfunction despite initial resuscitative measures. Primary indications for placement of an arterial line include continuous blood pressure monitoring, the need for frequent blood sampling, and serial measurements of $PaO_2$. When possible, the radial artery should be used for this purpose. It offers the advantages of a peripheral position and easy compressibility in the event of unsuccessful cannulation. Additionally, the nearby ulnar artery supplies collateral blood flow to the hand while the radial artery is cannulated. If the radial artery cannot be used, a line can be placed in other arteries, as listed in **Box 4.3**.

Catheter placement is guided by palpation of the artery. When the pulse is difficult to detect, ultrasound becomes an important aid for visualization of the target artery. Cannulation of the radial artery under ultrasound guidance is faster, requires fewer attempts, and is associated with fewer complications than the palpation method is.[15] Proper patient positioning for radial artery cannulation is illustrated in **Figure 4.9**.

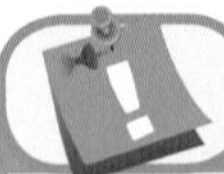

**TIPS AND TRICKS**

**Tips for Decreasing the Rate of Complications with Central Venous Catheterization**

Use maximal sterile barrier precautions—cap, mask, gown, gloves, and sterile drapes.

Use chlorhexidine-based solutions if available.

Do not allow inexperienced operators (<50 catheterizations) more than three attempts.

Whenever possible, place a subclavian central venous catheter, which is associated with the lowest rate of mechanical, infectious, and thrombotic complications.

Use ultrasonographic guidance routinely for internal jugular venous catheterization.

Do not use topical antibiotic ointments; they have not been shown to decrease the risk for catheter-related infections.

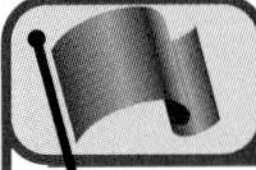

**RED FLAGS**

**Complications of Central Venous Catheterization**

Mechanical—5% to 19%

- Arterial puncture
- Arteriovenous fistula
- Pseudoaneurysm
- Atrial arrhythmias
- Ventricular arrhythmias
- Hematoma
- Catheter malposition
- Pneumothorax (subclavian, internal jugular)
- Embolism (air, thrombus, guidewire)
- Cardiac perforation producing tamponade
- Bladder aspiration (femoral)

Infection—5% to 26%

- Cutaneous infection
- Catheter-related bloodstream infection

Thrombosis—2% to 26%

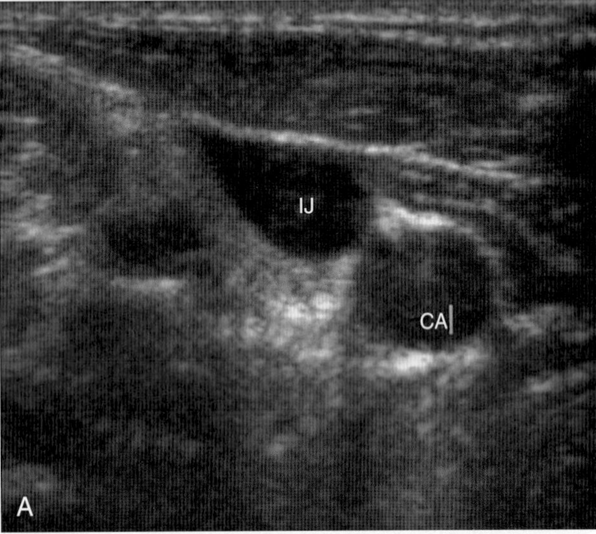


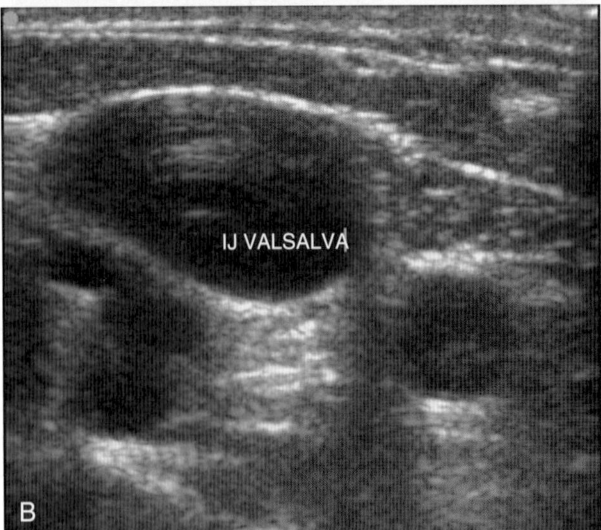


**Fig. 4.8** Ultrasonographic appearance of the internal jugular vein *(IJ)* at baseline (A) and when the patient performs a Valsalva maneuver (B). *CA*, Carotid artery.

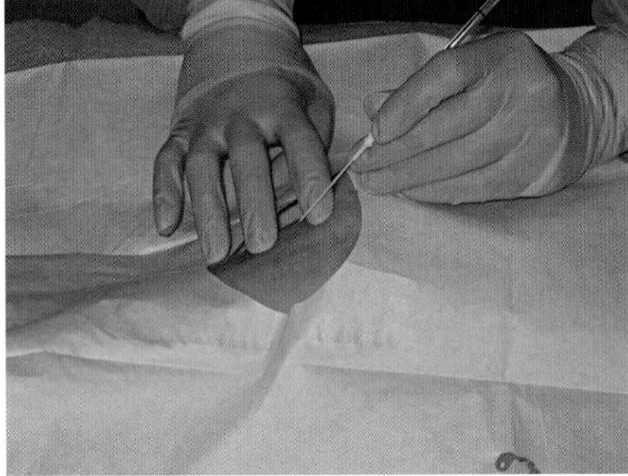

**Fig. 4.9** Proper patient positioning for cannulation of the radial artery.

## CENTRAL VENOUS PRESSURE

CVP is intravascular pressure in the central vena cava system, near its junction with the right atrium. Clinically, CVP is used as a marker of volume status and cardiac preload. Normal values for CVP range from 8 to 12 mm Hg. CVP can be estimated noninvasively by examining the internal jugular vein (as described in the physical examination section of this chapter), but bedside determinations have been shown to be inaccurate and unreliable.[16] Direct measurements, through a subclavian or internal jugular vein catheter, provide more reliable results. CVP can be measured via a femoral central venous catheter; however, values typically differ by 0.5 to 3 mm Hg from those obtained from the superior vena cava. In a patient who is not mechanically ventilated, CVP can be estimated noninvasively by visualizing the IVC with ultrasound (**Table 4.4**). For example, a normally sized IVC that collapses more than 50% correlates with a CVP between 0 and 5 mm Hg.[17]

**BOX 4.3 Arterial Cannulation: Insertion Sites, Possible Complications, Procedure Tips**

**Sites of Insertion**

Radial artery (most common and preferred)
Femoral artery
Brachial artery
Axillary artery
Ulnar artery
Dorsalis pedis artery

**Complications**

Thrombosis with arterial occlusion
Hematoma
Infection (catheter-related bloodstream infections)
Heparin-induced thrombocytopenia
Anemia (frequent blood sampling)

**Tips**

Avoid cannulation of the brachial artery, complications of which can be severe:

- Forearm ischemia
- Compartment syndrome
- Median nerve damage

A femoral arterial line has a lower rate of catheter malfunction and greater longevity but higher risk for infection.
Wear a sterile gown, gloves, and mask and place a drape.
Administer lidocaine without epinephrine for local anesthesia.
Flush the line frequently to maintain patency and prevent thrombosis.

**Table 4.4** Estimation of Right Atrial Pressure from Measurement of the Inferior Vena Cava

| SIZE OF IVC | IVC SIZE ON INSPIRATION | RA PRESSURE (mm Hg) |
|---|---|---|
| <1.5 cm (small) | Nearly total collapse | 0-5 |
| 1.5-2.5 cm (normal) | Decrease >50% | 5-10 |
| 1.5-2.5 cm | Decrease <50% | 10-15 |
| >2.5 cm | Decrease <50% | 15-20 |
| IVC and hepatic vein dilation | No change | >20 |

*IVC*, Inferior vena cava; *RA*, right atrial.

## PULMONARY ARTERY CATHETERIZATION

First described by Swan and colleagues in the early 1970s, pulmonary artery catheterization is considered the gold standard for circulatory monitoring in the critically ill. Circulatory measurements obtained with pulmonary artery catheterization include cardiac output, right ventricular ejection fraction, mixed venous oxygen saturation, and intrapulmonary vascular pressure. From these measurements, oxygen delivery, oxygen consumption, systemic vascular resistance, and left ventricular stroke index can be calculated. Because a pulmonary artery catheter gives clinicians the ability to measure oxygen delivery directly, it would seem to be an invaluable tool for circulatory monitoring. Unfortunately, routine use of this type of catheter remains controversial. Use of a pulmonary artery catheter has not been shown to decrease patient morbidity or mortality rates.[18] In fact, use of a pulmonary artery catheter may be detrimental. Complications of insertion include pneumothorax, ventricular arrhythmias, ventricular perforation, and pulmonary artery rupture. Until further evidence is published, pulmonary artery catheters should not be used in the ED for assessment and support of the circulatory system.

## ADDITIONAL CIRCULATORY MONITORING MODALITIES

The circulatory system can also be assessed with global, or tissue, markers of hypoperfusion. Methods of assessing global hypoperfusion in the ED include central venous oxygen saturation and serum lactate values. Under normal circumstances, cells extract 25% to 30% of the oxygen from the circulation. Therefore, blood returning to the central circulation has an oxygen saturation ranging from 70% to 75%. When the circulation fails to deliver adequate oxygen, cellular oxygen extraction is increased. This increase is reflected as decreased mixed venous oxygen saturation, measured via a pulmonary artery catheter. Mixed venous oxygen saturation values of less than 65% are associated with decreased perfusion and oxidative impairment of some vascular beds. Central venous oxygen saturation of less than 70%, measured intermittently or continuously via a central venous catheter, is a reliable surrogate for mixed venous oxygen saturation. Central venous oxygen saturation, as a global marker of hypoperfusion, was used in a landmark study that demonstrated a significant decrease in mortality rate in ED patients with sepsis in whom that marker was used.[19] Central venous oxygen saturation values should be obtained from either subclavian or internal jugular central venous catheters.

Serum lactate values are also used as global markers of hypoperfusion. With persistently impaired oxygen delivery, cells convert to anaerobic metabolism, which results in the accumulation of lactic acid. A lactate level higher than 2 mmol/L is considered an indicator of inadequate oxygenation. Abnormal lactate levels have numerous causes, but the clinician should always regard impaired tissue perfusion as the primary cause in an ED patient.

The trend in lactate values is the most clinically useful information. Increasing serial lactate levels portend a worse prognosis and indicate a persistent circulatory dysfunction. A 10% reduction in lactate concentration in serial samples may be a more clinically useful marker of resuscitation than central venous oxygen concentration.[20]

Tissue-specific monitors of hypoperfusion include gastric tonometry, sublingual capnometry, near-infrared spectroscopy, and tissue oxygen tension. These circulatory monitoring modalities detect hypoperfusion and impaired oxygen delivery in specific vascular beds. These promising modalities require further prospective investigation and are not used in the daily practice of emergency medicine. Available noninvasive methods for measuring cardiac output include esophageal Doppler ultrasonography, impedance plethysmography, and pulse-contour analysis. As with tissue-specific monitors of hypoperfusion, these noninvasive methods require further prospective analysis before widespread clinical application.

## TREATMENT OF CIRCULATORY DYSFUNCTION

Treatment goals for circulatory support are based on restoring adequate oxygen delivery. Methods of restoration consist of improving cardiac output, arterial oxygen content, and peripheral perfusion pressure. General ED therapies include supplemental oxygen, endotracheal intubation, intravenous fluids, vasoactive medications, and the use of mechanical support devices such as cardiac pacemakers. Regardless of the therapy chosen, it is important to recognize established end points of circulatory resuscitation. First and foremost, patients should exhibit clinical signs of improvement, such as improving mental status, increasing urine output, and normalization of vital signs. Additional end points of resuscitation are mean arterial blood pressure, serum lactate level, and central venous oxygen saturation. Mean arterial pressure represents true perfusion pressure; its measurement is superior to systolic blood pressure monitoring. Mean arterial pressure in patients with sepsis should be at least 65 mm Hg. There is no survival benefit to raising it beyond that level. As discussed earlier, serum lactate values should show a decreasing trend over serial measurements. Persistently elevated lactate values indicate inadequate and incomplete circulatory resuscitation. For patients with a central venous catheter, CVP and central venous oxygen saturation can be monitored. CVP should range from 8 to 12 mm Hg, whereas central venous oxygen saturation values should exceed 70%. The goals of resuscitation are summarized in **Box 4.4**.

### GENERAL TREATMENT PRINCIPLES

Patients with circulatory dysfunction require rapid assessment and simultaneous treatment:

1. Begin cardiac monitoring immediately to determine the patient's heart rate and rhythm regularity.
2. Provide supplemental oxygen to improve arterial oxygen saturation.
3. Maintain a low threshold for intubation. The respiratory muscles are avid consumers of oxygen, thereby limiting oxygen delivery to other vital organs. Early intubation and paralysis of respiratory muscles may be required in patients with ongoing circulatory compromise.
4. Establish peripheral intravenous access rapidly.
5. Obtain an electrocardiogram and a portable chest radiograph within the first minutes to evaluate for acute myocardial infarction and pneumothorax.
6. Perform ultrasonography early to look for myocardial dysfunction, pericardial effusion, hemoperitoneum, and abdominal aortic aneurysm in patients with persistent hypotension.

**BOX 4.4 Goals of Resuscitation**

**Clinical Signs**
Improved mental status
Improved capillary refill and skin perfusion

**Vital Signs**
Urine output of 0.5-1.0 mL/kg/hr
Mean arterial pressure >65 mm Hg
Heart rate <100 beats/min
Respiratory rate <20 breaths/min
Oxygen saturation >94%
Central venous pressure of 8-12 mm Hg (12-15 mm Hg if the patient is mechanically ventilated)

**Serum Markers of Hypoperfusion**
Normalization of serum lactate value
Central venous oxygen saturation >70%

### TRENDELENBURG POSITION

Hypotensive patients are often placed in the Trendelenburg position while resuscitative efforts, such as establishing intravenous access and administering fluids, are initiated. The Trendelenburg position was thought to increase venous return and thereby augment cardiac output. This assumption is incorrect because of the capacitance of the venous circulation. The Trendelenburg position does not promote venous return or increase cardiac output. Hypotensive patients should not be put in the Trendelenburg position. This position serves only to increase the risk for aspiration.

### INTRAVENOUS FLUID ADMINISTRATION

Acute circulatory failure should be treated initially with intravenous fluids. In the absence of left ventricular failure, rapid fluid therapy is provided to improve preload and augment cardiac output. For patients without preexisting cardiopulmonary disease, a 20- to 40-mL/kg bolus should be infused over a 10-minute period. In patients with existing cardiac disease, smaller volumes of fluid are infused (e.g., 250 to 500 mL over a 15-minute period). Regardless of the volume chosen, patients must be reassessed after every fluid bolus to determine whether additional treatment is needed.

The administration of colloid fluids during the initial circulatory resuscitation confers no mortality benefit.[21] An isotonic crystalloid solution should be the first-line intravenous fluid. Fluid therapy is continued until the end points of resuscitation are achieved or the patient demonstrates pulmonary edema or evidence of right heart dysfunction.

#### *Preload Responsiveness*

Before volume resuscitation is initiated in a critically ill patient, preload responsiveness should be assessed; that is, whether cardiac output is likely to improve with the administration of fluids. Depending on the underlying disease, cardiac output might not increase with volume infusion. Additionally, inappropriate administration of volume may be harmful (e.g., exacerbation of pulmonary edema leading to hypoxemia). Several techniques are available for assessment of preload responsiveness.

STATIC VERSUS DYNAMIC MEASUREMENTS Static and dynamic measurements are the two general methods for assessing preload responsiveness. Static measures are used as absolute cutoffs, and examples are CVP and PAOP.

Proponents of the use of CVP to assess preload responsiveness state that blood pressure will probably increase in a hypotensive patient with low CVP when a fluid bolus is given;

that is, the patient will be preload responsive. Conversely, blood pressure will not increase after volume infusion in a hypotensive patient with elevated CVP. These assumptions may be true for hypotensive patients, but the clinical utility of CVP is limited by several factors. CVP is affected by venous compliance, arrhythmias, right-sided heart disease, and alterations in intrathoracic pressure (e.g., as induced by mechanical ventilation). In addition, CVP depends on an appropriately selected reference point, and false results can be obtained if that point is zeroed incorrectly. The same limitations exist when considering PAOP to assess for preload responsiveness, and thus it should be used with caution.

Several studies have demonstrated that static measures are inaccurate in predicting preload responsiveness.[22,23] Nonetheless, the most recent Surviving Sepsis Campaign consensus guidelines recommend using static measurements such as CVP and PAOP to assess preload responsiveness and guide fluid resuscitation in septic patients.[24]

Given the controversies surrounding the use of CVP for assessment of preload responsiveness, we recommend the following:

- Patients with low CVP who are given a fluid challenge and show at least a 2–mm Hg increase in pressure probably have intravascular depletion and are preload responsive. Such patients require additional fluid administration to optimize preload and cardiac output.
- Normal or elevated CVP should not be interpreted as indicating adequate circulatory volume and cardiac preload. A method other than measurement of CVP should be used to assess preload responsiveness.

Dynamic assessments of preload responsiveness are believed to be more accurate than static assessments. Dynamic measures are derived from the interaction between the respiratory and cardiac systems during mechanical ventilation. Mechanical ventilation elevates intrathoracic pressure, which affects left ventricular preload and changes stroke volume in patients who are preload responsive. Patients who are not preload responsive do not have variations in stroke volume with mechanical ventilation. Stroke volume can be assessed with an arterial catheter or noninvasively by pulse oximeter plethysmographic waveform amplitude.[25]

Dynamic measures predict preload responsiveness as a percentage of change throughout the respiratory cycle. Examples of dynamic measurements for preload responsiveness include stroke volume variation, esophageal Doppler analysis, pulse pressure variation (PPV), the IVC distensibility index (DI), and the passive leg-raise maneuver. Dynamic assessment requires the patient to be mechanically ventilated (except for the passive leg-raise maneuver), to have ventilation at a set tidal volume (6 to 8 mL/kg), to have no spontaneous breaths, and to be in sinus rhythm. The most useful dynamic measures of preload responsiveness for the EP are the DI and PPV.

DISTENSBILITY INDEX The IVC is measured easily and reliably with ultrasound via the subcostal view. In mechanically ventilated patients, variations in intrathoracic pressure cause changes in IVC diameter; that is, increased diameter with a positive pressure breath and decreased diameter with expiration (**Fig. 4.10, *A* and *B***). This variability in diameter (the DI) is most pronounced when a patient is preload responsive. DI is defined as the difference between the maximum and minimum diameters divided by the minimum diameter × 100. A DI greater than 18% has 90% sensitivity and specificity for predicting preload responsiveness.[26] Because the IVC is easy to visualize and measure, the DI can be assessed following each fluid bolus. By continuously reassessing the DI, volume can be given up to the point at which a patient is no longer preload responsive.

Limitations of the DI include its unreliability in nonintubated patients and uncertainty about the optimal tidal volume and positive end-expiratory pressure during measurements. Nonetheless, because the DI is easy to measure and is reproducible, it remains a clinically valuable tool.

PULSE PRESSURE VARIATION PPV is another dynamic measure of preload responsiveness. PPV can be calculated with an arterial catheter or via pulse oximeter plethysmographic waveform analysis. PPV is calculated by taking the difference between the maximum and minimum pulse pressures during one respiratory cycle, dividing by the average of the two values (maximum and minimum), and then multiplying by 100 (**Fig. 4.11**). Values higher than 18% predict a hypotensive patient to be preload responsive; a volume challenge would probably increase stroke volume and cardiac

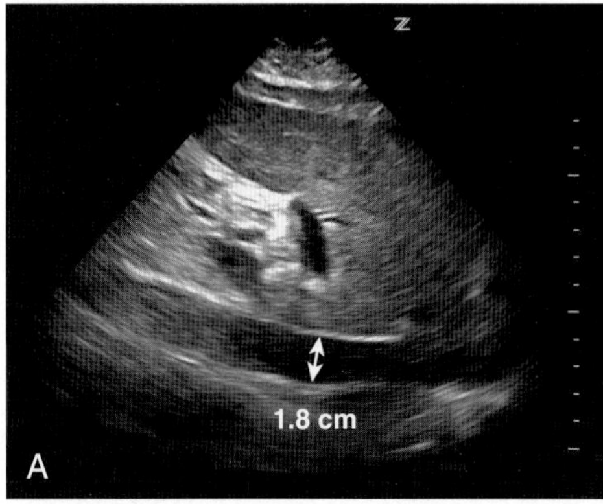


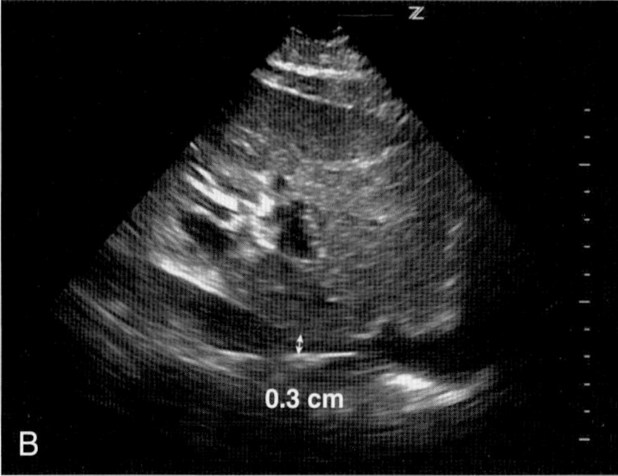


**Fig. 4.10 Sonographic demonstration of the inferior vena cava in a preload-responsive patient maintained on mechanical ventilation.** Notice the variation in diameter between a positive pressure breath (**A**) and expiration (**B**).

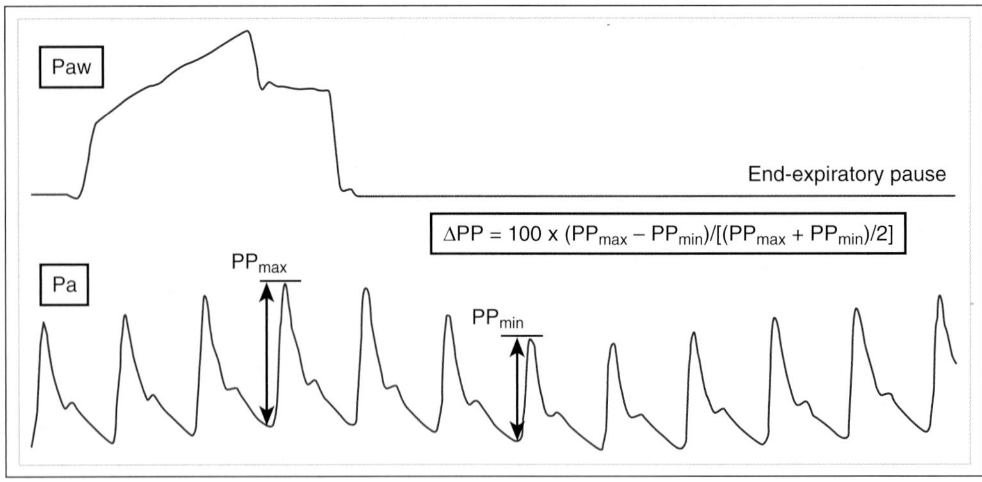


**Fig. 4.11 Determining pulse pressure variation as an index of preload responsiveness.** Arterial waveform tracings are used to detect pulse pressure variation.

**Table 4.5 Vasopressor Agents**

| AGENT | RECEPTOR ACTIVATION | CIRCULATORY EFFECTS | DOSAGE RANGE |
|---|---|---|---|
| Norepinephrine | $\alpha_1$ (primary)<br>$\beta_1$ (secondary) | Vasoconstriction<br>↑ Heart rate (HR) and contractility (small) | 1-30 mcg/kg/min |
| Dopamine | $DA_1$<br>$\beta_1$ (primary)<br>$\alpha_1$ | Vasodilation<br>↑ HR and contractility<br>Vasoconstriction | 1-5 mcg/kg/min<br>5-10 mcg/kg/min<br>10-20 mcg/kg/min |
| Vasopressin | $V_1$ (vascular)<br>$V_2$ (renal)<br>$V_3$ (pituitary) | Vasoconstriction<br>Antidiuretic effects<br>Adrenocorticotropic hormone secretion | 0.01-0.04 U/min |
| Epinephrine | $\alpha_1/\beta_2$<br>$\beta_1$ | Vasoconstriction<br>↑ HR and contractility | 1-10 mcg/kg/min |
| Phenylephrine | $\alpha_1/\alpha_2$ | Vasoconstriction | 40-180 mcg/kg/min |
| Dobutamine | $\beta_1$<br>$\beta_2$ | ↑ HR and contractility<br>Vasodilation | 2-20 mcg/kg/min |

Adapted from Holmes CL, Walley KR. The evaluation and management of shock. Clin Chest Med 2003;24:775-89.

output.[27] As mentioned previously, PPV has limitations when used to predict preload responsiveness (e.g., ventilation must be at a set tidal volume [6 to 8 m L/kg], no spontaneous breaths, sinus rhythm).

## VASOACTIVE THERAPY

Vasoactive medications are indicated when mean arterial pressure remains below 65 mm Hg despite a fluid challenge of 20 to 40 mL/kg and there is evidence that a patient is not preload responsive. Vasopressor agents help restore perfusion pressure and maintain cardiac output. These agents typically exert their effects through stimulation of α- and β-adrenergic receptors. The degree to which these receptors are stimulated depends on the agent. Common vasopressor agents used in emergency medicine are norepinephrine, dopamine, and vasopressin. Less commonly used agents are phenylephrine, epinephrine, and milrinone. The hemodynamic dose responses and dosage ranges of these agents are listed in **Table 4.5**. An important caveat is that a rise in blood pressure after administration of one of these drugs may not correlate with clinical improvement. Additional markers of hypoperfusion, such as the serum lactate level and central venous oxygen saturation, must be considered in the overall circulatory assessment. No studies have clearly supported the superiority of any vasopressor agent. The choice depends on the acute disease process and underlying comorbid conditions.

Patients with poor cardiac contractility may require inotropic support. Inotropic agents increase cardiac contractility through stimulation of $\alpha_1$ receptors, which results in rises in the intracellular calcium concentration. Dobutamine is the prototypic inotropic agent, but any vasopressor that stimulates $\beta_1$ receptors increases cardiac contractility. Dopamine, milrinone, and epinephrine are potent inotropic medications. Dobutamine can also cause peripheral vasodilation in hypovolemic patients. An additional vasopressor medication, such as norepinephrine, should be used in hypotensive patients requiring dobutamine for inotropic support.

## MECHANICAL CIRCULATORY SUPPORT

Support of the circulatory system may require cardiac pacing (**Box 4.5**), which can be performed transcutaneously or transvenously. Transcutaneous pacing is noninvasive and more commonly used in the ED. Proper pacer pad placement is crucial in this modality. The anterior pacer pad is placed close to the heart, typically at the location of the $V_3$ lead on an electrocardiogram; the posterior pad is placed between the spine and the inferior border of the left or right scapula. The subsequent steps in transcutaneous pacing are listed in **Box 4.6**.

Transvenous pacers are placed through a central venous catheter. The right internal jugular vein and the left subclavian vein are the preferred sites of cannulation. Attaining the proper position in the right ventricle can be difficult. Ultrasonography should be used to guide placement of the pacer. If ultrasonography is not available, the $V_1$ lead of an electrocardiograph machine should be attached to the cathode. Contact with the right ventricle is characterized by prominent ST-segment elevation. The ventricular rate is set the same as for transcutaneous pacing. When pacer output is adjusted, the pacing threshold for transvenous pacing is much less than that required for transcutaneous pacing, typically ranging between 1 and 2 mA. When the right ventricle is paced, the electrocardiogram should demonstrate a pacer spike followed by a QRS complex displaying a left bundle branch block pattern. Potential complications of emergency transvenous pacing are listed in **Box 4.7**.

**BOX 4.5 Indications for Temporary Cardiac Pacing**

Witnessed asystole
Hemodynamically significant bradycardia
Symptomatic second- or third-degree atrioventricular block
Complete atrioventricular dissociation with a ventricular rate lower than 50 beats/min
Termination of supraventricular or ventricular tachyarrhythmias

## SUMMARY

Assessment of the circulatory system is central to the evaluation of every ED patient. Assessment begins with a focused history, physical examination, noninvasive measurements of blood pressure and heart rate, and focused ultrasonography to identify causes of circulatory dysfunction. For many ED patients, additional circulatory assessment and monitoring are not needed. However, patients with evidence of circulatory dysfunction require rapid evaluation and support, as summarized in the following list (**Fig. 4.12**):

- Obtain peripheral venous access and administer isotonic crystalloid fluid boluses followed by frequent reassessment of blood pressure and preload responsiveness.
- Perform ultrasonography early in the evaluation of patients with severe circulatory compromise to exclude acute life-threatening conditions such as pericardial effusion, hemoperitoneum, and abdominal aortic aneurysm.
- Insert an arterial line for continuous blood pressure monitoring in patients who remain hypotensive despite initial administration of intravenous fluids.

**BOX 4.6 Steps and Tips for Transcutaneous Pacing**

**Step 1—Set the Rate**

For bradyarrhythmias, set the rate between 60 and 75 beats/min.
For overdrive pacing, set the rate to exceed the rate of the tachyarrhythmia.

**Step 2—Adjust the Output**

The pacing threshold for transcutaneous pacing typically ranges from 20 to 140 mA.
Increase the output (mA) until 100% of beats are captured.
Capture is indicated by a spike on the electrocardiogram followed by a wide QRS complex.
Set the output 5 to 10 mA above the threshold value.

**Step 3—Provide Analgesia**

Tip: Patients with emphysema or pericardial effusion or who are mechanically ventilated require higher pacing threshold values.

**BOX 4.7 Complications of Transvenous Pacing**

Arterial puncture
Hematoma
Pneumothorax
Atrial and ventricular arrhythmias
Myocardial perforation
Diaphragmatic stimulation

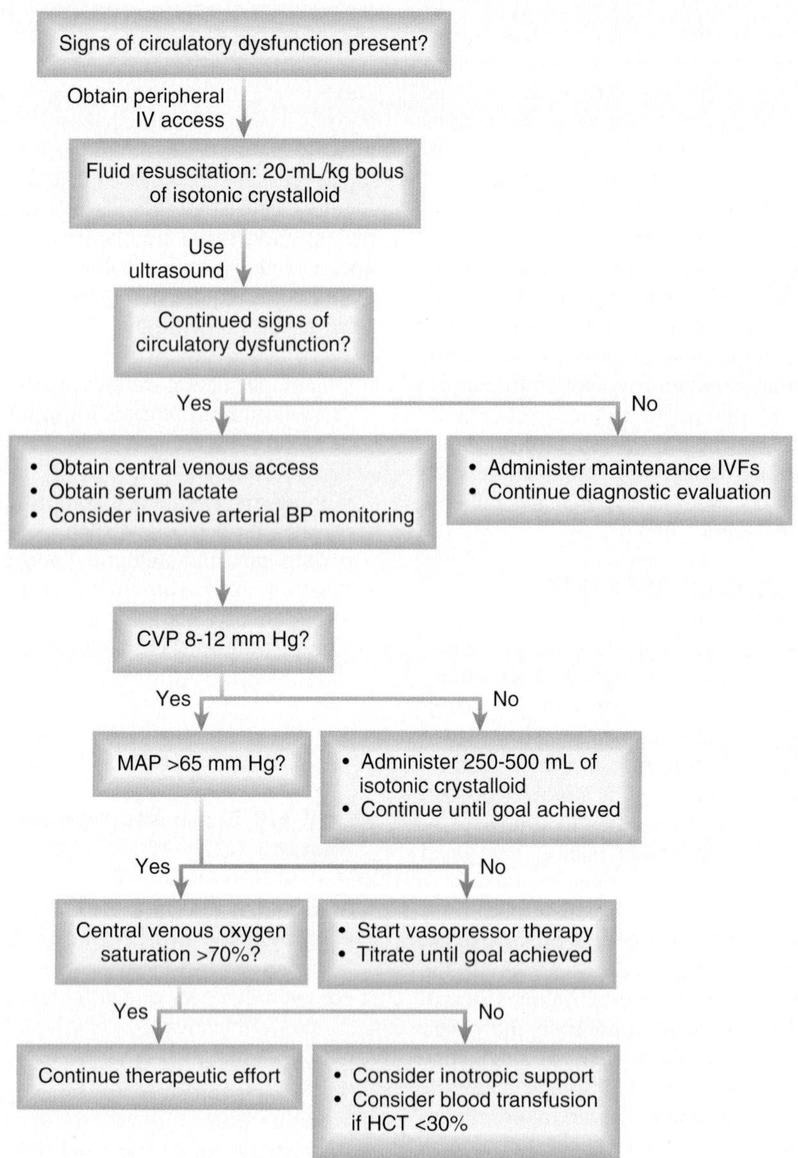


**Fig. 4.12 General algorithm for circulatory support.** *BP*, Blood pressure; *CVP*, central venous pressure; *HCT*, hematocrit; *IV*, intravenous; *IVFs*, intravenous fluids; *MAP*, mean arterial pressure.

- Use global markers of hypoperfusion, such as the serum lactate level and central venous oxygen saturation, to detect persistently impaired oxygen delivery.
- Begin a vasopressor agent in any patient with a mean arterial pressure of less than 65 mm Hg despite an adequate fluid challenge.

## REFERENCES

*References can be found on Expert Consult @ www.expertconsult.com.*

# Emergency Cardiac Ultrasound: Evaluation for Pericardial Effusion and Cardiac Activity

5

*Michael P. Mallin and Christine Butts*

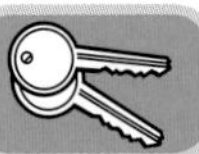

**KEY POINTS**

- Emergency cardiac ultrasound is performed by the emergency physician to assess for the presence of cardiac activity, determine whether a pericardial effusion is present, and answer other specific questions.
- Echocardiography can be used during cardiac arrest to guide resuscitation decisions.
- Emergency use of echocardiography is indicated for assessment of cardiac ejection fraction, wall motion abnormalities, and other critical findings that will direct acute diagnostic decision making.

## INTRODUCTION

Echocardiography has been the "gold standard" for cardiologists for decades. Over the past 20 years, emergency physicians have adopted point-of-care (POC) cardiac ultrasound to answer specific questions on the management of critical patients. Assessment for pericardial effusion and for cardiac activity have traditionally been the principal indications for emergency physicians, but indications for bedside echocardiography are growing rapidly.[1]

## WHAT WE ARE LOOKING FOR

The initial and best evidence-based indications include applications for tamponade, cardiac arrest, and acute heart failure. Rapidly developing areas of cardiac ultrasound include evaluation of hypotension, pulmonary embolism (PE), acute myocardial infarction, diastolic heart failure, and echocardiographically guided resuscitation (**Box 5.1**).[1,2]

## LITERATURE REVIEW

### ESTIMATION OF GLOBAL CARDIAC FUNCTION AND EJECTION FRACTION

Multiple studies have shown the ability of emergency physicians to accurately evaluate cardiac function and ejection fraction.[3,4] When compared with cardiologists, emergency physicians were found to have a correlation coefficient of 0.86 with cardiologists when assessing ejection fraction. Cardiologists had a similar coefficient of 0.84 among themselves.

### DIAGNOSIS OF PERICARDIAL EFFUSION

Emergency physicians have proved to be accurate in the diagnosis of pericardial effusion. Previous research has shown that emergency physicians have a sensitivity of 96%[5] to 100%[6] as compared with formal overreading by trained echocardiographers.

## HOW TO SCAN/SCANNING PROTOCOLS

### PROBE SELECTION

Classic echocardiography requires the use of a phased-array probe, sometimes referred to as the thoracic probe. These probes have a small footprint and are ideal for achieving visualization with a small acoustic window between ribs.

### ACOUSTIC WINDOWS

Bedside cardiac ultrasound is typically taught with the use of three separate acoustic windows and multiple orthogonal views within the windows. These acoustic windows include the parasternal, apical, and subcostal. Each window is then broken down into orthogonal views, including the parasternal long-axis, parasternal short-axis, apical four-chamber, apical two-chamber, apical long-axis, subcostal four-chamber, and subcostal long-axis views.

### PROBE ORIENTATION

Echocardiography places the probe marker on the right side of the ultrasound screen so that when the ultrasound machine is in the cardiac mode, the right-hand side of the screen indicates the side of the probe with the marker on it (this is opposite any other scanning mode).

### SPECIFIC VIEWS

#### *Parasternal Long Axis*

The parasternal long-axis view seen in **Figure 5.1** is obtained by placing the probe in the third to fourth intercostal space with the probe marker pointed toward the patient's right shoulder (**Figs. 5.2 and 5.3**). The long axis of the heart should be horizontal on the screen with the apex pointed to the left. If the apex is pointed up, the probe is too low and should be

**BOX 5.1 Traditional and Emerging Point-of-Care Cardiac Ultrasound Indications**

**Traditional Indications**
Tamponade
Cardiac standstill during cardiac arrest
Acute heart failure

**Emerging Indications**
Echocardiographically guided resuscitation
Undifferentiated hypotension
Pulmonary embolism
Acute myocardial infarction
Diastolic heart failure

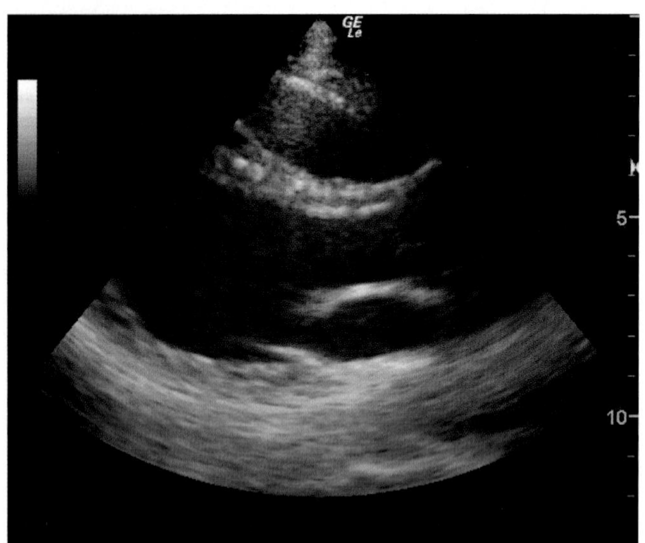


**Fig. 5.1** Parasternal long-axis view of a normal-appearing heart.

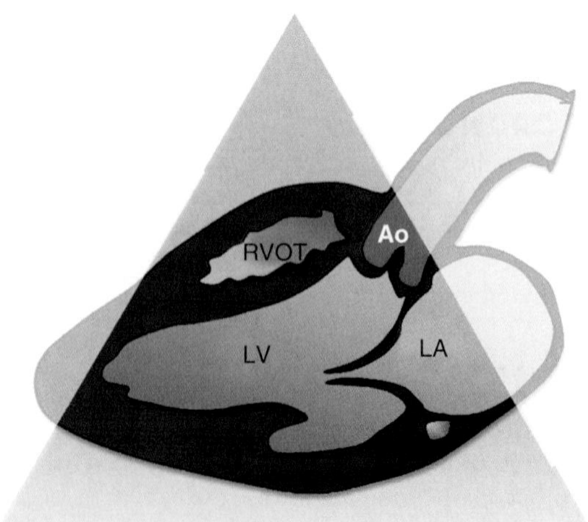


**Fig. 5.2** Parasternal long-axis diagram. *Ao*, Aorta; *LA*, left atrium; *LV*, left ventricle; *RVOT*, right ventricular outflow tract.

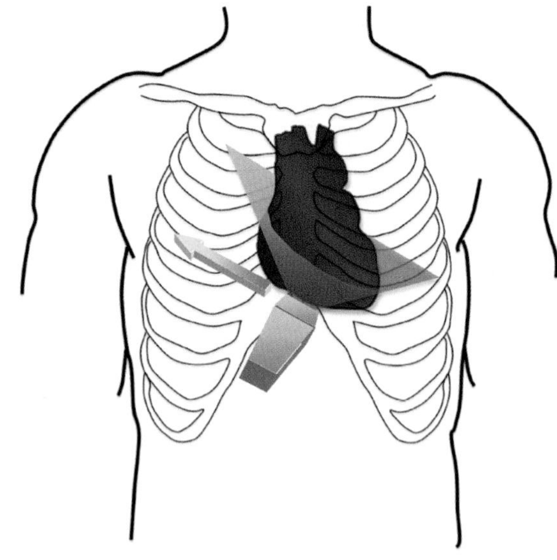

**Fig. 5.3** Probe orientation for the parasternal long-axis view.

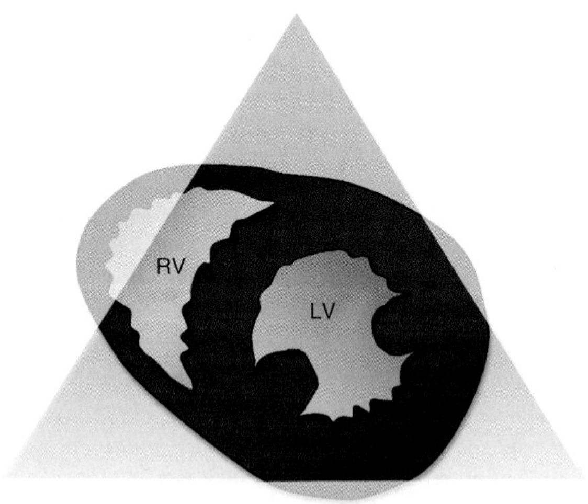


**Fig. 5.4** Parasternal short-axis diagram. *LV*, Left ventricle; *RV*, right ventricle.

moved up an interspace. This view allows visualization of the left ventricle, mitral valve, left atrium, right ventricular outflow tract, aortic valve, and aorta. The descending thoracic aorta is often visualized posterior to the left ventricle in transection.

## Parasternal Short Axis

The parasternal short-axis view is obtained by rotating the probe 90 degrees from the parasternal long-axis position so that the probe marker is pointed to the patient's left shoulder (**Figs. 5.4 and 5.5**). The ultrasound beam is now transecting the heart in its short axis. If the physician tilts the probe so that it is pointing to the base of the heart, the aortic valve is visualized along with the "inflow and outflow" of the right heart. This view includes the right atrium, right ventricular outflow tract, and pulmonic valve. As the probe is tilted more apically, the aortic valve is lost and a cross-sectional view of the mitral valve is obtained (**Fig. 5.6**). At this point the right ventricle becomes more apparent and takes a position as a

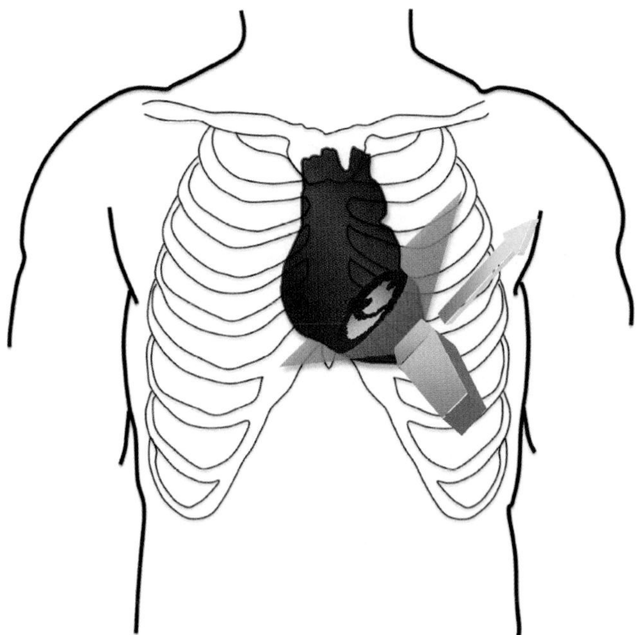

**Fig. 5.5 Probe orientation for the parasternal short-axis view.**

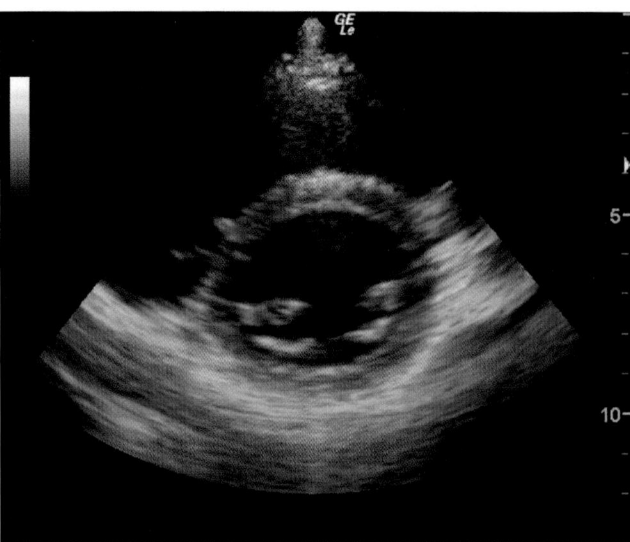

**Fig. 5.7 Parasternal short-axis view at the level of the papillary muscles.** This is an athletic heart with an enlarged right ventricle.

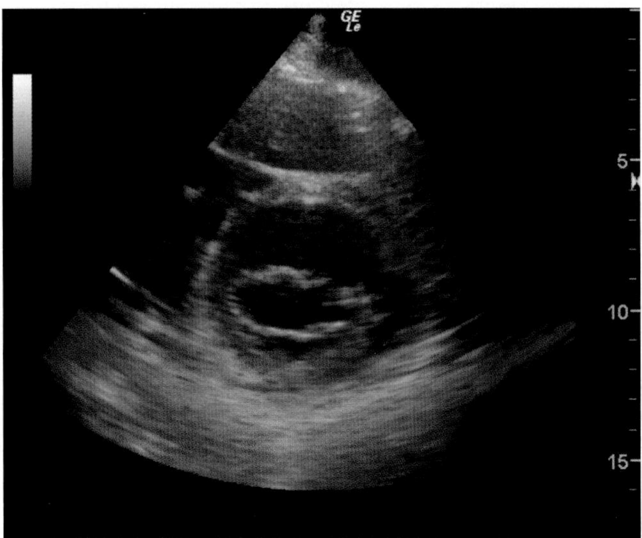

**Fig. 5.6 Parasternal short-axis view at the level of the mitral valve: the "fish mouth" view.**

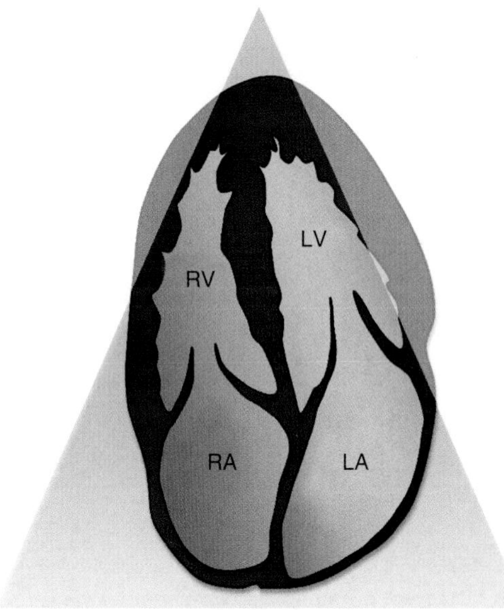


**Fig. 5.8 Diagram of the apical four-chamber view.** *LA*, Left atrium; LV, left ventricle; *RA*, right atrium; *RV*, right ventricle.

crescentic ventricle to the left and superficial to the mitral valve and left ventricle. Finally, as the probe is tilted more toward the apex, the mitral valve is lost and the muscular portion of the left ventricle is visualized. The posterior medial and anterior papillary muscles are visualized at this point, and the circular nature of the left ventricle can be appreciated (**Fig. 5.7**).

### Apical Four- and Two-Chamber Views

The apical window allows visualization of either all four chambers (**Figs. 5.8 and 5.9**) or just two chambers (the left atrium and ventricle) (**Fig. 5.10**). The apical windows are difficult to obtain in the emergency setting and often require the patient to be in the left lateral decubitus position, which is often impossible. The window is obtained by placing the probe at the location of maximal impulse with the probe marker pointed to the left axilla. The probe must be tilted so that the probe is pointed to the patient's right shoulder (**Fig. 5.11**).

The apical two-chamber view allows further evaluation of the left ventricle and mitral valve. The left atrial appendage can sometimes be see on the right side of the screen on the anterior side of the basal left ventricle.

### Subcostal Four-Chamber View

The subcostal four-chamber view (**Figs. 5.12 to 5.14**) is obtained by placing the probe just inferior to the xiphoid and applying pressure downward on the abdomen with the probe

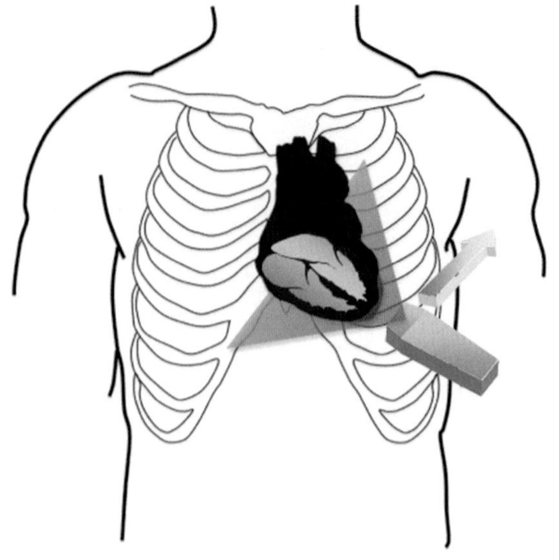

**Fig. 5.9 Probe orientation for the apical four-chamber view.**

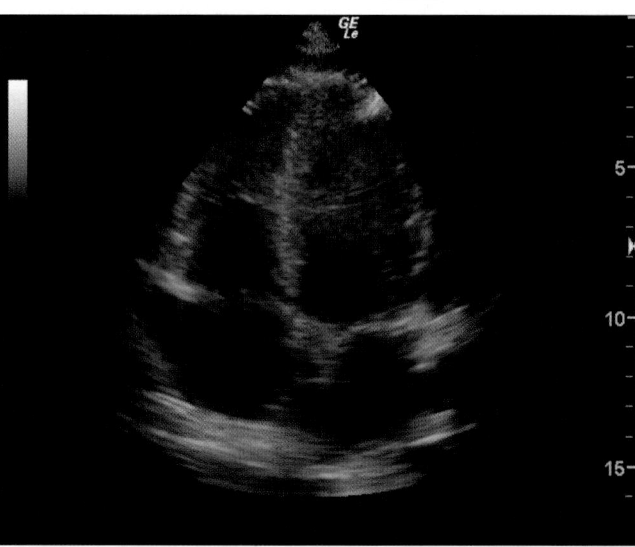

**Fig. 5.11 Apical four-chamber view.** Notice the size of the left ventricle in comparison with the right ventricle in this normal heart.

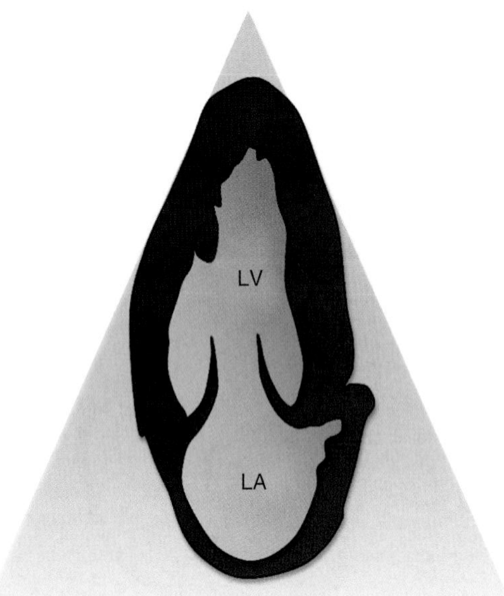


**Fig. 5.10 Diagram of the apical two-chamber view.** *LA*, Left atrium; *LV*, left ventricle.

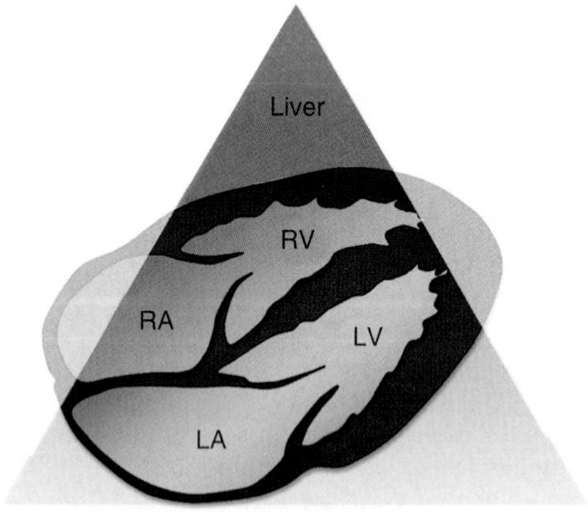

**Fig. 5.12 Subcostal four-chamber window.** Note the liver at the top of the ultrasound imaging window. *LA*, Left atrium; *LV*, left ventricle; *RA*, right atrium; *RV*, right ventricle.

horizontal. This view can be performed with either the curvilinear abdominal probe or the phased-array thoracic probe. The probe marker should be toward the patient's left in cardiac mode and toward the patient's right when using focused abdominal sonography for trauma (FAST) or abdominal protocols.

## NORMAL AND ABNORMAL FINDINGS

### PERICARDIAL EFFUSION

Evaluation of pericardial effusion is one of the first indications for cardiac ultrasound.[6] Identification of pericardial effusion (**Fig. 5.15**) is achieved by visualization of the heart in multiple views. The subcostal window is the most commonly taught site because of the FAST examination. An effusion will appear as an anechoic stripe of fluid surrounding the heart. This stripe is most commonly located between the right ventricle and the liver. Ideally, all three acoustic windows should be used when attempting to rule out pericardial effusion.

The critical complication of pericardial effusion is cardiac tamponade (**Fig. 5.16**). Physiologically, cardiac tamponade occurs when the pressure inside the pericardial sac becomes elevated above right ventricular diastolic filling pressure. This leads to decreased filling of the right ventricle in diastole and reduced preload and cardiac output. Echocardiographic signs of cardiac tamponade are the presence of right ventricular free wall collapse as seen in Figure 5.16. Alternatively, a more sensitive, but less specific finding is the presence of right atrial collapse during ventricular systole (atrial diastole).

### CARDIAC ARREST

POC cardiac echocardiography can be invaluable during cardiac arrest. Typical uses include evaluation for tamponade, hypovolemia, and suggestions of PE (clot, right ventricular

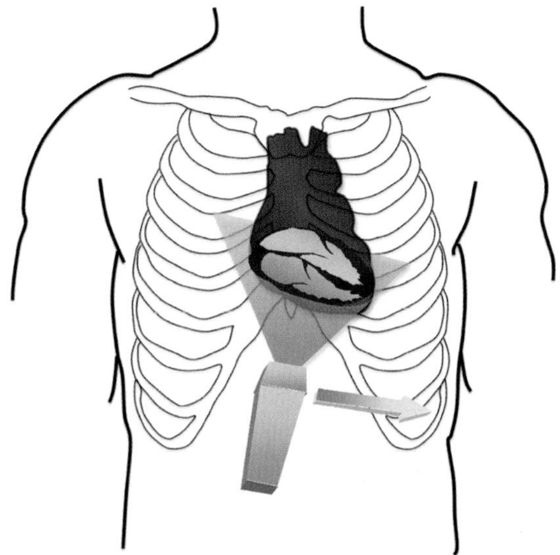

**Fig. 5.13 Probe orientation for the subcostal four-chamber window.** The probe is placed in the subxiphoid space with the probe marker oriented to the patient's left (cardiac mode) or to the patient's right (abdomen/focused abdominal sonography for trauma mode). The apex of the heart should be pointing to the right of the screen as seen in Figures 5.8 and 5.7.

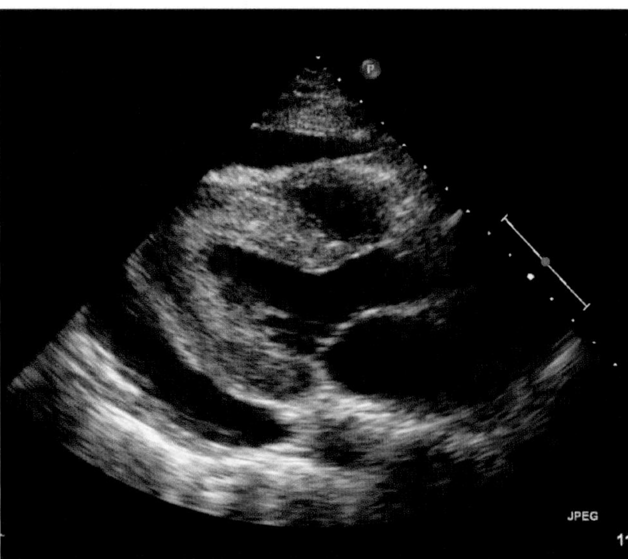

**Fig. 5.15 Pericardial effusion noted in the parasternal long-axis view.** Notice the location in reference to the descending thoracic aorta. Pericardial effusions track between the heart and the descending aorta, whereas pleural effusions can be seen posterior to the descending aorta.

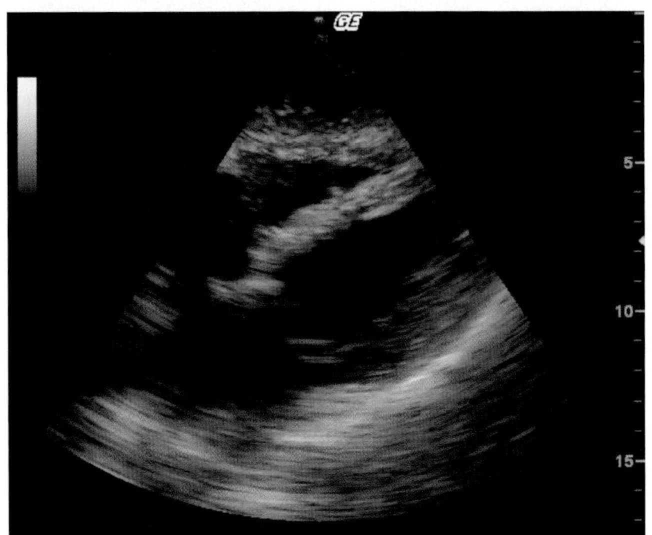

**Fig. 5.14 Subcostal four-chamber window.**

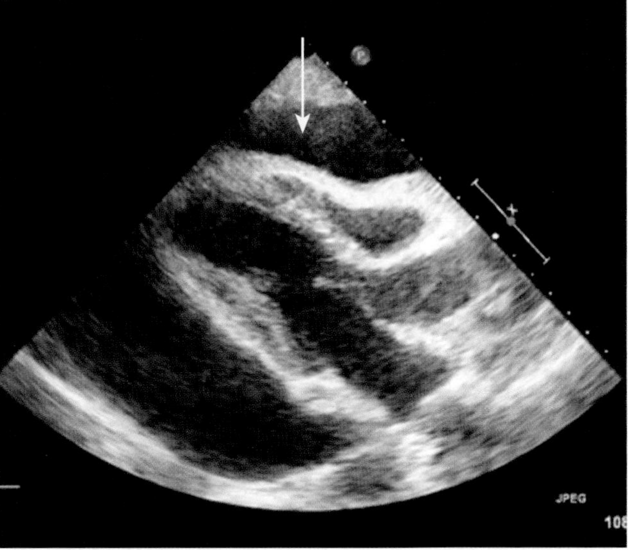

**Fig. 5.16 Pericardial effusion with tamponade.** Note the right ventricular free wall collapse in diastole *(arrow)*.

dilation); detection of aortic dissection; monitoring for pacer capture and the adequacy of compressions; and most important, evaluation for cardiac activity in patients with pulseless electrical activity (PEA) and asystole. Studies have shown cardiac standstill during arrest to be 100% predictive of mortality.[7] Furthermore, cardiac ultrasound has been used in place of a pulse check in pediatric populations because of the inherent difficulty of finding a pulse.[8] Typical algorithms use cardiac ultrasound to evaluate PEA and asystolic rhythms.[9] If cardiac standstill is present, further resuscitation is futile.[7]

## ACUTE HEART FAILURE

Emergency physicians have been shown to be accurate in estimating left ventricular ejection fraction (LVEF).[3] LVEF is most easily separated into three categories: reduced, normal, and hyperdynamic. Although echocardiographers often report actual percentages, we can think of normal LVEF as 55% to 75%, reduced as less than 55%, and hyperdynamic as greater than 75%. Some authors add a fourth category in which severely reduced LVEF is less than 30%. This distinction can be useful when discussing cardiac function with consultants.

The ejection fraction is typically estimated by visual inspection of the "squeeze" of the left ventricle, although it can also be measured with algorithms in the cardiac package of many emergency ultrasound machines.

### Pitfalls

Emergency cardiac ultrasound involves the use of clear indications and directed ultrasound of the heart to answer specific questions, as described in the "Introduction." Apart from these questions, a cardiologist should be consulted to aid in complex diagnosis and clinical decision making.

Normal systolic function does not rule out acute heart failure. Diastolic heart failure can occur in patients with a normal LVEF.

Diagnosis of cardiac tamponade by echocardiography can be complicated, and advanced echocardiographic techniques may be required, including Doppler evaluation. Stable patients may benefit from evaluation by a trained echocardiographer.

Technically, the bedside sonographer may encounter difficulty obtaining the full series of views as described earlier. Patient habitus or artifact from the lungs or ribs may present challenges. Placing the patient on the left side in a left lateral decubitus position may aid in better viewing the parasternal and apical windows. This position moves the heart closer to the anterior chest wall. In the subcostal window, asking the patient to breathe in deeply may move the heart closer to the transducer. Additionally, moving the transducer toward the patient's right, while still pointing toward the left side of the chest, may overcome artifact caused by the stomach or bowel by using the left lobe of the liver as an acoustic window.

## PULMONARY EMBOLISM

Although cardiac ultrasound cannot identify a pulmonary embolus,[10] several findings are suggestive of this diagnosis. Right ventricular dysfunction and dilation are typically visualized in the apical four-chamber window. Right ventricular dilation has been described in reference to the relative areas of the right and left ventricles at end-diastole. A right-to-left ventricular area ratio of greater than 0.66 has been shown to be 85% specific for PE.[11] Another finding is described as retained apical function in the setting of right ventricular free wall hypokinesis. This is called the McConnell sign and can be fairly specific for PE. McConnell et al. described this particular finding as being 94% specific for PE[11] (**Fig. 5.17**). An additional finding in acute PE is flattening of the interventricular septum. This is seen in the parasternal short-axis view and is due to either volume or pressure overload of the right heart (**Fig. 5.18**).[12]

## VOLUME STATUS

Assessment of the patient's condition and the presence of hypervolemia or hypovolemia can be complicated. Through direct visualization of chamber size and evaluation of the great vessels, this clinical conundrum can often be overcome.

Echocardiographic evaluation of volume status starts with global assessment of the ejection fraction and filling of the right and left sides of the heart. Reduced filling of both the right and left heart chambers implies reduced preload and hypovolemia. Conversely, the presence of dilated right and left heart chambers with a poor ejection fraction suggests hypervolemia. Finally, a dilated right ventricle with a contracted left ventricle and an elevated LVEF suggests a forward flow problem of the right heart, such as PE, right-sided myocardial infarction, or cor pulmonale.

Additionally, a body of research has led to evaluation of the inferior vena cava as a surrogate marker for central venous pressure and thus volume status.[13] The current recommendations are summarized in **Table 5.1**. The inferior vena cava should measured during both inspiration and expiration from the subcostal long-axis view as seen in **Figure 5.19**.

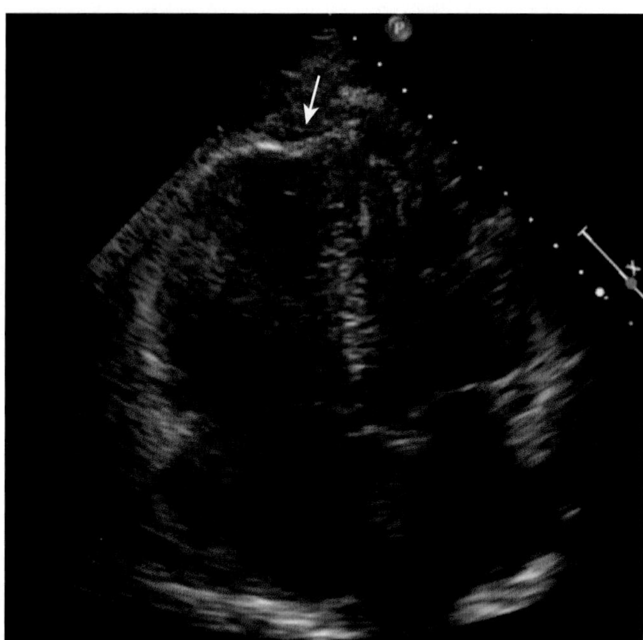

**Fig. 5.17 McConnell sign.** The apical contraction is denoted by the *arrow*.

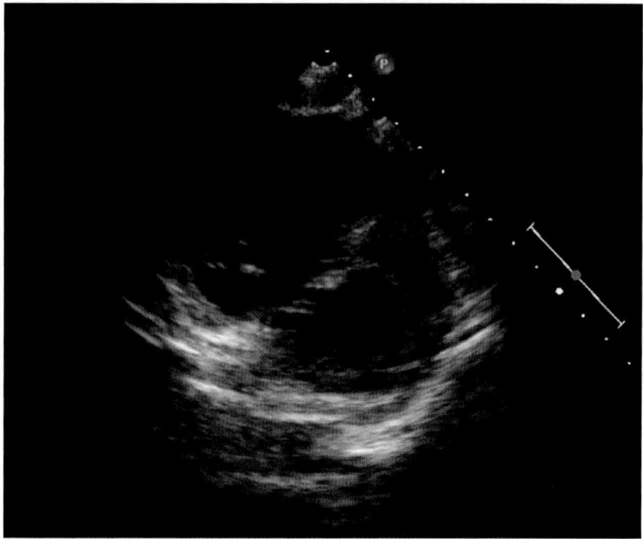

**Fig. 5.18 Parasternal short-axis view showing septal flattening associated with right-sided pressure or volume overload.**

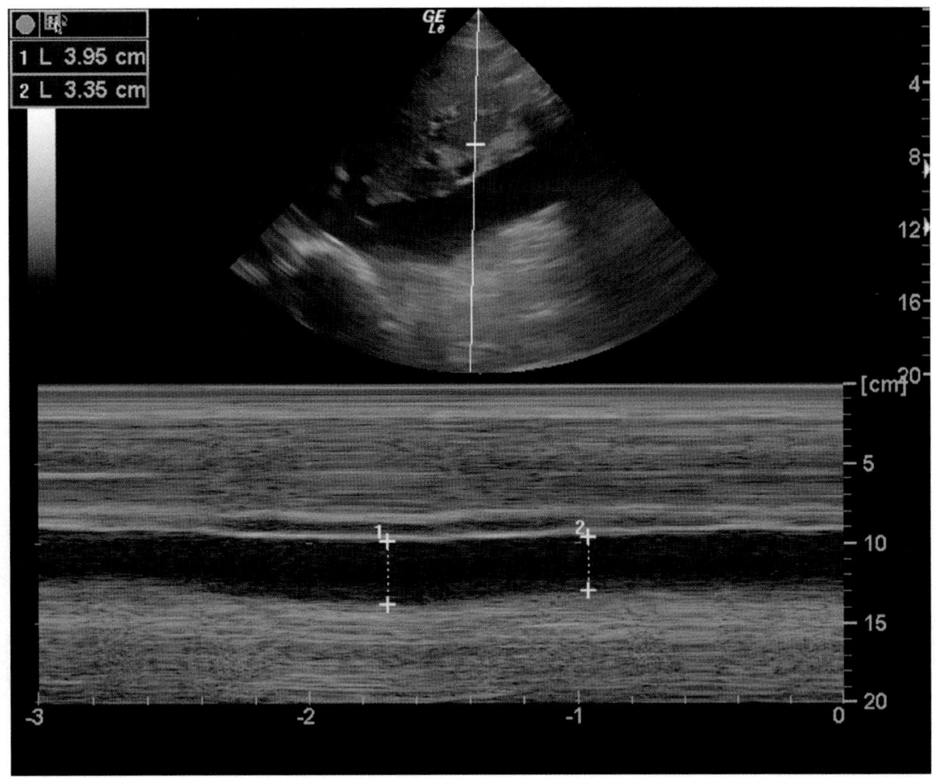


**Fig. 5.19** Subcostal long axis of the inferior vena cava used to estimate central venous pressure.

**Table 5.1** IVC Diameters and Respective Collapse Associated with CVP Estimates

| | IVC (CM) | COLLAPSE | CVP |
|---|---|---|---|
| Normal | <2.1 | >50% | 3 (0-5) |
| In between | <2.1/>2.1 | <50%/>50% | 8 (5-10) |
| High | >2.1 | <50% | 15 (10-20) |

*CVP*, Central venous pressure; *IVC*, inferior vena cava.

## SUGGESTED READINGS

Blaivas M, Fox J. Outcome in cardiac arrest patients found to have cardiac standstill on the bedside emergency department echocardiogram. Acad Emerg Med 2001;8:616-21.

Labovitz AJ, Noble VE, Bierig M, et al. Focused cardiac ultrasound in the emergent setting: a consensus statement of the American Society of Echocardiography and the American College of Emergency Physicians. J Am Soc Echocardiogr 2010;23:1225-30.

Mandavia D, Hoffner R, Mahaney K, et al. Bedside echocardiography by emergency physicians. Ann Emerg Med 2001;38:377-82.

Moore C, Rose GA, Tayal VS, et al. Determination of left ventricular function by emergency physician echocardiography of hypotensive patients. Acad Emerg Med 2002;9:186-93.

Perera P, Mailhot D, Riley D, et al. The RUSH exam: Rapid Ultrasound in SHock in the evaluation of the critically ill. Emerg Med Clin North Am 2010;28:29-56.

## REFERENCES

*References can be found on Expert Consult @ www.expertconsult.com.*

# 6 Ultrasound-Guided Vascular Access

*Andrew W. Shannon, Christine Butts, and Justin Cook*

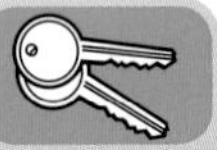

**KEY POINTS**

- The use of ultrasound for vascular access is now standard.
- Although bedside ultrasound improves the overall success of venous access and decreases complications, it is not without potential pitfalls.

## INTRODUCTION

Emergency physician expertise in the use of ultrasound for obtaining vascular access is widespread because of its clinical benefit. Patients may not have accessible superficial veins. Obesity and decreased intravascular volume further increase the challenges. Central venous access has known complications that include pneumothorax and injury to great vessels. Bedside ultrasound may decrease the complication rate by allowing direct, real-time visualization of vascular targets, decreasing the need for multiple attempts, and avoiding arterial injury.[1,2] The application of ultrasound for invasive and therapeutic procedures has become standard as reflected in the 2006 policy statement of the American College of Emergency Physicians on emergency ultrasound.[3] Over the past decade, wide acceptance of the benefits of ultrasound-guided vascular access has led to the recommendation that ultrasound guidance be used routinely in obtaining central vascular access.[4,5] Debate regarding the role of ultrasound has shifted to a focus on implementation of these recommendations and their cost-effectiveness.[6-9] Research is now largely focused on improving education and training techniques or documenting the adoption of ultrasound to augment central venous access in a wider variety of settings.[10,11]

## HOW TO SCAN AND SCANNING PROTOCOLS

Ultrasound-guided central venous access is accomplished with many of the same techniques as used by the traditional landmark approach. Patient positioning, informed consent, use of sterile technique with full draping, and selection of the anatomic site should be undertaken in the usual manner.

Either a two- or single-operator technique is acceptable.[12] A single operator will use the dominant hand to advance and aspirate the needle while manipulating the transducer with the opposite hand. In a two-operator procedure, the cannulating operator will concentrate on the needle and syringe, and the probe will be held steady by the second operator.

Two techniques are commonly accepted for achieving ultrasound-guided vascular access. In the *static* technique, ultrasound is used to identify vascular structures in relation to external landmarks, and then the ultrasound device is set aside and cannulation performed in the usual manner. The *dynamic* technique involves real-time, direct visualization of entry of the needle into the vein by ultrasound and seems to be preferable, particularly when the venous structures are small.[13] In this case, once the vein has been accessed (or a "flash" of blood is seen), the ultrasound device is set aside.

The probe most conducive to central venous access is a linear-array high-frequency (5- to 12-MHz) probe (**Fig. 6.1**). Care should be taken to identify the side of the probe bearing the indicator mark that corresponds to the on-screen indicator. This will allow the most intuitive positioning of the probe during venous access such that medial on the patient is medial on the screen of the machine as viewed by the operator when attempting cannulation (**Fig. 6.2**).

Once a site has been chosen, usually the internal jugular or femoral, it should be evaluated with ultrasound to identify the artery and the vein (**Fig. 6.3**). When compared with their accompanying veins, arteries appear thick walled, more circular, and pulsatile on ultrasound. Arteries do not compress with light pressure. Veins are more irregular in shape, sometimes appearing triangular rather than round, and compress with light pressure (see Videos 1 and 2). Use of color Doppler can also aid in identification (see Video 3).

Videos 1, 2, and 3 can be found on Expert Consult @ www.expertconsult.com.

It is often easiest to begin with the probe in a transverse orientation. In this view, the vessels appear in cross section as round or oval structures (see Fig. 6.3). The depth of the target vessel and its relationship to surrounding structures can be determined. The vein should then be centered on the screen. This allows an external landmark, the center of the transducer, to be established. Pressure over this area with a blunt object, such as a fingertip, can confirm the correct location. The needle should then be inserted at a 45-degree angle to the skin

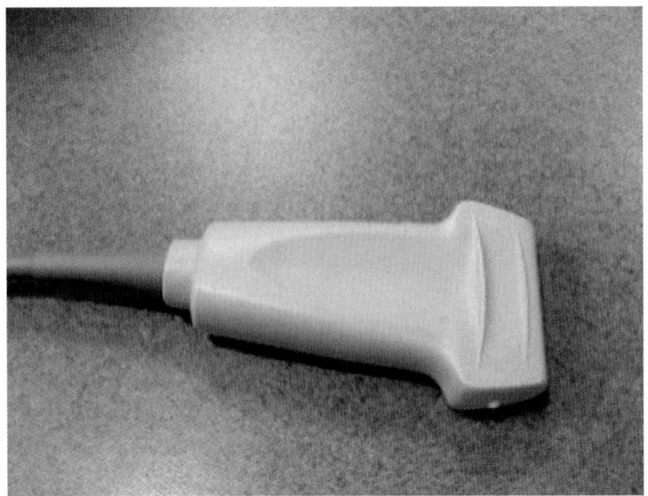

**Fig. 6.1 Image of a high-frequency, or linear, transducer.**

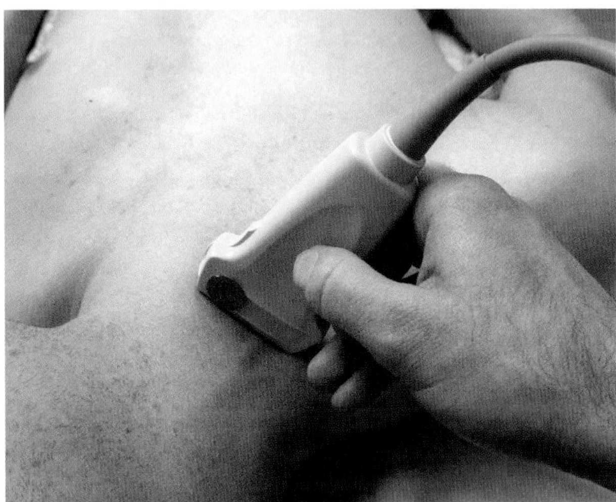

**Fig. 6.2 Position of the transducer to obtain a transverse image of the internal jugular vein.** Note that as the operator is standing at the patient's head, the indicator is pointing toward the patient's left. This ensures that when the operator is looking at the screen, the patient's left and the operator's left are the same. This minimizes confusion if the needle track needs to be adjusted.

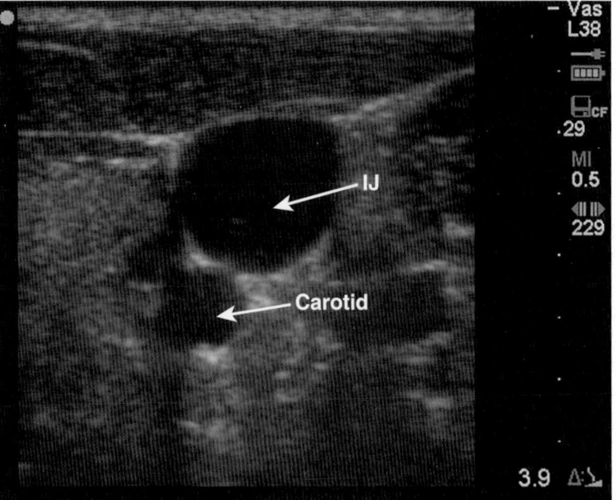


**Fig. 6.3 Transverse anatomy of the vessels of the neck.** In this image, the internal jugular (IJ) is seen lying on top of the carotid artery. The IJ is large and oval in shape. Direct pressure over it should cause slight collapse. The carotid remains stable in size, appearance, and compressibility. It is usually small, round, and noncompressible. Overlying the vessels is the sternocleidomastoid muscle.

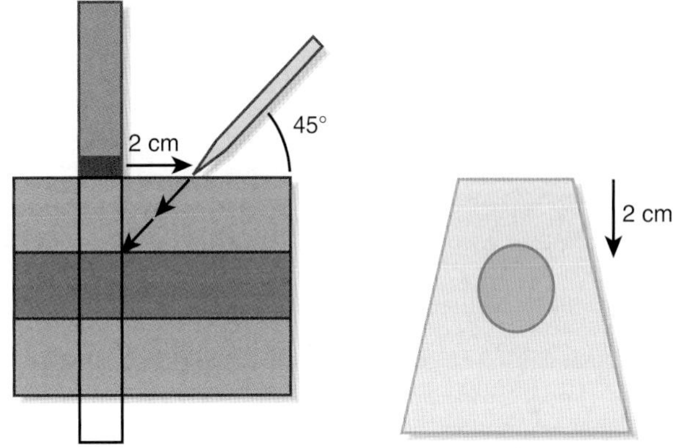


**Fig. 6.4 Demonstration of the method for judging the angle and placement of entry for ultrasound-guided vascular access.** Because the vessel is measured to be 2 cm below the surface, introducing the needle 2 cm from the transducer at an angle of 45 degrees will result in the correct trajectory to visualize the needle tip as it approaches the target vessel.

at a distance from the probe equal to the depth of the target vessel (**Fig. 6.4**). Immediately after entering the skin, the needle tip should be identified on the screen. It will appear as a hyperechoic (white) object within subcutaneous tissue. The needle tip should be followed with the transducer as it advances toward the vein. As the needle tip reaches the vein, the wall of the vessel will be seen to deform (see Video 4). A flash of blood in the syringe confirms that the needle has entered the vein (**Fig. 6.5**).

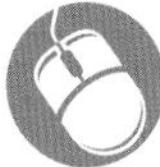

Video 4 can be found on Expert Consult @ www.expertconsult.com.

The longitudinal approach is somewhat more challenging to master but allows better visualization of the needle along its entire length. The longitudinal view is obtained by rotating the probe 90 degrees from the transverse position to line up in parallel with the course of the vein (**Fig. 6.6**). Extra care should be taken to differentiate venous from arterial vessels in this view and to avoid accidental migration of the probe. In this approach the needle should enter the skin at one end of the probe (**Fig. 6.7**)—and therefore the ultrasound screen—and be advanced in plane toward the underlying vein along the long axis (**Fig. 6.8**). Similar pressure deformity and indentation of the vessel wall should be noted before it is punctured, and a flash of blood should again be sought (see Video 5).

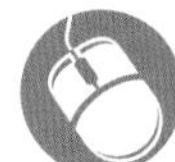

Video 5 can be found on Expert Consult @ www.expertconsult.com.

An oblique approach has been described in which the vessels are imaged with an orientation inbetween the

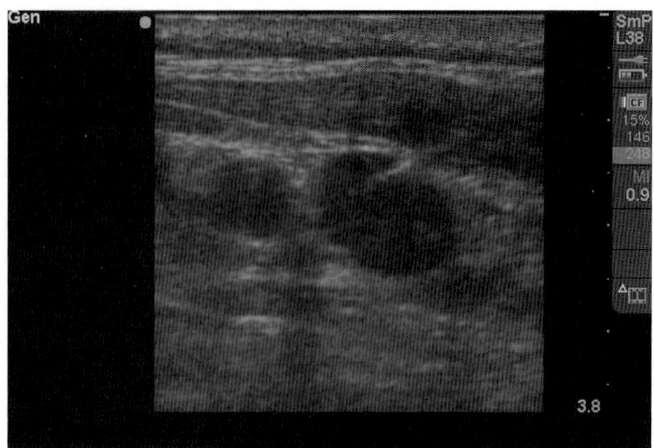

**Fig. 6.5 Image of a needle tip (seen as the hyperechoic structure on the right of the vessel) entering the internal jugular vein.** This image should correspond to a flash of blood seen in the syringe attached to the cannulating needle.

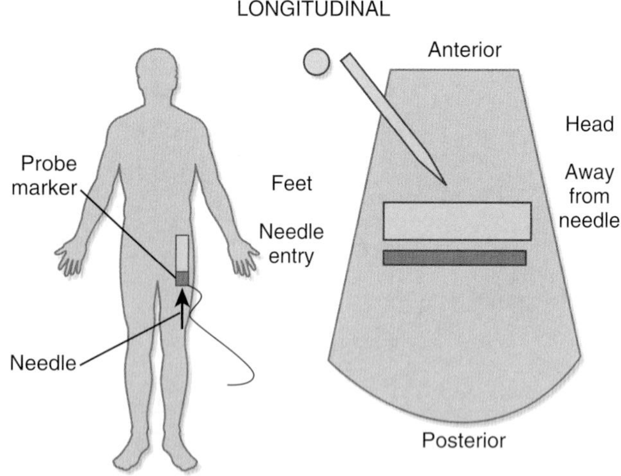


**Fig. 6.7 Schematic demonstrating the in-plane technique used for longitudinal or oblique placement of a catheter.** The indicator in the this image is pointing toward the patient's feet and the needle is inserted from this end. This causes the needle to appear from the left side of the screen as shown on the right of this figure. It can then be followed in plane as it advances toward the vessel.

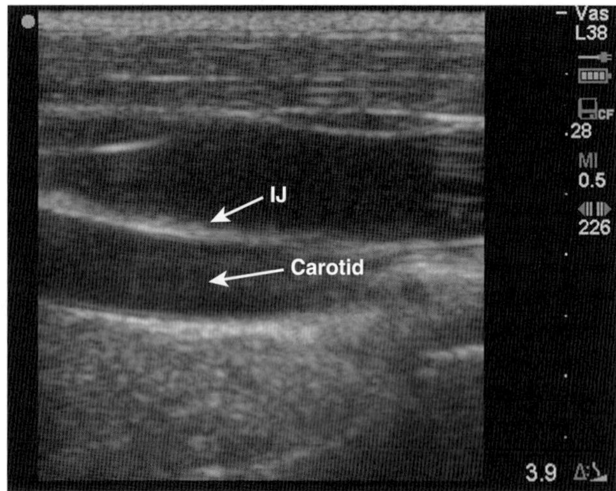


**Fig. 6.6 Image of the internal jugular (IJ) and carotid in longitudinal orientation.** Note how closely opposed these vessels are to one another. The IJ is the more superficial of the two and has thinner walls. Its size should vary with respiration and compression. The carotid artery is deep to the IJ, has thicker walls, and should not vary in size. At the left of the screen, a catheter or wire is seen within the lumen of the IJ.

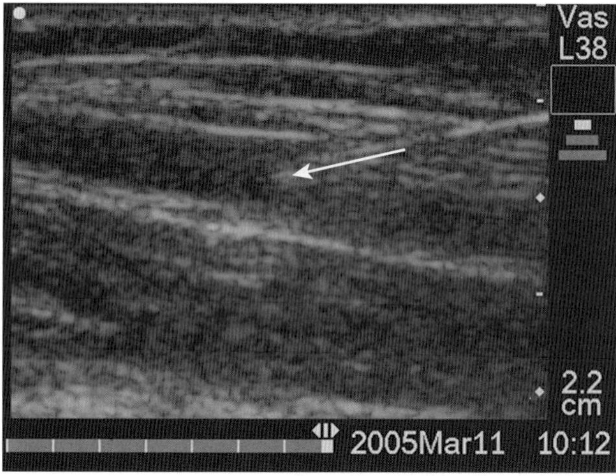


**Fig. 6.8 Image of a needle advancing toward the internal jugular in longitudinal orientation.** The needle is seen on the right of the figure as a hyperechoic object. It can be seen entering the vessel as shown by the *arrow*.

transverse and longitudinal views.[14] The probe is aligned obliquely over the vessel so that it appears between the structure typically seen in the transverse and longitudinal views. The needle can then be introduced from the end of the transducer and followed in plane as it advances toward the vessel.[15] The oblique approach combines the familiar view of the vessel with the reassurance of being able to view the length of the needle (see Videos 6 and 7).

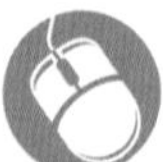

Videos 6 and 7 can be found on Expert Consult @ www.expertconsult.com.

Ultrasonography is also commonly used for peripheral approaches to intravenous access, particularly in patients with difficult access, such as those undergoing dialysis or chemotherapy.[16] The basilic vein is a usually a good option, even when other peripheral veins are unusable (**Fig. 6.9**). The extremity chosen should be positioned comfortably and a tourniquet applied to facilitate an initial ultrasound survey to identify candidate veins (**Fig. 6.10**). The operator localizes the vein (**Fig. 6-11**) and performs cannulation via the transverse or longitudinal approach, as described for central access. Because peripheral veins requiring ultrasound guidance for cannulation are often deeper structures, the use of longer catheters should be considered. It should also be appreciated that peripheral veins are much more likely to collapse with even light pressure from the ultrasound transducer.

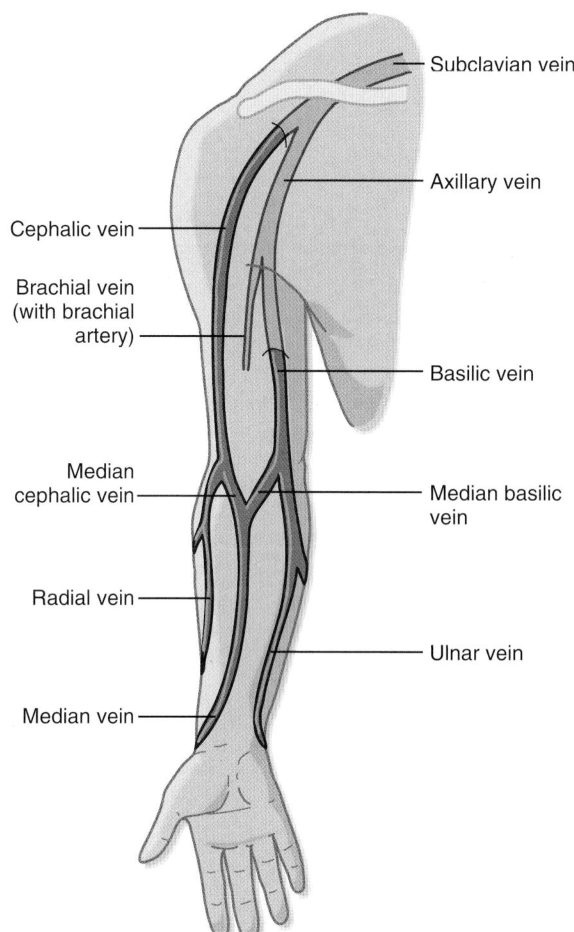


**Fig. 6.9 Schematic of the peripheral veins of the upper extremity.** The basilic vein is a frequent target of ultrasound-guided access because it is easy to find, relatively easy to access, and frequently available.

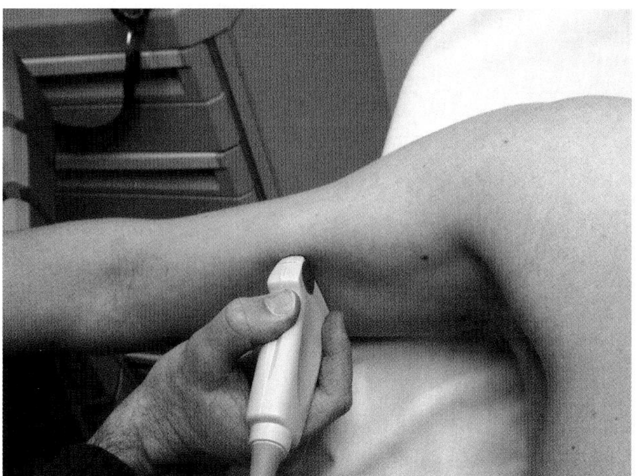

**Fig. 6.10 Image of a sonographer scanning the area of the basilic vein.** Note that the indicator is pointed toward the patient's right. This ensures that the image that is seen on screen is true to the surface anatomy. In other words, the orientation of the anatomy seen on screen is the same as the orientation encountered by the operator.

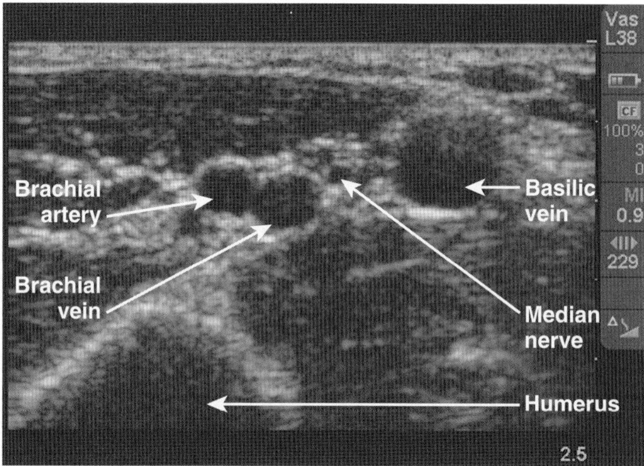


**Fig. 6.11 Transverse image of the basilic vein.** Note its close proximity to the brachial artery and vein.

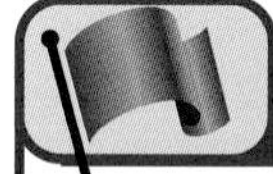

## RED FLAGS

Although bedside ultrasound improves the overall success of venous access and decreases complications, it is not without potential pitfalls.

When viewing vessels in the transverse orientation, only a small part of the needle can be visualized. Identifying and following the needle tip immediately after it enters the skin will avoid inadvertent arterial puncture. In the longitudinal orientation, the vein and artery are very closely opposed (see Fig. 6.4). Extra care should be taken to ensure that the vessel on screen is the target vessel.

Both the transverse and longitudinal orientations have limitations in localizing the needle tip. In the transverse orientation, the medial-to-lateral position of the tip can best be determined (**Fig. 6.12**), but the slope of the needle path may be difficult to appreciate. Conversely, in the longitudinal orientation, the slope can be appreciated, but the medial-to-lateral position may not be apparent (**Fig. 6.13**). A combination of these two approaches, or the oblique approach, may minimize these potential shortcomings.

It is also important to avoid reliance on any one aspect of the image to identify the structures. Variant vascular anatomy may make landmarks less reliable, and severe volume depletion may lead to a completely collapsed internal jugular vein with a compressible carotid. Multiple characteristics should be examined to confirm that the vessel in question is venous.

Even though visualization of the anatomy does make successful cannulation more likely, it is no guarantee. Inadvertent carotid puncture while using ultrasound guidance is well described, in particular as a result of a through-and-through venous puncture.[17,18] Prudence and careful technique are always appropriate.

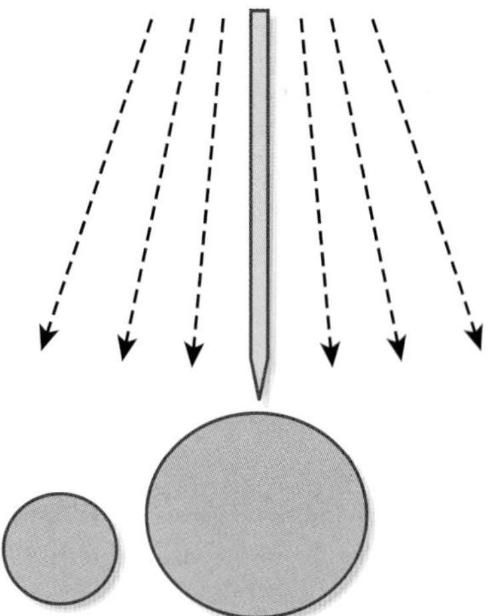


**Fig. 6.12 Schematic demonstrating the advantages of transverse orientation for vascular access.** In this orientation, the left-to-right (or medial-to-lateral) placement of the needle can be identified. However, the slope of the angle of the needle is out of the plane of this orientation and cannot easily be appreciated. Failure to appreciate this shortcoming may result in inadvertent arterial puncture.

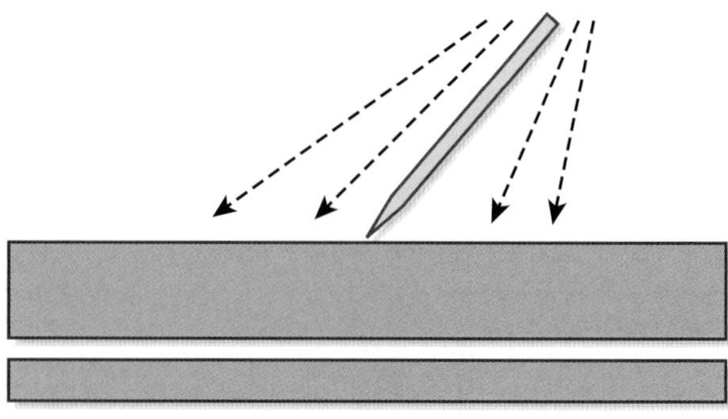


**Fig. 6.13 Schematic demonstrating the advantages of longitudinal orientation for vascular access.** In this orientation, the slope of the angle of the needle can be identified. However, the right-to-left (or medial-to-lateral) placement of the needle tip cannot easily be appreciated.

## SUGGESTED READINGS


1. Keyes LE, Frazee BW, Snoey ER, et al. Ultrasound-guided brachial and basilic vein cannulation in emergency department patients with difficult intravenous access. Ann Emerg Med 1999;34:711-14.
2. Leung J, Duffy M, Finckh A. Real-time ultrasonographically-guided internal jugular vein catheterization in the emergency department increases success rates and reduces complications: a randomized, prospective study. Ann Emerg Med 2006;48:540-7.
3. Phelan M, Hagerty D. The oblique view: an alternative approach for ultrasound-guided central line placement. J Emerg Med 2009;37:403-8.
4. Moon CH, Blehar D, Shear MA, et al. Incidence of posterior vessel wall puncture during ultrasound-guided vessel cannulation in a simulated model. Acad Emerg Med 2010;17:1138-41.


## REFERENCES

*References can be found on Expert Consult @ www.expertconsult.com.*

# Management of Cardiac Arrest and Post–Cardiac Arrest Syndrome

7

*William J. Brady, Peter P. Monteleone, Mark Sochor, and Robert E. O'Connor*

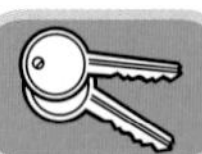

**KEY POINTS**

- The ultimate outcome of patients with cardiac arrest is frequently poor but can be improved by immediate bystander cardiopulmonary resuscitation, early defibrillation, and postresuscitation treatment.
- The classic ABC (airway, breathing, circulation) prioritization has changed to CAB to reinforce and prioritize early initiation of high-quality chest compressions and deemphasize early invasive airway management.
- Early defibrillation in patients with ventricular fibrillation and pulseless ventricular tachycardia is aided by various strategies, including automatic external defibrillators and improved provider awareness.
- Interruptions in chest compressions during cardiopulmonary resuscitation should be limited to maximize resuscitation; such interruptions can contribute to an unfavorable outcome.
- Postresuscitation care should include consideration of both induced hypothermia and urgent coronary reperfusion therapy.

## EPIDEMIOLOGY

In the United States, sudden cardiac death accounts for approximately 200,000 to 500,000 deaths per year, with nearly half of these events occurring outside the hospital. Regarding the primary inciting event, cardiac causes of sudden cardiac death are most common (**Fig. 7.1**). Even though individuals with established cardiac disease have a greater than 50% incidence of sudden death, only a minority of cardiac arrest incidents occur in this population. It is estimated that half of all deaths from cardiovascular disease are sudden and unexpected and occur soon after the onset of symptoms. Patient age at the time of cardiac arrest has two distinct peaks—infants younger than 6 months and adults 45 to 75 years of age. Most sudden deaths occur outside the hospital and are often unwitnessed.[1,2]

Despite comprehensive resuscitation programs and extensive research initiatives, survival rates in most American communities after out-of-hospital cardiac arrest range from 2% to 5%, and survival rates after in-hospital arrest range from 25% to 30%. Despite improvements in prehospital- and hospital-based management strategies and increased awareness in the lay public, cardiac arrest is still associated with extremely high mortality and a dismal neurologic outcome. Immediate, high-quality cardiopulmonary resuscitation (CPR) and effective defibrillation are rarely accomplished quickly enough to increase the likelihood of an improved outcome.

When resuscitation is successful, cardiac dysrhythmias remain a primary concern in the early phase of management of cardiac arrest. The four basic dysrhythmias encountered in cardiac arrest victims include pulseless ventricular tachycardia (VT), ventricular fibrillation (VF), asystole, and pulseless electrical activity (PEA). Pulseless VT and VF result in death unless treated aggressively and rapidly. Asystole, or effective absence of cardiac electrical activity, is the true cardiac arrhythmia (i.e., absence of any rhythm). PEA constitutes a diverse range of rhythms and related clinical scenarios. PEA is an electrical rhythm (i.e., the cardiac rhythm) with absence of discernible mechanical contraction of the heart and no detectable perfusion. The frequency of the dysrhythmias differs depending on the clinical setting (**Fig. 7.2**).

## GENERAL MANAGEMENT CONSIDERATIONS

The core concepts of management of cardiorespiratory arrest include the following goals: reversing any immediately treatable cause and ensuring the basics of circulatory and respiratory support. In the early phases of cardiac arrest, circulation is the most important issue and is addressed by performing high-quality, uninterrupted chest compressions and defibrillation for shockable rhythms.

Resuscitation rates in patients with out-of-hospital and in-hospital cardiac arrest remain poor despite significant advances in the medical sciences. Contemporary research and recommendations have demonstrated that basic life support (BLS) interventions are very important therapies that have a positive impact on outcome.[3] This same body of thought and investigation has suggested that advanced life support (ALS) treatments are of less value than originally thought.[3] In addition, studies have demonstrated that early access to ALS treatment may be of less importance than previously believed.[3,4] In the final phase of the Ontario Prehospital Advanced Life Support trial it was reported that in a community in which

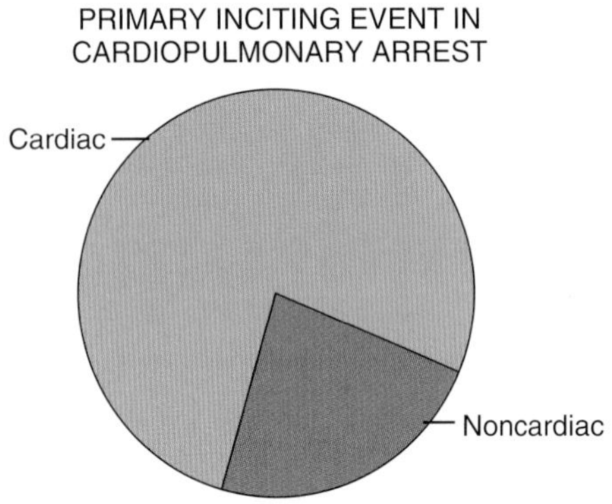

PRIMARY INCITING EVENT IN CARDIOPULMONARY ARREST

Cardiac

Noncardiac

**Fig. 7.1 Primary inciting event in cardiopulmonary arrest.** Sudden death may occur for a range of reasons, including medical and traumatic. Of the medical events, cardiac causes are the most frequently encountered; in fact, 75% of sudden death events are related to cardiac causes. In this setting, acute dysrhythmias are common, whether they represent the primary event (e.g., sudden ventricular fibrillation) or a secondary process related to the primary event (e.g., acute pulmonary edema with progressive hypoxemia and resultant bradycardia).

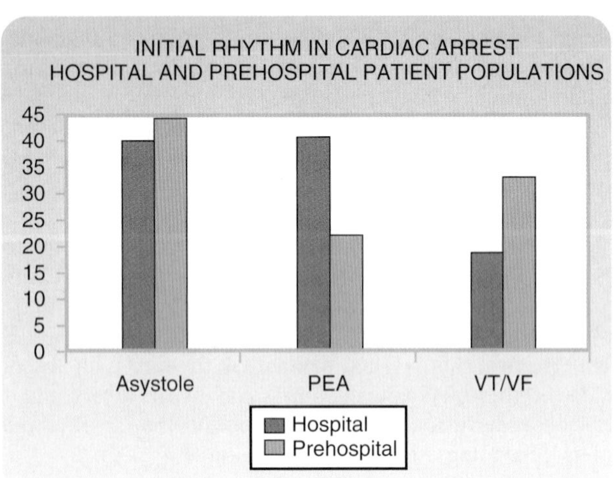


**Fig. 7.2 Cardiac arrhythmias encountered in cardiac arrest.** Note the preponderance of asystole in both groups, as well as increased rates of pulseless electrical activity (PEA) in the hospitalized patients and ventricular fibrillation and tachycardia (VT/VF) in the prehospital patients.

early CPR and early defibrillation are achieved, there is no survival benefit with the addition of prehospital ALS interventions.[3] ALS is of value, but it is limited and less valuable than BLS measures in the early phase of most cardiac arrest events.

The 2010 guidelines of the American Heart Association (AHA) further deemphasizes advanced interventions. The 2010 AHA Guidelines for Cardiopulmonary Resuscitation and Emergency Cardiovascular Care list five goals in the approach to cardiac arrest resuscitation: rapid activation of the emergency response team, effective and high-quality chest compressions, early access to defibrillation, effective ALS, and coordinated postresuscitation care.[5] Only one of these five goals addresses ALS interventions.

Critically, both BLS and ALS protocols and guidelines are important, but they are simply guides to management. Emergency physicians should use these protocols and guidelines as a framework to develop and implement the most appropriate management for their patients.

## CARDIOPULMONARY RESUSCITATION

CPR can be performed in two basic fashions. The traditional, or conventional, method includes chest compressions with ventilations; the newer and probably superior method is termed compression-only CPR and involves chest compressions only with avoidance of early airway management. Each of the management priorities in CPR—circulation, airway, and breathing (CAB)—must be addressed either in sequential fashion (limited personnel available) or simultaneously (multiple personnel available).

With respect to resuscitation in general and CPR in particular, it is important to note that *circulation* now precedes *airway* and *breathing*. Adequate circulation, largely achieved by appropriate chest compressions with limited interruption and early defibrillation for shockable rhythms, is a necessity throughout the resuscitation event and is particularly important in its early phase. Achieving an adequate airway with appropriate oxygenation and ventilation is an important intervention, but it appears to be less important than early and continuous adequate, uninterrupted chest compressions. Rhythm analysis, pulse determinations, and other periods without chest compression must be minimized so that perfusion can be sustained.

Numerous investigations have demonstrated that chest compressions are delayed, frequently interrupted, and of poor quality. Wik et al found that CPR was performed only 48% of the time when indicated and that when it was performed, the mean rate was just 64 compressions per minute, with an appropriate depth (at least 5 cm) attained in only 28% of cases.[6] Wang et al. and others reported that CPR was frequently interrupted for prolonged periods, anywhere from 1.8 to 7 minutes, to perform endotracheal intubation.[7,8]

One of the key components of the 2010 AHA guidelines[5] is the change from performing the ABCs (airway, breathing, circulation) to the CABs,[9] thus demonstrating how important compressions are relative to airway management and oxygenation—particularly early in cardiac arrest. Chest compression–only CPR has been proposed as an alternative method of basic resuscitation that is superior to traditional CPR with chest compressions and ventilations. The basic component of compression-only CPR is the performance of continuous, uninterrupted chest compressions of high quality. Compression-only CPR suggests that early management of the airway is not a priority.

Compression-only CPR has been shown to have similar efficacy to conventional CPR in terms of neurologically intact survival at 1 year in victims of witnessed cardiac arrest.[10] In patients with an initially shockable rhythm, Kellum et al. demonstrated an increased survival rate with neurologically intact status after receiving compression-only CPR.[11] The SOS-KANTO (Survey of Survivors After out-of Hospital Cardiac Arrest in the Kanto Area of Japan) trial reviewed 4068 patients with witnessed out-of-hospital cardiac arrests, 1151 of whom received bystander CPR. The 439 subjects who received hands-only CPR showed similar neurologic outcome at 30 days as did those who received conventional CPR (6% versus 4% of survivors); no benefit was seen with the addition of mouth-to-mouth ventilation.[12] In 2008 using the concept of minimally interrupted cardiac resuscitation, Bobrow et al.

demonstrated that cycles of 200 continuous compressions, followed by electrical defibrillation with immediate resumption of compressions before endotracheal intubation, resulted in an increased survival rate (1.8% versus 5.4%) in all patients. In the witnessed VF subgroup, the survival rate increased from 4.7% to 17.6%.[13]

When performing CPR, early emphasis on the airway and breathing components of CPR can hinder appropriate chest compressions and produce excessive ventilations. The concept of death by hyperventilation is based on overdistension of the thoracic cavity, which results in increased intrathoracic pressure. Increased intrathoracic pressure can impede venous return to the right side of the heart. Reduced venous return limits preload of the left ventricle, thereby resulting in diminished cardiac, cerebral, and vital organ perfusion. Excessive ventilation rates must be avoided; a ventilatory rate of 8 to 10 breaths/min is appropriate via either bag-mask ventilations or endotracheal tube.

## ELECTRICAL THERAPY

Electrical therapy—defibrillation and transcutaneous cardiac pacing—can be lifesaving when used in an appropriate and timely fashion. Early defibrillation improves survival rates, but only if accomplished within minutes. This therapy is appropriate only for pulseless VT and VF, and it has no indication in managing asystole or PEA rhythms.

Defibrillators exist in two basic styles—monophasic and biphasic. Most commercially available defibrillators (automatic and manual) are biphasic, although many monophasic models remain in use today. No defibrillator style, monophasic or biphasic, is associated with unequivocally higher rates of successful resuscitation or survival to hospital discharge. The biphasic defibrillator has achieved a higher rate of termination of pulseless VT and VF, but this early benefit has not translated into survival to hospital discharge with meaningful quality of life. When using a monophasic defibrillator, a 360-J shock should be applied; if a biphasic unit is in operation, the equivalent, device-specific maximal emergency should be applied. In either type of device, a single shock is delivered initially and in subsequent defibrillations.

Use of an automated external defibrillator (AED) is a lifesaving intervention when applied appropriately. Use of an AED by trained lay rescuers (the Public Access Defibrillation [PAD] program) has resulted in a markedly shorter time to defibrillation and an improved rate of resuscitation. AED use by nontrained rescuers in a PAD application has anecdotally demonstrated positive outcomes, but its use by untrained personnel requires additional investigation. The Targeted First Responder (TFR) application has also demonstrated significant success.

No conclusive data are available on the ideal timing of the initial defibrillation, regardless of the downtime. The AHA recommendation states that a patient in cardiac arrest with a shockable rhythm should undergo electrical defibrillation as soon as possible. Chest compressions should be initiated as soon as the defibrillator is located, applied, and activated.

The most recent analysis of the timing of initial defibrillation suggests that there is no benefit with delayed defibrillation, even in patients with prolonged downtimes. Simpson et al. performed a meta-analysis of the existing literature and noted that no benefit was found in delaying the first shock in patients with prolonged downtimes or unwitnessed arrest (or both).[14] The cumulative data demonstrated no benefit in providing chest compression before defibrillation versus immediate defibrillation and also no harm in performing CPR before the initial defibrillation. The 2010 AHA guidelines[5,9] also acknowledged that the literature does not support a chest compression–first approach, thus suggesting that clinicians should provide both therapies (chest compression and defibrillation) and base the time of the first defibrillation on analysis of the setting, personnel, and equipment parameters for individual cases.

The other primary form of electrical therapy used in managing cardiac arrest is transcutaneous cardiac pacing. Very early use of transcutaneous ventricular pacing can be considered, although conclusive supporting evidence is lacking. Transcutaneous pacing is much less effective after the loss of spontaneous circulation or prolonged cardiac arrest.[15,16] Transcutaneous pacing is a rapid, minimally invasive means of treating asystole and PEA bradyarrhythmias. Transcutaneous pacing electrodes are applied to the skin of the anterior and posterior chest walls, and pacing is initiated with a portable pulse generator. In an emergency situation, this type of pacing technique is easily and rapidly accomplished when compared with other methods of cardiac pacing.

## PHARMACOLOGIC THERAPY

Although numerous medications may be used in a resuscitation event, several "code drugs" are of potential importance, including epinephrine, vasopressin, atropine, amiodarone, lidocaine, magnesium, calcium, and sodium bicarbonate. Research into resuscitation after cardiac arrest has demonstrated that BLS interventions significantly contribute to favorable outcomes and that ALS treatments are less valuable than originally thought.[3,17] A review of the issue has suggested that the use of cardioactive medications can increase the rate of successful resuscitation but does not alter the ultimate survival rate or have an impact on neurologic status at discharge among survivors.[18]

Because these code drugs are still used with significant frequency by clinicians during resuscitation of patients in cardiac arrest, an understanding of these medications and their potential impact is essential. The code drugs are separated into several subcategories, including vasopressors (epinephrine and vasopressin), parasympatholytic drugs (atropine), antiarrhythmic agents (lidocaine and amiodarone), electrolytes (calcium and magnesium), buffer (sodium bicarbonate), and fibrinolytic medications.

The two primary vasopressor agents used in resuscitation are epinephrine and vasopressin. Epinephrine and vasopressin have demonstrated increased rates of return of spontaneous circulation (ROSC) but have not produced meaningful increases in survival to hospital discharge with intact neurologic status. Both vasopressors are indicated in all three cardiac arrest treatment scenarios, including pulseless VT and VF, PEA, and asystole. These medications can be used interchangeably in the cardiac arrest scenario; that is, use of one type of vasopressor does not preclude future use of the other agent in that same resuscitation. The vasopressor class of resuscitative agents can increase the rate of ROSC. To date, however, no single report has demonstrated an improvement in overall ultimate survival, with or without a measure of neurologic status, as a function of vasopressor application.

Atropine is a parasympatholytic drug that enhances both sinoatrial node automaticity and atrioventricular conduction via direct vagolytic action. In cardiac arrest, atropine can be considered in patients with both asystole and PEA, particularly those with bradydysrhythmic electrical activity. It is important to note that the AHA has removed atropine from all cardiac arrest algorithms.[5,9] Removal of atropine is based not on any negative impact on patient outcome but on a significant lack of benefit.[5,9] Atropine is still recommended in patients with compromising bradydysrhythmia with intact perfusion.[5,9,19,20]

Amiodarone and lidocaine are the primary antidysrhythmic agents used in cardiac arrest resuscitation scenarios. Amiodarone has a very broad range of mechanisms, including sodium and calcium blockade, antagonism of potassium efflux, and adrenergic blocking effects. In cardiac arrest, indications for its use include pulseless VT and VF unresponsive to CPR, defibrillation, and an initial vasopressor. Although amiodarone has demonstrated impressive results in terms of ROSC after cardiac arrest, it has not altered the ultimate outcome—meaningful survival to hospital discharge. Lidocaine is a well-known and widely used antidysrhythmic agent with limited efficacy in cardiac arrest. Unfortunately, lidocaine has demonstrated no alteration in outcomes of patients with out-of-hospital cardiac arrest secondary to pulseless VT and VF. Furthermore, when compared with amiodarone, lidocaine has been shown to have a less favorable rate of ROSC and an increased rate of asystole in general and following defibrillation. Like amiodarone, it may be used in patients with pulseless VT and VF unresponsive to initial therapies. At the present time, lidocaine is best considered an alternative to amiodarone for refractory pulseless VT and VF.

The electrolytes magnesium and calcium play a limited role in resuscitation. Magnesium should be used in patients with polymorphic VT (PVT) thought to be torsades de pointes (TdP). Possible secondary indications for magnesium include PEA cardiac arrest potentially resulting from hyperkalemia and cardiorespiratory arrest related to toxemia of pregnancy. Use of calcium should be limited to cardiac arrest involving excessive parenteral magnesium administration, hyperkalemia, and cardiotoxin ingestion.

Sodium bicarbonate is a potent buffer, but no evidence supports its widespread use for cardiac arrest. Sodium bicarbonate can adversely affect perfusion in certain vascular beds, unfavorably alter acid-base status at the tissue and cellular levels, and promote hyperosmolarity and hypernatremia. Sodium bicarbonate has several specific clinical scenarios in which it is potentially indicated: tricyclic antidepressant overdose (and other sodium channel blocking agents), severe acidosis (metabolic and respiratory), hyperkalemia, and prolonged cardiac arrest.

Acute thrombosis with or without embolization, either coronary or pulmonary, can cause cardiac arrest. Many investigators have considered the early use of fibrinolytic agents in the management of cardiac arrest with known or presumed acute thrombosis. Anecdotal reports describe the cases of adult patients who have been successfully resuscitated following the administration of a fibrinolytic agent when the condition leading to the arrest was acute myocardial infarction (AMI) or acute pulmonary embolism.[21] The 2010 AHA guidelines state that the evidence is insufficient to advocate the routine use of fibrinolytic agents during cardiac arrest but that its use should be considered on a case-by-case basis. Fibrinolytic agents are a level IIb recommendation in cardiac arrest secondary to pulmonary embolism.[5,9]

### THE AIRWAY

The AHA has moved away from the airway-first strategy with a reordering of the resuscitation alphabet from the ABCs to the CABs, thus highlighting the relative importance of circulation over airway management.[5,9] This change in strategy is based on the relative importance of circulation but also on the fact that airway interventions, particularly placement of an invasive airway, can interrupt continuous chest compressions and lessen the central nervous system (CNS), cardiac, and systemic perfusion produced by CPR. The airway should be managed invasively once appropriate chest compressions have been initiated and sustained and defibrillation has taken place. Management of the airway must not hinder appropriate chest compressions and other basic interventions. In cardiac arrest scenarios caused by a compromised airway or inadequate oxygenation and ventilation, or both, attention to invasive management of the airway is important.

## MANAGEMENT OF SPECIFIC DYSRHYTHMIAS

### VENTRICULAR FIBRILLATION AND PULSELESS VENTRICULAR TACHYCARDIA

VF and pulseless VT are discussed together because they occur in the same clinical settings and have similar mechanisms, causes, and modes of therapy. The only clinically significant classification system of VF concerns the amplitude of the chaotic waveform deflections. Regardless of the morphology of VF, without prompt therapy, VF invariably results in death.

VF is divided into two clinical types. It is considered primary in the absence of acute left ventricular dysfunction and cardiogenic shock, and it is noted in approximately 5% of patients with AMI. The majority of primary VF episodes occur within the first 4 hours of AMI, and 80% are seen within the initial 12-hour period of infarction. VF may represent abrupt reperfusion, but recurrent or ongoing ischemia is more likely. The overall prognosis for patients with primary VF does not differ from that in AMI patients without VF after a brief period of increased inpatient mortality. Secondary VF can occur at any time in the course of AMI; may be complicated by acute heart failure, cardiogenic shock, or both; and occurs in up to 7% of patients with AMI. Unlike primary VF, the prognosis for patients with secondary VF is poor, with in-hospital mortality approaching 60%, and long-term mortality beyond 5 years remains poor.

In contrast to VF, VT usually originates from a specific focus in the ventricular myocardium or in the infranodal conduction pathway. VT is defined as a rapid, wide regular QRS complex tachycardia originating from infranodal cardiac tissue. VT can be classified from several different perspectives, including the overall clinical findings (stable versus unstable), the hemodynamic state (presence or absence of a pulse), its temporal course (sustained versus nonsustained), and its morphology (monomorphic versus polymorphic). In sudden cardiac death, it is most appropriate to consider VT from the perspective of the overall clinical findings, with an emphasis on the temporal and hemodynamic factors. In this instance, VT is considered pulseless and sustained and thus unstable. Pulseless VT accounts for a minority of the rhythms seen in cardiac arrest and has the most favorable prognosis. This relatively infrequent occurrence results from an early appearance with rapid degeneration. If therapy is not initiated in arrest events, this rhythm rapidly decompensates into more malignant rhythms such as VF or asystole.

### Pathophysiology

These malignant dysrhythmias most often arise as a result of direct myocardial damage (i.e., AMI, myocarditis, cardiomyopathy), medication toxicity, or electrolyte abnormality. The pathophysiology usually involves either a reentry phenomenon or triggered automaticity. A reentry circuit within the ventricular myocardium is the most common source. The properties of a reentry circuit involve two pathways of conduction with differing electrical characteristics. The reentry circuits that provide the substrate for VT and VF generally occur in a zone of acute ischemia or chronic scarring. This dysrhythmia is usually initiated by an ectopic beat, although a number of other factors can be the primary initiating event, including acute coronary ischemia, electrolyte disorders, and dysautonomia. Triggered automaticity of a group of cells can result from various cardiac anomalies, including congenital heart disease, acquired heart ailments, electrolyte disorders, and medication toxicity.

One electrophysiologic model describes these ventricular dysrhythmias with respect to morphology and suggests that the three entities (VF, PVT, and monophasic VT [MVT]) are manifested across an electrophysiologic spectrum. This model notes that PVT differs from VF and MVT in frequency, amplitude, and variability, thus suggesting that MVT, PVT, and VF are states of electrical activity occurring across a spectrum of ventricular dysrhythmia. In this model, MVT is the most highly organized rhythm, whereas VF is the least; PVT represents an intermediate entity between the two end points of the spectrum.

### Clinical Presentation

VENTRICULAR FIBRILLATION VF results in a lack of spontaneous perfusion except in the rare case of a witnessed, recent onset in which the patient is able to cough, thereby enabling perfusion to continue for a short period. VF is diagnosed electrocardiographically (**Fig. 7.3**) in pulseless and apneic patients by the presence of lower amplitude and chaotic activity. The rate of the deflections is usually between 200 and 500 depolarizations per minute. Morphologically, VF is divided into coarse (Fig. 7.3, *A*) and fine (Fig. 7.3, *B* and *C*). Coarse VF tends to occur early after cardiac arrest; is characterized by high-amplitude, or coarse, waveforms; and has a better prognosis than fine VF does. With continued cardiac arrest the amplitude dampens, with a less dramatic appearance of the dysrhythmia and fine VF (Fig. 7.3, *B* and *C*) ultimately being produced. The R-on-T phenomenon can result in VF as noted in Figure 7.3, *D* and *E*.

Fine VF may be confused with asystole. If the sensing electrode is oriented perpendicular to the primary depolarization vector, the amplitude of the deflections is minimal, thus mimicking asystole. Such mimicking can have a negative impact on patient care if electrical defibrillation is not considered. This potential pitfall can easily be avoided if the dysrhythmia is viewed in at least two or three simultaneous or consecutive electrocardiographic leads. Fine VF has a significantly greater incidence of post-countershock asystole than coarse VF does. In this instance, aggressive resuscitation will probably improve the hemodynamic state and increase the opportunity for ROSC.

VENTRICULAR TACHYCARDIA VT is defined as three or more ventricular beats in succession with a QRS complex duration of greater than 0.12 second and a ventricular rate greater than 100 or 120 beats/min (**Fig. 7.4**). Most instances of VT are characterized by very rapid rates; however, patients may have slower versions of VT, particularly if using amiodarone.

From an electrocardiographic perspective (**Fig. 7.5**; also see Fig. 7.4), the morphology of the VT is of importance. MVT (Fig. 7.5, *A* and *B*) is identified when each consecutive waveform has a single morphology; that is, the beat-to-beat variation in QRS complex morphology is negligible. The rate is usually between 140 and 180 beats/min and very regular. MVT is the most common form of VT and is seen in 65% to 75% of patients with VT in the out-of-hospital setting (**Fig. 7.6**).[22,23] In patients with MVT, the cause of the dysrhythmia is usually myocardial scarring from a previous infarct.

PVT (see Fig. 7.4) is characterized by a frequently changing QRS complex (see Fig. 7-5, *C* and *D*). The QRS complex tends to be greater than 0.12 second with beat-to-beat variations in morphology and width. Significant variability in the R-R interval and QRS complex axis is present. Its rate is usually more rapid than that of MVT, with a range of 150 to 300 beats/min, and PVT accounts for 25% to 30% of cases of VT in patients with out-of-hospital cardiac arrest (see Fig. 7.6).[22,23]

The PVT subtype TdP (see Fig. 7.4) demonstrates polymorphous QRS complexes that vary from beat to beat (**Fig. 7.7**, *A* and *B*; also see Fig. 7.5, *D*). The variation is often quite pronounced and easily observed. TdP has a highly characteristic electrocardiographic pattern; the literal translation of the French term *torsades de pointes*—"twisting of the points"—elegantly describes the appearance of the QRS complex as it varies in amplitude and appears to rotate about the isoelectric baseline in a semisinusoidal fashion. Also required for electrocardiographic (and clinical) diagnosis of TdP is demonstration of abnormal repolarization as manifested by prolongation of the QT interval on the electrocardiogram when the patient is in a supraventricular rhythm (either before or after cardiac arrest) (Fig. 7.7, *B*).

### Management of Pulseless Ventricular Tachycardia and Ventricular Fibrillation

Resuscitative management of these two malignant dysrhythmias is similar. The basic approach (**Table 7.1**) includes CPR, with an emphasis on high-quality chest compressions, and electrical defibrillation. Once defibrillation has occurred, CPR is resumed for an additional 2 minutes. If the dysrhythmia persists on electrocardiographic analysis, a vasopressor is administered, either vasopressin or epinephrine. Epinephrine should be used in 1-mg doses, preferably administered via an intravenous or intraosseous line. If given by endotracheal tube

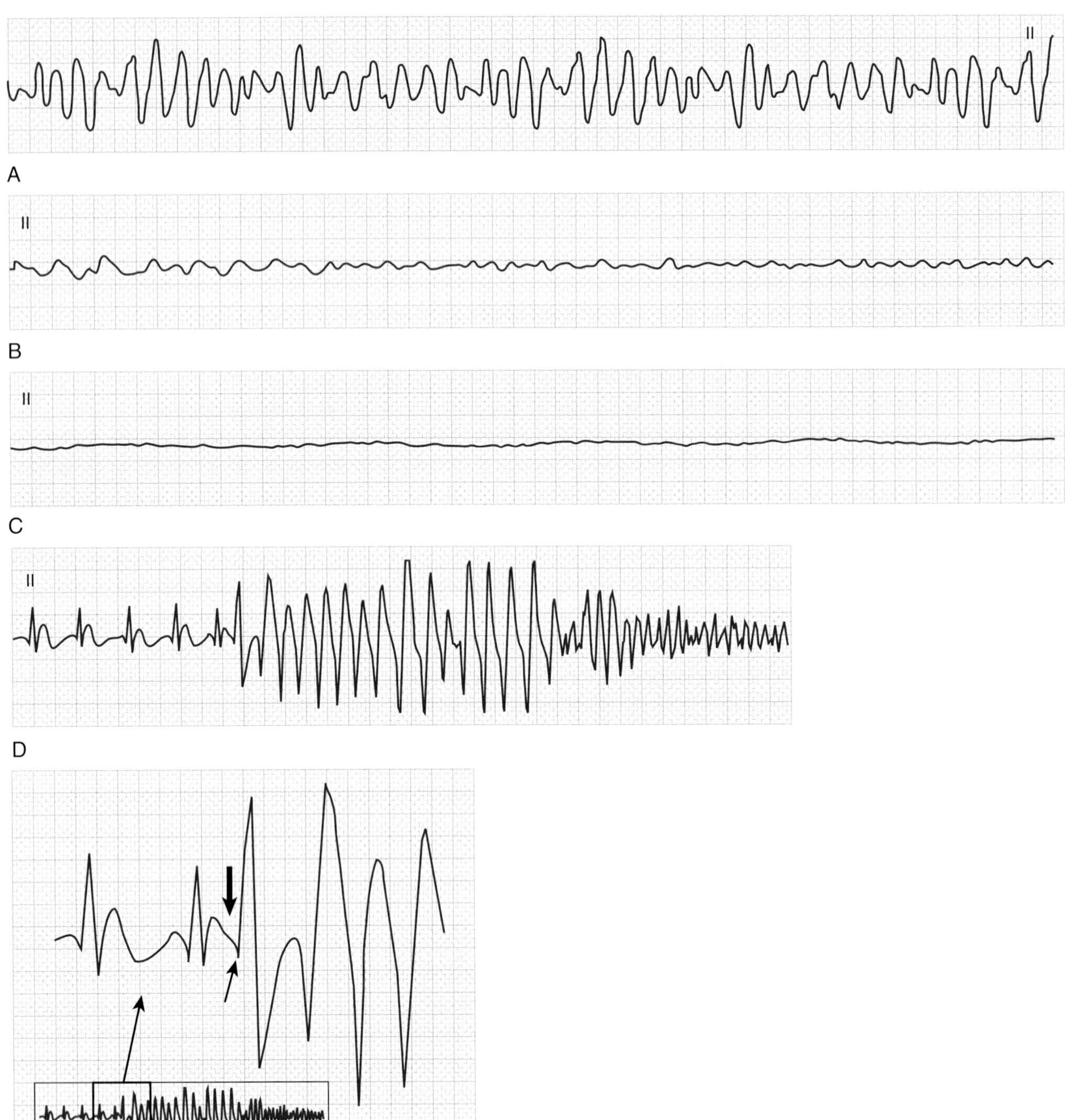


**Fig. 7.3 Ventricular fibrillation. A,** Coarse ventricular fibrillation. Note the large-amplitude deflections with no organized electrical activity. **B,** Ventricular fibrillation with low to intermediate deflections in amplitude; also, the absence of organized electrical activity is obvious. **C,** Very fine ventricular fibrillation. Note the apparent absence in this lead (lead II) of deflection. This rhythm may be incorrectly diagnosed as asystole if the patient is monitored solely with a single electrocardiographic lead. **D,** Sinus tachycardia with degeneration into ventricular fibrillation. Note the appearance of the R-on-T phenomenon, with the R wave of an early beat falling on the T wave of the preceding beat. The repolarization period of the electrocardiographic cycle is an electrically vulnerable period of the cardiac phase—insults, such as subsequent depolarizations, may cause the development of ventricular tachycardia or ventricular fibrillation. In this case, the patient has a short period of polymorphic ventricular tachycardia followed by coarse ventricular fibrillation. **E,** R-on-T phenomenon with the R wave *(thin arrow)* of an early beat falling on the T wave *(thick arrow)* of the preceding beat, followed by a short period of polymorphic ventricular tachycardia.

VENTRICULAR TACHYCARDIA

Ventricular tachycardia

Monomorphic ventricular tachycardia

Polymorphic ventricular tachycardia

Torsades de pointes PVT

Non–torsades de pointes PVT

**Fig. 7.4 Morphologic description of ventricular tachycardia (VT).** Morphologically, VT can be divided into monomorphic and polymorphic based on the nature of the QRS complex. Polymorphic VT (PVT) can be further subdivided into torsades de pointes (TdP) PVT and non-TdP PVT—this distinction considers not only the morphology of the QRS complex but also other electrophysiologic issues (the repolarization state as manifested by the QT interval); with TdP PVT, prolongation of the QT interval is noted—this determination obviously can only be made when the patient has an electrocardiogram exhibiting a supraventricular rhythm.

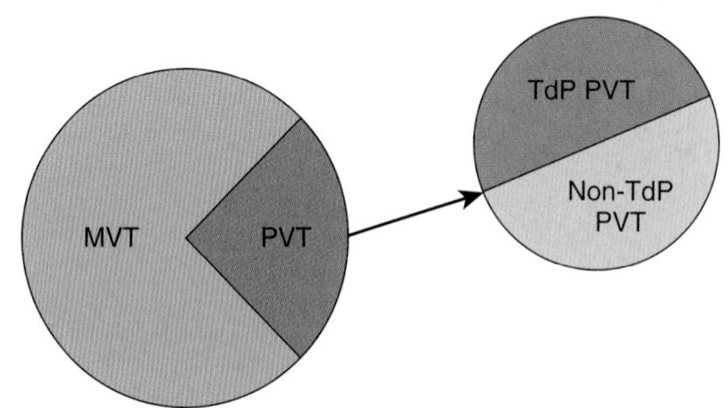


**Fig. 7.6 Morphologic subtypes of ventricular tachycardia (VT) in prehospital cardiac arrest patients.** In patients with polymorphic VT (PVT), both non–torsades de pointes (Non-TdP) and TdP versions are seen in approximately equal frequency. *MVT*, Monophasic ventricular tachycardia.

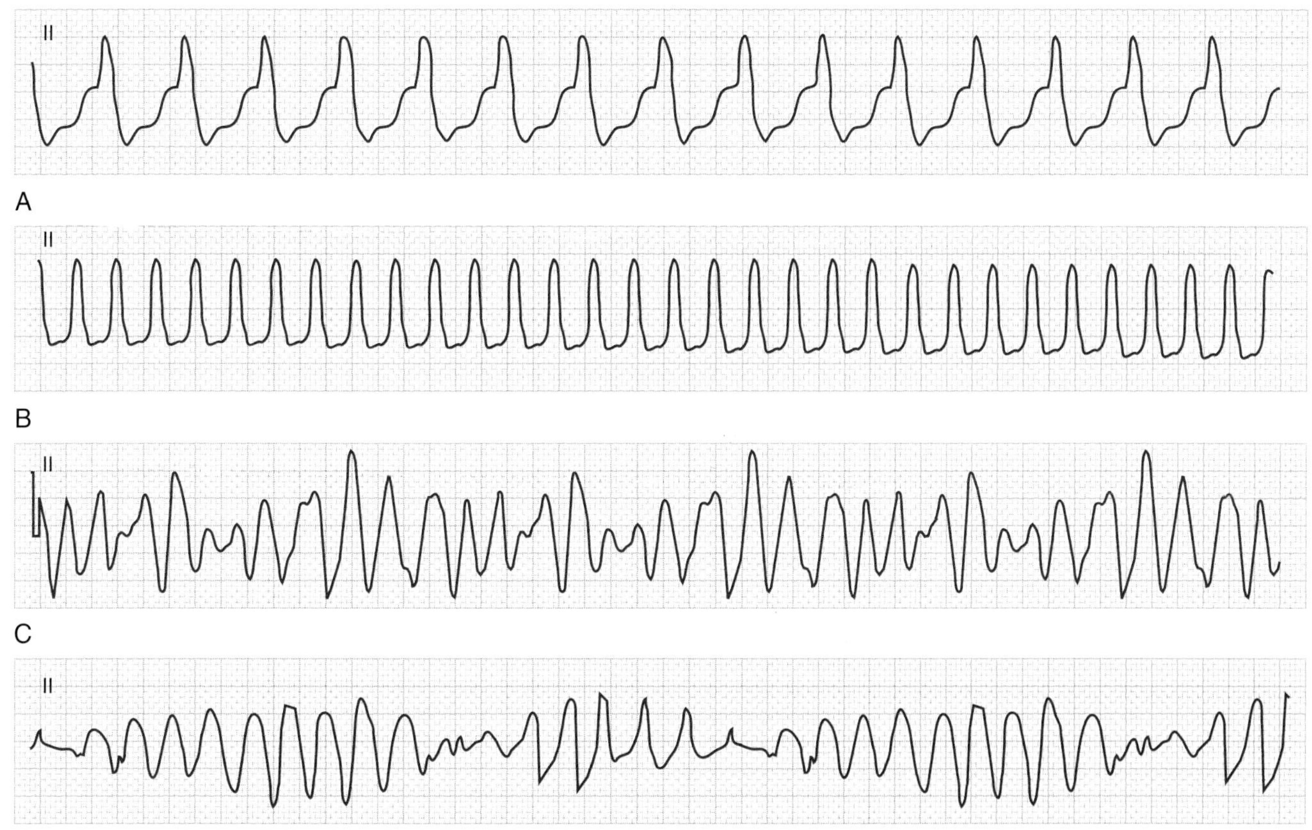


**Fig. 7.5 Ventricular tachycardia. A,** Monomorphic ventricular tachycardia. Note the very wide QRS complex and rate of approximately 150 beats/min. **B,** Monomorphic ventricular tachycardia. Note the very rapid rate of approximately 240 beats/min. **C,** Polymorphic ventricular tachycardia (PVT). The QRS complex is continually changing (potentially both in amplitude and morphology) in any single lead. The QRS complex also tends to be greater than 0.12 second with beat-to-beat variations in morphology and width being encountered; significant variability in the R-R interval and QRS complex axis is noted as well. **D,** PVT, torsades de pointes (TdP) type. Note the marked, beat-to-beat variation in QRS complex morphology occurring in a gradual pattern. The QRS complex ranges from small to large with an undulating pattern, as though it is "twisting about a point"—the TdP version of PVT. TdP PVT has a characteristic appearance—the QRS complex varies in amplitude and appears to rotate about the isoelectric baseline in a semisinusoidal fashion. Also required for the electrocardiographic (and clinical) diagnosis of TdP is demonstration of abnormal repolarization manifested by prolongation of the QT interval on the electrocardiogram when the patient is in a supraventricular rhythm.

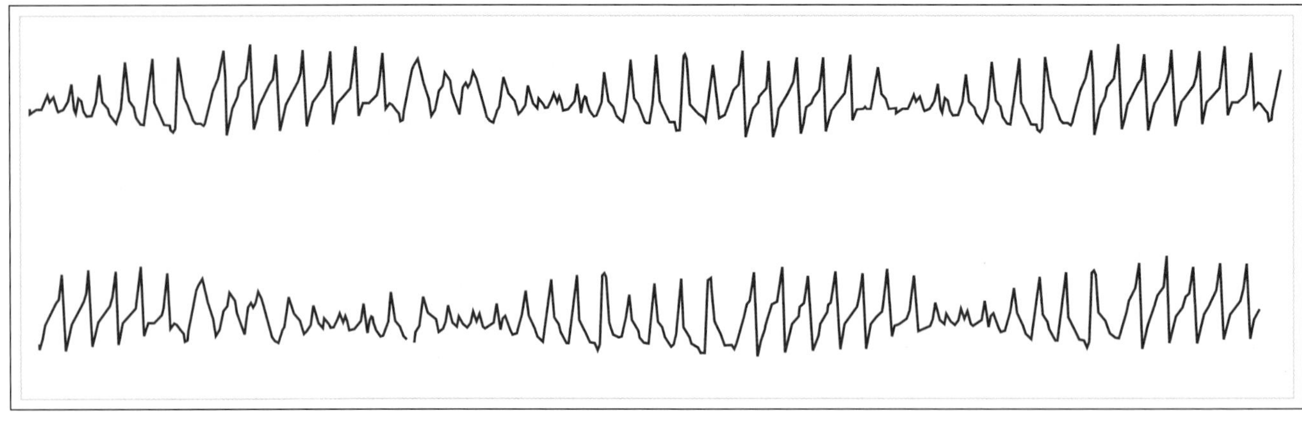

A

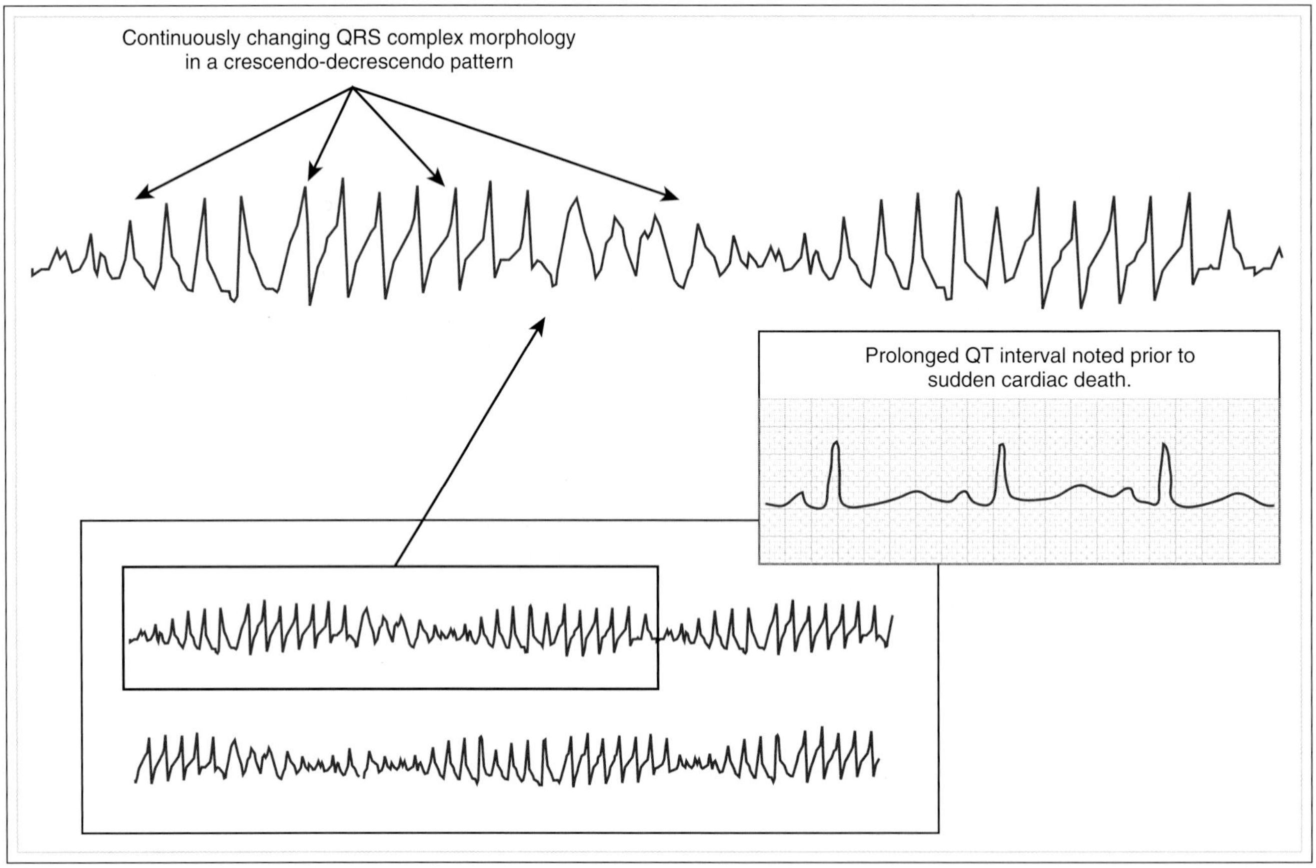

Continuously changing QRS complex morphology in a crescendo-decrescendo pattern

Prolonged QT interval noted prior to sudden cardiac death.

B

**Fig. 7.7** **A,** Torsades de pointes (TdP) polymorphic ventricular tachycardia. The appearance of the QRS complex is characteristic of this subtype of polymorphic ventricular tachycardia—in any single electrocardiographic lead it varies in both morphology and amplitude and appears to rotate about the isoelectric baseline in a semisinusoidal fashion. **B,** TdP polymorphic ventricular tachycardia. Note the polymorphous QRS complexes that vary from beat to beat. The variation is often quite pronounced, with marked variation easily observed in any single lead from one beat to the subsequent beat. TdP also demonstrates a highly characteristic electrocardiographic pattern; the literal translation of the French term *torsades de pointes*—"twisting of the points"—elegantly describes the appearance of the QRS complex as it varies in amplitude and appears to rotate about the isoelectric baseline in a semisinusoidal fashion. Also required for diagnosis is demonstration of abnormal repolarization as manifested by prolongation of the QT interval on the electrocardiogram when the patient is in a supraventricular rhythm (i.e., before arrest or after successful resuscitation and return of spontaneous circulation).

**Table 7.1 Ventricular Fibrillation and Pulseless Ventricular Tachycardia**

| TIME | TREATMENT PRIORITY | COMMENTS |
|---|---|---|
| Minute 0 | Chest compressions | Compressions should be performed at a rate of 100/min.<br>Initial compressions may improve shock efficacy by increasing the amplitude of ventricular fibrillation.<br>Pulse checks and rhythm analysis should be performed no more often than every 2 min.<br>Defibrillation should take place as soon as a device is available. |
| Minute 0-1 | Defibrillation, followed by chest compressions<br>IV access (if possible) | Because of the increased first shock conversion rate with biphasic energy and the importance of hands-off time, high-energy shock is recommended.<br>IV access should not interfere with chest compressions. |
| Minute 3 | Defibrillation, followed by immediate chest compressions<br>Vasopressin, 40 IU<br>Placement of an invasive airway (if possible) | Vasopressin or epinephrine may be given interchangeably initially.<br>Placement of an invasive airway should not interfere with chest compressions.<br>If an invasive airway is not possible at this time, noninvasive management of the airway is appropriate. |
| Minute 5 | Defibrillation, followed by immediate chest compressions<br>Amiodarone, 300 mg | CPR should take place over 2-min periods with intervening attempts at defibrillation.<br>Lidocaine is an acceptable alternative antiarrhythmic agent. |
| Minute 6 | Epinephrine, 1 mg | Medication is administered every 3-5 min for cardiac arrest; it should be realized that peak central levels may vary based on physiologic patient differences.<br>If vasopressin is given first, epinephrine is administered in all subsequent doses. |
| Minute 7 | Defibrillation, followed by immediate chest compressions | CPR should not be interrupted for periods longer than 15 seconds at a time. |
| Minute 9 | Defibrillation, followed by immediate chest compressions<br>Epinephrine, 1 mg | Other medications should be considered in patients with an identified underlying cause. |
| Minute 10 | Amiodarone, 150 mg | Amiodarone can be repeated in 5 min at half the initial dose. |

*CPR*, Cardiopulmonary resuscitation; *IV*, intravenous.

(ETT), a larger dose of two to three times the intravenous dose is recommended. Dosing through the ETT is not currently considered to be the most effective means of delivering the medication. Epinephrine should be readministered every 3 to 5 minutes during the resuscitation. In certain situations such as ingestion of a cardiotoxic drug, higher doses of epinephrine may be required, but this issue has not been explored. Vasopressin is administered via the intravenous or intraosseous routes at a dose of 40 international units (IU). In multiple studies of vasopressin alone or vasopressin versus epinephrine in prehospital and hospital-based populations, no significant difference has been found in survival to hospital discharge.[24-26] A single dose of vasopressin may be used as either the first or second vasopressor administered, and epinephrine can be used in a primary or secondary role.

After the administration of a vasopressor, CPR should be continued for 2 minutes, followed by a second defibrillation. If the VT or VF persists, amiodarone or lidocaine should be administered. Amiodarone is the preferred agent and should be considered in patients with pulseless VT or VF that is unresponsive to CPR, a vasopressor, and defibrillation. It is administered to a pulseless patient in a bolus dose of 300 mg intravenously, and it can be repeated with a second dose of 150 mg intravenously. Amiodarone has demonstrated a benefit over both placebo and lidocaine in this patient group. Even though rates of ROSC and survival to hospital admission were greater in amiodarone-treated patients, ultimate survival to hospital discharge was no different.[27,28]

PVT should be managed in similar fashion to pulseless MVT or VF. CPR, defibrillation, a vasopressor, and antidysrhythmic agents are appropriate therapeutic interventions. In two comparisons of MVT and PVT in prehospital patients with cardiorespiratory arrest, MVT occurred (60%) more often than PVT (15%) and TdP (15%).[22,23] Clinical outcomes were similar in both rhythm groups with similar therapies. Patients with the subset of TdP also fared as well as the non-TdP PVT and MVT groups.[22,23] If sustained, PVT is always unstable and requires immediate attention. Initial therapy is unsynchronized electrical cardioversion. Antiarrhythmic therapy is warranted, including the use of magnesium and amiodarone intravenously. Caution is advised because the rhythm frequently recurs.

## PULSELESS ELECTRICAL ACTIVITY

### Definition

PEA is indicative of a very serious underlying medical event, such as profound hypovolemia, massive myocardial infarction, large pulmonary embolism, significant electrolyte disorder, or cardiotoxic overdose. PEA features the unique combination of no discernible cardiac mechanical activity (i.e., a pulseless state) with persistent cardiac electrical activity (i.e., the cardiac rhythm). Essentially, any dysrhythmia other than VT or VF may be seen (**Figs. 7.8 and 7.9**).

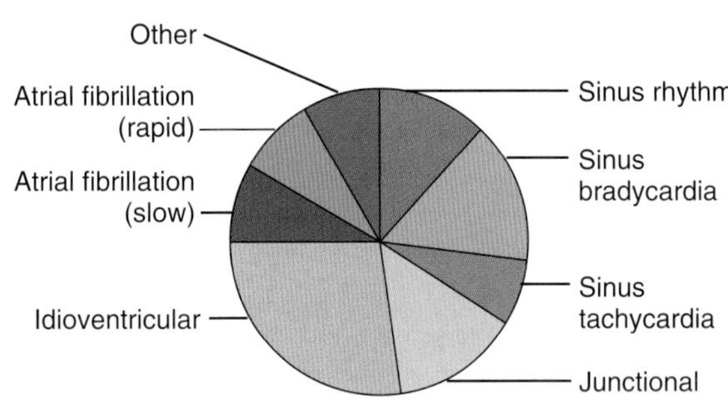


**Fig. 7.8 Electrical rhythm diagnoses in patients with pulseless electrical activity.**

### Pathophysiology

PEA must be separated into *pseudo* and *true* subtypes. Pseudo-PEA occurs when cardiac electrical activity (i.e., a cardiac rhythm) is present but a palpable pulse is absent and myocardial contractions are demonstrated by echocardiography or some other imaging modality. In true PEA, cardiac electrical activity in the form of a rhythm is noted, but absolutely no mechanical contraction of the heart is occurring.

It is important to distinguish the two subtypes of PEA. With pseudo-PEA, a significant pathophysiologic event has impaired the cardiovascular system's ability to perfuse. These cases usually involve profound hypovolemia as a result of hemorrhage, obstruction to forward flow secondary to massive pulmonary embolism, tension pneumothorax, or cardiac tamponade; hypocontractile states with poor vascular tone such as advanced anaphylactic or septic shock; or very rapid

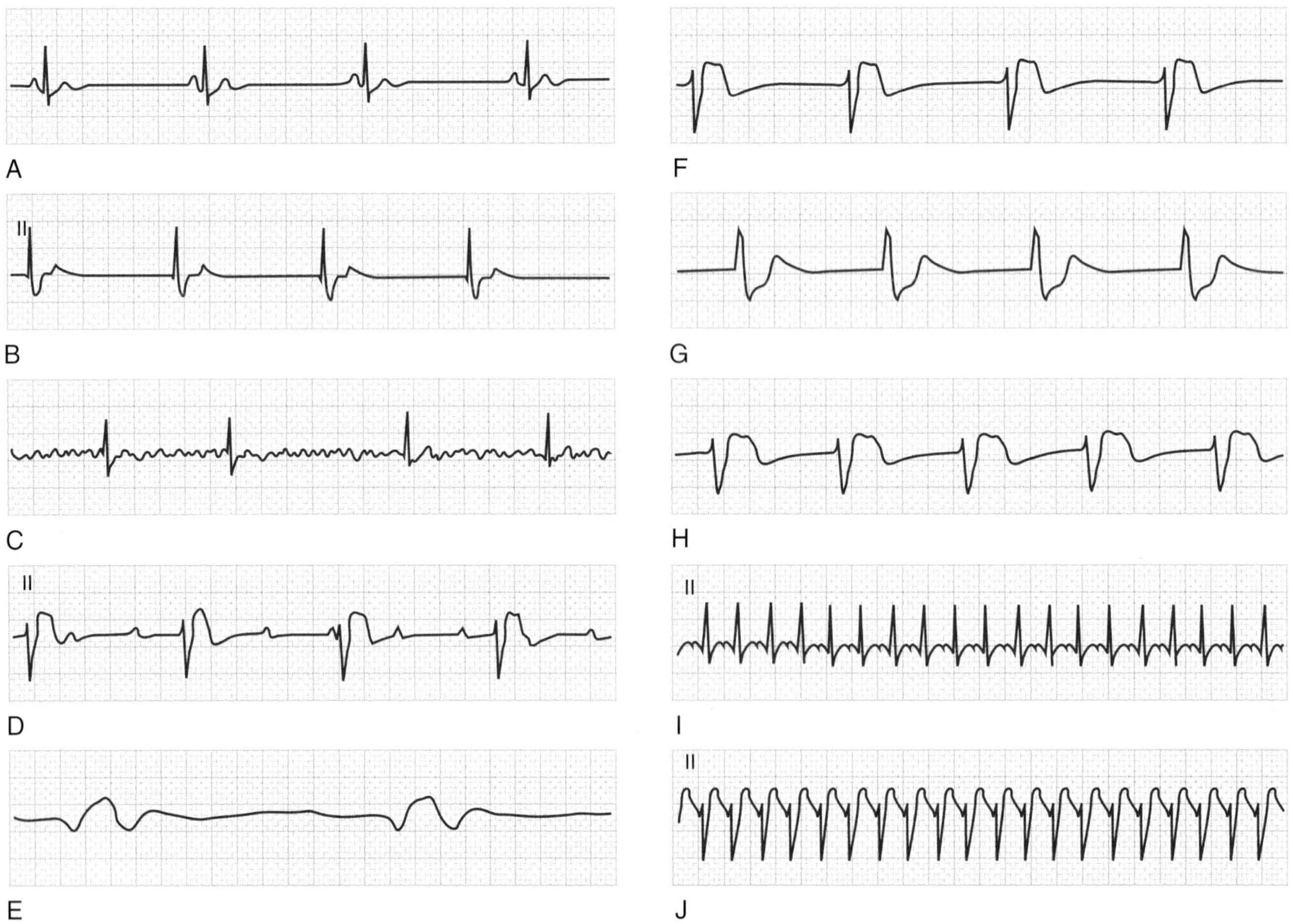

A B C D E F G H I J

**Fig. 7.9 Pulseless electrical activity (PEA).** This dysrhythmia requires the absence of detectable mechanical activity in the heart (i.e., absence of a pulse) with some form of organized electrical activity in the heart (i.e., a rhythm). Any dysrhythmia (other than ventricular fibrillation, ventricular tachycardia, or asystole) can be encountered in this cardiac arrest scenario. The most typical dysrhythmias seen in patients with PEA include both narrow– and wide–QRS complex bradycardias. **A,** Sinus bradycardia. **B,** Junctional bradycardia. **C,** Atrial fibrillation with slow ventricular response. **D,** Third-degree atrioventricular block. **E,** Idioventricular bradycardia. **F,** Idioventricular bradycardia. **G,** Idioventricular rhythm. **H,** Idioventricular rhythm. **I,** Sinus tachycardia. **J,** Sinus tachycardia with bundle branch block morphology.

tachydysrhythmia. Rhythms in these situations usually include tachycardias, predominantly sinus tachycardia or atrial fibrillation with rapid ventricular response. A directed therapeutic approach coupled with aggressive resuscitation will provide patients with pseudo-PEA with the best chance for survival.

True PEA occurs with primary electromechanical uncoupling of myocytes. From a cardiac electrical perspective, this uncoupling event is usually characterized by abnormal automaticity and disrupted cardiac conduction that results in the continued presence of a cardiac rhythm. Mechanically, this uncoupling is probably due to global myocardial energy depletion. Local myocardial tissue issues (hypoxia, acidosis, hyperkalemia, and ischemia) also contribute to this electromechanical dissociation. True electromechanical dissociation is seen in patients with prolonged cardiac arrest states, including metabolic, hypothermic, and poisoning sudden death scenarios. Another important subgroup of true PEA is characterized by patients with prolonged VF who are defibrillated to an electromechanical dissociation state with a broad QRS complex, bradycardic rhythm. In this instance, nearly complete exhaustion of energy substrate associated with profound hypoxia and acidosis accounts for this dismal scenario.

The PEA event usually starts with impaired perfusion and progresses to pseudo-PEA with continued cardiac contractions. Absence of a discernible pulse followed by loss of cardiac mechanical activity yields the development of true PEA.

### *Clinical Presentation*

Causes of PEA are numerous (see Table 7.1), spanning all of acute care medicine, and include profound hypovolemia, cardiac tamponade, large anterior wall myocardial infarction, tension pneumothorax, massive pulmonary embolism, severe sepsis, anaphylactic reaction with shock, significant electrolyte abnormality (e.g., disorders of potassium), pronounced metabolic acidosis, substantial cardiotoxin ingestion, and hypothermia. These conditions have a final common pathophysiologic denominator of severe hypovolemia (absolute or relative), marked obstruction to flow, profound hypocontractility, or any combination of the three. The PEA rhythm manifestations are numerous. The most frequent dysrhythmias seen in PEA include idioventricular, junctional, and sinus bradycardia (see Figs. 7.8 and 7.9). Some causes of PEA are reversible if recognized early and treated correctly in the initial phases of resuscitation. Hemorrhagic shock, pulmonary embolism, pericardial effusion, and tension pneumothorax can all lead to PEA and are potentially reversible.

The electrocardiographic rhythm may be a useful guide to the etiology and a key to successful resuscitation.[29] Rapid, narrow–QRS complex tachycardic manifestations are associated with a somewhat better opportunity for survival. Profound hypovolemia is the most frequently encountered event in patients with PEA. In an attempt to maintain cardiac output, the heart will increase its rate. This increased rate will usually be in the form of sinus tachycardia. In patients with atrial fibrillation, a rapid ventricular response will be present and create a manifestation that is probably a pseudo-PEA cardiac arrest.

Only 2% to 3% of patients with PEA as the initial or primary dysrhythmia in cardiac arrest survive to hospital discharge neurologically intact. Electrocardiographic variables may be predictive of successful resuscitation.[29,30] Rapid rhythm rates are much more frequently associated with ROSC than sinus bradycardia is. The width of the QRS complex is also potentially predictive of resuscitative outcome. Progressively wider QRS complexes are found in patients with a lower likelihood of restoration of spontaneous perfusion. In this risk prognostication application, an idioventricular rhythm is associated with a lower chance of resuscitation than is sinus bradycardia with a normal QRS complex duration. Other electrocardiographic findings encountered in PEA patients successfully resuscitated include the development of P waves and shortened QT intervals.

### *Management*

Management of a patient in PEA arrest should focus on standard resuscitation treatments and rapid identification and correction of reversible causes, but it is otherwise similar to the treatment of pulseless VT and VF (**Table 7.2**).

In the 2010 AHA guidelines, atropine was removed from the PEA and asystole algorithm. Atropine was removed not because of any harm induced but because of lack of efficacy.[5,9] The clinician at the bedside should use clinical judgment to determine whether atropine should be administered in this rhythm scenario. Epinephrine is recommended at a dose of 1 mg intravenously, repeated every 3 to 5 minutes during resuscitation. Vasopressin, 40 IU intravenously, can also be used once in the resuscitation event. Aggressive volume replacement with either crystalloid or colloid is recommended. Attention to the various causes and focused treatment of PEA is encouraged early in the resuscitation (see Table 7.1).

## ASYSTOLE

### *Definition*

Asystole is the absence of any and all cardiac electrical activity and usually results from failure of impulse formation in the primary (sinoatrial node) and default (atrioventricular node and ventricular myocardium) pacemaker sites. Asystole can also result from failure of propagation of impulses to the ventricular myocardium from atrial tissues.

### *Pathophysiology*

Patients with asystole have generally experienced prolonged cardiac arrest, probably initially manifested by either VT, VF, or PEA and ultimately degenerating to complete cessation of cardiac electrical activity. Asystole can be structurally mediated as a result of large myocardial infarction, neurally mediated as seen in aortic stenosis, or functionally mediated by cardiotoxin ingestion or metabolic poisoning. Regardless of the clinical event or mechanism responsible, patients with asystole demonstrate complete exhaustion of myocardial energy stores.

### *Clinical Presentation*

The AHA in the advanced cardiac life support (ACLS) teaching describes refractory asystole as "...the transition from life to death...." These patients have probably been in full cardiorespiratory arrest for prolonged periods. Patients with asystole as the initial or primary dysrhythmia most often do not survive. At best, 1% to 2% of patients with presumed asystole as the initial or primary dysrhythmia in cardiac arrest survive to hospital discharge and have a meaningful quality of life after arrest.

**Table 7.2** Etiologies, Pathophysiologic Events, and Specific Therapies for Cardiac Arrest with Pulseless Electrical Activity

| ETIOLOGY | PATHOPHYSIOLOGIC EVENT | POTENTIAL REVERSIBILITY | SPECIFIC THERAPY |
|---|---|---|---|
| Profound hypovolemia | Dehydration, hemorrhage | Yes | Volume resuscitation (crystalloid and colloid) |
| Cardiac tamponade | Obstruction to flow | Yes | Pericardiocentesis |
| Large acute myocardial infarction | Myocardial dysfunction | No | Volume resuscitation, inotropic and vasopressor support |
| Tension pneumothorax | Obstruction to flow | Yes | Chest decompression |
| Massive pulmonary embolism | Obstruction to flow | Yes | Fibrinolysis and embolectomy |
| Severe sepsis | Poor vascular tone, reduced contractility, increased capillary permeability | No | Volume resuscitation, inotropic and vasopressor support |
| Anaphylactic shock | Poor vascular tone, reduced contractility, increased capillary permeability | Yes | Volume resuscitation and inotropic and vasopressor support, particularly early administration of epinephrine |
| Significant electrolyte abnormality | Myocardial dysfunction | No | Target therapy |
| Pronounced metabolic acidosis | Myocardial dysfunction | No | Sodium bicarbonate, ventilation |
| Cardiotoxic ingestion | Myocardial dysfunction | No | Antidote |
| Hypothermia | Myocardial dysfunction | Yes | Rewarming therapy |
| Prolonged cardiac arrest | Myocardial malfunction | No | None |

Modified from Nolan JP, Neumar RW, Adrie C, et al. ILCOR consensus statement: post–cardiac arrest syndrome: epidemiology, pathophysiology, treatment, and prognostication. Resuscitation 2008;79:350-79; and Peberdy MA, Callaway CW, Neumar RW, et al. Part 9: post–cardiac arrest care: 2010 American Heart Association Guidelines for Cardiopulmonary Resuscitation and Emergency Cardiovascular Care. Circulation 2010;122:S768-86.

In asystole, the electrocardiogram demonstrates a flat line or nearly flat line (**Fig. 7.10**). Minimal undulations of the waveform resulting from electrocardiographic baseline drift can be seen. Several pitfalls must be avoided in the apparent asystolic manifestation, including monitor malfunction, disconnection of electrocardiographic leads, and fine VF with minimal amplitude in the imaging lead. The last potential error can be detected by confirming asystole with at least two leads oriented in perpendicular fashion (see Fig. 7.10).

### *Management*

Resuscitation should follow a similar algorithm as that for PEA (**Table 7.3**), with the notable exception of consideration of cardiac pacing. Even though several trials have not demonstrated a benefit of transcutaneous pacing in patients with asystolic arrest,[15,16] it is not unreasonable to consider a short course of cardiac pacing if performed very early in the resuscitation. A comment should be made on the choice of vasopressor. One large study demonstrated a short-term survival benefit of vasopressin with respect to epinephrine in these patients, and this benefit remained apparent at hospital discharge.[26]

## SPECIAL ARREST POPULATIONS AND SCENARIOS

### *Traumatic Injury*

Multiple traumatic causes can lead to cardiac arrest. The prognosis of patients with out-of-hospital cardiac arrest as a result of trauma is poor, particularly in the setting of blunt injury.[31]

In cases of traumatic arrest in which a clear etiology is not readily apparent, aggressive resuscitation is indicated, although the prognosis is bleak. General trauma management

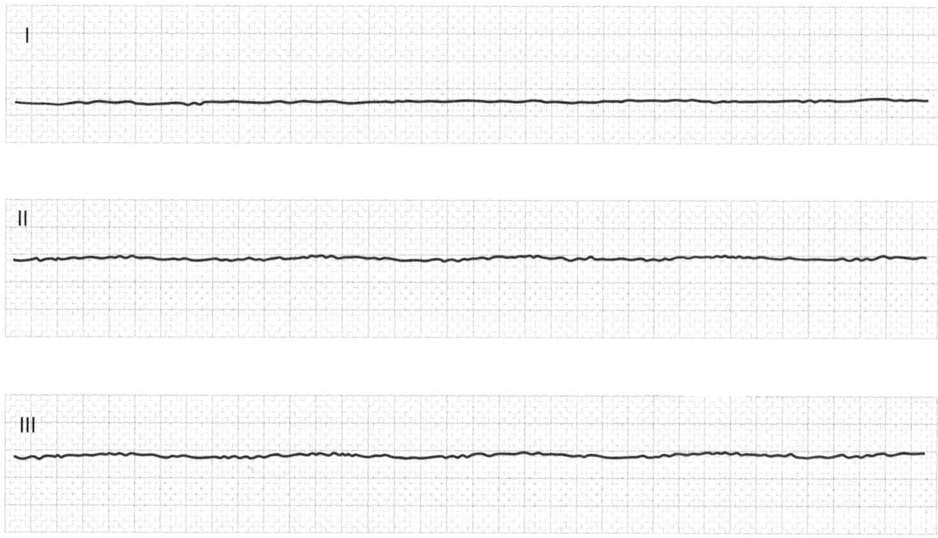


**Fig. 7.10 Asystole.** Note the proper determination of asystole in three simultaneous electrocardiographic leads. It is important to view any rhythm with at least two different electrocardiographic leads.

**Table 7.3 Pulseless Electrical Activity and Asystole**

| TIME | TREATMENT PRIORITY | COMMENTS |
|---|---|---|
| Minute 0 | Chest compressions | Compressions should be performed at a rate of 100/min.<br>Pulse checks and rhythm analysis should be performed no more frequently than every 2 min.<br>With a narrow-complex rhythm, assess for occult blood flow (i.e., pseudo-PEA). |
| Minute 1 | Chest compressions<br>IV or IO access<br>Vasopressor | Perform interventions but do not interrupt chest compressions for more than 15 sec after each 2-min cycle.<br>Early IV or IO access for drug administration is now preferred.<br>Vasopressin or epinephrine may be given interchangeably initially. |
| Minute 2 | Chest compressions<br>Placement of an invasive airway | Placement of an invasive airway is not a priority unless bag-mask ventilation is inadequate.<br>An invasive airway can be placed, but its placement should not interrupt chest compressions.<br>Atropine, 1 mg intravenously, can be given at this time if so desired, though its impact is minimal. |
| Minute 4 | Chest compressions<br>Vasopressor | Chest compressions should be interrupted only to change compressors (no longer than 15 sec).<br>If epinephrine was given initially, vasopressin can now be administered; epinephrine is then administered in all subsequent doses. |
| Minute 5 | Chest compressions<br>Supplemental medications | Underlying causes may necessitate the administration of adjunctive medications. |
| Minute 7 | Chest compressions<br>Vasopressor | Medication should be administered every 3-5 min for cardiac arrest; it should be realized that peak central levels may vary based on physiologic patient differences.<br>Atropine, 1 mg intravenously, can be given at this time if so desired. |
| Minute 10 | Chest compressions<br>Vasopressor | At 10 min the outcome-related implications should be weighed because survival to discharge decreases after this point without ROSC. |

*IO*, Intraosseous; *IV*, intravenous; *PEA*, pulseless electrical activity; *ROSC*, return of spontaneous circulation.

should be performed while specific therapy is aimed at the medical portion of the cardiorespiratory arrest. Standard ALS interventions aimed at management of the dysrhythmia should be pursued with the realization that the likelihood of successful resuscitation is minimal. Pulseless VT and VF should be defibrillated immediately on recognition. In most traumatic situations, the underlying etiology must be corrected for return of circulation to occur.[5,9] Medical therapies are unlikely to correct traumatized tissue and restore spontaneous circulation.

If definitive surgical intervention is available, resuscitative thoracotomy may be a reasonable intervention for a subset of trauma patients. This subset includes any traumatic arrest patient with the following features: witnessed arrest in the emergency department, arrest time less than 5 minutes with penetrating cardiac injury, arrest time less than 15 minutes with penetrating thoracic injury, or any exsanguinating abdominal vascular injury in which secondary signs of life are present (e.g., pupillary reflexes, spontaneous movement, organized electrocardiographic activity).[5,9,32] Thoracotomy allows internal cardiac massage and defibrillation, relief of pericardial tamponade, direct control of cardiac or thoracic hemorrhage, and cross-clamping of the aorta. Many of these interventions require a high degree of technical skill and should be attempted only by experienced providers; however, outcomes are predictably poor.

### Status Asthmaticus

More than 4000 deaths occur annually as a result of asthma. Two general scenarios in decompensated asthma patients most often account for the cardiac arrest. The first is the sudden onset of a severe exacerbation that rapidly worsens and progresses to full cardiorespiratory arrest. The second scenario involves patients with progressive bronchospasm that is unresponsive to maximal therapy. Progressive hypoxia and hypercapnia with metabolic and respiratory acidosis are responsible for the ultimate decline. At times in this setting, complications of therapy such as barotrauma account for the hemodynamic decline.

The mainstay of therapy in treating asthma-induced arrest is overcoming hypoxia and bronchoconstriction. In these cases, endotracheal intubation should be performed rapidly, and barotrauma (primarily pneumothorax) must be avoided. Decreasing tidal volumes to 5 to 6 mL/kg and reducing the ventilatory rate to 8 to 10 breaths/min can avoid excessive increases in lung volumes caused by breath stacking with prolonged expiratory phases. This technique is an extension of controlled hypoventilation, or permissive hypercapnia. If resuscitation is successful with return of spontaneous perfusion, sodium bicarbonate is administered intravenously to maintain the serum pH level greater than 7.15 to 7.20.

External compression of the thorax during the expiratory phase to maximize exhalation has been proposed,[33] but its use remains controversial and it will probably be difficult to coordinate during compressions. Needle or tube thoracostomy decompression should be performed if pneumothorax is detected or suspected. Bilateral decompression for refractory arrest is warranted given the potential for masking the lateralizing signs of pneumothorax.

Standard ALS strategies also apply to dysrhythmias. Epinephrine is likely to be the most useful of the standard drug therapies. Correction of profound acidosis via the empiric use of sodium bicarbonate may be necessary to achieve responsiveness to sympathomimetic agents. The addition of isoproterenol, aminophylline, terbutaline, and magnesium may be considered for improved bronchodilation, but their benefit in patients with asthma-induced cardiac arrest has not been reported, and they are unlikely to achieve success.

### Pregnancy

Causes of cardiac arrest specific to pregnant patients are maternal hemorrhage, toxemia, HELLP syndrome (hemolysis, elevated liver enzymes, and low platelet count), amniotic fluid emboli, and adverse effects of maternal care, including tocolytic and anesthetic therapies. Pregnancy also increases the likelihood of certain nonobstetric causes, including pulmonary embolism, septic shock, cardiovascular diseases such as cardiomyopathy and myocardial infarction, endocrine disorders, and collagen vascular disease. Traumatic causes of arrest should also be considered because of documented increased rates of abuse and homicide in pregnant women.

Cesarean delivery should be accomplished as soon as cardiac arrest is identified in a pregnant patient. The highest survival rates for infants older than 24 to 25 weeks' gestational age occurs in deliveries performed within 5 minutes of arrest of the mother. This intervention is most appropriately performed by a multidisciplinary team skilled in emergency obstetric surgery.[34]

Pregnant patients should be placed in the left lateral decubitus position. Displacement of the gravid uterus should be performed by elevating the right hip and lumbar region 15 to 30 degrees from the supine position. Manual displacement of the uterus by lifting it with two hands and directing it toward the upper left part of the patient's abdomen can be performed before blanket roll placement and afterward to optimize venous return.[34]

### Poisoning

Toxidromes may be masked in the setting of cardiac arrest because of prolonged hypoxia and hypoperfusion and thus complicate the selection of specific antidotes or therapies. Once poisoning is suspected, consultation with a medical toxicologist or poison control center should be sought if feasible.

In the setting of an unknown toxin or mixed ingestion, standard ALS algorithms are unlikely to be harmful and probably represent the most appropriate course of action. When specific antidotes are required, ACLS is insufficient. If a specific toxin is suspected based on the history or clinical signs, one should consider adding targeted therapies. It is also extremely important to remember that a single reported toxic ingestion is often accompanied by unreported accessory ingestions. Differential diagnoses and treatments must thus be kept broad when targeting treatment. When poisoning is suspected, prolonged resuscitation attempts might be warranted.

### Electrical Injury

The heart is particularly sensitive to electrical injury. Alternating current is likely to produce VT through a mechanism similar to the R-on-T phenomenon, whereas a lightning strike can produce asystole or VT through depolarization of the myocardium by a direct current shock.

ALS algorithms do not require modification for electrically induced cardiac arrest. The potential for successful resuscitation is higher than that for other causes of cardiac arrest given that these patients are typically younger and lack coexisting cardiopulmonary disease. Trauma and burn care is often required because they are common sequelae of electrical shock and lightning injury.

### Hypothermia

Severe hypothermia causes marked functional depression of all critical organ systems. Such dysfunction can lead to cardiovascular collapse but may also have a protective effect that allows successful resuscitation. Clinical judgment should prevail in the decision whether to attempt resuscitation. The often-quoted maxim—"one is not dead until he/she is warm and dead"—applies only in select situations and is not a blanket statement pertaining to all patients in cardiopulmonary arrest. The two basic types of patients who may actually benefit from rewarming therapy while in cardiorespiratory arrest include a full arrest patient who has very rapidly had a precipitous decline in body temperature (e.g., fall into a frigid lake in a very cold climate) and a profoundly hypothermic individual with signs of life in whom cardiorespiratory arrest has developed while in the emergency department. In other instances, resuscitation is futile and is therefore not recommended. If drowning occurs before hypothermia, the chances of resuscitation are markedly reduced. If the decision is made to attempt resuscitation in a patient with complete cardiopulmonary arrest and absence of signs of life, the patient should be orotracheally intubated and undergo CPR with chest compressions. Further efforts will then be guided by the core temperature, which should be measured as soon as possible. Needle-type electrodes, if available, are preferred for cardiac monitoring. For severe hypothermia with a core temperature lower than 30° C, aggressive active internal rewarming should be undertaken, including warmed, humidified oxygen and intravenous fluids, pleural or peritoneal lavage, and partial or complete cardiopulmonary bypass. A single attempt at defibrillation should be made for pulseless VT or VF. All ALS medications should be withheld. Both of these modifications are due to the likelihood that a hypothermic heart will remain unresponsive to subsequent shocks and medications are likely to accumulate and reach toxic levels.

For moderate hypothermia—body temperature of 30° C to 34° C—or once rewarming has raised the core temperature to 30° C, defibrillation should resume per ALS guidelines. Medications may be administered at standard doses, but the interval of administration should be increased. Active internal rewarming should be undertaken or continued. If the hypothermia is mild—temperature higher than 34° C—or when rewarming raises the core temperature to 34° C, standard ALS guidelines may be applied, including decisions regarding termination of resuscitation efforts. If rewarming efforts occur for longer than 45 minutes, volume expansion will probably be necessary because of vasodilation.

### *Submersion Injury and Near-Drowning*

Cardiac arrest after submersion is usually due to hypoxia as a result of suffocation, but it may also be secondary to head or spinal cord injury. For this reason, early intubation is suggested if feasible and should be performed with manual stabilization of the cervical spine. Aspiration of large volumes of fluid with submersion is rare, but increased inspiratory and positive end-expiratory pressure may be required to achieve adequate oxygenation because of pulmonary edema.

Routine ALS algorithms should be used for cardiac arrhythmias without modification. Electrolyte and acid-base disturbances are unlikely causes of cardiac arrest in the early manifestations of submersion injury and do not warrant empiric therapy. Correction of acidosis should be considered in patients who later deteriorate during observation. The prognosis depends on the duration of submersion and the severity and duration of hypoxia. Hypothermia and trauma are common confounders of submersion injury, and appropriate therapy should be applied.

## POSTRESUSCITATION PHASE

### POST–CARDIAC ARREST SYNDROME

Management of resuscitated cardiac arrest patients has undergone significant change in the past decade. The concept of post–cardiac arrest syndrome has been developed.[35,36] This syndrome, thought to occur in the initial 72 hours after ROSC, is a unique pathophysiologic entity found in patients who have been resuscitated from cardiorespiratory arrest. The primary considerations include CNS injury, myocardial dysfunction, systemic hypoperfusion with reperfusion-related damage, and the precipitating event. Brain injury from ischemia is responsible for many patient deaths, including approximately 70% of patients resuscitated after out-of-hospital arrest and 25% of individuals resuscitated after in-hospital arrest. The basic reasons for CNS injury include a limited tolerance for brain ischemia coupled with a unique response to reperfusion. Brain injury is an ongoing phenomenon, even after successful resuscitation, that usually results from a number of different pathophysiologic events. Injury can continue for 6 to 72 hours after the return of spontaneous perfusion despite adequate systemic blood pressure.

Mechanisms responsible for the CNS injury include the development of cerebral edema, dysfunctional circulation, disruption of the blood-brain barrier, and multiple small infarctions. Cerebral edema alters perfusion, hastens the production of inflammatory mediators, and produces cellular dysfunction. Dysfunctional circulation can occur at the microcirculatory level despite an intact macrocirculation. The cerebral edema and altered microcirculation disrupt the blood-brain barrier, whereas the altered perfusion produces ischemia and multiple small CNS infarctions. Three additional issues contribute to CNS injury: pyrexia, hyperglycemia, and seizure. The final common pathway of CNS injury is neuronal cell death with brain malfunction, poor neurologic recovery, and patient demise.

Myocardial dysfunction has a significant negative impact on survival, and it is both reversible and responsive to therapy. The myocardial dysfunction is not always due to infarction. Most often, myocardial stunning is responsible for the cardiac dysfunction and produces significant and profound reductions in cardiac output. Continued myocardial dysfunction results in respiratory compromise, impaired systemic perfusion, and worsening of multiorgan malfunction. Myocardial dysfunction is usually rapidly apparent after return of perfusion, thus requiring very close hemodynamic monitoring. As the exogenous catecholamines are metabolized once perfusion is restored, hypoperfusion becomes obvious. Hypoperfusion can be worsened by the use of sedative-hypnotic agents for the control of agitation and maintenance of unresponsiveness in a chemically paralyzed patient.

Increasing tachycardia and left ventricular end-diastolic pressure are seen within minutes of ROSC, whereas decreasing mean arterial pressure is not usually apparent for many hours after resuscitation. Hypotension is generally obvious at 4 to 6 hours, reaches a nadir at 8 hours, and classically recovers by 24 to 72 hours. This myocardial dysfunction creates additional tissue hypoxia and acidosis, intensifies the multiorgan injury, and contributes to a significantly increased risk for death.

Reperfusion-related injury results from the whole-body ischemia typical of cardiac arrest and produces a significant oxygen debt, depletion of energy substrates, and accumulation of waste products. The immunologic and coagulation systems are activated with the release of cytokines and endotoxins and complicated by fibrin deposition with microthrombosis. This component of injury is similar to sepsis syndrome and is manifested clinically by intravascular volume depletion, impaired vascular autoregulation, coagulopathies, ineffective oxygen delivery to tissues with inefficient tissue oxygen extraction, and increased susceptibility to infection.

Finally, the precipitating event must be considered for effective management of a postresuscitation patient. It is a major determinant of survival with a very broad range of potential events, involves both cardiac and noncardiac causes, and occurs over acute, acute-on-chronic, and chronic periods.

## POSTRESUSCITATION MANAGEMENT

Management considerations (**Figs. 7.11 and 7.12**) must address the following issues: CNS injury, myocardial dysfunction, systemic hypoperfusion, multiorgan failure, and the precipitating cause of the cardiac arrest. Multidisciplinary critical care support along with appropriate respiratory and hemodynamic support is vital. Two specific treatment considerations, therapeutic (induced) hypothermia and emergency coronary reperfusion, must be emphasized in these resuscitated patients.

Therapeutic hypothermia (TH), or induction of lower body temperatures in unresponsive patients resuscitated from cardiac arrest, is strongly encouraged in certain individuals. The AHA notes that "…therapeutic hypothermia in the resuscitated cardiac arrest patient can markedly improve outcome… both in terms of rates of survival and neurologic status."[35,36] TH is currently recommended for victims resuscitated after out-of-hospital cardiac arrest with initial rhythms of either pulseless VT or VF who remain unconscious. TH should also be considered in patients resuscitated from cardiac arrest associated with other initial rhythms (i.e., PEA and asystole) and in survivors of in-hospital cardiac arrest.[35,36] The actual beneficial mechanisms for TH are not fully known, but the basic accepted mechanism involves suppression of the chemical cascade associated with the total-body ischemia and reperfusion injury. These mechanisms probably involve a number of different protective processes, including a reduction in the metabolic rate, oxygen use, and CNS electrical activity. TH probably interrupts the injury process at many points in the pathophysiologic response to cardiac arrest and subsequent reperfusion. Regardless of the modes of action of this intervention, TH has been demonstrated to provide CNS protection, reduce the incidence of multiorgan failure syndrome, increase survival, and improve functional abilities. The outcome after cardiac arrest with our present abilities remains suboptimal. Use of TH can increase the rate of functional survival, but it is not a miracle cure.

Indications for TH include the following qualifiers: nontraumatic cardiac arrest, resuscitation with spontaneous perfusion, unresponsive status, and age between 18 and 75 years. Any set of indications for a clinical therapy is open to discussion and further consideration. Several qualifications are needed. First, primary cardiac arrest is the most appropriate indication for TH. Noncardiac causes of arrest such as sepsis, a CNS event, ingestion, trauma, and others are unlikely to benefit. Primary cardiac arrest, or an event related to cardiac arrhythmia that is due to a cardiac cause, is the most appropriate for TH. Certain other victims of noncardiac causes of arrest can be considered for TH. These potential additional indications include victims of a sudden event that when corrected does not leave a significant, lasting injury or process other than post–cardiac arrest syndrome. Consideration should be made for patients with sudden choking or hanging that leads to respiratory failure and subsequent cardiac arrest.

Second, resuscitated patients should be relatively stable in terms of the ABCs, which means that they are endotracheally intubated and undergoing mechanical ventilatory support with

PHASES OF POST–CARDIC ARREST SYNDROME

| Phase | | Goals | | | |
|---|---|---|---|---|---|
| | Immediate | Limit ongoing injury and provide organ support | | | Prevent recurrence |
| 20 minutes | Early | | | | |
| 6-12 hours | Intermediate | | Determine prognosis | | |
| 72 hours | Recovery | | | | |
| Disposition | Rehabilitation | Rehab | | | |

**Fig. 7.11** Phases of post–cardiac arrest syndrome with the primary management goals.

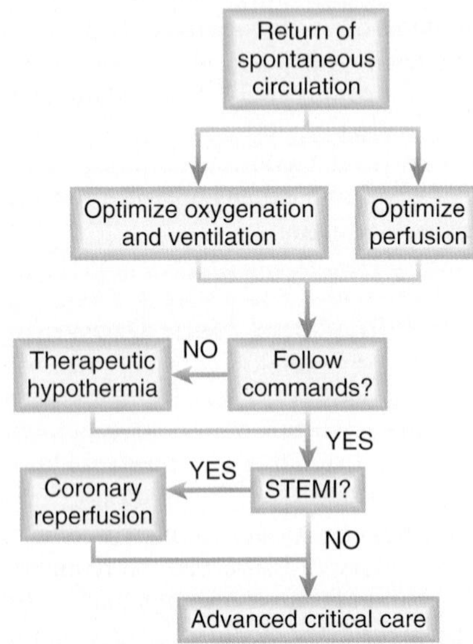


**Fig. 7.12 Resuscitative management of patients with post–cardiac arrest syndrome.** (Modified from Nolan JP, Neumar RW, Adrie C, et al. ILCOR consensus statement: post-cardiac arrest syndrome: epidemiology, pathophysiology, treatment, and prognostication. Resuscitation 2008;79:350-79; and Peberdy MA, Callaway CW, Neumar RW, et al. Part 9: post–cardiac arrest care: 2010 American Heart Association Guidelines for Cardiopulmonary Resuscitation and Emergency Cardiovascular Care Science. Circulation 2010;122:S768-86.)

intact perfusion. Significant difficulties with oxygen and ventilation must be addressed before the use of TH. Perfusion must be intact, whether spontaneously or supported by intravenous fluids, vasopressors, or inotropes, and it should be understood that significant difficulties in maintaining perfusion should delay the use of TH. Third, the patient must be unresponsive. Multiple different descriptors have been used to describe the patient's mental status, including unresponsive, comatose, or possessing a Glasgow Coma Scale score of 8 or less.

The last basic indication is age. The most appropriate patient is an adult. The most frequently listed age range is 18 to 75 years, thus removing all children and the extreme elderly from consideration. This age indication is at best a guide, and certain younger and older patients represent appropriate candidates for TH. A major consideration in these two excluded groups is that a primary cardiac etiology is less often the primary causative event in the development of cardiac arrest. Sepsis, trauma, ingestion, and other conditions are frequent causes of cardiac arrest in these two age groups and may exclude these candidates from consideration of TH. Clinician judgment with consideration of individual patient issues will be the most appropriate determinant of therapy with respect to the age extremes.

A thorough discussion of the process and technique of cooling is beyond the scope of this chapter. Highlights of TH include the following issues:

- Patients should be cooled as soon as possible after ROSC, ideally within 4 to 6 hours. Cooling should last for approximately 18 hours once the target temperature has been reached.
- The goal temperature is 32° C to 34° C.
- The patient is probably mechanically ventilated via an ETT.
- Pain medication and sedative agents are probably required for patient comfort and safety. Chemical paralytic agents are used with caution because seizures cannot be detected as easily.
- Shivering should be avoided if at all possible because of the related heat production, and appropriate treatment should be provided if it develops.
- Biometric surveillance should include an electrocardiogram, blood pressure, core temperature, oxygen saturation, and end-tidal $CO_2$ monitoring. Continuous electrocardiographic monitoring can also be considered. Laboratory studies should include electrolytes and serum glucose.
- The most appropriate cooling method is debatable. Two basic approaches have been advocated, but thus far neither therapy has proved to be superior. Rapid infusion of 2 L of chilled normal saline (4° C) represents the least challenging approach. The chilled saline is used in conjunction with cooling blankets and ice packs applied to the neck, armpits, groin, and other areas. The other technique, which is both more invasive and more expensive, involves the use of an intravascular cooling machine. This technique, once the intravascular catheter has been placed, is easier to use in terms of reaching the target temperature and maintaining this temperature.
- If instability develops, all cooling must be halted immediately and appropriate therapy initiated to address the current clinical situation.

It has been suggested that emergency coronary reperfusion, provided as soon as possible after ROSC from cardiac arrest, can not only improve survival but also increase the opportunity for more meaningful survival. Emergency coronary reperfusion can be achieved by fibrinolysis or percutaneous coronary intervention (PCI), with PCI being the preferred technique.

The primary indications for such an intervention included ST-segment elevation myocardial infarction (STEMI) and new-onset left bundle branch block. Patients who demonstrate one of these findings on electrocardiography, either before or after arrest, are candidates for emergency coronary reperfusion. The majority of cases of primary cardiac arrest are associated with acute coronary syndromes, and it would seem reasonable to assume that emergency coronary reperfusion in patients with ROSC would be associated with improved outcomes. The AHA issued a policy statement in 2010[37] supporting the use of immediate catheterization in survivors of cardiac arrest who demonstrate electrocardiographic evidence of STEMI: "Patients resuscitated from [out-of-hospital cardiac arrest] with STEMI should undergo immediate angiography and receive PCI as needed."

These two classic findings represent the primary indications for emergency coronary reperfusion. More recent investigation of this therapy has suggested that all patients suspected of having primary cardiac arrest can be considered for emergency coronary reperfusion. It is well known that the electrocardiogram is far from perfect in demonstrating evidence of AMI. Use of electrocardiography to determine which patients will benefit from emergency coronary reperfusion might potentially lead to some individuals missing out on such a benefit. The absence of ST-segment elevation after ROSC does not reliably rule out the presence of acute coronary artery occlusion.[37,38] There has been increasing support in the literature[39,40] for early coronary angiography in even these patients without ST-segment elevation.

The combination of TH and emergency coronary reperfusion offers very promising results. This combination of postresuscitative therapy has demonstrated survival rates approaching 50% with intact or nearly intact functional status, and both PCI and TH can be safely performed simultaneously.[41]

Finally, a multidisciplinary critical care team is strongly encouraged. Interventions such as TH, hemodynamic optimization, ventilation strategies, seizure management, serum glucose maintenance, and PCI are all recognized to be important considerations in these patients.

Medical centers that are well equipped, aggressive, and experienced in the use of post-arrest interventions are more likely to demonstrate the best outcomes. It has been suggested that outcomes in victims of cardiac arrest are better at facilities that care for at least 50 such cases per year.[37,42] Should postresuscitation care be regionalized? The Ontario Prehospital Advanced Life Support database demonstrates that transport time is not associated with outcome after cardiac arrest, thus suggesting that regionalization of this care might be appropriate.[43]

## REFERENCES

*References can be found on Expert Consult @ www.expertconsult.com.*

# 8 Trauma Resuscitation

*Trevor J. Mills*

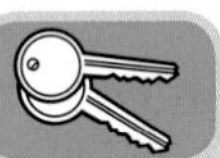

**KEY POINTS**

- The approach to trauma resuscitation is based on the assumption that all severely injured patients can initially be evaluated and treated with the same set of guidelines.
- Regardless of the specific injury, these guidelines focus on the broader concept of sustaining life by maximizing oxygenation, ventilation, and perfusion—the ABCs of trauma resuscitation.

## EPIDEMIOLOGY

Traumatic injury is a significant cause of death and disability worldwide, especially in the younger population. In the United States, unintentional injury is the leading cause of death in the age range between 1 and 44 years.[1] Approximately half of trauma-related deaths occur at the time of injury or before the patient reaches the hospital. Another 30% of traumatic deaths may occur in the first few hours after the event. It is this severely injured, but salvageable population that should be immediately evaluated and treated with the trauma resuscitation paradigm.

## PERSPECTIVE

In a traumatized patient, loss of the airway or respiratory failure (or both) may be due to direct injury to the head, face, oropharynx, neck, trachea, bronchi, chest, or lungs. Alternatively, secondary airway or respiratory compromise (or both) may be caused by injury that results in loss of muscle control or respiratory drive; aspiration of blood, tissue, teeth, or gastric contents; or air or fat emboli.

Shock in trauma patients is often due to hemorrhagic blood loss, but it may also be caused by damage to the heart, great vessels, or lungs or by hemodynamic compromise from fat emboli, ischemia, or neurogenic shock (**Box 8.1**).

## PRESENTING SIGNS AND SYMPTOMS

The American College of Surgeons and many emergency medical service systems have adopted algorithms based on clinical signs and symptoms for transport to a trauma center.[2] These signs and symptoms identify patients at high risk for injury and are based on early physiologic changes, anatomic criteria, or a mechanism with a high likelihood of significant injury (**Box 8.2**). Along with the trauma center criteria, in each of the major anatomic areas there are important clues to potentially life- and limb-threatening injures (**Table 8.1**).

Head injuries may result in a decreased level of consciousness leading to loss of airway protection or respiratory drive. Head injuries can also precipitate hemorrhagic shock as a result of the abundant vascular supply of the face and scalp. Because of their proportionally larger heads, children can lose a significant amount of blood with closed intracranial hemorrhage. For further specific evaluation and treatment of head injuries, see Chapter 73.

Injury to the face, including an unstable midface, or trauma to the oropharynx may cause direct airway compromise. Facial injuries can also lead to aspiration of blood, tissue, teeth, and bone. Early or prophylactic intubation should be considered if impending airway compromise is suspected or imminent.

High spinal injuries may lead to loss of airway control, loss of the respiratory drive, or hemodynamic instability as a result of spinal shock. Paralysis may also make evaluation of other injuries extremely difficult.

Thoracic injuries can result in direct tracheal, pulmonary, or cardiac damage and lead to significant intrathoracic hemorrhage or direct respiratory compromise.

Because the abdominal cavity can hold a large amount of blood, solid organ or vascular injury in the abdomen can easily result in hemodynamic collapse. Pelvic fractures are also a potential site of significant blood loss from uncontrolled venous bleeding.

Even isolated extremity injuries can result in arterial hemorrhage or considerable blood loss in the form of fracture-related hematomas. Fractures may cause delayed respiratory distress because of fat emboli.

A history of a significant injury mechanism, even without apparent injury, requires a thorough trauma evaluation. Examples include penetrating trauma to the head, neck, chest, abdomen, and proximal part of the extremities; significant

**BOX 8.1 Causes of Airway or Respiratory Compromise and Shock in Trauma Patients**

**Causes of Traumatic Airway or Respiratory Compromise**

Direct trauma to the face, oropharynx, neck, trachea, or pulmonary system resulting in obstruction of the airway or respiratory compromise

Indirect injury as a result of brain or spine injury (loss of drive), fat or air pulmonary emboli, or aspiration of blood or gastric contents

**Causes of Shock in Traumatized Patients**

Hemorrhagic shock

Injury to the heart (cardiac contusion, valve rupture, penetrating trauma)

Compression of the heart as a result of tamponade or tension pneumothorax

Cardiogenic shock (ischemia, arrhythmias)

Neurogenic or spinal shock

**BOX 8.2 Criteria for the Identification of Traumatized Patients with a High Probability of Injury Requiring Transport to a Trauma Center**

**Physiologic Criteria**

Glasgow Coma Scale score <14

Respiratory rate <10 or >29 breaths/min

Systolic blood pressure <90 mm Hg or the pediatric equivalent

**Anatomic Criteria (Injuries Need Only Be Suspected)**

Flail chest

Two or more long-bone fractures

Amputations proximal to the wrist or ankle

Penetrating trauma involving the head, neck, chest, abdomen, or extremity proximal to the elbow or knee

Limb paralysis

Pelvic fractures

Combination of significant trauma with burns

**Mechanism of Injury**

Ejection from a vehicle

Death of another person in the same vehicle

Pedestrian hit by a vehicle

High-speed motor vehicle collision

Falls of more than 20 feet

Rollover motor vehicle collision

Duration of extrication of the patient from entrapment of longer than 20 minutes

Motorcycle crash at a speed higher than 20 mph or with separation of the patient from the motorcycle

falls; rollover or high-speed motor vehicle collisions; and cyclists or pedestrians struck by a motor vehicle.

Some patient populations are more likely to have life-threatening injuries without obvious signs and symptoms. This group includes the elderly, the very young, patients with coagulopathies, and those with reduced physiologic reserve because of chronic disease or acute intoxication.

**Table 8.1** Signs of Significant Injuries in Trauma Patients

| ANATOMIC AREA | MOST THREATENING SIGNS |
|---|---|
| Head | Cerebrospinal fluid leak<br>Raccoon eyes<br>Battle sign<br>Hemotympanum<br>Anisocoria |
| Neck | Expanding hematoma<br>Thrill or murmur<br>Subcutaneous air<br>Trachea deviated from midline<br>Pulsatile hemorrhage |
| Spine | Paralysis<br>Paresthesias<br>Decreased rectal tone |
| Chest | Subcutaneous air<br>Multiple rib fractures<br>Sucking chest wound<br>Asymmetric chest rise |
| Abdomen | Abdominal wall bruising<br>Distended abdomen |
| Pelvis | Unstable pelvis<br>Large expanding hematoma<br>Blood at urethral meatus<br>Scrotal hematoma<br>Bone fragments in vaginal vault or rectum<br>High-riding prostate |
| Extremities | Pallor<br>Decrease in or absence of pulses<br>Weakness or paralysis |

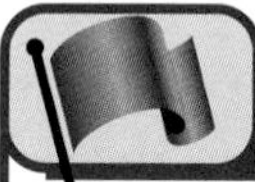

**RED FLAGS**

Early alterations in vital signs

Altered mental status

Patient at either extreme of age

Prolonged time on the scene or transport time (extrication of the patient or entrapment)

Weakness or paralysis

## DIFFERENTIAL DIAGNOSIS AND MEDICAL DECISION MAKING

Because trauma resuscitation is a "one size fits all comers" approach to the undifferentiated patient, there is no classic differential diagnosis. It is important to remember that a patient who arrives in traumatic shock may have a concurrent acute medical condition, such as acute myocardial infarction, hypoglycemia, or intoxication, that may confound the trauma evaluation.

### PRIMARY SURVEY

Medical decision making for a trauma patient involves use of the ABCDEF trauma resuscitation algorithm, with consideration for the patient's age, physiologic reserve, and underlying chronic conditions. (See the Red Flags box.)

Although performance of the primary survey should be fluid and may involve multiple individuals performing multiple actions simultaneously, the components of the primary survey can be broken down into six sequential steps: airway, breathing, circulation, disability, exposure, and fingers or Foley (ABCDEF) (see **Fig. 8-1** and Priority Actions box).

If an indication for intervention is discovered during the primary survey, treatment should be initiated and the primary survey restarted from the beginning (**Fig. 8.2**).

The primary survey starts as the patient enters the room by questioning the patient, evaluating for airway patency, and then directly visualizing the facial structures, neck, and oropharynx (A).

Breathing or ventilatory status can then be evaluated through visual examination of the neck and thorax, auscultation of all lung fields, and palpation of the chest. Palpation can provide clues to rib injury, open or sucking chest wounds, and subcutaneous air in the neck and chest. The respiratory rate, patient report of chest pain or shortness of breath, and pulse oximetry also contribute to this phase of the resuscitation (B).

Evaluation of circulatory status (C) involves a judgment of the patient's general appearance, heart rate and blood pressure, extremity pulses, and nail bed capillary refill. If the patient has not been connected to a continuous heart rate and blood pressure monitor, this step should be taken at this time.

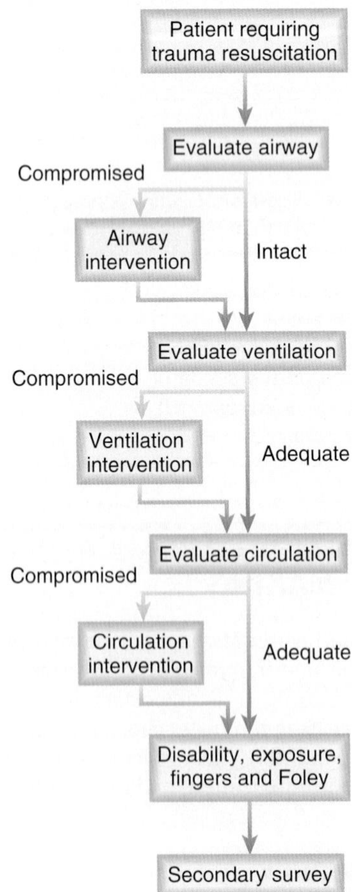


**Fig. 8.1 Approach to resuscitation after trauma.**

The next step is a brief neurologic examination (for disability—D). At this point, assessment for disability does not include a detailed neurologic examination but instead a look at the gross motor movement of all extremities and the patient's level of alertness. The most common tool for evaluating global neurologic function is the Glasgow Coma Scale (GCS) (**Table 8.2**).[3] Three systems are evaluated: eye opening, verbal response, and motor response. The closer that each function is to baseline, the higher the score for each system. A GCS score of 13 or higher correlates with mild brain injury, 9 to 12 with moderate injury, and 8 or less with severe brain

**Table 8.2 Glasgow Coma Scale Scoring***

| RESPONSE | SCORE |
|---|---|
| **Eye Opening** | |
| No eye opening | 1 |
| Eye opening to pain | 2 |
| Eye opening to verbal command | 3 |
| Eyes open spontaneously | 4 |
| **Verbal** | |
| No verbal response | 1 |
| Incomprehensible sounds | 2 |
| Inappropriate words | 3 |
| Patient confused | 4 |
| Patient oriented | 5 |
| **Motor** | |
| No motor response | 1 |
| Extension to pain | 2 |
| Flexion to pain | 3 |
| Withdrawal from pain | 4 |
| Patient localizes pain | 5 |
| Patient obeys commands | 6 |

*The best of each response is used for the individual score; scores are added for the total Glasgow Coma Scale score.

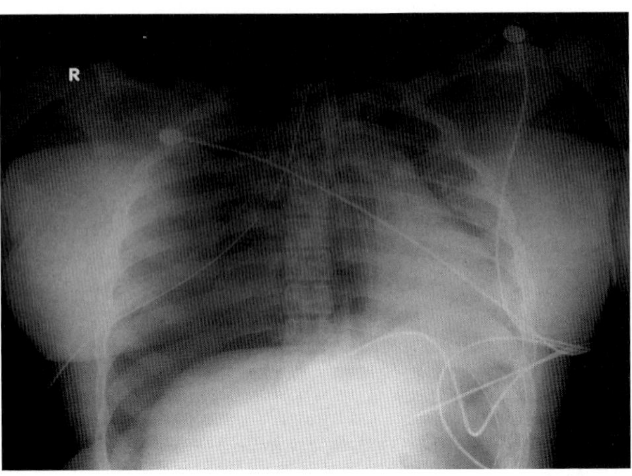


**Fig. 8.2** The patient whose radiograph is shown here initially improved with placement of a chest tube but later experienced decompensation. This case represents a good reason for the need to restart the ABCs (airway, breathing, circulation) of trauma resuscitation after any change in patient condition or after any intervention.

injury. A GCS score lower than 8 is an indication for immediate airway control. Thus, the GCS can help in evaluating the need for intubation, provide a marker for serial neurologic examinations, and promote clear communication with consultants regarding patient status.

Completion of the primary survey involves exposure of the entire patient (E) in a way that prevents hypothermia; coordinated in-line cervical spine immobilization should be maintained during this procedure.

The F (fingers and Foley) step of the primary survey involves consideration of placement of a Foley bladder catheter and orogastric tube, a rectal examination, and a bimanual vaginal examination. Even though there has been a trend away from the dogmatic approach to use of a rectal and Foley catheter for everyone who enters the trauma algorithms, these measures are still indicated in certain patients, especially those who are obtunded, have a high likelihood of bowel injury, or are hemodynamically unstable.

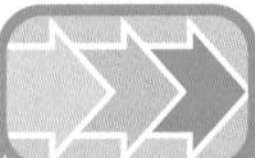

**PRIORITY ACTIONS**

**Primary Survey**

A = Airway control
B = Breathing: Maximize ventilation
C = Circulation: Stabilize hemodynamic status
D = Disability: Evaluate mental status and perform a neurologic examination
E = Exposure: Completely undress and examine the patient
F = Fingers and Foley: Perform orogastric, bladder catheter, vaginal, and rectal examinations

**Secondary Survey**

Head-to-toe physical examination
Focused abdominal sonography examination for trauma (FAST)
AMPLE (allergies, medications, past medical history, last meal, events of the injury)
Laboratory tests and radiology

## SECONDARY SURVEY

The secondary survey consists of an expanded history, a head-to-toe examination, focused sonography, and initiation of the standard trauma radiology and laboratory tests. If possible, the history should be taken from the patient or the prehospital personnel (e.g., emergency medical technicians) who delivered the patient to the hospital. The key points of the history can be remembered with use of the mnemonic AMPLE, which stands for allergies, medications, past medical history, last meal, and events of the injury.

The head-to-toe examination involves a second review of the airway and pulmonary examination, including an expanded physical examination to identify further injury.

In a hypotensive patient, because the abdominal cavity can conceal enough blood to be an immediate threat to life, part of the secondary survey is the focused abdominal sonography examination for trauma (FAST). FAST can be done in the resuscitation area. Because it is faster and less invasive to obtain, FAST has replaced diagnostic peritoneal lavage (**Table 8.3**).[4,5] Likewise, the more sensitive and specific computed tomography (CT) of the abdomen should wait until the end of the secondary survey because CT scanning may be time-consuming and takes the patient out of the resuscitation area.[6]

The advantage of a standardized approach to trauma radiology is that it can identify life-threatening injuries that may necessitate immediate attention. Significant cervical spine fractures may lead to airway compromise, loss of ventilatory drive, or spinal shock. The chest radiograph may identify a treatable condition, such as a large pneumothorax, hemothorax, or pulmonary contusion. Pelvic radiology can identify an open-book pelvic fracture, which may lead to hemorrhagic shock.

For many years, standard trauma series radiographs included plain films of the cervical spine, the chest, and the pelvis. Currently, the only standard plain film is the chest radiograph. The cervical spine radiograph has been replaced by CT of the cervical spine, but a rare exception is the use of screening films for penetrating trauma (**Fig. 8.3**). In the majority of trauma patients, the pelvic radiograph has been replaced by CT of the abdomen and pelvis with reconstructed images of the bony pelvis. In some patients, such as those who may need immediate pelvic binding to temporize hemorrhage or penetrating injury to the pelvis, a one-view pelvic radiograph in the trauma suite is still useful. Thus, the new standard trauma radiology series involves a chest radiograph and CT scans of the head, cervical spine, and abdomen and pelvis.[7] Chest CT is indicated for a widened mediastinum or if vascular injury is suspected. Early consideration of the need for CT angiography of the neck or extremities should be undertaken to minimize the load of contrast media.

**Table 8.3 Diagnostic Modalities Used for Abdominal Trauma**

| MODALITY | ADVANTAGES | DISADVANTAGES |
|---|---|---|
| Radiographs | Inexpensive<br>Easy to obtain and read<br>Good for identification of foreign objects and projectiles<br>May be useful as screening for free air before DPL | Very low sensitivity and specificity for injury in patients with blunt abdominal trauma |
| Computed tomography (CT) | High sensitivity<br>High specificity | Patient has to leave resuscitation area |
| Ultrasonography (US) | Easy and quick | Operator dependent<br>Variable sensitivity and specificity for organ injury |
| Diagnostic peritoneal lavage (DPL) | High sensitivity<br>High specificity | Operator dependent<br>Time-consuming<br>More invasive than CT or US<br>Significant complications (perforated bowel, bleeding, infection) |

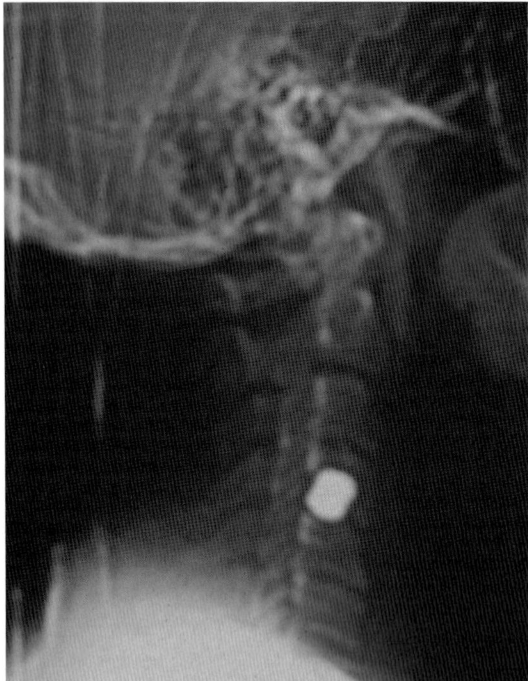

**Fig. 8.3** This case demonstrates the need for trauma series radiographs, even in patients with penetrating trauma. The radiograph shows that this patient sustained a gunshot wound to the shoulder without obvious injury to the neck.

Blood specimens for laboratory studies may be drawn during the initiation of intravenous (IV) access in the primary survey or can be obtained during the secondary survey. Laboratory tests should include a complete blood count, serum chemical analysis, coagulation studies (prothrombin time, partial thromboplastin time), and urinalysis. Two immediately available studies are the urine pregnancy test and fingerstick serum glucose measurement, and the results of either test can significantly change the course of the resuscitation. In the setting of altered mental status, a blood alcohol measurement and toxicology screen may also be useful. The serum lactate level can be monitored as a marker of tissue perfusion.[8,9]

After the primary and secondary surveys are completed and the patient is sufficiently resuscitated, the evaluation and treatment plan takes on a much more individualized course.[10]

## SPECIAL CIRCUMSTANCES

Depending on the specific patient's findings,[11] injuries, underlying diseases, and age, each injury may necessitate further radiologic studies (**Table 8.4**), observation, or surgical intervention.

## TREATMENT: PREHOSPITAL

As opposed to the "stay and play" approach to patients with cardiac arrest or pediatric respiratory arrest, where immediate emergency medical service intervention can improve patients' outcome, trauma patients should be transported with minimal delay (i.e., "scoop and run").

**Table 8.4 Additional Studies in Trauma Patients Dictated by Special Circumstances**

| TRAUMA PRESENTATION | ADDITIONAL STUDIES |
|---|---|
| Altered mental status, head trauma | Head computed tomography (CT)<br>Brain magnetic resonance imaging (MRI)<br>CT angiography of cerebral vascular system<br>See also Chapter 73 for detailed evaluation of head trauma |
| Chest wall trauma | Repeated chest radiography<br>Full upright posteroanterior and lateral chest radiographs<br>CT of the chest<br>Angiography<br>MRI of the chest<br>See also Chapter 78 for detailed evaluation of chest and thoracic trauma |
| Abdominal trauma | CT of the abdomen<br>Focused abdominal sonographic examination for trauma (FAST)<br>Diagnostic peritoneal lavage<br>See also Chapters 79 and 80 for detailed evaluation of abdominal trauma |
| Pelvis | Retrograde urethrography<br>Cystography<br>CT of the abdomen and pelvis |
| Extremity | Angiography |
| Neck, back, spine | CT or MRI of the cervical, thoracic, or lumbar spine |
| Obstetric | Ultrasonography<br>Fetal heart monitoring |

## TREATMENT: HOSPITAL

The key to maximizing the success of trauma resuscitation is early diagnosis and treatment of injuries. The extent of damage from many significant injuries can be reduced with early intervention, including cervical spine immobilization throughout the resuscitation.

For a severely injured patient, the primary airway intervention is orotracheal intubation by rapid-sequence induction. Indications for airway intervention include airway protection, expected clinical course, and the need for assisted ventilation or oxygenation (**Box 8.3**).

Alternative methods of orotracheal intubation include nasotracheal intubation, cricothyrotomy, laryngeal mask airway, retrograde intubation, and transtracheal jet insufflation. At a minimum, 100% oxygen should be administered via a nonrebreather mask to maximize tissue oxygenation.

After the airway is controlled, respiratory status is evaluated. Several alterations in ventilation mandate immediate intervention (**Table 8.5**).

After the airway and breathing are evaluated and stabilized, hemodynamic status should be evaluated. During trauma

**BOX 8.3 Indications for Airway Intervention**

Decreased level of consciousness (Glasgow Coma Scale score < 8)
Extreme agitation
Presence of or impending airway obstruction
Presence of or impending compromise of ventilation
Need for immediate surgical intervention
Hemodynamic instability

resuscitation, it is imperative that IV access be established immediately to facilitate rapid transfusion or administration of blood products (18-gauge or larger IV line). Ideal guidelines recommend a minimum of two working IV sites. Alternatives to large-bore peripheral IV access are intraosseous lines, central lines, and venous cutdown lines. In a hypotensive adult patient with trauma, an initial bolus of 2 L of warm normal saline or lactated Ringer solution is a reasonable starting point. In children, a 20-mL/kg bolus should be used. If the traumatized patient remains hypotensive after the initial bolus, transfusion of type O-negative or type-specific blood should be considered. A caveat to this statement is a patient who has sustained penetrating trauma to the chest or abdomen, in whom a short period of permissive hypotension (on the way to the operating room) may improve survivability by not disrupting an internal tamponade.[5] Recent military and trauma center practice has championed aggressive blood and fresh frozen plasma resuscitation in a 1 : 1 ratio in patients in hemorrhagic shock. When possible, manual pressure or military tourniquets should be used in conjunction with fluid or blood resuscitation to temporize hemorrhage.

Once the primary survey is completed and the patient is stabilized, the secondary survey is used to unveil the remaining injuries. Patients may then require specific care of individual injuries or specialty consultation as needed.

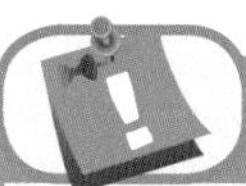

**TIPS AND TRICKS**

**Intubation**
Prepare the equipment.
Preoxygenate the patient with 100% $O_2$.
Evaluate the oropharynx.
Use an end-tidal $CO_2$ detector.
Have an alternative method available.

**Chest Tube Placement**
Extend the arm on the side of the chest tube above the head.
Use local anesthesia.
Have a cell saver in a pleural evacuation unit (Pleurovac) before patient arrival.

**Intravenous Access**
Place the access site away from injuries.
Consider an external jugular vein approach.
Consider femoral central venous access.

**Focused Abdominal Sonography for Trauma (FAST)**
Clamp a Foley catheter.
Perform serial examinations if the vital signs change.

**Table 8.5 Indications for Respiratory Intervention in Patients with Trauma**

| INDICATION | INTERVENTION |
|---|---|
| Tension pneumothorax | Needle decompression |
| Pneumothorax and hemothorax | Tube thoracostomy |
| Sucking chest wound | Tube thoracostomy, petroleum jelly (Vaseline) compression dressing |
| Pulmonary contusion with hypoxia | Intubation |

## FOLLOW-UP, NEXT STEPS IN CARE, AND PATIENT EDUCATION

All patients requiring trauma evaluation and treatment because of anatomic or physiologic trauma center criteria (see Box 8.2) must be admitted to the hospital. Patients who meet the mechanism criteria only and in whom thorough evaluation identifies no injuries may be candidates for discharge with careful warnings and comprehensive discharge planning.

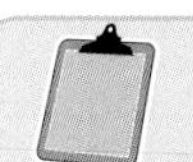

**DOCUMENTATION**

The following categories of information should appear in the documentation for every patient with trauma:

**History**
Prehospital history
Detailed mechanism (e.g., speed of the vehicle, height of the fall)
Circumstances (e.g., damage to the vehicle, type of weapon)
Timing of the event
Time until arrival at the emergency department
Concurrent medications
Drug or alcohol use
Past medical history
Last meal
Immunizations
Previous operations

**Physical Examination**
Primary survey and interventions
Head-to-toe examination

**Studies**
Emergency department interpretation of computed tomography scans and radiographs
Results of focused abdominal sonography examination for trauma (FAST)

**Medical Decision Making**
Reasons to pursue or not pursue a work-up for each injury
Consultation by surgical or other subspecialists

**Procedures**
Each procedure performed (document in full)

**Patient Instructions**
Discussion of injuries and potential outcomes with the patient or the patient's family (or both)

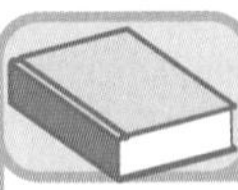

**PATIENT TEACHING TIPS**

Recovery from injuries takes time and frequently extensive rehabilitation.

Recidivism for certain injuries is common; consider referrals to specific programs according to circumstances.

Discuss prevention of further injury, wound care, cast care, and so on.

Alert the patient to warning signs for which immediate care should be sought.

## COMPLICATIONS

Patients with major trauma often have a long recovery period with a high risk for permanent deficits. Once stabilized, a team approach consisting of occupational therapy, physical therapy, nutrition, and mental health can help speed recovery and improve the long-term outcome.

## SUGGESTED READINGS

American College of Surgeons. Advanced trauma life support program for doctors. 8th ed. Chicago: American College of Surgeons; 2008.

Asimos AW, Gibbs MA, Marx JA, et al. Value of point of care blood testing in emergent trauma management. J Trauma 2000;24:1101-8.

Branney S, Moore EE, Cantrill SV, et al. Ultrasound based key clinical pathway reduces the use of hospital resources for the evaluation of blunt abdominal trauma. J Trauma 1997;42:1086-90.

Lavery RF, Livingston DH, Tortella BJ, et al. The utility of venous lactate to triage injured patients in the trauma center. J Am Coll Surg 2000;190:656-64.

Salim A, Sangthong B, Martin M, et al. Whole body imaging in blunt multisystem trauma patients without obvious signs of injury: results of a prospective study. Arch Surg 2006;141:468-73.

## REFERENCES

***References can be found on Expert Consult @ www.expertconsult.com.***

# Sonography for Trauma 9

*Christine Butts and Justin Cook*

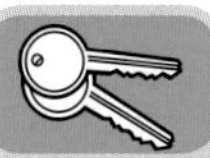

**KEY POINTS**

- Focused abdominal sonography for trauma (FAST) is sensitive and specific for the detection of intraperitoneal free fluid, but it has poor results when used in an attempt to localize solid organ injury.
- The indications for FAST have expanded to include the evaluation of patients with normotensive blunt trauma and penetrating trauma.
- FAST can be learned quickly by most emergency physicians, although its chief limitation is that it is operator dependent.

## FAST EXAMINATION

### INTRODUCTION

Ultrasound for the evaluation of trauma patients was one of the first applications of bedside ultrasound used by emergency physicians (EPs). The FAST examination (originally, focused abdominal sonography for trauma; currently, focused evaluation with sonography for trauma) was developed initially as a noninvasive modality for the initial triage of patients with hypotensive blunt abdominal or thoracic trauma. Its purpose was to rapidly identify patients with free intraperitoneal fluid or with pericardial effusion. However, over the past 20 years, FAST has evolved considerably to include the evaluation of patients after normotensive blunt trauma and penetrating trauma. Implementation of other bedside ultrasound advances has led to the development of E-FAST (or extended FAST). E-FAST involves evaluation of the inferior vena cava (IVC) for overall intravascular fluid status and assessment of the chest for pneumothorax and pleural effusion.

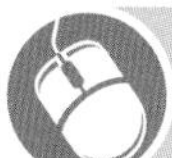

For more information on E-FAST, see www.expertconsult.com

### COMPARISON OF IMAGING MODALITIES FOR TRAUMA

Before the development of FAST, either computed tomography or diagnostic peritoneal lavage was the standard method for evaluating patients with abdominal trauma. Each of these modalities has distinct advantages and drawbacks.

FAST allows the EP to rapidly evaluate trauma patients at the bedside, frequently while other interventions are ongoing. It requires a minimum of training, is noninvasive, and can be repeated. In addition to evaluating the abdomen, ultrasound can be used to evaluate the pericardium and pleura. Another important advantage of this technique is that intravenous contrast material or ionizing radiation is not required, which allows safe use in a broad spectrum of patients, including pregnant women. FAST is not without limitations, however. Although it can be learned quickly by most, it is operator dependent. Achievement of the highest sensitivity relies on the sonographer obtaining adequate views, which can be hampered by patient habitus, bowel gas, or the presence of subcutaneous air. FAST is not as reliable for pinpointing the site of hemorrhage or for discerning solid organ injury. The retroperitoneum is also typically poorly visualized, and hemorrhage in this area may be missed.

### WHAT WE ARE LOOKING FOR

Following trauma, particularly blunt trauma, patients may be hemodynamically unstable because of bleeding from multiple sites. It can frequently be difficult to ascertain where the patient's injuries lie based on the history and physical examination alone. FAST was designed to identify possible sources of bleeding that result in instability. It relies on the premise that free fluid (blood) within the peritoneum will accumulate within the most gravity-dependent areas. These areas are the right upper quadrant between the liver and kidney (pouch of Morison), the right paracolic gutter, the left upper quadrant between the spleen and kidney, the potential space between the spleen and diaphragm, the left paracolic gutter, and the pelvis. FAST seeks to evaluate these areas quickly for the presence of free fluid. It also seeks to evaluate the pericardial sac for the presence of pericardial effusion and possible cardiac tamponade. The presence of cardiac activity or the status of overall cardiac function can also be assessed.

### LITERATURE REVIEW

Multiple studies have demonstrated the utility of FAST for the evaluation of patients after blunt abdominal trauma. One of the first studies to highlight FAST by EPs was performed by Ma and Mateer in 1995. This study evaluated ultrasound for detection of free fluid not only in the peritoneum but also in the pericardium, the retroperitoneal space, and the pleural cavity. The authors evaluated a total of 975 cavities and calculated a sensitivity of 90%, a specificity of 99%, and an accuracy of 99%.[1] This study demonstrated that with training, EPs are capable of identifying free fluid with high sensitivity and specificity.

Subsequent studies focusing on FAST have found variable results ranging from sensitivities of 79% to 100% and specificities of 95.6% to 100%.[2-5] Although calculated sensitivities and specificities have been variable across studies, one finding that seems consistent is that both sensitivity and specificity appear to increase in hypotensive patients.[6]

Conversely, a Cochran review published in 2005 found "insufficient evidence from RCTs [randomized controlled trials] to justify promotion of ultrasound-based clinical pathways in diagnosing patients with suspected blunt abdominal trauma."[7] These findings have been controversial, and a similar literature review by Melniker found "the FAST examination, adequately completed, is a nearly perfect test for predicting a 'Need for OR' in patients with blunt torso trauma."[8]

One finding that has appeared consistently in most studies is that although FAST is sensitive and specific for the detection of intraperitoneal free fluid, it has poor results when used in attempts to localize solid organ injury.[9,10]

Ultrasound has been shown to be a reliable study for the evaluation of traumatic pericardial effusions. Mandavia et al. found that EPs with training in echocardiography had a sensitivity of 96%, a specificity of 98%, and an overall accuracy of 97.5% for this indication.[11]

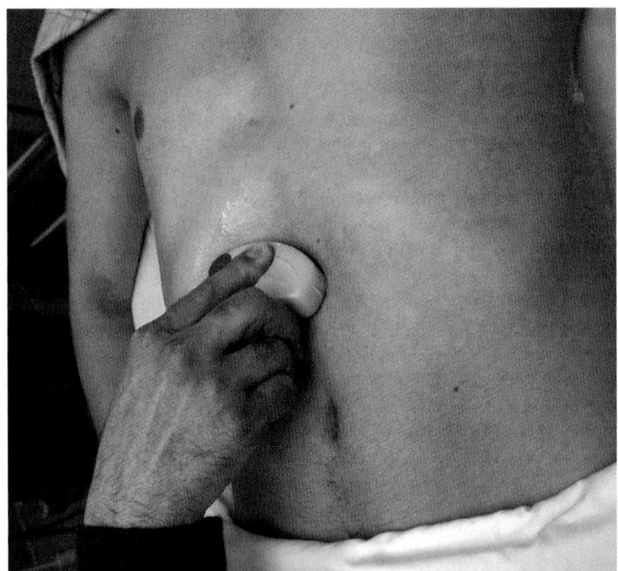

**Fig. 9.1 Proper placement of the transducer for a subxiphoid view of the heart.** Note that the sonographer is holding the transducer overhand and pushing downward into the subxiphoid space while pointing the transducer toward the left side of the chest.

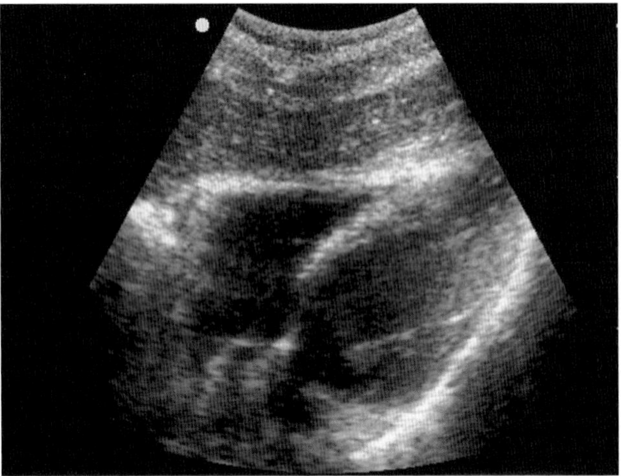

**Fig. 9.2 Subxiphoid view of the heart.** A four-chamber view of the heart surrounded by the hyperechoic (white) border of the pericardium is seen. At the top of the screen, the left lobe of the liver is adjacent to the right ventricle.

## HOW TO PERFORM A FAST EXAMINATION

FAST consists of ultrasound views of four primary areas, the right and left upper quadrants of the abdomen, the pelvis, and a view of the pericardium from the subxiphoid area.

A low-frequency transducer is typically used to ensure proper depth of penetration.

### SUBXIPHOID VIEW

To evaluate the subxiphoid view of the heart, the transducer is placed just below the subxiphoid process and aimed toward the patient's left shoulder (**Fig. 9.1**). It is frequently necessary to apply some pressure to the upper part of the patient's abdomen to enable the sonographer to look "up" into the patient's chest. It is also helpful to think of the transducer as a flashlight and imagine shining it toward the left side of the patient's chest. Another helpful tip for beginning sonographers is to increase the depth if at first the heart is not seen in full. A four-chamber view of the heart should be sought (**Fig. 9.2**). Specifically, the bright white (or hyperechoic) outline of the pericardium should be sought to evaluate for the presence of pericardial effusion.

### RIGHT UPPER QUADRANT

The right upper quadrant should be evaluated in both the coronal and transverse planes. To begin, the transducer is placed on the patient's midaxillary line between the 8th and 11th ribs (**Fig. 9.3**). This position should be adjusted as needed to overcome rib shadowing and to obtain the best image possible. Aiming the indicator toward the patient's head will yield a coronal image. The interface between the liver and kidney (pouch of Morison) and the potential spaces around this area should be thoroughly evaluated for the presence of free fluid (**Fig. 9.4**). This can be done by sweeping the transducer anteriorly and posteriorly. Moving the transducer superiorly a rib space or two will usually allow a view of the echogenic diaphragm curving over the dome of the liver. The area superior to the diaphragm, the costophrenic recess, can be evaluated for the presence of pleural fluid as well. Once a coronal image has been obtained, the transducer should be rotated so that the indicator points toward the patient's right to obtain a transverse view. Although such placement frequently provides an adequate view, it is often helpful to angle the transducer on a

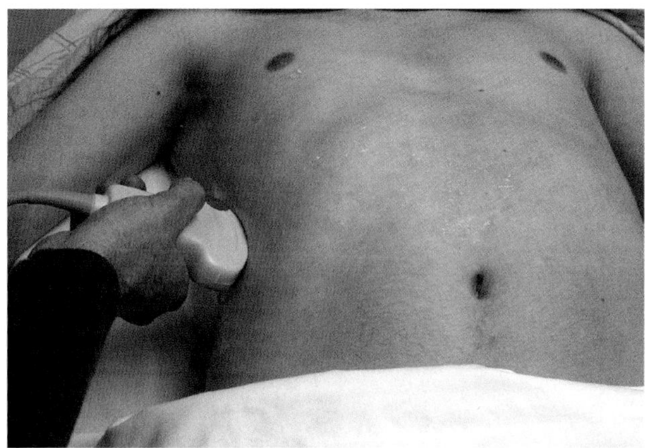

**Fig. 9.3 Placement of the transducer for evaluation of the right upper quadrant.** Note that the indicator on the transducer is pointing toward the patient's head. This will yield a coronal image. The transducer should be placed along the anterior midaxillary line between the 8th and 11th rib spaces.

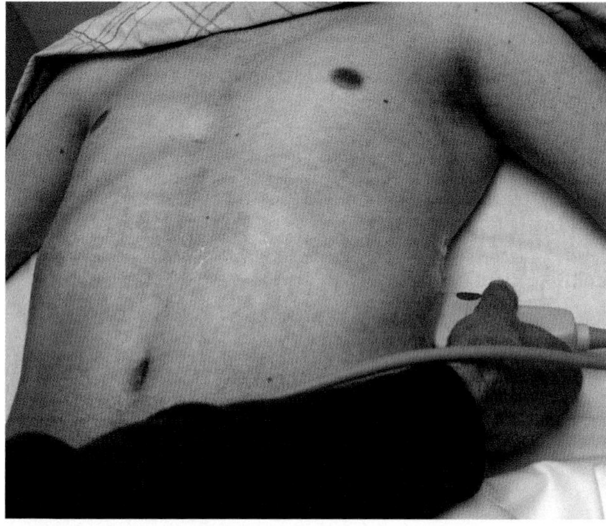

**Fig. 9.5 Placement of the transducer for evaluation of the left upper quadrant.** Note that the indicator on the transducer is pointing toward the patient's head, which will yield a coronal image. The transducer should be placed along the posterior midaxillary line between the 8th and 11th rib spaces.

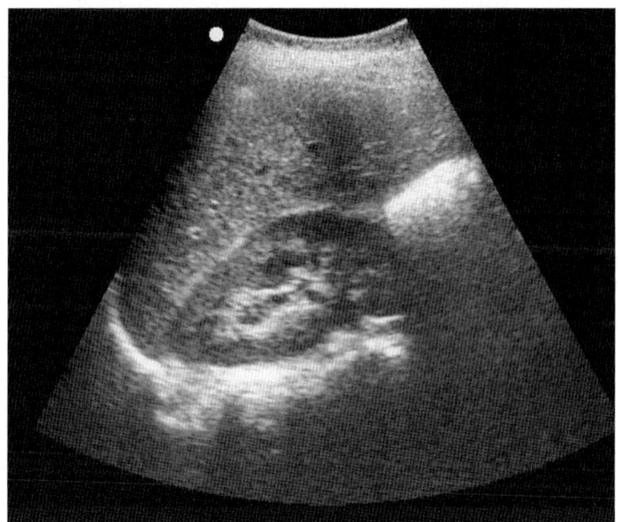

**Fig. 9.4 Normal right upper quadrant as viewed in a coronal orientation.** The liver is seen on the left of the image, with the kidney seen to the right and slightly inferior to the liver. The diaphragm is seen as a brightly echogenic arc on the far left of the image.

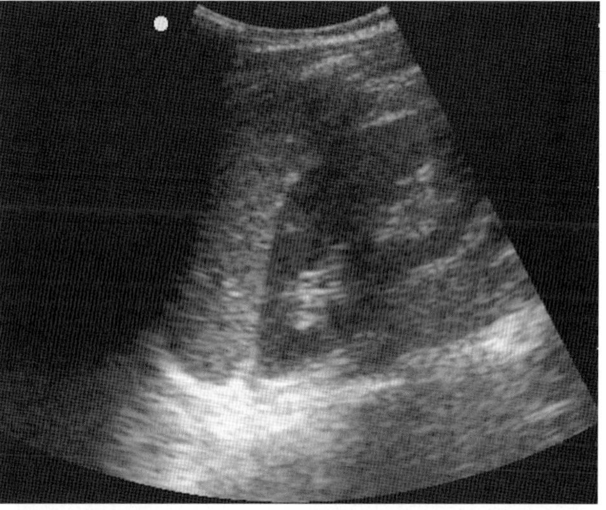

**Fig. 9.6 Normal left upper quadrant as viewed in a coronal orientation.** The spleen is seen on the left of the image, with the kidney lying to its right. At the bottom left of the image, a portion of the brightly echogenic diaphragm can be seen overlying the spleen.

slightly oblique plane so that it fits into the intercostal space and thus limits rib shadowing. Once the liver and kidney are seen, sweeping the transducer superiorly and inferiorly offers a full evaluation of areas in which free fluid may collect.

## LEFT UPPER QUADRANT

The left upper quadrant is evaluated in much the same manner as the right upper quadrant. One important distinction is that the left kidney is usually found in a more posterior and superior location. Therefore, to obtain a coronal image, the transducer is placed in the posterior midaxillary line between the 8th and 11th ribs (**Fig. 9.5**). The indicator should be pointing toward the patient's head. It is particularly important not only to evaluate the interface between the kidney and spleen but also to seek the interface between the spleen and diaphragm (**Fig. 9.6**). This aids in viewing the costophrenic recess for free pleural fluid, as well as the subphrenic recess, where free peritoneal fluid frequently collects. Again, once the coronal view has been obtained, the transducer should be swept anteriorly and posteriorly to fully assess the left upper quadrant. After the coronal plane has been viewed, the transducer should be rotated so that the indicator faces the patient's right. It may be helpful to place the transducer at a slight angle to avoid any artifact created by the ribs. Once the interface between the kidney and spleen is found, the transducer should be swept inferiorly and posteriorly to evaluate this region in full.

## PELVIS

The final component of the basic FAST examination is evaluation of the pelvis. The transducer should be placed just superior to the pubic symphysis. Beginning in the transverse plane, the indicator on the transducer should be facing toward the patient's right (**Fig. 9.7**). The bladder is easily identified in this orientation as a rectangularly shaped object filled with dark, anechoic urine, especially if the ultrasound can be performed before placement of a urinary catheter (**Fig. 9.8**). Although the bladder is generally identified quickly, the evaluation should proceed further and the bladder be used as an acoustic window to view the dependent portions of the pelvis. This can be done by tilting the transducer toward the patient's feet and back upward or more superiorly. The transducer can then be rotated toward the patient's head to view the same area in a sagittal orientation (**Fig. 9.9**). In this plane the bladder has a triangular appearance (**Fig. 9.10**). Complete evaluation of the potential spaces of the pelvis can be achieved by tilting the transducer from side to side.

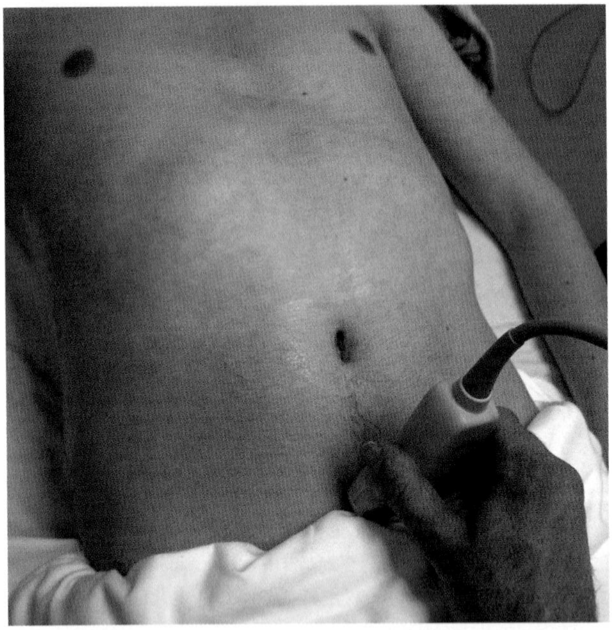

**Fig. 9.7 Placement of the transducer for evaluation of the pelvis in a transverse orientation.** Note that the indicator is pointing toward the patient's right. The transducer should be placed just superior to the pubic symphysis.

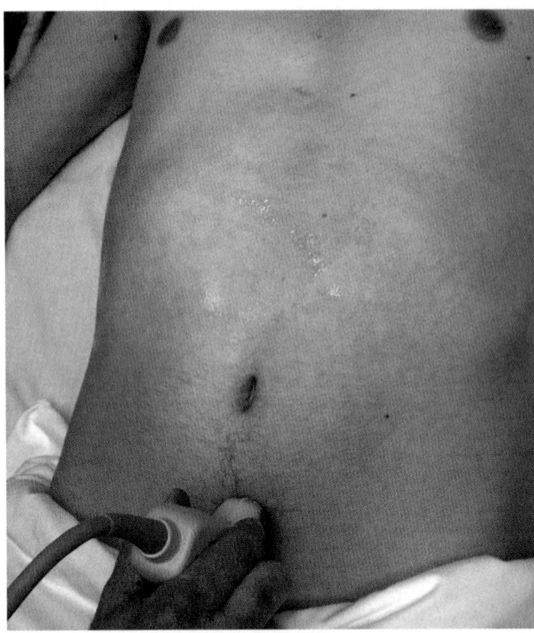

**Fig. 9.9 Placement of the transducer for evaluation of the pelvis in a sagittal orientation.** Note that the indicator is pointing toward the patient's head. The transducer should be placed just superior to the patient's pubic symphysis.

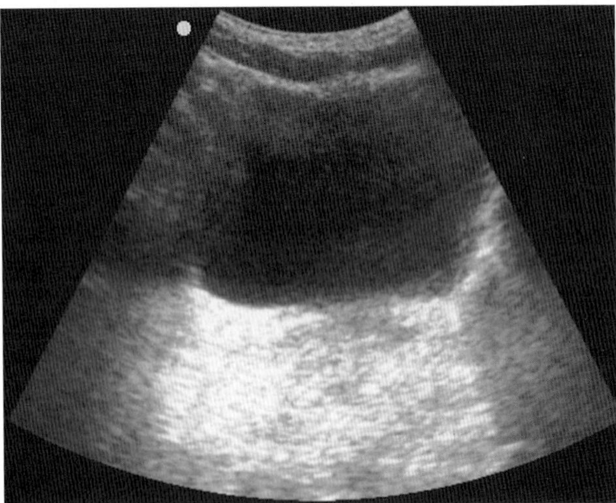

**Fig. 9.8 Normal pelvis as viewed in a transverse orientation.** In this image the bladder is clearly seen as a rectangularly shaped fluid collection. Its clearly defined walls distinguish it as the bladder as opposed to free fluid.

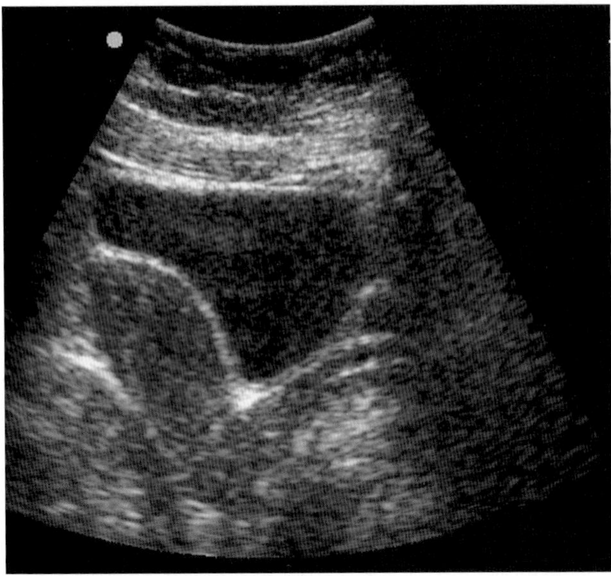

**Fig. 9.10 Normal pelvis as viewed in a sagittal orientation.** In this image the bladder is seen as a triangular fluid collection. Just deep to the bladder, the fundus of the uterus can be seen pushing into its posterior wall.

## NORMAL AND ABNORMAL FINDINGS

The primary purpose of FAST is to identify free fluid either within the peritoneum or within the pericardium. Free fluid, although it may accumulate in a number of dependent areas, is fairly reliable in its appearance. Fluid is identified as black on ultrasound, and most free fluid, in this case blood, will have a black appearance. Bleeding that has begun to form a clot is less fluid-like in its consistency and may appear as varying shades of gray.

When evaluating the subxiphoid view of the heart, the bright white, echogenic outline of the pericardium should be sought (see Fig. 9.2). Normally, the pericardium should closely abut the ventricle. Free fluid will be seen as a black collection between the pericardium and the ventricles of the heart (**Fig. 9.11**). Typically, fluid will first accumulate in the most dependent part of the pericardial sac and can thus be seen deep to the left ventricle. It should be noted that the amount of fluid seen may appear underwhelming on first inspection. It is important to realize that a smaller amount of fluid is needed to cause cardiac tamponade in a trauma patient. This is due to the rapid accumulation of free fluid within the pericardial sac, which quickly overcomes the ability of the fibers of the pericardium to stretch to accommodate increasing pressure.

In the right upper quadrant, free fluid most commonly accumulates in the area between the liver and kidney (pouch of Morison). Acute hemorrhage will be seen as an anechoic (black) stripe of varying size in this potential space (**Fig. 9.12**).

Free fluid in the left upper quadrant appears much the same as in the right upper quadrant. It may appear as an anechoic stripe between the spleen and kidney. However, the potential space between the spleen and the diaphragm is a common location for free fluid to accumulate and may be overlooked without careful evaluation (**Figs. 9.13 and 9.14**).

In the pelvis, free fluid will accumulate in the gutters surrounding the bladder (**Fig. 9.15**). The bladder can be distinguished from free fluid by noting the rectangular shape of the bladder. Free fluid is amorphous and will appear to seep into the gutters of the pelvis, whereas the bladder is either a rectangular (transverse) or triangular (sagittal) shape, depending on the imaging plane chosen.

## PITFALLS

The bedside sonographer may encounter both technical and diagnostic challenges while performing FAST.

Diagnostic challenges frequently arise from misuse or incorrect interpretation of the FAST examination. FAST was designed to evaluate the presence of free fluid and pericardial effusion and is most sensitive when used for this purpose, particularly in hypotensive blunt trauma patients. It does not

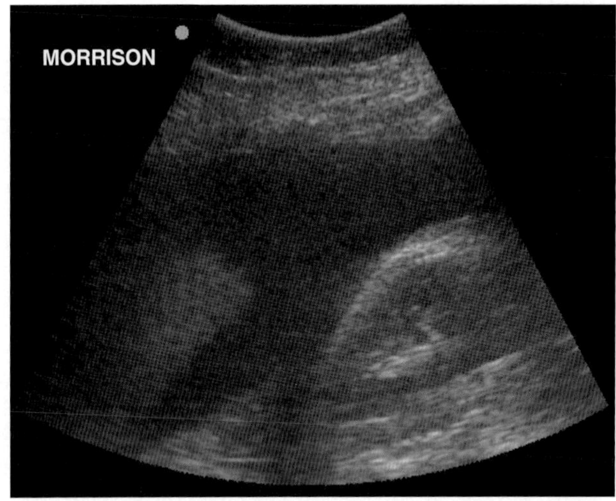


**Fig. 9.12 Right upper quadrant image demonstrating free fluid in the pouch of Morison.** This large amount of fluid is represented by the anechoic (black) area both surrounding the tip of the liver and in the space between the kidney and liver.

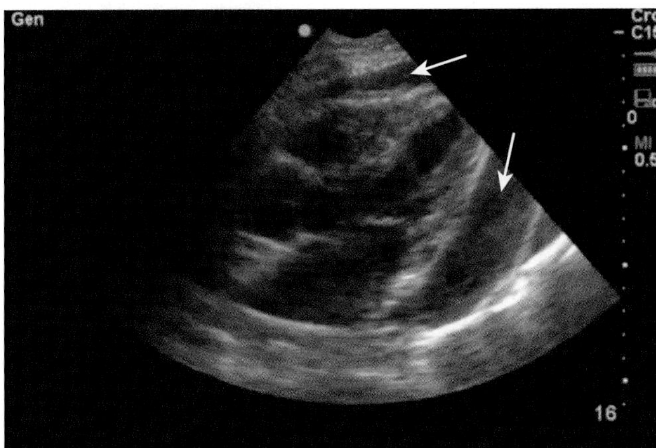


**Fig. 9.11 Subxiphoid image of the heart with a pericardial effusion demonstrated by the *arrow*.** The pericardium can be seen at the bottom of the image as a bright white boundary surrounding the dark fluid collection. This is a large pericardial effusion.

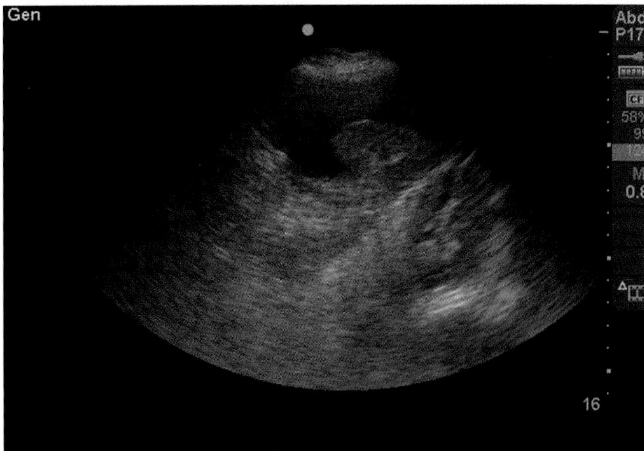


**Fig. 9.13 Transverse image of the left upper quadrant demonstrating an anechoic (black) fluid collection surrounding the spleen.** The kidney can be seen at the bottom right of the image.

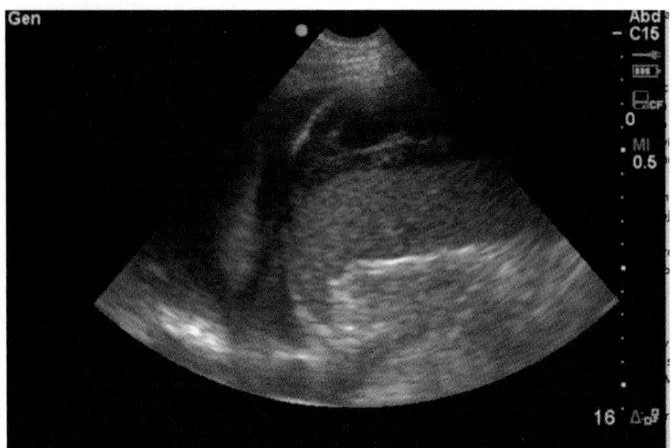


**Fig. 9.14 Coronal image of the left upper quadrant demonstrating an anechoic (black) free fluid collection between the spleen, on the right of the image, and the diaphragm, on the left of the image.**

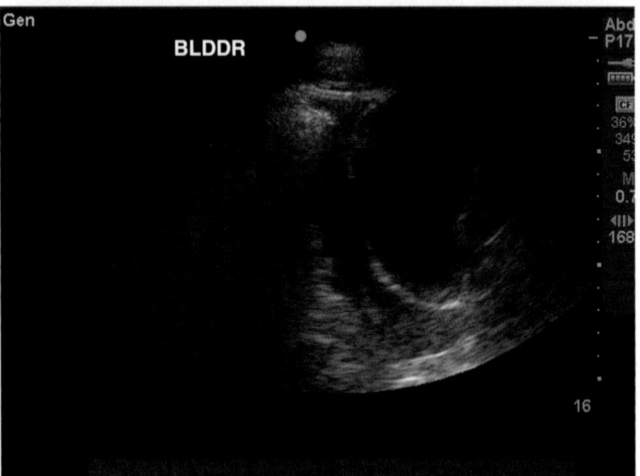


**Fig. 9.15 Pelvic image demonstrating free fluid overlying the bladder.** The bladder is seen as a well-defined fluid collection surrounded by echogenic walls at the right of the image. The free fluid is seen to the right of the bladder and is distinguished by its lack of clear boundaries. At the superior aspect of the free fluid, bowel loops are seen within it, a finding that further distinguishes it from the bladder.

fare as well when used to either diagnose the location of injury or rule out injury in normotensive or penetrating trauma patients.

The primary technical challenge faced by the sonographer is overcoming artifact. Subcutaneous air, bowel gas, or air in the stomach may make performing a complete FAST examination difficult.

Misidentification of normal structures may also cause falsely positive FAST findings. A full stomach, the IVC, and the gallbladder may appear similar to fluid collections. Knowledge of anatomy and experience with the normal appearance of the structures may minimize this mistake.

## SUGGESTED READINGS

Blaivas M, Lyon M, Sandeep D. A prospective comparison of supine chest radiography and bedside ultrasound for the diagnosis of traumatic pneumothorax. Acad Emerg Med 2005;12:844-9.

Ma OJ, Mateer JR, Ogata M, et al. Prospective analysis of a rapid trauma ultrasound examination performed by emergency physicians. J Trauma 1995;38:879-88.

Melniker LA. The value of focused assessment with sonography in trauma examination for the need for operative intervention in blunt torso trauma: a rebuttal to "emergency-ultrasound–based algorithms for diagnosing blunt abdominal trauma (review)," from the Cochrane Collaboration. Crit Ultra J 2009;1:73-8

Stengel D, Bauwens K, Sehouli J, et al. Emergency-ultrasound–based algorithms for diagnosing blunt abdominal trauma. Cochrane Database Syst Rev 2005;2:CD0044446.

## REFERENCES

*References can be found on Expert Consult @ www.expertconsult.com.*

# Procedural Sedation 10

*Steven A. Godwin and Beranton Whisenant*

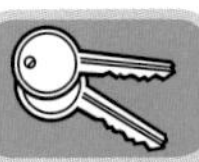

**KEY POINTS**

- Procedural sedation refers to the technique of administering sedatives or dissociative agents with or without analgesics to induce a state that allows the patient to tolerate unpleasant procedures while maintaining cardiorespiratory function.[1,2]
- Procedural sedation with analgesia in the emergency department is generally intended to create a depressed level of consciousness that allows the patient to maintain control of the airway and oxygenation without continuous assistance.
- Patients must be assessed before sedation to proactively identify potential difficulties associated with disease states and airway maintenance.
- When drugs are used in combination, their effects are more than additive, and this can be beneficial or can potentiate respiratory depression and cardiovascular instability.
- In patients with liver disease, the metabolism of drugs is altered in many ways and it is difficult to predict effects.
- In patients with a recent history of opiate and benzodiazepine overuse, propofol may offer advantages over other agents.

## DEFINITIONS

Procedural sedation, not including dissociative agents, represents a continuum of sedation ranging across defined levels of consciousness. These varying degrees of awareness have been termed *minimal sedation* (anxiolysis), *moderate sedation*, *deep sedation*, and *general anesthesia*. See **Table 10.1** for general definitions as defined by the Joint Commission. Because patients can move from one state or level of awareness to another without warning, serial assessment and close hemodynamic monitoring are advised.

## INDICATIONS FOR PROCEDURAL SEDATION AND ANALGESIA IN THE EMERGENCY DEPARTMENT

Patients often arrive at the emergency department (ED) with acute injuries or disorders that require timely intervention to reduce both the physical and the psychologic effects of pain, anxiety, disability, and life-threatening complications. Common indications that may require procedural sedation are listed in **Box 10.1**.

## PATIENT MONITORING

Because individual patient responses to sedatives and analgesics often vary, constant monitoring is essential to identify subtle changes in respiratory effort and hemodynamics. American College of Emergency Physician guidelines recommend that patients selected for procedural sedation and analgesia (PSA) undergo continuous cardiac monitoring, continuous pulse oximetry, and documented blood pressure checks every 5 minutes during the procedure and in the postprocedural period.[2] **Box 10.2** provides a list of objective physiologic parameters recommended for safe bedside monitoring. In addition, see **Table 10.2** for the six-point Ramsay sedation scale, which was initially validated in intensive care units for the assessment of sedation depth and later modified to correlate with the Joint Commission definitions of sedation.

### CAPNOMETRY (END-TIDAL CARBON DIOXIDE MONITORING)

Many PSA agents decrease tidal volume and the respiratory rate, thereby creating the potential for hypoventilation and apnea. In the majority of patients, pulse oximetry readings correlate well with arterial $O_2$ saturation values. Unfortunately, oximetry is ineffective in the early detection of hyperventilation-induced hypercapnia, particularly if patients are receiving supplemental oxygen. Growing evidence for the routine use of continuous capnography during procedural sedation has led to its increased clinical use in an attempt to identify hypoventilation and avoid unrecognized periods of apnea.[2] This monitoring technology may have its greatest benefit in patients whose ventilation status cannot be visualized (e.g., covered with a sterile sheet). Although clear evidence demonstrating differences in clinical outcomes with its use is not yet available, end-tidal $CO_2$ monitoring is probably useful in providing an added level of safety when performing PSA.

### PULSE OXIMETRY

Pulse oximetry readings may be misleading for a variety of reasons. The emergency physician must be aware of the pitfalls of this modality to correctly address changes in oxygenation (**Table 10.3**).[3,4]

### MONITORING DEPTH OF SEDATION

#### *Bispectral Index Monitoring*

Electroencephalographic (EEG) bispectral index monitoring has been studied for use in the ED as a means of avoiding hypercapnia and hypoxic events and to objectively determine the depth of sedation during PSA. The bispectral index is a

**Table 10.1** General Definitions Related to Anesthesia*

| PARAMETER | MINIMAL SEDATION | MODERATE SEDATION | DEEP SEDATION | GENERAL ANESTHESIA |
|---|---|---|---|---|
| Responsiveness | Normal response to verbal stimulation | Purposeful response to verbal or tactile sedation | Purposeful response after repeated or painful stimuli | Unarousable even with painful stimulation |
| Airway | Unaffected | No intervention required | Intervention may be required | Intervention often required |
| Spontaneous ventilation | Unaffected | Adequate | May be inadequate | Frequently inadequate |
| Cardiovascular function | Unaffected | Usually maintained | Usually maintained | May be impaired |
| Modified Ramsay sedation scale score | 1 | 2-4 | 5-7 | 8 |

*As defined by the Joint Commission.

**BOX 10.1 Indications for Procedural Sedation and Analgesia in the Emergency Department**

Fracture reduction and orthopedic procedures
Burn and wound débridement
Repair of lacerations, especially in children
Removal of foreign bodies
Elective and nonelective cardioversion
Insertion of a thoracostomy tube
Endoscopy
Awake intubation and mechanical ventilation
Radiologic studies in agitated or uncooperative patients

**BOX 10.2 Objective Physiologic Parameters for Patient Monitoring**

Vital signs: blood pressure, respiratory rate
Cardiac rhythm: cardiac monitor
Oxygenation: pulse oximetry
Clinical assessment of depth of sedation: modified Ramsey scale
Ventilatory effort: clinical examination and end-tidal $CO_2$ monitoring with continuous capnometry

statistical numeric value based on bispectral processing of the last 15 to 30 seconds of the harmonic and phase relationship of the frontal lobe EEG data. A score of 90 to 100 represents an awake state; 70 to 80, a moderate sedation state; 60 to 70, a deep sedation state; 40, general anesthesia; and 0, consistent with brain death. These scores can vary with the PSA used and in individual patients.[5] The use of combination PSA agents makes titrating to a predefined bispectral index value difficult because of the synergistic effect of the agents.[6,7] Evidence is insufficient to recommend the routine use of such monitoring in the ED.[2]

**Table 10.2** Ramsay Sedation Scale

| CLINICAL SCORE | LEVEL OF SEDATION ACHIEVED |
|---|---|
| 1 | Patient agitated, anxious |
| 2 | Patient cooperative, oriented, and tranquil |
| 3 | Patient responds to commands only |
| 4 | Brief response to light glabellar stimuli or loud auditory stimuli |
| 5 | Sluggish response to light glabellar tap or loud auditory stimuli |
| 6 | No response to light glabellar tap or loud auditory stimuli |

## PREPROCEDURAL CONSIDERATIONS AND RISK ASSESSMENT

The clinician must obtain and document a complete history and physical examination for a patient when administering sedative medications. This step is critical in determining whether the patient is an appropriate candidate for PSA.

The goal of PSA is to effectively alleviate the patient's anxiety, pain, and discomfort to the degree that best facilitates the safe performance of both painful and nonpainful procedures. PSA represents a dynamic continuum, with patients moving from one level of consciousness to the next without any clear point of transition. The predefined level of sedation should be determined on the basis of the patient's acute disease state, the nature and duration of the therapeutic intervention being planned, and sedation and analgesia goals such as pain control, anxiolysis, and amnesia. In the ED the preferred method of administration for most PSA agents is often intravenous. Some agents, including intramuscular ketamine and inhalational sedation with nitrous oxide, are equally effective when delivered by experienced personnel in the appropriate setting.

**Table 10.3 Pitfalls in Pulse Oximetry**

| | |
|---|---|
| Low perfusion states | Low cardiac output, vasoconstriction, or hypothermia |
| Motion artifact | The most common source of error |
| Nail polish | Black, green, and blue nail polish have the same light absorbency: 660 and 940 nm |
| Type of probe and location | Ear probes have rapid response time. Accuracy of reading dependent on patient's perfusion state and heart rate |
| Ambient light | Falsely low $O_2$ saturation with fluorescent and xenon surgical lamps |
| Dyshemoglobinemias: carboxyhemoglobin, methemoglobin | Overestimation of true $O_2$ saturation |
| Transient hypoxia consistent with patient's normal sleep patterns | Inherent disadvantage of oximetry with insignificant hypoxic episodes |

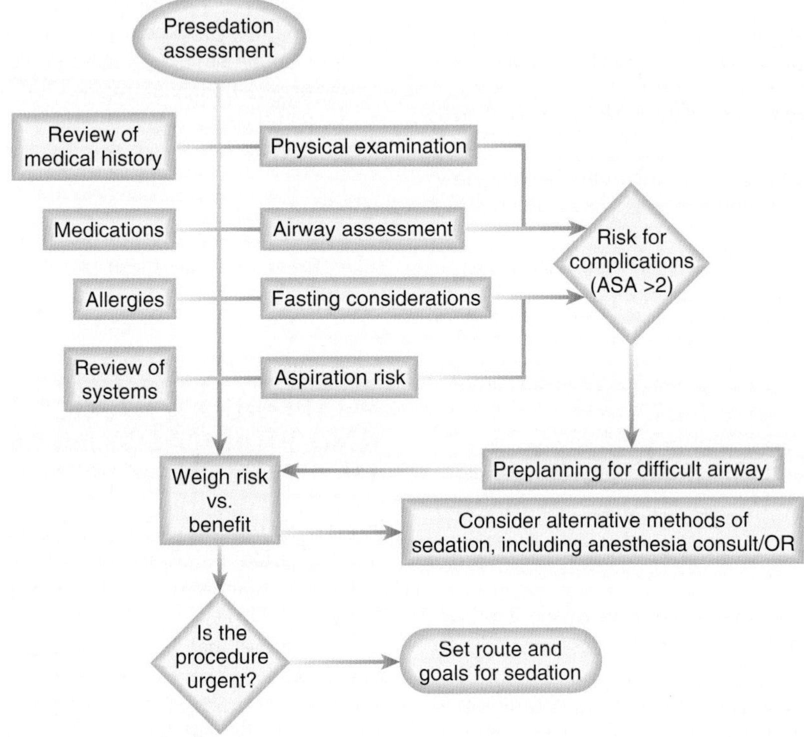


**Fig. 10.1 Algorithm for evaluation before sedation.** *ASA*, American Society of Anesthesiologists [score]; *OR*, operating room.

## GENERAL CONSIDERATIONS

- History: past medical history, anesthesia history, medications, allergies, review of systems, time of last meal
- Physical examination: vital signs (blood pressure, pulse rate, respiratory rate), pulse oximetry, airway assessment, cardiopulmonary and neurologic examinations
- Weighing risks against the benefits of performing PSA
- Urgency of performing PSA

## RISK ASSESSMENT

**Figure 10.1** presents an algorithm for evaluation before sedation.

### *Airway Evaluation*

Assessment of the patient for potentially difficult bag-mask ventilation because of facial, oral, or neck anomalies is important before administration of PSA. Use of the mnemonics MOANS and LEMONS has been described as an aid in identifying anatomic and clinical features that may pose potential difficulties in airway management should bag-mask ventilation or intubation become necessary (**Box 10.3**).[8]

### *Fasting Considerations*

No compelling evidence is available to support fasting in the emergency setting for either children or adults. The emergency physician may consider a patient's history of recent oral

**BOX 10.3 Use of the Mnemonics MOANS and LEMON for Preprocedural Airway Assessment for a Difficult Airway**

**MOANS: Difficult Bag-Mask Ventilation**

M: Mask seal—bushy beards, distorted lower facial contour

O: Obesity/obstruction—morbidly obese patients (because of increased redundant upper airway tissue) and patients with disorders that obstruct the upper airway

A: Age older than 55 years because of decreased muscular tone of the upper airway

N: No teeth, which creates difficulty in achieving an adequate mask seal

S: Stiff—patients with stiff noncompliant lungs, such as those with COPD, asthma, CHF, and pulmonary fibrosis

**LEMON: Difficult Intubations**

L: Look externally for physical features that may make intubation difficult—small mandible, large teeth, large tongue, short neck

E: Evaluate with the 3-3-2 rule:
- For mouth opening, 5 cm or at least 3 (patient's) fingerbreadths
- Thyromental distance of 5 cm or at least 3 fingerbreadths
- 2 fingerbreadths from the hyoid to the thyroid cartilage for evaluation of the position of the larynx in relation to the base of the tongue

M: Mallampati score—ability to visualize the posterior oropharynx with opening of the mouth

O: Obstruction—upper airway obstruction, stridor, odynophagia, and dysphagia

N: Neck mobility—immobilization because of cervical trauma, arthropathies

*CHF*, Congestive heart failure; *COPD*, chronic obstructive pulmonary disease.

intake when determining the appropriateness of the depth of sedation and the complexity of a procedure, especially in patients at higher risk for airway compromise and complications. Prudence and good clinical judgment are paramount.[2]

In addition, no strong evidence supports the use of gastric-emptying agents before sedation in either the pediatric or adult population.

### *Aspiration Risk*

Risk for aspiration is always a consideration in patients undergoing procedural sedation in the ED. The evidence suggests that these patients are at no increased risk for aspiration because of:

- Maintenance of protective reflexes during PSA
- Brevity of the procedures
- Lack of manipulation of the airway
- Depth of consciousness not meeting the level of general anesthesia

**BOX 10.4 Reversal Agents for Procedural Sedation and Analgesia (PSA)**

**Naloxone (Narcan)**

Opioid antagonist that is used for oversedation and respiratory depression with opioids:
- For partial reversal of oversedation of a PSA opioid agent, a dose of 0.1 to 0.4 mg can be used.
- For complete reversal of sedation, 2 mg should be given intravenously.
- Following reversal with naloxone, the patient should be observed for 90 minutes because of the risk for resedation.

**Flumazenil**

Reversal agent for benzodiazepine-induced oversedation and hypoventilation:
- Use 1 mg for complete reversal of PSA with midazolam.
- It has an onset of action of 1 to 2 minutes with a duration of 45 minutes.
- Caution should be used in patients who are long-term users of benzodiazepines because of the risk for acute withdrawal.

## PHARMACODYNAMICS AND PHARMACOKINETICS OF COMMON AGENTS

In view of the array of procedures requiring PSA in the ED and the varied underlying clinical disorders, an understanding of the pharmacology of individual agents is important. Such knowledge allows the provider to tailor sedation and analgesia to meet individual patients' needs. A number of agents are well suited to the ED environment because of their rapid onset of action, brief recovery period, and minimal untoward effects. It is difficult for a single agent to meet all the sedative and analgesic goals of an individual patient, and a combination of drugs is sometimes used. **Table 10.4** details the pharmacology of individual PSA agents,[9-15] and **Table 10.5** details the drug effects of commonly used combination pediatric regimens.[16,17] A list of reversal agents for PSA can be found in **Box 10.4**.

## REFERENCES

***References can be found on Expert Consult @ www.expertconsult.com.***

**Table 10.4 Pharmacodynamics and Pharmacokinetics of Common Sedation Agents**

| SHORT-ACTING PSA AGENTS | SUMMARY | PHARMACODYNAMICS AND PHARMACOKINETICS | RECOMMENDED SEDATIVE DOSE AND CLINICAL INDICATIONS | ONSET OF ACTION | RECOVERY PERIOD DURATION |
|---|---|---|---|---|---|
| Fentanyl | Synthetic opioid 100 times more potent than morphine<br>Analgesic agent<br>Minimal sedative effect<br>Use in combination with anxiolytic agent | Lipid soluble<br>Metabolized in liver to inactive metabolite<br>Side effects: hypotension, hypoxemia, apnea, vomiting, and rare episodes of chest wall rigidity reported when given over less than 2-min period | 0.5-1 mcg/kg every 1-2 min and titrate to desired level of sedation in combination with a sedative | Within 1 min | 30-60 min following single dose of 100 mcg |
| Midazolam | Potent anxiolytic, sedative, and amnesic properties<br>Useful for brief, painless ED procedures<br>Frequently used with opioid for analgesic effect | Binds to GABA receptors in CNS to exert anxiolysis<br>Drug effect is terminated by redistribution and hepatic metabolism to active metabolite<br>Active metabolite can accumulate and prolong sedation in patients who are elderly, have renal failure, and/or are taking protease inhibitors<br>Causes respiratory depression and hypotension<br>Should be used with caution in patients with COPD, cardiomyopathy, or hypovolemia | Adult: common dose regimen is 0.05-0.2 mg/kg IV<br>Decrease dose by 30-50% when combined with opioid | 30 sec to 1 min<br>Duration of action, 20 to 40 min | 20-40 min |
| Etomidate | Frequently used to facilitate performance of both painful and nonpainful procedures<br>Has sedative and hypnotic effects<br>Has minimal effect on cardiac and respiratory function | Exerts its sedative and hypnotic effects at GABA receptors by increasing the number and enhancing the functioning of these receptors<br>Is metabolized by the liver to a nonactive metabolite, but hepatic dysfunction does not affect the rapid recovery period<br>Side effects: myoclonus is the most unique side effect; also, nausea, vomiting, hiccups, superficial thrombophlebitis and/or apnea<br>Can cause hypoventilation and apnea when combined with an opioid or other anxiolytic agent<br>Mild (clinically insignificant) adrenocortical suppression after a single IV bolus | Adult: 0.2 mg/kg over 1-min period | <1 min | 5 min |
| Methohexital | Effective ultrashort-acting, rapid-recovery PSA agent of the barbiturate class<br>Most frequently used in the ED for short painful procedures such as orthopedic reduction | Rapidly produces state of unconsciousness and profound amnesia but has no analgesic properties<br>Is frequently combined with opioid for painful procedures<br>Side effects: most common are respiratory depression and apnea<br>Also has direct myocardial depressant effect and should not be used in hemodynamically unstable patients | Adult: 0.75- to 1-mg/kg IV bolus and can be titrated to 0.5 mg/kg at 3- to 5-min intervals to desired level of sedation | <1 min | 5-7 min |

*Continued*

**Table 10.4 Pharmacodynamics and Pharmacokinetics of Common Sedation Agents—cont'd**

| SHORT-ACTING PSA AGENTS | SUMMARY | PHARMACODYNAMICS AND PHARMACOKINETICS | RECOMMENDED SEDATIVE DOSE AND CLINICAL INDICATIONS | ONSET OF ACTION | RECOVERY PERIOD DURATION |
|---|---|---|---|---|---|
| Propofol | Ideal for procedures requiring brief periods of sedation<br>Rapid onset of action and rapid recovery make it an ideal PSA agent for use in ED<br>A preferred sedative for patients with brain injury | Produces its sedative-hypnotic effects by binding to and mediating upregulation of GABA receptors<br>Metabolized by extensive tissue redistribution and hepatic and extrahepatic metabolism<br>Coadministration with opioid slows metabolic clearance and prolongs recovery time<br>Side effects: respiratory depression, apnea, and hypotension; also, pain at injection site, hyperlipidemia, and pancreatitis | Adult: loading dose of 1 mg/kg over 1- to 2-min period, followed by continuous infusion at 1.5-4.5 mg/kg/hr or 0.5 mg/kg administered in 20-mg aliquots with titration to desired effect<br>Elderly patients: continuous infusion of 25 mcg/kg/min may be preferred without bolus injection to limit respiratory depression/hypotension | <1 min | 10 min |
| Dexmedetomidine | Highly selective $\alpha_2$-adrenergic agonist with sedative, anxiolytic, and analgesic properties<br>Induces natural sleep to exert its sedative-anxiolytic effects<br>Can be used to sedate patients who are insensitive to usual doses of benzodiazepines<br>Also used as effective PSA agent for nonpainful procedures | Acts on $\alpha_2$-adrenergic receptors in brain to regulate sleep and respiratory pattern | Adults: loading dose of 0.3-1 mcg/kg/min over 5- to 10-min period, followed by infusion at 0.5-1 mcg/kg/hr<br>Indications: patients at high risk for respiratory depression and airway obstruction, severe cervical trauma for short procedures, or awake fiberoptic intubation | Rapid | Short |
| Remifentanil | Provides excellent sedation and analgesia for brief ED procedures | Ester derivative of fentanyl with ultrashort-acting sedative and analgesic properties<br>Metabolized by esterases present in interstitial tissues and RBCs<br>Metabolism independent of hepatic or renal dysfunction<br>Side effect: respiratory depression that is responsive to verbal commands | Adult: infusion of 0.5 mcg/kg over 90-min period with continuous dosing of 0.25 mcg/kg as needed | <1 min | Rapid (3-15 min) |
| Pentobarbital | Used in ED for painless diagnostic procedures | Short-acting barbiturate agent with sedative and anticonvulsive properties<br>Exerts its sedative-hypnotic effects at GABA receptor site and is terminated by hepatic metabolism to inactive metabolite that is renally excreted<br>Side effects: hypotension, respiratory depression, and bronchospasm; use is contraindicated in patients with intermittent porphyria, COPD | Adults: loading dose of 100 mg by slow bolus that may be repeated every 1-3 min; maximum, 200-500 mg<br>Pediatric dose: 2-5 mg/kg; maximum, 100 mg | 3-5 min | 15-45 min when given IV; 1-2 hr when given IM |

**Table 10.4 Pharmacodynamics and Pharmacokinetics of Common Sedation Agents—cont'd**

| SHORT-ACTING PSA AGENTS | SUMMARY | PHARMACODYNAMICS AND PHARMACOKINETICS | RECOMMENDED SEDATIVE DOSE AND CLINICAL INDICATIONS | ONSET OF ACTION | RECOVERY PERIOD DURATION |
|---|---|---|---|---|---|
| Ketamine | Phencyclidine derivation with amnesic, sedative, analgesic properties<br>Agent of choice for pediatric patients | Dissociative effect is due to binding to NMDA receptors in CNS<br>Has bronchodilatory effect on bronchial smooth muscles and is useful in patients with bronchoconstriction<br>Side effects: most common adverse effect is emesis, which can be decreased with addition of midazolam<br>Emergence phenomena with vivid dreams, hallucinations, and recovery agitation | Adults: 1-mg/kg bolus injection followed by 0.25-0.5 mg/kg every 5-10 min as needed<br>Children: same dose as adults<br>IM dose: 3-4 mg/kg<br>Give glycopyrrolate, 0.2 mg, concomitantly for hypersalivation | IV: <1 min<br>IM: 5 min | 15-20 min |
| Nitrous oxide | Excellent agent for quick ED procedures | Blended solely with oxygen and has linear dose-response pattern<br>Advantage: does not requires vascular access<br>Side effects: emesis, dizziness, and headaches<br>Do not use in patients with bowel obstruction, pneumothorax | Gas mixture: 50:50 nitrogen and oxygen | 3-5 min | 3-5 min after cessation of gas |

*CNS*, Central nervous system; *COPD*, chronic obstructive pulmonary disease; *ED*, emergency department; *GABA*, γ-aminobutyric acid; *IM*, intramuscular(ly); *IV*, intravenous(ly); *NMDA*, *N*-methyl-D-aspartate; *PSA*, procedural sedation and analgesia; *RBCs*, red blood cells.

**Table 10.5 Pediatric Considerations for Procedural Sedation and Analgesia**

| COMBINED PSA REGIMENS | GENERAL COMMENTS | ONSET AND DURATION OF ACTION | SIDE EFFECTS |
|---|---|---|---|
| Propofol and fentanyl | This combination has rapid onset of action and rapid recovery period in comparison with other combinations<br>Significant clinical experience lacking in comparison with midazolam/fentanyl | Rapid onset (<1 min)<br>Rapid recovery (15 min) | Deep sedation with respiratory depression |
| Etomidate and fentanyl | Frequently used for painful procedures that require brief sedation | Short onset and duration of action | Hypoxic and respiratory depression frequent but short-lived |
| Midazolam and fentanyl | Has excellent safety profile when titrated for effect<br>Most commonly used PSA combination in ED | Short onset of action and relatively prolonged recovery time in comparison with other combination regimens | Hypoxic and respiratory depression<br>Prolonged recovery period with hangover effect lasting up to several hours because of active metabolite |
| Ketamine and midazolam | Very effective in producing excellent analgesia and sedation for more painful and anxiety-producing therapeutic procedures<br>Can be given as oral midazolam and IM ketamine, so IV access not necessary<br>Has excellent safety profile | Provides 15-20 min of dissociative sedation | More hypoventilation and hypoxia than with ketamine alone |
| Ketamine and propofol | Becoming popular combination<br>Synergy caused by opposing hemodynamic and respiratory effects<br>Greater provider satisfaction of sedation effect | Rapid onset of action and recovery time | Incidence of respiratory depression same as for propofol used alone |

*ED*, Emergency department; *IM*, intramuscular; *IV*, intravenous; *PSA*, procedural sedation and analgesia.

# 11 Resuscitation in Pregnancy

*Elizabeth M. Datner and Susan B. Promes*

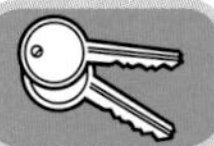

**KEY POINTS**

- Displace the gravid uterus off the great vessels either manually or with a left lateral tilt to avoid aortocaval compression.
- Gain intravenous access above the diaphragm.
- Preoxygenate with 100% oxygen before intubation in anticipation of a more rapid onset of hypoxemia.
- In a pregnant woman, hands for cardiopulmonary resuscitation, chest tubes, and defibrillator paddles should be placed higher on the chest wall.
- Cardioversion and defibrillation will not harm the fetus.
- When the uterus is palpable above the umbilicus and the mother is in cardiac arrest, perform cesarean section immediately.
- Continue cardiopulmonary resuscitation during and after perimortem cesarean section and consider therapeutic hypothermia in a comatose patient with return of spontaneous circulation.
- For an Rh-negative woman who has vaginal bleeding after trauma, administer Rh immunoglobulin (RhoGAM): a 50-mcg dose in the first trimester and a 300-mcg dose in the second or third trimester.
- In any pregnant woman at more than 24 weeks' gestation who suffers trauma to the abdomen, fetal monitoring should be initiated as soon as possible and be maintained for 4 to 6 hours.

## SCOPE

Resuscitation of a pregnant woman is an infrequent event. Cardiac arrest statistics are difficult to quantify, but cardiac arrest reportedly occurs in roughly 1 in 30,000 near-term pregnancies.[1] More recent data suggest an increase in maternal mortality from cardiac arrest, with frequency rates of 1 in 20,000.[2] In the event of cardiac arrest in a pregnant woman, two lives must be resuscitated. Quick, decisive management is paramount for the livelihood of the mother and her unborn child. Knowing exactly what to do and acting quickly ensure the best possible outcome for the mother and her unborn child.

## ANATOMY AND PHYSIOLOGY

What are generally considered abnormal vital signs in nonpregnant people may actually be within the normal range for a pregnant woman. In gravid females, the heart rate and respiratory rate are increased. In the second trimester, blood pressure is decreased by 5 to 15 mm Hg, but it returns to normal near term. Hypoxemia occurs earlier in pregnant patients because of diminished reserve and buffering capacity. Pregnant patients have a slight respiratory alkalosis—$P_{CO_2}$ of 30 mm Hg and pH of 7.43—that must be taken into account when interpreting arterial blood gas values. Central venous pressure decreases in pregnancy to a third-trimester value of 4 mm Hg.[3]

A pregnant woman has less respiratory reserve and greater oxygen requirements. The gravid uterus pushes up on the diaphragm, which results in reduced functional residual capacity. Minute ventilation and tidal volume rise, as does maternal oxygen consumption. The basal metabolic rate increases during pregnancy. The greater oxygen demands of the unborn child significantly alter the mother's respiratory physiology, and the mother hyperventilates to meet the demands of the fetus. A pregnant patient at baseline is in a state of compensatory respiratory alkalosis because of excessive secretion of bicarbonate. A pregnant woman's ability to compensate for acidosis is impaired. Other physiologic changes that may affect resuscitation are airway edema and friability, reduced chest compliance, and higher risk for regurgitation and aspiration.

As the uterus grows, it moves from the pelvis into the abdominal cavity, which pushes the contents of the abdominal cavity up toward the chest. In late pregnancy, the gravid uterus compresses the aorta and inferior vena cava and limits venous return to the heart. Stroke volume is decreased when a near-term pregnant woman is lying on her back and increased when the uterus is moved away from the great vessels. A woman in the second or third trimester of pregnancy should be placed in the left lateral tilt position, or the uterus should be manually displaced to the left to optimize cardiac output and venous return. During late pregnancy, cardiac output is increased. Pulmonary capillary wedge pressure remains unchanged, as does the ejection fraction.

Electrocardiographic changes, including left axis deviation secondary to the diaphragm moving cephalad and changing the position of the heart, are also present during pregnancy. Q waves are present in leads III and aVF, and flattened or inverted T waves are seen in lead III.

During pregnancy blood volume increases, which causes a dilution anemia. The average hematocrit value is 32% to 34%. White blood cell counts are higher than normal and platelet counts are lower in pregnancy. Blood urea nitrogen and serum creatinine values are lower than normal, as are cortisol values. The erythrocyte sedimentation rate is increased. Albumin and total protein levels are decreased. Fibrinogen levels double in pregnancy, so a patient with disseminated intravascular coagulation could have a normal fibrinogen level.

Pregnancy-related changes can be seen on radiographic studies. A chest radiograph of a pregnant woman shows an increased anteroposterior diameter, mild cephalization of the pulmonary vasculature, cardiomegaly, and a slightly widened mediastinum. Widening of the sacroiliac joints and pubic symphysis are apparent on imaging of the pelvis. Radiography should not be avoided in a pregnant woman because of concerns about radiation exposure of the fetus, which can simply be shielded. Ultrasonography can be used at the bedside to identify fluid in the abdomen, pelvis, and pericardium and to evaluate fetal activity and heart rate. Fetal well-being is closely linked to the well-being of the mother, so all studies indicated for diagnosis and treatment of the mother should be performed.

## DIFFERENTIAL DIAGNOSIS

Pregnant women are generally young and healthy. The rare cardiac arrest in a gravid female may be due to venous thromboembolism, severe pregnancy-induced hypertension, amniotic fluid embolism, or hemorrhage. In addition to such pregnancy-related problems, pregnant women are not exempt from common conditions that affect the general population. Trauma and sepsis may lead to cardiopulmonary failure and the need for maternal resuscitation. **Box 11.1** lists key etiologic factors leading to cardiac arrest in pregnant patients.[4]

### HEMORRHAGE

During routine vaginal delivery, the average blood loss is 500 mL. Excessive blood loss or postpartum hemorrhage complicates 4% of vaginal deliveries.[5] Common causes of hemorrhage around the time of delivery are uterine atony (excessive bleeding with a large relaxed uterus after delivery), vaginal or cervical tears, retained fragments of placenta, placenta previa, placenta accreta, and uterine rupture. Hereditary abnormalities in blood clotting may cause hemorrhage, so inquiries about excessive bleeding, known disorders, and family history are relevant in a patient with excessive bleeding.

### NONHEMORRHAGIC SHOCK

Causes of nonhemorrhagic obstetric shock—pulmonary embolism, amniotic fluid embolism, acute uterine inversion, and sepsis—are uncommon but are responsible for the majority of maternal deaths in the developed world.[6] These conditions must be diagnosed and treated expeditiously. Patients in whom pulmonary embolism is suspected should be administered heparin and then undergo diagnostic imaging. Although fibrinolytic agents are contraindicated in pregnancy, they have been used successfully in patients with life-threatening pulmonary embolism and ischemic stroke. Treatment of amniotic fluid embolism is supportive, the goals being to maintain maternal oxygenation and support blood pressure. Some case reports describe success with the use of cardiopulmonary bypass to treat women suffering from amniotic fluid embolism.

Acute uterine inversion can also cause shock. Cardiovascular collapse complicates approximately half the cases of acute uterine inversion. Classically, the extent of the shock is out of proportion to the blood loss noted. One theory to explain this observation is that a parasympathetic reflex causes neurogenic shock from stretching of the broad ligament or compression of the ovaries (or both) as they are drawn together. Uterine replacement combined with vigorous fluid resuscitation, including blood transfusion as required, should reverse the hypotension.[7]

**BOX 11.1 Major Causes of Cardiac Arrest During Pregnancy***

Venous thromboembolism
Pregnancy-induced hypertension
Sepsis
Amniotic fluid embolism
Hemorrhage:
- Placental abruption
- Placenta previa
- Uterine atony
- Disseminated intravascular coagulation

Trauma
Iatrogenic:
- Medication errors
- Allergic reactions to medications
- Anesthetic complications
- Oxytocin administration
- Hypermagnesemia

Preexisting heart disease:
- Congenital
- Acquired cardiomyopathy of pregnancy

*Listed in order of decreasing frequency.
From Mallampalli A, Powner DJ, Gardner MO. Cardiopulmonary resuscitation and somatic support of the pregnant patient. Crit Care Clin 2004;20:748.

### TRAUMA

Traumatic injuries occur commonly in pregnancy and are the leading cause of maternal death; they account for more than 46% of cases. Motor vehicle crashes, assaults, and falls are the most common causes of injuries. Pregnant women are at increased risk for domestic violence, and this possibility should be considered and the police notified when warranted.

Fetal outcome is affected when the mother becomes hypotensive or acidotic as a result of major injury. Maternal vital signs and physical symptoms do not predict fetal distress in women with minor trauma. Only cardiotocographic monitoring for a minimum of 4 to 6 hours is useful in predicting fetal outcome. After even apparently minor falls women should undergo fetal monitoring.

In pregnant women suffering blunt trauma, most fetal deaths occur as a result of placental abruption. Classic symptoms are abdominal cramps, vaginal bleeding, uterine tenderness, and hypovolemia (several liters of blood can accumulate in the uterus). None of these findings are sensitive and cannot be relied on, so monitoring is required.

## DIAGNOSTIC TESTING

### INTERVENTIONS AND PROCEDURES

A fundamental principle in treating pregnant women is that fetal well-being depends on maternal well-being. As with all patients in the emergency department (ED), resuscitation starts with the ABCs (airway, breathing, and circulation). One hundred percent oxygen should be administered to the mother early. Hypoxia should be treated aggressively in this patient population because when the mother is hypoxic, oxygen is shunted away from the fetus. Additionally, preoxygenation is important because apnea results in more rapid hypoxia in the setting of pregnancy. Rapid-sequence induction with precautions for aspiration is essential before intubation. Aggressive volume resuscitation, administration of vasopressors if needed, and close attention to the patient's body position are all very important in the treatment of hypotension in a pregnant patient. Fetal heart monitoring and, ideally, cardiotocographic monitoring should be initiated as soon as possible for patients in the second or third trimester of pregnancy.[8]

A commercially produced wedge called a Cardiff wedge is available to aid in the resuscitation of pregnant women. It can be placed under the woman's right side to support her back while she lies in the preferred left lateral tilt position. In the absence of a wedge, a human wedge can be used, with the patient being tilted on the bent knees of a kneeling rescuer. Pillows, towel rolls, and blanket rolls are readily available in EDs and accomplish the same purpose of angling the woman's back 30 to 45 degrees from the floor (**Fig. 11.1**). If for some reason the patient must lie on her back, as in the case for adequate cardiopulmonary resuscitation (CPR), a member of the health care team should manually displace the uterus to the left so that it does not rest on the great vessels.

The American Heart Association (AHA) basic life support guidelines should be followed with two modifications:

- Move the uterus off the great vessels.
- Adjust the hand position for CPR cephalad to account for displacement of the thoracic contents by the gravid uterus.

The AHA advanced cardiac life support (ACLS) guidelines for medications, intubation, and defibrillation for patients in cardiac arrest should be followed for gravid females with one simple exception—a change in placement of the defibrillation paddles and pads:

- Place one paddle below the right clavicle in the midclavicular line.
- Position the second paddle outside the normal cardiac apex so that it avoids breast tissue.[7]

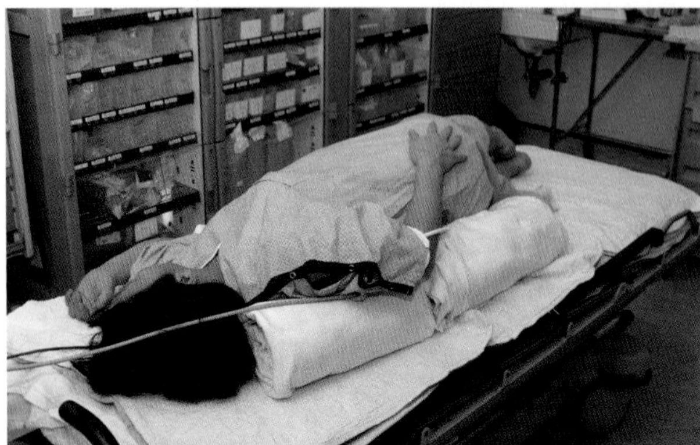

**Fig. 11.1 Blanket roll technique to tilt the patient.**

Defibrillation energy requirements remain the same (**Fig. 11.2**).[9] Defibrillation will not harm the fetus. ACLS medications should be used as needed. It is reasonable to remove external or internal fetal monitoring devices during electrical shock of the mother because of the possibility of creating an electrical arc to the monitoring equipment, but this is unlikely with the electrical current applied to the maternal thorax. **Box 11.2** lists the U.S. Food and Drug Administration categories for the various ACLS drug options during pregnancy.

In pregnant patients with trauma who are in need of a thoracostomy, the chest tube must be placed one or two intercostal spaces higher than normal to avoid diaphragmatic injury. An open supraumbilical approach should be used for diagnostic peritoneal lavage in a pregnant patient, with the gravid uterus palpable on abdominal examination.

If return of spontaneous circulation (ROSC) is achieved, effort must be directed at further hemodynamic stabilization. Post–cardiac arrest therapeutic hypothermia has been successful in the setting of early pregnancy and is recommended as for nonpregnant patients.[10] In a comatose post–cardiac arrest patient with ROSC, the patient should be cooled as soon as possible and within 4 to 6 hours to 32° C to 34.8° C for a 12-to 24-hour duration to gain the best possible neurologic outcome. If a perimortem cesarean section has not been performed because of gestational age less than 24 weeks, fetal monitoring should be performed during hypothermia in anticipation of bradycardia.[11]

### IMAGING

Ultrasonography is an important method for assessment of both the mother and fetus, but additional radiographic studies are often required. Shielding can ensure that exposure even with maternal head and chest computed tomography (CT) can be kept below the 1-rad (1000-millirad) limit. Intrauterine exposure to 10 rad (10,000 millirad) produces a small increase in childhood cancer; exposure to 15 rad creates a risk for mental retardation, childhood cancer, and a small head. A head or chest radiograph delivers less than 1 millirad to the shielded gravid uterus. A lumbar spine, hip, or kidneys-ureters-bladder radiograph delivers more than 200 millirad. A CT scan of the head delivers less than 50 millirad to the shielded uterus, and a chest CT scan provides an exposure of less than 1000 millirad. In sum, important radiographic studies of the head, neck, and chest can safely proceed if the uterus is shielded.

## FETOMATERNAL TRANSFUSION

After the 12th week of pregnancy, when the uterus rises above the pelvic rim and becomes susceptible to trauma, fetal blood can theoretically cross into the maternal circulation after significant trauma. A 50-mcg dose of Rh immunoglobulin (RhoGAM) is used when the mother is Rh negative. During the second and third trimesters a 300-mcg dose is administered, which protects against 30 mL of fetomaternal hemorrhage. A 16-week fetus has about a 30-mL volume of blood, so the entire blood volume is covered by the 300-mcg dose.

Pregnant patients in the second or third trimester who suffer major traumatic injury could theoretically have fetomaternal

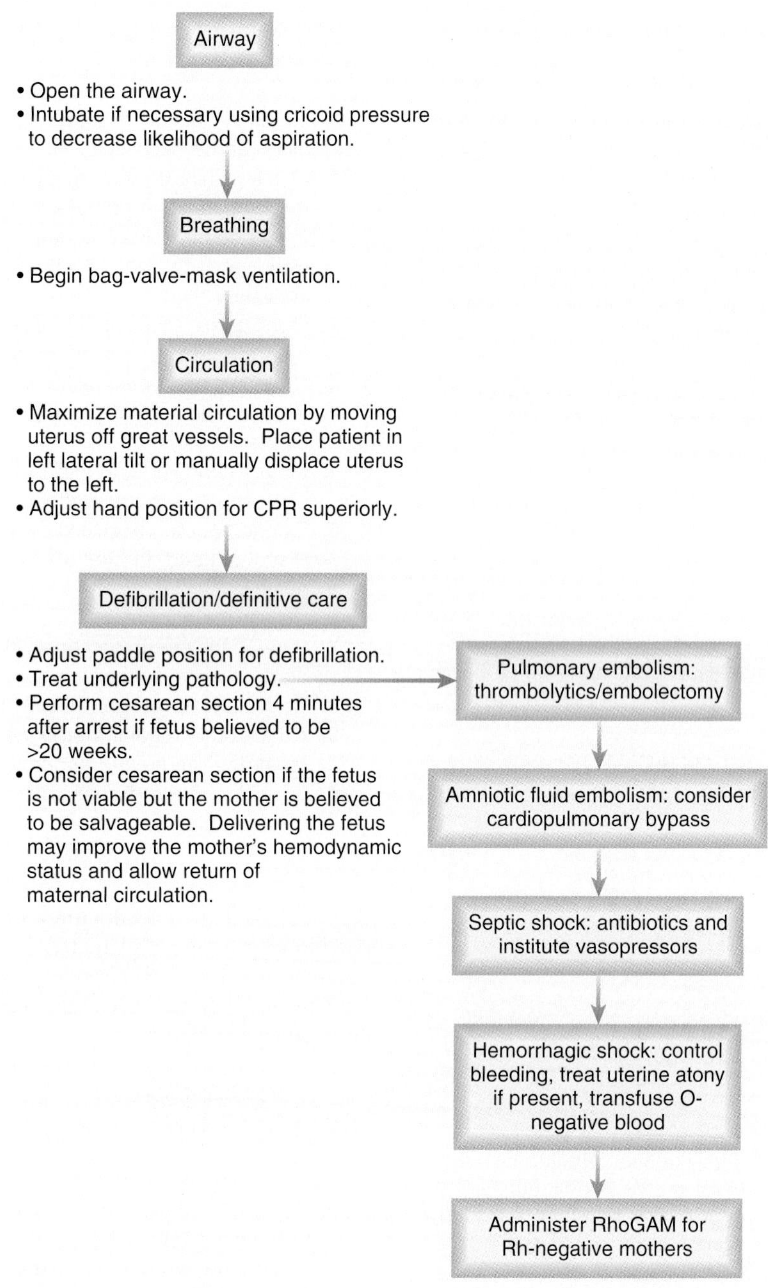


**Fig. 11.2 Algorithm for resuscitation of a pregnant patient.** *CPR,* Cardiopulmonary resuscitation.

transfusion that exceeds the coverage provided by the 300-mcg dose. This situation is rare and occurs in less than 1% of pregnant patients after trauma. In patients with major trauma and advanced pregnancy, the Kleihauer-Betke test should be considered, especially when significant vaginal bleeding is present. Rh immunoglobulin is effective when administered within 72 hours, so the test does not have to be performed in the ED.

## PERIMORTEM CESAREAN SECTION

The two goals of perimortem cesarean section are to improve the unstable hemodynamics of the mother and minimize morbidity and mortality in the child. If resuscitative efforts, including ACLS algorithms and alleviation of aortocaval compression, fail to improve maternal hemodynamics, perimortem cesarean section must be considered. The likelihood that perimortem cesarean section will result in a living and neurologically normal infant is related to the interval between onset of maternal cardiac arrest and delivery of the infant.[12,13] The gestational age of the neonate is also critical. If cesarean section is performed in the ED, it should be done rapidly. Time is of the essence. Fetal viability outside the uterus is best beyond 24 weeks' gestation, but it is not always possible to know the exact gestational age in the ED. On the basis of case reports, it is recommended that cesarean section be performed in the ED if the gestational age is believed to be more than

**BOX 11.2 Classification of Drugs Used During Pregnancy**

The U.S. Food and Drug Administration categories for the various advanced cardiac life support drug options during pregnancy are as follows:

**Category B**

***Definition***

Animal studies have revealed no evidence of harm to the fetus, although no adequate and well-controlled studies in pregnant women have been conducted.

*OR*

Animal studies have shown an adverse effect, but adequate and well-controlled studies in pregnant women have failed to demonstrate a risk to the fetus in any trimester.

***Agents***

Atropine
Magnesium

**Category C**

***Definition***

Animal studies have shown an adverse effect, and no adequate and well-controlled studies in pregnant women have been conducted.

*OR*

No animal studies have been conducted, nor have adequate and well-controlled studies in pregnant women been conducted.

***Agents***

Epinephrine
Lidocaine
Bretylium
Bicarbonate
Dopamine
Dobutamine
Adenosine

**Category D**

***Definition***

Adequate well-controlled or observational studies in pregnant women have demonstrated a risk to the fetus. The benefits of therapy may outweigh the potential risk. For example, the drug may be acceptable if needed in a life-threatening situation or for serious disease for which safer drugs cannot be used or are ineffective.

***Agent***

Amiodarone

20 weeks. At this stage of pregnancy, the fundus is likely to be palpable at or above the level of the umbilicus.

The child should be delivered within 5 minutes of maternal cardiac arrest, so the procedure should be initiated within 4 minutes of failed CPR of the mother. The procedure is summarized in **Box 11.3**. Maternal CPR should be maintained throughout the procedure to optimize blood flow to the uterus and the mother and should be continued after cesarean section. Once delivery is accomplished, ED personnel should be prepared to resuscitate the neonate. It is important to note

**BOX 11.3 Technique for Perimortem Cesarean Section**

*NOTE*: Have suction available for this procedure because bleeding can be excessive.

1. Ideally, while the emergency physician is preparing for the procedure, a catheter is placed in the bladder and the abdominal wall is prepared with povidone-iodine. However, do not delay the procedure for these activities.
2. Using a No. 10 scalpel, make a midline vertical incision from the umbilicus to the pubis along the linea nigra.
3. Once the peritoneal cavity is open, use bladder retractors and Richardson retractors to improve access to the uterus.
4. Make a short vertical incision in the lower uterine segment just cephalad to the bladder.
5. Extend the uterine incision cephalad with blunt scissors. Place a hand in the uterus to keep the baby from being cut.
6. Deliver the baby.
7. Suction the mouth and nose, cut and clamp the umbilical cord, and resuscitate the baby.
8. Document Apgar scores at 1, 5, and 10 minutes.
9. If the mother regains vital signs, remove the placenta and repair the uterus and abdominal wall.
10. Consider intramuscular injection of oxytocin into the bleeding uterus.

that published and anecdotal reports describe return of maternal blood pressure and maternal survival after perimortem cesarean section.[14] Successful resuscitation of a pregnant woman and her unborn child requires a coordinated team approach.

## CONCLUSION

In the setting of resuscitation, a pregnant woman poses challenges given the physiologic and anatomic changes associated with pregnancy. Remembering these normal adjustments that occur in gravid women is critical. Aortocaval compression must be avoided during resuscitation of a pregnant woman. Appropriately diagnosing the cause of the patient's medical problem while being mindful of the ABCs of resuscitation is a must. Thankfully, cardiac arrest is an uncommon event in pregnant women. When it occurs later in pregnancy, perimortem cesarean section may improve the outcome of the infant and mother if performed in a timely manner. As with all resuscitations, a team effort is mandatory, but possibly even more so in this setting because the emergency practitioner is caring for two patients whose lives are very tenuous and time is of the essence.

## REFERENCES

*References can be found on Expert Consult @ www.expertconsult.com.*

# Neonatal Cardiopulmonary Resuscitation 12

*Katherine Bakes and Ghazala Q. Sharieff*

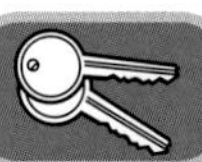

**KEY POINTS**

- In newborn resuscitation, simultaneous auscultative assessment of the heart rate and respirations should precede more advanced interventions.
- Because visual determination has been found to be unreliable, pulse oximetry with the minimal oxygen supplementation necessary to maintain adequate oxygen saturation should be used to assess newborns.
- Endotracheal intubation should be considered for tracheal suctioning of meconium, heart rates below 100 beats/min that do not respond to initial bag-valve-mask ventilation, prolonged bag-valve-mask ventilation or chest compressions, administration of medications, and other special considerations such as congenital diaphragmatic hernia and extremely low birth weight.
- If the heart rate remains below 60 beats/min despite respiratory support, chest compressions should be performed at a rate of at least 100 compressions per minute via the two-finger or chest-encircling technique. The chest-encircling technique is preferred for chest compressions. The ratio of compressions to ventilations should be 3:1, with 90 compressions and 30 breaths to achieve approximately 120 events per minute to maximize ventilation at an achievable rate. Each event will be allotted approximately ½ second, with exhalation occurring during the first compression after each ventilation.

## PERSPECTIVE

Approximately 10% of newborns require assistance after birth to achieve spontaneous breathing, and 1% need additional support. The likelihood of survival can be estimated from the gestational age and birth weight (**Fig. 12.1**).[1]

## SURVIVAL WITH COMORBID CONDITIONS

A 2001 study reviewing more than 700 neonatal intensive care unit admissions involving infants born at or before 25 weeks' gestation found that survivors (63%) had a high incidence of chronic lung disease (51%), high-grade retinopathy of prematurity (32%), intraventricular hemorrhage (44%), nosocomial infection (38%), and necrotizing enterocolitis (11%).[2]

In this same study, only 23% of survivors had no major morbidity, defined as chronic lung disease, necrotizing enterocolitis, at least grade 3 intraventricular hemorrhage, or at least grade 3 retinopathy of prematurity.

## ANATOMY

Anatomic considerations for the neonatal airway are similar to those discussed for pediatric patients (see Chapter 13), with the exception that the structures are even smaller and more anterior and superior, thus making visualization of the vocal cords an even greater challenge.

The neonatal chest wall is very flexible and can be notably distorted if vigorous inspiratory efforts are made; such distortion results in inadequate lung expansion and the potential need for positive pressure ventilatory support, particularly in premature infants who lack adequate surfactant production.

## PRESENTING SIGNS AND SYMPTOMS

"Yes" answers to the following three questions identify babies who do not require support after birth but can be dried, covered, and kept with the mother if desired.[3]

- Was the baby born after a full-term gestation?
- Is the baby breathing or crying?
- Does the baby have good muscle tone?

## INTERVENTIONS AND PROCEDURES: RESUSCITATION STEPS

**Figure 12.2** lists the steps in neonatal resuscitation.

If the answer to any of the three questions just listed is "no," the infant should receive the following in sequence, with 60 seconds allotted for completing and beginning ventilation if needed:

- Stabilization (warm, clear the airway, dry, stimulate)
- Ventilation
- Chest compressions
- Epinephrine, volume expansion, or both

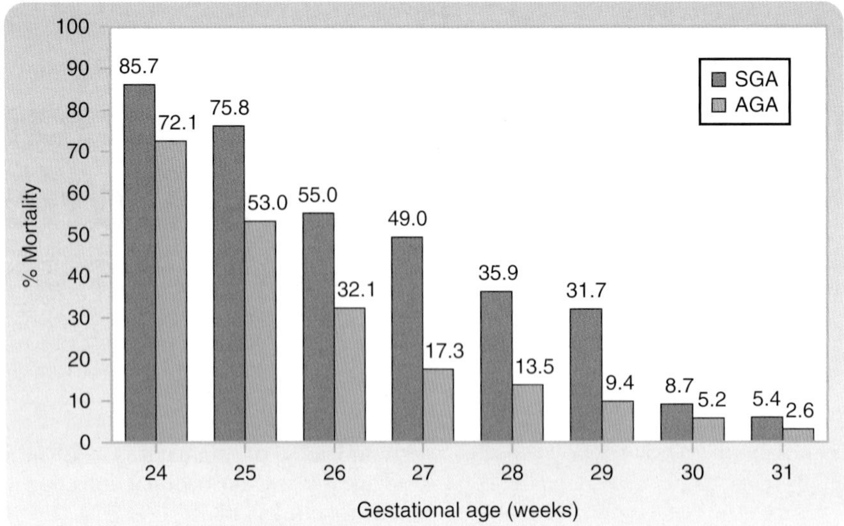


**Fig. 12.1 Percent mortality in infants who are small for gestational age (SGA) versus infants who are appropriate for gestational age (AGA) according to gestational age at birth.** The mortality rate of SGA infants was significantly higher than that of AGA infants in the 25th gestational week ($P = .015$) and from 26 to 29 weeks of gestation ($P < .01$). (From Regev RH, Lusky A, Dolfin T, et al. Excess mortality and morbidity among small-for-gestational-age premature infants: a population-based study. J Pediatr 2003;143:186-91.)

**Table 12.1 Apgar Scoring System**

| | Score | | |
|---|---|---|---|
| | **0** | **1** | **2** |
| Heart rate | Absent | <100 beats/min | >100 beats/min |
| Respiration | Absent | Slow, irregular; weak cry | Good; strong cry |
| Muscle tone | Limp | Some flexing of the arms and legs | Active motion |
| Reflex | Absent | Grimace | Grimace and cough or sneeze |
| Color | Blue or pale | Body pink; hands and feet blue | Completely pink |

Apgar scores are measured at 1 minute and 5 minutes after delivery. These scores are used to (1) predict which infants will require resuscitation and (2) identify infants who are at higher risk for neonatal mortality. A score of 7 or higher is reassuring (**Table 12.1**).

## AIRWAY

The American Heart Association (AHA) no longer recommends routine intrapartum oropharyngeal and nasopharyngeal suctioning because it has been shown to be associated with cardiopulmonary complications in healthy neonates. Oropharyngeal and nasopharyngeal suctioning should be reserved for newborns with obvious upper airway obstruction and associated respiratory distress.[3,4]

Meconium-stained amniotic fluid occurs in up to 20% of deliveries, and as many as 9% of infants with meconium-stained amniotic fluid experience meconium aspiration syndrome (MAS), which carries a modern-day mortality rate of up to 40%.[4]

MAS occurs when the fetus aspirates meconium before or during birth, which leads to obstruction of the airways, atelectasis, severe hypoxia, inflammation, acidosis, and infection.[5] The AHA guidelines regarding the management of a newborn with potential meconium aspiration make no distinction between thin and thick meconium because both have shown to lead to MAS.

In the absence of randomized controlled trials on routine tracheal suctioning of depressed infants born through meconium-stained amniotic fluid, the 2005 newborn resuscitation guidelines have not changed significantly. Thus, a nonvigorous newborn with meconium-stained amniotic fluid should not be suctioned on the mother's perineum. Avoiding such suctioning prevents undue stimulation, which would lead to breathing and aspiration of meconium before endotracheal suctioning.[6] Endotracheal intubation (ETI) and suctioning of meconium should be performed with a 10 French (F) to 14 F suction catheter and a meconium aspirator attached to an endotracheal tube. If intubation attempts are prolonged, bag-mask ventilation should not be delayed, especially when bradycardia is present.[4]

A vigorous neonate born with meconium-stained amniotic fluid does not require endotracheal suctioning for any level of meconium staining. Endotracheal suctioning has shown no benefit in this setting because the meconium has already caused irreversible damage to the lower airways. Vigorous is defined as having strong respiratory effort, good muscle tone, and a heart rate higher than 100 beats/min.[7]

## BREATHING

Methods to stimulate breathing in neonatal resuscitation are as follows:

- Rubbing the back/spine
- Flicking the soles of the feet
- Vigorously drying the skin

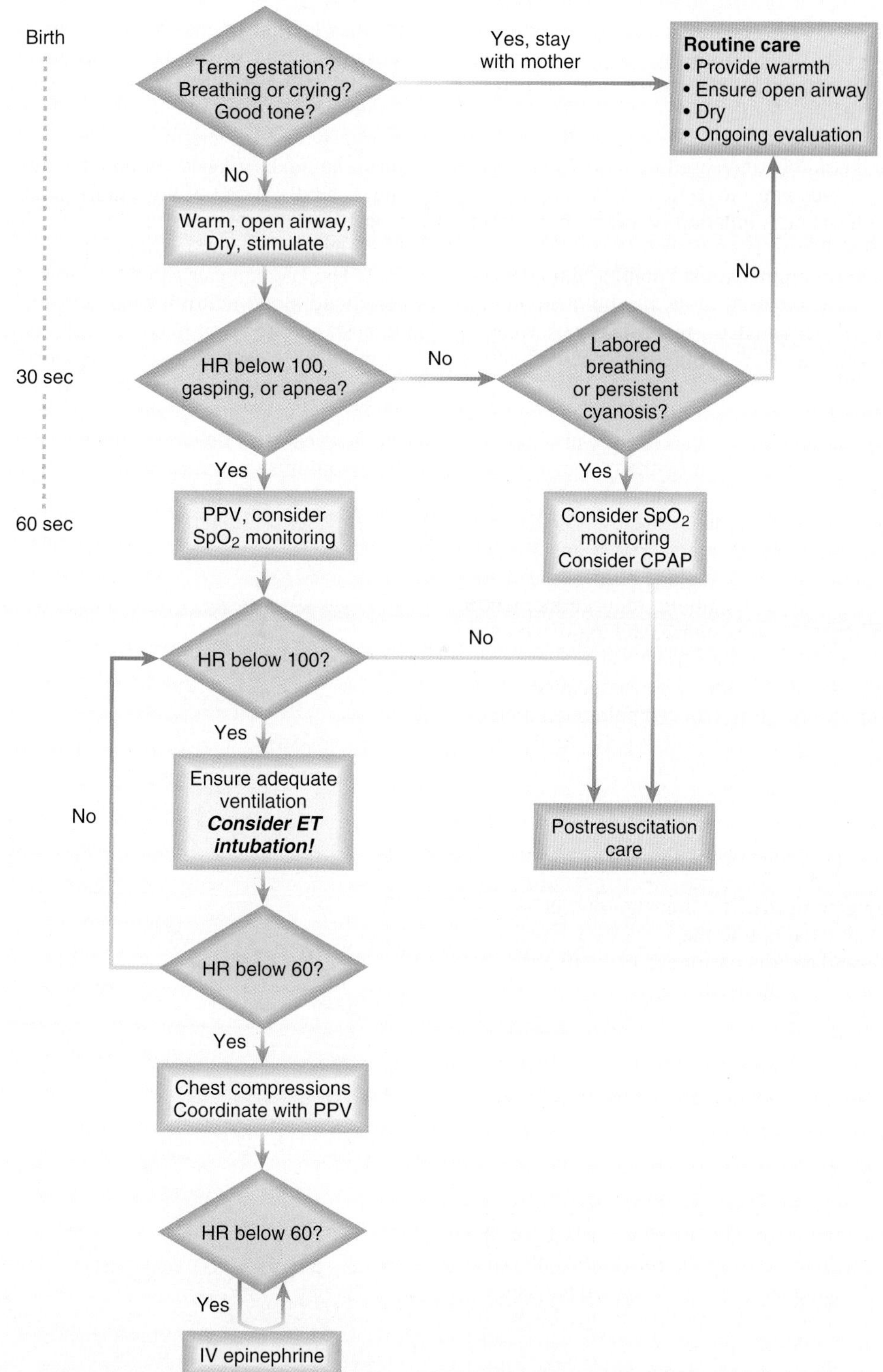


**Fig. 12.2 Newborn resuscitation algorithm.** *CPAP*, Continuous positive airway pressure; *ET*, endotracheal; *HR*, heart rate; *IV*, intravenous; *PPV*, positive pressure ventilation. (Modified from Kattwinkel J, Perlman JM, Aziz K, et al. Part 15: neonatal resuscitation: 2010 American Heart Association Guidelines for Cardiopulmonary Resuscitation and Emergency Cardiovascular Care. Circulation 2010;122:S909-19.)

If these measures are not stimulating an adequate change in heart rate, oxygenation, or activity, blow-by oxygen (blowing or wafting oxygen) should be administered.

Positive pressure ventilation (PPV) via a bag-valve-mask device at a rate of 40 to 60 breaths/min is indicated for the following situations[3,4]:

- The infant is apneic or gasping after warming, stimulation, and administration of blow-by oxygen.
- The heart rate remains lower than 100 beats/min after the preceding methods have been applied.
- The infant has persistent hypoxia.

Following pulse oximetry and titration of oxygen as needed, a term infant undergoing PPV should be started on room air and a preterm infant on a blend of air and oxygen. Starting PPV with 100% oxygen should be avoided because it is potentially harmful at the cellular level.

In a term infant, an initial inflation pressure of 20 cm $H_2O$ may be sufficient and could be increased to 30 to 40 cm $H_2O$ as needed to achieve adequate movement of the chest wall and elevation of the heart rate; inflation pressures in preterm infants should be 20 to 25 cm $H_2O$.

In the absence of meconium-stained amniotic fluid, laryngeal mask airways may be used in a newborn weighing more than 2000 g or delivered at more than 34 weeks' gestation and requiring assisted ventilation, but not chest compressions.[8]

Continuous positive airway pressure (CPAP) delivered via face mask immediately after delivery may be used in a neonate with respiratory effort but significant distress.[9] Devices that provide some level of CPAP include standard self-inflating bags, flow-inflating bags, and predetermined CPAP devices such as the Neopuff Infant Resuscitator (Fisher and Paykel, Auckland, NZ). Benefits of CPAP include reduced need for intubation, diminished work of breathing, reduced incidence of apnea, decreased inspiratory resistance, and improved oxygenation. Drawbacks include an increased risk for pneumothorax and those related to the risk associated with overdistention, which can result in reduced pulmonary perfusion, diminished cardiac output, and ultimately, ventilation-perfusion mismatch. The current AHA recommendations allow either CPAP or intubation to be used in infants requiring ventilatory support.[4]

Guidelines for ETI in neonatal resuscitation are as follows[3,4]:

- Tracheal suctioning is needed for nonvigorous newborns with meconium-stained amniotic fluid.
- Bag-valve-mask ventilation is prolonged or ineffective.
- Chest compressions are prolonged.
- Administration of medications by endotracheal tube is desired.
- Special considerations include conditions such as congenital diaphragmatic hernia or extremely low birth weight.

## CIRCULATION

It is recommended that assessment of the heart rate be performed via auscultation at the anterior surface of the chest. However, if palpation is used, the umbilical pulse should be used while recognizing that this method may underestimate the heart rate. If the heart rate remains below 60 beats/min despite respiratory support, chest compressions (on the lower third of the sternum and at a depth of one third the diameter of the chest) should be performed at a rate of at least 100 per minute with the two-finger or the preferred chest-encircling technique (**Fig. 12.3**). At this point, the ratio of chest compressions to breaths should be 3:1 unless a cardiac cause is suspected, in which case a 15:2 ratio should be considered.

If an intravenous (IV) line cannot be placed, an umbilical catheter can be used. The umbilical vein (UV) may be used for blood sampling, fluid or drug infusion, and monitoring of blood pressure and central venous pressure. Anatomically, there are typically two umbilical arteries (UAs) and one UV. The UV is usually in the 12-o'clock position and has a thinner wall and wider lumen than the UAs. The UV is often described as resembling a "smiley face." In emergency situations the UV is the preferred vessel to access because the UAs are often tortuous and difficult to cannulate. The umbilicus should be prepared with a bactericidal solution and draped, and a silk suture should be placed around the base of the umbilical stump. The distal end of the stump is cut off, and the vessels are occluded to prevent blood loss. A 3.5 to 5.0 F catheter is flushed with saline and inserted into the lumen of the desired vessel. The UV catheter should be advanced just to the point where good blood return is obtained (**Fig. 12.4**). Plain radiographs should be taken to confirm placement. Complications of umbilical catheters include hemorrhage, infection, air embolism, and perforation of a blood vessel.

Umbilical vein catheterization can reasonably be attempted up to 1 week after delivery, although the likelihood of cord patency diminishes with time.

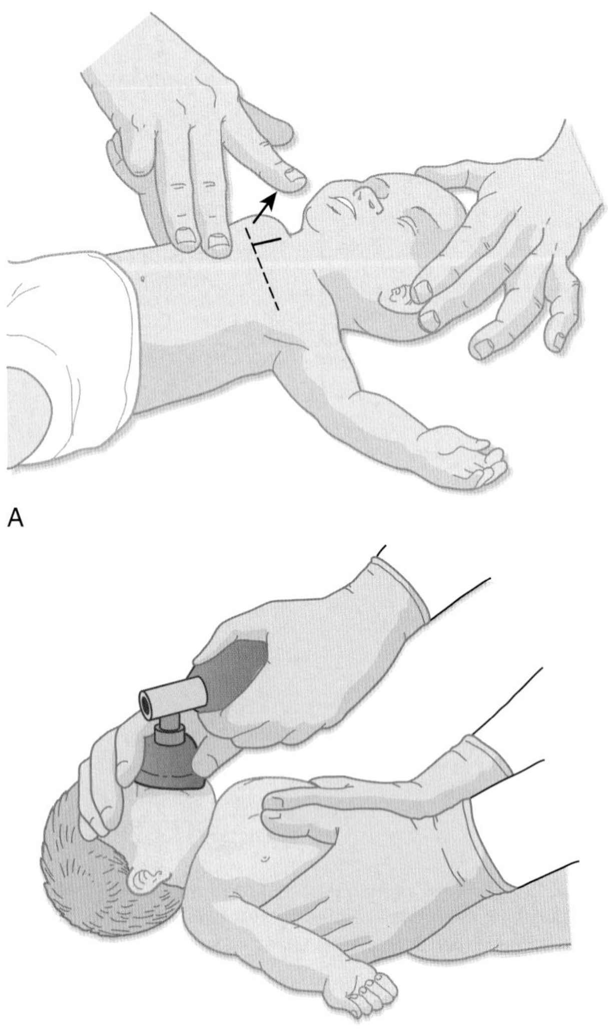


**Fig. 12.3 Two-finger (A) and chest-encircling (B) techniques.** A 3:1 ratio of compressions to ventilations should be used, which results in approximately 90 compressions and 30 ventilations per minute of cardiopulmonary resuscitation performed.

## MAINTENANCE OF TEMPERATURE

For a well term infant, temperature can be maintained with standard drying followed by swaddling and placement under warming lights or on the mother's warm skin.

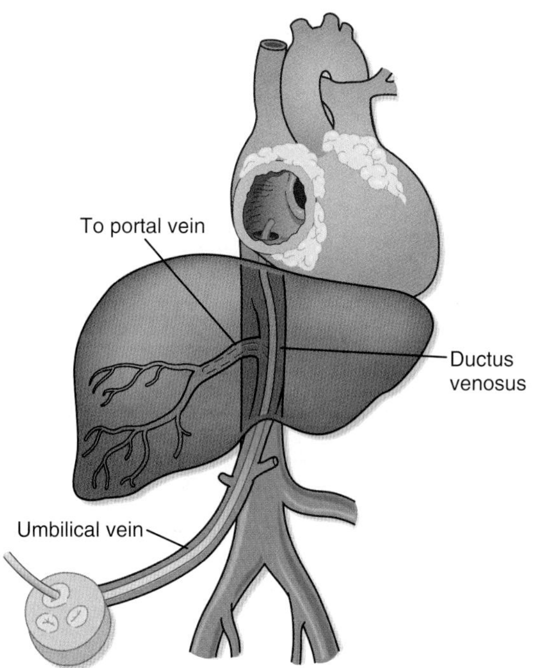


**Fig. 12.4 Umbilical vein catheterization.** The drawing illustrates passage of the catheter from the umbilical vein into the portal vein in the liver and then through the inferior vena cava to the right atrium. The tip of the catheter should be in the inferior vena cava, just at the entrance to the right atrium.

Very-low-birth-weight infants (<1500 g) require additional warming techniques. The AHA guidelines recommend wrapping the newborn in "food-grade heat-resistant plastic wrapping" and placing the newborn under radiant heat.

Some evidence indicates that induced hypothermia (33.5° C to 34.5° C) may decrease the rate of death or disability (or both) in asphyxiated newborns.[10] Using clearly defined protocols, infants born at greater than 36 weeks' gestation with suspected severe hypoxic-ischemic encephalopathy should be treated with therapeutic hypothermia within 6 hours. If these protocols are not in place, at the very least, hyperthermia should be strictly avoided.[3,4]

## RESUSCITATION MEDICATIONS AND VOLUME REPLACEMENT

The need for resuscitation medications is rare in the delivery room. Bradycardia is usually secondary to a primary respiratory cause. However, in the rare instance in which ventilatory support does not reverse the bradycardia, standard-dose IV epinephrine at 0.01 to 0.03 mg/kg of a 1 : 10,000 solution should be administered. Although IV administration is preferred, a higher dose of epinephrine, 0.05 to 0.1 mg/kg of a 1 : 10,000 solution, can be administered through the endotracheal tube until IV access has been established.

If volume replacement is necessary, isotonic crystalloid is recommended at 10 mL/kg, with repeated dosing as dictated by the clinical situation. Caution should be used when giving fluids because rapid newborn volume expansion has been associated with intraventricular hemorrhage (**Tables 12.2 and 12.3**). Glucose regulation is particularly important during the poststabilization period in an asphyxiated newborn, whose glycogen stores can be depleted rapidly. Although a target glucose level has not been established, a serum glucose level greater than 40 mg/dL should be maintained with the administration of 10% dextrose in water ($D_{10}W$).

**Table 12.2 Medications to Maintain Cardiac Output and for Postresuscitation Stabilization**

| MEDICATION | DOSE RANGE* | COMMENT |
|---|---|---|
| Inamrinone | 0.75-1 mg/kg IV/IO over 5 min; may repeat ×2; then 2-20 mcg/kg/min | Inodilator |
| Dobutamine | 2-20 mcg/kg/min IV/IO | Inotrope, vasodilator |
| Dopamine | 2-20 mcg/kg/min IV/IO | Inotrope, chronotrope, renal and splanchnic vasodilator in low doses, pressor in high doses |
| Epinephrine | 0.1-1 mcg/kg/min IV/IO | Inotrope, chronotrope, vasodilator in low doses, pressor in higher doses |
| Milrinone | 50-75 mcg/kg IV/IO over 10-60 min, then 0.5-0.75 mcg/kg/min | Inodilator |
| Norepinephrine | 0.1-2 mcg/kg/min | Inotrope, vasopressor |
| Sodium nitroprusside | 1-8 mcg/kg/min | Vasodilator, prepare only in $D_5W$ |

From 2005 American Heart Association Guidelines for Cardiopulmonary Resuscitation and Emergency Cardiovascular Care. Part 12: pediatric advanced life support. Circulation 2005;112(Suppl IV):IV-167-87.

*$D_5W$*, 5% dextrose in water; *IO*, intraosseously IV, intravenously.

*Alternative formula for calculating an infusion: Infusion rate (mL/hr) = Weight (kg) × Dose (mg/kg/min) × 60 (min/hr)] ÷ Concentration (mg/mL).

**Table 12.3 Medications for Pediatric Resuscitation and Arrhythmias**

| MEDICATION | DOSE | REMARKS |
|---|---|---|
| Adenosine | 0.1 mg/kg (maximum: 6 mg)<br>Repeat: 0.2 mg/kg (maximum: 12 mg) | Monitor the ECG<br>Rapid bolus IV/IO |
| Amiodarone | 5 mg/kg IV/IO; repeat up to 15 mg/kg<br>Maximum: 300 mg | Monitor the ECG and blood pressure<br>Adjust the administration rate to urgency (give more slowly when a perfusing rhythm present)<br>Use caution when administering with other drugs that prolong the QT interval (consider expert consultation) |
| Atropine | 0.02 mg/kg IV/IO<br>0.03 mg/kg ET*<br>Repeat once if needed<br>Minimum dose: 0.1 mg<br>Maximum single dose:<br>Child: 0.5 mg<br>Adolescent: 1 mg | Higher doses may be used with organophosphate poisoning |
| Calcium chloride (10%) | 20 mg/kg IV/IO (0.2 mL/kg) | Slowly<br>Adult dose: 5-10 mL |
| Epinephrine | 0.01 mg/kg (0.1 mL/kg 1:10,000) IV/IO<br>0.1 mg/kg (0.1 mL/kg 1:1000) ET*† <br>Maximum dose: 1 mg IV/IO; 10 mg ET | May repeat q3-5min |
| Glucose | 0.5-1 g/kg IV/IO | $D_{10}W$: 5-10 mL/kg<br>$D_{25}W$: 2-4 mL/kg<br>$D_{50}W$: 1-2 mL/kg |
| Lidocaine | Bolus: 1 mg/kg IV/IO<br>Maximum dose: 100 mg<br>Infusion: 20-50 mcg/kg/min | |
| Magnesium sulfate | 25-50 mg/kg IV/IO over 10-20 min; faster with torsades de pointes<br>Maximum dose: 2 g | |
| Naloxone | <5 yr or ≤20 kg: 0.1 mg/kg IV/IO/ET*‡<br>≥5 yr or >20 kg: 2 mg IV/IO/ET*‡ | Use lower doses to reverse respiratory depression associated with therapeutic opioid use (1-15 mcg/kg) |
| Procainamide | 15 mg/kg IV/IO over 30-60 min<br>Adult dose: 20-mg/min IV infusion up to total maximum dose of 17 mg/kg | Monitor ECG and blood pressure<br>Use caution when administering with other drugs that prolong the QT interval (consider expert consultation) |
| Sodium bicarbonate | 1 mEq/kg per dose IV/IO slowly | After adequate ventilation |

From 2005 American Heart Association Guidelines for Cardiopulmonary Resuscitation and Emergency Cardiovascular Care. Part 12: pediatric advanced life support. Circulation 2005;112(Suppl IV):IV-167-IV-187.

*$D_{10}W$*, 10% dextrose in water; *ECG*, electrocardiogram; *ET*, via endotracheal tube; *IO*, intraosseously; *IV*, intravenously.

*Flush with 5 mL of normal saline and follow with five ventilations.

†See text for neonatal ET dosing.

‡Not recommended in neonates.

Naloxone administration should generally be avoided in the resuscitation of a newborn at the time of delivery; instead, one should concentrate on support of breathing and the circulation. Administration of naloxone to mothers with known opioid addiction can have adverse outcomes and is not recommended by the AHA.[3]

Bicarbonate is not routinely recommended in the acute resuscitation of a newborn because of studies showing deleterious effects, including depression of myocardial function, intracellular acidosis, reductions in cerebral blood flow, and risk for intracranial hemorrhage.[11]

## REFERENCES

***References can be found on Expert Consult @ www.expertconsult.com.***

# Pediatric Resuscitation 13

*Ghazala Q. Sharieff and Katherine Bakes*

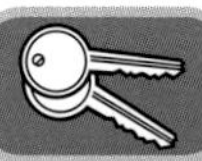

**KEY POINTS**

- Correct positioning is imperative for successful management of the anterior and cephalad pediatric airway.
- Outside the newborn period, use of a cuffed endotracheal tube in a child is acceptable.
- Children in full cardiorespiratory arrest who have an advanced airway should not receive more than 8 to 10 breaths per minute during resuscitation.
- "Push hard, push fast" with minimal interruptions between compressions is the recommendation for cardiopulmonary resuscitation.

## EPIDEMIOLOGY

Cardiac arrest in children most commonly stems from respiratory pathology, with pneumonia, asthma, bronchiolitis, and aspiration accounting for the most common causes. In pediatric in-hospital and out-of-hospital arrests, only 5% to 15% of patients will have pulseless ventricular tachycardia (VT) or ventricular fibrillation (VF). Although survival rates after in-hospital arrest have increased from 9% in the 1980s to 27% in 2006, the survival rate after out-of-hospital arrest has remained relatively constant at 6%.

Results from studies of pediatric in-patient cardiac arrest have shown that patients with VF or pulseless VT have a 34% survival rate to discharge whereas patients with pulseless electrical activity have a 38% survival rate. The worst outcomes occur in children with asystole, with only 24% of these children surviving to hospital discharge. Infants and children with a pulse but poor perfusion and bradycardia who require cardiopulmonary resuscitation (CPR) have the best survival to discharge (64%), thus suggesting that early intervention to prevent full cardiopulmonary arrest portends the best outcomes.

## BASIC PRINCIPLES OF CARDIOPULMONARY RESUSCITATION

Single-rescuer CPR providers should institute emergency medical service treatment after 1 minute of rescue breathing and compressions if the patient is younger than 8 years because the underlying cause is more likely to be respiratory than cardiac in this population. The American Heart Association (AHA) recommends "push hard and push fast" with compressions. Infants and children should have a compression rate of at least 100 per minute. In single-rescuer CPR, the compression-to-ventilation ratio should be 30 : 2. For health care providers or responders trained in CPR, the ratio is 15 : 2. In newborns, the compression-to-ventilation ratio should be 3 : 1. According to the pediatric advanced life support (PALS) guidelines, adequate compression depth is approximately one third to one half the anterior-posterior diameter of the patient's chest—4 cm in infants and 5 cm in children. In infants, the two-thumb method is preferred over the finger method for compressions. For optimal compressions, full recoil of the chest should take place after each compression, with a firm surface behind the victim.

The effectiveness of CPR is best judged by the presence of a femoral pulse with corresponding chest compressions. Interruptions in compressions have been shown to decrease the rate of return to spontaneous circulation and should be limited to less than 10 seconds for interventions such as placement of an advanced airway or defibrillation. Rhythm checks should be performed every 2 minutes (every five cycles of CPR). Once an advanced airway is in place, compressions and breaths should be performed continuously without interruption. Because of rescuer fatigue and the importance of proper compressions, it is ideal for the person performing compressions to be rotated every 2 minutes.

Foreign body removal maneuvers consist of a sequence of five back blows and five chest thrusts for infants and the Heimlich maneuver for children (**Fig. 13.1**). Blind finger sweeps should not be performed in children because a partial obstruction can be turned into a full obstruction if the foreign body is pushed further into the airway. Because of the pliability of the esophageal wall, foreign bodies in the esophagus can impinge on the trachea and result in airway obstruction. If the foreign body cannot be removed with basic life support maneuvers and the patient decompensates, the clinician can attempt to remove any visible foreign body with Magill forceps. Intubation may be required, and it may be possible to push the foreign body into a mainstem bronchus, most commonly on the right side. If this maneuver fails and the patient cannot be intubated, the last resort is either needle cricothyrotomy or a surgical airway. In a stable patient, bronchoscopy with maintenance of the patient's position of comfort is the treatment of choice.

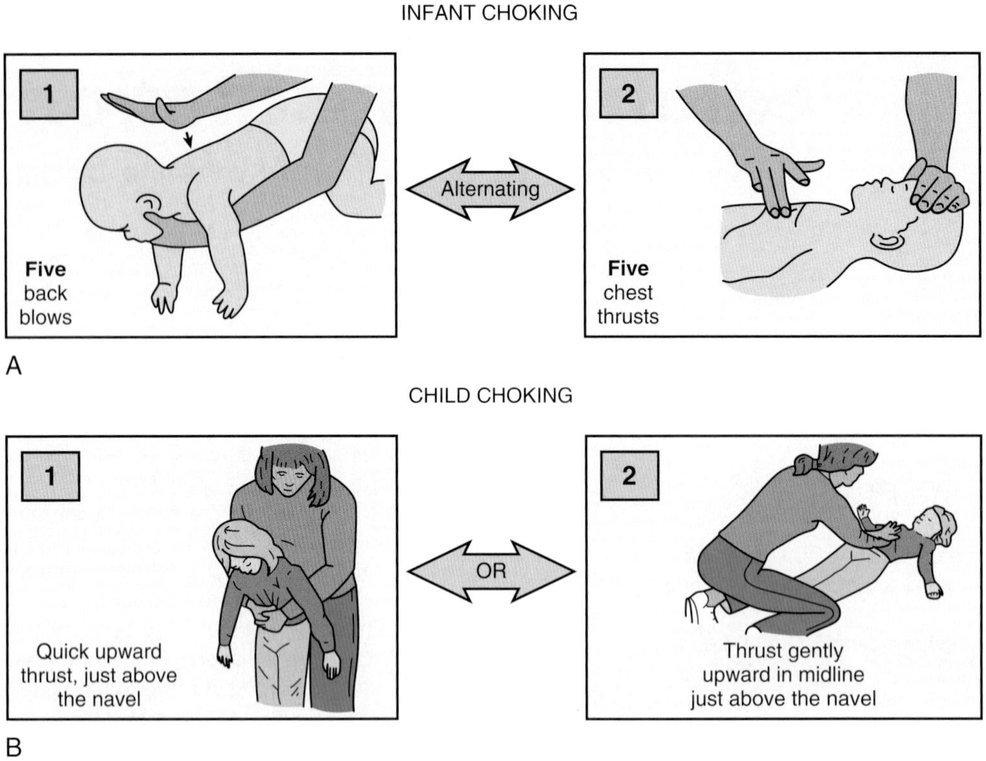

INFANT CHOKING

1 Five back blows — Alternating — 2 Five chest thrusts

A

CHILD CHOKING

1 Quick upward thrust, just above the navel — OR — 2 Thrust gently upward in midline just above the navel

B

**Fig. 13.1** Foreign body removal techniques in infants and children.

**BOX 13.1 Ways in Which a Child's Airway Differs Anatomically from an Adult's Airway**

The prominent occiput can cause airway obstruction and impede glottic visualization during intubation; a 1-inch towel roll should be placed below the shoulders
Dependence on nasopharynx patency; nasal airways should be avoided in children younger than 1 year because their larger adenoidal tissue can bleed
Copious secretions
Loose primary teeth
The relatively larger tongues can obstruct the airway and often necessitate an oral or nasal airway
The epiglottis is omega (Ω) shaped and floppy; a straight laryngoscope blade is used to lift the epiglottis out of view
The larynx is more anterior and cephalad
The cricoid is the narrowest portion of the airway
Small tracheal diameter and distance between rings, which makes tracheostomy or cricothyrotomy more difficult; the American Heart Association recommends needle cricothyrotomy for difficult airways (see text discussion of this modality)
Much shorter tracheal length (newborn, 4 to 5 cm; 18-month-old child, 7 to 8 cm)
The endotracheal tube may easily be dislodged; frequently reassess position of the tube
Greater airway resistance
Increased risk for aspiration and diaphragmatic dependence*

*Decompress the stomach to facilitate ventilation; a rough guide to nasogastric tube size is twice the endotracheal tube size.

## AIRWAY MANAGEMENT

Airway management in children can be anxiety provoking; the same preparation guidelines outlined in Chapter 1 should be followed. Signs of respiratory failure include an increased or decreased respiratory rate, nasal flaring, grunting, retractions, cyanosis, apnea, or altered mental status. Hypoxia, compromised airway protection, altered mental status, and impending respiratory failure are common indications for pediatric airway intervention. Because most pediatric cardiac arrests are secondary to respiratory failure, early airway intervention is crucial.

## ANATOMY

The pediatric airway differs significantly from the adult airway (**Box 13.1**), and some special techniques are helpful when intubating a child. An oral or nasal airway can assist in maintaining airway patency. Because of the large occiput in a young child, typically those younger than 1 year, a towel roll placed beneath the patient's shoulders often improves airway alignment. To visualize the very anterior pediatric airway, the operator must look up during intubation and may need to squat or raise the bed for adequate viewing. To see the glottic opening, a straight blade is recommended to lift up an infant's floppy omega-shaped epiglottis. Because of infants' small mouths, an assistant may need to pull the baby's cheek to the side to allow passage of the laryngoscope and endotracheal tube.[1,2]

## RAPID-SEQUENCE INTUBATION IN CHILDREN

The intubating time line and drugs of choice are listed in **Tables 13.1 and 13.2**. Postintubation assessment includes confirmation that the endotracheal tube is in correct position. First listen over the stomach and then over the axillae for breath sounds. A confirmatory device such as an end-tidal carbon dioxide monitor, a carbon dioxide chart (e.g., Pedi-Cap, which should change from purple to yellow with proper tube placement), or an esophageal detector should be used.[3,4] A nasogastric or orogastric tube should also be placed as soon as possible because any amount of gastric distention can make ventilation and oxygenation of a child difficult. A rough rule of thumb for nasogastric and orogastric tube size is two times the endotracheal tube size.

**Table 13.1** Paralytic Agents Commonly Used for Intubation in Children*

| AGENT | DOSE (MG/KG) | ONSET OF ACTION | DURATION OF ACTION (MIN) | COMMENTS |
|---|---|---|---|---|
| Succinylcholine | 1-2 | <1 min | <10 | Can cause bradycardia<br>DO NOT USE in children with chronic muscular disorders |
| Rocuronium | 1.0 | <1 min | 40-60 | Causes no change in potassium<br>Does not cause malignant hyperthermia |
| Vecuronium | 0.1 or 0.3 | 2-3 min or 60-90 sec | 30-40 or up to 100 | |

*Timed intubation: When using nondepolarizing agents, it is not necessary to induce anesthesia in the patient immediately. This permits a timed intubation in which the nondepolarizing agent is administered first and subclinical muscle relaxation is begun. Approximately 15 seconds later the induction agent is administered. Both agents then therapeutically overlap at about 30 to 45 seconds after the beginning of the procedure, which results in good intubating conditions.

**Table 13.2** Induction Agents for Intubation in Children

| DRUG | DOSE (MG/KG) | ONSET OF ACTION (SEC) | DURATION (MIN) | BLOOD PRESSURE RESPONSE | INTRACRANIAL PRESSURE RESPONSE | SIDE EFFECTS |
|---|---|---|---|---|---|---|
| Propofol | 1-2 | 10-20 | 3-14 | Decreases | Decreases | Antiepileptic effects<br>DO NOT USE in patients with soy or egg allergies |
| Etomidate | 0.3 | 20-30 | 7-14 | None | May decrease | Adrenal suppression, myoclonic jerks |
| Ketamine | IV: 1-2<br>IM: 4 | 15-60 | IV: 10-15<br>IM: 20-30 | Increases | Increases | Bronchial relaxation, myocardial depression |
| Thiopental | 3.0-5.0 | 20-30 | 3-5 | Decreases | Decreases | Antiepileptic effects<br>Can cause bronchospasm |
| Midazolam | 0.1-0.3 | 30-60 | IV: 30 | Decreases | May decrease | Antiepileptic effects |

*IM*, Intramuscularly; *IV*, intravenously.

**Table 13.3 Clinical Scenarios for Intubation and Recommended Induction Agents**

| CLINICAL SCENARIO | INDUCTION AGENTS |
|---|---|
| Isolated head injury | Propofol<br>Thiopental<br>Etomidate<br>? Do not use ketamine* |
| Status epilepticus | Thiopental<br>Propofol<br>Etomidate<br>Midazolam |
| Asthma | Ketamine<br>Etomidate<br>DO NOT USE thiopental |
| Respiratory failure | Ketamine<br>Etomidate<br>Propofol |

Adapted from a presentation by Sacchetti A. Boston: American College of Emergency Physicians Scientific Assembly; 2003.

*Several intensive care unit studies have shown that in intubated patients, ketamine does not increase intracranial pressure and may help maintain cerebral perfusion pressure. However, no emergency department studies have been performed to date.

**Table 13.4 Procedure for Rapid-Sequence Intubation in Children**

| | |
|---|---|
| Time to intubation 5 min | Start preoxygenation |
| Time to intubation 3 min | Give any premedication (atropine, lidocaine) |
| Intubation time | Push induction and paralytic agents |
| After the patient is relaxed | Intubate:<br>Apply cricoid pressure<br>Use the BURP (**b**ackward, **u**pward, and **r**ightward **p**ressure) technique* |
| Immediately after intubation | Release cricoid pressure<br>Secure the endotracheal tube<br>Place a nasogastric tube |

*Too much pressure can occlude the airway.

**BOX 13.2 Ways of Choosing Endotracheal Tube Size**

1. Estimate size according to the patient's age:
   - Newborns, 3.0 mm, or in large newborn, 3.5 mm
   - Up to 6 months, 3.5 to 4.0 mm
   - 1 year, 4.0 to 4.5 mm
   - Older than 1 year:
     - Uncuffed tube: 4 + (age ÷ 4)
     - Cuffed tube: 3.5 + (age ÷ 4). Cuffed tubes should not be used in neonates
2. Use a length-based resuscitation tape, such as the Broselow-Luten
3. Estimate according to the patient's finger:
   - The width of the child's little fingernail is used to estimate the internal diameter of the endotracheal tube
   - The width of the child's little finger is equal to the width of the whole endotracheal tube

## PHARMACOLOGIC AGENTS FOR RAPID-SEQUENCE INTUBATION IN CHILDREN

Potential combinations of agents for rapid-sequence intubation are listed in **Table 13.3**. Pretreatment with multiple agents is not recommended because placement of an advanced airway may be delayed. Atropine has recently been called into question for routine use in pediatric intubation, but it is recommended in infants younger than 1 year to avoid the bradycardia associated with airway manipulation in this population. The dose of atropine ranges from 0.01 to 0.02 mg/kg (minimum dose, 0.1 mg).

## PRINCIPLES OF ENDOTRACHEAL INTUBATION

Recommended endotracheal tube sizes are listed in **Box 13.2**. With the advent of high-volume, low-pressure cuffed endotracheal tubes, the dictum of using only uncuffed endotracheal tubes in children younger than 8 years has changed. It is not only acceptable but at times preferable (high peak pressure) to use a cuffed endotracheal tube in children. For an approximate guide to tube size, use 4 + (age ÷ 4) for uncuffed tubes and 3.5 + (age ÷ 4) for cuffed tubes. Cuff inflation pressure should be kept less than 20 to 25 cm $H_2O$. Cuffed endotracheal tubes are not recommended for use in neonates.[5,6]

**Table 13.4** summarizes the procedure for rapid-sequence intubation in children.

An incorrect endotracheal tube size can lead to an inability to ventilate if the tube is too small or result in airway trauma (e.g., subglottic edema) if the tube is too large. Easy formulas for estimating the depth of endotracheal tube placement are as follows:

3 × endotracheal tube size; for example, a 4.0-mm tube placed with the 12-cm mark at the gum line

10 + age in years = number of centimeters of the tube to the lips

For premature infants, the following estimations of tube depth based on body weight are helpful:

1 kg: 7 cm
2 kg: 8 cm
3 kg: 9 cm
4 kg: 10 cm

Approximate laryngoscope sizes are listed in **Table 13.5**. The Broselow-Luten resuscitation tape can also be used to select the weight-based appropriate size. It is important to remember that the actual blade size needed is determined by the individual patient's weight, body habitus, and anatomic variability. Preparation is essential; having laryngoscope blades available that are one size smaller and one size larger than anticipated prevents costly delays.

Once endotracheal tube placement is confirmed, the tube must be secured. The endotracheal tube can be dislodged very easily, particularly in young infants with small tracheal widths.

**Table 13.5** Choosing Laryngoscope Size and Type for a Child

| AGE OR WEIGHT | LARYNGOSCOPE SIZE | LARYNGOSCOPE TYPE |
|---|---|---|
| 2.5 kg | 0 | Straight |
| 0-3 mo | 1.0 | Straight |
| 3 mo-3 yr | 1.5-2.0 or 1.5 | Straight or curved Wisconsin |
| 3-12 yr | 2.0-4.0 | Straight or curved |

A cervical collar, even in the nontrauma setting, can minimize tube motion and dislodgement.

**Table 13.6** Recommended Laryngeal Mask Airway Sizes

| PATIENT AGE AND WEIGHT | SIZE |
|---|---|
| Neonates to 5 kg | 1 |
| Infants/children | |
| 5-10 kg | 1½ |
| 10-20 kg | 2 |
| 20-30 kg | 2½ |
| 30-50 kg | 3 |
| Adults | |
| 50-70 kg | 4 |
| 70-100 kg | 5 |
| >100 kg | 6 |

## BREATHING

### Bag-Valve-Mask Ventilation

Self-inflating, hand-squeezed resuscitators are commonly used in children because of the elasticity of the self-inflating bag, which allows independent refilling. Many of these bags have a pressure-limited pop-off valve, typically set at 30 to 35 cm $H_2O$ to prevent barotrauma. Sometimes higher pressure is required, depending on the child's pathophysiology. Correct mask sizing is vital for proper bag-valve-mask ventilation. The mask should fit snugly from the bridge of the nose to the cleft of the chin. A mask that is too large can place pressure on the eyes and cause vagal bradycardia. A mask that is too small will not allow adequate oxygenation and ventilation. The mask should be held with a "CE" grip—the holder's thumb and index finger grip the mask and the third, fourth, and fifth fingers are placed on the angle of jaw. It is important to avoid pushing on the soft tissue below the mandible, which can cause airway obstruction.

The rate of bagged breaths per minute is best controlled by having the operator say "squeeze-release-release" as the patient is being ventilated. This practice helps decrease the rapid rate of ventilation and resultant adverse effects of over-inflation. Patients in full arrest with an advanced airway in place should not receive more than 8 to 10 breaths/min via either a bag-valve-mask ventilator or an endotracheal tube. Complications of bag-valve-mask ventilation include gastric distention, pneumothorax, vomiting, aspiration, and hypoxia.

Appropriate bag size can be chosen as follows:

- For an infant or child up to 5 years of age: 450-mL bag
- For an older child: 750-mL or adult bag

To prevent confusion in resuscitation situations, neonatal 250-mL bags, which are inadequate for any child older than a newborn, should be well labeled and stocked in a separate area with other newborn resuscitation equipment.

### Initial Ventilator Settings

Initial ventilator settings are typically chosen through assessment of the height and weight of the patient and the underlying cause of the respiratory distress.

For children weighing less than 10 kg, a pressure-limited system should be used. The infant should be given sufficient oxygen to relieve cyanosis and maintain normal oxygen saturation (92% to 96%) or normal $PO_2$ (60 to 90 mm Hg). The following are recommended initial ventilator settings:

Rate: 20 to 60 breaths/min (goal $PaCO_2$, 35 to 45 mm Hg)
Fraction of inspired oxygen ($FIO_2$): 100% (wean slowly based on pulse oximetry)
Positive end-expiratory pressure (PEEP): 3 to 5 cm $H_2O$
Peak inspiratory pressure: 15 to 35 cm $H_2O$ (or sufficient to produce discernible chest wall movement)
Inspiratory time–to–expiratory time (I/E) ratio: 1:2 (inspiratory time of 0.4 to 0.7 second)

For children weighing more than 10 kg, a volume-limited system should be used. The following are recommended initial ventilator settings:

Volume: 10 to 15 mL/kg (if plateau pressure is greater than 35 mm $H_2O$ and for asthmatics, decrease to 6 to 8 mL/kg)
Rate: an for infant, 20 to 30 breaths/min; for a child, 15 to 20 breaths/min
$FIO_2$: 100% (wean slowly based on pulse oximetry)
PEEP: 3 to 5 cm $H_2O$
I/E ratio: 1:2

## THE DIFFICULT PEDIATRIC AIRWAY

### Failed Intubation

In the event that endotracheal intubation is unsuccessful, several options are available for airway rescue. The laryngeal mask airway (LMA) has the advantages of easy placement without the need for laryngoscopy and little cardiac effect during the insertion process. Disadvantages include the lack of airway protection from vomiting or aspiration of gastric contents, the requirement that the patient be unconscious or sedated for placement, and the fact that an LMA is not a definitive airway. Furthermore, in children less than 30 kg, higher ventilatory pressure may be required because the LMA can fold the epiglottis over and cause partial upper airway obstruction.

Approximate LMA sizes are listed in **Table 13.6**.

Complications of LMA placement are partial upper airway obstruction, coughing or bronchospasm, aspiration or regurgitation, airway trauma, lingual nerve palsy, vocal cord paralysis, hypoglossal nerve paralysis, hoarseness, stridor, and pharyngeal or mouth ulcers.

### Needle Cricothyrotomy (Jet Ventilation)

Needle cricothyrotomy should be used when endotracheal intubation is not successful. It is most often indicated in children younger than 10 to 12 years, in whom a surgical airway is technically difficult to perform. This chapter describes various oxygen setups that can be used in any emergency department to ventilate by needle cricothyrotomy without a jet ventilator attachment. The procedure for placing the needle is quite simple:

1. Identify the cricothyroid membrane; prepare with povidone-iodine solution if possible.
2. Use a 12- to 14-gauge angiocatheter attached to a syringe to puncture the cricothyroid membrane.
3. Direct the catheter at a 45-degree angle caudally (toward the patient's feet). Placement of normal saline in the syringe helps demonstrate when air is aspirated.
4. Remove the needle from the angiocatheter.

With these methods the child can be oxygenated, but ventilation ($CO_2$ exhalation) is limited.

### Methods of Ventilation

Once the angiocatheter is placed, one of the following methods may be chosen for ventilation:

- Attach the following items to the angiocatheter: a 3-mL syringe barrel, a 7.0 French (F) endotracheal tube adapter, and a bag-valve-mask ventilator. Turn the wall oxygen ($O_2$) up to 15 L and attempt to administer ventilation with the bag through the angiocatheter.
- Attach a 3.0 F endotracheal tube adapter directly to the angiocatheter and then a bag-valve-mask ventilator; turn the wall $O_2$ up to 15 L and attempt to administer ventilation with the bag and through the angiocatheter.
- Attach one prong of a nasal cannula to the angiocatheter and use the other prong for oxygen flow (1 second on for inspiration, 4 seconds off for expiration).
- Use an Enk Oxygen Flow Modulator Kit (Cook Medical).
- The QuickTrach kit (Rusch, Inc.) can also be used for cricothyrotomy.

## CIRCULATION

Volume resuscitation starts with 20 mL/kg of normal saline or lactated Ringer solution. In newborns, 10 mL/kg is a good starting point. Boluses may be repeated. In cases of hemorrhagic shock, if blood pressure does not improve after two or three boluses, packed red blood cells should be given at a dose of 10 mL/kg. The PALS formula for a blood pressure goal in children notes that the 5th percentile is 70 + (2 × age in years). Because this is only the 5th percentile, the preferred formula is 90 + (2 × age in years). Normal systolic blood pressure for term neonates is 60 mm Hg.

Shock results from inadequate blood flow and delivery of oxygen to meet the metabolic needs of the body. In children, the most common type of shock is hypovolemic.

**Table 13.7 Postresuscitation Medications**

| MEDICATION | DOSE RANGE |
|---|---|
| Inamrinone | 0.75-1 mg/kg IV/IO over 5-min period; may repeat twice, then 5-10 mcg/kg/min |
| Dobutamine | 2-20 mcg/kg/min IV/IO |
| Dopamine | 2-20 mcg/kg/min IV/IO |
| Epinephrine | 0.1-1 mcg/kg/min IV/IO |
| Milrinone | Loading dose: 50 mcg/kg IV/IO over 10- to 60-min period, then 0.25-0.75 mcg/kg/min |
| Norepinephrine | 0.1-2 mcg/kg/min |
| Sodium nitroprusside | Initially, 0.5-1 mcg/kg/min; titrate to effect up to 8 mcg/kg/min |

*IO*, Intraosseously; *IV*, intravenously.

Compensated shock is defined by the presence of tachycardia, cool extremities, prolonged capillary refill time, and weak peripheral pulses with normal systolic blood pressure. Decompensated shock occurs when hypotension, weak central pulses, and weak or absent peripheral pulses develop. **Table 13.7** lists the most commonly used medications for maintaining cardiac output and for postresuscitation stabilization.

## PERIPHERAL INTRAVENOUS LINES

The large peripheral veins, including the antecubital and saphenous veins, are good options in patients of all ages; a small, 20- to 24-gauge catheter may be necessary. Scalp veins and the external jugular veins are also excellent options if intravenous access in the extremities is difficult.

## INTRAOSSEOUS ACCESS

An intraosseous line should be considered when emergency access is necessary and peripheral vascular access cannot be obtained. The preferred site for placement of an intraosseous line is the anteromedial surface of the proximal end of the tibia 1 cm inferior and 1 cm medial to the tibial tubercle. Alternative sites are the distal end of the femur, the medial malleolus, the distal end of the humerus, and the anterior superior iliac crest. In older children and adults, attempts at intraosseous access may be made in the distal ends of the tibia and the radius and the ulna. In addition to commercially available intraosseous infusion needles (EZ-IO, BIG [Bone Injection Gun]), 15- and 18-gauge Jamshidi-type bone marrow aspiration needles are often used. Contraindications to placement of an intraosseous vascular line are a current attempt in the same area, cellulitis, fracture in the same bone, and osteogenesis imperfecta (relative contraindication).

The procedure for establishing intraosseous access in the anterior part of the tibia is as follows:

1. The skin over the anterior surface of the tibia is sterilized.
2. Starting 1 to 3 cm below the tibial tuberosity (to avoid damaging the growth plate), the needle is directed at a 90-degree angle to the medial surface of the tibia.

3. Once the cortex is passed, the operator must stop pushing to avoid forcing the needle through the other side of the bone.

The following signs help confirm that the needle is in the marrow cavity:

- A sudden decrease in resistance is felt as the needle passes through the cortex.
- The needle stands upright without support.
- When a syringe is attached to the needle, bone marrow may be aspirated. If this is not possible, an infusion flush should be used because it is common to be unable to aspirate marrow.
- Fluid infuses freely without signs of subcutaneous infiltration.

Any drug or fluid that can be administered intravenously can be infused rapidly through an intraosseous line. It should be noted that intraosseous lines are high-pressure systems; any fluid must be infused via either a pump or syringe. The aspirate can be sent for all laboratory studies except a complete blood count. Complications of intraosseous infusions are rare but include growth plate damage, osteomyelitis, compartment syndrome, tibial fracture, and skin necrosis.

### CENTRAL VENOUS ACCESS

Emergency indications for central venous access are an inability to establish peripheral venous or intraosseous access and monitoring of a hemodynamically unstable patient.

A 3 or 4 F percutaneous central venous catheter should be used in infants younger than 1 year and a 4 to 5.5 F catheter in children 1 year to 12 years of age. The subclavian, internal jugular, or femoral vein may be accessed with the percutaneous central venous catheter. The femoral vein is the easiest and safest central vein to cannulate in emergencies because of its large diameter and ability to be cannulated while CPR is in progress. The procedure is as follows:

1. The leg is slightly externally rotated and the area prepared and draped in sterile fashion.
2. The femoral vein is located medial to the femoral artery. In conscious patients, the area below the inguinal ligament, medial to the femoral artery, should be infiltrated with 1% lidocaine.
3. In children, the introducer needle is directed at a 30- to 40-degree angle to the skin, starting about 1 cm below the inguinal ligament and aiming toward the contralateral shoulder or umbilicus.
4. Once a flash of blood is obtained, the guidewire is threaded through the introducer.
5. The Seldinger technique is then followed to complete line placement.

## RESUSCITATIVE DRUGS

### EPINEPHRINE

The initial intravenous or intraosseous dose of epinephrine for patients in pulseless arrest who are older than neonates is 0.01 mg/kg (0.1 mL/kg) of a 1:10,000 standard epinephrine solution. All endotracheal doses are 0.1 mg (0.1 mL/kg) of a 1:1000 solution for pulseless arrest. Note that intravenous epinephrine and endotracheal epinephrine doses have the same number of milliliters; only the concentration of the drug changes. Little evidence exists that endotracheal administration improves outcomes. Though reasonable to perform when alternative access is not available, endotracheal administration should not delay establishing intravenous or intraosseous access. These doses may be administered every 3 to 5 minutes during arrest. Evidence suggests that high-dose epinephrine may worsen outcomes; consequently, PALS guidelines no longer recommend high-dose epinephrine except for special circumstances such as beta-blocker overdose.[7] For bradycardia, epinephrine may be given intravenously or intraosseously at 0.01 mg/kg (0.1 mL/kg) of a 1:10,000 solution or 0.1 mg/kg (0.1 mL/kg) of a 1:1000 solution via endotracheal tube.

### VASOPRESSIN

Although some adult studies have investigated the use of vasopressin for cardiac arrest, the pediatric literature to date does not provide clear evidence for its use in children. One pediatric study revealed that the use of vasopressin was associated with lower return of spontaneous circulation and a trend toward lower 24-hour and discharge survival.[7]

### ATROPINE

Atropine increases the heart rate and may help improve cardiac output. Atropine is indicated for symptomatic bradycardia associated with increased vagal tone or primary atrioventricular block after oxygenation-ventilation and epinephrine have been administered. It is also helpful in decreasing the vagolytic effects of airway manipulation in infants and children during intubation.

The recommended dose of atropine is 0.02 mg/kg, with a minimum dose of 0.1 mg (maximum single dose, 0.5 mg in children and 1.0 mg in adolescents); use of less than 0.1 mg may result in paradoxic bradycardia. The total of the two maximum doses should not exceed 1.0 mg in children or 2.0 mg in adolescents. The most efficacious dose of endotracheal atropine is unknown, but the currently recommended dose is 0.03 mg/kg.

### ELECTROLYTES

In infants and small children, the small reserve of endogenous glucose in the form of hepatic glycogen is readily exhausted during stress. In resuscitation settings, access to rapid and accurate bedside glucose testing is essential. Serum levels of glucose and lactate, its anaerobic end product, can be monitored during the resuscitation process. If needed, glucose can be given intravenously or intraosseously at a dose of 2 to 4 mL of 25% dextrose in water ($D_{25}W$) per kilogram. Peripheral vein sclerosis can occur in neonates if high glucose concentrations are used; therefore, $D_{10}W$ should be used in neonates (range, 2 to 10 mL).

Per the 2010 PALS update, routine administration of calcium is not recommended and has been shown to be associated with worse outcomes in pediatric CPR. Indications for administration of calcium are calcium channel blocker toxicity, hypocalcemia, hyperkalemia, and hypermagnesemia. Calcium chloride (10%) in a dose of 20 mg/kg (0.2 mL/kg) is the calcium solution of choice but can be administered only via an intraosseous or central line. Magnesium at a dose of 25 to 50 mg/kg (maximum, 2 g) may be used for hypomagnesemia or torsades de pointes.

According to the latest PALS consensus guidelines, routine administration of sodium bicarbonate is not recommended for pediatric arrest because it has been associated with decreased survival, but it may be indicated for cases of hyperkalemia or toxic ingestion (e.g., tricyclic antidepressants or other drugs with sodium channel–blocking effects). For specific indications, sodium bicarbonate can be given intravenously or intraosseously at a dose of 1 mEq/kg.

## ADENOSINE

Adenosine is a short-acting agent that slows conduction through the atrioventricular node and also acts to block reentry circuits. The treatment of choice for patients with stable supraventricular reentrant tachycardia, adenosine can be administered to unstable patients while preparing for cardioversion. The starting dose of adenosine is 0.1 mg/kg (maximum initial dose, 6 mg) given as centrally as possible and followed immediately by a 5-mL normal saline flush. The second dose is 0.2 mg/kg (maximum dose, 12 mg). Side effects include facial flushing, chest pain, bronchospasm, and anxiety. Because of the short half-life of adenosine, these effects resolve within 10 to 20 seconds.

## LIDOCAINE

Lidocaine is a class I antiarrhythmic agent that may be used in patients with VT and VF or symptomatic ventricular arrhythmias. The initial dose is a 1-mg/kg bolus (maximum dose, 100 mg), followed by a drip at 20 to 50 mcg/kg/min. The endotracheal tube dose is 2 to 3 mg/kg.

## AMIODARONE

Amiodarone is a class III antiarrhythmic agent that is now recommended for patients with VF and pulseless VT and should be administered as a 5-mg/kg bolus. The dose may be repeated up to a maximum of 15 mg/kg. Amiodarone can also be used for VT with a pulse or for supraventricular tachycardia (SVT) at a dose of 5 mg/kg infused over a 20- to 60-minute period. It is important to avoid concomitant use of amiodarone and procainamide because this combination can precipitate hypotension and QT prolongation.

## PROCAINAMIDE

Procainamide may also be used for VT with a pulse and for SVT. The dose is 15 mg/kg given over a period of 30 to 60 minutes. Amiodarone and procainamide should not be routinely administered together because the combination can precipitate hypotension and QT prolongation.

# INTERVENTIONS

Defibrillation is the immediate treatment for patients with witnessed pulseless VT or VF. If the time of arrest in unknown, CPR should be initiated for 2 minutes (five cycles) before attempts at defibrillation. "Stacked shocks" are no longer recommended. Instead, each shock should be followed by 2 minutes of CPR.

Synchronized cardioversion energy levels for SVT and unstable tachyarrhythmias are 0.5 to 1.0 J/kg, whereas unsynchronized cardioversion (defibrillation) for VF or pulseless VT starts at 2 J/kg. **Figure 13.2** illustrates an algorithm for potentially lethal arrhythmias. The new 2010 AHA guidelines recommend that the second and subsequent defibrillation attempts use 4 J/kg. A maximum of 10 J/kg may be attempted if the provider believes it to be warranted.

Management of pulseless electrical activity in children is similar to that in adults. The airway should be controlled, intravenous access obtained, and CPR initiated. Specific, treatable causes of pulseless electrical activity should be sought, including hypovolemia, hypoxemia, acidosis, hypothermia, hyperkalemia, tension pneumothorax, cardiac tamponade, ingestion of toxic substances, pulmonary embolism, and myocardial infarction. **Figure 13.3** outlines the cardiac arrest algorithm.

Airway management should be the initial focus in children with bradycardia because bradycardia is often secondary to respiratory compromise. Epinephrine is the initial drug of choice. Unlike adults, atropine is not typically the first-line agent for bradycardia in children. It may be used for bradycardia secondary to increased vagal tone, cholinergic drug toxicity, or atrioventricular block. In these situations, atropine may be used before epinephrine, but if no response is noted, epinephrine should be given. Pacer placement may be warranted if pharmacologic agents are not successful. The Broselow-Luten resuscitation tape relates the patient's length to weight and the appropriate drug dosages and equipment sizes.

If handheld paddles are being used, it is important not only to use the right size but also to position them correctly. The recommended paddle diameter for small children (less than 10 kg) is 4.5 cm; paddles up to 8 cm in diameter are used in larger children and adolescents. If only large paddles are available, they should be placed in the anteroposterior position. Regardless of position, a proper conducting medium must be used along with full paddle contact on the chest wall. The largest paddles or self-adhering electrodes that fit the child's chest and allow a 3-cm distance should be used. Electrode gel must be used on manually applied paddles.

Automatic external defibrillators (AEDs) are being used more commonly and may be effective. Some AEDs have pediatric dose attenuators, but if this device is unavailable, a standard AED should be used. According to the 2010 AHA guidelines published in the journal *Circulation*, in infants younger than 1 year, a manual defibrillator is recommended; if not available, the second choice is an AED with a pediatric dose attenuator. A standard AED may be used if neither a manual defibrillator nor an AED with a dose attenuator is available.

# REFERENCES

***References can be found on Expert Consult @ www.expertconsult.com.***

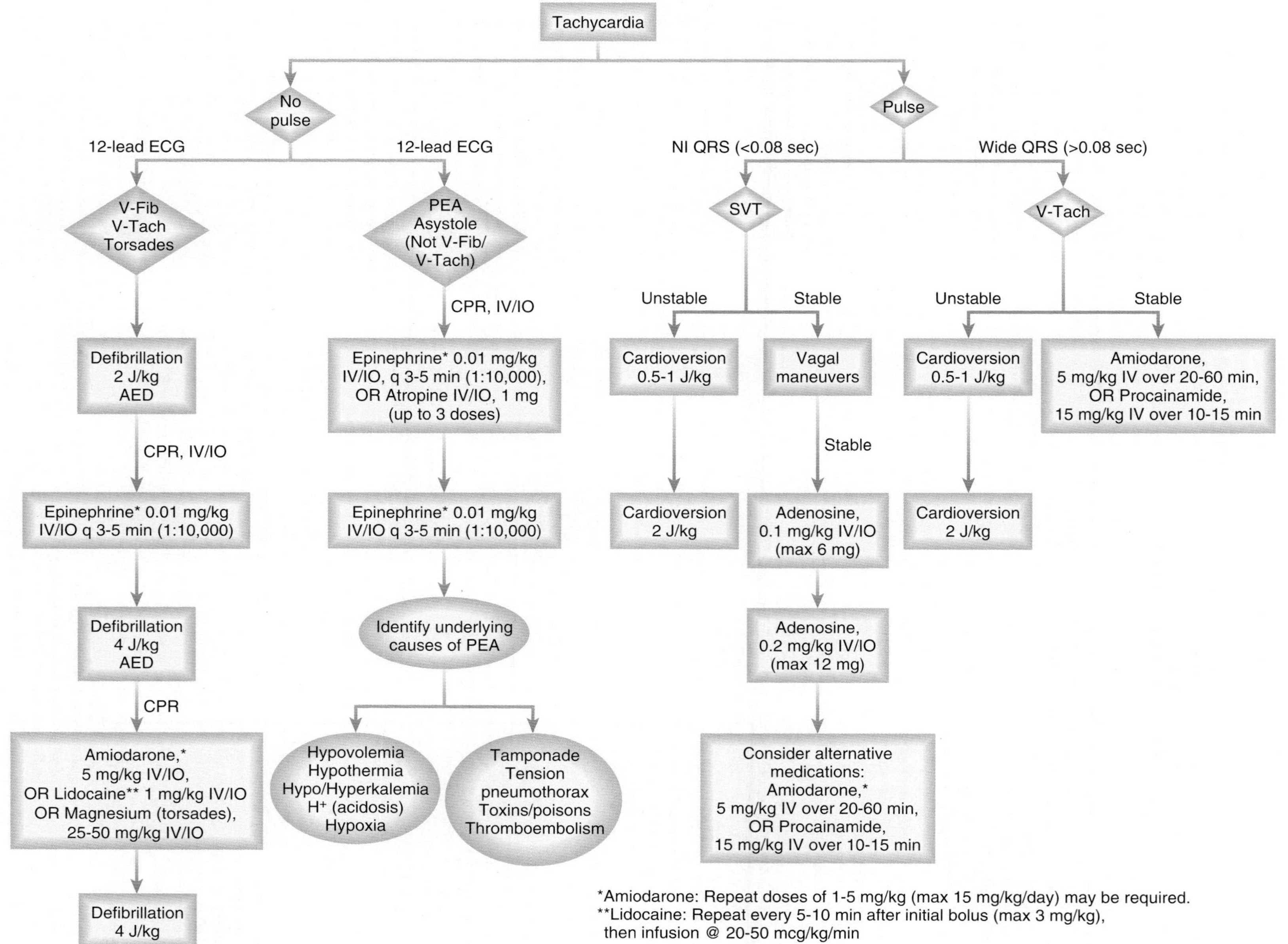


**Fig. 13.2 Tachycardia algorithm.** *AED*, Automatic external defibrillator; *CPR*, cardiopulmonary resuscitation; *ECG*, electrocardiogram; *IO*, intraosseously; *IV*, intravenously; *PEA*, pulseless electrical activity; *SVT*, supraventricular tachycardia; *V-Fib*, ventricular fibrillation; *V-Tach*, ventricular tachycardia. (Adapted from American Heart Association 2010 guidelines. Courtesy of Stephanie Doniger, MD, Children's Hospital, Oakland, CA.)

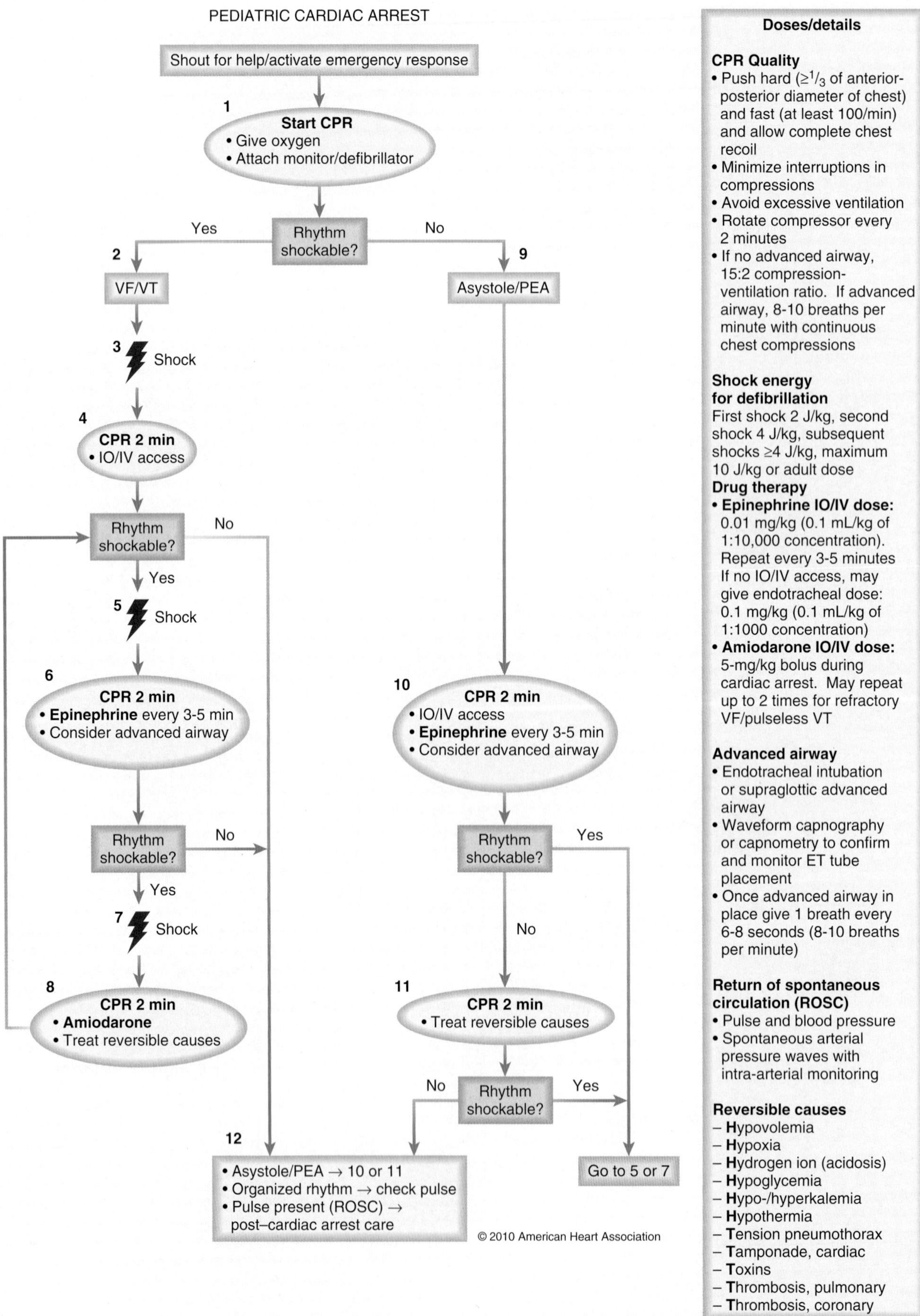


**Fig. 13.3 Pulseless arrest algorithm.** *CPR*, Cardiopulmonary resuscitation; *ET*, endotracheal; *IO*, intraosseous; *IV*, intravenous; *PEA*, pulseless electrical activity; *VF*, ventricular fibrillation; *VT*, ventricular tachycardia.

# General Approach to the Pediatric Patient 14

*Ghazala Q. Sharieff*

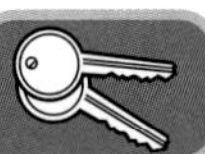

**KEY POINTS**

- Each stage of childhood development brings particular anatomic, physiologic, and developmental features that affect assessment and management.
- The emergency department must have the resources immediately available for stabilization of critically ill children. Written transfer agreements for specialized care are imperative.
- Parents or caregivers must be considered during every interaction with a child, especially if the child is seriously injured or ill. A child's anxiety and fear often reflect what the child feels or sees in the caregivers.
- Family presence during invasive procedures and resuscitation can be a positive experience for some caregivers, especially those treating children with chronic illnesses.

## GENERAL APPROACH

Children account for about 30% of all emergency department (ED) visits; of these, 80% are initially evaluated in a general rather than a pediatric ED.[1,2] Therefore, it is imperative that the general ED environment be not only child friendly but also child safe.

Children are triaged according to the same general guidelines as adults:

Level 1: Critically ill and need immediate attention
Level II: Emergency
Level III: Urgent
Level IV: Less urgent
Level V: Nonurgent

The pediatric assessment triangle (PAT), which consists of a 15- to 20-second evaluation of the patient's appearance, mental status, work of breathing, and circulation of the skin, should be performed before the physical examination. The PAT provides a rapid assessment of the child's oxygenation, ventilation, and perfusion and can help categorize the patient into a triage level. Normal vital signs by age are listed in **Table 14.1**. The PALS formula for blood pressure is 70 + (2 × age in years). It is important to note that this formula defines the 5th percentile for systolic blood pressure in children. Therefore, the preferred formula is 90 + (2 × age in years) because this is the 50th percentile for blood pressure. In the newborn period, normal systolic blood pressure is 60 mm Hg.

The following suggestions constitute a general approach to a child in the ED:

- Allow the parent or caregiver to stay with the child whenever possible.
- Ask what name to use for the child, and then address the child by name.
- Use nonmedical terminology when talking with the family, especially when discussing planned interventions, findings, and treatments. Use language that children will comprehend.
- Always provide privacy no matter how young the child.
- Observe the patient's level of consciousness, activity level, interaction with the environment and caregiver, position of comfort, skin color, respiratory rate and effort, and level of discomfort before touching the child. Compare the findings on evaluation with the parents' or caregivers' description of the child's normal behavior, such as eating and sleeping habits, activity level, and level of consciousness.
- Be honest with the child and parent or caregiver. Parents or caregivers require reassurance about and explanations of the situation and the anticipated plan of treatment.
- Acknowledge and compliment good behavior, and encourage and praise the child. Provide rewards such as stickers or books.
- Allow the child to make simple age-appropriate choices and to participate in the treatment plan. For example, ask the child which arm to use for measuring blood pressure.
- Encourage play during the examination and any procedures. Use diversion and distraction techniques, such as encouraging the child to blow bubbles and blow the hurt away. Ask the child to sing a favorite song, and sing along or have the parents or caregivers do so. Have the child picture a favorite place and describe it in detail with all five senses.
- Give the child permission to voice any feelings. Tell the child that it is okay to cry. Sympathy is essential.

Acknowledgment and thanks to Dr. Antonio E. Muniz for his work on the first edition.

- Assess for pain with age-appropriate assessment tools. Elicit from the parents or caregivers the child's typical response to pain.
- Be cautious about what you say in the presence of an awake or presumed unconscious child.

## GROWTH AND DEVELOPMENT

Although growth and development occur simultaneously, they are discrete and separate processes. Growth refers to an increase in the number of cells and leads to an increase in physical size. Development is the gradual and successive increase in ability or performance skills along a predetermined path, often referred to as developmental milestones or tasks (**Table 14.2**). Development is predominantly age specific and reflects neurologic, emotional, and social maturation. Although there is cross-cultural similarity in the sequence and timing of developmental milestones, cultures exert an all-pervasive influence on developing children.

**Table 14.1** Normal Vital Signs by Age

| AGE | RESPIRATORY RATE (BREATHS PER MINUTE) | HEART RATE (BEATS PER MINUTE) |
|---|---|---|
| <1 yr | 30-60 | 100-160 |
| 1-2 yr | 25-40 | 90-150 |
| 2-5 yr | 20-30 | 80-140 |
| 6-12 yr | 18-30 | 70-120 |
| >12 yr | 12-16 | 60-100 |

## THE FAMILY

The parents and other significant caregivers play a fundamental role in the child's health care experience.[3] Communicating effectively with the parents or caregivers is critical in obtaining an accurate history and consent for treatment.[3] When the child suffers from pain because of illness or injury, the parents or caregivers experience almost equal anxiety and emotional stress. The parent's or caregiver's reaction to the child's condition will directly affect not only how the child behaves but also the manner in which the medical team approaches the patient.

Innate parental or caregiver instincts may evoke powerful emotional reactions. Such reactions are affected by guilt, fear, anxiety, disbelief, shock, anger, and loss of control.[3] Abandoning a child to a stranger's care, not understanding what will occur next, and worrying about a child's condition leave caregivers feeling defenseless. Fear of the unknown, fear of separation, fear of the possibility of significant morbidity or death, and fear of a strange environment may add stress to the parents' or caregivers' attitudes about the illness or injury in their child. Parents' or caregivers' own anxiety and response to the event may negatively influence the ability to console the child, to understand information communicated by health care providers, to participate in decision making for the child's care, and to recall discharge instructions.[3]

Parents or caregivers in emotional shock from a child's acute illness or injury react differently. They may be very quiet, uncommunicative, withdrawn, and unaware of the presence of others. They may appear to ignore and may not answer questions. Alternatively, some parents or caregivers become very demanding, offensive, or rude. Such people, like parents or caregivers who react in other ways, need confident, competent care providers who are able to enlist them in the medical process.

**Table 14.2** Developmental Milestones

| AGE | MILESTONES |
|---|---|
| Newborn | *Prone*: Lies in flexed attitude, turns head from side to side, head lags on ventral suspension<br>*Supine*: Generally lies flexed with mildly increased muscle tone<br>*Visual*: Fixates to bright lights and close objects in line of vision, "doll's-eye" movement of eyes on turning of body<br>*Reflexes*: Moro, stepping and placing, grasping, rooting, startle, and Babinski<br>*Social*: Visual preference for human faces |
| 1 month | *Prone*: Legs are more extended; child holds chin up, turns head; head is lifted momentarily to plane of body on ventral suspension<br>*Supine*: Tonic neck posture predominates; is supple and relaxed, head lags on lifting to sitting position, has tight grasp<br>*Visual*: Follows moving object or person, watches a person<br>*Social*: Body movements in cadence with voice, smiles responsively, becomes alert in response to voice |
| 4 months | *Prone*: Lifts head and chest in vertical axis with legs extended, rolls front to back<br>*Supine*: Symmetric posture predominates, hands in midline, reaches and grasps objects and brings them to mouth<br>*Sitting*: No head lag on pulling to sitting position, head steady, enjoys sitting with full truncal support, tracks objects through 180-degree horizontal arc<br>*Standing*: When held erect, pushes with feet<br>*Adaptive*: When held erect, pushes with feet<br>*Reflexes*: Lacks Moro reflex<br>*Language*: Coos, says "aah"<br>*Social*: Laughs out loud, may show displeasure if social contact is broken, is excited at sight of food, waves at toys |

## FAMILY PRESENCE

Evidence now suggests that presence of the child's family during invasive procedures and resuscitation can be positive, especially in children with chronic illnesses.[4] Although many family members and health care providers support the concept of family presence, parents or caregivers are not frequently given the option to remain with the child during invasive procedures.[5] Many providers are concerned that family presence will impede care of the child, that it will be distracting to members of the team providing care, and that it will increase stress in the team.[5,6] Contrary to this belief, studies have shown that family members do not interfere with health care providers and that the family benefits in a variety of ways from the experience.[7-10] There is also evidence that children feel less stress when parents or caregivers are allowed to remain during procedures.[11] In addition, when institutions

**Table 14.2 Developmental Milestones—cont'd**

| AGE | MILESTONES |
|---|---|
| 6 months | *Prone*: Rolls over, may pivot<br>*Supine*: Lifts head, rolls over, makes squirming motions<br>*Sitting*: Sits unsupported but falls on hands, back is rounded<br>*Standing*: May support most of weight, bounces actively<br>*Adaptive*: Resists pull of a toy, reaches out for and grabs large objects, transfers object from hand to hand, grasps with radial palm, rakes at a pellet<br>*Motor*: Helps hold bottle during feeding<br>*Language*: Babbles, giggles, or laughs when tickled<br>*Social*: Responds more to emotions, enjoys looking at a mirror, responds to changes in emotional content, turns to a voice, clicks tongue to gain notice |
| 9 months | *Sitting*: Sits up alone with no support<br>*Standing*: Pulls to standing position<br>*Adaptive*: Grasps objects with thumb and forefinger, pokes at things with forefinger, picks up a pellet with assisted pincer movement, uncovers a hidden toy, attempts to retrieve a dropped object, releases object to other person<br>*Motor*: Crawls or creeps, walks holding onto furniture<br>*Language*: Makes repetitive sounds such as "mama" and "dada"; imitates speech<br>*Social*: Plays pat-a-cake or peek-a-boo, waves bye-bye, tries to find hidden objects, responds to name, begins to respond to "no" and to one-step commands |
| 1 year | *Motor*: Walks with one hand held, walks holding onto furniture, takes several steps; drinks from cup with help<br>*Adaptive*: Picks up a pellet with unassisted pincer movement of forefinger and thumb, releases a held object to other person on request or gesture, points to desired objects, tries to build tower of 2 cubes<br>*Language*: Has 3 simple words, understands approximately 10 words<br>*Social*: Plays simple games, makes postural adjustment to dressing, follows simple commands |
| 2 years | *Motor*: Walks up and down stairs with one hand held, jumps and runs well, stands on either foot alone for 1 second, climbs on furniture, kicks and throws ball<br>*Adaptive*: Handles spoon well, is able to turn doorknob, makes circular scribbling, imitates horizontal stroke, folds paper once imitatively, can build tower of 6 to 7 cubes, points to named objects or pictures<br>*Language*: Puts 3 words together, uses pronouns<br>*Social*: Listens to stories with pictures, turns pages of book, observes pictures, helps undress self, often tells immediate experiences, verbalizes toilet needs |
| 3 years | *Motor*: Goes up stairs while alternating feet, rides tricycle, stands momentarily on one foot<br>*Adaptive*: Can construct block tower of more than 9 cubes, makes vertical and horizontal strokes on paper but does not join them to make a cross, copies a circle, holds crayon with fingers<br>*Language*: Composes sentences of 3 to 4 words, has vocabulary of 900 words<br>*Social*: Knows own age and sex, counts 3 objects, knows first and last names, plays simple games, helps in dressing self, washes hands |
| 4 years | *Motor*: Hops on one foot, throws ball overhead, uses scissors to cut out pictures, climbs well, runs and turns without losing balance, stands on one leg for at least 10 seconds, catches bounced ball<br>*Adaptive*: Copies cross and square, draws people with 2 to 4 parts besides head, knows days of week<br>*Language*: Counts 4 pennies, tells a story, learns and sings simple songs, has vocabulary of more than 1500 words, easily composes sentences of 4 to 5 words, can use past tense, knows days of week, can ask up to 500 questions a day<br>*Social*: Plays with several children with beginning of social interaction and role-playing, goes to toilet alone |
| 5 years | *Motor*: Skips smoothly, can catch ball<br>*Adaptive*: Draws triangle from copy, names heavier of 2 weights, knows right and left hand, draws person with at least 8 details<br>*Language*: Names 4 colors, repeats sentences of 10 syllables, has vocabulary of more than 2100 words, counts 10 pennies, prints first name, tells age<br>*Social*: Dresses and undresses, asks questions about meanings of words, engages in domestic role-playing |

have incorporated family presence into their practice, staff members have remained supportive.[12] Family members who were present for procedures reported that they would do so again and that their grieving behavior was positively affected by the experience.[4]

Before a family member is offered the choice to be present during an invasive procedure, a health care provider must assess whether the person can cope with what will be experienced during the events. A family member who appears out of control or too emotional may be distracting and disruptive to the health care providers during the procedure. In this case, it may not be advisable to offer the opportunity for family presence. A designated member of the staff who functions to support the family and serve as a patient and caregiver advocate should stay with the family regardless of whether family members decide or are allowed to be present with the child.

The choice to remain present during invasive or resuscitation procedures must be made by the parent or caregiver.[13,14] If the parent or caregiver prefers to not stay with the child, ED personnel must respect that decision and continue to provide appropriate support and explanations.[14] If the parent or caregiver chooses to stay with the child, the health care team must ensure that this person is given a clear explanation of the procedure and expected responses.

Before escorting family members into the room of a child who is undergoing a procedure or resuscitation, the health care provider supporting them must prepare them for what they will see. Family members should be instructed about where they should stand while in the room, and if possible, they should have the opportunity to touch the child. The health care provider supporting the family should offer an ongoing account of activities in a gentle, calm, and directive voice. Should the resuscitation efforts or procedure not result in positive changes in the child's condition, the health care provider supporting the family must remember that his or her role is to support the family's presence and to avoid any derogatory comments.

## CONFIDENTIALITY AND CONSENT

Implied consent occurs when immediate therapy is required for a child who is critically ill. Direct consent is required when the necessary treatment is not an emergency. In a minor, such consent should be obtained from the parent or legal guardian. An emancipated minor is defined as one who lives apart from parents, is pregnant or a married or unmarried mother, is in college, is in the armed forces, or is self-supporting and managing his or her own financial matters. A mature minor is a patient who is a minor but has the intellect and maturity to make an informed, independent decision while understanding the risks and benefits of the recommended therapy. The age of maturity varies between states but in general ranges between 14 and 16 years of age.

Consent related to confidentiality issues is typically under the purview of state law. Treatment of sexually transmitted diseases, pregnancy-related conditions, and substance abuse concerns is an important issue that the emergency physician must be prepared to manage. Breach of confidentiality of these issues should only occur if physical or sexual abuse is a concern or if the child is homicidal or suicidal.

## REFERENCES

***References can be found on Expert Consult @ www.expertconsult.com.***

# Emergencies in the First Weeks of Life 15

*John Nelson Perret and Cristina M. Zeretzke*

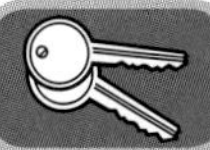

**KEY POINTS**

- Premature infants are at higher risk for most serious neonatal illnesses.
- Congenital heart and gastrointestinal anomalies are commonly manifested during the first month of life.
- A complete set of vital signs, including weight (undressed), is required for assessment and treatment of neonatal patients.
- The majority of neonates who have experienced an apparent life-threatening event have a normal appearance at the time of arrival at the emergency department.
- Laboratory work-up of infants after an apparent life-threatening event who have normal perinatal histories and normal findings on physical examination is most often unproductive.
- An echocardiogram may help distinguish between pulmonary and cardiac causes of cyanosis.
- **Figure 15.1** summarizes the initial evaluation and management of seriously ill infants in the emergency department.

In 2007 the infant (child <1 year old) death rate was 686.9 per 100,000 population. This death rate is not approached again until the sixth decade of life. Two thirds of the deaths that occur in the first year of life do so in the first month.[1]

Newborns are brought to the emergency department (ED) with a multitude of issues ranging from life-threatening conditions to benign findings. An understanding of age-appropriate norms can help the emergency physician (EP) identify infants with significant illness.

## THE NORMAL NEONATE

### WEIGHT

A normal neonate may lose up to 10% of birth weight during the first week of life. By the end of the second week, the infant should have returned to birth weight or a little above it. Weight gain from this point through the first month should be about 30 g (1 oz) per day. It is essential that the weight (undressed) of any neonate be measured accurately in the ED.

### FEEDING

The feeding schedules of neonates are quite variable, and the same child can exhibit significant variability within a 24-hour period. The average neonate eats between six and nine times a day. Intervals between feeding may range from 2 to 4 hours. Breastfed infants tend to eat more often than formula-fed infants.

### SLEEPING

Newborns sleep 16 to 18 hours per day, with almost equal amounts of day and night sleep. Awake periods are generally about 1 to 2 hours in duration.

### VITAL SIGNS

A normal neonatal pulse is in the range of 120 to 160 beats/min, but it rises if the child is stimulated. The heart rate slows during sleep.

The normal respiratory rate is between 40 and 60 breaths/min. Some irregularity and pauses of less than 20 seconds are normal in the neonatal period. Respiratory pauses should not be associated with any change in color or hypotonia. Because of this irregularity in respiratory rate, accurate measurements can be obtained only if breaths are counted for at least 30 seconds.

Measuring blood pressure in a newborn can be frustrating and time-consuming. A Doppler probe can facilitate the procedure. A systolic blood pressure of less than 60 mm Hg is abnormal in a neonate.

The core temperature in an infant is the same as that in an adult. Fever is generally recognized as a temperature higher than 38° C (100.4° F). Any temperature lower than 36.1° C (97° F) should raise concern for hypothermia. Because of limited thermoregulatory ability, neonates should be examined and treated in a warm ambient environment. See **Table 15.1** for normal neonatal vital signs.

## APNEA AND APPARENT LIFE-THREATENING EVENTS

### EPIDEMIOLOGY

General estimates suggest that between 0.5% and 6.0% of infants will experience an apparent life-threatening event (ALTE). A prospective Austrian study conducted from 1993 to 2001 revealed an incidence of 2.46 per 1000 live births.[2] In this study more than 60% of the events occurred in infants 2 months or younger.

### PATHOPHYSIOLOGY

ALTE is not a single disease entity but rather a constellation of signs and symptoms of numerous diseases that can have

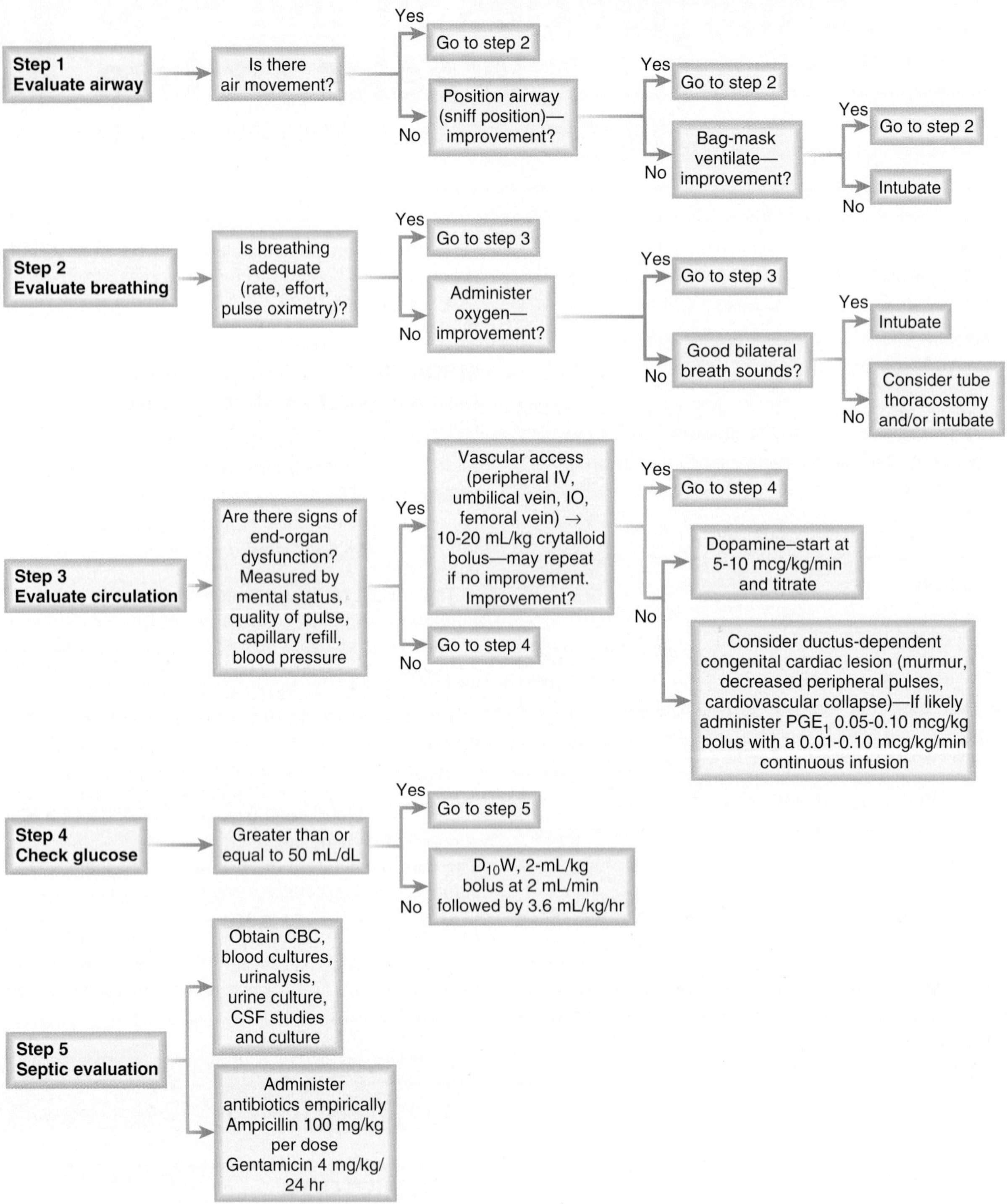


**Fig. 15.1 Initial evaluation and management of a seriously ill neonate.** *CBC*, Complete blood count; *CSF*, cerebrospinal fluid; *$D_{10}W$*, 10% dextrose in water; *IO*, intraosseous; *IV*, intravenous; *$PGE_1$*, prostaglandin $E_1$.

lethal consequences. The 1986 National Institutes of Health Consensus Development Conference on Infantile Apnea and Home Monitoring defined ALTE as "an episode that is frightening to the observer and is characterized by some combination of apnea (central or occasionally obstructive), change in color (usually cyanotic or pallid, but occasionally erythematous or plethoric), marked change in muscle tone (usually marked limpness), choking, or gagging."[3]

The conventional definition of apnea is absence of breathing for 20 seconds or for a shorter period if associated with clinical signs such as cyanosis, hypotonia, and bradycardia. Because periods of apnea of up to 30 seconds have been observed in normal, healthy, asymptomatic term and preterm infants, the duration of apnea does not seem to be as clinically important as apnea associated with signs and symptoms.[4] Apnea should be distinguished from the normal

**Table 15.1 Normal Vital Signs in Neonates**

| | |
|---|---|
| Heart rate | 120-160 beats/min |
| Respiratory rate | 40-60 breaths/min |
| Blood pressure | Systolic pressure > 60 mm Hg |
| Temperature | 36.1-38° C (97-100.4° F) |

**BOX 15.1 Historical Questions to Ask the Caregiver of an Infant Who Has Had an Apparent Life-Threatening Event or Apnea**

What was the appearance of the infant when found?
What was the infant doing when the episode occurred?
Were any interventions (cardiopulmonary resuscitation) necessary?
How long did the event last?*
Was the infant awake or asleep when the event occurred?
What was the infant's body position?
Was the infant alone in the bed?
When was the last time that the infant ate?
Was the infant sick or well in the time before the event?
Is there any history of trauma?
Is there a family history of sudden infant death syndrome or apparent life-threatening event?
What are the prenatal and perinatal histories?

*A trick that an emergency physician (EP) can use to help the caregiver answer this question is as follows: (1) the EP asks the caregiver to look at him or her, (2) the EP says "Go," and (3) the caregiver says "Stop" when he or she thinks that the time that has passed matches the time that the event ended.

periodic breathing of newborns, which is characterized by irregular breathing and episodes of pauses. This latter pattern is more commonly seen in premature infants during sleep. Although similarities exist, ALTE is now considered a different pathophysiologic entity from sudden infant death syndrome.

## PRESENTING SIGNS AND SYMPTOMS

The majority of neonates who have experienced an ALTE have a normal appearance at the time of arrival at the ED. Stratton et al. reported a prehospital study of 60 cases of ALTE in which 83% of the infants were asymptomatic by the time that emergency medical service personnel arrived.[5] A comprehensive history and a thorough physical examination should be performed. One study showed that the history and physical examination were helpful in diagnosing the cause of ALTE in 70% of cases.[6] The history should consist of a detailed description of the event, a prenatal and perinatal history, a review of systems, and a family history (especially child deaths, neurologic diseases, cardiac diseases, and congenital problems).

**BOX 15.2 Causes of Apparent Life-Threatening Events**

**Gastrointestinal**
Gastroesophageal reflux
Aspiration, choking, swallowing abnormalities
Volvulus
Intussusception
Infection

**Neurologic**
Seizure disorder
Infection
Congenital malformations of the brain (e.g., type II Chiari malformation)
Intraventricular hemorrhage
Neuromuscular disorders
Apnea of prematurity
Central hypoventilation syndrome (Ondine curse)
Brain tumors
Vasovagal reflex
Brainstem infarction
Drugs

**Respiratory**
Infection (respiratory syncytial virus, *Mycoplasma*, pertussis, croup)
Congenital airway abnormalities (Pierre Robin syndrome, laryngotracheomalacia)
Vocal cord abnormalities
Obstructive sleep apnea

**Cardiovascular**
Arrhythmias (long QT syndrome, Wolff-Parkinson-White syndrome)
Congenital heart disease
Myocarditis

**Metabolic or Endocrine**
Inborn errors of metabolism
Glucose and electrolyte disorders

**Other**
Sepsis
Medication or drug toxicity
Child abuse
Munchausen by proxy syndrome

**Box 15.1** lists essential historical questions in these cases. A detailed physical examination should pay particular attention to the neurologic, respiratory, cardiac, and developmental components. Evidence of child abuse should be sought, including a funduscopic examination for retinal hemorrhage.

## DIFFERENTIAL DIAGNOSIS AND MEDICAL DECISION MAKING

ALTEs and apnea are clinical manifestations that have many causes, as summarized in **Box 15.2**. The most common organ systems involved (in order of decreasing frequency)

**BOX 15.3 Low-Risk Criteria for Apparent Life-Threatening Events**

First event
Short self-correcting event
Occurred during feeding
Occurred in the awake state
Normal findings on physical examination
Older than 30 days
Understanding parents
Primary care follow-up arranged

are the gastrointestinal, neurologic, respiratory, cardiac, metabolic, and endocrine systems. The cause of ALTE in an individual patient is likely to be discovered only about 50% of the time.

Diagnostic testing is best guided by the history and physical examination. Laboratory tests have been shown to be contributory to the diagnosis only 3.3% of the time if the results of the history and physical examination were noncontributory.[6] An Israeli study concluded that diagnostic testing has low yield in infants with normal perinatal histories and normal findings on physical examination.[7]

## DISPOSITION

Historically it has been the practice that all infants with apnea or ALTE be admitted for observation. Some studies suggest that certain low-risk infant groups might be able to be discharged home from the ED.[8,9] **Box 15.3** lists low-risk criteria for ALTE. An infant meeting all the criteria in this box would have a very low probability of experiencing an adverse outcome. Otherwise, it is prudent to admit the infant for observation and in-patient evaluation by a pediatric specialist.

# EXCESSIVE CRYING AND IRRITABILITY

## EPIDEMIOLOGY

Crying peaks in infancy at 6 weeks of age with an average crying time of 3 hours per day. More of the crying time is clustered in the late afternoon and evening. Forty percent of these infants cry for 30 minutes or longer at one time, 75% of whom have the longest crying spells between 6 and 12 PM.[10] The prevalence of excessive crying varies between 1.5% and 11.9%, depending on the definition of excessive crying.[11]

## PATHOPHYSIOLOGY

Crying is a form of communication by the neonate. It signals some form of infant discomfort from hunger to lack of attention to other causes of pain, some that can be serious.

**BOX 15.4 Historical Questions to Ask the Caregiver of an Afebrile Infant with Acute and Excessive Crying**

Was the crying gradual or sudden in onset?
Is this the first episode?
How long has the child been crying?
Can the child be consoled?
Were there any potential inciting events (trauma, immunizations)?
Has the child been sick or had a fever?
Has any change in feeding pattern or stooling taken place?
Did the infant have any significant birth or perinatal problems?

## PRESENTING SIGNS AND SYMPTOMS

**Box 15.4** lists important questions to ask the caregiver of an afebrile infant with excessive crying. **Table 15.2** lists possible physical findings in these infants.

## DIFFERENTIAL DIAGNOSIS AND MEDICAL DECISION MAKING

The first differentiation that the clinician must make is whether the child is febrile (see the section "Fever"). In an afebrile infant the chronicity of the crying is important. Is the crying an acute single episode, or has it been an ongoing problem for some time?

The latter describes colic, which affects a large subgroup of excessively crying infants. Classically, colic has been described by the rule of threes—crying for 3 hours per day, for at least 3 days per week, for 3 weeks. Scores of theories concerning the etiology of colic have been proposed; such theories range from physiologic disturbances (cow's milk allergies, gastrointestinal reflux, hypocontractile gallbladder, and other gastrointestinal disturbances), to infant temperament and maternal response, to deficiencies in parenting practices.[12] No single cause has been identified.

No pharmacologic agent has been listed as being both safe and efficacious for the treatment of colic. Anticholinergic agents have been found to be more effective than placebo but are associated with apnea and should not be administered to infants younger than 6 months.[13] Many other interventions have been proposed for colic, such as having the infant in a car, specific ways to hold the infant, use of white noise, crib vibrators, and herbal teas. None have been shown to be particularly beneficial, however. The EP should reassure parents that there is no ideal treatment of colic, that their child is normal, that the infant will outgrow the colic, and that colic has no long-term sequelae.

A retrospective study involving 237 afebrile children younger than 1 year brought to the ED with the chief complaint of crying or fussiness revealed that 5.1% had a serious underlying etiology. The final diagnosis in the 237 patients was made by the history and physical examination alone in

**Table 15.2 Potential Abnormalities in Crying Infants Found on Physical Examination**

| | FINDINGS AND POSSIBLE DIAGNOSES |
|---|---|
| **Inspection** | |
| General | Ill appearance:<br>Sepsis, meningitis, other infectious process<br>Dehydration<br>Congenital heart disease (cardiogenic shock), supraventricular tachycardia<br>Volvulus, bowel perforation, incarcerated hernia, intussusception, appendicitis<br>Intracranial hemorrhage (traumatic/nontraumatic)<br>Hypoglycemia, inborn error of metabolism |
| Skin | Trauma, abscess, cellulitis |
| Eyes, ears, nose, throat | Corneal abrasion, foreign body, teething |
| Abdomen, genitourinary structures | Hernia, hair tourniquet on penis, paraphimosis |
| Extremities/clavicles | Fracture deformity (accidental/nonaccidental), digit hair tourniquet |
| **Palpation** | |
| Head | Trauma<br>Fontanelle: Dehydration, increased intracranial pressure |
| Chest | Clavicular fracture |
| Abdomen | Tenderness/peritoneal signs: Volvulus, bowel perforation, appendicitis, intussusception, incarcerated hernia |
| Genitourinary structures | Testicular torsion |
| Extremities/clavicles | Trauma, fracture, soft tissue infection |
| **Auscultation** | |
| Heart | Decreased pulses: Congenital heart disease, septic shock |
| Lungs | Murmur: Congenital heart disease<br>Tachycardia: Supraventricular tachycardia, congestive heart failure<br>Stridor: Upper airway obstruction<br>Wheezing: Airway foreign body, bronchiolitis<br>Rales: Pneumonia, congestive heart failure |
| Abdomen | Hypoactive/hyperactive or absence of bowel sounds: Volvulus, intussusception, appendicitis, incarcerated hernia |

66% of cases. Only 0.8% of the diagnoses were made by diagnostic evaluation alone. These authors concluded that afebrile crying infants younger than 1 month should undergo urinalysis.[14]

A suggested approach to the ED evaluation of an excessively crying child is presented in **Figure 15.2**.

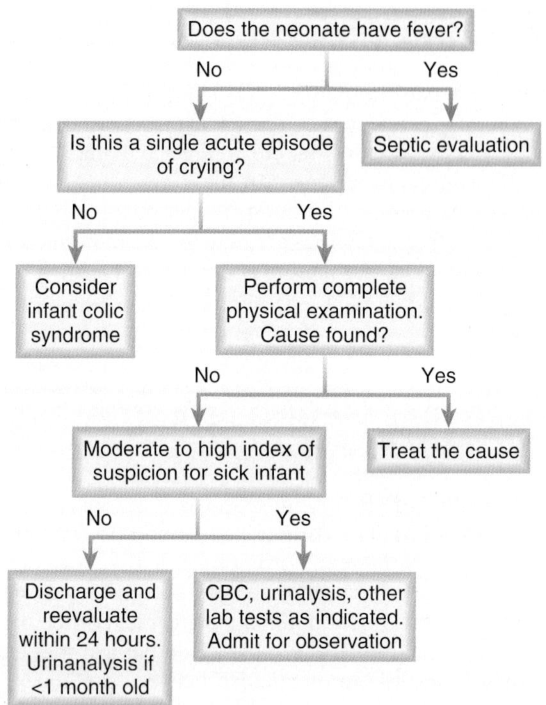


**Fig. 15.2 Evaluation of a crying neonate.** *CBC*, Complete blood count.

## TREATMENT

Treatment is determined by the underlying condition causing the crying.

## DISPOSITION

Afebrile crying infants may be discharged home if they are consolable, if they have a negative history and physical examination, and if the clinician has a low index of suspicion for a "sick" child.

# CYANOSIS

## PATHOPHYSIOLOGY

Cyanosis is the result of either deoxygenated hemoglobin or abnormal hemoglobin (methemoglobin). Cyanosis occurs with the presence of 4 to 5 g of deoxygenated (unsaturated or reduced) hemoglobin per 100 mL of blood. This is an absolute quantity and not a percentage of unsaturated hemoglobin. A cyanotic, polycythemic infant with a hemoglobin value of 18 g/100 mL might have no tissue hypoxia if the total amount of unsaturated hemoglobin is only 5 g/100 mL because the oxygen content of the blood would still be adequate. Conversely, an anemic infant with a hemoglobin value of 7 g/100 mL would have severe tissue hypoxia because at least 4 to 5 g/100 mL of the total is deoxygenated hemoglobin.

## PRESENTING SIGNS AND SYMPTOMS

Cyanosis in a neonate may be persistent or transient, central or peripheral (acrocyanosis). The EP can best evaluate cyanosis clinically by looking at the tongue and mucous membranes. Duskiness or blueness in these areas defines central cyanosis, a pathologic condition. In peripheral cyanosis, or acrocyanosis, the extremities are blue but the oral mucosa and tongue remain pink; this pattern is frequently a normal finding in a neonate but can be associated with pathologic oxygenation.

## DIFFERENTIAL DIAGNOSIS AND MEDICAL DECISION MAKING

An easy method of classifying cyanosis is by causative organ system (**Box 15.5**). The cardiac and respiratory systems are responsible for the large majority of cases of neonatal cyanosis. Distinguishing between these two categories can be difficult but is necessary for optimal management of the patient.

An echocardiogram is the most definitive test that can be performed in the ED to distinguish between pulmonary and cardiac causes of cyanosis. If unavailable, the next best test would be the hyperoxia-hyperventilation test (also called the 100% oxygen challenge test), and it is performed as follows:

1. Blood gas analysis is performed with the infant breathing room air.
2. The patient is then administered 100% oxygen, and the blood gas values are determined again.

If the hypoxia is secondary to pulmonary disease, $Pa_{O_2}$ usually rises to greater than 150 mm Hg with 100% oxygen. If the hypoxia is secondary to right-to-left cardiac shunting from congenital heart disease, the $Pa_{O_2}$ value does not rise significantly when the infant is receiving 100% oxygen. Occasionally, enough intrapulmonary right-to-left shunting occurs in lung disease to prevent a rise in $Pa_{O_2}$ with the simple administration of 100% oxygen. In these cases the infant can be manually ventilated with 100% oxygen, and $Pa_{O_2}$ rises if the source of cyanosis is in the lungs. In many instances these results are obtained clinically by the infant's response to oxygen during the initial resuscitation.

Though rare, methemoglobinemia is a possibility in a cyanotic neonate. This syndrome may be inherited or acquired. The acquired form is typically due to drugs and toxins such as nitrites, anesthetics, and aniline dyes, but it may occur as a result of diarrhea and acidosis.

**BOX 15.5 Causes of Neonatal Cyanosis**

**Respiratory**

***Upper Airway***

Choanal atresia
Macroglossia
Glossoptosis (secondary to micrognathia)
Laryngomalacia
Laryngeal web or cyst
Vascular anomalies (e.g., cystic hygromas, rings)
Subglottic stenosis (commonly secondary to intubation)
Foreign body

***Lower Airway***

Pneumonia
Bronchiolitis
Pulmonary edema
Atelectasis
Bronchopulmonary dysplasia

**Systemic**

Sepsis
Trauma
Poisons

**Cardiac**

Cyanotic congenital heart diseases
Transposition of the great vessels (most common neonatal)
Tetralogy of Fallot
Truncus arteriosus
Tricuspid atresia
Total anomalous pulmonary venous return
Ebstein anomaly

**Gastrointestinal**

Gastroesophageal reflux

**Neurologic**

Seizures
Central hypoventilation syndrome (Ondine curse)
Spinal muscular atrophy type I (Werdnig-Hoffmann)
Botulism
Congenital myopathies

**Hematologic**

Methemoglobinemia

## TREATMENT

The initial treatment of any neonate with cyanosis includes adequate supplemental oxygenation, ventilation, and an intravascular volume challenge with 10 to 20 mL/kg of normal saline (NS). If no response is seen to volume resuscitation, vasopressor support with dopamine, 5 to 20 mcg/kg/min, should be instituted.

If a cyanotic neonate continues to show signs of inadequate tissue oxygenation after the initial resuscitation, prostaglandin $E_1$ (alprostadil) should be given intravenously (IV) starting at 0.05 to 0.1 mcg/kg/min. Administration of prostaglandin is frequently associated with apnea, fever, and occasionally shock. The EP should be prepared to intubate the infant if such complications arise. One study has shown that aminophylline given as a 6-mg/kg bolus before the administration of prostaglandin $E_1$, followed by 2 mg/kg IV every 8 hours for 72 hours, significantly reduces apnea.[15]

Acquired methemoglobinemia is treated with methylene blue, 1 to 2 mg/kg IV as a 1% solution delivered over a 5-minute period.

## DISPOSITION

An acutely cyanotic infant will require admission to the hospital for evaluation and treatment. An infant with known cyanotic heart disease may be able to be discharged, but discharge should be done only in consultation with the infant's cardiology specialist.

# DIFFICULTY BREATHING

## PATHOPHYSIOLOGY

Difficulty breathing may arise from pathology in the heart, lungs, or central and peripheral nervous systems. Toxins and systemic illness, such as sepsis and acidosis, can cause breathing difficulty. Regardless of cause, immediate evaluation is required.

## PRESENTING SIGNS AND SYMPTOMS

Respiratory distress involves a spectrum of clinical findings from apnea, dyspnea, tachypnea, stridor, nasal flaring, grunting, chest retractions, wheezing, and rales to simple nasal congestion and periodic breathing. Tachypnea (fast breathing) should be distinguished from dyspnea (increased work of breathing) because lung pathology is more likely to be associated with dyspnea. Rapid, unlabored respirations are more likely to be seen in neonates with metabolic acidosis and cardiac pathology. Stridor is a symptom of upper airway obstruction from either intrinsic or extrinsic causes.

## DIFFERENTIAL DIAGNOSIS AND MEDICAL DECISION MAKING

A list of potential causes of respiratory distress that can occur anytime during the first 28 days is presented in **Box 15.6**. The majority of causes are pulmonary, cardiac, or infectious. Diagnostic testing includes a complete blood count, serum glucose measurement, metabolic profile, blood cultures, arterial blood gas measurements, urinalysis, urine culture, chest radiography, and electrocardiography.

The differential diagnosis of pulmonary causes of respiratory distress in a neonate can be divided into syndromes manifested in the first hours of life and those manifested anytime during the first 28 days. The former group includes transient tachypnea of the newborn, respiratory distress syndrome, persistent pulmonary hypertension of the newborn, and meconium aspiration syndrome. These conditions are not discussed further because they are almost certainly diagnosed and treated in the nursery, not the ED.

Pneumonia is the most common and most serious infectious cause of respiratory distress in the first 28 days of life. From a clinical perspective, neonatal pneumonia can be divided into early-onset and late-onset types (**Table 15.3**).

The clinical findings of neonates with pneumonia can be atypical. Signs of respiratory distress are generally present, but they may be absent. Gastrointestinal symptoms, such as vomiting, abdominal distention, and poor feeding, may predominate. General systemic signs such as lethargy, ill appearance, poor feeding, and jaundice may be the initial complaints. The classic radiographic appearance consists of bilateral alveolar densities with air bronchograms.[16] Hyperinflation of the lungs without evidence of infiltrate is a common early

**BOX 15.6 Etiologic Considerations in Infants with Difficulty Breathing**

**Respiratory System**

Infectious
- Pneumonia
- Bronchiolitis
- Laryngotracheitis
- Viral upper respiratory tract infection

Congenital structural
- Choanal atresia
- Laryngotracheomalacia
- Laryngeal webs
- Laryngeal cysts
- Laryngoceles
- Hemangiomas
- Foreign body

Acquired structural
- Pneumothorax
- Chest wall injury/rib injury

**Cardiovascular**

Congenital heart disease
- Cyanotic
- Noncyanotic

Hypovolemia

Anemia

**Metabolic**

Hypoglycemia

Acidosis

**Neurologic**

Central nervous system hemorrhage

Muscle disease

**Drugs**

**Sepsis**

**Table 15.3** Causes of Neonatal Pneumonia

| ONSET OF PNEUMONIA | BACTERIAL CAUSES | VIRAL CAUSES |
|---|---|---|
| Early | Group B streptococci (most common)<br>*Escherichia coli Klebsiella Staphylococcus aureus*<br>*Streptococcus pneumoniae*<br>*Listeria monocytogenes*<br>*Mycobacterium tuberculosis*<br>*Ureaplasma urealyticum* | Herpes simplex virus (most common)<br>Adenovirus<br>Enterovirus<br>Cytomegalovirus<br>Rubella |
| Late | *S. aureus*<br>*Streptococcus pyogenes*<br>*S. pneumoniaeE. coli*<br>*Klebsiella*<br>*Chlamydia trachomatis* | Respiratory syncytial virus (most common)<br>Rhinovirus<br>Adenovirus<br>EnterovirusInfluenza<br>Parainfluenza |

**BOX 15.7 Differential Diagnosis of Stridor in Neonates**

**Intrinsic Lesions**

***Larynx***
Laryngomalacia
Infection (laryngitis)
Vocal cord paralysis
Laryngeal web
Laryngocele or laryngeal cyst
Laryngotracheal esophageal cleft
Foreign body

***Trachea***
Tracheomalacia
Tracheal stenosis
Tracheoesophageal fistula
Subglottic hemangioma
Tracheal web

**Extrinsic Compression**
Vascular ring
Anomalous innominate artery
Mediastinal mass
Esophageal foreign body

**Other**
Macroglossia
Gastroesophageal reflux

finding with viral lower respiratory tract infections.[17] The chest radiograph may be normal in up to 15% of cases.[18]

Acyanotic cardiac conditions such as tachycardias, myocarditis, and ductus-dependent obstructive left-sided heart conditions (coarctation of the aorta, critical aortic stenosis, and hypoplastic left ventricle) may be accompanied by tachypnea. The tachypnea is often associated with diaphoresis during feeding. The left-sided obstructive lesions increase pulmonary blood flow secondary to left-to-right shunting. This will cause “wet lungs” (rales on physical examination and pulmonary congestion on chest radiograph). Other physical findings of left-sided obstructive heart disease are markedly diminished to absent peripheral pulses and signs of systemic hypoperfusion.

Laryngomalacia is the most common cause of stridor in infants. Stridor secondary to laryngomalacia starts soon after birth and is exacerbated by crying, agitation, and supine positioning. This disorder is generally benign and self-limited. The stridor worsens with upper respiratory tract infections and occasionally necessitates hospital admission for supportive care. Less than 10% of patients with laryngomalacia have significant respiratory or feeding problems that mandate epiglottoplasty or tracheotomy. Vocal cord paralysis is the next most common cause of neonatal stridor[19] and can be unilateral or bilateral. Unilateral cord paralysis generally requires conservative treatment, such as monitoring oxygen saturation and observing for aspiration secondary to an incompetent glottis.

See **Box 15.7** for the differential diagnosis of stridor in neonates. Inspiratory stridor indicates a lesion above the glottis such as laryngomalacia. Biphasic stridor usually points to a lesion at the level of the glottis or the subglottic area, such as vocal cord paralysis or subglottic stenosis. Expiratory stridor is caused by a lesion below the thoracic inlet, typically tracheomalacia. The stridor may result from a fixed narrowing that is not worsening or from progressive narrowing, which should alert the physician to urgent airway management action. A stridulous infant without severe distress should be examined by the EP. Radiographs of the chest and soft tissues of the neck are indicated. The definitive diagnostic test is direct laryngoscopy by a pediatric otorhinolaryngologist.

## TREATMENT AND DISPOSITION

The initial management of all newborns with difficulty breathing is to follow the ABCs (airway, breathing, circulation) of neonatal resuscitation.

Antibiotic coverage for early-onset pneumonia consists of ampicillin, 150 mg/kg IV every 12 hours if meningitis is suspected. If meningitis is not suspected, 50 to 100 mg/kg IV every 12 hours is adequate. Intravenous gentamicin is given according to gestational age and renal function. For infants born after 35 weeks of gestation, the dose is 4 mg/kg every 24 hours; for those born between 30 and 35 weeks of gestation, the dose is 3 mg/kg every 24 hours.[20] In neonates with late-onset neonatal pneumonia, some authorities would recommend administering vancomycin, 15 mg/kg IV every 12 hours with gentamicin, instead of ampicillin until the results of culture are available.[21] If herpes simplex virus pneumonia is suspected, acyclovir, 20 mg/kg IV every 8 hours (in infants with normal renal function), should be started.[22] All neonates with pneumonia should be admitted to the hospital.

In an infant with cardiovascular collapse from a ductus-dependent left-sided heart obstruction, the only nonoperative way to maintain adequate systemic perfusion is to keep the ductus arteriosus patent. This is done on an emergency basis by the administration of a continuous infusion of prostaglandin $E_1$ (alprostadil). The initial dose is 0.05 to 0.1 mcg/kg/min IV, with a maintenance dose titrated to the lowest dose effective in maintaining patency.[23] Treatment of a stridulous infant initially depends on the degree of respiratory distress. If respiratory distress is present, it is best to not manipulate the child too much unless emergency airway interventions are necessary. If possible, the EP should perform the physical examination of a stridulous infant in distress in the presence of an otorhinolaryngologist or pediatric surgeon who can obtain a surgical airway immediately in a controlled setting (operating suite). A neonate with stridor should be admitted to the hospital unless the EP is certain that the child is stable and the cause of the stridor is not progressing.

# FEVER

## SCOPE

Fever is defined as a rectal temperature of 38° C (100.4° F) or higher. The majority of febrile illnesses in infants are self-limited viral infections. Ten percent to 20% of febrile infants younger than 3 months have a serious bacterial infection (SBI), defined as bacterial meningitis, bacteremia, urinary tract infection, pneumonia, skin or soft tissue infection, bacterial enteritis, septic arthritis, or osteomyelitis. Bacteremia is twice as likely to occur in the first month of life as in the second month.[24]

**BOX 15.8 Septic Work-up for Febrile Infants Younger Than 28 Days**

Complete blood count with differential
Blood culture
Urinalysis—catheter or suprapubic
Urine culture
Lumbar puncture—cell count, glucose, protein, Gram stain, cerebrospinal fluid culture, herpes simplex virus polymerase chain reaction if suspected
Chest radiograph (if symptoms of respiratory infection present)
Stool for white blood cell count, culture, and sensitivity (if diarrhea present)
C-reactive protein/procalcitonin (consider)

## PATHOPHYSIOLOGY

A neonate's immature immune system lacks the ability to localize and contain infection; therefore, the newborn may not show specific signs of serious underlying disease. The birth process exposes the infant to an array of bacterial and viral pathogens. The most common bacterial pathogens in the first 28 days of life are group B streptococci and *Escherichia coli*. Other bacteria may be gram-negative (e.g., *Klebsiella, Enterobacter, Salmonella*) or gram-positive organisms (*Staphylococcus aureus, Enterococcus*, other streptococcal species, and *Listeria monocytogenes*). Herpes simplex virus and the enteroviruses can also cause febrile illness in neonates. Neonatal herpes can be a devastating illness, with only about half the cases caused by active maternal infection.

## PRESENTING SIGNS AND SYMPTOMS

A febrile neonate may look remarkably well or may be extremely toxic appearing.

## DIFFERENTIAL DIAGNOSIS AND MEDICAL DECISION MAKING

**Box 15.8** present a work-up for a febrile infant younger than 28 days.

Recent literature suggests that C-reactive protein levels can predict infection. The limitation to its use is that a period of up to 8 to 10 hours is required for synthesis, so it has a variable range of sensitivity (from 14% to 100%) in the first 24 hours. A cutoff of 70 g/L has been proposed, although it is a nonspecific marker for infection.[25] Procalcitonin also deserves mention as a possible marker for SBI. It is the prehormone of calcitonin and increases within 2 hours of an infection. Its sensitivity is 92.6% with a specificity of 97.5% if obtained outside the first 48 hours of life.[26]

## TREATMENT

Empiric antibiotic treatment of neonatal sepsis consists of either ampicillin and gentamicin or ampicillin and cefotaxime

**BOX 15.9 Empiric Antibiotic Therapy for Term Neonates Younger Than 7 Days with Fever**

Ampicillin, 75 mg/kg/day (150 mg/kg/day if meningitis is suspected) divided q8h
*and*
Gentamicin, 4 mg/kg/day, once-daily dosing
**OR**
Ampicillin, 75 mg/kg/day (150 mg/kg/day if meningitis is suspected) divided q8h
*and*
Cefotaxime, 100-150 mg/kg/day divided q8-12h

**BOX 15.10 Empiric Antibiotic Therapy for Term Neonates 8 to 28 Days Old with Fever**

Ampicillin, 100 mg/kg/day (200 mg/kg/day if meningitis is suspected) divided q6h
*and*
Gentamicin, 4 mg/kg/day, once-daily dosing
**OR**
Ampicillin, 100 mg/kg/day (200 mg/kg/day if meningitis is suspected) divided q6h
*and*
Cefotaxime, 150-200 mg/kg/day divided q6-8h

(**Boxes 15.9 and 15.10**). If neonatal meningitis is suspected, ampicillin and cefotaxime are preferred. Some authorities would add gentamicin as a third antibiotic for suspected meningitis when no organisms are seen on Gram stain of cerebrospinal fluid.[27] Herpes simplex virus infection should be strongly considered in febrile infants with seizures and abnormal cerebrospinal fluid results. Skin lesions and abnormal liver function values should further increase suspicion for this disorder. An infant with suspected herpes simplex virus infection should receive acyclovir, 60 mg/kg/day in three divided doses (20 mg/kg per dose). Acyclovir should be continued until the results of herpes simplex virus polymerase chain reaction are negative. Neonates with an identifiable viral infection (e.g., respiratory syncytial virus) have as high as a 7% chance of having a concomitant SBI.[28-31] Therefore, a septic evaluation should be performed in any child 1 to 28 days old with fever despite an identifiable viral infection. Antibiotics should be administered empirically to this group. Febrile neonates should be admitted to the hospital.

# VOMITING

## SCOPE

Vomiting is defined as forceful diaphragmatic and abdominal wall contraction with simultaneous relaxation of the stomach, gastroesophageal sphincter, and esophagus and closure of the gastric pylorus. Regurgitation, or "spitting up," is a nonforceful reflux of milk or gastric contents into the mouth. Regurgitation is generally a benign disorder but can occasionally be associated with gastroesophageal reflux disease and result in serious consequences such as apnea.

## PATHOPHYSIOLOGY

The appearance of the vomitus is important. Bilious vomit suggests obstruction below the ampulla of Vater. Undigested milk may simply be regurgitation but could be caused by gastrointestinal obstruction above the ampulla of Vater. Bloody vomitus requires a search for upper gastrointestinal bleeding.

## SIGNS AND SYMPTOMS

It is important to distinguish between bilious vomiting and nonbilious vomiting. If bilious vomiting is reported, it is assumed to be obstructive and a surgical emergency until proved otherwise. Studies have suggested that 20% to 50% of neonates with bilious emesis within the first week of life have a surgical condition.[32]

## DIFFERENTIAL DIAGNOSIS AND MEDICAL DECISION MAKING

Causes of vomiting can be divided into anatomic and nonanatomic categories (**Box 15-11**).

**BOX 15.11 Causes of Neonatal Vomiting**

**Anatomic Causes**

Esophagus, trachea, great vessels:
- Stricture
- Web
- Tracheoesophageal fistula
- Laryngeal cleft
- Double aortic arch

Stomach and duodenum:
- Pyloric stenosis
- Duodenal atresia (usually noted on the first day of life)

Small and large intestine:
- Volvulus secondary to malrotation
- Incarcerated hernia
- Hirschsprung disease (secondary to obstipation)
- Necrotizing enterocolitis

Genitourinary:
- Testicular torsion

**Nonanatomic Causes**

Infection:
- Septicemia
- Meningitis
- Urinary tract infection
- Gastroenteritis
- Otitis media?

Increased intracranial pressure:
- Cerebral edema
- Subdural hematoma
- Hydrocephalus
- Brain tumor

Congenital adrenal hyperplasia (salt-losing variety)
Inborn errors of metabolism
Renal disease

Volvulus from midgut malrotation can be manifested as a sudden onset of bilious vomiting, duodenal obstruction as a result of obstructing Ladd bands, or intermittent vomiting with failure to thrive. Most neonates with volvulus will appear to be well, but if necrosis of the gut or ischemia has begun, they may appear ill or in shock. Abdominal radiographs should be obtained if obstruction is a concern.

To make the diagnosis of volvulus secondary to midgut malrotation promptly, an upper gastrointestinal contrast-enhanced study is needed. The small intestine will have a “corkscrewing” appearance with the intestine rotated to the right side of the abdomen with midgut volvulus.

In dehydrated and toxic infants, a complete blood count, serum glucose and electrolyte measurements, and a septic evaluation should be performed.

A healthy-appearing infant with vomiting but appropriate weight gain and normal vital signs requires no diagnostic testing.

## TREATMENT

If the infant is moderately or severely dehydrated, 0.9% sodium chloride should be administered IV as a 20-mL/kg bolus. Oral rehydration may be tried in a mildly dehydrated infant. Nasogastric decompression is required for intestinal obstruction. Empiric therapy with ampicillin and gentamicin or ampicillin and cefotaxime should be administered for suspected sepsis.

In midgut malrotation with volvulus, management includes placement of a nasogastric tube, administration of broad-spectrum antibiotics (gentamicin, clindamycin, and ampicillin), and rapid fluid replacement with NS (20-mL/kg bolus) as needed.[33]

## FOLLOW-UP AND DISPOSITION

Infants with regurgitation may be managed as outpatients. Children younger than 28 days with true vomiting should be admitted to the hospital for further evaluation and treatment.

# DIARRHEA

## SCOPE

Diarrhea is defined as an increase in both the number and the looseness or wateriness of stools. Even in the neonatal period, diarrhea tends to be self-limited without significant morbidity.

## DIFFERENTIAL DIAGNOSIS AND MEDICAL DECISION MAKING

Viral infections are common, with rotavirus being the most frequent cause. Other viral causes of diarrhea are enterovirus, enteric adenovirus, and coronavirus. Bacterial diarrhea in neonates is caused by the same organisms found in other age groups, including *Salmonella, Shigella, Campylobacter, E. coli, Vibrio, Yersinia,* and *Clostridium difficile*.

*Salmonella* gastroenteritis is potentially dangerous in neonates because of its association with systemic sepsis. Bacteremia may occur in 30% to 50% of neonates infected with this organism. Diarrhea from *Salmonella* gastroenteritis is usually watery with mucus and may appear bloody. This organism is an enteroinvasive bacterium (i.e., it invades the intestinal mucosa), so a methylene blue smear of a stool specimen will reveal white blood cells. Necrotizing enterocolitis (NEC) is one of the more dangerous causes of neonatal diarrhea. It is classically seen in premature infants but can occur in term neonates. Its incidence is also higher in infants with congenital heart disease.[34] The diarrhea is typically bloody and is associated with other symptoms, such as decreased feeding, vomiting, ileus, and abdominal distention. If not treated, symptoms progress to bradycardia, hypothermia, apnea, hypotension, and death. Diagnostic radiographic findings are pneumatosis intestinalis (air in the bowel wall) and air in the portal vein. Intestinal perforation leads to pneumoperitoneum.

### TREATMENT

Neonates with *Salmonella* gastroenteritis should be treated with cefotaxime, 50 mg/kg IV every 12 hours. Treatment of NEC involves cessation of oral feeding, nasogastric decompression, intravenous fluids, and antibiotics (ampicillin, cefotaxime, clindamycin).

### FOLLOW-UP AND DISPOSITION

Neonates with suspected bacterial diarrhea or NEC should be admitted to the hospital.

## NEONATAL JAUNDICE

### EPIDEMIOLOGY

In almost all newborns, the bilirubin level reaches 2 to 3 mg/dL in the first few days of life. Neonatal jaundice occurs in up to 60% of term infants in the first week of life. Approximately 2% of newborns will reach levels of total serum bilirubin in excess of 20 mg/dL.

### PATHOPHYSIOLOGY

Hemoglobin degrades to form unconjugated bilirubin. This unconjugated (indirect) bilirubin is lipid soluble and binds to albumin. The bilirubin that is not bound to albumin can cross the blood-brain barrier and injure the brain (kernicterus). Albumin-bound unconjugated bilirubin is transported to the liver and converted to water-soluble conjugated bilirubin (direct bilirubin). Conjugated bilirubin is excreted into bile and then into the gut. Most bilirubin is eliminated from the gut in stool.

**BOX 15.12 Criteria for Physiologic Jaundice**

Jaundice occurring after 24 hours of life
Serum bilirubin level rising no faster than 0.5 mg/dL/hr or 5 mg/dL/day
Total bilirubin value not exceeding 15 mg/dL in a term neonate or 10 mg/dL in a preterm neonate
No evidence of acute hemolysis
Jaundice not persisting longer than 10 days in a term neonate or 21 days in a preterm neonate*

*Breastfed infants may remain jaundiced up to 2 weeks longer.

### SIGNS AND SYMPTOMS

Jaundice is most easily detected in the sclera, skin, and oral cavity.

### DIFFERENTIAL DIAGNOSIS AND MEDICAL DECISION MAKING

Jaundice can be normal (physiologic) or abnormal (nonphysiologic). Physiologic jaundice usually becomes visible on the second or third day of life. Jaundice in the first 24 hours of life is always abnormal. Physiologic jaundice is thought to be secondary to the higher breakdown of red blood cells in neonates and transient slowing of conjugation processes in the liver. It peaks at levels between 5 and 12 mg/dL on the third or fourth day of life and then starts to decline. Risk factors for higher levels of physiologic hyperbilirubinemia include a family history of neonatal jaundice, breastfeeding, bruising and cephalohematoma, maternal age older than 25 years, Asian ethnicity, prematurity, weight loss, and delayed bowel movement. **Box 15.12** lists the criteria for physiologic jaundice.

Breast milk jaundice develops after the seventh day of life and peaks during the second or third week. It is postulated that a glucuronidase in breast milk causes increased enterohepatic absorption of unconjugated bilirubin. Because of its late onset, breast milk jaundice is almost never a neurologic threat.

Laboratory tests are indicated in a jaundiced infant unless the EP is absolutely certain that the jaundice is physiologic. A total serum bilirubin measurement with direct and indirect fractions and a complete blood count are required. A Coombs test for autoimmune hemolysis is indicated if the maternal blood type is Rh negative and the infant's blood type is Rh positive or if the maternal blood type is O and the fetal blood type is A, B, or AB. A reticulocyte count is useful for evaluating hemolytic anemia. Because jaundice can be the initial manifestation of hypothyroidism, measurements of serum thyroid-stimulating hormone and thyroxine may be helpful. If the neonate appears ill—has lethargy, decreased feeding, temperature instability, or difficulty breathing—an evaluation for sepsis is indicated.

### TREATMENT

Early treatment of hyperbilirubinemia ensures adequate hydration and feeding. A breastfed infant should be fed more often to promote stooling and excretion of bilirubin. Further management of hyperbilirubinemia may involve phototherapy or exchange transfusion. Initiation of these therapies depends on several factors, including the total serum bilirubin level and the infant's birth weight and age. Some preterm infants are at higher risk for neurologic sequelae, which mandates a lower threshold for initiation of phototherapy.

The American Academy of Pediatrics (AAP) has issued practice guidelines for the treatment of neonatal jaundice.[35] One tool that the EP may find helpful is the website www.bilitool.org, in which parameters may be entered to determine the infant's risk based on the bilirubin level obtained. The following information is needed to estimate an infant's risk: (1) the infant's date of birth and time (to the hour), (2) the infant's gestational age, and (3) the time that the bilirubin level was obtained. After entering this information, the AAP guidelines will be listed and appropriate therapy recommendations will be displayed based on the level of risk.

## DISPOSITION AND FOLLOW-UP

Only well-appearing neonates with clearly physiologic or breastmilk jaundice and a serum bilirubin level below the guideline limits for phototherapy should be discharged. Close follow-up and monitoring should be arranged for such infants at the time of discharge. All other infants should be admitted for further testing and treatment.

# METABOLIC EMERGENCIES

## SCOPE

Metabolic emergencies account for a small percentage of disorders in neonates seen in the ED. This low incidence accounts for the difficulty recognizing and treating these emergencies. Adrenal insufficiency is one metabolic emergency in neonates that can be encountered in the ED and should be taken into consideration to reduce an infant's morbidity and mortality.[36]

## PATHOPHYSIOLOGY

Congenital adrenal hyperplasia (CAH) is the most recognized form of adrenal insufficiency in children and is sometimes identified as part of the initial newborn screening program. It is most commonly associated with the lack of 21-hydroxylase, an enzyme necessary for cholesterol metabolism and required to produce cortisol. This may result in virilization of females and be accompanied by an acute salt-wasting crisis. The male genitalia is not generally affected by CAH, thus making males more susceptible to underdiagnosis.

## PRESENTING SIGNS AND SYMPTOMS

Dehydration, hypotension, hypoglycemia, and shock are the most common signs seen in the ED. Neonates may also have fatigue, nausea, vomiting, or weight loss. Females may have an enlarged clitoris and fusion of the labial folds, and some females may be mistaken for males. This makes physical examination extremely important for this diagnosis, and close attention should be paid to the infant, with removal of the diaper and inspection of the genital area. The triad of hyponatremia, hyperkalemia, and hypoglycemia should alert the clinician to this possible diagnosis.

## TREATMENT

The first step is to restore volume with 0.9% NS in 20-mL/kg boluses. Following initial volume replacement, $D_5\frac{1}{4}$NS is administered at 1 to $1\frac{1}{2}$ times the maintenance rate. Cortisol replacement should be achieved by administration of hydrocortisone, 1 to 2 mg/kg IV for term infants and then 25 to 100 mg/m$^2$/day divided into three to four doses every 6 to 8 hours. Hyperkalemia is typically well tolerated and saline is usually all that is needed to lower the potassium level. Intravenous calcium gluconate, β-agonists, insulin, and glucose should be available for any potential cardiac arrhythmias.[37]

# CHILD ABUSE

Child abuse should be included in the topic of neonatal emergencies because it is a potential diagnosis in an infant with apnea, seizures, or altered mental status. If suspicion exists, non–contrast-enhanced computed tomography (CT) of the head should be performed, and if the patient is deemed stable, a skeletal survey should be considered. Any suspicion of child abuse should be reported to the Department of Children and Family Services immediately. The EP should also consider notifying the police because this provides protection for the child and the staff involved in the infant's care. Studies suggested for the initial work-up of child abuse include a complete blood count, coagulation profile, a chemistry panel, and liver function tests.

## SUGGESTED READINGS

Brand DA, Altman EI, Purtill R, et al. Yield of diagnostic testing in infants who have had an apparent life-threatening event. Pediatrics 2005;115:885–93.

Freedman S, Al-Harthy N, Thull-Freedman J. The crying infant: diagnostic testing and frequency of serious underlying disease. Pediatrics 2009;123:841.

## REFERENCES

***References can be found on Expert Consult @ www.expertconsult.com.***

# Emergencies in Infants and Toddlers 16

*Mark McIntosh and Todd Wylie*

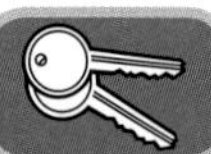

**KEY POINTS**

- Use a systematic approach to evaluate and manage infants and toddlers. Know common milestones and age-specific manifestation of illness, take an "AMPLIFIEDD" history, do a "head-to-toe" physical examination, and use the "head-to-toe" memory tool to generate an expanded differential diagnosis.
- Do not make the diagnosis of infantile colic on first episode of excessive crying. Remember Wessel's rule of 3.
- When the cause of illness in an infant or toddler is not obvious, the emergency practitioner should maintain a high level of suspicion for abuse, accidental toxin ingestion or exposure, intussusception, infection, and nonconvulsive seizure activity.

## PERSPECTIVE

More than 20% of emergency department (ED) visits are by pediatric patients, and a large proportion involve children 4 years or younger.[1,2] Common reasons for ED visits in this age group include traumatic injuries, fever, respiratory complaints, and gastrointestinal problems.[3-5] Although many of the disease processes are self-limited, it is imperative that the emergency practitioner (EP) identify infants and children at risk for progression to serious illness.

Knowledge of developmental milestones and age-specific manifestations of illness, in addition to taking a thorough history and physical examination, will greatly enhance the clinician's ability to diagnose and initiate appropriate therapeutic interventions. From early infancy to the toddler stage, remarkable developmental changes occur. Understanding the changes in language, motor, cognitive, and social skills is important to properly assess infants and toddlers (**Fig. 16.1**). Many of the common illnesses experienced are age related (**Table 16.1**), and early recognition of the signs and symptoms of the specific diseases that threaten infants and toddlers is an effective strategy. Taking an "AMPLIFIEDD" history (**Box 16.1**) and performing a "head-to-toe" physical examination allow the clinician to gather the clinical clues needed to generate a comprehensive differential diagnosis. Practitioners in the ED are encouraged to develop an expanded differential diagnosis by using their knowledge of anatomy to aid memory (**Table 16.2**).

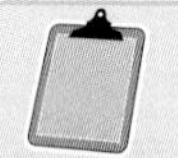

**DOCUMENTATION**

**Infant or Toddler in the Emergency Department**

Document consideration of life-threatening diagnoses.

Create a word picture of the child: minor or serious illness; for example:

- "Child is playful, interactive, and taking bottle or fluids well."
- "Well hydrated, nontoxic, and no evidence of trauma, sepsis, meningitis, or distress."
- "Alert, good tone, moving all extremities."
- "Child appropriately cries but can be consoled by caregivers."

This chapter demonstrates how to take a systematic approach to the evaluation of infants and toddlers in the ED to develop a comprehensive diagnostic and therapeutic plan by using three examples of different clinical manifestations: a crying infant, an infant or toddler with altered level of consciousness, and a vomiting infant or toddler.

## THE CRYING INFANT

*"Birds fly and babies cry"*

—Marc Weissbluth, pediatrician[6]

### PERSPECTIVE

One of the most challenging aspects of pediatric emergency care is managing an infant with the nonspecific symptom of acute, excessive crying. Infants are not able to vocalize complaints, and crying is the primary mode of communication until language development. According to Brazelton, most babies will cry between 1½ and 3 hours per day in the first 3 months of life, with the peak occurring at approximately 6 weeks.[7] By the time that parents bring their crying infant or

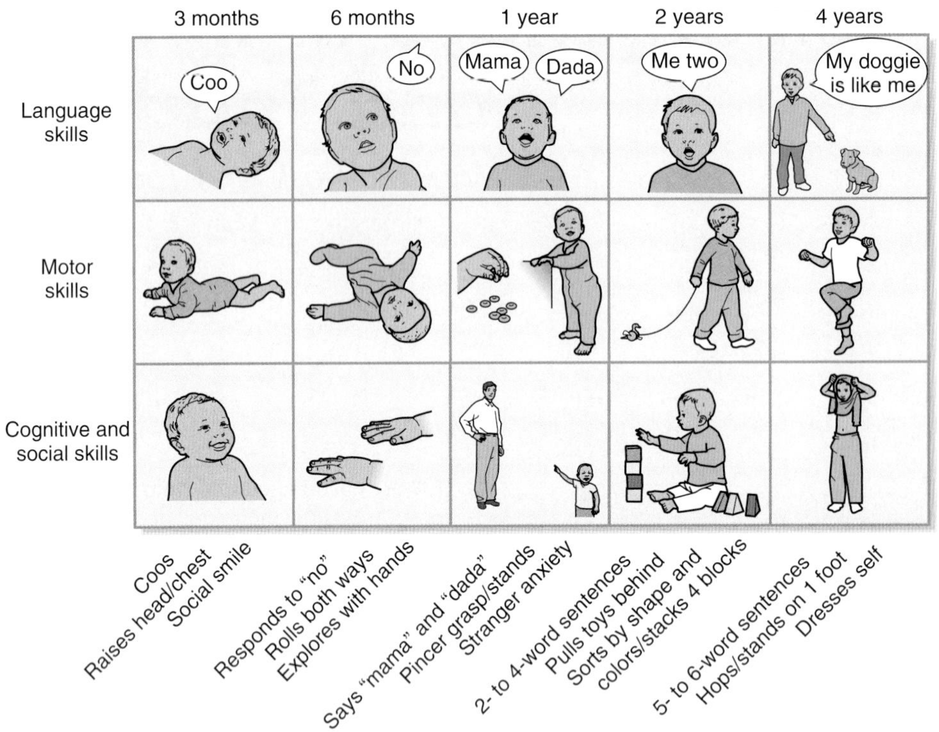


**Fig. 16.1 Easy-to-remember developmental milestones for the emergency department practitioner.**

**BOX 16.1 The "AMPLIFIEDD" History**

**A**llergies: to medications, environmental allergens
**M**edications: prescription, over the counter, natural remedies
**P**ast medical or surgical history:
- Birth history
- Congenital anomaly
- Chronic disease (e.g., inborn error of metabolism, endocrinopathy)
- Previous infections
- Surgeries

**L**ast "feed, pee, poop": Feeding, stool, and urine pattern; use of formula (dilution?)
**I**mmediate events (history of present illness and review of systems): *OLD CAARS*
- *O*nset: Rapid or gradual
- *L*ocation: Evidence of localized pain?
- *D*uration and progression of symptoms
- *C*haracterization of symptoms
- *A*lleviating factors of symptoms
- *A*ggravating factors of symptoms
- *R*ecurrence of symptoms: ever had similar manifestation?
- *S*everity and system review

**F**amily and social history
- Inherited disorders
- Day care: Who cares for child?

**I**mmunizations up to date?
**E**mergency medical service history: Elicit history of potential trauma, ingestion, abuse, or toxin exposure
**D**octor: Name of primary care physician or specialist for additional information and help
**D**ocuments: Obtain previous medical records

toddler to the ED, they are often exhausted from attempts to console the child. In such circumstances, the EP must be able to distinguish between relatively benign conditions, such as colic, and severe, life-threatening illnesses, such as meningitis. An orderly approach to infants with excessive unexplained crying will allow the EP to diagnose the occasional severe illness and provide guidance to the caregivers.

## EPIDEMIOLOGY

The prevalence of early excessive crying (e.g., >3 hours) in infants younger than 3 months has been estimated at 8% to 29%, but it may persist for months longer in up to 40% of these children.[8] However, there is no accurate estimate of the incidence of excessive crying secondary to illness because almost every disease process can be accompanied by the symptom of crying. As infants grow and expand their repertoire for expressing specific needs, excessive crying is less frequently voiced as a primary complaint by caregivers.

## PATHOPHYSIOLOGY

During the first few months of life, infants are expected to have variable periods of prolonged crying, which is normal behavior. However, crying is considered excessive when parents complain about it. Most paroxysmal episodes of crying have a behavioral etiology. In 1954 Wessel published his "rule of 3" for diagnosing colic: when an otherwise healthy infant between the ages of 3 weeks and 3 months cries more than 3 hours per day for more than 3 days per week.[9] However, if organic pathology is to be identified, the EP must recognize

**Table 16.1 Age-Related Differential Diagnosis for Various Chief Complaints (Overlap Can Occur)**

| | INFANTS | TODDLERS |
|---|---|---|
| **Respiratory Complaints** | | |
| Cough | Upper respiratory infection<br>Bronchiolitis<br>Croup<br>Pertussis<br>Pneumonia (viral or bacterial)<br>Tracheoesophageal fistula<br>Swallowing incoordination<br>Bronchogenic cyst<br>Vascular ring<br>Foreign body aspiration | Upper respiratory infection<br>Asthma<br>Croup<br>Postnasal drip<br>Pneumonia (viral or bacterial)<br>Foreign body aspiration<br>Allergy, anaphylaxis |
| Wheezing | Bronchiolitis<br>Reactive airways disease<br>Foreign body aspiration<br>Bronchopulmonary dysplasia<br>Tracheobronchomalacia<br>Gastroesophageal reflux<br>Congenital lobar emphysema<br>Vascular ring<br>Pulmonary edema (secondary to congenital heart disorders) | Asthma<br>Foreign body aspiration<br>Allergic reactions, anaphylaxis<br>Mediastinal mass (tumor or lymphadenopathy) |
| **Gastrointestinal Complaints** | | |
| Vomiting | Sepsis<br>Meningitis, encephalitis<br>Central nervous system mass<br>Head injury<br>Hydrocephalus<br>Posttussive emesis<br>Pneumonia<br>Gastroesophageal reflux disease<br>Gastroenteritis<br>Pyloric stenosis<br>Intussusception<br>Malrotation with volvulus<br>Incarcerated hernia<br>Hirschsprung disease<br>Peritonitis<br>Congenital adrenal hyperplasia<br>Urinary tract infection<br>Inborn errors of metabolism | Sepsis<br>Meningitis, encephalitis<br>Central nervous system mass<br>Head injury<br>Hydrocephalus<br>Appendicitis<br>Intussusception<br>Gastroenteritis<br>Incarcerated hernia<br>Peritonitis<br>Diabetic ketoacidosis<br>Neoplasm (Wilms tumor, neuroblastoma)<br>Urinary tract infection |
| Abdominal pain | Trauma (intentional and nonintentional)<br>Malrotation with volvulus<br>Intussusception<br>Gastroenteritis<br>Constipation<br>Incarcerated hernia<br>Malabsorptive diseases (celiac disease, lactase deficiency)<br>Hirschsprung disease<br>Hemolytic-uremic syndrome | Trauma (intentional and nonintentional)<br>Appendicitis<br>Intussusception<br>Gastroenteritis<br>Constipation<br>Diabetic ketoacidosis<br>Incarcerated hernia<br>Hemolytic-uremic syndrome<br>Neoplasm (Wilms tumor, neuroblastoma) |
| **Neurologic Complaints** | | |
| Seizures | Febrile seizure<br>Toxic ingestion<br>Hypoglycemia<br>Hyponatremia<br>Pyridoxine-dependent seizures<br>Meningitis<br>Encephalitis<br>Inborn errors of metabolism<br>Traumatic head injury<br>Myoclonic encephalopathy<br>Early infantile epileptic encephalopathy<br>Benign infantile seizures | Febrile seizure<br>Toxic ingestion<br>Hypoglycemia<br>Meningitis<br>Encephalitis<br>Traumatic head injury<br>Lennox-Gastaut syndrome<br>Childhood absence epilepsy<br>Partial benign epilepsy |

**Table 16.2** The "Head-to-Toe" Memory Tool

| "HEAD-TO-TOE" PHYSICAL EXAMINATION | POTENTIAL CLINICAL FINDINGS | GENERATE "HEAD-TO-TOE" DIFFERENTIAL DIAGNOSIS (EXAMPLES) |
|---|---|---|
| Head | Bulging fontanelle<br>Step-off, laceration, ecchymosis, hematoma<br>Ventriculoperitoneal shunt | Central nervous system infection<br>Meningitis<br>Encephalitis<br>Intracranial abscess<br>Closed head injury<br>Ventriculoperitoneal shunt malfunction<br>Central nervous system tumor<br>Cerebrovascular accident: ischemic or hemorrhagic<br>Seizure |
| Eyes | Icterus, conjunctival injection, cranial nerve deficit, retinal hemorrhage | Bile obstruction, hemolysis, foreign body or abrasion, shaken baby syndrome |
| Nose | Congestion | Upper airway distress (<6 mo) |
| Mouth | Poor dentition | Toxin ingestion or exposure<br>Oral infection |
| Neck | Mass | Thyroid or parathyroid disease<br>Adenitis |
| Chest<br>Pulmonary<br>Cardiac | Chest wall tenderness<br>Stridor, rales, rhonchi, wheezing, murmur, dysrhythmia | Trauma (e.g., child abuse)<br>Croup, tracheitis, pneumonia, bronchiolitis, asthma<br>Congenital heart disease, myocarditis, supraventricular tachycardia |
| Abdomen<br>Gastrointestinal tract<br>Liver<br>Pancreas<br>Kidney and urinary tract<br>Adrenal glands | Distention, tenderness, peritoneal signs, palpable mass | Gastroesophageal reflux, malrotation, pyloric stenosis, intussusception, hernia, appendicitis, Hirschsprung disease, constipation<br>Liver: inborn error<br>Pancreas: hypoglycemia, diabetic ketoacidosis<br>Urinary tract: electrolyte disorder, infection, torsion<br>Adrenal: congenital adrenal hyperplasia |
| Extremities | Deformity, tenderness, edema, induration, erythema | Fractures<br>Nonaccidental trauma<br>Accidental trauma<br>Osteomyelitis, septic arthritis, toxic synovitis<br>Rhabdomyolysis |
| Skin | Rash, petechiae | Abscess, cellulitis, omphalitis, mastitis, burn, anal fissure, sepsis |
| Neurologic | Weakness, decreased reflexes | Guillain-Barré syndrome, botulism |

that excessive crying has meaning and may be indicative of acute illness. In a study of 56 infants with an episode of excessive, prolonged crying without fever or cause identified by the parents, 61% had a serious final diagnosis.[10]

## PRESENTING SIGNS AND SYMPTOMS

The general appearance of the crying infant immediately helps the EP establish the severity of the illness (sick or not so sick?). A lethargic, ill-appearing, inconsolable infant mandates immediate consideration of sepsis, meningtis, increased intracranial pressure, or some other serious illness.

After the primary survey is complete and it is determined that no emergency intervention is indicated, the EP needs to elicit a comprehensive AMPLIFIEDD history (**Box 16.2**) from the primary caregiver. Clinical findings on the head-to-toe evaluation suggesting a potential cause of the excessive crying may include the following:

- Signs of head trauma, such as scalp contusions, ecchymoses and lacerations, hemotympanum, postauricular hematomas, or periorbital ecchymoses
- A bulging fontanelle indicative of increased intracranial pressure
- A sunken anterior fontanelle consistent with dehydration
- Fluorescein uptake indicating corneal abrasions
- Retinal hemorrhages raising concern for serious abuse
- An erythematous and bulging tympanic membrane signifying otitis media

**BOX 16.2 The AMPLIFIEDD History for a Crying Infant or Toddler**

**A**llergies
**M**edication (by mom or infant): Prescription, over the counter, natural remedies
**P**ast medical history
- Birth history: Prenatal-maternal illness or infections, illicit drug use
- Perinatal: Gestational age, complications, birth weight, infections in infant or mom
- Outpatient treatment or hospitalizations for illness or surgery
- Developmental milestones
- Appropriate weight gain
- Newborn screen: Identify abnormalities

**L**ast feed, pee, poop, sleep
- Feed: Diet, amount and frequency, correct formula preparation, recent changes, breast milk (maternal medications or drugs)
- Adequacy of urine output and characterization of stooling pattern
- Abnormal sleep pattern: Too much or too little

**I**mmediate events (history of present illness and review of systems): *OLD CAARS*
- *O*nset of crying (when did the crying begin?)
- *L*ocation: As the child develops a more expanded repertoire for communication and caretakers are able to intuit the child's behavior, localization of pain is possible
- *D*uration of crying
- *C*haracterization of crying: What does the cry sound like? Is it a cry of hunger, pain, or expression of a desire to be changed or cuddled?
- *A*ggravating factors: What factors exacerbate the crying (e.g., holding the child, manipulating an extremity)?
- *A*lleviating factors: What factors alleviate the crying (e.g., feeding, caretaker contact)?
- *R*ecurring factors: Is this episode acute and prolonged or a recurring event? If recurrent, establish the frequency and relationship to feeding and sleeping and ask about previous evaluations
- *R*eview of *S*ystems: Fever, trauma, rhinorrhea, cough, difficulty breathing, vomiting (bilious, projectile, feculent, bloody, or stomach contents only), diarrhea, blood in stool, rash, abnormal movement or spell-like behavior

**F**amily and social history
- Inherited disorders: Sickle cell disease, cystic fibrosis, immunodeficiency disorder, hemophilia, asthma
- Characterization of parental-infant interactions: Identify parental styles and management practices (include perceptions of extended family members)
- Birth order of child may influence parental interpretation of the meaning of crying
- Day care
- Smoking, use of illicit drugs, or excessive alcohol consumption in the household
- Exposure to other ill children or adults

**I**mmunizations: Nonstop crying episodes for longer than 3 hours can rarely occur with recent pertussis vaccination*
**E**mergency medical service history: Elicit history of potential trauma, abuse, or toxin exposure
**D**octor: Name of primary care physician or specialist for additional information and help
**D**ocuments: Obtain previous medical records

*Jefferson T, Rudin M, DiPietrantonj C. Systematic review of the effects of pertussis vaccines in children. Vaccine 2003;21:2003-14.

- Obstruction of the nares secondary to a foreign body
- Oral thrush or mucosal ulcers in the oropharynx often seen with stomatitis
- Exudative pharyngitis and fullness of the posterior pharynx suggesting peritonsillar or retropharyngeal abscesses
- Wheezing, rales, or rhonchi indicating a respiratory infection
- Palpation of a mass during the abdominal examination, which can be associated with pyloric stenosis, intussusception, or a tumor
- Diaper rash, anal fissure, or impacted stool on rectal examination
- Scrotal swelling consistent with an incarcerated hernia or testicular torsion
- Extremity tenderness, edema, or bruising concerning for a possible fracture
- Erythema, induration, and tenderness suggesting a soft tissue infection (cellulitis or abscess)
- Hair tourniquet on a toe or finger
- Rashes with potentially life-threatening causes (e.g., petechiae, purpura)

## DIFFERENTIAL DIAGNOSIS AND MEDICAL DECISION MAKING

A comprehensive history and systematic head-to-toe physical examination along with a period of ED observation are usually sufficient to differentiate acute illness or injury from a recurrent benign crying syndrome. It is important to remember that excessive crying may be the only behavioral change that the caregiver recognizes as an indicator of illness. Detection of subtle signs and symptoms will help identify high-acuity, low-frequency events. The practitioner should pay close attention to red flags in a young infant such as fever, failure to thrive, paradoxic irritability (crying with movement), vomiting, bloody stools, abnormal neurologic findings, and unexplained abnormal vital signs. A comprehensive differential diagnosis can be generated by using the head-to-toe memory tool (**Fig. 16.2** and **Box 16.3**).

Allow the history, physical examination, and observed behavior of the infant to guide a stepwise approach to

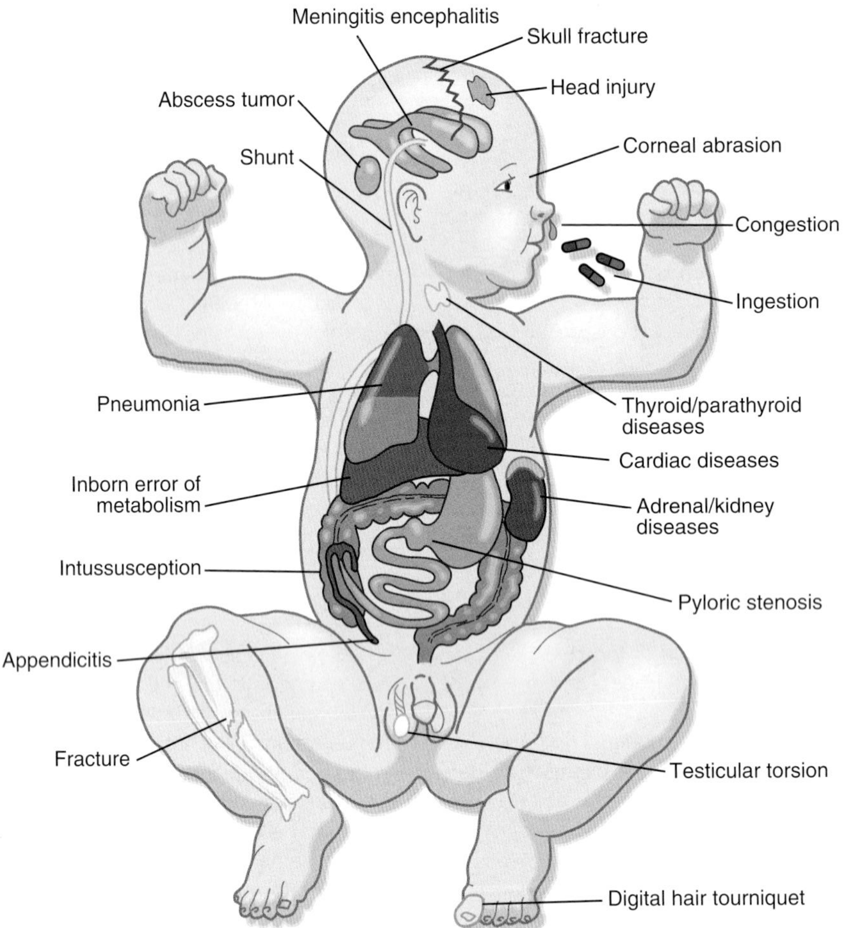


**Fig. 16.2 Head-to-toe differential diagnosis.**

**BOX 16.3 Differential Diagnosis of Crying (Head-to-Toe Memory Tool)**

**Head, Eyes, Ears, Nose, and Mouth**

*Head*: Meningitis, encephalitis, ventriculoperitoneal shunt malfunction or infection, closed head injury (skull fracture; epidural, subdural hematoma), cerebrovascular accident, tumor

*Eye*: Foreign body, corneal abrasion, glaucoma

*Ear*: Otitis media

*Nose*: Nasal congestion (distress in those <6 mo)

*Mouth*: Ingestion (drug toxicity such as carbon monoxide, methemoglobinemia), thrush, stomatitis

**Neck**

Mass, adenitis, torticollis, hyperthyroidism, hypothyroidism

**Chest**

*Chest wall*: Trauma

*Airway, lungs*: Pneumonia, bronchiolitis, hypoxia, hypercapnia, croup, tracheitis

*Cardiac*: Congenital heart disease, congestive heart failure, myocarditis, anomalous origin of the right coronary artery, supraventricular tachycardia

**Abdomen**

*Gastrointestinal tract*: Gastroesophageal reflux, aerophagia, pyloric stenosis, intussusception, malrotation with volvulus, inguinal hernia, gastroenteritis with dehydration, appendicitis, Hirschsprung disease, constipation, peritonitis

*Liver*: Inborn errors of metabolism

*Pancreas*: Hypoglycemia, diabetic ketoacidosis

*Kidney and urinary tract*: Electrolyte disorders, urinary tract obstruction, urinary tract infection, torsion of the testes or ovaries, hair tourniquet of the penis

*Adrenal*: Congenital adrenal hyperplasia

**Musculoskeletal**

Fracture or dislocation, osteomyelitis, septic arthritis, toxic synovitis, pain at injection site, pertussis vaccine reaction, hair tourniquet of a digit

**Skin**

Mastitis, omphalitis, burn, cellulitis, anal fissure, rash, insect or spider bite

**Neurologic**

Seizure activity, botulism

**Systemic**

Sepsis

**BOX 16.4 Diagnostic Tests to Consider in an Infant or Child with Inconsolable Crying**

**Radiographic**
Chest radiograph
Skeletal survey
Cranial, abdominal, pelvic computed tomography
Abdominal radiograph: Flat and upright
Abdominal ultrasound
Upper gastrointestinal series
Bone scan
Magnetic resonance imaging

**Diagnostic Procedures**
*Cerebrospinal fluid analysis and culture
Herpes polymerase chain reaction
*Fluorescein examination

**Laboratory Studies**
*Accu-Chek
*Complete blood count
*Serum electrolytes, calcium
*Urinalysis
*Blood and urine cultures
Serum ammonia
Lactate
Thyroid profile
Toxicologic screening
Erythrocyte sedimentation rate, C-reactive protein

**Cardiac Screening**
Electrocardiogram
Cardiac monitoring
Echocardiogram

*Routine tests to perform on a child with undifferentiated excessive crying.

diagnostic evaluation. A healthy-appearing infant who ceases crying before or soon after arrival at the ED rarely has a serious cause.[11] An infant who continues to cry will require diagnostic testing directed by careful consideration of the potential differential diagnosis (**Box 16.4**). For example, suspicion of child abuse should prompt a funduscopic examination and consideration of radiographic studies, including a skeletal survey, computed tomography (CT) of the head, and CT of the abdomen and pelvis. Evaluate cardiac problems with continuous cardiac monitoring, a 12-lead electrocardiogram, a chest radiograph, and an echocardiogram as indicated. Confirm gastrointestinal pathology with selective radiographic studies such as screening supine and upright abdominal radiographs, ultrasound, upper gastrointestinal series, or judicious use of CT scanning. Evaluate for infectious causes with a chest radiograph, cerebrospinal fluid analysis, and urinalysis. Serum electrolytes, ammonia level, serum pH, and lactate levels are useful to screen for an inborn error of metabolism. Use C-reactive protein, the erythrocyte sedimentation rate, bone scanning, and magnetic resonance imaging to evaluate potential musculoskeletal pathologies.

## TREATMENT AND DISPOSITION

The treatment plan and consultative services for excessive crying are determined by the underlying cause. An infant who ceases to cry and otherwise demonstrates no evidence of systemic illness may be discharged home with close follow-up. However, before discharge, carefully assess the caregiver's capacity to continue caring for the infant while recognizing that admission of the infant may provide a needed respite. In addition, minimize the risk for abuse by confirming that an adequate support system is available. If discharged home, provide clear instructions to return with any progression of symptoms.

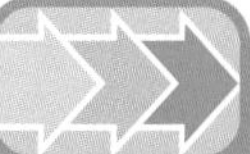

**PRIORITY ACTIONS**

Do not make a diagnosis of infantile colic on the first episode of excessive crying. Remember Wessel's rule of 3.[9]
Paradoxic irritability (crying with movement) and an acute onset of unexplained crying are red flags for serious illness.
Always undress the infant or child and document a rectal temperature.
Initiate a period of observation if the infant does not appear to be ill. Proceed with a further diagnostic work-up if the crying does not cease.
In a child who will be discharged home, document and review plans for followup and mandate return to the emergency department if the symptoms return or progress.

# ALTERED LEVEL OF CONSCIOUSNESS

## PERSPECTIVE

An infant or toddler with an altered level of consciousness may have a life-threatening illness that requires immediate recognition and treatment to prevent permanent central nervous system (CNS) dysfunction or death.

## EPIDEMIOLOGY

An altered level of consciousness in this age group is caused by nonstructural causes (e.g., infection, metabolic abnormalities, toxin ingestion) or primary structural disease of the CNS (e.g., hemorrhage, tumors). Physical abuse is the leading cause of serious head injury in young children. Shaken baby syndrome most often involves children younger than 2 years and can easily be misdiagnosed.[12]

## PATHOPHYSIOLOGY

A normal level of consciousness requires proper function and communication of the cerebral cortex and reticular activating system. Normal neuronal activity involves a multifaceted balance of water, electrolytes, metabolic substrates, and neurotransmitter concentrations within a tightly controlled environment of temperature, pH, and osmolality. Any alteration in this environment resulting from insufficient blood flow, electrolyte imbalance, lack of substrate, presence of toxins, abnormal concentration of metabolic waste products, or loss of temperature results in the final common pathway of CNS dysfunction and an altered level of consciousness.

**BOX 16.5 The AMPLIFIEDD History for an Infant or Toddler with Altered Level of Consciousness**

Allergies to medications, environmental allergens
Medications: prescriptions, over the counter, natural remedies
Past medical history: Birth history, congenital anomalies, chronic disease (e.g., inborn error of metabolism, endocrinopathy), infections, seizures
Last feed, pee, poop: Feeding, stool and urine pattern, use of formula (dilution?)
Immediate events (history of present illness and review of systems): *OLD CAARS*
- *O*nset: Rapid or gradual
- *L*ocation: Evidence of localized pain?
- *D*uration and progression of symptoms
- *C*haracterization of change in level of consciousness: Lethargy, irritability, excessive crying
- *A*lleviating factors: Can the child be consoled?
- *A*ggravating factors: Does movement of the child cause apparent discomfort (e.g., meningitis, peritonitis, injury)?
- *R*ecurrence of symptoms: Ever had similar findings?
- *S*ystem review: Trauma, seizure activity, fever, vomiting, diarrhea, recent infection, shortness of breath, change in behavior (e.g., colicky pain, paroxysmal crying), rash, irritability

Family and social history: Inherited disorders, day care, who cares for the child
Immunizations up to date?
Emergency medical system history: Elicit history of potential trauma, ingestion, abuse, or toxin exposure
Doctor: Name of primary care physician or specialist for additional information and help
Documents: Obtain previous medical records

## PRESENTING SIGNS AND SYMPTOMS

Always direct the initial evaluation toward identifying potential life-threatening conditions such as hypoxia, hypotension, extremes of temperature, hypoglycemia, seizure activity, and increased intracranial pressure, which require immediate intervention. Once these issues have been excluded, the EP should perform an AMPLIFIEDD history (**Box 16.5**). Investigate the risk for accidental or nonaccidental trauma, infection, ingestion, or toxin exposure while identifying signs or symptoms suggestive of systemic disease. Interview all available caretakers and emergency medical service personnel.

Following the primary survey, a head-to-toe evaluation should be performed. The EP should:

- Pay close attention to the pupillary response, which generally remain intact with metabolic insults but may be absent with structural lesions, toxin exposure, or severe asphyxia.
- Note the eye position (e.g., deviation of conjugate gaze away from brainstem lesions and toward cerebral lesions).
- Identify abnormalities in the respiratory pattern that may reflect CNS insults or metabolic conditions such as metabolic acidosis.
- Evaluate motor strength, tone, and reflexes, and characterize activity that may be consistent with seizures or abnormal posturing.
- Look for signs of trauma, such as scalp contusions and lacerations, hemotympanum, postauricular or periorbital hematomas, retinal hemorrhages, cerebrospinal fluid otorrhea, and a bulging anterior fontanelle suggestive of increased intracranial pressure.
- Note odors suggesting inborn errors of metabolism or other metabolic disorders (e.g., the smell of acetone in a child with diabetic ketoacidosis).
- Identify physical findings that indicate systemic infections involving the CNS (e.g., vesicular or purpuric rashes).
- Identify signs of other systemic disorders that have a negative impact on mental status, such as intussusception (e.g., abdominal mass, blood in the stool), hepatic disorders (e.g., jaundice, icterus), or cardiopulmonary disease (e.g., hypoxia, rales, hepatomegaly).

## DIFFERENTIAL DIAGNOSIS AND MEDICAL DECISION MAKING

A comprehensive differential diagnosis for alterations in consciousness in infants and toddlers can be generated with the head-to-toe memory tool (**Box 16.6**). Possible causes involve essentially every organ system. When the underlying cause of altered mental status is not obvious, a high level of suspicion should be maintained for abuse, accidental toxin ingestion or exposure, intussusception, infection, or nonconvulsive seizure activity.

Assess the ABCs of resuscitation—airway, breathing, and circulation—rapidly, initiate cardiorespiratory monitoring and pulse oximetry, and institute any necessary interventions immediately. Perform rapid bedside glucose testing as part of the primary survey. Consider antidotes for toxin exposure or poisoning (e.g., naloxone for opioid ingestion), and administer broad-spectrum antibiotics early if indicated.

Perform laboratory and radiographic testing via a systematic, comprehensive approach (**Box 16.7**). In a critically ill infant or toddler without a definitive diagnosis, routine testing for sepsis, trauma, and metabolic derangements should be supplemented with selective tests as dictated by progression of the clinical course, by the response to initial interventions, and by the history and physical findings.

## TREATMENT AND DISPOSITION

If a definitive diagnosis is not rapidly apparent in a child with an altered level of consciousness, institute supportive care to assist ventilation and maintain adequate circulation, and treat potentially life-threatening conditions such as sepsis or electrolyte abnormalities. When a cause is diagnosed, appropriate treatment should follow. Unless an easily recognizable and reversible cause is found, all children with an altered level of consciousness should be admitted to a pediatric intensive care unit.

**BOX 16.6 Differential Diagnosis of Altered Level of Consciousness in Infants and Toddlers Using the Head-to-Toe Memory Tool**

**Head and Mouth**

*Head*

- Seizure (postictal state)
- Infection: Meningitis, encephalitis, abscess, ventriculoperitoneal shunt malfunction or infection
- Closed head injury: Epidural, subdural, or intraparenchymal hematoma; concussion; cerebral edema
- Vascular: Ischemic or hemorrhagic infarction, subarachnoid hemorrhage, venous thrombosis
- Central nervous system tumor

*Mouth*: Toxin ingestion or exposure—sedatives, anticholinergics, tricyclic antidepressants, salicylates, alcohol, precipitant of methemoglobinemia, carbon monoxide, heavy metals

**Neck**

Hypothyroid, hyperthyroid, parathyroid (hypercalcemia, hypocalcemia)

**Chest**

*Pulmonary*: Respiratory failure, asphyxia, hypoxia secondary to pulmonary disease

*Cardiac*: Hypotension (congenital heart disease, dysrhythmias, congestive heart failure), anemia

**Abdomen**

*Gastrointestinal tract*: Intussusception, dehydration secondary to vomiting, diarrhea

*Liver*: Inborn errors of metabolism, Reye syndrome, hepatic encephalopathy

*Pancreas*: Hypoglycemia, diabetic ketoacidosis

*Kidney and urinary tract*

- Electrolyte disorders: Hyponatremia, hypernatremia, hypermagnesemia, hypomagnesemia, uremia, metabolic acidosis or alkalosis
- Infection: Pyelonephritis with urosepsis

*Adrenal gland*: Cortisol deficiency

**Other**

Sepsis, hypothermia, hyperthermia

**BOX 16.7 Laboratory and Radiographic Testing in Infants and Toddlers with Altered Level of Consciousness**

**Laboratory Testing**

***Routine***

Rapid bedside glucose
Bedside urine dip
Complete blood count
Electrolytes
Blood urea nitrogen and serum creatinine
Urinalysis

***Selective***

Blood gas analysis
Toxicology screening
Liver function testing
Serum ammonia, lactate (inborn errors of metabolism)
Plasma quantitative amino acids and acylcarnitine, quantitative urine organic acids (inborn errors of metabolism)
Serum osmolality (measured and calculated)
Blood and urine cultures
Cerebrospinal fluid analysis and culture
Ethanol level
Lead level
Serum cortisol measurement
Thyroid profile

**Radiographic Testing**

***Routine***

Chest radiograph

***Selective***

Cranial tomography
Abdominal ultrasonography
Abdominal computed tomography
Skeletal survey
Magnetic resonance imaging of the head
Barium or air contrast enema
Shunt series

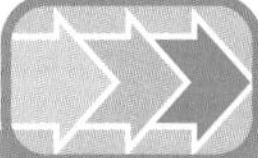

**PRIORITY ACTIONS**

**Infant or Toddler with Altered Level of Consciousness**

Perform rapid bedside glucose testing on arrival.

If the underlying cause is not clear, consider the following diagnoses: intussusception, accidental ingestion, environmental exposure, or nonaccidental trauma.

# VOMITING

## PERSPECTIVE

Vomiting in children is usually caused by a self-limited condition but may result from a severe, life-threatening illness. A systematic approach based on age-specific considerations is critical for making the appropriate diagnosis and treating infants and toddlers with vomiting. The EP should consider

**BOX 16.8 The AMPLIFIEDD History for an Infant or Toddler with Vomiting**

**A**llergies: To medications or foods ( protein intolerance to cow milk, soy, gluten)
**M**edication: Prescription, over the counter, natural remedies
**P**ast medical history
- Chronic or previous illness: Metabolic or endocrinopathy, recent unresolved illness
- Previous surgery suggesting abdominal adhesions, shunt infection, or obstruction
- Newborn screening: Identify abnormalities
- Appropriate developmental milestones?

**L**ast feed, pee, poop, sleep
- Feed: Diet, amount and frequency, correct formula preparation, recent changes, types of solids
- Pee and poop: Urine output and characterization of stooling pattern (diarrhea, blood, mucus)
- Sleep pattern: Waking with intermittent episodes of pain (intussusception)

**I**mmediate events (history of present illness and review of systems): *OLD CAARS*
- *O*nset of vomiting
- *L*ocation of pain (e.g., abdomen, head)
- *D*uration and frequency of vomiting: Estimate ongoing volume loss by quantifying number and quantity of vomiting or diarrheal episodes
- *C*haracterization of the emesis
  - Contents: Undigested gastric contents (reflux), bilious (postampullary obstruction), feculent (colonic obstruction), blood or coffeeground (gastritis, ulcer, Mallory-Weiss tear)
  - Force of vomiting: Projectile (pyloric stenosis), non-projectile (reflux, postfeeding regurgitation)
- *A*ggravating factors: What factors exacerbate the vomiting (early morning: central nervous system mass; feeding: food allergen, after ingestion of toxin)?
- *A*lleviating factors: What factors relieve the vomiting (keeping the child in an upright position: reflux)?
- *R*ecurrent: Similar episodes suggestive of recurring disorders (pyloric stenosis, cyclic vomiting, inborn error of metabolism, malrotation with intermittent volvulus)
- *S*ystems review: Inquire about fever, trauma, neurologic symptoms (headache, vertigo, visual symptoms), diarrhea (infectious gastroenteritis), ingestion of toxins

**F**amily and social history
- Infectious contacts, travel
- Characterization of caretaker-infant interactions: Identify risk for child abuse

**I**mmunizations up to date?
**E**mergency medical service history: Elicit history of potential trauma, ingestion, abuse, or toxin exposure
**D**octor: Name of primary care physician or specialist for additional information and help
**D**ocuments: Obtain previous medical records

**BOX 16.9 Key Objective Findings on Physical Examination for Assessing Dehydration**

The presence of two findings indicates greater than 5% dehydration; the presence of three or more findings indicates greater than 10% dehydration:
- Capillary refill > 2 seconds
- Dry mucous membranes
- Absent tears
- Abnormally lethargic or listless appearance

Adapted from Gorelick M, Shaw K, Murphy K. Validity and reliability of clinical signs in the diagnosis of dehydration in children. Pediatrics 1997;99(5):e6.

an expanded differential diagnosis in a child who comes to the ED with vomiting but no diarrheal illness.

## EPIDEMIOLOGY

Episodes of acute gastroenteritis in children younger than 5 years lead to 2 to 3 million physician visits annually.[13] The majority of these children have uneventful clinical courses.

## PATHOPHYSIOLOGY

Vomiting is coordinated by the vomiting center in the reticular formation of the medulla. This vomiting center integrates and responds to afferent pathways from higher cortical centers in the brain and to visceral afferents from receptors in the gastrointestinal tract and other organs. Specifically, the chemoreceptor trigger zone in the floor of the fourth ventricle monitors chemical abnormalities in the blood and cerebrospinal fluid. A basic understanding of these major pathways is essential for developing diagnostic and therapeutic strategies for infants and toddlers with vomiting.

## PRESENTING SIGNS AND SYMPTOMS

A review of the expansive list of potential causes of vomiting emphasizes the importance of developing an organized approach to achieve an accurate diagnosis. The EP should first elicit an AMPLIFIEDD history (**Box 16.8**) and perform a thorough head-to-toe physical examination focusing on the age of the infant or toddler. Evidence of bowel obstruction, peritonitis, and signs or symptoms suggestive of extraintestinal disease should be sought. Hydration status (**Box 16.9**) should be assessed. At the onset of the clinical encounter, the EP should clarify whether the child has had bilious or nonbilious vomiting because bilious emesis in infants implies intestinal obstruction until proved otherwise and requires immediate surgical consultation.[14]

Appearance and age-appropriate behavior should be assessed because a decrease in activity or level of consciousness may indicate serious illness. A bulging fontanelle suggests increased intracranial pressure from potential causes

**Table 16.3 Differential Diagnosis of Vomiting in Infants and Children Using the Head-to-Toe Memory Tool**

| | INFANTS | TODDLERS |
|---|---|---|
| Head | Meningitis, encephalitis<br>Central nervous system mass<br>Head injury<br>Hydrocephalus (e.g., shunt malfunction)<br>Otitis media<br>Spitting up | Meningitis, encephalitis<br>Central nervous system mass<br>Head injury<br>Hydrocephalus<br>Otitis media<br>Oral ingestion (overdose)<br>Cyclic vomiting<br>Psychogenic |
| Chest | Posttussive emesis secondary to reactive airways<br>Respiratory infection (pneumonia) | Posttussive emesis secondary to reactive airways<br>Respiratory infection (pneumonia) |
| **Abdomen** | | |
| Gastrointestinal tract | Gastroesophageal reflux disease<br>Gastroenteritis<br>Nutrient intolerance<br>Rumination<br>Obstruction:<br>Pyloric stenosis<br>Intussusception<br>Malrotation<br>Incarcerated hernia<br>Hirschsprung disease<br>Peritonitis | Peptic ulcer disease<br>Gastroenteritis<br>Obstruction:<br>Intussusception<br>Malrotation<br>Incarcerated hernia<br>Hirschsprung disease<br>Appendicitis<br>Meckel diverticulum<br>Peritonitis |
| Adrenals | Congenital adrenal hyperplasia | Adrenal insufficiency |
| Renal | Uremia<br>Obstruction<br>Urinary tract infection or pyelonephritis<br>Renal insufficiency | Uremia<br>Obstruction<br>Urinary tract infection or pyelonephritis<br>Renal insufficiency |
| Liver | Hepatitis<br>Inborn errors of metabolism | Hepatitis<br>Inborn errors of metabolism |
| Pancreas | Diabetic ketoacidosis<br>Pancreatitis | Diabetic ketoacidosis<br>Pancreatitis |
| Other | Sepsis | Sepsis |

such as meningitis, trauma, an intracranial mass, or intracranial bleeding. Retinal hemorrhages indicate nonaccidental trauma, and scleral icterus suggests hepatobiliary disease. An unusual odor may be the first clue to an inborn error of metabolism. Marked abdominal distention, peristaltic waves, increased bowel sounds, palpable masses, bloody stools, and guarding all point to an intraabdominal disorder. A thorough examination necessitates evaluation for torsion of the testes and the ambiguous genitalia associated with congenital adrenal hyperplasia. The skin should be examined for rashes indicative of an infectious cause. Unusual contusions or musculoskeletal injury may indicate nonaccidental trauma.

## DIFFERENTIAL DIAGNOSIS AND MEDICAL DECISION MAKING

The list of potential causes of vomiting in infants is extensive but can be conveniently organized according to age-related categories (**Table 16.3**). Many serious medical conditions may be initially manifested as vomiting, such as sepsis, meningitis, urinary tract infection, and hepatitis. These conditions must be differentiated from emergency surgical conditions such as an incarcerated hernia, intussusception, and malrotation with volvulus. Intussusception is the most common cause of intestinal obstruction in children 3 months to 5 years of age, whereas appendicitis is the most common condition requiring surgical intervention.[15,16]

The large number of potential causes of vomiting makes routine laboratory and radiographic evaluation impractical. The history and physical findings should direct the choice of testing for each patient. For most common conditions, laboratory testing is not indicated. A bedside blood glucose measurement should be performed in any child with altered mental status. Serum electrolytes should be measured in children with dehydration requiring intravenous rehydration. A serum bicarbonate level lower than 17 mEq/L appears to be the most useful laboratory value for predicting the likelihood of 5% dehydration.[17,18] Cerebrospinal fluid analysis should be performed if meningitis or encephalitis is suspected. Drug screening may be necessary to confirm an ingestion. Urinalysis, liver function tests, serum lipase, and ammonia measurements should be considered when the differential diagnosis is broadened.

Diagnostic imaging is also dictated by clinical findings. CT of the head should be performed for suspected closed-head injury, intracranial tumor, or hydrocephalus. Plain radiographs may be used to assess for bowel obstruction. An upper

**BOX 16.10 Oral Rehydration Therapy**

**Rehydration Phase**

Replace fluid deficit over a 4-hour period with rehydration solution (Rehydralyte, Pedialyte)

Administer oral rehydration therapy in frequent, small amounts: no more than 5 mL every 1 to 2 minutes via syringe, spoon, cup, or nasogastric tube

Goal: 50 mL/kg for mild dehydration, 100 mL/kg for moderate dehydration

Replace ongoing losses from diarrhea (10 mL/kg per watery stool) and vomiting (2 mL/kg per episode of emesis) with oral rehydration solution

Avoid nonphysiologic foods such as juice, tea, and cola during this phase

**Maintenance Phase**

Begin the realimentation phase with the goal of returning to unrestricted age-appropriate diet

Data from Practice parameter: The management of acute gastroenteritis in young children. American Academy of Pediatrics, Provisional Committee on Quality Improvement, Subcommittee on Acute Gastroenteritis. Pediatrics 1996;97:428-9.

gastrointestinal series is the preferred radiographic modality for diagnosing malrotation with volvulus.[19] Diagnostic ultrasonography is the modality of choice for diagnosing intussusception.[20] Ultrasonography and abdominal CT are used to investigate potential appendicitis when the diagnosis is in question. In children with equivocal findings for appendicitis, ultrasonography using the graded-compression technique should be performed, followed by focused abdominal CT if the ultrasonographic findings are normal.[21] Similarly, implement protocols for appropriate use of ultrasonography and CT for evaluation of intraabdominal pathology such as trauma, an intraabdominal mass, or nephrolithiasis.

## TREATMENT

Initial management of a vomiting infant or toddler should focus on hemodynamic stabilization. Persistent vomiting, severe dehydration, and electrolyte abnormalities necessitate treatment in parallel with other diagnostic testing. Rehydration is accomplished with 20-mL/kg intravenous boluses of isotonic saline, repeated as necessary. Additional treatment should be directed toward the underlying cause.

Immediately consult a surgeon for infants with bilious vomiting. Malrotation with volvulus is a surgical emergency requiring rapid response to prevent infarction of the bowel. Timely surgical consultation is also the standard of care for other conditions such as peritonitis and incarcerated hernia. In some cases the radiologist may successfully reduce the intussuscepted bowel with an air or contrast enema, although surgical backup is required for potential complications or treatment failure. Decompression with nasogastric suctioning is indicated for children with ileus or bowel obstruction.

Administration of an antiemetic may serve as a successful adjunct to suppress vomiting and allow oral rehydration. Intravenous and oral ondansetron (a selective serotonin [5-$HT_3$] receptor antagonist) has been used successfully in the ED for infants and children with vomiting secondary to gastroenteritis.[22-24]

Oral rehydration therapy should be administered to children with mild to moderate dehydration as a result of gastroenteritis (**Box 16.10**).[25] A metaanalysis of randomized control trials involving 1545 children younger than 15 years concluded that rehydration by the oral or nasogastric route is as effective if not better than intravenous rehydration.[26]

## DISPOSITION

An infant or toddler with a self-limited condition and no evidence of systemic illness or dehydration can be discharged. Provide clear plans for follow-up and instructions for outpatient oral rehydration to the parents or caregiver. Always confirm that the caretaker understands the need to return to the ED if the illness progresses.

Infants or children with persistent vomiting, abnormal electrolyte values, or a more complex diagnosis requiring further medical or surgical management should be admitted to the hospital.

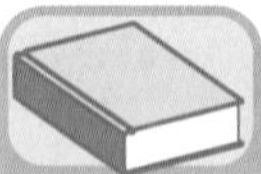

**PARENT TEACHING TIPS**

**Infant or Toddler in the Emergency Department**

Confirm that parents understand the diagnosis, treatment, followup plans, and any symptoms that warrant immediate return to the emergency department.

Reinforce that parents are always welcome to return to the ED with any concern.

## SUGGESTED READINGS

Brazelton T. Crying in infancy. Pediatrics 1962;29:579-88.

Steiner M, Dewalt D, Byerley J. Is this child dehydrated? JAMA 2004;291:2746-54.

Wessel M, Cobb J, Jackson E, et al. Paroxysmal fussing in infancy, sometimes called colic. Pediatrics 1954;14:421-35.

## REFERENCES

*References can be found on Expert Consult @ www.expertconsult.com.*

# Child with a Fever 17

*Jana L. Anderson, Christopher S. Kiefer, and James E. Colletti*

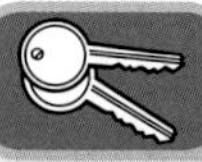

**KEY POINTS**

- A fever is defined as a temperature of 38.0° C (100.4° F) or higher measured rectally.
- Response to antipyretics is not a predictor of the presence of bacterial illness and therefore should not influence clinical decision making.
- The diagnostic evaluation of a febrile child is based on clinical findings, immunization status, and age of the child.
- The peripheral white blood cell count is unreliable in determining the presence or absence of bacterial illness and should not guide diagnostic and treatment decisions.

## PERSPECTIVE

Developing an accurate diagnostic impression, performing an appropriate work-up, and determining treatment and disposition for a febrile infant or child is not always a straightforward process. The diagnostic work-up varies dramatically based on the age of the child, clinical appearance, physical examination, maternal risk factors, and immunization status.

Fever is the most common chief complaint in children younger than 3 years seen in the emergency department (ED) (see Facts and Formulas box). Fever is defined as an elevation in temperature to 38.0° C (100.4° F) or higher. In young children, particularly those younger than 2 years, the temperature should be taken rectally because other methods such as tympanic and axillary are not as reliable or accurate.[1] Parental report of fever determined by touch is likely to be accurate regarding the presence of a fever.[2] A common misconception is that bundling a baby can account for an elevation in core temperature, but it cannot.[3] More than 20% of fevers seen in the ED will be fevers without a source and require risk stratification based on the child's age, appearance, and immunization status.

Infants are at particularly high risk for serious bacterial illnesses because of their minimal signs and symptoms, lack of immunity, maternal birth canal exposure, and difficulty in mounting a response to infections. To deal with this increased risk for infection, multiple protocols to evaluate a febrile infant have been developed (**Box 17.1**). As a general consensus, infants younger than 28 days with a temperature of 38.0° C should undergo a full sepsis evaluation, parenteral administration of antibiotics, and admission to the hospital.[4] A full sepsis evaluation includes a complete blood count (CBC) with differential, blood culture, and a catheterized urine sample sent for urinalysis, Gram stain, and culture. If symptoms are present, stool studies or a chest radiograph should be performed. A lumbar puncture with cell count and differential, Gram stain, and culture should be obtained. Antibiotics recommended are ampicillin, 50 mg/kg, and cefotaxime, 50 mg/kg. Ceftriaxone is not used in the neonatal period because of possible disconjugation of bilirubin. Neonatal herpes should also be considered as a cause of the fever, particularly in infants younger than 2 weeks. Frequently, the mother's history of maternal herpes is not known, nor does the child have any physical findings. If there is any concern, herpes polymerase chain reaction should be performed on cerebrospinal fluid and the child should be administered acyclovir (20 mg/kg). Overall, well-appearing febrile neonates have a 7% likelihood of having a serious bacterial infection, with the most common being a urinary tract infection.[5-7]

Infants 28 days to 2 to 3 months of age may be risk-stratified with the febrile infant protocol to help guide the evaluation of fever (**Figs. 17.1 and 17.2**). Many physicians use an age cutoff of 60 days or less to perform a full sepsis evaluation, although some physicians still perform a full sepsis evaluation in children up to 90 days of age.[8] These practice variations are seen in different settings: ED-based evaluation versus office-based evaluation and academic settings versus those in private practice.[9] If a young infant meets the low-risk criteria outlined in Box 17.1, the physician may send the infant home with no antibiotics and follow-up the next day (note that the Boston criteria do recommend antibiotic administration). If the physician has any reservation about the ability of the caregivers to follow-up or any social concerns, one should err on the side of caution and admit the child to the hospital. If the infant does not fall into the low-risk criteria outlined, parenteral antibiotics should be administered and the child admitted to the hospital. Parenteral antibiotics should be given only if a lumbar puncture has been performed. Antibiotics used in this age group are ceftriaxone, 50 mg/kg intravenously or intramuscularly, or cefotaxime, 50 mg/kg intravenously.

**BOX 17.1 Criteria Historically Used for Risk Stratification in Pediatric Fever**

**Rochester Criteria**

Previously healthy term infants without perinatal complications, younger than 3 months, and no soft tissue, ear, or skeletal infections

Nontoxic appearance

No previous use of antimicrobials

Lack of a focus of infection on examination

Peripheral white blood cell (WBC) count: 5000-15,000/μL

Band count: 1500/μL or higher

Stool WBC count: up to 5 WBCs per high-power field in infants with diarrhea

Spun urine: up to 10 WBCs per high-power field

**Philadelphia Criteria**

Infants 29 through 56 days of age with temperatures of 38.2° C or higher

***Observation Score***

Quality of cry (strong, whimpering, weak, high pitched)

Reaction to parent stimulation (cries briefly then stops, intermittent cry, continual cry)

State variation (awake, awake with stimulation, unarousable)

Color (pink, acrocyanotic, cyanotic)

Hydration (mucosal membranes: moist, slightly dry, dry)

Social responses (smile, brief smile, no smile)

***Diagnostic Testing***

WBC count: less than 15,000/mm$^3$

Spun urine: up to 10 WBCs per high-power field and absence of bacteria on bright-field microscopy

Cerebrospinal fluid with a WBC count of less than 8/mm$^3$ and a negative Gram stain from a nonbloody sample

Chest radiograph without an infiltrate

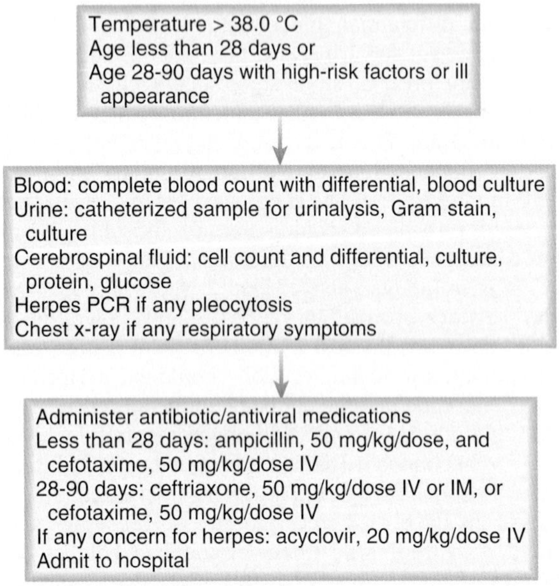

Temperature > 38.0 °C
Age less than 28 days or
Age 28-90 days with high-risk factors or ill appearance

↓

Blood: complete blood count with differential, blood culture
Urine: catheterized sample for urinalysis, Gram stain, culture
Cerebrospinal fluid: cell count and differential, culture, protein, glucose
Herpes PCR if any pleocytosis
Chest x-ray if any respiratory symptoms

↓

Administer antibiotic/antiviral medications
Less than 28 days: ampicillin, 50 mg/kg/dose, and cefotaxime, 50 mg/kg/dose IV
28-90 days: ceftriaxone, 50 mg/kg/dose IV or IM, or cefotaxime, 50 mg/kg/dose IV
If any concern for herpes: acyclovir, 20 mg/kg/dose IV
Admit to hospital

**Fig. 17.1 Approach to febrile infants 0 to 28 days of age or ill-appearing children 29 to 90 days of age.** *PCR*, Polymerase chain reaction.

The approach to fever evaluation in a 2- to 3-month-old to 3-year-old has changed dramatically over the past 10 years because of vaccine development and an increasing rate of vaccination.[10] An algorithm using an updated approach based on risk stratification is outlined in **Figure 17.3**. Before availability of the conjugated pneumococcal vaccine, a well-appearing child with a temperature of 39° C and no focus of infection would have blood drawn for a CBC and blood culture. The patient would have been administered a parenteral antibiotic if the white blood cell count was greater than 15,000/mm$^3$.[11] The concern was for occult bacteremia (OB) and possible progression of OB to meningitis. In 1987, the *Haemophilus influenzae* type B (Hib) vaccine was introduced and dramatically reduced the prevalence of OB secondary to Hib to the point of no longer being clinically pertinent.[12] The heptavalent pneumococcal conjugated vaccine (PCV-7) was introduced in the United States in 2000 and has recently been expanded to thirteen valent (PCV-13). PCV-13 is aimed at the most invasive strains of *S. pneumoniae* and is administered at 2, 4, 6, and 12 to 15 months. After one dose, the vaccine has 90% efficacy against vaccine serotypes. Although the recommended vaccination schedule for the pneumococcal vaccine includes four immunizations, it has been reported that two vaccinations induce satisfactory antibody responses and may therefore be protective.[13] It is thought that herd immunity may provide protection for older adults and unimmunized children.[14-16]

Lee et al. determined that at rates of pneumococcal bacteremia greater than 1.5%, obtaining a CBC, performing blood cultures, and administering antibiotics empirically was cost-effective.[17] Conversely, if the rate of pneumococcal bacteremia was less than 0.5%, strategies using empiric testing and antibiotics would no longer be cost-effective. Since the work of Lee et al. several investigations have determined the overall frequency of pneumococcal bacteremia to be well below 1%.[14,18,19] The rate of bacteremia may be low enough to support the evolving practice of not drawing blood for routine CBC and blood cultures in previously healthy febrile children between 2 and 36 months of age who have received at least one PCV-7 vaccination.[20] Evidence is mounting that the bacteremia rate and particularly the pneumococcal bacteremia rate have declined to the extent that empiric testing and treatment may no longer be necessary.

## PATHOPHYSIOLOGY

Fever is the host's adaptive response to an invading microorganism. The microorganism comes in contact with cells of the immune system, including macrophages and leukocytes, and such contact leads to the release of various cytokines, most notably interleukin-1, tumor necrosis factor, and interleukin-6. These cytokines circulate and come in contact

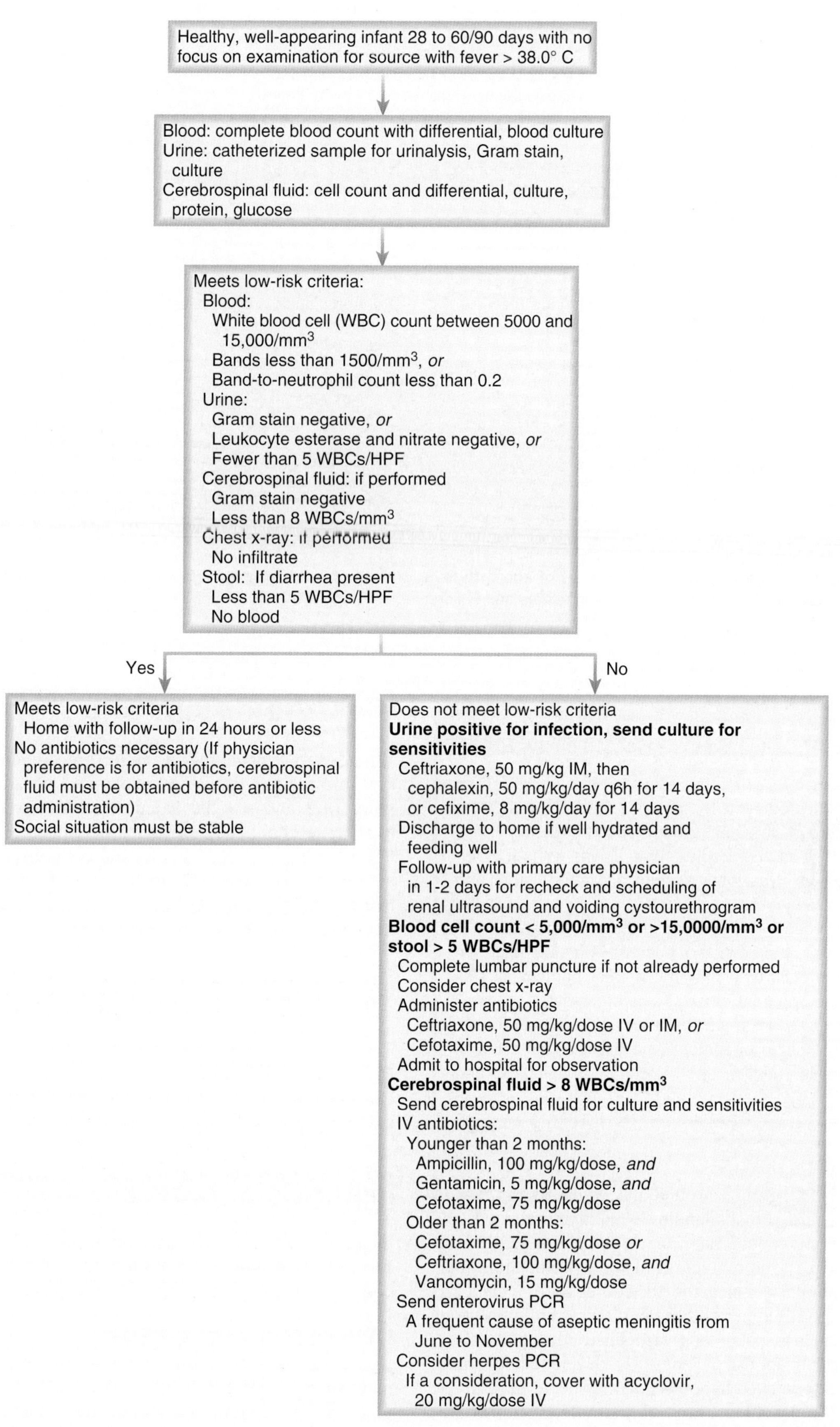


**Fig. 17.2 Approach to children 28 to 90 days old with fever and no source on initial evaluation.** *HPF*, High-power field; *PCR*, polymerase chain reaction. (Adapted from Baraff LJ. Management of fever without source in infants and children. Ann Emerg Med 2000;36:605; and Hoberman A, Wald ER, Hickey RW, et al. Oral versus initial intravenous therapy for urinary tract infections in young febrile children. Pediatrics 1999;104:79-86.)

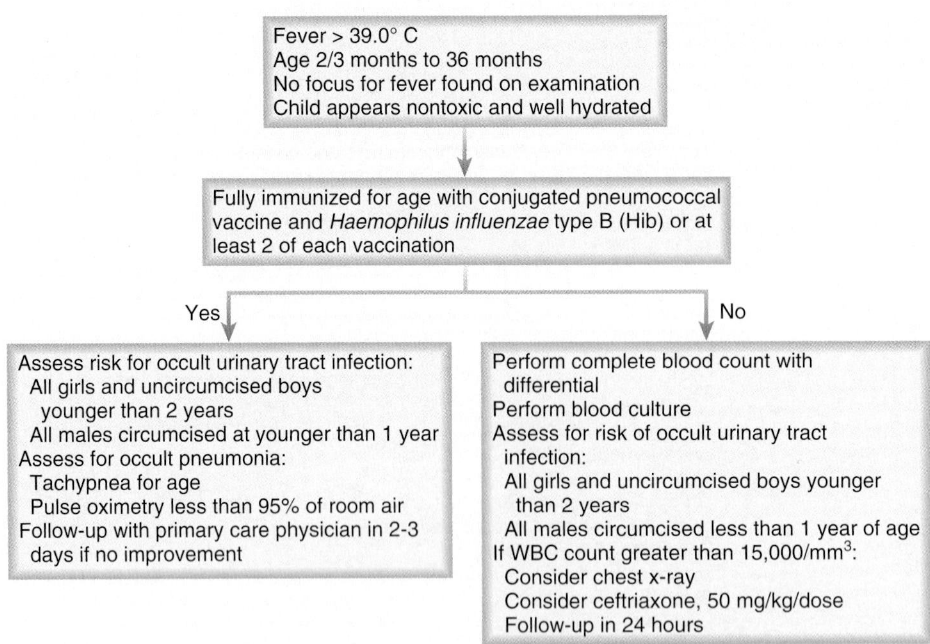


**Fig. 17.3 Approach to children 3 to 36 months of age with fever and no obvious source.** *WBC*, White blood cell. (Adapted from Baraff LJ. Management of fever without source in infants and children. Ann Emerg Med 2000;36:605.)

$SI = \frac{SV}{BSA}$ **FACTS AND FORMULAS**

*Fever*: for ages 0 to 2 months, a temperature of 38.0° C or higher measured rectally; for ages 2 to 36 months, a temperature of 39° C or higher measured rectally

*Fever without a source*: acute febrile illness without localizing signs or symptoms despite a careful history and physical examination

*Bacteremia*: presence of bacteria in the bloodstream

*Occult bacteremia*: presence of bacteria in the bloodstream of a febrile child who may not appear particularly sick and has no apparent other source of infection

*Serious bacterial illness*: accounts for 2% to 4% of fevers. Examples include pneumonia, cellulitis, septic arthritis, osteomyelitis, urinary tract infection, meningitis, and sepsis[21,22]

with neuronal cell groups around the edges of the brain's ventricular system. Prostaglandin $E_2$ is then released and binds to receptors on neurons in the hypothalamus and brainstem, which leads to upregulation of the hypothalamic thermostatic set-point.[23,24] Once the thermoregulatory center is reset, a higher body temperature is maintained through various mechanisms such as cutaneous vasoconstriction and shivering. The febrile response is not fully developed in young infants, and fever or even hypothermia may occur in response to infection. The physiologic limit of thermoregulation is estimated to be 41.1° C (106° F). According to McCarthy, children with a fever of this degree have a high rate of central nervous system insult.[1]

## PRESENTING SIGNS AND SYMPTOMS

When evaluating a febrile child, the clinician must obtain key information from the history and physical examination (**Box 17.2** and see the Documentation box). According to McCarthy et al., the sensitivity of clinical evaluation in an infant younger than 3 months and between 3 and 36 months of age is 78% and 89% to 92%, respectively.[1,25] After the history and physical examination, the source of fever remains inapparent in 20% of febrile children.[26,27]

## DIFFERENTIAL DIAGNOSIS

The differential diagnosis of acute pediatric fever is vast (**Box 17.3**). It is imperative to become familiar with the myriad causes of pediatric fever. The defining characteristics of each diagnosis can be found elsewhere in this text.

## DIAGNOSTIC TESTING

Diagnostic evaluation is based on the patient's age group.[11,26,28] **Figures 17.4 and 17.5** outline the indications for other common diagnostic tests in children with fever.[29-33]

### URINALYSIS AND CULTURE

Occult urinary tract infections occur in 2% to 3% of male infants younger than 1 year. Most of these infections occur in uncircumcised boys and infants younger than 6 months. Occult urinary tract infections occur in 8% to 9% of female children younger than 2 years.[26] Girls between 2 months and 2 years of age can be risk-stratified for urinary

**BOX 17.2 Physical Examination Findings in the Evaluation of a Febrile Infant or Child**

**Vital Signs**

**General Appearance**
Level of activity
Eye contact and tracking behavior
Tone
Consolability
Color

**Head, Ears, Eyes, Nose, and Throat**
Meningeal signs (may not be present in children younger than 1 year)
Otitis media (bulging tympanic membrane with decreased mobility)
Pharyngitis
Adenopathy

**Respiratory System**
Rate of respirations
Presence of increased work of breathing
Grunting
Nasal flaring
Retracting
Rales
Rhonchi
Wheezing
Stridor
Cough
Decreased breath sounds

**Cardiovascular System**
Pulse rate
Presence of a murmur

**Abdomen**
Tenderness
Distention
Guarding
Rebound
Organomegaly
Costovertebral angle tenderness

**Skin**
Rash

**Musculoskeletal System**
Point tenderness to palpation of bone or joints
Swelling
Erythema
Range of motion of joints
Gait and ability to ambulate

tract infection (see Fig. 17.4) with a sensitivity of 95% and specificity of 31%.[34]

Urine can be collected for testing in several ways. Bag collection is a noninvasive, convenient method, but it is not recommended because of a false-positive rate of nearly 85%.[25,35] Percutaneous bladder aspiration is another approach, but because this method is more invasive, it is also not the preferred approach except in male infants with severe phimosis.[29] Urethral catheterization is generally regarded as the preferred method of obtaining urine, and its sensitivity and specificity are reported to be 95% and 99%, respectively.[29] Once a catheterized urine specimen has been obtained, it should be sent for testing. A negative urinalysis and a negative Gram stain are not sufficient to exclude a urinary tract infection because up to 50% of patients with a urinary tract infection documented by urine culture have a false-negative urinalysis result. Therefore, it is important to obtain a urine culture in conjunction with urinalysis and a Gram stain.[29,35,36]

The utility of an elevated peripheral white blood cell count in evaluating a febrile child is debatable. It has been shown to be an inaccurate screen for bacteremia and meningitis in febrile infants.[37,38] The decision to administer antibiotics, to perform or withhold lumbar puncture, or to admit or discharge the patient should not be based solely on interpretation of the white blood cell count.[37,38]

## RADIOGRAPHY

Deciding when to perform a chest radiograph in a febrile child can be challenging. Nearly 7% of all febrile children younger than 2 years with a temperature higher than 38° C have pneumonia.[34] In an investigation by Bachur et al., occult pneumonia (defined as the presence of an infiltrate on a chest radiograph in a child without clear clinical evidence of pneumonia) was discovered in up to 26% of febrile children without a source and with a white blood cell count higher than 20,000/mm$^3$.[39-41] Several criticisms of this study have been raised, including the high degree of interobserver variability in interpretation of chest radiographs, failure to perform a peripheral white blood cell count in more than half the infants with a temperature of 38° C or higher, and performance of the majority of clinical assessments by physicians in training rather than by faculty physicians.[42-44] Nonetheless, data in the literature are sufficient to support the policy of the American College of Emergency Physicians, which outlines the indications for obtaining a chest radiograph in children younger than 3 years[29] (see Fig. 17.5).

## TREATMENT AND DISPOSITION

The clinician should administer appropriate dose of antipyretic early in the evaluation of a febrile child (acetaminophen, 15 mg/kg, or ibuprofen, 10 mg/kg). The response to antipyretics is not a useful determinant of the presence of bacterial illness and should not influence clinical decision making.[32] Treatment and disposition of infants younger than 90 days are outlined in Figures 17.1 and 17.2. For infants managed on an outpatient basis, tests performed in the ED occasionally come back positive after the patient has been discharged. If blood cultures are positive, the child should be admitted for evaluation of sepsis and parenteral administration of antibiotics, especially in the setting of persistent fever.[26] For positive urine cultures, the patient's symptoms affect disposition. In the setting of persistent fever, the child should be admitted to the hospital for evaluation of sepsis and parenteral administration of antibiotics. In an afebrile and well-appearing child, outpatient management with oral

**BOX 17.3 Differential Diagnosis of Acute Pediatric Fever**

**Common Viral Infections**

**Central Nervous System**
Meningitis
Encephalitis
Tumor
Brain abscess

**Head, Ears, Eyes, Nose, and Throat**
Otitis media
Pharyngitis
Retropharyngeal abscess
Peritonsillar abscess
Lateral pharyngeal wall abscess
Stomatitis
Influenza
Sinusitis
Parotitis
Cervical adenitis
Periorbital cellulitis
Orbital cellulitis or abscess

**Respiratory System**
Bronchiolitis
Croup
Epiglottitis
Pneumonia
Upper respiratory infection

**Cardiovascular System**
Myocarditis
Pericarditis
Endocarditis

**Genitourinary System**
Urinary tract infection
Tuboovarian abscess

**Gastrointestinal Tract**
Acute viral gastroenteritis
Bacterial enteritis
Appendicitis

**Focal Soft Tissue Infections**
Cellulitis

**Musculoskeletal System**
Osteomyelitis
Septic arthritis

**Rheumatologic Disorders**
Acute rheumatic fever
Juvenile rheumatoid arthritis
Henoch-Schönlein purpura

**Vasculitis**
Behçet syndrome

**Malignancy**
Leukemia
Lymphoma
Sarcoma

**Systemic Illness**
Bacteremia
Viremia
Sepsis
Kawasaki disease
Toxic shock syndrome
Rocky Mountain spotted fever
Meningococcemia

**Miscellaneous Disorders**
Toxicologic
- Anticholinergic toxidromes
- Salicylate overdose
- Amphetamine
- Cocaine

Endocrine
- Thyrotoxicosis

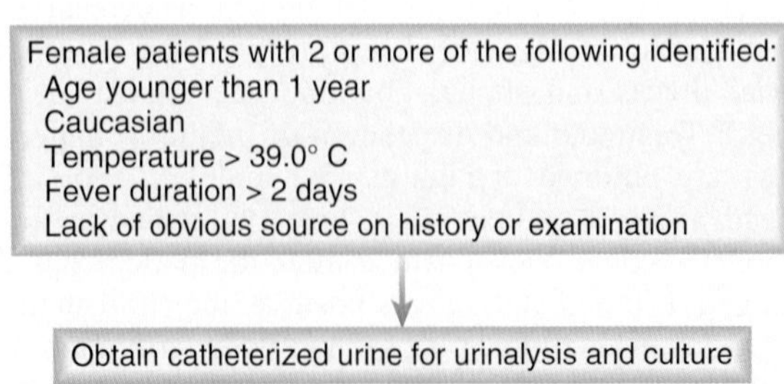


**Fig. 17.4 Indications to obtain a catheterized urine specimen in febrile female children arriving at the emergency department.** (Adapted from Gorelick MH, Shaw KN. Clinical decision rule to identify febrile young girls at risk for urinary tract infection. Arch Pediatr Adolesc Med 2000;154:386-90.)

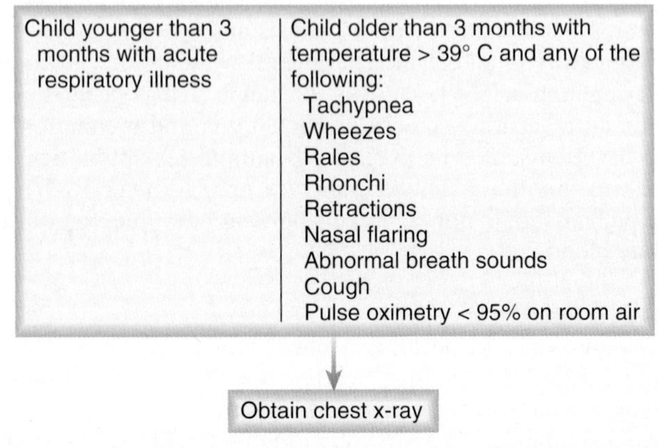


**Fig. 17.5 Indications for chest radiography in febrile pediatric patients arriving at the emergency department.** (Data from References 29 to 33.)

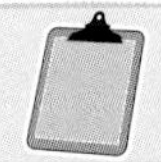

## DOCUMENTATION

**Key Historical Findings in the Evaluation of a Febrile Infant or Child**
Age of the child
Height and duration of the fever
Method of obtaining the temperature
Use, timing, and dose of antipyretics administered

**Caretaker's Report of Well-Being**
Level of activity
Consolability
Irritability
Lethargy
Playing
Smiling
Eating
Pitch of cry (a high-pitched cry may be indicative of a central nervous system infection)

**Hydration Status**
Fluid intake
Urinary output

**Respiratory Symptoms**
Cough
Work of breathing
Nasal flaring
Intercostal retractions
Grunting

**Gastrointestinal Symptoms**
Vomiting
Diarrhea
Abdominal pain

**Urinary Symptoms**
Dysuria
Frequency
Urgency
Hematuria

**Ear, Nose, and Throat Symptoms**
Earache
Sore throat

**Dermatologic Symptoms**
Rash

**Past Medical History**
Birth history
Length of gestation, mode of delivery, infections during pregnancy, antibiotics during pregnancy, mother's group B *Streptococcus* status
Immunization status
Underlying medical illnesses
Previous hospitalizations

**Social History**
Contact with ill persons
Day care
Recent travel

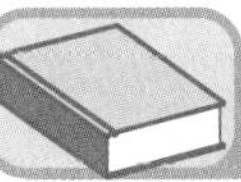

## PATIENT TEACHING TIPS

Explain to the caretaker that a fever in the absence of a serious bacterial illness is not harmful.
Explain how to take a temperature properly.
It is best to take the infant's or toddler's temperature rectally.
Hold the child belly down on your lap.
Lubricate the thermometer with water-soluble jelly.
Spread the buttocks and insert the lubricated thermometer approximately 1 inch into the rectum.

**Antipyretics**
Explain that many formulations of acetaminophen are available and that parents should base the dose of acetaminophen or ibuprofen on the weight of the child.

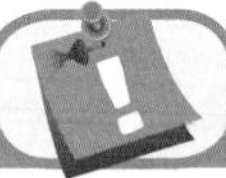

## TIPS AND TRICKS

Perform most of the physical examination with the child in the parent's lap.
Begin with less noxious components of the examination and proceed gradually to those that may be upsetting to the child (i.e., the pulmonary, cardiac, and neurologic components of the physical examination are performed before the abdominal, tympanic, and pharyngeal components).
Attempt to calm a fussy or uncooperative child through feeding, use of antipyretics, or aid of the child life team. For an apprehensive toddler, demonstrate examination of the particular body part on the parent holding the child before performing it on the child.

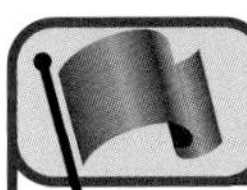

## RED FLAGS

Meningeal signs are not highly reliable in the first 12 to 16 months of life.
Remember to document the child's general appearance carefully.
Do not overly rely on the white blood cell count to determine the extent of evaluation in an infant.
In cases in which the reliability of the caregiver is in question, it is safer to admit the patient to the hospital. Indicators of unreliable follow-up are as follows:

- Young parents
- Parents without access to transportation
- Caretakers who do not believe that their child is ill[35]

Close (next day) and reliable follow-up is important.
Whenever possible, consult with the infant's pediatrician to obtain information regarding parental reliability, to discuss evaluation, and to arrange close follow-up.
In cases in which follow-up is uncertain, extensive evaluation and hospital admission are reasonable.

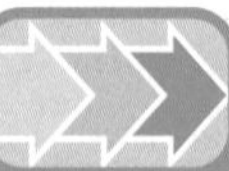

**PRIORITY ACTIONS**

Administer appropriate doses of antipyretics early in the patient's evaluation (acetaminophen, 15 mg/kg, or ibuprofen, 10 mg/kg).

When indicated, antibiotics should be administered as early in the patient's evaluation as possible.

Ensure close, reliable follow-up. When follow-up is uncertain, consider more extensive evaluation and hospital admission.

antibiotics is a reasonable plan. Follow-up studies, including repeated cultures of urine and blood, as well as voiding cystourethrography and renal ultrasound scanning, should be arranged.

In children 2 to 3 months to 36 months of age, the clinical impression and the patient's temperature guide management decisions. This approach is outlined in Figure 17.3. Toxic-appearing children with fever should be admitted to the hospital and treated. Well-appearing children with a temperature lower than 39° C should be treated with antipyretics and may be discharged. Laboratory testing should be withheld in these patients, and parents should be provided with instructions to return if their children have persistent fever or their condition deteriorates. In a well-appearing child with a temperature higher than 39° C, the guidelines for urine testing and chest radiography outlined in Figures 17.4 and 17.5 should be followed. Regardless of the management approach chosen, close outpatient follow-up should be ensured, and the patient's parents should be provided with clear instructions that describe when to return to the ED for reevaluation. **Box 17.4** provides information to provide to the parent. Fever is a common complaint in the ED in children younger than 36 months. The Hib and pneumococcal vaccines have reduced the incidence of OB and thus have altered the evaluation and management of febrile infants and children. This remains an evolving process, with the rate and degree of evolution yet to be determined.

**BOX 17.4 Information for the Parent: Goals for Care at Home**

1. Reduce the temperature
   - Appropriate dosing and intervals of administration of antipyretics based on information written on the label and the child's weight
2. Maintain hydration
   - Persistent or worsening vomiting and/or diarrhea
   - Signs of dehydration
     - Decreased urine output or tears
     - Sunken eyes
     - Dry diapers
3. Monitor for worsening or life-threatening illness and return immediately to the emergency department for:
   - Changes in level of alertness (lethargy, irritability, or inconsolability)
   - Signs of increased work of breathing (grunting; retracting; nasal flaring; rapid, shallow, or difficult respirations)
   - Bilious vomiting
   - Seizure
   - Purple or red rash
   - Persistent headache

## SUGGESTED READINGS

Baraff LJ. Management of infants and young children with fever without source. Pediatr Ann 2008;37:673-9.

Ishimine P. Fever without source in children 0 to 36 months of age. Pediatric Clin North Am 2006;53:167-94.

Ishimine P. The evolving approach to the young child who has fever and no obvious source. Emerg Med Clin North Am 2007;25:1087-115.

Joffe MD, Alpern ER. Occult pneumococcal bacteremia: a review. Pediatric Emerg Care 2010;26:448-54.

## REFERENCES

***References can be found on Expert Consult @ www.expertconsult.com.***

# Approach to the Pediatric Patient with a Rash 18

*Anna K. McFarlin, Tracy Leigh LeGros, and Heather Murphy-Lavoie*

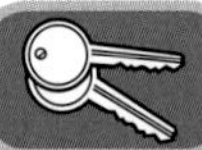

**KEY POINTS**

- Rashes with fever deserve special consideration, especially if the fever has been present for more than 5 days.
- Palpable petechiae and fever are associated with many types of bacteremia and should be treated with intravenous antibiotics immediately.
- Many pediatric exanthems are benign in children but potentially devastating to pregnant women and immunocompromised patients.
- Patients who are moderately to critically ill with evidence of rash should receive targeted empiric therapy.
- The mainstay of treatment of atopic dermatitis is topical corticosteroids.
- Diaper dermatitis present for more than 3 days is usually complicated by candidal infection.
- Staphylococcal scaled skin syndrome and toxic shock syndrome require antistaphylococcal antibiotics, hemodynamic stabilization, and supportive skin care.

## INTRODUCTION

Children are often brought to the emergency department with rashes ranging from the inconsequential (insect bites) to life-threatening emergencies (meningococcemia). When evaluating a rash, physicians should be systematic in the creation of an appropriate differential diagnosis, with early identification of possible life-threatening dermatologic conditions. Assessment of the distribution, morphology, and quality of the rash is of paramount importance. Detailed historical data regarding systemic symptoms and antecedent events are required. Please refer to Chapter 191 for the approach to undifferentiated rash. This chapter addresses dermatologic conditions most commonly diagnosed in pediatric patients.

## PATHOPHYSIOLOGY

The pathophysiology of rash in pediatric patients is broad and depends on the inciting etiologic agent. In this population, viral illnesses are most common. However, vasculitic reactions, primary and secondary bacterial infections, fungal infections, and chronic inflammatory states provide additional causes.

## PRESENTING SIGNS AND SYMPTOMS

### CLASSIC EXANTHEMS AND VIRAL RASHES

Historically, six infectious exanthems were originally described: measles or rubeola (first), scarlet fever (second), rubella (third), Dukes disease (fourth), erythema infectiosum (fifth), and exanthema subitum or roseola infantum (sixth).[1] The majority of childhood exanthems are nonspecific and cannot be accurately assigned to a discrete etiologic diagnosis. These exanthems are typically self-limited and resolve spontaneously within a week.[2] **Table 18.1** details these classic exanthems and viral rashes.

#### *Measles*

Measles is rarely seen in developed countries because of the widespread use of vaccination. However, measles continues to affect the populations of developing countries.[3,4] In 1997 it was the sixth leading cause of death worldwide; it is still the leading cause of blindness in African children.[5] The causative agent of measles is paramyxovirus, which has an incubation period of 7 to 12 days, and infection occurs most commonly in winter and spring.[1,6] Measles is contagious 3 days before and 5 days following onset of the rash. It begins with a prodrome of gradually increasing fevers (>40° C), headache, coryza, dry hacking cough, and an impressive bilateral conjunctivitis (the three C's). The prodrome occurs 2 to 4 days before the rash.[7] Koplik spots are clustered, white lesions ("grains of salt on a wet background") that may appear on the buccal mucosa opposite the second molars during the prodromal period (**Fig. 18.1**). They are pathognomonic if present.[7] The erythematous, nonpruritic, maculopapular rash first appears at the hairline and behind the ears and then spreads inferiorly. As the rash involves the trunk and extremities, the discrete macules coalesce. After 1 week the rash fades.[1,6] Diagnosis of measles is typically made clinically; however, laboratory diagnosis via serologic assay is available.[7,8] Treatment of measles is supportive. Administration of vitamin A is associated with a reduction in risk for mortality in children younger than 2 years, as well as a reduction in postmeasles pneumonia complications.[9] Complications of measles include

**Table 18.1 Classic Exanthems and Viral Rashes**

| DISEASE | SEASON | MORPHOLOGY | DISTRIBUTION | ASSOCIATED FINDINGS |
|---|---|---|---|---|
| Measles/rubeola (paramyxovirus) | Winter to spring | Erythematous, confluent, maculopapular | Begins at the hairline<br>Spreads inferiorly | Koplik spots<br>High fever<br>Cough, coryza, and conjunctivitis<br>Forchheimer spots |
| Scarlet fever (*Streptococcus pyogenes*) | Fall to spring | Generalized erythema with a sandpaper texture | Begins on the face and upper part of the trunk and spreads inferiorly | Pastia lines<br>Forchheimer spots<br>Strawberry tongue<br>Exudative pharyngitis<br>Abdominal pain<br>Rheumatic fever |
| Rubella (Rubivirus) | Late winter and early spring | Rose-pink, maculopapular | Spreads inferiorly | Lymphadenopathy<br>Arthralgias<br>Forchheimer spots |
| Erythema infectiosum (parvovirus B19) | Winter and spring | "Slapped cheek" appearance, lacy reticular rash | Erythematous cheeks<br>Reticular extremities | Rash waxes and wanes over weeks<br>Arthritis<br>Aplastic crisis |
| Roseola (human herpesvirus 6 and 7) | Spring | Rose-pink, maculopapular | Neck and trunk | Lymphadenopathy<br>Febrile seizures<br>Nagayama spots |
| Varicella (herpes zoster virus) | Later winter and early spring | Vesicles on an erythematous base, crusts | Begins on the face and trunk and spreads centripetally | Pruritus<br>Varicella-zoster |
| Hand-foot-and-mouth disease (Coxsackie A virus) | Late summer or early fall | Elliptical vesicles on an erythematous base<br>Oral vesicles<br>Erosions | Mouth, hands, and feet | Vesicles on the hands and feet and in the mouth |

blindness, pneumonia, laryngotracheobronchitis, otitis media, myocarditis, and encephalitis.[7,10]

### Scarlet Fever

Scarlet fever, an exotoxin-mediated illness caused by infection with *Streptococcus pyogenes*, occurs primarily in children younger than 10 years.[11] Scarlet fever is most often associated with streptococcal tonsillopharyngitis, although it can be seen following other streptococcal infections.[12] Its incidence is highest during the late fall to late winter, and the incubation period is 2 to 5 days.[12,13] Symptoms include an abrupt onset of fever, headache, malaise, and odynophagia with occasional vomiting and abdominal pain. This is followed by the appearance of a strawberry tongue and a bright red enanthem (oral rash) on the soft palate and uvula. These punctate, erythematous macules are called palatal petechiae or Forchheimer spots. The rash, which follows the fever by 1 to 2 days, is a generalized erythroderma with scattered pinpoint, erythematous blanching papules that have a sandpaper-like texture. Capillary fragility causes petechiae in the flexural surfaces (Pastia lines), and facial flushing with circumoral pallor is often apparent. The palms and soles are typically spared. The exanthem typically resolves in 5 days, followed 2 weeks later by postexanthematous desquamation, especially of the palms and soles.[1,11] The diagnosis is made clinically but can be confirmed by streptococcus-positive throat culture.[11] Penicillin remains the treatment of choice to prevent local suppurative complications and acute rheumatic fever.[13] Additional complications are rare but include sepsis, acute glomerulonephritis, pneumonia, pericarditis, hepatitis, otitis media, meningitis, and toxic shock syndrome (TSS) (**Fig. 18.2**).[11,14]

### Rubella

Rubella is a relatively mild illness caused by Rubivirus that is accompanied by a maculopapular rash. The incubation period is 12 to 23 days, with the period of infectivity extending from a few days before until 7 days following onset of the rash.[15] Rubella occurs most commonly in late winter and early spring.[15] The prodrome is mild, if present, and consists of malaise, pharyngitis, cough, low-grade fever, coryza, and a headache. A faint pink-red maculopapular rash subsequently appears, first on the face and then with rapid caudal spread. The rash typically resolves in 3 to 4 days.[15,16] The prodrome is common in adolescents and adults but is often absent in younger children. Other clinical findings include posterior cervical and occipital lymphadenopathy, Forchheimer spots, arthralgia, and neutropenia.[1,16] The diagnosis is made clinically but serologic tests are available.[16] Treatment of rubella is supportive. However, patients must avoid pregnant women (first 20 weeks of gestation) to prevent spontaneous abortion or congenital rubella syndrome.[15] Complications of rubella include arthritis, encephalitis, and thrombocytopenia.[15,17]

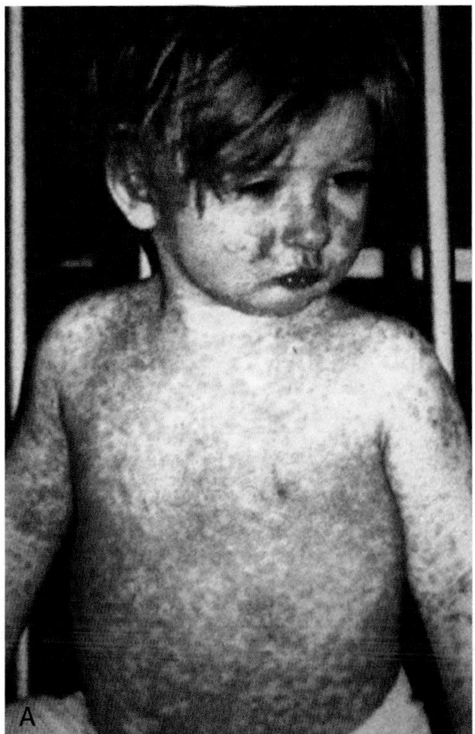

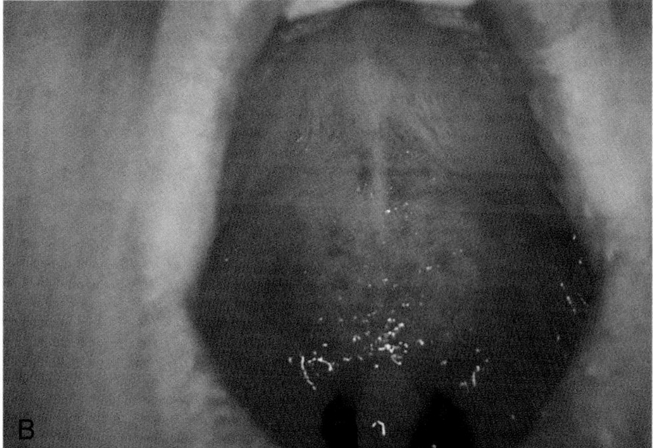

**Fig. 18.1** **A,** Measles. **B,** Forchheimer spots secondary to measles.

### Dukes Disease

Dukes disease (fourth disease) is a constellation of symptoms consistent with a viral syndrome. It is most likely not a distinct entity, but rather a collection of viruses that did not fall under the other diagnoses. These include coxsackie virus, echovirus, and enteroviruses. See the upcoming section on picornaviral exanthems.

### Erythema Infectiosum

Erythema infectiosum (fifth disease) is caused by human parvovirus B19 and typically affects school-age children. It has an incubation period of 1 to 2 weeks and occurs more frequently in winter and spring.[1,15,18] Children with this virus typically feel well. However, 10% of patients experience a prodrome consisting of low-grade fever, headache, sore throat, malaise, myalgia, and coryza.[1,18] This prodrome is followed by a bright, fiery red macular rash across the cheeks that gives the child a "slapped cheek" or sunburned appearance. This rash lasts 1 to 4 days and then progresses to a more generalized rash with a lacy reticular pattern, most prominent on the extremity extensor surfaces. The rash may then wax and wane for a month, with various stimuli increasing its intensity.[1,15] Once the rash appears, children are no longer infectious.[1] The diagnosis is made clinically, but serologic tests can be used. Treatment of erythema infectiosum is supportive, but parents must keep infected children away from pregnant women and those with hemolytic anemia. High-risk groups may be treated with intravenous immune globulin (IVIG).[15] Complications are rare but include symmetric arthritis of the hands, wrists, or knees and intrauterine infection and fetal death if the infection occurs during the first half of pregnancy. Children with hemolytic anemia and hemoglobinopathy (particularly sickle cell disease) are prone to transient aplastic crisis when infected with parvovirus.[18-21]

### Roseola Infantum (Exanthema Subitum)

Roseola is the most common viral exanthem in children younger than 3 years. It is called baby measles or 3-day fever, and the causative agents are human herpesviruses 6 and 7.[22,23] Roseola has an incubation period of 5 to 15 days.[15,24] It is characterized by high fever for 2 to 5 days in an otherwise well-appearing child. Following dissipation of the fever, a blanching, evanescent, pink maculopapular exanthem develops on the neck and trunk. The rash typically lasts approximately 1 to 2 days. Associated symptoms include mild coryza, cough, otitis media, headache, periorbital edema, and posterior cervical lymphadenopathy.[23-25] An enanthem of red papules (Nagayama spots) may be seen on the mucosa of the soft palate and uvula.[23,25] The diagnosis is made clinically and treatment is supportive.[15,24,26] Febrile seizures are a common complication. Other complications are uncommon but include thrombocytopenia, hepatitis, and encephalitis.[15,24,27]

### Varicella (Chickenpox)

The incidence of varicella has decreased 90% in the last 20 years with routine vaccinations.[28] Chickenpox, caused by varicella-zoster virus, is highly contagious, with a peak incidence in late winter and spring.[29,30] Children 2 to 8 years of age are primarily affected. After an incubation period of 10 to 21 days, the prodrome begins with malaise, low-grade fever, cough, coryza, anorexia, sore throat, and headache.[30,31] Within 1 to 2 days the skin eruption begins on the trunk and then spreads over the next week to the face (including the mucous membranes) and extremities (with sparing of the palms and soles). The lesions begin as red macules that quickly progress to discrete vesicles on an erythematous base (**Fig. 18.3**). The vesicles ("dew drops on a rose petal") rapidly evolve into pustules, which umbilicate and crust over in 5 to 10 days. These lesions are intensely pruritic and characteristically seen in all stages of development at once, with resolution in 7 to 10 days.[1,30] The infectivity period begins several days before onset of the rash and lasts until all the lesions are completely crusted.[31] The diagnosis is made clinically; however, a Tzanck preparation demonstrating multinucleated giant cells or other viral assays can be used for confirmation.[1,30] Treatment is usually supportive, with management of constitutional symptoms and pruritus and prevention of secondary infection.[1,30] Wet dressings, soothing baths, calamine lotion, and

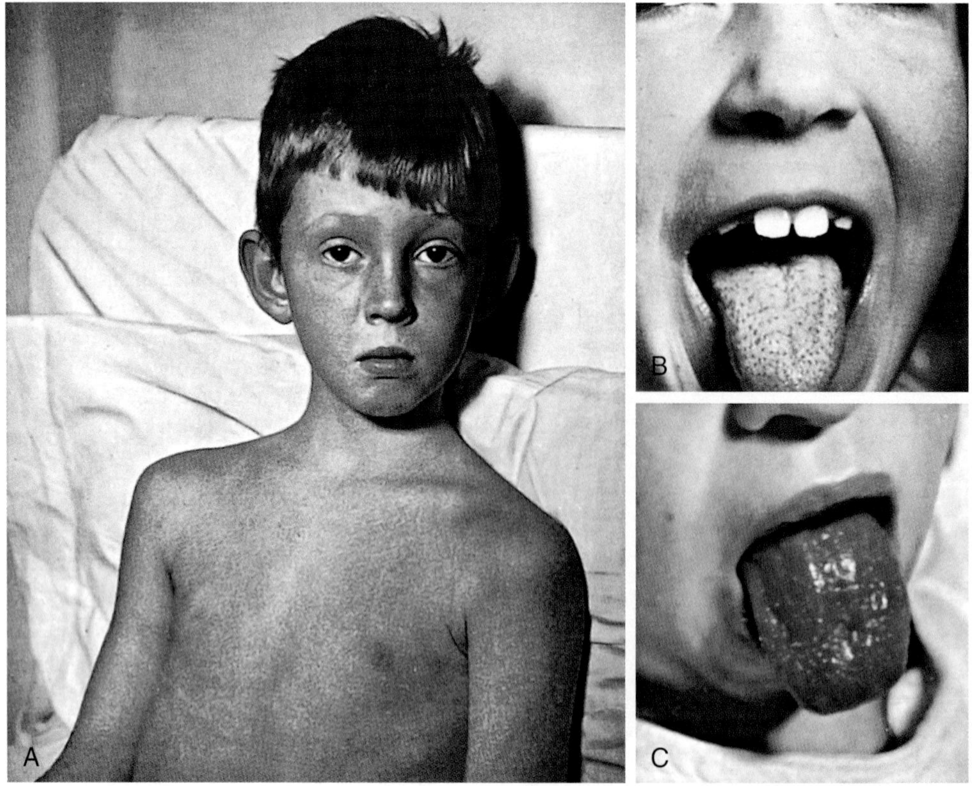

**Fig. 18.2 Scarlet fever. A,** Punctate, erythematous rash (second day). **B,** White strawberry tongue (first day). **C,** Red strawberry tongue (third day). (Courtesy Dr. Franklin H. Top, Professor and Head of the Department of Hygiene and Preventive Medicine, State University of Iowa, College of Medicine, Iowa City, IA; and Parke, Davis & Company's Therapeutic Notes. From Gershon AA, Hotez PJ, Katz SL. Krugman's infectious diseases of children. 11th ed. Philadelphia: Mosby; 2004.)

antihistamines may provide symptomatic relief. Acyclovir may be effective in treating varicella and preventing systemic complications in immunocompromised children. The role of acyclovir in otherwise healthy children remains unclear.[32,33] In normal, immunocompetent children, symptoms are mild and serious complications rare. Secondary bacterial infections should be treated with antibiotics directed at *Staphylococcus aureus* or group A β-hemolytic streptococci (cephalexin, amoxicillin-clavulanate, or dicloxacillin).[1] Mupirocin may be appropriate for minor, localized secondary infections. Other complications include pneumonia, vasculitis, and encephalitis.[34] Immunocompromised children and patients receiving chronic steroid treatment are more prone to extensive skin eruptions, varicella pneumonia, and severe constitutional symptoms.[35] Maternal infection (first trimester) can result in congenital varicella syndrome. Perinatal maternal infection can result in disseminated herpes of the neonate.[30,31] Perinatal varicella carries a mortality of up to 30%.[31]

### Picornaviral Exanthems

Picornaviruses are a family of RNA viruses that cause a variety of illnesses. Common viruses include coxsackieviruses, echoviruses, and enteroviruses. These are the most common summertime exanthems.[1,22] Disease expression ranges from exanthems (younger children) to aseptic meningitis (older children). The characteristic exanthem is typically morbilliform ("measlelike").[1] Associated symptoms include upper respiratory symptoms, conjunctivitis, fever, vomiting, and diarrhea. Complications include pericarditis, myocarditis, pleurodynia, parotitis, hepatitis, pancreatitis, and encephalitis.[1]

### Hand-Foot-and-Mouth Disease

This enteroviral exanthem is caused by Coxsackie A virus and enterovirus 71. It is characterized by oral vesicles, followed by vesicles on the hands and feet and may also include the buttocks.[15] Hand-foot-and-mouth disease has an incubation period of 3 to 6 days.[36] Patients are highly contagious 2 days before and 2 days following onset of the eruption. There is a brief prodrome consisting of low-grade fever, malaise, anorexia, and odynophagia. The oral lesions begin as small red macules that evolve into vesicles measuring 2 to 20 mm. These vesicles rupture rapidly and leave painful erosions. Children often refuse to eat or drink because of pain, and dehydration is a potential complication.[15,36] The lesions found on the hands and feet begin as macules and papules that evolve into flat-topped, elliptical vesicles with an erythematous base. The diaper area may be affected in infants.[1] The diagnosis is made clinically, and treatment is symptomatic. Anesthetic mouthwash may provide relief from painful oral ulcers.[15] Rare complications include myocarditis, pneumonia, meningoencephalitis, and aseptic meningitis. Infection during the first trimester of pregnancy may result in spontaneous abortion (see Table 18.1).[15]

## SKIN AND SOFT TISSUE INFECTIONS

These infections represent the most common bacterial, fungal, and viral infections of childhood. **Table 18.2** details these pediatric skin and soft tissue infections.

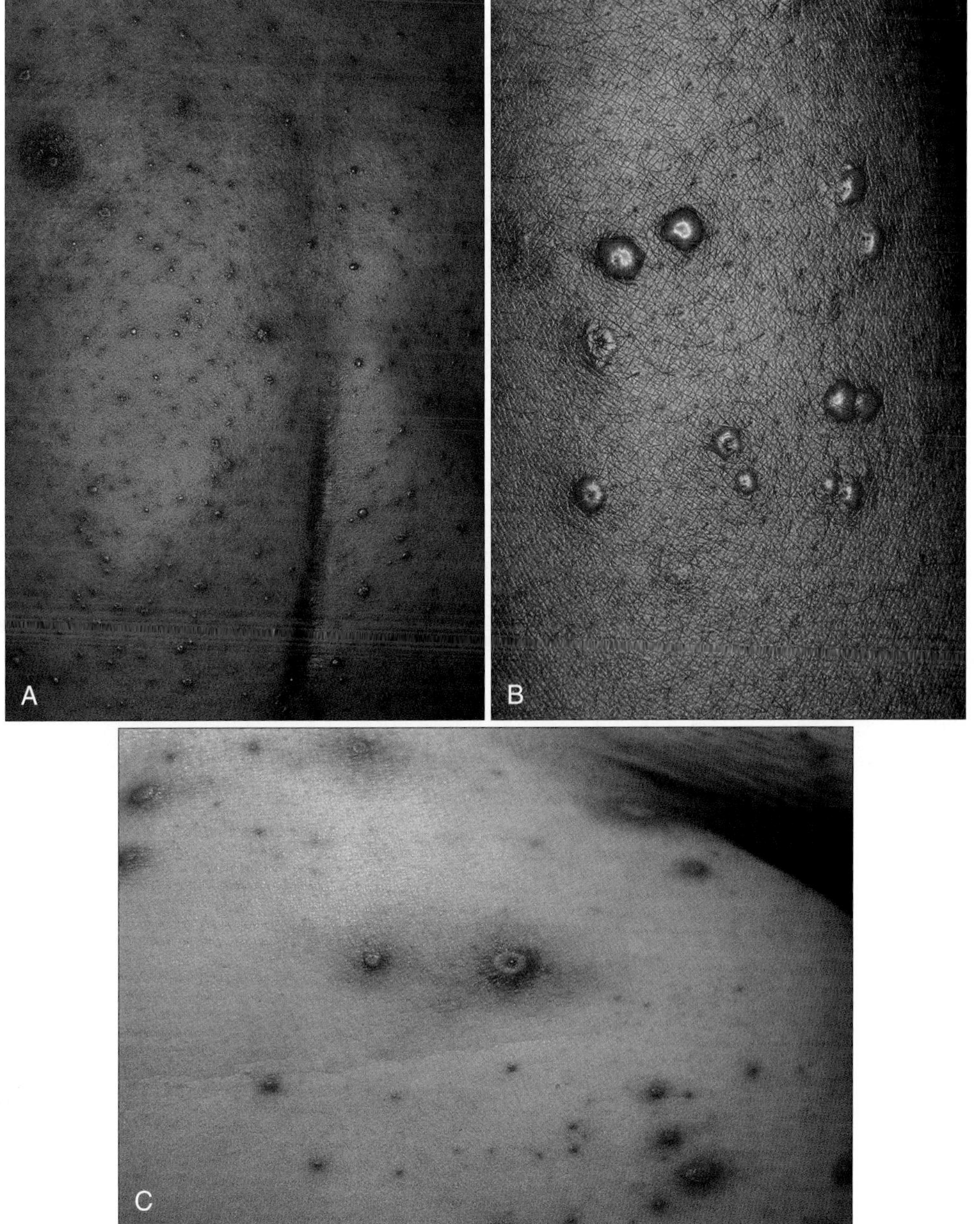

**Fig. 18.3 Varicella.** Widespread lesions are seen in different stages of development (**A**). Vesicles often develop central umbilication (**B**), and some lesions become pustular (**C**). (**A** and **B,** Courtesy Robert Hartman, MD.)

### *Impetigo*

Impetigo is a superficial bacterial skin infection typically caused by *S. aureus* or *S. pyogenes* and is the most common cutaneous infection in children.[1,32] Impetigo is most prevalent in children younger than 6 years and typically occurs in late summer and early fall secondary to microscopic breaks in the epidermal barrier.[12,37,38] Additional contributing factors include warm humid climates, overcrowding, and poor hygiene.[12] Impetigo is highly communicable.[37] Variants of impetigo include bullous impetigo and impetigo contagiosa. Bullous impetigo is seen most often in neonates and is caused by *S. aureus* phage group II. The lesions of bullous impetigo commonly occur in the periumbilical or perineal region in neonates and on the extremities in older children. The lesions are flaccid, thin-walled bullae that when ruptured leave shiny, rounded erythematous erosions with peeling edges ("coin lesions").[39,40] Associated lymphadenopathy is rare and the Nikolsky sign is negative. Impetigo contagiosa is the most common variant and is caused by *S. aureus* or group A β-hemolytic streptococci.[38] The rash begins as small painless erythematous macules, commonly near the nose and mouth, which then progress to small vesicles and pustules with erythematous margins. These lesions rupture easily and release a serous fluid, which dries to form a honey-colored crust.[38,39] Associated regional lymphadenopathy is common. Topical antibiotics, such as 2% mupirocin, are often effective for limited infections.[37,40,41] However, extensive lesions may be treated with 10 days of oral antibiotics directed at *Staphylococcus* and *Streptococcus*. Suggested antibiotics include cephalexin, amoxicillin-clavulanate, azithromycin,

**Table 18.2 Pediatric Skin and Soft Tissue Infections**

| | IMPETIGO | ERYSIPELAS | TINEA | MOLLUSCUM |
|---|---|---|---|---|
| Etiology | *Staphylococcus aureus*<br>*Streptococcus pyogenes* | Group A streptococci | *Microsporum canis*<br>*Trichophyton tonsurans* | Poxvirus |
| Age range | <6 yr | Infants<br>Young children<br>Elderly | 4-7 yr (capitus)<br>All ages | Young children |
| Season | Late summer<br>Early fall | All seasons | All seasons | All seasons |
| Morphology | Vesicles<br>Pustules<br>Thin-walled bullae | Shiny erythematous plaques<br>Blistering | Annular erythematous pruritic patches<br>Scaly/crusting pustules | Dome-shaped papules |
| Usual distribution | Face<br>Extremities<br>Periumbilical region<br>Perineal region | Face<br>Lower extremities | Scalp<br>Body<br>Groin<br>Feet | Face<br>Chest<br>Axilla<br>Upper extremities |
| Associated findings | "Coin lesions"<br>Honey-crusted lesions | Sharply demarcated borders | Hair loss<br>Kerion | Umbilicated papules |

dicloxacillin, and oxacillin.[32,37,39] The nose may serve as a reservoir of staphylococci, and children with recurrent impetigo may benefit from a course of intranasal mupirocin.[1] Though rare, poststreptococcal glomerulonephritis is the most significant complication of streptococcal impetigo.[12,38] Although systemic antibiotics help eliminate the cutaneous lesions of impetigo, they do not prevent poststreptococcal glomerulonephritis.[37] Other complications include local spread, cellulitis, regional lymphadenitis, staphylococcal scaled skin syndrome (SSSS), scarlet fever, rheumatic fever, and sepsis.[38]

### *Erysipelas*

Erysipelas is a distinctive form of cellulitis that affects mainly infants, young children, and the elderly.[22] It is caused by group A streptococci.[32,33] Erysipelas affects only the upper dermis, whereas the more classic cellulitis also involves the deep dermis and subcutaneous fat.[12,43] Erysipelas occurs most commonly on the face or lower extremities, although any area of the body may be affected.[43] The lesions appears as warm, tender, shiny, erythematous plaques with raised and sharply demarcated borders.[22,43] Rapid spread is the rule, and lesion blistering can occur. Associated signs and symptoms include high fever, chills, and anorexia.[22] The diagnosis is made clinically.[44] Treatment with penicillin plus clindamycin is recommended, and the combination may be associated with better outcomes than monotherapy.

### *Tinea*

*Tinea* is a general term used to describe a collection of skin mycoses, including tinea pedis (athlete's foot), tinea cruris (jock itch), tinea corporis (ringworm), and tinea capitis (scalp). These dermatophytes invade the dead keratin of skin, hair, and nails.[45] The most common offending fungi are *Microsporum canis* and *Trichophyton tonsurans*.[46,47] Tinea capitis is rarely seen past adolescence, whereas tinea pedis and cruris are usually seen in adolescents and adults.[46] Tinea corporis produces annular, erythematous, pruritic patches with a scaly leading edge.[45] Treatment of tinea corporis, cruris, and pedis includes topical antifungal preparations such as miconazole or clotrimazole for 2 to 4 weeks.[48] Tinea capitis is characterized by scaly discrete patches of alopecia. It is the most common dermatophytosis of childhood.[45] Most cases occur in children 4 to 7 years old, with a predilection for African Americans.[49] Clinical findings vary from scaling and patchy hair loss to pruritic papules, pustules, and crusting.[49] Occipital and posterior cervical adenopathy is usually present.[45] Additionally, "black dots," or short broken-off hairs, may be seen at the scalp surface.[47] A kerion (tender boggy abscess devoid of hair) occasionally develops as a severe inflammatory reaction to the fungus.[47,49] A Wood lamp can aid in the diagnosis of tinea capitis. Hairs infected with *Microsporum* will fluoresce blue-green. Wood lamp evaluation is not helpful in the diagnosis of tinea infections on hairless skin. Alternatively, direct KOH microscopy of skin scrapings can also be used for diagnosis.[45,47] Treatment of tinea capitis consists of 6 to 8 weeks of oral griseofulvin and a selenium sulfide shampoo twice weekly.[45,46] Treatment with griseofulvin mandates monitoring of liver function. Alternative treatment regimens consisting of terbinafine, itraconazole, and fluconazole may also be effective.[46] Contaminated hairbrushes, towels, pillows, and hats should be disinfected.

### *Molluscum Contagiosum*

Molluscum is a common childhood viral infection of the skin characterized by umbilicated papules. It is caused by a poxvirus and can occur at any age but is most common in young children and those with impaired cellular immunity.[50,51] Molluscum is contagious and seen frequently in swimmers, wrestlers, and sexually active persons. Those with atopic dermatitis and immunosuppression are especially susceptible.[50,51] The incubation period ranges from 2 to 8 weeks. The lesions are discrete skin-colored, dome-shaped papules 2 to 5 mm in diameter and usually umbilicated.[51,52] The lesions are typically painless and nonpruritic. They occur (alone or in groups) on

**Table 18.3 Pediatric Dermatitis**

| DERMATITIS | ATOPIC DERMATITIS | DIAPER DERMATITIS | SEBORRHEIC DERMATITIS |
|---|---|---|---|
| Etiology | Unknown | Inflammatory eruption<br>*Candida* infection | Chronic inflammatory disease |
| Age range | 95% by 5 yr | 6-9 mo | <6 mo<br>Postpubertal adolescents |
| Season | All seasons | All seasons | All seasons |
| Morphology | Vesicles<br>Scales/patches<br>Excoriation<br>Lichenification<br>Hyperpigmentation | Diaper dermatitis: confluent shiny erythema<br>*Candida* dermatitis: beefy-red patches | Salmon-colored rash<br>Greasy scales |
| Usual distribution | Young children: face, leg extensor surfaces, trunk<br>Older children: neck, flexural surfaces | Diaper dermatitis: spares intertriginous creases<br>*Candida* dermatitis: involves intertriginous creases | Sebaceous gland concentrations: scalp, face, diaper area |
| Associated findings | Dennie-Morgan lines<br>Allergic shiners<br>Palmar creases<br>Hertoghe sign<br>Periauricular fissures | Satellite lesions | Thick, adherent scales |

the face, chest, axilla, and upper extremities. The diagnosis is made clinically.[51] A single lesion may be treated with cryotherapy (liquid nitrogen) or by evisceration of the core with a comedone extractor, sterile needle, or scapel.[52] Treatment of multiple lesions includes the application of cantharidin, retinoic acid, or benzoyl peroxide.[51] If untreated, most lesions resolve spontaneously in less than a year.[51,52]

## DERMATITIS

*Dermatitis* is a general term used to refer to a collection of conditions producing a pruritic, inflammatory, noninfectious rash. **Table 18.3** outlines these pediatric dermatitis conditions.

### *Atopic Dermatitis*

Atopic dermatitis (AD), commonly referred to as eczema, is an inflammatory skin condition characterized by pruritus, erythema, vesicles, and scales. Once chronic, AD can also appear lichenified and hyperpigmented.[1,45] AD is more commonly diagnosed in children with a family history of atopy (allergic rhinitis, conjunctivitis, asthma, and atopic dermatitis).[1] Nearly 95% of patients in whom eczema is diagnosed are identified by 5 years of age.[1] The lifetime prevalence of AD is approximately 17%.[53] Although the exact cause is unknown, eczematous skin is postulated to have a decrease in skin lipids and thus altered water-binding capacity. This leads to marked skin dehydration, pruritus, and scratching, which results in the characteristic skin lesions.[53] In young infants, scaly, erythematous papules, patches, or vesicles commonly erupt on the face, the extensor surfaces of the legs, and less commonly the trunk. Approximately 50% of young infants in whom eczema is diagnosed have complete resolution of symptoms by 3 years of age. In older children, eczematous lesions tend to be found in the flexural surfaces and the neck. These lesions appear scaly and erythematous, often with crusts, excoriation, and lichenification. Of note, eczematous lesions in dark-skinned individuals frequently occur on extensor rather than flexural surfaces and are more papular and hyperpigmented in appearance. Treatment of AD includes behavioral changes, emollients, topical corticosteroids, and antihistamines.[1,53] Fragrances and bubble baths should be avoided. Mild, unscented moisturizing soaps (Dove, Aveeno) are preferred. Irritants such as overly hot water, synthetic fabrics, wool, stuffed toys, bleach, and fabric softeners should be avoided. Long-sleeved cotton shirts can protect the skin. Patients with AD should apply emollients (Aquaphor, Eucerin) after bathing while the skin is still moist to prevent flare-ups. Corticosteroids should be applied to areas of acute exacerbation to reduce and eliminate inflammation.[53] Ointments are preferred because they penetrate more efficiently and provide a more effective barrier against moisture loss than creams do. However, they may be less tolerable during the summer months. Low- to intermediate-potency steroids are recommended for the initial management of AD in older children and adolescents. Infants and young children should be treated with one of the lower-potency topical steroids (1% hydrocortisone). High-potency steroids are not usually required for the treatment of eczema except in regions with long-standing lichenified or intractable plaques.[1] Corticosteroids should be applied one to three times daily until the inflammation subsides. The least potent topical steroids should be applied to the face, axilla, and groin because these areas are especially prone to atrophy.[1] Pruritus can be treated with antihistamines (hydroxyzine or diphenhydramine). Localized infection should be treated with oral antibiotics effective against *S. aureus* (cephalexin, amoxicillin-clavulanate, or azithromycin).[1]

### Diaper Dermatitis

Diaper dermatitis is not one specific entity but incorporates all inflammatory eruptions occurring in the diaper area, including irritant diaper dermatitis and *Candida* diaper dermatitis. Diaper dermatitis has a prevalence of 7% to 35% and a peak incidence at about 6 to 9 months of age. Diaper dermatitis is triggered by the moist, occluded, macerated milieu of the diaper region. Other irritants include friction, diaper detergents, disinfectants, an alkaline pH, and fecal material.[54] Precipitating factors include infrequent diaper changes, insufficient bathing and cleansing, and especially occlusive diapers.[55] The rash typically begins over areas where friction is most pronounced, such as the buttocks, genitals, lower part of the abdomen, and inner aspect of the thighs. It begins as confluent shiny erythema with minimal scale that spares the intertriginous creases. Secondary infection with *Candida albicans* leads to progression of the eruption to a moist, beefy-red patch. Satellite lesions may be appreciated at the periphery.[56] Unlike simple irritant diaper dermatitis, *Candida* diaper dermatitis results in intertriginous involvement. *Candida* has been isolated in up to 80% of children with diaper dermatitis present for more than 3 days. Prevention and treatment of diaper dermatitis are typically achieved with simple measures to decrease irritation in the diaper region. Such measures include frequent diaper changes, the use of highly absorbent diapers, avoidance of cloth diapers, diaper-free periods, and avoidance of plastic or rubber diaper pants.[55] The diaper region should be cleansed gently with mild soap and dried completely. Use of barriers such as zinc oxide, petroleum, or talcum powder may help protect the skin from maceration. Candidal superinfection is treated with topical antifungal cream such as nystatin, clotrimazole, or miconazole.[57]

### Seborrheic Dermatitis (Cradle Cap)

Seborrheic dermatitis is a chronic inflammatory disease of unknown etiology with a bimodal distribution—infants younger than 6 months and postpubertal adolescents and young adults. It appears as a salmon-colored rash with overlying diffuse greasy yellow or white scales occurring in areas with high sebaceous gland concentration. Lesions are typically located on the scalp but may spread to involve the forehead, nasal folds, eyebrows, and diaper area. The lesions are not typically pruritic or painful.[1,58] Seborrheic dermatitis can be treated successfully with oatmeal baths and antiseborrheic shampoo (tar shampoo, selenium sulfide).[58] Ketoconazole has been shown to be effective. If the scales are particularly thick or adherent, loosening of the scales with warmed mineral oil and use of a fine-toothed comb before shampooing hasten clearing.[1] If the lesions are especially resistant to these treatments, corticosteroid preparations may be used.

## SEVERE PEDIATRIC RASHES

### Henoch-Schönlein Purpura

Henoch-Schönlein purpura (HSP) is a small-vessel vasculitis characterized by a purpuric rash, abdominal pain, arthritis, and hematuria.[59] It is usually seen in children between 3 and 10 years of age. HSP is often preceded by an upper respiratory infection or drug exposure.[59] The pathophysiology of HSP involves deposition of immunoglobulin A, C3, and immune complexes onto small vessels, which leads to systemic inflammation.[59] The HSP classic triad consists of purpura, abdominal pain, and arthritis. The purpura is palpable and most commonly found in a symmetric distribution over the buttocks and extensor surfaces of the legs. The abdominal pain is colicky and may be associated with nausea, vomiting, diarrhea, bloody stools, or intussusception.[59,60] Hematuria occurs in 10% to 20% of cases, and end-stage renal disease develops in approximately 1% of children.[59] The diagnosis of HSP is made clinically; however, a blood count, coagulation studies, chemistry panel, and urinalysis should be performed to exclude other diagnoses and evaluate renal function. HSP is a self-limited illness and treatment is supportive. Nonsteroidal antiinflammatory drugs (NSAIDs) may be used to reduce pain in the joints and soft tissue. The use of corticosteroids remains controversial.[59] Patients should be hospitalized if complications such as significant bleeding, intussusceptions, or renal failure develop.

### Meningococcemia

One of the most feared infections in the emergency department is meningococcemia caused by the bacterium *Neisseria meningitidis*. Although meningococcus is relatively rare in the United States, it is uniformly fatal, usually within 24 hours, if untreated.[61,62] This diagnosis must be considered in any child with fever, headache, and a rash. Meningococcemia may be manifested as a flulike illness with fever, myalgia, vomiting, and arthralgia. In up to two thirds of patients, the early, morbilliform ("measlelike") rash may mislead the physician into making the diagnosis of a viral exanthem.[63] The disease progresses quickly and exhibits more specific signs: nuchal rigidity, photophobia, altered mental status, and a petechial or purpuric rash. The rash most commonly involves the trunk and lower extremities; however, petechiae may also appear on the face, palms, and mucous membranes. As the infection proceeds, more extensive hemorrhagic lesions are seen on all body areas and progress to large ecchymotic areas.[62,63] Evaluation of patients with suspected meningitis should include blood cultures, serum chemistries, and a lumbar puncture with cerebrospinal fluid analysis and culture. If meningococcemia is suspected, antibiotics should be administered expeditiously (ceftriaxone or cefotaxime, plus vancomycin). Additional treatments include admission to the intensive care unit (ICU), fluid resuscitation, steroids, vasopressor agents, and prophylactic treatment of close contacts.[61-64]

### Staphylococcal Scalded Skin Syndrome

SSSS is a potentially life-threatening, toxin-mediated disease manifested by tender blistering and widespread desquamation. It usually occurs in children younger than 5 years.[11] The pathophysiology of this illness in children is postulated to be lack of antibodies against the toxin and reduced toxin excretion in comparison with adults.[63] The etiologic agent is exotoxin-producing *S. aureus* of phage group II.[11] The initial staphylococcal infection typically involves the nasopharynx, umbilicus, urinary tract, cutaneous wounds, conjunctiva, or blood. Symptoms of SSSS include a sudden onset of fever and irritability, followed by slight diffuse erythema (resembling a sunburn) and cutaneous tenderness (the infant does not want to be held). The rash initially affects the perioral and periorbital regions, neck, axilla, and groin. This is followed by the crusting exfoliative phase, which occurs around the mouth and eyes. Flaccid bullae also develop. Gentle traction on the affected skin results in epidermal separation (Nikolsky sign), which leaves a shiny, moist, red surface. The mucous membranes are not involved.[11,61,63] In newborns, the entire skin surface may be involved (Ritter disease). In SSSS, the cleavage plane for skin sloughing is epidermal. In toxic epidermal necrolysis (TEN), the cleavage plane is at the dermal-epidermal junction. Therefore, in SSSS only the epidermal layer is shed, thus resulting in less morbidity than that occurring with TEN.[63] The diagnosis is made clinically. Complications include sepsis and respiratory distress. Treatment is directed toward elimination of active *S. aureus* infection to eradicate toxin production. Patients are typically treated with a β-lactamase penicillin or clindamycin. Although antibiotics are recommended, it is unclear whether they measurably alter the course of the disease. Hospitalization for fluid and electrolyte management and for supportive skin care is indicated for most patients.

### Kawasaki Disease

Kawasaki disease (KD) is an acute, febrile, multisystem illness of unknown etiology that causes widespread vasculitis in young children. The incidence of KD peaks at about 9 to 11 months of age, with 80% of affected children being younger than 5 years.[63] The diagnosis of KD disease can be made if and five of the following criteria are present[65,66]:

- Temperature higher than 39° C is present for more than 5 days
- Bilateral conjunctival injection: without exudates
- Erythema of the oropharynx or lips: with fissures or strawberry tongue
- Acute cervical lymphadenopathy
- Polymorphous erythematous exanthem: morbilliform, scarlatiniform, or maculopapular (may have plaques or target lesions)
- Edema of the palms and soles: with desquamation occurring 2 to 3 weeks after onset of the illness

Patients with only four of these symptoms meet the criteria if coronary aneurysms are found on echocardiography. The most important clinical complication is coronary artery aneurysms, which may lead to myocardial ischemia and sudden death.[66,67] Other, less common complications include gallbladder hydrops, diarrhea, obstruction of the small bowel, arthritis, cystitis, pericarditis, myocarditis, valvulitis, and aseptic meningitis. All children with KD should be hospitalized. Management of KD is directed at reducing the risk for coronary artery aneurysm and thrombosis, which is achieved with high-dose aspirin and IVIG.[65,67,68]

### Toxic Shock Syndrome

Staphylococcal TSS is a potentially lethal disease characterized by acute fever, generalized erythroderma, and hypotension. It is due to a localized infection or colonization with a toxin-producing strain of *S. aureus*.[11] Although TSS is classically associated with menstruating girls using tampons, recent changes in the manufacturing and use of tampons have resulted in a decrease in the incidence of menstrual-associated TSS.[69] Currently, the incidence of nonmenstrual TSS exceeds that of menstrual TSS.[11,69] Symptoms characteristically begin with high fever, malaise, chills, headache, myalgia, vomiting, and diarrhea. Hypotension and multiorgan involvement follow rapidly. Cutaneous symptoms include a diffuse, blanching, macular eruption beginning on the trunk and spreading to the extremities. This is followed by desquamation, particularly on the palms and soles.[61,63] The mucous membranes are involved, and erythema and ulceration of the pharyngeal, oral, conjunctival, or vaginal mucosa may occur. Complications include refractory shock, acute renal failure, neurologic symptoms, disseminated intravascular coagulation, acute respiratory distress syndrome, and death.[11,63] The diagnosis is usually made clinically. However, *S. aureus* may be isolated from a localized infection.[69] Treatment of TSS includes hemodynamic stabilization of shock and management of multiorgan failure. Importantly, every attempt should be made to identify and treat the infection with local drainage, removal of infective material (tampon), and antistaphylococcal antibiotics.[11,32,63]

## TREATMENT

### CLASSIC EXANTHEMS AND VIRAL RASHES

The vast majority of these illnesses require only supportive care and surveillance for complications. Treatment of fever and constitutional symptoms with ibuprofen or acetaminophen is helpful. Vitamin A has been shown to reduce risk for mortality and complication in children with measles.[9] Treatment of scarlet fever is with penicillin.[13] Care of patients with varicella should include attention to pruritus, wound care, and prevention of secondary infections.[1,30] Immunocompromised children with varicella may benefit from acyclovir.[32,33] Patients with hand-foot-and-mouth disease benefit from soothing anesthetic mouth rinses.[15] All patients with viral illness must be kept away from pregnant women and immunocompromised individuals. All these illnesses have the potential for serious complications, and thus close monitoring for these adverse events is required.

### SKIN AND SOFT TISSUE INFECTIONS

The mainstay of treatment of impetigo is antibiotic therapy directed against *Staphylococcus* and *Streptococcus*. Agents include cephalexin, amoxicillin-clavulanate, azithromycin, dicloxacillin, and oxacillin.[33,37,39] Treatment of bacterial reservoirs with mupirocin may also be required. Erysipelas requires treatment with penicillin plus clindamycin. Tinea infections of the body, groin, and feet are treated with topical antifungal preparations (miconazole or clotrimazole) for 2 to 4 weeks.[48] Tinea capitis is treated with 6 to 8 weeks of oral griseofulvin and selenium sulfide shampoo, with periodic surveillance of liver function tests.[45,46] Molluscum infections may be left to resolve or, alternatively, treated by cryotherapy, excision, or application of chemicals.[51,52] Because all these illnesses have the potential for serious complications, close monitoring for adverse events is required.

### PEDIATRIC DERMATITIS

Treatment of atopic dermatitis is multidisciplinary in approach and includes behavior modification, emollients, topical steroids, and antihistamines. Diaper dermatitis is managed with measures aimed at decreasing regional irritation, including changes in diapering routine, use of barriers, and monitoring for candidal superinfection.[56,57] Seborrheic dermatitis is treated with oatmeal baths and antiseborrheic shampoos. Ketoconazole is also effective.[58]

### SEVERE PEDIATRIC RASHES

HSP is usually a self-limited disease, and treatment is supportive. Relief of pain symptoms with NSAIDs is helpful.[59] Meningococcemia is an overwhelming bacterial infection that requires ICU admission, early antibiotic therapy, fluid resuscitation, vasopressor support, and prophylaxis of close contacts. SSSS is also potentially life-threatening and mandates hospital admission, early antibiotic therapy, fluid and electrolyte management, and supportive skin care. All children with KD also require admission. Treatment with high-dose aspirin and IVIG is required, as well as surveillance for cardiovascular complications.[65,67,68] Treatment of TSS entails ICU admission, hemodynamic stabilization, removal of infective source material, and early antibiotic therapy.[23,32,63] All these illnesses have potentially devastating complications, and close and continual monitoring is therefore mandatory.

## FOLLOW-UP AND PATIENT EDUCATION

### CLASSIC EXANTHEMS AND VIRAL RASHES

The majority of these illnesses are self-limited or treated with simple measures. Appropriate follow-up for patients with these classic exanthems and viral rashes is with their pediatrician. The physician is a valuable resource for patient education, parent reassurance, and close monitoring of complications.

### SKIN AND SOFT TISSUE INFECTIONS

These illnesses are usually the result of common bacterial, fungal, or viral infections and should be monitored closely by the patient's pediatrician to ensure complete resolution, as well as provide family education regarding transmission and eradication of carrier states and identify any complications that may develop.

### DERMATITIS

These entities are common in most families and easily managed in concert with the patient's pediatrician. AD may benefit from dermatologic referral. All these conditions require serial evaluation for appropriate resolution and surveillance for complications.

### SEVERE PEDIATRIC RASHES

These illnesses have devastating complications and require not only close follow-up with a pediatrician but in many cases also specialist referral. HSP is generally self-limited. However, significant bleeding, intussusception, and renal failure do occur. Specialty consultation is warranted for end-organ damage in these patients. Meningococcemia has a multitude of potential sequelae associated with its resolution. The pediatrician should monitor these patients closely because they may benefit from neurologic consultation and specialist referral for end-organ damage. SSSS requires antibiotic therapy and wound care. The primary care physician is well equipped to oversee these therapies and monitor for complications. Patients with KD require admission to the hospital and close follow-up on discharge. Referral to a cardiologist for monitoring of cardiovascular sequelae may be coordinated through the pediatrician. TSS results in hypotensive shock and possible multisystem organ failure. Following resolution and discharge, these patients will require intensive, coordinated care by their pediatrician to ensure maximal recovery. Multiple specialists may be required.

## SUGGESTED READINGS

Boguniewicz M. Atopic dermatitis: beyond the itch that rashes. Immunol Allergy Clin North Am 2005;25:333-51.

Campbell M. Childhood rashes that present to the ED. Part I: viral and bacterial issues. Pediatr Emerg Med Pract 2007;4(3):1-24.

Campbell M. Childhood rashes that present to the ED. Part II: fungal, G. annulare, Kawasaki disease, insect related, and molluscum. Pediatr Emerg Med 2007;4(4).

Manders SM. Toxin-mediated streptococcal and staphylococcal disease. J Am Acad Dermatol 1998;39:383-98.

Pinna GS, Kafetzis DA, Tselkas OI, et al. Kawasaki disease: an overview. Curr Opin Infect Dis 2008;21:263-70.

Scott LA, Stone MS. Viral exanthems. Dermatol Online J 2003;9(3):4.

## REFERENCES

*References can be found on Expert Consult @ www.expertconsult.com.*

# Pediatric Cardiac Disorders 19

Nathan W. Mick

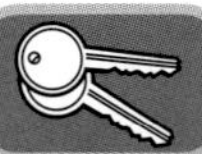

**KEY POINTS**

- Congenital heart disease is typically diagnosed in utero or before discharge from the newborn nursery, but delayed manifestations usually occur within the first 2 weeks of life when the ductus arteriosus closes.
- Congenital heart disease should be considered in a neonate who is in shock or has congestive heart failure or cyanosis.
- Subtle signs of cardiac disease in children include sweating, irritability, and poor feeding.
- Echocardiography is used for the diagnosis of structural congenital heart disease.
- Prostaglandin $E_1$ can be lifesaving in cases of ductal-dependent congenital heart disease.

## EPIDEMIOLOGY

The spectrum of congenital pediatric cardiac disorders includes structural congenital heart disease (CHD) and rhythm disturbances such as supraventricular tachycardia (SVT), long QTc syndrome, and congenital complete heart block.

Structural CHD occurs in approximately 8 in 1000 live births.[1] Most congenital lesions are diagnosed in utero or in the newborn nursery, but a significant proportion may not be manifested until 1 to 2 weeks of life, when the ductus arteriosus closes. In fact, a significant proportion of cases of CHD are diagnosed after hospital discharge. Normal findings on newborn evaluation does not rule out potentially significant and lethal lesions, and a high index of suspicion is critical to ensure timely diagnosis.[2] Many risk factors for the development of CHD have been identified (**Box 19.1**), including a family history of CHD, maternal diabetes (associated with ventricular septal defect [VSD], hypertrophic cardiomyopathy, and transposition of the great arteries [TGA]), and fetal drug exposure (e.g., Ebstein anomaly with maternal lithium therapy). Pediatric cardiac disease may be challenging because it may mimic more common illnesses, such as sepsis.

Rhythm disturbances are also important causes of pediatric cardiac disease and can occur in children with structural heart disease or in those with structurally normal hearts. SVT is the most common pediatric cardiac arrhythmia and includes atrioventricular nodal reentrant tachycardia (AVNRT), atrioventricular reentrant tachycardia (AVRT), and preexcitation conditions such as Wolf-Parkinson-White syndrome. Congenital complete heart block is associated with maternal connective tissue disease and the presence of anti-Ro/SSA and anti–La-SSB antibodies. Long QTc syndrome may be congenital or acquired; the congenital form is estimated to occur in 1 in 7000 to 10,000 live births.[3] Congenital long QTc syndrome may occur in an autosomal dominant form (Romano-Ward syndrome) or in an autosomal recessive form (Jervell and Lange-Nielsen syndrome) associated with sensorineural hearing loss.

## PATHOPHYSIOLOGY

Fetal circulatory anatomy is designed to transport oxygenated blood from the placenta to the systemic circulation while bypassing the lungs (**Fig. 19.1**). Fetal oxygenation occurs at the placenta, and blood is returned to the right atrium through the ductus venosus after bypassing the liver. Most of the oxygen-rich blood is shunted across the foramen ovale into the left atrium and is then delivered to the systemic circulation via the aorta. Some flow travels from the right atrium into the right ventricle and enters the pulmonary arteries. The pulmonary vasculature is constricted, and flow is shunted through the ductus arteriosus and mixes with blood in the aorta to supply the systemic circulation.

Birth results in a complex series of changes induced by expansion and oxygenation of the lungs. Oxygenation of the lungs leads to a marked decrease in pulmonary vascular resistance and a subsequent increase in pulmonary blood flow. Increasing pulmonary blood flow results in greater return of blood to the left atrium, which functionally closes the foramen ovale (the foramen may remain "probe patent" into adulthood). The decrease in pulmonary vascular resistance is coupled with an increase in systemic vascular resistance, and ductal flow reverses to become left to right. The blood traversing the ductus arteriosus is now highly oxygenated, a change that typically stimulates closure by 48 hours of life. In certain cases, the ductus arteriosus does not close until 1 to 2 weeks of life, and so-called ductal-dependent cardiac lesions may be manifested at this time (**Box 19.2**). The increased pressure and volume demands on the left ventricle stimulate growth of the left ventricle, and the decreased load on the right ventricle

**BOX 19.1 Risk Factors for the Development of Congenital Heart Disease**

Risk for congenital heart disease is increased with one affected parent or sibling and is three times greater if two close relatives have such disease.
Maternal diabetes is associated with hypertrophic cardiomyopathy, ventricular septal defect, and transposition of the great arteries.
Maternal phenytoin use is associated with aortic stenosis and pulmonic stenosis.
Maternal lithium use is associated with Ebstein anomaly.
Fetal alcohol syndrome is associated with atrial septal defect and ventricular septal defect.

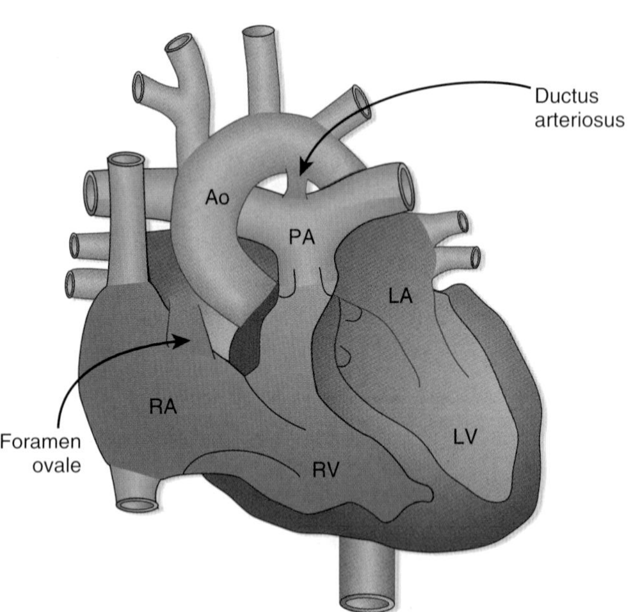


**Fig. 19.1 Normal fetal circulatory anatomy.** *Ao*, Aorta; *LA*, left atrium; *LV*, left ventricle; *PA*, pulmonary artery; *RA*, right atrium; *RV*, right ventricle.

**BOX 19.2 Congenital Heart Lesions That Depend on Patency of the Ductus Arteriosus**

**Right-to-Left Shunting Critical for Relief of Left-Sided Obstruction (Typically Present with Shock)**
Hypoplastic left heart syndrome
Total anomalous pulmonary venous return with obstruction
Critical coarctation of the aorta
Interrupted aortic arch
Congenital aortic stenosis

**Left-to-Right Shunting Critical for Relief of Right-Sided Obstruction (Typically Present with Cyanosis)**
Tetralogy of Fallot with severe right outflow tract obstruction
Tricuspid atresia
Pulmonic atresia
Ebstein anomaly

from decreased pulmonary vascular resistance results in a reduction in right ventricular mass.

## PRESENTING SIGNS AND SYMPTOMS

Infants with previously undiagnosed structural CHD are typically initially seen in the emergency department (ED) with shock, congestive heart failure (CHF), cyanosis, or a combination of these symptoms. Left-sided obstructive lesions such as hypoplastic left heart syndrome and coarctation of the aorta are manifested as shock as the ductus arteriosus closes and the blood supply to the systemic circulation dwindles. Shock can also be the initial sign of total anomalous pulmonary venous return (TAPVR) with obstruction. Evidence of poor perfusion, such as lethargy, mottled extremities, tachycardia, and tachypnea, is typically present. Sepsis and other noncardiac conditions (e.g., salt-wasting crisis in congenital adrenal hyperplasia) can cause similar findings. Shock may also be the manifestation of SVT or complete heart block that has become decompensated (**Table 19.1**).

CHF is a common manifestation of both structural heart disease and congenital rhythm disturbances. Although respiratory distress, tachypnea, and rales may be present, subtler signs such as poor feeding and hepatomegaly may be the only manifestations of CHF. Assessment of the liver's edge is a critical portion of the physical examination in these infants. Peripheral edema as a manifestation of CHF is rare in infants. Acyanotic heart diseases with large left-to-right shunts, such as congenital aortic stenosis, interrupted aortic arch, and coarctation of the aorta, are manifested as CHF because blood preferentially flows into the low-resistance pulmonary bed (**Box 19.3**). TAPVR and VSD can also be manifested as CHF as a result of volume overload of the right ventricle. Rhythm abnormalities such as sustained SVT and congenital complete heart block can likewise be manifested as CHF as a result of poor forward flow.

Cyanosis can be the first manifestation of CHD in infants, and severe lesions are typically diagnosed in utero or in the newborn nursery. Some lesions may escape detection, however, and first be recognized later in the neonatal period. Central

**Table 19.1 Differential Diagnosis of Shock in Infants**

| TYPE OF SHOCK | POSSIBLE CAUSES |
|---|---|
| Hypovolemic | Hemorrhage<br>Dehydration |
| Cardiogenic | Critical coarctation of the aorta<br>Interrupted aortic arch<br>Congenital aortic stenosis<br>Hypoplastic left heart syndrome<br>Arrhythmia<br>Myocarditis<br>Cardiac tamponade<br>Pulmonary embolism<br>Tension pneumothorax |
| Distributive | Sepsis<br>Spinal cord trauma<br>Anaphylaxis<br>Heavy metal poisoning |

cyanosis affecting the lips, mucous membranes, and trunk is due to decreased arterial oxygen saturation and is always pathologic. The differential diagnosis of central cyanosis is presented in **Table 19.2**. Peripheral cyanosis limited to the extremities or circumoral region is a normal newborn finding but can also be due to non-CHD causes such as sepsis, exposure to cold, and poor cardiac output.

**BOX 19.3 Differential Diagnosis of Congestive Heart Failure in Infants**

Critical coarctation of the aorta
Interrupted aortic arch
Congenital aortic stenosis
Hypoplastic left heart syndrome
Large ventricular septal defect
Truncus arteriosus
Unrecognized supraventricular tachycardia
Cardiac tamponade
Myocarditis

**Table 19.2 Differential Diagnosis of Central Cyanosis in Infants**

| | |
|---|---|
| **Cardiac Causes** | |
| Right-to-left shunting | Tetralogy of Fallot<br>Tricuspid atresia<br>Pulmonary atresia<br>Transposition of the great arteries with intact ventricular septum<br>Ebstein anomaly<br>Truncus arteriosus<br>Eisenmenger syndrome |
| **Pulmonary Causes** | |
| Right-to-left shunting | Persistent pulmonary hypertension of the newborn |
| Ventilation-perfusion mismatch | Transient tachypnea of the newborn<br>Congenital cystic adenomatoid malformation<br>Pneumonia<br>Congenital diaphragmatic hernia<br>Hyaline membrane disease<br>Pneumothorax<br>Pleural effusion<br>Hemothorax |
| Hypoventilation | Neonatal asphyxia<br>Intraventricular hemorrhage<br>Seizure<br>Encephalitis<br>Meningitis<br>Sedative agents<br>Botulism<br>Neonatal myasthenia<br>Croup<br>Bronchiolitis<br>Laryngotracheomalacia |
| **Hematologic Causes** | |
| Hemoglobinopathies | Carboxyhemoglobinemia<br>Methemoglobinemia |

Rhythm abnormalities such as SVT, long QTc syndrome, hypertrophic cardiomyopathy, and congenital complete heart block may be manifested as syncope, especially in older children. Syncope is a common pediatric finding and typically has a benign prognosis, although documentation of normal electrocardiographic (ECG) findings is important as a screen for more ominous causes of fainting. Though rare, sudden cardiac death as a first manifestation of long QTc syndrome occurs in 9% of affected children and may be an underappreciated cause of sudden infant death syndrome.[4]

Even though shock, CHF, cyanosis, and syncope are the common manifestation of CHD, the signs and symptoms that bring a pediatric patient to the attention of a health care provider may be more protean. CHD, either structural or arrhythmogenic, should be considered in a child with sweating during feeding, failure to thrive, irritability, chest pain (in older children), unexplained hypertension, or a new murmur. Murmurs are common in the pediatric age group and occur in up to 60% of newborns, the vast majority of whom have structurally normal hearts.[5] Most "innocent" murmurs of infancy and childhood are due to either peripheral pulmonary stenosis (PPS) or Still murmurs. PPS murmurs are grade 1 to 2 of 6, midsystolic, high-pitched ejection murmurs best heard over the pulmonary area. Still murmurs are grade 1 to 2 of 6, low-pitched systolic ejection murmurs best heard at the left lower sternal border; they vary with the heart rate and decrease in intensity with the Valsalva maneuver. Characteristics that differentiate between innocent and pathologic murmurs are presented in **Table 19.3**.

## DIFFERENTIAL DIAGNOSIS AND MEDICAL DECISION MAKING

### LESION-SPECIFIC PRESENTATIONS

#### *Lesions Manifested as Decreased Pulmonary Blood Flow*

TETRALOGY OF FALLOT The tetralogy of Fallot, the most common structural CHD occurring outside the neonatal period, consists of the following anatomic abnormalities: a

**Table 19.3 Differentiating Innocent Murmurs from Pathologic Murmurs**

| | INNOCENT | PATHOLOGIC |
|---|---|---|
| Grade (out of 6) | 1-2 | 3 or higher |
| Quality | Soft | Harsh or pansystolic |
| Second heart sound | Normally split | Single or fixed split |
| Other heart sounds | No clicks | Click present |
| Pulse findings | Normal | Decreased femoral pulses |
| Other abnormal findings | Absent | Present |

large VSD, varying degrees of right ventricular outflow tract obstruction, an overriding aorta, and right ventricular hypertrophy. Time of appearance is linked to the severity of right ventricular outflow tract obstruction and thus to the amount of pulmonary blood flow, with severe obstruction causing cyanosis in the newborn and earlier age of occurrence. Less severe obstruction (a "pink" tetralogy) may delay diagnosis, or an infant may be taken to the ED with "tet spells" in which the child becomes episodically more cyanotic as a result of worsening of the right ventricular outflow tract obstruction and decreased pulmonary blood flow.

Physical findings consist of right ventricular heave and a single second heart sound (no pulmonic valve component). A harsh systolic ejection murmur, a finding reflecting right ventricular outflow tract obstruction, may be present. The murmur characteristically softens as the severity of obstruction worsens and more blood is shunted across the VSD.

TRICUSPID ATRESIA Tricuspid atresia is characterized by complete absence of the tricuspid valve, a hypoplastic right ventricle, and the presence of a VSD. The size of the VSD determines the amount of pulmonary blood flow. Large VSDs may allow relatively normal pulmonary blood flow and delay detection. In these cases, because the left ventricle is the only functioning pumping chamber, fluid overload may occur, and affected infants and children may have heart failure and hepatomegaly. Infants with small VSDs are dependent on the ductus arteriosus for pulmonary blood flow and are seen in the neonatal period with cyanosis as the ductus arteriosus closes. Blood returning to the heart enters the right atrium and flows across the foramen ovale (which remains patent) to enter the systemic circulation. A murmur of pulmonic stenosis may be present if flow across the pulmonary valve is sufficient to be detected on auscultation.

PULMONARY ATRESIA Pulmonary atresia with an intact ventricular septum is associated with a hypoplastic right ventricle and is dependent on an atrial septal defect (ASD) and right-to-left shunting. Pulmonary blood flow depends on the ductus arteriosus, so affected patients are seen in the neonatal period with cyanosis as the ductus arteriosus closes. Physical examination typically demonstrates a single second heart sound (no pulmonic component), and if a murmur is present, it is typical of tricuspid regurgitation.

#### *Lesions Manifested as Increased Pulmonary Blood Flow*

TOTAL ANOMALOUS PULMONARY VENOUS RETURN TAPVR occurs as a result of embryologic failure of the pulmonary veins to form a connection to the left atrium. The pulmonary veins can dump into the superior vena cava (supracardiac connection), into the portal vein (infracardiac connection), or into the right atrium via the coronary sinus. Obstruction of any of these anomalous connections leads to pulmonary congestion, respiratory distress, and varying levels of heart failure. Cyanosis may develop because of the decrease in oxygenated blood returning to the heart. Physical findings may indicate heart failure, and TAPVR with obstruction is characterized by a fixed, widely split second heart sound.

TRUNCUS ARTERIOSUS Truncus arteriosus is defined as the presence of a single trunk arising from the heart that functions as both the aorta and the pulmonary artery. A single semilunar valve is present and overrides a VSD, thereby allowing complete mixing of systemic and pulmonary blood. As pulmonary vascular resistance falls after birth, more and more blood travels into the low-resistance pulmonary circuit, and heart failure develops. In affected infants in whom truncus arteriosus was not diagnosed in the newborn nursery, it is typically diagnosed when heart failure develops. Physical findings include a wide pulse pressure and a systolic ejection murmur representing increased flow across the semilunar valve. A single second heart sound may also be found.

TRANSPOSITION OF THE GREAT ARTERIES TGA is a common congenital defect in which the pulmonary and systemic circuits are arranged in parallel rather than in series. TGA may be associated with a VSD or ASD, but more commonly, no other defect is present, and mixing of oxygenated and deoxygenated blood occurs only at the ductus arteriosus. Infants with TGA are cyanotic at birth because of right-to-left shunting, and the cyanosis gets worse as the ductus arteriosus closes. If therapy to keep the ductus arteriosus open (see later) is not instituted promptly, hypoxemia, acidosis, and death quickly ensue. In TGA without an associated VSD or ASD, there may be no other telltale signs on physical examination. Children with TGA and an associated VSD or ASD may be seen later in the newborn period with heart failure, and a VSD murmur may be heard.

HYPOPLASTIC LEFT HEART SYNDROME Hypoplastic left heart syndrome involves a severely hypoplastic left ventricle and small, atretic mitral and aortic valves. The right ventricle is the default pumping chamber to both the lungs and the systemic circulation, and all systemic circulation crosses from the pulmonary artery through the ductus arteriosus to supply the body. Cyanosis from birth is the rule, and the lesions are typically diagnosed in utero or in the nursery. As the ductus arteriosus closes, all blood returning to the heart goes to the lungs, and heart failure develops as a result of volume overload. The pathway to the systemic circulation is also compromised, and shock develops. Physical findings include tricuspid and pulmonic murmurs because of increased flow. Hepatomegaly may be apparent as failure develops.

### ACYANOTIC STRUCTURAL CONGENITAL HEART DISEASE

#### *Coarctation of the Aorta*

Coarctation of the aorta refers to congenital narrowing of the aorta, most commonly at the level of the ductus arteriosus. Infants with coarctation have a normal oxygen saturation value and typically no cyanosis. When the ductus arteriosus is open, blood is able to bypass the obstruction, and few symptoms are present. As the ductus arteriosus closes, the systemic circulation may be compromised by the narrowed aorta. "Critical" coarctation occurs when the narrowing is severe, and these infants are brought to the ED when the ductus arteriosus closes and signs of shock appear. If the narrowing is less severe, the coarctation may be diagnosed later in life. Physical findings consistent with coarctation include normal or increased blood pressure in the upper extremities and decreased perfusion to the lower extremities. Four-extremity blood pressure should be measured in any child in whom the diagnosis of coarctation of the aorta is being entertained. Frequently, a harsh systolic ejection murmur is heard in the left axilla and back.

### *Congenital Aortic Stenosis*

Congenital aortic stenosis typically results when an aortic valve is congenitally bicuspid rather than tricuspid. Most infants with aortic stenosis are asymptomatic, and problems do not develop until later in life.[6] The condition may be diagnosed in affected children as part of an evaluation for a heart murmur. If the stenosis is severe, symptoms may develop in infancy. Typically, critical congenital aortic stenosis becomes apparent as the ductus arteriosus closes, and the findings consist of heart failure as a result of increased pulmonary blood flow and signs of systemic hypoperfusion. A murmur may not be appreciable because of poor cardiac output. Physical findings include signs of shock with poor peripheral perfusion.

## CONGENITAL RHYTHM DISTUBANCES

### *Supraventricular Tachycardia*

SVT is characterized by a narrow-complex elevated heart rhythm that is regular and generally above 220 beats/min. AVRT, including Wolff-Parkinson-White syndrome, and AVNRT are the two most frequent forms of SVT in children. AVRT is more common in infants and younger children, with AVNRT rising in frequency after 2 years of age. The majority of children with SVT have structurally normal hearts, although SVT is associated with CHD in about 25% of cases.[7] Infants may exhibit respiratory distress, poor feeding, and irritability, and the rhythm abnormality may not be recognized until heart failure develops. Older children may have syncope, chest pain, palpitations, or lightheadedness. Sudden cardiac death is rare with SVT unless an underlying structural heart disease is present. Physical findings include tachycardia, hypotension, and signs of heart failure.

### *Long QTc Syndrome*

Many patients with long QTc syndrome are asymptomatic, although syncope, palpitations, lightheadedness, or cardiac arrest may bring affected children to medical attention. Among those who have symptoms, a significant proportion have exercise-related complaints. Long QTc syndrome may actually cause some cases of sudden infant death syndrome. A family history of sudden cardiac death may be elicited. Autosomal recessive forms of congenital long QTc syndrome are associated with sensorineural hearing loss. Anderson syndrome is a rare autosomal dominant form of long QTc syndrome associated with hypokalemic periodic paralysis, facial dysmorphisms, and cardiac arrhythmias. Torsades de pointes is the classic rhythm abnormality occurring in long QTc syndrome, and the baseline ECG findings may consist of bradycardia or atrioventricular block. Physical examination may demonstrate signs of associated syndromic abnormalities.

### *Congenital Complete Heart Block*

Congenital complete heart block may be manifested at any time during childhood, although many cases are diagnosed in utero. The common finding is bradycardia. In infants in whom congenital complete heart block is diagnosed after birth, physical findings include cannon waves in the neck (as a result of atrial contraction against closed tricuspid valves) and signs of poor perfusion. A maternal history of connective tissue disease, particularly systemic lupus erythematosus, is sometimes present. Congenital complete heart block in older patients may be manifested as syncope or sudden cardiac death.

# DIAGNOSTIC TESTING

Evaluation of an infant in critical condition with suspected cardiac disease should focus on excluding noncardiac causes of the patient's symptoms while attempting to confirm a cardiac lesion. The distinction between sepsis and decompensated cardiac disease is often difficult, and it is advisable to rule out sepsis in critically ill children and begin treatment with empirically chosen antibiotics. In children with cardiac disease, polycythemia from chronic hypoxia may be noted. A thorough physical examination is critical to evaluate for sources of possible infection (indicating possible sepsis) or ambiguous genitalia (seen with salt-wasting crisis secondary to congenital adrenal hyperplasia).

## ELECTROCARDIOGRAM

A 12-lead ECG study should be performed on every infant and child in whom heart disease is suspected. If structural CHD is part of the differential diagnosis, a 15-lead ECG study (including leads $V_3R$, $V_4R$, and $V_7$) may give added information. Correct interpretation of pediatric ECG values can be challenging because most normal adult values are abnormal in the newborn period. Normal ECG parameters in children are presented in **Table 19.4**, whereas **Tables 19.5 and 19.6** list ECG findings associated with specific cardiac lesions.[8] SVT is typically manifested as a narrow-complex tachycardia with a regular rhythm. Heart rates are generally higher than 220 beats/min, and P waves may be visible. SVT with aberrant conduction (manifested as a wide-complex tachycardia) is rare in the pediatric population, and a wide-complex tachycardia should be considered ventricular in origin until proved otherwise. Long QTc syndrome is characterized by a QTc interval that is prolonged (>440 msec). Acquired causes of a prolonged QTc, such as electrolyte abnormality (hypocalcemia, hypokalemia, hypomagnesemia) and drug effect (erythromycin, trimethoprim, and others), should be ruled out.

## CHEST RADIOGRAPH

A chest radiograph is useful in the evaluation of suspected cardiac disease because it allows assessment of heart size, pulmonary vascular markings, and situs of the aortic arch. Heart size can help differentiate between a cardiac lesion and sepsis.[9] An enlarged heart may be seen with left-sided obstructive lesions such as congenital aortic stenosis, interrupted aortic arch, and critical coarctation of the aorta. Certain CHD lesions have specific radiographic findings, such as the egg-on-a-string pattern seen with TGA and the boot-shaped heart with the tetralogy of Fallot (**Fig. 19.2**). Structural CHD can be broken down into lesions that cause an increase in pulmonary blood flow and lesions that cause decreased pulmonary blood flow; the presence of increased pulmonary vascular markings on a radiograph can aid in diagnosis (**Box 19.4**). The aorta is normally left sided, and a right-sided aortic arch can be seen with the tetralogy of Fallot, TGA, and truncus arteriosus.

## HYPEROXIA TEST

Useful in distinguishing cardiac from pulmonary sources of cyanosis, the hyperoxia test hinges on the premise that supplemental oxygen does not increase $PaO_2$ in the presence of an intracardiac shunt to the same degree that it does with isolated pulmonary disease (see the Tips and Tricks box). A child with TGA or severe right ventricular outflow tract obstruction (i.e., tetralogy of Fallot, pulmonary atresia, tricuspid atresia) typically has $PaO_2$ values of less than 60 mm Hg during hyperoxia. In lesions such as truncus arteriosus, TAPVR, and hypoplastic left heart syndrome, which involve intracardiac mixing, $PaO_2$ values range between 75 and 150 mm Hg. It is critical to

**Table 19.4 Normal Pediatric Electrocardiographic Parameters**

| | | | Lead $V_1$ | | Lead $V_6$ | |
|---|---|---|---|---|---|---|
| AGE | HEART RATE (BEATS/MIN) | NORMAL QRS AXIS (MEAN) | MEAN R WAVE AMPLITUDE, mm (98th PERCENTILE) | MEAN S WAVE AMPLITUDE, mm (98th PERCENTILE) | MEAN R WAVE AMPLITUDE, mm (98th PERCENTILE) | MEAN S WAVE AMPLITUDE, mm (98th PERCENTILE) |
| 0-7 days | 95-160+ | +30 to −180 (+110) | 13.3 (25.5) | 7.7 (8.8) | 4.8 (11.8) | 3.2 (9.6) |
| 1-3 wk | 105-180 | +30 to +180 (+110) | 10.6 (20.8) | 4.2 (10.8) | 7.6 (16.4) | 3.4 (9.8) |
| 1-6 mo | 110-180 | +10 to +125 (+70) | 9.7 (19) | 5.4 (15) | 12.4 (22) | 2.8 (8.3) |
| 6-12 mo | 110-170 | +10 to +125 (+60) | 9.4 (20.3) | 6.4 (18.1) | 12.6 (22.7) | 2.1 (7.2) |
| 1-3 yr | 90-150 | +10 to +125 (+60) | 8.5 (18) | 9 (21) | 14 (23.3) | 1.7 (6) |
| 4-5 yr | 65-135 | 0 to +110 (+60) | 7.6 (16) | 11 (22.5) | 15.6 (25) | 1.4 (4.7) |
| 6-8 yr | 60-130 | −15 to +110 (+60) | 6 (13) | 12 (24.5) | 16.3 (26) | 1.1 (3.9) |
| 9-11 yr | 60-110 | −15 to +110 (+60) | 5.4 (12.1) | 11.9 (25.4) | 16.3 (25.4) | 1.0 (3.9) |
| 12-16 yr | 60-110 | −15 to +110 (+60) | 4.1 (9.9) | 10.8 (21.2) | 14.3 (23) | 0.8 (3.7) |
| >16 yr | 60-100 | −15 to +110 (+60) | 3 (9) | 10 (20) | 10 (20) | 0.8 (3.7) |

**Table 19.5 Physical, Chest Radiographic, and Electrocardiographic Findings in Children with Congenital Heart Disease**

| CONDITION | PHYSICAL FINDINGS | CHEST RADIOGRAPHIC FINDINGS | ELECTROCARDIOGRAPHIC FINDINGS |
|---|---|---|---|
| Truncus arteriosus | SEM, wide pulse pressure, single $S_2$ | Increased PBF | Biventricular hypertrophy, LAE |
| Transposition of the great arteries | None | Normal or increased PBF | RVH |
| Total anomalous pulmonary venous return | Fixed split $S_2$ | Increased PBF, small heart | RVH |
| Hypoplastic left heart syndrome | TS, PS murmur | Increased PBF | RVH |
| Tricuspid atresia | ±PS murmur | Decreased PBF | LVH, RAE |
| Pulmonary atresia | ±TR murmur, single $S_2$ | Decreased PBF, large heart | LVH |
| Tetralogy of Fallot | PS murmur, single $S_2$ | Decreased PBF, boot-shaped heart | RVH |
| Coarctation of the aorta | SEM, pulse differential between upper and lower extremities | Rib notching late | LVH |
| Aortic stenosis | SEM | Increased PBF | LVH |

±, Sometimes present, sometimes not; *LAE*, left atrial enlargement; *LVH*, left ventricular hypertrophy; *PBF*, pulmonary blood flow; *PS*, pulmonic stenosis; *RAE*, right atrial enlargement; *RVH*, right ventricular hypertrophy; $S_2$, second heart sound; *SEM*, systolic ejection murmur; *TR*, tricuspid regurgitation; *TS*, tricuspid stenosis.

understand that some pulmonary lesions cause right-to-left shunting (persistent pulmonary hypertension of the newborn) or severe ventilation-perfusion mismatch (meconium aspiration syndrome, pneumonia) and the $PaO_2$ value may not rise above 150 mm Hg with hyperoxia.

**TIPS AND TRICKS**

**The Hyperoxia Test**

Have the patient breathe 100% oxygen for 10 minutes (hyperoxia), and then draw a postductal blood sample for arterial blood gas analysis.

Pulmonary disease is suggested if $PaO_2$ with 100% oxygen is greater than 150 mm Hg.

If the $PaO_2$ value is below 150 mm Hg during hyperoxia, a cyanotic cardiac lesion should be suspected.

**Table 19.6 Electrocardiographic Findings in Children with Congenital Rhythm Disturbances**

| CONDITION | FINDINGS |
|---|---|
| Supraventricular tachycardia | Regular R-R interval<br>Heart rate > 220 beats/min<br>Narrow QRS complex |
| Long QTc syndrome | QTc interval > 440 msec<br>Resting electrocardiogram may show bradycardia or atrioventricular block |
| Congenital complete heart block | Atrioventricular dissociation, bradycardia |

## ECHOCARDIOGRAPHY

Echocardiography is the definitive test for suspected structural heart disease. Any infant with central cyanosis, cardiac enlargement on chest radiography, a suspicious murmur, or a pulse differential across the ductus arteriosus or whose $PaO_2$ fails to rise with the hyperoxia test should be evaluated with echocardiography. This modality also allows evaluation of heart function and pericardial fluid in those with acquired conditions such as myocarditis. Echocardiography should likewise be considered in the evaluation for suspected SVT because a significant proportion of cases are associated with structural CHD.

**BOX 19.4 Lesion-Specific Manifestations Based on Pulmonary Blood Flow**

**Congenital Lesions Causing Increased Pulmonary Blood Flow or Left-to-Right Shunting**

Total anomalous pulmonary venous return
Tricuspid atresia
Transposition of the great arteries
Truncus arteriosus
Hypoplastic left heart syndrome
Isolated atrial septal defect
Isolated ventricular septal defect

**Congenital Lesions Causing Decreased Pulmonary Blood Flow or Right-to-Left Shunting**

Tetralogy of Fallot
Tricuspid atresia
Pulmonary atresia

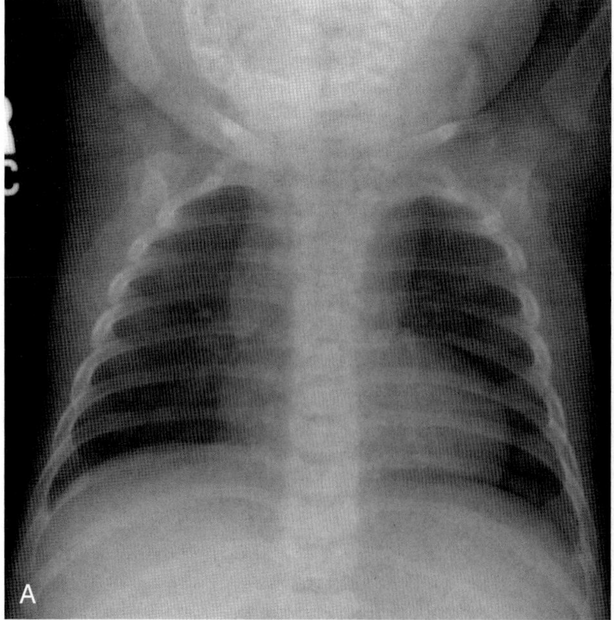


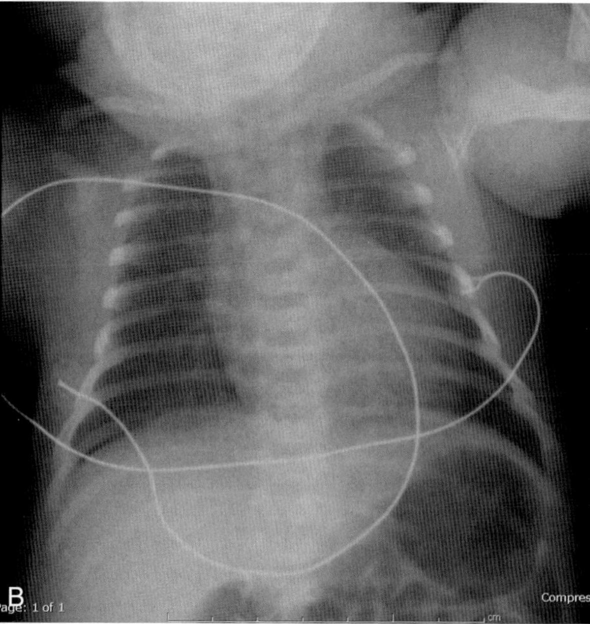


**Fig. 19.2 Classic chest radiographic findings in children with congenital heart disease. A,** Tetralogy of Fallot (boot-shaped heart). **B,** Transposition of the great vessels (egg-on-a-string pattern). (From Multimedia Library, Children's Hospital Boston. **A,** Available at http://www.childrenshospital.org/cfapps/mml/index.cfm?CAT=media&MEDIA_ID=1420; **B,** Available at http://www.childrenshospital.org/cfapps/mml/index.cfm?CAT=media&MEDIA_ID=1355.)

## TREATMENT

### INTERVENTIONS

Initial management of an infant or child with suspected cardiac disease who appears in extremis should focus on cardiopulmonary support, establishment of intravenous (IV) access, and appropriate monitoring. Intubation may be required, and rapid-sequence intubation should be considered the method of choice for management of the pediatric airway. Because the signs and symptoms of decompensated pediatric cardiac disease and sepsis are similar, empirical treatment with broad-spectrum antibiotics (ampicillin, 100 to 200 mg/kg/day, and gentamicin, 5 to 6 mg/kg/day, *or* ceftriaxone, 100 mg/kg if the child is older than 28 days) should be started after appropriate specimens for blood, urine, and cerebrospinal fluid culture are obtained. If the shock does not respond to fluid resuscitation (normal saline, 20 mL/kg intravenously to a total of 60 mL/kg), inotropes such as dopamine (start with 5 mcg/kg/min and titrate to effect) or dobutamine (0.5 mcg/kg/min) may be added.

If a neonate is in shock and does not promptly improve with IV fluid administration, CHD may be present; a neonatologist should be called and prostaglandin $E_1$ treatment should be considered, even presumptively. Prostaglandin $E_1$ infusion can be lifesaving in infants with ductal-dependent pulmonary or systemic blood flow. The infusion should be started at 0.1 mcg/kg/min and increased or decreased according to clinical response. Side effects include flushing, diarrhea, fever, and apnea. Many such patients require intubation, especially those being transferred to another hospital.

### TET SPELLS

Hypercyanotic tet spells typically occur in infants with uncorrected tetralogy of Fallot and should be treated with supplemental oxygen, morphine (0.1 mg/kg), and knee-chest positioning. Bicarbonate administered as a 1-mEq/kg bolus should also be considered to relieve the acidosis common in tet spells. If these measures fail, in consultation with a pediatric cardiologist consideration can be given to phenylephrine infusion (0.1 mcg/kg/min titrated to effect) to increase systemic vascular resistance and drive more blood flow across the right ventricular outflow tract obstruction.

### SUPRAVENTRICULAR TACHYCARDIA

Treatment of SVT depends on the clinical stability of the child. If signs of decompensation (hypotension, poor perfusion) are present, immediate synchronized cardioversion at 0.5 to 1 J/kg should be performed. In a more stable child, vagal maneuvers (i.e., application of ice to the face, Valsalva maneuver) may be attempted. Once IV access is obtained, adenosine (0.1 mg/kg to a maximum dose of 6 mg) should be administered via rapid IV bolus if vagal maneuvers fail. If no response is seen after the first dose, the second dose should be 0.2 mg/kg to a maximum of 12 mg, administered in the same manner.

### LONG QTc SYNDROME

The mainstay of therapy in patients in whom congenital long QTc syndrome is diagnosed is beta-blocker therapy, which should be given in consultation with a pediatric cardiologist (**Box 19.5**). Treatment of torsades de pointes associated with long QTc syndrome should consist of cardioversion (0.5 to 1 J/kg) if the patient is unstable. Magnesium sulfate (25 to 50 mg/kg intravenously) is the antiarrhythmic agent of choice for the treatment of torsades.

**BOX 19.5 Management Approach for Congenital Long QTc Syndrome**

If the first electrocardiogram (ECG) shows QTc > 440 msec, a second ECG should be performed. Results of the second ECG dictate actions to be taken, as follows:

- Normal QTc: No action needed.
- QTc of 440 to 500 msec: Evaluation (ECG screening of family, genetic testing, Holter monitoring). Also, beta-blocker therapy should be considered.
- QTc > 500 msec: Evaluation as above and initiation of beta-blocker therapy.

## NEXT STEPS IN CARE: ADMISSION AND DISCHARGE

Any child in extremis with a new diagnosis of CHD should be admitted to an intensive care unit in a hospital with pediatric cardiology services until stabilized. Children who are less ill may be managed on an appropriately monitored floor. Outpatient management may be appropriate for children in whom structural heart disease is suspected on the basis of a murmur but who have no other symptoms.

Patients with SVT who are asymptomatic, who have no signs of heart failure, and in whom the SVT converted to a normal sinus rhythm in the ED can be considered for outpatient management if appropriate follow-up with a pediatric cardiologist can be arranged. Patients with symptomatic long QTc syndrome (resuscitated arrest, torsades de pointes) should be admitted to a monitored bed. Most other cases can be managed with outpatient pediatric cardiology follow-up. A child with congenital complete heart block, when diagnosed, should be admitted to a monitored setting because of the risk for hemodynamic compromise.

## SUGGESTED READINGS

Brickner ME, Hillis LD, Lange RA. Congenital heart disease in adults: first of two parts. N Engl J Med 2000;342:256.

Brickner ME, Hillis LD, Lange RA. Congenital heart disease in adults: second of two parts. N Engl J Med 2000;342:334.

Hoke TR, Donohue PK, Bawa PK, et al. Oxygen saturation as a screening test for critical congenital heart disease: a preliminary study. Pediatr Cardiol 2002;23:403.

Schwartz PJ, Stramba-Badiale M, Segantini A, et al. Prolongation of the QTc interval and the sudden infant death syndrome. N Engl J Med 1998;338:1709.

VanRoekens CN, Zuckerberg AL. Emergency management of hypercyanotic crises in tetralogy of Fallot. Ann Emerg Med 1995;25:256.

## REFERENCES

***References can be found on Expert Consult @ www.expertconsult.com.***

# Pediatric Genitourinary and Renal Disorders

# 20

*Suzanne Lippert and N. Ewen Wang*

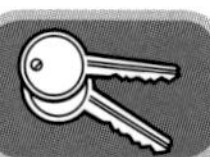

**KEY POINTS**

- Children often cannot differentiate between abdominal pain and groin pain—a complete physical examination is therefore necessary.
- The pathophysiology, clinical findings, and treatment of paraphimosis, testicular torsion, and priapism are similar in both the pediatric and adult population. They are emergencies that require immediate intervention.
- The most common cause of acute renal failure in children is hemolytic-uremic syndrome.
- Poststreptococcal glomerulonephritis is the most common cause of acute glomerulonephritis. IgA nephropathy is the most commonly diagnosed cause of glomerulonephritis in adolescents.
- One third of patients with Henoch-Schönlein purpura have renal involvement. This disorder is the most common form of vasculitis in childhood and is usually characterized by the triad of abdominal pain, arthritis, and purpura.

## DEVELOPMENTAL BASIS OF GENITOURINARY TRACT PATHOLOGY

The male genital organs originate within the abdominal cavity and then migrate externally during fetal development. Delays in testicular migration explain much of the pathology of scrotal masses. The testes, attached to their blood supply, drag their peritoneal covering (known as the tunica vaginalis) through the inguinal canal and into the scrotal sac.

The left testicle usually completes migration before the right testicle, thus explaining the increased frequency of right-sided inguinal hernias and undescended right testicles. Impediments to migration cause cryptorchidism. Failure of the peritoneal space to close after testicular migration can lead to hydroceles and inguinal hernias. Failure of fixation of the testes within the scrotal sac allows testicular torsion to occur. Differences in venous return make left-sided varicoceles much more common than right-sided ones.

Posterior urethral valves represent a disturbance in urethral development in males that is the leading cause of lower urinary tract obstruction in neonates. One third of patients with posterior urethral valves progress to end-stage renal disease, and 10% to 15% of children who require renal transplantation have posterior urethral valves.

## DEVELOPMENTAL ANATOMY OF THE KIDNEYS

The full complement of nephrons is present at birth, although newborn nephrons are heterogeneous in glomerular size and proximal tubule length. Anatomy and function mature postnatally. Although fetal urine is excreted into the bladder by 10 to 11 weeks of gestation, the ability to conserve and excrete sodium, concentrate urine, and reabsorb substrates such as glucose evolves to maturity over the first 2 years of life. In utero, the glomerular filtration rate (GFR) is minimal secondary to placental function; at birth, the GFR is 10% of adult values and matures by 12 to 24 months of age. Therefore, an increase in an infant's creatinine to "normal" adult ranges can indicate pathology.

# Genitourinary Disorders

## CRYPTORCHIDISM (UNDESCENDED TESTIS)

By birth, the testes have usually descended from the abdominal cavity into the scrotum; only 3% to 5% of full-term newborns have an undescended testicle. Although spontaneous descent does occur in the first year of life, 0.8% of males are still affected at 12 months of age, and spontaneous descent becomes increasingly unlikely after 6 months. With a careful physical examination, 80% of undescended testes are palpable, most commonly in the inguinal canal. Children with undescended testes are at higher risk for torsion, trauma, and malignancy.

## CLINICAL PRESENTATION AND DIAGNOSIS

Children with undescended testes are ideally identified by careful physical examination before any complications occur. The differential diagnosis of testes that are not palpable includes undescended, retractile, and absent testes. Children younger than 1 year should be examined while they are relaxed in a warm bath because the testes can be retracted during

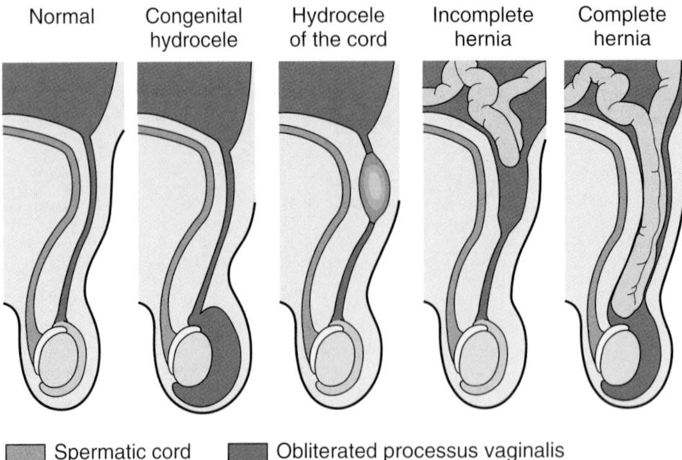


**Fig. 20.1 Abnormalities of the processus vaginalis.** (From Zitelli BJ, Davis HW. Atlas of pediatric physical diagnosis. 5th ed. Philadelphia: Mosby; 2007. Fig. 17-133.)

examination. Children older than 1 year whose testes are not palpable during routine physical examination should be evaluated by a urologist. Histologic deterioration of the testes, presumably secondary to increased ambient temperature, can begin as early as 6 to 12 months and is correlated with infertility, even in cases of unilateral undescended testes. Abdominal pain in children with undescended testes should prompt emergency evaluation for intraabdominal torsion.

### TREATMENT

The optimal time for surgical intervention is between 6 and 12 months.

## HYDROCELE

A hydrocele **(Fig. 20.1)** is a collection of fluid that accumulates within the layers of the tunica vaginalis and may or may not communicate with the peritoneal space. Hydroceles are often present at birth and occur most frequently on the right side because of delayed migration of the right testicle. Noncommunicating hydroceles in older children and adolescents should prompt examination for epididymitis, orchitis, trauma, tumor, or testicular torsion.

### CLINICAL PRESENTATION AND DIAGNOSIS

Hydroceles are usually painless. Physical examination reveals enlargement of the scrotum that may transilluminate because of its cystic structure. Ultrasonography is necessary to exclude acute pathology if the infant or child appears to be in pain. The majority of hydroceles not associated with inguinal hernia tend to resolve spontaneously between 12 and 24 months of age.

### TREATMENT

Hydroceles associated with an inguinal hernia, those that communicate with the peritoneal space, or those that occur or persist after 2 years of age require outpatient surgical repair.

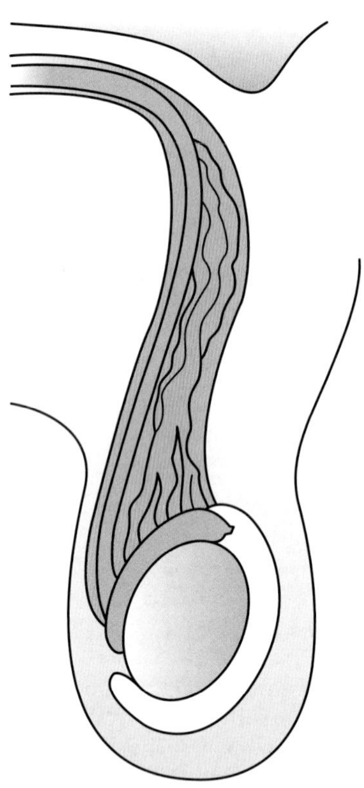

**Fig. 20.2** Varicocele. (From Zitelli BJ, Davis HW. Atlas of pediatric physical diagnosis. 5th ed. Philadelphia: Mosby; 2007. Fig. 14-44.)

## VARICOCELE

A varicocele is a collection of spermatic venous varicosities in the scrotum caused by incomplete drainage of the pampiniform plexus **(Fig. 20.2)**. They are rare in children younger than 10 years. Varicoceles most commonly develop between 10 and 15 years of age and have an incidence of approximately 15% in males.[1,2] The majority (85% to 95%) of varicoceles are left sided, the result of spermatic venous incompetence secondary to drainage of the left spermatic vein into the renal vein at a right angle.

**Table 20.1 Age-Based Differential Diagnosis of Pediatric Scrotal Masses and Pain**

| DIAGNOSIS | AGE AT ONSET | PAIN | POSITION OF TESTES, TENDERNESS | SYSTEMIC SYMPTOMS | COMMENT |
|---|---|---|---|---|---|
| Testicular torsion* | All ages; peak onset at 12-18 yr | 60% sudden onset; diffuse tenderness | High-riding horizontal lie | Vomiting common; dysuria and fever uncommon | |
| Testicular appendix torsion | Prepuberty; average age 10 yr | Acute or gradual; focal tenderness | Normal lie; blue dot | Vomiting, dysuria, and fever uncommon | |
| Epididymoorchitis | >16 yr | Gradual; posterior tenderness | Normal lie | Vomiting uncommon; dysuria and fever common | Adolescent etiology: STD |
| Hydrocele | Most common during first year of life | Painless | Normal lie | None | Usually resolves by age 12 mo |
| Inguinal hernia (incarcerated hernia, strangulated hernia*) | Most common during first year of life | Pain with incarceration or strangulation | Normal lie | Vomiting, abdominal pain with incarceration or strangulation | Occurs 10 times more frequently in males than in females; right-sided more common |
| Varicocele | 10-15 yr | Painless, mild discomfort, "pressure or fullness" | Normal lie | None | Associated with infertility; right-sided varicocele should prompt evaluation for tumor causing IVC compression |
| Testicular tumor | Rare; most occur in patients <3 yr old | Painless | Normal lie, nontender mass | None unless advanced tumor | |

*IVC*, Inferior vena cava; *STD*, sexually transmitted disease.
*Emergency condition.

## CLINICAL PRESENTATION AND DIAGNOSIS

Right-sided varicoceles should prompt an evaluation for intraabdominal pathology such as thrombosis or a tumor causing compression of the inferior vena cava.[3] Similarly, sudden onset of a left-sided varicocele should raise suspicion for renal cell carcinoma with obstruction of the left renal vein. The differential diagnosis of varicoceles and other scrotal masses is outlined in **Table 20.1**.

Varicoceles can cause mild discomfort and may lead to infertility in adult males. They are usually diagnosed on routine physical examination and are characterized by a full hemiscrotum without skin changes and a classic "bag of worms" finding on palpation.

## TREATMENT

A varicocele is generally an incidental finding in adolescence and is not an emergency. Referral to outpatient urology is appropriate.

# TESTICULAR TORSION

The pathophysiology, clinical findings, and treatment of testicular torsion in the pediatric population is similar to that in adults. Detailed discussion of torsion can be found in Chapter 111.

# INGUINAL HERNIA

An inguinal hernia occurs when an intraabdominal organ, usually intestine, herniates into a patent processus vaginalis (see Fig. 20.1). An incarcerated hernia refers to an intestinal loop that is not reducible. A strangulated hernia results when the blood supply to the intestinal loop is obstructed and bowel ischemia ensues.

## EPIDEMIOLOGY AND PATHOPHYSIOLOGY

Inguinal hernias occur in 15 of every 1000 live births. The incidence in premature and low-birth-weight infants is much higher (approximately 30%), whereas the incidence in males is three to four times higher than that in females. They are most commonly identified during the first year of life, with a peak in diagnosis during the first month.

Indirect hernias are more common on the right side (60%) because of later testicular descent into the scrotum. If a left-sided hernia exists, there is a strong possibility that an occult right-sided hernia is present. A family history of hernia, prematurity, or undescended testicle is associated with inguinal hernias.

### CLINICAL PRESENTATION

Incarceration is more common with small hernias and occurs frequently during the first 6 months of life, less commonly after 2 years of age, and rarely after the age of 5. Strangulation and perforation can occur within 2 hours of decreased blood flow. Incarceration occurs more frequently in females; however, it is the ovaries, not the intestines, that herniate and become incarcerated.

### TREATMENT

Given the high frequency of incarceration in the first year of life, hernias found on routine examination without symptoms should be referred for surgical repair. Approximately 90% of complications can be avoided if surgery is performed within the first month after diagnosis.

## IDIOPATHIC SCROTAL EDEMA

Idiopathic scrotal edema is manifested as painless erythema and induration of the scrotum. More than 75% of cases occur in boys younger than 10 years. Two thirds of cases are unilateral.

### CLINICAL PRESENTATION

Patients may complain of pruritus. Edema and erythema may extend to the phallus, groin, and abdomen. The testes and epididymis will have no palpable masses, and systemic symptoms are rare.

### TREATMENT AND DISPOSITION

Idiopathic scrotal edema is a diagnosis of exclusion. If acute pathology has been excluded, patients can be discharged home with outpatient follow-up. Most cases resolve spontaneously within a few days and do not require specific treatment. The recurrence rate is 21%.

## CARCINOMA

Testicular and scrotal cancer accounts for 1% of solid tumors in children. The incidence is increased in patients with bilateral cryptorchidism.

### CLINICAL PRESENTATION AND DIAGNOSIS

On examination, a painless unilateral mass can be palpated separately from the testis; there may also be a sensation of fullness, tugging, or increased weight in the scrotum associated with testicular enlargement. A reactive hydrocele is present in 7% to 25% of patients and may lead to a delay in diagnosis. Further examination reveals a firm mass, either smooth or nodular, that does not transilluminate. Lymphadenopathy, petechiae, abdominal masses, hepatosplenomegaly, or gynecomastia may be present. Lymphoma and leukemia can metastasize to the testicles and be manifested similarly.

A complete blood count, urinalysis, urine test for human chorionic gonadotropin (produced by germ cell tumors), and testicular ultrasound images should be obtained.

### TREATMENT

Management consists of prompt urologic and oncologic consultation for biopsy and staging.

## PHIMOSIS

Phimosis is a constriction of the penile foreskin that results in an inability to retract the prepuce over the glans. A fully retractable foreskin is present in 4% of newborns, 50% of 1-year-olds, 80% of 2-year-olds, and 90% of 4-year-olds. In the remaining cases, the foreskin may not be retractable until puberty.[4]

### CLINICAL PRESENTATION

Although most cases of phimosis in children are physiologic, symptoms may include pain, hematuria, and in severe cases, urinary obstruction. Adolescents may complain of pain on erection secondary to tension on the foreskin from glandular adhesions. Phimosis can also result from trauma, infection, chemical irritation, and poor hygiene or as a complication of circumcision. Severe stenosis or obstructive uropathy can result from chronic symptomatic phimosis.

### TREATMENT

Because the ability to retract the foreskin is age related, parents should not forcefully retract the prepuce. Good hygiene should be taught. If the child has signs of urinary outlet obstruction, dilation of the meatus by gentle use of forceps is warranted.

Steroid preparations (0.05% to 5% betamethasone cream two to four times daily or 1% hydrocortisone cream two to three times daily) have been used with varying success.[5] Severe phimosis may mandate incision of the dorsal inner foreskin by a urologist.

## PARAPHIMOSIS

Paraphimosis is a urologic emergency in which the foreskin of an uncircumcised male is retracted behind the glans penis and acts as a constricting band **(Fig. 20.3)**. The resulting venous and lymphatic congestion precludes returning the foreskin to its normal position, threatens arterial blood flow to the glans penis, and can result in penile necrosis, gangrene, or infarction of the glans over a period of hours to days. In infants and young boys, paraphimosis most commonly results after cleaning by a caretaker.

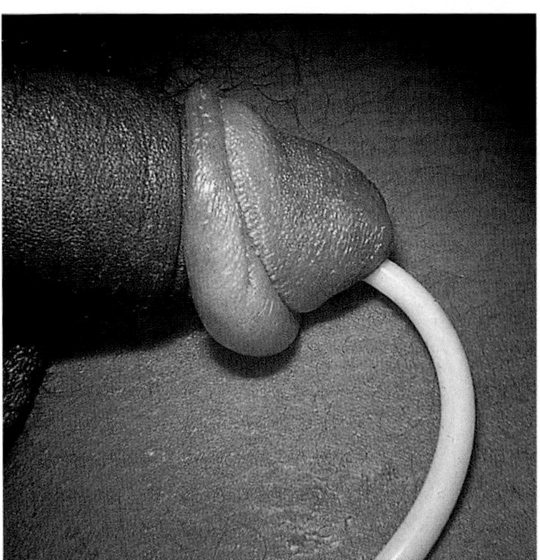

**Fig. 20.3 Paraphimosis in a catheterized patient with an edematous prepuce proximal to the glans.** (From Zitelli BJ, Davis HW. Atlas of pediatric physical diagnosis. 5th ed. Philadelphia: Mosby; 2007.)

## CLINICAL PRESENTATION

Paraphimosis is accompanied by penile pain and swelling and must be differentiated from balanoposthitis, tourniquet syndrome, and the generalized edema seen with renal, cardiac, or liver failure. Irritable and inconsolable male infants should be examined for evidence of paraphimosis. Urinary obstruction can be a late finding.

## TREATMENT

Emergency reduction of the foreskin back over the glans penis is the primary management of paraphimosis and should be attempted in the emergency department (ED). In the case of ischemic changes in the glans, practitioners should undertake immediate reduction and consultation with urology. Adequate analgesia is essential and, depending on the age and discomfort of the patient, can include topical medications, dorsal penile nerve block, or procedural sedation. Manual compression and reduction of the foreskin should be attempted first and can be aided by the application of ice or granulated sugar to decrease the swelling. Additional procedures include retraction with noncrushing Babcock forceps placed in the four quadrants of the foreskin or more invasive procedures that can be undertaken in consultation with urology, such as aspiration of the glans penis and a dorsal slit procedure.

# BALANITIS AND BALANOPOSTHITIS

Balanitis is an infection of the glans penis, whereas balanoposthitis is an infection of the foreskin in addition to the glans. Balanitis occurs in approximately 3% of boys, usually between 2 and 5 years of age, especially if they are uncircumcised.[6]

## CLINICAL PRESENTATION AND DIAGNOSIS

Balanitis and balanoposthitis can be caused by trauma; by irritation such as contact dermatitis from urine, soaps, powders, and ointments; or by infection. Causative agents of infectious balanoposthitis include group A streptococci (GAS), anaerobic bacteria, *Candida*, and sexually transmitted infections such as gonorrhea and chlamydial infection. Most children with GAS balanoposthitis have a characteristic moist balanoposthitis caused by a nonretractable prepuce, often in conjunction with a current or recent GAS infection at another site.[7] Signs of group A β-hemolytic streptococcal infection include pain, intense fiery redness, and a moist, glistening transudate or exudate under the prepuce. Streptococcal infection can be diagnosed by rapid antigen detection and culture.

Gonorrhea and chlamydial infection without frank urethral discharge are unusual in preschool children; however, after puberty, gonorrhea may be detected in the absence of urethral discharge.[8] In severe cases, cellulitis can extend down the penile shaft. Palpable inguinal adenopathy is often present.

## TREATMENT AND DISPOSITION

Noninfectious balanoposthitis should be managed with careful attention to hygiene, use of warm water sitz baths, and avoidance of causative agents. Treatment of infectious balanoposthitis should be tailored to the particular infection: minor, polymicrobial infection can be treated with topical mupirocin or bacitracin; GAS infection should be treated with 10 days of ampicillin, amoxicillin, a cephalosporin, or clindamycin. Children with sexually transmitted infections should be admitted to the hospital and evaluated for sexual abuse.

Indications for admission include severe infection and urinary retention.

# MEATAL STENOSIS

Meatal stenosis is narrowing of the urethral meatus, usually secondary to recurrent episodes of subclinical meatitis. It can be caused by ammonia diaper irritation in circumcised boys and by recurrent balanoposthitis in uncircumcised boys. Acquired meatal stenosis more commonly occurs in circumcised boys because the foreskin in uncircumcised boys acts as a protective cover for the meatus. Congenital meatal stenosis is rare.

## CLINICAL PRESENTATION AND DIAGNOSIS

Obstructive symptoms occur occasionally, including hesitancy, straining, urgency, frequency, and postvoid dribbling. An abnormal urinary stream may be seen, but urinary retention is rare. An erythematous swollen meatus is noted, often with purulent discharge. Radiographic studies are seldom necessary.

## TREATMENT

Treatment of purulent meatitis includes sitz baths and the administration of oral antibiotics (e.g., cephalexin) for 7 days.

Urinary retention is an indication for urology consultation and hospital admission; otherwise, prompt outpatient follow-up is sufficient.

## URETHRAL STRICTURE

In the United States, most cases of urethral stricture are acquired by infection and trauma. Gonococcal urethritis or infection resulting from an indwelling Foley catheter are the most common infection-related causes. In developing countries, sexually transmitted urethritis is the most common cause. Trauma can result in urethral stricture secondary to pelvic fracture and straddle injury.

## CLINICAL PRESENTATION AND TREATMENT

Clinically, the patient has difficulty passing urine. Slowing, spraying, or dribbling of the urine stream may be noted. When patients with this condition are seen in the ED, outpatient management, including prophylactic antibiotics, is appropriate. Urethrography or voiding cystourethrography should be performed before dilation of the stricture if this procedure is necessary.

## URETHRAL FOREIGN BODY

A urethral foreign body in older boys may have been inserted for sexual purposes. Most objects are palpable if they are in the anterior urethra. Retained foreign body should be included in the differential diagnosis of a male with signs and symptoms of recurrent urinary tract infection and no urogenital abnormalities. Most foreign bodies can be removed endoscopically.

## URETHRAL PROLAPSE

Prolapse of the urethra is most common in young African American girls (**Fig. 20.4**). The prolapsed mucosa is visible and may be irritated, congested, and hemorrhagic. Though quite alarming on physical examination, it is not associated with sexual abuse. Treatment consists of sitz baths three times a day.

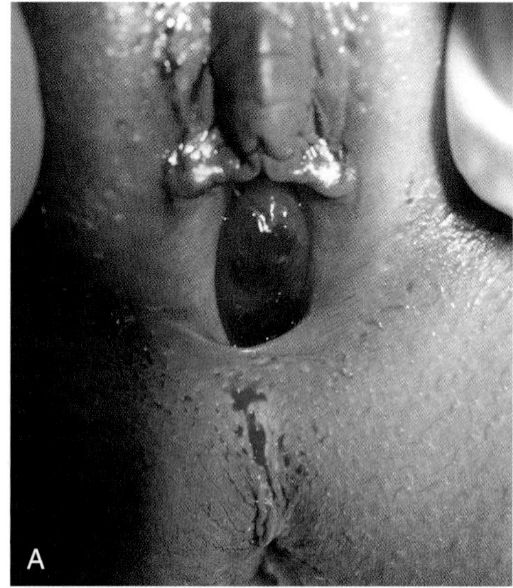


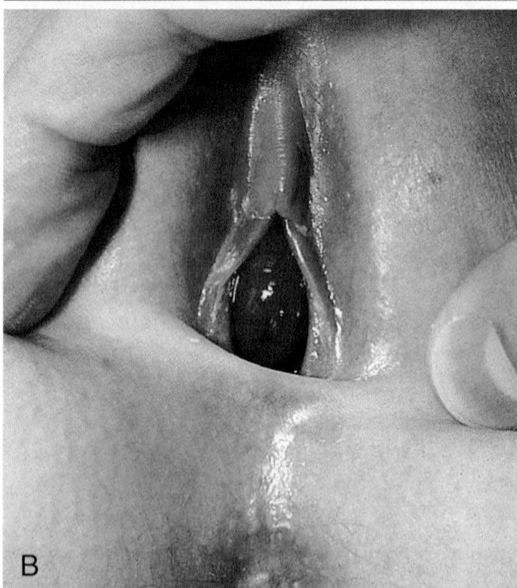


**Fig. 20.4** Two examples of urethral prolapse. **A,** Urethral prolapse in a 4-year-old girl who had bloody spotting on her underwear. **B,** Urethral prolapse. (**A**, From Behrman RE, Kliegman RM, Jenson HB. Nelson's textbook of pediatrics. 18th ed. Philadelphia: Saunders; 2007. Fig. 544-10; **B**, from Zitelli BJ, Davis HW. Atlas of pediatric physical diagnosis. 5th ed. Philadelphia: Mosby; 2007. Fig. 14-50.)

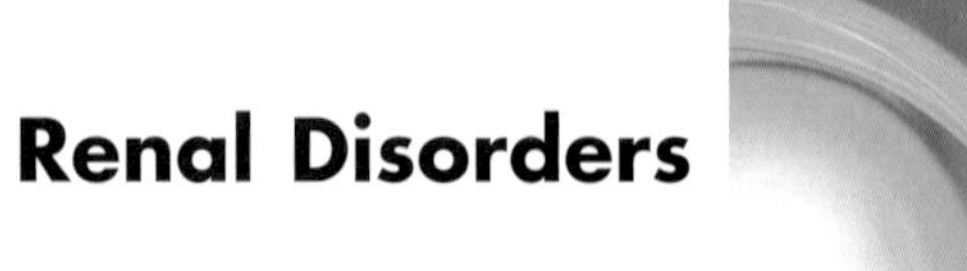

# Renal Disorders

## NEPHROTIC SYNDROME

Nephrotic syndrome is the clinical manifestation of a variety of primary and secondary glomerular disorders characterized by the following findings:

- Hypoproteinemia (serum albumin <3 g/dL)
- Marked proteinuria (>40 g/m$^2$/hr in a 24-hour period)
- Edema
- Hyperlipidemia (predominantly triglycerides and cholesterol)

## PATHOPHYSIOLOGY

Nephrotic syndrome is classified as *primary*, defined as nephrotic syndrome without systemic disease, or *secondary*, defined as nephrotic syndrome in the presence of systemic disease. Ninety percent of children with nephrotic syndrome have the primary syndrome, the most common of which is minimal change disease (idiopathic nephrotic syndrome).

Idiopathic nephrotic syndrome is classified by its response to corticosteroids, with the majority being steroid responsive and approximately 20% being unresponsive to steroids. Lack of response to steroids portends a poor prognosis and a 50% risk for progression to end-stage renal failure.

## EPIDEMIOLOGY

The incidence of nephrotic syndrome in children younger than 16 years is 2 to 7 per 100,000 per year, and the prevalence is 15 cases per 100,000. Boys are more likely to be affected than girls. The typical age at onset of primary nephrotic syndrome is 18 months to 6 years. Children with nephrotic syndrome at an age older than 5 years are more likely to have the secondary form. Neonates are most likely to have the congenital (Finnish) type, which is steroid resistant and generally fatal. In adolescents, nephrotic syndrome is most often associated with a primary or secondary form of an underlying nephritis.

## CLINICAL PRESENTATION

The usual initial sign in a child with nephrotic syndrome is edema. The edema starts with early-morning periorbital swelling, often misattributed to a cold or allergies. As the edema spreads to the abdomen, trunk, and extremities, children have increasing difficulty fitting into their pants and shoes. Parents can mistake this for weight gain. The child otherwise appears well, although ascites, pleural effusion, or pulmonary edema may be present. Ascites and an edematous intestinal wall can be manifested as abdominal pain, nausea, vomiting, or diarrhea.

## COMPLICATIONS

Complications include infection, hypercoagulability, hypovolemia, respiratory distress, and acute renal failure.

### INFECTION

Increased susceptibility to infection results from disease-mediated impairment of the immune system, as well as treatment with immunosuppressive therapy, both of which may mask the typical signs of infection. The most common bacterial infection is peritonitis, although cellulitis, pneumonia, sepsis, and meningitis are also seen. Infection with encapsulated bacteria, such as *Escherichia coli, Haemophilus influenzae*, and *Streptococcus pneumoniae*, is the main cause of death in children with nephrotic syndrome.

### HYPERCOAGULABILITY

Hypercoagulability occurs in 3% of patients with nephrotic syndrome. Thromboembolic events can involve the arteries and veins, most commonly the pulmonary arteries, renal veins, and deep leg veins. A sudden onset of gross hematuria or renal failure should prompt investigation for renal vein thrombosis.

Because prednisone exerts an antiheparin effect, practitioners should not attempt deep venous punctures on children treated with steroids unless no alternative exists.

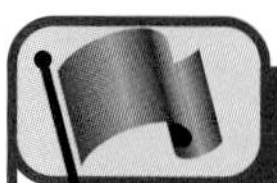

**RED FLAGS**

Do not attempt deep venous punctures in children who have nephrotic syndrome and are receiving chronic prednisone therapy because they are at increased risk for thromboembolic events.

### RESPIRATORY DISTRESS

Pleural effusions, pulmonary edema, and massive ascites can cause respiratory distress.

## TREATMENT

The goals of ED management are restoration of volume, treatment of symptomatic edema, and evaluation for and treatment of infectious complications. Patients in shock should be treated by isotonic hydration consisting of a 20-mL/kg bolus per hour until they are normotensive. If the patient is clinically dehydrated with hemoconcentration but not in shock, a trial of orally administered sodium-deficient fluids at twice the maintenance dose is preferable to intravenous solutions. Small amounts of oral hydration fluid should be administered frequently to avoid vomiting caused by an edematous gut.

If the patient is well hydrated and exhibits symptomatic edema or anasarca, diuretics may be warranted but should be used judiciously because these children have decreased circulating volume and are prone to thromboembolic events. Intravenous or oral administration of furosemide, 1 to 2 mg/kg/24 hr divided into two doses, can be used. Loop diuretics are most effective, but additional diuretics such as hydrochlorothiazide or spironolactone may be administered if the response is inadequate. Diuretics are not effective with albumin concentrations of less than 1.5 g. Albumin infusions may be necessary before administration of diuretics (0.5 to 1 g/kg given as 25% salt-deficient albumin, followed by 0.5 to 1 mg/kg of furosemide).

Although patients may arrive in shock from intravascular volume depletion alone, sepsis should be excluded. Any child with nephrotic syndrome and an unexplained fever must be considered to have a bacterial infection until proved otherwise. Because persons receiving steroid therapy may not demonstrate abdominal pain or typical signs of infection, diagnostic paracentesis is necessary to exclude bacterial peritonitis in children with abdominal pain or fever in the setting of ascites. Treatment with cephalosporins or ampicillin (with or without gentamicin) is recommended. Prophylactic antibiotics are not necessary unless infection is suspected, and material should be collected for culture.

The mainstay of treatment of nephrotic syndrome is steroid therapy. Generally, patients initially receive prednisone, 2 mg/kg/24 hr (maximum, 60 mg/24 hr) divided into two or three doses. Approximately 90% of patients with idiopathic nephrotic syndrome respond to steroid therapy by the end of a 4-week course, with response defined as trace or negative amounts of urine protein for 3 days. Failure to respond to steroid treatment increases the likelihood of a cause other than minimal change disease.

## DISPOSITION

### ADMISSION CRITERIA

- Any infant with nephrotic syndrome
- Any patient with respiratory distress or shock
- Nephrotic patients with infections, unexplained fever, refractory edema, renal insufficiency, dehydration, abdominal complaints, or hemoconcentration greater than 50%
- Patients with newly diagnosed nephrotic syndrome to complete the evaluation and educate the parents about outpatient management

## FOLLOW-UP FOR PATIENTS WITH NONNEPHROTIC PROTEINURIA

Very few patients with dipstick proteinuria have renal disease. In the absence of edema, hypertension, oliguria, or hematuria, urinalysis repeated in 2 to 4 weeks is recommended.

# HEMOLYTIC-UREMIC SYNDROME

Hemolytic-uremic syndrome is the most common cause of acute renal failure in children, with an incidence of 1 to 10 cases per 100,000 children younger than 5 years. The mean age at diagnosis is 3 years, and the diagnosis becomes increasingly unlikely after 5 years of age. Caucasian children are more often affected than others, and there is no gender preference.

## PATHOPHYSIOLOGY

Hemolytic-uremic syndrome is defined by the presence of the classic triad of microangiopathic hemolytic anemia (MAHA), thrombocytopenia, and acute renal failure (**Box 20.1**).

In contrast to the adult form of the disease (thrombotic thrombocytopenic purpura), the microthrombi of hemolytic-uremic syndrome are usually confined to the kidneys. Thrombotic thrombocytopenic purpura has a predominantly neurologic manifestation, a higher mortality rate, and a better response to plasmapheresis and fresh frozen plasma. Renal involvement is the defining feature of hemolytic-uremic syndrome.

The usual cause of epidemic hemolytic-uremic syndrome is the verotoxin-producing strain of *Escherichia coli* serotype O157:H7, although it can be caused by *Shigella* organisms that produce a similar toxin. Transmission is through person-to-person contact or ingestion of contaminated food, such as unpasteurized dairy products or undercooked beef. The verotoxin binds to and destroys the colonic mucosa, thereby leading to bloody diarrhea.

**BOX 20.1 Hallmarks of Hemolytic-Uremic Syndrome**

Acute renal failure
Microangiopathic hemolytic anemia
Fever
Thrombocytopenia

## CLINICAL PRESENTATION

The epidemic form begins with a prodrome of nausea, vomiting, watery diarrhea, crampy abdominal pain, and occasionally fever. Bloody stools typically develop on the second or third day of symptoms. Usually between 5 and 10 days after the prodromal gastroenteritis, there is a sudden onset of pallor, listlessness, irritability, and oliguria because of development of the classic triad (MAHA, thrombocytopenia, renal failure). Additional signs on clinical examination may include dehydration, edema, hypertension, petechiae, hepatosplenomegaly, jaundice, and neurologic manifestations (obtundation, hemiparesis, seizures, brainstem dysfunction).

Gastrointestinal complications such as toxic megacolon, ischemic colitis, intussusception, and perforation are also possible. Pancreatic insufficiency from microinfarction in the pancreas can lead to permanent insulin-dependent diabetes mellitus.

## DIAGNOSTIC TESTING

Hemolytic-uremic syndrome is diagnosed clinically by symptoms coupled with consistent laboratory findings. The presence of MAHA is necessary to establish the diagnosis. The peripheral blood smear demonstrates signs of a microangiopathic process: teardrop cells, helmet cells, spherocytes, and burr cells.

A complete blood count may show leukocytosis, profound anemia (with hemoglobin levels of 5 to 9 g/dL), and mild to moderate thrombocytopenia (platelet counts are generally around 40,000/mm$^3$).

C-reactive protein levels may be elevated. The coagulation profile is usually normal, and although serum fibrin split products might be elevated, fulminant disseminated intravascular coagulation is rare. Chemistry abnormalities include hyponatremia, hyperkalemia, azotemia, metabolic acidosis, hyperbilirubinemia, low total protein as a result of proteinuria, and elevated lactate dehydrogenase. Urinalysis often shows hematuria, proteinuria, and pyuria. Granular and hyaline casts are seen in the urine sediment.

Specific serologic testing for antibodies to the lipopolysaccharide of *E. coli* O157:H7 is necessary because routine stool cultures may not always detect the bacteria or verotoxin.

## TREATMENT AND DISPOSITION

Severe anemia, defined as a hemoglobin concentration lower than 6 g/dL, requires transfusion of packed red blood; platelet transfusion is recommended only with active bleeding or in preparation for a required invasive procedure.

Indications for dialysis in children with hemolytic-uremic syndrome are similar to those with renal failure: signs and symptoms of uremia, azotemia, severe fluid overload, and electrolyte disturbances not responsive to medical therapy. Rehydration should be done slowly to avoid fluid overload.

Hypertension is generally responsive to the administration of calcium channel blockers, labetalol, captopril, hydralazine, or in refractory cases, nitroprusside. Seizures will respond to benzodiazepines and phenytoin; however, hyponatremic seizures do occur and should be evaluated for and treated with hypertonic 3% saline. Plasmapheresis or fresh frozen plasma infusion has no proven efficacy for diarrhea-associated hemolytic-uremic syndrome but may be useful for recurrent, inherited, drug-induced, or idiopathic hemolytic-uremic syndrome, especially in those with neurologic involvement. The role of antibiotics remains controversial. One theory is that antibiotics may enhance the release of verotoxin from the bacteria; therefore, they are not generally recommended. Antimotility agents should be avoided because they may cause toxic megacolon.

Patients require admission and pediatric nephrology consultation. The prognosis is poor in patients who have nondiarrheal forms of the disease, are younger than 1 year, or have prolonged anuria, hypertension, or severe central nervous system disease. In general, mortality is less than 5%, and an additional 5% will have long-term consequences of end-stage renal disease or stroke.

## ACUTE GLOMERULONEPHRITIS

Acute glomerulonephritis refers to a spectrum of inflammatory renal disorders characterized by hematuria and proteinuria.

### PATHOPHYSIOLOGY

The most common form of acute glomerulonephritis in children occurs 1 to 3 weeks after a throat or skin infection with group A β-hemolytic streptococci. The humoral immune response to the infection leads to the deposition of antibodies, activation of complement, and ultimately, inflammation within the glomeruli. The latency period for both the pharyngeal and cutaneous forms can be as long as 6 weeks. Anuria and renal failure occur in 2% of patients.

### CLINICAL PRESENTATION

The signs and symptoms of acute glomerulonephritis are presented in **Box 20.2**.

The diagnosis is usually made in the ED based on the patient's history. The typical patient is a 5- to 6-year-old boy who is brought to the ED 1 to 2 weeks after a preceding streptococcal infection or 3 to 6 weeks after the onset of pyoderma. The patient has had a sudden onset of brown, tea-colored, or grossly bloody urine; decreased urine output; and edema involving the face, periorbital areas, and extremities. On examination, hypertension (both systolic and diastolic) may be found. Some children may be asymptomatic except for the change in urine color. Rarely, patients with advanced disease may have congestive heart failure, hypertensive encephalopathy, or other life-threatening complications of renal failure.

**BOX 20.2 Signs and Symptoms of Acute Glomerulonephritis**

Hematuria (gross or microscopic)
Dysmorphic red blood cells and red blood cell casts
Proteinuria
Hypertension
Edema
Renal insufficiency

### DIAGNOSTIC TESTING

Urinalysis is the single most important test in categorizing glomerulonephritis. Proteinuria is almost always more than 2+ on the dipstick, which indicates that the measured protein is not merely secondary to hematuria. In 60% of cases, red blood cell casts are seen on microscopic analysis. Hyaline granular casts and pyuria are common. Urine culture should always be performed.

Serologic testing can confirm streptococcal infection. Antistreptolysin O titers are elevated in 90% of cases, peak at 10 to 14 days, and return to normal after 3 to 4 weeks; antihyaluronidase titers peak at 3 to 4 weeks. In patients with skin infections, anti–DNAse-B antibodies can be measured.

### TREATMENT AND DISPOSITION

The key to a successful outcome is early diagnosis in the ED and treatment of life-threatening emergencies such as hyperkalemia, hypertension, and congestive heart failure. Management of patients with nephritis is primarily supportive, with restricted fluid and sodium intake. Antibiotics are required for ongoing infectious processes.

Any child who is oliguric or hypertensive should be hospitalized and scheduled for nephrology consultation. Otherwise, discharge from the ED is reasonable, with instructions for a low-sodium diet and close follow-up with the pediatrician. The family should be advised to monitor the patient's urine output and weight and observe for signs of congestive heart failure or hypertension. In general, the prognosis is excellent. Approximately 80% to 90% of these children recover without any persistent renal abnormalities except for microscopic hematuria, which may persist for up to 18 months.

## IgA NEPHROPATHY

IgA nephropathy, also known as Berger disease, is the type of glomerulonephritis most commonly diagnosed in adolescence.[9] This disease accounts for up to 25% of cases of glomerulonephritis in Asia and Europe and up to 10% in the United States.

### CLINICAL PRESENTATION AND DIAGNOSIS

The classic finding is hematuria or proteinuria with a preceding upper respiratory infection. The diagnosis is confirmed by a renal biopsy specimen with deposition of IgA in the mesangium.

### TREATMENT AND DISPOSITION

Gross hematuria resolves spontaneously within days without serious sequelae in 85% of patients. Because the prognosis is good in most patients without significant proteinuria or renal dysfunction, treatment is not usually needed. However, proteinuria, hypertension, or renal insufficiency portends a poor prognosis and should be managed in consultation with nephrology.

## HENOCH-SCHÖNLEIN PURPURA WITH RENAL INVOLVEMENT

Henoch-Schönlein purpura is the most common form of small-vessel vasculitis in childhood. Most patients have the triad of abdominal pain, arthritis, and purpura. A third of the patients have renal involvement, 80% of whom will have asymptomatic hematuria. The populations most affected are school-age children and young adults, and it occurs more commonly in Caucasians and males. One third to three fourths of patients have a preceding respiratory infection.

## CLINICAL PRESENTATION

Usually occurring within the first month of illness, renal involvement develops in approximately one third of patients, with progression to end-stage renal disease in less than 1%. Predictors of a poor prognosis include late onset of renal involvement in older children and massive proteinuria; 20% of such cases result in end-stage renal failure. Approximately 50% of patients in whom nephritic syndrome with Henoch-Schönlein purpura develops will progress to end-stage renal disease within 10 years.

The diagnosis is made clinically and not based on laboratory studies.

## TREATMENT

Prednisone, 1 to 2 mg/kg/day for 2 weeks (max 60 mg/day), with tapering of the dose over a 2-week period, has been shown to improve gastrointestinal and joint symptoms and lessen the severity of nephritis. About one third of affected patients will have a recurrence of at least one symptom. Fortunately, most patients recover quickly in several weeks with supportive treatment.

# RENAL TUBULAR ACIDOSIS

The normal response to acidemia is to reabsorb all the filtered bicarbonate and to increase excretion of hydrogen, primarily by excreting ammonium ions in urine.

Renal tubular acidosis occurs when the renal tubules are unable to perform these functions. Accumulation of ammonium ions and subsequent metabolic acidosis can cause growth retardation, kidney stones, bone disease, and progressive renal failure.

Four subtypes of renal tubular acidosis are recognized:

Type 1—distal (classic form)
Type 2—proximal (bicarbonate wasting)
Type 3—a combination of types 1 and 2
Type 4—hyperkalemic (rare in children)

Types 1 and 2 are encountered most frequently in children. The diagnosis of all types requires a serum electrolyte panel and urinalysis with urine pH.

## TYPE 1 RENAL TUBULAR ACIDOSIS

Distal renal tubular acidosis results from a defect in the tubular transport of hydrogen in the distal nephron. The most common form in children is hereditary, but it can be a complication of systemic diseases seen more commonly in adults such as Sjögren syndrome, lupus erythematosus, and hyperparathyroidism. Patients have failure to thrive, anorexia, vomiting, and dehydration. Hyperchloremic metabolic acidosis and hypokalemia may be seen. Hypercalciuria can be manifested as rickets, nephrocalcinosis, nephrolithiasis, and renal failure. Urine pH usually exceeds 6.5.

The classic diagnostic test for distal renal tubular acidosis is an acid load from ammonium chloride; however, this is a tedious test that can generate severe acidosis. Distal renal tubular acidosis can be permanent, but children may outgrow it by the time that they are of school age. Treatment is focused on correction of the acidosis with sodium bicarbonate or sodium citrate, which may also prevent kidney stone formation. Target serum $HCO_3$ levels should be between 20 and 22 mEq/L in infants and between 22 and 26 mEq/L in children.

## TYPE 2 RENAL TUBULAR ACIDOSIS

Proximal renal tubular acidosis is the most common form found in children. Because approximately 85% to 90% of bicarbonate reabsorption occurs in the proximal tubules, proximal renal tubular acidosis is characterized by an alkaline urine (usually pH >7), loss of bicarbonate in urine, and mildly reduced serum bicarbonate concentration.

Proximal renal tubular acidosis can result from inherited disorders (hereditary fructose intolerance, Wilson disease, cystinosis, Fanconi syndrome, Lowe syndrome), exposure to medications (chemotherapy agents, acetazolamide, sulfonamides), anatomic abnormalities (obstructive uropathy, reflux), or exposure to heavy metals. Treatment consists of alkaline therapy with citrate solutions (Bicitra, Polycitra) or sodium bicarbonate. Potassium supplements may also be required because the added sodium load of the sodium bicarbonate may increase potassium loss in the distal tubule.

# URINARY RETENTION

Urinary retention is defined as failure to urinate for more than 12 hours. More than 90% of all newborns void within the first 24 hours of life and 99% within the first 48 hours. In male children, posterior urethral valves are the most common cause of retention. Other causes include urethral polyps, urethral stricture, urethral diverticulum, meatal stenosis, and fecal impaction. In female infants, the differential diagnosis includes prolapsing ureterocele, urethral prolapse, and foreign bodies. Infections, medications, spinal cord abnormalities, and sexual abuse can cause retention in both male and female children. Diagnostic tests in the ED include blood urea nitrogen, creatinine, and urinalysis.[10]

## REFERENCES

*References can be found on Expert Consult @ www.expertconsult.com.*

# Pediatric Gynecologic Disorders 21

*Jennifer F. Anders*

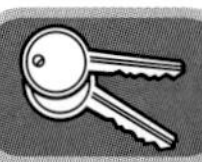

**KEY POINTS**

- Prepubertal girls have thin, sensitive vaginal mucosa that is easily irritated.
- If speculum examination is necessary in a young girl, examination under anesthesia should be considered.
- Parents of young girls taken to the emergency department because of gynecologic complaints are often worried about the possibility of sexual abuse but may not verbalize their concern until appropriate questions are asked.
- Most pediatric gynecologic complaints are not related to abuse.
- Most sexually abused children have no abnormalities on examination.
- Emergency department evaluation of possible sexual abuse should focus on identification of patients who require urgent treatment, urgent collection of evidence, or protective custody.

## EPIDEMIOLOGY

Gynecologic concerns are common but nonetheless anxiety producing in prepubertal girls. Vulvovaginitis is the most common gynecologic problem affecting prepubertal girls and is responsible for the largest number of health care visits. Pediatric sexual abuse affects more than 100,000 children a year, and many of these girls will be taken to the emergency department (ED) for initial evaluation. Many parents going to the ED have spoken or unspoken concerns about sexual abuse that need to be addressed.

## PATHOPHYSIOLOGY

Pediatric gynecologic problems differ from those of adult women chiefly because the vaginal mucosa is thin, dry, and easily irritated in the absence of estrogen. This makes prepubertal girls more sensitive to a variety of chemical, physical, and microbiologic irritants. The normal hymen looks thin, with an average opening of about 4 mm. However, there is great variability in normal hymenal shape, ranging from imperforate to multiple small fenestrations to oval, round, or stellate openings (**Fig. 21.1**). Abnormal findings that may correlate with vaginal penetration include lacerations of the hymen or a thickened hymen with rolled edges. These findings are extremely difficult to differentiate from normal variations, and photos should always be taken if sexual abuse is suspected. Neonates have swollen labia and thick, moist vaginal epithelium for several weeks after birth, but most prepubertal girls have smooth pink vaginal mucosa and a pale vulva that barely covers the clitoris.

## PRESENTING SIGNS AND SYMPTOMS

The chief complaints of children with gynecologic problems include vaginal discharge or bleeding, itching or rubbing of the genitals, dysuria or refusal to void, or a foul genital odor noted by caregivers. The initial differential diagnosis can be guided by the predominant complaints (**Box 21.1**).

A calm, professional, thoughtful approach is essential to allow parents to discuss their concerns, enable a physical examination, and appropriately treat the patient. Vulvovaginitis, for example, can cause vaginal discharge or bleeding, itching or pain, urinary retention, abnormal appearance noted by caregivers, and concerns about possible sexual abuse.

The approach to pediatric gynecologic problems must take into account the developmental and psychologic state of the patient. Children zealously guard autonomy over their bodies. In addition, little girls are socialized to hide their genitals and will resist examination for various reasons throughout developmental stages—it is important to help them overcome their fear, embarrassment, or anxiety. It is helpful, when attempting to make the child comfortable with the examination, to speak directly to the child in language appropriate for her age (see the Tips and Tricks box). In teaching hospitals, try to coordinate care so that the examination is performed only once.

**TIPS AND TRICKS**

**Promoting Body Safety While Accomplishing the Necessary Genital Examination**

State to the child that you are a doctor or nurse.

Perform the nonthreatening aspects of the physical examination first (listen to the heart and palpate the abdomen).

Review and respect privacy and safe-touching rules.

Stand back and let the parent or other caregiver help the child with undressing.

**Sample Conversation**

"Hi, my name is Dr. Smith. I need to check you." (Begin with nonthreatening parts of the physical examination [even if not necessary]—listen to the heart and palpate the abdomen.)

"Has anybody talked to you about your private parts? Most of the time, no one is allowed to look at or touch your private parts. But your parents or doctor can look if you need help. This is a time when a doctor needs to check because you are hurting."

"Mommy is going to be right here with you. Mommy will help you take your pants off, and then I will look at the outside."

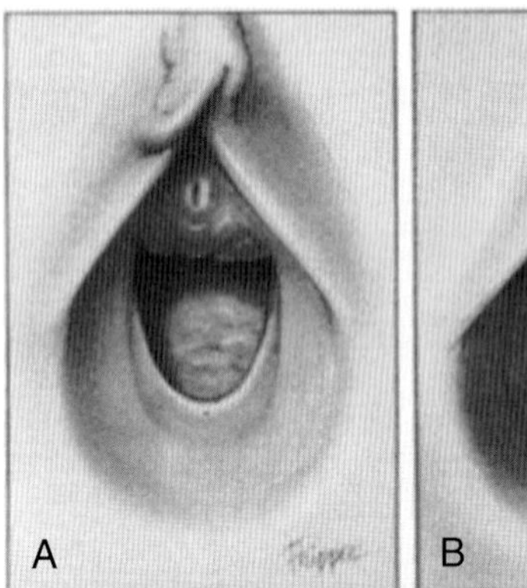


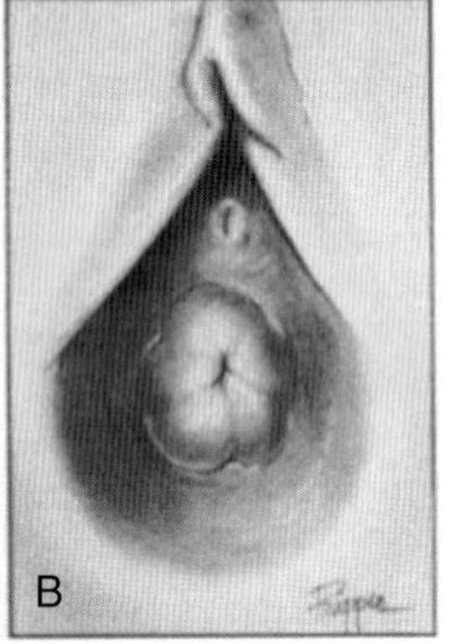


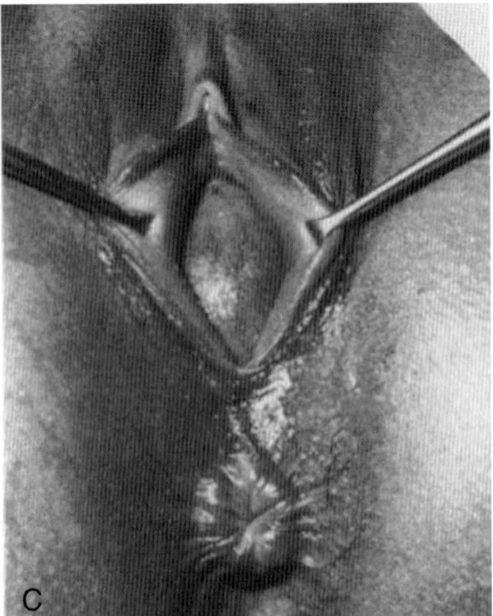


**Fig. 21.1 Types of hymens in prepubertal girls. A,** Posterior rim of a crescentic hymen. **B,** Fimbriated or redundant hymen. **C,** Imperforate hymen. (From Pokorny SF. Configuration of the prepubertal hymen. Am J Obstet Gynecol 1987;157:950.)

**BOX 21.1 Differential Diagnosis of Gynecologic Disorders in Children**

**Discharge**
Physiologic leukorrhea in newborns and early puberty
Foreign body
Sexually transmitted infection
Sexual abuse

**Pain or Itching**
Nonspecific vulvovaginitis (chemical or physical irritants)
Group A *Streptococcus* infection
*Shigella* infection
Pinworm (*Enterobius vermicularis*) infestation
Foreign body
Genital warts
Behçet syndrome
Lichen sclerosus et atrophicus
Sexual abuse

**Bleeding**
Trauma
Urethral prolapse
Foreign body
Lichen sclerosus et atrophicus
Sexual abuse
Endocrine abnormalities
Genital warts
Genital tumor
Withdrawal bleeding (newborn)

## SEXUAL ABUSE

ED evaluation of possible sexual abuse should focus on identifying patients who require urgent treatment, urgent collection of evidence, or protective custody (**Fig. 21.2**). Open-ended questions by the emergency practitioner (EP) will allow the parents to voice their concerns about possible molestation (this should be done away from the child). When interviewing the patient, history taking should be limited to open-ended questions phrased in child-appropriate language, such as "How did you get this ouchie?" Do not make suggestions that the child may follow in an attempt to please. Do not direct, lead, or ask questions with embedded information because such information can appear in the child's later responses. Formal interviewing and complete examination are best minimized in the ED and instead carried out by trained personnel. ED providers should be aware of local resources and if possible refer children to a designated child sexual abuse evaluation center.

If abuse is alleged within the past 72 hours, collection of evidence should be undertaken as soon as possible. In studies of forensic evidence collection in prepubertal sexual assault cases, the majority of usable evidence is found on clothing and linen. In one large study of prepubertal sexual assault victims, no swabs were positive for blood after 13 hours or for semen or sperm after 9 hours.[1]

A brief physical examination of the vulva, vagina, and anal area should be undertaken, as described previously. The chief

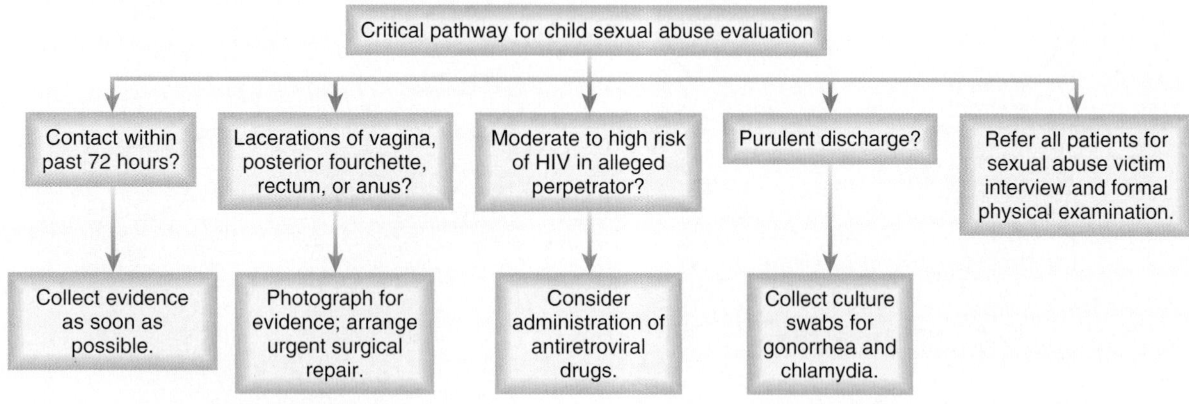


**Fig. 21.2 Algorithm showing the critical pathway for evaluation of pediatric sexual abuse.** *HIV*, Human immunodeficiency virus.

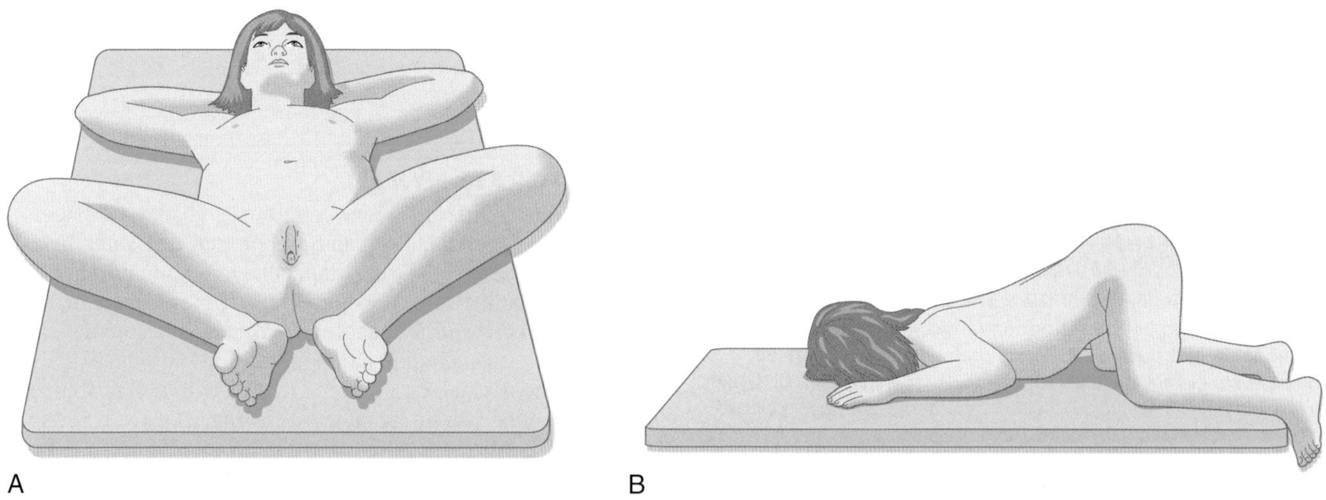


**Fig. 21.3 Pediatric gynecologic examination positions. A,** Frog-leg position. **B,** Knee-chest position.

purpose of the initial physical examination is to discover injuries in need of urgent treatment (vaginal lacerations, anal tears) or injuries that may change over a short period and require documentation. Bruises or petechiae may fade quickly, and the ED description of the fresh injuries may be important evidence in legal proceedings. If possible, photographs should taken for legal evidence. Areas of perineal erythema, abrasion, lacerations, bruising, and petechiae, as well as the shape or tears of the hymen, should be described in writing and pictured in drawings.

However, most children who have been molested have no physical findings related to abuse. The absence of physical findings should not be used to negate any statement or suspicions. All concerns must be thoroughly, supportively, and objectively explored by a trained interviewer.

## GENITAL EXAMINATION

Infants and young toddlers can usually be examined easily if positioned supine in the frog leg position (**Fig. 21.3**). Prepubertal girls can be examined in either the supine or the prone position. If the child is cooperative, she can lie in the supine position with the feet together and the knees bent and placed apart in the frog-leg position. Visualization can be improved by applying labial traction in two directions—both apart and apart and down (**Fig. 21.4**).

Some children may be more comfortable hugging their knees to their chest (knee-chest position); labial traction will also be necessary when using this position. In a variation of the knee-chest position, the child rises on her hands and knees and then puts her head down on the examination table (see Fig. 21.3, *B*).

If the child is uncooperative, it is a matter of clinical judgment whether the importance of the examination is worth the stress caused by it. Referral to a child sexual abuse center or examination under anesthesia should be considered.

The EP should avoid directly touching the sensitive mucosa.

## DIFFERENTIAL DIAGNOSIS AND MEDICAL DECISION MAKING

### LABIAL ADHESIONS

In prepubertal girls, a small section or the entire labia majora may be fused in the midline (**Fig. 21.5**). Labial adhesion is a self-limited condition and the labia will open with estrogenization at puberty. Though usually asymptomatic, some girls with labial adhesions may have an increased propensity for urinary tract infections. Occasionally, labial adhesions will

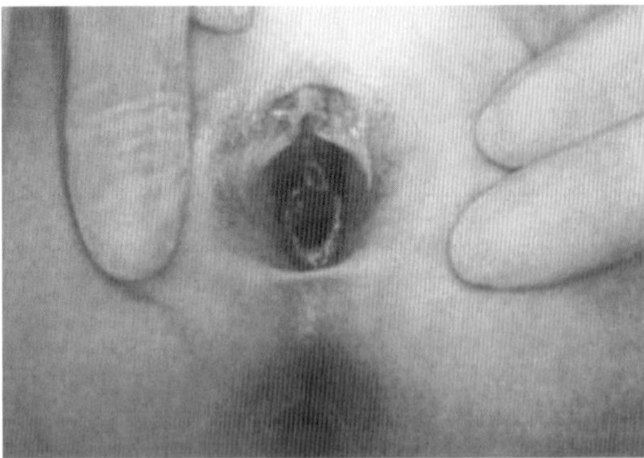

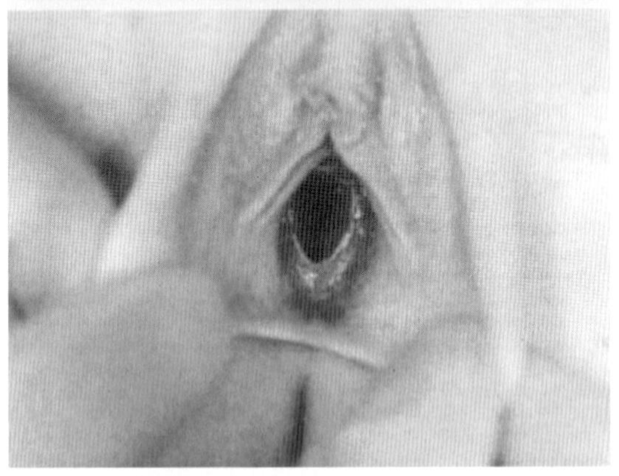

**Fig. 21.4 Examination of the vulva, hymen, and anterior vagina by gentle lateral retraction *(above)* and gentle gripping of the labia and pulling anteriorly *(below).*** (From Emans SJ. Office evaluation of the child and adolescent. In: Emans SJ, Laufer MR, Goldstein DP, editors. Pediatric and adolescent gynecology. 4th ed. Philadelphia: Lippincott-Raven; 1998.)

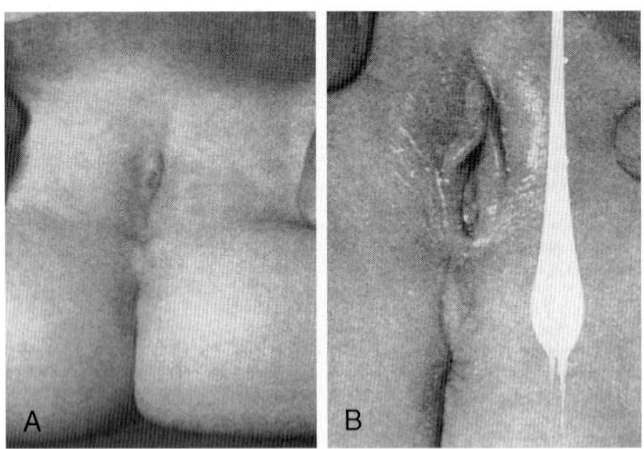


**Fig. 21.5 A,** Labial adhesions in a 2½-year-old girl. Two tiny openings exist—one beneath the clitoris and another near the middle line of fusion. **B,** Appearance of the same child after 10 days of local application of estrogen ointment. (From Dewhurst CJ. Gynaecological disorders of infants and children. Philadelphia: Davis; 1963.)

be noted in the ED because they obscure the urethral meatus and make bladder catheterization difficult or impossible. In these cases, management options include a clean-catch midstream urine collection, a bagged urine specimen, or suprapubic aspiration.

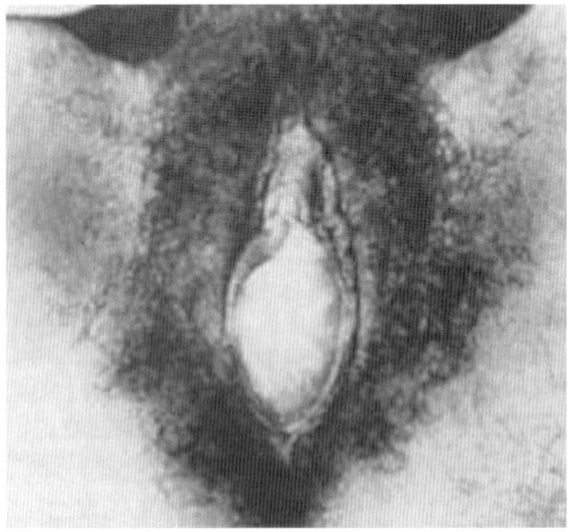

**Fig. 21.6 Imperforate hymen distended by hematocolpos.** (From Baramki TA. Treatment of congenital anomalies in girls and women. J Reprod Med 1984;29:376.)

## IMPERFORATE HYMEN

Imperforate hymen is a rare condition and may be encountered at any age. Neonates and prepubertal girls may have a bulging hymen noted during diaper changing or bathing. More classically, pubertal or postpubertal girls are evaluated for abdominal pain and absence of menses despite the development of breasts and pubic hair. Findings on physical examination may be normal, or a bulging hymen with a dark (bloody) fluid collection behind it may be seen (**Fig. 21-6**). Ultrasonography will confirm the diagnosis of hydrometrocolpos (a fluid- and blood-filled uterus and vagina). A similar finding may be present with a transverse vaginal septum, but in this condition the hymen is patent.

## VAGINAL DISCHARGE WITHOUT ASSOCIATED SYMPTOMS

Physiologic leukorrhea is a manifestation of the effect of estrogen on the vaginal mucosa. Otherwise asymptomatic discharge may be seen in neonates and begins again 1 to 2 years before menarche. Many girls or their parents will complain of a white or yellowish discharge found on the girl's underwear. Unlike vulvovaginitis, no irritation or pain is present. In sexually active girls, wet preparations and cultures may be necessary to rule out sexually transmitted infection. After infancy and before early puberty, the EP should consider the possibility of a foreign body in girls with a complaint of vaginal discharge, even without other symptoms.

## VULVOVAGINITIS

Vulvovaginitis (vaginal discharge with irritation and itching) is a common condition in prepubertal girls. Common complaints include vaginal discharge, itching, redness, dysuria, and bleeding (**Fig. 21-7**). The prepubertal vaginal mucosa is thin, dry, and very sensitive to minor irritants. Poor hygiene, tight clothing, perfumes and bubble baths, and overzealous wiping are common causes of vulvar irritation and inflammation.

In addition, a variety of infectious agents can cause vulvovaginitis. Pinworm (*Enterobius vermicularis*) infestation

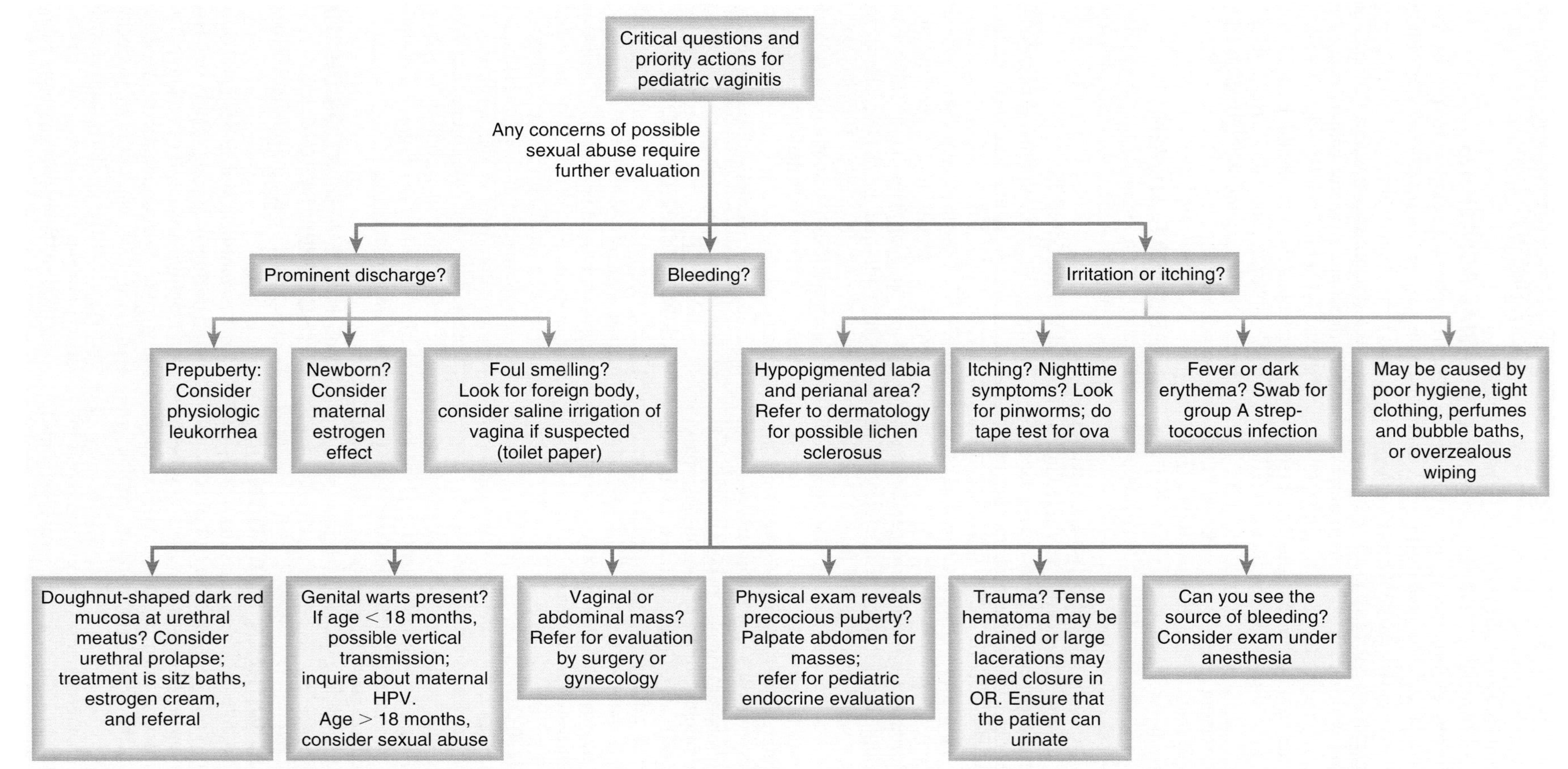


**Fig. 21.7 Algorithm showing critical questions and priority actions for pediatric vaginitis.** *HPV*, Human papillomavirus; *OR*, operating room.

should be suspected in girls with pronounced itching, particularly at night. Vulvovaginitis may be caused by group A β-hemolytic streptococcal infection and should be suspected when the vulvar area is beefy red or if the patient has systemic signs of streptococcal infection (fever, scarlatina rash). A retrospective study found that 21% of prepubertal girls with vulvovaginitis were culture positive for group A streptococcal infection.[2] Streptoccocal infection is more likely in older girls (school age) and in those with recent exposure to other children with streptoccocal pharyngitis. Rarely, *Shigella* can cause a similar infectious vaginitis. Yeast does not thrive in the dry mucosa of prepubertal girls, and vaginal candidiasis is extremely rare.

The EP should inquire about contact with individuals who have infectious pharyngitis or diarrhea and send culture swabs from the vagina for analysis when suspicion exists. The swabs should be moistened with nonbacteriostatic saline before sampling to reduce the patient's discomfort.

Rarely, vulvovaginitis may be caused by sexual abuse or sexually transmitted infection. If a sexually transmitted infection is suspected, culture specimens for gonorrhea (plated on chocolate agar) and *Chlamydia* (Dacron swab in viral transport medium) should be obtained, in addition to DNA probe testing if warranted (in many areas, DNA probe testing is not admissible in court).

Vulvar itching and bleeding can be caused by genital warts. If warts are seen on examination, it may be an indication of sexual abuse, but genital warts could result from nonsexual contact with common warts. Vertical transmission of genital human papillomavirus infection from the birth canal may give rise to condyloma acuminatum after a period of several months.

Lichen sclerosus et atrophicus is an autoimmune condition marked by thinned and bleeding labia. The classic finding is a figure-of-eight pattern of hypopigmentation and skin breakdown around the labia and anus. Often mistaken for trauma from sexual abuse, this condition is potentially disfiguring. The patient should be referred to a dermatologist for evaluation and initiation of treatment, which usually consists of potent topical steroids or testosterone cream.

### VAGINAL FOREIGN BODIES

Patients with vaginal foreign bodies may have complaints of itching, pain, and bloody or foul-smelling vaginal discharge. Toilet paper is overwhelmingly the most common type of a vaginal foreign body. Insertion of other objects may be the result of exploratory play in very young, developmentally delayed, or sexually abused girls. The possibility of sexual abuse should be considered in girls with vaginal foreign bodies other than toilet paper.[3,4]

### VAGINAL BLEEDING WITHOUT IRRITATION

Precocious menarche is defined as cyclic bleeding before the age of 8 years. Precocious puberty should be suspected when vaginal bleeding is accompanied by breast swelling or growth of pubic hair. Most precocious puberty is idiopathic but may occasionally be a sign of hormone production by ovarian or pituitary tumors.

Urethral prolapse is characterized by dysuria and blood in the patient's underwear or on toilet paper. It is most commonly seen in prepubertal African American girls. Examination reveals a doughnut-shaped eversion of dark red mucosa at the urethral meatus, which may cover the vaginal introitus.

## TREATMENT

### LABIAL ADHESIONS

If treatment of labial adhesion is necessary, an estrogen-containing cream may be applied to the fused area. In more than 90% of cases, the adhesions will be released within a few weeks of treatment; however, fusion often recurs. After release of adhesions, a barrier cream such as Vaseline or zinc oxide should be applied to the labia several times a day to prevent recurrence. Parents should be told that topical estrogen is easily absorbed and may cause vaginal hyperpigmentation or breast swelling, which should resolve after discontinuation of the cream.

### IMPERFORATE HYMEN

Referral should be made to a gynecologist for incision of an imperforate hymen or resection of a transverse septum.

### VULVOVAGINITIS

Treatment of vulvovaginitis should be tailored to the underlying cause. For the majority of girls with nonspecific vulvovaginitis, sitz baths and education about hygiene will suffice. Girls with severe dysuria or urinary retention may be able to urinate in the tub during a sitz bath (see the Patient Teaching Tips box). Streptococcal infection can be treated with oral penicillin, clindamycin, or a macrolide antibiotic for 10 days. *Shigell*a infection can be treated with amoxicillin or trimethoprim-sulfamethoxazole. Pinworm infestation is easily treated with chewable mebendazole and a repeat dose in 2 weeks. Children with genital warts should be referred to dermatology or pediatric gynecology services for treatment.

### VAGINAL FOREIGN BODIES

Vaginal foreign bodies will often be visible on physical examination without the use of a speculum and can be removed under direct visualization or by irrigation. To perform irrigation, instruct the patient to sit on a bedpan or an absorbent pad. Insert a small catheter or feeding tube several centimeters into the vagina and flush warm saline solution through a large syringe until confident that no further foreign body remains. If unable to remove the foreign body by irrigation in the ED or if a speculum examination is required, it is advisable to schedule an examination under anesthesia and treatment by a pediatric gynecologist.

### VAGINAL BLEEDING OR DISCHARGE WITHOUT IRRITATION

Treatment of physiologic leukorrhea consists of only reassurance.

In a patient believed to have precocious menarche, the EP should document staging of pubertal development and palpate for abdominal masses. If an abdominal mass is palpated, ultrasonography or abdominal computed tomography should be performed. Girls with signs of precocious puberty should be referred to their primary care physician or a pediatric endocrinologist.

Urethral prolapse will generally reduce itself if left alone. Conservative treatment with sitz baths should be initiated in the ED, with primary care follow-up to consider the need for estrogen cream or surgical excision in recalcitrant cases.

## TRAUMA

Straddle injuries involving the vulva and vagina result from falls onto playground equipment, bicycles, or furniture. Although straddle injuries require sensitive handling, they are no more likely than other traumatic injuries to be the result of sexual abuse. If the history does not correlate with the findings on physical examination, further investigation for child abuse is indicated. Frequent findings with straddle injury include abrasions or bruising of the labia, lacerations of the labia or posterior fourchette, tears of the vagina and hymen, and vulvar hematoma.[5] If the extent of the internal injury is at all in question, referral to a pediatric gynecologist or pediatric surgeon for examination under anesthesia should be considered. Other indications for referral include tense vulvar hematomas, which may require drainage to avoid tissue necrosis, and lacerations requiring surgical closure. For minor trauma not requiring further referral, ensure that the patient is able to urinate before she is discharged from the ED.

## NEWBORN VAGINAL DISCHARGE AND BREAST SWELLING

Maternal estrogen is the cause of most newborn gynecologic complaints. Physiologic leukorrhea appears as a white or cream-colored vaginal discharge. Newborn girls often have a smear of blood on their diaper, the result of endometrial sloughing after withdrawal of maternal estrogen. Parents occasionally mistake a peach-colored smear of urate crystals on the diaper for blood. Urate crystals are commonly seen in the first several days of life, most often in breastfed babies who are mildly dehydrated.

Maternal estrogen can also cause noticeable swelling of the breast buds in both male and female infants. Expression of milk on palpation (witch's milk) is possible, but manipulation of the swollen tissue should be discouraged because it may cause infection. The swelling should be examined carefully for signs of infection; it should be mobile and without redness, warmth, or undue tenderness.

Neonatal mastitis is a potentially serious bacterial infection that requires aggressive work-up and treatment like any other infection in this age group. Treatment consists of antistaphylococcal antibiotic coverage. Neonatal mastitis can develop into an abscess requiring incision and drainage. Consultation with a pediatric surgeon should be considered if an incision near the breast bud is required because damage to the breast bud can lead to a poor cosmetic outcome of the breast in later life.

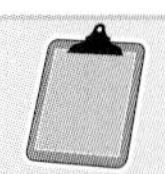

### DOCUMENTATION

**History**—Duration of symptoms; description of any discharge, odor, itching, pain, dysuria, bleeding, enuresis, or urinary retention; history of genital or urinary problems or trauma.

**Physical examination**—Breast and pubic hair development; abdominal palpation for a mass; genital examination, including color (red or pale), discharge, odor, open sores, bleeding, lacerations, petechiae, bruising, and tears of the mucosa, hymen, posterior fourchette, and anal area; visualization of vaginal masses or foreign bodies; and if necessary, rectal examination to palpate masses or large foreign bodies.

**Studies**—As indicated: urinalysis with microscopy and culture, bacterial culture, tape test for pinworm eggs, gonorrhea/*Chlamydia* cultures.

**Medical decision making**—Concern or lack of concern for abuse; ability of the child to tolerate a gynecologic examination.

**Procedures**—Success of foreign body removal or suspicion of a retained foreign body; documentation of the timing of collection of sexual abuse evidence and transfer of the evidence to the police.

**Photos**—Photos should be taken of any abnormal findings or if there is a question of sexual abuse.

**Patient instructions**—Discussion of hygiene, education about warning signs of a retained vaginal foreign body; record the follow-up plan (phone or visit) for any cultures; if sexual abuse is suspected, document referral to child protection services and the sexual abuse evaluation center.

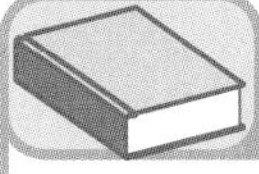

### PATIENT TEACHING TIPS

**Patient Discharge Information for Vulvovaginitis**

It is normal for little girls to have sensitive skin in the vagina; this is nature's way of saying that they are not ready to be touched there.

Child should undergo a sitz bath twice a day for 3 to 5 days—sit for 5 minutes in 2 inches of plain water.

If the child will not urinate because of pain or anxiety, try encouraging her to urinate while in the bath water.

Avoid irritants—bubble bath, lotions, perfumed toilet paper.

Wear loose-fitting, cotton clothing and underwear.

Practice proper hygiene—wipe gently from front to back after using the toilet.

Take a complete course of antibiotic treatment for infections when indicated.

## BREAST DISORDERS IN OLDER CHILDREN

Both male and female children and adolescents may experience some degree of breast bud swelling in early puberty, before the growth spurt and development of adult body hair. The physical examination should include palpation and a description of the breast swelling, a description of any axillary and pubic hair, and—in male patients—palpation of the testicles.

Normal breast tissue should be rubbery, firm, smooth, mobile, and somewhat tender. Gynecomastia can be exceptionally distressing for boys, who should be told that this is a normal male response to hormonal surges and is not evidence of any developmental or sexual abnormality. In most cases it resolves after sexual maturity. Rarely, boys with marked gynecomastia may need referral for cosmetic surgery.

A breast mass in teenage girls is uncommon but causes considerable psychologic distress. Although breast cancer is extraordinarily rare in adolescents, it is usually the prime concern of young girls with a breast mass. Most adolescent breast masses are cystic and caused by fibrocystic breast disease, as in adults. Fibroadenomas are the most common solid masses seen in teenagers. Most adolescent girls with a breast mass should be referred to their primary physician for reexamination later in the menstrual cycle. Suspected abscesses may be drained by needle aspiration or treated conservatively with antistaphylococcal antibiotics. If imaging is necessary, ultrasonography is most helpful to differentiate cystic from solid masses and support needle aspiration of fibrocystic disease or abscesses.

## FOLLOW-UP, NEXT STEPS IN CARE, AND PATIENT EDUCATION

Nearly all children with gynecologic and breast problems can be treated as outpatients and referred to their primary care physician for follow-up. Newborns with mastitis and fever may require hospital admission for evaluation of sepsis and intravenous antibiotic administration.

Older children may require admission for treatment under anesthesia for drainage of tense vulvar hematomas, repair of lacerations, incision of an imperforate hymen, or removal of foreign bodies. Available surgical services vary, but care can be provided by pediatric general surgery, gynecology, or rarely urology services. All prepubertal girls requiring internal pelvic examination should be referred to a pediatric specialty center for examination under anesthesia.

Suspicion of child sexual abuse mandates referral to child protective services and an experienced evaluation center. In cases of suspected abuse in which the home environment is not safe, children may require admission to the hospital or discharge to temporary foster care to ensure their safety pending investigation by child protective services.

## REFERENCES

***References can be found on Expert Consult @ www.expertconsult.com.***

# Pediatric Abdominal Disorders 22

*Russ Horowitz*

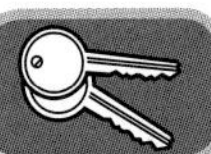

**KEY POINTS**

- The most common cause of intestinal obstruction in patients younger than 6 years is intussusception.
- Henoch-Schönlein purpura is a vasculitis that causes abdominal pain, purpura, and arthritis. Renal involvement is present in up to 50% of cases and is manifested as microscopic hematuria and proteinuria.
- Bilious emesis in infants is suggestive of highly morbid conditions such as malrotation with volvulus, necrotizing enterocolitis, sepsis, or small bowel obstruction.
- In up to 90% of children younger than 2 years with appendicitis, the appendix has perforated by the time of diagnosis. These patients will be found to have generalized peritonitis and shock more often than older children or adults with appendicitis.

## EPIDEMIOLOGY

Abdominal pain is a common complaint in children. Up to 25% of children will experience discomfort severe enough to interfere with activity, and annually, one in every seven children in the United States will visit a physician because of abdominal complaints, yet most will have no organic cause identified. Between 2% and 4% of all pediatric outpatient visits are related to abdominal complaints.[1-3] Discerning the presence of serious underlying disease can be challenging. This chapter describes several of the most significant pathologic abdominal conditions in pediatric patients.

## ABDOMINAL MASSES

Obstructive uropathy and renal cysts are the most likely causes of abdominal distention in infancy. Abdominal tumors are slow growing and usually recognized incidentally (e.g., when a parent or physician feels an abdominal mass). The two most common malignancies are Wilms tumor and neuroblastoma. The majority of affected children are younger than 5 years. Wilms tumor arises from the renal parenchyma and in most cases is asymptomatic. Neuroblastoma develops from the adrenal gland or along the sympathetic chain and may thus be manifested as either a midline or flank mass. It is an aggressive malignancy and has often metastasized at diagnosis. Ultrasonography and computed tomography (CT) are useful for investigation of abdominal lesions. A pediatric surgeon and oncologist should be consulted early for management of abdominal tumors.

## GASTROINTESTINAL BLEEDING

As a general rule, gastrointestinal (GI) bleeding is not usually as severe in children as in adults. In particular, the vast majority of cases of neonatal GI bleeding are benign. The first step in evaluation is to confirm that the suspicious material found in the stool or diaper is actually blood by performing a guaiac filter test for occult blood. Children routinely consume both foods (watermelon) and liquids (antibiotics such as cefdinir, fruit punch, and other juices) that turn the stool red, which may falsely lead both parents and health care workers to believe that GI blood loss is occurring. The benign pink or orange urate crystals in the urine of some neonates and young children are sometimes mistaken for blood when seen in diapers. Urinary tract infections and urethral prolapse may also result in deposition of blood in the diaper that could be confused with GI blood.

Upper GI bleeding produces dark brown, black, or simply heme-positive stool. However, because of the fast transit time in neonates, some upper GI bleeding may be bright red. The most common cause is swallowed maternal blood, acquired either during delivery or as a result of breastfeeding from irritated or cracked nipples.

Esophageal varices are rare in children. In contrast to adults, in whom primary hepatic disease is the leading cause, the most likely cause of varices in children is splanchnic and portal vein obstruction. Varices may develop secondary to umbilical vein catheterization, dehydration, sepsis, or omphalitis. Less common causes are hepatic parenchymal conditions such as biliary cirrhosis secondary to biliary atresia, cystic fibrosis, $\alpha_1$-antitrypsin deficiency, and hepatitis. Early onset of inflammatory bowel disease occurs in the teenage years and is uncommon in younger children.

Perirectal skin breakdown and external rectal fissures both produce blood-streaked stool and are easily identifiable on

**BOX 22.1 Meckel Diverticulum—the Rule of 2s**

2% of the population are affected.
2% of patients with Meckel diverticulum experience a complication.
2 inches is the usual length.
2 feet from the ileocecal valve is the usual location.
2 times as common in males as females.

physical examination. Sitz baths and stool softeners are useful in treating rectal fissures.

Emergency department (ED) management of GI bleeding is directed at fluid and blood resuscitation.

## MECKEL DIVERTICULUM

A Meckel diverticulum is the most common omphalomesenteric remnant. The most frequently observed finding is painless rectal bleeding, which occurs as a result of ulceration of the diverticulum or neighboring mucosa by the ectopic tissue. The ectopic tissue is gastric in origin in more than 80% of cases, but it may be pancreatic as well. Symptoms usually occur within the first 2 years of life, and in the majority of affected individuals it is diagnosed by 20 years of age (**Box 22.1**). A Meckel diverticulum can act as a lead point in intussusception. The diagnostic study of choice is a radiolabeled bleeding study called a Meckel scan. Definitive therapy is surgical excision.

## INTUSSUSCEPTION

Intussusception occurs when one loop of intestine invaginates into another. Intussusception of the mesentery can also occur and result in edema and vascular congestion. It is the most common cause of intestinal obstruction in children younger than 6 years. The ileocolic region is most often involved. Intussusception is usually manifested in children 6 to 18 months old, with a peak occurrence at 10 to 12 months. The vast majority of cases in children younger than 3 years are idiopathic. One etiologic theory is that inflammation of Peyer patches within the intestine acts as a lead point for the intussusception. In children older than 5 years, a true lead point is found more than 75% of the time. Lead points include polyps, lymphoma, Meckel diverticulum, surgical adhesions, and mucosal inflammation secondary to vasculitis.

Intussusception is often preceded by a viral illness, and the patient may have a low-grade fever at the time of evaluation. Symptoms consist of vomiting and episodic, crampy abdominal pain. Initially, children return to baseline between episodes, but as the condition persists, they may become lethargic. Screaming episodes lasting up to 10 to 15 minutes with hip and knee flexion are routine. The episodes increase in frequency and duration over time, with subsequent shortening of asymptomatic intervals.

The classic triad of symptoms—vomiting, abdominal pain, and "currant jelly" stools—is seen in less than one third of patients. However, more than 75% have two of these findings. Early on, stools test guaiac negative. If bowel ischemia ensues, frank blood mixed with mucus gives the stool a currant jelly appearance.

Some children have only lethargy, which can delay the diagnosis. The most commonly confused entity is constipation because of the similar pattern of colicky abdominal pain. These two conditions can easily be differentiated with a plain abdominal radiograph.

The history is the best guide to the diagnosis of intussusception. On abdominal palpation the right lower quadrant may be empty because the cecum has rotated out of its standard position. The actual intussusception may be palpated as a sausage-shaped mass in the right upper quadrant. Normal physical findings should not dissuade the examiner from proceeding with investigation because most children appear normal between episodes. No laboratory studies are available to confirm the diagnosis, and guaiac test–positive stool is a late finding. Abdominal radiographic findings are most often normal, but a mass may be seen in the right upper quadrant.

Intussusception can be reliably diagnosed with ultrasound.[4] Enemas are both diagnostic and therapeutic. Intussusceptions that cannot be reduced by enema must be reduced surgically. Up to 10% of cases recur, most often within 24 hours. After reduction, the child must be admitted to the hospital for a 24-hour observation period.

Children with a history and physical findings suspicious for intussusception must be evaluated quickly because the passage of time increases both the edema and the difficulty of achieving reduction. A pediatric surgeon should be contacted before the child undergoes attempted enema reduction in case of failure or perforation. Ileoileal intussusceptions may be difficult to visualize and reduce via enema unless there is significant reflux of contrast material. Such intussusceptions are associated with Henoch-Schönlein purpura (HSP), in which the vasculitis acts as a lead point.[5]

## HENOCH-SCHÖNLEIN PURPURA

HSP is a vasculitis that predominantly affects the capillaries and small vessels. It occurs most commonly in school-age children, with the classic triad consisting of abdominal pain, purpura, and arthritis. Elevations of immunoglobulin A (IgA) are detectable in the blood, along with immune complex deposition in the skin and glomeruli. There is no known etiology, but HSP has often been found to occur after upper respiratory infections. Recurrences are seen in up to 50% of cases.

Abdominal pain occurs in half the patients and is most frequently colicky in nature. Intussusception should be strongly considered in children with guaiac test–positive or frankly bloody stools accompanied by severe pain. The subtype of intussusception associated with HSP is often ileoileal, which is difficult to visualize and reduce with a contrast enema. CT is the imaging modality of choice for ileoileal intussusception associated with HSP, and reduction must often be achieved surgically.

The rash associated with HSP is petechial, purpuric, and usually located on the buttocks and lower extremities. It is seen in dependent areas, so the scrotum and hands may also be affected. In younger children, the rash is displayed on the dorsal surfaces of the extremities, trunk, and head. The lesions are palpable and appear and progress like common bruises.

Arthritis occurs in two thirds of patients and most often involves the large joints of the lower extremities. The knees and ankles may be edematous and tender to palpation or with movement. Joint pain may be so severe that it interferes with ambulation.

Renal involvement occurs in 25% to 50% of patients and is usually manifested as microscopic hematuria and proteinuria.

The diagnosis of HSP is based on the characteristic rash and accompanying symptoms. The results of a complete blood count and clotting studies are normal.

Nonsteroidal antiinflammatory drugs are the traditional therapy for the arthralgias observed with HSP. Use of corticosteroids for the management of abdominal pain and renal involvement is controversial.[6,7] Outpatient management is usually sufficient, although substantial joint or abdominal discomfort may require inpatient admission. Severe abdominal pain, especially in conjunction with guaiac test–positive or grossly bloody stools, merits an evaluation for intussusception.

## GASTROESOPHAGEAL REFLUX

Gastroesophageal reflux (GER) is caused by a loose esophageal sphincter with retrograde passage of food into the esophagus. It is usually manifested in the first few weeks after birth as emesis during or soon after the cessation of feeding. The emesis may be blood streaked but should never be bilious. Some children in whom GER is eventually diagnosed may have previously been incorrectly labeled as having colic, feeding difficulties, or formula intolerance.

Symptoms of GER range from small "wet burps" to discomfort during feedings with arching of the back. One particularly severe form of reflux is the Sandifer syndrome, in which the child has opisthotonic movements and unusual head and neck positioning. The head movements may be an attempt to reduce pain by elongating the esophagus and protecting the airway from aspiration. Complications of GER include failure to thrive, apnea, laryngospasm, and aspiration pneumonia. Reflux esophagitis may be the culprit in children with guaiac test–positive stools or iron deficiency anemia. In most cases, GER resolves spontaneously by 1 year. The diagnosis is most often made from a careful history. Esophageal pH probe, nuclear milk scan, barium swallow study, and direct feeding under fluoroscopic observation are all diagnostic options.

Nonpharmacologic interventions are frequently sufficient to relieve the majority of cases of GER. Smaller-volume feedings with breaks for burping are often helpful. Caregivers should be instructed to keep children semiupright for 30 to 45 minutes after feedings. Thickening of feedings with cereal reduces crying and improves symptoms.

Ranitidine, a histamine blocker, reduces gastric acid and aids mucosal healing. Metoclopramide stimulates esophageal and gastric motility, thereby decreasing the volume of gastric contents that may reflux. GER that is severe and resistant to medical therapy may require surgical intervention with a Nissen fundoplication. This procedure involves wrapping and surgically fixing a portion of the stomach around the esophagus.

## PYLORIC STENOSIS

Pyloric stenosis results from idiopathic hypertrophy of the antrum of the stomach. The male-to-female ratio is 5 : 1, and familial occurrence is present in up to 50% of patients. It is usually diagnosed in children at 2 to 5 weeks of age and rarely after 3 months. They feed normally at first but later experience vomiting in the midst of or soon after feeding. The emesis begins as mild and small and then progresses to voluminous and projectile. It is never bilious, although it may be blood streaked. The patient appears to vomit the entire bottle and then refeeds ravenously. After eating, peristaltic waves may be visible across the abdomen. If the condition continues, the child loses weight and becomes dehydrated, with sunken eyes, loose skin, and lethargy. Electrolyte analysis shows a hypochloremic, hypokalemic metabolic alkalosis. As the child continues to vomit, hydrogen and chloride are expelled. The kidneys attempt to maintain normal pH by eliminating potassium and hydrogen ions.

The differential diagnosis includes GER, overfeeding, and gastritis. Careful examination may detect the pylorus or "olive," especially in a thin, dehydrated child with prolonged illness. Pyloric stenosis is identified with either ultrasonography or an upper GI series. Ultrasonography is the preferred modality because in addition to its high rate of accuracy, no radiation exposure is involved. Ultrasonographic diagnosis is made by visualization of a thickened pylorus. An upper GI radiographic series will demonstrate a "string sign" as the contrast agent squeezes through a narrowed pylorus.

Surgery is the treatment of choice for pyloric stenosis. However, diagnosis of this disorder does not represent a surgical emergency. ED management consists of rehydration and correction of electrolyte status before surgical intervention.

## MALROTATION WITH VOLVULUS

Early in normal embryonic development, the intestine rotates around the superior mesenteric artery. The duodenum and cecum become widely displaced and fixed into position by peritoneal attachments called Ladd bands. They are loosely connected by a broad mesentery. In cases of malrotation, the cecum and duodenum do not separate but remain closely aligned. They are only loosely fixed into position, and the mesentery does not fan outward. This narrow stretch of mesentery, which contains the superior mesenteric artery, crosses over the duodenum. It can easily twist on itself and cause duodenal obstruction and arterial compression. The result is ischemia with the potential for intestinal necrosis within 1 to 2 hours.

The common manifestation is an acute onset of abdominal pain with bilious emesis. Abdominal distention may or may not be present, depending on the anatomic level of the obstruction. Affected children are usually seen in the first year of life, with the majority of cases occurring within the first week to month. Older children may have a history of intermittent episodes of vomiting and abdominal pain that suddenly become more severe. Bloody stools should raise the level of concern for bowel ischemia and impending gangrene. Patients are often quite ill and may be in shock at initial evaluation.

The differential diagnosis of bilious emesis in infants includes a short list of highly morbid conditions (**Box 22.2**).

**BOX 22.2 Differential Diagnosis of Bilious Emesis and Associated Radiographic Findings**

Small bowel obstruction: air-fluid levels
Necrotizing enterocolitis: pneumatosis intestinalis
Malrotation: small bowel overlying the liver and absence of distal bowel gas
Sepsis: possible ileus

Data from Long FR, Kramer SS, Markowitz RI, et al. Radiographic patterns of intestinal malrotation in children. Radiographics 1996;16:547-56.

**BOX 22.3 Special Considerations in Children with Suspected Appendicitis**

Vomiting may be the first sign.
Children may not experience anorexia and may actually request food.
Most young children have experienced perforation at the time of diagnosis.
Children younger than 2 years often have generalized symptoms such as irritability and tachypnea.
Thin appendiceal walls and loose omentum make perforation more likely and serious in children.
Ultrasonography is useful in the evaluation of children and prevents exposure to radiation.

In addition to malrotation, sepsis, small bowel obstruction, and necrotizing enterocolitis (NEC) must be considered.

A loop of small bowel overlying the liver may be visible on plain abdominal radiographs. Distal bowel gas is limited or absent. The "double bubble" sign can be visualized on an upright film; it is produced by a dilated stomach and duodenum. An upper GI radiographic series, the diagnostic study of choice, demonstrates abnormal anatomy with a coiled spring appearance of the jejunum in the right upper quadrant.[8]

All children with bilious emesis need immediate evaluation by a surgeon. Malrotation with midgut volvulus is a surgical emergency because bowel infarction can occur rapidly.

## NECROTIZING ENTEROCOLITIS

NEC is generally a disease of premature infants and is usually diagnosed in the intensive care unit. However, up to 10% of infants with NEC are born at full term, so initial evaluation in the ED is a possibility. Signs and symptoms range from feeding intolerance and vomiting to pneumatosis intestinalis (air within the intestinal wall), perforation, shock, and disseminated intravascular coagulation. Most affected newborns experience vomiting, which may or may not be bilious. The clinical findings may be limited to guaiac test–positive stools and feeding intolerance, but in severe cases, infants have massively distended, rigid abdomens in the setting of shock. Gas within the biliary tract is present in 10% to 30% of cases. With improved survival of premature infants, children may seen in the ED with sequelae of NEC, such as strictures, obstruction, fistulas, and short gut syndrome.

## APPENDICITIS

Appendicitis is typically accompanied by diffuse or periumbilical abdominal pain. Within 8 to 24 hours, vomiting begins, and the pain migrates to the right lower quadrant. Abdominal pain, vomiting, and fever are the classic symptom triad for the disease. Although the pain precedes other symptoms in adult studies, such may not be the case in many children with appendicitis. Up to one third of pediatric cases do not follow this order of symptoms, and vomiting is often reported as the first sign. Fever is routinely low grade; a temperature higher than 39° C reduces the likelihood of appendicitis, except in cases of perforation.

The position of the appendix dramatically affects the location of the pain and symptoms. A normally placed appendix produces discomfort at the McBurney point. A low-lying pelvic appendix may irritate the sigmoid colon and mimic enteritis with diarrhea. A retrocecal appendix may produce flank or posterior pain and may be confused with pyelonephritis or septic arthritis of the hip.

Movement increases the discomfort (e.g., bumps in the car ride to the hospital, walking, jumping) such that patients may walk hunched over, limp, have a shuffling gait, or put weight preferentially on the left leg. Although anorexia is a classic finding, children can be enticed by their favorite foods and may even want to eat.

Examinations should be gentle, and the right lower quadrant should be palpated last to allow evaluation of reportedly nontender regions and to gain the patient's confidence. Bowel sounds are usually normal or hypoactive. An external genital examination must be performed to exclude testicular disorders and incarcerated hernia.

Appendicitis is particularly difficult to identify early in the course of the illness and in the very young (**Box 22.3**).[9] Approximately 90% of patients younger than 2 years with appendicitis have a perforated appendix at the time of diagnosis. Children have a thinner appendiceal wall and a less well-developed omentum. Therefore, rupture occurs more readily and results in more diffuse bacterial dissemination. Pediatric cases of appendiceal perforation have more severe and diffuse peritonitis than do adult cases. Although the mortality from appendicitis has improved dramatically, the rate of perforation has not changed significantly in the past few decades.

A complete blood count showing leukocytosis and a left shift is supportive of the diagnosis, but many children have normal white blood cell (WBC) counts.[10] Most patients with appendicitis have an elevated WBC count in the range of 11,000 to 15,000 cells/mm$^3$. An appendix in close proximity to the ureter can produce sterile pyuria and mild hematuria. A positive urine Gram stain response and the presence of leukocyte esterase and nitrites can help differentiate a true urinary tract infection from inflammatory hematuria secondary to appendicitis.

In the case of perforation, the pain initially resolves but then becomes more generalized with peritoneal symptoms. It may be most severe in both lower quadrants as the purulent material settles. Young children may simply have nonspecific symptoms such as fussiness, inconsolable crying, irritability, and grunting respirations. Once perforation occurs, the child may have poor perfusion, tachycardia, high fever (>39° C), and even septic shock. Bowel sounds are then absent; the abdomen is rigid with rebound tenderness and involuntary guarding. The WBC count is dramatically elevated with a significant left shift.[10]

A fecalith is visible on plain abdominal radiographs in 8% to 10% of patients with appendicitis. A number of other findings can be seen on plain films, including scoliosis concave toward the right side, a sentinel loop overlying the appendix indicating an area of inflammation, air within the appendix, a mass in the right lower quadrant (more often in cases of abscesses), and loss of the psoas shadow on the right.

Ultrasonography is a useful tool for evaluating children with concerns for appendicitis. The classic finding known as the "target sign" is a fecalith inside a large, inflamed appendix. In obese children, visualization and diagnosis become more challenging. The sensitivity and specificity of ultrasonography exceed 90%, but ruptured appendices are notoriously difficult to identify. No diagnosis can be made if the appendix is not visualized. Ultrasonography is helpful in differentiating appendicitis from other causes of abdominal pain, such as ovarian cysts, but cannot exclude conditions such as mesenteric adenitis. CT has a sensitivity and specificity higher than 95% and may be used in cases with a broad differential diagnosis or when the findings on ultrasound are equivocal or it is unavailable.[11] Abdominal CT is helpful in diagnosing inflammatory bowel disease and mesenteric adenitis. Admission for serial abdominal examinations is warranted for a child with a compelling history and physical examination findings but equivocal laboratory findings.

A surgeon should be involved early in the ED evaluation of a child with suspected appendicitis because imaging may be avoided in classic cases. Pain must be addressed, and numerous studies have shown that narcotics do not affect the diagnostic accuracy of the examination. Surgeons may choose to evaluate the patient before analgesia is given, but pain medication should not be withheld indefinitely pending surgical assessment. Signs of shock should be addressed aggressively, and children with suspected rupture should receive broad-spectrum antibiotic coverage.

## HIRSCHSPRUNG DISEASE

Hirschsprung disease is caused by the absence of ganglion cells in the myenteric plexus of the colon. Without ganglion cells, that segment is under constant contraction. The proximal region dilates to compensate, with resultant constipation. Patients have complaints of chronic constipation, abdominal distention, and vomiting. Physical examination demonstrates palpable stool in the abdomen with a tight anal sphincter, but absence of stool in the rectal vault. Hirschsprung disease has a 4:1 male preponderance. In 80% of affected patients it is diagnosed within the first year of life. The most serious complications are toxic megacolon, perforation, and enterocolitis. A dilated colon, fecal impaction, and air-fluid levels are visible on abdominal radiographs. The diagnosis is made from the finding of aganglionosis on biopsy or anal manometry. A barium enema without bowel preparation shows a narrowed colonic segment and a dramatically dilated proximal segment. In uncomplicated cases, outpatient surgical evaluation is indicated. Resection of the aganglionic segment is curative.

The vast majority of cases of constipation are functional and tied to behavioral and psychologic causes. Pathologic causes are rare and, in addition to Hirschsprung disease, include cystic fibrosis and hypothyroidism.

## BILIARY TRACT DISEASE

Gallstones are an unusual condition in healthy children. The most common type, pigment stones, usually develop in children with underlying hemolytic conditions such as sickle cell disease and hereditary spherocytosis. Cholesterol stones are more prevalent in adolescent girls, obese children, patients with cystic fibrosis, and those who depend on total parenteral nutrition. Because of the large percentage of pigment stones, up to 50% of cases of cholelithiasis in children are visible on abdominal radiographs, in contrast to 10% to 15% of cases in adults.

Acalculous cholecystitis (inflammation of the gallbladder in the absence of gallstones) is more common in children than cholelithiasis is. Causes include Kawasaki disease; bacterial infections such as typhoid, shigellosis, and scarlet fever; and viral infections such as hepatitis.

Acute cholangitis usually occurs in children with a history of biliary surgery, as used for the management of choledochal cysts and biliary atresia. The clinical picture is similar to that in adults and consists of right upper quadrant pain, fever, and vomiting. Treatment is inpatient admission for therapy with broad-spectrum antibiotics such as ampicillin, gentamicin, and metronidazole.

## MILK PROTEIN ALLERGY

Milk protein allergy is manifested as blood-streaked, mucous stools in young infants exposed to cow's milk–based formulas. Significant flatus and mild discomfort with feeding may be noted. However, most children appear nontoxic and otherwise well. Edema, inflammation, and discrete ulcerations are present in the intestinal mucosa. This condition is best described to occur with consumption of milk protein but may develop with any formula, including soy. Treatment is to change to a formula with a different protein source. The symptoms should resolve within 1 week of complete withdrawal of the offending agent.[12]

## REFERENCES

***References can be found on Expert Consult @ www.expertconsult.com.***

# 23 Pediatric Trauma

*Katherine Bakes and Ghazala Q. Sharieff*

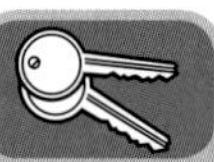

**KEY POINTS**

- Trauma is the leading cause of death in children.
- Pediatric trauma victims have worse outcomes than adult victims do.
- Head trauma is the leading cause of death and disability from pediatric trauma, followed by thoracic and abdominal trauma.
- Children with life-threatening injuries may have little or no external evidence of trauma.
- Pediatric resuscitation equipment should be stored in an easily accessed, clearly labeled area in the emergency department.
- Pediatric medication dosing and treatment algorithms should be posted in the emergency department, and Broselow-Luten resuscitation tapes should be available.

## EPIDEMIOLOGY

The report of the Institute of Medicine's Committee on Future of Emergency Care, released in June 2006, identified a lack of pediatric emergency services as a significant problem facing the health care system in the United States.[1] Trauma is the leading cause of death and disability in children and young adults.[2]

## PATHOPHYSIOLOGY

The anatomic characteristics of children predispose them to more significant injuries than adults would experience from similar trauma. The severity of pediatric head injury is related to the immature brain myelination, thin skulls, and larger head-to-body ratios in children. The bones and connective tissues of children are more pliable than those of adults, which can lead to potentially severe internal injuries with minimal external evidence of thoracoabdominal trauma. Because children have a greater ratio of surface area to volume, force can more easily be transferred to internal organs. Multiple trauma is common in children as a result of the smaller distance between vital structures. The sympathetic tone of a child is better than that of an adult, so a child's blood pressure may be maintained despite large volume loss. Once a critical percentage of blood volume is lost (25%), a child's blood pressure can drop precipitously, partly because of the inability of pediatric patients to change cardiac contractility and their dependence on the compensatory mechanisms of increased peripheral vascular resistance and heart rate. It should be noted that posttraumatic pediatric hypotension may also be an indicator of head injury rather than hemorrhage.[3]

## APPROACH AND MANAGEMENT

The ABCs of resuscitation (airway, breathing, circulation) should first be used to identify the loss of an airway or respiratory failure (or both). Direct injuries to the airway (oropharynx, trachea, or bronchi) are not the only cause of airway failure. An expanding neck hematoma or aspirated foreign body can have similar effects.

Breathing difficulty in children may be the sequelae of insults to the chest wall, lungs, heart, great vessels, or abdomen, as well as neurologic or muscular injuries. It may also result from the loss of ventilatory musculature, as with a cervical spine injury or respiratory muscle fatigue. Young children may have disordered ventilation secondary to gastric distention because considerable air is gulped into the stomach during crying.[4]

Circulation can be assessed in children through an evaluation of mental status, skin color and temperature, heart sounds, pulses, and capillary refill. Shock should be identified and treated immediately. Children differ from adults in several critical ways. The leading cause of cardiac arrest in children is hypoxemia. Normal blood pressure may be maintained in children sustaining trauma despite severe injury and massive blood loss (up to 25%). Shock in the setting of trauma should be presumed to be secondary to blood loss and be treated by restoration of volume. Two intravenous (or intraosseous) lines of the largest bore possible should be established immediately. Two boluses of crystalloid solution, 20 mL/kg each, should be administered. If shock persists, packed red blood cells should be transfused at 10 mL/kg and repeated as necessary. Other causes of shock, such as tension pneumothorax, pericardial tamponade, neurogenic shock, hypoxemia, metabolic derangements, and toxidromes, should be sought and treated concomitantly with restoration of volume.

**Table 23.1** AVPU Scale

| CATEGORY | APPROPRIATE RESPONSE | INAPPROPRIATE |
|---|---|---|
| **A**lert | Normal interaction for age | Lethargic, irritable |
| **V**erbal | Responds to name | Confused, unresponsive |
| **P**ainful | Withdraws from pain | Nonpurposeful movement or sound without localization of pain |
| **U**nresponsive | No response to verbal or painful stimuli | |

**PRIORITY ACTIONS**

A = Airway control—bag-valve-mask ventilation, endotracheal intubation
B = Breathing—maximize ventilation
C = Circulation—stabilize hemodynamic status
D = Disability—evaluate mental status and perform a neurologic examination
E = Exposure—completely undress and examine the patient
F = "Fingers and Foleys"—selective nasogastric or orogastric tube, bladder catheter, vaginal and rectal examinations
Secondary survey: Head-to-toe physical examination and AMPLE history (allergies, medications, past medical history, last meal, and events leading up to the patient's arrival in the emergency department)
Laboratory studies and radiographs

Disability must be assessed thoroughly. Mental status is evaluated with the Glasgow Coma Scale (GCS) or an AVPU (alert, verbal, painful, unresponsive) scale (**Table 23.1**). An age-appropriate examination should be performed to evaluate for neurologic deficits.

Exposure of the body immediately after the ABCs have been addressed is imperative in all pediatric trauma patients. Emergency personnel should briefly expose and roll (with precautions) the patient to assess for initially unapparent injuries, such as a puncture wound in the posterior aspect of the chest in a victim of assault. Because of the increased ratio of surface area to volume in children and a propensity for hypothermia, blankets and warmed intravenous fluids should be used to maintain normothermia. Whenever feasible, family presence, which has been shown to not impede pediatric trauma resuscitation, should be accommodated during resuscitation to comfort the child.[5] The emergency practitioner should communicate with the child during the examination.

After exposure, the secondary survey should be performed. An AMPLE history (allergies, medications, past medical history, last meal, and events leading up to the patient's arrival in the ED) is obtained, followed by a complete head-to-toe examination. Particular attention should be paid to the eyes, ears, mouth, axillae, hands, and genitals. The utility of rectal examination has recently been called into question. In particular settings where questionable neurologic deficits are present or rectal or urogenital trauma is evident, a rectal examination may prove useful. It should be selective to avoid unnecessary emotional stress in the child.[6] In an unconscious intubated patient, an orogastric or nasogastric tube and Foley catheter should be placed. As part of the secondary survey, initial radiographs and laboratory studies should be selectively ordered to further investigate any history and physical findings.

Younger children, particularly infants, have little functional ventilatory reserve.[7] Time is therefore of the essence in restoring oxygenation, ventilation, and circulation. The ABCs of resuscitation should be repeated if there is any change in the patient's status.

The most common life- and limb-threatening injuries in children are those to the head, chest, and abdomen. In each of these areas, there are subtle but important clues to such injures (**Box 23.1**).

**BOX 23.1 Overview of Pediatric Trauma Management**

Attend to the ABCs of resuscitation (airway, breathing, circulation) first. Connect the patient to a cardiac and oxygen saturation monitor; administer oxygen or secure the airway as needed.
Obtain intravenous or intraosseous access.
If the patient is hypotensive or tachycardic, administer normal saline in a 20-mL/kg bolus.
Roll the patient, perform a secondary survey, and recheck the vital signs.
If shock persists, additional intravenous access should be obtained (at least two large-bore intravenous lines), and a second 20-mL/kg bolus of normal saline should be administered.
Abdominal and thoracic ultrasonography, radiography, and laboratory studies should be performed as indicated.
If shock persists, transfuse packed red blood cells at 10 mL/kg, and continue evaluation for and treatment of life-threatening injuries.

## DIAGNOSTIC TESTING

### PRIMARY AND SECONDARY SURVEYS

Primary and secondary surveys should be performed in children just as in adults. Particular modalities of testing are discussed in depth in later sections on specific systems and injuries. In a child with multiple trauma or severe injury, basic tests must be ordered as part of the primary and secondary surveys. Cardiac and oxygen saturation monitoring should be instituted. Plain radiographs of the cervical spine, chest, and pelvis should be obtained and reviewed immediately at the bedside. A bedside focused assessment with sonography for trauma (FAST) should be performed to evaluate for free fluid in the abdomen or pericardium. Laboratory studies include an immediate bedside glucose test, a complete blood count, serum chemistry analysis, coagulation studies, urinalysis, blood typing and cross-matching, blood gas measurements, and a pregnancy test. Further radiologic testing (e.g., computed tomography [CT], angiography, magnetic resonance imaging [MRI]), as well as more in-depth laboratory testing (e.g., hepatic function tests, screening for toxins or drugs, pancreatic enzyme measurements), may be ordered as indicated.

There are some pediatric-specific issues in the management of trauma. With younger patients, small tubes should be used for laboratory testing to avoid iatrogenic blood loss. The clinician should be aware that the hematocrit does not drop immediately in a child with acute blood loss before receiving isotonic volume resuscitation. For minimally injured patients, such as those with isolated extremity fractures or low-risk head or abdominal trauma, no laboratory studies are needed. In patients requiring an observation period, tracking the hematocrit or hemoglobin may be useful in combination with clinical reassessment. Toxidromes must be considered, especially in a patient with altered mental status, if the circumstances of the event are suspicious or when the patient is a teenager.

The ALARA (as low as reasonably achievable) principle should be applied to minimize exposure to radiation. The clinician should limit the number of CT scans performed and should make size-based adjustments to the radiation scanning parameters.[8] Some investigators have questioned the need for portable radiographs of the cervical spine, chest, and pelvis to screen for injury in all trauma patients.[4] As with trauma triage, it is advisable to err on the side of caution. These studies should be performed in all seriously injured patients or if the status of the spine, chest, or pelvis is at all uncertain. A more focal radiologic screening examination, as indicated by the history and findings on physical examination, may be considered in stable patients with normal mental status. Children younger than 2 years in whom child abuse is suspected must undergo a skeletal radiographic survey to diagnose occult or remote injuries.

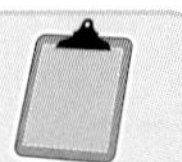

**DOCUMENTATION**

The following information should be documented:

**History**

Prehospital history

Detailed mechanism of the injury (e.g., speed of the vehicle, height of the fall)

Circumstances of the injury (e.g., damage to the vehicle, type of weapon)

Timing of the even

Time until arrival at the emergency department

Concurrent medications

Patient's access to medications or exposure to drugs or toxins

Past medical history

Last meal

Immunizations

Previous surgeries

Inconsistencies in the history between witnesses, particularly when child abuse is suspected

**Physical Examination**

Primary survey and interventions

Head-to-toe physical examination

**Laboratory Studies**

Emergency department interpretation of radiographs

Laboratory studies ordered and their results

Results of focused abdominal sonography for trauma or diagnostic peritoneal lavage

**Medical Decision Making**

Reasons to pursue or not pursue a work-up for each injury

Timing of consultation of surgical or other subspecialists

**Procedures**

Each procedure in full

**Patient Instructions**

Discussion of injuries and potential outcomes with the patient, patient's family, or both

## PEDIATRIC HEAD TRAUMA

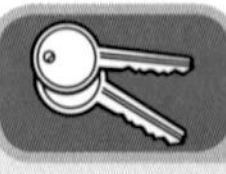

**KEY POINTS**

- Head trauma is responsible for 80% of pediatric trauma deaths.
- Cervical immobilization is required if head injury is suspected.
- The AVPU scale can be used in children as an alternative to the GCS score.
- Significant alterations in a child's mental status should prompt early airway management and immediate CT of the brain.
- Declining mental status with suspected intracranial injury requires immediate neurosurgical evaluation or transfer of the patient to a facility with neurosurgical capability.

### SCOPE AND OUTLINE

Head injury is the leading cause of death and is responsible for 80% of pediatric trauma deaths. Annually in the United States, 500,000 emergency department (ED) visits and almost 100,000 hospital admissions are due to pediatric head trauma. The leading causes of head trauma are falls, motor vehicle collisions, bicycle accidents, auto-pedestrian accidents, diving injuries, sporting accidents, and child abuse.

### PATHOPHYSIOLOGY

Children have relatively larger heads than adults do. A child's skull is thinner and less rigid than an adult's, and infants and younger children have open or soft sutures, which can help decompress elevations in intracranial pressure. As a result, parenchymal injury may occur in the absence of a skull fracture.

## CLINICAL PRESENTATION

Major intracranial injuries may be immediately apparent from the patient's depressed level of consciousness or confusion or from abnormal neurologic findings. Significant injuries may be present in a patient with completely normal neurologic findings. Early recognition and treatment of mild or moderately severe head injury in a child are as important as recognition and treatment of serious injuries (see Red Flags: Warning Signs box). An epidural hematoma in a mildly confused victim of a car accident can have dire consequences. It is important to screen for injuries to other systems and to aggressively treat a child with a head injury. Strict attention should be paid to maintaining oxygenation and cerebral perfusion in a head-injured child to avoid secondary injury.

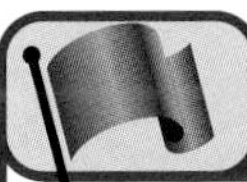

**RED FLAGS**

**Warning Signs of Intracranial Injury in Children with Head Trauma**

Prolonged loss of consciousness
Multiple seizures
Persistent vomiting
Amnesia
Lethargy
Irritability
Large cephalohematoma or clinical skull fracture
Abnormal neurologic findings

## APPROACH AND MANAGEMENT

A physical examination should be performed with attention to any neurologic findings. Obvious external head and neck trauma may be an indicator of serious injury, although severe internal injury often exists with minimal or no external signs. The GCS or AVPU scale may be used to assess mental status. An age-appropriate neurologic examination may reveal deficits requiring further testing and treatment. The clinician should have a low threshold for managing the airway of a pediatric trauma patient with altered mentation.

## DIAGNOSTIC TESTING

The goal of diagnostic testing in children in whom intracranial injury is suspected is to identify those with injuries that will require intervention before the condition worsens. A secondary goal is to avoid unnecessary testing and admission, both to prevent overutilization of resources and to avoid unnecessary exposure to radiation. The most commonly used and most widely available options for the evaluation of children with head injuries are plain radiography of the skull, CT of the head, and observation with serial examinations.

# CERVICAL SPINE INJURY

## SCOPE AND OUTLINE

Spinal cord injuries are uncommon in children and account for less than 2% of injuries found in pediatric trauma patients. Motor vehicle collisions represent the most common mechanism for this injury, and death is usually secondary to brain injury.

## PATHOPHYSIOLOGY AND ANATOMY

Mechanisms of fractures of the cervical spine in children are similar to those in adults, although children have a higher risk for ligamentous injuries (**Box 23.2 and Fig. 23.1**). Because the pediatric cervical spine is hypermobile, a traumatic injury can cause transient severe ligamentous disruption and lead to brief sensory or motor deficits or electric shocks with rapidly clearing weakness. The initial rapid resolution of symptoms represents realignment of structures with the counterforce of the injury such that the cord is drawn back into its anatomic position. Unfortunately, this phase can be followed by delayed neurologic deficits precipitated by cord edema after this stretch injury. The delay can be quite significant, with deficits appearing up to 4 days after the inciting event.

Fortunately, documented cases of this type of injury, known as spinal cord injury without radiographic abnormality (SCIWORA), tend to not be subtle in a preverbal child and result from impressive multiple-trauma mechanisms such as falls from extreme heights and motor vehicle accidents involving a high-risk mechanism. In a verbal older child, SCIWORA can initially be manifested as mild transient neurologic

**BOX 23.2 Unique Characteristics of the Pediatric Cervical Spine**

Incomplete ossification of the posterior elements
Physiologic C1-C2 widening
Predental space should not exceed 5 mm in children (3 mm in adults)
Pseudosubluxation at C2-C3 and C3-C4 (see Fig. 23.1)
Hypermobility or ligamentous laxity of the intervertebral ligaments
Horizontal orientation of the facet joints, which allows increased mobility and leads to:
- Loss of normal lordosis
- Pseudosubluxation of C2 on C3
- Spinal cord injury without radiographic abnormalities

Accentuated prevertebral soft tissue spaces, which should not exceed two thirds of the C2 body
Portions of the vertebra are radiolucent or wedge-shaped up to 8 years, which leads to widened disk spaces and anterior wedging
Anatomic fulcrum in children younger than 8 years between C1 and C3:
- Most injuries occur in the upper cervical spine
- After age 8, the anatomic fulcrum is between C5 and C6

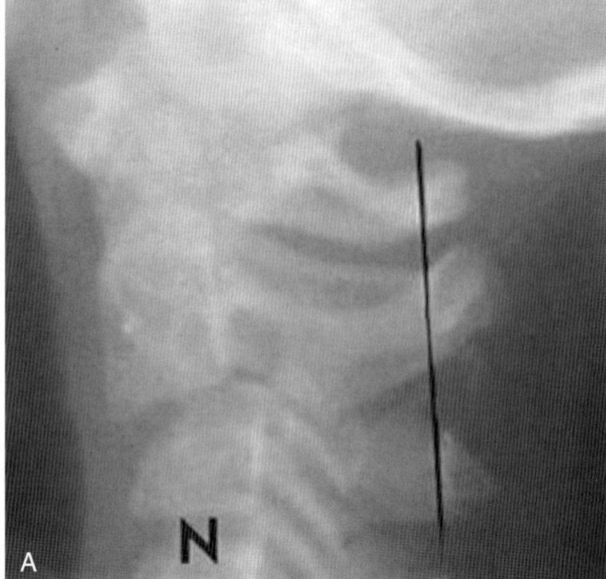


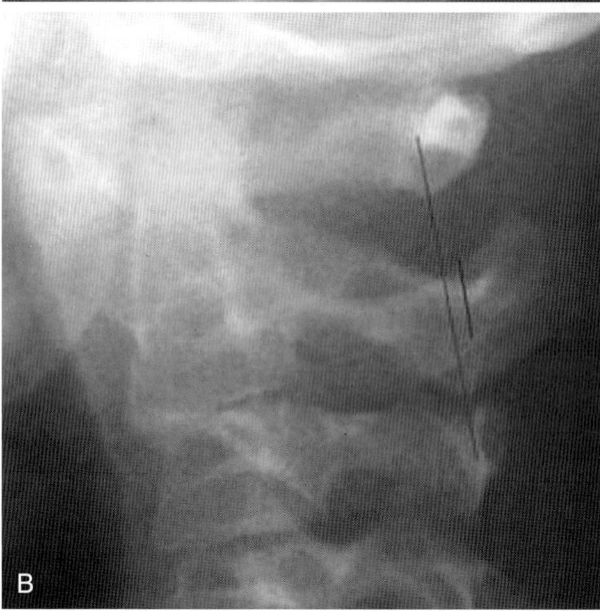


**Fig. 23.1 Radiographs showing pseudosubluxation of the cervical spine.** The clinician should draw a line through the cortices of the spinous processes of C1 and C3. If the cortex of the spinous process of C2 is more than 1.5 mm off this line (line of Swischuk), a fracture or ligamentous injury should be suspected. **A,** Normal cervical spine with pseudosubluxation. Note that the line of Swischuk is straight but the anterior and posterior spinal lines have step-offs. **B,** The cortex of the spinal process of C2 is less than 1.5 mm off the line of Swischuk.

complaints. Heightened awareness of this phenomenon is needed so that the treating physician can take the necessary steps for diagnosis and treatment.

## DIAGNOSTIC TESTING

### PLAIN RADIOGRAPHS

The two studies most widely used to predict cervical spine injury, the Canadian C-Spine Study and the National Emergency X-Radiography Utilization Study, did not target the pediatric population.[9] Though still requiring prospective validation, the Pediatric Emergency Care Applied Research Network (PECARN) recently published an eight-variable model for predicting pediatric cervical spine injury: altered mental status, focal neurologic findings, neck pain, torticollis, substantial torso injury, congenital conditions predisposing to cervical spine injury, diving, and high-risk motor vehicle crash. The presence of one or more of these factors was 98% sensitive and 26% specific for cervical spine injury[10] (**Boxes 23.3 and 23.4**).

Flexion and extension radiographs of the cervical spine are not used in the acute management phase of children in the ED.

**BOX 23.3 PECARN Data: Indications for Cervical Spine Radiography in Children**

Altered mental status
Focal neurologic deficit
Complaint of neck pain (age > 2 years)
Torticollis
Conditions known to predispose to cervical spine injury*
Substantial injury to the torso (clavicles, abdomen, flanks, back including the spine, and pelvis)
High-risk motor vehicle crash (head-on collision, rollover, ejection from a vehicle, death in the same crash, or speed > 55 mph)
Diving mechanism

From Leonard JC, Kupperman N, Olsen C, et al, for The Pediatric Emergency Care Applied Research Network. Factors associated with cervical spine injury in children after blunt trauma. Ann Emerg Med 2011;58:145-55.
*PECARN*, Pediatric Emergency Care Applied Research Network.
*Down syndrome, Klippel-Feil syndrome, achondrodysplasia, mucopolysaccharidosis, Ehlers-Danlos syndrome, Marfan syndrome, osteogenesis imperfecta, Larsen syndrome, juvenile rheumatoid arthritis, juvenile ankylosing spondylitis, renal osteodystrophy, rickets, history of CSI or cervical spine surgery.

**BOX 23.4 Tips for Reading Cervical Spine Radiographs in Children**

Look for compression or widening of the intervertebral spaces.
Widening of the prevertebral soft tissue space should not be greater than one third to one half the width of the adjacent vertebral body in C1-C4 and not greater than a full vertebral body width for C5-C7.
Radiographs may be repeated with adequate inspiratory breath and neck positioning (not in flexion).

### COMPUTED TOMOGRAPHY

Evidence is mounting that patients with a high-risk mechanism of injury, such as a fall from a height or a high-speed motor vehicle collision, should undergo CT evaluation of the cervical spine.

### MAGNETIC RESONANCE IMAGING

To exclude the possibility of SCIWORA, any history of transient neurologic dysfunction requires extended observation or MRI, even if findings on plain radiography are normal.

## TREATMENT AND DISPOSITION

Immobilization with a cervical collar is required for any child with a cervical injury. When such an injury is diagnosed, emergency consultation with a pediatric spine surgeon and admission of the patient to the hospital are mandatory. Though still somewhat controversial, there is no evidence to recommend the use of high-dose methylprednisolone in the treatment of pediatric spinal cord lesions with neurologic deficits after blunt trauma.[9]

# PEDIATRIC THORACIC TRAUMA

**KEY POINTS**

- Respiratory distress or hypoxemia should prompt a thorough radiographic evaluation.
- Gastric decompression should be performed early in any child with respiratory distress or hypoxemia.

## PERSPECTIVE

Trauma involving the chest is the second leading cause of death from trauma in children. The majority of cases are the result of blunt mechanisms. Associated injury is the most important mortality factor. The death rate from isolated chest trauma in children is 5%, whereas that from abdominal and chest trauma is 20% and that from trauma involving the head, chest, and abdomen is 39%.[11]

## ANATOMY AND PATHOPHYSIOLOGY

The thorax of a child is smaller and more compliant than that of an adult. Because children's bones are less dense and less rigid, less force is required for intrathoracic injury. Associated abdominal, pelvic, and head injuries are relatively common, and the clinician should suspect concomitant abdominal injuries in victims of chest trauma until proved otherwise. Infants and toddlers depend on diaphragmatic breathing, and therefore respiratory depression can develop if mobility of the diaphragm is impaired. In children, the ratio of oxygen consumption to mass is high and functional residual capacity is lower, thereby putting them at risk for sudden respiratory failure and rapid oxygen desaturations with little to no warning.

## CLINICAL PRESENTATION

Patients with major thoracic injuries frequently have significant chest pain, respiratory distress, disordered chest and abdominal movement, hypoxemia, or hemodynamic compromise. They may also exhibit chest deformity, flail chest, crepitus, decreased breath sounds, or sucking chest wounds.

**BOX 23.5 Most Common and Most Lethal Injuries Involving the Chest in Children**

**Most Common**
Pulmonary contusion
Rib fractures
Pneumothorax
Hemothorax
Cardiac injury
Great-vessel injury
Diaphragmatic injury

**Most Lethal**
Great-vessel injury
Cardiac injury
Hemothorax
Rib fracture

**BOX 23.6 Indications for Computed Tomography of Chest in Pediatric Trauma**

Wide mediastinum on a chest radiograph
Thoracic spine fracture
Superior rib fracture
Abnormal lung fields
Unexplained hypotension or hypoxemia
New cardiac murmur or carotid bruit
Asymmetric pulses or blood pressure

Thoracic injuries account for 5% to 12% of admissions to pediatric trauma centers,[12] but many children evaluated for chest trauma in the ED have much more subtle findings (**Box 23.5**). Children with chest pain, dyspnea, altered mental status, tachypnea, retractions, hypoxemia, shock, multiple-system trauma, or concern because of a high-risk mechanism should be evaluated for thoracic trauma. Injuries may occur in isolation or in combination with other thoracic or extrathoracic problems. Significant injuries may be present with little or no external evidence.

## DIAGNOSTIC TESTING

### CHEST RADIOGRAPHY

A chest radiograph is the most useful test in the evaluation of suspected chest trauma, although it is not as sensitive as CT scanning for many diagnoses, such as rib fracture, sternal fracture, pneumothorax, hemothorax, pulmonary contusion, and great-vessel injury. A chest radiograph should be obtained to confirm endotracheal position, identify intrathoracic causes of hypotension, exclude pneumothorax in patients with suggestive signs or symptoms (e.g., respiratory distress, crepitus, tenderness), or evaluate for external evidence of thoracic trauma.[13]

### COMPUTED TOMOGRAPHY OF THE CHEST

The best test to define the extent of intrathoracic injury is CT. For evaluation of great-vessel injury, CT angiography has largely replaced angiography (**Box 23.6**).

## SPECIFIC INJURIES

### RIB FRACTURES

Rib fractures are less common in children than in adults. The compliance of a child's rib cage allows transfer of strong force to the internal organs before fracture. Half of significant intrathoracic injuries in children occur without a rib fracture. Mortality rises with the number of fractures. Rib fracture, particularly posterior and multiple ones in a young infant, should raise suspicion for nonaccidental trauma. Flail rib segments, or three or more ribs broken in a segmental fashion, can lead to serious respiratory compromise. The clinician should manage pain aggressively, and early intubation should be considered in a child with flail chest or multiple rib fractures. Otherwise, treatment is supportive. In addition to parenteral pain medication, intercostal nerve block and epidural anesthesia can be effective.

### PULMONARY CONTUSION

Pulmonary contusion occurs in up to 71% of children with thoracic injuries.[14] Because of the increased compliance of the rib cage in children, force is transferred directly to the lung parenchyma. Parenchymal hemorrhage and edema lead to alveolar collapse and disorders of gas exchange. Contusions large enough to impair respiratory function may occur without any external signs of trauma. Contusions may be immediately visible on chest radiographs or have a delayed appearance. The radiographic appearance of a pulmonary contusion ranges from minimal hazy opacity to a diffuse, dense infiltrate. The sensitivity of chest radiography for detection of pulmonary contusion was 67% in one study that used CT of the chest as the "gold standard." Contusions not visible on chest radiographs were not clinically significant and did not require a change in management.[15] Treatment of pulmonary contusion consists of pain control, pulmonary toilet, and mechanical ventilation when appropriate.

### PNEUMOTHORAX

Though spontaneous at times, pneumothorax occurs primarily in children as a result of trauma. Signs and symptoms are pain, dyspnea, hemoptysis, tachypnea, retractions, hypoxemia, decreased breath sounds, and tympany. The clinician should also consider pneumothorax in the setting of chest wall abrasion, contusion, laceration, wound, or deformity. Auscultatory lung examination is unreliable because the small chest cavity in children transmits breath sounds easily even in the presence of pneumothorax. Because of the mobile pediatric mediastinum, tension pneumothorax can result in rapid cardiovascular and ventilatory collapse.

The primary screening examination is a chest radiograph, performed with the patient supine if the cervical spine has not been determined to be uninjured. It is an insensitive test for pneumothorax, with some estimates of sensitivity as low as 20% to 60%.[16] An upright chest radiograph should be performed if possible. CT of the chest is extremely sensitive for the detection of pneumothorax, even very small ones that may need no intervention. Abdominal CT may demonstrate pneumothorax, but patients with pneumothorax detected only by this modality uncommonly need tube thoracostomy (**Table 23.2**).[14] In adults, bedside ultrasonography has been shown to be comparable in specificity but more sensitive than chest radiography for the detection of traumatic pneumothorax.[17]

**Table 23.2 Treatment of Pneumothorax**

| SIZE | TREATMENT |
|---|---|
| More than 20% of the pleural space | Tube thoracostomy |
| Less than 20% of the pleural space | High-flow oxygen<br>Observation<br>Second chest radiograph in 3-6 hr<br>Tube thoracostomy if mechanical ventilation or air transport is required |

Data from Weissberg D, Refaely Y. Pneumothorax: experience with 1,199 patients. Chest 2000;117:1279–85.

### DIAPHRAGMATIC INJURY

Injury to the diaphragm may result from either penetrating trauma or, more commonly, a major blunt injury to the abdomen, such as a fall from a height, a crush injury, or a high-speed motor vehicle collision. Diaphragmatic injury is uncommon in children and occurs in about 3% of victims of blunt abdominal trauma. Patients may be asymptomatic, may have chest or abdominal pain, or may initially be seen with respiratory failure and shock.

The diagnosis of diaphragmatic injury is difficult. If significant abdominal contents have herniated into the thorax, the diaphragmatic injury may be diagnosed on screening chest radiography. Overall, sensitivity rates for both chest radiography and chest CT are not good. Sensitivity rates for CT of the chest in detecting blunt diaphragmatic rupture have been reported to be 42% to 90%. One study found that diaphragmatic injury was correctly diagnosed on admission in only 50% of patients admitted to a level I trauma center.[18] Diagnostic peritoneal lavage (DPL) may have some utility in detecting diaphragmatic injury, although it is performed less frequently today than previously. Its sensitivity has been reported to be 80% in a selected population, although it is not specific. Because of the pressure differential between the abdomen and thorax, any missed defect in the diaphragm will continue to enlarge until it is repaired surgically.

### CARDIAC CONTUSION

A patient with a cardiac contusion may complain of chest pain or palpitations. External findings are sternal fracture, rib fracture, chest contusion, and sometimes no signs of trauma. The most common dysrhythmia is sinus tachycardia. The patient is unlikely to have complications if the findings on electrocardiography (ECG) are normal and the troponin level is normal over a 6- to 12-hour period of observation. In one study of pediatric blunt cardiac injury, no hemodynamically stable patient with a normal sinus rhythm subsequently demonstrated a cardiac arrhythmia or cardiac failure.[19] Use of any changes on ECG, including sinus tachycardia, bradycardia, conduction delays, and atrial or ventricular dysrhythmias, can provide a sensitivity of 100%, a specificity of 47%, and a negative predictive value of 90% for the detection of complications related to blunt cardiac injury that require treatment.

Several prospective series have demonstrated that if admission ECG displays normal sinus rhythm, the risk for development of cardiac complications related to blunt cardiac injury is extremely small.[20,21]

### COMMOTIO CORDIS

Commotio cordis resulting from blunt chest trauma that caused cardiac arrest has been reported to occur in children. The clinician should apply the normal pediatric advanced life support algorithm for treatment. Commotio cordis may or may not respond to treatment.

### TRAUMATIC ASPHYXIA

Traumatic asphyxia is unique to children. Findings include cervical and facial petechiae or cyanosis with vascular engorgement and subconjunctival hemorrhage. The syndrome is secondary to blunt, compressing thoracic trauma with airway obstruction and retrograde high pressure in the superior vena cava. Central nervous system injuries, pulmonary contusions, and intraabdominal injuries are commonly associated with thoracic injuries. Despite the dramatic manifestation of traumatic asphyxia, the overall prognosis is good for patients who arrive at the ED with normal vital signs.

## DISPOSITION

Children with significant thoracic trauma are admitted to the hospital after the trauma surgery team has been consulted. In centers where pediatric trauma care is unavailable, transfer to a pediatric trauma center is recommended. A child with an isolated rib fracture and a small pneumothorax who is stable on chest radiography after 4 to 6 hours of observation or in whom a suspected myocardial contusion has been ruled out may be discharged. Any child with suspected child abuse should receive a thorough evaluation and be considered for hospital admission. Police and child protective services should be contacted to investigate, and hospital social workers should be involved.

# PEDIATRIC ABDOMINAL TRAUMA

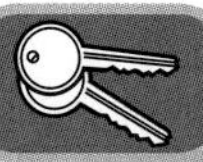

**KEY POINTS**

- Abdominal trauma is the third leading cause of traumatic death in children.
- Most intraabdominal injuries are the result of blunt trauma.
- Missed intraabdominal injuries are a leading cause of preventable death.
- Children in whom intraabdominal injury is suspected are admitted to a pediatric trauma center.
- Most injuries to solid organs are managed nonoperatively.

## PERSPECTIVE

Motor vehicle accidents are the leading cause of abdominal trauma, although falls, sports accidents, and child abuse account for a significant number of injuries. Children struck by motor vehicles or who as motor vehicle passengers are not properly restrained or are ejected are at increased risk. Blunt trauma accounts for 90% of all pediatric injuries.[22] Missed intraabdominal injury in the setting of blunt abdominal trauma is a leading cause of preventable mortality and morbidity in children.

## ANATOMY AND PATHOPHYSIOLOGY

The abdomen of a child is smaller than that of an adult, so forces are distributed over a smaller area. Children have less adipose tissue than adults do, and the muscular layers of the child's abdomen are thinner and weaker. External forces are transmitted efficiently to abdominal organs. In children found to have intraabdominal injuries, multiple-organ injury is common. Injuries to solid organs, such as the liver, spleen, pancreas, and kidneys, may result in significant hemorrhage. Hollow viscus injuries rarely result in hemodynamic compromise and are more challenging to diagnose in the ED. Injury to the inferior ribs, lumbar spine, or pelvis should raise suspicion for intraabdominal injury.

## CLINICAL PRESENTATION

Children with abdominal injuries may exhibit abdominal pain, vomiting, distention, or abdominal tenderness; however, they may also have none of these findings. Intraabdominal injuries should be strongly suspected in children with altered mental status, hemodynamic instability, respiratory distress, or injury to multiple systems. Head injuries, fractures, and even significant soft tissue injuries should be considered distracting injuries in children. A thorough abdominal evaluation should be performed in children suspected of sustaining abdominal trauma. It is important to remember that significant intraabdominal injury can occur in children without any external evidence of trauma. An example is a child who sustains a handlebar injury to the abdomen at normal bicycling speed. Such a child may have a completely transected pancreas and torn duodenum and yet have no external signs of trauma.

Abdominal trauma in children is a challenge to evaluate and manage, even in the setting of hard evidence of intraabdominal injury (e.g., positive FAST findings). Most children with blunt trauma do not have intraabdominal injury, and most of those with solid organ injury do not require surgery. Serious injuries commonly occur in the setting of high-risk mechanisms, but they also occur in what may initially be reported as minor trauma. Identification of injuries in preverbal children or those who do not have normal mental status is difficult. A high index of suspicion is required, even in a stable patient. The clinician should pay particular attention to injuries from an automobile lap belt or bicycle handlebar.

In a patient with free fluid in the abdomen, the physician should start with a bolus of crystalloid solution. If the patient is stabilized and does not have other threats to life or limb,

CT of the abdomen and pelvis should be performed immediately to identify and grade the injury.

## DIAGNOSTIC TESTING

### LABORATORY VALUES

Routinely ordering a full "trauma panel" of laboratory tests is not recommended for a child with abdominal trauma.[23] In a hypotensive patient, blood typing plus cross-matching is the most important laboratory test to order early. In patients with a low risk for intraabdominal injury, urinalysis may be the only test with relatively high diagnostic yield. Few consistent data are available to support a recommendation for which laboratory tests to order for screening of children with low- to moderate-risk trauma for the presence of intraabdominal injury. In children with blunt abdominal trauma, Holmes et al. recently validated a six-variable prediction rule (94% sensitive and 37% specific) for indentifying intraabdominal injuries: low age-adjusted systolic blood pressure, abdominal tenderness, elevated hepatic enzymes (aspartate transaminase > 200 U/L or alanine transaminase > 125 U/L), urinalysis with more than five red blood cells per high-power field, initial hematocrit lower than 30%, and the presence of a femoral fracture.[24]

### FOCUSED ABDOMINAL ULTRASONOGRAPHY FOR TRAUMA

The sensitivity of FAST in pediatric trauma is 55% to 82%.[25-28] Its utility is higher in unstable patients. The finding of free fluid on FAST in stable pediatric patients rarely leads to operative management. The vast majority of children with such findings are observed and discharged with some restrictions in activity and appropriate return precautions. For this reason, an argument can be made that abdominal ultrasonography is less useful in pediatric trauma. One study found that using ultrasonography as a triage tool can reduce the cost of pediatric abdominal evaluation.[29] Ultrasound allows the clinician to quickly identify significant intraperitoneal fluid that would require further evaluation and possible laparotomy. In this study, children with positive ultrasonographic findings who showed a response to initial fluid resuscitation underwent abdominal CT, and unstable patients underwent laparotomy. This approach allowed a major reduction in the number of CT scans performed. It has also been suggested but not proved that FAST, aside from being a screening tool, is sufficient for evaluation of the majority of children sustaining blunt abdominal trauma.

### COMPUTED TOMOGRAPHY

Abdominal CT should be performed in any stable patient in whom intraabdominal injury is suspected or to type and grade the injury in a patient with a positive FAST finding. Intravenous administration of a contrast agent is sufficient, and oral administration is not necessary (**Box 23.7**).[30] CT findings allow the inpatient trauma service to select the appropriate level of inpatient care and monitoring for the patient.[31] Although CT is excellent for evaluating solid organ injury, it is less sensitive for mesenteric, intestinal, and diaphragmatic injuries. If these latter injuries are suspected, further evaluation, such as admission to the hospital, serial abdominal examinations, and laboratory tests, are indicated.[32] There are drawbacks to the routine performance of CT in any child in whom intraabdominal injury is suspected after trauma. CT is expensive, requires transport away from the direct caregiving environment, and may necessitate sedation of the child. In addition, computed risk estimates now suggest that CT may impose a higher lifetime risk for radiation-induced cancer in children than in adults.[33] Use of the six-variable prediction rule by Holmes et al. (described earlier) has the potential to reduce unnecessary CT examinations by 30%.

**BOX 23.7 Indications for Computed Tomography of the Abdomen in Pediatric Trauma**

- Abdominal pain
- Distracting injury accompanied by suspicion of abdominal trauma
- Altered mental status
- Hemodynamic instability without an identifiable source
- Abdominal tenderness
- Seat belt sign
- Inferior rib fractures
- Thoracolumbar spine fractures
- Pelvic fractures
- Gross hematuria

### DIAGNOSTIC PERITONEAL LAVAGE

Although it has fallen out of favor with the increasing availability of CT and ultrasonography, DPL still plays a role in the management of abdominal trauma. This procedure has excellent sensitivity for intraabdominal injury and may be of value in unstable pediatric trauma patients with suspected intraabdominal injury. DPL is also useful in the evaluation of children with penetrating injury to the abdomen, particularly in stable patients in whom a bowel injury is suspected that would not be well evaluated with either FAST or CT of the abdomen.

## SPECIFIC INJURIES

Penetrating injuries to the abdomen must be evaluated by a surgeon. If the wound is suspected of violating the abdominal fascia, surgical exploration is the standard of care.

Blunt injuries to the abdomen may cause a variety of internal damage, and a high index of suspicion is therefore required in their evaluation.

The seat belt sign refers to ecchymoses, abrasions, or erythema caused by restraint by the seat belt across the abdomen during a motor vehicle accident.[34] Its presence carries an increased risk for intraabdominal injuries, particularly to the intestines and pancreas. Proper, age-appropriate restraint of a child in an automobile is extremely important. Proper seat belt use does not increase the risk for injury, but use of just a lap belt does change the spectrum of injury.[35] Other injuries associated with the use of lap belts are facial fractures and lumbar spine fractures termed Chance fractures.

Solid organ injuries include injuries to the liver, spleen, kidneys, and pancreas. Findings on FAST may or may not be positive in the presence of a solid organ injury. Injuries that are the result of blunt trauma are increasingly being managed nonoperatively in stable patients. In unstable patients, resuscitation with crystalloid solution followed by the administration of blood is attempted. If the patient's condition stabilizes, nonoperative management may still be appropriate, as determined by the pediatric trauma surgeon who has seen and evaluated the patient. Unstable patients in whom FAST demonstrates free fluid in the abdomen go directly to surgery. Even if nonoperative management is the plan, admission to a pediatric trauma center, usually to an intensive care unit for at least the first 24 hours, is required.

Hollow viscus injury may occur with penetrating or blunt trauma. In penetrating trauma, enterotomy may occur when a missile or sharp object passes directly through the intestine. In blunt trauma, a portion of a viscus, such as the sigmoid or the duodenum, may be crushed against the retroperitoneum and could rupture. A portion of a viscus may rupture from sudden increases in intraabdominal pressure or may be torn by being swung forcefully on the mesentery with a sudden deceleration.

Mesenteric injuries may also occur with similar mechanisms. FAST findings are frequently normal in the setting of hollow viscus or mesenteric injury. CT has better sensitivity but may still miss significant hollow viscus injuries because free fluid in the abdomen or air in the peritoneum may not be visualized immediately. Even with a high index of suspicion and admission of the patient for serial examination and observation, these injuries will sometimes be missed. Patients with hollow viscus injuries are treated in the operating room, as are unstable patients with mesenteric injuries. A stable patient with a mesenteric injury may be admitted to the hospital and observed rather than undergo exploratory laparotomy.

Injuries to the bladder and urethra are uncommon in children. A child with gross hematuria and no CT evidence of kidney injury should undergo retrograde urethrography to evaluate for rupture of the bladder or a torn urethra. Injuries to the urinary collecting system require emergency evaluation by a pediatric urologist.

## DISPOSITION

Children with abdominal trauma who are suspected of having intraabdominal injury and in whom the results of ED evaluation are otherwise negative for injury are generally admitted to the hospital for observation. Children without other indications for admission and in whom abdominal CT findings are normal may be considered for discharge from the ED if they are free of pain, tolerate a regular diet, and have a responsible adult parent or guardian.

## REFERENCES

***References can be found on Expert Consult @ www.expertconsult.com.***

# 24 Pediatric Traumatic Brain Injury

*Danny G. Thomas*

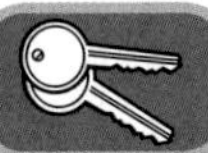

**KEY POINTS**

- Traumatic brain injury is a common pediatric problem, with mild injury being the predominant form.
- Abuse must be considered a mechanism of injury in preverbal children. Children younger than 2 years are at increased risk for skull fractures.
- Among pediatric patients with a Glasgow Coma Scale score of 14 or higher, a small number have significant intracranial injury. Guidelines can be used to identify those who are at very low risk for injury and minimize the use of computed tomography.
- Concussion is an important diagnosis to make in the emergency department setting. Appropriate discharge instructions (i.e., rest, restriction of activity, awareness of symptoms) may decrease morbidity.

## EPIDEMIOLOGY

An estimated 615,000 traumatic brain injuries (TBIs) occur each year in patients younger than 19 years; this figure accounts for 26% of pediatric hospitalizations and 15% of all pediatric deaths.[1] Children 0 to 4 years of age and older adolescents 15 to 19 years of age are most likely to sustain a TBI. Mild traumatic brain injury (mTBI), or concussion, represents the predominant form of acquired brain injury and accounts for 75% to 90% of all instances.[2,3]

## PATHOPHYSIOLOGY

The mechanisms of pediatric TBI are similar to those in adults, with falls being the most common cause. However, child abuse must be considered as an occult mechanism of head injury in preverbal children because abusive head trauma remains the most common cause of traumatic death in infancy. Findings in such patients may be subtle, with nonspecific symptoms (vomiting, fussiness) and no history of trauma. Clinicians must maintain a high index of suspicion for inflicted injury in young children. In older adolescents, sports are a common cause of concussive injury, and return to sports should be addressed in the discharge instructions.

As in adults, the pathophysiology of pediatric head trauma is related to the degree of force. With moderate force, injury can occur to the brain parenchyma, which primarily results in nonoperative lesions, or can involve vascular structures, which typically results in operative lesions.

Patients younger than 2 years are at higher risk for skull fractures, with the most common type being linear fractures. In infants, fractures may occur even after short falls (≤3 to 4 feet). The majority of fractures have an overlying hematoma or swelling; only 15% to 30% are associated with an intracranial injury.[4] In general, linear skull fractures heal without incident. Rarely, in children with open fontanelles (<2 years old) and fractures with greater than 3-mm separation, a tear in the dura allows pulsation of cerebrospinal fluid (CSF) or herniated meninges, which impedes fracture healing and extends the fracture over time.[5] This may become apparent months to years after the initial injury and usually requires surgical correction. Depressed skull fractures with greater than 5 mm of depression generally require surgical correction. Basilar skull fractures have classic findings on physical examination (raccoon eyes, Battle sign, hemotympanum) and may be associated with cranial nerve palsies (facial palsy, nystagmus, diplopia, and facial numbness), CSF rhinorrhea or otorrhea, and hearing loss.

## PRESENTING SIGNS AND SYMPTOMS

As with adults, the most predictive early indicator of outcome following head trauma is the initial Glasgow Coma Scale (GCS) score.[6] The GCS has been modified for preverbal children (**Table 24.1**). A GCS score lower than 12 defines severe TBI. A GCS score of 13 to 15 represents mild to moderate TBI.

## MEDICAL DECISION MAKING

Clinical decision making has been geared toward reducing the mortality associated with TBI. The greatest improvements in mortality occur when deterioration is prevented in those with minor head injury.

Neuroimaging has been used to identify patients at risk for deterioration following TBI, but clinicians working with pediatric populations must balance the utility of neuroimaging with the risks associated with radiation and sedation (children may require sedation to obtain a computed tomography [CT] scan). Studies suggest that the theoretic risk for fatal brain tumors increases as age at time of intracranial imaging decreases, and even though complications of sedation are rare, many children experience prolonged recovery and delayed

**Table 24.1 Modified Glasgow Coma Scale**

| | | |
|---|---|---|
| Best eye response | 1 | No response |
| | 2 | To pain only |
| | 3 | To verbal stimuli |
| | 4 | Spontaneous |
| Best verbal response | 1 | No response |
| | 2 | Moaning |
| | 3 | Inappropriate words (cries only to painful stimuli) |
| | 4 | Confused (irritable and crying) |
| | 5 | Oriented (coos and babbles) |
| Best motor response | 1 | No response |
| | 2 | Extension in response to pain (decerebrate) |
| | 3 | Flexion in response to pain (decorticate) |
| | 4 | Withdraws from pain |
| | 5 | Localizes pain |
| | 6 | Obeys commands (spontaneous movement) |

side effects.[7] Studies have found that approximately 6% of children with minor head injury have abnormal findings on CT and, more important, that less than 1% require neurosurgical intervention.[8] When compared with the adult population, pediatric patients are more likely to be seen in the ED following very mild injury, thus further lowering the pretest probability of significant intracranial injury.

Given this tendency, many studies have sought to identify criteria that would guide the use of neuroimaging in pediatric populations. A recent study by the Pediatric Emergency Care Applied Research Network (PECARN) assessed 42,000 pediatric patients to develop a decision rule.[9] For children 2 years or younger, they found that patients with abnormal mental status, non–frontal scalp hematoma, loss of consciousness, a severe mechanism of injury, and a palpable skull fracture and those who were not "acting normally" per parent could be accurately predicted to have significant intracranial injury. For patients older than 2 years, they found abnormal mental status, loss of consciousness, significant vomiting, severe mechanism of injury, clinical signs of basilar skull fracture, and severe headache predicted significant intracranial injury (**Fig. 24.1**). Use of these clinical guidelines would significantly reduce unnecessary intracranial imaging.

Observation is an alternative to neuroimaging in patients with mild injury. A retrospective Canadian study of approximately 17,000 pediatric patients older than 8 years found that delayed deterioration (>6 hours) occurred in no patients with a normal GCS score.[10] Pediatric patients are often evaluated several hours after their injury; continued observation within the department or at home would be an acceptable alternative to emergency imaging in low-risk patients.

For patients with mTBI or concussion, emergency department (ED) clinicians in general have not focused on the morbidity associated with this injury and may not recognize their ability to improve patient outcomes. It has been shown that accurate assessment of the severity of the injury and consequent outpatient guidance and management may decrease recovery time, reduce the risk for secondary complications, and improve outcomes. mTBI or concussion can also be challenging to diagnose. Patients with polytrauma or other significant injury may not be screened for the subtle findings associated with concussion, which can result from any blow to the head or an indirect force through the neck or to the body. The immediate symptoms of concussion are the result of trauma-induced alterations in neurologic function and include amnesia (retrograde or anterograde), altered consciousness (loss of consciousness, dazed, stunned, confused), migrainelike symptoms (headache, nausea, photophobia or phonophobia, visual changes, dizziness or balance problems), cognitive symptoms (difficulty concentrating or remembering), and changes in personality. These immediate symptoms are typically short-lived and are associated with a normal findings on physical examination and neuroimaging. Clinicians in the ED are in a unique position to diagnose mTBI and initiate proper management to minimize the adverse outcomes of concussion.

## TREATMENT

With severe or moderate injury, initial pediatric management is similar to adult management. The primary focus is to protect the airway, maintain hemodynamic stability, and identify patients with more significant intracranial injury. Patients with severe TBI require early consultation with a pediatric neurosurgeon or transport to a pediatric trauma center (or both). Early surgical intervention and initiation of intracranial pressure monitoring have been shown to improve long-term outcomes.

## ADMISSION AND DISCHARGE

The majority of patients with mTBI or concussion are reassured and discharged home. For these patients, appropriate diagnosis, patient education, and outpatient management may decrease recovery time, reduce the risk for secondary complications, and improve outcomes.[11] Pediatric patients with normal neuroimaging findings but persistently abnormal GCS scores, severe vomiting, or unremitting headache should be admitted to the hospital for observation and hydration.

Determining concussion severity and recovery is critical because returning patients to physical activities too soon following concussion can lead to disabling and even life-threatening outcomes such as second impact syndrome, which is the sudden onset of cerebral edema after a second (even minor) concussion. Historically, however, evaluation and management of victims of concussion have been inconsistent. To add to the confusion, more than 25 concussion grading systems exist, each with their own ranking of concussion severity and management recommendations. Unfortunately, these clinical grading systems are not validated and have not allowed clinicians, patients, or families to recognize the spectrum of postconcussive symptoms.

The Centers for Disease Control and Prevention has recently changed its recommendations for acute concussion management from the use of grading scales to use of the Acute Concussion Evaluation (ACE) (see ACE and ACE-Care Plan, available at www.cdc.gov). The ACE is a paper evaluation form that was designed to provide a diagnostic framework for

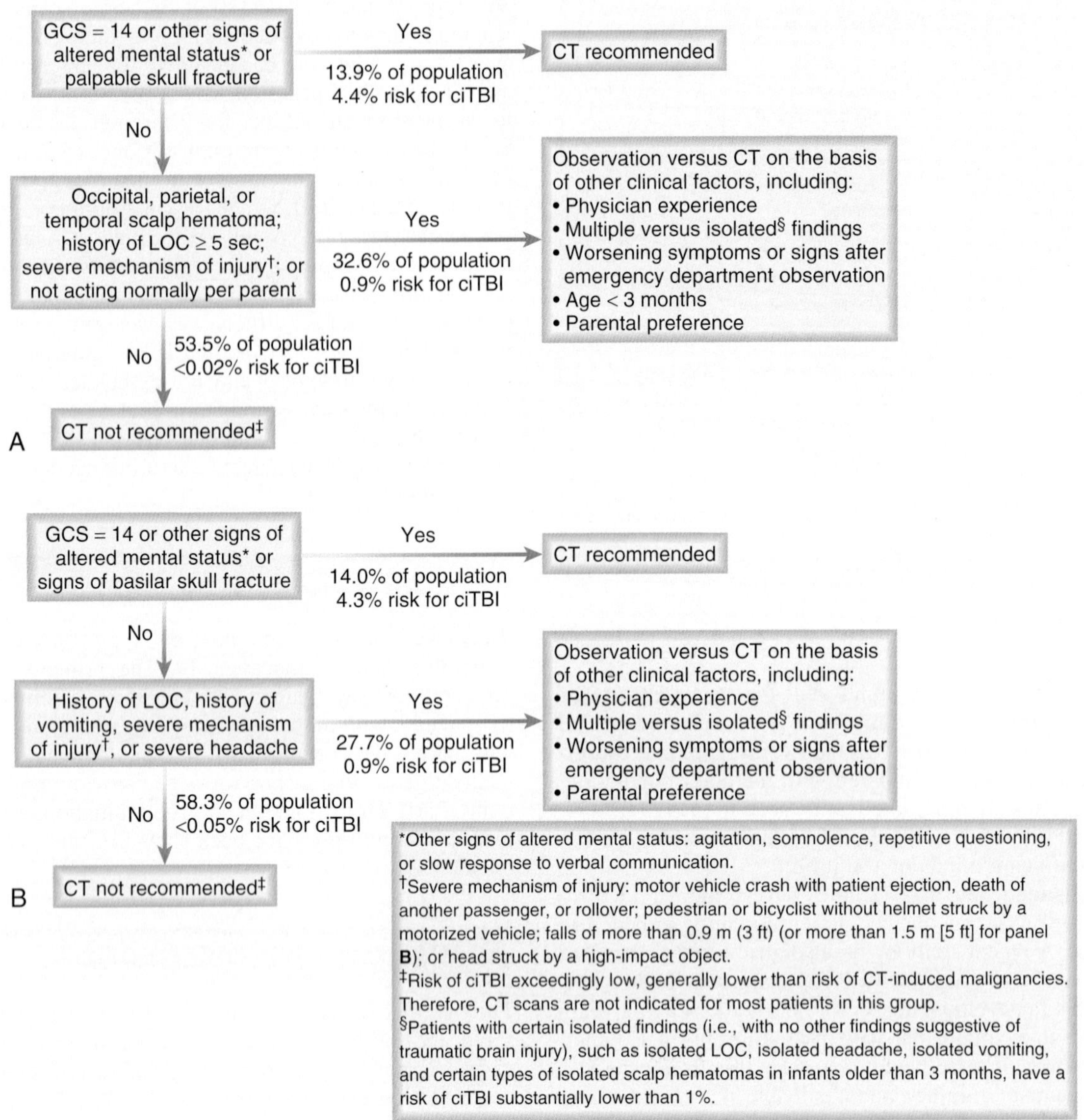


**Fig. 24.1** Suggested computed tomography (CT) algorithm for children younger than 2 years (**A**) and for those aged 2 years and older (**B**) with Glasgow Coma Scale (GCS) scores of 14 to 15 after head trauma. (From Kuppermann N, Holmes JF, Dayan PS, et al. Lancet 2009;374:1160-70.) ciTBI, clinically important traumatic brain injury; LOC, loss of consciousness.

clinicians in the outpatient setting to define concussion and characterize the patient's symptoms.[12] Rather than focus on grading assessments of concussion severity, the ACE provides a standardized tool to aid in identifying mTBI in primary care settings. Unlike grading systems that provide set return-to-play decisions (e.g., those with grade 1 concussion may return to play in 15 minutes), the ACE offers an ACE-Care Plan, a set of best-practice discharge instructions that strongly recommend rest and endorse the "Stepwise Return to Play" (**Box 24.1**). The ACE-Care Plan also offers extensive information regarding return to school and work to minimize overexertion and improve recovery. The ACE and ACE-Care Plan represent a transition from passive management to active evaluation of concussion and intervention to decrease secondary injury.

Most patients with mTBI will recover within the first 7 to 10 days. In others, postconcussive syndrome will develop, a constellation of neurocognitive symptoms (including headaches, fatigue, sleep problems, changes in personality, photophobia, hyperacusis, dizziness, and deficits in short-term memory and problem solving) that may persist for days to weeks. Athletes who suffer multiple concussions are more likely to be plagued with postconcussive symptoms. School performance may be affected in these children, and some may need specific accommodation plans. Patients at high risk for complications related to mTBI (e.g., athletes, those with previous concussions or personal history of migraines) should be evaluated by a concussion specialist.[13]

Occasionally, patients with postconcussive syndrome return to the ED for subsequent problems. In patients with waxing and waning postconcussive symptoms or migraine headache, emergency imaging is not necessary except to exclude alternative diagnoses. Postconcussive symptoms respond well to

**BOX 24.1 Stepwise Return to Play**

1. Rest until asymptomatic (no signs or symptoms at rest or with exertion)
2. Light aerobic activity (e.g., walking, stationary bike)
3. Sport-specific activity (e.g., running in soccer, skating in hockey)
4. Noncontact training drills
5. Full-contact practice training
6. Game play

If symptoms recur during any step, the patient should return to step 1. If asymptomatic, the patient may advance to the next step every 24 hours.

Adapted from McCrory P, Meeuwisse W, Johnston K, et al. Consensus statement on concussion in sport—the 3rd International Conference on Concussion in Sport, held in Zurich, November 2008. J Clm Neurosci 2009;16:755-63.

standard migraine treatment (nonsteroidal antiinflammatory drugs, intravenous fluids, antiemetics). These patients should be referred to a concussion specialist for follow-up.

## SUGGESTED READINGS

Bazarian JJ, Blyth B, Cimpello L. Bench to bedside: evidence for brain injury after concussion—looking beyond the computed tomography scan. Acad Emerg Med 2006;13:199-214.

Kuppermann N, Holmes JF, Dayan PS, et al, for the Pediatric Emergency Care Applied Research Network (PECARN). Identification of children at very low risk of clinically-important brain injuries after head trauma: a prospective cohort study. Lancet 2009;374:1160-70.

McCrory P, Meeuwisse W, Johnston K, et al. Consensus statement on concussion in sport—the 3rd International Conference on concussion in sport, held in Zurich, November 2008. J Clin Neurosci 2009;16:755-63.

## REFERENCES

*References can be found on Expert Consult @ www.expertconsult.com.*

# 25 Pediatric Orthopedic Emergencies

*Russ Horowitz*

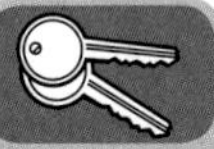

**KEY POINTS**

- Ligaments are stronger than bones in young children.
- The history should be consistent with the injury and the developmental stage of the child.
- Children are poor at localizing pain and often refer symptoms to neighboring joints. The pathologic site in knee pain may be the hip.
- Growth plate injuries are subtle but have the potential to lead to growth arrest.
- Radiographs of the contralateral side are useful as comparison views for the investigation of subtle fractures.

Pediatric musculoskeletal trauma and infections are a major cause of morbidity, including growth arrest, limb deformity, chronic pain, and arthritis. Investigation of pediatric orthopedic injuries and conditions requires knowledge and understanding of the unique childhood bony anatomy. To maximize normal growth and development, the emergency physician should be mindful of physeal injuries, bone-remodeling potential, and unique pediatric orthopedic conditions.

## RADIAL HEAD SUBLUXATION

Radial head subluxation, or nursemaid's elbow, is a common injury that affects children between the ages of 6 months and 5 years. It results from hyperextension with subluxation of the radial head and acute interposition of the annular ligament into the radiocapitellar joint. A history of longitudinal traction may not be obtained because the caretaker may not be aware of a particular event or may feel guilty about causing the child's injury. A concern about wrist or shoulder injury may be reported because inadvertent manipulation of the injured elbow caused pain.

### PRESENTING SIGNS AND SYMPTOMS

Children refuse to use the affected arm and hold it close to the body and in slight flexion. They do not appear to be in particular distress but may be fearful that examination will elicit pain. There is no tenderness with palpation or bony or soft tissue abnormality. Radiographs are unnecessary unless another particular injury is suspected. Edema and tenderness are present with supracondylar fractures.

A number of reduction techniques are used, including the hyperpronation method and the supination-flexion method. The hyperpronation method has proved more effective and appears to be less traumatic.[1] With the arm held in extension, the wrist is hyperpronated and a click is sometimes heard. In the supination-flexion approach the examiner places the thumb of one hand over the radial head and provides countertraction. Next, while holding the wrist, the elbow is pulled into extension. The final phase is supination and flexion at the elbow. Most children return to full functioning within 15 minutes, and the child should be observed until full range of motion is regained.

When multiple reductions fail, radiography should be considered. In a child with failed reduction and negative radiographic findings, a sling or posterior splint is necessary with close orthopedic follow-up.

## FRACTURES

Trauma to immature and incompletely ossified bones results in unique pediatric orthopedic injuries, including torus, greenstick, bowing, and physeal fractures. These patterns do not occur in dense adult bone. Because the radiographic findings of some of these abnormalities are incredibly subtle, comparison views are particularly helpful. Trauma that would result in sprains and strains in structurally mature individuals causes the thick periosteum to be torn from the bony cortex and resultant avulsion fractures. Ligamentous tears are uncommon in children because their ligaments are stronger than the neighboring bones.

Children's bones are apt to bend with a fracture on only one side of the periosteum. Callus formation and remodeling are extensive in pediatric injuries and contribute to the faster healing found in children. The goal of reduction should always be nearly perfect alignment, and growing bones have a dramatic potential for spontaneous correction.

Pediatric bones are less dense and therefore more prone to compression or bending when an axial load is applied. Falls onto an outstretched arm may result in torus or buckle fractures (**Fig. 25.1**). Greenstick fractures are incomplete, with the cortex remaining intact on one surface. To obtain complete

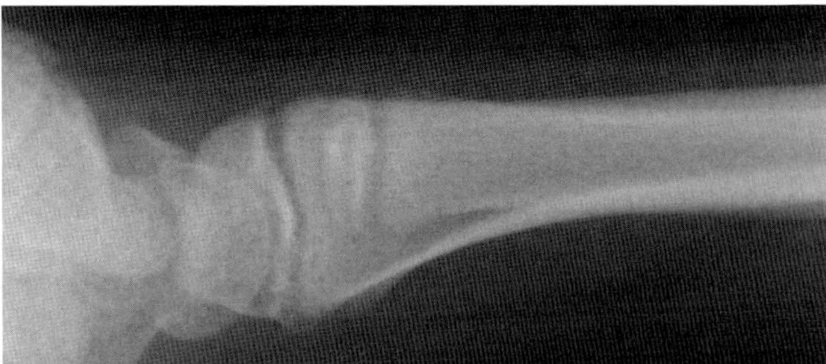

**Fig. 25.1** Torus fracture of the distal end of the radius.

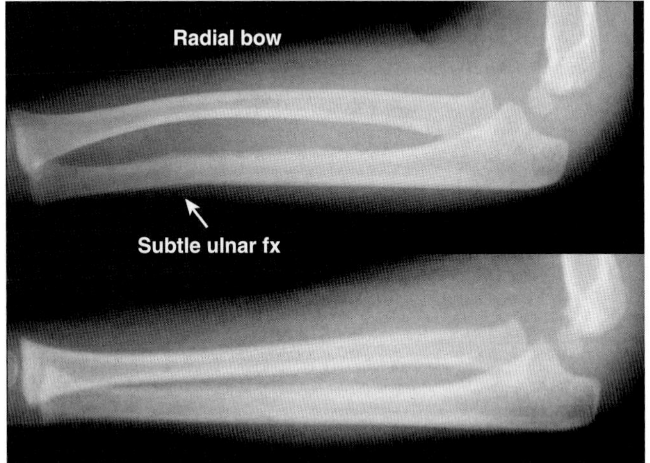


**Fig. 25.2** Radial bowing fracture with the normal contralateral side shown for comparison.

reduction, completion of the fracture is necessary. Bowing fractures result when the force is insufficient to cause a complete break but results in deformation of the osseous structure (**Fig. 25.2**). Cosmetic deformity and functional abnormality will result without complete reduction. Repair is often difficult because both cortices remain intact.

The physis or growth plate is a weak area of cartilage present in developing bone. Trauma that causes strains or joint dislocations in skeletally mature individuals frequently results in growth plate fractures in children. Anatomic alignment of such fractures is critical for optimal growth.

## SALTER-HARRIS CLASSIFICATION OF FRACTURES

The most commonly used system to identify physeal injuries is the Salter-Harris classification. Fractures are categorized as types I through V, with the higher numbers having the greater risk for growth abnormalities. All such injuries require pediatric orthopedic follow-up.[2]

Type I fractures result from a longitudinal force through the physis that splits the epiphysis from the metaphysis. Radiographs may reveal a widened growth plate. Identification can be difficult, particularly when the displacement is minimal, and a fracture should be suspected in children with tenderness along the physis even in the absence of radiologic findings. Type I fractures rarely result in growth disturbances and can be treated effectively with immobilization.

Type II fractures, the most common type, occur when a piece of the metaphysis remains attached to the epiphysis

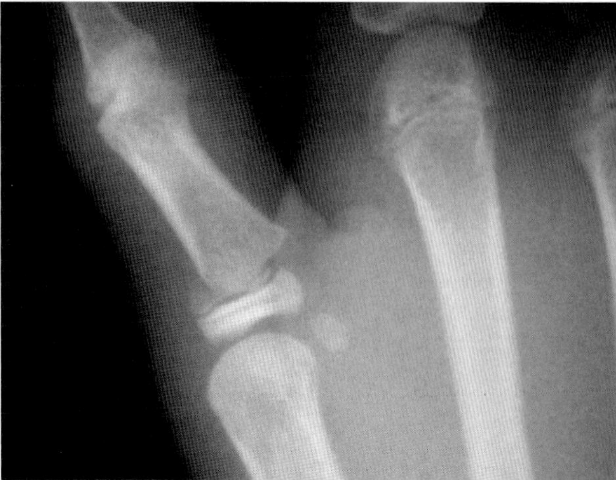

**Fig. 25.3** Type II Salter-Harris fracture at the metacarpophalangeal joint of the thumb.

(**Fig. 25.3**). They require splinting and generally carry a good prognosis. Types III and IV are intraarticular fractures that also involve the growth plate. In a type III injury, the fracture line extends through the epiphysis into the physis. In type IV, the fracture passes through the epiphysis, physis, and metaphysis. Types III and IV carry a risk for growth retardation, altered joint mechanics, and functional impairment and thus require urgent orthopedic evaluation. Type V fractures are compression injuries and are difficult to visualize on radiographs. The diagnosis is often made retrospectively following a case of growth arrest.

## TODDLER'S FRACTURES

Toddler's fractures are nondisplaced oblique or spiral fractures through the distal end of the tibia. Questioning may not reveal any significant injury, just that the child might refuse to bear weight after a day playing at the park. Findings on physical examination can range from entirely benign to diffuse tenderness along the tibial shaft. The absence of edema and ecchymosis is commonplace and not surprising. Gentle twisting of the lower part of the leg may elicit pain as the fracture plane is opened. Radiographic findings are subtle, and multiple views, including anteroposterior (AP), lateral, and oblique images, may be necessary. In the event of negative findings, a bone scan may be considered.

If the symptoms persist, one may choose to repeat the films in 7 to 10 days to look for new subperiosteal bone formation. Immobilization is sufficient to promote healing. When the child limps and radiographic findings are negative, a fracture or injury in another location should be considered. Varied pathology, including appendicitis, toxic synovitis, septic arthritis, foot and ankle fractures, soft tissue injuries, and abuse (**Box 25.1**), may all be manifested as a limp in a toddler.

## SUPRACONDYLAR FRACTURES

Supracondylar fractures are the most frequent elbow fractures in children and often occur in children 3 to 10 years of age. The most common mechanism is a fall onto an outstretched hand with the elbow hyperextended.

Classification of the types of supracondylar fractures is based on the extent of the injury: type I is nondisplaced (**Fig. 25.4**), type II is displaced posteriorly with an intact cortex

**BOX 25.1 Fractures Suggesting Abuse***

Multiple fractures, especially in various stages of healing
Fracture patterns inconsistent with the history
Fractures coexistent with soft tissue injuries consistent with abuse
Metaphyseal chip fractures
Lower-extremity fractures in nonambulatory children
Spiral fractures of the humerus
Multiple depressed skull fractures
Rib fractures, especially multiple posterior fractures

Data from Belfer RA, Klein BL, Orr L. Use of the skeletal survey in the evaluation of child maltreatment. Am J Emerg Med 2001;19:122-4.
*A skeletal survey should be done in all cases of suspected abuse.

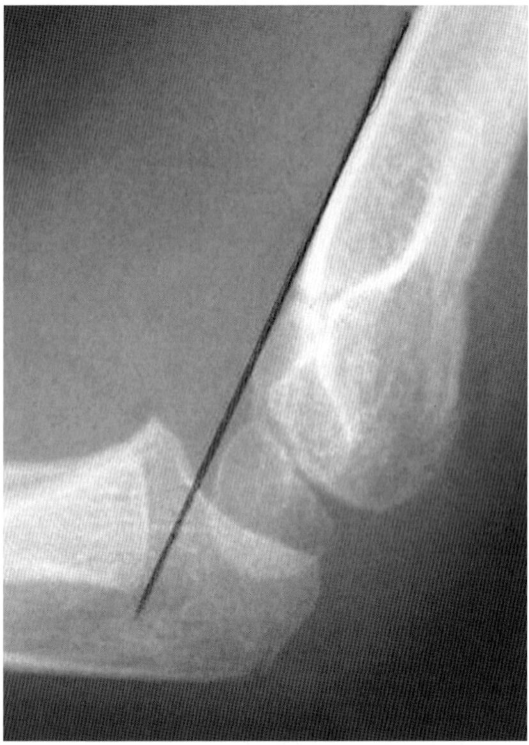

**Fig. 25.4 Type I supracondylar fracture.** The anterior humeral line does not intersect with the capitellum. A subtle fracture is visible along the anterior surface of the humerus.

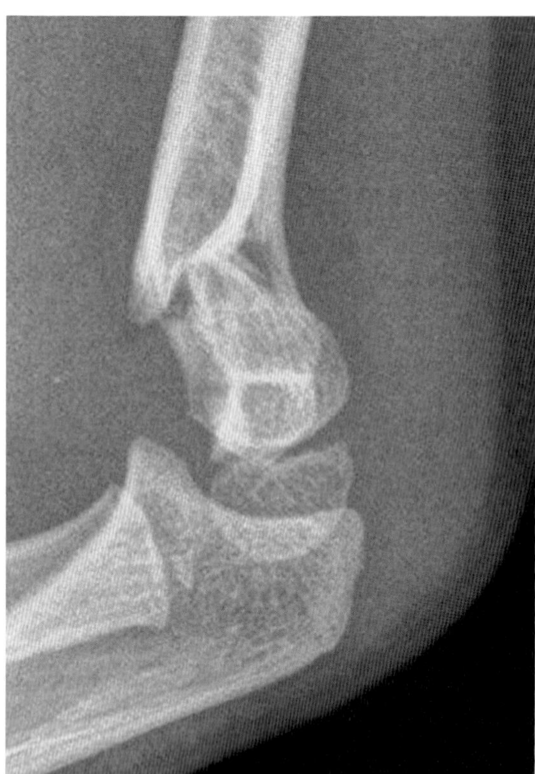

**Fig. 25.5 Type II supracondylar fracture.**

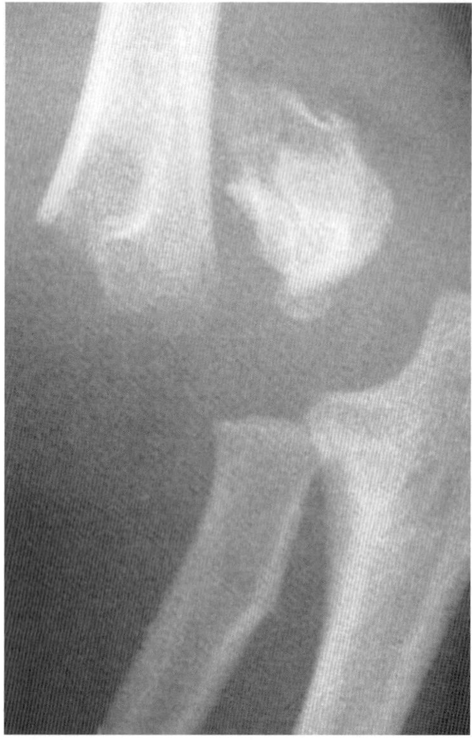

**Fig. 25.6 Type III supracondylar fracture.**

(**Fig. 25.5**), and type III is completely displaced with no cortical contact (**Fig. 25.6**). Type I injuries are managed by immobilization for 4 to 6 weeks. Treatment of type II injuries is based on the extent of the damage, and an orthopedist should be consulted. More severe cases require admission, reduction, and internal fixation, but milder cases may be treated as type I injuries. All type III fractures require closed reduction with pinning in the operating room.

Radiographic findings may be subtle, particularly in type I injuries (**Box 25.2**). When a fracture line cannot be visualized easily, other findings may assist in making the diagnosis. A posterior fat pad or joint effusion located dorsal to the distal end of the humerus at the level of the olecranon fossa is always pathologic and evidence of a fracture. An anterior fat pad is normal unless it is lifted up and squared off inferiorly into a "sail sign." A line drawn along the anterior surface of the humerus should intersect the capitellum in its middle third. Posterior displacement of the distal end of the humerus will cause the line to fall further anteriorly or miss the capitellum entirely.

**BOX 25.2 Radiographic Evidence of Supracondylar Fractures**

Direct fracture visualization
Posterior fat pad
Sail sign
Joint effusion
Malalignment of the anterior humeral line

With more severe injuries, the difficulty is not in making the diagnosis but rather recognition and reduction of complications. Morbidity includes range-of-motion abnormalities, neurovascular compromise, and long-term deformities. A thorough examination and documentation of neurovascular status, pain control, and stabilization are mandatory. The limb should be splinted in the deformed position. Motor and sensory function of the median, ulnar, and radial nerves is at risk. Direct vascular injury is uncommon, but because a potential for compartment syndrome does exist, examinations should be repeated frequently and recorded.[3]

## SLIPPED CAPITAL FEMORAL EPIPHYSIS

A slipped capital femoral epiphysis affects boys twice as commonly as girls. In most children the condition is diagnosed early in their growth spurt, with boys being affected at 13 to 15 years and girls at 11 to 13 years of age (because of girls' earlier onset of pubertal development). Obesity is a risk factor, but slipped capital femoral epiphysis develops in many average-sized children.

### PRESENTING SIGNS AND SYMPTOMS

Pain and limp are the most common reasons for seeking care in the emergency department, and symptoms may have been present for weeks to months. Pain, which can range from dull and intermittent to severe and persistent, can be present in the hip or referred to the knee, groin, or anterior aspect of the thigh. Sometimes a history of trivial trauma prompts medical evaluation. Physical examination reveals a hip in flexion with mild external rotation. Range of motion is limited, especially full flexion, medial rotation, and internal rotation.

### DIAGNOSTIC TESTING

Radiographic studies should include both AP and frog-leg views because an AP view alone may miss the diagnosis. On the AP view of a normal hip, a line drawn along the superior margin of the femoral neck cortex should transect the epiphysis by a small margin. With a slipped capital femoral epiphysis, the line passes outside the epiphysis or just at the superior edge. Contralateral images or full pelvic views are helpful; however, up to 25% of cases of slipped capital femoral epiphysis are bilateral.

### TREATMENT

Diagnosis of slipped capital femoral epiphysis necessitates urgent orthopedic evaluation. Management is surgical and consists of placing screws through the femoral neck into the epiphysis. Delay in diagnosis or management may lead to avascular necrosis and long-term disability.

## LEGG-CALVÉ-PERTHES DISEASE

Legg-Calvé-Perthes disease is characterized by avascular necrosis and resorption of the femoral head. Its onset occurs in children between 4 and 9 years of age, and it is more common in overweight boys. Although the definitive etiology is unknown, research has focused on clotting abnormalities and increased blood viscosity.

### PRESENTING SIGNS AND SYMPTOMS

The disease is initially clinically silent and may come to medical attention incidentally as a result of trauma. The onset of symptoms is usually insidious. Pain may be present in the hip or be referred to the hip, knee, anterior aspect of the thigh, or groin. Tenderness is rarely present, and symptoms include an antalgic gait with decreased hip abduction and medial rotation.

### DIAGNOSTIC TESTING

AP and frog-leg views of the pelvis allow optimal visualization of the femoral head. Disease findings include widening of the articular cartilage, subchondral fractures, irregularity, and flattening of the epiphysis.

### TREATMENT AND DISPOSITION

Treatment includes pain management with nonsteroidal anti-inflammatory drugs (NSAIDs) and referral to a pediatric orthopedic surgeon. The majority of children with this disease do well with observation and nonsurgical intervention.[4]

## SEPTIC ARTHRITIS

Septic arthritis is a true medical emergency that requires early intervention to prevent permanent joint destruction. The joint space is invaded by microbes as a result of hematogenous seeding, local spread from neighboring infection, or direct inoculation from trauma or surgical infection. Bacterial enzymes cause direct tissue destruction. Synovial edema, increased synovial fluid production, and pus increase intraarticular pressure, which causes damage to vessels and articular cartilage. Commonly involved organisms are *Staphylococcus aureus* and assorted *Streptococcus* species. Group B streptococci and *Escherichia coli* are important causes in neonates, and gonococcal arthritis should be a serious consideration in sexually active adolescents.

### PRESENTING SIGNS AND SYMPTOMS

Children suffering from septic arthritis are frequently ill appearing with a fever of 104° F (40° C) or higher, limited range of motion in the affected joint, and pain and swelling.[5] The pain is constant and increases with movement. In the case of septic arthritis of the hip, the child lies in a position of comfort with the hip slightly flexed, abducted, and externally rotated. An infected knee will be erythematous, edematous, warm, and tender to palpation.

### DIAGNOSTIC TESTING

Plain radiographs, a complete blood count, erythrocyte sedimentation rate, C-reactive protein, and blood culture are necessary in the evaluation of children with suspected septic arthritis. Radiologic findings include joint space widening, soft tissue swelling, and displacement of adjacent fat pads. Comparison views may be helpful because a difference of only a few millimeters from the teardrop of the acetabulum to the medial metaphysis of the femoral neck may be significant. In young children, lack of ossification limits the usefulness of radiographs, and ultrasonography provides more detail.

A convincing clinical or laboratory picture justifies joint aspiration for fluid analysis, including protein, glucose, Gram stain, and culture. Joint fluid yields a positive culture in approximately 50% to 75% of cases. Blood culture is much less effective and is positive in approximately one third of cases.

### TREATMENT

Definitive therapy is intravenous administration of antibiotics and surgical drainage of purulent material from the joint. Because the potential for joint destruction is great and the yield of Gram stain is low, empiric antibiotic therapy in the emergency department is indicated. Coverage should include an antistaphylococcal agent, either a β-lactamase–resistant penicillin, clindamycin, or a first-generation cephalosporin. Gram-negative coverage should also be considered for neonates.

## TOXIC SYNOVITIS

Toxic, or transient, synovitis is a benign, self-limited inflammatory condition. A postinfectious inflammatory response has been suggested as the possible cause, but no definitive etiology has been determined. It affects children 3 to 10 years of age, and its findings mimic those of septic arthritis. The joints most often involved include the hip and knee. Fever is rarely present, but when it does occur, it is usually low grade.

### PRESENTING SIGNS AND SYMPTOMS

Although patients will sit in a position of comfort and complain with movement of the limb, the affected joint has full range of motion.[5] This is in stark contrast to septic arthritis, in which the child appears systemically ill, is in significant pain, and cannot move the affected join through full range of motion.[6]

**Table 25.1 Septic Arthritis versus Toxic Synovitis**

| FINDINGS | SEPTIC ARTHRITIS | TOXIC SYNOVITIS |
|---|---|---|
| Fever (° C) | ≥38.5 | <38.5 |
| Complete blood count (cells/mm$^3$) | ≥12,000 | <12,000 |
| C-reactive protein (mg/dL) | ≥2.0 | <2.0 |
| Erythrocyte sedimentation rate (mm/hr) | ≥40 | <40 |

Data from Kocher MS, Zurakowski D, Kasser JR. Differentiating between septic arthritis and transient synovitis of the hip in children: an evidence-based clinical prediction algorithm. J Bone Joint Surg Am 1999;81:1662-70.

### DIAGNOSTIC TESTING

The white blood cell count, erythrocyte sedimentation rate, and C-reactive protein findings are usually normal or slightly elevated, consistent with an inflammatory process.[5] Radiographs are often normal or may reveal a mild effusion with joint space widening. Because sufficient overlap exists in some manifestations of septic joint and toxic synovitis, synovial fluid is necessary to make the diagnosis (**Table 25.1**). When obtained, synovial fluid is sterile.

### TREATMENT

Treatment is directed at relief of symptoms with NSAIDs on an outpatient basis. Pain usually lasts 3 to 4 days but may persist for a few weeks. Children return to full activity with no associated morbidity.

## REFERENCES

***References can be found on Expert Consult @ www.expertconsult.com.***

# Eye Emergencies 26

Kriti Bhatia and Rahul Sharma

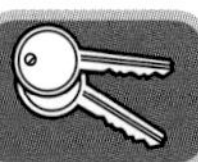

**KEY POINTS**

- Eye emergencies can be classified into three major types: the red eye, the painful eye, and visual loss.
- Nausea and vomiting may be the only symptoms of acute angle-closure glaucoma, especially in elderly patients.
- Topical anesthetics should not be prescribed for a painful eye disorder because their use may lead to corneal ulcers.
- Close follow-up with an ophthalmologist should be recommended for most eye emergencies.

## EPIDEMIOLOGY

Approximately 2% of emergency department (ED) visits involve complaints associated with the eye or vision.[1] Eye injuries account for 3.5% of all occupational injuries in the United States, and about 2000 U.S. workers injure their eyes each day.[2] Eye emergencies can be categorized as the red eye, the painful eye, and visual loss. This chapter discusses the various disorders that fall into each category. **Table 26.1** summarizes the differential diagnosis and priority actions to be taken for any patient arriving at the ED with an eye complaint.

## PHYSIOLOGY

Light passes through the cornea and then through an opening in the iris, the pupil. The iris is responsible for controlling the amount of light that enters the eye by dilating and constricting the pupil. This light then reaches the lens, which refracts the light rays onto the retina. The anterior chamber is located between the lens and the cornea and contains aqueous humor, which is produced by the ciliary body. This fluid maintains pressure and provides nutrients to the lens and cornea. It is reabsorbed from the anterior chamber into the venous system through the canal of Schlemm. The vitreous chamber, located between the retina and the lens, contains a gelatinous fluid called vitreous humor. Light rays pass through the vitreous humor before reaching the retina. The retina lines the back of the eye and contains photoreceptor cells called rods and cones. Rods help vision in dim light, whereas cones aid light and color vision. The cones are located in the center of the retina in an area called the macula. The fovea is a small depression in the center of the macula that contains the highest concentration of cones. The optic nerve is located behind the retina and is responsible for transmitting signals from the photoreceptor cells to the brain (**Fig. 26.1**).

The extraocular muscles (**Fig. 26.2**) help in stabilization of the eye. Six extraocular muscles assist in horizontal, vertical, and rotational movement. These muscles are controlled by impulses from cranial nerves III, IV, and VI, which tell the muscles to relax or contract.

# GLAUCOMA

## EPIDEMIOLOGY

More than 3 million Americans suffer from glaucoma, the leading cause of preventable blindness in the United States.[3] The term *glaucoma* refers to a group of disorders that damage the optic nerve and thereby lead to loss of vision. The two main classifications of glaucoma are open angle and angle closure. Acute angle-closure glaucoma is more common in white persons and women. Its peak incidence occurs between the ages of 55 and 70.[4] African Americans, patients older than 65 years, and people with diabetes and ocular trauma are at increased risk for open-angle glaucoma. Differentiation between the two types of glaucoma lies in the mechanism of obstruction of outflow, as described later. Intraocular pressure (IOP) is determined by the rate of aqueous humor production relative to its outflow and removal. Normal IOP is between 10 and 20 mm Hg. This discussion focuses mainly on acute angle-closure glaucoma.

When the angle of the anterior chamber is reduced, outflow of aqueous humor is blocked, which results in elevated IOP and ultimately visual compromise. Patients with a shallow anterior chamber, hyperopic (farsighted) eyes, and eyes with lens abnormalities such as cataracts are more prone to acute angle-closure glaucoma. Pupillary dilation, caused by events such as presence in a dark room, is the most significant event that can cause an acute attack of glaucoma because the flaccid iris can be pushed against the trabecular meshwork and result in obstruction.

## PRESENTING SIGNS AND SYMPTOMS

Patients with acute angle-closure glaucoma may have a sudden onset of headache or eye pain. Occasionally, nausea and vomiting from vagal stimulation can be the dominant symptoms. Shortly after the onset of pain, blurry vision or halos in the visual field may occur.

**Table 26.1 Differential Diagnosis and Priority Actions for Eye Complaints in the Emergency Department**

| | |
|---|---|
| **Eye Pain?** | |
| Does the patient have any changes in vision, history of trauma, or associated neurologic complaints? | Separate the causes into traumatic and atraumatic.<br>Perform a complete eye examination, including assessment of visual acuity, slit-lamp examination, and measurement of intraocular pressure (IOP). |
| **Decreased Visual Acuity?** | |
| Does the patient have any risk factors for central retinal vessel occlusion or glaucoma?<br>Is there any history of recent infection or trauma?<br>Does the patient also have a headache or any associated neurologic complaints? | Perform a complete eye examination, including assessment of visual acuity, slit-lamp examination, and measurement of IOP, as well as a neurologic examination. |
| **Eye Trauma?** | |
| Does the patient have any evidence of increased IOP or decreased visual acuity? | Consider computed tomography of the orbits with possible emergency lateral canthotomy and immediate ophthalmologic consultation. |
| **Red Eye?** | |
| Is any evidence of infection, trauma, a foreign body, or a systemic illness present? | Perform a complete eye examination, including assessment of visual acuity and IOP measurement, and treat with appropriate medications (see Table 26.2). |

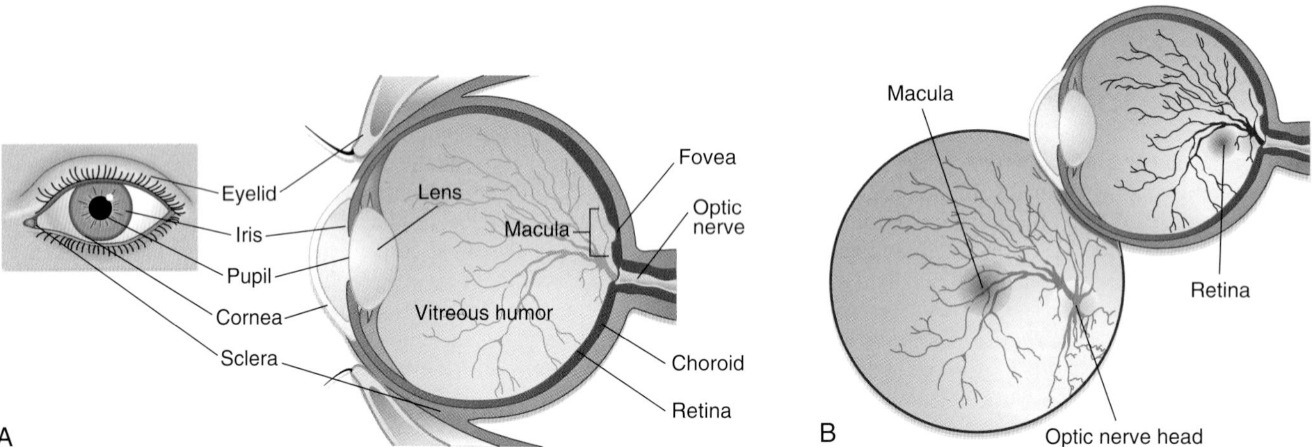


**Fig. 26.1 Anatomy of the eye (A) and retina (B).**

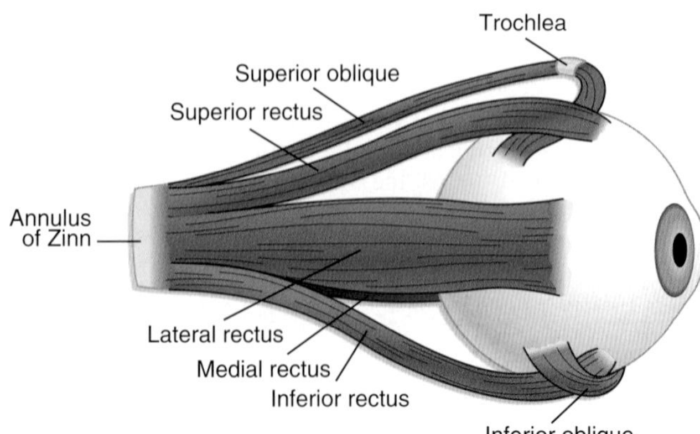


**Fig. 26.2 Extraocular muscles.** (Courtesy Ted Montgomery, OD. Available at www.tedmontgomery.com/the_eye/.)

The classic physical findings are unilateral eye injection, especially at the limbus; a nonreactive, midsize pupil; shallow anterior chamber; corneal edema or haziness; and high IOP (often 60 to 90 mm Hg). If the attack has been prolonged, ischemia of the ciliary body reduces aqueous humor production with a resultant decrease in IOP. This process is especially important because the ultimate damage depends on the duration of the attack rather than the severity of the elevation in pressure.

With open-angle glaucoma, development of the disease is usually insidious, bilateral, slowly progressive, and painless.

## MEDICAL DECISION MAKING

Visual acuity should be recorded in both eyes. Examination of the eye should include a search for the classic signs of glaucoma already described, including a middilated pupil in the affected eye and corneal haziness. A slit lamp should be used to estimate the depth of the anterior chamber. If this depth is less than one fourth the corneal thickness, the anterior chamber angle is very narrow. It is important to measure anterior chamber depth in both eyes; a shallow angle in only one eye argues against acute angle-closure glaucoma. IOP is usually measured with a tonometer; the cornea is flattened, and pressure is determined by measurement of the force needed to flatten it, as well as measurement of the area flattened.

## TREATMENT

Acute angle-closure glaucoma is an ophthalmologic emergency. Because outcome depends on the duration of elevated IOP, treatment should be initiated promptly. Therapy is geared toward decreasing aqueous production, increasing aqueous outflow, and reducing vitreous volume to lower IOP.

Initial treatment includes a topical, nonselective beta-blocker such as 0.5% timolol to reduce aqueous production. Topical beta-blockers are absorbed and can cause systemic effects. Intravenous administration of a carbonic anhydrase inhibitor such as acetazolamide, 500 mg, will also rapidly reduce aqueous humor production. Intravenous mannitol will create an osmotic gradient between the vitreous and blood and thereby cause a reduction in vitreous volume, so it may be useful for severe cases. Tonometry can be performed frequently, even every 15 minutes, to assess progress.

Topical 2% pilocarpine is used to help reopen the angle. Miotics such as the direct-acting parasympathomimetic agent pilocarpine might be less effective at very high IOP because the iris is relatively ischemic and therefore less responsive. Sometimes pilocarpine is used after IOP has been reduced to less than 40 mm Hg. Pilocarpine will therefore be more effective as the initially high pressures are reduced with the initial beta-blocker drops and acetazolamide. Topical 1% prednisolone acetate may sometimes be added to reduce inflammation. For ongoing treatment, topical 2% pilocarpine and prednisolone acetate may be administered every 6 hours and oral acetazolamide two times per day. Sedatives and antiemetics may be administered as needed. When the inflammation has been reduced sufficiently, the patient will be taken for iridotomy by the ophthalmologist.

## DISPOSITION

Disposition of the patient is determined in conjunction with the consulting ophthalmologist. Indications for admission include intractable nausea and vomiting and need for careful monitoring to administer systemic agents.

# CENTRAL RETINAL ARTERY OCCLUSION

## EPIDEMIOLOGY

Retinal artery occlusion affects less than 1 per 100,000 persons annually.[5,6] It is most commonly caused by an embolus from the carotid artery that lodges in a distal branch of the ophthalmic artery. Central retinal artery occlusion most commonly affects elderly patients and men. Although most emboli are formed from cholesterol, they may also be calcific, fat, or bacterial from cardiac valve vegetations.

## PATHOPHYSIOLOGY

The visual complaints and deficits resulting from retinal artery disease are caused by ischemia. In addition to the embolic causes already described, low-flow states and vasospasm may have the same visual consequences.

## PRESENTING SIGNS AND SYMPTOMS

Sudden, painless visual loss is the classic manifestation of central retinal artery occlusion. Sometimes patients report transient visual loss before complete compromise. The visual loss is usually profound. Examination can often elicit an afferent pupillary defect (when light is shined into the abnormal eye, the pupil of the affected eye paradoxically dilates instead of constricting). Funduscopic examination typically demonstrates a pale retina with a cherry-red spot at the fovea (**Fig. 26.3**). Complete evaluation involves auscultation of the carotid arteries for bruits, palpation of the temporal artery for tenderness, and cardiac auscultation and palpation of the pulse to detect atrial fibrillation.

## DIFFERENTIAL DIAGNOSIS

Sudden, painless visual loss can also result from central retinal vein occlusion, temporal arteritis, ischemic optic neuropathy, amaurosis fugax, retinal detachment, or vitreous hemorrhage. If the loss of vision is accompanied by pain, arterial dissection should be part of the differential diagnosis. The presence of a headache, temporal artery tenderness, and an elevated erythrocyte sedimentation rate (ESR) suggests temporal arteritis. Amaurosis fugax, or unilateral transient obstruction of a retinal artery, does not cause visual loss lasting longer than 15 minutes. Ischemic optic neuropathy causes optic disk pallor and elevation. Retinal detachment and vitreous hemorrhage

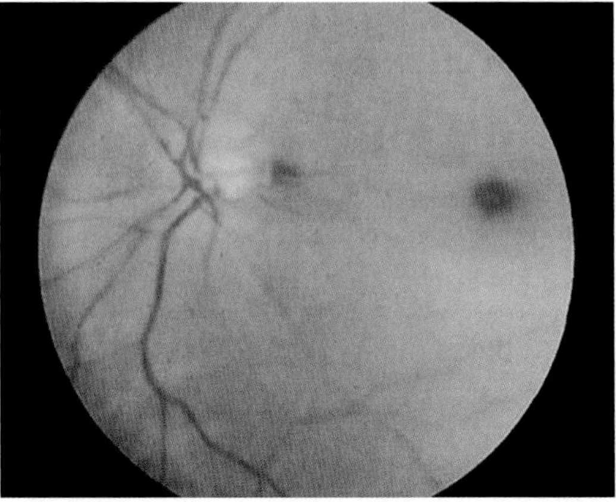

**Fig. 26.3 Central retinal artery occlusion.** (Courtesy Ted Montgomery, OD. Available at www.tedmontgomery.com/the_eye/.)

result in visual disturbances such as floaters in addition to the loss of vision—the occurrence of which is variable with a detached retina. Vitreous hemorrhage causes absence of the normal red reflex of the fundus. A neurologic etiology such as a cerebral infarct must also beconsidered.

## TREATMENT

Treatment must be initiated immediately because the visual loss is generally irreversible after 2 hours of ischemia. Regardless, the outcome is generally poor. Several approaches may be used. Intermittent globe massage can be performed in an effort to dislodge the clot and propel it distally: moderate pressure is applied for 5 second and then released for 5 seconds, and the cycle is repeated. The use of anterior chamber paracentesis for visual loss is based on the principle that decreased IOP allows better perfusion of the retinal artery and may propel the clot distally. Acetazolamide can be administered intravenously for the same purpose. Inhaled carbogen (mixture of 95% oxygen and 5% carbon dioxide) can be used to dilate the vasculature and thereby increase retinal $Po_2$.

Other treatment options are intraarterial thrombolysis and hyperbaric oxygen; however, studies have shown limited improvement in visual outcome with early administration of both these treatment modalities.[7-10] One retrospective study found that even with thrombolysis, vision did not improve to better than 20/300 in the affected eye.[7] Another study investigated the outcomes of 32 patients with central retinal artery occlusion, 17 of whom underwent fibrinolysis.[6] This study found that all but six of the treated patients reported improvement in their visual compromise but that only five of the untreated patients had any improvement. In this study, patients with a duration of symptoms of up to 24 hours were treated.

Patients with sudden visual loss are admitted to the hospital so that the underlying cause can be sought.

# CENTRAL RETINAL VEIN OCCLUSION

## EPIDEMIOLOGY

Patients older than 50 years who have cardiovascular disease, hypertension, glaucoma, venous stasis, hypercoagulable conditions, collagen vascular diseases, or diabetes are at risk for central retinal vein occlusion.[1]

## PATHOPHYSIOLOGY

Two types of retinal vein occlusion are distinguished, ischemic and nonischemic. The ischemic type is also known as hemorrhagic retinopathy, and the nonischemic type is also called venous stasis retinopathy. The manifestations and physical findings differ according to the type of occlusion involved.

## PRESENTING SIGNS AND SYMPTOMS

Typically, patients with ischemic retinal vein occlusion report an acute and relatively profound decrease in visual acuity.

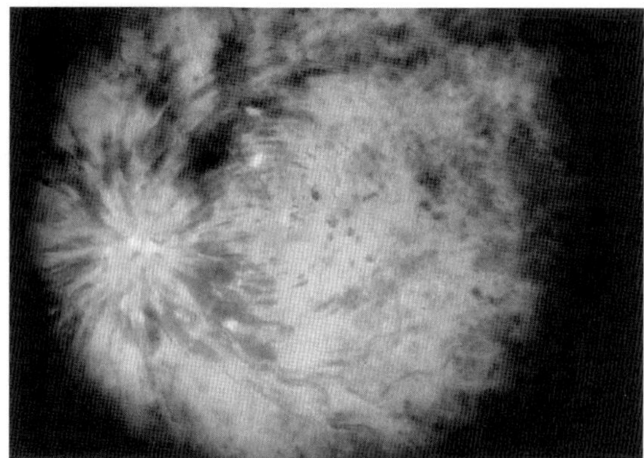

**Fig. 26.4 Central retinal vein occlusion.** (From Noble J. Textbook of primary care medicine. 3rd ed. St. Louis: Mosby; 2001.)

Those with the nonischemic type have progressively blurry vision that is worse in the morning. An afferent pupillary defect is found in the ischemic type. Funduscopic examination shows an edematous optic disk and macular, dilated retinal veins, retinal hemorrhage, and cotton-wool spots. Sometimes these findings are called the "blood and thunder" appearance of the fundus (**Fig. 26.4**).

## DIFFERENTIAL DIAGNOSIS

The processes that must be considered when assessing a patient with possible central retinal vein occlusion are the same as those for central retinal artery occlusion. Branch retinal vein occlusion may also occur distal to an arteriovenous crossing, with hemorrhage developing distal to the occlusion site.

## MEDICAL DECISION MAKING

No specific diagnostic test can identify central retinal vein occlusion. The diagnosis is based on the clinical history and physical examination, which exclude other processes that also cause painless visual loss.

## TREATMENT

No effective therapeutic regimen exists for central retinal vein occlusion. The emergency physician (EP) should arrange for immediate ophthalmologic consultation. A search for a cause should be performed to protect the contralateral eye from the same problem. The prognosis largely depends on the type of retinal venous occlusion. Nonischemic vein occlusion, unless the macular involvement is extensive, offers a better outcome than the ischemic type does. Spontaneous resolution may occur in some cases.

Although no specific treatment is available, a number of interventions have been proposed and practiced.[11,12] However, these interventions have not been based on evidence of efficacy. Laser photocoagulation, for example, cauterizes leaking vessels with the aim of halting further visual loss. This procedure can be especially helpful for branch retinal vein occlusion. With nonischemic vein occlusion, attempts to reduce macular edema can be helpful. The reduction is accomplished with the administration of topical corticosteroids. Studies have been conducted to determine the benefit of steroids in treating both forms of retinal vein occlusion. Jonas et al.[11] conducted a prospective, comparative, nonrandomized clinical interventional study to evaluate the visual outcomes in 32 patients with central retinal vein occlusion after intravitreal administration of triamcinolone acetate. The study included patients with both the ischemic and nonischemic forms of retinal vein occlusion. These researchers found that the medication resulted in temporary (up to 3 months) improvement in visual outcome but also raised IOP. Anticoagulants are not recommended because they may propagate hemorrhage.

# OPTIC NEURITIS

## EPIDEMIOLOGY

Optic neuritis is inflammation of the optic nerve, and visual loss is due to focal demyelination of the optic nerve. Most affected patients are between 15 and 40 years of age. This disorder can be associated with numerous diseases, including sarcoidosis, systemic lupus erythematosus, measles, leukemia, syphilis, and alcoholism; however, it is most commonly associated with multiple sclerosis. In fact, in up to a third of patients with optic neuritis, multiple sclerosis is eventually diagnosed, and approximately two thirds of patients with multiple sclerosis have optic neuritis. Optic neuritis can also be idiopathic.

## PATHOPHYSIOLOGY

Optic neuritis results from an autoimmune reaction that ultimately causes demyelinating inflammation. In idiopathic and multiple sclerosis–related optic neuritis, lesions are characterized by areas of loss of the myelin sheath with preservation of axons. In acute disease, remyelination may occur. In chronic disease, because of the accumulation of scar tissue, the process becomes irreversible. The lesions in multiple sclerosis–associated optic neuritis are pathologically the same as those in the brain.

## PRESENTING SIGNS AND SYMPTOMS

Symptoms of optic neuritis are generally unilateral. Patients complain of pain, especially with eye movement. Visual loss, which can range from minimal loss to complete loss of light perception, usually occurs over a number of hours or days. Patients may also experience dulling of color vision, worse vision after exertion or exposure to steam, brief light flashes, and central scotoma. An afferent pupillary defect is always present. Funduscopic examination may show disk pallor, swelling, or elevation. However, because up to two thirds of cases are retrobulbar, the fundus can appear normal.

## DIFFERENTIAL DIAGNOSIS AND MEDICAL DECISION MAKING

Any condition that causes visual disturbance along with eye pain must be considered in the differential diagnosis of optic neuritis. Orbital cellulitis can cause this clinical picture but does not include an afferent pupillary defect; furthermore, inspection alone should allow differentiation between the two diseases. Glaucoma can also cause the combination of ocular pain and visual impairment. Physical examination, including assessment of pupil size and reactivity, as well as corneal inspection, allows distinction between glaucoma and optic neuritis.

Unilateral ocular pain with visual compromise should always raise clinical suspicion for optic neuritis. If no afferent pupillary defect is found on physical examination, another diagnosis is almost ensured. Although imaging is usually not indicated, magnetic resonance imaging (MRI) provides adequate visualization of the optic nerve.

## TREATMENT AND DISPOSITION

Ophthalmologic and neurologic consultation should be obtained if optic neuritis is suspected. Approximately 31% of patients with optic neuritis have a recurrence within 10 years of the initial episode.[13] The goals of treatment are to restore visual acuity and prevent propagation of the underlying disease process. The Optic Neuritis Treatment Trial was a randomized, 15-center clinical trial involving 457 patients that was performed to evaluate both the benefit of corticosteroid treatment of optic neuritis and the relationship of this entity to multiple sclerosis. Use of intravenous steroids in conjunction with oral steroids reduced the short-term risk for the development of multiple sclerosis as determined by MRI evaluation. No long-term immunity from or benefit for multiple sclerosis was reported, however. The study concluded that although intravenous steroids have only minimal, if any effect on the patient's ultimate visual acuity, they do expedite recovery from optic neuritis. Use of oral steroids alone is associated with a higher recurrence rate of optic neuritis. The dosage regimen recommended on the basis of the study results was methylprednisolone, 250 mg intravenously every 6 hours for 3 days, followed by prednisone, 1 mg/kg/day orally for 11 days.[14]

# RETINAL DETACHMENT

Retinal detachment is a true ophthalmologic emergency. Unfortunately, it is also relatively common and affects 1 in 300 people. Before the introduction of and improvement in a number of treatment modalities, this entity was uniformly blinding. Early diagnosis and treatment are imperative for preservation of vision. Retinal detachment may be associated with vascular disorders, congenital malformations, metabolic disarray, trauma, shrinking of the vitreous, myopia, degeneration, and less commonly, diabetic retinopathy and uveitis. It is generally more common in older patients. Three different types of retinal detachment are recognized, each associated with different conditions.

## PATHOPHYSIOLOGY AND ANATOMY

The retina has two layers, the inner neuronal layer and the outer pigment epithelial layer (the choroid). Retinal detachment refers to separation of the two layers. *Rhegmatogenous* retinal detachment, the most common of the three types, is caused by a tear or hole in the neuronal layer, which leads to extrusion of fluid from the vitreous cavity into the potential space between the two retinal layers. It is more common in patients older than 45 years and those with severe myopia. When caused by trauma, this type of detachment can affect any age group. *Exudative* retinal detachment is caused by leakage of fluid or blood from within the retina itself. Predisposing factors for this type include hypertension, vasculitis, and central retinal venous occlusion. *Traction* retinal detachment results from the formation and subsequent contraction of fibrous bands in the vitreous.

## PRESENTING SIGNS AND SYMPTOMS

Retinal detachment can occasionally be asymptomatic. More commonly, patients complain of flashes of light, floaters, or fine dots or cobwebs in their visual fields. Generally, a new onset of floaters associated with flashing lights is indicative of retinal detachment unless proved otherwise. Visual acuity correlates with the extent of macular involvement and can be minimally changed to severely decreased. The loss of vision is usually sudden in onset and starts peripherally, with propagation to the central visual field. The visual loss is commonly described as a filmy, cloudy, or curtainlike appearance. Visual field cuts relate to the location of the retinal detachment, and an afferent pupillary defect occurs if the detachment is large enough. Retinal detachment is painless. On examination, the detached retina may appear gray or translucent or may seem out of focus (**Fig. 26.5**). Retinal folds may be seen. The visual field defects are variable, depending on the involvement of the retina and macula. Bedside ED ultrasonography has been shown to be helpful in confirming the presence of retinal detachment.[15] Left untreated, all cases of retinal detachment progress to involve the macula and result in complete loss of vision in the affected eye.

## DIFFERENTIAL DIAGNOSIS AND MEDICAL DECISION MAKING

Vitreous hemorrhage, which results from bleeding into either the preretinal space or the vitreous cavity itself, can be difficult to distinguish from retinal detachment. Complaints with this disorder range from floaters or cobwebs in the visual field to severe, painless loss of vision. Vitreous hemorrhage without concomitant retinal detachment should not, however, cause an afferent pupillary defect. Ophthalmoscopy usually demonstrates discoloration (ranging from reddish to black) with fundal structural details difficult to discern. Therapy for vitreous hemorrhage consists of bed rest with head elevation followed by possible interventional procedures such as laser photocoagulation and cryotherapy.

All macular disorders can cause painless visual loss. They are manifested as loss of central vision with preservation of peripheral vision, as well as findings of retinal abnormalities. A careful history and physical examination can exclude macular degeneration as a cause of central visual loss. Funduscopic examination in individuals with age-related macular degeneration shows the presence of drusen—small, yellow masses scattered on the retina. A gray-green subretinal neovascular membrane may also be seen. Inflammatory processes involving the retina often cause inflammatory proteins to fill the vitreous, thus making it appear cloudy.

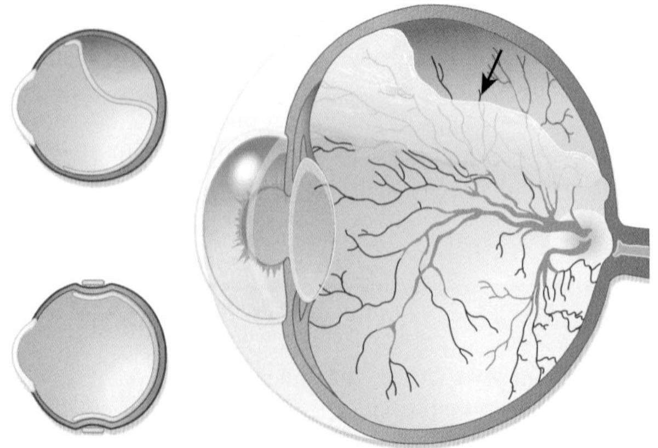

**Fig. 26.5 Retinal detachment.** (Courtesy Ted Montgomery, OD. Available at www.tedmontgomery.com/the_eye/.)

## TREATMENT

The sooner that treatment of retinal detachment is initiated, the greater the chance of visual preservation and recovery. After detachment, retinal ischemia ensues because of loss of the choroidal blood supply. Patients with suspected or confirmed retinal breaks or detachments require emergency ophthalmologic consultation. Contrary to traditional belief, not all detachments are managed surgically. Laser photocoagulation or cryotherapy is frequently used to create small burns around the area of detachment to prevent further leakage of fluid between the retinal layers. Intraocular gas is sometimes used to tamponade the tear. These procedures are approximately 95% effective in halting the disease process.[16] Surgical intervention may be needed to repair the tear and simultaneously remove the traction forces on the retina. The modality of treatment is at the discretion of the consulting ophthalmologist.

# TEMPORAL ARTERITIS

Temporal arteritis, an inflammatory condition that results from a generalized vasculitis of medium and large arteries, typically affects patients older than 50 years. This condition is also called giant cell arteritis. It has a female preponderance. Temporal arteritis occurs in as many as 1 in every 2000 people. Although mortality is not affected by the condition, it can cause blindness. Up to 75% of patients with visual compromise as a result of temporal arteritis would eventually experience contralateral visual impairment if not treated. Temporal arteritis is commonly, though not uniformly associated with polymyalgia rheumatica.

## PATHOPHYSIOLOGY

Vessels affected by giant cell arteritis are infiltrated with lymphocytes, plasma cells, and multinucleated giant cells in patches or segmental patterns. A cell-mediated immune response is thought to account for the vascular changes seen with this disorder. Inflammation of branches of the ophthalmic artery, especially the posterior ciliary artery, leads to ischemic optic neuritis, which compromises vision. The central retinal artery is also often affected. Inflammation of the temporal artery causes the classic headache associated with this diagnosis.

## PRESENTING SIGNS AND SYMPTOMS

Unilateral headache, jaw or tongue claudication, constitutional symptoms, including anorexia and malaise, and visual impairment are common initial symptoms of temporal arteritis. Occasionally, the visual loss is preceded by amaurosis fugax. In one series of patients, visual loss was unilateral in 46%, sequential in 37%, and simultaneously bilateral in 17%.[17] Patients with polymyalgia rheumatica may also complain of pain and stiffness in the shoulders or hips.

Examination may demonstrate tenderness and decreased pulsations over the involved temporal artery. Funduscopic findings may be normal or consist of optic disk edema or pallor, scattered cotton-wool spots, flame-shaped retinal hemorrhages, and distended retinal veins. An afferent pupillary defect may be present. When vision is evaluated, horizontal field defects and involvement of the extraocular muscles are often detected.

## DIFFERENTIAL DIAGNOSIS AND MEDICAL DECISION MAKING

In patients who do not have visual complaints, a differential diagnosis for headache must be investigated. Migraines, tension headaches, and subarachnoid hemorrhage may mimic temporal arteritis. Palpation of the temporal artery along with a careful history, including questions about jaw symptoms, may allow distinction. Because temporal arteritis is a medical emergency associated with high morbidity if not recognized and treated promptly, it must be definitively excluded on the basis of the history and physical or laboratory findings before the patient's symptoms are attributed to another entity. Acute angle-closure glaucoma is also high on the differential diagnosis list, regardless of whether visual symptoms are present. Occasionally, headache can be the dominant symptom of glaucoma. In glaucoma, however, physical examination should find a middilated, nonreactive pupil with corneal haziness and a shallow anterior chamber.

Although temporal arteritis can rarely be accompanied by a normal ESR, this parameter is almost always elevated. The upper limit of normal ESR increases with age. A rough approximation of the upper limit of normal for men is age in years divided by 2. For women it is age in years plus 10, with the sum divided by 2, or half the age in years plus 5. Elderly patients with new-onset headaches, visual loss, and an elevated ESR should always be treated for temporal arteritis. Generally, the ESR is higher than 80 mm/hr in individuals with temporal arteritis. Temporal biopsy confirms the presence of the disease. Early in the course of the disease, however, biopsy findings may be normal. Ultrasound has been proposed as a possible diagnostic modality for temporal arteritis, but studies have yielded conflicting results. Further investigation is necessary before a definitive conclusion can be drawn about its standard use.

## TREATMENT

Treatment of temporal arteritis should never be delayed to await the results of biopsy because outcome is contingent on early medical treatment. Initial treatment should consist of prednisone, 60 to 80 mg, or high-dose intravenous methylprednisolone. The exact duration and regimen of steroid therapy are determined on a case-by-case basis. Generally, treatment is continued until the symptoms improve and the ESR begins to normalize. It has also been suggested that methotrexate, infliximab, and aspirin may also halt progression of the visual symptoms, but further studies are necessary to establish practice patterns.[18]

# ORBITAL CELLULITIS AND PERIORBITAL CELLULITIS

Without proper treatment, orbital cellulitis causes blindness and death in approximately 20% of patients. Because venous drainage of the orbital regions occurs through communicating vessels into the brain via the cavernous sinus, infection can progress rapidly with devastating consequences. Differentiation of orbital from periorbital (preseptal) cellulitis can be difficult but is important because the outcomes of the two entities—and therefore their treatments—are different.

## ANATOMY AND PATHOPHYSIOLOGY

Orbital cellulitis is inflammation of any of the tissues within the orbit posterior to the orbital septum, whereas preorbital cellulitis is confined to the tissues anterior to the septum. Making this distinction is extremely important for management. Because of the gravity of the potential consequences of orbital cellulitis and the fact that most cases of orbital cellulitis have a concomitant periorbital component, the EP evaluating an infected, erythematous orbit should always assume that the patient has orbital cellulitis until it can be definitively excluded.

Approximately 75% of cases of orbital and periorbital cellulitis have identifiable antecedent causes. Sinusitis is the most common predisposing condition. Because the inferior, medial, and superior walls of the orbit lie adjacent to the sinuses, it is easy to understand how extension of infection may occur. The ethmoid sinus is most commonly involved. Infection after trauma or surgery with direct inoculation of pathogens and hematogenous spread from other sources of bacteremia are other methods of acquiring the infection. The pathogen involved is contingent on the mode of infection. Aerobic, non–spore-forming organisms are most frequently the culprits. Anaerobic organisms tend to be causative when infection results from chronic sinusitis.

## PRESENTING SIGNS AND SYMPTOMS

Patients with infection limited to the periorbital tissues typically have erythema, edema, and warmth of the external eye tissues. Though generally unilateral, the infection can be

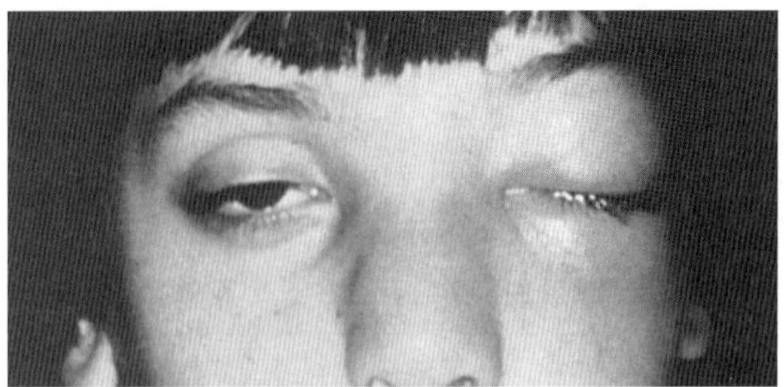

**Fig. 26.6 Orbital cellulitis.** (From Long SS, Pickering LK, Prober CG, editors. Principles and practice of pediatric infectious diseases. 2nd ed. Philadelphia: Churchill Livingstone; 2003.)

bilateral. Constitutional symptoms, including fever and malaise, may be present. The presence of ocular pain, ophthalmoplegia, and pain with extraocular movement suggests orbital involvement. Patients with orbital infection may also have decreased visual acuity and pupillary paralysis. Elevated IOP, preseptal (periorbital) cellulitis, conjunctival injection, and proptosis may additionally be present (**Fig. 26.6**).

## DIFFERENTIAL DIAGNOSIS AND MEDICAL DECISION MAKING

The signs of periorbital infection can be similar to those of allergic periorbital swelling, especially when the involvement is bilateral. With an allergic reaction, cobblestoning may be noted on the interior aspect of the upper lid, and the condition should improve with the administration of diphenhydramine or another antihistamine. It can be difficult to distinguish orbital cellulitis from subperiosteal and orbital abscesses and even from cavernous sinus thrombosis, which carries a dismal prognosis. With subperiosteal abscesses, the globe is often displaced by the abscess; the displacement should be obvious on inspection. Orbital abscesses are located in postseptal tissues. They may cause obvious pus, significant ophthalmoplegia, and exophthalmos, as well as globe displacement. Cavernous sinus thrombosis typically starts unilaterally and progresses to contralateral involvement. Examination should detect dilation of the episcleral vessels and venous engorgement of the fundus; the pupil may be fixed and dilated. Depending on the time course, orbital neoplasm with associated inflammation may cause similar symptoms.

In many cases it may be possible to exclude orbital involvement on the basis of the history and physical examination alone. If there is any doubt or another entity or complication such as abscess is suspected, computed tomography (CT) is the diagnostic modality of choice. It is not necessary to use intravenous contrast material. MRI is another acceptable mode of diagnosis.

## TREATMENT AND DISPOSITION

In adults, preorbital infection should be treated with oral antibiotics, and close outpatient follow-up should be arranged. An antibiotic that provides coverage for staphylococci, streptococci, and Enterobacteriaceae is appropriate. Orbital cellulitis should be treated with broad-spectrum intravenous antibiotics, the patient should be admitted to the hospital, and consideration should be given to incision and drainage if imaging reveals a collection. Because of the increased incidence of community-acquired methicillin-resistant *Staphylococcus aureus*, empiric coverage for this pathogen may also be considered. For periorbital infection in children, the threshold for admission to the hospital should be lower. Patients with mild periorbital cellulitis can be discharged with arrangements for extremely close outpatient follow-up. For patients with more involved cases, including any underlying comorbid conditions, admission for observation should be considered.

## THE RED EYE

An injected, red eye signals an inflammatory reaction. Fortunately, most inflammation is self-limited and can be treated on an outpatient basis. The specific cause, treatment, course, and prognosis, as well as the impact on vision, depend on the underlying cause (**Table 26.2**).

This discussion focuses on conjunctivitis, the diagnosis in 30% of patients seen in the ED with ocular complaints and the most common cause of red eye.[19] When the cornea is involved as well, the process is called keratoconjunctivitis.

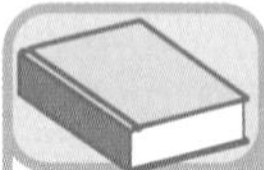

**PATIENT TEACHING TIPS**

A patient with a red eye should seek evaluation by a primary care physician because this disorder has several benign and serious causes.

If the pain worsens, visual acuity decreases, a discharge appears, or a fever develops, the patient should immediately return to the emergency department for reevaluation.

Patients at high risk for eye problems (e.g., those with diabetes) should be encouraged to obtain yearly eye examinations. More information for patients with diabetes is available from the American Diabetes Association (www.diabetes.org).

## PATHOPHYSIOLOGY AND ANATOMY

An eye appears red because of dilation of blood vessels. Ciliary injection, caused by dilation of branches of the anterior ciliary arteries, indicates inflammation of the cornea, iris, or ciliary body. Conjunctival injection results from dilation of the more posterior, superficial conjunctival vessels. Because of the conjunctiva's more superficial location, vascular dilation causes more dramatic injection there than in the ciliary body.

Conjunctivitis refers to inflammation of the mucous membrane that lines the anterior sclera and inner eyelids. The conjunctiva is a key player in maintaining lubrication of the eye. Infection can result in scarring and abnormal tear formation in the affected eye.

Conjunctivitis can have a viral, bacterial, fungal, toxic, chemical, or allergic cause. The clinical findings and treatment differ with the underlying etiology. Sometimes it may be difficult to determine the underlying cause.

**Table 26.2** Treatment of Eye Inflammation (Red Eye) According to Cause

| FEATURE | CONJUNCTIVITIS | SCLERITIS | ACUTE ANGLE-CLOSURE GLAUCOMA | ACUTE ANTERIOR UVEITIS | SUPERFICIAL KERATITIS | TRAUMATIC IRITIS | FOREIGN BODY |
|---|---|---|---|---|---|---|---|
| Ocular pain | Mild | Moderate to severe | Moderate to severe | Moderate | Moderate to severe | Moderate to severe | Moderate to severe |
| Visual acuity | Usually normal | May be reduced | Severely reduced | Mildly reduced | Moderately to severely reduced | Mildly reduced | May be reduced |
| Cornea | Clear | Clear | Hazy | Can be hazy | Hazy | Can be hazy | Clear or abrasion |
| Pupil | Normal | Normal<br>Constricted if uveitis present | Dilated, unreactive to light | Constricted with poor response to light | Normal<br>Constricted if uveitis present | Constricted, weakly dilating | Normal if no globe penetration |
| Discharge | Yes | No | No | Minimal | Not usual, except with infectious cause | No | Not usual unless superinfection present |
| Hyperemia | Diffuse | Focal or diffuse | Diffuse | Diffuse | Diffuse | Perilimbal | Focal or diffuse |
| Intraocular pressure (IOP) | Normal | Normal | Increased | Usually normal but can increase if not treated | Normal | Can be increased | Normal |
| Treatment | Pain medications<br>Antibiotics if bacterial, antiviral if herpes, ocular decongestants if allergic<br>Supportive care with artificial tears if viral | Pain medications; steroid therapy in consultation with an ophthalmologist<br>Eye shield to protect the eye | Decrease in IOP, pain medications | Pain medications, steroid therapy in consultation with an ophthalmologist, cycloplegics | Antibiotics if superinfection present, pain medications | Cycloplegics and steroids in consultation with an ophthalmologist | Pain medications, removal of foreign body, check/update tetanus status, antibiotics if corneal abrasion present |

## PRESENTING SIGNS AND SYMPTOMS

Generally, bilateral conjunctivitis signifies an infectious or allergic cause. However, such is not always the case. Viral infection is the most common cause of conjunctivitis. Adenovirus infection, which is highly contagious, is extremely common. Other viral causes include coxsackievirus and enteroviruses. Patients have significant injection, itching, irritation, and watery discharge. They may have accompanying preauricular adenopathy. Patients often have associated mild systemic symptoms because the conjunctivitis occurs in concert with a viral syndrome. Epidemic keratoconjunctivitis, which may result in the development of pseudomembranes, is caused by adenovirus types 8 and 19; this is the classic pink eye. Patients are contagious for up to 2 weeks.

Herpes simplex conjunctivitis is manifested as unilateral conjunctival injection with a clear discharge. Patients complain of a foreign body sensation and photophobia. With gross inspection alone it may be impossible to distinguish herpes simplex from other viral causes. Patients may have facial or lid vesicles. This infection can spread rapidly and cause corneal damage, which is seen as a dendritic pattern on fluorescein examination. Depending on the location, size, and depth of corneal involvement, patients may have decreased visual acuity.

Herpes zoster ophthalmicus is caused by activation of the virus along the ophthalmic branch of the trigeminal nerve. A vesicular rash is present along the involved dermatome and results in forehead and upper eyelid lesions. Lesions on the tip of the nose, called the Hutchinson sign, signify involvement of the nasociliary branch of the fifth cranial nerve. The presence of the Hutchinson sign indicates a much higher likelihood of ocular involvement (76% risk versus a 34% risk in the absence of such lesions). Fluorescein examination may show punctate, ulcerated, or dendritic corneal lesions (**Fig. 26.7**).

Patients with bacterial conjunctivitis have conjunctival erythema, a foreign body sensation, purulent drainage, and morning crusting of the eye. They do not usually experience photophobia or loss of visual acuity. The most common causative organisms are *Staphylococcus, Streptococcus*, and *Haemophilus* (although with immunization this last pathogen is being seen decreasingly).

Gonococcal infection generally results in unilateral conjunctival injection, copious purulent discharge, and edema and erythema of the lids. The infection is sudden in onset and progresses rapidly.[19] Patient populations usually affected are infants, health care workers, and sexually active young adults. The amount of discharge helps distinguish gonococcal infection from other bacterial pathogens. Patients may have associated urethral discharge or arthritis.

*Pseudomonas aeruginosa* infection should be suspected in patients who are immunosuppressed or wear contact lenses. Usually, a sticky, mucopurulent, yellow-green discharge is present. The cornea should be inspected carefully for ulceration because corneal perforation with progression of the infection is a major concern with this organism.

Fungal pathogens that cause conjunctivitis include *Actinomyces, Aspergillus, Candida, Coccidioides*, and *Mucor* (in diabetic patients). These organisms should be considered in any immunosuppressed patient, as well as any individual who has sustained eye trauma involving vegetable matter. Examination may show a corneal infiltrate with underlying endothelial plaque and hypopyon, which is the presence of pus cells in the anterior chamber.

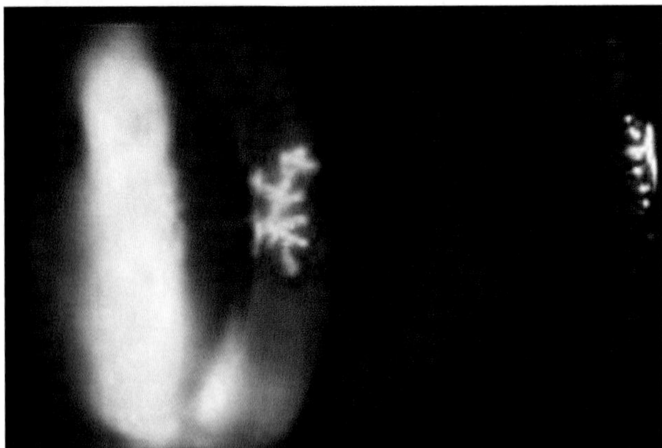

**Fig. 26.7 Herpes zoster ophthalmicus.** (Available from www.emedicine.com.)

Chlamydial conjunctivitis is fairly common, especially in sexually active young adults. It is also a frequent cause of neonatal conjunctivitis. Patients may have associated gonococcal disease and should thus be asked about urethral discharge and arthritis. Patients with chlamydial conjunctivitis have a scant seropurulent eye discharge and fair to moderate conjunctival injection. Preauricular adenopathy is occasionally associated with this disorder.

Allergic conjunctivitis gives rise to significant pruritus and chemosis. Generally, an associated clear discharge is present in varying amounts. Cobblestoning may be seen on the inner eyelids.

## DIAGNOSIS

The diagnosis of conjunctivitis is based on the history, physical examination, and appropriate exclusion of other causes of red eye. It is important, in the correct setting, to perform a thorough examination to rule out both other causes of red eye and potential complications of conjunctivitis such as corneal ulceration. When particularly virulent pathogens are a consideration, Gram stain and cultures may be necessary. Because the diagnosis of viral conjunctivitis can be made clinically, viral culture and laboratory investigation are not necessary.[20]

## TREATMENT AND DISPOSITION

Some basic tenets should be followed in the treatment of conjunctivitis, with separate consideration for the specific cause as detailed later.

Frequently, treatment is supportive. Cold compresses help alleviate the swelling and lid discomfort. Broad-spectrum antibiotic drops are used for bacterial conjunctivitis and often to prevent superinfection with other organisms. Erythromycin is appropriate for uncomplicated cases. A fluoroquinolone that provides coverage against *Pseudomonas* should be given to contact lens wearers. Topical corticosteroids should be prescribed only after consultation with an ophthalmologist and should never be used in a patient with suspected or confirmed herpes infection. Artificial tears alleviate keratitis and photophobia.

### ADENOVIRUS

Adenovirus infection requires supportive care consisting of cool compresses, decongestants, and lubricants, as well as topical antibiotics to prevent superinfection. Because of the high transmissibility of adenovirus, care should be taken to prevent contamination of the other eye and those of others. Cases of adenovirus conjunctivitis can be managed on an outpatient basis.

### HERPES SIMPLEX CONJUNCTIVITIS

Ophthalmologic consultation is indicated immediately for patients with herpes simplex conjunctivitis. The ophthalmologist may consider mechanical débridement. Topical antivirals such as 3% vidarabine and 1% trifluridine are prescribed in consultation with an ophthalmologist. Up to 97% of patients have been shown to heal within 2 weeks following trifluridine therapy.[4] Topical prophylactic antibiotics and cycloplegia are also used.

### HERPES ZOSTER OPHTHALMICUS

The EP should consult an ophthalmologist about a patient with herpes zoster ophthalmicus. Systemic antiviral agents are indicated early in the disorder. Early treatment with antiviral therapy within 72 hours of onset of the rash has been shown to reduce acute pain and ocular complications.[21] Corticosteroid therapy may be considered in consultation with the ophthalmologist.

### UNCOMPLICATED BACTERIAL CONJUNCTIVITIS

Supportive care with warm compresses and lubricants should be given as needed for bacterial conjunctivitis. Topical antibiotics should be prescribed. The multiple choices include erythromycin, 10% sulfacetamide, 0.3% gentamicin, polymyxin B–neomycin-bacitracin (Neosporin), and ciprofloxacin. Use of neomycin solutions is associated with a relatively high incidence of hypersensitivity. Coverage against *Pseudomonas* should be included for contact lens wearers.

### GONOCOCCAL CONJUNCTIVITIS

Gonococcal conjunctivitis should be considered a systemic condition. Affected patients require emergency ophthalmologic consultation, and hospital admission is usually indicated. Treatment involves topical and parenteral antibiotic therapy and frequent eye irrigation to prevent corneal perforation. In some situations, patients are given one dose of ceftriaxone intramuscularly and are then discharged after receiving topical antibiotics, instructions for eye rinsing, and arrangements for close follow-up.

### CHLAMYDIAL CONJUNCTIVITIS

Like gonococcal infection, chlamydial conjunctivitis requires systemic therapy. Treatment involves oral and topical antibiotics. In neonates, systemic therapy is effective for concomitant pneumonitis.

### FUNGAL CONJUNCTIVITIS

For a patient with fungal conjunctivitis, the EP should consult with an ophthalmologist about prescribing an appropriate topical agent, such as a 5% suspension of natamycin. Patients with this eye disorder require close follow-up.

### ALLERGIC CONJUNCTIVITIS

Patients with allergic conjunctivitis need supportive care with compresses, artificial tears, and ocular decongestants. Diphenhydramine therapy can also be effective.

## CORNEAL ABRASIONS

Corneal abrasions, one of the most common ocular injuries, account for 10% of ED visits related to ocular complaints. They result from scraping away of the corneal epithelium by contact with a foreign body or application of a moving force, such as rubbing over a closed lid. Most corneal abrasions heal spontaneously without long-term sequelae; on occasion, however, scarring and permanent epithelial damage ensue. Corneal abrasions are more common in contact lens wearers.

## PATHOPHYSIOLOGY

Corneal abrasions are defects in the corneal surface that are typically limited to the epithelial layer. Sometimes the bulbar conjunctiva is also affected. Severe injuries can involve the deeper, thicker stromal layer of the cornea.

## PRESENTING SIGNS AND SYMPTOMS

Common complaints of patients with corneal abrasions include photophobia, foreign body sensation, pain, and tearing. Conjunctival injection and blepharospasm may or may not be seen. Depending on the location and size of the abrasion, patients may also complain of decreased visual acuity. Fluorescein examination demonstrates the abrasion as a staining defect (**Fig. 26.8**). If a linear abrasion is noted, the EP should search carefully for a retained foreign body on the inner side of the upper eyelid. Corneal ulceration should be excluded with a slit-lamp examination, especially in contact lens wearers. A topical anesthetic should be administered to facilitate the examination.

**TIPS AND TRICKS**

- Perform a slit-lamp examination before fluorescein examination to prevent false-positive results of assessment for corneal abrasions.
- Apply local anesthetic (e.g., tetracaine) to facilitate a slit-lamp examination.
- A cotton-tipped applicator can be used to evert the upper eyelid.
- Never send a patient home with topical anesthetic eyedrops, which can raise the risk for further injury.

## DIFFERENTIAL DIAGNOSIS

All entities that cause eye pain should be included in the differential diagnosis for corneal abrasion. Because erythema and changes in visual acuity may or may not be present, the differential diagnosis has to be tailored to the individual case. Examination and measurement of IOP should eliminate glaucoma as a cause of the symptoms. Slit-lamp examination demonstrates cells and flare in the anterior chamber in a patient with iritis. Lack of infiltrate and ulcer morphology exclude corneal ulcers. The EP should look carefully for a foreign body to eliminate it as a cause of the complaints.

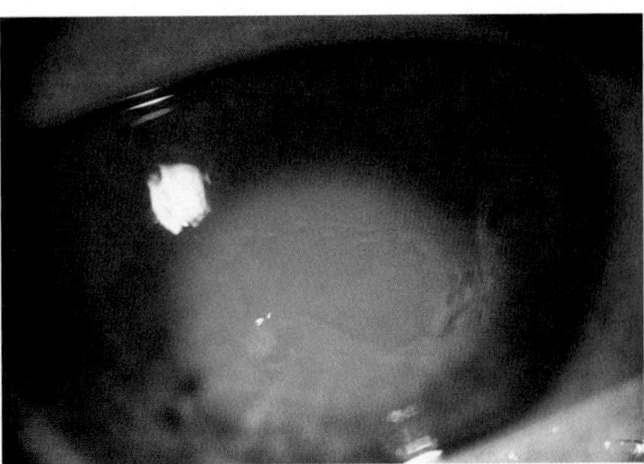

**Fig. 26.8 Corneal abrasions.** (From Goldman L, Ausiello D, editors. Cecil medicine. 23rd ed. Philadelphia: Saunders; 2007.)

## TREATMENT

Providing comfort for the patient is the goal of treatment of corneal abrasion. Although topical antibiotics may be administered to facilitate evaluation, patients should never be discharged with such medications. Continued use of topical ocular anesthetics may cause injury through loss of the protective reflexes and drying of the eye. Systemic analgesia should be prescribed as needed. Studies have suggested that topical nonsteroidal antiinflammatory drugs also provide relief and may reduce the need for oral narcotic agents. A cycloplegic agent such as homatropine provides relief from photophobia and blepharospasm.

The practice of routinely prescribing topical antibiotics for corneal abrasions to prevent corneal ulceration is not clearly based on evidence, although some studies have suggested that it is beneficial. For example, a prospective study investigating the incidence of corneal ulceration in close to 35,000 patients in whom corneal abrasions were diagnosed demonstrated that none of the patients who received antibiotics had ulceration. Contact lens wearers should be treated with agents that provide coverage against *Pseudomonas*. Eye patching should be avoided, especially in contact lens wearers and patients whose abrasions were cause by organic material, because it may encourage infection. Evidence suggests that patching may be harmful, but current data are not available. Patients with abrasions should discontinue contact lens wear during the healing period.

Tetanus prophylaxis has been a long-standing component of the treatment of corneal abrasions, but evidence suggests that this practice is not routinely indicated. In the absence of infection, corneal perforation, or devitalized tissue, no benefit is seen with the routine administration of a tetanus booster. However, current Centers for Disease Control and Prevention guidelines recommend a tetanus booster within 5 years if the event causing the corneal abrasion involved a dirty vector such as vegetable matter and within 10 years if the corneal injury was caused by a clean, uncontaminated vector.[22,23] Corneal abrasions heal within 3 to 5 days, and patients can be discharged with arrangements for close outpatient follow-up.

# CORNEAL ULCERS

Generally, corneal ulcers are infectious in etiology. A corneal ulcer is an ophthalmologic emergency because the diagnosis carries a risk for permanent visual impairment and eye perforation. Risk factors for corneal ulcer include eye trauma, known infection, contact lens wear, and immunosuppression.

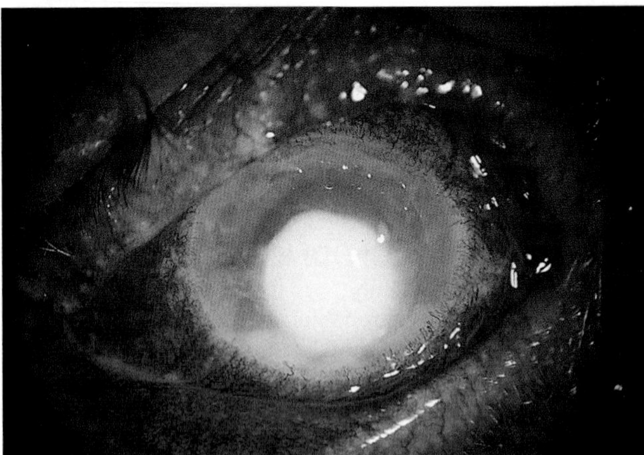

**Fig. 26.9 Corneal ulcers.** (From Auerbach PS, editor. Wilderness medicine. 5th ed. Philadelphia: Mosby; 2007.)

## PATHOPHYSIOLOGY

Even seemingly minor trauma involving the cornea can create a break, which serves as a port of entry for bacteria. Conditions such as lack of lubrication and malnutrition make the cornea more susceptible to injury.

## PRESENTING SIGNS AND SYMPTOMS

Corneal ulcers cause significant eye pain, ciliary injection, tearing, foreign body sensation, blurry vision, and photophobia. Eyelid swelling and purulent drainage may be present. Depending on the location and extent of the lesion, visual acuity may be decreased. Inspection may show eyelid swelling and erythema. Large ulcers can be seen as round or oval white spots on the cornea with the naked eye. Fluorescein and slit-lamp examinations demonstrate a corneal defect, usually with sharply demarcated borders and a gray appearance of the infiltrated ulcer base. On examination of the anterior chamber, hypopyon or a flare consistent with iritis is often seen. With the exception of the classic dendritic lesions that occur with herpes simplex virus infection, no pathognomonic signs or symptoms can be used to diagnose the cause of the ulcer seen on examination (**Fig. 26.9**).

## DIFFERENTIAL DIAGNOSIS

The same conditions that must be considered in the differential diagnosis for patients with corneal abrasions must be considered for those with corneal ulcers.

## TREATMENT AND DISPOSITION

Immediate ophthalmologic consultation should be obtained for a patient with a corneal ulcer. Some ophthalmologists advocate discharge with follow-up the next day. A cycloplegic agent such as homatropine is given for comfort. Frequent topical antibiotic therapy should be prescribed. The typical regimen involves administration of the drops every 1 to 2 hours until the follow-up appointment the next day.

# OCULAR FOREIGN BODIES

Corneal foreign bodies are generally superficial and do not cause long-term morbidity. However, if allowed to remain in place for a long enough time, infection, tissue necrosis, and scarring may occur.

## PATHOPHYSIOLOGY

Objects, especially those projected with considerable force, may become embedded in the corneal epithelium or deeper into the stroma. The associated irritation triggers a cascade of events, including vascular dilation, which is manifested as conjunctival injection and lid edema.

## PRESENTING SIGNS AND SYMPTOMS

Typical symptoms of an ocular foreign body include pain, photophobia, tearing, conjunctival injection, and a foreign body sensation. Examination may show conjunctival injection, a visible foreign body, a corneal epithelial defect, and corneal edema. White blood cell mobilization may occur and can be detected as anterior chamber flare and the presence of cells. Visual acuity can be decreased. Metallic foreign bodies can cause visible rust rings (**Fig. 26.10**).

## DIFFERENTIAL DIAGNOSIS

Conditions that may mimic corneal abrasion and corneal ulceration must also be considered in patients with an ocular foreign body. Application of topical anesthesia blunts or obliterates the pain and photophobia associated with superficial corneal processes. This response can be helpful in distinguishing among the various eye disorders.

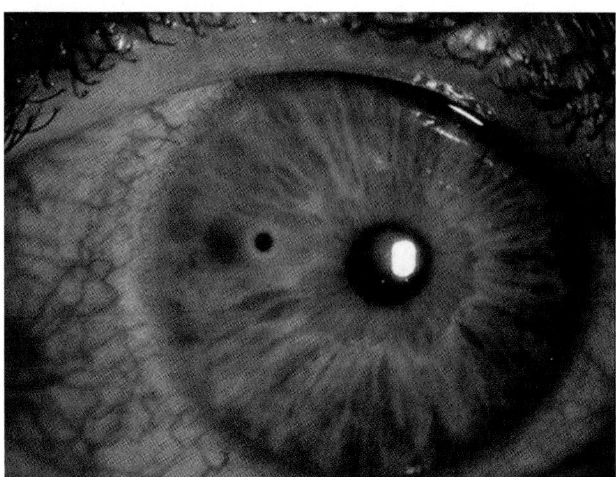

**Fig. 26.10 Rust ring seen after removal of a metallic foreign body.** (Courtesy Ted Montgomery, OD. Available at www.tedmontgomery.com/the_eye/.)

## DIAGNOSIS

The diagnosis of an ocular foreign body is based on the history and physical findings. If there is concern about a foreign body that is not visible, especially an intraocular foreign body, a CT scan should be obtained. MRI is contraindicated if it is possible that the foreign body is metallic. Ultrasonography can be used to visualize a superficial foreign body, but this modality is limited by the type of particle, as well as possible obscuration of findings by processes such as subconjunctival hemorrhage. A Seidel test should be performed to look for corneal rupture if deep projection is suspected. The lids should be everted and a possible lodged foreign body sought.

## TREATMENT AND DISPOSITION

Treatment consists first of removal of the foreign body. Topical anesthesia should be provided and a cycloplegic agent considered. Superficial foreign bodies are removed with a spud or needle. A cotton-tipped applicator should be used with great caution because its large surface area may result in abrasion. The foreign body should be removed under magnification with a slit lamp. The EP should approach the foreign body with the removal device held parallel to the surface of the eye to avoid inadvertent perforation. Retained rust rings after removal of a metallic foreign body must be removed with a rust ring drill; an ophthalmologist should be consulted for this maneuver.

After removal of the foreign body, the patient should be given topical antibiotics. Patching of the eye for comfort is not necessary and is strictly contraindicated in those with severe corneal injury because it may foster infection. Pain control should be adequate, and arrangements should be made for prompt follow-up.

# INTRAOCULAR FOREIGN BODY

More than three fourths of intraocular foreign bodies enter the eye through the cornea. Suspicion of such a foreign body is based on patient complaints, as well as the history. Injuries associated with mechanical grinding, drilling, and hammering should raise the possibility of an intraocular foreign body. Intraorbital and intracranial injury should always be considered in patients with an intraocular injury.

The extent and process of the eye damage depend on the object involved and the area penetrated. Because of gravity, the inferior aspect of the eye is more commonly injured. The composition of the object involved affects local tissue reaction. Inert substances such as glass cause less reaction than organic materials do. Metallic and magnetic substances are most common.

The signs and symptoms also vary according to the factors just described. Patients often complain of discomfort or pain deep within the eye. The presence of obvious abnormalities on inspection, such as conjunctival injection, is variable. Visual acuity is also contingent on the area involved. Careful slit-lamp and funduscopic examinations should be performed to search for the object. An abnormally shaped pupil is suspicious for rupture of the globe.

CT is the imaging modality of choice if it is necessary to search for the injury or to more closely ascertain its specifics. Ultrasonography can be helpful with relatively superficial objects. Plain radiographs cannot distinguish between intraocular and extraocular positions of a foreign body. MRI cannot be used if there is any suspicion that the foreign body may be metallic.

## DIFFERENTIAL DIAGNOSIS

If the eye with the foreign body appears normal externally, inspection alone excludes several painful eye disorders, such as iritis. Application of topical anesthetics should not affect the pain caused by an intraocular foreign body—in contrast to the pain associated with a corneal foreign body or abrasion. A careful examination can exclude glaucoma as the cause of the patient's symptoms.

## TREATMENT

Consultation with an ophthalmologist should be sought immediately. The patient should not eat or drink, and antibiotics and pain medications should be administered. Tetanus status should be updated as necessary. Generally, intraocular foreign bodies are removed surgically. The technique and approach are chosen by the ophthalmologist. Patients with an intraocular foreign body should be admitted to the hospital.

# OCULAR BURNS

Ocular burns, which include burns involving the sclera, conjunctiva, cornea, and lids, can be damaging to visual integrity, as well as cosmesis. Burns may be chemical, thermal, or related to radiation exposure. The method and extent of damage vary with the cause.

## PATHOPHYSIOLOGY

Burns cause tissue damage by denaturing and coagulating cellular proteins and by leading to vascular ischemia. Thermal burns usually cause superficial epithelial destruction, but deep penetration can occur. Radiation injury causes punctuate keratitis, which is extremely painful. Patients with radiation ocular burns report exposure to sun lamps, tanning booths, high altitudes, or welder's arcs. Acidic burns cause coagulation necrosis, which serves as a barrier and limits the extent of penetration. Alkaline chemicals can cause devastating injury. Such a chemical causes liquefaction necrosis, which continually penetrates and dissolves tissue until the chemical is removed. At pH values greater than 11.5, the damage is generally irreversible.

## PRESENTING SIGNS AND SYMPTOMS

Patients usually complain of eye pain and limited visual acuity. Examination in the acute phase often shows corneal cloudiness and scleral whitening. The eye may be erythematous or whitened. Findings consistent with anterior chamber reaction, chemosis, and vascular engorgement may be present. Radiation burn or ultraviolet keratitis causes intense pain, tearing, photophobia, blepharospasm, and a foreign body sensation. Physical findings include punctate lesions on the corneal epithelium, conjunctival injection, and decreased visual acuity. Thermal burns are almost always limited to the corneal epithelium.

## DIFFERENTIAL DIAGNOSIS

A history of exposure usually leads to a clear diagnosis. Radiation burns are not always so clear-cut because symptoms develop 6 to 10 hours after exposure to the light source. Other conditions to consider are iritis, glaucoma, corneal ulcer, corneal abrasion, and a retained foreign body. Slit-lamp and fluorescein examinations allow differentiation among the various entities.

## DIAGNOSIS

The type of chemical burn can be diagnosed by determination of the pH of the affected eye. Findings depend on the concentration of the chemical and the duration of exposure to it. Most burns can be diagnosed from the history alone. Radiation burns can be a bit more challenging to diagnose because of extreme patient discomfort. Providing adequate topical analgesia should enable examination.

## TREATMENT AND DISPOSITION

The most important component in the treatment of chemical burns is copious irrigation. Eye irrigation should be started immediately—with no waiting even for measurement of visual acuity. After irrigation for 30 minutes, the pH should be checked. The EP should not withhold irrigation or delay its initiation even if the patient underwent prehospital irrigation. Irrigation should continue until a normal pH is recorded. Once a normal pH is obtained, the measurement should be repeated 10 to 15 minutes later to confirm neutrality. Topical anesthetics and manual lid retraction may be necessary for proper irrigation. Any particles should be removed from the fornices with a cotton swab.

After adequate irrigation, complete examination of the eye, including slit-lamp examination and determination of visual acuity, should be performed. Patients with minor burns can be discharged home with topical antibiotics, oral analgesics, and cycloplegics as necessary with arrangements for follow-up in 24 hours. An ophthalmologist should be consulted for all but the most minor ocular burns. Severe burns may cause secondary glaucoma, which is treated in consultation with the ophthalmologist. Patients with severe burns require admission for monitoring, including IOP measurements, and adequate analgesia.

Most thermal burns, which are relatively minor and restricted to the lid and corneal epithelium, can be treated the same as corneal abrasions. Initial irrigation may provide relief. Topical antibiotics, oral pain medications, and cold compresses should be provided. Patients can be discharged with outpatient follow-up. An ophthalmologist should be consulted for more severe burns.

Radiation burns are treated with cycloplegic agents and topical antibiotics. Eye patching can be considered for comfort, and oral pain medications should be prescribed. *Topical anesthetics delay healing and can lead to corneal ulcer formation.* Follow-up in 24 hours should be arranged.

## RETROBULBAR HEMATOMA

Retrobulbar hematoma is bleeding in the potential space surrounding the globe. It results from blunt trauma, as well as from retrobulbar injection and operative intervention. This entity can compromise vision, so immediate recognition and intervention are warranted. Bleeding typically results from injury to the infraorbital artery or one of its branches. Accumulation of blood results in an increase in pressure, which ultimately compresses blood vessels and other structures. The compression leads to optic nerve and central retinal artery ischemia. With trauma, concomitant orbital wall fractures serve to decompress the hemorrhage, thereby sparing vision.

### PRESENTING SIGNS AND SYMPTOMS

Severe eye pain, nausea, vomiting, diplopia, and decreases in both visual acuity and eye movement are common complaints at initial evaluation of a patient with retrobulbar hematoma. Physical findings include proptosis, decreased ocular motility, visual loss, elevated IOP, and hemorrhagic chemosis. An afferent pupillary defect is common (**Fig. 26.11**).

### DIAGNOSIS

Clinical examination suggests the diagnosis. If the diagnosis is in doubt, CT can be performed to demonstrate the hematoma.

### TREATMENT

The rate of development of retrobulbar hematoma dictates the treatment. If the condition develops over minutes, the eye must be decompressed immediately via lateral canthotomy (**Fig. 26.12**). Orbital CT demonstrates the hematoma; however, treatment should not be delayed while waiting for imaging to be performed. If the process is slower and develops over a period of hours, conservative management can be effective and consists of head elevation, ice packs to reduce swelling, intravenous acetazolamide and mannitol, and topical beta-blockers. Progress is monitored through serial measurements of IOP and pupillary reactivity. An ophthalmologist should be notified for consultation as soon as the diagnosis is suspected. Patients with retrobulbar hematoma are admitted to the hospital to monitor progress.

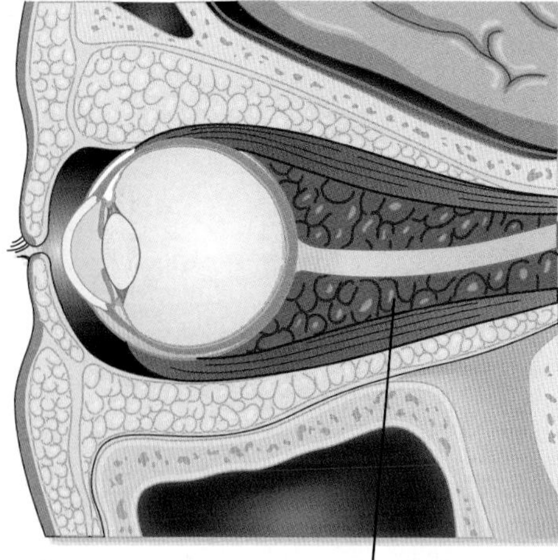


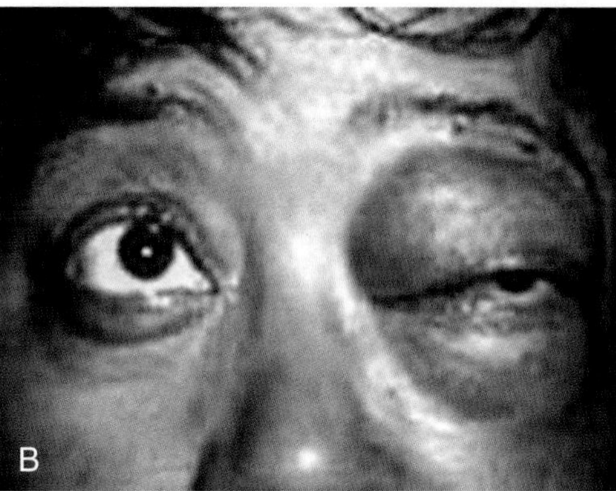


**Fig. 26.11** **A and B, Retrobulbar hematoma.** (**B,** from Pacific University: Online Optometry Education. Available at http://www.opt.pacificu.edu/ce/catalog/10310-SD/Trauma%20Pictures/Retrobulbar%20Heme.jpg.)

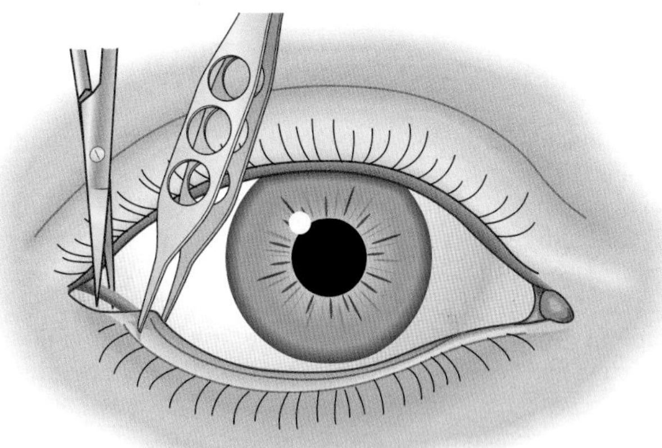

**Fig. 26.12** **Lateral canthotomy.**

## HYPHEMA

Accumulation of blood in the anterior chamber is called hyphema. Traumatic hyphema, which can occur from both blunt and penetrating mechanisms, is generally caused by a ruptured iris root vessel. Hyphemas range from minimal blood seen only with the slit lamp to the "eight ball" or total hyphema with blood that has clotted. Spontaneous hyphemas are most commonly associated with sickle cell disease and the neovascularization of diabetes. Even small hyphemas can signal significant injury.

### PRESENTING SIGNS AND SYMPTOMS

Patient symptoms and findings on examination correlate with the size of the hyphema. Typically, patients complain of eye

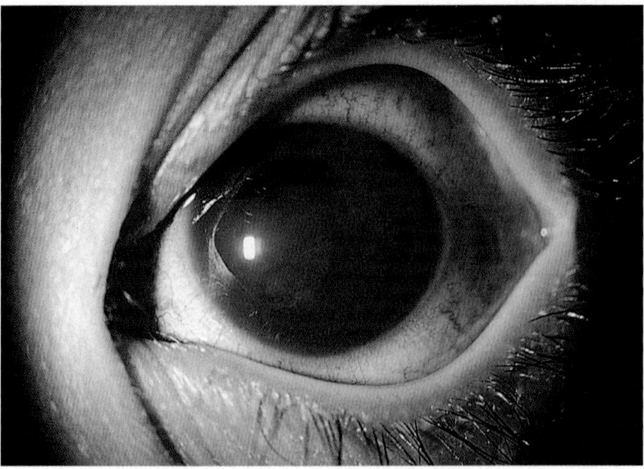

**Fig. 26.13 Hyphema.** (From Auerbach PS, editor. Wilderness medicine. 5th ed. Philadelphia: Mosby; 2007.)

pain, decreased visual acuity, and photophobia. If the patient is upright, the hyphema usually layers out in the inferior portion of the anterior chamber. Depending on the size of the hyphema, it can be seen with either the naked eye or a slit-lamp examination. If the hyphema is large, IOP can be elevated. IOP is elevated in approximately 27% of patients acutely but is usually mild and self-limited. Pressures greater than 35 mm Hg with durations greater than 5 to 14 days are more likely to be associated with optic atrophy.[20] Generally, no afferent pupillary defect is present (**Fig. 26.13**).

## DIAGNOSIS

The diagnosis is made by visualization of blood in the anterior chamber.

## TREATMENT AND DISPOSITION

All patients with hyphemas should be seen by an ophthalmologist. The goal is to stop damage to the visual process by preventing or curbing elevations in IOP. The patient's head should be elevated to allow inferior settling of the red blood cells. Such settling will prevent clogging of the trabecular meshwork. The pupil should be dilated to avoid "pupillary play"—movements of the iris to accommodate changing light conditions; this step should be taken in consultation with the ophthalmologist. Dilation does not block drainage of aqueous humor in normal eyes. Topical beta-blockers should be used to lower IOP. Topical $\alpha$-agonists, topical carbonic anhydrase inhibitors, and systemic acetazolamide or mannitol may also be considered. Adequate analgesia should be given, with care taken to avoid aspirin and other antiplatelet agents.

Surgery may be necessary if the elevated IOP is refractory to medical therapy or to remove a large clot. Patients with hyphemas larger than 50%, decreased vision, increased IOP, and sickle cell disease should all be considered for admission.[24] In consultation with an ophthalmologist it may be determined that a patient with an extremely small hyphema can receive outpatient management. The major complication of hyphema is rebleeding after 2 to 5 days when the initial clot loosens, which results in potentially severe elevations in IOP. The reported incidence of rebleeding is between 6% and 33%.[20]

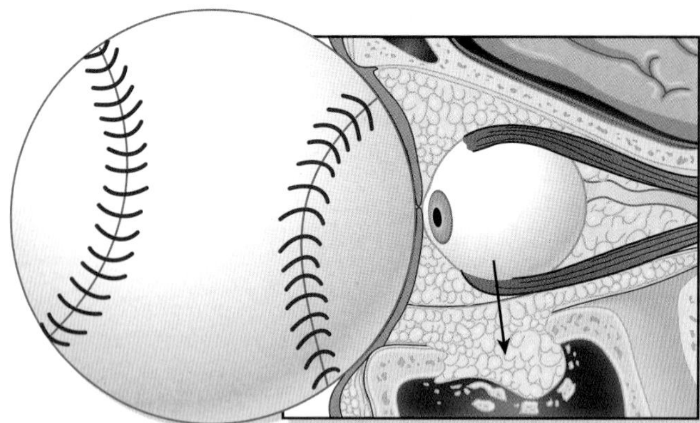

**Fig. 26.14 Orbital wall or blow-out fracture.**

## ORBITAL WALL OR BLOW-OUT FRACTURES

Blunt force to the orbital region can raise intraorbital pressure, relief of which is accomplished by fracture of the orbital walls. A fracture of the orbital wall should always be suspected when a patient has soft tissue swelling following trauma to the globe The inferior and medial walls are most frequently involved. The orbital contents slip into the corresponding sinus: the maxillary sinus for inferior wall fractures and the ethmoid sinus for medial wall fractures. Concomitant facial injuries should be sought in a patient with an orbital wall or blow-out fracture (**Fig. 26.14**).

## PRESENTING SIGNS AND SYMPTOMS

The signs and symptoms in patients with an orbital wall or blow-out fracture can be highly variable and range from mild swelling and ecchymosis to impairment of vision. Patients may exhibit tenderness with palpation of the orbit. Subcutaneous orbital emphysema can often be found by examination. Inferior wall fractures can cause entrapment of the inferior rectus and inferior oblique muscles and orbital fat. Patients may have restricted upward gaze and diplopia, anesthesia of the ipsilateral cheek and upper lip, and ptosis. Epistaxis and diplopia can be seen with medial wall fractures. On rare occasion, orbital emphysema can cause a mass effect in which the optic nerve is compressed and blindness ensues.

## DIAGNOSIS

A Waters view radiograph can show indirect signs of fracture: a cloudy sinus, a bulge extending from the orbit into the maxillary sinus (the teardrop sign), or an air-fluid level in the maxillary sinus. CT is the diagnostic study of choice because it demonstrates the fracture, as well as other injuries. The use of bedside ultrasound has also shown to be helpful in the identification of orbital wall fractures.[25]

### TREATMENT AND DISPOSITION

Indications for surgical repair include muscle entrapment and cosmetic deformity with significant enophthalmos. Immediate surgery is not necessary. Surgery is delayed to allow abatement of the swelling and a better examination. The preferred time frame for operative repair is 10 to 14 days, which optimizes the balance between reduced swelling and absence of scar tissue formation. Administration of prophylactic antibiotics for an orbital wall or blow-out fracture without evidence of sinus infection is controversial. Data are inadequate for a definitive recommendation, as review of 214 studies to examine this very question found.[26,27]

## RUPTURED GLOBE

Globe rupture involves a full-thickness defect in the cornea, sclera, or both. Penetrating mechanisms are almost always involved. Rarely, enough force is generated by a blunt injury that transmission of the force results in eventual rupture. Ruptures are most common at the insertions of the intraocular muscles or at the limbus, where the sclera is thinnest.[28] This entity is a true ophthalmologic emergency and always requires surgical intervention.

Sharp objects and objects traveling at considerable velocity have the potential to perforate the globe directly. Any projective injury can cause globe rupture. Significant blunt force can result in compression of the globe with resultant increases in IOP sizable enough to tear the sclera. Such injuries typically occur where the sclera is the thinnest, such as at muscle insertion sites or sites of previous surgery.

### PRESENTING SIGNS AND SYMPTOMS

Patients with globe rupture complain of eye pain and decreased visual acuity. Because this entity is associated with a high rate of concomitant orbital floor fractures, patients may report diplopia. Rupture may not be easily apparent on examination. A shallow anterior chamber on slit-lamp examination, hyphema, and an irregular (teardrop) pupil are possible findings. A Seidel test can identify wound leaks from the anterior chamber.

### DIAGNOSIS

Diagnosis is not always easy. The history and physical findings described lead to the diagnosis. Though not always indicated, CT can detect occult tears, as well as retained foreign bodies. Plain radiographs may show foreign bodies.

### TREATMENT AND DISPOSITION

Direct pressure should never be applied to a globe that is suspected or confirmed to be ruptured because of the risk for extrusion of intraocular contents. Although a lower than normal IOP is a good indication of rupture, tonometry should not be performed in patients with suspicion of globe rupture. A protective eye shield should be placed, and an ophthalmologist should be contacted immediately. The patient's tetanus status should be checked and updated if necessary, and a dose of prophylactic antibiotics should be given to prevent endophthalmitis. Because skin flora is typically involved in infections of a ruptured globe, cefazolin or ciprofloxacin plus clindamycin is a good choice. Adequate antiemetics should be given to prevent Valsalva maneuvers. Surgery is performed expeditiously, and all patients with globe rupture are admitted to the hospital.

## TRAUMATIC IRITIS

Blunt ocular trauma can contuse and irritate the iris, with resultant ciliary spasm. Symptoms usually start 1 to 4 days after the injury.

### PRESENTING SIGNS AND SYMPTOMS AND DIAGNOSIS

Eye pain and photophobia are the most common patient complaints with traumatic iritis. Patients report impaired vision. Evaluation shows perilimbal conjunctival injection, cells and flare in the anterior chamber, and a constricted, weakly dilating pupil.

### TREATMENT AND DISPOSITION

Treatment involves administration of a long-acting cycloplegic agent such as 5% homatropine, a topical steroid chosen in consultation with an ophthalmologist, and oral analgesics. Patients can be discharged with arrangements for ophthalmologic follow-up.

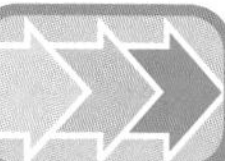

**PRIORITY ACTIONS**

- Determine whether the patient's complaint is monocular or binocular.
- Determine whether the complaint is related to trauma.
- Ask whether the patient wears contact lenses or glasses.
- Check the patient's visual acuity.
- Determine whether vision is monocular or binocular.
- Involve an ophthalmologist in the treatment of a patient with an eye complaint as soon as possible if there is reasonable suspicion of a vision-compromising process, such as acute angle-closure glaucoma or central retinal artery occlusion.

### REFERENCES

*References can be found on Expert Consult @ www.expertconsult.com.*

# 27 Ear Emergencies

Thomas Morrissey and John B. Lissoway

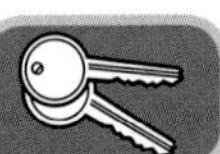

**KEY POINTS**

- Ears are exquisitely sensitive organs. Treating pain is important in caring for patients with ear problems and will facilitate performance of the examination.
- Simple otitis externa can be treated with topical medications and débridement.
- Many cases of uncomplicated otitis media resolve spontaneously. Watchful waiting with use of a "rescue" antibiotic prescription has been shown to decrease unnecessary antibiotic use and improve patient and parent satisfaction.
- Subtle malalignments or malformations after repair of ear trauma can have profound cosmetic consequences.
- Pain from the teeth, pharynx, or temporomandibular joint or from cranial or cervical neuropathies can be referred to the ear.
- Hearing loss must be categorized as conductive or sensorineural. Conductive lesions can often be diagnosed clinically. Sensorineural hearing loss requires urgent referral to an otolaryngologist to improve the chance for recovery of hearing.

## PATHOPHYSIOLOGY

Anatomically, the ear is divided into three areas. The *external ear* extends outward from the tympanic membrane and serves to guide sound waves into the "business end" of the ear. Its external location places it at high risk for traumatic injuries, environmental exposure, obstruction, and infection. The *middle ear* extends inward from the tympanic membrane to the oval and round windows. It transfers mechanical energy from the outside world, through the ossicles in the middle ear, to the inner ear, where it is translated into signals that the brain interprets as sound. The enclosed nature of the middle ear predisposes it to accumulation of fluid, infection, and barotrauma. The *inner ear* is composed of the structures responsible for sound transduction and balance (organ of Corti, cochlea, vestibule [saccule and utricle], and semicircular canals). Dysfunction of this portion of the ear accounts for some visits to the emergency department (ED), but treatment options are limited and consist mostly of patient education, prognostication, limitation of further damage, and appropriate ear, nose, and throat (ENT) referral. The ear is surrounded by the middle cranial fossa superiorly, the mastoid air cells posteriorly, the cranial vault medially, and the temporomandibular joint and parotid glands anteriorly. Evaluation of these structures is a necessary part of the ear examination.

## EAR PAIN

Ear pain may be referred from or occur as a result of infections, trauma, or a foreign body affecting the ear.

### INFECTIONS

Ear pain is commonly caused by infection. Any portion of the ear can become infected. The disease state is categorized by the portion of the ear that is primarily affected.

#### *Otitis Externa*

Infections of the outer ear canal most often begin when breakdown of the natural barriers allow infectious organisms to gain a foothold. This commonly occurs in the summer months, when warm weather and frequent water sports lead to excessive ear moisture, which washes out the cerumen and alkalinizes the normally acidic environment—hence the term *swimmer's ear*. Cotton swab trauma can be the inciting event, especially in diabetic patients.

The most common pathogens are *Pseudomonas aeruginosa* (frequently found in pools) and *Staphylococcus aureus*. Less common causes include chemical or contact dermatitis and fungal infections. The spectrum of disease ranges from mild (with minimal pain and inflammation of the canal) to severe (complete canal occlusion and exquisite pain). Further extension results in an invasive or systemic disease state called necrotizing external otitis (formerly malignant otitis externa; see later).

The diagnosis of external otitis is made from the history and findings of pain, pruritus, canal irritation, and edema on physical examination. Thick greenish discharge suggests *Pseudomonas*, whereas golden crusting implicates *S. aureus*. Other colored or black discharge may indicate fungal infections, of which *Candida* and *Aspergillus* are the most commonly isolated species.[1] Small abscesses in the external ear canal can cause obstruction. These abscesses often require incision and drainage, as well as standard treatment of otitis externa.

### Treatment

Treatment consists of débridement or aural toilet and antibiotics. Despite a relative lack of controlled studies, the American Academy of Otolaryngology–Head and Neck Surgery Foundation has released clinical practice guidelines based on evidence available as of 2005 (**Fig. 27.1**; also see the Patient Teaching Tips box).[2] Briefly, these guidelines are as follows:

1. Distinguish acute external otitis from other causes of otalgia, otorrhea, and inflammation. Diagnostic criteria include rapid onset (2 to 3 days) and a duration of less than 3 weeks. Symptoms include otalgia, itching, or fullness. Signs include tenderness of the pinna or tragus or visual evidence of canal erythema, edema, or otorrhea.
2. Assess for factors that may complicate the disease or treatment (e.g., perforation of the tympanic membrane or eustachian tubes, immunocompromising states, previous radiotherapy). These factors raise the level of treatment needed and heighten suspicion for more invasive disease states such as necrotizing otitis externa (see later). These guidelines pertain to patients older than 2 years with normal states of health.
3. Pay attention to assessment and treatment of pain! Mild to moderate pain usually responds to acetaminophen or a nonsteroidal antiinflammatory drug alone or in combination with an opioid.
4. Topical preparations are first-line agents for the treatment of acute uncomplicated otitis externa. Reserve systemic therapy for immunocompromised patients or extension of disease beyond the ear canal. Topical therapy produces drug concentrations 100 to 1000 times that available with systemic administration and can thus overwhelm resistance mechanisms. No clear evidence points to the superiority of one particular treatment. Antiseptic and acidifying agents (e.g., aluminum acetate and boric acid) appear to work as well as antibiotic-containing solutions (e.g., solutions that contain cortisone and Neosporin or a fluoroquinolone). Corticosteroids in the drops decrease the duration of pain by approximately 1 day.[3]
5. Make sure that the patient can instill the drops correctly. Edema can prevent the drops from entering the canal. Debris or detritus should be removed or irrigated out. Placement of a compressed cellulose or ribbon gauze wick in the canal will enable the drops to penetrate, but placement can be painful. Within 1 to 2 days the canal edema should subside, and the wick falls out or can be removed (**Fig. 27.2**).
6. If you cannot be sure that the tympanic membrane is intact, use a nonototoxic, pH-balanced preparation such as ofloxacin and ciprofloxacin-dexamethasone.
7. Educate and reassess your patients. Pain should decrease significantly in 1 to 2 days and resolve by 4 to 7 days. Failure to improve may indicate more invasive disease (e.g., necrotizing otitis), inability of drops to reach the canal (wick needed), or noncompliance with therapy.

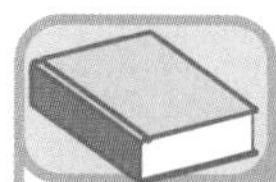

**PATIENT TEACHING TIPS**

**Otitis Externa**

Most patients with otitis externa can be managed as outpatients. Follow-up in 1 to 2 days is indicated if a wick is placed for treatment, if oral antibiotic therapy is started, or if the pain does not begin to resolve in 24 to 36 hours.

Patients should discontinue use of the drops after full resolution of their symptoms. Continued use of antibiotics (especially neomycin) can predispose to changes in the environment of the ear canal and foster fungal infections or sensitivity reactions.

Patients must avoid getting water in the ear during the healing process. Cotton balls soaked in petroleum jelly work well as earplugs. Any water that gets into the ear can be removed by gentle blow-drying.

Patients with evidence of significant immunocompromise or failure to improve in 1 to 2 days should be considered for admission to the hospital to be evaluated for more extensive disease.

Drying the ear after swimming or showering helps prevent otitis externa. Placing drops of acetic acid (vinegar) and rubbing alcohol in the ear two or three times a week during periods of heavy water exposure (summer vacation) helps dry the ear and restore the acidic environment that protects against otitis externa.

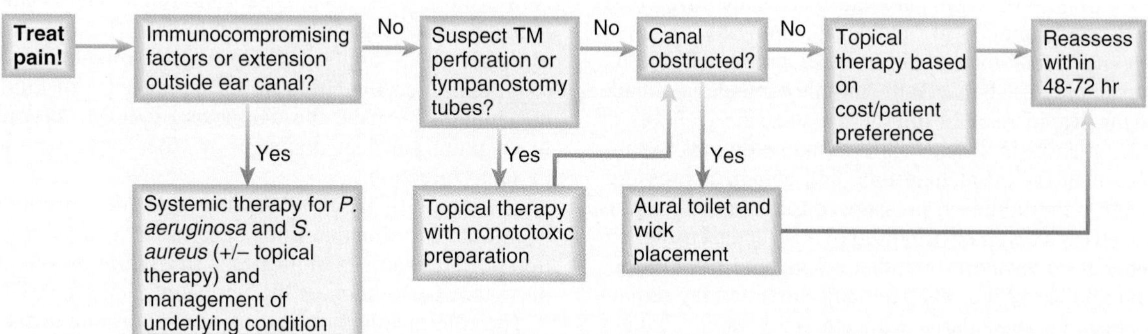


**Fig. 27.1 Algorithm for the treatment of acute otitis externa.** *TM*, Tympanic membrane. (Adapted from Rosenfeld RM, Brown L, Cannon CR, et al. Clinical practice guideline: acute otitis externa. Otolaryngol Head Neck Surg 2006;134;S4-23.)

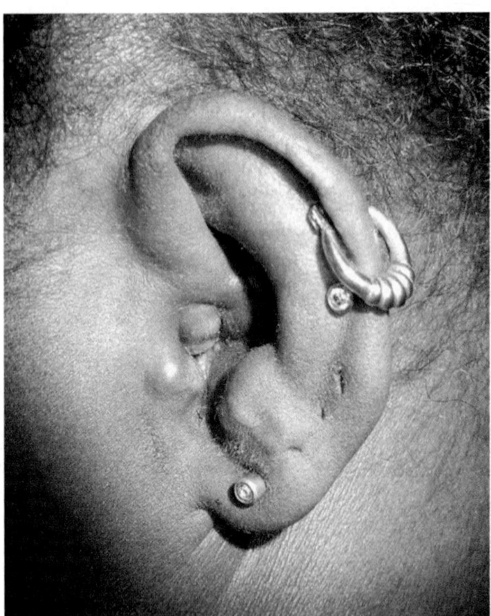

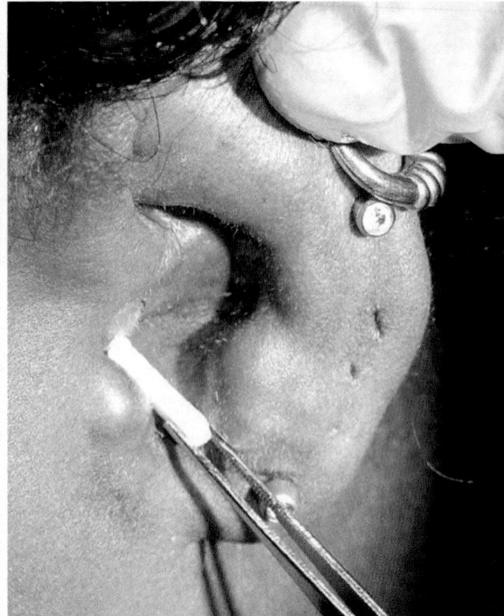

**Fig. 27.2** Edema from otitis externa may cause obstruction. Placement of a wick or gauze ribbon will allow the drops to penetrate the external ear canal.

### *Otitis Media (Acute and Chronic)*

Accumulation of fluid in the middle ear (medial to the tympanic membrane) is termed *otitis media.* Fluid collections can be clinically sterile, as in barotrauma-mediated effusions or chronic otitis media with effusion, or can result from infectious causes (*acute otitis media* [AOM]). Infection-mediated effusions may be serous (usually viral in origin) or suppurative (primary or secondary bacterial infection). The common link between all these processes is eustachian tube dysfunction. The eustachian tube acts as a vent and conduit between the middle ear and posterior pharynx in which air pressure between the middle ear and ambient air is equalized and fluid can drain from the middle ear cavity. After infections (primarily upper respiratory infections [URIs]), edema can cause blockage of the tube. Air is easily absorbed through the middle ear tissues, thereby leading to a relative negative pressure in the middle ear. This negative pressure draws fluid into the enclosed cavity. Native or invasive bacteria can work their way into this enclosed area and proliferate.[4,5] Common bacterial pathogens are the same as those frequently found in sinus infections and include *Streptococcus pneumoniae*, nontypeable *Haemophilus influenzae*, and *Moraxella catarrhalis*. Currently, approximately 60% to 70% of *S. pneumoniae* species are covered by the polyvalent pneumococcal vaccine (Pneumovax).[6,7]

Barotrauma refers to the rapid development of relative differences in pressure between the middle ear and the outside environment. Rapid rises in middle ear pressure (relative to the outside, such as in ascent while flying or diving) usually forces air out of the eustachian tube and equalizes pressure. A relative drop in middle ear pressure (during descent) that is not equalized (as a result of collapsed or obstructed eustachian tubes) generates a vacuum force that draws fluid from tissues into the middle ear space. The resultant effusion may remain sterile or become secondarily infected. Very rapid changes in pressure can even cause direct trauma to the tympanic membrane, including rupture or hemorrhage within the layers of the membrane itself.

*Acute otitis media* is primarily a disease of children. In early childhood the eustachian tubes are not angled downward and do not drain well spontaneously. The relatively small tube size and higher frequency of URIs in children 6 to 24 months old lead to the highest incidence of otitis media in this age group. Another increase in the incidence of otitis media occurs at 5 to 6 years, which coincides with entrance into school and a higher frequency of URIs. The craniofacial abnormalities seen with some developmental disorders (e.g., Down syndrome) also predispose to the development of middle ear effusions.

Otitis media is one of the most common reasons for pediatric physician visits, with estimates that $5 billion is spent as direct or indirect costs annually. A significant proportion of cases are probably misdiagnosed, and guidelines have been issued to ensure proper diagnosis and thus curb wasting of resources.[8] "Visualization of the tympanic membrane with identification of a middle ear effusion and inflammatory changes is necessary to establish the diagnosis with certainty."[8] Effusions are signified on physical examination by bulging of the tympanic membrane, bubbles or fluid levels behind the membrane, loss of the light reflex (opacification or cloudiness of the membrane), and (most definitively) loss of tympanic membrane mobility on pneumatic insufflation. Newer modalities, such as acoustic reflectometry and tympanometry, also demonstrate middle ear effusions but are not available in many EDs. Tympanic membrane injection (common in crying children) or the presence of fluid alone is not enough to make the diagnosis of AOM. Accompanying fever, pain, purulent drainage, or other systemic signs point to acute infection.

Chronic otitis media is defined as (1) the chronic presence of middle ear effusion in the absence of acute signs of infection or (2) chronic complications from otitis media, including persistent perforation of the tympanic membrane.

The role of infectious organisms in chronic otitis media is unclear. It was originally thought to be a noninfectious entity, but studies have shown the presence of bacteria (and bacterial DNA, mRNA, and proteins) in a biofilm model of chronic otitis media.[9] Current guidelines offer the option of a trial of antibiotics (typically amoxicillin) or watchful waiting as treatment.[8]

### Treatment

American physicians have historically treated otitis media with antibiotics, whereas European physicians are typically less likely to do so. A 2005 study compared immediate antibiotic treatment with watchful waiting for *nonsevere* otitis media.[10] In the watchful waiting group, 66% of children had complete resolution of symptoms with no antibiotic treatment, no adverse outcomes, cost savings, and similar patient satisfaction.

Treatment options and recommendations by the American Academy of Pediatrics for acute otitis media include the following[8]:

1. Pain management must be addressed in patients with AOM. Particular attention should be paid to pain management in the first 24 hours of any treatment regimen.
2. Observation without the use of antibacterial agents is an option for the first 2 to 3 days in selected children[11] (**Table 27.1**). The child must be otherwise healthy and in a sound social environment with an adult capable of watching the child closely and returning to the physician if the condition deteriorates.
3. If antimicrobial treatment is chosen, the first-line agent should be amoxicillin, 80 to 90 mg/kg/day. With treatment failures or cases in which broader β-lactamase coverage is desired, amoxicillin, 90 mg/kg, with clavulanate, 6.4 mg/kg, in two divided doses can be used. Penicillin-allergic patients (non–type 1) can be treated with a third-generation cephalosporin (cefdinir, cefpodoxime, cefuroxime, or ceftriaxone). For patients with severe type 1 penicillin allergy, alternative treatments include azithromycin, clarithromycin, erythromycin-sulfisoxazole, and sulfamethoxazole-trimethoprim. Treatment is aimed at common pathogens, including *S. pneumoniae*, nontypeable *H. influenzae*, and *M. catarrhalis*. *Mycoplasma* species can also cause otitis media and are often responsible for blister formation on the tympanic membrane (bullous myringitis). Multiple virus species can cause otitis media and are obviously unaffected by antibiotics.
4. Failure of response in 2 to 3 days should prompt initiation of or a change in antibiotic treatment. If amoxicillin fails, alternatives include amoxicillin-clavulanate, cephalosporin (ceftriaxone), macrolides, and sulfa preparations.

**Table 27.1 Acute Otitis Media Treatment Guidelines**

| AGE | CERTAIN DIAGNOSIS OF ACUTE OTITIS MEDIA | UNCERTAIN DIAGNOSIS |
|---|---|---|
| <6 mo | Antibacterial therapy | Antibacterial therapy |
| 6 mo to 2 yr | Antibacterial therapy | Severe illness: antibacterial therapy<br>Nonsevere illness: observation option* |
| ≥2 yr | Severe illness: antibacterial therapy<br>Nonsevere illness: observation option* | Observation option* |

From Johnson NC, Holger JS. Pediatric acute otitis media: the case for delayed antibiotic treatment. J Emerg Med 2007;32:279-84.

*Observation: defer antibiotic treatment for 48 to 72 hours.

Some authorities have suggested a compromise between meeting patients' expectations and decreasing the inappropriate overuse of antibiotics.[12,13] Patients can be given a "rescue" prescription, which they should have filled only if no improvement occurs in 2 to 3 days.

Chronic otitis media is not typically an emergency. The American Academies of Family Physicians, Pediatrics, and Otolaryngology–Head and Neck Surgeons have recently issued guidelines to direct the diagnosis and treatment of otitis media with effusion; they are summarized as follows:

1. Pneumatic otoscopy should be used to identify the presence of effusion.
2. The history and physical examination (to search for acute signs and symptoms of inflammation or infection) should be used to distinguish this disorder from AOM.
3. Otitis media with effusion should be managed with watchful waiting for 3 months in children who are not at risk for speech, language, or other learning disabilities.
4. Hearing tests (referral to an otolaryngologist) should be performed if the disease lasts longer than 3 months or earlier if any language, learning, or hearing problems are suspected.
5. Antihistamines and decongestants are ineffective and should not be used as treatment; antimicrobial agents and steroids do not have long-term efficacy and should not be used for routine management.

Middle ear effusions in adults should be able to be explained clinically (e.g., after URI) and should resolve within a few weeks. Any other circumstances require otolaryngologic

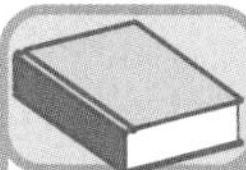

**PATIENT TEACHING TIPS**

**Otitis Media**

Most patients with otitis media can be treated as outpatients.

If antibiotic therapy is chosen, patients should be counseled to take the entire course of antibiotic therapy.

Watchful waiting with a rescue prescription can be chosen for healthy-appearing patients older than 2 years. Parents should be educated about signs of worsening infection, including pain and fever.

Patients should follow up with their primary physicians or return to the emergency department if no improvement occurs in 1 to 3 days.

Patients should be warned of the signs and symptoms of intratemporal and intracranial complications (headache, neck stiffness, vomiting, altered mental status).

Patients should also be apprised of the risks associated with otitis media with effusion and must be sure to follow up with their primary physicians to alleviate the risk for hearing deficits.

referral to evaluate for other nasopharyngeal disease, such as an obstructing tumor.

### Necrotizing (Malignant) Otitis Externa

Necrotizing otitis externa (formerly known as malignant otitis externa) is aggressive extension of infection from the auditory canal to the skull base and other nearby bony structures. This complication occurs nearly exclusively in immunocompromised hosts, with elderly diabetic patients accounting for most of the affected population. It can be the initial complaint in patients with undiagnosed diabetes, and all patients with progressive ear infection need prompt evaluation for diabetes. The emergence of widespread human immunodeficiency virus infection now puts children at risk for a condition that was once almost exclusively an adult disease.[14]

Necrotizing otitis externa may be difficult to distinguish from simple otitis externa in the early stages, but exquisite otalgia and otorrhea unresponsive to topical measures point to the former diagnosis. The pain often extends to the temporomandibular joint and gets worse with chewing. Granulation tissue is frequently seen at the inferior portion of the canal where the cartilage and bone meet, at the site of the fissures of Santorini. Inflammation of bony structures as a result of the osteomyelitis can cause nerve palsies (facial nerve most frequently involved). Progression of the infection inward can lead to catastrophic complications such as brain or epidural abscess, sinus thrombophlebitis, and meningitis. Evaluation with computed tomography (CT) or magnetic resonance imaging (MRI) can show the extent of the invasive process and may be helpful in evaluating for intracranial complications, but arranging for such an evaluation should not delay initiation of treatment.

More than 95% of cases of necrotizing otitis externa are caused by *P. aeruginosa*, and antibiotic therapy should be aimed at this organism. Since the introduction of semisynthetic penicillins, antipseudomonal cephalosporins, and antipseudomonal fluoroquinolones, mortality from this disorder has decreased from 50% to 10%. Empiric treatment with ciprofloxacin, 400 mg intravenously every 8 hours, is reasonable. Alternative treatments are an antipseudomonal penicillin (e.g., ticarcillin-clavulanate [Timentin], 3.1 g intravenously every 6 hours) and cephalosporins (e.g., ceftazidime, 1 to 2 g every 8 hours). Recently, resistance of *P. aeruginosa* to ciprofloxacin has been reported to be as high as 33%. Resistance is related to widespread use of quinolones for the treatment of URIs, topical preparations for otitis media and externa, and inadequate treatment courses in patients with malignant otitis externa.[15]

### Ramsay Hunt Syndrome

The combination of ear pain, ipsilateral facial paralysis, and vesicular lesions characterize Ramsay Hunt syndrome, also known as herpes zoster oticus. This reactivation of latent varicella-zoster infection in the geniculate ganglion with spread to the eighth cranial nerve (and frequently cranial nerves V, IX, and X) results in both auditory and vestibular dysfunction.[16]

Physical examination usually demonstrates vesicular lesions in the ear canal, but the variable course and innervation of the nervous structures may lead to involvement of the anterior aspect of the tongue, soft palate, pinna, and face. Because of the proximity of the ear to the eye, evaluation for ocular involvement is necessary. The disease tends to be self-limited and mortality is extremely rare, but deficits in nerve function and facial paralysis are common, and patients with such paralysis are much less likely to recover than those with Bell palsy.

Treatment is aimed at shortening the duration of the outbreak and controlling symptoms. Acyclovir and steroids are often used, but no clear prospective studies have been undertaken. In light of the known safety and effectiveness of anti–varicella-zoster or anti–herpes simplex drugs, acyclovir (800 mg five times per day) or famciclovir (500 mg three times per day) should be strongly considered, along with added prednisone.[17] Aggressive analgesia is frequently needed for pain control. Vestibular symptoms can be treated with meclizine or diphenhydramine. Cranial nerve VII palsies can occur and lead to an inability to close the eye, which can cause drying and abrasions. Use of a moisturizer or lubricant ophthalmic ointment (Lacri-Lube) or other measures to moisten and protect the eye are often needed.

### Mastoiditis

All cases of otitis media are accompanied by some subclinical fluid collection in the mastoid air cells, often seen on CT. Further blockage of the communicating spaces by mucosal edema and inflammation generates pus under pressure in the mastoid air spaces and results in what we know as clinically significant mastoiditis. Left untreated, the chronic inflammation results in abscess formation and resorption of trabecular bone.

This process can further extend outward or inward. Outward extension leads to subperiosteal abscess formation. This development is associated with the classic findings for mastoiditis: tenderness and erythema over the mastoid process, outward bulging of the pinna, loss of the postauricular crease, and fluctuance behind the ear. Inward extension leads to potentially catastrophic complications such as erosion into the cranial vault, meningitis, and brain abscess formation.

Mastoiditis is a clinical diagnosis, and physical findings should prompt CT evaluation to delineate the extent of the process. Treatment consists of supportive care and resuscitation, administration of antibiotics, and otolaryngologic or ENT consultation for surgical drainage. Antibiotic coverage should initially be broad spectrum and include coverage against common otitis media pathogens, anaerobes, and *Pseudomonas* and *Bacteroides* species.

## TRAUMA

External ear trauma can be classified into contusions and ecchymoses; seromas and hematomas; and lacerations, tears, and avulsions. Fluid collections and anatomic disruptions require directed attention because of the propensity for necrosis or disfigurement if managed inappropriately.

*Blunt trauma* can cause blood to collect in the fascial plane between the cartilage and the perichondrium. The cartilage is an avascular structure that derives its nutritional support from the blood supply of the perichondrium, and separation of the two starves the cartilage. Furthermore, neocartilage formation in the fluid collection space leads to scarring and deformation (cauliflower ear). Fluid collections can be drained by either needle aspiration or open evacuation. For cosmetic purposes, collections that form lateral (external) to the cartilage layer can be drained through a medial approach. A gentle compression dressing can then be applied by packing the ear canal with dry cotton and packing the rest of the auricle with a conforming material (gauze or foam). A gauze roll and an elastic bandage can then be carefully wrapped around the head to compress the entire bandage in place while avoiding overly tight placement, which could cause ear necrosis. Follow-up within 24 hours is needed to check for reaccumulation of fluid, which would need to be redrained.

*Lacerations* and *avulsions* need special repair techniques because of the cosmetic importance of ears. As with all facial wound repairs, minimal débridement (to minimize tissue loss) and alignment of visually eye-catching anatomic lines are key to aesthetic repair. Through-and-through lacerations of the pinna necessitate alignment and repair of the underlying cartilage. The use of deep sutures should be minimized (usually one or two), and small absorbable sutures should generally be used. The overlying skin can then be closed to realign the pinna rim first, followed by closure of the remainder of the defect. Similar technique should be used for earlobe clefts, which commonly occur after abrupt traction on earrings causes either a partial or complete tear of the earlobe. Compression packing should be applied to prevent reaccumulation of fluid. Complex disruptions with significant tissue loss can be managed conservatively, with referral for plastic or reconstructive repair at a later date to maximize the chance for a good cosmetic outcome.

## FOREIGN BODY

Direct visualization of any foreign body in an ear is critical to identification of the object and aids in the choice of removal method. A small amount of lidocaine or mineral oil instilled into the ear anesthetizes or immobilizes most insects in the ear canal within about a minute.

Methods of foreign body removal are as follows:

- *Irrigation*: An intravenous catheter without a needle (18 to 20 gauge) can be used with a 10- to 20-mL syringe. Irrigating the superior portion of the canal seems to provide the best results. The force generated is well below that needed to perforate a normal tympanic membrane. Materials that swell when wet (vegetables, cellulose, wood) should not be removed by this method because of the risk for further swelling.
- *Forceps*: Small forceps (alligator forceps) can be used to grasp objects. Use of an ENT scope and speculum greatly facilitates the process (**Fig. 27.3**).
- *Cyanoacrylate*: A small amount of cyanoacrylate (e.g., Super Glue) can be applied to the blunt end of a cotton-tipped applicator and held against the impacted object for about 60 seconds to glue the foreign body to the applicator and allow gentle removal of it. This method should not be attempted in a moving, uncooperative patient.
- *Right-angle probe*: A small probe can sometimes be worked behind the object and used to pull it forward. This works best for loose or pliable objects.

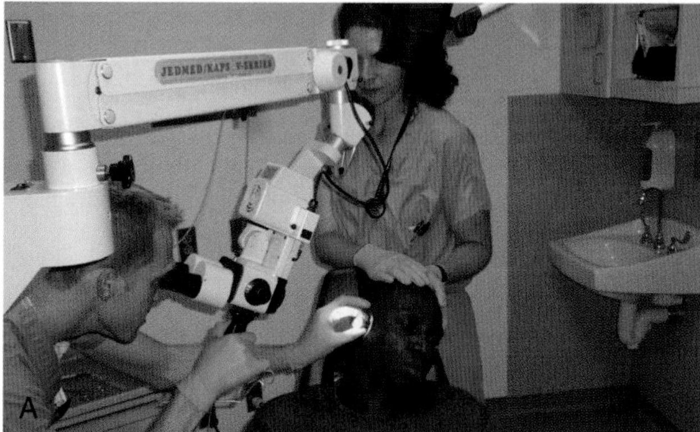


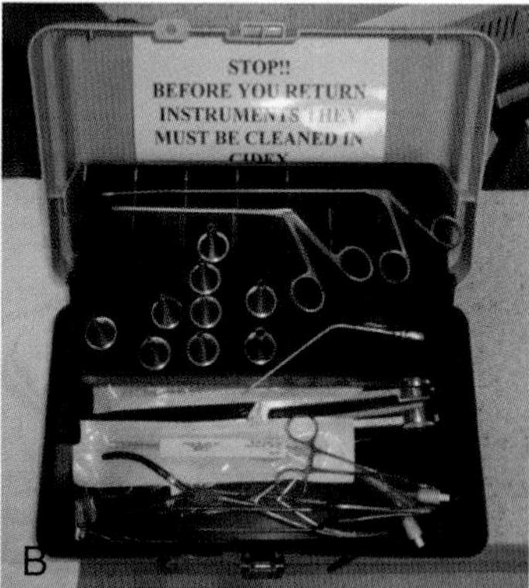


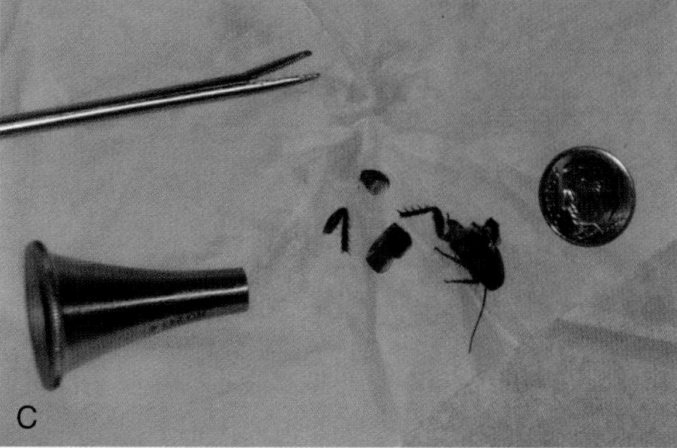


**Fig. 27.3** An ear, nose, and throat scope (**A**) frees up both hands for removal of foreign bodies. A selection of different-sized reflective speculua and forceps (**B**) greatly facilitates extraction of foreign bodies (bug; **C**).

- *Suction*: A flanged end of thin plastic tubing (or a premade suction device) can sometimes be used to grasp smooth, regularly shaped objects (beads) or pieces of insects for removal.

If removal of a foreign body from the ear canal is difficult or impossible, in most cases the patient can be treated with pain and anxiety medications and followed up in an otolaryngologic clinic in 12 to 24 hours. Exceptions to this statement are lodged button batteries (risk for caustic damage from leakage) and signs of advanced infection (redness, fever, uncontrollable pain); such cases require otolaryngologic consultation in the ED.

*Cerumen*, or earwax, is a naturally occurring substance that cleans, protects, and lubricates the external auditory canal. Excessive accumulation of cerumen is one of the most common reasons that patients seek medical care for ear-related reasons. When associated with symptoms, it is recommended that clinicians use ceruminolytic agents (triethanolamine, docusate sodium, saline), irrigation, or manual removal to treat a patient with impacted cerumen.[18]

## SUDDEN HEARING LOSS

Anatomically and physiologically, the hearing process consists of two parts. Conduction refers to the mechanical transmission of sound waves from the external environment through the outer and middle ear to the round window. The sensorineural component refers to transduction of sound waves to electrical (neural) impulses and delivery of these impulses to the brain, where they can be interpreted as sound. Hearing can be impaired by dysfunction in either or both of these pathways. The first step in evaluating hearing complaints (and the primary guide to treatment) is to ascertain the location and extent of the hearing loss. The history and physical examination provide nearly all the information needed to guide ED treatment of hearing loss. The history must include details about the timing of hearing loss, laterality, previous episodes, associated symptoms (tinnitus, vertigo, or pain), preceding events (diving, plane rides, trauma), potential placement of a foreign body, environmental noise exposure, and potential ototoxic drugs.

Tuning fork tests provide the best clues to distinguish between conductive and sensorineural hearing loss. The key component of the test is to compare how well the ear hears conduction through bone versus conduction through air. A 512-Hz fork should be used. The *Weber test* compares the two ears with each other (**Fig. 27.4**). A vibrating fork is placed midline on the top of the head or between the front top teeth (some patients find this intolerable). The patient is asked which ear hears the vibrations better. Because outside sounds (from air conduction) suppress the perception of vibratory conduction, an ear with a conductive hearing defect will "hear" the fork vibrating through bone "louder" than the other ear will. So if the fork is heard louder in one ear, either that ear has a conductive deficit or the other ear has a neural deficit (**Table 27.2**).

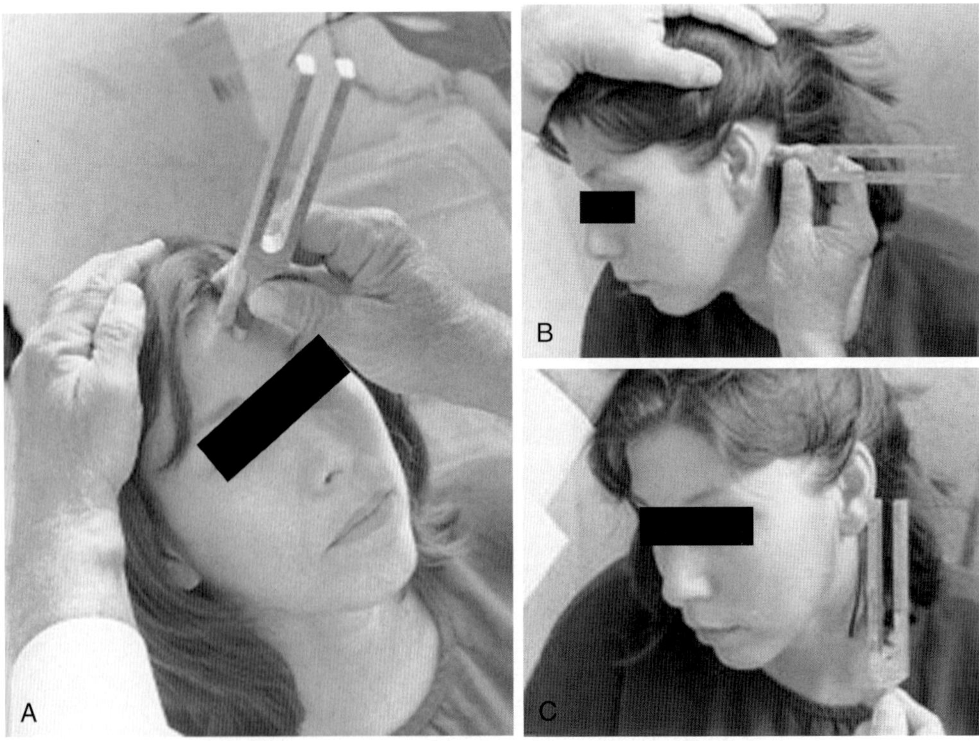


**Fig. 27.4** The Weber test compares hearing in the two ears with each other. A vibrating tuning fork is held midline against the patient's forehead (**A**). The patient is asked whether one ear hears the fork more loudly. Unequal perception of sound indicates a conductive deficit in the loud ear or a neural deficit in the quiet ear. The Rinne test compares air and bone conduction in each ear independently. A vibrating tuning fork is held against the mastoid process (bone conduction; **B**) until the vibrations can no longer be heard. The still-vibrating tip is then moved near the canal opening to see whether the patient can still hear the vibration through air conduction (**C**). Longer or louder hearing through air conduction is normal. Longer or louder hearing through bone conduction indicates a conductive hearing deficit.

**Table 27.2 Interpretation of the Weber and Rinne Tests**

| | WEBER WITHOUT LATERALIZATION | WEBER LATERALIZES RIGHT | WEBER LATERALIZES LEFT |
|---|---|---|---|
| Rinne both ears: AC > BC | Normal | S/N loss in the left ear | S/N loss in the right ear |
| Rinne left ear: BC > AC | – | Combined loss: conduction and S/N loss in the left ear | Conduction loss in the left ear |
| Rinne right ear: BC > AC | – | Conduction loss in the right ear | Combined loss: conduction and S/N loss in the right ear |

*AC*, Air conduction; *BC*, bone conduction; *S/N*, sensorineural.

**Table 27.3 Lesions That Cause Hearing Loss**

| | DESCRIPTION OF PATHOLOGY | ONSET/COURSE | ACTIONS OR TREATMENT | PROGNOSIS |
|---|---|---|---|---|
| **Conductive Lesion** | | | | |
| Foreign body | Mass in external canal blocks sound conduction | Acute onset associated or not with pain, drainage, or odor | Removal. Evaluate for infection. Evaluate for TM perforation | Excellent |
| Otitis externa | Edema and detritus obstruct external canal | Rapid onset. Pain, edema, swelling. Drainage, odor often present | Aural toilet to remove debris. Topical (± oral) antibiotics. Evaluate for necrotizing otitis | Excellent if treated appropriately |
| Exostosis | Bony growths obstruct canal. Often seen with prolonged exposure to cold water (divers) | Slow insidious onset. No pain or drainage unless causes complete obstruction | Evaluate for infection. Reassure patient. Refer to ENT | Good |
| Tympanosclerosis | TM scarring from perforations or infections. Decreased mobility impairs sound conduction | Slow onset following perforations, trauma or infections | ENT referral. Reassurance | Variable |
| Perforated TM | Disruption of TM integrity results in impaired transmission of sound to ossicle | Acute onset. May follow direct trauma or sudden barotrauma. May have sudden relief from pain if caused by otitis media | Treat infectious causes. Counsel on importance of keeping water out of ear canal. ENT referral | Good |
| Sterile effusion (barotrauma) | Fluid in middle ear dampens conduction through ossicles | Often following flight, diving, or URI. Bubbles can cause intermittent pain | Decongestants. Evaluate for infection. Follow-up | Excellent |
| Acute otitis media | Pus (or fluid) in middle ear dampens conduction through ossicles | Acute to subacute onset, often following URI. Often associated with pain ± fever | Antibiotics (unless viral cause suspected), decongestants, pain control | Excellent if treated appropriately |
| Cholesteatoma | Trapped stratified squamous epithelial mass in middle ear. Interferes with ossicle conduction | Slow onset. Often history of previous perforations or chronic infections | ENT referral | Variable. May destroy ossicles or erode into surrounding structures |
| Glomus tumor | Vascular tumor occupies middle ear space. Interferes with ossicle conduction | Slow onset. May be associated with rushing pulsatile sensation | ENT referral | Variable |
| Cancer | Squamous cell most common. Obstructs external canal | Slow onset. Often noticed first by others. Painless unless occlusion causes otitis externa | ENT referral. Evaluate for secondary infection | Variable |

*Continued*

**Table 27.3 Lesions That Cause Hearing Loss—cont'd**

| | DESCRIPTION OF PATHOLOGY | ONSET/COURSE | ACTIONS OR TREATMENT | PROGNOSIS |
|---|---|---|---|---|
| **Sensorineural Lesion** | | | | |
| Perilymph fistula (inner ear barotrauma) | Disruption of round or oval window allows leakage of perilymph into middle ear | Sudden onset of hearing loss often with tinnitus and vertigo. Frequently follows straining or abrupt change in pressure. Turning in direction of fistula exacerbates symptoms | Complete bed rest. Elevate head of bed and avoid increases in CSF pressure. Severe symptoms or noncompliance may require hospitalization. ENT consultation for possible oval or round window patch | Variable |
| Viral cochleitis | Cochlear inflammation. Often following URI | Rapid onset. Often following URI | Steroids often used (no good data) | Variable |
| Presbycusis | Age-related hearing loss. May be related to previous chronic noise exposure | Slow onset. Usually symmetric. High frequencies most affected. Tinnitus may occur | Hearing aid may help with both hearing loss and tinnitus | Variable |
| Acoustic neuroma | Benign schwannoma of 8th cranial nerve | Slow onset. Usually unilateral. May exhibit tinnitus, vertigo. May exhibit facial hyperesthesias or twitching | May require surgical excision if symptoms debilitating | Variable |
| Ototoxic agents | Direct toxicity to inner ear structures | Variable onset. High frequency most affected. Exposure to ototoxic drugs. May have associated tinnitus | Stop use of offending agent | Variable. Hearing loss at time of stopping offending agent is usually permanent |
| Multiple sclerosis | Multiple demyelinating lesions interfere with nerve conduction | Often other associated neurologic findings. May wax and wane | Standard multiple sclerosis treatment (steroids, cytotoxic agents) | Variable |
| Stroke/CVA | Focal ischemic lesion of auditory nerve or auditory cortex | Sudden onset. Often associated with other neurologic deficits | Treat CVA risk factors (ASA, anticoagulants, glycemic control, BP control) | Variable |
| Meningitis | Infection enters inner ear through CNS-perilymph connection. Damages organ of Corti | Follows clinical picture of meningitis | Treat infection. Steroids may limit inflammation and damage | Variable |
| Meniere disease (endolymphatic hydrops) | Abnormal homeostasis of inner ear fluids (clinical diagnosis; definitive diagnosis made histologically) | Episodic spells of vertigo. Associated sensation of fullness, tinnitus, and SNHL or auditory distortion. Low-frequency ranges most affected | Reduce salt, caffeine, nicotine (vasoconstrictors) intake. Consider diuretics, antihistamines, anticholinergics. ENT referral | Variable |
| Chronic noise exposure | Direct mechanical damage to cochlear structures and hair cells | Slow onset. Usually high frequency most affected | Prevention measures (earplugs). Stop exposure | Usually permanent |
| Skull trauma | Interruption of cranial nerve VIII, ossicle disruption, or shearing effects on organ of Corti | Sudden onset after trauma | ENT consultation for possible surgical repair | Variable: ossicle disruption has better prognosis than nerve or organ of Corti damage |
| Autoimmune causes | Vascular or neuronal inflammatory changes | Bilateral asymmetric SNHL. May be fluctuating or progressive. Often other systemic autoimmune findings | Outpatient autoimmune evaluation. Steroids and cytotoxic agents may slow progression | Variable |

*ASA*, Acetylsalicylic acid; *BP*, blood pressure; *CNS*, central nervous system; *CSF*, cerebrospinal fluid; *CVA*, cerebrovascular accident; *ENT*, ear, nose, and throat; *SNHL*, sensorineural hearing loss; *TM*, tympanic membrane; *URI*, upper respiratory infection.

The *Rinne test* evaluates each ear independently (see Fig. 27.4). Normally, air conduction is more sensitive than bone conduction, and one should be able to hear a vibrating fork longer through the air than through bone. The handle of a vibrating fork is placed on the mastoid process of the side being evaluated. The vibrating end is then held near the ear canal. Normally functioning ears hear the air conduction louder and longer than the bone conduction. Perception of sound better through bone conduction indicates a conductive deficit. Lack of hearing either bone or air conduction points to sensorineural hearing loss (see Table 27.2).

## TREATMENT

Treatment options for hearing loss are limited in the ED environment and are governed by the physical findings (**Table 27.3**).

Perforation of the tympanic membrane causes conductive hearing deficits, with losses being greater in the low-frequency range. Traumatic perforations usually occur in the pars flaccida (the portion inferior to the malleolar fold). Perforations generally heal spontaneously but require urgent referral to an otolaryngologist for follow-up. Larger perforations are more likely to require specialist interventions such as patching. All patients with perforations need clear counseling about the importance of keeping the affected ear clean and dry.

Fluid collections in the middle ear dampen the vibrations of the ossicles and decrease the transmission of sound waves, thereby resulting in a relative conductive hearing deficit. Acute middle ear fluid collections may respond to decongestants alone. If evidence of infection (otitis media) is present, antibiotics may be added to the treatment regimen. Solid masses may be seen behind the tympanic membrane but are not usually treatable in the ED. All patients with chronic fluid collections and masses require referral to an otolaryngologist because studies have indicated a connection between increased duration of middle ear disease and extent of sensorineural hearing loss.[19,20]

Sensorineural hearing loss may stem from several causes, but there are few emergency treatment options. The patient can be counseled about the variable recovery rate, and some prognosis may be given on the basis of the suspected cause of the lesion. Viral causes and inflammatory or autoimmune causes may respond to steroid treatment started in the first few days. Steroids have been regarded as standard therapy for sensorineural hearing loss suspected to be of viral etiology, although no controlled trials have shown significant benefit.[21,22] Steroids should be prescribed with caution, and care must be taken to rule out infections, which may worsen with steroid treatment. Steroids should be given only if prompt follow-up is ensured. Antiviral agents (acyclovir, famciclovir, valacyclovir) are also commonly prescribed because of the possible role of herpes simplex virus type 1 as an etiologic agent in sensorineural hearing loss. No clear evidence has, however, shown a better outcome with steroids plus antiviral agents than with steroids alone.[23-25]

Patients with suspected perilymph fistulas need absolute bed rest with head elevation to avoid raising intracranial pressure (and increasing flow of cerebrospinal fluid through the fistula). Some patients may require admission and sedation for this goal to be achieved.

Other causes of sensorineural hearing loss are not likely to be identified in the ED. These cases need expedited follow-up with an otolaryngologist for MRI and audiometry. Many patients receive relief from reassurance that their hearing loss is not a life-threatening event, but the emergency practitioner should be cautious and not give an overly optimistic picture because hearing often does not return after this type of hearing loss.

## REFERENCES

***References can be found on Expert Consult @ www.expertconsult.com.***

# 28 Dental Emergencies

*Kip Benko*

**KEY POINTS**

- Adults have 32 permanent teeth. Children have 20 primary teeth.
- A tooth consists of (1) the enamel, which is the outermost, hard protective layer; (2) the underlying elastic and porous dentin, which cushions the tooth during mastication and carries nutrients from the pulp to the enamel; (3) the pulp, which contains the neurovascular supply of the tooth; and (4) the cementum and the periodontal ligament, which anchor the tooth into alveolar bone.
- Use of bupivacaine in the form of a dental nerve block is an effective means of providing relief from severe odontalgia. A dental block should also be performed before manipulation of any significantly traumatized tooth.
- Radiographs are not usually necessary for most dental complaints, but they can be useful when one must search for a tooth fragment, an avulsed or intruded tooth, or a mandibular fracture.
- Any exposed dentin or pulp of an acutely fractured tooth should be covered. The covering aids in pain control and may prevent the need for a root canal.
- Subluxated or luxated teeth should be splinted if significantly loosened to prevent aspiration and maximize potential viability.
- Avulsed teeth should be placed in a storage medium immediately by emergency medical services or emergency department personnel to maximize potential viability.

## EPIDEMIOLOGY

The incidence of dental complaints in emergency departments (EDs) appears to be rising, which may reflect the increasing use of EDs as primary care facilities.[1] Injuries involving the younger population are most often secondary to falls or accidents, whereas those in older age groups are most often secondary to motor vehicle accidents, falls, or assaults.[2] Traumatic dental injuries usually involve the permanent anterior dentition, but adult dentoalveolar injuries are frequently associated with fractures of the mandible and face. Patients who have fractures of both the mandibular condyle and body are more likely to have related tooth injury than are patients with either isolated body or condylar fractures.[2]

## STRUCTURE AND FUNCTION

### THE STOMATOGNATHIC SYSTEM

The muscles of mastication are responsible for opening and closing the mouth and are those most frequently associated with temporomandibular disorders (TMDs). The clinician should be knowledgeable about the position of the muscles to perform an examination properly and to recognize the origin of certain painful conditions. The muscles that close the mouth are those most often associated with TMDs; these muscles are the masseter, the temporalis, and the medial pterygoid (**Fig. 28.1**).[3] Contraction of this group of muscles bilaterally serves to move the condyle superiorly and posteriorly, which causes the mouth to close. The muscles that open the mouth are the anterior digastric, posterior digastric, mylohyoid, geniohyoid, and infrahyoid muscles (**Fig. 28.2**). The lateral pterygoid muscles are responsible for anterior translation and lateral movement of the mandible (**Fig. 28.3**). Unilateral contraction causes lateral movement away from the side of the muscle contraction, whereas bilateral contraction causes protrusion of the mandible.

Each side of the mandible consists of the horizontal body and ascending ramus, which are connected by the angle. The bodies of the mandible are connected by the symphysis in the midline. The ascending ramus gives rise to two processes superiorly, the condylar process and the coronoid process (**Fig. 28.4**). The mandibular condyle, along with the mandibular fossa and the articular eminence of the temporal bone, make up the temporomandibular joint (TMJ). The TMJ provides both hinge and gliding actions. Between the mandibular condyle and the articular eminence lies the meniscus, a fibrous collagen disk. A ligamentous joint capsule surrounds the TMJ and serves to limit condylar movement. TMJ pain may be caused by a number of conditions, both traumatic and nontraumatic.

### TEETH

#### *Names*

The adult dentition normally consists of 32 teeth, of which 8 are incisors, 4 are canines, 8 are premolars, and 12 are molars.

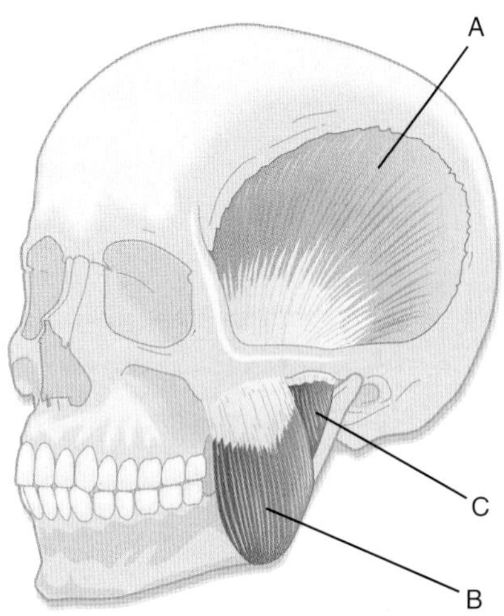

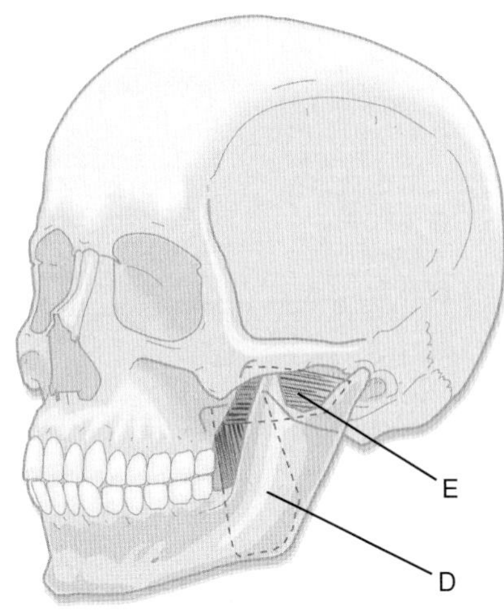


**Fig. 28.1 Muscles responsible for closing and excursive mandibular movements.** Sagittal skull views illustrate the anatomic positions of the following muscles: *A,* Temporalis; *B,* superficial masseter; *C,* deep masseter; *D,* medial pterygoid; *E,* lateral pterygoid. (From King R, Montgomery M, Redding S, editors. Oral-facial emergencies—diagnosis and management. Portland, OR: JBK Publishing; 1994.)

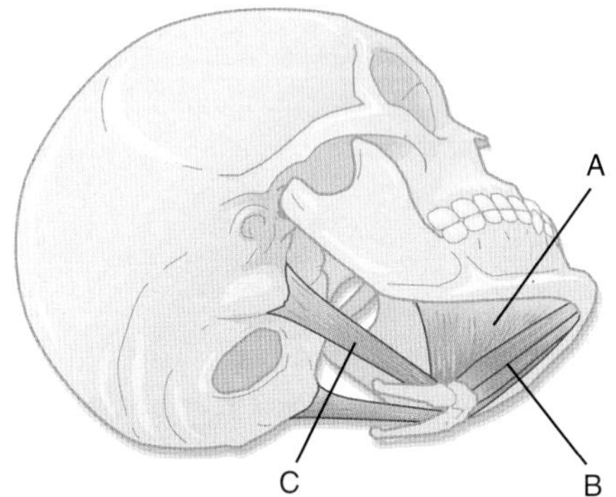

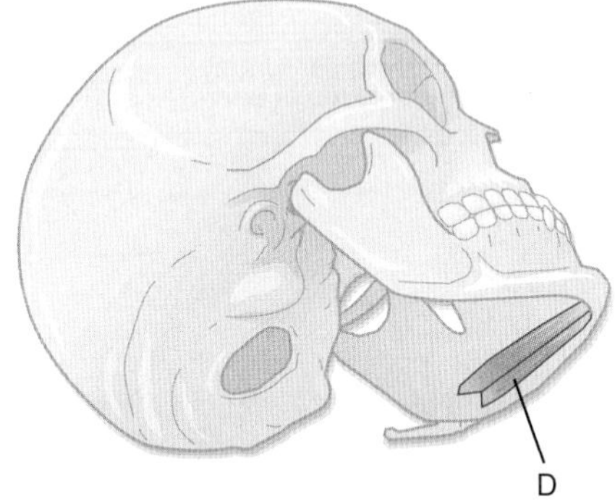


**Fig. 28.2 Muscles responsible for mandibular opening.** Oblique skull views illustrate the anatomic positions of the following muscles: *A,* Mylohyoid; *B,* anterior belly of the digastric; *C,* posterior belly of the digastric. *D,* geniohyoid. (From King R, Montgomery M, Redding S, editors. Oral-facial emergencies—diagnosis and management. Portland, OR: JBK Publishing; 1994.)

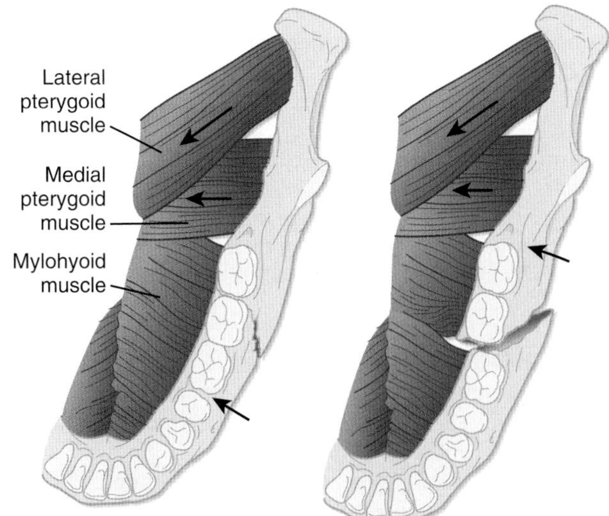


**Fig. 28.3 Axial view of the floor of the mandible.** *Arrows* indicate the direction of pull of the lateral pterygoid, medial pterygoid, and mylohyoid muscles. The view on the right shows how contraction of the pterygoids displaces a fracture. (From Eisele D, McQuone S, editors. Emergencies of the head and neck. St. Louis: Mosby; 2000.)

From the midline to the back of the mouth on each side are a central incisor, a lateral incisor, a canine (eye tooth), two premolars, and three molars, the last of which is the troublesome wisdom tooth (**Fig. 28.5**).

### Numbers

The adult teeth are numbered sequentially from 1 to 32, with the No. 1 tooth being the right upper wisdom tooth and the No. 16 tooth being the left upper wisdom tooth. The left lower wisdom tooth is No. 17, and the right lower wisdom tooth is No. 32.

### Identification of Teeth

Numerous classification and numbering systems of the teeth have been devised; however, it is probably best for emergency practitioners (EPs) to simply describe the location and type of tooth in question, for example, "the upper (or maxillary) right second premolar" or "the left lower (or mandibular) canine." This approach removes any question when the EP is discussing a case with a consultant.

The primary teeth, or "baby teeth," are also best described by determining which tooth is involved, not by its official classification. A full complement of primary teeth consists of 20 teeth: 8 incisors, 4 canines, and 8 molars. The earliest

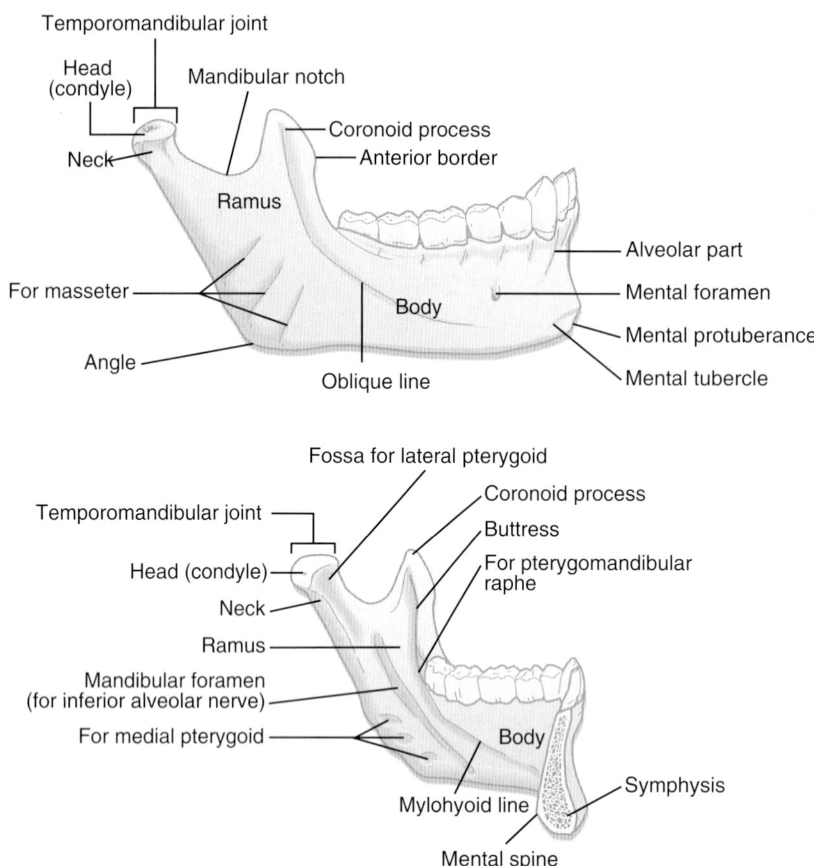


**Fig. 28.4 Anatomy of the mandible.** *Top,* View from a lateral (buccal) perspective. *Bottom,* View from a medial (lingual) perspective. (Redrawn from Grant JC. Grant's atlas of anatomy. 5th ed. Baltimore: Williams & Wilkins; 1962.)

primary teeth to erupt are the central incisors, usually at 4 to 8 months. Children usually have a full complement of teeth by the time that they are 3 years old (**Table 28.1**).

### Anatomy

A tooth consists of the central pulp, the dentin, and the enamel (**Fig. 28.6**). The pulp contains the neurovascular supply of the tooth, which delivers nutrients to the dentin, a microporous system of microtubules. The dentin makes up the majority of the tooth and cushions it during mastication. The white, visible portion of a tooth, the enamel, is the hardest part of the body. A tooth may also be described in terms of its coronal portion (crown) or its root. The crown is covered in enamel, and the root is anchored in alveolar bone by the periodontal ligament and cementum.

The following terminology is used to describe the different anatomic surfaces of the tooth:

*Facial*: The part of the tooth that faces the opening of the mouth. This surface is visible when someone smiles. This is a general term applicable to all the teeth.
*Labial*: The facial surface of the incisors and canines.
*Buccal*: The facial surface of the premolars and molars.
*Oral*: The part of the tooth that faces the tongue or palate. This is a general term applicable to all the teeth.
*Lingual*: Toward the tongue; the oral surface of the mandibular teeth.
*Palatal*: Toward the palate; the oral surface of the maxillary teeth.
*Approximal/interproximal*: The contacting surfaces between two adjacent teeth.
*Mesial*: The interproximal surface facing anteriorly or closest to the midline.
*Distal*: The interproximal surface facing posteriorly or away from the midline.
*Occlusal*: Biting or chewing surface of the premolars and molars.
*Incisal*: Biting or chewing surface of the incisors and canines.
*Apical*: Toward the tip of the root of the tooth.
*Coronal*: Toward the crown or the biting surface of the tooth.

## THE PERIODONTIUM

The periodontium is the attachment apparatus. It consists of the gingival and periodontal subunits, which maintain the integrity of the entire dentoalveolar unit. The gingival subunit consists of gingival tissue and junctional epithelium. The periodontal subunit consists of the periodontal ligament, the alveolar bone, and the cementum of the root of the tooth (see Fig. 28.6). The gingival sulcus is the space between the attached gingiva and the tooth. The mucobuccal fold is that area of mucosa where the attached gingiva gives rise to the looser buccal mucosa. The mucobuccal fold is the area penetrated when most dental nerve blocks are performed.

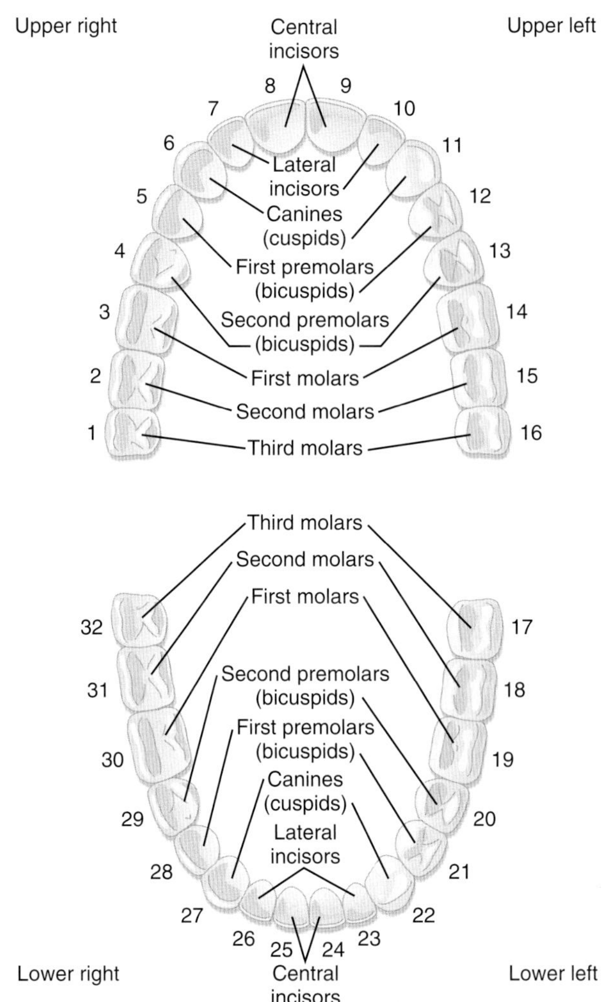


**Fig. 28.5** Adult dentition.

**Table 28.1** Tooth Names

| TOOTH DESIGNATION | NAME OF TOOTH | APPEARANCE IN THE MOUTH |
|---|---|---|
| **Baby (Primary) Teeth** | | |
| A | Central incisor | 4-14 mo |
| B | Lateral incisor | 8-18 mo |
| C | Canine tooth | 14-24 mo |
| D | First molar | 10-20 mo |
| E | Second molar | 20-36 mo |
| **Adult (Permanent) Teeth** | | |
| 1 | Central incisor | 5-9 yr |
| 2 | Lateral incisor | 6-10 yr |
| 3 | Canine tooth | 8½-14 yr |
| 4 | First premolar (bicuspid) | 9-14 yr |
| 5 | Second premolar (bicuspid) | 10-15 yr |
| 6 | First molar (6-yr molar) | 5-9 yr |
| 7 | Second molar (12-yr molar) | 10-15 yr |
| 8 | Third molar (wisdom tooth) | 17-25 yr |

## PRESENTING SIGNS AND SYMPTOMS

The patient's signs and symptoms can be elicited by means of a thorough history. If the patient has sustained trauma, it is important to ascertain the following information:

1. When did the incident occur? This is important in the evaluation of avulsed permanent teeth because the decision to reimplant a tooth is based largely on the duration of the avulsion.
2. Were any teeth found at the scene?
3. Did the patient have any symptoms suggestive of tooth aspiration, such as coughing or choking at the scene?
4. Has the patient been using alcohol or any other sedatives or recreational drugs that may have made aspiration more likely?
5. Does the patient have amnesia, which may suggest loss of consciousness?
6. Does the patient complain of pain? Do the teeth feel as though they are touching normally? Is the pain associated with occlusion? Mandibular fractures typically worsen with jaw movement, and patients complain that their bite is off. Pain from TMJ injuries is often referred to the ear. Fractured teeth frequently hurt more with the inspiration of air or contact with cold substances.

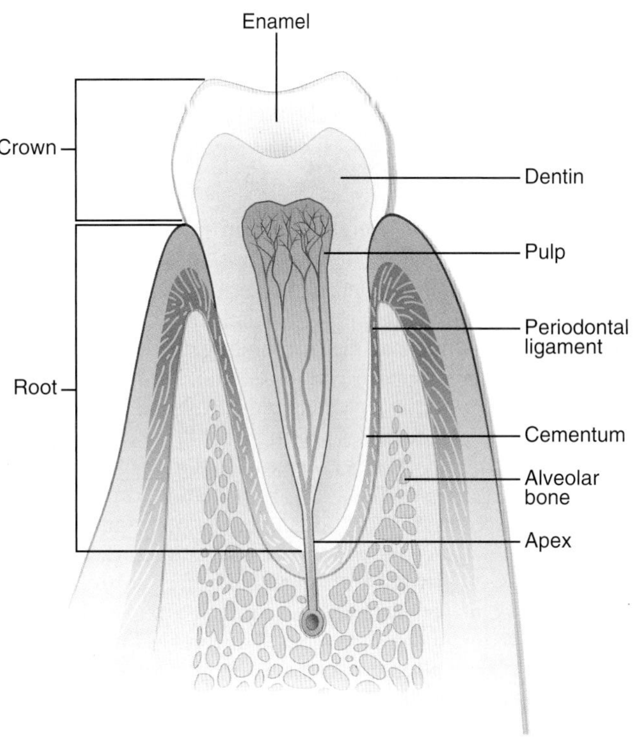


**Fig. 28.6** Dental anatomy.

Luxated or subluxated teeth hurt during mastication or chewing.

7. Did the patient take any over-the-counter analgesics or apply any substances to decrease the pain? Over-the-counter topical anesthetics can cause sterile abscesses when applied directly to the pulp.[3]
8. Is the tooth a permanent or a primary tooth? Avulsed primary teeth are managed differently from avulsed permanent teeth.
9. Does the patient have a history of bleeding disorders or allergies?

Additional historical information must be obtained if the complaint does not involve trauma:

1. Has the patient had any recent dental work? Dry sockets, for example, occur several days after a tooth has been extracted.
2. Does the patient have a history of poor dentition or multiple caries?
3. Is the patient having difficulty opening the mouth, which suggests a TMJ problem?
4. Has the patient had any difficulty swallowing? Has a change in voice or any shortness of breath occurred? Has any swelling developed? These symptoms suggest a possible deep space infection or hematoma.
5. Is the patient immunocompromised? Deep space infections spread rapidly to the mediastinum and cavernous sinus in an immunocompromised patient.
6. Does the patient have a coagulopathy secondary to aspirin, warfarin, or other anticoagulants or symptoms or a history suggestive of a bleeding disorder?
7. Was the time course of the problem insidious or rapid? Has the patient had symptoms of infection, such as fever, chills, or vomiting?
8. Does the patient have a history of rheumatic fever or valvular disease, such as mitral valve prolapse?[4] Does the patient have artificial joints, valves, or shunts? These may predispose to endocarditis or infection of the implant or shunt if dental infection is present.

## DIFFERENTIAL DIAGNOSIS

Trauma to the teeth usually consists of fracture, subluxation (loose but nondisplaced tooth), luxation (loose displaced tooth), intrusion, or complete avulsion. Lacerations of the oral soft tissues can be challenging to find, and therefore good lighting is essential. Trauma to the surrounding maxillofacial structures and mandible must also be considered. The final diagnosis is determined primarily by a meticulous physical examination, with radiography sometimes serving a confirmatory role.

Nontraumatic dental emergencies usually result from poor oral hygiene, recent dental instrumentation, or infection. Uncomplicated tooth pain (odontalgia) is often pulpitis, and further diagnostic testing is not necessary in the ED. The other consideration is periodontal or pulpal infection or abscess. Nonodontogenic sources may cause referred pain to the dentition. Referred pain from the sinuses or the TMJ must also be considered, especially for pain that cannot be localized (**Table 28.2**). A patient who has recently undergone dental instrumentation or extraction may be seen in the ED with dry socket, hematoma, or hemorrhage.

**Table 28.2 Differential Diagnosis of Orofacial Pain**

| | |
|---|---|
| Odontogenic pain | Dental caries<br>Reversible pulpitis<br>Irreversible pulpitis<br>Pulpal necrosis and abscess<br>Tooth eruption<br>Pericoronitis<br>Postrestorative pain<br>Postextraction discomfort<br>Postextraction alveolar osteitis<br>Bruxism<br>Cervical erosion<br>Deep space odontogenic infection<br>Deep space hematoma<br>Alveolar osteitis<br>Periapical abscess<br>Dentoalveolar abscess<br>Oral hemorrhage |
| Periodontal pathology | Gingivitis<br>Periodontal disease<br>Periodontal abscess<br>Acute necrotizing gingivostomatitis |
| Orofacial trauma | Dental fractures: subtle enamel cracks, Ellis fractures<br>Dental subluxation, luxation, intrusion, avulsion<br>Facial fractures<br>Alveolar ridge fractures<br>Soft tissue lacerations<br>Traumatic ulcers<br>Mandible/maxilla fracture<br>Mucosa/tongue lacerations |
| Infection | Oral candidiasis<br>Herpes simplex, types 1 and 2<br>Varicella-zoster, primary and secondary<br>Herpangina<br>Hand-foot-and-mouth disease<br>Sexually transmitted diseases<br>Mycobacterial infections<br>Mumps |
| Malignancies | Squamous cell carcinoma<br>Kaposi sarcoma<br>Lymphoma<br>Leukemia<br>Graft-versus-host disease<br>Melanoma |
| Other causes | Cranial neuralgia<br>Stomatitis and mucositis: uremia, vitamin deficiency, other<br>Erythema migrans<br>Pyogenic granuloma<br>Ulcerative disease: lichen planus, cicatricial pemphigoid, pemphigus vulgaris, erythema multiforme<br>Crohn disease<br>Behçet syndrome |

Adapted from Tintinalli JE, Kelen GD, Stapczynski JE, editors. Emergency medicine: a comprehensive study guide. 5th ed. New York: McGraw-Hill; 2000.

## INTERVENTIONS AND PROCEDURES

### PHYSICAL EXAMINATION

Simple observation and discussion with the patient can often provide clues to the diagnosis. The EP should pay attention to changes in voice, muffling, drooling, and other signs of airway involvement. External inspection may disclose injuries such as mandibular dislocations and fractures, which often result in asymmetry, swelling, or deformity of the face. Abscesses or deep space infections will cause swelling over the involved space, although such swelling can be subtle; therefore, the face should be viewed from multiple angles. Opening of the mouth should be smooth and complete, with no limitations or hesitations. Erythema, warmth, or drainage is indicative of possible abscess, cellulitis, or hematoma formation. The face should be palpated for fractures, tenderness, and crepitus. The entire mandible and midface should be palpated with particular attention to the maxilla, zygomas, mandibular condyles, and coronoid processes. The TMJ should be palpated throughout its range of motion. No clicks, pops, or pain should occur as the joint moves.

During palpation of the anterior portion of the neck, particular attention should be paid to the area along and beneath the length of the mandibular body. The oral cavity should be examined for any bleeding, swelling, tenderness, fractures, abrasions, or lacerations, and each tooth should be percussed and accounted for. A tongue blade should be used to assess the entire mucobuccal fold region. The EP should palpate the cheek and the floor of the mouth with the thumb of a gloved hand inside the patient's oral cavity. Each tooth should be percussed with a tongue blade for sensitivity and palpated with gloved fingers for mobility. Blood in the gingival crevice (the area where the gingiva meets the enamel) suggests a traumatized tooth or a fractured jaw (see Fig. 28.13, *B*). The teeth should meet symmetrically and evenly during biting, and the patient should be able to exert firm pressure on a tongue blade when biting with the molars. An inability to crack a tongue blade bilaterally when it is twisted between the molars (the tongue blade test) suggests a mandibular fracture (**Fig. 28.7**).

## CONTROL OF HEMORRHAGE

Bleeding from the oral cavity is common and often associated with trauma and dental procedures. The EP is frequently the first clinician to see the problem when it occurs in a delayed manner. First, the EP should ascertain whether the bleeding is from recent dental instrumentation or was spontaneous. Spontaneous bleeding from the oral cavity that is not secondary to recent instrumentation or trauma suggests advanced periodontal disease or a systemic process.

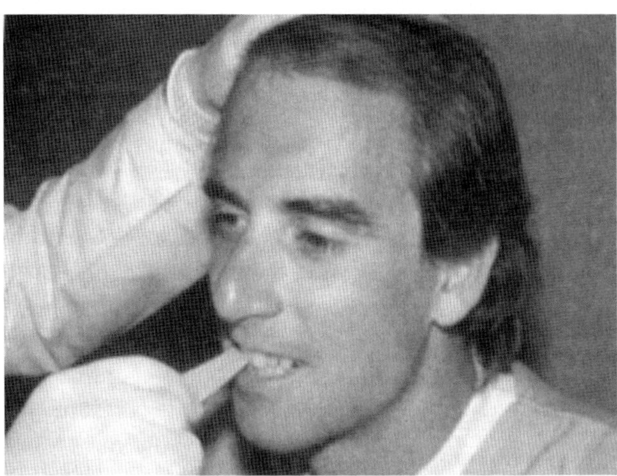

**Fig. 28.7** Tongue blade test.

Bleeding from the gingiva after scaling or other routine dental procedures can usually be controlled with direct pressure. Gingival bleeding that persists suggests a coagulopathy, alcoholism, medications, and other causes. Much more common than gingival bleeding is postextraction bleeding, usually from the molars. Patients with such problems usually arrive at the ED after normal office hours and after they have failed to stop the bleeding at home. The EP has a number of options to stop the bleeding. A systematic approach should be taken, as follows:

1. Apply direct pressure. Any excessive clot should be removed and the area anesthetized with local infiltration of lidocaine or bupivacaine with epinephrine. The epinephrine provides vasoconstriction, and the anesthetic enables the patient to bite harder. Anesthetic without epinephrine should generally be avoided because the amide anesthetics are vasodilators and may increase the bleeding. Next, insert dental roll gauze or a dental tampon into the space that was left by the extracted tooth. Dental roll gauze fits nicely into the extraction space and thus helps increase direct pressure. Use a folded-up 2- × 2-inch gauze pad if dental rolls are unavailable. Cover the dental roll gauze with 2- × 2-inch gauze pads and have the patient bite firmly on it for 10 to 15 minutes. It also helps to soak the dental rolls in epinephrine or phenylephrine.
2. If the bleeding persists, insert a hemostatic agent (Celox, HemCon, Surgicel, Gelfoam) into the socket. Both of the chitin-derived dressings (Celox, HemCon) have been shown to decrease bleeding better than direct pressure does, as well as to control bleeding in patients taking anticoagulants. If Gelfoam or Surgicel is used, the surrounding cusp of gingiva may require closure with a fast-absorbing suture to ensure that the dressing remains seated. Instruct the patient to bite down on gauze placed over the dressing. If HemCon or Celox is used or if not enough gingival tissue is available for closure, simply place the coagulating agent into the socket and have the patient bite down into gauze placed over the bleeding socket.
3. Topical thrombin, which can usually be obtained from the operating room, is also very effective in stopping oozing blood, but it is very expensive. Simply spraying topical thrombin onto the site and then having the patient bite into gauze generally work well.
4. Low-temperature cautery is also very effective, although it can be destructive to tissue if not used carefully. Battery-operated thermal cautery units, which are often used for nail trephination, are available in many EDs. Anesthetize the gingiva before using the cautery.
5. If the preceding measures are not effective in controlling bleeding, call a specialist. It is also reasonable to consider the use of fresh frozen plasma or platelets if a coagulopathy is determined to be present.

If the bleeding can be controlled, the patient may be discharged and instructed to not eat or drink anything for several hours and then to have only cold liquids and soft foods.

## MANAGEMENT OF PAIN

Severe tooth pain (odontalgia), as anyone who has experienced it knows, can be debilitating. Frequently, the quickest relief is found in the ED. The ability to perform dental nerve blocks is valuable and rewarding.

The use of bupivacaine in dental block anesthesia affords the patient the luxury of 8 to 12 hours of relative comfort until follow-up with a dentist is possible. Likewise, the use of narcotics is minimized because the patient's pain has been relieved. Topical anesthesia in the form of 20% benzocaine or 5% lidocaine is also a valuable aid because both agents decrease the pain of intraoral injection. It behooves the EP to be able to use them properly.[5]

## DIAGNOSTIC TESTING

A panoramic facial radiograph (Panorex) and a Towne view are probably the most useful and cost-effective radiographs for evaluating mandibular trauma in the ED.[6] A panoramic radiograph of the mandible shows the mandible in its entirety and demonstrates fractures in all regions, including the symphysis.[6] Occasionally, however, such a radiograph can miss overriding anterior fractures; if these fractures are probably present, computed tomography (CT) is indicated. The Towne view allows better visualization of the condyles than a panoramic radiograph does. A coronal CT scan is more definitive and is often used for preoperative evaluation, but it is seldom necessary for the diagnosis of isolated mandibular trauma. CT should be performed if multiple facial fractures are suspected or if the initial radiographic findings for the mandible are equivocal and clinical suspicion is high.[6,7] If the patient is immobilized, mandibular films or CT scanning may be obtained. Mandibular films may miss the symphysis, and if the clinician is concerned about a symphyseal fracture, either occlusal films or a CT scan should be obtained.

Dental abscesses or infections are best treated by antibiotics, incision and drainage, or both. Although panoramic radiographic views can visualize sizable periapical abscesses, their routine use in the ED is not warranted because their results would not change the treatment and disposition of the patient.[3] Bite-wing radiographs, obtained in the dentist office, are the standard for diagnosing small periapical abscesses and caries. Deep space infections of the head and neck are often difficult to localize by physical examination, and CT scanning has become the modality of choice to delineate collections of abscess or cellulitis of the face and neck.[8]

# TREATMENT AND DISPOSITION

## TRAUMA

### *Fractured Teeth*

Injury to the maxillary central incisors accounts for between 70% and 80% of all tooth fractures. The morbidity associated with dental fractures can be significant and includes failure to erupt, abscess formation, loss of space in the dental arch, change in color of the tooth, ankylosis, and root resorption. The following principles apply to the ED evaluation and management of dental trauma:

1. Identify all fracture fragments and mobile teeth, and note whether a mandibular fracture is open or closed. Radiographs should be taken if fragments have intruded into the mucosa or alveolar bone. Perform chest radiography if there is any concern about aspiration of a tooth or tooth fragment.
2. The dentition is much more easily manipulated if the patient is not in significant discomfort. Tooth infiltration and dental block anesthesia should be part of the EP's armamentarium. Narcotic and nonnarcotic alternatives, though helpful after treatment is completed, do not usually offer the patient enough comfort to allow the performance of most dental manipulations.
3. Administer a tetanus booster if indicated.

ED management of fractured teeth depends on the extent of fracture with regard to the pulp, the extent of development of the apex of the tooth, and the age of the patient.[9] Many classification systems are used for describing injured dentition, such as the Ellis system; however, most dentists and maxillofacial surgeons do not use this nomenclature. The most easily understood method of classification is based on a description of the injury.[10]

CROWN FRACTURES Crown fractures may be divided into complicated and uncomplicated categories. Uncomplicated crown fractures involve the enamel alone or the enamel and dentin in combination.

*Uncomplicated crown fractures through the enamel only* are not usually sensitive to forced air, temperature, or percussion and generally pose no real threat to the dental pulp. ED treatment is not necessary but may consist of smoothing the sharp edges with an emery board if they are significantly bothersome to the patient. The patient should be reassured that the dentist can restore the tooth with bonding composites and resins. Follow-up is important because pulp necrosis and color change can occur, though rarely (0% to 3% of cases) (**Figs. 28.8 and 28.9**).[11]

*Uncomplicated fractures that extend through the enamel and dentin* are at higher risk for pulp necrosis and need more aggressive treatment (**Fig. 28.10**; also see Fig. 28.8). The risk for pulp necrosis in these patients is 1% to 7% but increases as time until treatment extends beyond 24 hours.[12] Affected patients usually have sensitivity to forced air, percussion, and extremes of temperature. Physical findings are notable for the yellowish tint of the dentin in contrast to the white hue of the enamel. Fractures that are close to the pulp reveal a slight pink coloration. Dentin is porous, which allows oral flora to pass into the pulp chamber and thereby possibly facilitates inflammation and infection. This process occurs predominantly after 24 hours but may do so earlier if the fracture is closer to the pulp. Patients younger than 12 years have a higher pulp-to-dentin ratio than adults do and are therefore at higher risk for pulp contamination. Dentin fracture in a younger patient should be treated more aggressively, and the patient should be seen by a dentist within 24 hours.[12]

The two primary reasons to treat dental fractures in the ED are (1) to cover the exposed dentin and prevent inflammation and infection and (2) to provide relief of pain. If a tooth is properly covered in the ED, a dentist can later rebuild it with modern composites. A tooth nerve block should be performed before covering the tooth. Dressings that may be considered for covering tooth fractures include calcium hydroxide paste, zinc oxide paste, zinc oxide eugenol, glass ionomer composites, and cyanoacrylates.[13-15] Some emergency medicine texts support the use of glass ionomer cements in the ED; however,

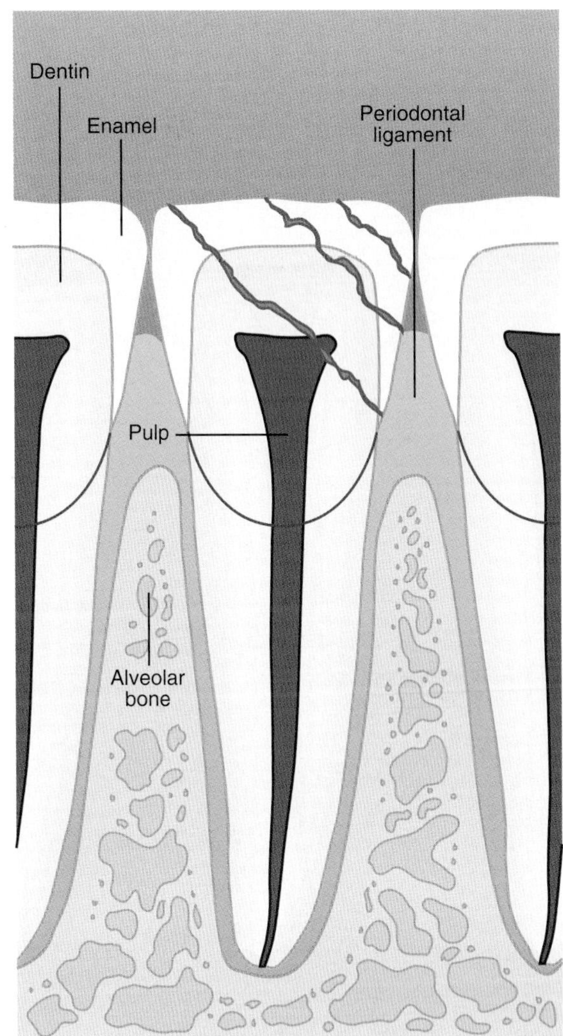

Fig. 28.8 Dental fractures.

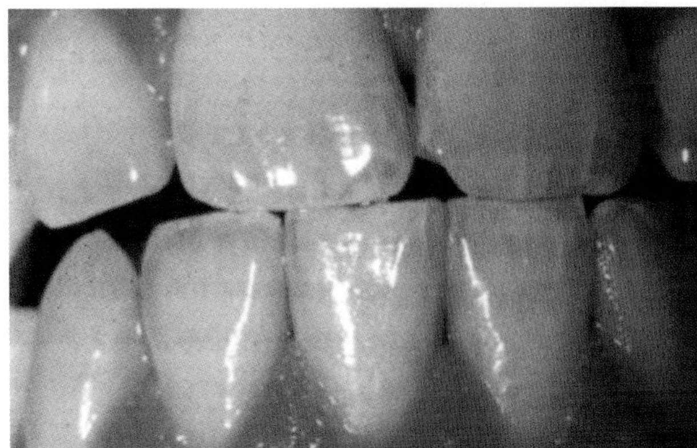
Fig. 28.9 Enamel fractures.

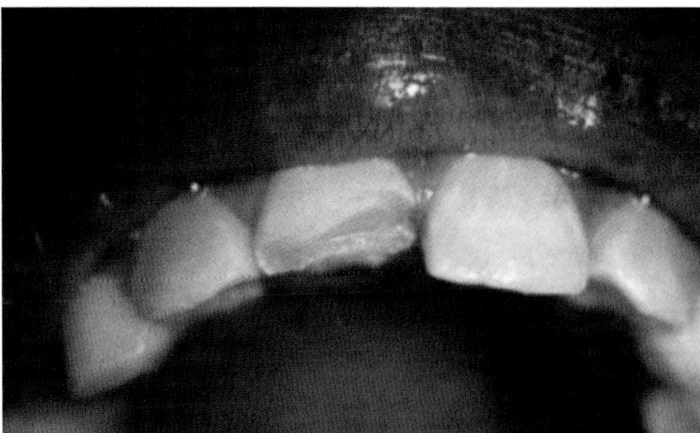
Fig. 28.10 Dentin fracture.

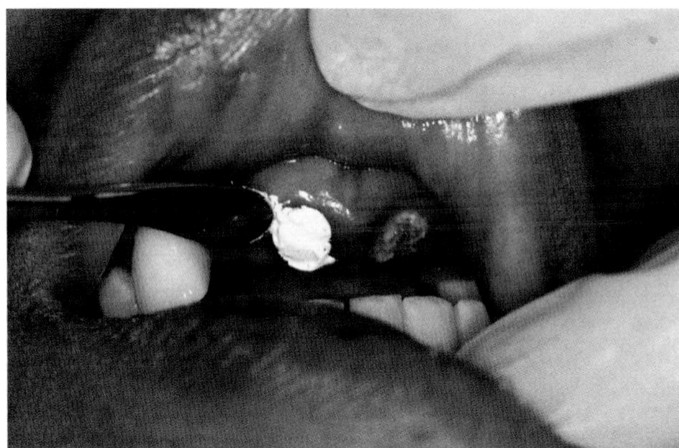
Fig. 28.11 Calcium hydroxide paste.

this issue is controversial in the dental community. The ease of use, affordability, and inherent properties of calcium hydroxide paste make it an attractive option in the ED. It is watertight, dries on contact with saliva, is durable, and is pH compatible (**Fig. 28.11**). Composites that are applied with a bonding light are beyond the scope of most emergency medicine practice. Bone wax is sometimes used but is not recommended because it is slightly porous and cannot be used as a base in rebuilding the tooth. Skin adhesives have been used in fracture repair, but they last only a short time inside the mouth and cannot be used as a base in tooth restorations. Their use will probably become more commonplace if their durability improves and clinical studies corroborate their usefulness.

Many patients sustaining deep dentin fractures eventually require a root canal or other definitive endodontic therapy; however, timely application of an appropriate dressing in the ED can prevent contamination and necrosis of the pulp and might prevent the need for a root canal. Even if it does not save the pulp, such a dressing will eliminate the majority of the pain because the dentin is no longer exposed to air. The EP should make sure to remind the patient that anterior tooth trauma may disrupt the neurovascular supply and possibly result in pulp necrosis, change in color, or root resorption.

*Complicated fractures of the crown involving the pulp* are true dental emergencies (**Fig. 28.12**; see Fig. 28.8). They lead to pulp necrosis at least 10% to 30% of the time, even with rapid, appropriate dental treatment.[11] Such fractures are distinguished by the pink-red tinge of the pulp. They are usually severely painful, but lack of sensitivity occasionally occurs secondary to disruption of the neurovascular supply of the tooth. Immediate management involves referral to a dentist, endodontist, or oral surgeon. These fractures generally require pulpectomy (complete pulp removal) or, in the case of

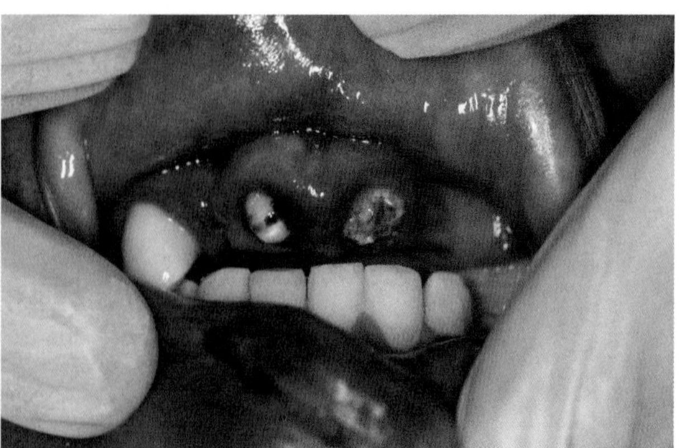

**Fig. 28.12** Pulp fracture.

primary teeth, pulpotomy (partial pulp removal) as definitive treatment.[12,16,17] The longer the pulp is exposed, the greater the chance for abscess development or pulp necrosis. If a dentist cannot see the patient immediately, the EP should relieve the pain with a supraperiosteal injection and cover the pulp with one of the dressings described previously. If bleeding is brisk, it can usually be controlled by having the patient bite onto a gauze pad soaked with epinephrine or phenylephrine. Alternatively, injecting a small amount of lidocaine with epinephrine into the pulp will stop the bleeding and poses no threat to the tooth because the pulp needs to be removed regardless.

If the exposure was prolonged, many authorities and dentists would advocate antibiotic prophylaxis with penicillin or clindamycin, although the effectiveness of this approach has never been proved.[18] With regard to antibiotic prophylaxis for dental fractures, it is important to remember the following assumptions: it is uncertain when many patients will be able to secure follow-up, and delayed fracture care and poor gingival health raise the risk for pulp necrosis and, potentially, the development of an abscess. Therefore, although it has not been proved that antibiotics are useful in patients with dentin or pulp fractures, such treatment should be considered if the patient has the previously mentioned risk factors or if the consulting dental professional has requested them.

### Luxation and Subluxation

With subluxation, a tooth is mobile but not displaced, whereas a luxated tooth has been removed, either completely or partially, from its socket. Luxation injuries are further categorized as follows:

*Extrusive luxation*: The tooth is displaced in a direction toward the crown (**Fig. 28.13**).

*Intrusive luxation*: The tooth is forced apically toward the root of the tooth; it may be associated with crushing or fracture of the apex of the tooth (**Fig. 28.14**).

*Lateral luxation*: The tooth is displaced facially, mesially, lingually, or distally (**Fig. 28.15**).

*Complete luxation:* The tooth is completely avulsed out of its socket (**Fig. 28.16**).

Teeth that are minimally mobile and minimally displaced do well with conservative management alone. A traumatized tooth will firm up as the alveolar ligament binds to the alveolar bone. The patient should be instructed to eat only a soft diet for 1 to 2 weeks and to follow up with a dentist as soon as possible.

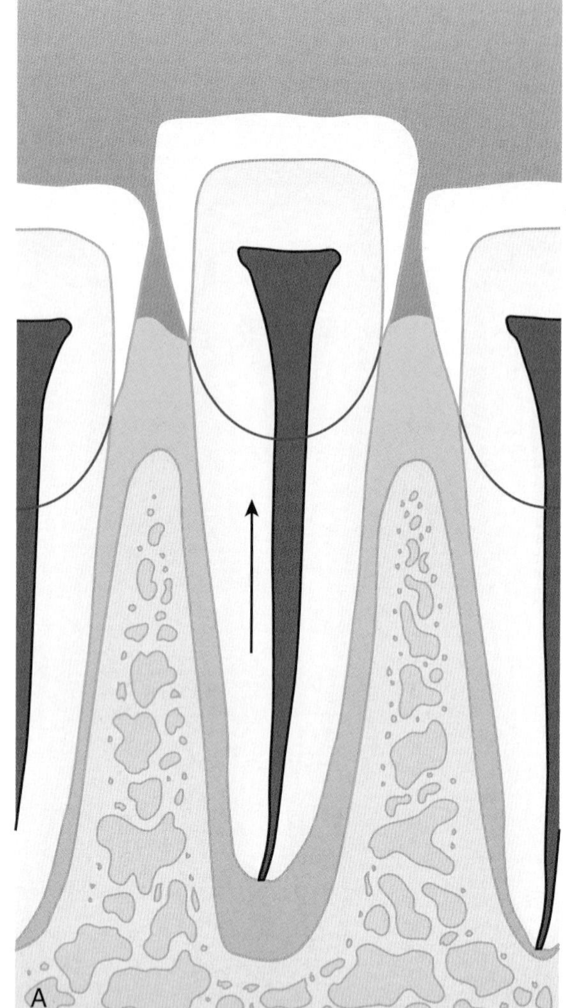



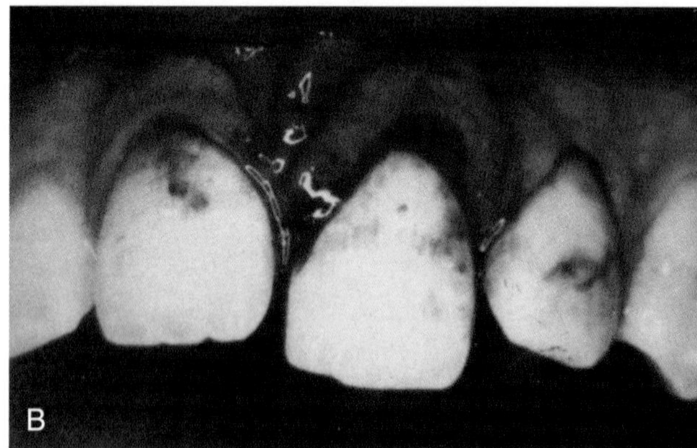



**Fig. 28.13** A and **B,** Extrusive luxation. Blood is apparent in the gingival sulcus in **B**.

Grossly mobile teeth, however, require some form of stabilization in the ED. Fixation is best accomplished by a dental professional with enamel bonding materials or wire splinting, which are not usually practical in the ED. Many different techniques are available to the EP, although one must

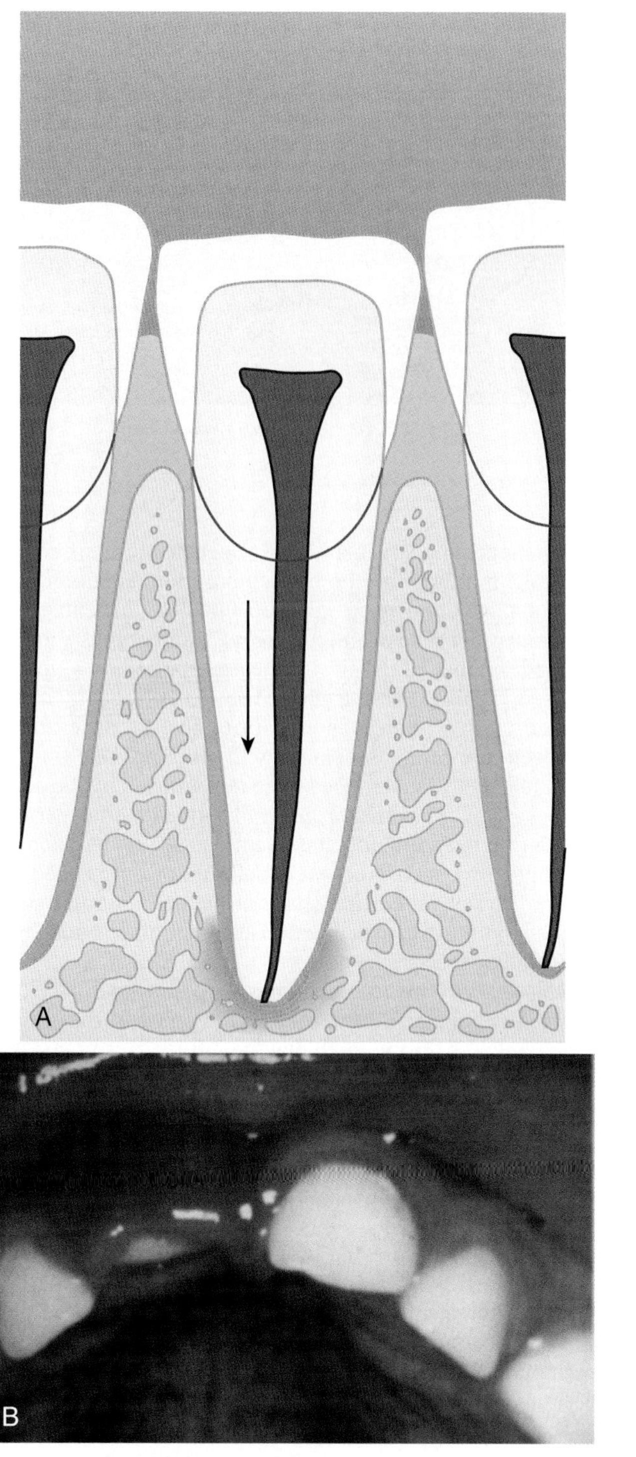


Fig. 28.14 A and B, Intrusive luxation.

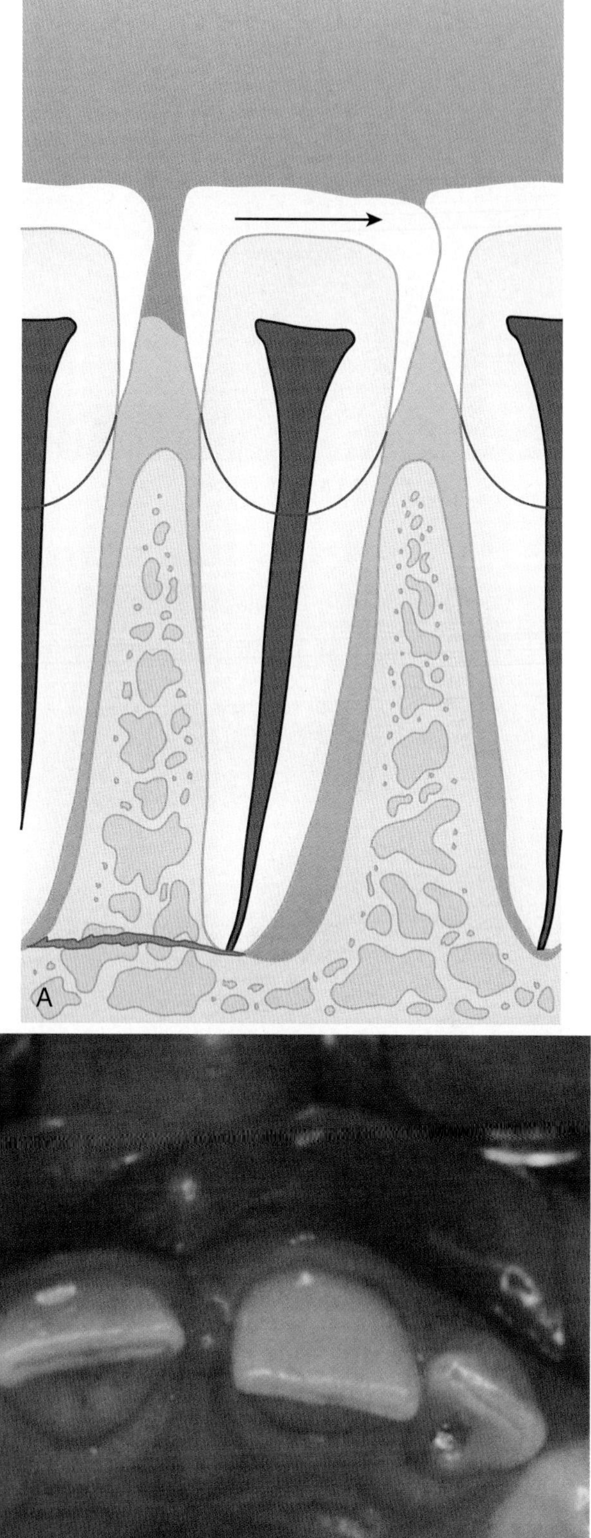


Fig. 28.15 A and B, Lateral luxation.

be aware of the concern for aspiration of teeth or even the splint if the splinting technique fails.

Temporizing splinting techniques available for use by EPs include periodontal paste and self-cure composites. At this time, tissue glues do not have the durability properties required to firmly splint teeth, but this situation may change and tissue glue in combination with splinting wire may eventually be a good option.

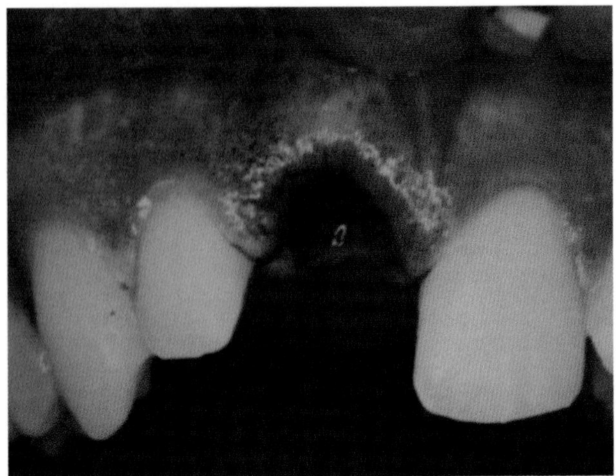

**Fig. 28.16** Avulsion.

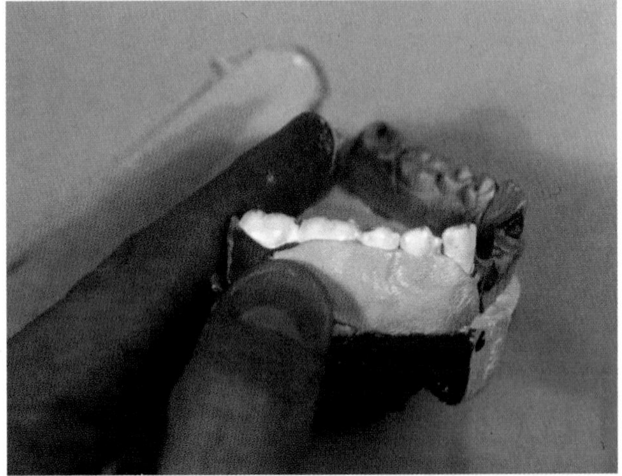

**Fig. 28.17** Periodontal paste.

Coe-Pak, a commercially available form of periodontal paste, is a very sticky dressing that becomes firm after application (**Fig. 28.17**). Periodontal paste is also very useful as a primary treatment of gingival and palatal lacerations, with the caveat that the paste must be removed by a dental professional. Self-cure composite is another reasonable splinting option in the ED. Self-cure composite does not require etching acids or bonding lights and is easy to use (**Fig. 28.18**). The disadvantage of self-cure composite is that it is rigid and inflexible and tends to pop off with slight movement of the teeth before the patient sees a dentist. Both splinting techniques are easily removed by a dentist or oral surgeon during formal restoration.

Teeth that are luxated in the horizontal or axial planes or teeth that are slightly extruded can be splinted with the preceding techniques. Teeth do not need to be in perfect alignment before the patient is discharged from the ED.

### *Intrusion and Avulsion*

Intruded teeth have been forced into the alveolar bone and often cause disruption of the attachment apparatus or fracture

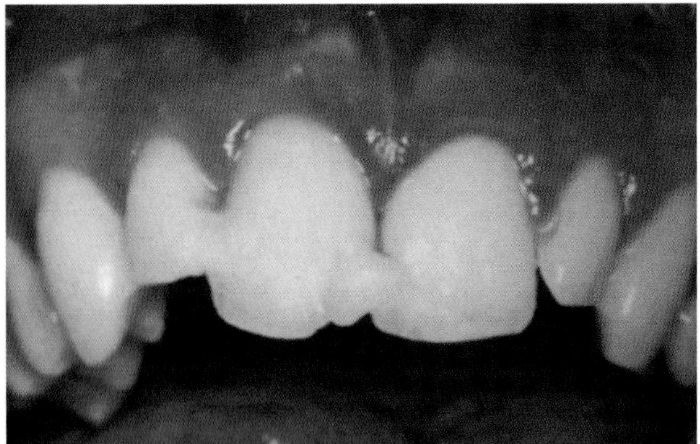

**Fig. 28.18** Self-cure composite.

of the supporting alveolar bone. Such teeth are frequently immobile and therefore do not require immobilization in the ED, but they often need later treatment by a dentist or an endodontist because of pulp necrosis. Radiographs should be obtained in the ED if it is uncertain whether a tooth is fractured, avulsed, or intruded. The dentist should manage intruded teeth within 24 hours if possible because intruded adult teeth are often associated with alveolar bone fractures. Permanent teeth usually need to be repositioned by the dentist, whereas primary teeth are generally given a trial period to erupt on their own before interventions are undertaken. The EP should always consider the possibility of an intruded tooth if there is a new abnormal space in the dentition because an intruded tooth can cause infection and craniofacial abnormalities if undiagnosed.

Avulsed teeth are true dental emergencies and provide an opportunity for the EP to make a difference in the outcome of the patient. Missing teeth may be intruded, aspirated, fractured, swallowed, or embedded in the oral mucosa. A panoramic radiograph, facial films, or a chest radiograph should be considered to look for fragments of fractured teeth or a missing tooth. Management of avulsed teeth depends on multiple factors, including patient age, periodontal health, and duration of time since avulsion. Primary teeth are not replaced because they can fuse to the underlying alveolar bone and cause craniofacial abnormalities or infection and may also interfere with normal eruption of the permanent teeth. Parents should be reassured that prosthetic teeth can be worn until the permanent teeth erupt, if desired, although this is not typically necessary.

Time since avulsion is the most important determinant in the decision whether to reimplant an avulsed tooth. Generally, the longer the tooth is out of its socket, the higher the incidence of periodontal ligament necrosis and subsequent reimplantation failure.[18] Periodontal ligament cells usually die within 1 to 2 hours if not placed in an appropriate transport medium.[19,20] Many studies have been conducted on the various storage media used to keep the cells of the periodontal ligament viable. Milk, Hank's balanced salt solution, EMT Toothsaver, Save a Tooth (commercial formulations of Hank's solution), saliva, water, and Gatorade have all been studied. Cell culture formulations have been developed that cause periodontal ligament cells to not only remain viable but also proliferate; however, they are not practical for ED use. To date, warmed milk and warmed Hank's solution (generic or commercial formulation) are best for prehospital and ED use.[20] They each preserve the periodontal ligament for at least 4 to 8 hours, although reimplantation should take place as rapidly as reasonably possible.

The tooth should be placed in some sort of storage medium immediately after avulsion if possible because even 5 to 10 minutes of exposure to air will begin to cause desiccation and death of periodontal ligament cells. Saline is less optimal than the media mentioned earlier but should be used before water or saliva if it is the only option.[21] The tooth should be reimplanted into the socket at the scene by paramedics, but if they are unable to do so, the tooth should be reimplanted as soon as possible in the ED. Preparation of the socket, including suctioning and irrigation, can take place while the tooth is soaking in the storage medium. The patient's tetanus status should be updated as necessary and the patient discharged home on a soft diet. Many dental professionals recommend antibiotics effective against mouth flora (penicillin or clindamycin) to decrease inflammatory resorption of the root after fractures or avulsions.[12,14,17] This, however, has never been proved to be necessary or beneficial. Treatment with antibiotics should be tailored to the individual patient after discussion with the consultant who will see the patient later.

The prognosis of a reimplanted tooth depends on many factors, the most critical being the time until reimplantation. The age of the patient, the stage of development of the root (younger is better), and the overall health of the gingiva are also important. It is always better to keep a native tooth if possible, and that should be the goal of an EP confronted with an avulsed or fractured tooth. A tooth that has been reimplanted often loses the majority of its neurovascular supply and undergoes pulp necrosis, but the periodontal ligament attaches and the tooth will remain a functional unit, thereby obviating an implant or a prosthesis. Complications that can be expected after reimplantation include some resorption of the root and some discoloration of the tooth. These issues can be managed by the follow-up dentist.

### Alveolar Bone Fractures

Trauma to the anterior teeth may result in fractures of the alveolar ridge, which is the tooth-bearing portion of the mandible or maxilla. Alveolar ridge fractures often occur in multitooth segments and vary in the number of teeth involved, the amount of mobility present, and the amount of displacement of the affected segment. Dental bite-wing radiographs obtained in the dental office confirm the diagnosis, and facial films or a panoramic radiograph may show a fracture line apical to the roots of the involved teeth.

Treatment consists of rigid splinting of the affected segment, which should be performed urgently by an oral surgeon or dentist. It should ideally be done within 24 hours, but the urgency depends on the extent, mobility, and displacement of the affected segment. The role of the EP is to diagnose the injury, identify any avulsed or fractured teeth, and preserve as much of the alveolar bone and surrounding mucosa as possible. Alveolar bone that is lost, débrided, or missing is difficult for the specialist to repair properly.[14] Patients with alveolar ridge fractures, if nonmobile with good hemostasis, may be discharged with next-day follow-up, but most will require admission or transfer for repair.

### Alveolar Osteitis (Dry Socket)

Dry socket pain is severe and frequently requires intervention other than oral pain medication. Alveolar osteitis is associated with severe postextraction pain that occurs when alveolar bone becomes exposed and inflamed. It typically occurs when a clot that is present after a tooth extraction becomes dislodged or prematurely dissolves, most commonly 2 to 4 days after a tooth extraction. The cause of disruption of the clot is not completely agreed on but is thought to be secondary to locally increased fibrinolytic activity.[22] The examination is unremarkable with the exception of the missing clot, which is not always obvious to the untrained eye. Smoking, drinking from a straw, periodontal disease, hormone replacement therapy, and being a female are all risk factors predisposing a patient to dry socket.[22] This complication occurs after 2% to 5% of all extractions, although the rate increases if the extraction was especially traumatic or involves an impacted mandibular third molar.[3,11,22]

Patients with dry socket usually have little response to nonsteroidal antiinflammatory drugs or narcotics but experience immediate relief from a dental nerve block. After a dental block, the socket can be irrigated, suctioned, and packed appropriately. The socket may be packed with gauze impregnated with eugenol or a local anesthetic. Gauze tends to dry out and loosen, so it generally needs to be replaced in 24 to 36 hours. The socket may also be packed with a slurry of hemostatic gauze and eugenol (or lidocaine). The hemostatic gauze acts as a matrix to hold the anesthetic in place. Commercial paste for dry sockets (Dry Socket Paste, Alvogyl) can also be applied to the socket. Commercial pastes have the advantage of ease of use, but as with gauze, they will most likely need to be replaced at least once before complete epithelialization of the socket takes place.

Antibiotics can be given to patients with alveolar osteitis, but this is not a common practice, and dry socket heals completely once the socket has been covered. Antibiotics should be prescribed only after consultation with the patient's dentist or oral surgeon.[11]

## DENTAL INFECTIONS

Dental infections run the gamut from minor, easily managed infections, to abscesses, to severe, life-threatening deep space infections that require airway management and operative intervention. Dental infections seen in the ED are most commonly secondary to pulp infection or inflammation or to periodontal disease. Disease of the periodontium is usually a chronic condition, but over time, abscesses develop and require emergency treatment.

Diseases of the pulp can be secondary to trauma or operations, but clearly the most common cause is bacterial invasion after carious destruction of the enamel. As enamel is destroyed, carious development progresses rapidly through the dentin and into the pulp chamber and causes an inflammatory reaction known as pulpitis. If the erosion caused by bacteria is large enough to drain the developing inflammation, the patient may remain asymptomatic for a long time. When the drainage becomes blocked, the process progresses to the pulp and periapical space and results in exquisite tenderness. Periapical abscesses follow the path of least resistance, which may be through the alveolar bone and gingiva and into the mouth or into the deep structures of the neck. If the infection has progressed apically through the alveolar bone and localized swelling and tenderness at the base of the tooth are present, incision plus drainage in the ED is indicated. Antibiotics effective against oral flora should be prescribed.

In the ED differentiation between periapical abscesses and pulpitis is very difficult, and dental bite-wing radiographs are seldom available. Therefore, some physicians begin antibiotic therapy in patients who have not undergone recent dental instrumentation but complain of tooth pain and exhibit tenderness with percussion. Routine administration of antibiotics for tooth pain that is caused by pulpitis, instrumentation, or a localized abscess is not recommended by the dental societies, and a study in the emergency medicine literature suggests that the use of antibiotics for undifferentiated dental pain is not necessary.[23,24] Antibiotics have been recommended for odontogenic infections that have spread outside the immediate periapical area or have associated systemic signs, such as fever, swelling, and trismus. Supraperiosteal infiltration (tooth nerve block) should be performed in most cases, not only to provide immediate and long-acting relief but also because it reduces the need for narcotic analgesics even after the anesthetic has worn off.

Periodontal disease, unlike pulpal disease, is usually asymptomatic unless accompanied by an abscess or ulcerations. *Periodontal disease* is infection of the gingiva, periodontal ligament, or alveolar bone, which essentially make up the attachment apparatus of the tooth. *Gingivitis* is inflammation of the gingiva caused by bacteria; in advanced cases, the gingiva may be reddened, painful, and inflamed. In chronic disease, abscess formation occurs as organisms become trapped in the periodontal pocket. The purulent collection generally drains through the gingival sulcus. However, it can become invasive and involve the supporting tissues, alveolar bone, and the periodontal ligament (periodontitis). Periodontal abscesses that are not draining adequately through the gingival sulcus should be drained in the ED. Antibiotics should be prescribed, and saline rinses are encouraged to promote drainage, but chlorhexidine rinses can be substituted for saline in those with more severe disease.

Pericoronitis usually occurs when the wisdom teeth erupt and the gingiva overlying the erupting teeth becomes traumatized and inflamed. The gingiva overlying the crown may entrap bacteria and occasionally become infected, but the patient generally has pain from inflamed gingival tissue. Rarely, however, the localized infection can spread to deeper tissues, such as the pterygomandibular or submasseteric space. Clinically, patients with spread of pericoronal infection are found to have trismus secondary to irritation of the masseter and pterygoid muscles. If the pericoronal infection is localized, saline rinses and oral antibiotics are prescribed with dental follow-up in 24 to 48 hours.

### Deep Space Infections of the Head and Neck

It is not unusual for odontogenic infections to spread to the various potential spaces in the head and neck. The initial signs and symptoms are varied but usually consist of pain, swelling, difficulty swallowing or speaking, trismus, fever, and chills.

Certain teeth allow infections to spread to particular deep spaces in the head and neck, but rapid spread of these infections can make localizing the exact space difficult. Maxillary extension is likewise possible and can spread to several different spaces and potentially to the cavernous sinus.

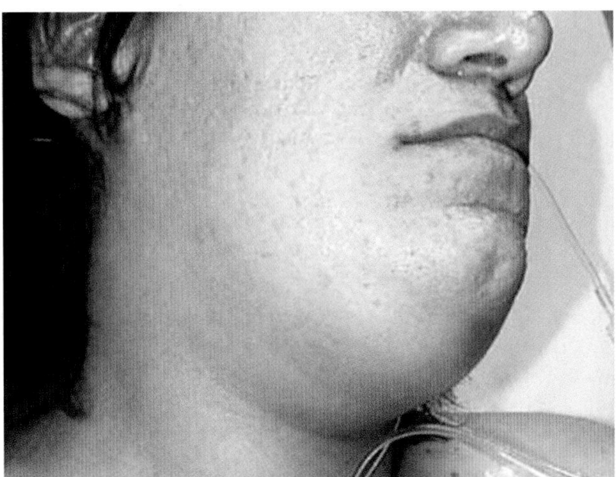

**Fig. 28.19** Ludwig angina.

Cavernous sinus involvement is generally associated with periorbital cellulitis, as well as meningeal signs or a change in mental status.

Deep space infections can rapidly become severe and life-threatening. The submandibular space connects to the sublingual space, and bilateral involvement of the sublingual spaces can result in a condition known as Ludwig angina, an airway-compromising deep space infection that may require airway intervention (**Fig. 28.19**).

Management of complicated odontogenic head and neck infections focuses primarily on airway management, surgical drainage, and antibiotics. CT has become the imaging modality of choice for deep space infections of the head and neck and should be used to localize and delineate collections of abscess or cellulitis that cannot be precisely determined by physical examination.[8] Airway intervention should be performed early if there is any question of compromise. The EP should administer antibiotics intravenously and obtain surgical consultation early in evaluation and treatment of the patient.

The bacteria usually isolated from deep space infections of the head and neck typically consist of mixed *Staphylococcus* and *Streptococcus* or mixed aerobic and anaerobic flora. Almost half the isolates from odontogenic infections are resistant to β-lactam antibiotics.[25] Drugs of choice include penicillin G plus metronidazole or extended-spectrum penicillins such as ampicillin-sulbactam, ticarcillin-clavulanate, and piperacillin-tazobactam. These combination antibiotics are effective against β-lactamase–producing bacteria, as well as common oral anaerobes such as *Bacteroides fragilis*. Clindamycin is an effective choice for penicillin-allergic patients, but it should be combined with a cephalosporin such as cefotetan or cefoxitin for resistant organisms. It is prudent to remember that antibiotics are adjunctive therapy only and not a substitute for surgical therapy.

## REFERENCES

***References can be found on Expert Consult @ www.expertconsult.com.***

# Pharynx and Throat Emergencies 29

*H. Gene Hern, Jr.*

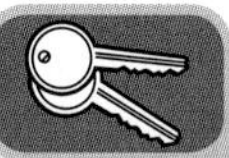

**KEY POINTS**

- Viruses cause most cases of pharyngitis, but the modified Centor score represents a scoring system that can increase detection of group A β-hemolytic streptococcal pharyngitis.
- Consider corticosteroids in patients with pharyngitis for symptomatic relief of tonsillar hypertrophy.
- Unilateral pain and swelling may indicate peritonsillar abscess (consider ultrasound).
- Consider epiglottitis in circumstances in which the findings on physical examination do not match the patient's pain and other symptoms. Visualize the epiglottis to rule out the disease.
- Ludwig angina is characterized by bilateral submandibular swelling, fever, and an elevated or protruding tongue.
- Lemierre syndrome, a suppurative thrombophlebitis located within the internal jugular vein, is a complication of nearby infections in the pharynx or mastoid space.
- Retropharyngeal abscesses in children younger than 6 years are due to infected lymph nodes and in adults are due to local or hematogenous spread. They require imaging to make the diagnosis because examination findings are notoriously unreliable in this population.

## OROPHARYNGEAL COMPLAINTS

### EPIDEMIOLOGY

Upper respiratory complaints are the most common reason that patients seek medical care. Pharyngitis is diagnosed in more than 10 million patients per year. Millions of dollars are spent not only on medications and medical visits but also to arrange child care and sick leave for patients unable to go to work or school. Even though most causes of throat pain are benign and self-limited, a number of causes of sore throat may be severe and life-threatening.

The oropharynx plays a vital role in the health of every patient. Not only is it the needed entry point for food and nutrition, but oxygen and carbon dioxide must also move through the oropharynx every minute to maintain metabolic homeostasis. Any disease process that interferes with the function of the oropharynx has the potential to cause significant morbidity and perhaps mortality.

### PATHOPHYSIOLOGY

The structure of the oropharynx also provides multiple types of complications from pharyngeal emergencies. The most obvious potential complication from diseases of the airway is airway compromise. Restrictive spaces such as the hypopharynx and larynx (with the narrow vocal cords and superior epiglottis) provide ample opportunity for even mild inflammation or edema to significantly alter normal airflow through this region. In addition, the proximate location of the great vessels of the carotid artery and internal jugular veins provide fertile ground for infections or complications from airway procedures such as drainage of peritonsillar abscesses. The fascial planes in the oropharynx reach toward vital structures, which when infected may have disastrous results. The deep fascial planes track posteriorly toward the vertebral column, inferiorly into the mediastinum, and superiorly near the cavernous sinus, thus providing opportunities for cervical vertebral osteomyelitis, mediastinitis, or cranial nerve problems.

### ANATOMY

The pharyngeal anatomy resembles an inverted cone, with the narrowest part at the point where it attaches to the esophagus at the level of the cricoid cartilage and the widest part attaching to the base of the skull. It is a muscular and fibrous tube located immediately behind the nasal cavity and mouth and has many functions. The pharynx connects anteriorly and superiorly with the nasal cavity to allow movement of air into the lungs though a continuously open passage. At its midpoint, the pharynx connects with the oral cavity for passage of nutrition and hydration into the esophagus. Inferiorly, it connect with the esophagus posteriorly and the larynx inferiorly and allows the complex selection of food and air to travel to different organ systems. The pharynx has abundant immunologic tissue to help fight infection—the palatine tonsils, adenoids, and lingual tonsils—which may predispose the host to dangerous circumstances (e.g., airway compromise) if the inflammatory response is too dramatic.

## ACUTE PHARYNGITIS AND TONSILLITIS

An inflammation of the oropharynx, pharyngitis is predominantly an infectious disease. Pharyngeal pain and dysphagia are some of the more common complaints in outpatient clinics and emergency departments (EDs) alike. Though mostly a benign disease, occasionally the immunologic response to the infection causes severe complications both in immediate proximity to the tissues of the airway and also systemically. The local inflammation may give rise to straightforward complications such as otitis media, but more dramatic complications such as dehydration, tissue edema, and airway compromise may also occur.

Pharyngeal irritation and inflammation produce throat pain that is worsened by swallowing. Occasionally, this pain may radiate to the ears or feel pressure-like because the eustachian tubes may also be blocked or swollen. The tonsils and pharynx may be erythematous with or without tonsillar enlargement, exudates, petechiae, or lymphadenopathy. Subtle variations or systemic symptoms may be present to aid in the diagnosis, but exact determination of the specific clinical cause of the pharyngitis from clinical criteria alone is notoriously difficult.

## PATHOPHYSIOLOGY

Viruses cause most cases of pharyngitis. Even the most common cause of bacterial pharyngitis in children, group A β-hemolytic *Streptococcus* (GAβHS), is responsible for only 30% of cases of pharyngitis. In adults, *Streptococcus* species account for 23% of cases, with *Mycoplasma* (9%) and *Chlamydia* (8%) species also being significant.[1] Recently, *Fusobacterium necrophorum*, known to be a factor in Lemierre syndrome, has been show to be a causal agent in as many as 10% of cases of pharyngitis in young adults.[2]

## PRESENTING SIGNS AND SYMPTOMS

### VIRAL

In addition to the characteristic pharyngeal pain and dysphagia, viral causes of pharyngitis may also produce low-grade fevers, cough, rhinorrhea, myalgias, or headaches. Viral causes may produce exudates as well, although cervical adenopathy is less common. Common viral causes include rhinoviruses, adenoviruses, Epstein-Barr virus (EBV), herpes simplex virus (HSV), and influenza and parainfluenza viruses. Less common viruses that may cause pharyngitis include respiratory syncytial virus, cytomegalovirus, and primary human immunodeficiency virus (HIV).

Pharyngitis in young adults may be due to infectious mononucleosis, an infection caused by EBV. It is often characterized by thick tonsillar exudates or membranes, as well as other systemic symptoms and signs. Splenomegaly (50%) is frequently present and generalized lymphadenopathy is usually present. Palatal petechiae and periorbital edema may likewise be seen.

Also a disease of young adults, HSV infection may produce a painful and characteristic pharyngitis. HSV pharyngitis is typically accompanied by painful vesicles on an erythematous base. These vesicles occur in the pharynx, lips, gums, or buccal mucosa. Fever, lymphadenopathy, and tonsillar exudates may also be present and last for 1 to 2 weeks. HSV pharyngitis may be either a primary infection or reactivation of a previous infection. In addition, bacterial superinfection of affected tissues may occur.

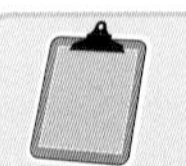

**DOCUMENTATION**

- Visualization of the airway, including patients with suspected epiglottitis or supraglottitis
- Work of breathing and use of accessory muscles
- Patient's ability to take fluids by mouth
- Discussion (and understanding) with the patient and family of the need for close observation and what symptoms to return for arranged follow-up

### BACTERIAL

The most common cause of bacterial pharyngitis in children is GAβHS. It is less frequently implicated in patients older than 15 years. During epidemics, the incidence may double. Characteristic symptoms include tonsillar exudates, high fevers (temperature > 38.3° C), tender cervical adenopathy, and pharyngeal erythema. Headache, nausea, and abdominal pain may also be found. GAβHS pharyngitis usually lacks the traditional symptoms of viral infections (cough, rhinorrhea, myalgias). It occasionally produces a fine sandpaper-like rash that is termed scarlet fever.

Pharyngitis caused by *Mycoplasma pneumoniae* occurs in crowded conditions, may be associated with epidemics, and typically produces a mild pharyngitis. Symptoms include exudates and a hoarse voice, and it may also be associated with lower respiratory symptoms such as cough and occasionally dyspnea.

*Chlamydia pneumoniae* pharyngitis resembles *Mycoplasma* pharyngitis in its occurrence in epidemic and crowded conditions. This pharyngitis is classically described as severe and persistent with tenderness in the deep cervical lymph nodes and occasional associated sinusitis.

Gonococcal and *Chlamydia trachomatis* pharyngitis have varying manifestations from exudative to nonexudative, mildly symptomatic to severely symptomatic, and transient or persistent. These infections result from orogenital sexual transmission, and asymptomatic carriers exist and may unknowingly spread the disease.

*F. necrophorum*, known to be a factor in Lemierre syndrome, frequently causes pharyngitis in young adults and is a common causative agent of recurrent pharyngitis as well.

## DIFFERENTIAL DIAGNOSIS AND MEDICAL DECISION MAKING

### VIRAL

Diagnostic testing for viral pharyngitis is limited to only a few different specific causes. EBV infection may be diagnosed with a few different tests. The peripheral blood smears of up to 75% of patients with EBV demonstrate atypical mononuclear cells. An EBV monospot test may be positive in up to 95% of adults and 90% of children, but the test may not be positive during the first few days of illness. EBV IgM antibodies develop in 100% of patients but may also initially be negative.

Herpes pharyngitis is diagnosed by serologic tests, herpes culture, or cytopathologic tests from lesion scrapings. Primary HIV pharyngitis may be diagnosed with serologic tests such as Western blot and enzyme-linked immunosorbent assay. New rapid HIV tests using buccal swabs have also been shown to be effective in an ED setting.

### BACTERIAL

Diagnostic testing for GAβHS is a subject of some controversy. Although the diagnosis of GAβHS infection is important in preventing many serious complications of streptococcal pharyngitis, including rheumatic fever, accurate diagnosis of GAβHS pharyngitis is notoriously difficult. The only valid method of diagnosing acute GAβHS infection involves acute and chronic antistreptolysin O titers. However, this method is far from practical in the emergency setting. Throat cultures have a sensitivity of nearly 90% for detecting *Streptococcus pyogenes* in the pharynx, but their accuracy may vary, depending on recent antibiotic use and culture and collection techniques.

Rapid diagnostic testing for GAβHS detects antigens via varying techniques, including latex agglutination, enzyme-linked or optical immunoassay, and DNA luminescent probes. Specificities are reported to be greater than 90% with sensitivities between 60% and 95%.[3] A positive test appears to be a reliable indicator of the presence of GAβHS in the pharynx, but a number of factors must be considered. Some patients with a positive test may be asymptomatic carriers, and rapid tests may be negative in patients with low bacterial counts.

In addition to cultures and rapid streptococcal tests, a number of authors have proposed clinical criteria to aid in the diagnosis of GAβHS pharyngitis. The most well known are the Centor criteria and the McIssac modifications of these criteria. The modified Centor score gives one point each to temperature higher than 38° C, swollen tender anterior cervical nodes, tonsillar swelling or exudates, absence of upper respiratory tract symptoms (e.g., cough, coryza), and age between 3 and 15 years. If the patient is older than 45 years, a point is subtracted. If the score is 1 or less, no further testing or treatment is warranted. For scores of 2 to 3, further testing may be indicated, such as cultures or rapid streptococcal tests. For scores of 4 or higher, no further testing is required and all patients may receive antibiotics for GAβHS pharyngitis (**Box 29.1**).[4,5]

In two recent guidelines (from the Infectious Diseases Society of America [IDSA] and the American Society of Internal Medicine [ASIM]), slightly different approaches to patients with pharyngitis have been proposed. In children the guidelines are similar and call for the use of a rapid test in all children; those with a positive test are treated, those with a negative test undergo a throat culture, and those with a positive culture result are treated. The guidelines have suggested different approaches to adults with pharyngitis, however. The IDSA guidelines propose treating all adults in a fashion similar to their pediatric recommendations.[6] The ASIM guidelines, though, allow two additional approaches for adults, including performing a rapid test on all adults with a Centor score of 2 or 3 and treating those with a positive test result, as well as empirically treating all patients with a score of 4 or higher. The final approach endorsed by the ASIM suggests testing no adults but treating all adults with a Centor score of 3 or 4 empirically.[7] A recent analysis comparing the different recommendations found that an approach using throat cultures had a sensitivity of 100%; approaches using rapid treptococcal tests involving clinical criteria alone had sensitivities of approximately 75%. Furthermore, the specificity of clinical criteria alone was below 50%, thus suggesting that many adults were prescribed antibiotics for pharyngitis unnecessarily.[8]

Diagnostic testing for other causes of bacterial pharyngitis requires either culture on special media (Thayer-Martin agar for gonococcal infection) or specialized antigen or serologic testing. *Mycoplasma* infection may be detected by culture, serologic testing, or rapid antigen testing. Antigen detection may also be used for chlamydial infection, as well as culture or serologic testing.

**BOX 29.1 Clinical Diagnosis of Streptococcal Pharyngitis**

The modified Centor criteria constitute a scoring system that can increase detection of group A β-hemolytic streptococcal pharyngitis. One point each is assigned to the following features:

- Temperature > 38° C
- Swollen, tender anterior cervical nodes
- Tonsillar swelling or exudates
- Absence of symptoms of upper respiratory tract infection (e.g., cough, coryza)
- Age between 3 and 15 years (if the patient is older than 45 years old, a point is taken off)

If the score is 1 or less—no treatment.

For scores of 2 to 3, further testing may be indicated, such as cultures or rapid streptococcal tests.

For scores of 4 or greater, no further testing is required and all patients may receive antibiotics for group A β-hemolytic streptococcal pharyngitis.

## DIFFERENTIAL DIAGNOSIS

In addition to the infectious causes of pharyngitis mentioned in this chapter, a number of other infectious and noninfectious causes must be considered in the differential diagnosis of patients with pharyngitis. Among dangerous infections, deep space infections such as retropharyngeal abscesses, peritonsillar abscesses, and epiglottitis must be considered. Noninfectious but potentially serious diseases in the differential diagnosis include drug or allergic reactions, foreign body or caustic ingestion, angioedema, and chemical or thermal burns.

## TREATMENT

Fortunately, most cases of pharyngitis are acute and self-limited. Supportive care with analgesics and antipyretics and perhaps topical anesthetics (lozenges or sprays) helps in alleviating the symptoms. However, even most infectious causes of pharyngitis rarely cause serious complications.

Among viral causes, few allow specific treatment. HSV infection may be treated with acyclovir, famciclovir, or valacyclovir, all of which produce similar earlier resolution of symptoms but do not eradicate the etiologic agent. Infectious mononucleosis has no effective antiviral agent, but some important aspects of disposition remain important. Patients suspected of having infectious mononucleosis should be advised against contact sports for 6 to 8 weeks because of concern for potential serious splenic injury. Patients with infectious mononucleosis in whom tonsillar edema and hypertrophy severely limit adequate oral hydration secondary to dysphagia may receive corticosteroids (dexamethasone, 6 to 10 mg intramuscularly) to aid in relief of symptoms.

Of all bacterial causes, GAβHS is the most common and most often studied. Regardless of the diagnostic strategy used, antimicrobial therapy directed at streptococcal species will probably be very effective. There are two main reasons to treat GAβHS pharyngitis—to improve symptoms and decrease complications. Patients who receive antibiotics during the first 2 to 3 days of symptoms are likely to improve 1 to 2 days faster than those not taking antibiotics. In terms of complications, the most feared complication of GAβHS infection is acute rheumatic fever. Antibiotic treatment within the first 9 days of infection decreases the rate of rheumatic fever after GAβHS infection. However, the incidence of acute rheumatic fever has fallen drastically in the last few decades such that the number needed to treat to prevent one case of rheumatic fever has risen from 63 to now more than 4000. This is due to the amount of antibiotics prescribed for GAβHS infection over the years, as well as the presence of less virulent strains of bacteria and improved living conditions. Antibiotic use also limits transmission to others and the amount of suppurative complications, including peritonsillar abscesses, retropharyngeal and other deep space infections, otitis, and mastoiditis. Use of antibiotics has no effect on the incidence of poststreptococcal glomerulonephritis.

Penicillin remains an effective choice for GAβHS pharyngitis. Benzathine penicillin, 1.2 million units, or a 10-day course of penicillin VK, 500 mg orally twice per day, both effectively treat pharyngitis and reduce symptoms. The intramuscular route may be more effective in treating streptococcal pharyngitis secondary to compliance issues but is associated with more severe allergic reactions. Alternative regimens include macrolide antibiotics (e.g., erythromycin, azithromycin) and clindamycin. Oral cephalosporins have been shown to result in slightly improved cure rates when compared with penicillins and may be taken over a shorter course (5 days).

Mycoplasmal pharyngitis may be treated with a course of macrolide antibiotics or tetracycline or doxycycline. *C. pneumoniae* pharyngitis is treated for 10 days with doxycycline, trimethoprim-sulfamethoxazole, or a macrolide. *C. trachomatis* pharyngitis may require repeated courses or prolonged use of antibiotics. *F. necrophorum* is susceptible to penicillin or clindamycin.

Corticosteroids, in conjunction with antibiotics, decrease the duration of symptoms in patients with pharyngitis without increasing complications. Steroids are particularly useful in patients with profound tonsillar hypertrophy and edema or in patients with severe dysphagia and mild dehydration. By reducing the inflammatory response, steroids allow patients to swallow without significantly reducing the pain sooner.

## DISPOSITION

Patients with pharyngitis usually have full resolution of their symptoms without difficulty. However, life-threatening complications do occur. Infectious mononucleosis may lead to airway obstruction, epiglottitis, deep space infections, and distant or systemic disorders such as splenic injury, thrombocytopenia, or hemolytic anemia. Complications of GAβHS pharyngitis include deep space infections, toxic shock syndrome, peritonsillar abscesses and autoimmune-related glomerulonephritis, rheumatic fever, and erythema nodosum. Patients in whom airway compromise is at all a concern should be admitted to the hospital for observation and personnel with advanced airway skills alerted for the potential need for a surgical airway.

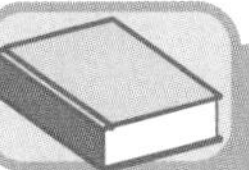

**PATIENT TEACHING TIPS**

When to take antibiotics
When to take pain medicine
Return for
- Increased difficulty breathing
- Increased difficulty swallowing
- Worsening pain
- Confusion or changes in thinking
- Worsening fever

# PERITONSILLITIS, PERITONSILLAR CELLULITIS, AND ABSCESS

## EPIDEMIOLOGY AND PATHOPHYSIOLOGY

Peritonsillar cellulitis and peritonsillar abscess exemplify the continuum of peritonsillar infections best characterized as peritonsillitis. Peritonsillar infections represent the most common deep infection of the head and neck region. These infections occur more frequently in teenagers and young adults, but they can develop at any age. The infection begins most commonly when tonsillitis spreads beyond the boundary of the tonsillar capsule and invades the potential space between the lateral aspect of the tonsillar capsule and the superior constrictor muscle of the pharynx. The local spread of infection begins as cellulitis but progresses to abscess formation if left untreated. Predisposing factors include chronic tonsillitis, dental infections, smoking, and infectious mononucleosis. Peritonsillitis can occur in patients who have previously undergone complete tonsillectomy.

## PRESENTING SIGNS AND SYMPTOMS

### SYMPTOMS

Symptoms of peritonsillitis begin with the symptoms of tonsillitis and progress over a few days to increasing pain and unilateral symptoms. Patients with peritonsillitis often complain of dysphagia, odynophagia, drooling, trismus, and referred otalgia on the affected side. In addition, patients will describe changes in voice (hoarseness or a "hot potato" voice) as a result of decreased movement of the palate. Patients may report recurrent bouts of pharyngitis or trials of antibiotics without resolution of symptoms.

### SIGNS

On physical examination the patient may have trismus, which may prevent clear visualization of the pharynx but may respond to benzodiazepines. Erythematous mucosa and purulent exudates may be present. The distinguishing features of a peritonsillar abscess include unilateral swelling and displacement of the infected tonsil and frequently the soft palate toward the midline with resultant deviation of the uvula to the contralateral side. Peritonsillar abscesses are generally unilateral and can occur in the superior pole of the tonsil.

## DIFFERENTIAL DIAGNOSIS

The differential diagnosis of peritonsillitis includes infectious mononucleosis, cervical adenitis, tubercular granuloma, internal carotid artery aneurysms, and neoplasms. Obviously, infectious causes will be manifested in a more rapid manner than chronic granulomas, masses, or aneurysms. Pulsatile masses or findings that do not suggest an acute infectious cause must be evaluated with other imaging techniques to elucidate the cause of the symptoms.

## DIAGNOSTIC TESTING

Plain radiographs do not aid in the diagnosis or treatment of uncomplicated cases of peritonsillitis. Although it is often difficult to distinguish peritonsillar cellulitis from peritonsillar abscess,[9] a number of modalities can aid in diagnosis. For patients who cannot lie down or who are unable to cooperate with needle aspiration, intraoral ultrasound is a useful test.[10] Computed tomography (CT) is helpful in delineating the extent and scope of the abscess, but it may be difficult for the patient to lie supine during the study.

## TREATMENT

Pending airway obstruction requires emergency aspiration of a peritonsillar abscess. For less urgent conditions the classic recommendation was incision and drainage. Needle aspiration, with or without ultrasound guidance, provides a diagnosis, induces less pain, and is easier to perform than traditional incision and drainage. Approximately 10% of needle-aspirated abscesses require repeated aspiration.[9]

Patients should receive antibiotics (penicillin or clindamycin) and steroids for relief of the pain and swelling, regardless of whether the abscess is drained. One strategy if the peritonsillitis is thought to be cellulitis or if the aspiration reveals no purulence is to start antibiotic and steroid treatment and assess the patient in 24 hours to see whether the symptoms are improving or another aspiration is required.

## DISPOSITION

Most patients with peritonsillitis can be treated safely and discharged home with antibiotics, steroids, and close follow-up in 24 to 48 hours. For patients with severe dehydration or severe trismus requiring intravenous hydration, a brief inpatient stay may be required. Any patient with tissue edema and potential airway compromise must be admitted to the hospital for observation and potential aggressive airway management.

# EPIGLOTTITIS AND SUPRAGLOTTITIS

## EPIDEMIOLOGY AND PATHOPHYSIOLOGY

Inflammation and edema of the epiglottis may result in rapid and life-threatening airway obstruction if not identified and treated effectively. In addition, the tissues immediately adjacent to the epiglottis (arytenoids, false vocal cords, and pharyngeal wall) may also become edematous and result in a similar infection known as supraglottitis. The signs and symptoms of the two diseases may be remarkably similar, although their populations may be somewhat different. Until introduction of the *Haemophilus influenzae* type B (Hib) vaccine in the mid-1980s, epiglottitis was a disease of children. The annual incidence decreased dramatically to a very low 0.3 to 0.6 per 100,000 children.[11] Adult epiglottitis appears to be on the rise. One study showed a 31% rise in the incidence of adult epiglottitis over an 18-year period.[12] Incidence rates for adults cluster near 3 per 100,000, with a case fatality rate reported to be as high as 7%. The lower overall bacteremia rates in adults than in children suggest that adults may have more viral causes, as well as other noninfectious causes. Noninfectious causes include trauma, ingestion of caustic substances, or thermal injuries from illicit drug inhalation. Of organisms recovered in blood cultures, Hib still predominates, but *Streptococcus* and *Staphylococcus* species may be isolated as well.

## PRESENTING SIGNS AND SYMPTOMS

### CHILDREN

Epiglottitis in children produces a dramatic progression from a relatively well child to a toxic-appearing one. Eighty-five percent of patients are sick for less than 24 hours. Affected children appear anxious, may be sitting forward in a tripod position, and may have difficult clearing secretions (**Table 29.1**).

### ADULTS

Adults with epiglottitis have a mean age of between 42 and 50 years. Unlike children, adults are usually seen after 2 to 3 days of symptoms. Adults exhibit odynophagia and throat pain rather than the drooling and stridor of pediatric patients. This difference is thought to be due to the larger and more rigid trachea and lack of generous lymph tissue in adults. The pharyngeal pain may be disproportionate to the clinical findings. Fever is frequently absent in adults until the later stages. Additionally, epiglottitis or supraglottitis is frequently misdiagnosed in adults as streptococcal pharyngitis, only to have the true diagnosis made later (**Table 29.2**).

**Table 29.1** Symptoms of Epiglottitis or Supraglottitis in Children

| | FREQUENCY (%) | |
|---|---|---|
| SYMPTOM | AGE < 2 YR | AGE > 2 YR, < 18 YR |
| Fever | 100 | 99 |
| Difficulty breathing | 97 | 94 |
| Irritability | 89 | 94 |
| Change in voice or cry | 82 | 96 |
| Stridor | 92 | 88 |
| Retractions | 88 | 78 |

**Table 29.2 Symptoms of Epiglottitis or Supraglottitis in Adults**

| SIGNS AND SYMPTOMS | FREQUENCY (%) |
|---|---|
| Muffled voice | 54-79 |
| Pharyngitis | 57-73 |
| Fever | 54-70 |
| Anterior neck tenderness | 79 |
| Dyspnea | 29-37 |
| Drooling | 22-39 |
| Stridor | 12-27 |

## DIFFERENTIAL DIAGNOSIS

The differential diagnosis for epiglottitis includes other pharyngeal diseases, from the straightforward such as pharyngitis and peritonsillar abscess to the life-threatening such as retropharyngeal abscess and Ludwig angina. If the symptoms are consistent with the physical findings, the diagnosis of pharyngitis or peritonsillar abscess may be appropriate. However, if the symptoms are out of proportion to the findings on examination, the more dangerous diseases must be excluded. Other life-threatening conditions include angioedema, aspiration of a foreign body, laryngospasm, and ingestion of a caustic substance. One rare disease that is occasionally confused with epiglottitis is adult botulism. The blockade of cholinergic nerve transmission characteristically produces an inflamed and painful pharynx, and the muscular paralysis may produce a muffled voice, which may be confused with epiglottitis.

## MEDICAL DECISION MAKING

Patients with any sign of respiratory distress (drooling, aphonia, or stridor) should be moved to a critical care room and plans made for obtaining a surgical airway if needed. Any attempt at direct laryngoscopy to visualize the epiglottis should occur only if the personnel and equipment are available to secure a surgical airway (cricothyrotomy or tracheostomy).

A lateral radiograph of patients with suspected epiglottitis has high sensitivity approaching 90% when compared with direct laryngoscopy. Findings on a lateral radiograph may include an edematous and thickened epiglottis (thumb shaped) (**Fig. 29.1**), disappearance of the vallecula, swelling of the epiglottic folds or arytenoids, or edema of the retropharyngeal spaces. Adults with normal radiographic findings and suspected epiglottitis must undergo laryngoscopy, either direct or indirect. In no pediatric patients should an attempt be made to visualize the epiglottis in the ED. Pediatric patients should be taken to the operating room for direct laryngoscopy while surgical staff members are present to obtain a surgical airway, if needed.

## TREATMENT

All patients with suspected epiglottitis should be treated with extreme caution because they may suddenly progress to complete airway obstruction without warning. Endotracheal intubation must be performed under direct visualization either with a laryngoscope or with a fiberoptic bronchoscope/laryngoscope. At all times, equipment and personnel for emergency cricothyrotomy must be present.

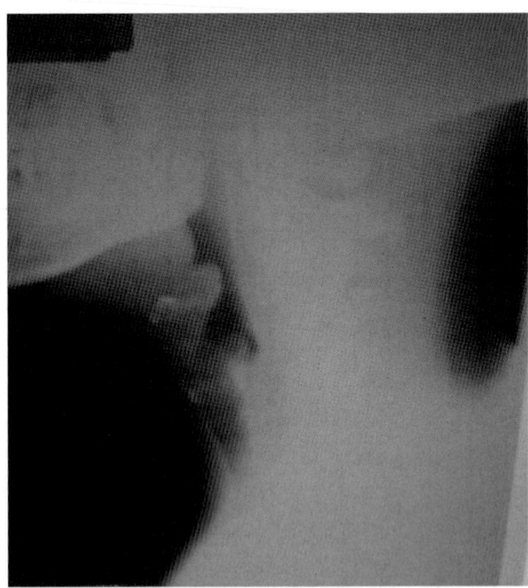

**Fig. 29.1 Classic radiograph of epiglottitis with the thumb sign indicating a swollen epiglottis.**

Patients should receive broad-spectrum antibiotics that include coverage against *H. influenzae*, as well as other common bacterial pathogens. Ampicillin-sulbactam and ceftriaxone are both acceptable first-line agents. Steroids and racemic epinephrine have not been conclusively proved to be of benefit in these patients.

## DISPOSITION

All patients suspected of having epiglottitis or supraglottitis should be admitted to the hospital. Adults without respiratory distress (drooling, stridor, or dyspnea) may be admitted without intubation and observed, but in a carefully monitored setting. The vast majority of children with suspected epiglottitis should be intubated in the operating room and then admitted to the intensive care unit (ICU) for intravenous antibiotics. Rarely, a child with epiglottis may not require intubation. However, this is done only in consultation with the pediatric anesthesiologist and intensivist after they have evaluated the patient. Children with epiglottis who are not intubated should always be admitted to an ICU setting because of their very high potential for rapid deterioration.

# LUDWIG ANGINA

## EPIDEMIOLOGY AND PATHOPHYSIOLOGY

First described in 1836, Ludwig angina is a fast-spreading, potentially lethal infection of the submandibular, sublingual, and submental spaces. These spaces effectively function as one unit, and infection can easily spread between them. True Ludwig angina involves all of the submandibular spaces; however, serious and life-threatening infections can occur with infection of only some of the spaces. Before the advent of antibiotics and surgical decompression, mortality with this disease approached 50%, but it is now commonly reported to be less than 10%.[13]

Approximately 80% of cases involve patients with odontogenic disease. Patients with infection or recent extraction of the second or third molars are particularly at risk because the roots of these teeth extend below the mylohyoid ridge. Abscesses located in this region can easily perforate the lingual plate of the mandible, thereby allowing direct spread of infection to the submandibular spaces. Other predisposing conditions include deep lacerations or trauma to the floor of the mouth, mandibular fractures, and salivary calculi.

## PRESENTING SIGNS AND SYMPTOMS

Patients with Ludwig angina appear ill and anxious. Males predominate over females by a ratio of 3:2. The classic symptoms include tooth pain (79%), swelling of the neck or chin (71%), dysphagia (52%), neck pain (33%), respiratory symptoms (dyspnea, tachypnea, stridor) (27%), and dysarthria (18%).

Physical findings in almost all patients include bilateral submandibular swelling, fever, and an elevated or protruding tongue (**Figs. 29.2 through 29.4**). Trismus is found in approximately half of all patients. Complications of Ludwig angina can be disastrous, with infection spreading to the mediastinum, pericardium, or pleural cavity, as well as the lungs and great vessels.

## DIFFERENTIAL DIAGNOSIS AND MEDICAL DECISION MAKING

The differential diagnosis in a patient with suspected Ludwig angina should also include Lemierre syndrome (septic thrombophlebitis of the superior internal jugular vein), which is distinguished from Ludwig angina by the unilateral nature of the infection. Tumors in the floor of the mouth can be distinguished from Ludwig angina by their tendency to exhibit much slower growth. Mandibular abscesses are generally unilateral and produce less swelling of the floor of the mouth.

## DIAGNOSTIC TESTING

Because Ludwig angina is predominantly a clinical diagnosis, diagnostic testing commonly delineates the extent of infection, not whether it is present. Soft tissue lateral neck radiographs may be helpful in showing edema of the soft tissues and air in the soft tissue spaces. If the patient is able to lie supine for a short while, helical CT may be helpful in delineating progression of the abscess and allow more accurate surgical débridement (**Fig. 29.5, *A* and *B***). If the safety of the patient lying supine is at all in question, the airway must be secured first. At all times the utmost caution is required in these patients, and securing the airway will probably involve the joint capabilities of anesthesia, otorhinolaryngologic, and

**PRIORITY ACTIONS**

Move patients with potential airway compromise to code rooms.

Prepare for an emergency airway procedure:
- Intubation
- Fiberoptic intubation
- Surgical cricothyrotomy

In pediatric patients with possible epiglottitis, laryngoscopy should not be attempted until personnel skilled in emergency airway techniques are present.

Initiate antibiotic therapy early in patients with serious infections.

Perform appropriate imaging of patients for serious infections such as retropharyngeal abscess or supraglottitis when their pain is out of proportion to the findings on examination.

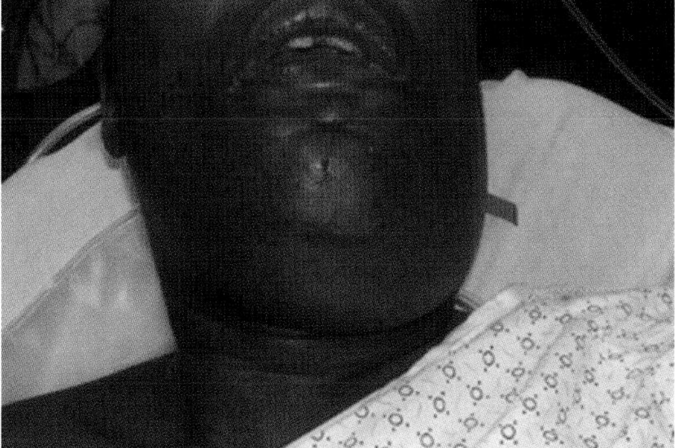

**Fig. 29.2 Submandibular swelling in a patient with Ludwig angina.**

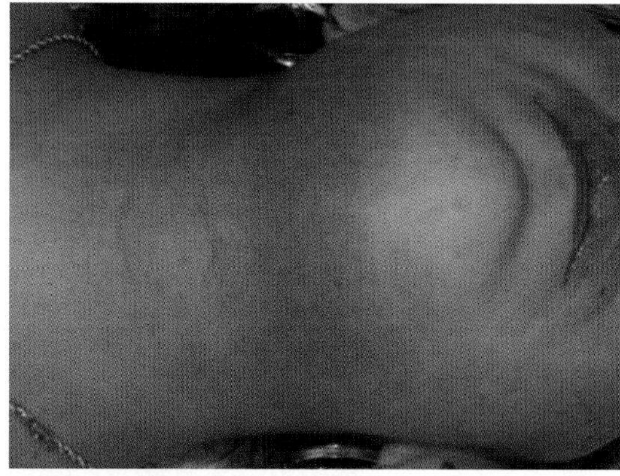

**Fig. 29.3 Submandibular redness and swelling in a patient with Ludwig angina.**

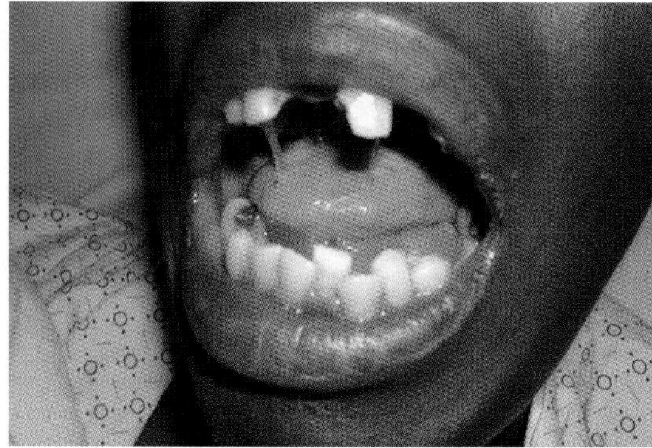

**Fig. 29.4 Raised floor of the mouth in a patient with Ludwig angina.**

general surgical colleagues. No airway maneuvers may be attempted until the equipment and personnel capable of obtaining a surgical airway are present at the bedside.

## TREATMENT

Treatment of patients with Ludwig angina predominantly involves three issues: protection of the airway though nasal (fiberoptic), oropharyngeal, or surgical techniques; administration of antibiotics; and surgical débridement. The antibiotic selected should have broad-spectrum coverage because up to 50% of patients have polymicrobial involvement. Although *Streptococcus, Staphylococcus*, and *Bacteroides* are the organisms commonly cultured, other species have included *Klebsiella, H. influenzae, Proteus*, and *Pseudomonas* species. Once the airway is protected, 50% will resolve with only antibiotics.

## DISPOSITION

All patients with Ludwig angina should be admitted to an ICU for further monitoring and fluid resuscitation should the clinical picture deteriorate into one of bacteremia and sepsis. ICU observation is required for those with the rare milder cases who are not immediately intubated, because progression to airway compromise and obstruction may be rapid.

# LEMIERRE SYNDROME

## PATHOPHYSIOLOGY

A particularly dangerous and intractable complication of nearby infections, Lemierre syndrome is a suppurative thrombophlebitis located within the internal jugular vein. This dangerous but fortunately rare complication of nearby infections in the pharynx or mastoid may produce septic emboli.

Lemierre syndrome is often caused by the organism *F. necrophorum*, a gram-negative anaerobe that produces endotoxin and is also responsible for many cases of acute and recurring pharyngitis, as well as peritonsillar abscesses.[14] *F. necrophorum* can colonize the upper respiratory, gastrointestinal, and genitourinary tracts. Other organisms that may also cause this particular variant of septic thrombophlebitis include *Bacteroides melaninogenicus, Eikenella corrodens*, and non–group A streptococci.

## PRESENTING SIGNS AND SYMPTOMS

The signs and symptoms of Lemierre syndrome may mimic those of other localized infections and include fever, swelling, tenderness, and pain with range of motion of the neck. It does, however, include the additional feature of obstruction of normal blood flow in the affected internal jugular vein, which may cause unilateral swelling, edema, and induration in the tissues on the affected side, regardless of whether they actually infected.

## DIFFERENTIAL DIAGNOSIS AND MEDICAL DECISION MAKING

When considering Lemierre syndrome, one must also consider Ludwig angina or other deep space infections in the neck and parapharyngeal tissues. Whether from odontogenic, lymphatic, or other sources, deep space infections in the neck and pharynx must be taken very seriously.

## DIAGNOSTIC TESTING

Lemierre syndrome is a diagnosis that when suspected requires confirmatory testing to document involvement of the

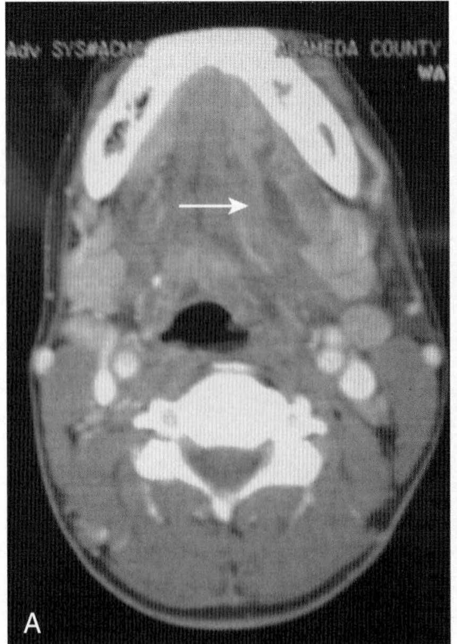


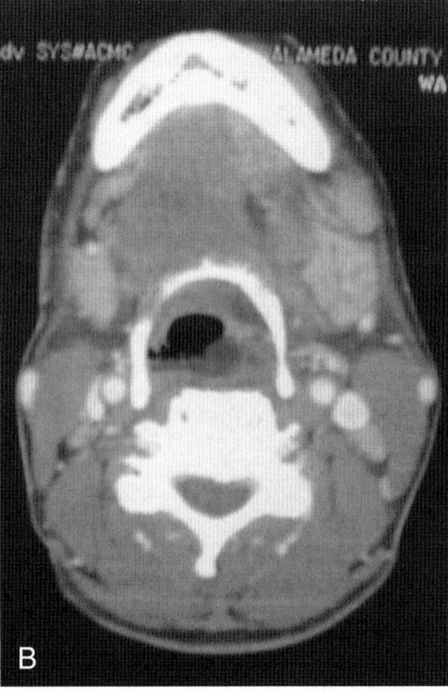


**Fig. 29.5** **A,** Computed tomography (CT) scan of Ludwig angina showing infection in the submandibular spaces (*arrow*). **B,** CT scan of Ludwig angina showing infection in the submandibular spaces.

internal jugular vein. Soft tissue lateral neck radiographs may be helpful in showing edema of the soft tissues and air in the soft tissue spaces, but they lack the specific information on vein involvement needed to make the diagnosis of Lemierre syndrome. The diagnosis is made most commonly via a contrast-enhanced CT scan of the neck. In addition, magnetic resonance imaging (MRI) may also delineate the extent of involvement of the jugular vein. Both these modalities will also provide information about the surrounding anatomy, including distortion of nearby tissues and localized pockets of infection that must be drained. Other tests that may aid in the diagnosis of Lemierre syndrome include duplex ultrasonography, retrograde venography, and gallium scanning. If there is any question about the safety of the patient lying supine, the airway must be secured first.

## TREATMENT

Treatment of Lemierre syndrome must include both heparin and antibiotics. The thrombus provides a nidus of ongoing infection and, subsequently, septic emboli. The anticoagulation effectively limits progression of the thrombosis and, in turn, limits the development of further septic emboli. The initial choice of antibiotics should be broad spectrum. Prolonged high-dose broad-spectrum antimicrobial therapy is recommended because of the high risk for septic emboli and endocarditis. Close consultation with an infectious disease specialist would be helpful in such cases.

## DISPOSITION

Patients with Lemierre syndrome clearly need to be admitted to the hospital, and consultation with a vascular surgeon may be helpful if thrombectomy is being considered.

# RETROPHARYNGEAL ABSCESS

## PATHOPHYSIOLOGY

Even though retropharyngeal abscesses predominantly occur in the pediatric population, adults may also be affected. Pediatric patients possess prominent lymph nodes in the retropharyngeal area, which can become infected and progress to cellulitis and abscess formation. These nodes atrophy by 6 years of age, and the incidence of retropharyngeal abscess drops precipitously.

The cause of retropharyngeal abscesses in the nonpediatric population differs greatly from the local lymph node infections in the age group younger than 6 years. The cause of adult retropharyngeal abscesses ranges from extension of other pharyngeal infections (e.g., parotitis, peritonsillar abscess, tonsillitis, Ludwig angina, dental infections) to instrumentation and other trauma (fishbones or dental instruments) to hematologic spread of systemic infections.[15]

Microbiologic testing of retropharyngeal abscesses reveals a diverse array of causative bacteria. Although the preponderance of abscesses are polymicrobial (up to 86%), some species predominate. The majority of aerobic pathogens include *Streptococcus* and *Staphylococcus* species, and *Bacteroides, Fusiform*, and *Peptostreptococcus* species dominate the anaerobic isolates. Tuberculous and fungal causes must also be considered.

## PRESENTING SIGNS AND SYMPTOMS

Patients will have a sore throat, as well as any number of other symptoms, including dysphagia, drooling, odynophagia, neck pain, and a muffled voice. The dysphonia frequently sounds like a duck quack (cri du canard). Patients may complain of a feeling of a lump in their throat and may prefer to lie supine or with their neck extended to keep the swelling in their posterior pharynx from compressing their upper airway. In the pediatric population, many case series have reported the mean age as being 3 years. It is uncommon for children in this age group to describe these symptoms, and the more common complaints are related to feeding, fever, and stridor.[16]

On physical examination only a minority of adult patients (37%) will have visible swelling of the posterior pharynx.[17] Other physical findings might include cervical lymphadenopathy, torticollis, and trismus. Palpation of the neck or moving the larynx and trachea side to side (tracheal "rock" sign) may induce pain. Pain and other symptoms out of proportion to the findings on physical examination require further diagnostic testing and evaluation.

## DIFFERENTIAL DIAGNOSIS AND MEDICAL DECISION MAKING

Other possible diagnoses to consider in these patients include other pharyngeal infections such as pharyngitis, peritonsillar abscess, and infectious mononucleosis. Abrasions or caustic burns involving the posterior pharynx might produce similar symptoms of dysphagia and odynophagia. Other causes of retropharyngeal swelling and pain may include cervical fracture, hematoma, or other causes of tissue edema such as tendonitis. Finally, distinguishing between a true abscess and pharyngeal cellulitis may be difficult and might be accomplished only with imaging techniques.

## DIAGNOSTIC TESTING

Imaging of retropharyngeal abscesses involves two main types of radiologic tests, plain lateral neck radiographs and CT scans. Early studies of normal lateral radiographs suggest that the upper limit of normal for the retropharyngeal spaces is 7 mm at C2 and 22 mm at C6. Anything beyond 7 mm is considered pathologic in both children and adults. In addition, retropharyngeal abscesses will displace the larynx and esophagus anteriorly. If there is still a question about the extent of involvement or the distinction between cellulitis and abscess, CT of the neck (**Fig. 29.6**) or MRI (**Fig. 29.7**) will easily elucidate the exact anatomic extension of the abscess. Of course, patients must be stable enough to lie flat in the supine position for the time needed to complete the study. In addition, intraoral ultrasound is another modality with great potential for distinguishing between abscess and cellulitis.[18]

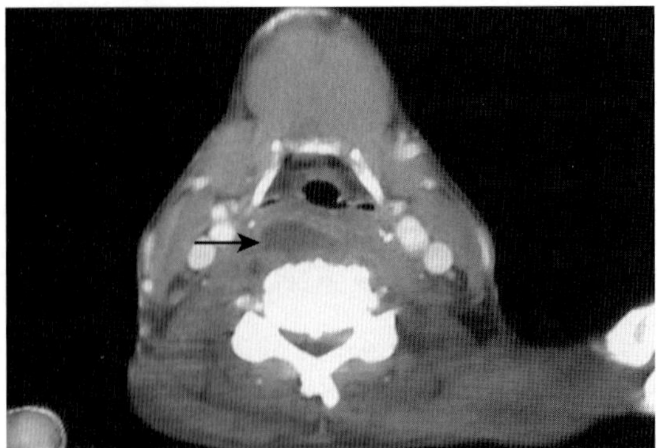

**Fig. 29.6 Computed tomography scan of a retropharyngeal abscess *(arrow)*.**

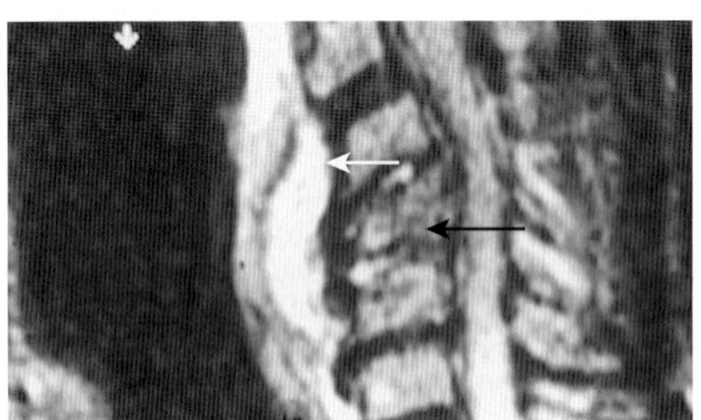

**Fig. 29.7 Magnetic resonance imaging of a retropharyngeal abscess *(white arrow)*.** Note extension into the vertebral bodies (osteomyelitis) *(black arrow)*.

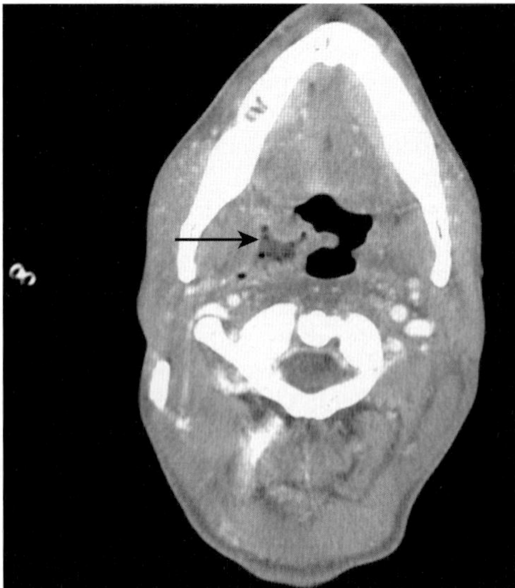

**Fig. 29.8 Computed tomography scan of a retropharyngeal abscess *(arrow)* extending laterally and inferiorly.**

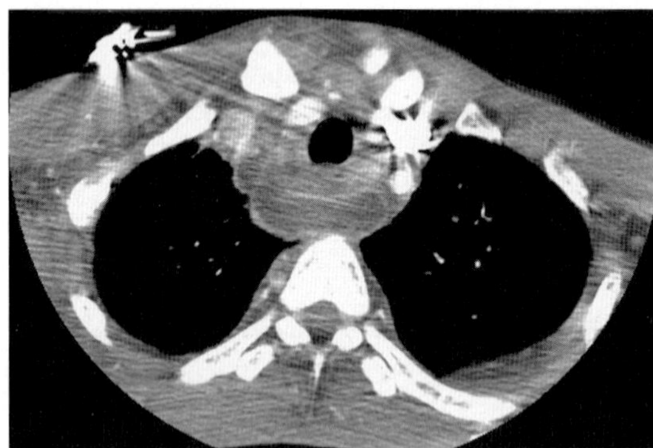

**Fig. 29.9 Computed tomography scan showing inferior extension of a retropharyngeal abscess into the mediastinum.**

## TREATMENT AND DISPOSITION

Retropharyngeal infections require broad-spectrum intravenous antibiotics. The antibiotics must cover anaerobes, as well as gram-positive and gram-negative species. Although most retropharyngeal abscesses require surgical drainage, selected cases may occasionally be managed with intravenous antibiotics alone.[19] Even if surgical drainage is deferred, admission to a monitored bed after thorough airway evaluation is required.

Complications from retropharyngeal abscesses include spread of infection inferiorly or laterally (**Fig. 29.8**) into the mediastinum (**Fig. 29.9**), pericardium, and nearby vascular structures. Osteomyelitis (see Fig. 29.7), transverse myelitis, and epidural abscesses have also been reported.

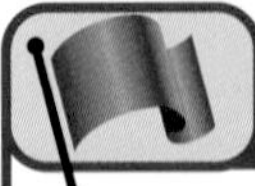

**RED FLAGS**

- Do not miss the diagnosis of acute epiglottitis or supraglottitis. It is more sudden in children than in adults.
- Do not give ampicillin to patients with suspected infectious mononucleosis because an uncomfortable rash develops.
- Do not miss abscesses. Use ultrasonography or computed tomography to diagnose peritonsillar abscesess. Retropharyngeal abscesses are difficult to diagnose unless considered and imaged.
- When the pharyngeal pain is out of proportion to the findings on physical examination, exclude more serious causes such as epiglottitis and deep space infections.

## SUGGESTED READINGS


Aliyu SH, Marriott RK, Curran MD, et al. Real-time PCR investigation into the importance of *Fusobacterium necrophorum* as a cause of acute pharyngitis in general practice. J Med Microbiol 2004;53:1029-35.

Bisno AL. Acute pharyngitis. N Engl J Med 2001;344:205-11.

Frantz TD, Rasgon BM. Acute epiglottitis: changing epidemiologic patterns. Otolaryngol Head Neck Surg 1993;109:457-60.

Lyon M, Blaivas M. Intraoral ultrasound in the diagnosis and treatment of suspected peritonsillar abscess in the emergency department. Acad Emerg Med 2005;12:85-8.

Spires JR, Owens JJ, Woodson GE, et al. Treatment of peritonsillar abscess. A prospective study of aspiration vs incision and drainage. Arch Otolaryngol Head Neck Surg 1987;113:984-6.


## REFERENCES

***References can be found on Expert Consult @ www.expertconsult.com.***

# Maxillofacial Disorders 30

*Laura J. Bontempo*

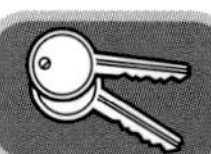

**KEY POINTS**

- Temporomandibular joint dislocation is usually readily reduced in the emergency department after the patient has been pretreated with analgesic and antispasmodic agents.
- Epistaxis may be the initial complaint of a patient with a more serious systemic illness, such as a clotting disorder.
- When visible blood loss from the nasopharynx has been stopped, the clinician should examine the posterior oropharynx for ongoing occult blood loss.
- Posterior epistaxis accounts for about 10% of nasal hemorrhages and can result in large volumes of blood loss.
- Any abnormal neurologic or ocular physical findings in a patient with rhinosinusitis mandate further investigation to assess for central nervous system extension of the disease.

## TEMPOROMANDIBULAR DISORDERS

### EPIDEMIOLOGY

The temporomandibular articulations are unique within the body in that they are bilateral joints that are nearly continuously in use. Consequently, the temporomandibular joint (TMJ) is subject to both pain and dislocation. Discomfort of the TMJ was previously referred to as TMJ pain dysfunction syndrome. However, because it was realized that more than just the actual joint can be the source of a patient's discomfort, the term has evolved to *temporomandibular disorder* (TMD). TMD is defined as craniofacial pain that involves the TMJ, masticatory muscles, and associated head and neck musculoskeletal structures.[1] It is roughly estimated that more than 10 million people in the United States alone have symptomatic TMD.[2] Most of those affected are women.

TMJ dislocation is an uncommon disorder, with one case series reporting 37 occurrences in 700,000 patient visits.[3]

### PATHOPHYSIOLOGY

TMD is probably due to excessive strain on the muscles of mastication with resultant strain on the capsular ligaments of the TMJ.[4] The result is that the mandibular condyle does not articulate properly in its joint. The patient feels pain and senses an occlusal disturbance.

Patients with TMJ dislocation are unable to close their mouth. With normal function, when the mandible is open, the mandibular condyle moves anteriorly and inferiorly. When the mandible closes, the condyle moves posteriorly and superiorly and returns to its original location (**Fig. 30.1**). TMJ dislocation results when the mandibular condyle moves anterior to the temporal eminence (the anterior portion of the mandibular fossa) (see Fig. 30.1). Once the dislocation occurs, the muscles of mastication spasm, which results in trismus and inability of the patient to return the mandibular condyle to its anatomic position. The dislocation usually results from excessive opening of the mouth, such as occurs with yawning or laughing. TMJ dislocation can also be the result of trauma, seizure, or dystonic drug reactions.

### PRESENTING SIGNS AND SYMPTOMS

Unilateral pain in the region of the TMJ and clicking or crepitance that is exacerbated by chewing are the classic complaints of a patient with TMD (**Box 30.1**). The dull or throbbing pain is localized to the preauricular region or to the muscles of mastication and typically worsens with movement of the mandible, such as when eating or talking. Pain may be most severe in the morning if bruxism is an issue.[5] If a click is present, the patient hears it when jaw opening is initiated. The pain may also radiate to the neck, ears, mandible, or temporal region.

Physical examination should include evaluation of the muscles of mastication by intraoral and external palpation. Palpation may reveal muscular spasm and tenderness. Palpation of the TMJ or muscles of mastication may reproduce the patient's symptoms and trigger significant pain. The patient may have great pain with any attempt at jaw range of motion. Physical findings are also notable for reduced jaw opening and possible lateral deviation of the jaw.

An inability to close the mouth following extreme jaw opening, such as yawning, is the classic manifestation of TMJ dislocation. If the dislocation is unilateral, the mandible will deviate away from the side of the dislocation (**Box 30.2**).

### DIFFERENTIAL DIAGNOSIS AND MEDICAL DECISION MAKING

When considering the diagnosis of TMD, the emergency practitioner must rule out odontogenic causes. If an intraoral cause remains possible after a carefully performed history and physical examination, the patient should be referred to a dentist

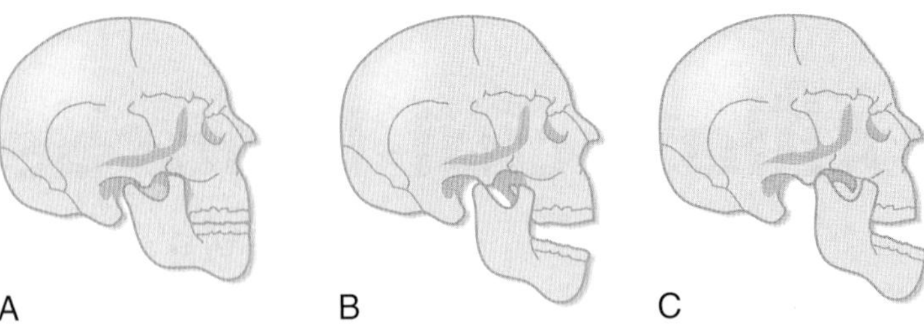


**Fig. 30.1** Anatomic drawing of the mandible in open **(A)**, closed **(B)**, and dislocated **(C)** positions.

**BOX 30.1 Signs and Symptoms of Temporomandibular Disorder**

Dull or throbbing facial pain
Unilateral pain more common than bilateral
Pain localized to the jaw or temporomandibular joint
Ear pain or fullness
Decreased mouth opening
Clicking sounds from the temporomandibular joint

**BOX 30.2 Signs and Symptoms of Temporomandibular Joint Dislocation**

Inability to close the mouth
Jaw deviation if the dislocation is unilateral

for a full dental evaluation. This evaluation can be done concurrently with the start of TMD treatment. Less common mimics, including jaw tumors and trigeminal neuralgia, should also be considered.

Central nervous system (CNS) disorders must be ruled out in the evaluation of a patient with symptoms suggestive of TMD. The clinician must be especially careful to address this possibility when the patient's complaints include CNS-related symptoms such as headache and vertigo. A detailed neurologic examination must be performed. Except for possible hyperesthesia immediately around the TMJ, patients with TMD should have no abnormal neurologic findings.

When evaluating a patient for a possible TMJ dislocation, the emergency practitioner must rule out a dystonic medication reaction or a mandibular fracture, both of which can be manifested in similar fashion. In patients with a history of trauma, panoramic radiographic evaluation of the mandible, a TMJ radiographic series, or computed tomography (CT) of the mandible should be performed to assess for a fracture before attempting reduction.

## TREATMENT

### TEMPOROMANDIBULAR DISORDERS

Management of TMD is primarily directed at improving the patient's comfort, which is accomplished with analgesia, muscle relaxation, and behavioral modifications. In the absence of trauma, there is no indication for emergency imaging of the TMJ.

Pain should be addressed with antiinflammatory agents (e.g., ibuprofen, 600 mg by mouth every 6 hours, or naproxen, 500 mg by mouth every 12 hours) and narcotic pain medications (e.g., oxycodone, 5 to 10 mg by mouth every 6 hours as needed). Warm compresses should also be applied to the TMJ region for 15 minutes three times per day. Benzodiazepines are used to relieve masseter muscle spasm (e.g., diazepam, 5 mg by mouth every 8 hours as needed). Behavioral modifications include minimizing masseter muscle use through a soft diet and cessation of gum chewing. Reassurance is important because up to 40% of patients will experience resolution of their TMD symptoms with little or no treatment (**Box 30.3**).[6]

If bruxism is suspected, dental follow-up should be arranged, and a bite appliance can be considered. To date, experimentation with the use of botulinum toxin to reduce masseter muscle contractility and strength has yielded mixed results.[7]

**BOX 30.3 Treatment of Temporomandibular Disorder**

Nonsteroidal antiinflammatories
Benzodiazepines for muscle relaxation
Mandibular rest (no gum chewing, teeth clenching, fingernail biting)
Reassurance

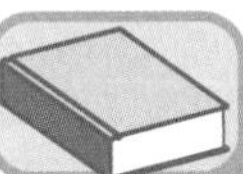

**PATIENT TEACHING TIPS**

**Temporomandibular Disorders**

Take antiinflammatory and pain medications as prescribed.
Apply warm compresses in front of your ear for 15 minutes 3 times per day.
Benzodiazepines may have been prescribed to control muscle spasm. These drugs may cause sedation.
Eat only soft foods until the symptoms resolve.
Avoid chewing gum.
See your dentist for follow-up to evaluate whether bruxism is the cause of your condition.
Many cases resolve spontaneously and very few require aggressive treatment.
See your doctor or return to the emergency department if your pain is not controlled or if you are unable to fully open or close your mouth, which may indicate a dislocation of your jaw.

### TEMPOROMANDIBULAR DISLOCATION

TMJ reduction is performed in the emergency department (ED) and is usually readily accomplished. Controlling the

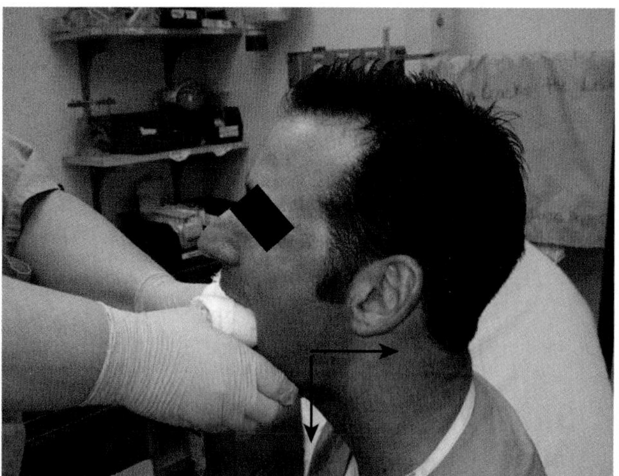

**Fig. 30.2** Proper technique for reduction of a dislocated temporomandibular joint.

patient's pain and masseter spasm facilitates the procedure. Analgesics (e.g., morphine, 5 mg intravenously as needed) and antispasmodics (e.g., diazepam, 5 to 10 mg intravenously titrated to the patient response) should be administered before reduction is attempted. Atraumatic TMJ dislocations do not require imaging.

Once the patient is comfortable, the clinician faces the patient and grasps the mandible inferiorly with the fingers of both hands. The clinician's thumbs should be heavily wrapped in gauze for protection and then placed on the occlusive surfaces of the mandibular molars. Downward pressure is applied to move the mandibular condyle inferior to the temporal eminence. The mandible is then pushed posteriorly (**Fig. 30.2**). Once the condyle is posterior to the temporal eminence and pressure is released, the condyle returns to its anatomic position in the mandibular fossa. At the time of reduction, the masseter muscles may contract forcefully and cause the patient to inadvertently clench the jaw. The clinician must be aware of this possibility and ensure that the thumbs are guarded during the procedure and remove the thumbs from the occlusive surface of the molars as quickly as possible. If this method does not work, both thumbs may be placed simultaneously on the dislocated side and the reduction reattempted.[8]

In an effort to minimize risk to the practitioner, an extraoral approach to TMJ reduction was proposed by Chen et al. in 2007.[9] The physician faces the patient and places a thumb on the palpable coronoid process that is displaced anteriorly. The fingers of that hand are placed on the mastoid process for stability. On the nondislocated side, the thumb is placed on the zygoma and the fingers hold the mandible angle. The nondisplaced side of the mandible is pulled anteriorly while concomitant pressure is applied posteriorly to the displaced coronoid process. Although this approach is less successful than the traditional approach, there is no risk of injury to the practitioner.

When reduction of the TMJ has been accomplished, the patient needs to avoid excessive mouth opening to prevent recurrent dislocation and may be discharged home. Postreduction pain can be treated with analgesics and antispasmodics. Advising a soft diet for 2 weeks will also minimize the patient's discomfort. The patient should be evaluated by an oromaxillofacial surgeon within 2 weeks.

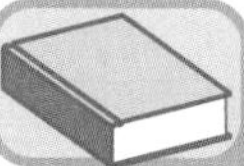

**PATIENT TEACHING TIPS**

**Temporomandibular Joint Dislocation**

Avoid excessive mouth opening, including laughing and yawning, to prevent recurrence of the dislocation.

Take pain medications and muscle relaxants as prescribed. These drugs may cause sedation.

Eat a soft diet for 2 weeks.

Follow up with an oromaxillofacial surgeon within 2 weeks.

Return to the emergency department if your pain is not controlled or if you are unable to fully close your mouth, which may indicate a recurrent dislocation.

# EPISTAXIS

## EPIDEMIOLOGY

The incidence of epistaxis is unknown, but it is estimated to occur in up to 60% of all individuals. The vast majority of these episodes are self-limited and only 6% require medical attention.[10] Epistaxis affects both adults and children, with a higher incidence in children younger than 10 years and adults older than 35 years.[11]

The anterior nasal septum is the source of bleeding in 90% of patients with epistaxis; the posterior nasal septum and lateral nasal wall account for 10% of cases of nasal bleeding. Posterior nasal hemorrhage is more common in the elderly population.

## PATHOPHYSIOLOGY

The nasal mucosa is a highly vascular area, and any disruption of the mucosa can result in bleeding. Although epistaxis can be caused by trauma, this is not the most common cause. Bleeding more commonly results from upper respiratory infections (URIs), a dry environment, nasal foreign bodies, allergic rhinitis, nasal mucormycosis, topical nasal medications (including antihistamines and corticosteroids), and drugs taken intranasally such as cocaine (**Box 30.4**). Additionally, epistaxis may be the initial symptom of a primary or secondary systemic bleeding disorder. One study found that 45% of patients with bleeding severe enough to warrant hospitalization had an associated systemic disorder that may have contributed to the epistaxis.[12]

The relationship of hypertension to epistaxis is controversial. It is unclear whether elevated blood pressure is the cause or the effect of epistaxis; therefore, hypertension alone is not known to be an independent risk factor for nasal hemorrhage.[13-15]

The Kiesselbach plexus is located at the anterior portion of the nasal septum and is the source of bleeding in patients with anterior epistaxis. The plexus is supplied by branches of the

**BOX 30.4 Risk Factors for Epistaxis**

Alcoholism
Allergic rhinitis
Anticoagulant use
Barotrauma
Blood dyscrasia
Diabetes mellitus
Endometriosis
Intranasal drug use
Intranasal medication use
Intranasal neoplasm
Low-humidity environment
Nasal foreign body
Nasal polyps
Platelet inhibitor use
Pregnancy
Recent otorhinolaryngologic surgery
Septal deviation or perforation
Sinusitis
Trauma, including nose picking
Upper respiratory tract infection

internal and external carotid arteries via the sphenopalatine, ethmoidal, and superior labial arteries. Another name for the Kiesselbach plexus is the Little area. The posterior nasal septum and lateral nasal wall are supplied by the sphenopalatine artery, which is the source of bleeding for posterior epistaxis.

Functionally, epistaxis is considered anterior when the site of bleeding can be visualized in the anterior portion of the nasopharynx. Posterior nasal hemorrhage cannot be directly visualized and occurs in the posterior or lateral parts of the nose.

## PRESENTING SIGNS AND SYMPTOMS

Epistaxis may be manifested as minor bleeding with small quantities of blood dripping from the nares or as major bleeding with the patient vomiting blood. Approximately 90% of cases of epistaxis are anterior and the bleeding source is unilateral. Many patients, however, have blood flowing from both nares because blood from the unilateral bleeding source travels around the septum posteriorly and exits on the other side.

Patients with epistaxis may arrive at the ED with various home treatments in progress. All foreign bodies (cotton, tissues, tampons) should be removed from the nose after the patient arrives to better assess the location and quantity of bleeding.

Important historical elements include the duration of the bleeding, laterality, estimated blood loss, recent trauma, and other associated symptoms.

Obtaining a detailed history is often the key to determining the cause of the patient's epistaxis. The clinician must know whether the patient has recurrent epistaxis, easy bruising, or other sources of bleeding, such as when shaving or brushing the teeth, or is taking a platelet inhibitor or anticoagulant medication. The past medical history is important in a patient who has hepatic disease, atherosclerosis, Osler-Weber-Rendu disease (hemorrhagic telangiectasia), diabetes mellitus, or cancer with ongoing chemotherapy treatment because each of these conditions is a risk factor for epistaxis.[16] Women are more prone to epistaxis during pregnancy.

Trauma, nose picking, recent otorhinolaryngologic surgery, nasal foreign body, URI, nasal polyps, and exposure to a low-humidity environment all predispose to epistaxis and should be addressed in the patient's history. The family medical history may reveal recurrent epistaxis in multiple family members. In the absence of a hereditary bleeding disorder, such a history suggests familial idiopathic epistaxis. A social history must also be obtained to identify alcoholism, intranasal drug use, or domestic violence.

Physical examination of a patient with epistaxis must focus on the nasopharynx and oropharynx; however, a complete examination is helpful. A skin examination may reveal ecchymoses or petechiae (suggestive of a systemic bleeding disorder), spider angiomas or caput medusa (suggestive of hepatic disease), or signs of trauma. Cardiac examination may demonstrate an irregular heartbeat and should prompt the clinician to inquire further about anticoagulant medications.

Concurrent with examining the nasal mucosa, the posterior oropharynx must also be evaluated. The nares may be occluded with nasal packing or clotted blood but continue to have significant blood loss into the oropharynx. The patient swallows this blood, and without a careful examination, the ongoing loss may not be evident until hematemesis or hemodynamic instability develops.

Alternatively, a patient may have a chief complaint of hemoptysis. If a patient has low-volume nasal bleeding with blood flowing posteriorly into the oropharynx, coughing up gross blood may be the initial symptom of epistaxis.

## DIFFERENTIAL DIAGNOSIS AND MEDICAL DECISION MAKING

Mechanical causes of epistaxis, such as trauma, nose picking, nasal foreign bodies, and nasogastric or nasotracheal intubation, directly disrupt the nasal mucosa. Blood dyscrasias, hepatic disease, platelet inhibitors, and anticoagulant medications result in decreased blood clotting and predispose the host to bleeding. Infectious causes include sinusitis, rhinitis, mucormycosis, and URIs that result in nasal congestion and vasodilation.[16] In women, both endometriosis and pregnancy must be considered as causes of epistaxis. Environmental factors also play a role in the incidence of epistaxis. Visits to the ED for the treatment of epistaxis are more common in the winter months.[11] This has been proposed to be due to lower ambient humidity and subsequent drying of the nasal membranes during the winter season. Barotrauma can also incite epistaxis.

Recurrent, refractory unilateral epistaxis merits investigation for a possible neoplastic etiology, especially with abnormal findings on neurologic examination.

In patients with larger-volume hemorrhage, hematemesis may be the initial complaint. Once the emesis has been controlled, examination of the oropharynx shows blood entering superiorly from the nasal cavity. The clinician can then work to localize the source of bleeding in the nose without being misled into investigating a gastrointestinal source.

## TREATMENT

In the prehospital setting or if the patient has to wait before being seen in the ED, the patient can apply direct pressure to the area by squeezing the soft tissue portion of the nose with the fingers. The nares are successfully compressed when a change in the patient's voice is heard.

Standard supplies for the treatment of epistaxis include suction with a Frazier tip, nasal speculum, bayonet forceps, cotton-tipped applicators, silver nitrate cautery sticks, packing

**BOX 30.5 Treatment of Epistaxis**

| Vasoconstrictors | Analgesics |
|---|---|
| 4% cocaine | 4% cocaine |
| Epinephrine (1:1000) | 4% lidocaine |
| Oxymetazoline | |
| Phenylephrine | |

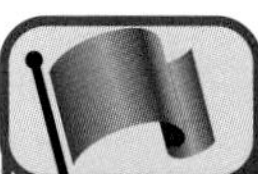

**RED FLAGS**

**Epistaxis**

Epistaxis may be the initial manifestation of a primary or secondary blood dyscrasia.

Occluded nares may mask ongoing bleeding.

Hematemesis may be the initial complaint in patients with large-volume bleeding.

An antihypertensive agent (i.e., beta-blocker) can mask the early stages of hemorrhagic shock by limiting tachycardia.

material, nasal tampons or balloons, gelatin foam (Gelfoam) or oxidized cellulose (Surgicel), a posterior nasal balloon with syringe, and a good light source. Universal precautions should be followed at all times. The clinician must also wear eye protection because of the risk for ocular exposure during management of the epistaxis.

In the absence of massive epistaxis, the initial step is to evacuate intranasal clots and apply a topical vasoconstrictor and analgesic to the mucosa (**Box 30.5**). This can be achieved by soaking cotton pledgets in a combined vasoconstrictor and topical analgesic solution. If cotton is not available, rolled 2- × 2-inch gauze can be used. The analgesic is added to improve patient comfort during any necessary interventions once vasoconstriction has occurred. These medications are left in contact with the mucosa for 5 to 10 minutes.

After removal of the pledgets, the nasal cavity and oropharynx are inspected. If the source of bleeding is identified in the nose and the oropharynx is dry, anterior epistaxis has been confirmed. For anterior epistaxis in which vasoconstriction has mostly controlled the bleeding, chemical cautery with silver nitrate is an excellent first choice. The silver nitrate cautery stick is moistened and applied directly to the area of bleeding from peripheral to central and from superior to inferior. This method minimizes the quantity of blood that comes between the cautery stick and the nasal mucosa. Septal damage from silver nitrate can occur. For this reason, the cautery stick should not be in contact with the nasal mucosa for more than 15 seconds, and bilateral septal coagulation should be avoided. Bilateral coagulation can lead to septal ischemia, necrosis, and perforation.

Another approach to anterior epistaxis is to apply a topical hemostatic packing agent, such as gelatin foam or oxidized cellulose, directly to the bleeding area. These products will be absorbed or degrade and do not require removal.

If neither of the preceding measures is successful, direct compression of the mucosa through packing the anterior nasal cavity is necessary. This can be accomplished with nonadherent ribbon gauze packing or a nasal tampon or balloon. Preformed nasal tampons and nasal balloons are now widely available and are easily inserted. The tampon or balloon is lubricated with a water-based lubricant and then directed posteriorly into the nasal cavity. The tampon should be placed gently but firmly and quickly into the nasal cavity. If it is inserted too slowly, the first part may expand from contact with blood before insertion is complete, which makes further insertion more difficult for both the patient and clinician. If after insertion the tampon is not fully expanded, saline or a vasoconstrictive agent (see Box 30.5) can be dripped into the nasal cavity until expansion is achieved. If a balloon is used, it will need to be inflated with saline or air, depending on the model used. If nonadherent ribbon gauze is to be used instead, the technique is to insert the packing in an accordion pattern from posterior to anterior and inferior to superior. If the septum bows to the contralateral side after packing, packing the other side may be necessary. Pain medication may be needed to alleviate the discomfort from nasal packing. The packing should remain in place for 1 to 3 days.

Bleeding from posterior epistaxis is more challenging to control. By definition, the bleeding site is not readily visualized, thus making compression and treatment more difficult. The most rapid method for controlling posterior epistaxis is insertion of a posterior balloon device. Typically, this device has a double-balloon design, one balloon to tamponade the posterior nasal cavity and the other for the anterior nasal cavity. After the device is lubricated, it is inserted into the nasal cavity to its hub. The posterior balloon is inflated and the hub is then drawn out away from the nose until resistance is met. Resistance indicates that the posterior balloon has set in the posterior nasal cavity and is not in the pharynx. Next, the anterior balloon is inflated. The quantity of saline required to fill each balloon varies by device but is typically 7 to 10 mL for the posterior balloon and 15 to 30 mL for the anterior balloon.[16]

If a posterior balloon device is not available, a Foley catheter can be used in its place. A 12- to 14-French catheter with a 30-mL balloon is used. The catheter is inserted through the nose until the noninflated balloon can be seen in the posterior oropharynx. The balloon is then inflated with 10 mL of saline, and the catheter is slowly withdrawn from the nose until resistance is met. While traction is maintained, the anterior nasal cavity is packed with ribbon gauze. The catheter is secured by placement of a padded umbilical clamp or other equivalent device around the catheter at the point where it exits the nostril. Securing the catheter properly is extremely important. If the catheter is allowed to migrate posteriorly, the inflated balloon descends into the oropharynx and possibly the trachea and obstructs the airway. Using a Foley catheter for control of posterior epistaxis is only a temporary technique, and the catheter should be exchanged for a safer double-balloon device as soon as possible.

For patients with massive epistaxis, use of nasal tampons and balloons is the fastest way to minimize or stop the bleeding. Bilateral anterior tampons or balloons are placed and then the oropharynx examined. If active bleeding continues into the oropharynx, one tampon or balloon is removed and replaced with a posterior balloon device. If significant bleeding continues, the second tampon or balloon is removed and a second posterior balloon inserted. Immediate otorhinolaryngologic consultation is then necessary. Bilateral posterior balloons should be in place for the minimal amount of time possible. Fluid resuscitation is then begun for any patient with significant blood loss or signs of shock.

Laboratory tests have a limited role in patients with epistaxis. Patients with low- or moderate-volume anterior bleeding who have no known blood dyscrasia and who are not taking anticoagulant medications do not require any laboratory studies.[12]

If, however, the patient's history or physical examination raises concern for a systemic cause of the epistaxis, studies should be ordered as appropriate for the clinician's specific suspicions. Such studies may include a prothrombin time, activated partial thromboplastin time, coagulation factor levels, bleeding time, vitamin K level, and liver function tests.[16] In patients exhibiting signs of shock, the hematocrit should be checked to obtain a starting value with which to compare serial measurements. Additionally, blood typing and screening may be necessary for a possible transfusion.

Otorhinolaryngologic consultation is not routinely necessary and should be reserved for refractory epistaxis, for which endoscopy for direct visualization and cauterization, surgical vessel ligation, or embolization may be necessary.[11]

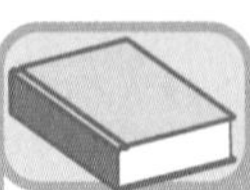

**PATIENT TEACHING TIPS**

**Epistaxis**

Avoid nose blowing, bending over, and straining.
Be sure to open your mouth when you sneeze.
Avoid any activity that puts you at risk for nasal injury.
Use humidifiers and saline nasal spray to help keep the interior of your nose moist.
Take pain medications as needed.
Do not take aspirin or aspirin products.
Follow up with an otorhinolaryngologist in 24 to 72 hours.
Take your antibiotics as prescribed. It is important that you continue to take antibiotics as long as your nasal packing or balloon is in place.
Do not put anything into your nose.
If bleeding recurs, compress your nose by squeezing the bottom half of it with your thumb and index finger. Hold this compression for 10 minutes. If bleeding continues beyond this time, see your doctor or return to the emergency department.
See your doctor or return to the emergency department if a fever or rash develops.

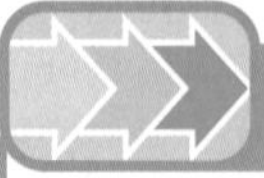

**PRIORITY ACTIONS**

Epistaxis

Apply a topical vasoconstrictive agent to the nasal mucosa.
Examine the nasopharynx and the posterior oropharynx to localize the source of bleeding.
Chemical cautery should be used with caution and bilateral septal cautery should be avoided to minimize the risk for septal injury.
Ensure that a posterior nasal balloon is properly secured to avoid airway occlusion.

## FOLLOW-UP AND NEXT STEPS IN CARE

A hemodynamically stable patient with anterior epistaxis in whom hemostasis has been achieved and maintained should be discharged home. The patient is instructed to avoid nose blowing, bending over, straining, closed-mouth sneezing, and any activity that raises the risk for nasal trauma. In dry environments, humidifiers and saline nasal spray are recommended to help keep the nasal mucosa moist. Pain medications are prescribed as needed for patient comfort; however, aspirin products should be avoided. Any patient with anterior packing or recurrent epistaxis must be evaluated by an otorhinolaryngologist in 24 to 72 hours.

Patients with nasal packing or balloons should be treated with antistaphylococcal antibiotics to minimize the risk for sinusitis and toxic shock syndrome.[17] Drug choices include amoxicillin–clavulanate potassium, 875 mg two times per day, and cephalexin, 500 mg four times per day. The packing should be left in place for 1 to 3 days and antibiotics continued until the packing is removed. Nasal packing containing antibiotics is also available; these products have been shown to inhibit the growth of nasal flora and may supplant the need for additional systemic antibiotics.

Patients with posterior epistaxis require admission to the hospital. If a posterior balloon were to become dislodged and migrate posteriorly, airway compromise could occur. Additionally, such a patient may have a drop in $PaO_2$ and a rise in $PaCO_2$ after placement of posterior packing. Bradycardia and other cardiac dysrhythmias have also been reported. The mechanism of these events is unclear.

# SINUSITIS

## EPIDEMIOLOGY

Sinusitis is an inflammatory disease of the paranasal sinuses, and rhinitis is an inflammatory disease of the membranes lining the nose. Because sinusitis without associated rhinitis is rare, the term *rhinosinusitis* is now the accepted nomenclature for this disease complex.[18-22] In much of the current literature, however, the terms *sinusitis* and *rhinosinusitis* are used interchangeably.

Rhinosinusitis is estimated to affect one in seven adults in the United States and has a significant impact on missed workdays and health care costs.[23,24] It is a complication of URI in 5% to 10% of children and 0.5% to 2% of adults. The actual number of people affected by rhinosinusitis may be significantly higher than reported because of the multitude of over-the-counter sinus medications available.

Over the past decade, five major expert organizations have generated guidelines on the definitions and treatments of rhinosinusitis and its subtypes.[18-22] There is variation among many of the guidelines' definitions and recommendations. The information presented in this chapter reflects the areas of greatest consensus among the expert groups.

*Rhinosinusitis* is the parent term for several subtypes of disease. In acute rhinosinusitis (ARS), symptoms last 4 weeks or less; recurrent ARS is defined as three or more episodes of ARS within 1 year, with resolution of symptoms between

**Table 30.1 Clinical Forms of Rhinosinusitis Based on Duration of Symptoms**

| TYPE | DEFINITION |
|---|---|
| Acute | Symptoms present < 4 wk |
| Chronic | Symptoms present > 12 wk |
| Recurrent | >3 acute episodes within 1 yr |

**BOX 30.6 Diagnostic Criteria for Acute Rhinosinusitis**

| Primary Diagnostic Indicators | Other Suggestive Symptoms |
|---|---|
| Nasal congestion, obstruction, or blockage | Hyposmia or anosmia |
| Purulent anterior or posterior rhinorrhea | Cough |
| Facial pain or pressure | Dental pain |
| | Ear pain or pressure |
| | Fatigue |
| | Halitosis |
| | Headache |

episodes; and chronic rhinosinusitis requires symptoms for 12 weeks or longer[18-22] (**Table 30.1**).

## PATHOPHYSIOLOGY

There are four pairs of paranasal sinuses: frontal, maxillary, sphenoid, and ethmoid. Maxillary sinusitis is the most common, followed by ethmoid, frontal, and then sphenoid sinusitis.

Each sinus drains through an ostium, which communicates with the nose. The frontal, maxillary, and anterior ethmoid sinuses empty into the medial meatus, between the middle and inferior turbinates. This region is termed *the ostiomeatal complex*. Obstruction of this complex is a critical step in the development of rhinosinusitis.

Each sinus is lined with ciliated epithelium and mucous goblet cells. Healthy sinuses have relatively few mucus-producing goblet cells, and the cilia beat the mucus toward the ostium of the sinus. The patent ostium allows the free flow of mucus and air from the sinus to the nose. When an ostium is occluded, air and mucus no longer flow freely, new mucus-producing cells develop, and mucostasis results.[25]

## PRESENTING SIGNS AND SYMPTOMS

The diagnosis of ARS is based on three signs or symptoms: nasal congestion, obstruction, or blockage; anterior or posterior purulent rhinorrhea; and facial pain or pressure.[18-22] Other suggestive symptoms support the diagnosis but serve only as adjuncts (**Box 30.6**).

A detailed history to determine the duration, severity, and course of the symptoms is the only readily available tool to differentiate acute viral rhinosinusitis from acute bacterial rhinosinusitis[18-22,26] (see Fig. 30.2). It can be challenging to differentiate early rhinosinusitis from URI because viral URIs are the most common event precipitating rhinosinusitis and the two may be present concurrently.

The signs and symptoms of chronic rhinosinusitis include those of ARS plus a decreased sense of smell.[18-22] The symptoms are often more vague and less severe and, by definition, must be present for 12 weeks or longer.

Physical examination will reveal nasal mucosal erythema and edema leading to nasal obstruction. Purulent secretions may also be seen in the nose or the posterior oropharynx. Purulent secretions have the highest positive predictive value for rhinosinusitis of any physical finding.[27] The nasal cavities must also be thoroughly inspected for foreign bodies, especially in children.

Sinus tenderness to percussion may be present on examination, although this finding is neither sensitive nor specific. Transillumination of the frontal and maxillary sinuses is also neither sensitive nor specific, and it is not possible to differentiate a fluid-filled sinus from a congenitally small sinus after a single evaluation. The clinician must examine the oral cavity for evidence of a dental infection, which can be the source of maxillary sinusitis. Periorbital edema may also be found.

## DIFFERENTIAL DIAGNOSIS AND MEDICAL DECISION MAKING

The diagnosis of ARS is clinical, and in the absence of specific concerns raised by the history and physical examination, no imaging or laboratory tests are warranted. Nasal cultures may be considered during outpatient care in the event of treatment failure.[18] Evaluation for systemic disorders predisposing to rhinosinusitis, such as cystic fibrosis or immunodeficiency, can be done on a nonemergency basis.

The infectious organisms causing rhinosinusitis are most commonly viral, then bacterial, then fungal. The most common viruses are rhinovirus, parainfluenza virus, and influenza virus. The most common bacterial pathogens of ARS and recurrent ARS in an immunocompetent host are *Streptococcus pneumoniae*, *Haemophilus influenzae*, and *Moraxella catarrhalis*. Rhinosinusitis pathogens more commonly found in immunocompromised hosts are *Pseudomonas aeruginosa, Rhizopus, Aspergillus, Candida, Histoplasma, Blastomyces, Coccidioides*, and *Cryptococcus*. *P. aeruginosa* is also a common pathogen in patients with cystic fibrosis.[28]

The pathogens of chronic rhinosinusitis include those of acute bacterial rhinosinusitis plus group A streptococci, *Staphylococcus aureus, P. aeruginosa*, and fungi.

Noninfectious causes include congenital diseases that inhibit ciliary function, such as cystic fibrosis and Kartagener syndrome; autoimmune diseases, such as Wegener granulomatosis and sarcoidosis; anatomic obstruction, such as from nasal polyps, nasal tumors, or foreign bodies; and facial trauma that directly disrupts sinus drainage.[28]

Any abnormality found on neurologic or ocular examination in a patient with rhinosinusitis must raise concern for CNS extension of the disease and warrants imaging. CT or magnetic resonance imaging should include the brain, orbits, or sinus (or any combination of these structures), depending on clinical suspicion.

Acute or chronic frontal rhinosinusitis can lead to erosion through the frontal bone and a resultant subperiosteal abscess known as Pott puffy tumor. In addition to signs and symptoms of rhinosinusitis, patients with this disorder have a severe localized headache, swelling of the forehead, fever, and possibly orbital abnormalities. These infections are most commonly polymicrobial. Frontal sinusitis can also lead to osteomyelitis. Complications of frontal sinusitis are most common during the second and third decades of life.

Intracranial complications of rhinosinusitis, such as an intracranial abscess, meningitis, epidural abscess, subdural empyema, and cavernous sinus thrombosis, are serious sequelae of the disease. Disease can progress intracranially through direct extension or via thrombophlebitis of the diploic veins. Any focal neurologic deficits found on examination must raise concern for intracranial extension of rhinosinusitis. Patients with subdural empyema exhibit systemic toxicity, nuchal rigidity, and photophobia, as well as cranial nerve deficits. The emergency practitioner must maintain a high index of suspicion. A review of patients found that headache and fever without other neurologic abnormalities were the most common manifestations of early intracranial complications of rhinosinusitis.

Pansinusitis leads to orbital sequelae in 60% to 80% of patients. Preseptal cellulitis is the most common complication. Clinical findings suggestive of preseptal cellulitis are periorbital edema without any associated change in vision or limitation of ocular mobility. Orbital cellulitis, orbital subperiosteal abscesses, and orbital abscesses are other complications of pansinusitis; they are manifested as periorbital edema, proptosis, orbital pain, and limitations in ocular mobility.

## TREATMENT

Treatment of ARS is primarily based on reducing the obstruction of the ostiomeatal complex and thereby relieving the patient's discomfort.

Intranasal corticosteroids are known to decrease nasal inflammation and may therefore improve ostial patency. These agents have very few identified side effects and are effective in reducing symptoms even as monotherapy.[29] Mometasone nasal spray, 200 mcg in each nostril twice daily, may be used.[29,30]

Topical and oral α-adrenergic decongestants are often prescribed for patients with rhinosinusitis to induce vasoconstriction and reduce nasal mucosal swelling, thereby improving ostial patency and sinus drainage. No controlled clinical trials, however, have examined the efficacy of these agents,[28] and the recommendations by the five expert panels are widely disparate.[18,20,21] There is no evidence that decongestants are harmful in patients with rhinosinusitis, and therefore the decision regarding their use is left to the clinician. Topical sprays, such as oxymetazoline, two sprays in each nostril every 12 hours, or oral decongestants, such as pseudoephedrine, 60 mg every 6 hours, should be considered on the basis of the risk-to-benefit profile of the individual patient. Decongestant nasal sprays should not be used for longer than 5 days because of the risk for rebound nasal congestion (rhinitis medicamentosa).

Antihistamines are a useful adjunct for patients whose rhinosinusitis has an allergic cause. Diphenhydramine, 25 to 50 mg every 6 hours, loratadine, 10 mg daily, or fexofenadine, 180 mg daily, may all be used. No studies have indicated that antihistamines play a role in nonallergic rhinosinusitis.[20]

Saline nose drops prevent crusting of nasal secretions and facilitate elimination of these secretions. Physiologic saline and hypertonic saline sprays both increase mucociliary clearance and increase nasal airway patency.[31,32] Saline nose drops, normal or hypertonic, may be a useful adjunct to aid in relieving the symptoms of rhinosinusitis.

Guaifenesin is an expectorant that decreases sputum viscosity. It has been shown to improve the ease of sputum expectoration in patients with respiratory infections but has not been demonstrated to aid in the management of rhinosinusitis (**Box 30.7**).

The vast majority of cases of ARS are caused by viruses, with only 0.5% to 2.0% estimated to have a bacterial cause.[33] For this reason, antibiotic treatment should be initiated only in patients for whom the clinician has high suspicion of acute bacterial rhinosinusitis (**Table 30.2**).

First-line antibiotic therapy is amoxicillin. If the incidence of β-lactamase–positive *S. pneumoniae, H. influenzae*, or *M. catarrhalis* infection is high in the area of patient care, adults should be treated with amoxicillin–clavulanate potassium. Alternative first-line agents are certain second- and third-generation cephalosporins. Third- or fourth-generation quinolone antibiotics are also appropriate agents for adult acute bacterial rhinosinusitis. Azithromycin or clarithromycin are additional treatment choices, but the local resistance patterns of *S. pneumoniae* and *H. influenzae* must first be assessed. The clinician should tailor the choice of antibiotic to the specific resistance patterns of the practice environment. See **Box 30.8** for doses and duration of treatment.

**BOX 30.7 Treatment of Acute Rhinosinusitis**

Intranasal corticosteroids
Decongestants
Antihistamines if an allergic cause is suspected
Saline nasal spray
Antibiotics only if the signs and symptoms are consistent with acute bacterial rhinosinusitis

**Table 30.2 Differentiating Acute Viral from Acute Bacterial Rhinosinusitis**

| VIRAL | BACTERIAL |
|---|---|
| Symptom duration < 10 days | Symptom duration ≥ 10 days |
| Worst symptoms at days 2-3 | Increasing symptoms 5 days after onset |
| Improving symptoms after day 3 | Worsening symptoms after initial improvement |
| | Severe symptoms (high fever, unilateral facial or tooth pain, periorbital swelling, orbital cellulitis) |

**BOX 30.8 Antibiotic Choices for Acute and Chronic Rhinosinusitis**

Amoxicillin, 45 mg/kg per dose PO every 12 hr; adult dose, 500 mg twice daily*
Amoxicillin–clavulanate potassium, 875 mg PO twice daily
Cefuroxime, 500 mg PO twice daily
Cefpodoxime, 400 mg PO twice daily
Levofloxacin, 500 mg PO daily
Gatifloxacin, 400 mg PO daily
Azithromycin, 500 mg once then 250 mg daily for 4 additional days
Clarithromycin, 500 mg PO twice daily
If protracted or severe course, consider anaerobic coverage:
- Clindamycin, 450 mg every 8 hr for 14 days
- Metronidazole, 500 mg every 8 hr

*Avoid in areas with high β-lactam resistance.
*PO,* By Mouth.

Previously, sulfamethoxazole-trimethoprim was a popular antimicrobial agent for the treatment of rhinosinusitis; however, as resistance to it has increased, its clinical utility has become limited.[20]

Acute bacterial rhinosinusitis should be treated with antibiotics for 10 to 14 days (except azithromycin, as noted previously). The patient should be reassessed 3 to 5 days after antibiotic treatment has begun. If no improvement is seen, concern for resistant organisms is raised, and a change in antibiotics should be considered. Chronic rhinosinusitis is treated with a 21-day course of antibiotics, although data supporting the optimum duration of treatment are minimal.[22,23]

ARS for is treated for 10 days, unless otherwise noted. Chronic rhinosinusitis is treated for a minimum of 21 days.

Any patient with evidence of ocular or intracranial extension of sinus disease requires immediate otorhinolaryngologic, ophthalmologic, or neurosurgical consultation (or any combination of the three). Broad-spectrum intravenous antibiotic therapy, such as with a third-generation cephalosporin and vancomycin, must be started.[21] However, because many of these complications require surgical intervention, the choice of antibiotic should be made in conjunction with the surgical service. A patient with this complication must be admitted to the hospital.

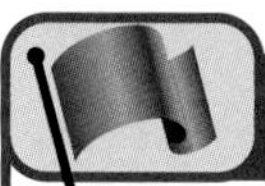

**RED FLAGS**

**Rhinosinusitis**
Abnormal finding on neurologic examination
Abnormal findings on ocular examination
Nuchal rigidity
Systemic toxicity

## SUGGESTED READING

Chen YC, Chen CT, Lin CH, et al. A safe and effective way for reduction of temporomandibular joint dislocation. Ann Plast Surg 2007;58:105-8.
Meltzer EO, Hamilos DL. Rhinosinusitis diagnosis and management for the clinician: a synopsis of recent consensus guidelines. Mayo Clin Proc 2011;86:427-43.
Viehweg TL, Roberson JB, Hudson JW. Epistaxis: diagnosis and treatment. J Oral Maxillofac Surg 2006;64:511-18.

## REFERENCES

***References can be found on Expert Consult @ www.expertconsult.com.***

# Esophageal Disorders 31

Todd A. Guth

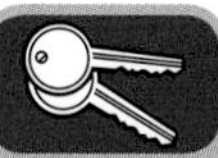

**KEY POINTS**

- Esophagitis is inflammation or infection of the esophagus and can be caused by reflux of gastric contents, infectious organisms, corrosive agents, or direct contact with swallowed pills.
- *Candida* species, cytomegalovirus, and herpes simplex virus are the most common organisms that infect the esophagus of an immunosuppressed patient.
- The most dangerous esophageal foreign body is a disc (button) battery, which can cause a chemically induced perforation in as little as 4 hours.
- Esophageal perforation may initially be manifested as nonspecific chest symptoms. The condition can rapidly progress to mediastinitis, overwhelming sepsis, and death.
- Esophageal motility disorders represent a heterogeneous group of conditions that result from derangement in peristalsis of the esophagus and abnormal functioning of the lower esophageal sphincter.

## REFLUX ESOPHAGITIS

### EPIDEMIOLOGY

Gastroesophageal reflux disease (GERD) describes a constellation of symptoms or complications that result from reflux of gastric contents into the esophagus. Even though approximately 40% of adults in the United States suffer from symptoms of heartburn at least once per month, the overall prevalence of GERD is just 14%.[1,2] GERD represents a spectrum of disease from nonerosive to erosive esophagitis and finally Barrett esophagus.[3] Common complications of GERD include esophageal strictures and the development of esophageal adenocarcinoma. Within the United States, the incidence of esophageal adenocarcinoma is increasing at an alarming rate of 4% to 10% per year.[4]

### PATHOPHYSIOLOGY

A number of conditions and lifestyle choices increase the risk for reflux esophagitis (**Box 31.1**). The primary pathophysiologic mechanism contributing to the development of GERD is an incompetent lower esophageal sphincter (LES). Inability of the LES to prevent reflux of stomach contents is influenced by esophageal anatomy, impaired gastrointestinal motility, acid hypersecretion, and increased abdominal pressure. Patients with a higher incidence of hiatal hernias, low LES pressure confirmed by manometry, and increased levels of reflux confirmed by esophageal pH monitoring have been shown to experience more severe GERD symptoms.[5]

The entire esophageal lumen is lined with stratified squamous epithelium, which is susceptible to injury by acidic gastric contents. Gastric acid, bile, or pepsin that passively regurgitates into the esophagus can irritate the mucosa and may cause erosions and ulcerations. In cases of persistent reflux, a metastatic columnar lining may replace the normal stratified squamous epithelium; this premalignant condition is called Barrett esophagus. Studies have demonstrated a clear relationship between Barrett esophagus and the development of esophageal adenocarcinoma.

### PRESENTING SIGNS AND SYMPTOMS

The most common symptom of reflux esophagitis is "heartburn," or the epigastric, retrosternal burning sensation that typifies GERD. Heartburn often radiates to the back and neck and may be described as burning, pressure, squeezing, or sharp pain. With severe GERD, patients may demonstrate diaphoresis, dyspnea, nausea, and vomiting. The entire symptom complex may be clinically indistinguishable from cardiac ischemia.

Heartburn is more severe when patients are supine, bend forward, wear tight clothing, or consume large meals. The pain may last from minutes to hours and may resolve spontaneously or with antacids. Patients with nocturnal symptoms often complain of "water brash," which is the bitter, metallic taste of regurgitated gastric contents noted on arising from sleep. Approximately 80% of patients with GERD have primarily nocturnal symptoms that are exacerbated by being supine.[6] Patients with daytime symptoms have postprandial heartburn and fullness even when upright. GERD can cause chronic cough, recurrent throat clearing, and wheezing as a result of aspiration of gastric contents from the esophagus into the trachea and larynx.[7] A complaint of dysphagia in the setting of GERD is an ominous sign that should prompt endoscopic evaluation for underlying strictures or adenocarcinoma.

### DIFFERENTIAL DIAGNOSIS AND MEDICAL DECISION MAKING

GERD is a clinical diagnosis elicited by a detailed and directed history of the present illness. GERD should be diagnosed only after other life-threatening causes of chest pain have been convincingly excluded (**Box 31.2**). Providers must consider

**BOX 31.1 Conditions and Lifestyle Choices That Increase Risk for Reflux Esophagitis**

**Esophageal Anatomy**
Hiatal hernia
Esophageal strictures or rings

**Impaired Gastrointestinal Motility**
Achalasia
Diabetic gastroparesis
Scleroderma
Medications (anticholinergic drugs, narcotics)

**Acid Hypersecretion**
Foods (peppermint, chocolate, fatty foods)
Smoking and nicotine
Gastrinoma

**Increased Abdominal Pressure**
Obesity
Pregnancy

**BOX 31.2 Differential Diagnosis for Reflux, Infectious, and Pill Esophagitis**

Acute coronary syndrome
Pulmonary embolism
Pneumothorax
Pneumomediastinum
Peptic ulcer disease
Gastroesophageal reflux disease
Aortic dissection
Pericarditis
Pneumonia
Pancreatitis
Biliary tract disease
Esophageal perforation
Dyspepsia
Esophageal motility disorders

the potential life threats and serious medical conditions that can be manifested in a similar fashion to GERD. A thorough history is the most important consideration in the differentiation diagnosis of patients with GERD-like symptoms. The initial history should be obtained in concert with immediate electrocardiography. Physical examination, laboratory testing, and radiographic imaging aid only in the exclusion of alternative diagnoses. Cardiac stress testing may be required in certain patient populations. A reported clinical response to antacids should not be used to make the presumptive diagnosis of GERD in the emergency department (ED).

## TREATMENT

Lifestyle modifications may reduce symptoms by decreasing the frequency and amount of gastric reflux. Examples of low-cost, low-risk recommendations are summarized in the Patient Teaching Tips box in this section of the chapter.[8]

Acid-suppressive medications are indicated in patients without adequate relief from lifestyle modifications. The two most commonly used drugs for the treatment of GERD are $H_2$ receptor antagonists (H2RAs) and proton pump inhibitors (PPIs). Acid-suppressive medications do not prevent reflux; they improve GERD symptoms by suppressing production of acid in the stomach and raising the pH of the refluxed material.

H2RAs have similar efficacy with equivalent dosing schedules (**Table 31.1**). These agents have previously been recommended as first-line therapy; however, a Cochrane review suggests that PPIs relieve heartburn better than H2RAs do in patients treated without specific diagnostic testing.[9] These

**Table 31.1 Equivalent Dosages for Histamine $H_2$ Receptor Antagonists**

| DRUG | RECOMMENDED DOSE |
|---|---|
| Cimetidine | 400 mg twice daily<br>*OR*<br>800 mg at bedtime |
| Ranitidine | 150 mg twice daily<br>*OR*<br>300 mg at bedtime |
| Famotidine | 20 mg twice daily<br>*OR*<br>40 mg at bedtime |
| Nizatidine | 150 mg twice daily<br>*OR*<br>300 mg at bedtime |

medications should be used for 2 to 4 weeks before any reassessment of symptoms. Recurrence is a common problem in patients with reflux, and therefore many patients require long-term maintenance therapy.

Success rates with PPIs approach 90%, and all agents have equal efficacy at appropriate doses (**Table 31.2**). Once-daily dosing before breakfast is sufficient for the control of mild to moderate GERD; twice-daily dosing should be considered for those with severe or refractory symptoms. Gastroprokinetic agents (cisapride) and coating agents (sucralfate) are less effective than PPIs but may be useful in selected patients as second-line agents.

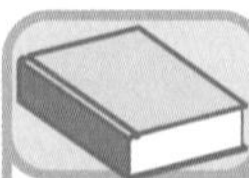

**PATIENT TEACHING TIPS**

**Gastroesophageal Reflux**

**Dietary Avoidance**
Avoid foods that are acidic
- Citrus foods
- Tomatoes
- Spicy foods
- Carbonated beverages

Avoid foods that cause reflux
- Fatty foods
- Coffee, tea, and caffeinated beverages
- Chocolate
- Peppermint

**Lifestyle Modifications**
Smoking cessation
Weight reduction
Reduction in meal size
Reduction in alcohol consumption
Elevation of the head of the bed
No eating within 3 hours of bedtime

## NEXT STEPS IN CARE

Admission to an inpatient or observation unit is indicated when life-threatening causes of the patient's complaints cannot be excluded in the ED. The vast majority of patients in whom clinically suspected GERD is diagnosed in the ED can be sent home with outpatient follow-up. Emergency physicians can initiate presumptive acid-suppressive therapy;

**Table 31.2 Equivalent Dosages for Proton Pump Inhibitors**

| DRUG | RECOMMENDED DOSE |
|---|---|
| Omeprazole | 20 mg before breakfast<br>*OR*<br>20 mg twice daily* |
| Lansoprazole | 30 mg before breakfast<br>*OR*<br>30 mg twice daily* |
| Rabeprazole | 20 mg before breakfast<br>*OR*<br>20 mg twice daily* |
| Pantoprazole | 40 mg before breakfast |
| Esomeprazole | 20 mg or 40 mg before breakfast |

*Second doses should be taken before dinner.

however, patients must understand the need for follow-up for confirmation of the diagnosis and additional management.

Further diagnostic evaluation, including endoscopy, pH monitoring, manometry, and referral to a gastroenterologist, may be indicated for patients with persistent symptoms. Patients with known reflux esophagitis should be admitted to the hospital for suspected esophageal perforation, significant bleeding, obstruction, volume depletion, or intractable pain. Emergency upper endoscopy is indicated if life-threatening complications are suspected in patients demonstrating dysphagia, odynophagia, upper gastrointestinal bleeding, or weight loss.[10]

# INFECTIOUS ESOPHAGITIS

## EPIDEMIOLOGY

Infection of the esophageal mucosa, known as infectious esophagitis, may result from a variety of organisms in an immunocompromised host. Esophageal infections are more commonly observed in patients with acquired immunodeficiency syndrome, cancer, neutropenia, or diabetes mellitus or in those taking chronic immunosuppressive medications, especially corticosteroids.[11] *Candida* species are by far the most common cause of infectious esophagitis, although cytomegalovirus (CMV), varicella-zoster virus, and herpes simplex virus (HSV) represent common viral causes of the condition.[12]

## PATHOPHYSIOLOGY

Infectious esophagitis results from direct invasion of the infectious agent into esophageal tissue. Immunosuppression from any condition can lead to esophageal infections, although patients infected with advanced human immunodeficiency virus and those with lymphoma and leukemia receiving chemotherapy are at highest risk. Prevention of adherence of esophageal pathogens is an important pathophysiologic defense. Impairment of salivation, impairment of esophageal motility, and reduction in gastric acid production can result in opportunistic infections. Injury to the esophageal mucosa from radiation treatment also increases the risk for infection.[12]

## PRESENTING SIGNS AND SYMPTOMS

Candidal esophagitis may be manifested as retrosternal pain, dysphagia, or odynophagia. Other symptoms of esophageal candidiasis are nausea, vomiting, fever, abdominal pain, and anorexia. Oral candidiasis (thrush) is not consistently present in patients with endoscopically confirmed candidal esophagitis. Systemic candidal infections may be seen in cases of significant immunosuppression.

HSV esophagitis is manifested as severe odynophagia, dysphagia, nausea, and vomiting. Oropharyngeal ulcerations and white exudates may indicate HSV infection, although oral lesions are neither sensitive nor specific enough to confirm a definitive diagnosis. HSV esophagitis is frequently severe enough to warrant admission for pain control.

## DIFFERENTIAL DIAGNOSIS AND MEDICAL DECISION MAKING

Pain or difficulty swallowing is the hallmark of infectious esophagitis; however, many infections may be asymptomatic or have other associated symptoms. Infectious esophagitis should be considered in immunocompromised patients at risk for opportunistic infections. Given the similar spectrum of signs and symptoms, the differential diagnosis of infectious esophagitis includes the same life threats and serious conditions as reflux esophagitis (see Box 31.2).

## TREATMENT

In patients in whom infectious esophagitis is suspected, empiric treatment of *Candida* should be initiated. Esophageal candidiasis requires systemic therapy; topical agents are ineffective. Treatment should begin with fluconazole, 100 to 200 mg daily for 2 to 3 weeks; this regimen is efficacious in 80% to 90% of cases. Esophagitis caused by HSV or CMV needs to be confirmed by biopsy and requires systemic antiviral therapy.

## NEXT STEPS IN CARE

All cases of infectious esophagitis require consultation with infectious disease and gastroenterology specialists to arrange for expedited testing. Patients with significant symptoms in whom infectious esophagitis is suspected need to be admitted to facilitate diagnosis by upper endoscopy. Suspicion of a systemic infection mandates hospital admission.

Biopsies, cultures, and other related testing may be deferred to the inpatient setting. Outpatient management should be reserved for stable patients for whom urgent follow-up has been scheduled with a primary care or subspecialty physician. Treatment failures with fluconazole will probably be the result of either primary infection or coinfection with HSV, CMV, or other viral or bacterial organisms.

## PILL ESOPHAGITIS AND CAUSTIC ESOPHAGEAL INJURY

### EPIDEMIOLOGY

Pill esophagitis refers to damage to the esophageal mucosa by prolonged direct contact with a caustic agent. A variety of medications have been reported to cause esophageal injury, but the majority of cases involve potassium chloride, quinidine, emepronium bromide (Cetiprin), alendronate sodium (Fosamax), nonsteroidal antiinflammatory drugs, vitamin supplements, or antibiotics.[13] Caustic injury to the esophagus results from the accidental or intentional ingestion of extremely acidic or alkaline agents. Caustic injuries are reported to have an estimated incidence of approximately 10,000 cases per year in the United States.[14]

### PATHOPHYSIOLOGY

Bisphosphonates, a notorious cause of pill esophagitis, cause esophageal injury as a result of nonspecific irritation secondary to contact between the pill and the esophageal mucosa.[13] Following ingestion of a caustic substance, the extent of tissue injury and destruction depends on the physical properties and concentration of the ingested agent, the duration of contact, and the amount ingested.

Acidic agents produce coagulation necrosis, which creates burns that limit tissue damage. In contrast, alkaline agents produce liquefaction necrosis, which continues to cause tissue damage as long as the offending substance is in contact with the tissue. Esophageal erosions from pill irritation or caustic ingestion can progress to ulcerations and ultimately to perforation in rare cases. The most concerning long-term complications from damaging caustic ingestions are stricture formation and esophageal malignant transformation.

### PRESENTING SIGNS AND SYMPTOMS

Symptoms begin shortly after the patient takes the medication or ingests the agent and include nausea, vomiting, severe retrosternal pain, odynophagia, and difficulty handling secretions. Patients are more likely to experience pill esophagitis if they take their medications with minimal fluid, while recumbent, or immediately before bedtime. Ingestion of strong acidic or strong alkaline substances can produce serious injury and significant symptoms, whereas agents such as bleach, detergent, and ammonia cause only mild injury and symptoms.

### DIFFERENTIAL DIAGNOSIS AND MEDICAL DECISION MAKING

A presumptive diagnosis of pill esophagitis or caustic ingestion can be made when the history and the signs and symptoms are clear. For confusing or atypical findings, the same differential diagnosis for GERD listed in Box 31.2 must be investigated. If other esophageal disease is suspected (e.g., strictures, perforation), additional testing is indicated. Upper endoscopy is the most sensitive method of detecting pill-induced mucosal injury and assessing the extent of caustic injury following the ingestion of a corrosive agent. The timing of endoscopy is still under debate, but most medical centers perform the procedure early to define the extent of esophageal injury.[13]

### TREATMENT

Analgesics and coating agents may provide temporary symptomatic relief of pill esophagitis. Conversion of the offending medication to a liquid preparation often prevents recurrence. Another preventive measure is drinking water before and with medication, preferably in a fully upright position. Frequently, the use of sucralfate may promote healing of the injured mucosa.

Induced emesis, gastric lavage, and charcoal are not indicated in the setting of caustic ingestion. Dilution of the substance with water is a reasonable treatment option. Deferment of oral intake, aggressive supportive management, and high vigilance for esophageal perforation are necessary in the setting of serious esophageal damage.

### NEXT STEPS IN CARE

Most patients with pill esophagitis may be discharged with analgesics and follow-up. Patients unable to swallow secondary to severe odynophagia or a suspected stricture must be admitted for intravenous hydration, pain control, and gastroenterology consultation. Most patients with serious caustic ingestions will need admission to the hospital for emergency endoscopy. The ultimate disposition of the patient depends on the extent of injury.

## ESOPHAGEAL FOREIGN BODIES AND FOOD IMPACTION

### EPIDEMIOLOGY

Ingestion of a foreign body and food impaction are relatively common causes of ED visits. Esophageal foreign bodies are most commonly seen in children (80%) between 1 and 4 years of age.[15] A significant proportion of adults with esophageal foreign bodies are prisoners, suffer from psychiatric illness, or have recurrent episodes of intentional foreign body ingestion. A wide range of ingested foreign bodies have been reported, and they can be conceptually grouped into the most threatening and most common foreign bodies (**Box 31.3**). The most dangerous esophageal foreign body in children is a disc (button) battery, which has shown a greater than sixfold increase in serious complication or fatalities from 1985 to 2009.[16]

### PATHOPHYSIOLOGY

Foreign objects tend to lodge in one of four areas of anatomic narrowing in the esophagus: the upper esophageal sphincter, the aortic crossover, the left mainstem bronchus crossover,

**BOX 31.3 Most Threatening and Most Common Esophageal Foreign Bodies**

| Most Threatening | Most Common |
|---|---|
| ***In Children*** | ***In Children*** |
| Disc batteries | Coins |
| Bones | Marbles |
| Needles | Buttons |
| Other sharp objects | Toys |
| ***In Adults*** | ***In Adults*** |
| Disc batteries | Food boluses |
| Bones | Bones |
| Packets of illicit drugs | Dentures |
| Toothpicks | Oral piercings |

**BOX 31.4 Differential Diagnosis for Esophageal Foreign Bodies**

| In Children | In Adults |
|---|---|
| Perforation | Perforation |
| Abrasion or laceration | Abrasion or laceration |
| Airway foreign body | Spasm |
| Esophagitis | Esophagitis |
| Epiglottitis | Diverticulum |
| Globus hystericus | Malignancy |
| Reactive airways disease | Myocardial infarction |
| | Globus hystericus |

and the LES. The upper sphincter is the most common site of impaction in children (75%), and the LES is the most common location in adults (70%).[17] Foreign bodies in the upper esophageal sphincter may compress the airway and cause respiratory distress. Erosions from a foreign body or perforation from an ingested sharp object can result in mediastinitis and injury to adjacent structures such as the great vessels and trachea.

Although food impaction can occur in patients with a normal esophagus, both adult and pediatric patients often have an underlying esophageal abnormality. Abnormal areas of esophageal narrowing that predispose individuals to foreign body impaction include strictures, malignancies, dysmotility disorders (achalasia), and scleroderma.[18,19]

## PRESENTING SIGNS AND SYMPTOMS

Children and adults with esophageal foreign bodies may have an acute onset of drooling or respiratory distress. Other common symptoms associated with esophageal foreign bodies are retrosternal pain, dysphagia, coughing, gagging, wheezing, anorexia, and refusal to drink fluids. Unwitnessed ingestions account for approximately 40% of esophageal foreign bodies in children.[20] Parental suspicion of an ingested object may prompt ED evaluation, even in an asymptomatic child. The vast majority of ingested objects will pass spontaneously; however, dangerous objects such as button batteries and sharp objects must be removed, even in asymptomatic patients.

Adults with esophageal impaction after a known ingestion generally have symptoms of dysphagia, foreign body sensation, chest pain, and vomiting. Impaction commonly involves a large, poorly chewed food bolus such as a piece of meat. Patients with complete obstruction of the esophagus are unable to swallow, drool, and have episodes of retching in an attempt to dislodge the obstruction.

## DIFFERENTIAL DIAGNOSIS AND MEDICAL DECISION MAKING

**Box 31.4** lists the differential diagnosis for esophageal foreign bodies. If a report of an ingested object is obtained from the patient, the diagnostic considerations are relatively straightforward. In both children and adults in whom a history of ingestion is unclear, more comprehensive assessment of the patient's symptoms to include cardiac ischemia, infectious causes, and motility disorders should be considered. A high index of suspicion for an ingested foreign object must be maintained in children younger than 4 years because the history of ingestion is often absent and verbalization of symptoms is problematic.

## TREATMENT

A diagnostic algorithm for the evaluation of a suspected esophageal foreign body is presented in **Figure 31.1**. Foreign bodies found to be in the stomach will probably pass through the remainder of the gastrointestinal tract without intervention. Oral fluid challenges should be attempted when a foreign body is not identified on plain radiographs. Inability to tolerate fluids should prompt further evaluation with computed tomography or endoscopy.

Endoscopy is the preferred method for definitively removing or advancing an esophageal foreign body, especially when the presence or nature of the foreign body is uncertain. Endoscopy allows direct visualization of sharp or otherwise dangerous foreign objects that pose a significant risk for perforation. Although endoscopy is costly and requires the availability of a specialty consultant, this technique can be performed in the ED and may prevent hospital admission.

Foreign bodies may also be guided into the stomach by bougienage, or advancement of a rubber dilator from the oropharynx into the esophagus. Removal of the foreign body may be attempted by passing a urinary catheter distal to the object under fluoroscopic guidance, inflating the balloon, and using the inflated distal catheter to withdraw the object. Foreign body advancement via bougienage and removal with a urinary catheter should be attempted only by skilled operators; complications include airway compromise and esophageal perforation. When reserved for relatively low-risk foreign bodies such as coins, these techniques have reported success rates of approximately 95% without serious complications.[20] It should be recognized that removal of foreign bodies by bougienage is considered by many to be quite controversial.

Glucagon, nitroglycerin, and benzodiazepines have commonly been used to relax the LES and promote advancement of the foreign body in the esophagus. No convincing trials,

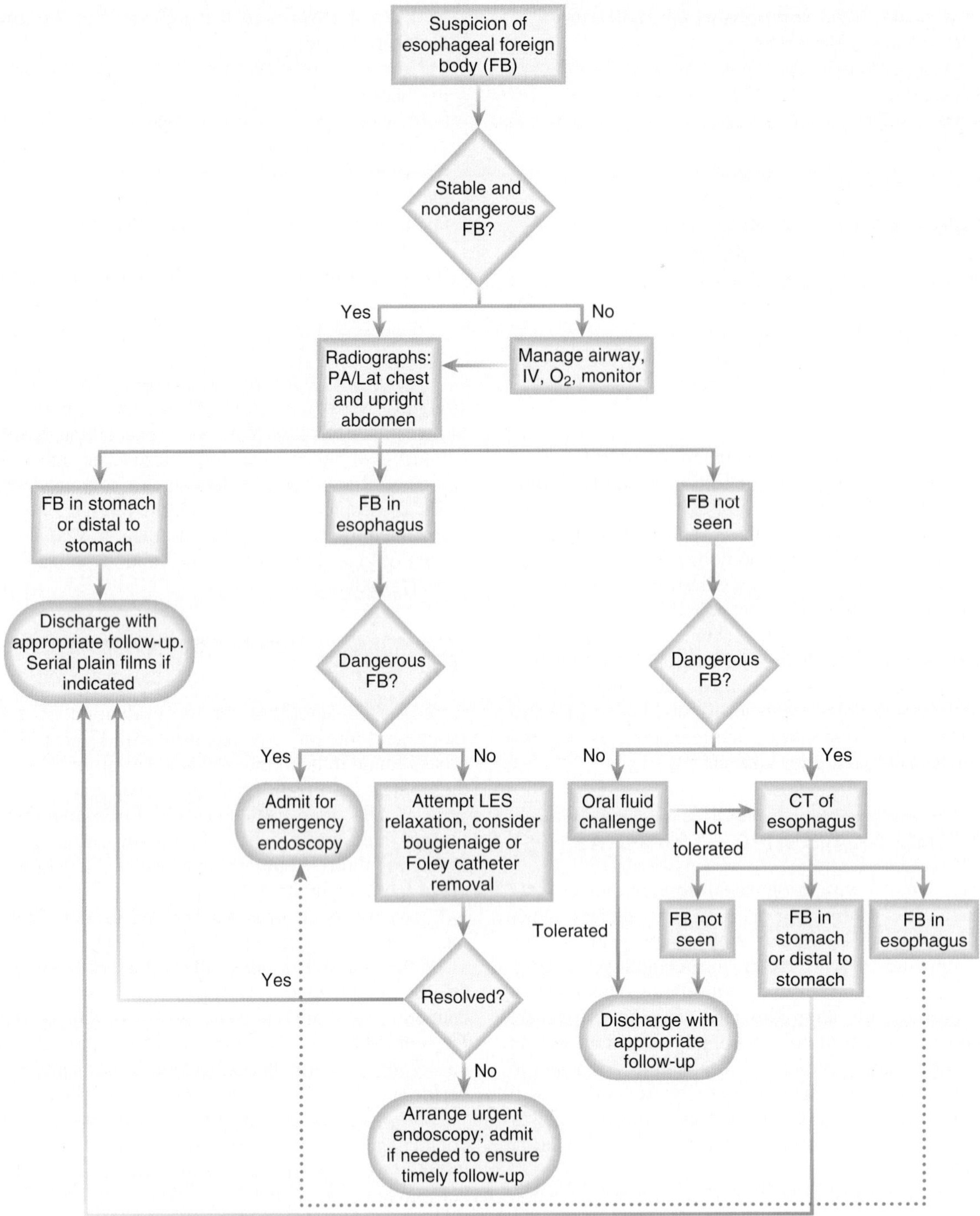


**Fig. 31.1 Diagnostic algorithm for the evaluation of a suspected esophageal foreign body.** *CT*, Computed tomography; *IV*, intravenous line; *Lat*, lateral; *LES*, lower esophageal sphincter; *PA*, posteroanterior.

however, have demonstrated that these medications improve the resolution of esophageal foreign bodies.[21] Glucagon commonly causes vomiting, which poses an increased risk for aspiration. Use of these medications often serves only to delay involvement of a consultant for definitive removal of the foreign body. The addition of a gas-forming agent or oral meat tenderizer is also not recommended because of an increased risk for perforation.

## NEXT STEPS IN CARE

Patients with dangerous foreign bodies such as disc batteries and sharp objects should undergo emergency endoscopy. The opportunity for safe removal of an esophageal button battery is approximately 2 hours, with delay in diagnosis or removal of the battery contributing to catastrophic outcomes.[16] Patients with unresolved but low-risk foreign bodies should be referred

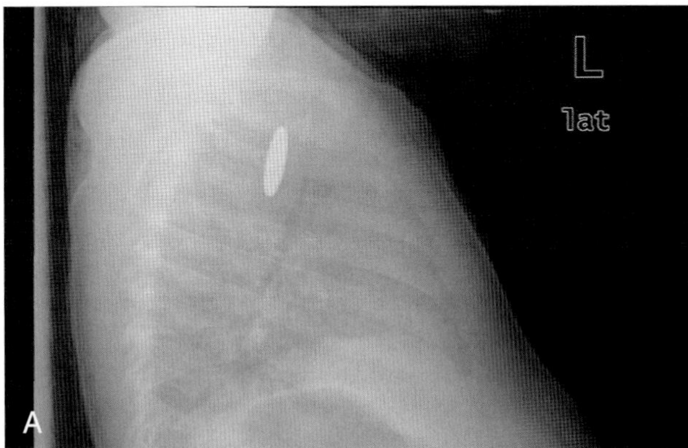


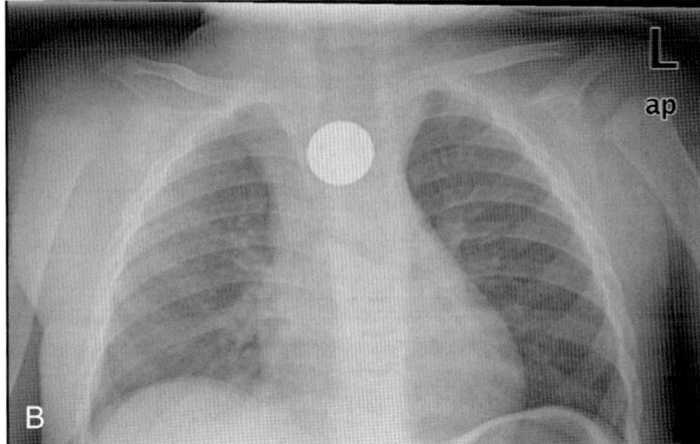


**Fig. 31.2** **A** and **B,** Chest radiographs demonstrating a coin in the esophagus (coronal lie).

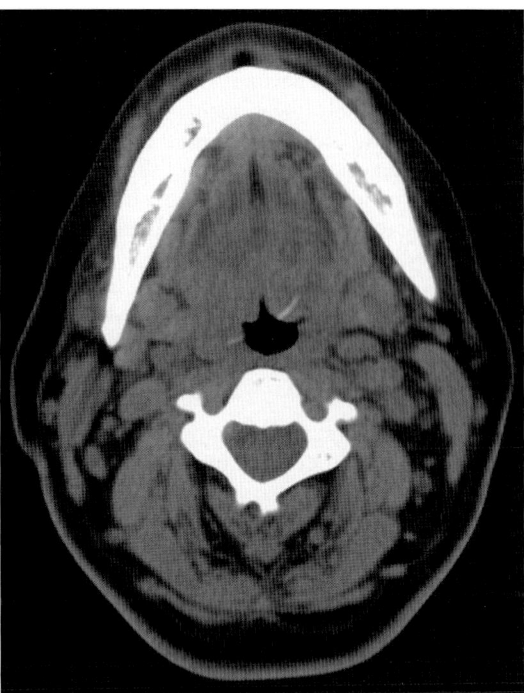

**Fig. 31.3 Computed tomography scan of the esophagus demonstrating an impacted foreign body: a fish bone was impacted in the hypopharynx.** (Courtesy of E. Wolf, MD, Montefiore Medical Center, Bronx, NY.)

for endoscopy within 24 hours if they are able to tolerate oral fluids. Stable patients with nondangerous foreign bodies can be observed for several hours without harm.

Adults with foreign bodies that resolve with observation should be referred for outpatient evaluation of potential structural or neuromuscular diseases of the esophagus. Children with resolved foreign bodies may be discharged for follow-up with a primary care provider. A swallowed coin in the esophagus (**Fig. 31.2**) and a fishbone in the hypopharynx (**Fig. 31.3**) are common esophageal foreign bodies.

# ESOPHAGEAL PERFORATION

## EPIDEMIOLOGY

Esophageal perforation is defined as a transmural communication between the upper gastrointestinal tract and the mediastinum. Perforation leads to a rapidly progressive chemical and infectious mediastinitis that can result in sepsis and death. Iatrogenic perforations may occur at any anatomic location and account for up to 60% of all cases; they carry a mortality rate of approximately 20%.[22]

Boerhaave syndrome, or spontaneous esophageal perforation, is most commonly the result of forceful retching or vomiting. Other conditions associated with this syndrome are childbirth, coughing, seizures, asthma exacerbations, and the Valsalva maneuver. Even with treatment, this entity has a mortality rate approaching 30%.[23]

## PATHOPHYSIOLOGY

Esophageal perforations occur as a result of injury to the esophageal wall through direct trauma, tumor growth, or caustic erosion. Most cases of Boerhaave syndrome occur in the left posterolateral portion of the esophagus because of the relatively thin muscularis layer and lack of external structural support in this area.

## PRESENTING SIGNS AND SYMPTOMS

Esophageal perforation is classically accompanied by mild, nonspecific symptoms that lead to misdiagnosis initially in more than half the patients. Pain is the initial symptom in 70% to 90% of cases, although variability in location makes this symptom difficult to interpret. Pain may be felt in the chest, neck, abdomen, or upper part of the back and may be increased with deep breathing or swallowing.[24] Other common symptoms are dyspnea, odynophagia, vomiting, and hematemesis.

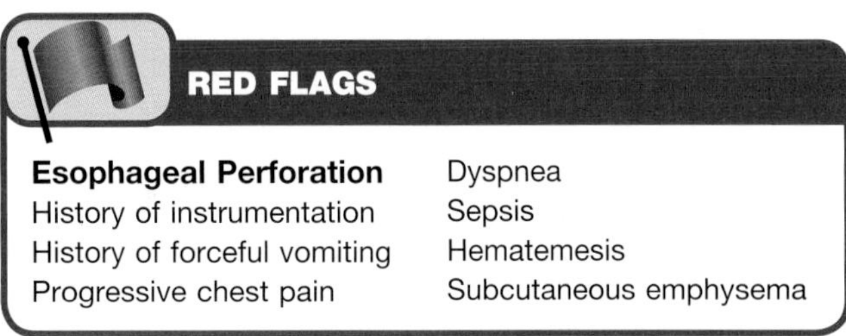

**RED FLAGS**

**Esophageal Perforation**

| | |
|---|---|
| History of instrumentation | Dyspnea |
| History of forceful vomiting | Sepsis |
| Progressive chest pain | Hematemesis |
| | Subcutaneous emphysema |

The clinical findings depend on the location of the perforation and the delay between perforation and evaluation. Delayed evaluation for esophageal perforation will be complicated by findings of septic shock: fever, tachypnea, tachycardia, and hypotension. Physical examination may reveal subcutaneous emphysema of the neck or upper part of the chest in approximately 60% of patients. Hamman crunch is a classic but uncommon auscultatory finding attributed to mediastinal emphysema.

## DIFFERENTIAL DIAGNOSIS AND MEDICAL DECISION MAKING

Given the variable findings in patients with esophageal perforation, misdiagnosis and delay in treatment are unfortunately typical. The initial symptoms, like many other esophageal disorders, can be consistent with myocardial infarction, peptic ulcer disease, pancreatitis, aortic dissection, and pneumothorax. A diagnostic algorithm for the evaluation of suspected esophageal perforation is presented in **Figure 31.4**. Chest radiographs often demonstrate nonspecific findings such as pleural effusions or perhaps pneumomediastinum. Contrast-enhanced fluoroscopic swallow studies should be performed in patients who can sit erect and tolerate liquids (**Figs. 31.5 and 31.6**). Computed tomography of the esophagus is an alternative method of confirming the presence but not necessarily the location of a suspected perforation (**Fig. 31.7**). Again, pleural effusions and pneumomediastinum are common findings.

## TREATMENT

Severe sepsis can develop quickly in patients with esophageal perforation, especially those with a delayed diagnosis or evaluation. Aggressive resuscitation with early surgical consultation is mandatory. The ED practitioner should obtain intravenous access and administer broad-spectrum antibiotics effective against gram-positive, gram-negative, and anaerobic organisms. Acceptable empiric regimens include piperacillin/tazobactam (Zosyn), 3.375 g intravenously (IV), or ceftriaxone, 2 g IV, plus metronidazole (Flagyl), 500 mg IV, or clindamycin, 900 mg IV. A nasogastric tube should be inserted to decompress the stomach and reduce further mediastinal contamination (see also Chapter 46).

Early surgical intervention improves the odds of survival in patients with esophageal rupture, with the best results achieved if primary closure is performed within 24 hours. An increasing body of evidence suggests that esophageal stenting and nonoperative management may be useful in selected cases.[25] In nonoperative management, drainage of pleural fluid collections with tube thoracostomy, continued nasogastric suction, and bypass of the esophagus with gastric tube placement or total parenteral nutrition are common adjunctive therapies.

## NEXT STEPS IN CARE

All patients in whom the diagnosis of esophageal perforation is suspected or confirmed should be admitted to a monitored or intensive care unit under the care of a thoracic surgeon or a general surgeon experienced in esophageal repair.

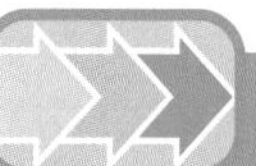

**PRIORITY ACTIONS**

**Esophageal Perforation**

Address airway compromise.
Check the electrocardiogram on arrival.
Establish intravenous access.
Provide supplemental oxygen.
Apply a telemetry monitor.
Obtain a chest radiograph.
Consult a thoracic surgeon.
Administer antibiotics.
Perform gastric decompression (nasogastric tube).
Confirm decompression by fluoroscopy or computed tomography.

# ESOPHAGEAL MOTILITY DISORDERS

## EPIDEMIOLOGY

Esophageal motility disorders represent a spectrum of disorders caused by abnormal coordination of peristalsis and relaxation of the esophageal sphincters. Effective characterization of these disorders has only recently been achieved after manometric and fluoroscopic measurements became more widely available. Five distinct disorders have been described: achalasia, diffuse esophageal spasm, nutcracker esophagus, ineffective esophageal motility, and disorders of LES relaxation.[26] The best-defined esophageal motility disorder, achalasia, is rare with an incidence of 1 per 100,000 population.

## PATHOPHYSIOLOGY

Esophageal motility disorders result from a number of different pathophysiologic mechanisms that result in functional aberrations of the esophagus. Anatomically and radiographically, the esophagus usually appears normal. Achalasia results from degeneration of the plexus myentericus, which causes an impairment in relaxation of the LES and abnormal peristaltic contractions of the esophagus.[27] The other motility disorders are less well understood and are believed to be caused by an impairment in the normally coordinated muscle contractions that occur with swallowing.

## PRESENTING SIGNS AND SYMPTOMS

Dysphagia is the hallmark symptom of esophageal motility disorders. Dysphagia occurs with both solid foods and liquids, in contrast to causes of mechanical obstruction, which are

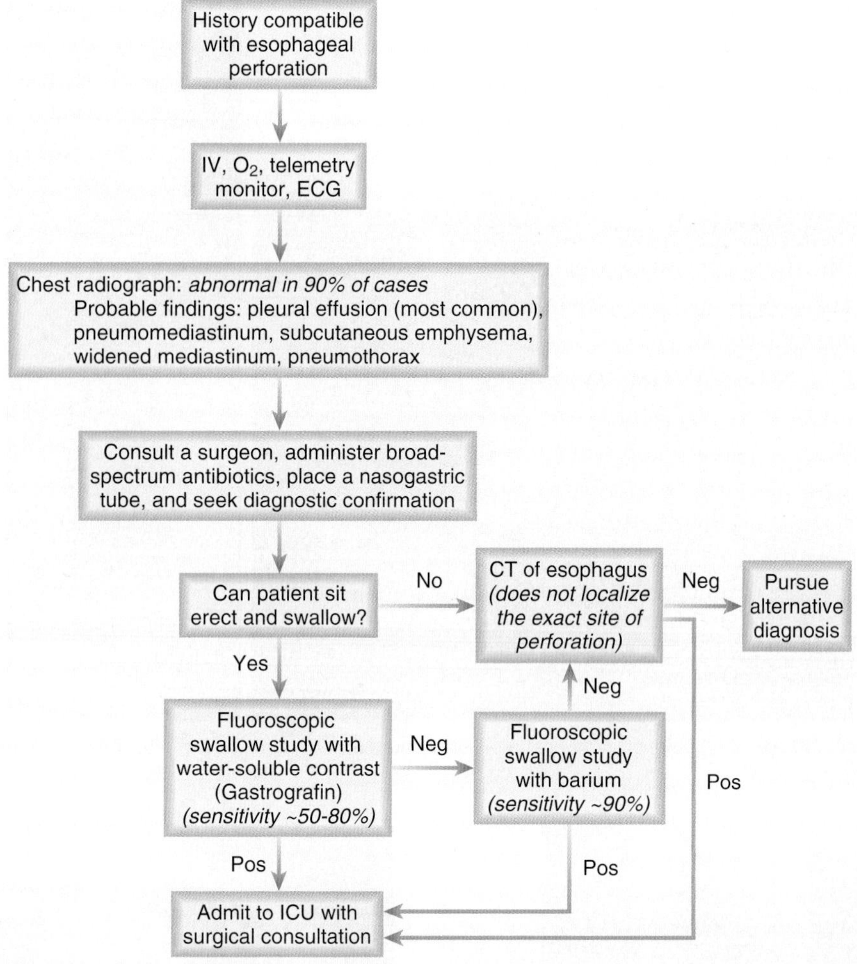


**Fig. 31.4 Diagnostic algorithm for the evaluation of suspected esophageal perforation.** *CT*, Computed tomography; *ECG*, electrocardiogram; *ICU*, intensive care unit; *IV*, intravenous line; *Neg*, negative; *Pos*, positive.

typically associated with difficulties only with solids. Similar to other esophageal disorders, the associated symptoms of heartburn, odynophagia, chest pain, and dyspnea are common in esophageal motility disorders. Regurgitation of previously swallowed, undigested food material is typical of advanced achalasia. Patients with diffuse esophageal spasm or nutcracker esophagus (resulting from disordered propagation of peristalsis) can have severe chest pain and dysphagia mimicking cardiac ischemia.

## DIFFERENTIAL DIAGNOSIS AND MEDICAL DECISION MAKING

Esophageal motility disorders can be diagnosed only with manometric measurements of the esophagus. Emergency medicine physicians need to be aware that esophageal motility disorders exist and can be suspected clinically; however, they cannot be definitively diagnosed in the ED. Other life-threatening and serious causes of dysphagia, chest pain, and heartburn should be considered first. The same considerations for the broad differential diagnosis presented in Box 31.2 should be investigated.

## TREATMENT

Therapies for esophageal motility disorders are as poorly defined as the disorders themselves. Treatment options for achalasia focus on reduction of LES pressure. Botulinum toxin injections, myotomy, and dilation of the LES have been use to treat achalasia with mixed success. Smooth muscle relaxant medications, such as calcium channel blockers, and benzodiazepines have also been used anecdotally to treat achalasia and other esophageal motility disorders without clear benefit.[28]

## NEXT STEPS IN CARE

Patients with cardiac risk factors and no known diagnosis of an esophageal motility disorder are often admitted to the hospital for observation. Most patients can be discharged from the ED for follow-up with a primary care physician in the absence of serious or concerning symptoms. Patients with persistent symptoms will ultimately need to be referred to a specialist in esophageal motility disorders for manometric testing.

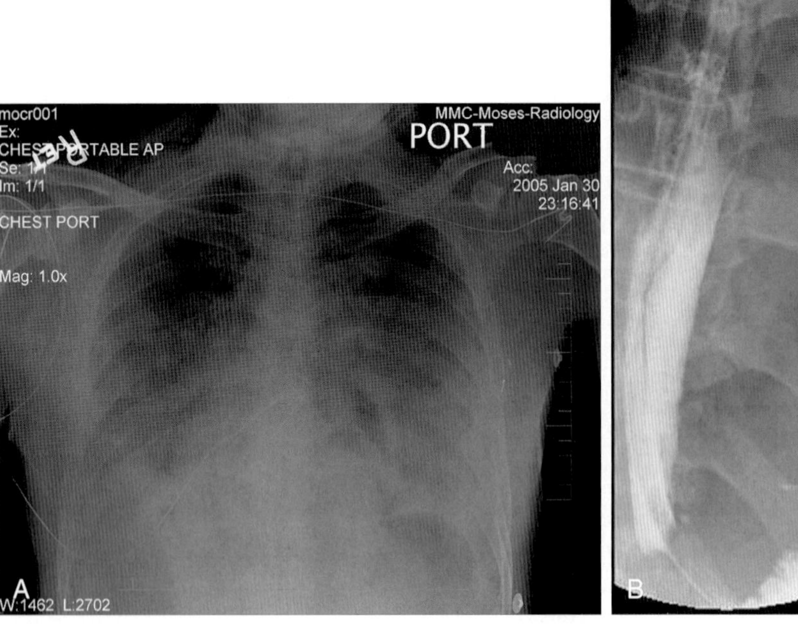


**Fig. 31.5** **A** and **B,** Chest radiographs demonstrating pneumomediastinum and bilateral pleural effusions. (Courtesy of E. Wolf, MD, Montefiore Medical Center, Bronx, NY.)

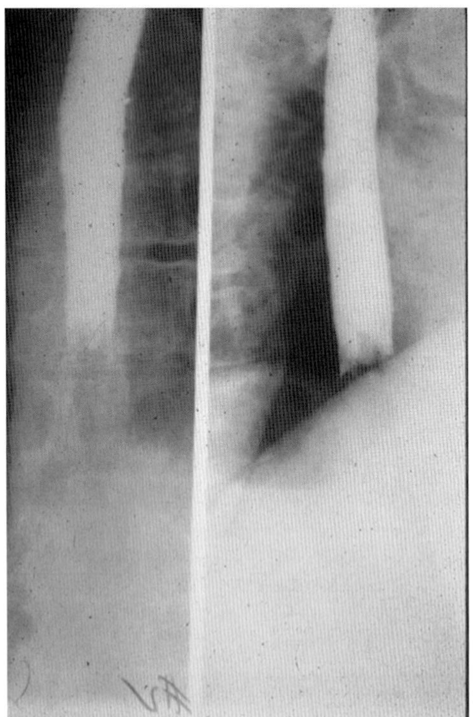

**Fig. 31.6 Fluoroscopic swallow study showing extravasation of contrast agent (as seen from the left side of the film).** (Courtesy of E. Wolf, MD, Montefiore Medical Center, Bronx, NY.)

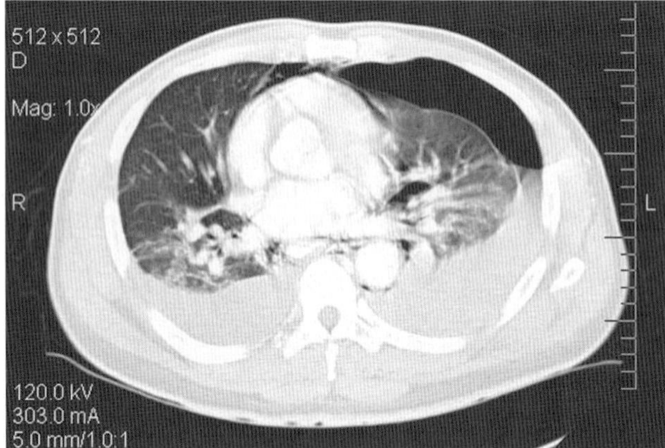


**Fig. 31.7 Esophageal computed tomography scan demonstrating typical fluid collections in the setting of perforation.**

## SUGGESTED READINGS

Kahrilas PJ. Gastroesophageal reflux disease. N Engl J Med 2008;359:1700-7.

Litovitz T, Whitaker N, Clark L, et al. Emerging battery-ingestion hazard: clinical implications. Pediatrics 2010;125:1168-77.

Pace F, Antinori S, Repici A. What is new in esophageal injury (infection, drug-induced, caustic, stricture, perforation)? Curr Opin Gastroenterol 2009;25:372-9.

Sepesi B, Raymond DP, Peters JH. Esophageal perforation: surgical, endoscopic, and medical management strategies. Curr Opin Gastroenterol 2010;26:379-83.

van Pinxteren B, Sigterman KE, Bonis P, et al. Short-term treatment with proton pump inhibitors, $H_2$-receptor antagonists and prokinetics for gastro-oesophageal reflux–like symptoms and endoscopy negative reflux disease. Cochrane Database Syst Rev 2010;11:CD002095.

## REFERENCES

*References can be found on Expert Consult @ www.expertconsult.com.*

# Diseases of the Stomach 32

*Danielle M. Ware-McGee and Natasha Wheaton*

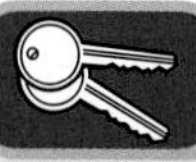

**KEY POINTS**

- Dyspepsia, gastritis, peptic ulcer disease, and gastric carcinoma represent a progressive spectrum of illness.
- *Helicobacter pylori* is the causative agent of 90% of duodenal ulcers and 60% of gastric ulcers; it is a precursor to gastric carcinoma and is the only bacterium listed as a class I carcinogen.
- In the absence of *H. pylori*, use of nonsteroidal antiinflammatory drugs is the cause of peptic ulcer disease in up to 60% of patients.
- The findings associated with acute dyspepsia and acute coronary syndrome are often indistinguishable in the emergency department. The primary diagnostic goal of the emergency physician is to exclude acute coronary syndrome through risk stratification and appropriate testing.
- In a hemodynamically stable patient with peptic ulcer disease without perforation, first-line treatment consists of a 6-week trial of a proton pump inhibitor.
- Serologic testing for *H. pylori* is more cost-effective than empiric treatment without testing.
- All emergency department patients with dyspepsia require referral for outpatient evaluation for serologic testing or endoscopy (or both) to exclude malignant disease.

## EPIDEMIOLOGY

*Dyspepsia* refers to chronic or recurrent pain of gastroduodenal origin centered in the upper part of the abdomen. Dyspepsia affects 25% to 40% of people in industrialized nations, who regularly experience pain accompanied by any or all of the following associated symptoms: bloating, fullness, early satiety, nausea, anorexia, heartburn, regurgitation, and belching.[1] Patients experiencing dyspepsia with endoscopic evidence of gastric mucosal inflammation are said to have *gastritis*, and those with ulcerations of the stomach or duodenal lining have *peptic ulcer disease* (PUD). Dyspepsia, gastritis, PUD, and the long-term complication *gastric carcinoma* represent a progressive spectrum of illness.

Dyspepsia accounts for 2% to 5% of annual visits to primary care physicians in the United States, and more than 1 billion health care dollars is spent on prescription medications for this disorder each year.[1] PUD chronically affects large portions of the U.S. population and leads to impressive health expenditures because many affected patients leave the workforce. More than 7000 American deaths are attributed to PUD each year, largely as a result of perforation and gastrointestinal (GI) bleeding.

In up to 60% of patients in whom dyspepsia is diagnosed, the results of endoscopic evaluation are nondiagnostic.[1] The remaining 40% generally have one of three causative diagnoses: PUD, gastroesophageal reflux disease, or gastric cancer.[2] The broad differential diagnosis of recognized causes of PUD is summarized in **Table 32.1**.

Duodenal ulcers occur three to four times more frequently than gastric ulcers worldwide, with men being affected more commonly than women for both ulcer types. The male-to-female ratio for duodenal ulcer (4 : 1) is higher than that for gastric ulcer (2 : 1). Such distributions are observed mainly in the developing countries of Africa and Asia. In westernized societies, the distribution of both ulcer types between the sexes has become more equal over the past few decades, although the mechanisms underlying these epidemiologic changes are unknown.[3]

PUD is the most common cause of upper GI bleeding in the United States and accounts for 27% to 40% of all cases.[4] Patients with PUD who are at highest risk for upper GI bleeding include alcoholics, chronic users of nonsteroidal antiinflammatory drugs (NSAIDs), and patients with renal dysfunction.

## PATHOPHYSIOLOGY

The stomach is anatomically subdivided into three parts: the fundus, the corpus (body), and the antrum (**Fig. 32.1**).[5] This subdivision reflects differences in function. The stomach functions as a reservoir for ingested meals, as well as the site of food agitation with gastric secretions—the first step in digestion (see Fig. 32.1). The acidic fluid is secreted by parietal cells in the fundus and body of the stomach under the control of hormones secreted by endocrine cells in the antrum. Acid secretion is controlled by the complex interaction of gastrin from G cells and histamine from

**Table 32.1 Differential Diagnosis of Peptic Ulcer Disease**

| | |
|---|---|
| Cardiovascular | Acute myocardial infarction<br>Dissecting aneurysm<br>Angina pectoris<br>Pericarditis<br>Ischemic bowel disease |
| Gastrointestinal | |
| Esophageal | Gastroesophageal reflux disease<br>Erosive esophagitis<br>Esophageal spasm<br>Esophageal stricture<br>Schatzki ring<br>Esophageal cancer |
| Stomach | Gastritis<br>Gastroparesis<br>Gastric lymphoma/carcinoma |
| Other | Biliary tract disease<br>Cholelithiasis<br>Pancreatitis<br>Pancreatic carcinoma<br>Infiltrative disorders—sarcoidosis and Crohn disease<br>High small bowel obstruction<br>Subphrenic abscess<br>Early appendicitis<br>Hypercalcemia<br>Hyperkalemia |

From Ferri FF. Ferri's clinical advisor 2007: instant diagnosis and treatment. St. Louis: Mosby; 2006.

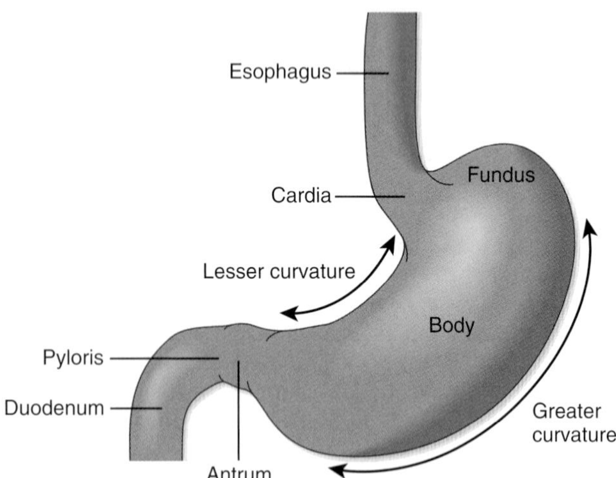


**Fig. 32.1 Divisions of the stomach.** (From Zuidema G. Shackelford's surgery of the alimentary tract. 4th ed. Philadelphia: Saunders; 1995.)

enterochromaffin-like cells. Somatostatin further regulates these cells by inhibition (**Fig. 32.2**).

PUD results from a complex interplay of factors that disrupt the delicate balance between the production of protective barrier agents, such as bicarbonate-rich mucus, and the hypersecretion of acid from parietal cells. Recognition of *Helicobacter pylori* as the causative agent of 90% of duodenal ulcers and 60% of gastric ulcers has led to a paradigm shift in the understanding and management of PUD.[6]

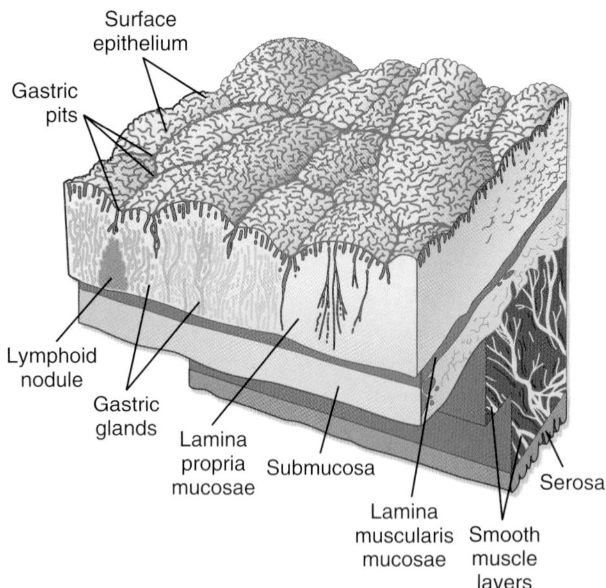


**Fig. 32.2 Surface of the gastric mucosa.** (From Zuidema G. Shackelford's surgery of the alimentary tract. 4th ed. Philadelphia: Saunders; 1995.)

## INFECTIOUS CAUSES

*H. pylori*, a gram-negative, helix-shaped bacterium, infects at least 50% of the population worldwide and is recognized as an important risk factor for the development of PUD and ultimately gastric adenocarcinoma and lymphoma. Infection is probably acquired in childhood and, in the absence of antimicrobial therapy, persists for life with an estimated lifetime risk for PUD of 15%.[7-9] Risk factors for the acquisition of *H. pylori* include sharing of a bed in childhood, large number of siblings, lower socioeconomic status, and lack of a fixed hot water supply.[6,19] Although it is still unclear whether transmission occurs person to person, three different mechanisms for such transmission have been postulated: fecal-oral, through saliva, and by vomitus.[6,9]

*H. pylori* causes acute dyspepsia characterized by epigastric pain, nausea, vomiting, and halitosis. Symptoms usually last several weeks and then disappear, although the organism loiters within the stomach. Gastritis persists throughout life in various locations; it shifts from an antrum-predominant pattern to a corpus-predominant pattern or pangastritis.[10] The chronic phase of the disease is usually benign, but in susceptible individuals, complications such as gastric or duodenal ulcers may arise.

If sufficiently virulent, *H. pylori* gastritis leads to destruction of the gastric mucosa, which can ultimately result in the development of intestinal metaplasia or eventually carcinoma. The rate of gastric acid secretion declines, thereby fostering conditions beneficial to colonization of the gastric lumen by fecal organisms. *H. pylori* eventually disappears because the organism is ill-equipped to compete with a growing number of other organisms and is unable to thrive on metaplastic cells in the absence of hyperacidic conditions. Despite its eventual demise, the initial invasion of the stomach lumen by *H. pylori*

**BOX 32.1 Nonsteroidal Antiinflammatory Drug–Induced Risk Factors for Peptic Ulcer Disease**

Previous peptic ulcer disease
Age older than 65 years
History of complications of peptic ulcer disease
Concurrent use of steroids
Concurrent use of other anticoagulants
High dose of nonsteroidal antiinflammatory drugs or prolonged use
Significant comorbid diseases (coronary artery disease, chronic kidney disease)

From Dincer D, Duman A, Dikici H, et al. NSAID-related upper gastrointestinal bleeding: are risk factors considered during prophylaxis? Int J Clin Pract 2006;60:546-8.

**BOX 32.2 Drugs Associated with Peptic Ulcer Disease**

Nonsteroidal antiinflammatory drugs
Potassium chloride
Bisphosphonates
Mycophenolate
Floxuridine
Crack cocaine*
Amphetamines*

*Associated with a higher rate of perforation.

incites conditions that favor the evolution of non-cardia–associated gastric cancer.[6]

Though most common, *H. pylori* is not the sole infectious cause of PUD. *Helicobacter heilmannii*, another spiral nonspirochetal bacterium transmitted via domestic animals and monkeys, has been associated with *H. pylori*–negative duodenal ulcers. It is much rarer than *H. pylori*, is less pathogenic, and can easily be differentiated by routine histology. Treatment strategies similar to those for *H. pylori* are successful in eradicating this organism.[10]

Additional infectious agents include cytomegalovirus (CMV), herpes simplex virus type 1, (HSV-1) and syphilis. CMV was first associated with peptic ulcers in renal transplant recipients and is the only organism to be significantly associated with peptic ulceration in persons positive for human immunodeficiency virus. The ulcers in these patients are usually gastric and numerous. The diagnosis is confirmed by the finding of intranuclear inclusion bodies or CMV DNA (or both) in the gastric mucosa on biopsy specimens taken from the base of the ulcer. HSV-1–induced ulcers are generally located in the antrum and often occur in immunocompetent individuals.[10]

## DRUG-RELATED CAUSES

In the absence of *H. pylori*, use of NSAIDs is the cause of PUD in up to 60% of patients.[10] Because gastroduodenal damage does not occur in all patients taking NSAIDs, it is important to identify those at increased risk (**Box 32.1**). Factors associated with higher rates of NSAID-related GI complications are a previous history of PUD or hemorrhage, age older than 65 years, prolonged use of high-dose NSAIDs, use of more than one NSAID, concomitant use of corticosteroids or anticoagulants, and serious comorbid illness such as cardiovascular, renal, or hepatic impairment, diabetes, or hypertension.[11] Many other drugs are associated with PUD and are listed in **Box 32.2**.

Crack cocaine and methamphetamines have been linked to PUD, as well as a higher rate of gastric perforation thought to be secondary to vasoconstriction and resulting local tissue ischemia. Additionally, tobacco and alcohol can further precipitate gastritis and PUD.[11]

## ZOLLINGER-ELLISON SYNDROME

Zollinger-Ellison syndrome (ZES) is an uncommon cause of PUD but should be considered in patients with refractory, atypically located, or numerous ulcers, especially in the absence of *H. pylori* or NSAID use.[10,12] The ulcers in patients with ZES are caused by a gastrin-secreting tumor, or *gastrinoma*.

The incidence of ZES in the United States ranges from 0.1% to 1% in patients with PUD. The most common functional pancreatic tumors in patients with multiple endocrine neoplasia type 1 (MEN-1) are gastrinomas, and approximately 20% of patients with ZES also have MEN-1. The mean age at diagnosis is 50 years, but patients with ZES range in age from 7 to 90 years. Patients with both MEN-1 and ZES become symptomatic at an earlier age, with PUD usually developing in the third decade of life. The male-to-female ratio of patients with ZES ranges from 2 : 1 to 3 : 2.[10,12]

Patients with ZES commonly have symptoms of PUD such as epigastric pain, nausea, and vomiting. Alternatively, severe diarrhea may be the only symptom. Perforated ulcer remains a common complication; approximately 7% of patients with ZES are initially seen with perforation of the jejunum.[12]

Evaluation for ZES includes measurement of fasting serum gastrin and basal gastric acid secretion with a secretin stimulation test. Imaging fails to demonstrate the tumor in up to 50% of cases; nonetheless, computed tomography, magnetic resonance imaging, radionuclide octreotide scanning, endoscopic ultrasonography, and the selective arterial secretin injection test are recommended for potential localization.[12]

All patients with sporadic gastrinoma who have resectable metastatic disease should undergo exploratory laparotomy for potential curative resection. Surgery may be the most effective treatment of metastatic gastrinoma if the tumor can be excised completely.

## IDIOPATHIC ULCERS

Once all known causes are excluded, a group of peptic ulcers remain that are then considered idiopathic. The etiology of idiopathic PUD is poorly understood but is thought to include a genetic predisposition, altered acid secretion, rapid gastric emptying, defective mucosal defense mechanisms, psychologic stress, and smoking.[10] Management of idiopathic peptic ulcers is challenging because these ulcers are more resistant to standard therapy and are associated with more frequent complications. Patients who relapse may require long-term maintenance proton pump inhibitor (PPI) therapy.[10]

## PRESENTING SIGNS AND SYMPTOMS

Dyspepsia refers to a group of symptoms attributed to various pathologic conditions of the upper GI tract, including epigastric pain, bloating, nausea, anorexia, fullness, early satiety, regurgitation, and belching.[1,13,14]

Classically, duodenal ulcer pain is described as a gnawing, hungerlike pain in the epigastrium with occasional but generally mild radiation to the back. The pain typically improves just after eating and worsens 2 to 5 hours after meals. Duodenal ulcer pain tends to be more pronounced in the early morning hours (11 PM to 2 AM) because of peak acid levels in the stomach at that time. Peptic ulcers have similar findings, although classically the pain intensifies with food intake, in contrast to duodenal ulcers. The pain in patients with untreated PUD tends to occur in clusters, with intermittent pain lasting weeks to months and asymptomatic periods between flares.

Several red flags should be considered when taking a history from patients with dyspepsia. These red flags increase the risk for gastric carcinoma as the cause of the patient's symptoms and include age older than 45 years, unintentional weight loss, persistent vomiting, progressive dysphagia, odynophagia, unexplained anemia or iron deficiency, hematemesis, palpable abdominal mass, family history of GI cancer, and previous gastric surgery or jaundice (see the Red Flags box).[14] Several ethnic groups also have a higher disease prevalence, including Afro-Caribbean, Hispanic, Asian, and Native American populations.[14,16,17]

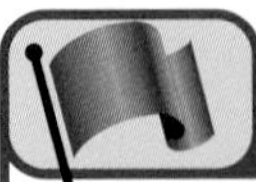

**RED FLAGS FOR PELVIC ULCER DISEASE**

Age older than 45 years
Dysphagia
Anorexia/early satiety
Persistent vomiting
Jaundice
Palpable abdominal mass
Family history of gastric cancer
Previous pelvic ulcer disease
Unexplained weight loss
Indications of significant gastrointestinal bleeding (e.g., anemia, melena)

Patients should be screened for historical features suggestive of disease progression and complications, including perforation, pyloric outlet obstruction, and hemorrhage. A change in the character of pain from vague, epigastric discomfort to severe, localized pain, especially with radiation to the back, can indicate perforation. Additionally, unremitting pain that was previously well controlled with food or antacids also suggests progression of disease.

Acute, severe, diffuse abdominal pain with or without referred shoulder pain may indicate recent perforation. Although nausea can be associated with dyspepsia, vomiting is less common; early pyloric stenosis should be considered if vomiting is a prominent feature.

Hemorrhage from upper GI bleeding may be manifested as syncope, melena, or hematemesis; consequently, GI bleeding should be considered in the differential diagnosis of patients with vague presyncope or syncope, especially those with risk factors for PUD.

Unstable vital signs suggest the possibility of massive GI bleeding in the setting of PUD. The overall appearance of the patient may be noteworthy for cachexia, which is concerning for underlying malignancy. Skin should be examined for jaundice and pallor, which is concerning for anemia.

Abdominal findings in the setting of uncomplicated PUD are generally normal or may be significant only for mild epigastric pain. Peritoneal findings suggest perforation.[18]

## DIFFERENTIAL DIAGNOSIS AND MEDICAL DECISION MAKING

The primary goal of emergency department (ED) evaluation of dyspepsia is to localize the source of the symptoms to the upper GI tract by excluding other life-threatening diagnoses, most notably acute coronary syndrome. Atypical acute coronary syndrome may have similar manifestations as PUD, especially in elderly, diabetic, and female patients. An electrocardiogram and cardiac markers should be evaluated in an all ED patients with a new onset of dyspepsia.

Other organ-specific conditions in the differential diagnosis include pulmonary disease (lower lobe pneumonia, embolism), pancreatitis, biliary disease, inflammatory bowel disease, irritable bowel syndrome, gastroparesis, mesenteric ischemia, and abdominal wall pathology, including abscess, rectus hematoma, or musculoskeletal pain. Systemic and metabolic diseases that should be considered include sarcoidosis, thyroid disease, parathyroid disease, hyperkalemia, and hypercalcemia. The broad differential diagnosis of dyspepsia is summarized in Table 32.1.

A rare though serious infectious source of epigastric pain is phlegmonous gastritis caused by a bacterial infection of the stomach. This infection of mixed gram-positive cocci and gram-negative rods occurs in the setting of previous gastric pathology, including PUD, gastritis, gastric surgery, or carcinoma. These patients are very ill appearing, and treatment includes aggressive resuscitation, early antibiotics, and admission to the intensive care unit.

Although laboratory tests are not required in routine cases of chronic, recurrent dyspepsia, they are necessary in the evaluation of patients with a first episode of dyspepsia or a change in symptoms to exclude complications of disease progression or alternative cardiac, pulmonary, or GI conditions on the differential. A complete blood count, comprehensive metabolic panel, lipase, and cardiac enzymes should be evaluated. Imaging is not generally indicated unless perforation with free air (upright chest radiograph) or biliary disease (right upper quadrant ultrasound) is a concern.

## MEDICAL TREATMENT

For patients in whom acute coronary syndrome can be excluded in favor of a diagnosis of gastritis or PUD, empiric treatment strategies and referral for diagnostic testing are appropriate.

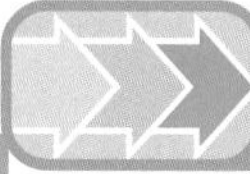

**PRIORITY ACTIONS**

Keep the differential diagnosis of dyspepsia broad. Investigate potential life threats, especially atypical acute coronary syndrome.

Search for red flags suggestive of disease progression or gastric carcinoma by findings on the history, physical examination, or laboratory testing.

Hemodynamically unstable patients mandate prompt resuscitation, intensive care unit monitoring, and gastroenterology consultation.

All patients with acute, severe epigastric pain should have an upright chest radiograph to exclude free air secondary to perforation.

Perform a digital rectal examination with Hemoccult testing to assess for occult or fresh blood in the stool.

Perform serial examinations of patients with dyspepsia to exclude the possibility of the development of perforation and to assess the benefit of therapeutic interventions.

For acute pain management in the ED, start with oral liquid antacids (e.g., Maalox, 30 to 60 mL orally) mixed with viscous lidocaine, 15 to 20 mL orally. The addition of an anticholinergic, antispasmodic agent such as Donnatal has no role in treatment. $H_2$ blockers may be initiated in the ED, although the onset of action after both oral and parenteral administration of these agents is too slow to provide immediate pain relief. Parenteral $H_2$ blocker therapy (e.g., Pepcid, 20 mg intravenously) may be most useful for patients with suspected ZES who will be admitted to the hospital. Parenteral narcotic analgesics should be administered to patients with pain uncontrolled by oral agents or to those in whom perforation or hemorrhage is suspected (i.e., oral medications are contraindicated).

In hemodynamically stable patients whose symptoms are not severe enough to warrant admission, three options are available for the management of dyspepsia not related to NSAIDs. The first option is a single, short-term trial of empiric antiulcer therapy with a PPI in a setting in which the patient has reliable follow-up.[19] Cytoprotective agents such as sucralfate suspension may prevent further injury to the gastric mucosa and provide immediate relief of symptoms. Regardless of response, all such trials should be stopped after about 6 weeks and an evaluation performed if symptoms recur; further investigation is warranted earlier if the symptoms do not respond in 2 weeks. The second option is a definitive endoscopic evaluation, especially in patients with red flags by history, physical examination, or laboratory evaluation. The urgency for definitive diagnosis stems from a risk that gastric ulcers harbor malignancy in this population. The third option is noninvasive testing for *H. pylori* via serum antibody screening followed by outpatient prescription of antibiotics in *H. pylori*–positive subjects. For most low-risk patients, referral to a primary care physician for *H. pylori* testing plus initiation of symptomatic PPI therapy in the ED is the preferred option.[13,20]

Patients with known *H. pylori* disease who are either treatment naïve or were inadequately treated should start a regimen of either a bismuth-metronidazole-tetracycline combination plus a PPI or a PPI plus clarithromycin and either metronidazole or amoxicillin.[21] When *H. pylori* is a consideration, endoscopy should be delayed for 4 to 8 weeks after discontinuation of antibiotics, PPI, and bismuth so that infection status can be more reliably assessed at biopsy.

Communicate with the patient's primary provider if serologic testing was performed or empiric therapy for *H. pylori* was started so that the outpatient provider can arrange further diagnostic evaluation. Additionally, confirm with patients that they understand the treatment plan, the seriousness of the diagnosis, and which lifestyle modifications would aid in healing. Specifically, patients should be educated about the negative effects of smoking, excessive alcohol use, failure to follow up, and noncompliance with medication. Finally, patients should decrease or avoid the use of NSAIDs.[19] If NSAID therapy must continue, the addition of a PPI will allow most duodenal and gastric ulcers to heal in timely fashion.[10,19] Patients with healed NSAID-induced ulcers are among those at highest risk for further gastroduodenal injury and serious complications such as perforation and bleeding; strict return precautions should be provided for these patients.[11]

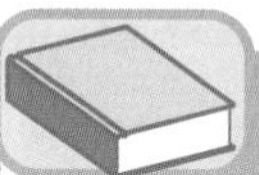

**PATIENT TEACHING TIPS**

Refer to a primary care provider and gastroenterologist to ensure follow-up and to tailor a cohesive treatment plan to fit the individual patient.

Educate patients about the dangers of smoking, excessive use of alcohol and caffeine, and medication noncompliance.

Provide information about various smoking cessation aids and programs.

Stress the importance of abstaining from the use of nonsteroidal antiinflammatory drugs.

Provide well-written, clear, concise anticipatory discharge instructions. Every patient should leave the emergency department understanding the dangers of worsening pain, hematemesis, melena, or hematochezia.

## SURGICAL TREATMENT

Surgery is rarely necessary given that medical therapies for PUD are so effective. Indications for elective surgical treatment of PUD are (1) protracted and failed medical therapy and (2) suspicion of malignancy.[22] For the rare nonhealing benign gastric ulcer, resection is indicated for the management of symptoms and prevention of malignancy.

Profuse bleeding was a previous indication for surgery, but endoscopic therapy (whether by electrocautery, heater probe, or injection sclerotherapy) controls bleeding in the majority of cases (**Fig. 32.3**).[22] Surgery is indicated for cases in which bleeding is not controlled with endoscopy or is recurrent.

When surgery is being considered, some well-established risk factors increase the likelihood of a fatal outcome, including the presence of severe comorbid conditions, perforation longer than 24 hours in duration, and the presence of hypotension on initial evaluation. Conservative management consisting of nasogastric suction, circulatory support, and antibiotics should be used in elderly patients with these risk factors.[22]

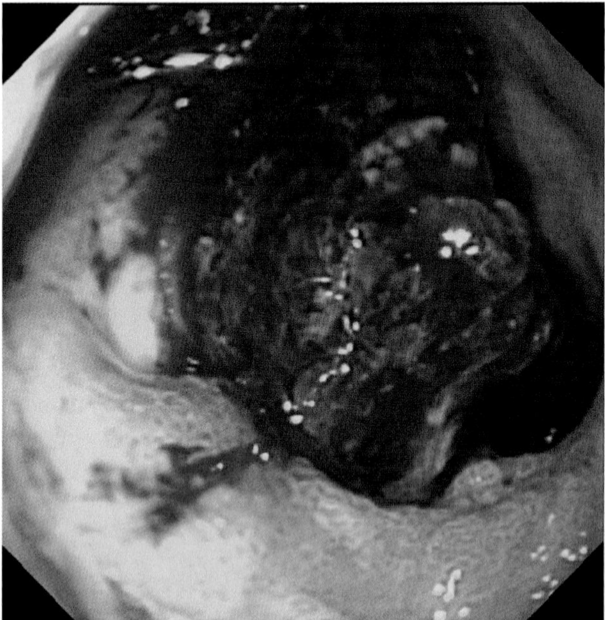

**Fig. 32.3 Endoscopic appearance of a duodenal bulb ulcer with a fresh adherent clot.** (From Feldman M, Friedman LS, Brandt LJ, editors. Sleisenger & Fordtran's gastrointestinal and liver disease: pathophysiology/diagnosis/management. 8th ed. Philadelphia: Saunders; 2006.)

## SEQUELAE OF PEPTIC ULCER DISEASE

### GASTRIC CANCER

Gastric cancer is the second most common cause of cancer-related death worldwide. It is the third most common cancer in southeastern Europe and South America, and globally it is the fourth most common form of cancer.[23] In comparison with the rest of the world, Western Europe and the United States have a relatively low incidence of gastric cancer; the highest incidence of gastric cancer is reported in Japan, China, and South America.[4] Gastric cancer rates remain quite high in some subgroups of African Americans, Hispanics, and Native Americans. In the United States, the mean age at diagnosis is 48 years, and the male-to-female ratio is 1 : 1.[23]

Although certain well-established genetic factors predispose one to gastric cancer, such as blood type A, the main causative agents are environmental.[24] *H. pylori* infection promotes apoptosis in infected cells, thereby starting a metaplastic path of destruction. Inhibition of E cadherin synthesis by *H. pylori* is also associated with the development of gastric cancer. The International Agency for Research on Cancer has classified *H. pylori* as a class I carcinogen, the only bacterial agent with this distinction.[23]

The prognosis of patients with gastric cancer is poor, with 5-year survival rates of less than 25%.[23] The improved survival seen in Japanese populations has been attributed to identification of earlier-stage lesions by aggressive screening programs. Such screening programs are less common in the United States. ED patients with suspected dyspepsia and red flags must undergo urgent outpatient follow-up for endoscopic screening for gastric malignancy (**Fig. 32.4**).

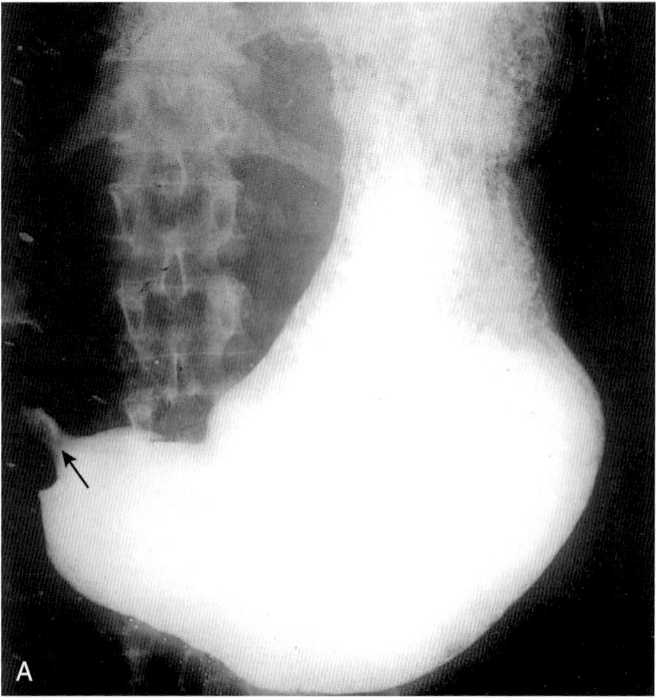



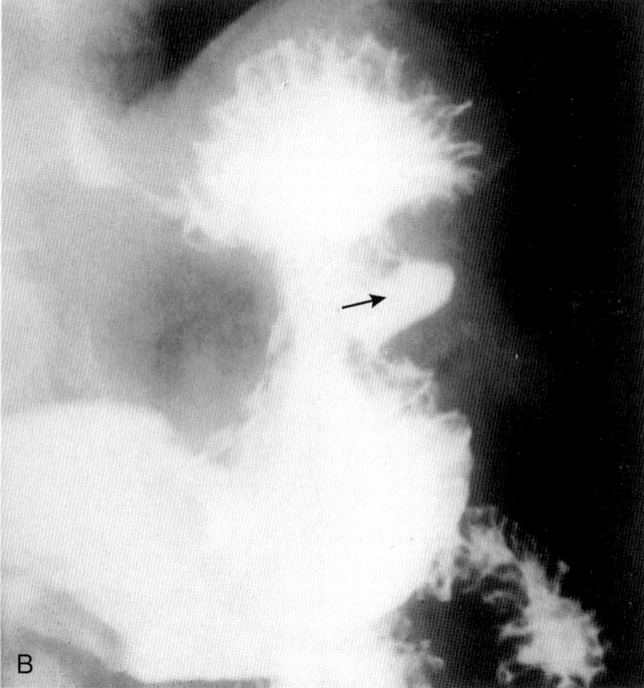



**Fig. 32.4 Radiologic and endoscopic examples of gastric cancer. A,** Pyloric (gastric outlet) obstruction *(arrow)*. **B,** Large greater curve ulcer within a mass *(arrow)*.

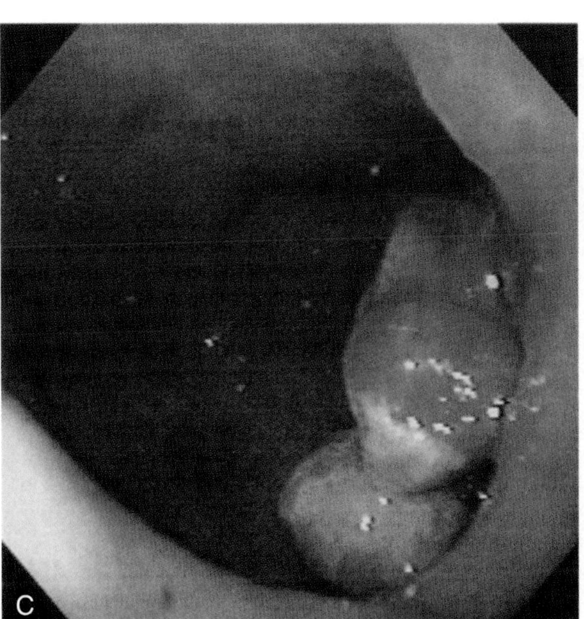


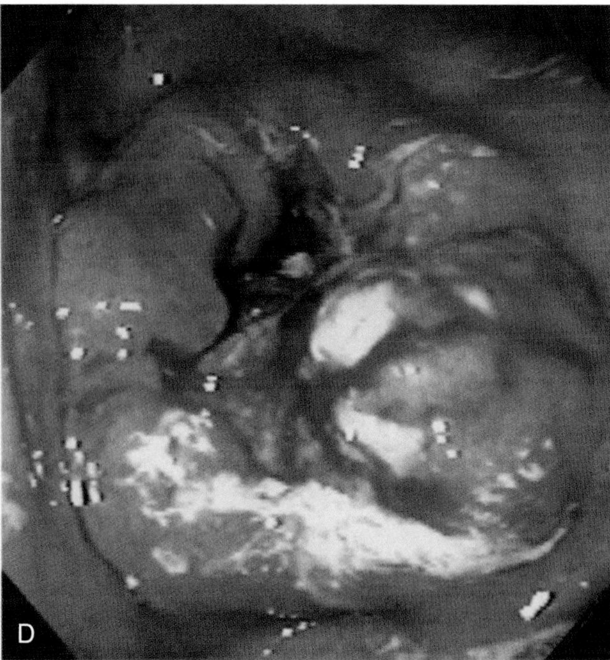


**Fig. 32.4, cont'd** **C,** Polypoid gastric cancer. A trilobed polyp is apparent at the angularis. **D,** Exophytic gastric cancer. A circumferential masslike lesion involves the gastric body and is collapsing the antrum. (From Feldman M, Friedman LS, Brandt LJ, editors. Sleisenger & Fordtran's gastrointestinal and liver disease: pathophysiology/diagnosis/management. 8th ed. Philadelphia: Saunders; 2006.)

## GASTRIC OUTLET OBSTRUCTION

Chronic peptic ulcers in either the stomach or duodenum may cause scarring and impair gastric emptying, a condition known as gastric outlet obstruction (**Fig. 32.5**). In adults, PUD is the major cause of benign gastric outlet obstruction—more than 95% of cases are associated with duodenal or pyloric channel ulceration. Resolution of gastric outlet obstruction after the eradication of *H. pylori* has been demonstrated in several studies. Symptomatic improvement can be seen a few weeks after the start of antimicrobial therapy for *H. pylori*, and the benefits seem to persist on long-term follow-up.[25]

Treatment of gastric outlet obstruction should start with pharmacologic eradication of *H. pylori*, even when the stenosis is considered to be fibrotic or when some gastric stasis is present. If such noninvasive treatment is unsuccessful, NSAID use may be the underlying cause.[25] Dilation or surgery should be reserved for patients who show no response to medical therapy.

ED patients with signs or symptoms of gastric outlet obstruction should be admitted for gastroenterology consultation, hydration, and further management.

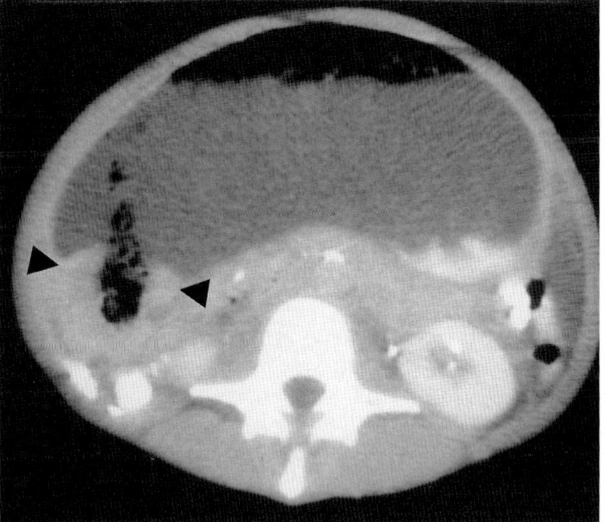

**Fig. 32.5 Gastric outlet obstruction—cancer of the antrum.** A markedly distended stomach with an air-fluid level is seen on computed tomography. In this case a mass in the distal end of the antrum is apparent *(arrowheads).* (From Grainger RG, Allison DJ, Dixon AK, editors. Grainger & Allison's diagnostic radiology: a textbook of medical imaging. 4th ed. St. Louis: Churchill Livingstone; 2001.)

## REFERENCES

***References can be found on Expert Consult @ www.expertconsult.com.***

# 33 Gastrointestinal Bleeding

*Sheryl L. Heron and Patricia Baines*

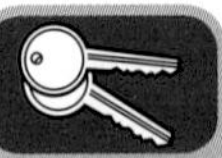

**KEY POINTS**

- Morbidity and mortality from gastrointestinal bleeding increase significantly if aggressive resuscitation is not initiated immediately in the emergency department.[1,2]
- Assessment and management of gastrointestinal bleeding depend on the site of the hemorrhage—that is, whether the bleeding is from an upper or lower gastrointestinal tract source.
- Gastroenterology consultation should be obtained immediately to arrange for diagnostic and therapeutic endoscopy or colonoscopy for cases of active bleeding.
- Causes of gastrointestinal bleeding in children vary considerably with age; most cases are benign and self-limited, although Meckel diverticulum, midgut volvulus, and intussusception can result in massive rectal bleeding.

## SCOPE

Demographic risk factors for patients with gastrointestinal (GI) bleeding include older age, male gender, and the use of alcohol, tobacco, aspirin, or nonsteroidal antiinflammatory drugs (NSAIDs).[3] Risk for bleeding is significantly higher in elderly patients who have recently started a regimen of NSAIDs or regular-dose aspirin than in long-term users of these agents.[4] Additional independent risk factors are unmarried status, cardiovascular disease, difficulty performing activities of daily living, use of multiple medications, and use of oral anticoagulants.[5]

Intensive resuscitation in the emergency department (ED) significantly decreases mortality in patients with *hematemesis* (vomiting blood), *hematochezia* (red bloody stools), or *melena* (black tarry stools).[2] Application of the predictive mnemonic BLEED (ongoing *b*leeding, *l*ow systolic blood pressure, *e*levated prothrombin time, *e*rratic mental status, unstable comorbid *d*isease) at the initial ED evaluation can predict hospital outcomes in patients with acute upper or lower GI hemorrhage.[6] Although the incidence of peptic ulcer bleeding has decreased, the decline in incidence has occurred only in patients younger than 70 years,[7] and mortality from multiorgan failure, cardiopulmonary conditions, or terminal malignancy has remained constant.[1]

Lower GI bleeding (LGIB) afflicts 20 to 27 of every 100,000 persons annually in the United States.[8] The rate of LGIB increases more than 200-fold from the third to the ninth decade of life, with 25% to 35% of all cases occurring in elderly patients. It is one of the common medical emergencies that can become life-threatening in elderly patients.[9,10] Risk stratification for LGIB by Strate et al. has identified seven predictors of severe bleeding: heart rate higher than 100 beats/min, systolic blood pressure lower than 115 mm Hg, syncope, nontender abdominal examination, gross rectal bleeding, aspirin use, and more than two comorbid conditions. Patients with more than three risk factors have an 84% risk for severe bleeding, defined as transfusion of more than 2 units of red blood cells.[11-13]

Pediatric GI bleeding is fairly common worldwide; however, the incidence of severe GI bleeding in U.S. children is very low.[14] LGIB is a more common complaint in the practice of general pediatrics, and it accounts for 10% to 15% of referrals to a pediatric gastroenterologist.[15-17] In most children, bleeding is not life-threatening and ceases spontaneously, with only supportive care being required.[16,17] The age of the child guides the clinician toward specific diagnoses.[16,18]

## PATHOPHYSIOLOGY

### UPPER GASTROINTESTINAL BLEEDING

Upper GI bleeding (UGIB) is defined as bleeding from a source proximal to the ligament of Treitz, which is located at the junction of the duodenum and jejunum. UGIB accounts for three quarters of cases of GI tract hemorrhage, with duodenal and gastric ulcers being the specific sources in more than half of patients with an upper tract cause.

Hematochezia is generally a symptom of LGIB but may be associated with brisk upper tract hemorrhage. UGIB sources are identified in 11% of patients in whom LGIB was initially suspected.[3] Melena most commonly results from bleeding proximal to the jejunum and should be considered a marker of UGIB.

Variceal hemorrhage is the most serious complication of portal hypertension and occurs in one third of patients with esophageal varices.[3] It is more common in patients with Child B and C cirrhosis.[21] The extent of severe bleeding depends on portal pressure, variceal size, and variceal wall thickness.[22] Esophageal varices should be suspected in any alcoholic with unexplained anemia or obvious GI bleeding.

One study noted a decline in the frequency of peptic ulcer disease in patients with UGIB and reported that the

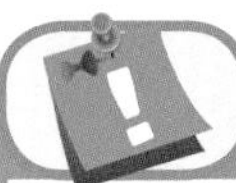

**TIPS AND TRICKS**

Patients with upper gastrointestinal bleeding should be instructed to avoid nonsteroidal antiinflammatory drugs (NSAIDs).[19,20] Studies have shown that the risk for recurrent bleeding is significantly higher in long-term users of NSAIDs or regular-dose aspirin, especially if patients are elderly. For short-term users of NSAIDs or aspirin, cotreatment with proton pump inhibitors (but *not* with histamine $H_2$ blockers) may reduce the risk for bleeding to less than the risk in nonusers.[4]

proportion of bleeding ulcers with a nonvisible vessel is now 20%, which is less than previously reported.[23] Such decline may be related to improved treatment of *Helicobacter pylori* infection.

In children, the pathophysiology of the bleeding is determined by the specific causes of hemorrhage for each age group.[24]

### LOWER GASTROINTESTINAL BLEEDING

LGIB refers to bleeding that originates from an intestinal source distal to the ligament of Treitz. The majority of patients with hematochezia bleed from a colonic source. Diverticular disease, angiodysplasia, and neoplasm are the leading causes of LGIB in adults. Anal fissure and hemorrhoids are the most benign causes of LGIB. Approximately 10% of all patients will never have a source identified, and up to 40% of patients with LGIB have more than one potential bleeding source.[11]

Comorbid illnesses and decreased physiologic reserve make elderly patients more vulnerable to the adverse consequences of acute blood loss and prolonged hospitalization.[10,25] Specifically, hematochezia is more commonly associated with syncope, dyspnea, altered mental status, stroke, falls, fatigue, and acute anemia in older patients. Poor prognostic indicators also include continued bright red rectal bleeding, excessive transfusions, orthostasis, shock, and altered mental status on admission.[9]

Ulcerative colitis accounts for the majority of cases of massive LGIB in young adults in the second or third decade of life. Diverticulosis and arteriovenous malformation are found in older adults.[15]

The independent risk factors listed earlier are useful prognostic indicators, and outcomes are poorer in patients with either upper or lower tract bleeding.[5] Specifically, use of over-the-counter NSAIDs may represent an important cause of peptic ulcer disease and ulcer-related hemorrhage in those with UGIB.[4,26]

Although most causes of LGIB in children are self-limited and benign, it is imperative to consider Meckel diverticulum, midgut volvulus, and intussusception in appropriate age groups.[15]

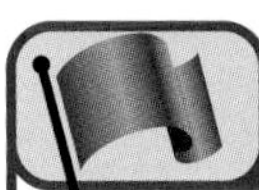

**RED FLAGS**

Use of nonsteroidal antiinflammatory drugs
Coagulopathies
Long-term alcohol use
Neoplasms
Previous aortic surgery
Recent nosebleeds

Data from Swaim M, Wilson J. GI emergencies: rapid therapeutic responses for older patients. Geriatrics 1999;54:20.

## CLINICAL PRESENTATION

Patients with GI bleeding can be rapidly assessed by their reported volume of blood loss and initial hemodynamic status. Massive hemorrhage is associated with signs or symptoms of hemodynamic instability, including tachycardia (heart rate greater than 100 to 120 beats/min), systolic blood pressure less than 90 to 100 mm Hg, symptomatic orthostasis, syncope, ongoing bright red or maroon hematemesis, transfusion requirements in the first 24 hours, and inability to stabilize the patient.[27]

Vital signs and postural changes should be assessed in patients who appear sufficiently stable. An increase of 20 beats/min or more in pulse or a decrease of 20 mm Hg in systolic blood pressure between the supine and upright positions indicates loss of more than 20% of blood volume in normal adult patients.[9] Tachycardia, low blood pressure, reduced urine output, and conjunctival pallor in patients with GI bleeding are signs that mandate immediate volume replacement. Hypovolemic shock implies at least a 40% loss of blood volume. Note that abnormalities in vital signs, especially postural vital sign, are unreliable in pediatric and elderly patients.

The history should focus on the quantity, frequency, and duration of bleeding (differentiating between melena and hematochezia) to characterize the nature of the GI bleeding. Comorbid status, including other GI disorders, anticoagulant use, syncope, weight loss, alcohol intake, and cardiovascular disease, should be assessed.

In addition to continuous monitoring of vital signs, physical examination should include assessment of mental status, skin (for jaundice or pallor), and pulmonary and cardiovascular compromise (especially in the elderly because of ischemia from blood loss), as well as a thorough abdominal examination for distension, tenderness, or masses. Digital rectal examination and testing of stool for gross or occult blood should be performed in patients with suspected GI bleeding.

Complaints associated with LGIB include hematochezia or melena, although patients may have additional findings, such as anemia, light-headedness, hypovolemia, weakness, malaise, chest pain, and dyspnea. It is important to note that patients with LGIB may be asymptomatic and have complaints seemingly unrelated to intestinal bleeding (e.g., fatigue, weight loss); dramatic findings consisting of massive rectal bleeding in acutely ill and unstable patients are less common.[28]

Delayed black tarry stools may occur from a source of bleeding in the small bowel or ascending colon and may not be noted by the patient until several days after the bleeding has stopped.[29]

A thorough history and complete physical examination are important for evaluation of a child with GI bleeding. Bright red blood that coats but is not mixed with stool suggests an anorectal source. Hematochezia indicates bleeding from the distal part of the small bowel or proximal part of the colon. Bloody diarrhea usually suggests colonic bleeding. Currant-jelly stools are indicative of the vascular congestion and hyperemia seen with intussusception.

Food allergy may lead to GI bleeding from food-induced colitis and could result in dehydration in infants younger than 3 months.[17] Anal fissures are common in infants and produce red streaks or spots of blood in the diaper.[15] Other causes of dark stool are iron, charcoal, flavored gelatin, red fruits, bismuth, and food dyes. Maternal blood swallowed by neonates during delivery may be diagnosed with the Apt test.[17]

## DIFFERENTIAL DIAGNOSIS

The most common causes of UGIB in adults are listed in **Box 33.1**, and causes of LGIB in adolescents and adults are listed in **Box 33.2**.

The exact cause of the GI bleeding is less important to the emergency physician (EP) than differentiation between upper and lower tract sources.

An aortoenteric fistula may have developed in a patient with massive LGIB and recent surgery.[9]

### DIFFERENTIAL DIAGNOSIS FOR PEDIATRIC GASTROINTESTINAL BLEEDING

**Table 33.1** lists the differential diagnosis for UGIB and LGIB according to patient age. Ingestion of maternal blood is the most common cause of suspected GI bleeding in neonates; blood is swallowed during either delivery or breastfeeding (from a fissure in the mother's breast). Other causes of GI bleeding in neonates include bacterial enteritis, milk protein allergies, intussusception, anal fissures, lymphonodular hyperplasia, and erosions of the esophageal, gastric, and duodenal mucosa.

Mucosal injuries presumably result from a dramatic rise in gastric acid secretion and laxity of the gastric sphincters in infants. Maternal stress in the third trimester has also been proposed to increase maternal gastrin secretion and enhance infantile peptic ulcer formation.

Some drugs have been implicated in neonatal GI bleeding, including NSAIDs, heparin, and tolazoline, which are used for persistent fetal circulation. Indomethacin, administered to

**BOX 33.1 Causes of Upper Gastrointestinal Bleeding**

**More Common**
Peptic ulcer disease
Gastritis
Esophagitis
Varices
Mallory-Weiss tears

**Less Common**
Gastric cancer
Dieulafoy lesion
Portal gastropathy
Gastric antral vascular atresia

From Maltz C. Acute gastrointestinal bleeding. Best Pract Med 2003:1-23. Available at http://merck.microdex.com/index.asp?page=bpm_brief&article_id=BPM01GA08.

**BOX 33.2 Causes of Lower Gastrointestinal Bleeding**

**Adolescents**
Upper gastrointestinal bleeding
Inflammatory bowel disease
Polyps
Meckel diverticulum
Infectious diarrhea
Anal fissures
Hemorrhoids

**Adults**
Upper gastrointestinal bleeding
Diverticulosis
Angiodysplasia
Cancer
Ischemic bowel disease
Polyps
Inflammatory bowel disease
Infectious diarrhea
Foreign body

From Akhtar AJ. Lower gastrointestinal bleeding in elderly patients. J Am Med Dir Assoc 2003;4:320-2.

**Table 33.1 Causes of Gastrointestinal (GI) Bleeding in Children by Age**

| AGE GROUP | CAUSES OF UPPER GI BLEEDING | CAUSES OF LOWER GI BLEEDING |
|---|---|---|
| Neonates | Hemorrhagic disease of the newborn<br>Swallowed maternal blood<br>Stress gastritis<br>Coagulopathy | Anal fissure<br>Necrotizing enterocolitis<br>Malrotation with volvulus |
| Infants (1 mo-1 yr) | Esophagitis<br>Gastritis | Anal fissure<br>Intussusception<br>Gangrenous bowel<br>Milk protein allergy |
| Infants (1-2 yr) | Peptic ulcer disease<br>Gastritis | Polyps<br>Meckel diverticulum |
| Children (2-12 yr) | Esophageal varices<br>Gastric varices | Polyps<br>Inflammatory bowel disease<br>Infectious diarrhea<br>Vascular lesions |

From Arensman R, Abramson L. Gastrointestinal bleeding: surgical perspective. EMedicine 2004. Available at www.emedicine.com/ped/topic3027.htm.

maintain a patent ductus arteriosus in neonates, may cause GI bleeding through intestinal vasoconstriction and platelet dysfunction. Maternal medications can also cross the placenta and incite GI problems in the developing fetus and neonate on delivery. Aspirin, cephalothin, and phenobarbital are well-known causes of coagulation abnormalities in neonates. Stress ulcers in newborns are associated with dexamethasone, which is used for fetal lung maturation.

Rarer causes of GI bleeding in a neonate are volvulus, coagulopathies, arteriovenous malformations, necrotizing enterocolitis (especially in preterm infants), Hirschsprung enterocolitis, and Meckel diverticulitis.[14]

In infants, GI mucosal lesions and irritations are the most common causes of bleeding and include esophagitis, gastritis, duodenitis, ulcers, colonic polyps, and anorectal disorders. Intussusception is a common and important cause of GI bleeding in this age group. The incidence of intussusception is greatest in infants aged 3 months to 1 year, but it can occur in children up to 5 years of age. Approximately 80% of all cases of intussusception occur in infants younger than 2 years.

Other causes of infantile GI bleeding are infectious diarrhea, midgut volvulus, Meckel diverticulum, arteriovenous malformation, and GI duplication. Rare causes include foreign body ingestion, variceal disease, irritable bowel disease, and acquired thrombocytopenia.

Older children may have any of the preceding conditions, but duodenal ulcer, Mallory-Weiss tear, and nasopharyngeal bleeding are important causes of bleeding in this age group. Less common causes are gastritis or ulcers induced by salicylates or NSAIDs, Henoch-Schönlein purpura, ingestion of caustic substances, hemolytic-uremic syndrome, inflammatory bowel disease, and vasculitis. In adolescents older than 12 years, the most common causes of UGIB are duodenal ulcers, esophagitis, gastritis, and Mallory-Weiss tears.[14]

## DIAGNOSTIC TESTING

### NASOGASTRIC ASPIRATION

Historically, nasogastric aspiration has been used to determine whether the bleeding originated from the upper GI tract in patients with melena—a bloody aspirate confirmed an upper tract source, whereas an aspirate testing negative for blood represented either resolved bleeding or a more distal site of hemorrhage. In some studies, however, nasogastric aspiration was noted to be insensitive for detection of UGIB in patients *without* active hematemesis, and a negative result provided little information about the cause of the bleeding.[30,31] The routine use of gastric aspiration and lavage in patients arriving at the ED with GI bleeding is not supported.[32] Aspirates testing positive for blood confirm only that the bleeding is proximal to the pylorus, and patients must undergo endoscopy for further differentiation.

A nasogastric aspirate containing more than 1 L of fresh blood or inability to obtain a clear aspirate through lavage with more than 1500 mL of saline should alert the physician to massive UGIB that requires immediate gastroenterologic or surgical intervention. In patients with frank hematemesis and brisk persistent hematochezia, the information provided by nasogastric aspiration may be lifesaving.[33]

### UPPER ENDOSCOPY

Esophagogastroduodenoscopy (EGD) is now the diagnostic test of choice for establishing the source of UGIB. The overwhelming majority of existing data suggest that early endoscopy is a safe and effective procedure in all risk groups.[34,35] Patients without active hematemesis may benefit from immediate upper endoscopy by a gastroenterologist to confirm the site of bleeding rather than undergoing the potential additional discomfort and morbidity associated with placement of a nasogastric tube. Endoscopy is both diagnostic and therapeutic in many cases.[36] One study noted that live-view video capsule endoscopy (VCE) accurately indentifies high- and low-risk patients in the ED with UGIB. The use of VCE to risk-stratify these patients significantly reduced time to performance of emergency EGD and therapeutic intervention.[37]

### TAGGED RED BLOOD CELL STUDIES

An advanced modality for detecting of the source of GI bleeding is radionuclide imaging, such as radioisotopic imaging with technetium Tc 99m sulfur colloid– or technetium pertechnetate–labeled red blood cells. Technetium Tc 99m red blood cell imaging is a useful test in the management of acute GI bleeding, particularly if the bleeding has been occurring for more than 3 hours and other modalities have failed to identify a source. A limitations of this test is poor detection of bleeding in the foregut, with the highest sensitivity noted for bleeding in the colon.[38] A technetium Tc 99m sulfur colloid–labeled red blood cell study requires active bleeding at a rate of more than 0.1 mL/min for visualization. Radionuclide imaging has not been widely tested in the ED setting and is still reserved for inpatient use at most institutions.

### ARTERIOGRAPHY

Angiography is appropriate for initial testing of patients with massive bleeding.[39] When the bleeding cannot be identified and controlled by endoscopy, intraoperative enteroscopy or arteriography may help localize the bleeding source and facilitate segmental resection of the bowel.[40] Mesenteric angiography can detect bleeding at a rate of 0.5 mL/min or greater.[41] Either angiography or angiographic computed tomography may be used to identify aortoenteric fistulas.

Intraarterial injection of vasopressin or other vasoconstrictors at the site of bleeding can control hemorrhage; embolization is an option when intraarterial injection is unsuccessful.[42,43]

### DISTAL COLONIC IMAGING

Colonoscopy has high diagnostic yield and a low rate of perforation in patients with LGIB. It is best performed after colonic cleansing and in patients with slow bleeding. Proctosigmoidoscopy is used in patients with mild rectal bleeding to determine whether stool above the rectum contains blood. Barium enema is not useful in the acute setting but can be ordered after an acute bleeding episode has resolved.[44]

The optimal timing for colonoscopic intervention for LGIB is still unclear.[10] More recent literature defines urgent colonoscopy as taking place within 12 hours.[45] Evidence suggests that earlier colonoscopy leads to more diagnostic and therapeutic opportunities[45] and reduces hospital length of stay.[10,12,45]

## MULTIDETECTOR COMPUTED TOMOGRAPHY TECHNOLOGY

Multidetector computed tomography (MDCT) can be used to evaluate both acute and obscure (recurrent or persistent) GI tract bleeding. Initial experience indicates that MDCT angiography is a promising first-line modality that is time efficient and sensitive and allows accurate diagnosis or exclusion of active GI hemorrhage. The potential for an impact on the evaluation and treatment of patients with acute GI bleeding is notable.[46,47]

## LABORATORY TESTING

Initial laboratory studies include a complete blood cell count, coagulation studies, and blood typing and crossmatching for patients with active bleeding or unstable vital signs. Serial hematocrit measurements are more useful than one isolated test, although marked changes in hematocrit typically lag behind actual blood loss. A blood chemistry panel, liver profile, and lipase measurement should be performed. Stool evaluation for leukocytes, bacteria, ova, parasites, and *Clostridium difficile* should be considered in patients with bloody diarrhea.[17] Electrocardiograms and cardiac enzyme testing are necessary for patients at risk for early coronary artery disease or those older than 50 years to screen for ischemia secondary to blood loss.

## PROCEDURES

Proper technique for the safe placement and use of nasogastric tubes and gastroesophageal balloon tamponade tubes (e.g., Blakemore-Sengstaken tube) is discussed in Chapter 46.

## TREATMENT

**Figure 33.1** presents an algorithm for the treatment of GI bleeding. Insert two 18-gauge or larger intravenous lines and administer 0.9% normal saline or lactated Ringer solution on arrival of the patient.[41] Quickly evaluate the patient's hemodynamic status and determine the extent of blood or fluid resuscitation necessary. Standard resuscitative measures for the management of shock should precede or occur in parallel with definitive diagnostic testing. Management should otherwise be directed toward the underlying source of bleeding. Note that in 80% of cases, LGIB spontaneously stops.[25]

If the patient is hemorrhaging, consult a gastroenterologist and surgeon. Upper endoscopy is the diagnostic and therapeutic procedure of choice for acute UGIB. Surgery is indicated for patients with active bleeding when medical therapy proves

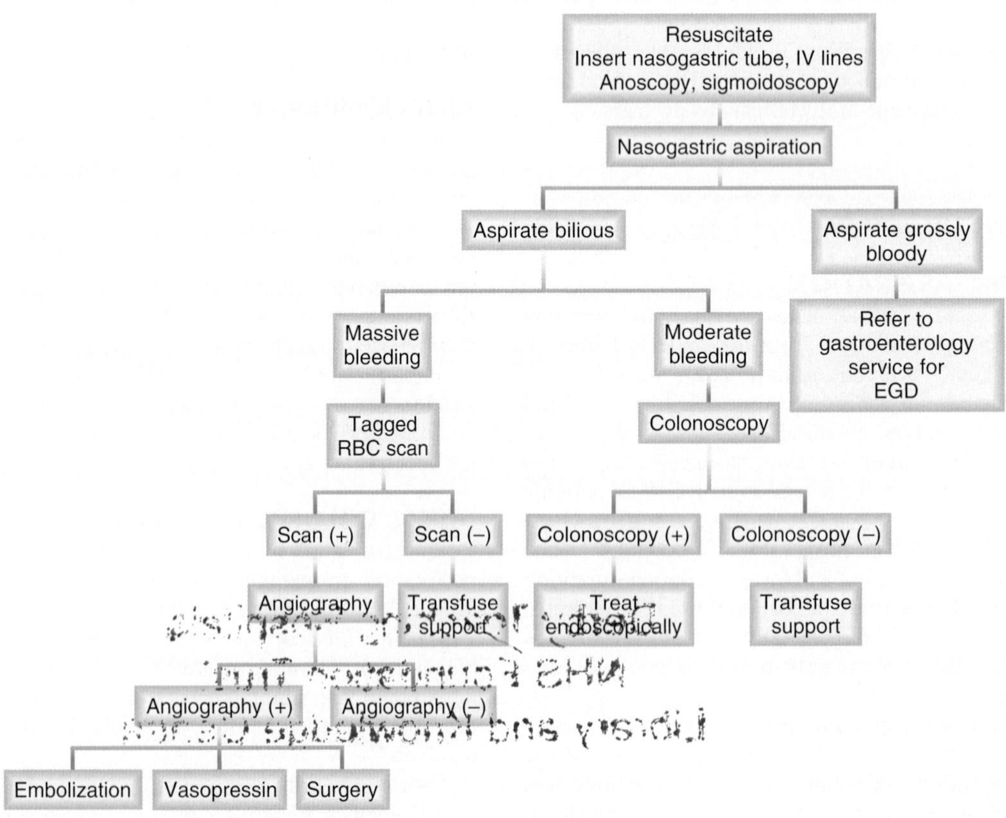


**Fig. 33.1 Management of lower gastrointestinal hemorrhage.** *EGD*, Esophagogastroduodenoscopy; *IV* intravenous; *RBC*, red blood cell; *(+)*, positive test result; *(–)*, negative test result. (Adapted from Hoedema RE, Luchtefeld MA. The management of lower gastrointestinal hemorrhage. Dis Colon Rectum 2005;48:2010-24.)

ineffective and continued hemorrhage requires more than 5 units of blood within the first 4 to 6 hours.[28,29,41,48] Bowel resection may be required for pronounced LGIB.

In the absence of consultants, massive esophageal hemorrhage as a result of variceal bleeding may be temporarily treated with the placement of a gastroesophageal balloon tamponade device (Blakemore-Sengstaken tube). Although this is an uncommon procedure, EPs in remote practice locations should be familiar with the indications for and proper use of such potentially lifesaving devices.

Octreotide acetate is a synthetic analogue of somatostatin that should be administered intravenously to all patients with suspected UGIB from esophageal varices to induce splanchnic vasoconstriction and a reduction in portal hypertension. The loading dose is 50 mcg intravenously, followed by infusion of 25 to 50 mcg/hr for 5 days.

Comorbid condition, such as coagulopathies, hyperkalemia, and cardiac ischemia, should be identified and treated. The EP should consider the administration of fresh frozen plasma, platelets, recombinant factor VIIa (NovoSeven), or desmopressin (DDAVP) as appropriate.

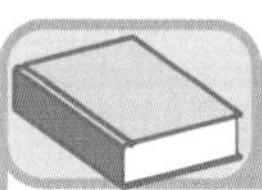

### PATIENT TEACHING TIPS

Patients should stop drinking alcohol and seek an alcohol cessation program immediately if needed.

Patients who take nonsteroidal antiinflammatory agents should receive concomitant therapy with a proton pump inhibitor.

Patients with gastric ulcers should be reexamined 6 to 8 weeks after the initial bleeding episode.

Patients should maintain daily intake of synthetic bulk-forming agents.

Surveillance colonoscopy should be performed every 3 years in patients with colon polyps and adenomatous changes or every 5 years in those with hyperplastic polyps.

Data from Swaim M, Wilson J. GI emergencies: rapid therapeutic responses for older patients. Geriatrics 1999;54:20.

## DISPOSITION

Most patients seen in the ED with GI bleeding should be admitted for further evaluation and treatment. Patients who require transfusions, have severe anemia or continued bleeding, or are unstable should be admitted to the intensive care unit. Admission to a hospital ward is reserved for stable patients with melena or a history of resolved bleeding with normal physical findings and no significant comorbidity. Stable patients with melena and symptoms of suspected or known cardiac disease must be admitted to a telemetry unit.

Patients with normal physical findings, trace heme-positive stool, and stable vital signs may be sent home with close follow-up. Patients with reported hematochezia but normal-appearing stool and no evidence of hemodynamic compromise may be managed as outpatients with arrangements for urgent colonoscopy and primary care referral.[41]

Patients who have anal fissures, hemorrhoids, or other rectal causes of bleeding can be discharged with conservative therapy and reassurance. A detailed discussion of the management of anorectal disorders can be found in Chapter 41.

Patients should be instructed to return to the ED if they experience signs and symptoms of recurrent bleeding, fatigue, chest discomfort, dyspnea, or near-syncope.[49]

## SUGGESTED READINGS


Manning-Dimmitt LL, Dimmitt SG, Wilson GR. Diagnosis of gastrointestinal bleeding in adults. Am Fam Physician 2005;71:1339-46.

Peter D, Dougherty J. Evidence based emergency medicine: evaluation of the patient with gastrointestinal bleeding: an evidence based approach. Emerg Med Clin North Am 1999;17:239-61.

Pitera A, Sarko J. Just say no: gastric aspiration and lavage rarely provide benefit. Ann Emerg Med 2010;55:365-6.

Spiegel BM. Endoscopy for acute upper GI tract hemorrhage: sooner is better. Gastrointest Endosc 2009;70:236-9.


## REFERENCES

*References can be found on Expert Consult @ www.expertconsult.com.*

Derby Teaching Hospitals
NHS Foundation Trust
Library and Knowledge Centre

# 34 Mesenteric Ischemia

*Kelly P. O'Keefe and Tracy G. Sanson*

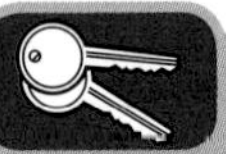

**KEY POINTS**

- Severe abdominal pain out of proportion to the findings on physical examination should always raise suspicion for mesenteric ischemia, especially in elderly patients.
- The presence of hypotension, atrial fibrillation, severe cardiovascular disease, or recent myocardial infarction increases the likelihood of mesenteric ischemia.
- No serum marker is sensitive or specific enough to establish or exclude the diagnosis of bowel ischemia.
- Bloody diarrhea is a late finding that indicates mucosal sloughing—do not wait for the appearance of hematochezia or melena to make the diagnosis of mesenteric ischemia.
- Patient survival improves with early mesenteric angiography or surgical intervention (or both).

## PERSPECTIVE

Mesenteric ischemia results from lack of adequate blood flow to and oxygenation of the mesentery and intestines. The clinical course consists of rapid progression from bowel ischemia to infarction, sepsis, and usually death. The incidence of acute mesenteric ischemia is increasing because of an aging population and the prolonged survivability of patients with severe cardiovascular disease and other significant medical conditions.

Four types of mesenteric ischemia must be considered: acute mesenteric ischemia, nonobstructive mesenteric ischemia (NOMI), mesenteric vein thrombosis, and chronic mesenteric ischemia (or mesenteric angina). The most deadly of these is acute mesenteric ischemia, which results from sudden obstruction of blood flow to the intestines and has a mortality rate approaching 90%.

## EPIDEMIOLOGY

Mesenteric ischemia accounts for 0.1% of all hospital admissions and 1% of emergency department (ED) visits for abdominal pain in geriatric patients. Cases of mesenteric vein thrombosis are more difficult to estimate accurately but have been reported at 2 per 100,000 admissions over a period of 20 years at one center.[1-3]

The overall mortality associated with mesenteric ischemia is between 60% and 93% but rises precipitously once bowel wall infarction has occurred. Mortality remains greatest for acute mesenteric ischemia resulting from obstruction or embolic phenomena. Patients with an early manifestation of NOMI have mortality rates of 50% to 55%, whereas patients with mesenteric vein thrombosis have a 15% mortality at 30 days.[1-3] Those affected by chronic mesenteric ischemia have a more prolonged course, are relatively protected by dual blood supply, and present the physician with more numerous chances for intervention.

## PATHOPHYSIOLOGY

Any patient with advanced age, atherosclerosis, thromboembolic disease, atrial fibrillation, and processes leading to chronic low-flow states is at risk for the development of arterial mesenteric ischemia (**Tables 34.1 and 34.2**).[1,2,4,5] Mesenteric venous obstruction carries its own separate risk factors, which are similar to those for venous thrombosis anywhere in the body.

Acute mesenteric ischemia is a result of the precipitous onset of hypoperfusion caused by occlusive or nonocclusive obstruction of either arterial or venous blood flow. Acute hypoperfusion occurs in 65% of cases and carries a mortality rate exceeding 60%. Occlusive arterial obstruction is most commonly caused by embolic or thrombotic obstruction of the superior mesenteric artery (SMA). NOMI is often due to vasoconstriction of the splanchnic system. Occlusive venous obstruction occurs with thrombosis or segmental strangulation. Mesenteric venous thrombosis is the main cause of mesenteric ischemia in younger patients without cardiovascular disease.

Acute arterial embolism causes a dramatic cessation of blood flow, with rapid progression from ischemia to infarction. As the bowel wall necroses, contamination with intraluminal bacteria leads to peritonitis, sepsis, and toxin-mediated hypotension.

Nonocclusive infarction, which represents 25% of all cases of acute ischemia, is most often caused by splanchnic hypoperfusion and vasoconstriction. Risk factors for nonocclusive disease include advanced age, acute myocardial infarction (AMI), acute cardiac decompensation, and heart failure.

**Table 34.1 Risk Factors for Ischemic Bowel Diseases***

| RISK FACTOR | ARTERIAL THROMBOSIS | EMBOLUS | MESENTERIC VEIN THROMBOSIS | NONOBSTRUCTIVE MESENTERIC ISCHEMIA |
|---|---|---|---|---|
| Advanced age | + | + | + | + |
| Atherosclerosis | + | | | |
| Aortic dissection | + | | | |
| Low cardiac output | + | + | | + |
| Congestive heart failure | | | | + |
| Shock | | | | + |
| Severe dehydration | + | | + | |
| Cardiac arrhythmias, especially atrial fibrillation | | + | | + |
| Severe cardiac valvular disease | | + | | |
| Recent myocardial infarction | + | | | + |
| Intraabdominal malignancy | | | + | |
| Abdominal trauma | | | + | |
| Intraabdominal infection | | | + | |
| Intraabdominal inflammatory conditions | | | + | |
| Parasitic infection (ascariasis) | | | + | |
| Hypercoagulable states (venous thrombosis) | | | + | |
| Sickle cell anemia | | | + | |
| Recent cardiac surgery | + | + | | + |
| Recent abdominal surgery | | | + | |
| Vascular aortic prosthetic grafts proximal to the superior mesenteric artery | | + | | |
| Hemodialysis | | | | + |
| Vasculitis | + | | + | |
| Drugs that cause constriction | | | | |
| Digitalis | | | | + |
| Cocaine | | | | + |
| Amphetamines | | | | + |
| Pseudoephedrine | | | | + |
| Vasopressin | | | +† | + |
| Estrogen therapy | | | + | |
| Pregnancy | | | + | |
| Decompression sickness | | | + | |
| Blast lung caused by systemic air embolism | | + | | |

Data from references 1, 2, 4, and 5.

*A plus sign (+) indicates that the factor is a risk for the disease subtype.

†Especially after sclerotherapy.

**Table 34.2 Incidence of Ischemic Bowel Diseases**

| DISEASE | INCIDENCE (%)* |
|---|---|
| Superior mesenteric artery (SMA) embolism: The SMA is susceptible to embolism because of large vessel caliber and a narrow angle of departure from the aorta. The proximal SMA is most commonly obstructed within 6-8 cm of the aorta. | 50 |
| Nonocclusive ischemia | 25 |
| SMA thrombosis | 20 |
| Mesenteric venous thrombosis | 5 |

*Percentage of all cases of acute mesenteric ischemia.

Diuretics contribute to a decrease in splanchnic perfusion in patients with profound heart disease, whereas medications such as digoxin and alpha-blockers cause regional vasoconstriction and may add to a low-flow state. Cocaine can cause splanchnic vasoconstriction and should be suspected as a cause of mesenteric ischemia in younger patients.

Bowel perfusion is generally preserved during periods of hypotension; therefore, NOMI represents failure of the normal autoregulatory systems.[2,6,7] Patients with chronic renal failure may have bowel ischemia after hemodialysis, probably from hypoperfusion, which promotes preferential shunting of blood from the splanchnic circulation to preserve flow to the cardiac and cerebrovascular systems.

Although acute mesenteric vein thrombosis accounts for a small proportion of cases of ischemic bowel disease (5% to 10%), the ease of diagnosis with computed tomography (CT) has allowed identification of a greater number of patients with venous thrombosis. Symptoms are even less specific than those of arterial obstruction and are manifested over a longer period before bowel infarction occurs. Thrombus secondary to hypercoagulable states develops first in the smaller vessels and later progresses into the larger veins; clots associated with cirrhosis, neoplasm, or local injury (operative, trauma) start at the site of obstruction and evolve distally.[4]

Thrombotic arterial ischemia occurs late in the course of severe mesenteric atherosclerotic disease and involves the three major sources of intestinal blood supply: the celiac artery, the SMA, and the inferior mesenteric artery (IMA). Symptoms are typically manifested when two of the three vessels are significantly stenosed or completely obstructed.

A review of the anatomy of arterial blood flow to the intestines is helpful in understanding the pathophysiology of mesenteric ischemia.

The celiac artery arises anteriorly from the abdominal aorta at the level of the 12th thoracic vertebra. The celiac artery branches into the common hepatic, splenic, and left gastric arteries. These vessels supply their corresponding organs with significant redundancies, so ischemia in these areas is rare.

The SMA comes off the aorta 1 cm below the celiac artery and terminates as the ileocolic artery. This latter vessel supplies the majority of the blood delivered to the small intestine, as well as some flow to the pancreas, right colon, and transverse colon.

The IMA originates from the aorta 7 cm distal to the SMA. It provides blood to the distal transverse colon, descending colon, and rectum.

There is a significant array of collateral blood vessels and flow patterns. The small intestine is especially vulnerable to ischemia, however, because the terminal arterioles enter the intestinal wall without collateral pathways.[4] Splanchnic blood flow requirements vary continuously but can account for up to 35% of cardiac output.

Venous drainage of the system occurs via the superior mesenteric vein, which empties into the portal vein.

## PRESENTING SIGNS AND SYMPTOMS

### CLASSIC PRESENTATION

Soon after ischemia begins, patients have complaints of severe abdominal pain that is clearly out of proportion to the findings on physical examination, such as a soft abdomen that is not very tender to palpation. The description and location of the pain vary over time. As the disease progresses, infarction develops and the symptoms may temporarily remit. Over the next several hours, bowel necrosis leads to signs of peritonitis: the abdomen becomes rigid, distended, and very painful with decreased bowel sounds. The intestinal mucosa begins to slough, and rectal bleeding occurs. At this point the stool contains occult blood in 60% of patients. The bowel may perforate, as signaled by findings of hypotension and sepsis.

Clues to diagnosis of the various ischemic bowel diseases are as follows:

- Acute abdominal pain followed by rapid and forceful evacuation of the bowels (vomiting or diarrhea) strongly suggests an embolic phenomenon in the SMA.
- Long-standing abdominal pain (weeks to months), which is then followed by acute worsening, suggests intestinal angina and SMA thrombosis.
- Patients with risk factors for NOMI may have unexplained abdominal distention or gastrointestinal bleeding; pain is totally absent in up to 25% of these patients, and unexplained distention may herald infarction.

Chronic mesenteric ischemia, or "intestinal angina," refers to a pattern of pain typically brought on after eating that is usually episodic and recurrent, is sometimes constant, and lasts for up to 3 hours at a time. Mesenteric arterial atherosclerotic disease is generally the cause of chronic mesenteric ischemia, with a process similar to that of coronary artery disease and resultant angina pectoris.

Colonic ischemia occurs much less frequently than small bowel ischemia. Colonic ischemia often resolves spontaneously and without sequelae but can lead to significant morbidity and, in some cases, death.

### VARIATIONS IN PRESENTATION

In patients with NOMI, the severity and location of pain vary, which complicates early diagnosis. A heightened level of suspicion is necessary for patients with significant risk factors.

Mesenteric vein thrombosis may be totally asymptomatic and might be diagnosed as an incidental finding in patients

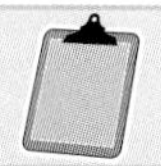

**DOCUMENTATION**

Onset, severity, and duration of symptoms
Presence of melena or hematochezia
Presence or absence of risk factors
Vital signs: evidence of shock, sepsis
Findings of cardiac, full abdominal, genitourinary, and rectal examinations
Emergency department course: times of discussions with consultants, discussions with family, code status, availability of testing, treatments, delays

undergoing CT of the abdomen for reasons other than abdominal pain. Blockage of the IMA may be silent because of adequate collateral circulation.

Patients with mesenteric atherosclerosis may have symptoms of abdominal angina, classically manifested as postprandial pain. As a result, fear of eating, early satiety, weight loss, and altered bowel habits develop. This syndrome occurs in up to 50% of patients in whom thrombotic mesenteric ischemia eventually develops.[2]

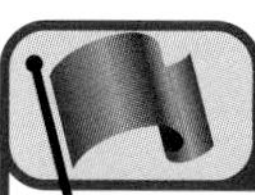

**RED FLAGS**

Pain out of proportion to the findings on physical examination
Presence of one or more risk factors
Pain not responsive to narcotics
Rectal bleeding (late finding)

## DIFFERENTIAL DIAGNOSIS

Few diagnoses portend a more serious course and risk for mortality than mesenteric ischemia does. Patients at risk for AMI are generally also at risk for aortic disease. Other items in the differential diagnosis are listed in **Box 34.1**.

**BOX 34.1 Differential Diagnosis of Ischemic Bowel Disease***

Abdominal aortic aneurysm: rupture or expansion
Perforated ulcer or viscus
Ruptured ectopic pregnancy (woman of childbearing age)
Incarcerated or strangulated hernia
Septic shock
Intussusception
Volvulus
Salpingitis or tuboovarian abscess
Torsion of the ovary or testicle
Appendicitis
Pelvic mass or torsion
Pancreatitis
Diverticulitis
Ruptured ovarian cyst
Renal colic
Biliary colic
Also consider atypical manifestations of:
- Inferior wall myocardial infarction
- Pulmonary embolism
- Pneumonia
- Diabetic ketoacidosis
- Acute glaucoma

*Differential diagnoses are listed in order of urgency.

## DIAGNOSTIC TESTING

### ANGIOGRAPHY AND COMPUTED TOMOGRAPHIC ANGIOGRAPHY

Mesenteric angiography provides direct visualization of the vasculature and remains a valuable method of evaluation in patients with suspected bowel ischemia (**Table 34.3**). Angiography is both sensitive (74% to 100%) and specific (100%); the test also differentiates between occlusive and nonocclusive disease. Patients who undergo angiography in timely fashion have better survival; mortality rates of 70% to 90% are observed when bowel infarction has occurred.[4]

**Table 34.3 Angiographic Findings in Ischemic Bowel Disease**

| DISEASE | FINDINGS |
|---|---|
| Superior mesenteric artery (SMA) embolus | Filling defects with obstruction of distal flow<br>Secondary vasoconstriction |
| Nonobstructive mesenteric ischemia | Narrowing of the origins of SMA branches<br>Irregularities in SMA branches<br>Spasm of the mesenteric arcades<br>Impaired filling of the intramural vessels |
| SMA thrombus | Occlusion of the proximal SMA<br>Secondary distal vasoconstriction<br>Absence of collateral flow |
| Superior mesenteric vein (SMV) thrombus | Thrombus with partial or complete occlusion<br>Failure to visualize the SMV or portal vein<br>Slowness or absence of filling of the mesenteric veins<br>Failure of the arterial arcades to empty<br>Prolonged blush in the involved segment |

Data from Burns BJ, Brandt LJ. Intestinal ischemia. Gastroenterol Clin North Am 2003;32:1127-43.

CT angiography (CTA) is largely replacing standard angiography because it is more readily available and more quickly accomplished. A metaanalysis published in 2010 confirmed CTA as the first-line imaging modality because of its high sensitivity (93%) and specificity (96%).[8] CTA is clearly more advantageous in the ED; interventional radiology (IR) involvement later offers additional treatment advantages in the perioperative or observational inpatient phases.

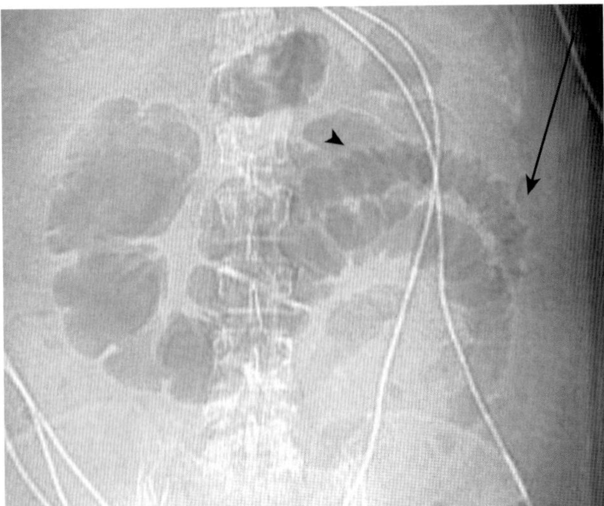

**Fig. 34.1 Thumbprinting in a patient with superior mesenteric vein thrombosis and bowel ischemia *(arrowhead).*** A normal concave pattern of the small bowel and convex thumbprinting with wall thickening *(long arrow)* are seen. (From Hendrickson M, Narpast TR. Abdominal surgical emergencies in the elderly. Emerg Med Clin North Am 2003;21:937-69.)

Standard angiography allows local administration of thrombolytic or vasodilatory therapy concomitant with the diagnostic procedure, thereby improving mortality. The emergency physician (EP) must weigh the diagnostic and therapeutic advantages of CTA or standard angiography against concerns for dye administration in patients susceptible to renal insufficiency (almost every patient with mesenteric ischemia), availability of an interventional radiologist, stability of the patient, and delays in surgical intervention (**Fig. 34.1**). In all cases of suspected mesenteric ischemia, the surgeon should be contacted for involvement before or simultaneously with the ordering of advanced diagnostic testing, with the caveat that any delay in diagnosis and operative intervention increases mortality.

With the exception of contrast-enhanced CT scans for mesenteric vein thrombosis, all other imaging tests are fraught with error and lead to diagnostic delays. Standard CT should not be considered an alternative to CTA or standard angiography for the definitive diagnosis of mesenteric ischemia. Once the diagnosis is considered seriously, all testing and consultation should be arranged in parallel rather than sequentially.

### COMPUTED TOMOGRAPHY

Early CT findings of acute arterial ischemia are poorly sensitive and nonspecific; late findings identify disease in patients with prolonged ischemia and probable necrosis (**Table 34.4**). CT is the imaging test of choice only for mesenteric vein thrombosis, for which it has a diagnostic accuracy of 90%.[6] Angiography may be avoided when the diagnosis of SMV thrombosis is confirmed by standard CT, although it may still be used for catheter placement and local papaverine infusion.

### OTHER IMAGING MODALITIES

Magnetic resonance angiography (MRA) with gadolinium enhancement is useful for evaluation of the proximal celiac trunk and SMA. MRA less accurately identifies disease of the IMA, peripheral vessel disease, and NOMI. The findings are similar to those with CT. In the future, rapid MRA may replace angiography for the diagnosis of ischemic bowel disease.

**Table 34.4 Computed Tomography Findings in Ischemic Bowel Disease**

| DISEASE | FINDINGS |
|---|---|
| Arterial ischemia: | |
| Early | No specific findings |
| Late | Bowel wall thickening<br>Luminal dilation<br>Pneumatosis<br>Mesenteric and portal venous gas |
| Mesenteric vein thrombosis | Lack of opacification of the mesenteric veins after intravenous administration of a contrast agent<br>Central lucency in the superior mesenteric vein lumen<br>Congestion of collateral veins<br>Thickened mesentery<br>Bowel wall thickening |

Data from Burns BJ, Brandt LJ. Intestinal ischemia. Gastroenterol Clin North Am 2003;32:1127-43.

Duplex ultrasonography can assess flow and thrombosis in the SMA or the portal vein. Ultrasonography is frequently limited by the patient's symptoms, condition, and abdominal distention. It is accurate only for evaluation of proximal vessel disease; false-negative results are common in cases of NOMI or distal disease.

Plain radiographs have no role in the evaluation of acute ischemic disease but are frequently ordered to quickly assess for the presence of processes such as a perforated viscus and free air. Plain film findings are usually normal early in the course of illness. Late findings suggest mucosal edema and hemorrhage and include bowel wall thickening, ileus, and thumbprinting, which describes the appearance of bowel wall edema, as though a thumb had been pressed into the bowel wall and caused an indentation. Pneumatosis intestinalis, the presence of gas in the bowel wall, may also be seen. Air in the portal venous system may likewise be seen (**Fig. 34.2**). Late findings are associated with a poor prognosis.

## LABORATORY STUDIES

No laboratory studies are confirmatory of mesenteric ischemia. Delaying diagnostic imaging by waiting for laboratory results decreases survival. Laboratory abnormalities are nonspecific and occur late in disease (**Box 34.2**)[4,7,9]; their absence in no way rules out acute ischemia.[5,9]

An elevated serum amylase level is commonly noted with bowel infarction and sometimes leads to an incorrect diagnosis of pancreatitis. The EP should beware of the presence of elevated amylase when the serum lipase value is normal. Diffuse elevation of liver enzymes is seen with hepatic involvement and ischemia.

Levels of ischemia-modified albumin increase in AMI, as well as in several other vascular diseases; their potential role in early diagnosis remains undefined.[10]

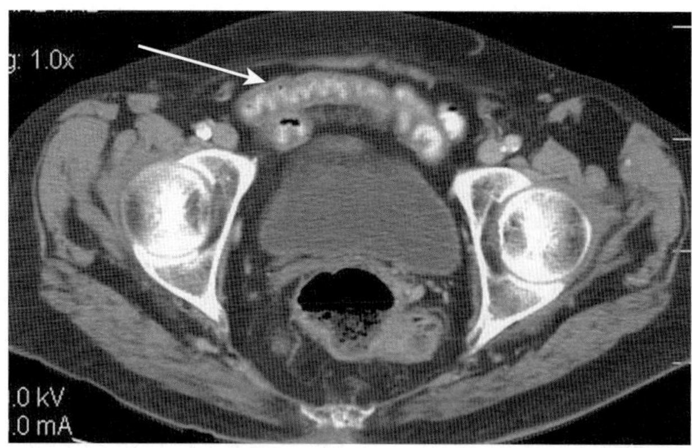

**Fig. 34.2 Pneumatosis intestinalis.** A computed tomography scan shows intramural gas (*arrow*) in the bowel wall caused by bowel infarction from a superior mesenteric artery embolus. (From Hendrickson M, Narpast TR. Abdominal surgical emergencies in the elderly. Emerg Med Clin North Am 2003;21:937-69.)

**BOX 34.2 Laboratory Abnormalities in Late-Stage Mesenteric Ischemia**

Leukocytosis (white blood cell count > 15,000 cells/mm$^3$)
Metabolic acidemia
Elevated serum lactate
Elevated D-dimer
Elevated serum and peritoneal amylase (with normal lipase)
Bacteremia

**TIPS AND TRICKS**

Suspect the disease, especially in the elderly.
Do not delay obtaining imaging or consultation while waiting for laboratory test results.
Rectal findings are often normal.
An elevated serum amylase value may suggest bowel infarction, *not* pancreatitis.
A patient with a history of deep vein thrombosis is at risk for superior mesenteric vein thrombosis, which tends to develop less acutely than other causes of ischemia.
Bowel ischemia promotes acidosis, lethargy, and confusion in the elderly; altered mental status complicates up to 30% of cases.

## TREATMENT

Early surgical consultation is a high priority in patients with suspected mesenteric ischemia. Initial ED management should include volume resuscitation, treatment of contributing cardiac abnormalities (dysrhythmias, heart failure, hypotension), and administration of broad-spectrum antibiotics (**Box 34.3**). Administration of antibiotics decreases the infectious complications of bowel infarction when they are given early to patients with suspected ischemia.[6] The most difficult process for the EP is to see past the present crisis and perform a complete and thorough evaluation of the patient; atrial fibrillation with a rapid ventricular response is a common finding, but hypotension and the altered mental status attributed to it may actually be due to the resultant mesenteric ischemia and sepsis. Look for and pay attention to the other findings pointing to coexisting diagnosis.

**BOX 34.3 Emergency Department Treatment**

Fluid resuscitation and oxygen supplementation; treat shock as indicated
Apply telemetry monitoring and obtain an electrocardiogram
Broad-spectrum antibiotics to cover bowel flora
Nasogastric tube and Foley catheter
Address comorbid conditions with specific treatment
Surgery consultation as soon as the diagnosis is strongly suspected

Blood tests and radiographs might be ordered to exclude other causes during the wait for surgical consultation and angiography. Placement of a nasogastric tube reduces abdominal distention and may improve the symptoms; nothing should be given by mouth. Blood typing and cross-matching should be performed in the expectation that the patient will undergo surgery. Central venous pressure monitoring may be useful to ensure adequate volume resuscitation in critically ill patients.

Surgical exploration is mandatory when peritonitis is present to remove necrotic bowel and restore blood flow via arterial bypass or embolectomy. A second-look procedure is generally performed 12 to 24 hours after the first operation to evaluate for additional loss of bowel (**Fig. 34.3**).

When peritonitis and gastrointestinal bleeding are not present, thrombolytic agents or vasodilators (papaverine), or both, are useful measures that may avoid surgery. Thrombolytics given within 12 hours of the onset of symptoms may completely resolve a partially obstructing or distal thrombus.

Vasospasm may become irreversible if not addressed early; it can lead to bowel necrosis even after surgical embolectomy or thrombolysis. Papaverine is infused locally at 30 to 60 mg/hr for vasodilation via an IR-placed angiography catheter for all causes of ischemic bowel disease. Papaverine is routinely and safely administered from the preoperative period to several days after surgery. Vasodilation may be used as monotherapy in patients with minor emboli or those who have major emboli but for whom surgery poses a high risk. Reperfusion of vascular structures distal to the obstruction must be demonstrated by angiography.

Placement of intravascular stents is successful in selected cases of SMA thrombosis. Mesenteric vein thrombectomy is similarly useful in certain cases of mesenteric vein thrombosis.

Anticoagulation is routinely administered postoperatively to patients with mesenteric vein thrombosis. Immediate heparinization after surgery decreases the chance of thrombus recurrence from 25% to 13%, prevents disease progression, and reduces mortality from 50% to 13%.[11] With the absence of peritonitis, anticoagulation may be used in lieu of surgery. If deemed successful after close observation, anticoagulation therapy is generally continued for 3 to 6 months.

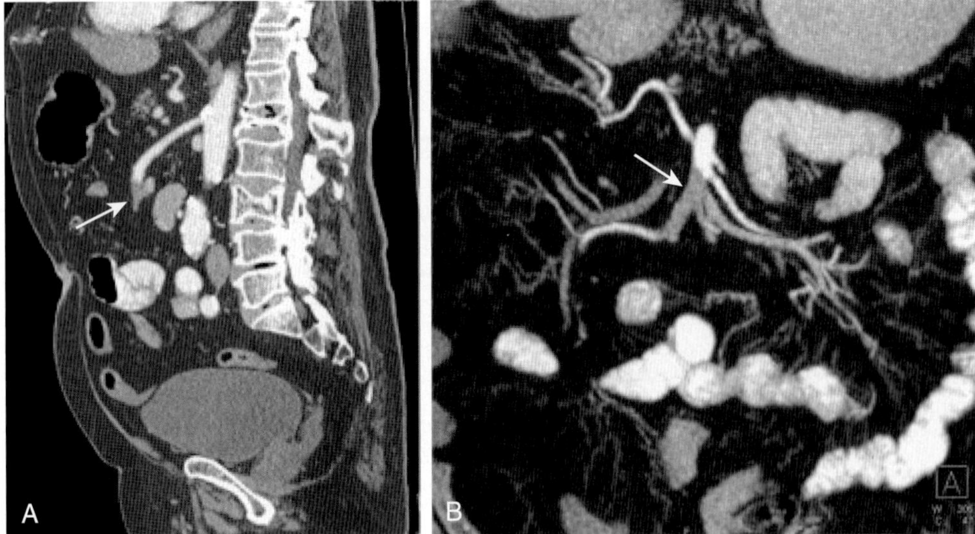

**Fig. 34.3 Eighty-year-old man with acute abdominal pain.** A sagittal multiplanar reconstruction (**A**) and coronal maximum intensity projection (**B**) show a large thrombus in the middle of the superior mesenteric artery *(arrow);* this was embolic, presumably from a cardiogenic source. Surgical embolectomy was performed. (From Horton KM, Fishman EK. CT angiography of the mesenteric circulation. Radiol Clin North Am 2010;48:331-45, viii.)

Additional therapeutic possibilities currently being explored include the use of heparin-binding epithelial growth factor–like growth factor to protect the intestines and other organs from ischemic injury, percutaneous transluminal angioplasty of the SMA, tolazoline and nitroglycerin as local intraarterial infusions, and prostaglandin $E_1$ infusions in patients with NOMI.[12-16]

## FOLLOW-UP, NEXT STEPS IN CARE, AND PATIENT EDUCATION

Critical care admission is required for all patients with ischemic bowel disease regardless of whether they are to undergo surgical or medical management.

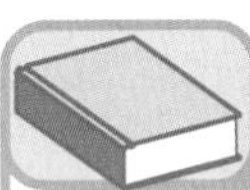

### PATIENT TEACHING TIPS

Have an early discussion with the patient and family regarding the severity of the illness, need for an aggressive approach to diagnosis and treatment, and high mortality.

Determine the patient's and the family's desire for full resuscitation efforts given the mortality rate associated with mesenteric ischemia.

## SUGGESTED READINGS

Bjorck M, Wanhainen A. Nonocclusive mesenteric hypoperfusion syndromes: recognition and treatment. Semin Vasc Surg 2010;23:54-64.

Horton KM, Fishman EK. CT angiography of the mesenteric circulation. Radiol Clin North Am 2010;48:331-45.

Menke J. Diagnostic accuracy of multidetector CT in acute mesenteric ischemia: systematic review and meta-analysis. Radiology 2010;256:93-101.

## REFERENCES

*References can be found on Expert Consult @ www.expertconsult.com.*

# Diverticulitis 35

Kelly P. O'Keefe and Tracy G. Sanson

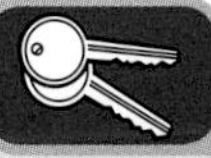

**KEY POINTS**

- Diverticulitis is an acute inflammatory process caused by injury and bacterial proliferation in an existing diverticulum.
- Patients with diverticular disease may be seen in the emergency department with inflammation manifested as abdominal pain or, less commonly, with hematochezia.
- Consider complicated disease (perforation of a diverticulum or abscess formation) and surgical consultation in patients who have peritoneal findings on examination.

## PERSPECTIVE

A *diverticulum* is a saclike protrusion from the wall of the intestines that commonly occurs in the large bowel; *diverticula* is the plural form. *Diverticulosis* connotes the presence of diverticula. *Diverticulitis* refers to a symptomatic inflammatory process involving these structures, which may be characterized as simple (uncomplicated) or complicated. Diverticular hemorrhage is a complication that usually occurs without evidence of inflammatory changes (i.e., without diverticulitis) and represents the most common cause of massive lower gastrointestinal bleeding.

## EPIDEMIOLOGY

The prevalence of diverticulosis is related to age and ranges from 5% at 40 years to 65% by 85 years of age. Approximately 70% of patients with diverticula are asymptomatic, whereas the remainder of patients experience at least one major complication. Twenty percent have diverticulitis and 10% have episodes of bleeding from their diverticula.[1] Diverticulitis accounts for 6% of emergency department (ED) visits for acute abdominal pain in the elderly and occurs more frequently than appendicitis in this age group.[2]

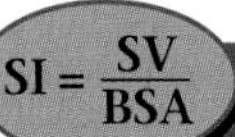


**FACTS AND FORMULAS**

Sixty-five percent of patients 85 years or older have diverticular disease.

## PATHOPHYSIOLOGY

### DIVERTICULOSIS

Diverticula are thought to arise from defects in the muscularis layer of the intestines (**Fig. 35.1**) and are related to abnormalities in muscle tone and increased intraluminal pressure; saclike protrusions eventually form at points of weakness. If stool is caught in these sacs, it becomes inspissated and hardened and causes abrasions of the mucosa that lead to inflammation, although the same end result can occur from pressure differentials alone without the presence of trapped fecal material.

Diverticula generally form at a site of focal weakness in the wall of the bowel, such as the location of blood vessel penetration (vasa recta). The mucosal and submucosal layers herniate through the muscular layer of the intestine, with only a covering of serosa remaining. This leads to an inherent weakness in the diverticular sac relative to the normal bowel. Only thinned layers of mucosa protect blood vessels, which are subject to stretching and thinning of their media, thereby predisposing to weakness and rupture of the vascular tissue.

The left side of the colon is the most common site for diverticulosis in patients with westernized diets and lifestyle. Right-sided diverticula occur more frequently in certain Asian populations. Right-sided diverticula have a higher rate of hemorrhage because of anatomic differences in their development.[3] Small bowel diverticula occur most commonly in the duodenum, where they are predominantly asymptomatic. About 20% of small bowel diverticula occur in the jejunum or ileum; complications develop in these diverticula at rates three times greater than in duodenal diverticula.[4]

A low-fiber diet and constipation may contribute to the development of diverticular disease. High-fiber diets that prevent constipation clearly lead to fewer relapses of diverticulitis and less frequent complications. Lack of physical activity and advanced age are both believed to increase the incidence of the disease. Men and women are affected equally.

### DIVERTICULITIS

Diverticulitis arises from the initial microperforation of a diverticulum (**Table 35.1**).[5] The process starts with blockage of the colonic opening of the diverticulum or by direct contact with food and fecal particles lodged in the affected portion of the bowel. Increased intraluminal or direct local pressure causes erosion of the diverticular wall, which leads to inflammatory changes, focal necrosis, and eventually perforation. The process is generally mild and limited by local pericolic fat and mesentery. Virtually all cases of diverticulitis involve perforation of the intestines, with the course of the resultant

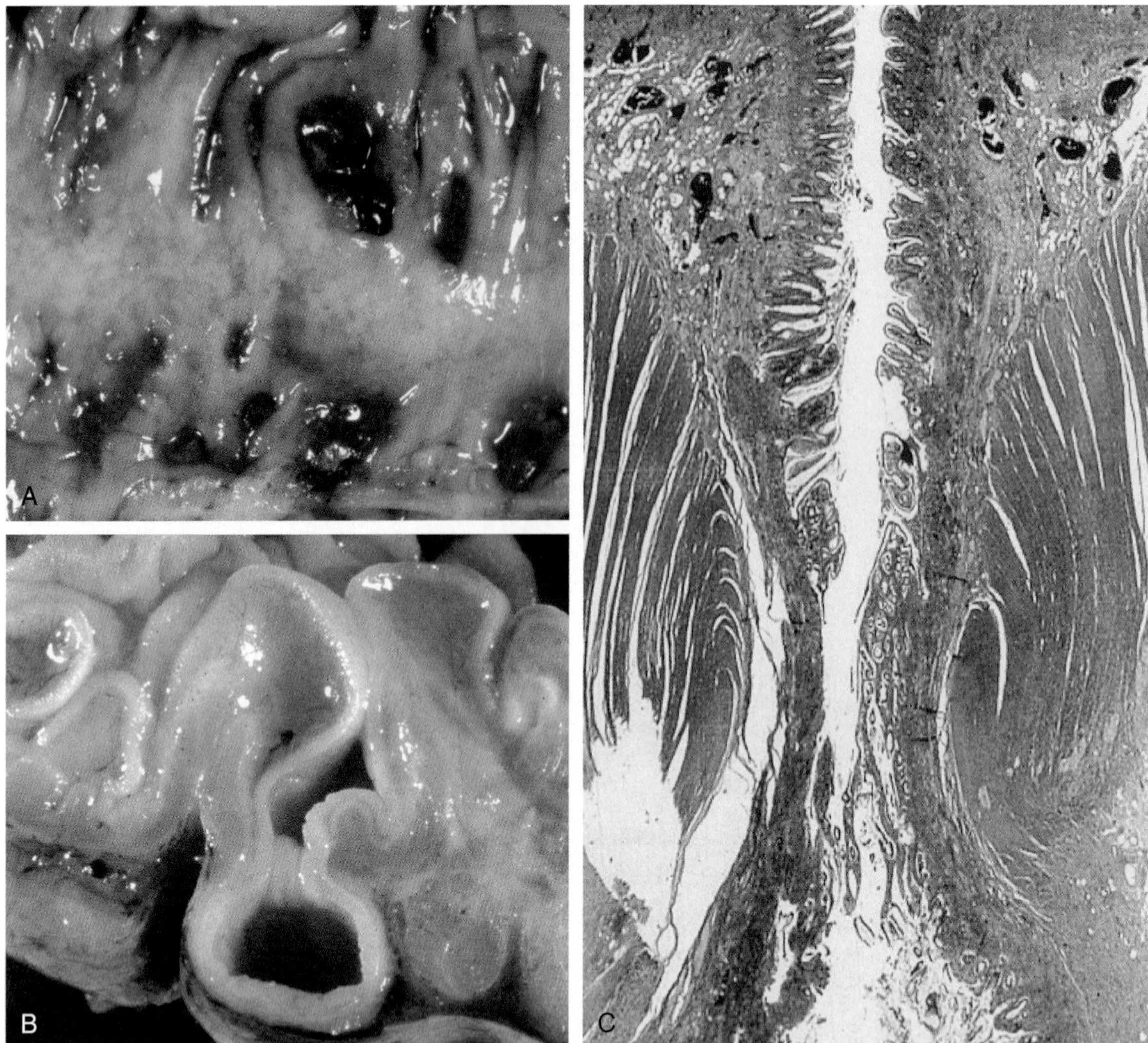


**Fig. 35.1 Sigmoid diverticular disease. A,** Stool-filled diverticula are regularly arranged. **B,** Cross section showing an outpouching of mucosa beneath the muscularis propria. **C,** Low-power photomicrograph of a sigmoid diverticulum showing protrusion of the mucosa and submucosa through the muscularis propria. (From Kumar V, Abbas AK, Fausto N, Aster J. Robbins and Cotran pathologic basis of disease, professional edition. 8th ed. Philadelphia: Saunders; 2009.)

**Table 35.1 Classification of the Severity of Colonic Diverticulitis**

| STAGE | DEFINITION |
|---|---|
| 1 | Small, confined pericolic abscesses |
| 2 | Larger purulent collections |
| 3 | Generalized suppurative peritonitis |
| 4 | Fecal peritonitis |

Adapted from Hinchey EG, Schaal PGH, Richards GK. Treatment of perforated diverticular disease of the colon. Adv Surg 1978;12:85-109.

illness determined by the extent of this perforation. Complicated diverticulitis refers to regional spread of the inflammatory process by the formation of larger abscesses, a fistula with adjacent organs, or peritonitis (**Fig. 35.2**).[1,5] Patients with purulent peritonitis have a mortality rate of 6%, which rises to 35% when fecal soilage of the peritoneal cavity occurs. Patients with diverticular disease occasionally have segmental colitis of the sigmoid colon, probably from fecal stasis or localized ischemia. The effects can be mild or may resemble those of inflammatory bowel disease.[1]

## PRESENTING SIGNS AND SYMPTOMS

### HISTORY AND PHYSICAL EXAMINATION

A focused history and physical examination are important in making the diagnosis of diverticular disease. Essential historical elements are bowel habits, diet, elucidation of classic symptoms, and previous occurrence. Physical examination should assess for hemodynamic stability, the presence of peritonitis, and occult or obvious hemorrhage. Complete abdominal, genitourinary, and rectal examinations must be documented.

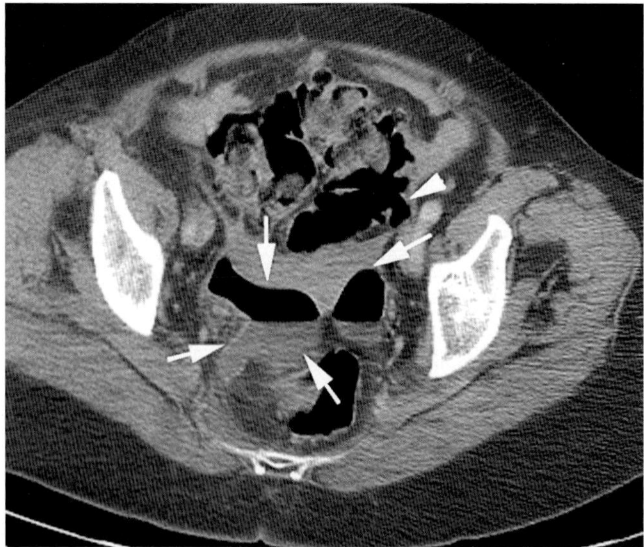

**Fig. 35.2 Computed tomography scan of diverticulitis with a large pelvic abscess containing an air-fluid level *(arrows)* indicating a communicating abscess.** Note the diverticulum outlined by air *(arrowhead)*. (From Adam A. Grainger & Allison's diagnostic radiology. 5th ed. Philadelphia: Churchill Livingstone; 2008.)

**BOX 35.1 Differential Diagnosis for Suspected Diverticulitis**

The following diagnoses should be considered in order of urgency:

- Abdominal aortic aneurysm: rupture or expansion
- Mesenteric ischemia
- Perforated ulcer
- Ruptured ectopic pregnancy
- Incarcerated or strangulated hernia
- Salpingitis, tuboovarian abscess
- Ovarian or testicular torsion
- Appendicitis
- Pelvic mass torsion
- Ischemic colitis
- Inflammatory bowel disease
- Pancreatitis
- Ruptured ovarian cyst
- Renal colic
- Biliary colic
- Also atypical manifestations of inferior wall myocardial infarction, pulmonary embolism, pneumonia, diabetic ketoacidosis, and acute glaucoma

The classic manifestation of diverticulitis involves several days of worsening left lower quadrant abdominal pain. Low-grade fever commonly develops but is not uniformly present. Patients typically reports similar past episodes of pain and fever. Other common symptoms are nausea, vomiting, constipation (50%), and diarrhea (40%). Urinary symptoms (dysuria, urgency, frequency) caused by local inflammation of the bladder occur in only 10% of patients. Fever is often absent in elderly patients, and a rectal temperature may be required for detection of fever in this population. Dementia, polypharmacy, and other causes of chronically altered mental status may complicate diagnostic accuracy; imaging should be used liberally in these patients. Signs of peritonitis may be minimal or absent in even the most fully competent and communicative older patient.

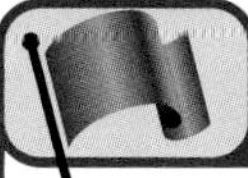

**RED FLAGS**

Hospitalize patients with signs and symptoms of systemic illness, even without clear peritonitis.

Consider risk factors for abdominal aortic aneurysm and mesenteric ischemia.

Rectal findings can be negative or normal in a patient with episodic diverticular bleeding.

## DIFFERENTIAL DIAGNOSIS

**Box 35.1** presents the differential diagnosis for suspicion of diverticulitis.

## DIAGNOSTIC TESTING

### LABORATORY TESTS

Leukocytosis is noted in only half of patients with diverticulitis. Disease severity, advancing age, and underlying health status affect the white blood cell count; it may not be elevated in elderly patients or the chronically ill even with significant acute disease. Similarly, hemoglobin levels may not accurately reflect the severity of recent diverticular bleeding. Urinalysis should be performed to evaluate any urinary symptoms; abnormalities may reflect inflammatory changes, infection, or contamination via colovesicular fistula formation. Blood cultures should be obtained with any suspicion of sepsis.

Additional laboratory testing is helpful in excluding other processes. Standard tests for the evaluation of abdominal pain should be ordered when indicated, including a complete blood count, metabolic panel, liver function tests, and lipase. An elevated serum lipase value should reliably diagnose acute pancreatitis. Typing and crossmatching of blood should be performed in patients with hematochezia or signs of a surgical abdomen. Coagulation tests are indicated for bleeding patients, for those taking anticoagulant medications, and for critically ill patients at risk for disseminated intravascular coagulopathy. A pregnancy test is required for any woman of childbearing age who complains of abdominal pain.

### IMAGING

Plain radiographs of the chest and abdomen are useful to evaluate for the presence of other processes but do not assist in the diagnosis of diverticular disease. Free air is occasionally present in patients with a perforated diverticulum. Evidence of ileus or obstruction may be seen with complicated disease.

Computed tomography (CT) of the abdomen and pelvis is the test of choice for confirming the diagnosis of diverticulitis, assessing its severity and complications, and directing intervention. CT findings for and complications of diverticular disease are listed in **Box 35.2**.

Contrast enema studies are less expensive than CT and are better able to evaluate the lumen of the colon. They are generally performed with water-soluble agents rather than barium given the high likelihood of perforation in patients with

**BOX 35.2 Computed Tomography in Diverticulitis**

**CT Features of Acute Diverticulitis***

Increased soft tissue density with pericolic fat changes (98%)
Colonic diverticula (84%)
Bowel wall thickening (70%)
Soft tissue fluid collections or abscess (35%)

**Complications of Diverticulitis Found on CT**

Peritonitis (diffuse inflammatory changes, scattered loculated fluid collections)
Fistula formation
Bowel obstruction
Diverticular disease is indistinguishable from carcinoma of the colon in up to 10% of patients

*Data from Young-Fadok T, Pemberton JH. Clinical manifestations and diagnosis of colonic diverticular disease. UpToDate March 2005. Available at www.uptodate.com.

**BOX 35.3 Treatment: Antibiotics for Diverticulitis**

Antibiotic therapy should be directed against the usual colonic flora, particularly gram-negative rods and anaerobes (especially *Escherichia coli* and *Bacteroides fragilis*). Suitable regimens are as follows:

- Piperacillin-tazobactam
- Ticarcillin-clavulanate
- Ampicillin, gentamicin, and metronidazole
- Imipenem-cilastin or other carbapenems
- Ampicillin-sulbactam (outpatient)
- Quinolone and metronidazole (outpatient)
- Sulfamethoxazole-trimethoprim and metronidazole (outpatient)
- Cefazolin and metronidazole (outpatient)*
- Ceftriaxone and metronidazole

*Clindamycin is an acceptable alternative to metronidazole for the coverage of anaerobes.

diverticulitis. Contrast enema studies provide little information, however, about complications of diverticular disease.

Compression ultrasonography is a relatively new diagnostic procedure for diverticular disease. Ultrasonography may be used to serially assess fluid collections or to assist in the transrectal or transvaginal drainage of abscesses. The "pseudokidney" sign (thickening of the bowel wall that mimics the appearance of a kidney) may represent acute diverticulitis and aid in rapid diagnosis by ultrasound. This finding, however, is not specific to diverticular disease.[6]

Colonoscopy and flexible sigmoidoscopy have limited roles in evaluating diverticulitis in the acute setting. All patients with diverticulitis should be referred for outpatient colonoscopy when their acute illness has subsided. These modalities allow direct visualization of the colonic lumen and biopsy of any lesions. Colonoscopy remains an important initial diagnostic procedure for patients with acute diverticular bleeding.

## TREATMENT

The majority of patients with acute, uncomplicated diverticulitis respond to bowel rest and antibiotics (**Box 35.3**).[6] The remaining patients require various levels of intervention ranging from percutaneous drainage of abscesses to laparoscopic or other surgical procedures. The surgical mortality rate ranges from 1% to 5%, depending on comorbid conditions and the severity of disease.

Fluid resuscitation is needed in patients with dehydration, peritonitis, complicated disease, and significant bleeding. Patients with evidence of peritonitis or other disease complications require surgical consultation and admission. Patients with complicated disease should take nothing by mouth. Nasogastric decompression should be used in patients with symptomatic ileus.

Pain medication is necessary in most patients with acute diverticulitis. Narcotic analgesics may slow recovery because they promote constipation; patients should be warned to limit the use of these medicines or use adjunctive bulk laxatives. Patients with significant pain should be admitted to the hospital. Titration of pain medication should begin in the ED as indicated by the patient's reported pain scale, not based on the timing of examination by the consultant surgeon. Fentanyl is easily titrated in parenteral doses of 25 to 50 mcg, is short acting, and causes minimal histamine release or hemodynamic instability.

## CONSULTATION

Surgical consultation should be obtained immediately for patients with peritonitis or a vascular catastrophe. Consultants should be notified early in the treatment of elderly or immunocompromised patients, as well as for patients with clear indications of complicated disease. Twenty-five percent of patients with a new diagnosis of diverticulitis have complicated disease and require surgical intervention. Patients with uncomplicated disease may require only follow-up with a surgeon on an outpatient basis. One third of these patients eventually require surgery.[6]

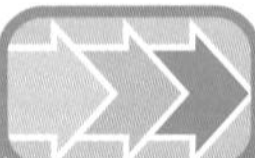

**PRIORITY ACTIONS**

Establish intravenous access for the management of diverticulitis.
Obtain a pertinent history and perform a physical examination, including rectal and genitourinary examination.
Consider life-threatening conditions in the differential diagnosis.
Obtain surgical consultation for any patients with evidence of peritonitis.
Arrange for radiographic and laboratory analysis.

## COMPLICATIONS

Intestinal obstruction is a rare complication of diverticular disease and generally arises from the small bowel rather than the large bowel. Obstructions result from chronically diseased bowel and adhesion formation. Recurrent attacks of acute disease can cause strictures and narrowing of the lumen of the colon as well, but subsequent complete obstruction of the large bowel is uncommon.

Overall complications from diverticulosis of the small bowel are unusual when compared with those from disease of the colon. Rarely reported problems include massive gastrointestinal hemorrhage from an arteriovenous malformation located in the submucosa of a jejunal diverticulum, a diverticulum-induced ileoabdominal fistula, and cases of small bowel obstruction with volvulus.[4,7-9]

Duodenal diverticula have been associated with a higher rate of common bile duct stones identified on endoscopic retrograde cholangiopancreatography.[10,11] This finding may be due to higher rates of bacterial contamination in the biliary system in patients with small bowel diverticula.[12] Rarely, congenital intraluminal diverticula may lead to recurrent abdominal pain and obstructive symptoms.

Jejunoileal diverticula occur in 1% of the population and may cause malabsorption from chronic bacterial overgrowth. Other symptoms include early satiety, bloating, and chronic upper abdominal discomfort.

Colonic diverticular bleeding is generally manifested as painless hematochezia that is self-limited. The amount can be voluminous, with the blood being maroon or bright red. Because bleeding commonly occurs without other signs of inflammation, the abdominal findings may be unremarkable. Only 5% of patients with diverticular bleeding have massive, hemodynamically significant gastrointestinal hemorrhage. These patients are typically older than 60 years and have comorbid conditions.

Ninety percent of all diverticular fistulas arise from the sigmoid portion of the colon. Classically involved organs are the bladder, vagina, skin, and noncontiguous bowel. Colovesicular fistulas occur more commonly in men than in women because of interposition of the uterus between the colon and bladder; fistulas involving the ureter or fallopian tubes are unusual. Enterovascular fistulas may lead to gas in the mesenteric and hepatic portal veins, and septic thrombophlebitis (pylephlebitis) may occur as well.

## FOLLOW-UP, NEXT STEPS IN CARE, AND PATIENT EDUCATION

Patients with uncomplicated diverticulitis can be considered for discharge on the basis of hydration status, ability to tolerate oral fluids, pain level, comorbid conditions, immune function, home support, age, reliability of follow-up, and ability to obtain antibiotics and take them as required. Those with high fevers and significant leukocytosis should be admitted because of the potential for bacteremia or undetected complications. Patients with complex underlying medical diseases should undergo a period of inpatient observation if there is any concern that the disease may progress to perforation or sepsis.

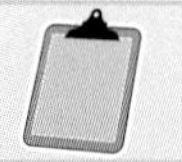

### DOCUMENTATION

Duration of symptoms, onset, severity
Previous occurrence, history of diverticulosis
Melena or hematochezia
Risk factors, bowel habits
Vital signs
Findings on cardiac, abdominal, genitourinary, rectal, and vascular examination
Document multiple repeated examinations
Emergency department course: times of consultations, discussions with family and consultants, availability of testing, delays
Document and address other potentially lethal diagnoses (abdominal aortic aneurysm, mesenteric ischemia)

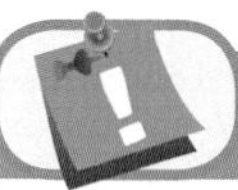

### TIPS AND TRICKS

Signs of serious disease or peritonitis may be masked in elderly patients.
Right-sided diverticulitis is often confused with appendicitis.
Patients with signs of localized peritonitis require hospital admission.

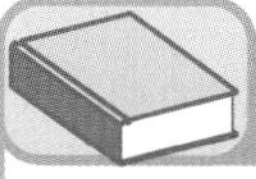

### PATIENT TEACHING TIPS

Return for worsening pain, fever, vomiting, bloody stool
Treatment of constipation: avoid frequent narcotic use
Complications of disease: abscess, perforation, fistula, bleeding
Need for antibiotic treatment
Complications of pain medications (constipation)
Dietary considerations: high-fiber diet shown to decrease complications associated with diverticular disease
Candidates for outpatient treatment should be restricted to consumption of clear liquids for several days; the diet should be advanced cautiously as tolerated

## SUGGESTED READINGS

Bauer VP. Emergency management of diverticulitis. Clin Colon Rectal Surg 2009;22:161-8.
Peterson MA. Disorders of the large intestine. In Marx J, Hockberger R, Walls R, editors. Rosen's textbook of emergency medicine: concepts and clinical practice. 7th ed. Philadelphia: Mosby; 2009.
Touzios JG, Dozois EJ. Diverticulosis and acute diverticulitis. Gastroenterol Clin 2009;38:513-25.
Young-Fadok T, Pemberton JH. Treatment of acute diverticulitis. UpToDate September 2010. Available at www.uptodate.com.

## REFERENCES

***References can be found on Expert Consult @ www.expertconsult.com.***

# 36 Inflammatory Bowel Disease

*James Ahn*

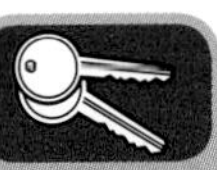

**KEY POINTS**

- Acute exacerbations of inflammatory bowel disease are characterized by abdominal pain, nausea, vomiting, diarrhea, and gastrointestinal bleeding.
- Life-threatening complications include bowel obstruction, hemorrhagic shock, toxic megacolon, malabsorption, abscess formation, and sepsis.
- Treatment with analgesics, intravenous hydration, antiemetics, and electrolyte replacement should occur in parallel with appropriate diagnostic imaging and laboratory studies.
- Antibiotics, steroids, and immunosuppressant therapies can be used in conjunction with specialty consultation.
- Hypersensitivity reactions may result from long-term immunomodulator and antiinflammatory therapies.
- Patients receiving immunosuppressant therapy have increased susceptibility to opportunistic infections.

## PERSPECTIVE

Approximately 1 million people in the United States suffer from inflammatory bowel disease (IBD). The two major forms of IBD are Crohn disease and ulcerative colitis (UC). The incidence of both disease processes is similar, although Crohn disease appears to be increasing.[1] Each disease may relapse and remit, with exacerbations that often require emergency care and hospitalization.

IBD has a familial predilection, with an absolute risk of 7% among first-degree relatives.[2,3] Up to a fifth of patients with IBD have an affected first-degree family member. Ashkenazi Jewish populations continue to have the highest documented incidence per capita of any group in the world. Hispanic and African American populations have a lower incidence of IBD than the Caucasian population does.[4]

The age at onset of IBD is bimodal. The greatest numbers of new cases are diagnosed in patients 15 to 35 years of age. Classically, a second peak is observed during the sixth decade of life.[5] Advances in diagnostic testing have probably contributed to an overall rise in the number of new cases of IBD, as well as to the identification of the disease in younger patients.

## PATHOPHYSIOLOGY

### CROHN DISEASE

#### *Pathology*

Crohn disease is characterized by segmental, transmural, granulomatous inflammatory changes that can occur anywhere along the gastrointestinal tract from the mouth to the perianal area. Disease of the terminal ileum is present in 80% of patients with Crohn disease, and 50% of patients have ileocolitis. Approximately 33% and 20% of patients demonstrate only ileal and colonic involvement, respectively. The finding of skip lesions between areas of normal bowel and cobblestoning of the intestinal mucosa is classic for Crohn disease. Chronic inflammation commonly leads to bowel stenosis.

#### *Epidemiology*

The yearly incidence of Crohn disease is between 3 and 14 cases per 100,000 people in North America, with a disease prevalence of 26 to 201 cases per 100,000. The incidence rate of Crohn disease has risen steadily, with the highest incidence found in North America and Northern Europe. Crohn disease is more common in Caucasian and Latino people in the United States than in African Americans, Native Americans, and Asian Americans. Women have a 20% to 30% higher incidence than men do.

The cold chain hypothesis suggests that the rise in incidence of Crohn disease has been associated with the development of home refrigeration techniques. Bacteria that thrive in refrigerated foods, such as *Yersinia* and *Listeria*, are thought to play a role in stimulation of the immune and inflammatory responses that ultimately lead to Crohn disease.[6] Exacerbations of Crohn disease may be worsened during periods of higher physiologic or mental stress.[7] Other environmental factors such as cigarette smoking, use of nonsteroidal antiinflammatory drugs (NSAIDs), increased refined sugar intake, increased dietary fat, and decreased fiber intake have been linked to the development of Crohn disease.[8-11]

Genetic mutations and chromosomal variants have also been linked to the development of Crohn disease. Specific alterations in the *NOD2* gene are associated with a 20-fold increase in the likelihood of Crohn disease with ileal predilection.[12-15] Patients with Crohn disease may also be HLA-B27 positive.

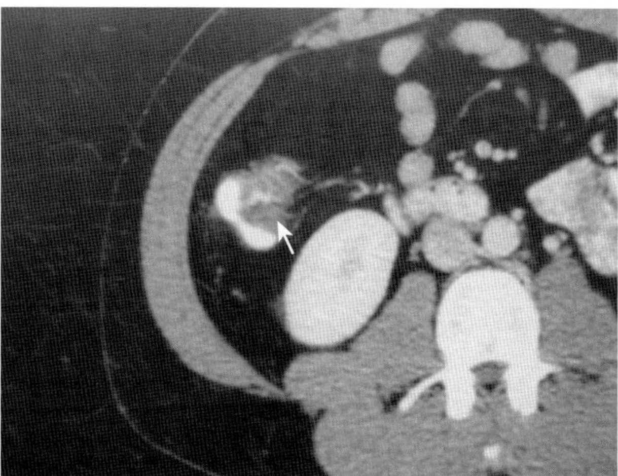

**Fig. 36.1 Computed tomography scan showing terminal ileitis *(arrow)* in a patient with Crohn disease.**

### *Clinical Presentation*

Patients with Crohn disease typically have abdominal pain, fever, diarrhea, and weight loss. Because Crohn disease involves the entire gastrointestinal tract, patients may suffer from oral ulcers, odynophagia, dysphagia, and symptoms of gastric outlet obstruction. Sinus tracts may develop and lead to common complications such as abscesses and fistula formation. Patients with Crohn disease can also have gastrointestinal bleeding, though to a lesser extent than patients with UC. Other complications include bowel obstruction, fissures, malignancy, malabsorption, malnutrition, and hypocalcemia.

Crohn disease is associated with an increased risk for demyelinating diseases, as well as a higher incidence of inflammatory processes such as asthma, arthritis, bronchitis, psoriasis, and pericarditis.[16,17] Approximately 20% of patients with Crohn disease experience one or more of the following extraintestinal manifestations of disease during their lifetimes: ankylosing spondylitis, uveitis, episcleritis, hepatitis, cholelithiasis, pancreatitis, primary sclerosing cholangitis, cholangiocarcinoma, nephrolithiasis, and erythema nodosum (**Fig. 36.1; Box 36.1**).

## ULCERATIVE COLITIS

### *Pathology*

UC is a recurring inflammatory disease confined to the mucosal layer of the colon and rectum only. Areas of inflammation are continuous, not segmental; patients commonly experience ascending disease from the rectum to the colon. Isolated rectal involvement is present in a minority of patients.

## EPIDEMIOLOGY

The yearly incidence of UC is relatively constant—in the United States it is 8 per 100,000 people, with a disease prevalence of 246 cases per 100,000 people.[18,19] The etiology of this disease is unknown, although certain risk factors have been identified. UC is most commonly found in North American and Northern European Caucasian populations. In addition, similar to Crohn disease, development of UC has been linked to the use of NSAIDs, increased refined sugar intake, increased dietary fat, and decreased fiber intake.[9-11] However, cigarette smoking appears to lessen the risk for development of UC.[20]

**BOX 36.1 Differential Diagnosis: Colitis**

Inflammatory bowel disease:
- Crohn disease
- Ulcerative colitis
- Indeterminate colitis

Infectious colitis:
- *Shigella*
- *Amoeba*
- *Giardia*
- *Escherichia coli* O157:H7
- *Yersinia*
- *Campylobacter*
- *Entamoeba histolytica*
- Viral infections
- Mycotic infections

Pseudomembranous colitis (*Clostridium difficile*):
Diverticulitis
Sarcoidosis
Tuberculosis
Proctitis (including sexually transmitted causes):
Collagenous colitis
Irritable bowel syndrome
Food intolerance

### *Clinical Presentation*

Although UC has variable findings, bloody, purulent, and mucoid diarrhea is considered to be the classic manifestation. Fever, weight loss, dehydration, anemia, and hypoalbuminemia are common. Patients may be categorized as having mild disease (60%), moderate disease (25%), or severe disease (15%). Severe disease is defined as six or more bowel movements per day.

Significant lower gastrointestinal bleeding is the most common complication, with 3% of patients with UC having massive hemorrhage. Patients may also have toxic megacolon as a complication of fulminant colitis. Toxic megacolon causes a loss of colonic muscular tone that results in luminal diameters larger than 6 cm—pathologic changes that increase the risk for perforation and mortality. Long-term complications of UC include bowel strictures and the development of colon cancer.

Patients with UC may have extraintestinal complications such as concurrent arthritis, uveitis, erythema nodosum, pyoderma gangrenosum, and progressive liver disease (**Fig. 36.2; Table 36.1**).

# DIAGNOSTIC TESTING

## IMAGING MODALITIES

Most cases of IBD diagnosed in the emergency department (ED) are found via computed tomography (CT) of the abdomen in patients with severe, unexplained abdominal pain. A presumptive diagnosis of IBD can be based on typical CT findings coupled with the appropriate signs and symptoms. CT enterography has been shown to have 100% sensitivity and 95% specificity for detection of small bowel lesions associated with Crohn disease.[21] CT enterography is superior to

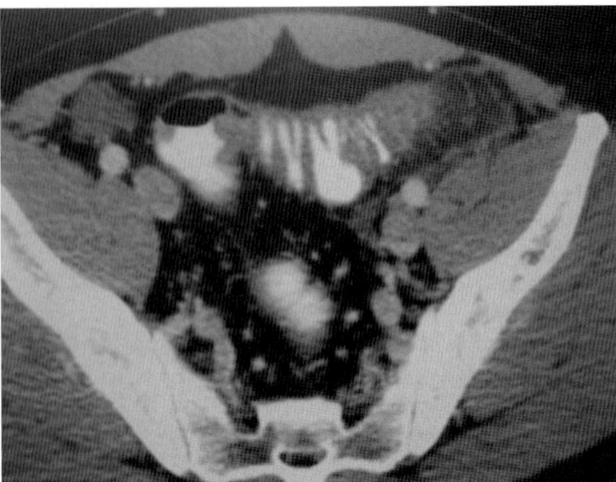

**Fig. 36.2 Computed tomography scan showing colonic wall thickening in a patient with ulcerative colitis.**

standard CT of the abdomen and pelvis in patients with a high pretest probability of Crohn disease (i.e., first-degree family members of patients with IBD). Confirmation of the diagnosis is made by histologic examination of tissue biopsy specimens obtained via inpatient endoscopy or surgery.

Patients seen in the ED with an exacerbation of known IBD do not always require CT. Plain films are generally sufficient to exclude complications such as bowel obstruction and rare perforations. CT should be used to identify abscesses or other intraabdominal disease in patients with peritoneal findings or sepsis.

Other imaging modalities are best used outside the ED. Barium and air-contrast radiographic studies frequently demonstrate classic radiographic evidence of IBD; they are useful tests for obese patients who exceed the weight limit for standard CT scanners. Upper and lower endoscopy allows direct visualization and biopsy of suspected lesions. Technology that enables patients to swallow endoscopic cameras as capsules represents a promising, minimally invasive method to visualize the bowel mucosa.

### LABORATORY TESTS

Laboratory studies have limited value in the ED evaluation of IBD. Most tests serve to exclude complications or alternative diagnoses. A complete blood count can provide a baseline hemoglobin level. Leukocytosis is a nonspecific finding in patients with chronic IBD; marked elevations in the white blood cell count may correlate with new abscess formation, toxic megacolon, sepsis, or corticosteroid therapy. A serum chemistry panel is needed to exclude hypokalemia, hypocalcemia, and electrolyte imbalances in patients with severe vomiting and diarrhea. Hypoalbuminemia is often detected with liver function tests. The erythrocyte sedimentation rate and C-reactive protein levels add little value for guiding ED therapy.

Serologic markers may be used to differentiate Crohn disease from UC. The presence of p-ANCAs (perinuclease-staining antineutrophil cytoplasmic antibodies) is sensitive and predictive of UC, whereas detection of ASCA (anti—*Saccharomyces cerevisiae* antibodies) markers probably predicts Crohn disease. These serologic tests are not indicated for use in the ED.

**Table 36.1 Features of Crohn Disease and Ulcerative Colitis**

| FINDING | CROHN DISEASE | ULCERATIVE COLITIS |
|---|---|---|
| **Location** | | |
| Colonic | Common | Common |
| Rectal | Common | Common |
| Extracolonic | Common | Never |
| Ileal | Common | Never |
| **Signs and Symptoms** | | |
| Fever | Common | Common |
| Diarrhea | Common | Common |
| Vomiting | Variable | Occasional |
| Abdominal pain | Common | Variable |
| Hematochezia | Variable | Common |
| Weight loss | Common | Common |
| Perianal disease | Common | Never |
| **Pathologic Findings** | | |
| Continuity | Discontinuous | Continuous |
| Inflammation | Transmural | Mucosal |
| Oral ulcers | Variable | Never |
| Fissures | Common | Never |
| Fistulas | Variable | Rare |
| Cobblestoning | Common | Never |
| Strictures | Common | Rare |
| **Laboratory Findings** | | |
| Perinuclease-staining antineutrophil cytoplasmic antibody (p-ANCA) positivity | Uncommon | Common |
| Anti-*Saccharomyces cerevisiae* antibody (ASCA) positivity | Common | Uncommon |

## TREATMENT

### GENERAL MANAGEMENT

Exacerbations of IBD are often marked by significant pain, fever, diarrhea, gastrointestinal bleeding, anorexia, and dehydration; severity is most pronounced in patients with chronic disease who seek treatment in the ED because of exacerbations. Management of symptoms should be done in parallel with diagnostic testing. Analgesics, antiemetics, and intravenous hydration should be administered on arrival of the

| Condition | Treatment |
|---|---|
| Colitis or ileocolitis | Oral 5-ASA drug or metronidazole and/or ciprofloxacin —*Continued activity*→ Prednisone —*Continued activity or steroid dependence*→ Immunomodulator —*Continued activity*→ Surgery or infliximab |
| Ileitis | Prednisone —*Continued activity*→ Immunomodulator —*Continued activity*→ Surgery or infliximab |
| Fistula | TPN or immunomodulator or infliximab —*Failure to close*→ Surgery |
| Abscess | Antibiotics, drainage, and resection |
| Obstruction due to inflammation | IV fluids, nasogastric suction, parenteral steroids —*Failure to respond*→ Surgery |
| Obstruction due to scarring | IV fluids, nasogastric suction —*Failure to respond*→ Surgery |
| Perianal disease | Antibiotics and surgical drainage |
| Disease in remission | Maintenance with oral 5-ASA drugs or immunomodulators |

**Fig. 36.3 Treatment algorithm for Crohn disease.** *5-ASA*, 5-Aminosalicylic acid; *IV*, intravenous; *TPN*, total parenteral nutrition. (From Goldman L, Ausiello D, editors. Cecil's textbook of medicine. 22nd ed. Philadelphia: Saunders; 2003.)

| Condition | Treatment |
|---|---|
| Proctitis | 5-ASA enemas or 5-ASA suppositories or oral 5-ASA drugs or corticosteroid enemas —*Continued activity*→ Prednisone or immunomodulators —*Continued activity*→ Colectomy |
| Mild to moderate pancolitis | Oral 5-ASA drugs —*Continued activity*→ Prednisone —*Continued activity or steroid dependence*→ Immunomodulators or colectomy |
| Severe or fulminant pancolitis | Parenteral steroids —*Continued activity*→ Cyclosporine or colectomy |
| Disease in remission | Maintenance with oral 5-ASA drugs |

**Fig. 36.4 Treatment algorithm for ulcerative colitis.** *5-ASA*, 5-Aminosalicylic acid. (From Goldman L, Ausiello D, editors. Cecil's textbook of medicine. 22nd ed. Philadelphia: Saunders; 2003.)

patient. In the setting of refractory emesis or bowel obstruction, nasogastric tube decompression may provide substantial relief. Identification and treatment of electrolyte imbalances, concurrent infections, and hemorrhage should precede hospital admission.

Immunomodulator, antiinflammatory, and antibiotic agents should be given in consultation with the patient's gastroenterologist. Because these medications often require long-term administration and dose adjustments, complex drug regimens are typical. Treatment algorithms for Crohn disease and UC are summarized in **Figures 36.3 and 36.4**.

## COMMON MEDICATIONS

Sulfasalazine is a first-line oral agent used for the treatment of mild to moderate IBD. Colonic bacteria cleave the drug into 5-aminosalicylic acid (5-ASA) and sulfapyridine. 5-ASA acts directly on intraluminal lesions without systemic absorption. Although its mechanism of action is still unclear, 5-ASA probably inhibits leukocyte chemotaxis, as well as prostaglandin and leukotriene production. Sulfapyridine is a toxic by-product responsible for a variety of dose-related adverse effects (nausea, vomiting, diarrhea, headache, abdominal pain, arthralgias) and hypersensitivity reactions (rash, bone marrow suppression, fever, pancreatitis, liver disease, nephrotoxicity). Sulfasalazine at doses of 4 g or more per day should produce a clinical response within 3 to 4 weeks. Oral, enema, and suppository preparations of sulfasalazine are available.

Oral steroids improve mild to moderate IBD symptoms within days to weeks and are used in patients who do not improve with 5-ASA agents. Prednisone, 40 mg/day, is an acceptable starting dose; equivalent parenteral administration should be reserved for severe disease or for patients who cannot tolerate oral medications. Long-term corticosteroid therapy at a low maintenance dose is often required. Patients with small bowel obstruction secondary to terminal ileitis may have a response to early treatment with steroids, thereby reducing the need for surgical intervention (**Fig. 36.5**).

Patients with Crohn disease can benefit from maintenance therapy with azathioprine or its active metabolite 6-mercaptopurine (6-MP). These immunomodulator drugs inhibit lymphocytic proliferation and subsequent activation of the inflammatory cascades. Their onset of action is 3 to 5 months in most cases. 6-MP is reserved for patients with disease refractory to other medications. Adverse effects include pancreatitis, leukopenia, hepatitis, and lymphoma. Methotrexate is another immunosuppressant that is used for Crohn disease refractory to 6-MP or in patients exhibiting Crohn disease–related arthritis. Adverse effects of methotrexate include leukopenia, anemia, thrombocytopenia, hepatobiliary complications, pericarditis, and thrombosis.

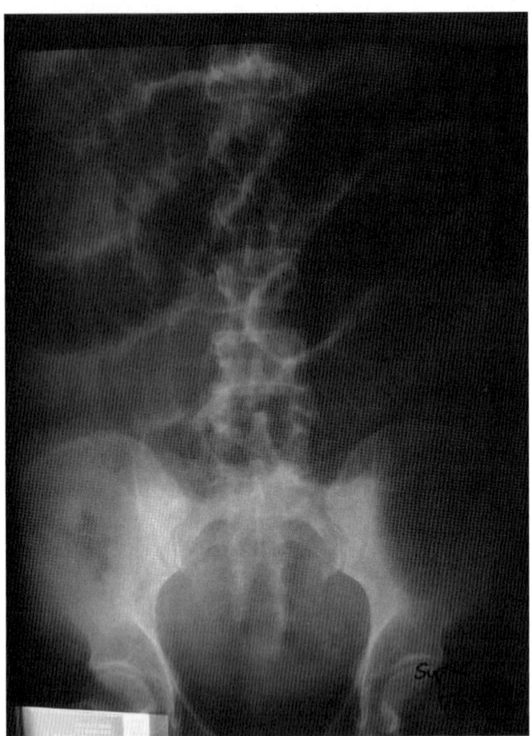

**Fig. 36.5 Plain radiograph showing small bowel obstruction as a result of terminal ileitis.**

Infliximab (Remicade) is an inhibitor of tumor necrosis factor that is administered intravenously for the control of severe, refractory Crohn disease. Complications of infliximab therapy are sepsis, hepatotoxicity, pneumonia, lupuslike syndrome, hypersensitivity reactions, lymphoma, leukopenia, and demyelinating disease. Infliximab, as well as cyclosporine, may be beneficial in the treatment of patients awaiting surgical intervention. Because of the strong immunosuppressant nature of certain IBD therapies, a high index suspicion for opportunistic infections must be maintained.

Antibiotics may be needed to treat patients with Crohn disease. Antibiotics are indicated for active Crohn disease and pouchitis; promising results have been shown for fistulizing Crohn disease.[22-25] The antibiotics most commonly used are a combination of metronidazole and ciprofloxacin. The utility of these agents for UC has not been proved.

### SURGERY

Seventy-five percent of patients with Crohn disease require surgery within the first 20 years after diagnosis. Emergency consultation should be obtained for patients with complications of IBD-related surgery or for patients with suspected life-threatening complications, including massive hemorrhage, abscess formation, obstruction, toxic megacolon, and perforation. Intravenous hydration, nasogastric decompression, and broad-spectrum antibiotic therapy should be given in preparation for surgery.

## DISPOSITION

Hospital admission is required for moderate to severe exacerbations of IBD. Patients with severe dehydration, systemic infection, abscesses, or potentially life-threatening complications such as hemorrhage, toxic megacolon, perforation, and bowel obstruction must be managed as inpatients. Discharge should be reserved for patients with mild disease in whom oral hydration and pain control are easily attained. Changes in medication and disposition should be decided in consultation with a gastroenterologist.

## SUGGESTED READINGS

Podolsky DK. Inflammatory bowel disease. N Engl J Med 2002;347:417-29.

Rothfuss KS, Strange EF, Herrlinger KR. Extraintestinal manifestations and complications in inflammatory bowel diseases. World J Gastroenterol 2006;12:4819-31.

## REFERENCES

***References can be found on Expert Consult @ www.expertconsult.com.***

# Constipation 37

*Kathleen S. Schrank*

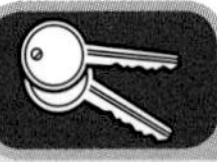

**KEY POINTS**

- Constipation has a variety of meanings to patients. Ask about pain, stool frequency, stool hardness, and difficulty with passage.
- Dangerous conditions such as early bowel obstruction can mimic functional constipation, especially in the elderly. Red flags include severe pain, vomiting, fever, gastrointestinal bleeding, acute onset without an obvious cause (e.g., opiate use), peritoneal signs, and significant systemic symptoms.
- In most patients, constipation has a functional, nonemergency cause that is often related to medications or lifestyle habits such as dietary fiber intake, fluid intake, and toileting.
- The treatment goal for uncomplicated constipation consists of initial cleansing, a maintenance plan, and preventive lifestyle changes.
- A wide range of underlying conditions, such as malignancy and systemic disorders, can cause constipation. Primary care follow-up is warranted.

## PERSPECTIVE

Constipation is a common symptom causing visits to the emergency department (ED) and rarely requires extensive ED evaluation or hospital admission. Associated signs and symptoms determine the optimal ED approach to evaluation and management. Although the majority of these patients will have chronic functional constipation, identifying which patients have serious underlying pathology is of greatest concern for the emergency physician (EP).

### EPIDEMIOLOGY

Constipation is common at all ages, with the reported prevalence ranging from 2% to 27%,[1] depending on the definition used. Prevalence is higher in women than in men (approximately 2:1), perhaps related to an increased prevalence of pelvic floor dyssynergy in women.[2] Prevalence is higher in the elderly: in those older than 84 years, self-reported rates are 25.7% in men and 34.1% in women,[3] and up to 74% of elderly nursing home residents are taking laxatives daily.[2] The condition is much less common in populations with non-Western diets containing more bulk. Although many people do not seek medical attention for their constipation, this condition is estimated to result in almost $7 billion in medical costs in the United States each year.[3]

## PATHOPHYSIOLOGY

Constipation is often multifactorial, with disordered movement of stool through the colon and anorectum. Oral intake, hydration, and general mobility affect colonic function. Numerous anatomic and structural entities, gastrointestinal (GI) disorders, medications, and systemic disorders may secondarily lead to constipation (**Boxes 37.1 to 37.4**) by altering intraluminal contents, fluid balance, intestinal contractions, or neuromuscular coordination. However, the majority of patients have primary *chronic functional constipation* that falls into one or more of three categories. Many actually have normal intestinal transit time; their constipation is perceptual and related to habits. Others have slow transit times because of overall colonic slowing (pancolonic inertia) or sigmoid spasm (left colonic hypermotility with uncoordinated segmental contractions and poor propulsion). An important but underrecognized group has pelvic floor dyssynergy (obstructive defecation), an acquired behavioral condition that begins with chronically ignoring the urge to defecate. Disordered defecatory function of the pelvic floor muscles and sphincters eventually produces difficulty expelling stool, even if soft. Hormonal contributions are unclear, but constipation is common in pregnancy[4] and before menstruation. Contrary to past thinking, chronic laxative abuse does not cause chronic constipation.[5] High rates in the elderly are not due to aging itself but to concomitant conditions or medications.[6]

## PRESENTING SIGNS AND SYMPTOMS

To the physician, the term *constipation* usually means a reduced frequency of bowel movements (less than three per week in Western culture) or difficult passage of hard stool (or both). To the patient, *constipation* may mean frequency reduced to less than daily, decreased volume per defecation, passage of hard stool, difficulty passing stool, straining, a feeling of incomplete evacuation, abdominal pain, rectal pain,

**BOX 37.1 Gastrointestinal Causes of Constipation**

Anal fissure
Anal stricture
Anorectal (pelvic) dyssynergy
Chronic poor toileting habits
Diverticular disease
Functional constipation
Hemorrhoids
Hernias (incarcerated)
Inflammatory bowel disease
Intussusception
Irritable bowel syndrome
Obstructing lesion
Perirectal or perianal abscess
Rectal pain from any cause
Rectocele
Strictures and adhesions
Tumors and neoplasms
Volvulus

inability to defecate when desired or without a laxative, abdominal distention or bloating, or any combination thereof. An individual's perception of what is "normal" is also highly variable and often deeply ingrained, with many convinced that less than one stool per day is a serious problem.

A formal consensus definition is therefore used by gastroenterologists, and the label of chronic functional constipation requires two or more of the following occurring for at least 3 months of the past year: straining for at least 25% of defecations, lumpy or hard stools in 25% or more of defecations, sensation of incomplete evacuation in 25% or more of defecations, sensation of anorectal obstruction or blockage in 25% or more of defecations, manual maneuvers to facilitate passage (digital evacuation or support of the pelvic floor) in 25% or more of defecations, or fewer than three defecations per week.[7] A practical pediatric definition is delay or difficulty in defecation present for 2 or more weeks.[8]

Abdominal bloating and mild diffuse abdominal discomfort are common with functional constipation. Vomiting, severe pain, fever, and GI bleeding indicate more serious causes. Passage of hard stool may produce rectal bleeding, but the quantity should be small. Straining may cause dizziness, a vagal reaction, or both.

With functional constipation, the findings on physical examination should be normal other than palpation of abundant stool on abdominal or rectal examination (or both) and perhaps mild discomfort on abdominal palpation.

**BOX 37.2 Systemic Causes of Constipation**

**Central Nervous System and Neurogenic Disorders**
Amyotrophic lateral sclerosis
Autonomic neuropathies
Cerebral palsy
Chagas disease
Cerebrovascular accident
Delirium
Dementia
Hirschsprung disease
Intestinal pseudoobstruction
Multiple sclerosis
Myotonic dystrophy
Neurofibromatosis
Parkinson disease
Shy-Drager syndrome
Spinal cord lesions:
- Cauda equina syndrome
- Meningomyelocele
- Spinal cord injury

Trauma to the nervi erigentes

**Endocrine and Metabolic Disorders**
Adrenal insufficiency
Amyloidosis
Celiac disease
Cushing syndrome
Cystic fibrosis
Diabetes
Glucagonoma
Hypercalcemia
Hyperparathyroidism
Hypokalemia
Hypomagnesemia
Hypophosphatemia
Hypothyroidism
Multiple endocrine neoplasia type 2B
Panhypopituitarism
Pheochromocytoma
Porphyria
Pregnancy
Uremia

**Psychiatric Disorders**
Anorexia and bulimia
Chronic psychoses
Defecation avoidance
Depression

**Lifestyle and Nutritional Problems**
Dehydration from any cause
Immobility
Inadequate dietary intake, especially fiber
Inadequate toileting opportunities

**Collagen Vascular Disorders**
Dermatomyositis
Systemic lupus erythematosus
Systemic sclerosis

**Other**
Intraabdominal abscess
Pelvic mass
Pelvic trauma

**BOX 37.3 Medications That Cause Constipation**

**Analgesics**
Narcotics
Nonsteroidal antiinflammatory drugs

**Anticholinergics**
Antidepressants
Antihistamines
Antiparkinsonian agents
Antipsychotics
Antispasmodics

**Cation-Containing Agents**
Aluminum (antacids, sucralfate)
Barium sulfate
Bismuth
Calcium (antacids, supplements)
Iron

**Other**
Anticonvulsants
Antihypertensives (diuretics, clonidine)
Calcium channel blockers
Ganglionic blockers
Nicotine
Serotonin type 3 receptor antagonists
Vinca alkaloids

**BOX 37.4 Additional Considerations in Infants and Children**

**Anorectal Disorders**
Anal stenosis
Anteriorly displaced anus
Imperforate anus
Intussusception at anal canal
Skin tags

**Neuromuscular Disorders**
Cerebral palsy
Down syndrome
Ganglioneuromatosis
Gastroschisis
Hirschsprung disease
Hypoganglionosis
Intestinal neuronal dysplasia
Intestinal pseudoobstruction
Meningomyelocele
Myotonic dystrophy
Neurofibromatosis
Prune belly syndrome
Spina bifida

**Metabolic and Endocrine Disorders**
Celiac disease
Cystic fibrosis

**Other**
Behavioral/defecation withholding
Maternal drugs
Sexual abuse history
Cow's milk protein intolerance

## DIFFERENTIAL DIAGNOSIS AND MEDICAL DECISION MAKING

Constipation is a symptom that may be secondary to a myriad of other causes, but it most often represents chronic functional constipation. Boxes 37.1 to 37.4 list the various causes of secondary constipation—GI and systemic disorders, medications, and additional causes in children.

Evaluation in the ED is focused on distinguishing potentially serious cases that warrant immediate inpatient care via a careful history (what the patient means by the term *constipation*, bowel history, and potential underlying causes, especially medications) and examination (particularly vital signs, abdominal examination, perirectal inspection, and rectal examination). With chronic symptoms, it is important to ask what precipitated today's ED visit. New-onset constipation suggests new medications, sudden lifestyle changes, anal sphincter spasm and pain, or more serious conditions, including mass lesions and intestinal obstruction.

Signs of obvious systemic abnormalities, volume depletion, infection, peritonitis, ileus, and obstruction are important to identify early. In patients with functional constipation, abdominal examination should find only mild discomfort at most. Excessive colonic stool can often be palpated. Unlike a solid mass, stool should indent somewhat on palpation. Serial abdominal examinations are invaluable in uncertain cases. Fecal impaction, abnormal sphincter tone, and potential sources of bleeding or rectal pain may be detected on perirectal and rectal examination. Anoscopy (with topical anesthetic applied before the examination) is appropriate in patients with rectal complaints.

Red flags for a more serious acute condition include severe pain, vomiting, fever, GI bleeding, acute onset, persistent tachycardia, hypotension, and peritoneal signs. Elderly patients warrant higher clinical suspicion for worrisome causes, particularly if febrile, and extraabdominal infections may be manifested as general failure to thrive or constipation. In adults older than 50 years, anemia, weight loss, acute change in bowel habits, GI bleeding, and a family history of colon cancer or inflammatory bowel syndrome (IBS) are "alarm" findings of possible underlying malignancy or IBS and warrant early referral for endoscopy or radiographic studies.[9]

In ED patients in whom clinical suspicion for serious pathology is low, appropriate studies are limited to basic chemistry panels (including calcium) and a complete blood count. Suspicion of an obstruction, fecal impaction, ileus, megacolon, or perforation should prompt plain abdominal films (flat and upright); serial plain films may assist in diagnosing early obstruction when the initial evaluation is unclear. Emergency computed tomography (CT) scans are appropriately limited to situations suggesting obstruction, intraabdominal abscess, complicated hernia, or diverticulitis. Early surgical consultation is appropriate for probable obstruction or peritonitis.

## CONSIDERATIONS BY PATIENT AGE

### *Neonates*

Neonates have an increased risk for serious underlying illness or anatomic abnormalities, such as Hirschsprung disease, intestinal pseudoobstruction, imperforate anus, or hypothyroidism.

### Children

Functional constipation is more common in boys, frequently at the time of toilet training or initial school entrance, when children withhold defecation for psychosocial reasons. A vicious cycle of difficult passage of hard stool leads to more withholding, which causes harder stool and more difficult passage. Fecal soiling (encopresis) is a common result and frequent initial symptom.

### Adolescents

Constipation is more common in adolescent girls than boys, with the predominant symptom being straining to initiate defecation. Typically, this is a functional problem arising from chronic suppression of the urge to defecate for psychosocial reasons. An underlying eating disorder or surreptitious opiate use should also be considered.[10]

### Adults

Usually, adults have a chronic functional cause, including IBS. Extreme functional constipation (two or fewer stools per month) is almost exclusively seen in young women.

### Elderly Institutionalized Patients

Mental confusion, immobility, poor oral intake, limited toileting opportunities, and medications all contribute to a high prevalence of chronic constipation and high risk for fecal impaction. Impaction is the most common cause of fecal incontinence and may lead to stercoraceous ulceration or perforation of the colon.[11]

## CONSIDERATIONS BY CAUSE

### Anatomic and Structural Causes

Examination may reveal anatomic or muscular anomalies or masses (neoplasm, fecaloma, abscess, hernia, closed or trapped loop of bowel, rectocele) that may cause blockage. Other structural causes are painful rectal disorders, intussusception, volvulus, and adhesions. Lower spinal cord injury may produce constipation or incontinence (or both); with high cord injuries the colonic reflexes usually remain intact, although digital rectal stimulation is often needed to initiate defecation.

### Medications

An accurate and complete list of medications (prescription, nonprescription, and alternative) should be established because so many cause or exacerbate constipation. Classic scenarios include elderly patients taking multiple prescription drugs, recreational users of opiates, and patients with acute painful injuries who were prescribed opiates without stool softeners.

### Systemic Illnesses

A long list of metabolic, endocrine, and neurogenic disorders may secondarily produce constipation. These conditions are usually obvious from the history, physical examination, and basic laboratory studies, so extensive diagnostic searches are rarely appropriate in the ED setting.

### Functional Constipation

In the vast majority of patients, constipation has an idiopathic functional cause related to psychosocial stressors, unintentionally learned rectal dysfunction, and lifestyle habits such as dietary fiber intake, fluid intake, and toileting. About 25% of patients have a component of pelvic dyssynergy. IBS is a common functional dysmotility disorder characterized by intermittent abdominal pain, distention, and variable diarrhea or constipation with no structural lesions found; concomitant upper GI symptoms and pelvic dyssynergy are common.[12,13]

Diagnosis is inexact because no specific diagnostic tests are available, but the constipation usually responds to bulk agents. Similarly, the label of chronic functional constipation is a clinical one, but exact diagnosis is not needed in the ED setting.

## TREATMENT

Intravenous fluid repletion with correction of electrolyte disturbances is the mainstay of initial management in sicker patients. Suspected *mechanical obstruction* or *perforation* warrants immediate surgical consultation and admission. Intravenous fluids and analgesics are warranted, whereas laxatives are contraindicated. Patients with nausea or vomiting need antiemetics. Those with obstruction or ileus may benefit from nasogastric suctioning, plus an intravenous gastric acid blocker to prevent metabolic alkalosis. Large bowel obstruction may require early colonoscopy with decompression.

Patients with *pseudoobstruction* warrant inpatient care unless they are known to have chronic intermittent pseudoobstruction with only a mild exacerbation of their constipation. For acute megacolon from colonic pseudoobstruction, the prokinetic neostigmine is a standard therapy, but this is usually ordered by the gastroenterologist and followed by decompressive colonoscopy.[14] Prokinetic agents are contraindicated in patients with obstruction, perforation, or peritonitis.

Fecal impaction may complicate long-standing constipation, particularly in nursing home residents or opiate users. Initial cleansing in milder cases may be done safely with large-volume oral polyethylene glycol (PEG), which is done in many nursing homes. Others usually require initial digital disimpaction, as discussed later, followed by PEG cleansing and then a maintenance plan. ED time constraints may prompt admission to an observation unit for initial cleansing.

For patients with *uncomplicated constipation*, the starting point in the ED focuses on volume repletion and electrolyte correction as needed, followed by a bowel regimen appropriate for the level of fecal loading, plus any treatment specific to contributing causes. The EP should also consider whether pelvic floor dyssynergy is a probable component that the patient should discuss with a primary care physician. The clinician should keep in mind the problem that bothers the patient the most (infrequency, straining, or hard stool) and that the patient's expectations often include prescription "cures" and an unrealistic goal of rapidly becoming "normal." Patient education is vital.

The plan for bowel care includes:

- Initial cleansing (usually laxatives, both oral and rectal)
- Maintenance plan (increase fluid and fiber intake, consideration of laxatives or softeners)
- Behavioral modification (diet, toilet habits, exercise)
- Other interventions tailored to the suspected underlying cause or causes

Most patients are sent home with a management plan and education, but initial cleansing in the ED or observation unit and serial reexamination should be considered if a suspicion remains about a more serious underlying cause or if the patient may not be able to perform the initial steps (or has no reliable caretaker to do so). A myriad of products are available for constipation **(Table 37.1).**[15] Selection should focus on efficacy, safety, and cost, as well as patient preference.

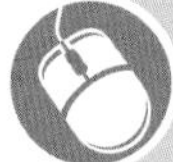

See Table 37.1 Therapeutic Agents for Constipation in Adults, online at www.expertconsult.com

If ED cleansing is necessary, time constraints prompt the use of stimulant laxatives per rectum, either suppositories (glycerin or bisacodyl) or enemas (tap water or phosphate). A topical anesthetic gel will decrease defecatory pain. Digital disimpaction may speed the process but is generally reserved as a last resort. Digital stimulation (several gentle rotations of a gloved, well-lubricated finger within the rectum) may loosen up fecal concretions and stimulate spontaneous defecation; this may be repeated after a 10-minute pause. If no response is seen, the lumps will need to be gently broken up and removed by finger. In spinal cord or elderly patients, the pulse and blood pressure should be monitored during disimpaction for changes secondary to vagal stimulation or autonomic dysreflexia.[16]

Outpatient treatment should start with osmotic laxatives such as PEG to be taken at home or just bulk agents, prune juice, or dried prunes if the constipation is mild. A stimulant laxative (e.g., glycerin suppository) is to be taken if the simpler treatment fails.[17] Strong evidence supports the use of PEG, moderate evidence supports lactulose and psyllium, and little evidence exists for or against other agents.[18,19] In the elderly, all laxative categories may cause some bloating, flatulence, or abdominal pain.[20]

*Bulk agents* are the first-line maintenance treatment of functional constipation with a normal or slow transit time. Bulk agents increase fecal water content and stool volume, reduce transit time, and improve stool consistency. Bran fiber (25 g/day) in foods may be adequate and must be accompanied by increased fluid intake. Fiber may cause increased gas (bloating, flatulence), but this is less likely if intake is increased gradually.

The *stool softeners* sodium and calcium docusate decrease surface tension and allow stool to mix with fluids but do not induce defecation. These agents are not good for long-term use because of tachyphylaxis, but they are very useful in the short term while taking constipating medications (e.g., opiates) or for patients who should avoid straining.

*Lubricant agents* penetrate and soften stool. Mineral oil can be given orally or by enema. Because it may be aspirated and cause lipoid pneumonia, it should not be used in patients with esophageal dysmotility, dysphagia, or gastroesophageal reflux.

*Osmotic laxatives* are hyperosmotic agents that generally provide excellent relief of constipation and may be used in small doses for the long term if needed. A large volume of PEG is used for procedural preparation or initial cleansing of large fecal loads, but most cases of constipation respond to one packet (17 g) daily, which may be continued as a maintenance dosage; PEG without electrolytes is more palatable. Lactulose and sorbitol (given orally or as enemas) are nonabsorbable sugars degraded by colonic bacteria to acids that increase stool acidity and osmolarity and thereby lead to accumulation of fluid in the colon to speed defecation. Lactulose is excellent for long-term use in small doses but should be avoided in most diabetics. Corn syrup is used in infants.[8]

*Stimulant laxatives* are the most rapidly acting agents and are taken either orally or per rectum (faster). They are likely to cause some cramping. Saline cathartics exert osmotic effects to increase intraluminal water content. Though relatively nonabsorbable, magnesium preparations should be avoided in patients with renal failure because they may cause hypermagnesemia or fluid retention. Castor oil is hydrolyzed to ricinoleic acid, which stimulates intestinal secretion and motility. Bisacodyl causes fluid accumulation and increased motor activity. Anthraquinones (cascara, senna) are converted to active states by intestinal microorganisms and increase fluid and electrolyte accumulation in the distal end of the bowel; melanosis coli may result from long-term use but is benign and reversible. Stimulants are not generally recommended for frequent long-term use.

*General measures* often help:

- Higher intake of fluids (≥2 L daily) and fiber
- Greater physical mobility and exercise (brisk daily walk)
- Dedicated and unhurried time for defecation

Dietary fiber sources are primarily bran and grains, but dried fruits, pulp-rich citrus juices, many vegetables, and even popcorn contribute fiber. Retraining bowel habits may help; patients must allow an unhurried time (20 minutes or so) to use the toilet, especially after a meal (breakfast is ideal) to take advantage of the gastrocolic reflex, and they should respond to the urge to defecate. Contributing medications require careful review of their necessity, planned duration of use, and alternatives. For drugs that must be continued, increased fiber and the addition of stool softeners may suffice, with daily PEG or lactulose added if needed. Bulk agents may affect the bioavailability of some drugs. The EP must communicate clearly to the patient that the constipation is a side effect of medications that needs to be discussed with the primary care provider.

Concomitant treatment of underlying causes and contributors is essential. Treatment of painful rectal problems improves overall bowel function. Although they are not generally prescribed in an ED setting, other treatments are available.[19] Lubiprostone is a bicyclic fatty acid that activates GI chloride channels to increase intestinal fluid secretion and effectively treats chronic functional constipation.[21] Even in the elderly, pelvic floor dyssynergy may respond well to physical therapy, behavioral modification, and biofeedback training.[22,23] Surgery may relieve specific defects, such as rectoceles, and is the mainstay for treatment of Hirschsprung disease.[9]

## FOLLOW-UP CARE AND PATIENT EDUCATION

### ADMISSION

Indications for admission are limited to patients with obstruction, pseudoobstruction, severe electrolyte disturbances, or other serious causes of secondary constipation. An observational stay may be appropriate for those with an inability to safely perform initial bowel cleansing at home or those with moderate clinical suspicion of another underlying cause (e.g., those with persistent abdominal pain or low-grade fever without obvious cause).

## FOLLOW-UP

Follow-up primary care visits are adequate discharge planning for most patients. Those with obvious structural causes (e.g., hemorrhoids, rectoceles) or high suspicion for causes such as spinal cord pathology, Hirschsprung disease, and other conditions, warrant specialty referral. Outpatient studies of colorectal structure (e.g., colonoscopy) are appropriate for those older than 50 years as cancer screening and are necessary for patients of any age with alarming signs or symptoms (acute and unexplained onset, weight loss, bleeding, iron deficiency anemia). However, structural studies do not provide an assessment of functional constipation, and few patients need functional studies; clinical response to treatment and further needs are better judged with ongoing primary care.

## PATIENT EDUCATION

Patient education is crucial. Patients are often frightened and disturbed by symptoms that the physician may take lightly; reassurance and discussion are invaluable. As appropriate, the EP should explain that cancer or other serious disease is highly unlikely but that compliance with follow-up remains essential. The patient should be taught about "normal" bowel function, general measures to improve symptoms, and reasonable goals. The EP and nurse must also ensure that patients know how to use the items recommended, especially suppositories or enemas.[24]

## COMPLICATIONS AND PITFALLS

Although constipation is straightforward in most patients, certain potential pitfalls need to be avoided. Determination of exactly what the patient means by the word *constipation* is important, as are realistic goals for those with chronic constipation. Reassurance and patient education with specific treatment and follow-up instructions are essential in functional constipation cases, particularly in adults to avoid missing an opportunity for outpatient screening with early diagnosis of an underlying malignancy. Failure to recognize obstruction is often avoidable with serial reexaminations over a 4- to 6-hour period and by observing the patient after food intake. Unrecognized fecal impaction can lead to GI bleeding, mucosal ulceration, or even perforation; negative findings on rectal examination do not rule out a higher impaction, so plain radiographs are appropriate if suspicious. Overly aggressive digital disimpaction may lead to bacteremia; not all reachable stool pellets need to be removed at a single time when follow-up with PEG will clear the rest. Fever in an elderly patient is not explained by constipation. In children, a careful perirectal and rectal examination is difficult, but otherwise it is easy to overlook an anal fissure. In women of childbearing age (including perimenopausal), a pregnancy test is necessary, especially before consideration of a CT scan or outpatient radiographic colonic study.

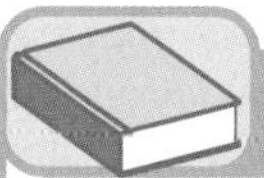

**PATIENT TEACHING TIPS**

**Functional Constipation**

**General Concepts**

Goals: bowel movements three or more times per week, pain free, with minimal straining.

Daily bowel movements are not needed.

The long-term prognosis is excellent and serious diseases such as cancer are not likely, but outpatient follow-up is always important to see how you are doing and whether other tests may be needed.

If constipation is long-standing, return to "normal" bowel habits may take several weeks.

Keep a bowel diary (brief description of food and fluid intake, bowel movements, problems) for 1 to 2 weeks to review with your primary care doctor.

**Recommended Medications and Laxatives**

Follow the plan recommended by your physician today.

Short-term use of strong laxatives for the next few days is OK for initial cleansing, but avoid long-term use unless your primary care doctor advises you to do so.

Small daily doses of osmotic laxatives such as lactulose or polyethylene glycol may be needed for a few weeks, along with bowel retraining.

**Healthy Bowel Habits**

Visit the toilet every day after the meal of your choice (breakfast is best), and sit for 15 to 20 minutes:

Relax, do not hurry, and do not strain.

Try for about the same time every day.

Do respond to the urge to defecate.

Drink at least 2 L of fluids (without caffeine or alcohol) daily to stay well hydrated.

Gradually increase your fiber intake (bran, high-fiber cereals, fruits, vegetables, or nonprescription fiber products such as psyllium) to about 25 g/day.

Note whether milk or milk products aggravate your symptoms.

Regular exercise (walking) may help stimulate improved bowel movements.

## SUGGESTED READINGS

Bouras EP, Tangalos EG. Chronic constipation in the elderly. Gastroenterol Clin North Am 2009;38:463-80.

Brandt LJ, Prather CM, Quigley EM, et al. Systematic review on the management of chronic constipation in North America. Am J Gastroenterol 2005;100(Suppl 1):S5-21.

Constipation Guideline Committee of the North American Society for Pediatric Gastroenterology, Hepatology and Nutrition. Evaluation and treatment of constipation in infants and children: recommendations from the North American Society for Pediatric Gastroenterology, Hepatology and Nutrition. J Pediatr Gastroenterol Nutr 2006;43(3):e1-13.

Rao SS. Dyssynergic defecation and biofeedback therapy. Gastroenterol Clin North Am 2008;37:569-86.

Youssef NN, Sanders L, Di Lorenzo C. Adolescent constipation: evaluation and management. Adolesc Med Clin 2004;15:37-52.

## REFERENCES

***References can be found on Expert Consult @ www.expertconsult.com.***

# Hernias 38

*Chandra D. Aubin*

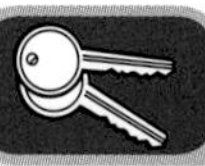

**KEY POINTS**

- Smaller defects in the abdominal wall are more likely to be manifested as incarcerated or strangulated hernias.
- Reduction of a hernia should not be attempted if strangulation is suspected.
- Hernias with signs or symptoms suggestive of bowel obstruction or ischemia are true surgical emergencies and require immediate consultation for operative repair.
- Manual reduction can be aided by placement of the patient in a supine or Trendelenburg position, application of ice to the hernia site before reduction, and administration of analgesics or anxiolytics, or both.
- Postoperative complications of herniorrhaphy include wound infection, seroma, hematoma, ileus, small bowel obstruction, recurrence of the hernia, erosion of preperitoneal mesh into intraabdominal organs, fistula formation, genitourinary trauma, and chronic pain secondary to nerve injury.

## EPIDEMIOLOGY

Herniorrhaphy (also known as hernioplasty, or surgical repair of a hernia) is a common procedure in the United States. Approximately 800,000 inguinal hernia repairs were performed in the United States in 2003; mesh was used in 90% of the cases.[1]

Of groin hernias, inguinal hernias (96%) are much more common than femoral hernias (4%). The male-to-female ratio for inguinal hernias is 9:1, and that for femoral hernias is 1:4. In elderly women, femoral hernias are as common as inguinal hernias. The incidence of strangulation increases with advancing age.

Operative mortality for a strangulated hernia is 5% to 10% in patients older than 80 years, as compared with 3% for elective repair in that age group. Mortality increases to 19% when bowel necrosis is present.

The incidence of postoperative intraabdominal hernias is increasing because of the higher number of Roux-en-Y gastric bypass procedures performed each year; postoperative hernias are observed in 2.5% to 4.5% of patients undergoing bariatric surgery.

Incisional hernias of the abdominal wall occur in up to 11% of all other postoperative patients and in as many as 23% of patients with postoperative wound infections. Trocar site hernias after laparoscopic surgery are reported in up to 6% of patients. Parastomal hernia formation occurs in 28% of ileostomies and 48% of colostomies. Morbidity depends on the location and contents of the hernia, as well as the development of incarceration or strangulation.

## PATHOPHYSIOLOGY

Hernias are congenital or acquired defects in the abdominal wall that allow protrusion of intraabdominal contents through the pathologic opening. The characteristic finding consists of pain and swelling at the hernia site. Intraabdominal hernias, which can occur spontaneously or after surgery or trauma, are caused by defects in the diaphragm, mesentery, or ligamentous structures.

Incarcerated hernias are those in which abdominal contents have become trapped in the opening (i.e., nonreducible). Bowel incarceration can be manifested as pain, vomiting, or frank obstruction.

Strangulated hernias involve a compromise of the blood supply to the hernia contents. Strangulation can be manifested as fever, ischemia, or necrosis of the hernia contents and, occasionally, erythema or necrosis of the skin overlying the hernia. Smaller defects in the abdominal wall are more likely to be manifested as incarceration or strangulation.

Reduction—replacement of the hernia contents back into the abdominal cavity—is the immediate treatment of a hernia. Reduction of a hernia is accomplished by gentle pressure over the area of herniation. Reduction is assisted by use of the supine or Trendelenburg position, application of ice, analgesia, and procedural sedation to relax the musculature of the abdominal wall. Reduction should not be attempted if necrosis of the hernia contents is suspected. Definitive hernia treatment is surgical repair.

## NOMENCLATURE

**Table 38.1** and **Box 38.1** summarize the nomenclature of hernias, and **Figures 38.1 to 38.13** illustrate some of the hernia types.

**Table 38.1 Nomenclature of Hernias**

| | |
|---|---|
| **Groin Hernias** | |
| Inguinal hernia (Fig. 38.1) | Physical examination cannot accurately distinguish between indirect and direct inguinal hernias |
| Indirect | Occurs through the inguinal canal<br>Inguinal canal contents include the ilioinguinal nerve, genital branch of the genitofemoral nerve, spermatic cord in men (vas deferens, testicular artery, and vein), and round ligament in women |
| Direct | 65% of inguinal hernias are indirect<br>Weakness of the aponeurosis of the transversus abdominis and transversalis fascia in the Hesselbach triangle (the medial border of which is the lateral aspect of the rectus abdominis, the superior border is the epigastric artery, and the inferior border is the inguinal ligament) |
| Femoral hernia | Occurs through the femoral canal, inferior to the inguinal ligament, medial to the femoral vein<br>More common in elderly, parous women |
| Sportsman's hernia | Syndrome of persistent groin pain in athletes; probably caused by recurrent or persistent groin strain, osteitis pubis, or a nonpalpable hernia<br>More common in kicking sports |
| **Abdominal Wall Hernias** | |
| Anterior (Fig. 38.2) | |
| Epigastric hernia | Occurs through the linea alba, the midline between the xiphoid line and umbilicus |
| Umbilical hernia | Caused by an abnormally large or weak umbilical ring<br>Umbilical hernia usually closes spontaneously in infancy but does not heal in adulthood<br>Rarely incarcerates in children<br>Worsened by pregnancy, obesity, or cirrhosis with ascites |
| Spigelian hernia (Figs. 38.3 and 38.4) | Lateral ventral hernia through the spigelian zone: transversalis fascia between the lateral margin of the rectus abdominis muscle, medial margins of the external and internal obliques, and the transversus abdominis muscles<br>Accounts for 1-2% of all hernias |
| Ventral or incisional hernia (Fig. 38.5) | Trocar sites:<br>Difficult to recognize on physical examination<br>Dangerous cause of early postoperative small bowel obstruction<br>Can be the Richter type (incarceration of one intestinal wall)<br>Iliac crest bone graft sites<br>Parastomal hernias |
| Traumatic | Caused by blunt or penetrating trauma<br>"Handlebar" hernia:<br>Can occur in any location on the abdominal wall from a fall on a bicycle handlebar with tear of the abdominal wall muscles<br>Has also been reported in the thorax from a tear of the intercostal muscles (similar hernias have been reported as a result of severe coughing) |
| Congenital abdominal wall defects | Surgical emergencies in neonates:<br>Immediate management: cover the abdominal contents with warm moist saline-soaked gauze, insert a nasogastric tube, administer intravenous fluids and antibiotics, obtain surgical consultation<br>Types:<br>Gastroschisis: intact umbilical cord, evisceration of the bowel through a defect usually to the right of the cord; no membrane covering<br>Omphalocele: herniation of the bowel, liver, and other organs into the intact umbilical cord; membrane present unless ruptured |
| Posterior (lumbar) hernias (Fig. 38.6) | Bounded superiorly by the 12th rib, inferiorly by the iliac crest, posteriorly by the erector spinae muscles, and anteriorly by the posterior border of the external oblique muscle<br>Types:<br>Inferior or Petit: just superior to iliac crest (point up)<br>Superior or Grynfeltt: just below the 12th rib, inverted triangle (point down) |
| **Diaphragmatic Hernias** | |
| Congenital hernia (Fig. 38.7) | Eventration: thin diaphragm with normal but widely spaced muscle fibers<br>Posterolateral: through the foramen of Bochdalek<br>Anterior, retrosternal, or parasternal: through the foramen of Morgagni (Figs. 38.8 and 38.9)<br>Peritoneopericardial |
| Acquired hernia | Hiatal: sliding or fixed<br>Paraesophageal<br>Acquired eventration: caused by phrenic nerve injury and paralysis<br>Traumatic (Fig. 38.10) |

**Table 38.1 Nomenclature of Hernias—cont'd**

| | |
|---|---|
| **Pelvic Wall and Floor Hernias** | |
| Sciatic hernia (Fig. 38.11) | Protrusion of the peritoneal sac and contents through the greater or lesser sciatic foramen |
| Obturator hernia (Fig. 38.12) | Protrusion of preperitoneal fat or intestine through the obturator foramen |
| Perineal hernia | Protrusion of a viscus through the pelvic floor (rare) |
| Prolapse | Weakness of the pelvic floor muscles can cause a cystocele, rectocele, and uterine or rectal prolapse |
| **Intraabdominal Hernias** | |
| Spontaneous | |
| Transmesenteric hernia | Through the sigmoid mesocolon, broad ligament, or falciform ligament |
| Transomental hernia | Hernia beneath a mesenteric or peritoneal fold (no disruption of the peritoneum)<br>Locations:<br>Epiploic foramen of Winslow (Fig. 38.13)<br>Paraduodenal<br>Superior ileocecal fossa<br>Internal supravesicular |
| Postoperative | Transmesenteric and transomental hernias are most common, especially after Roux-en-Y procedures<br>May occur through the falciform ligament from a trocar puncture during laparoscopic cholecystectomy<br>Retroanastomotic—may occur behind the anastomosis |

**BOX 38.1 Eponyms Associated with Hernias**

Richter hernia (partial enterocele): Herniation of only the anterior surface of the intestinal wall through the hernia defect; accounts for 10% of strangulated hernias

Amyand hernia: Acute appendicitis in the sac of an inguinal hernia

Garengeot hernia: Acute appendicitis in the sac of a femoral hernia

Littre hernia: Strangulated Meckel diverticulum in a hernia sac

Maydl hernia: Internal hernia with double-loop strangulation

Chilaiditi syndrome: Symptomatic interposition of the intraabdominal contents between the liver and diaphragm; can become incarcerated

Canal of Nuck: The portion of the processus vaginalis that accompanies the round ligament through the inguinal canal in women; may contain hernia contents or, rarely, hydrocele in women

Romberg-Howship sign: Lancinating pain along the inner side of the thigh to the knee or down the leg to the foot caused by compression of the obturator nerve in cases of incarcerated obturator hernia

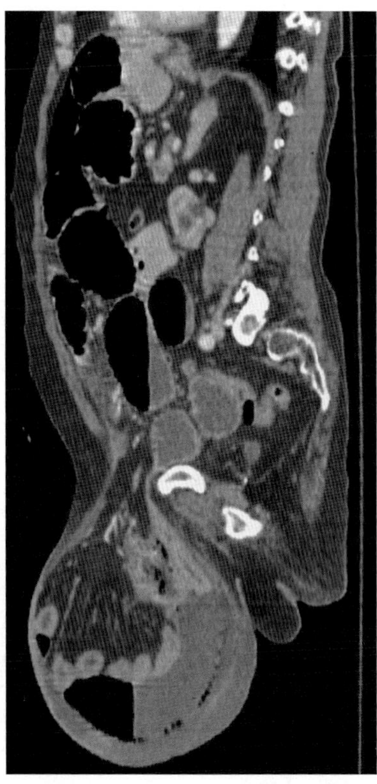

**Fig. 38.1** Infarcted inguinal hernia.

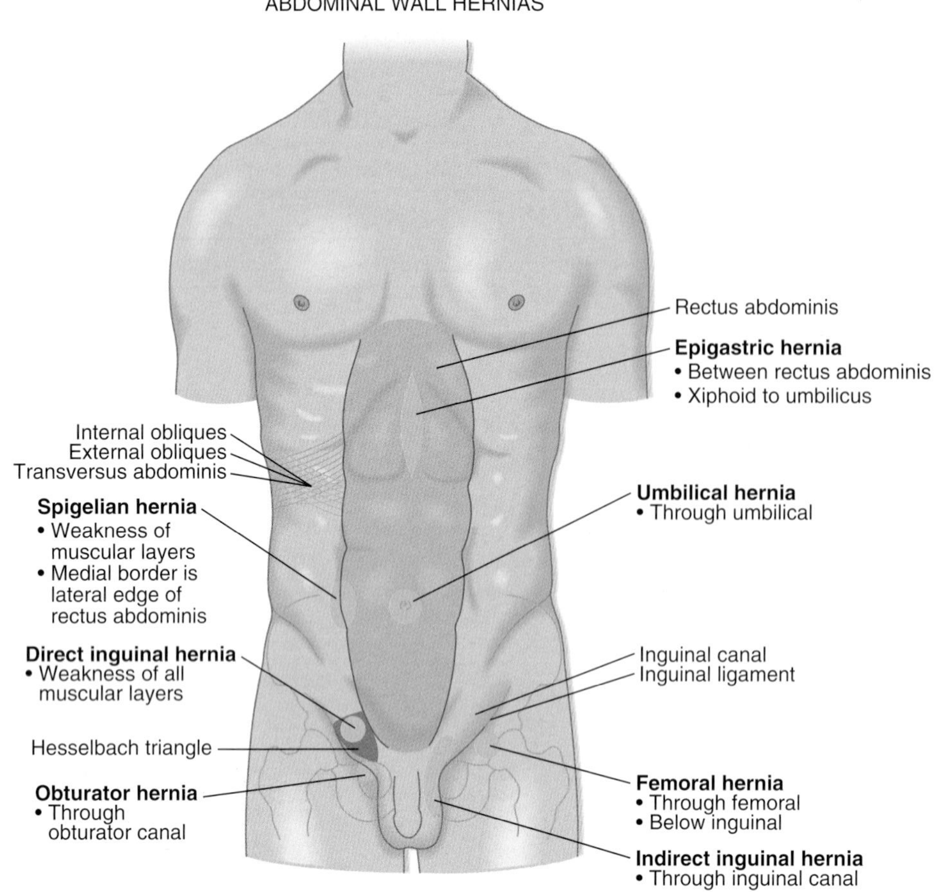


**Fig. 38.2 Anterior abdominal wall hernia.**

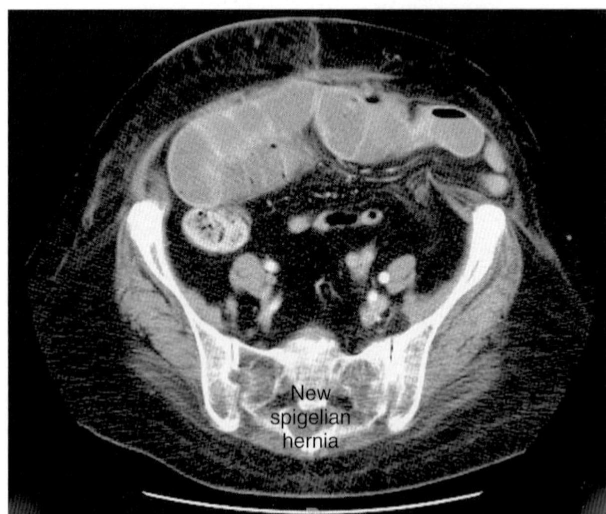


**Fig. 38.3 Spigelian hernia.**

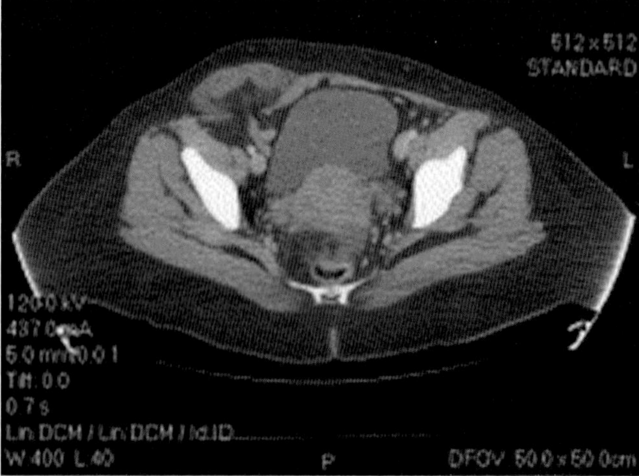


**Fig. 38.4 Computed tomography scan of a spigelian hernia in an adult woman with right lower quadrant pain.** (From Mull AC, Hurtado TR. Right lower quadrant pain in an adult woman. Am J Emerg Med 2011;29:132.e1-2.)

## PATHOPHYSIOLOGY

In comparison with controls, patients in whom incisional or recurrent hernias develop may exhibit abnormal synthesis of type I and type III collagen.[2] A higher incidence of incisional hernia formation is seen in patients with wound infection, obesity, and multiple comorbid conditions. The use of synthetic mesh and "tension-free" repair techniques has reduced rates of hernia recurrence.

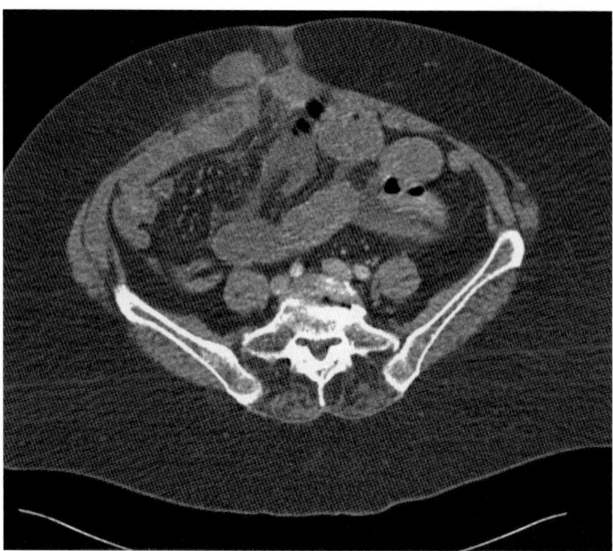

**Fig. 38.5** Ventral hernia with small bowel obstruction.

## PRESENTING SIGNS AND SYMPTOMS

The classic manifestation of an abdominal wall hernia is pain and swelling at the hernia site. Symptoms are more pronounced with increased intraabdominal pressure, such as occurs with standing, coughing, and straining. Occasionally, patients report an acute onset of symptoms after heavy lifting or during sports. Many patients observe that the swelling ("lump" or "knot") resolves when they are supine or pressure is applied over the area.

Inguinal hernias can be manifested as scrotal pain, a groin mass, or swelling. Incarcerated hernias typically feature a painful lump or knot on the abdominal wall or in the scrotum. The hernia is very tender to palpation and is not reduced by gentle pressure. If small bowel is incarcerated in the hernia sac, the patient may exhibit nausea and vomiting. Incarcerated omentum or preperitoneal fat may give rise to only a localized painful mass.

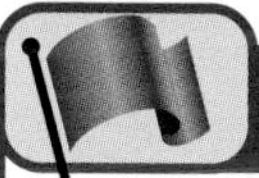

**RED FLAGS**

Symptoms that suggest hernia complications (obstruction, incarceration, or strangulation) are as follows:

- Diffuse rather than localized pain and tenderness with guarding or rebound
- Nausea or vomiting
- Markedly tender, nonreducible hernia
- Fever
- Erythema or necrosis of the skin overlying the hernia

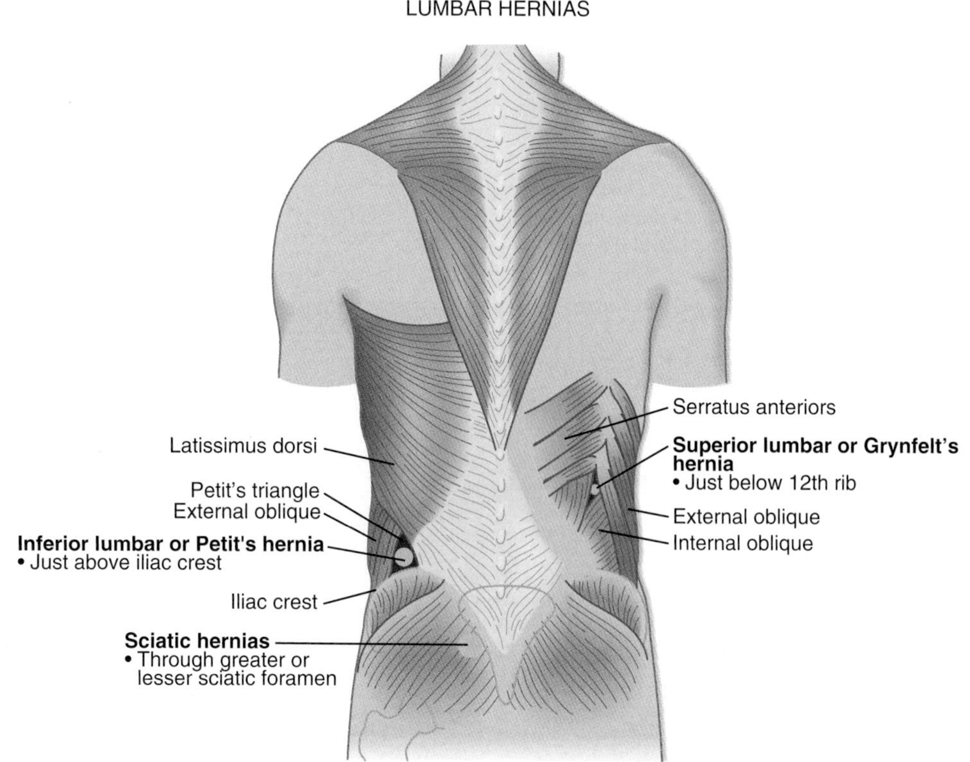


**Fig. 38.6** Locations of lumbar hernias.

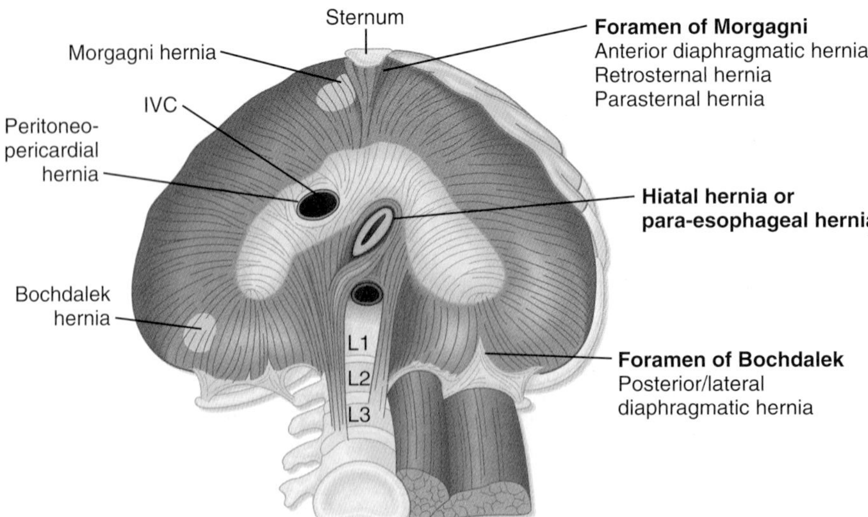


**Fig. 38.7 Locations of diaphragmatic hernias.** *IVC*, Inferior vena cava.

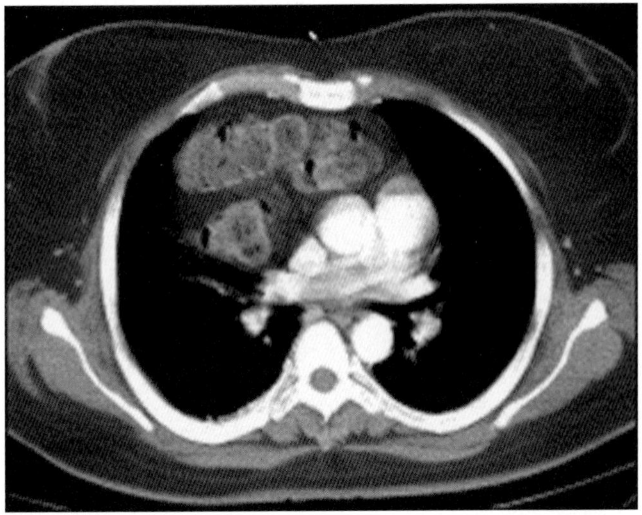

**Fig. 38.8 Morgagni-type diaphragmatic hernia manifested as an abnormal cardiac silhouette.** (From Daneshvar S, Shriki J, Sohn H, et al. Morgagni-type diaphragmatic hernia presenting as an abnormal cardiac silhouette. Am J Med 2010;123:e11-2.)

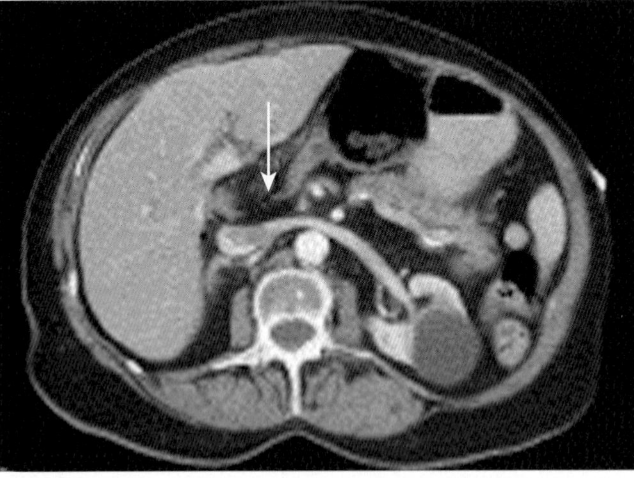

**Fig. 38.9 Morgagni-type diaphragmatic hernia manifested as an abnormal cardiac silhouette *(arrow)*.** (From Daneshvar S, Shriki J, Sohn H, et al. Morgagni-type diaphragmatic hernia presenting as an abnormal cardiac silhouette. Am J Med 2010;123:e11-2.)

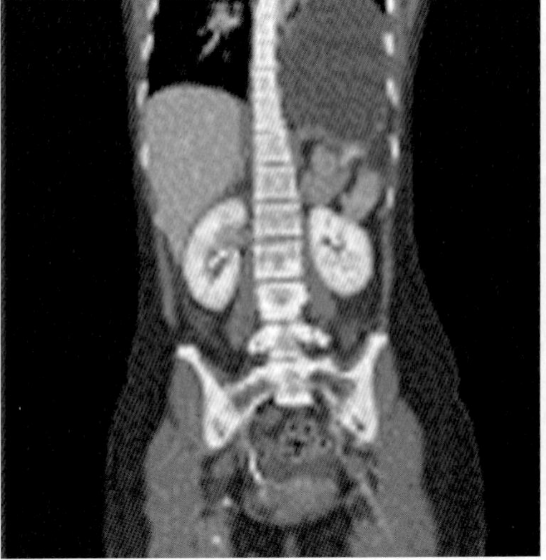

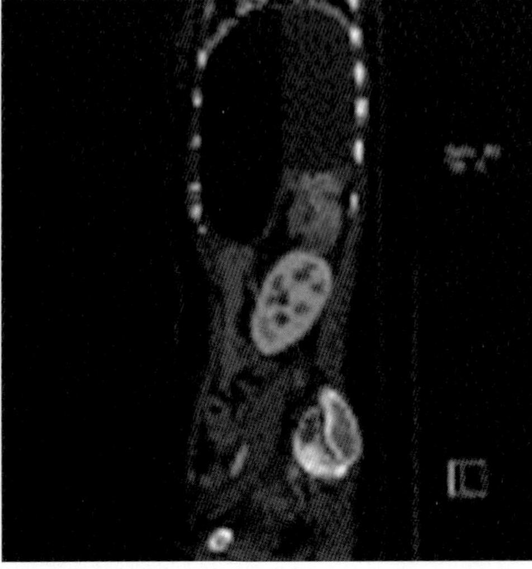

**Fig. 38.10 Computed tomographic scan of a diaphragmatic hernia.** (From Yang YM, Yang HB, Park JS, et al. Spontaneous diaphragmatic rupture complicated with perforation of the stomach during Pilates. Am J Emerg Med. 2010;28:259.e1-3.)

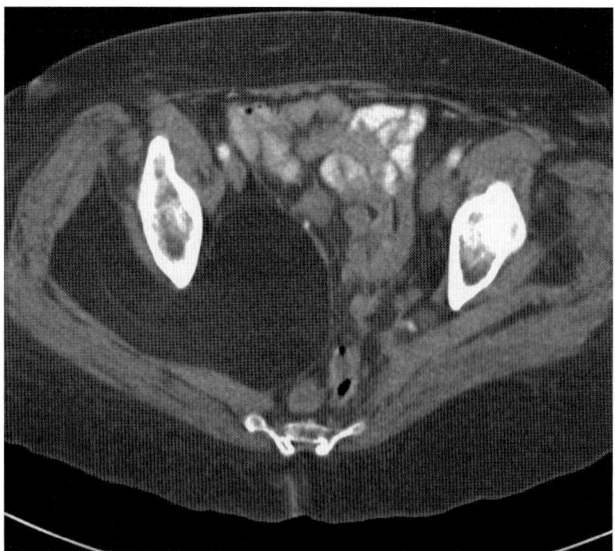

**Fig. 38.11 Sciatic lipoma.**

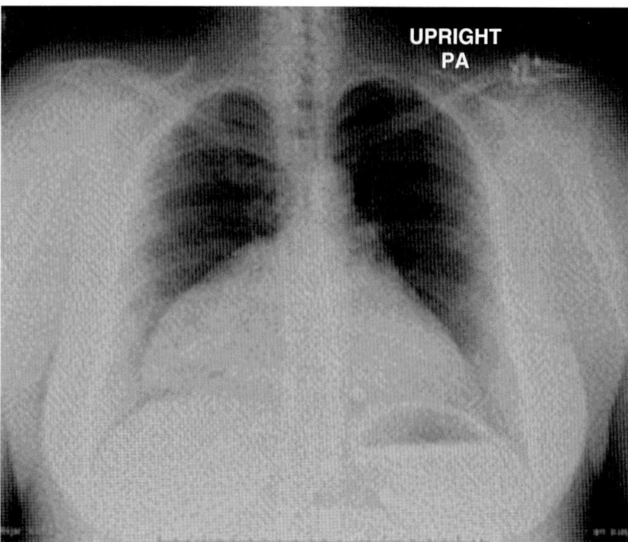


**Fig. 38.13 Internal hernia through the foramen of Winslow.** In a single contrast-enhanced axial computed tomographic image through the abdomen, the foramen of Winslow is seen with loops of ileum and colon herniating through it. The bowel demonstrates "beaking" as it passes through the foramen. *PA*, Posterior. (From Manna SA, Tynan J, Warburton R, et al. Answer to the case of the month #161. Internal hernia through the foramen of Winslow. Can Assoc Radiol J 2010;61:113-6.)

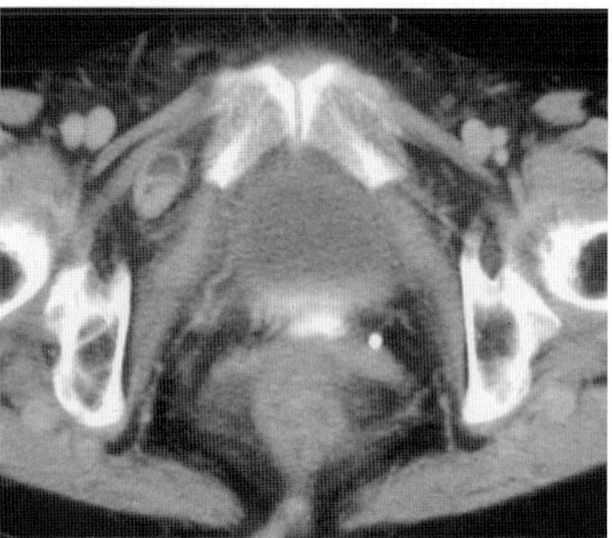

**Fig. 38.12 Obturator hernia with bowel obstruction.**

As the incarceration persists over time, swelling of the hernia contents eventually compromises the blood supply and strangulation ensues. The signs and symptoms vary with the contents of the hernia. Patients with incarcerated intestine leading to intestinal ischemia or necrosis may have fever and peritonitis. Prolonged incarceration with necrosis of the hernia contents may cause erythema or necrosis of the skin overlying the hernia.

Long-standing hernias may feature very large defects in the abdominal wall. In general, larger defects are less likely to be manifested as strangulation. A large hernia may be chronically incarcerated or nonreducible. With time, fibrous adhesions develop and prevent spontaneous reduction when the patient is supine.

Less typical findings include ill-defined abdominal pain, nausea, and vomiting but without an obvious mass on the abdominal wall. This manifestation is more likely to occur with intraabdominal hernias, in obese patients, or in patients who are unable to give an adequate history.

The incidence of postoperative internal hernias is rising because of the increase in bariatric operations in the United States, particularly Roux-en-Y gastric bypass.[3] Postoperative complications of hernia repair include wound infection, seroma or hematoma, ileus or small bowel obstruction, recurrence of the hernia, and in rare cases, erosion of preperitoneal mesh into intraabdominal organs with associated fistula formation.[4] Complications of inguinal hernia repair are chronic pain as a result of nerve disruption or entrapment and, rarely, testicular ischemia.

Traumatic diaphragmatic disruption from penetrating trauma should be suspected when the trajectory of a gunshot wound or the location of a stab wound potentially crosses the diaphragm. Though rare, diaphragmatic disruption can occur after significant blunt trauma and is more common on the left side. Traumatic diaphragmatic disruption is difficult to diagnose in the acute stage because of nonspecific signs, but it should be suspected when the patient has a proximate injury and pain out of proportion to the physical findings. Standard imaging techniques, including chest and abdominal computed tomography (CT), may miss small diaphragmatic injuries, and laparoscopy, thoracoscopy, or surgical exploration may be required.

Diaphragmatic disruption has also been described after forceful coughing or vomiting. Delayed manifestations of diaphragmatic hernias consist of chest pain, dyspnea, or abnormal findings on chest radiography or CT (with or without abdominal symptoms). The use of multidetector CT scanning has improved the detection of diaphragmatic hernias.

## DIFFERENTIAL DIAGNOSIS AND MEDICAL DECISION MAKING

The differential diagnosis of abdominal wall hernias includes other masses involving the abdominal wall, such as lipomas and rectus sheath hematomas. Abdominal wall or intraabdominal hernias should be considered a potential cause in patients with signs and symptoms of small bowel obstruction. In patients who have previously undergone abdominal surgery, either open or laparoscopic, careful examination of the incisions,[5] trocar sites,[6] and parastomal areas[7] should be performed to detect masses or abdominal wall defects. To facilitate detection of the hernia, the examiner should hold the tips of the fingers over the incision while the patient coughs or strains.[8]

Inguinal hernias should be considered in the evaluation of patients with scrotal pain or swelling. Detection of inguinal hernias is improved by examination of the patient in a standing position and insertion of the examiner's finger into the inguinal canal through the loose skin of the scrotum. This technique allows direct palpation of the inguinal ring. Having the patient cough or strain allows the examiner to palpate the hernia bulging against the examining finger. Other causes of scrotal pain, masses, or swelling are testicular torsion, tumor, orchitis, epididymitis, lipoma, hydrocele, and varicocele.[9]

Congenital anatomic fistulas of the urachus or omphalomesenteric duct can be manifested in children or adults as umbilical pain, swelling, a mass, erythema, or discharge and can be confused with an umbilical hernia.

Obturator or other rare pelvic floor hernias should be considered in the differential diagnosis of patients with chronic atypical pelvic pain; CT should be performed.

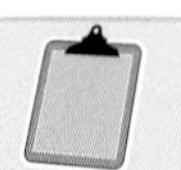

### DOCUMENTATION

- Physical examination
- Ultrasound, especially for scrotal hernias
- Computed tomography when internal hernia, small bowel obstruction, intestinal ischemia, or necrosis is a concern
- Rarely magnetic resonance imaging or laparoscopy

In the majority of cases, physical examination alone enables the identification of abdominal wall or inguinal hernias. When physical examination is not sufficient, ultrasonography, CT, and occasionally magnetic resonance imaging can assist in the identification of hernias and serve to further delineate their contents.

Ultrasonography is the imaging modality of choice in the evaluation of scrotal swelling or masses because it allows differentiation of the testicles, spermatic cord, hydrocele, or varicocele separately from the hernia contents. This modality can assist in the diagnosis of abdominal wall hernias through identification of bowel loops within the hernia sac. Color flow Doppler imaging can detect the presence or absence of blood flow in some cases, thereby aiding in the diagnosis of strangulation.[10]

CT can be used to identify intraabdominal and abdominal wall hernias (as well as delineate the contents of the hernia sac) and signs of ischemia, perforation, or abscess formation. Plain abdominal films have limited utility in the diagnosis and evaluation of hernias. Laparoscopy may be necessary to assist in the diagnosis of difficult cases when the findings of other modalities are unrevealing.

## PEDIATRIC CONSIDERATIONS

Omphalocele occurs in 2 to 3 per 10,000 births. Historically, gastroschisis occurred less frequently than omphalocele, but recent trends show an increase in the incidence of gastroschisis worldwide (and in the United States). Gastroschisis occurs more commonly with younger maternal age and is associated with fewer congenital anomalies than omphalocele is. Ultrasonography has led to more frequent prenatal diagnosis, but cesarean delivery has not been shown to improve outcomes over vaginal delivery in infants with abdominal wall defects.

Congenital diaphragmatic hernias occur in 1 in 2500 births. The mortality rate is high because of pulmonary hypoplasia and the development of pulmonary hypertension. Ultrasonography allows prenatal diagnosis and identification of infants with the potential for a poor prognosis. The prognosis worsens when the liver is located intrathoracically and total lung volume is less than total head volume. In utero repair of diaphragmatic hernias has been performed, although better outcomes than those with conventional treatment have not been observed.[11]

Percutaneous placement of a fetal endoluminal tracheal occlusion balloon may improve survival by preventing egress of the pulmonary fluid needed to stimulate lung growth.[12] This treatment is still controversial because of a higher incidence of preterm labor. Stabilization of infants with congenital diaphragmatic hernia consists of intravenous fluid resuscitation, insertion of a nasogastric tube, intubation with gentle ventilation or permissive hypercapnia (to avoid barotrauma), and surgical consultation. The use of nitric oxide and surfactant has not been demonstrated to improve outcomes in infants with congenital diaphragmatic hernias.

Late manifestations of congenital diaphragmatic hernia have been described in children and adults. Cases typically involve respiratory difficulty, and tension gastrothorax has also been reported. Unrecognized diaphragmatic hernias can be exacerbated by pregnancy and be manifested as incarceration and bowel obstruction, in addition to respiratory distress.

Indirect inguinal and umbilical hernias are extremely common in children—parents may bring an infant or child to the emergency department when the lump or bulge is first noted. Incarceration or strangulation is uncommon but can occur. The clinical findings in children are similar to those in adults. Physical examination of the scrotum and groin is mandatory in the evaluation of crying or vomiting infants. Ultrasonography is used more often than CT for the evaluation of hernias in children.

## TREATMENT

### HOSPITAL

Reduction of the hernia is attempted by applying slow gentle pressure over the hernia contents and directing the contents toward the defect in the abdominal wall. Reduction can be facilitated by placing the patient in a supine or Trendelenburg position and administering analgesia, which may decrease intraabdominal pressure and relax the abdominal musculature. Some authorities advocate placing a cool pack of ice over the area to decrease swelling and provide slow continuous pressure. Procedural sedation should be used when the patient exhibits significant tenderness and anxiety.

**TIPS AND TRICKS**

To reduce a hernia through a small defect, it may be wise to pull on the hernia instead of pushing. Imagine a balloon trying to pass through a small hole—direct pressure on the balloon flattens the mass rather than pushing it through the hole. Instead, pressure applied at the defect in the abdominal wall (the base of the hernia) with accompanying traction on the herniated contents can narrow the sac and facilitate passage. The emergency physician should apply horizontal pressure with the tips of the fingers to narrow the base of the herniated contents while gently pulling the herniated mass. Pulling on the hernia from the base may be more successful than pushing.

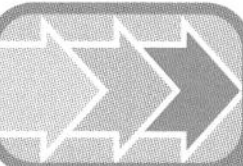

**PRIORITY ACTIONS**

Analgesia, fluid resuscitation, attempts at manual reduction of the hernia, and procedural sedation should be used as necessary.

Complications of persistent hernia incarceration include small bowel obstruction, bowel ischemia, or necrosis of the hernia contents.

Surgical consultation should be obtained for possible operative intervention in cases of persistent incarceration, small bowel obstruction, bowel ischemia or necrosis.

Reduction should not be attempted when the patient has signs of peritoneal irritation, fever, or erythema or necrosis of the skin overlying the hernia. These signs signal the possibility of necrotic bowel, reduction of which could lead to diffuse peritonitis and abscess formation. When bowel ischemia or necrosis is suspected, antibiotics that cover intraabdominal pathogens should be administered and surgical consultation obtained.

Patients with signs of volume depletion or sepsis should receive fluid resuscitation with normal saline. Urine output should be monitored via catheter placement to help to guide fluid replacement. A nasogastric tube should be placed in patients with signs of bowel obstruction.

The current surgical trend is toward laparoscopic repair of most hernias.[13] Laparoscopic repair of incisional hernias tends to decrease perioperative pain and recovery time and has complication and recurrence rates similar to those with open repair.[14] Laparoscopic inguinal hernia repair has a slightly higher incidence of bladder and vascular injury than open repair does.[15]

Postoperative complications of hernia repair include bowel injury, hemorrhage, wound infection, and recurrence. The use of prosthetic mesh has decreased hernia recurrence, although mesh is problematic when wound infection occurs. Late complications of the use of prosthetic mesh for hernia repair consist of fibrosis and erosion into adjacent structures, including bowel and bladder, and occasionally fistula formation.[16]

Other complications of inguinal hernia repair are entrapment of the genitofemoral or ilioinguinal nerves, persistent pain syndromes, and in male patients, injury to the vas deferens and testicles with resultant alterations in fertility.[17] Repair of abdominal wall hernias can injure cutaneous nerves and give rise to persistent abdominal wall pain syndromes.[18]

## FOLLOW-UP, NEXT STEPS IN CARE, AND PATIENT EDUCATION

Hernias with signs or symptoms suggestive of bowel obstruction or ischemia are true surgical emergencies that require immediate consultation.

Emergency repair of incarcerated or strangulated hernias is associated with higher morbidity and mortality than is the case with elective repair, especially in elderly patients or those with multiple medical comorbid conditions.[19] Complications include a higher incidence of bowel ischemia and necrosis, wound infection and dehiscence, intraabdominal compartment syndrome, sepsis and respiratory compromise, and hernia recurrence.[20]

Patients with easily reducible hernias may be discharged for surgical follow-up and elective hernia repair. Repair is generally recommended for symptomatic hernias in otherwise healthy patients. Patients who have multiple medical problems and for whom surgery poses a high risk may not be suitable candidates for elective hernia repair, especially when the fascial defect is large and less likely to become incarcerated. The decision about the timing of hernia repair should be made by the patient in conjunction with the primary care physician and the surgeon. Elective repair of symptomatic hernias in elderly patients should be considered.[21]

Unrepaired hernias may gradually enlarge over time, and some become incarcerated. Patients with incarcerated hernias that cannot be reduced should be admitted for urgent surgical reduction and repair because some hernias progress to ischemia of the hernia contents.

**DOCUMENTATION**

Presence or absence of a palpable hernia mass or fascial defect with estimation of size

Presence or absence of erythema or necrosis of the overlying skin

Presence or absence of fever, signs of small bowel obstruction

Presence or absence of guarding or rebound

Name of consultant, time of consultation

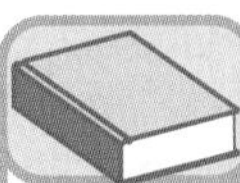

### PATIENT TEACHING TIPS

A hernia is a defect in the abdominal wall that allows the intestines or abdominal fat to bulge through the opening. Hernias do not typically heal spontaneously and may enlarge over time. They may be repaired by surgery.

Sometimes the contents of the hernia may become trapped or incarcerated, which is potentially dangerous because the blood supply to the contents of the hernia may be cut off. You should return to the emergency department if your hernia suddenly becomes larger or more painful or if fever, nausea, vomiting, or redness over your hernia develops; if any of those things happen, your hernia would need to be treated right away.

## SUGGESTED READINGS

INCA Trialists Collaboration. Operation compared with watchful waiting in elderly male inguinal hernia patients: a review and data analysis. J Am Coll Surg 2011;212:251-9.e1-4.

Maish MS. The diaphragm. Surg Clin North Am 2010;90:955-68.

Monkhouse SJ, Morgan JD, Norton SA. Complications of bariatric surgery: presentation and emergency management—a review. Ann R Coll Surg Engl 2009;91:280-6.

Montgomery JS, Bloom DA. The diagnosis and management of scrotal masses. Med Clin North Am 2011;95:235-44.

## REFERENCES

***References can be found on Expert Consult @ www.expertconsult.com.***

# Appendicitis 39

*Rita A. Manfredi and Claudia Ranniger*

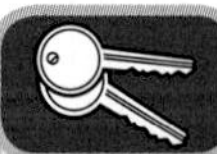

**KEY POINTS**

- Appendicitis is the most common abdominal surgical emergency in the United States.
- Physical signs and symptoms vary with the location of the appendix.
- Children, pregnant women, and elderly patients may exhibit subtle clinical findings.
- No single diagnostic test can reliably confirm or exclude appendicitis.
- Early surgical consultation should not be delayed for diagnostic testing.
- Protocols involving ultrasound and then computed tomography can decrease radiation exposure in patients requiring diagnostic imaging.
- Narcotic analgesia does not interfere with diagnostic accuracy.
- Prophylactic antibiotic therapy, properly timed, decreases postoperative infection rates.

## PERSPECTIVE

Appendicitis is the most common cause of acute abdominal pain that requires surgical intervention. Failure to diagnose acute appendicitis is one of the leading causes of malpractice claims for emergency physicians. Appendicitis should be included in the differential diagnosis for any patient evaluated in the emergency department (ED) for abdominal pain.

## EPIDEMIOLOGY

About 1% of patients seeking care in the ED for abdominal pain have appendicitis, and missed diagnosis and subsequent morbidity continue to occur. The lifetime risk for appendicitis is approximately 9% in men and 7% in women.[1] The classic "textbook" manifestation of appendicitis—right lower quadrant pain, abdominal rigidity, and migration of pain from the periumbilical area to the right lower quadrant—is the exception rather than the norm. Symptoms are frequently atypical, and subtle findings are common. Delayed diagnosis results in a higher risk for perforation, which increases morbidity and mortality. When the diagnosis is delayed, about 20% of appendicitis cases perforate.

## ANATOMY

The appendix is a tubular structure that arises from the cecum and consists primarily of smooth muscle and an abundance of lymphoid tissue. The average adult appendix can reach a length of 10 cm with a luminal width of 6 to 7 mm. Innervation from sympathetic and vagus nerves accounts for referred pain to the umbilicus when inflammatory changes are present. The location of the appendix (retrocecal, 65%; pelvic, 31%; subcecal, 2%) determines the clinical findings and risk for the development of perforated appendicitis.[2]

## PATHOPHYSIOLOGY

Acute appendicitis develops as a result of luminal obstruction, which promotes bacterial overgrowth and distention. Obstruction of the appendiceal lumen is commonly caused by fecal stasis and fecaliths; other obstructive masses include lymphoid hyperplasia, vegetable matter, fruit seeds, intestinal worms, inspissated radiographic barium, and tumors (e.g., carcinoid). Luminal obstruction creates a closed space in which bacterial overgrowth leads to the accumulation of fluid and gas. Organisms are typically polymicrobial, with a predominance of anaerobic and gram-negative species.[2]

As the appendix distends, normal circulatory supply is impaired and the inflammatory changes worsen. Ischemia, infarction, and perforation can ensue. Progression of an inflamed appendix from gangrene to perforation is variable, with a mean duration of abdominal symptoms of between 2 days (gangrene) and 3 days (perforation).

## CLINICAL PRESENTATIONS

### CLASSIC

The pain of acute appendicitis starts as diffuse, poorly localized, periumbilical discomfort (*visceral pain*) that localizes to the McBurney point in the right lower quadrant over a period of 12 to 24 hours (*peritoneal pain*). The McBurney point is located one third of the distance from the right anterior superior iliac crest to the umbilicus. The appendix is located within 5 cm of the McBurney point in only 50% of patients.

Once the pain is perceived in the right lower quadrant, sudden movements cause severe discomfort consistent with localized peritonitis. Associated symptoms often include anorexia, nausea, and vomiting. Diarrhea is uncommon, although patients may report an increasing urge to defecate (the "downward urge"). Bowel movements or the passage of flatus does not relieve the pain, however.

Up to 50% of patients have a normal body temperature on initial arrival at the ED.[3] Patients with significant inflammation prefer to remain still in an effort to minimize peritoneal irritation. The right leg may be flexed at the hip to further decrease peritoneal stretch (see **Table 39.1**, Special Maneuvers That Suggest Appendicitis, online at www.expert.consult.com). Palpation of the abdomen generally reveals localized right lower quadrant tenderness. Rebound tenderness, voluntary and involuntary guarding, and rigidity may be observed, depending on the extent of appendiceal inflammation.

*Physical signs and symptoms vary with the location of the appendix.* If the appendix is *retrocecal*, pain and tenderness may localize to the flank and not to the right lower quadrant. A *retroileal* appendix in men or boys may irritate the ureter with resulting radiation of pain to the testicle. The gravid uterus of a pregnant patient was previously thought to displace the appendix superiorly as the pregnancy progresses and cause right upper quadrant or flank pain. However, recent studies suggest that this conventional belief may be incorrect and that the location of the appendix may be similar in pregnant and nonpregnant patients.[4,5] A *pelvic* appendix may irritate the bladder or rectum and result in dysuria, suprapubic pain, or a more pronounced urge to defecate. If the appendix is low lying, isolated rectal tenderness may be the only sign.[2]

## VARIATIONS

### Children

Appendicitis is the most common condition requiring emergency abdominal surgery in children. Up to 8% of children seen in the ED with abdominal pain have appendicitis. In the very young, appendicitis is quite uncommon because the appendix is funnel shaped and less prone to obstruction. Symptoms of appendicitis in this age group are nonspecific and mimic those of gastroenteritis, viral syndrome, and intussusception. The incidence of appendicitis rises with age, but the likelihood of perforation is highest in infants. Neonatal appendicitis has a high mortality rate. Almost 100% of children younger than 2 years have a perforated appendix at the time of diagnosis. In children 3 to 5 years of age the perforation rate is 71%, and in children 6 to 10 years of age the rate is 40%. Appendicitis most frequently occurs in patients between 10 and 20 years old.

Children with appendicitis commonly exhibit fever and vomiting. These two signs, along with abdominal distention, are most often seen in infants. A lethargic, irritable baby with grunting respirations may be a typical manifestation in this age group. Toddlers are more likely to have vomiting and fever followed by pain. In school-age children, vomiting and abdominal pain are the more frequent symptoms.[6] When the diagnosis is unclear, one should avoid diagnosing acute gastroenteritis in young children without diarrhea.

In the vast majority of children, the diagnosis of appendicitis is made only after perforation occurs, possibly because of a child's inability to describe the pain or the physician's misattribution of symptoms to other childhood diseases or to gastroenteritis. As a result of perforation, worsening peritonitis in children might be manifested as lethargy, inactivity, and hypothermia.[7]

Adolescent girls are a subset of the pediatric population that deserves special attention in the evaluation of acute appendicitis. The etiology of right lower quadrant pain in prepubertal and postpubertal girls includes ovarian torsion, ovarian cyst, intrauterine pregnancy, and ectopic pregnancy. A urine pregnancy test followed by pelvic ultrasonography may be helpful in distinguishing ovarian pathology from appendicitis.[6]

### Elderly

Elderly patients are often initially seen late in the course of the disease and are three times more likely than the general population to have perforated appendicitis. The elderly have a higher incidence of early perforation (up to 70%) because of the anatomic changes in the appendix that occur with age, such as thinner mucosal lining, decreased lymphoid tissue, a narrowed appendiceal lumen, and atherosclerosis.[8] A definitive diagnosis is often difficult to make because of associated comorbid conditions and the possibility of immunosuppression. Appendicitis accounts for 7% of abdominal pain in the elderly. Geriatric patients most commonly have an atypical manifestation and delay seeking medical intervention.[9] In patients older than 70 years, the mortality rate is higher than 20% because of diagnostic and therapeutic delays.[10] The majority of older patients with acute appendicitis are afebrile and do not have leukocytosis. When the clinical, laboratory, and imaging findings are equivocal, a low threshold for surgical consultation and inpatient observation must be considered for elderly patients with abdominal pain.

### Pregnant Women

Appendicitis is the most common extrauterine surgical emergency during pregnancy. Diagnosis of appendicitis in pregnancy is difficult because the appendix migrates upward as the uterus enlarges, so the location of pain or tenderness is variable. Early symptoms of appendicitis, particularly nausea and vomiting, are common in pregnancy. Leukocytosis is also a normal finding in pregnancy and does not aid in the differentiation of appendicitis, although an increase in band cells implies the presence of infection.

Pregnancy appears to have a protective effect on the development of appendicitis, especially in the third trimester.[2] A fetal loss rate of up to 5% is seen in patients with unruptured appendicitis. Maternal death from appendicitis is extremely rare; however, perforation and subsequent peritonitis cause fetal mortality to rise to 30% and maternal mortality to 2%. The use of ultrasonography may differentiate obstetric causes of abdominal pain from appendicitis without the need for imaging studies that involve radiation, such as computed tomography (CT). Once the diagnosis of appendicitis has been made in a pregnant patient, urgent surgical exploration should be performed.[11]

### Nonpregnant Women

Gynecologic causes of lower abdominal pain often mimic appendicitis.[10] Up to 45% of women who appear to have appendicitis on clinical examination are found to have a normal appendix at surgery. The highest percentage of misdiagnosis occurs in women of childbearing age.

## DIFFERENTIAL DIAGNOSIS

When a patient complains of abdominal pain, suspicion for appendicitis, whether high or low, should be present in the

**BOX 39.1 Differential Diagnosis of Acute Appendicitis**

**Women**
Pelvic inflammatory disease and salpingitis
Ruptured ovarian cyst
Ovarian and adnexal torsion
Endometriosis
Ectopic pregnancy
Tuboovarian abscess

**Men**
Testicular torsion
Epididymitis and orchitis

**Men and Women**
Nephrolithiasis
Urinary tract infection and pyelonephritis
Diverticulitis
Inflammatory bowel disease (terminal ileitis in Crohn disease)
Infectious enteritis and colitis
Incarcerated hernia
Mesenteric adenitis

**Elderly Patients**
Diverticulitis
Mesenteric ischemia
Vascular disease

clinician's thought. The differential diagnosis for acute appendicitis is extensive and includes all causes of an acute abdomen (**Box 39.1**). Given that atypical manifestations in children, pregnant women, and the elderly are not uncommon, a high index of suspicion and early surgical consultation are critical.[12]

## DIAGNOSTIC TESTING

*No single diagnostic test can reliably confirm or exclude the diagnosis of appendicitis.* Diagnostic testing should not delay surgical consultation for patients with worrisome findings on examination. The surgeon should be engaged immediately (before laboratory testing or imaging) for a patient with an acute abdomen or when appendicitis is the most likely clinical diagnosis (**Box 39.2**).

The goals of testing are to improve accuracy and speed of diagnosis, exclude alternative causes of abdominal pain, and reduce the rate of appendectomies performed in patients who have a normal appendix (negative appendectomy rate).

**BOX 39.2 Diagnostic Considerations**

**Laboratory Testing**
Exclude pregnancy in women of childbearing age.
The combination of an elevated white blood cell count and C-reactive protein has a high positive predictive value in patients in whom appendicitis is suspected.
Urinalysis results may be abnormal in up to 50% of patients with appendicitis.

**Imaging Studies**

***Computed Tomography***
Abdominal-pelvic and focused appendiceal study protocols are available.
Use oral, rectal, or intravenous administration of contrast agents as needed; discuss with the radiologist.

***Ultrasonography***
Ultrasound is the preferred modality for children, pregnant women, and nonpregnant women in whom concern for pelvic disease is high.
A diagnostic strategy of ultrasound and then computed tomography may decrease radiation exposure in patients with an uncertain diagnosis.

***Plain Radiographs***
Plain films are not indicated for evaluation of appendicitis.
They are useful to exclude pneumoperitoneum, bowel obstruction, and foreign body.

***Magnetic Resonance Imaging***
Consider in patients in whom computed tomography is contraindicated and other studies are nondiagnostic.

### LABORATORY TESTING

Elevations in the white blood cell (WBC) count, percentage of bands, absolute neutrophil count, and C-reactive protein (CRP) level have each been associated with a greater likelihood of appendicitis. Taken individually, these tests have poor predictive value.[7] In combination, elevated WBC and CRP values have been associated with positive likelihood ratios between 7 and 23 for the prediction of appendicitis in both children and adults.[13,14] The likelihood of appendicitis when both WBC and CRP values are in the normal range is low.[15,16] However, CRP and WBC values vary with age and the duration of symptoms; patients who are seen early in the disease process may have a normal CRP level.

Scoring systems that include historical data, physical findings, and laboratory markers have been developed to assist in differentiating appendicitis from other sources of abdominal pain. However, the sensitivity and specificity of these systems are not sufficient to predict the presence or absence of appendicitis with adequate reliability. These tools are more frequently used to risk-stratify patients who may need further diagnostic testing or observation.[17-21]

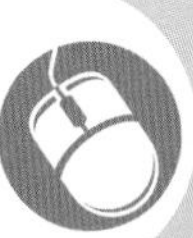

**See additional information on this topic, Table 39.2, Common Appendicitis Scoring Systems, and Table 39.3, Interpretation of Common Appendicitis Scoring Systems,**
online at www.expertconsult.com.

It is imperative that pregnancy be excluded early in the assessment of a woman of childbearing age by checking a urine or serum quantitative human chorionic gonadotropin level.

An abnormal urinalysis result must be interpreted with caution in a patient with suspected appendicitis and a low likelihood of cystitis. Abnormal urinalysis results (including more than 4 red blood cells [RBCs] per high-power field [HPF], more than 4 WBCs per HPF, or proteinuria greater than 0.5 g/L) are observed in 36% to 50% of patients with acute appendicitis.[22] These findings are more common in women, in patients with perforated appendicitis, and in patients in whom the appendix is located near the urinary tract. No upper limit of urinary WBC or RBC counts has been defined for appendicitis.

## IMAGING

### Plain Radiographs

Plain abdominal radiography is *not* indicated for the evaluation of potential appendicitis. Barium-enhanced imaging (via oral or rectal administration) demonstrates equally poor sensitivity because of nonfilling of the appendix and therefore has no role in the diagnosis of acute appendicitis. Plain radiography should be performed only to exclude suspected pneumoperitoneum, bowel obstruction, or foreign body.

### Helical Computed Tomography

High-resolution helical CT is the diagnostic test of choice for suspected appendicitis (**Fig. 39.1**). CT findings in appendicitis include an appendiceal diameter greater than 7 to 10 mm, wall enhancement, wall thickening greater than 3 mm, and periappendiceal fat stranding.[23,24] The reported sensitivity and specificity of helical CT for appendicitis in adults range between 91% and 96% and 90% and 95%, respectively.[25-28]

The use of CT as a diagnostic tool for suspected appendicitis has grown explosively in recent years, with adult imaging rates in the United States reported to be greater than 90%.[29-31] CT imaging is correlated with a significant decrease in the negative appendectomy rate to less than 9%.[29,32,33] The highest benefit of CT in reducing the negative appendectomy rate is appreciated in adult women.[30,31] In the elderly, who often have atypical symptoms, the use of helical CT aids in early diagnosis and has reduced the rate of perforated appendicitis from 72% to 51%.[9]

Intravenous, rectal, or oral administration of a contrast agent to enhance CT imaging in patients with suspicion of appendicitis is controversial. Variations in patient population, contrast protocol, scanner resolution, and radiation dosing all contribute to reported diagnostic accuracy. Contrast agent administered enterally or intravenously enhances the appendiceal wall, lumen, and periappendiceal fat, thereby improving visualization of adjacent intraperitoneal organs. An intravenously administered contrast agent can provide valuable information in patients with little visceral fat but may cause allergic reactions or exacerbate renal insufficiency.[34] An enterally administered contrast agent is particularly useful in the identification of perforation, but oral administration of a contrast agent may exacerbate nausea, and 1 to 2 hours is required for the contrast agent to traverse the gut before imaging. Newer-generation multislice CT systems have improved image resolution, even without contrast enhancement. Judicious use of non–contrast-enhanced protocols may reduce diagnostic delays and avoid potential contrast agent–related morbidity.[35-37]

Radiation exposure may be limited by using a focused appendiceal (right lower quadrant) CT study. Such protocols may be desirable for children and pregnant women, in whom large radiation exposure is a concern, but other intraabdominal disease may be missed.

In children, the sensitivity of helical CT for appendicitis with contrast enhancement is 92% to 100% and the specificity is 87% to 100%.[7,28,36] The relative paucity of intra-abdominal fat in children decreases the visualization of periappendiceal inflammatory changes, and contrast-enhanced protocols should be used to maximize diagnostic yield.

### Ultrasonography

Graded compression ultrasonography is conducted by applying pressure at and around the point of maximum abdominal tenderness. Ultrasonographic findings highly associated with appendicitis include an enlarged, tender appendix greater than 6 mm in diameter with enhancing (hyperechoic) surrounding fat.[24] Other signs include an inability to compress the appendix, the presence of periappendiceal fluid, and hypervascularity (**Fig. 39.2**). Formal ultrasonography for appendicitis has demonstrated sensitivities of 78% to 87% and specificities of 81% to 93% in nongravid adults.[25-28] Accuracy is reduced by a thick abdominal wall and intestinal tract; consequently, ultrasonography is best used in thin patients and in children. It is the initial imaging test of choice in pregnant women and children, in whom one wishes to avoid radiation exposure. Ultrasonography is of added benefit when lower abdominal pain may be of pelvic etiology in women of childbearing age.

In children, the sensitivity and specificity of ultrasonography for the diagnosis of appendicitis range from 78% to 100% and 88% to 98%, respectively.[28,36]

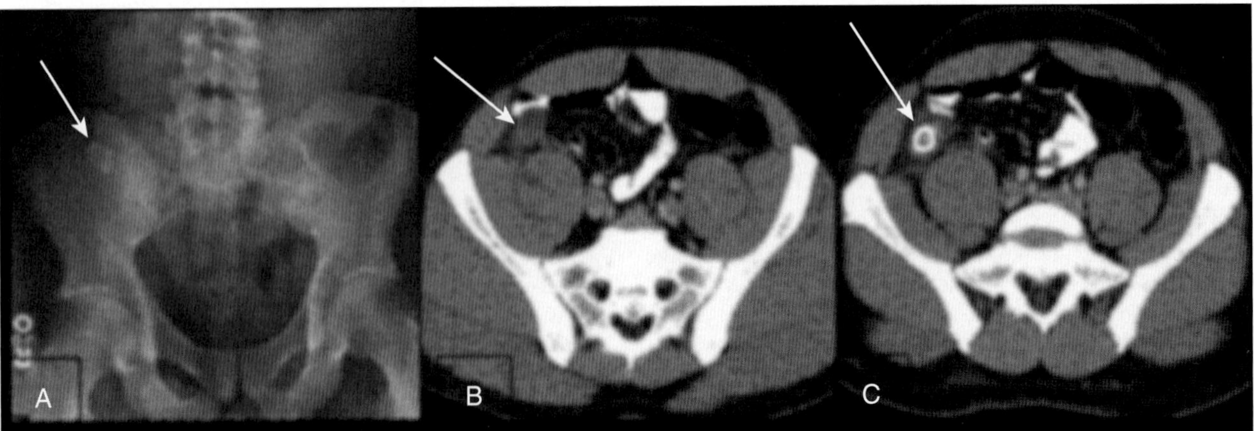


**Fig. 39.1 Plain abdominal radiography and computed tomography demonstrating appendicitis. A,** The plain film shows an appendiceal fecalith *(arrow)* overlying the iliac crest. Computed tomography with oral contrast enhancement demonstrates an enlarged, fluid-filled appendix (*arrow*, **B**) and a fecalith with periappendiceal inflammation (*arrow*, **C**).

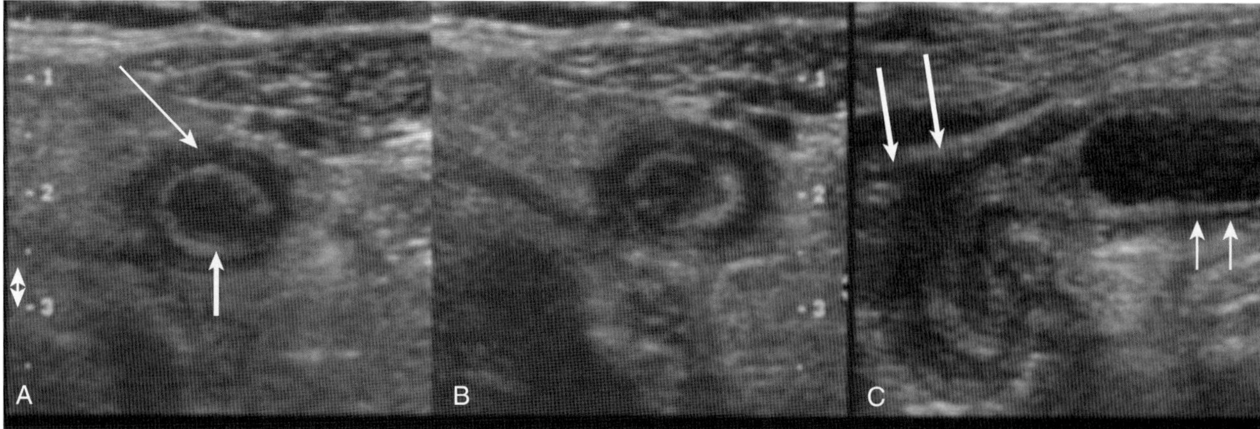


**Fig. 39.2 Transabdominal ultrasonography in a 37-year-old woman with pelvic pain. A,** Cross-sectional view of a dilated appendix *(large arrow)* with periappendiceal fluid *(small arrow)*. **B,** Compression yields minimal change in appendiceal diameter and causes significant pain. **C,** A longitudinal view of the appendix *(small arrows)* and its origin at the cecum *(large arrows)*.

Emergency sonography is compelling because it does not require radiation exposure and can be performed rapidly at the bedside by the clinician. However, large variations in sensitivity (65% to 96%), probably related to operator experience, reduce its current utility as a reliable diagnostic tool.[38,39]

### Combined Ultrasound and Computed Tomography Protocols

CT is more sensitive and specific for the diagnosis of appendicitis than ultrasound is in both adult and pediatric populations, and the accuracy of ultrasound is highly operator dependent. However, concern regarding radiation exposure—especially in children—has led to the implementation of protocols involving ultrasound and then CT in which only patients with negative or nondiagnostic findings on ultrasound undergo CT. This serial diagnostic approach has been applied to both adults and children, with sensitivities and specificities ranging from 94% to 100% and 86% to 94%, respectively.[7,40-42] Concerns that delays in definitive therapy associated with serial imaging protocols could cause an increase in the rate of perforated appendicitis have not been validated.

### Magnetic Resonance Imaging

Findings on magnetic resonance imaging (MRI) in patients with appendicitis consist of a thickened appendiceal wall, a dilated lumen filled with high-intensity material, and periappendiceal enhancement on T2-weighted images. The utility of MRI in diagnosing appendicitis is curtailed by its limited availability, higher cost, and longer image acquisition time. MRI may be appropriate in patients in whom radiation exposure is contraindicated and ultrasonography is nondiagnostic.[43,44]

## TREATMENT

Early surgical consultation should be obtained whenever appendicitis is suspected (**Box 39.3**). Delays in surgery raise the risk for appendiceal perforation, peritonitis, and sepsis. Children, pregnant women, and elderly patients with abdominal pain have especially atypical manifestation and are at higher risk for perforation. Surgical consultation should not be delayed for testing, and testing should be undertaken only when the clinical diagnosis is in question.

**BOX 39.3 Emergency Department Treatment of Patients with Suspected Appendicitis**

Immediate resuscitation with isotonic fluids
Advise the patient to abstain from oral intake
Early surgical consultation (do not delay for diagnostic testing)
Parenteral antibiotics to reduce the risk for perioperative infections
Pain control with narcotic analgesia
Nausea control with parenteral medications

Intravenous administration of isotonic crystalloid should be initiated as indicated, particularly if prolonged vomiting, anorexia, or fever has been reported. In anticipation of surgery, the patient should be advised not to eat or drink.

Control of pain and nausea is both medically rational and humane. Narcotic administration has not been shown to affect the sensitivity of the physical examination in either adults or children or delay the time to diagnostic decision making, although adequately powered studies in children are lacking.[45-48] Analgesia with morphine sulfate, hydromorphone, or fentanyl is appropriate. An antiemetic, such as ondansetron, promethazine, prochlorperazine, or metoclopramide, may also be required.

Prophylactic administration of antibiotics has been shown to reduce perioperative infection rates in both simple (nonperforated) and complicated (perforated or gangrenous) appendicitis.[49,50] Their administration should be timed in consultation with the surgeon so that high antibiotic tissue levels coincide with the surgical procedure. The antibiotics should be effective against both skin flora and common appendiceal pathogens, including *Escherichia coli, Klebsiella, Proteus*, and *Bacteroides* species (**Table 39.4**).

## DISPOSITION

Patients in whom the findings are a concern despite normal laboratory and imaging results should be admitted for observation and serial abdominal examinations (**Box 39.4**). Patients with undifferentiated abdominal pain, low risk for

**Table 39.4 Options for Preoperative Antibiotics in Patients Suspected of Having Appendicitis**

| | | |
|---|---|---|
| Adults | Uncomplicated (nonperforated) | Cefoxitin or cefotetan |
| | Perforated or gangrenous appendicitis | A carbapenem<br>Ticarcillin-clavulanate<br>Piperacillin-tazobactam<br>Ampicillin-sulbactam<br>A fluoroquinolone (ciprofloxacin, levofloxacin), metronidazole |
| Children | | Ampicillin, gentamicin, metronidazole<br>Ampicillin, gentamicin, clindamycin<br>A carbapenem<br>Ticarcillin-clavulanate<br>Piperacillin-tazobactam |

**BOX 39.4 Disposition of Patients with Undifferentiated Abdominal Pain**

Admit for observation if:
- Suspicion for appendicitis or another urgent intraabdominal process is high despite negative test results.
- Poor follow-up is likely.
- Oral intake is impaired.

Discharge home if:
- Good follow-up can be arranged and there are no impediments to obtaining care.
- The patient is able to tolerate oral fluids.

Discharge considerations:
- Instruct the patient to return to the emergency department for increasing pain, fever, nausea, vomiting, or anorexia.
- Do not prescribe narcotic analgesics.
- Do not prescribe antibiotics.

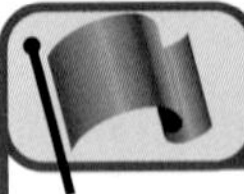

**RED FLAGS**

In geriatric or female patients with right lower quadrant pain, the misdiagnosis rate can be as high as 40%.

In the pediatric age group, misdiagnosis of appendicitis approaches 50%.

The incidence of diarrhea in children younger than 3 years with acute appendicitis is 33%.

appendicitis, and negative diagnostic evaluation results may be considered for discharge if their clinical symptoms improve and they are able to tolerate oral fluids. Arrangements should be made for close follow-up for such patients, who should be given specific instructions to return to the ED if their symptoms worsen. Antibiotics should not be prescribed for discharged patients with undifferentiated abdominal pain. Narcotic analgesics may mask disease progression and are not recommended.

**TIPS AND TRICKS**

If a patient is discharged with the diagnosis of acute abdominal pain, ensure that the plan for that patient is clear and specific. Ask the patient or caregiver to repeat the explained plan. Be sure to include the time and place of the repeat abdominal examination.

Check that the β-human chorionic gonadotropin level is determined in all female patients of childbearing age.

Be certain that the imaging study demonstrates a *normal* appendix to exclude the diagnosis. Caution should be used when attributing pain to an ovarian cyst or uterine fibroid discovered on ultrasound.

**DOCUMENTATION**

Include the following elements in your documentation:
- Initial physical examination and serial abdominal examinations
- Differential diagnosis of the patient's abdominal pain
- Discussions with consultants, patient, and family members

If a patient with unexplained abdominal pain is discharged, explain why you concluded that the patient did not have acute appendicitis. Include laboratory results, imaging studies, serial examinations, and consultations.

Document in the discharge instructions when the patient with unexplained abdominal pain should undergo a repeat abdominal evaluation: 8, 12, 24, or 36 hours.

## SUGGESTED READINGS

Adibe OO, Amin SR, Hansen EN, et al. An evidence-based clinical protocol for diagnosis of acute appendicitis decreased the use of computed tomography in children. J Pediatr Surg 2011;46:192-6.

Bundy DG, Byerley JS, Liles EA, et al. Does this child have appendicitis? JAMA 2007;298:438-51.

Hlibczuk V, Dattaro JA, Jin Z, et al. Diagnostic accuracy of noncontrast computed tomography for appendicitis in adults: a systematic review. Ann Emerg Med 2010;55:51-9.

Howell JM, Eddy OL, Lukens TW, et al. Clinical policy: critical issues in the evaluation and management of emergency department patients with suspected appendicitis. Ann Emerg Med 2010;55:71-116.

Vissers RJ, Lennarz WB. Pitfalls in appendicitis. Emerg Med Clin North Am 2010;28:103-8.

## REFERENCES

*References can be found on Expert Consult @ www.expertconsult.com.*

# Bowel Obstructions 40

*Keith Boniface*

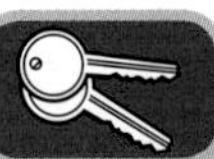

**KEY POINTS**

- Complete small bowel obstructions are at high risk for strangulation and typically require surgical treatment.
- Partial small bowel obstructions are at lower risk for strangulation and are generally managed nonoperatively.
- Closed-loop bowel obstructions have a higher likelihood of concomitant vascular compromise and strangulation.
- Strangulation may lead to bowel wall necrosis, perforation, peritonitis, sepsis, and death. Fever in a patient with bowel obstruction suggests strangulation and perforation.
- Plain radiographs can be used initially to evaluate cases of suspected bowel obstruction. Computed tomography may be necessary to confirm the diagnosis when plain radiographic findings are nondiagnostic. Computed tomography can exclude the diagnosis of closed-loop obstruction.
- Obstructions that complicate the first 30 days after laparotomy are often managed nonoperatively, whereas obstructions that occur after laparoscopy generally require surgery.

## PERSPECTIVE

Bowel obstructions develop from mechanical blockage of normal intestinal transit. Blockages may result from intraluminal matter (e.g., foreign bodies), intramural wall thickening (tumors, hernia, inflammation), or extraluminal compression (hernias, masses, adhesions). Bowel proximal to the obstruction progressively dilates, which leads to pain, obstipation (inability to pass flatus), and vomiting. Dehydration and electrolyte abnormalities ensue. As the bowel wall becomes edematous, increasing pressure causes collapse of the capillary bed and subsequent tissue ischemia, a condition known as strangulation. Strangulation may lead to bowel wall necrosis, perforation, peritonitis, sepsis, and death. Patients with small bowel obstruction have a 5% to 42% incidence of strangulation, which carries a mortality of 20% to 37%.[1]

Obstruction can be partial, with some intestinal contents allowed to progress through the area of narrowing, or complete. A patient with complete obstruction has a low likelihood of spontaneous resolution and a high likelihood of bowel strangulation, whereas a patient with partial obstruction can typically be managed nonoperatively because of the lower risk for bowel strangulation. The central dilemma in caring for patients with small bowel obstruction is to identify those at risk for strangulation to ensure timely surgical intervention.

## PATHOPHYSIOLOGY

Bowel obstructions can be divided into simple obstructions (bowel occlusion at one location with an intact blood supply) and closed-loop obstruction (occluded loop of bowel at two adjacent points, which may or may not involve a vascular pedicle). Closed-loop obstructions are most commonly caused by entrapment of bowel in a hernia (incarceration) or, less commonly, by volvulus. Closed-loop bowel obstructions have a higher likelihood of concomitant vascular compromise and strangulation, thus warranting a more aggressive management approach.

Large bowel obstructions are at increased risk for perforation if a closed-loop obstruction is present or if the ileocecal valve is functional (preventing proximal decompression into the small bowel). The most likely sites of perforation are at the cecum (especially if the diameter is larger than 10 cm) or at the site of a primary tumor.

Volvulus, or axial twisting of the bowel, represents a special category of closed-loop obstruction. Volvulus occurs most commonly at either the cecum or the sigmoid colon and much less frequently at the transverse colon, small bowel, or stomach. Sigmoid volvulus, which is responsible for 50% to 75% of all cases of colonic volvulus, is more common in elderly and institutionalized patients. Cecal volvulus is found in younger patients, who may have an anatomic predisposition because of abnormal fixation of the right colon.

## CLINICAL PRESENTATION

Bowel obstructions are manifested as colicky abdominal pain that precedes the onset of nausea and vomiting, abdominal distention, constipation, and obstipation. Proximal small bowel obstructions tend to have minimal distention and an early onset of intractable vomiting because the bowel proximal to the obstruction has minimal capacity to distend. Conversely, distal small bowel obstructions are characterized by abdominal distention, colicky abdominal pain, and obstipation before the onset of vomiting. Large bowel obstruction may be preceded by changes in stool caliber and progressive abdominal distention when it is caused by a slow-growing tumor, or it may be sudden in onset in the setting of volvulus.

Physical examination may detect signs of volume depletion, tachycardia, and hypotension. Fever suggests strangulation and perforation. The abdomen is variably distended and tympanitic, depending on the level of obstruction. Scars from previous surgery can provide valuable clues to the cause of the obstruction. Bowel sounds tend toward high-pitched rushes of "tinkling" borborygmi; a silent abdomen is an ominous sign of perforation and peritonitis. Tenderness may be present, but localized tenderness and peritoneal signs indicate perforation. The examination should include a search for hernias.

A digital rectal examination should be performed to exclude stool impaction in the elderly. Occult blood may be detected in cases of strangulated obstruction, intussusception, or an obstructing mass. A rectal mass may be identified as the cause of large bowel obstruction.

## DIFFERENTIAL DIAGNOSIS

Many abdominal disorders may cause a functional ileus that can be mistaken clinically for bowel obstruction.

Potential causes of mechanical small or large bowel obstruction are summarized in **Box 40.1**.

**BOX 40.1 Causes of Mechanical Bowel Obstruction**

**Causes of Small Bowel Obstruction**
Adhesions
Inflammatory bowel disease
Neoplasms
Hernias
Abscess
Intussusception
Foreign bodies

**Causes of Large Bowel Obstruction**
Neoplasms
Volvulus
Diverticulitis
Metastatic cancer (extrinsic compression)
Stricture
Hernia
Fecal impaction
Adhesions

## DIAGNOSTIC TESTING

### LABORATORY TESTING

Laboratory abnormalities are not diagnostic of bowel obstruction but instead may indicate complications of obstruction. A complete blood count may demonstrate leukocytosis with a left shift in a patient with strangulation; serum chemistry evaluations may show dehydration, hypokalemia, and acid-base disturbances. The serum lactate concentration can be elevated in the setting of strangulation, but its measurement is neither sensitive nor specific.[2]

### RADIOGRAPHS

Plain supine and upright radiographs of the abdomen are the most commonly ordered initial diagnostic study for bowel obstruction because of their widespread availability and the low cost of radiographic evaluation (**Fig. 40.1**).

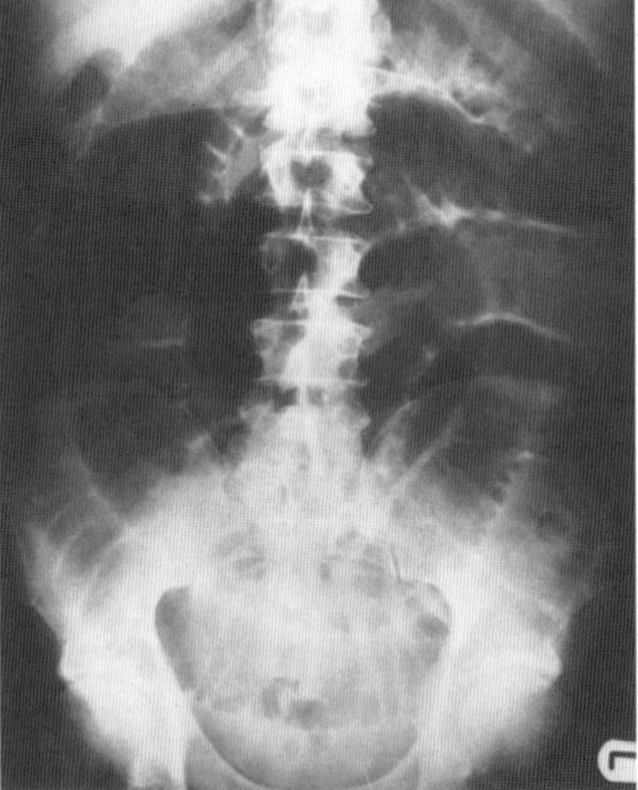

**Fig. 40.1 Supine radiograph showing very distended small bowel identified by its central position, multiple loops, and valvulae conniventes.** (From Adam A, Dixon AK, Grainger & Allison's diagnostic radiology. 5th ed. Philadelphia: Churchill Livingstone; 2008.)

Small bowel obstruction appears on radiographs as air-fluid levels and dilated loops of bowel. Air in the distal part of the colon and rectum implies early or partial small bowel obstruction. As the obstruction progresses, small bowel dilation and air-fluid levels become more prominent, and the distal end of the bowel decompresses and collapses.

Ileus is distinguished from mechanical obstruction by the presence of air-fluid levels at uniform height across an upright image of the abdomen; with obstruction, air-fluid levels are classically found at variable heights.

Plain radiography is less useful for closed-loop obstructions, which are detected only by the subtle finding of a paucity of intestinal gas in the region of an often fluid-filled closed loop.

Sigmoid volvulus is characterized by a massively distended loop of large bowel arising out of the pelvis, sometimes

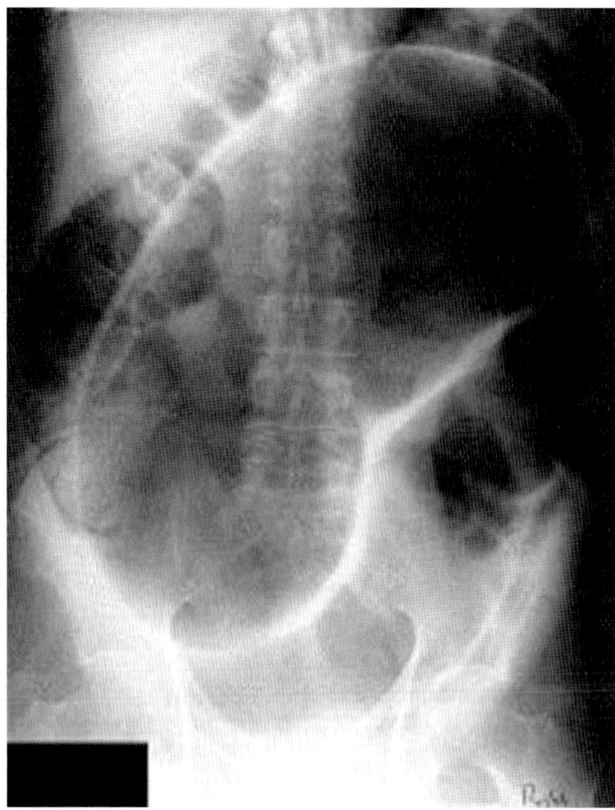

**Fig. 40.2 Sigmoid volvulus.** Note U-shaped, massively dilated, and ahaustral sigmoid. (From Kahi CJ, Rex DK. Bowel obstruction and pseudo-obstruction. Gastroenterol Clin North Am 2003;32: 1229-47.)

described as a "bent inner tube," with accompanying proximal large bowel dilation. (The large bowel is identified by widely spaced haustral markings that do not completely traverse the bowel lumen.) A competent ileocecal valve prevents decompression into the small bowel, thereby leading to massive dilation of the large bowel (**Fig. 40.2**).

Cecal volvulus appears as a coffee bean–shaped loop of bowel projecting from the right lower quadrant into the upper part of the abdomen, often with a collapsed distal large bowel and accompanying small bowel dilation that can be mistaken for a primary small bowel obstruction.

Large bowel obstruction resulting from mechanical causes must be differentiated from pseudoobstruction, a colonic motility disorder that is treated nonoperatively. Enemas of a water-soluble contrast agent (WSCA) (used instead of barium to avoid chemical peritonitis in the setting of perforation) can differentiate obstruction from pseudoobstruction. A contrast agent enema improves the sensitivity and specificity for mechanical obstruction from 84% and 72% to 96% and 98%, respectively, by using a criterion standard of laparotomy findings and clinical follow-up.[3] In addition, a contrast agent enema is helpful in confirming the diagnosis of sigmoid and cecal volvulus, with a tapering "bird's beak" appearance at the end of the column of contrast agent as it reaches the base of the colonic twist.

Studies evaluating the effectiveness of plain radiography in diagnosing obstruction are limited by their methodology. Researchers have used combinations of discharge diagnosis, surgical reports, enteroclysis, and clinical follow-up as criterion standards. A review of these studies shows that plain radiographs are of limited value because they are diagnostic in only 50% to 60% of cases[4] and have a reported sensitivity of just 46% to 76%.[5] A study of plain radiographs interpreted by gastrointestinal radiologists had a sensitivity of 66%; 21% of radiographic studies reported as showing normal bowel were actually images of obstructions.[6] Despite the limitations related to false-negative interpretations, plain radiography is still recommended as the initial test of choice for the evaluation of possible bowel obstruction because the classic radiographic findings, when present, are useful for quickly confirming the diagnosis.

Computed tomography (CT) has supplanted the emergency department (ED) use of contrast-enhanced radiography to confirm suspected bowel obstruction when initial plain radiographs are nondiagnostic (typically in cases of low-grade or intermittent obstruction).

## COMPUTED TOMOGRAPHY

CT of the abdomen is commonly used for the diagnosis of bowel obstruction (1) to confirm a clinically suspected obstruction not identified on a plain radiograph; (2) to determine the level, severity, and cause of the obstruction; (3) to characterize a closed-loop obstruction; (4) to demonstrate signs of strangulation[7]; and (5) to identify alternative causes of acute abdominal pain when obstruction is not present.

CT has a sensitivity of 64% to 100% and a specificity of 71% to 100% for the diagnosis of bowel obstruction.[8] Signs of small bowel obstruction on CT consist of small bowel dilation to a caliber of 2.5 cm or greater with a distinct transition zone and a collapsed distal bowel lumen. The "small bowel feces sign"—the presence of intraluminal particulate material in dilated small bowel—can be helpful in confirming the diagnosis of small bowel obstruction.[9] CT correctly identifies the cause of obstruction in 73% to 95% of patients.[10]

A completely fluid-filled closed-loop obstruction is more easily diagnosed with CT than with plain radiography. Characteristics of closed-loop obstruction include a C- or U-shaped configuration of the dilated loops, a radial distribution of the dilated loops toward the site of obstruction, a radial distribution and engorged mesenteric vessels toward the site of obstruction (the "beak and whirl" sign), and the presence of two collapsed bowel lumens adjacent to the site of obstruction.[1]

Intravenous contrast-enhanced CT has a sensitivity for the diagnosis of strangulation of 56% to 85% and a specificity exceeding 90%.[1,11,12] Strangulation is suggested by a characteristic configuration of the obstructed loop, bowel wall thickening and reduced contrast enhancement, mesenteric vascular changes, gas in the bowel wall, and the presence of free peritoneal fluid. Combinations of clinical, laboratory, and radiographic features have been used in an attempt to identify patients with strangulation who need urgent surgery. One study suggested that the presence of any three of six variables (duration of pain longer than 4 days, abdominal guarding, C-reactive protein level higher than 75 mg/L, white blood cell count greater than 10,000/mm$^3$, presence of more than 500 mL of intraabdominal fluid on CT, or reduced wall contrast enhancement on CT) had a sensitivity of 68% for resection of small bowel.[13] Another study found that the presence of two of four clinical criteria (tachycardia, leukocytosis, fever, and tenderness) increased the specificity of the CT criteria.[14]

CT enteroclysis (delivery of contrast agent to the small bowel via a tube so that it bypasses the pylorus) combines the anatomic information provided by CT with the intraluminal detail of enteroclysis. Although this technique is more labor-intensive because of the need to intubate the small bowel, it may play a role in the future evaluation of small bowel obstruction.[15] CT enteroclysis is a useful test for confirming the diagnosis of superior mesenteric artery syndrome, a rare cause of proximal small bowel obstruction that occurs after rapid weight loss.

Orally administered WSCA can help distinguish partial small bowel obstruction from complete obstruction. Two separate metaanalyses have shown that identification of oral contrast agent in the colon 4 to 24 hours after administration predicts the success of conservative management with a pooled positive likelihood ratio of 25 to 40 and that the absence of contrast agent predicts failure of conservative therapy with a pooled negative likelihood ratio of 0.03 to 0.04.[16,17]

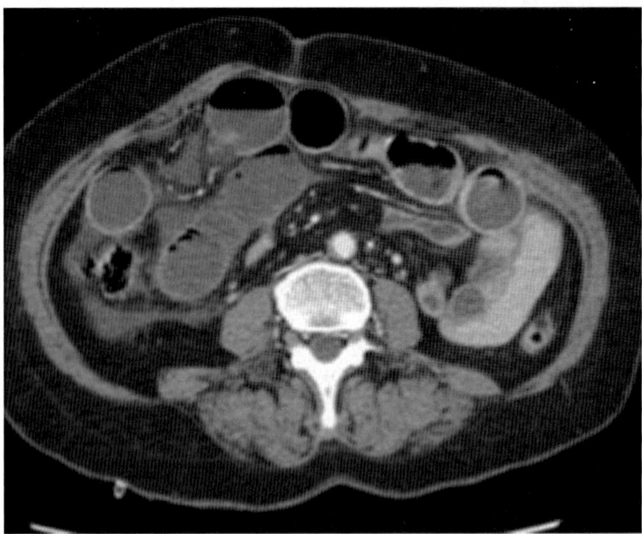

**Fig. 40.3 Computed tomography scan showing small bowel obstruction, proximal jejunum collapse, fluid distension in the ileum, and evidence of peritoneal fluid.** Ischemia and infarction of the intestine are related to the obstruction. (From Romano S, Bartone G, Romano L. Ischemia and infarction of the intestine related to obstruction. Radiol Clin North Am 2008;46:925-42.)

## TREATMENT

### CONSERVATIVE MANAGEMENT OF SMALL BOWEL OBSTRUCTION

"Don't let the sun set on a bowel obstruction." This adage has guided surgeons since the advent of operative therapy for this condition inasmuch as clinical and radiographic predictors of strangulation were poor before the advent of CT. In the modern era, however, nearly half of all patients with acute small bowel obstruction improve with conservative therapy.[18] The mainstay of nonoperative treatment is gastric decompression via nasogastric suctioning. The nasogastric tube is easy to insert, requires no fluoroscopic guidance to place, and reduces the risk for aspiration pneumonia by effectively relieving the gastric distention. Nasointestinal (long) tubes that cross the pylorus are not recommended for ED use.

Small bowel obstructions caused by postoperative adhesions in the first 30 days after laparotomy complicate up to 10% of procedures. These early adhesions represent inflammatory reactions, unlike the fibrous adhesions that develop later in the postoperative course. Obstructions occurring in the early postlaparotomy period can usually be managed nonoperatively because more than 85% resolve spontaneously.[19] Conversely, early postlaparoscopic small bowel obstructions generally require surgery because they are typically caused by herniation of bowel through the peritoneal defect made by the trochar.[20]

Oral contrast agents have been postulated to have a therapeutic role in resolving small bowel obstructions because WSCAs are hyperosmolar and draw water into the small bowel lumen while decreasing bowel wall edema, but studies have demonstrated conflicting results. A metaanalysis of four trials demonstrated no significant difference between WSCAs and placebo in successful nonoperative management of acute small bowel obstruction; however, hospital stay was shorter in patients given WSCAs than in patients receiving placebo.[16]

### SURGICAL MANAGEMENT OF SMALL BOWEL OBSTRUCTION

Surgical excision of an obstructive lesion and assessment of bowel viability are mandated for all cases of suspected bowel strangulation. Viability is assessed by visual inspection of the decompressed bowel during surgery; in questionable cases, fluorescein injection and subsequent fluorescence of the intestines confirm viability. Complete small bowel obstructions and closed-loop obstructions pose higher risks for strangulation and are therefore managed more aggressively with surgical intervention. A trial of nasogastric decompression is reasonable for partial small bowel obstructions.

Laparoscopic treatment of small bowel obstruction appears to be appropriate for carefully selected patients.[21] The most significant complication of laparoscopy is iatrogenic perforation of bowel, which occurs in 1% to 16% of patients. Between 8% and 40% of cases initially planned as laparoscopic procedures are converted to laparotomy intraoperatively. Prospective studies are needed to further compare the risks and benefits of laparoscopic and open surgery for acute small bowel obstruction (**Fig. 40.3**).

### MANAGEMENT OF LARGE BOWEL OBSTRUCTION

Large bowel obstruction can be divided into four types according to treatment options: mechanical obstruction as a result of cancer, sigmoid volvulus, cecal volvulus, and pseudoobstruction. Mechanical large bowel obstruction is treated surgically, with resection and primary anastomosis in most cases of right and transverse colon carcinoma. For carcinoma of the left colon, either initial decompression followed by staged resection or immediate resection (with or without primary anastomosis) is performed. Palliative treatment of obstruction secondary to disseminated or recurrent carcinoma includes creation of a colostomy (or ileostomy for right-sided masses) proximal to the obstruction, corticosteroids, placement of a self-expanding stent, and chemotherapy.

Sigmoid volvulus is initially treated by nonoperative decompression, followed by elective surgery to prevent recurrence after colonoscopy excludes the possibility of carcinoma.

Decompression can be performed via rigid or flexible endoscopic detorsion of the twisted segment.[22] Endoscopy is contraindicated in patients with suspected intestinal necrosis. A rectal tube may be left in place before surgery to facilitate further decompression and prevent recurrence during hospitalization.

Cecal volvulus is managed surgically, with most surgeons choosing a right colectomy as definitive therapy. Cecopexy, or manual detorsion and subsequent correction of the underlying hypermobile right colon, is associated with a high rate of recurrent volvulus.[23]

Pseudoobstruction can initially be managed nonsurgically with a combination of decompression, colonoscopy, and promotility agents, including neostigmine.[24] Medications that slow colonic motility should be discontinued, and suspected infectious causes should be treated appropriately. Surgical management is indicated when conservative therapy fails or in cases of suspected colonic ischemia, perforation, or sepsis. Because of the large number of potential causes of pseudoobstruction, inpatient management with surgical and gastroenterologic consultation is recommended.

## DISPOSITION

Surgical consultation is indicated for all patients with partial or complete bowel obstruction. Such patients require hospital admission for resuscitation, decompression, serial abdominal examination, and possibly operative therapy.

## SUGGESTED READINGS

Abbas S, Bissett IP, Parry BR. Oral water soluble contrast for the management of adhesive small bowel obstruction. Cochrane Database Syst Rev 2007;3:CD004651.

Maglinte DDT, Heitkamp DE, Howard TJ, et al. Current concepts in imaging of small bowel obstruction. Radiol Clin North Am 2003;41:263-83.

## REFERENCES

***References can be found on Expert Consult @ www.expertconsult.com.***

# 41 Anorectal Disorders

*John M. Boe*

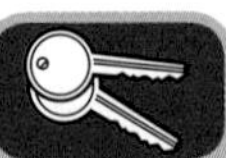

**KEY POINTS**

- Structures proximal to the dentate line are insensate, but tissue external to this boundary can be painful when damaged by trauma, infection, or inflammation.
- An anoscope should be used to directly visualize the internal anatomy if abnormalities are suspected.
- Internal hemorrhoids cannot be distinguished from normal rectal tissue by digital rectal examination. Anoscopy is required to visualize suspected internal hemorrhoids.
- Thrombosed external hemorrhoids are treated with an elliptical incision rather than a linear incision and drainage.
- Fissures that are not properly treated may become chronic and develop the classic triad consisting of sentinel pile, deep ulcer, and enlarged anal papillae.
- Pain that subsides between bowel movements is classic for anal fissures.
- Any patient with suspected rectal perforation because of a foreign body (insertion or removal) should undergo proctosigmoidoscopy performed by a gastroenterologist or colorectal surgeon before discharge.

## PERSPECTIVE

The anorectum marks the end of the digestive tract as it transitions from the endodermal tissues of the colon and intestine to the ectodermal tissues of the skin (**Fig. 41.1**). The rectum is the portion of the digestive tract that extends distally from the rectosigmoid junction at approximately the level of the S3 sacral vertebral body to the dentate line. At the dentate line, the endodermal tissue transitions to ectodermal tissue. The first 1 to 2 cm is considered the anal canal. This tissue, the anoderm, is squamous in origin but contains no hair follicles or sweat glands. At the anal verge, this tissue transforms to more normal external skin marked by hair follicles, apocrine glands, and subcutaneous tissue.

Just proximal to the dentate line, the tissue of the rectum takes on a pleated appearance and forms the rectal ampulla. These pleats create multiple crypts and the anal valves with their insertion at the dentate line. Proximal to the crypts are the columns of Morgagni, where the epithelium of the anoderm transitions to that of the rectum.

Because of the varying embryonic origins of the anorectal region, the vasculature and innervation demonstrate distinct areas of function. The superior, middle, and inferior hemorrhoidal arteries supply blood to the anorectum; they arise, respectively, from the inferior mesenteric, internal iliac, and internal pudendal arteries. Likewise, venous drainage of the rectum is divided between the superior hemorrhoidal vein (which drains into the portal system) and the inferior hemorrhoidal vein (which drains into the caval system).

Sensory perception of the rectum is supplied by the pudendal nerve, which arises from pelvic branches of the S3 and S4 nerve roots. Structures proximal to the dentate line are insensate, whereas tissue distal to this boundary can be painful when damaged by trauma, infection, or inflammation.

Fecal continence is maintained by motor innervation that arises from the S2 to S4 nerve roots. Defecation is the result of concomitant parasympathetic and sympathetic simulation, as well as voluntary contraction of the abdominal muscles.

## EXAMINATION

To examine the anorectum, the emergency physician (EP) places the patient in the lateral decubitus position (Sims position) or a knee-to-chest position on the examination table (**Fig. 41.2**). The anorectal skin, hygiene, and any anatomic abnormalities are inspected. The EP has the patient bear down (Valsalva maneuver) to accentuate any prolapse of the rectum or internal hemorrhoids. The skin of the anorectum is spread to identify fissures that may be hidden in the folds. A 360-degree digital rectal examination is performed, with note being made of the prostate in males and the cervix in females. The sample of stool on the withdrawn glove is assessed for gross or occult blood. If abnormalities are suspected, an anoscope is used to directly visualize the internal anatomy.

# ANORECTAL ABSCESS

## PATHOPHYSIOLOGY

Anorectal abscesses are caused primarily by infection of obstructed anal glands, ducts, and crypts. Abscesses are polymicrobial and involve both anaerobic and aerobic bacteria. Other causes of anorectal abscess are immunosuppression, atypical infection (e.g., tuberculosis, actinomycosis, lymphogranuloma venereum), inflammatory bowel disease (Crohn disease), trauma (e.g., foreign body), surgery (e.g., anorectal, genitourinary, and gynecologic procedures), malignancy (e.g., rectal carcinoma, leukemia, lymphoma), radiation, and anal fissures. Anorectal abscesses are classified according to location. The four main types are perianal (most common), ischiorectal, intersphincteric, and supralevator (least common) (**Fig. 41.3**).

## PRESENTING SIGNS AND SYMPTOMS

General complaints in patients with anal abscesses are pain, swelling, and occasionally fever. Signs and symptoms of a perianal abscess are a tender, erythematous, fluctuant mass at the anal verge and pain that worsens with sitting or defecating. The patient is usually afebrile. If large, an ischiorectal abscess may be manifested as a lateral perianal swelling. The patient has severe buttock pain but typically little to no cutaneous findings. Fever and leukocytosis are also present.

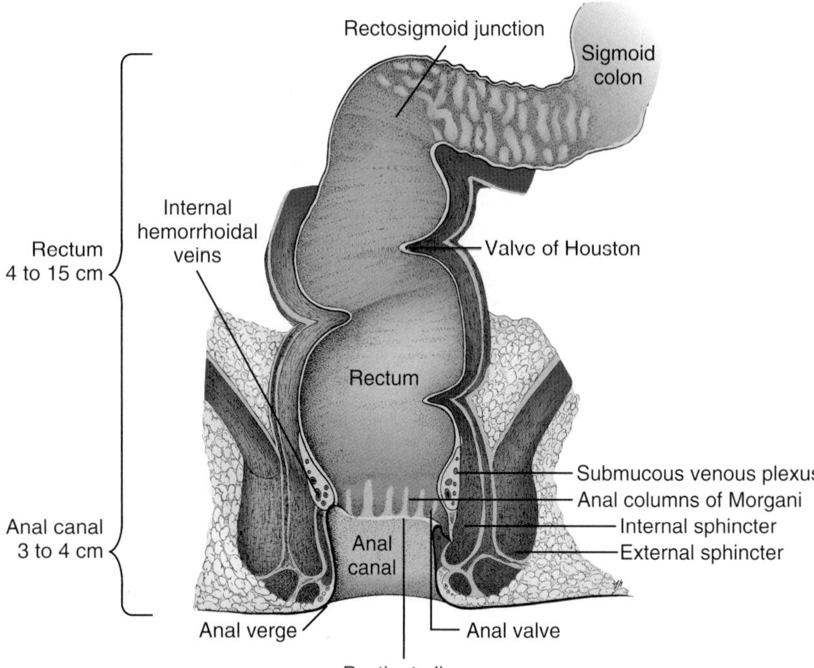


**Fig. 41.1 Anatomy of the terminal gastrointestinal tract.** (From Roberts JR, Hedges JR. Clinical procedures in emergency medicine. 5th ed. Philadelphia: Saunders; 2009.)

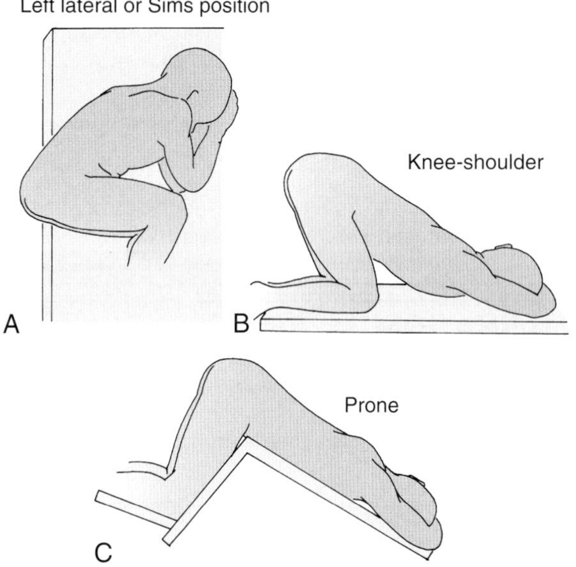


**Fig. 41.2 A-C,** Positions for performing anoscopy. (From Hill II GJ. Outpatient surgery. 3rd ed. Philadelphia: Saunders; 1988.)

With an intersphincteric abscess, there is constant rectal pressure and the patient has severe rectal pain with sitting or straining. An erythematous, painful rectal mass is present, along with fever and leukocytosis.

The signs and symptoms of supralevator abscess are severe rectal or gluteal pain with no external skin signs, urinary retention, fever, and leukocytosis. A tender mass is detected on rectal or vaginal examination.

## DIFFERENTIAL DIAGNOSIS

The differential diagnosis for anal abscess consists of strangulated internal or thrombosed external hemorrhoid, anal fistula, anal fissure, sentinel pile, gonococcal proctitis, and rectal duplication in infants.

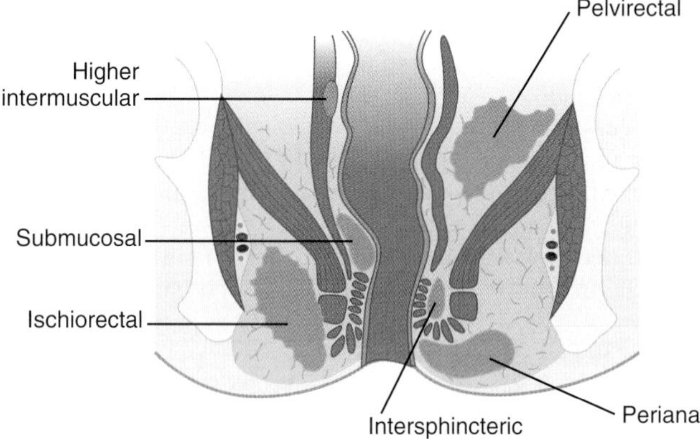


**Fig. 41.3 Common locations of anorectal abscesses.**

## DIAGNOSTIC TESTING AND EXAMINATION

- Classic history and physical examination findings
- Abdominal examination to evaluate for intraabdominal involvement
- Perianal examination to evaluate for perianal abscess and cellulitis
- Rectal examination to evaluate for deeper abscesses
- Vaginal examination to evaluate for deeper abscesses
- Bedside glucose measurement to evaluate for diabetes mellitus
- Abdominal and pelvic computed tomography (CT) or ultrasonography to identify deep abscesses when suspected

## TREATMENT

### PERIANAL ABSCESS

Patients who do not have a complicating disorder and whose perianal abscess (**Fig. 41.4**) measures 10 cm or smaller may

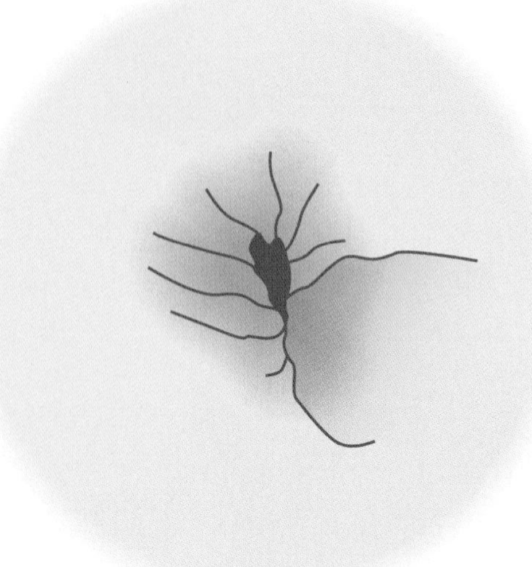

**Fig. 41.4 Perianal abscess.**

be treated by incision and drainage in the emergency department (ED). Elliptical or cruciate incisions are recommended for better drainage, and procedural sedation may be required. Postincision care consists of sitz baths, stool softeners, and a high-fiber diet.

Abscesses in immunocompromised patients (e.g., diabetes, human immunodeficiency virus [HIV] infection, transplantation, chemotherapy) should be treated in the operating room under general anesthesia.

Antibiotics should be prescribed only if surrounding cellulitis is present or the patient is immunocompromised.

### ISCHIORECTAL ABSCESS

Superficial ischiorectal abscesses may be drained in the ED (although the recurrence rate is high). Deeper abscesses, however, must be drained in the operating room. If signs of systemic involvement (fever or leukocytosis) are present, intravenous (IV) antibiotics should be used at the time of drainage, and oral antibiotics should be added to the postincision care regimen.

### INTERSPHINCTERIC ABSCESS

Patients with an intersphincteric abscess should undergo urgent drainage in the operating room and be administered IV antibiotics.

### SUPRALEVATOR ABSCESS

Emergency surgery should be performed in the operating room for any patient with a supralevator (muscle) abscess. IV antibiotics should be used.

## DISPOSITION

Patients with a simple perianal abscess that has been drained in the ED can be discharged. Arrangement should be made for packing changes, wound checks, or both in the ED or with the patient's primary care physician in 48 hours. Surgical consultation should be obtained for patients with all other anorectal abscesses.

# CRYPTITIS

## PATHOPHYSIOLOGY

The anal crypts are small pockets of epithelium located between the anal papillae at the proximal end of the anal canal (the mucocutaneous junction). These crypts have tiny glands that secrete a small drop of mucus as the sphincter muscles contract to ease the passage of stool. Cryptitis occurs when these crypts become inflamed and the mucosal lining of their roofs becomes denuded. Possible causes of cryptitis are as follows:

- Repeated watery stools that can cause trauma or deposits in the crypts
- Direct trauma from large, hard stools
- Inflammation from adjacent structures
- External sources of infection, such as parasites or foreign bodies

If left untreated, cryptitis can lead to perirectal abscess, anal fissure, or anal fistula.

## PRESENTING SIGNS AND SYMPTOMS

The signs and symptoms of cryptitis are anal pain (rectalgia), which is described as burning or dull in nature and exacerbated with bowel movements, as well as anal spasm, pruritus, and occasionally bleeding.

## DIFFERENTIAL DIAGNOSIS

The differential diagnosis for cryptitis includes hemorrhoids, anal fissure, anorectal abscess, and proctitis.

## DIAGNOSTIC TESTING AND EXAMINATION

- Palpation of hypertrophied (indurated) papillae adjacent to the crypt
- Classic "pearl of pus" beading from the crypt at the dentate line on anoscopy

## TREATMENT

Treatment of cryptitis consists of bulk laxatives to promote well-formed stools and decrease trauma, as well as warm sitz baths. Patients with advanced disease should receive outpatient surgical referral for excision of the gland.

# ANAL FISSURE

## PATHOPHYSIOLOGY

An anal fissure, also called fissure in ano, is a superficial linear tear of the anoderm that begins at or just below the dentate line and extends distally toward the anal verge. Anal fissures are the most common cause of painful rectal bleeding; they are also the most common cause of rectal bleeding in infants.

Ninety-nine percent of fissures in men and 90% of fissures in women are in a posterior midline location. Posterior midline anal fissures are typically caused by the passage of large, hard stool through a tight anus. The posterior midline is affected most because of weaker skeletal muscle and the acute angle of the rectum on the anus posteriorly.

Anterior midline fissures are most common in postpartum women. Anal fissures in other areas can be caused by receptive anal intercourse or insertion of foreign bodies or may be manifestations of conditions such as Crohn disease, cancer, tuberculosis, HIV infection, and syphilis.

Fissures that are not properly treated may become chronic and develop the classic triad consisting of sentinel pile, deep ulcer, and enlarged anal papillae. The ulcerating fissure causes edema and irritation of the surrounding tissue. Proximally, the result is hypertrophied papillae. Distally, the result is the formation of sentinel pile—fibrotic tissue that may be confused with an external hemorrhoid. The sentinel pile may eventually develop into a skin tag.

### PRESENTING SIGNS AND SYMPTOMS

In infants, anal fissures are signified by small amounts of bright red blood on the stool or diaper. Children with anal fissures have painful defecation and "constipation" because of refusal to defecate because of pain.

Adults describe a sharp, cutting, or burning pain with defecation that can persist as a nagging, dull pain for several hours but usually subsides between bowel movements. A small amount of bright red blood may be noted on the stool or toilet paper. Sphincter spasm may also occur and cause further pain.

### DIFFERENTIAL DIAGNOSIS

The differential diagnosis of anal fissure includes hemorrhoids, proctitis, cryptitis, perianal abscess, and primary syphilis (chancre).

### DIAGNOSTIC TESTING AND EXAMINATION

Diagnosis of an anal fissure must be made by physical examination, which should be done very carefully to avoid further spasm and pain. Application of a topical anesthetic such as lidocaine jelly may be necessary to facilitate the examination. Gentle retraction of the buttocks and perianal skin with the patient bearing down may expose the distal end of the fissure. The sentinel pile may also be visualized in this manner.

Because of the severe pain and spasm, the patient may not be able to tolerate a digital rectal examination. If such an examination is performed, the surrounding hypertrophic papillae may be palpated.

If the fissure is not located in the midline, the differential diagnosis and consequent testing must be expanded to include more serious conditions such as cancer, HIV disease, Crohn disease, sexually transmitted diseases, and tuberculosis.

### TREATMENT

Medical treatments that are most common and most effective for anal fissures are as follows:

- Warm sitz baths for 15 minutes three times per day
- A high-fiber diet
- Oral analgesics (narcotics increase constipation and should thus be avoided)
- Topical anesthetics such as lidocaine jelly
- Topical 0.2% nitroglycerin ointment, which may reduce sphincter spasm but is associated with higher recurrence rates
- Topical calcium channel blockers (e.g., nifedipine, diltiazem), which are also associated with higher recurrence rates

Chronic fissures for which medical treatment fails are often repaired successfully through a lateral internal sphincterotomy, which is performed by a surgeon. Patients with nonmidline fissures should be referred for further diagnostic testing, including ulcer biopsy and anal cultures.

## ANAL FISTULA

### PATHOPHYSIOLOGY

Anal fistula, also called fistula in ano, is considered a chronic variant of a poorly healed anorectal abscess. Fistulas are tracts between the anal canal (or rectum) and the skin that are lined with epithelial or granulation tissue. Although anal fistulas typically arise from an anorectal abscess, they can also be associated with inflammatory bowel disease, malignancies, infection (sexually transmitted diseases, actinomycosis, tuberculosis, and diverticulitis), anal fissures, or foreign bodies.

### PRESENTING SIGNS AND SYMPTOMS

The signs and symptoms of anal fistulas are a blood-tinged, malodorous discharge and rectal pain that improves with an increased discharge. An abscess may be located at the opening of the fistula. The fistula can be palpated as a cord leading to the sphincter.

### DIFFERENTIAL DIAGNOSIS

The differential diagnosis of anal fistula consists of abscess, hemorrhoid, anal fissure, and gonococcal proctitis.

### DIAGNOSTIC TESTING AND EXAMINATION

- Anal and rectal examinations with classic findings
- Abdominal and pelvic CT demonstration of a fistula tract
- Transanal ultrasonography (with or without hydrogen peroxide injected into the tract)

### TREATMENT

Treatment of anal fistulas consists of surgical excision to eliminate the fistula, prevent recurrent disease, and preserve sphincter function. Stable patients may be referred for urgent outpatient surgical consultation.

## ANORECTAL FOREIGN BODIES

### PATHOPHYSIOLOGY

The structure of the rectum and distal end of the colon predisposes a foreign body to migrate cephalad after insertion. A delay in evaluation may also allow the development of edema, which further complicates removal of a foreign body. Foreign bodies with smooth contours and a diameter near that of the rectum or colon may become "vacuum-locked" in place, with attempts at removal causing collapse of the rectum or colon distal to the object.

## PRESENTING SIGNS AND SYMPTOMS

Although anorectal foreign bodies are often the subject of humor and medical lore, ED management of an anorectal foreign body is actually quite rare. Because of the social stigma involved, patients are reluctant to come to the ED and are often not forthcoming about their actual complaint. The patient has frequently attempted to remove the foreign body before seeking medical attention, thereby potentially causing further damage or complicating removal.

Although the majority of patients give an accurate history,[1] some have vague complaints of abdominal pain or an unlikely story about how the object became lodged in the rectum. In the ED, every effort must be made to ascertain the type, shape, number, and composition of a retained foreign body, as well as how long it has been in the anorectum, before removing it.

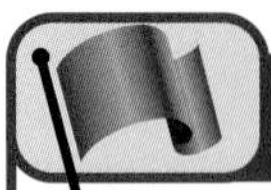

**RED FLAGS**

**Foreign Bodies**
Type: glass, food, metallic, sharp
Shape
Number of objects present
Time of insertion (delays in treatment promote edema)

## DIFFERENTIAL DIAGNOSIS

Objects lodged in the anorectum may have been self-inserted, inserted as a result of sexual assault, iatrogenically inserted (e.g., rectal thermometer), or swallowed.

## DIAGNOSTIC TESTING AND EXAMINATION

The shape, composition, surface, contour, and orientation of a foreign body influence the ultimate method of removal. Most foreign bodies can be classified as low lying and therefore palpable in the rectal ampulla or as high lying, at or proximal to the rectosigmoid junction.[2]

Examination and diagnostic testing should include the following:

- Thorough palpation of the abdomen (to identify masses, peritonitis)
- Flat and upright radiographs of the abdomen
- Digital rectal examination (if the object is not sharp by patient report and does not appear sharp on radiographs)

Anoscopy to visualize the foreign body should be considered.

## TREATMENT

Treatment of an anorectal foreign body is based on the results of abdominal and rectal examination, as well as plain radiographs (**Fig. 41.5**). Patients with palpable, low-lying foreign bodies can undergo conscious sedation and local anesthesia for attempted removal in the ED. Patients with high-lying foreign bodies or risk for perforation should be managed operatively.

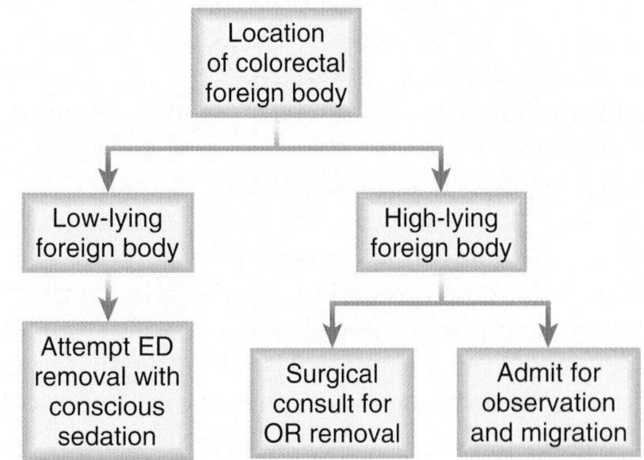


**Fig. 41.5 Treatment algorithm for a colorectal foreign body.** *ED*, Emergency department; *OR*, operating room.

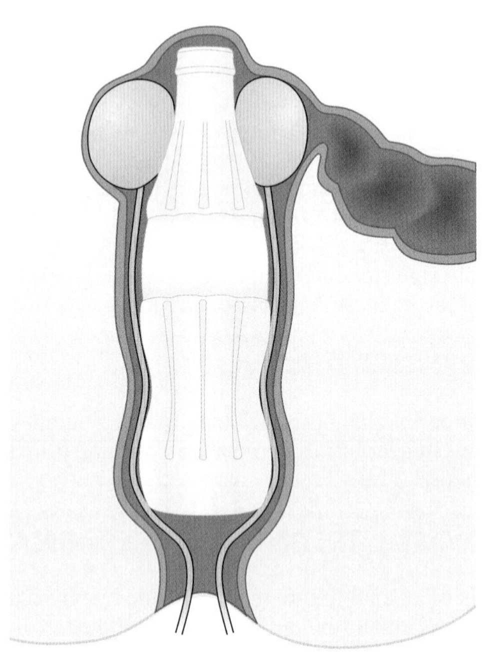

**Fig. 41.6 Use of two Foley catheter balloons to aid in removal of a rectal foreign body.**

### FOLEY CATHETER REMOVAL OF ANORECTAL FOREIGN BODIES

A Foley catheter can be used to break the suction caused by insertion of an object with a diameter similar to that of the colon or rectum; the procedure is as follows (**Fig. 41.6**):

1. Place the patient in the lithotomy position.
2. Pass one or more Foley catheters beyond the foreign body.
3. Insufflate air to break the suction.
4. Inflate the Foley balloons.
5. While grasping the foreign body and applying gentle traction with either hands or forceps, slowly remove the catheter or catheters with moderate pressure.

## DISPOSITION

A patient who underwent successful removal of a low-lying foreign body may be discharged from the ED. For any patient with suspected rectal perforation, proctosigmoidoscopy should be performed by a gastroenterologist or colorectal surgeon before disposition.

# HEMORRHOIDS

## PATHOPHYSIOLOGY

The hemorrhoidal plexuses provide a vascular cushion to the area surrounding the anus. The hemorrhoidal vessels are one of three layers of submucosal tissue that support the anal canal and aid in continence and defecation. As this tissue deteriorates and weakens, the hemorrhoidal veins may prolapse or may become engorged or thrombosed.

The internal hemorrhoidal veins are located above the dentate line. Their blood supply is derived from the superior hemorrhoidal plexus, and drainage is into the portal system by way of the superior rectal veins and the inferior mesenteric vein. They also communicate with the external hemorrhoidal veins. Internal hemorrhoids are covered by transitional or columnar epithelial mucosa without pain fibers. They are nearly always in the same positions: left lateral (9 o'clock), right posterolateral (5 o'clock), and right anterolateral (2 o'clock) (**Fig. 41.7**). They are classified into four categories according to severity (**Table 41.1**).

The external hemorrhoidal veins are located below the dentate line. Their blood supply is derived from the inferior hemorrhoidal plexus, with drainage into the iliac and pudendal venous systems. They are covered by anoderm (modified squamous epithelium) with sensory nerve endings that contain pain receptors.

## PRESENTING SIGNS AND SYMPTOMS

The most common symptom of hemorrhoids is painless bleeding with defecation (blood on stool or toilet paper). If the hemorrhoid is thrombosed, strangulated, or prolapsed, pain with defecation also occurs. The lesion is detected as a curvilinear mass at the anus.

Prolapsed hemorrhoids also cause discharge of mucus and pruritus ani. A thrombosed external hemorrhoid appears as a dark blue, firm, tender mass distal to the anal verge. A prolapsed, strangulated internal hemorrhoid appears as a purplish tender mass covered by mucosa and emerging from the anal verge. A strangulated internal hemorrhoid is often associated with a thrombosed external hemorrhoid.

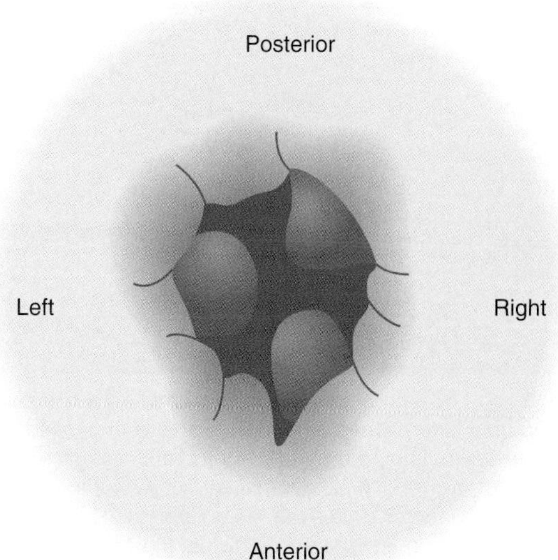


**Fig. 41.7** **Common positions of internal hemorrhoids.**

## DIFFERENTIAL DIAGNOSIS

The differential diagnosis for hemorrhoids consists of anal fissure, rectal prolapse, perianal condyloma, abscess, fistula, rectal varices, tumors, and manifestations of inflammatory bowel disease.

## DIAGNOSTIC TESTING AND EXAMINATION

The diagnostic criteria for hemorrhoids are as follows:

- Prolapse of hemorrhoids is noted on rectal examination when the patient bears down.
- Internal hemorrhoids are not palpable, so anoscopy is required to visualize them.

## TREATMENT

As a rule, most hemorrhoids should be treated conservatively, as follows:

- Warm sitz baths for 15 minutes three times per day
- Increase in dietary fiber
- Stool softeners and bulk laxatives (those causing liquid stool, which could lead to cryptitis, should be avoided)
- 0.2% topical nitroglycerin ointment to treat pain by decreasing sphincter spasm
- Topical anesthetics and steroid creams, though controversial, provide anecdotal pain relief
- Judicious use of narcotics (stool softeners should also be used if narcotics are prescribed)

**Table 41.1** **Classification of Internal Hemorrhoids**

| SEVERITY (DEGREE) | FINDINGS |
|---|---|
| First | No prolapse; painless bleeding |
| Second | Prolapse with straining and spontaneous reduction<br>Mild discomfort and bleeding |
| Third | Prolapse with straining, which requires manual reduction<br>Some throbbing pain, itching, bleeding, and mucus discharge |
| Fourth | Permanent prolapse that cannot be reduced<br>Pain and bleeding common<br>Potential for thrombosis and strangulation |

Acutely thrombosed external hemorrhoids can be excised in the ED (**Fig. 41.8**). Rather than performing simple incision and drainage, the EP should excise the roof of the thrombosed hemorrhoid as an ellipse. Excision of thrombosed hemorrhoids should never be performed in the ED in children or in adults who are immunocompromised or pregnant, in patients receiving anticoagulation therapy, and in patients with portal hypertension.

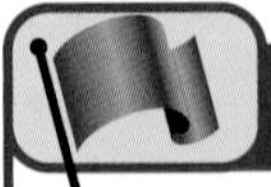

**RED FLAG**

Excision of a nonthrombosed hemorrhoid should never be attempted.

### EXCISION PROCEDURE

Thrombosed external hemorrhoids can be excised as follows (**Fig. 41.9**):

1. Put the patient in a prone or left lateral decubitus position.
2. If a single provider is performing the procedure without an assistant, tape the buttocks as shown in **Figure 41.10**.
3. With a 27-gauge needle, infiltrate bupivacaine with epinephrine into the overlying skin and the skin underneath the clot.
4. Make an elliptical incision in the overlying skin (distal to the anal verge).
5. Excise the clot or clots through this opening.
6. To control bleeding, place a small piece of gauze or absorbable gelatin sponge (Gelfoam) into this opening and cover with a pressure dressing.

The patient should remove the dressing in 6 hours, at the time of the first sitz bath.

## DISPOSITION

Most patients with hemorrhoids can be discharged home. Immediate surgical consultation should be obtained for patients with strangulated fourth-degree internal hemorrhoids or bleeding hemorrhoids and severe anemia.

Patients with second-degree, third-degree, or nonstrangulated fourth-degree internal hemorrhoids should be referred to an outpatient surgeon for possible sclerotherapy, rubber band ligation, infrared coagulation, or excisional hemorrhoidectomy.

Patients who have undergone ED excision of thrombosed external hemorrhoids should be referred for follow-up with a surgeon.

# HIDRADENITIS SUPPURATIVA

## PATHOPHYSIOLOGY

Perianal hidradenitis suppurativa is a disease of the skin and subcutaneous tissue that arises from occlusion of the apocrine glands with keratin. It tends to be chronic, recurrent, and primarily localized to areas with the highest density of apocrine sweat glands (groin, axilla, and mammary regions). Sequelae include inflammation, infection, and eventual rupture of the gland with secondary cellulitis of the

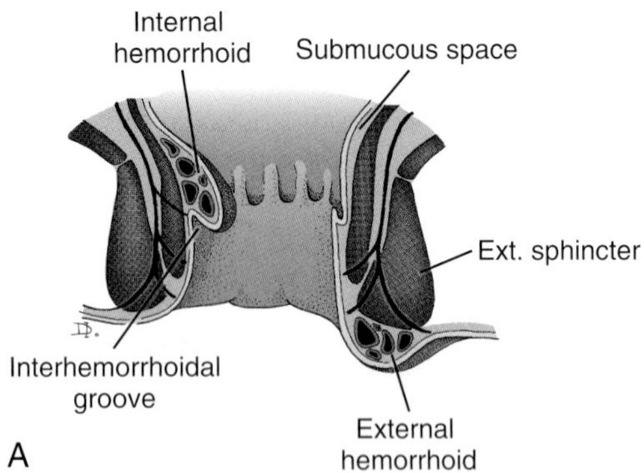


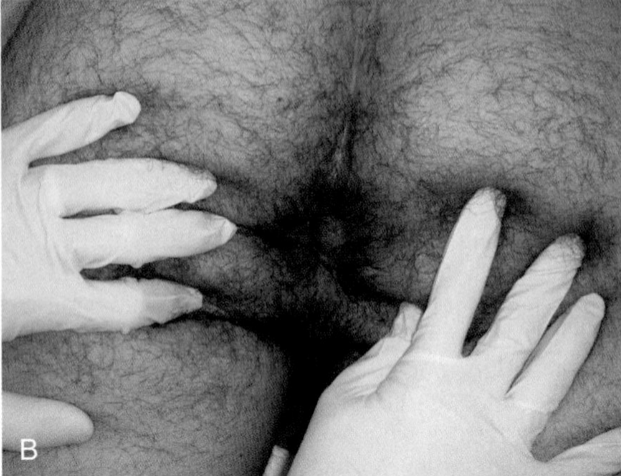


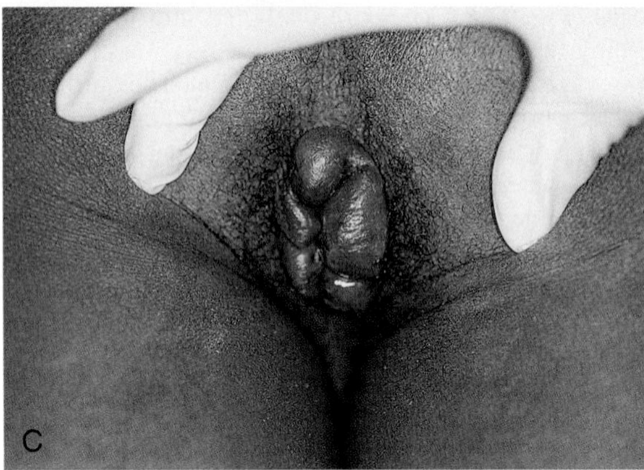


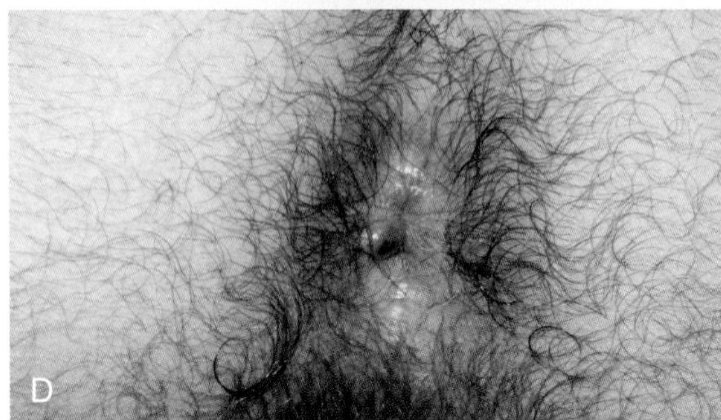


**Fig. 41.8** **A,** Location of internal and external hemorrhoids. **B,** Thrombosed external hemorrhoid. **C,** Partially prolapsed thrombosed internal hemorrhoid. **D,** Ruptured small external hemorrhoid. (**A,** from Hill II GJ. Outpatient surgery. 2nd ed. Philadelphia: Saunders; 1980. **B-D,** from Roberts JR, Hedges JR. Clinical procedures in emergency medicine. 5th ed. Philadelphia: Saunders; 2009.)

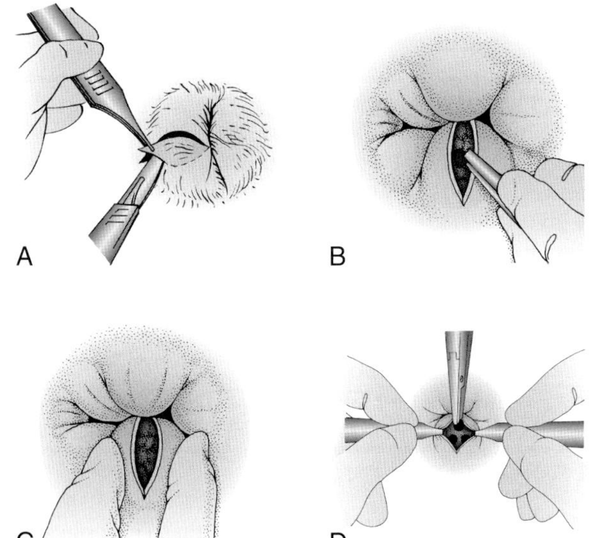


**Fig. 41.9 Schematic of the technique for excision of thrombosed external hemorrhoids. A,** For the unroofing technique, make an elliptical or triangular incision to remove a piece of the overlying skin. To prevent skin tags, do not use a simple linear incision. **B,** Blood clots may extrude spontaneously, but remove the remaining ones with forceps or express them with the fingers (**C**). **D,** Frequently, multiple clots are present, and they should all be removed. Ask an assistant to provide exposure with forceps if necessary. (From Roberts JR, Hedges JR. Clinical procedures in emergency medicine. 5th ed. Philadelphia: Saunders; 2009.)

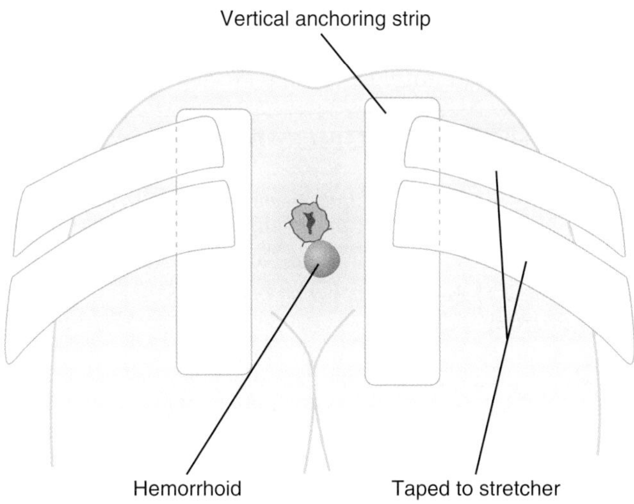


**Fig. 41.10 Diagram for taping the buttocks.**

surrounding tissue. The disease ultimately leads to the formation of chronic draining sinuses.[3]

## PRESENTING SIGNS AND SYMPTOMS

Patients with the early stages of perianal hidradenitis suppurativa typically have a painful boil in the perianal region. Classically, the abscess is deep and round without any central necrosis or fluctuance. The patient may describe similar episodes that resolved spontaneously. Later, more chronic stages of the disease may be manifested as open draining fistulas and sinuses (**Box 41.1**).

**BOX 41.1 Characteristics of Hidradenitis Suppurativa**

Age at onset: puberty
Female-to-male ratio: 3:1
Associated conditions: acne, comedones, obesity, hirsutism
Sites affected (in descending order of frequency): axillary, inguinal, perianal and perineal, mammary and inframammary, buttock, pubic region, chest, scalp, retroauricular, eyelid

## DIFFERENTIAL DIAGNOSIS

The differential diagnosis of perianal hidradenitis suppurativa consists of carbuncles, lymphadenitis, infected sebaceous cysts, noninflamed cysts, other infectious processes (abscesses, fistulas), and Crohn disease.

## TREATMENT

Medical treatment of perianal hidradenitis suppurativa consists of weight loss, smoking cessation (if applicable), and the use of antibiotics. Clindamycin, 300 mg twice daily, has been shown to be effective in suppression,[3-5] but the disease often returns when use of the antibiotics ceases; topical clindamycin cream is similarly effective. Retinoids may also be tried. Acitretin, 25 mg daily, decreases keratin production and has been shown to reduce the number of outbreaks. Hormonal therapy may also be effective; finasteride was shown to induce remission in a small case study.[3]

Surgical drainage provides only short-term relief because the condition has a 100% recurrence rate.[4,5] Radical excision of the inflamed apocrine tissue carries a recurrence rate of 25%.[5]

## DISPOSITION

All patients with perianal hidradenitis suppurativa should be referred to a dermatologist for long-term management.

# PILONIDAL DISEASE

## PATHOPHYSIOLOGY

Pilonidal disease is a common disorder that generally affects young adults—those between the ages of 15 and 24 years—with a 3:1 male preponderance. Pilonidal disease often causes a considerable amount of suffering, inconvenience, and time away from work. An estimated 40,000 to 70,000 patients are treated annually, mostly as outpatients.[6] Approximately 50% of patients with this condition are initially seen by an EP with an acute pilonidal abscess.[7]

The term *pilonidal* is a combination of the words *pilus,* meaning "hair," and *nidus,* meaning "nest." The condition is believed to arise from hairs in the natal cleft that because of their location, grow inward rather than outward. The shafts of these hairs penetrate the skin, thereby leading to a condition of chronic inflammation and eventual infection. Chronic infection results in the formation of sinus tracts and recurrent disease.

### PRESENTING SIGNS AND SYMPTOMS

The initial signs and symptoms of pilonidal disease are usually pain and swelling in the sacrococcygeal region with inability to sit on one side of the buttocks or perhaps an inability to tolerate a sitting position at all. Systemic involvement is rare. Physical examination generally demonstrates either a tender fluctuant mass over the coccyx or sacrum or a larger area of inflammation with multiple draining tracts.

### DIFFERENTIAL DIAGNOSIS

Other diseases manifested as an infection or fistula must be excluded, such as rectal or perirectal abscess, Crohn disease, and hidradenitis suppurativa.

### DIAGNOSTIC TESTING AND EXAMINATION

The classic clinical signs and symptoms of pilonidal disease are sufficient for diagnosis. Imaging is not useful for a typical manifestation of this condition.

### TREATMENT AND DISPOSITION

Treatment is both medical and surgical. ED treatment generally consists of incision and drainage of the abscess. Simple incision plus drainage results in healing in 58% of patients within 10 weeks; of these patients, 40% have no further symptoms and 20% experience only minor symptoms.[8] Antibiotics should be prescribed to treat any secondary cellulitis. In one study, metronidazole, 500 mg orally four times per day for 14 days, resulted in more rapid healing than did no antibiotics.[8]

Patients with pilonidal disease can be discharged from the ED with arrangements or instructions for follow-up with a surgeon.

## PROCTALGIA FUGAX

### PATHOPHYSIOLOGY

Proctalgia fugax is severe, episodic anal pain. The disorder is poorly understood and difficult to treat. The pathophysiology of this condition is unclear, although it is believed to be caused by spasm of either the anal sphincter or the muscles of the pelvic floor.

### PRESENTING SIGNS AND SYMPTOMS

Proctalgia fugax is usually characterized by sudden episodes of intense pain around the anal ring that can occur at any time and may last from 20 minutes to several hours. Typically, the pain occurs at night and often awakens the patient. The sensation may be associated with an urge to pass stool or flatus. Some patients may experience only one episode in their lifetime. The lifetime prevalence of this condition is 14%.[9]

### DIFFERENTIAL DIAGNOSIS

Other conditions that commonly cause rectal pain should be considered in the differential diagnosis of proctalgia fugax, such as anal fissure, hemorrhoids, perirectal abscess, and proctitis.

### TREATMENT AND DISPOSITION

No specific treatment exists for proctalgia fugax. Anecdotal evidence supports the use of warm baths, topical treatment with glyceryl trinitrate, benzodiazepines, topical anesthetics,[9] and botulinum toxin.[10] Hot packs or direct anal pressure has also been recommended.[11]

Patients with recurrent disease should be referred to a gastroenterologist.

## PROCTITIS

### PATHOPHYSIOLOGY

Proctitis is defined as inflammation of the rectal mucosa. It can involve actual loss of mucosal cells, as well as damage to the endothelium of the small arterioles supplying the mucosa. The condition may improve spontaneously, depending on the cause, or may progress with resulting tissue ischemia, mucosal friability, bleeding, ulcers, strictures, and fistula formation. Causes of proctitis are listed in **Box 41.2**.

### PRESENTING SIGNS AND SYMPTOMS

The signs and symptoms of proctitis include fecal urgency, sensation of rectal fullness, rectalgia, pruritus, rectal bleeding (spotting), and a mucoid or purulent rectal discharge. The patient may also describe a change in bowel habits (diarrhea or constipation) and abdominal pain. Ulcers, vesicles or pustules, and strictures may be found on rectal examination.

### DIFFERENTIAL DIAGNOSIS

The differential diagnosis of proctitis consists of anal fistula, anal fissure, rectal foreign body, diverticulosis, and vulvovaginitis.

### DIAGNOSTIC TESTING AND EXAMINATION

Anoscopy in a patient with proctitis identifies erythema, friability, bleeding, edema, ulcers, and vesicles; rectosigmoid-

**BOX 41.2 Causes of Proctitis**

- Autoimmune inflammatory bowel disorders
- Crohn disease
- Ulcerative colitis
- Radiation
- Sexually transmitted disease–related infections: gonorrhea, chlamydia, syphilis (usually secondary), herpes simplex virus types 1 and 2, lymphogranuloma venereum, amebiasis (oral-anal inoculation)
- Non–sexually transmitted disease–related infections: *Campylobacter, Entamoeba histolytica, Salmonella, Clostridium difficile*
- Trauma
- Idiopathic

oscopy demonstrates similar findings. The following laboratory tests should be performed:

- Stool: culture and testing for ova, parasites, fecal leukocytes, and *Clostridium difficile* toxin
- Gonorrhea and chlamydia cultures and Gram stain of anorectal swabs
- Venereal Disease Research Laboratory or rapid plasma reagin test if syphilis is suspected

## TREATMENT

Most cases of proctitis can be treated medically. The underlying cause, if known, should also be treated. All forms of the disorder may benefit from the following measures:

- Sitz baths
- Antispasmodic agents
- Low-residue diet
- Stool softeners

# PRURITUS ANI

Pruritus ani is a recurrent and unpleasant itching sensation in the anal canal or perianal, perineal, vulvar, scrotal, or buttock areas. Approximately 1% to 5% of the population seeks medical attention for this condition during their lifetime. More men than women experience the disorder, which is more common in the fifth and sixth decades of life.[12] Because of the social stigma involved, many patients attempt self-treatment before seeking care. The condition is often poorly understood and improperly treated by health care providers.

## PATHOPHYSIOLOGY

In 50% of cases of pruritus ani, the cause is unknown. Potential causes (especially malignancy) must be excluded before the symptoms can be classified as idiopathic (**Table 41.2**).

## PRESENTING SIGNS AND SYMPTOMS

Patients typically describe an itching sensation that is worse at night and during the summer months. As the patient scratches, the perianal skin is further irritated and the condition worsens. Physical findings vary with the duration of the condition and include:

- Erythema
- Whitening or cracking of the perianal skin
- Bleeding in severe cases

## DIFFERENTIAL DIAGNOSIS

See Table 41.2.[13] Fecal contamination of the perianal skin is the most common cause of pruritus ani.

## DIAGNOSTIC TESTING AND EXAMINATION

Evaluation should include a careful history of potential exposures, examination of the perianal skin, digital rectal examination, anoscopy, and directed testing to exclude specific suspected causes.

**Table 41.2 Differential Diagnosis of Pruritus Ani**

| | |
|---|---|
| Anorectal disease | Fissures<br>Proctitis<br>Hemorrhoids<br>Abscess<br>Fistula<br>Malignancy |
| Dermatologic disease | Lichen planus<br>Lichen sclerosis<br>Lichen atrophicus<br>Eczema<br>Psoriasis<br>Seborrhea |
| Infectious disease | *Candida albicans* dermatophytes<br>*Staphylococcus aureus*<br>*Corynebacterium minutissimum*<br>Group A β-hemolytic streptococci<br>Human papillomavirus<br>Herpes simplex<br>*Enterobius vermicularis*<br>*Sarcoptes scabiei*<br>Pinworms |
| Medications | Colchicine<br>Quinidine<br>Mineral oil<br>Neomycin |
| Systemic disease | Diabetes mellitus<br>Renal failure<br>Lymphoma |
| Foods | Tomatoes<br>Citrus fruits<br>Nuts<br>Chocolate<br>Coffee<br>Tea<br>Cola<br>Beer |
| Irritants | Fecal contamination<br>Excess moisture<br>Soap<br>Aggressive anal wiping<br>Scented toilet paper |

Data from Jones DJ. ABC of colorectal disease: pruritus ani. BMJ 1992;305:575-7.

## TREATMENT

Most cases of pruritus can be treated conservatively with the following measures:

- Gentle cleansing and attention to hygiene of the perianal skin
- Modifications in diet and medications
- Brief courses of topical steroids (long-term steroid therapy should be avoided because it may thin the perianal skin and further exacerbate the condition)
- An oral antipruritic medication such as hydroxyzine or diphenhydramine

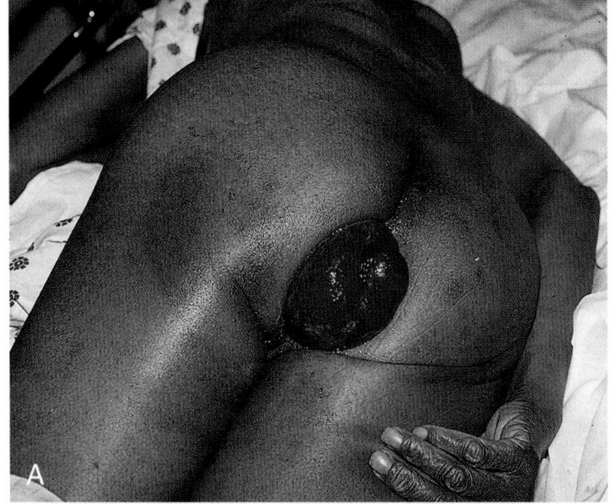


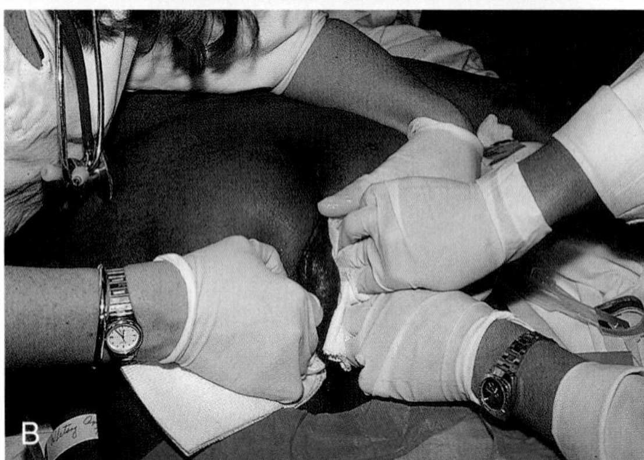


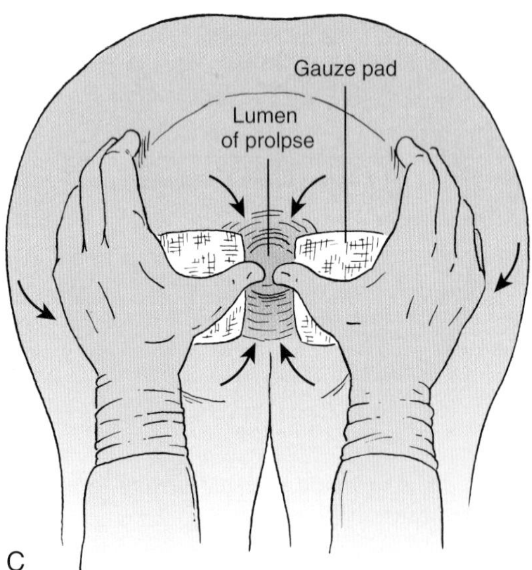


**Fig. 41.11 Rectal prolapse. A,** Complete rectal prolapse or procidentia. **B,** Reduction of the prolapsed rectum. **C,** Diagram of the reduction technique. (From Roberts JR, Hedges JR. Clinical procedures in emergency medicine. 5th ed. Philadelphia: Saunders; 2009.)

- Daily application of topical capsaicin cream (0.006%), which has been shown to be effective in reducing or eliminating symptoms[14,15]

The patient should also be referred to the primary care physician for evaluation of chronic symptoms, biopsy, and other testing.

# RECTAL PROLAPSE

## PATHOPHYSIOLOGY

Rectal prolapse or procidentia is a circumferential protrusion of all layers of the rectum through the anus (**Fig. 41.11,** ***A***). The cause is largely unclear, although the condition seems to be more common in elderly women with a female-to-male preponderance of 6:1. Predisposing factors include pelvic floor laxity, pelvic floor neuropathy, persistent straining, chronic constipation, rectal tumors, and disfunction of the anal sphincter.

## PRESENTING SIGNS AND SYMPTOMS

Actual protrusion of the rectum is the most common manifestation. Other symptoms may include anorectal pain or discomfort during defecation, sensation of incomplete evacuation, rectal and urinary incontinence, and rectal bleeding or discharge.

## DIFFERENTIAL DIAGNOSIS

The EP should differentiate this condition from external hemorrhoids, prolapsed internal hemorrhoids, rectal tumors, and uterine prolapse.

## DIAGNOSTIC TESTING AND EXAMINATION

Imaging is not necessary in making the diagnosis of rectal prolapse. Colonoscopy should be performed in all patients after reduction to clarify the diagnosis and further define the anatomy.

## TREATMENT AND DISPOSITION

Every effort should be made to reduce the prolapsed rectum in the ED to prevent the complications of strangulation, ischemia, ulceration, or perforation. Various methods have been described for reduction, including ice packs, injection of diluted epinephrine, and manual reduction under conscious sedation or general anesthesia (Fig. 41.11, *B*). Applying ordinary granulated table sugar to the prolapsed tissue, a technique borrowed from veterinary medicine, has been used successfully to quickly reduce the edema and aid in reduction.[16]

## SUGGESTED READINGS

Fry RD. Hemorrhoids, fissures, and pruritus ani. Surg Clin North Am 1994;74:1289-92.

Slade D, Powell B, Mortimer P. Hidradenitis suppurativa: pathogenesis and management. Br J Plast Surg 2003;56:451-61.

Vincent C. Anorectal pain and irritation. Prim Care 1999;26:53-66.

## REFERENCES

***References can be found on Expert Consult @ www.expertconsult.com.***

# Liver Disorders 42

*Richard Paula*

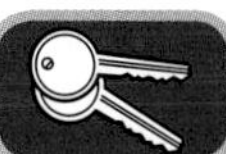

**KEY POINTS**

- Causes of jaundice are best categorized by the fraction of measured bilirubin implicated in disease—unconjugated or conjugated hyperbilirubinemia.
- The possibility of cerebral edema should be considered in patients with advanced liver disease and nausea, vomiting, and changes in mental status.
- As a result of the uncertain relationship of measured serum ammonia and cerebral ammonia concentration, patients with known or suspected hepatic encephalopathy should be treated for hyperammonemia regardless of the measured level.
- The prevalence of spontaneous bacterial peritonitis is high in cirrhotic patients, with rates of 3.5% in those with no symptoms to 30% in patients who seek treatment in a hospital for any reason and undergo paracentesis.
- Hepatitis B virus immune globulin effectively prevents transmission of hepatitis B virus if administered within 72 hours of exposure; it should be given for any high-risk exposure.
- Pyogenic liver abscesses are best treated with a combination of antibiotics and percutaneous drainage. Antibiotics alone are insufficient treatment.

## EPIDEMIOLOGY

Chronic liver disease accounts for 70,000 hospitalizations annually in the United States and is one of the top 10 leading causes of death. Almost half of the 40,000 deaths per year in the United States are related to alcohol abuse. Although the majority of deaths are due to chronic liver disease and cirrhosis, 2000 deaths per year are associated with fulminant hepatic failure.[1] Many of these patients die while awaiting liver transplantation. Hepatitis B and hepatitis C infections account for 40% of chronic liver disease, although many of these cases are exacerbated by concomitant alcohol abuse.

Liver disease is debilitating and deadly because the liver is intimately involved in many physiologic functions. The liver (1) synthesizes coagulation factors, cholesterol, bile, and glycogen; (2) conjugates bilirubin; and (3) detoxifies exogenous chemicals such as alcohol, as well as endogenous metabolic by-products such as ammonia. Loss of any of these functions significantly impairs homeostasis.

## Common Signs and Symptoms of Liver Disease

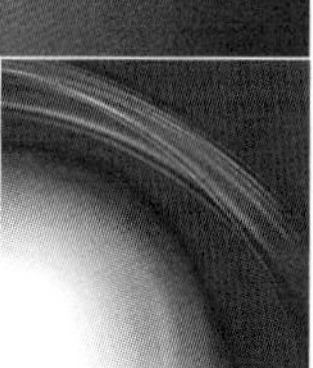

### JAUNDICE

The most common and immediately apparent evidence of liver disease is jaundice, which is often manifested without any other symptoms.

Jaundice begins to appear when the serum bilirubin level reaches 3 mg/dL in white persons and at higher levels in darker-skinned persons. Jaundice does not require treatment in adults as it does in neonates, but instead, the cause of jaundice in adults should be investigated.

Causes of jaundice are often categorized according to the type of bilirubin implicated in disease, unconjugated or conjugated hyperbilirubinemia. In context with associated symptoms, knowledge of the fractionations of bilirubinemia aids in narrowing the differential diagnosis.

Pancreatic and biliary cancer associated with jaundice may be manifested as pain.[2] Patients with cirrhosis from chronic hepatitis are likely to describe painless jaundice but also complain of fatigue, pruritus, and constitutional symptoms. Patients who are acutely ill with jaundice, nausea, emesis, and fever should be tested for causes of acute hepatitis; similar manifestations without fever occur in toxic ingestions.

### NAUSEA

Nausea is a common extrahepatic symptom that may complicate hepatitis, toxic liver injury, cholestasis, and many other causes of acute or chronic liver disease. Management of nausea is sometimes the sole reason that a patient with acute hepatitis requires hospital admission.

Particular attention should be given to patients with known liver disease who have nausea, emesis, and changes in mental status; the emergency physician should consider the possibility of cerebral edema, especially in patients with advanced liver disease.

### NEUROPSYCHIATRIC SIGNS AND SYMPTOMS

Changes in mental status in the setting of liver disease should be treated aggressively. The degree of encephalopathy is directly correlated to the degree of liver dysfunction. Patients with a sudden change in mental status and acute hepatic insufficiency usually have an advanced stage of disease that will frequently progress to acute, fulminant liver failure.

Cerebral edema often occurs in tandem with encephalopathy because of elevated ammonia levels; immediate treatment with ammonia-clearing agents (e.g., lactulose) is required. Note that lactulose is less effective in treating mental status changes associated with acute liver failure than in treating those associated with chronic disease. Caregivers of patients with chronic hepatic insufficiency often titrate lactulose dosing in accordance with cognitive function.

## HEPATOMEGALY

In patients with hepatomegaly, the liver becomes significantly enlarged and easily palpable as a result of sudden edema from hepatitis or the appearance of fatty infiltrates with alcohol binging. If the enlargement is significant enough to cause portal hypertension, the spleen is often enlarged and palpable as well. As the liver scars and hepatocytes are replaced by fibrous tissue in cirrhosis, the organ shrinks and eventually becomes small and nodular. The presence or absence of hepatomegaly on examination is an unreliable estimate of liver function and should not be used to exclude a particular diagnosis.[3,4]

## RASH

Many patients with liver disease complain of skin irritation. Hepatitis has been associated with livedo reticularis, a lacy, erythematous rash caused by capillary spasm. Dermatitis caused by autoimmune hepatitis that promotes jaundice has an intense pruritic component. Patients with liver disease may be unable to control scratching, and infections develop in the self-induced excoriations. Finally, patients may complain of a "rash" that represents ecchymosis secondary to coagulopathy; such bruising without reported trauma should raise concern for advanced liver disease.

# Signs and Symptoms of Advanced Liver Disease

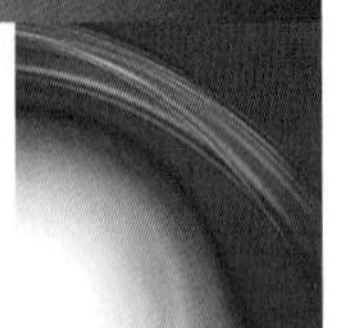

## ENCEPHALOPATHY

Changes in mental status may occur with either acute or chronic liver disease. The pathophysiology of hepatic encephalopathy is not completely understood, but it is clear that pronounced encephalopathy is associated with poor outcomes. Although many chemical markers have been implicated as the cause of hepatic encephalopathy, most studies identify two important factors, γ-aminobutyric acid (GABA) and ammonia ($NH_3$).

Serum GABA levels are elevated in patients with cirrhosis. Administration of a GABA receptor antagonist (flumazenil) results in transient but significant improvements in cirrhotic patients' mental status.

The second and more easily measurable toxicity results from an increased ammonia concentration. The serum ammonia concentration rises as liver function declines, with intermittent fluctuations occurring in chronically ill patients. Many factors affect ammonia production, including changes in diet, constipation, hepatorenal syndrome, and gastrointestinal bleeding. Ammonia readily crosses the blood-brain barrier, and in patients with hepatic encephalopathy, ammonia causes cerebral toxicity, which promotes mental status decline and eventually coma.[5-7]

Ammonia is clearly toxic, and in animal models, ammonia infusions alone have been directly linked to the development of cerebral edema. In the setting of acute liver failure, ammonia levels higher than 200 mcg/dL are strongly associated with the development of cerebral edema and herniation.[8-10] In patients with advanced liver disease and cirrhosis, however, mental status may not correlate directly with measured ammonia levels. Ammonia tends to accumulate in the brain, and although blood levels may be normal, the patient may still have enough ammonia in cerebrospinal fluid to induce encephalopathy.

Because of the uncertain relationship of the measured serum ammonia and cerebral ammonia concentration, patients with known or suspected hepatic encephalopathy should be treated for hyperammonemia regardless of measured serum levels. No convincing evidence suggests that arterial sampling for measurement of ammonia is superior to venous measurements.[7]

### TREATMENT

Emergency department (ED) management of hepatic encephalopathy consists of appropriate airway control and resuscitation, followed by the administration of ammonia-lowering agents. Lactulose (15 to 45 mL once or twice daily) is the most common treatment of choice in the United States, although sodium benzoate has been shown to be equally effective and less expensive.[11] Lactulose is a nonabsorbable disaccharide that decreases intestinal transit time through a direct cathartic effect, thus lowering intestinal bacterial loads. Lactulose also lowers intestinal pH, which favors competitive non–ammonia-producing bacteria. Lactulose may be given orally, by nasogastric tube, or in severely obtunded patients, as a retention enema.[12]

Neomycin is a poorly absorbed aminoglycoside used as secondary treatment to further reduce intestinal bacterial counts. Even though it is poorly absorbed, neomycin does cause systemic toxicity and should be used only when lactulose is ineffective. Mannitol (0.5 to 1 g/kg) effectively reduces cerebral edema and improves survival in patients with hepatic encephalopathy secondary to acute liver failure.[8,13]

The following therapies have been shown to be ineffective and should be avoided: hyperventilation,[8,14] corticosteroids,[8,13] and terlipressin.[15]

## ASCITES

Ascites is the abnormal accumulation of peritoneal fluid, a common feature in patients with advanced liver disease. The exact pathogenesis of ascites has not been established, but multiple theories focus on the interaction of the liver with various other organ systems. The combination of portal hypertension and decreased albumin production contributes significantly to the accumulation of ascitic fluid.

Ascites associated with cirrhosis has a poor prognosis. One episode of ascites has a 3-year mortality rate of 50%, and recurrent ascites has the same 50% mortality at 1 year.[16,17] Comorbid conditions contribute to mortality, including the development of hepatocellular carcinoma, gastrointestinal hemorrhage, coma, and infection.

One important infectious cause of death in patients with ascites is spontaneous bacterial peritonitis (SBP). The prevalence of SBP in cirrhotic patients is high, with rates of 3.5% in asymptomatic patients to 30% in patients who seek treatment in a hospital for any reason and undergo paracentesis.[18,19]

Paracentesis for the relief of tense ascites has been shown to improve cardiac function.[20] Reduction of intraabdominal hypertension and resolution of an effective abdominal compartment syndrome improve venous return to the heart.[21]

Patients with symptomatic ascites require paracentesis. Given the high rate of occult SBP in these patients, peritoneal fluid should always be sent for analysis. Previously, it was thought that large-volume paracentesis was associated with complications and should be avoided, but this common misperception has been disproved. Large-volume (>5 L) paracentesis is safe and is associated with shorter hospitalization than is the case with diuretic therapy in patients with refractory ascites.[22,23]

Complications of paracentesis are rare, even in thrombocytopenic patients. Most complications involve bleeding or persistent leakage from the puncture site and occur within 24 hours. Patients with such complications should be admitted to the hospital for observation.[24,25]

Controversy exists regarding volume expansion with colloids in conjunction with paracentesis. Studies have not demonstrated any short-term improvements in mortality or morbidity with the use of plasma expanders, although some alterations in renal function, such as elevations in blood urea nitrogen and decreased sodium levels (both of which are associated with a worse prognosis), have been observed. Albumin is the least expensive, safest, and usually most effective colloid for intravascular volume expansion and should be used in patients with paracentesis volumes of 5 L or larger.[26-28]

Paracentesis is improved when ultrasonography is used to identify ascites and guide the paracentesis. In one study, paracentesis performed under ultrasonographic guidance was successful in 95% of patients as opposed to 65% of procedures without such guidance.[29]

Outpatient treatment of ascites should center on dietary sodium restriction in combination with diuretics. Management by a primary care physician includes frequent checks of potassium and sodium levels, both of which have been implicated in morbidity in these patients. Patients with recurrent ascites should be referred for surgical evaluation for a possible transjugular intrahepatic portosystemic shunt procedure.

## SPONTANEOUS BACTERIAL PERITONITIS

Symptoms of SBP are often vague. Although abdominal pain and fever are common, both may be absent. Patients may complain only of increased fatigue, myalgia, worsening ascites, or decline in mental status.

SBP is thought to be caused by translocation of intestinal flora, although this long-held premise is now under question. Previously, SBP was almost entirely associated with gram-negative bacteria, mostly *Escherichia coli*; a growing number of patients with SBP now have gram-positive organisms.[30]

The diagnosis is confirmed by culture of peritoneal fluid aspirated during paracentesis. SBP is likely if peritoneal fluid neutrophil counts are greater than 250 cells/μL. Peritoneal fluid lactate levels may be even more accurate.[26,27]

Patients with suspected SPB should have as much fluid drained as possible. Empiric antibiotic treatment should begin as soon as the diagnosis is considered. SBP in cirrhotic patients carries a mortality rate of 20% to 40%, with a 1-year survival rate of just 40%.[26] Treatment should begin with a third-generation cephalosporin, such as ceftriaxone or cefotaxime. Quinolones should not be used because bacterial resistance to these agents is high and will worsen if the incidence of gram-positive infections continues to rise. Failure rates have been increasing regardless of which antibiotic regimen is used—it is often necessary to tailor individual therapy to the organisms found on culture.[31]

## CIRRHOSIS

Continued liver injury results in irreparable damage with permanent loss of liver function and subsequent chronic disease states. Cirrhosis is the common end point of many chronic liver diseases characterized by the replacement of functioning hepatocytes with physiologically inactive fibrotic tissue. Patients with cirrhosis may have any number of symptoms or clinical conditions related to end-stage liver disease.

## PORTAL HYPERTENSION

Portal hypertension occurs when intraportal pressure is elevated 10 mm Hg above normal throughout the portal system. The cause is multifactorial, and the disorder can occur with conditions other than cirrhosis.

Parasitic infections are an extremely common cause of reversible portal hypertension in developing countries. Parasites, commonly those responsible for schistosomiasis, cause chronic inflammatory states in the portal sinusoids that lead to granuloma formation and fibrosis.

Portal hypertension develops in patients with cirrhosis because of increased intrahepatic resistance to greater portal flow. Numerous cellular disorders occur simultaneously in cirrhotic patients with increased portal pressure. Lack of intrahepatic vasodilation is caused by fibrocyte deposition and decreased nitric oxide production within the liver. Increased portal flow results from higher cardiac output and splanchnic flow associated with extrahepatic nitric oxide production. The greater pressure causes deposition of peritoneal fluid and redirection of blood flow. As these forces coincide, blood is rerouted around the liver to compensate. Collateral flow increases as portal pressure rises; pressures greater than 12 mm Hg promote the formation of *varices*—chronically dilated veins in the collateral bed that shunt blood flow away from the liver. Varices occur in the following locations:

*Abdominal wall*: Varices involving the abdominal wall are called caput medusae, so named for their serpentine appearance. They arise from dilation of the abdominal wall and umbilical veins.

*Rectum:* Hemorrhoids represent a form of rectal varices. They are often friable and subject to significant bleeding.

*Esophagus:* Esophageal varices are a common source of gastrointestinal bleeding in patients with portal hypertension. Bleeding may be massive and difficult to control because of concomitant coagulopathy.

## HYPONATREMIA

Cirrhotic patients have impaired excretion of free water. Low sodium levels, found in a third of all patients with cirrhosis, contribute to ascites, frequent falls, and cognitive decline. Hyponatremia is associated with a decreased response to diuretic therapy and a poor prognosis.[32] In 2009 the U.S. Food and Drug Administration approved the novel drug tolvaptan for the treatment of hyponatremia; tolvaptan acts as a vasopressin antagonist. As with any new pharmaceutical class, data are limited, but the early results are promising.[33]

## HEPATORENAL SYNDROME

Hepatorenal syndrome exists as a chronic debilitating state or as a rapidly progressive and terminal condition. This syndrome occurs when kidney function declines in the setting of liver failure. All patients with cirrhosis have some degree of renal insufficiency; most continue to decline slowly, whereas others progress rapidly to renal failure.

Hepatorenal syndrome is diagnosed in a patient with cirrhosis who also has a rise in creatinine levels to more than 1.5 mg/dL in conjunction with a serum sodium level lower than 130 mEq/L. SBP, acute alcoholic hepatitis, and hypotension are common precipitants of this syndrome. Although hepatorenal syndrome frequently develops in patients being treated for SBP, some evidence has shown that administering albumin as a component of SBP management reduces the likelihood of development of this syndrome.

Liver transplantation is the only therapy that has been shown to reduce mortality in patients with fulminant hepatorenal syndrome.[34]

# Infectious Causes of Liver Disease

## HEPATITIS A VIRUS

Hepatitis A virus (HAV) is a single-stranded RNA enterovirus in the disease-producing family Picornaviridae, which also includes poliovirus. Also known as epidemic hepatitis because of its ability to spread swiftly and suddenly, HAV infects an average of 60,000 individuals annually worldwide. Transmission is fecal-oral, as in settings such as day care, or through sexual contact. It may also be transmitted by contaminated water or food sources; shellfish is a common vector, although seemingly innocuous food sources, such as imported lettuce, have been implicated in outbreaks as well.[35,36]

### SYMPTOMS, SIGNS, AND DIAGNOSTIC TESTING

Incubation may be as long as 30 days. Symptoms include anorexia, nausea, emesis, diarrhea, fever, and eventually jaundice. Serum IgM titers are diagnostic of HAV infection.

### TREATMENT AND PROGNOSIS

Treatment of HAV infection is supportive. Most infections are subclinical, and full recovery is expected in more than 99.5% of those infected. A vaccine is commercially available for HAV and is recommended for persons traveling to endemic areas. HAV immune globulin may be used up to 2 weeks after exposure; it is generally reserved for high-risk patients, such as those with preexisting infectious hepatitis (other than HAV), elderly patients, and immunocompromised individuals.

### DISPOSITION

Patients infected with HAV may need to be admitted to the hospital for parenteral control of vomiting and administration of fluids. Liver function values are often markedly elevated, although this finding is not an indication for admission.

## HEPATITIS B VIRUS

Hepatitis B virus (HBV) is a double-stranded DNA virus that has a cross-species reservoir. It infects human, ducks, and squirrels. HBV is transmitted person to person through sexual contact, blood exposure, transfusion, and perinatal vertical transmission. It is highly virulent—infection may be caused by a small number of virions. HBV is easily passed through contaminated needles, either from needle sharing among drug abusers or through occupational exposure in health care workers.

More than 1 million individuals have chronic HBV infection in the United States, and approximately 500 million are infected worldwide. From 1990 to 2004, the overall incidence of reported acute HBV infection declined 75% through vaccination efforts, from 8.5 to 2.1 per 100,000 persons.[37-39]

### SYMPTOMS AND SIGNS

Acute infection with HBV causes anorexia, nausea, emesis, diarrhea, fever, and eventually jaundice. Serum levels of alanine transaminase (ALT) and aspartate transaminase (AST) may both rise to greater than 10,000 U/L and cause constitutional symptoms that precede the appearance of jaundice.

### DIAGNOSTIC TESTING

HBV infection can be defined as acute, chronic, or carrier. If the patient has not been immunized against HBV and has not previously shown signs of the disease, the presence of hepatitis B surface antigen and expected symptoms confirms the diagnosis of acute infection.

## TREATMENT AND PROGNOSIS

The prognosis of patients with HBV infection varies widely, although most individuals (90% to 95%) recover completely. Up to 10% of patients enter a chronic infectious state and are at risk for cirrhosis and hepatocellular carcinoma. Approximately 2% die of fulminant hepatic failure.

Multiple drug regimens exist for the treatment of HBV, most notably peginterferon alfa-2b with or without lamivudine. Such regimens have never been shown to be effective in the acute setting, and recommendations are to withhold treatment until evidence of ongoing viral replication is present.

HBV immune globulin (HBV-IG) effectively prevents transmission if given within 72 hours of exposure and should be administered to patients after high-risk exposure. Centers for Disease Control and Prevention guidelines recommend administration of HBV-IG and HBV vaccine to unvaccinated health care workers exposed to patients known to have HBV and administration of HBV-IG to persons with unknown HBV status after high-risk exposure. Nonoccupational postexposure prophylaxis should follow similar recommendations (e.g., sexual assault or coincident with human immunodeficiency virus postexposure prophylaxis).

## DISPOSITION

Patients with HBV infection may require admission for parenteral control of vomiting and administration of fluids. Evidence of possible hepatic failure is reflected in prolongation of the prothrombin time (PT), which should be measured if HBV infection is suspected. Liver function values are often markedly elevated, but this finding is not an indication for admission.

# HEPATITIS C VIRUS

An RNA virus that is extremely complex and diverse, hepatitis C virus (HCV) has at least six distinct genotypes and 50 subtypes. This genetic diversity complicates development of a vaccine against it. HCV infection is the leading reason for liver transplantation; chronic infection commonly causes cirrhosis and hepatocellular carcinoma.[38] Transmission occurs through sexual contact and sharing needles with infected individuals.

HCV transmission peaked in the United States in the 1980s before its discovery, with an estimated 250,000 new cases per year in that decade. Infection rates have dropped to approximately 40,000 annually. Carriers with chronic HCV infection number almost 3 million.[40] The prevalence of HCV in trauma patients is 15% to 20%.[41,42]

## DIAGNOSIS

Unlike acute infection with HAV or HBV, acute HCV infection is much more likely to pass without symptoms—up to 80% of infected persons are asymptomatic. HCV can produce a flulike illness that is easily ignored. It is ultimately diagnosed with anti-HCV antibody screening, which is confirmed by polymerase chain reaction for HCV RNA.

## TREATMENT AND PROGNOSIS

HCV is much more destructive than either HAV or HBV. Approximately 15% of infected persons fully recover, but cirrhosis develops in 15% and hepatocellular carcinoma eventually develops in 5%. HCV accounts for 50% of cases of cirrhosis diagnosed in the United States.

Treatment with various drug regimens is available, although none are recommended for use in the ED in patients with suspected infection. Viral replication must be verified and serotyped to guide treatment. Neither vaccine prophylaxis nor postexposure prophylaxis is currently available.

## DISPOSITION

Patients infected with HCV may have to be admitted to the hospital for parenteral control of vomiting and administration of fluids. Evidence of possible hepatic failure is reflected in prolongation of the PT, which should be measured if HCV infection is suspected. Liver function values are often markedly elevated, but this finding is not an indication for admission.

# AMEBIASIS

Amebic liver infections are of growing concern in the United States, although the infection is much more prevalent in the developing world. Amebiasis affects 50 million persons worldwide and is estimated to cause 50,000 to 100,000 deaths per year.[43]

Amebiasis is frequently manifested as colitis. It is unknown what percentage of cases progress to abscess formation, although approximately one third of patients with abscesses have prodromal nausea, emesis, diarrhea, and bloating.[44,45] Solitary abscess formation is common in patients with amebic abscesses, as opposed to the multiple foci often seen in those with pyogenic abscesses. Amebic abscesses have a predilection for males, with a 10 : 1 ratio of infection; such gender bias is not seen with pyogenic abscesses.

## DIAGNOSIS

Most patients in the United States in whom amebic liver abscess is diagnosed are seen in the southwestern states and are males of Mexican origin.[46] The symptoms may mimic those of cholecystitis, with right upper quadrant abdominal pain, fever, chills, and nausea. In one series, 20% of patients with amebiasis had isolated pulmonary complaints.[46]

Abscesses are easily seen on ultrasonography. The ultrasonographic appearance in combination with acute symptoms makes the diagnosis in at least two thirds of patients.[45,47,48] Computed tomography (CT) is sensitive as well and should be used when the diagnosis is in question.

Tests for *Entamoeba histolytica*–specific antibodies should be performed if an amebic abscess is suspected.

## TREATMENT AND PROGNOSIS

Metronidazole remains the first-line treatment (a high-dose schedule consisting of 750 mg three times daily for 10 days provides a 90% cure rate).[49] Aspiration has traditionally been recommended for abscesses larger than 5 cm, although the results of studies examining this practice are equivocal.[50,51]

## DISPOSITION

Patients with amebic abscesses smaller than 5 cm are at low risk for rupture. If they are able to tolerate oral fluids and medications, such patients should be discharged after high-dose metronidazole therapy is started and appropriate follow-up is arranged.

When the diagnosis of amebic abscess cannot be confirmed in the ED by serologic testing, the patient should be admitted to exclude potential pyogenic abscesses.

# PYOGENIC LIVER ABSCESSES

Liver abscesses in the United States and worldwide are most often due to amebiasis, although pyogenic abscesses represent a more serious condition. Pyogenic abscesses were diagnosed in 3000 patients per year in one European study.[52]

Patients with pyogenic abscesses are more ill, have multiple abscesses, and suffer a worse prognosis than do those with amebic abscesses. Unlike those with amebic abscesses, approximately 50% of patients have multiple pyogenic abscesses, either from hematogenous spread (as a result of infections such as diverticulitis) or through direct extension from suppurative cholangitis (now thought to be the most common cause).

Bacterial causes of pyogenic abscess are diverse and include *E. coli, Klebsiella, Staphylococcus aureus,* and various anaerobes.

Patients with pyogenic abscesses are much less likely to have the classic symptoms of liver abscesses seen with amebic infections, such as right upper quadrant pain, fever, nausea, and vomiting.

## DIAGNOSIS

Because the causes of pyogenic abscesses are so varied, the abscesses are not manifested in a uniform fashion. Right upper quadrant tenderness and hepatomegaly are noted in approximately 50% of cases.[53] Patients commonly show signs of systemic disease, such as fever, malaise, weight loss, and anorexia.

Liver function values may or may not be elevated and should not be used to exclude the diagnosis. Ultrasonography and CT are both excellent imaging modalities, with sensitivities of 85% and 95%, respectively.[53,54]

## TREATMENT AND PROGNOSIS

Pyogenic liver abscesses are treated with a combination of antibiotics and drainage. Catheter drainage and needle aspiration produce similar success rates of 60% to 90%, although these two options have not been compared directly. The largest published trials have demonstrated success rates exceeding 95% with ultrasound-guided aspiration without catheter placement followed by broad-spectrum intravenous antibiotics (to cover gram-positive, gram-negative, and anaerobic organisms).[55,56] Antibiotic therapy without abscess drainage is generally unsuccessful.

## DISPOSITION

Even with appropriate therapy, the mortality rate in patients with pyogenic abscesses is 5% to 10%. Any patient with a suspected pyogenic abscess must be admitted to the hospital.

# PARASITIC INFECTIONS

The most common parasitic infections of the liver are schistosomiasis (which commonly affects the portal and mesenteric circulation) and clonorchiasis (found in the biliary tree). Both parasitic infections are very common outside the United States—an estimated 1 in 30 persons worldwide are infected with *Schistosoma*, and 25% of all Asian immigrants to the United States are infected with *Clonorchis sinensis*. These parasites cause portal hypertension in a large percentage of patients in developing countries and often go undetected for years because of lack of symptoms.

## DIAGNOSIS

Patients with parasitic infections exhibit symptoms based on the number of parasites causing infection. Those with a smaller number of organisms are asymptomatic or may have only malaise and diarrhea. With higher numbers of parasites, more constitutional symptoms are present, such as fever, chills, and weight loss.

ED patients with hepatobiliary symptoms after travel to Asia should be considered at high risk for parasitic infection. Ultrasonography and CT may show indirect signs of infection, such as biliary stones and dilation; these imaging methods are not helpful for identifying the organisms themselves.[57]

## TREATMENT AND PROGNOSIS

Praziquantel is effective for both clonorchiasis and schistosomiasis, with cure rates of 60% to 95%.[58] Reversal of portal hypertension is observed in 95% of children and 85% of adults with these parasitic diseases.[59]

## DISPOSITION

Patients with suspected acute parasitic disease should be admitted to the hospital because of a significant risk for mortality from *Schistosoma japonicum*. Chronic infection may be managed with supportive care and outpatient follow-up.

# Noninfectious Liver Disorders

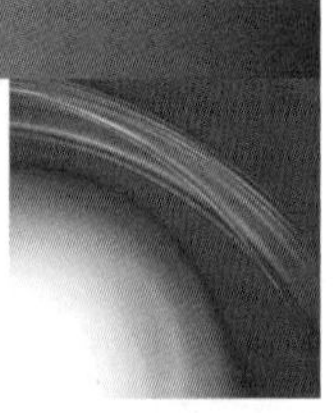

# ALCOHOLIC LIVER DISEASE

Alcohol consumption is responsible for half of all chronic liver disease in the United States.[1] Alcohol may poison the liver acutely or may damage hepatocytes through repeated insult, with permanent destruction of hepatic architecture and the eventual development of cirrhosis. Alcohol consumption causes accumulation of fat in the liver that displaces hepatocytes; the accumulation is normally reversible, but if the liver is subject to repeated insult, the accumulation of fat slowly becomes permanent. Chronic fatty liver is subject to inflammatory changes that induce scarring and permanent replacement of functional hepatocytes with lipocytes and fibrous tissue. The smaller numbers of hepatocytes cannot handle the physiologic requirements of the body. This pathologic progression is significantly accelerated by coexisting HCV or HBV infection.[60] Women are much more prone to alcohol-induced hepatic injury.[61]

Acute hepatitis secondary to alcohol consumption is termed *alcoholic hepatitis* or *alcoholic steatohepatitis.* Steatohepatitis, so named from the overwhelming fatty infiltration seen with alcohol metabolism, is associated with impairment of liver function. Acute alcoholic hepatitis is common in heavy, chronic, binge-type alcohol users.

## DIAGNOSIS

Patients with alcoholic hepatitis often admit to heavy alcohol use and may appear jaundiced or complain of dark urine. Constitutional symptoms are common—weakness, nausea, emesis, and malaise. Patients often display signs of chronic liver insufficiency, including asterixis and spider angiomas.

## TREATMENT AND PROGNOSIS

Treatment is mostly supportive, although as with other forms of liver disease, both coagulopathy and changes in mental status should be treated aggressively. The mortality rate in hospitalized patients with alcoholic hepatitis is approximately 10%.[62] Higher mortality is observed when patients have concomitant encephalopathy and coagulopathy; immediate liver transplantation may be required for their survival.

Corticosteroid use in hospitalized patients with alcoholic hepatitis is controversial. During the 1980s and early 1990s, a number of published studies proclaimed significant reductions in mortality with the use of corticosteroids (particularly convincing was one study of the use of prednisolone in 1992[63]). However, a carefully performed metaanalysis published in 1995 that examined 12 controlled trials did not find any benefit.[64] The use of corticosteroids should be reserved for inpatient units and not be initiated in the ED.

## DISPOSITION

Admission to the hospital is necessary for patients with acute alcoholic hepatitis because of high mortality rates and a significant need for transfusion, vasopressors, and aggressive resuscitation.

## AUTOIMMUNE LIVER DISORDERS

The two major immunologic causes of liver disease are autoimmune hepatitis and primary biliary sclerosis. Patients with immune-related liver disease are mostly female and show signs of autoimmune disease, as well as liver disease. The clinical signs regularly include myalgia, polyarthritis, rash, and findings consistent with other autoimmune disorders, such as Sjögren syndrome and systemic lupus erythematosus.

Patients with autoimmune liver disorders have progressive disease and a survival rate of 10% to 50% at 5 years if untreated. As the disease advances, the patient exhibits signs of liver insufficiency similar to those in other patients with chronic liver disease.[65,66]

### BOX 42.1 Drugs That Cause Liver Disease

**Anesthetics**
Halothane
Enflurane
Isoflurane

**Antimicrobials**
Sulfonamides
Dapsone
Pyrazinamide
Ketoconazole
Isoniazid
Rifampin

**Anticonvulsants**
Phenytoin
Valproic acid
Carbamazepine
Felbamate

**Analgesics**
Acetaminophen
Diclofenac
Sulindac
Etodolac
Oxaprozin

**Miscellaneous**
Nicotinic acid
Labetalol
Flutamide
Disulfiram
Propylthiouracil
Nefazodone

From Lewis J. Drug-induced liver disease. Med Clin North Am 2000;84:1275-311.

These diseases are difficult to detect and differentiate from other forms of chronic liver disease—such differentiation is not a goal of ED care.

Management of patients with autoimmune liver disorders is complicated by the immunosuppressive drugs used for treatment (prednisone and azathioprine are most commonly prescribed). When caring for patients in the ED, the clinician must consider complications of immunosuppressive therapy and administer stress-dose corticosteroids when required.

The prognosis has improved with liver transplantation, which provides a 10-year survival rate of 75%; recurrence is seen in 42% of patients.[67]

## DRUG-INDUCED LIVER DISEASE

Many pharmaceutical and naturally occurring substances can cause catastrophic liver injury (**Box 42.1**). The manifestation of drug-induced liver disease varies from benign jaundice to fulminant hepatic failure. Almost 40% of cases of acute hepatic failure in the United States are caused by drug-induced injury; almost half of these cases are due to acetaminophen alone.[68,69]

# Care of Patients with Liver Transplants

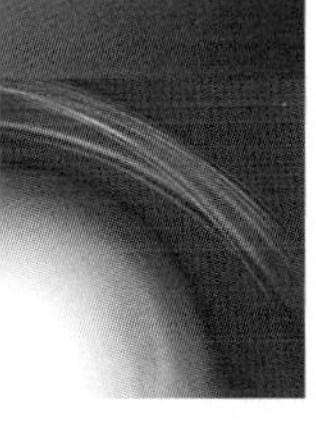

More than 36,000 patients living in the United States have undergone liver transplantation.[70] Transplantation patients come to the ED with common complaints, such as fever and abdominal pain, which are associated with high morbidity in this population. Almost 70% of liver transplant recipients who seek care in an ED require hospitalization.[71]

Transplant recipients are immunosuppressed, and any fever must be taken seriously. Serious febrile illnesses associated with liver transplantation are bacteremia and pneumonia; otitis media is common. Immunosuppressive medications also raise the risk for viral and fungal infections.

## INFECTIOUS COMPLICATIONS

The most common serious infection seen in the first few months after transplantation is cytomegalovirus, which is manifested as fever, arthralgias, and malaise. Other viral infections, such as herpes simplex virus, varicella-zoster virus, and herpes zoster virus, are also common but are not as serious as cytomegalovirus.[70] Infections with fungi such as *Candida* should also be suspected.

Serious infections may be present in the absence of fever or leukocytosis. Half of liver transplant recipients with the eventual diagnosis of a serious infection had neither a fever nor an elevated white blood cell count.

## MECHANICAL COMPLICATIONS

Liver transplant recipients are subject to vascular or structural problems surrounding and within the transplant. Hepatic artery stenosis and hepatic artery thrombosis are each present in approximately 10% of liver transplant recipients, frequently because of rejection. Either stenosis or thrombosis of the hepatic artery can be manifested as abdominal pain, and both are accurately detected with ultrasonography.[71] Timely discussion with a transplant team and early use of angiography are recommended because of the need for a rapid decision on corrective treatment.

The portal system may also be affected; ultrasonography should be used to evaluate the portal system at the time that the arterial system is examined because another 10% of liver transplant recipients have portal vein or hepatic vein thrombosis. Magnetic resonance venography is needed to confirm suspected portal or hepatic vein thrombosis.

Finally, the biliary tree is also affected by stenosis or ischemia in approximately 10% of patients and is diagnosed by ultrasonography or angiography.[72]

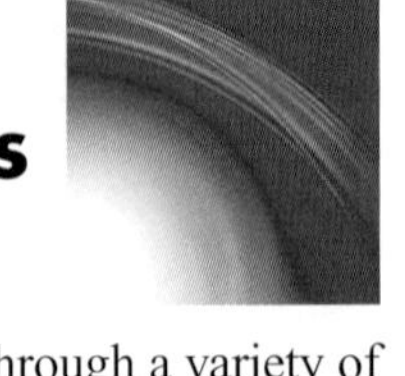

# Liver Function Tests

Liver function may be measured indirectly through a variety of laboratory tests. Laboratory abnormalities are neither specific nor sensitive and can therefore be misleading; however, certain abnormalities can help guide the astute physician toward further diagnostic testing in search of a specific diagnosis.

## ALANINE TRANSAMINASE AND ASPARTATE TRANSAMINASE

Both ALT and AST, which are called transaminases, are concentrated intrahepatocyte enzymes (although AST exists in

**Table 42.1 Causes of Hyperbilirubinemia**

| TYPE | CAUSE | CLINICAL FEATURES AND BIOCHEMICAL ABNORMALITIES |
|---|---|---|
| Unconjugated hyperbilirubinemia | Hemolysis | Decreased hemoglobin and haptoglobin levels<br>Increased reticulocyte count |
| | Gilbert syndrome | None |
| | Hematoma reabsorption | Increased creatine kinase and lactic dehydrogenase levels |
| | Ineffective erythropoiesis | — |
| Conjugated hyperbilirubinemia | Bile duct obstruction | Preceded by a marked increase in transaminase levels<br>Presence of suggestive symptoms (right upper quadrant pain, nausea, fever) |
| | Hepatitis (various causes) | Concomitant moderate to marked increase in transaminase levels |
| | Cirrhosis | Transaminase levels may be normal or only slightly increased<br>Presence of other physical and instrumental signs of chronic liver disease |
| | Autoimmune cholestatic diseases (primary biliary cirrhosis, primary sclerosing cholangitis) | Marked increase in ALP levels with normal or mildly increased transaminase levels<br>Presence of other autoimmune diseases or associated diseases (e.g., inflammatory bowel disease) |
| | Total parenteral nutrition | Increased ALP and $\gamma$-glutamyltransferase levels |
| | Drug toxins | Concomitant increase in ALP levels |
| | Vanishing bile duct syndrome | Can be associated with drug reactions or occur with orthotopic liver transplantation |

From Giannini E, Testa R, Savarino V. Liver enzyme alteration: a guide for clinicians. CMAJ 2005;172:367-79.
*ALP*, Alkaline phosphatase.

**Table 42.2 Guide to Interpretation of Hepatic Function Panel Results**

| | PROBABLE TEST RESULTS | | | | | | | |
|---|---|---|---|---|---|---|---|---|
| SUSPECTED HEPATIC DISORDER | TOTAL PROTEIN | ALBUMIN | AST | ALT | AST/ALT RATIO | ALP | TOTAL BILIRUBIN | DIRECT BILIRUBIN |
| Acute hepatitis | ⇄ | ⇄ | ↑↑ to ↑↑↑ | ↑↑ to ↑↑↑ | <1 | ⇄ to ↑ | ↑↑ to ↑↑↑ | ↑↑ to ↑↑↑ |
| Acute alcoholic hepatitis | ⇄ | ⇄ | ↑ to ↑↑ | ↑ | 1 to >2 | ⇄ to ↑ | ↑↑ to ↑↑↑ | ↑↑ to ↑↑↑ |
| Chronic hepatitis | ↑ to ↑↑ | ↓ to ↓↓ | ↑ to ↑↑ | ↑ to ↑↑ | <1 to 1 | ⇄ to ↑ | ↑ to ↑↑ | ↑ to ↑↑ |
| Chronic alcoholic disease | ↑ to ↑↑ | ↓ to ↓↓ | ↑ to ↑↑ | ↑ to ↑↑ | >1 | ⇄ to ↑ | ↑ to ↑↑ | ↑ to ↑↑ |
| Diffuse intrahepatic cholestasis | ⇄ to ↑↑ | ⇄ to ↓↓ | ↑ to ↑↑ | ↑ to ↑↑ | 1 | ↑↑ to ↑↑↑ | ↑ to ↑↑ | ↑ to ↑↑ |
| Extrahepatic obstruction | ⇄ to ↑↑ | ⇄ to ↓↓ | ↑ to ↑↑ | ↑ to ↑↑ | 1 | ↑↑ to ↑↑↑ | ↑ to ↑↑ | ↑ to ↑↑ |
| Focal intrahepatic disease | ⇄ to ↓↓ | ⇄ to ↓↓ | ↑ to ↑↑ | ↑ to ↑↑ | 1 | ↑↑ to ↑↑↑ | ⇄ | ⇄ to ↑ |

Modified from Burke M. Liver function: test selection and interpretation of results. Clin Lab Med 2002;22:377-90.

*ALP*, Alkaline phosphatase; *ALT*, alanine transaminase; *AST*, aspartate transaminase; ⇄, within reference limits; ↑, slightly increased; ↓, slightly decreased; ↑↑, moderately increased; ↓↓, moderately decreased; ↑↑↑, markedly increased; ↓↓↓, markedly decreased.

measurable quantities elsewhere in the body as well). Any hepatocyte necrosis elevates these enzymes. The often quoted 2:1 ratio of AST to ALT in patients with alcoholic liver disease is not supported by the literature.[73,74]

Chronic disease states such as HCV, alcoholic cirrhosis, and autoimmune hepatitis are often associated with persistent elevations in ALT and AST, although normal values should not be used to exclude the possibility of disease. More than 15% of patients with biopsy-proven chronic HCV disease have transaminase elevations.[75]

## ALKALINE PHOSPHATASE AND γ-GLUTAMYLTRANSFERASE

Both alkaline phosphatase (AP) and γ-glutamyltransferase (GGT) are markers of cholestasis. However, AP is present at significant levels in many other organ systems—bone, intestine, and placenta. AP values are elevated in normal pregnancy and with metastatic disease involving bone (e.g., prostate cancer). Children also have physiologically normal elevations in AP during growth. GGT is much more highly concentrated in the liver and can be used in conjunction with AP to determine whether an abnormality is intrahepatic or extrahepatic.

## PROTHROMBIN TIME

The PT measures the activity of certain clotting factors in both the intrinsic and extrinsic pathways. The liver is the primary site for manufacture of these clotting factors, and decreases in synthesis by an impaired liver can be inferred from a prolonged PT. Vitamin K is a cofactor in clotting factor synthesis, and medications that block its absorption, such as warfarin, prolong PT values.

## BILIRUBIN

Bilirubin exists in two distinct forms, conjugated (direct) and unconjugated (indirect). Bilirubin is a by-product of hemoglobin metabolism. Unconjugated bilirubin is present in serum bound to albumin in a water-insoluble state. It is transported to the liver, where it is conjugated with glucuronide in preparation for excretion into bile.

Understanding this process of bilirubin metabolism helps focus the differential diagnosis of patients with hyperbilirubinemia or jaundice, or with both (**Tables 42.1** and **42.2**). Unconjugated hyperbilirubinemia results from increased production of bilirubin (hemolysis) or from decreased uptake in the liver (as seen in various inherited conditions). Conjugated hyperbilirubinemia results from loss of excretory capacity, which can occur as a result of intrahepatic diseases (e.g., drug reactions, hepatitis, cirrhosis) or biliary obstruction. Obstructive jaundice is due to a lesion that blocks the excretion of bile through the biliary ducts, either proximally at the hepatic duct or more distally at the common bile duct.[73,76]

## SUGGESTED READINGS

Burke M. Liver function: test selection and interpretation of results. Clin Lab Med 2002;22:377-90.

Cardenas A. Hepatorenal syndrome: a dreaded complication of end-stage liver disease. Am J Gastroenterol 2005;100:460-7.

Evans LT. Spontaneous bacterial peritonitis in asymptomatic outpatients with cirrhotic ascites. Hepatology 2003;37:897-901.

Knox T, Olans L. Liver disease in pregnancy. N Engl J Med 1996;335:569-76.

Polson J, Lee WM. American Association for the Study of Liver Disease: AASLD position paper: the management of acute liver failure. Hepatology 2005;41:117997.

## REFERENCE

*References can be found on Expert Consult @ www.expertconsult.com.*

# 43 Pancreatic Disorders

*Mitchell C. Sokolosky*

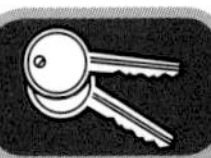

**KEY POINTS**

- Pancreatitis is an inflammatory condition of the pancreas that results from premature activation of pancreatic enzymes and autodigestion of the gland.
- Gallstones and alcohol use are the most common causes of acute pancreatitis.
- Elevations in serum pancreatic enzyme values help confirm the diagnosis in suspected cases.
- Computed tomography scans are not usually indicated on admission unless needed to exclude other serious causes of abdominal pain.
- The spectrum of illness ranges from mild (edematous) to severe (necrotizing) disease.
- Most patients with acute pancreatitis require hospitalization for supportive care and have a benign course.
- Necrotizing pancreatitis carries significant rates of morbidity and mortality, especially if infection is present.

## EPIDEMIOLOGY

More than 200,000 patients with acute pancreatitis are admitted to U.S. hospitals each year.[1] Eighty percent of these patients suffer from mild disease and demonstrate an overall mortality rate of just 1%. Approximately 20% of patients have severe necrotizing pancreatitis, however, which has a mortality rate of up to 25%.[2,3] The estimated incidence of pancreatitis in the United States is 79.8 per 100,000.[4] Men are affected more commonly than women, and the condition develops in most patients between 40 and 60 years of age.[5]

## PATHOPHYSIOLOGY

The pancreas is a retroperitoneal organ with a primary role in digestion; it exhibits both exocrine (i.e., pancreatic enzymes) and endocrine (i.e., insulin and glucagon) functions. *Pancreatitis* is an inflammatory condition of the pancreas that arises from premature activation of pancreatic enzymes and results in autodigestion of the gland. The exact pathogenesis of this disease is unclear. Both acute and chronic forms exist.

*Acute pancreatitis* is most often caused by gallstones or alcohol use. Gallstone pancreatitis occurs secondary to obstruction of the common bile or pancreatic duct. Alcohol or its metabolic by-products are thought to act as a direct toxin to the pancreas, and the effects are usually dose dependent. Other less common causes are hyperlipidemia, hypercalcemia, medications, toxins, trauma, surgery, sphincter of Oddi dysfunction, invasive diagnostic procedures (endoscopic retrograde cholangiopancreatography), and hereditary causes. Approximately 20% of cases are idiopathic, with occult microlithiasis thought to be the underlying cause in half of them.[6] Acute pancreatitis can be classified histologically as edematous or necrotizing, which corresponds to clinically mild or severe disease, respectively. Risk factors for severe disease include older age (>55 years), obesity (body mass index > 30 kg/m$^2$), and pleural effusions or infiltrates (or both).[7] Pancreatic necrosis (nonviable tissue) is associated with significant morbidity and mortality, especially if infection is present. Complications from pancreatitis include pseudocyst and abscess formation.

*Chronic pancreatitis* is often a progressive disorder with irreversible lesions, such as glandular fibrosis, distortion of the pancreatic duct, and strictures. Long-standing alcohol abuse is the most common cause of chronic pancreatitis.

Standard definitions and terminology for acute pancreatitis (**Table 43.1**) have been proposed to establish an exact vocabulary among institutions and within the literature.[8]

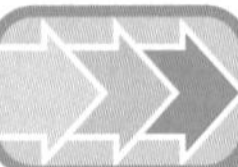

**PRIORITY ACTIONS**

1. Provide aggressive intravenous hydration to treat or prevent hypovolemia.
2. Provide appropriate parental narcotics for pain control.
3. Consider computed tomography if concerned about other possible serious causes of abdominal pain, such as a perforated ulcer.
4. Consider admission to the intensive care unit for patients with organ failure.
5. Start broad-spectrum antibiotics for clinical evidence of sepsis.

**Table 43.1 Definitions of Acute Pancreatitis Terminology**

| | |
|---|---|
| Acute pancreatitis | Acute inflammation of the pancreas |
| Mild acute pancreatitis | Minimal organ dysfunction responsive to fluid administration |
| Severe acute pancreatitis | One of the following: local complications (pancreatic necrosis, pancreatic pseudocyst, pancreatic abscess), organ failure, ≥3 Ranson criteria, APACHE II score ≥ 8 |
| Acute fluid collections | Fluid collection in or near the pancreas, without a defined wall, occurring early in the course of disease |
| Acute pseudocyst | Fluid collection containing pancreatic secretions, with a defined wall |
| Pancreatic necrosis | Nonviable pancreatic tissue diagnosed by contrast-enhanced computed tomography |
| Pancreatic abscess | Collection of purulent material in or near the pancreas |

*APACHE II*, Acute Physiology and Chronic Health Evaluation, version 2.

**BOX 43.1 Nonpancreatic Causes of Elevations in Serum Amylase**

Abdominal aortic aneurysm
Anorexia nervosa, bulimia
Appendicitis
Burns
Cerebral trauma
Drugs (azathioprine, sulfonamides, tetracycline, furosemide, valproic acid)
Hepatitis
Idiopathic hyperamylasemia
Intestinal obstruction
Ketoacidosis
Macroamylasemia
Mesenteric infarction
Ovarian cysts
Perforated bowel
Peritonitis
Pneumonia
Renal failure
Ruptured ectopic pregnancy
Salivary diseases
Salpingitis

## PRESENTING SIGNS AND SYMPTOMS

### CLASSIC

Acute pancreatitis is manifested as severe, upper abdominal pain that may radiate to the back. The onset of pain is rapid, typically over a period of an hour or less. The pain is constant and is often worsened by lying flat and partially relieved by sitting up. Nausea and vomiting are typically present. Fever and anorexia may or may not be present. Jaundice is rare. Findings on examination vary with the severity of disease. Abdominal examination usually demonstrates a soft, tender epigastrium without peritoneal signs. Guarding or rebound tenderness suggests more severe disease. Distention may be present secondary to concomitant ileus.

### VARIATIONS

Painless pancreatitis may be encountered in the postoperative period after major surgery or in association with peritoneal dialysis or legionnaires disease. Though rare, ecchymoses in the flanks (Grey Turner sign) or in the periumbilical area (Cullen sign) from intraabdominal hemorrhage suggest severe disease. Diaphragmatic irritation from an inflamed pancreatic tail may produce hiccups and pleural effusions. Patients with necrotizing pancreatitis may arrive at the emergency department (ED) in shock or coma.

## DIFFERENTIAL DIAGNOSIS

The differential diagnosis for pancreatitis includes peptic ulcer disease with or without perforation, gastritis, biliary colic, acute cholecystitis, aortic dissection, mesenteric ischemia, myocardial infarction, and renal colic.

## DIAGNOSIS

Diagnosis of acute pancreatitis requires two of the following three features: (1) characteristic abdominal pain, (2) elevated serum pancreatic enzymes, and (3) characteristic findings on computed tomography (CT).[7]

## DIAGNOSTIC TESTING

### LABORATORY TESTS

No biochemical marker is considered the "gold standard" for diagnosis or assessment of the severity of acute pancreatitis.[9] Serum amylase and lipase measurements remain important diagnostic tests for acute pancreatitis. Other useful prognostic tests are a complete blood count; measurements of blood urea nitrogen and serum electrolyte, creatinine, glucose, and triglyceride levels; and liver function tests.

Total serum *amylase* has a reported sensitivity of 83% and specificity of 88% for acute pancreatitis.[10] Amylase levels rise within 6 to 12 hours of onset and usually remain elevated for 3 to 5 days. A normal amylase value would generally exclude the diagnosis of acute pancreatitis except in cases involving hyperlipidemia, acute exacerbations of chronic pancreatitis, or markedly delayed manifestations (in which case amylase levels may have normalized). Acute pancreatitis should not be excluded on the basis of a normal or mildly elevated amylase value when clinical suspicion of this diagnosis is high. Serum amylase values cannot be used to estimate the severity or determine the cause of acute pancreatitis. Nonpancreatic causes of elevated serum amylase levels are listed in **Box 43.1**.

The serum *lipase* level is more sensitive (92%) and specific (96%) than total amylase for acute pancreatitis.[10] Lipase has

**BOX 43.2 Nonpancreatic Causes of Serum Lipase Elevation**

Acute cholecystitis
Acute renal failure
Bone fracture
Crush injury
Diabetic ketoacidosis
Extrahepatic biliary obstruction
Fat embolism
Intestinal infarction
Intestinal obstruction
Liver diseases
Mumps
Pancreatic hyperenzymemia
Peptic ulcer disease
Perforated bowel
Postcholecystectomy syndrome
Type I or IV hyperlipoproteinemia

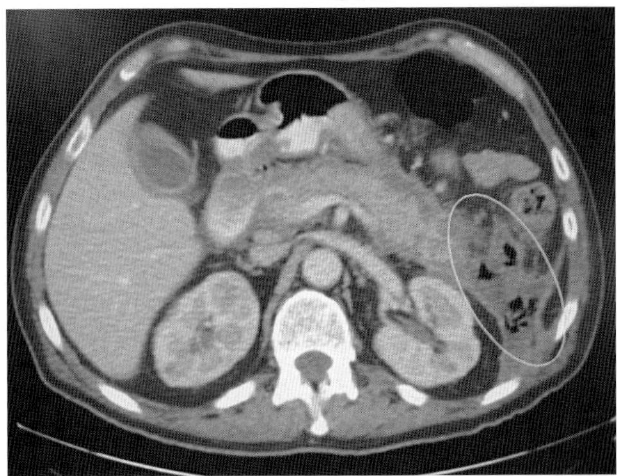

**Fig. 43.1** Necrotic portions of the pancreas *(circled)* with gas suggest infection.

greater sensitivity in patients with acute alcoholic pancreatitis. It is useful in delayed clinical manifestations because the serum lipase value stays elevated longer than the serum amylase value does. However, serum lipase is not as specific for acute pancreatitis as once thought. The value is elevated in as many disorders as the amylase value (**Box 43.2**). As with serum amylase values, serum lipase values cannot be used to estimate the severity or determine the cause of acute pancreatitis.

Controversy exists whether measurements of serum amylase, serum lipase, or both should be ordered in a patient in whom pancreatitis is suspected. Within 24 hours after the onset of symptoms, both enzyme values have high sensitivity and specificity for acute pancreatitis. Simultaneous evaluation of these two serum enzymes has not been shown to increase overall diagnostic accuracy, and the extent of elevation in pancreatic enzyme levels does not correlate with the severity of disease. The serum lipase value is thought to have higher diagnostic accuracy because it remains elevated longer than serum amylase does.

A uniform threshold has not been established for serum amylase or lipase for the diagnosis of acute pancreatitis, but most of the published literature has reported thresholds of two to four or more times the upper limit of normal. However, the diagnosis of acute pancreatitis should not rely solely on elevations in serum enzymes above the arbitrary limit of normal laboratory levels but instead should be made on the basis of the onset of clinical symptoms because the sensitivities of these enzyme values change with the timing of their measurements.[10]

The *urinary dipstick test* for detecting pancreatic amylase in urine has demonstrated a sensitivity of 97%. This test for amylase may therefore be a useful point-of-care screening test for acute pancreatitis in the ED but is currently not in widespread use.[11]

*C-reactive protein* (CRP) is the best available serum marker for assessing the severity of acute pancreatitis.[4] A threshold level greater than 150 mg/L is now accepted as a proven predictor of severity. However, CRP levels must be monitored after hospital admission because it takes 48 to 72 hours for the value to peak, thus making it less useful in the ED.

*Hemoconcentration* secondary to volume depletion has been identified as an early marker of pancreatic necrosis. In one study, an admission hematocrit value of 47% or higher and failure of the value to decrease at 24 hours after admission were associated with the development of pancreatic necrosis.[12] An increase in *serum alanine transaminase* levels to higher than 150 IU/L is suggestive of gallstone pancreatitis.[13] A lower value does not exclude the diagnosis, however.

Measurement of isoamylases, immunoreactive trypsinogen, macroamylases, or elastase has no role in the routine management of acute pancreatitis in the ED.[14]

## IMAGING

*Plain abdominal radiographs* are rarely useful except to exclude other causes of abdominal pain such as perforation and obstruction. Positive findings in acute pancreatitis include the presence of a sentinel loop (an area of focal ileus) or a colon cutoff sign (a paucity of colonic air distal to the splenic flexure caused by functional spasm of the descending colon secondary to pancreatic inflammation). Pancreatic calcifications can be seen on radiographs in patients with chronic pancreatitis.

*CT* of the abdomen can aid in the diagnosis of acute pancreatitis and its complications, as well as assess the severity of disease. Most ED patients with acute pancreatitis do not require a CT scan at admission unless it is needed to exclude other serious causes of acute abdominal pain, such as a perforated ulcer. Contrast-enhanced CT of the abdomen is considered the best available test for the noninvasive diagnosis of pancreatic necrosis.[15] Necrosis may develop several days after admission and should be suspected in patients with clinical evidence of increased severity. Affected portions of the necrotic pancreas do not show normal contrast enhancement on CT (**Fig. 43.1**). Non–contrast-enhanced CT will not aid in the diagnosis of pancreatic necrosis but may be considered in patients with renal insufficiency to provide other useful information. CT can diagnose complications such as pseudocysts (**Fig. 43.2**), phlegmon, and abscesses.

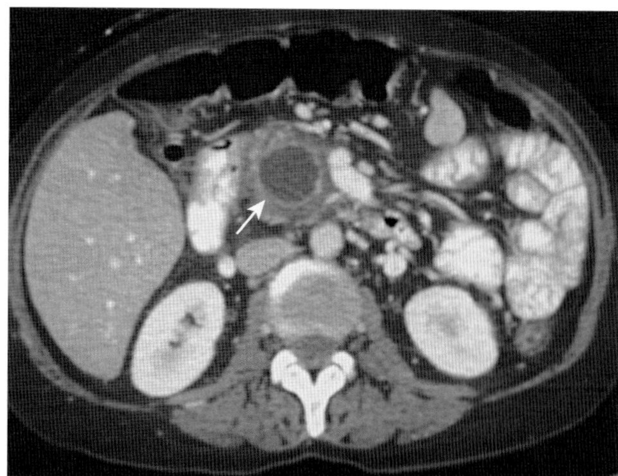

**Fig. 43.2** Computed tomography can diagnose complications such as pseudocysts *(arrow)*.

*Ultrasonography* has a limited role in the diagnosis of pancreatitis. Findings positive for acute pancreatitis include a diffusely enlarged, hypoechoic pancreas. Ultrasonography is very useful for imaging the biliary tract and diagnosing gallstones.

*Magnetic resonance imaging* (MRI) has been used in the diagnosis and management of acute pancreatitis. This modality is superior to CT in its categorization of fluid collections, necrosis, abscess, hemorrhage, and pseudocysts.[16] Disadvantages include the lack of availability of MRI when urgently needed and the difficulty of caring for critically ill patients undergoing MRI.

### Criteria for Determining Severity

The two most important markers of severity in acute pancreatitis are the presence of organ failure because of the systemic release of local inflammatory mediators (i.e., shock, pulmonary insufficiency, renal failure, gastrointestinal bleeding) and pancreatic necrosis.[7]

Contrast-enhanced CT of the abdomen is considered the best available test for determining the severity of disease, particularly after 2 to 3 days of illness.[17] A CT Severity Index Score can be calculated on the basis of CT findings, with a score of 6 or higher indicating severe disease (**Table 43.2**).[18]

**Table 43.2 Computed Tomography Severity Index Score for Pancreatitis***

| GRADE† | CT FINDINGS | SCORE |
|---|---|---|
| A | Normal pancreas | 0 |
| B | Focal or diffuse enlargement of the pancreas, contour irregularities, heterogeneous attenuation, no peripancreatic inflammation | 1 |
| C | Grade B plus peripancreatic inflammation | 2 |
| D | Grade C plus a single fluid collection | 3 |
| E | Grade C plus multiple fluid collections or gas | 4 |

| PERCENT NECROSIS PRESENT ON CT | SCORE |
|---|---|
| 0 | 0 |
| <33 | 2 |
| 33-50 | 4 |
| >50 | 6 |

*Severity Index Score = Grade score + Percent Necrosis score. Maximum score = 10; severe disease = 6 or higher.

†Severity of the acute inflammatory process.

Though not as accurate as the CT system, scoring systems that include clinical criteria may also be used to estimate severity but have a limited role in the ED because of either timing or the complexity of the data elements. The most commonly used clinical scores for determining the severity of acute pancreatitis are the Ranson criteria (**Box 43.3**) and the second version of the Acute Physiology and Chronic Health Evaluation (APACHE II).

The Ranson score is based on 11 prognostic signs.[19] Five of the signs are measured on admission, and six are measured 48 hours later, thus making it less useful in the ED setting. Mortality estimates are based on the number of signs present. Mortality is less than 0.9% when three or fewer signs are present; it is 100% when more than six signs are noted.

The APACHE II score is based on 12 physiologic variables, age, and previous health.[17] The APACHE II score is probably the best clinical predictor of the severity of acute pancreatitis.[20] A severity score can be assessed on admission and recalculated daily. (A calculator is available at www.sfar.org/scores2/apache22.html.) An APACHE II score higher than 8 indicates severe disease. However, the complexity of the APACHE II score limits its usefulness in the ED setting. An APACHE III score, developed to improve accuracy, does not appear to be more useful than APACHE II in differentiating mild from severe disease.[21]

The "harmless acute pancreatitis score" takes a completely new approach and attempts to predict mild disease instead of severe pancreatitis. This simple clinical algorithm assesses three variables (no rebound tenderness or guarding, normal hematocrit, normal creatinine) to identify patients who have a benign course 98% of the time. This information may quickly aid the physician in determining the appropriate level of care for admission if warranted.[22]

## TREATMENT

No specific treatment is available for pancreatitis other than supportive care. Supplemental oxygen, aggressive intravenous hydration, pain management, and monitoring are the mainstays of treatment. Supplemental oxygen is vital for treating and preventing hypoxemia. Aggressive intravenous hydration consisting of fluid boluses to establish hemodynamic stability followed by appropriate maintenance fluids is of critical importance in treating and preventing hypovolemia. Hypovolemia occurs secondary to vomiting, decreased oral intake, diaphoresis, third-space losses, and inflammatory-mediated increased vascular permeability. Hypovolemia compromises the pancreatic microcirculation and can contribute to the development of pancreatic necrosis. Nasogastric tubes are not indicated in all patients but may be helpful in those with significant vomiting or in whom enteral feeding is indicated. Anticholinergic agents, once given to decrease gastric secretions, are no longer recommended. Endoscopic retrograde cholangiopancreatography is usually indicated within 24 to 48 hours of arrival in patients with severe pancreatitis secondary to gallstones (Box 43-3).

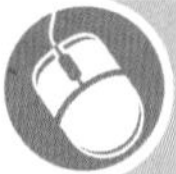

See Box 43-3, Ranson Criteria and Score, online at www.expertconsult.com.

Narcotic analgesia is often needed to control the pain of acute pancreatitis. Controversy exists over which narcotic to use. Morphine has historically been avoided because of the potential to cause spasm of the sphincter of Oddi and subsequent worsening of symptoms.[23] Meperidine is often used in place of morphine, but no conclusive evidence supports the use of meperidine rather than other narcotics.[24] In fact, meperidine has several disadvantages, including the potential formation of neurotoxic metabolites, muscle fibrosis if given intramuscularly, and a short duration of action. Administration of adequate doses of narcotic analgesia is probably more important than the particular narcotic used.

Management of necrotizing pancreatitis usually involves admission to a higher level of care (step-down unit or intensive care unit) because of the associated increased morbidity and mortality. The use of prophylactic antibiotics to prevent infection in patients with pancreatic necrosis is no longer recommended.[7] Antibiotics are indicated for septic patients while an investigation for the source of infection is undertaken. Carbapenems are acceptable empiric choices.[25] Infected necrotizing pancreatitis is considered uniformly fatal without intervention and should be suspected in patients with clinical evidence of sepsis. Urgent surgical consultation should be obtained if infection is suspected because aggressive surgical débridement (necrosectomy) may be necessary.[9] CT-guided fine-needle aspiration may be necessary to establish the diagnosis in suspicious cases. Drainage options for patients with pancreatic necrosis who will not undergo surgery (poor surgical candidates or patients whose infection is well contained) are expanding and include both percutaneous therapy (interventional radiology) and endoscopic therapy. Treatment of sterile necrosis remains supportive.

## DISPOSITION

Most patients with acute pancreatitis require hospital admission for supportive care and have a benign course. Patients with acute necrotizing pancreatitis usually require admission to either a step-down or intensive care unit for closer monitoring and treatment. The presence of organ failure is one of the indications for considering admission to an intensive care unit. Patients with tachycardia, oliguria, and inadequate pain control may benefit from management in a step-down unit. Mild cases of pancreatitis may be managed on an outpatient basis if the pain is controlled and the patient is tolerating liquids. Patients who are discharged home require proper follow-up and written discharge instructions. Alcoholic patients with pancreatitis are encouraged to stop drinking and seek detoxification treatment.

## PANCREAS TRANSPLANT COMPLICATIONS

Acute rejection can occur immediately or at any point during the course of the patient's life. Patients who have undergone pancreatic transplantation are maintained on immunosuppressive agents and thus are at risk for a variety of infectious complications. Vascular thrombosis of the pancreatic portal vein is a very early complication typically seen within 24 to 48 hours of transplantation and is thought to be due to the relatively low-flow state of the pancreatic graft. Transplantation pancreatitis occurs to some degree in all patients postoperatively within 48 to 96 hours and is usually transient and mild.[26]

Other complications vary with the specific surgical technique performed (i.e., bladder-drained or enteric-drained transplant). Complications of bladder-drained pancreas transplantation include urinary tract infections, hematuria, sterile cystitis, urethritis, balanitis, and metabolic acidosis (because of the bladder excreting large volumes of alkaline pancreatic secretions). Reflux pancreatitis secondary to reflux of urine through the ampulla into the pancreatic ducts can mimic acute rejection but usually resolves after Foley catheterization. The most serious complication of bladder-drained pancreatic transplantation is a urine leak from breakdown of the duodenal segment and is usually seen in the first 2 to 3 weeks postoperatively. A high index of suspicion is required to make the diagnosis because the symptoms usually include nonspecific abdominal pain and elevated pancreatic enzymes. Voiding cystography or CT aids in making the diagnosis. The most serious complication of enteric-drained pancreatic transplantation is leak and intraabdominal abscess, which usually occur 1 to 6 months postoperatively. Patients generally have abdominal pain, fever, and leukocytosis. CT aids in making the diagnosis. Treatment includes broad-spectrum antibiotics and surgical consultation.

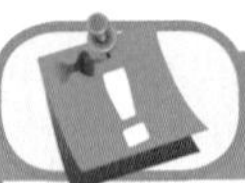

**TIPS AND TRICKS**

The diagnosis of acute pancreatitis should not rely solely on elevations of serum enzymes above the arbitrary limits of normal laboratory levels; instead, it should be based on the onset of clinical symptoms because the sensitivities of these enzyme values change with the timing of their measurements.[10]

## REFERENCES

***References can be found on Expert Consult @ www.expertconsult.com.***

# Biliary Tract Disorders 44

Julie J. Cooper

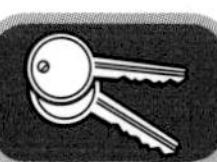

**KEY POINTS**

- Risk factors for the development of gallstone disease include female gender, increasing age, obesity, rapid weight loss, and underlying liver disease.
- The majority of patients with gallstone disease are asymptomatic. Symptomatic complications include biliary colic, acute cholecystitis, choledocholithiasis, cholangitis, and acute pancreatitis.
- A high index of suspicion should be maintained for acute cholangitis in the chronically ill, elderly, or diabetic patients with sepsis of unknown source.
- Ultrasound is the initial diagnostic study of choice in patients with suspected gallstone disease. Cholecystoscintigraphy is the most sensitive test for cholecystitis, and magnetic resonance cholangiopancreatography is the most sensitive test for bile duct stones.

## CHOLELITHIASIS AND ACUTE CHOLECYSTITIS

### EPIDEMIOLOGY

Cholelithiasis affects 20 to 25 million Americans, which represents 10% to 15% of the adult population. Although most gallstones are clinically silent, 20% of people harboring stones experience biliary symptoms at some time; 1% to 2% of patients each year experience complications and require surgical removal of the gallbladder. In the United States, cholecystectomy is the most common elective abdominal surgery, with approximately 750,000 procedures performed per year. Complications of cholelithiasis include acute cholecystitis, ascending cholangitis, acute pancreatitis, and adenocarcinoma of the gallbladder, which result in a combined mortality of 5000 to 10,000 deaths per year (**Box 44.1**).

### PATHOPHYSIOLOGY

Bile is primarily composed of cholesterol, lecithin, bile salts, bilirubin, and electrolytes (i.e., calcium, carbonate, phosphate). Once these solutes exceed their solubility, they form crystals. Crystals trapped in biliary mucus produce sludge and aggregate to form stones. Cholesterol is the primary constituent in 60% to 80% of all gallstones. Calcium bilirubinate salts predominate in another 10% to 20% of stones; cholesterol and calcium bilirubinate are present in relatively equal quantities in the remainder of calculi. Biliary stasis is thought to play a significant role in stone formation.[12]

Although bile itself is normally sterile, any alterations in biliary motility lead to an increased risk for bacterial infection. The organisms implicated in cholecystitis are generally bowel flora and include *Escherichia coli, Klebsiella,* enterococci, and anaerobes.[13]

### PRESENTING SIGNS AND SYMPTOMS

Gallstones can be manifested as a spectrum of disease and may be divided into asymptomatic, symptomatic, and complicated gallstone disease. Only 15% to 20% of stones become symptomatic, between 1% and 3% per year. Approximately 66% of patients have a recurrent episode of biliary colic within 2 years, and about one in six have a complication of gallstone disease[13] (**Table 44.1**).

### DIFFERENTIAL DIAGNOSIS AND MEDICAL DECISION MAKING

Patients with suspected complications of gallstone disease should be evaluated for alternative diagnoses, as well as complications of gallstones such as pancreatitis and cholangitis. Laboratory evaluation for all these patients should include a complete blood count, basic serum chemistries, liver function tests, serum amylase and lipase, and urinalysis. A urine pregnancy test should always be performed in women of childbearing age.

Laboratory test results in patients with symptomatic cholelithiasis should be normal except for a mild elevation in serum alkaline phosphatase. Alkaline phosphatase is synthesized by the biliary tract epithelium but is also found in bone. γ-Glutamyltransferase (GGT) is another enzyme secreted by the biliary epithelium that may be elevated in patients with biliary obstruction.

### DIAGNOSTIC IMAGING FOR CHOLELITHIASIS AND CHOLECYSTITIS

Ultrasonography is the preferred first-line modality for evaluating potential biliary stones (**Fig. 44.1**). A metaanalysis of studies demonstrated that ultrasound has a sensitivity of 97% and specificity of 95% for the diagnosis of cholelithiasis.[17] Common findings on ultrasonography are hyperechoic stones with hypoechoic shadowing, biliary sludge, and stone mobility with changes in patient positioning (**Fig. 44.2**). Pericholecystic fluid (**Fig. 44.3**), gallbladder wall thickening (>3 mm), common bile duct dilation (>6 mm), and intrahepatic and extrahepatic biliary ductal dilation are highly suggestive of acute cholecystitis.

Cholecystoscintigraphy or hepatobiliary iminodiacetic acid (HIDA) scanning is a more sensitive test for diagnosing acute cholecystitis. In this nuclear medicine study, a radioactive tracer is injected peripherally and allowed to circulate to the liver, where it is excreted in bile. In the absence of disease, the gallbladder is visualized within 1 hour of injection (**Fig. 44.4**). Nonvisualization of the gallbladder within 4 hours after injection indicates either cholecystitis or cystic duct obstruction

## BOX 44.1 Risk Factors for the Development of Cholelithiasis

**Gender**

Women have twice the incidence and prevalence of gallstones.

Estrogen stimulates low-density lipoprotein receptors and increases the uptake of cholesterol; higher cholesterol content in bile is associated with greater risk for gallstone formation.[1]

After menopause, the incidence of gallstone disease in women and men is comparable.

**Ethnicity**

The incidence of cholelithiasis is highest in North American Indians (especially Pima Indians), followed by South American Indians and Mexican Americans.

Black Africans have the lowest incidence and prevalence of gallstone disease.[1]

**Age**

Gallstone prevalence increases after 40 years of age.[1]

**Obesity**

Obesity is associated with increased cholesterol secretion into bile.[2]

**Rapid Weight Loss**

Low-calorie diets and rapid weight loss are associated with the development of gallstones in 30% to 71% of persons.

Weight loss exceeding 1.5 kg/wk, after bariatric surgery in particular, increases the risk for stone formation.[1,3]

**Total Parenteral Nutrition**

Loss of enteric stimulation of the gallbladder in the absence of eating leads to gallbladder stasis.

Total parental nutrition (TPN) increases the risk for biliary sludge, gallstone disease, and acalculous cholecystitis.

After 4 weeks of TPN, gallbladder sludge develops in half of patients and after 6 weeks in all. The sludge resolves within 4 weeks of resuming oral intake.[4]

**Family History**

Occurrence of gallstone disease within families can be a product of genetic and shared environmental factors.[5]

The frequency is increased in monozygotic (12%) as opposed to dizygotic twins (6%).[6]

Genetic effects account for 25%, shared environmental effects for 13%, and unique environmental effects for 62% of the phenotypic variance in gallstone production.[7]

**Chronic Diseases**

The overall prevalence of gallstones in patients with cirrhosis is 25% to 30% (double that in the general population).[8]

Crohn disease causes ileal malabsorption of bile acids. These acids normally solubilize cholesterol and bilirubin to be excreted. An inadequate amount of bile acid means that increased cholesterol and bilirubin are available to form stones.[9]

Cystic fibrosis is also associated with bile acid malabsorption and gallstones.

**Medications**

Octreotide is used for the treatment of acromegaly and carcinoid syndrome; it affects biliary motility and sphincter of Oddi function. Cholelithiasis develops in more than 50% of patients receiving octreotide. The majority are asymptomatic.[10]

Ceftriaxone is secreted unmetabolized into bile, where it reaches high concentrations and produces biliary sludge.[11]

**Table 44.1** Symptoms of Gallstone Disease and Its Complications

| DISEASE | PATHOPHYSIOLOGY | SYMPTOMS |
|---|---|---|
| Biliary colic | Transient gallstone impaction at the cystic duct or ampulla of Vater | Intermittent RUQ pain associated with nausea or vomiting.<br>Pain in the epigastrium or radiating to the right scapular tip.<br>Episodes last 30 min to several hours with days or months between episodes. |
| Acute cholecystitis | Inflammation of the gallbladder caused by obstruction of the cystic duct<br>May occur in the presence or absence of bacterial superinfection | Patients appear ill and cannot take deep breaths. They have constant pain that lasts 30-60 min and worsens with movement.<br>Persistent common bile duct impaction usually promotes vomiting.<br>Physical examination demonstrates RUQ tenderness with voluntary guarding and a positive Murphy sign (arrest of inspiration during deep palpation over the gallbladder). |
| Emphysematous cholecystitis | Infection with gas-producing bacteria such as *Escherichia coli, Clostridium perfringens*, and anaerobic streptococci | Symptoms are similar to those with acute cholecystitis.<br>Gas may be seen on abdominal plain films or CT.<br>Male diabetics are most commonly affected. |
| Chronic cholecystitis | Persistent inflammation and fibrosis of the gallbladder with poor motor and absorptive function | Patients are usually asymptomatic but may report multiple previous attacks of colic.<br>Porcelain gallbladder develops from chronic inflammation and may progress to carcinoma. |
| Acalculous cholecystitis | Probably related to biliary stasis in the setting of critical illness and altered gastrointestinal motility | Seen in patients with traumatic injuries, burns, and critical illness, as well as in those receiving total parenteral nutrition.<br>The mortality for this disorder is twice as high as that for acute calculous cholecystitis.[14] |
| Gallbladder perforation | Stones erode through an inflamed and necrotic gallbladder wall<br>Stones may travel into the peritoneal cavity or cause adhesions between nearby structures. Bile peritonitis may develop | More than half of patients with gallbladder perforation have fever and a palpable RUQ mass.[15]<br>Mortality in these patients is 30%.[16] |

*CT*, Computed tomography; *RUQ*, right upper quadrant.

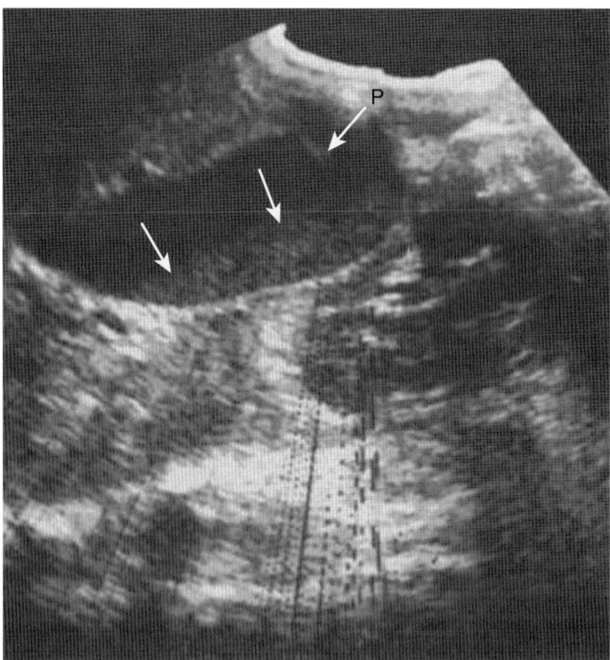


**Fig. 44.1 Ultrasonogram demonstrating biliary sludge *(arrows).*** *P*, Polyp. (From Berk RN, Ferrucci Jr JT, Leopold GR. Radiology of the gallbladder and bile ducts: diagnosis and intervention. Philadelphia: Saunders; 1983. p. 206.)

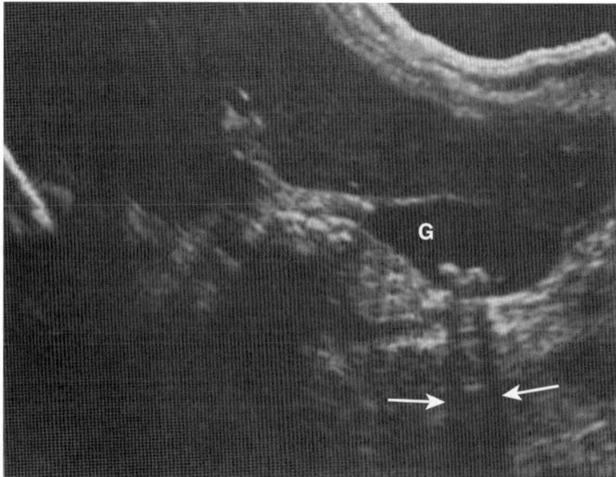


**Fig. 44.2 Cholelithiasis shown by ultrasonography *(arrows).*** *G*, Gallbladder. (From Berk RN, Ferrucci Jr JT, Leopold GR. Radiology of the gallbladder and bile ducts: diagnosis and intervention. Philadelphia: Saunders; 1983. p. 255.)

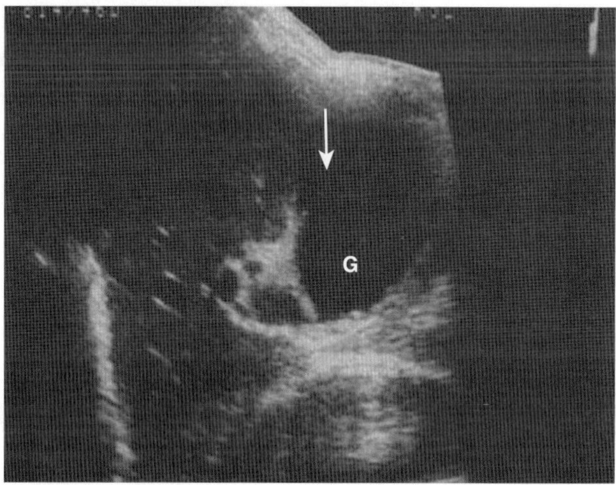


**Fig. 44.3 Ultrasonogram demonstrating pericholecystic fluid *(arrow).*** *G*, Gallbladder. (From Berk RN, Ferrucci Jr JT, Leopold GR. Radiology of the gallbladder and bile ducts: diagnosis and intervention. Philadelphia: Saunders; 1983. p. 213.)

(**Fig. 44.5**). In a retrospective review of 170 patients evaluated in the emergency department (ED) because of right upper quadrant (RUQ) pain, cholecystoscintigraphy had a diagnostic sensitivity of 86% for acute cholecystitis as compared with 48% for ultrasonography. In another study, the results of cholecystoscintigraphy were positive in 87% of patients in whom the initial ultrasonographic findings were negative.[18]

Computed tomography (CT) is less sensitive than ultrasonography for the diagnosis of acute biliary disease.[19] CT may offer valuable information about the surrounding anatomy if confounding clinical signs or symptoms are present, if ultrasonography does not demonstrate calculus, or if an alternative diagnosis is as likely as biliary disease (**Fig. 44.6**). A retrospective study of 123 patients who underwent both CT and RUQ ultrasonography demonstrated a sensitivity of only 39% for CT in detecting biliary disease.[19] Ultrasonography had a sensitivity of 83% in that study and suggested the correct diagnosis in seven of eight patients in whom the CT findings led to misdiagnosis (**Fig. 44.7**). **Figure 44.8** presents a summary of the diagnostic and treatment algorithm for right upper quadrant pain.

## TREATMENT

### MEDICAL MANAGEMENT

Initial ED management of all patients with suspected complications of gallstone disease should include nothing by mouth, intravenous fluids, analgesics, and antiemetics as needed. For those without contraindications to nonsteroidal antiinflammatory drugs (NSAIDs), ketorolac (Toradol), 60 mg intramuscularly (IM) or 30 mg intravenously (IV), is an effective parenteral treatment of biliary colic. Opiate analgesia starting at 0.1 mg/kg of morphine or its equivalent is appropriate for patients in whom NSAIDs do not provide adequate effect. Nausea and vomiting are treated with metoclopramide (Reglan), 10 mg IV, or ondansetron (Zofran), 4 mg as an orally disintegrating tablet, IM, or IV.

Empiric antibiotics should cover *E. coli, Klebsiella, Streptococcus faecalis*, and anaerobic organisms. An acceptable combination regimen consists of a third- or fourth-generation cephalosporin (e.g., ceftazidime) plus metronidazole. An alternative would be a combination of a β-lactam antibiotic and a β-lactamase inhibitor such as piperacillin and tazobactam or ampicillin and sulbactam.[13]

Medical therapy for chronic gallstone disease may include oral bile acids or extracorporal shock wave lithotripsy (ESWL). Oral bile acids dissolve cholesterol gallstones. The most commonly used agent is ursodeoxycholic acid, which is a primary bile acid of bears. It both dissolves cholesterol gallstones and reduces biliary cholesterol secretion.[20] ESWL fragments gallstones with external shock waves. These stones are then more amenable to dissolution with oral bile acids. The major complications are biliary colic and problems stemming from the expulsion of smaller gallstones, such as acute pancreatitis.[21]

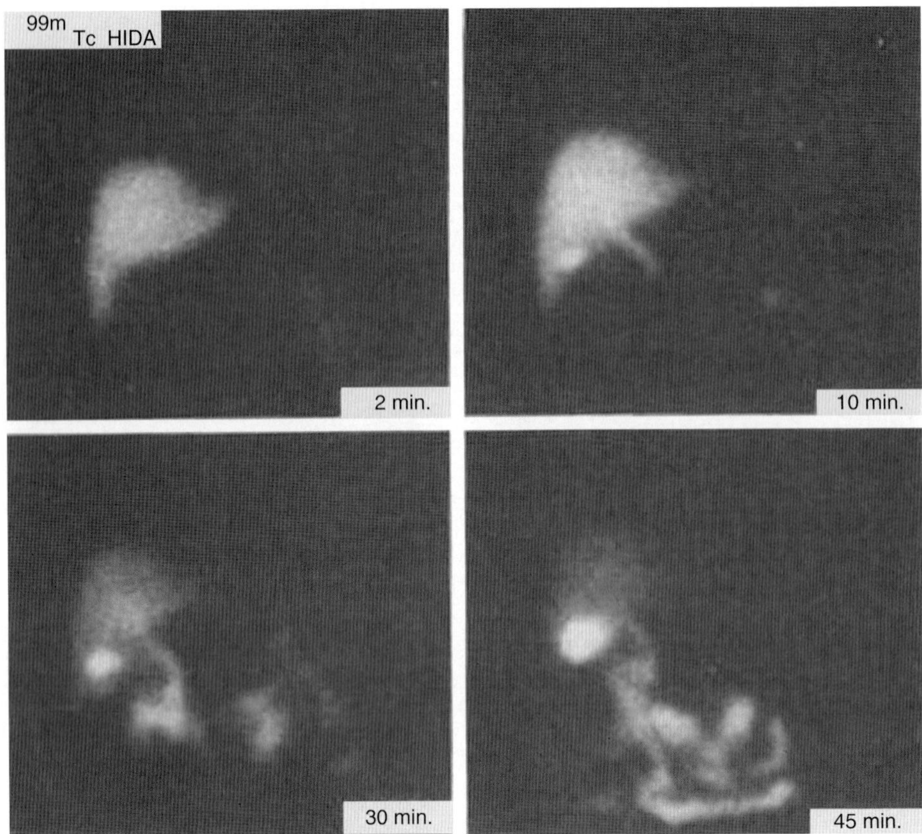


**Fig. 44.4 Normal cholecystoscintigrams.** (From Berk RN, Ferrucci Jr JT, Leopold GR. Radiology of the gallbladder and bile ducts: diagnosis and intervention. Philadelphia: Saunders; 1983. p. 265.)

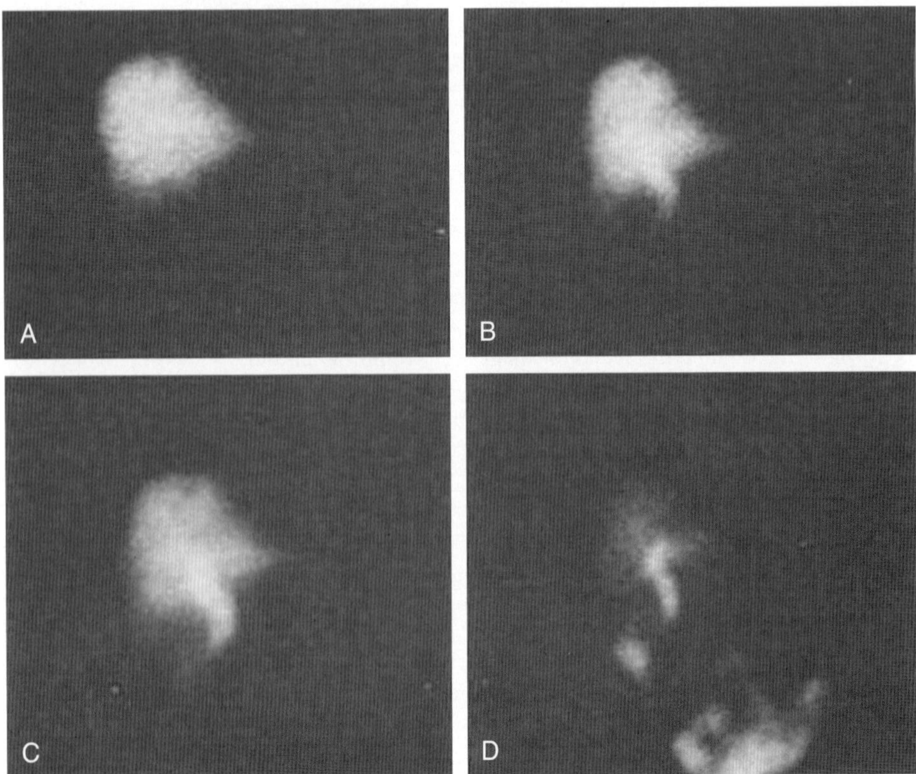


**Fig. 44.5 A** to **D,** Abnormal cholecystoscintigrams. (From Berk RN, Ferrucci Jr JT, Leopold GR. Radiology of the gallbladder and bile ducts: diagnosis and intervention. Philadelphia: Saunders; 1983. p. 273.)

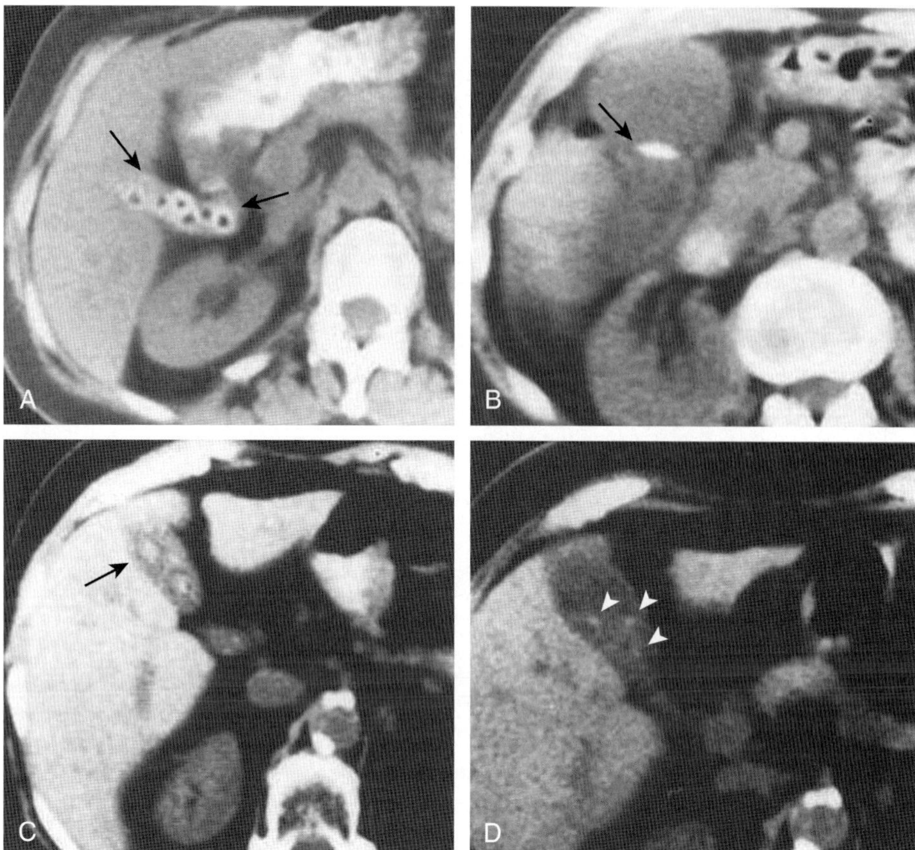


**Fig. 44.6** **A** to **D,** Computed tomography scans showing cholelithiasis (*arrows* and *arrowheads*) in four different patients. (From Berk RN, Ferrucci Jr JT, Leopold GR. Radiology of the gallbladder and bile ducts: diagnosis and intervention. Philadelphia: Saunders; 1983. p. 215.)

## SURGICAL MANAGEMENT

Laparoscopic cholecystectomy is the mainstay of surgical treatment of symptomatic gallstones. When compared with open cholecystectomy, laparoscopic surgery is associated with decreased postoperative pain; decreased hospital length of stay; decreased risk for mortality, cardiopulmonary complications, and wound infections, but also with an increased risk for bile duct injuries.[22,23] Cholecystectomy is also the treatment of choice for acute cholecystitis. Although the timing of surgery in this context has been debated, early cholecystectomy within a few days of initial evaluation is probably associated with lower morbidity and mortality.[24] Patients who are critically ill or have acute contraindications to cholecystectomy can be temporized with percutaneous cholecystostomy for drainage pending definitive management.

The most common immediate complication of cholecystectomy is bile leakage, which is treated by endoscopic retrograde cholangiopancreatography (ERCP) with stent placement.[25] Stent placement decreases outflow resistance and allows spontaneous closure of the leak, usually within a few days. Postoperative cholecystectomy patients with recurrent abdominal symptoms should be evaluated for retained stones along with choledocholithiasis, pancreatitis, abscess, or bile leak.

## FOLLOW-UP, NEXT STEPS IN CARE, AND PATIENT EDUCATION

Patients with biliary colic may be discharged home if their symptoms can be adequately controlled with oral medications, complications have been excluded with blood tests and appropriate imaging, and they are able to arrange follow-up with a surgeon. Patients should be discharged with an adequate supply of analgesic and antiemetic medications and strict return precautions for intractable pain or vomiting, fever, or jaundice. Those with suspected cholecystitis should be admitted to the hospital for intravenous antibiotics and definitive imaging studies with surgical consultation.

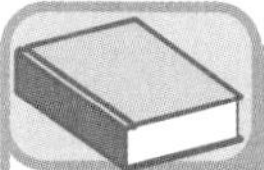

### PATIENT TEACHING TIPS

**Biliary Colic**

Avoid high-fat foods.

Use prescribed pain and nausea medications as needed.

Return to the emergency department if you have intractable pain, vomiting, fever, or chills.

Make a follow-up appointment with a surgeon.

### DOCUMENTATION

Presence of fever, changes in stool color, vomiting

Personal or family history of gallstones

Presence of the Murphy sign or jaundice on physical examination

Improvement in pain, tolerance of oral fluids, and patient teaching before discharge

Return precautions, referral to a surgeon

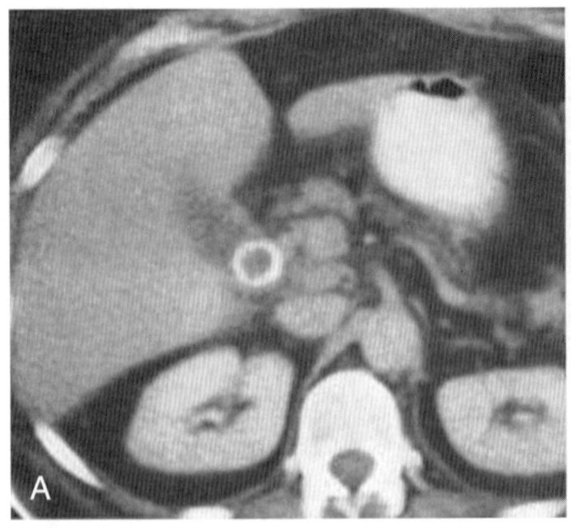


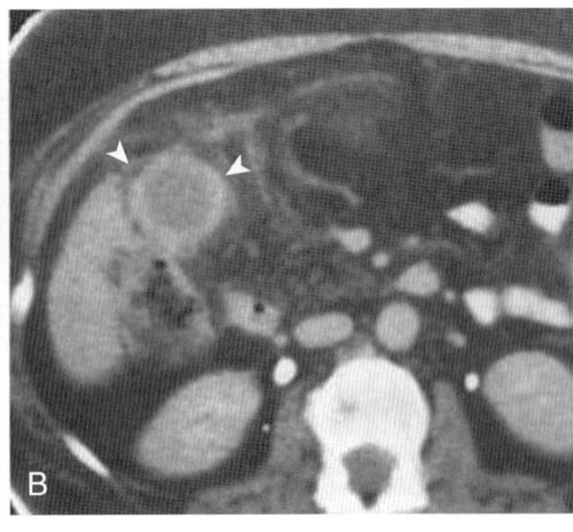


**Fig. 44.7** **A** and **B,** Cholelithiasis with cholecystitis *(arrowheads)* on computed tomography. (From Berk RN, Ferrucci Jr JT, Leopold GR. Radiology of the gallbladder and bile ducts: diagnosis and intervention. Philadelphia: Saunders; 1983. p. 255.)

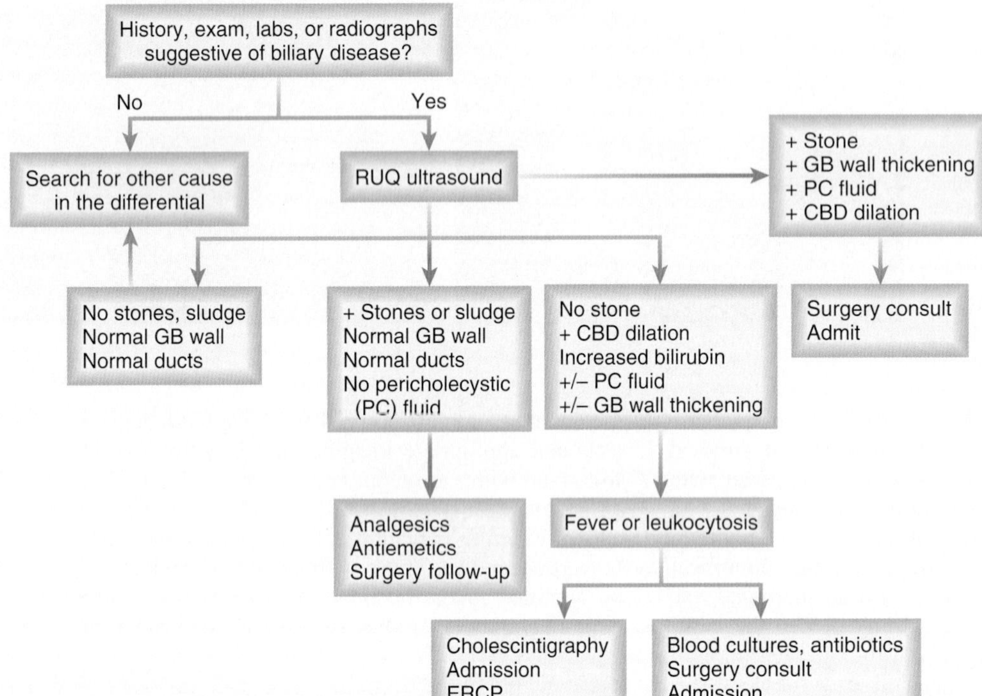


**Fig. 44.8** **Treatment algorithm for right upper quadrant (RUQ) pain.** *CBD*, Common bile duct; *ERCP*, endoscopic retrograde cholangiopancreatography; *GB*, gallbladder; *RUQ*, right upper quadrant; +, with; –, without; ±, with or without.

# CHOLEDOCHOLITHIASIS AND CHOLANGITIS

## EPIDEMIOLOGY

Approximately 80% of cases of cholangitis are caused by obstructing gallbladder stones, with a reported mortality of 5%.[26]

## PATHOPHYSIOLOGY

*E. coli, Klebsiella, Streptococcus, Clostridium*, and *Bacteroides* are the common bacterial organisms inciting cholangitis. Infection usually spreads in a retrograde fashion from the intestines because of obstruction. The resulting damage to the biliary ductal epithelium causes fibrosis and ductal loss. This sequence of events may also be seen without biliary obstruction in patients who have undergone sphincteroplasty or biliary anastomosis to the duodenum (sump syndrome).[15]

Infection by the Chinese liver fluke (*Clonorchis sinensis*) with secondary bacterial infection can cause cholangitis. Patients with acquired immunodeficiency syndrome may have cholangitis with or without obstruction. The infectious organisms associated with this and other immunodeficiency disorders are cytomegalovirus, *Cryptosporidium, Cryptococcus*, and *Candida albicans*.[27,28] Neonates may have cholangitis secondary to cytomegalovirus or reovirus type III. Cholangitis may also be seen in patients with failing liver transplants as a result of graft incompatibility or hepatic arterial thrombosis.[29] Rejection leading to cholangitis is likewise seen in patients who have undergone allogeneic bone marrow transplantation.[30] Progressive biliary ductal necrosis eventually leads to cirrhosis (**Table 44.2**).

## DIFFERENTIAL DIAGNOSIS AND MEDICAL DECISION MAKING

The differential diagnosis of choledocholithiasis and cholangitis encompasses the previously discussed differential diagnosis of RUQ pain and gallstone disease.

Laboratory evaluation may help distinguish biliary colic and cholecystitis from choledocholithiasis. In choledocholithiasis, more than 90% of patients will have elevations in serum alkaline phosphatase and GGT levels.[33] Obstruction of the common bile duct will lead to elevation of total and conjugated serum bilirubin, although most ductal stones result in serum bilirubin levels lower than 15 mg/dL because the biliary obstruction that they cause is intermittent. Serum transaminase levels may be elevated, rarely with profound elevations of greater than 2000 IU/L mimicking acute hepatitis.[32]

Transabdominal ultrasound has low sensitivity (25% to 60%) for the detection of bile duct stones, but it has a very high specificity.[32] Stones within the common bile duct are difficult to visualize on ultrasonography, but greater than 6-mm dilation of the common bile duct suggests the presence of a calculus. CT imaging also has low sensitivity for bile duct stones but can demonstrate biliary dilation and exclude other causes of biliary obstruction such as tumor. Magnetic resonance cholangiopancreatography and ERCP can detect stones with comparable accuracy (**Fig. 44.9**).[34]

## TREATMENT

Initial management of cholangitis is typically medical with empiric antibiotics. Multiple antibiotic regimens are acceptable, and emergency physicians should follow institutional preferences and local resistance patterns when choosing antibiotics. Accepted regimens are combination therapy with an extended-spectrum cephalosporin, metronidazole, and ampicillin; single-agent or combination fluoroquinolones; and ureidopenicillins alone or with metronidazole.[35] Although fluoroquinolones are thought to have greater biliary penetration, they do not change the mortality associated with this disease.[36] Unless concomitant signs of infection are present, patients with primary sclerosing cholangitis do not experience improvement with antibiotics.

ERCP with sphincterotomy is the treatment with the lowest mortality.[37] Percutaneous transhepatic cholangiography (PTC) with drainage is a consideration for patients in whom ERCP fails.[38] Emergency common bile duct exploration with T-tube placement can be performed either by open means or laparoscopically.[32] If emergency ERCP or PTC cannot be arranged in the ED, surgical consultation should be obtained.

## FOLLOW-UP, NEXT STEPS IN CARE, AND PATIENT EDUCATION

Patients with infectious cholangitis should be admitted to the hospital for biliary drainage in consultation with gastroenterology or surgery (or both).

**Table 44.2** Signs and Symptoms of Choledocholithiasis and Cholangitis

| DISEASE | PATHOPHYSIOLOGY | SIGNS AND SYMPTOMS |
|---|---|---|
| Choledocholithiasis | Obstruction of the common bile duct by a gallstone that either migrates from the gallbladder or (less commonly) forms primarily in the duct<br>Obstruction of the pancreatic duct can cause acute gallstone pancreatitis | Manifestations are similar to those of biliary colic, but jaundice may develop. |
| Cholangitis | Inflammation of the bile ducts<br>May be caused by infection (bacterial, viral, tuberculin) or autoimmune reaction | The Charcot triad of fever, jaundice, and RUQ pain is neither sensitive nor specific.[31]<br>The addition of obtundation and hypotension to the triad constitutes the Reynold pentad.<br>Patients with infectious cholangitis are usually older, appear ill, and may not complain of RUQ pain. Younger patients with diabetes can also have nonspecific complaints. |
| Acute gallstone pancreatitis | Increased pancreatic ductal pressure, possibly with biliopancreatic reflux, that occurs when the bile duct stone passes or becomes impacted at the ampulla of Vater | Patients typically have a sudden onset of unrelenting upper abdominal pain that radiates to the back in about 50% of cases.[32] |
| Primary sclerosing cholangitis (PSC) | Immune-mediated progressive fibrosis of the intrahepatic or extrahepatic biliary ducts (Fig. 44.9) | More than 70% of patients with PSC have concomitant inflammatory bowel disease, and elevated alkaline phosphatase is found on routine screening.[15]<br>The majority of patients with PSC are asymptomatic until signs of cirrhosis develop.<br>Common symptoms are RUQ pain, jaundice, pruritus, weight loss, and fatigue. |

*RUQ*, Right upper quadrant.

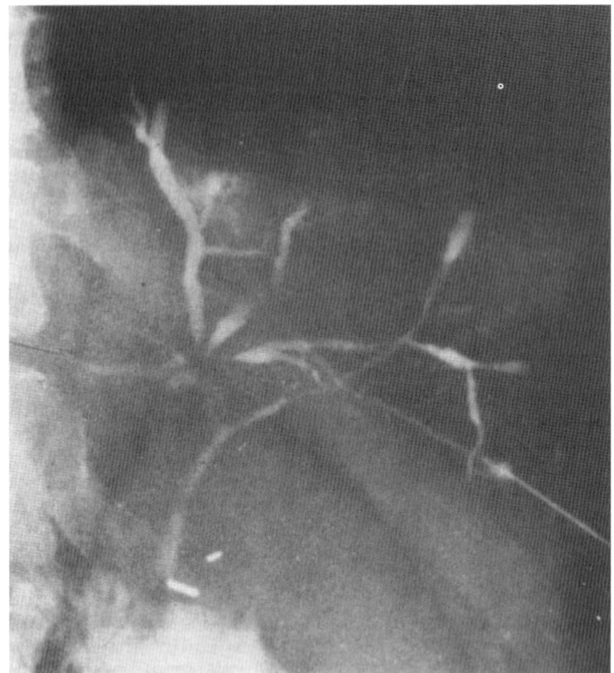

**Fig. 44.9 Primary sclerosing cholangitis demonstrated on endoscopic retrograde cholangiopancreatography.** (From Berk RN, Ferrucci Jr JT, Leopold GR. Radiology of the gallbladder and bile ducts: diagnosis and intervention. Philadelphia: Saunders; 1983. p. 320.)

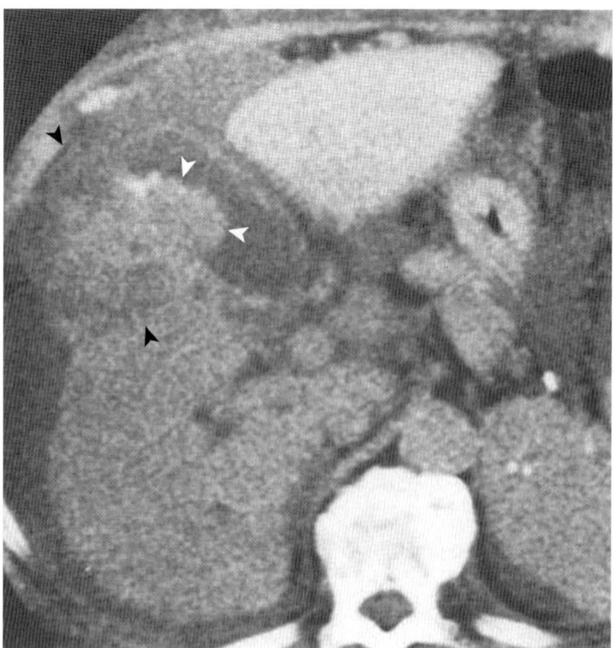

**Fig. 44.10 Computed tomography scan showing gallbladder carcinoma *(arrowheads).*** (From Berk RN, Ferrucci Jr JT, Leopold GR. Radiology of the gallbladder and bile ducts: diagnosis and intervention. Philadelphia: Saunders; 1983. p. 256.)

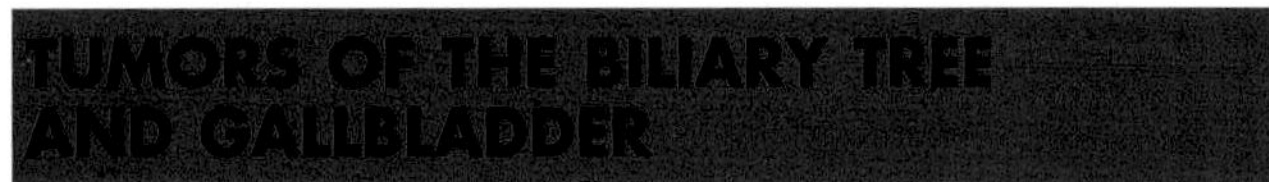

# TUMORS OF THE BILIARY TREE AND GALLBLADDER

## EPIDEMIOLOGY

Tumors of the biliary tree are relatively rare and range from benign tumors such as adenoma and papilloma to carcinoma of the gallbladder and cholangiocarcinoma. Because gallbladder carcinoma is closely associated with underlying gallbladder disease and chronic stasis, patient populations at risk for gallstone disease are also at higher risk for gallbladder carcinoma (see Box 44.1).[39] The overall 5-year survival rate in patients with gallbladder cancer is approximately 12%.[40]

## PATHOPHYSIOLOGY

Papillomas and adenomas are benign tumors of the gallbladder. Papillomas are small, usually multiple tumors that contain cholesterol esters and are not precancerous lesions. Adenomas, semisolid masses found at the fundus, are normally solitary. Both tumors are asymptomatic and can be distinguished from gallstones ultrasonographically because of their fixed position with movement of the patient.

Carcinoma of the gallbladder is an uncommon malignancy associated with chronic cholecystitis and porcelain gallbladder (**Fig. 44.10**). It is most commonly an adenocarcinoma that arises in the fundus or neck. Physical examination usually demonstrates jaundice in an elderly patient, RUQ pain, and weight loss. An abdominal mass may be palpable.

Cholangiocarcinoma refers to malignancy anywhere from the intrahepatic ducts to the common bile duct. It is an adenocarcinoma that spreads along and through the duct wall, with extension to the lymph nodes, peritoneum, gallbladder, and liver in 50% of patients. Associations with primary biliary cirrhosis (PBC), primary sclerosing cholangitis, ulcerative colitis, and *C. sinensis* infestation have been documented. One study found that the risk for bile duct carcinoma significantly decreases 10 years after cholecystectomy.[41]

## PRESENTING SIGNS AND SYMPTOMS

Patients are most commonly seen in the ED with painless jaundice and pruritus, symptoms that suggest an obstructing mass in the distal biliary tree. Pain is present in only one third of patients and is generally mild.[15] Those with malignancy have associated malaise and weight loss. Hepatomegaly without splenomegaly is often noted. Fever is uncommon, but if present, concurrent cholangitis should be considered.

## DIFFERENTIAL DIAGNOSIS AND MEDICAL DECISION MAKING

A thorough search for the cause of jaundice in an older patient should be initiated in the ED and will likely necessitate admission for further imaging studies. Liver function tests show elevations in serum bilirubin and alkaline phosphatase.

Ultrasonography and CT demonstrate intrahepatic biliary ductal dilation in jaundiced patients but may not show the actual mass. Depending on the tumor's location along the biliary tree, the common duct may be normal or may be dilated proximal to the mass.

Both ultrasonography and CT have a sensitivity of 60% to 70% for detecting carcinoma[42]; when results are positive, they usually show a mass in the lumen. Spread via the venous and lymphatic systems prevents early detection, and metastasis is present at the time of diagnosis in 50% of cases.[43] The 1-year survival rate after diagnosis is approximately 14%.[44]

## TREATMENT

Treatment of cancers of the biliary tree depends on the subtype of tumor and the extent of spread. Any combination of surgery, chemotherapy, and radiation therapy may be indicated.

## FOLLOW-UP, NEXT STEPS IN CARE, AND PATIENT EDUCATION

Patients with jaundice and findings suspicious for a tumor should be admitted to a medical service for ERCP and biopsy.

# PRIMARY BILIARY CIRRHOSIS

## EPIDEMIOLOGY

PBC progressively destroys the intrahepatic bile ducts (**Fig. 44.11**). The disease is found in all races, with a 90% female preponderance. PBC is diagnosed in patients 20 to 80 years of age, although the majority of cases are found in patients 40 to 60 years old. A genetic predisposition is likely because family members of patients with PBC have a higher prevalence of mitochondrial antibodies associated with the disease. A medical history of an autoimmune disorder such as rheumatoid arthritis, systemic lupus erythematosus, or mixed connective tissue disease has an association with PBC.[13]

## PATHOPHYSIOLOGY

The etiology of this disease is unknown, but the final mechanism involves immune-mediated biliary duct destruction via cytotoxic T cells. Viruses, bacteria, and defective immune regulation have been theorized to incite this cascade.

## PRESENTING SIGNS AND SYMPTOMS

Patients are normally asymptomatic but may experience pruritus. Chronic RUQ pain is an infrequent complaint, and jaundice is not an early feature of this disease. Patients may remain asymptomatic for many years after ductal destruction has begun, but for those with symptoms and jaundice, the average survival time without treatment is 7 years.

## DIFFERENTIAL DIAGNOSIS AND MEDICAL DECISION MAKING

The most common laboratory abnormality is an elevation in serum alkaline phosphatase and GGT. Total serum cholesterol is usually elevated and the serum bilirubin value only mildly elevated (generally less than 2 mg/dL).[15] Complications of the disease result from liver cirrhosis (i.e., ascites, bleeding esophageal varices, coagulopathy). The diagnosis is suggested

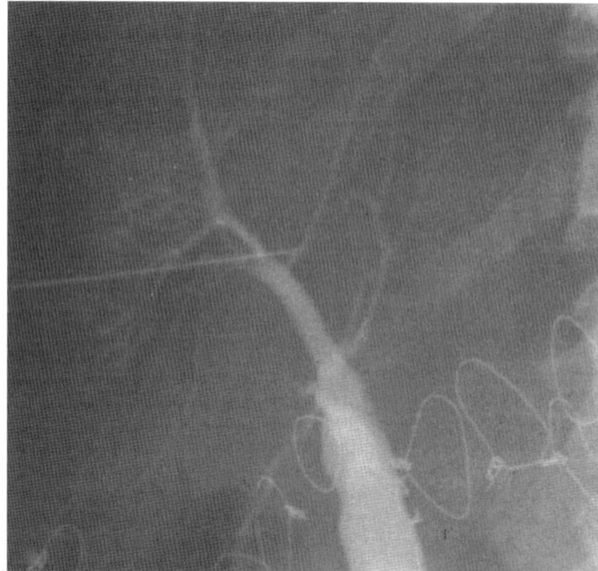

**Fig. 44.11 Primary biliary cirrhosis demonstrated by endoscopic retrograde cholangiopancreatography.** (From Berk RN, Ferrucci Jr JT, Leopold GR. Radiology of the gallbladder and bile ducts. diagnosis and intervention. Philadelphia: Saunders; 1983. p. 320.)

by antimitochondrial antibodies in the serum and confirmed by liver biopsy.

## TREATMENT

Treatment is initially aimed at controlling itching and steatorrhea. Vitamin D and calcium supplements are necessary because of the bile deficiency. The only drug shown to improve mortality in patients with PBC is ursodeoxycholic acid. Hepatic transplantation is the best treatment option to extend life, with a 5-year survival rate of 60% to 70%.[45]

## FOLLOW-UP, NEXT STEPS IN CARE, AND PATIENT EDUCATION

Patients with cirrhotic complications should be considered for transplantation. Those in whom complications are diagnosed early or who have a serum total bilirubin value of 9 mg/dL or higher should be transferred to a transplant center.[15]

## SUGGESTED READINGS

Attasaranya S, Fogel E, Lehman G. Choledocholithiasis, ascending cholangitis and gallstone pancreatitis. Med Clin North Am 2008;92:925-60.

Kalimi R, Gecelter GR, Caplin D, et al. Diagnosis of acute cholecystitis: sensitivity of sonography, cholescintigraphy, and combined sonography-cholescintigraphy. J Am Coll Surg 2001;193:609-13.

Schiff ER, Sorrell MF, Maddey WC, editors. Schiff's diseases of the liver, vol 1. 8th ed. Philadelphia: Lippincott-Raven; 1999.

## REFERENCES

*References can be found on Expert Consult @ www.expertconsult.com.*

# 45 Emergency Biliary Ultrasonography

*Bart S. Brown, Beatrice Hoffmann, and Vicki E. Noble*

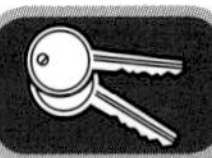

**KEY POINTS**

- Hepatobiliary disease has a high prevalence and is a common cause of abdominal symptoms in patients seeking care in the emergency department.
- Biliary infections represent up to 25% of the causes of intraabdominal sepsis in the elderly.
- Poor sensitivity of the clinical and laboratory data for cholecystitis creates a large demand for hepatobiliary imaging.
- Ultrasound is the initial imaging modality of choice in evaluating the biliary tract for suspected infection or obstruction.
- Focused hepatobiliary ultrasound is a skill that can be effectively learned by emergency department physicians and performed rapidly at the patient's bedside.
- Focused hepatobiliary ultrasound is a dynamic process that can be facilitated by proper patient positioning, inspiratory maneuvers, and Doppler evaluation.
- Beside ultrasound is a useful adjunct for the detection of ascites in patients with hepatic disease and can provide procedural guidance for paracentesis.

## INTRODUCTION

Hepatobiliary disease is a common cause of abdominal pain in patients evaluated in the emergency department. Cholelithiasis is present in 20 to 25 million of Americans, which represents 10% to 15% of the adult population.[1] Cholecystectomy has become the most common elective abdominal surgery performed in the United States.[2] Significant clinical symptoms, however, do not develop in the majority of patients (up to 80%) with gallstones.[3] Both the prevalence and the complication rate of cholelithiasis increase with age. Biliary infection is a common cause of abdominal sepsis in the elderly.

Ultrasound is the initial imaging modality most commonly used for hepatobiliary evaluation in cases of suspected cholecystitis and biliary obstruction. Timely comprehensive sonographic evaluation is not always available in the emergency setting, and an increasing number of emergency providers use point-of-care biliary sonography to rapidly evaluate symptomatic patients for the presence of cholelithiasis and its complications.

Evaluation of elderly patients with suspected biliary sepsis is frequently complicated by altered mental status. In contrast to younger patients, sepsis from ascending cholangitis may be accompanied by atypical or vague clinical findings. Focused ultrasound is a valuable tool that can quickly evaluate the hepatobiliary tract and expedite appropriate treatment and disposition when signs of biliary infection are found.

Bedside ultrasound is also a useful adjunct to the emergency physician for certain patients with chronic hepatic disease. Ultrasound can quickly evaluate for the presence of ascites and provide procedural guidance for paracentesis.

## REVIEW OF LITERATURE ON EVALUATION FOR CHOLECYSTITIS

Clinical findings and laboratory data lack acceptable sensitivity to rule out cholecystitis,[4] which has led to the need for abdominal imaging to aid in determining the patient's disposition. Commonly used imaging modalities to evaluate for cholecystitis and its complications are ultrasound, computed tomography (CT), and cholescintigraphy or hepatobiliary iminodiacetic acid (HIDA) scanning. The sensitivity and specificity of ultrasound for the detection of cholelithiasis can approach 100% for providers with significant ultrasound experience.[5] CT is much less sensitive than ultrasound for detecting cholelithiasis and misses up to 25% of gallstones.[6] HIDA scanning has been reported to have high sensitivity for acute cholecystitis, but it does not provide an adequate structural evaluation of the hepatobiliary system. HIDA scanning also has limited availability in many locations and is not a practical screening modality in the emergency department setting. These distinctions make ultrasound the imaging modality of choice for the initial evaluation of patients with right upper quadrant pain and suspected cholecystitis.[7]

Emergency physicians have demonstrated the ability to effectively learn to perform point-of-care bedside hepatobiliary ultrasonography.[8] Studies on emergency physician–performed biliary sonography have demonstrated sensitivities and specificities of up to 92% and 87% for the detection of cholelithiasis.[9,10]

## BILIARY DUCT EVALUATION

Transabdominal ultrasound is the initial imaging modality used to evaluate for suspected choledocholithiasis and obstruction of the biliary ducts. In the western world, gallstones are the most common cause of both biliary obstruction and cholangitis.[11,12] Even with the most advanced equipment, the sensitivity of ultrasound in detecting choledocholithiasis is still essentially dependent on the examiner's proficiency and can range between 22% and 100%.[5,11,13-15] Specific data on the accuracy of emergency medicine physicians' performance in detecting choledocholithiasis are not yet available and need further investigation. The overall specificity of transabdominal sonography for detection of common bile duct (CBD) stones is usually very high and ranges between 95% and 100%.[11]

## BILIARY SEPSIS

In patients older than 65 years, cholecystitis and cholangitis each account for 12% of the causes of intraabdominal sepsis, or 24% of the total causes of intraabdominal sepsis combined.[16] Bedside ultrasound can be used to detect this common entity and expedite the initiation of appropriate antibiotics and consultation if signs of biliary infection or obstruction are identified.

## HOW TO SCAN, PROBE SELECTION, AND MACHINE SETTINGS

Bedside hepatobiliary imaging is most often performed with a lower-frequency (2- to 5-MHz) curvilinear probe (**Fig. 45.1**). The lower frequencies typically provide the most appropriate penetration relative to the depth of the structures of interest. In young or very thin patients with superficially located structures of interest, use of a higher-frequency probe may provide better image resolution. A phased-array probe can limit the amount of rib shadowing when intercostal imaging is required.

After selecting the abdominal preset, the gain should be adjusted accordingly. The depth needs to be optimized to see the structures of interest and the area posterior to them without creating needless dead space beyond them. Tissue harmonic imaging has been demonstrated to enhance the visibility of lesions and diagnostic confidence in abdominal imaging, particularly in areas containing echogenic tissue such as fat, calcium, or air.[17] The tissue harmonics feature should be used when assessing the gallbladder because it typically reduces artifact interference and facilitates imaging. The sonographer should also be comfortable with the color and power Doppler functions, which can be used to distinguish the biliary ducts and gallbladder from adjacent vascular structures.

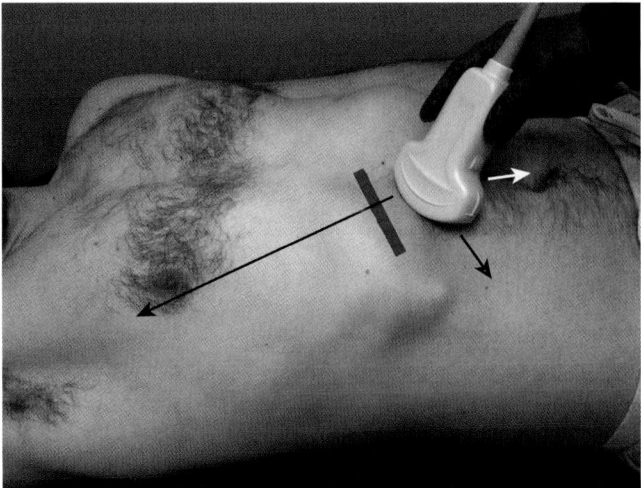

**Fig. 45.1 Position for initial placement of the transducer.** The probe is placed below the subcostal margin *(blue line)* at the intersection with a line running from the right shoulder to the umbilicus *(black arrows)* and angled at about 45 degrees. The probe marker points to the right of the patient *(white arrow)*.

## PATIENT POSITIONING

Imaging begins with the patient in a supine position, but it should be acknowledged that repositioning the patient is required in many cases to obtain the views needed. Rolling the patient to the left lateral decubitus position can help displace the bowel and reduce interference from bowel gas. In some cases, rolling a patient to a semiprone position or having the patient stand up may further facilitate image acquisition. If possible, the patient should elevate the right arm above the head to improve the sonographic accessibility of the inferior liver and for transthoracic scanning.

## INSPIRATORY TECHNIQUES

Having patients hold their breath after a full inspiration is also a useful technique. This pushes the liver inferiorly and may aid in displacing the overlying bowel. The liver also provides a friendly imaging window. However, breath-holding can increase air in the antrum, pylorus, and duodenum, which can interfere with the ability to visualize the gallbladder. In general, in the beginning of the examination it is often better to place the probe over the anatomic area of interest and review structures of interest as they are pushed in and out of the sonographic field via the normal respiratory cycle. Once the patient initiates breath-holding, air swallowed into the antrum will quickly move with peristalsis and may obscure areas of interest.

## SYSTEMATIC SCANNING APPROACH

Significant anatomic variability, interference from adjacent bowel, and variations in the amount or overlying tissue can make localization of the gallbladder a difficult task. Gallbladder imaging is best approached as a dynamic process, and the sonographer should be prepared to try different imaging windows and repositioning of the patient as needed to obtain the appropriate images.

The authors suggest the following systematic approach:

1. The patient is placed in a supine position with the right arm raised above the head. To begin the examination, the

sonographer should imagine a line that connects the patient's umbilicus and right shoulder. The probe is placed immediately below the intersection of this line with the right inferior costal margin. The probe is placed parallel to the rib in about 45 degrees of angulation (see Fig. 45.1).

2. If the liver and aspects of the gallbladder are not in the visual field, the probe is fanned cephalad and caudal. If the gallbladder is still not visualized, the probe should be moved slowly along the inferior costal margin while repeating the fanning motion upward and downward and moving the probe laterally and medially.
3. If no liver tissue or gallbladder can be visualized along this inferior margin, the probe is moved one intercostal space up and placed in the same position where the line between the umbilicus and right shoulder intersects with now the last intercostal space. The probe is angled 60 to 90 degrees (**Fig. 45.2**). Next, the fanning maneuver is repeated and the probe moved within this intercostal space medially and laterally. The process is repeated in next intercostal space if needed.

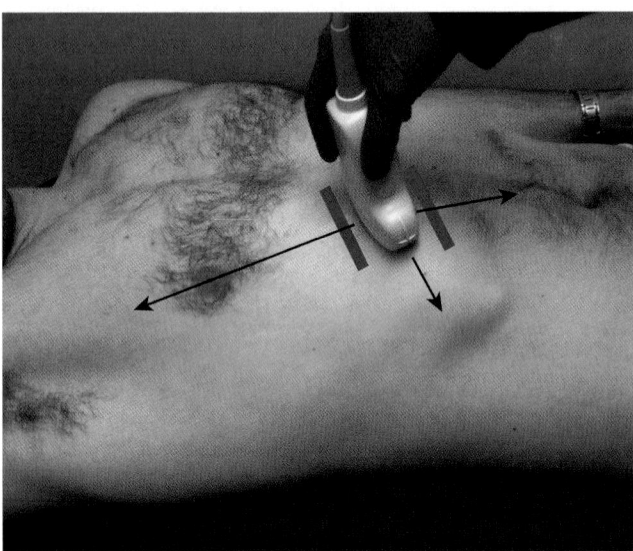

**Fig. 45.2** The probe is placed in the next intercostal margin *(blue lines)* at the intersection with the right shoulder–umbilicus axis *(black arrows)* and angled perpendicularly or slightly caudally. The probe marker points to the right of the patient *(white arrow)*.

4. If unsuccessful, the transducer is placed in a modified focused abdominal sonography for trauma (FAST) view. Instead of angling down to the retroperitoneal location of the kidney, the transducer is angled up toward the tip of the liver, and the lateral margin of the liver is scanned until the gallbladder is located.
5. If unsuccessful after steps 1 to 4, the patient is placed in the left lateral decubitus position and steps 1 to 4 are repeated.
6. Finally, if feasible, have the patient stand up, which often drops the liver and gallbladder more caudally and makes them more accessible for sonography.

## GALLBLADDER EVALUATION

After locating the gallbladder, the probe is rotated clockwise and counterclockwise as needed to obtain a longitudinal (long-axis) view (**Fig. 45.3**). Next, the probe is moved medially and laterally to evaluate the entire gallbladder in long axis. A normal gallbladder has echogenic walls with an anechoic internal cavity. The gallbladder should be thoroughly evaluated for the presence or absence of cholelithiasis. Special attention should be paid to the gallbladder neck for impacted stones.

Following long-axis evaluation, the probe is rotated 90 degrees to the patient's right (the indicator is rotated 90 degrees counterclockwise), which will give a transverse or short-axis view of the gallbladder (see Fig. 45.3). The probe should be angled or moved cephalad and caudad to evaluate the entire gallbladder. The gallbladder is scanned from the fundus to the neck. Again, particular attention should be directed to the gallbladder neck. Air artifact can obscure small stones in this area.

The next step should be to measure the thickness of the gallbladder wall (**Fig. 45.4**). Transmission of ultrasound waves through the fluid-filled gallbladder leads to enhancement of the posterior gallbladder wall, and posterior enhancement can result in overestimation of wall thickness. Hence, measurements are obtained at the anterior wall. Thickness of the anterior wall greater than 3 mm is considered abnormal.[18] One should be aware that isolated increased gallbladder wall thickness is not a sensitive finding for detecting acute inflammation because it can be caused by multiple disease processes (e.g., chronic cholecystitis, ascites, hepatitis).[19] Next, the area encompassing the gallbladder should be evaluated for the

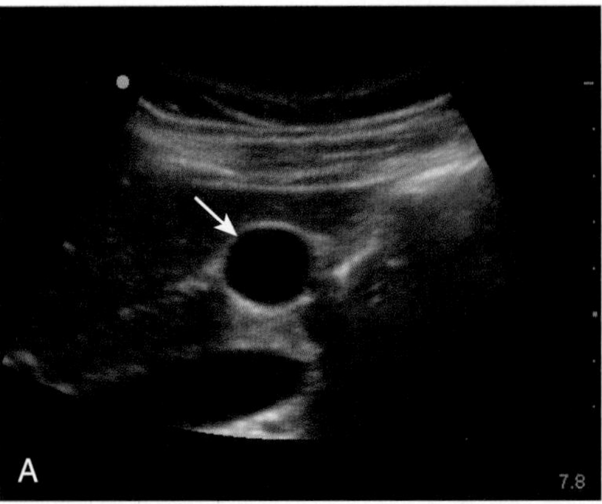



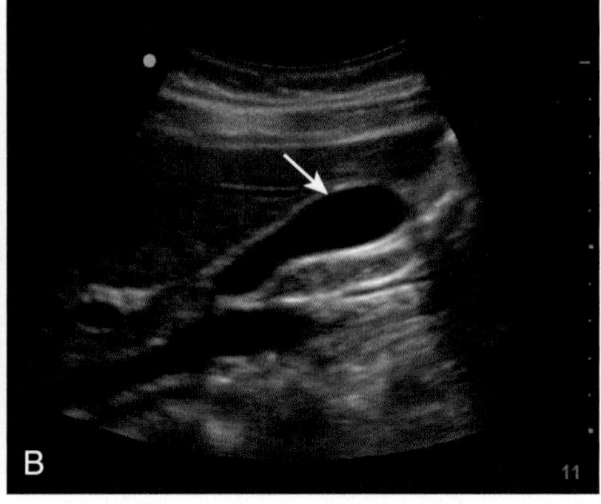



**Fig. 45.3** Image of the gallbladder in transverse (A) and longitudinal (B) views.

presence of pericholecystic fluid. This finding will appear as anechoic areas adjacent to the gallbladder. Pericholecystic fluid with septations, internal echoes, or thick walls may suggest perforation of the gallbladder with abscess formation.[18]

Finally, one should evaluate for a sonographic Murphy sign, which is defined as reproducible tenderness when transducer pressure is applied with the gallbladder in direct view. Correct evaluation for the Murphy sign includes repeating this maneuver on both the left and right sides next to the gallbladder, but with the gallbladder out of the visual field. With a true Murphy sign, tenderness or discomfort in areas away from the gallbladder should be significantly less.[18]

## COMMON BILE DUCT

### *Locating the Common Bile Duct*

The CBD is approximately 4 cm long and intimately associated with the portal vein and hepatic artery in the portal triad. Several approaches can be used to locate this structure. First, one can attempt to find the portal triad. The CBD is located ventral to the portal vein and lacks flow with Doppler imaging. One method to locate the portal triad is to follow the intrahepatic portal vein branches to the liver hilum and main portal vein. The CBD can also be found when following the neck of the gallbladder or the main lobar hepatic fissure toward the hepatic hilum. If the proximal portion of the CBD is difficult to assess, the distal part can be located when scanning the pancreatic head and the duct can then be traced back along the portal vein.

### *Evaluation of the Common Bile Duct*

Once located, the sonographer should interrogate the portal triad with color Doppler to distinguish the CBD from the vessels. The hepatic artery and the portal vein should demonstrate flow, whereas the CBD will not (**Fig. 45.5**). In patients with sluggish portal flow, the sensitivity of the color or power Doppler settings should be adjusted until the vessels can be distinguished from the CBD. This should be carefully evaluated with a steady hand because motion artifact may produce the illusion of flow with more sensitive Doppler settings. Once the CBD is identified, it should be measured inner wall to inner wall in the transverse plane (**Fig. 45.6**).

CBD diameter sizes of 1 mm per decade of life and CBD measurements of up to 1 cm following cholecystectomy have traditionally been accepted as normal.[20] Measurements of CBD diameter accepted as normal range from 6 to 8 mm, with 7 mm commonly recognized as the upper limit of normal CBD size.[21,22]

More recent studies, however, do not correlate with the extent of traditionally expected increases in size in elderly and postcholecystectomy patients. A large study of patients older than 60 years found that mean bile duct size increases from

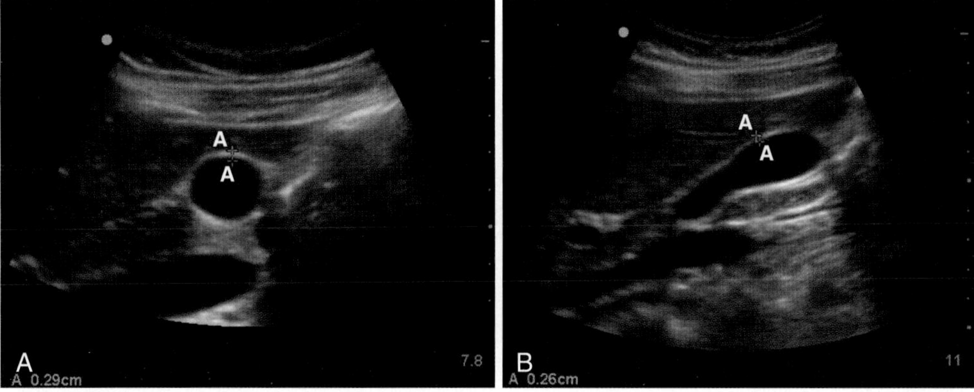


**Fig. 45.4 Measuring gallbladder wall thickness.** Wall thickness is measured at the anterior wall of the gallbladder in transverse (preferred, **A**) or longitudinal (**B**) view.

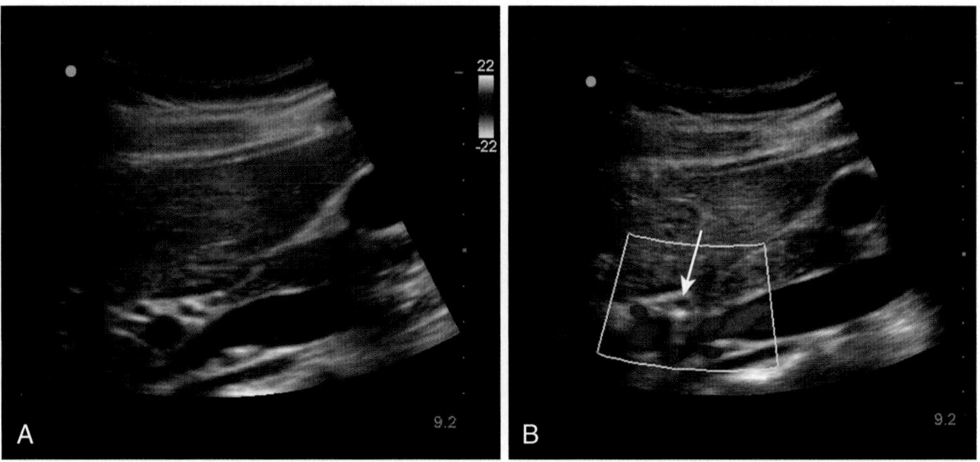


**Fig. 45.5 Common bile duct (CBD) in transverse view (A) showing no flow with Doppler (B, *white arrow*).**

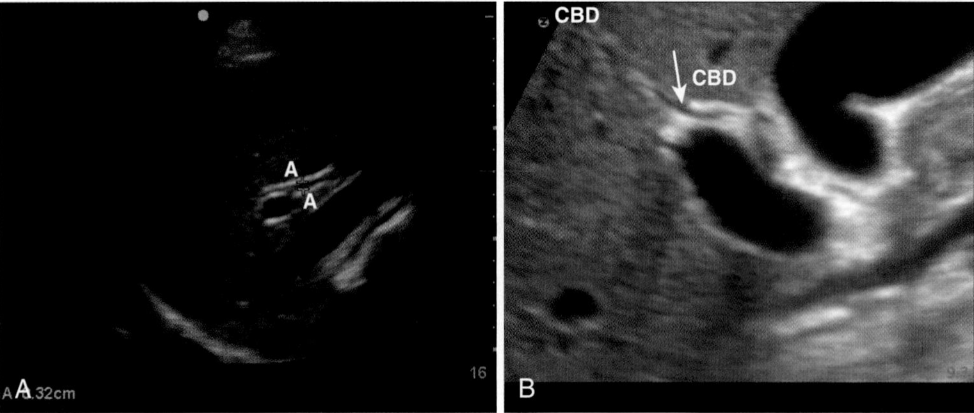


**Fig. 45.6** **A,** Common bile duct (CBD) measurement is performed from inside to inside wall. **B,** Using the zoom-in function can be helpful to visualize small CBDs *(arrow)*.

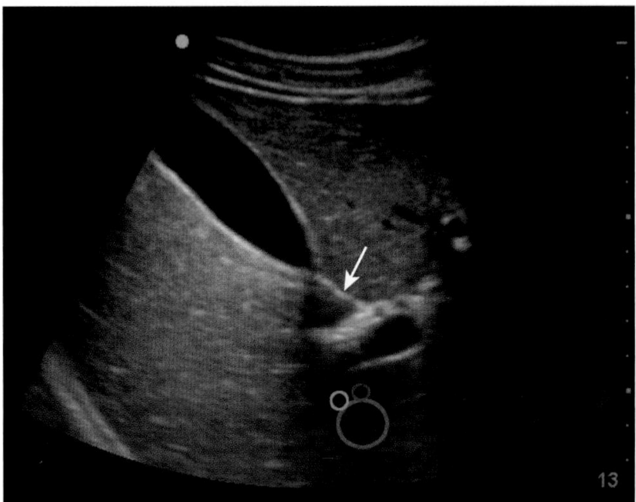


**Fig. 45.7** **Main lobar fissure.** The main lobar fissure *(arrow)* is an echogenic, fibrous structure that can be used as a landmark to connect the gallbladder to the portal triad. The portal triad is seen in transverse view with the portal vein *(blue circle)*, hepatic artery *(red circle)*, and common biliary duct *(green circle)*.

3.6 ± 0.26 mm at 60 years of age to 4 ± 0.25 mm in patients older than 85. Interestingly, 98% of ducts were less than 7 mm in diameter.[23] Additionally, two large studies of patients undergoing cholecystectomy revealed postsurgical mean CBD diameters of 3.96 mm and 6.1 mm, respectively.[24,25]

## MAIN LOBAR FISSURE

The gallbladder and the hepatic hilum are connected by the hepatic main lobar fissure (**Fig. 45.7**). Sonographically, it appears as a bright echogenic structure, relative to the adjacent liver, because of its fibrous content. It is a useful landmark that can be followed away from the gallbladder to locate the portal triad. Conversely, it can be traced from the portal triad to locate obscure gallbladders.

## COMMON OBSTACLES AND TIPS

### *Obesity*

Obesity often increases the depth needed to reach the structures of interest, which decreases the quality of the images. For obese patients, one should consider using a lower-frequency probe or changing to lower-frequency settings to increase tissue penetration.

### *Bowel Gas*

The acoustic mismatch that occurs when bowel gas is encountered creates artifacts that prevent the user from visualizing distal structures. If bowel gas interferes with the sagittal imaging technique mentioned earlier, the transducer can be moved laterally to a near-coronal or coronal imaging plane (step 4 above). From this location, the liver can be used as an acoustic window to locate the gallbladder. Imaging from a coronal plane may be complicated by interference from rib shadowing. Having the patient take several sips of water, if possible, may also help displace gas in the small bowel within the upper gastrointestinal tract. After waiting 15 to 30 minutes, peristalsis may create changes in the bowel gas and better imaging windows may be found.

### *Postprandial Patients*

Postprandial patients typically have a contracted gallbladder, which makes evaluation of wall thickness unreliable (**Fig. 45.8**). Contracted gallbladders can also be more difficult to locate.

# IMAGES—NORMAL AND ABNORMAL

## CHOLELITHIASIS

Gallstones tend to be rounded, mobile structures found in a dependent position. They have a highly reflective surface, which leads to visualization of a curved echogenic surface and shadowing posterior to the gallstone (**Fig. 45.9**). An attempt should be made to confirm that the gallstones identified are mobile and not impacted.

## ACUTE CHOLECYSTITIS

Components of the focused sonographic examination for suspected cholecystitis are listed in **Box 45.1**. Because no single sonographic finding is diagnostic of cholecystitis, the ultrasound findings must be interpreted in conjunction with the clinical picture and laboratory data. The absence of cholelithiasis combined with a negative sonographic Murphy sign has a negative predictive value of 95%. When cholelithiasis is identified, its positive predictive value is increased in the

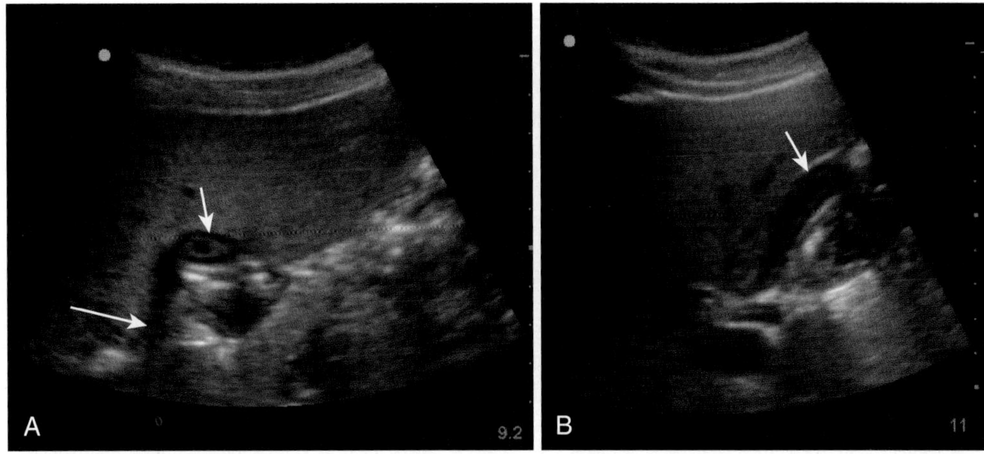


**Fig. 45.8** Contracted gallbladder *(arrows)* in a postprandial patient in transverse (**A**) and longitudinal (**B**) views. The *long arrow* in **A** points to an edge artifact.

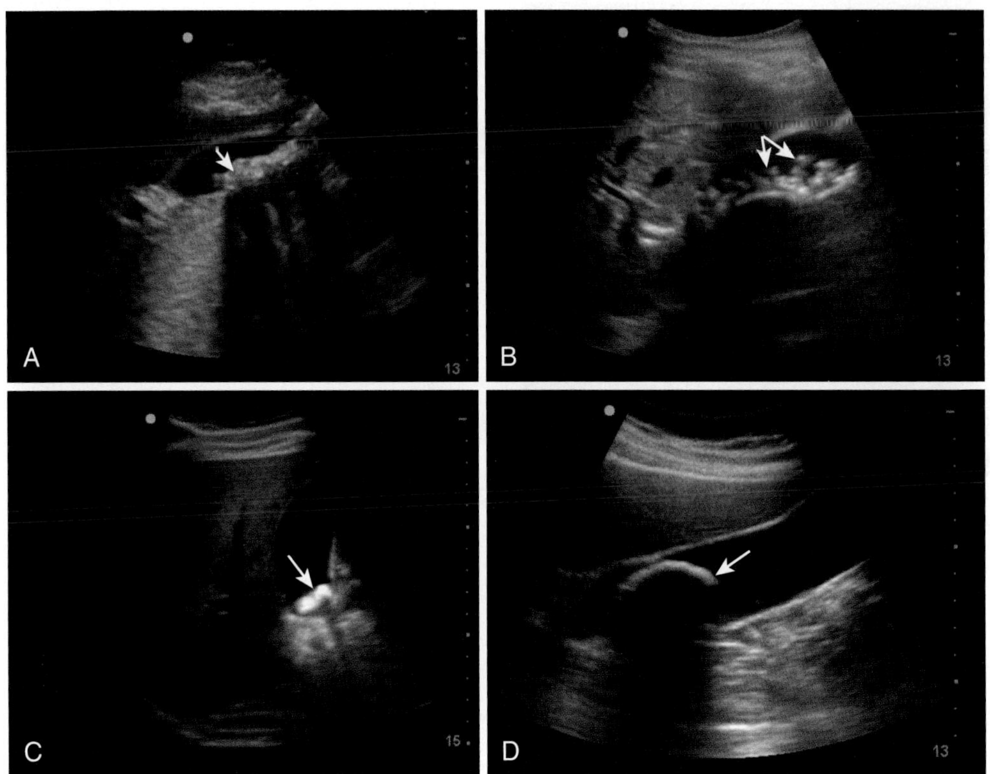


**Fig. 45.9 Examples of cholelithiasis (A to D) depicting the different appearances of gallstones *(arrows)*.**

presence of gallbladder wall thickening (95%) or a positive sonographic Murphy sign (92.2%).[26] Pericholecystic fluid is also a common finding in patients with acute cholecystitis (**Fig. 45.10**).

### *Cholecystitis Variants*

Emphysematous cholecystitis occurs when the gallbladder is infected with a gas-producing organism. Focal areas of gas and its characteristic appearance of small, hyperechoic areas with reverberation artifacts can be identified *within* the gallbladder wall (**Fig. 45.11**). This can be difficult to differentiate from overlying bowel in some cases. Less than 10% of cases

**BOX 45.1 Components of Focused Hepatobiliary Sonography for Suspected Cholecystitis**

Evaluate for cholelithiasis
Measure the anterior gallbladder wall
Measure the common bile duct
Evaluate for pericholecystic fluid
Evaluate for a sonographic Murphy sign

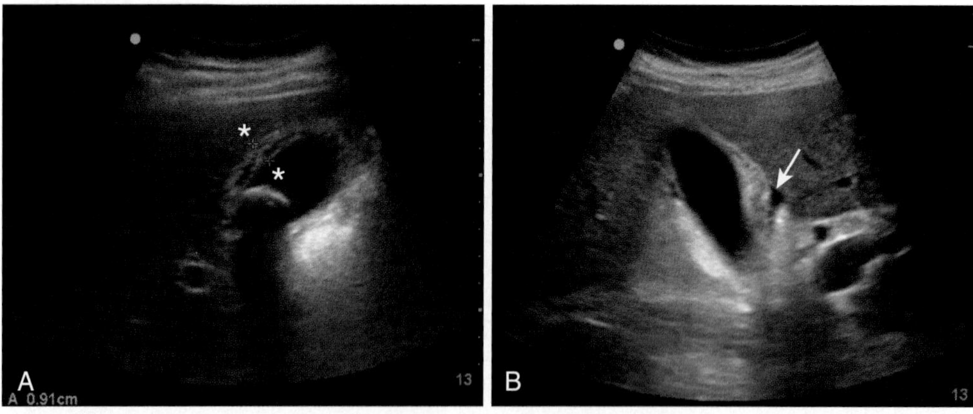


**Fig. 45.10 Acute calculous cholecystitis. A,** Gallstone with posterior shadowing and anterior wall thickening (measured to be 9.1 mm with the calipers; *stars* indicate the ends of the calipers measuring the gallbladder wall). **B,** Acute cholecystitis with pericholecystic fluid *(arrow)*. A gallstone was impacted in the gallbladder neck.

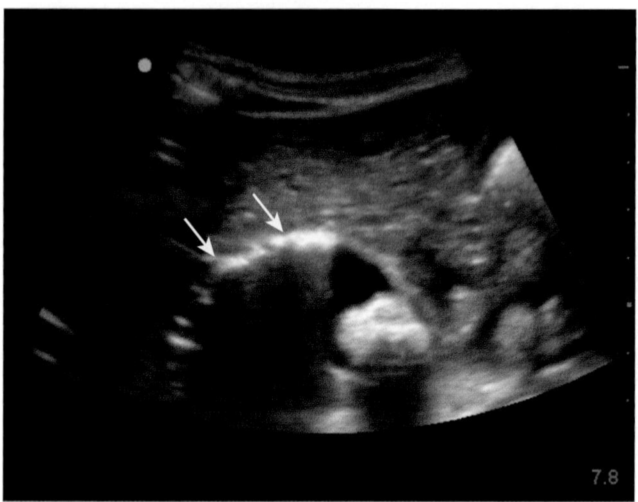


**Fig. 45.11 Emphysematous cholecystitis.** Gas can be seen in the anterior wall of this patient *(arrows)* with emphysematous cholecystitis. The acoustic mismatch of gas produces a brightly echogenic image followed by irregular "dirty"-appearing shadowing.

of cholecystitis occur without cholelithiasis (acalculous cholecystitis).[27] Debilitated or critically ill patients are most commonly affected (**Fig. 45.12**). Occasionally, a gallbladder abscess can develop (**Fig. 45.13**).

### *Wall-Echo-Shadow Sign*

The wall-echo-shadow (WES) sign (**Fig. 45.14**) describes cholecystitis cases in which ultrasound reveals a thickened gallbladder wall closely followed by a hyperechoic line (representing the gallstone surface) and shadowing distal to it. In cases with minimal to no appreciable intervening bile, the WES sign can be difficult to differentiate from adjacent bowel, but the nature of the acoustic shadowing can help differentiate it. Gallstones have surfaces that are strongly reflective of ultrasound waves, thereby leading to a "clean" acoustic shadow, in contrast to the irregular shadowing produced by the scattering of ultrasound waves when bowel gas is encountered.

## INTRAHEPATIC BILIARY DUCT DILATION AND COMMON BILE DUCT STONES

Dilation of the intrahepatic biliary ducts (**Fig. 45.15**) suggests ductal obstruction, although it is not diagnostic of a specific etiology. Obstruction has multiple causes, including choledocholithiasis (most common in the western world; **Fig. 45.16**), biliary duct stricture, ductal edema (as seen with Mirizzi syndrome), and compression from pancreatic masses.

When dilation of the CBD is found, the duct should be followed as far medially as possible to search for choledocholithiasis. Scanning through the liver may also reveal intrahepatic ductal dilation. Sensitivity is significantly dependent on operator performance and ranges from 25% to 100%.[5]

## CHOLANGITIS

Cholangitis is due to a combination of infection and complete or partial biliary obstruction. Choledocholithiasis is the most common cause. Focused ultrasound is a sensitive modality for detection of cholelithiasis and biliary ductal dilation. Identification of these findings should be correlated to the clinical picture. Biliary ductal dilation is not specific for choledocholithiasis and cholangitis, and ultrasound lacks universal high sensitivity for detecting choledocholithiasis, the main cause of cholangitis.

## LIVER MASSES

Although use of ultrasound for evaluation of liver masses is beyond the scope of emergency medicine, observation of liver masses with bedside imaging is not uncommon. Common benign liver masses are hemangiomas (**Fig. 45.17**) and adenomas. Metastatic disease is the most frequent cause of malignant liver masses, and hepatocellular carcinoma is the most common primary malignant liver tumor. The sonographic features of hepatic masses depend on both the composition of the liver mass and secondary factors, such as associated edema, hemorrhage, and necrosis. The findings often mimic a target lesion (**Fig. 45.18**).

Identification of a liver mass should prompt appropriate referral for further work-up. Liver cysts can also be encountered, and the findings can be quite impressive in patients with polycystic liver disease, which is often combined with kidney disease (**Fig. 45.19**).

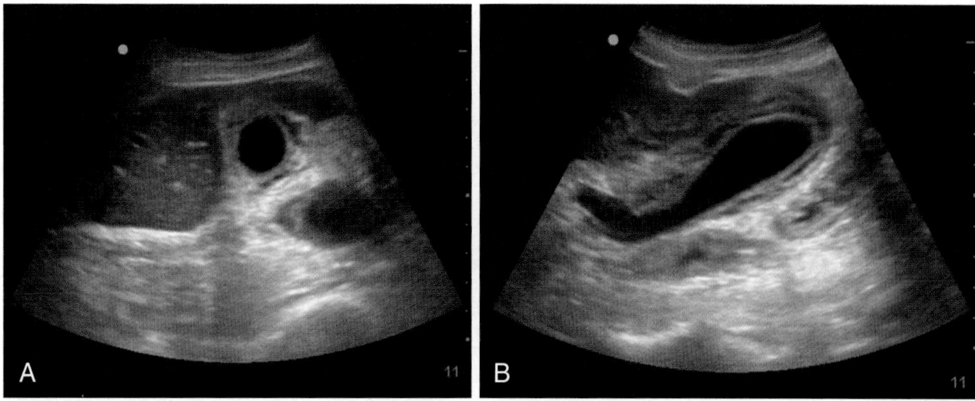


**Fig. 45.12 Acalculous cholecystitis.** This patient arrived at the emergency department with a history of pneumonia and a lung abscess with severe sepsis. Abdominal ultrasound showed significant gallbladder wall edema and thickening. No gallstones were found in this patient. Transverse (**A**) and longitudinal (**B**) views of the gallbladder are shown.

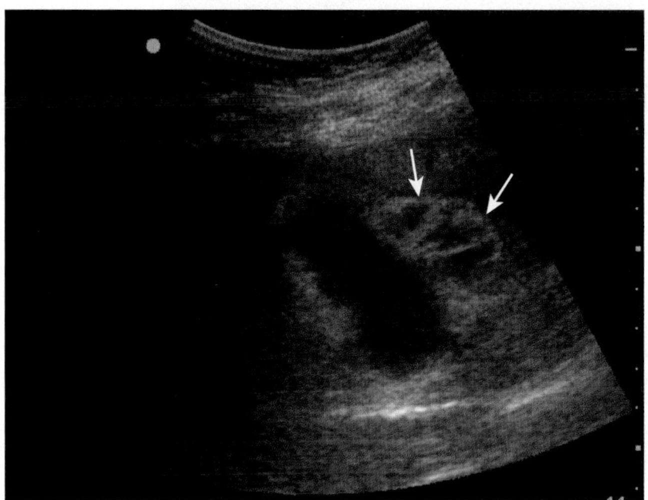

**Fig. 45.13 Gallbladder abscess.** This patient had marked abdominal pain and fever for several days. Ultrasound in the emergency department showed an irregular, complex fluid collection with internal septations adjacent to the gallbladder *(arrows)*.

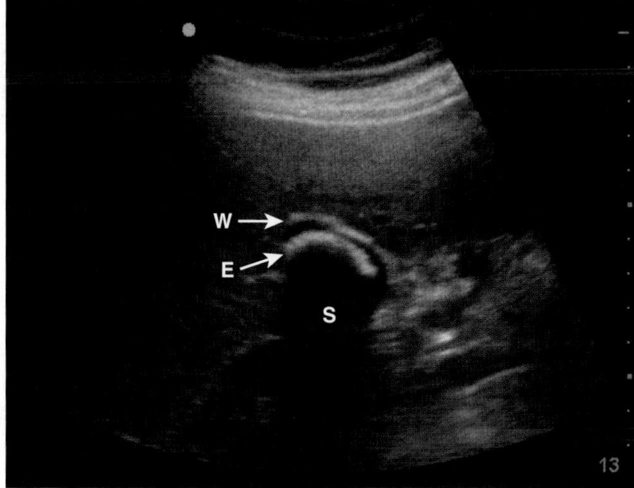


**Fig. 45.14 WES sign.** The WES sign stands for "wall-echo-shadow." The echogenic gallbladder wall (W) is followed by a trace amount of biliary fluid and then by a curved, echogenic surface of a large gallstone (E) followed by posterior shadowing (S). In some cases the intervening biliary fluid may not be appreciated.

## HEPATITIS AND CIRRHOSIS

The most common sonographic features of acute hepatitis are increased liver size and decreased echogenicity of the liver (because of increased fluid content as a result of inflammation and edema).

Chronic liver disease and other conditions that elevate portal venous pressure can produce sonographic findings that can mimic acute cholecystitis. Gallbladder wall thickening and ascites are common findings. Ascites may be mistaken for pericholecystic fluid. As the disease progresses, the liver will eventually become hyperechoic in comparison with healthy liver tissue with tissue changes manifested as multiple liver nodules surrounded by echogenic fibrotic tissue. As the cirrhosis progresses, the liver typically decreases in size. Occasionally, a transjugular intrahepatic portosystemic shunt can be detected in patients with portal hypertension (**Fig. 45.20**).

## NORMAL VARIANTS

Polyps appear sonographically as fixed, pedunculated structures adherent to the gallbladder wall that are unchanged by patient positioning. Gallstones are typically mobile and settle to dependent areas of the gallbladder cavity unless they are impacted. Gallbladder polyps do not normally cause posterior shadowing (**Fig. 45.21**). Gallbladder folds are commonly encountered normal variants that appear as a bright echogenic line within the gallbladder lumen. A fold at the fundus is commonly seen and is termed a *phrygian cap* (**Fig. 45.22**). A fold may appear to divide the gallbladder into two sections.

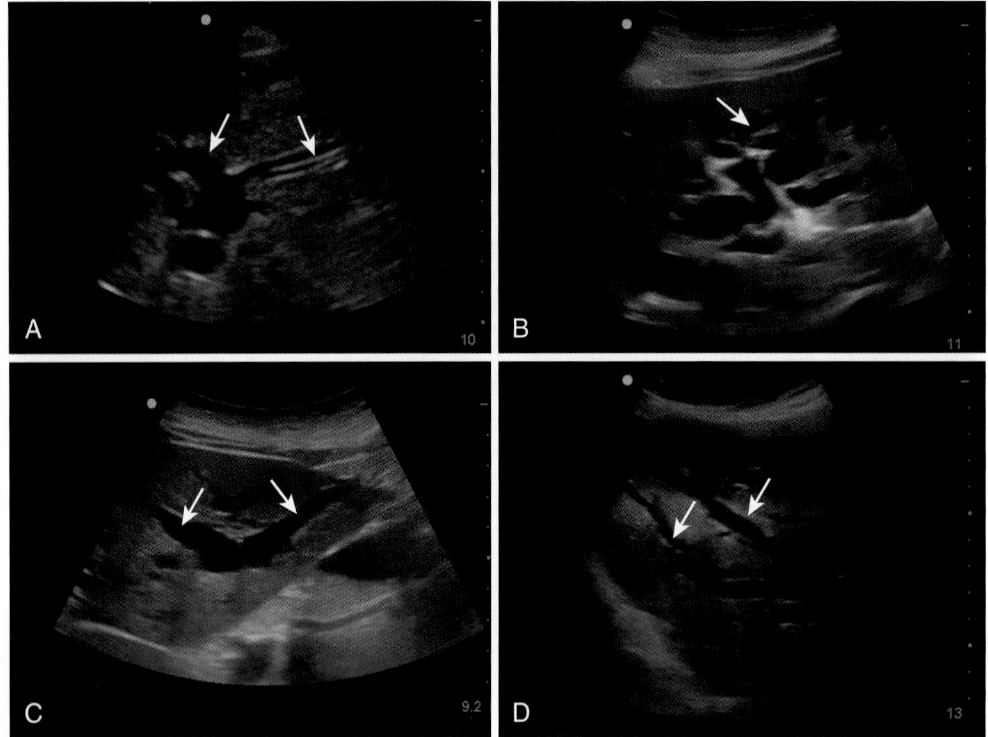


**Fig. 45.15 Appearance of intrahepatic biliary duct dilation. A-D,** Multiple areas of intrahepatic ductal dilation *(arrows)* can be seen. Intrahepatic biliary ducts have echogenic walls and typically contain anechoic bile within. Color Doppler can be used to differentiate bile ducts (no flow) from vessels (see Fig. 45.16). Prominent dilation of major biliary ducts is sometimes described as a "staghorn" appearance (**C**).

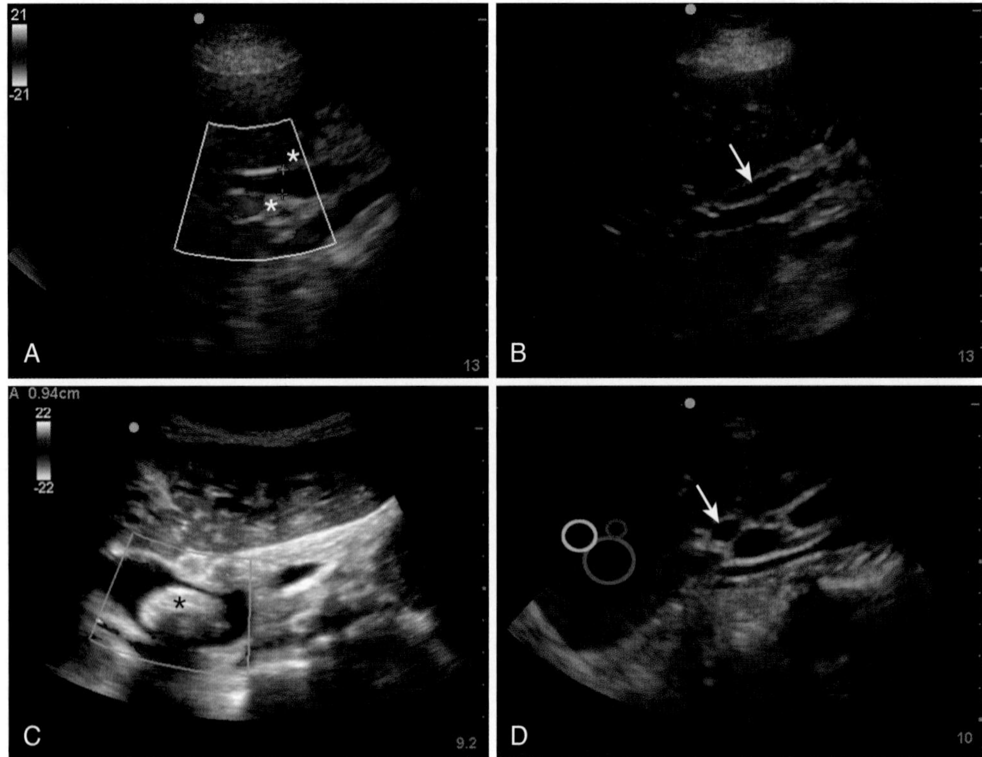


**Fig. 45.16 Common bile duct dilation and choledocholithiasis. A,** Semilongitudinal view of a dilated common bile duct (CBD) (measured at 9.4 mm; *stars* indicate the ends of the calipers measuring the common bile duct) Long axis (**B**) and short axis (**D**) of the dilated proximal CBD. The portal triad consisting of the portal vein *(blue circle)*, hepatic artery *(red circle)*, and dilated common biliary duct *(green circle)* is seen in **D** in transverse view. **C,** Color Doppler image of the distal CBD (no internal flow is seen) with a large stone and posterior shadowing *(asterisk)*.

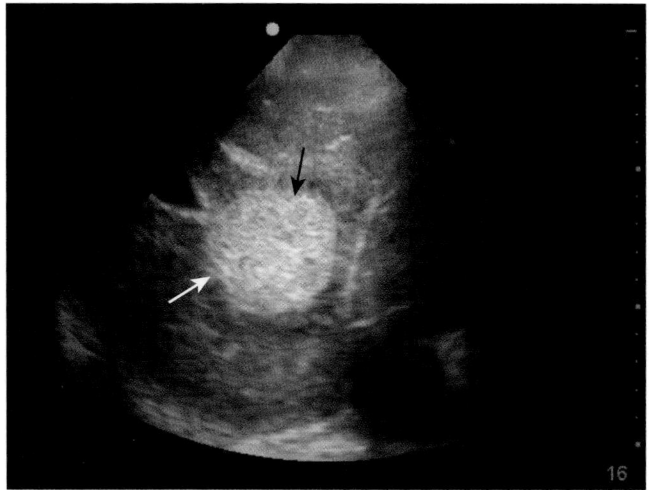


**Fig. 45.17 Hemangioma.** A round, sharply demarcated hyperechoic liver mass *(arrows)* can be seen in the right lobe of the liver.

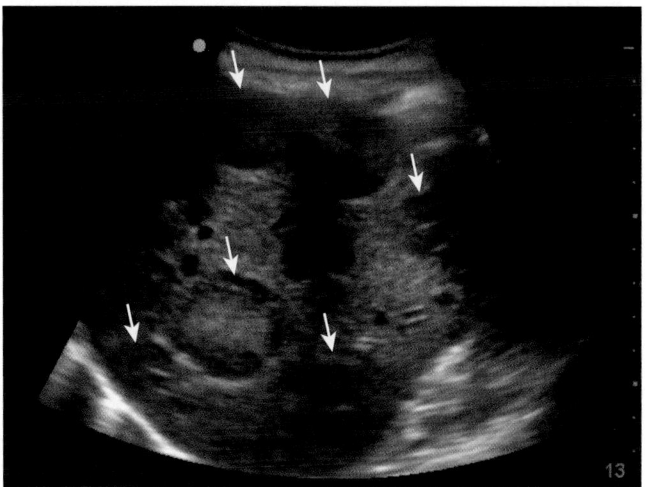


**Fig. 45.18 Liver metastasis.** This 38-year-old patient experienced weakness and 1 week of abdominal pain 2 years after breast cancer treated with radical mastectomy and chemotherapy. Emergency department ultrasound shows multiple liver metastases *(arrows)* with the appearance of "target lesions." Because of differing vascularity, tissue edema, internal hemorrhage, and areas of necrosis, metastatic liver tumors may have multiple sonographic features. The appearance often mimics a target lesion.

Careful imaging of the gallbladder in multiple planes can decrease the likelihood of misdiagnosis.

Adenomyomatosis is a common benign condition with a reported incidence of 2.8% to 5% that leads to hyperplastic changes and thickening of the gallbladder wall.[28] It is usually asymptomatic, however. In the majority of cases it is associated with chronic biliary inflammation, most commonly gallstones in 25% to 75% but also cholesterolosis in 33% and pancreatitis. Cholesterol crystals precipitate in the bile trapped in Rokitansky-Aschoff sinuses and cause a quite a distinct sonographic ring-down artifact (**Fig. 45.23**). Duplicated gallbladder, intrahepatic gallbladder, and congenital absence of the gallbladder are all uncommon variants that may be encountered.

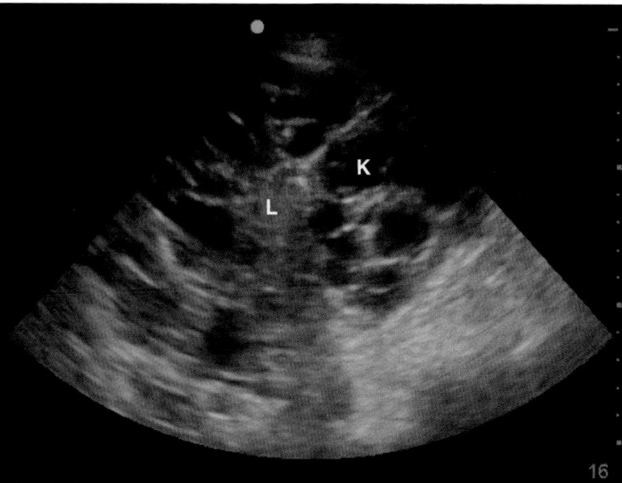


**Fig. 45.19 Polycystic liver and kidney disease.** Multiple cysts can be seen in both the liver (L) and the right kidney (K).

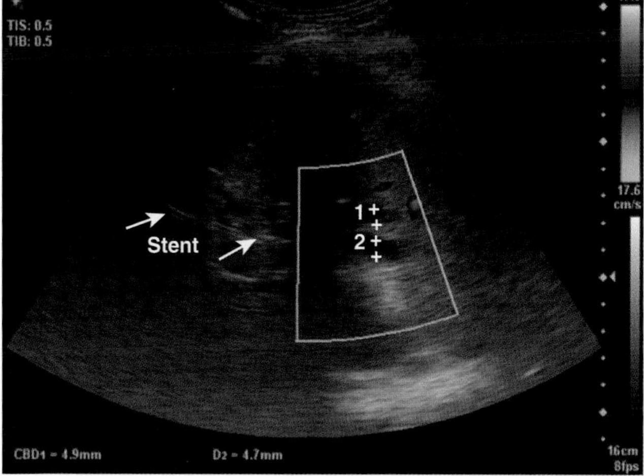


**Fig. 45.20 Transjugular intrahepatic portosystemic shunt (TIPS).** A TIPS catheter can be seen coursing through the liver tissue *(arrows)*. The echogenic walls are separated by an anechoic lumen.

## GALLBLADDER SLUDGE AND GRAVEL

Gravel is a variant of cholelithiasis that has a distinct ultrasound appearance identified as multiple small individual dependent stones (**Fig. 45.24**). Sludge produces a homogeneous, hyperechoic area in the gallbladder that does not produce shadowing. Sludge is viscous and settles to the dependent portion of the gallbladder, but it may take longer to settle than larger stones (**Fig. 45.25**).

## HOW TO INCORPORATE EVALUATION OF SUSPECTED CHOLECYSTITIS INTO PRACTICE

Findings should be correlated with the clinical and laboratory picture. The absence of cholelithiasis on focused hepatobiliary imaging makes the diagnosis of cholecystitis much less

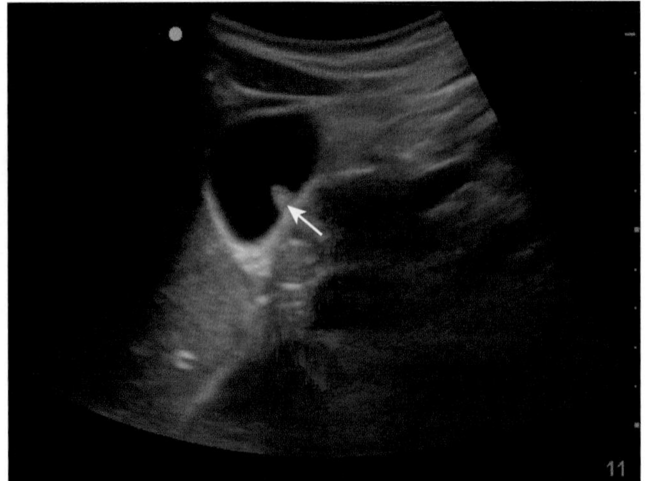

**Fig. 45.21 Gallbladder polyp.** A pedunculated gallbladder polyp *(arrow)* can be seen protruding from the gallbladder wall. Polyps do not typically produce shadowing unless they are calcified.

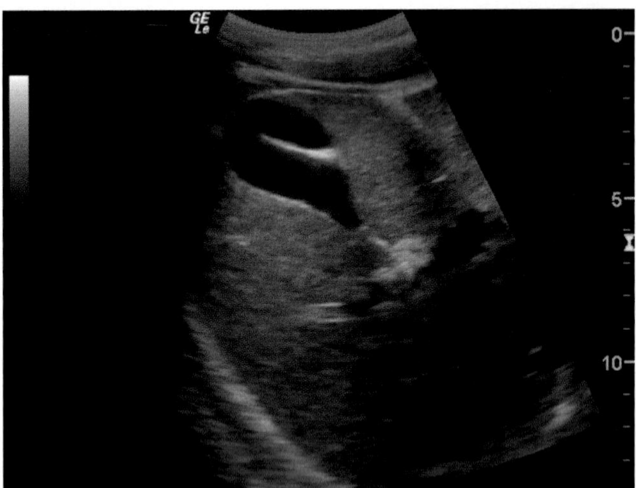

**Fig. 45.22 Gallbladder fold.** The echogenic line partially transecting the middle of the gallbladder lumen is a gallbladder fold.

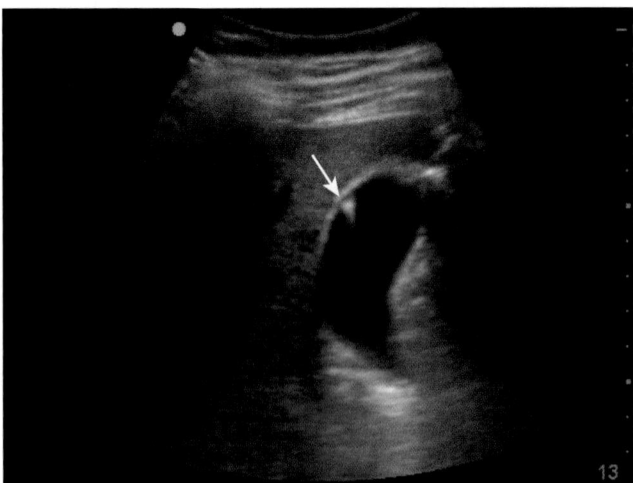

**Fig. 45.23** Adenomyomatosis of the gallbladder wall with the classic appearance of a ring-down artifact caused by cholesterol crystal precipitation in the Rokitansky-Aschoff sinuses.

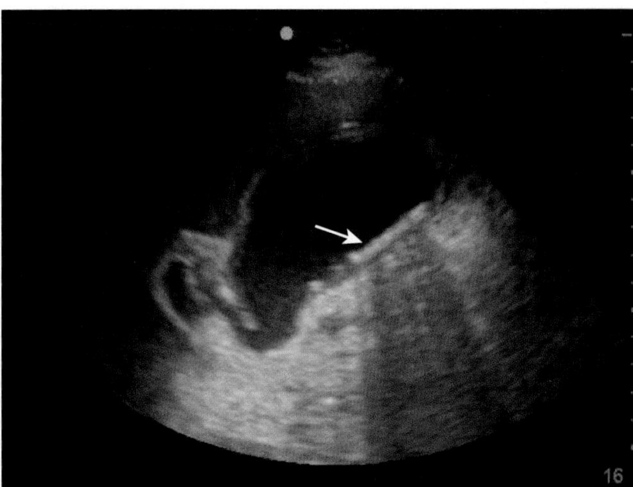

**Fig. 45.24 Gallstone "gravel."** The term *gallstone gravel* can be used when multiple shadowing gallstones *(arrow)* are seen in the dependent portion of the gallbladder. In this patient, acute cholecystitis developed.

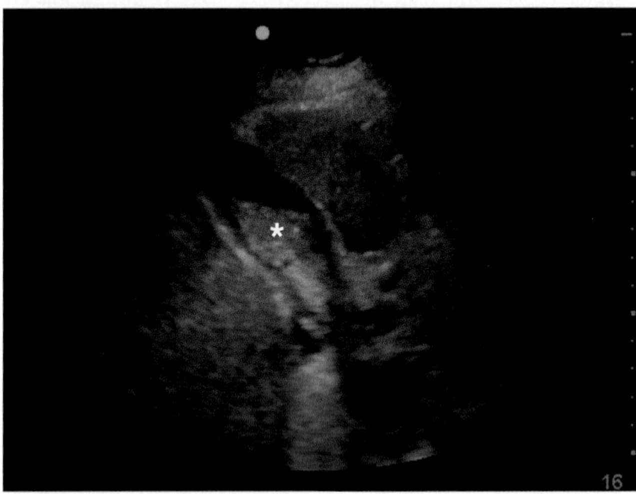

**Fig. 45.25 Gallbladder sludge.** Gallbladder sludge *(asterisk)* can be seen to layer in the dependent portion of the gallbladder. Note that sludge does not produce shadowing like stones typically do.

likely, and other diagnoses should be entertained. Patients with ultrasound findings suggestive of cholecystitis should be administered antibiotics and undergo surgical consultation. If cholelithiasis is seen without other evidence of cholecystitis, the patient's laboratory findings and clinical picture should be reviewed. Patients with resolution of pain and without laboratory abnormalities should have close follow-up arranged. Patients with persistent pain or laboratory abnormalities concerning for cholecystitis should undergo appropriate consultation and possibly a HIDA scan.

## BILIARY SEPSIS

Biliary infection is a common cause of sepsis, and its incidence increases with age. Findings on bedside ultrasound, when suggestive of cholecystitis or cholangitis, can reduce time to appropriate antibiotic administration. Consultation to arrange biliary decompression can be expedited as well.

## EVALUATION OF JAUNDICED PATIENTS AND THOSE WITH SUSPECTED BILIARY OBSTRUCTION

In patients with jaundice, focused ultrasound can help differentiate obstructive from nonobstructive causes. Dilation of the CBD and intrahepatic ducts indicates outflow obstruction of the biliary tracts and an obstructive etiology. Identification of biliary obstruction in the setting of acute infection should prompt the physician to consider urgent decompression of the biliary tract.

Discovery of a dilated CBD should prompt the sonographer to follow the CBD as far medially as possible. The most common cause of biliary obstruction is choledocholithiasis, for which transabdominal ultrasound has a specificity of up to 95%.[11] It should be noted, however, that ultrasound is not a specific modality for distinguishing the cause of biliary obstruction with the isolated finding of CBD dilation. Further imaging is often required.

## ASCITES EVALUATION AND ULTRASOUND-GUIDED PARACENTESIS

Bedside ultrasound can rapidly identify ascites and visualize the relationship of pockets of ascites to adjacent bowel and other abdominal structures. If paracentesis is required, ultrasound allows the user to choose a location that maximizes the chance for a successful procedure while minimizing the chance of damage to nearby structures.

## REFERENCES

***References can be found on Expert Consult @ www.expertconsult.com.***

# 46 Gastrointestinal Devices, Procedures, and Imaging

*Kerin A. Jones*

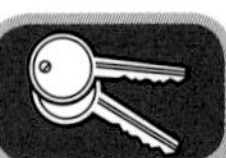

**KEY POINTS**

- Nonfunctional feeding tubes can be safely replaced in the emergency department with a commercial tube or by making a few simple alterations to a standard Foley catheter to prolong its longevity.
- Gastroesophageal balloon tamponade tubes are used only for life-threatening variceal bleeding that is refractory to standard, first-line endoscopic and pharmacologic treatment. There is no absolute contraindication to the use of such tubes as a heroic, lifesaving measure.

## NASOGASTRIC TUBES

The Salem Sump tube is the most commonly used nasogastric tube (NGT) in the emergency department (ED). The Salem Sump is a double-lumen tube with multiple distal suction eyes. The second lumen allows venting during suction, which prevents invagination and subsequent gastric injury. Indications for its use include gastric evacuation or decompression, diagnostic aspiration of gastric contents, and infusion of therapeutic agents. Intermittent suction may be set at a pressure of less than 120 mm Hg.[1] A Levin tube is a single-lumen tube with multiple distal openings for suction, referred to as "eyes." The Levin tube's relatively large internal diameter makes it ideal for rapid decompression or drug infusion. Intermittent suction may be set at a level lower than 40 mm Hg. A Levin tube has the same uses as the Salem tube except that it may not be used for long-term gastric evacuation.[1]

### INDICATIONS AND CONTRAINDICATIONS

**Box 46.1** lists the indications for and contraindications to the use of NGTs in the ED.

### INSERTION PROCEDURE

Inserting an NGT may cause the patient to cough, vomit, retch, or sneeze. Because traumatic epistaxis is common, protective apparel should be worn when placing an NGT—gloves, gown, and mask. The patient should be placed in either an upright or Fowler position.

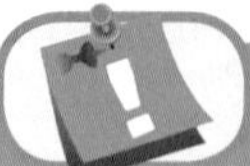

**TIPS AND TRICKS**

**Inserting a Nasogastric Tube**

Warming the tube will make it more pliable and easier to advance along the curvature from the nasopharynx into the oropharynx.

Flexing the patient's neck can help direct the tube from the oropharynx into the esophagus.

If choking, gagging, or muffling of the voice occurs, withdraw the tube to the oropharynx only. Do not remove the tube completely, or it must be repassed through the nasopharynx into the oropharynx, which is usually the most difficult and painful part of the procedure.

The tube can coil within the patient's mouth; if problems occur when placing or verifying placement of the tube, always check the mouth.

In an unconscious patient, elevating the jaw will move the trachea anteriorly, a maneuver that can relieve pressure on the esophagus and make it easier to pass the tube.[2]

A lubricated, soft nasopharyngeal airway may be inserted if neither naris appears to be amenable to placement of the larger, more rigid nasogastric tube (NGT). The nasopharyngeal airway may be used to dilate the nasal passage for a few minutes and then removed to allow another attempt at placing the NGT. Alternatively, a smaller NGT may be passed through the nasopharyngeal airway into the esophagus.

#### *1. Estimation of Tube Length*

To place the drainage eyes in the proper location in the stomach (**Fig. 46.1**), the length of tube to be inserted can be estimated by adding the following three measurements together[3]:

a: Measurement from the patient's xiphoid process to the earlobe
b: Measurement from the earlobe to the tip of the nose
c: 15 cm

#### *2. Nares Patency Check, Anesthesia, and Vasoconstriction*

Patency of the nares should be checked before placing an NGT. This can be done by direct visualization or by having

**BOX 46.1 Indications for and Contraindications to the Use of Nasogastric Tubes**

**Indications**

In gastrointestinal bleeding, to monitor blood loss, which may help differentiate upper from lower tract sources of bleeding

In intubated patients, to decrease risk for pulmonary aspiration, treat gastric distention, and deliver medications

Decompression of intestinal obstruction

Treatment of paralytic ileus, intractable vomiting

Treatment of gastric outlet obstruction and distention

In trauma patients, to evaluate for transdiaphragmatic hernia when the nasogastric tube is seen above the diaphragm on a chest radiograph

Rightward deviation of the tube may be seen on a chest radiograph in patients with aortic dissection

**Relative Contraindications**

Facial fractures: trauma patients with suspected cribriform plate or midfacial fractures are susceptible to intracranial placement of nasogastric tubes

Severe coagulopathy

Ingestions likely to cause upper gastrointestinal perforation, such as alkali and highly volatile substances

Esophageal strictures

Recent bariatric surgery

the patient sniff or blow out of each nostril with the other naris occluded. Topical anesthetic spray or ointment should be used to decrease the discomfort and gagging associated with tube placement. The more patent nostril should be used for the procedure.

PRETREATMENT MEDICATIONS Placement of an NGT is one of the most painful routine procedures performed in the ED. In nonemergency situations it is best practice to treat the patient with nasal vasoconstrictors and anesthetics before placing the tube.[4]

Vasoconstrictors may be used 3 to 5 minutes before the procedure to decrease traumatic bleeding. Phenylephrine (Neo-Synephrine 0.5%) or oxymetazoline (Afrin 0.05%) is typically used. Vasoconstrictors must be used with caution in hypertensive patients.

Application of lidocaine before inserting an NGT has been shown to significantly decrease pain during the procedure.[5-7] Lidocaine can be delivered as viscous, nebulized, or atomized preparations. Application of viscous lidocaine to the nasal passage combined with lidocaine spray applied to the posterior pharynx has been shown to be superior to other forms of anesthetics when placing an NGT or transnasal bronchoscope.[6,8] However, no definitive study or review article has determined the best concentration, form, or dose of lidocaine to use.[7]

LIDOCAINE OPTIONS

- Viscous lidocaine—5 to 10 mL of 2% lidocaine applied to an adult nasal passage 0 to 5 minutes before NGT placement combined with lidocaine spray applied to the posterior pharynx.[6,8,9] Introduce 3 mL of 2% viscous lidocaine into the nostril and then have the patient snort the medication.

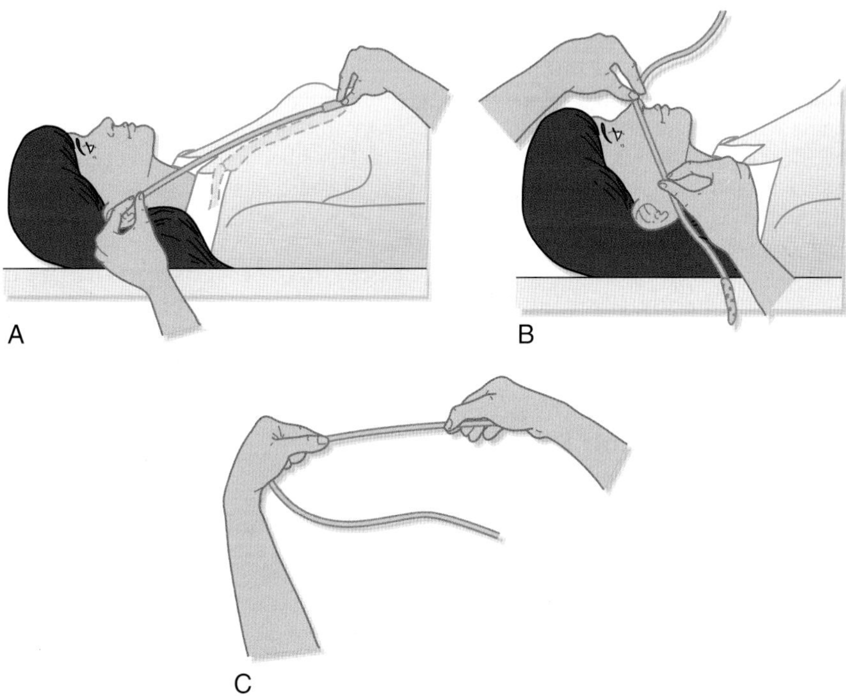


**Fig. 46.1** To estimate the length of nasogastric tube to be inserted, add together the measurement from the patient's xiphoid process to the earlobe (**A**), plus the measurement from the earlobe to the tip of the nose (**B**), plus 15 cm (**C**). (From Samuels LE. Nasogastric and feeding tube placement. In: Roberts JR, Hedges JR, editors. Clinical procedures in emergency medicine. 4th ed. Philadelphia: Saunders; 2004. pp. 794-816.)

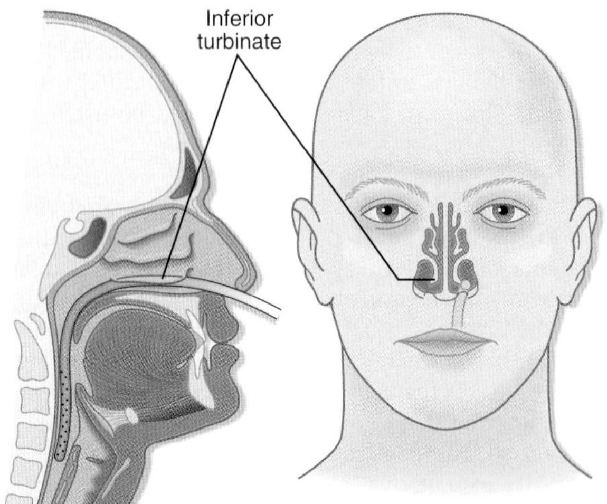


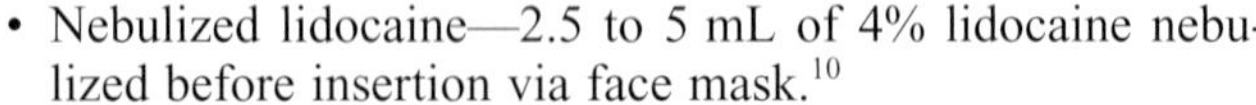

Fig. 46.2 The nasogastric tube is passed parallel to the floor of the nose posteriorly and usually passes inferior to the inferior turbinate. The tube should not be directed cephalad. (From Samuels LE. Nasogastric and feeding tube placement. In: Roberts JR, Hedges JR, editors. Clinical procedures in emergency medicine. 4th ed. Philadelphia: Saunders; 2004. pp. 794-816.)

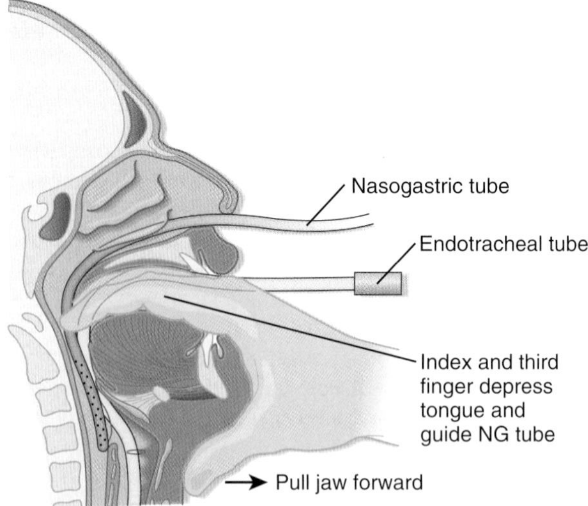


**Fig. 46.3 Digital placement of a nasogastric (NG) tube in a paralyzed, sedated, intubated patient.** (From Samuels LE. Nasogastric and feeding tube placement. In: Roberts JR, Hedges JR, editors. Clinical procedures in emergency medicine. 4th ed. Philadelphia: Saunders; 2004. pp. 794-816.)

- Nebulized lidocaine—2.5 to 5 mL of 4% lidocaine nebulized before insertion via face mask.[10]
- Atomized lidocaine—1.5 mL of 4% lidocaine or two puffs of 10% lidocaine atomized to the nasal passage.[6,11]

### 3. Lubrication of the Tube

Once the naris has been pretreated with the vasoconstrictor and anesthetic agents, a water-soluble lubricant is applied to the distal aspect of the tube.

### 4. Insertion of the Tube

The tube is inserted into the naris along the floor of the nose inferior to the lower turbinates. The tube should be inserted at close to a 90-degree angle with the face and directed parallel to the floor of the nose (posteriorly), not cephalad (**Fig. 46.2**). Gentle pressure should be used to advance the tube past the nasopharynx and into the oropharynx. Once the tube is in the posterior pharynx, the patient is asked to swallow or take a sip of water to aid in smooth passage of the tube into the esophagus. The tube is then quickly advanced to the premeasured length to minimize discomfort. Care should be taken to not use excessive force when placing an NGT to avoid mucosal injury.

### Alternative Approaches with Difficult Tube Insertions

In comatose, paralyzed, or sedated patients, an NGT may be placed under direct visualization with the use of a laryngoscope and McGill forceps. The tube is inserted via the nose into the nasopharynx. The mouth is opened, and a laryngoscope is used to directly visualize the hypopharynx. With Magill forceps, the NGT is grasped and inched into the esophagus under direct visualization.

Alternatively, digital placement of an NGT can be accomplished in a paralyzed, sedated, and intubated patient. The emergency physician places the second and third fingers in the posterior pharynx of the patient and depresses the tongue. The tube is passed through the nose into the posterior pharynx with the fingers in the pharynx to direct the tube into proper location (**Fig. 46.3**).[2]

### Verifying Tube Placement

Radiographic verification is the most sensitive test to detect proper placement, but it is not necessary to meet the standard of care. Methods that are normally used to verify tube placement at the bedside are as follows:

- Insufflation of air causing or resulting in borborygmi (gurgling) sounds heard over the epigastrium verifies that the tube is in the stomach.
- Aspiration of gastric fluid; a pH less than 4 is correlated with a 95% likelihood that the tip of the tube is in the stomach.
- In a conscious patient, normal clear speech without coughing is suggestive of proper tube placement.[12]

### Securing the Nasogastric Tube

The NGT is taped in place once proper tube insertion is verified. Silk tape is torn into a butterfly configuration, with one end of the tape placed on the nose and the torn ends of the tape wrapped around the tube in opposite directions. Tincture of benzocaine can be used on the skin before placement of the tape to more securely adhere both the tube and tape.

## COMPLICATIONS

Placement of an NGT has a complication rate between 0.5% and 1.5%. Common complications are as follows[13]:

- Epistaxis
- Tracheal or bronchial placement
- Pneumothorax
- Intracranial placement
- Esophageal or pharyngeal perforation
- Gastric or duodenal rupture
- Esophageal obstruction or rupture

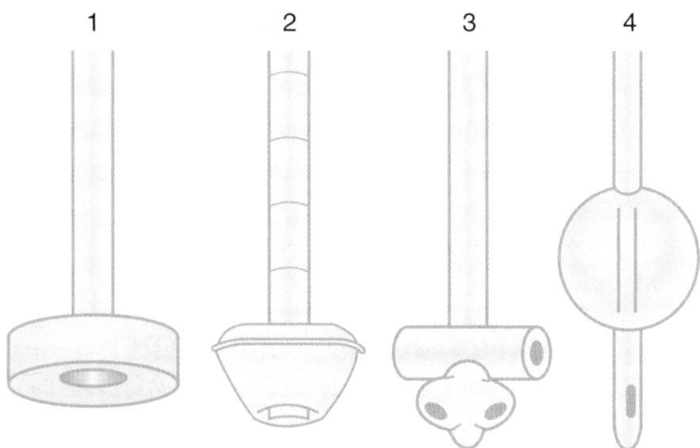


**Fig. 46.4 Types of gastrostomy tubes.** *1,* Polyurethane catheter with a collapsible foam flange (CORPAK MedSystems, Wheeling, IL). *2,* Silicone catheter (American Endoscopy, Bard Interventional Products, Billerica, MA). *3,* Latex catheter with a movable external bolster and an internal mushroom- or de Pezzer–type flange on the end (American Endoscopy). *4,* Balloon (Foley) catheter (Wilson-Cooke Co., Winston-Salem, NC). (From Samuels LE. Nasogastric and feeding tube placement. In: Roberts JR, Hedges JR, editors. Clinical procedures in emergency medicine. 4th ed. Philadelphia: Saunders; 2004. pp. 794-816.)

- Gastrothorax and tension gastrothorax
- Pulmonary aspiration; the NGT may induce a hypersalivation response, a depressed cough reflex, or mechanical or physiologic impairment of the glottis[14-16]

## TRANSABDOMINAL FEEDING TUBES

Feeding tubes are placed to provide long-term nutritional support. They are classified both by the location of their terminal lumen and by the method of placement. Gastrostomy tubes have a terminal lumen located within the stomach and are now typically placed via a percutaneous endoscopic technique; they are thus called PEG (percutaneous, endoscopically placed gastrostomy) tubes (**Fig. 46.4**). Several manufacturers make various types of PEG tubes. The other most frequently encountered feeding tube is a J tube, or jejunostomy tube. Such tubes are longer, smaller-caliber tubes that terminate in the jejunum. Unlike a gastrostomy tube, a J tube does not have an inflated balloon on its terminal end.

The classic open surgical gastrostomy procedure is less commonly performed than the percutaneous techniques. Percutaneous tubes can be placed by a gastroenterologist via endoscopy or by a radiologist via fluoroscopy. Fewer complications are seen with radiographically placed tubes than with tubes placed either by an open technique or endoscopically (**Fig. 46.5**).[17,18]

### MAJOR COMPLICATIONS OF TRANSABDOMINAL FEEDING TUBES

Serious complications seen with transabdominal feeding tubes almost always require hospitalization and gastroenterology or surgery consultation (or both). Intestinal complications include obstruction, perforations, gastrointestinal (GI) bleeding, volvulus, and gastric outlet obstruction. Serious infections include bacteremia, pulmonary aspiration, sepsis, peritonitis, advanced local cellulitis, and necrotizing fasciitis.[19-22] Other complications of gastrostomy tubes are

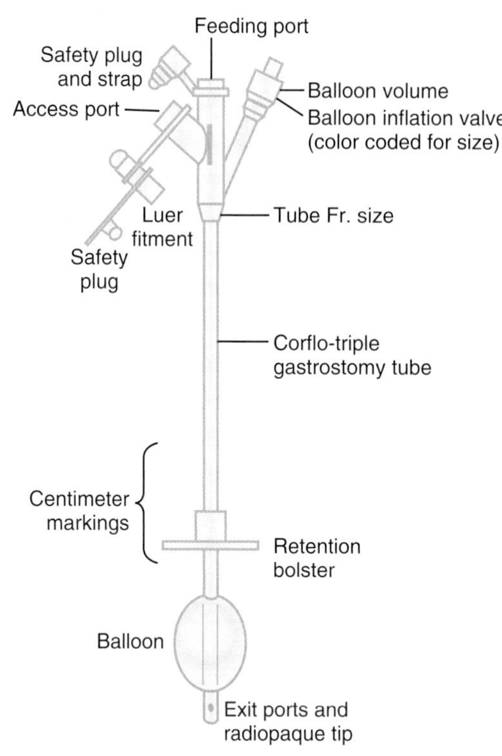


**Fig. 46.5 User-friendly gastrostomy tube from CORPAK MedSystems (Wheeling, IL).** The tube is packaged with lubricant, a prefilled syringe for inflating the balloon, and an extension set. The color-coded inflation valve indicates tube size (12F to 24F). The silicone tube uses a retention balloon and a movable bolster, similar in design to a Foley catheter. Note that the retention bolster is designed to prevent inward migration of the tube and is not to be an anchoring device sutured to the skin. (From Samuels LE. Nasogastric and feeding tube placement. In: Roberts JR, Hedges JR, editors. Clinical procedures in emergency medicine. 4th ed. Philadelphia: Saunders; 2004. pp. 794-816.)

prolapse with and without intestinal obstruction, extraluminal position of the tube, and fistula formation.[23] Patients may also demonstrate minor and major electrolyte abnormalities and, rarely, pneumothorax.

### REPLACING A TUBE

Transabdominal feeding tubes must be replaced (**Fig. 46.6**) for many reasons, including expulsion, malfunction, leakage, tube deterioration resulting in cracks or fissures, and aneurysmal dilations of the tube. It is important that a patient's tube be correctly identified with respect to type, size, and manufacturer before an attempt at replacement. A dislodged tube should be replaced as quickly as possible to maintain patency of the feeding tube tract. When replacing a feeding a tube it is important to clarify whether the terminal end was in the stomach versus the jejunum. After placement, the anchoring balloon in the replacement tube should be inflated in G tubes but never in J tubes.

### REMOVING A NONFUNCTIONAL TUBE

If the nonfunctioning PEG tube was placed under fluoroscopic guidance by a radiologist, it can usually be removed by deflation of the balloon and gentle retraction. Some devices have

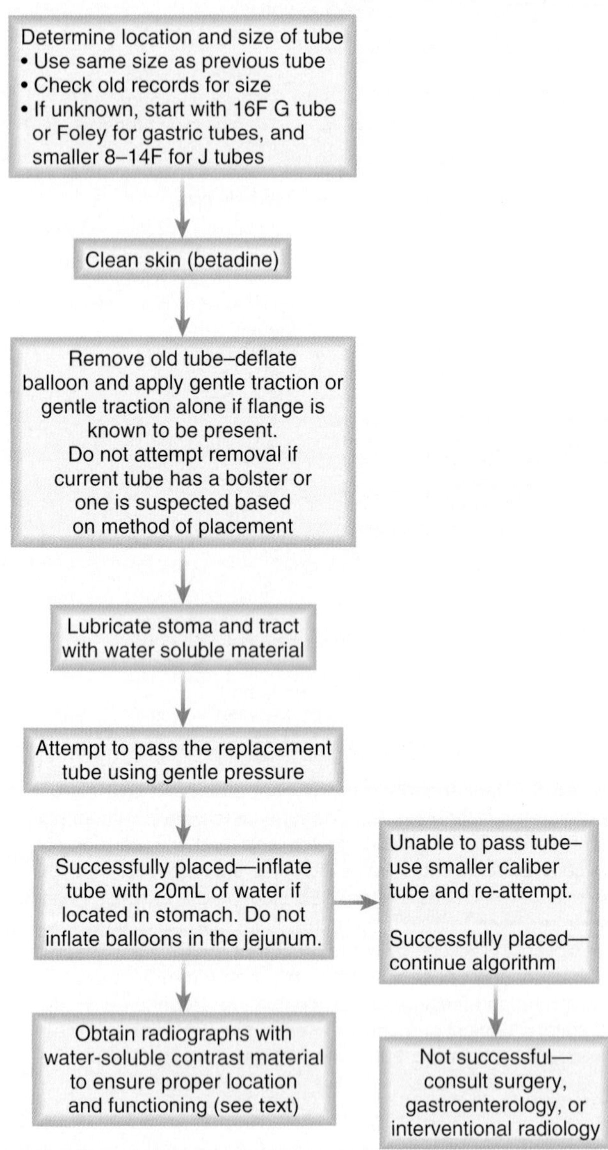


**Fig. 46.6** **Steps for replacing a transabdominal feeding tube.**

a flange rather than a balloon, and these flanges usually collapse with slow, gentle traction. If the tube was placed by a gastroenterologist or a surgeon, it may have an anchoring device or an internal component that prevents the tube from becoming dislodged from the gastrostomy tract. Such a tube cannot be removed by gentle traction alone; the internal component must be removed endoscopically. If resistance is met when attempting removal, a gastroenterologist, interventional radiologist, or surgeon should be consulted.

As an alternative method, the tube is lifted off the abdominal wall skin to allow the tube to be cut as close to the skin as possible. The internal component is then pushed into the GI tract so that it is free to pass through the intestines and be eliminated rectally. Most internal components pass within 2 weeks. There have, however, been reported cases of intestinal obstruction, perforation, and rarely death with this method.[24,25] The internal component is less likely to pass without complications in children than in adults.[26] If this technique is used, reliable patient follow-up is needed for serial abdominal radiographs. Radiographs should be taken within 1 week to monitor the progress of the component through the GI tract. If the internal component has not passed within 1 to 2 weeks, impaction has probably occurred, and endoscopic removal should be considered. Primary endoscopic removal is also advised in patients with intestinal obstruction, pseudoobstruction, pyloric stenosis, intestinal stricture, history of irradiation, and inflammatory bowel disease.[27]

## FOLEY CATHETERS VERSUS COMMERCIAL FEEDING TUBE PRODUCTS AS REPLACEMENTS

Both commercially available feeding tubes and Foley catheters can be used to replace a dislodged feeding tube. Commercial feeding tubes are more expensive than Foley catheters. Studies have found that a silicone Foley catheter with a retention disk and ring has the same efficacy and complication rate as a commercially available replacement gastrostomy tube. The retention disk and ring are used to prevent distal migration of the tube into the GI tract.[28] However, many institutions do not stock silicone Foley catheters.

### *Foley Catheters Used as Replacement Feeding Tubes*

A few simple modifications to a standard Foley catheter can maximize its longevity as a feeding tube, as well as reduce the chance of complications. When using a Foley catheter to replace a feeding tube, an external bolster, or anchor, is fashioned to prevent ingress of the tube into the ostomy and distal migration into the GI tract. An external bolster may be constructed by cutting a 3-cm section from a large rubber catheter. The outer bolster should be secured approximately 1 cm from the skin to prevent trapping of moisture and maceration.[29] Its construction is as follows:

1. Cut a 3-cm section from the proximal segment of a Foley catheter to be used as a bolster, the end without the balloon. A silicone catheter is preferred over a latex one (**Fig. 46.7, A**).
2. Fold this segment in half and make a diagonal cut on each side of the fold to create a diamond-shaped opening in the middle of each side of the 3-cm segment of tubing. Cut the holes slightly smaller than the tube to be inserted and used as the feeding tube to ensure a snug fit of the bolster on the replacement tube (see Fig. 46.7, *B* and *C*).
3. Insert a hemostat through the two holes created in the bolster.
4. Grab the proximal end of the replacement tube with the hemostat and pull the tube through the bolster (see Fig. 46.7, *D*).
5. Advance the bolster to its proper location about 1 cm above the skin of the abdomen (see Fig. 46.7, *E*).[28,30]

### *Verifying Tube Location*

No standard method for verifying tube placement has been established. The safest and best practice is to obtain radiographic confirmation when a feeding tube is replaced.[31] Radiographic confirmation should be obtained in the following circumstances:

- With replacement of a recently placed feeding tube (less than 3 months) because the tract may not be mature
- When tube replacement was difficult

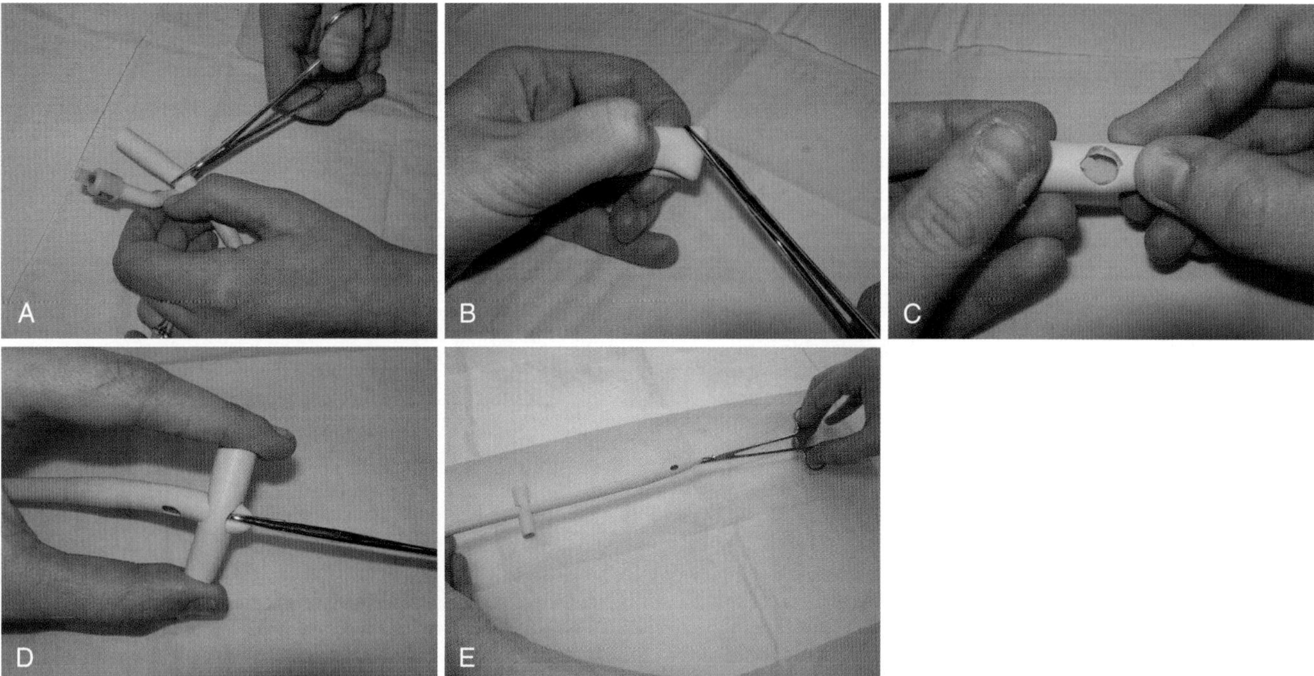


**Fig. 46.7 Modifying a Foley catheter for use as a replacement feeding tube.**

- When gastric material cannot be aspirated after placement
- When the patient is unable to communicate about symptoms such as pain with tube placement and use

Radiographic confirmation can be accomplished with fluoroscopy or by injection of water-soluble contrast material into the tube followed by plain radiography. Typically, 20 to 30 mL of contrast material is injected into the tube via a catheter tip syringe. An abdominal film should be obtained within 1 to 2 minutes. Generally, a flat-plate abdominal view is sufficient to verify tube placement. If insertion of the tube was very difficult or malposition is suspected, a two-view abdominal film may be required to ensure proper tube location. Proper location of the replaced tube is indicated by (1) ease of injection of the contrast material and (2) visualization of the gastric and intestinal walls as they are outlined by the contrast material. If extravasation of the dye is seen outside the stomach or intestine, tube malposition is verified.

Recently, two newer verification techniques have been described in small studies. The first uses air insufflation through the replacement tube to verify proper placement. Once the tube is replaced, a total of 240 mL of air is insufflated through the tube with a 60-mL syringe. The tube is considered properly replaced if it can be seen clearly within an air-distended stomach on a plain radiograph.[32] The second technique was described in a small study with 10 subjects. Ultrasound was used to visualize the new tube as it was placed in the established tract. After insertion, color Doppler was applied over the catheter tip while it was gently oscillated to enhance visualization[11] (**Fig. 46.8**).

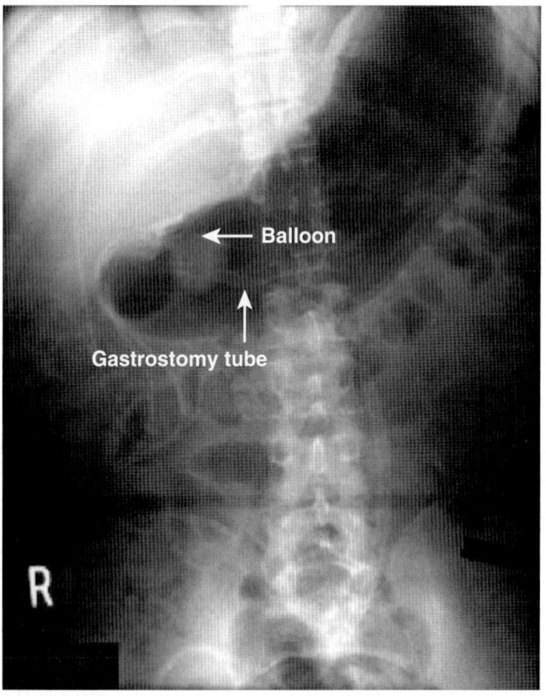


**Fig. 46.8 Anteroposterior abdominal radiograph after a percutaneous, endoscopically placed gastrostomy tube with injection of 240 mL of air.** The tube can be seen projecting left of the midlumbar spine with a loop to the right and crossing the greater curvature of the stomach. The stomach is distended with air, and the balloon, near the tip of the tube, is noticeably outlined with air within the lumen of the stomach. (From Burke DT, El Shami A, Heinle E, et al. Comparison of gastrostomy tube replacement verification using air insufflation verus Gastrografin. Arch Phys Med Rehabil 2005;87:1530-3.)

## CLOGGED FEEDING TUBES

Larger-diameter feeding tubes are less likely than smaller tubes to become clogged. A tube can become obstructed if kinking occurs or the lumen is clogged with debris. A recently placed or reinserted tube is prone to kinking. A kink can be treated by withdrawing the tube a few centimeters and then advancing it again. Contrast-enhanced radiographs should be obtained whenever significant tube manipulation has occurred to evaluate for patency and proper location. A persistently clogged tube needs to be removed and replaced.

If a feeding tube is clogged by debris, the following approaches can be used to unclog the tube:

- Milk the external part of the tube backward in an attempt to expel the debris.
- Irrigate with small aliquots of carbonated beverages.
- Irrigate with small aliquots of warm water at high pressure; use a small syringe (5 to 10 mL) with manual injection.

Instrumentation of the tube with either a Fogarty arterial embolectomy catheter or a nasal foreign body catheter can also be attempted. The length of the feeding tube external to the abdomen should be measured and the Fogarty catheter inserted only to this length. An instrument should *never* be inserted past the abdominal wall skin. The balloon on the catheter can be inflated in the tube if an obstruction is encountered and then further advanced to probe the entire length of the external tube. The catheter should not be withdrawn with the balloon inflated because this action might cause removal of the feeding tube. In a 10 French (10F) or 12F tube, a No. 4 embolectomy catheter should be used; a 14F tube requires a No. 5 embolectomy catheter.[33]

If a feeding tube has been unclogged by force or instrumentation, water-soluble contrast–enhanced radiographs should be obtained to verify proper tube placement, as well as to evaluate for tube perforation.

## GASTROESOPHAGEAL BALLOON TAMPONADE

Variceal bleeding is a leading cause of significant morbidity and mortality in patients with cirrhosis. Sengstaken and Blakemore first described the use of a double-balloon tamponade system to control variceal bleeding in 1950. Sengstaken-Blakemore (SB) tubes are not advocated as primary or secondary therapy for cirrhotic patients; they are used as rescue therapy for life-threatening variceal bleeding.

Two gastroesophageal balloon tubes are in general use. The SB tubes have three lumens—a gastric balloon, an esophageal balloon, and a gastric aspiration port. The Minnesota tube has a fourth lumen for esophageal aspiration.

The indication for gastroesophageal balloon tamponade (GEBT) is severe, acute variceal bleeding that is refractory to available first-line interventions such as sclerotherapy and vasoconstrictor therapy. Relative contraindications are esophageal strictures, recent esophageal surgery, and decreased level of consciousness without airway protection. A patient with a decreased level of consciousness should always be intubated before insertion of an SB tube.

### PROCEDURE

The following equipment is needed:

- Gloves and personal protective equipment
- GEBT tube
- NGT if the tamponade tube does not have an esophageal aspiration lumen
- Traction device
- Manometer or sphygmomanometer
- Y-tube connector
- Emesis basin
- Water-soluble lubricant
- Suction device with connectors
- Tubing to connect to suction
- Clamps or nonserrated hemostats
- Silk sutures
- Tape and gauze

The procedure is as follows[2]:

1. If needed, intubate the patient before placement of the tube.
2. Check the balloons for patency and leaks before use: use 100-mL increments of air to inflate the gastric balloon, and check the pressure with a sphygmomanometer after each increment. These pressure measurements should be recorded for each 100-mL increment of air and will be used to compare pressure readings once the tube has been inserted (step 12). The pressure in the gastric balloon should not increase more than 15 mm Hg with insufflation of each 100 mL of air.
3. If an NGT is to be inserted, tie a suture around it and the GEBT tube to secure them together. The tip of the NGT should be located 3 to 4 cm proximal to the esophageal balloon.
4. Lubricate the tube or tubes with a water-soluble lubricant.
5. Position the patient either upright angled at 45 degrees or in the left lateral decubitus position.
6. Anesthetize the posterior pharynx or nasopharynx with topical anesthetic spray or nebulized lidocaine (or both; see previous discussion on NGT insertion).
7. Place an NGT and evacuate the stomach before placing a GEBT tube to decrease the chance of emesis and aspiration. Once the gastric contents have been evacuated, remove the NGT.
8. Deflate all balloons and either clamp the ends of the tubes or place plugs in each lumen if provided by the manufacturer.
9. Pass the tube to a minimum level of 50 cm as marked on the tube.
10. Connect suction to the gastric and esophageal lumens to check for contents and to decrease the likelihood of aspiration.
11. Confirm proper tube placement with radiographs even if gastric contents or blood is evacuated. The tip of the tube or balloon should be located below the diaphragm if properly placed.
12. Remove the clamps or plugs and inflate the gastric balloon slowly with 100-mL increments of air. Check the pressure of the gastric balloon after each injection; with each 100 mL of air insufflated, the pressure should not be more than 15 mm Hg higher than the pressure measurements previously obtained for the same volume of air (step 2). If the pressure rises by more than 15 mm Hg, the balloon may be located in the esophagus and not in the stomach. If this occurs, deflate the balloon and obtain

another radiograph to ensure proper tube location before resuming air insufflation. Generally, 400 to 500 mL of air must be insufflated to obtain the proper pressure; check the manufacturer's recommendation for the tube being used.

13. Once proper pressure is obtained, clamp or plug the lumens of the gastric balloon and the air inlet.
14. Gently pull back on the GEBT tube until it snugs up against the diaphragm and applies pressure at the gastroesophageal junction.
15. Secure the GEBT tube to the traction device to be used while applying a small amount of tension to the GEBT tube to keep constant pressure on the lower esophageal sphincter. The traction devices may be an orthopedic trapeze apparatus or another device provided by the manufacturer.
16. If the tube was passed nasally, place the sponge rubber cuffs provided by the manufacturer into each nostril or pad the nostrils with gauze to prevent pressure ulcers.
17. Once the tube is properly placed and secured, lavage the stomach with room-temperature water to assess for active bleeding. Attach the gastric lumen to high-pressure, intermittent suction.
18. If blood continues to be aspirated from the gastric lumen, the esophageal balloon can be inflated to a minimum pressure level to control the bleeding or to the maximum pressure advised by the manufacturer (typically 30 to 45 mm Hg). Clamp or plug the lumen of the esophageal balloon once a desired pressure level is obtained.
19. Frequent manometer readings of the esophageal balloon should be obtained to decrease the risk for complications.
20. If bleeding continues, the most likely source is gastric; tension on the gastric balloon may be increased gradually to help control the bleeding.
21. Obtain radiographs any time that the position of the tube comes into question.
22. Once the bleeding is controlled, attempts should be made to decrease the pressure in the esophageal balloon by increments of 5 mm Hg every 3 hours until a pressure of 25 mm Hg is reached (or as recommended by the manufacturer). Typically, a pressure of 25 mm Hg can be maintained for 12 to 24 hours if the bleeding is controlled.
23. If the esophageal balloon requires inflation at pressures greater than 30 mm Hg, the balloon should be deflated every 6 hours for 5-minute intervals to prevent complications such as mucosal ischemia and necrosis.
24. To prevent vomiting and aspiration, the esophagus must be emptied continuously even if the esophageal balloon is not inflated. The gastric balloon will preclude passage of secretions into the stomach. Aspirate with either an esophageal aspiration port in a Minnesota tube or an NGT with its tip located in the esophagus next to the GEBT tube. The volume of oral and esophageal secretions can total up to 1500 mL/day.
25. Once the GEBT tube is properly inserted and bleeding has been controlled, the tube should not be disturbed for 12 to 24 hours.

**BOX 46.2 Complications of Gastroesophageal Balloon Tamponade**

**Major Complications**

Aspiration pneumonia (most common)
Airway obstruction
Asphyxiation
Esophageal mucosal ischemia and necrosis
Esophageal perforation
Duodenal rupture
Tracheobronchial rupture
Mediastinitis
Migration of the balloon causing one of the preceding complications

**Minor Complications**

Pressure necrosis of the nose and lips
Gastroesophageal ulceration
Emesis
Epistaxis
Oral and tongue pressure necrosis
Lacerations

26. If bleeding cannot be controlled, further therapies are indicated, such as emergency surgery, endoscopic interventions, or angiographic embolization.

## COMPLICATIONS

Use of the GEBT tube is associated with many minor and major complications (**Box 46.2**). Such tubes should be used only when life-threatening bleeding occurs and other available modalities have failed. Approximately 8% to 16% of patients treated with GEBT tubes have a major complication, with reported mortality rates of 3%.[34-36]

## SUGGESTED READINGS

Jacobson G, Brokish PA, Wrenn K. Percutaneous feeding tube replacement in the ED—are confirmatory x-rays necessary? Am J Emerg Med 2009;27:519-24.
Kadakia SC, Cassaday M, Shaffer RT. Comparison of Foley catheter as a replacement gastrostomy tube with commercial replacement gastrostomy tube: a prospective randomized trial. Gastrointest Endosc 1994;40:188-93.
Kuo YW, Yen M, Fetzer S, et al. Reducing the pain of nasogastric tube intubation with nebulized and atomized lidocaine: a systematic review and meta-analysis. J Pain Symptom Manage 2010;40:613-20.
McCormick PA, Burroughs AK, McIntyre N. How to insert a Sengstaken-Blakemore tube. Br J Hosp Med 1990;43:274-7.

## REFERENCES

*References can be found on Expert Consult @ www.expertconsult.com.*

# 47 Complications of Bariatric Surgery

*Robert F. Poirier*

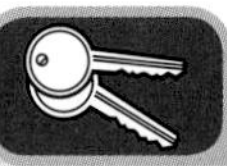

**KEY POINTS**

- Laparoscopic Roux-en-Y gastric bypass is the most commonly performed bariatric procedure in the United States.
- Pulmonary embolism (30% to 40%) is the most common cause of death after bariatric surgery, followed by cardiac events (25%) and anastomotic leaks (20%). Dumping syndrome, wound infections, strictures, and stomal ulcerations are common complications.
- Acute gastric distention is a rare but potentially deadly early postoperative complication that requires decompression.
- A nasogastric tube could perforate the pouch site in patients who have recently undergone surgery.
- Abdominal pain without vomiting in the early postoperative weeks might represent a small bowel obstruction or internal hernia.
- Laparoscopic adjustable gastric banding (LAGB) is the most commonly performed bariatric procedure in Europe and is becoming more common in the United States.
- Acute anterior or posterior gastric band slippage is the most common complication of LAGB requiring emergency treatment (band deflation).
- LAGB has the lowest morbidity and mortality of all currently performed bariatric procedures.

## EPIDEMIOLOGY

The prevalence of morbid obesity has risen more than fourfold since 1986.[1] Currently, 1.7 billion people worldwide are considered obese and approximately 60% of the U.S. population is overweight. In excess of 100 billion dollars is spent annually on obesity health care–related costs.

To be considered morbidly obese, one must have either a body mass index (BMI) greater than 40 kg/m$^2$ or a BMI of 35 to 40 kg/m$^2$ with comorbid conditions.[2] More than 15 million Americans currently have BMI levels that make them eligible for bariatric surgery.[3] In the United States only about 1% of eligible patients undergo bariatric surgery.

Morbid obesity promotes the development of diabetes mellitus, hypertension, dyslipidemia, cardiovascular disease, gastroesophageal reflux, asthma, and obstructive sleep apnea. Premature death from obesity now rivals the mortality rates related to smoking, with more than 300,000 deaths attributable to obesity per year.[4]

Bariatric surgery is the most effective and durable treatment to achieve weight loss and its associated comorbidity. Five-year mortality is reduced 89% in severely obese patients who undergo weight loss surgery.[5,6] Fifteen-year survival increases by one third in patients who undergo bariatric surgery in comparison with those who do not. New laparoscopic surgical techniques have contributed to the growing demand for and acceptance of bariatric surgery. Approximately 4925 bariatric procedures were performed in 1990, as compared with an estimated 220,000 in 2008. Bariatric surgery is now the second most common abdominal operation in the United States.

Women are more likely than men to choose bariatric surgery. It is estimated that men make up 36% of the morbidly obese population in the United States, although they account for less than 20% of patients choosing weight loss surgery each year. The typical demographic profile of a bariatric surgery patient is a woman 35 to 49 years of age with private insurance who belongs to a higher socioeconomic class.

Recent trends suggest that higher-risk, older patients are undergoing bariatric procedures with greater frequency; surprisingly, they demonstrate postoperative morbidity and mortality rates similar to those in the general population.[7] Rates of perioperative complications, reoperation, hospital readmission, and emergency department (ED) visits have been falling. The rates for these indicators are highest with gastric bypass followed by sleeve gastrectomy and lowest for laparoscopic adjustable gastric banding (LAGB).[8] Overall, in-hospital mortality rates are between 0.05% and 0.2%, and 30-day mortality rates have been reported to range between 0.05% and 2%.

Complications of bariatric surgery are common and are generally initially treated in the ED. Up to 20% of patients are admitted for a postoperative complication within 1 year of the bariatric procedure; this rate increases to 40% within 3 years. The potential postoperative complications of the various bariatric procedures have predictable timing and clinical manifestations.[9]

## TYPES OF BARIATRIC SURGERY: ROUX-EN-Y AND GASTRIC BANDING

The two most common types of bariatric surgery in the United States are the Roux-en-Y gastric bypass (RYGBP) (54%) and adjustable gastric banding (39%). Adjustable gastric banding continues to rapidly gain in popularity since initial federal approval in 2001.[7]

Caloric restriction and malabsorption are the principal means of weight loss. In the United States, weight loss procedures that combine both restrictive and malabsorptive components are the most popular. RYGBP, biliopancreatic diversion (BPD), and BPD with duodenal switch are examples of techniques that involve both malabsorption and restriction. In Europe, the preference is for purely restrictive bariatric procedures.

## MALABSORPTION

Surgical techniques that induce malabsorption were the first attempted. Malabsorptive techniques were thought to be the most effective method of achieving rapid and sustained weight loss. Surgeons initially connected the proximal jejunum to a distal portion of the ileum or ascending colon in a procedure known as jejunoileal bypass (**Fig. 47.1**). This technique resulted in severe diarrhea, dangerous metabolic derangements, arthropathy, renal calculi, gallstones, liver disease, and short bowel syndrome. Gastric bypass has been shown to be a more effective malabsorptive procedure with fewer side effects than those associated with jejunoileal bypass. Malabsorptive procedures still in current use include laparoscopic RYGBP, BPD, duodenal switch, and isolated intestinal bypass.

## RESTRICTION

Purely restrictive procedures are less effective than malabsorptive techniques.[6] Restrictive surgeries act by reducing oral intake through induction of early satiety. However, some areas of the stomach easily dilate over time, which causes gradual increases in perceived hunger and subsequent food intake. Restrictive procedures are more successful when the lesser-curve gastric pouch is 15 mL or smaller.[4] Restrictive weight loss procedures such as vertical banded gastroplasty and isolated partial gastrectomy (sleeve gastrectomy) have fallen out of favor. LAGB is the most common, poses the least risk, and is the most effective restrictive technique currently performed.[10]

## ROUX-EN-Y GASTRIC BYPASS

The RYGBP procedure creates a gastric pouch from the proximal portion of the lesser curvature of the stomach that can hold about 15 to 30 mL of fluid and food (**Fig. 47.2**). A portion of the distal end of the small bowel is connected to this pouch to create a concurrent malabsorptive process. Historically, RYGBP was an open procedure, but currently the majority are performed laparoscopically.

Early postoperative complications of RYGBP include obstruction of the bypassed small bowel segment, obstruction of the Roux limb, anastomotic leak, and gastrointestinal (GI) or intraperitoneal bleeding. Pulmonary embolism, a rare postoperative complication, remains the most common cause of postoperative death, followed by complications resulting from anastomotic leaks. Other complications include pneumonia, myocardial infarction, renal failure secondary to rhabdomyolysis, and nutritional deficiencies.

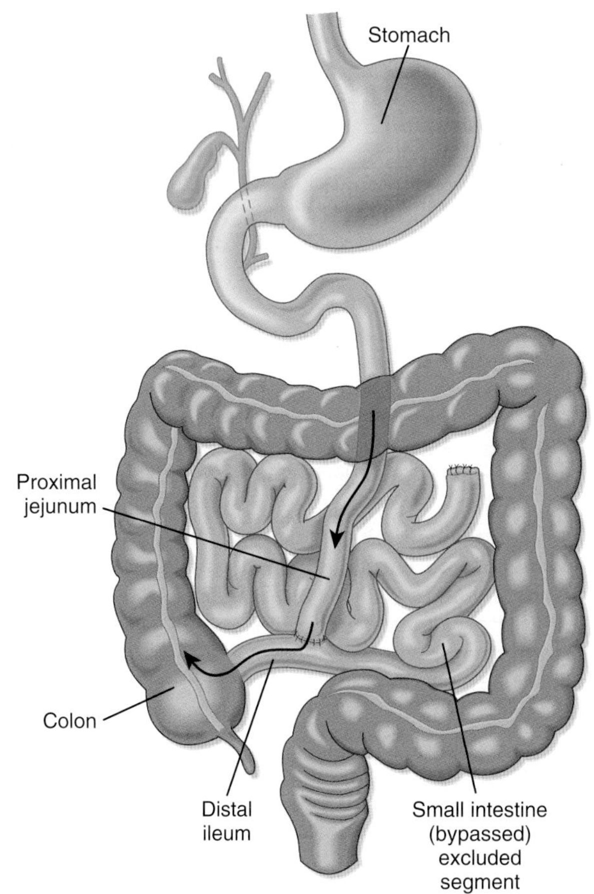


**Fig. 47.1 Jejunoileal bypass.**

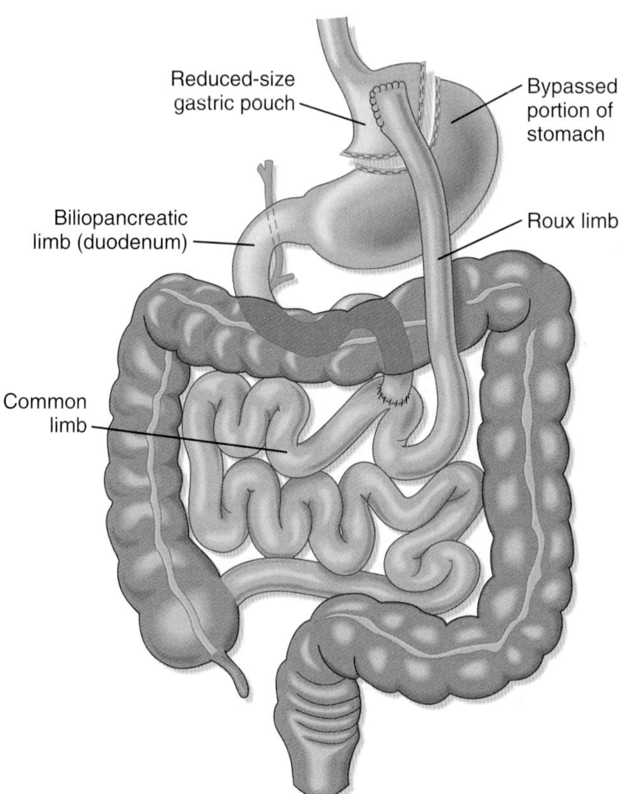


**Fig. 47.2 Roux-en-Y gastric bypass.**

Late complications generally involve both anatomic and systemic complications. Anatomic complications include esophageal reflux, chronic abdominal pain, internal hernias, ulcers, stricture, stenosis, and bowel obstruction. Systemic complications are manifested mostly as nutritional deficiencies.[11] Clinical manifestations include anemia (iron deficiency), osteopenic fractures (calcium deficiency), fatigue and lower extremity edema (protein-calorie malnutrition), chronic pain and proximal muscle weakness (vitamin D deficiency), visual deficits (vitamin A deficiency), and vague neurologic symptoms (thiamine, folate, and vitamin $B_{12}$ deficiencies).

### *Complications of Open versus Laparoscopic Procedures*

Wound infections and incisional hernias are more common with open bariatric procedures (7% and 9%, respectively) than with laparoscopic procedures (3% and 0.5%, respectively). Patients who have undergone laparoscopic gastric bypass have a slightly higher rate of small bowel obstruction, anastomotic stomal stenosis, internal hernias, and GI hemorrhage. Pulmonary embolism, pneumonia, and anastomotic leaks have similar incidences after both open and laparoscopic procedures. Stomal stenosis manifested as postprandial epigastric pain and vomiting of undigested food is thought to be more common after laparoscopic RYGBP because a mechanical stapler is used instead of the hand-sewn methods with open RYGBP. Endoscopy often both diagnoses and treats this complication.

### *Specific Clinical Presentations*

Persistent, severe vomiting can be caused by anastomotic strictures. Strictures can usually be treated by endoscopic balloon dilation but occasionally require surgical revision. Some episodes of nausea and vomiting are common during the immediate postoperative period, but if the vomiting persists, an anastomotic stricture may have formed.

Obstruction of the Roux limb requires percutaneous decompression. Patients with such an obstruction experience nausea, vomiting, abdominal pain, and distention. Diagnosis may require computed tomography (CT).

The occurrence of acute fever and tachycardia within weeks of a Roux-en-Y procedure suggests an anastomotic leak with or without abscess formation. The symptoms are often subtle but can include dyspnea, unexplained sepsis, changes in mental status, and restlessness. Peritoneal signs are often lacking. Because abdominal examination of morbidly obese patients is unreliable, the diagnosis is best accomplished through imaging studies. CT of the abdomen and pelvis with oral and intravenous (IV) administration of a contrast agent is the modality of choice. If the patient is unable to undergo CT because of the weight limitations of the CT table, an upper GI radiographic series should be obtained. The false-negative rate is high (up to 44%) with CT and other imaging studies for the evaluation of anastomotic leaks. Laparoscopy should be considered in cases of negative imaging but high pretest probability of an anastomotic leak.[12,13]

Esophageal reflux occurs infrequently after this procedure but may represent damage to the lower esophageal sphincter or impaired gastric emptying secondary to a distal obstruction. Overfilling of the pouch, operative vagal nerve injury, or stomal stricture can lead to gastroesophageal reflux disease (GERD). Educating patients to avoid overeating, chew food properly, use acid suppression medication, and eat small frequent meals reduces the incidence of GERD.

Diarrhea with malodorous flatulence may result from a short Roux limb and usually resolves spontaneously. Persistent diarrhea after weight stabilization, however, should raise suspicion of bacterial overgrowth in the bypassed tract.

Dumping syndrome consisting of abdominal cramping, nausea, vomiting, and diarrhea can be seen immediately postoperatively and may last up to 12 to 18 months. Noncompliance with diet is the most common and preventable cause. Treatment includes rehydration, electrolyte correction, and education of the patient regarding diet.

Constipation may result from decreased fiber intake.

Cholelithiasis may develop during the period of initial rapid weight loss. Biliary colic and cholecystitis are high on the differential diagnosis list for abdominal pain in patients with ongoing reductions in weight. Prophylactic cholecystectomy was often performed during open RYGBP. The transition to laparoscopic surgery for most RYGBP procedures has led to a decrease in prophylactic cholecystectomy and thus an increase in cholelithiasis rates.

Bleeding may occur at any anastomotic site but is most common and dangerous in the gastrojejunostomy area. It often results in melena, hematemesis, hematochezia, or hypotension (or any combination of these findings) secondary to upper GI bleeding. Upper endoscopy is the most reliable way to confirm blood loss from this site. Bleeding at other anastomotic sites (jejunojejunostomy and the transected gastric remnant) is usually self-limited and managed nonoperatively.[11] Stomal ulcers can occur 2 to 4 months after surgery and are identified by endoscopy. Many can be treated on an outpatient basis with proton pump inhibitors or sucralfate.

## LAPAROSCOPIC ADJUSTABLE GASTRIC BANDING

The LAP-BAND (Allergan, Inc., Irvine, CA) is an adjustable device that is laparoscopically secured around the upper portion of the stomach (**Fig. 47.3**). The band is connected by a tube to a port implanted under the skin. Surgeons may adjust the extent of constriction (restriction) of the LAP-BAND by injecting saline into the subcutaneous port. Increased restriction limits food intake; adjustments can be made in response to adverse symptoms or patient preference, thereby allowing some control over the weight loss process. Operative risks for LAGB are less than those for RYGBP.

In 2007 the Food and Drug Administration (FDA) approved a second gastric banding device called the Realize Adjustable Gastric Band. The Heliogast and Midband adjustable gastric bands are available only outside the United States and have not been approved by the FDA. All gastric banding devices work similarly. In 2011 the U.S. FDA approved expanding the use of gastric banding surgery for an additional 27 million American patients with mild obesity (BMI of 30 to 35 kg/m$^2$) who have one obesity-related health condition (e.g., hypertension, diabetes mellitus).

### *Complications*

LAGB is generally performed as outpatient surgery. Immediate postoperative vomiting is usually caused by gastric wall edema under the band. Inflation of the band during surgery increases the likelihood of gastric wall edema. IV hydration is required until the edema subsides. Maintenance of nothing

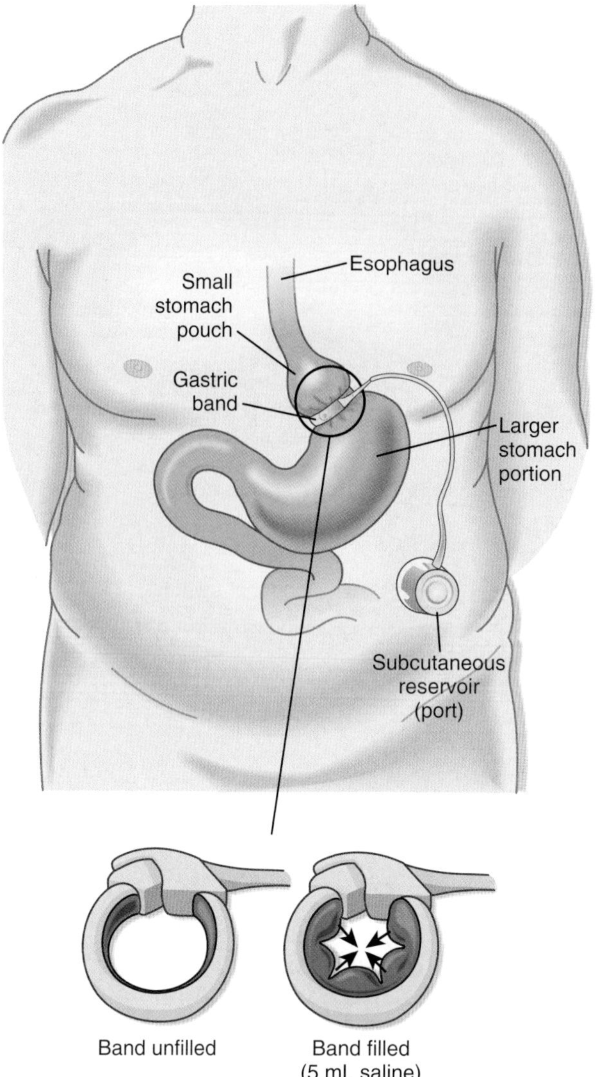


**Fig. 47.3 Laparoscopic adjustable gastric banding.**

by mouth (NPO) and IV steroids are thought to increase the resolution rate.

Immediate postoperative vomiting or dysphagia may also be due to gastroesophageal obstruction caused by proximal band slippage (1% to 3%). Gastric dilation and food intolerance may develop. Gastric necrosis and perforation may result from band migration at any time. A GI swallow study using fluoroscopy is the preferred method of diagnosing band migration, but a two-view upper GI contrast study or abdominal radiograph may capture the position of the radiolucent band. An abdominal CT scan may also demonstrate movement of the band. Band slippage is the most common LAGB complication occurring early to late in the postoperative period. Band slippage rates are decreasing, however, with new placement techniques.

Any patient with signs of obstruction after LAGB should undergo immediate deflation of the band. Emergency physicians can deflate an adjustable gastric band by accessing the subcutaneous anterior abdominal port (see Fig. 47.3). A noncoring Huber needle should be used to remove the amount of saline injected during the previous two adjustments. The patient should know this volume of saline, but if not, one can aspirate all the saline in the reservoir. Fluoroscopy or ultrasound may be required if the port cannot be accessed easily. A GI swallow study and surgical consultation should be obtained after any band deflation. Symptoms should resolve over a couple of days after deflation. Surgery is often required to definitively repair gastric band slippage.

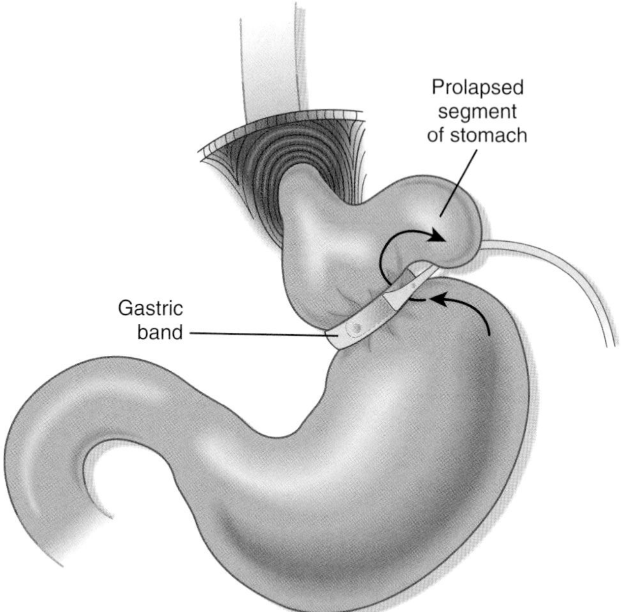


**Fig. 47.4 Gastric prolapse.**

Gastric stoma obstruction by food, swelling, or hematoma can be an early or late complication. Partial obstruction can be treated conservatively with hydration and NPO status. Complete obstruction often requires band deflation and surgery to reposition the band.

Band erosion can occur in up to 4% of patients over time. The band can erode and migrate silently into the stomach. Peritonitis is often absent, but GI bleeding and bowel obstruction can occur. Port site infections may be the first sign of band erosion, and endoscopy is the best method to diagnose band erosion. Upper GI studies and CT scans can assist in making the diagnosis as well. Removal of the band and repair of the stomach are required.

Gastric injury as a result of stomach perforation occurs rarely. One to 2 days following band placement an acute abdomen may develop. IV fluids, broad-spectrum antibiotics, NPO status, and surgical consultation with subsequent repair of the stomach are required.

Gastric necrosis of the stomach wall is a late complication that often results from ischemia caused by a combination of gastric prolapse—the part of the stomach below the band herniates up through the device (**Fig. 47.4**) and pressure from the band. Patients appear ill, with an acute abdomen. Upper GI studies or CT scans show an overly distended gastric pouch. Patients require emergency surgery to remove the band and repair the stomach wall.

Esophageal and gastric pouch dilation occurs when the band is too tight or patients are not compliant with their diet. The symptoms are similar to those seen with gastric slippage. Upper GI contrast studies make the diagnosis. Treatment is

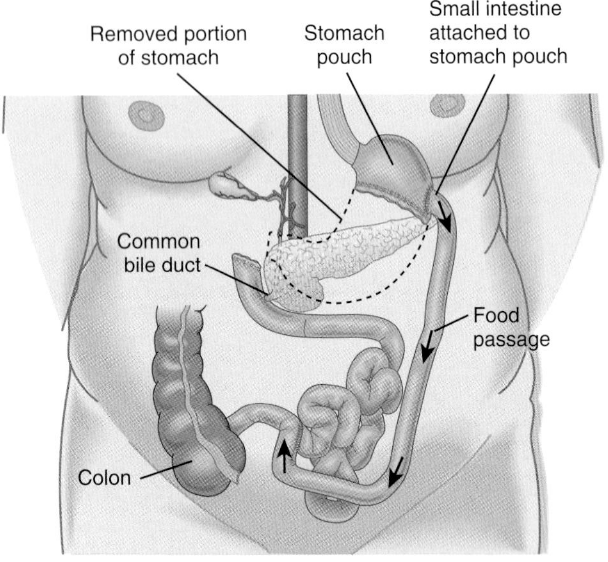


**Fig. 47.5 Biliopancreatic diversion.**

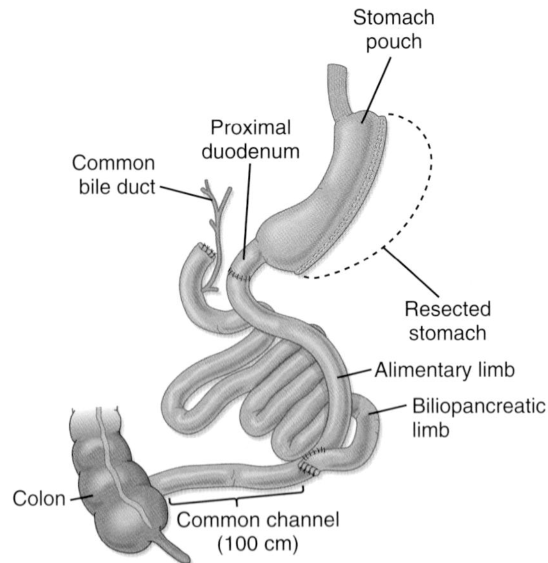


**Fig. 47.6 Duodenal switch.**

band deflation and close follow-up with the bariatric physician. Prolonged dilation can result in chronic esophageal dysmotility, severe achalasia, and GERD, which is not always reversible (13%) with band deflation and removal.[14]

Device malfunction can cause port infections, tube leakage, tube disconnection, and skin ulceration. Plain radiographs, abdominal CT scans, and upper endoscopy may all aid in the diagnosis of gastric erosion and device malfunction.

Recent controversies have arisen regarding the long-term complications of gastric banding. Few long-term studies have been performed, but a recent 14-year study (1995 to 2009) of gastric band surgery showed high complication and reoperation rates. Reoperation because of complications was reported to occur in 30% of patients, band removal was needed in 12%, and weight regain began after 5 years of follow-up.[15] Still, gastric banding has been shown to have a lower mortality rate than other bariatric surgeries, is less invasive, and is reversible.

## BILIOPANCREATIC DIVERSION

BPD is popular in Italy (**Fig. 47.5**). The procedure involves a distal gastrectomy that leaves a 250-mL stomach capacity with a drastic intestinal bypass. Half of the jejunum and ileum are disconnected and reconnected near the terminal ileum. This procedure is particularly effective for severely obese patients (BMI > 50 kg/m$^2$), in whom it causes significant weight loss and reduced morbidity. Less bacterial overgrowth occurs in the bypassed intestine because it is continuously exposed to bile and pancreatic enzymes. Serious complications can result, however, particularly the metabolic abnormalities and nutritional deficiencies seen after aggressive malabsorptive procedures. Hepatic dysfunction can develop in 2% of patients undergoing BPD.

## DUODENAL SWITCH AND SLEEVE GASTRECTOMY

The duodenal switch procedure is similar to BPD, but the jejunum is connected to the proximal duodenum rather than the ileum (**Fig. 47.6**). This operation is also known as the biliopancreatic diversion–duodenal switch (BPD-DS) procedure. It is considered an improvement on BPD alone because the length of the small intestine is increased to 100 cm, which allows better absorption of nutrients.

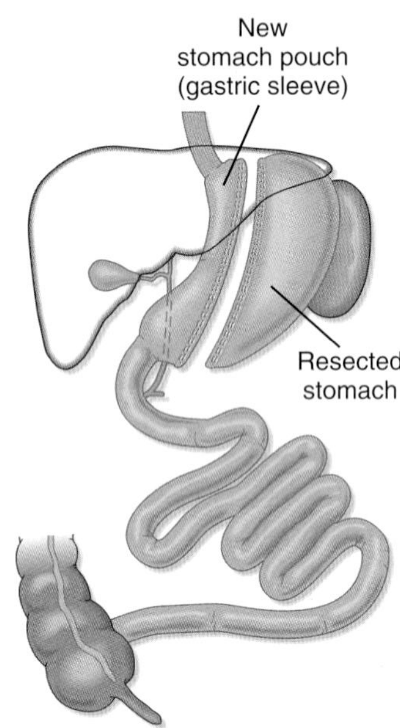


**Fig. 47.7 Sleeve gastrectomy.**

A linear (sleeve) gastrectomy in which a restrictive pouch of the lesser curvature is left is also performed during the duodenal switch. BPD-DS with sleeve gastrectomy allows gastric emptying to be somewhat regulated through preservation of a functioning pylorus. The risk for dumping syndrome is subsequently reduced.

Some surgeons prefer to perform only a sleeve gastrectomy in high-risk patients (**Fig. 47.7**). This simple restrictive procedure avoids intestinal bypass and anastomoses of the GI tract. Side effects such as nutritional deficiencies are rare because only mild malabsorption results from sleeve gastrectomy alone.

## COMPLICATIONS OF BARIATRIC SURGERY

### GENERAL COMPLICATIONS

Serious complication rates are lower in hospitals with a high volume of bariatric surgery procedures.[16]

#### *Pulmonary Embolism*

Pulmonary embolism is the leading cause of death after bariatric surgery. Although the postoperative incidence of deep vein thrombosis (DVT) and pulmonary embolism is only 2%, almost one third of affected patients die. The incidence of DVT and pulmonary embolism has not diminished despite the use of pneumatic compression stockings, low-molecular-weight heparin, and various other prophylactic measures. Early postoperative ambulation may be the most important preventive measure in the bariatric population. Lower extremity duplex Doppler ultrasonography for DVT and helical pulmonary CT scanning for pulmonary embolism are the preferred diagnostic studies. If weight limitations prevent performance of a CT scan, ventilation-perfusion scintigraphy should be considered.

#### *Wound Infections, Seromas, and Dehiscence*

Wound infections occur in 10% to 15% of patients undergoing open procedures and in 3% to 4% of those treated by laparoscopic techniques. Seromas commonly occur in up to 40% of patients. Although the wound infections may appear superficial, deep extensions may be present in the morbidly obese. Patients with wound infections and fever should undergo contrast-enhanced CT of the abdomen to exclude deep infections.

#### *Intraperitoneal Fluid Collections and Peritonitis*

Intraperitoneal fluid collections, abscesses, and peritonitis occur in less than 2% of patients undergoing bariatric procedures. Anastomotic leaks are the most common cause of fluid collections in the early postoperative period. Clinical signs are often subtle, and the diagnosis cannot be made by physical examination alone. Patients may have low-grade fevers, tachycardia, and mild tachypnea. Early surgical consultation should be obtained to facilitate the most efficient evaluation and treatment because life-threatening sepsis may ensue. The poor cardiopulmonary reserve of morbidly obese patients may allow rapid clinical deterioration. Some institutions advocate CT-guided aspiration during initial imaging.

#### *Incisional Hernia*

Incisional hernias occur in up to 9% of patients after open RYGBP. Rarely are incisional hernias seen in those who undergo laparoscopic procedures. Physical examination alone confirms the diagnosis.

#### *Gallstones*

The incidence of cholelithiasis is 1% to 3% after bariatric surgery. Rapid weight loss is known to promote the formation of gallstones, and most surgeons perform prophylactic cholecystectomy in patients with known cholelithiasis. The distorted anatomy after gastric bypass often precludes successful endoscopic retrograde cholangiopancreatography. Symptomatic biliary disease in patients who have undergone a Roux-en-Y procedure usually requires surgical intervention or percutaneous drainage.

**BOX 47.1 Top 10 Complications of Bariatric Surgery**

1. Dumping syndrome
2. Vitamin and mineral deficiencies
3. Nausea and vomiting
4. Staple line failure
5. Infection
6. Bowel obstruction and anastomotic stenosis
7. Gastric and stomal ulceration
8. Bleeding
9. Iatrogenic splenic injury
10. Perioperative death (pulmonary embolism, sepsis, myocardial infarction)

From Abell TL, Minocha A. Gastrointestinal complications of bariatric surgery: diagnosis and therapy. Am J Med Sci 2006;331:214-8.

### PROCEDURE-SPECIFIC COMPLICATIONS

**Box 47.1** lists the most common GI complications of bariatric surgery.[12]

#### *Anastomotic (Staple Line) Leak*

Anastomotic leaks most often occur in the immediate postoperative period, although some leaks are not apparent until weeks after surgery. GI leaks are one of the most serious and potentially deadly complications of gastric bypass surgery. The incidence is up to 6% in patients after first procedures, but it rises 5-fold to 10-fold in patients who undergo revision of the initial procedure. Leaks are difficult to diagnose because of initial nonspecific signs and symptoms: low-grade fever, abdominal tenderness, tachypnea and respiratory insufficiency, tachycardia, left shoulder pain, anxiety, and a feeling of impending doom. An upper GI radiographic series or abdominal CT scan sometimes confirms the diagnosis by demonstrating extravasation of the oral contrast agent (Gastrografin). However, an upper GI series or CT scan often misses the leak. Many bariatric surgeons question the need for confirmatory studies and believe that patients should be taken to the operating room for laparoscopic examination when tachycardia greater than 120 beats/min and symptoms indicative of a leak are present.[17] The most common site of the leak is the gastrojejunostomy anastomosis. Interventional or surgical management is required. Early antibiotic therapy is recommended.

#### *Acute Gastric Distention*

Acute gastric distention is a rare, potentially deadly, early postoperative complication. Patients may have pain, nausea, vomiting, abdominal distention, bloating, hiccups, tachycardia, shortness of breath, or referred left shoulder pain. Abdominal plain films or abdominal CT scans usually demonstrate a large air-fluid level in a dilated stomach. Obstruction or edema at the enteroenterostomy site is often the cause of this complication and is best evaluated by CT. Treatment includes percutaneous fine-needle decompression, drainage via a gastrectomy tube, or surgery for cases of recurrence or rupture. A nasogastric tube should not be used because of possible perforation.

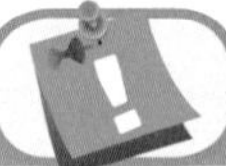

**TIPS AND TRICKS**

Consult the bariatric surgeon or gastroenterologist (if endoscopy is required) early for patients who have previously undergone bariatric surgery.

Do not place a nasogastric tube in patients who have undergone gastric bypass without consultation from the bariatric surgeon. Blind placement of such a tube may result in perforation of the pouch site, particularly in the immediate postoperative period.

Laparoscopy is often required for definitive diagnosis of internal hernias and anastomotic leaks.

Small gastric pouches limit the amount of oral contrast agent that patients can ingest for a computed tomography scan. If contrast is required, patients should be told to sip as much contrast agent as they feel comfortable taking over a 3-hour period before imaging. The scan is then performed, regardless of the amount of contrast ingested.[12]

### *Stomal Stenosis and Anastomotic Strictures*

The incidence of anastomotic strictures occurring at the gastrojejunostomy site varies from 2% to 11%. Patients often have progressive postprandial, epigastric pain and vomiting. Patients are initially unable to tolerate solid foods, with characteristic progression to poor tolerance of liquids over time. Findings on plain radiography and CT of the abdomen are usually unremarkable. Upper endoscopy both diagnoses and treats this condition. Repeated endoscopic balloon dilation of the stricture is often required. Fluoroscopically guided balloon dilation is an alternative treatment.

### *Stomal Ulceration*

Stomal ulceration causes severe dyspepsia, burning retrosternal pain, and vomiting. Abdominal plain films, CT scans, and other upper GI radiographic studies are not useful in diagnosing this complication. Endoscopy is the diagnostic modality of choice. Proton pump inhibitors treat stomal ulceration, and antibiotics are prescribed if the patient is found to have coinfection with *Helicobacter pylori*.

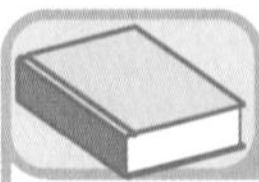

**PATIENT TEACHING TIPS**

The American Society for Bariatric Surgery's website has excellent educational resources (www.asbs.org).

The patient should return to the hospital if nausea, vomiting, or a fast heart rate develops.

Blood glucose levels can fluctuate widely after weight loss surgery and require close monitoring.

Patients must adhere strictly to the postoperative diet instructions to prevent potential complications.

### *Small Bowel Obstruction and Internal Hernia*

Abdominal pain without vomiting in the early postoperative weeks might represent small bowel obstruction or an internal hernia. Small bowel obstructions and internal hernias are difficult to differentiate and have a combined incidence of 5% within the first postoperative month. Small bowel obstructions are more common after open bariatric surgery because of adhesion formation; internal hernias are more common after laparoscopic surgery. The Roux limb or pancreaticobiliary limb may herniate through the potential spaces created during surgery. Patients have nonspecific symptoms, including abdominal cramping, periumbilical pain, and nausea. Vomiting is uncommon because only minimal secretions are present in the small gastric pouch. Abdominal plain films are nondiagnostic because dilated loops of bowel are not commonly seen. Upper GI studies and abdominal CT are often unable to distinguish between obstruction and hernia. Surgeons may perform laparoscopy early to prevent potential bowel strangulation.

### *Dumping Syndrome*

Dumping syndrome occurs in almost half of patients undergoing gastric bypass. Typical symptoms are bloating, abdominal cramping, nausea, diaphoresis, and lightheadedness; the symptoms are more pronounced after eating food with high concentrations of refined sugar. The effects are self-limited and diminish as patients becomes more selective with their diet.

## DISPOSITION

Patients who go to the ED because of systemic or GI symptoms after bariatric surgery often have a postoperative complication that mandates hospital admission. They generally need CT, an upper GI radiographic series, endoscopy, or any combination of these imaging modalities. Discharge should be considered only for patients who have been evaluated in consultation with a surgeon or gastroenterologist (or both), who have stable vital signs and minimal pain, and who can easily tolerate oral fluids.

## SUGGESTED READINGS

Edwards ED, Jacob BP, Gagner M, et al. Presentation and management of common post–weight loss surgery problems in the emergency department. Ann Emerg Med 2006;47:160-6.

Ellison SR, Ellison SD. Bariatric surgery: a review of the available procedures and complications for the emergency physician. J Emerg Med 2008;34:21-32.

Tanner BD, Allen JW. Complications of bariatric surgery: implications for the covering physician. Am Surg 2009;75:103-12.

Trus TL, Pope GD, Finlayson RG. National trends in utilization and outcomes of bariatric surgery. Surg Endosc 2005;19:616-20.

## REFERENCES

*References can be found on Expert Consult @ www.expertconsult.com.*

# Asthma 48

*Rita K. Cydulka and Craig G. Bates*

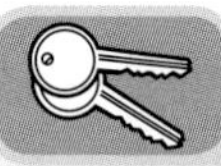

**KEY POINTS**

- Asthma is a chronic inflammatory condition that can be controlled.
- Indications of inadequate control of asthma include frequent use of short-acting β-agonist agents, wheezing, coughing, and nighttime symptoms.
- Emergency department treatment of asthma exacerbation includes a targeted history and physical examination, aerosolized β-agonist agents, and systemic steroids with objective measures of response to therapy. Anticholinergic agents should be used in the emergency department for patients with a severe exacerbation.
- At discharge, controller medications should be prescribed in addition to rescue medications for patients with chronic persistent asthma. Patients should follow up with a primary care physician or asthma specialist within several weeks.

## PERSPECTIVE

Asthma is a chronic inflammatory disorder characterized by increased responsiveness of the airways to multiple stimuli. Many cells and cellular elements, such as mast cells, eosinophils, T lymphocytes, macrophages, neutrophils, and epithelial cells, play a role in development of the inflammatory response.[1] The inflammation causes recurrent episodes of wheezing, breathlessness, chest tightness, and coughing, particularly at night or in the early morning. These episodes are associated with airflow obstruction that is reversible either spontaneously or with treatment. Although patients appear to clinically recover completely, evidence suggests that some asthmatic patients have chronic airflow limitation. The recognition that asthma is a chronic inflammatory disorder of the airways has significant implications for the diagnosis, management, and potential prevention of acute exacerbations.

## EPIDEMIOLOGY

Asthma affects approximately 4% to 5% of the population in the United States.[2] Although it is the most common chronic disease of childhood, with a prevalence of 5% to 10%, it also affects 7% to 10% of the elderly. Epidemiologic studies suggest that asthma is underdiagnosed and undertreated in all age groups. Part of the problem is that the transient nature of asthma allows many patients to tolerate intermittent respiratory symptoms before seeking medical care. Another important factor resulting in underdiagnosis of asthma is the sometimes nonspecific nature of the symptoms.

About half of cases of asthma develop before 10 years of age and another third before 40 years. The 2 : 1 male-to-female preponderance of asthma in childhood equalizes by 30 years of age.[3] The average asthmatic patient has 15 days of restricted activity each year and spends 5.8 days in bed. Approximately 2 million emergency department (ED) visits, 484,000 hospitalizations, and more than 4000 deaths per year are attributed to asthma. In the United States alone, the estimated direct and indirect cost of asthma in all age groups was $56 billion in 2007.[4]

## PATHOPHYSIOLOGY

All asthmatic patients have hyperresponsive airways that narrow when exposed to various stimuli: allergic, infectious, pharmacologic, environmental, occupational, exercise related, and emotional.

Allergic asthma occurs when inhaled allergens bind to immunoglobulin E molecules bound to mast cells in the lining of the tracheobronchial tree. During the early response, various mediators are released and cause greater vascular permeability, mucosal edema, and contraction of bronchial smooth muscle. A second wave of reaction, the late response, is seen hours to days later; it involves accumulation of inflammatory cells in the bronchial mucosa, thus perpetuating the reaction. The release of mediators and regulation of the inflammatory process in asthma are complex, redundant, and self-perpetuating.[5]

Although several theories attempt to explain the pathophysiologic changes that occur in nonallergic asthma, none adequately explain all clinically observed phenomena. Research suggests that even patients without atopy have pathophysiology similar to that in atopic patients.[5] Respiratory infections, particularly viral infections, may precipitate bronchospasm. Viruses cause mucosal inflammation and lower the firing threshold of the subendothelial vagal receptors, which results in enhanced airway reactivity that may last up to 8 weeks, even in nonasthmatic persons. Pharmacologic agents, such as aspirin and nonsteroidal antiinflammatory compounds, coloring agents, and beta-blockers, also induce acute asthma. In addition, sulfating agents, which are used widely as food preservatives and antioxidants in pharmaceutical products, can exacerbate asthma.

A large variety of occupational dust and fumes may provoke acute airway obstruction. Patients with occupational asthma classically report a cyclic history; they are symptom free during weekends, vacations, and on arrival at work. Exercise may also stimulate an asthma attack. Exercise-induced bronchospasm is usually noted within 5 to 20 minutes after the completion of exercise and is related to thermal changes in the respiratory tree. Exercising in a cold, dry environment causes a more marked response than does exercising in a warm, humid environment. Finally, endocrine factors, such as variations in progesterone and estradiol levels, also influence asthma exacerbations, probably through modification of vagal efferent activity.

Most patients with asthma seem to display an exaggerated bronchoconstrictive response to a variety of exogenous and endogenous stimuli, and inflammation plays a key role. The final common pathway is as follows[1]:

- Airway narrowing
- Bronchial wall edema
- Bronchial smooth muscle contraction
- Mucosal plugging
- Enhanced airway reactivity and remodeling of the airway wall, which results in increased airway resistance
- Decreased forced expiratory volumes and flow rates
- Lung hyperinflation
- Increased work of breathing
- Ventilation-perfusion mismatch

## PRESENTING SIGNS AND SYMPTOMS

When evaluated in the ED, many patients relay a history of asthma, but some do not. Patients with a severe asthma attack may be in obvious respiratory distress, with rapid breathing and loud wheezing, but patients with mild exacerbation may exhibit coughing and end-expiratory wheezing. The classic symptoms of asthma consist of the triad of dyspnea, wheezing, and coughing, but physical findings during an asthma exacerbation can be variable. Early symptoms include a sensation of chest constriction and coughing. As the exacerbation progresses, wheezing becomes apparent, expiration becomes prolonged, and use of the accessory respiratory muscles may become evident. Patients may sit upright or lean forward in an attempt to decrease the work of breathing. Use of the accessory muscles of inspiration indicates diaphragmatic fatigue, whereas the appearance of paradoxic respirations reflects impending ventilatory failure. Alteration in mental status heralds respiratory arrest.

### VARIATIONS IN PRESENTING SIGNS AND SYMPTOMS

Patients with asthma exacerbations may simply exhibit coughing or have a feeling of chest tightness. At the other end of the spectrum are patients with a "silent chest," which reflects very severe airflow obstruction and air movement insufficient to promote a wheeze.

A subset of asthmatic patients experience a sudden onset of severe symptoms. These individuals tend to respond rapidly to treatment but appear to be at significant risk for a fatal outcome.[6-9]

## DIFFERENTIAL DIAGNOSIS

Wheezing, coughing, and dyspnea may be cause by many common conditions, including pneumonia, bronchitis, croup, bronchiolitis, chronic obstructive pulmonary disease, congestive heart failure, pulmonary embolism, allergic reactions, and upper airway obstruction from edema or a foreign body. Less common conditions with similar symptoms are cystic fibrosis, hypersensitivity pneumonitis, carcinoid syndrome, and exposure to odors, dust, and gas. A careful history and physical examination should help differentiate asthma from these other conditions.

## DIAGNOSTIC TESTING

As for all patients who come to the ED for care, a directed history and physical examination should be performed. Key historical points should be elicited, such as the duration and onset of the current attack, identification of precipitating causes, type and amount of medications used before arrival at the ED, response to previous therapy, including current or previous use of corticosteroids, frequency of ED visits and hospitalizations, previous need for intubation or ventilation, history of concurrent medications and allergies, and history of concurrent medical problems. At some point during the patient's ED stay, effort should be made to evaluate both the severity of the obstruction and the adequacy of ongoing asthma control (**Table 48.1**).

The physical examination should focus on observing respiratory effort and use of accessory muscles and listening for wheezing or other abnormal breath sounds and prolongation of the expiratory phase. Although wheezing results from movement of air through narrowed airways, the intensity of the wheeze may not correlate with the severity of airflow obstruction. Tachycardia and tachypnea are usually present in patients with acute asthma, but vital signs normalize very quickly as the airflow obstruction is relieved.[10] Therefore, a normal heart rate and respiratory rate are not reliable indicators of the degree of relief from obstruction.

Bedside spirometry provides a rapid, objective assessment of patients and helps both indicate the effectiveness of and guide therapy. Sequential measurements assist emergency physicians in assessing the severity of the problem and determining the response to therapy. Although forced expiratory volume in 1 second ($FEV_1$) and the peak expiratory flow (PEF) rate measure the extent of large airway obstruction, patient cooperation is essential for these tests to be reliable. When possible, management decisions should be guided by a patient's personal best PEF rate or $FEV_1$ value or, if unknown, a percentage of the predicted value in addition to other physiologic and historical factors.[1]

Pulse oximetry is a useful and convenient method for accessing oxygenation and monitoring oxygen saturation during treatment. Analysis of arterial blood gases is not indicated in the majority of patients with mild to moderate asthma

**Table 48.1 Classification of Asthma Severity: Clinical Features Before Treatment**

| | SYMPTOMS | NIGHTTIME SYMPTOMS | LUNG FUNCTION |
|---|---|---|---|
| Step 4: Severe persistent | Continual symptoms<br>Limited physical activity<br>Frequent exacerbations | Frequent | $FEV_1$ or PEF < 60% of predicted value<br>PEF variability > 30% |
| Step 3: Moderate persistent | Daily symptoms<br>Daily use of inhaled short-acting $\beta_2$-agonist<br>Exacerbations affecting activity<br>Exacerbations > 2 times per week; may last days | >1 time per week | $FEV_1$ or PEF > 60% but <80% of predicted value<br>PEF variability > 30% |
| Step 2: Mild persistent | Symptoms > 2 times per week but >1 time per day<br>Exacerbations may affect activity | 3-4 times per month | $FEV_1$ or PEF ≥ 80% of predicted value<br>PEF variability 20%-30% |
| Step 1: Mild intermittent | Symptoms < 2 times per week<br>Asymptomatic and normal PEFR between exacerbations<br>Exacerbations brief (from a few hours to a few days; intensity may vary) | ≤2 times per month | $FEV_1$ or PEF ≥ 80% of predicted value<br>PEF variability < 20% |

Adapted from National Institutes of Health, National Heart, Lung and Blood Institute, National Asthma Education and Prevention Program. Expert Panel Report 3: guidelines for the diagnosis and management of asthma. NIH Publication No. 08-4051. Bethesda, MD: U.S. Department of Health and Human Services; August 2007.

*$FEV_1$*, Forced expiratory volume in 1 minute; *PEF*, peak expiratory flow; *PEFR*, peak expiratory flow rate.

exacerbation, but it is helpful if there is concern for hypoventilation with carbon dioxide retention and respiratory acidosis. Patients with the latter problems almost always have clinical evidence of severe attacks or spirometry demonstrating PEF or $FEV_1$ less than 25% of the predicted value.[11,12] Practitioners should be aware that a normal or slightly elevated $Paco_2$ (e.g., 42 mm Hg or higher) indicates extreme airway obstruction and fatigue and may herald the onset of acute ventilatory failure.[11,12]

Routine radiography is unnecessary but is indicated if the possibility of pneumothorax, pneumomediastinum, pneumonia, or other medical conditions is a concern. In up to one third of asthmatic patients requiring admission, an abnormality is demonstrated on chest radiographs.[13]

A routine complete blood cell count is not indicated and would probably show modest leukocytosis secondary to the administration of $\beta_2$-agonist therapy or corticosteroid treatment. In patients taking theophylline before ED evaluation, a serum theophylline level should be determined. A routine electrocardiogram is also unnecessary; electrocardiographic abnormalities noted include right ventricular strain, abnormal P waves, and nonspecific ST-T wave abnormalities, which resolve with treatment. Older patients, especially those with coexisting heart disease, should undergo cardiac monitoring during treatment. Asthma severity index scores have failed to predict outcome better than clinical judgment does.

Use of exhaled nitric oxide measurements and other serum and urine markers for detection of the severity of the asthma exacerbation is currently under investigation.[14-17]

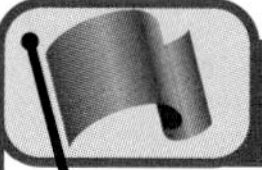

**RED FLAGS**

A silent chest indicates severe obstruction.

Do not wait for arterial blood gas confirmation to aggressively treat ventilatory or respiratory failure.

Listen to the patient—the patient will frequently be able to assess the severity of the exacerbation.

## TREATMENT

The goal of treatment of acute asthma in the ED is to rapidly reverse the airflow obstruction with repetitive or continuous administration of inhaled $\beta_2$-agonists, ensure adequate oxygenation, and relieve inflammation. The National Asthma Education and Prevention Program Expert Panel has developed guidelines for emergency treatment of asthma (**Fig. 48.1**),[1] as have other organizations around the world. Prehospital treatment with oxygen and $\beta_2$-agonists is usually initiated. The following types of medications have been shown to be effective for the treatment of acute asthma: $\beta_2$-agonists, anticholinergics, and glucocorticoids (**Table 48.2**).[1] Magnesium should be considered in patients with severe obstruction. Current evidence does not support the use of heliox (helium-oxygen mixture) or ketamine, even when the aforementioned medications fail to relieve bronchospasm. Mast cell–stabilizing agents, methylxanthines, and leukotriene modifiers are currently reserved for maintenance therapy only.

### PHARMACEUTICALS

#### *$\beta_2$-Agonist Agents*

$\beta_2$-Agonists are the preferred initial rescue medications for acute bronchospasm. In addition to bronchodilation, these drugs inhibit the release of mediators and promote mucociliary clearance.[1]

The most common side effect of $\beta_2$-agonist drugs is skeletal muscle tremor. Patients may also experience nervousness, anxiety, insomnia, headache, hyperglycemia, palpitations, tachycardia, and hypertension. Despite earlier concerns about the potential cardiotoxicity of these agents, clinical experience has not revealed significant problems. Arrhythmias and

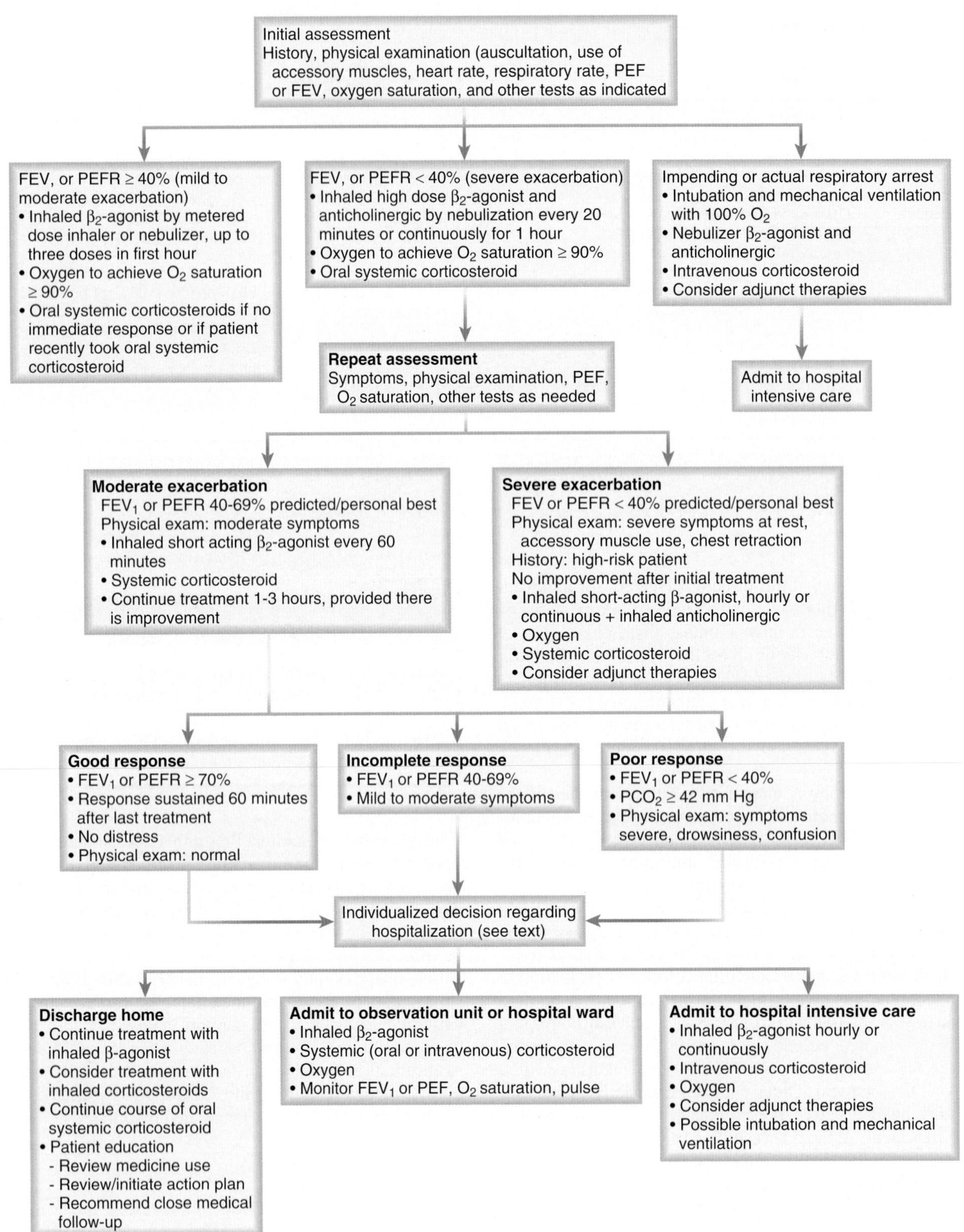


**Fig. 48.1 Management of asthma exacerbations: emergency department– and hospital-based care.** *$FEV_1$*, Forced expiratory volume in 1 second; *PEF*, peak expiratory flow; *PEFR*, peak expiratory flow rate. (Adapted from National Institutes of Health, National Heart, Lung and Blood Institute, National Asthma Education and Prevention Program. Expert Panel Report 3: guidelines for the diagnosis and management of asthma. NIH Publication No. 08-4051. Bethesda, MD: U.S. Department of Health and Human Services; August 2007.)

**Table 48.2 Medications Used to Treat Asthma Exacerbations**

| | DOSAGES | | |
|---|---|---|---|
| **MEDICATION** | **ADULT DOSE** | **CHILD DOSE*** | **COMMENTS** |
| **Short-Acting Inhaled $\beta_2$-Agonists** | | | |
| Albuterol | | | |
| Nebulizer solution (5.0 mg/mL, 2.5 mg/3 mL, 1.25 mg/3 mL, 0.63 mg/3 mL) | 2.5-5 mg every 20 min for 3 doses, then 2.5-10 mg every 1-4 hr as needed, or 10-15 mg/hr continuously | 0.15 mg/kg (minimum dose, 2.5 mg) every 20 min for 3 doses, then 0.15-0.3 mg/kg up to 10 mg every 1-4 hr as needed, or 0.5 mg/kg/hr by continuous nebulization | Only selective $\beta_2$-agonists are recommended<br>For optimal delivery, dilute aerosols to a minimum of 3 mL with gas flow of 6-8 L/min |
| MDI (90 mcg per puff) | 4-8 puffs every 20 min up to 4 hr, then every 1-4 hr as needed | 4-8 puffs every 20 min for 3 doses, then 1-4 hr inhalation maneuver<br>Use spacer/holding chamber | As effective as nebulized therapy if patient is able to coordinate |
| Bitolterol | | | |
| Nebulizer solution (2 mg/mL) | See albuterol dose | See albuterol dose<br>Thought to be half as potent as albuterol on a milligram basis | Use has not been studied for severe asthma exacerbations<br>Do not mix with other drugs |
| MDI (370 mcg per puff) | See albuterol dose | See albuterol dose | Use has not been studied for severe asthma exacerbation |
| Levalbuterol (*R*-albuterol) nebulizer solution (0.63 mg/3 mL, 1.25 mg/3 mL) | 1.25-2.5 mg every 20 min for 3 doses, then 1.25-5 mg every 1-4 hr as needed, or 5-7.5 mg/hr continuously | 0.075 mg/kg (minimum dose, 1.25 mg) every 20 min for 3 doses, then 0.075-0.15 mg/kg up to 5 mg every 1-4 hr as needed, or 0.25 mg/kg/hr by continuous nebulization | 0.63 mg of levalbuterol is equivalent to 1.25 mg of racemic albuterol in both efficacy and side effects |
| Pirbuterol MDI (200 mcg per puff) | See albuterol dose | See albuterol dose<br>Thought to be half as potent as albuterol on a milligram basis | Use has not been studied for severe asthma exacerbations |
| **Systemic (Injected) $\beta_2$-Agonists** | | | |
| Epinephrine 1:1000 (1 mg/mL) | 0.3-0.5 mg every 20 min for 3 doses SC | 0.01 mg/kg up to 0.3-0.5 mg every 20 min for 3 doses SC | No proven advantage of systemic therapy over aerosol |
| Terbutaline (1 mg/mL) | 0.25 mg every 20 min for 3 doses SC | 0.01 mg/kg every 20 min for 3 doses, then every 2-6 hr as needed SC | No proven advantage of systemic therapy over aerosol |
| **Anticholinergics** | | | |
| Ipratropium bromide | | | |
| Nebulizer solution (0.25 mg/mL) | 0.5 mg every 30 min for 3 doses, then every 2-4 hr as needed | 0.25 mg every 20 min for 3 doses, then every 2 to 4 hr | May mix in same nebulizer with albuterol<br>Should not be used as first-line therapy; should be added to $\beta_2$-agonist therapy |
| MDI (18 mcg per puff) | 4-8 puffs as needed | 4-8 puffs as needed | Dose delivered from MDI is low, and its use has not been studied for asthma exacerbations |
| Ipratropium with albuterol | | | |
| Nebulizer solution (each 3-mL vial contains 0.5 mg ipratropium bromide and 90 mcg albuterol) | 3 mL every 30 min for 3 doses, then every 2-4 hr as needed | 1.5 mL every 20 min for 3 doses, then every 2-4 hr | Contains EDTA to prevent discoloration<br>This additive does not induce bronchospasm |
| MDI (each puff contains 18 mcg ipratropium bromide and 90 mcg albuterol) | 4-8 puffs as needed | 4-8 puffs as needed | |

Continued

**Table 48.2 Medications Used to Treat Asthma Exacerbations—cont'd**

| | *Dosages* | | |
|---|---|---|---|
| **MEDICATION** | **ADULT DOSE** | **CHILD DOSE*** | **COMMENTS** |
| **Systemic Corticosteroids†** | | | |
| Prednisone, methylprednisolone, prednisolone | 40-80 mg/day in 1 or 2 divided doses until PEF reaches 70% of predicted value or patient's personal best | 1 mg/kg (maximum, 60 mg/day) in 2 divided doses until PEF reaches 70% of predicted value or patient's personal best | For outpatient "burst," use 40-60 mg in a single dose or 2 divided doses for adults (children: 1-2 mg/kg/day; maximum, 60 mg/day) for 3-10 days |

*EDTA*, Ethylenediaminetetraacetic acid; *MDI*, metered dose inhaler; *PEF*, peak expiratory flow; *SC*, subcutaneously.

*Children younger than 12 years.

†*Note*: No advantage has been found for higher-dose corticosteroids for severe asthma exacerbations, nor does intravenous administration have any advantage over oral therapy, provided that gastrointestinal transit time or absorption is not impaired. The usual regimen is to continue the frequent multiple daily doses until the patient achieves a forced expiratory volume in 1 second or PEF of 50% of the predicted value or the patient's personal best—which usually occurs within 48 hours—and then to lower the dosage to twice daily. Therapy after a hospitalization or ED visit may last 3 to 10 days. For corticosteroid courses lasting 1 week or less, there is no need to taper the systemic corticosteroid dose. For slightly longer courses (e.g., up to 10 days), there is probably no need to taper, especially if patients are concurrently taking inhaled corticosteroids. If the follow-up systemic corticosteroid therapy is to be given once daily, one study indicates that it may be more clinically effective to give the dose in the afternoon at 3 PM, with no increase in adrenal suppression.[18]

evidence of myocardial ischemia are rare, especially in patients without a previous history of coronary artery disease.

Aerosol therapy with $\beta_2$-agonist drugs produces excellent bronchodilation with minimal systemic absorption and few side effects. Aerosol delivery may be achieved with a metered dose inhaler (MDI) with a spacing device or a compressor-driven nebulizer.[19] A spacing device attached to the inhaler can improve drug deposition when patient technique is inadequate. Even with optimal technique only a maximum of 15% of the dose of the drug is retained in the lungs, regardless of the aerosol method used. Since 2008, dry-powder delivery devices and MDIs using hydrofluoroalkane as propellant have replaced chlorinated fluorocarbon–driven devices. Aerosol treatments may be administered every 15 to 20 minutes or on a continuous basis.[20] Subcutaneous administration of terbutaline or epinephrine may be used in patients unable to coordinate aerosolized or MDI treatments or to tolerate aerosolized medications.[21]

Intravenous $\beta_2$-agonist infusions offer no advantage over aerosolized or MDI-delivered agents and carry potential risk.[22]

Salmeterol xinafoate is indicated only as maintenance therapy, should never be used more frequently than twice per day, and is to be avoided for the treatment of acute exacerbations.[1]

### Corticosteroids

Corticosteroids, highly effective drugs for asthma exacerbation, are a cornerstone of treatment.[23] They are thought to produce beneficial effects by restoring $\beta_2$-agonist responsiveness and reducing inflammation. Onset of the antiinflammatory effects of corticosteroids is delayed at least 4 to 8 hours after intravenous or oral administration.

Data indicate that corticosteroids, administered within 1 hour of arrival in the ED, reduce the need for hospitalization of a patient with an asthma exacerbation.[23] Although evidence for what constitutes the optimal dose for acute asthma is lacking, experts agree that an initial 40- to 60-mg dose of prednisone or an intravenous 60- to 125-mg bolus of methylprednisolone in patients unable to tolerate oral medications is usually adequate. No advantage has been demonstrated for higher doses.[24] Additional doses should be given every 4 to 6 hours until significant subjective and objective improvement is achieved. Patients who are being discharged home after ED treatment should be prescribed a 3- to 10-day nontapering "burst" of oral steroids, such as prednisone, 40 to 60 mg/day, or its equivalent.

Current recommendations favor inhaled corticosteroids for maintenance of all patients with mild persistent asthma or more severe asthma.[1] Therefore, consideration should be given to discharging any patient with mild persistent or more severe asthma with maintenance inhaled corticosteroid therapy in addition to the burst of oral steroids.[25]

### Anticholinergics

Aerosolized ipratropium bromide, 0.5 mg, should be administered to patients with a severe exacerbation of asthma. Ipratropium is a synthetic quaternary derivative that is available as both a nebulized solution and in an MDI (18 mg per puff) and is well tolerated (see Table 48.2). Clinical trials indicate that adding ipratropium to $\beta_2$-agonist agents offers mild additional improvement in bronchodilation and significantly decreases the need for hospitalization.[26] Side effects include dry mouth, thirst, and difficulty swallowing. Less commonly, tachycardia, restlessness, irritability, confusion, difficulty in micturition, ileus, blurring of vision, and an increase in intraocular pressure are noted.

At discharge, addition of tiotropium to the patient's current inhaled corticosteroid dose is comparable to the addition of salmeterol—both are more effective in achieving disease control than is doubling the inhaled corticosteroid dose.[27]

### *Magnesium*

Intravenous magnesium sulfate is indicated for the management of acute, very severe asthma, such as a patient with an $FEV_1$ less than 25% of predicted, but not in those with mild or moderate asthma exacerbation.[28-30] The dose is 1 to 2 g intravenously delivered over a 30-minute period. Inhaled magnesium may also be a helpful adjunct in the treatment of a severe exacerbation.[31,32] Magnesium is not a substitute for standard therapy regimens.

### *Heliox, Ketamine, and Halothane*

Helium is not indicated for use in patients with mild or moderate asthma exacerbation, although several studies have demonstrated its effectiveness for very severe asthma.[33] Several investigators have reported success with ketamine[34,35] and halothane in patients in whom all other treatment modalities have failed. Controlled trials substantiating these claims are lacking.

### *Mast Cell Modifiers*

Neither cromolyn nor nedocromil, both modulators of mast cell mediator release and eosinophil recruitment, is indicated for the treatment of acute bronchospasm.

### *Leukotriene Modifiers*

Leukotriene modifiers improve lung function, diminish symptoms, and reduce the need for short-acting $\beta_2$-agonists.[1] They are recommended as an alternative to low-dose inhaled corticosteroid therapy in patients with mild persistent asthma and as steroid-sparing agents with inhaled corticosteroids in those with moderate persistent asthma. Several leukotriene modifiers—montelukast, zafirlukast, and zileuton—are currently available as oral tablets for the treatment of asthma. Although intravenous montelukast has been demonstrated to cause rapid bronchodilation when used as adjuvant therapy for acute asthma in a single trial, recommending its use for the treatment of acute bronchospasm in the ED would be premature.[36] Montelukast, zafirlukast, and zileuton have been associated with neuropsychiatric side effects.

### *Theophylline*

Although theophylline is no longer considered a first-line treatment of acute asthma,[37] some patients who come to the ED for treatment may be using it at home. Some data suggest that this agent has an antiinflammatory mechanism of action. When used in combination with inhaled $\beta_2$-agonists, theophylline appears to increase the toxicity—but not the efficacy—of treatment. The most common side effects of theophylline are nervousness, nausea, vomiting, anorexia, and headache. At plasma theophylline levels greater than 30 mcg/mL, there is a risk for seizures and cardiac arrhythmias.

## MECHANICAL VENTILATION

When it appears that a patient needs more than the aforementioned treatments, noninvasive positive pressure ventilation may be attempted. Data showing that bilevel positive airway pressure reduces the need for intubation and mechanical ventilation are lacking.[38-40]

If the patient begins to exhibit signs of acute ventilatory failure with progressive hypercapnia and acidosis or becomes exhausted or confused, intubation and mechanical ventilation are needed to prevent respiratory arrest. Mechanical ventilation can eliminate the work of breathing and enable the patient to rest. It does not relieve the airflow obstruction. Direct, controlled oral intubation by an experienced physician is preferred.

The potential complications of mechanical ventilation in asthmatic patients are numerous: barotrauma, hemodynamic impairment, mucous plugging leading to increased airway resistance, atelectasis, and pulmonary infection. Air trapping and increased residual volume (intrinsic positive end-expiratory pressure) may be partially avoided with controlled mechanical hypoventilation or permissive hypoventilation.[39,40] This form of mechanical ventilation is achieved by using a reduced respiratory rate and low inspiratory volume and pressure and allowing adequate time for the expiratory phase. One can achieve the goal of ventilatory support—maintenance of adequate arterial oxygen saturation (90% or greater)—without concern about "normalizing" the hypercapnic acidosis. All patients requiring mechanical ventilation should be admitted to an intensive care unit.

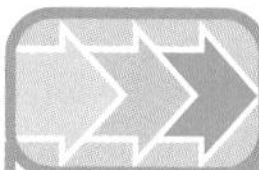

**PRIORITY ACTIONS**

1. Ensure adequate oxygenation.
2. Reverse airflow obstruction with $\beta_2$-agonists.
3. Relieve inflammation by prescribing oral systemic corticosteroids.
4. Monitor response to therapy with serial assessments.

## DISPOSITION

Disposition decisions for patients after treatment of asthma exacerbation are rarely straightforward. A number of subjective and objective factors should be considered, as follows:

- Does the patient feel that the wheezing and air exchange have improved?
- Does auscultation confirm improvement or lack thereof?
- Has a significant improvement in $FEV_1$ or PEF been noted?
- What is the patient's health care history?
- Is the patient usually compliant with care plans and medication regimens?
- Does the patient have access to prompt follow-up?
- Does the patient usually require hospitalization after an exacerbation?

Unfortunately, a formula for successful discharge without risk for early relapse does not yet exist, and up to 25% of patients treated in the ED for asthma return within 3 weeks.[41-44]

Because some degree of residual airflow obstruction, airway lability, and inflammation persists after treatment and discharge from the ED, a postdischarge treatment plan must be formulated.

Addition of a short, nontapering course of oral steroids to the scheduled use of a $\beta_2$-agonist bronchodilator reduces relapse rates in discharged patients. Patients with chronic asthma who are not using controller medications at home should be prescribed and educated about the daily use of either inhaled corticosteroids or leukotriene modifiers, in addition to their rescue medications.[45] Data indicate that relying on the primary care physician to prescribe these controllers at follow-up is inadequate.[25]

Current guidelines suggest that patients with a good response to treatment, as demonstrated by complete resolution of symptoms and a PEF or $FEV_1$ value greater than 70% of predicted, can be safely discharged home. Patients with a poor response to treatment, as defined by persistent symptoms, a PEF or $FEV_1$ value less than 50% of predicted, and persistent wheezing and dyspnea at rest, should be admitted. Many patients with an incomplete response to treatment, as defined by some persistence of symptoms and a PEF or $FEV_1$ value between 50% and 70% of predicted, may be discharged home safely, provided that they have no risk factors for death from asthma.[1] Patients who do not show adequate improvement over several hours because they are in the late phase of the exacerbation and those with significant risk factors for death from asthma should be admitted to either an observation unit or the hospital. Most patients have an incomplete response to treatment and fall into this "gray zone" of disposition decisions.

Studies indicate that the majority of asthmatic patients admitted to an observation unit where strict care protocols are followed can be successfully treated and discharged.[45]

Early follow-up care is indicated to monitor resolution of the exacerbation and to review the long-term medication and care plans for the ongoing management of asthma. High relapse rates despite the routine use of steroids strongly suggest the need for follow-up within days of the ED visit. Ideally, education of the patient begins in the ED, and a written plan of action that addresses both routine treatment and care of worsening symptoms is developed either in the ED or at follow-up. ED personnel should provide basic education about asthma and help connect the patient with a primary care provider or asthma specialist while providing discharge instructions. Review of the patient's discharge medication, evaluation of inhaler technique, and instruction on the use of peak flow monitoring are just some of the issues that emergency physicians can teach and emphasize.

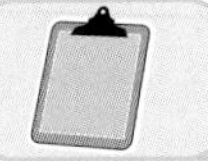

### DOCUMENTATION

**History**

Asthma control and severity

Previous severe exacerbations (need for intubation or intensive care unit admission)

Risk factors:

- Two or more hospitalizations or more than three emergency department visits in the past year
- Use of more than two canisters of short-acting β-agonists per month
- Poor perception of bronchospasm
- Medication noncompliance
- Illicit drug use
- Major psychosocial problems or psychiatric disease
- Comorbid conditions, such as cardiovascular disease or other chronic lung disease

**Examination**

Vital signs and oxygen saturation

Cardiopulmonary examination

**Emergency Department Course**

Monitor response to therapy with serial assessments

## SUGGESTED READINGS

National Institutes of Health, National Heart, Lung and Blood Institute, National Asthma Education and Prevention Program. Expert Panel Report 3: guidelines for the diagnosis and management of asthma. NIH Publication No. 08–4051. Bethesda, MD: U.S. Department of Health and Human Services; August 2007.

Rodrigo GJ, Castro-Rodriguez JA. Anticholinergics in the treatment of children and adults with acute asthma: a systematic review with meta-analysis. Thorax 2005;60:740-6.

Rowe BH, Spooner C, Ducharme FM, et al. Early emergency department treatment of acute asthma with systemic corticosteroids. Cochrane Database Syst Rev 2001;1:CD002178.

Rowe BH, Spooner CH, Ducharme FM, et al. Corticosteroids for preventing relapse following acute exacerbations of asthma (Cochrane Review). In: The Cochrane Library. Oxford: Update Software; 2004.

## REFERENCES

***References can be found on Expert Consult @ www.expertconsult.com.***

# Chronic Obstructive Pulmonary Disease

49

*Craig G. Bates and Rita K. Cydulka*

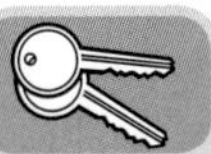

**KEY POINTS**

- Chronic obstructive pulmonary disease (COPD) is a chronic lung disease with significant societal costs; its prevalence is probably underestimated.
- Acute exacerbations of COPD are usually triggered by respiratory irritants or infections that initiate an inflammatory cascade.
- Emergency department evaluation of potential acute exacerbations must include evaluation for other life-threatening causes of dyspnea such as cardiac ischemia, pneumonia, pulmonary embolism, and congestive heart failure.
- Emergency department management of COPD exacerbation includes oxygen, inhaled bronchodilators, antibiotics, corticosteroids, and in serious cases, noninvasive positive pressure ventilation or intubation.

## PERSPECTIVE

Chronic obstructive pulmonary disease (COPD) is a heterogeneous disease that encompasses clinical entities such as emphysema and chronic bronchitis.[1] Although a variety of guidelines have addressed the definition and diagnosis of COPD, a major issue is that most guidelines include a combination of clinical terms and anatomic pathology, which limits their utility for emergency physicians (EPs). The American Thoracic Society defines COPD as a disease state characterized by the presence of airflow obstruction as a result of chronic bronchitis or emphysema. Chronic bronchitis is defined as the presence of a chronic productive cough for 3 months in each of 2 successive years in a patient in whom other causes of chronic cough have been excluded. Emphysema is defined as abnormal permanent enlargement of the air spaces distal to the terminal bronchioles accompanied by destruction of their walls without obvious fibrosis.[2] A potentially more useful definition for EPs comes from the Global Initiative for Chronic Obstructive Lung Disease (GOLD), which states that COPD is a disease state characterized by airflow limitation that is not fully reversible.[3] The limitation in airflow is usually both progressive and associated with an inflammatory response of the lungs to noxious particles or gases, such as tobacco smoke in particular. This definition encompasses chronic bronchitis, emphysema, bronchiectasis, and to a lesser extent, asthma and acknowledges that most patients with COPD have a combination of these different diseases.

## EPIDEMIOLOGY

Lack of agreement among definitions of COPD, combined with delayed diagnosis in many patients, makes estimates of prevalence difficult. In 2008, 13.1 million U.S. adults (aged 18 and older) were estimated to have COPD,[4] but close to 24 million U.S. adults have evidence of impaired lung function, thus indicating underdiagnosis of COPD.[5]

COPD accounted for 1.5 million emergency department (ED) visits and 726,000 hospitalizations in 2000.[6] In 2010, the cost to the nation for COPD was projected to be approximately $49.9 billion, including $29.5 billion in direct health care expenditures, $8.0 billion in indirect morbidity costs, and $12.4 billion in indirect mortality costs.[7] COPD was the third leading cause of death in the United States in 2007 with 124,477 victims, more than half of whom were female.[8] Of note, the prevalence of COPD in women has doubled in the past few decades but has remained stable in men.

In industrialized countries, 80% to 90% of the risk for COPD is from cigarette smoking. Tobacco smoke is the major risk factor for the development of COPD, but only 15% of smokers experience COPD. Other factors associated with the development of COPD, in addition to smoking, are occupational dust, chemical exposure, and air pollution.

## PATHOPHYSIOLOGY

### CHRONICALLY COMPENSATED CHRONIC OBSTRUCTIVE PULMONARY DISEASE

The lung reacts to irritants such as tobacco smoke by increasing the number of macrophages and neutrophils in the airways, lung interstitium, and alveoli. In susceptible individuals, these inflammatory cells release proteases that if left unchecked, eventually break down lung parenchyma and stimulate mucus secretion. Cells that normally secrete surfactant and protease inhibitors are replaced by mucus-secreting cells. At the alveolar and bronchiolar level there is loss of elastic recoil caused by tissue destruction, as well as collapse and narrowing of the smaller airways because of loss of surfactant-producing cells. At the bronchial level, irritants cause pooling of mucus and resultant colonization by bacteria.

### ACUTE EXACERBATIONS

Acute exacerbations of COPD are usually triggered by an event, such as an infection or other respiratory irritant, that starts an inflammatory cascade. In more than 75% of patients with acute exacerbations an infectious agent is found.[9] In addition, it is likely that up to 50% of acute exacerbations are bacterial in nature.[10] Other important triggers for exacerbation are oxidative stress, lower temperatures,[11] and medications. Beta-blockers, sedatives, and narcotics are the medications that most frequently contribute to exacerbations. Regardless of the specific trigger or triggers, inflammatory mediators cause bronchoconstriction and pulmonary vasoconstriction.

Another aspect of the pathophysiology of acute exacerbation is the potential for acute respiratory acidosis. When high levels of inspired oxygen are administered during management of a COPD exacerbation, the vasoconstriction that normally shunts blood away from inadequately ventilated areas is reversed, thereby leading to worsening ventilation-perfusion mismatch and acute rises in the arterial $CO_2$ concentration. Contrary to previous dogma, the hypoxic drive in this process has no significant role.

The overall clinical picture during acute exacerbations of COPD is caused by bronchospasm, inflammation, and mucus hypersecretion, which results in airway narrowing, worsening ventilation-perfusion mismatch, and hypoxemia. The work of breathing increases during an exacerbation as a result of greater airway resistance and hyperinflation. This increase creates a higher oxygen demand by the respiratory muscles, which further contributes to the physiologic stress on the patient.[12] The limitation in expiratory airflow is not significantly increased during acute exacerbations, and the majority of the pathophysiologic manifestations result from ventilation-perfusion mismatch.[13]

## PRESENTING SIGNS AND SYMPTOMS

### CLASSIC

The signs and symptoms in a chronically compensated patient depend largely on the stage of the patient's disease. Very early in the course of the disease, patients often do not carry the diagnosis of COPD and have subtle findings, such as mild exertional dyspnea and a chronic cough that is frequently identified as a "smoker's cough."

Acute exacerbations produce signs and symptoms that represent the impact on multiple body systems. See **Table 49.1** for the signs and symptoms of both chronically compensated COPD and acute exacerbations of COPD.

### VARIATIONS

Because COPD encompasses a wide range of severity of disease, it has a variety of different manifestations. The biggest variations are to be found at the extremes of disease.

Early in the course of the disease, patients may simply have a persistent cough without notable dyspnea. It is important to identify such patients and secure follow-up care. Patients may also note a dry cough that is triggered by deep breaths and may or may not be associated with wheezing and dyspnea. This symptom suggests an episode of bronchitis that could be an exacerbation of underlying lung disease in at-risk patients.

Patients in the late stages of COPD pose a new set of challenges. Those with significant airway obstruction may not

**Table 49.1 Signs and Symptoms of Chronic Obstructive Pulmonary Disease (COPD)**

| TYPE OF COPD | SYMPTOMS | SIGNS |
|---|---|---|
| Chronically compensated COPD | | |
| Earlier stages of disease (not likely to have a COPD diagnosis yet) | Mild to moderate exertional dyspnea<br>Chronic cough, frequently with small-volume hemoptysis | Mild tachypnea<br>Wheezing with forced expiration |
| Later stages of disease | Increasing exertional dyspnea | Prolonged expiratory phase (pursed-lip breathing)<br>Increasing tachypnea<br>End-expiratory wheezing with normal breathing<br>Use of accessory respiratory muscles<br>Weight loss caused by both reduced caloric intake and increased caloric demands from work of breathing<br>Plethora from secondary polycythemia<br>Barrel chest (predominantly emphysematous disease)<br>Decreased breath sounds globally (predominantly emphysematous disease)<br>Coarse crackles or rhonchi from increased secretions (predominantly bronchitic disease) |
| Acute exacerbations | Dyspnea at rest<br>Exertional dyspnea that inhibits normal activities<br>Increase in coughing frequency and/or change in appearance of sputum<br>Apprehension | Tachypnea at rest<br>Use of accessory respiratory muscles<br>Diffuse expiratory wheezing at all times<br>Tachycardia<br>Cyanosis<br>Altered mental status |

generate enough air movement to wheeze and have a "silent chest." Such patients need aggressive management to avoid progressive respiratory failure. Patients with a significantly enlarged chest from emphysematous changes may be difficult to auscultate. Finally, patients with severe hypoxemia or hypercapnia (or both) may have primarily symptoms of altered mentation.

## DIFFERENTIAL DIAGNOSIS

The differential diagnosis of acute dyspnea is quite large. Because many of these conditions are life-threatening, it is critical to differentiate between them so that appropriate treatment can be initiated.

The EP must resist the temptation to automatically diagnose COPD as the sole cause of dyspnea in a patient with a history of COPD. Patients with COPD frequently have serious comorbid conditions that may be unrecognized and play a role in their ED visit. It is also important for the EP to continue to keep an open mind to the possibility of alternative diagnoses, particularly if the patient is not showing the expected response to standard treatment of COPD.

### ASTHMA

Asthma and COPD coexist in some patients, and both diseases involve the presence of airway obstruction, with some key differences. In the ED setting the key point is that the initial stabilizing actions for severe manifestations of either disease do not vary greatly.

### CONGESTIVE HEART FAILURE

Congestive heart failure (CHF) can pose a significant diagnostic challenge for EPs because it can be manifested similar to other causes of acute dyspnea and also coexists with other chronic causes of dyspnea such as COPD. Patients with a history of both conditions and acute dyspnea may have exacerbations of one or even both conditions at the same time.

Historical elements are minimally helpful in discriminating among patients. Although studies indicate that the presence of orthopnea (likelihood ratio [LR] = 2.0) and dyspnea with exertion (LR = 1.3) is more commonly associated with CHF, both symptoms are common in either disease.[14]

Physical examination can be of some assistance in clarifying the differentiation between CHF and COPD. The presence of jugular venous distention is helpful in pointing toward CHF, and evidence has shown that hepatojugular reflux is probably more reliable.[15] To check hepatojugular reflux, the EP puts the head of the bed at 45 degrees and presses on the upper part of the patient's abdomen for 10 seconds. The result is positive if the venous pulsations rise at least 3 cm over baseline. Wheezing can be present with both CHF and COPD and therefore does not have high diagnostic certainty.

The chest radiograph is most useful in patients with evidence of significant interstitial edema. Absence of this finding does not rule out CHF, however, because patients with chronic lung disease are less likely to have the classic chest radiographic findings of CHF.[15]

The brain natriuretic peptide (BNP) assay shows great promise in assisting in making the diagnosis of CHF. In one study it was more accurate than any other single variable (including the history, physical examination, chest radiographs, and electrocardiogram) in determining whether CHF was present.[16] It is most helpful if the value is very high (>500 pg/mL) or very low (<100 pg/mL).[17,18] A number of disease states other than CHF can cause elevation of the BNP value; in particular, the presence of COPD with associated cor pulmonale elevates the BNP value to a lesser degree than does left-sided failure.[19] Be aware that obesity can falsely decrease a BNP value.[20]

### PULMONARY EMBOLISM

The diagnosis of pulmonary embolism (PE) must be considered in any dyspneic patient, particularly when risk factors for venous thromboembolism are present. There is evidence that 25% of patients with a severe COPD exacerbation of unknown origin actually have PE.[21,22] Key risk factors include older age, recent surgery or trauma, previous venous thromboembolism, hereditary thrombophilia such as factor V Leiden, malignancy, smoking, and use of estrogen-containing hormone replacement therapy. The classic manifestation of PE—pleuritic chest pain, dyspnea, tachycardia, and hypoxia—is not frequently encountered in the ED, but at least one of these elements is almost always present. Some historical clues to possible PE are a sudden onset of symptoms and syncope or near syncope in combination with the risk factors listed previously.

Physical examination offers no clues to the diagnosis of PE in 28% to 58% of patients.[23] The diagnosis is based on a combination of the initial clinical impression of a patient's risk level and the results of additional testing such as pulmonary imaging. Patients with significant underlying asthma or COPD are frequently not good candidates for ventilation-perfusion scans because preexisting ventilation and perfusion abnormalities will reduce the utility of the test by increasing the likelihood of an intermediate-probability result. D-dimer testing may be of some assistance in patients with a sufficiently low pretest probability, as determined by various clinical decision rules in the literature. The EP must be aware of the many disease processes that cause false-positive results and make the utility of D-dimer assay questionable in many acutely ill patients. It is of highest utility in a population that is at low risk for PE and has a lower severity of symptoms, and it is unlikely to include patients with an exacerbation of COPD.

### ACUTE CORONARY SYNDROME

Dyspnea can be the main complaint in patients with acute coronary syndromes. Among elderly patients with a diagnosis of acute coronary syndrome in the Global Registry of Acute Coronary Events (GRACE), dyspnea was the dominant symptom in 49.3%.[24] An electrocardiogram should be obtained in all patients seen in the ED with significant dyspnea. Patients with underlying coronary artery disease may have elevations in cardiac biomarkers simply from cardiac myonecrosis secondary to hypoxia. Clinical judgment will guide further cardiac evaluation.

### PNEUMOTHORAX

COPD is a risk factor for spontaneous pneumothorax, and the primary diagnostic tool is the chest radiograph. The EP should also look for clinical clues, such as asymmetric chest wall excursion and asymmetry in breath sounds or, in more severe cases, tracheal deviation and hemodynamic instability.

### PNEUMONIA

Pneumonia commonly coexists with a COPD exacerbation. Clues such as the presence of fever and asymmetric rales on chest auscultation are helpful, but the chest radiograph remains the most useful tool for this diagnosis. The EP should be wary of the accuracy of temperatures taken orally in patients with tachypnea.[25]

## DIAGNOSTIC TESTING

### HISTORY

The history should focus on determining the severity of disease to predict critical outcomes, such as the need for admission and mechanical ventilation. Key historical elements include fever, changes in sputum production, hemoptysis, exercise tolerance, orthopnea, current medications, and compliance with medications. The EP should remember to consider key elements of the differential diagnosis while taking the history and should remain alert for alternative causes of the patient's dyspnea. The presence of symptoms such as chest pain and leg swelling and clarification of how acute in onset the symptoms were will help include or exclude other life-threatening diseases. Important historical questions to ask patients with possible COPD for the purpose of risk stratification are listed in **Box 49.1**.

### PHYSICAL EXAMINATION

On entering the room, the EP should observe the patient's overall level of distress and body position. Patients with significantly increased work of breathing or in the tripod position should undergo immediate and aggressive intervention.

The patient's respiratory rate should then be assessed; very high or very low respiratory rates are ominous. Next, the patient's use of accessory muscles and the proportion of the expiratory phase during breathing should be evaluated. The expiratory phase will lengthen in direct proportion to the degree of airway obstruction. The length of the patient's sentences provides a simple method of determining the severity of the illness and can be used for more objective reassessment after treatment is initiated.

Assessment of the patient's overall mental status should follow. Before being spoken to, does the patient appear awake and alert or drowsy? When asked questions, does the patient respond quickly and do the answers make sense? Mental status is an important clue to the level of hypoxia or hypercapnia present.

Next, the EP should observe movement of the chest wall. Is it symmetric? Is there evidence of abdominal breathing, or are retractions present? On auscultation, are wheezes, rales, or rhonchi apparent, and where are they located? The EP should be wary of a "silent chest," which implies poor air movement. Wheezing can occur as a result of CHF, and asymmetric auscultation findings suggest other diagnoses, such as pneumothorax and pneumonia.

The remainder of the physical examination should focus on findings that suggest alternative diagnoses. The EP should seek signs of CHF, such as gallop rhythms, jugular venous distention, and symmetric lower extremity edema. Asymmetric lower extremity edema and calf tenderness would suggest deep vein thrombosis.

**BOX 49.1 Important Historical Questions for Risk Stratification of Patients with Chronic Obstructive Pulmonary Disease**

How many times have you visited the emergency department in the past year? When was the last time?
How many times have you been admitted to the hospital in the past year? When was the last time?
Have you ever been intubated or placed on bilevel positive airway pressure ventilation?
Do you use oxygen at home? If so, how many liters per minute and how many hours per day?
Are you taking prednisone on a regular basis?
Does this feel like your usual exacerbation of chronic obstructive pulmonary disease?
How bad does this attack seem to you?

### IMAGING AND LABORATORY TESTING

#### *Chest Radiographs*

Chest radiographs should be obtained in all patients with anything but a very mild acute exacerbation of COPD. Evidence has shown that clinical criteria are unreliable in accurately predicting the need for radiography.[26] The chest radiograph provides valuable information about alternative diagnoses, such as pneumonia, CHF, pneumothorax, and aortic dissection.[3]

#### *Pulse Oximetry*

Pulse oximetry provides a simple and noninvasive method of monitoring hypoxemia in patients with exacerbations of COPD. Pulse oximeters provide accurate estimates of $Pa{O_2}$ (arterial partial pressure of oxygen), as long as the $Sa{O_2}$ (arterial oxygen saturation) value is greater than approximately 90%; with an $Sa{O_2}$ value below this level, the hemoglobin-oxygen dissociation curve becomes quite steep and the correlation is far less reliable. Evidence indicates that an $Sa{O_2}$ value of 92% correlates with a $Pa{O_2}$ value of greater than 60 mm Hg.[27]

#### *Arterial Blood Gas Analysis*

Arterial blood gas (ABG) measurements are not routinely required for COPD exacerbations, although they can be helpful in patients with altered mental status, severe distress, or acidosis. ABG analysis can be helpful for estimating the severity of exacerbations or predicting the future need for mechanical ventilation or bilevel positive airway pressure (BiPAP).[28] Patients with simultaneous hypoxemia and hypercapnia are at greatest risk for the development of respiratory failure. It is important to remember that the decision to initiate mechanical ventilation should be based on clinical grounds and not be delayed to obtain ABG results. ABG values can provide clues to questions about issues such as patient fatigue but can never replace the decision-making ability of an experienced EP.

Venous blood gas values may be used to screen for hypercapnia. Although correlation between arterial and venous pH is good, agreement for $P{CO_2}$ (partial pressure of carbon dioxide) is only fair. Data indicate that venous $P_{CO_2}$ is 5.8 mm Hg higher than arterial $P_{CO_2}$, but the confidence interval was wide and the correlation was not consistent. This same study indicated that when a cutoff of 45 mm Hg is used, venous blood gas measurements are 100% sensitive and 57% specific in detecting hypercapnia.[29]

### *Spirometry*

Unlike the case with asthma, spirometry is not of significant utility in assessing acute exacerbations of COPD. Spirometry in patients with COPD is most useful in the primary care setting to monitor disease progression over time. Its use in diagnosing or assessing acute exacerbation is not recommended by either the American College of Physicians or the American College of Chest Physicians. Forced expiratory volume in 1 second ($FEV_1$) is only weakly correlated with $P_{CO_2}$ and pH and has no correlation with arterial $P_{O_2}$ in acute exacerbations.[30] Although many ED studies use spirometry to track clinical changes in patients with COPD, it is important to realize that doing so may provide an incomplete picture of patient status.

### *Additional Laboratory Testing*

No data support or refute the use of routine laboratory testing such as a complete blood count or serum chemistry panels in patients with exacerbations of COPD. The need will be dictated mainly by the potential alternative diagnoses, such as CHF or pneumonia. A serum chemistry panel is helpful if an ABG measurement has been ordered. ABG analysis provides a more reliable bicarbonate measurement for clarifying the acuity of respiratory acidosis and in addition assists in diagnosing other acid-base disorders that may be present. A serum chemistry panel should also be ordered in patients complaining of vomiting or weakness and in patients who are taking diuretics or have a history of renal failure. Because of the frequently significant comorbid conditions present in patients with COPD who are sick enough to require admission, laboratory tests for cardiac biomarkers and BNP are often indicated. Other indications for testing are discussed in the section on differential diagnosis.

## INTERVENTIONS, PROCEDURES, AND TREATMENT

ED goals for treating acute exacerbations of COPD are as follows:

- Rule out other life-threatening causes of dyspnea.
- Ensure adequate oxygenation and ventilation.
- Manage reversible airway obstruction.
- Treat any infectious component of the exacerbation.
- Determine appropriate patient disposition.
- Provide a discharge plan of care that will minimize the risk for recurrences.

A concise summary of the ED management of acute exacerbations of COPD can be found in **Table 49.2**, and key indicators of severe disease are described in the Red Flags box. The rest of this section supplies additional detail on the different components of management.

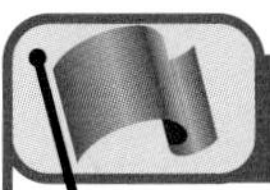

**RED FLAGS**

Worse than the patient's typical exacerbation of chronic obstructive pulmonary disease
Significant hypoxia (i.e., $Sa_{O_2} < 92\%$) with a typical home $O_2$ flow rate
Drowsiness or confusion—probable secondary to hypoxia or hypercapnia
Silent chest—indicative of poor air movement and potential impending respiratory failure

## OXYGEN

Appropriate use of supplemental oxygen is a key component of management of COPD exacerbations. Oxygen has a number of benefits during exacerbations, including relief of pulmonary vasoconstriction, decrease in right heart workload, and reduction of myocardial ischemia. The effects on the heart allow an increase in oxygen delivery to tissues above and beyond simple rises in hemoglobin oxygen saturation.

The challenge is to maintain appropriate oxygenation while not provoking acute $CO_2$ retention. For most patients, targeting an oxygen saturation value of just over 92% (a reasonable surrogate for a $P_{O_2}$ value of 60 mm Hg) provides a good balance between these two issues.[3] Whether this saturation value is maintained with oxygen administered via nasal cannula or a Venturi-type mask is not important as long as the saturation values are closely monitored to avoid delivering too little or too much oxygen.

There is good evidence in the prehospital setting that carefully titrated oxygen delivery results in reduced mortality, hypercapnia, and respiratory acidosis in patients experiencing an acute exacerbation of COPD.[31]

## INHALED MEDICATIONS

After oxygen, inhaled $\beta_2$-agonists and anticholinergics are the primary treatment modality for COPD exacerbations because there is usually a small reversible component of the airflow obstruction.

The prototypic $\beta_2$-agonist for COPD is albuterol, delivered either by nebulizer or by metered dose inhaler (MDI) with a spacer. Side effects include tremor, palpitations, tachycardia, headache, mild hypokalemia, nausea, and vomiting. Evidence has shown that the two delivery methods are probably comparable but that severely dyspneic patients may tolerate nebulized medications better.[32] Albuterol can be given continuously via nebulizer or intermittently. The American Thoracic Society guidelines advise that $\beta_2$-agonists may be used every 30 to 60 minutes but that more frequent use or continuous administration is well tolerated and may have some benefit. However, the literature on continuous administration of $\beta_2$-agonists in the treatment of COPD is limited. Decreasing the treatment interval from 60 to 20 minutes has not been shown to improve $FEV_1$, but patients with a lower starting $FEV_1$ value appear to have more benefit with shorter treatment intervals.[33] It is important to realize the limitations of the $FEV_1$ value in assessing acute exacerbations; the EP should instead rely on the overall clinical picture to guide treatment. Evidence suggests that 2.5 to 5 mg per dose is adequate for the management of COPD exacerbation.[34]

**Table 49.2 Basic Approach to Acute Exacerbations of Chronic Obstructive Pulmonary Disease**

| INTERVENTION | COMMENTS AND CAUTIONS |
|---|---|
| Initiate $O_2$ to maintain saturation >90% | Observe closely for $CO_2$ retention |
| Initiate continuous cardiac monitoring and pulse oximetry | |
| Albuterol, 2.5-5 mg via nebulizer | Can give continuously (10-15 mg/hr) or q20-60min<br>Alternatively, give 4-10 puffs via MDI with spacer |
| Ipratropium, 0.5 mg via nebulizer | Little data on frequency of administration—typically given once during emergency department visit<br>Can mix with albuterol nebulizer<br>Alternatively, give 4-6 puffs via MDI with spacer |
| Prednisone, 60 mg orally, or methylprednisolone (Solu-Medrol), 125 mg intravenously | Oral and intravenous routes probably equivalent in patients who are well enough to tolerate oral administration; however, little data on this issue |
| Administer antibiotics | Many options—common choices include macrolides such as azithromycin (plus ceftriaxone if being admitted) or quinolones such as moxifloxacin<br>Local resistance patterns and patient's previous antibiotic use are important considerations |
| Consider NIPPV in seriously ill patients who do not yet need intubation | NIPPV is most effective in reducing need for intubation if initiated early |
| Chest radiograph | Seek out alternative diagnoses<br>Perform as soon as possible in course because can be done without disrupting lifesaving care |
| Electrocardiography | Most useful for patients with chest pain, arrhythmias, severe exacerbations<br>Strongly consider for all patients |
| Directed laboratory testing | ABG analysis if severe disease, altered mental status, significant hypoxia, suspected acidosis<br>Theophylline level as appropriate<br>Electrolytes if renal failure, vomiting, weakness<br>BNP if differential diagnosis unclear<br>D-dimer as appropriate |
| Further diagnostic imaging | Pulmonary embolism protocol; CT if differential diagnosis in doubt |
| Determination of disposition | If good response to therapy with mild exacerbation, consider discharge home<br>For patients with moderate exacerbations, consider admission to observation unit if available<br>Patients with severe illness and/or multiple significant comorbid conditions will probably need hospital admission—use likelihood of need for ventilatory support to guide decision for ICU versus floor<br>Patients requiring NIPPV should be admitted to a closely monitored setting, which in most hospitals means at least a stepdown-level bed |

*ABG*, Arterial blood gas; *BNP*, brain natriuretic protein; *CT*, computed tomography; *ICU*, intensive care unit; *MDI*, metered dose inhaler; *NIPPV*, noninvasive positive pressure ventilation.

Ipratropium bromide, a quaternary anticholinergic compound, is delivered either by nebulizer or by MDI with a spacer. Side effects include tremor and dry mouth. Both ipratropium bromide and albuterol have comparable clinical effects, and when used together, these two agents improve clinical outcomes and shorten ED length of stay.[35]

Long-acting inhaled anticholinergics, such as tiotropium, have no place in the acute management of COPD. This agent has demonstrated better efficacy than ipratropium taken four times daily for the chronic management of COPD.[36]

## CORTICOSTEROIDS

Administration of corticosteroids in the ED, followed by an outpatient course of treatment, improves oxygenation and airflow and decreases the rate of treatment failures.[37,38] The current literature supports a longer course of treatment than is traditionally done for asthma. Tapering the dosage over a period of 7 to 14 days most likely sufficiently balances the risks associated with corticosteroid use with the advantage of decreased treatment failures. No evidence has shown that a corticosteroid course longer than 14 days confer added benefits. Despite common practice, no strong clinical evidence has indicated that courses shorter than 14 days require a tapering dose.

Administration of corticosteroids in the ED has not been shown to affect the rate of hospitalization. This finding is probably due to the approximate 6-hour delay before the onset of action of corticosteroids.[39] Nevertheless, it is important to administer these medications in the ED as soon as possible and before transferring the patient to an inpatient unit because doing so will probably decrease the overall length of stay in the hospital.

In patients who can tolerate oral intake, there is probably no advantage to intravenous administration of corticosteroids, but data specifically addressing this clinical question are limited.

## ANTIBIOTICS

The use of antibiotics for acute exacerbations of COPD is recommended in all current guidelines despite some conflicting evidence regarding their efficacy. Two large systematic reviews showed an overall benefit to antibiotic use, with greater efficacy in more severe exacerbations.[28,40] Antibiotics shorten the duration of the exacerbation and accelerate recovery of peak expiratory flow rates.

The choice of antibiotic has been studied with particular concern about recent increases in β-lactamase–producing strains of bacteria. There is evidence that newer extended-spectrum quinolones achieve better clinical outcomes at lower overall cost than does nonquinolone therapy in patients at high risk for treatment failure (severe underlying lung disease, more than four exacerbations per year, COPD duration > 10 years, elderly, and significant comorbid illnesses).[41] There is also evidence that newer antibiotics, such as macrolides, quinolones, and amoxicillin-clavulanate, are associated with lower hospitalization and clinical failure rates while costing less overall than older antibiotics such as cephalosporins and trimethoprim-sulfamethoxazole.[42] When selecting an antibiotic, factors such as previous antibiotic treatment in the past 3 months, severity of illness, and community resistance patterns must be taken into account.

The ideal duration of antibiotic treatment is not clear. Data suggest that 5 days of antibiotic treatment is probably sufficient,[43] but studies on the optimal duration of treatment with extended-spectrum macrolides and quinolones are lacking.

## METHYLXANTHINES

Despite a number of guidelines that still recommend their use, methylxanthines such as aminophylline are of no significant benefit to patients with acute exacerbations of COPD and should not be used.[44] It is useful, however, to measure methylxanthine drug levels in patients who are already taking them on an outpatient basis.

## NONINVASIVE POSITIVE PRESSURE VENTILATION

Noninvasive positive pressure ventilation (NIPPV) involves the application of positive pressure ventilation via face mask and is associated with significantly fewer complications than is the case with endotracheal intubation and mechanical ventilation. NIPPV can be applied in one of two modes, continuous positive airway pressure (CPAP) or BiPAP. Both modes can have oxygen bled into the system.

CPAP delivers a continuous level of positive pressure throughout the respiratory cycle and is analogous to positive end-expiratory pressure (PEEP) in mechanical ventilation. CPAP improves respiratory mechanics by increasing mean airway pressure, improving functional residual capacity, and opening underventilated and collapsed alveoli. The overall effect is to enhance gas exchange and oxygenation. CPAP is usually initiated at a low level and titrated upward to a typical maximum of 15 cm $H_2O$ to allow adequate oxygenation with as low an $FIO_2$ (fraction of inspired oxygen) value as possible.

BiPAP provides different levels of positive airway pressure for inspiration (IPAP) and expiration (EPAP). This is analogous to pressure support and PEEP in mechanical ventilation. BiPAP provides the same benefits of continuously applied positive pressure as CPAP does but also theoretically reduces the work of breathing by providing a pressure boost for inspiration. BiPAP can be time-triggered to a certain number of breaths per minute or flow-cycled to allow the patient to trigger the device. IPAP is generally started at approximately 8 cm $H_2O$ and titrated upward to a typical maximum of 20 cm $H_2O$. EPAP is generally started at approximately 4 cm $H_2O$ and titrated upward to a typical maximum of 15 $H_2O$. The settings should be balanced to allow physiologic tidal volumes (5 to 7 mL/kg) and maximal oxygenation with a minimum $FIO_2$ while still maintaining patient comfort.

To be successful candidates for NIPPV, patients must be alert, breathing spontaneously, and able to cooperate with instructions (**Box 49.2**). This modality can be used with extreme care in patients with mild decreases in level of consciousness.[45] A good rule of thumb is that patients who cannot constantly keep their head up independently will not probably succeed with NIPPV. Adequate staffing levels, continuous monitoring of the heart rate and pulse oximetry, and intermittent blood pressure measurements are essential for safe and successful use of NIPPV. NIPPV is most likely to be successful when a partnership exists among the patient, nursing staff, respiratory therapist, and physician that involves effective communication in all directions before and during the initiation of treatment. It is also most likely to be successful if initiated early in the patient's stay in the ED.

As with mechanical ventilation, the EP must be alert for hemodynamic changes and desaturations that may indicate loss of mask seal, intrinsic PEEP (also called auto-PEEP), pneumothorax, and patient intolerance. Gastric distention with resultant restriction of diaphragmatic excursion or vomiting is another potential complication of NIPPV.

Contraindications to NIPPV are altered mental status, impaired airway protection mechanisms, apnea, cardiovascular instability, and pneumothorax. In addition, any craniofacial abnormality (e.g., previous surgery, trauma) that impairs the ability to obtain a reliable mask seal would preclude NIPPV.

**BOX 49.2 Indications for Use of Noninvasive Positive Pressure Ventilation (NIPPV)**

NIPPV should be considered in patients with the following clinical features as long as the contraindications previously discussed are not present:

- Difficulty maintaining oxygen saturation greater than 90% with a nonrebreather mask
- Moderate to severe dyspnea
- Respiratory rate greater than 25 breaths/min
- Moderate respiratory acidosis (pH of 7.30 to 7.35)
- Sufficient alertness to hold one's own head upright and follow commands

**BOX 49.3 General Criteria for Intubation in Patients with Acute Exacerbations of Chronic Obstructive Pulmonary Disease**

Severe dyspnea with the use of accessory muscles
Respiratory rate greater than 35 breaths/min
Life-threatening hypoxemia ($Po_2 < 40$ mm Hg or $Po_2/Fo_2 < 200$)
Severe acidosis (pH < 7.25) and hypercapnia ($Pco_2 > 60$ mmHg)
Respiratory arrest
Somnolence or significant impairment in mental status
Cardiovascular complications (hypotension, shock, heart failure)
Other complications (metabolic abnormalities, sepsis, pneumonia, pulmonary embolism, barotrauma, massive pleural effusion)
Failure of noninvasive positive pressure ventilation

In patients with COPD, NIPPV has been shown to significantly decrease both the need for intubation and overall patient mortality and to generate significant improvements in pH, $Pco_2$, and respiratory rate.[46,47] The delivery method (CPAP versus BiPAP) has not been shown to make a significant difference in outcomes.

## ENDOTRACHEAL INTUBATION AND MECHANICAL VENTILATION

The decision to intubate a patient with COPD is based largely on clinical judgment and experience. Some patients obviously need intubation (respiratory arrest, decline with NIPPV), but in other patients the need is far less apparent. As mentioned previously, ABG values can assist in the decision to intubate, but the ultimate decision must always be based on clinical assessment. Intubation decisions should not be delayed in critically ill patients to wait for ABG results. General guidelines are available to assist in this decision-making process, but they are just tools that will not make the final decision, and some of the guidelines are vague; they are listed in **Box 49.3**.[3]

Once the EP has determined that a patient with COPD requires intubation, a few special considerations should be borne in mind. In general, the largest tube that can fit safely between the vocal cords should be used (8 to 8.5 in men, 7.5 to 8 in women) to decrease overall airway resistance. The EP must also carefully consider the expected difficulty of intubation before administering paralytic agents. Effective bag-valve-mask ventilation can be difficult in patients with COPD because of higher airway resistance and lung hyperinflation. Other potential comorbid conditions such as obesity can also make intubation difficult. Patients with COPD are commonly difficult to preoxygenate adequately, a feature that significantly reduces the time available for direct laryngoscopy. Even in a patient who is known to require intubation, NIPPV combined with supplemental oxygen can be helpful in maximizing the effectiveness of preoxygenation. Consider an "awake" look with a combination of topical anesthesia of the airway and light sedation before using full rapid-sequence intubation, particularly in patients in whom intubation may be difficult. Ketamine in initial doses of 0.5 to 1 mg/kg intravenously has some properties that make it an attractive option in this situation because it preserves the airway protection reflexes and also has bronchodilation properties. Additional doses can be given as necessary. Ketamine can stimulate the sympathetic nervous system, so it should be used with caution in patients with significant coronary artery disease. Other options include benzodiazepines and propofol, but these agents often cause respiratory depression at sedative doses. A full discussion of these issues is outside the scope of this chapter.

**Table 49.3 Causes and Treatment of Hypotension After Initiation of Positive Pressure Ventilation in Patients with Chronic Obstructive Pulmonary Disease**

| CAUSE | TREATMENT |
|---|---|
| Tension pneumothorax | Needle decompression with a large-bore Angiocath |
| Reduced venous return from auto-PEEP (positive end expiratory pressure) | Remove the patient from ventilator<br>Squeeze the chest<br>Adjust the ventilator settings to allow sufficient exhalation time between breaths<br>Fluid boluses to augment preload |
| Reduced sympathetic drive | Use smaller doses of sedative medications and fluid boluses to augment preload; rarely is the use of vasopressors is needed |

The best treatment is anticipation of potential issues—many patients requiring intubation for exacerbations of chronic obstructive pulmonary disease will require preintubation consideration for all these conditions. All patients being intubated should have a fluid bolus ready for rapid administration through a freely flowing intravenous line if needed.

Management of hypotensive episodes in patients recently intubated for COPD is the same as that for other intubated patients, but some causes are more common in COPD. Note that patients with NIPPV can exhibit similar issues. See **Table 49.3** for additional information.

## DISPOSITION AND FOLLOW-UP

The decision to admit or discharge a patient with exacerbation of COPD is multifactorial and involves issues that may not be clinical. The response to ED management is the most useful indicator of disposition. EPs must consider whether the patient will be able to receive the maintenance care necessary at home; that is, outpatient management will almost certainly fail in a patient with an oxygen requirement who was not already receiving oxygen. Clinicians must also estimate the probable clinical course: is this patient showing a clear trend toward improvement, or is the course in doubt? The availability of rapid and reliable follow-up care can allow safe discharge of potentially sicker patients. Unfortunately, the absence of such care is more frequently encountered in the ED environment; patients whose social issues, such as limited access to care, put them at high risk for a return ED visit should be admitted.

Finally, it is important to emphasize to patients with COPD that they should promptly seek medical attention for

**BOX 49.4 Risk Factors for Relapse Within 2 Weeks of an Emergency Department (ED) Visit**

Evidence has shown that the following factors place patients at higher risk for relapse within 2 weeks after an ED visit[49]:

- Number of ED or clinic visits in the past year (>5 visits)
- Amount of limitation in activity before arrival
- Initial respiratory rate higher than 16 breaths/min
- Patients who were taking oral corticosteroids before arriving at the ED

worsening respiratory symptoms. Patients who wait longer than 24 hours before seeking medical attention are more than twice as likely to require admission regardless of what home care was administered.[48]

Patients at higher risk for relapse need more careful discharge planning that includes reliable follow-up (**Box 49.4**).

## SUGGESTED READINGS

Kim S, Emerman CL, Cydulka RK, et al. MARC Investigators: prospective multicenter study of relapse following emergency department treatment of COPD exacerbation. Chest 2004;125:473-81.

Quon BS, Gan WQ, Sin DD. Contemporary management of acute exacerbations of COPD: a systematic review and metaanalysis. Chest 2008;133:756-66.

Ram FSF, Rodriguez-Roisin R, Granados-Navarrete A, et al. Antibiotics for exacerbations of chronic obstructive pulmonary disease. Cochrane Database System Rev 2011;1:CD004403.

Scala R, Naldi M, Archinucci I, et al. Noninvasive positive pressure ventilation in patients with acute exacerbations of COPD and varying levels of consciousness. Chest 2005;128:1657-66.

Walters JAE, Gibson PG, Wood-Baker R, et al. Systemic corticosteroids for acute exacerbations of chronic obstructive pulmonary disease. Cochrane Database Syst Rev 2009;1:CD001288.

## REFERENCES

***References can be found on Expert Consult @ www.expertconsult.com.***

# 50 Lung Infections

*David S. Howes and Joseph F. Peabody*

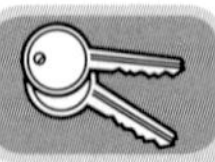

**KEY POINTS**

- A wide variety of infectious agents, including bacteria, viruses, and fungi, cause pneumonia.
- Diagnosis and treatment of pneumonia are determined by assessment of patient risk factors, other elements of the history, diagnostic studies, and physical examination.
- Special care must be taken to identify patients at risk for health care–associated pneumonia or unusual or resistant organisms.
- Chest radiography is an important diagnostic tool that can offer valuable clues to the etiology. Other laboratory and sputum studies may also be useful.
- Because the causative agent is typically not known at initial evaluation, timely institution of carefully selected empiric antibiotic therapy is paramount.
- Age, comorbid diseases, and clinical and laboratory data guide disposition decisions for a patient with pneumonia, such as admission to an intensive care unit.
- Isolation measures such as droplet precautions should be initiated immediately for patients with acute febrile respiratory illnesses.

## EPIDEMIOLOGY

Pneumonia is one of the most common infectious diseases encountered in the emergency department (ED), with more than 1.5 million visits for this infection annually.[1] When combined with influenza, pneumonia ranks as the sixth leading cause of death in the United States and the most common cause of infection-related mortality.[2-5]

Pneumonia is typically defined as an infection of the lung parenchyma with associated symptoms of cough, fever, and abnormal breath sounds on physical examination. Usually an infiltrate is seen on chest radiographs.

Because of the many potential pathogens causing this disease, a thorough history and physical examination are very important in guiding selection of the appropriate empiric antibiotic coverage in patients with pneumonia.

## PATHOPHYSIOLOGY

The lungs are constantly exposed to potential pathogens by both organisms in inspired air and those living in the oropharynx and upper respiratory tract. As a result of multiple layers of defense, the lower respiratory tract usually remains sterile. Many protective mechanisms—the cough and gag reflexes, upper airway particle filtration, proper mucociliary clearance, and humoral and cellular immunologic defenses at the alveolar level—play an important role in guarding the lungs against infection.

Pneumonia typically occurs when the protective defenses just described are breached and the lungs are exposed to a heavy inoculation of organisms or to very virulent organisms. The lung's defenses can be impaired at multiple levels. Aspiration can result when altered levels of consciousness secondary to a neurologic insult or alcohol or drug intoxication impair the gag reflex. The upper airway defenses are often bypassed by endotracheal tubes or tracheostomy. Smoking and chronic lung disease can impair mucociliary function. Bronchial obstruction secondary to tumor or lymphadenopathy can lead to obstruction and pneumonia. Immunologic impairment as a result of infection with human immunodeficiency virus (HIV), chemotherapy, splenectomy, or advanced age also predisposes to pneumonia. The elderly are particularly vulnerable because of impairments at many of these levels and a higher incidence of comorbid conditions[5] (**Fig. 50.1**).

## PRESENTING SIGNS AND SYMPTOMS

The classic symptoms of pneumonia are fever, cough, purulent sputum, and shortness of breath. Patients may also have several nonrespiratory symptoms such as sweats, chills, confusion, headache, fatigue, abdominal pain, nausea, and myalgias. Infants may have decreased oral intake, lethargy, and apnea. Patients of advanced age are less likely to have typical symptoms, instead often exhibiting only weakness or altered mental status.

A goal-directed, comprehensive history is very important in the evaluation of a patient with pneumonia. Historical clues such as risk for aspiration, recent travel, animal or environmental exposure, HIV status or risk, alcoholism, and comorbid illnesses can point toward specific causes and guide the proper choice of initial empiric therapy (**Table 50.1**).[6,7] Special

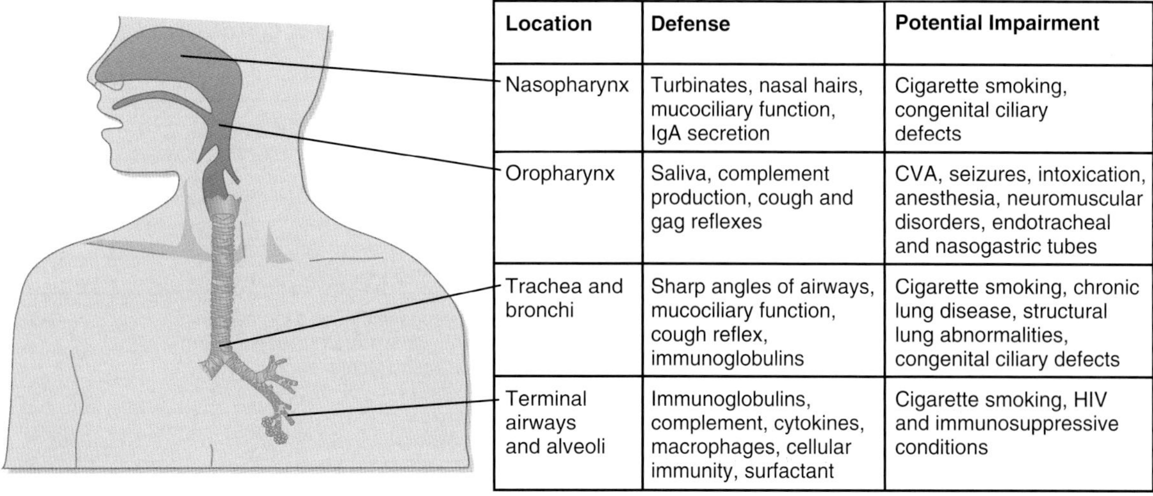

| Location | Defense | Potential Impairment |
|---|---|---|
| Nasopharynx | Turbinates, nasal hairs, mucociliary function, IgA secretion | Cigarette smoking, congenital ciliary defects |
| Oropharynx | Saliva, complement production, cough and gag reflexes | CVA, seizures, intoxication, anesthesia, neuromuscular disorders, endotracheal and nasogastric tubes |
| Trachea and bronchi | Sharp angles of airways, mucociliary function, cough reflex, immunoglobulins | Cigarette smoking, chronic lung disease, structural lung abnormalities, congenital ciliary defects |
| Terminal airways and alveoli | Immunoglobulins, complement, cytokines, macrophages, cellular immunity, surfactant | Cigarette smoking, HIV and immunosuppressive conditions |

**Fig. 50.1 Host defenses against infection.** *CVA*, Cerebrovascular accident; *HIV*, human immunodeficiency virus; *IgA*, immunoglobulin A. (Modified from Donowitz G, Mandell G. Acute pneumonia. In: Mandell GL, Bennett JE, Doline R, editors. Mandell, Douglas, and Bennett's principles and practice of infectious disease. 6th ed. Philadelphia: Saunders; 2005. pp. 819-41.)

**Table 50.1 Epidemiologic Conditions Related to Specific Pathogens in Patients with Selected Community-Acquired Pneumonia**

| CONDITION | COMMONLY ENCOUNTERED PATHOGENS |
|---|---|
| Alcoholism | *Streptococcus pneumoniae,* oral anaerobes |
| Chronic obstructive pulmonary disease and/or smoking | *S. pneumoniae, Haemophilus influenzae, Moraxella catarrhalis, Legionella* spp., *Chlamydia pneumoniae* |
| Poor dental hygiene | Oral anaerobes |
| Aspiration/lung abscess | Oral anaerobes |
| Exposure to bats or to soil enriched with bird droppings | *Histoplasma capsulatum* |
| Exposure to birds | *Chlamydia psittaci,* avian influenza (poultry exposure) |
| Exposure to rabbits | *Francisella tularensis* |
| Exposure to farm animals or parturient cats | *Coxiella burnetii* (Q fever) |
| Human immunodeficiency virus infection: | |
| Early | *S. pneumoniae, H. influenzae, Mycobacterium tuberculosis* |
| Late | Above plus *Pneumocystis jiroveci (carinii), Cryptococcus, Histoplasma* |
| Travel to or residence in the southwestern United States | *Coccidioides* spp. |
| Travel to or residence in Asia | *Burkholderia pseudomallei,* severe acute respiratory syndrome |
| Influenza active in the community ("flu season") | Influenza, *S. pneumoniae, Staphylococcus aureus, H. influenzae* |
| Structural lung disease (e.g., bronchiectasis) | *Pseudomonas aeruginosa, Burkholderia cepacia, S. aureus* |
| Injection drug use | *S. aureus,* skin anaerobes, *M. tuberculosis, S. pneumoniae* |
| Endobronchial obstruction | Anaerobes, *S. pneumoniae, H. influenzae, S. aureus* |
| Recent hospitalization or nursing home residence | Drug-resistant *S. pneumoniae*, gram-negative bacilli, *S. aureus* |
| In the context of bioterrorism | *Bacillus anthracis* (anthrax), *Yersinia pestis* (plague), *F. tularensis* (tularemia) |

Modified from File T, Niederman M. Antimicrobial therapy of community-acquired pneumonia. Infect Dis Clin North Am 2004;18:993-1016.

care should be taken to identify patients at risk for health care–associated pneumonia (HCAP), such as recent health care and antibiotic exposure, which could predispose them to multidrug-resistant pathogens and alter treatment choices.[8]

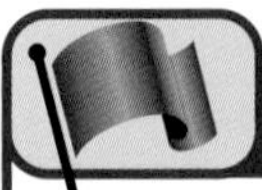

**RED FLAGS**

Look for key clues in the history and physical findings that would suggest pneumonia caused by an unusual or resistant organism.

Identify patients at risk for health care–associated pneumonia.

Maintain high suspicion for aspiration pneumonia in the elderly and in patients with altered mental status or a recent cerebrovascular accident.

**Table 50.2 Etiology of Community-Acquired Pneumonia**

| PATHOGEN | PREVALANCE (%) |
|---|---|
| *Streptococcus pneumoniae* | 20-60 |
| *Haemophilus influenzae* | 3-10 |
| *Staphylococcus aureus* | 3-5 |
| Gram-negative bacilli | 3-10 |
| Miscellaneous (includes *Moraxella catarrhalis*, group A streptococci, and *Neisseria meningitidis*, each accounting for 1-2% of cases) | 3-5 |
| *Legionella* spp. | 2-8 |
| *Mycoplasma pneumoniae* | 1-6 |
| *Chlamydia pneumoniae* | 4-6 |
| Viruses | 2-15 |
| Aspiration | 6-10 |

From Niederman M. Review of treatment guidelines for community acquired pneumonia. Am J Med 2004;117;52S.

## PATHOGENS

Community-acquired pneumonia is often defined as pneumonia in a patient who has not been hospitalized and has not resided in a long-term care facility for more than 14 days before the appearance of symptoms.[3] With the growing prevalence of mixed-organism infections, drug-resistant pathogens, and patients with comorbid illnesses, this definition has become somewhat more complicated. Guidelines from the American Thoracic Society (ATS), Centers for Disease Control and Prevention, and Infectious Diseases Society of America (IDSA) now address the treatment of patients at increased risk for pseudomonal infection, those with significant comorbid conditions, and those at risk for infection with drug-resistant *Streptococcus pneumoniae*.

The most common etiologic agent causing pneumonia is *S. pneumoniae*, which is responsible for about two thirds of all cases (**Table 50.2**).[3] Other bacterial pathogens that are often isolated are *Mycoplasma pneumoniae, Chlamydia pneumoniae, Haemophilus influenzae*, and *Legionella pneumophila* (often called "the atypical organisms"). Community-acquired pneumonia is also caused by several viruses, including influenza, parainfluenza, and respiratory syncytial virus (RSV). Other pathogens, such as *Pseudomonas aeruginosa*, drug-resistant *S. pneumonia*, and methicillin-resistant *Staphylococcus aureus* (MRSA), should additionally be considered in patients who have had recent health care exposure or have recently taken broad-spectrum antibiotics. Multiple other organisms may be considered based on a history of specific exposures, travel, and lung or immunosuppressive diseases.

## SPECIAL POPULATIONS

### CHILDREN

Pneumonia and acute bronchiolitis are the most common lower respiratory tract infections in children. They are caused by a variety of viruses and bacteria, with the prevalence varying by age group[9,10] (**Table 50.3**). As in adults, *S. pneumoniae* is the predominant organism causing pneumonia except in newborns, in whom group B streptococci and gram-negative bacilli dominate. *H. influenzae* type B remains an important bacterial pathogen causing pneumonia in the developing world. It has nearly been eliminated in the United States through immunization practices. Pneumococcal vaccines also appear to be lowering the incidence of invasive pneumococcal disease and pneumonia, but more data are needed.[11] Many viruses, mainly influenza, parainfluenza, and RSV, can also cause pneumonia in children. Most children with pneumonia have cough, fever, and abnormal lung findings. Signs of tachypnea and increased work of breathing are often present and may be the only signs of disease in infants.[9]

Acute bronchiolitis is typically caused by RSV or parainfluenza viruses and predominantly affects children younger than 2 years. It can be difficult to distinguish from pneumonia because the clinical features are similar. Bronchiolitis is seasonal, with frequent occurrence in the winter and early spring months. Affected infants typically exhibit sneezing, rhinorrhea, coughing, wheezing, fever, and even respiratory distress. Chest examination typically demonstrates diffuse fine crackles and expiratory wheezes. Grunting respirations, cyanosis, retractions, and use of accessory muscles are signs of respiratory distress. Antibiotics are not usually indicated in patients with acute bronchiolitis, and treatment is primarily supportive. Bronchodilator therapy with nebulized albuterol or racemic epinephrine may be effective.

Pertussis (whooping cough) is a respiratory tract infection worthy of special mention. Caused by the organism *Bordetella pertussis*, it typically affects young children and adolescents. The incidence of the disease has markedly decreased because of immunization. Pertussis is manifested in three distinct stages. The first (catarrhal) stage consists of a mild cough, conjunctivitis, and coryza lasting up to 2 weeks. The second stage consists of severe paroxysms of coughing, often followed by strong inhalations of air, which produces the

**Table 50.3 Typical Pathogens in Pediatric Pneumonia and Recommended Treatment**

| AGE OF CHILD | USUAL PATHOGENS (IN GENERAL ORDER OF PREDOMINANCE) | EMPIRIC ANTIBIOTIC TREATMENT RECOMMENDED | |
|---|---|---|---|
| | | OUTPATIENT | INPATIENT |
| Birth-3 wk | Group B streptococci<br>Gram-negative enteric bacteria<br>Viral causes | Most require inpatient therapy | IV ampicillin and IV gentamicin with or without IV cefotaxime |
| 3 wk-3 mo | *Chlamydia trachomatis*<br>Viral causes<br>*Streptococcus pneumoniae*<br>*Bordetella pertussis* (rare)<br>*Staphylococcus aureus* (rare) | PO erythromycin or PO azithromycin | (Admit if hypoxia, respiratory distress, or sepsis present)<br>IV erythromycin<br>Add IV cefotaxime for signs of sepsis |
| 3 mo-5 yr | Viral causes<br>*S. pneumoniae*<br>*Mycoplasma pneumoniae* (less likely) | PO amoxicillin | IV ceftriaxone or IV cefotaxime |
| 5-18 yr | Viral causes<br>*M. pneumoniae*<br>*S. pneumoniae* | PO erythromycin, azithromycin, or clarithromycin<br>Consider PO doxycycline if patient > 8 yr | IV erythromycin or IV azithromycin<br>Add IV ceftriaxone or IV cefuroxime for sepsis, lobar infiltrate, or effusion |

From McIntosh K. Community acquired pneumonia in children. N Engl J Med 2002;346:429-37.
*IV*, Intravenous; *PO*, oral.

characteristic "whoop." This stage can last up to 4 weeks. The third (convalescent) stage consists of a chronic cough. The disease is important to identify because multiple complications can occur, such as complete airway obstruction, secondary pneumonia, seizures, and encephalitis. Treatment is with oral erythromycin or azithromycin. Close contacts of the patient should receive prophylactic antibiotics.[9]

## PATIENTS INFECTED WITH HUMAN IMMUNODEFICIENCY VIRUS

Pneumonia is one of the most common serious bacterial illnesses affecting patients infected with HIV. In addition to the common community-acquired pathogens, patients with HIV are more susceptible to opportunistic infections with *Pneumocystis carinii*, pulmonary tuberculosis, and recurrent bacterial pneumonia. Antibiotic chemoprophylaxis, highly active antiretroviral therapy, and preventive vaccines appear to be significantly improving the incidence and the morbidity and mortality of pneumonia in patients with HIV.[12]

## ASPIRATION PNEUMONIA

Aspiration of oral or gastric contents can occur in the setting of altered mental status or dysfunctional swallowing reflexes secondary to neurologic impairment such as stroke. Aspiration is typically "silent," and therefore a high index of clinical suspicion is needed for making the proper diagnosis. Aspiration can lead to chemical pneumonitis and bacterial aspiration pneumonia more than 60% of the time.[5] Abscesses and empyema can occur in more advanced cases. The pathogens involved are typically those found in the oropharynx. Patients who have recently been hospitalized or who reside in nursing homes may be colonized with *S. aureus* or gram-negative bacilli, which can cause aspiration pneumonia. Treatment with clindamycin or piperacillin-tazobactam is generally indicated.

## INFLUENZA

Influenza is one of the most common and most serious viral infections causing pneumonia. Influenza usually has a seasonal occurrence, typically from December to April. Bacterial superinfections can occur with pneumonia caused by influenza, most commonly with *S. pneumoniae* or *S. aureus*. Rapid identification tests are available to assist in diagnosis. Antiviral therapy with amantadine or rimantadine (for influenza A) or oseltamivir (for influenza A and B) may lessen the symptoms and quicken recovery if started within 48 hours of the onset of illness. In spring 2009 a novel influenza A virus (H1N1) spread globally and resulted in the first influenza pandemic since 1968, with infection occurring outside the usual influenza season in many parts of the world.[13] The pandemic put nearly all health care and public health institutions to the test and offered valuable lessons in emergency preparedness, virus detection, antiviral treatment, and immunization.

## COMMUNITY-ACQUIRED METHICILLIN-RESISTANT *STAPHYLOCOCCUS AUREUS*

MRSA is usually considered a nosocomial pathogen and accounts for 20% to 40% of all cases of HCAP and ventilator-associated pneumonia (VAP).[14] A new variant with a different genetic makeup, community-acquired MRSA, has been observed to cause cases of severe and rapidly progressing community-acquired pneumonia. It is typically seen in young and previously healthy patients, often with preceding influenza-like illnesses. Chest radiographs generally reveal multilobar cavitating infiltrates. Currently, intravenous vancomycin or linezolid is recommended, but the optimal treatment regimen has yet to be determined and may eventually include a combination of antibiotics with antibacterial and antitoxin mechanisms of action.[1]

## EVALUATION AND DIAGNOSTIC TESTING

Patients with pneumonia should undergo a complete initial assessment of vital signs, including pulse oximetry and evaluation of the respiratory rate.

### CHEST RADIOGRAPHS

Most authorities agree that chest radiographs (posteroanterior and lateral if possible) should be obtained in all patients with suspected pneumonia. Radiographs help confirm the diagnosis of pneumonia and provide possible clues to the causative agent (**Table 50.4**). Radiographs will also demonstrate associated conditions, such as lung abscess, bronchial obstruction, and pleural effusion (**Figs. 50.2 to 50.4**). Computed tomography may be necessary for further evaluation of complex infiltrates with pleural effusions, suspected masses, or abscesses. Typical radiologic patterns are expected with certain infections (see Table 50.4). It is important to remember that multiple factors, such as age, immune status, hydration status, and underlying lung disease, can alter the radiographic appearance of pneumonia.[15]

### SPUTUM STUDIES

Sputum Gram stain and culture should be performed only if a good-quality specimen can be obtained, transported, and processed appropriately. Sputum studies should be strongly considered for severe pneumonia, for suspected MRSA, in

**Table 50.4 Etiologic Agents of Pneumonia and Common Radiographic Patterns**

| RADIOGRAPHIC PATTERN | PATHOPHYSIOLOGY | TYPICAL PATHOGENS |
|---|---|---|
| Lobar or multilobar infiltrate with air bronchograms | Edema fluid/inflammatory reaction in alveoli occurring initially in the periphery of the lung<br>Larger bronchi usually remain patent and cause air bronchograms | Bacterial pneumonias (*Streptococcus pneumoniae, Klebsiella, Legionella*) |
| Interstitial infiltrates | Edema and inflammatory cellular infiltrate in interstitial tissue surrounding small airways and vessels | *Mycoplasma pneumoniae, Pneumocystis jiroveci (carinii),* viral pneumonias |
| Bronchopneumonia | Diffuse patchy infiltrates and peribronchial thickening secondary to large and intermediate airway involvement | *Staphylococcus aureus*, gram-negative organisms, fungi |
| Abscesses | Abscess cavity, isolated or within areas of consolidation | *S. aureus, Pseudomonas*, anaerobes |
| Cavitary masses | Inflammation and necrosis of lung parenchyma | *Mycobacterium tuberculosis, Nocardia, Aspergillus, Actinomyces* |

From Tarver R, Teague S, Heitkamp D, et al. Radiology of community acquired pneumonia. Radiol Clin North Am 2005;43:497-512.

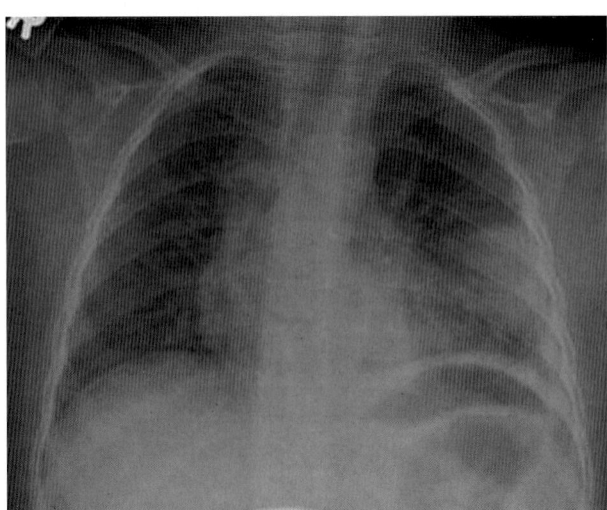

**Fig. 50.2** Chest radiograph of a 33-month-old child showing a left lower lobe infiltrate and a small effusion.

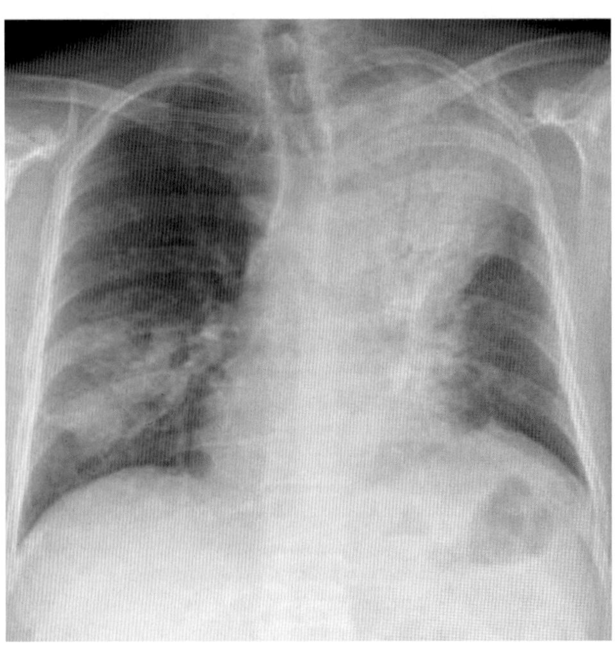

**Fig. 50.3** Chest radiograph of an adult with extensive lobar infiltrate and air bronchograms.

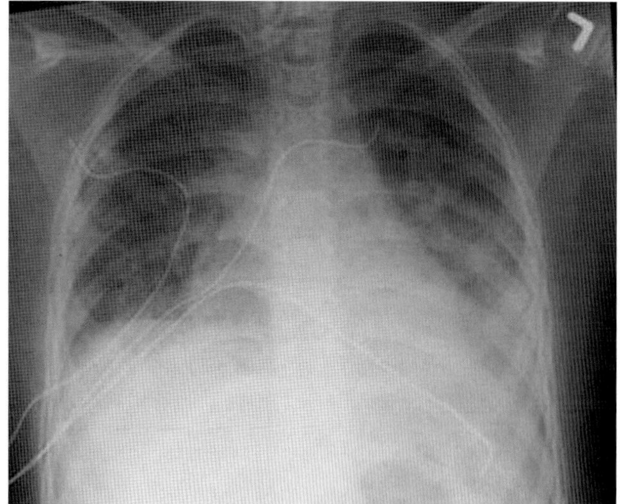

**Fig. 50.4 Chest radiograph of a child showing an interstitial infiltrate.**

patients with radiographs consistent with *Mycobacterium tuberculosis*, and in patients who are critically ill.[16,17] Sputum cultures should routinely be ordered in cases of suspected hospital-acquired pneumonia, HCAP, and VAP.[18] In the ED setting, sputum studies may be particularly useful in rapid testing for influenza or RSV in peak seasons to help select appropriate antiviral therapy and avoid unnecessary antibiotic use.

### BLOOD CULTURES

In a 2005 study of 414 ED patients with pneumonia, Kennedy et al. found that blood culture results rarely altered antibiotic therapy decisions. Resistant organisms requiring a broadening of antibiotic therapy were identified in only 1% of patients.[19] In a 2009 American College of Emergency Physicians clinical policy statement, the committee concluded that routine use of blood cultures has low yield and rarely leads to a change in management or outcome. A more patient-tailored approach has been suggested, with blood cultures being reserved for higher-risk groups such as those admitted to intensive care units (ICUs) with severe pneumonia, immunocompromised status, or significant comorbid conditions.[20]

### OTHER STUDIES

A complete blood count and basic serum chemistry studies are typically performed in patients admitted with pneumonia. The blood count can identify disorders such as lymphopenia (possibly indicating HIV infection), neutropenia, and anemia and thus help guide appropriate therapy. Electrolyte and glucose abnormalities are often found in patients with pneumonia, and testing for them may provide prognostic information. Measurement of blood urea nitrogen and serum creatinine is important in determining the level of nursing care and appropriate antibiotic dosing for each patient. Urinary studies such as antigen testing for *Legionella* and *S. pneumoniae* may be useful. Bronchoscopy may be considered in patients with HIV, patients who are immunosuppressed, and patients in whom an unusual infection is suspected. Two newer serum biomarkers, C-reactive protein and procalcitonin, may be useful in predicting patients at risk for increased 30-day mortality. In addition, serial measurements of procalcitonin may be useful for guiding the duration of antibiotic therapy.[1,21] Thoracentesis may be necessary if a pleural effusion is present and freely flowing. Ultrasonography may be beneficial in identifying free-flowing effusions and to guide sampling of the fluid for cell count, cultures, pH, and fluid analysis.[17]

## TREATMENT

After decisions regarding respiratory, hemodynamic, and ventilatory support, the most important decision in treating patients with pneumonia is selection of timely and appropriate initial antibiotic therapy. Multiple factors, such as suspected causes, severity of illness, recent antibiotic therapy, patient disposition, antibiotic allergies, and comorbid illnesses, contribute to the selection of optimal antimicrobial therapy.

As already described, the ATS and IDSA have issued detailed guidelines for the treatment of community-acquired pneumonia. Several studies have demonstrated lower mortality in hospitalized patients treated with guideline-recommended antimicrobial regimens.[6] In a 2004 study of 420 patients with pneumonia, Mortensen et al.[22] found significantly lower 30-day mortality in patients who received antimicrobial therapy in concordance with the ATS or IDSA guidelines.

The recommendations in the guidelines are summarized in **Box 50.1**. The guidelines group recommendations according to the site of therapy (outpatient, inpatient, or ICU), severity of disease, comorbid illnesses, and risk for resistant organisms or *Pseudomonas aeruginosa*.

Ideally, antibiotic therapy should be started in the ED as soon as possible after the diagnosis is made. Because pneumonia accounts for approximately 1.7 million hospitalizations per year with an estimated annual cost of more than $9 billion, improving pneumonia care has become a focus of the Joint Commission on Accreditation of Healthcare Organizations and the Centers for Medicare and Medicaid Services.[20] Several defined quality measures (core measures) have been identified, including the use of evidence-based antibiotic choices, timely antibiotic administration, appropriate use of blood cultures before administration of antibiotics, and administration of pneumococcal and influenza vaccines for appropriate patients. Although the validity of some of the measures are questioned by some authorities, these data are publicly reported and adherence with the measures is often a priority for institutions.

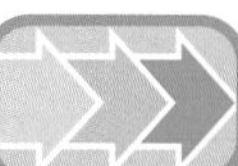

**PRIORITY ACTIONS**

Provide immediate supplemental oxygen or ventilatory assistance (or both) to patients with suspected pneumonia as needed.

A mask should be placed over the face of any patient with suspected pneumonia to prevent spread of disease to other patients waiting for evaluation.

Antibiotic therapy should ideally be initiated in the emergency department as soon as possible after the diagnosis is made.

**BOX 50.1 Recommended Empiric Antibiotics for Community-Acquired Pneumonia**

**Outpatient Treatment**

1. Previously healthy and no use of antimicrobials within the previous 3 months:
   - A macrolide (strong recommendation; level I evidence)
   - Doxycycline (weak recommendation; level III evidence)
2. Presence of comorbid conditions such as chronic heart, lung, liver, or renal disease; diabetes mellitus; alcoholism; malignancies; asplenia; immunosuppressing conditions or use of immunosuppressing drugs; or use of antimicrobials within the previous 3 months (in which case an alternative from a different class should be selected):
   - A respiratory fluoroquinolone (moxifloxacin, gemifloxacin, or levofloxacin [750 mg]) (strong recommendation; level I evidence)
   - A β-lactam plus a macrolide (strong recommendation; level I evidence)
3. In regions with a high rate (>25%) of infection with high-level (MIC = 16 mcg/mL) macrolide-resistant *Streptococcus pneumoniae*, consider use of the alternative agents listed above in No. 2 for patients without comorbid conditions (moderate recommendation; level III evidence)

**Inpatients, Non-ICU Treatment**

A respiratory fluoroquinolone (strong recommendation; level I evidence)

A β-lactam plus a macrolide (strong recommendation; level I evidence)

**Inpatients, ICU Treatment**

A β-lactam (cefotaxime, ceftriaxone, or ampicillin-sulbactam) plus either azithromycin (level II evidence) or a respiratory fluoroquinolone (strong recommendation; level I evidence) (for penicillin-allergic patients, a respiratory fluoroquinolone and aztreonam are recommended)

**Special Concerns**

If *Pseudomonas* is a consideration:

- An antipneumococcal, antipseudomonal β-lactam (piperacillin-tazobactam, cefepime, imipenem, or meropenem) plus either ciprofloxacin or levofloxacin (750 mg)

**or**

- The above β-lactam plus an aminoglycoside and azithromycin

**or**

- The above β-lactam plus an aminoglycoside and an antipneumococcal fluoroquinolone (for penicillin-allergic patients, substitute aztreonam for above β-lactam) (moderate recommendation; level III evidence)

If community-acquired methicillin-resistant *Staphylococcus aureus* is a consideration, add vancomycin or linezolid (moderate recommendation; level III evidence)

From Mandell LA, Wunderink RG, Anzueto A, et al. Infectious Diseases Society of America/American Thoracic Society consensus guidelines on the management of community-acquired pneumonia in adults. Clin Infect Dis 2007;44:S27-S72.

*ICU*, Intensive care unit; *MIC*, minimal inhibitory concentration.

## HEALTH CARE–ASSOCIATED PNEUMONIA

In the current era of shorter hospital stays and expanded home and long-term care facility treatment, the emergency physician frequently encounters patients at risk for HCAP. In 2005, a joint committee of the ATS and IDSA published an additional set of guidelines for the evaluation and treatment of HCAP. They also apply to hospital-acquired pneumonia and VAP. The guidelines emphasize that HCAP can be caused by a wide variety of bacteria, including multidrug-resistant pathogens, gram-negative organisms, and MRSA, and is often polymicrobial. It is recommended that sputum cultures be performed in all such patients, before antibiotic therapy if possible. The recommendations for initial empiric antibiotic therapy are summarized in **Table 50.5**. The commission also recognized the variability in bacterial pathogens from one institution to another and recommended that local microbiologic data be taken into account when selecting antibiotic therapy.[18]

## FOLLOW-UP, NEXT STEPS IN CARE, AND PATIENT EDUCATION

Several validated prediction tools can be used to identify patients with pneumonia who are at increased risk for complications and would benefit from inpatient or ICU treatment. These tools evaluate important patient characteristics, such as age, vital signs, radiographic and laboratory data, and comorbid illnesses, and identify patients at increased risk for 30-day mortality.

In 1997 the Pneumonia Patient Outcomes Research Team (PORT)[23] published a prediction rule to identify patients at low risk for death from pneumonia within 30 days; it is now known as the PORT criteria or the Pneumonia Severity Index. A 2005 comparison of three prediction guidelines by Aujesky et al.[24] found the Pneumonia Severity Index to be most accurate in identifying low-risk and high-risk patients with pneumonia. The system was developed through analysis of data from thousands of patients with community-acquired pneumonia and was validated in more than 50,000 patients. Patients are divided into five classes based on increasing risk for mortality. Class I (mortality, 0.1% to 0.4%) is assigned on the basis of an age of 50 years or younger and key information from the history and physical examination. Other classes are identified with a point system calculated from the presence of historical data and physical and laboratory findings (**Box 50.2**).[23]

Class I and class II patients are considered to have very low risk (30-day mortality, <1%) and can probably be treated as outpatients. Many patients in class III (30-day mortality, <2.8%) might also be candidates for outpatient treatment. Patients in class IV or class V are at much higher risk (30-day mortality, 8.5% to 31.1%) and should probably be admitted to the hospital.[23,24]

**Table 50.5 Initial Empiric Antibiotic Therapy Recommendations for Health Care–Associated Pneumonia**

| SITUATION | POTENTIAL PATHOGENS | RECOMMENDED ANTIBIOTIC |
|---|---|---|
| No known risk factors for multidrug-resistant pathogens,* early onset (<5 days' hospitalization) | *Streptococcus pneumoniae, Haemophilus influenzae*, methicillin-resistant *Streptococcus aureus* (MRSA), antibiotic-sensitive gram-negative organisms (*Escherichia coli, Klebsiella, Enterobacter, Proteus, Serratia*) | Ceftriaxone<br>*OR*<br>Advanced fluoroquinolone<br>*OR*<br>Ampicillin-sulbactam<br>*OR*<br>Ertapenem |
| Late-onset disease (≥5 days' hospitalization) or risk factors present for multidrug-resistant pathogens* | As above plus:<br>*Pseudomonas*<br>*Klebsiella* (extended-spectrum β-lactamase [ESBL])<br>*Acinetobacter* (ESBL)<br>MRSA<br>*Legionella* | Antipseudomonal cephalosporin (cefepime, ceftazidime)<br>*OR*<br>Antipseudomonal carbapenem (imipenem or meropenem)<br>*OR*<br>Piperacillin-tazobactam plus antipseudomonal fluoroquinolone (ciprofloxacin or levofloxacin)<br>*OR*<br>Aminoglycoside (amikacin, gentamicin, tobramycin) plus linezolid or vancomycin† |

From American Thoracic Society. Guidelines for the management of adults with hospital-acquired, ventilator-associated, and healthcare-associated pneumonia. Am J Respir Crit Care Med 2005;171;388-416.

*Risks include antimicrobial therapy in the preceding 90 days, current hospitalization of 5 days or longer, high frequency of antibiotic resistance in the institution or community, hospitalization for 2 days or more in the preceding 90 days, residence in a nursing home or extended care facility, home infusion therapy, long-term dialysis within 30 days, home wound care, family member with multidrug-resistant pathogens, and immunosuppressive diseases or therapy.

†If MRSA is a risk factor or has a high incidence locally.

**BOX 50.2 Summary of Risk Class Assignment for Patients with Pneumonia Based on the Pneumonia Severity Index (PORT Criteria)**

**Step 1**

Does the patient have one or more of the following features?

- Age > 50 years
- Neoplastic disease
- Congestive heart failure
- Cerebrovascular disease
- Renal disease
- Liver disease
- Altered mental status
- Pulse > 125 beats/min
- Respiratory rate > 30 beats/min
- Systolic blood pressure < 90 mm Hg
- Temperature < 35° C or > 40° C

*No: Assign to risk class I.*

*Yes: Go to Step 2.*

**Step 2**

Assign points to the patient's risk score according to the presence of the following characteristics:

| CHARACTERISTIC | POINTS ASSIGNED |
|---|---|
| **Age** | |
| Men | Age in years (1 point for each year) |
| Women | Age in years (1 point for each year) − 10 |
| Nursing home residency | +10 |
| **Coexisting Illnesses** | |
| Neoplastic disease | +30 |
| Liver disease | +20 |
| Congestive heart failure | +10 |
| Cerebrovascular disease | +10 |
| Renal disease | +10 |
| **Physical Findings** | |
| Altered mental status | +20 |
| Respiratory rate > 30 breaths/min | +20 |
| Systolic blood pressure < 90 mm Hg | +20 |
| Temperature < 35° C or > 40° C | +15 |
| Pulse > 125 beats/min | +10 |
| **Laboratory and Radiographic Findings** | |
| Arterial pH < 7.35 | +30 |
| Blood urea nitrogen > 30 mg/dL | +20 |
| Sodium < 130 mmol/L | +20 |
| Blood glucose > 250 mg/dL | +10 |
| Hematocrit < 30% | +10 |
| $Pao_2$ < 60 mm Hg or pulse oximetry value < 90% | +10 |
| Pleural effusion | +10 |

**Step 3**

Use the total points accumulated in step 2 to assign the patient to the corresponding risk class, as follows:

- ≤70—class II
- 71-90—class III
- 91-130—class IV
- >130—class V

Data from Fine M, Auble T, Yealy D, et al. A prediction rule to identify low-risk patients with community acquired pneumonia. N Engl J Med 1997;336:243-50; and Aujesky D, Auble T, Yealy D, et al. Prospective comparison of three validated prediction rules for prognosis in community-acquired pneumonia. Am J Med 2005;118:384-92.

*PORT,* Pneumonia Patient Outcomes Research Team.

The British Thoracic Society has also published a prediction tool, CURB-65, to identify patients at high risk for 30-day mortality. Confusion, elevated blood urea nitrogen, elevated respiratory rate, low systolic or diastolic blood pressure, and age older than 65 years are the high-risk variables identified. A simplified version (CRB-65) allows prediction based on clinical variables alone (eliminating blood urea nitrogen) and may be useful in the outpatient setting. A score of 2 or higher predicts increased risk for mortality, and these patients should probably be admitted. ICU admission should be considered for those with a score of 3 or higher.[1]

It must be emphasized that these prediction rules are only guidelines. Many other factors, such as unique comorbid conditions, psychosocial factors, ability to take oral medications, and patient and caregiver reliability, must also be considered in the decision to admit or discharge the patient. Patients demonstrating signs of shock or respiratory distress should be treated in an ICU setting.

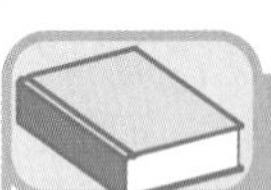

**PATIENT TEACHING TIPS**

Encourage outpatients to finish their course of antibiotics, even if they start to feel better earlier, because not finishing the full course of medicine could lead to incomplete treatment of the infection and clinical relapse.

Because most respiratory infections are spread by means of respiratory droplets, patients with pneumonia should be told to wash their hands frequently, not share utensils or cups, and cover their mouth when coughing to prevent spread of the infection to close contacts. Patient may wish to wear a mask over their mouth and nose when around others who have chronic lung disease or are immunosuppressed.

Patient should be encouraged to return to the emergency department if they experience worsening of symptoms or increasing shortness of breath.

## SUGGESTED READINGS

American College of Emergency Physicians Clinical Policies Subcommittee (Writing Committee) on Critical Issues in the Evaluation and Management of Adult Patients Presenting to the Emergency Department With Community-Acquired Pneumonia. Clinical policy: critical issues in the evaluation and management of adult patients presenting to the emergency department with community-acquired pneumonia. Ann Emerg Med 2009;54:704-31.

Niederman M. Recent advances in community-acquired pneumonia: inpatient and outpatient. Chest 2007;131:1205-15.

Slaven E, Santanilla J, DeBlieux P. Healthcare-associated pneumonia in the emergency department. Semin Respir Crit Care Med 2009;30:46-51.

## REFERENCES

***References can be found on Expert Consult @ www.expertconsult.com.***

# Pneumothorax 51

*David E. Manthey and Bret A. Nicks*

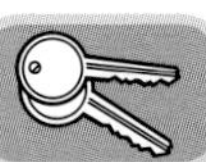

**KEY POINTS**

- Primary pneumothoraces (spontaneous or traumatic) occur in patients without clinically apparent lung disease.
- Chronic obstructive pulmonary disease is the most common cause of secondary pneumothorax.
- Physical examination may miss a pneumothorax occupying up to 27% of lung volume.
- Standard posteroanterior and lateral chest radiographs are the only routine examination needed because expiratory films add little to diagnostic accuracy.
- Ultrasound's lung point sign has an overall sensitivity of 66% and a specificity of 100%.
- Treatment of pneumothorax is based on its cause, size and stability, symptoms, and the presence or absence of underlying lung disease. Treatment options include observation, catheter aspiration, and tube thoracostomy.

## EPIDEMIOLOGY

Primary spontaneous pneumothorax occurs at a rate of 10 to 18 cases per 100,000 population per year in men and 5 cases per 100,000 in women. It has a peak incidence in young adults (20 to 30 years).

Secondary pneumothoraces make up one third of spontaneous pneumothoraces and occur with underlying pulmonary disease. Of note, chronic obstructive pulmonary disease (COPD) is the most common cause of secondary spontaneous pneumothorax. Recurrences are common, so prevention of recurrence is indicated after the first episode.

Patients with a spontaneous pneumothorax have a 30% recurrence rate within 2 years after air evacuation only; patients who have experienced two pneumothoraces have about an 80% chance of a recurrent pneumothorax.

## PATHOPHYSIOLOGY

### PNEUMOTHORAX

The pleural space lies between the parietal and visceral pleura and is normally negatively pressured at −5 mm Hg with fluctuations of 6 to 8 mm Hg between inspiration and expiration. With loss of the normal negative pressure, the affected lung collapses. Primary spontaneous pneumothorax occurs when a subpleural bleb, most commonly in the lung apex, ruptures into the pleural space. In secondary spontaneous pneumothorax, rupture of the visceral pleura and alveolar barrier is most commonly due to the underlying pulmonary disease process.

#### *Open Pneumothorax*

Open chest wounds become symptomatic when the diameter of the chest wall defect approaches two thirds the size of the trachea. At this point, air preferentially enters the pleural cavity during inspiration (negative intrathoracic pressure) via the chest wall defect instead of the trachea, which leaves the lungs without oxygenation or ventilation.

#### *Tension Pneumothorax*

Tension pneumothorax occurs when a one-way valve develops in the injured lung and allows entry of air into the pleural space during inspiration without being able to escape during expiration. Tension physiology occurs when the increased intrathoracic pressure (15 to 20 mm Hg) limits the return of venous blood flow from the body to the right heart and compresses the great vessels and pericardium. Compression of the affected lung causes hypoxia and arterial constriction, which shunts blood flow mostly to the contralateral lung and decreases the magnitude of preload to the left atrium.

## PRESENTING SIGNS AND SYMPTOMS

### PNEUMOTHORAX

Classically, the symptoms of primary spontaneous pneumothorax are a sudden onset of ipsilateral, pleuritic chest pain and associated dyspnea. The pain typically begins at rest and is worsened with deep inspiration. It may eventually become a dull persistent ache that does not vary with respiration. Profound dyspnea is rare in the absence of tension pneumothorax or underlying parenchymal disease. Sinus tachycardia is the most common physical finding, with other classic signs such as decreased breath sounds, hyperresonance to percussion, unilateral enlargement of the hemithorax, absence of tactile fremitus, and decreased excursion volumes occurring less frequently. Symptoms may resolve in 24 hours without resolution of the pneumothorax. Many patients (45%) may delay seeking medical care for 48 hours. The severity of symptoms does not necessarily correlate with the size of the pneumothorax.

The ability of auscultation to detect hemothorax, pneumothorax, or hemopneumothorax associated with penetrating trauma had a sensitivity of 58%, a specificity of 98%, and a positive predictive value of 98% in one study.[1] Auscultation can miss up to 600 mL of hemothorax, a pneumothorax occupying up to 28% of lung volume, and a combined hemopneumothorax of up to 800 mL and 28%.[1] Physical examination alone is not sensitive enough to exclude the diagnosis of pneumothorax.

### OPEN PNEUMOTHORAX

Patients with an open pneumothorax have significant dyspnea and a history of a penetrating wound to the thorax. Physical examination will reveal a chest wound that produces an audible, sucking air movement sound on inspiration and may bubble on expiration. Findings of a pneumothorax will also be present.

### TENSION PNEUMOTHORAX

Patients with tension pneumothorax exhibit extreme dyspnea, hypotension, and cyanosis. Physical findings are hyperresonance, hyperinflation, absence of breath sounds on the affected side, and deviation of the trachea (at the sternal notch) away from the affected side. Tachycardia is often present and is defined as a pulse greater than 120 beats/min. Patients with tachycardia should undergo immediate tube thoracostomy (or needle thoracostomy if a chest tube is not immediately available) without waiting for a confirmatory radiograph.

### SECONDARY PNEUMOTHORACES

Patients with pneumothoraces secondary to underlying lung disease may experience extreme dyspnea as a result of deflation of one lung and limited capacity and function of the remaining lung. Classically, symptoms do not resolve without intervention. Because of the underlying lung disease (most commonly COPD), lung findings may be abnormal, with hyperinflation and decreased lung sounds being noted.

## DIAGNOSTIC TESTING AND MEDICAL DECISION MAKING (TABLE 51.1)

### RADIOGRAPHY

The primary evaluation tool is the standard posteroanterior chest radiograph to look for loss of lung markings in the periphery and a pleural line that runs parallel to the chest wall but does not extend outside the chest cavity. A lateral radiograph contributes to the diagnosis in 14% of cases.[2] There is no evidence that an expiratory radiograph adds any value even with small apical pneumothoraces.[3] The sensitivity for flat anteroposterior chest radiography, versus computed tomography (CT) as the "gold standard," has been found to be 75.5%

**Table 51.1 Differential Diagnosis of Pneumothorax**

| | |
|---|---|
| Pulmonary embolism | Perform a risk stratification based on the Wells or Charlotte criteria.<br>If the result of stratification is not low probability or the D-dimer test result is positive, proceed to computed tomography–pulmonary angiography.<br>A chest radiograph may show infarcted lung. |
| Pleurisy | Look for an underlying disease process (connective tissue, pneumonia).<br>Pleura-based diseases (pneumonia, tumor, effusion) often have radiographic findings. |
| Pneumonia | Chest radiography will be helpful.<br>Clinical examination and the history may suggest pneumonia because of cough (uncommon with pneumothorax), upper respiratory symptoms, fever, or immunosuppression. |
| Pericarditis | Look for an underlying disease process.<br>Check the electrocardiogram (ECG) for classic but not common PR-segment depression and/or widespread ST-segment elevation.<br>Does position affect the pain (less with leaning forward, more with lying back)?<br>Consider ultrasonography to diagnose effusion. |
| Myocardial infarction | Assess for appropriate risk factors.<br>Evaluate with an ECG and cardiac marker measurements if suspicious.<br>ECG findings associated with a pneumothorax include axis deviation, decreased voltage, and T-wave inversion. |
| Aortic dissection | Interscapular back pain with a tearing sensation is typical.<br>Check the chest radiograph for a widened mediastinum, apical capping, left-sided pleural effusion, blurring of the aortic knob, or displacement of the trachea or esophagus to the anatomic right.<br>Consider checking bilateral arm pressures.<br>Look for a neurologic deficit or end-organ ischemia. |
| Musculoskeletal pain | Is the pain reproducible with palpation and use of the muscle group?<br>Does the patient have a history consistent with muscle injury?<br>Are the findings on chest radiography and ECG normal? |
| Pneumomediastinum | Is subcutaneous emphysema present on physical examination?<br>Is mediastinal, pericardiac, or prevertebral air found on the chest radiograph?<br>Does it typically occur during a Valsalva maneuver or exertion? |

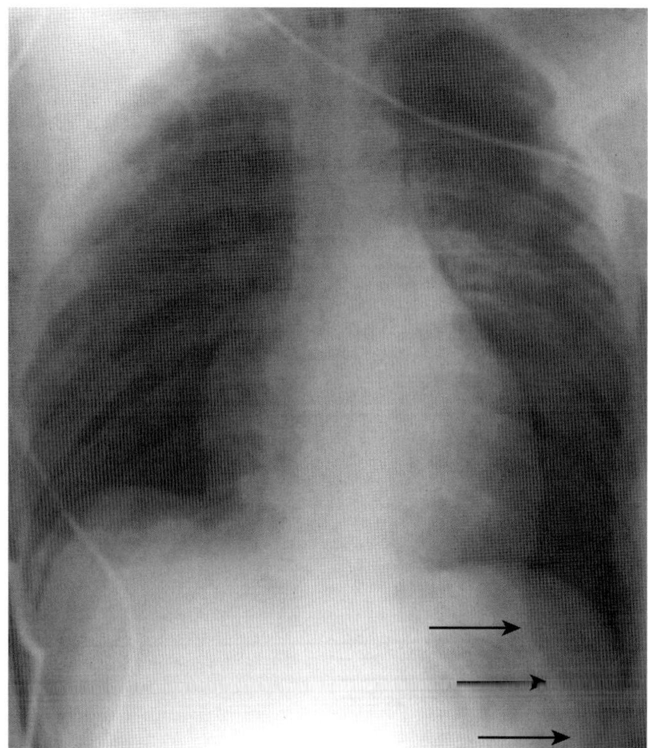

Fig. 51.1 Deep sulcus sign.

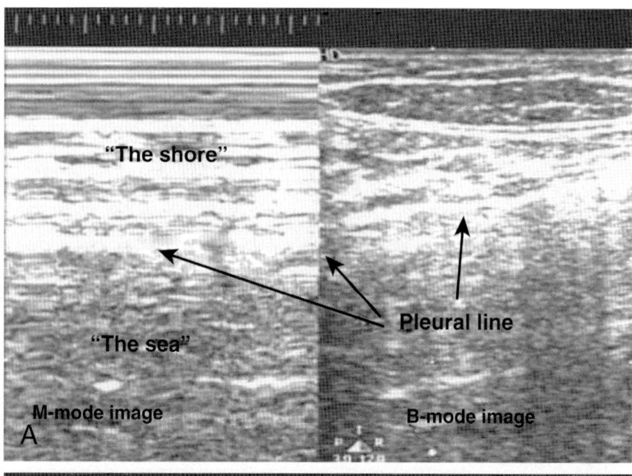


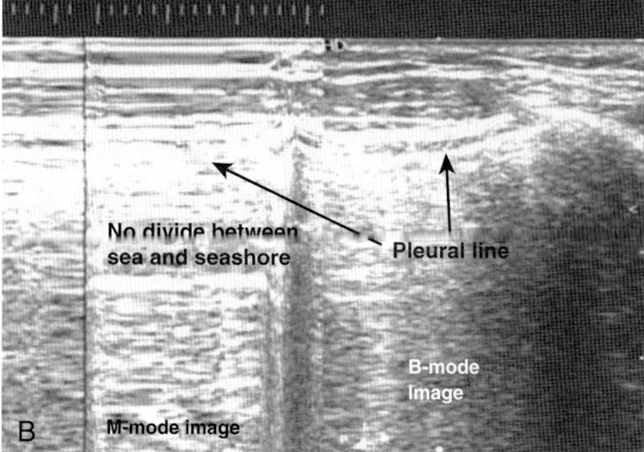


**Fig. 51.2 Ultrasonograms of abnormal (A) and normal (B) pleura with M-mode and B-mode imaging.** (Courtesy Christopher L. Moore, MD, Yale University School of Medicine.)

(95% confidence interval [CI], 61.7% to 86.2%), and the specificity is 100% (95% CI, 97.1% to 100%).[4]

Shift of the mediastinum away from a pneumothorax on a chest radiograph can be a normal phenomenon that occurs without tension physiology. In critically ill patients in whom a radiograph can be taken only in the supine position, the emergency physician (EP) should look for the presence of a deep sulcus sign—a deep lateral costophrenic angle on the ipsilateral side (**Fig. 51.1**). Diaphragmatic depression or ipsilateral transradiancy (fewer lung markings, clearer image) may also be seen.[5]

Large bullae can be mistaken for a pneumothorax. With a pneumothorax, the pleural line runs parallel to the chest wall, whereas bullae more commonly have a medially concave appearance and are limited to a single lobe. A chest CT scan can help differentiate these entities. Pleural adhesions may alter the appearance of the pneumothorax by tethering the lung to the chest wall. Clothing, hair, and skin folds may appear as visceral pleural lines but often continue beyond the chest wall.

In most cases, an upright radiograph is sufficient to identify a pneumothorax. If not, EPs should consider additional modalities if they strongly suspect a pneumothorax, particularly if the patient is unstable, if underlying lung disease is present (and thus no reserve if a pneumothorax is missed), or if the patient is being treated with positive pressure ventilation.

## ULTRASONOGRAPHY

Normal lung shows a shimmering echogenic stripe of both the parietal and visceral pleura on ultrasonography. A sliding sign at the pleural stripe can be seen with movement of the visceral pleura in relation to the parietal pleura. The "seashore analogy" refers to movement of the lung (ocean) against the stationary chest wall (shore). A comet tail reverberation can be seen distal to the pleura when no pneumothorax is present. The sliding sign of the pleural stripe and the comet tail reverberation are lost with a pneumothorax because of intrapleural air[6] (**Fig. 51.2**). Doppler mode may be of some help in detecting this movement. Multiple other reasons can account for loss of the sliding, including atelectasis, mainstem intubation, acute respiratory distress syndrome, pleural adhesions, and pulmonary contusion, thus limiting specificity for pneumothorax in some cases.

Deep to this pleural line, vertical artifacts called B lines may be seen. They originate at the pleural line, align vertically, continue the entire depth of the screen without any fading, and move with breathing. The finding of B lines rules out the presence of a pneumothorax, but the absence of B lines does not signify the presence of a pneumothorax.[7]

The lung point sign has a specificity approaching 100% for pneumothorax and is determined by the absence of lung sliding and B lines. The probe is moved gradually toward the lateral lower aspect of the chest.[8] The goal is to identify lung sliding and B lines suggesting the "point" at which the lung is adherent to the pleura again (**Fig. 51.3**). A large pneumothorax may not display this point, thus diminishing the sensitivity of the lung point sign.

The sensitivity of ultrasound detection of pneumothorax has been found to be 98.1% (95% CI, 89.9% to 99.9%) and

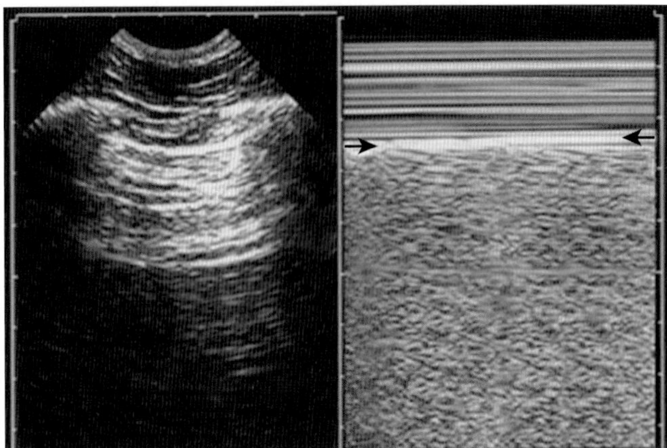

**Fig. 51.3 Lung point sign.** (Courtesy Christopher L. Moore, MD, Yale University School of Medicine.)

the specificity was 99.2% (95% CI, 95.6% to 99.9%), which makes it more sensitive than a flat-plate anteroposterior radiograph.[4] The use of ultrasonography as part of the extended focused assessment with sonography for trauma (eFAST) examination has been suggested in unstable patients with suspected pneumothorax.

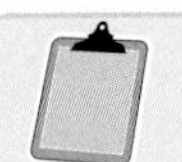

**DOCUMENTATION**

Document the presence of underlying lung disease to establish the primary versus secondary status of the pneumothorax.

In the case of primary pneumothorax, document whether it was traumatic.

Document the estimated size of the pneumothorax and method of intervention.

If the patient is being discharged, document follow-up and discussion of reasons to return.

## COMPUTED TOMOGRAPHY

CT is more accurate than radiography for the detection of pneumothoraces; it detects between 25% and 40% of pneumothoraces after lung biopsy that were not visualized on postprocedure chest radiographs.[9] Up to 50% of traumatic pneumothoraces may be occult. CT can detect other problems, such as pulmonary blebs, vascular abnormalities, contusions, infiltrates, and tumors. CT is recommended in uncertain or complex cases such as symptomatic high-risk patients with suspected occult pneumothorax, those who have underlying lung disease, patients undergoing positive pressure ventilation, or those just completing lung biopsy.

## DETERMINING THE SIZE OF THE PNEUMOTHORAX

Foremost, the degree of clinical symptoms is more important than the size of the pneumothorax in determining the appropriate therapy. Chest radiography underestimates the size of pneumothoraces because it is a two-dimensional view of a three-dimensional abnormality.

U.S. guidelines suggest measurement from the apex of the lung to the cupula of the thoracic cavity on an upright

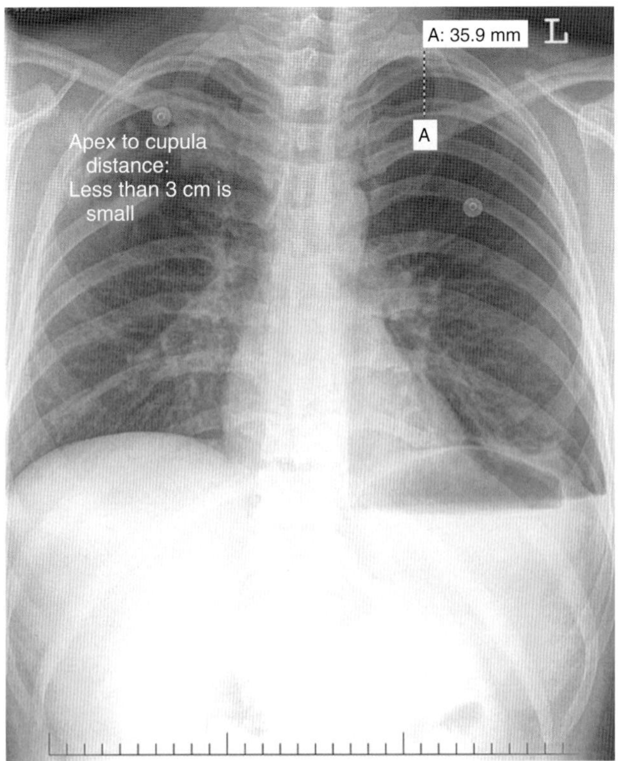


**Fig. 51.4 Apex-to-cupula measurement performed in a patient with a left-sided pneumothorax.**

posteroanterior radiograph (**Fig. 51.4**). Less than 3 cm is considered small. British guidelines (2010) suggest the interpleural distance at the level of the hilum (**Fig. 51.5**). A 2-cm distance correlates with an approximate 50% pneumothorax by volume.[10]

CT-directed size classification allows grading of occult pneumothoraces. Minuscule refers to air collections less than 1 cm thick that appear on fewer than five contiguous 10-mm slices. Anterior pneumothoraces are air collections more than 1 cm thick that appear on five or more contiguous 10-mm slices and do not extend to the midcoronal line (**Fig. 51.6**). Anterolateral pneumothoraces extend to the midcoronal line or beyond.

# TREATMENT

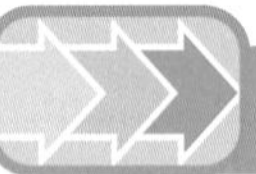

**PRIORITY ACTIONS**

1. Administer oxygen.
2. Determine whether tension pneumothorax physiology exists. If present, proceed to tube thoracostomy without delay for imaging.
3. Close an open pneumothorax with a three-sided dressing.
4. Obtain posteroanterior and lateral chest radiographs.
5. Determine the size of the pneumothorax.
6. Assess the patient for underlying lung disease, adhesions, and other complications.

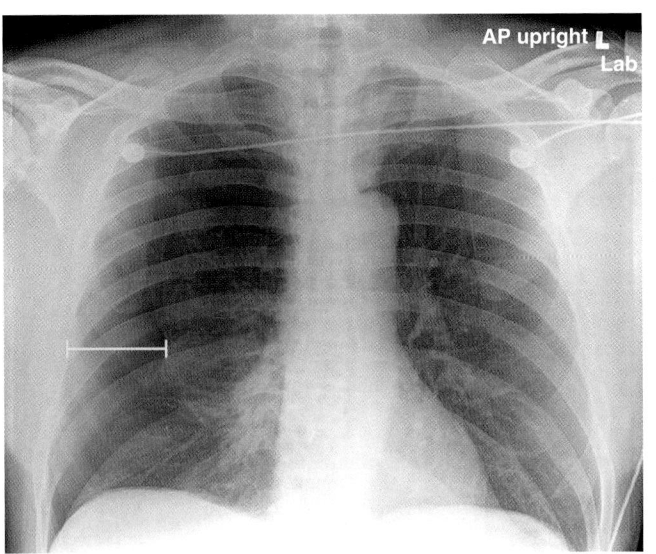


**Fig. 51.5 Intrapleural space measured at the hilum in a patient with a right-sided pneumothorax.** *AP*, Anteroposterior.

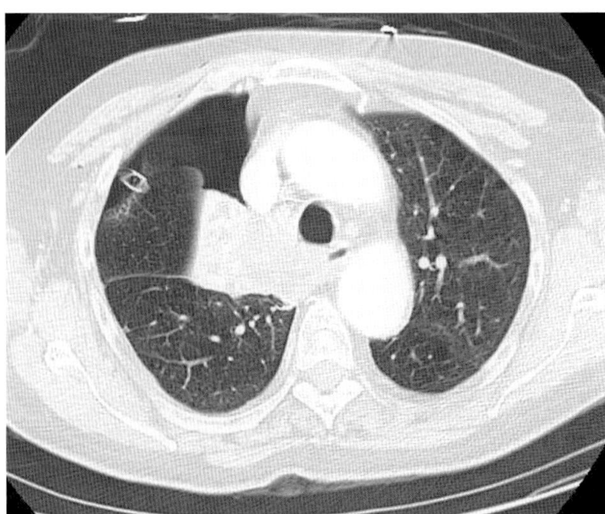

**Fig. 51.6 Computed tomography scan of the chest showing an anterior pneumothorax and a chest tube.**

## PREHOSPITAL MANAGEMENT

### Tension Pneumothorax

Emergency needle aspiration is usually performed by emergency medical services personnel when tension pneumothorax is suspected. In an ED setting, placement of a chest tube more reliably and more definitively addresses the problem in a relatively short time.

### Open Pneumothorax

An open pneumothorax should be taped on three sides with material that will be airtight. An airtight seal can be accomplished with petrolatum gauze (Xeroform) or the aluminum foil of the gauze packaging. Securing only three sides prevents the development of tension pneumothorax by allowing escape of air from the pleural space via this one-way valve.

## HOSPITAL MANAGEMENT

Oxygen should be administered to all patients with a pneumothorax because it helps in resorption of the pneumothorax and increases oxygenation of the available alveoli in the noncollapsed lung. The untreated resorption rate is 1% to 2% per day, and the rate increases fourfold with the administration of 100% oxygen.[11]

The stability of the patient, the severity of the symptoms, the current size of the pneumothorax, the change in size over time, the cause of the pneumothorax (primary, secondary, traumatic), and the severity of the underlying lung disease must all be considered in the decision whether to intervene in a patient with pneumothorax.

A stable patient with pneumothorax has been described as one who has a respiratory rate of less than 24 breaths/min, a heart rate between 60 and 120 beats/min, normal blood pressure, oxygen saturation greater than 90% when breathing room air, and the ability to speak in full sentences between breaths.[12]

**Figures 51.7 and 51.8** present algorithms to assess the need for intervention in patients with primary spontaneous pneumothorax or traumatic pneumothorax, respectively. Patients with bilateral pneumothoraces are treated by aspiration or chest tube placement.

Patients with secondary pneumothoraces should be admitted to the hospital. A patient who is not at risk for large air leaks and has a small pneumothorax can be treated by aspiration via a small-bore catheter. A clinically unstable patient or a stable patient with a large pneumothorax should be treated with a chest tube.

Chest tube sizes for patients with spontaneous pneumothoraces are recommended as follows. Catheter (simple) aspiration seems to be as effective as chest tube treatment in patients with a small pneumothorax. Aspiration of more than 2.5 L of air suggests an air leak and may require a small-bore chest tube. Clinically stable patients with a large pneumothorax are treated by aspiration via a small-bore catheter (14 to 16 gauge) or with a 14 French (14F) chest tube. Clinically unstable patients with a large primary pneumothorax should be treated by tube thoracostomy. A larger (14F to 28F) chest tube should be used for patients requiring positive pressure ventilation and those at risk for large pleural air leaks (bronchopleural fistula). With traumatic pneumothoraces, a 28F to 36F chest tube should be used because of the risk for associated hemothorax.

Postprocedure monitoring and radiographs should be obtained to assess the success of the intervention and the position of the chest tube.

### Heimlich Valve

A Heimlich valve is a one-way valve that can be attached to the end of a chest tube. Suction has not been proved to aid in reexpansion or the outcome of a pneumothorax, and it is not recommended. Instead, a water seal or Heimlich valve is used.[13] A Heimlich valve allows the patient to ambulate unrestricted. It should not be used in patients with underlying lung disease or other medical problems that prevent them from tolerating a recurrence of the pneumothorax. Complications of this method include obstruction of the valve with fluid and disconnection.

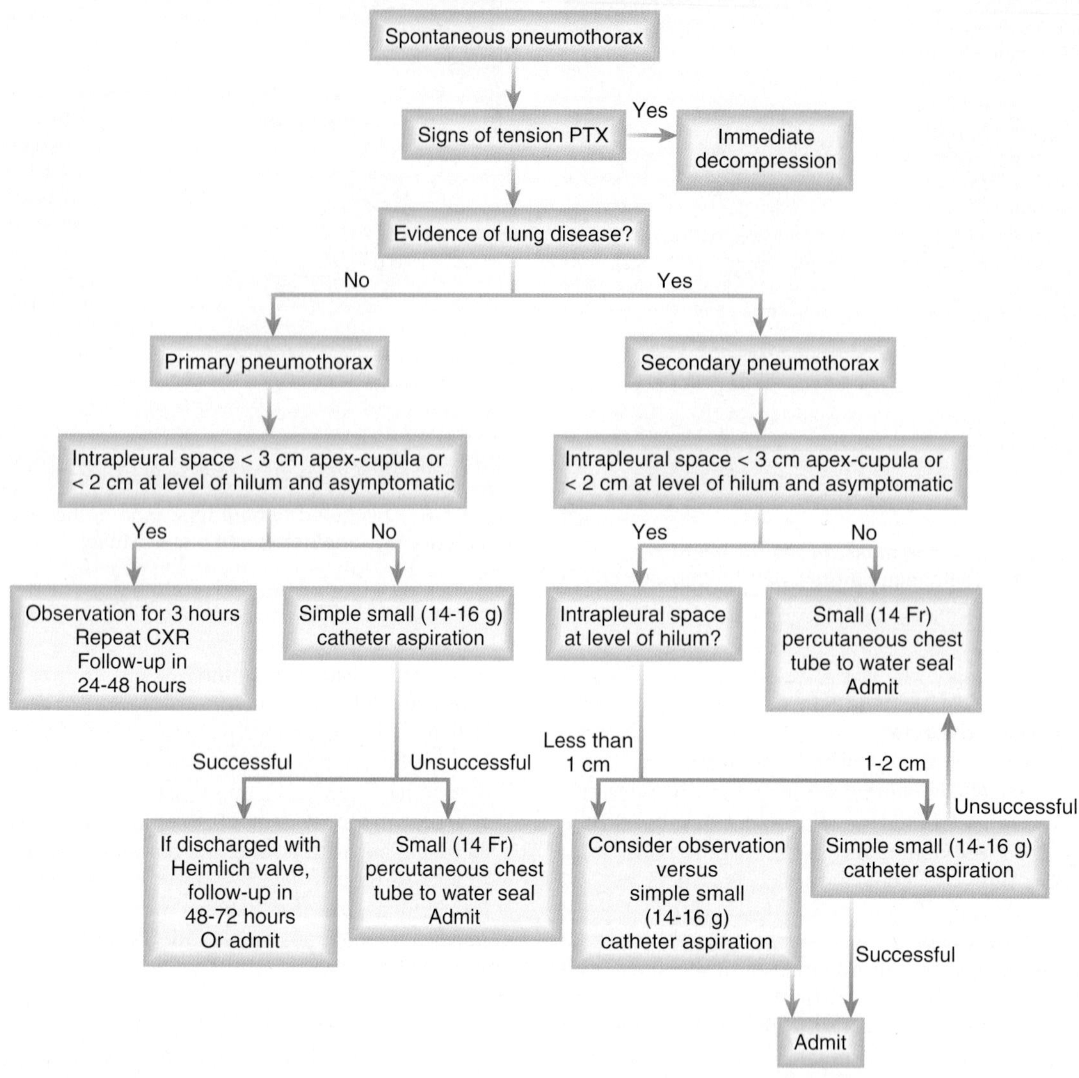


**Fig. 51.7 Algorithmic approach to the treatment of primary spontaneous pneumothorax.** *CXR*, Chest radiograph.

### Consultation

Decisions regarding catheter aspiration versus chest tube treatment for a pneumothorax should include the input of the physician who will continue care, either in the hospital or on an outpatient basis.

Any patient with a persistent air leak after tube thoracostomy, a history or findings of pleural adhesions, recurrent pneumothoraces, or secondary pneumothoraces should be discussed with the chest surgeon to determine optimal care. Such care may include video-assisted thoracic surgery or pleurodesis.

## FOLLOW-UP, NEXT STEPS IN CARE, AND PATIENT EDUCATION

### DISPOSITION

The disposition of patients with pneumothorax is detailed in the algorithms in Figures 51.7 and 51.8. A patient with a primary spontaneous pneumothorax who has been treated by observation or catheter aspiration can be discharged if the pneumothorax does not increase over a period of 3 to 6 hours and the symptoms do not worsen. For a patient discharged with a primary spontaneous pneumothorax without intervention, follow-up should occur in the next 24 to 48 hours to document stability or resolution of the pneumothorax.

In patients with a secondary (associated with underlying lung disease) spontaneous pneumothorax, the treatment algorithm is altered by the underlying lung disease. Clinically stable patients, regardless of the duration of symptoms, should not be monitored in the ED or treated with catheter aspiration and discharged. They should all be admitted to the hospital for observation, simple aspiration, or tube thoracostomy.[13]

### COMPLICATIONS

Complications of pneumothorax include those related to hypoxia, hypercapnia, and hypotension. Reexpansion lung injury is rare but most commonly occurs after reexpansion of

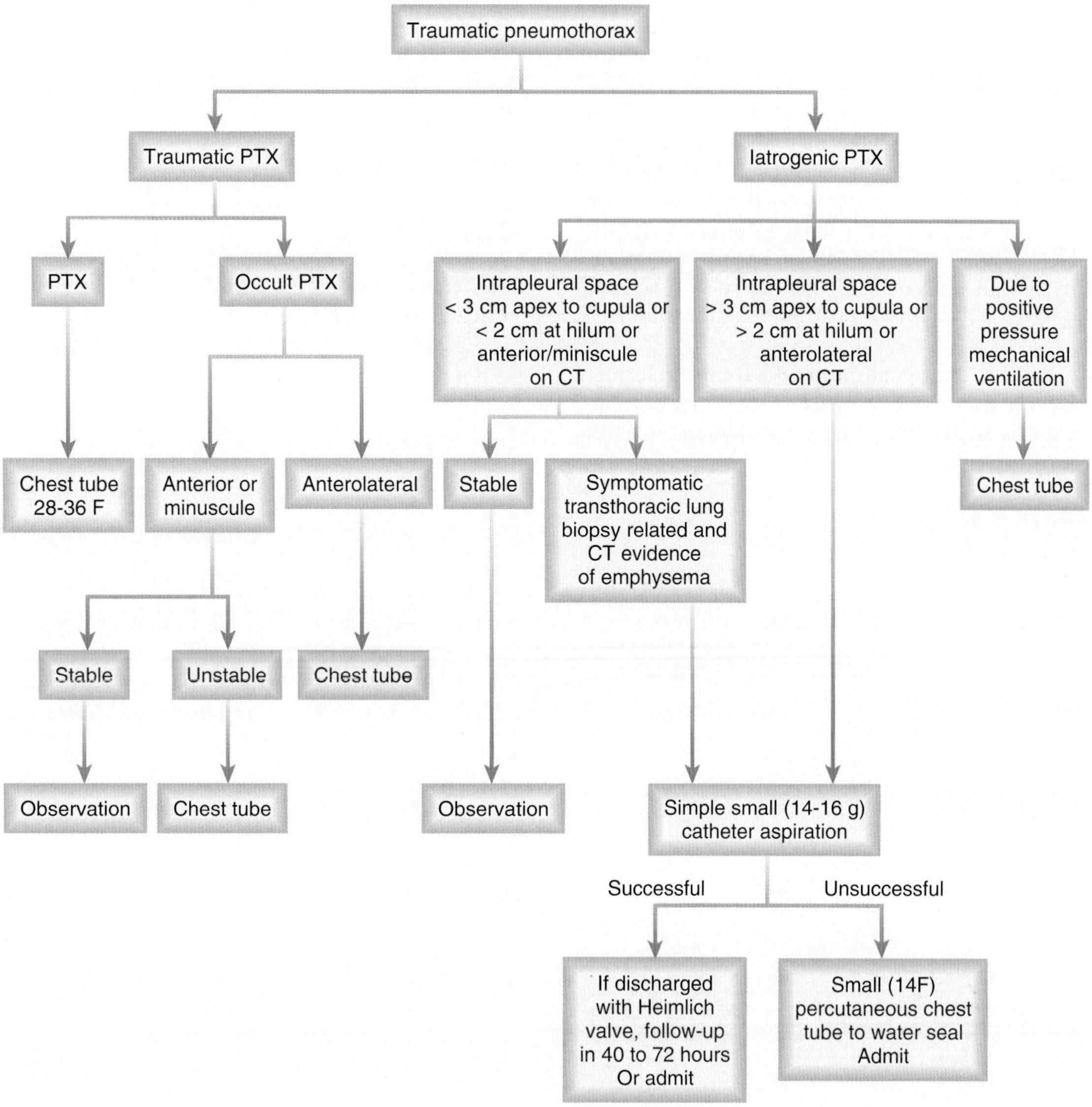

- Traumatic pneumothorax
  - Traumatic PTX
    - PTX
      - Chest tube 28-36 F
    - Occult PTX
      - Anterior or minuscule
        - Stable
          - Observation
        - Unstable
          - Chest tube
      - Anterolateral
        - Chest tube
  - Iatrogenic PTX
    - Intrapleural space < 3 cm apex to cupula or < 2 cm at hilum or anterior/miniscule on CT
      - Stable
        - Observation
      - Symptomatic transthoracic lung biopsy related and CT evidence of emphysema
        - Simple small (14-16 g) catheter aspiration
    - Intrapleural space > 3 cm apex to cupula or > 2 cm at hilum or anterolateral on CT
      - Simple small (14-16 g) catheter aspiration
        - Successful
          - If discharged with Heimlich valve, follow-up in 40 to 72 hours Or admit
        - Unsuccessful
          - Small (14F) percutaneous chest tube to water seal Admit
    - Due to positive pressure mechanical ventilation
      - Chest tube

**Fig. 51.8 Algorithmic approach to the treatment of traumatic pneumothorax.** *CT*, Computed tomography; *PTX*, pneumothorax.

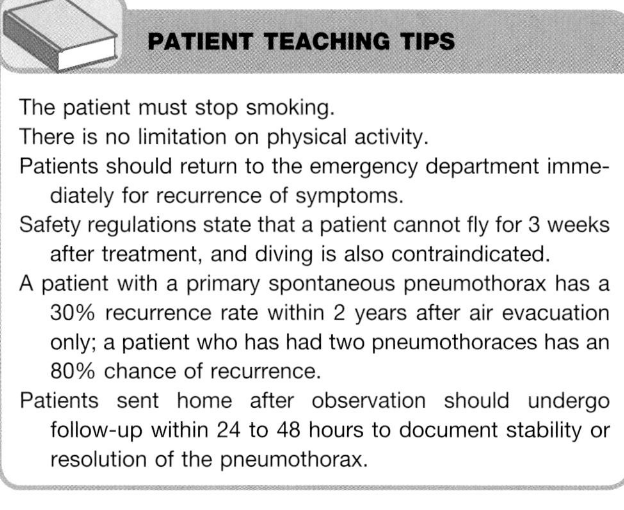

**PATIENT TEACHING TIPS**

The patient must stop smoking.

There is no limitation on physical activity.

Patients should return to the emergency department immediately for recurrence of symptoms.

Safety regulations state that a patient cannot fly for 3 weeks after treatment, and diving is also contraindicated.

A patient with a primary spontaneous pneumothorax has a 30% recurrence rate within 2 years after air evacuation only; a patient who has had two pneumothoraces has an 80% chance of recurrence.

Patients sent home after observation should undergo follow-up within 24 to 48 hours to document stability or resolution of the pneumothorax.

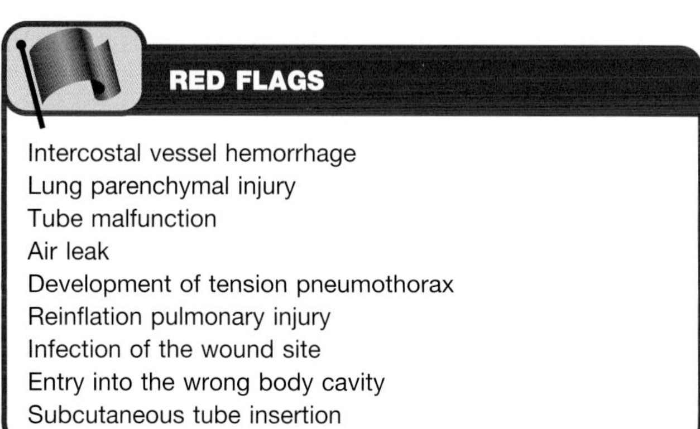

**RED FLAGS**

Intercostal vessel hemorrhage

Lung parenchymal injury

Tube malfunction

Air leak

Development of tension pneumothorax

Reinflation pulmonary injury

Infection of the wound site

Entry into the wrong body cavity

Subcutaneous tube insertion

a large pneumothorax. Risk factors appear to include collapse of the lung for longer than 72 hours, a large pneumothorax, rapid reexpansion, and use of negative pleural pressure suction greater than 20 cm $H_2O$.[14]

Persistent air leaks occur when the volume of air escaping into the pleural space is greater than the volume of air being removed by the drainage device. This complication is more common with a pneumothorax secondary to underlying lung disease. Typically, such air leaks resolve spontaneously within a week (in 75% of patients with a primary pneumothorax and in 61% with a secondary pneumothorax). If an air leak persists beyond 7 days, surgical intervention should be considered.

Complications that can occur during chest tube placement or catheter aspiration include intercostal vessel damage and hemorrhage, lung parenchymal injury, and tube malfunction.

## SUGGESTED READINGS

Haynes D, Baumann MH. Management of pneumothorax. Semin Respir Crit Care Med 2010;31:769-80.

MacDuff A, Arnold A, Harvey J. Management of spontaneous pneumothorax: British Thoracic Society Pleural Disease Guideline 2010. Thorax 2010;65:ii18-31.

Volpicelli G. Sonographic diagnosis of pneumothorax. Intensive Care Med 2011;37:224-32.

## REFERENCES

***References can be found on Expert Consult @ www.expertconsult.com.***

# Pleural Effusion 52

*Bret A. Nicks and David E. Manthey*

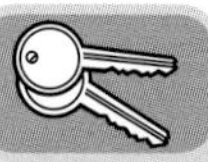

**KEY POINTS**

- Pleural effusion is the manifestation of an underlying disease process.
- The most common cause of pleural effusion in developed countries is congestive heart failure.
- Pulmonary embolism should be considered in patients with pulmonary effusions of uncertain etiology.
- Therapeutic thoracentesis is indicated in the emergency department for relief of acute respiratory or cardiovascular distress.
- Diagnostic thoracentesis should be performed in the emergency department to diagnose immediately life-threatening conditions in toxic-appearing patients.

## EPIDEMIOLOGY

Because pleural effusions are harbingers of underlying disease, their precise incidence is difficult to determine. The incidence in the United States is estimated to be at least 1.5 million cases annually.[1] In industrialized countries worldwide, the incidence approaches 320 cases per 100,000 people—with heart failure, bacterial pneumonia, cirrhosis, malignancy, and pulmonary embolism representing the most common causes. The morbidity and mortality associated with pleural effusion are directly related to cause, stage of disease at the time of diagnosis, and biochemical findings in the pleural fluid. Because pleural effusions are manifestations of underlying diseases, age, sex, race, and socioeconomic status reflect the variation in incidence of the causative disease state or disorder.

## PATHOPHYSIOLOGY

Under normal physiologic conditions, the parietal and visceral pleurae are in close apposition, with only a small potential space between them. This potential space contains a small amount of pleural fluid (1 mL) to minimize friction from continuous movement of the appositional lining. The accumulation of pleural fluid (whether osmotic or hydrostatic in nature) can usually be explained by either increased pleural fluid formation or decreased pleural fluid absorption, or both.

Pleural effusions caused by an increase in pleural fluid formation can be further subdivided into elevation in hydrostatic pressure (e.g., congestive heart failure), decreased colloid osmotic pressure (e.g., cirrhosis, nephrotic syndrome), increased capillary permeability (e.g., infection, neoplasm), passage of fluid through openings in the diaphragm (e.g., ascites), or reduction of pleural space pressure (e.g., atelectasis). An effusion caused by decreased pleural fluid absorption can be qualified further as either lymphatic obstruction or elevation of systemic venous pressure resulting in impaired lymphatic drainage (e.g., superior vena cava syndrome).

The presence of fluid in the normally negative pressure environment of the pleural space has a number of consequences for respiratory physiology. Pleural effusions produce a restrictive ventilatory defect and also decrease total lung capacity, functional residual capacity, and forced vital capacity. They may cause ventilation-perfusion mismatches and, when large enough, compromise cardiac output.[2]

The classic work of Light et al.[3] in 1972 demonstrated that 99% of pleural effusions could be classified into these two general categories, transudative and exudative (**Box 52.1**). A basic difference is that transudates generally reflect a systemic process whereas exudates usually signify underlying local pleuropulmonary disease.[3]

## PRESENTING SIGNS AND SYMPTOMS

In many cases, pleural effusions are asymptomatic when discovered. Physical findings of pleural effusions are unlikely to be manifested until an effusion exceeds 300 mL. Dyspnea, the most common symptom associated with pleural effusion, is related more to distortion of the diaphragm and chest wall during respiration than to hypoxemia. Less commonly, symptoms of pleural effusions consist of a mild, nonproductive cough and chest pain. Pleuritic chest pain indicates inflammation of the parietal pleura because the visceral pleura is not innervated. In many patients, drainage of pleural fluid alleviates the symptoms despite limited improvement in gas exchange. Findings on lung examination such as decreased breath sounds, dullness to percussion, pleural friction rub, egophony, and reduced tactile fremitus have all been described.[1,2] Auscultation alone can miss up to 600 mL of fluid in the lung.[4-6]

**BOX 52.1 Light Criteria for Classification of Pleural Effusions**

In 1972, Light et al.[3] developed the currently accepted benchmark for classifying pleural fluid, as follows:

- Pleural fluid protein–to–serum protein ratio > 0.5 : 1
- Pleural fluid lactate dehydrogenase (LDH)–to–serum LDH ratio > 0.6 : 1
- Pleural fluid LDH greater than two thirds the upper limit of normal for serum LDH (a cutoff value of 200 IU/L was used previously)

Pleural fluid is classified as an exudate if it meets any of the aforementioned criteria. Conversely, if all three characteristics are absent, the fluid is classified as a transudate. These researchers achieved a diagnostic sensitivity of 99% and specificity of 98% for classification of an exudate.

**BOX 52.2 Signs and Symptoms of Effusion***

Dyspnea
Cough (dry, nonproductive)
Chest pain (pleuritic or nonpleuritic)
Chest wall discomfort
Decreased breath sounds
Dullness to percussion
Egophony, tactile fremitus
Pleural friction rub
Disease-specific signs and symptoms may include:
  Orthopnea
  Paroxysmal nocturnal dyspnea
  Fever
  Night sweats

*A detailed past medical history may uncover the cause of the effusion.

The emergency physician should assess for the cause of the effusion. If a patient complains of fever, weight loss, and a progressively worsening cough with associated dyspnea, an oncologic or infectious cause is likely. Constant chest wall pain may reflect chest wall invasion by bronchogenic carcinoma or malignant mesothelioma. Pleuritic chest pain suggests either pulmonary embolism or an inflammatory pleural process. An effusion can mimic the classic symptoms of acute coronary syndrome, such as chest pain, dyspnea, and shoulder pain (**Box 52.2**).

## DIFFERENTIAL DIAGNOSIS AND MEDICAL DECISION MAKING

A pleural effusion is frequently identified during evaluation of the underlying chief complaint of the patient. Because the etiology of pleural effusion is myriad, a thorough history and physical examination may narrow the differential diagnosis substantially. **Box 52.3** lists the common causes of pleural effusion. Frequently, effusion is identified on physical examination or with basic chest radiography, but additional imaging modalities, including radiography, ultrasonography, and computed tomography (CT), may identify the cause and provide additional insight about the effusion.[1,3,6]

**BOX 52.3 Causes of Pleural Effusions**

**Transudates**
Atelectasis (early)
Congestive heart failure
Cirrhosis
Glomerulonephritis
Hypoalbuminemia
Myxedema
Nephrotic syndrome
Peritoneal dialysis
Pulmonary embolism
Superior vena cava syndrome

**Exudates**

***Infectious***
Bacterial infection
Bronchiectasis
Fungal infection
Lung abscess
Parasitic infection
Traumatic hemothorax
Tuberculosis
Viral illness

***Malignancies***
Lymphoma
Mesothelioma
Primary lung cancer
Pulmonary metastasis

***Connective Tissue Disease***
Rheumatoid arthritis
Systemic lupus erythematosus

***Abdominal/Gastrointestinal***
Esophageal rupture
Pancreatic disorders
Subphrenic abscess

***Other***
Atelectasis (chronic)
Chylothorax
Drug reactions (amiodarone)
Postpartum state
Pulmonary infarction or embolism
Uremia

$SI = \frac{SV}{BSA}$ **FACTS AND FORMULAS**

Auscultation alone can miss effusions of up to 600 mL.
Effusions of approximately 400 mL are routinely visible on upright chest radiographs.
Bedside ultrasonography is effective for visualizing and characterizing effusions.
Ultrasound-guided thoracentesis should be performed when available.

## DIAGNOSTIC CONSIDERATIONS

### RADIOGRAPHY

Erect posteroanterior and lateral chest radiographs are still the most important initial tools in the diagnosis of a pleural effusion. On upright and lateral decubitus films, loss of the costophrenic angle is seen. With increasing size of the pleural effusion, the hemidiaphragm is obscured (**Fig. 52.1**), and a mass effect with shift of the mediastinum away from the affected side is noted. If a film is taken with the patient supine, one may see only a nonspecific haze over the affected hemithorax because the fluid layers posteriorly. To confirm that the fluid is free flowing, lateral decubitus films with the affected side down are often obtained. With very large effusions, the affected side may remain opacified, thus rendering the decubitus film unhelpful. In adults the minimum amount of fluid required for identification of effusion on an upright film is approximately 400 mL, whereas lateral decubitus films (with the affected side down) may detect as little as 50 mL of fluid. A lateral decubitus film with the affected side up may facilitate evaluation of the underlying lung for atelectasis, a mass, or infiltrates along the lateral portion of the lung.[5,6]

Mediastinal shift contralateral to the effusion (observed with effusions > 1000 mL) with concomitant displacement of the trachea is an important clue to obstruction of a lobar bronchus by an endobronchial lesion, possibly because of malignancy or, less commonly, obstruction by a foreign body.

Subpulmonic effusions are an uncommon manifestation of pleural effusions seen when fluid accumulates between the lower lung lobe and diaphragm. The fluid collection may mimic an elevated hemidiaphragm in upright imaging (**Fig. 52.2**). Upward of 400 mL of fluid can collect in the subpulmonic region before the posterior costophrenic sinus is filled. Evidence of an elevated hemidiaphragm with steep lateral peaks, obscured pulmonary vessels below the level of the diaphragm on a lateral projection, or a flat appearance of the posterior aspect of the hemidiaphragm on a lateral projection is suggestive of a subpulmonic effusion.[6]

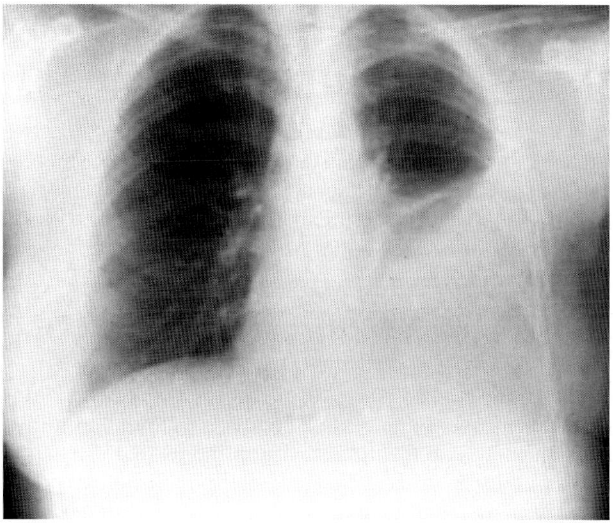

**Fig. 52.1** Large parapneumonic effusion on an upright chest radiograph.

### ULTRASONOGRAPHY

Ultrasonography is effective for visualizing an effusion and determining whether the fluid is free flowing or loculated (**Fig. 52.3**).[7-9] In a prospective study, Piccoli et al.[8] compared ultrasonography, physical examination, and radiography in patients with suspected effusions. Findings on physical examination and radiography were in agreement 76% of the time, with a kappa value of 0.52. When compared with chest ultrasonography, physical examination showed a sensitivity of 69% and a specificity of 77%. Ultrasonography may help distinguish a large solid chest mass from an effusion and can be used to guide thoracentesis. Ramnath et al.[10] suggested early use of ultrasonography to identify complicated effusions (loculations or organization) because patients whose effusions were

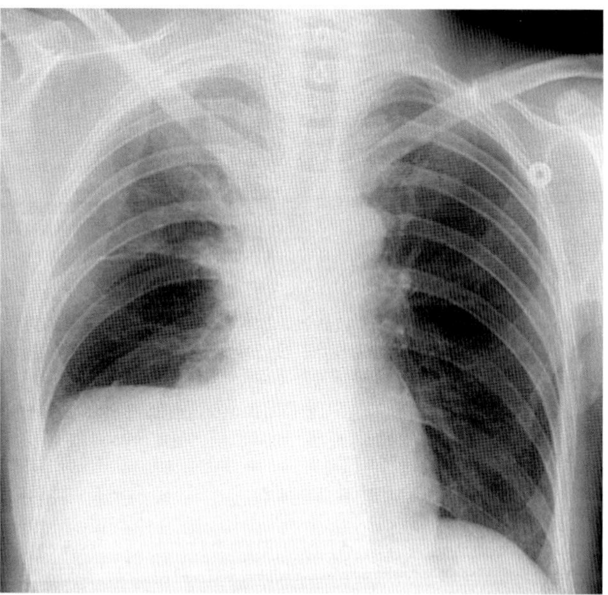

**Fig. 52.2** A subpulmonic effusion may mimic the surface of the diaphragm without blunting the costophrenic angle.

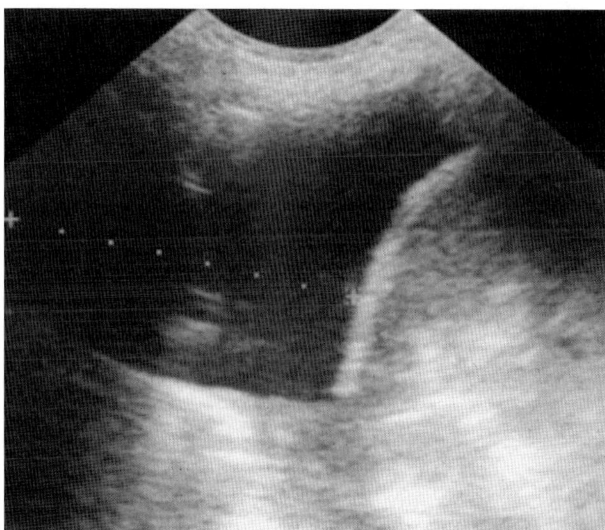

**Fig. 52.3** Upright bedside ultrasonogram of a large pleural effusion.

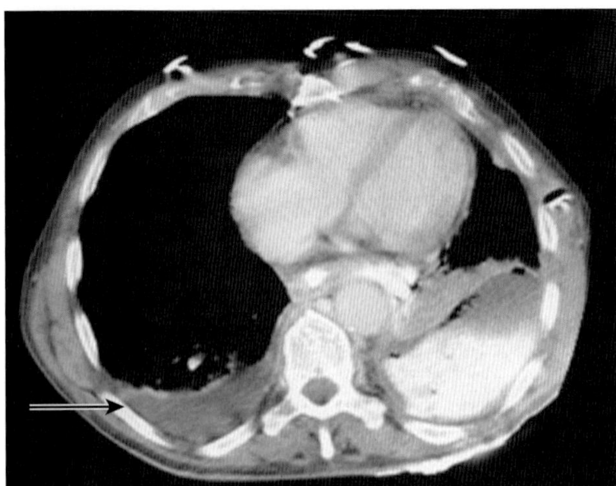

**Fig. 52.4** A pleural effusion *(arrow)* seen on chest computed tomography.

**BOX 52.4 Fluid Analysis of Pleural Effusions**

**Exudates**

Protein content > 3 g/dL
High lactate dehydrogenase (LDH) content
Pleural fluid–to–serum LDH ratio > 0.6 : 1
Pleural fluid–to–serum protein ratio > 0.5 : 1

**Differential Clues**

Gross blood in pleural fluid suggests tumor, trauma, or infarction.
Pleural fluid amylase elevation is associated with pancreatic disease, esophageal rupture, or malignancy.
Pleural fluid pH is normally higher than 7.30; a pH lower than 7.2 suggests an infectious process such as empyema.
Consider pulmonary emboli as the cause of loculated pleural effusions, particularly if the pleural fluid predominantly contains lymphocytes.

treated aggressively by decortication had significantly shorter hospital stays than did those whose effusions were treated with tube thoracostomy alone. The same study showed that in children with effusions but no ultrasonographic evidence of organization, outcomes in those receiving treatment consisting of intravenous antibiotics and drainage were similar to outcomes in those undergoing aggressive treatment such as thoracoscopy or decortication. The major advantage of ultrasonography over conventional radiography is its ability to differentiate between solid and liquid components, thereby assisting in identification of pleural fluid loculations.

## COMPUTED TOMOGRAPHY

CT is rarely needed to diagnose a pleural effusion but may identify an underlying mass. In adults the presence of parietal pleural thickening on contrast-enhanced CT is a specific but insensitive indicator of an exudate. Cross-sectional imaging more clearly distinguishes anatomic compartments such as the pleural space from lung parenchyma (**Fig. 52.4**). Chest CT is likely to be valuable in making management decisions for complicated effusions because it can distinguish empyema from lung abscess, detect pleural masses, outline loculated fluid collections, and identify additional problems such as contusions, blebs, and infiltrates.[6]

## PLEURAL FLUID ANALYSIS

Ideally, evaluation of a pleural effusion should begin with diagnostic thoracentesis and proceed to classification of the pleural fluid as either a transudate or an exudate. The currently accepted benchmark for classifying pleural fluid, developed by Light et al.,[3] is shown in Box 52.1. A number of later studies used modifications of the Light criteria but had poorer diagnostic accuracy.[11]

Normal pleural fluid pH has been estimated to be approximately 7.64. A pH below 7.30 suggests the presence of an inflammatory or infiltrative process,[12] such as parapneumonic effusion, empyema, malignancy, connective tissue disease, tuberculosis, or esophageal rupture. According to the current American College of Chest Physicians consensus statement on the treatment of parapneumonic effusions, pH is the preferred pleural fluid chemistry test for classifying the category of a parapneumonic effusion for subsequent management (**Box 52.4**).[13,14] Additional testing considerations for pleural fluid include cholesterol, glucose, amylase, and adenosine deaminase.[11,13,14]

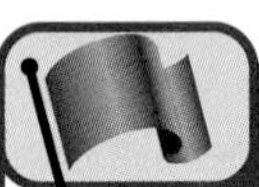

**RED FLAGS**

Failure to establish a working differential diagnosis or identify the underlying cause
Failure to initiate prompt source management for an underlying infectious cause
Failure to identify and manage tension physiology caused by large effusions on an emergency basis

# TREATMENT

Acute medical management of pleural effusions is based on both therapeutic and diagnostic considerations. In the emergency department (ED), therapeutic thoracentesis is indicated for relief of acute respiratory or cardiovascular distress. Diagnostic thoracentesis should be used in the ED to diagnose immediately life-threatening conditions in toxic-appearing patients. Circumstances outside these situations should not necessitate emergency thoracentesis, but appropriate monitoring and further medical management are essential. **Table 52.1** summarizes findings dictating the appropriateness of intervention.[13]

## APPROACH TO UNILATERAL PLEURAL EFFUSION

Thoracentesis should be performed for new and unexplained pleural effusions when sufficient fluid is present to allow a safe procedure. Conventional wisdom holds that if a 10-mm layer of fluid is visible on a radiograph, sufficient fluid is present for thoracentesis to be successful. Treatment of the underlying disorder is generally all that is required for effusions caused by renal, cardiac, or rheumatologic diseases.

**Table 52.1 Management of Patients with Parapneumonic Effusions**

| PLEURAL ANATOMY | PLEURAL FLUID MICROBIOLOGY | PLEURAL FLUID CHEMICAL ANALYSIS | PERFORM DRAINAGE? |
|---|---|---|---|
| Minimal effusion: <10 mm on lateral decubitus radiograph; No loculations | Unknown culture and Gram stain results | Unknown pH | No |
| Small to moderate effusion: >10 mm but <½ the hemithorax on lateral decubitus radiograph; No loculations | Negative culture and Gram stain results | pH > 7.20 | No |
| Large effusion: >½ the hemithorax or associated loculations or pleural thickening | Positive culture or Gram stain results | pH < 7.20 | Yes |
| Other | Purulent | pH < 7.0 | Yes |

## APPROACH TO PLEURAL EFFUSION ASSOCIATED WITH MALIGNANCY

Malignancy-induced pleural effusions should undergo therapeutic thoracentesis as needed. If effusions are undiagnosed, cytologic evaluation is required for patients with oncologic risks. Completion of evaluation may require CT assessment and subsequent tissue biopsy.

## APPROACH TO PARAPNEUMONIC PLEURAL EFFUSIONS

Parapneumonic effusion and empyema are treated initially with empiric antibiotics according to the patient's age and the probable organisms and sensitivities commonly present in the community. Parapneumonic effusion usually progresses through three stages. The exudative stage is associated with capillary leak during the first 3 days; the fibrinopurulent stage is associated with bacterial invasion of the pleura between days 3 and 7; and the organizational stage is characterized by fibroblast growth, occurring for 2 to 3 weeks, if the effusion is not treated properly. Lack of early diagnosis and drainage of empyema, especially in younger children, may worsen the course of disease. In a hospitalized patient with a complicated parapneumonic effusion, antibiotics are administered intravenously and a thoracostomy tube is left in place until the patient is afebrile and improving clinically. Oral antibiotics are frequently continued for weeks after these procedures.[1,13]

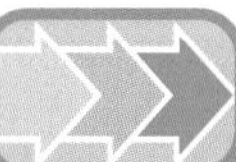

**PRIORITY ACTIONS**

Identify the cause of the pleural effusion.
Therapeutic thoracentesis is recommended for symptomatic patients.
Assess respiratory status before and after any intervention.
Inform patients about the complications associated with pleural effusions and thoracentesis.

## THORACENTESIS: THE IDEAL APPROACH

Thoracentesis is an elective procedure requiring informed consent. Sterile technique and procedural experience lower the incidence of complications.

Drainage of a pleural effusion is indicated for the following reasons:

- Diagnostic fluid or cellular analysis
- Therapeutic relief of symptomatic dyspnea
- Evaluation of complicated parapneumonic effusions or empyema

### POSITIONING

Ideally for thoracentesis, the patient should sit on the edge of the bed, lean forward slightly, and rest on an adjustable table. If the patient cannot sit up because of hemodynamic status, mental status, or the presence of tubes and indwelling lines, thoracentesis can be performed with the patient supine. In this case, the patient should turn onto the side with the effusion and move to position the back at the edge of the bed.

### PROCEDURAL APPROACH

Diagnostic thoracentesis is used to determine the cause of a pleural effusion, and therapeutic thoracentesis is performed to relieve symptoms of respiratory distress. Therapeutic thoracentesis may be repeated if indicated, but more definitive therapy such as sclerosis is usually needed to treat recurrent symptomatic pleural effusions. If more than 1.0 to 1.5 L of fluid is removed at one time, reexpansion pulmonary edema (RPE) and postthoracentesis shock should be anticipated in the postprocedural period. Supplemental oxygen should be provided because postthoracentesis decreases in arterial oxygenation have been reported. The magnitude and duration of this decline roughly correlate with the amount of fluid removed. If removal of a large volume of fluid is anticipated, concurrent fluid resuscitation should be considered to blunt postthoracentesis shock. Depending on the causative process, reaccumulation of pleural fluid may occur.

After appropriate positioning, the patient is prepared in standard sterile fashion. The effusion can be identified along the posterior infrascapular line by either clinical examination (auscultation and percussion) or bedside ultrasonography. Ultrasonography is recommended because it identifies not only the level of effusion but also the subdiaphragmatic organs that should be avoided and the depth of the fluid pocket.[7,8] As the angiocatheter is advanced, the neurovascular bundles located on the inferior aspect of the ribs should be avoided. Aspiration of fluid can continue until enough fluid is obtained for diagnostic purposes or therapeutic relief.

Needle thoracentesis is adequate for both diagnostic evaluation and therapeutic management of most parapneumonic pleural effusions. When the effusion has progressed to the fibrinopurulent or organizational stage, needle thoracentesis is often inadequate. Thoracoscopy offers the advantages of visual evaluation of the pleura, direct tissue sampling, and therapeutic intervention such as dissecting loculations and pleurodesis. Appropriate consultation for medical thoracoscopy and video-assisted thoracoscopy is indicated in these circumstances.

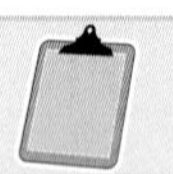

**DOCUMENTATION**

Identify the size and location of the effusion.
Consider the cause and duration of the effusion.
Discuss the appropriate intervention and associated risks.
Assess respiratory function before and after any intervention.
Document repeated physical examination and vital signs during the postprocedural period.
Ensure appropriate outpatient follow-up or inpatient evaluation.

## CONTRAINDICATIONS

Procedural contraindications to pleurocentesis or thoracostomy are listed in **Box 52.5**. Absolute contraindications include coagulopathy, known adhesions, and a history of pleurodesis. If the patient is symptomatic and coagulopathic, correction of coagulopathy and ultrasonographic guidance are recommended to minimize bleeding risks. Pleurodesis, or the introduction of a chemical or medication (talc, tetracycline, or bleomycin sulfate) into the chest cavity, triggers an inflammatory reaction over the surface of the lung and inside the chest cavity that causes the pleurae to adhere to each other and prevents or reduces further accumulation of pleural fluid. Thoracentesis should be avoided in patients at increased risk for adverse reactions as a result of unstable angina or arrhythmia or known medical noncompliance, including lack of established outpatient care. Relative contraindications include mechanical ventilation because of an increased risk for lung collapse and difficulty with positioning. In intubated patients, use of ultrasonography or CT for thoracentesis or postponing the procedure is recommended if the indication is not urgent. Patients with known bullous lung disease are at increased risk for postprocedural pneumothorax. Placement of the thoracentesis needle through a concurrent chest wall infection should be avoided because the pleural space may become seeded. A postprocedure radiograph should always be obtained to assess for pneumothorax.[13,15]

**BOX 52.5 Contraindications to Thoracentesis**

**Absolute Contraindications**
Adhesions, pleurodesis
Coagulopathy
Dysrhythmia
Known medical noncompliance or lack of established outpatient care

**Relative Contraindications**
Bullous disease
Concurrent chest wall infection
Mechanical ventilation

## COMPLICATIONS

Adverse outcomes associated with pleural effusions can be characterized as iatrogenic or pathologic. Thoracentesis can predispose patients to pneumothorax, acute RPE, shock, subsequent fluid reaccumulation, bleeding, infection, and solid organ injury. If untreated, the parapneumonic effusion can progress to fibrinopurulent empyema, which frequently requires surgical intervention.

If the patient complains of increasing respiratory distress within the first hour after thoracentesis, RPE or pneumothorax may be occurring, and an emergency chest radiograph should be obtained. RPE is a syndrome associated with hypotension and hypoxemia. It is thought to be a result of combined alveolar-capillary membrane disruption initiated by distention, reperfusion-mediated injury, and increased pulmonary flow. Risk factors include previous atelectasis and rapid reexpansion of the lung parenchyma. Typically, a patient with significant RPE becomes symptomatic within 15 minutes to 2 hours after rapid reexpansion of the lung. Treatment is based on adequate oxygenation and circulation, generally with positive end-expiratory pressure. Concern about the potential for RPE after thoracentesis is important because mortality in patients with this condition is consistently 15% to 20% despite mechanical ventilation.[16,17]

## FOLLOW-UP, NEXT STEPS IN CARE, AND PATIENT EDUCATION

In many cases, small pleural effusions are identified during evaluation of the patient's chief complaint. Although not all effusions require immediate drainage, when thoracentesis is performed, stable patients with a clear etiology and well-established care plan may be discharged after an appropriate observation period of 3 to 6 hours. Patients with large-volume evacuation or exudative effusions or those who require further evaluation and stabilization should be admitted to the hospital.[13,16]

Close outpatient follow-up and management are required for all patients evaluated for pleural effusion, regardless of whether they underwent thoracentesis, to further address the underlying cause and monitor the effusion.

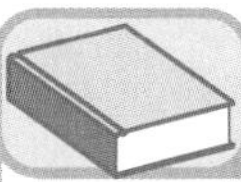

## PATIENT TEACHING TIPS

Pleural effusions represent an underlying disease process that must be addressed.

Possible complications of pleural effusions include pneumothorax, respiratory failure secondary to massive fluid reaccumulation, septicemia, bronchopleural fistula, and pleural thickening.

Follow-up is recommended for all patients undergoing thoracentesis. Some experts recommend serial chest radiographs to ensure clearing. Some perform computed tomography after plain radiographs show clearing.

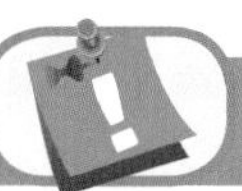

## TIPS AND TRICKS

Establish bedside ultrasonography as part of assessment for pleural effusions.

Consider pulmonary embolism with an uncertain pleural effusion etiology.

Ultrasound-guided thoracentesis enhances visualization and minimizes complications.

Complicated pleural effusions may require surgical intervention.

“Two-test” and “three-test” rules for pleural fluid analysis exist but are not as specific as the Light criteria.

## SUGGESTED READINGS

Neustein SM. Reexpansion pulmonary edema. J Cardiothorac Vasc Anesth 2007;21:887-91.

Sahn SA. The value of pleural fluid analysis. Am J Med Sci 2008;335:7-15.

Sartori S, Sombesi P. Emerging roles for transthoracic ultrasonography in pleuropulmonary pathology. World J Radiol 2010;2:83-90.

Thomsen TW, DeLaPena J, Setnik GS. Thoracentesis. N Engl J Med 2006;355:e16.

## REFERENCES

***References can be found on Expert Consult @ www.expertconsult.com.***

# 53 Lung Transplant Complications

*Michael K. Abraham and Robert L. Rogers*

**KEY POINTS**

- All lung transplant recipients with respiratory complaints should be assessed for the possibility of rejection and parenchymal lung infection. In most cases, assessment leads to admission to the hospital.
- Rejection and pulmonary infection are frequently indistinguishable. The clinical manifestation of pneumonia and lung allograft rejection may be subtle, and admission is required to address both entities.
- Lung rejection is common and can occur anytime after transplantation.
- Transplanted lungs are highly susceptible to pneumonia. Cytomegalovirus pneumonia is the most common opportunistic pulmonary infection after lung transplantation.

## SCOPE

A lung transplant recipient may seek care in the emergency department (ED) as a result of complications related to the surgical procedure, infections, or medication interactions. The main worry when dealing with transplant patients is to identify the threat for lung allograft rejection and begin treatment if necessary. To complicate matters, potent immunosuppressive regimens may mask serious or life-threatening infectious diseases in organ transplant recipients. This chapter provides information to arm the emergency physician (EP) with the knowledge necessary to take care of this complex group of patients.

More than 1500 lung transplants are performed each year in the United States; worldwide, approximately 3000 were performed in 2009.[1] Survival rates had been rising in recent years because of technologic advances in surgical technique and immunobiology, but they seem to have reached a plateau. The current survival rate 1 year after transplantation is 79%.[1] Multiple conditions necessitate lung transplantation, including cystic fibrosis, end-stage chronic obstructive lung disease, and interstitial lung disease (**Box 53.1**).[2] The primary reason for bilateral lung transplantation is chronic obstructive pulmonary disease.[3]

The number of patients who have undergone solid organ transplantation increases every year. In 2008 alone, 27,281 organ transplantations were performed in the United States.[2] This figure represents a large number of patients who might seek medical care in an ED. In addition, current survival rates are rising. In 1998, 1-, 3-, and 5-year survival rates were 70.7%, 54.8%, and 42.6%, respectively, for lung transplant recipients. In 2009, the rates were 79%, 63%, and 52%.[1] Although survival rates for lung transplantation lag behind those for other solid organ transplantations, enhancements in immunotherapy will probably continue to advance.[4,5]

## COMPLICATIONS RELATED TO THE SURGICAL PROCEDURE

The type of transplant (single lung, double lung, combined heart and lung, lobar) depends on the recipient's disease and the particular transplant center where the procedure is performed.[6] Single-lung transplantation requires a lateral thoracotomy incision, and double-lung transplantation requires a double thoracotomy ("clamshell") incision. The heart may be transplanted along with one or both lungs. In some cases, a lobar segment of donor lung is transplanted. The surgical procedure includes anastomosis of the pulmonary arteries, veins, and bronchus.

## EMERGENCY DEPARTMENT PRESENTATION

Patients who have undergone lung transplantation should be considered high risk when seen in an ED for evaluation. Because many patients live far from the facility where their surgery was performed, they are likely to go the nearest ED when problems arise. In a retrospective review of 131 lung and heart-lung transplant patients who visited an ED, the most common complaints were fever (37%), shortness of breath (13%), gastrointestinal symptoms (10%), and chest pain (9%).[6,7]

ED manifestations of lung transplant recipients are commonly related to complications of the surgical procedure and immunosuppression. Disease unrelated to the transplant may also be present.

**BOX 53.1 Reasons for Lung Transplantation**

Emphysema/chronic obstructive pulmonary disease
Cystic fibrosis
Idiopathic pulmonary fibrosis
Primary pulmonary hypertension
$\alpha_1$-Antitrypsin deficiency
Lung retransplantation (rejection, graft failure)
Sarcoidosis
Bronchiectasis
Pulmonary fibrosis
Occupational lung disease

From United Network for Organ Sharing, 2007. Available at www.unos.org.

**BOX 53.2 Clinical Findings of Acute Lung Allograft Rejection**

Nontoxic-appearing patient
Leukocytosis
Dry, nonproductive cough
Fever
Shortness of breath
Hypoxia
Abnormal chest radiograph findings
Abnormal lung physical examination findings

## DIFFERENTIAL DIAGNOSIS

Patients who have undergone lung transplantation may come to the ED with myriad complaints. Among the most important complications are acute or chronic allograft rejection and infections. To make matters more complex, the required use of immunomodulating agents may diminish or mask objective findings. In addition to rejection and infection, patients in the early postoperative period are at risk for mechanical complications such as bronchial dehiscence. It is important to ascertain the procedure that was performed and the technique that was used. Patients who have received single-lung transplants are at risk for infection, cancer, and other complications in both the transplanted and the native lung.[8]

### REJECTION

Lung allograft rejection is one of the most feared life-threatening complications of lung transplantation; in some cases, the emergence of rejection necessitates retransplantation. The majority of transplant recipients experience at least one episode of rejection. Patients who experience repeated episodes of allograft rejection are at increased risk for chronic rejection (bronchiolitis obliterans syndrome).[9-11]

The clinical findings in patients with lung allograft rejection can be nonspecific or even silent[12] (**Box 53.2**). Patients may report a dry cough, subjective fevers, varying degrees of shortness of breath, or any combination of these symptoms. Episodes of rejection cannot be distinguished from pulmonary infection on clinical grounds alone.[9] The important point for EPs to remember is that the symptoms of allograft dysfunction or rejection may be subtle. Patients may not appear ill or seem to have anything more than a viral upper respiratory tract infection.[13,14]

During the first 6 months after transplantation, chest radiographs may show pleural effusions, interstitial edema, or perihilar infiltrates. Episodes of rejection occurring after this time tend to not lead to abnormalities on the chest radiograph. Normal chest film findings do not rule out the presence of underlying rejection. In the ED, chest radiographs may help in the evaluation of entities that would require immediate therapy, such as pneumothorax or a large pleural effusion.[13,14]

Lung allograft rejection is not usually diagnosed in the ED. Typically, patients are admitted and must undergo fiberoptic bronchoscopy and biopsy for diagnosis. Treatment of suspected lung transplant rejection begins with clinical suspicion. In all cases of suspected rejection, the patient's pulmonologist or lung transplant surgeon should be contacted. This potentially life-threatening entity should be treated before the results of bronchoscopy become available. The biopsy indicates the presence and degree of tissue rejection and inflammation. The complex and histologically directed scale of rejection is beyond the scope of this chapter. The main ED treatment for patients with rejection is high-dose intravenous corticosteroids. Patients are usually given intravenous methylprednisolone at a dose of 0.5 to 1.0 g/day for 3 days, with the first dose given in the ED. If rejection is present, the symptoms should resolve rapidly. The therapy is then switched to oral corticosteroids. It is essential that rejection be diagnosed and treated in the ED in consultation with the patient's transplant physician.[9] Other interventions for acute rejection include methotrexate, muromonab-CD3, antithymocyte globulin, total lymphoid irradiation, and extracorporeal photopheresis.[15-18]

### INFECTIOUS COMPLICATIONS

Despite or possibly as a result of advances in immunosuppression, infection is a common complication after any solid organ transplantation, particularly of the lung.[19-21] Because of the lung parenchyma's interaction with the environment, the most common infection is pneumonia, but any opportunistic infection can occur.

Infectious complications after organ transplantation have been studied extensively and are related to multiple factors, the most important being the time since transplantation. Infections in organ recipients can be broken down into three periods (**Fig. 53.1**).

During the first month after transplantation, nosocomial infections predominate. Wound infections, urinary tract infections, pneumonia, and vascular access infections are common in this period. Opportunistic infections, such as those caused by *Pneumocystis* and *Nocardia* species, do not usually occur in the first month after transplantation.[22] Infections that emerge 1 to 6 months after solid organ transplantation include many of the opportunistic infections, such as those caused by *Pneumocystis carinii* and *Listeria monocytogenes*. In addition,

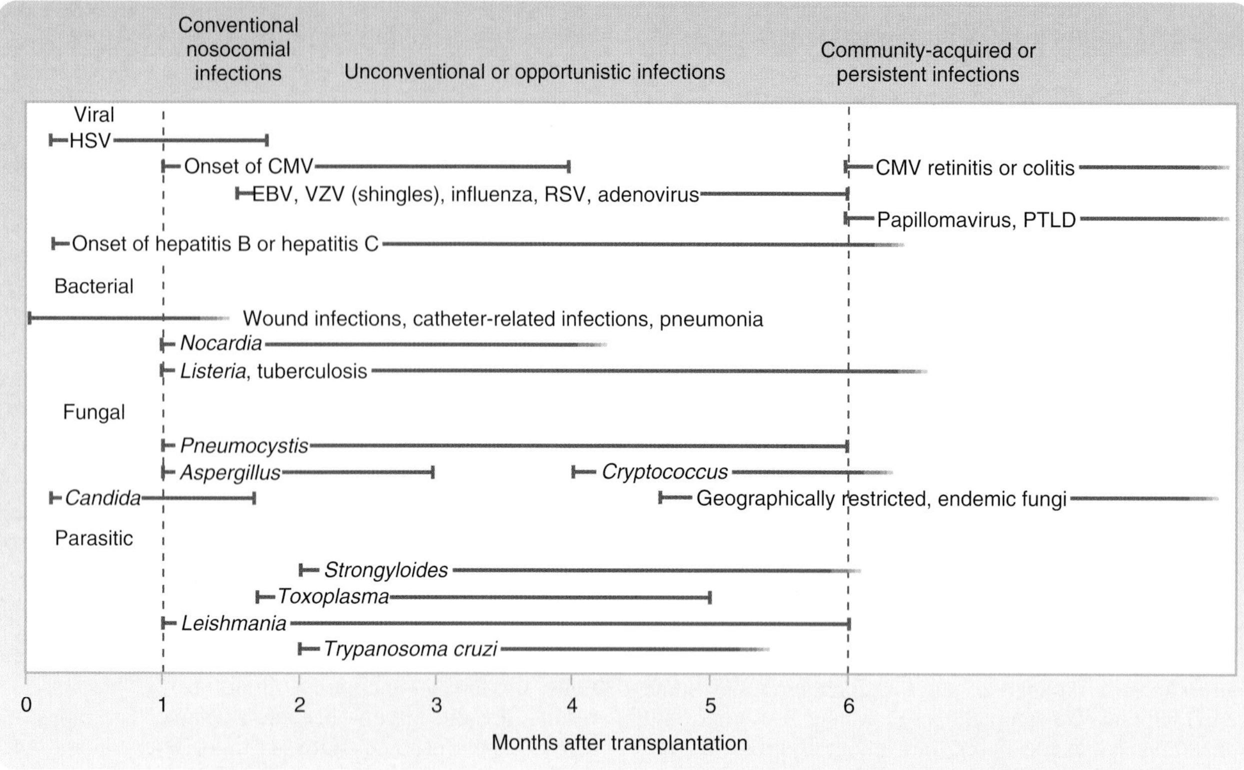


**Fig. 53.1 Time course and probable diseases in patients with lung transplants: infection, acute rejection, and chronic rejection.** *CMV*, Cytomegalovirus; *EBV*, Epstein-Barr virus; *HSV*, herpes simplex virus; *PTLD*, posttransplantation lymphoproliferative disorder; *RSV*, respiratory syncytial virus; *VZV*, varicella-zoster virus.

immunomodulating viruses (particularly cytomegalovirus [CMV]) become important pathogens. Epstein-Barr virus, hepatitis B virus, hepatitis C virus, and human immunodeficiency virus can also produce infection during this time frame.[22]

Viral infections that emerge after the first month following transplantation may be associated with chronic or progressive infection and may cause significant injury to the affected transplanted organ. Patients who experience chronic or recurrent bouts of organ rejection are invariably exposed to higher and prolonged periods of immunosuppressive therapy and thus tend to be vulnerable to these opportunistic pathogens.[1]

## PULMONARY INFECTIONS

The lungs are particularly vulnerable to infection after solid organ transplantation. The highest risk for posttransplantation pulmonary infection occurs in lung transplant recipients. Pulmonary infections are the most common infectious complication in heart and lung transplant recipients[19-21] and the least common in kidney transplant recipients.[23] Multiple factors explain this higher incidence of lung infections (**Box 53.3**).

Organisms that commonly cause pulmonary infection in the postoperative period are gram-negative organisms (nosocomial) and *Staphylococcus aureus*. Community-acquired bacterial pneumonia tends to occur later in the posttransplantation period.[16] Causative organisms include *Haemophilus influenzae, Streptococcus pneumoniae*, and *Legionella* species. Most cases of bronchiolitis obliterans syndrome are caused by *Pseudomonas aeruginosa*. Patients with this syndrome commonly have recurrent episodes of purulent bronchitis and pneumonia.[21] Other infections to consider are fungal pneumonia and tuberculosis (**Table 53.1**).

**BOX 53.3 Factors Contributing to Risk for Pulmonary Infections in Lung Transplant Recipients**

Impairment in cough because of lung denervation
Narrowing of the bronchial anastomosis
Disruption of pulmonary lymphatics
Impairment of the mucociliary "escalator"
Passive transfer of occult pneumonia from the donor

From Kotloff R, Ahya V, Crawford S. Pulmonary complications of solid organ and hematopoietic stem cell transplantation. Am J Respir Crit Care Med 2004;170:22-48.

Pulmonary infections in transplant patients may not cause the symptoms seen in other outpatients who have not received a transplant. As stated earlier, the symptoms may be subtle and may be as simple as a dry cough and mild upper respiratory tract discomfort. Fever in a patient receiving immunosuppressive treatment is a worrisome sign and may be the only manifestation of a serious underlying lung infection such as pneumonia. Many lung transplant recipients do not look that ill initially or do not have fulminant symptoms of pneumonia when first evaluated (**Fig. 53.2**).

**Table 53.1 Differential Diagnosis of Fever and Pulmonary Infiltrates in Organ Transplant Recipients According to the Abnormality on Chest Radiographs and Rate of Progression of the Illness**

| RADIOGRAPHIC ABNORMALITY | CAUSE: ACUTE ILLNESS* | CAUSE: SUBACUTE OR CHRONIC ILLNESS* |
|---|---|---|
| Consolidation | Bacteria (including *Legionella*)<br>Thromboembolism<br>Hemorrhage<br>Pulmonary edema | Fungi<br>*Nocardia asteroides*<br>Tumor<br>Tuberculosis<br>Viruses<br>Drug reactions<br>Radiation exposure<br>*Pneumocystis carinii* |
| Peribronchovascular abnormality | Pulmonary edema<br>Leukoagglutinin reaction<br>Bacteria<br>Viruses (influenza) | Viruses<br>*P. carinii*<br>Irradiation<br>Drug reactions<br>Occasionally *N. asteroides*, tumor, fungi, tuberculosis |
| Nodular infiltrate† | Bacteria (including *Legionella*)<br>Pulmonary edema | Fungi<br>*N. asteroides*<br>Tuberculosis<br>*P. carinii* |

Adapted from Shreeniwas R, Schulman LL, Berkmen YM, et al. Opportunistic bronchopulmonary infections after lung transplantation: clinical and radiographic findings. Radiology 1996;200:349-356

**Acute illness* develops and requires medical attention in less than 24 hours. *Subacute* or *chronic illness* develops over a period of several days to a week.

†A *nodular infiltrate* is one or more focal defects greater than 1 $cm^2$ in area on chest radiographs with well-defined borders and surrounded by aerated lung. Multiple tiny nodules are seen in a wide variety of disorders (e.g., cytomegalovirus, varicella-zoster virus infection) and are not included here.

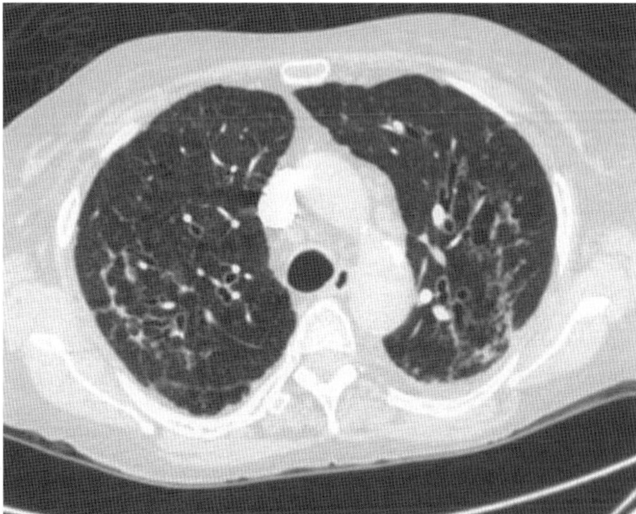

**Fig. 53.2 Computed tomography (CT) scan of the chest showing an atypical infection.** This is a CT scan of the chest with intravenous contrast enhancement in a bilateral lung transplant recipient. The patient came to the ED with a complaint of shortness of breath. The patient's plain chest radiograph was interpreted as normal. The CT scan was negative for pulmonary embolism but shows diffuse inflammation. Bronchoscopy performed as an inpatient procedure was positive for *Pseudomonas aeruginosa* infection.

When a lung transplant recipient is being evaluated in an ED, pulmonary infection must be highest on the differential diagnosis, and the patient's pulmonary or transplant physician should be contacted. Any suspicion of a pulmonary infection warrants the administration of broad-spectrum antibiotics that cover common community-acquired pathogens and health care–associated pathogens, including *Pseudomonas* species. In most cases, patients in whom pulmonary infection is suspected are admitted to the hospital or transferred to another facility where they will probably undergo fiberoptic bronchoscopy.

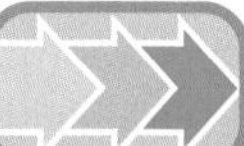

**PRIORITY ACTIONS**

Do not assume that patients with allograft rejection or pneumonia will manifest obvious symptoms.

Admit patients to the hospital if rejection or infection is suspected.

Discuss every lung transplant recipient seen in the emergency department with the patient's pulmonary physician or lung transplant surgeon.

Institute therapy with broad-spectrum antibiotics if pulmonary symptoms are present or pneumonia is suspected.

Treat suspected rejection with high-dose intravenous corticosteroids in conjunction with consultation.

**BOX 53.4 Clinical Findings in Cytomegalovirus Disease**

| | |
|---|---|
| Fever | Cough |
| Malaise | Dyspnea |
| Myalgia | Unexplained leukopenia |

## CYTOMEGALOVIRUS INFECTION

CMV causes one of the most important and lethal infections in solid organ recipients.[23] This virus, referred to as the "troll of transplantation," is the second most common infection in lung transplant recipients after bacterial pneumonia.[24] The overall likelihood of CMV infection in a lung transplant recipient is approximately 50% and is related to the CMV status of the donor and recipient.[25]

CMV infection generally occurs 1 to 3 months after transplantation. Any episode of acute rejection raises the patient's risk for continued CMV infection because of the immunosuppression required. The clinical findings may range from asymptomatic viremia to overwhelming sepsis and multiorgan failure. True clinical disease may be manifested as a mononucleosis-like syndrome with fever, malaise, and leukopenia (**Box 53.4**). There may also be organ-specific involvement in the lungs (pneumonitis), gastrointestinal system (colitis and hepatitis), and central nervous system. Over time, CMV infection leads to a high level of immunosuppression and the subsequent development of chronic allograft dysfunction and possibly failure.[23,26,27]

Pneumonitis is the most common manifestation of CMV disease after lung transplantation.[28] Clinically, CMV pneumonitis may look like acute rejection. Patients with either acute lung allograft rejection or CMV pneumonitis may have low-grade fever, a nonproductive cough, and shortness of breath. Further inpatient work-up (i.e., bronchoscopy) is generally required to distinguish the cause. CMV pneumonitis is diagnosed through serologic testing and the results of bronchoscopy, discussion of which is beyond the scope of this chapter. As many as 10% to 15% of patients with CMV pneumonitis are asymptomatic initially. A prodrome consisting of fever, malaise, and myalgias frequently precedes the onset of pneumonitis (cough and dyspnea). The disease may appear as opacities, nodules, or lobar infiltrates on chest radiographs.[29,30]

Treatment of CMV infection may start in the ED. The diagnosis of CMV infection may not be established on initial evaluation, but a presumptive diagnosis is frequently made and empiric therapy started. Standard treatment of CMV infection consists of a 2- to 3-week course of intravenous ganciclovir.[31] In some cases, ganciclovir is combined with CMV hyperimmune globulin. These therapies are usually started after the patient has been admitted.[31]

All lung transplant recipients seen in an ED within the vulnerable period of 1 to 3 months after surgery should be evaluated carefully for CMV disease. It should be assumed that any lung transplant recipient who underwent transplantation less than 3 months previously and who has fever, cough, or other suspicious findings may have active CMV disease. In many cases, therapy is started in the ED in consultation with the patient's physician.

## MEDICAL COMPLICATIONS

Patients who have undergone single-lung transplantation are at increased risk for bronchogenic carcinoma in their native lung.[32] Venous thromboembolism (VTE) is a potential complication of any surgery, and lung transplantation increases the risk 8% to 29% over other forms of organ transplantation.[33] Thus, the diagnosis of VTE and pulmonary embolism should be entertained when the initial complaint is shortness of breath or chest pain.

Patients who undergo long-term immunosuppression are at risk for posttransplant lymphoproliferative disorder (PTLD). Its prevalence is higher in lung transplant recipients than in other solid organ transplants.[34] PTLD is typically manifested as non-Hodgkin lymphoma, which results from infection with Epstein-Barr virus, and nodules or masses can be seen on the chest film.[35]

# DIAGNOSTIC TESTING

Diagnostic imaging in the ED is usually limited to plain film chest radiography and, occasionally, computed tomography (CT). EPs should maintain a low threshold for obtaining a CT scan of the chest in lung transplant recipients. CT has been shown to be far superior to chest radiography in detecting subtle cases of pneumonia in transplant patients.[36]

# IMMUNOSUPPRESSIVE THERAPY

Because transplant recipients undergo long-term immunosuppressive therapy, they are prone to multiple drug side effects, drug-drug interactions, and higher risk for opportunistic infections. EPs must use caution when prescribing any new medication to transplant patients in the ED because potentially serious drug side effects and drug-drug interactions may result. It is best to discuss medication issues with the patient's physician or a pharmacist.

Medications commonly used in lung transplant patients are calcineurin inhibitors (e.g., cyclosporine), cell cycle inhibitors, and corticosteroids. Their side effects are listed in **Table 53.2**. Most patients are maintained on a combination of these classes of medications.

Many commonly used medications may interfere with drugs used for long-term immunosuppression. Medications known to increase the blood levels (and thus toxicity) of certain medications include cyclosporine (Neoral) and tacrolimus (Prograf). In particular, erythromycin, doxycycline, and azole antifungal agents (ketoconazole, fluconazole, itraconazole) all raise serum concentrations of cyclosporine and tacrolimus. In contrast, other medications, such as isoniazid, rifampin, and rifabutin, lower the blood levels of these two immunosuppressants and may put the patient at risk for organ rejection. Sulfonamides, ganciclovir, and acyclovir potentiate the bone marrow toxicity of azathioprine and mycophenolate mofetil.[37-40]

# TREATMENT AND DISPOSITION

All patients with suspected lung transplant rejection or infection should be admitted to the hospital for further diagnostic

**Table 53.2 Drugs Commonly Used in Solid Organ Transplant Recipients**

| DRUG | MECHANISM OF ACTION | ADVERSE EFFECTS |
|---|---|---|
| Corticosteroids (prednisone) | Inhibits expression of genes encoding proinflammatory cytokines | Cushingoid features, infection, hypertension, edema, osteoporosis, bone necrosis, psychiatric disease |
| Azathioprine | Inhibitor of purine synthesis | Leukopenia, thrombocytopenia, anemia, hepatotoxicity, increased risk for malignancy |
| Mycophenolate (CellCept) | Inhibits purine synthesis | Nausea, vomiting, diarrhea, dyspepsia, leukopenia, anemia |
| Cyclosporine (Sandimmune, Neoral); causes renal vasoconstriction and ischemia | Calcineurin inhibitor (impairs T-cell function) | Nephrotoxicity (acute or chronic renal failure, renal vasoconstriction), infections, hypertension, hyperkalemia, increased lipids and glucose, gout, hypomagnesemia, tremor, encephalopathy, thrombotic thrombocytopenic purpura (TTP), hirsutism, gingival hyperplasia, hepatotoxicity |
| Tacrolimus (FK-506, Prograf) | Calcineurin inhibitor | Same as cyclosporine except much less risk for TTP |
| Sirolimus | Inhibits cell proliferation (T cells) | Infections, thrombocytopenia, anemia, leukopenia, hyperlipidemia, edema, diarrhea, headaches |
| Cyclophosphamide | Interferes with B-cell and T-cell proliferation and function | Leukopenia, hemorrhagic cystitis, bladder cancer, syndrome of inappropriate antidiuretic hormone secretion |
| OKT3-monoclonal (used to treat rejection) | Targets $CD3^+$ T cells and impairs their function<br>Transiently activates T cells | "Cytokine release syndrome" (fever, tachycardia, hypotension), pulmonary edema, aseptic meningitis |
| ATGAM-polyclonal | Bind to peripheral lymphocytes | Anaphylaxis, serum sickness, fever, rash |
| Interleukin-2 (IL-2) receptor antibodies (daclizumab, basiliximab) | Bind to IL-2 receptor | Rare hypersensitivity syndrome |

**BOX 53.5 Key Pitfalls in Evaluation of Lung Transplant Recipients**

Relying on a normal chest radiograph to exclude underlying pulmonary infection and/or rejection
Failure to discuss evaluation and treatment options with the patient's physician
Failure to appreciate that symptoms of lung allograft rejection may be subtle

testing and evaluation. The importance of appreciating the subtle nature of these complications cannot be overemphasized. It is wise to seek consultation with the patient's pulmonary physician or surgeon. A safe way to evaluate any lung transplant recipient seen in the ED is to assume that infection or rejection is present until proved otherwise (**Box 53.5**).

Lung transplant recipients are maintained on multiple immunosuppressive medications that interfere with many commonly used medications, such as antibiotics. EPs should never take it on themselves to add a drug to a transplant recipient's regimen or alter the dose of an immunosuppressant without first consulting with the patient's physicians.

By understanding the subtleties of rejection and pneumonia and the importance of drug side effects and interactions in lung transplant recipients, the EP will be in a better position to take care of this complex group of patients in the ED.

## SUGGESTED READINGS


Chakinala MM, Trulock EP. Acute allograft rejection after lung transplantation: diagnosis and therapy. Chest Surg Clin North Am 2003;13:525-42.

Christie JD, Edwards LB, Kucheryavaya AY, et al. The registry of the International Society for Heart and Lung Transplantation: twenty-seventh official adult lung and heart-lung transplant report—2010. J Heart Lung Transplant 2010;29:1104-18.

Hachem RR. Lung allograft rejection: diagnosis and management. Curr Opin Organ Transplant 2009;14:477-82.

Zaas DW. Update on medical complications involving the lungs. Curr Opin Organ Transplant 2009;14:488-93.


## REFERENCES

*References can be found on Expert Consult @ www.expertconsult.com.*

# Chest Pain 54

*Matthew Strehlow and Jeffrey Tabas*

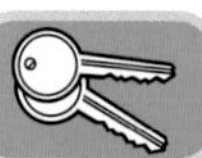

**KEY POINTS**

- Observation and repeated testing are extremely valuable in a patient with chest pain in whom the diagnosis is unclear.
- Rapid ruling out of acute myocardial infarction can be performed with serial cardiac marker testing once an appropriate interval after symptom onset has elapsed (8 hours for troponin I or T), although shorter intervals may be acceptable if immediate stress testing is performed.
- Normal cardiac marker values do not exclude unstable angina.
- Consider life-threatening diagnoses other than acute myocardial infarction in patients with chest pain, including aortic dissection, which is frequently missed and often manifested atypically.

## EPIDEMIOLOGY

Every year 6.2 million people are seen in U.S. emergency departments (EDs) with complaints of chest pain, which accounts for roughly 6% of ED visits and is the second most common reason for such visits. The differential diagnosis of chest pain ranges from benign causes, such as muscle strain, to the immediately life-threatening ones, such as acute coronary syndrome, pulmonary embolism, and aortic dissection. Although the focus in patients with chest pain remains appropriately on life-threatening causes, a majority of patients have benign or indeterminate diagnoses after ED evaluation. In one study of ED patients with symptoms consistent with acute cardiac ischemia, only 8% had acute myocardial infarction (AMI) and 9% had unstable angina.[1] Another investigation of patients evaluated in the ED for nontraumatic chest pain found that AMI was diagnosed in 4%, unstable angina or stable coronary disease in 7.5%, and pulmonary embolism or aortic dissection in less than 1%.[2] Given the potentially lethal nature of conditions manifested as chest pain and the lack of sensitivity or specificity, in many instances, of the history and physical examination, the emergency physician (EP) must have an organized approach, a complete differential diagnosis, and a thorough understanding of assessment and management of this common complaint.

## PATHOPHYSIOLOGY

In the differential diagnosis of patients with chest pain, one must consider the five groups of structures in the thorax: cardiac (heart and pericardium), pulmonary (lungs and pleura), gastrointestinal (esophagus and upper abdominal contents), vascular (aorta and great vessels), and musculoskeletal (chest wall). Chest discomfort is experienced through three distinct pathways, as follows:

*Visceral pain*, from internal structures such as the heart, lungs, esophagus, and aorta, may be difficult for the patient to define or localize. It is experienced as discomfort or a vague sensation and is often difficult to pinpoint.

*Somatic pain*, from chest wall structures and the parietal pleura, is often easier to describe and localize. Somatic pain may be sharp or stabbing and exacerbated by movement or position.

*Referred pain*, from irritation or inflammation of the upper abdominal contents, is a form of visceral pain that may be perceived in the chest wall, shoulder, or upper part of the back.

A differential diagnosis based on anatomic structures within the chest is presented in **Box 54.1**.

## PRESENTING SIGNS AND SYMPTOMS

Most patients with nontraumatic chest pain warrant high triage priority and an early electrocardiogram (ECG) (recommended within 10 minutes) to evaluate for AMI. Patient stabilization, evaluation of the history, physical examination, and diagnostic and therapeutic interventions proceed simultaneously. As assessment continues, interventions are refined (**Box 54.2**). Importantly, the history and physical findings alone are often inadequate to definitively establish or exclude life-threatening diagnoses.

The EP should keep the following points and issues in mind during assessment of a patient with chest pain:

- Use the term *discomfort* as opposed to *pain* to facilitate communication.
- Do not ascribe partially reproducible pain to a musculoskeletal cause. Pain arising from inflammation of the pericardium (secondary to AMI or pericarditis) or inflammation of the pleura (pulmonary embolism, pneumonia, or pleurisy) can be partially reproduced by palpation.
- Chest pain that is completely pleuritic (present only on inspiration) or completely reproducible significantly decreases suspicion for cardiac causes and raises suspicion for pulmonary or musculoskeletal causes. Partially pleuritic (worse with inspiration) or partially reproducible chest pain has much less predictive value.

**BOX 54.1 Differential Diagnosis of Chest Pain**

**Heart**
Myocardial infarction
Unstable angina
Pericarditis
Myocarditis
Valvular disease (especially aortic stenosis)

**Lungs**
Pneumonia, other infections
Pneumothorax
Pulmonary embolism
Exacerbation of chronic obstructive pulmonary disease or asthma
Tumor

**Chest Wall**
Costochondritis (Tietze disease)
Contusion
Rib fracture
Muscle strain or tear
Varicella zoster

**Aorta**
Dissection
Aneurysm
Aortitis

**Gastrointestinal**

***Esophagus***
Esophagitis (e.g., candidal)
Gastroesophageal reflux disease
Spasm (nutcracker esophagus)
Foreign body
Rupture (Boerhaave syndrome)

***Upper Part of the Abdomen***
Cholecystitis
Pancreatitis
Duodenal ulcer
Hepatic disease
Biliary disease
Subphrenic abscess

**BOX 54.2 Approach to Patients with Chest Pain**

**Initial Assessment (<10 Minutes)**
- ABCs: airway, breathing, and circulation
- Patient appearance
- Vital signs, $O_2$ saturation
- Electrocardiogram
- Directed history and physical examination

If the patient appears ill, the history raises concerns, vital signs are abnormal, or the electrocardiogram shows evidence of ischemia, the following actions should be taken:
- Establishment of intravenous access
- Cardiac monitoring
- $O_2$ administration if low $O_2$ saturation or shortness of breath is present
- Immediate subsequent assessment (as follows)

**Subsequent Assessment**
- Aspirin, 325 mg orally (unless ischemia is excluded or aspirin is contraindicated)
- Complete history and physical examination
- Radiographic, laboratory, and further electrocardiographic evaluation as indicated

- Substantial evidence suggests that responses to treatments such as sublingual nitroglycerin or a "gastrointestinal cocktail" do not differentiate the etiology of the chest pain.
- Do not overestimate the value of low-risk features when high-risk features are present (i.e., pain that is completely pleuritic but radiates to the left arm should still raise concern for possible acute coronary syndrome).
- The history and physical examination of patients with nonspecific chest pain are inadequate to justify discharge without further evaluation.

# ACUTE CORONARY SYNDROME

## EPIDEMIOLOGY

Several risk stratification systems have been proposed for acute coronary syndrome. These systems have been shown to help in risk stratification, thereby enabling triage decisions. They have never been shown to improve the ability to formulate discharge decisions in comparison with practitioner judgment. The American College of Cardiology and the American Heart Association have published criteria to determine a patient's risk for coronary artery disease and adverse outcomes from acute coronary syndrome.[3] These guidelines are cumbersome and more appropriately applied to patients with documented disease than to undifferentiated ED patients. A simplified approach to stratifying risk is to determine whether the patient has definite acute coronary syndrome, probable acute coronary syndrome, or possible acute coronary syndrome, as follows[4]:

- Patients with definite acute coronary syndrome are those with (1) changes diagnostic of ischemia or infarction on an ECG, (2) diagnostic elevation of serum cardiac markers, or (3) evidence of new heart failure or shock directly attributable to an acute ischemic event.
- Patients with probable acute coronary syndrome are those in whom suspicion for acute coronary syndrome is high but definitive criteria are lacking. An example is a patient with a classic history for acute coronary syndrome or whose cardiac marker values are slightly elevated but still below the diagnostic cutoff and who does not have clear ECG evidence of ischemia.
- Patients with possible acute coronary syndrome constitute the majority of patients with chest pain. They have atypical histories, their ECG findings are normal or unchanged from previous studies, or suspected alternative causes are triggering their symptoms.

This chapter is focused on patients with possible acute coronary syndrome. After chest radiography, a substantial proportion of such patients require further testing and observation, such as serial cardiac biomarker testing or other tests to evaluate for alternative diagnoses.

The challenge for the EP lies in determining when and which patients with possible acute coronary syndrome can be safely discharged home. At this time no definitive answer exists. A critical error, however, is failure to identify features that warrant further evaluation. Characteristics such as advanced age, known coronary artery disease, diabetes, pain similar to that of a previous myocardial infarction, worsening of typical angina, pressurelike or squeezing discomfort, and radiation of pain to the neck, left shoulder, or left arm have all been shown to increase the likelihood of AMI.

## PRESENTING SIGNS AND SYMPTOMS

The classic manifestation of AMI is discomfort that feels like an elephant sitting on one's chest; radiates to the left shoulder, arm, or jaw; and is associated with shortness of breath, nausea, or diaphoresis. Patients may describe their discomfort with a clenched fist against their chest, a finding known as the Levine sign. Physical examination demonstrates tachycardia, diaphoresis, and if the infarction has compromised left ventricular function, findings of acute heart failure such as hypoxia, tachypnea, elevated jugular venous pulsations, and bilateral rales. The classic manifestation in patients with unstable angina is a sense of discomfort or pressure that is similar to that of AMI but transient in nature. Patients with unstable angina experience similar associated symptoms typically brought on by exertion and relieved with rest or nitroglycerin. In practice, these classic findings are the exception, not the norm.

Risk factors for coronary artery disease predict a patient's risk for the development of ischemic heart disease over a period of many years but are only moderately predictive of acute coronary syndrome in the ED. Most important, it is well established that a lack of cardiac risk factors by itself does not place a patient at low risk for acute cardiac events.

Historical and examination features that raise or lower the likelihood of acute coronary syndrome are described in **Box 54.3** and **Table 54.1**. It is important to remember that the presence of lower-likelihood features does not exclude the diagnosis of acute coronary syndrome. One study of patients with AMI found that 22% had sharp or stabbing pain and 13% had partially pleuritic pain.[5]

The physical examination should be thorough, and findings suggestive of an alternative diagnosis may be helpful but are often not adequately specific to exclude acute coronary syndrome. For example, in 7% of patients with AMI, the pain is fully reproduced by palpation.[5]

**BOX 54.3 Clinical Features of Patients with Chest Pain That Raise the Likelihood of Acute Myocardial Infarction**

**Features with a High Likelihood Ratio (>2.0)**
Age > 60 years (2.2)
Diabetes (2.4)
Radiation of pain to either or both arms, the shoulder, or the jaw (3.0)
Findings of congestive heart failure (3.0)
Similarity to previous acute myocardial infarction or angina (4.0)
Ischemia noted on electrocardiography (from 5 to 50)

**Features with a Moderate Likelihood Ratio (1.5 to 2.0)**
History of smoking (1.5)
Family history of premature cardiac death (1.5)
History of myocardial infarction (2.0)
Chest pain as the chief complaint (2.0)
Nausea or vomiting (2.0)
Sweating (2.0)
Male gender (1.6)

**Table 54.1 Features of Chest Pain That Lower the Likelihood of Acute Myocardial Infarction***

| FEATURE | FREQUENCY IN PATIENTS WITH ACUTE ISCHEMIA (%) |
|---|---|
| Pleuritic pain | 13 |
| Pain that is reproducible with palpation or movement | 7 |
| Sharp, stabbing pain | 22 |
| Pain that lasts seconds or is constant for 24 hours or longer[3] | NA |

*NA*, Not available
*Likelihood ratio of approximately 0.3.

## DIAGNOSTIC TESTING

In adult patients with chest pain or acute coronary syndrome equivalents, an ECG is recommended within 10 minutes of ED arrival. Thirty percent to 50% of patients with AMI have diagnostic ECG findings, 40% to 70% have nonspecific ECG findings, and 1% to 10% have normal ECG findings. Nonspecific or unchanged ECG findings do not affect the likelihood of acute coronary syndrome; although a normal ECG does not exclude acute coronary syndrome, it significantly decreases the likelihood. Comparing the ECG with previous or serial ECGs can improve sensitivity and specificity. A right-sided ECG is recommended in all patients with inferior ST changes, and a posterior lead ECG is recommended if ST depression is present in septal leads $V_1$ through $V_3$. The ECG helps guide not only diagnosis but also therapy decisions (i.e., the presence of ST-segment elevation in AMI is a primary criterion for thrombolytic therapy). As with all tests, it is imperative that the ECG findings be interpreted in context.

An understanding of cardiac biomarkers is pivotal to excluding possible AMI in the ED. Currently, AMI is defined as the rise and fall of serum cardiac biomarkers in the presence of at least one of three other findings: ischemic symptoms, a pattern of progressive ischemic changes on ECG, or imaging evidence of a new regional wall motion abnormality.

**Table 54.2 Characteristics of Cardiac Marker Levels After Myocardial Infarction (MI)***

| CARDIAC MARKER | TIME OF RISE (HOURS AFTER MI) | TIME OF PEAK (HOURS AFTER MI) | TIME OF RETURN TO BASELINE (AFTER MI) | TIME OF SECOND MEASUREMENT (HOURS AFTER MI) |
|---|---|---|---|---|
| Myoglobin | <3 | 4-9 | <24 hr | — |
| Creatine kinase—MB form (CK-MB) | 3-8 | 9-30 | 1-3 days | 6-10 |
| CK-MB subforms | 1-3 | 4-6 | 18-24 hr | 6-10 |
| Troponin T | 2-6 | 10-24 | 10-15 days | 8-12 |
| Troponin I | 2-6 | 10-24 | 7-10 days | 8-12 |

*The American College of Emergency Physicians recommends an initial measurement of cardiac markers and a second measurement at the given intervals for rapid exclusion of MI in low- to moderate-risk patients. It is unclear whether a second measurement is needed if the time between symptom onset and the patient's arrival at the ED exceeds the recommended interval for the second measurement. See Fesmise FM, Decker WW, Diercks DB, et al. Clinical policy: critical issues in the evaluation and management of adult patients with non–ST-segment elevation acute coronary syndromes. Ann Emerg Med 2006;48:270-301.

Current guidelines recommend the use of cardiac troponins for the evaluation of all patients with suspected acute coronary syndrome. Troponins, regulatory proteins found in cardiac muscle, are composed of three subunits: I, T, and C. Cardiac subunits I and T are genetically distinct from the skeletal muscle forms, and no cross-reactivity occurs on immunoassays. Within 2 to 8 hours of AMI, troponin levels are abnormal and remain so for 7 to 10 days (**Table 54.2**). Detectable troponin but at a value below the diagnostic cutoff for AMI still portends a higher risk for adverse outcomes.[6] Nonspecific elevations, especially of troponin T, can occur with renal dysfunction, pulmonary embolism, septic shock, decompensated heart failure, myocardial contusion, pericarditis, and myocarditis. Cardiac troponins are more sensitive and specific than creatinine kinase, MB fraction (CK-MB), and myoglobin for cardiac muscle damage, and contemporary troponin assays identify the majority of AMIs within 3 hours, thus limiting the utility of CK-MB and myoglobin.

CK-MB is an enzyme present at higher percentages in cardiac muscle than in skeletal muscle, and it is relatively specific for cardiac muscle damage. False-positive results occur in patients with renal failure and in those with large amounts of skeletal muscle injury, such as seen with rhabdomyolysis. The CK-MB index improves the specificity of the biomarker by comparing the ratio of CK-MB with total CK. Levels higher than 5% are consistent with AMI, whereas those from 3% to 5% are indeterminate. CK-MB is detectable in blood 3 to 8 hours after myocardial infarction and returns to normal within 48 to 72 hours (see Table 54.2). The CK-MB subforms CK-MB1 and CK-MB2 rise earlier than CK-MB and are detectable 1 to 3 hours after injury, with a sensitivity of 92% achieved at 6 hours. Unfortunately, laboratory testing for CK-MB1 and CK-MB2 is not widely available.

Myoglobin is a heme protein in skeletal and cardiac muscle whose levels rise rapidly within 2 to 4 hours and return to normal within 24 to 36 hours. Its utility is limited by inadequate sensitivity and specificity, and its measurement is primarily used in combination with that of CK-MB and troponin as a point-of-care "triple-marker" assay. Studies have demonstrated that specificity can be improved through evaluation of the rate of myoglobin elevation (delta myoglobin) over a 1- to 2-hour period. It is recommended that delta myoglobin cutoff values of 25% to 40% be used to indicate abnormality. Other cardiac markers are being investigated, and their roles are being determined.

Recommendations based on the best available evidence and consensus argue against using a single cardiac marker value within 6 hours of the onset of symptoms to exclude AMI. For patients initially seen more than 6 to 8 hours after onset of the most recent episode of pain, a single negative cardiac marker value is often adequate to exclude AMI (but not unstable angina) in those with possible acute coronary syndrome. A period of observation that includes repeated ECG and serum CK-MB and troponin measurements can be used to rapidly rule out AMI at 6 and 8 hours after the onset of symptoms, respectively (see Table 54.2). Some evidence shows that a more accelerated testing approach is appropriate when such testing is followed immediately by stress imaging. In fact, one investigation found that it was safe to test patients with chest pain on an exercise treadmill immediately without initially determining cardiac marker values. The patients involved in this study, however, were at extremely low risk, with normal or nearly normal ECG findings, no evidence of heart failure, and the ability to exercise, and they were found to have only a 1% rate of AMI.[7]

## OBSERVATION UNITS AND PROTOCOLS

Increases in resource utilization, cost, and medicolegal concerns associated with patients evaluated in the ED for chest pain have led to the advent of rapid assessment protocols and chest pain units. These strategies aim to lower admission rates and cost of care while minimizing the inappropriate discharge of patients with unrecognized acute coronary syndrome. Approaches vary widely in these strategies, and most published methodologies involve immediate stress testing of low- to moderate-risk patients after a period of observation with serial ECGs and cardiac marker testing. Protocol-driven strategies increase the number of patients evaluated, accelerate the rate of evaluation, lower the number of missed events, and may save overall costs.

After a period of observation, repeated cardiac marker testing, and either continuous or intermittent ECG monitoring, patients in whom the ECG findings are unremarkable and cardiac biomarker results are negative undergo stress testing. Guidelines recommend that the stress test be performed within 72 hours of ED discharge; a majority of published reports describe stress testing before discharge.[3]

The most common adjunctive test is the continuous ECG treadmill stress test (TST). Patients with normal TST results under these circumstances have been found to have acceptably low rates of missed ischemia and adverse events. Unfortunately, a reasonable percentage of patients are poor candidates for an ECG TST (18% in one study) because of either an inability to ambulate at a moderate (2.5 mph) pace or the presence of confounding baseline ECG findings, such as left ventricular hypertrophy, left bundle branch block, ventricular-paced rhythm, or preexcitation syndrome. ECG TSTs also have a 5% to 25% nondiagnostic rate, depending on the patient population and protocol used. Patients in whom the ECG TST cannot be used must undergo stress imaging studies. Patients with nondiagnostic or abnormal ECG TST results should undergo further evaluation, which usually requires admission.

Although the percentage of low-risk chest pain patients in whom acute coronary syndrome is diagnosed during their hospital evaluation is low, 0.5% to 5%, the admission rate of patients who have been evaluated in a chest pain unit ranges from 10% to 50%. Patients discharged after a rapid assessment protocol or evaluation in a chest pain unit should receive outpatient follow-up soon.

## TREATMENT

Patients with possible acute coronary syndrome should receive aspirin. In patients with ongoing ischemic symptoms, nitrates may be given. Nitrates have never been shown to improve outcomes in patients with acute coronary syndrome, and recently, the response to nitrates has been shown to lack predictive value in the diagnosis of acute coronary syndrome. Their use in these low-likelihood patients should be weighed against the risk for hypotension or even headache. Analgesics such as morphine are given to patients with discomfort unresponsive to nitrates. Controversy surrounds the use of β-adrenergic receptor blockers. Currently, routine administration of intravenous beta-blockers in the prehospital setting or ED is not recommended.[8] Therapies such as heparin, clopidogrel, and glycoprotein IIb/IIIa inhibitors have been shown to be of benefit primarily in patients with definite acute coronary syndrome and therefore should not be used in this low-likelihood group.[4]

## DISPOSITION

It is important to acknowledge that the clinician cannot obtain perfect sensitivity in the assessment of patients with any disease. An analysis of multiple studies on acute coronary syndrome found that clinicians missed fewer AMIs when they admitted more patients.[9] Clearly, there is a limit to this strategy, although evidence does suggest that providing resources to increase the number of patients undergoing evaluation may reduce the proportion of acute coronary syndrome that is missed. This appears to be a cost-effective approach but depends on multiple factors that may be outside the clinician's and even the institution's control. Even when clinicians are confident of an alternative diagnosis, subsequent adverse cardiac events may occur, with a 2.8% rate documented in one large study.[10] The acceptable "miss rate" depends on the following factors:

- Risk aversion of the clinician
- Risk aversion of the patient
- Resources available
- Perceived risk of litigation for an adverse outcome even when the care is appropriate

Even patients with chest pain who undergo thorough evaluation that yields unremarkable findings experience a low but meaningful rate of adverse events. On the basis of these considerations, clinicians must decide the level of acceptable risk for missed acute coronary syndrome while realizing there is a finite rate of adverse outcomes. It is best for the EP to explain these risks to the patient, clearly document the reasoning, clearly document the patient's understanding, provide appropriate discharge instructions, and document the recommendations for follow-up.

## AORTIC DISSECTION

Aortic dissection is a tear in the intimal lining of the aorta. It is a distinct entity from a dilated aortic aneurysm, which involves pathologic dilation of the intima, media, and adventitia and can result from traumatic aortic injury. The reported incidence is 2.9 cases per 100,000 patients per year, which corresponds to roughly 5000 new adult cases per year in the United States. Missing or incorrectly diagnosing this condition can be fatal, especially if anticoagulation or fibrinolysis is initiated. Risk factors for aortic dissection include hypertension, Marfan disease, pregnancy, valvular disease, syphilis, and cocaine use.

## PRESENTING SIGNS AND SYMPTOMS

The classic manifestation of aortic dissection is acute (with maximum intensity at onset), severe, tearing chest pain that radiates to the back in patients with a history of hypertension. On examination, patients may exhibit pulse deficits or an aortic insufficiency murmur. Unfortunately, the classic manifestation is the exception and the clinical spectrum is broad (**Table 54.3**). Symptoms frequently mimic more common disorders, and the clinician must maintain a high index of suspicion.[11]

No single finding or combination of findings has been determined to be sensitive or specific enough to direct the evaluation for aortic dissection. Given that the diagnosis is frequently missed, the EP should have a low threshold for evaluating patients for aortic dissection when it is part of the differential diagnosis. Aortic dissection should be considered in a patient with any of the following features:

- Severe chest pain
- Pain that occurs in more than one anatomic distribution (chest and back, chest and abdomen)
- Pain accompanied by a focal neurologic complaint

**Table 54.3 Frequency of Symptoms and Physical Findings in Patients with Aortic Dissection**

| FEATURE | FREQUENCY (%) |
|---|---|
| **Symptoms** | |
| Pain | 95 |
| Severe or worst ever | 90 |
| Abrupt onset | 85 |
| Location in chest | 75 |
| Location in chest and back or back alone | 50 |
| Tearing or ripping | 50 |
| Syncope | 10 |
| **Physical Findings** | |
| Hypertension | 50 |
| Aortic insufficiency murmur | 30 |
| Pulse deficit (pulse differences in the four extremities) | 15 |
| Hypotension | 5 |

## DIAGNOSTIC TESTING

Chest radiography alone is insufficient to exclude aortic dissection. However, normal findings on chest radiography significantly decrease the level of suspicion—as long as they are truly normal; only 12% of chest radiographs in patients who do have aortic dissection are retrospectively considered normal.[11] In 78% of patients with aortic dissection, chest radiography demonstrates either a widened mediastinum or abnormal aortic contour. If possible, the EP should inform the radiologist that aortic dissection is under consideration to direct examination of the radiograph toward the pertinent abnormalities.

The following features are found on the chest radiographs of patients with aortic dissection:

- Wide mediastinum or abnormal aorta (in 78% of cases)
- Normal mediastinum and aorta (12.5%)
- Wide paraspinal shadow
- Pleural effusion
- Tracheal shift
- Calcification displacement
- "Lump" distal to vessels

ECG findings are neither sensitive nor specific for the diagnosis. In fact, as many as one in six patients with aortic dissection have evidence of ischemia or AMI on an ECG—presumably resulting from occlusion of the coronary vessels by an intimal flap or thrombosis—and 70% have normal or nonspecific findings.

Helical computed tomography and echocardiography provide definitive testing for aortic dissection. Either

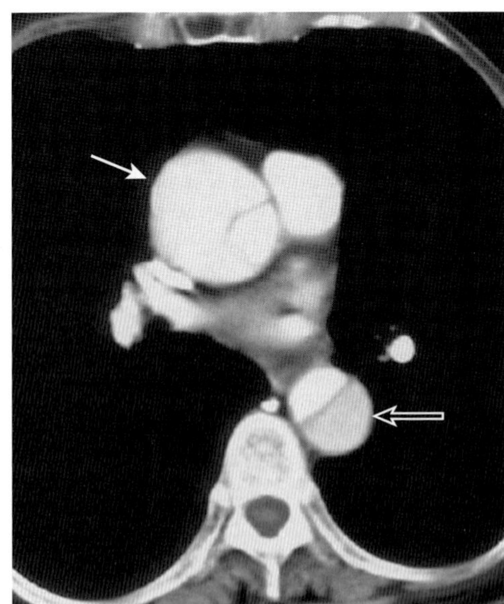

**Fig. 54.1 Computed tomography scan in a patient with aortic dissection.** The *solid arrow* at the ascending aorta and the *outlined arrow* at the descending aorta show the large area of a false lumen.

diagnostic test is 95% to 100% sensitive; echocardiography is preferred when the patient is unstable because it can be performed in the critical care setting. Transthoracic echocardiography is extremely sensitive in detecting abnormalities of the aortic root and ascending aorta, whereas the transesophageal approach is required to exclude involvement of the arch or descending aorta (**Fig. 54.1**).

## TREATMENT

The goal of initial ED treatment of patients with aortic dissection is to decrease shearing stress on the aorta with negative inotropic and chronotropic agents, such as intravenous beta-blockers or calcium channel blockers. Further blood pressure control can be achieved with intravenous nitroprusside or nitroglycerin. Desired values are a heart rate of 50 to 60 beats/min and a systolic blood pressure of 100 to 110 mm Hg.

## DISPOSITION

Once aortic dissection is confirmed, ED medical management proceeds in parallel with emergency surgical evaluation, and if surgery is deemed appropriate, arrangements for intervention should not be delayed.

# COCAINE-ASSOCIATED CHEST PAIN

The U.S. Department of Health and Human Services reported in 2002 that 33 million people 12 years and older (14.4% of the U.S. population) reported using cocaine at least once in their lifetimes. Cocaine abuse is not limited to a specific subset of the population and is frequently seen in ED patients, as demonstrated by an urban ED report that 2% of the institution's patients 60 years and older tested positive for cocaine.[12]

## PATHOPHYSIOLOGY

Chest pain, the most common complaint of ED patients with cocaine-associated visits, results from myocardial ischemia, trauma, pulmonary damage, and probably nonspecific vasospasm. Cocaine raises the risk for myocardial ischemia via multiple factors, including α-adrenergic receptor–mediated coronary vasoconstriction, platelet aggregation, direct myocardial toxicity, accelerated atherosclerosis, and increased myocardial oxygen demand. Therefore, acute coronary syndrome may be present in individuals who would otherwise be considered to have a very low risk for the disorder.

## PRESENTING SIGNS AND SYMPTOMS

Inquiry should be made about recent cocaine use in all patients seen in the ED with chest pain. Patients who have used cocaine recently often have significant elevations in blood pressure in addition to their chest pain. They may be jittery and somnolent at the same time after having binged on crack cocaine. Studies have documented the incidence of AMI in patients with cocaine-associated chest pain to be approximately 6%. One study found that patients with cocaine-associated AMI were young (mean age, 38 years), tobacco smokers (91%), and nonwhite (72%) and had used cocaine within the proceeding 24 hours (88%).[13] Nevertheless, a significant proportion of patients with cocaine-associated chest pain are older, and their risk for myocardial ischemia, though greatest in the first hours after the drug use, remains elevated for at least 2 weeks after discontinuation of the drug.

## MEDICAL DECISION MAKING AND DIFFERENTIAL DIAGNOSIS

The chest pain or dyspnea associated with cocaine use may stem from a variety of causes. In addition to acute coronary syndrome, aortic dissection has been reported to be associated with cocaine use.[14] The barotrauma induced by smoking crack cocaine results from deep inhalation followed by the Valsalva maneuver or severe coughing and leads to pneumothorax, pneumomediastinum, and pneumopericardium. Pulmonary diseases associated with smoking cocaine include noncardiogenic pulmonary edema, pneumonia, asthma, interstitial lung disease, bronchiolitis obliterans–organized pneumonia, parenchymal hemorrhage, and pulmonary vascular disease. Musculoskeletal trauma may also occur.

## DIAGNOSTIC TESTING

The initial evaluation of a patient with chest pain is the same regardless of whether cocaine is involved. The EP should order laboratory testing of blood, an ECG, and chest radiography for similar indications. The ECG findings do not depend on whether the AMI is cocaine related. In both those with and those without cocaine-related AMI, ECG findings are normal in 1% to 10%, nondiagnostic but abnormal in 30% to 50%, and diagnostic in 50% to 60%. Nonspecific abnormalities and normal variations often found in young persons, such as J-point elevation and left ventricular hypertrophy, are common.

Testing for the myocardial markers troponin and CK-MB is the cornerstone of evaluation for AMI in patients with cocaine-associated chest pain. Troponins are the markers of choice because unlike CK-MB, they are not affected by recent cocaine use. The extent to which skeletal muscle breakdown from cocaine use affects the diagnostic accuracy of CK-MB measurement has not been established.

Stress testing in patients with cocaine-associated chest pain after appropriately timed myocardial marker testing to evaluate for AMI is considered safe. The utility of exercise ECGs, myocardial perfusion, or stress echocardiography may be limited, however, given the low rate of reversible coronary artery lesions in these patients (2% to 14%) and the significant false-positive rate.

## TREATMENT AND DISPOSITION

Initial management (cardiopulmonary monitoring and aspirin) of patients with cocaine-associated chest pain is similar to that for patients with typical chest pain. In addition, the use of short-acting benzodiazepines, such as lorazepam, 1 mg intravenously repeated as necessary, in combination with nitroglycerin is recommended to counteract the sympathomimetic effects of cocaine. Hypertension usually responds to the preceding treatments. Additional blood pressure control is occasionally required because of suspicion for end-organ damage. β-Adrenergic blockade raises the theoretic concern of worsening hypertension as a result of vasospasm from unopposed α-adrenergic stimulation; however, little evidence supports this potential complication. Finally, for patients with evidence of cardiac ischemia or infarction, cardiac catheterization is beneficial and is preferred over thrombolytics, which should be used with caution.

There is some controversy regarding the disposition of patients with cocaine-associated chest pain. The EP should maintain a low threshold in evaluating for aortic dissection if the symptoms are severe and persistent. For patients in whom the findings are unremarkable—no ECG evidence of ischemia, no elevation in serial cardiac markers, and symptoms that resolve with treatment during observation—many authorities would argue that discharge is safe. Preliminary evidence has shown that this population is at low risk for subsequent complications. Until this issue is studied systematically, however, whether patients with cocaine-associated chest pain should be admitted for further evaluation is unclear.

## REFERENCES

***References can be found on Expert Consult @ www.expertconsult.com.***

# 55 Acute Coronary Syndrome

*David F.M. Brown*

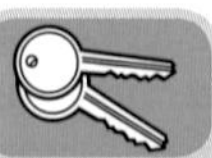

**KEY POINTS**

- Acute coronary syndrome (ACS) occurs as a spectrum of diseases that includes unstable angina pectoris, non–ST-segment elevation myocardial infarction, and ST-segment elevation myocardial infarction.
- ACS is classically manifested as chest tightness or pressure with associated dyspnea, nausea, and diaphoresis.
- ACS is diagnosed through a careful history and analysis of the 12-lead electrocardiogram.
- Treatment of the spectrum of ACS involves oxygen, aspirin, beta-blockers, nitrates, and anticoagulants.
- Patients with evidence of myocardial infarction also benefit from clopidogrel and glycoprotein IIb/IIIa receptor inhibitors.
- Patients with ST-segment elevation myocardial infarction require early revascularization therapy with either fibrinolysis or primary percutaneous coronary intervention.
- Immediate complications of ACS include congestive heart failure, cardiogenic shock, and rhythm disturbances, both tachyarrhythmias and bradyarrhythmias.

## EPIDEMIOLOGY

Ischemic heart disease occurs as a result of coronary artery disease and does not discriminate on the basis of gender, ethnicity, or race. Ischemic heart disease remains the leading cause of death in the United States and is responsible for more than half a million deaths annually—despite the marked advances over the past 5 decades in prevention as well as diagnosis and treatment of coronary artery disease. Advances include a reduction in smoking rates; improvements in the management of diabetes, hypertension, and hyperlipidemia; use of aspirin and other antiplatelet agents as both primary and secondary prevention; and improvements in the acute management of acute coronary syndrome (ACS). The last factor has evolved significantly, beginning with the advent of cardiac monitoring and the development of external cardiac defibrillators in the 1950s and progressing to widespread use of external cardiac massage and cohorting of patients with ACS within coronary care units in the 1960s. Pharmacologic developments in the management of ACS began with the use of beta-blockers and aspirin and advanced rapidly to include more sophisticated antiplatelet and anticoagulant agents.

The 1980s brought the widespread use of fibrinolytic therapy and ushered in the reperfusion era of therapy for ACS. Also in the 1980s, coronary angiography was first performed in the setting of acute myocardial infarction (MI) and demonstrated occlusion of the infarct-related artery (IRA), and mechanical interventions were subsequently developed to open the artery, beginning with balloon angioplasty and evolving to more sophisticated techniques such as stenting, thrombectomy, and atherectomy. All these advances have led to a significant decline in the overall age-adjusted mortality of patients with ischemic heart disease, primarily because of a diminution in both the incidence and case fatality rate of acute MI.

Nonetheless, the burden of ACS remains significant both from a health care perspective and from an economic perspective. More than 1 million acute MIs occur in the United States annually, and 20% of affected patients die before reaching the hospital, primarily from arrhythmias during the first hours of symptoms.[1] Many survivors of acute MI are left with impaired cardiac function, which adversely affects their ability to perform activities of daily living and their quality of life. Approximately 6 million emergency department (ED) visits in the United States are made annually for the evaluation of chest pain, and as many as one in three of these patients are ultimately found to have ACS.[2] The annual cost of providing care for patients with ACS, both immediately and then later for those who survive, is more than $100 billion.[3] Finally, despite advances in diagnostic techniques, 2% to 5% of patients with acute MI are discharged from the ED because their disease is not identified.[4] These "missed MI" patients represent the highest mean payments for emergency medicine–related medical malpractice claims.

## DEFINITIONS

Angina pectoris or, simply, angina is defined as transient and episodic discomfort in the chest occurring as a result of myocardial ischemia. Chronic stable angina can be reproduced with a specific level of physical or emotional stress and reliably resolves with rest, relief of the stress, or nitroglycerin therapy.

Unstable angina pectoris (UAP) is defined as angina of new onset that occurs at rest or in a crescendo pattern (with longer duration or intensity or with increasingly less exertion). If the angina is occurring at rest, it must be of at least 20 minutes' duration to be characterized as unstable. Pathophysiologically, UAP is characterized by the presence of unstable coronary atherosclerotic plaque with thrombosis and partial obstruction of the involved coronary artery but without myocardial cell death. In contrast, chronic stable angina is generally related to fixed stable atherosclerotic lesions without rupture or thrombosis. Variant (or Prinzmetal) angina also occurs at rest but is due to coronary vasospasm rather than unstable coronary atherosclerotic plaque. It may be manifested as ST-segment elevation on an electrocardiogram (ECG) and mimic ST-segment elevation myocardial infarction (STEMI) but generally responds to nitroglycerin with resolution of the acute ECG abnormalities.

Myocardial infarction is defined as myocardial necrosis. Clinical criteria for the presence of an acute, evolving, or recent MI, which have been laid out jointly by the American College of Cardiology and the European Society of Cardiology, focus on any evidence of myocardial cell death. The exact definition of an acute or evolving MI is a rise above the upper limit of normal and subsequent fall in levels of cardiac biomarkers specific for myocardial necrosis (troponin or the MB fraction of creatine kinase MB [CK-MB]) along with at least one of the following[5]:

- Symptoms consistent with ACS
- ECG evidence of myocardial ischemia, specifically, ST-segment elevation or depression or T-wave inversions
- Development of pathologic Q waves on the ECG
- Percutaneous coronary artery intervention

Myocardial infarction is further classified as STEMI and non–ST-elevation MI (NSTEMI). STEMI is present when the patient has (1) cardiac biomarkers for necrosis as previously defined and (2) new or presumed new ST-segment elevation in two or more contiguous ECG leads. The cutoff point for ST-segment elevation is 0.1 mV.[6] Contiguous leads are defined in the chest leads as $V_1$ through $V_6$ and in the frontal plane as the sequence aVL, I, inverted aVR, II, aVF, and III. Patients who meet the clinical criteria for STEMI and left bundle branch block (LBBB) and are not old or who have ECG evidence of an isolated true posterior MI are also considered, for treatment algorithm purposes, to have STEMI. NSTEMI is present when the patient meets the criteria for MI as previously defined but exhibits no evidence of ST-segment elevation, new LBBB, or ECG evidence of an isolated posterior wall MI.

Acute coronary syndrome is the clinical manifestation of acute myocardial ischemia resulting from the presence of unstable coronary plaque. Accordingly, ACS is represented by the full spectrum of STEMI, NSTEMI, and UAP, which comprise a continuum of similar clinical and pathophysiologic features. STEMI and NSTEMI are differentiated by the findings on a 12-lead ECG, whereas UAP is identical to NSTEMI except that the cardiac biomarkers remain normal in the former. Given that a laboratory result is the only distinguishing feature between patients with UAP and those with NSTEMI, patients are treated identically on arrival by the initial health care provider.

## PATHOPHYSIOLOGY

The pathophysiology of acute myocardial ischemia is related to an imbalance between myocardial oxygen supply and demand. Specifically, myocardial ischemia occurs when coronary perfusion is insufficient to meet myocardial oxygen consumption needs. Myocardial oxygen needs depend on the heart rate, afterload conditions, and contractility of the myocardium. Insufficient coronary perfusion is generally due to atherosclerosis involving the coronary arteries. In patients with chronic stable angina, fixed atherosclerotic lesions partially obstruct flow of blood to the myocardium; when demand for oxygen increases (e.g., because of exercise), flow may become insufficient to meet the demand, and myocardial ischemia and anginal symptoms occur.

The pathophysiology of ACS begins when an atherosclerotic plaque within a coronary artery becomes unstable as a result of plaque rupture or hemorrhage into the plaque. The atherosclerotic plaque need not be causing critical stenosis before becoming unstable. Plaque rupture or hemorrhage exposes the lipid-rich core of the plaque and the basement membrane proteins of the blood vessel wall. As part of the resultant inflammatory cascade, platelets adhere to the core of the ruptured plaque and start to release platelet agonists—adenosine diphosphate, thrombin, and epinephrine. These agonists induce platelet activation, which is characterized by the expression of 50,000 to 80,000 glycoprotein (GP) IIb/IIIa receptors on the surface of each platelet. Fibrinogen, freely circulating in the bloodstream, is a bivalent molecule with binding sites on each end that are specific for the GP IIb/IIIa receptor. Fibrinogen thus facilitates platelet aggregation because each strand cross-links two platelets. The resultant platelet-fibrinogen web is further stabilized by thrombin, which is released by activated platelets and by activation of the coagulation cascade. Thrombin cross-links and modifies fibrinogen to the more stable fibrin.

As the platelet-fibrin aggregation grows, it traps red and white blood cells moving through the coronary artery, and a thrombus forms. At the same time, the inflammatory process leads to the release of vasoactive mediators, which may induce vasospasm, further compromising coronary blood flow. If this process leads to complete occlusion of the epicardial coronary artery at the site of plaque rupture, STEMI will result. If the thrombus is partially obstructing coronary blood flow and generating microemboli to smaller coronary arterioles, which in turn may become obstructed or exhibit spasms, NSTEMI (if myocardial cell death has occurred as shown by a rise in cardiac biomarkers) or UAP (if biomarkers remain normal) results.

Much less commonly, ACS may be due to primary vasospasm rather than primary plaque rupture. Generally the result of sympathetic overstimulation by endogenous epinephrine or serotonin, coronary vasospasm may lead to platelet activation and thrombus formation, even in the absence of underlying coronary artery atherosclerosis. Coronary vasospasm is more likely to cause UAP than MI.

## PRESENTING SIGNS AND SYMPTOMS

### HISTORY

Patients with ACS classically have chest discomfort in the substernal (precordial) area. Typically, this discomfort is described as pain, pressure, or tightness and may begin at rest or during exertion. It may also be located in the left or right anterior portion of the chest and may radiate to the shoulder, neck, jaw, arm, or back. Characteristically, the duration of discomfort ranges from several minutes to an hour. It is rare for the discomfort related to ACS to last only seconds or to persist continuously for hours. Associated symptoms that may be present are dyspnea, nausea, vomiting, diaphoresis, weakness, dizziness, and fatigue.

### ATYPICAL PRESENTATIONS

The emergency physician (EP) should beware of atypical manifestations of ACS, which are common and portend a markedly worse clinical outcome. The quality of the chest discomfort cannot be relied on to exclude ACS. Patients with discomfort that is sharp or stabbing in quality or is pleuritic, palpable, or positional in nature make up a significant minority of patients with ACS. Furthermore, any of the associated symptoms listed previously can occur either alone or together without chest discomfort and still represent ACS. Findings of this type (without chest discomfort) are referred to as an *anginal equivalent* and require the same clinical management as cases manifested more classically. Other atypical manifestations include isolated back, neck, jaw, or arm discomfort; epigastric pain or burning; indigestion; isolated dyspnea; and generalized weakness. Elderly patients are particularly likely to have atypical symptoms, in particular, weakness and altered mentation. Other populations in whom ACS is likely to be manifested atypically are women, nonwhite patients, and diabetic patients. In all these groups ACS is much more likely to be misdiagnosed initially than in the overall population.

### PHYSICAL FINDINGS

Physical examination is often unrevealing in patients with ACS because most of the findings are related to complications of ACS. The vital signs should be evaluated carefully and monitored for evidence of arrhythmia, respiratory compromise, and cardiogenic shock. Jugular venous distention, rales, and a third heart sound ($S_3$) are signs of congestive heart failure complicating ACS. When these signs are coupled with altered mental status and hypotension, cardiogenic shock is likely.

Physical findings can also help suggest an alternative diagnosis. For example, fever and signs of consolidation on lung examination are suggestive of pneumonia rather than ACS, whereas unilateral absence of breath sounds suggests pneumothorax as the most likely diagnosis. Although chest wall tenderness is suggestive of a musculoskeletal etiology, ACS should not be excluded as a diagnosis solely on the basis of chest discomfort that is reproducible on palpation.

## DIFFERENTIAL DIAGNOSIS AND MEDICAL DECISION MAKING

The differential diagnosis in patients with ACS includes a host of other diseases that can be manifested as chest pain or dyspnea: stable angina, pericarditis, myocarditis, pulmonary embolism (PE), aortic dissection, pneumonia, pleurisy, pneumothorax, Boerhaave syndrome, esophageal reflux, esophageal spasm, gastritis, biliary colic, pancreatitis, peptic ulcer disease, musculoskeletal pain, and herpes zoster. One of the historical features that tends to favor a diagnosis of ACS is chest pressure or tightness rather than a sharp pain, which is more commonly associated with pericarditis, pleurisy, pneumothorax, PE, and aortic dissection. In addition, the chest discomfort in patients with ACS tends to gradually worsen, unlike the pain associated with PE or aortic dissection, which is generally worst at the onset and then persistently severe. Pain of a pleuritic nature tends to favor PE, pleurisy, or pneumothorax, whereas pain that is worse on palpation tends to suggest a chest wall musculoskeletal cause. Discomfort that is positional in nature tends to favor pericarditis or gastrointestinal causes rather than ACS. However, it is very important to remember that a significant percentage of patients with ACS have pleuritic, positional, or palpable chest pain and that these historical features cannot be used to exclude the diagnosis.[7]

Although the differential diagnosis of chest discomfort is long and includes entities from several different organ systems, some bear special mention because of the risk that they pose to patients. In each patient with chest discomfort, the EP should consider and reasonably exclude aortic dissection, PE, pneumonia, pneumothorax, and Boerhaave syndrome. This does not mean that these diagnoses must be excluded by definitive diagnostic techniques. They may be reasonably excluded on the basis of the history and physical findings, but this thought process should be documented clearly in the medical record.

## DIAGNOSTIC TESTING

### ELECTROCARDIOGRAM

The 12-lead ECG is the most important diagnostic test for patients with suspected ACS. In addition to providing diagnostic information, the ECG can be used to assess progression of the syndrome and response to therapeutic interventions. In addition, ECG findings determine treatment pathways and assist with disposition decisions. The ECG in patients with suspected ACS should be carefully and systematically analyzed for evidence of ST-segment elevation, ST-segment depression, T-wave inversion, and pathologic Q waves as signs of myocardial ischemia or infarction. Also, the rate, rhythm, and intervals, along with QRS morphology, should be studied for evidence of complications of ACS. Finally, evidence of noncardiac causes of chest pain should be sought on the ECG, in particular, findings suggestive of PE and pericarditis.

It important to remember that many patients with confirmed ACS have normal or nondiagnostic findings on the ECG. Even in patients with acute MI, the ECG findings can be normal in a small percentage of cases. In addition, the ECG represents only one static point in time, and ACS is a dynamic process. Hence, a single nondiagnostic ECG cannot be relied on to exclude the diagnosis of ACS, and the history elicited from the patient remains more important than findings on the ECG, particularly when they are negative or nondiagnostic. Nonetheless, specific ECG findings of myocardial ischemia or infarction are often present and are very helpful in determining treatment and disposition.

#### *Electrocardiographic Findings in ST-Segment Elevation Myocardial Infarction*

The initial ECG abnormality that occurs in patients with epicardial coronary artery occlusion is peaked hyperacute T waves in the distribution supplied by the IRA. T waves become tall and sharply peaked within minutes of occlusion of the IRA (**Fig. 55.1**, *A*). Peaked T waves may also be seen in patients with hyperkalemia, pericarditis, early repolarization, and LBBB. In the next several minutes, ST-segment elevation becomes evident on the ECG (see Fig. 55.1, *B*). To be diagnostic, the ST-segment elevation must be at least 1 mm above the baseline; this is generally considered the TP segment.

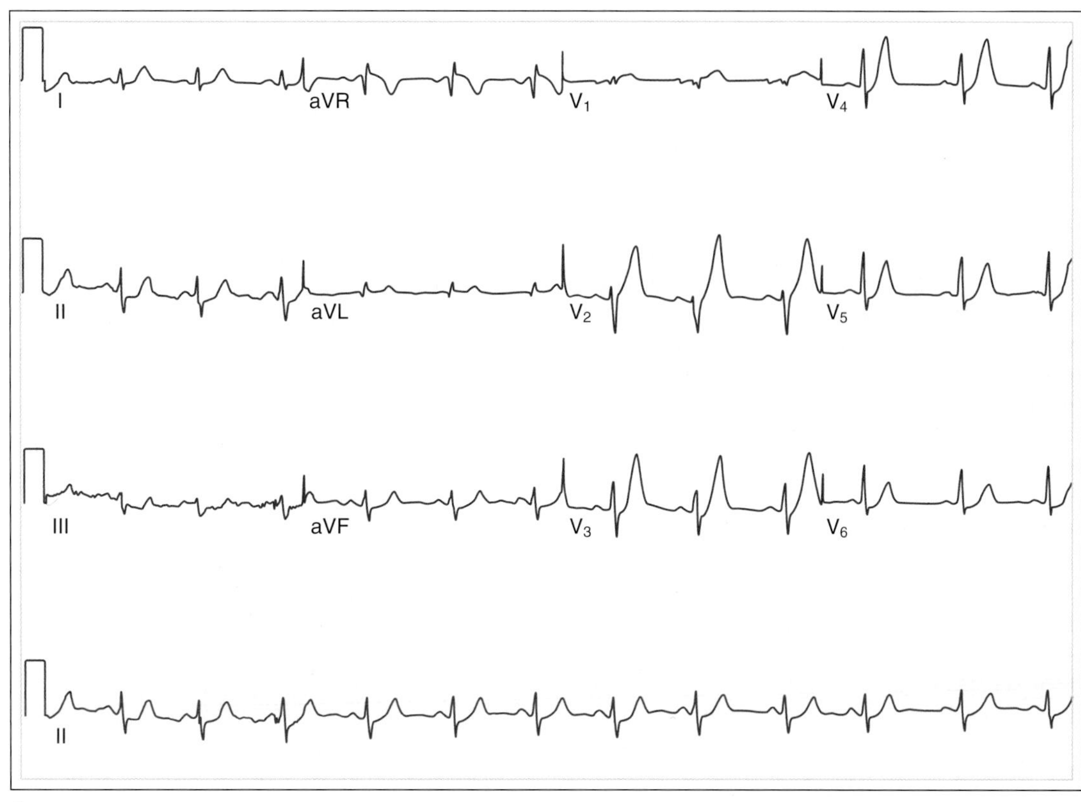


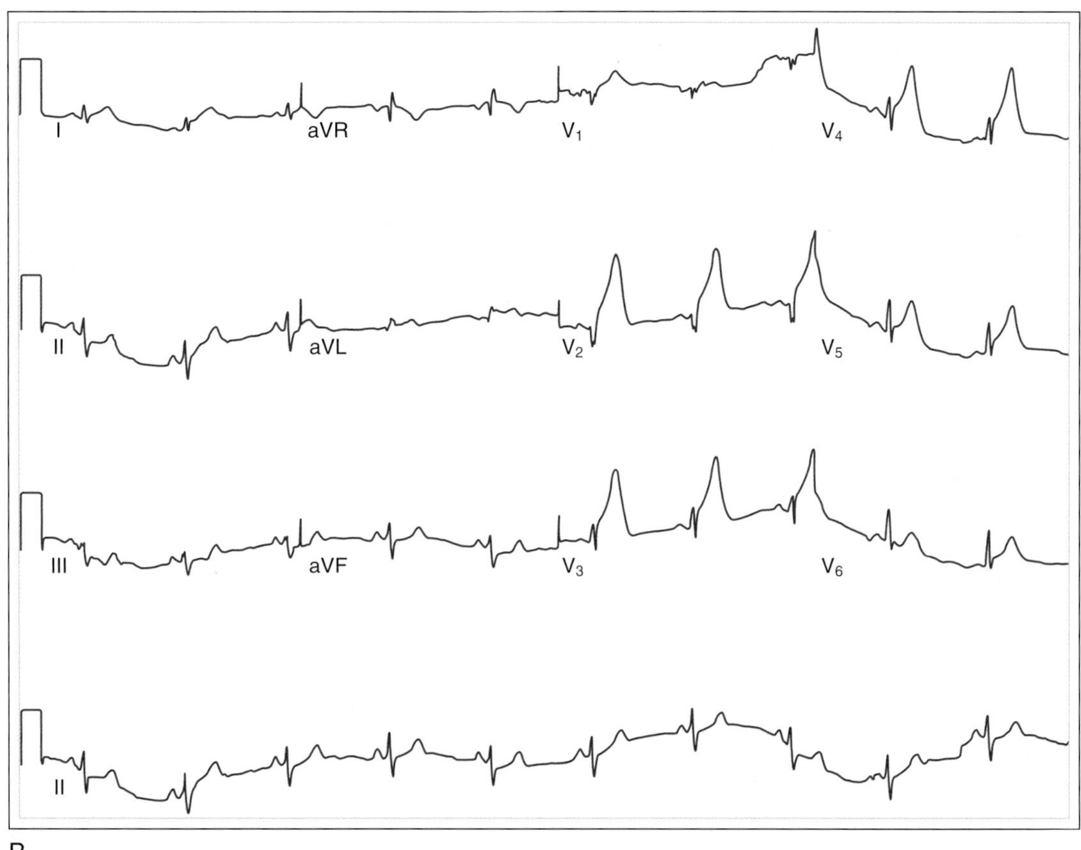


**Fig. 55.1** **A,** An initial electrocardiogram (ECG) obtained shortly after the onset of symptoms shows hyperacute peaked T waves in leads $V_2$ through $V_5$, consistent with early anterior transmural injury current. **B,** A second ECG obtained several minutes later shows hyperacute T waves and ST-segment elevation in the precordial leads along with ST-segment elevation in leads 1 and aVL, consistent with acute anterolateral myocardial infarction secondary to proximal occlusion of the left anterior descending coronary artery.

Most typically, this ST elevation is convex or domed, though less commonly it may be straight or, rarely, concave. Concave ST-segment elevations are more characteristic of other conditions associated with ST-segment elevation (**Box 55.1**).

In addition to the clinical situation, a factor distinguishing STEMI from other conditions is the dynamic nature of the ST-segment changes with STEMI; serial ECGs commonly show waxing and waning ST-segment elevation. Hours to days later, the ST segments return toward baseline, the T waves invert, and pathologic Q waves develop in areas of the ECG that correspond to the IRA. The location of the ST elevations and other findings on the ECG generally correspond to the anatomic location of the myocardium and the associated IRA. Anterior infarctions exhibit ST elevation in leads $V_1$ through $V_4$ (**Fig. 55.2**). Findings in leads $V_1$ and $V_2$ indicate involvement of the septum. MIs with these findings are caused by occlusion of the left anterior descending (LAD) coronary artery. When additional ST elevations are seen in leads $V_5$, $V_6$, I, and aVL, the location of the LAD occlusion is probably proximal to the first diagonal branch, which causes an anterolateral infarction (see Fig. 55.1, *B*). Inferior infarctions are characterized by ST elevations in leads II, III, and aVF (**Fig. 55.3, *A***) and are due most commonly to right coronary artery (RCA) occlusion. Reciprocal ST depressions may be present in leads I and aVL.

**BOX 55.1 Differential Diagnosis of ST-Segment Elevation on Electrocardiography**

ST-segment elevation myocardial infarction
Pericarditis
Benign early repolarization
Left bundle branch block
Left ventricular hypertrophy
Left ventricular aneurysm
Paced ventricular rhythms
Prinzmetal angina
Hyperkalemia
Hypothermia with Osborne waves
Intracranial hemorrhage
Brugada syndrome
Normal variant

Inferior MIs are associated with concomitant right ventricular infarction, which can be evident on right-sided ECG leads, particularly in $RV_4$ and $RV_5$ (see Fig. 55.3, *B*). Inferior MIs are also frequently associated with posterior wall involvement, which is seen on the ECG as ST depressions in leads $V_1$ through $V_3$ and, on occasion, early R-wave progression with tall R waves in leads $V_1$ through $V_3$ (**Fig. 55.4**).

Isolated posterior MIs, the rarest of transmural MIs, are the most easily misdiagnosed because the 12-lead ECG may show ST depressions in $V_1$ through $V_3$ and sometimes $V_4$ and $V_5$, often with tall R waves in $V_1$ through $V_3$ but without evidence of ST elevations (**Fig. 55.5**). This situation can be confused with anterior wall ischemia. Clues on the ECG to the diagnosis of isolated posterior wall MI include horizontal (rather than sloping) ST depressions with prominent R waves and tall upright T waves in leads $V_1$ through $V_3$. Occasionally, isolated posterior wall MIs are manifested as a nondiagnostic 12-lead ECG (**Fig. 55.6, *A***), with small pathognomonic ST-segment elevations evident only when extended ECG leads are placed inferior to the tip of the left scapula ($V_8$) and in the left paraspinal line at the same level ($V_9$) (see Fig. 55.6, *B*). Posterior wall MIs are the result of occlusion of the posterior descending coronary artery or the posterior left ventricular branch,

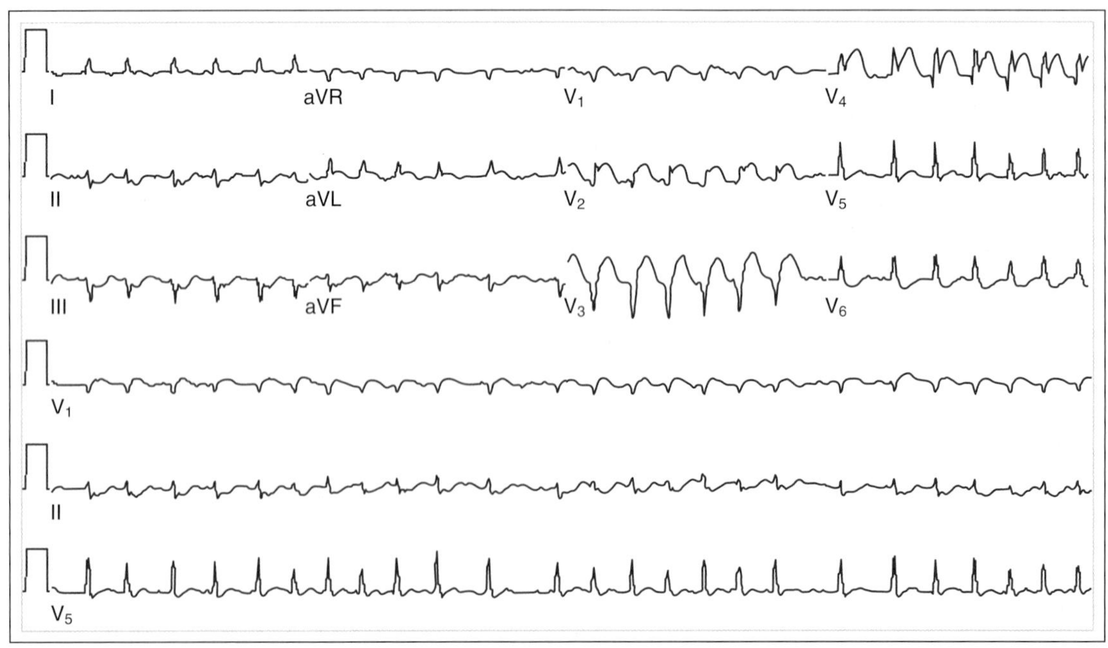


**Fig. 55.2** A 12-lead electrocardiogram shows ST-segment elevation in leads $V_1$ through $V_4$, consistent with acute anteroseptal myocardial infarction. Note that rapid atrial fibrillation is also present.

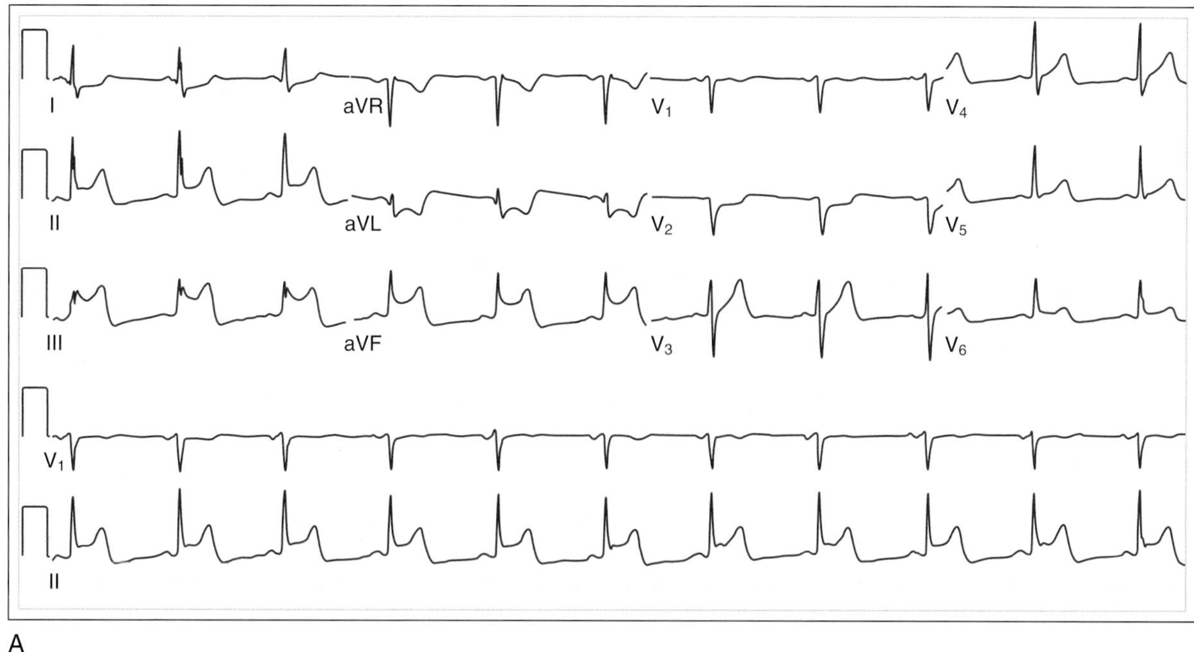


A

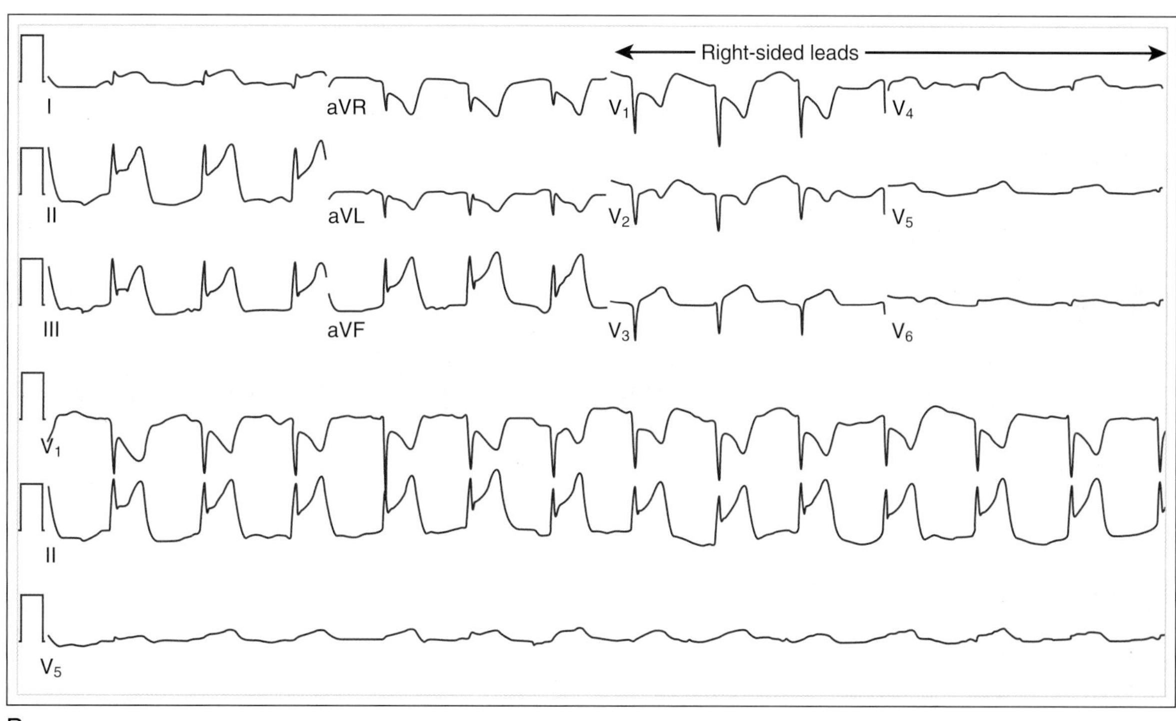


B

**Fig. 55.3** **A,** A 12-lead electrocardiogram shows ST elevation in leads II, II, and aVF, consistent with acute inferior myocardial infarction (MI). Note the reciprocal ST depressions in leads I and aVL. **B,** The right-sided precordial leads in a patient with acute inferior ST-segment elevation MI show ST-segment elevation in leads $RV_4$ and $RV_5$, consistent with concomitant right ventricular infarction.

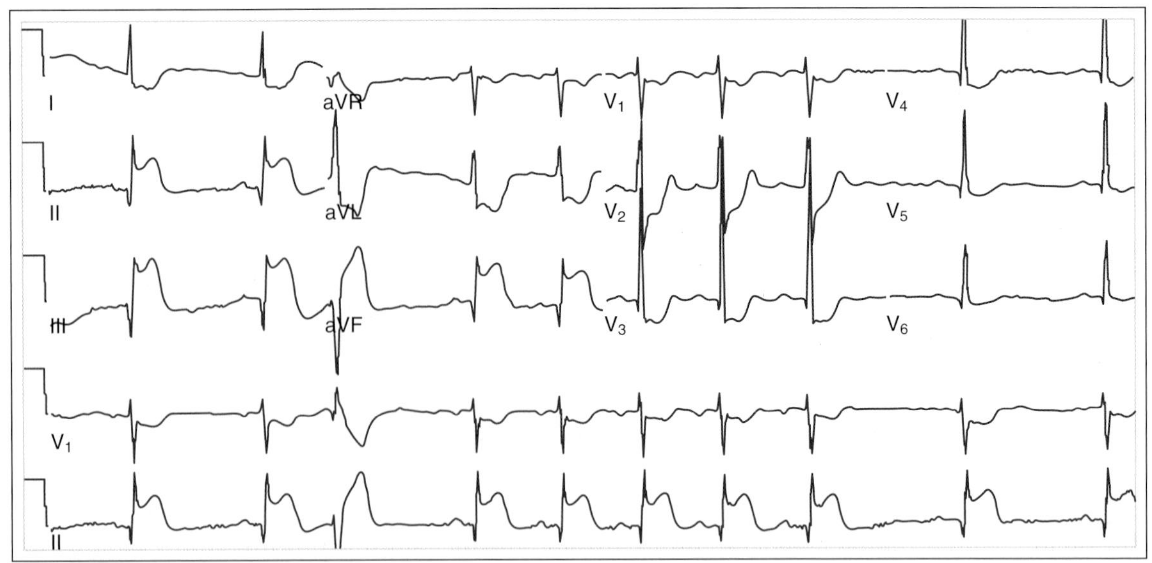


**Fig. 55.4** A 12-lead electrocardiogram shows ST elevation in leads II, III, and aVF with ST depressions and prominent R waves in $V_1$ through $V_3$, consistent with acute inferoposterior myocardial infarction. Note the sinus arrhythmia and premature ventricular beat.

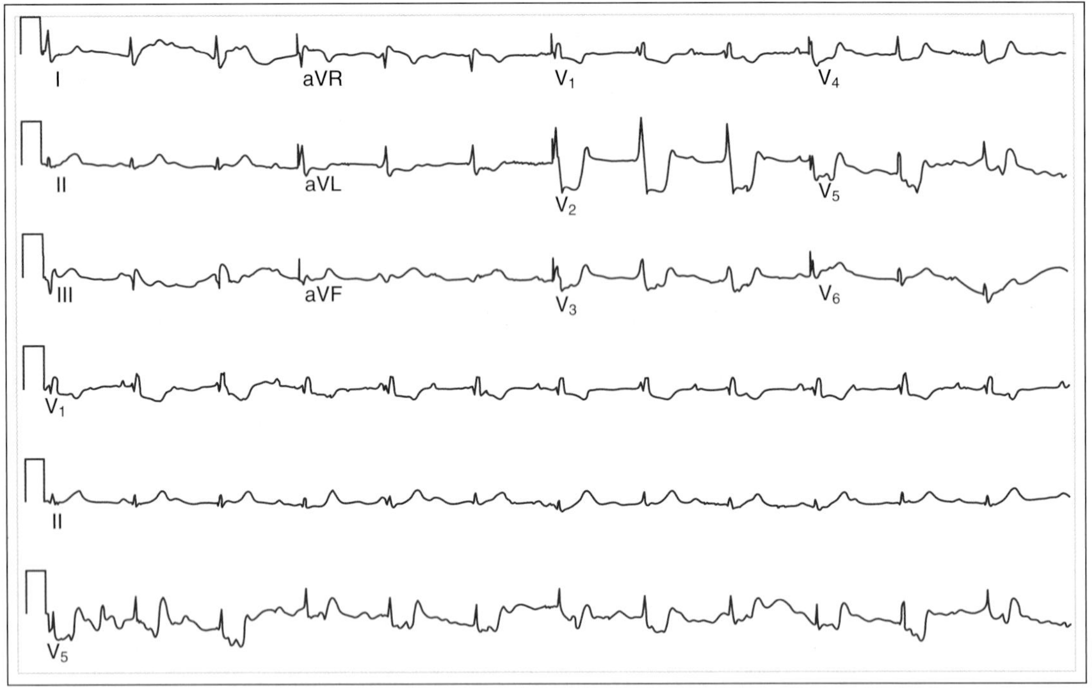


**Fig. 55.5** A 12-lead electrocardiogram shows ST depressions in leads $V_1$ through $V_4$ with prominent R waves in $V_1$ and $V_2$, consistent with isolated acute posterior myocardial infarction. Note that a complete heart block is also present.

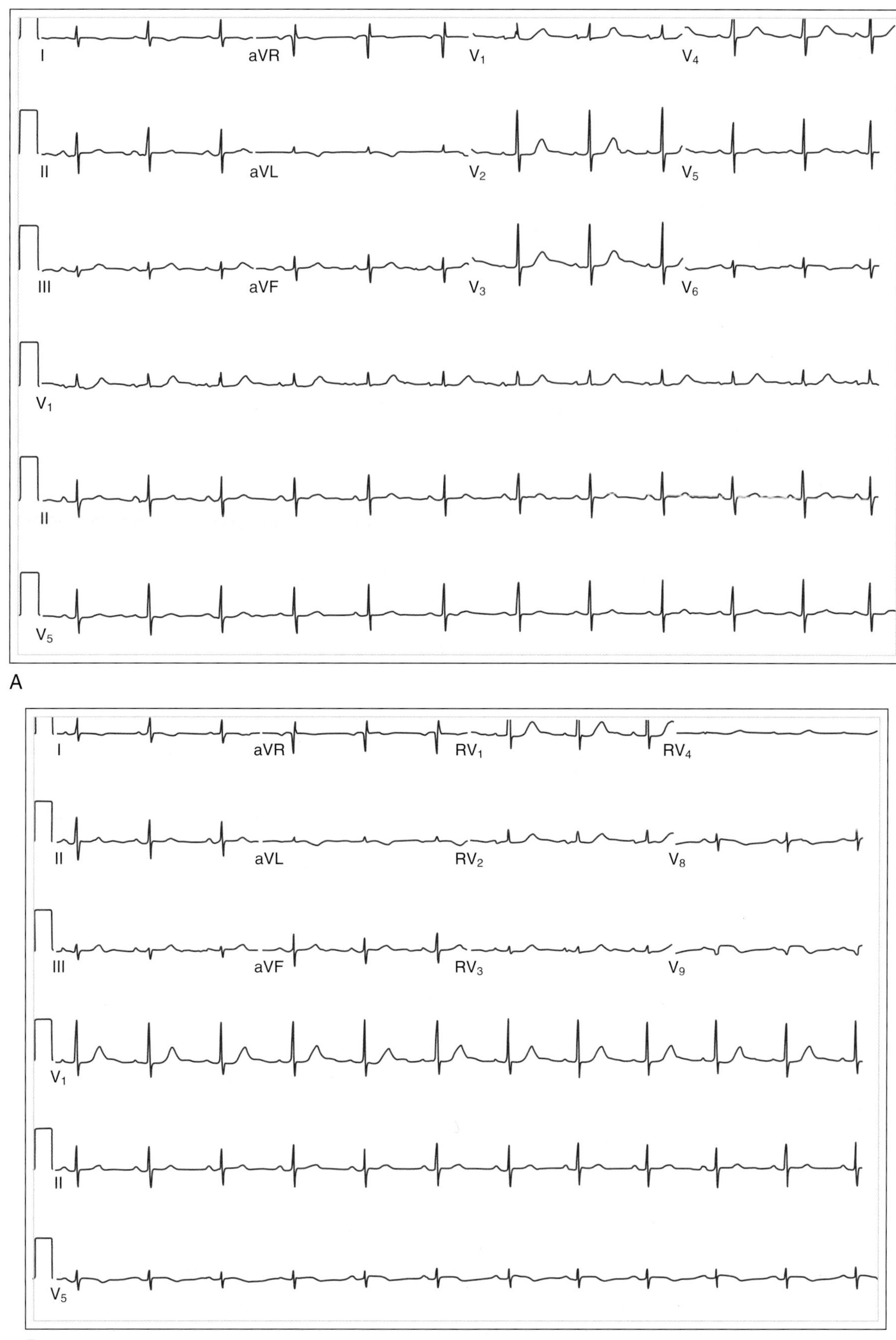


**Fig. 55.6** **A,** A 12-lead electrocardiogram (ECG) in a patient with chest pain is notable only for prominent R waves in the precordial leads with early R-wave progression. **B,** Extending the ECG to include right-sided and posterior leads demonstrates ST elevations in leads $V_8$ and $V_9$, consistent with isolated acute posterior myocardial infarction.

either of which can arise from the RCA (more commonly) or the left circumflex coronary artery.

Lateral wall MIs, characterized by ST-segment elevation in some or all of leads I, aVL, $V_5$, and $V_6$, may be associated with anterior MI as previously described or with inferior or posterior MI or may occur in isolation. This is because the lateral wall of the heart is variably supplied with blood by the LAD, the RCA, and the left circumflex artery. Isolated lateral wall MIs are most commonly associated with left circumflex artery occlusion; the ECG may show reciprocal ST depressions in leads II, III, and aVF (**Fig. 55.7**).

### *Electrocardiographic Findings in Non–ST-Segment Elevation Acute Coronary Syndrome*

In the clinical setting of NSTEMI, the ECG may be normal or unchanged from baseline, although more commonly it will show ST-segment depressions, T-wave abnormalities, or both in the area of the ECG representing the area of ischemia or infarction in the heart (**Fig. 55.8**). As mentioned, ST-segment depressions in the precordial leads may also represent true posterior wall transmural infarction. In addition, ST depressions may also represent reciprocal changes, with STEMI occurring in another location; this is most commonly seen in the lateral leads in patients with an inferior STEMI or in the inferior leads in patients with a lateral STEMI (see Fig. 55.7). T-wave inversions are nonspecific findings, particularly when seen in isolation (without ST-segment depressions), but they do suggest ACS in the right clinical setting, especially when comparison with previous tracings shows that the findings are new. Note that T waves are normally inverted in leads aVR and $V_1$ and are variably inverted in leads III, aVF, aVL, and $V_2$.

One important subgroup of T-wave inversions occurs in the precordial leads. The changes may be symmetric deep T-wave inversions (**Fig. 55.9,** ***A***) or more subtle biphasic T-wave changes. This pattern, referred to as Wellen syndrome, represents an unstable lesion in the LAD. Without prompt appropriate treatment, this lesion may lead to an anterior STEMI (see Fig. 55.9, *B*). The differential diagnosis of inverted T waves includes not only ACS but also left ventricular hypertrophy, LBBB, pericarditis, myocarditis, pulmonary embolism, Wolfe-Parkinson-White syndrome, ischemic or hemorrhagic stroke, hypokalemia, and a persistent juvenile pattern. These findings may also be normal variants. Occasionally, patients with chronically inverted T waves are found to have new upright T waves in the setting of chest pain or anginal equivalent. This finding, referred to as pseudonormalization of the T waves, is highly suggestive of ACS.

## CARDIAC BIOMARKERS

Numerous cardiac biomarkers become elevated in the setting of myocardial cell death and are thus indicators of MI. The most sensitive and specific of these biomarkers at present are troponins, which are detectable in serum 4 to 10 hours after the onset of MI. Consequently, a single "negative" troponin value cannot be used to exclude MI. In addition to troponins, CK-MB and myoglobins are also useful and widely used. However, none of the cardiac biomarker measurements currently available represent an adequate test for unstable angina (without MI). For a complete discussion of cardiac biomarkers, see Chapter 54.

## OTHER TESTS

Cardiac ultrasonography, nuclear imaging, and stress testing can be very important in confirming the diagnosis of ACS

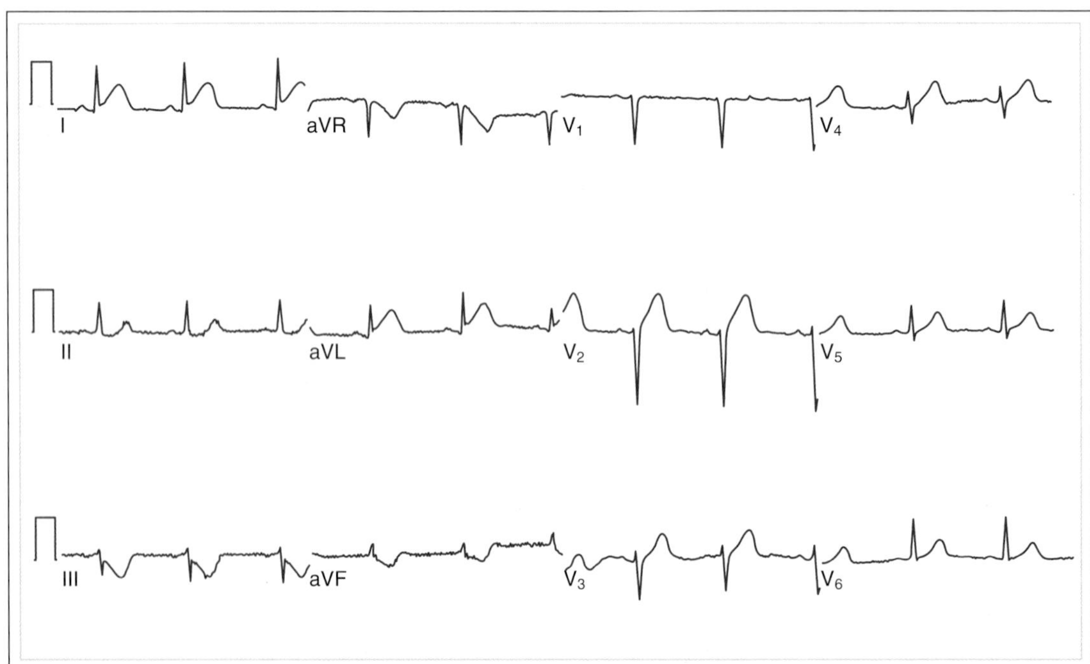


**Fig. 55.7** A 12-lead electrocardiogram shows ST-segment elevations in leads I and aVL, consistent with acute lateral wall ST-segment elevation myocardial infarction. Note the reciprocal ST depressions in leads III and aVF.

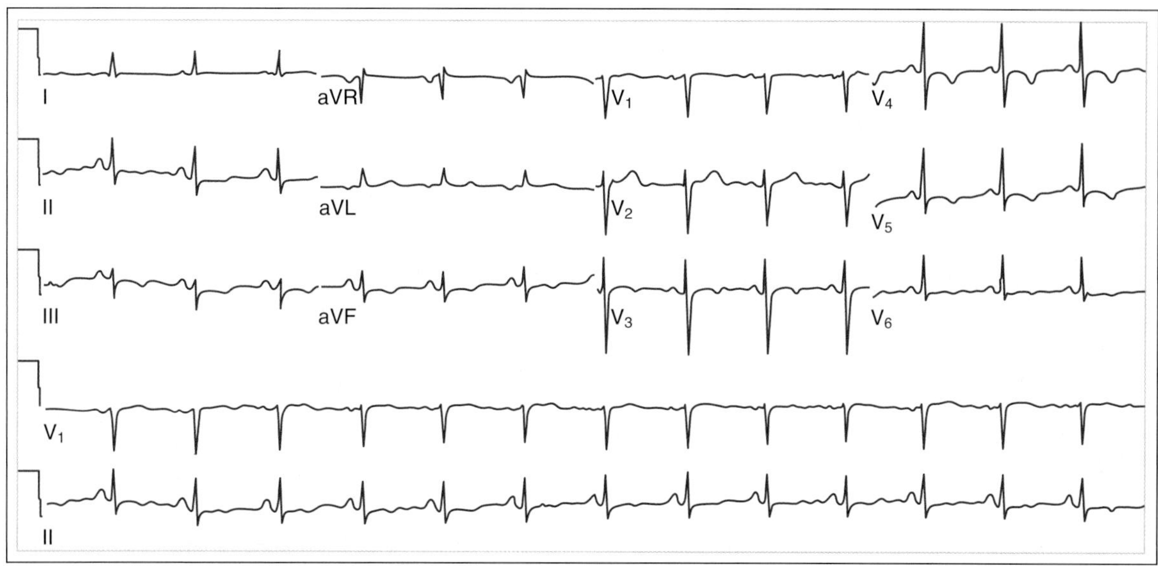


**Fig. 55.8** A 12-lead electrocardiogram shows T-wave inversions in leads $V_3$ through $V_6$ and ST-segment depressions with T-wave inversions in leads II, III, and aVF, consistent with non–ST-segment elevation acute coronary syndrome.

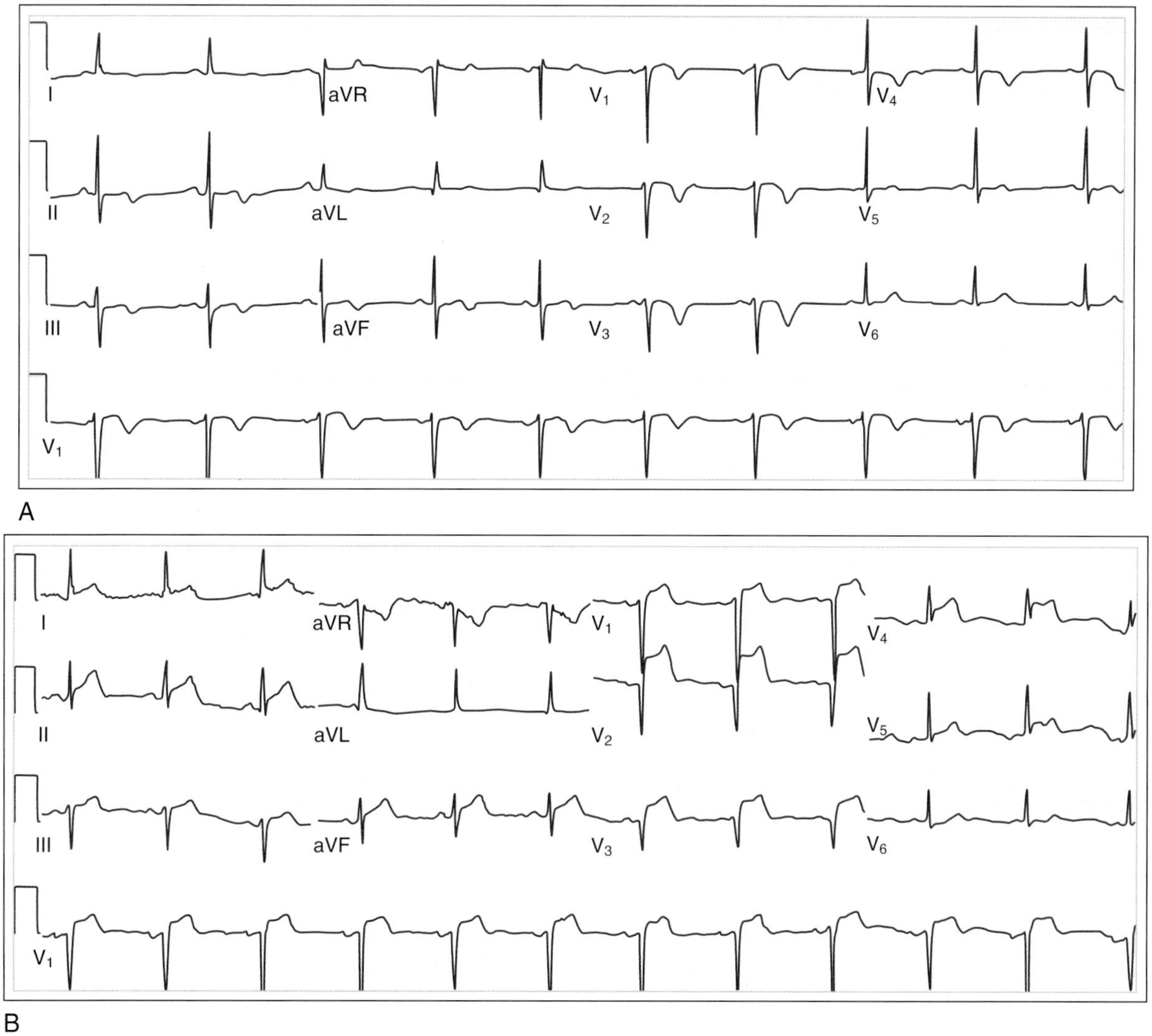

A

B

**Fig. 55.9** **A,** 12-lead electrocardiogram (ECG) in a woman with resolved chest pain. The deep symmetric precordial T-wave inversions represent Wellen syndrome. **B,** ECG from the same patient obtained 30 minutes later, now with recurrent chest pain. Note the anterior ST-segment elevation consistent with acute occlusion of the left anterior descending coronary artery.

or in suggesting an alternative cause of the symptoms. Most recently, contrast-enhanced multidetector computed tomography of the coronary arteries has been shown to have a role in the evaluation of patients with chest pain. These tests are discussed in detail in Chapter 56.

Findings on chest radiography are usually normal or unchanged from baseline in patients with ACS. However, the chest film can be useful to assess for other causes of chest pain, including pneumothorax, pneumonia, Boerhaave syndrome, and to a lesser degree, aortic dissection. In addition, chest radiography is valuable when ACS is complicated by congestive heart failure.

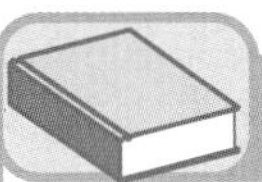

**PATIENT TEACHING TIPS**

Recognize chest pain and anginal equivalents as an indicator of potential acute coronary syndrome.

Call 911 for new-onset symptoms or those that do not resolve promptly with cessation of exertion or the use of sublingual nitroglycerin.

Do not ascribe symptoms to gastrointestinal or other noncardiac causes.

Diet, exercise, and smoking cessation should be encouraged for all patients.

For patients with a history of acute coronary syndrome, carrying an accurate medication list and a copy of the baseline electrocardiogram can be useful.

## TREATMENT

### PREHOSPITAL MANAGEMENT

Patients who activate the 911 system because of signs and symptoms associated with ACS should be assessed by paramedics, if available. Those exhibiting hemodynamic or respiratory compromise should be transported by an advanced life support unit. All patients should receive the following:

- Cardiac monitoring and, if possible, a prehospital 12-lead ECG
- Supplemental oxygen with pulse oximetry monitoring
- Intravenous access
- Aspirin, administered orally in the absence of known allergy
- Nitroglycerin administered sublingually in the absence of contraindications for ongoing chest pain

The prehospital staff should alert the receiving ED of the transport, and if evidence of STEMI is seen on the 12-lead ECG, this should be communicated to the ED staff specifically. In some communities, identification of STEMI in the prehospital setting will result in transport to a hospital capable of performing percutaneous coronary intervention (PCI), even if not the closest facility. Additionally, in some health care systems, prehospital identification of STEMI will allow immediate activation of cardiac catheterization laboratory personnel.

### HOSPITAL MANAGEMENT

**Figures 55.10 and 55.11** present treatment algorithms for STEMI and non–ST-segment acute coronary symptoms.

Treatment of ACS is time sensitive and aimed at improving myocardial tissue oxygen supply, reducing myocardial oxygen demand, protecting ischemic myocardium, restoring coronary blood flow, and preventing reocclusion of the artery. Specific therapy depends on where along the spectrum of disease the individual case lies. Generally, unless contraindicated, all patients receive aspirin, oxygen, beta-blocker therapy, nitrates, and antithrombin therapy. Use of other antiplatelet agents depends in part on the clinical situation, whereas revascularization strategies are used only in patients with STEMI.

#### *Platelet Inhibitors*

Aspirin remains the cornerstone of therapy across the spectrum of ACS. It is highly cost-effective and remains one of a few drugs with a mortality benefit in patients with ACS. In patients with STEMI, aspirin independently reduces mortality by approximately 23%.[8] Aspirin is an antiplatelet agent that irreversibly inactivates platelet cyclooxygenase and also reduces the formation of prostacyclin by endothelial cells. It should be administered in the ED orally (chewed and swallowed) or rectally; the standard dose is 162 to 325 mg. The EP should take care to avoid using enteric-coated preparations in the acute treatment of ACS. The only true contraindication to aspirin in patients with ACS is a history of severe allergic reaction.

Clopidogrel is one of several currently available thienopyridines, a class of drugs that inhibits adenosine diphosphate–mediated platelet aggregation. These drugs are more potent platelet inhibitors than aspirin is. Ticlopidine, another drug in this class, is not generally used because of its slow onset of action and concerns about its adverse effects, which include neutropenia and, rarely, agranulocytosis. Prasugrel, a more potent thienopyridine recently approved for use in patients with ACS, may play an increasing important role in the future, but at present clopidogrel remains the most commonly used drug in this class. Clopidogrel has been shown to improve clinical outcomes in patients with non–ST-segment elevation ACS, particularly in those who undergo PCI.[9,10] Clinical benefit is demonstrable within 24 hours of dosing, but it has been associated with a small increase in bleeding in those who undergo coronary artery bypass grafting (CABG) within 5 days of discontinuation of clopidogrel.[9] The traditional loading dose of clopidogrel has been 300 mg orally, but 600 mg appears to be equally safe and may be more efficacious. Clopidogrel (300 to 600 mg orally) should be administered to all patients with ACS and documented aspirin allergy, as well as to those in whom a noninterventional approach is planned.[11] Clopidogrel should also be administered to patients with non–ST-segment elevation ACS in whom emergency CABG is deemed unlikely[11]; this may best be determined in consultation with a cardiologist. For patients with STEMI, clopidogrel, 300 mg, is indicated as an adjunct to fibrinolytic therapy.[12] In patients with STEMI who will undergo PCI, it is reasonable to administer clopidogrel, 300 to 600 mg, in the ED, provided that transfer to the catheterization laboratory is not delayed as a result.

GP IIb/IIIa receptor blockers inhibit the final common pathway of platelet aggregation, namely, the cross-linking of two platelets by one strand of fibrinogen, a bivalent molecule with two binding sites specific for the GP IIb/IIIa receptor. As

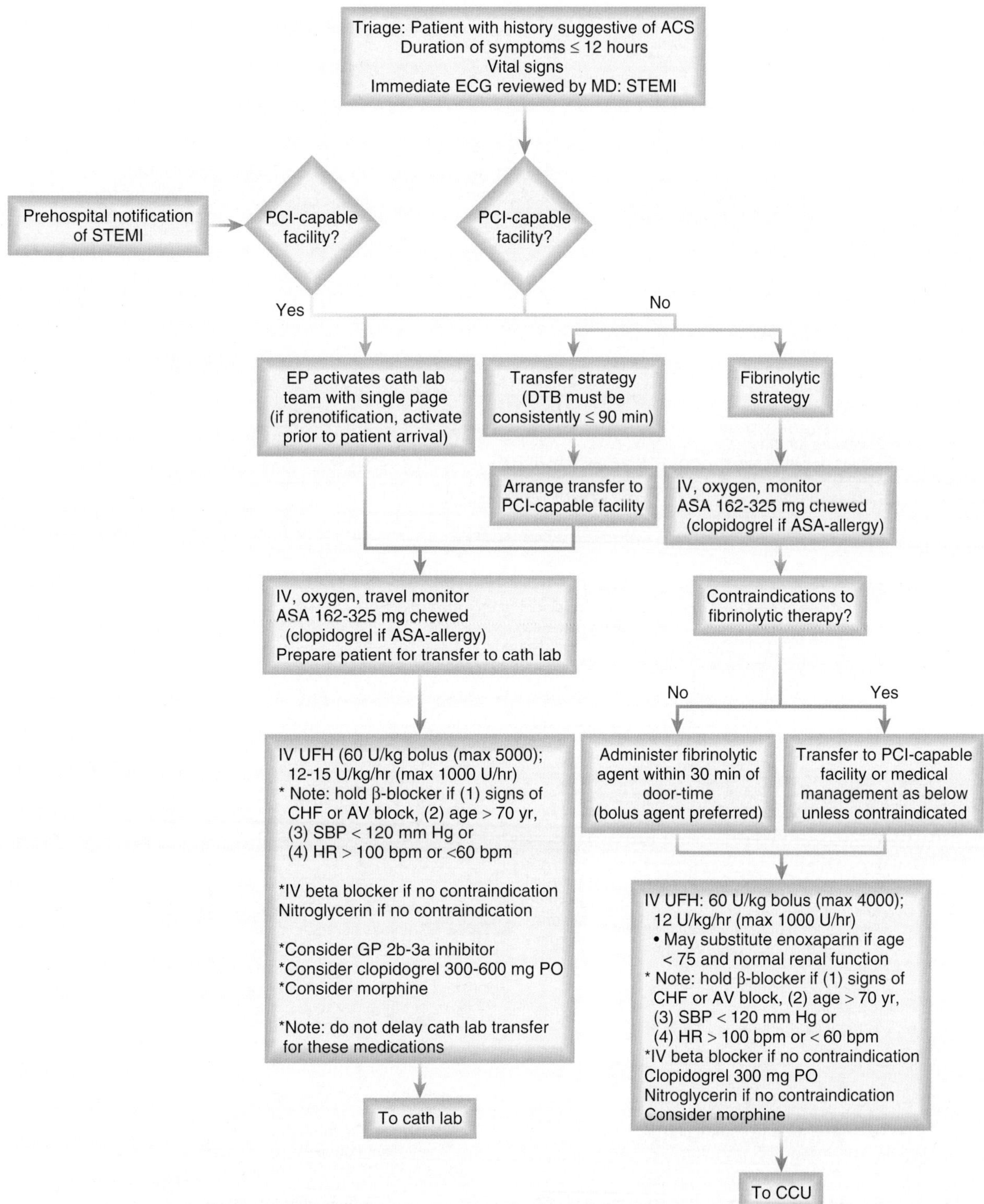


**Fig. 55.10 Assessment and treatment algorithm for ST-segment elevation myocardial infarction (STEMI).** *ACS*, Acute coronary syndrome; *ASA*, acetylsalicylic acid; *AV*, atrioventricular; *bpm*, beats per minute; *cath lab*, catheterization laboratory; *CCU*, cardiac care unit; *CHF*, congestive heart failure; *DTB*, door-to-balloon time; *ECG*, electrocardiogram; *EP*, emergency physician; *GP*, glycoprotein; *HR*, heart rate; *IV*, intravenous/intravenous line; *PCI*, percutaneous coronary intervention; *PO*, orally; *SBP*, systolic blood pressure; *UFH*, unfractionated heparin.

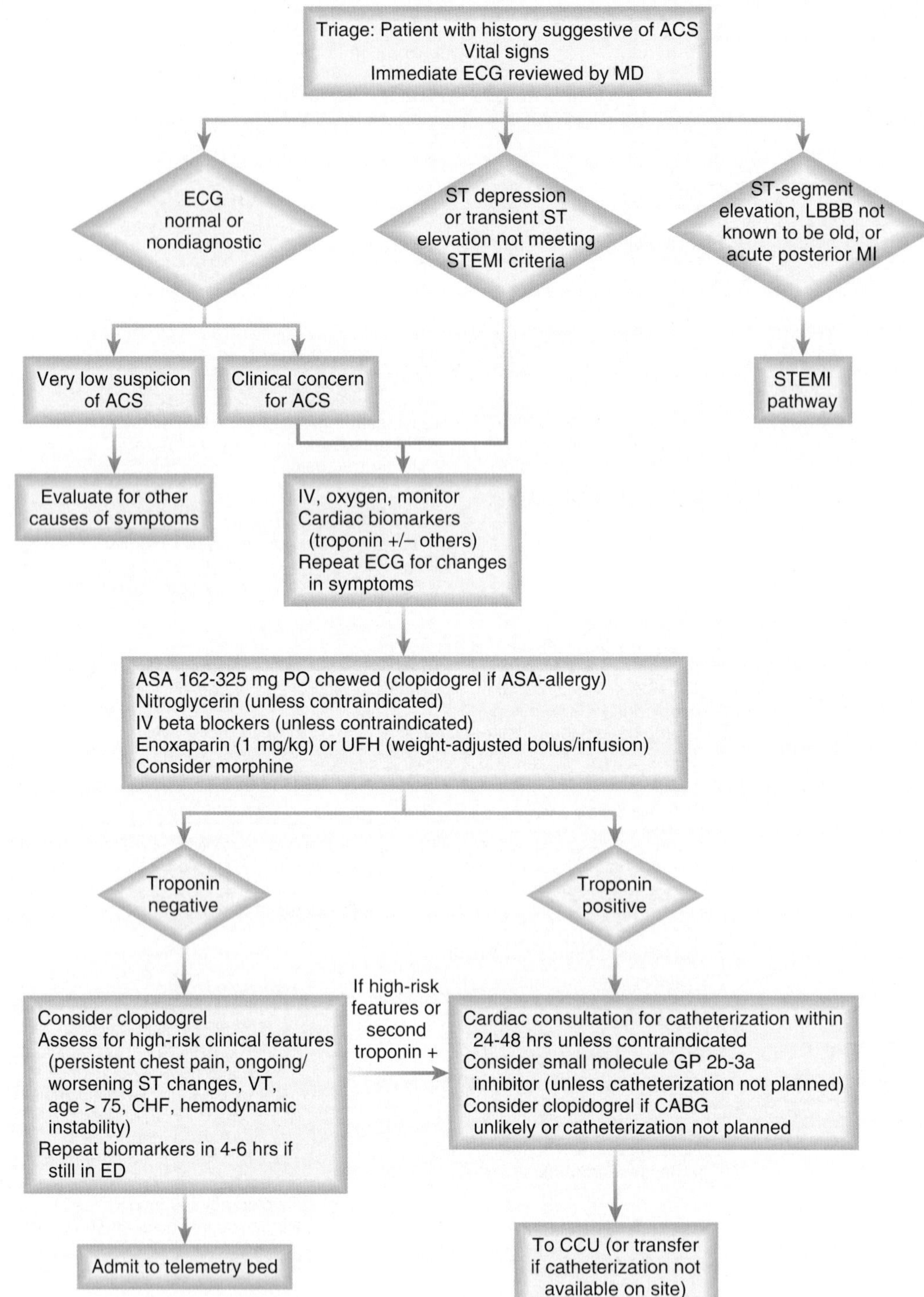


**Fig. 55.11 Assessment and treatment algorithm for non–ST-segment elevation myocardial infarction.** *ACS*, Acute coronary syndrome; *ASA*, acetylsalicylic acid; *CABG*, coronary artery bypass grafting; *CCU*, cardiac care unit; *CHF*, congestive heart failure; *ED*, emergency department; *ECG*, electrocardiogram; *GP*, glycoprotein; *IV*, intravenous/intravenous line; *LBBB*, left bundle branch block; *MI*, myocardial infarction; *STEMI*, ST-segment elevation myocardial infarction; *UFH*, unfractionated heparin; *VT*, ventricular tachycardia.

already mentioned, activated platelets have 50,000 to 80,000 receptors on their cell surfaces, so in the absence of GP IIb/IIIa inhibitors, a complete platelet-fibrinogen web can develop rapidly. With proper dosing, however, platelet inhibition of greater than 85% can be attained. For this reason, GP IIb/IIIa inhibitors are the most potent platelet inhibitors currently available. Nonetheless, GP IIb/IIIa inhibitors have been shown to provide benefit only to the subgroup of patients with ACS who undergo PCI.

Three GP IIb/IIIa inhibitors are currently available in the United States: abciximab, eptifibatide, and tirofiban. Abciximab, the first agent developed, is a unique chimeric monoclonal antibody to the GP IIb/IIIa receptor. It binds to the receptor by steric hindrance in a noncompetitive fashion and has a long half-life, with antiplatelet effects persisting for 24 hours after discontinuation of infusion. Eptifibatide and tirofiban, referred to as "small-molecule GP IIb/IIIa inhibitors," are derived from the poisonous venom of two different vipers and bind competitively to the receptor. As a result, both can prevent fibrinogen from initially binding to the GP IIb/IIIa receptor and also displace bound fibrinogen from the receptor. These drugs are cleared renally and have shorter half-lives, with their antiplatelet effects persisting for several hours after discontinuation of infusion.

GP IIb/IIIa inhibitors have been shown to provide benefit to patients with ACS treated by PCI. Some data also show benefit in troponin-positive patients who test positive for troponins, but not in patients who test negative or who are managed medically. Consequently, current recommendations for the use of this class of drugs are as follows[11]: GP IIb/IIIa inhibitors should be administered, along with aspirin and a heparin preparation, to patients with ACS in whom PCI is planned, even when clopidogrel is also given. However, the best available evidence suggests that no benefit is seen when GP IIb/IIIa inhibitors are administered in the ED versus delayed provisional use in the cardiac catheterization laboratory.[13,14] Furthermore, delaying this decision to the time of catheterization may reduce the likelihood of medication administration error, as well as the incidence of adverse effects and overall cost. With this in mind, the decision to use these drugs in the ED setting should be made with caution and limited to patients who have a compelling history of ACS, test positive for troponins, have no contraindication to cardiac catheterization, and are expected to have a delay in prompt interventional treatment.

### Beta-Blocking Agents

Beta-blockers are an important first-line therapy for patients with ACS. These agents act by reducing the effects of catecholamines on the heart—they slow the heart rate, reduce myocardial contractility, and thereby lower myocardial demand for oxygen. They are also potent antiarrhythmic agents and lessen the likelihood of ventricular and atrial tachyarrhythmias. However, they have also been shown, when given intravenously to patients with STEMI, to increase risk for the development of cardiogenic shock, which counterbalances the salutary effects of beta-blockers and results in no overall mortality benefit.[15] Thus beta-blockers should be administered intravenously with caution in the ED setting to patients with STEMI and specifically withheld, per the most recent American College of Cardiology and American Heart Association guidelines for STEMI, in the following settings[16]:

- Age greater than 70 years
- Signs of heart failure or heart block
- Heart rates lower than 60 or greater than 100 beats/min
- Systolic blood pressure less than 120 mm Hg

Oral administration of beta-blockers may be preferable in the ED across the spectrum of ACS, but this remains to be determined in clinical trials. When intravenous use is deemed appropriate, several different agents are available, including metoprolol, atenolol, propranolol, and the ultrashort-acting esmolol. Metoprolol is most commonly used; it is administered in 5-mg increments by slow intravenous "push" up to a total of 15 mg. This can be followed by 25 to 50 mg given orally. Atenolol is the longest acting and thus is not generally the best choice for ED use.

Propranolol is not selective for $\beta_1$-adrenergic receptor blockade but has been used effectively for many years. It can be administered intravenously in 1-mg increments titrated to the desired effect. Esmolol is ultrashort acting and must be administered by intravenous bolus followed by continuous infusion. Its ED utility is generally limited to patients in whom it is strongly suspected that beta-blockers will not be tolerated, such as those with chronic obstructive pulmonary disease or asthma.

### Nitrate Preparations

Nitrates may be administered in a number of forms to patients with ACS. Most commonly, sublingual tablets containing 0.3 or 0.4 mg of nitrate are given first, followed by intravenous, oral, or transdermal preparations as tolerated and as needed for ongoing symptoms. It is important to remember that although they do reduce symptoms of chest pain, nitrates have not been shown to reduce mortality. Because they may cause hypotension, it is important to administer nitrates judiciously in the ED. In addition, nitrates are contraindicated in the setting of acute right ventricular infarction, hypotension, critical aortic stenosis, and use of phosphodiesterase inhibitor drugs (e.g., sildenafil) within 24 to 48 hours.

### Oxygen

Supplemental oxygen should be administered to all patients with ACS, even if the initial oxygen saturation value is normal. This step is particularly important in patients treated with nitrates, which cause pulmonary arterial dilation and thereby impair the ability of the lung to autoregulate pulmonary blood flow. Treatment with oxygen reduces the areas of the lungs that are poorly oxygenated, thus giving less opportunity for shunting and resultant hypoxia.

### Anticoagulants

Anticoagulant (or antithrombin) therapy is indicated for patients with ACS who have no contraindications to its use. These agents are particularly useful in patients with recurrent anginal symptoms, "positive" cardiac biomarker values, or ischemic changes on the ECG. Available agents include unfractionated heparin (UFH), low-molecular-weight heparin (LMWH), fondaparinux, and direct thrombin inhibitors (DTIs). The heparins (UFH and LMWH) work by activating antithrombin III, which in turn inhibits thrombin and factor Xa. LMWH can also directly inhibit factor Xa. Fondaparinux inhibits factor Xa as its principal mechanism of anticoagulation, and DTIs, as their name suggests, act directly on thrombin. The net result of therapy with all the drugs in this class is to prevent the conversion of fibrinogen to fibrin, thereby avoiding clot propagation. These drugs are contraindicated in patients with active bleeding. In addition, heparin and LMWH are contraindicated in patients with a known history of heparin-induced thrombocytopenia.

UFH has a synergistic salutary effect on ischemic outcomes when combined with aspirin in patients with ACS, particularly those with MI. Several LMWH preparations have shown efficacy in patients with ACS, but only enoxaparin has demonstrated an improvement over UFH. Therefore, enoxaparin is the LMWH of choice for the treatment of ACS. Current guidelines recommend the administration of UFH or enoxaparin to patients with ACS in conjunction with antiplatelet therapy.[11] For non–ST-segment elevation ACS, enoxaparin (1 mg/kg given subcutaneously twice daily) is the preferred agent unless urgent CABG is planned.[11] UFH is dosed as an intravenous bolus of 60 U/kg (maximum, 4000 units), followed by an infusion at 12 U/kg/hr (maximum, 1000 U/hr).[6,11] UFH use must be monitored by serial prothrombin time determinations; such monitoring is not necessary in patients treated with enoxaparin. Either drug should be discontinued immediately in patients with evidence of bleeding or if thrombocytopenia develops.

Fondaparinux is a relative newcomer to the class of anticoagulant drugs. It is a pentasaccharide molecule that represents the terminal five saccharide moieties of heparin. Principally a factor Xa inhibitor, this agent is administered as a subcutaneous injection, with dose reductions required in patients with renal insufficiency. Fondaparinux already has indications for the treatment of venous thromboembolic disease, and data suggest that it is similar to enoxaparin in terms of safety and efficacy for the treatment of non–ST-segment elevation ACS.[17] Current published guidelines recommend fondaparinux as an acceptable alternative to UFH or enoxaparin in patients with non–ST-segment elevation ACS.[11]

DTIs offer theoretic advantages over heparins in that they do not work through the intermediary antithrombin III to inhibit thrombin. Nevertheless, no convincing data have shown that DTIs provide clinical benefits over UFH or LMWH in ED patients with ACS. Because of this and their high cost, current ED use of the presently available DTIs—argatroban, hirudin, and bivalirudin—should be limited to patients with a history of heparin-induced thrombocytopenia.

### *Morphine*

Morphine sulfate is an opioid analgesic that has fallen out of favor for the treatment of ACS. There is no compelling evidence in favor of its use, and reports suggest that its sedative effects are associated with an increased risk for respiratory compromise and aspiration. In addition, this agent may cause hypotension through arterial and venous dilation. Morphine has a small role in managing pain that is refractory to other antiischemic therapy and in reducing anxiety in patients in whom anxiety is a prominent feature. It may be delivered intravenously in 3- to 5-mg increments.

### *Angiotensin-Converting Enzyme Inhibitors*

Angiotensin-converting enzyme (ACE) inhibitors have a limited role in the treatment of patients with ACS. This class of drugs, which causes afterload reduction, includes captopril, lisinopril, and enalapril. The principal acute adverse effect is hypotension. It is clear that ACE inhibitors are beneficial in the subset of patients with acute or preexisting left ventricular dysfunction. They are also useful as adjunctive therapy for patients with STEMI that is being treated with fibrinolytic therapy. However, no compelling data support the use of ACE inhibitors in the ED, and it is reasonable to defer their administration to the inpatient setting. If they are initiated in the ED, it is preferable to start with a low dose and increase it as tolerated by the blood pressure. Renal function should be monitored during the initial phases of therapy with ACE inhibitors.

### *Revascularization Therapy*

Patients with STEMI who arrive at the ED within 12 to 24 hours of the onset of symptoms require urgent revascularization therapy. It can be accomplished mechanically with primary PCI or pharmacologically with fibrinolytic therapy. Although fibrinolytic therapy remains the most common strategy worldwide, use of primary PCI for STEMI has been growing rapidly in the United States and has been deemed a preferable approach in terms of safety and efficacy. If a primary PCI strategy is chosen, the IRA must be opened within 90 minutes of patient arrival at the health care system to achieve maximal efficacy.[5] This interval includes time spent at the initial hospital if transfer to a PCI-capable facility is necessary. If the "door-to-balloon" target time of 90 minutes cannot be routinely achieved, a fibrinolytic strategy is preferable, particularly for patients who are seen early (within 3 hours of symptom onset).[5]

For patients in cardiogenic shock or those with contraindications to fibrinolytic therapy, primary PCI should be performed as soon as possible. In addition, patients in whom fibrinolytic therapy fails, as evidenced by ongoing anginal symptoms and ST-segment elevations continuing an hour or more after therapy, should be referred for rescue PCI, which should be performed as soon as possible. Patients with STEMI who undergo primary PCI should also receive aspirin, clopidogrel, and UFH. It is reasonable to administer a GP IIb/IIIa inhibitor to these patients as well, and abciximab is the preferred agent in this setting. However, current evidence suggests that this decision can be safely deferred to the time of catheterization and PCI,[13] which may allow the drug to be given more safely.

It is important to emphasize that none of these adjunctive therapies should delay transfer of the patient from the ED to the cardiac catheterization laboratory, which is the first priority. A number of validated strategies should be used to decrease door-to-balloon time.[18] Those that specifically affect the ED are (1) empowering the EP to activate the entire cardiac catheterization laboratory team with a single phone call; (2) increasing, when possible, the capacity to obtain prehospital ECG tracings in patients with chest pain and activation of the catheterization laboratory team while the patient is still en route to the hospital; and (3) providing prompt feedback from a multidisciplinary quality improvement team to all clinical providers involved in care of the patient.[18]

Fibrinolytic therapy remains an important treatment option for patients with STEMI, particularly those who go to community hospitals that do not have the capability of performing PCI. Rapid initiation of treatment is the standard of care, with a target goal "door-to-needle" time of less than 30 minutes. Fibrinolytic therapy is indicated for patients who have symptoms consistent with ACS within 12 hours of symptom onset, meet ECG criteria (**Box 55.2**), and do not have an absolute contraindication to the therapy (**Box 55.3**). The presence of relative contraindications (**Box 55.4**) must be weighed against the risk of treatment delay if primary PCI is not readily available. Advanced age alone is *not* a contraindication, and although elderly patients treated with fibrinolytic therapy do have a higher incidence of hemorrhage, they also have a significantly higher mortality rate, which can be mitigated with therapy.

**BOX 55.2 Electrocardiographic Criteria for Fibrinolytic Therapy**

ST-segment elevation of 0.1 mV or greater in two or more contiguous leads
Left bundle branch block not known to be old
ST-segment depressions and prominent R waves in leads $V_1$ through $V_4$

**BOX 55.3 Absolute Contraindications to Fibrinolytic Therapy**

Previous history of intracranial hemorrhage
Known malignant intracranial neoplasm
Known cerebrovascular lesion (e.g., arteriovenous malformation)
Suspected aortic dissection
Active bleeding (excluding menses) or known bleeding diathesis
Significant closed-head or facial trauma within the previous 3 months
Ischemic stroke within the previous 3 months (except if within 3 hours)

**BOX 55.4 Relative Contraindications to Fibrinolytic Therapy**

History of chronic, severe, poorly controlled hypertension
Uncontrolled hypertension at initial evaluation (systolic blood pressure higher than 180 mm Hg or diastolic blood pressure higher than 110 mm Hg)
Previous ischemic stroke more than 3 months earlier
Traumatic or prolonged (>10 minutes) cardiopulmonary resuscitation or major surgery within less than 3 weeks
Recent (within 2 to 4 weeks) internal bleeding
Noncompressible vascular punctures
Pregnancy
Active peptic ulcer
Current use of anticoagulants

Several fibrinolytic agents are available. They include streptokinase, which is not fibrin specific and is administered as an intravenous infusion of 1.5 million units delivered over a 1-hour period, and tissue plasminogen activator (t-PA), which is fibrin specific and administered as a bolus followed by two separate weight-adjusted infusions. Considerable data suggest that the bolus-administered fibrinolytic agents reteplase (recombinant plasminogen activator [r-PA]) and tenecteplase are safer and easier to use than the infused fibrinolytic drugs and have equivalent clinical efficacy; cost are similar to that for t-PA. Both these newer agents are highly fibrin specific, and bolus administration lends itself to prehospital use if that is a consideration. r-PA is administered as a double bolus of 10 units intravenously at time 0 and again at 30 minutes; weight adjusting is not necessary. Tenecteplase is administered in a weight-tiered fashion as a single bolus of 30 to 50 mg based on known or estimated patient weight.

All patients with STEMI treated with fibrinolytic therapy should also receive aspirin and clopidogrel. Beta-blockers should be given with caution and perhaps should be limited in the ED setting to oral use in appropriate patients as discussed earlier. If a fibrin-specific agent is administered, UFH should be given in a bolus dose of 60 U/kg (maximum, 4000 units) and as an infusion of 12 U/kg/hr (maximum, 1000 U/hr). Enoxaparin can be safely and effectively substituted for UFH in patients with normal renal function who are younger than 75 years.[19] If streptokinase is administered, either heparin preparation should be withheld.

Combination pharmacologic treatment of STEMI has attracted considerable interest. The most promising combination has been half-dose fibrinolytic therapy coupled with a GP IIb/IIIa inhibitor, which has been demonstrated to provide better angiographic outcomes in the IRA at 90 minutes. However, large-scale clinical trials have failed to show a mortality benefit of this combination, although they have suggested that it achieves reductions in the risk for recurrent MI and the need for rescue angioplasty.[20] At present, combination therapy, because it is more expensive and cumbersome to administer, should be considered for use only in facilities whose remote locations make transfer of a patient for rescue PCI very difficult.

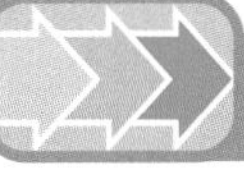

**PRIORITY ACTIONS**

1. Immediate 12-lead electrocardiogram for all patients with chest pain or anginal equivalent
2. Administration of aspirin to patients with acute coronary syndrome, the only contraindication being a true aspirin allergy
3. Prompt revascularization for patients with ST-segment elevation myocardial infarction ("door-to-needle" time of less than 30 minutes or "door-to-balloon" time of less than 90 minutes)
4. Early recognition and treatment of electrical and mechanical complications of acute coronary syndrome
5. Admission to a telemetry unit or coronary care unit for all patients with acute coronary syndrome

## FOLLOW-UP AND NEXT STEPS IN CARE

All patients with ACS should be admitted to a hospital bed equipped with cardiac monitoring. In some institutions, patients with negative initial troponin test values and nondiagnostic ECG findings who are deemed to be at low risk for ACS may be admitted to ED- or cardiology-based chest pain observation units, where the remainder of the diagnostic and therapeutic evaluation may take place. In most hospitals, however, patients with suspected ACS are admitted as inpatients and generally to a cardiac intensive care unit. Cardiac consultation is indicated. Patients with STEMI who are managed with primary PCI go directly from the ED to the cardiac catheterization laboratory and thereafter to a cardiac intensive care unit.

Complications of ACS that are manifested acutely include congestive heart failure or cardiogenic shock (because of a large infarction or acute valvular incompetence) and rhythm disturbances (ventricular fibrillation, atrial fibrillation, and atrioventricular nodal block, among others). In patients with STEMI, particularly those with delayed revascularization and those who are revascularized with fibrinolytic therapy, myocardial rupture of the infarcted portion of the left ventricle can occur, generally in the period 1 to 5 days after infarction, and result in an acute ventricular septal defect with flash pulmonary edema or free wall rupture with tamponade. The most important longer-term complication is chronic congestive heart failure, development of which is dependent on several things, including the extent of the index MI and the speed and success of revascularization, as well as the degree of underlying heart disease and preexisting left ventricular dysfunction, ischemic in origin or otherwise. Ventricular tachyarrhythmia may also be a long-term complication of patients with ACS.

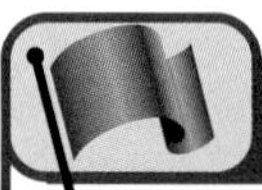

**RED FLAGS**

Many patients with acute coronary syndrome, particularly the elderly, have atypical manifestations.

Normal electrocardiographic findings do not exclude acute coronary syndrome.

A single set of "negative" cardiac biomarkers does not exclude acute myocardial infarction.

Recognize that patients with ST-segment elevation myocardial infarction who are transferred for primary percutaneous coronary intervention may not be revascularized within the recommended treatment window; consider fibrinolysis for these patients instead.

Avoid nitrates and intravenous beta-blockers in situations in which their use is contraindicated.

## SUGGESTED READINGS

Anderson JL, Adams CD, Antman EM, et al. ACC/AHA 2007 guidelines for the management of patients with unstable angina/non ST-elevation myocardial infarction: a report of the American College of Cardiology/American Heart Association Task Force on Practice Guidelines (Writing Committee to Revise the 2002 Guidelines for the Management of Patients With Unstable Angina/Non ST-Elevation Myocardial Infarction). Circulation 2007;116:e148-304.

Antman EM, Hand M, Armstrong PW, et al. 2007 Focused update of the ACC/AHA 2004 Guidelines for the Management of Patients With ST-Elevation Myocardial Infarction: a report of the American College of Cardiology/American Heart Association Task Force on Practice Guidelines: developed in collaboration with the Canadian Cardiovascular Society endorsed by the American Academy of Family Physicians: 2007 Writing Group to Review New Evidence and Update the ACC/AHA 2004 Guidelines for the Management of Patients With ST-Elevation Myocardial Infarction, Writing on Behalf of the 2004 Writing Committee. Circulation. 2008;117:296-329.

Bradley E, Herrin H, Wang Y, et al. Strategies to reduce the door-to-balloon time in acute myocardial infarction. N Engl J Med 2006;355:2308-20.

Chen ZM, Pan HC, Chen YP, et al. Early intravenous then oral metoprolol in 45,852 patients with acute myocardial infarction: randomised placebo-controlled trial. Lancet 2005;366:1622-32.

## REFERENCES

***References can be found on Expert Consult @ www.expertconsult.com.***

# Cardiac Imaging and Stress Testing 56

*Ryan T. Geers, John Deledda, and Andra L. Blomkalns*

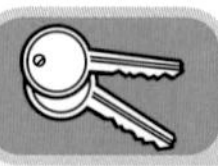

**KEY POINTS**

- Cardiac imaging and stress testing are key components of any comprehensive patient evaluation for possible acute coronary syndromes or coronary heart disease.
- Exercise or pharmacologic stress testing is used to risk-stratify patients and determine the presence of stress-induced ischemia.
- Rest myocardial perfusion imaging assesses for ischemia during symptoms at the time of evaluation, whereas stress testing evaluates for stress-induced (exercise or pharmacologic) ischemia.
- Rest myocardial perfusion imaging can be a useful tool for risk stratification and diagnosis in patients with active or recent chest discomfort (<2 hours).
- Echocardiography can be used to assess global cardiac function and may be performed with the patient at rest or with stress.
- Electron beam computed tomography is gaining momentum as an imaging technology that is potentially useful in the emergency department environment.
- Several chest pain unit protocols using various combinations of cardiac biomarkers, imaging modalities, stress testing, and time courses of evaluation have proved successful in many environments.
- Individual institutions and their emergency departments should develop their own custom protocols to best care for patients in that community given the resources available, personnel, and practice patterns.

## BACKGROUND AND SCOPE

The diverse group of patients with symptoms of chest discomfort remains a significant challenge for the emergency physician (EP). High-risk patients with classic angina and young, low-risk patients with atypical symptoms represent only a fraction of those with chest discomfort seem in the everyday emergency department (ED) setting. Frequently, patients have one or two risk factors and some but not all of the classic ischemic symptoms, and the findings on an electrocardiogram (ECG) are nondiagnostic. These patients carry up to a 10% chance of significant cardiac disease and need appropriate risk stratification and diagnostic evaluation.[1] As EPs, our goal is not to diagnose the condition of coronary heart disease but, rather, to stratify patients' risk and identify those at risk for imminent cardiac ischemia and poor outcomes.

EPs use several methods and modalities to evaluate this very heterogenous patient group, each of which has benefits and limitations. Aside from a comprehensive history and physical examination, standard adjuncts include an ECG, serial cardiac biomarker measurements, and some choice of cardiac imaging. The ECG, though often considered the principal diagnostic tool in cardiac evaluation, is the most basic and rapid way to image the heart. Elevations in available cardiac biomarkers indicate the end result of ischemic myocardium and signify myocardial necrosis or cell death. Cardiac imaging indirectly reflects cardiac anatomy and tissue function with the goal of revealing occult cellular ischemia at risk for cell death. Cardiac imaging can be performed with the patient at rest or under physical or pharmacologic stress. Some of the factors to be considered for the appropriate choice of imaging modality include patient selection, exposure to radiation (**Table 56.1**), and availability of resources, technology, and personnel to perform the study and interpret the results.[2] The goal of this chapter is to familiarize the reader with common cardiac imaging modalities used in the ED for the evaluation of this difficult and high-risk population.

This chapter focuses on the most common and established cardiac imaging modalities of echocardiography and myocardial perfusion nuclear imaging. An example of how these modalities might be incorporated into an ED patient evaluation protocol is also presented. Finally, we briefly highlight the new and promising cardiac imaging capabilities of computed tomography (CT) and magnetic resonance imaging (MRI).

## ELECTROCARDIOGRAM

An ECG should be obtained within 10 minutes of a patient's arrival at the ED.[3] Though often considered to be the most important diagnostic and prognostic tool available, ECGs rather primitively indicate only gross electrical derangements caused by dead or dying muscle tissue. Serial ECGs during progression or regression of a patient's symptoms can be helpful, similar to procuring prior ECGs from a previous medical visit.

Common errors in reading ECGs include distinguishing between true posterior and right ventricular ischemia. A true

**Table 56.1 Approximate Radiation Exposure with Common Imaging Studies as Part of Cardiac Evaluation**

| STUDY | MEAN EFFECTIVE DOSE (MILLISIEVERTS) |
|---|---|
| Chest radiograph | 0.02 |
| Echocardiogram | 0 |
| Myocardial perfusion imaging | 15 |
| Ventilation-perfusion ($\dot{V}/\dot{Q}$) scan | 1.2-2 |
| Computed tomographic (CT) angiography of the chest (noncoronary) | 15 |
| CT angiography (coronary) | 8-15 |
| Percutaneous coronary intervention | 7-15 |

Adapted from Fazel R, Krumholz HM, Wang Y, et al. Exposure to low-dose ionizing radiation from medical imaging procedures. N Engl J Med 2009;361:849-57.

posterior infarction is suggested by marked ST depression, upright T waves, and tall R waves in the anterior leads ($V_1$ to $V_3$). This can be further confirmed by data acquired from posterior leads ($V_7$ to $V_9$) placed on the patient's back. Because of the opposite direction of reading the ECG current, these leads ($V_7$ to $V_9$) will show ST-segment elevation with posterior ischemia. If unable to get posterior leads, flipping the regular ECG to view $V_1$ to $V_3$ upside down through the ECG paper can demonstrate what $V_7$ to $V_9$ would show. In comparison, the right ventricle lies on the anterior and inferior surface of the heart. This area is best reflected through right-sided leads in which the precordial leads are placed from the sternum to the right side of the patient's chest ($V_1$ to $V_6$). ST-segment elevation in leads $V_3$ to $V_4$ indicates right ventricular involvement. Right ventricular involvement is commonly associated with inferior infarctions. These infarcts can be volume dependent, and such patients require careful use of nitrates and perhaps even small fluid boluses to maintain hemodynamic stability.

## CHEST ROENTGENOGRAM

Though not usually considered to be a cardiac imaging modality, the chest radiograph is an important diagnostic tool in the evaluation of patients with chest pain. Probably the most useful function of the chest radiograph lies in identifying or suggesting alternative diagnoses for the patient's symptoms. Chest radiographs are safe and result in relatively low radiation exposure (0.02 millisievert) when compared with the cardiac-specific modalities (see Table 56.1). Pneumothorax or pneumonia can be identified on a chest radiograph. Mediastinal widening, apical capping of pleural fluid, tracheal deviation, or displacement of intimal calcium from the outer vessel wall may indicate aortic dissection. An enlarged cardiac silhouette may signify the presence of a pericardial effusion or, if seen together with pulmonary congestion, congestive heart failure. Pulmonary emboli may be accompanied by focal oligemia, wedge-based densities, or enlarged pulmonary arteries on chest radiographs. Every patient with chest discomfort should have a chest radiograph taken before additional evaluation.

## EXERCISE TREADMILL TESTING

Graded exercise testing is a popular method of cardiac stress testing in both the inpatient and outpatient settings. Many of the early ED accelerated diagnostic protocols used this test after initial risk stratification via cardiac biomarkers and the ECG.[4-8] This was the beginning of chest pain unit protocols and the ability to appropriately risk-stratify ED patients with chest pain within 6 to 12 hours. Outcomes at 6 to 12 months have been found to be similar with very few adverse events between patients admitted to the hospital and those cared for in an ED chest pain unit setting. Although exercise treadmill testing has a lower positive predictive value (great proportion of false-positive results) than some other more contemporary myocardial perfusion imaging (MPI) modalities, its use still diminishes unnecessary admissions.[9]

Selection criteria for exercise testing are more restrictive than those for other imaging modalities. Patients must be able to walk on a treadmill, and findings on the ECG should be normal or show no new changes. Agents such as dobutamine, dipyridamole, adenosine, or regadenoson can be used in lieu of exercise. Although exercise testing is slowly being supplanted by studies offering more detailed functional information, it is still a major tool in many centers (**Fig. 56.1**).

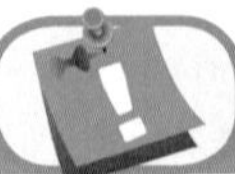

**TIPS AND TRICKS**

Meet the patient's expectations by explaining the process and time requirements for a comprehensive risk stratification protocol.

Even after a negative rest protocol result, be sure to emphasize to the patient the need to pursue further stress testing and risk factor modification.

Determine the patient's ability to exercise before sending the patient for an exercise study. Many patients cannot exercise sufficiently for adequate results and ultimately need pharmacologically induced stress to maintain their heart rate in the appropriate range.

## ECHOCARDIOGRAPHY

### REST ECHOCARDIOGRAM

Two-dimensional rest echocardiography enables real-time visualization of the anatomy and physiology of the heart and thereby provides an abundant amount of diagnostic information in patients seen in the ED. The procedure itself is safe, painless, and without radiation. In some patients with chest pain, a rest echocardiogram is a sensitive bedside test that can be an important tool in guiding diagnosis, therapeutic interventions, and final disposition of the patient.

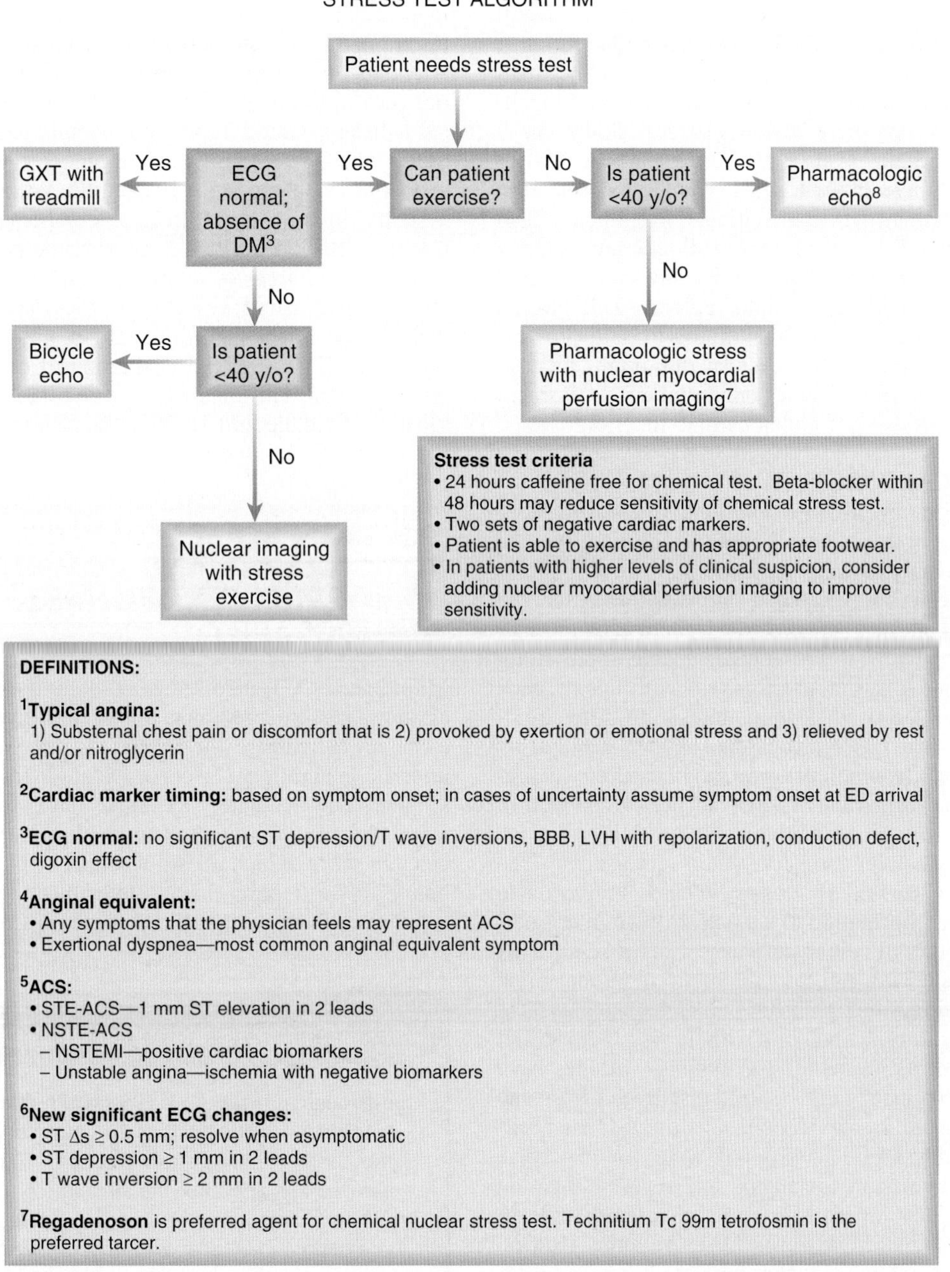


**Fig. 56.1 Stress test algorithm.** *ACS*, Acute coronary syndrome; *BBB*, bundle branch block; *DM*, diabetes mellitus; *ECG*, electrocardiogram; *echo*, echocardiography; *ED*, emergency department; *GTX*, graded exercise test; *LVH*, left ventricular hypertrophy; *NSTE*, non–ST-segment elevation; *NSTEMI*, NSTE myocardial infarction; *STE*, ST-segment elevation; *y/o*, years old.

Echocardiography is a comprehensive diagnostic tool for a number of conditions, including cardiac ischemia, acute pulmonary embolism, pericardial effusion, aortic dissection, pericarditis, hypertrophic cardiomyopathy, mitral valve prolapse, and aortic stenosis (**Box 56.1**).

Rest echocardiography has an important role in risk stratification of patients in the ED with potential myocardial ischemia. In a healthy heart, increases in heart rate and myocardial contractility are seen with cardiac stress. In patients with myocardial ischemia, segmental changes can be seen with rest echocardiography, including decreased wall thickness during stress, a decrease or no change in the ejection

**BOX 56.1 Conditions Detected by Echocardiography**

Cardiac ischemia
Hypertrophic cardiomyopathy
Aortic dissection
Pericarditis
Mitral valve prolapse
Aortic stenosis
Acute pulmonary embolism
Pericardial effusion

fraction, and regional wall motion abnormalities. The diagnostic accuracy of rest echocardiography depends on several factors, including proximity in time to the patient's symptoms, size of the myocardium affected, depth of the ischemic myocardial tissue, and limitations of the specific-generation technology being used. For these reasons, several studies have reported widely varying positive predictive (31% to 100%) and negative predictive (57% to 98%) values for detecting myocardial ischemia in the acute setting.[10] Preliminary data indicate a potential ED use of echocardiographic contrast agents, which are absorbed by healthy myocardium and thereby more able to identify subtle regional wall motion abnormalities.[11] Finally, EPs are continuing to gain prowess in bedside ultrasonography. However, at this point, focused cardiac ultrasound by EPs includes only a binary assessment (normal versus depressed) of global cardiac function.[12]

### STRESS ECHOCARDIOGRAM

Stress echocardiography provides additional diagnostic capability in detecting inducible wall motion abnormalities in patients who may have normal wall motion at rest. A stress echocardiogram can be performed immediately after the patient undergoes physical stress through the use of a treadmill or bike. Alternatively, if the patient is unable or unwilling to undergo exercise, pharmacologic stress with agents such as dobutamine can be used. Dobutamine is an adrenergic-stimulating agent that raises myocardial oxygen demand by increasing contractility, blood pressure, and heart rate. Dobutamine stress echocardiography (DSE) has performed well in providing excellent negative predictive value (NPV) for the diagnosis of obstructive coronary artery disease.[13-15] The greatest diagnostic benefit of stress echocardiography is to provide prognostic information in patients with an intermediate pretest probability of having coronary artery disease. This may include patients with some combination of coronary risk factors (hypertension, smoking history, diabetes) and atypical angina, patients with typical angina without risk factors, and patients with abnormal baseline ECG findings. Studies have shown that these patients can be safely discharged from the ED with outpatient follow-up if the results of DSE are negative. In one ED study, DSE had NPVs of 98.8% for all cardiac events (hospital admission for angina and revascularization procedure) and 99.6% for hard cardiac events (cardiac death and nonfatal myocardial infarction).[7] In several other studies, the NPV of DSE in patients undergoing ED chest pain protocols ranged from 91% to 96% for cardiac events at 6 months.[13-15]

## MYOCARDIAL PERFUSION IMAGING

MPI involves the injection of a radioisotope such as thallous chloride Tl 201 (thallium) or technetium Tc 99m radiopharmaceuticals and imaging of its uptake and diffusion through cardiac tissue. One important advantage of Tc 99m is that unlike Tl 201, it distributes to areas of highest myocardial perfusion and does not redistribute to other areas over time. This property allows the practitioner to inject the patient with the radionuclide agent during or proximate to the patient's symptoms at rest and obtain the images several hours later.

MPI has gained wide acceptance for the diagnosis of myocardial ischemia in a variety of patient populations traditionally difficult to diagnose, such as women, asymptomatic diabetic patients, patients with existing ECG abnormalities such as left bundle branch block, and patients with severe renal disease. Gated single-photon emission computed tomography (SPECT) with an attenuation correction has made MPI even more valuable in the ED setting. With multihead SPECT systems, imaging can often be completed in less than 10 minutes. Also with SPECT, inferior and posterior abnormalities and small areas of infarction can be identified, as well as the occluded blood vessels and the mass of infarcted and viable myocardium. Several landmark trials have shown a high NPV for MPI in the ED evaluation of chest discomfort.[16-18] Although thallium imaging is more established, the diffusion kinetics of technetium Tc 99m makes it more desirable in the ED setting.

## ELECTRON BEAM COMPUTED TOMOGRAPHY AND COMPUTED TOMOGRAPHIC CORONARY ANGIOGRAPHY

Multidetector CT, also known as "ultrafast" CT or CT angiography, has emerged as a highly sensitive means by which to detect calcium in the atherosclerotic lesions of coronary arteries. In addition, CT coronary angiography using 64-slice scanners can accurately visualize the coronary arteries in a large majority of patients. The results are typically given as a calcium score, which does not reflect a potential acute thrombus. CT also imparts the additive advantage of being able to visualize other potentially significant conditions, such as

$SI = \frac{SV}{BSA}$ **FACTS AND FORMULAS**

The myocardium takes up technetium 99m proportional to blood flow; unlike thallium 201, technetium 99m is redistributed minimally after injection. This feature allows delayed imaging after the initial radioisotope injection.

Perfusion defects signify areas of acute ischemia, acute infarction, or old scar and hence have to be interpreted cautiously in patients with a preexisting history of acute coronary syndrome or coronary artery disease.

Radiation exposure with different cardiac imaging techniques varies widely and should be a consideration in the most appropriate choice for each patient. Such exposure is particularly important in patients who undergo multiple or repeated studies. See Table 56.1.

Contemporary 64-slice computed tomography (CT) scanners generate images with the spatial resolution of 0.4 mm and a temporal resolution of 83 to 165 msec. Although traditional coronary angiography has a spatial resolution of 0.15 mm and a temporal resolution of 0.33 sec, CT angiography can yield sufficient diagnostic data in many patients. To facilitate adequate imaging for CT angiography, patients may undergo beta-blocker therapy to achieve a heart rate of approximately 60 beats/min.

pulmonary embolism and aortic dissection ("triple rule out").[19] Both these modalities show promise in the risk stratification of low- to moderate-risk patients with chest pain.[20,21] Possible limitations include availability of this technology and radiologists or cardiologists to read these studies in real time. The previous requirement of lowering the patient's heart rate grows less necessary with advanced multislice and source technologies. The results from ongoing studies will help determine the optimal role of CT in cardiac evaluation.[22]

### PATIENT TEACHING TIPS

Patients experiencing chest discomfort with or without the classic associated symptoms should call their emergency response system (i.e., 911) instead of driving to the nearest hospital.

To provide appropriate risk stratification, chest discomfort evaluation protocols may take several hours to finish.

A right-sided infarction and posterior infarction are separate clinical entities identified by separate and specific electrocardiographic findings.

Even after a negative rest imaging evaluation result, the patient should arrange for further risk assessment and stress imaging with a primary care physician or cardiologist.

Therapeutic lifestyle modifications and attention to modifiable cardiac risk factors should be part of any evaluation protocol.

The patient should keep copies of the imaging records, including a copy of the latest electrocardiogram, in a personal health file. These records can be tremendously useful to other physicians if further emergency cardiac evaluation is required.

## MAGNETIC RESONANCE IMAGING

Current research continues to explore new and hopefully more effective imaging strategies for the evaluation of patients with chest discomfort in the ED. MRI can be used to determine both myocardial perfusion and regional wall motion abnormalities, including transient stunning after an ischemic event. Several studies have shown its utility in the diagnosis of acute coronary syndrome, and recent clinical trials have demonstrated its potential value in identifying atherosclerotic lesions and vulnerable plaque.[23,24] We currently believe that limited availability and high cost preclude MRI from becoming a standard, acceptable modality until further studies demonstrate a decisive advantage over nuclear imaging or echocardiography.[25]

## EXAMPLE OF A CHEST PAIN UNIT PROTOCOL THAT USES RISK STRATIFICATION AND CARDIAC IMAGING

Each institution should develop cardiac evaluation protocols based on the risk profile of its population and the availability of imaging modalities and in collaboration with emergency medicine, radiology, and cardiology physicians. Specific protocols and imaging modalities vary among locations and institutions. **Figure 56.2** shows an example of a chest pain unit protocol at a large urban center.

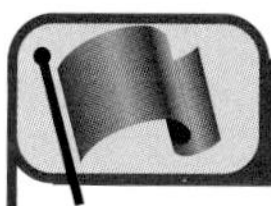

### RED FLAGS

For nuclear imaging, the best results are obtained if the radionuclide is injected while the patient is experiencing symptoms or is undergoing exercise or pharmacologic stress.

Many protocols for stress testing preclude proximate caffeine ingestion. Make sure to note the patient's prior caffeine intake and to have the patient avoid the inadvertent ingestion of any caffeine-containing product (regular or decaffeinated coffee, tea, soft drinks, and chocolate) during the initial evaluation phase.

Know the difference in the electrocardiographic findings of an inferior, right ventricular, and posterior infarction.

The pharmacy or nuclear medicine department regulates the supply of any nuclear imaging agent. If these agents are unused for a time, they expire and must be discarded. Additional preparation or acquisition of fresh agent may cause the work-up of an individual patient to be delayed.

Even if the cardiac imaging and evaluation results are negative, alternative diagnoses such as aortic dissection, peptic ulcer disease, and pulmonary embolism should be considered. Patients should leave the emergency department with some idea about what may be causing their symptoms.

Two nuclear imaging studies, such as a technetium Tc 99m sestamibi scan and a ventilation-perfusion ($\dot{V}/\dot{Q}$) lung scan, cannot be performed within the same 24-hour period. If the differential diagnosis includes pulmonary embolism, alternative and complementary imaging modalities may have to be used.

Exercise and pharmacologic stress studies require that the patient's heart rate rise to appropriate levels. The emergency physician should be cautious about starting beta-blocker therapy in patients who will undergo stress studies in the emergency department. Although beta-blockade is a standard treatment in patients with myocardial ischemia, it can hamper the physician's ability to perform risk stratification for low-risk patients because it results in nondiagnostic stress evaluations.

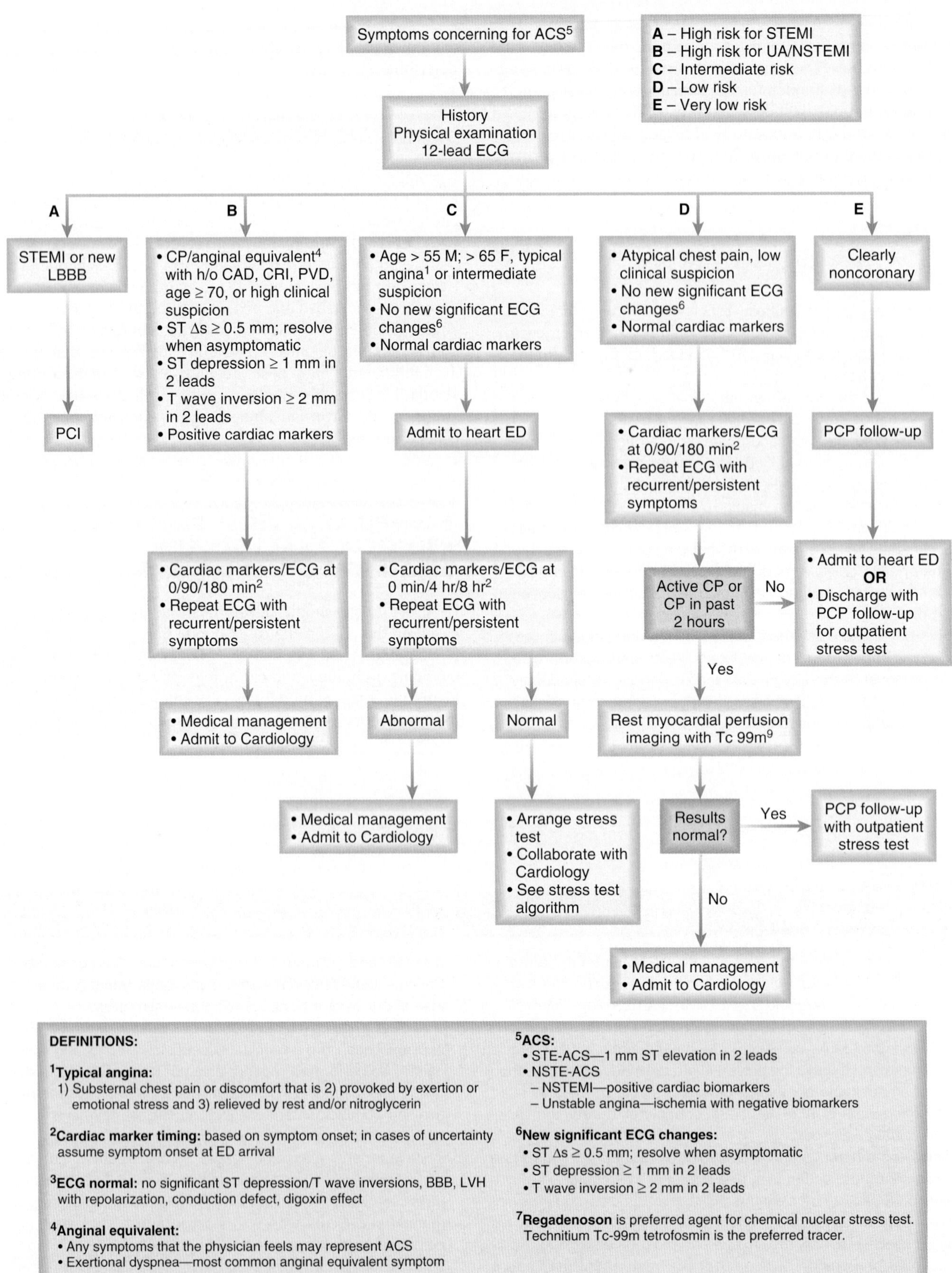


**Fig. 56.2 Evaluation of patients for acute coronary syndrome (ACS).** *CAD*, Coronary artery disease; *CP*, chest pain; *CRI*, chronic renal insufficiency; *ECG*, electrocardiogram; *ED*, emergency department; *h/o*, history of; *LBBB*, left bundle branch block; *NSTE*, non–ST-segment elevation; NSTEMI, non–ST-segment elevation myocardial infarction; *PCP*, primary care physician; *PVD*, peripheral vascular disease; *STE*, ST-segment elevation; *STEMI*, ST-segment elevation myocardial infarction; *UA*, unstable angina.

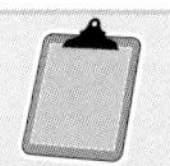

**DOCUMENTATION**

A description of the patient's symptoms should include onset, duration, severity, location, quality, context, associated symptoms, and modifying factors.

Documentation of a past family history of early coronary heart disease or acute coronary syndromes provides useful risk stratification information.

A social history of smoking or the use of cocaine should be documented.

Nuclear imaging documentation should include the patient's last episode of chest discomfort, particularly whether a radiopharmaceutical was injected during the chest discomfort.

The clinician needs to justify an extended period of evaluation by documenting the need for further risk stratification and observation.

## SUMMARY

Cardiac imaging is an important component in the evaluation of patients seen in the ED with chest discomfort. Astute clinicians should understand the benefits and limitations of each modality and should incorporate appropriate imaging into the framework of the institution, its resources, and its physician collaborators.

## REFERENCES

***References can be found on Expert Consult @ www.expertconsult.com.***

# 57 Congestive Heart Failure

*Joshua M. Kosowsky*

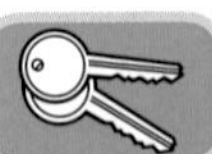

**KEY POINTS**

- Acute decompensated heart failure can be manifested as volume overload, acute diastolic dysfunction, and low cardiac output.
- Identifying and addressing the precipitants of the decompensation are as important as treating the decompensation itself.
- Biomarkers such as B-type natriuretic peptide and the inactive N-terminal fragment of B-type natriuretic peptide can assist in making the diagnosis, but it is important to understand the limitations of these tests.
- In patients with volume overload, diuretics remain the cornerstone of therapy.
- Not all patients with acute decompensated heart failure are significantly volume-overloaded; overaggressive diuresis risks hypotension and worsening renal function.
- Nitrates are first-line therapy for patients in whom an acute reduction in cardiac preload and afterload is desired.
- Inotropic therapy should not be routinely instituted unless the patient is in cardiogenic shock.
- For patients in respiratory distress, noninvasive support (continuous positive airway pressure or bilevel positive airway pressure) may reduce the need for endotracheal intubation.

## EPIDEMIOLOGY

With the aging of the U.S. population and improved survival after myocardial infarction, the prevalence of heart failure is on the rise.[1] At the same time, advances in medical therapy are allowing patients with heart failure to live longer. In 2008, 5.7 million Americans were estimated to have heart failure, with approximately 670,000 new cases diagnosed that year. Heart failure contributes to nearly 300,000 deaths per year, and costs associated with the treatment of heart failure exceed $30 billion annually. Heart failure accounts for nearly 1 million inpatient admissions per year and represents the primary reason for hospitalization in the growing elderly population. Approximately four of every five patients hospitalized for heart failure initially come to the emergency department (ED) for treatment.

Evidence-based literature for ED management of heart failure lags behind that of other emergency conditions, such as acute coronary syndrome and stroke. The number of large, randomized controlled clinical trials is small, and most practice guidelines, such as those from the Heart Failure Society of America and the European Society of Cardiology, rely heavily on consensus statements.[2,3] A recent American Heart Association scientific statement highlighted the significant gaps in knowledge and the lack of evidence-based approaches to the management of heart failure in the ED.[4] In contrast, data from the Acute Decompensated Heart Failure National Registry (ADHERE) and the Acute Heart Failure Global Survey of Standard Treatment (ALARM-HF) registry have provided important insight into the clinical characteristics and actual patterns of care of these patients.[5,6]

**BOX 57.1 Causes of Heart Failure**

Coronary artery disease
Hypertension
Valvular disease
Idiopathic cardiomyopathy
Alcoholic cardiomyopathy
Toxin-related cardiomyopathy (e.g., from doxorubicin)
Postpartum cardiomyopathy
Hypertrophic obstructive cardiomyopathy
Tachyarrhythmia-induced cardiomyopathy
Infiltrative disorders (e.g., amyloid)
Congenital heart disease
Pericardial disease
Hyperkinetic states (anemia, arteriovenous fistula, thyroid disease)

In addition to the paucity of controlled clinical trial data, there remains confusion about terminology. Heart failure refers to the clinical syndrome that can result from any structural or functional cardiac disorder that impairs the ability of the ventricle to fill with or eject blood. Causes of chronic heart failure are numerous and diverse (**Box 57.1**), but in the United States the majority of cases arise as a consequence of coronary artery disease and long-standing hypertension. The term *acute heart failure* is reserved for the presence of acute signs and symptoms of heart failure in an individual without previously known structural or functional cardiac disease. Examples of acute heart failure are massive ST-segment elevation myocardial infarction, acute papillary muscle rupture, and fulminant myocarditis. Much more commonly, a patient comes to the ED with worsening symptoms of known chronic heart failure, in common parlance a "heart failure exacerbation." The term *acute decompensated heart failure* (ADHF) has been adopted to describe this phenomenon, whereby a patient with an established diagnosis of heart failure

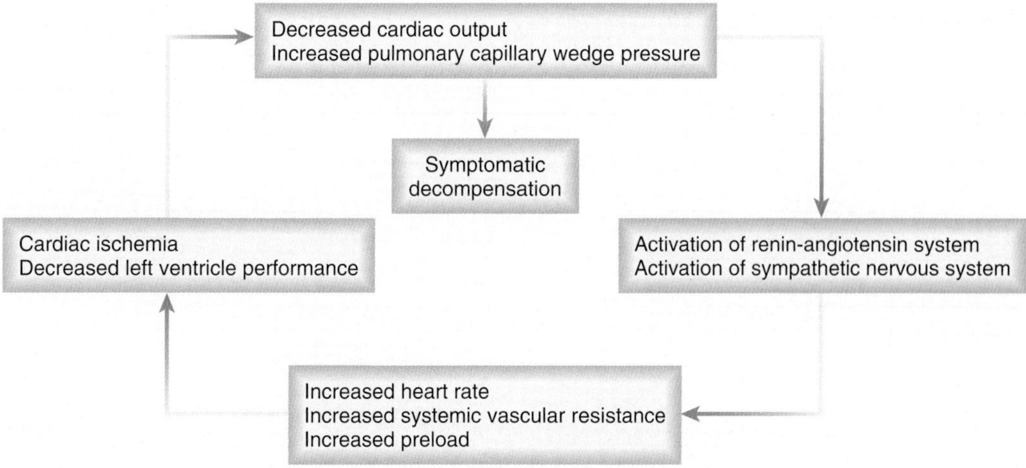


**Fig. 57.1 Pathophysiology of heart failure.**

**BOX 57.2 Common Precipitants of Acute Decompensate Heart Failure**

Medication noncompliance, dietary indiscretion
Myocardial ischemia or infarction
Cardiac arrhythmia (e.g., atrial fibrillation)
Pulmonary and other infections
Administration of inappropriate medications
Anemia
Alcohol withdrawal
Thyrotoxicosis

experiences increasing signs and symptoms of the disease after a period of relative stability.

## PATHOPHYSIOLOGY

In patients with chronic heart failure, inadequacy of cardiac function sets in motion a common set of compensatory mechanisms based on the Frank-Starling relationship and characterized by elevated sympathetic tone, fluid and salt retention, and ventricular remodeling. These adaptations can allow heart failure to remain stable (or "compensated") for a time but also provide the final common pathway for decompensation—a downward spiral that can accelerate in response to a particular precipitant or stress (**Fig. 57.1**). High circulating levels of aldosterone, vasopressin, epinephrine, and norepinephrine can become maladaptive when tachycardia and vasoconstriction compromise intrinsic left ventricular (LV) performance and worsen myocardial oxygen balance. Deteriorating LV function can result in further neurohormonal activation and self-perpetuation of this adverse cycle. Acute decompensation can develop over a period of minutes, hours, or days and can range in severity from mild symptoms of volume overload or decreased cardiac output to frank pulmonary edema or cardiogenic shock.

Although ADHF represents a final common pathway, it is generally triggered by one or more specific precipitants (**Box 57.2**). Noncompliance with medications or dietary restrictions and myocardial ischemia are believed to be the most common causes of clinical cardiac decompensation. Other cardiovascular precipitants are arrhythmia (atrial fibrillation in particular), acute valvular dysfunction, and hypertensive crisis, but ADHF can also arise as a consequence of noncardiac conditions such as infections, anemia, alcohol withdrawal, uncontrolled diabetes, and thyroid disease.

## PRESENTING SIGNS AND SYMPTOMS

The heterogeneity of the signs and symptoms in patients with ADHF reflects, to some extent, the relative contributions of volume overload, acute diastolic dysfunction, and low cardiac output (**Table 57.1**). Volume overload, which usually occurs in the setting of medication noncompliance or dietary indiscretion (or both), is classically associated with gradually worsening congestive symptoms. Acute diastolic dysfunction can occur in the setting of myocardial ischemia, tachyarrhythmia, or uncontrolled hypertension and is typically manifested as flash pulmonary edema. Nearly half of all patients admitted to the hospital for ADHF have mild or no impairment in systolic function.[5] Overt manifestations of low cardiac output (i.e., hypoperfusion) are not generally seen except in patients with advanced LV dysfunction.

Most patients with ADHF have some degree of dyspnea. However, ADHF can closely mimic many other cardiac, respiratory, and systemic diseases. Historical features such as a history of orthopnea, paroxysmal nocturnal dyspnea, or peripheral edema make the diagnosis of ADHF more likely. The most valuable single piece of historical information to elicit from patients is a previous history of heart failure, myocardial infarction, or coronary artery disease. For example, patients evaluated in the ED because of acute dyspnea are approximately six times more likely to have ADHF if they have previously experienced heart failure (**Table 57.2**).[7]

Older patients may lack the typical signs and symptoms of heart failure because they are obscured by the aging process itself or by the presence of coexisting medical conditions.

**Table 57.1 Syndromes of Acute Decompensated Heart Failure**

| | SYSTEMIC VOLUME OVERLOAD | ACUTE DIASTOLIC DYSFUNCTION | LOW-OUTPUT FAILURE |
|---|---|---|---|
| **Frequency** | High | High | Low |
| **Onset** | Gradual | Rapid | Gradual |
| **Characteristics** | Congestive | Congestive/ischemic | Poor perfusion |
| **Example** | Diuretic noncompliance | Hypertensive crisis | End-stage cardiomyopathy |

**Table 57.2 Sensitivity, Specificity, and Positive Likelihood Ratio of Selected Clinical Findings Associated with Acute Decompensated Heart Failure**

| | SENSITIVITY (%) | SPECIFICITY (%) | POSITIVE LIKELIHOOD RATIO (:1) |
|---|---|---|---|
| **Past Medical History** | | | |
| Heart failure | 60 | 90 | 4.4 |
| Myocardial infarction | 40 | 87 | 3.1 |
| Coronary artery disease | 52 | 70 | 1.8 |
| **Symptoms** | | | |
| Paroxysmal nocturnal dyspnea | 41 | 84 | 2.6 |
| Orthopnea | 50 | 77 | 2.2 |
| Edema | 51 | 76 | 2.1 |
| **Signs** | | | |
| Third heart sound | 13 | 99 | 11 |
| Abdominojugular reflux | 24 | 96 | 6.4 |
| Jugular venous distention | 39 | 97 | 5.1 |
| Peripheral edema | 50 | 78 | 2.3 |
| Rales | 60 | 78 | 2.8 |
| Wheezing | 22 | 58 | 0.52 |
| **Diagnostic Findings** | | | |
| Atrial fibrillation | 26 | 93 | 3.8 |
| Pulmonary venous congestion | 54 | 96 | 12.0 |
| Cardiomegaly | 74 | 78 | 3.3 |

Modified from Wang CS, FitzGerald JM, Schulzer M, et al. Does this dyspneic patient in the emergency department have congestive heart failure? JAMA 2005;294:1944-56.

Nonspecific symptoms such as weakness, lethargy, fatigue, anorexia, and light-headedness may actually be manifestations of decreased cardiac output. Abdominal or epigastric discomfort can be a manifestation of low output or, more commonly, hepatic congestion.

Vital signs provide a sense of the severity of illness and can suggest etiologic factors for decompensation. Hyperthermia or hypothermia may indicate sepsis or thyroid disease. In the absence of rate-controlling pharmacologic agents, tachycardia is nearly universal in patients with decompensated heart failure. Bradycardia should raise concern for high-degree atrioventricular block, hyperkalemia, drug toxicity (digoxin, calcium channel blocker, beta-blocker), or severe hypoxia. Hypertension is commonly seen in patients with both systolic and diastolic dysfunction. Hypotension may represent baseline blood pressure (BP) in patients with end-stage cardiomyopathy but otherwise raises concern for shock, whether cardiogenic or otherwise.

The diagnostic utility of the physical examination has been well studied in the setting of chronic heart failure but less so for ADHF. It should be recognized that in ADHF, physical findings may be misleading because of the rapidly evolving clinical situation. Generally speaking, jugular venous distention, abdominojugular reflux, pedal edema, and an audible third heart sound are specific but insensitive indicators of heart failure, whereas the presence of pulmonary rales has only moderate specificity for heart failure (see Table 57.2).[7]

## DIFFERENTIAL DIAGNOSIS AND MEDICAL DECISION MAKING

The differential diagnosis in patients with acute respiratory distress is broad and includes ADHF, asthma, chronic obstructive pulmonary disease (COPD), pneumonia, pulmonary embolism, and multiple systemic diseases, including sepsis.

Even before patients reach the hospital, ADHF is associated with significant morbidity and mortality, including malignant arrhythmias and prehospital cardiac arrest. With few exceptions, the safety and efficacy of prehospital interventions have been poorly studied. Prehospital therapy for decompensated heart failure should be undertaken with caution in light of the relatively high number of inaccurate diagnoses made in the field. In as many as 50% of patients with assumed heart-associated respiratory distress, a different condition is diagnosed once they arrive at the hospital. Despite these concerns, evidence suggests that prehospital therapy for presumed heart failure can prevent serious complications and improve survival, particularly for critically ill patients. For example, prehospital use of continuous positive airway pressure (CPAP) in patients with acute pulmonary edema may avert the need for endotracheal intubation.[8]

Nitroglycerin appears to be the safest and most effective of the prehospital medications used for presumed pulmonary edema.[9] The role of other medications for heart failure in the prehospital setting is less clear. Early administration of furosemide appears to have very little benefit and may result in short-term complications. Prehospital use of morphine sulfate for presumed pulmonary edema has been associated with a higher rate of endotracheal intubation, particularly in patients whose condition turns out to have been misdiagnosed in the field.

## EMERGENCY DEPARTMENT EVALUATION

The approach to patients with ADHF begins with stabilization of respiratory and hemodynamic status and rapid exclusion or treatment of reversible life-threatening conditions. Clinical evaluation and empiric therapy begin simultaneously and consist of supplemental oxygen, cardiac monitoring, pulse oximetry, and intravenous access. Patients with clinical signs of exhaustion or hypoxia despite supplemental oxygen require respiratory support via either invasive or noninvasive means. Those with hypotension, obtundation, cool extremities, or other signs of poor perfusion should be presumed to be in or near cardiogenic shock and be managed accordingly. An electrocardiogram (ECG) should be obtained early to exclude ST-segment elevation myocardial infarction. Once the initial resuscitation is under way, further efforts should be made to establish the diagnosis of ADHF and identify an underlying cause of the acute decompensation.

## DIAGNOSTIC STUDIES

### LABORATORY TESTS

The majority of patients with complaints suggestive of ADHF will require laboratory testing. A complete blood count is useful for ruling out anemia as an alternative cause of the dyspnea or as a precipitant of ADHF. An elevated white blood cell count may suggest the presence of an infectious process, especially if bands are present; however, this finding has not been well studied in patients with suspected ADHF. Serum chemistry analysis is important for assessing renal function and overall fluid and electrolyte balance, particularly in patients already receiving diuretic therapy and likely to require additional diuresis.

### MARKERS OF CARDIAC ISCHEMIA

Elevations in cardiac troponin levels may be found in up to one third of patients with ADHF and can identify patients with a worse short-term prognosis. In any individual case, it remains a clinical determination whether elevations in biomarkers (1) reflect an acute coronary syndrome (i.e., unstable plaque causing ischemia and myocardial cell death and leading to worsening heart failure) or (2) simply reflect the severity of the heart failure (i.e., myocardial cell death with or without underlying ischemia). Information from the history (e.g., onset of symptoms, comparison with previous episodes) and from the ECG may be helpful in this regard.

### B-TYPE NATRIURETIC PEPTIDE AND NT-PROBNP

B-type natriuretic peptide (BNP) is a counterregulatory hormone produced by cardiac myocytes in response to increased end-diastolic pressure and volume, as occurs in the setting of heart failure. ProBNP is released into the circulation and cleaved into biologically active BNP and an inactive N-terminal fragment, NT-proBNP, which has a half-life three to six times that of BNP. Plasma levels of BNP and NT-proBNP correlate with the degree of LV overload, severity of clinical heart failure, and both short- and long-term cardiovascular mortality.

Plasma levels of BNP and NT-proBNP have been shown to be useful in distinguishing between cardiac and noncardiac causes of dyspnea.[10,11] Acutely dyspneic patients with plasma BNP levels lower than 100 pg/mL or NT-proBNP levels lower than 300 pg/mL are very unlikely to have ADHF (90% to 99% sensitivity), whereas those with BNP levels higher than 500 pg/mL or NT-proBNP levels higher than 1000 pg/mL are very likely to have ADHF (87% to 95% specificity). Intermediate levels must be interpreted in the clinical context (**Fig. 57.2**).

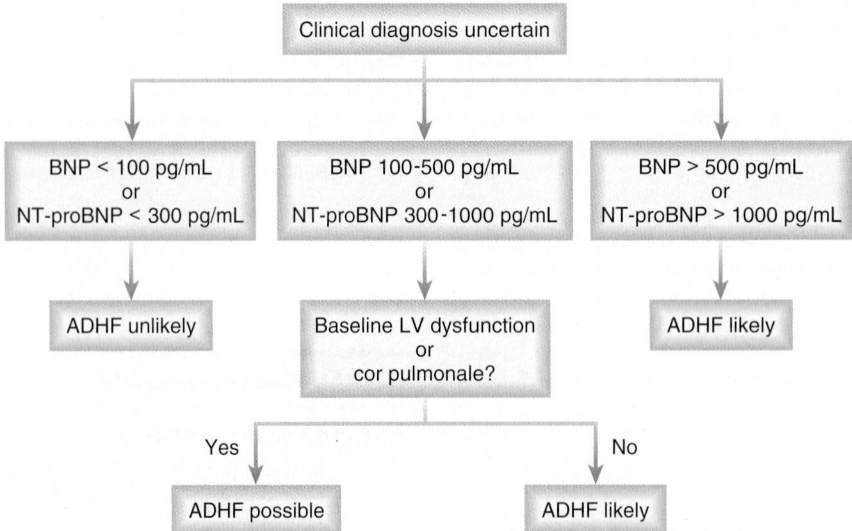


**Fig. 57.2 Interpretation of natriuretic peptide levels.** *ADHF*, Acute decompensated heart failure; *BNP*, B-type natriuretic peptide; *NT-proBNP*, inactive N-terminal fragment of BNP.

Interpretation of BNP levels must take into account baseline LV dysfunction and other known or suspected conditions associated with left or right ventricular pressure overload that may result in elevations in BNP. Patients with advanced age or renal insufficiency tend to have higher BNP and NT-proBNP levels, whereas those with a high body mass index tend to have lower levels. Although BNP and NT-proBNP measurements retain discriminatory power in these subpopulations, the optimal cutoff points for diagnosing ADHF may vary. The duration of symptoms also plays a role; for example, in the setting of acute pulmonary edema, these levels may not yet be elevated.

In general, emergency physicians (EPs) are about 80% accurate in distinguishing between cardiac and noncardiac causes of dyspnea on clinical grounds. Supplementing clinical acumen with routine BNP or NT-proBNP measurement does increase diagnostic accuracy overall, but as demonstrated in the Breathing Not Properly Multinational Study, the improvement is rather marginal.[12] For example, in clear-cut cases, very high or very low values are unlikely to have an effect on diagnosis, whereas in less clear-cut cases, intermediate results are more likely.

BNP and NT-proBNP levels also carry modest prognostic information.[13] Although levels at admission correlate only modestly with short-term outcomes, discharge levels are strong independent predictors of death or readmission.

## ELECTROCARDIOGRAPHY

The ECG is likely to be abnormal in patients with heart failure. Signs of preexisting conditions such as hypertrophy, myocardial infarction, or dilated cardiomyopathy may be present. Atrial fibrillation or other arrhythmias may be detected. A large proportion of heart failure exacerbations are accompanied by cardiac ischemia, which may be detectable on an ECG.

## CHEST RADIOGRAPHY

A chest radiograph should be obtained in all patients with suspected ADHF to assess for pulmonary congestion and assist in the differential diagnosis of other lung diseases. Findings on chest radiographs in patients with ADHF include cardiomegaly, vascular redistribution (e.g., cephalization, fullness of the hilar vessels), interstitial edema, and pulmonary edema. Pleural effusions in patients with heart failure tend to be bilateral or localized to the right side. Although the presence of pulmonary congestion is associated with a very high likelihood of ADHF, it should be noted that as many as one in five patients with ADHF do not have evidence of congestion on chest radiographs. In individuals with underlying pulmonary emphysema, congestion may appear atypical or not at all, and patients with long-standing congestive heart failure (CHF) may have scant radiographic evidence of congestion because of well-developed pulmonary lymphatics. Cardiomegaly may be absent in patients with acute heart failure, particularly in those with preserved LV systolic function.

## CARDIAC ECHOCARDIOGRAPHY

Echocardiography is considered the "gold standard" for assessing the status of LV function, distinguishing between systolic and diastolic failure, and identifying regional wall motion abnormalities. Perhaps more important in the ED setting, echocardiography can assist in diagnosing or excluding potentially reversible causes of acute cardiac decompensation, such as pericardial tamponade, massive pulmonary embolism, ruptured chordae tendineae, and ruptured ventricular septum. As a practical matter, emergency echocardiography is not generally required in most instances of ADHF, particularly if a patient has a history of heart failure and a clear precipitant for decompensation.

## PULMONARY ARTERY (SWAN-GANZ) CATHETERIZATION

Invasive hemodynamic monitoring is not usually necessary for the diagnosis and management of ADHF, and its routine use is not recommended. In the absence of pulmonary disease or disproportionate right heart failure, clinical estimation or measurement of right atrial pressure usually correlates with left-sided filling pressures. When compared with standard clinical management, hemodynamically guided therapy is not associated with improvement in short- or long-term outcome. Conversely, right heart catheterization remains a reasonable option in patients with cardiogenic shock or when a patient's hemodynamic status is uncertain after careful clinical evaluation and initial therapy.

### OTHER DIAGNOSTIC MODALITIES

Elevated end-tidal $CO_2$ concentrations and reduced peak expiratory flow rates are more commonly seen exacerbations of COPD than of ADHF. However, in neither case is a cutoff value available that can be used to accurately distinguish between cardiac and respiratory causes of dyspnea. Another noninvasive means proposed for aiding in the diagnosis of ADHF is impedance cardiography, in which real-time estimates of cardiac output and pulmonary capillary wedge pressure are derived via dynamic measurement of thoracic bioimpedance. Although the technology has been available for some time, data on the overall utility of this diagnostic tool in the ED setting are limited.

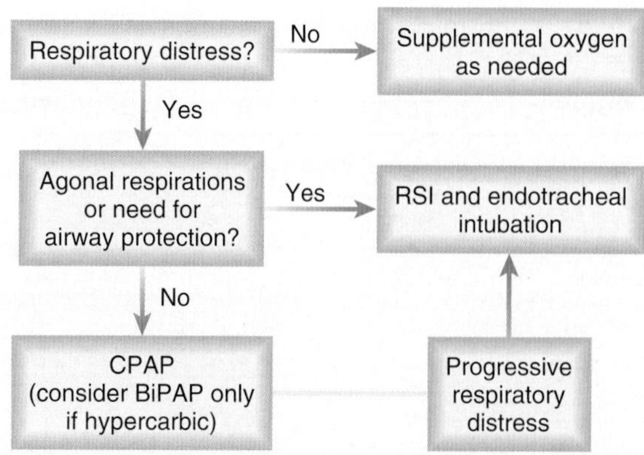


**Fig. 57.3 Algorithm for ventilatory support of patients with acute decompensated heart failure.** *BiPAP*, Bilevel positive airway pressure; *CPAP*, continuous positive airway pressure; *RSI*, rapid-sequence intubation.

## TREATMENT

### PRIORITIES OF TREATMENT

All patients with ADHF who are in respiratory distress should receive supplemental oxygen and be positioned upright, if possible, to improve respiratory dynamics and maximize oxygen delivery to vital organs. Practice guidelines recommend the early application of monitors, such as pulse oximetry, noninvasive BP, and continuous cardiac monitoring, to provide early warning of further decompensation.

Although most patients in respiratory distress can be managed with supplemental oxygen and noninvasive ventilatory support (see the next section), the presence of agonal respirations or profoundly depressed mental status mandates endotracheal intubation. In general, airway management should be accomplished with rapid-sequence intubation because prolonged attempts at intubation risk worsening hypoxia, further cardiac decompensation, and cardiopulmonary arrest. Keeping the patient in an upright position as long as possible before intubation may assist in maximizing preoxygenation. Most induction agents (thiopental, fentanyl, and midazolam) are associated with a significant risk for hypotension in patients with ADHF, whereas induction with etomidate is generally considered safe.

#### *Noninvasive Respiratory Support*

For patients with respiratory distress in whom intubation is not immediately required, noninvasive respiratory support via CPAP or bilevel positive airway pressure (BiPAP) should be instituted (**Fig. 57.3**). Although the decision to initiate noninvasive respiratory support may depend on a variety of factors, the presumption is that the earlier therapy is instituted, the greater the likelihood of averting intubation. Success also depends on appropriate patient selection. Patients with unstable cardiac rhythms or cardiogenic shock are generally believed to not be candidates for a noninvasive approach. Likewise, in the setting of severe myocardial ischemia or infarction, full ventilatory support may be preferable to decrease myocardial oxygen demand.

CPAP improves lung mechanics by recruiting atelectatic alveoli, improving pulmonary compliance, and reducing the work of breathing. At the same time, particularly in patients with heart failure, CPAP improves hemodynamics by reducing preload and afterload, thereby enhancing LV performance. Pooled data from several randomized, controlled clinical trials suggest that the use of CPAP (at 5 to 10 mm Hg) in patients with respiratory distress caused by ADHF reduces the frequency of endotracheal intubation and may be associated with lower mortality.[14]

BiPAP adds to the physiologic advantages of CPAP during expiration by providing differential positive pressure during inspiration, thereby providing direct assistance with ventilation. However, at present, little evidence suggests an advantage of BiPAP over CPAP in patients with ADHF and pure hypoxemic respiratory failure.

In patients with progressive respiratory failure despite noninvasive support, endotracheal intubation and mechanical ventilation should be instituted.

### PHARMACOLOGIC THERAPY

The twin objectives of pharmacologic therapy for ADHF are relief of pulmonary congestion and improvement in systemic tissue perfusion. Strategies to achieve these goals involve reducing preload and enhancing LV function while aiming to maintain or even improve myocardial oxygen balance (**Table 57.3**).

#### *Diuretics*

Diuretics constitute the mainstay of therapy for patients with volume overload. Although their use is widely recommended as initial therapy for most patients with ADHF, it should be noted that until very recently this practice had not been evaluated in any large, prospective trial. Evidence from in vitro and in vivo experiments suggests that the direct vascular effects of diuretics may also contribute to their mechanism of action. However, studies comparing the acute effects of diuretics and nitrates have tended to emphasize the more favorable overall hemodynamic effects of the latter group (see the next section).

Depending on a patient's clinical condition and previous use of diuretics, an initial intravenous (IV) dose of

**Table 57.3 Pharmacologic Therapy for Acute Decompensated Heart Failure**

| THERAPY | ACTIONS | INDICATIONS | CAUTIONS OR ADVERSE EFFECTS | DOSING |
|---|---|---|---|---|
| Oxygen | Improvement in systemic and myocardial oxygen balance | Hypoxia and/or dyspnea | Respiratory depression (chronic obstructive pulmonary disease) | Titrate to pulse oximetry |
| Morphine | Relief of anxiety | Pulmonary edema | Respiratory depression<br>Hypotension | 2- to 4-mg intravenous boluses |
| Furosemide | Preload reduction | Volume overload | Hypotension<br>Prerenal azotemia | Start with a 20- to 40-mg (or daily oral dose) intravenous bolus |
| Nitroglycerin | Preload and afterload reduction<br>Antiischemic | Dyspnea<br>Myocardial ischemia | Hypotension<br>Tolerance | Start at 10-20 mcg/min intravenously (IV) and titrate upward |
| Nitroprusside | Afterload reduction | Severe hypertension<br>Refractory pulmonary edema | Hypotension<br>Myocardial ischemia<br>Cyanide toxicity | Start at 0.1-0.2 mcg/kg/min IV and titrate upward |
| Nesiritide | Preload and afterload reduction | Dyspnea | Hypotension<br>?Impact on renal function<br>Mortality | 2-mcg/kg bolus, 0.01 mcg/kg/hr |
| Dobutamine | Positive inotropy<br>Afterload reduction | Low-output heart failure<br>Refractory pulmonary edema | Tachycardia<br>Arrhythmia<br>Hypotension<br>Bronchoconstriction | Start at 2.5 mcg/kg/min IV and titrate upward |
| Milrinone | Positive inotropy<br>Afterload reduction | Low-output heart failure<br>Refractory pulmonary edema | Arrhythmia<br>Hypotension | Give a 50-mcg/kg bolus over a 10-min period; then start at 0.375 mcg/kg/min IV and titrate upward |

furosemide, 20 to 200 mg, is typically administered. For patients already receiving diuretic therapy, a common strategy is to begin with the usual daily dose given as an IV bolus. A recently published multicenter, prospective, double-blind, randomized trial comparing a strategy of low-dose furosemide (equivalent to the patient's previous oral dose) versus high-dose furosemide (2.5 times the previous oral dose) in 308 patients with ADHF found no significant differences in patients' global assessment of symptoms or in the change in renal function over the first 72 hours.[15] A high-dose strategy was associated with greater diuresis, but median length of hospital stay was not significantly different. In the same trial, patients randomized to bolus IV therapy (every 12 hours) or the same dose of furosemide delivered via continuous IV infusion had no significant difference in outcome.

It is important to recognize that not all patients with ADHF are substantially volume-overloaded. For example, patients with acute diastolic dysfunction may benefit more from redistribution of circulating volume (e.g., with a vasodilator) than from diuresis per se. The indiscriminate use of diuretics carries the risk for overdiuresis, with detrimental effects on systemic perfusion in general and renal function in particular.

Although not all patients with ADHF require bladder catheterization, monitoring of urinary output is important in any patient in whom diuresis is a chosen as a treatment strategy.

### *Nitrates*

Nitrates are recommended for the treatment of ADHF, whether of ischemic or nonischemic origin. At low doses, nitroglycerin induces venodilation (preload reduction); at higher doses, nitroglycerin also causes arterial dilation (afterload reduction). Significantly, in patients with severe underlying LV dysfunction, afterload reduction appears to predominate over preload reduction, even with moderate doses of nitroglycerin.

Nitrates have been shown to be both safe and effective for the treatment of ADHF, particularly in the context of acute pulmonary edema.[16] When compared with placebo therapy in the Vasodilation in the Management of Acute Congestive Heart Failure (VMAC) trial, IV nitroglycerin resulted in better dyspnea scores, but the study was not powered to demonstrate differences in morbidity or mortality.[17]

Single doses of sublingual nitroglycerin (0.4 mg) can be given repeatedly every 5 to 10 minutes to provide adequate BP. In the hospital setting, however, continuous IV administration of nitroglycerin is more convenient and allows titration to specific clinical or hemodynamic end points (typically starting at 10 to 20 mcg/min and ranging up to 200 mcg/min). The hemodynamic effects of transdermal nitroglycerin are comparable with those of IV nitroglycerin, but this route of administration is less amenable to titration and may be less effective in patients with poor skin perfusion.

The hypotension induced by standard nitrate therapy is generally mild and transient. Severe or persistent hypotension should raise suspicion for hypovolemia, stenotic valvular disease such as aortic stenosis, cardiac tamponade, right ventricular infarction, or recent use of sildenafil (Viagra). If these conditions are known or suspected, nitrates should be avoided or used with extreme caution. Nitrate therapy may not be particularly effective in patients with massive peripheral edema. In such cases, aggressive diuretic therapy is more likely to be of benefit.

Sodium nitroprusside is recommended for patients with marked systemic hypertension, severe mitral or aortic valvular regurgitation, or pulmonary edema not responsive to standard nitrate therapy. Nitroprusside profoundly dilates resistance vessels and thereby rapidly reduces BP and afterload. Typically, nitroprusside is started at a dose of 0.1 to 0.3 mcg/kg/min, and the dose is increased as needed to improve clinical and hemodynamic status while maintaining systolic BP above 90 mm Hg or mean arterial pressure above 65 mm Hg. In patients with renal insufficiency, long-term use of nitroprusside carries the potential for cyanide toxicity as metabolites of the agent accumulate.

### Nesiritide

Nesiritide (recombinant BNP) is the only pharmacologic therapy for dyspnea associated with ADHF that has been approved by the U.S. Food and Drug Administration (FDA) in recent years. Like other natriuretic peptides, nesiritide has intrinsic vasodilatory as well as mild diuretic and natriuretic properties when administered in supraphysiologic doses (2-mcg/kg bolus, followed by continuous infusion at 0.01 mcg/kg/hr).

A number of trials have shown nesiritide to be more effective than placebo in improving hemodynamic parameters in patients with ADHF, but it is less clear what, if any, clinically important outcomes are improved. In the VMAC trial, pulmonary capillary wedge pressure was lower in patients receiving nesiritide than in those receiving nitroglycerin, but dyspnea scores at 3 and 24 hours were not significantly different between the two randomized groups.[17] Studies have yet to show differences in more durable outcomes, such as of length of hospital stay and hospital costs.

Pooled data from several trials have suggested an association between nesiritide and adverse events, specifically, worsening renal function and death.[18,19] In contrast, in a more recent multicenter trial, nesiritide demonstrated no excess adverse effects on either renal function or mortality in patients with ADHF. However, in this same trial, nesiritide failed to meet primary efficacy end points with respect to improvement in dyspnea or 30-day outcomes when compared with placebo.[20]

### Angiotensin-Converting Enzyme Inhibitors

The beneficial effects of angiotensin-converting enzyme (ACE) inhibitors in patients with chronic heart failure have been appreciated for more than 2 decades. Though not formally recommended by consensus guidelines for the treatment of ADHF, small studies have demonstrated their safety and efficacy as treatment of ADHF.

ACE inhibitors are contraindicated in the context of pregnancy, hyperkalemia, or a history of ACE inhibitor–induced angioedema. Unlike nitrates, most ACE inhibitors have a relatively prolonged duration of action, thus making their dosage less easily titratable.

### Inotropic Therapy

Outside the setting of cardiogenic shock (see later), inotropic therapy is not recommended for the routine management of ADHF. Although short-term inotropic therapy may improve hemodynamic performance and acute symptoms, the impact on outcomes is considerably less sanguine. One of the largest randomized placebo-controlled trials ever conducted in patients with ADHF, the Outcomes of a Prospective Trial of Intravenous Milrinone for Exacerbations of Chronic Heart Failure (OPTIME-CHF), showed no difference in mortality or readmission rate in patients receiving inotropic therapy but significantly higher rates of adverse events, particularly sustained hypotension and new atrial arrhythmias.[21]

Nevertheless, in patients with severe signs and symptoms of low-output failure or no response to standard therapy, short-term treatment with inotropic agents may be considered. The goals of therapy must be considered carefully in the context of the patient's risk for arrhythmia.

Digoxin has a very limited role in the ED management of heart failure. The inotropic effects of digoxin are modest and unpredictable, and they are delayed for at least 90 minutes after intravenous loading.

### Morphine

Morphine, one of the oldest drugs still in use for the treatment of ADHF, remains an important adjunct for treating the anxiety and discomfort associated with pulmonary edema. The predominant hemodynamic effects of morphine appear to be mediated through the central nervous system. Morphine can be administered safely to most patients at low IV doses (2 to 4 mg); however, because of its sedative properties and potential to depress respirations, caution should be exercised in administering morphine to patients with chronic pulmonary insufficiency or suspected acidosis. Although a number of retrospective studies have shown an association between administration of morphine to patients with ADHF and higher rates of adverse events, it is not clear that this link is causative.

### Investigational Drugs

Over the past decade, a number of newer drugs ranging from various receptor antagonists to calcium sensitizers and novel peptides have been investigated for the treatment of ADHF. Despite early promise with many of these agents, none have been shown in a prospective, placebo-controlled, randomized clinical trial to meet a primary clinical end point with respect to the treatment of ADHF.

In the EVEREST trial, tolvaptan, a vasopressin antagonist, improved short-term signs and symptoms in patients hospitalized with ADHF and receiving standard therapy, but this was not a primary end point of the long-term study.[22] Tolvaptan was, however, approved by the FDA in 2009 for the treatment of hyponatremia associated with heart failure, among other hypervolemic states.

Relaxin, a natural peptide structurally similar to insulin that has unique vasodilator properties, is currently in phase III trials as a potential treatment option for ADHF.

#### *Beta-Blockers*

Long-term beta-blocker therapy affords an important survival benefit for patients with systolic heart failure. In contrast, administration of beta-blockers to patients with acute systolic dysfunction has been associated with life-threatening clinical deterioration. For this reason, institution of beta-blocker therapy is not recommended in the setting of ADHF, and long-term beta-blocker therapy is generally administered cautiously or at a reduced dose.

### ULTRAFILTRATION

A novel approach to the problem of volume overload involves ultrafiltration of peripheral blood to remove excess fluid and electrolytes. Though typically reserved for patients with significant renal failure or volume overload unresponsive to diuretics, evidence from the Ultrafiltration vs IV Diuretics for Patients Hospitalized for Acute Decompensated CHF (UNLOAD) trial demonstrated that as an alternative to diuretic therapy, ultrafiltration results in greater fluid loss and lower rates of rehospitalization.[23] In the ED, a major limitation of this approach is the feasibility of securing the necessary equipment and intravenous access.

## SPECIAL CIRCUMSTANCES

### CARDIOGENIC SHOCK

Heart failure with cardiogenic shock can be the initial manifestation of acute ST-segment elevation myocardial infarction. Although mortality remains high in this setting, referral for emergency cardiac catheterization and revascularization is of proven benefit. Noncardiac causes of shock, such as hypovolemia, sepsis, poisoning, and massive pulmonary embolism, must also be considered.

Aside from addressing reversible causes of shock, the overarching goal in treating patients with cardiogenic shock should be to restore and maintain perfusion of vital organs. Patients who are initially seen in shock with normal BP or only mild hypotension often have a favorable response to dobutamine (starting at 2 to 3 mcg/kg/min). When compared with dopamine, dobutamine is associated with a lower incidence of arrhythmias, less peripheral vasoconstriction, and more consistent reduction in LV filling pressure for a comparable rise in cardiac output. Dopamine is required for patients who have severe hypotension (systolic BP of approximately 70 to 80 mm Hg) in the presence of volume overload or after bolus administration of saline. At moderate doses (4 to 5 mcg/kg/min), dopamine improves cardiac output without causing excessive systemic vasoconstriction. If the patient can be stabilized with dopamine, dobutamine can then be added and the dose of dopamine lowered, with the goal of reducing myocardial oxygen demand. In extreme cases, norepinephrine can be added to increase systolic pressure to acceptable levels (≈80 mm Hg). However, because of the adverse effects on renal and mesenteric perfusion, use of high-dose dopamine or norepinephrine should be considered only as a temporizing measure until definitive therapy can be substituted.

It is important for the EP to distinguish patients with acute cardiogenic shock from those with low BP or other signs of systemic hypoperfusion in the setting of preexisting severe or end-stage systolic heart failure. Assessment and treatment of these patients can be extremely challenging, and optimal management may require the involvement of a heart failure specialist. Attempts to aggressively treat these patients can lead to rapid decompensation. Frequently, the key to management is identifying the cause of the decompensation.

### ATRIAL FIBRILLATION

Atrial fibrillation is seen in approximately one third of patients with ADHF. Although loss of synchronized atrial contractions is of minimal hemodynamic significance in patients with normal ventricular function, in those who have abnormal LV systolic or diastolic function, loss of the atrial kick can have profound consequences. This is particularly evident when atrial fibrillation is accompanied by a rapid ventricular response, thereby reducing filling time.

When assessing a patient with rapid atrial fibrillation and ADHF, it is often difficult to attribute cause and effect. New-onset rapid atrial fibrillation may be the precipitant of ADHF, but more commonly, rapid atrial fibrillation is a response to worsening heart failure (e.g., via neurohormonal activation). This distinction can sometimes be difficult to make clinically, but regardless, attention must be paid, to some degree, to managing both conditions.

Management of atrial fibrillation in the context of ADHF should focus on treating the underlying precipitants of decompensation (e.g. volume overload) while also controlling the ventricular rate. However, caution should be exercised in the use of a beta-blocker or calcium channel blocker for rate control because of the potential negative inotropic effects. Digoxin, diltiazem, and amiodarone are considered acceptable agents for rate control, even in patients with LV systolic dysfunction. Cardioversion, whether electrical or chemical, is a reasonable treatment alternative for truly unstable atrial fibrillation, but sinus rhythm may not be achieved or maintained if the underlying heart failure is not addressed.

### RENAL DYSFUNCTION

In part because of common preconditions such as diabetes and hypertension and in part because of the effects of diuretics and low cardiac output on renal function, heart failure and renal insufficiency frequently coexist. Approximately 1 in 5 patients with ADHF have creatinine levels higher than 2.0 mg/dL. In patients with ADHF, preexisting renal insufficiency is associated with greater morbidity and mortality, and worsening of renal function over the course of treatment is associated with poorer outcomes.

In patients undergoing hemodialysis, heart failure is the most common reason for ED visits. Not surprisingly, ADHF is frequently a result of volume overload between dialysis treatments. Although hemodialysis is the obvious treatment of choice for these patients, it may not always be immediately available, and supplemental oxygen, CPAP, and nitrates are generally effective in stabilizing patients until hemodialysis can be performed.

## FOLLOW-UP AND NEXT STEPS IN CARE

The vast majority of patients with ADHF evaluated in the ED are admitted to the hospital.[5] Discharge from the ED without adequate treatment may be associated with recurrent visits and short-term morbidity and mortality. ADHF is often a dynamic entity: one patient may appear dramatically ill at initial evaluation but respond rapidly to treatment, whereas another patient may experience serious complications after a period of apparent stability. For any individual patient, identifying and addressing the precipitant of the decompensation is critical to making the correct disposition.

The Heart Failure Society of America has established criteria for discharging patients with heart failure from the ED (**Box 57.3**). However, these guidelines have not been prospectively studied. It should be noted that previously published criteria from the U.S. Agency for Health Care Policy and Research failed to account for more than 30% of 30-day mortality.[24] Thus, although published guidelines can assist with triage, the significant rate of morbidity mandates that clinical judgment be incorporated into the decision-making process.

For patients with ADHF admitted to the hospital, inpatient mortality is approximately 4%, and the median length of stay exceeds 4 days.[5] In those admitted with advanced stages of heart failure, inpatient mortality approaches 10%. Clinical correlates of major complications or death during hospitalization include hypotension; tachypnea; ECG abnormalities; hyponatremia; renal insufficiency; elevations in troponin, BNP, and NT-proBNP; and poor initial diuresis. However, even patients without any of these risk factors have measurable rates of in-hospital morbidity and mortality. A risk stratification tool derived from the ADHERE registry has been developed to help clinicians determine the risk for mortality in patients with ADHF (**Fig. 57.4**).[25]

For a patient discharged home from the ED, consultation with the patient's primary care physician or cardiologist is important. For example, it is likely that the patient's outpatient medication regimen will require adjustment to prevent a return to the ED. In some studies, intensive outpatient

**BOX 57.3 Heart Failure Society of America Recommendations for Discharge of Emergency Department Patients with Heart Failure**

**Admission is recommended for:**

Severe acute decompensated heart failure:
- Hypotension
- Worsening renal function
- Altered mental status

Dyspnea at rest

Arrhythmia with hemodynamic compromise, including new-onset atrial fibrillation

Acute coronary syndrome

**Admission should be considered for:**

Worsening congestion (pulmonary or systemic)

Significant electrolyte disturbance

Associated comorbid conditions:
- Pneumonia
- Pulmonary embolism
- Diabetic ketoacidosis
- Transient ischemic attack, cerebrovascular accident

New-onset heart failure

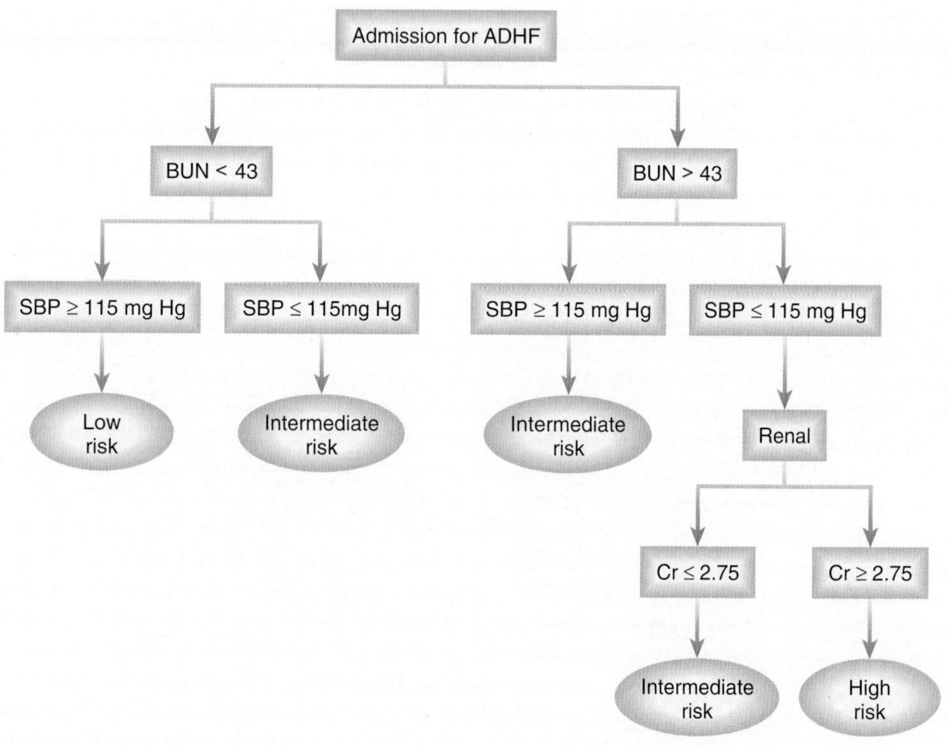


**Fig. 57.4 Risk stratification of patients hospitalized for acute decompensated heart failure (ADHF).** *BUN*, Blood urea nitrogen; *Cr*, [serum] creatinine; *SBP*, systolic blood pressure.

follow-up has been shown to be successful in preventing recurrent ED visits and hospitalizations.

## OBSERVATION UNITS

ED observation units have been advanced as a safe and cost-effective means of treating a subset of ADHF patients, thereby avoiding the need for hospital admission. Admission to an observation unit allows the ED physician to assess a patient's response to diuretic (or other) therapy over time. Although interest in this field is growing, no randomized studies have been performed to date to substantiate the use of such units.[26]

## REFERENCES

***References can be found on Expert Consult @ www.expertconsult.com.***

# Bradyarrhythmias 58

Sarah A. Stahmer

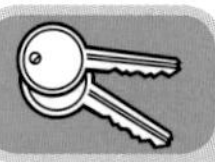

**KEY POINTS**

- Look at the patient first and then the heart rhythm. A "slow heart rate" is relative to the patient's age, clinical condition, and comorbid conditions.
- Determine whether the cause is extrinsic or intrinsic to the conduction system.
- Assess the functionality of the key elements of the conduction system: sinoatrial and atrioventricular nodes and the infranodal conduction system.
- Know the vascular supply of the conduction system to determine the significance of bradyarrhythmias and conduction blocks in the setting of acute myocardial infarction.
- Identify risk for failure of the conduction system and the "backup"; for example, a stable escape rhythm, atropine, or a pacemaker.

## EPIDEMIOLOGY

Bradycardia is a frequent finding in clinical practice, and its significance is dependent on the underlying cause and clinical effects. The baseline heart rate in an individual patient is determined predominantly by the balance between the parasympathetic and sympathetic nervous systems, and a "normal" heart rate has been defined arbitrarily as 60 to 100 beats/min at rest. The heart rate will vary depending on age, physical condition, and time of observation. Normal ranges for a healthy asymptomatic individual will vary from 46 to 93 beats/min in men and 51 to 95 beats/min in women during the day to rates as low as 40 beats/min at night.[1] The heart rate should fluctuate with respiration, the Valsalva maneuver, and other vagal influences confirming normal autonomic control of the sinus node. Bradycardia is a frequent finding in trained athletes, in whom heart rates lower than 40 beats/min are often observed at rest.[2] Bradycardias of clinical significance increase in frequency with age and in the setting of illnesses or medications affecting the heart and its conduction system.

## PATHOPHYSIOLOGY

Bradyarrhythmias are the result of either (1) extrinsic factors slowing the normally functioning sinus node and conduction pathways or (2) failure of the sinus node and conduction pathways because of intrinsic causes of degeneration of the conduction system.

### EXTRINSIC CAUSES

Clues to an extrinsic cause of a bradyarrhythmia are a history of a new cardioactive medication, conditions that activate vagal tone, and extreme electrolyte imbalances, specifically potassium (**Table 58.1**). The associated rhythms are typically those that are due to dysfunction of the sinus or atrioventricular (AV) node:

- Sinus bradycardia, arrest (**Figs. 58.1 to 58.3**)
- Type I second-degree AV nodal block (**Fig. 58.4**)
- Third-degree heart block (see Fig. 58.6)

### INTRINSIC CAUSES

Certain conditions result in failure of elements of the conduction system because of aging, ischemia or infarction, surgical trauma, or infiltration (**Table 58.2**). The latter cause encompasses a large group of conditions that include infectious and rheumatologic diseases.[3-5] The associated rhythms are typically those that indicate failure of one element of the conduction system rather than failure to generate a rhythm:

- Second-degree AV block (either type I or type II) (**Fig. 58-5**; also see Fig. 58.4)
- Third-degree heart block (**Fig. 58.6**)
- Associated fascicular or bundle branch blocks (see Fig. 58.5)

### RELATIVE BRADYCARDIA

Relative bradycardia is the presence of a heart rate that is inappropriately slow for the clinical findings. Though often caused by coexisting beta-blocker therapy or age-related blunting of sinus node automaticity, it is also a diagnostic feature of a number of infectious disorders. Relative bradycardia is most useful in differentiating infectious diseases that resemble each other; for example, legionnaires' disease from *Mycoplasma* pneumonia and psittacosis or Q fever from tularemia pneumonia.[3]

## PRESENTING SIGNS AND SYMPTOMS

Cardiac output is dependent on the patient's stroke volume and heart rate. Bradycardias are symptomatic only to the extent that they affect cardiac output, which is a product of the heart rate and stroke volume. In the setting of a normal stroke volume, heart rates as low as 20 to 30 beats/min can sustain a reasonable cardiac output. A heart rate of 40 beats/min may be physiologically normal for some individuals, whereas a rate of 60 beats/min may be inadequate for patients with conditions that compromise stroke volume, such as cardiomyopathies, bleeding, or sepsis.

**Table 58.1 Extrinsic Causes of Bradyarrhythmias**

| | COMMON | UNCOMMON |
|---|---|---|
| Drugs | Class Ia antiarrhythmic agents<br>Class Ic antiarrhythmic agents<br>Beta-blocking agents<br>Calcium channel blockers<br>Class III antiarrhythmic agents<br>Amiodarone and sotalol<br>Digoxin<br>Cholinergic agents<br>$\alpha_2$-Agonists<br>Opioids<br>Sedative-hypnotics<br>Organophosphates<br>Tricyclic antidepressants | Lithium<br>Phenothiazines<br>Reserpine<br>Amantadine<br>Chloroquine<br>Phenytoin<br>Carbamazepine<br>Clonidine<br>Physostigmine<br>Cimetidine<br>Propoxyphene<br>Thioridazine |
| Situational reflex | Neurocardiogenic syncope<br>Maxillofacial reflex<br>Micturition syncope<br>Oculocardiac reflex<br>Cough syncope | Pain syncope<br>Defecation syncope<br>Vomiting<br>Swallow syncope |
| Metabolic | Hypokalemia<br>Hyperkalemia<br>Hypothyroidism | Hypermagnesemia<br>Hypercalcemia |
| Ischemia and infarction | Inferior wall ischemia or infarction is associated with bradycardia and/or atrioventricular nodal conduction delays that are due to abnormal sensitivity to parasympathetic stimulation and are responsive to atropine | — |
| Other | Obstructive sleep apnea<br>Hypothermia<br>Hypoxia | — |

From Ford M. Clinical toxicology. Philadelphia: Saunders; 2001. pp. 23-5.

Symptoms of low cardiac output are due to hypoperfusion of vital organs and muscle tissue. Mild reductions in cardiac output usually cause exertional fatigue and dyspnea. Greater reductions in cardiac output can produce signs and symptoms of cerebral ischemia, congestive heart failure, mesenteric ischemia, and renal insufficiency. Complete heart block with slow escape rhythms or bradycardia in the setting of profound reductions in stroke volume can manifest as syncope, pulmonary edema, and cardiogenic shock.

Alternatively, a profound bradycardia that does not result in hemodynamic compromise does not need to be treated but should be considered an important diagnostic clue. The classic example is a patient with intracranial hemorrhage and Cushing reflex, which will be manifested as hypertension and often profound bradycardia. In this case the bradycardia is a sign of elevated intracranial pressure, and treatment should focus on reducing it.

## DIFFERENTIAL DIAGNOSIS AND MEDICAL DECISION MAKING

The key to diagnosis and treatment is accurate interpretation of the 12-lead electrocardiogram (ECG). Though not a comprehensive review of all bradycardic rhythms, the following are those commonly encountered.[6-8]

### SINUS BRADYCARDIA

For the diagnosis of sinus bradycardia, P waves must be present at a heart rate of less than 60 beats/min. The morphology of the P wave must be consistent with a sinus beat (upright in leads I and II), and each P wave must be followed by a QRS complex with a fixed PR interval.

### SICK SINUS SYNDROME

Sick sinus syndrome consists of a group of diseases characterized by dysfunction of the sinus node that can have a variety of appearances on an ECG. The most common ECG finding is severe, inappropriate sinus bradycardia. Another frequently encountered form is sinus arrest with a prolonged period (>2.5 seconds) and no atrial activity. The final form of sick sinus syndrome is tachycardia-bradycardia

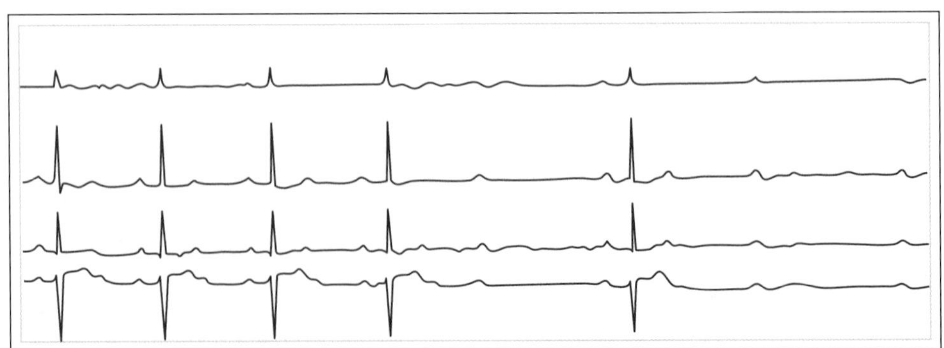

**Fig. 58.1 Rhythm strip of a patient with a bradycardia that is due to a hypervagal response.** The initial portion of the strip shows a sinus rhythm with progressive slowing to the point of sinus arrest. In addition, there is progressive prolongation of the PR interval, which indicates that atrioventricular node conduction is affected as well. This finding suggests that the cause is "external" and affecting both the sinoatrial and atrioventricular nodes and not intrinsic disease of either node.

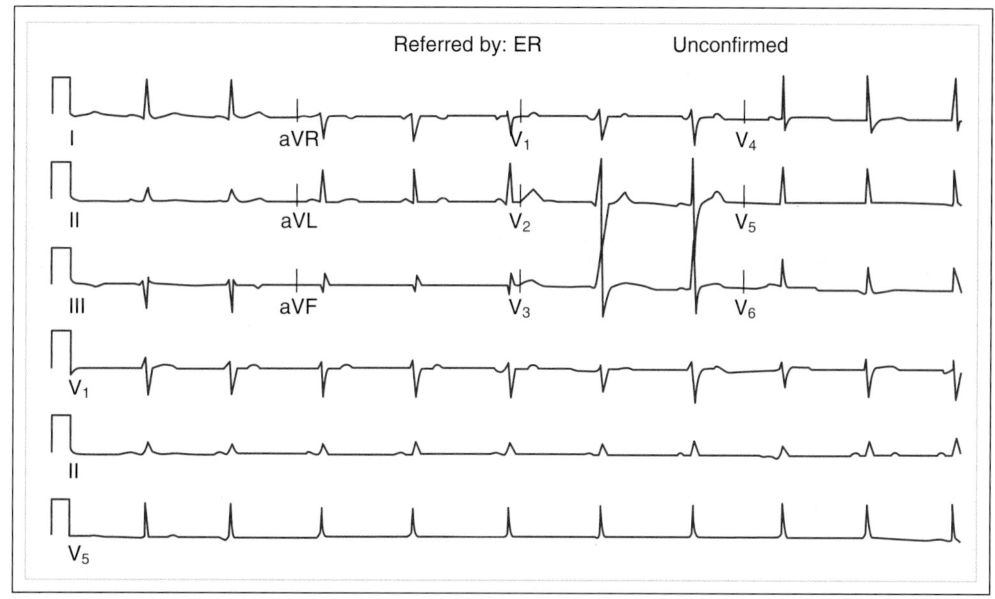


**Fig. 58.2 Sinus bradycardia with a ventricular response rate of 59 beats/min.** There is a P wave for every QRS complex and normal PR Intervals

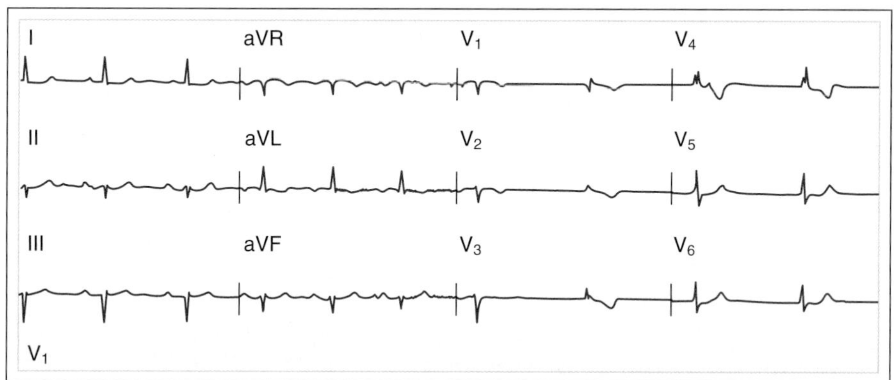


**Fig. 58.3 Sick sinus syndrome.** This syndrome has many variants, but all have the common feature of abrupt dysfunction of the sinus node. This electrocardiogram shows a normal sinus rhythm with abrupt absence of P waves.

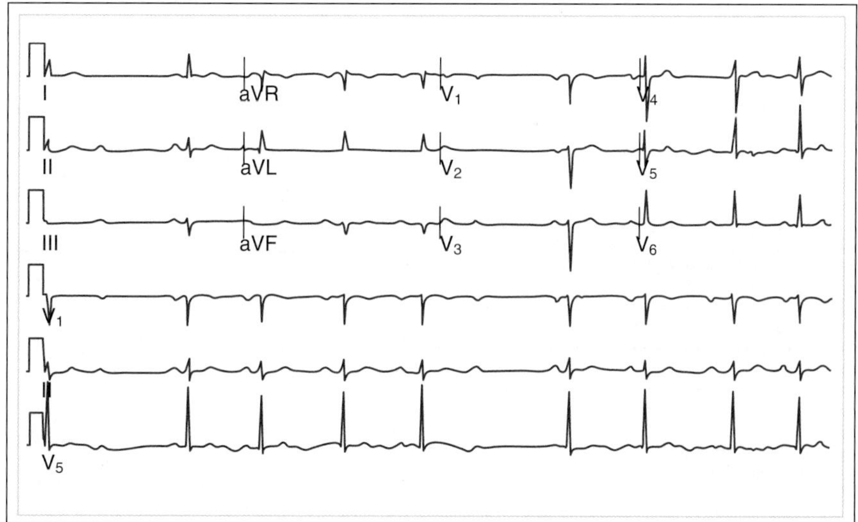


**Fig. 58.4 Mobitz type I second-degree heart block.** This is sinus rhythm at 70 beats/min with a slower ventricular rate because of a progressive delay in atrioventricular (AV) nodal conduction and, finally, a dropped beat. Note that the PR interval after the dropped beat is shorter than the PR interval just before the dropped beat. The hallmark feature of this type of second-degree AV block is the presence of a normal sinus rhythm with a progressive delay in AV nodal conduction.

**Table 58.2 Intrinsic Causes of Bradyarrhythmias**

| | |
|---|---|
| Ischemia and infarction | Inferior wall MI—sinus bradycardia, type I second-degree heart block, third-degree heart block<br>Anterior wall MI—type II second-degree heart block, third-degree heart block |
| Infection | Viral—varicella, mononucleosis, hepatitis, mumps, rubella, rubeola<br>Bacterial—endocarditis, diphtheria, Lyme disease<br>Parasitic—Chagas disease |
| Malignancy | Lymphoma, sarcoma |
| Rheumatologic | Systemic lupus erythematosus, rheumatoid arthritis, Reiter syndrome, systemic sclerosis |
| Other | Sarcoid, amyloid, Lev disease (spread of fibrosis and calcification from the adjacent cardiac skeleton), Lenègre disease (idiopathic fibrotic degeneration of the His-Purkinje system) |

*MI*, Myocardial infarction.

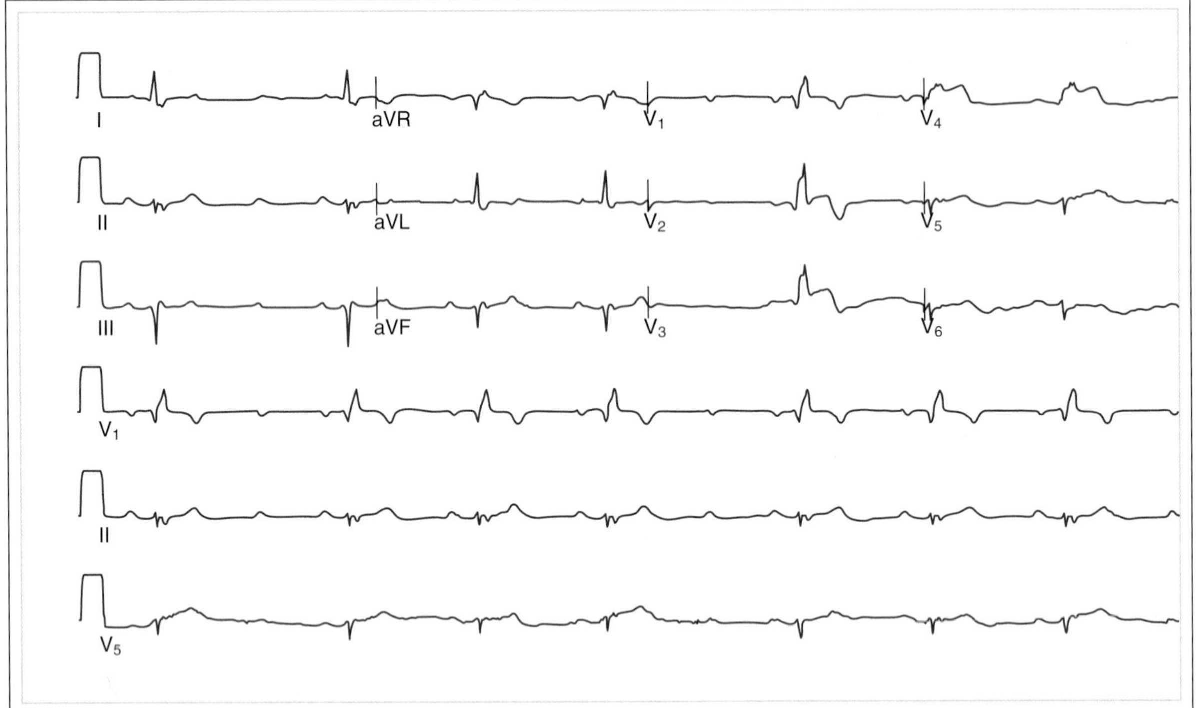


**Fig. 58.5 Mobitz type II second-degree atrioventricular block.** Careful review of this electrocardiogram shows a sinus rhythm with a left anterior fascicular block and a right bundle branch block. Importantly, there is evidence of an anterior wall infarct with ST-segment elevation in the anterior leads. This demonstrates a significant complication of anterior wall infarcts involving the septum, with necrosis of the right bundle branch and left anterior fascicle and intermittent failure of the left bundle branch.

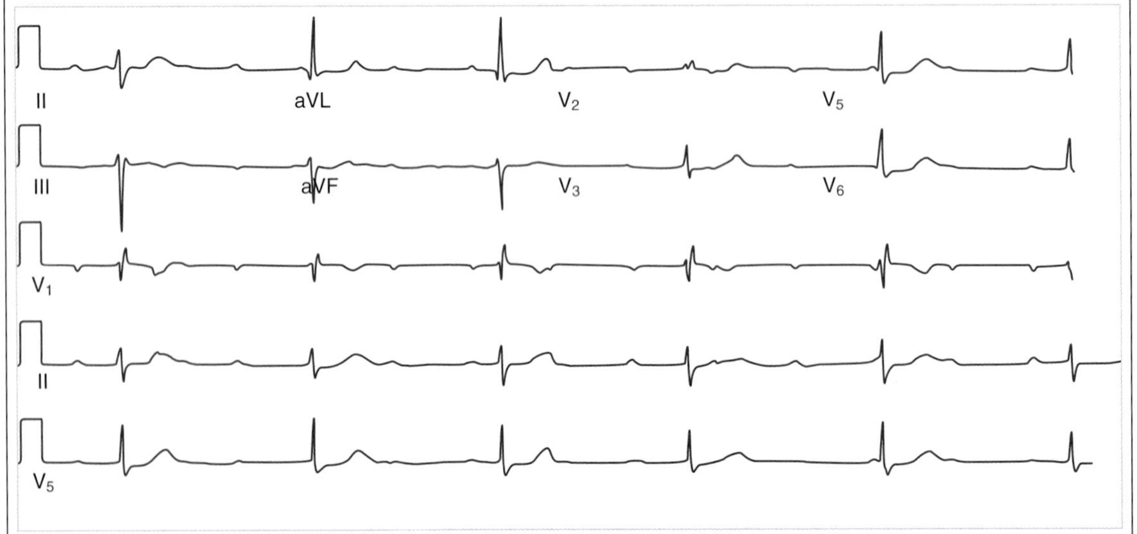


**Fig. 58.6 Complete atrioventricular block.** This electrocardiogram shows an underlying sinus rhythm that is regular at approximately 80 to 90 beats/min. The ventricular escape rhythm is slow and regular with no apparent relationship between the P waves and the QRS complexes.

syndrome, which is characterized by alternating periods of severe bradycardia interrupted by paroxysms of supraventricular tachycardia, usually atrial fibrillation.

## SECOND-DEGREE HEART BLOCK

These heart blocks will be manifested as bradycardia only if the sinus rhythm is slow or a significant percentage of the sinus beats are not conducted.[9]

### *Type I Second-Degree Atrioventricular Block*

The key ECG feature of a Mobitz type I second-degree AV block (i.e., a Wenckebach block) is progressive lengthening of the PR interval leading to a dropped QRS complex. The PR interval of the first-conducted QRS complex after a nonconducted beat has the shortest or a relatively normal PR interval. These blocks are usually indicative of a medication effect, AV node disease, or ischemia, but the rhythm is rarely the source of the instability[10] (**Fig. 58.7**; also see Fig. 58.4).

### *Type II Second-Degree Atrioventricular Conduction Block*

Diagnosis of a Mobitz type II heart block is determined by the presence of an intact sinus pacemaker with intermittent failure of conductance to the ventricles. This is due to failure of either the bundle of His or one of the Purkinje fibers. This rhythm is indicative of significant disease of the infranodal conducting system and is likely to progress to a complete heart block. These blocks are often due to myocardial ischemia and are symptomatic (see Fig. 58.5).

## THIRD-DEGREE ATRIOVENTRICULAR BLOCK

This rhythm should be considered first in a patient with bradyarrhythmia because it is always clinically significant, often hemodynamically compromising, and unstable (**Fig. 58.8**; also see Fig. 58.6). The ventricular rate is typically very slow, but the actual rate varies according to the inherent rate of the escape rhythm. In this rhythm there is evidence of independent activity because of no connection between the atria and ventricles. It is important to "march out" the P waves to see if they are regular because some are most likely buried within or are part of the QRS complex or T wave. It should be apparent that there is no fixed relationship between the P waves and the QRS complexes. The QRS complexes can be narrow or wide, depending on the location of the escape pacemaker. Junctional escape pacemakers are faster (50 to 60 beats/min), narrow, and relatively stable in comparison with a ventricular escape rhythm, which is slow (30 to 40 beats/min), wide, and unstable. Often, the most helpful feature of the ECG for this rhythm is that the QRS complexes should be absolutely regular. This is a rhythm initiated by a slower pacemaker exhibiting spontaneous automaticity that has "escaped" the influence of the overriding sinus rhythm. Escape rhythms fire automatically at their inherent rate and are regular. Any irregularity in the escape rhythm suggests a high-grade incomplete AV block or an inherently unstable escape rhythm.

## BRADYCARDIA ASSOCIATED WITH A WIDE QRS COMPLEX

Bradyarrhythmia associated with a "new" widening of the QRS complex suggests a cause that results in diffuse slowing of depolarization and conduction and that usually implicates agents that block the fast sodium channels or their ability to repolarize. This bradycardia is typically seen in patients with poisoning from agents such as tricyclic antidepressants, in patients with hypothermia, or in those with hyperkalemia (**Figs. 58.9 and Fig. 58.10**).

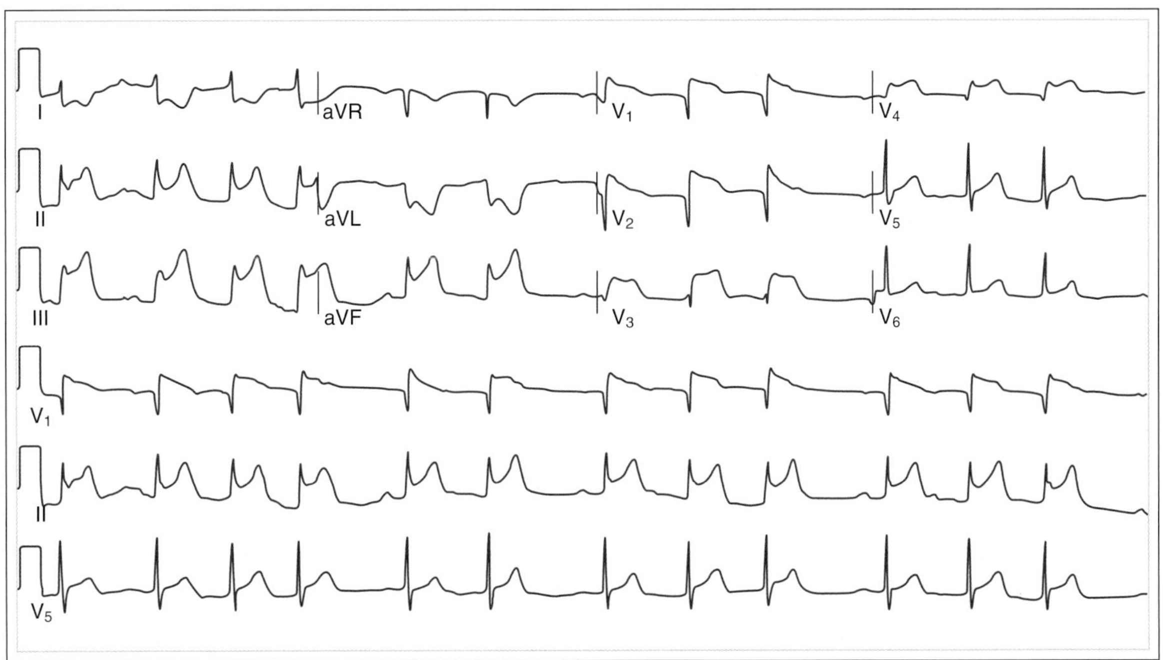


**Fig. 58.7** This electrocardiogram shows diffuse ST elevations involving both the inferior and anterior walls. The ventricular rate is irregular, which indicates that the rhythm is originating from the sinus node and is not an escape rhythm. Though not the typical pattern of a Mobitz type I second-degree heart block, the progressive lengthening of the PR intervals suggests that the block is occurring at the level of the atrioventricular node. This conduction disturbance may be responsive to atropine.

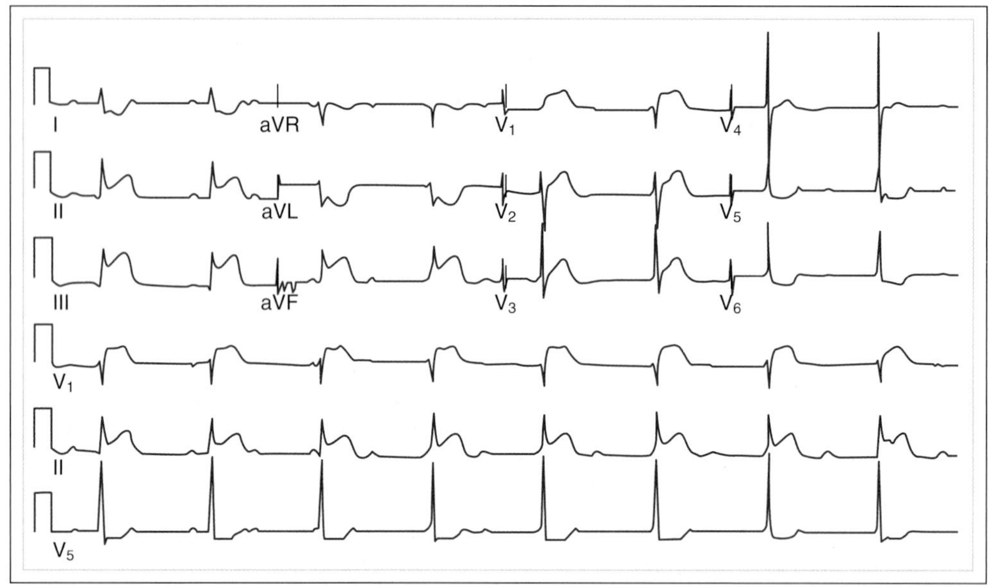


**Fig. 58.8 Acute myocardial infarction and third-degree atrioventricular block.** The sinus rhythm is regular and slow. The lead II rhythm strip shows that there is no fixed relationship between the P waves and the QRS complex. The ventricular response is also regular and narrow, thus suggesting a junctional escape rhythm in the setting of an inferior wall myocardial infarction. The block is at the level of the atrioventricular node and may be responsive to atropine.

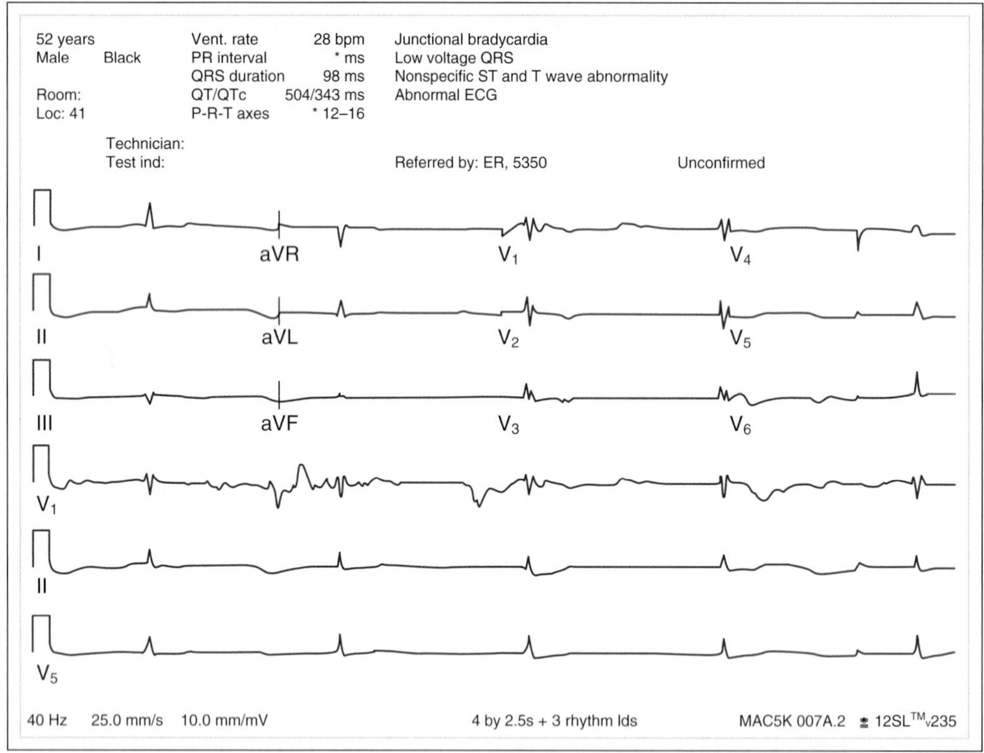


**Fig. 58.9 Hyperkalemia.** This electrocardiogram (ECG) is from a 52-year-old man who complained of generalized weakness in the previous week. The ECG shows a very slow rhythm that is regular and has a wide QRS complex. No obvious P waves are present, and the morphology of the QRS complexes is not typical for a right or left bundle branch block. The differential diagnosis includes sinus arrest with an escape rhythm and electrolyte abnormalities. After treatment with intravenous calcium gluconate, insulin, and 5% dextrose in water, the heart returned to a normal sinus rhythm with a narrow QRS complex. The patient's serum potassium value was found to be 7.1 mEq/L.

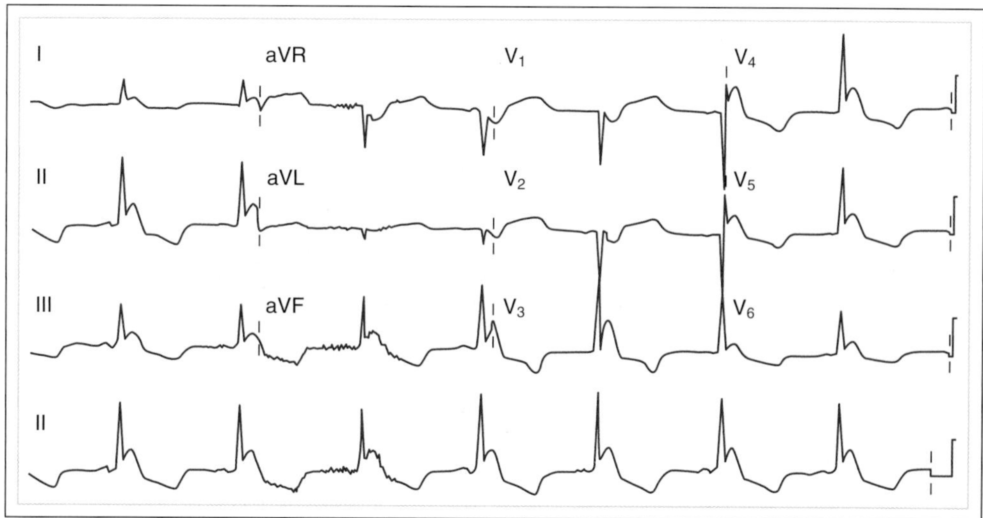


**Fig. 58.10 Electrocardiogram showing sinus bradycardia with Osborn waves distorting the QRS complexes.** These are classic findings in patients with clinically significant hypothermia. Treatment consists of rewarming and monitoring the patient's condition via telemetry.

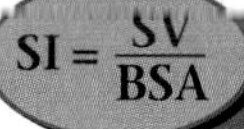


**FACTS AND FORMULAS**

Sinus bradycardia (adults): Sinus rhythm < 60 beats/min.

Junctional escape rhythm: Ventricular response rate of 40 to 60 beats/min. No P waves. Regular narrow QRS (unless preexisting BBB present).

Idioventricular rhythm: Ventricular response rate of 30 to 45 beats/min. No P waves. Regular wide QRS (usually does not appear as a typical right or left BBB pattern).

Type I second-degree heart block: Sinus rhythm with progressive PR prolongation and a nonconducted beat. The PR interval of the conducted beat following the blocked beat is the shortest interval in the sequence. The QRS complex is usually narrow.

Type II second-degree heart block: Normal sinus rhythm with fixed PR intervals. Random sinus beats are not conducted to the ventricle. The QRS complex is often wide.

Third-degree heart block: Sinus rhythm with P waves visible. The ventricular response rate is regular but slower than the atrial rate with no visible relationship between the P waves and QRS complexes. The QRS rate and width are dependent on the site of the escape rhythm. The junctional escape rate is 40 to 60 beats/min and the QRS complex is narrow. The ventricular escape rhythm is 30 to 45 beats/min and the QRS complex is wide.

*BBB*, Bundle branch block.

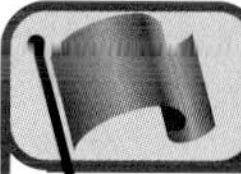

**RED FLAGS**

Bradycardia is relative. When cardiac stroke volume is normal, perfusion (e.g., blood pressure and cerebral perfusion) can be perfectly adequate even with ventricular response rates in the 30s. When a patient is symptomatic with a bradyarrhythmia, it is often multifactorial in etiology and attention must be paid to optimizing the stroke volume with fluids, reversing the ischemia, or adding inotropic agents in addition to increasing the heart rate.

Bradycardia not associated with hypotension or signs of hypoperfusion may be normal.

Bradycardia not associated with hypotension or signs of hypoperfusion may be an important clue to potentially serious conditions such as elevated intracranial pressure, electrolyte disturbances, or cardiac toxicity from medications.

Bradycardias associated with a wide QSR complex should be reviewed carefully for the presence of a complete heart block or medication or electrolyte effects.

Bradycardia or conduction disturbances in the setting of acute myocardial infarction should be looked for and recognized as a potential clinically significant complication.

## TREATMENT

### PREHOSPITAL CARE

Respiratory disorders and myocardial ischemia are often associated with bradycardia, and prehospital care should focus on optimizing oxygenation, ventilation, and blood pressure and on relieving ischemia if present. Treatment of bradycardia is indicated only for patients who have a bradycardia that is inappropriate for the clinical condition and the patient is symptomatic (**Fig. 58.11**).

1. Optimize oxygenation (supplemental oxygen) and/or ventilation (continuous positive airway pressure) if needed.
2. Establish intravenous access.
3. Place the patient on telemetry and obtain a 12-lead ECG if possible.

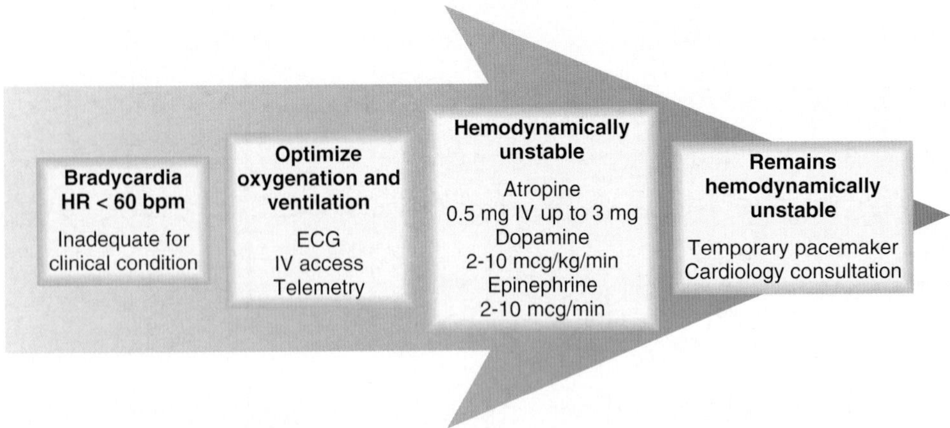


**Fig. 58.11 Treatment flow chart detailing initial stabilization of patients with bradycardia.** *ECG*, Electrocardiogram; *HR*, heart rate; *IV*, intravenous/intravenously.

4. If the absolute ventricular response rate is the probable cause of the hemodynamic instability, the following interventions may be helpful:
   a. Atropine, 0.5 mg intravenously (IV) up to 3 mg, may be effective for sinus bradycardia, Mobitz type I second-degree AV block, and third-degree heart block.
   b. Glucagon, 1 mg IV, may be effective for beta-blocker and calcium channel blocker toxicity.
   c. Calcium gluconate, 10 mL of a 10% solution IV, may be effective for calcium channel blocker toxicity or hyperkalemia.

## HOSPITAL CARE

On arrival at the hospital, a slow heart rate will be readily identified while obtaining triage vital signs. The patient should be assessed rapidly for conditions that would cause the bradycardia through a screening examination for respiratory distress, medication toxicities, or myocardial ischemia. Once identified, disease-specific treatment plans will usually treat the bradycardia as well. Mainstays of management include the following:

1. Optimize oxygenation and ventilation.
2. Establish intravenous access and administer bolus intravenous fluid if the patient is hypotensive without signs of congestive heart failure.
3. Obtain a 12-lead ECG and rhythm strip.
4. Interventions:
   a. The patient remains hemodynamically compromised by the heart rate:
      - Sinus bradycardia, type I second-degree heart block, third-degree heart block:
        - Atropine, 0.5 mg IV up to 3 mg; atropine dosing should be aimed at obtaining the lowest heart rate that will optimize perfusion. In the setting of myocardial ischemia, the clinician must carefully balance the priority of maintaining perfusion to vital organs without exacerbating the myocardial ischemia.
        - Glucagon, 1 mg IV, may be effective for beta-blocker and calcium channel blocker toxicity.
        - Calcium gluconate, 10 mL of a 10% solution IV, may be effective for calcium channel blocker toxicity or hyperkalemia.
        - Temporary pacemaker.
      - Type II second-degree heart block, third-degree heart block (particularly with a wide QRS complex):
        - Atropine is unlikely to work when the location of the block is in infranodal tissue (e.g., the bundle of His or more distal conduction system) because the blockade is less likely to be reversed with anticholinergic medication. These blocks are preferably treated with temporary pacing or β-adrenergic support as temporizing measures while the patient is being prepared for permanent transvenous pacing.
        - Dopamine hydrochloride can be effective in hypotensive, bradycardic patients and can be titrated to more selectively target the heart rate or vasoconstriction. Initial dosing in an unstable patient should start at 2 to 5 mcg/kg/min and be titrated to optimize blood pressure.
        - Epinephrine is a catecholamine with α and β activity and may increase the heart rate and support the blood pressure. The infusion can be initiated at 2 to 10 mcg/min and titrated to patient response. Use of vasoconstrictors requires that the recipient be assessed for adequate intravascular volume and volume status supported as needed.
        - Temporary pacing.
   b. The patient is not hemodynamically compromised by the heart rate:
      - Sinus bradycardia, type I second-degree heart block:
        - Treat the underlying cause—myocardial infarction (MI), myocardial ischemia.
        - Discontinue the offending medication.
        - Optimize electrolytes and volume status.
      - Type II second-degree heart block, third-degree heart block:
        - Temporary pacemaker.
        - Cardiology consultation.

- Treat the underlying cause—MI, myocardial ischemia.
- Optimize electrolytes and volume status.

### CONSULTATION

Cardiology consultation is recommended for bradyarrhythmias that require pacemaker support and those that are due to failure of the infranodal conduction system or occur in the context of MI. Temporary cardiac pacing (TCP) can be an effective bridge to permanent pacemaker placement. The limited data on the effectiveness of TCP in patients with symptomatic bradycardia show that it is comparable with atropine and dopamine when hospital survival is used as an outcome.[11] Its clinical utility is limited by the fact that it is poorly tolerated by awake patients and capture may be unreliable over time. It is reasonable to initiate TCP in unstable patients who do not respond to oxygen, fluids, and pharmacologic interventions as noted earlier. The decision regarding implantation of a pacemaker depends on the underlying cause and the likelihood that the AV block will be permanent. Many conditions affecting the conduction system will predictably resolve, such as electrolyte abnormalities, medication effects, hypothermia, and inferior wall MI, and will require at most TCP. Conversely, pacemaker implantation is indicated, even without hemodynamic instability, for conditions that are likely to progress and place the patient at risk for failure of the conduction system.[12,13]

Bradycardias caused by intrinsic disease of the myocardial conduction system are typically type II second-degree heart blocks and third-degree heart block and will usually require permanent pacemaker placement. Type I second-degree heart blocks rarely result in clinically significant bradycardia, but pacemaker therapy is warranted in patients who progress to complete heart block that does not respond to pharmacologic interventions.

MI is associated with significant bradyarrhythmia 25% to 30% of the time.[14] The underlying mechanism is either direct ischemic injury to the sinus node, AV node, or conduction system or exaggerated vagally mediated reflexes. The bradyarrhythmias and conduction blocks associated with inferoposterior infarcts are commonly due to vagal reflexes, are responsive to atropine, and are usually transient[15,16] (see Figs. 58.7 and 58.8). Sinus bradycardia and AV nodal blockade in the context of an inferior wall MI have been attributed to a higher density of cardiac afferent receptors in the inferoposterior portions of the heart. For hemodynamically compromising bradycardias, atropine is an excellent initial therapy, particularly in the first 6 hours. Doses should be administered in 0.5-mg increments with a maximum dose of 0.04 mg/kg or 3 mg. Doses lower than 0.5 mg should be avoided because of the risk for a paradoxic bradycardic response. When atropine is ineffective, transcutaneous or transvenous pacing is indicated. It is uncommon for type I second-degree and third-degree heart block to be the primary cause of hypotension in a patient with acute MI. Hypotension is usually due to poor stroke volume from the MI, and therapeutic effort should focus on restoring blood flow to the myocardium.

The conduction blocks associated with anterior infarcts typically involve the septum and the bundle branches that run through it. These blocks are not responsive to atropine and generally require permanent pacemaker support. Conduction blocks are typically those that are due to type II second-degree heart block or third-degree heart block. The anterior circulation perfuses the septum containing the His-Purkinje fibers. Ischemia and infarction of the septum may result in failure of one of the fascicles to conduct, usually the right bundle and left anterior fascicle, which lie in the anterior portion of the septum. Fascicular failure alone does not result in bradycardia as long as there is one functioning fascicle in sinus rhythm. Bradycardia may occur with either intermittent failure of the one remaining fascicle to conduct or failure of the bundle of His, which results in a type II second-degree heart block or third-degree heart block. Treatment is placement of a permanent pacemaker.[12,13]

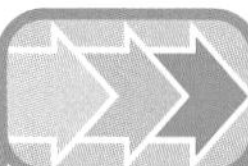

**PRIORITY ACTIONS**

1. Determine whether the patient is hemodynamically compromised by the bradyarrhythmia. If the patient is hypotensive, determine whether it is due to the absolute heart rate or associated conditions that will cause a relative bradycardia to be symptomatic, such as volume loss or left ventricular dysfunction.
2. Establish intravenous access.
3. If it is determined that the absolute ventricular response rate is inappropriate for the clinical condition, the following interventions may be helpful:
   - Atropine, 0.5 mg intravenously up to 3 mg, may be effective for sinus bradycardia, Mobitz type I second-degree heart block (particularly in the setting of inferior wall myocardial infarction)
   - Glucagon, 1 mg intravenously, for beta-blocker and calcium channel blocker toxicity
   - Calcium gluconate, 10 mL of a 10% solution intravenously, for calcium channel blocker toxicity
4. Indications for temporary transcutaneous pacemaker placement include the following:
   - Symptomatic bradycardia unresponsive to pharmacologic therapy
   - Mobitz type II second-degree block
   - Third-degree heart block

## FOLLOW-UP, NEXT STEPS IN CARE, AND PATIENT EDUCATION

### ADMISSION

Admission for patients with bradycardia is dependent on the underlying cause, the extent to which the bradycardia is clinically significant, and whether interventions require in-hospital monitoring, treatment, or both.

### PROGNOSIS

The prognosis varies with the cause of the bradyarrhythmia. Bradyarrhythmias secondary to extrinsic causes are reactive and usually recoverable once the offending agent or condition is removed. Intrinsic causes often suggest disease of the cardiac conduction system and require permanent pacing. Rarely is a recognized bradyarrhythmia a primary cause of death.

### DOCUMENTATION

Bradyarrhythmias are a symptom, not a disease. Frequently, the underlying cause is clearly identified, and documentation is fairly simple—for example, the patient is experiencing effects of a new blood pressure medication. When the cause is less clear, the documentation must clearly include or exclude variables that must be considered in the work-up and treatment:

- Determine the clinical significance of the bradycardia. Did the patient pass out or complain of chest pain, exertional fatigue, or dyspnea? Precipitating factors such as nausea, head turning, tight ties, and new medications are important clues to the underlying cause.
- Does the patient have underlying cardiac disease, specifically left ventricular dysfunction, that would contribute to a bradyarrhythmia being symptomatic?
- The medical history should include a detailed medication list and recent dosing history.
- The physical examination may provide clues to the cause of the bradycardia:
  - Lethargy and hypertension—elevated intracranial pressure
  - Dialysis catheter or shunt—hyperkalemia
  - Obesity and sonorous breathing—sleep apnea
- The electrocardiogram and frequently multiple electrocardiograms, particularly when the patient reports symptoms, often specify the diagnosis.

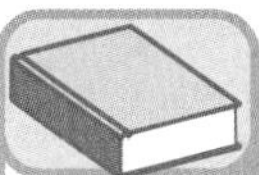

### PATIENT TEACHING TIPS

Patients have the ability to exacerbate symptoms in specific conditions that cause bradycardia and thus should be given guidelines to avoid doing so if possible. These generally fall into the category of extrinsic causes of bradycardia:

- Patients with cough, micturition, and bradycardia or syncope should be advised to seek treatment to minimize triggers and to have access to support rails. Patients should lie down when lightheaded and should call 911 for persistent or particularly severe symptoms.
- Patients with carotid sinus hypersensitivity should avoid wearing tight ties and buttoned collars.
- Patients with documented sensitivity to medications that affect the sinus node or the atrioventricular node (or both) should report this fact when being prescribed any new medications.

## PITFALLS

Bradycardia is readily identified because of the heart rate being an essential component of triage and monitoring of vital signs. The diagnosis is dependent on accurate interpretation of the ECG in the context of the patient's overall medical findings. Treatment "failures" are often due to the clinician's focus on the bradyarrhythmia without consideration of the underlying cause. When the bradycardia is not causing hemodynamic instability, it does not need to be "treated" but remains an important clue to underlying conditions, such as medication effects, elevated intracranial pressure, pulmonary hypertension, or cardiac ischemia.

## REFERENCES

***References can be found on Expert Consult @ www.expertconsult.com.***

# Tachydysrhythmias 59

*Keith A. Marill*

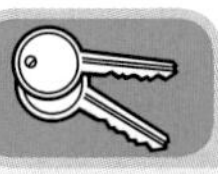

**KEY POINTS**

- Tachydysrhythmia may be due to intrinsic cardiologic disease or external stimulation.
- Noncardiologic causes, such as hypoxia, inadequate perfusion, metabolic derangements, or toxicity from medications or other agents, should always be considered.
- The higher the tachycardic heart rate, the greater the likelihood of instability.
- Patients with ventricular tachycardia may not necessarily appear unstable.
- If there is uncertainty, wide QRS complex tachycardia should be assumed to be ventricular in origin.
- The most effective treatment of ventricular tachycardia is electrical cardioversion. However, antidysrhythmic medications may also be necessary to prevent recurrence.
- All ostensibly healthy young patients with syncope should be assessed for valvular disease, left ventricular hypertrophy, Wolff-Parkinson-White syndrome, abnormal QT interval or T-wave morphology, and Brugada syndrome.

## EPIDEMIOLOGY

Heart rhythms with rapid rates, or tachydysrhythmias, have a range of causes and associated incidences, morbidities, and mortality. Atrial fibrillation (AF) occurs in up to 5% of people older than 65 years. Conversely, sustained ventricular tachycardia (VT) is rare and accounts for less than 0.1% of emergency department (ED) visits. Morbidity ranges from temporary lightheadedness to syncope and deterioration, ventricular fibrillation (VF), or embolization and subsequent permanent disability as a result of ischemic stroke. Mortality from atrial tachydysrhythmias is generally low. Mortality from VT is approximately 5%, and that from VF ranges from 80% to greater than 90%, depending on the clinical circumstances.[1] A particular exception to the low mortality associated with atrial tachydysrhythmias is AF or flutter with rapid ventricular excitation via a bypass tract, such as in Wolff-Parkinson-White (WPW) syndrome.[2]

## PATHOPHYSIOLOGY AND MECHANISMS

Tachycardia is defined as a rhythm with at least three consecutive heartbeats occurring at a rate higher than 100 beats/min. The primary mechanisms for tachycardia are enhanced automaticity, reentry, and triggered beats. Sometimes a combination of these mechanisms is required for both initiation and maintenance of the tachydysrhythmia.

The normal progression of depolarization in the heart begins with the sinus node, followed by the atria, the atrioventricular (AV) node, the His-Purkinje system, and the ventricles. Sinus and AV nodal tissue depolarization is mediated primarily by calcium channels, and depolarization of the other cardiac tissue is mediated by sodium channels. Repolarization is mediated predominantly by potassium channels.

Automaticity is a characteristic of cardiac tissue wherein the cells depolarize at a periodic rate according to the tissue subtype. Sinus node tissue normally has the fastest intrinsic rate, and thus the sinus node serves as the pacemaker for the heart. Abnormal tachycardia occurs when other foci or circuits supersede the sinus node rate.

Enhanced automaticity occurs when the normal periodicity of cells is accelerated. Such acceleration may be either a normal physiologic response to increased sympathetic tone or fever or a pathologic response to an overdose of a medication such as digoxin or theophylline, a stimulant such as an amphetamine or cocaine, or other extrinsic factors. An automatic tachycardia occurs when an ectopic focus of tissue develops a heart rate greater than the sinus rate and paces the heart.

Reentry refers to a microscopic or macroscopic circular pattern of myocardial depolarization. A wave of excitation passes around the circuit and depolarizes the cells until it arrives at the beginning, and the process repeats itself. Reentry can occur if the circuit is sufficiently long or there is a slow-conducting portion that allows enough time for cells to have recovered from their refractory period before the wave of excitation returns (**Fig. 59.1**). The reentrant rhythm becomes the cardiac pacemaker if it is sufficiently fast to outpace the sinus node.

Tachydysrhythmias can also be initiated or triggered by small depolarizing ion movements that occur during or after normal cellular repolarization. These ion movements are termed early afterdepolarizations (EADs) and delayed afterdepolarizations (DADs), respectively. They can trigger a new wave of excitation in myocardial tissue before the normal sequence of depolarization from the sinus node. Unlike early beats secondary to enhanced automaticity, these beats have a close correlation with the preceding beat and its repolarization phase. Some tachydysrhythmias use multiple dysrhythmic mechanisms (e.g., an EAD may initiate a reentrant tachycardia).

## PRESENTING SIGNS AND SYMPTOMS

Patients with tachydysrhythmias may be entirely asymptomatic or may have a range of symptoms. They may be lightheaded or may experience palpitations, chest discomfort, shortness of breath, transient syncope, or sudden death.

Signs of tachycardia include a rapid pulse and heart sounds. An irregularly irregular pulse is often detectable in patients with AF and atrial flutter or atrial tachycardia (AT) with variable AV conduction. VT may be associated with retrograde ventriculoatrial conduction, or AV dissociation may be present. In patients with VT and AV dissociation, signs of dissociation may be difficult to discern but can include variable intensity of the first heart sound and arterial or jugular venous pulsations. Tachycardia can lead to congestive heart failure (CHF) secondary to inadequate diastolic filling, myocardial ischemia, or other mechanisms. If CHF occurs, typical signs such as jugular venous distention, rales on pulmonary auscultation, and dependent edema may be present.

The primary findings to assess in the diagnosis of a patient with a tachycardiac electrocardiogram (ECG) are as follows:

- The presence, periodicity, and morphology of the P waves
- The relationship of the P waves, if any, to the QRS complexes
- The morphology of the QRS complexes and other waves as compared with a previous tracing if available

The response of the ECG tracing to vagal maneuvers and other therapies such as adenosine infusion may also uncover the underlying rhythm diagnosis.

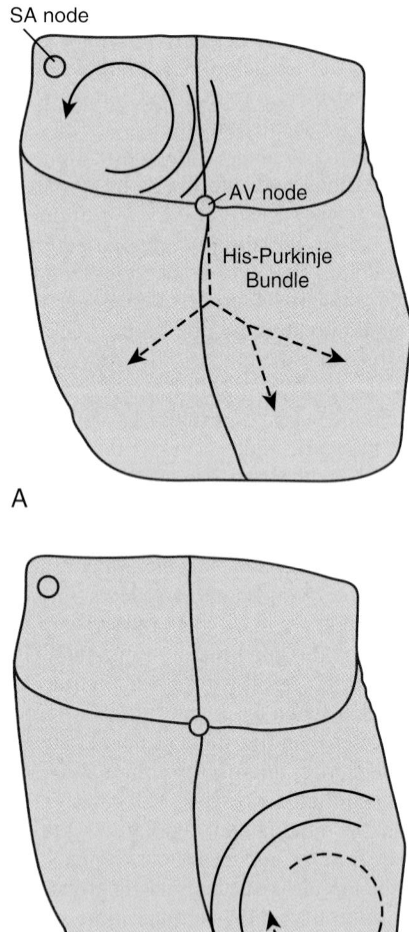


**Fig. 59.1 Schematic diagrams of cardiac conduction depicting the four heart chambers and the sinoatrial (SA) and atrioventricular (AV) nodes.** Normal His-Purkinje conduction is represented by *dotted lines*, with *arrows* representing conduction through the bundle branches below the AV node. Reentrant waves of cardiac depolarization are represented by *semicircular lines with arrows*. Conduction through atrial or ventricular myocardial tissue is shown by *arcs* representing wavelets emanating from the source of excitation. **A,** Typical atrial flutter. **B,** Ventricular tachycardia.

## DIFFERENTIAL DIAGNOSIS

A variety of noncardiologic conditions can cause syncope and other symptoms that may suggest a tachydysrhythmia. Inadequate oxygenation of vital organs may be due to anemia, hemoglobin malfunction, or respiratory failure. Metabolic derangements include hypoglycemia, hyperthyroidism, dehydration, and fever. A hyperadrenal state secondary to acute excitement or agitation or, uncommonly, to pheochromocytoma can lead to sinus tachycardia. Neurologic events such as a seizure or cerebrovascular accident can cause tachycardia and altered consciousness, which can be confused with a primary tachydysrhythmia. Intoxication with stimulants and anticholinergics can manifest similarly. Overdose with prescription medications such as antihypertensive agents can result in tachycardia and hypotension.

Primarily nondysrhythmic cardiopulmonary conditions should also be considered in the differential diagnosis. Valvular disease, particularly that involving the aortic site, can lead to tachycardia, chest discomfort, or inadequate cardiac output with subsequent syncope. Hypertrophic obstructive cardiomyopathy can cause inadequate cardiac output if the subaortic hypertrophy obstructs cardiac outflow, and pulmonary embolism can lead to pulmonary vasospasm and obstruction to flow. Conditions leading to tamponade, such as pericardial effusion and tension pneumothorax, compromise cardiac output by impairing diastolic filling.

## TREATMENT

The primary emergency therapies for tachydysrhythmias include medications to slow electrical conduction or to increase the cellular refractory period in the AV node or other groups of cardiac cells (**Table 59.1**). The goal of therapy is to terminate and suppress the abnormal rhythm or to slow the response in the remainder of the heart. Electrical therapy, including synchronized cardioversion and defibrillation, is used in potentially or frankly unstable patients. Electrical therapy has the advantages of high efficacy and safety, but shocks are painful and do not prevent recurrence of the tachydysrhythmia. Patients with higher heart rates, regardless of the underlying rhythm, have compromised diastolic filling and cardiac output. These patients should be treated more aggressively with early electrical therapy. The emergency physician (EP) should understand and use antidysrhythmic medications but should minimize the use of multiple agents in a single patient. Use of multiple drugs increases the likelihood of drug interactions and compromised cardiac output.

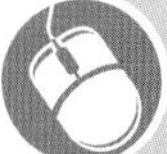

See Table 59.1, Select Tachydysrhythmia Medications, online at www.expertconsult.com

## SPECIFIC TACHYCARDIAS

Primary tachycardiac conditions can be divided most simply into those of supraventricular and ventricular origin (**Box 59.1; Fig. 59.2**; see also Fig. 59.1). Supraventricular tachycardia (SVT) must involve tissue above the ventricles but may also involve ventricular tissue in a tachycardiac circuit, whereas VT involves only ventricular tissue below the AV node. The remainder of the chapter deals with the diagnosis and treatment of specific tachycardiac conditions.

**BOX 59.1 Major Tachydysrhythmias**

**Supraventricular Tachycardias**

- Irregular
  - Atrial fibrillation
  - Multifocal atrial tachycardia
- Regular
  - Sinus tachycardia
  - Atrial flutter
  - Atrial tachycardia
  - Atrioventricular tachycardia
  - Atrioventricular nodal reentrant tachycardia
  - Junctional tachycardia

**Ventricular Tachycardias**

- Monomorphic ventricular tachycardia
- Polymorphic ventricular tachycardia
  - Normal QT interval
  - Prolonged QT interval
    - Acquired versus congenital

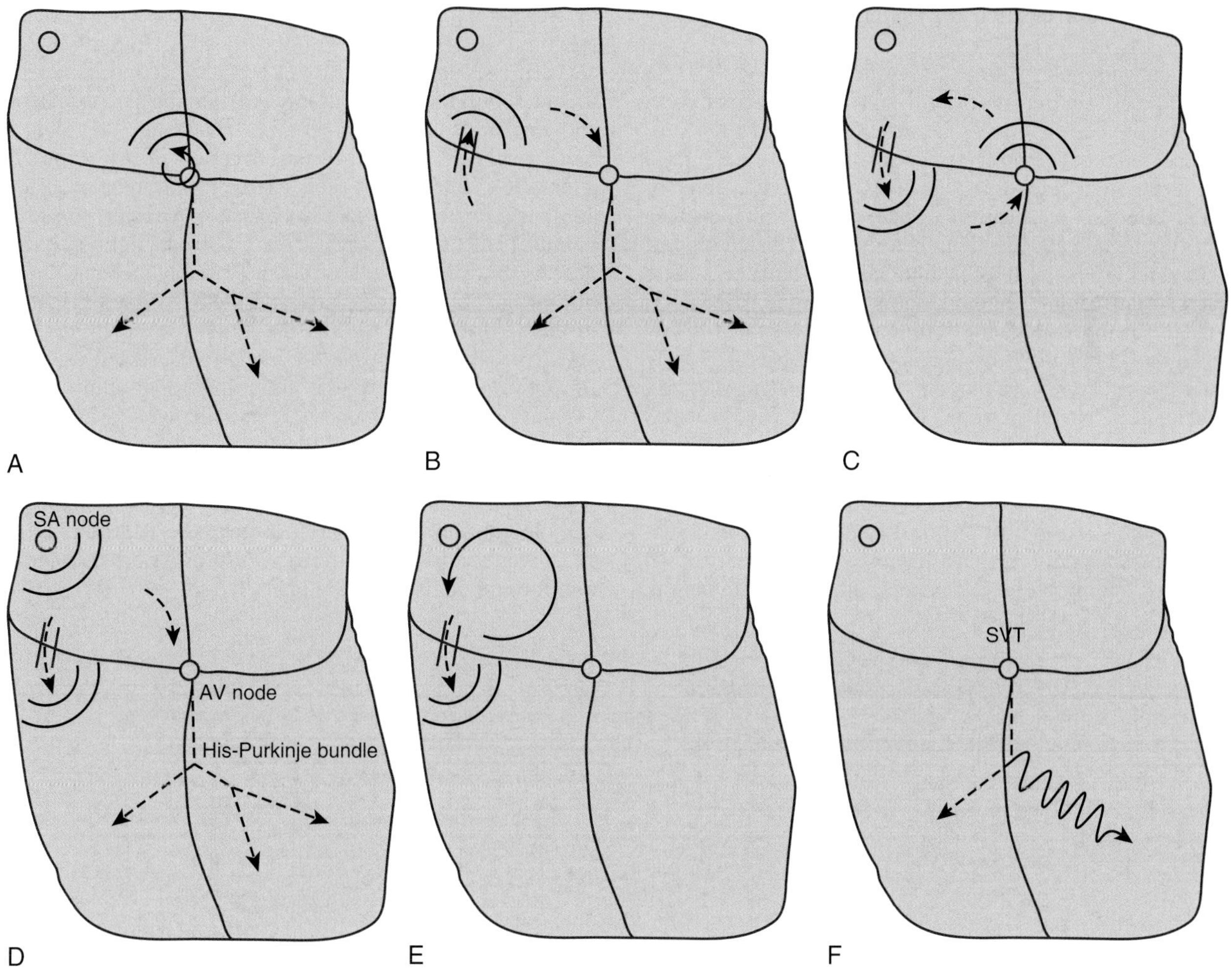

**Fig. 59.2** **A,** Atrioventricular (AV) nodal reentrant tachycardia. **B,** AV reentrant tachycardia (orthodromic). **C,** AV reentrant tachycardia (antidromic). **D,** Normal sinus rhythm and Wolff-Parkinson-White syndrome. **E,** Atrial fibrillation or flutter with rapid conduction via the accessory pathway. **F,** Supraventricular tachycardia (SVT) with aberrancy. *SA*, Sinoatrial.

## SUPRAVENTRICULAR TACHYCARDIAS

### *Irregular Supraventricular Tachycardias*

ATRIAL FIBRILLATION The most common cause of an irregularly irregular heartbeat, AF is particularly common in the elderly, as well as in patients with preexisting cardiopulmonary disease. The mechanism is rapid, quasiperiodic, chaotic reentry within the atria. Consequently, the AV node is bombarded with atrial excitation waves at a high irregular rate. Conduction of signals through the AV node is limited by the refractory period of the nodal tissue. The AV node cannot conduct until the cells have recovered from depolarization and are ready to fire again. This determines the rate of the irregular ventricular response to AF.

The clinician can usually diagnose AF at the bedside by feeling the pulse, listening to the heart sounds, and observing a single-lead cardiac monitor. The ECG may show fine or coarse irregular undulations of the baseline and an absence of regular P waves. The QRS complex is usually normal; however, if the ventricular response is rapid, the QRS complex may be transiently widened because of intermittent aberrant conduction through the His-Purkinje system (**Fig. 59.3**). This finding, termed the Ashman phenomenon, can occur when areas of the His-Purkinje tissue have a longer refractory period than the AV node does. Such bursts of wide QRS complex tachycardia can be confused with nonsustained VT, but on close inspection the rhythm remains irregularly irregular.

The most common treatment issue for patients with AF in the emergency setting is control of the ventricular rate. Depending on the function of the patient's AV node, the ventricular rate may range up to approximately 150 beats/min in adults. Ventricular rates this fast allow insufficient time for diastolic filling of the heart. The rate can be slowed with a variety of agents that act to lengthen the refractory period of the AV nodal tissue, such as calcium channel blockers,[3] beta-blockers,[4] magnesium,[5] digoxin, and amiodarone. Digoxin is less useful in the emergency setting because it takes a few hours to work, but the other agents must be used carefully because they can decrease blood pressure to varying degrees. The calcium channel blocker diltiazem usually provides excellent rate control with minimal loss of blood pressure. Beta-blockers may cause a greater loss of blood pressure and must be used with caution in patients with CHF or pulmonary disease. There is no indication for the administration of adenosine in patients with AF. The diagnosis should be made on the basis of findings from the history, physical examination, and ECG. Furthermore, adenosine, which only transiently blocks AV nodal conduction, would have no lasting therapeutic benefit.

If a patient with AF has a rapid ventricular response and associated hypotension, emergency cardioversion should be considered. It is unusual for AF alone to cause hypotension, so the possibility of additional causative conditions that can be corrected, such as dehydration, occult hemorrhage, and the metabolic conditions previously mentioned, should also be considered. Nevertheless, cardioversion can be accomplished by electrical, chemical, or combined therapies. For a patient with cardiovascular instability, emergency direct current cardioversion (DCCV) is most effective and safe. The patient should be sedated if clinical circumstances allow and treatment begun at 100 J with a biphasic or monophasic pulse. A short-acting benzodiazepine such as midazolam is often the first choice for sedation because it is safe and effective and has amnestic properties as well. The defibrillator should be set to the synchronized mode to synch ronize the pulse, if possible, with the QRS deflection, even though the QRS waves occur irregularly. If the initial shock is unsuccessful, the energy of the pulse can be escalated as needed.

Cardioversion can also be accomplished chemically when circumstances allow. Agents that slow conduction or increase the refractory period of atrial tissue are used to break the reentrant microcircuits within the atria. Vaughn-Williams class III and class I medications that can accomplish this goal include ibutilide, amiodarone, procainamide, propafenone, and flecainide.[6,7] These agents can terminate AF alone and increase the likelihood of cardioversion of AF with subsequent DCCV. However, their use entails some risk. There is an approximately 2% to 5% chance of causing torsades de pointes (TdP) after the infusion of ibutilide, amiodarone, and procainamide because these agents variably increase the duration of the depolarized phase and the associated QT interval in the ventricles, as well as the atria. The newly developed agent vernakalant may be less likely to cause TdP because of its action in blocking the ultrarapid potassium channels located primarily in the atria. Hypokalemia and hypomagnesemia raise the risk for TdP. Pretreatment with magnesium may be protective in some circumstances, even in patients with normal serum electrolyte levels.[8] Propafenone and flecainide can slow conduction, exacerbate heart failure, and cause ventricular dysrhythmias. Cardioversion also carries a risk for embolic stroke.

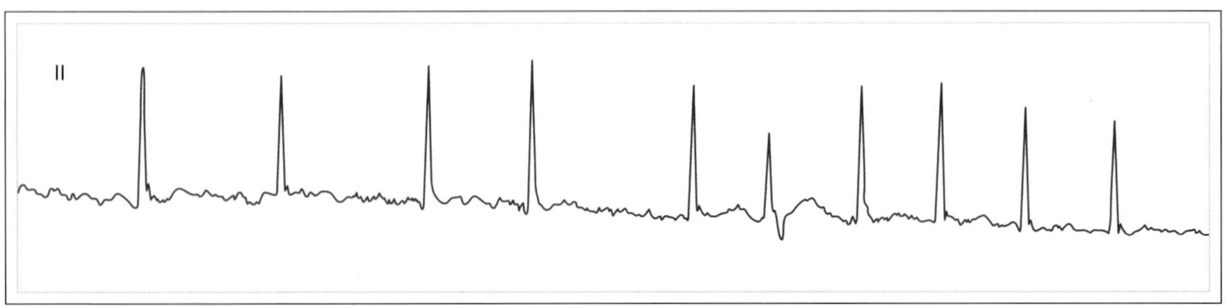


**Fig. 59.3 Electrocardiogram showing atrial fibrillation with no clear P waves and an irregularly irregular ventricular response.** Note that the QRS complex is widened in a single beat after a relatively short R-R interval. This is the Ashman phenomenon, which occurs because the His-Purkinje system is still partly refractory to excitation.

AF is associated with unsynchronized, quivering motion of the atrial wall. As a result, there is stasis of blood in the atria and a risk for spontaneous clot formation. AF is an important cause of embolic stroke, with the embolism emanating from the left atrium or its appendage. Long-term anticoagulation with warfarin has been found to reduce the likelihood of embolic stroke, particularly in patients with risk factors, including previous stroke, valvular heart disease, hypertension, diabetes, CHF, and age older than 65 years.

In the acute setting, clot may form within 48 hours after the onset of AF. Cardioversion of AF may cause a new clot to embolize into the systemic circulation. If the patient can clearly discern when he or she is in AF, symptoms have begun within the preceding 1 to 2 days, and the patient is not at high risk for stroke, it is generally safe to perform cardioversion without anticoagulation.[9] However, if there is any uncertainty about the time of onset of the tachydysrhythmia or if it occurred more than 48 hours ago, the patient should not undergo immediate cardioversion. Instead, the cardiology service should be consulted and transesophageal echocardiography performed to search for atrial clot formation, or cardioversion should be deferred until adequate anticoagulation has been established.[10] The only exception would be cardiovascular instability secondary to AF, which requires emergency DCCV. Continuation of anticoagulation should also be considered for 4 weeks after cardioversion because there may be some delay in return of normal atrial contraction.

The disposition of patients with AF depends on a number of factors, including age, comorbid illnesses and social and outpatient medical support, adequacy of control of the ventricular rate, plans for cardioversion, and the state of anticoagulation.[11] If the patient requires ongoing adjustment of medications to control a rapid ventricular response, attempted cardioversion is planned, or new anticoagulation is initiated, hospitalization should be considered. The EP should make this decision in concert with the patient and the consulting cardiologist.

MULTIFOCAL ATRIAL TACHYCARDIA Multifocal AT (MFAT) is a relatively uncommon tachydysrhythmia that primarily affects older patients with chronic lung diseases such as chronic obstructive pulmonary disease, and it appears to be related to the administration of methylxanthine.[12] Its mechanism is uncertain, but MFAT is thought to occur as a result of DADs in atrial tissue triggering ectopic beats. The diagnosis is made on the basis of the following ECG criteria: at least three consecutive P waves with different morphologies, variable P-P and PR intervals, and a heart rate greater than 100 beats/min. Treatment of MFAT is centered on treating the underlying pulmonary disease and possible hypoxia. Antidysrhythmic agents are poorly effective in slowing the atrial rate or the ventricular response or in terminating MFAT. Nevertheless, a carefully administered trial of a calcium channel blocker or amiodarone is reasonable. Generally, beta-blockers should be avoided in patients with any evidence of bronchospasm. Magnesium therapy, particularly in combination with potassium replacement, may slow the rate or terminate the tachydysrhythmia. Patients usually require admission to treat the pulmonary disease.

### *Regular Supraventricular Tachycardias*

SINUS TACHYCARDIA Sinus tachycardia may be due to a wide variety of physiologic, pathologic, or pharmacologic causes. If necessary, treatment is usually directed toward the underlying cause. In some settings, such as CHF or acute myocardial infarction (MI), treatment of sinus tachycardia with beta-blockers may improve cardiac hemodynamics and outcome. Sinus tachycardia is often part of the differential diagnosis of other regular tachydysrhythmias. Identifying characteristics of sinus tachycardia are (1) regularly occurring identical P waves with a leftward inferior axis in the frontal plane and (2) gradual onset and offset of the tachycardiac rate.

ATRIAL FLUTTER Atrial flutter can occur as a result of a variety of cardiopulmonary and metabolic derangements, often in association with atrial dilation. Patients with atrial flutter also tend to experience AF, but atrial flutter is less common overall. The mechanism of atrial flutter is a macroreentrant circuit in the right atrium (see Fig. 59.1, *A*). The most common variant of atrial flutter is termed typical atrial flutter and involves a counterclockwise wave of roughly circular excitation when viewed from a position facing the front of the patient. The flutter pathway is constrained in the inferior portion of the circular loop by anatomic structures, and it travels between the tricuspid annulus anteriorly and the inferior vena cava and coronary sinus posteriorly. This segment of the pathway, the isthmus, contains the relatively slower-conducting tissue in the reentrant loop. Atypical atrial flutter most commonly travels over the same pathway, but in the opposite direction.

The rate of atrial flutter waves ranges from 250 to 350 beats/min. The diagnosis is made from the ECG tracing, which demonstrates typical sawtooth-shaped flutter waves at the appropriate rate, generally most prominent in the inferior limb leads (II, III, and aVF) and lead $V_1$. The flutter waves tend to be identical and to recur regularly, and there is no isoelectric or flat ECG segment between the waves (**Figs. 59.4 and 59.5**). As in AF, the refractory period of the AV node usually controls the ventricular response to atrial flutter. The

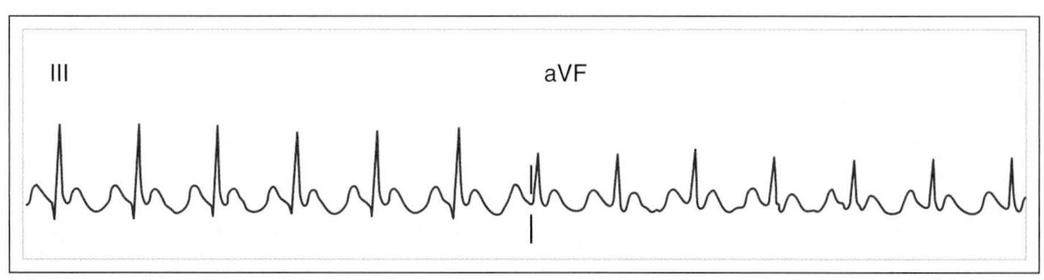


**Fig. 59.4 Electrocardiogram showing atrial flutter with 2:1 conduction and a regular ventricular rate of 150 beats/min.**

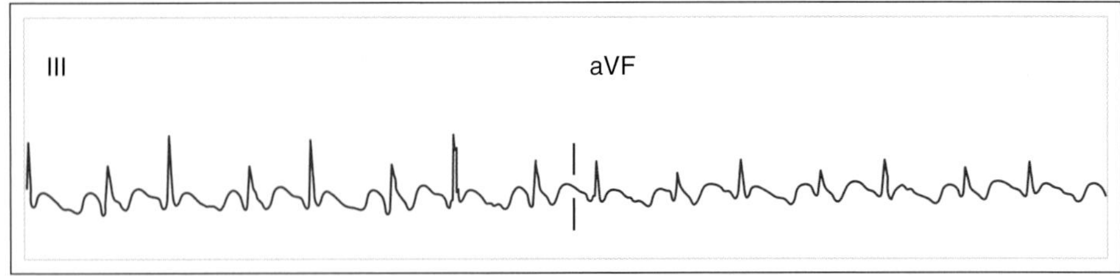


**Fig. 59.5 Electrocardiogram showing atrial flutter at approximately 260 beats/min with regularly irregular 3:2 conduction (3 flutter waves per 2 QRS complexes).** Note the variable flutter-to–QRS conduction interval (Wenckebach pattern) and alternating QRS complex morphology. These findings suggest that the heart rate is on the cusp of the refractory period of both the atrioventricular node and the His-Purkinje system.

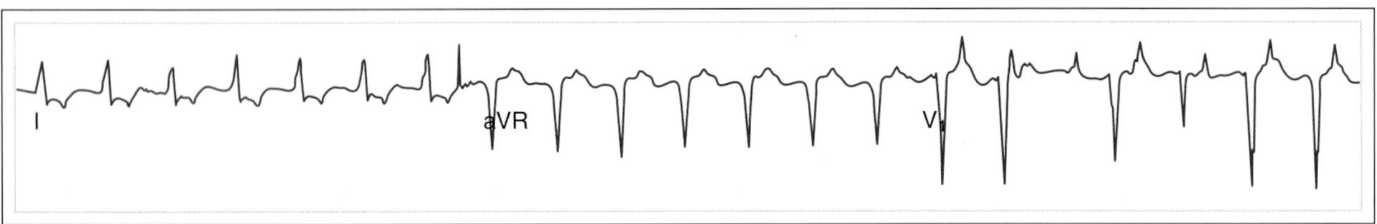


**Fig. 59.6 Electrocardiogram showing atrial tachycardia at a rate of 163 beats/min with a first-degree heart block and mostly 1:1 atrioventricular (AV) conduction with a single nonconducted beat (see lead $V_1$).** The abnormal rightward P-wave axis in lead I is not consistent with sinus rhythm. The rhythm is too slow for atrial flutter, and dropped beats would not be expected with a reentrant rhythm involving the AV node and ventricles.

most common response is 2:1 AV conduction; however, higher, lower, or variable ratios of conduction are also possible. The ratio of conduction depends on the atrial flutter rate, the health of the AV node, and any modifying physiologic, metabolic, or pharmacologic factors. Because atrial flutter is most commonly manifested as flutter waves at 300 beats/min, 2:1 AV conduction, and a ventricular response rate of 150 beats/min, atrial flutter should be the first diagnosis considered in all patients with a regular tachycardia at 150 beats/min. It is important to remember, however, that pharmacologic agents can slow the rate of atrial flutter and decrease or increase AV nodal conduction, thereby altering the usual characteristics.

Management of atrial flutter is similar to that for AF but can be a bit more difficult. Agents that lengthen the refractory period of the AV node tend to gradually decrease the ventricular response rate to AF. In the setting of atrial flutter, the decrease in the ventricular response rate with the same agents may be stepwise and incremental and thus more difficult to control. Furthermore, concomitant slowing of the atrial flutter waves may paradoxically allow greater efficiency of AV nodal conduction. For example, slowing flutter from 280 to 180 beats/min could lead to augmentation of the ventricular response from 2:1 conduction at 140 beats/min to 1:1 conduction at 180 beats/min.

Control of the ventricular rate in patients with atrial flutter can usually be achieved with a calcium channel antagonist such as diltiazem, a beta-blocker, or digoxin. Both electrical cardioversion and chemical cardioversion have a high success rate. Synchronized DCCV should start at 50 J, and the shock should be repeated with higher energy if the first is ineffective. Chemical cardioversion can be achieved with a variety of agents, including class III antidysrhythmics such as ibutilide and amiodarone, class I agents such as procainamide, and the beta-blocker esmolol. Rate control should generally be achieved before attempted chemical cardioversion. These agents can slow the atrial flutter rate with adverse enhancement of the conduction ratio as previously described, or in the case of procainamide or quinidine, the agent's vagolytic properties may independently enhance AV nodal conduction.

Cardioversion of atrial flutter is associated with thromboembolism, although the association is probably weaker than that with cardioversion of AF.[10] For this reason, cardioversion of atrial flutter should probably not be undertaken in the ED unless the indication is an emergency because of cardiovascular instability, the combined duration of atrial flutter and AF is less than 48 hours, the patient has been adequately anticoagulated before arrival in the ED, or the patient is newly anticoagulated without evidence of atrial thrombi on transesophageal echocardiography. The decision to hospitalize patients with atrial flutter involves weighing issues similar to those described for AF.

ATRIAL TACHYCARDIA Regular AT is a relatively uncommon tachydysrhythmia. It may be due to cardiopulmonary disease with dilated atria and a reentrant mechanism; toxicity from digoxin, methylxanthines, or adrenergic agents with increased automaticity; or other causes. AT is distinguished from atrial flutter by separate identifiable P waves with an intervening isoelectric baseline and a rate lower than 200 beats/min (**Fig. 59.6**). Sometimes the P waves have an abnormal upward or rightward axis, or the onset of tachycardia is abrupt. These characteristics would distinguish the rhythm from sinus tachycardia. Finally, as discussed later, unlike reentrant atrial rhythms that involve the AV node, AT would not be expected to terminate with agents that slow AV nodal conduction. As with atrial flutter, decreasing AV nodal conduction

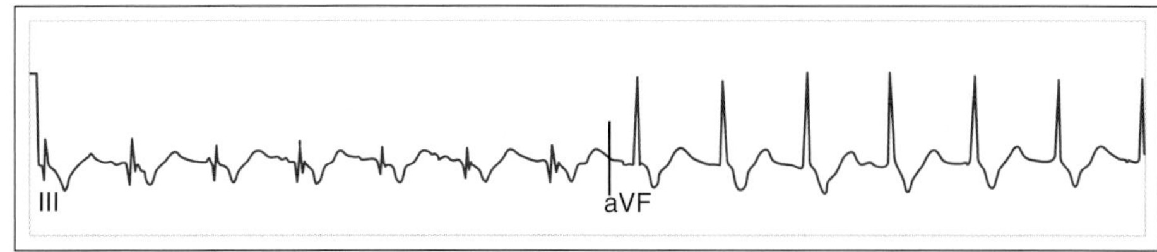


**Fig. 59.7 Electrocardiogram showing atrioventricular reentrant tachycardia (AVRT) with retrograde P waves (inverted in the inferior leads) following the QRS complexes.** This strip demonstrates the more common orthodromic conduction variant of AVRT. The ventricles are depolarized normally, and then the signal travels up through the bypass tract to depolarize the atria from bottom to top.

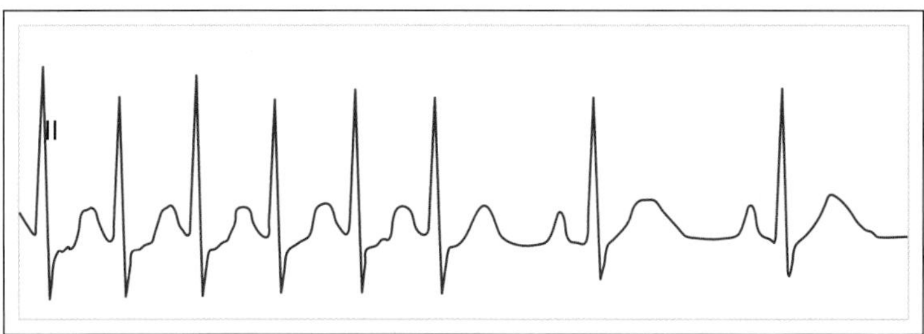


**Fig. 59.8 Electrocardiogram showing atrioventricular nodal reentrant tachycardia at 180 beats/min with spontaneous termination to normal sinus rhythm.** During tachycardia, retrograde atrial depolarization occurs simultaneously with ventricular depolarization. Thus, retrograde P waves are buried within the QRS complexes.

dynamics might slow the ventricular response to the rhythm and facilitate the diagnosis. It would not generally terminate the rhythm because the origin of the tachycardia is contained entirely within the atria.

Treatment of AT begins with assessment of the underlying causes. Digoxin toxicity should be suspected if AT is accompanied by high-grade AV block. Tachycardia in patients with digoxin toxicity results from altered intracellular calcium dynamics and increased excitability, whereas high-grade AV block results from enhanced vagal tone. When there is no evidence of underlying toxicity, ventricular rate control and electrical or chemical cardioversion for AT should be approached as for AF and flutter. If the patient shows evidence of drug toxicity or uncontrolled pulmonary disease or has new tachycardia, admission for further treatment should be considered.

REENTRANT SUPRAVENTRICULAR TACHYCARDIA The nomenclature of reentrant SVTs can be confusing. They are often termed paroxysmal because of their abrupt onset, or they may simply be called SVT. More precisely, they consist of two major subtypes of SVT, AV reentrant tachycardia (AVRT) and AV nodal reentrant tachycardia (AVNRT). Reentrant SVTs are moderately common in both children and adults and most frequently are not associated with other cardiopulmonary disease.

Mechanistically, the two major subtypes of reentrant SVT are distinguished by the route of the reentrant pathway. AVRT uses a macroreentrant circuit with atrial and ventricular segments and connecting segments that involve the AV node and an accessory conducting tract, or rarely, two accessory conducting tracts (see Fig. 59.2, *B* and *C*). The AV nodal segment usually serves as the necessary slow-conducting portion of the reentrant circuit.

Many patients have at least two discrete segments that can conduct the input wave of excitability from the right atrium into the AV node. The conducting properties of these inputs may differ, and frequently both a fast-conducting input or pathway and a relatively slow-conducting one are present. Usually, conduction to the AV node is via the fast pathway. AVNRT uses a small macroreentrant circuit consisting of the AV node, right atrial tissue, and connecting fast and slow pathway segments to form a full circle of conduction (see Fig. 59.2, *A*).

Within each subtype of reentrant SVT, the direction of the wave of excitation can vary. In AVRT, the wave of excitation most commonly proceeds down the AV node and normally through the His-Purkinje system, and it returns in a retrograde direction up the accessory tract to the atria to complete the circuit; this pathway is termed orthodromic conduction (see Fig. 59.2, *B*). Antidromic conduction occurs when the wave of excitation proceeds in the opposite direction, down the accessory pathway, and returns in retrograde fashion up the AV node (see Fig. 59.2, *C*). In this case, conduction down the His-Purkinje system and normal, nearly simultaneous excitation of the ventricles do not occur. Rather, the ventricles are activated from the terminus of the accessory tract, and the wave of excitation must propagate across the ventricular myocardium similar to excitation from a premature ventricular contraction (PVC). Consequently, it takes longer to excite the entire ventricular muscle mass, and the corresponding QRS wave is widened with antidromic conduction.

Reentrant SVTs are usually easily diagnosed from the ECG. The most common finding is a narrow QRS complex tachycardia at rate of 120 to 250 beats/min. The atria are activated in a retrograde direction from the AV node or an accessory tract. In AVRT, retrograde P waves that are inverted in $V_1$ and the inferior leads may be observed just after the QRS complex (**Fig. 59.7**). In AVNRT, retrograde excitation of the atria is often simultaneous with ventricular excitation, and retrograde P waves are not observed because they are hidden or buried within the QRS complex (**Fig. 59.8**). In this case, P waves appear to be absent.

Reentrant SVT may be manifested as a wide QRS complex primarily for two reasons. Normal rapid conduction down the His-Purkinje system leads to nearly simultaneous excitation and depolarization of the ventricular myocardium and a narrow QRS complex on the ECG. If the left or right bundle of the Purkinje system fails to conduct, the QRS complex is widened and displays bundle branch block (BBB) morphology (see Fig. 59.2, *F*). This can occur as a result of intrinsic conduction system disease and chronic BBB, or the failure may be rate dependent and occur only during tachycardia. The other reason for a widened QRS complex is AVRT with antidromic conduction antegrade down the accessory pathway (see Fig. 59.2, *C*). This path does not use the His-Purkinje system, and a widened QRS complex without typical BBB morphology would be expected.

Particularly in children, reentrant SVTs are usually well tolerated. Patients with more rapid heart rates are more prone to cardiovascular instability, including hypotension and presyncope. Patients may also feel palpitations, dyspnea, and chest pain, which can be due to myocardial ischemia.

From an ED perspective, it is not usually important to distinguish AVRT from AVNRT. The acute treatment and prognosis for the two conditions are the same. Vagal maneuvers[13] should be attempted or drugs administered to slow conduction and increase the refractory period through the AV nodal tissue so that the node is refractory to excitation and conduction when the reentrant wave approaches it. Agents such as adenosine and calcium channel blockers act directly on the nodal tissue, whereas other interventions, such as vagal maneuvers, digoxin, and beta-blockers, may alter vagal or adrenergic tone (**Box 59.2**). Adenosine may be the optimal agent because it is highly effective and safe with an ultrashort (9-second) half-life in serum. Rapid clearing, however, can be a disadvantage if the tachydysrhythmia is recurrent. In this case, the calcium channel blocker verapamil may be useful because it is equally effective for termination and may prevent recurrent episodes.[14] Verapamil should not be used in infants, however, because of the risk for cardiovascular collapse.[15]

Physiologic maneuvers that increase vagal tone, such as immersion of the face in iced water, massage of the carotid bulb, and the Valsalva maneuver, may also be effective but have the same potential disadvantage of recurrence of the tachycardia. Iced water immersion may be more effective and better tolerated in children. Carotid massage should not be attempted in adults until a carotid bruit has been ruled out by auscultation. As for other supraventricular tachydysrhythmias, synchronized DCCV should be reserved for patients who demonstrate cardiovascular instability. Most patients can be discharged home after termination of reentrant SVT. Hospitalization should be considered for those whose tachydysrhythmia is recurrent or associated with cardiovascular instability.

**BOX 59.2 Treatment of Reentrant Supraventricular Tachycardia**

| Medications | Physiologic |
|---|---|
| Adenosine | Vagal maneuvers: |
| Verapamil, diltiazem | Valsalva maneuver |
| Metoprolol | Carotid massage |
| Procainamide | Iced water immersion |
| Amiodarone | **Electrical Treatment** |
| Digoxin | Synchronized cardioversion |

PREEXCITATION (WOLFF-PARKINSON-WHITE) SYNDROME When a patient has an accessory pathway of myocardial fiber connecting the atria and ventricles with evidence of antegrade conduction down this pathway, the patient has preexcitation, or WPW, syndrome. The syndrome is uncommon, is usually diagnosed in children or young adults, and is most commonly not associated with other cardiopulmonary disease. Patients may be in normal sinus rhythm or have a variety of supraventricular tachydysrhythmias, including AVRT in 80% of cases, AF in 15% to 30%, and atrial flutter in 5%. Approximately 85% of AVRT episodes have an orthodromic direction of activation, and 15% are antidromic.

The diagnosis can be made while the patient is in normal sinus rhythm if the following characteristics are observed on the ECG: (1) shortened PR interval (<120 msec), (2) widened QRS complex beyond 120 msec, and (3) atypical initiation of the QRS complex with a delta-wave morphology (**Fig. 59.9**). Associated ST-T wave abnormalities are often present, with the T wave inverted with respect to the delta wave and QRS complex. These three diagnostic abnormalities are easily understood from an electrophysiologic perspective (see Fig. 59.2, *D*).

In normal sinus rhythm, the wave of excitation can propagate down both the AV node and the accessory pathway. Because the accessory pathway does not contain slow-conducting tissue, the wave traverses the accessory pathway and reaches the ventricular myocardium before traversing the AV node. The shortened PR interval and early delta wave upstroke of the QRS wave are due to preexcitation of the

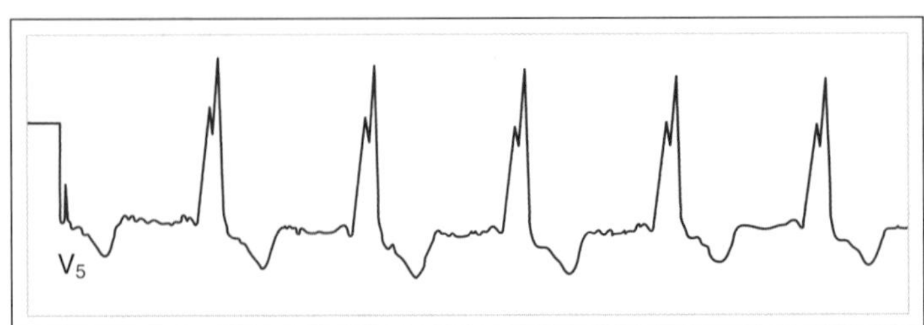


**Fig. 59.9 Electrocardiogram showing Wolff-Parkinson-White (WPW) syndrome with normal sinus rhythm.** Note the shortened PR interval, widened QRS wave with slurred upstroke, and abnormal inverted T wave. These findings in lead $V_5$ are diagnostic of WPW syndrome with an accessory conduction tract, probably in the left lateral position.

ventricle via the accessory pathway. Eventually, the atrial excitation wave also traverses the AV node, and once this occurs, it will move rapidly through the specialized rapid-conducting His-Purkinje system. In the meantime, the wave that has traversed the accessory pathway propagates slowly through the ventricular myocardium because it does not use the Purkinje fibers for rapid transmission. Consequently, the QRS deflection arrives early with a delta wave, but the latter portion normalizes as a result of the influence of normal AV nodal conduction. Because of the atypical pattern of ventricular depolarization, repolarization changes in the form of ST-T abnormalities are expected.

Patients with WPW syndrome are predisposed to AVRT, as well as to AF and atrial flutter, which often demonstrates a rapid ventricular response. The pathway of conduction of the AF wavelets from the atria to the ventricles depends on the relative refractory period of the accessory pathway with respect to the AV node. The slow-conducting cells of the AV node have a long refractory period, and the refractory period of the accessory conducting tissue is usually shorter. Consequently, the AV node remains refractory when the accessory pathway tissue is repolarized and ready for conduction. In WPW syndrome, AF usually conducts down the accessory pathway with a rapid ventricular response rate that is determined by the refractory period of the accessory conducting tissue (**Fig. 59.10**; also see Fig. 59.2, *E*). Similar to the situation with normal sinus rhythm, the ventricles are activated from the ectopic accessory pathway terminus, and an irregularly irregular tachycardia with a wide QRS complex results.

Perhaps the greatest concern regarding patients with WPW syndrome is their higher risk for sudden cardiac death. This risk is inversely associated with the minimum refractory period of the accessory conducting tissue.[2] The mechanism of sudden cardiac death is thought to most commonly be AF with accessory tract conduction and a dangerously high ventricular response rate that causes ischemia and electrical instability and degenerates to VF.

It is important to remember that like the AV node and other cardiac tissue, accessory pathways have dynamic electrophysiologic properties that may vary with the hormonal, physiologic, or pharmacologic milieu. However, in this respect, accessory pathway tissue behaves more like myocardium and less like AV nodal tissue, which is highly sensitive to vagal stimulation. Depending on the current milieu, conduction in many patients with WPW syndrome may variably occur primarily down the accessory pathway or the AV node in normal sinus rhythm, and this variation even occasionally occurs in AF (**Fig. 59.11**).

Treatment of AF with rapid ventricular response in patients with WPW syndrome must be approached differently. The usual treatment of AF is to administer agents that increase the refractory period of the AV node and slow AV nodal conduction. Because conduction is primarily down the accessory pathway in WPW syndrome, treatment must be directed toward lengthening the refractory period of the accessory pathway tissue, not the AV node. Paradoxically, agents that block AV nodal conduction, such as beta-blockers, calcium channel blockers, adenosine, and digoxin, may also cause vasodilation, decrease contractility, or have other effects that reflexively increase adrenergic tone or stimulate and enhance accessory pathway conduction. For this reason, these agents should not be used.

The preferred pharmacologic agents for patients with WPW syndrome and AF with a rapid ventricular response are the class IA antidysrhythmic agent procainamide[16] and, possibly, class III medications such as amiodarone and sotalol. These antidysrhythmics are used to decrease the ventricular response rate, and they may also terminate AF. Nevertheless, they have multiple potential dangers and must be used with caution. All these antidysrhythmic agents can decrease blood pressure. When administered intravenously, amiodarone blocks AV nodal conduction, so the concerns already described with other AV nodal blocking agents may be applicable.[17] The safest and most effective treatment for patients with WPW

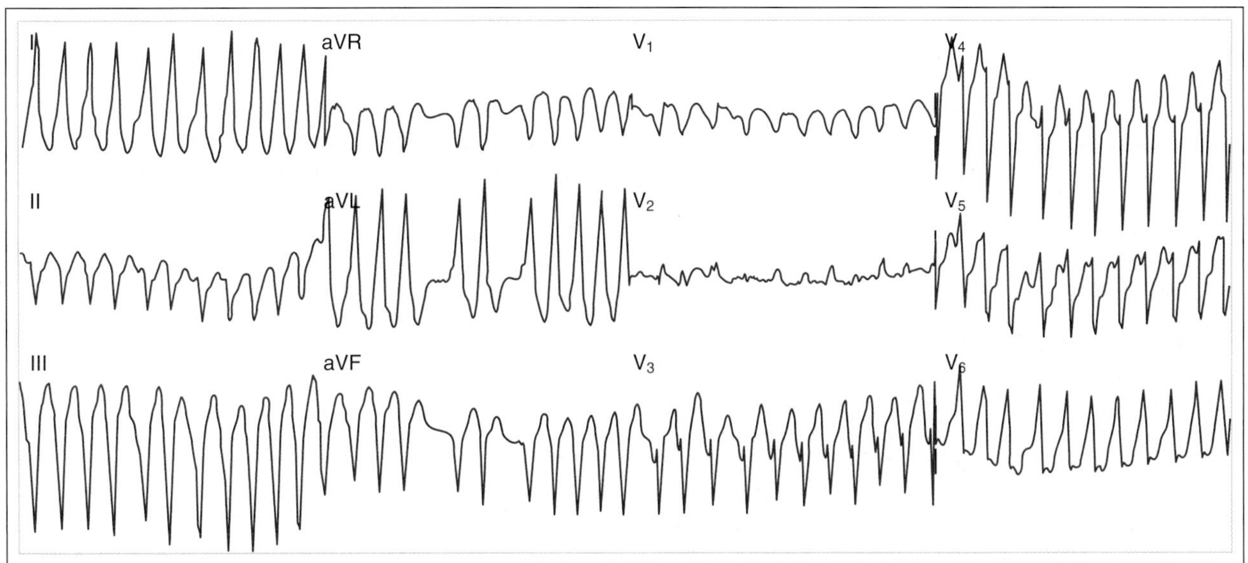


**Fig. 59.10 Electrocardiogram showing atrial fibrillation with wide QRS complexes and a rapid variable ventricular response rate consistent with Wolff-Parkinson-White syndrome.** The grossly irregularly irregular rhythm distinguishes this condition from ventricular tachycardia. This is a dangerous condition that requires immediate attention and treatment. The risk for conversion to ventricular fibrillation and cardiovascular collapse is inversely associated with the length of the shortest R-R interval.

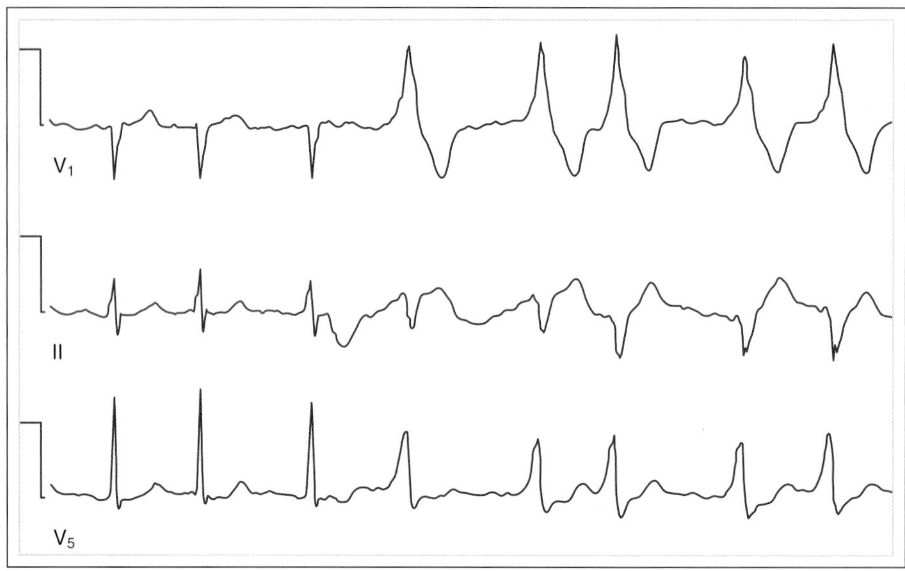


**Fig. 59.11 Electrocardiogram showing atrial fibrillation in a patient with Wolff-Parkinson-White syndrome and variable conduction down the atrioventricular node and His-Purkinje system with a resulting narrow QRS complex, as well as down the accessory pathway with a slurred upstroke, wide QRS complex.** The slow ventricular response rate suggests that this accessory pathway has a relatively long refractory period and a more benign prognosis.

syndrome and AF with a rapid ventricular response is synchronized DCCV. The EP should consider using DCCV with sedation before administering antidysrhythmics to patients with a ventricular response greater than 150 beats/min or borderline low blood pressure.

For patients with WPW syndrome, the principles of treatment of AVRT are similar to those for AF. AV nodal blocking agents should not be used to treat presumed antidromic wide QRS complex AVRT because the underlying rhythm could be misdiagnosed as atrial flutter or tachycardia with accessory pathway conduction. AV nodal blocking agents could be used to treat orthodromic AVRT with a narrow QRS complex, but subsequent AF with rapid accessory pathway conduction remains a potential concern. It may be wiser to use the class IA or class III antidysrhythmics described previously or to proceed directly to DCCV.

Patients with WPW syndrome and rapid antegrade bypass tract conduction are at higher risk than other patients with SVT for cardiovascular decompensation. In particular, patients with recurrent unstable tachycardias should be admitted to the hospital. Nevertheless, the decision to admit or discharge most patients should be made individually in consultation with the cardiologist.

JUNCTIONAL TACHYCARDIA Junctional tachycardia is an uncommon dysrhythmia associated with toxic stimulation of the AV node by digoxin, methylxanthines, or other stimulants or with cardiac disease such as inferior MI, acute rheumatic fever, or myocarditis. The most common mechanism is enhanced automaticity of the nodal tissue. The heart sounds are usually regular. In patients with simultaneous antegrade ventricular and retrograde atrial activation, the right atrium may contract against a closed tricuspid valve and thereby lead to large cannon jugular venous waves. The ECG appearance is a narrow complex tachycardia up to a rate of approximately 130 beats/min without synchronous preceding P waves. P waves may be present with evidence of AV dissociation. Alternatively, retrograde nodal-to-atrial conduction with abnormal P waves and a superior axis occurring after the QRS deflection may be seen. P waves may be absent if atrial depolarization occurs simultaneously with ventricular depolarization.

Digoxin toxicity is an important cause of junctional tachycardia. In particular, digoxin toxicity should be suspected when the rapid ventricular response to AF becomes regular during digoxin treatment. Diagnosis and treatment should focus on identifying and addressing the underlying cause, including reversal of toxicity, if any. Digoxin immune Fab fragments (Digibind) may be necessary for the cardiovascular instability associated with digoxin toxicity, and DCCV should be avoided if possible. Most patients require admission until the underlying disease or toxicity is resolved.

## VENTRICULAR TACHYCARDIAS

### *Premature Ventricular Contractions and Nonsustained Ventricular Tachycardia*

PVCs are common. They can occur chronically with no associated cardiac disease or can develop in association with acute cardiopulmonary or metabolic derangements. Some specific causes include:

- Cardiac ischemia, which may be due to local coronary artery disease or systemic hypoxia
- Heart failure with increased myocardial stretching
- Inflamed myocardium
- Electrolyte imbalance
- A vast array of medications and toxins

There is a spectrum of frequency of ventricular ectopy. PVCs may occur singly in isolation, or a PVC may occur every second or third beat, an arrhythmia termed bigeminy or trigeminy, respectively. Three or more ventricular beats in a row at a rate greater than 100 beats/min is defined as VT. If the consecutive ventricular beats resolve spontaneously or terminate within 30 seconds, the VT is nonsustained (NSVT).

All the major dysrhythmic mechanisms described, including enhanced automaticity, triggered beats, and reentry, may be involved in the development of PVCs and NSVT. Irregular cardiac contractions interspersed with a regular rhythm can be heard on cardiac auscultation or felt on examination of the pulse. However, the diagnosis is usually made by examining the ECG tracing. The QRS deflections are wide because the ectopic ventricular beats generally do not use the specialized Purkinje conduction system, and the T wave is usually large and inverted with respect to the QRS complex. No premature P wave precedes the ventricular beat, but there may be a visible or hidden inverted retrograde P wave following it. Patients may be asymptomatic, or they may feel palpitations and discomfort from the ectopic beats. If the frequency of ectopic ventricular beats or the rate of NSVT is sufficiently high, hemodynamic compromise with hypotension, presyncope, or CHF may be present.

Chronic ventricular ectopy does not generally require emergency treatment, and suppression of chronic ventricular ectopy after MI does not lower the mortality.[18] Patients with chronic PVCs may be at variably higher risk for sudden death, depending on other clinical factors, but even so, it is often unclear whether the increased risk is directly attributable to the ectopy or to the underlying cardiac disease. EPs must commonly manage new ventricular ectopy in association with acute MI or other severe systemic disease. The greatest concern is that PVCs may induce sustained VT or VF. Theoretically, this could occur if the ectopic ventricular depolarization occurs during the vulnerable period or upstroke of the T wave of the preceding beat (R-on-T phenomenon).

The risk for VF and sudden death is elevated during acute MI, but this risk is not decreased with routine suppressive class I antidysrhythmic therapy.[19] Conversely, beta-blockade with metoprolol may not affect the occurrence of PVCs or NSVT but does lower the rate of VF and death.[20] Suppression of new ventricular ectopy should be considered if the PVCs or tachydysrhythmias are symptomatic and contributing to hemodynamic instability or the patient has already experienced sustained VT or VF. The first priority is to search for reversible causes of ventricular ectopy, such as hypoxia; potassium, magnesium, or other electrolyte imbalance; or drug toxicity. After reversible causes are addressed, the most commonly used agents include beta-blockers, amiodarone, lidocaine, and procainamide. The class I effect of myocardial sodium channel blockade may be particularly prominent for lidocaine in an ischemic and acidotic local cellular environment. Evidence suggests that amiodarone may be effective when lidocaine fails.[21] The antidysrhythmics should be given as a loading dose followed by a sustained infusion, and the patient should be monitored closely for adverse effects and admitted to a cardiac care unit.

### *Monomorphic Ventricular Tachycardia*

VT is considered sustained if it is continuous for at least 30 seconds. If the QRS complex has primarily a single morphology, the VT is monomorphic, whereas if the QRS complex varies, the VT is polymorphic. Monomorphic VT is an uncommon condition that underlies the chief complaint in approximately 1 in every 10,000 ED visits. The mechanism in the majority of cases is reentry within the ventricular myocardium, where the slow-conducting segment of the reentrant loop is associated with a scar from a previous MI (see Fig. 59.1, *B*). The scar tissue serves to enable and fix the location of the VT circuit within the myocardium. Other causes of monomorphic VT that are less commonly encountered in the ED are dilated cardiomyopathy, hypertrophic cardiomyopathy, previous surgical repair of congenital heart disease with a myocardial scar, arrhythmogenic right ventricular dysplasia, right ventricular outflow tract VT, and fascicular tachycardia.

Patients with VT may experience palpitations, lightheadedness, chest discomfort, dyspnea, or more progressive cardiovascular compromise. The heart sounds and pulse are regular and rapid. Approximately half the patients have separate atrial activity with AV dissociation, evidence of which can occasionally be detected on physical examination as variable intensity of the first heart sound or arterial or jugular venous pulsations. The ECG tracing demonstrates a regular wide QRS complex tachycardia without preceding P waves. Nonetheless, it can be difficult to differentiate VT from SVT with a wide QRS complex because of aberrant or antegrade accessory pathway conduction. The next section addresses this issue specifically. Ultimately, the diagnosis can be most accurately determined when synthesizing combined information from the medical history, physical examination, and ECG.

Treatment of monomorphic VT depends on the patient's cardiovascular status. The patient's condition can be categorized as pulseless, unstable, or stable. Pulseless VT should receive the same treatment as VF: immediate chest compressions and initial shock using unsynchronized 200 J with a biphasic or monophasic waveform as soon as defibrillation is available.

Patients are unstable if they have a pulse but also symptoms of lightheadedness, chest pain, dyspnea, other signs of inadequate perfusion of vital organs, or frank hypotension. Patients with unstable VT should undergo cardioversion using synchronized 100 J with a biphasic or monophasic waveform. An awake patient should receive presedation as long as it would not significantly delay DCCV.

Patients with stable VT may initially be treated with medical or electrical therapy. The primary principle of treatment with class I or III antidysrhythmic agents is to prolong the refractory period of the ventricular myocardium so that the cells remain refractory when the reentrant wave of excitation returns. Amiodarone is recommended by the American Heart Association, and procainamide and sotalol can be used as alternatives when cardiac output seems to be clinically preserved. Lidocaine is no longer recommended for this purpose. Unfortunately, neither amiodarone nor lidocaine immediately increases the refractory period of normal myocardium after intravenous administration. Both are unlikely to terminate VT within 20 minutes of treatment.[22] However, amiodarone may become more effective in both terminating and preventing VT over the ensuing hours after administration.[21] Procainamide and racemic sotalol do prolong the refractory period soon after administration and are more likely to terminate VT. However, procainamide blocks cardiac sodium channels, and the *l* isomer of sotalol is a beta-blocker; thus, both agents can cause a decrease in cardiac contractility and subsequent hemodynamic instability. Intravenous sotalol is not currently available in the United States. Other agents that have been used in this situation are pure beta-blockers and magnesium. Neither has been proved to be effective, however, and pure beta-blockers may cause hypotension.

The safest and most effective treatment of stable monomorphic VT remains DCCV. Initial DCCV should be particularly considered in patients with ventricular rates greater than 150 beats/min because they are at higher risk for compromised cardiac output and hemodynamic collapse. Cardioversion using synchronized 100 J with a biphasic or monophasic waveform should be performed after appropriate sedation. If the patient already has an internal implantable cardioverter-defibrillator (ICD), overdrive pacing or synchronized cardioversion may be performed by the device automatically or manually at the bedside by the electrophysiologist. Suppressive treatment with antidysrhythmic agents should be considered if the VT is recurrent. Over a period of hours, intravenous amiodarone or procainamide is likely to be the most effective of the agents currently available in the United States. If procainamide is used, it should be loaded slowly over a period of approximately 1 hour and the patient monitored closely for hypotension. Generally, infusion of multiple antidysrhythmics should be avoided because it might increase the likelihood of adverse effects. Most patients with monomorphic VT should be admitted for observation and further treatment.

**BOX 59.3 Diagnosing Regular Wide QRS Complex Tachycardia: Predictors Suggestive of Ventricular Tachycardia**

**Past Medical History**

Previous ventricular tachycardia
Previous myocardial infarction
Age > 35 years
Male sex

**Physical Findings**

Variable first heart sound or jugular venous pulsation

**Electrocardiographic Findings**

Frontal axis −90 to −180 degrees
QRS interval > 140 msec (right bundle branch block) or >160 msec (left bundle branch block) or RS interval > 100 msec
Positive or negative concordance across the precordial leads
Wide QRS morphology grossly different from the QRS morphology in sinus rhythm
Atrioventricular dissociation (including fusion or capture beats)

**Findings on Diagnostic Intervention**

No response to a 12-mg bolus of adenosine

WIDE QRS COMPLEX TACHYCARDIA: DIFFERENTIATING SUPRAVENTRICULAR FROM VENTRICULAR TACHYCARDIA Wide QRS complex tachycardia may be due to an SVT with aberrant His-Purkinje conduction or antegrade conduction down an accessory pathway or be due to VT. Diagnosis of the underlying mechanism is important for a number of reasons. The optimal short- and long-term treatment and prognosis may vary considerably, depending on the mechanism involved. The history, physical examination, and ECG findings can be used to make the diagnosis (**Box 59.3**). In the ED, the pretest probability favors VT by a ratio of 2 : 1 to 3 : 1.

No single historical factor has been found to be both sensitive and specific for diagnosing VT. Nevertheless, age older than 35 years and male sex are sensitive for VT, and a previous history of MI or coronary artery bypass graft surgery, recent angina, or CHF is a specific predictor of VT.[23] The primary underlying theme for all these predictors is a greater likelihood of coronary artery disease and previous infarction with scar formation. In fact, the strongest single historical predictor of VT is a history of MI, which has a positive likelihood ratio of 13 : 1 to 20 : 1 and a negative likelihood ratio of 0.36.[23,24]

A number of approaches may be used to diagnose wide QRS complex tachycardia from the physical examination. Perhaps the first and most important principle to remember is that apparent hemodynamic stability does not rule out VT. AV dissociation is present about half the time in patients with VT.[25] When it is present, the atria are contracting independently of the ventricles, so the atria may either contract during ventricular diastole and assist cardiac output or contract against closed valves during ventricular systole with a large retrograde venous pulsation. The EP can assess for beat-to-beat variation of the first heart sound or systolic blood pressure or for large cannon jugular venous waves. Unfortunately, even under controlled experimental conditions, none of these findings are both sensitive and specific.[26] In clinical conditions in which about half the patients have some form of retrograde ventricular-atrial conduction, these tests for physical evidence of AV dissociation can approach a sensitivity for VT of only approximately 50% at best.

Vagal maneuvers, such as carotid sinus massage or the Valsalva maneuver, can be performed to increase vagal tone and alter AV nodal conduction. Depending on the type of SVT, vagal maneuvers could terminate a reentrant rhythm involving the AV node or temporarily decrease the ventricular response to a purely atrial rhythm such as atrial flutter. Termination of wide QRS complex tachycardia with vagal maneuvers would suggest a supraventricular rhythm because most forms of VT are not responsive. Temporary slowing of the ventricular response to an atrial tachydysrhythmia could be diagnostic.

A similar principle of brief increased refractoriness of the AV node underlies the use of adenosine to diagnose and treat wide QRS complex tachycardia. The combined response to a 12-mg bolus of adenosine—either termination of the tachycardia or transient ventricular slowing—has a sensitivity of 90% and a specificity of 98% for an underlying SVT.[27] Considered in reverse fashion, "nonresponse" to a 12-mg bolus of adenosine would have a positive likelihood ratio of about 9 and a negative likelihood ratio of 0.03 for VT. This test is useful for diagnosis, but is it safe?

The primary safety concern is the administration of adenosine to patients with atrial flutter and antegrade accessory pathway conduction, which might cause subsequent transient acceleration of this conduction and the ventricular response. This and other destabilizing scenarios have been reported after the administration of adenosine to patients with wide QRS complex tachycardia secondary to SVT and VT. Adenosine should never be given to patients with a rapid, irregularly irregular wide QRS complex tachycardia because it may actually be AF with accessory pathway conduction, and acceleration of the ventricular response has been reported in this situation as well. Nonetheless, the adverse affects previously described after adenosine administration to patients with regular wide QRS complex tachycardia are rare. Multiple consecutive case series have found no greater rate of adverse effects with adenosine than with other antidysrhythmic medications.[27,28] Adenosine should be used as a diagnostic and therapeutic agent for regular wide QRS complex tachycardia when the history, physical examination, and ECG findings suggest a supraventricular origin. The EP should ensure that the adenosine is used properly—administered as a 12-mg rapid bolus dose followed immediately by a normal saline bolus flush, with a cardioverter-defibrillator immediately available in the event of destabilization.

A number of ECG findings can be used to diagnose wide QRS complex tachycardia. Possible differentiating characteristics include the heart rate, frontal axis of the QRS deflection, concordance across the precordial leads, QRS duration, morphology of the QRS complex, AV dissociation, and capture or fusion beats. On average, wide QRS complex tachycardia secondary to SVT has a faster heart rate than that secondary to VT.[25] This difference has been slightly augmented in the recent past with the use of ICDs. A patient with VT may have already received an ICD, which is preferentially programmed to treat rapid VT, usually greater than 160 to 180 beats/min. It cannot be programmed to treat slower VT because of the risk for inappropriate pacing or shocks for sinus tachycardia. Nevertheless, there is still too much overlap in the heart rate of patients with SVT and VT to use it as a firm differentiating factor. Regardless of the underlying rhythm, higher heart rates are associated with compromised cardiac output because of inadequate diastolic filling and greater electrical instability. Immediate DCCV should be considered for patients with rapid wide QRS tachycardia, regardless of the presumed etiology.

Because of the common ectopic left ventricular origin of the rhythm in VT, abnormal upward and rightward propagation of the excitation wave may be seen. In fact, the QRS axis may point to any of the four quadrants in VT, but an upward and rightward QRS axis is highly unusual for SVT. This finding, defined by a negative QRS deflection in leads I and aVF, is insensitive (24%) but highly specific (100%) for VT (**Fig. 59.12**).[29] An abnormal QRS vector that points toward or away from all of the precordial leads simultaneously is also indicative of VT. A QRS deflection that is primarily positive in all of the precordial leads is defined as positive concordance. The finding of primarily negative QRS deflections in all precordial leads is defined as negative concordance. Each of these findings is also insensitive (10%) but specific (85%) for VT.[29]

On average, the duration of initial depolarization as recorded by the QRS wave is longer with VT than with wide QRS complex SVT. A QRS duration greater than 140 msec with a right BBB (RBBB) pattern or a QRS duration greater than 160 msec with a left BBB (LBBB) pattern is insensitive but more than 90% specific for VT.[29] Brugada et al.[30] modified this concept and found that an RS interval greater than 100 msec in the precordial leads has a sensitivity of 66% and a specificity of 98% for VT (**Fig. 59.13**). Unfortunately, the high specificity of these findings is not applicable if the patient has received a medication that widens the QRS complex, such as a class I antidysrhythmic.

QRS morphology may be helpful, particularly if an old ECG is available. QRS morphology with tachycardia similar to a previous BBB morphology noted in sinus rhythm may suggest, but does not prove SVT.[31] The distinction of RBBB versus LBBB is itself not helpful, but various morphologic variants within these two categories can at least be theoretically helpful.[24,25,30]

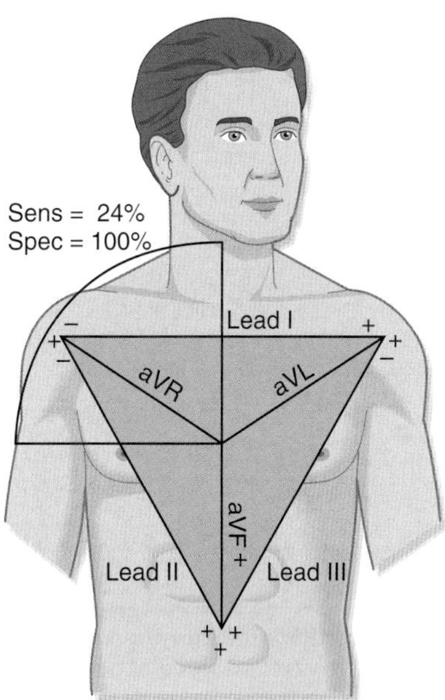


**Fig. 59.12 Diagram of the chest with the six electrocardiographic limb leads superimposed.** Depolarization of the QRS complex can be viewed as primarily positive in one of four quadrants, and the right upward quadrant is specifically identified in this diagram. Normal QRS depolarization is most commonly in the direction of the left lower quadrant. When the QRS complex points to the right upward quadrant, it is highly abnormal and suggestive of ventricular tachycardia. *Sens,* Sensitivity; Spec, specificity.

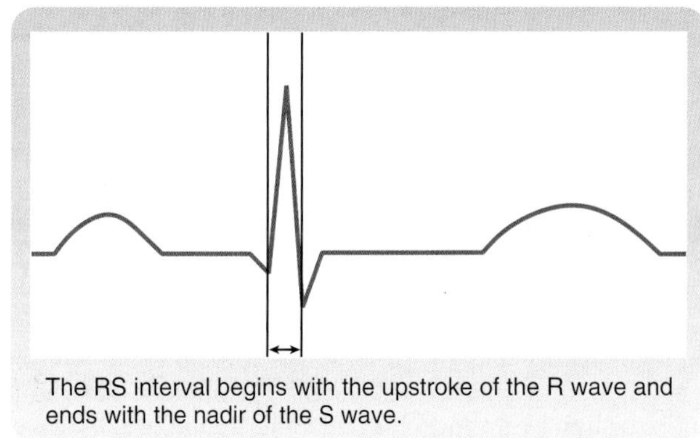


**Fig. 59.13 How to measure the RS interval *(double arrow).*** The RS interval begins with the upstroke of the R wave and ends with the nadir of the S wave.

When present, the most definitive evidence of VT is AV dissociation. In SVT an atrial contraction is associated with each ventricular beat. AV dissociation is defined by atrial activity that is separate and independent of ventricular contractions (**Fig. 59.14**). AV dissociation is present in about half of VT episodes, and it can be seen on the ECG in half of these cases, or about one quarter of all VT episodes. Thus, AV dissociation has a sensitivity of about 25% and specificity approaching 100% for VT. Dissociated P waves should be sought in the $V_1$ rhythm strip, where they are usually most

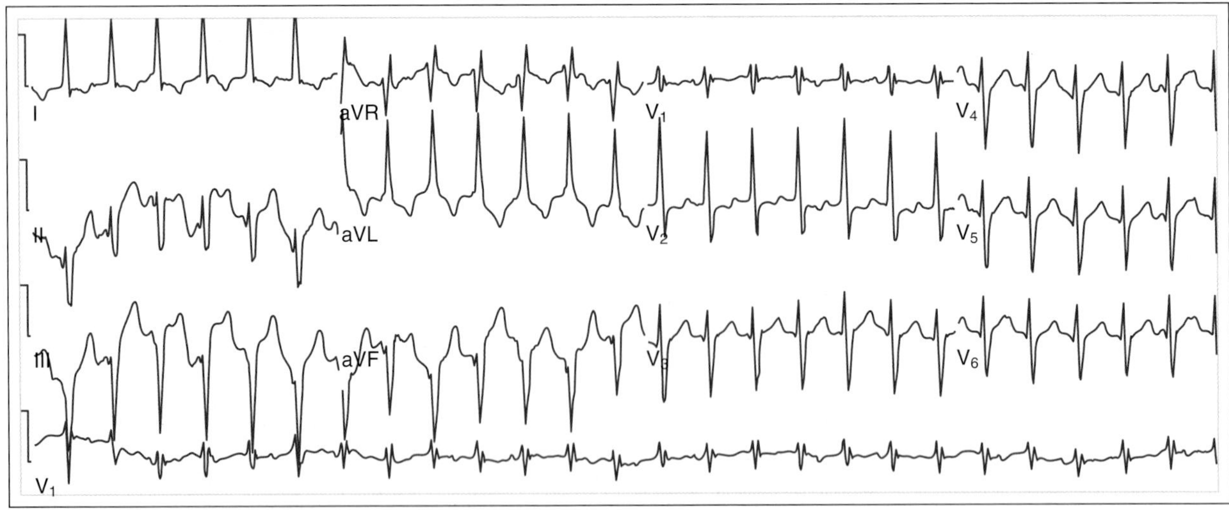


**Fig. 59.14 Electrocardiogram showing ventricular tachycardia with atrioventricular dissociation.** Although the QRS complexes are relatively narrow, there is clear evidence of atrioventricular dissociation in the $V_1$ rhythm strip.

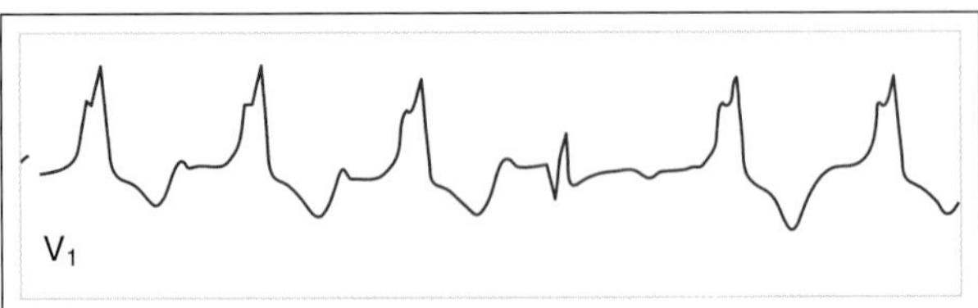


**Fig. 59.15 Electrocardiogram showing ventricular tachycardia with a single capture beat.**

easily seen. The key is to find two candidate P waves. One can then look an equal distance on each side of these two waves for a third deflection. If three consecutive deflections are found that "march out," they are probably P waves; such identification can be confirmed by marching out more on the ECG. Fusion beats represent fusion of supraventricular excitation mediated by the His-Purkinje system and local ventricular excitation. Capture beats signify complete ventricular depolarization by a supraventricular signal and usually have a narrow QRS complex. Both these phenomena also suggest AV dissociation and VT (**Figs. 59.15 and 59.16**).

Severe hyperkalemia can also cause wide QRS complex tachycardia. Clues to this diagnosis include a history of renal failure or other medical causes of hyperkalemia and an ECG with very wide and bizarre QRS complexes (**Fig. 59.17**). Once the condition is diagnosed, it should be confirmed with a serum potassium measurement and treated with intravenous calcium, insulin, glucose, and bicarbonate. Patients who overdose with cyclic antidepressants or other sodium channel blocking agents may have a wide QRS complex tachycardia. An important clue to this diagnosis on the ECG is right axis deviation of the terminal 30 msec of the QRS complex. Patients with suspected overdose should be treated with a continuous intravenous sodium bicarbonate infusion. Patients with acute respiratory distress secondary to pulmonary disease and with an underlying BBB may appear to have a primary tachydysrhythmic condition. Addressing the airway, with intubation if necessary, may slow the heart rate, expose the P waves, and clarify the rhythm.

Finally, in a significant proportion of cases it may not be possible to make a definitive ED diagnosis. In some cases of VT the bundle branches may be used as part of the reentrant limb, thereby mimicking aberrant conduction, and excitation of the ventricles via an accessory pathway may give an ECG appearance of VT. When the diagnosis is in doubt, the safest approach is to sedate the patient, perform DCCV, and leave the definitive diagnosis for the electrophysiologist.

### Polymorphic Ventricular Tachycardia

Polymorphic VT is defined as VT with varying QRS wave morphology (**Fig. 59.18**). A specific type of polymorphic VT characterized by sinusoidal variation of the QRS deflection occurs in patients with a long QT interval during sinus rhythm (**Fig. 59.19**). This tachydysrhythmia is termed torsades de pointes (TdP), or "twisting of the points" (**Fig. 59.20**). There are a number of causes of polymorphic VT and TdP, which itself is an important cause of sudden cardiac death. Fortunately, this tachydysrhythmia is rare.

Polymorphic VT in the setting of a normal QT interval is most often associated with acute cardiac ischemia. It is a rare but important indicator of ongoing ischemia. The most important treatment is revascularization therapy. Pending revascularization, suppression of the dysrhythmia can be attempted with lidocaine or amiodarone.

Polymorphic VT in association with a long QT interval can be due to a congenital or acquired cause. The mechanisms involved in initiation and propagation of this form of polymorphic VT termed TdP are not entirely understood. Prolongation of the QT interval itself may not cause TdP but may lead to secondary phenomena that initiate TdP. Such phenomena are increased QT dispersion and EADs. QT dispersion refers to the maximum variation in the QT interval observed in the 12 leads on the ECG tracing. If the QT interval and corresponding refractory period of the myocardium have increased heterogeeity, partial and abnormal depolarization of cells may occur, particularly after an EAD with subsequent loss of synchrony. Spiral reentrant waves can result, but the prolonged QT interval may determine the geometry and appearance of polymorphic VT as opposed to frank VF.

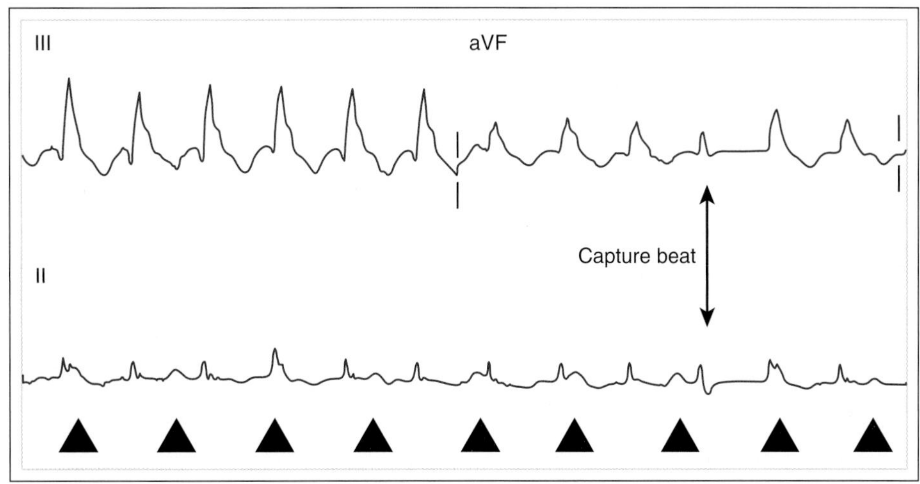


**Fig. 59.16 Electrocardiogram showing ventricular tachycardia with evidence of atrioventricular dissociation and independent atrial activity *(arrowheads)*.** Note that a single atrial beat partly captures the ventricles *(arrow)*, and there is probably fusion with the ongoing ventricular cycle.

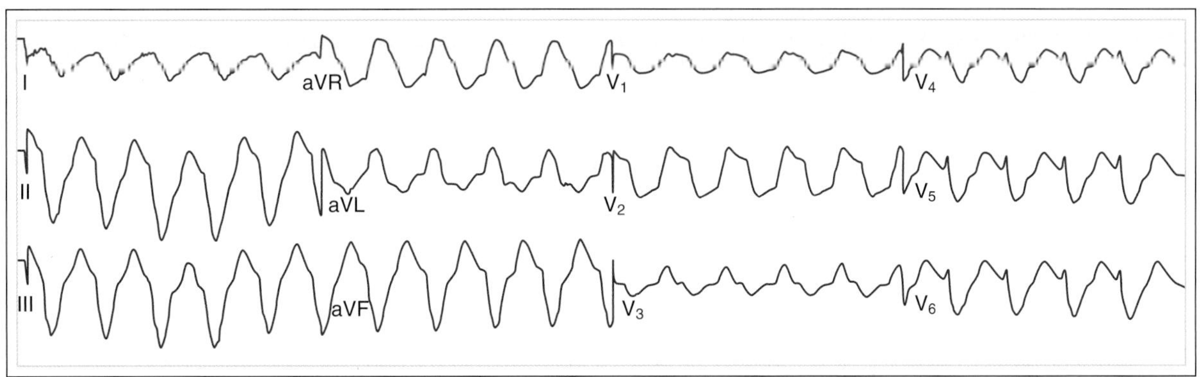


**Fig. 59.17** A 50-year-old man was found lying down with lethargy and shortness of breath. He was a hemodialysis patient who had missed dialysis for a week. His serum potassium level was 8.4 mEq/L. Note the marked wide and bizarre QRS complexes with a right upward frontal plane axis on his electrocardiogram.

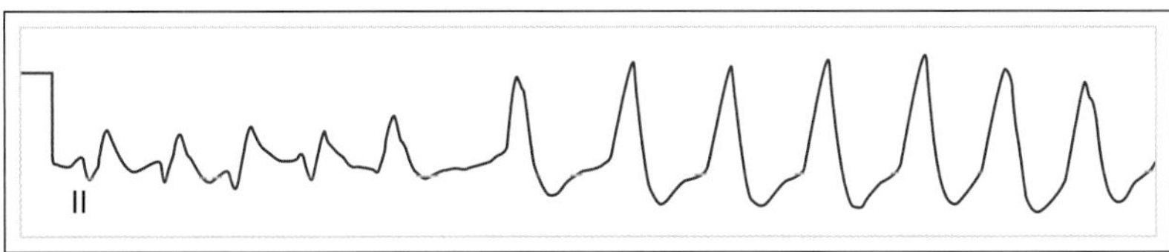


**Fig. 59.18** When the electrocardiogram shows polymorphic ventricular tachycardia (VT), the setting and the underlying QT interval should be considered. When this condition occurs in association with a normal QT interval, acute ischemia is often present, and treatment is focused on the ischemic process. When undulating polymorphic VT occurs in association with a prolonged QT interval in sinus rhythm, the diagnosis is torsades de pointes.

Cellular repolarization and the QT interval vary as a function of the preceding heart rate. Thus, the measured QT interval is corrected for the heart rate, most commonly with the Bazett formula. After puberty, on average, women have a slightly longer QT interval than men do (**Table 59.2**), and a variety of medications can prolong the QT interval. Patients with a prolonged QT interval are asymptomatic unless TdP or another tachydysrhythmia develops, which may be manifested as syncope or sudden cardiac death.

Congenital long QT syndrome with TdP is due to a growing number of known ion channelopathies (**Table 59.3**). The most common defects lead to deficient potassium channel conduction and augmentation of sodium channel conduction, which cause a prolonged QT interval. Other genetic abnormalities associated with polymorphic VT and sudden cardiac death are rare calcium channel defects, ion channel defects leading to a shortened QT interval, and Brugada syndrome, which is attributed primarily to premature inactivation of sodium channel conduction. As with hemoglobinopathies, there appear to be a wide variety of defects associated with myocardial conducting channels and their supporting proteins, and they are associated with varying risk for tachydysrhythmias and mortality.

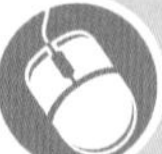

See Table 59.3, Known Genetic Tachydysrhythmias, online at www.expertconsult.com

The possibility of congenital long QT interval should be considered in all patients with palpitations, presyncope, syncope, or seizures. What were the circumstances of the event, and has the patient previously had similar events? Did the onset of symptoms occur during rest, sleep, or activity or after the patient was startled (see Table 59.3)? How long did the symptoms last, and were there any associated symptoms of chest pain or shortness of breath? Many of these conditions exhibit autosomal inheritance, although new mutations are common. The family history should be assessed for recurrent syncope and sudden death.

In a patient with sinus rhythm, the physical findings are usually normal. However, analysis of the QT interval and T-wave morphology on the ECG is critical. Different channelopathies tend to be associated with specific T-wave abnormalities. Assess for the morphology of Brugada syndrome, an RBBB pattern in the precordial chest leads with associated downsloping ST-segment elevation (**Fig. 59.21**). Search for evidence of other cardiologic causes of syncope, including

**Table 59.2 Suggested QTc Values* for Diagnosing QT Prolongation**

| | QTc Values by Age Group or Gender | | |
|---|---|---|---|
| | **1-15 YR** | **MEN** | **WOMEN** |
| Normal | <0.44 | <0.43 | <0.45 |
| Borderline | 0.44-0.46 | 0.43-0.45 | 0.45-0.47 |
| Prolonged (top 1%) | >0.46 | >0.45 | >0.47 |

*The QTc values ($sec^{1/2}$) are derived from the measured QT interval in seconds divided by the square root of the R-R interval in seconds.
From Moss AJ. Measurement of the QT interval and the risk associated with QTc interval prolongation: a review. Am J Cardiol 1993;72: 23B-25B.

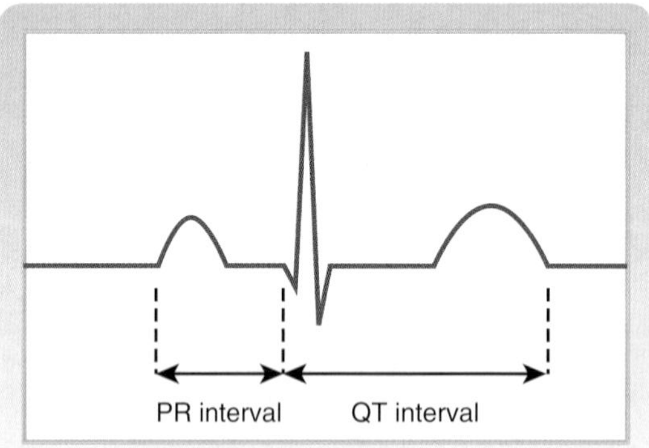


**Fig. 59.19 Defining the QT interval.** The QT interval starts at the beginning of the Q wave—or the R wave if no Q wave is present—and ends when the T wave returns to the baseline.

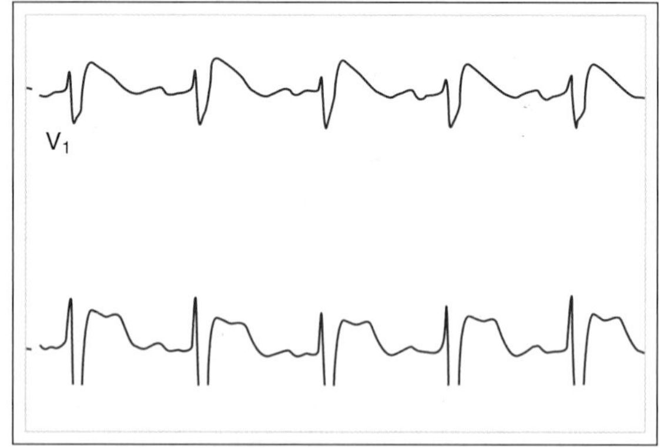


**Fig. 59.21 Electrocardiographic tracings from septal precordial leads with an incomplete right bundle branch block and downsloping ST-segment elevation consistent with Brugada syndrome.**

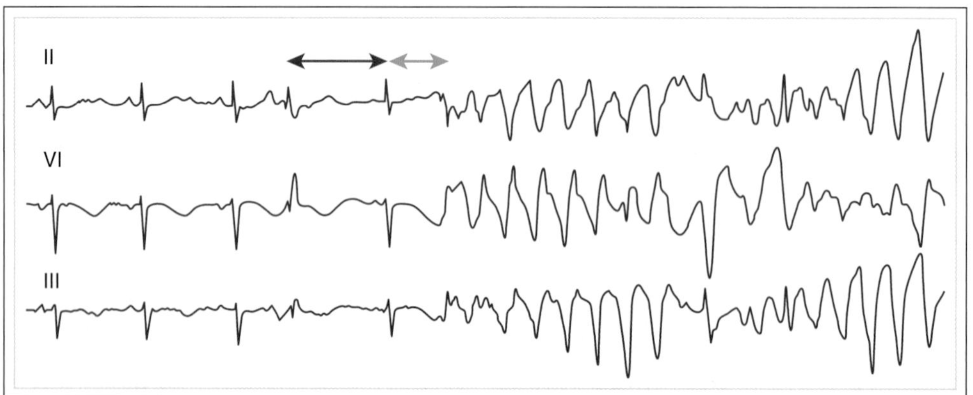


**Fig. 59.20 Three-lead electrocardiogram tracing demonstrating normal sinus rhythm with a prolonged QT interval and torsades de pointes.** Note the classic long-short pattern of initiation. A premature ventricular contraction *(left arrowhead of the red arrow)* causes a subsequent long R-R interval *(red arrow)*. The long R-R interval causes a particularly long QT interval in the next beat *(green arrow)*. This beat with a long QT interval is particularly susceptible to depolarization during the vulnerable relative refractory period of the T wave and initiation of torsades de pointes as shown.

preexcitation and WPW syndrome, ventricular hypertrophy, aortic valvular disease, and other tachydysrhythmias or bradydysrhythmias. Serum electrolytes, including potassium, calcium, and magnesium, should be measured, and treatment should be administered as needed.

Acquired long QT syndrome is due to toxicity from medications that either prolong the QT interval or block the metabolism of QT-prolonging agents (**Box 59.4**). Medications that prolong the QT interval act by altering ion channel flow, such as by disrupting the outward potassium repolarizing current. Women are more prone to acquired long QT syndrome, perhaps in part because of their longer baseline QT interval. Acute symptoms are similar to those in the congenital form of disease.

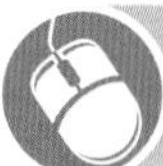

See Box 59.4, Causes of Acquired Long QT Syndrome, online at www.expertconsult.com

Treatment of TdP involves immediate unsynchronized defibrillation if the patient is unstable or pulseless. An initial energy of 200 J should be used for biphasic defibrillation or 360 J for a monophasic waveform. Synchronized DCCV is not usually recommended because of the variability of the QRS waveform and potential failure to synchronize. Magnesium should be administered to terminate TdP and possibly to prevent recurrences. Increasing the heart rate reduces the QT interval. The heart rate can be increased by external or internal pacing or with the administration of isoproterenol. Class I and III antidysrhythmic agents are generally contraindicated because they may further prolong the QT interval and increase QT dispersion. Removal of the offending agent should be considered in patients with acquired QT prolongation, although this step is not usually feasible. Patients with polymorphic VT and TdP require admission to a monitored unit for further evaluation and treatment.

## SUMMARY

ED disposition of a patient with a tachydysrhythmia depends on the diagnosis, if known; symptoms of cardiovascular instability, including presyncope, chest pain, or shortness of breath during tachycardia; the patient's underlying cardiovascular health; and the patient's social support and medical follow-up. Patients with known recurrent supraventricular tachydysrhythmias that are well tolerated hemodynamically can usually be discharged with close follow-up. Generally, patients with a new-onset, undiagnosed, or ventricular tachydysrhythmia should be admitted.

The long-term and definitive care of patients with dysrhythmias has advanced remarkably. Definitive catheter ablation can be performed on selected patients with AF, atrial flutter, AVT, AVNRT, and VT. ICDs are commonly implanted in patients with ventricular tachydysrhythmias or a low ejection fraction after MI. Patients may also require adjunctive oral antidysrhythmic therapy to minimize ICD shocks. The EP should expect to see more patients with intracardiac devices and advanced treatments in the future. Optimal ED care of these patients will require sound understanding of the clinical issues, familiarity with new technologies, and close collaboration with cardiology colleagues.

## REFERENCES

***References can be found on Expert Consult @ www.expertconsult.com.***

# 60 Pericarditis, Pericardial Tamponade, and Myocarditis

*Amal Mattu and Joseph P. Martinez*

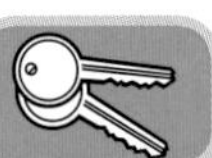

**KEY POINTS**

- The classic symptom of acute pericarditis is sharp, pleuritic retrosternal chest pain that radiates to one or both trapezius ridges and changes with body position.
- The hallmark electrocardiographic findings in patients with pericarditis include diffuse ST-segment elevation with PR-segment depression in the same leads.
- High-dose aspirin or a nonsteroidal antiinflammatory drug with the addition of colchicine is effective treatment of most cases of acute pericarditis.
- Steroids should be avoided in the early treatment of first-time pericarditis because their use may actually increase the chance of recurrence.
- Large pericardial effusions often cause severe tachypnea and dyspnea; however, oxygen saturation levels are usually normal.
- Jugular venous distention is typical in patients with pericardial tamponade, but it may be absent in those with hypovolemia or if the tamponade developed rapidly.
- The hallmark echocardiographic finding in patients with pericardial tamponade is the presence of a large effusion with diastolic collapse of the right heart chambers.
- The classic manifestation of acute myocarditis includes low-grade fever, tachypnea, and tachycardia out of proportion to the fever.

## EPIDEMIOLOGY

Although the greatest concern in patients with chest pain is usually vascular causes of chest pain—acute coronary syndrome, pulmonary embolism, and aortic dissection—other less common, but potentially deadly illnesses must be considered, including pericarditis, pericardial tamponade, and myocarditis.

Acute pericarditis is often subclinical, so its incidence is uncertain. However, rough estimates range from 2% to 6%,[1] and this disorder may be responsible for as many as 1 in every 1000 hospital admissions.[2] Although acute pericarditis is not usually deadly, it can be painfully disabling if not treated appropriately.

Pericardial tamponade is a potentially deadly result of pericardial effusion. Such an effusion can develop from pericardial inflammation or cardiac trauma. Unfortunately, the early features of tamponade can mimic those of other diseases and lead to initial misdiagnosis.

Acute myocarditis is relatively uncommon, but it is a devastating condition that can occur and progress quickly, with little warning. The initial findings can vary from mild, viral-type symptoms to fulminant cardiogenic shock.

## PERICARDITIS

### PATHOPHYSIOLOGY

The pericardium is the layer of tissue surrounding the heart. It consists of two layers, a serous inner layer (visceral pericardium) and a fibrocollagenous outer layer (parietal pericardium). The pericardium completely encloses the ventricles and the right atrium; a portion of the left atrium remains outside the sac. A thin layer of plasma fluid (usually 15 to 30 mL) separates the visceral and parietal pericardial layers and acts as a lubricant. The main function of the pericardium appears to be provision of ligamentous stability to withstand forces against the heart. It also provides some shielding for the heart. Despite these apparent functions, however, the majority of patients who undergo pericardiectomy do not appear to suffer any decrease in cardiac performance or other ill effects.

Pericarditis refers to inflammation of the layers of the pericardium. It has many possible causes (**Box 60.1**), but in most cases the cause is unknown. In the majority of these idiopathic cases the presumed cause is viral, although most attempts to prove a viral cause have low yield. The most common viral cause is coxsackievirus B. The most common cause of pericarditis worldwide is tuberculosis.[3]

### PRESENTING SIGNS AND SYMPTOMS

#### CLASSIC

Chest pain is the typical complaint of patients with acute pericarditis. Classically, the chest pain is sharp, retrosternal, and pleuritic, and it radiates to one or both trapezius ridges

**BOX 60.1 Causes of Pericarditis**

Viral infections
- Coxsackievirus B (most common)
- Coxsackievirus A
- Echovirus
- Human immunodeficiency virus
- Influenza virus
- Epstein-Barr virus
- Adenovirus
- Varicella virus

Bacterial infections
- *Staphylococcus*
- *Pneumococcus*
- *Mycoplasma*
- *Streptococcus*
- *Meningococcus*
- Tuberculosis
- *Salmonella*
- *Haemophilus*
- *Rickettsia*

Parasitic infections
- Toxoplasmosis
- Amebiasis

Fungal infections
- *Histoplasma*
- *Aspergillus*
- *Blastomyces*

Connective tissue diseases
- Systemic lupus erythematosus
- Rheumatoid arthritis
- Sarcoidosis
- Amyloidosis
- Scleroderma

After myocardial infarction (MI)
- Early post-MI pericarditis
- Delayed (4 to 6 weeks) pericarditis (Dressler syndrome)

Malignancies
- Primary: mesothelioma, angiosarcoma
- Metastatic (more common): breast, lung, melanoma, lymphoma, leukemia

Radiation therapy

Thoracic aortic dissection

Medications
- Hydralazine
- Procainamide
- Methyldopa
- Penicillin
- Cromolyn sodium
- Dantrolene
- Methysergide
- Anticoagulants (heparin, warfarin)

Cardiac trauma

Cardiac surgery

because the phrenic nerve, which traverses the pericardium, innervates these muscles.[4] Typically, the pain also changes with body position: it improves when the patient sits up and leans forward and worsens when the patient lies supine.

The physical examination of patients with acute pericarditis is usually nondiagnostic. Although some researchers report the presence of a friction rub in up to 85% of patients at some point in the course of the disease,[5] the presence of a friction rub at the time of initial evaluation is unreliable. When a friction rub is present, it is best heard at the left sternal border at end-expiration with the patient leaning forward. The rub is usually described as consisting of three components that correspond to atrial systole, ventricular systole, and rapid diastolic filling. A friction rub is thought to be caused by rubbing of the inflamed layers of the pericardium against each other.

## TYPICAL VARIATIONS

The typical findings in patients with acute pericarditis may not always be present. Although chest pain is the most common symptom, patients sometimes have dyspnea as the primary complaint. When chest pain is present, it is not always positional or pleuritic, and it may not always radiate to the trapezius ridge. Patients may also complain of cough, upper respiratory symptoms, nausea, or vomiting, which may mislead the physician to an alternative diagnosis. Patients with bacterial infections are likely to have complaints of fever, and patients with tuberculous pericarditis are likely to report a chronic cough, weight loss, and night sweats.

Although the presence of a triphasic friction rub is classic, it actually occurs in only half of patients with pericarditis.[6] The physical findings may also be notable for hypotension and jugular venous distention in the presence of pericardial tamponade (discussed later).

## DIFFERENTIAL DIAGNOSIS AND MEDICAL DECISION MAKING

A thorough differential diagnosis of a patient with chest pain is described in Chapter 54. However, the most important initial consideration should always be the deadly causes of chest pain: pericarditis, acute coronary ischemia or infarction, thoracic aortic dissection, and pulmonary embolism. **Table 60.1** lists some historical and physical examination features that are helpful in distinguishing among these conditions. Distinction among these causes of chest pain is critical in terms of treatment; patients with pulmonary embolism or myocardial infarction often require treatment with anticoagulants and thrombolytics, medications that can be deadly in patients with acute pericarditis or aortic dissection.

The diagnosis of acute pericarditis is based primarily on the clinical findings. In many cases an electrocardiogram (ECG) is helpful in confirming the diagnosis. Sound knowledge of the ECG findings in patients with acute pericarditis is critical, as well as some findings that help in diagnosing pericarditis versus myocardial infarction (see Table 60.1). Classically, pericarditis evolves through four ECG stages as described in **Table 60.2**. The first stage of acute pericarditis, characterized by diffuse ST-segment elevation and PR-segment depression or downsloping (**Fig. 60.1**), is the most common stage encountered in the emergency department (ED). The ST segments should be concave upward; a convex upward ("tombstone")

**Table 60.1 Differential Diagnosis of Acute Pericarditis**

| | ACUTE PERICARDITIS | ACUTE MYOCARDIAL ISCHEMIA OR INFARCTION | AORTIC DISSECTION | PULMONARY EMBOLISM |
|---|---|---|---|---|
| Chest pain description | Sharp, pleuritic, positional | Pressure, squeezing, tightness | Sharp, maximal intensity at onset | Sharp, pleuritic, abrupt onset |
| Chest pain radiation | Trapezius ridge | Usually to the left arm, jaw, neck, or shoulder; may also radiate to the right side | Straight to midscapular area of the back | Not typical |
| Response to nitroglycerin | Not typical | Improves | Not typical | Not typical |
| Vital signs | Tachycardia and fever common | Fever not typical; blood pressure and heart rate are variable | Hypertension common | Occasionally low-grade fever, tachycardia and hypoxia common |
| Other physical examination findings | Friction rub common during course, though less common on initial evaluation | Fourth heart sound is "classic" in cases of cardiac ischemia; third heart sound if heart failure present | Occasional pulse deficits | Occasional leg swelling or tenderness if embolus originated in the legs |
| Electrocardiographic findings | (See Table 60.2) Early: diffuse ST-segment elevation and PR-segment depression<br>Absence of reciprocal ST-segment depression<br>Sinus tachycardia common; bradycardia and atrioventricular (AV) blocks uncommon | ST-segment elevation or depression typically in an anatomic distribution corresponding to the involved coronary vessel<br>Tachycardia or bradycardia and AV blocks not uncommon | Left ventricular hypertrophy if chronic hypertension present<br>Variable ST-segment or T-wave changes<br>Sinus tachycardia common | Sinus tachycardia common; bradycardia and AV blocks uncommon<br>Large emboli often associated with T-wave inversions, most commonly in right precordial leads and less commonly in inferior leads<br>ST-segment elevation possible but uncommon |
| Chest radiography findings | Usually normal; cardiomegaly if large pericardial effusion present | Cardiomegaly if chronic left ventricular hypertrophy present; evidence of heart failure may be present | Cardiomegaly common if chronic left ventricular hypertrophy present; wide mediastinum common | Usually normal; most common abnormalities are elevated hemidiaphragm, atelectasis, small pleural effusion |
| Cardiac biomarkers | Levels usually normal; mild elevations not uncommon | Elevations typical in myocardial infarction | Levels normal | Large emboli occasionally associated with mild elevations in troponin or brain natriuretic peptide |

**Table 60.2 Electrocardiographic Stages of Acute Pericarditis**

| | |
|---|---|
| Stage I | Diffuse ST-segment elevation and PR-segment depression (except in leads $V_1$ and aVR) |
| Stage II | Resolution of the ST-segment and PR-segment changes<br>T-wave flattening in the same leads |
| Stage III | T-wave inversions in the same leads |
| Stage IV | Normalization of electrographic abnormalities |

morphology virtually excludes the diagnosis of pericarditis and rules in acute myocardial infarction. ST-segment depression may be present in leads aVR and $V_1$ in a patient with pericarditis but is unlikely to be present in any of the other 10 leads. In fact, the presence of ST-segment depression in any of the other 10 leads should be considered the "reciprocal" changes of acute myocardial infarction.

These four stages generally progress over the course of days to weeks. The ECG changes in the second and third stages usually occur in the same leads in which abnormalities in the initial stage occurred.

Although the abnormalities noted on an ECG are typically described as "classic" for acute pericarditis, physicians should

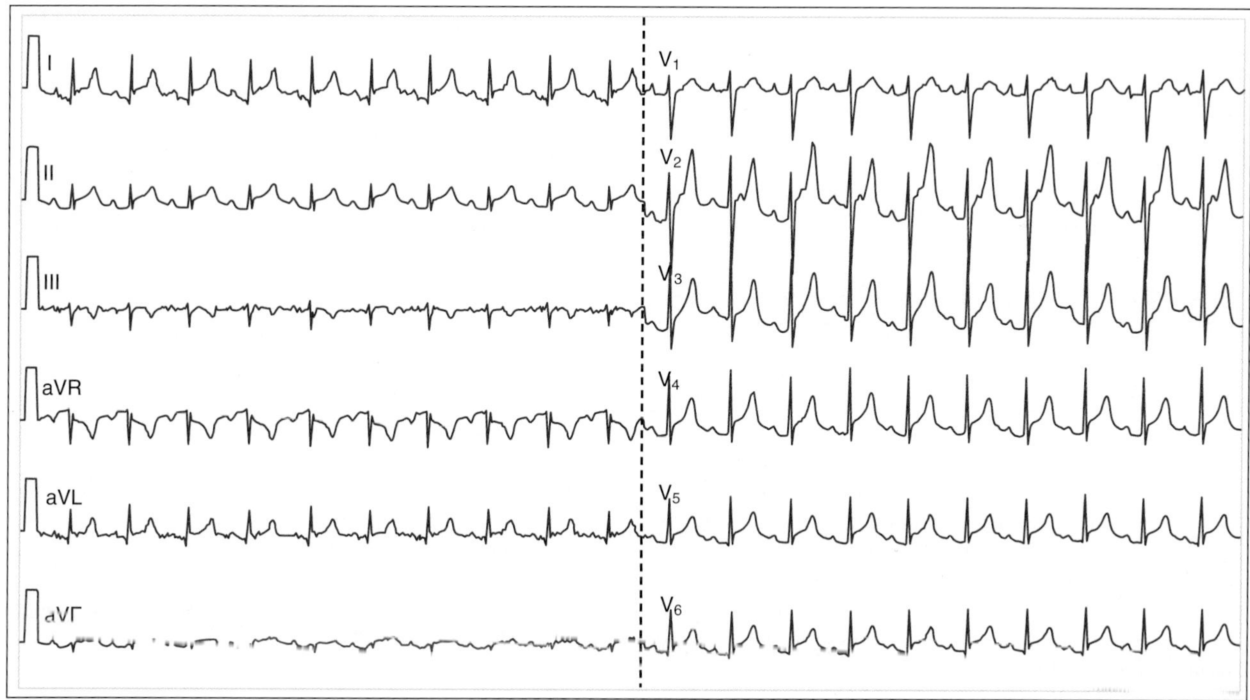


**Fig. 60.1 Acute pericarditis.** The electrocardiogram demonstrates diffuse ST-segment elevation with PR-segment depression in multiple leads.

be aware that these findings are typical only for acute viral pericarditis. Other forms of pericarditis less commonly cause PR-segment depression and occasionally cause less pronounced ST-segment elevation. In these cases, the diagnosis must be based purely on the clinical rather than the ECG findings.

Laboratory studies are rarely helpful in the diagnosis of acute pericarditis. Patients may have an elevated white blood cell count because of pain or infection (or both). Other serum markers of inflammation, including the erythrocyte sedimentation rate and C-reactive protein value, are often elevated, but such elevations are nonspecific. Cardiac biomarkers may be minimally elevated but should not demonstrate the rise and fall typical of myocardial infarction. Chest radiography is also rarely helpful in the diagnosis of acute pericarditis; it is used mainly to evaluate for alternative causes of chest pain (e.g., pneumonia, aortic dissection).

Echocardiography can be useful in distinguishing between acute pericarditis and acute myocardial infarction. Echocardiograms in patients with pericarditis lack the focal wall motion abnormalities that are typical of echocardiograms in those with myocardial infarction. Echocardiography is also useful to look for evidence of pericardial effusion, a potential complication of acute pericarditis (see later). If a large pericardial effusion is present, pericardiocentesis (ultrasonographically guided in a stable patient) can be performed to obtain fluid for testing for infections and cytologic analysis.

## TREATMENT

Treatment of patients with acute pericarditis should be targeted at the underlying cause. The majority of patients with viral, rheumatologic, posttraumatic, or idiopathic pericarditis are effectively treated with high-dose aspirin (2 to 4 g daily) or nonsteroidal antiinflammatory drugs (NSAIDs). Ibuprofen is effective in most cases and has fewer side effects than other NSAIDs; the pain usually improves significantly within days with ibuprofen therapy. If the patient's symptoms persist, an alternative NSAID is indicated. Indomethacin is often used for severe cases because of its stronger antiinflammatory effect, although it should be avoided in patients with a history of ischemic heart disease because it may decrease coronary blood flow.[4,7] Evidence now suggests that addition of colchicine (1.0 to 2.0 mg for the first day and then 0.5 to 1.0 mg/day for 3 months) to the standard regimen is effective in hastening the resolution of acute symptoms and also preventing recurrence rates, regardless of the cause of the pericarditis.[8] Colchicine is also effective in cases of recurrent pericarditis.[9,10] The use of corticosteroids is generally reserved for recurrent cases of pericarditis that are unresponsive to aspirin or NSAIDs plus colchicine. Initiation of steroids early in the course of first-time pericarditis may actually be an independent risk factor for recurrence.[8]

Patients with bacterial or other nonviral infectious causes of pericarditis should be treated aggressively with antimicrobial therapy. Large infected pericardial effusions require drainage as well. Management of neoplastic causes of pericarditis should be targeted at treating the underlying malignancy. Patients with uremic pericarditis require urgent hemodialysis.

## FOLLOW-UP AND NEXT STEPS IN CARE

The majority of patients with acute pericarditis can be treated as outpatients, with the symptoms generally resolving within 2 weeks. Outpatient management is suitable for patients with mild symptoms, hemodynamic stability, and ability to tolerate oral medications. Reasonable indications for admission include fever or suspicion of a bacterial cause of the pericarditis, immunosuppression, pericarditis associated with trauma, presence of a moderate to large pericardial effusion, and hemodynamic instability. A history of active anticoagulant use is generally considered a poor prognostic factor and warrants hospital admission as well.[4]

# PERICARDIAL TAMPONADE

## PATHOPHYSIOLOGY

Trauma or inflammation of the pericardium can cause fluid to accumulate within the intrapericardial space. Normally, the pericardium is capable of stretching and accommodating 2 L of fluid or more when the fluid accumulates very slowly.[11] However, if the fluid accumulates more rapidly than can be accommodated by the distensibility of the pericardium, especially in the case of trauma, in the presence of fibrotic pericardium, or if the volume of pericardial fluid is excessive, significant intrapericardial pressure results and can produce pericardial tamponade.

Pericardial tamponade develops when intrapericardial fluid produces sufficient pressure to compress the cardiac chambers. Compression of the chambers impairs ventricular diastolic filling and stroke volume. Initial compensatory mechanisms, especially tachycardia, may temporarily sustain cardiac output. However, as pericardial fluid continues to increase, the compensatory mechanisms begin to fail, and diminished cardiac output, hypotension, and full cardiovascular collapse ensue.

The typical causes of pericardial tamponade include any disorder that results in acute or chronic pericardial inflammation, as well as conditions in which a patient sustains penetrating trauma to the heart or cardiac surgery. The conditions previously noted to cause pericarditis are common precipitants of pericardial tamponade. The composition of the intrapericardial effusion varies according to the precipitating cause; in bacterial pericarditis, for example, the effusion is often pus, and in cardiac trauma or cardiac surgery, it is often blood and clots. Regardless of the composition of the effusion, the physiology that leads to pericardial tamponade and the immediate treatment are similar.

## PRESENTING SIGNS AND SYMPTOMS

### CLASSIC

The typical symptoms associated with a large pericardial effusion are nonspecific. Malaise, generalized weakness, ascites, and edema are common in patients with subacute or chronic effusions as a result of poor cardiac function.[12] Many other symptoms are related to compression of adjacent mediastinal structures by the effusion. Dyspnea and cough are common and may be due to displacement or compression of bronchial structures or lung tissue by the effusion. Dyspnea on exertion is common as well and results from impairment of venous return and cardiac output. Patients often report a sense of dysphagia, which is due to esophageal compression. Hiccups may occur as a result of esophageal compression and involvement of the phrenic and vagus nerves. Hoarseness may result from compression of the recurrent laryngeal nerve.[12]

Physical findings are also often nonspecific. Tachycardia and tachypnea are common. Despite the presence of tachypnea and dyspnea, however, oxygen saturation levels are usually normal because the effusion itself does not impair alveolar air exchange. Lung sounds are generally normal as well. Findings of hypoxia or focal abnormalities on lung examination should suggest a superimposed pulmonary condition or an alternative diagnosis. Fever is common if the underlying cause is infectious. Pericardial friction rubs are reportedly common if the underlying cause is inflammatory,[13] although diminished heart sounds are also frequent because of reduced cardiac function and attenuation of their transmission by the effusion.

When a pericardial effusion produces pericardial tamponade, additional findings are notable. Decreased cardiac function produces hypotension and shock. Jugular venous distention is typically present because of impaired venous return. Pulsus paradoxus (drop in systolic blood pressure of greater than 10 mm Hg during normal inspiration) is also typical, although its presence has limited specificity for pericardial tamponade. Several other conditions that are associated with hypotension or dyspnea (or both) can also produce pulsus paradoxus, including massive pulmonary embolism, hemorrhagic shock, and obstructive lung disease.[12] Death is usually preceded by pulseless electrical activity.[14]

### TYPICAL VARIATIONS

Although the symptoms and physical findings already noted are common, certain conditions may produce unexpected findings in the presence of pericardial tamponade. Patients who have severe hypothyroidism or uremia or who take atrioventricular nodal blocking agents (e.g., calcium channel blockers, beta-blockers, digoxin) may have a relative bradycardia. Jugular venous distention is typical in pericardial tamponade as well, but it is often absent in patients who are hypovolemic or in whom the pericardial tamponade developed very quickly (e.g., after cardiac trauma). Overt hypotension may be absent as well in patients with a history of severe antecedent hypertension.[12,15]

## DIFFERENTIAL DIAGNOSIS AND MEDICAL DECISION MAKING

A complete differential diagnosis of hypotension and shock is beyond the scope of this chapter. However, the emergency physician (EP) should always consider other typical causes of hypotension, especially those that similarly produce jugular venous distension: massive pulmonary embolism, large left ventricular myocardial infarction with cardiogenic shock, right ventricular myocardial infarction, acute aortic or mitral valve insufficiency, and superior vena cava syndrome.

The primary means of diagnosing pericardial tamponade is via two-dimensional echocardiography. A pericardial effusion is easily seen in most patients on subcostal or parasternal views (**Fig. 60.2**). An echo-free space should be visible throughout the cardiac cycle when the pericardial effusion is at least 25 mL.[3] The presence of a pericardial effusion in combination with hypotension and echocardiographic

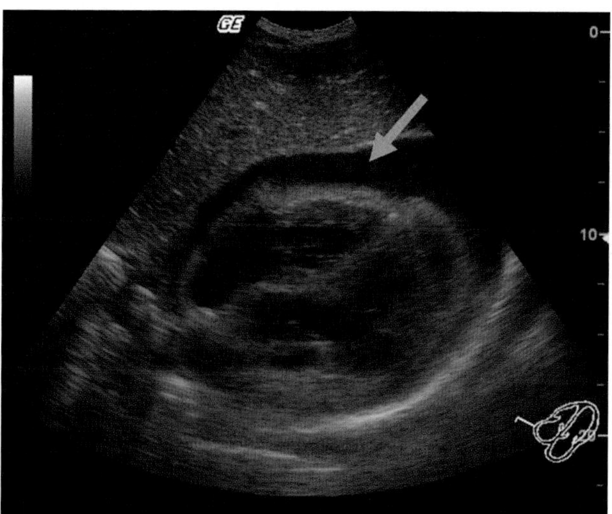

**Fig. 60.2 Large pericardial effusion.** The ultrasonogram is a subcostal four-chamber view of the heart that demonstrates a large pericardial effusion (*arrow*). The patient also had dynamic changes consistent with pericardial tamponade—right atrial and right ventricular diastolic collapse. (Courtesy Dr. Brian Euerle, Director of Emergency Ultrasound, Emergency Medicine Residency, University of Maryland School of Medicine.)

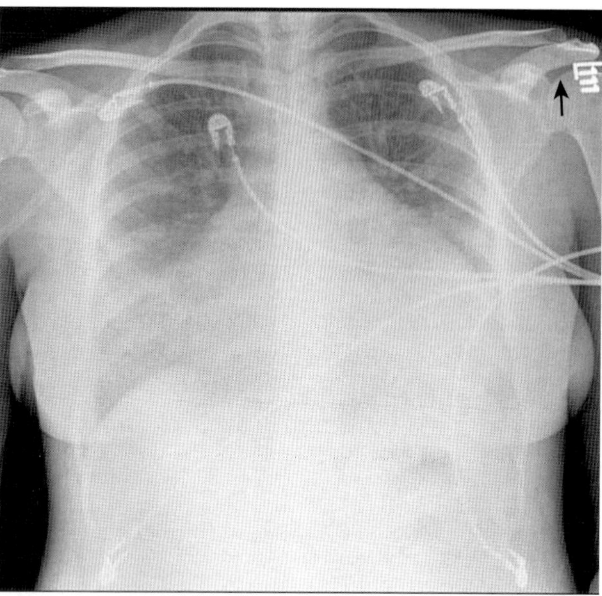

**Fig. 60.3 Large pericardial effusion.** The chest radiograph demonstrates massive cardiomegaly, a nearly universal finding in patients with large pericardial effusions.

evidence of early diastolic right ventricular collapse and late diastolic right atrial collapse is diagnostic of pericardial tamponade. In approximately 25% of cases, the left atrium also demonstrates collapse, a very specific sign of tamponade. The left ventricle rarely demonstrates collapse except in specific conditions such as localized postoperative tamponade.[12] Other echocardiographic findings that may be found in patients with pericardial tamponade are a dilated inferior vena cava without inspiratory collapse and beat-to-beat swinging of the heart within the pericardial fluid (when the effusion is large).[3]

Other imaging studies can be helpful in evaluating these patients as well. Computed tomography (CT) and magnetic resonance imaging are very accurate in detecting pericardial effusions, in addition to diagnosing alternative conditions. However, they should not be used in patients with borderline or overt hemodynamic instability because of the need to remove such patients from the ED for the procedures. Chest radiography is primarily used to evaluate the patient for alternative diagnoses as well, such as pneumonia or pulmonary edema. In patients with a large pericardial effusion, cardiomegaly is a nearly universal finding (**Fig. 60.3**). The chest radiograph is particularly helpful in this setting if previous radiographs are available that demonstrate a normal-sized heart. Previous radiographs that show the massive cardiomegaly to be new are highly suggestive of a large pericardial effusion.

The ECG can be helpful in the diagnosis of large pericardial effusions. The most common abnormality is tachycardia, especially in the presence of tamponade. Low voltage is common as well and is caused by attenuation of the electrical impulse as it passes through the effusion before reaching the ECG electrodes. Although low voltage is nonspecific, the presence of new low voltage (in comparison with previous ECGs) is much more specific for large pericardial effusions. The third "classic" ECG abnormality is electrical alternans. Electrical alternans refers to beat-to-beat variation in amplitudes of the ECG complexes (**Fig. 60.4**) and is attributed to "swinging" of the heart back and forth within the pericardial fluid. Electrical alternans is present in less than one third of cases of pericardial tamponade. Although none of these three findings individually is completely diagnostic of large pericardial effusions, the combination of all three is very highly specific.

## TREATMENT

Initial management of patients with pericardial tamponade should focus on the typical ABCs of resuscitation (airway, breathing, circulation). Certain caveats should be made, however. Although the primary pathophysiologic abnormality underlying hemodynamic compromise in patients with pericardial tamponade is ventricular filling, the benefit of volume infusion to improve filling is controversial. Animal studies have shown variable results with respect to the hemodynamic benefit of volume infusion,[12,16] which may improve systemic perfusion only in patients with hypovolemia. Strong supporting data in humans are lacking, however. In patients with traumatic pericardial tamponade, large-volume infusions may actually precipitate further deterioration.[17] Strong evidence supporting specific inotropic agents is lacking as well, although theoretically agents that reduce the elevated vascular resistance,[12] such as dobutamine and milrinone, would seem ideal. Mechanical ventilation should generally be avoided except in patients with respiratory failure; the positive airway pressure associated with mechanical ventilation decreases venous return and cardiac output.

Treatment of pericardial tamponade is drainage of the intrapericardial fluid (pericardiocentesis). Drainage is best

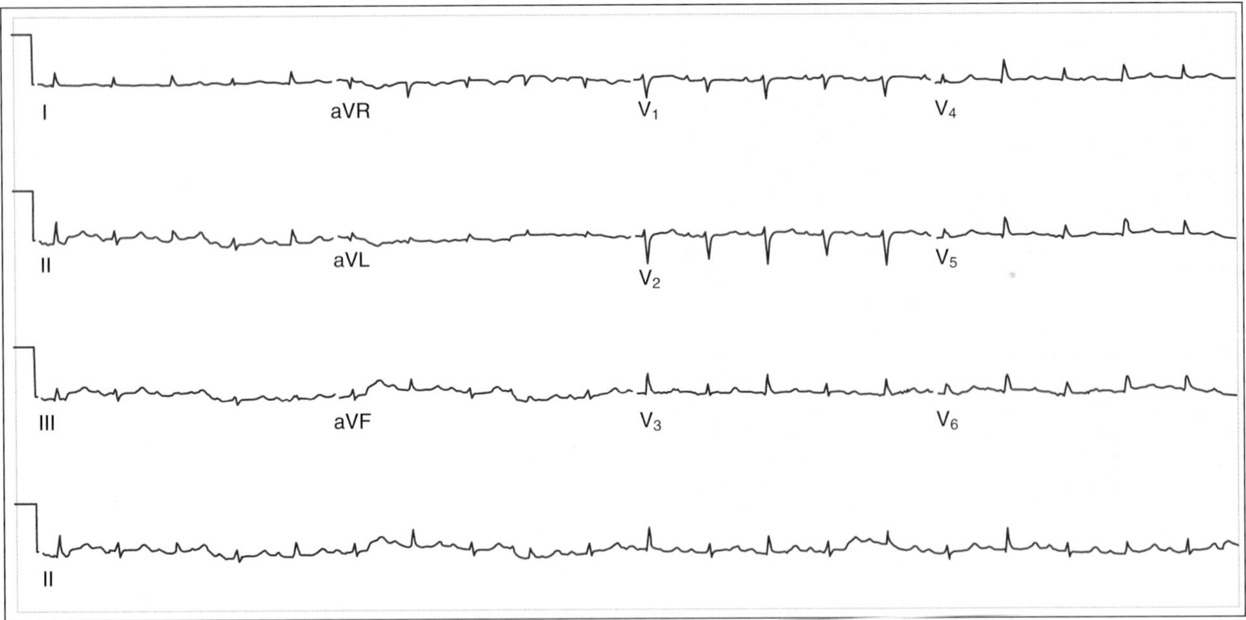


**Fig. 60.4 Large pericardial effusion.** The electrocardiogram demonstrates the three classic findings in a patient with a large pericardial effusion: sinus tachycardia, low voltage, and electrical alternans.

performed via needle aspiration under echocardiographic, CT, or fluoroscopic guidance. In patients who exhibit rapid cardiac decompensation or are in cardiac arrest, the EP should perform emergency pericardiocentesis without waiting for imaging guidance. The procedure is performed with a 16- or 18-gauge needle, most commonly inserted into the left paraxiphoid area of the chest. The needle is pointed downward at an approximately 30-degree angle to the chest to bypass the left costal margin and is aimed toward the left shoulder. The needle should be inserted and advanced slowly until the pericardium is penetrated and fluid is aspirated. Use of a sheathed needle can facilitate the process—once the pericardium has been penetrated, the core of the needle can be removed with the sheath left in the pericardial space to assist in further removal of fluid.[12] Some researchers have advocated attaching ECG leads to the hub of the needle so that when the pericardium is penetrated, an injury pattern (i.e., ST-segment elevation) will be noted.[18] However, a recent review recommends against this practice because of the likelihood of misleading results.[12]

In patients with acute cardiac decompensation, aspiration of even 10 to 20 mL of blood should be sufficient to produce some hemodynamic improvement. However, once full cardiac arrest has occurred, pericardiocentesis has a limited success rate. Potential complications of pericardiocentesis include puncture or laceration of the cardiac chambers, injury to coronary vessels, pneumothorax, ventricular dysrhythmias, pneumopericardium, and delayed infection.[19] These complications are more common in the setting of emergency pericardiocentesis, which is sometimes performed without imaging guidance.

Because pericardiocentesis is less likely to be successful in patients with clotted hemopericardium, surgical drainage will be necessary. Surgical drainage is also required in patients in whom intrapericardial bleeding is present (e.g., postoperative pericardial tamponade, traumatic pericardial tamponade, pericardial tamponade with aortic dissection). In these patients, pericardiocentesis is temporizing at best; in conjunction with surgical drainage, definitive repair of the bleeding sites is essential. Additional therapy should focus on treating the underlying cause of the pericardial inflammation that led to pericardial tamponade.

## FOLLOW-UP AND NEXT STEPS IN CARE

Patients with pericardial tamponade should be admitted to an intensive care setting for definitive therapy and close hemodynamic monitoring. If surgical therapy is indicated, emergency surgical consultation is mandatory. When surgical therapy is not planned, cardiology consultation is most appropriate for the performance of pericardiocentesis under echocardiographic guidance. Nephrology consultation is also appropriate for urgent hemodialysis in patients with uremia.

# MYOCARDITIS

## PATHOPHYSIOLOGY

Myocarditis is an inflammatory condition that causes myocardial damage, usually because of infectious, immunologic, or toxin-mediated conditions (**Box 60.2**). Myocarditis can be manifested as mild constitutional symptoms, moderate cardiopulmonary symptoms, or fulminant cardiopulmonary decompensation leading to death. In the majority of adult cases, the myocardial damage is believed to be caused by autoimmune processes that are often triggered by viral or other infections,[20] whereas in neonates and infants, injury to myocytes is believed to occur more often because of direct injury by the pathogen itself.[21]

Approximately 10% of postmortem examinations demonstrate some degree of histologic evidence of myocarditis. However, most of the patients were not clinically symptomatic

**BOX 60.2 Causes of Myocarditis**

Viral infections (most common)
- Coxsackievirus (most common virus)
- Echovirus
- Human immunodeficiency virus
- Influenza virus
- Parainfluenza virus
- Epstein-Barr virus
- Adenovirus
- Varicella virus
- Cytomegalovirus
- Herpesvirus
- Rabies virus
- Poliovirus
- Hepatitis A, B, C, or D virus
- Rubella virus
- Mumps virus
- Rubeola virus

Bacterial infections
- *Staphylococcus*
- *Borrelia* (Lyme disease)
- *Legionella*
- *Corynebacterium diphtheriae*
- Tuberculosis
- *Mycoplasma*
- *Streptococcus*
- *Meningococcus*
- *Chlamydia* (*pneumoniae* and *psittaci*)
- *Enterococcus*

Parasitic infections
- Toxoplasmosis
- Trypanosomiasis
- Trichinosis
- Echinococcosis
- Chagas disease

Medications/toxins
- Methyldopa
- Penicillin
- Hydrochlorothiazide
- Sulfamethoxazole
- Lithium
- Doxorubicin
- Cyclophosphamides
- Zidovudine
- Acetaminophen
- Lead
- Arsenic
- Carbon monoxide
- Cocaine
- Ethanol
- Interleukin-2
- Anabolic steroids
- Radiation therapy

Connective tissue diseases
- Systemic lupus erythematosus
- Rheumatoid arthritis
- Dermatomyositis
- Sarcoidosis

Miscellaneous
- Giant cell arteritis
- Kawasaki disease
- Cardiac transplant rejection
- Peripartum state

before death.[22] Conversely, in patients in whom myocarditis is diagnosed clinically, only one third have histologic findings consistent with the disease. Even in cases that progress to dilated cardiomyopathy, only 40% of patients have microscopic evidence of myocarditis. Consequently, the actual incidence of myocarditis is unknown.[23]

## PRESENTING SIGNS AND SYMPTOMS

### CLASSIC

The clinical manifestations of myocarditis usually begin days to weeks after the acute infection, especially when viruses are implicated as the cause. However, only 50% of patients report a recent upper respiratory or gastrointestinal viral type of infection.[23] The initial symptoms are nonspecific and constitutional in nature: low fever, fatigue, malaise, myalgia, and arthralgia. These mild symptoms are often the reason for initial misdiagnosis or delays in proper diagnosis of this condition. Cardiopulmonary symptoms, especially mild dyspnea and chest pain, are common as well. The chest pain can be pleuritic, sharp, and positional, much like pericarditis, or substernal and squeezing, much like typical ischemic pain. Patients with congestive heart failure may report more significant dyspnea, as well as cough, orthopnea, paroxysmal nocturnal dyspnea, and edema. Less commonly, patients may initially be seen after a syncopal episode, usually the result of a bradydysrhythmia.

The physical findings are often notable for low-grade fever, tachypnea, and tachycardia. Classically, the patient has "tachycardia out of proportion to the fever"—extreme tachycardia without obvious hypovolemia or high fever (**Fig. 60.5**). Patients may also experience bradycardia if a high-grade atrioventricular block develops (**Fig. 60.6**). Evidence of congestive heart failure is frequently present as well: jugular venous distention, bibasilar rales on lung examination, a third heart sound ($S_3$) on cardiac examination, and peripheral edema. Patients with advanced or fulminant myocarditis may arrive at the ED in full cardiogenic shock.

### TYPICAL VARIATIONS

Pediatric patients tend to have early, nonspecific symptoms, including fever, viral upper respiratory symptoms, and poor feeding. In more severe cases, the infant or neonate may exhibit severe tachycardia, tachypnea, sweating while feeding, respiratory distress, and cyanosis or other signs of poor perfusion. Tachydysrhythmias and bradydysrhythmias, especially those involving a high-grade atrioventricular block, are

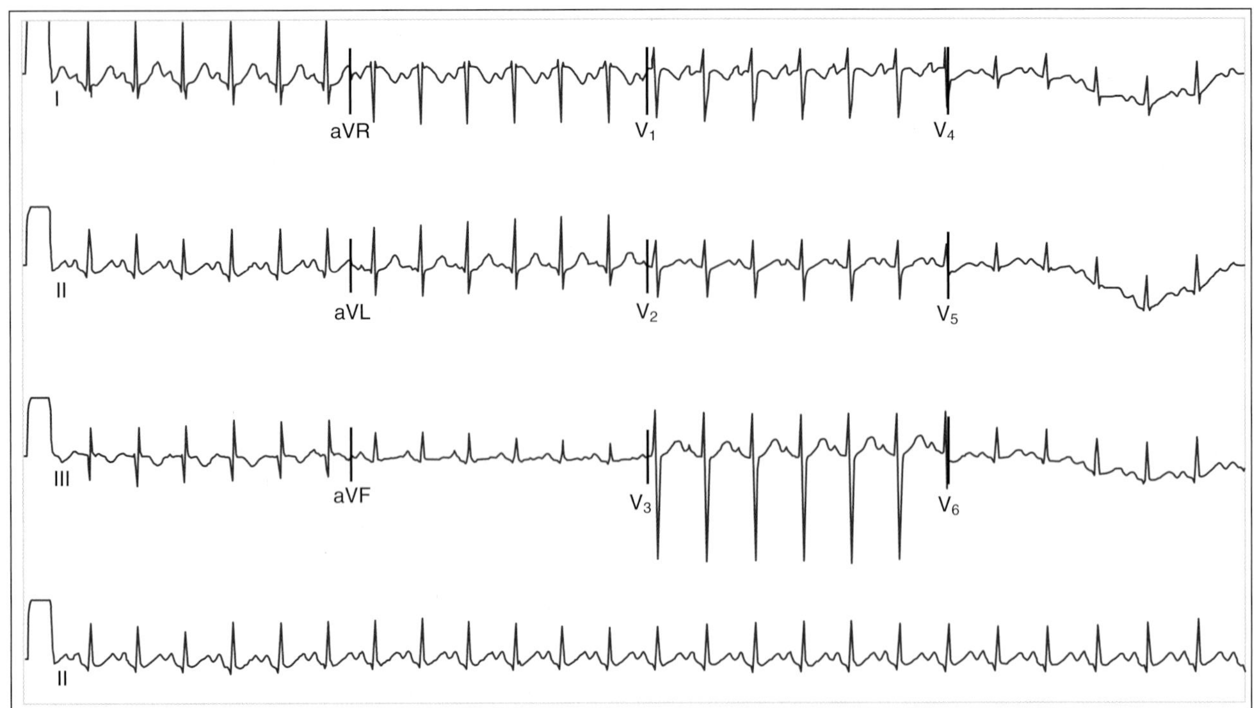


**Fig. 60.5** Sinus tachycardia (rate of 150 beats/min) in a patient with myocarditis.

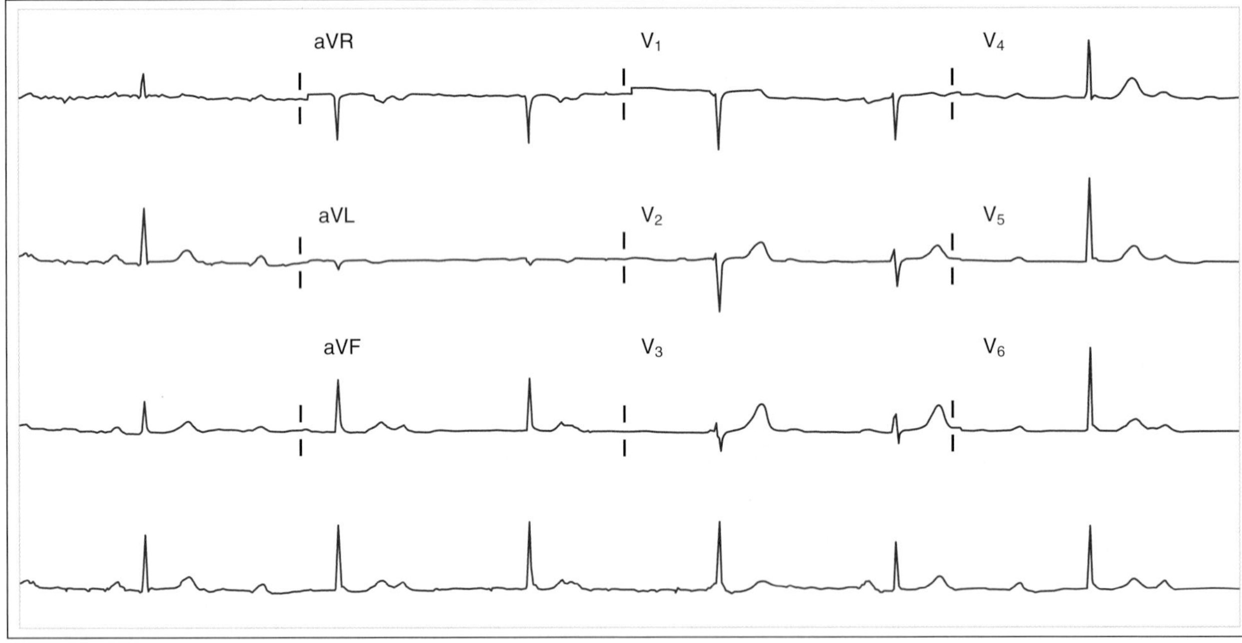


**Fig. 60.6** Sinus rhythm with atrioventricular (AV) dissociation and a high-grade AV block in a patient with myocarditis.

common as well. Severe myocarditis in the very young is often also manifested as pulmonary edema, cardiogenic shock, and multiorgan hypoperfusion.

## DIFFERENTIAL DIAGNOSIS AND MEDICAL DECISION MAKING

The differential diagnosis of myocarditis is extremely broad because of the nonspecific nature of the initial findings. Patients who are initially seen with cardiopulmonary symptoms have a slightly more limited differential diagnosis, but initial consideration should as always be focused on the most deadly diseases that produce chest pain or dyspnea: acute coronary syndrome, aortic dissection, pulmonary embolism, acute pericarditis or pericardial tamponade, esophageal rupture, cardiogenic pulmonary edema, and pneumonia.

The initial diagnostic evaluation should be prompted by clinical suspicion. The finding of cardiopulmonary complaints, unexplained tachycardia, or evidence of congestive heart failure on examination in young patients should prompt consideration of myocarditis. An ECG and chest radiograph are appropriate initial tests in these patients. Despite the absence of a specific or single diagnostic ECG abnormality, the majority of patients with myocarditis have at least some abnormality noted on the ECG. The most common abnormalities are sinus tachycardia (see Fig. 60.5) and nonspecific ST-segment or T-wave changes. Other abnormalities that may occur in patients with myocarditis are conduction abnormalities (new fascicular blocks, new bundle branch blocks, and atrioventricular blocks), atrial or ventricular tachydysrhythmias and bradydysrhythmias, overt ischemic changes (T-wave inversions, ST-segment changes), and Q-wave formation. The ischemic changes are often indistinguishable from those seen with true cardiac ischemia or myocardial infarction. If the pericardium is also involved (myopericarditis), PR-segment depression with concurrent ST-segment elevation may be found. If a pericardial effusion develops, low voltage may occur. The ECG findings are rarely completely normal.

Findings on plain chest radiographs are often frequently in mild or early cases of myocarditis. However, most patients with cardiopulmonary complaints have some radiographic signs of congestive heart failure: cardiomegaly, pulmonary vascular redistribution, interstitial edema, and frank pulmonary edema. Pleural effusions may be present as well.

Laboratory studies typically ordered in the ED include evaluation of markers of inflammation and cardiac biomarkers. Inflammatory markers, such as the white blood cell count, erythrocyte sedimentation rate, and C-reactive protein value, are expected to be elevated, but unfortunately, such elevations are nonspecific. Measurements of markers are sometimes used to monitor the course of the disease after the diagnosis is made. Cardiac biomarkers, including troponin and creatinine phosphokinase values, are also sometimes elevated. The initial elevations in cardiac biomarkers are frequently indistinguishable from those expected with acute myocardial infarction. Serial measurements of cardiac biomarkers can be helpful, however, because the levels do not tend to rise and fall as quickly with myocarditis as with myocardial infarction.

Echocardiography may also be helpful in the ED, especially when there is confusion in distinguishing between myocarditis and acute coronary syndrome. Echocardiography in patients with acute coronary syndrome (with active ischemia) usually demonstrates focal wall hypokinesis. Patients with myocarditis can also have focal hypokinesis, but they are more likely to have diffuse hypokinesis and multichamber dilation as well.[23] In addition, the echocardiogram can demonstrate evidence of complications, such as pericardial effusion or intracardiac thrombus.

Endomyocardial biopsy is usually considered the "gold standard" for the diagnosis of myocarditis. Evidence of microscopic myocardial inflammation with various levels of necrosis is generally used to diagnose and categorize stages of myocarditis.[23,24] However, biopsy is not feasible in the ED. Additionally, recent reports have questioned the sensitivity and specificity of the test.[23,25]

Other tests that can be ordered by the EP are viral cultures, blood cultures, and other immunologic studies. These tests are rarely helpful in the acute setting but may of use to inpatient physicians during the hospital course.

## TREATMENT

Close attention should be paid to the ABCs of resuscitation because patients with fulminant myocarditis can decompensate rapidly. The mainstay of treatment of myocarditis is primarily supportive with a focus on hemodynamic support and management of complications. Congestive heart failure and hypoxia should be treated as usual, with high-flow oxygen, preload and afterload reduction, and diuretics. The patient's fluid status must also be monitored closely because of the risk for congestive heart failure. Bradydysrhythmias should be managed as usual. Patients with high-degree atrioventricular blocks often require pacemaker placement. Tachydysrhythmias should generally be managed as usual, although preference should be given to titratable medications because drugs with negative inotropic effects can precipitate unpredictable hemodynamic collapse in these patients with myocarditis, whose status is tenuous. Intramural thrombi noted on echocardiography should be treated with anticoagulation. The benefit of prophylactic anticoagulation is uncertain, especially given the risk that these patients have for hemopericardium. Additional myocardial workload reduction can be accomplished through fever reduction and correction of anemia.[23]

Patients in shock should be treated aggressively. Adequate perfusion should be achieved in hypotensive patients through the use of vasopressors (e.g., dopamine, norepinephrine) and positive inotropic agents (e.g., dobutamine). Ventricular assist devices, intraaortic balloon counterpulsation, and cardiopulmonary bypass have been used successfully in some patients during the wait for clinical improvement or cardiac transplantation.[23]

Antiviral therapy may be helpful during the patient's hospital course if a viral cause of the myocarditis has been determined. Other therapies should be focused on the determined underlying condition (e.g., Lyme carditis, toxin-induced myocarditis). Immunosuppressive medications have been used successfully in some patients in the later stages of illness, but this experience appears to be anecdotal only.[26] The use of corticosteroids lacks good evidence of benefit as well. High-dose intravenous gamma globulin has been used successfully in some pediatric patients, with improvement in ventricular function at 1 year.[23]

## FOLLOW-UP AND NEXT STEPS IN CARE

Patients in whom myocarditis is suspected should be admitted to the hospital. Cardiac monitoring should be started to assess for the development of dysrhythmias, and close hemodynamic monitoring is indicated as well. Critical care, infectious disease, and cardiology consultants should be involved in the care plans for these patients. Because patients with severely decompensated cardiac conditions may require cardiac transplantation, appropriate surgical consultants should also be involved in the care of patients with severe myocarditis.

## REFERENCES

*References can be found on Expert Consult @ www.expertconsult.com.*

# 61 Cardiac Valvular Disorders

*Pierre Borczuk*

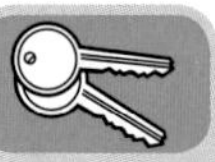

**KEY POINTS**

- In patients evaluated in the emergency department for chest pain, dyspnea, syncope, arrhythmia, or shock, the possibility of valvular heart disease should be considered.
- Emergency echocardiography is essential in elucidating whether acute valvular pathology is responsible for hemodynamic collapse in a patient with cardiogenic shock.
- An asymptomatic patient with a grade 2/6 systolic murmur needs no further work-up.
- Diastolic murmurs are always pathologic and require echocardiography.
- Endocarditis prophylaxis is recommended only for dental procedures and no longer needed for gastrointestinal or genitourinary procedures.

## EPIDEMIOLOGY

Many medical conditions can affect the cardiac valves, including congenital heart disease, infectious or rheumatic causes, and complications of ischemic heart disease. However, in the United States, because of the aging population, degenerative valve disease is the most common cause of valvular pathology. This inflammatory damage to cardiac valves, though of much later onset than rheumatic heart disease and pathologically similar to atherosclerosis, has become an increasingly common cause of valvular heart disease (VHD) in developed nations. In contrast, on a global basis, rheumatic heart disease still remains a major causative agent of VHD.

The American Heart Association/American College of Cardiology has published guidelines for assessment, diagnostic testing, and medical and surgical treatment of VHD.[1] However, there are still many practice guidelines that are based on observational studies instead of randomized controlled trials. Recent trends in care include identifying subgroups of asymptomatic patients who may benefit from surgical intervention, valvular repair rather than replacement, and minimally invasive or percutaneous options.

## PATHOPHYSIOLOGY AND PRESENTING SIGNS AND SYMPTOMS

Of the four heart valves, three are tricuspid (aortic, pulmonic, and tricuspid) and one is bicuspid (mitral). Failure of normal function of these valves is due to lesions that make them incompetent and allow backward flow (regurgitation) or to lesions that decrease orifice size and cause restriction of flow (stenosis). In addition, combinations of these lesions may occur within the same valve, and multiple valves may be involved (commonly the aortic and mitral valves with rheumatic heart disease). Cardiac murmurs result from (1) increased blood flow across a normal or abnormal valve orifice, (2) turbulent flow across a narrow or irregular orifice into a dilated blood vessel or cardiac chamber, or (3) backward flow across an incompetent valve or other cardiac defect. However, most systolic murmurs are related to a physiologic increase in blood velocity and are not pathologic.

Physical examination establishes where the murmur occurs within the cardiac cycle and its location, duration, and intensity. Murmurs are classified as systolic, diastolic, and continuous. Systolic murmurs are further subclassified into holosystolic (pansystolic), midsystolic, early systolic, and late systolic. Clicks can be heard from the snapping shut of diseased valves. Diastolic and continuous murmurs are nearly always pathologic and require investigation, even in the absence of symptoms. Although many systolic murmurs merit investigation, especially those associated with symptoms, the majority of systolic murmurs do not signify valvular disease.[2] A summary of the typical findings in the major valvular abnormalities is presented in **Table 61.1**.

A heart affected by valvular pathology has the ability to compensate over time, and symptoms are commonly absent for decades. Emergency physicians need to be able to identify when certain valvular lesions have progressed to the point that they are clinically important and responsible for the patient's symptom complex. Shortness of breath, arrhythmias, and heart failure are common reasons why patients with VHD seek treatment at an ED. Other clinical scenarios include valve infection, myocardial infarction with papillary muscle dysfunction, and failure of a prosthetic device, which can cause rapid heart failure and shock. It should be kept in mind that valvular pathology is in the differential diagnosis of patients with congestive heart failure, shock, and angina. The clinician should perform a careful cardiac examination with attention

**Table 61.1 Characteristics of Common Cardiac Murmurs**

| VALVE PATHOLOGY | MURMUR | LOCATION | VALSALVA EFFECT |
|---|---|---|---|
| Aortic stenosis | Systolic crescendo-decrescendo | Base to neck | Decreases |
| Aortic regurgitation | Diastolic decrescendo | Left sternal border | Decreases |
| Mitral stenosis | Diastolic rumble | Apex | Decreases |
| Mitral regurgitation | Holosystolic | Apex to axilla | Decreases |
| Mitral valve prolapse | Midsystolic click, late crescendo-decrescendo | Apex to axilla | Increases |
| Tricuspid regurgitation | Holosystolic | Left sternal border | Decreases |

to pulses, quality, and murmur types and locations. Does the patient with an aortic stenosis murmur have symptoms of angina pectoris, syncope, or heart failure? Are signs of embolic phenomena present in a patient with fever and a prosthetic heart valve? It is important to identify patients with severe aortic stenosis before using certain medications with preload effects because these drugs can cause significant hypotension.

Patients with midsystolic murmurs, grade 2 or less, and no associated findings or symptoms do not need any further work-up other than a history and physical examination. Aortic sclerosis is the most common defect found in these patients and requires no other intervention. However, patients with holosystolic murmurs, grade 3 murmurs, and diastolic or continuous murmurs should undergo further work-up with echocardiography.[3] Some of these patients may eventually need cardiac catheterization if valve repair is planned. In patients with cardiopulmonary symptoms, detection of any new murmur warrants further investigation. The lack of a murmur in a patient with prosthetic heart valves may be pathologic and also requires further evaluation.

Clues about the significance of the VHD can be gleaned from chest radiography and electrocardiography (ECG). One may note valvular calcifications, asymmetric chambers sizes, and prosthetic valves. ECG may reveal signs of left atrial enlargement with tall or biphasic P waves, as well as left ventricular hypertrophy (LVH) or atrial fibrillation (AF).

## DIFFERENTIAL DIAGNOSIS AND MEDICAL DECISION MAKING

Valvular causes must be kept in mind in patients with chest pain, shortness of breath, arrhythmia, syncope, or shock. Patients with fever and new heart murmurs may have infectious endocarditis. An aortic insufficiency (AI) murmur in a patient with chest pain would lead to a diagnostic work-up for aortic dissection. Patients sustaining blunt trauma may rarely have traumatic aortic injury and, though rare, acute traumatic valvular injury as well.

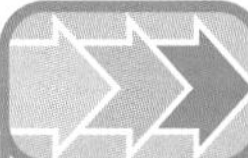

**PRIORITY ACTIONS**

A new diastolic murmur in a patient with chest or back pain should raise suspicion for aortic dissection and requires urgent testing and consultation, as well as control of the heart rate and blood pressure.

Patients with valvular heart disease may become hemodynamically unstable with rapid atrial fibrillation and require cardioversion.

Infectious endocarditis should be considered in all patients with a prosthetic valve and fever. Blood cultures and empiric antibiotics are indicated.

Beside echocardiography should be performed in patients with shortness of breath who have recently undergone prosthetic valve replacement to rule out pericardial tamponade.

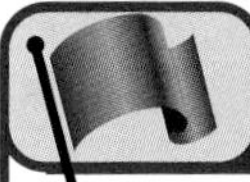

**RED FLAGS**

A careful murmur examination should be performed in patients with chest pain. Individuals with severe aortic stenosis are dependent on preload to maintain systolic blood pressure, and treatment with nitrates can cause severe hypotension.

Patients in cardiogenic shock from acute mitral regurgitation, aortic regurgitation, or prosthetic valve dysfunction may not have an appreciable murmur and require emergency echocardiography. These conditions are treated surgically and will require cardiac surgery consultation.

Emergency physicians need to recognize that the absence of a murmur or mechanical heart sound is pathologic in a patient with mechanical heart valve prosthesis.

Be vigilant in patients with a bicuspid valve and chest pain because of an increased risk for aortic dissection in these individuals.

## SPECIFIC VALVE LESIONS

### AORTIC STENOSIS

Aortic stenosis (AS) is the third most common form of cardiovascular disease in the Western world after hypertension and coronary artery disease. The most common causes of AS are calcification of a normal tricuspid valve and a congenital bicuspid aortic valve. Calcific degeneration of the aortic valve results from an inflammatory process similar to atherosclerotic vascular disease; it begins with intimal injury, such as

**Table 61.2** Aortic Stenosis—Severity of Disease

| SEVERITY | MEAN GRADIENT (mm Hg) | VALVE AREA (cm²) | JET VELOCITY (m/sec) |
|---|---|---|---|
| Mild | <25 | >1.5 | <3 |
| Moderate | 25-40 | 1-1.5 | 3-4 |
| Severe | >40 | <1 | >4 |

calcification from the base of the cusps to the leaflets, which impairs motion, and progresses through fusion of valve leaflets and stenosis of the aortic valve orifice. When rheumatic heart disease is the culprit, the aortic valve commonly exhibits both stenosis and regurgitation and is usually associated with concomitant mitral valve disease.

The degree of aortic valve disease is based on several factors[4] (**Table 61.2**). Such assessment may be inaccurate and underestimate valve area and jet velocity in patients with impaired cardiac output. Progression of AS is usually quite slow, with symptoms taking decades to become manifested in most cases. An average 0.1-cm² decrease in valve area occurs per year.[5] The left ventricle is faced with systolic pressure overload and compensates through hypertrophy of the left ventricular (LV) wall. Normal chamber volume is maintained, but with increased wall thickness. The hypertrophic wall may lead to decreased coronary blood flow, even in the absence of stenosis and angina. Diastolic dysfunction and heart failure symptoms may also be present. These patients are dependent on forceful atrial contraction to maintain elevated LV end-diastolic pressure (LVEDP) to overcome the obstruction to outflow. Therefore, individuals who have AF and AS may suffer hemodynamic consequences from loss of the atrial kick.

Auscultation reveals a systolic murmur associated with diminished and delayed carotid pulses (parvus et tardus), a sustained LV impulse on palpation, and a decreased or absent aortic component of the second heart sound ($S_2$). Parvus et tardus may not be readily apparent in the elderly because of decreased compliance of the aging arterial vessels. Chest radiography may show normal heart size (remember concentric LVH) with rounding of the LV border. ECG can show LVH with a repolarization abnormality, which is seen in 85% of patients with severe AS. Echocardiography is indicated every year for patients with severe AS to assess the severity of the AS, wall thickness, and LV function. Exercise stress testing may lead to complications in patients with symptomatic AS and should not be performed.[6]

Asymptomatic patients with AS have the same life expectancy outcome as age-matched controls. Once symptoms appear, the average survival is 2 to 3 years, with a risk for sudden death (<1% per year). Angina develops in 35% of patients, syncope in 15%, and congestive heart failure or dyspnea in 50%.

No medical treatment has been shown to decrease progression of disease in the leaflets, although statins are currently being studied. Significant care should be taken when treating these patients with preload-reducing agents (nitrates) because the sudden decrease in preload can cause severe hypotension, which in turn can lead to decreased coronary flow and worsen ischemia and shock. Cardiac catheterization is indicated in patients who have a discrepancy between the clinical complex and the results of echocardiography. Patients in whom cardiac surgery is planned need to undergo cardiac catheterization to assess the need for a concomitant coronary artery bypass grafting (CABG) procedure. The average mortality in patients who undergo aortic valve replacement (AVR) is 3% to 4% and, when associated with a CABG procedure, 5.5% to 6.8%. Percutaneous valvuloplasty is the use of a balloon to fracture calcium deposits in the leaflets. It results in immediate improvement in valve gradients; however, restenosis occurs in 6 to 12 months, and it is therefore not recommended for definitive treatment. This procedure has been used as a temporizing measure in patients who are not initially AVR candidates. Procedures are now available that allow percutaneous AVR in such patients.[7]

## AORTIC REGURGITATION

Multiple conditions can cause aortic regurgitation (AR); the most important for the emergency department (ED) physician are aortic dissection, trauma, and endocarditis.[8] Patients with congenital bicuspid valves are also at risk for both AI and dissection. Rheumatic heart disease is still the most common cause of AR worldwide. Cardiac examination in patients with AR reveals a murmur during diastole, more low pitched and associated with a widened pulse pressure and displaced LV impulse. Eponyms associated with AR include Corrigan pulse (rapid rising pulse that falls rapidly), Quincke pulse (capillary pulsations at the base of the nail when pressure is applied at the tip), and the Duroziez sign (to-and-fro murmur over the femoral arteries).

Patients with acute AI have a sudden large regurgitant blood volume. Because the heart has not had time to compensate, large rises in LVEDP and left atrial pressure and a decrease in stroke volume occur.[9] Patients are seen in shock, with hypotension and pulmonary edema. If the LVEDP and aortic pressure gradients are close enough, decreased coronary blood flow and myocardial ischemia can develop. This low gradient may make it impossible to hear a murmur. Emergency bedside echocardiography with color flow Doppler imaging is necessary to establish the diagnosis.

Medical management of acute AI should be directed toward reducing afterload and increasing contractility. Combinations of nitroprusside and dobutamine may augment forward flow and reduce regurgitant volume and LVEDP. Intraaortic balloon pump treatment is contraindicated because it increases regurgitant volume as it inflates during diastole. Ideally, patients with acute AR have a lesion that is surgically amenable and medical management is only a bridge to definitive therapy.

In patients with chronic AI the left ventricle has had time to compensate to the increased volume by increasing both LV end-diastolic volume and LV wall compliance. This allows accommodation of the increased regurgitant volume without significantly increasing chamber pressure. Stroke volume is increased to make up for the backward flow volume.

Echocardiography is essential in the diagnostic management of patients over time. Patients who have AI, normal LV function, and no symptoms do not need any medical treatment. Valve replacement is recommended in patients with severe AR or LV dysfunction, regardless of whether they are symptomatic. Medical therapy with vasodilating drugs (nifedipine, hydralazine, angiotensin-converting enzyme inhibitors) is reserved for patients with severe AR who are not surgical candidates or as short-term treatment before valve replacement. Beta-blockers will theoretically increase time during diastole and worsen the amount of regurgitant volume. The rate of progression from an asymptomatic patient with normal LV function to an asymptomatic patient with LV dysfunction is 3.5% per year. Once LV dysfunction is detected on ultrasound, most patients will become symptomatic in 2 to 3 years.

## MITRAL STENOSIS

The normal mitral valve has an area of 4 to 5 cm$^2$, and symptoms usually begin when the valve area becomes less than 2.5 cm$^2$. Mitral stenosis (MS) nearly always results from previous rheumatic fever. In fact, a history of rheumatic fever can be elicited in up to 60% of patients with MS. A period of 20 to 40 years may transpire between the occurrence of rheumatic fever and the onset of symptoms, and another 10 years may elapse before these symptoms become disabling.[10] The ratio of women to men with MS is 2:1. MS can also result from severe degenerative calcification, especially in the elderly. Dyspnea is the cardinal symptom of significant MS. Shortness of breath may not develop in patients with milder MS until AF with rapid ventricular response or pregnancy occurs or it is precipitated by exercise or infection.

Because the main problem in MS is obstruction to blood flow, no medical therapy is available that will relieve this obstruction. The principal treatment is surgical repair or valve replacement. Beta-blockers will cause bradycardia and increase diastolic filling time and may benefit patients in whom symptoms develop secondary to tachycardia. Anticoagulation is indicated in patients with MS and AF because systemic embolization occurs in 10% to 20% of patients with MS.

Percutaneous mitral balloon valvotomy in the hands of skilled operators can be the procedure of choice in patients with moderate to severe MS who are symptomatic (significant MR and left atrial thrombus are contraindications to this procedure).[11] Open surgical commissurotomy and mitral valve replacement are other alternatives for mitral valve treatment.

## MITRAL REGURGITATION

Causes of mitral regurgitation (MR) can be split into organic and functional categories. Organic causes include mitral valve prolapse (MVP), rheumatic fever, endocarditis, and certain medications (most recently the use of diet supplements). The most common functional cause of MR is secondary LV dilation leading to a dilated annulus. Other functional causes include ruptured chordae tendineae, ruptured papillary muscle, and infective endocarditis. Patients with MR may exhibit a holosystolic murmur in association with a first heart sound ($S_1$) that is soft or absent and, frequently, a normal second heart sound ($S_2$).

Patients with acute MR have acute volume overload on the left atrium and left ventricle and, given lack of time for compensation, both decreased cardiac output and increased pulmonary congestion. The role of medical therapy is limited to stabilizing the patient's hemodynamics before surgery. Diminishing MR, increasing forward flow, and improving pulmonary congestion can all be accomplished by afterload reduction with nitroprusside (if the patient can tolerate it) or an inotropic medication (dobutamine). An intraaortic balloon pump can also be used as a temporizing measure before definitive treatment. Therapy for acute papillary muscle rupture is emergency valve repair or replacement.

Clinically, however, most patients will have chronic MR. The heart will compensate by increasing LV size (the usual mechanism for chronic volume overload). This increased size allows a higher volume at lower pressure. The duration of this asymptomatic chronic phase is about 6 to 10 years.[12] Patients with ischemic cardiomyopathy can be treated with beta-blockers and angiotensin-converting enzyme inhibitors. AF rate control is also important. In patients with severe MR who are symptomatic, as well as in asymptomatic patients with severe MR and an ejection fraction of 30% to 60%, surgical therapy is indicated and includes mitral valve repair or replacement.

## MITRAL VALVE PROLAPSE

MVP is defined as billowing of the leaflets into the left atrium with or without associated MR. Current estimates of MVP based on newer diagnostic criteria suggest that less than 2.5% of the population is affected. Familial causes may represent a manifestation of connective tissue disease. Patients with MVP may experience chest pain, anxiety, palpitations, and dyspnea. Physical examination reveals a midsystolic click, frequently in association with a late systolic murmur.[13] Patients suspected of having MVP should arrange follow-up with a cardiologist or primary care physician and will probably undergo echocardiography. Patients with MVP who have had a transient ischemic attack or cerebrovascular attack should be treated with daily acetylsalicylic acid.[14]

## ENDOCARDITIS AND RHEUMATIC FEVER PROPHYLAXIS

Recently, guidelines for the prophylaxis of infective endocarditis have undergone changes based on working group review. No randomized controlled trial examining the efficacy of prophylaxis before procedures has ever been conducted. In fact, endocarditis is more likely to be related to random bacteremia with daily activities than to specific dental, gastrointestinal, or genitourinary procedures. Therefore, prophylaxis would prevent only a very small number of cases. Because antibiotics have side effects, in many scenarios the risk exceeds any possible prophylactic benefit. High-risk events include dental procedures that involve the gingiva. Prophylaxis would be recommended in (1) patients with prosthetic valves or prosthetic material, (2) patients with a history of endocarditis, (3) patients with valve disease and a transplanted organ, and (4) high-risk patients with congenital heart disease. Antibiotic prophylaxis is not recommended for gastrointestinal or genitourinary procedures or for respiratory procedures.

Patients who have previously had rheumatic fever are at higher risk for the development of another episode of rheumatic fever. Because antibiotics have been shown to prevent recurrent attacks, prophylaxis with penicillin or an antibiotic of the macrolide class is recommended.

## PROSTHETIC VALVE DISORDERS

Valve repair and replacement surgery are common procedures that have been significantly refined over the past 40 years, and approximately 100,000 prosthetic valves are implanted in patients in the United States and 300,000 worldwide. Prosthetic heart valves are divided into two broad classes, mechanical and biologic. Mechanical valves have evolved considerably since their introduction in 1965 with the Starr-Edwards ball valve. Shortly thereafter, in 1969, disk valves were introduced with the Björk-Shiley valve. Problems involving strut malfunction led to discontinuation of this valve in the United States in 1986. Bileaflet valves, including the St. Jude valve, which was introduced in 1977, are the most commonly implanted mechanical valves today.

Biologic valves are used in patients in whom long-term systemic anticoagulation is less desirable, and their use must be balanced against the need for reoperation because these valves will degenerate over the years. The most common biologic valve in the United States is the Carpentier-Edwards valve. Valves in the mitral position are at higher risk for thrombus formation than are valves in the aortic position, and some clinicians will treat bioprosthetic valves in the mitral position with warfarin.

A lateral chest radiograph can help in identifying a prosthetic valve. An imaginary line is drawn from the cardiac apex to the carina. Valves above this line are aortic and pulmonic, whereas valves below this line are mitral and tricuspid (**Fig. 61.1**).

Early complications after valve replacement include pericardial effusion with tamponade (pericardial inflammation and bleeding, which is exacerbated by anticoagulation), perioperative myocardial infarction, Dressler syndrome, AF, and early endocardial infection. Late prosthetic valve complications include AF, thromboembolic phenomena, endocarditis, valve malfunction as a result of thrombus or tissue ingrowth (pannus formation), and mechanical hemolytic anemia. Valve complications should be considered in any patient with a prosthetic valve who has symptoms of dyspnea, syncope, angina, or fever or has neurologic signs or symptoms. Absence of a murmur does not rule out prosthetic valve dysfunction. Cardiology consultation and admission for further evaluation are warranted. In patients with mechanical heart valves and reversal of the international normalized ratio (INR) who have previously had thromboembolism, cessation of warfarin therapy is associated with a 10% to 20% annual risk for recurrent thromboembolism. Therefore, the risk is relatively small for reversal if brief (days), and these risk-benefit decisions must be individualized: Because its onset of action of vitamin k is delayed, its use should be avoided because it will only lead to a prolonged time for achieving a therapeutic INR once warfarin is reinstituted.

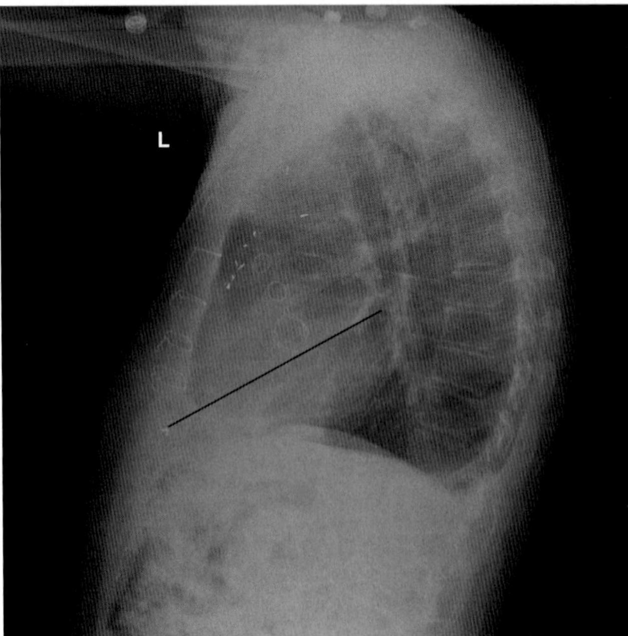


**Fig. 61.1 Imaginary line technique for identification of prosthetic valves.** An imaginary line is drawn from the carina to the apex. An aortic valve rests above this line (as in the radiograph shown), whereas a mitral valve would appear below the line.

## TREATMENT

In all patients with VHD, the goals of the emergency physician are to (1) determine whether valvular abnormality is the cause of the signs and symptoms, (2) optimize the hemodynamic status of patients who have suffered acute decompensation, (3) remember that certain subgroups of patients may need prophylaxis for endocarditis, and (4) make the appropriate consultations with cardiology and surgery.

Patients with new heart murmurs should undergo focused physical examination, ECG, and chest radiography. The outpatient arena is usually the venue for asymptomatic patients. Innocent murmurs will not need any further evaluation, whereas other murmurs will require outpatient echocardiography; communication with the patient's primary care physician or cardiologist (or both) is essential.

It is critical to consider VHD as a cause of the symptoms in all patients with shock, dyspnea, chest pain, syncope, or other symptoms that that are consistent with worsening heart failure or arrhythmia. Echocardiography is recommended for all symptomatic patients in whom the findings on evaluation are consistent with valvular abnormality, as are hospital admission and cardiology consultation. It may be difficult to establish a valvular cause of cardiogenic shock based on physical examination only, and these patients will require emergency echocardiography.

Management of patients with acute valvular decompensation requiring stabilization and hemodynamic support is similar to that for any critically ill patient and begins with airway management. Assessment of circulation includes examination of the pulse, blood pressure, and systemic oxygen delivery. Skin color, temperature, capillary refill time, and measurement of serum lactate and B-type natriuretic peptide should be performed. Maneuvers should then be undertaken to improve cardiac output to meet systemic oxygen demand. Treating shock in patients with acute valvular disorders requires a thorough understanding that maximizing cardiac output and systemic oxygen delivery does not necessarily mean increasing blood pressure. Similarly, patients with pulmonary congestion may not all benefit from a significant reduction in circulating volume or preload. In general, patients who are hypotensive should benefit from volume infusion unless they exhibit overt signs or symptoms of pulmonary edema. However, in patients with MR, greater preload or volume may result in an increase in mitral orifice size and thus in regurgitant volume. In patients in whom an acute coronary syndrome is a possibility, emergency diagnostic cardiac catheterization may be appropriate. An intraaortic balloon pump may also be useful to a failing heart. A bedside ED echocardiogram demonstrating a pericardial effusion will hasten the work-up for aortic arch dissection.

## DISPOSITION

Medical and surgical management of patients with VHD is based on symptomatology and echocardiographic measurements. Therefore, patients seen in the ED with symptoms and findings on physical examination, ECG, and chest radiography consistent with valvular dysfunction need an expedited work-up and should be admitted to the hospital for echocardiography and cardiology evaluation. Patients in cardiogenic shock will need intensive care unit management, and if a valvular cause is strongly being considered, such management should occur at an institution with the capability of cardiac surgery because emergency valve surgery may be needed. Prosthetic valve endocarditis should be considered in all patients with artificial valves who exhibit fever, congestive heart failure, or thromboembolic phenomena. Antibiotics need to be instituted empirically after adequate blood is obtained for culture.

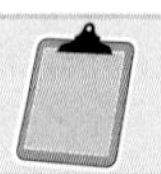

### DOCUMENTATION

Intensity (grade 1-6 out of 6), timing during the cardiac cycle, location, and radiation are the principal ways to characterize a cardiac murmur.

Comment on heart size and chamber enlargement on the chest radiograph and whether left ventricular hypertrophy is present on the electrocardiogram.

Document the rationale if transfer is required for urgent cardiology or cardiothoracic surgery consultation.

Document risk-benefit discussions with patients and consultants when reversing anticoagulation in patients with mechanical prosthetic valves.

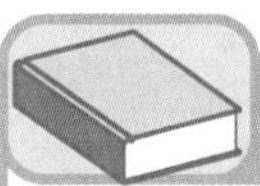

### PATIENT TEACHING TIPS

Murmurs are the sound that blood makes as it moves through the heart, and most of these sounds are normal and do not represent disease.

An ultrasound of your heart is the way that the doctor determines whether the heart valve is leaking (regurgitation) or whether its opening is narrowed (stenosis).

In most situations, people with heart murmurs and no other symptoms do not need any treatment. Some categories of heart murmurs will require monitoring with ultrasound to evaluate for progression of disease.

Chest pain, fainting, shortness of breath, and palpitations are symptoms that require evaluation by a physician and possible cardiology referral.

## REFERENCES

*References can be found on Expert Consult @ www.expertconsult.com.*

# 62 Endocarditis

*Osman R. Sayan and Wallace A. Carter*

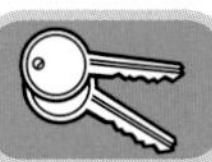

**KEY POINTS**

- Endocarditis is an inflammation of the endothelial lining of the heart. It is usually focal and commonly occurs at points of endocardial injury. The mitral and aortic valves are the most common sites of involvement.
- Most sites of endocardial injury become seeded with bacteria during episodes of transient bacteremia and thus develop into infective endocarditis.
- The initial symptoms are often vague—low-grade fever, malaise, and weakness.
- Manifestations can vary from direct structural cardiac injury to conduction system disturbances, embolic phenomena, and cardiogenic or septic shock.
- Suspicion of infective endocarditis should be raised by the presence of well-known risk factors, such as acquired or congenital valvular or structural heart disease, a prosthetic valve, implanted medical devices, injection drug use, and a previous history of endocarditis.
- Laboratory testing is often not useful for the emergency physician, but at least three sets of blood cultures performed over time are critical for the diagnosis of infective endocarditis, as well as for guiding subsequent therapy.
- The most useful initial diagnostic test is echocardiography.
- In an acutely ill patient, prompt resuscitation, antibiotics, and surgical consultation are imperative.
- In a stable patient with subacute disease, time until initiation of antibiotic therapy is less critical than performance of serial blood cultures.
- Nearly all patients with infective endocarditis require hospital admission. Only the most stable patients with no complications in whom the diagnosis of infective endocarditis is being entertained but not confirmed may be discharged with very close follow-up care.
- Despite medical advances, the overall mortality for both native valve and prosthetic valve infective endocarditis still ranges from 20% to 25%.[1]
- Prevention of disease is most important. In 2007 the American Heart Association issued revised guidelines for antibiotic prophylaxis in patients at risk for endocarditis.

## EPIDEMIOLOGY

Endocarditis is an inflammation of the endothelium, or inner lining, of the heart or heart valves (or both). The disrupted endothelium is very susceptible to seeding with infectious agents such as bacteria, viruses, and fungi, a condition known as infective endocarditis (IE). Recognized by medical science for more than 400 years, IE remains an illness that is difficult to diagnose and treat and still results in significant morbidity and mortality.

Over the last 30 years, published reports regarding the overall incidence of IE have conflictingly cited both a stable incidence and a rising incidence.[1-3] Mortality ranges from 5% to 50% or higher. The reason for such variation in the statistics is that IE is a diverse and evolving disease entity—one that is strongly influenced by the characteristics of both the human and microbial populations being studied (**Table 62.1**).

In the developed world, IE has undergone a remarkable transformation over the last century. In the developing world, however, it has remained rather unchanged. Much of this difference is a result of the influence of advances in health care (e.g., antibiotics, disease prevention, medical devices, the resulting longevity of populations), as well as the complications that arise from these advances (e.g., nosocomial infections and resistant organisms).[4,5]

Unfortunately, the tremendous advances made in health care have not translated into the gains that we have seen in other infectious diseases in the last 50 to 80 years. Untreated, IE has a mortality of nearly 100%. When treated, however, IE is still associated with a mortality rate of 20% to 25%.[5] The overall incidence of IE in the developed world has remained unchanged.[1] Why has the advent of antibiotics, advanced critical care and surgical techniques, and medical devices such as prosthetic valves not made a difference in this statistic? There are several reasons.

First, with a low prevalence, no pathognomonic signs or symptoms, and no single diagnostic front-line test, IE remains difficult to diagnose. Therefore, many cases are missed or diagnosed only when the disease is advanced. Second, despite the effective control of rheumatic heart disease in the developed world, new risk factors have arisen to fill the void. Degenerative heart disease in the growing elderly population has replaced rheumatic fever as the major cause of valvular disease. The same intravascular medical devices that have improved survival for patients (e.g., valvular prosthetics, cardiac pacemakers, long-term indwelling vascular catheters)

**Table 62.1 Statistics for Infective Endocarditis (IE) in the Developed World**

| | |
|---|---|
| Median age of IE patients in the preantibiotic era | 30-40 yr |
| Median age of IE patients in the antibiotic era | 47-69 yr |
| Mean male-to-female ratio | 1.7-2.0:1 |
| Incidence of community-acquired native valve IE (western Europe/ United States) | 1.7-6.2 cases per 100,000 person-years |
| Incidence of IE in persons with known mitral valve prolapse | 100 cases per 100,000 person-years |
| Incidence of IE in injection drug users | 150-2000 cases per 100,000 person-years |
| Prosthetic valve IE | 7-25% of all cases of IE |
| Overall mortality for both native and prosthetic valve IE | 20-25% |
| Mortality with viridans group streptococci and *Streptococcus bovis* IE | 4-16% |
| Mortality with enterococci IE | 15-25% |
| Mortality with Q fever IE | 5-37% |
| Mortality with *Staphylococcus aureus* IE | 25-47% |
| Mortality with *Pseudomonas aeruginosa*, Enterobacteriaceae, or fungal IE | >50% |

Adapted from Mylonakis E, Calderwood SB. Infective endocarditis in adults. N Engl J Med 2001;345:1318-30.

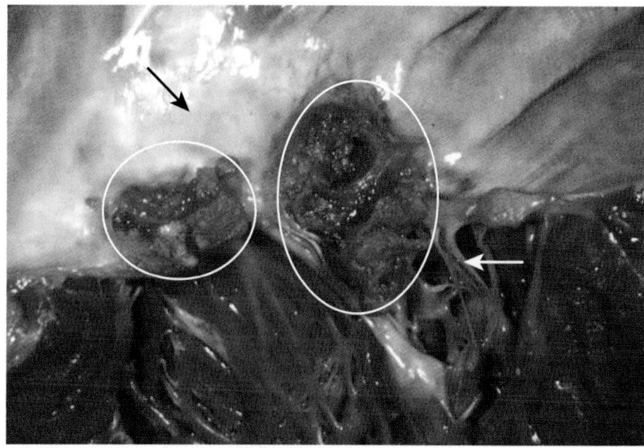

**Fig. 62.1 Large vegetations *(circles)* at the edge of this mitral valve *(black arrow)*.** Chordae tendineae *(white arrow)* connect the mitral valve to papillary muscles in the left ventricle. (Courtesy Charles C. Marboe, MD.)

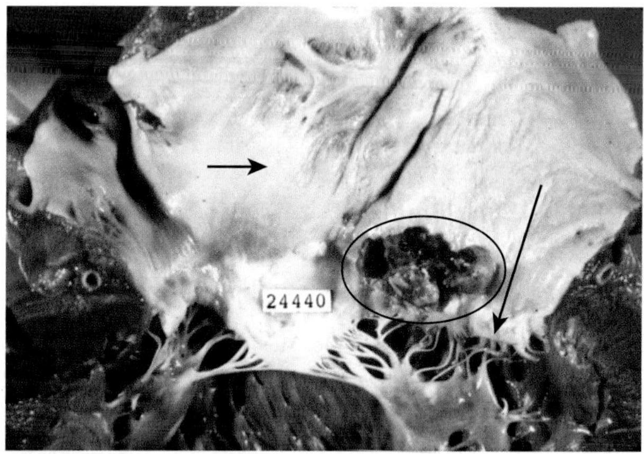


**Fig. 62.2 Large vegetation *(circle)* in a patient with endocarditis.** The *short arrow* indicates the endocardial surface of the dilated left atrium, and the *long arrow* indicates the edge of the mitral valve and chordae tendineae. (Courtesy Charles C. Marboe, MD.)

predispose them to the development of IE (regardless of whether they have had IE in the past). Third, the number of patients at risk for IE has increased—the elderly, patients receiving critical care, and immunocompromised patients (because of acquired immunodeficiency syndrome, diabetes mellitus, end-stage renal disease, chemotherapy, and other reasons). Risky social behavior, such as body piercing and injection drug use, is practiced more today than in the early 20th century. Finally and most concerning of all, burgeoning antibiotic resistance is making treatment of IE more challenging and sometimes unachievable.[6]

Because prevention and early diagnosis are the keys to reducing the morbidity and mortality associated with IE, emergency physicians (EPs) must play an important role in this process. Vigilance is key. EPs must consider the diagnosis when patients with risk factors for IE are seen in the emergency department (ED) with subtle symptoms. EPs must provide education to patients who are at high risk for IE and must provide prophylaxis for IE when warranted.

## PATHOPHYSIOLOGY

The term *endocarditis* literally means inflammation of the inner lining or endothelium of the heart or lining of heart valves (or both). Local or systemic stressors, such as trauma, blood-borne contaminants (e.g., talc from injection drug use), inflammation, and abnormal blood turbulence, induce injury to the endothelium. Clinically relevant endocarditis results from the formation of a fibrin and platelet cap on the area of altered surface endothelium. Most commonly, a sterile cap forms at a site of endothelial injury. IE occurs when microbes adhere to these sites of sterile endothelial injury during transient periods of bacteremia, fungemia, or viremia. Colonization occurs, followed by microbial multiplication and growth of each cap into a vegetation (**Figs. 62.1 and 62.2**). Because of their direct contact with the bloodstream, these infections cause a continuous, albeit low-level presence of microbes in the blood. The clinical manifestations of endocarditis are quite varied as a result of immunologic, infectious, and embolic processes. It is this variation in manifestations that often makes endocarditis difficult to identify.

## MICROBIOLOGY OF INFECTIVE ENDOCARDITIS

Although the microbiology of IE can predict the course of a patient's illness and guide therapy, the actual infecting organism is rarely known to the EP. The EP needs to know the microbes that cause IE (**Box 62.1**) and the local resistance patterns to make sound choices regarding empiric antibiotic treatment regimens. This section discusses the organisms most commonly associated with IE.[6] Certain patient characteristics and clinical scenarios are associated with particular microorganisms (**Table 62.2**). These scenarios may guide the EP's choice of empiric antibiotics; specific regimens are discussed later in this chapter (see Table 62.4).

**BOX 62.1 Microorganisms That Cause Infective Endocarditis (Approximate Percentage)**

**Most Common**

*Staphylococcus aureus* (31%)
Viridans group streptococci (17%)
Enterococci (11%)
*Staphylococcus epidermidis* (11%)

**Less Common**

*Streptococcus bovis* (7%)
*Streptococcus pneumoniae* and other streptococci (5%)
*Pseudomonas aeruginosa* (<3%)
Culture-negative bacteria (12%):
- *Abiotrophia* spp.
- *Bartonella* spp. (usually *henselae* or *quintana*)
- *Brucella* spp. (usually *melitensis* or *abortus*)
- *Chlamydia* spp. (usually *psittaci*)
- *Coxiella burnetii* (Q fever)
- HACEK group of gram-negative bacteria*
- *Legionella* spp.
- *Tropheryma whippelii*

Fungi (2%)

**Haemophilus* species, *Actinobacillus actinomycetemcomitans*, *Cardiobacterium hominis*, *Eikenella corrodens*, and *Kingella kingae*.
Adapted from Baddour LM, Wilson WR, Bayer AS, et al, for the Committee on Rheumatic Fever, Endocarditis, and Kawasaki Disease; Council on Cardiovascular Disease in the Young; Councils on Clinical Cardiology, Stroke, and Cardiovascular Surgery and Anesthesia; American Heart Association; Infectious Diseases Society of America. Infective endocarditis: diagnosis, antimicrobial therapy, and management of complications. A statement for healthcare professionals from the Committee on Rheumatic Fever, Endocarditis, and Kawasaki Disease, Council on Cardiovascular Disease in the Young, and the Councils on Clinical Cardiology, Stroke, and Cardiovascular Surgery and Anesthesia, American Heart Association: endorsed by the Infectious Diseases Society of America. Circulation 2005;111:e394-434; and Murdoch DR, Corey GR, Hoen B, et al, for the International Collaboration on Endocarditis—Prospective Cohort Study (ICE-PCS) Investigators. Clinical presentation, etiology, and outcome of infective endocarditis in the 21st century. Arch Intern Med 2009;169:463-73.

### BACTERIA

#### *Viridans Group Streptococci*

*Streptococcus viridans*, formerly a species name, is actually a group of gram-positive cocci. This group has been the most common cause of IE, although more recent case series have shown that *Staphylococcus aureus* may now be more common.[6,7] These streptococci usually seed previously damaged cardiac tissue. The clinical findings are usually more insidious, however, with patients experiencing malaise, weakness, and low-grade fever.

#### Staphylococcus aureus

Studies have now identified *S. aureus* rather than the viridans group of streptococci as the most common cause of IE.[1,7] *S. aureus* can infect normal valvular endothelium—that is, endothelium without antecedent damage or disease—and usually causes aggressive valve destruction. It is associated with injection drug use, as well as with prosthetic valve endocarditis that occurs more than 1 month after surgery.

Over the last decade, the story of *S. aureus* and *S. aureus* IE has become increasingly complicated with the emergence of methicillin-resistant *S. aureus* (MRSA), as well as the subsequent identification of community-associated (CA-MRSA) and hospital-associated (HA-MRSA) subtypes. CA-MRSA has a tendency to affect previously healthy individuals but has a drug sensitivity pattern more favorable than that of HA-MRSA. HA-MRSA tends to affect the infirm (hospitalized, nursing home, elderly, preterm, and immunocompromised patients) and has a limited sensitivity pattern. A review of cases of native valve IE caused by these organisms reveals a higher mortality rate with HA-MRSA (37%) than with methicillin-sensitive *S. aureus* and CA-MRSA (23% and 13%, respectively).[8]

#### Staphylococcus epidermidis

*S. epidermidis* is an organism associated with prosthetic valve endocarditis, especially that occurring within 1 month of surgery. The course of IE attributable to this organism is usually aggressive.

#### Streptococcus bovis

Infective endocarditis caused by *S. bovis* occurs more commonly in the elderly and often originates from a gastrointestinal (GI) source. It is commonly associated with GI polyps, inflammatory bowel disease, and GI malignancy.

#### Streptococcus pneumoniae

*S. pneumoniae* is an aggressive organism that frequently causes an acute, fulminant illness. It can infect normal heart valves, most often the aortic valve, with a high risk for the development of perivalvular abscesses or pericarditis. Pneumococcal endocarditis can occur in association with pneumococcal pneumonia and meningitis in a grouping called the Austrian triad.

#### *Enterococci*

Enterococci are normal flora of the GI tract and, occasionally, the anterior urethra. IE caused by one of these organisms usually runs a subacute course, but cure is often difficult because of the bacteria's intrinsic resistance to antibiotics. The

**Table 62.2** Characteristics of Patients with Infectious Endocarditis and Associated Microorganisms

| CHARACTERISTIC | ORGANISM | COURSE/FACTS* |
|---|---|---|
| Community-acquired IE involving a native valve | Viridans group streptococci | Indolent gram-positive bacteria<br>Most common cause of native valve endocarditis<br>Usually seeds damaged cardiac tissue |
| | *Staphylococcus aureus* | Aggressive gram-positive bacterium<br>Some new case series identify *S. aureus* as the new most common cause of IE<br>Can seed normal valves |
| Prosthetic valve IE < 1 mo after surgery | *Staphylococcus epidermidis* | Aggressive gram-positive bacterium |
| Prosthetic valve IE > 1 mo after surgery | *S. aureus* | Aggressive gram-positive bacterium |
| Elderly patient | Enterococci | Gram-positive bacteria<br>Usually a subacute manifestation<br>Difficult to treat because of intrinsic antibiotic resistance<br>GI flora<br>Typically affects older men after genitourinary manipulation or middle-aged women after obstetric procedures |
| Elderly patient with a GI process | *Streptococcus bovis* | Gram-positive bacterium<br>Can be aggressive<br>Associated with inflammatory bowel disease, colonic polyps, colon cancer |
| Injection drug user | *S. aureus* | Aggressive gram-positive bacterium<br>Most common cause of tricuspid valve IE<br>Usually multiple-valve involvement<br>Often oxacillin resistant |
| | Viridans group streptococci | Indolent gram-positive bacteria<br>Usually cause left-sided IE in injection drug users |
| | *Pseudomonas aeruginosa* | Aggressive gram-negative bacterium<br>Usually multiple-valve involvement |
| | Fungi | Patient usually very ill<br>Large vegetations often embolize<br>Surgical intervention commonly needed |
| Patient is critically ill, is being treated in an intensive care unit, or is immunocompromised | Fungi | Patient usually very ill<br>Rare<br>Large vegetations often embolize<br>Surgical intervention commonly needed |
| | *P. aeruginosa* | Aggressive gram-negative bacterium<br>Rare<br>Usually multiple-valve involvement |

*GI*, Gastrointestinal; *IE*, infective endocarditis.

*Data from Baddour LM, Wilson WR, Bayer AS, et al, for the Committee on Rheumatic Fever, Endocarditis, and Kawasaki Disease; Council on Cardiovascular Disease in the Young; Councils on Clinical Cardiology, Stroke, and Cardiovascular Surgery and Anesthesia; American Heart Association; Infectious Diseases Society of America. Infective endocarditis: diagnosis, antimicrobial therapy, and management of complications. A statement for healthcare professionals from the Committee on Rheumatic Fever, Endocarditis, and Kawasaki Disease, Council on Cardiovascular Disease in the Young, and the Councils on Clinical Cardiology, Stroke, and Cardiovascular Surgery and Anesthesia, American Heart Association: endorsed by the Infectious Diseases Society of America. Circulation 2005;111:e394-434.

relapse rate is high after standard therapy. Typically, this problem occurs in older men after genitourinary manipulation and in middle-aged women after obstetric procedures.

## Pseudomonas aeruginosa

A rare cause of IE, *P. aeruginosa* is an aggressive gram-negative bacterium. IE caused by this organism usually complicates the course of critically ill patients and injection drug users.

## *Culture-Negative Bacteria*

The culture-negative bacteria group infrequently causes IE. These bacteria are characterized as culture negative because they either grow slowly in routine media, require special media to grow, or cannot be cultured. If clinical suspicion exists, the clinician must ask that blood cultures be held for a prolonged incubation period (14 to 21 days), request special culture media, or use the serologic and polymerase chain reaction assays available for some of these bacteria. A list of culture-negative bacteria is provided in Box 62.1.

The HACEK bacteria (*Haemophilus* species, *Actinobacillus actinomycetemcomitans, Cardiobacterium hominis, Eikenella corrodens*, and *Kingella kingae*) are normal bacteria that commonly colonize the human oropharynx.

### FUNGI

Fungi are rarely a cause of endocarditis, but fungal IE has high mortality. *Candida* species are responsible for most cases of fungal IE. *Aspergillus* species are also seen. Fungal IE tends to occur in patients with cardiac abnormalities, medical devices (prosthetic valves, long-term indwelling vascular catheters), some level of compromised immunity (human immunodeficiency virus, malignancy, organ transplantation), and injection drug use.[9] Fungal IE usually produces large vegetations and is an indication for surgical intervention.

**BOX 62.2 Risk Factors for Infective Endocarditis**

Acquired or congenital valvular and structural heart disease, including mitral valve prolapse, rheumatic heart disease, and hypertrophic cardiomyopathy
Prosthetic valves, including bioprosthetic devices
Implantable medical devices (cardiac pacemakers, long-term indwelling vascular catheters, implantable defibrillators)
Injection drug use
Poor dental hygiene
Long-term hemodialysis
Diabetes mellitus
Previous history of endocarditis
Immunocompromised states

Adapted from Mylonakis E, Calderwood SB. Infective endocarditis in adults. N Engl J Med 2001;345:1318-30.

## PRESENTING SIGNS AND SYMPTOMS

IE can vary greatly in the severity of its manifestations. Depending on the extent of the injury, location of the injury, microorganism involved, and comorbid conditions in the patient, IE can be an insidious chronic or subacute disease or an aggressive, rapidly debilitating process. Recent prospective cohort data from an international multicenter study have revealed that the acute manifestation is becoming more common—perhaps because of the increasing prevalence of *S. aureus* IE.[7]

The diagnosis of IE is challenging in both its insidious and acute forms. When the findings are subtle, a more benign diagnosis, such as a nonspecific viral syndrome, may be blamed for the illness. When the manifestation is acute and critical, a diagnosis in accordance with the syndrome (e.g., congestive heart failure [CHF], sepsis, heart block, stroke) may be made—with failure to identify the underlying cause (endocarditis). In both scenarios there is continued morbidity and possibly mortality.

EPs must maintain high clinical suspicion in situations associated with IE. Patients at high risk for IE are listed in **Box 62.2**. In such patients, sepsis, embolization, or cardiac failure or shock should warrant an evaluation for endocarditis. By understanding the pathophysiology of this disease, the clinician can predict the signs and symptoms that might be seen with IE.

### CLASSIC TRIAD

The triad consisting of fever, heart murmur, and anemia has classically been ascribed to the diagnosis of IE. Unfortunately, the sensitivity and specificity of these findings for endocarditis are poor. The clinician must combine these findings with high-risk patient characteristics (see Box 62.2).

### ORGAN-SPECIFIC CLINICAL FINDINGS

Most commonly, patients with IE have symptoms of malaise and fatigue in the setting of a low-grade fever. Most of this probably reflects the immunologic response to constant bacteremia. Patients may complain of generalized weakness with anorexia and weight loss. Without high clinical suspicion, a nonspecific viral syndrome may often be diagnosed.

#### *Vascular Signs and Symptoms*

Septic embolization of the vasa vasorum (blood vessels that feed large blood vessels) can lead to the development of mycotic aneurysms in any of the body's larger arteries. Patients can exhibit pain, lightheadedness, altered mental status, and even syncope from the vascular insufficiency or hemorrhage that may occur at any of the sites of involvement.

The signs and symptoms that may be seen with involvement of specific vascular sites are as follows:

- Central nervous system (CNS) arteries—headache, focal neurologic deficits, confusion
- Sinus of Valsalva—pleuritic chest pain, muffled heart tones
- Hepatic artery—right upper quadrant pain, hematemesis
- Splenic artery—abdominal pain, intraabdominal hemorrhage
- Renal arteries—flank pain, hematuria
- Intestinal arteries—abdominal pain, intraabdominal hemorrhage, melena, hematochezia.

#### *Cardiac Signs and Symptoms*

Cardiac symptoms of IE include chest pain, shortness of breath, lightheadedness, and even syncope. These symptoms can result from a variety of heart-specific processes.

Valvular damage can lead to valvular insufficiency (and murmur), which may progress to CHF and even frank cardiogenic shock, especially with left-sided valve involvement. With right-sided valve endocarditis, right heart failure with hepatosplenomegaly and peripheral edema might be evident.

Intracardiac abscess formation causes clinical compromise in a number of ways, depending on the cardiac structure involved. Erosion into the conduction system can lead to all manner of heart blocks, including complete heart block. Involvement of the valvular annulus can result in valvular incompetence and heart failure or may lead to erosion into the pericardial space and cardiac tamponade. Cardiac wall abscess can give rise to septal or free wall rupture or to valvular compromise as a result of papillary muscle rupture.

Embolization of endocarditis vegetations to the coronary arteries can cause diffuse myocarditis via diffuse seeding of the myocardium. Myocardial infarction may occur through direct intraluminal embolization and coronary artery occlusion or through embolic seeding of the coronary vasa vasorum and the formation of coronary mycotic aneurysms.

### Pulmonary Signs and Symptoms

Pulmonary complaints need not be present in patients with IE. Common pulmonary symptoms are dyspnea and cough. Pulmonary complaints related to embolization may accompany right-sided IE—tricuspid or pulmonic valve endocarditis. Patients may have pneumonia secondary to pulmonary septic emboli. Ventilation-perfusion mismatching may develop as a result of pulmonary embolization. Left-sided endocarditis can lead to pulmonary congestion secondary to cardiac failure and acute pulmonary edema.

### Neurologic and Psychiatric Signs and Symptoms

Endocarditis can be accompanied by myriad neurologic and psychiatric signs and symptoms. They can be a result of the systemic effects of hypotension and sepsis or a direct result of focal CNS embolization. Clinical findings may include confusion, complex changes in behavior, headache, seizure, stroke, or coma. The diagnosis of IE can be hard to make because of the large list of differential diagnoses for these symptoms.

### Ophthalmologic Signs and Symptoms

The eye is not immune to endocarditis. Both embolic and immune phenomena can affect the optic nerves, ophthalmic vessels, conjunctivae, and retina. Initial complaints may include painless conjunctival hemorrhages, visual field cuts, and even monocular blindness. Emboli can cause infarction of the ophthalmic or retinal vessels and lead to loss of vision. Hemorrhages with pale cotton-wool centers known as Roth spots can be visualized on the retina (**Fig. 62.3**). EPs should be aware that these spots are not pathognomonic for IE but rather, if seen, should raise suspicion for this disease. Painless subconjunctival hemorrhages (**Fig. 62.4**), or petechiae involving the conjunctivae, can also be present and again are not specific.

### Hematopoietic Signs and Symptoms

Weakness and fatigue can result from anemia, which can be associated with IE. Usually, the anemia is normocytic and mild. IE can also stimulate an immune response marked by leukocytosis and splenomegaly.

### Gastrointestinal Signs and Symptoms

Nausea and vomiting are very nonspecific symptoms. In a patient with IE, these symptoms may accompany complications such as myocardial infarction, pulmonary edema, and processes that increase intracranial pressure. Abdominal pain in patients with IE may be a manifestation of a nonspecific ileus, mesenteric ischemia from mesenteric emboli, or mycotic aneurysms of the splanchnic vasculature.

### Renal Signs and Symptoms

Emboli to the kidneys can result in abscess formation, ischemia, and infarction. The resultant flank pain, pyuria, or hematuria (or any combination of the three) may easily be misdiagnosed as urolithiasis or pyelonephritis. Hematuria can also be a manifestation of glomerulonephritis from immune complex deposition related to IE.

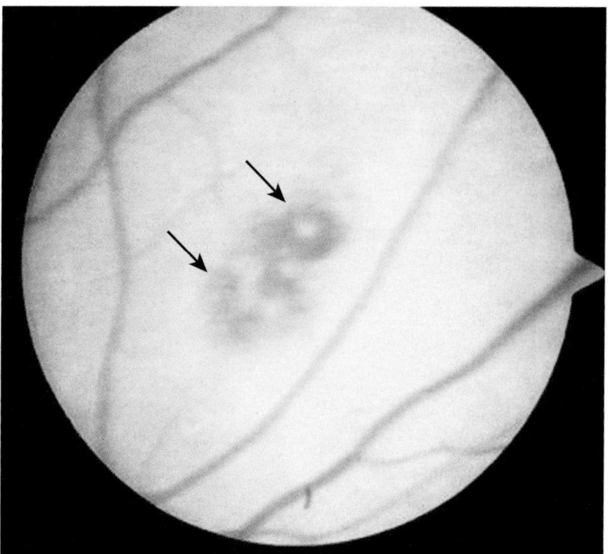

**Fig. 62.3 Roth spots.** Septic microemboli to the retinal arteries result in infarction. The ischemic cotton-wool centers are surrounded by hemorrhagic halos *(arrows)*. These spots are not pathognomonic for endocarditis. (From Mandell GL, Bennett JE, Dolin R, editors. Principles and practice of infectious diseases. 6th ed. Philadelphia: Churchill Livingstone; 2005.)

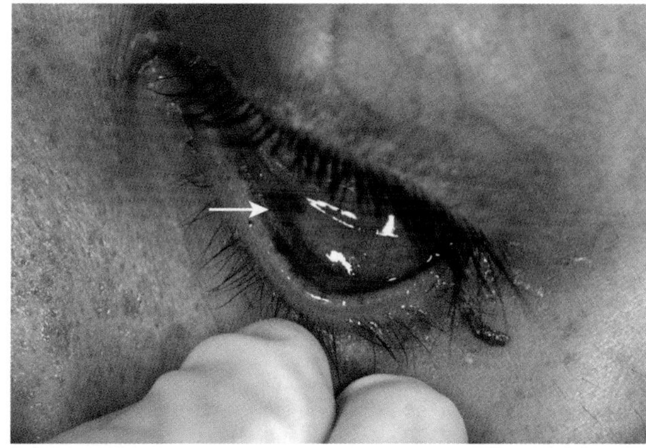

**Fig. 62.4 Subconjunctival hemorrhages *(arrow)* in patient with viridans group streptococcal endocarditis.** (Courtesy Marc E. Grossman, MD, FACP.)

### Dermatologic Signs and Symptoms

The skin can give great clues to the presence of IE. Classic findings are Janeway lesions, Osler nodes, and splinter hemorrhages.

Janeway lesions are small, painless hemorrhages with a macular or slightly nodular character (**Fig. 62.5**). They are found on the thenar and hypothenar eminences of the palms and soles. The histologic findings are generally consistent with septic microemboli. Bacteria have been cultured from these lesions. Janeway lesions are usually present for days to

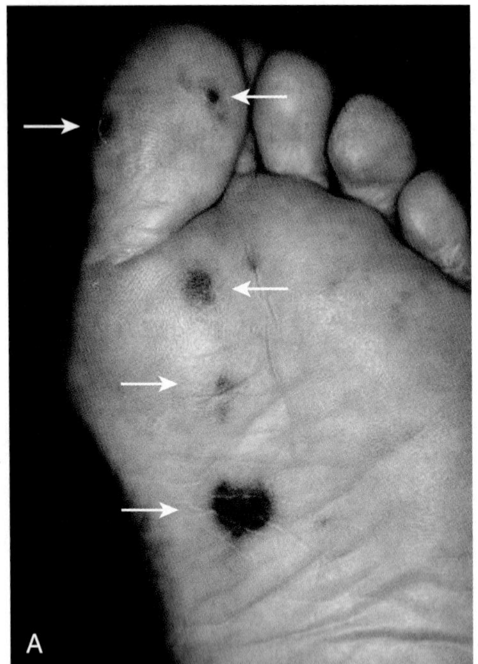


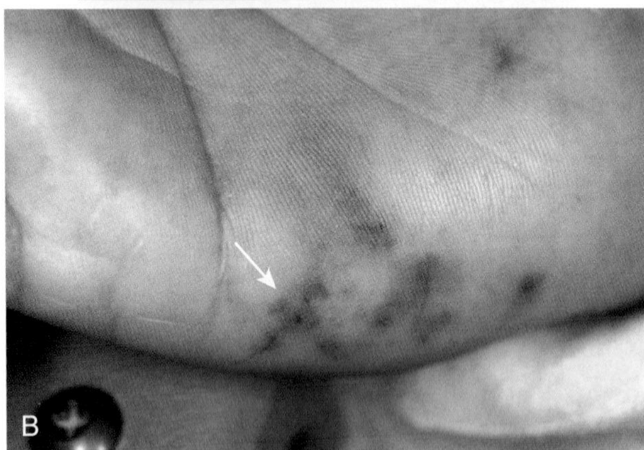


**Fig. 62.5 Janeway lesions.** These nontender, often hemorrhagic lesions *(arrows)* are most commonly associated with *Staphylococcus aureus* endocarditis. They result from septic microembolization. The lesions are usually macular to slightly nodular and involve the soles (**A**) and the thenar and hypothenar eminences of the palms (**B**). (From Mandell GL, Bennett JE, Dolin R, editors. Principles and practice of infectious diseases. 6th ed. Philadelphia: Churchill Livingstone; 2005; **B,** courtesy Marc E. Grossman, MD, FACP.)

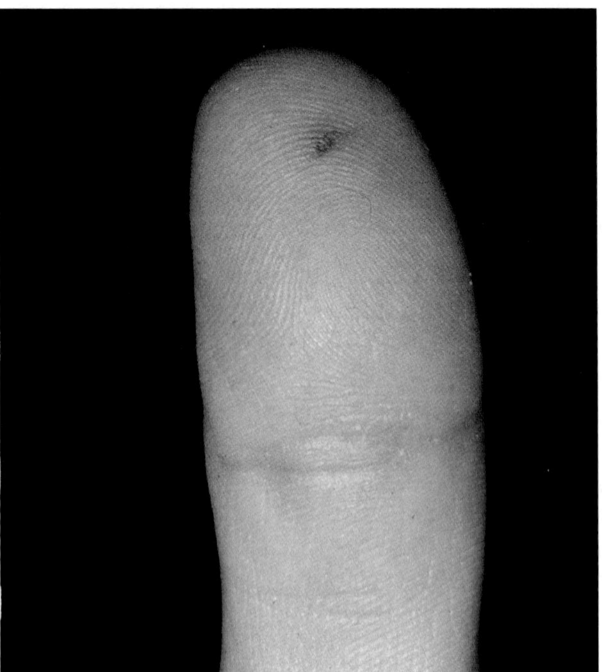

**Fig. 62.6 Osler nodes.** (From Cohen J, Powderly WG, editors. Infectious diseases. 2nd ed. Philadelphia: Mosby; 2004.)

weeks before healing. They are most often associated with acute IE from *S. aureus*.

Osler nodes are small, tender, red to purple nodules. They are most often found on the pulp of the distal phalanges of the fingers and toes, the soles, and the thenar and hypothenar eminences of the palms (**Fig. 62.6**). Preceding the appearance of the nodes, patients often experience neuropathic pain. Although these nodes were initially believed to be purely immunologic in nature, reports have now isolated bacteria from them. It has been postulated that early microembolization with microabscess formation is followed by an immune-mediated hypersensitivity vasculitis. Osler nodes can appear at any point in the course of IE and can last a few hours to several days. They tend to be associated with subacute IE.

Splinter hemorrhages are linear petechiae visible on the nail beds of affected patients (**Fig. 62.7**). They do not blanch when pressure is applied to the nail and are seen better if a bright light is shone directly onto the distal tip of the digit.

## DIFFERENTIAL DIAGNOSIS AND MEDICAL DECISION MAKING

### DIFFERENTIAL DIAGNOSIS

Because of the many clinical manifestations of IE, the list of differential diagnoses is overwhelmingly large. Broad areas include infectious and febrile illnesses, as well as cardiovascular, neurologic, psychiatric, GI, renal, dermatologic, and immunologic disorders (**Box 62.3**). Most interestingly, IE can lead to manifestations that are diagnoses; the EP must think past that initial diagnosis and identify IE as the underlying cause. For example, a cerebrovascular accident or myocardial infarction may be secondary to the embolization or mycotic aneurysms of IE; this fact is important because therapy must also focus on treating the IE.

The most common illness in the differential diagnosis list for IE is febrile illness of any source. Viral syndromes, pneumonia, and urinary tract infections may cause fever, weakness, behavioral abnormalities, and even hemodynamic instability.

The most life-threatening entities are aortic catastrophes, myocardial infarction (with or without acute valve failure), complete heart block, massive pulmonary embolism, cerebrovascular accident, and sepsis.

As mentioned frequently in this chapter, high clinical suspicion guided by knowledge of risk factors (see Box 62.2) is the key to including IE in this long, complex list of differential diagnoses.

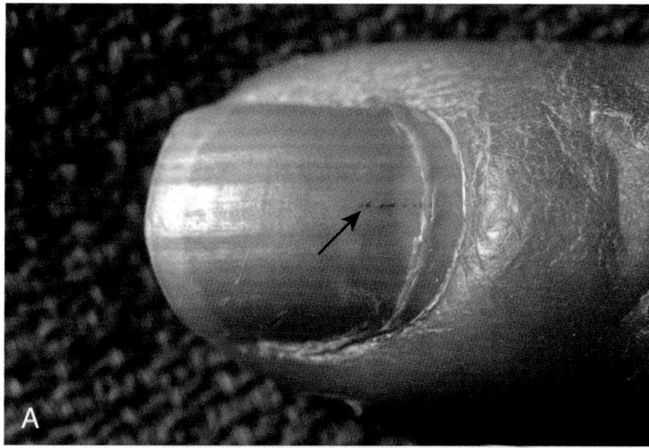


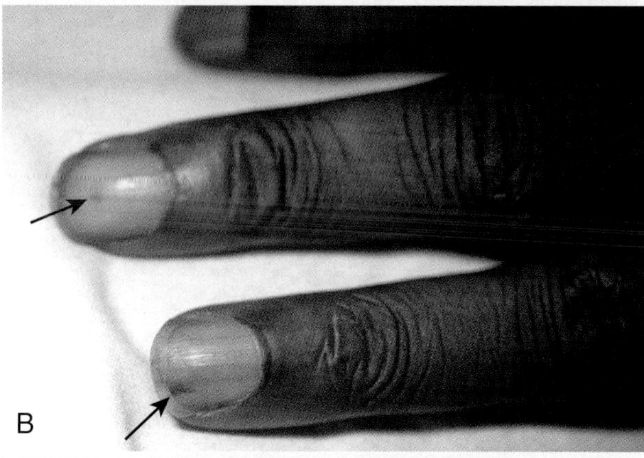


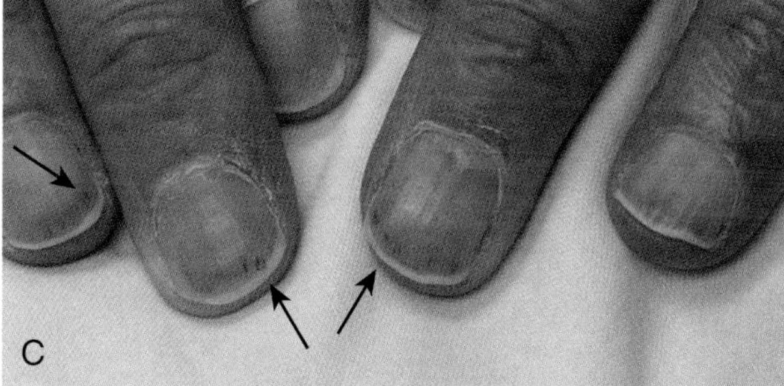


**Fig. 62.7 Splinter hemorrhages.** These lesions appear as narrow, red to reddish brown hemorrhages beneath the nails that tend to run in the direction of nail growth. Most commonly caused by trauma, splinter hemorrhages are associated with endocarditis and may represent vessel damage from vasculitis or microemboli. (**A** and **B,** Courtesy Marc E. Grossman, MD, FACP; **C,** used with permission from Johns Hopkins University and obtained online from www.vasculitis.med.jhu.edu/typesof/polyangiitis.html/.)

**BOX 62.3 Partial Differential Diagnosis for Infective Endocarditis**

- Aortic catastrophes
- Cardiac tamponade
- Central nervous system abscess
- Cerebrovascular accident
- Complete heart block
- Delirium of any cause
- Epilepsy
- Hematologic disorders (e.g., anemia, platelet disorders)
- Infarction
  - Bowel
  - Central nervous system
  - Intestinal
  - Liver
  - Myocardial, acute
  - Renal
  - Spleen
- Infection
  - Chronic (e.g., tuberculosis, human immunodeficiency virus)
  - Intraabdominal
  - Respiratory (e.g., pneumonia)
  - Urinary tract (e.g., pyelonephritis)
  - Viral
- Intestinal vascular insufficiency
- Malignancy
- Meningitis
- Mental illness (e.g., depression, psychosis)
- Pericarditis, acute
- Pulmonary edema, acute
- Pulmonary embolism
- Rheumatic fever, acute
- Rheumatologic and immunologic disorders (e.g., vasculitides)
- Rupture
  - Arterial aneurysm
  - Myocardial wall
- Septic shock
- Toxidromes or medication-related disorders
- Urolithiasis
- Valvular dysfunction, acute

## MEDICAL DECISION MAKING

Contributing to the complexity of IE is the fact that there is neither a single rapid test to diagnose the disorder nor any routine ancillary test that hints at the diagnosis. Some physical findings might clue the EP to this diagnosis, but they are nonspecific. For the EP, the most important tool for diagnosing IE is clinical suspicion. Elements of the history known to identify patients at high risk for endocarditis must trigger this suspicion and lead the EP to focus on physical findings typical of endocarditis. When suspicious for IE based on the history and physical findings, the EP must order serial blood cultures and an echocardiogram to confirm the diagnosis. A diagnostic algorithm is presented in **Figure 62.8**.

The most accepted diagnostic schema for IE is the modified Duke criteria (**Box 62.4**).[10] Unfortunately for the EP, this approach relies heavily on blood culture and echocardiography, the results of which are rarely available to EPs at the outset of care. With recent efforts to bring ultrasonography skills to the ED bedside, echocardiography may become more readily available as an initial evaluation tool, but for now, the procedure requires cardiology consultation and is often not available during the first few hours of care.

According to the modified Duke criteria (see Box 62.4), an echocardiogram positive for IE along with presence of three minor criteria would allow the EP to actually make a "definite diagnosis" of IE in the ED. In all other cases, an echocardiogram positive for IE enables the diagnosis to be "possible IE" as the clinician awaits the results of blood cultures or serologic analysis. It must be emphasized, however, that normal

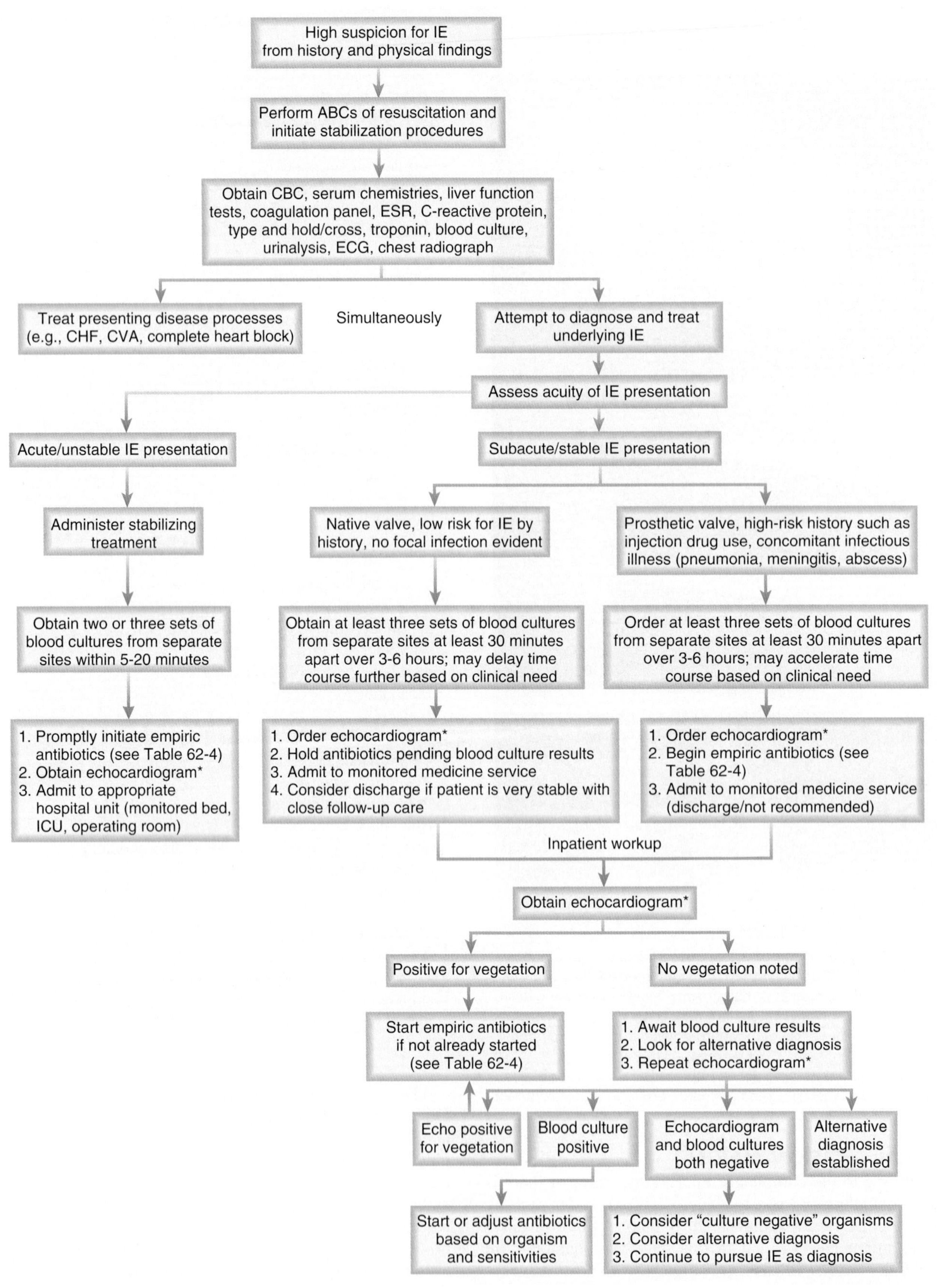


**Fig. 62.8 Diagnostic algorithm for the emergency department management of patients in whom infective endocarditis (IE) is suspected.** *Echocardiography can be performed via either the transthoracic (TTE) or transesophageal (TEE) technique. TEE is more invasive but is more sensitive for detecting vegetations and complications of IE, such as perivalvular abscesses; it is recommended for prosthetic valves; for situations in which optimal visualization by TTE will be difficult, such as emphysema and morbid obesity; for high suspicion of IE but normal TTE findings; and for high suspicion of a complication of IE, such as perivalvular abscess. Normal findings with either technique do not exclude IE if clinical suspicion is high. Echocardiograms can be repeated in an attempt to identify problems such as vegetations and abscesses that may not be noted initially. *ABCs*, Airway, breathing, and circulation; *CBC*, complete blood count; *CHF*, congestive heart failure; *CVA*, cerebrovascular accident; *ECG*, electrocardiogram; *ESR*, erythrocyte sedimentation rate; *ICU*, intensive care unit.

**BOX 62.4 Modified Duke Diagnostic Criteria for Infective Endocarditis**

**Stratification of Patients**

The modified Duke diagnostic criteria stratify patients with suspected infective endocarditis (IE) into one of three categories as follows; the major and minor criteria are listed below.

A **diagnosis of "definite" endocarditis** is made in a patient with *one* of the following:

- Histologic and/or microbiologic evidence of infection at surgery or autopsy
- 2 major criteria
- 1 major criterion and 3 minor criteria
- 5 minor criteria

A **diagnosis of "possible" endocarditis** is made in a patient with *one* of the following:

- 1 major criterion and 1 minor criterion
- 3 minor criteria

A **diagnosis of endocarditis is "rejected"** in a patient with *one* of the following:

- Negative findings at surgery or autopsy in a patient who received antibiotic therapy for ≤4 days
- A firm alternative diagnosis
- Resolution of illness with antibiotic therapy for ≤4 days
- Failure to meet the criteria for "possible" endocarditis

**Major Criteria**

***Blood Culture Results Positive for Infective Endocarditis***

1. Typical microorganisms causing IE from two separate blood cultures in the absence of a primary focus:
   - Viridans group streptococci
   - *Streptococcus bovis*
   - HACEK group of bacteria*
   - Community-acquired *Staphylococcus aureus* or *Enterococcus*
2. Persistently positive blood culture results, defined as recovery of a microorganism consistent with IE from *one* of the following:
   - Blood culture specimens obtained more than 12 hours apart
   - All of 3 *or* a majority of 4 or more separate blood culture specimens, the first and last of which have been obtained at least 1 hour apart
3. Single positive blood culture result for *Coxiella burnetii* or anti–phase 1 immunoglobulin G antibody titer > 1:800.

***Evidence of Endocardial Involvement***

1. Positive echocardiographic results for IE:
   - *Transesophageal echocardiography* recommended in patients who have prosthetic valves, who have been rated as having at least "possible IE" by clinical criteria, or who have complicated IE (paravalvular abscess).
   - *Transthoracic echocardiography* recommended as the first test in other patients.

   The definition of a positive echocardiographic result is presence of one of the following:
   - Oscillating intracardiac mass on a valve or supporting structures, in the path of regurgitant jets, or on implanted material in the absence of an alternative anatomic explanation
   - Abscess
   - New partial dehiscence of a prosthetic valve
2. New valvular regurgitation. An increase or change in a preexisting murmur is not sufficient evidence.

**Minor Criteria**

*Predisposition*: Predisposing heart condition or intravenous drug use

*Fever*: Body temperature > 38.0° C (100.4° F)

*Vascular phenomena*: Major arterial emboli, septic pulmonary infarcts, mycotic aneurysms, intracranial hemorrhage, conjunctival hemorrhages, Janeway lesions

*Immunologic phenomena*: Glomerulonephritis, Osler nodes, Roth spots, rheumatoid factor

*Microbiologic evidence*: Positive blood culture result but not meeting the major criteria as noted above (excluding a single positive culture result for coagulase-negative staphylococci and organisms that do not cause endocarditis) *OR* serologic evidence of active infection with an organism consistent with IE.

**Haemophilus* species, *Actinobacillus actinomycetemcomitans, Cardiobacterium hominis, Eikenella corrodens*, and *Kingella kingae*.

Data from Li IS, Sexton DJ, Mick N, et al. Proposed modifications to the Duke criteria for the diagnosis of infective endocarditis. Clin Infect Dis 2000;30:633-8.

echocardiographic findings would not eliminate the diagnosis of IE, especially in the setting of high clinical suspicion (high-risk patient, strongly suggestive findings). Evaluation should continue until the diagnosis of IE is "rejected" according to the modified Duke criteria. This often means establishment of an alternative diagnosis or the finding of sterile blood cultures after appropriate incubation procedures (proper media and incubation times) and resolution of the illness.

## DIAGNOSTIC TESTING

Many diagnostic tests are available to help the EP evaluate and manage patients with possible IE. Many of these tests assist in identifying the complications of this disease process.

### LABORATORY TESTS

Though not diagnostic when performed alone, some laboratory tests can be useful in diagnosing endocarditis and managing patients in the ED.

The complete blood cell count is less useful than one might think. Leukocytosis is present only in some cases. Normochromic normocytic anemia may be seen.

An elevated erythrocyte sedimentation rate or C-reactive protein value can be a good though nonspecific clue. Both findings are markers for an ongoing inflammatory process and are nearly always present in patients with IE.

Urinalysis often shows proteinuria and sometimes hematuria. Proteinuria may occur as a result of the immunologic effects of endocarditis. Chronic infection or inflammation leads to the formation of immune complexes and their deposition in the glomeruli. Depending on the duration of this illness, the patient may have glomerulonephritis and renal insufficiency.

Renal function can be affected in patients with IE. A serum creatinine measurement is not useful for the diagnosis of IE, but it is for its management. Antibiotic dosing and the use of intravenous contrast–enhanced computed tomography (CT) are dependent on a patient's renal function.

Less useful for the EP but part of the modified Duke criteria for IE are serologic tests. Rheumatoid factor may occasionally be found in patients with IE, particularly those with long-standing, indolent cases. Serologic assays can detect the presence of bacteria such as *Coxiella, Brucella, Bartonella, Legionella*, and *Chlamydia*. Polymerase chain reaction testing for specific DNA or RNA from blood, urine, or surgically excised tissue can be performed when the potential pathogen is slow growing or cannot be cultured by conventional methods.[11]

## MICROBIOLOGY

Perhaps the most useful test for the diagnosis and management of IE is serial blood cultures. Unfortunately, the results of cultures are often not available to the EP. Three sets of blood culture specimens should ideally be collected before the initiation of antibiotics at intervals of least 30 minutes and over a period of 3 to 6 hours. There is little increased culture yield beyond three sets of blood cultures as long as they are obtained before the administration of antibiotics.

IE results in a constant, low-grade bacteremia. Therefore, it is not necessary to obtain blood culture specimens only during temperature spikes. Serial blood culture specimens obtained over a period of hours to days (in the absence of antibiotic therapy) should all yield positive results as long as at least 10 mL of blood per culture bottle is collected. In the interest of identifying endocarditis caused by more fastidious organisms, it is recommended that blood cultures be held for 14 to 21 days before being labeled negative.

The EP must remember that antecedent antibiotic treatment can also result in negative blood culture results, so the history should include questions about such treatment.[11] In a stable patient with a history of antecedent antibiotic therapy, serial blood culture specimens should be collected over a longer time (even days) before initiation of antibiotic therapy for IE.

The caveat to the timing of serial blood sampling for culture is that withholding antibiotics should be the strategy in a stable patient who has no other indications for antibiotics. In an unstable or acutely ill patient, the three sets of blood culture specimens should be obtained over a period of 5 to 20 minutes and then antibiotics given as early as possible.

## ELECTROCARDIOGRAPHY

Acquisition of an electrocardiogram (ECG) is often prompted by abnormalities in vital signs, initial symptoms, or clinical instability. If the EP suspects IE, an ECG must be performed. Abnormalities found on the ECG can be caused by endocarditis, but as with other findings for this diagnosis, these abnormalities are nonspecific. The pathologic findings that can be associated with endocarditis are acute myocardial infarction (secondary to coronary artery involvement), complete heart block, atrioventricular block, and bundle branch blocks. Infarction can occur as a result of direct embolization to the coronary arteries or coronary mycotic aneurysm formation. Conduction abnormalities can arise from direct extension of infection to the conduction system. Most commonly, the ECG in patients with endocarditis is normal or reveals a sinus tachycardia.

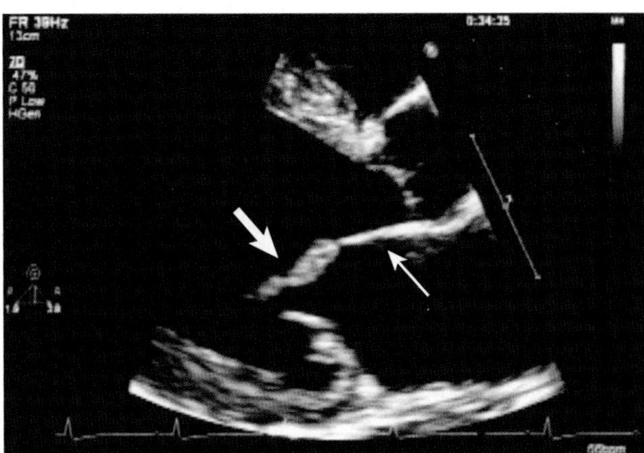

**Fig. 62.9 Valvular vegetations.** This parasternal long view on a transthoracic echocardiogram shows a large vegetation *(thick arrow)* on the mitral valve *(thin arrow)*. The *large arrow* is in the left ventricle and the *thin arrow* is in the left atrium. (Courtesy Mark Goldberger, MD.)

## ECHOCARDIOGRAPHY

Echocardiography is the most important diagnostic tool available to the EP for the early identification of endocarditis and must be performed rapidly in all cases of suspected IE.[6,12] It is one of the major criteria for the diagnosis of IE according to the modified Duke criteria (see Box 62.4 for echocardiographic findings that are diagnostic of IE[10]) (**Fig. 62.9**). In addition, echocardiography allows assessment of disease severity, complications, prognosis, and the need for surgical therapy. It is therefore a critical component in the initial assessment of a patient suspected of having IE.[12,13]

### *Transthoracic Echocardiography*

Easily done at the bedside, transthoracic echocardiography (TTE) is recommended as the initial imaging modality. It can identify valvular damage and valvular vegetations, as well as assess cardiac function and pulmonary pressure. Its limitations lie in the assessment of patients with a prosthetic valve or intracardiac hardware.

### *Transesophageal Echocardiography*

Although it requires more preparation and is more invasive than TTE, transesophageal echocardiography (TEE) has greater sensitivity and specificity (**Table 62.3**). It can visualize smaller vegetations, as well as myocardial involvement such as abscesses and prosthetic valve vegetations. TEE is recommended for patients with the following findings:

- The TTE result is negative, but clinical suspicion for IE is high.
- The TTE result is positive, but there is concern for the presence of a high-risk complication of IE, such as large or mobile vegetations, significant valvular insufficiency, or a suggestion of perivalvular extension.
- The TTE result is suboptimal because of, for example, morbid obesity, mechanical ventilation, emphysema, or chest wall deformity.
- Prosthetic valves are in place.

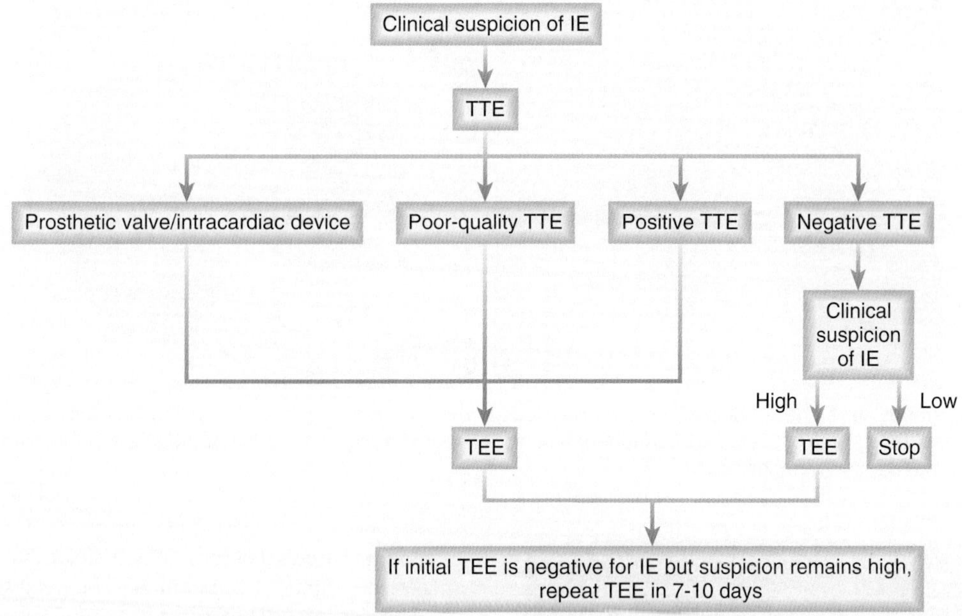


**Fig. 62.10 Algorithm for the role of echocardiography in the diagnosis of infective endocarditis (IE).** *TEE*, Transesophageal endocardiography; *TTE*, transthoracic echocardiography. (Modified from Habib, G, Hoen B, Tornos P, et al, for the ESC Committee for Practice Guidelines [CPG]. Guidelines on the prevention, diagnosis, and treatment of infective endocarditis [new version 2009]: the Task Force on the Prevention, Diagnosis, and Treatment of Infective Endocarditis of the European Society of Cardiology [ESC]. Eur Heart J 2009;30:2369-413.)

**Table 62.3 Comparison of the Sensitivity and Specificity of Transthoracic and Transesophageal Echocardiography for the Diagnosis of Cardiac Vegetations**

| | | Sensitivity | | Specificity | |
|---|---|---|---|---|---|
| | **No. Patients** | **TTE** | **TEE** | **TTE** | **TEE** |
| Shapiro et al., 1994 | 64 | 60% | 87% | 81% | 91% |
| Erbel et al., 1988 | 96 | 63% | 100% | 98% | 98% |
| Shively et al., 1991 | 66 | 44% | 94% | 98% | 100% |

From Evangelista A, Gonzalez-Alujas MT. Echocardiography in infective endocarditis. Heart 2004;90:614-7.

In patients with high clinical suspicion for IE, a normal echocardiographic result is not sufficient to discontinue diagnostic assessment or treatment. TTE or TEE should be repeated within 7 to 10 days. TTE or TEE can be used subsequently to assess the response to treatment or progression of the disease. Please see **Figure 62.10** for the echocardiography algorithm.[6,12]

## RADIOGRAPHY

Chest radiographs are obtained routinely in most patients with cardiopulmonary symptoms, fever, or both. No specific finding on the chest radiograph is pathognomonic for IE. Multiple bilateral pulmonary infiltrates might be a clue that septic emboli may be present (**Fig. 62.11,** ***A***).

CT is an excellent tool for the evaluation of symptoms that may be associated with IE. The discovery of ischemic or infectious foci or abscesses, especially multiple lesions, should raise suspicion for a septic focus, such as IE. Contrast-enhanced CT is preferred for differentiating mass lesions with necrotic centers from abscesses.

Chest CT may better identify multiple septic emboli, effusions, or pulmonary abscesses (see Fig. 62.11, *B*). Brain CT for the evaluation of patients with neurologic or neuropsychiatric symptoms may demonstrate ischemic or infectious foci. Contrast-enhanced abdominopelvic CT might identify ischemia or infarction of the intestines, liver, spleen, or kidneys (**Fig. 62.12**).

For identifying the presence of mycotic aneurysms or peripheral embolization, conventional angiography remains the "gold standard," although screening may be undertaken with CT angiography or magnetic resonance angiography.

## LUMBAR PUNCTURE

Lumbar puncture is not helpful in making the diagnosis of IE but is mandatory for diagnosing meningitis. Headache, neck stiffness, fever, alteration in mental status, or any combination of these symptoms should make one think of the diagnosis of meningitis. Independent of IE or a complication of IE, the diagnosis of meningitis—especially bacterial meningitis—must be made expeditiously. Lumbar puncture allows the EP to make the diagnosis of meningitis, initiate treatment, and ultimately, identify the causative organism.

# TREATMENT

## RESUSCITATION

Emergency treatment always begins with the cardinal ABCs of resuscitation—airway, breathing, and circulation. Patients with issues in any of these areas must be stabilized by the

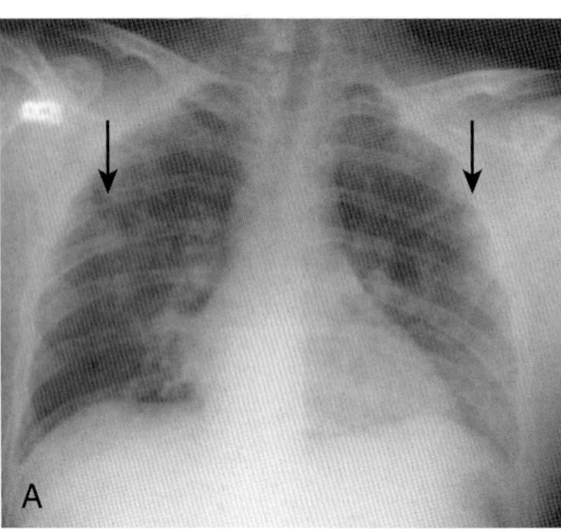

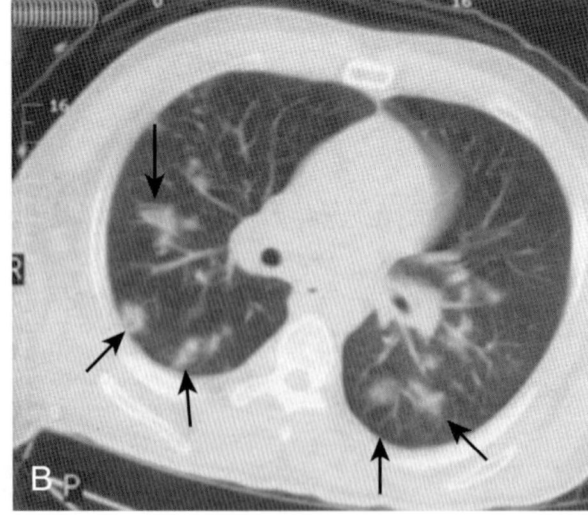


**Fig. 62.11 Septic emboli. A,** A chest radiograph shows two nodular densities *(arrows)*. In this case they are foci of infection from embolization of infected vegetations. **B,** This non–contrast-enhanced computed tomography scan of the chest demonstrates multiple small infiltrates *(arrows)* caused by septic embolization.

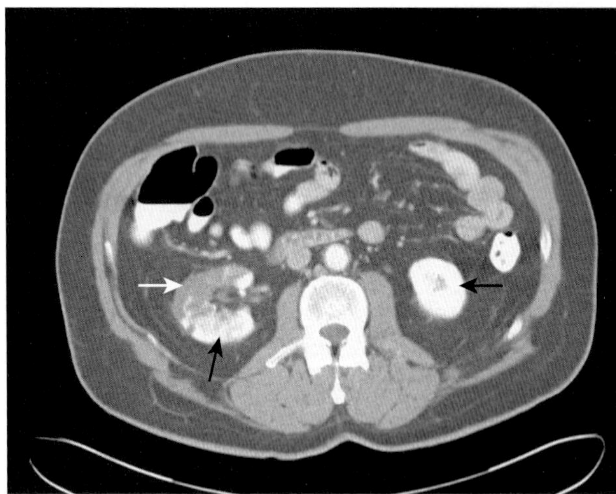

**Fig. 62.12 Renal infarction.** A contrast-enhanced abdominopelvic computed tomography scan demonstrates patchy uptake of intravenous contrast agent by the right kidney. Gray areas *(white arrow)* within the anterolateral aspect of the midpole of the right kidney represent infarction caused by septic emboli from infective endocarditis. This contrasts with the rather homogeneously white, well-perfused left kidney and posterior aspect of the right kidney *(black arrows)*. (Courtesy Jeffrey Newhouse, MD.)

usual methods. Supplemental oxygen or endotracheal intubation (or both) should be used as needed. Circulatory instability as a result of either cardiogenic or septic shock should be corrected with volume or pressor support, or both. Refractory cardiogenic shock may require the use of an intraaortic balloon counterpulsation device (contraindicated in patients with aortic insufficiency) or emergency heart surgery.

## EMPIRIC ANTIBIOTIC THERAPY

Antibiotics are the keystone of treatment of IE, and selection of the proper regimen depends on the causative organism. Identification of the specific organism and its resistance pattern allows a properly tailored antibiotic regimen that minimizes the overuse of extended-spectrum agents. With this in mind, EPs should make every effort to obtain serial blood specimens for culture before starting antibiotic treatment. Three sets (aerobic and anaerobic) of blood culture specimens should be obtained. The sets should ideally be collected at least 30 minutes apart and over a period of 3 to 6 hours.

The urgency for empiric antibiotic therapy varies by patient subgroup. In stable patients with subacute manifestations and native valves who have signs and symptoms most consistent with a viral syndrome, antibiotic therapy can be withheld for hours and even days to allow proper culture results to be obtained. Patients with the same stable, subacute findings and viral syndrome–type symptoms but with a prosthetic valve or a history of injection drug use should be admitted to the hospital and receive appropriate empiric antibiotic therapy after the 3- to 6-hour collection of serial blood culture specimens. In a patient with a concomitant infectious process such as meningitis, pneumonia, or abscess and in whom the diagnosis of IE is being entertained, the serial blood culture specimens should still be collected but over a shorter time frame to allow sooner initiation of appropriate empiric antibiotic therapy to cover both the identified infection and the possible IE. Finally, in a patient with an acute, unstable manifestation of suspected IE, empiric antibiotics should not be withheld for collection of serial blood culture specimens. Three specimens can be collected over a 5- to 20-minute period to allow expeditious antibiotic treatment.

Unfortunately for the EP, the causative organism is rarely known because culture results are often not available yet. As with many infections, the EP must choose an empiric regimen. So how does the EP choose the empiric regimen? A group of organisms are known to cause IE (see Box 62.1). Certain of these organisms are more common, depending on the clinical scenario (see Table 62.2). Armed with this knowledge, the EP can tailor the empiric antibiotic regimen to the clinical scenario presented. Examples of such scenarios are native valve involvement, prosthetic valve involvement, injection drug use, history of allergy to antibiotics, prolonged hospitalization, admission to the intensive care unit, and a high prevalence of resistant organisms (**Box 62.5**). All these factors would influence the antibiotic regimen chosen.

Should the empiric regimen include antibiotics that cover all possible organisms and all resistance patterns? Actually, because many patients with IE have stable, subacute manifestations, the EP is not forced to achieve a perfect match of

**BOX 62.5 Clinical Scenarios to Help Tailor an Empiric Antibiotic Regimen for a Patient with Suspected Infective Endocarditis**

Important factors in choosing an antibiotic are as follows:

- Acuity of findings
- Native valve endocarditis
- Prosthetic valve endocarditis
- Endocarditis in an injection drug user
- Recent or current use of antibiotics
- Recent hospitalization
- Antibiotic allergies
- Renal function
- Relapse of previously treated endocarditis
- Regional prevalence of certain organisms and resistance patterns

organism and antibiotic. Changes can be made in 2 to 3 days, when the organisms and resistance patterns become known. In contrast, for unstable, acute cases, EPs should maximize coverage to ensure that they account for all possibilities of organism and resistance. Morbidity and mortality could be influenced by failure to properly treat early.

Initial antibiotic therapy should always be parenteral and bactericidal.[1] Because of growing antibiotic resistance, combination therapy with two or more agents should be used. Recommended empiric antibiotic regimens are listed in **Table 62.4**.

For complex cases, it is advisable to seek the expertise of an infectious disease specialist. In addition, patients with confirmed IE require prolonged antibiotic administration and will probably be discharged with a long-term central intravenous catheter such as a Groshong catheter or peripherally inserted central catheter.

**Table 62.4 Empiric Antibiotic Regimen for Presumed Infectious Endocarditis*†‡**

| | |
|---|---|
| Suspected native valve IE with a subacute manifestation§ | Penicillin G, 200-400 U/kg (normal adult dose, 12-20 million U/day) IV divided q4h, or ampicillin, 200 mg/kg/day (normal adult dose, 12 g/day) IV divided q4h<br>*plus*<br>Nafcillin or oxacillin, 200 mg/kg/day (normal adult dose, 12 g/day) IV divided q4h<br>*plus*<br>Gentamicin, 1 mg/kg IV or IM q8h (adjust for peak serum concentration of 3-4 mcg/mL and trough of <1 mcg/mL)¶ |
| Suspected native valve IE with the following characteristics:<br>Patient with penicillin allergy<br>*or*<br>Acute manifestation<br>*or*<br>History of injection drug use<br>*or*<br>From a region with a high incidence of IE caused by *Staphylococcus aureus*, especially oxacillin-resistant *S. aureus* | Vancomycin, 15 mg/kg IV q12h (adjust for 1-hr peak serum concentration of 30-45 mcg/mL and trough of 10-15 mcg/mL)¶<br>*plus*<br>Gentamicin, 1 mg/kg IV or IM q8h (adjust for peak serum concentration of 3-4 mcg/mL and trough of <1 mcg/mL)¶ |
| Suspected prosthetic valve IE | Vancomycin, 15 mg/kg IV q12h (adjust for 1-hr peak serum concentration of 30-45 mcg/mL and trough of 10-15 mcg/mL)¶<br>*plus*<br>Gentamicin, 1 mg/kg IV or IM q8h (adjust for peak serum concentration of 3-4 mcg/mL and trough of <1 mcg/mL)‖<br>*plus*<br>Rifampin, 20 mg/kg/day (normal adult dose, 900 mg/day) PO divided q8h** |

Data from Baddour LM, Wilson WR, Bayer AS, et al, for the Committee on Rheumatic Fever, Endocarditis, and Kawasaki Disease; Council on Cardiovascular Disease in the Young; Councils on Clinical Cardiology, Stroke, and Cardiovascular Surgery and Anesthesia; American Heart Association; Infectious Diseases Society of America. Infective endocarditis: diagnosis, antimicrobial therapy, and management of complications. A statement for healthcare professionals from the Committee on Rheumatic Fever, Endocarditis, and Kawasaki Disease, Council on Cardiovascular Disease in the Young, and the Councils on Clinical Cardiology, Stroke, and Cardiovascular Surgery and Anesthesia, American Heart Association: endorsed by the Infectious Diseases Society of America. Circulation 2005;111:e394-434.

*Empiric therapy must be designed on the basis of clinical and epidemiologic clues.

†The duration of therapy varies with the microorganism and its drug sensitivities, the presence of prosthetic devices, and the response to therapy.

‡The pediatric dose should not exceed the normal adult dose.

§Penicillin G or ampicillin is added to this regimen because nafcillin/oxacillin and gentamicin may not be adequate coverage of enterococci.

‖Aminoglycosides such as gentamicin should not be given as single daily doses.

¶Doses of vancomycin and gentamicin should be adjusted for reduced renal function, as well as measured serum concentration values.

**Rifampin increases the warfarin requirement for anticoagulation.

*IE*, Infectious endocarditis; *IM*, intramuscularly; *IV*, intravascularly; *PO*, orally.

### CARDIAC PACING

Any hemodynamically unstable patient with a complete heart block, irrespective of cause, warrants at least temporary cardiac pacing. In the setting of IE, in which a high-degree heart block is unlikely to be a temporary condition, a transvenous pacemaker is preferable to transthoracic pacing.

### ANTICOAGULATION

Anticoagulation is not indicated for patients with endocarditis. It prevents neither the formation nor the embolization of vegetations. In the setting of native valve IE, anticoagulation should be avoided because it affords no benefit and might cause harm by converting CNS infarcts from bland to hemorrhagic.

Understanding the risks associated with anticoagulation in the setting of IE, what does the EP do with patients who would normally require anticoagulation? An excellent example would be a patient with IE and an anticoagulation-requiring prosthetic valve. The recommendation is that anticoagulation should be continued, barring the presence of acute hemorrhage, CNS infarction or hemorrhage, or a mycotic aneurysm. Any complaint that may result from these issues should be fully investigated to best inform decisions regarding anticoagulation. CT of the brain should be performed in any patient with possible CNS involvement. Any patient with unexplained abdominal or flank pain should undergo contrast-enhanced abdominal CT to evaluate for the presence of a mycotic aneurysm. Visual complaints warrant a complete funduscopic examination. If contraindications are identified, temporary discontinuation of anticoagulation is appropriate even in patients with a prosthetic valve.[1,13,14] In these circumstances, close consultation with the appropriate specialty services is recommended.

Patients taking warfarin should be switched to intravenous, unfractionated heparin in the event that cardiac surgery is required.

Aspirin has not been shown to prevent embolic events but is probably associated with an increased risk for bleeding. It therefore has no role in early management of IE.[15]

### SURGICAL THERAPY

There are both early and late indications for surgical intervention in the management of IE. Keeping this fact in mind, the EP should obtain early cardiothoracic surgery consultation if any early indications for surgery exist. The only true indication for early, emergency surgical intervention is severe CHF or cardiogenic shock secondary to valvular insufficiency. Intraaortic balloon counterpulsation devices can be used to temporize all forms of cardiogenic shock except that caused by aortic valve insufficiency. In the case of aortic valve incompetence, valve replacement becomes imperative. The presence of an annular or aortic abscess (with or without a conduction system disturbance), a sinus or aortic true or false aneurysm, or paravalvular leak of a prosthetic valve warrants surgical intervention but need not be performed as an emergency procedure if the patient is otherwise stable.

Other potential indications for surgery in patients with IE are failure of antibiotic therapy, vegetations larger than 10 mm on echocardiography, fungal endocarditis, early prosthetic valve endocarditis (within the first 2 months after surgery), and recurrent embolization despite medical therapy.[14]

### REMOVAL OF MEDICAL HARDWARE

Blood culture specimens should be obtained via any long-term indwelling intravascular catheter. These devices should then be removed. Decisions to remove prosthetic valves or pacemaker wires are complex and should be made in consultation with cardiology, cardiothoracic surgery, or infectious disease specialists (or all three).

## FOLLOW-UP, NEXT STEPS IN CARE, AND PATIENT EDUCATION

All patients with suspected or confirmed IE should be admitted to the hospital. The EP might consider discharge from the ED if the following conditions are all met: low risk for IE (native valves, immunocompetent, no injection drug use, no comorbid conditions), a stable or subacute manifestation, nondiagnostic findings on TTE, and very well-defined follow-up. Such patients may undergo TEE as an outpatient, and the serial blood culture results can be followed by their personal physicians.

Otherwise, the disposition of all other patients with potential or confirmed IE is driven by the following factors:

- Need for further evaluation (diagnosis or extent of involvement not certain)
- Severity of the illness
- Need for surgical or mechanical support (e.g., mechanical ventilation, intraaortic balloon counterpulsation device)
- Need for intravenous antibiotic therapy
- Reliability of the patient
- Availability of close follow-up

Immediate operative care should be strongly considered if the surgical criteria are met. Patients in critical condition who do not require surgery should be admitted to the intensive care unit. Most other patients with presumed IE can be admitted to a medical service with cardiac monitoring for further evaluation, initiation of intravenous antibiotic therapy, and arrangement for further outpatient care.

## NONBACTERIAL THROMBOTIC ENDOCARDITIS

Endocarditis is not always associated with infection. In some disease states, vegetations composed of bland, platelet-fibrin aggregates may adhere to the endocardium. Eventually, fibrosis of these lesions occurs. These vegetations are usually sterile but may become seeded with infectious organisms. Illnesses associated with nonbacterial thrombotic endocarditis (NBTE) include malignancies, severe burns, hypercoagulable states (e.g., antiphospholipid syndrome and disseminated intravascular coagulopathy), uremia, and connective tissue diseases such as systemic lupus erythematosus.[16]

It stands to reason that the clinical manifestations of NBTE are related mainly to embolic phenomena and, occasionally, to valvular dysfunction. Without infectious vegetations, the generalized immune response and the localized destruction and infectious seeding of other organs do not occur. The primary indication for surgical intervention in patients with NBTE is valvular dysfunction, although surgery may be performed to prevent embolic events.

## ENDOCARDITIS PROPHYLAXIS

For more than 50 years, the American Heart Association (AHA) has set forth recommendations in an effort to prevent IE. Antimicrobial regimens were recommended for planned, potentially contaminated procedures (dental, respiratory, GI, and genitourinary) in an effort to prevent IE in at-risk populations. Unfortunately, these guidelines lacked good evidence to support their efficacy and were so complex that their implementation was difficult. In April 2007, the AHA released new guidelines in an effort to address these issues.[17]

Rather than provide prophylaxis to patients at risk for the development of IE, the 2007 guidelines have changed to recommend that antimicrobial prophylaxis be administered only to patients at highest risk for an adverse outcome from IE (**Box 62.6**), thereby greatly reducing the group of eligible patients. The procedures for which prophylaxis is recommended are listed in **Box 62.7** and antimicrobial regimens in **Table 62.5**.

EPs may encounter difficulty managing the expectations of patients who were previously recommended to receive IE prophylaxis but now are not. The rationale for the changes is the lack of scientific evidence to support the claim that IE prophylaxis is actually effective. In fact, the bacteremia resulting from daily activities such as toothbrushing and eating is more likely to result in IE than is the bacteremia associated with dental procedures. Therefore, even if 100% effective, prophylaxis probably prevents only an extremely small number of cases of IE. The cost of prophylaxis is borne financially[18] and through adverse drug reactions. As a result, the AHA is now emphasizing maintenance of optimal oral health and

**BOX 62.6 AHA Recommendations for Prevention of Infective Endocarditis**

Cardiac conditions associated with the highest risk for an adverse outcome from endocarditis for which antibiotic prophylaxis is recommended are as follows:

- Prosthetic cardiac valves
- Previous infective endocarditis
- Congenital heart disease (CHD)*
  - Unrepaired cyanotic CHD, including palliative shunts and conduits
  - Completely repaired congenital heart defect with prosthetic material or device, whether placed by surgery or by catheter intervention, during the first 6 months after the procedure†
  - Repaired CHD with residual defects at the site or adjacent to the site of a prosthetic patch or prosthetic device (which inhibits endothelialization)
- Cardiac valvulopathy in a cardiac transplantation recipient

Adapted from Wilson W, Taubert KA, Gewitz M, et al. Prevention of infective endocarditis: guidelines from the American Heart Association. A guideline from the American Heart Association Rheumatic Fever, Endocarditis, and Kawasaki Disease Committee, Council on Cardiovascular Disease in the Young, and the Council on Clinical Cardiology, Council on Cardiovascular Surgery and Anesthesia, and the Quality of Care and Outcomes Research Interdisciplinary Working Group. J Am Dent Assoc 2007;138:739-45, 747-60.

*Except for the conditions listed here, antibiotic prophylaxis is no longer recommended for any other form of CHD.

†Prophylaxis is recommended because endothelialization of prosthetic material occurs within 6 months after the procedure.

**BOX 62.7 Emergency Department Procedures Requiring Antimicrobial Prophylaxis Against Infective Endocarditis in High-Risk Patients**

Patients at high risk for an adverse outcome from infective endocarditis (see Box 62.6) should receive antimicrobial prophylaxis (see Table 62.4) for the following procedures:

**Dental Procedures**

- All dental procedures that involve manipulating gingival tissue or the periapical region of teeth or perforating the oral mucosa.

The following procedures and events do not need prophylaxis: routine anesthetic injections through noninfected tissue, taking of dental radiographs, placement of removable prosthodontic or orthodontic appliances, placement of orthodontic brackets, shedding of deciduous teeth, and bleeding from trauma to the lips or oral mucosa.

**Otorhinolaryngologic/Respiratory Procedures**

- Any surgical procedure that involves an incision in respiratory mucosa (e.g., peritonsillar abscess incision and drainage, cricothyroidotomy, tracheotomy, tonsillectomy and/or adenoidectomy)
- Bronchoscopy with a procedure that involves an incision in respiratory mucosa

**Minor Surgical Procedures**

- Any surgical procedure that involves infected skin, skin structure, or musculoskeletal tissue (e.g., incision and drainage of an abscess)

NOTE: Prophylaxis for gastrointestinal procedures is no longer recommended.

NOTE: Prophylaxis for genitourinary procedures is recommended only if the patient is known to have enterococcal colonization or urinary tract infection at the time of instrumentation.

Modified from Wilson W, Taubert KA, Gewitz M, et al. Prevention of infective endocarditis: guidelines from the American Heart Association. A guideline from the American Heart Association Rheumatic Fever, Endocarditis, and Kawasaki Disease Committee, Council on Cardiovascular Disease in the Young, and the Council on Clinical Cardiology, Council on Cardiovascular Surgery and Anesthesia, and the Quality of Care and Outcomes Research Interdisciplinary Working Group. J Am Dent Assoc 2007;138:739-45, 747-60.

**Table 62.5 Antibiotic Prophylaxis Regimens for Dental Procedures*†**

| PATIENT | ANTIBIOTIC AGENT | SINGLE DOSE TO BE ADMINISTERED 30-60 MIN BEFORE THE PROCEDURE | |
|---|---|---|---|
| | | ADULTS | CHILDREN |
| Can take oral medications | Amoxicillin | 2 g PO | 50 mg/kg PO |
| Cannot take oral medication | Ampicillin | 2 g IM or IV | 50 mg/kg IM or IV |
| | *OR* | | |
| | Cefazolin or ceftriaxone | 1 g IM or IV | 50 mg/kg IM or IV |
| Is allergic to penicillins and able to take oral medication | Cephalexin‡§ | 2 g PO | 50 mg/kg PO |
| | *OR* | | |
| | Clindamycin | 600 mg PO | 20 mg/kg PO |
| | *OR* | | |
| | Azithromycin or clarithromycin | 500 mg PO | 15 mg/kg PO |
| Is allergic to penicillins and unable to take oral medication | Cefazolin or ceftriaxone§ | 1 g IM or IV | 50 mg/kg IM or IV |
| | *OR* | | |
| | Clindamycin | 600 mg IM or IV | 20 mg/kg IM or IV |

Adapted from Wilson W, Taubert KA, Gewitz M, et al. Prevention of infective endocarditis: guidelines from the American Heart Association. A guideline from the American Heart Association Rheumatic Fever, Endocarditis, and Kawasaki Disease Committee, Council on Cardiovascular Disease in the Young, and the Council on Clinical Cardiology, Council on Cardiovascular Surgery and Anesthesia, and the Quality of Care and Outcomes Research Interdisciplinary Working Group. J Am Dent Assoc 2007;138:739-45, 747-60.

*IM*, Intramuscularly; *IV*, intravenously; *PO*, orally.

*If a resistant *Enterococcus* species or resistant *Staphylococcus aureus* is suspected, consultation with an infectious disease specialist should be considered.

†These regimens may be used for ear/nose/throat, respiratory, and contaminated skin/musculoskeletal procedures as well.

‡Other first- or second-generation oral cephalosporins in appropriate doses can be substituted for cephalexin.

§Cephalosporins should not be used in patients with a history of anaphylaxis, angioedema, or urticaria in association with penicillin or penicillin-related drugs.

hygiene as the means to reduce the incidence of IE related to daily activities, as well as dental procedures.[17]

## ACKNOWLEDGMENT

We are indebted to Dr. Ahmet R. Sayan (cardiology) for his critical appraisal of this manuscript.

## SUGGESTED READINGS

Baddour LM, Wilson WR, Bayer AS, et al, for the Committee on Rheumatic Fever, Endocarditis, and Kawasaki Disease; Council on Cardiovascular Disease in the Young; Councils on Clinical Cardiology, Stroke, and Cardiovascular Surgery and Anesthesia; American Heart Association; Infectious Diseases Society of America. Infective endocarditis: diagnosis, antimicrobial therapy, and management of complications. A statement for healthcare professionals from the Committee on Rheumatic Fever, Endocarditis, and Kawasaki Disease, Council on Cardiovascular Disease in the Young, and the Councils on Clinical Cardiology, Stroke, and Cardiovascular Surgery and Anesthesia, American Heart Association: endorsed by the Infectious Diseases Society of America. Circulation 2005;111:e394-e434.

Habib G, Hoen B, Tornos P, et al, for the ESC Committee for Practice Guidelines (CPG). Guidelines on the prevention, diagnosis, and treatment of infective endocarditis (new version 2009): the Task Force on the Prevention, Diagnosis, and Treatment of Infective Endocarditis of the European Society of Cardiology (ESC). Eur Heart J 2009;30:2369-413.

Li IS, Sexton DJ, Mick N, et al. Proposed modifications to the Duke criteria for the diagnosis of infective endocarditis. Clin Infect Dis 2000;30:633-8.

Murdoch DR, Corey GR, Hoen B, et al, for the International Collaboration on Endocarditis—Prospective Cohort Study (ICE-PCS) Investigators. Clinical presentation, etiology, and outcome of infective endocarditis in the 21st century. Arch Intern Med 2009;169:463-73.

Mylonakis E, Calderwood SB. Infective endocarditis in adults. N Engl J Med 2001;345:1318-30.

Wilson W, Taubert KA, Gewitz M, et al. Prevention of infective endocarditis: guidelines from the American Heart Association. A guideline from the American Heart Association Rheumatic Fever, Endocarditis, and Kawasaki Disease Committee, Council on Cardiovascular Disease in the Young, and the Council on Clinical Cardiology, Council on Cardiovascular Surgery and Anesthesia, and the Quality of Care and Outcomes Research Interdisciplinary Working Group. J Am Dent Assoc 2007;138:739-45, 747-760.

## REFERENCES

***References can be found on Expert Consult @ www.expertconsult.com.***

# Management of Emergencies Related to Implanted Cardiac Devices 63

*Daniel Cabrera and Wyatt W. Decker*

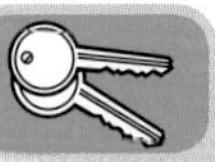

**KEY POINTS**

- Chest compressions should not be performed on patients with an implanted left ventricular assist device who are in cardiac arrest because the device may shear the aorta.
- Major failure of an implanted left ventricular assist device is extremely serious but not catastrophic; patients' minimal but present cardiac function gives time for temporizing maneuvers.
- Patients who have had a cardioverter-defibrillator implanted and experience multiple shocks per day are deemed to be in electrical storm and should be managed very aggressively for ischemia and electrolyte abnormalities.
- A magnet changes most pacemakers to a continuous, preset rate, usually about 80 beats/min. When a magnet is moved away from a pacemaker, the device returns to the previously programmed, baseline function. Implantable cardioverter-defibrillators may need to be reprogrammed after exposure to a magnet.

## INTRODUCTION

The use of implantable devices to support the electrical function of the heart has become widespread since they were first described in the early 1950s.[1] Most recently, the use of ventricular assist devices has become more common in the scenario of an increasing number of patients with severe congestive heart failure (CHF).[2]

Currently, millions of patients in the United States have such implants, and they seek care in emergency departments (EDs) because of complications related to these devices and the conditions that led to the implantation.[3]

This chapter focuses on general concepts and the approach to and management of emergencies related to permanently implanted cardiac devices, specifically, pacemakers (PMs), implantable cardioverter-defibrillators (ICDs), and left ventricular assist devices (LVADs).

## IMPLANTABLE CARDIOVERTER-DEFIBRILLATORS

An ICD is the first line of therapy for prevention of sudden cardiac death, which is commonly the result of ventricular fibrillation (VF) or ventricular tachycardia (VT).[4] The first internal defibrillator was implanted in 1980 by Mirowski and Mower. Since then, the technology and indications have grown enormously. More than 120,000 devices are implanted in the United States every year.[5] Given this scenario, emergency physicians (EPs) face a growing number of patients with increasing complexity who are arriving at EDs with ICD-related complaints.

### GENERAL CONCEPTS OF FUNCTION

Current ICDs correspond to third-generation devices, which are small (40 mL) and reliable and contain sophisticated electrophysiologic analysis algorithms. They can store and report a large number of variables, such as electrocardiograms (ECGs), defibrillation logs, energies, lead impedance, and battery charge.[6] ICDs are usually implanted in the left infraclavicular area via a transvenous technique.

The ICD unit consists of a case containing the battery, circuitry, and pulse generator; a right ventricular apex lead for sensing and defibrillation; and an atrial lead. Current devices for biventricular pacing can be equipped with a coronary venous lead. The diagnostic and treatment functions are configured during placement of the device, along with determination of the defibrillatory threshold (DFT) necessary for the specific patient.[6,7] Typically, the ICD is set to deliver energies 5 to 10 J above the DFT. According to these specifications, the battery life of the modern lithium-silver-vanadium device is approximately 8 years but depends largely on the frequency of the shocks delivered. Most of the devices are equipped with a patient alert system that prevents clinically significant battery-related complications.[7]

The algorithmic criteria for delivering a shock are based largely on the rate, duration, polarity, and waveform of the signal sensed. When the ICD detects atrial and ventricular electrical signals that fulfill the preprogrammed criteria for VT or VF, the device decides the appropriate tier of treatment, which can be:

- Antitachycardia pacing, generally for monomorphic tachycardias
- Low-energy defibrillation (±2 J synchronized with the R wave)
- High-energy defibrillation in which the shocks are delivered as a biphasic wave

These treatments can be felt by the patient as sensations varying from discomfort to frank pain.[6]

Approximately 50% of the patients will experience an ICD discharge in the first 2 years of use. To lower the incidence of ventricular and supraventricular arrhythmias, a considerable proportion of these patients receive adjunctive pharmacologic therapy, usually with amiodarone, sotalol, and statins.[8]

After the ICD delivers a shock, three scenarios are possible: successful defibrillation, continuation of the VT or VF, or conversion to another rhythm—usually pulseless electrical activity (PEA) or asystole. After an efficacious shock, the patient's heart returns to a previous stable rhythm. If the patient continues in VT or VF, the device delivers five more rescue shocks, after which it reanalyzes the waveform.[6,7] In case of postdefibrillation (or primary) bradycardia or asystole, the ICD can display antibradycardiac features similar to those of a VVI PM.

Up to 25% of patients can experience an inappropriate shock, defined as a shock delivered for a rhythm different from sustained VT or VF. The most common causes of inappropriate shocks are supraventricular tachycardias (e.g., atrial fibrillation, paroxysmal supraventricular tachycardia, sinus tachycardia), which are read as VT.[6] Another common cause is misreading of T waves as part of the QRS complex, thereby duplicating the sensed rate. Occasionally, the leads can suffer mechanical damage, such as insulation defects or lead fracture, and such damage can cause electronic noise to be mistakenly detected as VT or VF. These problems are partially solved in modern "noncommitted" apparatuses, which can reanalyze the appropriateness of the rhythm after charging but before shocking.[7]

Currently, no evidence has shown that the electromagnetic fields from daily life artifacts can interfere significantly with defibrillators. However, it is recommended that patients with ICDs avoid placing their cell phones closer than 15 cm to the device and avoid long exposure to metal detectors or antitheft devices.[7] Some medically related sources of interference such as electrocauteries can cause significant malfunction; therefore, interrogation of the device after exposure is recommended.[9] Magnetic resonance imaging (MRI) is contraindicated in patients with ICDs given the risk for mechanical torque, thermal injury, and deprogramming.

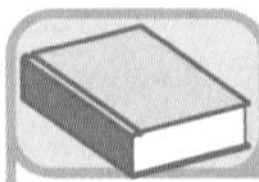

**PATIENT TEACHING TIPS**

**Implantable Cardioverter-Defibrillator**

The occurrence of more than one shock makes urgent medical attention mandatory; the patient should call 911.

If the ICD is firing, the patient must avoid driving.

The patient should always carry the identification card for the ICD, as well as contact information (emergency phone number) for the treating cardiologist.

Pain or swelling in the pocket area could be a sign of infection; the patient should seek medical care as soon as possible.

It is recommended that a cell phone not be placed closer than 15 cm from the ICD and that the patient not linger in metal detectors or antitheft devices.

**TIPS AND TRICKS**

**Implantable Cardioverter-Defibrillator**

The ICD does not prevent but only treats ventricular fibrillation or tachycardia. Always look for reversible causes: ischemia, hypokalemia, hypomagnesemia, proarrhythmic drugs.

If the ICD does not deactivate when a magnet is placed over it, try to place the magnet in the opposite corner of the ICD, or if the patient is very obese, use two magnets.

Always assume that the ICD is permanently disabled after being exposed to a magnet.

The most common cause of death in a patient with an ICD is pulseless electrical activity.

Always look for mechanical lead complications (fracture or dislodgement) on the chest radiograph, especially after the patient has experienced trauma or has undergone cardiopulmonary resuscitation.

Patients receiving multiple shocks may require at least mild anxiolysis.

ST abnormalities on the electrocardiogram are attributable to ICD shocks only if they occur soon after the shock event.

In patients with cardiorespiratory symptoms, it is always advisable to interrogate the device to obtain information regarding dysrhythmias, both supraventricular and ventricular.

## INDICATIONS FOR PLACEMENT OF AN IMPLANTABLE CARDIOVERTER-DEFIBRILLATOR

The major and commonly accepted indications for use of an ICD are summarized in **Box 63.1**. In recent years the indications and uses have expanded such that the current published guidelines have been outpaced.[10] Multiple trials showing a significant reduction in sudden cardiac death have been followed by publications with similar results regarding primary prevention in selected populations with structural heart disease and a low ejection fraction, as well as in other populations with specific cardiac abnormalities.

## APPROACH TO COMPLICATIONS RELATED TO THE IMPLANTATION PROCEDURE

During the early days of ICDs, with their large abdominal cases and pericardial leads, the morbidity and mortality associated with the procedure were considerable. With later use of the transvenous technique, the perioperative mortality rate for ICD placement is less than 0.8%.[4] Nevertheless, infectious, lead-related, thromboembolic, and mechanical complications can occur.

The rate of pocket or lead infection has been reported to be between 2% and 7%.[11] The most common pathogens are cutaneous flora, usually *Staphylococcus aureus* and *Staphylococcus epidermidis*. During the first year after ICD implantation, infections related to the device are primarily due

**BOX 63.1 Commonly Accepted Indications for Placement of an Implantable Cardioverter-Defibrillator**

**Class I**

Structural heart disease and episode of sustained VT
Syncope of unknown source with inducible VT or VF in electrophysiologic studies
Patients with LVEF < 35% (NYHA class II or III)
Patients with LVEF < 40% because of previous myocardial infarction with inducible VT or VF in electrophysiologic studies

**Class II**

Unexplained syncope with LV dysfunction
Sustained VT
Hypertrophic cardiomyopathy with associated with risk factors for sudden cardiac death
Arrhythmogenic right ventricular dysplasia with associated risk factors for sudden cardiac death
Patients with long QT syndrome and syncope or VT while receiving treatment
Nonhospitalized patients waiting for a heart transplant
Patients with Brugada syndrome and an episode of syncope or VT
Patients with catecholaminergic polymorphic VT and an episode of syncope or VT while receiving treatment
Patients with cardiac sarcoidosis, giant cell myocarditis, or Chagas disease

*LV*, Left ventricular; *LVEF*, left ventricular ejection fraction; *NYHA*, New York Heart Association; *VF*, ventricular fibrillation; *VT*, ventricular tachycardia.

to the procedure; after that period they are probably due to secondary seeding. From a clinical perspective, common infectious signs and symptoms in patients with ICDs are notoriously absent and patients may have only vague complaints. Infections of the case and leads have a wide incidence of about 1% to 12%. Diagnosis of a delayed hardware infection requires a high index of suspicion given the absence of a confirmatory ancillary test. Almost without exception, suspected or proven hardware infections require contact with the patient's primary electrophysiologist, hospital admission, long-term intravenous antibiotic therapy, and potential removal of the device.[7,11]

Modern lead systems are extremely reliable but are still prone to fracture, malposition, dislodgment, and damage to the insulation. These defects commonly lead to electrical noise that can precipitate inappropriate shocks. In the evaluation of a patient with suspected lead malfunction, a chest radiograph is required for confirmation of proper positioning and integrity of the leads.[4,7,11] Contacting the implant team for replacement of the lead is the only alternative possible for hardware failure. Problems related to the battery, pulse generator, and circuitry are extraordinarily rare.

Thromboembolic complications can be seen in as many as 30% of patients with ICDs; they usually involve the cephalic and subclavian veins and do not generally lead to ICD malfunction. Affected patients exhibit unilateral arm swelling, pain, discoloration, and paresthesias, which require evaluation with ultrasonography, venography, or computed tomography. Standard treatment with heparin and warfarin usually results in a good outcome.[11]

The many mechanical complications related to placement may be manifested early or in delayed fashion. A considerable number of patients experience some degree of tricuspid regurgitation, with approximately 10% of cases being clinically significant. In addition, there is a theoretic risk for fibrosis of the apical lead, which could increase the DFT and make the shocks ineffective. Later manifestations with life-threatening mechanical complications, such as cardiac perforation, cardiac tamponade, hemothorax, pneumothorax, and air embolism, are very rare.[11]

**BOX 63.2 Clinical Findings in Patients with Problems Related to Functioning of Implantable Cardioverter-Defibrillators**

Cardiac arrest
Unstable with ongoing shocks and arrhythmias
Electrical storm
Stable and complaining about a recent isolated shock
Stable and complaining about other cardiorespiratory symptoms

## APPROACH TO PROBLEMS RELATED TO FUNCTION AND DYSFUNCTION

In a patient with complaints related to functioning of the ICD, the EP must consider that the majority of such patients have severe structural heart disease with a poor ejection fraction and that most of them are in end-stage CHF.[7] They can have a myriad of symptoms; however, these symptoms can be approached systematically (**Box 63.2**). Evaluation of a patient with an ICD must start by placing the patient in a monitored setting with external defibrillator capacity.[8,12]

### *Cardiac Arrest*

Causes of death in this population are PEA after VT or VF (29%), defibrillation failure (26%), primary PEA (16%), and refractory VT or VF (13%).[12] When a patient is seen in VT- or VF-related cardiac arrest, the most likely scenario is that VT or VF occurred and the ICD correctly sensed and delivered the shocks but failed to achieve defibrillation. It is critical for the EP to recognize and treat correctable causes of VT and VF. Common causes in this population are ongoing ischemia, electrolyte disturbances (especially hypokalemia and hypomagnesemia), and the arrhythmic effect of drugs.[4] Many such patients have non–VT/VF-associated cardiac arrest in the context of end-stage CHF; in these cases, disabling the device could be helpful in the resuscitative efforts. Disabling can be accomplished by placing a magnet over the surface of the case pocket. It is very important to remember that after a magnet is placed over the device, it must be assumed that the device is permanently disabled and reprogramming is needed. Standard advanced cardiac life support (ACLS) protocols must be followed both for VT/VF- and non–VT/VF-related causes of cardiac arrest, the only difference being that the external defibrillator paddles and patches should not be placed directly over the ICD case.

### Unstable with Ongoing Shocks

Management of an unstable patient must be based on the functioning of the ICD. Basically, this situation may represent two scenarios:

- Inappropriate shocks leading to hemodynamic compromise
- Refractory VT with a pulse and delivery of multiple appropriate shocks

Patients can experience cardiovascular collapse caused by repetitive inappropriate shocks secondary to true or misdiagnosed supraventricular tachycardias. In such cases, treatment must start by decreasing the rate of the tachycardia with the usual pharmacologic treatment (e.g., beta-blockers, calcium channel blockers). If these measures fail, the next step is to disable the ICD. A considerable proportion of patients arrive at the ED in unstable bradycardia; in this setting the VVI function of the device will be helpful, but prompt recognition of the cause (commonly end-stage CHF) and standard ACLS treatment are mandatory.[7]

Those with sustained VT with a pulse and appropriately shocked by the device represent an in extremis population. The most critical intervention is the delivery of higher-energy shocks with an external defibrillator (regardless of whether the ICD is disabled) and rapid correction of the cause of the VT.[7,8]

Both populations require mandatory electrophysiologic consultation and interrogation of the device.

### Electrical Storm

Electrical storm is commonly defined as more than two therapies (antitachycardia pacing or shocks) delivered in a 24-hour period.[13] It is believed to affect about 10% of patients with ICDs[7] and is a common complaint in these patients.[8] Classically, such patients are rather stable but complain of several shocks delivered in the preceding hours. The significance of electrical storm is that it is usually a herald of life-threatening acute pathology, commonly acute cardiac ischemia, hyperkalemia, and decompensated CHF, thus placing these patients at immediate high risk for death.

Management starts with standard stabilization and cardiac monitoring followed by correction of any obvious abnormalities, evaluation for mechanical failure, device interrogation, electrophysiologic consultation, and aggressive management of CHF and acute ischemia.

### Stable with a Recent Isolated Shock

The most important first step is to determine whether the shocks were appropriate.[4] The patient should be placed in a monitored setting where the heart rhythm can be recorded, followed by a chest radiograph to evaluate for possible hardware failure (e.g., lead fracture) and basic laboratory tests to look for ischemia or electrolyte disturbances. Any signs or symptoms around the moment of the shock (e.g., chest pain, shortness of breath, chest trauma) should be noted. It is also important to inquire about new drugs or changes in dosage (especially for amiodarone). Arrhythmias discovered during monitoring, as well as metabolic causes of VT or VF, must be treated in the usual fashion.

Occasionally, patients complain of hearing a beep from the device. Some models can emit a beep in the event of battery discharge or another cause of malfunction. Stable patients with an isolated shock require interrogation of the ICD so that the underlying rhythms can be evaluated and the ICD can be reprogrammed.[4] The decision for hospital admission is usually made jointly by the EP and the electrophysiologist based on the appropriateness of the shock, the availability of follow-up, and the overall clinical status of the patient. Patients who have experienced isolated appropriate shocks but have no change in cardiopulmonary status, no evidence of ischemia, and no electrolyte abnormalities can be discharged from the ED for follow-up with an electrophysiologist.[14]

### Stable with Other Cardiorespiratory Symptoms

Patients can come to the ED with cardiorespiratory complaints not clearly related to ICD functioning, such as chest pain, shortness of breath, and dizziness. Evaluation and interrogation of the ICD are advisable to ensure that the symptoms are not related to device malfunctioning. Further management is focused on the patient's complaint once information from the device has been gathered.

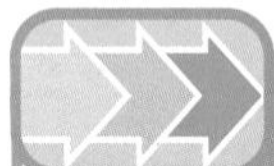

**PRIORITY ACTIONS**

**Implantable Cardioverter-Defibrillator**

Patients with ICD-related complaints must have prompt transport by emergency medical services to the closest emergency department.

Always place a patient with an ICD in a monitored bed.

In the case of a disabled or malfunctioning ICD, the defibrillator patches must be placed in the anteroposterior position during monitoring and away from the ICD pocket.

Gather focused clinical and technical information about the device, and contact the electrophysiologist taking care of the patient.

Obtain an anteroposterior chest radiograph and measurements of cardiac biomarkers and serum electrolytes.

The patient will most probably need admission to a unit with a monitored bed.

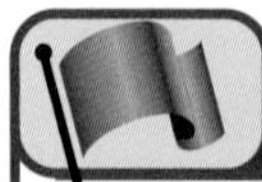

**RED FLAGS**

**Implantable Cardioverter-Defibrillator**

- Multiple shocks probably represent electrical storm, which confers high risk for an adverse outcome in the patient.
- Chest pain before ICD discharge can be a sign of ischemia leading to ventricular tachycardia or ventricular fibrillation.
- Amiodarone and class I antidysrhythmic agents raise the defibrillatory threshold, and recent changes in the dose or interactions with other medications can cause failure of ICD defibrillation.
- A history of syncope may represent successfully treated ventricular tachycardia or fibrillation.

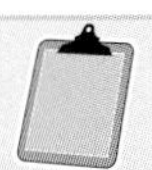

**DOCUMENTATION**

**Implantable Cardioverter-Defibrillator**

Primary indication for the automatic ICD
Number of treatments (shocks) received in the last 24 hours
Consultation with electrophysiology
Result of interrogation of the automatic ICD

## LEFT VENTRICULAR ASSIST DEVICES

LVADs were initially developed more than 25 years ago as intermediate treatments to "bridge" patients to heart transplantation. In this chapter the discussion pertains particularly to permanent devices such as the WorldHeartNovacor, HeartMate VE, and HeartMate XVE.

Currently, more than 5 million Americans are estimated to suffer from heart failure with an aggregate 5-year survival rate of 50%.[15] The high mortality and poor quality of life in patients with late-stage heart failure has led to further study and proposed uses for LVADs; the device has now been approved as a therapy for candidates waiting for a heart transplant (bridge therapy) and for patients with end-stage heart failure who are not candidates for heart transplantation because of age or other medical comorbid conditions, known as destination therapy.[16] Currently, nearly a thousand patients have undergone implantation of an LVAD as destination therapy for severe heart failure,[17] but an estimated 30,000 to 60,000 patients per year could be eligible for the procedure.[18]

### GENERAL CONCEPTS OF FUNCTION

LVADs are battery-operated, mechanical or electric pumps that are surgically implanted to help maintain and augment the pumping ability of the heart. Increasing problems with limited organ availability for transplantation and greater numbers of patients with heart failure have expanded the use of these devices.

Conceptually, the device consists of a stroke-volume generator pump, an outflow tract efferent from the left ventricle, an inflow tract afferent to the ascending aorta, and a battery support system. The pump mechanism is implanted into the upper part of the abdomen or lower part of the thorax, and a skin-tunneled driveline connects with the exterior to permit electrical connections and pneumatic venting.

Originally, most models consisted of mechanical pumps, which were diaphragm oscillators that generated pulsatile blow flow through the outflow tract. Current devices work on axial pump flow in which electromagnetic centrifugal or rotatory engines generate nonpulsatile flow; this translates to no pulse or a very faint pulse when examining such patients. These newer axial flow pumps confer several benefits such smaller pumps and drivelines, fewer moving parts, and more efficient use of energy. Among their disadvantages are the requirement for systemic anticoagulation and the lack of a backup method (e.g., the hand-operated pump in older models) when device failure occurs.[19]

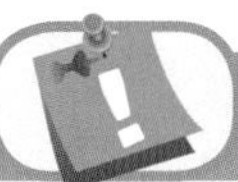

**TIPS AND TRICKS**

**Left Ventricular Assist Device**

Assume that the patient has severe right ventricular failure and almost no left ventricular reserve.
Be aware of the type-specific devices common in the local population.
Stock troubleshooting manuals and batteries in the emergency department for devices common in the local population.
Exercise caution with the amount of fluid used for volume resuscitation.
In patients with axial flow pump devices, absence of a peripheral pulse is expected.

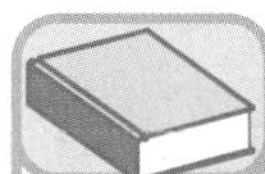

**PATIENT TEACHING TIPS**

**Left Ventricular Assist Device**

The patient must be aware of the type of device implanted and must carry contact information for the implanting surgical team.
The patient must carry backup batteries and the manual pump for the implanted device.
The patient should avoid long periods with the device on battery power.

### INDICATIONS FOR PLACEMENT OF A LEFT VENTRICULAR ASSIST DEVICE

Indications for LVAD placement can be categorized according to therapeutic goals (**Box 63.3**). Patients awaiting cardiac transplantation and those with New York Heart Association class IV heart failure (and who are ineligible for transplantation) are candidates for LVAD implantation. The Randomized Evaluation of Mechanical Assistance for the Treatment of Congestive Heart Failure (REMATCH) trial compared patients with optimal medical management alone and those with medical management and implantation of a HeartMate VE LVAD. The study, conducted over a period of 2 years, showed a relatively lower risk for death (48%) during the follow-up period in the LVAD group than in the medical management group.[16] The Food and Drug Administration approved the LVAD device in 2002 as destination therapy for patients with heart failure. Further follow-up has continued to show better survival in LVAD recipients, as well as improved quality of life.[20]

**BOX 63.3 Categories of Indications for Placement of a Left Ventricular Assist Device**

Bridge to recovery (e.g., severe left ventricular dysfunction secondary to a reversible cause such as myocarditis)
Bridge to transplantation
Destination therapy (patients with end-stage congestive heart failure who are not candidates for transplantation)

**BOX 63.4 Categories of Complications of Left Ventricular Assist Devices**

Thromboembolic and bleeding events
Infections
Minor device failure (e.g., battery dysfunction)
Major device failure (e.g., outflow tract disconnection, pump failure)

## APPROACH TO PROBLEMS RELATED TO FUNCTION AND DYSFUNCTION

As growing numbers of patients are undergoing LVAD implantation, it will be important for EPs to understand the major complications of these devices. Problems with LVADs can be divided into four broad categories (**Box 63.4**).

Hardware malfunction is not uncommon and can occur at a combined rate of about 0.87 events per patient per year.[21] The incidence of life-threatening hardware failure can be as high as 7.8% during the implantation period, often related to pump or inflow valve problems.[22,23] Because these patients are in extremis, it is paramount for the EP to know that chest compressions should almost never be performed in patients with an LVAD because the trauma from the compressions can shear the outflow tract from the aorta and cause massive hemorrhage. ACLS protocols can otherwise be followed during resuscitation of patients with an LVAD.

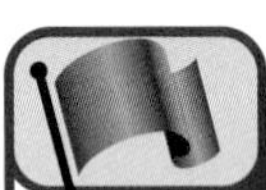

**RED FLAGS**

**Left Ventricular Assist Device**

Local pain in the pocket or driveline may herald infection.
Signs and symptoms of right-sided heart failure can indicate device malfunction.
Look for evidence of thromboembolic disease, and proceed with standard management.

### *Thromboembolic and Bleeding Events*

Patients usually require systemic anticoagulation with an international normalized ratio of 2.5 to 3.0 and aspirin for antiinflammatory purposes. Those experiencing thromboembolic complications such as a cerebrovascular accident and peripheral embolism will benefit from standard treatments. Of note, there is no clear evidence related to the use of thrombolysis in this population; however, the risks appear to outweigh the benefits, and close discussion and planning among emergency medicine, thoracic surgery, and neurology are essential.

In patients who are bleeding, the cardiovascular team must be contacted before reversal of anticoagulation. Caution must be exercised in volume resuscitation of such patients given the tenuous function of the ventricles. Management does not differ significantly from that for the regular population.

### *Infections*

Infectious complications of the LVAD components are common, about 6 per 1000 device-days.[24] The signs and symptoms can be deceiving given the paucity of classic infections. Pain located near the case or driveline is often a sign of hardware infection. Patients in whom such infections are suspected must be admitted to the hospital for intravenous antibiotic therapy under the care of the implantation team. Frequently, débridement and mobilization of the components (e.g., the driveline) must be performed.

### *Minor Device Failure*

Minor device failure is a broad category related to malfunction of the hardware apart from the pump. Commonly, the patient has a nonfunctioning device secondary to a discharged battery or an external circuitry error.[22] In older mechanical models, the pumping function of the LVAD can be supported manually until the battery or the control panel can be replaced. Before discharge from the hospital all patients undergoing LVAD implantation and their family members are taught how to disengage the device and attach a hand pump to continue blood flow through the LVAD. The hand pump should be carried with the patient at all times. Information about how to engage the hand pump system can be found on websites for each of the devices.[17]

Current models have the ability to alert patients when electrical and battery issues are diagnosed, which usually leads to an ED visit. In both situations just described, the implantation team should be contacted to evaluate the device. Usually, these issues do not lead to explantation of the device.

### *Major Device Failure*

A life-threatening emergency, major device failure is caused by outflow or inflow disconnections, flow valve problems, or pump failure, and patients are commonly initially seen in cardiogenic shock or cardiac arrest.[22] The catastrophic nature of such an event requires prompt and aggressive cardiac life support and emergency consultation with the cardiovascular surgical team. The use of vasoactive drugs and intraaortic balloon pump support constitute the basis of management.

Troubleshooting of device failure by nonexperienced physicians is extremely complicated and discouraged. Patients with an LVAD characteristically have a severely low but measurable ejection fraction. The remnant systolic function is often enough to keep the patient alive until temporizing measures can be instituted. Aggressive management of cardiogenic shock and immediate involvement of the implantation team are mandatory.

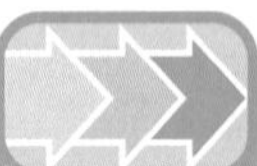

**PRIORITY ACTIONS**

**Left Ventricular Assist Device**

Institute continuous cardiac monitoring in all patients.
Do not start chest compression in patients with cardiac arrest who have a left ventricular assist device in place.
Start manual pumping in patients with hardware failure.
Contact the implantation team as soon as feasible.

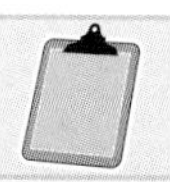

**DOCUMENTATION**

**Left Ventricular Assist Device**
Document the type of device.
Document consultation with the implantation team.

## PACEMAKERS

In 1952 a PM became the first electronic implantable device when it was used to treat a patient with a high-degree block. A few years later, PM use became widespread for treating myriad conditions, from sick sinus rhythm to cardiac resynchronization.[1] Now, millions of Americans have an implanted PM, with an estimated 425 new PMs per 100,000 people per year.[25]

### GENERAL CONCEPTS OF FUNCTION

A PM has two basic components: a pulse generator (which also contains analyzing hardware and firmware) and the lead or leads. Conceptually, the device senses the intrinsic activity of the heart, atrial or ventricular, and after processing the information with the preprogrammed algorithm, decides if it is necessary to initiate a myocardial depolarization.

PMs have evolved and become more complex in recent years. A five-digit code system to describe function was developed by North American Society of Pacing and Electrophysiology and the British Pacing and Electrophysiology Group.[26] It explains the sensing and pacing abilities and the expected actions (**Table 63.1**). Currently, the most common pacing modes are AAI, VVI, and DDD.

**Table 63.1 North American Society of Pacing and Electrophysiology and the British Pacing and Electrophysiology Group Pacemaker Code**

| POSITION | ACTION | DESCRIPTION |
|---|---|---|
| I | Chamber(s) paced | A = Atrium<br>V = Ventricle<br>D = Dual<br>O = None |
| II | Chamber(s) sensed | A = Atrium<br>V = Ventricle<br>D = Dual<br>O = None |
| III | Response to sensing | T = Triggered<br>I = Inhibited<br>D = Dual<br>O = None |
| IV | Programmability | P = Simple<br>M = Multi<br>C = Communicating<br>R = Rate modulation<br>O = None |
| V | Antitachydysrhythmia functions | P = Pacing<br>S = Shock<br>D = Dual<br>O = None |

It is of cardinal importance that EPs understand the representation of the PM activity on the surface ECG. The triggering activity of the device is able to be visualized as a spike (also known as an artifact) on the ECG. These spikes will usually precede the atrial or ventricular activity. Older models are commonly monophasic and produce a conspicuous electrical spike on the surface tracing; however, modern devices are biphasic, which produces an artifact that is considerably smaller and can sometimes be very difficult to appreciate. In this scenario, recording of the ECG at higher amplitude (i.e., to increase to size of the QRS complex) may be helpful to appreciate the artifact. In cases in which failure to pace is suspected (see later), it may be helpful to place a magnet over the PM case, which will turn the device into an asynchronous mode, commonly VV, and make assessment easier. Extreme caution is necessary in patients who are dependent on the PM.

The surface ECG will show a left bundle branch block as the electric stimulus is arising from the right ventricle. It is important to remember that the QRS complex will be discordant from the ST segment.

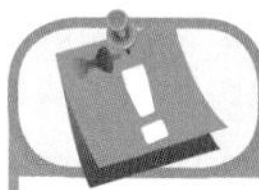

**TIPS AND TRICKS**

**Pacemaker**
Understand pacemaker nomenclature (see Table 63.1).
Look for the presence of pacemaker spikes on the electrocardiogram; they can be very subtle or, rarely, not visible.
The presence of a bundle branch block pattern on the electrocardiogram should alert the clinician to the possibility of a paced rhythm.
Know how and when to use a magnet.

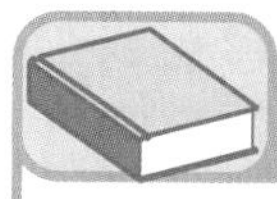

**PATIENT TEACHING TIPS**

**Pacemaker**
Discuss the importance of regularly scheduled checkups for the device, as well as the patient.
Warn of possible interference with device by medical imaging and procedures.
Highlight the importance of carrying device information all the time.

### INDICATIONS FOR PLACEMENT OF A PACEMAKER

There are many indications for PM placement, some of which are widely accepted whereas others are more controversial. Common indications include patients with high-degree atrioventricular block, symptomatic blocks, and sick sinus rhythm. Recent years have seen an increase in the use of dual-chamber PMs for cardiac resynchronization in patients with heart failure. **Box 63.5** contains a summary of class I indications for PM placement.[27]

## APPROACH TO COMPLICATIONS RELATED TO THE IMPLANTATION PROCEDURE

The complications related to placement of a PM are similar to those described for ICDs; the most significant are infections, thromboembolic disease, and tricuspid valve regurgitation.

Infections have an incidence of about 1.9 events per 1000 device-years.[28] Signs and symptoms such as malaise, pocket pain, or swelling may indicate infection. It is recommended that blood be collected for culture and broad-spectrum antibiotics be initiated with a focus on cutaneous flora. Admission and consultation with the primary electrophysiologist are recommended.

Thromboembolic disease is manifested similar to other causes, including pain, swelling, vein distention, and shortness of breath. Treatment does not differ from that for standard venous thromboembolism and rests on the use of anticoagulants. The decision to perform lead change or explantation is not an emergency, and it is usually done at the discretion of the implantation team.[29]

The incidence of tricuspid regurgitation after PM placement is relatively low. Fifty percent of these patients will have right heart failure, whereas others may remain asymptomatic. Valve replacement or annuloplasty is sometimes required.[30]

**BOX 63.5 Class I Indications for Placement of a Pacemaker**

1. Third-degree and advanced second-degree atrioventricular (AV) block at any anatomic level and associated with any of the following conditions:
   a. Bradycardia with symptoms (including heart failure) presumed to be due to AV block (level of evidence: C)
   b. Arrhythmias and other medical conditions requiring drugs that result in symptomatic bradycardia
   c. Documented periods of asystole of 3.0 seconds or longer or any escape rate less than 40 beats/min in awake, symptom-free patients (levels of evidence: B, C)
   d. After catheter ablation of the AV junction (levels of evidence: B, C). No trials have assessed outcome without pacing, and pacing is virtually always planned in this situation unless the operative procedure is modification of the AV junction
   e. Postoperative AV block that is not expected to resolve after cardiac surgery (level of evidence: C)
   f. Neuromuscular diseases characterized by an AV block, such as myotonic muscular dystrophy, Kearns-Sayre syndrome, Erb dystrophy (limb-girdle), and peroneal muscular atrophy, with or without symptoms, because of the potential for unpredictable progression of AV conduction disease (level of evidence: B)
2. Second-degree AV block regardless of the type or site of block and with associated symptomatic bradycardia (level of evidence: B)

## APPROACH TO PROBLEMS RELATED TO FUNCTION AND DYSFUNCTION

PM emergencies can be broadly divided into the following categories (**Box 63.6**):

1. Failure to capture, in which the pulse generator is sending an appropriate electrical impulse but it is not resulting in a heartbeat
2. Failure to pace, in which the device is not generating an electrical impulse
3. Failure to sense, in which the pacemaker is firing inappropriately despite a normal cardiac rhythm
4. Pacemaker-induced tachycardia

The manifestation of PM-related emergencies varies from asymptomatic (e.g., found to be defective on a routine ECG) to full cardiac arrest. Intermediate findings, including palpitations, anxiety, and light-headedness, are common.

Patients with suspected PM malfunction should be connected to a cardiac monitor and undergo evaluation with a 12-lead ECG. This latter step will be of key importance in assessing the cardiac rhythm and identifying any malfunction. It is also recommended that a chest radiograph be obtained for evaluation of mechanical lead problems (e.g., fracture, dislodgment). General laboratory evaluation is likewise warranted given that electrolyte abnormalities and ischemia may increase the depolarization threshold of the myocardium and lead to failure to capture (see the next section).

The majority of PMs are equipped with a magnetic switch that will put the device into synchronized pace mode at a set rate (typically 80 or 100 beats/min). A ring magnet made for this purpose should be held over the pulse generator. Although device-specific magnets are available, any PM magnet will usually suffice. In patients with symptomatic native bradycardia, placement of a magnet may be lifesaving, and it should be maintained until the permanent PM is repaired or a temporary transvenous PM has been placed.

### *Failure to Capture*

Failure to capture is defined as the PM being able to sense and deliver an electric stimulus but the electric current fails to elicit myocardial depolarization. Classically, PM spikes are present, but no atrial or ventricular activity follows (**Fig. 63.1**). Potential causes include lead dislodgment or malposition[31] and inflammation at the electrode tip; as mentioned previously, a chest radiograph can assist in assessing lead location and damage. Similar to the previous scenario, the patient will have symptoms of the underlying disease. Standard ACLS management is recommended, in addition to consideration of a transcutaneous PM in patients dependent on a PM.

**BOX 63.6 Categories of Pacemaker Emergencies**

Failure to pace
Failure to capture
Failure to sense
Pacemaker-induced tachycardia

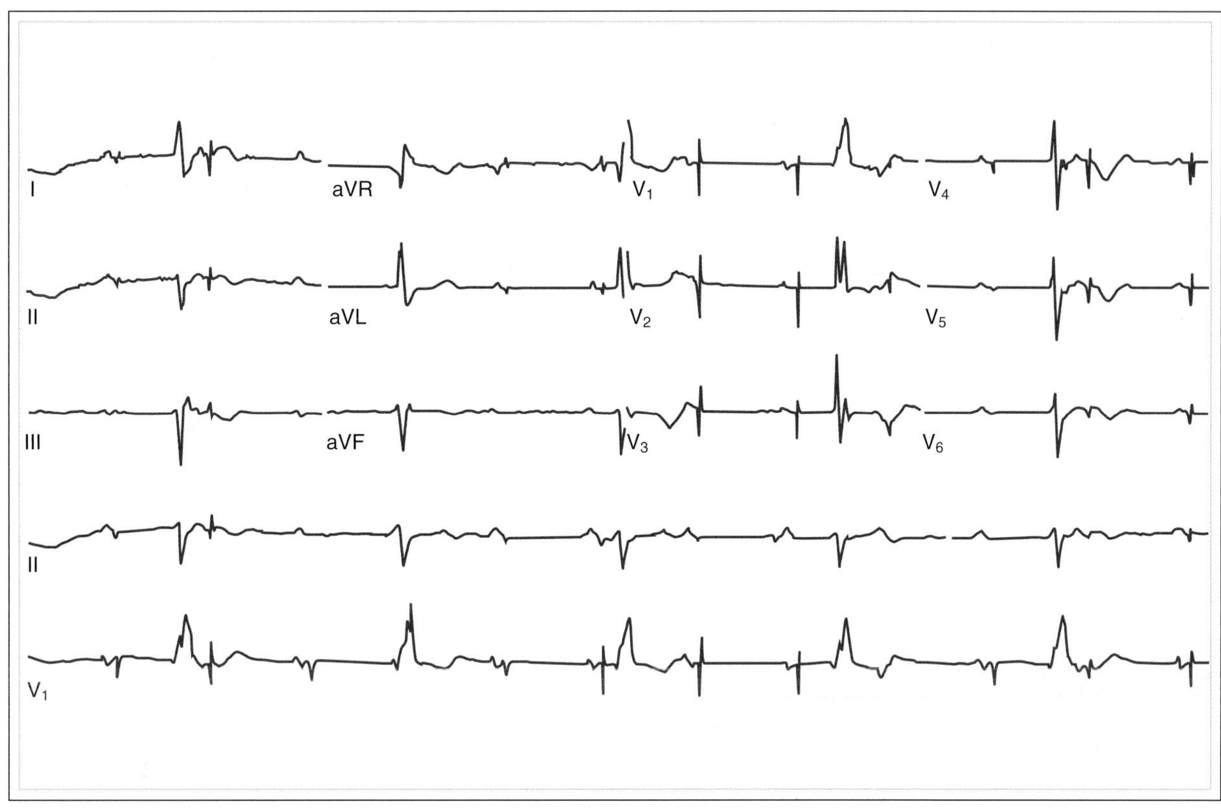


**Fig. 63.1 Electrocardiogram depicting failure to sense and failure to capture.**

### Failure to Pace

This type of failure is characterized as the PM being able to adequately sense but does not deliver an electric stimulus when it should do so. In failure to pace, PM spikes are absent from the ECG despite an abnormal or slow native rhythm. Causes include lead fracture, battery depletion, failure of the pulse generator, and most commonly, oversensing.[31,32] Frequently, the scenario is defined as the sensing element of the PM being confused by other electrical signals such as muscular electrical activity, electrical noise, or ventricular signals. The device inappropriately recognizes these signals as atrial in nature and decides to inhibit the delivery of an electric impulse. Failure of the pulse generator can result from an internal malfunction, blunt trauma, and a number of iatrogenic causes, including MRI, radiation therapy, and electrocautery.[31,33]

Patients will have signs and symptoms related to the underlying disease, commonly with bradycardic rhythms and high atrioventricular blocks. Management consists of standards ACLS bradycardia management followed by interrogation and reprogramming of the PM.[31,32] Use of a magnet may be helpful in converting the device into an asynchronous mode, thereby potentially bypassing the effect of oversensing.

### Failure to Sense

Failure to sense occurs when the PM delivers an electric stimulus regardless of appropriate native cardiac activity. It can be caused by lead dislodgment, lead fracture, development of scar tissue at the site of the lead contact, battery depletion, or an unusually low-amplitude cardiac signal. Evaluation of this type of PM failure is very difficult because the ECG will give limited information.

Patients will have the signs and symptoms of CHF. In patients with no obvious trigger to CHF exacerbation, the possibility of PM undersensing must be considered. Device interrogation is highly recommended because information will be obtained about functioning of the device and will potentially be helpful in reprogramming the PM with the necessary new settings.[32]

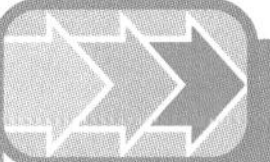

**PRIORITY ACTIONS**

**Pacemaker**

Assess patients for the ABCs of resuscitation (airway, breathing, circulation), and intervene as appropriate.

Initiate monitoring of the cardiac rhythm and obtain a 12-lead electrocardiogram.

Assess patients for the four primary pacemaker malfunctions:

- Failure to capture
- Failure to pace
- Failure to sense
- Pacemaker-induced tachycardia

Use a magnet to assess for failure to pace.

### Pacemaker-Induced Tachycardia

Rarely, patients will experience PM-induced tachycardia, also known as runaway PM syndrome. This condition is seen most

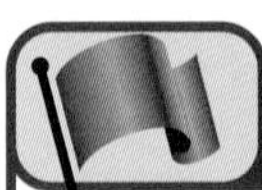

**RED FLAGS**

**Pacemaker**

Look for neck and upper extremity venous distention as a sign of superior vena cava syndrome.

Look for the classic findings of the Beck triad—distended neck veins, muffled heart sounds, and hypotension—in a patient with cardiac tamponade caused by perforation of the myocardium by a lead, especially with recently placed devices.

Pacemaker-induced tachycardia is a rare complication that may respond to placement of a magnet over the pacemaker.

often with older, dual-chamber PM models. The cycle is initiated by atypical conduction through the heart, such as a retrograde P wave that falls immediately after the preprogrammed refractory period and sets up a reentry circuit in which the PM fires rapid ventricular beats in response to a perceived atrial beat. As PMs have become more sophisticated, this condition has become far less common.[323] A magnet is the first-line intervention for PM-associated tachycardia because it may break the rhythm. Should this approach fail in an unstable patient, external pacing and, ultimately, lead exposure and cutting may be needed.

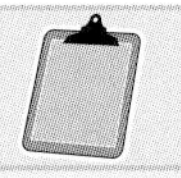

**DOCUMENTATION**

**Pacemaker**

Document the date of insertion, make, and model of the pacemaker (if available; this information is often carried by the patient).

Document key rhythm strips.

Document response to any interventions, especially a rhythm strip with a magnet in place.

## SUGGESTED READINGS

Chan TC, Cardall TY. Electronic pacemakers. Emerg Med Clin North Am 2006;24:179-94, vii.

DiMarco JP. Implantable cardioverter-defibrillators. N Engl J Med 2003;349:1836-47.

Gehi AK, Mehta D, Gomes JA. Evaluation and management of patients after implantable cardioverter-defibrillator shock. JAMA 2006;296:2839-47.

John R. Current axial-flow devices—the HeartMate II and Jarvik 2000 left ventricular assist devices. Semin Thorac Cardiovasc Surg 2008;20:264-72.

## REFERENCES

***Reference can be found on Expert Consult @ www.expertconsult.com.***

# Syncope 64

*James Quinn*

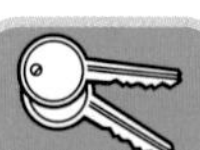

**KEY POINTS**

- Syncope is a symptom, not a diagnosis.
- Patients with cardiac syncope have a 6-month mortality rate in excess of 10%.
- If the diagnosis can be made, the disposition will be based on that diagnosis.
- When the patient's symptoms have resolved and the cause is unclear, risk stratification can help in making decisions on disposition.
- Risk factors in emergency department patients include abnormal electrocardiographic findings, including any rhythm abnormalities detected during monitoring. Other risk factors include a history of cardiac disease (especially congestive heart failure) and absence of a prodrome, which places patients at risk for unfavorable cardiac outcomes. Those with persistently abnormal vital signs, shortness of breath, or a low hematocrit are also at higher risk for other adverse outcomes.

## EPIDEMIOLOGY

It is estimated that 1 in 4 people will faint during their lifetime and that 6 in 1000 people per year will suffer from the symptom of syncope. Syncope is responsible for 1% to 2% of all emergency department (ED) visits, and the cost of hospitalization for syncope approaches $2 billion annually.[1-4]

Syncope is defined as a transient loss of consciousness that does not require resuscitative efforts and subsequent return to the patient's baseline neurologic condition. Loss of consciousness associated with neurologic deficits or persistent alteration in the level of consciousness is, strictly speaking, not properly described as syncope; although such events are commonly referred to as syncope in the literature, in this chapter they are termed apparent syncope.

## PATHOPHYSIOLOGY

Syncope comes from the Greek word *synkoptein*, meaning "to cut short." Hippocrates was the first to use the term and describe the symptom.[5] Syncope has many causes, but the pathophysiology of the final pathway is the same: hypoperfusion of the cerebral cortex and reticular activating system, which after 8 to 10 seconds of interrupted perfusion causes loss of consciousness; a shorter period results in lightheadedness or dizziness and is referred to as near syncope.

## PRESENTING SIGNS AND SYMPTOMS

The symptoms of syncope can be dramatic. Patients may or may not have a warning, or prodrome, and frequently suffer a fall and have associated trauma. Those with a prodrome frequently experience lightheadedness, diaphoretic warmth, nausea and vomiting, or any combination of these symptoms. Those witnessing the event often fear that the patient has died or was dead for a short period, thus making it an emotionally charged and anxiety-provoking event.

## CLASSIFICATION OF SYNCOPE

The American College of Physicians lists four major prognostic categories of syncope: neurally mediated, orthostatic, neurogenic, and cardiac; actually, a fifth category ("syncope of unknown cause") is recognized because in most cases the cause of the syncope remains unknown even after extensive investigation.[6,7]

### NEURALLY MEDIATED SYNCOPE

Neurally mediated syncope is syncope associated with inappropriate vasodilation, bradycardia, or both as a result of inappropriate vagal or sympathetic tone.[8] It is a benign type of cardiovascular syncope that is often associated with a sensation of increased warmth and may be accompanied by preceding lightheadedness (prodrome) along with sweating and nausea. A slow, progressive onset suggests the subcategory vasovagal syncope. Sweating and nausea do not occur with orthostatic hypotension, which is another cause of syncope preceded by lightheadedness.[5]

Neurally mediated or vasovagal syncope may occur after exposure to an unexpected or unpleasant sight, sound, or smell; fear or other emotional distress; severe pain; or surgical procedure. It may also occur in association with prolonged standing or kneeling in a crowded or warm place or after exertion. As a result, the vagus nerve is stimulated, which causes reflex bradycardia and vasodilation.

Situational syncope occurs during or immediately after coughing, micturition, defecation, or swallowing via a similar mechanism. Carotid sinus syncope can be associated with neck pressure (shaving, tight collar) or head turning resulting in stimulation of the carotid sinus in the neck.

### ORTHOSTATIC SYNCOPE

Orthostatic syncope occurs in individuals with documented postural hypotension associated with syncope or symptoms of presyncope.[4] In cases of orthostatic syncope, measurement of blood pressure is recommended, first after the patient is supine for 5 minutes and then after the patient is able to stand for 1 to 3 minutes. A decrease of more than 20 mm Hg in systolic pressure is considered abnormal, as is a drop in pressure below 90 mm Hg independent of the development of symptoms.[9]

Because orthostatic hypotension occurs in asymptomatic individuals, vital signs are neither particularly sensitive nor specific. In fact, positive orthostatic changes have been documented in up to 40% of asymptomatic patients older than 70 years and in 25% of those younger than 60 years. Similarly, a notable number of children who are asymptomatic have been documented to have orthostatic hypotension.[5,10]

The most common cause of orthostatic syncope is intravascular volume loss, which may be due to dehydration or bleeding. Orthostatic syncope is not always benign because many patients with serious causes can have this symptom.[11]

### NEUROLOGIC SYNCOPE

Neurologic causes of apparent syncope include seizures, transient ischemic attacks, migraine headaches, subarachnoid hemorrhage, and subclavian steal syndrome. Confusion after apparent syncope that lasts more than 5 minutes, tongue biting, incontinence, and epileptic aura suggest a seizure. A significant differential in blood pressure between the two arms suggests subclavian steal or dissection. For neurologic causes to be considered true syncope, they must by definition be transient in nature and result in a return to baseline neurologic function. Thus, loss of consciousness with persistent neurologic deficits or altered mental status is not true syncope. In fact, according to this criterion very few neurologic events (especially strokes or subarachnoid hemorrhage) meet the definition of syncope.

Most cases involving neurologic causes of syncope are easily predicted. In general, when these patients have symptoms suggesting a specific disease process, the need for intervention based on neurologic symptoms is usually obvious. It is not recommended that a routine neurologic work-up be performed in all patients with syncope unless related neurologic symptoms are present. It has been determined that routine neurologic testing and investigation, such as computed tomography (CT), is not cost-effective in patients without neurologic symptoms.[12]

### CARDIAC-RELATED SYNCOPE

Cardiac-related syncope is clearly the most dangerous class of syncope, and it can be a harbinger of sudden death. Because patients with documented cardiac syncope have a 6-month mortality rate of greater than 10%, timely and thorough evaluation is warranted.[13]

Syncope in this class can be caused by many types of arrhythmias (benign and malignant), valvular and ischemic heart disease, and cardiomyopathies. Although it is clear that patients with known cardiac disease and syncope have a significantly increased incidence of cardiac-related death, cardiac disease may not be recognized in many patients with cardiac syncope, and persons with a history of cardiac disease may appear to be very stable. Therefore, depending on the history and age of the patient, a relatively aggressive search for cardiac problems may be necessary. However, the urgency of these investigations and whether they should be done in the ambulatory or inpatient setting (e.g., monitoring) are unclear.

### SYNCOPE OF UNKNOWN CAUSE

Syncope of unknown cause is the largest category of syncope, with estimates as high as 40%, even with extensive work-up.[1] Some studies have found that after evaluation in the ED, physicians are uncertain of the cause of the syncope more than 50% of the time.[14] As a result, many serious cases are initially classified in this category, which causes a dilemma for emergency physicians who must decide whether to admit or discharge these patients. It is this largest group of patients who present the greatest challenge for physicians.

## RECOMMENDED DIAGNOSTIC TESTS

Ongoing or related symptoms associated with syncope should direct the ED investigation. CT is not indicated for all patients, but one should not ignore associated symptoms, for which a complete work-up should be performed[7] (e.g., CT in patients with associated headache or abdominal pain, urine pregnancy tests in females, ultrasonography in pregnant women, troponin assay and CT angiography in patients with chest pain and dyspnea).

A routine electrocardiogram (ECG) is almost always indicated, as are rhythm strips and monitoring while the patient is in the ED. Any nonsinus rhythms or new changes on the ECG should be a concern. Routine basic laboratory tests in asymptomatic patients are not recommended, and their use should be guided by the history and physical examination. Recent work has focused on the value of brain natriuretic peptide (BNP) as a predictor of risk in patients with syncope.[15] BNP may have some utility but requires further consideration before becoming a recommended test. In particular, the value of a single reading and the timing of drawing blood in relation to the event require further work. In addition, although it makes sense that BNP may be helpful because it is a predictor of congestive heart failure (CHF) and structural heart disease, it remains unclear whether it provides any greater value over taking a good history, especially given the added cost of the test.[16]

## PROGNOSIS

Perhaps the best investigation of the prognosis of patients with syncope was done by Soteriades et al., who used data from the Framingham study.[13] This study assessed the risk for death in a prospective cohort of 7814 patients over a 17-year period. The results were dramatic. Those with documented heart disease and syncope had twice the mortality rate of patients without syncope, and patients with syncope with a neurologic cause were 50% more likely to die. People with syncope of unknown cause also had a significantly increased risk for death of 30%, whereas those with neurally mediated (vasovagal) syncope had a lower risk. The study clearly shows that the increased risk for death in this group requires further scrutiny, as does ED disposition and management.

Other studies suggest that cardiac-related syncope represents 5% to 40% of the causes of syncope and is associated with a significant increase in mortality. ED management of patients with cardiac symptoms such as chest pain in addition to syncope is obvious; however, of most concern are asymptomatic patients with syncope.

The absence of cardiac symptoms is not reassuring because patients can have serious "silent symptoms" (silent myocardial infarction and silent arrhythmia, such as Brugada syndrome[17]) that may not be obviously associated with syncope on initial evaluation. Such patients may not have a history of cardiac disease, and syncope may be the first symptom. Patients with cardiac symptoms and syncope clearly need thorough and timely evaluation and thus in most cases require emergency hospitalization.[18]

Physicians evaluating patients with syncope who are asymptomatic and without a clear cause are faced with the following questions:

1. Is the syncope a symptom indicating that known underlying heart disease is active, unstable, and related to the episode?
2. Is the syncope a symptom of occult underlying heart disease?
3. Is the syncope a symptom of an occult noncardiac life-threatening process (e.g., pulmonary embolism, occult bleeding, transient ischemic attack, subarachnoid hemorrhage)?

To maximize the sensitivity of detecting underlying disease, physicians frequently admit low-risk patients for further evaluation, although the cost-effectiveness and value of such decisions are often questioned.[19] It is this group of asymptomatic patients with syncope who are most likely to benefit from risk stratification strategies to guide disposition decisions.

## ACUTE RISK STRATIFICATION IN THE EMERGENCY DEPARTMENT

Martin et al. developed the first risk stratification scheme for patients evaluated in the ED for syncope.[20] The stratification was premised on 1-year prognosis for death or cardiac morbidity. Four predictors of death at 1 year were found: age older than 45 years, history of ventricular dysrhythmias, history of CHF, and abnormal findings on an ECG. A similar study found that an abnormal ECG and history of structural heart disease (primarily CHF) predicted mortality but that a much higher age cutoff (older than 65 years) could predict death at 1 year.[3]

Sarasin et al. developed a risk score for ED patients with syncope.[21] The score was based on three factors associated with increased risk for an arrhythmia: abnormal findings on an ECG, age older than 65 years, and a history of any cardiac disease (primarily CHF).

Finally, Quinn et al. derived and validated a decision rule that addresses short-term risk (7 days) to better determine immediate risk in patients in the ED.[2,22] Again, a history of CHF and abnormal findings on an ECG were the most important predictors. The decision rule considered all patients with syncope and also determined that shortness of breath, hematocrit higher than 30, and systolic blood pressure greater than 90 mm Hg were important risk factors. Age older than 75 years was found to be sensitive but nonspecific in this cohort and not useful as a predictor.

Others have tried to validate this work with variable success.[23-25] The key to studies being able to most closely validate the work is using the proper ECG definition, which includes not only new changes on the ECG but also any nonsinus rhythms that are found not only on the ECG but also during monitoring throughout the patient's ED stay.[26]

Other important prospective risk stratification studies are from Italy. The OESIL study found that age older than 65 years, history of cardiovascular disease, syncope without a prodrome, and ECG abnormalities were risk factors.[3] The EGSYS study found an abnormal ECG, history of heart disease, absence of a prodrome, supine status, palpitations, and effort-related syncope to be risk factors.[27] Finally, the STePS study found ECG abnormalities, concomitant trauma, absence of a prodrome, and male gender to be short-term risks.[28]

Age as a risk factor deserves specific mention because physicians often admit patients with syncope just because of age. For almost all diseases, older people die sooner than younger people, and health problems in general increase with age. Recommending that all people older than 45 years (or even those older than 65 or 75 years) be admitted because this factor predicts 1-year death is impractical. Although it may be sensitive as a predictor, age by itself is a poor discriminator; many younger people have significant illness that puts them at even greater risk. This was demonstrated in a study of the short-term outcomes of asymptomatic patients who had syncope of unknown cause and were older than 50 years; all had benign outcomes.[14] Furthermore, comparison of age solely as a risk versus other risk factors has shown that risk factors perform better than age alone.[29]

In summary, advanced age is a risk, but no practical age cutoff for risk has been established, and it should be considered with other risk factors. In particular, almost every study on risk factors has found that an abnormal ECG, including abnormalities detected on cardiac monitoring, is important, as is a history of cardiac disease, specifically CHF. The lack of a prodrome or vagal symptoms is also important in every study, but one study that looked at its subjective nature found that physicians had poor agreement on the presence of vagal symptoms.

## IMPROVED DIAGNOSTIC STRATEGIES IN THE EMERGENCY DEPARTMENT

Some investigators have reported that diagnostic and prognostic ability improve with more invasive testing such as echocardiography. This makes sense in that this procedure may identify patients with structural heart disease and a limited ejection fraction; however, another study found that patients who would benefit from echocardiography could be identified by their history and physical examination and that this procedure may not be cost-effective.[30] Another group in the United Kingdom found that risk stratification could be improved by

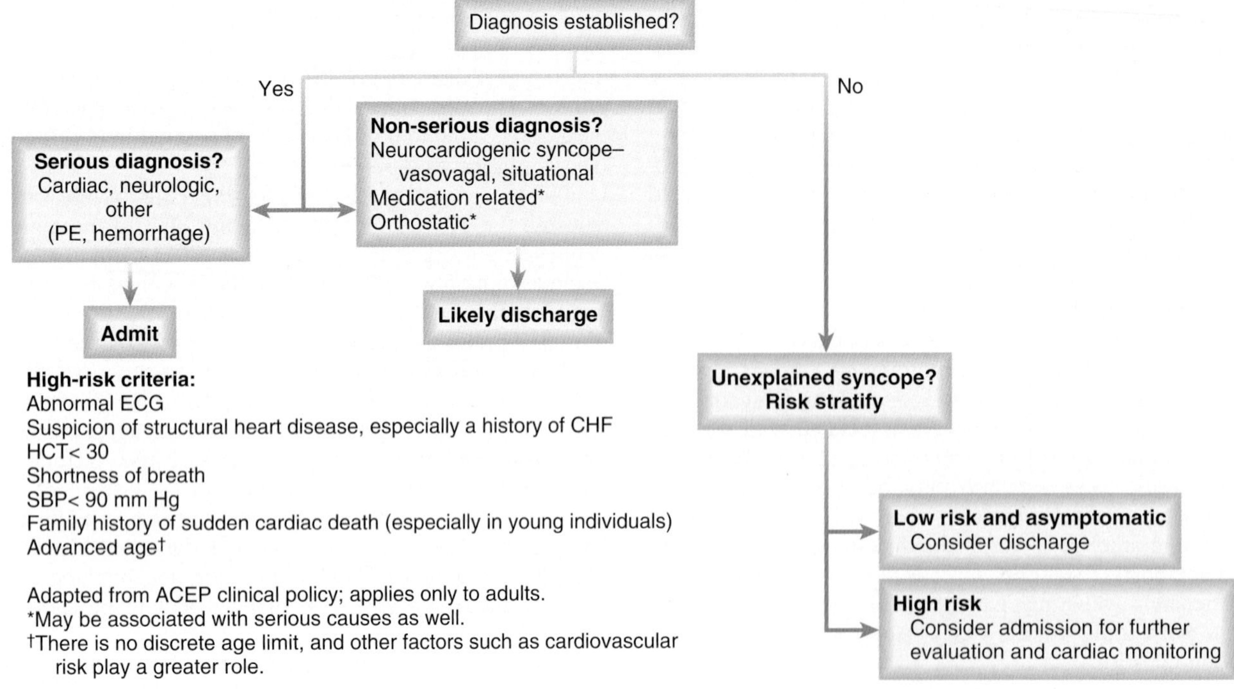


**Fig. 64.1 Emergency department evaluation of syncope.** *ACEP*, American College of Emergency Physicians; *CHF*, congestive heart failure; *ECG*, electrocardiogram; *HCT*, hematocrit; *PE*, pulmonary embolism; *SBP*, systolic blood pressure.

implementing a protocol of more aggressive strategies such as tilt-table testing and echocardiography but noted that such strategies may not be cost-effective or practical in the ED.[31] An Italian group thought that diagnosis could be improved just with more aggressive history taking and physical examination.[32]

Because echocardiography and other invasive tests are not routinely available in the ED 24 hours per day, investigators have started to use observation units to avoid inpatient admission for a select group of intermediate-risk patients evaluated in the ED.[33] There appears to be some promise for syncope observation units, with the goal being to move more low- and intermediate-risk syncope patients from the traditional inpatient work-up to a more structured and efficient observation or outpatient work-up.

## GUIDELINES FOR ADMISSION AND DISPOSITION

Many specialty societies have devised consensus guidelines for admission to the hospital that have focused on the best available data.[34,35] The American College of Emergency Physicians recommends that patients with evidence of cardiac and neurologic causes of syncope, as well as other serious outcomes diagnosed in the ED, be admitted to the hospital. Admission is also recommended for patients with undifferentiated syncope who have risk factors for adverse outcomes (**Fig. 64.1**).

Physicians may consider for discharge asymptomatic, well-appearing patients and those with a negative work-up for associated symptoms. One should remember that many studies show increased risk in patients with nonsinus rhythms, abnormalities on the ECG, a history of CHF (or other significant heart disease), shortness of breath, anemia, persistently low blood pressure, and advanced age. Patients with these risk factors, even though they are asymptomatic and appear to be well, have a high risk for adverse outcomes and should be considered for admission to the hospital, observational status, or aggressive outpatient investigation.

## REFERENCES

***References can be found on Expert Consult @ www.expertconsult.com.***

# Aortic Dissection 65

Nima Afshar

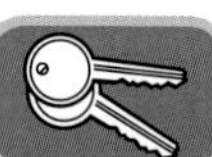

**KEY POINTS**

- Aortic dissection is deadly and difficult to diagnose. It is suspected less than half the time at initial evaluation.
- Ninety percent of patients with aortic dissection have sudden, severe, or unrelenting pain in the chest or upper part of the back, or in both areas.
- When a patient has chest pain with a pulse deficit or any acute neurologic deficit, aortic dissection is the most likely diagnosis.
- D-dimer is a sensitive biomarker for ruling out dissection. Computed tomographic angiography is the study of choice for making the diagnosis.
- Systolic blood pressure in patients with aortic dissection should be maintained at less than 120 mm Hg regardless of the patient's baseline blood pressure unless symptoms or signs of organ malperfusion are present. Beta-blockers are the first-line antihypertensives.

## EPIDEMIOLOGY

Aortic dissection is longitudinal cleavage of the aortic wall by blood, which creates a false lumen that may propagate. The disease was first described in detail by Morgagni in 1761. In 1955, with the advent of cardiopulmonary bypass, DeBakey successfully repaired a dissected descending aorta, thereby providing the first cure. The proximal aorta was first repaired and medical management was established in the 1960s, thus setting the stage for the modern approach to this disease.

A patient in the emergency department (ED) whose proximal aorta has dissected has about a 2% chance of dying every hour during the first 12 hours and almost a 50% chance of dying within 48 hours without surgical treatment.[1,2] Unfortunately, this disease is often difficult to diagnose. A study involving three academic EDs found that the diagnosis was suspected during the initial encounter in only 43% of cases.[3]

The incidence is 3 per 100,000 people per year.[4,5] A typical large urban ED sees several cases per year.[3] About 1 in 350 patients evaluated in an ED for chest pain has aortic dissection.[4-6]

Sixty percent of aortic dissections involve the ascending aorta, either alone or with other parts of the aorta; they are referred to as type A in the now standard Stanford classification. The 40% that do not involve the ascending aorta are Stanford type B (**Fig. 65.1**). This distinction has important prognostic and therapeutic implications.

## THE YOUNG PATIENT

About 7% of patients with aortic dissection are young (<40 years) and usually have no history of hypertension or other known medical problems.[7] These patients nearly always have occult structural cardiovascular disease.

The most important structural vascular disease is Marfan syndrome, which has a prevalence of 1 in 10,000 and occurs in all races. Marfan syndrome accounts for half of aortic dissections in patients younger than 40 years.[7] It is caused by an autosomal dominant mutation in the gene for a type of fibrillin, a protein that makes up part of the elastic fibers in connective tissue of the aorta, lens, and periosteum. Patients are typically tall with long digits, scoliosis, pectus excavatum, and visual problems because of lens dislocation (**Fig. 65.2, *A* to *C***). Most important, however, thoracic aneurysms invariably develop early in life, usually in the ascending aorta. If their aneurysms are not repaired, most patients will die of aortic dissection or rupture.

Other young patients without a history of severe hypertension who are nevertheless at risk for dissection are those with bicuspid aortic valves and those experiencing acute insults such as cocaine use and trauma. A family history of aortic aneurysms and dissection, beyond syndromes usually associated with aortic pathology, is a newly recognized risk factor seen in 10% to 20% of patients with dissection.[8]

## PATHOPHYSIOLOGY

The aorta dissects by two possible mechanisms (**Fig. 65.3**). The classic mechanism is an intimal tear, which is generally transverse and extends through the very thin tunica intima into the tunica media. Under pulsatile force, blood enters a layer of the media and dissects longitudinally and usually in a distal direction. The other major mechanism is rupture of the vasa vasorum, usually of a penetrating branch within the tunica media, with consequent bleeding into the media. Progression then occurs in the same fashion, either with or without secondary tearing through the intima into the aortic lumen. The aorta generally tears near tethering points, where the vessel undergoes the greatest flexion stress during cardiac contractions. Thus the most common location for initiation of dissection is the first few centimeters of the ascending aorta, the next most common being the origin of the descending aorta just distal to the left subclavian artery.

Major complications of aortic dissection, in order of risk for mortality, are (1) rupture through the thin remaining outer wall; (2) proximal propagation, which can cause coronary occlusion, acute aortic regurgitation, or cardiac tamponade (or any combination of such complications); and (3) occlusion or dissection of branch arteries.

Those who suffer dissection are predisposed to it by a weakened aorta, specifically, degeneration of the tunica media, or suffer a hemodynamic or traumatic insult, or both (**Table 65.1**).[7-9] Medial degeneration can be secondary to chronic hypertension, hereditary diseases of elastin (Marfan syndrome) or collagen (Ehlers-Danlos syndrome), hereditary structural abnormalities (bicuspid aortic valve and aortic coarctation), chronic inflammation, and aneurysm of any cause, which increases wall tension according to Laplace's law.

Hemodynamic stress on the aorta is produced by hypertension and shear force (dP/dt)*, or the force of blood ejected from the left ventricle. A hypercontractile, tachycardic heart produces the greatest shear force. These factors may contribute to the initiation of dissection and strongly determine whether a dissection propagates. Exacerbations of hypertension, cocaine intoxication, and third-trimester pregnancy are examples of states that can cause hemodynamic stress on the aorta and result in dissection.

Traumatic causes include medical procedures, such as aortic catheterization and cardiac surgery, and deceleration

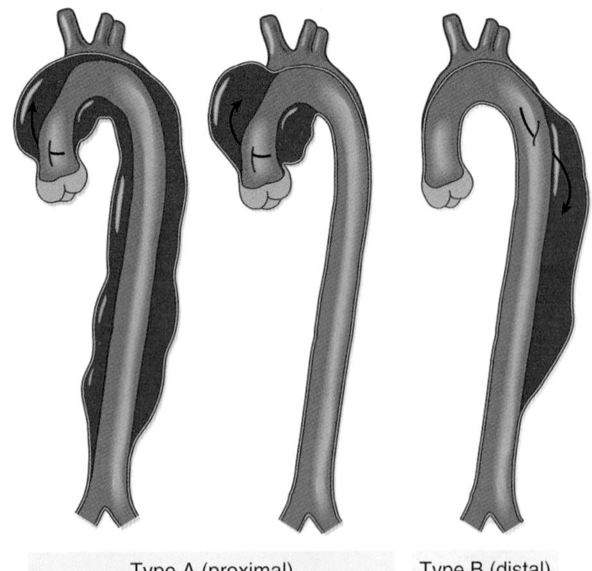


**Fig. 65.1 Classification of aortic dissection.** Types A and type B represent the two subtypes of dissection under the Stanford classification system. Subtypes of the older DeBakey classification system are types I, II, and III. (From Zipes DP, Libby P, Bonow RO, et al, editors. Braunwald's heart disease: a textbook of cardiovascular medicine. 7th ed. Philadelphia: Saunders; 2005.)

$$* \frac{dP}{dt} = \frac{\text{Change in pressure (mm Hg)}}{\text{Change in time}}$$

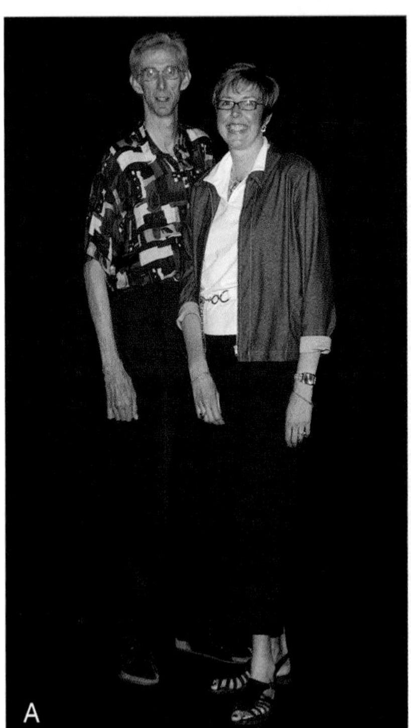


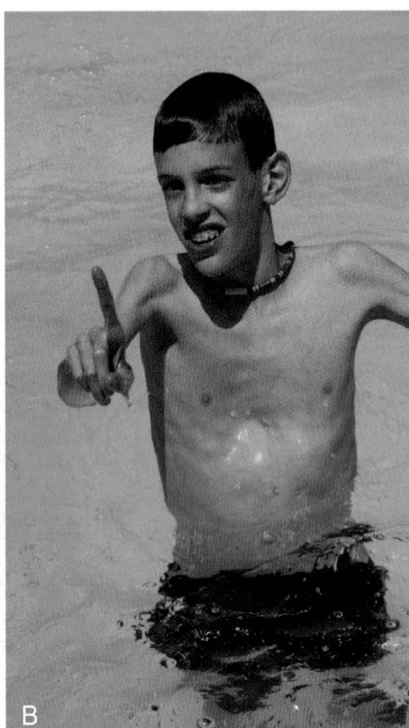


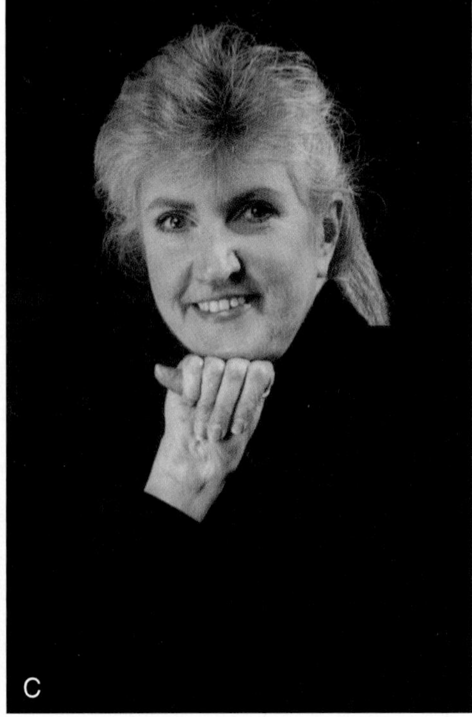


**Fig. 65.2** These patients with Marfan syndrome have long extremities and digits, tall stature, and pectus carinatum. (Photographs courtesy National Marfan Foundation.)

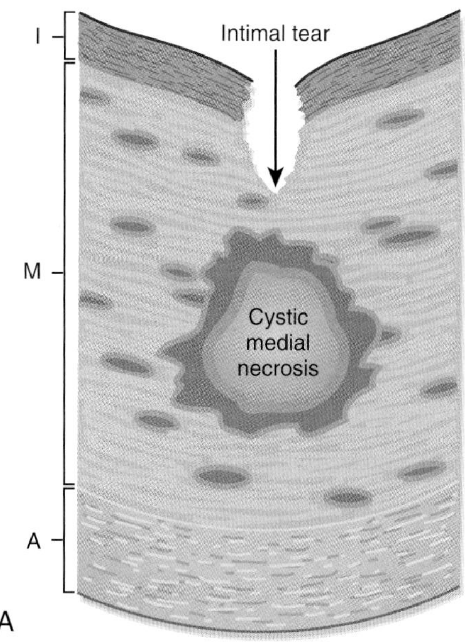


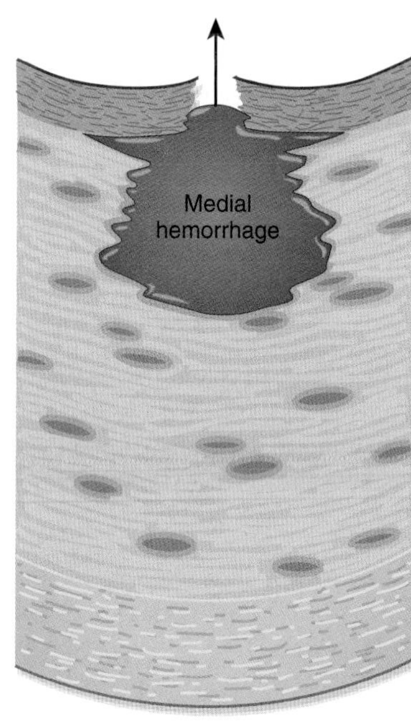


**Fig. 65.3 Two mechanisms of aortic dissection. A,** Intimal tear. **B,** Rupture of the vasa vasorum. *A*, Adventitia; *I*, intima; *M*, media. (From Zipes DP, Libby P, Bonow RO, et al, editors. Braunwald's heart disease: a textbook of cardiovascular medicine. 7th ed. Philadelphia: Saunders; 2005.)

**Table 65.1 Risk Factors for Aortic Dissection**

| RISK FACTORS | PREVALENCE (%) |
|---|---|
| **Common Factors** | |
| Hypertension | 70 |
| Family history of aortic dissection or aneurysm | 10-20 |
| Aortic aneurysm (known) | 13 |
| Previous aortic dissection | 5 |
| Marfan syndrome | 5 (50% in patients < 40 yr) |
| Aortic valve disease: atrioventricular replacement, bicuspid aortic valve | 9 |
| Iatrogenic: cardiac surgery, cardiac catheterization | 4 |
| **Uncommon Factors** | |
| Cocaine or methamphetamine use | |
| Pregnancy | |
| Weight lifting | |
| Ehlers-Danlos syndrome—vascular type | |
| Coarctation of the aorta | |
| Chronic inflammation<br>Giant cell (temporal) arteritis<br>Takayasu arteritis<br>Tertiary syphilis | |
| Trauma | |

Data from references 7-9.

events (e.g., falls, motor vehicle collisions), although in blunt trauma, aortic rupture is far more common than dissection.

## PRESENTING SIGNS AND SYMPTOMS

Dissection of the aorta is usually extremely painful, so acute pain is a chief complaint in nearly 95% of cases (**Table 65.2**).[7,10-14] Aortic pain is sudden and maximal at onset, with its intensity often proportional to the length of dissection. The location of pain is midline and, classically, correlates with the location of dissection: dissection of the ascending aorta results in chest pain, dissection of the arch results in neck or jaw pain, and dissection of the descending aorta results in back and sometimes abdominal pain. Thus the pain may migrate as the dissection propagates. However, there is considerable variability in symptoms and major overlapping of symptoms in type A and type B dissections.[3,9]

The typical patient is 50 to 70 years old with a history of poorly controlled hypertension. He (2 : 1 male-to-female ratio) has intense chest or back pain (or both) and is likely to describe it as sharp rather than tearing. The pain does not respond to nitroglycerin. The patient is not dyspneic unless suffering from one of the cardiac complications of dissection.

The patient appears to be in obvious pain and often has elevated blood pressure (see Table 65.2). On cardiac examination the emergency physician (EP) may hear a fourth heart sound ($S_4$) because of left ventricular hypertrophy. The patient must be examined for two life-threatening

**Table 65.2 Symptoms, Signs, and Findings in Patients with Aortic Dissection**

| | PREVALENCE (%) |
|---|---|
| **History** | |
| Pain | |
| Any | 94 |
| Sudden | 90 |
| Severe | 90 |
| Migrating | 25 |
| Tearing/ripping | ≈35 |
| Chest pain | 67 |
| Back pain | 50 |
| Abdominal pain | 25 |
| Syncope | 12 |
| **Physical Findings** | |
| High blood pressure | 50 |
| Hypotension or shock | 15 |
| Diastolic murmur | 33 |
| Pulse deficit | 30 |
| Focal neurologic deficit | 15 |
| **Study Results** | |
| Chest radiograph | |
| Wide mediastinum | ≈60 |
| Abnormal aortic contour | ≈60 |
| Normal | 15 |
| Electrocardiography | |
| Myocardial infarction (ST elevation or new Q waves) | 5 |
| Myocardial ischemia (ST depression or T-wave inversion) | 15 |

Data from references 7, 10-14.

complications of type A dissection with retrograde propagation: aortic regurgitation and cardiac tamponade. Aortic regurgitation occurs audibly in a third of cases and is manifested as a decrescendo early diastolic murmur, best heard at the left lower sternal border with the patient sitting up, leaning forward, and holding breath at end-expiration; peripheral pulses can be bounding if the pulse pressure is wide. Cardiac tamponade may be manifested as distant heart sounds, but more often tachycardia and jugular venous distention occur and are followed by hypotension; the pulsus paradoxus should be 10 mm Hg higher, and bedside ultrasound will reveal a pericardial effusion.

Peripheral pulses should also be examined. If the false lumen is occluding one of the subclavian arteries, a focal, palpably weak pulse is usually present, a finding specific for aortic dissection.[11] Blood pressure should be measured in both arms—a difference of 20 mm Hg or greater between extremities should alert the EP to the possibility of subclavian occlusion. It must be remembered, though, that nearly 20% of hypertensive patients have a blood pressure differential of at least 10 mm Hg between extremities.[15] Lower extremity pulses should also be evaluated because frank ischemia of the lower extremities occurs in nearly 10% of cases of aortic dissection.[13]

A thorough neurologic examination should be performed. Fifteen percent of patients with aortic dissection have a focal neurologic deficit, and in the setting of severe acute chest or abdominal pain, this finding is also highly specific for the disease.[11] Potential neurologic deficits in patients with aortic dissection include stroke secondary to carotid occlusion, spinal cord syndromes as a result of spinal or intercostal arterial occlusion, and peripheral neuropathy caused by neuronal ischemia or compression of a peripheral nerve by the false lumen.

## ALTERNATIVE PRESENTATIONS

### *Abdominal Pain*

Abdominal pain is one of the complaints in about 25% of patients with aortic dissection and is the primary complaint in 5% of patients[13]; such patients invariably have dissection of the descending aorta. The pain is usually midline but can be referred to the flank, frequently on the left. The pain is typically out of proportion to the physical findings.

### *Painless Dissection*

About 6% of patients with aortic dissection do not have pain. Half of these patients have previously undergone cardiovascular surgery, which potentially disrupts the thoracic nerves. One third have syncope, 20% have heart failure, and more than 10% have stroke.[14] There are numerous reports of patients with painless spinal cord syndromes as well.[1] In these difficult cases, picking up clues such as a diastolic murmur, pulse deficit, and an abnormal mediastinum on chest radiography is critical to making the correct diagnosis.

## DIFFERENTIAL DIAGNOSIS AND MEDICAL DECISION MAKING

Aortic dissection is often manifested as chest pain (in up to 75% of cases in recent large studies). In any patient with chest pain, the EP must think of three difficult diagnoses that are life-threatening: acute coronary syndrome, pulmonary embolism, and aortic dissection. Acute coronary syndrome often causes a pressurelike pain that is more crescendo than sudden; electrocardiography (ECG) frequently shows ischemic changes, and in the absence of complete coronary occlusion, the pain is usually responsive to nitroglycerin. In fact, one distinguishing feature of both pulmonary embolism and aortic dissection is that in the first several hours of either, the pain typically does not resolve. With pulmonary embolism, the pain is generally pleuritic and associated with significant pulmonary symptoms or signs. Other diagnoses to consider are pericarditis or cardiac tamponade, spontaneous pneumothorax, and esophageal rupture.

In one prospective study, the absence of aortic pain (sudden and severe), a pulse or blood pressure differential, and mediastinal or aortic widening on chest radiography had a

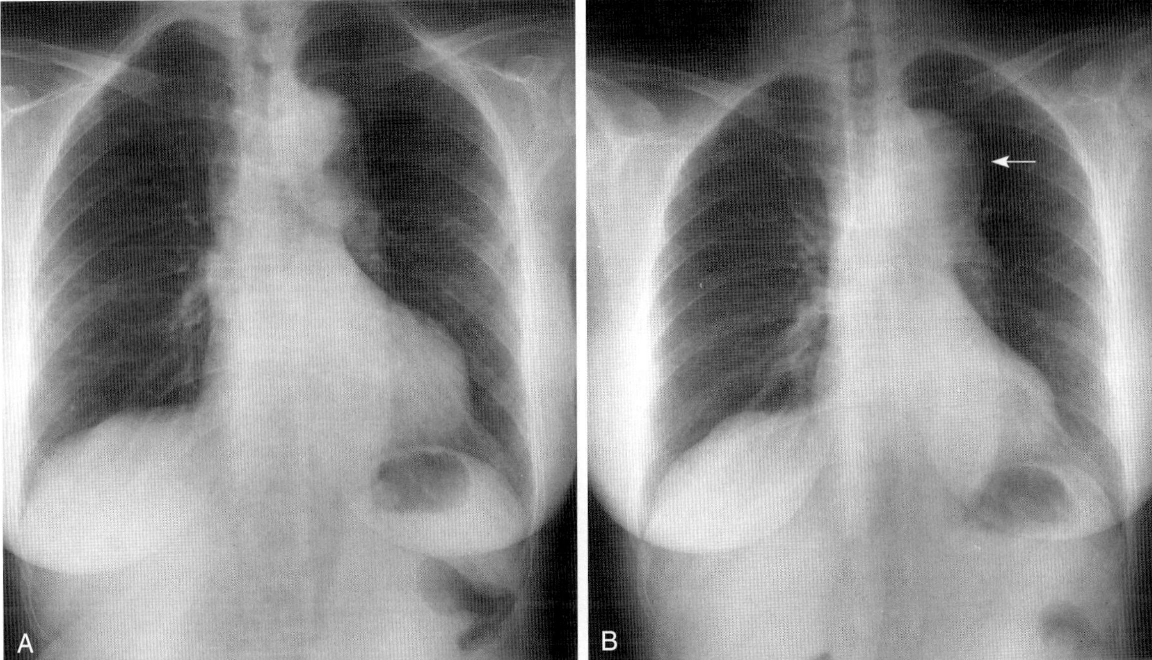


**Fig. 65.4 Chest radiographs of aortic dissection. A,** Chest radiograph from 3 years previously showing that the patient's cardiac structures are normal. **B,** Current chest radiograph of the same patient showing interval enlargement of the aortic knob *(arrow)*. (From Zipes DP, Libby P, Bonow RO, et al, editors. Braunwald's heart disease: a textbook of cardiovascular medicine. 7th ed. Philadelphia: Saunders; 2005.)

sensitivity of 96% for ruling out the diagnosis of aortic dissection. Conversely, the presence of a pulse deficit or a focal neurologic deficit, with positive likelihood ratios of 47 and 33, respectively, markedly raised the probability of aortic dissection.[11]

## PATIENTS WITH UNDIFFERENTIATED CHEST PAIN

In patients with aortic dissection, aspirin should be avoided because it could cause excessive surgical bleeding and may raise the risk for aortic rupture. Nitroglycerin, in the absence of beta-blockade, should also be avoided because it could cause reflex tachycardia. Because acute coronary disease is far more common than dissection, many patients with undifferentiated chest pain receive aspirin or nitroglycerin (or both) at the initial encounter from either paramedics or ED caregivers. However, if the patient's findings strongly suggest aortic dissection, it is prudent to wait until after imaging studies have ruled out the diagnosis before initiating these therapies. Anticoagulation should be avoided if dissection is even being considered.

## CHEST RADIOGRAPHY

The chest radiograph classically shows a wide mediastinum, predominantly on the right in patients with dissection of the ascending aorta and on the left with dissection of the descending aorta (**Fig. 65.4**). The physician's subjective impression, rather than formal measurements, is the best indicator of whether the mediastinum is wide. A widened mediastinum is not a sensitive indicator of aortic dissection. It probably occurs in about 60% of cases, but some reports note a widened mediastinum in less than 20%.[3,10] Other abnormalities of the aorta, such as inward displacement of intimal calcification and a double aortic shadow, may be observed. Pleural effusion may also occur, usually on the left.

## D-DIMER

After the history, physical examination, ECG, and chest radiography, the clinician must decide whether aortic dissection is a reasonable possibility (**Fig. 65.5**). If so, additional testing is required.

Numerous small studies have demonstrated that the serum biomarker D-dimer is useful for excluding the diagnosis. A meta-analysis that included seven studies with a total of 300 patients with dissection found that D-dimer—at the 500-ng/mL cutoff value commonly used for excluding pulmonary embolism—is 97% sensitive for acute aortic dissection.[16] D-dimer is probably inadequately sensitive in patients with subacute manifestations and those with pure intramural hematoma. In acute manifestations in which the pretest probability of dissection is low, it is reasonable to use D-dimer to exclude the diagnosis and forego further testing.

If the pretest probability is not low, the manifestation is subacute, or D-dimer levels are elevated, an advanced imaging study is required (**Table 65.3**). All of the modalities described are highly sensitive (98% to 100%) and specific (95% to 98%) and thus in most cases will definitively rule in or rule out dissection.[17]

## COMPUTED TOMOGRAPHY

The diagnostic study of choice is computed tomographic (CT) angiography of the aorta (**Fig. 65.6**). It is immediately available in most EDs and can be interpreted quickly by a radiologist. It is highly sensitive for dissection, especially as CT

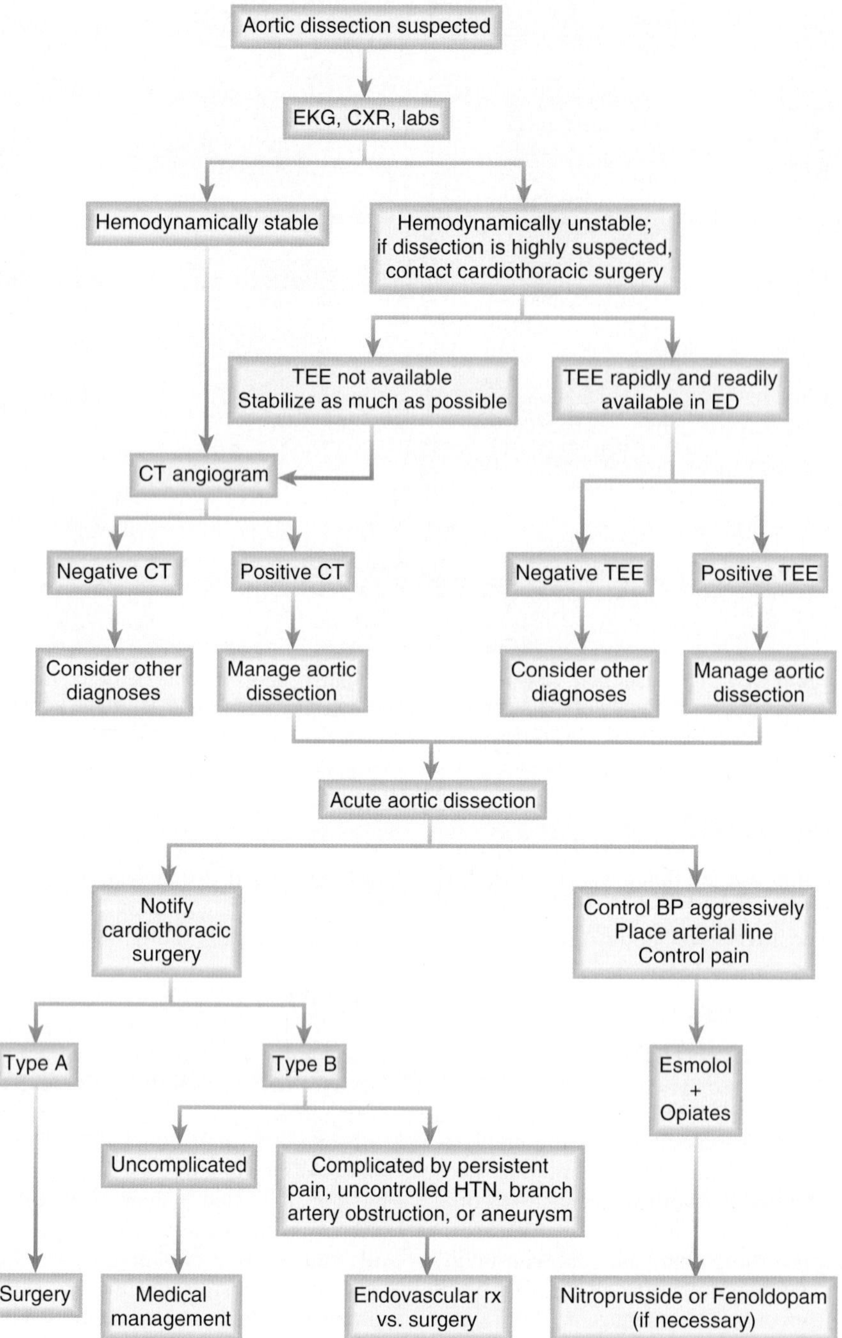


**Fig. 65.5 Algorithm for the diagnosis and treatment of aortic dissection.** *BP,* Blood pressure; *CT,* computed tomography; *CXR,* chest radiograph; *ECG,* electrocardiography; *ED,* emergency department; *HTN,* hypertension; *labs,* laboratory tests; *TEE,* transesophageal echocardiography.

technology advances—in fact, a 2005 study reported that multidetector CT scanning was 100% accurate in patients with suspected acute aortic disease.[18] Moreover, when its results are negative for dissection, CT scanning frequently shows alternative serious disease to explain the patient's symptoms. In the ED, CT scanning is more readily available than transesophageal echocardiography (TEE) or magnetic resonance imaging (MRI), and most patients (even if somewhat clinically unstable) are able to undergo CT scanning to enable the diagnosis to be made.

## TRANSESOPHAGEAL ECHOCARDIOGRAPHY

Generally performed by a cardiologist, TEE is an alternative technique in patients with renal failure, which is a relative contraindication to CT scanning (**Fig. 65.7**). TEE is as sensitive as CT scanning for type A aortic dissection but may be slightly less sensitive for type B lesions[19]; TEE has the advantage of assessing the aortic valve and pericardial space for complications of type A dissection. It may also detect focal ventricular wall motion abnormalities suggesting myocardial ischemia as the cause of the patient's symptoms. Finally,

**Table 65.3 Advanced Imaging Studies for Aortic Dissection**

| STUDY | SENSITIVITY (%) | ADVANTAGES | DISADVANTAGES |
|---|---|---|---|
| Computed tomography | 93-100 | Immediately and widely available; rapid results<br>Technology improving—sensitivity now near 100%<br>Alternative diagnoses often made | Uses a large amount of contrast agent<br>Often misses the site of intimal tear |
| Transesophageal echocardiography | 88-98 | Safe: done at the bedside, no contrast agent or radiation exposure<br>Identifies intimal tears: aids surgical planning<br>Can diagnose tamponade, aortic regurgitation, heart failure, and often, myocardial ischemia | Requires skilled operator—may create delay<br>Blind spots: proximal arch and distal aorta |
| Magnetic resonance imaging | 95-100 | Highly accurate<br>No contrast agent or radiation exposure<br>Alternative diagnoses often made | Slow: patient far from emergency department for prolonged period<br>Expensive, often unavailable |
| Aortography | 87 | Able to image or treat coronary arteries, so may be the study of choice in patients with ST elevation | Invasive, uses a large amount of contrast agent<br>Time-consuming |

Data from references 17-19.

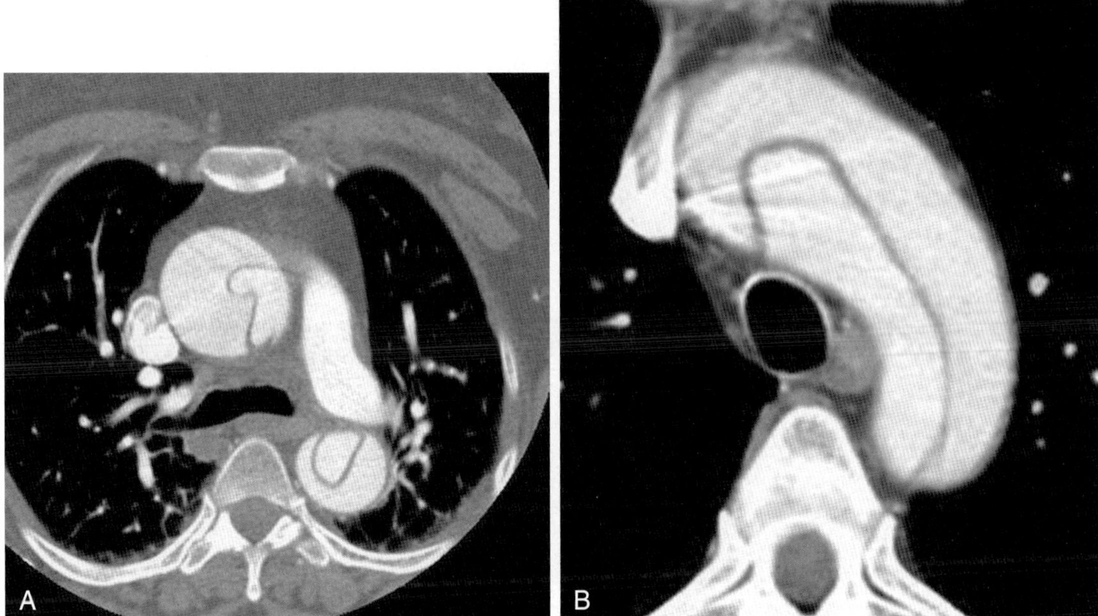


**Fig. 65.6 Computed tomography scans of aortic dissection.** The first axial scan (**A**) shows aortic dissection, demonstrated as serpiginous radiolucencies in the ascending and descending aorta. The second scan (**B**) shows dissection of the aortic arch. (Courtesy Leslie Quint, University of Michigan.)

unlike CT scanning, TEE usually identifies the exact location of the intimal tear and assesses overall cardiac function, which aids in operative planning and risk assessment. The downside of TEE, especially during off hours, is the difficulty performing TEE on an emergency basis. Nonetheless, cardiothoracic surgeons may request the study even when dissection has already been diagnosed.

## MAGNETIC RESONANCE IMAGING

MRI is useful in stable patients with renal failure (gadolinium contrast is not required), especially when a type B dissection is suspected or TEE cannot be performed. However, MRI is slow and the patient must remain in the MRI suite, usually far from the ED, which can be risky in the setting of a potentially life-threatening disease.

## ANGIOGRAPHY

Conventional angiography of the aorta is invasive and rarely needed for the diagnosis of aortic dissection. A possible exception is rare patients with ST-segment elevation myocardial infarction (MI) in whom aortic dissection is still a concern.

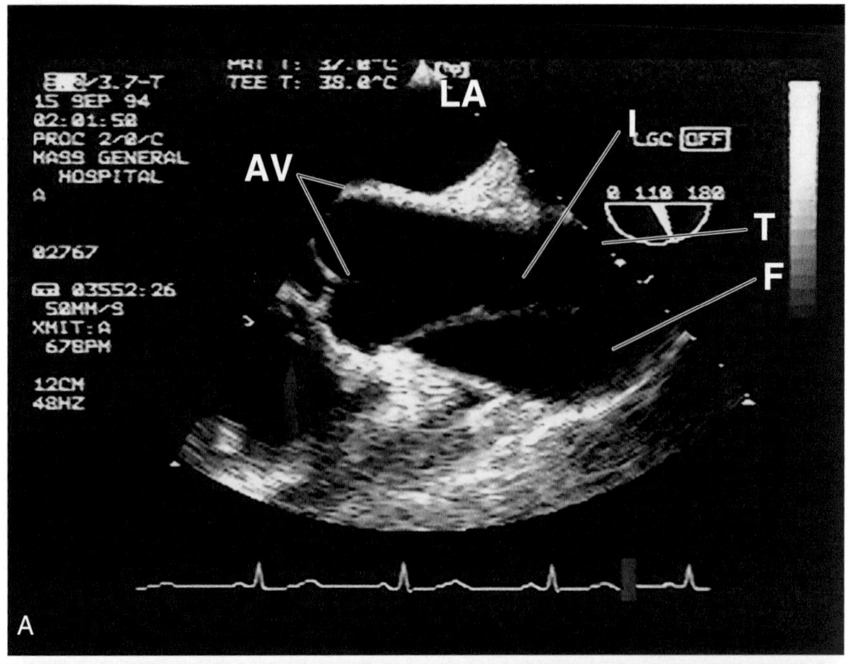


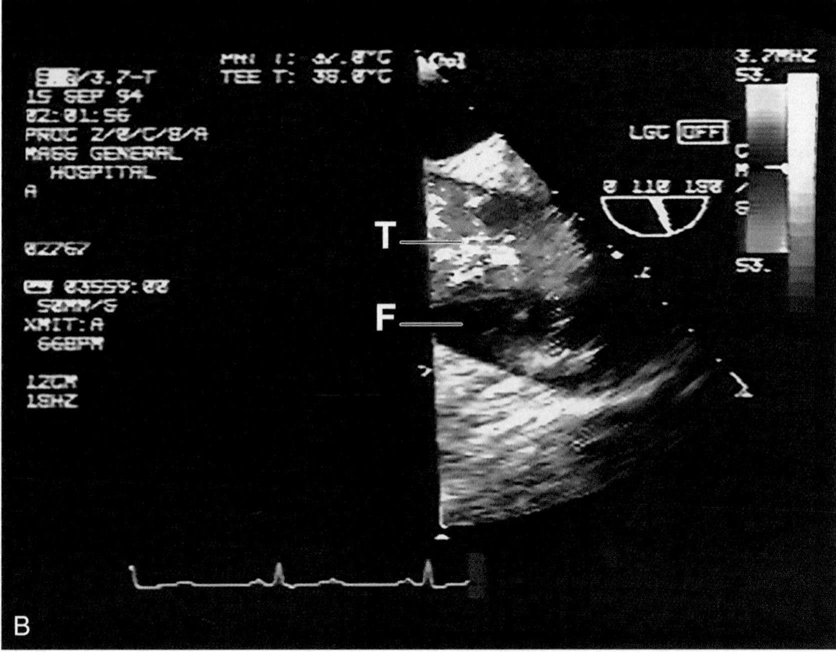


**Fig. 65.7 Transesophageal echocardiograms of the proximal ascending aorta in long-axis view in a patient with proximal aortic dissection. A,** The left atrium (LA) is closest to the transducer. The aortic valve (AV) is seen on the left in this view, with the ascending aorta extending to the right. Within the proximal aorta is an intimal flap (I) that originates just at the level of the sinotubular junction above the right sinus of Valsalva. The true lumen (T) and the false lumen (F) are separated by the intimal flap. **B,** The addition of color flow Doppler imaging in the same view confirms the presence of two distinct lumens. The true lumen (T) fills completely with brisk blood flow *(bright blue)*, whereas minimal retrograde flow *(dark orange)* is seen in the false lumen (F). (From Zipes DP, Libby P, Bonow RO, et al, editors. Braunwald's heart disease: a textbook of cardiovascular medicine. 7th ed. Philadelphia: Saunders; 2005.)

In such cases, the interventional cardiologist may perform angiography of the aorta as part of the cardiac catheterization procedure, thereby ruling out dissection without delaying coronary angiography and potential revascularization. However, even in this time-sensitive situation, many cardiologists prefer CT scanning because cannulation of a dissected aorta is not without risk.

## ELECTROCARDIOGRAPHY

Findings on ECG are usually unremarkable even though the patient reports severe pain. This incongruence is a red flag. Nonspecific findings on ECG in a patient with severe chest pain should alert astute clinicians to consider aortic dissection.

Patients at risk for aortic dissection may have long-term, poorly controlled hypertension. Therefore, ECG might reveal

**Table 65.4 Intravenous Antihypertensive Drugs for the Treatment of Aortic Dissection**

| MEDICATION | MECHANISM | PHARMACOKINETICS | DOSING | NOTES |
|---|---|---|---|---|
| **Cardiac Inhibitors** | | | | |
| Esmolol | Beta ($\beta_1$)-blocker | Onset: <1 min<br>Duration: 10-20 min<br>Metabolism: blood | Load 500 mcg/kg, then 25 to 50 mcg/kg/min by drip; titrate by 25-50 mcg/kg/min every 5-10 min<br>Maximum: 200 mcg/kg/min | Drug of choice<br>Effectively reduces shear force<br>Highly titratable |
| Labetalol | Beta ($\beta_1/\beta_2$)- and alpha ($\alpha_1$)-blocker (7:1 $\beta:\alpha$ ratio) | Onset: 2-5 min<br>Peak effect: 5-15 min<br>Duration: 2-4 hr<br>Metabolism: mostly blood (no dose change with liver or kidney disease) | Bolus of 20 mg<br>Then give further boluses of 40-80 mg q10min<br>*or*<br>Start drip at 1-2 mg/min and titrate<br>Maximum total dose: 300 mg | Beta- and alpha-blockade may obviate a second agent<br>Also has $\beta$2-agonist activity, which limits negative effect of nonspecific $\beta$-adrenergic antagonism on the lungs<br>Not as titratable as esmolol |
| Diltiazem | Calcium channel blocker<br>Negative chronotropy >> negative inotropy<br>Vasodilation | Onset: 3 min<br>Duration: 1-3 hr<br>Metabolism: probably in the liver (no dose change) | Bolus of 0.25-0.35 mg/kg over 2 min. May repeat. Then 5- to 15-mg/hr drip | Use when beta-blockers are contraindicated<br>Blood pressure reduction occurs via vasodilation |
| **Vasodilators** | | | | |
| Nitroprusside | Nitric oxide–mediated vasodilation | Onset: seconds<br>Duration: 2 min<br>Metabolism: blood (but toxic metabolites excreted by kidney) | Start drip at 0.3-0.5 mcg/kg/min and titrate<br>Maximum: 3 mcg/kg/min—larger doses confer high risk for cyanide toxicity | Extremely potent; highly titratable<br>Vasodilators cause reflex tachycardia; should be started only after cardiac inhibition established<br>When used in those with chronic kidney disease, higher risk for renal failure and cyanide toxicity |
| Fenoldopam | Dopamine agonist<br>Vasodilation: renal and peripheral arteries<br>Natriuresis | Onset: 5 min<br>Peak effect: 15 min<br>Duration: 30-60 min<br>Metabolism: liver (no dose change) | Start drip at 0.1 mcg/kg/min; titrate by 0.05-0.1 mcg/kg/min every 15 min<br>Maximum: 0.8 mcg/kg/min; higher doses associated with adverse effects | Enhances renal perfusion; ideal in those with acute or chronic renal failure<br>Attenuates renal failure during aortic cross clamping; preferred by some surgeons<br>Much slower-acting than nitroprusside |

Data from references 22, 23.

left ventricular hypertrophy with high-amplitude QRS complexes and typical ST-T strain patterns. Low-amplitude QRS complexes or electrical alternans may occur in the presence of cardiac tamponade.

A minority of patients are found to have ischemic changes on ECG, which can be due to demand ischemia or partial occlusion of a coronary artery. About 5% of aortic dissections completely occlude a coronary artery, predominantly the right coronary artery. The occlusion usually causes an ST-segment elevation myocardial injury pattern in the inferior leads. With any MI, especially an inferior one, the EP should ideally assess the mediastinum and aorta on a chest radiograph before anticoagulants are given and especially before thrombolysis is begun. The patient should be asked specifically about pain radiating to the back, which is uncommon with MI.

## TREATMENT

The main goal of ED care is to identify the disease and then manage the patient's blood pressure and heart rate to minimize aortic shear force. The goal for systolic blood pressure is 100 to 120 mm Hg,[20] and the goal for the heart rate is a rate lower than 60 beats/min.[21] Note that the blood pressure goal is independent of the patient's baseline blood pressure, unlike the approach to most hypertensive emergencies. Therefore, the clinician must watch for signs of iatrogenic end-organ malperfusion. Very short-acting antihypertensives should be used and administered as drips to precisely titrate the dose to effect.

**Table 65.4** summarizes the intravenous hypertensive agents used for treatment of aortic dissection.[20,22,23] Beta-blockers are the first-line antihypertensive agents in patients with aortic dissection because they most effectively reduce both blood pressure and shear force (in patients with significant asthma, diltiazem can be used instead). The ideal beta-blocker is esmolol because of its short half-life and thus its titratability. If blood pressure control with beta-blockers is limited by bradycardia or a plateau effect, a second antihypertensive agent may be needed, invariably a vasodilator.

The standard second-line agent is nitroprusside, which is extremely short-acting and universally effective. Fenoldopam, a highly selective dopamine agonist, is another option. To avoid reflex tachycardia (which increases shear force), vasodilators should be started only after the heart rate has been controlled pharmacologically.

A minimum of two peripheral intravenous lines will be needed, along with an arterial line for continuous blood pressure monitoring. If possible, the arterial line should be placed in the right radial artery so that it is less likely to be affected by the dissection occluding the upstream artery.

The EP must remember that because aortic pain is very severe, adequate analgesia with intravenous opioids should be provided. Opioids help reduce blood pressure.

For any thoracic aortic dissection the clinician should consult a cardiothoracic surgeon immediately. Cardiology consultation may be needed as well, either for admission of a patient with type B dissection or for preoperative TEE, if needed, in a patient with type A dissection.

Type A aortic dissection generally requires emergency thoracic surgery because the mortality rate in patients who do not undergo surgery increases hourly and is 50% to 80% at 1 month. Typically, the surgeon excises the segment of aorta containing the intimal tears and replaces it with a graft, often with some dissected aorta left in place. The aortic valve frequently needs to be replaced as well. With surgery, survival of patients with type A dissection is improved remarkably, to greater than 95% at 1 year.[24] Recently, some experts have advocated nonsurgical management for patients with subacute manifestations or a history of aortic valve replacement (both confer a better prognosis) and for patients with acute stroke or severe comorbid conditions (both confer a worse surgical prognosis).[20]

Type B dissection is usually treated medically, with a 90% survival rate at 1 month. Type B dissection that is complicated by persistent pain, uncontrolled hypertension, branch artery obstruction, or aneurysm has traditionally required surgery. However, endovascular stent placement and balloon fenestration have become therapeutic options; malperfusion syndromes can be reversed in the vast majority of cases, and the false lumen can often be obliterated, thus reducing the chance of aneurysm development and other future complications.[25] Mortality appears to be substantially lower (10% to 15%) with stenting than with surgery (25% to 35%) for complicated type B dissection.[26]

## FOLLOW-UP, NEXT STEPS IN CARE, AND PATIENT EDUCATION

All patients with newly diagnosed aortic dissection should be admitted to the intensive care unit. Patients with type A dissection may go to the operating room first. In the ED, these patients need intensive care unit–level management and should be in a resuscitation bay with a 1 : 1 nurse-to-patient ratio to ensure adequate monitoring of blood pressure and response to therapy (see the Red Flags box).

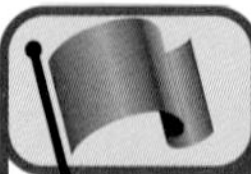

### RED FLAGS

- One third of patients seen in the emergency department with aortic dissection do not have chest pain.
- Aortic dissection occurs more commonly in winter, even in temperate climates.
- Forty percent of patients with dissection have a normal mediastinal width on chest radiographs.
- Beware of pseudohypotension, which is a low blood pressure reading caused by occlusion of an extremity by a dissected vessel wall.
- Detection of ischemia on an electrocardiogram does not rule out aortic dissection. Always consider dissection in a patient with inferior ST-segment elevation myocardial infarction; most ascending aortic dissections involve the right aortic wall, and occasionally the right coronary artery will be occluded.
- Appropriate medical management of confirmed dissection involves dropping systolic blood pressure to 100 to 120 mm Hg regardless of the starting blood pressure.

## REFERENCES

*References can be found on Expert Consult @ www.expertconsult.com.*

# Abdominal Aortic Aneurysm 66

*Danielle M. Ware-McGee and Melissa Marinelli*

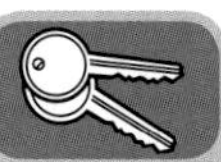

**KEY POINTS**

- The word *aneurysm* is derived from a Greek word meaning "widening." It has further been defined as permanent and irreversible localized dilation of a vessel.1
- Abdominal aortic aneurysm (AAA) refers to pathologic widening of the aorta, and AAAs continue to be a significant cause of morbidity and mortality; early diagnosis is the key to reducing mortality.
- The risk for rupture relates linearly to the maximum cross-sectional diameter of the aneurysm, and 4.5 to 5 cm is the generally accepted size when intervention should occur.
- Elective repair of nonruptured AAAs lowers mortality significantly and warrants a high level of vigilance by health care providers to diagnose this condition in its potentially curative stages.
- Many risk factors promote the development of AAAs, but the most important are smoking, male gender, and family history.
- The two current operative approaches for repair of AAAs are open surgery and endovascular repair; the better approach for individual patients depends on several clinical variables and specific patient characteristics.

## EPIDEMIOLOGY

Finding a unifying definition for abdominal aortic aneurysm (AAA) that encompasses the various classification schemes related to their size, shape, and location is an arduous task. Simplistically, most AAAs occur infrarenally and are defined as an aortic diameter greater than 3 cm, mostly measured in the anteroposterior dimension.[1-3] Although normal aortic diameter differs between the sexes, it is not substantial enough to warrant changing the size limit of 3 cm that is currently used to characterize a small AAA.[3] Finally, it is important to note that dilation of an aneurysm encompasses the three layers of the vascular wall; otherwise, the dilation is a *pseudoaneurysm*.[1] For the commonly accepted descriptions and locations of most aneurysms, please see **Box 66.1**.

At present, AAA is the thirteenth leading cause of death in the United States. Once an AAA ruptures, death is a certainty in more than 65% of cases,[1] with some studies reporting mortality rates as high as 90%, thus highlighting the necessity for rapid surgical repair.[4] Low rates of postmortem examination and the high likelihood that some of these deaths have been erroneously attributed to cardiac causes severely hamper gathering true estimates of the prevalence of and mortality associated with ruptured AAAs.[2] Elective repair of an AAA lowers the mortality to less than 5%, so there is an obvious benefit to diagnosing and treating these aneurysms before they rupture.[4,5] Given that this disease affects 4% to 7% of adults 65 years or older, the onus increasingly falls on physicians to accomplish this task as the population ages.[4]

## PATHOPHYSIOLOGY

There is abundant research on identification of risk factors that potentiate the development and growth of AAAs (**Box 66.2**). Besides male gender, age, and hypertension, every study on the subject of AAAs singles out long-term tobacco smoking as the most important risk factor.[2] AAAs develop in tobacco smokers more than four times more frequently than in lifelong nonsmokers.[1] Lederle et al.[6] compared the relative risk for different diseases in long-term cigarette smokers and found that risk for the development of AAAs is fivefold higher than that for cerebrovascular disease and threefold higher than that for coronary artery disease.[1] Smoking not only raises the risk for the development of AAAs but also increases the annual growth rate of existent AAAs, with some studies reporting a rate of 2.83 mm/yr in smokers versus 2.53 mm/yr in nonsmokers.[1,7] However, the exact means by which smoking enhances aneurysm formation remains a mystery.

In addition to tobacco smoking, there are other risk factors. Atherosclerosis is so highly associated with the development and expansion of AAAs that the American Heart Association (AHA) guidelines on the treatment of AAAs mandate that blood pressure and fasting serum lipid values be strictly monitored and controlled in patients with AAAs.[3] The AHA also recommends that smoking cessation interventions be provided to patients with a personal or family history of aneurysms.[3] Despite the importance of atherosclerosis, additional factors are probably present because not every patient with atherosclerosis has an AAA.[1]

Many authorities cite a possible causal link between the development of AAAs and chronic obstructive pulmonary disease (COPD). Researchers blame tobacco smoking–induced elastin degradation for this proposed association.[3] A review of the literature notes that patients with COPD undergoing long-term treatment with corticosteroids have a much

**BOX 66.1 Aneurysm Classification—Description versus Location**

**Description**

Fusiform aneurysms are circumferential with respect to the artery.

Saccular aneurysms affect only part of the circumference.

Inflammatory aneurysms demonstrate extensive perianeurysmal and retroperitoneal fibrosis, as well as dense adhesions to neighboring organs, which frequently causes ureterohydronephrosis.

**Location**

Juxtarenal aneurysms arise distal but in very close proximity to the renal arteries.

Pararenal aneurysms originate from one or both renal arteries.

Suprarenal aneurysms affect the superior mesenteric and celiac arteries.

Type IV thoracoabdominal aneurysms are suprarenal aneurysms that extend upward to the crus of the diaphragm.

**BOX 66.2 Risk Factors for the Development of Abdominal Aortic Aneurysms**

Smoking
Male gender
Age
Family history—especially male first-degree relatives
Hypertension
Dyslipidemia

higher AAA expansion rate than do COPD patients not taking steroids.[3] Hence, steroid use and coexisting disease are more likely to be responsible for the high prevalence of AAAs in patients with COPD.[3] Finally, from a genetic standpoint, several screening studies suggest that male first-degree relatives of people with COPD are most at risk. Female first-degree relatives appear to be at similar risk, but the data are less certain.[3] Familial aneurysms differ from nonfamilial aneurysms mainly in that they may develop at an earlier age.[3] Existing genetic polymorphisms probably account for the familial clustering of AAAs, but this clustering could also result from exposure to common environmental factors, such as tobacco smoke.[1]

Histologically, AAAs develop as a result of a complex interplay of immunologically mediated proteases and antiproteases that cause destruction of elastin and collagen in the arterial wall. Recent research has focused on the role of matrix metalloproteinases (MMPs) in the degradation of elastin and collagen, the main proteins involved in AAA growth and rupture, respectively. In early aneurysm formation, elastic fibers are lost, fragmented, or attenuated, which contributes to development of the actual wall of the aneurysm.[1,8] Once the concentration of medial elastin is severely decreased, the collagen-rich adventitial tissue constitutes the artery's last mode of resistance, and once completely degraded, rupture inevitably ensues.[1,8] The natural history of all arterial aneurysms encompasses gradual or sporadic growth in their diameter (or both) and accretion of mural thrombus.[3] These features contribute to rupture, thromboembolic ischemic events, and compression or erosion of adjacent structures, three of the most common complications of AAAs.[3]

**Table 66.1** Variations in Clinical Findings in Patients with Abdominal Aortic Aneurysms

| CLASSIC TRIAD | MOST COMMON FINDINGS | INFLAMMATORY ANEURYSM CLINICAL FINDINGS |
|---|---|---|
| Abdominal pain | Younger patients tend to be symptomatic earlier | Triad of chronic abdominal pain, weight loss, and elevated erythrocyte sedimentation rate |
| Pulsatile abdominal mass | Steady, aggravating back pain and hypogastric pain are the most common symptoms | These patients usually have concurrent peripheral vascular disease and coronary artery disease |
| Shock | Pain is usually unaffected by position or movement | These patients are more symptomatic at initial evaluation |
| Only 50% of patients have this triad | Pain can radiate to the scrotum, groin, buttocks, or legs | These patients tend to have more of a retroperitoneal inflammatory reaction |

## PRESENTING SIGNS AND SYMPTOMS

AAA continues to be such a difficult diagnosis because of vague and variable symptoms (**Table 66.1**), which carry large differential diagnoses. Vague symptoms such as back or abdominal pain often herald this diagnosis in its early (virtually asymptomatic) and potentially curative stages. The symptoms may masquerade as those of renal colic, diverticulitis, or gastrointestinal hemorrhage, thereby leading to a fatal misdiagnosis.[3] Commonly, patients with nonruptured AAAs are seen only after suffering complications such as various thromboembolic events or after thorough evaluation for chronic vague abdominal and back pain.[3]

Nonruptured aneurysms are sometimes found incidentally. An astute clinician can find them on physical examination. Palpation of AAAs is safe and has not been reported to precipitate rupture.[3] Abdominal palpation is moderately sensitive for the detection of AAAs that meet the size criteria necessary for surgical intervention, but even large aneurysms may be difficult to palpate, especially in obese patients. However, in the case of AAAs that are small or have already ruptured, physical examination alone is not nearly precise enough.[3]

When aneurysms rupture, the extent of shock varies according to the location and size of the rupture and the amount of delay before the patient is examined.[1] AAAs that rupture anterolaterally dramatically violate the peritoneal cavity and are most often associated with sudden death. Patients with ruptured AAAs who reach a physician tend to have ruptures involving the posterolateral wall in the retroperitoneal space. Some of these patients are fortunate enough that their bodies temporarily tamponade a small tear so that they suffer relatively small initial blood loss.[1] A few of these patients with contained ruptures may even exhibit flank ecchymosis, a physical finding known as the Grey Turner sign.[3] However, AAAs are not contained for long, and even these patients suffer the deleterious effects of a larger rupture if they fail to seek medical attention early or if the physician fails to recognize the signs of impending rupture.[1]

## DIFFERENTIAL DIAGNOSIS AND MEDICAL DECISION MAKING

As a result of the variable manifestations of AAAs just mentioned, the differential diagnosis is broad. **Table 66.2** lists the differential diagnostic entities for AAA, along with priority actions for each. The correct diagnosis of AAA, regardless of whether it is ruptured, hinges on maintaining a high level of suspicion and pursuing an appropriate work-up.

Before the 1970s, standard plain radiographs were the only means by which to monitor the expansion rate of aneurysms. However, plain films are useful for this purpose only when the aneurysm has mural calcifications, which can be easily seen on radiographs. Additionally, the film may show obscuration of the psoas margin by a soft tissue mass and, possibly, extension of mural calcification into a periaortic soft tissue mass, thus hinting at a possible ruptured aneurysm.[3] It is not the current standard of care to use plain radiographs for surveillance of AAAs, but quite a few such lesions are initially discovered as incidental findings on plain abdominal films obtained for other purposes.[3]

Ultrasonography is an excellent choice for diagnosing AAAs for several reasons (**Fig. 66.1,** *A*). First, it is an easy, inexpensive, and accurate diagnostic modality that can evaluate the aorta in the transverse, longitudinal, and anteroposterior dimensions. For these reasons, it is ideal for initial evaluation, surveillance, and population screening with a sensitivity ranging from 92% to 99% and a diagnostic specificity of nearly 100%.[3] In addition, ultrasonography provides the

**Table 66.2 Differential Diagnosis of Abdominal Aortic Aneurysm and Priority Actions**

| ALTERNATIVE DIAGNOSIS | PRIORITY ACTIONS AND COMMENTS |
|---|---|
| Myocardial infarction | Pursue a thorough cardiac work-up, and if the diagnosis is in doubt, be sure to consult both cardiothoracic surgery and cardiology specialists before initiating thrombolytic or anticoagulant therapy. |
| Ischemic bowel | Assuming that the patient has no clinical signs of rupture and is hemodynamically stable, obtain a CT scan to allow a definitive diagnosis. |
| Acute appendicitis | If patient is hemodynamically stable, obtain both an immediate surgical consultation and a CT scan. |
| Gastrointestinal bleeding | This diagnosis is not usually subtle and is fairly easy to make at the bedside with a rectal examination or nasogastric lavage; be wary of an aortoenteric fistula. |
| Pancreatitis | Though a relatively common diagnosis and one that usually requires medical treatment only, pancreatitis is still a life-threatening condition. Be sure to obtain a serum lipase measurement to screen for this diagnosis. |
| Bowel obstruction | If bowel obstruction is a concern, an acute abdominal radiographic series will aid in quick diagnosis. |
| Peptic ulcer disease, perforated ulcer | Upright bedside chest radiography to evaluate for free air should be a routine part of the work-up for an AAA to quickly rule out or rule in peptic ulcer disease and perforated ulcer. |
| Cholelithiasis | On the basis of the patient's clinical symptoms, it may be prudent to order a hepatic function test at initial evaluation. |
| Diverticulitis | If the abdominal examination raises enough concern for diverticulitis, immediate surgical consultation is mandatory; if the patient is hemodynamically stable enough for CT, the diagnosis is made easily. |
| Gastritis | Though part of the differential diagnosis for AAA, gastritis is more of a diagnosis of exclusion after life-threatening possibilities have been evaluated or treated. |
| Cauda equine, epidural abscess, vertebral osteomyelitis | Consider obtaining an erythrocyte sedimentation rate measurement, magnetic resonance imaging, and neurosurgical consultation. |
| Urinary tract infection (females), pyelonephritis, nephrolithiasis | Urinalysis and CT are useful in differentiating these possibilities. |
| Musculoskeletal pain | Often a diagnosis of exclusion. |

*AAA,* Abdominal aortic aneurysm; *CT,* computed tomography.

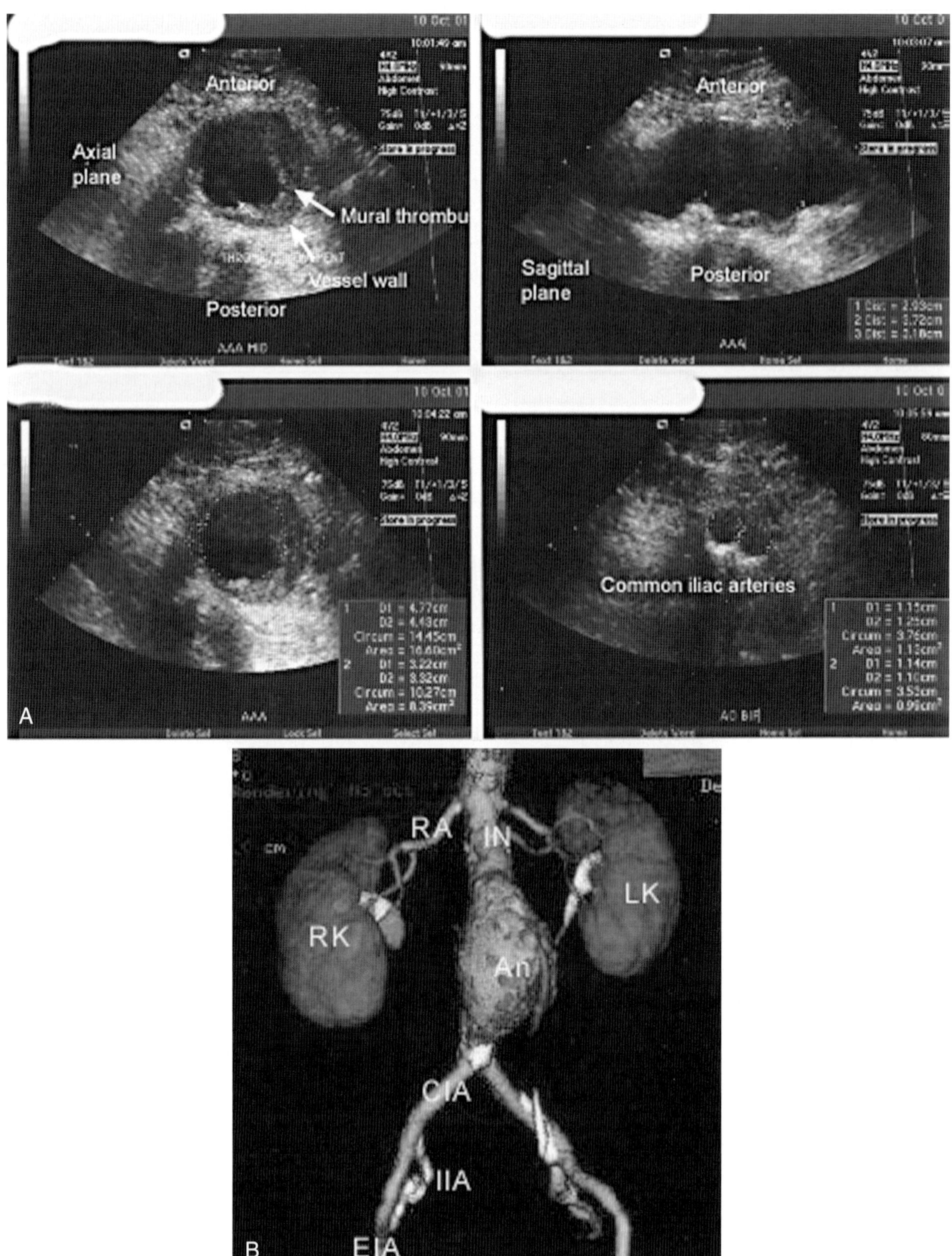


**Fig. 66.1** **A,** Ultrasonography demonstrating an abdominal aortic aneurysm. Note the posterior mural thrombus within the aneurysm sac. **B,** Three-dimensional computed tomography scan illustrating the presence of an infrarenal abdominal aortic aneurysm (An). *CIA*, Common iliac artery; *EIA*, external iliac artery; *IIA*, internal iliac artery; *IN*, infrarenal neck; *LK*, left kidney; *RA*, renal artery; *RK*, right kidney. (From Townsend CM, Beauchamp RD, Evers BM, et al, editors. Sabiston textbook of surgery: the biological basis of modern surgical practice. 17th ed. Philadelphia: Saunders; 2004.)

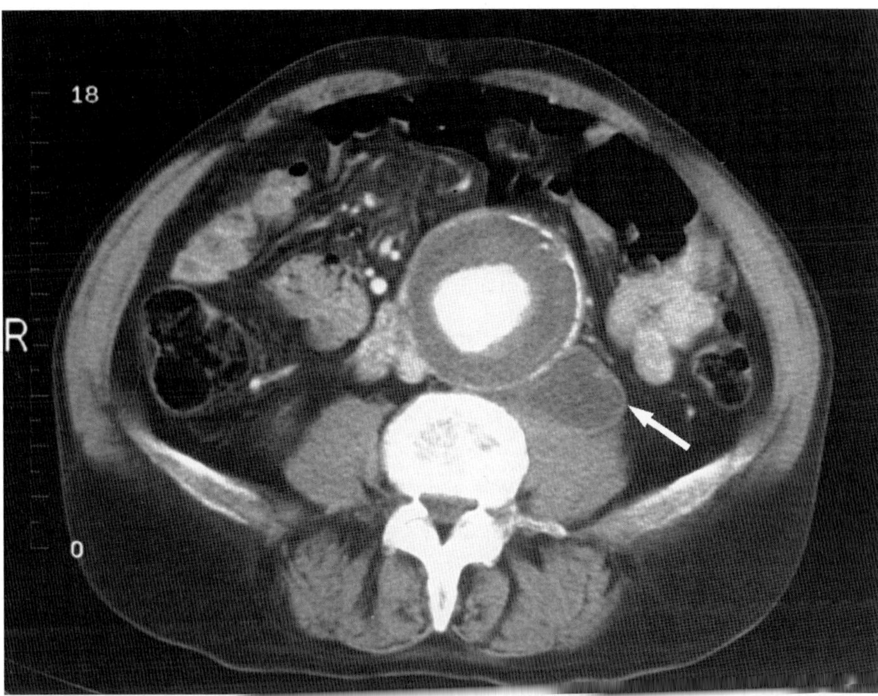


**Fig. [illegible] Computed tomography scan of a ruptured abdominal aortic aneurysm with calcification of the aortic wall and intraluminal thrombus.** The patent lumen enhances with the administration of contrast material, but the periaortic hematoma *(arrow)* does not. (Courtesy Richard Rensio, MD; from Marx JA, Hockberger RS, Walls RM, editors. Rosen's emergency medicine: concepts and clinical practice. 6th ed. Philadelphia: Mosby; 2006.)

emergency physician with a rapid, accurate mode of bedside assessment of a hypotensive patient with a suspected AAA who is too unstable to leave the emergency department (ED) for computed tomography (CT), magnetic resonance imaging (MRI), or magnetic resonance angiography (MRA). However, ultrasonography does have its limitations. Despite its efficacy in ascertaining the size of infrarenal aortic aneurysms, it is unreliable for imaging pararenal, juxtarenal, and suprarenal aneurysms and for imaging the common and internal iliac arteries for aneurysms.[3] Spiral CT scans of the abdomen and pelvis with three-dimensional reconstruction are far superior to ultrasonography for this purpose and are most physicians' first choice for diagnostic purposes (Fig. 66.1, *B*).[3] Before the advent of CT, transcatheter arteriography was the "gold standard" for the preoperative assessment of AAAs despite its inability to determine the exact size of an aneurysm in the presence of a mural thrombus.[3] CT has several advantages over this technique; it is cheaper, less invasive, carries a lower radiation dose, and provides information about the aorta and surrounding structures simultaneously. MRI and MRA can provide the same information as CT and can do so without the use of nephrotoxic agents. MRI and MRA are viable, albeit more costly and time-consuming options for patients with contraindications to iodinated contrast dye who are stable enough to leave the ED for an extended period.

Serial CT scans can be used preoperatively to give the vascular team charged with repairing the AAA several pieces of important information, especially if endovascular repair is being considered. CT can adequately visualize the proximal neck (the transition between the normal and aneurysmal aorta) and map out any dangerous venous anomalies that would make access difficult.[1] CT can also measure the thickness of a mural thrombus and display the presence of blood within a thrombus.[1] Blood within the thrombus is known as the crescent sign and has been highly touted by some as a reliable sign of impending rupture.[1,3,9] Another important marker of aneurysm rupture is extravasation of contrast material. Finally, CT can demonstrate a contained rupture by showing clear evidence of draping of the posterior aspect of the aorta over the adjacent vertebral body; sometimes concomitant vertebral body erosion may be seen (**Fig. 66.2**).[9]

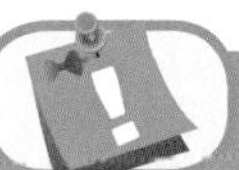

**TIPS AND TRICKS**

At baseline, women have slightly smaller normal aortic diameters than men do (1.9 versus 2.3 cm); however, this difference in normal aortic diameter between the sexes is not substantial enough to warrant changing the upper limit of 3 cm that is used to characterize a small abdominal aortic aneurysm (AAA).

Patients who undergo emergency surgery for AAAs and are found to have intact, symptomatic aneurysms still have a mortality of 20% to 25% versus 5% for those undergoing elective repair.

In stable patients with abdominal or back pain in whom AAA is high on the differential diagnosis, the emergency physician should choose the type of computed tomography (CT) scan that allows diagnosis of the most likely cause; rapid abdominal CT without oral contrast enhancement may be most beneficial.

Currently, many researchers are actively investigating markers of rupture other than size. Much research revolves around the use of MMPs. These zinc- and calcium-dependent enzymes are produced by smooth muscle and inflammatory cells, and several of these proteinases may participate in AAA formation. McMillan and Pearce[10] found that the amount of circulating MMP-9 is significantly higher in patients with AAAs. Lindholt et al.[11] then noted an impressive association with the size and expansion rate of these aneurysms, which prompted many to theorize that serum levels of MMP may soon become a standard part of physicians' diagnostic arsenal.[1]

An approach to the diagnosis and management of AAAs is shown in **Figure 66.3**.

## TREATMENT

Any patient in whom a ruptured AAA or a symptomatic intact AAA is diagnosed needs emergency surgical intervention. Volume resuscitation and cross-matching of large amounts of blood should be undertaken immediately (see Fig. 66.3). Vascular surgery consultation should be sought as soon as the diagnosis is made.

The single most compelling reason to repair AAAs is to prevent fatal rupture. Besides rupture, other rare complications also mandate emergency repair, such as distal embolization and fistulous connections between the aorta and adjacent

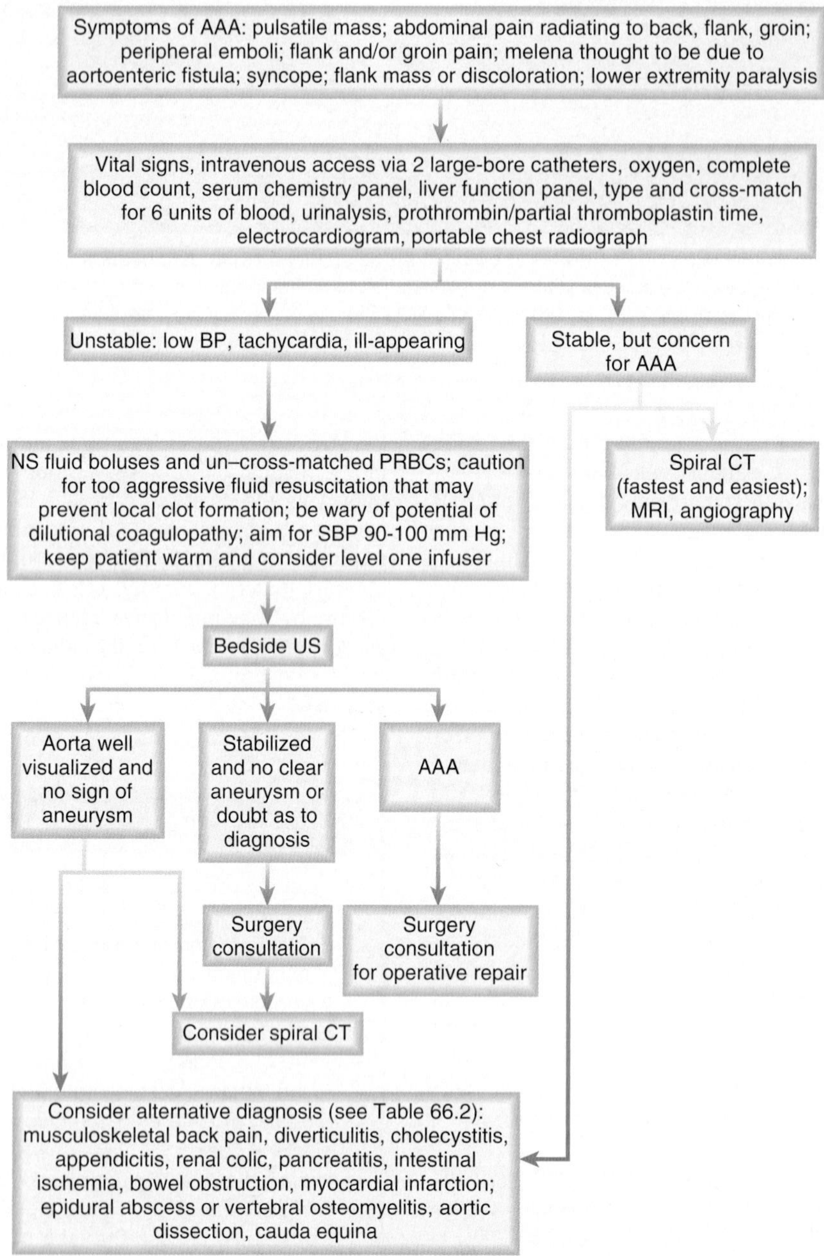


**Fig. 66.3 Algorithm for the diagnosis and treatment of abdominal aortic aneurysms (AAAs).** *BP*, Blood pressure; *CT*, computed tomography; *MRI*, magnetic resonance imaging; *NS*, normal saline; *PRBCs*, packed red blood cells; *SBP*, systolic blood pressure; *US*, ultrasonography.

structures.[2-4] Once an AAA is identified, the obvious next step is to identify its size via ultrasonography, CT, MRI, or MRA to discern whether immediate intervention or periodic surveillance is warranted. One prospective but nonrandomized study demonstrated that observation alone is safe until an aneurysm undergoes a growth spurt or attains a threshold diameter of 5.0 cm.[3,12] Aneurysms with a diameter of this size or larger weaken the aortic wall, which is then at higher risk for rupture.[3] Estimates place the risk for rupture at 1% to 3% per year for AAAs measuring up to 5 cm, 11% per year for 5- to 7-cm aneurysms, and nearly 20% per year for aneurysms larger than 7 cm.[9] Several studies have confirmed the linear association between AAA diameter and annual expansion rate. An observed rate of growth that surpasses these estimates is indicative of a "growth spurt" that may necessitate early elective aneurysm repair. Katzen et al.[4] defined this "growth spurt" as an increase of 1 cm/yr. In addition, if the patient is a woman with smaller native vessels, one must remember that the relative size representing aneurysmal disease may be less than the conventional range of 5 to 5.5 cm.[3]

Prospective randomized trials comparing early intervention with expectant observation for infrarenal AAAs measuring 4.0 to 5.4 cm in diameter were conducted in the United Kingdom and by the U.S. Department of Veterans Affairs during the past decade.[13,14] Elective surgical treatment was delayed in patients in the nonoperative cohort in each trial until their aneurysms exceeded 5.4 cm on serial imaging studies.[3] On the basis of data regarding gender differences in the United Kingdom trial, a guidelines subcommittee of the American Association for Vascular Surgery and the Society for Vascular Surgery now recommends a diameter of 4.5 to 5.0 cm as the appropriate threshold for elective repair of asymptomatic infrarenal aortic aneurysms in women.[3,15] The general consensus regarding suprarenal, pararenal, or type IV thoracoabdominal aortic aneurysms is that because of the higher risk for surgical complications with these aneurysms, elective intervention should be considered at a slightly larger diameter than with infrarenal aortic aneurysms.[3]

A caveat in successful watchful waiting is patient cooperation. Valentine et al.[16] studied 101 patients with aneurysms less than 5.0 cm in diameter and did not find ruptures in patients who adhered to their follow-up program but did find a 10% rupture rate in patients who complied poorly. If continued surveillance is planned, lifestyle and dietary modification should be encouraged. As mentioned earlier, patients who smoke should be strongly encouraged to stop smoking and use any and all available smoking cessation aids, and they should undergo rigorous monitoring and treatment of blood pressure and cholesterol levels, as currently recommended for patients with atherosclerosis.[3]

Once an aneurysm has met the criteria for repair, the vascular surgeon can choose between open and endovascular repair when determining the operative approach. The most important factor determining the utility of either approach is patient selection. Generally, open surgical repair is appropriate for younger, low-risk patients, whereas endovascular repair is preferred for older, higher-risk patients[4] (**Box 66.3**). Studies have shown lower 30-day mortality for endovascular repair (roughly 1.2%) than for open surgery (4.6%).[4] Further study is required to determine whether either affords a long-term survival advantage. It is quite clear that both approaches decrease the risk for death from AAA rupture.[4]

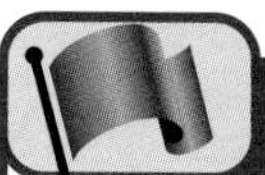

**RED FLAGS**

- The rate of abdominal aortic aneurysms (AAAs) in tobacco smokers is more than four times that in lifelong nonsmokers.
- Estimates place the risk for rupture at 1% to 3% per year for AAAs 4 to 5 cm in diameter, at 6% to 11% per year for those 5 to 7 cm, and nearly 20% per year for those larger than 7 cm.
- Patients usually complain of pain that is steady and aggravating in nature, lasts for hours to days, and is unaffected by movement or position.
- The triad of chronic abdominal pain, weight loss, and elevated erythrocyte sedimentation rate may signal the presence of an inflammatory aneurysm.
- One complication of AAA is rupture into the bowel, commonly involving the duodenum, and exsanguination is the usual fatal result, but slow leaks may be manifested as melena and masquerade as peptic ulcer disease.
- Patients who stabilize with fluid resuscitation should be monitored closely because they are at high risk for rapid [illegible].

Elective repair has resulted in a drastic reduction in mortality in comparison with emergency intervention because patients undergoing elective AAA repair are not suffering the catastrophic physiologic demands of sudden, rapid, high-volume loss at the time of repair. Additionally, they have had time to undergo a thorough preoperative evaluation. A number of studies have demonstrated that the mortality rate for open aortic aneurysm repair can be reduced to less than 2% in settings in which approximately 5% to 15% of patients undergo preliminary coronary artery intervention.[17] Numerous studies have also been performed to elicit risk stratification methods to help the surgeon identify markers that herald higher morbidity and mortality risks in patients requiring intervention. Multiple studies have shown that the mortality rate with elective operations is so much lower than that with ruptured aneurysms that octogenarians should be offered surgical repair. Generally, AAA repair should be offered regardless of age.[3,19,20]

**BOX 66.3 Five Preoperative Risk Factors That Predict Mortality**

**Risk Factors**

Age older than 76 years
Serum creatinine value higher than 190 μmol/L
Hemoglobin value below 9 g/dL
Loss of consciousness
Electrocardiographic evidence of ischemia[18]

**Mortality**

Mortality rate of 100% with 3 or more risk factors
Mortality decreases to 48% with 2 risk factors
Mortality decreases to 28% with 1 risk factor
Mortality decreases to 18% in patients without risk factors

Study results do not agree regarding the extent to which race influences outcome. Some suggest that race plays no role, whereas others suggest that the mortality rate with elective AAA repair is higher in African Americans.[3,21,22] Surprisingly, gender has proved to be influential. According to larger, population-based data sets in various states and countries, the mortality rate with both elective and ruptured aneurysm repair may be as much as 50% higher in women than in men.[3]

With regard to emergency repair of ruptured AAAs, mortality depends on the hemodynamic status of patients at the time of surgery. In contrast to the decreased mortality associated with elective repair, no improvement in the mortality of patients with operatively managed ruptured aneurysms has been reported during the past decades, and it remains 30% to 70%.[1] Clinical variables that have been found to significantly influence the mortality rate after ruptured aneurysm repair are presented in **Box 66.4**.

### FUTURE THERAPY

Given the delineation of the role that MMPs play in aneurysm development and rupture, a fair amount of research has been undertaken in an effort to find inhibitors of these proteases and the utility of such agents in the treatment of small asymptomatic AAAs. Tetracyclines are potentially effective treatment for this purpose. Protracted administration of doxycycline has been associated with reduced plasma MMP-9 levels, but the long-term effects of this medication on the rate of aneurysm growth have yet to be determined.[1,3] Interestingly, 3-hydroxy-3-methylglutaryl coenzyme A reductase inhibitors have been found to decrease the expression of MMP in addition to their effects on cholesterol. Perhaps in time, statins will prove to be useful adjuncts to the prevention and treatment of AAAs.[1,3] Finally, nonsteroidal antiinflammatory drugs and beta-blockers are being studied as possible medical treatments to prohibit the development of AAAs or inhibit their expansion rate.[1,3]

**BOX 66.4 Variables That Significantly Increase the Mortality Rate in Patients After Repair of Ruptured Abdominal Aortic Aneurysms[3]**

Low initial hematocrit
Hypotension that requires resuscitation
Cardiac arrest
High Acute Physiological and Chronic Health Evaluation (APACHE) score
Advanced age

From Hirsch AT, Haskal ZJ, Hertzer NR, et al. ACC/AHA 2005 practice guidelines for the management of patients with peripheral arterial disease (lower extremity, renal, mesenteric, and abdominal aortic): a collaborative report from the American Association for Vascular Surgery/Society for Vascular Surgery, Society for Cardiovascular Angiography and Interventions, Society for Vascular Medicine and Biology, Society of Interventional Radiology, and the ACC/AHA Task Force on Practice Guidelines (Writing Committee to Develop Guidelines for the Management of Patients With Peripheral Arterial Disease): endorsed by the American Association of Cardiovascular and Pulmonary Rehabilitation; National Heart, Lung, and Blood Institute; Society for Vascular Nursing; TransAtlantic Inter-Society Consensus; and Vascular Disease Foundation. Circulation 2006; 113:e463-654.

## FOLLOW-UP, NEXT STEPS IN CARE, AND PATIENT EDUCATION

### ADMISSION AND DISCHARGE

Any patient in whom a ruptured AAA or a symptomatic intact AAA is diagnosed needs emergency surgical intervention. Treatment will continue in the surgical intensive care unit if the patient survives the operative repair.

The disposition of asymptomatic patients in whom the diagnosis is made incidentally depends on the size of the aneurysm, and such patients should be referred for possible elective repair or screening. An asymptomatic patient with an aneurysm larger than 5.5 cm should be referred to a surgeon immediately and should undergo preoperative testing.

### COMPLICATIONS

As mentioned, AAAs are the thirteenth leading cause of death in the United States. Consequently, they are also associated with several other complications. First, as many as 13% of patients with aortic aneurysms have multiple aneurysms elsewhere,[3] with some studies finding that more than 20% of patients with thoracic aortic aneurysms have concomitant AAAs.[3] Thus, a patient in whom an aneurysm is discovered at any level should undergo a thorough examination of the entire aorta.[3] A less common complication is aortocaval fistula. The overall prevalence of aortocaval fistula is 3% to 6% of all ruptured aortic aneurysms.[1] The clinical features of patients with an acute aortocaval fistula usually consist of lower extremity swelling, engorged veins, and high-output cardiac failure.[9] In fact, the development of high-output congestive heart failure with the perception of continuous abdominal noise is pathognomonic of an aortocaval fistula.[1]

Other, even more rare complications of AAA can develop. One is rupture into the bowel, usually involving the duodenum.[9] Exsanguination is the fatal result, but slow leaks may be manifested as melena and masquerade as peptic ulcer disease.[9] The incidence of this complication is very low, and it is found less than 0.1% of the time at autopsy. However, the incidence rate of aortoduodenal fistula following previous repair is 0.5% to 2.3%.[9] Exceptionally large or inflammatory aortic aneurysms can occasionally be associated with early satiety or gastric outlet symptoms because of duodenal compression. Finally, infectious or mycotic aneurysms are worthy of mention. Such an aneurysm may arise by one of two means. It may occur secondary to infection of a preexisting aneurysm,[3] or the aortic wall itself may become infected and give rise to the development of an aneurysm, usually saccular in nature.[3] Primary aortic infections are most commonly caused by *Staphylococcus* and *Salmonella*.[3,23] Tuberculosis has also been found to be responsible for infection of aortic pseudoaneurysms.[3]

### PATIENT EDUCATION

Lifestyle modification is essential in the treatment of AAAs, as well as in limiting their progression; patients must be instructed to stop smoking and must be given help to do so. Many patients can avoid the complications of AAA rupture by developing long-lasting relationships with a primary care provider and adhering to their prescribed surveillance programs. Diameter is the best predictor of AAA rupture, and the follow-up interval depends on size. The risk for rupture of

AAAs according to diameter is as follows: less than 4 cm, 0% per year; 4.0 to 5.5 cm, 0.6% to 1% per year; 5.5 to 5.9 cm, 4.4% per year; 6.0 to 6.9 cm, 10.2% per year; and 7 cm or greater, 32.5% per year. In patients with an AAA, the aorta is believed to increase 0.5 cm in diameter every year, and these patients will eventually need surgery. As a result, the recommended screening intervals for patients with smaller baseline AAA diameters are as follows: less than 3.5 cm, 36 months; 4.0 cm, 24 months; 4.5 cm, 12 months; and 5 cm, 3 months. Patients should be educated about the early clinical signs of the rare but deadly complications of aortocaval and aortoenteric fistulas so that they can seek immediate medical attention. If discharged after an incidentally found aneurysm, close follow-up should be arranged as detailed earlier, and the patient should be cautioned to return if abdominal, back, or flank pain occurs.

## SUGGESTED READING

Assar AN, Zarins CK. Ruptured abdominal aortic aneurysm: a surgical emergency with many clinical presentations. Postgrad Med J 2009;85:268-73.

## REFERENCES

***References can be found on Expert Consult @ www.expertconsult.com.***

# 67 Aortic Ultrasound

*Vanessa Maria Piazza, Christine Butts, and Justin Cook*

**KEY POINTS**

- Bedside ultrasound has emerged as a powerful tool for the diagnosis and disposition of patients with a suspected abdominal aortic aneurysm (AAA) or rupture of an AAA.
- Ultrasound has improved time to diagnosis and time to disposition in patients requiring operative intervention.
- The abdominal aorta must be seen in its entire length to rule out an AAA.

## INTRODUCTION

An abdominal aortic aneurysm (AAA) can be a challenging diagnosis to make and a deadly diagnosis to miss. Patients may be asymptomatic until rupture, or they may have vague complaints such as chronic abdominal or back pain. Frequently, these symptoms are misdiagnosed as less deadly processes, such as renal colic.[1,2] Once ruptured, time to diagnosis is the biggest determinant of survival.[3] Commonly relied on methods of diagnosis, such as computed tomography (CT), may delay care and result in patient decompensation. Bedside ultrasound has emerged as a powerful tool in the diagnosis and disposition of patients with a suspected AAA or rupture of an AAA. When used properly, bedside ultrasound improves the time to diagnosis and survival.[4]

## WHAT WE ARE LOOKING FOR

Because the signs and symptoms of an AAA may be vague and nonspecific, bedside ultrasound of the aorta is indicated in the following clinical scenarios: abdominal pain, back pain, flank pain, unexplained hypotension, syncope, cardiac arrest, or known history of an aneurysm.[5,6] The goal of bedside ultrasound is to measure the size of the abdominal aorta and exclude the presence of an AAA. When rupture of an AAA is suspected, the peritoneum should also be evaluated with focused abdominal sonography for trauma (FAST) to search for free fluid.

## SUPPORTING EVIDENCE

A large amount of research has confirmed bedside ultrasound to be a useful and lifesaving tool in the emergency department (ED). Tayal et al. conducted a prospective study of the accuracy and outcome of bedside ultrasound for the diagnosis of AAA by emergency physicians. They evaluated 125 patients suspected of having an AAA with bedside ultrasound. Twenty-nine patients were found to be positive for AAA, for a positive predictive value of 93% and a negative predictive value of 100%. The sensitivity was 100% with a specificity of 98% for 10 of the 27 patients found to have an AAA, and disposition was immediate to the operating room without a confirmatory study.[3,7]

Another emergency medicine study performed in 2005 evaluated 238 patients who arrived at the ED with symptoms suggestive of a ruptured AAA. Third-year emergency medical residents, trained according to guidelines from the American College of Emergency Physicians, performed all ultrasound examinations. Thirty-six aortic abnormalities were diagnosed with a sensitivity of 100% and specificity of 100% for this end point in comparison with "gold standard" diagnostic testing.[8]

Knaut et al. assessed the accuracy of measurements taken by emergency physicians via ultrasound versus measurements taken by CT. They found that in all cases, their measurements approximated those found on CT within 1.41 cm or less.[9]

Plummer et al. randomized patients to ultrasound versus standard-of-care diagnostics and compared time to diagnosis and to the operating room. Ultrasound improved time to diagnosis (5.4 versus 83 minutes) and improved time to disposition for patients requiring operative intervention (90 versus 12 minutes).[4]

## SCANNING PROTOCOLS

Bedside ultrasound of the aorta can be completed in 2 to 3 minutes. To rule out the presence of an aneurysm, the entire length of the abdominal aorta from the diaphragmatic hiatus to the aortic bifurcation should be evaluated in both the longitudinal and transverse planes. A low-frequency transducer should be selected for this examination. A 2- to 5-MHz curvilinear transducer will be the best choice for most patents because it offers adequate depth and resolution. A phased-array or microconvex transducer can also be used.

The examination begins just below the patient's xiphoid process. With the indicator pointing toward the patient's right, the transducer should be facing straight down to the patient's back (**Fig. 67.1**). Although the aorta may be identified immediately, some effort is frequently required to orient the sonographer to the anatomy. The easiest landmark to identify initially is the vertebral body. It is seen as a hyperechoic (white) arc casting a dark acoustic shadow, usually near the bottom of the screen. Just above the vertebral body, two circular, anechoic (black) vessels should be seen (**Fig. 67.2**). The aorta lies to the patient's left and the inferior vena cava (IVC) lies to the patient's right. The IVC is oval shaped and compressible and has thinner walls. The aorta is round, noncompressible, thicker walled, and pulsatile. A measurement should be taken in this transverse orientation, from outer wall to outer wall in both the anterior-posterior and side-to-side planes (**Fig. 67.3**). While maintaining contact with the skin, the transducer should be moved caudally to follow the course of the aorta. From this point, the branches of the aorta can be seen, and the first branch is the celiac trunk. Caudally, the superior mesenteric artery may also be seen, followed by the bifurcation of the celiac trunk, which is often referred to as the "seagull sign" (**Fig. 67.4**). As the examination proceeds caudally, a second measurement should be taken midway between the xiphoid process and the umbilicus. Theoretically, this should be near the origin of the renal arteries. The measurement should be taken in the transverse orientation, from outer wall to outer wall and in both the anterior-posterior and side-to-side planes.

The examination continues caudally until the aorta is seen to bifurcate into the common iliac arteries just above the xiphoid process. Once this bifurcation is identified, a third measurement should be taken just above this location in the same manner described previously. The examination concludes with evaluation of the aorta in the longitudinal, or sagittal, plane. Beginning again just caudal to the xiphoid process, the transducer is now placed with the indicator

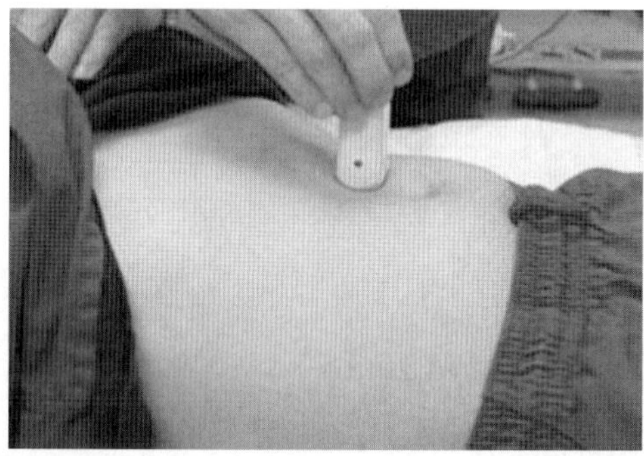

**Fig. 67.1 Ultrasound of the aorta in a transverse orientation.**

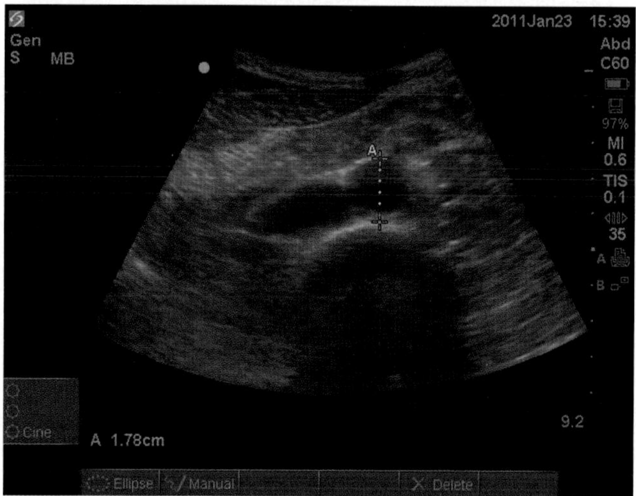


**Fig. 67.3 Measurement of a normal aorta as seen in a transverse orientation.**

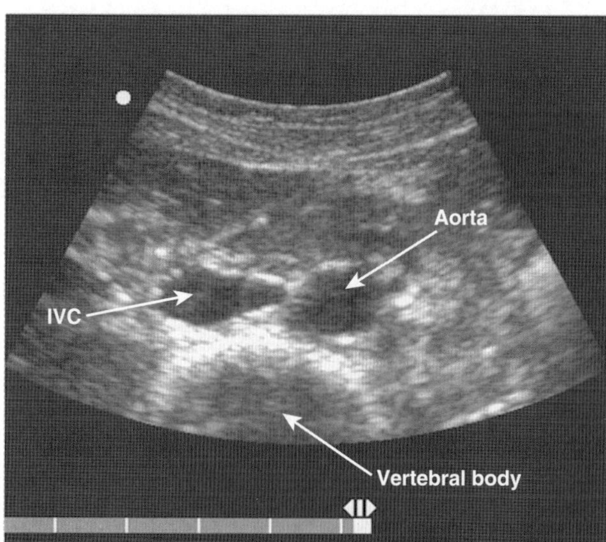


**Fig. 67.2 Normal anatomy of the aorta in a transverse orientation.** Note the hyperechoic (white) arc of the vertebral body at the bottom of the screen. The aorta is seen just above, to the patient's left, with the inferior vena cava (IVC) lying to the patient's right.

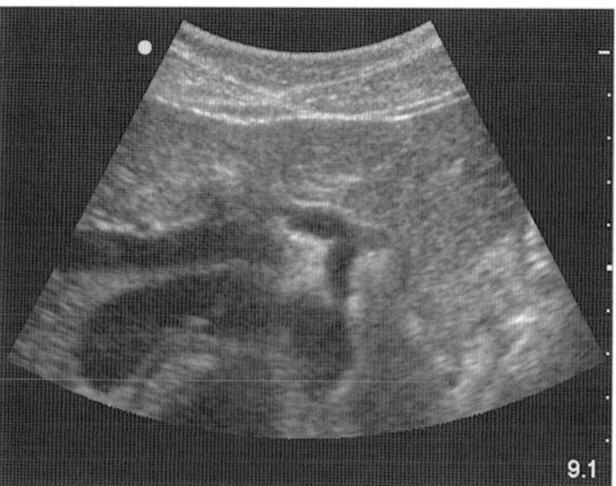


**Fig. 67.4 Normal anatomy of the aorta at the level of the celiac trunk.** The vertebral body is again seen at the bottom of the screen with the inferior vena cava lying just above it to the patient's right. The aorta is just to the patient's left, and the celiac trunk can be seen branching off the aorta; it appears as a seagull with its wings extended (the "seagull sign").

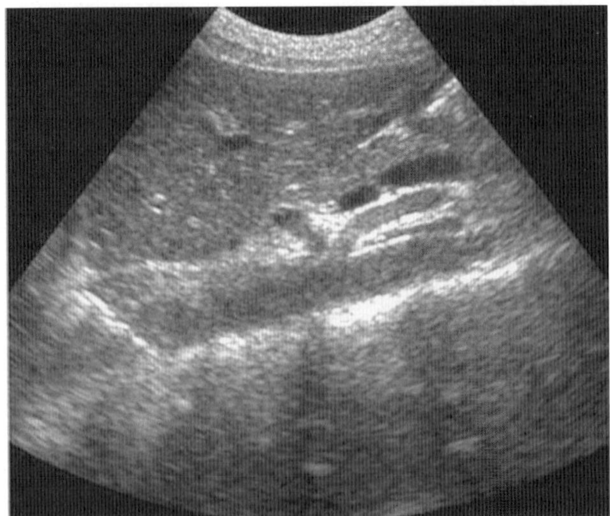

**Fig. 67.5 Normal anatomy of the aorta in a longitudinal or sagittal orientation.** The celiac trunk can again be seen as the first branch, with the superior mesenteric artery just beyond it.

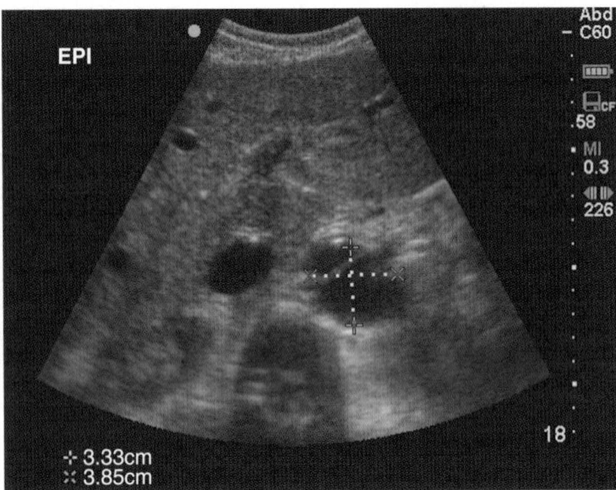


**Fig. 67.6 Transverse image of an abdominal aortic aneurysm.** Note the measurements of 3.35 × 3.85 cm. The inferior vena cava is seen to the patient's right of the aorta, and the vertebral body is seen below the two vessels. Note also that there appears to be an echogenic flap within the aorta, possibly representing an aortic dissection.

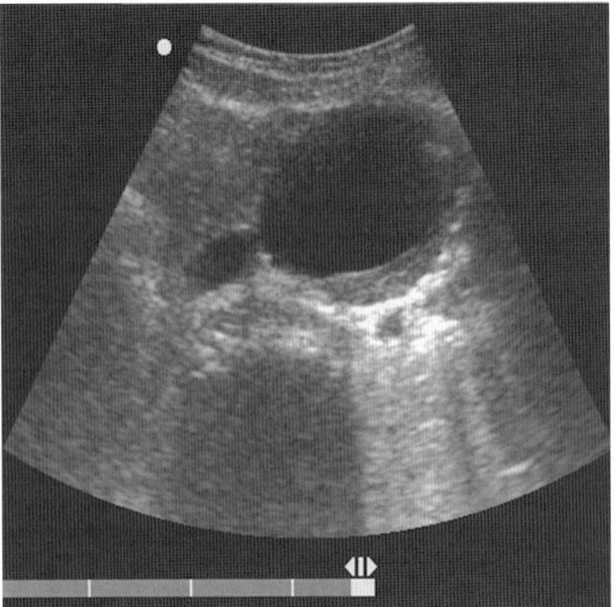

**Fig. 67.7 Large aortic aneurysm in a transverse orientation.** Note the hypoechoic (dark gray) crescent-shaped area along the wall of the aorta, which represents mural thrombus. The inferior vena cava is seen to the patient's right, and both vessels lie above the vertebral body.

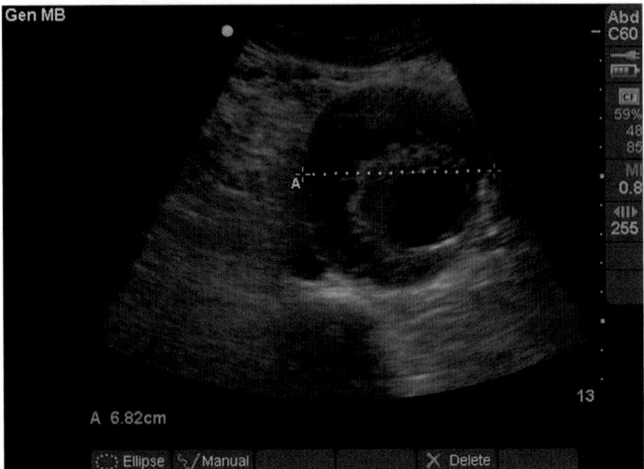


**Fig. 67.8 Another example of a large aortic aneurysm in transverse orientation.** Again, a large mural thrombus is seen around the periphery of the vessel.

directed toward the patient's head. It is frequently necessary to move the transducer slightly toward the patient's left side to visualize the aorta (**Fig. 67.5**). The aorta is distinguished from the IVC as described previously. This longitudinal view of the aorta allows additional information and frequently details suspected abnormalities. Measurements of the diameter of the aorta should not be done in this plane. Underestimation of the diameter may occur if the beam is off center, known as the "cylinder" artifact.

## ABNORMAL FINDINGS

An AAA is defined as an aortic diameter greater than 3 cm or greater than 50% of normal. This diagnosis can easily be made with simple measurements of aortic diameter (**Fig. 67.6**). Frequently, mural thrombus is seen within the lumen of an AAA as a result of decreased blood flow at the periphery of the vessel (**Figs. 67.7 and 67.8**). Thrombus is seen as a hypoechoic (dark gray) crescent along the wall of the aneurysm. The type of aneurysm may also be apparent by examining the aorta in multiple dimensions. A fusiform aneurysm will be dilated in a uniform manner around the circumference of the vessel, whereas a saccular aneurysm is a focal dilation of one aspect of the vessel. If an aneurysm is found, the peritoneum should be evaluated for the presence of free fluid with a FAST examination (**Fig. 67.9**).

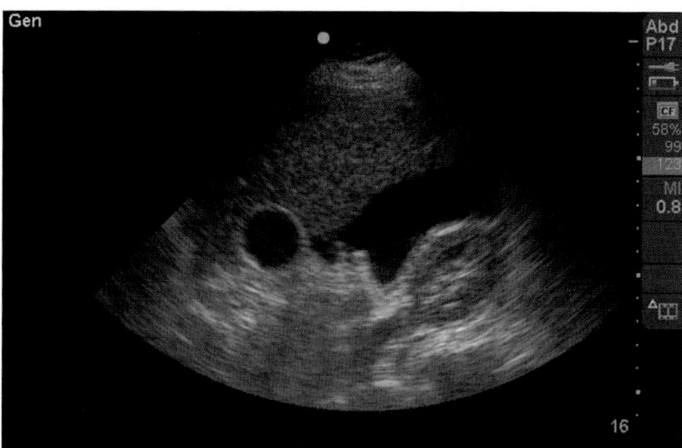


**Fig. 67.9 Image of the right upper quadrant with anechoic (black) free fluid seen surrounding the liver.** Abdominal aortic aneurysms most commonly rupture into the retroperitoneal space; however, the peritoneum should be evaluated for free fluid if rupture is suspected.

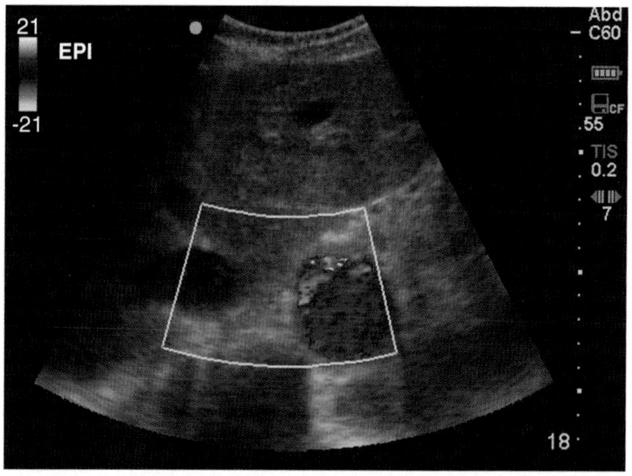

**Fig. 67.10 Example of the use of color flow Doppler to locate the aorta.** In this image the color flow box is placed over the area where the aorta is suspected to lie, and pulsatile flow is demonstrated.

## PITFALLS

Frequently, a beginning sonographer has difficulty identifying and following the abdominal aorta. Patient habitus and the presence of bowel gas may result in a large amount of hazy gray scatter artifact. To initially identify the aorta, a helpful first step is increasing the overall depth of the image. Some patients may require a depth of 30 cm to "see" far enough into the abdomen. The vertebral body makes a helpful landmark because it typically stands out among the other structures in the abdomen. Careful evaluation of the image for pulsations or use of the color flow box may help in initially identifying the aorta (**Fig. 67.10**).

Once the aorta has been identified, another common pitfall is an inability to follow the aortic course to its bifurcation because of bowel gas and body habitus.[10] To overcome this challenge, application of steady pressure from the subxiphoid area to the umbilicus will frequently cause bowel gas to disperse enough to allow a sufficient image. Additionally, the patient can be placed in either the right or left decubitus position to help displace abdominal gas.

Once technical difficulties have been overcome, the sonographer should be mindful to avoid diagnostic errors. Bedside ultrasound seeks to identify the presence of an aneurysm and is most sensitive when used for this purpose. Because the aorta is a retroperitoneal organ, it most often ruptures into this space, thus making diagnosis difficult. Although free fluid may be seen within the peritoneum as described earlier, this is a rare location for rupture. Rupture of an AAA should be assumed in any patient with an aneurysm and evidence of acute decompensation (e.g., hypotension). The abdominal aorta must be seen in its entire length to rule out an AAA.[10] Aneurysms are frequently focal and confined to a relatively small portion of the vessel, so evaluation of only portions of the aorta may result in overlooking a significant aneurysm.

## SUGGESTED READINGS

Costantino TG, Bruno E, Handly N, et al. Accuracy of emergency medicine ultrasound in the evaluation of abdominal aortic aneurysm. J Emerg Med 2005;29:455-60.

Kuhn M, Bonnin RL, Davey MJ, et al. Emergency department ultrasound scanning for abdominal aortic aneurysm: accessible, accurate, and advantageous. Ann Emerg Med 2000;36:219-23.

Perera P, Mailhot T, Mandavia D. The RUSH exam: rapid ultrasound in shock in the evaluation of the critically ill. Emerg Med Clin North Am 2010;28:29-56.

Plummer D, Clinton J, Matthew B. Emergency department ultrasound improves time to diagnosis and survival in ruptured AAA (abstract). Acad Emerg Med 1998;5:147.

Tayal VS, Graf CD, Gibbs MA. Prospective study of accuracy and outcome of emergency ultrasound for abdominal aortic aneurysm over 2 years. Acad Emerg Med 2003;10:867-71.

## REFERENCES

*References can be found on Expert Consult @ www.expertconsult.com.*

# 68 Peripheral Arterial Disease

*Christopher Ross and Theresa Schwab*

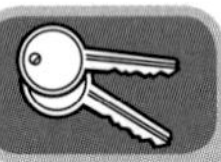

**KEY POINTS**

- Intermittent claudication is the earliest clinical manifestation of pathologically significant peripheral arterial disease.
- The ankle-brachial index can help confirm clinical suspicion of occlusive arterial disease.
- Ischemic rest pain signals critical, limb-threatening disease.
- The classic manifestation of acute arterial occlusion is described by the six "P's": pain, polar (cold), paresthesia, paralysis, pallor, and pulselessness.
- Treatment of nonischemic peripheral arterial disease consists of modification of risk factors, exercise programs, and medications aimed at platelet inhibition.
- Prompt initiation of therapy is the most important aspect of the treatment of acute limb ischemia, and patients should receive a heparin bolus followed by an infusion, ideally even before diagnostic testing is begun.
- Treatment of ischemic peripheral arterial disease depends on whether the extremity is viable (angiography to assess the extent of disease), nonviable (primary amputation), or threatened (immediate surgical intervention required).

## EPIDEMIOLOGY

The most common term used to describe atherosclerotic vascular disease of the lower extremities is *peripheral arterial disease* (PAD). In North America and Europe, it is estimated that 27 million individuals are affected by PAD. In a significant proportion of patients the disease is occult but is nevertheless an important indicator of significant cardiovascular events.[1,2] Systemic atherosclerotic disease with damage to end-organs other than the heart continues to be associated with high morbidity and mortality,[3] and surprisingly little research is being done on it.

By 50 years of age the prevalence of PAD is 2% to 3%, and it rises to 20% in those older than 75 years.[4] The clinical findings of PAD in patients older than 50 years is as follows: 10% to 35% have classic claudication, 20% to 50% are asymptomatic, 40% to 50% have atypical leg pain, and the remaining 1% to 2% have critical ischemia.[5,6] Women have a relative risk of 0.7 in comparison with men. African American subjects have the highest risk for PAD (2.5) relative to the white population, followed by Hispanic subjects (1.5).

**Box 68.1** lists the risk factors for PAD.[6] They are similar to the risk factors that promote the development of coronary atherosclerosis. The risk factor with the highest correlation to PAD is cigarette smoking. When compared with nonsmokers, smokers have a 1.7- to 5.6-fold increase in the development and progression of atherosclerosis in the peripheral vasculature.[7] In patients with symptomatic PAD, smoking increases this risk 8 to 10 times.[8] Risk increases in a powerful dose-dependent manner according to the number of cigarettes smoked per day and the number of years of smoking. Diabetes increases the risk for PAD, 3.5 times in men and 8.6 times in women.[9] Diabetic patients are also 7 to 15 times more likely to require amputation. The Framingham Heart Study found that risk for the development of intermittent claudication was 2.5-fold and 4-fold higher in men and women, respectively, who had hypertension and that this risk was proportional to the severity of the hypertension.[9] Genetic predisposition represents an important risk factor for atherosclerosis, and such predisposition accounts for as much as 50% of the risk in some studies.[10] Patients who have PAD also have a high incidence of coronary heart disease (CHD), and in general, patients have a two to four times higher incidence of CHD and cerebrovascular disease if PAD is also present.[7]

## PATHOPHYSIOLOGY

Atherosclerosis was originally thought to be primarily lipoprotein accumulation but is now better understood, fundamentally, as chronic inflammatory disease of the arterial system.[11] The inflammatory process leads to plaque disruption and thrombosis, and the plaques that are vulnerable are characterized by a large lipid core, a thin fibrous cap, and inflammatory cells at the thinnest portion of the cap surface (**Fig. 68.1**).[12] Plaque rupture has been shown to be critical in the development of acute coronary syndromes, but the importance of this event in patients with PAD is not known at this time.

**BOX 68.1 Risk Factors for Lower Extremity Peripheral Arterial Disease**

Age 70 years and older
Age 50 to 69 years with a history of smoking or diabetes
Age younger than 50 years with diabetes and one other atherosclerotic risk factor (smoking, dyslipidemia, hypertension, or hyperhomocysteinemia)
Leg symptoms with exertion (suggestive of claudication) or ischemic rest pain
Abnormal lower extremity pulse findings
Known atherosclerotic coronary, carotid, or renal artery disease

Data from Hirsch AT, Haskal ZJ, Hertzer NR, et al. American Association for Vascular Surgery/Society for Vascular Surgery; Society for Cardiovascular Angiography and Interventions; Society for Vascular Medicine and Biology; Society of Interventional Radiology; ACC/AHA Task Force on Practice Guidelines: ACC/AHA 2005 guidelines for the management of patients with peripheral arterial disease (lower extremity, renal, mesenteric, and abdominal aortic): a collaborative report from the American Associations for Vascular Surgery/Society for Vascular Surgery, Society for Cardiovascular Angiography and Interventions, Society for Vascular Medicine and Biology, Society of Interventional Radiology, and the ACC/AHA Task Force on Practice Guidelines (Writing Committee to Develop Guidelines for the Management of Patients With Peripheral Arterial Disease): summary of recommendations. J Am Coll Cardiol 2006;47:1239-312.

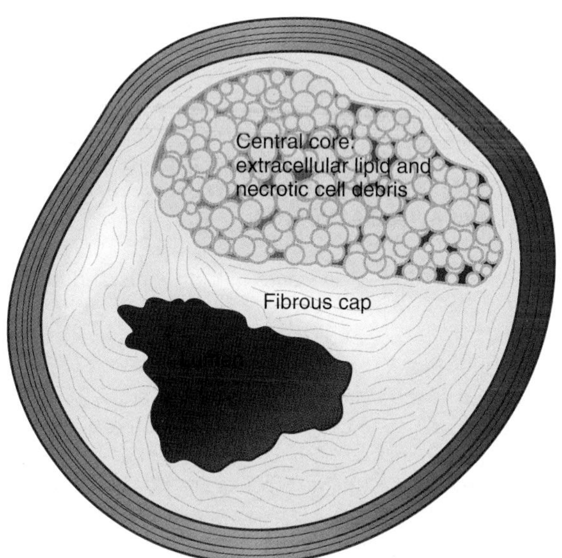


**Fig. 68.1 Cross section of a human artery with advanced atherosclerotic plaque.** The fibrous cap is a layer of smooth muscle cells and fibrous tissue that separates the necrotic core of the plaque from the lumen.

The vascular smooth muscle cell is important in the development of atherosclerosis. Once activated, the cell migrates into the intima and begins to proliferate and secrete matrix proteins and enzymes. This step has been shown to be important in the development of stenosis both in the atherosclerotic vessel and in vessels that have been stented.[13] In addition, the vessel often constricts rather than dilates, thereby narrowing the lumen even more.[14] Progression of PAD can result from worsening local atherosclerotic disease or a superimposed embolic, thrombotic, inflammatory, traumatic, or vasospastic event.

## THROMBOEMBOLISM

More than 80% of arterial emboli originate in the heart and travel to the extremities, the lower extremities being much more frequently affected than the upper ones. Emboli typically lodge in places with acute narrowing of the artery, such as an atherosclerotic plaque or a point where the vessel branches. The frequencies with which emboli lodge in various areas are as follows[15]: femoral arteries, 28%; arm vessels, 20%; aortoiliac vessels, 18%; popliteal arteries, 17%; and visceral vessels, 9%.

Because of the size of most emboli, the femoral and popliteal arteries are involved more often than the larger aortic and iliac vessels. Atrial fibrillation can lead to thrombosis of the left atrium and is present in 60% to 75% of patients with embolic events. Valvular heart disease (aortic and mitral) accounts for approximately 5% to 10% of cases of thromboembolic disease. The amount of tissue destruction depends on the size of the vessel, the extent of obstruction, and the amount of collateral circulation available to compensate. Once the embolus has lodged in the vessel wall, further propagation can occur either distally or proximally via thrombosis, which can further exacerbate the ischemia.

## ATHEROEMBOLISM

Debris from atherosclerotic plaque can break off in proximal vessels and give rise to atheroemboli. Atheroemboli are less likely to produce symptoms of acute arterial occlusion. The atheroembolus is usually irregularly shaped and nondistensible, thus leading to incomplete occlusion with secondary ischemic atrophy. One exception is blue toe syndrome, in which atheroemboli cause complete occlusion of the digital arteries in the foot. In patients with simultaneous evidence of both venous and arterial embolism, a patent foramen ovale should be considered.

## INFLAMMATION

Irradiation, drugs, trauma, or bacterial or fungal invasion can result in an inflammatory arterial injury. Infectious causes lead to direct invasion of the vessel wall and are usually related to intravenous drug abuse, infective endocarditis, or generalized sepsis.

## TRAUMA

Blunt injury to vessel walls can result in disruption of the intima, which can then cause obstruction and thrombosis. Usually, it takes hours to days for complete occlusion to become manifested. Arterial lacerations can be partial or complete, and either type can cause distal ischemia and infarction. Partial arterial lacerations continue to bleed because of the intact portion of the vessel, and such bleeding can result in hematoma formation outside the vessel and thrombosis within the vessel. The hematoma can cause progressive pain, deformity, nerve compression, and subsequent vascular compromise. Complete arterial lacerations actually bleed very little acutely because of spasm of the transected ends. Eventually, however, the spasm relaxes, which can lead to delayed bleeding, and the thrombus on the distal side may separate and move distally.

### VASOSPASM

Abnormal vasomotor responses in distal small arteries can cause ischemic symptoms without tissue loss.

### ARTERIOVENOUS FISTULAS

Sometimes there may be communication between the arterial and venous systems, which can cause vascular distention, tortuosity, aneurysm formation, and alterations in hemodynamics that are favorable for the development of thrombosis. The fistulas result in elevation of the local venous system, which can lead to skin breakdown in the form of dermatitis and ulceration.

## PRESENTING SIGNS AND SYMPTOMS

The clinical signs and symptoms of PAD may be nonspecific and be manifested in a variable fashion according to degree and location of the atherosclerotic disease, as well as the presence of other previously described pathologic processes, such as thromboemboli, atheroemboli, inflammation, trauma, and vasospasm. The clinical spectrum ranges from a nonspecific systemic illness to a catastrophic event such as an ischemic leg. The gastrointestinal tract is an often-overlooked area of involvement that has been shown to be involved in about a fifth of cases. Patients may complain of nausea, vomiting, abdominal pain, melena, or hematochezia. Stools may be heme positive, and intestinal ischemia can progress to infarction in some cases. Skin manifestations are the most common finding in patients with PAD and appear in approximately a third of cases.[16] Livedo reticularis is a red-blue netlike mottling of the skin and represents embolization to the skin. Such mottling is generally seen on the legs, buttocks, and thighs and rarely involves the arms.

Key components of the vascular review of symptoms and family history are listed in **Box 68.2**. Physical findings in patients with PAD are listed in **Box 68.3**. Despite general relationships between PAD and the site of pain, the history and physical examination are not reliable for the detection of lower extremity PAD. Relying solely on the presence of classic claudication will miss up to 90% of cases.[5,6] Physical examination can also be unreliable. For instance, an abnormal femoral pulse has high specificity and positive predictive value but low sensitivity for large-vessel disease. The best single discriminator is an abnormal posterior tibial pulse.[17]

**BOX 68.2 Key Findings in the Vascular Review of Systems**

- Any exertional limitation of the lower extremity muscles or any history of walking impairment (fatigue, aching, numbness, or pain). The primary site or sites of discomfort in the buttock, thigh, calf, or foot should be recorded along with the relationship of such discomfort to rest or exertion
- Any poorly healing or nonhealing wounds on the legs or feet
- Any pain at rest localized to the lower part of the leg or foot and its association with the upright or recumbent positions
- Postprandial abdominal pain that is reproducibly provoked by eating and is associated with weight loss

### ACUTE ARTERIAL OCCLUSION

Patients with acute arterial occlusion commonly complain of a sudden onset of pain and coldness distally, on the side of the occlusion (**Fig. 68.2**). As the ischemia progresses, the classic findings of acute arterial occlusion become evident, as described by the six "P's": pain, polar (cold) sensation, paresthesia, paralysis, pallor, and pulselessness. As the peripheral nerves become ischemic, paresthesias, numbness, and then paralysis develop sequentially. The sensory peripheral nerves are affected first, with decreases in proprioception and light touch, and then the larger pain and motor fibers become involved and give rise to a loss of sensation, weakness, and paralysis. Paralysis is usually a bad prognostic sign for reversibility of the ischemia. Signs of ischemia can be seen distal to the level of arterial occlusion. During the first 8 hours after the ischemic insult, the extremity looks pale because of the spastic nature of the arterial tree surrounding the region. Twelve to 24 hours after the injury, the extremity may become cyanotic and mottled. As arterial flow ceases, venous drainage also slows or stops, thereby leading to profound stasis, which further aggravates the damage. On careful examination, the cold part of the extremity can easily be demarcated from its

**BOX 68.3 Key Components of the Vascular Physical Examination in a Patient with Possible Peripheral Arterial Disease**

- Measurement of blood pressure in both arms and notation of any interarm asymmetry
- Palpation of the carotid pulses and notation of carotid upstroke and amplitude and the presence of bruits
- Auscultation of the abdomen and flank for bruits
- Palpation of the abdomen and notation of the presence of aortic pulsation and the maximum diameter of the aorta
- Palpation of pulses at the brachial, radial, ulnar, femoral, popliteal, dorsalis pedis, and posterior tibial sites
- Auscultation of both femoral arteries for the presence of bruits
- Assessment of pulse intensity, which should be recorded numerically as follows: 0, absent; 1, diminished; 2, normal; 3, bounding
- Inspection of the feet for evaluation of color, temperature, and integrity of the skin and intertriginous areas and recording of the presence of ulceration
- Documentation of the presence of symmetry, edema, and venous distention of the lower extremities
- Recording of additional findings suggestive of severe peripheral arterial disease, including distal hair loss, trophic skin changes, and hypertrophic nails

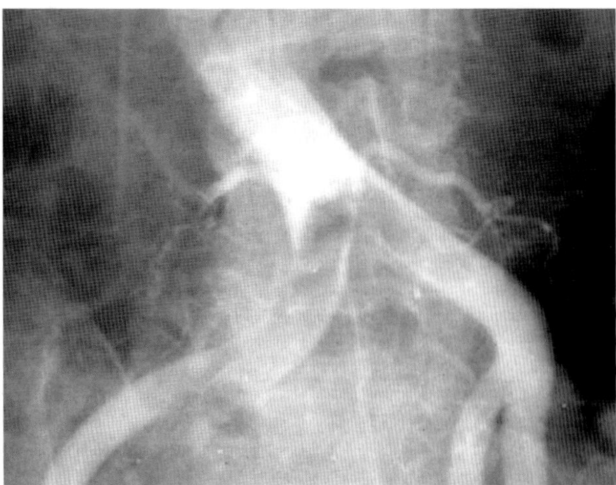

**Fig. 68.2 Large saddle clot at the bifurcation of the aorta at the iliac vessels.** This clot not only can cause symptoms by itself but can also embolize more distally.

warmer proximal portion. The ischemia is unlikely to be reversible if the affected limb is paralyzed.

## INTERMITTENT CLAUDICATION

The primary symptom of lower extremity atherosclerotic disease is intermittent claudication. Claudication, from the Latin word for "limp," is defined as reproducible discomfort of a defined group of muscles that is induced by exercise and relieved with rest. It results from an imbalance in the blood flow needed to meet the metabolic demands of the tissue. Intermittent claudication has three major clinical features: it is consistent and reproducible from day to day, symptoms resolve within a couple of minutes after cessation of exercise, and discomfort occurs again at the same distance once the patient resumes the activity. The symptoms usually occur gradually and may be absent or minimal, even in those with significant disease. The pain may also be felt in the thigh, hip, and buttock as the level of obstruction moves proximally. If many of the vessels are involved, the most distal muscle group is affected first, followed by proximal migration as the patient continues to walk. The pain is primarily unilateral at onset but may be bilateral if distal aortic occlusion occurs. Progressive arterial insufficiency causes a collateral circulation to develop, which will allow the patient's symptoms to not progress despite worsening of the culprit artery. As described, there is a relationship between the site of pain and the site of arterial disease, as follows: foot (tibial and peroneal artery), calf (superficial femoral artery or popliteal artery), thigh (common femoral artery or aorta and iliac artery), and buttocks and hips (aorta and iliac artery).

## REST PAIN

Ischemic pain at rest can be a symptom of severe to critical limb ischemia. The pain typically occurs at night when the patient is supine, and the patient may awaken from sleep with pain in the toes or forefoot. The pain is generally worse in a single extremity and is relieved by dependency. The patient may either stand up or hang the legs over the edge of the bed for relief. In this scenario, physical examination may show marked pallor with elevation of the legs, marked rubor with dependency, and delayed venous filling times. Usually by the time that rest pain occurs, severe arterial insufficiency is present in multiple arterial segments.

After rest pain, progression of disease causes necrosis of tissue, generally between two toes. Eventually, the ulcers may coalesce or progress to dry gangrene over the tips of the toes or at pressure points. Peripheral gangrene arising from an arterial cause may be difficult to differentiate from that with a venous cause. A patient with arterial ischemia exhibits severe ischemic changes followed by edema because the limb is kept in a dependent position. With venous gangrene, however, the edema occurs first, before the onset of frank ischemic changes.

**BOX 68.4 Categories of Acute Limb Ischemia**

**Viable:** The extremity is not immediately threatened. The patient does not complain of ischemic rest pain, no neurologic deficit is present, and the capillary circulation in the skin appears to be adequate. Physical examination demonstrates pulses with either palpation or a Doppler flowmeter.

**Threatened viability:** Reversible ischemia has occurred, and the extremity is salvageable without major amputation if the arterial obstruction is relieved promptly. Affected patients have ischemic rest pain with mild transient or incomplete neurologic symptoms. The pulses are not detected with a Doppler flowmeter.

**Nonviable (major, irreversible ischemic change):** Major amputation of the affected limb is frequently required. Affected patients have profound sensory loss and muscle paralysis, absence of capillary flow, or evidence of more advanced ischemia (muscle rigor or marbled skin). No pulses can be palpated or detected with a Doppler flowmeter.

# DIFFERENTIAL DIAGNOSIS AND MEDICAL DECISION MAKING

The clinician will often need to determine whether the patient's symptoms are related to peripheral neuropathy or ischemic disease. Patients with neurologic disease usually have bilateral leg pain that is not relieved by dependency, as well as neurologic signs such as decreased deep tendon reflexes and loss of touch and vibratory sensation. With ischemia, the sensory peripheral nerves are affected first and result in decreases in proprioception and light touch; the larger pain and motor fibers then become involved, which leads to loss of sensation, weakness, and subsequently paralysis.

Once the clinician is convinced that the patient's symptoms are related to PAD, the first priority is to determine whether the symptoms represent PAD without occlusion (nonischemic) or whether ischemic PAD is present. The next step is to determine whether the extremity is viable, threatened, or nonviable (**Box 68.4**). When arterial blood flow is insufficient to meet the metabolic demands of resting muscle or tissue,

**BOX 68.5 Causes of Acute Arterial Occlusion**

**Embolus**

***Cardiac Source***

Atrial fibrillation
Myocardial infarction
Endocarditis
Valvular disease
Atrial myxoma
Prosthetic valves

***Arterial Source***

Aneurysm
Atherosclerotic plaque
Paradoxic embolus

**Thrombosis**

Vascular grafts
Atherosclerosis
Thrombosis of an aneurysm
Entrapment syndrome
Hypercoagulable state
Low-flow state

**Trauma**

Blunt
Penetrating
Iatrogenic

**BOX 68.6 Ankle-Brachial Index Measurements**

Measurements must be obtained properly for accuracy and reliability and be done in the following sequence:

1. Arm systolic pressure should always be measured with a Doppler flowmeter because measurement by auscultation can be inaccurate.
2. Pressure must be recorded in both arms and both tibial arteries at the ankle.
3. Systolic pressure is measured at the point at which flow is first detected, not at the point at which it is lost during inflation.
4. The absolute levels of blood pressure and the ankle-brachial index are then measured.

limb-threatening ischemia results. This is the most common indication for emergency arterial reperfusion. The selected group of patients requires immediate assessment of their vascular system. Arteriography provides the most useful information in the setting of acute arterial occlusion because in addition to providing information on anatomy, it can distinguish between embolism and thrombosis. Embolism has a sharp cutoff of contrast agent with a reverse meniscus sign; thrombosis usually has a more tapered cutoff. Diffuse atheromatous disease is also usually found around a thrombotic occlusion.

## ACUTE ARTERIAL OCCLUSION

Acute arterial occlusion (critical limb ischemia) is defined as a sudden decrease in limb perfusion that causes a potential threat to limb viability in patients seen within 2 weeks of the acute event.[18] Acute arterial occlusion can be the result of emboli from a distant source, thrombosis of a previously patent artery, or direct trauma to an artery (**Box 68.5**).

## BLUE TOE SYNDROME

Blue toe syndrome is a commonly seen condition characterized by the sudden appearance of a cool, painful, cyanotic toe or forefoot. It generally occurs in the presence of a palpable peripheral pedal pulse and warm forefoot. This syndrome is usually due to embolic occlusion of the digital arteries as a result of atheroemboli from proximal arterial sources. It is not typically due to local atherosclerotic disease. Identification of the embolic source and treatment of the diseased segment are required.

## ANKE-BRACHIAL INDEX

Because blood flow is diminished, the most common sensor used is the Doppler flowmeter. Calculation of the ankle-brachial index (ABI) is an accurate way to diagnose PAD. The ABI is a simple and relatively inexpensive test to confirm the clinical suspicion of occlusive arterial disease, and it provides a measure of the severity of the peripheral vascular disease.[19] The ABI is calculated by measuring systolic blood pressure with a Doppler probe in the brachial, posterior tibial, and dorsalis pedis arteries. The highest of the measurements in the ankle and foot is divided by the highest in the upper extremity. The ABI in normal individuals is 1.0 or greater; values higher than 1.3 usually indicate a calcified vessel that is noncompressible. An ABI of less than 0.9 has 95% sensitivity (100% specificity) for PAD and is associated with 50% or greater stenosis in one or more major vessels (**Box 68.6**).

## IMAGING

### Duplex Ultrasonography

The term *duplex ultrasonography* refers to B-mode real-time imaging and pulsed Doppler analysis of the velocity of flowing blood in arteries and veins. Arterial duplex ultrasonography provides a "road map" of stenosis of the arteries of the lower extremities. The sensitivity of duplex ultrasonography in detecting occlusions and stenosis is 95%, with a specificity of 98%.[20] The utility of performing duplex ultrasonography in the emergency department is limited because most decisions about patient care are based on the history and physical findings.

### Computed Tomographic Angiography

Computed tomographic angiography (CTA) is a vascular imaging technique that can be used to assess many vascular diseases rapidly and safely. Multidetector computed tomography can provide very high-quality resolution in comparison with the single-detector scanners from the not-so-distant past. CTA has the following advantages over regular angiography: (1) the images can be reconstructed from multiple angles and in multiple planes, (2) soft tissues and other anatomic structures are better identified, and (3) the technique is less invasive with fewer complications and lower cost.[1,21] CTA does, however, expose patients to radiation and potentially nephrotoxic dye loads. Because PAD is commonly multifocal, both arterial inflow and runoff should be imaged in their entirety. Studies have shown 100% concordance of CTA with angiography, as well as better visualization of other portions of distal vessels that are not seen with traditional angiography.[1,21]

### Magnetic Resonance Angiography

Magnetic resonance angiography (MRA) of the peripheral vasculature can be performed quickly and accurately. MRA has two distinct advantages over CTA: its contrast agents are not nephrotoxic, and images are obtained without exposure to radiation. The quality of MRA is now so good that it has virtually surpassed angiography for evaluating stable patients with PAD to determine what type of intervention is most appropriate.[22] MRA can assess not only vessel occlusion and stenosis but also the arterial wall for evidence of atherosclerosis.[23] MRA investigations require prolonged study times and transport from the emergency department, thus limiting their usefulness in emergency situations.

### *Diagnostic Angiography*

Catheter-based angiography yields images of the vascular lumen. Any condition that requires luminal evaluation for diagnosis or characterization is best assessed with this technique. Catheter-based angiography is very important in the evaluation of atherosclerotic, thrombotic, and embolic occlusions because it provides access for some definitive modalities and is indispensable before most percutaneous and surgical procedures related to lower extremity atherosclerotic disease. The contrast materials used today are much safer and more tolerable than previous agents. One adverse effect of contrast administration, renal toxicity, has not been reduced by use of low-osmolality agents. Contrast agent–induced renal impairment can be decreased by identifying patients at risk for renal impairment, attempting to correct comorbid conditions, limiting the amount of contrast agent given, and ensuring appropriate hydration of the patient.

In digital subtraction angiography (DSA), the image is acquired, converted with an image intensifier, transferred to a monitor, and saved in digital format. DSA is a computer-assisted radiographic technique that subtracts images of bone and soft tissue to permit viewing of the cardiovascular system. Structures that do not change during injection are canceled out, which results in the "disappearance" of structures such as bone, soft tissues, and air. Improved hardware, software, and speed of the techniques combined with better outcomes from interventions mean that DSA is heavily relied on for vascular disease. The need for lower concentrations of iodinated contrast agents or the use of nonnephrotoxic agents also makes it a more desirable imaging technique than regular angiography.[24] The major attributes of DSA that contribute to its importance are high resolution, ability to selectively evaluate individual vessels, and ability to access direct physiologic information from the tissues. Despite the diagnostic paradigm shift away from angiography, DSA is a cornerstone technology in PAD intervention and will probably remain so for the foreseeable future.[19]

## TREATMENT

The spectrum of PAD ranges from asymptomatic to critical limb ischemia, and coronary artery disease and other atherosclerotic vascular disorders may coexist with PAD. Indications for urgent intervention are (1) incapacitating claudication that interferes with work or lifestyle and (2) limb salvage in persons with limb-threatening ischemia, as manifested by rest pain, nonhealing ulcers, or infection or gangrene.

Prompt initiation of therapy is the most important aspect of the treatment of acute limb ischemia. Patients should immediately receive a heparin bolus followed by an infusion to prevent clot propagation and inhibit thrombosis distal to the lesion, where low flow or stasis is present. Heparin should be administered before diagnostic testing is performed.[25,26] Subsequent therapy depends on whether the extremity is viable, threatened, or nonviable.

### PATIENTS WITH VIABLE EXTREMITIES

Patients found to have an ischemic but viable extremity on clinical examination should undergo urgent arteriography. Once the anatomy has been defined, vascular surgeons can determine whether surgical or intraarterial thrombolytic therapy is needed. One study reported limb salvage rates of approximately 70% with both thrombolytic therapy and surgical intervention in this patient population.[27] The important thing for the emergency physician to remember is that thrombolytic therapy is limited by the length of time needed to dissolve the thrombus and the severity of the ischemia. Thrombolytics are given at the site of occlusion through the catheter used for angiography. This method has been shown to have a better outcome with fewer bleeding complications than is the case with intravenous administration. Both urokinase and tissue plasminogen activator have been studied and appear to be similar in outcome measures. Patients who have had ischemic symptoms for less than 14 days and are treated with thrombolytics have better amputation-free survival and shorter hospital stays than do those who undergo surgery; patients with ischemic symptoms for longer than 14 days have a better outcome with surgical intervention. In addition, in patients who have received thrombolytic therapy and eventually require surgical intervention, the magnitude of the surgical procedure is less than in patients who have not received thrombolytics.

The surgeon and interventional radiologist help determine the optimal therapy for a patient with limb ischemia and a viable extremity according to (1) the location and length of the lesion, (2) the cause (embolus versus thrombus), (3) the duration of symptoms, and (4) the suitability of the patient for surgery. In general, smaller, more distal emboli are best treated with thrombolytics, whereas a large embolus at a more proximal location is best treated by embolectomy[27] (**Figs. 68.3 and 68.4**).

### PATIENTS WITH THREATENED EXTREMITIES

Patients with threatened extremities should undergo immediate surgical revascularization.[25] The vast majority of such patients have had an embolic event. Irreversible changes, including necrosis, may occur within 4 to 6 hours of the initial insult, thus leaving a fairly small therapeutic window. The small amount of time available makes thrombolytic therapy of limited utility[27,28] (**Figs. 68.5 and 68.6**).

Surgery usually reveals an embolus that can be removed by embolectomy. After embolectomy, most surgeons perform intraoperative arteriography to assess distal blood flow. If small distal emboli are found after embolectomy, intraoperative thrombolytic therapy may be considered. If the ischemia has been prolonged, compartment syndrome may result once blood flow is restored. Therefore, oral anticoagulation should be instituted after the procedure to prevent subsequent embolization.[26]

### PATIENTS WITH NONVIABLE EXTREMITIES

If clinical evaluation of a patient's extremity reveals nonviability, amputation should proceed promptly.[25] Angiography is not normally required to make this diagnosis, and the clinical findings dictate the level of amputation. In general, surgeons

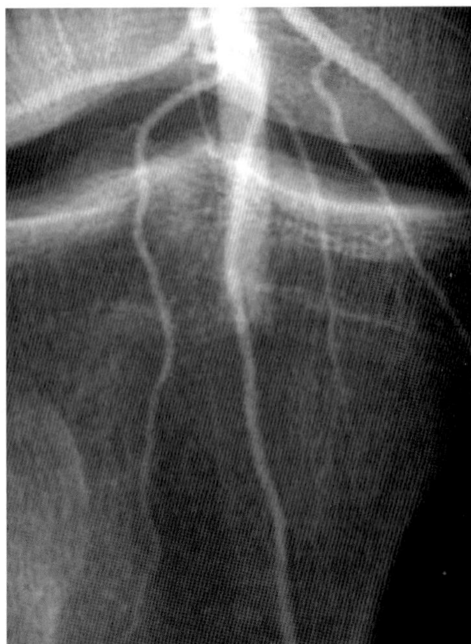

**Fig. 68.3 Popliteal artery with a sharp cutoff of the contrast material in a patient with a painful, acutely ischemic leg.** See Figure 68.4.

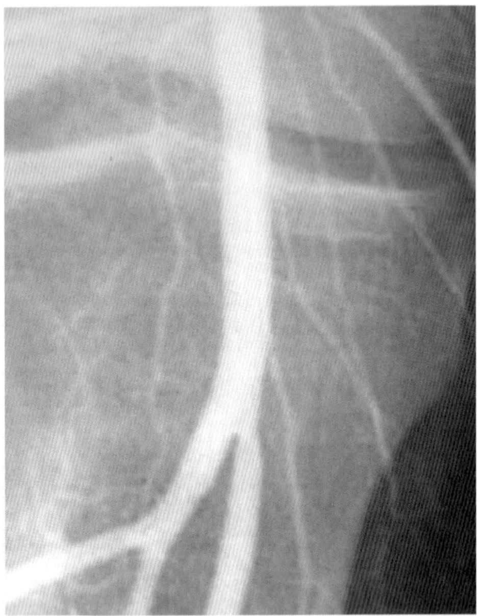

**Fig. 68.4 Leg of the same patient as in Figure 68.3 after administration of a thrombolytic agent.** Note the resumption of normal flow distal to the previous obstruction.

try to preserve as many joints as possible to decrease the work of ambulating with a prosthesis. If amputation is not performed in an expedient manner, the patient may have complications such as sepsis, acute renal failure, rhabdomyolysis, hyperkalemia, and cardiovascular collapse.

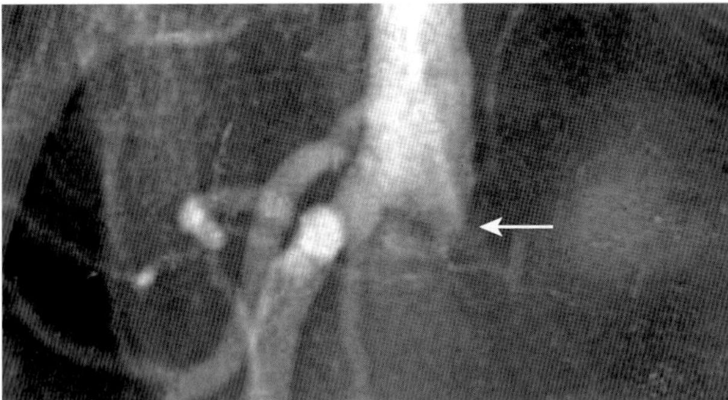

**Fig. 68.5 Angiogram of a patient with embolic disease at the proximal femoral artery as it bifurcates to the deep femoral system *(arrow)*.** Note the abrupt cutoff of contrast material. See Figure 68.6.

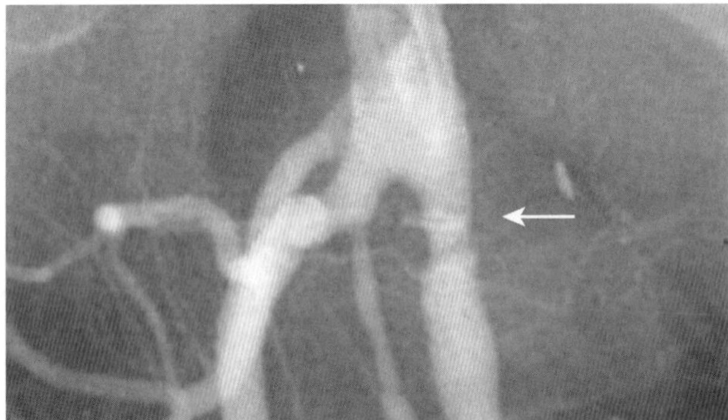

**Fig. 68.6 Angiogram of the same patient as in Figure 68.5 after thrombectomy.** Note the resolution of flow and absence of visible clot *(arrow)*.

## NONISCHEMIC PERIPHERAL ARTERIAL DISEASE

Patients who have nonischemic PAD should be referred for follow-up with vascular surgery. Initial therapy should include institution of an exercise program and risk factor modification, along with antiplatelet therapy.[29]

## FOLLOW-UP, NEXT STEPS IN CARE, AND PATIENT EDUCATION

Vascular diseases are common, and prompt treatment can diminish disability and death. Individual health can be preserved (better functional status and survival) and public health goals achieved (e.g., diminished rates of amputation, fewer cardiovascular ischemic events and death) by establishing an accurate vascular diagnostic assessment and treatment plan. Patients with nonischemic PAD can be discharged with instructions for risk factor modification and follow-up with a vascular surgeon. Any patient with signs of ischemic PAD should be admitted to the hospital as part of evaluation and treatment.

Of patients in whom PAD develops in association with symptoms of intermittent claudication, 70% to 80% will have stable symptoms at 5 years, with the remaining 10% to 20%

having worsening claudication. Five percent to 10% will require revascularization in the subsequent 5-year period. Over the same interval, about 1% to 2% of patients will have critical leg ischemia, some of whom will require amputation.[6,30] Predictors of progression include cigarette smoking, diabetes, high cholesterol, and hyperlipidemia.[31] It should be noted that there is both wide geographic and wide ethnic variation in the outcome of PAD. White persons are more likely to undergo aortoiliac surgery and less likely to need lower extremity amputation than other ethnic groups are.[32] This discrepancy cannot be explained by the higher prevalence of risk factors in other ethnic groups.

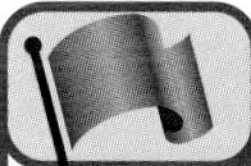

**RED FLAGS**

- Risk for peripheral arterial disease increases in a powerful dose-dependent manner with the number of cigarettes smoked per day and the number of years of smoking.
- Ischemic fissures, decubitus ulcers of the ankles and heels, and ischemic ulcers correlate with arterial insufficiency.
- More than one third of patients with embolic disease have skin manifestations, thus making them the most common physical finding.
- In contrast to patients with ischemia pain, those with peripheral neuropathy usually have bilateral leg pain that is not relieved by dependency, as well as neurologic signs such as decreased deep tendon reflexes and loss of touch and vibratory sensation.
- Attempts at limb salvage in a patient with hard neurologic findings indicative of prolonged ischemia may endanger the life of the patient because of the severe metabolic changes that occur after revascularization.
- Acute extremity ischemia is associated with high rates of limb loss (30%) and hospital morbidity and mortality (20%).

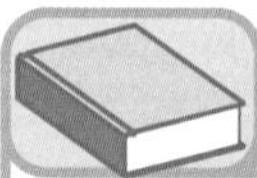

**PATIENT TEACHING TIPS**

- Physicians must educate patients on the importance of pain as a symptom of significant arterial disease and the need for immediate evaluation to save a limb.
- Modification of risk factors, especially smoking, can not only arrest progression of the disease but may also, in some cases, reverse some of the clinical effects.
- Patients with peripheral arterial disease must also undergo testing for associated coronary artery disease because of the close association of the two disease processes.

## REFERENCES

*References can be found on Expert Consult @ www.expertconsult.com.*

# 69 Hypertensive Crisis

*Philip Shayne and Catherine A. Lynch*

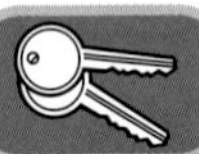

**KEY POINTS**

- Hypertension is a common, serious disease that is often undertreated.
- Hypertensive urgency or emergency is the presence of elevated risk for or actual end-organ dysfunction caused by the elevated blood pressure. Severely elevated blood pressure itself does not create an emergency.
- A hypertension evaluation is, primarily, the assessment of key organ systems.
- Hypertensive emergencies are decompensated processes requiring immediate stabilization.
- Hypertensive urgencies occur in patients with underlying target organ disease and no evidence of current compounded dysfunction but who have higher risk for near-term complications.
- Severely elevated blood pressure alone does not usually require aggressive therapy.
- Therapy should be determined by the underlying pathology.
- Frequently, the most important intervention is establishing good primary care.

## EPIDEMIOLOGY

Worldwide, as many as 1 billion people suffer from hypertension, and about 7.5 million deaths per year are attributed to hypertension.[1] Approximately 28.9% of individuals in the United States, or 85 million, are affected by hypertension.[2,3] Less than two thirds of U.S. adults with hypertension are aware of their condition, less than half are currently undergoing treatment of it, and only 30% have their blood pressure under control, yet of those seen in hypertensive crisis, it has been previously diagnosed in most of them and they have inadequate blood pressure control.[4] Although hypertensive crisis develops in only 1% of patients with hypertension, some studies have found that hypertensive emergencies account for 28% of all patient visits to the emergency department (ED) for medical complaints, 21% of which were hypertensive urgencies and 6.4% were hypertensive emergencies.[5] Preeclampsia (pregnancy-induced hypertension with proteinuria) occurs in 7% of pregnancies and most frequently in primigravidas.[4] Uninsured populations, who receive a disproportionate amount of their care in EDs, have a higher prevalence and poorer control of elevated blood pressure. In inner-city public EDs, as many as 20% of the adult population have been found to have blood pressure higher than 140/90 mm Hg.[5-7] As an important cardiovascular, cerebrovascular, and renal failure modifiable risk factor, a modest 5–mm Hg decrease in the population is estimated to reduce stroke mortality by 9% and cardiovascular deaths by 12%.[8]

## PATHOPHYSIOLOGY

Hypertension is multifactorial and includes genetic and environmental causes, and the causes of hypertensive crises are poorly understood.[9] Hypertension coincides with elevated peripheral vascular resistance (PVR) and normal to low cardiac output.[10] The mechanism of the disease is probably an imbalance in autoregulation of the renin-angiotensin system. Malignant-accelerated hypertensive crises are thought to be due to an abrupt increase in PVR caused by humoral vasoconstrictors leading to endothelial injury, vascular permeability, activation of the coagulation cascade, and necrosis of arterioles.[11,12] Other hypertensive crises occur when the elevated blood pressure of patients with hypertension exacerbates injury to target organs; it often results in a pathologic feedback loop, which further elevates the blood pressure and exacerbates the damage.

## PRESENTING SIGNS AND SYMPTOMS

Hypertensive disease occurs in organ systems in which injury to arterioles leads to ischemic damage or hemorrhage. These target organs include the brain, heart, blood vessels, and kidneys (**Box 69.1**). Therefore, the clinical history and physical examination must include an evaluation of these organ systems.

**BOX 69.1 Common Symptoms of Hypertension**

**Neurologic**
Headache
Visual changes
Altered mental status
Seizures
Nausea

**Cardiovascular**
Chest pain
Back pain
Dyspnea

**Renal**
Oliguria
Anuria
Proteinuria

**BOX 69.2 Hypertensive Emergencies**

**Primary**
Hypertensive encephalopathy
Accelerated-malignant hypertension

**Secondary**

***Cerebrovascular Accidents***
Thromboembolic stroke
Hemorrhagic stroke
Subarachnoid hemorrhage

***Cardiovascular Crises***
Myocardial infarction
Acute coronary syndromes
Cardiogenic pulmonary edema
Aortic dissection
Uncontrollable arterial bleeding

***Renal Crises***
Acute renal failure
Glomerular nephritis
Severe hypertension after kidney transplantation

***Other Emergencies***
Preeclampsia or eclampsia
Perioperative hypertension
Catecholamine excess

## DIFFERENTIAL DIAGNOSIS

Persistently elevated blood pressure can trigger or exacerbate crises in these target organs. Rapid and progressive target organ damage secondary to severely elevated blood pressure defines a hypertensive emergency.[13,14] Less commonly, hypertension is the primary crisis. Increasing systemic pressure causes an inflammatory endovasculitis; further damage and aggravation as a result of adrenergic stimulation and vasoconstriction accelerate the elevated blood pressure. The multiorgan disease resulting from an overwhelmed autoregulatory function is called malignant-accelerated hypertension. Inflammatory changes in the cerebral vasculature produce a serious alteration in mental status termed hypertensive encephalopathy. Primary and secondary hypertensive emergencies that must be included in the initial differential diagnosis are listed in **Box 69.2**.

### HYPERTENSIVE ENCEPHALOPATHY

The triad of severe hypertension, altered mental status, and (often) papilledema characterizes hypertensive encephalopathy, and it may be accompanied by lethargy, confusion, headache, visual disturbances, and seizures. Somnolence, stupor, and nausea or vomiting may also occur. Retinopathy may or may not be present. The mechanism of the disease is loss of autoregulation as a result of the cerebral overperfusion caused by profound hypertension; when the hypertension is controlled, the patient's mental status improves. Persistent overperfusion results in vasodilation and increased permeability of cerebral blood vessels, which in turn leads to the development of cerebral edema. If not adequately treated, hypertensive encephalopathy can progress to cerebral hemorrhage, coma, and death.

Hypertensive encephalopathy is most likely to occur in previously normotensive individuals who experience a rapid rise in blood pressure, such as children with acute glomerulonephritis and young women with preeclampsia or eclampsia. Because chronically hypertensive patients usually experience a more gradual rise in blood pressure, cerebrovascular decompensation is less likely. Hypertensive encephalopathy produces characteristic findings on computed tomography (CT). Scans show a posterior leukoencephalopathy that predominantly affects the white matter of the parietooccipital regions bilaterally. CT is useful in excluding other causes of altered mental status such as intracranial bleeding.

### ACCELERATED-MALIGNANT HYPERTENSION

Accelerated-malignant hypertension occurs most commonly in young African American males with underlying renal parenchymal disease or renovascular disease. It is most commonly found in patients with long-standing hypertension and usually occurs without encephalopathy.[10] When endothelial vasodilator responses are overwhelmed, further hypertension and endothelial damage occur and lead to inflammatory vasculopathy. Marked elevation in blood pressure and characteristic eyeground findings make the diagnosis. Flame-shaped hemorrhages develop around the optic disk because of the high intravascular pressure, and soft exudates are caused by ischemic infarction of the nerve fibers secondary to occlusion of the supplying arterioles. Common symptoms include headache (85%), visual blurring (55%), nocturia (38%), and weakness (30%). Laboratory evidence includes azotemia, proteinuria, hematuria, hypokalemia, and metabolic alkalosis. Papilledema is considered the sine qua non of malignant hypertension. Accelerated hypertension is used to describe the same condition (hemorrhages and exudates) without papilledema. Because the absence of papilledema does not connote a different clinical prognosis or therapy, the term *accelerated-malignant hypertension* is now recommended.

## CEREBROVASCULAR HYPERTENSIVE CRISIS

Hypertension frequently complicates the management of patients with cerebrovascular accidents (CVAs). After a CVA patients generally have focal neurologic deficits that are somewhat predictable based on the territory of the brain affected. A thorough neurologic examination can elucidate clues about the vessel in which flow has been disrupted either by occlusion or by hemorrhage. Ischemic strokes result from three major categories: thrombotic, embolic, and hypoperfusion. Compromised blood flow produces cell death at the center of the ischemic region and reversibly damaged neurons in the periphery, also known as the penumbra. The penumbra's viability depends on its perfusion. Hemorrhagic stroke is caused by either intracranial or subarachnoid bleeding. Intracranial pressure (ICP) increases and cerebral perfusion pressure (CPP) is reduced at the site of the hematoma. Therefore, maintaining cerebral perfusion is key in both types of CVA, and an understanding of cerebrovascular physiology is helpful in determining the best treatment strategy.

Cerebral blood flow (CBF), a function of CPP, is equal to mean arterial pressure (MAP) minus ICP (CPP = MAP − ICP). The process of vasoconstriction and vasodilation of the cerebral vasculature maintains a steady CBF. However, cerebral autoregulation fails at approximately 25% above or below the patient's usual MAP. In addition, changes in ICP or brain injury can result in loss of the brain's ability to autoregulate blood flow. Increased ICP, commonly seen with hemorrhage or edema, decreases CPP and makes the brain more vulnerable to changes in MAP. In normal individuals, CBF remains fairly constant at MAP values of approximately 60 mm Hg up to 150 mm Hg. When MAP decreases to less than the lower limits of autoregulation, the brain becomes hypoperfused and cerebral hypoxia develops, with symptoms such as dizziness, nausea, and syncope. In chronically hypertensive individuals, the lower limit of autoregulation increases, and autoregulation might fail at MAP values that are well tolerated in nonhypertensive individuals. This suggests that chronically hypertensive patients cannot tolerate a rapid return to "normal" blood pressure and that MAP should be acutely decreased by no more than 20% to 25%.

## CARDIOVASCULAR HYPERTENSIVE CRISIS

Hypertensive emergencies involving the heart and great vessels include congestive heart failure, acute coronary syndromes, and aortic aneurysm or dissection. Blood pressure is frequently elevated in patients with acute pulmonary edema, particularly when a high-output state is the cause, such as volume overload with renal failure, thyrotoxicosis, or severe anemia. Transient diastolic dysfunction, which may or may not be a direct result of the elevated blood pressure, also causes acute pulmonary edema with hypertension and congestive heart failure. Symptoms include tachypnea, tachycardia, pulmonary rales, jugular venous distention, and an $S_3$ gallop.

Acute coronary syndromes are also frequently accompanied by hypertension. Reducing myocardial work by lowering blood pressure and the heart rate has been demonstrated to decrease infarct size in patients not receiving thrombolytic therapy. Classically, patients have symptoms of chest pain, dyspnea, diaphoresis, nausea, and light-headedness.

Acute aortic dissection is thought to occur as a result of aortic dilation or high blood pressure superimposed on a structural weakness of the arterial wall causing a tear in the intimal layer. Pulsatile pressure extends the dissection by separating the layers of the arterial wall. Historical series report a mortality of 1% to 2% per hour. The stresses that extend the dissection are thought to be related as much to the aortic pulse wave or pulse pressure (the difference between systolic and diastolic pressure over time) as it is to MAP. Heart rate, myocardial contractility, and MAP all contribute to increased pulse pressure. Affected patients include elderly persons with hypertension or atherosclerotic disease and individuals with connective tissue disorders. Hallmark symptoms are acute, severe retrosternal pain radiating to the back or intrascapular pain. Patients may have pulse deficits, neurologic symptoms, or ischemic symptoms in involved organs such as the gut, kidney, or heart.

$SI = \frac{SV}{BSA}$ **FACTS AND FORMULAS**

Mean arterial pressure (MAP) = (Systolic pressure + [2 × Diastolic pressure])/3

Cerebral perfusion pressure (CPP) = MAP − Intracranial pressure (ICP)

Pulse pressure (dp/dt) = (Systolic pressure − Diastolic pressure)/Heart rate

## RENOVASCULAR HYPERTENSIVE CRISIS

The kidney is unique in being both a target organ and the cause of many hypertensive emergencies. Hypertension causes 30% of cases of end-stage renal disease, which makes it the second most common cause after diabetes. Nephrosclerosis may develop in chronically hypertensive patients after 10 to 15 years and is manifested as damage to the medial layer of capillaries, reduced kidney size, and nonnephrotic levels of proteinuria without hematuria. By contrast, malignant hypertension damages the intimal layer of the renal capillary bed and may result in enlarged kidneys, cellular urinary sediment, hematuria, and severe proteinuria.

Severe hypertension in a young patient raises the possibility of intrinsic acute renal disease, such as glomerulonephritis. IgA nephropathy has surpassed poststreptococcal glomerulonephritis in frequency, and Henoch-Schönlein purpura is the most likely cause of acute glomerular disease in children.

Renal artery stenosis is present in only 1% of unselected hypertensive patients but is seen in 4% of blacks and 32% of whites who have severe hypertension (diastolic blood pressure > 125 mm Hg with retinopathy). It is also more common in patients with a rapidly progressive course. Occasionally, devastating acute renal failure may occur as a result of intrarenal vasculitis. This is common in the setting of scleroderma and may be responsive to angiotensin-converting enzyme inhibitors (ACEIs).

## CATECHOLAMINE EXCESS

The most familiar drugs found to cause hypertension in EDs today are sympathomimetic drugs such as phenylephrine, cocaine, and methamphetamine. Tyramine can induce a hypertensive crisis in patients taking a monoamine oxidase inhibitor, and hypertension can complicate withdrawal syndromes from alcohol, benzodiazepines, clonidine, and beta-blockers. Pheochromocytoma can cause intermittent hypertensive crisis and may be responsible for many clinical findings besides hypertension, such as headache, sweating, palpitations, pallor, nausea, and rarely, seizures. Some patients with pheochromocytoma may have paroxysms of low blood pressure as well.

### HYPERTENSION IN PREGNANCY

Third trimester emergencies are addressed separately in Chapter 121. Emergencies include eclampsia and preeclampsia. Pregnant women between 20 weeks' gestation and 2 weeks postpartum who have any degree of hypertension (≥140/90 mm Hg) or an increase of more than 30/15 mm Hg above their baseline blood pressure, accompanied by peripheral edema and proteinuria, have preeclampsia. Hypertension is important mainly as a symptom of the underlying disorder rather than as a cause. Preeclampsia is essential to recognize because it can progress suddenly to eclampsia, defined by the occurrence of convulsions. Additional symptoms include headache, visual changes, epigastric pain, oliguria, facial and extremity edema, and HELLP syndrome (hemolysis, elevated liver enzymes, and low platelet count). Eclampsia can rapidly progress to coma or death. Magnesium infusion is more effective than other anticonvulsants in this setting. Because definitive treatment consists of delivery of the fetus, the emergency physician (EP) usually collaborates with an obstetrician early in the patient's course through the department.

## MEDICAL DECISION MAKING

EPs evaluate and treat hypertension in a variety of contexts ranging from compliant patients with well-controlled blood pressure, to asymptomatic patients with increased blood pressure, to critically ill patients with increased blood pressure and acute target organ deterioration. Many patients with severely elevated blood pressure have a combination of long-standing, poorly treated hypertension and acute aggravating conditions such as pain, anxiety, or intoxication. Though a major public health risk, elevated blood pressure is rarely a crisis in the ED. Evidence-based national guidelines exist for the evaluation and treatment of hypertension,[15,16] but there is no good evidence to guide the acute treatment of a patient with severely elevated blood pressure. Instead, the EP relies on an understanding of the disease process, its associated complications, and the health care support available to the patient.

Patients often have elevated blood pressure and nonspecific symptoms. The EP must make a prospective decision about the cause of the symptoms to determine management of the blood pressure. If a hypertensive patient's chest pain is possibly anginal, immediate parenteral control might be necessary. However, if the EP determines that the pain is not cardiovascular in origin, the same patient might not need immediate treatment of the elevated blood pressure. Findings on assessment of the patient determine the need for treatment.

The concept of hypertensive urgency, which refers to markedly elevated, asymptomatic blood pressure requiring rapid intervention, is no longer widely used. Most patients without acute, progressive target organ disease can have their severely elevated blood pressure managed on an outpatient basis. However, certain patients are at higher risk for near-term complications from their uncontrolled hypertension. This group includes the elderly or frail and especially those with a history of previous end-organ disease (e.g., history of stroke, heart failure, renal insufficiency). These patients do require increased vigilance and possibly aggressive intervention.

## DIAGNOSTIC TESTING

The nature, severity, and management of hypertensive crises are determined by clinical evaluation. When a patient with markedly elevated blood pressure is seen in the ED, accurate measurement of blood pressure is the first step. Blood pressure that is initially elevated in the ED frequently decreases spontaneously by the time that a second reading is obtained.[17,18] Any intervention should be based on the composite of several repeated blood pressure measurements. To obtain an accurate measurement, the patient should be seated with the arm at the level of the heart and at least 80% of the arm circumference covered with the cuff bladder. Pressure is evaluated in both arms. Blood pressure measurement with an automated cuff may be inaccurate in patients with atrial fibrillation and other heart rhythm irregularities. Appropriate pain management and relief of the underlying cause (e.g., hypoxia, bladder distention) may resolve the hypertension. Certain medications, over-the-counter preparations, or illicit drugs may transiently exacerbate hypertension (**Box 69.3**).

**TIPS AND TRICKS**

- Elevated triage blood pressure readings often spontaneously improve without treatment. Always recheck abnormal readings.
- An initially elevated blood pressure might resolve with proper cuff size or treatment of pain, urinary retention, or hypoxia.
- If no emergency is anticipated and immediate parental therapy is not required, patients should be given a dose of the medications that they were supposed to have taken so that some effect has occurred if and when they are ready to be discharged.
- Become comfortable with a small number of parental agents; in most instances any one will work.
- Elicit a history of use of cocaine or other sympathomimetic drugs.

**BOX 69.3 Medications That Can Elevate Blood Pressure or Interfere with the Effectiveness of Antihypertensive Agents**

Oral contraceptives
Steroids
Nonsteroidal antiinflammatory drugs
Nasal decongestants
Cold remedies
Appetite suppressants
Tricyclic antidepressants
Monoamine oxidase inhibitors

If the patient's blood pressure is persistently elevated, elicitation of the history should start with an assessment of symptoms that might be consistent with target organ compromise. Details include the duration and severity of preexisting hypertension, success with previous blood pressure regimens, and any history of target organ disease (cardiovascular, cerebrovascular, renovascular, and great vessel). Physical examination should be directed toward identifying signs of target organ damage. Funduscopic examination showing retinal hemorrhage or papilledema is sufficient to diagnose accelerated-malignant hypertension. The cardiovascular examination focuses on identifying signs of heart failure (e.g., increased jugular venous pressure, pulmonary rales, and $S_3$ heart sound). The neurologic examination assesses the level of consciousness, visual fields, and the presence of focal motor and sensory deficits.

The patient's symptoms direct the EP's diagnostic evaluation. For example, dyspnea or signs of heart failure are an indication for a chest radiograph, and neurologic findings are an indication for CT of the head. Box 69.1 summarizes some common symptoms and their associated end-organs. Few studies have assessed the prognostic value of laboratory testing in asymptomatic patients with severely elevated blood pressure.[19] However, asymptomatic patients with blood pressure persistently higher than 180/110 mm Hg warrant a brief assessment of target organ function (**Fig. 69.1**). Because renal failure is silent, measurement of serum creatinine or urinalysis (or both) for evidence of renal failure or nephritis is reasonable. An electrocardiogram (ECG) is useful in assessing the baseline level of left ventricular hypertrophy, ischemia, or infarction. The presence of left ventricular hypertrophy on an ECG carries a poor prognosis and necessitates a more vigilant

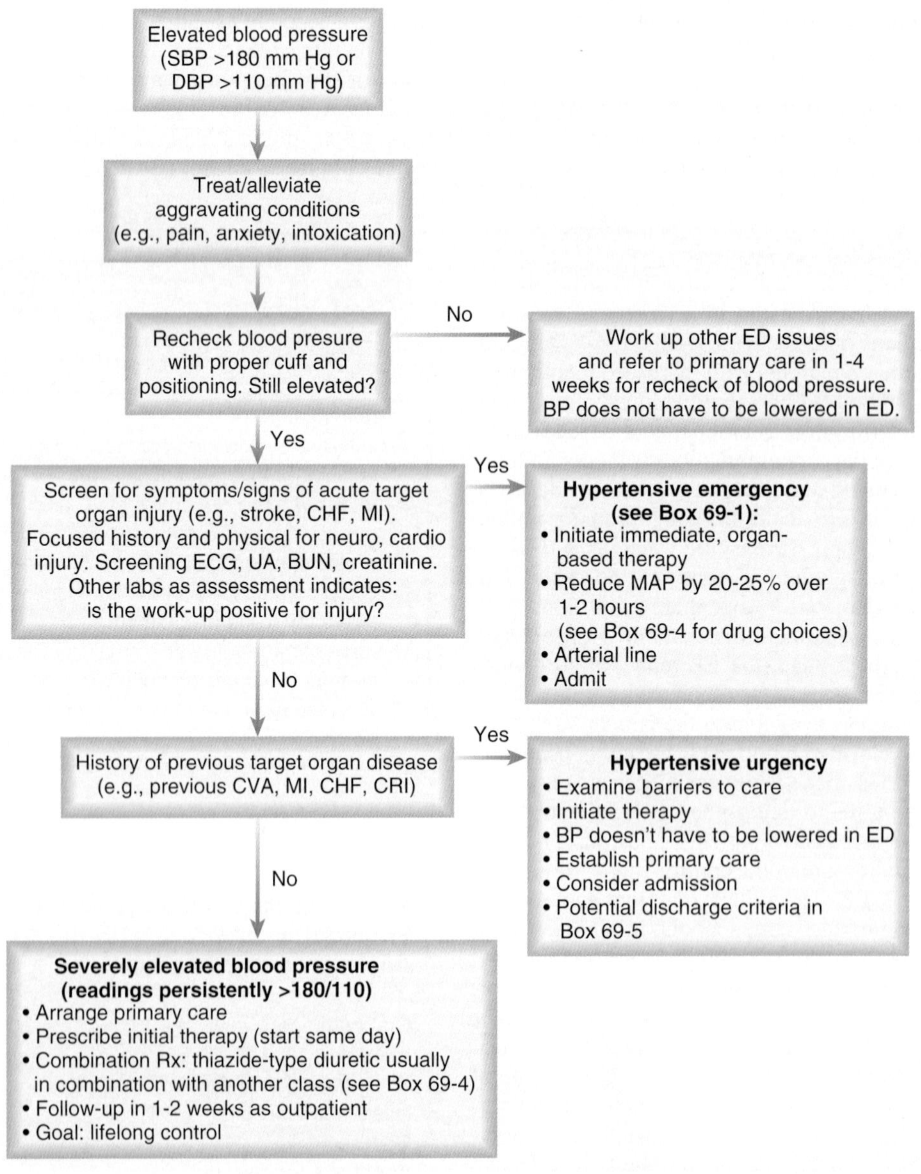


**Fig. 69.1 Management of patients with severely elevated blood pressure (BP).** *BUN*, Blood urea nitrogen; *CHF*, congestive heart failure; *CRI*, chronic renal insufficiency; *CVA*, cerebrovascular accident; *DBP*, diastolic BP; *ECG*, electrocardiogram; *ED*, emergency department; *MAP*, mean arterial pressure; *MI*, myocardial infarction; *Rx*, therapy; *SBP*, systolic BP; *UA*, urinalysis.

follow-up. When renovascular disease or hypercortisolism is suspected to be a cause of the hypertension, serum should be drawn to determine plasma renin activity and aldosterone levels before administering medications. A urine screen for cocaine and amphetamines may help confirm extrinsic causes of the elevated blood pressure. The value of obtaining a chest radiograph or a complete blood count in patients in the ED without relevant symptoms is likely to be low.

## TREATMENT

### PREHOSPITAL MANAGEMENT

To date, the role of prehospital treatment of hypertension or hypertensive emergencies is minimal. Hypertension complicating angina or pulmonary edema should be treated with nitrates (other medications are not time critical if transport time is brief). Emergency medical service providers should not lower blood pressure in patients with a possible stroke because of the possibility of extending the ischemic region.

### HOSPITAL MANAGEMENT

Ideally, ED management of hypertensive crises would entail the administration of fast-acting, rapidly reversible medications that can easily be titrated to the desired effect of a 20% decrease in MAP. No single agent is optimal in all cases of hypertensive crisis. The agent of choice and the manner of administration depend on the severity of the blood pressure abnormality, the severity and type of end-organ dysfunction present, and the clinical findings.

### HYPERTENSIVE EMERGENCY

The goal of therapy in patients in hypertensive crisis is a 20% to 25% reduction in MAP over a period of 1 to 2 hours. The ideal drug for treating hypertensive emergencies would easily titrate blood pressure through rapid onset, rapid maximal effect, and rapid offset.[5,20-22] These characteristics are found only in parenteral agents. **Table 69.1** summarizes the most commonly used medications and doses.

Nitroprusside is the classic agent for the treatment of patients with hypertensive emergencies. Nitroprusside decreases both preload and afterload without significant reflex tachycardia through arteriovenous vasodilation. It has a quick onset of action, and its effect lasts for only 2 to 5 minutes after use of the drug is discontinued. Hemodynamics must be monitored closely to prevent inadvertent hypotension. Thiocyanate toxicity may occur if the drug is administered for more than 48 to 72 hours, particularly in patients with renal failure. It is contraindicated in pregnancy. Because no oral form is available, the patient must be switched to a different antihypertensive once control is achieved. Despite the many benefits of nitroprusside, other agents are often better suited for individual hypertensive crises.

Nicardipine is a rapidly acting parenteral calcium channel blocker. It has a predictable and smooth onset of action, but it is relatively long acting. Esmolol is a beta-blocking agent that is both rapid in onset and of short duration, thus making it easy to titrate. Labetalol, an easily titratable medication, combines alpha- and beta-blockade, which makes it more potent than esmolol. Comparatively, labetalol maintains a more consistent CPP and has a longer half-life. This enables the administration of miniboluses instead of a constant infusion but makes it more difficult to titrate downward. Caution is advised when administering beta-blockers to patients with asthma, chronic obstructive pulmonary disease, acute congestive heart failure, cocaine abuse, or other contraindications to beta-blockade. Fenoldopam is a parenteral dopaminergic receptor blocking agent with an excellent efficacy and safety profile. Fenoldopam holds some promise as being equivalent to nitroprusside in efficacy without the rare side effects associated with nitroprusside's cyanide moiety and perhaps with less overshoot hypotension, but it is costly. Other options include enalaprilat, a parenteral ACEI, and phentolamine, a pure alpha-blocking agent.

### CEREBROVASCULAR CRISIS

Blood pressure control should be undertaken with caution in patients with cerebrovascular hypertensive emergencies.[23] Parenteral drugs that have a short half-life, are easily titrated, and have minimal effect on the cerebral vasculature are ideal. Because labetalol does not dilate cerebral capacitance vessels, it is theoretically attractive in patients with intracerebral disorders. Caution should be used with direct vasodilators such as nitroprusside in patients with focal brain injury because they can extend an area of ischemia. Although nicardipine is safe and widely used, other calcium channel blockers have been linked to a rise in ICP and are therefore not favored in patients with brain injury.

Treatment of elevated blood pressure in the setting of ischemic CVAs is controversial. When systemic blood pressure is reduced, cerebral autoregulation may fail, thereby extending the ischemic penumbra surrounding the infarct and leading to extension of the stroke. Alternatively, infarction may lead to edema, elevated ICP, and a further reduction in CBF. The current American Stroke Association guidelines recommend lowering blood pressure in patients with stroke only when MAP is greater than 130 mm Hg or systolic blood pressure is greater than 220 mm Hg.[23]

Theoretically, treatment of elevated blood pressure in patients with hemorrhagic CVAs and subarachnoid hemorrhage should be more aggressive than in patients with ischemic strokes. The rationale is to decrease the risk for ongoing bleeding from ruptured small arteries and arterioles; however, the relationship between rebleeding and systemic blood pressure is unproven.[24] As with ischemic CVAs, overly aggressive treatment of hypertension may worsen brain injury by decreasing CPP when ICP is increased. The American Stroke Association guidelines for blood pressure control in patients with hemorrhagic stroke are similar to those for ischemic stroke: blood pressure should be lowered only when MAP is greater than 130 mm Hg or systolic blood pressure is greater than 220 mm Hg. Nimodipine, an oral calcium channel blocker, may be administered to decrease the incidence of vasospasm and rebleeding after subarachnoid hemorrhage, but the drug is not recommended for blood pressure control.

### CARDIOVASCULAR CRISIS

Nitroglycerin (NTG) is favored for the treatment of severe hypertension complicating cardiac ischemia. NTG is a direct vasodilator that affects the venous more than the arterial vasculature. NTG dilates the coronary arteries and, in contrast to nitroprusside, promotes a favorable redistribution of blood flow to ischemic areas. Beta-blockers are also effective and

**Table 69.1 Parenteral Drugs for Treatment of Hypertensive Emergencies**

| DRUG | DOSE* | ONSET OF ACTION | DURATION OF ACTION | ADVERSE EFFECTS† | SPECIAL INDICATIONS |
|---|---|---|---|---|---|
| **Vasodilators** | | | | | |
| Sodium nitroprusside | 0.25-10 mcg/kg/min as IV infusion‡ (maximal dose for 10 min only) | Immediate | 1-2 min | Nausea, vomiting, muscle twitching, sweating, thiocyanate and cyanide intoxication | Most hypertensive emergencies; caution in patients with high intracranial pressure or azotemia |
| Nicardipine hydrochloride | 5-15 mg/hr IV | 5-10 min | 1-4 hr | Tachycardia, headache, flushing, local phlebitis | Most hypertensive emergencies except acute heart failure; caution in patients with coronary ischemia |
| Fenoldopam mesylate | 0.1-0.3 mcg/kg/min as IV infusion | <5 min | 30 min | Tachycardia, headache, nausea, flushing | Most hypertensive emergencies; caution in patients with glaucoma |
| Nitroglycerin | 5-100 mcg/min as IV infusion‡ | 2-5 min | 3-5 min | Headache, vomiting methemoglobinemia, tolerance with prolonged use | Coronary ischemia |
| Enalaprilat | 1.25-5 mg every 6 hr IV | 15-30 min | 6 hr | Precipitous fall in pressure in high-renin states; response variable | Acute left ventricular failure; avoid in patients with acute myocardial infarction |
| Hydralazine hydrochloride | 5-20 mg IV<br>10-50 mg IM | 10-20 min<br>20-30 min | 3-8 hr | Tachycardia, flushing, headache, vomiting, aggravation of angina | Eclampsia |
| Diazoxide | 50-100 mg as IV bolus repeated or as 15- to 30-mg/min infusion | 2-4 min | 6-12 hr | Nausea, flushing, tachycardia, chest pain | Now obsolete; used when intensive monitoring not available |
| **Adrenergic Inhibitors** | | | | | |
| Labetalol hydrochloride | 20-80 mg as IV bolus every 10 min or as 0.5- to 2.0-mg/min IV infusion | 5-10 min | 3-6 hr | Vomiting, scalp tingling, burning in throat, dizziness, nausea, heart block, orthostatic hypotension | Most hypertensive emergencies except acute heart failure |
| Esmolol hydrochloride | 250-500 mcg/kg/min for 1 min, then 50-100 mcg/kg/min for 4 min; may repeat sequence | 1-2 min | 10-20 min | Hypotension, nausea | Aortic dissection, perioperative |
| Phentolamine | 5-15 mg IV | 1-2 min | 3-10 min | Tachycardia, flushing, headache | Catecholamine excess |

Modified from Lenfant C, Chobanian AV, Jones DW, et al. Seventh report of the Joint National Committee on the Prevention, Detection, Evaluation, and Treatment of High Blood Pressure (JNC 7): resetting the hypertension sails. Hypertension 2003;41:1178-9.

*These doses may vary from those in the *Physicians' Desk Reference* (51st edition).

†Hypotension may occur with all agents.

‡Requires a special delivery system.

recommended therapy for acute coronary syndromes. The goal of treatment in patients with acute coronary syndromes is reduction of blood pressure to normal if evidence of ischemia persists.[25] However, careful blood pressure reduction requires intensive patient monitoring; overly vigorous lowering of blood pressure may worsen the ischemia because coronary perfusion depends on diastolic blood pressure.

Most critical cases of congestive heart failure are treated with a combination of NTG, furosemide, and an ACEI. For patients with pulmonary edema and hypertension, sublingual NTG should be initiated while preparing intravenous NTG. Captopril should be administered orally or sublingually or enalaprilat administered intravenously. If systemic fluid overload is present, intravenous furosemide should be administered. However, up to 25% of patients with heart failure and severely elevated blood pressure may have "dry failure" in which pressure natriuresis makes them fluid depleted. Further diuresis may exacerbate the process and continue to stimulate the renin-angiotensin axis. The decision should be based on clinical judgment of whole-body fluid status. Although beta-blockers have been found to improve survival in patients with chronic congestive heart failure, use in patients with acute pulmonary edema may precipitate immediate worsening because of their negative inotropic effects and bradycardia. Intravenous nesiritide improves hemodynamic function and symptoms in patients with decompensated heart failure and has a modest antihypertensive effect,[26] but it has not been well studied in the setting of hypertensive crisis.

With aortic dissection, progression of the vascular injury is dependent not only on the elevated blood pressure but also on the aortic ejection velocity or tachycardia-induced sheer forces. Therefore, a rate-controlling agent such as esmolol should be initiated before starting nitroprusside to avoid the effects of reflex tachycardia.[27] Alternatively, labetalol, nicardipine, or fenoldopam has been suggested as possible substitutes for nitroprusside. Labetalol achieves its maximal effect within minutes and then remains effective for several hours, thus allowing titration with small boluses and avoiding the constant monitoring and increased cost required with nitroprusside. Nicardipine and fenoldopam are vasodilators that would require the intensive monitoring needed with nitroprusside but are less toxic alternatives.[28]

### RENOVASCULAR CRISIS

When compared with nitroprusside, fenoldopam may improve outcomes in patients with hypertension and acute renal failure. Even though malignant hypertension may precipitate acute renal failure by injuring the kidney's microvasculature, this causal chain is often reversed with chronic renal failure when long-term renal damage is manifested as severe hypertension. Because this distinction cannot be made in the ED, all these patients should have their blood pressure lowered. Both nitroprusside and labetalol are excellent choices in this setting. Although ACEI drugs definitely improve the prognosis of patients with chronic hypertension and mild proteinuria, they should be used cautiously in hyperkalemic patients with acute uremia. Nitroprusside may cause thiocyanate poisoning over a period of several days in patients with renal failure; it should be used only it briefly or if the patient will undergo dialysis soon.

Treatment with an ACEI may reverse high blood pressure dramatically in patients with unilateral renal artery stenosis, but it may provoke acute renal failure and severe hyperkalemia in patients with bilateral stenosis, particularly if they are taking supplemental potassium or a potassium-sparing diuretic. This complication can be completely reversed by discontinuing the ACEI.

### CATECHOLAMINE EXCESS

Patients with severe hypertension secondary to pheochromocytoma are treated with the pure alpha-blocker phentolamine administered intravenously. It may be accompanied by a beta-blocker if needed for tachycardia. Administration of beta-blockers alone in the setting of any sympathomimetic (e.g., cocaine) may leave the alpha receptors "open," with subsequent worsening of the hypertension.[29] Thus, an attractive alternative to beta-blockers is labetalol, a beta-blocker with some alpha-antagonist properties. However, the alpha- and beta-blockade with labetalol may not be equally effective.[30] Additionally, benzodiazepines are useful adjuncts in patients with cocaine-induced catecholamine excess. They decrease both the central and peripheral sympathomimetic outflow stimulated by cocaine, thereby lowering the heart rate, psychomotor hyperactivity, and blood pressure.

### HYPERTENSION IN PREGNANCY

The mainstay of antihypertensive treatment of pregnant patients in hypertensive crisis in many institutions is hydralazine administered intravenously in boluses of 5 to 10 mg every 20 to 30 minutes. This is in addition to magnesium therapy for control of seizures. If the hypertension is refractory to hydralazine, second-line agents are diazoxide and beta-blockers. Calcium channel blockers have been studied in pregnant patients with chronic hypertension, but they may not be effective in treating proteinuric hypertension.

## CONSULTATION

Hypertensive emergencies require admission to a monitored setting. These patients generally require emergency involvement of an appropriate specialist for management of a neurologic, cardiovascular, or renovascular crisis. Close blood pressure monitoring, preferably with an arterial line, is indicated. Patients with preeclampsia or eclampsia require emergency obstetric consultation.

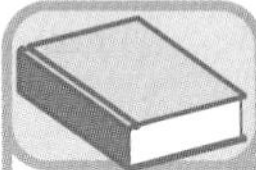

**PATIENT TEACHING**

Uncontrolled hypertension causes profound and irreversible internal injuries over the long term, many of which are asymptomatic.

Transient blood pressure elevation is rarely dangerous, and management decisions must be based on evidence of extended hypertension.

There are many medications with different convenience and side effect profiles that the primary care provider can substitute to find a good match.

Adherence to a medication regimen is essential for healthy living.

Chest pain, difficulty breathing, severe and new headaches, and focal numbness or weakness are possible signs of heart or brain injury and should be evaluated by a doctor immediately.

## NEXT STEPS IN CARE AND ADMISSION

All hypertensive patients with evidence of end-organ dysfunction require hospitalization for management of their blood pressure, treatment of their organ dysfunction, and consultation with appropriate specialists.

Most patients with elevated blood pressure are not in crisis. Very few asymptomatic patients with markedly increased blood pressure will experience a near-term adverse event. Very high blood pressure might be seen in chronically hypertensive patients as a consequence of discontinuing previous therapy or as a result of other easily reversible causes, such as anxiety, pain, drug use, or change in diet.[31,32] No evidence

**BOX 69.4 Initial Drug Choices for Hypertension**

Use unless contraindicated. Start with a low dose of a long-acting once-daily drug and titrate the dose; low-dose combinations might be appropriate.

**Uncomplicated Hypertension**
Diuretics
Beta-blockers

**Diabetes Mellitus (Type 1) with Proteinuria**
Angiotensin-converting enzyme (ACE) inhibitors

**Heart Failure**
ACE inhibitors
Diuretics

**Isolated Systolic Hypertension (Older Person)**
Diuretics preferred
Long-acting dihydropyridine calcium antagonist

**Myocardial Infarction**
Beta-blockers (without intrinsic sympathomimetic activity)
ACE inhibitors (with systolic dysfunction)

has shown that the absolute level of a patient's blood pressure warrants immediate or aggressive treatment. Rather, in patients with asymptomatic, elevated blood pressure and no evidence of target organ disease, the most important intervention is to ensure proper follow-up. The goal should be lifelong control of the blood pressure.

When the elevated blood pressure may be the artifact of a systemic process such as pain or infection, the best strategy is to refer the patient for reevaluation of the blood pressure once the primary problem has resolved. If the patient has discontinued the blood pressure medications, the regimen should be restarted, barriers to compliance evaluated, and a primary care physician contacted to ensure reevaluation in a week. The hypertension guidelines recommend a thiazide-type diuretic as an initial agent, usually in combination with a drug from another class.[15,33] The second agent may be from a number of categories and is best chosen in accordance with any compelling indications in the patient's history (**Box 69.4**).

In principle, in individuals without a previous measurement of elevated blood pressure, the blood pressure needs to be rechecked at another visit before the diagnosis of hypertension can be made. However, in individuals with readings persistently higher than 180/110 mm Hg in the ED, the latest national guidelines recommend that combination therapy be started immediately (same day).[15] In the best scenario, the EP contacts a primary physician for the patient, who then selects an initial antihypertensive agents or agents and provides follow-up within about a week.

An intermediate group of patients has severely elevated blood pressure and known target organ disease but no active decompensation. An example is a severely hypertensive patient with a previous history of myocardial infarction or stroke. Immediacy arises because a patient with known target organ disease may be considered at higher risk for a hypertension-related adverse event in the short term. However, there is no good evidence base for the best management of these patients. A treatment strategy should be initiated in the ED, although blood pressure does not necessarily need to be

**BOX 69.5 Discharge Criteria for "Hypertensive Urgency"**

1. Likely to be compliant with established primary care
2. Known to have hypertension
3. Reversible precipitating cause (e.g., medication noncompliance, adverse drug effect)
4. Able to resume a previously effective medication regimen
5. Can be seen for follow-up within 7 days.

lowered during the visit. These patients do require an increased level of vigilance. It may be reasonable to treat them as outpatients, although some may need to be held for short-term observation if their medication compliance or blood pressure monitoring is uncertain; the decision depends on clinical judgment (see **Box 69.5**).

In practical terms, hypertensive emergencies require an immediate (within 1 to 2 hours) decrease in blood pressure, hypertensive urgency requires initiation of a strategy to decrease and monitor blood pressure over a 24- to 48-hour period, and uncontrolled severe hypertension requires therapy to decrease blood pressure within 1 week. Stratification within these categories involves careful clinical evaluation and understanding of target organ disease and treatment strategies.

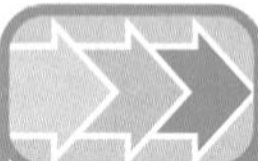

**PRIORITY ACTIONS**

**Severely Elevated Blood Pressure**

Recheck the patient's blood pressure with the correct method in both arms.
Evaluate and treat aggravating conditions (e.g., pain, anxiety, intoxication).
Evaluate for evidence of target organ damage.
Elicit a history of target organ disease.
Administer therapy based on the underlying pathology.
Reevaluate continuously for signs of response to therapy or deterioration.

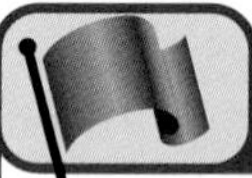

**RED FLAGS**

Diagnosing a hypertensive emergency when one does not exist. Patients with hypertensive emergencies have evidence of acute end-organ dysfunction.
Reducing blood pressure too quickly or to too low a level in patients with chronic hypertension whose autoregulation curve has been reset can lead to cerebral or cardiac ischemia.
Lowering a patient's blood pressure acutely without an urgent indication.
Failing to diagnose hypertension or preeclampsia in pregnant patients with blood pressures higher than 140/90 mm Hg or with an increase in blood pressure of more than 30/15 mm Hg.
Neglecting to match the antihypertensive agent to the clinical scenario.

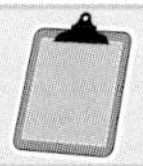

## DOCUMENTATION

Be sure that any elevated blood pressure is noted and addressed.

Be sure to document any change in blood pressure with treatment.

Document possible causes of the elevated blood pressure.

List any past medical history of target organ disease.

List current antihypertensives and any recent changes in medications or noncompliance.

Document the presence or absence of end-organ dysfunction found during assessment of the patient's elevated blood pressure.

Document patient counseling for medications, reasons to return, and primary care follow-up.

## SUGGESTED READINGS

Chobanian AV, Bakris GI, Black HR, et al. The seventh report of the Joint National Committee on Prevention, Detection, Evaluation, and Treatment of High Blood Pressure: the JNC 7 report. JAMA 2003;289:2560-72.

Decker WW, Goodwin SA, Hess EP, et al. Clinical policy: critical issues in the evaluation and management of adult patients with asymptomatic hypertension in the emergency department. Ann Emerg Med 2006;47:237-49.

Gilmore RM, Miller SJ, Stead LG. Severe hypertension in the emergency department patient. Emerg Med Clin North Am 2005;23:1141-58.

Karras DJ, Ufberg JW, Heilpern KL, et al. Elevated blood pressure in urban emergency department patients. Acad Emerg Med 2005;12:835-43.

Varon J. Treatment of acute severe hypertension: current and newer agents. Drugs 2008;68:283-97.

## REFERENCES

***References can be found on Expert Consult @ www.expertconsult.com.***

# 70 Pulmonary Embolism

D. Mark Courtney

## KEY POINTS

- Appropriate testing for pulmonary embolism (PE) requires both an understanding of the pretest probability for each individual patient and knowledge of the characteristics of the diagnostic test used at your specific institution.
- A pretest probability of less than 10% with a negative D-dimer result that has a sensitivity of at least 95% is sufficient to rule out PE in most clinical circumstances.
- Right heart strain on an echocardiogram or electrocardiogram, decreased oxygen saturation, elevated brain natriuretic peptide, and elevated troponin may predict a worse short- and long-term outcome in patients in whom PE is diagnosed.
- Treatment of PE consists of heparin and initiation of warfarin to prevent additional clot formation.
- Treatment of shock associated with PE includes intravenous fluid, vasopressors, respiratory support, and thrombolytic therapy.
- PE represents a spectrum of severity determined by the size of the clot and baseline cardiopulmonary disease.
- The probability of mortality increases steeply once right ventricular dysfunction and hypotension occur.
- Diagnosis of PE as a cause of shock requires consideration of PE as a potential cause and a stepwise approach to simultaneous testing and resuscitation.

## EPIDEMIOLOGY

The annual incidence of diagnosed pulmonary embolism (PE) is approximately 1.5 new cases per 1000 persons and is relatively similar among Western populations.[1] Dyspnea and chest discomfort are the most typical symptoms of PE, and these chief complaints are responsible for between 9 and 10 million annual patient visits to U.S. emergency departments (EDs).[2] Physicians evaluate large numbers of patients for PE because the symptoms can be vague and severity may range from asymptomatic to shock and subsequent cardiac arrest.[3]

The widespread availability of D-dimer and computed tomography (CT) testing for PE, as well as medical-legal concerns of missing the diagnosis, continues to result in dramatic increases in testing relative to the last decade. In some settings it is not uncommon for 1% to 3% of all adult ED patients to undergo some testing for PE. Physicians have become aware that patients without what was previously thought to be "classic" risk factors (hypercoagulability, trauma, and immobility) may still have PE. In addition, the aging demographics of the U.S. population will continue to drive the need to evaluate for PE in the ED because increased age is a strong independent risk factor for PE. To deal with these challenges, the practicing physician has three aims:

1. Recognize the potential for PE to exist in the appropriate settings
2. Perform the optimal test based on pretest probability and specific test characteristics
3. Be capable of estimating the prognosis for each patient after the diagnosis is made and institute appropriate therapy

## PATHOPHYSIOLOGY

PE is part of the continuum of venous thromboembolism (VTE), which most often starts with deep vein thrombosis (DVT) in the leg. Patients with DVT often have concurrent PE when evaluated with imaging tests, and many patients with PE have concurrent DVT. Treatment is similar for both. Risk factors for VTE include the triad described by Virchow: injury, venous stasis, and hypercoagulability. These conditions are most commonly thought of as occurring at the level of the venous endothelium, but it is helpful to also think of them as occurring at the level of the patient. For instance, overall injury to the patient (trauma), stasis of the patient (immobility), and hypercoagulability of the patient (malignancy and known thrombophilic conditions) all result in elevated risk. **Table 70.1** lists several risk factors for VTE. Understanding risk factors is critical to recognizing the potential for PE to exist.

An embolus in the pulmonary vasculature may result in a large bilateral central clot with severe obstruction of flow (so-called saddle embolism), a medium clot in the lobar or segmental branches, or a small clot in the peripheral vasculature. Embolism involving the pulmonary vasculature activates the process of local inflammation and thereby leads to vasoconstriction and some degree of pulmonary hypertension with resultant symptoms of dyspnea and possibly chest pain.

**Table 70.1 Risk Factors for Pulmonary Embolism**

| RISK FACTORS | SPECIFIC NOTES |
|---|---|
| Previous history of PE or DVT | Inquire about the setting and circumstance of the previous VTE |
| Recent trauma or surgery | In general, trauma requiring admission or surgery requiring general anesthesia within the previous month. Recent long-bone trauma or surgery may especially increase the risk |
| Cancer | In general, patients with currently treated cancer or palliative care. Remotely treated and inactive cancer probably does not increase the probability of PE |
| Age | Risk significantly increases above the age of 50 to 60 years |
| Oral contraceptives | Especially third-generation formulations |
| Hormone replacement therapy | Contemporary patients are less commonly receiving hormone replacement |
| Pregnancy | Risk increases along with the duration of pregnancy; it peaks at term and then decreases over a period of 4 to 6 weeks postpartum |
| Immobility | Includes casts and splints, as well as permanent limb or generalized body immobility |
| Factor V Leiden mutation | Most common in northern European populations. A heterozygous carrier state exists in 3% to 7% of many samples. Homozygous mutation is less common and confers three times greater risk for VTE relative to the normal genotype |
| Antiphospholipid antibody syndrome | Very potent risk factor that is associated with large and recurrent PE. It may be associated with anticardiolipin antibodies, CVA, MI, and first-trimester miscarriages |
| Prothrombin mutation | |
| Hyperhomocysteinemia | Can occur as a result of inadequate folate and vitamin B intake, as well as with a genetic mutation in methyltetrahydrofolate reductase |
| Deficient levels of clotting factors | Protein C, protein S, antithrombin III |
| Congestive heart failure | |
| Chronic obstructive pulmonary disease | |
| Air travel | Primary risk with travel of more than 5000 km (3100 miles) and concurrent other risk factors |
| Obesity | Elevated at a body mass index higher than 25 and even greater risk if higher than 29 |

*CVA*, Cerebrovascular accident; *DVT*, deep vein thrombosis; *MI*, myocardial infarction; *PE*, pulmonary embolism; *VTE*, venous thromboembolism.

## PRESENTING SIGNS AND SYMPTOMS

Dyspnea and chest pain are the most common findings in patients with PE. Brief, resolved chest pain in the absence of any shortness of breath or any respiratory signs or symptoms is not a typical manifestation. Other symptoms that can be associated with PE include syncope, cough, flank pain, abdominal pain, and even fever (**Box 70.1**). The severity of symptoms in a given patient is a function of two factors: the baseline cardiopulmonary status of the patient and the size of the clot[4] (**Fig. 70.1**). This is why large clots are occasionally tolerated fairly well in young patients with no cardiopulmonary disease whereas a much smaller clot burden may result in hypotension, hypoxemia, and deterioration in patients with preexisting cardiopulmonary disease. Older patients often have a worse clinical course and outcome with PE, largely as a consequence of having worse cardiopulmonary status at baseline rather than simply being elderly.

Shock may be a primary sign of PE. Patients may not be able to provide a history of symptoms or risk factors for PE and may not be sufficiently stable to allow imaging outside the ED, yet consideration of empiric treatment of PE with anticoagulation may be warranted. A rapid bedside evaluation to search for clues to non-PE diagnoses can be done promptly and is described in **Figure 70.2**. A potential pitfall is to attribute shock to a primary

**BOX 70.1 Symptoms That May Be Present in Patients in Whom Acute Pulmonary Embolism Is Diagnosed**

Dyspnea
Pleuritic chest pain
Substernal chest pain
Syncope
Cough
Anxiety
Hemoptysis
Dizziness, lightheadedness

cardiac etiology despite an electrocardiogram (ECG) with no significant ischemic changes and no significant dysrhythmia and a chest radiograph with no evidence of pulmonary vascular congestion or cardiomegaly. If patients can be stabilized, imaging with CT should be done. If not, emergency bedside echocardiography to look for signs of massive PE (right ventricular dilation and hypokinesis, septal shift to the left, tricuspid regurgitation) should be done as an alternative means of heightening certainty of the diagnosis of PE.

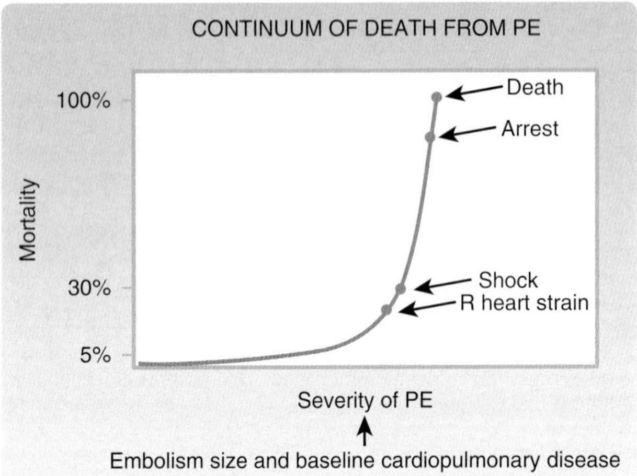


**Fig. 70.1** The degree of severity of symptoms in a given patient is a function of two factors: (1) the baseline cardiopulmonary status of the patient and (2) the size of the clot. *PE*, Pulmonary embolism; *R*, right. (Adapted from Wood KE. Major pulmonary embolism: review of a pathophysiologic approach to the golden hour of hemodynamically significant pulmonary embolism. Chest 2002;121:877-905.)

The other end of the spectrum is the diagnosis of PE in patients with relatively mild symptoms. Despite the fact that patients may have PE with normal oxygen saturation, no known risk factors, and no pulmonary symptoms, this combination is uncommon. Strict attention to details such as oxygen saturation after walking, physician-obtained respiratory rate, examination of the legs, and serial assessment may help either reassure physicians that patients have such a low probability of PE that testing is unwarranted or provide evidence to justify an evaluation for PE.

## DIFFERENTIAL DIAGNOSIS AND MEDICAL DECISION MAKING

Because of the vague yet common nature of dyspnea and chest pain, the differential diagnosis is broad. However, a targeted diagnostic approach should be used rather than a "chest pain work-up" in an attempt to test for every diagnosis possible without regard to the pretest probability or negative consequences of overtesting. This is particularly important for PE because tests are not 100% sensitive or specific and the consequences of a false-positive diagnosis may include 6 months of oral anticoagulation with high direct and indirect costs to the patient and society. This is especially true in young patients with limitations in activity, as well as in older patients at risk for falls, medication interaction, and bleeding. **Table 70.2** lists potential alternative diagnoses in ED patients evaluated for PE and clues to assist in rapid decision making. It is not

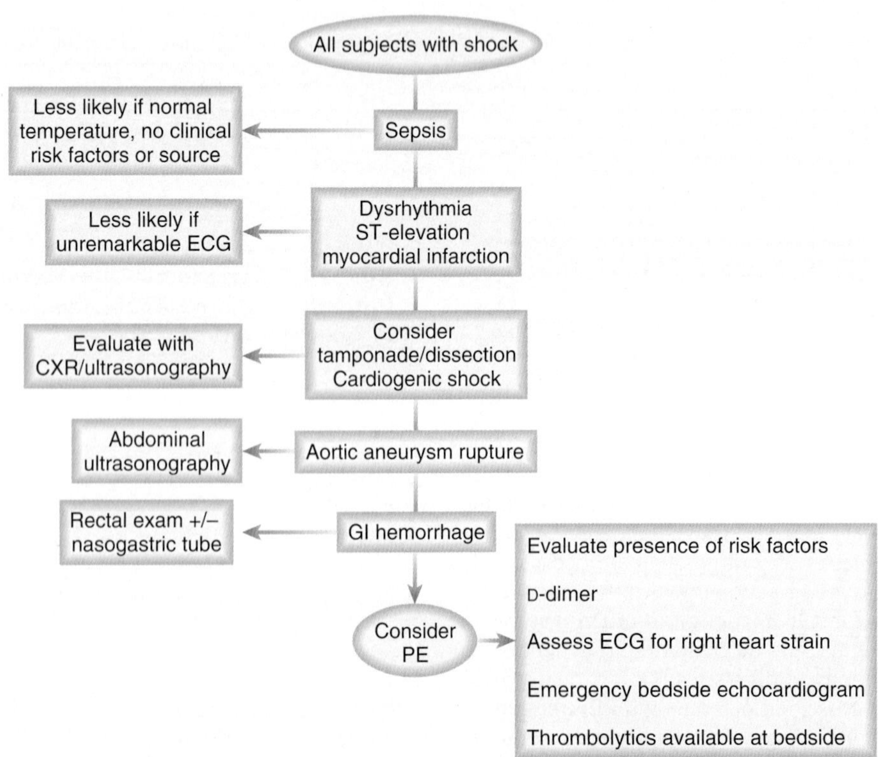


**Fig. 70.2 Stepwise approach to undifferentiated shock with consideration of pulmonary embolism (PE) as a possible cause.** *CXR*, Chest x-ray; *ECG*, electrocardiogram; *GI*, gastrointestinal.

surprising that many of these conditions are common entities such as pneumonia, bronchitis, asthma, musculoskeletal pain, gastroesophageal reflux or spasm, and anxiety or panic attack. Many of the most threatening alternative diagnoses can initially be evaluated with a chest radiograph, an ECG, bedside cardiac ultrasound, and cardiac enzyme testing during the first hour in the ED.

It is most helpful to think of PE as a continuum of cardiopulmonary stress as shown in Figure 70.1. Even in normotensive patients, in-hospital or 30-day mortality in those with diagnosed PE is approximately 8% to 13%.[5-9] This mortality in PE patients without shock is greater than that for acute myocardial infarction.[10] When early signs of right heart dysfunction occur, mortality begins to curve upward. This is followed by compensated shock, which may initially respond to intravenous fluid. Later, as left-sided filling is decreased because of septal shift into the left ventricle, as well as decreased filling of the left atrium, overt shock is present and mortality is in excess of 30%. If untreated, cardiac arrest ensues, with pulseless electrical activity being the most likely first rhythm.[11,12]

**Table 70.2 Other Diagnoses That Should Be Considered Along with Pulmonary Embolism**

| DIAGNOSIS | MEANS OF RAPIDLY OBTAINING CLUES |
|---|---|
| **Potential Threats to Life** | |
| Myocardial ischemia, cardiogenic shock, dysrhythmia, congestive heart failure | ECG/CXR |
| Pneumothorax | CXR |
| Cardiac tamponade | Bedside cardiac ultrasound |
| Pneumonia | CXR |
| Esophageal rupture | CXR |
| Pulmonary malignancy (metastatic or primary) | CXR, history |
| Asthma | Examination, history |
| Aortic dissection | History |
| Pericarditis | ECG |
| **Non–Life-Threatening** | |
| Bronchitis | History |
| Chest wall pain | History |
| Pleuritis, pleurisy | History |
| GERD, esophageal spasm, peptic ulcer disease | History |
| Panic attack | History |

*CXR*, Chest x-ray; *ECG*, electrocardiogram; *GERD*, gastroesophageal reflux disease.

## DIAGNOSTIC TESTING

Pretest probability is the probability that the physician believes to be present before any test results are obtained. It is typically calculated by either a scoring system or the physician's own "gestalt" estimation. Despite the fact that debate exists over the relative accuracy of using gestalt versus a structured means of assessing pretest probability, the American College of Emergency Physicians practice guideline of 2003 recommended pretest probability assessment in patients being evaluated for PE.[13]

The main structured pretest probability system with the longest track record of use and investigation is the Canadian score derived by Wells et al., which results in a score for an individual patient that can be used to estimate ranges of pretest probability[14] (**Table 70.3** and **Fig. 70.3**). Widespread clinical application of this scoring system can be challenging because of difficulty in physician recall[15] and the fact that it provides a range of probability rather than an exact estimate. An alternative to these structured pretest probability systems is unstructured or implicit estimation systems whereby physicians arrive at their own pretest probability based on their experience and overall integration of clinical information for a unique patient. This is commonplace but imprecise and subject to wide variability.[16] Recent data from a large multicenter study of ED patients in the United States found that several variables not in the Wells score may be significantly associated with the outcome of PE in ED patients who are tested. These variables are noted in Figure 70.3 and may be important in addition to the Wells score in formulating overall pretest probability.[17]

The most typical approach to testing for PE is to determine whether the pretest probability is sufficiently low (Wells score ≤ 4 or physician's gestalt of "low risk") and then to use a sensitive D-dimer blood test that detects the presence of fibrin breakdown products (see Fig. 70.3). If D-dimer is normal in

**Table 70.3 Components of the Wells Score**

| WELLS SCORE | POINTS |
|---|---|
| Alternative diagnosis less likely | 3 |
| Signs and symptoms of DVT | 3 |
| History of PE or DVT | 1.5 |
| Surgery or immobilization within 1 mo | 1.5 |
| Pulse > 100 beats/min | 1.5 |
| Hemoptysis | 1 |
| Cancer | 1 |
| **With a score of 4 or less, the pretest probability is 5% or less; with a score higher than 4, the pretest probability is greater than 5%.** | |

Other factors to consider include estrogen use (oral contraceptive pill or hormone replacement therapy), thrombophilic condition, pleuritic nature of the chest pain if present, family history of PE or DVT, and oxygen saturation lower than 95%.
*DVT*, Deep vein thrombosis; *PE*, pulmonary embolism.

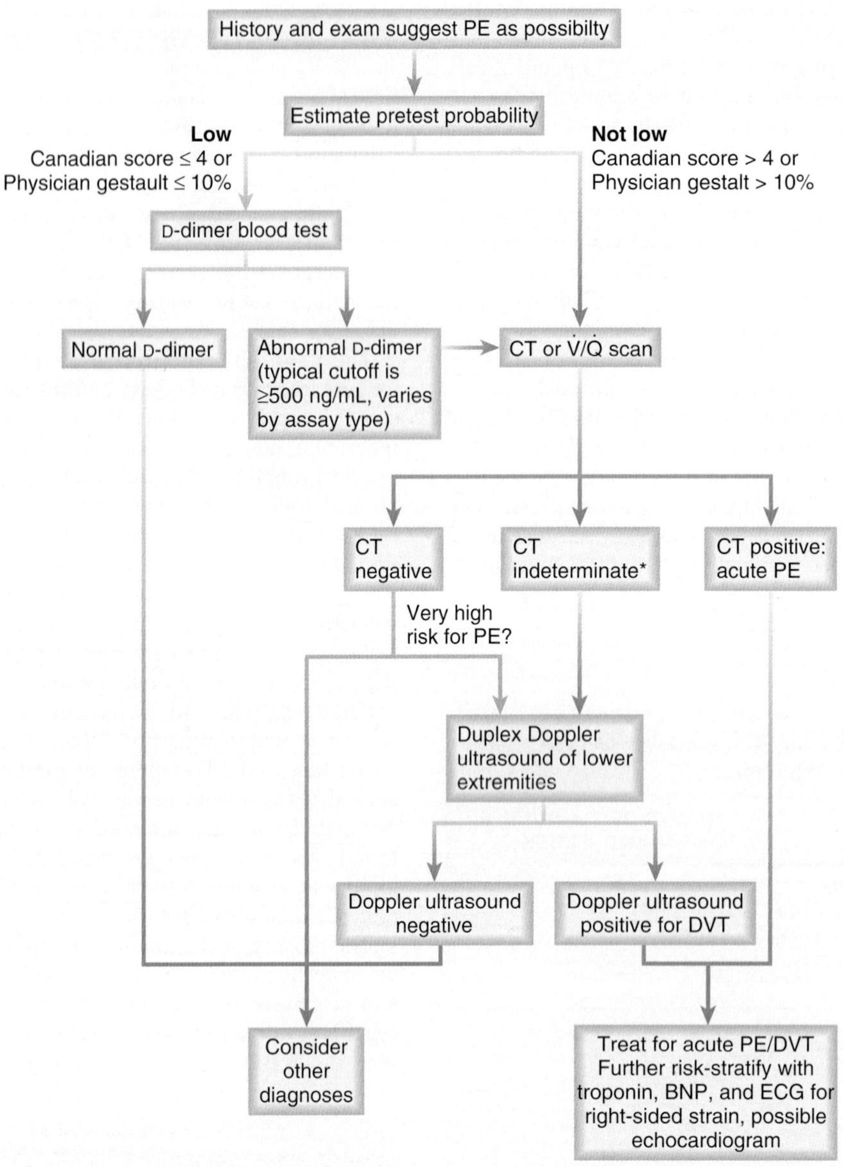


**Fig. 70.3 Typical algorithmic approach to ruling out pulmonary embolism (PE).** *BNP*, B-type natriuretic peptide; *CT*, computed tomography; *DVT*, deep vein thrombosis; *ECG*, electrocardiogram; *V̇/Q̇*, ventilation-perfusion.

these low-risk patients, the posttest probability of PE is below a sufficient test threshold (<1% to 2%), and PE can be considered to be sufficiently excluded in these patients.[18,19] Typically, two types of D-dimer tests are available for ED testing: (1) quantitative tests, including enzyme-linked immunosorbent assay or immunoturbidimetric tests, which are considered to be abnormal at a particular cutoff, typically ≥500 ng/mL, and (2) qualitative whole blood agglutination or immunofiltration tests, which yield a binary result of positive or negative. Benefits of the quantitative tests include higher sensitivity. Benefits of the qualitative tests include rapid results because of bedside testing. **Table 70.4** describes how the two different types of D-dimer tests may be used to rule out PE. These are estimates of diagnostic test performance, and individual tests will vary in their actual sensitivity, specificity, and likelihood ratio, thus emphasizing the importance of clinician knowledge of the specific test at their institution.

Unfortunately with these tests, 20% to 40% of positive results may be falsely positive because of the low specificity of these blood tests. These patients require confirmation of the presence or absence of PE with an imaging test, usually a CT scan of the pulmonary arteries or a ventilation-perfusion (V̇/Q̇) scan. If imaging tests are negative in these low-risk patients, PE can be considered to be sufficiently excluded.

The decision to test for PE should always assume that if D-dimer is positive, more definitive tests would be undertaken. It is therefore important to consider the possible consequences of radiation exposure, contrast reaction, and volume overload

**Table 70.4 Comparison of Two Different Types of D-Dimer Tests**

| Pretest probability | 10% or less | 5% or less |
|---|---|---|
| Type of D-dimer | Quantitative: ELISA or turbidimetric test | Qualitative: whole blood agglutination or immunofiltration tests |
| Approximate sensitivity | 94% | 85%* |
| Approximate specificity | 55% | 60% |
| Likelihood ratio with a negative result | 0.1 | 0.25 |
| Probability of PE after a negative test (posttest probability) | ≤1.2% | ≤1.3% |

*ELISA*, Enzyme-linked immunosorbent assay; *PE*, pulmonary embolism.
*Low sensitivity makes this test unfavorable.

**BOX 70.2 Pulmonary Embolism Rule-Out Criteria**

If all the criteria below are met, the probability of PE is below a test threshold of 1.8% and testing may be more harmful than beneficial.

- Age < 50
- Pulse < 100 beats/min
- Oxygen saturation > 94%
- No hemoptysis
- No clinical evidence of DVT
- No hormone use
- No recent surgery or trauma
- No past history of PE or DVT

*DVT*, Deep vein thrombosis; *PE*, pulmonary embolism.

from the osmotic effects of contrast agents; concerns in pregnant patients; and the overall safety of leaving the ED when initiating testing for PE.

For these reasons, as well as the significant negative impact that a false-positive diagnosis may have for the patient because of months of anticoagulation, attempts to reduce testing in very low-risk settings have been proposed. One such method is the PE rule-out criteria shown in **Box 70.2**.[18,20] It was derived from a multicenter U.S. sample and provides simple, easy-to-apply clinical criteria that when satisfied, indicate that the baseline probability of PE is below a test threshold (<1.8%) and testing in this setting may be more likely to lead to patient harm than benefit. This is only an attempt to support clinician judgment when the probability of PE is already very low and it is not intended to replace or dictate individual patient-based decision making. Patients who meet the PE rule-out criteria but for other reasons are thought to need testing for PE should undergo the standard evaluation.

CT has largely supplanted the use of $\dot{V}/\dot{Q}$ scans because of the perception that they produce a binary positive/negative result, as well as the fact that other chest pathology may be seen with CT.[21] The sensitivity and specificity of chest CT angiography have improved with the advent of multidetector CT with higher spatial resolution and lower image acquisition time. Overall, well-accepted sensitivity and specificity data are lacking because of diverse differences in the equipment used, image acquisition technique, and image interpretation, but spiral CT is generally regarded to have greater than 90% sensitivity and specificity. One systematic review based on 3500 patients in 15 studies reported a pooled negative predictive value of 99.1% and a likelihood ratio for a negative result of 0.07. Newer CT scan machines with 128 detector systems and sophisticated image postprocessing will become more commonplace and improve the diagnostic accuracy of current imaging. Even with these newer machines, motion artifact, inadequate contrast bolus timing, and varied experience of readers may result in a surprising level of indeterminate or nondiagnostic results.[22] Pretest probability assessment and D-dimer testing will still be important to avoid unnecessary radiation exposure and possible false-positive CT results in a large number of patients who have a very low likelihood of PE.

$\dot{V}/\dot{Q}$ scanning is an alternative to CT for patients with contrast allergy or renal insufficiency and for pregnant patients. It is important to remember that patients who are found to be at high risk by pretest probability assessment and have low or indeterminate $\dot{V}/\dot{Q}$ scans cannot be assumed to have PE ruled out. These patients need anticoagulation and further testing—typically, duplex Doppler ultrasound of the lower extremities.

Controversy exists regarding the optimal approach in pregnant patients. The estimated radiation dose from CT of the chest is low (7 to 14 millisieverts), and with shielding of the abdomen and pelvis, only a small fraction of this dose would be expected to be received by the fetus. It would be expected to be significantly lower than the threshold of teratogenicity. However, no prospective longitudinal data exist to clearly know what the optimal strategy should be or what the long-term risk is. $\dot{V}/\dot{Q}$ scans have been used over a long period in pregnant patients and are thought to provide minimal to no risk to the fetus. However, the need for experienced technicians and experienced nuclear medicine physicians may limit the availability of $\dot{V}/\dot{Q}$ scans. Regardless of what imaging method is available or chosen, it is important to minimize the amount of potential radiation received by the fetus. Discussion with the patient, obstetrician, radiologist, and family needs to occur at the outset even before tests are ordered and should include comment on the probability of disease, extremely low probability of radiation-associated negative effects, and potential morbidity with undiagnosed PE. Tests should be performed if appropriate concern exists for PE. The use of D-dimer is problematic in pregnant patients because the likelihood of a false-positive D-dimer result increases with progression of the pregnancy. It has been advocated that an elevated cutoff for quantitative D-dimer in a low-risk patient may be adequate to rule out PE. However, no prospective management trials exist to clarify a potential role of D-dimer in pregnancy. If used in early pregnancy, when the likelihood of a false-positive result is at its lowest, it may be adequate to rule out PE if the patient is low risk and the result is normal. Patients who are otherwise low risk should not be automatically assumed to have a high pretest probability just because they are pregnant.

## TREATMENT

The defining characteristic of the emergency medicine physician is simultaneous treatment and evaluation. Oxygen should be given to patients suspected of having PE. Correction of local hypoxemia assists in decreasing reflexive vasoconstriction in the pulmonary vasculature. Patients who are thought to be at high risk for PE and have a high pretest probability should be considered candidates for empiric treatment with anticoagulation while awaiting the results of tests, provided that they have no contraindications. Low-molecular-weight heparin (LMWH) has become standard therapy despite being more costly than unfractionated heparin. It has benefit in achieving appropriate anticoagulation rapidly without the need to monitor coagulation levels, and it is also associated with a less likelihood of heparin-induced thrombocytopenia with thrombosis. Some studies have suggested that LMWH may have somewhat higher efficacy in terms of time to thrombus resolution and recurrence in patients with DVT.[23] Unfractionated heparin is still a safe and effective treatment and may be especially useful if a shorter term of anticoagulation with the ability to rapidly cease anticoagulation is desired. Unfractionated heparin and LMHW do not act to break down existing thrombus but rather act to decrease thrombus propagation and extension. Endogenous mechanisms of antithrombin and plasmin activation are responsible for gradually effecting thrombus breakdown. The dose of enoxaparin, the most commonly used LMHW, is 1 mg/kg subcutaneously every 12 hours. The dose of unfractionated heparin is typically a 80-U/kg bolus intravenously and then an 18-U/kg/hr intravenous infusion.

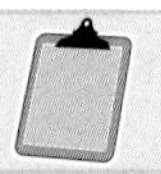

### DOCUMENTATION

**History**
Risk factors as listed in Table 70.1 and Figure 70.3

**Physical Examination**
Does the patient look ill?
Cardiac status (blood pressure, arrhythmias, right heart strain)
Respiratory and airway status
Should include repeated examinations while the patient is in the emergency department

**Studies**
Laboratory tests, results, delays in obtaining studies

**Medical Decision Making**
Pretest probability, risk factors, and decision to pursue testing
Anticoagulation decisions and reasoning

**Treatment**
Anticoagulation, fibrinolytics, and times given

## RISK STRATIFICATION

It is critical to assess the likelihood for further deterioration. Figure 70.1 demonstrates the increase in mortality that occurs gradually with right heart strain and then more steeply with shock. It is possible to gather data in the ED to estimate the likelihood of right heart strain and early shock. The ECG is the starting point, and the presence of T-wave inversion in leads $V_1$ to $V_4$, incomplete or complete right bundle branch block, an S wave in lead I, a Q wave in lead III, and an inverted T wave in lead III may all be evidence of right heart strain. Pulse oximetry is an important predictor of 30-day mortality in normotensive ED patients with PE when less than 95% on room air.[7] Other means of risk stratification include brain natriuretic peptide (BNP) and troponin blood testing. Though not specific for PE and not helpful in establishing the diagnosis, these factors are being seen in emerging studies to predict a more complicated course both in the hospital and several months later. The most accepted means of risk stratification is the echocardiogram. Though often not available on an emergency basis in many EDs, it is a rapid means of identifying right heart strain (**Box 70.3**).

## TREATMENT OF PATIENTS WITH CONFIRMED PULMONARY EMBOLISM AND SHOCK

In a practice guideline statement the American College of Emergency Physicians recommended fibrinolytic therapy for hemodynamically unstable patients with confirmed PE as a class B recommendation.[13] (Class B represents a moderate level of certainty.) Despite controversy over the use of thrombolytics and mortality in patients with PE and shock, in selected samples it seems clear that fibrinolytic therapy has been associated with improved perfusion and better right heart function. Catheter-based techniques of thrombus fragmentation, as well as surgical embolectomy, are alternatives to pharmacologic fibrinolysis. These techniques are unlikely to be available outside dedicated interventional radiology and cardiovascular surgery centers and are highly operator dependent. No evidence has shown that they are superior to pharmacologic approaches.

**BOX 70.3 Signs of Severe Pulmonary Embolism on Echocardiography**

Right heart dysfunction
RV hypokinesis
RV dilation
Tricuspid regurgitation
Elevated pulmonary artery pressure
Impediments to LV output
Septal shift
Decreased LV filling

*LV*, Left ventricular; *RV*, right ventricular.

When the use of fibrinolytics has been studied in patients without overt shock but with right ventricular dysfunction, they have been associated with decreased need to escalate therapy with vasopressors, as well as reduced rates of intubation or additional thrombolytic treatment.[24] The Food and Drug Administration–approved on-label use of fibrinolytic therapy for PE is alteplase, 15 mg as an intravenous bolus and then 85 mg intravenously over a 2-hour period (heparin infusion should be stopped during alteplase administration). Other off-label dosing regimens have been described, including a 15-mg bolus with an 85-mg infusion over a 90-minute period, which has been used in the near-arrest setting.[25] In conclusion, it is accepted that fibrinolytic therapy is appropriate in patients with confirmed PE and shock. Identification of PE as a cause of shock can be aided by a stepwise approach to diagnosis with consideration of other causes of shock (see Fig. 70.2). If shock is present and no right heart abnormalities are seen on echocardiography, PE is a very unlikely explanation for the shock.

## FOLLOW-UP, NEXT STEPS IN CARE, AND PATIENT EDUCATION

Most patients with a new diagnosis of acute PE will be admitted to the hospital for initiation of anticoagulation and serial evaluation of oxygen saturation, blood pressure, and overall functional capacity. Patients with minimal cardiopulmonary comorbidity, normal oxygen saturation, and no evidence of hypotension are typically discharged shortly after warfarin anticoagulation is initiated, and trends outside the United States have included outpatient treatment of low-risk PE patients. In either case, patients continue home self-treatment with LMWH for several days until the outpatient international normalized ratio is above 2.0, at which point they may stop taking LMHW and continue warfarin.

Patients with low oxygen saturation (less than 95%), right heart strain on an echocardiogram or ECG, elevated BNP, or elevated troponin should be observed closely for deterioration. The decision for intensive care unit management should be based on the level of specialized care that patients need (**Box 70.4**).

Patients with a history of previous PE present several challenges. Recurrent PE, defined as an acute clot in a new or different anatomic location, should be treated as acute PE, and if patients are no longer taking anticoagulation agents, they need treatment as stated earlier. In contrast, a persistent or chronic clot is not uncommonly seen in the same areas as previous PE and may look radiographically distinct from acute PE on CT. If patients are appropriately anticoagulated and do not have other indications for admission, they may be discharged from the ED, provided that no other inpatient evaluation for the symptoms is warranted. However, patients with no new clot visualized on CT may be suffering from chronic venous thromboembolic syndrome, a condition in which pulmonary hypertension and chronic vascular changes in the lung can lead to chronic disabling dyspnea and other symptoms that may prompt ED evaluation. Depending on oxygenation and functional status, these patients should be admitted or, if discharged, referred for outpatient echocardiography and pulmonary consultation, but no specific therapy as yet exists for this condition, which may affect 1% to 3% of all patients with PE (**Box 70.5**).

**BOX 70.4 Indications for Intensive Care Unit Management of Patients with Pulmonary Embolism**

Shock
Mental status: acutely decreased and not improving
Respiratory effort: poor or worsening
Cardiac ischemia
Troponin elevation
Worsening electrocardiographic findings
Oxygen requirement: high
Worsening overall clinical course:
- Pulse increasing
- Blood pressure decreasing
- Oxygen saturations decreasing
- Recurrent syncope

**BOX 70.5 Future Trends in the Diagnosis, Prognosis, Treatment, and Disposition of Patients with Pulmonary Embolism**

Electronic decision support aids to provide more accurate point-of-care pretest probability
Effective risk stratification for short- and long-term adverse events
Improved understanding of thrombophilic states
Outpatient or emergency department observation-based treatment of selected low-risk new patients with pulmonary embolism
Oral rapid-acting anticoagulation medications as alternatives to warfarin and low-molecular-weight heparin
Fibrinolytic therapy for patients at high risk for immediate and delayed adverse events

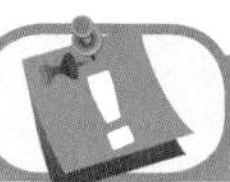

**TIPS AND TRICKS**

The combination of normal oxygen saturation, no known risk factors, and no pulmonary symptoms is very uncommon.
A targeted diagnostic approach should be used rather than a "chest pain work-up" in an attempt to test for every diagnosis possible without regard to the pretest probability or negative consequences of overtesting.
Many of the most threatening alternative diagnoses can initially be assessed with a chest radiograph, electrocardiogram, bedside echocardiogram, and cardiac enzyme testing during the first hour.
Patients who are otherwise at low risk should not be automatically assumed to have a high-risk pretest probability just because they are pregnant.
Patients with a history of pulmonary embolism and no new clot on computed tomography may be suffering from chronic venous thromboembolic syndrome, a condition in which pulmonary hypertension and chronic vascular changes in the lung can lead to chronic disabling dyspnea.

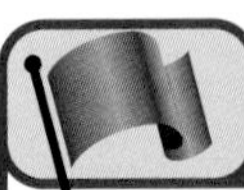

### RED FLAGS

Mortality in patients who have PE without shock is greater than that in those with acute myocardial infarction.

Physician gestalt is useful only when the probability of PE is already very low; therefore, patients who meet the PE rule-out criteria but for other reasons are thought to need testing for PE should undergo the standard evaluation.

Patients at high risk by pretest probability assessment and have low or indeterminate $\dot{V}/\dot{Q}$ scans cannot be assumed to have PE ruled out.

Patients with a high pretest probability are candidates for empiric treatment with anticoagulation agents while awaiting test results, provided that they have no contraindications.

Unfractionated heparin and LMWH do not act to break down existing thrombus but rather act to decrease thrombus propagation and extension.

The ACEP practice guideline recommends fibrinolytics for unstable patients with confirmed PE as a class B recommendation.

Patients without overt shock but with right ventricular dysfunction who are treated with fibrinolytics have a lower need for vasopressors and intubation.

If shock exists and no right heart abnormalities are seen on echocardiography, PE is a very unlikely explanation for the shock.

Patients with low oxygen saturation (less than 95%), right heart strain on echocardiography or electrocardiography, elevated BNP, or elevated troponin should be observed closely.

*ACEP*, American College of Emergency Physicians; *LMWH*, low-molecular-weight heparin; *PE*, pulmonary embolism; $\dot{V}/\dot{Q}$, ventilation-perfusion.

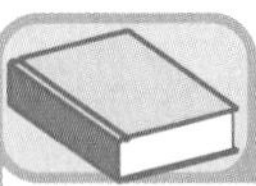

### PATIENT TEACHING TIPS

The decision to test for pulmonary embolism should always assume that if screening tests such as the D-dimer blood test are positive, more definitive tests will be undertaken. It is critical to explain this to patients so that they are not surprised and displeased when many of them have a false-positive D-dimer result and need to stay in the emergency department for imaging.

In pregnant patients, a detailed discussion with the patient, radiologist, obstetrician, and the patient's family should occur at the outset even before tests are ordered and should include the probability of disease, the extremely low probability of radiation-associated negative effects, and the potential morbidity with undiagnosed pulmonary embolism.

## REFERENCES

***References can be found on Expert Consult @ www.expertconsult.com.***

# Venous Thrombosis 71

D. Mark Courtney

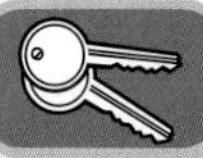

**KEY POINTS**

- Distinction between symptoms of chronic venous disease and acute deep vein thrombosis (DVT) can be difficult. Careful attention to the time course of symptoms as reported by the patient and scrutiny of the medical record may reveal that the symptoms are less likely to be acute.
- The D-dimer blood test can be useful in the evaluation of potential DVT. Just as with pulmonary embolism, its use and interpretation need to take into account the pretest probability of disease.
- Many patients may not have classic, obvious risk factors for DVT but may still have the disease.
- The lack of 24-hour availability of duplex ultrasound, the imaging method of choice for DVT, requires a clear estimate of the probability of disease, the likelihood and timing of follow-up, and consideration of the risks and benefits of temporary empiric anticoagulation.
- Follow-up of patients is critical for monitoring the anticoagulation effects of warfarin, evaluation of progression of symptoms, and determination of the duration of anticoagulation.

## EPIDEMIOLOGY

Deep vein thrombosis (DVT) is a common diagnosis that may be seen in emergency department (ED) patients with minimal to no symptoms or with obvious findings on examination. DVT most typically arises in the lower part of the leg and may exist in combination with or as a precursor to pulmonary embolism (PE). Together, DVT and PE are termed venous thromboembolism (VTE). Understanding VTE as a single disease is useful because risk factors, urgency in establishing a diagnosis, and treatment are similar for both PE and DVT. The annual incidence of DVT has been estimated to be 92 cases per 100,000 persons, and the rate steadily advances with increased age (32/100,000 in persons younger than 55 years, 282/100,000 in those 65 to 74 years of age, and 553/100,000 in those 75 years or older).[1]

## PATHOPHYSIOLOGY

DVT can occur in both young and old patients and may result in both acute and chronic morbidity. It may be acute and life- or limb-threatening (PE, total iliofemoral obstruction) or can lead to chronic and debilitating complications (postphlebitic syndrome, venous stasis and ulceration, recurrent DVT).

Typical DVT risk factors are summarized by the Virchow triad: trauma, stasis, and hypercoagulability. These risk factors are the same as for PE (**Table 71.1**). However, 25% to 50% of patients with DVT may have no identifiable risk factor known at the time of evaluation.

The timing of development of DVT is difficult to know, but it typically starts with small asymptomatic abnormalities in flow at the level of the endothelium. It may be precipitated by venous valve dysfunction or immobility, both of which decrease the normal function of the venous-muscle pump system for return of blood from the legs.

DVT can also develop in the pelvic veins (typically associated with comorbid pelvic or gynecologic conditions) or upper extremity (typically with venous catheters), but by far most cases of DVT diagnosed in the ED are in the legs.

Understanding the venous anatomy of the leg is crucial for interpreting risk and diagnostic tests. The most obvious and concerning cases of DVT occur in the proximal deep system. In order from distal to proximal, the proximal deep veins are the popliteal, femoral, deep femoral, common femoral, and finally the external iliac. Occasionally, the femoral vein is referred to as the superficial femoral vein, which results in confusion because it is a deep vein and clots there should be treated as DVT. Thrombosis may develop in the distal deep system (the calf), and these veins are the anterior tibial, the posterior tibial, and the peroneal. These are deep veins and thrombosis here is DVT, but management of isolated distal DVT is somewhat less certain than that for proximal DVT. Finally, the superficial venous system of the leg can be subject to thrombosis and superficial thrombophlebitis, but this is managed differently from thrombosis in the deep system. These veins are the lesser and greater saphenous and the perforating veins. This is not DVT, and isolated thrombosis here is not typically treated with systemic anticoagulation.

The morbidity associated with venous thrombosis is not just due to subsequent embolization. Even with anticoagulation there is the possibility of injury to the endothelium and venous valve system, both of which can result in chronic venous stasis and recurrent clots.

## PRESENTING SIGNS AND SYMPTOMS

Patients can have a variety of symptoms that may include fullness, cramping, achiness, or vague pain in the calf or posterior part of the leg. They may also report swelling. It is important to distinguish between unilateral symptoms, which may be more likely to be due to DVT, and bilateral symptoms, which may be more likely to be a consequence of some other disease process. The exception would be the rare case of obstruction of the inferior vena cava or simultaneous bilateral DVT. Signs on examination may include edema, redness, and tenderness, particularly in the posterior aspect of the calf or the upper part of the leg.

Swelling may be minimal or extensive and involve the entire extremity. It can be challenging to distinguish chronic symptoms of venous stasis from acute DVT based on a single examination. Therefore, a careful history to establish the time course of the findings in the leg is critical, and examination of the past medical record can be highly valuable.

Use of examination alone to determine the presence or absence of DVT is problematic. Classic teaching is that the accuracy of physical examination alone for the diagnosis of DVT is 50%. This is a bit of a generalization, but it is clear that findings may be subtle, patients may not have detectable tenderness or edema early in the course or spectrum of disease

**Table 71.1 Known Risk Factors for Acute Deep Vein Thrombosis**

| RISK FACTORS | SPECIFIC NOTES |
|---|---|
| Previous history of PE or DVT | Inquire about the setting and circumstances of the previous VTE |
| Recent trauma or surgery | In general, trauma requiring admission or surgery requiring general anesthesia within the previous month. Recent long-bone, vascular, or trauma surgery may especially increase the risk |
| Cancer | In general, patients with currently treated cancer or palliative care |
| Central or long-term vascular catheters | |
| Age | Risk significantly increases above the age of 50 to 60 years |
| Oral contraceptives | Especially third-generation formulations |
| Hormone replacement therapy | Currently less common than in the past |
| Pregnancy | Risk increases along with the duration of pregnancy; it peaks at term and then decreases over a period of 4 to 6 weeks postpartum |
| Immobility | Includes casts or splints, as well as permanent limb or generalized body immobility, including that from general hospitalization |
| Factor V Leiden mutation | Most common in northern European populations. The heterozygous carrier state exists in 3% to 7% of many samples. A homozygous mutation is less common and confers three times greater risk for VTE relative to the normal genotype. |
| Antiphospholipid antibody syndrome | Very potent risk factor. Associated with large and recurrent PE. May be associated with anticardiolipin antibodies, stroke, myocardial infarction, and frequent first-trimester miscarriages |
| Prothrombin mutation | |
| Hyperhomocysteinemia | Can occur as a result of inadequate folate and B vitamin intake, as well as a genetic mutation in methyltetrahydrofolate reductase. The degree of elevation in risk is controversial |
| Deficient levels of clotting factors | Protein C, protein S, antithrombin III |
| Congestive heart failure | May result from generalized immobility or vascular stasis |
| Chronic obstructive pulmonary disease | May result from generalized immobility |
| Air travel | Primary risk with travel in excess of 5000 km (3100 miles) and concurrent other risk factors. The degree of elevation in risk is controversial |
| Obesity | The degree of elevation in risk is controversial |

severity, and some patients may be nearly asymptomatic. The often mentioned, but rarely understood or performed Homan sign—calf pain elicited by passive dorsiflexion of the ankle—is insensitive, nonspecific, and useless.

## DIFFERENTIAL DIAGNOSIS AND MEDICAL DECISION MAKING

Many other diseases may be accompanied by pain, swelling, and tenderness of the leg. **Box 71.1** presents a differential diagnosis of conditions that should be considered.

Clinicians often have a difficult time distinguishing between cellulitis and DVT. The pain, swelling, erythema, and unilateral nature of cellulitis may be clinically similar to findings in patients with DVT, and the two conditions can even coexist. A break in the skin, fever, or warmth may more strongly suggest cellulitis. However, distinguishing between the two may be impossible without objective testing for DVT.

Compartment syndrome can be manifested as pain and swelling in the leg and is an emergency, time-dependent diagnosis. Extreme pain, exquisite tenderness in the compartment, coolness of the extremity, and in later stages, diminished pulses and decreased sensation may all indicate this diagnosis. It is most common in the context of trauma to the leg from either penetrating, blunt, or fracture mechanisms. If being considered, it must be assessed by measuring compartment pressures and, if appropriate, emergency orthopedic or traumatic surgery consultation. Trauma of this significance can be associated with concomitant DVT and compartment syndrome, so if compartment pressures are normal, testing for DVT can and should proceed.

Many of the other conditions in the list of differential diagnoses are easier to differentiate from DVT by close attention to the time course and other symptoms as revealed from a careful patient history. Overall edematous conditions are listed (congestive heart failure, renal failure, liver failure), but they are commonly associated with gradual or recurrent episodes of bilateral edema. The possible important exception is a patient with congestive heart failure who has undergone coronary artery bypass grafting with removal of the saphenous vein. These patients may, if asked, report that they always have some asymmetry in their swelling and leg size.

Baker cyst rupture or inflammation is a common cause of pain behind the knee and even in the calf. It may be very painful and can result in redness and swelling. An acute onset associated with bending over or being on flexed knees suggests this diagnosis, but confirmation is often achieved with an ultrasound study that is otherwise negative for DVT.

**BOX 71.1 Differential Diagnosis of Leg Swelling**

Deep vein thrombosis
Cellulitis
Baker cyst rupture or inflammation
Congestive heart failure
Renal failure
Liver failure
Inferior vena cava compression
Musculoskeletal trauma
Polyarteritis nodosa
Erythema nodosum
Myositis
Tendinitis
Lymphedema
Superficial thrombophlebitis
Compartment syndrome
Necrotizing fasciitis

## DIAGNOSTIC TESTING

### PRETEST PROBABILITY

Just like any possible diagnosis in the ED for which further testing is considered, the first step should be an assessment of what the pretest probability of disease is.[2,3] This can be done easily by using a clinical decision model such as that derived and validated by Wells et al.[4] to stratify patients as low risk or high risk for having DVT (**Table 71.2**). It has been also advocated by some authors that experienced clinicians may empirically use clinical gestalt to estimate the probability of DVT as low or not low. In either case, documentation on the medical record should clearly indicate the physician's pretest probability estimate for DVT and what the supporting evidence for this may be from the history and examination.

**Table 71.2 Wells Model for Estimating the Pretest Probability for Deep Vein Thrombosis**

| CLINICAL VARIABLE | SCORE |
|---|---|
| Active cancer (treatment ongoing, within the previous 6 months, or palliative) | 1 |
| Paralysis, paresis, or recent plaster immobilization of the lower extremities | 1 |
| Bedridden for 3 days or more or surgery requiring general anesthesia in the last 3 mo | 1 |
| Localized tenderness along the deep venous system | 1 |
| Swelling of the entire leg | 1 |
| Calf swelling measured to be 3 cm greater than other leg (at 10 cm below the tibial tuberosity) | 1 |
| Pitting edema in the symptomatic leg | 1 |
| Collateral superficial veins (nonvaricose) | 1 |
| Previous deep vein thrombosis | 1 |
| Alternative diagnosis at least as likely as deep vein thrombosis | −2 |
| **A score of 1 or less indicates that deep vein thrombosis is not likely.** | |

Adapted from Wells PS, Anderson DR, Rodger M, et al. Evaluation of D-dimer in the diagnosis of suspected deep-vein thrombosis. N Engl J Med 2003;349:1227-35.

## ULTRASONOGRAPHY

Venous duplex ultrasonography is noninvasive, not associated with radiation exposure, and accurate in detecting proximal DVT. It has become the first-line imaging test for DVT. When performed by a certified sonographer and interpreted by a radiologist or other credentialed expert, it has a sensitivity and specificity of approximately 95% for proximal thrombosis. Ultrasonography does present some problems, however, including limited availability at night in many institutions, operator variability, occasional difficulty in visualization because of body habitus, and at times interobserver disagreement regarding distal DVT. Nonetheless, it is the imaging test of choice for most ED clinicians, and absence of DVT on ultrasonography should be reassuring that no DVT requiring emergency treatment is present. The question of whether to include visualization of the infrapopliteal veins and the clinical significance of isolated distal DVT are controversial.[5,6]

### *Ultrasound Performed by Emergency Department Clinicians*

A limited study compared ultrasound of the common femoral and popliteal veins performed by emergency physicians versus formal duplex ultrasound performed by certified ultrasonographers in radiology or vascular departments.[7-10] A sensitivity of 89% to 100% and a specificity of 75% to 91.9% were reported. However, the extent of operator training and the specific protocols used have varied widely among published studies.[11] One study prospectively investigated the performance of ED-based ultrasound by a heterogeneous mix of 56 emergency physicians with varied levels of ultrasound experience and found a summary sensitivity of 70%, which is low for the evaluation of a disease with significant potential morbidity.[11] Not surprisingly, sonographers with the most experience had the most accuracy in this study. It remains to be seen what the best method is to train emergency medicine ultrasonographers for evaluation of DVT and what the overall diagnostic performance would be when done outside academic centers or institutions without ultrasound fellowships and dedicated training. In the future this may be a cost-effective and safe option as this modality evolves. Presently, a clearly negative result of a limited scan performed by a properly trained emergency physician suggests the absence of DVT in the proximal leg veins. If the results are positive or equivocal or involve patients with a high probability, confirmatory studies by the radiology or vascular service should be performed.

### *Additional or Follow-up Ultrasonography*

There can be significant confusion and disagreement between the emergency medicine physician consultant and the literature over the need for additional ultrasonographic studies in patients with negative ultrasound findings. Some suggest that if the initial ultrasound visualized only the proximal system, a second ultrasound as an outpatient is needed. However, studies have found this practice to yield a very low rate of disease. A more common and feasible strategy would be to refer patients with equivocal findings in the distal system or those with a high pretest probability of DVT for additional studies done as an outpatient. Integration of the ultrasound results with pretest probability and D-dimer testing as indicated later can limit confusion on this issue.

## VENOGRAPHY

Venography has been the historical "gold standard" for the diagnosis of DVT, but as with pulmonary angiography, this invasive and painful test is now rarely performed. Complications include contrast reaction, contrast nephropathy, vascular injury, and the possibility of subsequent DVT in previously nonthrombosed vessels.

### *Runoff Venography After Chest Computed Tomography for Pulmonary Embolism*

When computed tomography (CT) of the chest is performed as part of imaging for possible PE, some institutions also use a delayed imaging protocol that visualizes the pelvis and legs to assess for the presence of DVT. This may add a marginal value of about 2% to the overall sensitivity of this testing strategy. However, many sites do not use this protocol because of radiation exposure, cost, time needed to read the images, and less than optimal interobserver agreement on the venography aspect of the study. In general, this is a hospital- and radiology-specific decision with no conclusive evidence in the literature on its value. CT venography done independent of a PE protocol study is not typically performed because of the alternative nonradiating and noninvasive nature of duplex ultrasonography.

## D-DIMER TEST

The D-dimer test is a blood-based assay that uses antibodies to the D-dimer protein to measure the presence or level of circulating D-dimer. D-dimer is a breakdown product of fibrin, and elevated levels are associated with elevated fibrin or clot somewhere in the body. Unfortunately, elevated D-dimer can occur in a variety of conditions other than acute PE and DVT, most notably malignancy, pregnancy (particularly later trimesters), chronic inflammatory conditions, recent surgery, infection, stroke, myocardial infarction, and even advanced age. For many versions of this test, levels below 500 ng/mL are considered negative, but this may vary by laboratory and assay used.

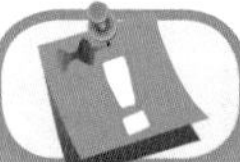

**TIPS AND TRICKS**

**Testing for Deep Vein Thrombosis**

Physical examination alone is unreliable for the diagnosis of deep vein thrombosis (DVT), but duplex ultrasonography is noninvasive and the diagnostic imaging method of choice.

In patients deemed unlikely to have DVT by a Wells DVT score of 1 or less or an empiric unstructured estimate of the probability of DVT of less than 10%, DVT may be essentially ruled out by a quantitative negative D-dimer blood test.

In patients with DVT deemed to be likely by a Wells DVT score of 2 or greater or an empiric unstructured estimate of probability of greater than 10%, negative findings on duplex ultrasound should be followed by either a negative D-dimer test or a negative additional ultrasound as an outpatient before the diagnosis is excluded.

## COMBINING OF PRETEST PROBABILITY, D-DIMER TESTING, AND DUPLEX ULTRASONOGRAPHY

This integrated strategy has been advocated as a way to optimize the speed of evaluation, cost, need for imaging, and safety. Similar to the risk stratification and D-dimer approach to PE testing, it starts with physician estimation of the probability of disease in a symptomatic ED patient. If DVT is determined to be "unlikely" by the Wells DVT score (1 or less), a D-dimer test that is negative is reassuring to stop ED testing for DVT and consider other diagnoses.[12] If D-dimer is positive, ultrasound is the next step, with results guiding further decision making. One approach for those who are not "DVT unlikely" still uses D-dimer but mandates that all patients, regardless of the D-dimer result, undergo ultrasonography, and D-dimer is then used to guide who needs follow-up in 1 week for an additional ultrasound. This integrated strategy is shown in **Figure 71.1**.

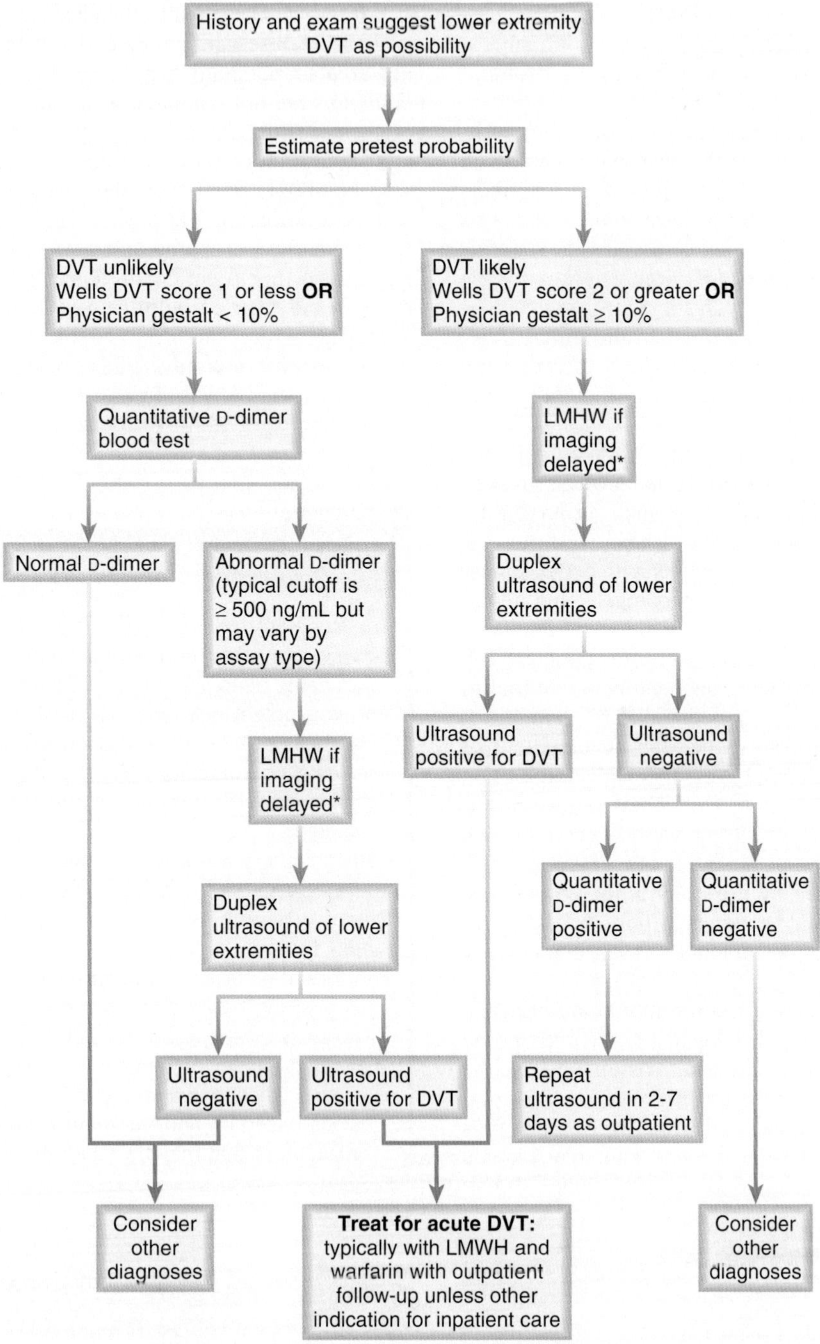


**Fig. 71.1 Pretest probability–based diagnostic algorithm for the evaluation of potential deep vein thrombosis (DVT) in emergency department patients.** *LMWH*, Low-molecular-weight heparin.

## TREATMENT

Subcutaneous injection of low-molecular-weight heparin (LMWH, including enoxaparin, dalteparin, and others) is the standard of care used to treat acute DVT and provide rapid therapeutic anticoagulation until the effects of oral warfarin are sufficient to result in therapeutic anticoagulation (usually 4 to 7 days). The goal of long-term warfarin treatment is to prevent recurrence of DVT or PE, which is achieved by targeting the international normalized ratio (INR) to a level between 2.0 and 3.0 during the treatment period. Therapeutic anticoagulation may also lower the risk for postphlebitic syndrome,[13] in addition to the risk for recurrent VTE.

Unfractionated heparin administered via continuous infusion is used less often now than in the past, but it can be an option if there is a potential need to rapidly stop the effects of anticoagulation at a later time in care. Other than this unique situation, LMWH has become the first choice for anticoagulation in patients with acute VTE, largely because of the ease of administration, its efficiency in achieving anticoagulation, and the potential reduced bleeding. In the initial treatment of DVT, once-daily dosing appears to be as effective and safe as twice-daily dosing, but the frequency may vary with the agent used.

The duration of warfarin treatment may vary by patients. Typically, it is taken for 3 to 6 months. Patients with provoked DVT (from a specific temporary event such as an injury, surgery, or pregnancy) are more likely to have warfarin discontinued at 3 to 6 months than are patients with active cancer or unprovoked idiopathic VTE. Some oncologists and hematologists recommend daily LMWH for oncology patients with VTE rather than transition to warfarin, and some patients with nontemporary risk factors for VTE, such as incurable malignancy, may be maintained on an anticoagulation regimen for life. Both LMWH and warfarin reduce the development of additional thrombosis but do not have a mechanism of action that dissolves or lyses the existing clot. The natural fibrinolytic system accomplishes this task to a varied degree in each individual patient, depending on many factors. Pharmacologically, lysis can be facilitated by use of thrombolytic agents, but at present such treatment is indicated only for extensive limb-threatening thrombosis not amenable to vascular surgery and other rare instances.

Other anticoagulants, such as direct thrombin inhibitors and factor Xa inhibitors, have been developed and are undergoing additional testing in large trials. These anticoagulants have the advantage of rapid time to therapeutic effect and ease of oral dosing and appear to be equally effective as LMHW plus warfarin, but they are not easily reversed and may incur a significant increase in cost relative to warfarin alone.

## DISPOSITION

Most patients with acute DVT who have the ability to self-administer subcutaneous injections of LMHW, continue warfarin anticoagulation as an outpatient, have a means of determining the INR, and have additional follow-up arranged can be discharged from the ED. Of course, if other conditions are thought to be present that mandate inpatient testing or treatment, patients are admitted for inpatient care. Patients who are thought to have concomitant PE based on clinically significant signs or symptoms may require testing for this condition and admission for monitoring of oxygen saturation and the degree of pulmonary symptoms, but pharmacologic treatment remains the same for PE and DVT. The counterintuitive practice pattern whereby patients are typically discharged from the ED with uncomplicated DVT but often admitted for uncomplicated PE is subject to ongoing debate, with some experts advocating for outpatient care of PE in patients who do not have an oxygen requirement and are otherwise at low risk for adverse events. In the absence of randomized trials or large-scale observational data, this debate lingers as an evolving area of potential health services research. In any case, clinicians are not mandated to order pulmonary angiography or chest CT in patients without pulmonary or chest symptoms and should not embark on a quest to find PE in every patient who has DVT. Such a strategy would be costly, expose the patient to radiation and other potential risks such as contrast reaction and nephropathy, and would not change management. Explaining this to patients requires deliberate, clear communication but may be helpful in reducing subsequent anxiety as they learn more about VTE in the outpatient setting. Finally, follow-up must be emphasized as being important. The clinical course of acute DVT is impossible to predict, even with appropriate anticoagulation treatment.

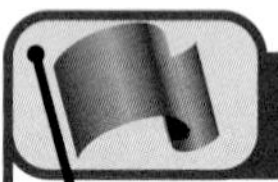

**RED FLAGS**

- The superficial femoral vein is actually part of the deep venous system, and thrombosis there should be treated as acute deep vein thrombosis (DVT).
- Age is a potent risk factor for DVT, as it is for pulmonary embolism. Although advanced age is not part of the Wells prediction model for DVT, it should be considered when estimating the probability for DVT and the need for imaging.
- Patients taking warfarin may still have DVT or extension of DVT despite a therapeutic international normalized ratio.
- Do not "rule out" DVT solely on the basis of the absence of risk factors.
- The role of emergency department–based ultrasonography is evolving but is operator dependent, and most protocols examine only portions of the proximal deep venous system. Specific training and experience are needed. Caution may be warranted in formulating treatment decisions based on findings that may not have optimal visualization or that may be equivocal.

## SPECIAL CASES RELATED TO TREATMENT OR DISPOSITION DECISIONS

### SUPERFICIAL THROMBOPHLEBITIS

Painful inflammation of superficial veins because of thrombus is called superficial thrombophlebitis. Because it possible for DVT to be present with superficial thrombophlebitis, it is not unreasonable to consider ultrasound evaluation in these patients. If deep venous involvement is not present, a thrombus in the superficial vein is not generally thought to pose a threat for significant embolization, but appropriate follow-up and return instructions are needed because in a minority of these patients, DVT or worsening of their superficial disease may eventually occur.

Outpatient treatment of superficial thrombophlebitis usually consists of nonsteroidal antiinflammatory medications, heat, and compression. The pain may persist for weeks, and the condition may recur.

## ISOLATED CALF DEEP VEIN THROMBOSIS

Treatment of isolated calf DVT with anticoagulants is controversial. Advocates of treatment cite the not-insignificant risk for proximal propagation and potential subsequent PE.[6] Opponents argue that isolated calf DVT is less likely to be associated with clinically significant PE.[5] A period of several days to a week of outpatient treatment with 325 mg of aspirin daily and ultrasound repeated within 1 week may be an option in these patients if discussed with the patient and primary physician.

## PHLEGMASIA CERULEA DOLENS

Extensive iliofemoral thrombosis may rarely produce an enlarged, doughy, painful blue leg, a condition called phlegmasia cerulea dolens. Greatly increased hydrostatic pressure from occluded venous flow results in impressive edema. The edema elevates tissue pressure, which ultimately impedes arterial flow and produces ischemic conditions and cyanosis. If the obstruction is not relieved, venous gangrene may ensue, with loss of limb and high mortality. Unfractionated heparin should be started, and because the patient's intravascular volume is depleted as a result of third spacing, fluid resuscitation should also be administered. This is a time-dependent emergency, and if available, vascular surgery should be consulted for consideration of thrombectomy. Alternatively, systemic thrombolytic therapy with tissue plasminogen activator is a potential strategy if vascular surgery is unavailable or operative risks are deemed to be too high.

## POSTPHLEBITIC SYNDROME

Venous thrombosis may eventually result in chronic valvular incompetence through inflammatory damage, partial recanalization with the presence of residual clot, or simple vessel distention producing loss of coaptation of valves. With loss of normal valve function, blood return from the lower extremity depends on higher venous pressure. This pressure distends the veins and becomes painful. Depending on the extent of valvular damage, the discomfort may be mild or highly disabling. Patients commonly suffer from some degree of chronic edema and skin changes, which can progress to ulceration. Patients with severe forms of this disorder may not be able to stand or walk for significant periods and are unable to exercise. Such disability may be career changing and can occur in young, otherwise healthy individuals.

## REFERENCES

*References can be found on Expert Consult @ www.expertconsult.com.*

# 72 Lower Extremity Venous Ultrasonography

*James Q. Hwang and Vicki E. Noble*

**KEY POINTS**

- Lower extremity ultrasound is the primary modality used to diagnose or exclude deep vein thrombosis (DVT).
- Clinician-performed bedside ultrasound can be accurate in detecting DVT when compared with radiology-performed examination.
- Two-point compression lower extremity ultrasound is a simplified approach that consists of compression of the common femoral vessels in the groin and the popliteal vessels in the popliteal fossa.
- Compressibility of veins via gray-scale B-mode ultrasound is the most important criterion for assessing DVT.
- Current practice guidelines recommend that proximal lower extremity ultrasound be repeated in 5 to 7 days after an initial negative two-point compression result to rule out propagation of unseen distal DVT.

## EPIDEMIOLOGY

About 250,000 cases of deep vein thrombosis (DVT) are diagnosed each year. Failure to recognize and appropriately manage DVT can increase risk for the development of postthrombotic syndrome (disabling leg symptoms caused by venous reflux or ulceration) or pulmonary embolism (PE).[1-4]

DVT may develop in the lower or upper extremities. Although up to 18% are located in the upper extremities,[5] the majority arise from the lower extremities. In the lower extremities, DVT is referred to as proximal when it is found in the popliteal veins or higher and as distal when it is located in the calf.

## PERSPECTIVE

Unfortunately, the diagnosis of DVT cannot be made on clinical signs and symptoms alone. The location of swelling and pain does not correlate with the location or extent of the clot, and symptoms localized to the calf may have an etiology in more proximal veins.[6] Clinical signs have been analyzed statistically and found to be of little value in reliably determining the presence or absence of DVT.[7] The differential diagnosis for leg pain and swelling includes lymphedema, chronic venous insufficiency, infection (cellulitis), aneurysm, pseudoaneurysm, Baker cyst, and other musculoskeletal causes. Diagnosis of DVT depends on the clinician's pretest probability assessment and a combination of several noninvasive diagnostic tools (lower extremity ultrasound, D-dimer, or both). The exact diagnostic path or algorithm pursued depends somewhat on local availability and expertise. When available, lower extremity ultrasound is the primary modality used to diagnose or exclude DVT. The lower extremity ultrasound may be a proximal lower extremity examination, a whole-leg examination, or an abbreviated, two-point compression examination. If proximal lower extremity ultrasound is performed, current practice guidelines recommend that ultrasound of the proximal veins be repeated 5 to 7 days after an initial negative result to safely exclude clinically suspected DVT.[8,9] This recommendation stems from the observation that up to 20% of cases of distal DVT may propagate into the proximal veins.[10,11] A systematic review and metaanalysis published in 2010 found that after a negative whole-leg study, anticoagulation may be withheld safely without the need for a repeated ultrasound examination.[12]

Despite the numerous benefits of lower extremity sonography, many emergency providers continue to be unable to obtain lower extremity ultrasound after hours, on weekends, and on holidays. Clinician-performed two-point compression lower extremity ultrasound is now considered an appropriate method for assessing lower extremity DVT in the emergency department (ED) and is one of the 11 core emergency ultrasound applications.[13,14] Emergency providers who perform two-point compression lower extremity sonography have demonstrated scan times of less than 4 minutes per patient and time savings of more than 2 hours in terms of time to patient disposition.[15,16] When ultrasound is not available, providers may be forced to administer low-molecular-weight heparin and either keep the patient in the ED overnight or coordinate an outpatient study for the patient the following day. Although the risk for bleeding in these situations is low, boarding the patient in the ED or relying on patient-initiated follow-up is less than ideal. Given ever-increasing patient volumes and ED crowding, the value of clinician-performed two-point compression lower extremity ultrasound cannot be overstated.

## EVIDENCE-BASED REVIEW

Radiology-performed lower extremity duplex ultrasound has reported sensitivities of 91% to 96% and specificities of 98% to 100%.[17,18] Multiple studies have demonstrated that clinician-performed two-point compression bedside ultrasound can be accurate in detecting DVT when compared with radiology-performed examinations.[19-22] In a systematic review, Burnside et al. found an overall sensitivity of 95% and specificity of 96% for detection of lower extremity DVT by emergency physician–performed ultrasound.[19] The authors caution that the six studies included in their analysis were limited by small sample size and by emergency physicians with high levels of ultrasonographic expertise, thus leaving their estimates at risk for being overly optimistic. A prospective study by Kline et al. in the same year assessed a more diverse range of clinician sonographers with more limited training in ultrasonography and found a sensitivity of 70% and specificity of 89%.[20] They concluded that ultrasound performed by providers with limited training in compression ultrasonography of the lower extremity had intermediate diagnostic accuracy that may be improved by pretest probability assessment. A more recent prospective study by Crisp et al. included a large, heterogeneous group of emergency providers with variable levels of ultrasonographic experience but found the test results to be similar to those from the Burnside review with a sensitivity of 100% and specificity of 99%.[21]

It is important to note that clinician-performed lower extremity sonography focuses on compressibility and typically does not include color flow Doppler or pulsed wave spectral Doppler beyond its use to localize or distinguish between vessels. Compressibility of veins with gray-scale B-mode ultrasound is the most important criterion and is widely accepted as being highly accurate.[7] Color flow Doppler and pulsed wave spectral Doppler provide additional information and may be particularly useful when uncertainty exists or when assessing for pelvic DVT. Even though Doppler imaging has utility, it can be limited by the following: nonocclusive thrombus, the presence of collateral flow, and sonographer skill. Some studies have found that Doppler adds little to the information obtained by compression ultrasound for the detection of proximal DVT.[22] In a prospective study by Biondetti et al., vein compressibility alone was compared with contrast-enhanced venography and found to have an overall sensitivity of 87% and a specificity of 100%.[23] Because six of the seven false-negative examinations resulted from isolated distal DVT, the sensitivity of compression-only ultrasound for detecting proximal DVT was noted to be 98%. It is reasonable that clinician-performed lower extremity ultrasound studies consist only of compression.

### TWO-POINT COMPRESSION VERSUS WHOLE-LEG COLOR DUPLEX ULTRASOUND

Two-point compression lower extremity ultrasound is a simplified approach that consists of compression of the common femoral vessels in the groin and the popliteal vessels in the popliteal fossa. The concept behind this abbreviated approach stems from the idea that clot usually involves multiple or whole venous segments. Several studies have shown that few cases of proximal DVT occur without involving either the common femoral vein (CFV) or the popliteal vein (PV), or both, and that isolated thrombus in the superficial femoral vein (SFV) is rare.[24-27] In a study of limited compression ultrasound in patients with symptomatic DVT, Pezzullo et al. found a 54% reduction in examination time (9.7 minutes) while still maintaining high accuracy and patient safety.[26] To the contrary, Frederick et al. prospectively studied 721 symptomatic patients and determined after 755 examinations that DVT limited to a single vein occurs with sufficient frequency that the lower extremity ultrasound cannot be abbreviated without resultant loss of diagnostic accuracy.[28] To that end, in a retrospective study of 2704 lower extremity ultrasound examinations, Maki et al. found that acute DVT was isolated to the SFV in 22.3% of patients with DVT.[29] They concluded that abbreviated imaging studies that evaluate only the CFV and PV could fail to detect up to 20% of proximal DVT and recommended interrogation of the SFV. The question of whether two-point compression can be performed in place of full-length examination remains controversial. In clinical situations in which radiology-performed, whole-leg sonography is not available, there is little controversy; clinicians should proceed with performing two-point compression lower extremity ultrasound. One solution to the vexing problem of missed SFV clots is to perform "two-region" compression ultrasound—that is, perform compression in the groin region from the greater saphenous junction through the bifurcation of the superficial and deep femoral veins and perform compression in the popliteal region from the PV to the trifurcation of the distal calf veins. This "two-region" approach has not been studied as a specific technique, although previous research would seem to support it as a compromise approach.

The value of whole-leg color duplex ultrasound is dependent on the significance of identifying distal DVT. The clinical relevance plus need to treat distal DVT is a controversial topic that continues to be debated. Proponents of full-length lower extremity examination point to a randomized trial by Lagerstedt et al. in which the usefulness of long-term anticoagulation (for 3 months) was assessed in patients with distal DVT. The authors found that those who did not receive long-term anticoagulation therapy had a significantly higher recurrence rate than those who did (8 of 28 patients versus 0 of 23 patients; $P < .01$).[30] This study suggests that calf vein thrombi are important, should be sought in symptomatic patients, and when found, should be treated with long-term anticoagulation. Although the American College of Chest Physicians is in agreement with these findings,[31] there is no universally accepted consensus on the management of distal DVT.[32] Proponents of full-length examination often point to literature in which a proximal progression rate of up to 20% has been observed.[10,11] Righini et al. contend that there is considerable uncertainty over the natural history of distal DVT and, in particular, over the rate of extension to proximal veins.[33] The authors argue that if identifying and treating distal DVT do not improve patient outcomes, whole-leg color duplex ultrasound is of less clinical utility. Previous trials have demonstrated that it is safe to withhold anticoagulation in patients with suspected venous thrombosis and negative serial proximal ultrasound results even though some patients have calf vein thrombi.[34] In a more recent, prospective, randomized multicenter study, Bernardi et al. compared serial two-point ultrasonography plus D-dimer testing with whole-leg color-coded Doppler ultrasonography for diagnosing suspected symptomatic DVT.[35] Although the two-point protocol missed

65 cases of isolated calf DVT, the long-term outcomes for the two groups were similar, thus suggesting that searching for distal clots may be unnecessary.

### ONE LEG VERSUS BOTH LEGS

The question of whether lower extremity ultrasound examination should include only the symptomatic extremity or both lower extremities is a controversial topic. Proponents of scanning both legs point to literature demonstrating that unsuspected contralateral DVT and bilateral DVT are not uncommon and occur in up to 30% of cases.[36,37] By interrogating both legs, a baseline study for future comparison can be obtained that may help differentiate acute from chronic venous thrombosis. Opponents of the bilateral lower extremity approach point to literature that describes the likelihood of finding clot solely in the asymptomatic leg to be as low as 0% to 1%.[38] A retrospective study by Strothman et al. found that unilateral scanning would decrease examination times by 21% and could potentially increase total reimbursement for symptomatic venous scans by 9% when compared with routine bilateral duplex scanning.[37] Supporters of single-leg studies note that treatment of DVT is typically the same regardless of whether DVT is found to be unilateral or bilateral. Because treatment with systemic anticoagulation is not altered and the potential for significant time and cost savings is real, many question the necessity of bilateral lower extremity imaging in all patients. As per the American College of Radiology–American Institute of Ultrasound in Medicine (ACR-AIUM) practice guidelines for the performance of peripheral venous ultrasound examinations, compression sonography may be unilateral (depending on the patient's signs and symptoms and the clinical indication), but spectral Doppler, when performed, must at a minimum include spectral waveforms from both lower extremities.[39]

## HOW TO SCAN

Lower extremity ultrasound is performed with the ultrasound machine positioned on the right side of the patient. Most ultrasound machines have different settings, and if available, the vascular or venous lower extremity setting should be selected. Room lighting should be decreased as much as possible to reduce the amount of gain required and help optimize the image. Typically, a linear probe with a frequency of 8 to 10 MHz is used (**Fig. 72.1**). For larger patients or those with significant edema, a probe with a lower frequency of 5 to 8 MHz may be used. Transducers with a curved footprint may make compression and assessment of vessel collapse more challenging. The probe should be held with the transducer marker pointing toward the patient's right side or, in an equivalent manner, pointing toward the sonographer's left side. The patient is positioned in the supine position with the head of the bed elevated 30 to 45 degrees, or alternatively, the head of the bed may be elevated in the reverse Trendelenburg position. Placing the patient in this position distends the lower extremity vessels and allows easier visualization and assessment. Color flow Doppler and pulsed wave spectral Doppler may be used to help distinguish or localize vessels when visualization through soft tissue is poor. The depth and focal zones should be adjusted accordingly to optimize the image.

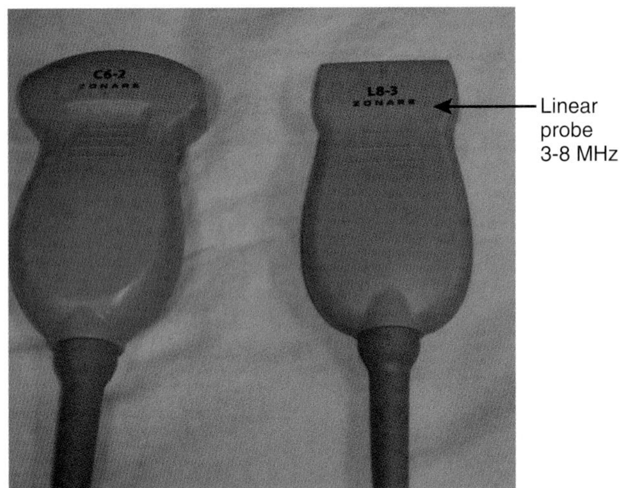


**Fig. 72.1** Linear probe with a frequency of 3 to 8 MHz. Compression with a curved footprint transducer may be more challenging.

Compressibility is determined by applying direct pressure over the vein with the probe and assessing for coaptation of the vessel walls. It is important to note that firm pressure is often required and that the appropriate amount of downward pressure is typically achieved when the walls of the adjacent artery begin to deform. Compressibility is normal when coaptation of the vessel walls and complete obliteration of the intravascular space are seen. Anything short of this is concerning for DVT. With the amount of pressure required, some have questioned whether lower extremity ultrasound could potentially dislodge a thrombus and result in PE. Only one case report of PE resulting from compression sonography has been published.[40] In general, compression sonography is regarded as safe, and gentle compression is advised. In situations in which thrombus can be directly visualized or is noted to be free floating, compression is not generally indicated. Another key point is the importance of applying pressure evenly and not at an angle; otherwise, the probe may roll off the vessel. A frequent initial challenge of performing lower extremity ultrasound is keeping the vessel in the middle of the viewing screen as pressure is applied. The probe is marched one probe width or approximately 1 to 2 cm at a time down the lower extremity. Acute DVT is diagnosed when the vein is found to be noncompressible. In some instances, thrombus may be directly visualized, but it is important to note that acute DVT tends to be less echogenic than chronic thrombus (**Figs. 72.2 to 72.6**). Acute DVT may also expand the vessel lumen or appear as a color void on color flow Doppler (**Fig. 72.7**).

Compression sonography of the lower extremity begins just below the inguinal ligament, where the CFV is identified medial to the common femoral artery (**Figs. 72.8 to 72.10**). Within a few centimeters below the inguinal ligament, the most proximal branch of the CFV may be seen—the greater saphenous vein (GSV). The GSV runs medial and superficial as the probe is moved caudad away from the inguinal ligament (**Figs. 72.11 and 72.12**). Compression of the proximal GSV at its junction with the CFV is important because thrombus in this location is considered DVT and requires treatment. As the probe is marched caudad, the CFV then divides into the SFV

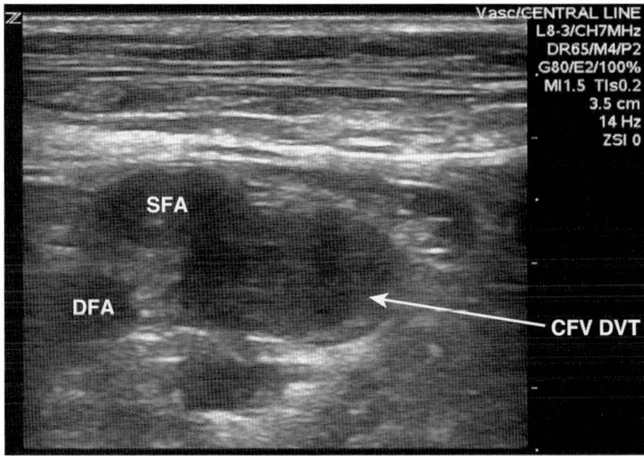


**Fig. 72.2 Noncompressible and hyperechoic deep vein thrombosis (DVT) in the right common femoral vein (CFV).** *DFA,* Deep femoral artery; *SFA,* superficial femoral artery.

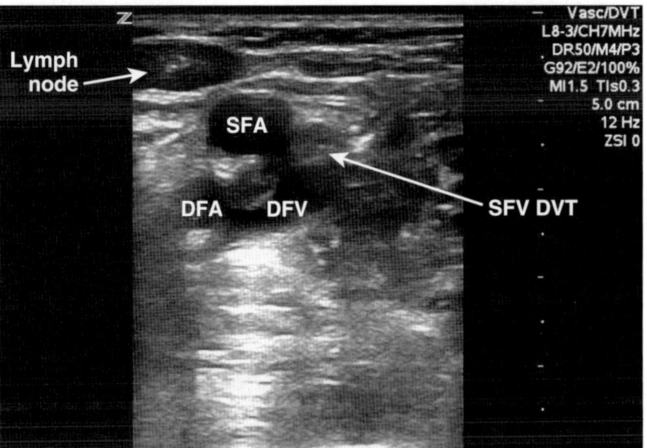


**Fig. 72.3 Hyperechoic deep vein thrombosis (DVT) in the right superficial femoral vein (SFV) and right deep femoral vein (DFV).** A lymph node is seen superficial to the vessels. *DFA*, Deep femoral artery; *SFA*, superficial femoral artery.

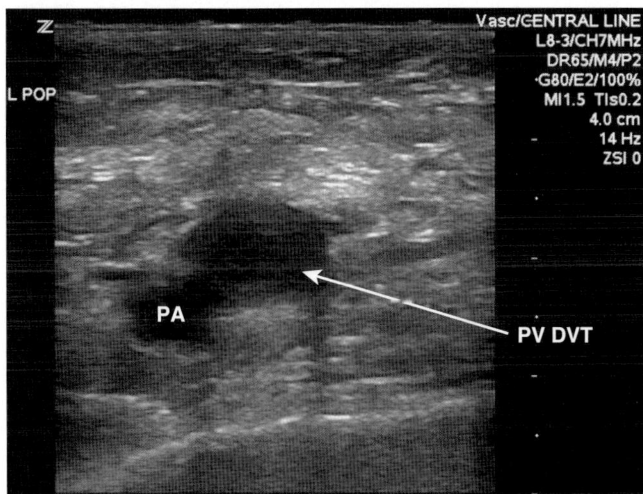


**Fig. 72.4 Noncompressible and hyperechoic deep vein thrombosis (DVT) in the popliteal vein (PV).** *PA*, Popliteal artery.

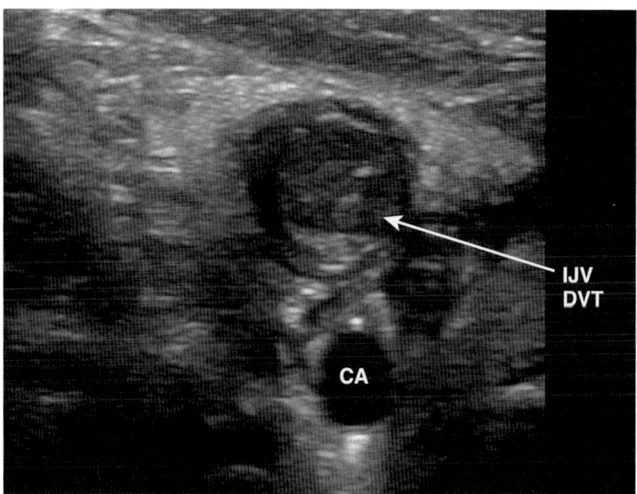


**Fig. 72.5 Noncompressible and hyperechoic deep vein thrombosis (DVT) expanding the lumen of the internal jugular vein (IJV).** *CA,* Carotid artery.

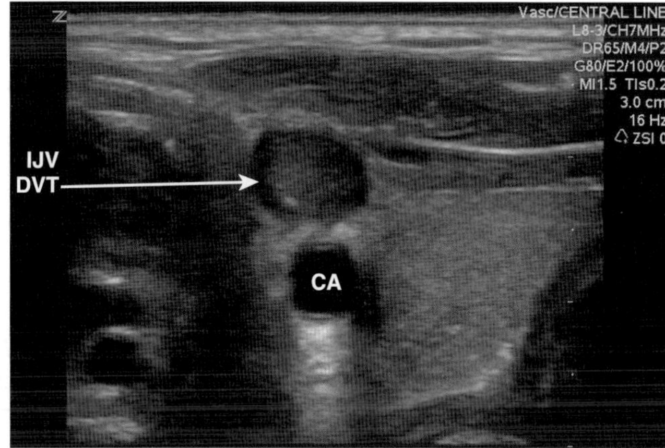


**Fig. 72.6 Noncompressible and hyperechoic deep vein thrombosis (DVT) in the internal jugular vein (IJV).** *CA,* Carotid artery.

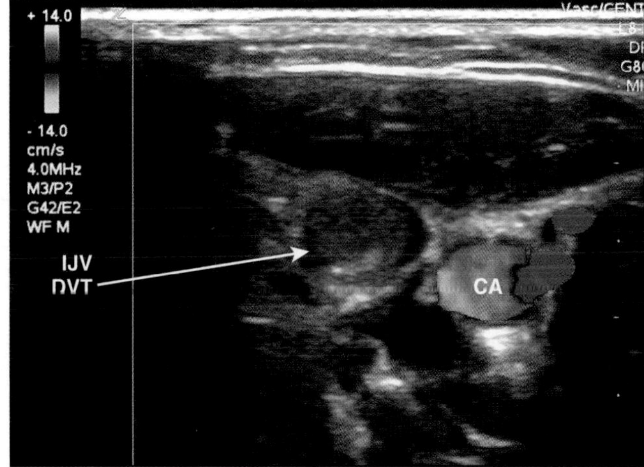


**Fig. 72.7 Noncompressible and hyperechoic deep vein thrombosis (DVT) in the internal jugular vein (IJV) with color flow Doppler.** *CA,* Carotid artery.

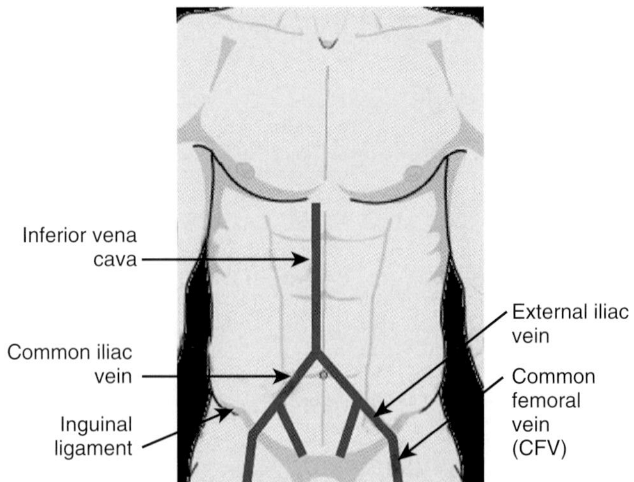


**Fig. 72.8 Compression sonography of the lower extremity begins just below the inguinal ligament at the CFV.**

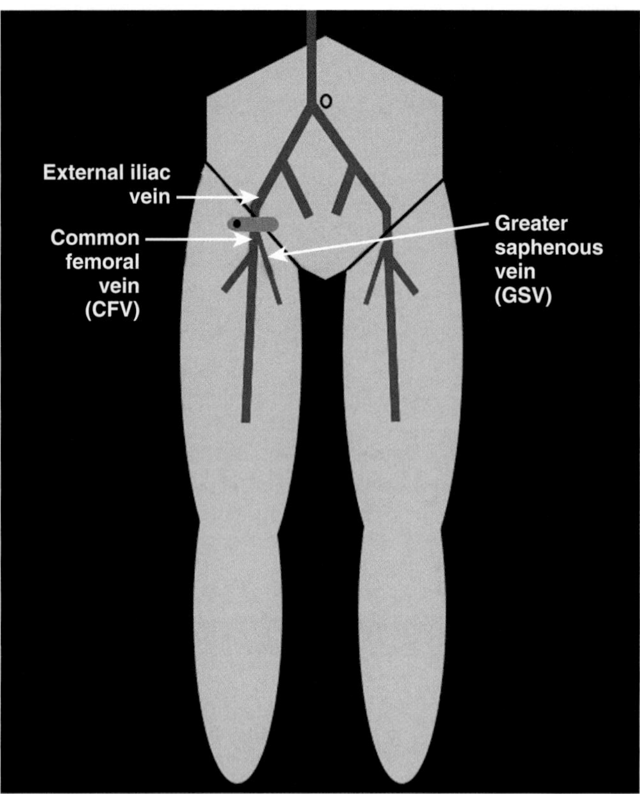


**Fig. 72.11 The GSV is the most proximal branch of the CFV and runs medial and superficial.**

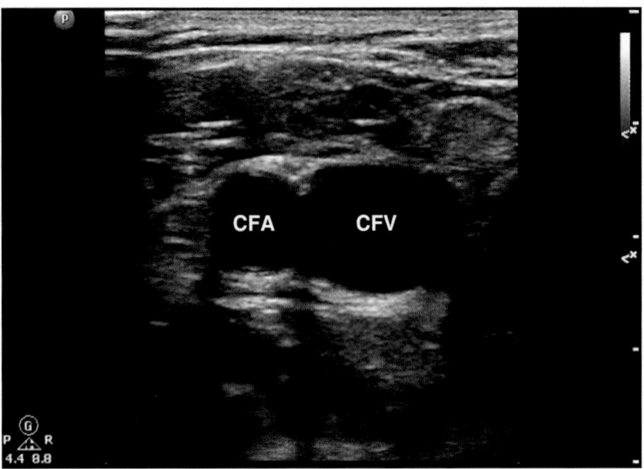


**Fig. 72.9 Right lower extremity.** The common femoral vein (CFV) is identified medial to the common femoral artery (CFA).

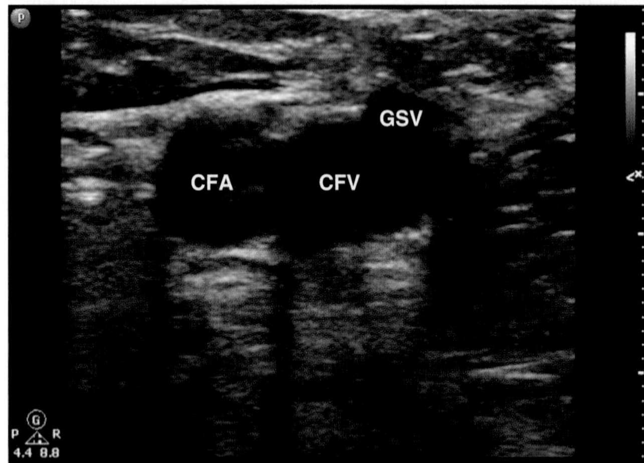


**Fig. 72.12 The greater saphenous vein (GSV) is the most proximal branch of the common femoral vein (CFV) and runs medial and superficial.** *CFA*, Common femoral artery.

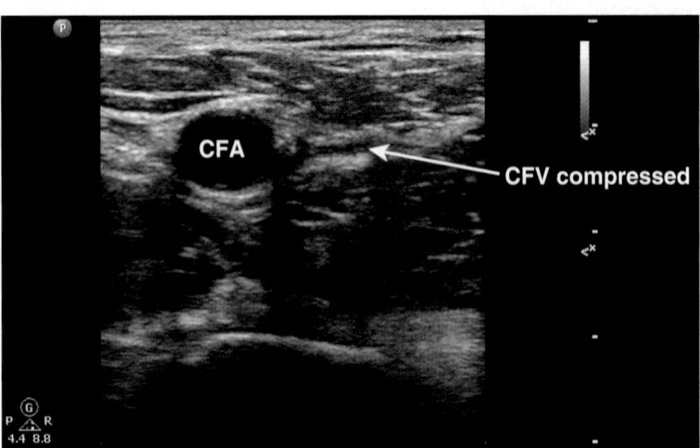


**Fig. 72.10 Right lower extremity.** Normal compression of the common femoral vein (CFV) with complete obliteration of the intravascular space. *CFA,* Common femoral artery.

and the deep femoral vein (DFV) (**Figs. 72.13 and 72.14**). It is important to recognize that the SFV is part of the deep venous system and not a superficial vein despite its name. There is considerable duplication of the lower extremity venous system, with multiple femoral veins occurring at a frequency of up to 20% to 30%.[7,41] Compression sonography of the first few centimeters of the SFV and DFV should be performed, and once completed, the scan then proceeds down behind the knee in the popliteal fossa. To obtain access to the popliteal fossa, the

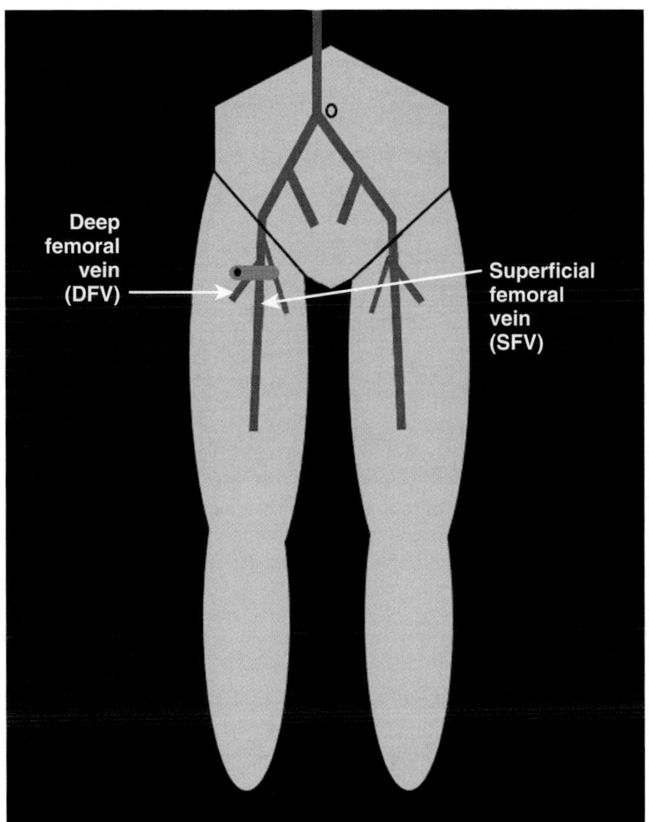


**Fig. 72.13** The common femoral vein (CFV) divides into the SFV and the DFV.

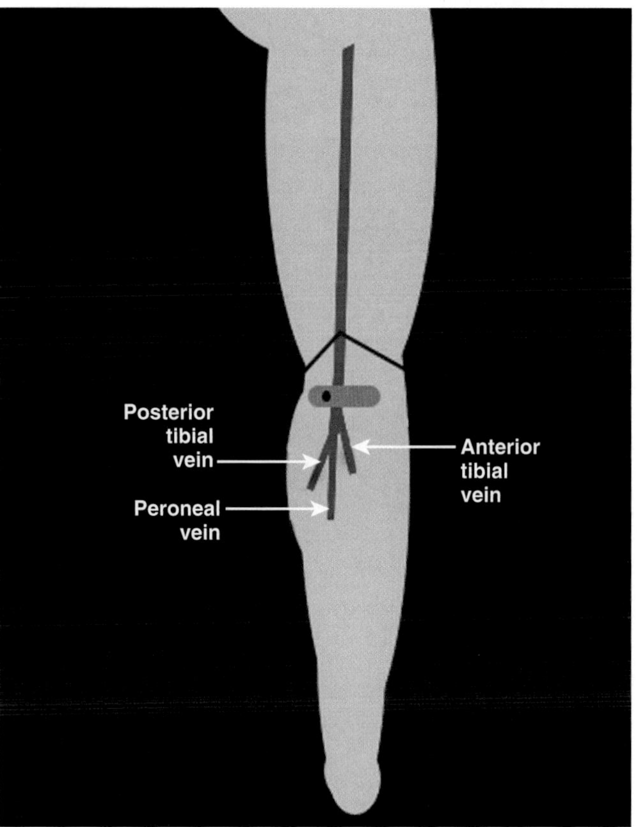


**Fig. 72.15** The popliteal vein divides into the anterior tibial vein, peroneal vein, and posterior tibial vein.

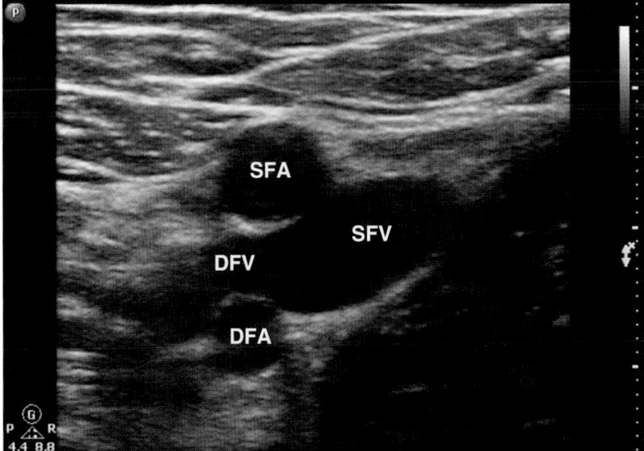


**Fig. 72.14** The common femoral artery divides into the superficial femoral artery (SFA) and the deep femoral artery (DFA). The common femoral vein divides into the superficial femoral vein (SFV) and the deep femoral vein (DFV).

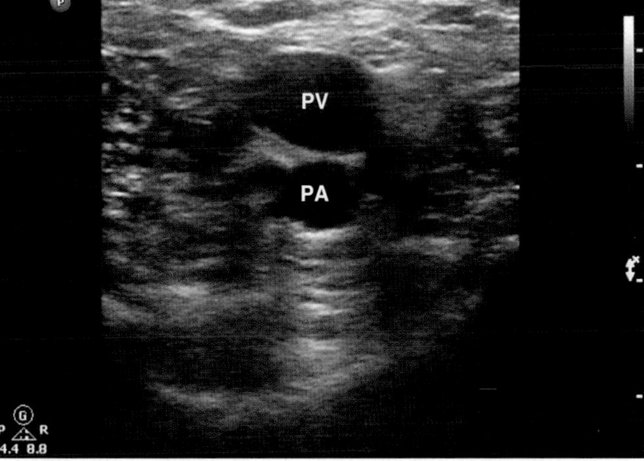


**Fig. 72.16** The popliteal vein (PV) is more posterior than the popliteal artery (PA), and because the probe is placed posteriorly in the popliteal fossa, the PV appears more superficial on the viewing screen.

lower extremity is flexed and externally rotated. Alternatively, the patient may be positioned in either a decubitus position with the study side up or in a prone position with the knee flexed 20 to 30 degrees. The PV is more posterior than the popliteal artery. Because the probe is placed posteriorly in the popliteal fossa, the PV appears more superficial on the viewing screen (i.e., at the top in the near field) (**Figs. 72.15 to 72.17**). The probe is placed behind the knee, high in the popliteal fossa, and compression is performed. The probe is then marched caudad along the PV until it trifurcates into the anterior tibial vein, posterior tibial vein, and peroneal vein (**Fig. 72.18**). It is important to scan the most proximal portions of these calf veins because thrombus in any of these locations is considered DVT and warrants anticoagulation. Although the

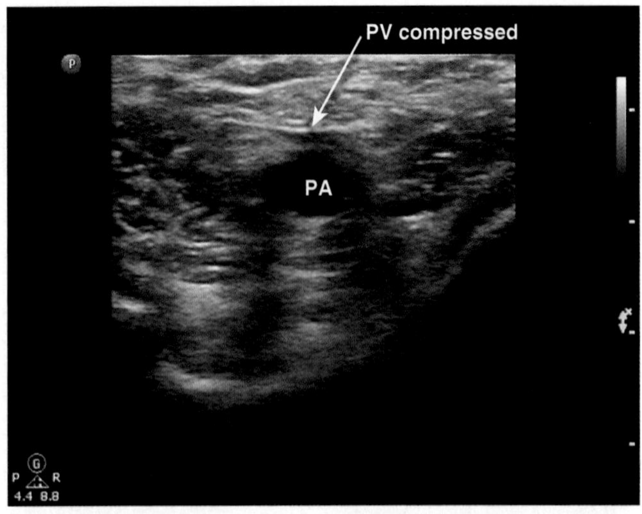


**Fig. 72.17 Normal compression of the popliteal vein (PV) with complete obliteration of the intravascular space.** *PA*, Popliteal artery.

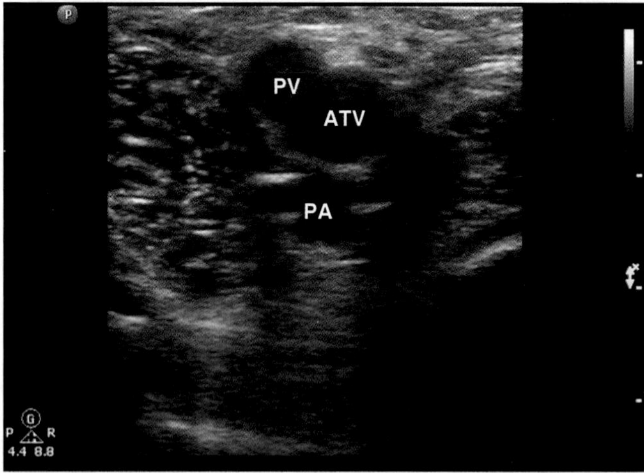


**Fig. 72.18 The popliteal vein (PV) divides into the anterior tibial vein (ATV), peroneal vein, and posterior tibial vein (the peroneal vein and posterior tibial vein are not visualized).** *PA*, Popliteal artery.

venous system is relatively straightforward in the proximal end of the lower extremity, there is considerable variability below the popliteal fossa and in the calf. As per the ACR-AIUM practice guidelines, interrogation of the calf veins is not required.[39] Even with the most careful and detailed examination of the calf veins it can be difficult to be certain that all of the possibly duplicated veins are free of thrombus.

## HOW TO INCORPORATE INTO PRACTICE

Clinician-performed lower extremity ultrasound can be performed in any patient with suspected DVT. As stated previously, the diagnosis of DVT depends on pretest probability assessment and a combination of several noninvasive diagnostic tools. In a certain subset of patients, D-dimer combined with clinical assessment may be used to eliminate or safely reduce the number of patients needing further noninvasive testing.[32,42] Even with the use of such algorithms, D-dimer testing can exclude only less than half of patients with suspected DVT.[43] With focused education and training,[14] emergency providers may perform lower extremity ultrasound accurately and safely integrate bedside sonography into their specific DVT evaluation algorithms. Providers must remember that current practice guidelines recommend that proximal lower extremity ultrasound be repeated in 5 to 7 days after an initial negative result.[8,9] Emergency providers should recognize that patient follow-up can be an issue and limitation. In a prospective observational study assessing patient follow-up after negative lower extremity bedside ultrasound, McIlrath et al. found that only 28% of patients obtained a follow-up ultrasound examination to rule out propagation of unseen distal DVT.[44]

## SUGGESTED READINGS

American Institute of Ultrasound in Medicine, American College of Radiology, Society of Radiologists in Ultrasound. Practice guideline for the performance of peripheral venous ultrasound. J Ultrasound Med 2011;30:143-50.

Bernardi E, Camporese G, Buller HR, et al. Serial 2-point ultrasonography plus D-dimer vs whole-leg color-coded Doppler ultrasonography for diagnosing suspected symptomatic deep venous thrombosis: a randomized controlled trial. JAMA 2008;300:1653-9.

Burnside PR, Brown MD, Kline JA. Systematic review of emergency clinician–performed ultrasound for deep venous thrombosis. Acad Emerg Med 2008;15:493-8.

Crisp JG, Lovato LM, Jang TB. Compression ultrasonography of the lower extremity with portable vascular ultrasonography can accurately detect deep vein thrombosis in the emergency department. Ann Emerg Med 2010;56:601-10.

Dean AJ, Ku BS. Deep venous thrombosis. In: Hoffman B, editor. Ultrasound guide for emergency physicians. http://www.sonoguide.com/dvt.html; 2008 Accessed 20.04.12.

Johnson SA, Stevens SM, Woller SC, et al. Risk of deep venous thrombosis following a single negative whole-leg compression ultrasound: a systematic review and meta-analysis. JAMA 2010;303:438-45.

## REFERENCES

***References can be found on Expert Consult @ www.expertconsult.com.***

# Traumatic Brain Injury (Adult) 73

*Tomer Begaz*

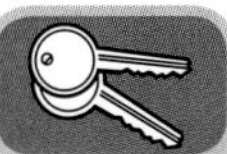

**KEY POINTS**

- Emergency treatment of traumatic brain injury is aimed at rapidly identifying surgically correctable lesions and preventing secondary insults such as hypoxemia and hypotension.
- Triage to a neurosurgical trauma center is recommended for patients with intracerebral hemorrhage or persistent altered mental status.
- Early computed tomography is used to identify intracranial hemorrhage in patients with a significant mechanism of injury, history of altered mental status, or risk factors such as anticoagulant therapy.
- Osmotic agents such as mannitol or hypertonic saline are important first-line therapies for patients with elevated intracranial pressure.
- Hyperventilation should be avoided except as a temporizing measure in patients with impending herniation.
- A significant proportion of patients with mild head injury will have persistent postconcussive symptoms. All head-injured patients should be counseled about this possibility and be given appropriate outpatient referral.
- Athletes suffering from concussion should return to play only after completing a supervised stepwise rehabilitation program.

## EPIDEMIOLOGY

Traumatic brain injury (TBI) is one of the leading causes of morbidity and mortality worldwide, with more than 100,000 deaths annually in the United States alone. In addition, an estimated 2 million individuals suffer permanent, life-altering disabilities each year from these injuries. TBI has resulted in a greater number of years of productive life lost than either heart disease or stroke. The most common causes of TBI are falls, motor vehicle collisions, and assault.

## PATHOPHYSIOLOGY

Hemorrhage or edema following TBI leads to rapid increases in intracranial pressure (ICP). Initially, cerebrospinal fluid (CSF) can be shunted out of the skull via the ventricles and cisterns. However, after severe TBI, this capacity is quickly overcome, and a rapid rise in ICP with compromised cerebral blood flow and cerebral ischemia ensues. Ultimately, the brain tissue itself may be forced downward across the rigid tentorium or out of the base of the skull itself, thereby resulting in a herniation syndrome and rapid death. Systemic hypoxia and hypotension occur with high frequency in patients with TBI and are associated with increased mortality (**Fig. 73.1**).

## PRESENTING SIGNS AND SYMPTOMS

### GLASGOW COMA SCALE SCORE

An altered level of consciousness in the setting of trauma is the primary indicator of TBI requiring an advanced level of care. The Glasgow Coma Scale (GCS) score is the method most commonly used to quantify level of consciousness. In particular, changes in the GCS score over time are highly predictive of outcome, thus mandating repeated assessments both in the field and in the emergency department (ED).

### CLINICAL FINDINGS

In addition to the GCS score, the initial clinical examination should include assessment for pupil reactivity and symmetry, focal sensorimotor deficits, and cerebellar abnormalities. A thorough cranial examination should be performed to identify external evidence of trauma, potential skull fracture, or evidence of basilar skull fracture. Signs of basilar skull fracture include periorbital (raccoon eyes) or retroauricular (Battle sign) ecchymosis, hemotympanum, and CSF otorrhea and rhinorrhea. In the setting of TBI, any fluid leaking from the nose or ears should be suspected to be CSF. Because of the high coincidence of cervical spine fractures in the setting of severe TBI, the cervical spine should be examined carefully and imaged liberally as clinically indicated.

Historical features that should raise suspicion for serious intracranial injury include a history of loss of consciousness or posttraumatic amnesia, severe headache, vomiting, and confusion. Patients taking anticoagulant medications and those with bleeding disorders are at higher risk for intracranial hemorrhage and should be imaged liberally.

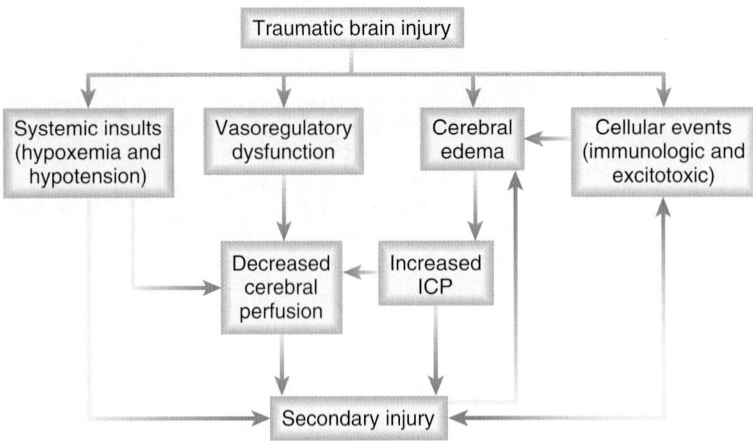


**Fig. 73.1 Algorithm showing the pathophysiologic mechanisms of traumatic brain injury.** *ICP*, Intracranial pressure.

## DIFFERENTIAL DIAGNOSIS AND MEDICAL DECISION MAKING

### IMAGING

Non–contrast-enhanced computed tomography (CT) is the initial imaging study of choice in the evaluation of patients with TBI. Plain radiographs are neither sensitive nor specific in identifying intracranial lesions or skull fracture and are therefore not recommended as a diagnostic study. CT has excellent sensitivity in detecting the presence of intracranial hemorrhage, a mass effect such as ventricular compression or midline shift, and the presence of significant cerebral edema. CT also has the advantage of being widely available and rapid. See **Box 73.1** for examples of CT findings in patients with TBI.

Other modalities used to diagnose TBI include magnetic resonance imaging (MRI), functional imaging, brain acoustic monitoring, and bispectral electroencephalography. MRI is superior to CT in identifying cerebral edema and diffuse axonal injury. In addition, analysis sequences allow sensitive detection of acute hemorrhage, particularly in the brainstem and posterior fossa, where CT is less sensitive. However, application of MRI in the management of TBI has been limited because of the lack of uniform availability, the increased time needed for administration and patient isolation during the procedure, and the added challenges of resuscitation and ventilator management within the strong magnetic field. For this reason, MRI is used more commonly in the subacute or chronic phases or in patients whose signs and symptoms are not well explained by the findings on CT. Functional imaging with positron emission tomography, single-photon emission CT, xenon-enhanced CT, and MRI-based imaging may also be useful later in a patient's course to assess cerebral blood flow and oxygenation, which has prognostic value in predicting functional outcomes but is unlikely to be useful in the acute resuscitation and management of patients with TBI in the ED. Finally, newer modalities such as brain acoustic monitoring and bispectral electroencephalography appear to be useful in the detection of TBI because of prognostic ability rivaling that of CT and the ability to provide continuous data. Future investigations should focus on the utility of these modalities in the ED setting.

**BOX 73.1 Findings on Computed Tomography in Individuals with Traumatic Brain Injury**

Acute hemorrhage appears hyperdense on computed tomography (CT) scans, with the shape and location of hemorrhage suggesting the underlying pathology. *Epidural hematomas* are classically lentiform (lens shaped) because of their relationship to arterial injury, with the higher pressure compressing the brain parenchyma **(Fig. 73.2)**. *Subdural hematomas* are more commonly crescent shaped, with blood from torn veins tracking along the surface of the brain beneath the dura mater **(Fig. 73.3)**. *Intraparenchymal hemorrhage* can exist as a discrete hematoma or as multiple smaller foci throughout a contused area of brain **(Fig. 73.4)**. In addition to focal areas of hemorrhage, cerebral contusions typically involve cerebral edema, which may progress markedly over a period of several days. Skull fractures may be seen on plain radiographs, but more important is the potential for injury to the underlying brain parenchyma or the existence of intracranial hemorrhage **(Fig. 73.5)**. *Subarachnoid hemorrhage* appears as hyperdensities within the ventricles, along the falx and tentorium, and around the circle of Willis **(Fig. 73.6)**. One of the most elusive diagnoses is *diffuse axonal injury*, in which the findings on CT are often much less impressive than the degree of obtundation. Small, punctate hemorrhages along the gray-white interface at the cortical periphery suggest this diagnosis, although the initial scan may be completely normal.

## TREATMENT

### GENERAL

The approach to patients with suspected TBI is directed toward reversal of physiologic derangements and avoidance of secondary insults, early triage to a facility with appropriate resources, and expedited neurosurgical care.

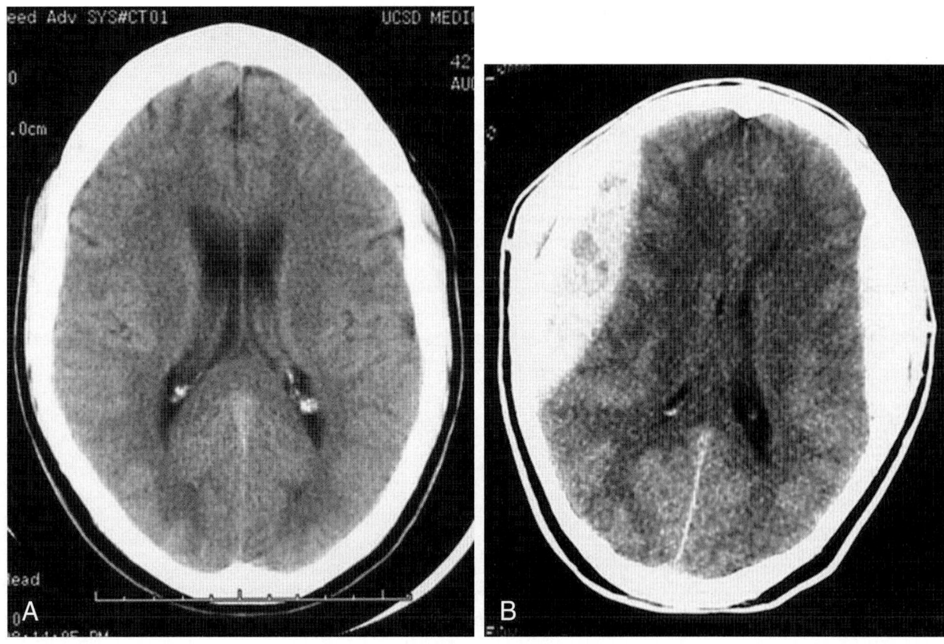


**Fig. 73.2** **A,** Normal head computed tomography (CT) scan at the same level as **B**. **B,** Bilateral epidural hematomas on a head CT scan.

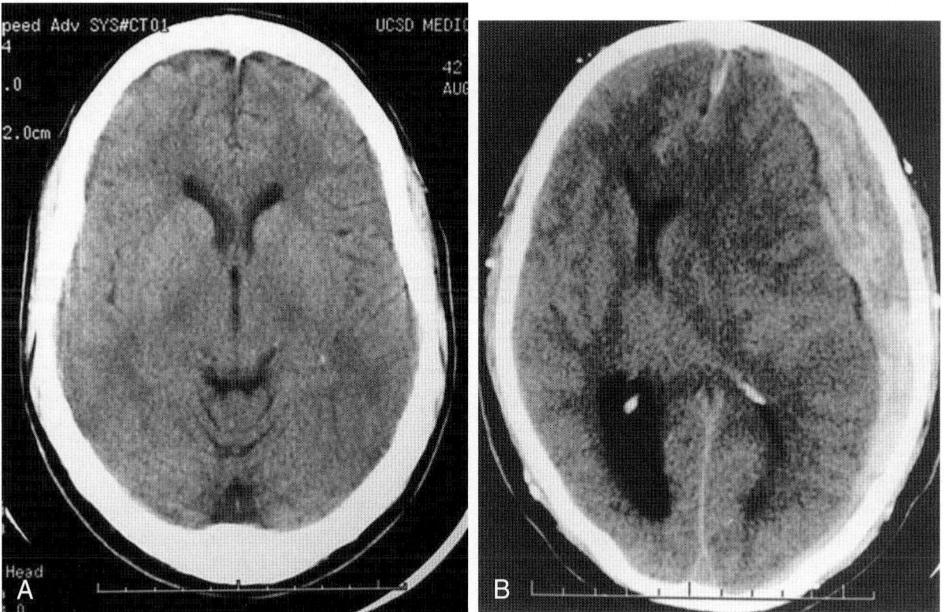


**Fig. 73.3** **A,** Normal head computed tomography (CT) scan at the same level as **B**. **B,** Large subdural hematoma with a midline shift and compression of the ventricles on a head CT scan.

## PREHOSPITAL MANAGEMENT

Half of all patients who die of TBI do so within the first few hours after their injury.

Prehospital assessment of patients with TBI should include rapid airway evaluation, continuous pulse oxygen saturation monitoring, frequent measurement of blood pressure, determination of GCS scores, and pupillary evaluation.[1] Prehospital intubation should be avoided in patients who are spontaneously breathing and maintaining greater than 90% oxygen saturation.[2] Prehospital airway management may be necessary in patients with a GCS score lower than 9 or those unable to maintain oxygen saturation greater than 90% with supplemental oxygen. If prehospital endotracheal intubation is performed, confirmation of placement should be done with auscultation and end-tidal capnography. Even mild hyperventilation should be avoided in all cases with the exception of patients who have evidence of herniation or acute neurologic deterioration. Hypotension should be treated with isotonic fluids, although protocols involving prehospital hypertonic saline administration are reasonable for patients with GCS scores lower than 9. Rapid transport is a priority, ideally to a facility with immediately available imaging and neurosurgical care.

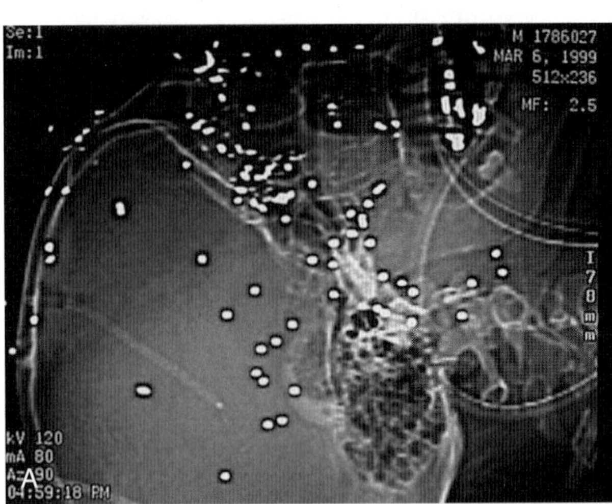


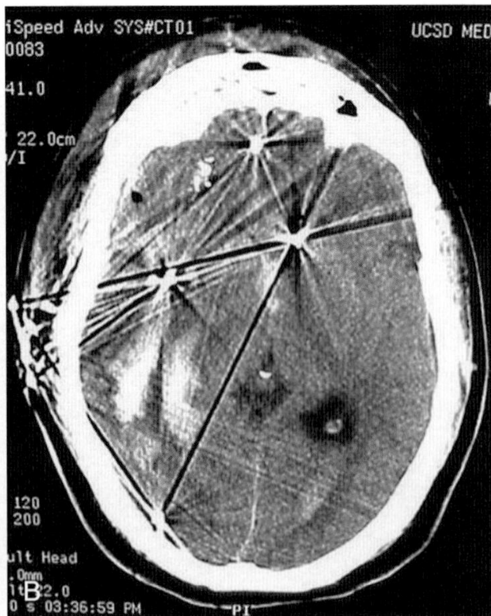


**Fig. 73.4** **A,** Plain film showing multiple metallic fragments from a shotgun blast involving the eye socket. **B,** Head computed tomography scan of the same patient showing intracerebral hemorrhage.

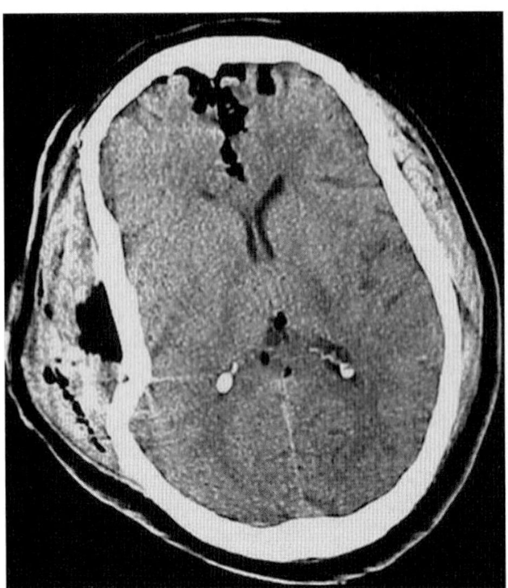

**Fig. 73.5 Depressed skull fracture with intracerebral air on a head computed tomography scan.**

**Fig. 73.6 Traumatic subarachnoid hemorrhage on a head computed tomography scan.**

## AIRWAY AND BREATHING

Trauma data registries have shown increased mortality in TBI patients with hypoxemia.[3] This association has led to an aggressive approach to airway management in patients with severe TBI, including oxygen supplementation and early intubation. All patients with TBI should undergo pulse oximetry monitoring and administration of supplemental oxygen to correct the hypoxemia ($PaO_2 < 60$ mm Hg or oxygen saturation < 90%).

In patients with severe TBI, endotracheal intubation is critical. Indications for endotracheal intubation include a GCS score lower than 9, airway protection when airway protective reflexes are in question, hypoxia refractory to supplementary oxygen, and agitated or combative patients who cannot comply with a rapid and thorough assessment, including CT.[4]

Rapid-sequence intubation (RSI) is the recommended strategy for securing the airway in patients with TBI because of its ability to produce optimal intubation conditions and minimize the adverse effects of laryngoscopy on the injured brain. The most serious risk associated with RSI is the potential for apnea and hypoxia during paralysis. Aggressive preoxygenation and early use of adjunctive airway measures can minimize hypoxic insults.

Patients with TBI may be sensitive to the increases in ICP associated with RSI, and some experts recommend neuroprotective adjuncts to traditional RSI medications. Preadministration of lidocaine at a dose of 1.5 to 2 mg/kg may blunt the rise in ICP associated with laryngoscopy and intubation. Coadministration of 2.5 to 3 mcg/kg of fentanyl with the induction agent may prevent the tachycardia and hypertension

**BOX 73.2 Example of a Neuroprotective Induction Strategy for Individuals with Traumatic Brain Injury**

1. Preoxygentate with 100% $O_2$.
2. Administer lidocaine, 1.5 to 2 mg/kg.
3. Administer a defasciculation dose of a nondepolarizing neuromuscular blocking agent (e.g., rocuronium, 0.1 mg/kg, or pancuronium, 10 mcg/kg).
4. Administer fentanyl, 2.5 to 3 mcg/kg.
5. Induce with etomidate, 0.3 mg/kg.
6. Paralyze with succinylcholine, 1.5 to 2 mg/kg.

associated with tracheal intubation.[5] Finally, a small dose of a nondepolarizing neuromuscular agent, such as pancuronium, before administration of succinylcholine can protect against fasciculations, which may lead to a rise in ICP. The "defasciculation" dose is typically one tenth of the full paralytic dose of the agent. **Box 73.2** presents a sample neuroprotective RSI strategy. It should be noted that although all the aforementioned adjuncts to RSI in patients with TBI are reasonable considerations, they should be implemented as part of a streamlined approach to TBI patients. The higher priority is rapid and safe intubation that avoids hypoxia and aspiration. If implementation of these adjuncts to traditional RSI results in delay or complications, all theoretic benefit is lost. Therefore, it is also reasonable to use traditional RSI in TBI patients without adjunctive medications.[6]

The postintubation ventilation strategy significantly influences outcomes in patients with TBI. This reflects the adverse effects of positive pressure ventilation on cardiac output, hypocapnic cerebral vasoconstriction, and retrograde cerebral transmission of intrathoracic pressure via the jugular venous system, all of which can lead to cerebral hypoperfusion and ischemia. $PaCO_2$ should be maintained as close to normal as possible, within the range of 30 to 39 mm Hg.[7] Hyperventilation does decrease ICP, but it does so by causing cerebral vasoconstriction and results in decreased cerebral blood.[8] Transient hyperventilation, to a $PaCO_2$ in the range of 30 to 35 mm Hg, is therefore reserved as a temporizing measure in the setting of acute deterioration as a means of avoiding herniation. Serial arterial blood gas analysis or $PETCO_2$ monitoring should be performed after intubation to ensure proper ventilation because traditional pulse oximetry monitoring reflects only oxygenation status.

## CIRCULATION

Systemic hypotension has been associated with increased mortality in studies of TBI. Although the normal brain can maintain cerebral blood flow despite a range of mean arterial pressure levels, this ability appears to break down following TBI. In addition, intracranial hypertension requires higher mean arterial pressure to maintain adequate cerebral perfusion pressure. Every effort should be made to avoid hypotension in TBI patients and maintain systolic blood pressure lower than 90 mm Hg at all times if possible.

The use of pressors is generally discouraged in the initial resuscitation of multiple-trauma victims. Thus, the main focus of therapy is volume replacement with intravenous fluids and blood products. Albumin and nonprotein colloids have no role in the initial resuscitation of patients with TBI.[9] Hypertonic saline solutions appear to have osmotic properties that may lower ICP and decrease cerebral edema. However, outcome data have been disappointing,[10] and at this time the initial resuscitation fluid of choice remains standard crystalloid (lactated Ringer or 0.9% saline solution).

## AVOIDING CEREBRAL HERNIATION

The development of unilateral papillary dilation, hemiparesis, or deterioration in the level of consciousness is very concerning for the devastating complication of cerebral herniation. Heroic measures are in order. Aside from definitive neurosurgical management, the emergency physician should perform two interventions in this setting: hyperosmolar therapy and hyperventilation.

Patients with cerebral herniation should receive mannitol, 0.25 to 1 g/kg in bolus form, repeated every 4 to 6 hours.[3,11] Mannitol is an osmotic diuretic that can decrease brain edema, reduce blood viscosity, and cause a transient increase in circulating volume that improves cerebral blood flow and oxygenation. Hypertonic saline at concentrations of 7.2% to 23.4% has been studied as an alternative or adjunct to mannitol with favorable results. This is a promising therapy that has been beneficial in multiple small studies,[12-15] but at the time of this writing, evidence has not yet reached the level to change practice guidelines, and we therefore still recommend mannitol as the first-line hyperosmolar therapy.

Hyperventilation temporarily lowers ICP as a result of cerebral vasoconstriction. As stated earlier, the decrease in ICP seen with hyperventilation comes at the price of an even greater compromise in cerebral blood flow, which ultimately results in cerebral ischemia. Impending herniation is the one clinical setting in which transient hyperventilation, to a $PaCO_2$ value of 30 to 35 mm Hg, should be initiated as a temporizing measure until hyperosmolar therapy takes effect or surgical decompression can be performed.

## SEIZURE PROPHYLAXIS

Seizures in patients with TBI have a constellation of effects, including elevated ICP, hypoxia, hypercapnia, and massive release of excitatory neurotransmitters, all of which result in secondary insults to an already injured brain. Seizures should be treated immediately with benzodiazepines. There is no evidence that early seizure prophylaxis decreases the likelihood that a delayed seizure disorder will develop, but prophylaxis does decrease the likelihood of early seizures (within the first 7 days after injury). The decision to empirically administer seizure prophylaxis should weigh the likelihood of seizures against the possible side effects of medication. There is currently no consensus regarding which patients should receive prophylaxis, but it is reasonable to consider administration in high-risk patients. Patients at high risk for seizures include those with a GCS score lower than 10, cerebral contusion or hematoma, depressed skull fracture, and penetrating injury.[3] The first-line agent for seizure prophylaxis is phenytoin.

### STEROIDS IN PATIENTS WITH TRAUMATIC BRAIN INJURY

Corticosteroids do not improve outcome in TBI patients, and their use is associated with harmful complications. Steroids should not be administered as treatment of TBI.

## MILD TRAUMATIC BRAIN INJURY

### OVERVIEW

Current practice in EDs and trauma centers focuses on identifying TBI patients who require emergency neurosurgical intervention or close monitoring. However, about two thirds of patients with TBI in the United States sustain mild injury and are discharged home after a brief observation period. Mild TBI is generally defined as blunt injury to the head with resulting symptoms (which may or may not include loss of consciousness) and a GCS score higher than 13. For the emergency physician there are three important components of the management of every patient with mild TBI: when to image, disposition planning, and discharge instructions.

### IMAGING

As discussed earlier, the modality of choice for the initial imaging of patients after TBI is non–contrast-enhanced CT. The prevalence of CT abnormalities is about 5% in patients arriving at the hospital with a GCS score of 15 and increases significantly with a lower initial GCS score.[11] Approximately 1% of all patients with mild TBI ultimately require neurosurgical intervention. Several clinical decision rules designed to help clinicians decide which patients with mild TBI require imaging have been validated. Their recommendations differ because of variations in definitions and study populations. That said, certain features are consistently associated with intracranial pathology, such as older age, vomiting, focal neurologic deficit, and persistent alteration in level of consciousness. Recent consensus guidelines have been developed to guide imaging decisions and are summarized in **Box 73.3**.

## FOLLOW-UP, NEXT STEPS IN CARE, AND PATIENT EDUCATION

### DISPOSITION

Patients suffering TBI who have abnormalities on head CT or persistent alteration in mental status should be admitted to a hospital with neurosurgical capability and be closely monitored for deterioration (**Fig. 73.7**). There is good evidence that patients with head injury who have normal findings on head CT and neurologic examination can be safely discharged from the ED without an extended observation period.[16,17] It must be noted that the studies that came to this conclusion excluded certain populations, in particular, patients with bleeding disorders and those taking anticoagulant medications. Therefore, the data are insufficient to be certain that this recommendation is safe in these patients.[18] We recommend a more careful approach to patients with acquired or inherited bleeding diatheses: either close observation in the hospital or discharge in the care of responsible caregivers who can watch the patient closely for signs of deterioration and have rapid access to return to the hospital for reevaluation. It is reasonable to include patients and their families in this decision and have an open discussion of the uncertainty in our understanding of the risk for deterioration in patients with TBI.

### PATIENT TEACHING

The most important consideration when counseling patients sent home from the ED is to communicate the signs and symptoms of an evolving intracranial process, especially in patients who have not undergone CT imaging. Such signs and symptoms include worsening headache, persistent

**BOX 73.3 Consensus Guidelines to Direct Imaging Decisions**

A non–contrast-enhanced head computed tomography (CT) scan *is indicated* in head trauma patients with loss of consciousness or posttraumatic amnesia if one or more of the following is present:

- Glasgow Coma Scale score lower than 15
- Vomiting
- Age older than 60 years
- Drug or alcohol intoxication
- Deficits in short-term memory
- Physical evidence of trauma above the clavicle
- Posttraumatic seizure
- Headache
- Focal neurologic deficit
- Coagulopathy

A non–contrast-enhanced head CT scan *should be considered* in head trauma patients with no loss of consciousness or posttraumatic amnesia if one or more of the following is present:

- Focal neurologic deficit
- Vomiting
- Severe headache
- Age 65 years or older
- Physical signs of a basilar skull fracture
- Glasgow Coma Scale score lower than 15
- Coagulopathy
- Dangerous mechanism of injury
  - Ejection from a motor vehicle
  - Striking of a pedestrian
  - A fall from a height of more than 3 feet or 5 stairs

Adapted from Jagoda AS, Bazarian JJ, Bruns JJ, et al. Clinical policy: neuroimaging and decision making in adult mild traumatic brain injury in the acute setting. Ann Emerg Med 2008;52:714-48.

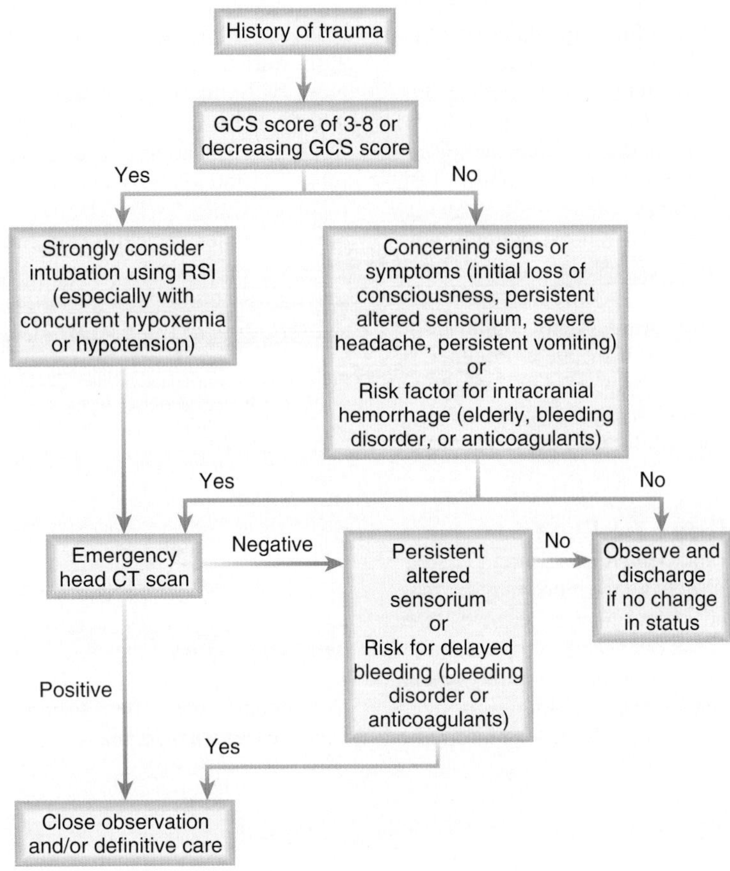


**Fig. 73.7 Algorithm depicting the differential diagnosis of traumatic brain injury.** *CT*, Computed tomography; *GCS*, Glasgow Coma Scale; *RSI*, rapid-sequence induction.

**Table 73.1 Stepwise Progression of Rehabilitation After Concussion**

| REHABILITATIVE STAGE | FUNCTIONAL EXERCISE AT EACH STAGE OF REHABILITATION | OBJECT OF EACH STAGE |
|---|---|---|
| 1. No activity | Complete physical and cognitive rest | Recovery |
| 2. Light aerobic exercise | Walking, swimming, or stationary cycling while keeping the intensity at <70% of the maximum predicted heart rate; no resistance training | Increase the heart rate |
| 3. Sport-specific exercise | Skating drills in ice hockey, running drills in soccer; no head impact activities | Add movement |
| 4. Noncontact training drills | Progression to more complex training drills, such as passing drills in football and ice hockey; may start progressive resistance training | Exercise, coordination, and cognitive load |
| 5. Full-contact practice | Following medical clearance, participation in normal training activities | Restore athlete's confidence; coaching staff assesses functional skills |
| 6. Return to play | Normal game play | |

If symptoms recur during any step, the patient should return to step 1. If asymptomatic, the patient may advance to the next step every 24 hours.

Adapted from McCrory P, Meeuwisse W, Johnston K, et al. Consensus statement on concussion in sport: the 3rd international conference on concussion in sport held in Zurich, November 2008. J Athl Train 2009;44:434-48.

vomiting, confusion, and balance problems. Any of these findings should prompt return to the ED for immediate reevaluation and consideration of appropriate imaging studies.

It is also important to communicate to patients the possibility of *postconcussive syndrome* (PCS). This syndrome of persistent neurologic, behavioral, and cognitive symptoms develops in a substantial proportion of patients with mild TBI. Symptoms include headache, memory impairment, difficulty concentrating, anxiety, and depression. Of all patients with mild TBI, about 50% at 3 months and 15% at 1 year[19,20] will have persistent PCS. Even though no specific treatments are available for PCS, early psychosocial intervention appears to reduce postconcussion symptoms and limit the emergence of persistent problems. Awareness can help validate symptoms that might otherwise not be attributed to the traumatic incident and lead to referral for neurorehabilitation or psychologic services or support groups.

## CONCUSSION AND RETURN TO PLAY

The term *concussion* refers to short-lived impairment of neurologic function after trauma. Such impairment may or may not involve loss of consciousness and typically resolves over a sequential course, although postconcussive symptoms may be prolonged.[21] A primary concern of emergency physicians and trainers is *second-impact syndrome*, which has been reported in athletes who return to play while still symptomatic from a concussion and sustain another head injury. These athletes, despite having mild symptoms and sustaining apparently mild second injuries, are at risk for the rapid development of brain swelling, herniation, and death. Additionally, athletes who sustain repeated concussions are at higher risk for long-term cognitive deficits. A stepwise progression of rehabilitation after concussion is recommended before return to play (**Table 73.1**), ideally supervised by an experienced athletic trainer or health care provider.

## SUGGESTED READINGS

Brain Trauma Foundation. Guidelines for the management of severe head injury 3rd edition. J Neurotrauma 2007;24(Suppl 1):S1-106.

Jagoda AS, Bazarian JJ, Bruns JJ, et al. Clinical policy: neuroimaging and decision making in adult mild traumatic brain injury in the acute setting. Ann Emerg Med 2008;52:714-48.

McCrory P, Meeuwisse W, Johnston K, et al. Consensus statement on concussion in sport: the 3rd international conference on concussion in sport held in Zurich, November 2008. J Athl Train 2009;44:434-48.

## REFERENCES

***References can be found on Expert Consult @ www.expertconsult.com.***

# Imaging of the Central Nervous System 74

*Andrew D. Perron and Carl A. Germann*

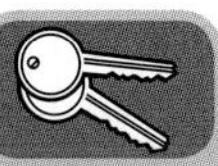

**KEY POINTS**

- The emergency physician needs to be able to accurately interpret and act on certain findings on computed tomography (CT) because many disease processes require immediate action.
- Even with a brief educational intervention, emergency physicians can significantly improve their ability to interpret cranial CT scans.
- Use the mnemonic "blood can be very bad" (where blood = blood, can = cisterns, be = brain, very = ventricles, and bad = bone) to quickly and thoroughly review a cranial CT scan for pathology.
- Magnetic resonance imaging offers excellent anatomic resolution and provides greater discrimination of various soft tissues than CT does.

## PERSPECTIVE

Imaging of the central nervous system (CNS) has assumed a critical role in the practice of emergency medicine for the evaluation of intracranial emergencies, both traumatic and atraumatic. A number of studies have revealed a deficiency in the ability of emergency physicians (EPs) to interpret head computed tomography (CT) scans.[1-6] However, a number of these same studies also show that with even brief educational effort, EPs can gain considerable proficiency in cranial CT scan interpretation.[2,3] This is important because in many situations the EP must interpret and act on head CT results in real time without assistance from other specialists such as neurologists, radiologists, or neuroradiologists.[7,8] Advantages of using these technologies for diagnosing CNS pathology in the emergency department (ED) include widespread availability at many institutions, speed of imaging, patient accessibility, and sensitivity in detecting many emergency pathologic processes.

## COMPUTED TOMOGRAPHY

### BASIC PRINCIPLES

The fundamental principle behind radiography is the following statement: x-rays are absorbed to different degrees by different tissues. Dense tissues such as bone absorb the most x-rays and hence allow the fewest to pass through the body part being studied to reach the film or detector. Conversely, tissues with low density (e.g., air, fat) absorb almost none of the x-rays, and most pass through to the film or detector. Conventional radiographs are two-dimensional images of three-dimensional structures; they rely on a summation of the density of tissues penetrated by x-rays as they pass through the body.

With CT scanning, an x-ray source and detector, situated 180 degrees across from each other, move 360 degrees around the patient while continuously detecting and sending information about the attenuation of x-rays as they pass through the body. Very thin x-ray beams are used to minimize the degree of scatter or blurring that limits conventional radiographs. In CT a computer manipulates and integrates the acquired data and assigns numeric values on the basis of subtle differences in x-ray attenuation. Based on these values, a gray-scale axial image is generated that can distinguish between objects with even small differences in density.

### ATTENUATION COEFFICIENT

The tissue contained within each image unit (called a pixel) absorbs a certain proportion of the x-rays that pass through it (e.g., bone absorbs a lot, air almost none). The ability to block x-rays as they pass through a substance is known as attenuation. For a given body tissue, the amount of attenuation is relatively constant and is known as that tissue's attenuation coefficient. In CT, these attenuation coefficients are mapped to an arbitrary scale of between −1000 Hounsfield units (HU) (air) and +1000 HU (bone) (**Box 74.1**). This scale is the Hounsfield scale (in honor of Sir Jeffrey Hounsfield, who received a Nobel Prize for his pioneering work with this technology).

### WINDOWING

Windowing allows the CT scan reader to focus on certain tissues within a CT scan that fall within set parameters. Tissues of interest can be assigned the full range of blacks and

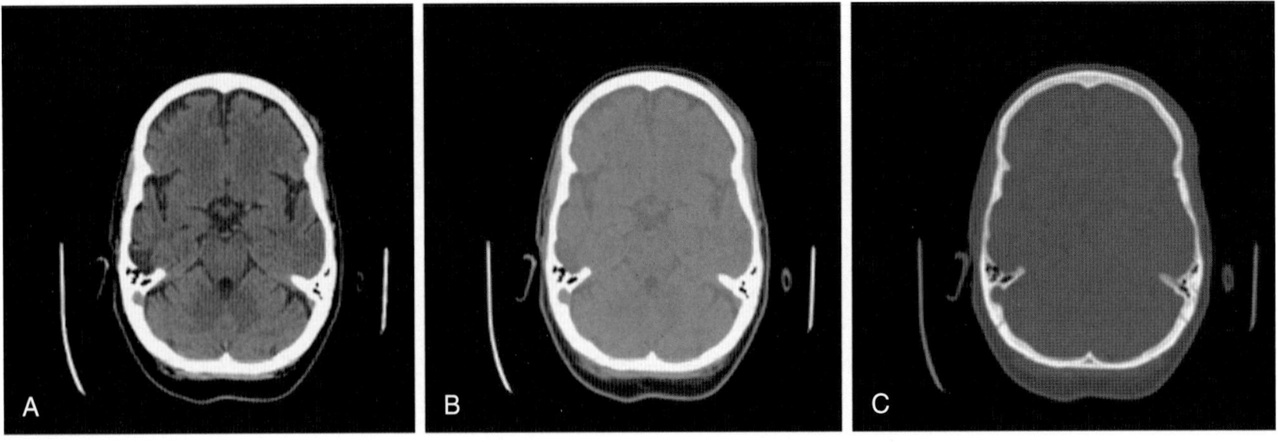


**Fig. 74.1** **CT scan windowing. A,** Brain. **B,** Blood. **C,** Bone.

**BOX 74.1 Appearance and Density of Tissues on Cranial Computed Tomography**

**Appearance**

Black → → → → → → → → → → White

−1000 HU → → → → → → → → +1000 HU

Air, fat, CSF, white matter, gray matter, acute hemorrhage, bone

**Important Densities**

Air = −1000 HU

Water = 0 HU

Bone = +1000 HU

*CSF*, Cerebrospinal fluid; *HU*, Hounsfield units.

whites rather than a narrow portion of the gray scale. With this technique, subtle differences in tissue densities can be maximized. The image displayed depends on both centering of the viewing window and the width of the window. Most CT imaging includes windows that are optimized for brain, blood, and bone (**Fig. 74.1**).

## ARTIFACT

CT of the brain is subject to a few predictable artifactual effects that can potentially inhibit the ability to accurately interpret the images. Besides motion and metal artifact (self-explanatory), the two most common effects are called beam hardening and volume averaging. It is important to understand these artifactual effects and to be able to identify them because they can mimic pathology, as well as obscure actual significant findings.

Beam hardening is a phenomenon that causes an abnormal signal when a relatively small amount of hypodense brain tissue is immediately adjacent to dense bone. The posterior fossa, where extremely dense bone surrounds the brain, is particularly subject to this phenomenon. It appears as either linear hyperdensities or hypodensities that can partially obscure the brainstem and cerebellum. Although beam hardening can be reduced with appropriate filtering, it cannot be eliminated.

Volume averaging (also called partial volume artifact) arises when the imaged area contains different types of tissue (e.g., bone and brain). For that particular image unit, the CT pixel produced will represent an average density for all the structures contained within it. In the instance of brain and bone, an intermediate density will be represented that may have the appearance of blood. As with beam hardening, certain techniques can minimize this type of artifact (e.g., thinner slices, computer algorithms), but it cannot be eliminated, particularly in the posterior fossa.

## NORMAL NEUROANATOMY AS SEEN ON HEAD COMPUTED TOMOGRAPHY

As with radiologic interpretation of any body part, working knowledge of normal anatomic structures and location is fundamental to the clinician's ability to detect pathologic variants. Paramount in head CT interpretation is familiarity with the various CNS structures, ranging from parenchymal areas, such as the basal ganglia, to vasculature structures, cisterns, and ventricles. Additionally, knowing the neurologic function of these regions of the brain helps when correlating CT results with findings on physical examination.

Although detailed knowledge of cranial neuroanatomy and its CT appearance is clearly in the realm of the neuroradiologist, familiarity with a relatively few structures, regions, and expected findings allows sufficient interpretation of most head CT scans by the EP. **Figures 74.2 through 74.5** demonstrate key structures of a normal head CT scan.

### IDENTIFYING CENTRAL NERVOUS SYSTEM PATHOLOGY ON CRANIAL COMPUTED TOMOGRAPHY

As long as one is systematic in the search for pathology, any number of techniques can be used when reviewing head CT images. Some recommend a "center-out" technique in which the examiner starts from the middle of the brain and works outward. Others advocate a "problem-oriented" approach in which the clinical history directs the examiner to a particular portion of the scan. In the author's experience, both these approaches are of limited utility to clinicians who do not frequently review scans. A preferred method, one that has been demonstrated to work in the ED, is to use the mnemonic

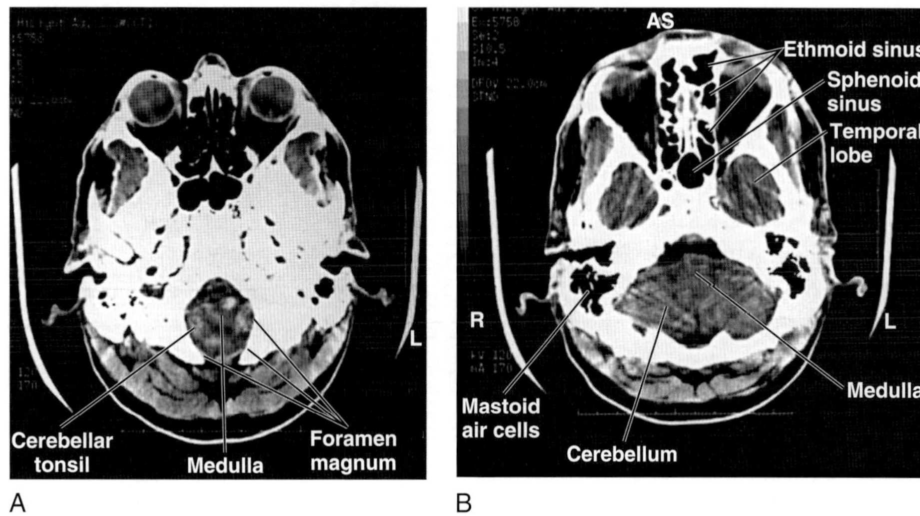


**Fig. 74.2 Head CT—normal anatomy. A,** Posterior fossa. **B,** Low cerebellum.

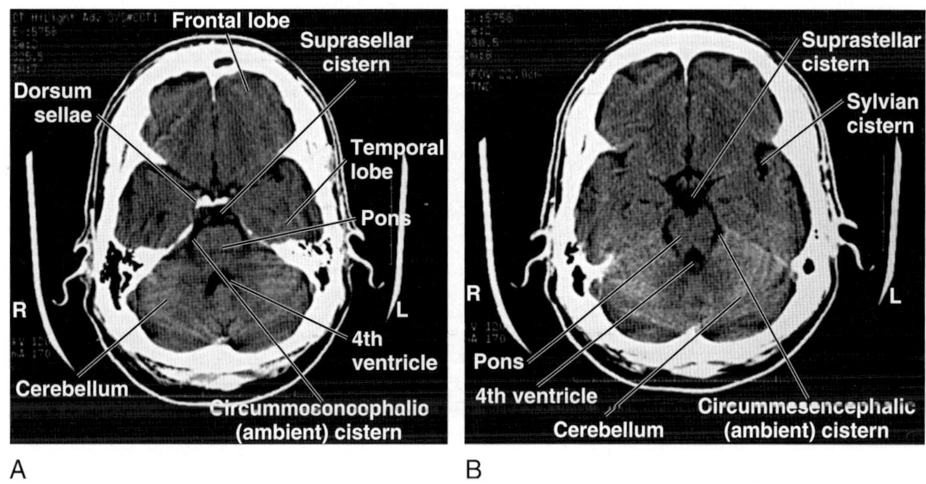


**Fig. 74.3 Head CT—normal anatomy. A,** High pons. **B,** Cerebral peduncles.

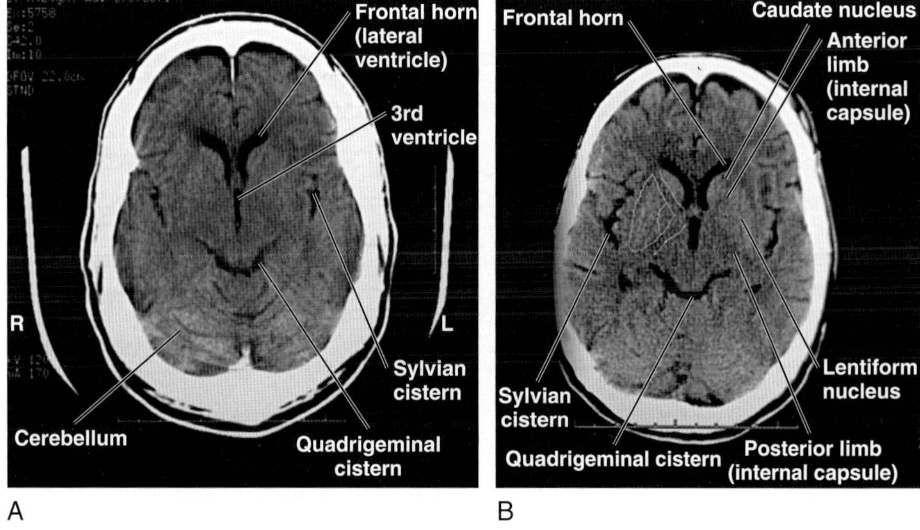


**Fig. 74.4 Head CT—normal anatomy. A,** High midbrain level. **B,** Basal ganglia region.

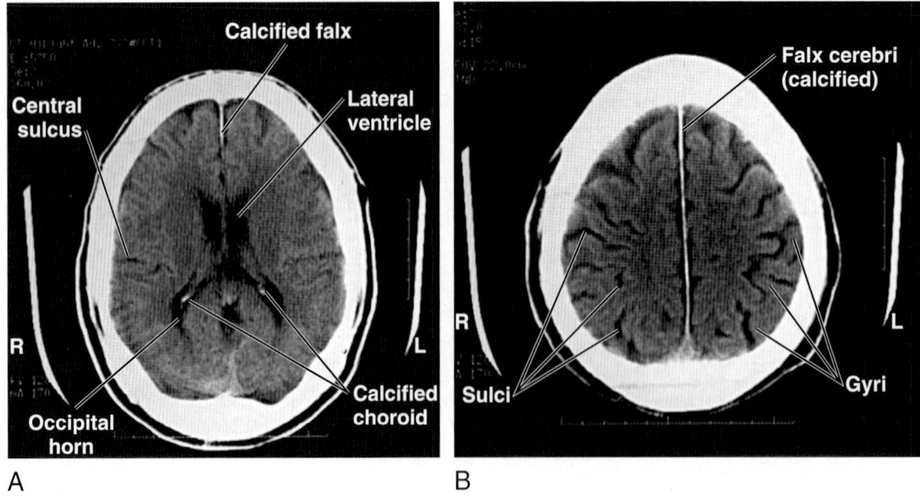


**Fig. 74.5 Head CT—normal anatomy. A,** Lateral ventricles. **B,** Upper cortex.

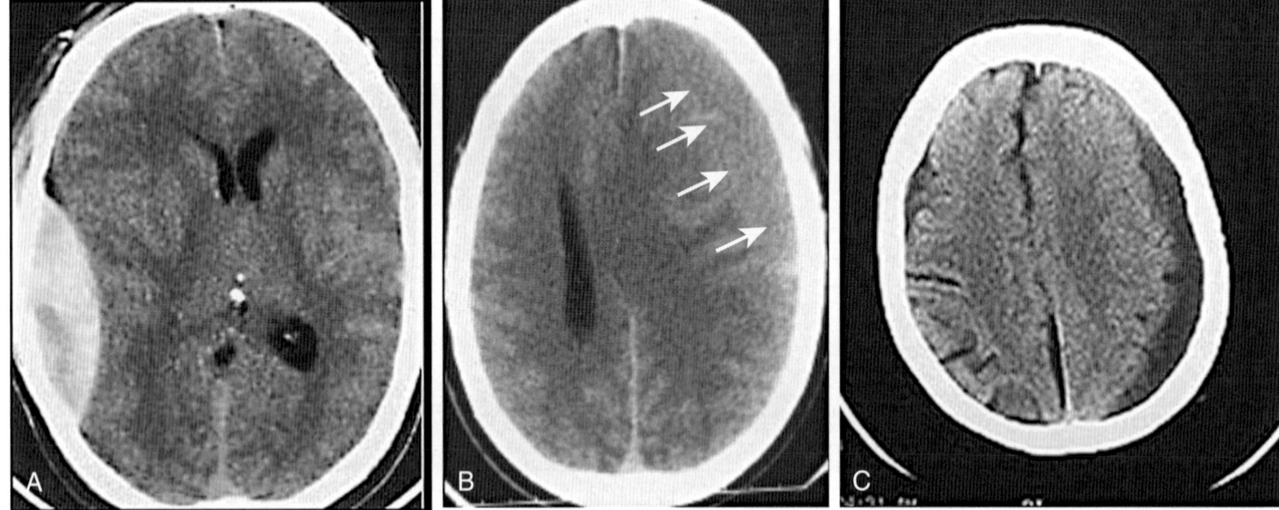


**Fig. 74.6 CT scan appearance of central nervous system hemorrhage. A,** Acute. **B,** Subacute; *arrows* identify subtle brain-blood interface. **C,** Chronic.

"blood can be very bad" (**Box 74.2**).[2] In this mnemonic, the first letter of each word prompts the clinician to search a certain portion of the CT scan for pathology.

## Blood

The appearance of blood on a head CT scan depends primarily on its location and amount. Acute hemorrhage will appear hyperdense (bright white) on cranial CT images. This is attributed to the fact that the globin molecule is relatively dense and hence effectively absorbs x-ray beams. Acute blood is typically in the range of 50 to 100 HU. As the blood becomes older and the globin molecule breaks down, it will lose this hyperdense appearance, beginning at the periphery and working in centrally. On CT scans, blood will become isodense relative to brain tissue at 1 to 2 weeks, depending on clot size, and will become hypodense relative to brain tissue at approximately 2 to 3 weeks (**Fig. 74.6**).

Precise localization of the blood is as important as identification of its presence (**Fig. 74.7**). Epidural hematomas, subdural hematomas, intraparenchymal hemorrhage, and subarachnoid hemorrhage each have a distinct appearance on CT, as well as different causes, complications, and associated conditions.

EPIDURAL HEMATOMA Epidural hematoma most frequently appears as a lens-shaped (biconvex) collection of blood, usually over the brain convexity. An epidural hematoma will not cross a suture line because the dura is tacked down in these areas. Epidural hematomas arise primarily (85%) from arterial laceration as a result of a direct blow, with the middle meningeal artery being the most common source. A small proportion, however, come from other injured arteries and can even be venous in origin.

SUBDURAL HEMATOMA Subdural hematoma appears as a sickle- or crescent-shaped collection of blood, usually over the cerebral convexity. Subdural hematomas can also be seen as isolated collections that appear in the interhemispheric

**BOX 74.2 The "Blood Can Be Very Bad" Mnemonic***

Blood—Acute hemorrhage appears hyperdense (bright white) on computed tomography. The globin molecule is relatively dense and effectively absorbs x-ray beams. As the blood ages, the globin molecule breaks down and loses its hyperdense appearance, beginning at the periphery. Precise localization of the blood is as important as identification of its presence.

Cisterns—Cerebrospinal fluid collections in the brain. The four key cisterns must be examined for blood, asymmetry, and effacement (representing increased intracranial pressure):

- Circummesencephalic—Cerebrospinal fluid ring around the midbrain; it is the first to be effaced with increased intracranial pressure
- Suprasellar (star-shaped)—Location of the circle of Willis; this is a frequent site of aneurysmal subarachnoid hemorrhage
- Quadrigeminal—W-shaped cistern at the top of the midbrain; it is effaced early by rostrocaudal herniation
- Sylvian—Between the temporal and frontal lobes; this is the site of traumatic and distal midcerebral aneurysm and subarachnoid hemorrhage

Brain—Examine for:

- Symmetry—The sulcal pattern (gyri) is well differentiated in adults and symmetric side to side.
- Gray-white differentiation—The earliest sign of cerebrovascular aneurysm is loss of gray-white differentiation; metastatic lesions are often found at the gray-white border.
- Shift—The falx should be midline, with the ventricles evenly spaced to the sides; it can also have a rostrocaudal shift, as evidenced by loss of cisternal space; unilateral effacement of the sulci signals increased pressure in one compartment; bilateral effacement signals globally increased pressure.
- Hyperdensity/hypodensity—Increased density with blood, calcification, intravenous contrast media; decreased density with air or gas (pneumocephalus), fat, ischemia (cerebrovascular aneurysm), tumor.

Ventricles—Pathologic processes cause dilation (hydrocephalus) or compression or shifting; hydrocephalus is usually first evident with dilation of the temporal horns (normally small and slitlike); the examiner must assess the "whole picture" to determine whether the ventricles are enlarged because of lack of brain tissue or increased cerebrospinal fluid pressure.

Bone—Highest density on computed tomography; diagnosis of skull fractures can be confusing because of the presence of sutures in the skull; compare with the other side of the skull for symmetry (suture) versus asymmetry (fracture); basilar skull fractures are commonly found in the petrous ridge (look for blood in the mastoid air cells)

*Blood = blood; Can = cisterns; Be = brain; Very = ventricles; Bad = bone.

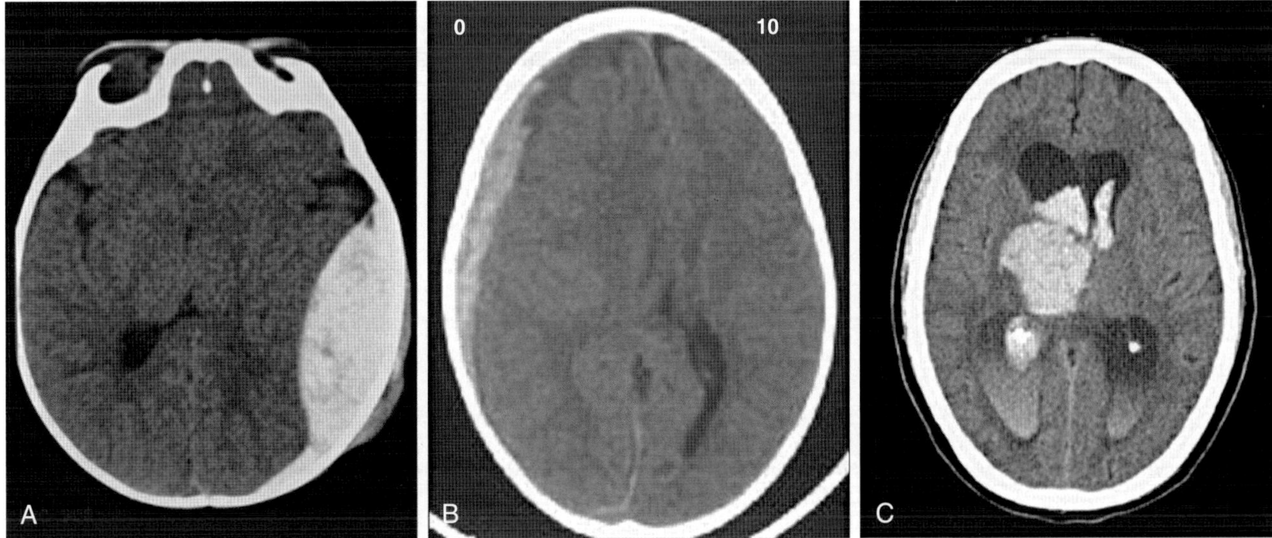


**Fig. 74.7 CT appearance of blood in patients with hematoma. A,** Epidural hematoma. **B,** Subdural hematoma. **C,** Intraparenchymal and intraventricular hematomas.

fissures or along the tentorium. As opposed to epidural hematomas, subdural hematomas will cross suture lines because there is no anatomic limitation to blood flow below the dura. A subdural hematoma can be either acute or chronic. Although both result primarily from disruption of surface or bridging vessels, the magnitude of impact damage is usually much higher with acute lesions. Thus, they are frequently accompanied by severe brain injury, which contributes to a much poorer overall prognosis than seen with epidural hematoma.

Chronic subdural hematoma, in contrast, usually follows a more benign course than acute subdural hematoma does. Attributed to slow venous oozing after even a minor closed

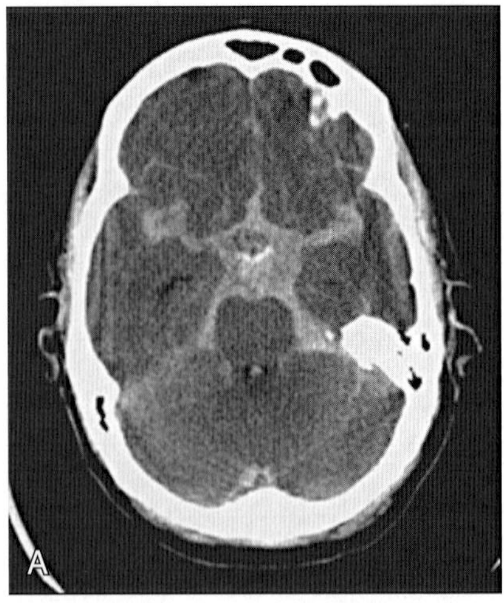


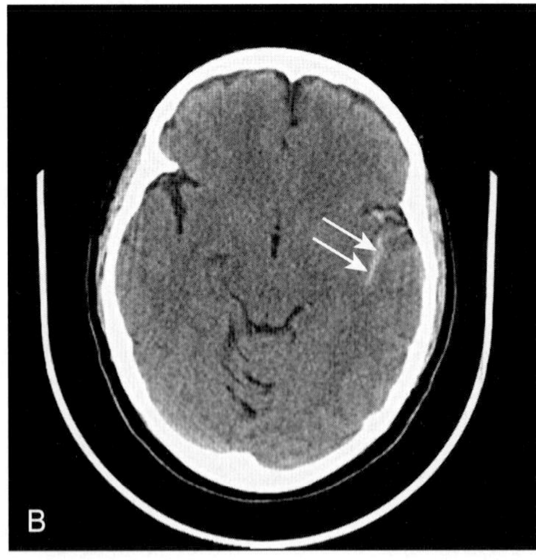


**Fig. 74.8 CT appearance of subarachnoid hemorrhage. A,** Blood filling the suprasellar cistern. **B,** Blood filling the sylvian cistern *(arrows)*.

head injury, the clot can accumulate gradually, which allows the patient time to compensate. Because the clot is frequently encased in a fragile vascular membrane, however, these patients are at significant risk for rebleeding after additional minor trauma. The CT appearance of a chronic subdural hematoma depends on the length of time since the initial bleeding. A subdural hematoma that is isodense with respect to brain tissue can be very difficult to detect on CT, and in these cases contrast enhancement may highlight the surrounding vascular membrane.

INTRAPARENCHYMAL HEMORRHAGE Cranial CT can reliably identify intraparenchymal (or intracerebral) hematomas as small as 5 mm. They appear as high-density areas on the CT scan, usually with much less mass effect than their apparent size would indicate. Traumatic intraparenchymal hemorrhages may be seen immediately following an injury, or they can appear in delayed fashion, after sufficient time for swelling has elapsed. Additionally, contusions may enlarge and coalesce over first 2 to 4 days. Traumatic contusions most commonly occur in areas where sudden deceleration of the head causes the brain to impact on bony prominences (e.g., temporal, frontal, occipital poles).

In distinction to traumatic lesions, nontraumatic hemorrhagic lesions caused by hypertensive disease are typically seen in elderly patients and occur most frequently in the basal ganglia region. Hemorrhage from such lesions may rupture into the ventricular space, with the additional finding of intraventricular hemorrhage on CT. Posterior fossa bleeding (e.g., cerebellar) may dissect into the brainstem (pons, cerebellar peduncles) or rupture into the fourth ventricle. Besides hypertensive causes, intraparenchymal hemorrhage can be caused by arteriovenous malformations, bleeding from or into a tumor, amyloid angiopathy, or aneurysms that happen to rupture into the substance of the brain rather than into the subarachnoid space.

INTRAVENTRICULAR HEMORRHAGE Intraventricular hemorrhage can be traumatic in origin or secondary to intraparenchymal hemorrhage or subarachnoid hemorrhage with ventricular rupture. Identified as a white density in the normally black ventricular spaces, it is associated with a particularly poor outcome in cases of trauma (although this may be more of a marker than a causative issue). Hydrocephalus can be the end result regardless of the cause. Cerebrospinal fluid (CSF) is produced in the lateral ventricles at a rate of 0.5 to 1 mL/min, and such production will occur regardless of intraventricular pressure. A block at any point in the CSF pathway (lateral ventricles → foramen of Monro → third ventricle → aqueduct of Sylvius → fourth ventricle → foramina of Luschka and Magendie → cisterns → arachnoid granulations) will result in hydrocephalus and the potential for herniation.

SUBARACHNOID HEMORRHAGE Subarachnoid hemorrhage is defined as hemorrhage into any subarachnoid space that is normally filled with CSF (e.g., cistern, brain convexity). The hyperdensity of blood in the subarachnoid space is frequently visible on CT imaging within minutes of the onset of hemorrhage (**Fig. 74.8**). Subarachnoid hemorrhage is most commonly aneurysmal (75% to 80%), but it can also occur with trauma, tumor, arteriovenous malformations, and dural malformations. As a result of arachnoid granulations becoming plugged with red blood cells or their degradation products, hydrocephalus complicates approximately 20% of cases of subarachnoid hemorrhage.

The ability of a CT scanner to demonstrate subarachnoid hemorrhage depends on a number of factors, including the generation of scanner, the time since the initial bleeding, and the skill of the examiner. According to some studies, CT is 95% to 98% sensitive for subarachnoid hemorrhage in the first 12 hours after the ictus.[9-11] This sensitivity is reported to decrease as follows:

90% to 95% at 24 hours
80% at 3 days
50% at 1 week
30% at 2 weeks

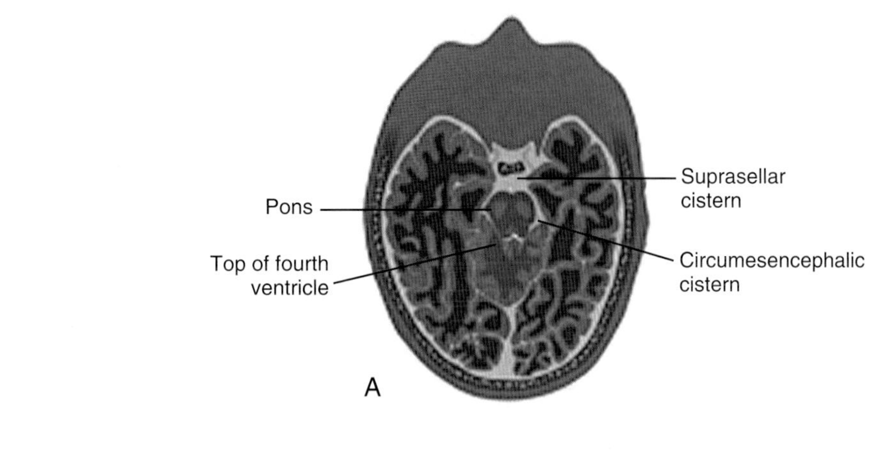


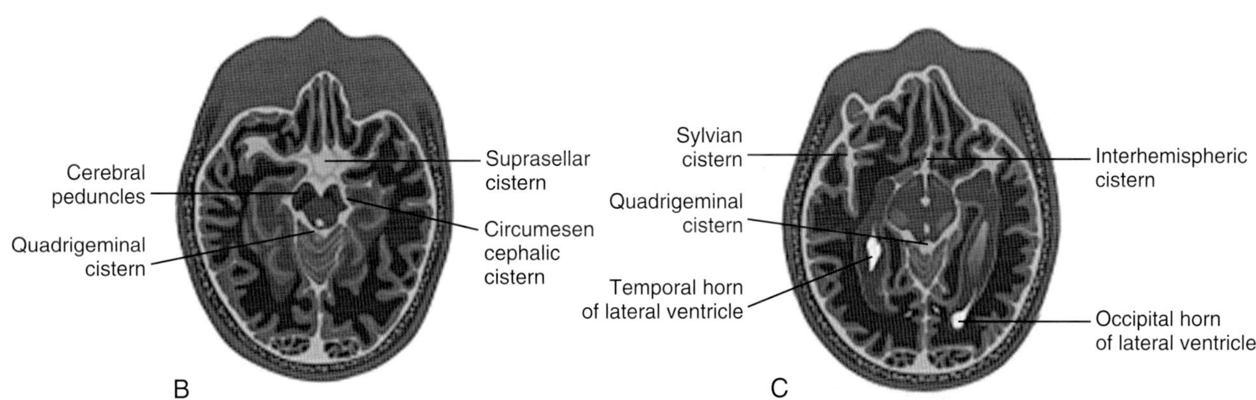


**Fig. 74.9 Three important cerebrospinal fluid cisterns. A,** Cisterns viewed at the high pontine level. **B,** Cisterns viewed at the level of the cerebral peduncles. **C,** Cisterns viewed at the high midbrain level.

EXTRACRANIAL HEMORRHAGE The presence and significance of extracranial blood and soft tissue swelling on CT imaging are often overlooked. The examiner should use this finding to lead to subtle fractures that can be identified in areas of maximal impact (and hence maximal soft tissue swelling). This will also direct the examiner to search the underlying brain parenchyma in these areas for parenchymal contusions, as well as to areas opposite maximal impact to search for contrecoup injuries.

### *Cisterns*

Cisterns are potential spaces that form where CSF pools as it works its way up to the superior sagittal sinus from the fourth ventricle. Of the numerous named cisterns (and some with multiple names), the EP needs to be familiar with four key cisterns to identify increased intracranial pressure, as well as the presence of blood in the subarachnoid space (**Fig. 74.9**). These cisterns are as follows:

- Circummesencephalic—Hypodense CSF ring around the midbrain; most sensitive marker for increased intracranial pressure; will become effaced first with increased pressure and herniation syndromes
- Suprasellar—Star-shaped hypodense space above the sella and pituitary; location of the circle of Willis and hence an excellent location for identifying aneurysmal subarachnoid hemorrhage
- Quadrigeminal—W-shaped cistern at the top of the midbrain; can be a location for identifying traumatic subarachnoid hemorrhage, as well as an early marker of increased intracranial pressure and rostrocaudal herniation (**Fig. 74.10**)
- Sylvian—Bilateral CSF space located between the temporal and frontal lobes of the brain; another good location to identify subarachnoid hemorrhage, whether caused by trauma or aneurysmal leakage (particularly distal middle cerebral artery aneurysms)

### *Brain*

Normal brain parenchyma has an inhomogeneous appearance where the gray and white matter interface. Because cortical gray matter is denser than subcortical white matter, the cortex will appear lighter on CT imaging. Many disease processes are unilateral (e.g., cerebrovascular aneurysm, tumor, abscess), and thus particular attention should be paid to side-to-side symmetry on the scan. Gyral and sulcal patterns should be symmetric (**Fig. 74.11**). It is also important to examine the brain parenchyma for the following:

- Gray-white differentiation—The earliest sign of an ischemic cerebrovascular aneurysm will be loss of gray-white

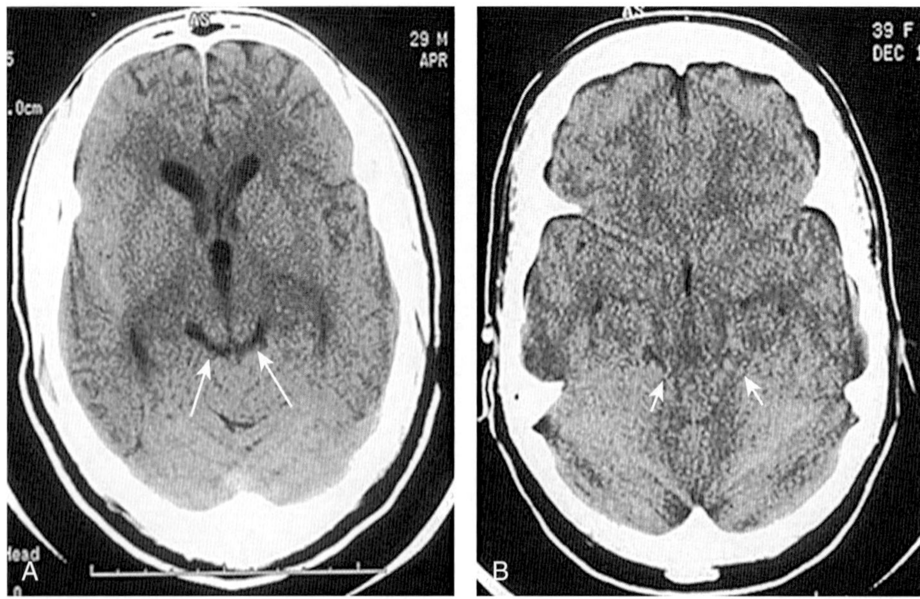


**Fig. 74.10 CT appearance of increased intracranial pressure as noted by compression of the quadrigeminal cistern *(arrows)*.** **A,** Normal intracranial pressure. **B,** Elevated intracranial pressure.

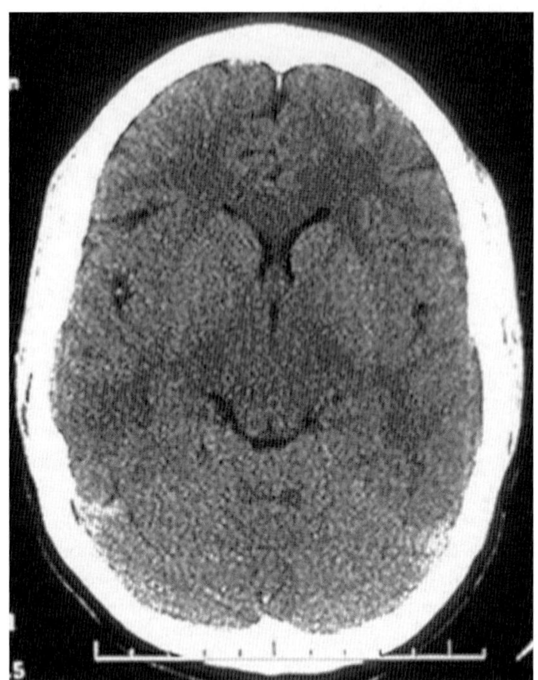

**Fig. 74.11 CT appearance of a normal brain.**

differentiation. Tumors can also obscure this interface, particularly when associated edema is present (hypodensity).

- Shift—The falx should be midline and the ventricles evenly spaced to the sides. With rostrocaudal herniation the midline will be preserved, but this will usually be evidenced by loss of cisternal spaces. Unilateral effacement of the sulci signals increased pressure in one compartment. Bilateral effacement signals globally increased pressure.
- Hyperdensity/hypodensity—Brain will take on increased density with blood, calcification, and intravenous contrast media. It will take on decreased density with air (pneumocephalus), water, fat, and ischemia (cerebrovascular accident). Tumor may result in either increased or decreased density on CT imaging, depending on the type of tumor and amount of edema.

## SPECIFIC BRAIN PARENCYMAL LESIONS

*Tumor* Brain tumors usually appear as hypodense, poorly defined lesions on non–contrast-enhanced CT. It is estimated that 70% to 80% of brain tumors will be apparent on plain scans without the use of an intravenous contrast agent. The calcification and hemorrhage associated with a tumor can cause it to have a hyperdense appearance. Tumors should be suspected on a non–contrast-enhanced CT scan when significant edema is associated with an ill-defined mass. This vasogenic edema is due to loss of integrity of the blood-brain barrier, which allows fluid to pass into the extracellular space. Edema, because of the increased water content, appears hypodense on CT (**Fig. 74.12**).

Intravenous contrast material can help define brain tumors. Contrast media will leak through the incompetent blood-brain barrier into the extracellular space surrounding the mass lesion and result in a contrast-enhancing ring. Once a tumor is identified, the clinician should make some determination of the following information: location and size—intraaxial (within the brain parenchyma) or extraaxial; and degree of edema and mass effect—for example, herniation may be impending because of swelling.

*Abscess* A brain abscess appears as an ill-defined hypodensity on non–contrast-enhanced CT. A variable amount of edema is usually associated with such lesions, and like tumors, they frequently demonstrate ring enhancement with the addition of an intravenous contrast agent.

*Ischemic Infarction* Strokes are classified as either hemorrhagic or nonhemorrhagic. Nonhemorrhagic infarctions can be seen as early as 2 to 3 hours following ictus, but most will

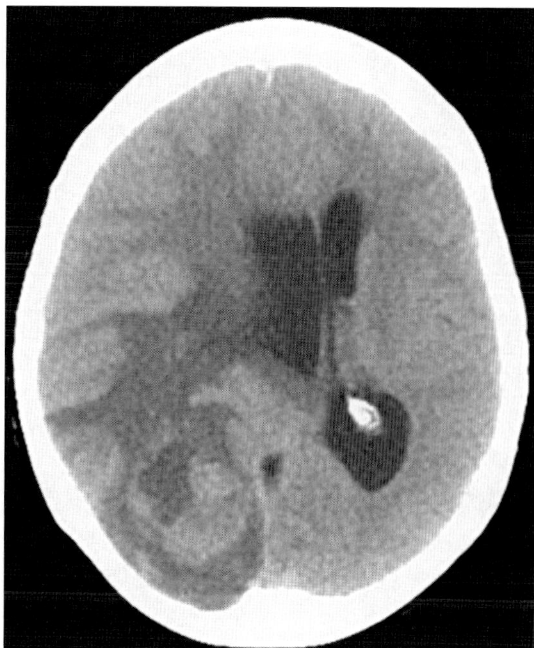

**Fig. 74.12 CT appearance of tumor with edema and a midline shift.**

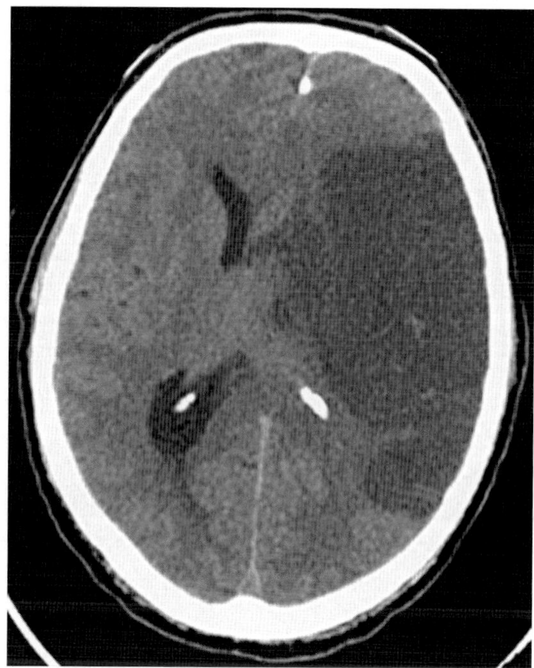

**Fig. 74.13 CT appearance of a large left middle cerebral artery stroke.** The hypodense brain is the infarcted region. Note the midline shift from left to right.

not begin to be clearly evident on CT scans for 12 to 24 hours. The earliest change seen in areas of ischemia is loss of gray-white differentiation as a result of influx of water into the gray matter. Because gray matter is metabolically more active than white matter, the gray cells are affected first, become edematous, and take on the CT appearance of white matter. This loss of gray-white differentiation may initially be a subtle finding but will become more pronounced, with peak findings becoming evident between 3 and 5 days (**Fig. 74.13**).

Any vascular distribution can be affected by ischemic lesions (e.g., middle cerebral artery, posterior inferior cerebellar artery). One specialized type of stroke frequently identified on CT imaging is a lacunar infarction, which consists of small, discrete nonhemorrhagic lesions usually secondary to hypertension and found in the basal ganglia region. They are often clinically silent.

### Ventricles

Pathologic processes can cause either dilation (hydrocephalus) or compression or shifting of the ventricular system (**Fig. 74.14**). Additionally, hemorrhage can occur into any of the ventricles and result in the potential for obstruction of flow and subsequent hydrocephalus. The term *communicating hydrocephalus* is used when CSF freely egresses from the ventricular system with blockage at the level of the arachnoid granulations. The term *noncommunicating hydrocephalus* is used if obstruction occurs anywhere along the course of flow from the lateral ventricles through egress from the fourth ventricle. Hydrocephalus is frequently first evident with dilation of the temporal horns, which are normally small with a slitlike morphology.

When examining the ventricular system for hydrocephalus, the clinician needs to consider the entire picture of the brain because the ventricles can be large for reasons other than increased pressure (e.g., atrophy). If the ventricles are large, the clinician should investigate whether other CSF spaces in the brain are large (e.g., sulci, cisterns). This can be a result of loss of brain volume rather than an increase in ventricular size. Conversely, if the ventricles are large but the brain appears "tight" with sulcal and cisternal effacement and loss of sulcal space, the likelihood of hydrocephalus is high.

### Bone

As demonstrated earlier, bone has the highest density on CT (+1000 HU). Consequently, depressed or comminuted skull fractures can usually be easily identified on CT; however, small linear (nondepressed) skull fractures and fractures of the skull base may be more difficult to find (**Fig. 74.15**). Additionally, diagnosing fractures can be confusing because of the presence of sutures in the skull.

Fractures may occur at any portion of the skull. The presence of a fracture should increase the index of suspicion for other intracranial injury. If intracranial air is seen on CT, this indicates that the skull and dura have been violated at some point (**Fig. 74.16**). Basilar skull fractures are most commonly found in the petrous ridge (the dense pyramidal-shaped portion of the temporal bone). Because of the density of this bone, the fracture line may not be easily identified in this area. The clinician should not only search for such a fracture line but also pay close attention to the normally aerated mastoid air cells that are contained within this bone. Any blood in the mastoid air cells means that a skull base fracture is likely. Analogous to the mastoid air cells, the maxillary, ethmoid, and sphenoid sinuses should be visible and aerated; the presence of fluid in any of these sinuses in the setting of trauma should

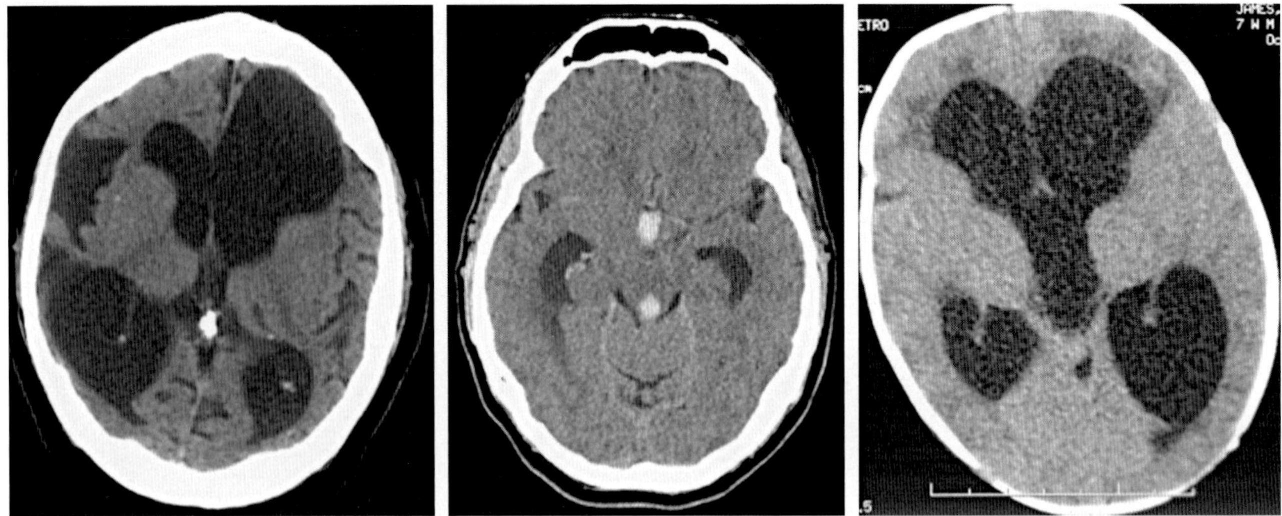

**Fig. 74.14 CT appearance of abnormal ventricles.**

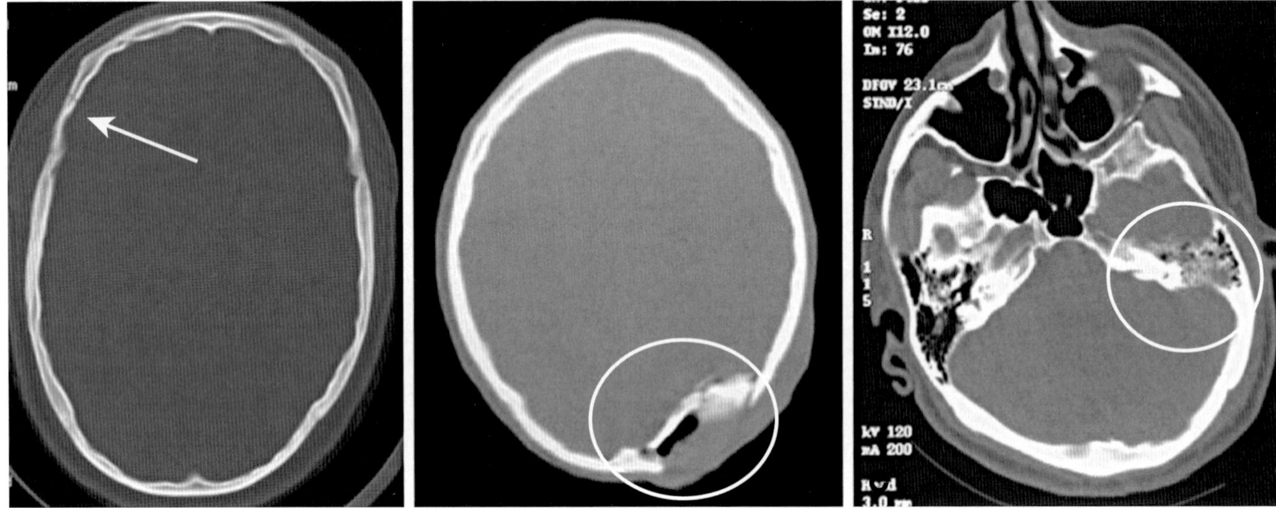


**Fig. 74.15 CT appearance with bone pathology. A,** Linear skull fracture (*arrow*). **B,** Depressed, comminuted skull fracture (*circle*). **C,** Basilar skull fracture (*circle*).

also raise suspicion for a skull fracture. In nontraumatic cases, fluid in the mastoids may indicate mastoiditis, and fluid in the sinuses may indicate sinusitis.

## MAGNETIC RESONANCE IMAGING

### BASIC PRINCIPLES

Unlike CT, magnetic resonance imaging (MRI) technology does not use ionizing radiation. Instead, images are created via magnetic fields and radiowaves. First, a strong magnetic field causes alignment of the magnetic poles of hydrogen nuclei (protons). The hydrogen nucleus is targeted because of its abundance in water and fat. A brief radiofrequency stimulus is then applied to the area being studied and causes a disruption in the magnetic alignment of the protons. The protons then return to their baseline state, during which they emit a signal that forms the image. The frequency of the radiowave emitted is related to the density and location of the proton and discriminates one tissue from another. For example, certain radiofrequency pulse sequences may be used to acquire clearer images of dense tissue, blood vessels, or other fluid-filled structures.

Although many MRI techniques exist, the two basic types of imaging sequences are T1 and T2. T1 and T2 images demonstrate the local tissue relaxation time that follows a radiowave pulse and thus reflect the three-dimensional molecular environment that surrounds each proton. For example, brain tissue contains intracellularly bound water and has shorter T1 and T2 times than do tissues with larger amounts of extracellular water, such as most neoplasms. (**Figs. 74.17 and 74.18**). T1 is a measure of the proton's ability to exchange energy with its surroundings. In other words, T1 is a measure of how quickly the tissue can become magnetized. T1-weighted

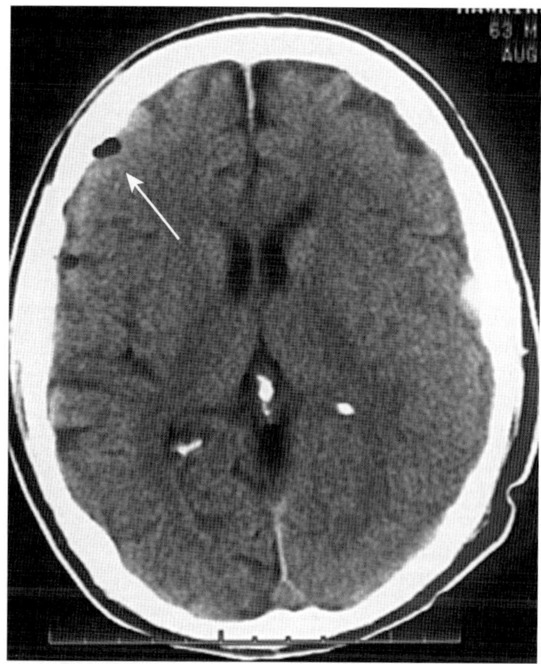


**Fig. 74.16** CT appearance of intracranial air *(arrow)*.

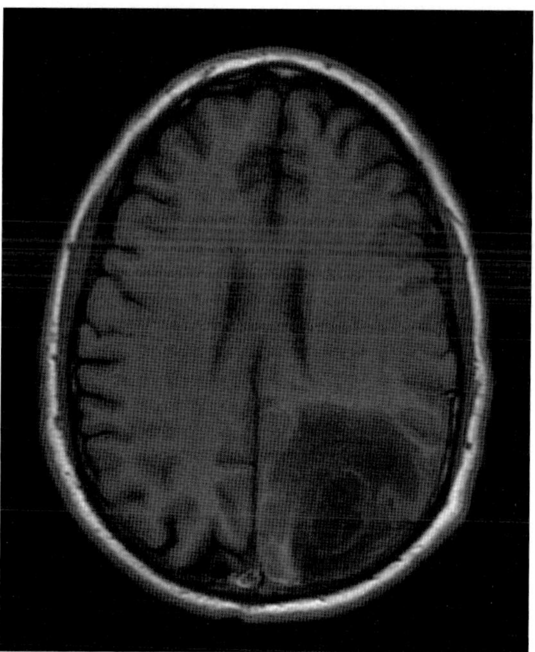

**Fig. 74.17** MRI—T1-weighted image without gadolinium contrast enhancement.

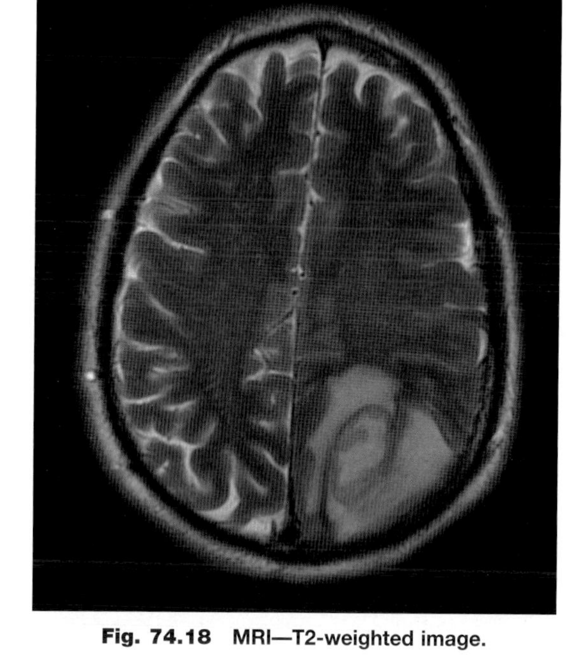

**Fig. 74.18** MRI—T2-weighted image.

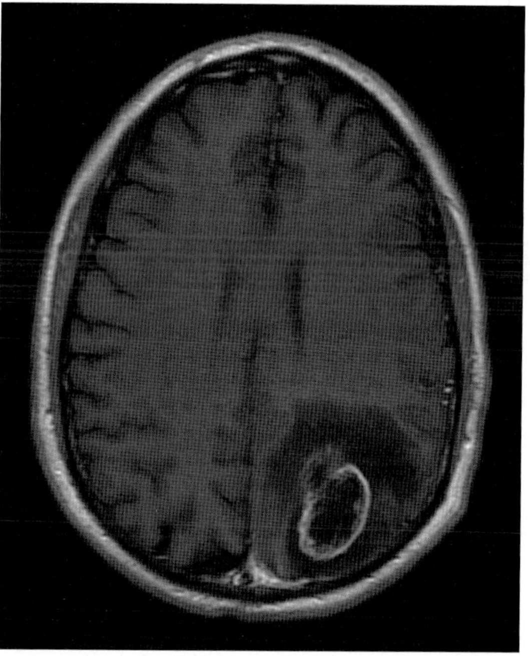

**Fig. 74.19** MRI—T1-weighted image with gadolinium contrast enhancement.

images show fat as a white or bright signal, whereas water or CSF is dark. T2 measures how quickly tissue looses magnetization. On a T2-weighted image, fat is dark, and blood, edema, and CSF appear white. Contrast dye such as gadolinium may also be used to enhance organs and accentuate pathology by shortening the T1 and T2 relaxation times of the hydrogen nuclei (**Fig. 74.19**).

Other commonly used radio wave pulse sequences include STIR (short time of inversion recovery) and FLAIR (fluid-attenuated inversion recovery). STIR sequencing is used to emphasize differences in T1 images and accentuate tissue with high water content while suppressing fat signal. STIR images are especially useful in spinal and joint imaging. For example, suppressed signal from bone marrow and surrounding fat allows bone tumors to be visualized more clearly. The FLAIR technique suppresses the T1 signals generated by fluid to better identify adjacent tissue abnormalities (**Fig. 74.20**). FLAIR is useful for differentiating

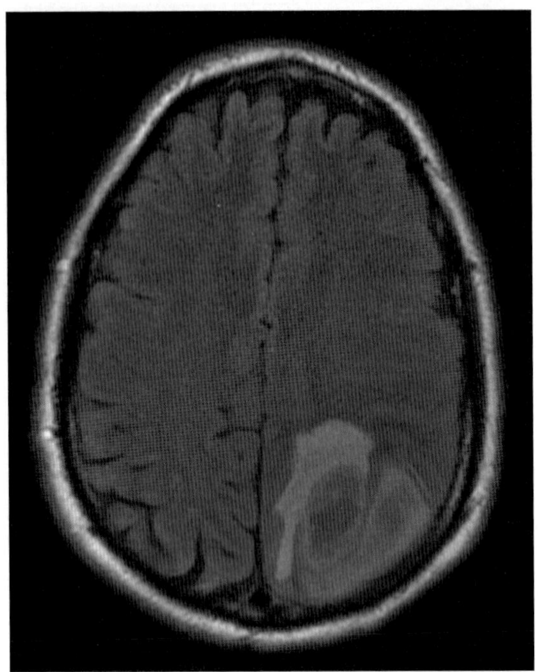

**Fig. 74.20 MRI—T2-weighted image with a fluid-attenuated inversion recovery technique.**

periventricular and spinal cord edema from CSF. The signal from CSF is nulled and appears darker in water-suppressed images.

## MAGNETIC RESONANCE IMAGING VERSUS COMPUTED TOMOGRAPHY

In general, MRI offers excellent anatomic resolution and provides greater discrimination of various soft tissues than CT does. For example, MRI provides clear images of the CNS and stationary soft tissues such as the shoulder or knee joints. In addition, many diseases are characterized by an increase in localized water content, for which MRI is sensitive in detecting. MRI is more sensitive than CT for diagnosing inflamed tissue secondary to cerebral ischemia, infection, or malignancy. MRI and CT are both sensitive in detecting acute hemorrhage; however, MRI is much more sensitive in detecting subacute or chronic hemorrhage, which may be less apparent on CT.

Disadvantages of MRI include cost, artifact because of patient motion, and inability to bring metallic objects into the room. MRI requires a cooperative patient but may induce claustrophobia in some patients. Finally, MRI often requires more time to perform than CT does, and immediate access to life support equipment is frequently limited.

## REFERENCES

***References can be found on Expert Consult @ www.expertconsult.com.***

# Spine Trauma and Spinal Cord Injury 75

*Michelle Lin and Swaminatha V. Mahadevan*

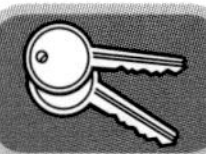

## KEY POINTS

- Patients with spinal pain and spine fractures should receive a thorough neurologic examination to look for spinal cord injury.
- Spine fractures are associated with a high incidence of concurrent noncontiguous spine fractures and spinal cord injuries.
- The National Emergency X-radiography Utilization Study criteria or the Canadian Cervical-Spine Rule criteria can be used to identify low-risk patients who do not need cervical spine imaging.
- Imaging with plain films versus computed tomography of the cervical spine should be based on the pretest probability of a significant injury and the irradiation risk with computed tomography.
- Spinal shock, or transient physiologic transection of the spinal cord as a result of trauma, is different from neurogenic shock, which is physiologic sympathectomy of the upper spinal cord leading to peripheral vasodilation.
- Patients with a spinal cord injury caused by blunt trauma are often given high-dose corticosteroids within 8 hours of injury, although such therapy is controversial.

## EPIDEMIOLOGY

The estimated annual cost of spine injuries, including inability to work and health care costs, exceeds $5 billion in the United States.[1]

In the emergency department (ED), all trauma victims are screened for vertebral fractures, ligamentous disruptions, and spinal cord injuries because of the potentially devastating neurologic consequences of overlooking these injuries. Patients with a delayed diagnosis of spinal fracture are 7.5 times more likely to sustain secondary neurologic deficits.[2] Neurologic deficits from spinal cord injury may be subtle and can easily be missed if not specifically evaluated. Adding to these difficulties, plain film radiographs of the spine, though an adequate screening tool for other fractures, can miss 23% to 42% of cervical spinal fractures[3,4] and 13% to 50% of lumbar fractures.[5,6]

## PATHOPHYSIOLOGY

In the setting of spinal trauma, the bone, ligaments, spinal cord, and vascular structures may be injured. Anatomically, the vertebral bony spine can be divided into structural columns. The cervical spine is traditionally divided into two columns—anterior and posterior. The *anterior column* consists of the load-bearing vertebral bodies, intervertebral disks, anterior longitudinal ligament, and posterior longitudinal ligament (**Fig. 75.1**). The *posterior column* consists of the more posterior structures, including the pedicles, laminae, and transverse and spinous processes (**Fig. 75.2**).

In contrast, the thoracic and lumbar vertebral spines are divided into three columns based on the modified Denis model—anterior, middle, and posterior (**Fig. 75.3**). The *anterior column* consists of the anterior longitudinal ligament, the anterior two thirds of the vertebral body, and the intervertebral disk. The *middle column* consists of the posterior longitudinal ligament, the posterior third of the vertebral body, and the intervertebral disk. Any disruption of the middle column predisposes a patient to significant spinal cord injury because the middle column abuts the spinal canal. The *posterior column* consists of the remaining posterior structures.

The C1 and C2 vertebrae are anatomically unique (**Fig. 75.4**). C1 (atlas) is a ring-link structure without a vertebral body. It articulates superiorly with the occipital condyles. This articulation allows 50% of normal neck flexion and extension. C2 (axis) projects the dens superiorly to articulate with C1. The transverse ligament tethers the dens to the anterior arch of C1. This atlantoaxial articulation allows 50% of normal neck rotation left and right.

The spinal cord spans from the foramen magnum to the L1 level, whereupon the spinal cord tapers into the conus medullaris and cauda equina, a collection of peripheral lower lumbar and sacral nerve roots. Because the spinal cord is thickest in the cervical spine, there is relatively less spinal canal space in the cervical levels than in the thoracic or lumbar spine. Thus spinal cord injuries occur more frequently with cervical spine trauma than with thoracic or lumbar spine trauma. The neurologic dermatomes can help localize the injury (**Table 75.1**).

The vertebral arteries branch off the subclavian arteries and course superiorly within the transverse foramina of C2 to C6. These arteries then merge to form the basilar artery.

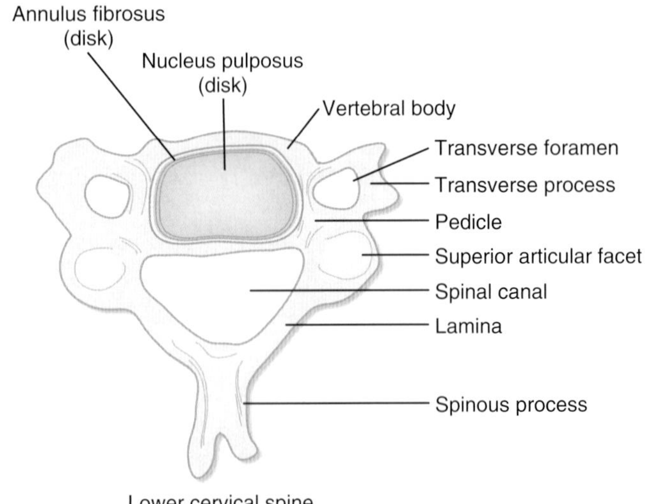


**Fig. 75.1 Bony anatomy of a typical lower cervical vertebra (C3-C7): superior axial view with the anterior aspect oriented upward and the posterior aspect oriented downward.**

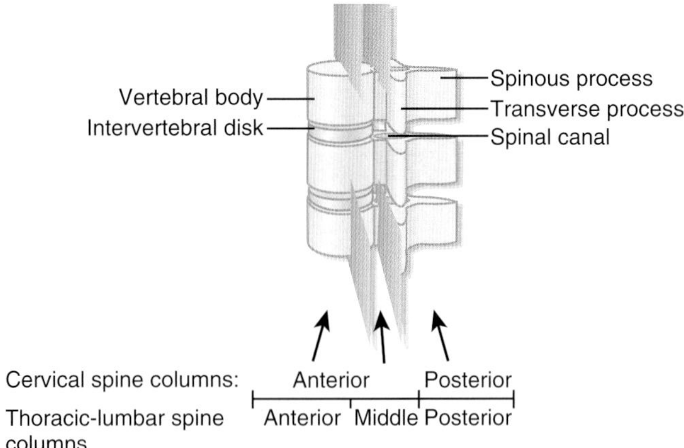


**Fig. 75.3 Schematic diagram illustrating the lateral view of the anatomic columns of the cervical and thoracic/lumbar spine.** Note that the cervical spine's anterior column is composed of the same structures as the thoracic/lumbar spine's anterior and middle columns.

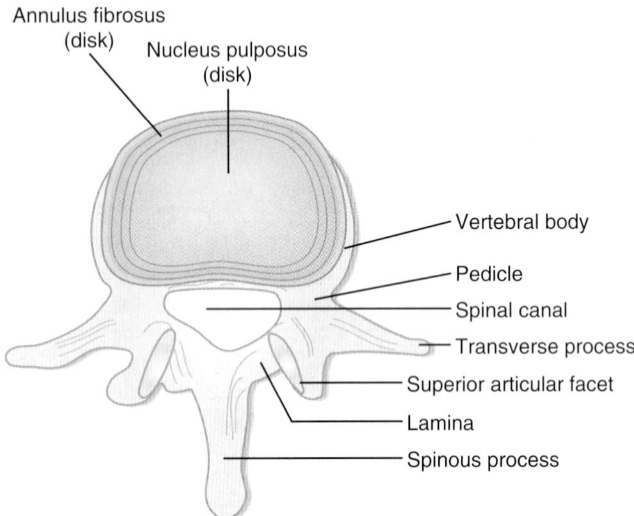


**Fig. 75.2 Bony anatomy of a typical thoracic and lumbar vertebra (T1-L5): superior axial view with the anterior aspect oriented upward and the posterior aspect oriented downward.**

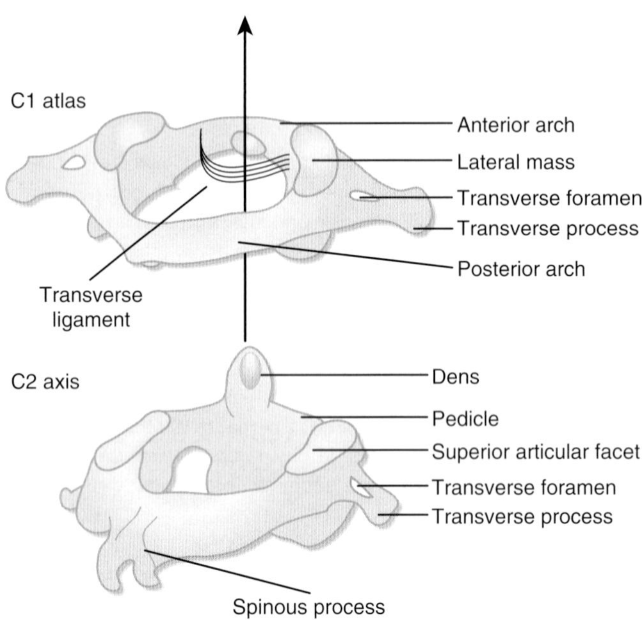


**Fig. 75.4 Bony anatomy of the upper cervical spine (C1 and C2): posterolateral view.** The C1 lateral masses articulate with the occipital condyles. The C2 dens projects cephalad, articulates with the C1 anterior arch, and is stabilized by the C1 transverse ligament.

## PRESENTING SIGNS AND SYMPTOMS

Patients with vertebral fractures usually have significant midline spinal tenderness on palpation. High-risk findings include spinal soft tissue swelling, ecchymosis, and step-off misalignment of the spine. Pain radiating along a dermatomal distribution suggests an associated radiculopathy. Thoracic spine fractures are uncommon because the articulating ribs provide stability to the spinal column; however, the thoracolumbar junction (encompassing the T10 to L2 vertebral levels) is commonly injured because the spine curvature changes from the kyphotic thoracic spine to the lordotic lumbar spine.

Patients with spinal cord injuries may have a spectrum of findings ranging from subtle neurologic deficits to grossly obvious paralysis. Spinal cord injuries should be suspected in any trauma victim who complains of neck or back pain, especially pain exacerbated by movement. Neurologic symptoms suggesting spinal cord injury include numbness, tingling, paresthesias, focal weakness, and paralysis. Other worrisome symptoms include urinary or fecal incontinence and urinary retention. Unconscious patients and those with impaired consciousness secondary to intoxication may harbor occult spinal cord injuries. Physical examination should focus on the spine and areas where associated injuries may occur (**Tables 75.2 to 75.4**).

**Table 75.1 Individual Spinal Sensory Dermatomes, Motor Function, and Reflex Arcs**

| SPINAL LEVEL | SENSORY DISTRIBUTION | MOTOR FUNCTION | REFLEX |
|---|---|---|---|
| C2 | Occiput | | |
| C3 | Thyroid cartilage | | |
| C4 | Suprasternal notch | Spontaneous respiration | |
| C5 | Infraclavicular area | Shoulder shrugging | Biceps |
| C6 | Thumb | Elbow flexion | Triceps |
| C7 | Index finger | Elbow extension | |
| C8 | Little finger | Finger flexion (with T1) | |
| T4 | Nipple line | | |
| T10 | Umbilicus | | |
| L1 | Inguinal ligament | Hip flexion (with L2) | |
| L2 | Medial thigh | Hip flexion | |
| L3 | Medial thigh | Hip adduction | |
| L4 | Medial foot | Hip abduction | Patellar |
| L5 | Web space between big toe and second toe | Foot dorsiflexion | |
| S1 | Lateral foot | Foot plantar flexion (with S2) | Achilles |
| S2 | Perianal area (with S3, S4) | Foot plantar flexion | |
| S3-4 | Perianal area | Rectal sphincter tone | |

**Table 75.2 Physical Examination Findings Associated with Vertebral Fractures and Spinal Cord Injuries**

| INJURY | PHYSICAL EXAMINATION AREA | ASSOCIATED FINDINGS |
|---|---|---|
| Vertebral fracture | Spine | Tenderness of the neck and/or back. Examine the entire spine because vertebral fractures may occur in multiples. |
| | Neurologic | See spinal cord injury below. |
| | Chest | *Thoracic spine fractures*: Check for chest tenderness, unequal breath sounds, and arrhythmia, which are suggestive of an associated intrathoracic injury or myocardial contusion. |
| | Abdomen/pelvis | *Thoracolumbar and lumbar spine fractures*: Check for abdominal or pelvic tenderness. For instance, up to 50% of patients with a transverse process fracture[7] and 33% of patients with a Chance fracture[8] have concurrent intraabdominal pathology. A transverse area of ecchymosis on the lower abdominal wall (seat belt sign) increases the chance of an abdominopelvic injury. |
| | Extremity | *Thoracolumbar and lumbar spine fractures*: Check for calcaneal tenderness because 10% of calcaneal fractures are associated with a low thoracic or lumbar fracture. Mechanistically, these areas are fractured as a result of axial loading. |
| Spinal cord injury | Neurologic, motor (anterior column) | Assess motor function on a scale of 0 to 5 (see Table 75.3). *Motor level* is defined as the most caudal segment with at least 3/5 strength. Injuries to the first eight cervical segments result in tetraplegia (previously known as quadriplegia); lesions below the T1 level result in paraplegia. |
| | Neurologic, sensory (spinothalamic tract) | Assess sensory function via pinprick and light touch on the following scale: 0 = absent; 1 = impaired; 2 = normal. The *sensory level* is defined as the most caudal segment of the spinal cord with normal sensory function. The highest intact sensory level should be marked on the patient's spine to monitor for progression. |
| | Neurologic, sensory (dorsal column) | Assess vibratory sensory function on a scale of 0 to 2 by using a tuning fork over bony prominences. Assess position sense (proprioception) by flexing and extending the great toe. |
| | Neurology, deep tendon reflex | On a scale of 0 to 4, assess the deep tendon reflexes in the upper (biceps, triceps) and lower (patellar, Achilles) extremities (see Table 75.4). |
| | Anogenital | Assess rectal tone, sacral sensation, signs of urinary or fecal retention or incontinence, and priapism. Also check the anogenital reflexes: an *anal wink* (S2-S4) is present if the anal sphincter contracts in response to stroking the perianal skin area. The *bulbocavernosus reflex* (S3-S4) is elicited by squeezing the glans penis or clitoris (or pulling on an inserted Foley catheter), which results in reflexive contraction of the anal sphincter. |
| | Head-to-toe examination | A spinal cord injury may mask a patient's ability to perceive and localize pain. Imaging of high-risk areas, such as the abdomen, and areas of bruising or swelling may be required to exclude occult injuries. |

**Table 75.3** Graded Assessment of Motor Function

| GRADE | ASSESSMENT ON PHYSICAL EXAMINATION |
|---|---|
| 0 | No active contraction |
| 1 | Trace visible or palpable contraction |
| 2 | Movement with gravity eliminated |
| 3 | Movement against gravity |
| 4 | Movement against gravity and resistance |
| 5 | Normal power |

*Spinal shock* is a neurologic phenomenon resulting from physiologic transection of the spinal cord. It results in flaccid paralysis and loss of reflexes below the level of the spinal cord lesion. Spinal shock is temporary, commonly lasting for 24 to 48 hours, although it can persist for weeks. Patients suffering from spinal shock may appear (clinically) to have a complete spinal cord injury only to "miraculously" recover once the spinal shock has passed. Termination of spinal shock is identified by return of segmental reflexes; anogenital reflexes are the earliest to recover.

*Neurogenic shock* may occur in patients with cervical or high thoracic spinal cord injuries. It is a neurocardiovascular phenomenon resulting from impairment of the descending sympathetic pathways in the spinal cord. As a result, vasomotor tone is lost and visceral and peripheral vasodilation and hypotension ensue. Diminished sympathetic innervation to the heart also occurs and results in relative bradycardia despite the presence of hypotension.

## DIFFERENTIAL DIAGNOSIS AND MEDICAL DECISION MAKING

### INDICATIONS FOR CERVICAL SPINE IMAGING

In the year 2000, in the hope of reducing the number of low-risk patients undergoing cervical spine plain film radiography, a multicenter study by the National Emergency X-radiography Utilization Study (NEXUS) group validated a set of five low-risk criteria for determining which patients do not require radiographic imaging if all the criteria are met (**Box 75.1**). This clinical decision tool demonstrated a sensitivity of 99.6% and a specificity of 12.9% for detecting clinically significant cervical spine fractures. It was thus extrapolated that 4309 (12.6%) of the 34,069 patients enrolled could have avoided plain film radiography.[9]

Following development of the NEXUS criteria, the Canadian Cervical-Spine Rule (CCR) was developed (**Fig. 75.5**). The validated sensitivity and specificity for this decision rule were 99.4% and 45.1%, respectively.[10]

The CCR study excluded the following subjects: patients younger than 16 years; patients with an abnormal Glasgow Coma Scale score, abnormal vital signs, injuries more than 48 hours old, penetrating trauma, paralysis, and history of vertebral disease; patients seen previously for the same injury;

**Table 75.4** Graded Assessment of Deep Tendon Reflexes

| GRADE | ASSESSMENT ON PHYSICAL EXAMINATION |
|---|---|
| 0 | Reflexes absent |
| 1 | Reflexes diminished but present |
| 2 | Normal reflexes |
| 3 | Reflexes increased |
| 4 | Clonus present |

**BOX 75.1 NEXUS Low-Risk Criteria for a Cervical Spine Injury**

A patient does not require cervical spine radiographic imaging if all five of the following low-risk conditions are met:

1. No posterior midline neck pain or tenderness
2. No focal neurologic deficit
3. Normal level of alertness
4. No evidence of intoxication
5. No clinically apparent, painful distracting injury*

From Hoffman JR, Mower WR, Wolfson AB, et al. Validity of a set of clinical criteria to rule out injury to the cervical spine in patients with blunt trauma. N Engl J Med 2000;343:94-9.

*NEXUS*, National Emergency X-radiography Utilization Study.

*Defined as a condition thought by the clinician to be producing pain sufficient to distract patients from a second (neck) injury.

and pregnant patients. Because these cases were not studied, the CCR guidelines should not be applied to such patients.

### CHOOSING THE IMAGING MODALITY TO EVALUATE THE CERVICAL SPINE (Fig. 75.6)

When patients have at least one high-risk criterion for a spinal fracture, imaging begins with either plain films or computed tomography (CT) scans. The pros and cons of both imaging approaches are listed in **Table 75.5**.

Patients with symptoms suggestive of a spinal cord injury should undergo CT and magnetic resonance imaging (MRI) of suspicious areas of the spine. Although plain films and CT do not directly reveal spinal cord injuries, they may supply indirect evidence of such injuries. *Spinal cord injury without radiographic abnormality* (SCIWORA) is a traumatic myelopathy in which no abnormalities can be identified on plain films or CT.

#### *Computed Tomography*

With increasing evidence in the literature showing that CT is much more sensitive (98%) than plain film radiography (53%) in detecting cervical spine fractures, future recommendations will probably recommend cervical spine CT as the first-line diagnostic approach for most patients because of the neurologic significance of a missed cervical spine injury.[11] Conventional radiography is especially difficult to interpret in the high cervical spine (occiput, C1, C2) and cervicothoracic

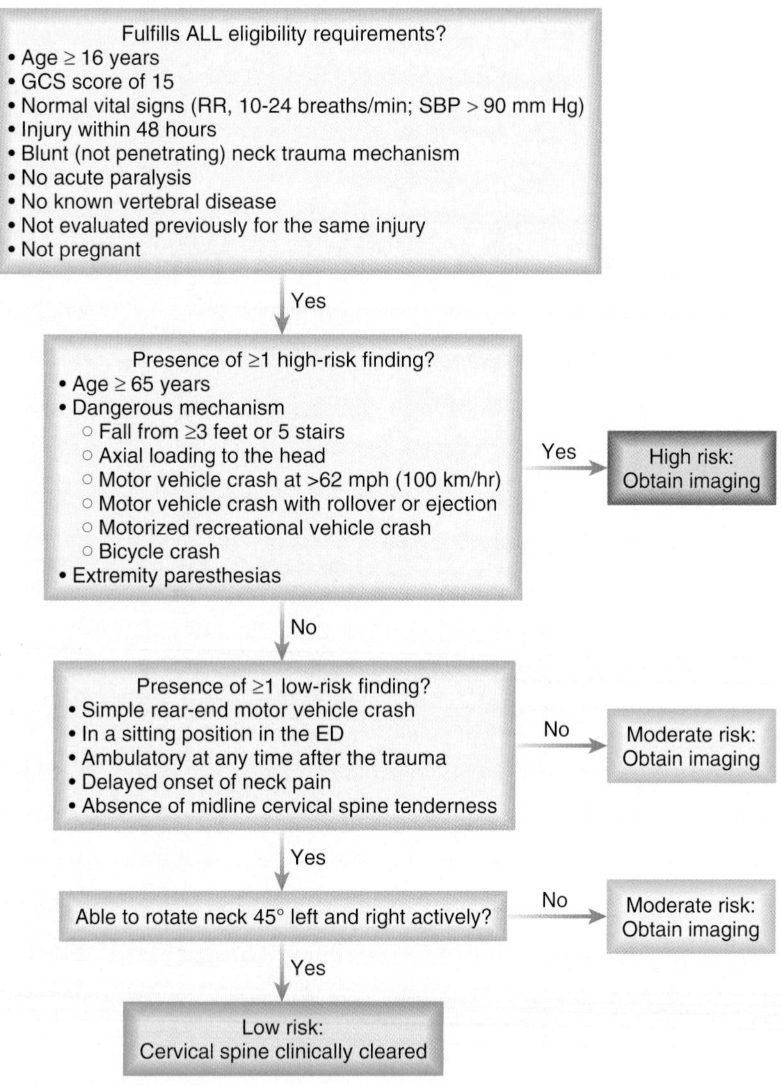


**Fig. 75.5 Canadian Cervical-Spine Rule (CCR) algorithm for clinical clearance of the cervical spine.** The *green box* signifies a low-risk, negative work-up and clinical cervical spine clearance. *Orange boxes* signify a moderate-risk condition, and the *red box* signifies a high-risk condition, both of which require plain film radiography. *ED*, Emergency department; *GCS*, Glasgow Coma Scale; *RR*, respiratory rate; *SBP*, systolic blood pressure. (Data from Stiell IG, Clement CM, McKnight RD, et al. The Canadian C-Spine Rule versus the NEXUS low-risk criteria in patients with trauma. N Engl J Med 2003;349:2510-8.)

junction (C6, C7, T1), where coincidentally most cervical spine fractures occur.[12] It is important to obtain sagittal CT reconstructions, in addition to the traditional axial views, to adequately assess spinal alignment.

Cost analyses have shown that cervical spine CT scans are actually less expensive than conventional radiography in high-risk patients. These studies factored personnel time, delays in patient management while obtaining films, and the neurologic sequelae of initially missing a cervical spine injury. Cost savings are especially evident if the patient is already undergoing CT imaging of other body parts, such as head scanning for a closed head injury. With multidetector scanners being more readily available, an additional cervical spine scan would add less than 5 minutes of scan time at a relatively small cost.[13]

The risk for cancer from irradiation serves as the major deterrent against universally performing CT in all patients with neck trauma. It is estimated that up to 2% of cancers in the United States are attributable to CT studies.[14] The thyroid gland, breast tissue, and lens are exposed to especially high levels of radiation in cervical spine CT, thus placing the patient at high risk for the development of thyroid cancer, breast cancer, and cataracts. Patients receive an effective dose of 0.2 millisievert (mSv) and 6 mSv for cervical spine plain films and CT, respectively. In contrast, the effective dose of a posteroanterior and lateral chest radiograph is just 0.1 mSv.[15] The overall lifetime carcinogenic risk from CT imaging, however, varies depending on the patient's age at the time of irradiation. Younger patients have greater risk, partly because they have more years of life left for the development of cancer.

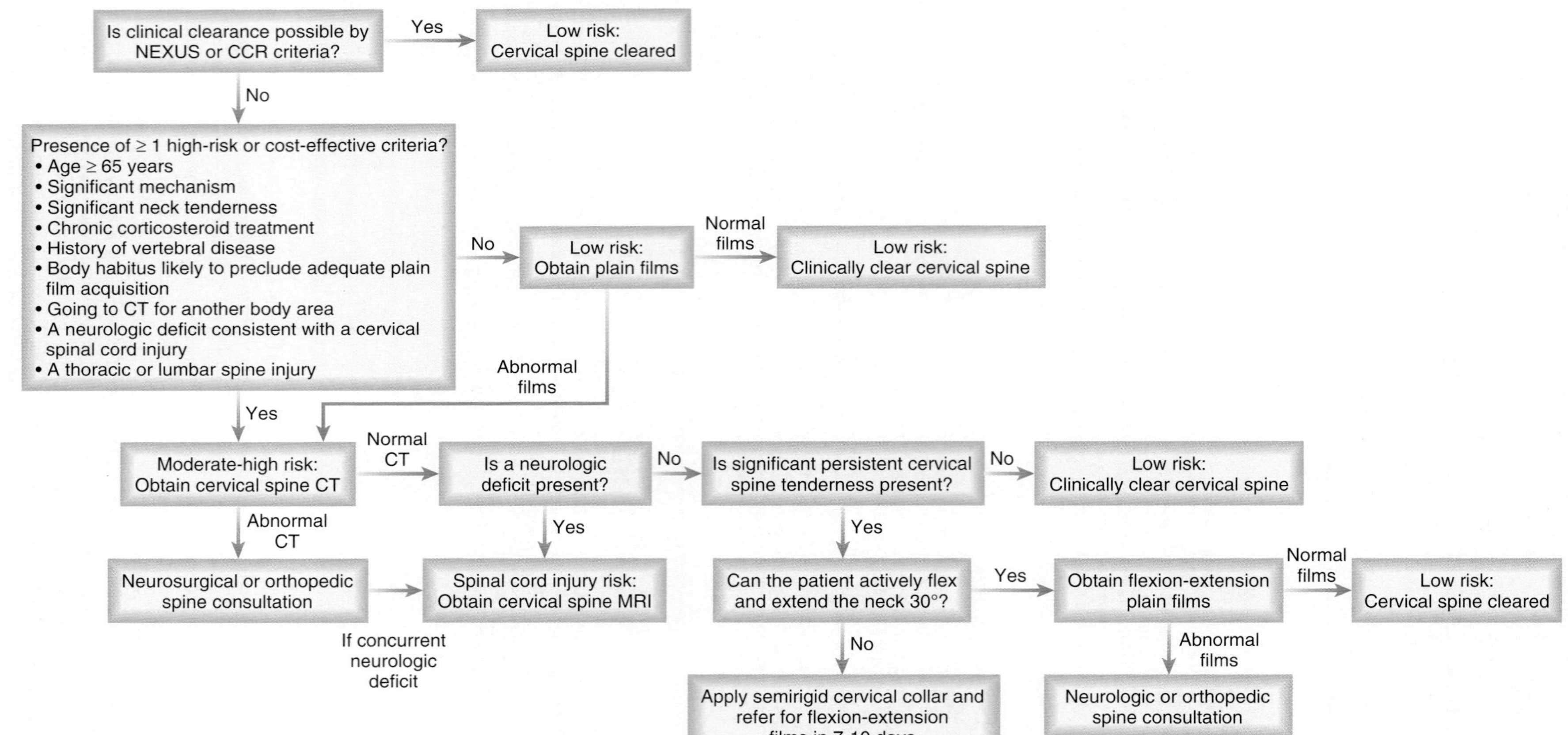


**Fig. 75.6 Diagnostic algorithm for a patient with neck pain resulting from blunt trauma.** *CCR*, Canadian Cervical-Spine Rule; *CT*, computed tomography; *MRI*, magnetic resonance imaging; *NEXUS*, National Emergency X-radiography Utilization Study.

**Table 75.5 Advantages and Disadvantages of Plain Film Imaging and Computed Tomography of the Cervical Spine**

| | PLAIN FILM RADIOGRAPHY | COMPUTED TOMOGRAPHY |
|---|---|---|
| Advantages | Less irradiation of the thyroid, breast, and lens<br>Can be performed at the bedside | 98% sensitivity in detecting fractures<br>More cost-effective than plain films<br>Less delay in patient management, especially if the patient is already going to CT scanner for imaging of another body part |
| Disadvantages | Only 53% sensitivity in detecting fractures<br>Three-view films are inadequate >50% of the time, especially films of the cervicocranial and cervicothoracic junction<br>Inefficient use of radiology personnel, who are often repeating films because of image inadequacy<br>A suspicious fracture or one detected on plain films requires additional evaluation by CT for confirmation and further delineation | More irradiation of the thyroid, breast, and lens<br>Requires the patient to be hemodynamically stable because of being transported out of the emergency department to the CT scanner |

Furthermore, children are more radiosensitive. If irradiated after 40 years of age, the risk reaches its nadir, with an estimated lifetime attributable risk for death from cancer of less than 0.2%.[14]

Because of such concerns for radiation exposure, low-risk patients should undergo conventional radiography. Only patients with radiographic evidence of an injury on plain films should subsequently undergo CT scanning. For moderate- to high-risk patients, cervical spine CT should be the first-line imaging modality, especially for patients scheduled for CT scanning of another body part.

### *Flexion-Extension Plain Film Radiography*

A normal cervical CT image adequately excludes a cervical spine fracture but cannot sufficiently evaluate ligamentous instability. In patients who have sustained significant flexion, extension, or rotational injury to the neck and have persistent neck pain, ligamentous stability should be assessed within 10 days either in the ED or by a neurosurgeon or orthopedic spine specialist.

In the ED, patients who are awake and alert and can actively flex and extend their neck 30 degrees may undergo flexion-extension plain film radiography to evaluate for spinal stability. Vertebral body subluxation or focal widening of the spinous processes suggests an unstable ligamentous injury. Because no serious adverse outcomes have resulted from voluntary neck movement by an awake, alert patient without neurologic deficits, manual manipulation of the patient's neck should be avoided during flexion-extension radiography.

Many acutely injured patients have such severe associated cervical muscle spasms that they have limited neck mobility. As a result, flexion-extension films are often inadequate, and these patients should be immobilized in a semirigid cervical collar (e.g., a Philadelphia or Miami J collar) and undergo delayed flexion-extension plain film radiography after 7 to 10 days, when the cervical muscle spasm diminishes.

### *Magnetic Resonance Imaging*

MRI is the best available modality for detection and characterization of spinal cord injury, but it is less sensitive than CT for cervical spine fractures. In an acute trauma patient with potential spinal injury, indications for emergency MRI include (1) complete or incomplete neurologic deficits suspicious for a spinal cord injury, (2) deterioration of spinal cord neurologic function, and (3) signs of unstable ligamentous injury. Abnormal MRI findings may include the presence of spinal canal compromise, disk herniation, and spinal cord edema or hemorrhage.

## OLDER AND OSTEOPENIC PATIENTS

Patients older than 65 years old and those taking corticosteroids on a long-term basis are probably osteopenic. They can sustain spinal fractures with mild trauma, such as a fall from a standing position, and often exhibit minimal associated pain. Specifically, patients older than 65 years have an increased risk for cervical spine fracture (relative risk of 2.09).[16] In addition, acute back pain in chronic corticosteroid users is correlated with 99% specificity for a spinal compression fracture.[17] Thus, imaging should be performed in these potentially osteopenic patients in the setting of neck or back pain.

## CLINICAL CLEARANCE OF THE CERVICAL SPINE

Not all patients require cervical spine imaging. To clinically clear a cervical spine, the patient's neck should be reevaluated for tenderness. First, unfasten the cervical collar. Next, palpate the posterior aspect of the patient's neck while applying the other hand to the patient's forehead to prevent spontaneous and reflexive head lifting. In the absence of significant midline tenderness, remove your hands and instruct the patient to actively lift the head off the gurney and place the neck through a range of motion by looking right, left, caudad, and cephalad. Do not assist the patient.

If the patient is able to move spontaneously and easily without pain or neurologic symptoms, the patient's neck is considered to be "clinically cleared" and the collar may be removed.

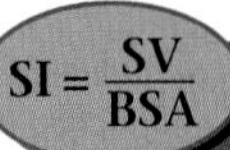


**FACTS AND FORMULAS**

Ten percent of spinal fractures have a second noncontiguous fracture along the vertebral spine.

Ten percent of patients with a calcaneal fracture have an associated thoracic or lumbar fracture.

The most commonly fractured cervical spine level is C2, especially in the elderly.

Approximately 20% of computed tomography–confirmed burst fractures in the thoracic and lumbar spine appear as wedge fractures on plain film radiography.[18]

High-dose methylprednisolone is administered as a 30-mg/kg bolus and then as a 5.4-mg/kg/hr infusion for 24 hours (if started within 3 hours of injury) or for 48 hours (if started within 8 hours of injury).

Consider early endotracheal intubation in spinal cord injury patients with a negative inspiratory force of less than –25 cm $H_2O$ or a vital capacity of less than 15 mL/kg.

## CLASSIC FRACTURE PATTERNS (Tables 75.6 to 75.8; Figs. 75.7 to 75.9)

### CERVICAL SPINE INJURIES

Based on the NEXUS study of 818 patients with cervical spine injury, fractures occurred most commonly at the level of C2 (24% of all fractures), C6 (20%), and C7 (19%). Anatomically, the most commonly fractured part of the cervical spine was the vertebral body, which accounted for 30% of fractures at the C3 to C7 levels. It was more common than fractures of the spinous process (21%), lamina (16%), and articular process (15%). Subluxations occurred most commonly at the C5-C6 (25%) and C6-C7 (23%) levels.[19]

### THORACIC AND LUMBAR SPINE INJURIES

Similar to patients undergoing cervical spine assessment, low-risk patients may selectively be cleared clinically without radiographic imaging. Although no large studies of thoracic and lumbar spine injuries equivalent to the NEXUS and CCR

**Table 75.6 Classic Upper Cervical Spine Injury Patterns (C1-C2)***

| INJURY | MECHANISM | STABILITY | FIGURE | COMMENTS |
|---|---|---|---|---|
| Atlantooccipital dislocation | Flexion | Unstable | 75.7, *A* | Often instantly fatal<br>More common in children because of small, horizontally oriented occipital condyles<br>Dislocation can be anterior (most common), superiorly distracted, or posterior |
| Anterior atlantoaxial dislocation | Flexion | Unstable | 75.7, *B* | Associated with rupture of the transverse ligament<br>Most commonly occurs in patients with rheumatoid arthritis and ankylosing spondylitis from ligament laxity<br>Widening of the predental space seen on lateral plain films |
| Jefferson fracture (C1 burst fracture) | Axial compression | Unstable | 75.7, *C* | 33% with associated C2 fracture<br>Low incidence of neurologic injury because of a wide C1 spinal canal<br>Usually involves fractures of both the anterior and posterior C1 arches, often with 3 or 4 fracture fragments<br>*Complication*: transverse ligament rupture, especially if the C1 lateral masses are ≥7 mm wider than expected (MRI recommended); vertebral artery injury (CT angiography recommended) |
| C1 posterior arch fracture | Extension | Stable | 75.7, *C* | An associated C2 fracture (occurs 50% of time) makes a posterior arch fracture unstable<br>On plain films, no displacement of lateral masses on the odontoid view and no prevertebral soft tissue swelling, unlike a Jefferson burst fracture |
| C2 dens fracture | Flexion | Variable | 75.7, *D* | *Type I (stable)*: Avulsion of the dens with an intact transverse ligament<br>*Type II (unstable)*: Fracture at the base of the dens; 10% have an associated rupture of the transverse ligament—MRI provides a definitive diagnosis of ligament rupture<br>*Type III (stable)*: Fracture of the dens extending into the vertebral body |
| Hangman's fracture (C2 spondylolisthesis) | Extension | Unstable | 75.7, *E* | Bilateral C2 pedicle fractures<br>At risk for disruption of the PLL, C2 anterior subluxation, and C2-C3 disk rupture<br>Low risk for spinal cord injury because of C2 anterior subluxation, which widens the spinal canal |
| Extension teardrop fracture | Extension | Unstable | 75.7, *F* | Small triangular avulsion of the anteroinferior vertebral body at the insertion point of the ALL<br>Occurs most frequently at the C2 level but can occur in the lower cervical spine<br>*Complication*: central cord syndrome as a result of the ligamentum flavum buckling during hyperextension<br>Requires CT differentiation from a very unstable *flexion* teardrop fracture (see "flexion teardrop fracture" in Table 75.7) |

*ALL*, Anterior longitudinal ligament; *CT*, computed tomography; *MRI*, magnetic resonance imaging; *PLL*, posterior longitudinal ligament.
*Listed in progressive order from the occiput, to C1, to C2.

projects have been conducted, recommendations can be extrapolated from the relevant literature.

Based on the NEXUS criteria, patients with (1) significant back pain or tenderness, (2) clinical evidence of drug- or alcohol-related intoxication, (3) lower extremity neurologic deficits, (4) Glasgow Coma Scale score lower than 15, or (5) a distracting injury cannot be cleared clinically for a thoracic or lumbar fracture. Patients with alcohol intoxication, for example, should not be cleared clinically until they are sober and found to fulfill no other high-risk criteria.

Furthermore, based on the CCR criteria and the American Healthcare Research and Quality "red flag" indications for imaging, injured patients who are (1) older than 65 years with any degree of back pain or tenderness, (2) are receiving

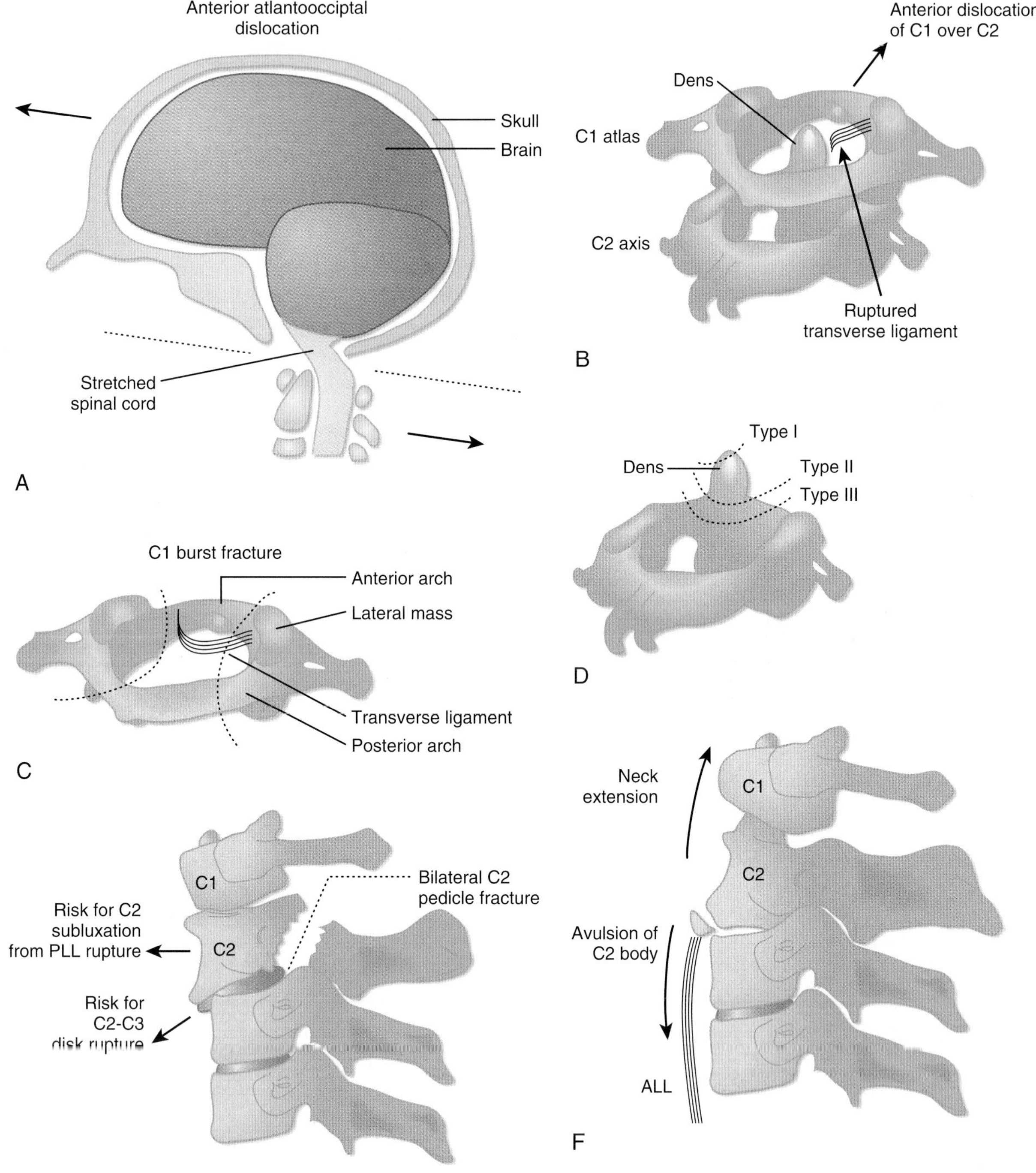


**Fig. 75.7** **A,** Cross-sectional sagittal view of anterior atlantooccipital dislocation with associated spinal cord injury. **B,** Posterolateral view of anterior atlantoaxial dislocation from rupture of the transverse ligament. **C,** Posterolateral view of a C1 Jefferson burst fracture through the anterior and posterior arch and an isolated C1 posterior arch fracture. **D,** Posterolateral view of the three types of C2 dens fractures. **E,** Sagittal view of a hangman's fracture with bilateral C2 pedicle fracture. *PLL,* Posterior longitudinal ligament. **F,** Sagittal view of a C2 extension teardrop fracture. *ALL,* Anterior longitudinal ligament.

**Table 75.7 Classic Lower Cervical Spine Injury Patterns (C3-C7)**

| INJURY | MECHANISM | STABILITY | FIGURE | COMMENTS |
|---|---|---|---|---|
| Articular mass fracture | Flexion-rotation | Stable | 75.8, *A* | Associated with transverse process and vertebral body fractures<br>Uncommon |
| Burst fracture | Axial compression | Stable | 75.8, *B* | Compressive fracture of the anterior and posterior vertebral body<br>Intact ALL and PLL<br>*Complication*: spinal cord injury because of a retropulsed vertebral body fragment (especially anterior cord syndrome) |
| Clay shoveler's (spinous process) fracture | Flexion | Stable | 75.8, *B* | Spinous process fracture from forceful neck flexion<br>Most commonly occurs in the lower cervical levels, usually C7<br>Not associated with neurologic injury |
| Extension teardrop fracture | Extension | Unstable | 75.7, *F* | Most commonly occurs at C2<br>See Table 75.6 |
| Facet dislocation, bilateral | Flexion | Unstable | 75.8, *C* | Significant anterior displacement (>50%) of the spine when bilateral inferior facets displace anterior to the superior facets below<br>At risk for injuring the disk, vertebral arteries, and spinal cord |
| Facet dislocation, unilateral | Flexion-rotation | Stable | 75.8, *D* | Usually causes 25-50% anterior displacement of the spine<br>*Complication*: vertebral artery injury (CT angiography recommended) |
| Flexion teardrop fracture | Flexion and axial loading | Unstable | 75.8, *E* | One of the most unstable fractures in the lower cervical spine because it involves both columns<br>Fracture and anterior displacement of the anteroinferior vertebral body (appears similar to an extension teardrop fracture except that it is much more unstable)<br>Unique findings for flexion (versus extension) teardrop fractures include same-level fractures and displacement of posterior structures<br>Rupture of both ALL and PLL complexes<br>Usually occurs at C5 or C6<br>Can result from diving into shallow water or a football tackling injury<br>Often associated with spinal cord injury and tetraplegia |
| Subluxation, anterior | Flexion | Unstable | 75.8, *F* | Anterior slipping of a vertebra over another<br>Ruptured PLL such that the anterior and posterior vertebral lines are disrupted<br>*Complication*: vertebral artery dissection (CT angiography recommended)<br>May be evident only during flexion views by conventional radiography when the interspinous distance widens and the vertebral body subluxates anteriorly |
| Transverse process fracture | Lateral flexion | Stable | 75.8, *A* | *Complication*: vertebral artery injury because it travels within the transverse foramina (CT angiography recommended); associated cervical radiculopathy and brachial plexus injuries in 10% of cases |
| Wedge fracture | Flexion | Stable | 75.8, *G* | Compression fracture of only the anterosuperior vertebral body end plate<br>Disruption of the anterior vertebral line<br>Intact posterior vertebral body and posterior vertebral line |

*ALL*, Anterior longitudinal ligament; *CT*, computed tomography; *PLL*, posterior longitudinal ligament.

chronic corticosteroid therapy, or (3) have a history of vertebral disease should undergo radiography.

Classic patterns of thoracic and lumbar spine injuries are shown in Table 75.8.

## CLASSIFICATION OF SPINAL CORD INJURIES

### COMPLETE INJURY

A spinal cord injury is classified as physiologically complete if the patient has no demonstrable motor or sensory function below the level of injury. During the first few days following injury, this diagnosis cannot be made with certainty because of the possibility of concurrent spinal shock.

### INCOMPLETE INJURY

A spinal cord injury is incomplete if motor function, sensation, or both are partially present below the level of the injury. Signs of an incomplete injury may include (1) the presence of any sensation or voluntary movement in the lower extremities or (2) evidence of sacral sparing. Signs of sacral sparing include perianal sensation, voluntary anal sphincter contraction, and voluntary great toe flexion.

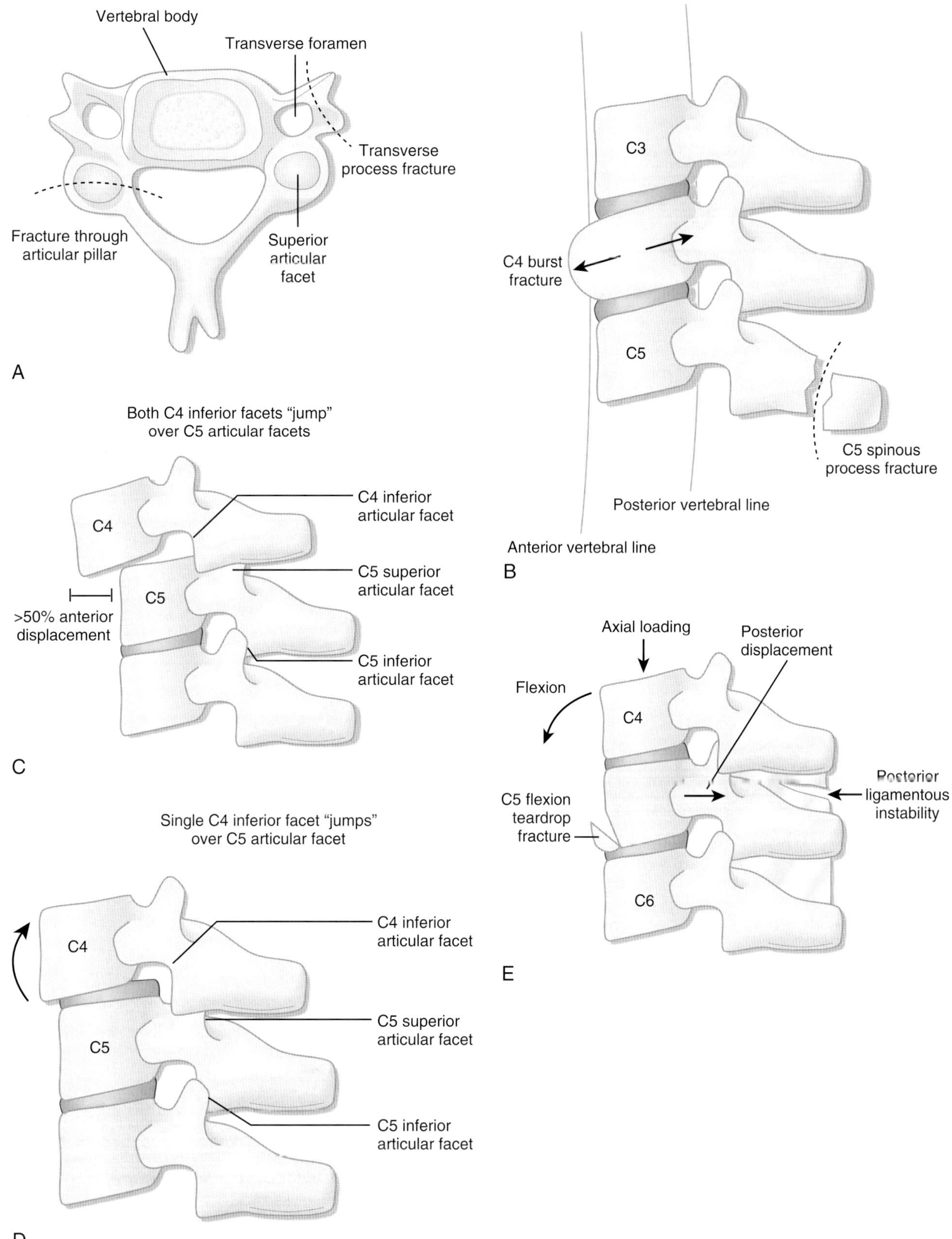


**Fig. 75.8 A,** Superior axial view of an articular pillar fracture and transverse process fracture. **B,** Sagittal view of a C4 burst fracture and C5 clay shoveler's (spinous process) fracture. **C,** Sagittal view of bilateral C4 facet dislocation. **D,** Sagittal view of unilateral C4 facet dislocation. **E,** Sagittal view of a C5 teardrop fracture.

*Continued*

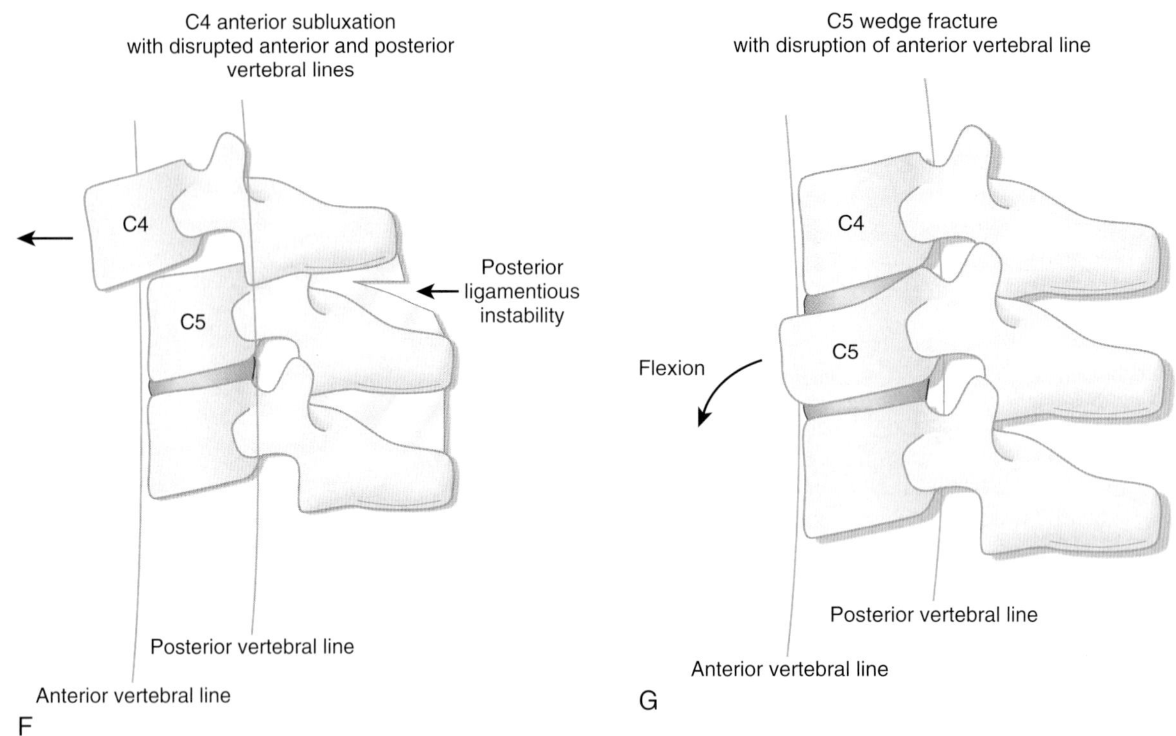


**Fig. 75.8, cont'd** **F,** Sagittal view of C4 anterior subluxation. **G**, Sagittal view of a C5 wedge fracture.

**Table 75.8** Classic Thoracic and Lumbar Spine Injury Patterns

| INJURY | MECHANISM | STABILITY | FIGURE | COMMENTS |
|---|---|---|---|---|
| Wedge fracture | Flexion | Stable, usually | 75.8, *G* | Most common fracture in the thoracic spine<br>Isolated anterior column fracture<br>Disruption of the anterior vertebral line with an intact posterior vertebral line (classic)<br>Maintain a low threshold to obtain spine CT for differentiation of a wedge from a burst fracture (up to 22% of burst fractures appear to have an intact posterior vertebral line) |
| Burst fracture | Axial loading | Variable | 75.8, *B* | Fracture of the anterior and middle columns<br>Disruption of the anterior and posterior vertebral lines (classic)<br>65% have associated spinal cord injury because of middle column compromise |
| Chance fracture | Flexion-distraction | Unstable | 75.9, *A* | Fracture through the anterior, middle, and posterior columns, progressing from posterior to anterior<br>Usually located at the T12-L2 junction<br>Classically caused by a lap belt hyperflexion mechanism in a motor vehicle collision<br>33-89% associated with intraabdominal injury<br>Spinal cord injury is uncommon because of the distraction mechanism |
| Transverse process fracture | | Stable | 75.9, *B* | Most common fracture in the lumbar spine<br>Classically has a vertical fracture orientation<br>A horizontal transverse process fracture orientation suggests a distraction injury (Chance fracture)<br>More than 50% of transverse process fractures are missed by conventional radiography and detected on spine CT<br>Clinically insignificant, but a risk factor for other injury patterns<br>50% associated with an intraabdominal injury<br>30% associated with a pelvic fracture (especially an L5 transverse process fracture)<br>L2 transverse process fracture is associated with renal artery thrombosis |
| Fracture-dislocation | Compression or distraction | Unstable | 75.9, *C* | Significant spinal misalignment and vertebral column discontinuity<br>Fracture through the anterior, middle, and posterior columns<br>Extremely high incidence of spinal cord injury |

*CT*, Computed tomography.

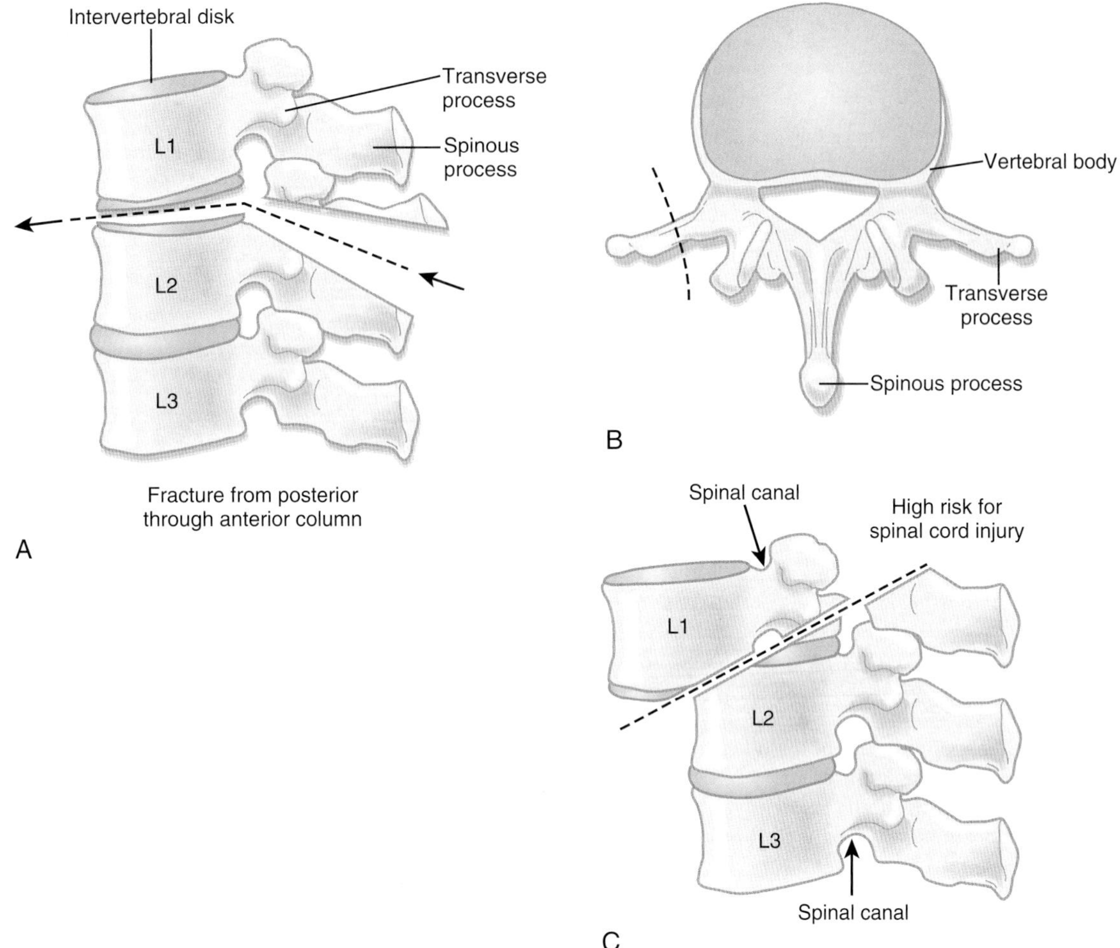


**Fig. 75.9** **A,** Sagittal view of an L2 Chance (flexion-distraction) fracture. **B,** Superior axial view of a transverse process fracture in a typical lumbar spine. **C,** Sagittal view of an L1-L2 fracture-dislocation injury, which is at high risk for a spinal cord injury because of discontinuity of the spinal canal.

Specific incomplete spinal cord injuries include central and anterior cord syndromes, Brown-Séquard syndrome, and conus medullaris syndrome. Patients with these syndromes have certain characteristic patterns of neurologic injury with distinct findings on physical examination.

## CENTRAL CORD SYNDROME

Central cord syndrome is the most common spinal cord syndrome and is usually due to neck hyperextension. Trauma to the central portion of the cord results in injury to the medially located corticospinal motor tracts of the upper extremities. As a result, the upper extremities are predictably and disproportionately weaker than the lower extremities. Many patients exhibit bladder dysfunction (e.g., urinary retention) and varying degrees of sensory loss. Elderly patients are more at risk for central cord syndrome because of underlying cervical spondylosis, a thickened ligamentum flavum, or both.

## ANTERIOR CORD SYNDROME

Anterior cord syndrome results from blunt or ischemic injury to the anterior spinal cord. Affected patients have a complete and usually bilateral motor deficit below the level of the injury along with loss of pain and temperature sensation a few levels below the lesion. Typically, posterior column function is preserved.

## BROWN-SÉQUARD SYNDROME

Brown-Séquard syndrome is a rare hemicord injury that is usually associated with penetrating trauma. Patients have crossed sensory and motor deficits: ipsilateral loss of motor function and position sense below the level of the lesion and contralateral loss of pain and temperature sensation one to two levels below the injury.

## CONUS MEDULLARIS SYNDROME

Conus medullaris syndrome results from injury to the spinal cord with occasional involvement of the lumbar nerve roots. It results in areflexia of the bladder, bowel, and lower extremities. Patients may exhibit perianal numbness. Motor and sensory deficits in the lower limbs vary.

## CAUDA EQUINA SYNDROME

Although cauda equina syndrome is not a direct spinal cord injury because the cauda equina is composed entirely of peripheral nerves (lumbar, sacral, and coccygeal nerve roots),

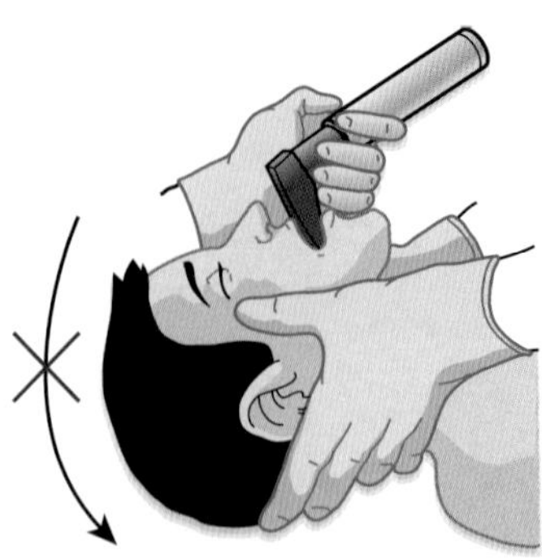

**Fig. 75.10 In-line cervical spine immobilization during endotracheal intubation.** Standing to the patient's side, the assistant uses both hands to stabilize the neck to prevent hyperextension.

it still requires emergency neurosurgical intervention. Clinical findings include asymmetric sensory loss, weakness of the lower extremities, urinary retention or incontinence, decreased rectal tone, and saddle anesthesia.

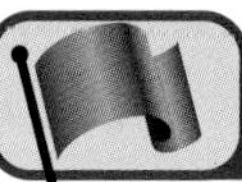

**RED FLAGS (PITFALLS)**

Failure to identify occult injuries in hypoesthetic areas. For example, in a patient with a midthoracic sensory level deficit, occult intraabdominal injuries may be hidden because the abdomen may be insensate.

Failure to consider a spinal cord injury in a patient with normal radiographic and computed tomographic (CT) findings.

Failure to repeat plain films or obtain CT imaging when plain film radiographs of the cervical, thoracic, or lumbar spine are inadequate.

Failure to exclude other causes of hypotension in a trauma patient before assuming that it is neurogenic shock. A search for occult blood loss should first be done.

Failure to consider a distracting injury, particularly fractures, as a reason for a patient's ability to localize neck and back pain.

## TREATMENT

Prehospital and ED management should include protection of the spine and spinal cord until injuries can be identified or excluded. A rigid backboard should typically be removed promptly from beneath cooperative patients because a calm person can maintain spinal column neutrality. Extended use of a rigid backboard is associated with complications such as back pain, respiratory impairment, aspiration, and decubitus ulcers.

### IN-LINE IMMOBILIZATION OF THE CERVICAL SPINE

During the initial resuscitation phase of trauma victims, patients with a potential cervical spine injury may require endotracheal intubation before a definitive diagnosis can be made. By preventing neck hyperextension during direct laryngoscopy, in-line cervical spine immobilization during intubation maintains cervical spine neutrality (**Fig. 75.10**).

### NEUROGENIC SHOCK

Neurogenic shock results from a sympathectomy-induced reduction in blood pressure, heart rate, cardiac contractility, and cardiac output. Overly vigorous fluid resuscitation can be hazardous because of compromised cardiac output. Judicious use of vasopressors such as phenylephrine hydrochloride, dopamine, and norepinephrine is often indicated. Significant bradycardia should be treated hemodynamically with atropine.

Systolic blood pressure lower than 80 mm Hg is rarely due to neurogenic shock alone, and other causes of shock, primarily from hemorrhage, must be excluded. It should never be assumed that hypotension is due to spinal shock until hemorrhage is excluded.

### CORTICOSTEROID THERAPY FOR SPINAL CORD INJURY

Though controversial, treatment of blunt spinal cord injury with high-dose methylprednisolone is common. This therapeutic recommendation is based on the findings of the National Acute Spinal Cord Injury Study (NASCIS), which demonstrated improved neurologic function in patients receiving high-dose corticosteroids within 8 hours of injury. Improved neurologic function, however, was defined as a modest gain in motor scores but not functional improvement. In NASCIS, a loading dose of 30 mg/kg of methylprednisolone administered over a 15-minute period was followed by an infusion of 5.4 mg/kg/hr and continued for 24 hours (in patients treated within 3 hours of injury) or 48 hours (in patients treated 3 to 8 hours after injury).[20,21] No benefit was found when steroids were administered more than 8 hours after injury.

Steroid therapy is not indicated for penetrating injuries and has not been adequately studied in children younger than 13 years or in patients with cauda equina or spinal root injury.

Finally, systemic corticosteroid therapy is not benign. Complications of steroid therapy include gastrointestinal hemorrhage and wound infection in patients treated with corticosteroid infusions for 24 hours and higher rates of severe sepsis and severe pneumonia in those treated for 48 hours. The use of steroids for blunt traumatic spinal cord injury is far from the standard of care.[22] More research is needed to verify or refute this controversial therapy.

### SURGICAL MANAGEMENT OF SPINAL CORD INJURY

Timely reduction of the displaced spinal column plus decompression of the spinal cord has been associated with recovery from otherwise devastating spinal cord injuries.[23] The optimal timing of surgery following a spinal injury remains controversial. Some argue for immediate surgery, whereas others advocate delayed surgery because of the initial posttraumatic swelling. The sole absolute indication for immediate surgery is progressively worsening neurologic status in patients with spinal fracture-dislocations who initially have incomplete or absent neurologic deficits.[24]

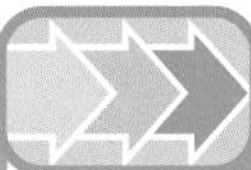

**PRIORITY ACTIONS**

Provide pain control.
Maintain full spinal precautions until the spine can be cleared radiographically or clinically.
If intubating a trauma patient, an assistant should provide in-line cervical spine immobilization until the cervical spine can be assessed more definitively at a later time.
Perform a careful initial neurologic examination, especially in patients who are about to undergo sedation or neuromuscular blockade.
If a spinal fracture is suspected or detected, evaluate for associated injuries:

- For the cervical spine, examine for associated head and facial injuries.
- For the thoracic spine, examine for rib fractures and pulmonary, cardiac, diaphragmatic, and mediastinal injuries.
- For the lumbar spine, examine for intraabdominal injuries, pelvic fractures, and calcaneal fractures.
- For all spinal levels, examine for spinal cord injury.

Obtain urgent spine imaging if a fracture or spinal cord injury is suspected.
Obtain emergency magnetic resonance imaging of the spine if a spinal cord injury is suspected.
Consider administering corticosteroids if an adult patient has sustained blunt spinal trauma and exhibits neurologic deficits within 8 hours of injury.

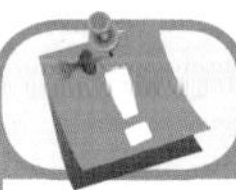

**TIPS AND TRICKS**

Prolonged immobilization on a rigid backboard is uncomfortable for the patient and places the patient at risk for aspiration and early pressure sores. Aim to remove the backboard as soon as possible and ideally within 2 hours of patient arrival. A standard hospital gurney provides adequate thoracic and lumbar stability.
Perform serial neurologic examinations on patients with suspected or known spinal injuries to document neurologic improvement or deterioration. Neurologic deterioration involving the cervical and upper thoracic levels may require empiric endotracheal intubation for impending respiratory failure.
Once a spinal injury is detected, carefully reexamine the entire cervical, thoracic, and lumbar spine. Obtain plain films or computed tomography scans of any levels with pain or tenderness because of the high risk for a second spinal injury.
When performing "clinical clearance" of a patient's cervical spine or obtaining flexion-extension cervical spine plain films, do not passively range the neck for the patient. This may cause an iatrogenic spinal injury. Pain with active movement will prevent the patient from overranging the neck.

In a series of patients with traumatic central cord syndrome, those who underwent early surgery (<24 hours after injury) and had an underlying disk herniation or fracture-dislocation exhibited significantly greater overall motor improvement than did those who underwent late surgery (>24 hours after injury).[25] Unfortunately, early decompressive surgery does not uniformly improve outcome following spinal cord injury.

## FOLLOW-UP, NEXT STEPS IN CARE, AND PATIENT EDUCATION

Most patients with traumatic spinal fractures are admitted to the hospital because they fulfill at least one of four admission criteria: (1) intractable pain, (2) fracture involvement of more than one column, (3) a functionally unstable fracture pattern, and (4) the presence or potential for development of a spinal cord injury.

Patients who can be discharged home include those with normal neurologic function and (1) an isolated, stable posterior column fracture (spinous process, transverse process) in the cervical, thoracic, or lumbar spine or (2) a stable wedge fracture in the thoracic or lumbar spine.

Patients with confirmed or suspected spinal cord injury should be scheduled for early consultation with a neurosurgeon or orthopedist. This may require transfer of the patient to a spine specialty center.

The level of the spinal cord injury, associated neurologic deficits, and other traumatic injuries will determine whether the patient should be admitted to the intensive care unit, neurosurgical observation unit, or general ward. Circular beds, rotating frames, and serial inflation devices are used to protect the patient from pressure sores.

Discharged patients without a fracture or spinal cord injury require only conservative management. Discharged patients with a stable spinal fracture require only conservative management with or without an immobilization device, such as a cervical collar or thoracolumbar sacral orthosis back brace. Soft collars and back braces are not recommended because they predispose patients to stiffness of the neck and back, respectively.

Discharged patients with persistent neck pain who are still at risk for an unstable ligamentous injury should wear a semirigid cervical collar (e.g., Philadelphia or Miami J collar) for 7 to 10 days until adequate flexion-extension plain films can be obtained. Discharge instructions should include information about the warning signs of spinal cord injury.

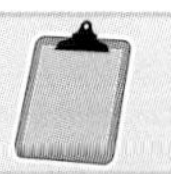

**DOCUMENTATION**

Document neck and back tenderness, along with the neurologic examination, in all trauma patients.
In spinal cord injury patients, mark the initial level of sensory deficit to monitor progression of the patient's neurologic status.
For patients with neurologic deficits, perform and document the bulbocavernosus reflex and sacral-sparing examination to assess for spinal shock.

## SUGGESTED READINGS


1. Bracken MB, Shepard MJ, Holford TR, et al. Administration of methylprednisolone for 24 or 48 hours or tirilazad mesylate for 48 hours in the treatment of acute spinal cord injury. Results of the Third National Acute Spinal Cord Injury Randomized Controlled Trial. National Acute Spinal Cord Injury Study. JAMA 1997;277:1597-604.
2. Hoffman JR, Mower WR, Wolfson AB, et al. Validity of a set of clinical criteria to rule out injury to the cervical spine in patients with blunt trauma. N Engl J Med 2000;343:94-9.
3. Stiell IG, Clement CM, McKnight RD, et al. The Canadian C-Spine Rule versus the NEXUS low-risk criteria in patients with trauma. N Engl J Med 2003;349:2510-8.


## REFERENCES

***References can be found on Expert Consult @ www.expertconsult.com.***

# Facial Trauma 76

*John H. Burton and Karen Nolan Kuehl*

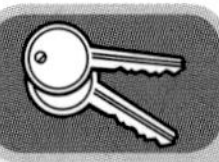

**KEY POINTS**

- Treatment of all facial injuries should initially be directed toward maintaining the airway and stabilizing life-threatening injuries.
- Facial computed tomography is routinely performed to visualize facial fractures; however, plain radiographs may be sufficient in patients with isolated facial injury and a low index of suspicion for a midface fracture or concomitant intracranial injuries.

## PERSPECTIVE

A person's face is the focal point of conversation and social interaction. Within the face is embodied each person's mode of expression and communication. The face also has a receptive importance, with many special sensory functions of the body located within the facial structures. It is not surprising that facial disfigurement harbors the potential for both physical impairment and long-term psychologic sequelae.[1,2]

Death from facial trauma is rare, and the severity of facial injuries is often perceived by the patient to be out of proportion to the actual injury. The goal of the emergency physician (EP) is to secure the airway, identify the injury, preserve appearance, and consult with the appropriate surgeon to determine further treatment and follow-up.[3] Although zygomatic and nasal fractures may occur in isolation, any fracture of the frontal bone and maxilla must raise suspicion for the possibility of associated facial fractures, intracranial injury, and concomitant cervical spine injury.[4-7] Proper diagnosis and recognition of zygoma and nasal pathology are essential for maintenance of adequate cosmetic and physiologic function. Trauma involving the mandible, the strongest facial bone, may result in fracture or dislocation. Fifty percent of mandibular fractures occur at two or more locations because of its pseudoring shape. Detection of one fracture site should always prompt a search for a second fracture.[8]

## GENERAL ANATOMY

The major bones of the face create the defining features and include the frontal, nasal, zygoma, maxilla, mandible, and temporal bones. The orbit consists of the maxilla, zygoma, frontal, sphenoid, orbital, and lacrimal bones (**Fig. 76.1**).

The face is conventionally divided into thirds: upper, middle, and lower. The borders of each third are loosely defined by branches of the trigeminal nerve, which provides sensory innervation to the face. Identification of the exiting foramen for the distributing branches of the trigeminal nerve (cranial nerve V) is crucial when providing local nerve anesthesia (**Fig. 76.2**).

The facial nerve (cranial nerve VII) intricately courses through the parotid duct and provides parasympathetic innervation, special sensory function to the tongue and soft palate, and general motor function to the 44 muscles of facial expression. Deep facial lacerations between the tragus and lateral canthus may jeopardize the integrity of the facial nerve. Any damage to the facial nerve distal to the stylomastoid foramen can result in facial nerve dysfunction, commonly referred to as Bell palsy.

The parotid duct lies in a plane with the tragus and inferior corner of the nasal vestibule. Competency of the parotid duct must be considered in patients with deep lacerations in this region of the face (**Fig. 76.3**).[9]

The external carotid artery is the major vascular supply to the face. This vessel provides extensive collateral supply to the midline tissues through anastomosis (**Fig. 76.4**).[10]

## APPROACH TO MULTITRAUMA PATIENTS WITH FACIAL INJURIES

The degree of tissue distortion following facial trauma should not dissuade the EP from addressing the initial treatment priorities in patients. Though uncommon, facial trauma can be a life-threatening insult, and the EP must address life-threatening injuries before evaluating the obvious facial injury. The mere presence of a facial fracture, particularly one involving the midface, greatly increases the risk for traumatic brain injury.[11,12] The energy required to fracture the midface is often transmitted to the neurocranium, and such fractures are associated with a high incidence of brain death. In general, patients with facial fractures who do not survive have higher injury severity scores and lower Glasgow Coma Scale scores and consist of an older population. Other typical concomitant injuries include pulmonary contusions, abdominal injuries, and cervical spine injuries.[13] The emergence of motor vehicle air bags has decreased patient mortality. However, increased concern is warranted for injuries to the orbits, globes, facial

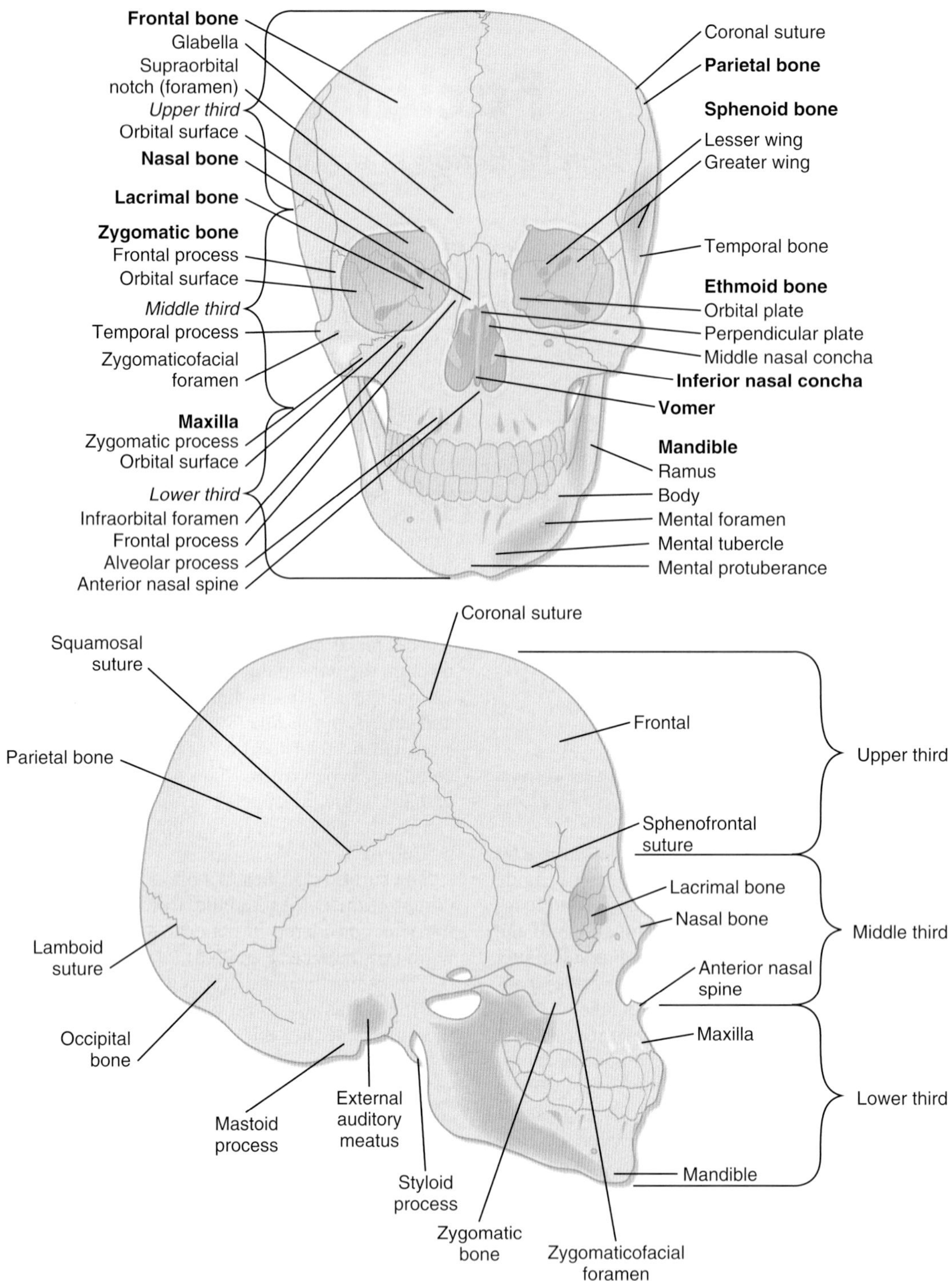


**Fig. 76.1 Facial bones and essential structures of the facial anatomy.**

soft tissues, and temporomandibular joints, as well as cervical fractures of the posterior arches of C1 and C2.

The blood supply to the face consists of a complex system involving branches of the internal and external carotid arteries with several anastomoses between them. The majority of the facial vascular supply is via the internal maxillary artery, which originates from the external carotid. The internal maxillary artery passes between the Le Fort fracture lines and can be dissected with severe midface trauma.

Treatment of bleeding must begin with inspection of the airway and maintenance of its patency. Local hemorrhage may be controlled with posterior nasal packing or insertion of a Foley catheter into the nasopharynx and inflation with air. The catheter should be gently pulled anteriorly in an attempt to close the posterior choana. Temporary external reduction of fractures may also provide stabilization of arterial injuries. Finally, surgical ligation of the external carotid artery or transcatheter arterial embolization of the maxillary artery can be

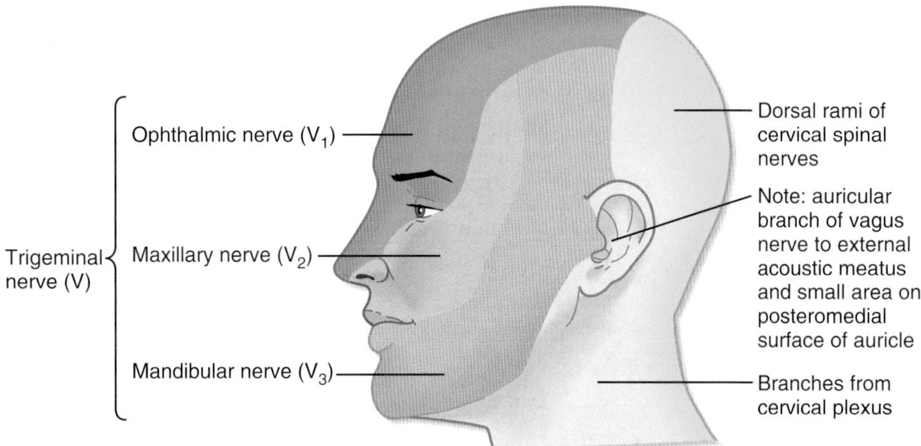


**Fig. 76.2** Anatomic location and distribution of the trigeminal nerve.

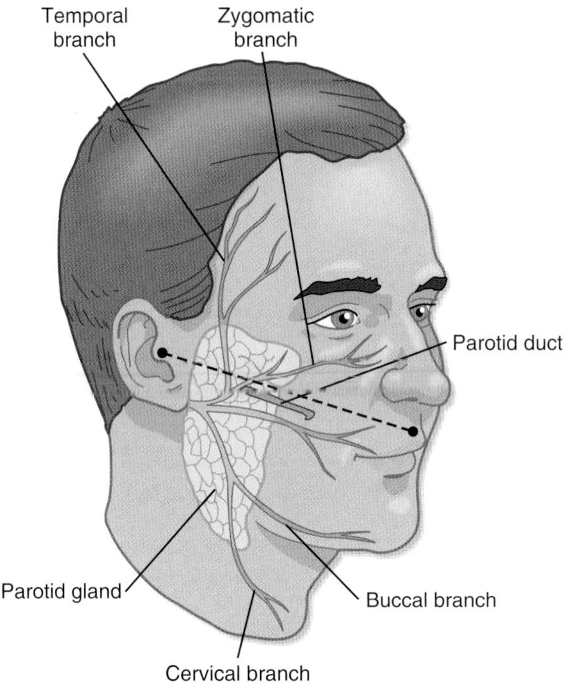


**Fig. 76.3** Location of the parotid duct complex.

performed to effect hemostasis.[14] Less obvious sources of serious blood loss must be monitored (scalp lacerations, nasal fractures, mandibular fractures) because persistent bleeding may lead to hypovolemia.[15]

# FRONTAL SKULL INJURIES

## PATHOPHYSIOLOGY

The force necessary to fracture the frontal bone is commonly the result of a motor vehicle accident in which the forehead strikes the dashboard or steering wheel. Assault with a blunt object is also a common injury mechanism.

## ANATOMY

The frontal bone is the only constituent of the forehead; the prominent protuberance is called the glabella. Within the frontal bone resides the frontal sinus, which communicates with the nasopharynx via the frontonasal canal. The anterior bone of the frontal sinus is thicker than the posterior aspect. The intracranial dura mater is adherent to the posterior frontal sinus wall. Cutaneous innervation of the frontal bone is supplied by the superior orbital nerve, a branch of the trigeminal nerve.

## TREATMENT

Frontal sinus fractures are usually diagnosed by computed tomography (CT). Displaced anterior wall fractures require either immediate repair or delayed reconstruction. Conversely, frontal bone fractures that involve the posterior wall of the sinus are associated with cerebrospinal fluid (CSF) rhinorrhea; the patient will require urgent consultation with a neurosurgeon and admission to the hospital.[16] Ocular trauma or sudden loss of vision associated with a frontal bone injury requires immediate ophthalmologic consultation.

## FOLLOW-UP, NEXT STEPS IN CARE, AND PATIENT EDUCATION

Anterior frontal sinus fractures without any concomitant injuries are not life-threatening; the patient can be discharged with close consultant follow-up to maintain an adequate cosmetic result. Although antibiotics have not been shown to decrease the incidence of meningitis associated with a CSF leak and frontal bone fracture, antibiotic therapy should be based on the consultant's preference.

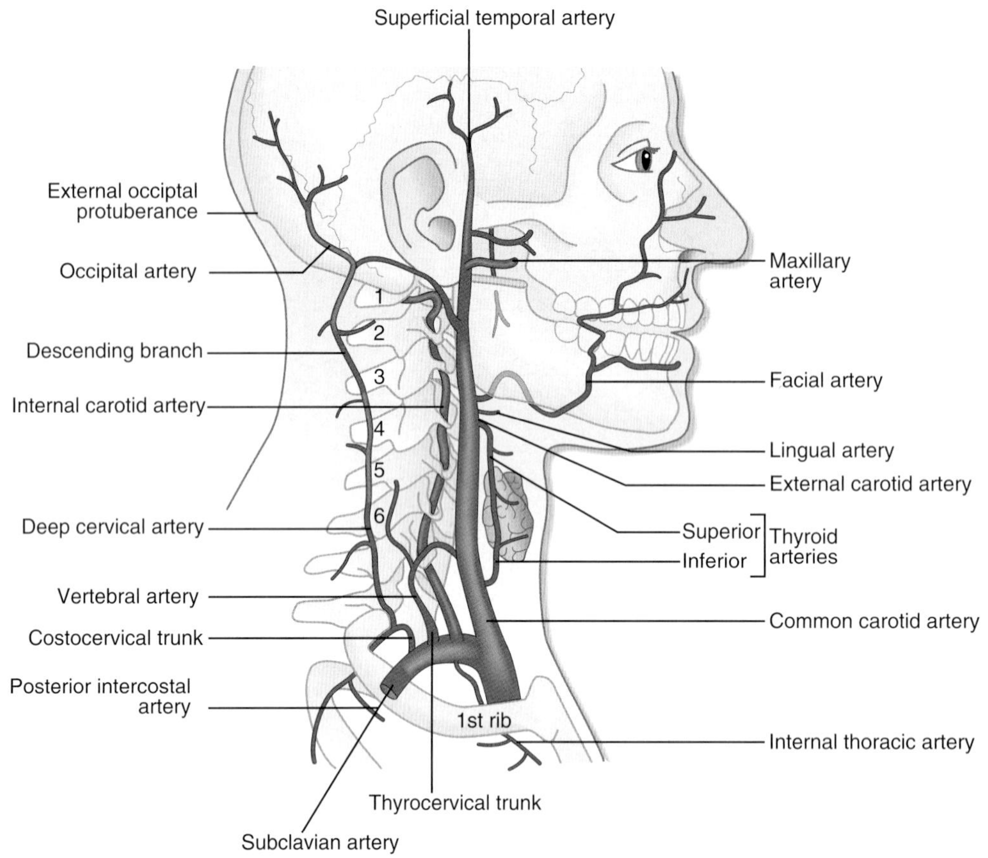


**Fig. 76.4 Vascular supply to the face and skull.**

# BLUNT OPHTHALMIC AND ORBITAL TRAUMA

## PATHOPHYSIOLOGY

Trauma to the eye can result from falls, motor vehicle accidents, and direct blows from an assault or a projectile object (hockey puck, baseball). Serious eye injury has been shown to most commonly be associated with midface fractures.[17,18] Ocular trauma can be divided into two broad categories: direct trauma to the globe and trauma to the orbit. Direct globe trauma ranges in severity from a benign corneal abrasion to rupture of the globe. Orbital trauma involves injuries such as benign contusions and fractures with complications to surrounding structures, including the globe and extraocular muscles.

Orbital fractures are classified as "impure" when the fracture line involves the orbital rim or as "pure" in the case of a fracture with no rim involvement. Compression of the optic nerve (ocular neuropathy) can be caused by displacement of a fracture, increased pressure from a retrobulbar hemorrhage, or optic nerve hemorrhage.[19] Each of these processes has the potential to lead to rapidly progressive visual loss and is an ophthalmologic emergency.

The mechanism of orbital blowout fractures was investigated by Waterhouse et al. via the same principles as Le Fort a century earlier (see later).[20] Waterhouse investigated the two possible mechanisms for an orbital blowout fracture, the hydraulic and buckling theories. The hydraulic mechanism occurs when the vector of the force directed onto an uninjured globe is transmitted to the fixed orbital walls; it results in a large fracture of the inferior or medial orbital wall, or both (**Fig. 76.5**). This mechanism is commonly associated with herniation of the orbital contents through the fractured orbital wall, hence the term *blowout*. The buckling mechanism, in contrast, occurs when a traumatic force is directed to the inferior orbital rim and causes only the inferior floor of the orbit to buckle, or fracture, with no associated herniation of the orbital contents.

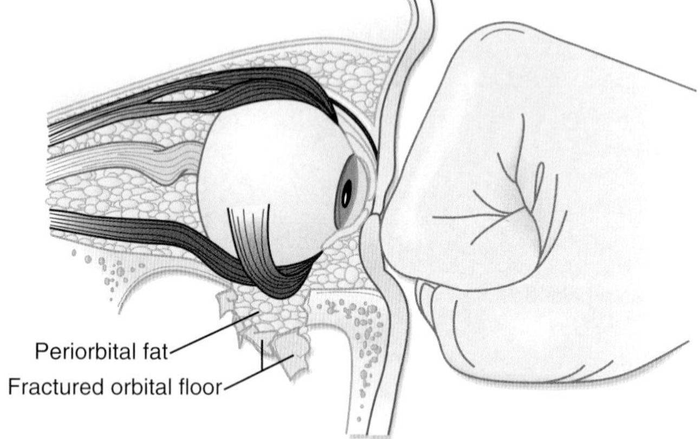


**Fig. 76.5 Mechanism and structures involved in an orbital blowout fracture.**

Herniation of the orbital contents—fatty connective tissue, inferior rectus, and inferior oblique muscles—occurs at the weakest portions of the orbit, specifically, the orbital floor and the anteromedial wall. With increased pressure on the globe, any defect in these bony structures may lead to herniation of the orbital contents and resultant muscular entrapment.

## ANATOMY

The globe resides within a cone-shaped socket composed of seven bones of varying thickness. The thinnest bony portion of the socket is the orbital floor. The globe is protected from trauma by the thick superior rim of the frontal bone and the inferior rim of both the maxilla and zygoma. The orbital rim possesses a smooth contour with occasional notching that is symmetric when encountered. Any asymmetric step-off of this rim is indicative of a potential rim fracture.

The eye is cushioned by a retrobulbar fat pad encasing the globe. The extraocular muscles complete the orbital anatomy by surrounding the globe and enabling eye movement. Herniation of any orbital contents through the inferior or medial walls will result in protrusion of these structures, in whole or in part, into the maxillary or ethmoidal sinus, respectively. The inferior rectus and inferior oblique muscles, both innervated by cranial nerve III, lie adjacent to the inferior and medial orbital floors and are the most commonly affected extraocular muscles with a blowout injury.

## PRESENTING SIGNS AND SYMPTOMS

Patients with a history of facial trauma should undergo complete evaluation of the eye and the encasing orbit. Initial inspection may reveal periorbital ecchymosis and edema, discrepancy in eye level, or enophthalmos. Enophthalmos is consistent with an orbital blowout fracture. Anesthesia of the ipsilateral cheek and upper lip is indicative of inferior orbital nerve impingement.

Key points in the patient's history include the following:

- Binocular diplopia (blurring of vision when both eyes are open) is indicative of an ocular muscle imbalance between the two eyes as a consequence of muscle entrapment, contusion, or displacement of the globe secondary to edema from surrounding structures.
- Monocular diplopia (blurring of vision when only one eye is open) is often indicative of lens dislocation, hyphema, or partial globe rupture.
- Flashing lights, or floaters, can be consistent with a retinal tear, retinal detachment, or vitreous hemorrhage.
- Any loss of perception of light or identification of colors or the presence of central scotomata without association with pain is indicative of optic neuropathy. Absence of light perception following an orbital fracture is a poor prognostic indicator for recovery of vision.
- Rapid loss of vision in one eye associated with edema, proptosis, and tension on palpation should heighten suspicion for the presence of a retrobulbar hematoma.
- Pain with eye movement is commonly associated with an orbital fracture.

The eye examination should begin with palpation of the orbital rims. The rims should be evaluated for crepitus, a step-off deformity, subcutaneous emphysema, and decreased sensation in the distribution of the inferior and superior orbital nerves.

Pupil size, shape, and light reflex must be examined to assess optic nerve status. Full ocular muscle function is evaluated by slow, directed passive range of motion. Upward gaze palsy with vertical diplopia is consistent with dysfunction of the inferior rectus muscle and suggests entrapment from an orbital blowout fracture. Enophthalmos is common when a large amount of tissue herniates through an orbital floor defect into the adjacent maxillary sinus.

The EP must evaluate both eyes for visual acuity. This examination may be facilitated by using a Snellen eye chart or pocket card or by asking the patient to read the text of a newspaper or other print. Visual impairment should prompt immediate consultation for the suspected injury. If the patient's injury allows proper positioning and cooperation, a slit-lamp examination is warranted to fully evaluate the conjunctiva, lens, iris, sclera, cornea, and anterior chamber of the globe. Intraocular pressure can be measured. However, if the globe has possibly been ruptured, intraocular pressure assessment should be deferred to an ophthalmologist.

## DIAGNOSTIC CRITERIA AND TESTING

If the pretest probability of orbital or ocular damage is low or if CT is not available, a Waters view radiograph of the midface is a screening tool for fracture or resultant blood in the sinus, subcutaneous emphysema, depression of the bony fragments, or the "hanging teardrop" sign whereby herniated globe structures may be visualized in the maxillary sinus roof. If suspicion of orbital or ocular injury is high, particularly when concomitant intracranial or facial injuries are suspected, CT is required to elucidate the extent of the identified injury. This examination should include views of the head, as well as axial and coronal cuts of the midface and orbits.

## TREATMENT

Management of blowout fractures is complicated.[21] The presence of an orbital fracture with findings of herniation on clinical or radiographic examination requires immediate surgical consultation to guide the treatment plan. Immediate indications for surgical intervention include muscular entrapment with gaze restriction or acute enophthalmos. Contraindications to surgery include globe rupture, hyphema, and retinal tears. These injuries should prompt emergency ophthalmologic consultation. An ophthalmologist should also be contacted for patients with evidence of lens dislocation, laceration of the cornea or sclera, or rapid loss of visual acuity.

Patients with an isolated blowout fracture may be discharged home with follow-up arranged within 2 weeks to assess for resolution of the swelling. If entrapment is present at follow-up, the patient would require open reduction of the fracture. Even patients with a blowout fracture may have their symptoms improve over a 10-day to 2-week period and may not require surgical intervention.

An increase in retrobulbar pressure from a hematoma or emphysema can lead to acute and permanent loss of vision. Lateral canthotomy can be a vision-saving intervention in this context. This simple procedure is intended to relieve pressure on the optic nerve and, ultimately, preserve the patient's vision through resolution of the optic nerve traction and ischemia. Immediate ophthalmologic consultation should be obtained to perform the lateral canthotomy; when a consultant is unavailable or if a lengthy response time is anticipated, the procedure should be undertaken by the EP.

Local anesthetic without epinephrine is injected into the lateral canthus. An incision is made in the canthus with a pair of fine, sharp scissors. The incision is made in the canthus at the juncture of the upper and lower eyelids between the globe and the orbital rim. Expulsion and drainage of the hematoma should ensue through the incision site.

## FOLLOW-UP, NEXT STEPS IN CARE, AND PATIENT EDUCATION

Pain should be controlled as deemed appropriate and antibiotic administration initiated if sinus integrity has been disrupted as evidenced by subcutaneous emphysema or radiographic findings. Prophylactic antibiotics are no longer recommended.

# ZYGOMA INJURY

## PATHOPHYSIOLOGY

Zygoma fractures are the result of an anterolateral force applied to the midface by falls, deceleration injuries, or assault by blunt objects, including a fist. The zygoma is a thick bone. A direct blow to the zygoma may not necessarily result in a fracture but instead may transmit the force to adjacent weaker areas of the orbit and maxilla and cause a complex fracture. Inward and downward displacement of the zygoma in relation to its articulating surfaces results in the classic zygomaticomaxillary complex fracture, also called a tripod or malar fracture (**Fig. 76.6**).[22] Comminuted fractures of the zygoma are associated with penetrating trauma, such as gunshot wounds.

## ANATOMY

The term *zygoma* is derived from the Greek word *zygon*, meaning a yoke or crossbar by which two draft animals are hitched to a plow. The zygoma forms the lateral buttress of the face, inferior and lateral orbital rim, and a portion of the orbital floor. Thus a zygoma fracture, by definition, is an orbital floor fracture.

The zygoma articulates with four bones: the maxilla, temporal bone, frontal bone, and greater wing of the sphenoid. For this reason, a zygomaticomaxillary complex fracture—typically referred to as a tripod fracture—is technically a misnomer.

The zygoma forms part of the superior and lateral aspect of the maxillary sinus, and disruption may lead to subcutaneous air. Numerous muscles attach to the zygoma, the most prominent being the masseter, which consequently results in inward and downward displacement of a zygomaticomaxillary complex fracture and trismus.

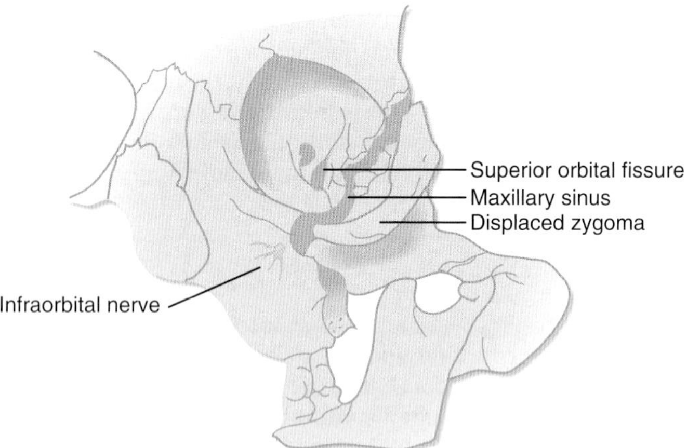


**Fig. 76.6 Zygomaticomaxillary complex fracture, also known as a tripod or malar fracture.**

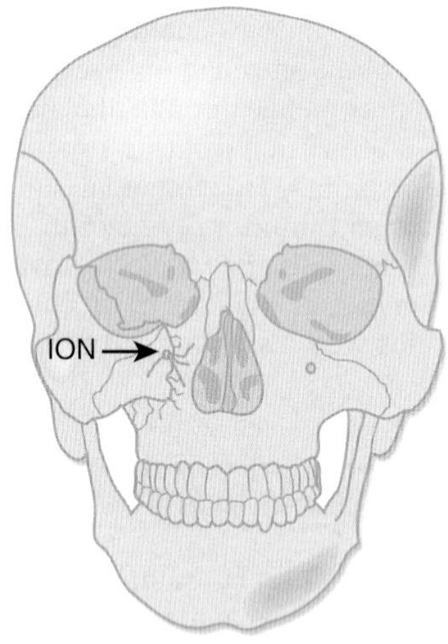


**Fig. 76.7 Relationship of the infraorbital nerve (ION) and foramen to a zygomaticomaxillary complex fracture.**

## PRESENTING SIGNS AND SYMPTOMS

Common symptoms with fracture of the zygoma include the following:

- Pain over the affected area
- Difficulty opening the jaw secondary to the origin of the masseter (trismus)
- Paresthesia in the distribution of the inferior orbital nerve (**Fig. 76.7**)
- Binocular diplopia as a result of entrapment of intraocular muscles

The initial physical examination typically reveals severe edema of the zygoma area with possible inferior displacement of the lateral canthus, periorbital edema, and subconjunctival hemorrhage. The face should be evaluated from the superior and inferior aspects to discern any flattening of the cheek relative to the contralateral side. The zygoma should be palpated for evidence of a step-off of the inferior orbital rim, crepitus of the zygoma, or subcutaneous emphysema.

Intraoral examination of the zygoma is accomplished by placing a gloved finger along the superior and lateral aspect of the maxillary molars. If this area is tender or if the finger is unable to pass under the arch, a fracture of the zygoma is likely.

A complete ocular examination should be performed to evaluate for entrapment of muscles and possible orbital fracture. Ten percent to 20% of zygoma injuries will be associated with ocular injury.

## DIAGNOSTIC CRITERIA AND TESTING

If a nondisplaced, isolated zygoma fracture is suspected, a "jug-handle," submentovertex plain radiographic view may be sufficient for diagnosis. Otherwise, a Waters view constitutes an adequate screening radiographic study for a more complicated fracture. If the Waters view reveals a zygomaticomaxillary complex fracture or if ocular muscle entrapment is suspected, facial CT scans are required for more complete evaluation of the injury.

## TREATMENT

Initial management of patients with zygomaticomaxillary complex fractures should include prompt diagnosis and exclusion of ocular muscle entrapment or intracranial injuries. If subcutaneous emphysema is present, antibiotics should be initiated immediately; amoxicillin is an effective first-line agent.[23]

## FOLLOW-UP, NEXT STEPS IN CARE, AND PATIENT EDUCATION

Patients with an isolated arch fracture can be discharged with appropriate follow-up. However, patients with greater than 2-mm displacement will typically require open reduction. In contrast, patients with a zygomaticomaxillary complex fracture, any injury with impairment of vision, or substantial concomitant injuries will require admission to the hospital with surgical consultation for consideration of open reduction and internal fixation.

# MAXILLARY AND MIDFACE INJURIES

## PATHOPHYSIOLOGY

### LE FORT CLASSIFICATION

Maxillary fractures resulting from severe blows to the head have traditionally been classified according to the Le Fort classification scheme established by René Le Fort in 1901. Le Fort was a French surgeon who induced trauma in 35 cadaveric heads by striking them with a bat or smashing them against a table edge. Next, Le Fort boiled the heads to remove the soft tissue and documented the fracture lines. In his classic treatise on the subject, Le Fort illustrated three predictable midface fracture lines. These injuries rarely occur in isolation, but they are often used as a reference to describe maxillary trauma (**Fig. 76.8**).

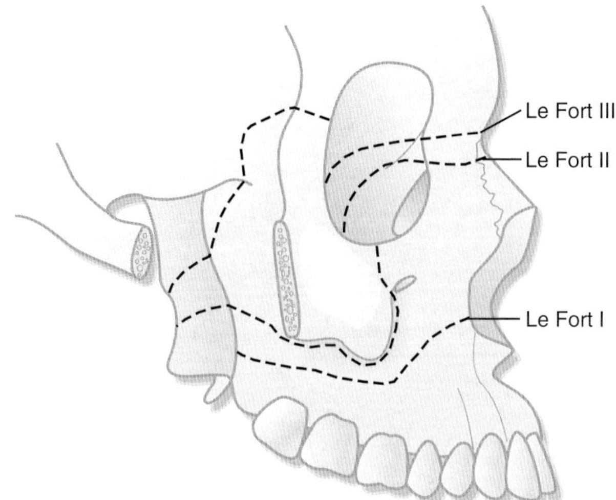


**Fig. 76.8 Fracture lines of the midface as described by Le Fort.**

#### *Le Fort I (Transverse)*

This midface fracture is the result of lateral force applied to the face. The Le Fort I fracture line extends horizontally above the roots of the teeth and involves only the maxilla. A step-off deformity of the upper palate will be present (if not complete). Rocking of the teeth will lead to motion of the midface, with a sensation similar to that of a loose denture.

#### *Le Fort II (Pyramidal)*

This injury is the result of extreme force directed to the nose and midface and results in separation of the midface from its articulating structures. The Le Fort II fracture line extends through the inferior orbital rim and over the nasal ridge and separates the upper palate and nose from the remainder of the face.

#### *Le Fort III (Craniofacial Disjunction)*

A Le Fort III is the most severe type of facial fracture. The facial fracture line is horizontal and extends through the nasal bone and laterally through the orbits. This injury results in separation of the facial bones from the base of the skull.

## ANATOMY

The maxilla is primarily innervated by the inferior alveolar nerve, which emerges from the inferior orbital foramen. Clues to evidence of a midface fracture may include paresthesias in the region of the inferior alveolar nerve.

The nose is a highly vascularized structure within the maxilla. Severe epistaxis associated with a maxillary injury can lead to airway obstruction. Therefore, hemostasis is essential in the approach to maxillary injuries.

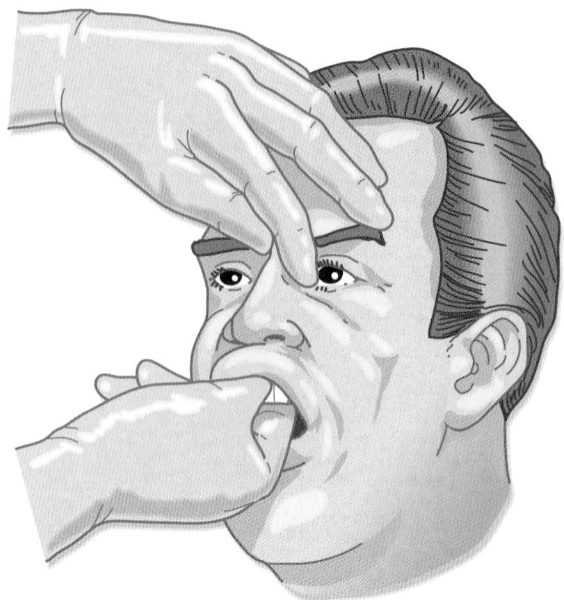

**Fig. 76.9 Examination of the midface for instability.**

## PRESENTING SIGNS AND SYMPTOMS

Initial evaluation of a patient with a maxillary injury depends on its severity; findings include severe edema, malocclusion, periorbital ecchymosis, facial asymmetry, a long or "donkey" face, and enophthalmos. Palpation of the maxillary structures may reveal crepitus and abnormal mobility of the structures. Anesthesia over the cheek implies disruption of the inferior orbital nerve.

The EP should place one hand on the patient's forehead to stabilize the head while grasping the upper palate by the anterior teeth with the other hand. Gentle back-and-forth pressure should be applied while palpating the midface for movement (**Fig. 76.9**). If motion of the midface structures is detected with this technique, further classification of the extent of the injury should be performed by localization of the nasal ridge or inferior orbital rims with the other hand. If CSF rhinorrhea is suspected, testing the fluid for glucose or the halo sign may be undertaken; however, both these assessments have a high false-positive rate and are considered unreliable. If a fracture is highly suspected or if CT is planned, manipulation of the midface offers little benefit and may cause increased bleeding.[24]

## DIAGNOSTIC CRITERIA AND TESTING

In patients with a high index of suspicion for a facial fracture, neurologic deficit, or severe facial distortion or in those who are undergoing CT evaluation for any reason other than midface trauma, CT of the facial bones with fine axial and coronal cuts should be the initial imaging study.

If no other significant injuries are present and the findings on clinical examination are ambiguous for a facial fracture, a Waters plain radiographic facial view is an excellent screening examination. If plain radiography reveals an obvious fracture or opacification of a maxillary sinus, CT is warranted and should be performed in follow-up or at the time of the initial encounter, as dictated by the needs of the patient and preference of the surgical consultant.

## TREATMENT

Before a thorough evaluation of the maxilla is undertaken, the EP must first stabilize the patient and ensure that the airway is preserved. Airway compromise is more common with Le Fort II and III fractures but may also be seen with Le Fort I injuries.

Airway obstruction is often secondary to uncontrolled bleeding. Therefore, attempts at hemostasis should be undertaken early in the evaluation. Assessment of facial fracture bleeding should be completed during the "circulation" component of the ABCDE (airway, breathing, circulation, disability, exposure) evaluation technique advocated by the advanced trauma life support protocol. Early oral endotracheal intubation may be required and allows more aggressive control of bleeding.

Nasopharyngeal intubation should be avoided with midface injuries. A surgical airway (e.g., cricothyrotomy) may be necessary because of anatomic damage or excessive bleeding. Placement of an orogastric tube will allow assessment of swallowed blood, which can provide valuable information in a multitrauma patient with developing tachycardia, hypotension, or both.

If hemostasis of the nares cannot be achieved, a Foley catheter should be carefully advanced into the nasopharynx and inflated with air (overinflation may result in septal necrosis). The catheter should be gently pulled anteriorly in an attempt to close the posterior choana. Once the catheter is in place, the nasal cavity can be packed with gauze or nasal tampons for control of anterior epistaxis. The physician must be careful when advancing any tube through the nares because violation of the anterior cranial base can allow passage of the catheter into the cranium. If bleeding is not controlled with Foley catheters and packing, embolization of bleeding vessels with possible surgical exploration and ligation of vessels should occur. Emergency consultation with ear, nose, and throat (ENT), plastic surgery, and interventional radiology services should be considered early if the patient requires angiography. Regardless of the severity of bleeding, all patients with facial fractures should be reevaluated for hemorrhage every 30 minutes for a period of up to 6 hours.[25]

## FOLLOW-UP, NEXT STEPS IN CARE, AND PATIENT EDUCATION

Antibiotic prophylaxis for basilar skull fractures has not been shown to decrease the risk for meningitis.[26] However, prophylactic antibiotic regimens may still be used in an attempt to prevent translocation of mouth and sinus flora.[27]

Evidence of a basilar skull fracture or pneumocephalus requires prompt neurosurgical consultation. Maxillary fractures often require surgical repair to restore normal occlusion and facial stabilization, and thus consultation and follow-up with an oromaxillofacial or plastic surgeon is important. Patients with demonstrated or suspected Le Fort II or Le Fort III injuries require hospital admission for stabilization and management.

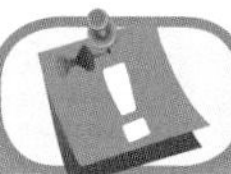

TIPS AND TRICKS

Identification of the exiting foramen for the distributing branches of the trigeminal nerve is crucial when providing regional anesthesia.

Severe epistaxis may be controlled with a Foley catheter advanced into the nasopharynx, inflated, and retracted against the nasopharynx as a posterior nasal pack.

Upward gaze palsy with vertical diplopia is consistent with dysfunction or entrapment of the inferior rectus muscle and suggestive of an orbital blowout fracture.

Pain with eye movement is indicative of an orbital fracture.

Intraoral examination of the zygoma is accomplished by placing a gloved finger along the superior and lateral aspect of the maxillary molars.

Any palpation of subcutaneous air in the face is indicative of sinus disruption with a midface fracture

Antibiotic prophylaxis for basilar skull fractures has not been shown to decrease the risk for meningitis.

Treatment of eyebrow lacerations does not require shaving the brow hairs. Additionally, sutures should be placed parallel to the hair follicles.

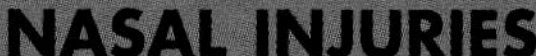

# NASAL INJURIES

## PATHOPHYSIOLOGY

Nasal bone fractures are commonly the result of sports-related trauma, assault, and motor vehicle crashes. The force required to fracture the nasal bone ranges from 16 to 66 kPa, the least of any facial bone.[28] Simple deviated nasal fractures are the result of a lateral force against the nasal prominence. More complex nasoorbitoethmoid fractures are due to a stronger force directed toward the bridge of the nose with displacement of the bone segments posteriorly. This type of fracture is frequently associated with other facial and brain injuries.

## ANATOMY

The nasal bone consists of two small wedge-shape bones that are fused in the midline and protrude from the frontal process of the maxilla laterally and frontal bone superiorly. The upper portion of this paired structure is significantly thicker than the lower segments, thereby leading more commonly to fractures of the latter. The external nose is composed of cartilaginous and fatty tissue and has an intricate blood supply from distal branches of the internal and external carotid arteries.

## PRESENTING SIGNS AND SYMPTOMS

Patients with nasal trauma have complaints of tenderness, edema, epistaxis, and periorbital ecchymosis. Palpation of the area can reveal crepitus, hypermobility, and deformity of the nasal septum.

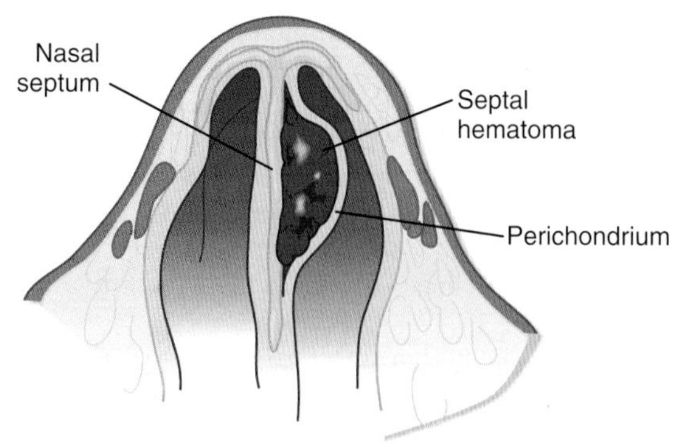


**Fig. 76.10 Septal hematoma.**

Each naris must be inspected carefully with a nasal speculum to evaluate for a septal hematoma. A sepal hematoma is a collection of blood between the mucoperichondrium or mucoperiosteum of the nasal septum and septal cartilage. A septal hematoma appears as a purple, bulging oval structure on the nasal septum that invades the midline (**Fig. 76.10**). Failure to promptly identify and treat a septal hematoma can lead to necrosis of the septum and potentially a saddle nose deformity.

A nasoorbitoethmoid fracture should be suspected in patients with flattening of the bridge of the nose or telecanthus (an increase in the distance between the medial portions of the eyes). Patients may have evidence of ocular injury and CSF rhinorrhea. Additionally, disruption of the lacrimal apparatus is not uncommon with more severe nasal injuries.

## DIAGNOSTIC CRITERIA AND TESTING

Plain radiography is of limited value in patients with simple nasal trauma and has no clinical implication in management. Patients can be reassured that radiographs may be obtained at follow-up if any cosmetic deformity persists and surgical repair is required. If the physician is concerned that a nasoorbitoethmoid fracture is present, axial and coronal CT of the face is necessary.

## TREATMENT

The EP should not attempt reduction of closed nasal fractures. Given the extensive edema that generally ensues before the patient arrives at the emergency department (ED), the EP will be unable to approximate realignment of the nasal septum.[29] Epistaxis should be dealt with during the clinical evaluation. Analgesia should be adequately addressed during the patient's visit and at follow-up.

## FOLLOW-UP, NEXT STEPS IN CARE, AND PATIENT EDUCATION

Patients with known or suspected nasal fractures or septal displacement should be referred to an otolaryngologist or plastic surgeon within 1 week of their injury for reevaluation and planning of management. Patients may also be educated that if no deformity is apparent after the swelling has subsided, ENT follow-up is unnecessary. Children with nasal fractures should be seen in follow-up within 4 days because of rapid bone healing. Patients should be instructed to avoid blowing their nose given that subcutaneous emphysema may ensue as a result of displacement of air across the injured nasal structures.

Emergency consultation for consideration of nasal reduction is indicated if the nasal pyramid is deviated greater than half the width of the nasal bridge or if an open septal fracture has occurred. Open nasal fractures require immediate attention because cartilage necrosis may ensue if the exposed cartilage is not covered within 24 hours. Nasoorbitoethmoid fractures require a multidisciplinary approach, including oromaxillofacial, plastic, and neurosurgical consultation.

If a septal hematoma is identified, immediate evacuation is required. The nasal passage on the affected side is prepared via topical anesthesia and injection of lidocaine into the anterior septum. The hematoma is initially drained with a large-bore needle at the inferior aspect. The needle track is then enlarged with a No. 15 surgical blade. Next, the anterior nares are tightly packed bilaterally in an attempt to reappose the septal mucosa. Patients with septal hematoma should routinely be prescribed a course of antibiotics and otolaryngologic follow-up arranged within 4 days to assess the injury for evidence of reaccumulation of the hematoma. On discharge, patients need to be educated that any reaccumulation of septal hematoma will require emergency reevacuation. In addition, these patient need to be educated to avoid blowing their nose.

# LOWER FACE INJURIES

## PATHOPHYSIOLOGY

The location of mandibular fractures has some correlation to the insult received.[30] High-velocity forces directed to the chin result in symphysis or condylar fractures (or both), and a high proportion of these injuries result in comminuted fractures. In contrast, assault-related injuries are more commonly associated with fractures of the angle and ramus. The location of trauma impact does not necessarily correlate with the location of the fracture site because the force of the impact can be transmitted to a distant area.

Dislocations of the mandible can be due to trauma, excessive mouth opening (yawning), seizure, or a dystonic reaction from medication. The mandible dislocates anteriorly and then superiorly, with spasm of the jaw muscles preventing realignment. Unilateral dislocation causes deviation of the mandible away from the affected side. Bilateral dislocation results in an open jaw and underbite appearance.

## ANATOMY

The mandible is a horseshoe-shaped bone and appears similar to the letter L from a lateral view (**Fig. 76.11**). It has 16 tooth sockets innervated by the inferior alveolar nerve. The mandible articulates with the temporal bone bilaterally via a ginglymoarthrodial (hinge and sliding) joint to form the temporomandibular joint. The arterial supply to the mandible is via branches of the maxillary artery.

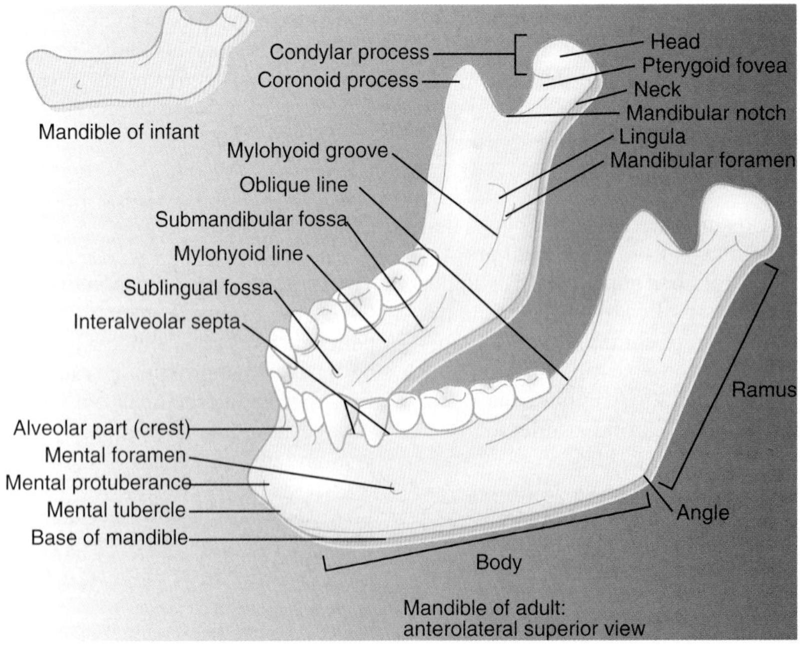


**Fig. 76.11 Anatomy of the mandible.**

The temporomandibular joint consists of the mandibular condyle process and the mandibular fossa of the temporal bone interspaced with a cartilaginous disk and surrounded by a joint capsule. If the jaw is opened slightly, the hinge action predominates as the condylar process rotates within the socket. However, as the jaw is opened wider, the mandibular condyles glide forward to the articular tubercle of the temporal bone. Overextension of the joint results in anterior dislocation of the mandibular condyle process and subsequent spasm in the masseter and pterygoid muscles, which prevents normal mouth closure.

## PRESENTING SIGNS AND SYMPTOMS

Typical initial symptoms of a mandibular injury include mandibular pain, abnormal jaw motion, malocclusion, and paresthesia of the ipsilateral lower lip secondary to disruption of the mandibular nerve. Patients often state that their "bite is off," a sign of displacement or malocclusion of the mandible or maxilla. If the patient reports pain in the preauricular area, fracture of the condyle is frequently present.

Examination of the mandible should begin with visual inspection for edema, deviation with passive range of motion, and a "widened face," an indication of a bilateral condylar fracture. The EP should palpate the outside of the face to ensure preservation of the smooth contour of the mandible. During the intraoral examination, clues to a mandibular fracture include ecchymosis of the floor of the mouth and mucosal tears. Any obvious separation of the lower teeth or step deformity is pathognomonic for fracture.

The EP inspects the temporomandibular joint by first performing an otoscopic examination for signs of perforation of the external ear canal or hemotympanum. A Battle sign is indicative of perforation of the glenoid fossa by a fractured condyle. Next, the examiner's fingers are placed in the external canal, and the patient is instructed to open and close the mouth. Tenderness or crepitus elicited with this examination is indicative of a condylar fracture.

If the clinical findings are misleading, one can perform the tongue blade test, which has been demonstrated by Alonso and Purcell to have high sensitivity in screening for mandibular fractures.[31] The test is performed by placing a wooden tongue blade between the molars (**Fig. 76.12**). The patient is instructed to bite down, and the examiner exerts a twisting motion in an effort to crack the wooden blade between the patient's teeth. If the EP is unable to crack the blade between the patient's teeth during the twisting motion—because of pain or malocclusion—a positive test is confirmed with subsequent enhanced suspicion for a mandibular fracture.

## DIAGNOSTIC CRITERIA AND TESTING

Initial radiographs should include lateral and posteroanterior views and a Towne view of the mandible (if Panorex is unavailable). If the index of suspicion for a condylar fracture is high despite normal radiographic findings, CT with fine cuts of the condyle will be necessary to definitively rule out a fracture. If evidence of an avulsed tooth is present on clinical examination, a chest radiograph should be obtained to evaluate for aspiration.

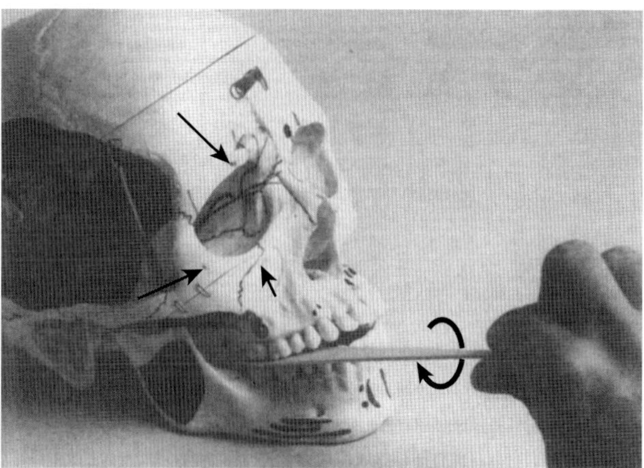

**Fig. 76.12 Performance of the tongue blade test to assess for a mandibular fracture.**

## TREATMENT

Initial management of a mandibular fracture should ensure that the patient can maintain a patent airway without difficulty. Pain relief may then be obtained with nonsteroidal antiinflammatory drugs and narcotic agents. Because of the potential for wound infection from mouth flora, patients with open mandibular fractures should be treated with oral or intravenous penicillin. Clindamycin is an excellent choice for penicillin-allergic patients. Stabilization of a displaced mandibular fracture can be achieved with a Barton bandage.

When traumatic temporomandibular joint dislocation is encountered, the EP must obtain a dental panoramic study to consider the presence of a concomitant condylar fracture. If no indication of fracture is present, an attempt at reduction of the mandible in the ED may be undertaken with provision of intravenous benzodiazepines, as well as occasional procedural sedation and analgesia, to relax the muscles of mastication.

To perform reduction, the EP's thumbs are wrapped in gauze (to prevent injury). The EP faces the patient and places the thumbs on the posterior molars of the patient's mandible; the remaining fingers are wrapped around the inferior border of the mandible. Force is directed down on the thumbs as the symphyseal area is raised toward the EP. If reduction is unsuccessful, the patient may require general anesthesia. After reduction of an acute dislocation, the patient should be placed on a soft diet and instructed not to open the mouth wide for 7 days.

## FOLLOW-UP, NEXT STEPS IN CARE, AND PATIENT EDUCATION

Any patient with an open or unstable mandibular fracture requires admission for occlusion fixation or mandibular wiring. Patients with stable fractures may be discharged home and instructed to maintain a soft diet, and prompt outpatient follow-up should be arranged with an otolaryngologist or oral surgeon. Edentulous patients usually require admission to the hospital and internal fixation because they do not have teeth to assist in stabilizing the fracture. Phone consultation with an oromaxillofacial or plastic surgeon is essential to formulate an appropriate treatment plan.

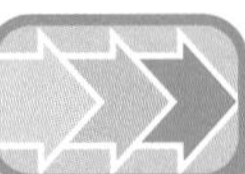

**PRIORITY ACTIONS**

Suspicious mechanism of injury? Is the patient being physically abused? Unwitnessed head, neck, and facial injuries, particularly in women, should raise concern for interpersonal violence.

- Obtain a history with only the patient in the room, and ask directed questions concerning the mechanism of injury and patient circumstances.
- Contact appropriate resources if the patient confirms a history of physical abuse.

Typical concomitant injuries in a patient with facial trauma include contusions, intracranial pathology, and abdominal and cervical spine injuries.

- In patients with severe facial injuries, consider elevating the head of the bed to reduce facial soft tissue swelling and possible airway compromise.
- Reassess the patient for hemorrhage from a facial fracture on arrival and at 30-minute intervals up to 6 hours.

Is the patient experiencing sudden loss of vision or eye pain? Increased retrobulbar pressure from a hematoma or emphysema can lead to acute and permanent loss of vision.

- Lateral canthotomy can be a vision-saving intervention.
- Loss of the perception of light or the ability to identify colors without associated eye pain is indicative of optic neuropathy.
- Emergency consultation with an ophthalmologist and computed tomography of the orbits and globes are required when considering optic nerve impingement.

Pain with eye movement? Does the patient have muscle entrapment?

- Perform computed tomography of the maxilla and orbit when considering a blowout fracture of the orbit.

Loss of sensation in the nerve distribution?

- Superior orbital nerve: consider a superior orbital rim or frontal bone fracture.
- Inferior orbital nerve: consider a zygoma, inferior orbital rim, or maxillary fracture.
- Mandibular nerve: consider a mandibular fracture.

Does the patient have malocclusion? Consider a mandibular or maxillary fracture.

- The tongue blade test is useful as a clinical screening examination for mandible fractures.

Lacerations through the vermilion border require extra attention to detail with surgical closure. Slight misalignment at the time of wound closure may result in substantial cosmetic implications.

Competency of the parotid duct must be considered with all deep cheek lacerations.

Do not attempt to realign a fractured nose in the emergency department.

Does the patient have a septal hematoma?

- A septal hematoma requires immediate evacuation, application of a wound dressing, prophylactic antibiotics, and close follow-up for wound care.

Does the patient have an otohematoma?

- Otohematomas should be drained and an adherent pressure dressing applied to prevent reaccumulation.

Is the patient's tetanus immunization up to date?

- Prophylactic antibiotics should be considered in patients with grossly contaminated wounds, open fractures, and joint wounds; in immunocompromised patients; with delayed wound closure; with high-velocity gunshot wounds; and in patients at high risk for endocarditis.

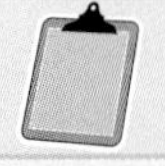

**DOCUMENTATION**

A detailed cranial nerve examination should be documented with special attention paid to the following:

- Ocular movements
- Sensory examination of the face
- Visual acuity
- Cervical spine "cleared" by clinical or radiographic criteria
- Absence of septal hematoma with a history of nasal trauma

## SUGGESTED READINGS

Dean NR, Ledgard JP, Katsaros J. Massive hemorrhage in facial fracture patients: definition, incidence, and management. Plast Reconstr Surg 2009;123:680-90.

Howes DS, Dowling PJ. Oral facial emergencies: triage and initial evaluation of the oral facial emergency. Emerg Med Clin North Am 2000;18:371-8.

Parry M. Maxillofacial trauma—developments, innovations, and controversies. Injury 2009;40:1252-9.

## REFERENCES

*References can be found on Expert Consult @ www.expertconsult.com.*

Derby Teaching Hospitals
NHS Foundation Tr..t
Library and Knowledg... ...tre

# Penetrating Neck Trauma 77

Niels K. Rathlev and Ron Medzon

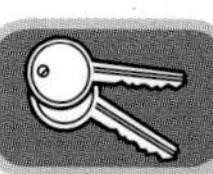

**KEY POINTS**

- Thorough vascular and esophageal evaluation is required, even with minor neck wounds, if any abnormalities are evident on examination or radiographs.
- Radiographs do not rule out esophageal injury.
- Early airway management is crucial, with orotracheal intubation being the initial method of choice.
- A thorough neurologic examination is essential in all patients with neck trauma.
- "Hard signs" of vascular injury include bruit, thrill, expanding or pulsatile hematoma, pulsatile or severe hemorrhage, pulse deficit, and central nervous system ischemia.
- The "gold standard" for diagnosing vascular injury is conventional angiography.
- Admission criteria include signs and symptoms of organ damage and penetration of the platysma muscles.

## EPIDEMIOLOGY

The incidence of injuries to the critical airway and the vascular, gastrointestinal, skeletal, and neurologic organs depends on the location and mechanism of injury. In the case of interpersonal violence, the distance between the assailant and victim and the type of weapon must be established. In total, 44% of injuries to critical organs involve vascular structures. This is a major source of morbidity and mortality (**Table 77.1**).[1]

## PERSPECTIVE

In the Vietnam War, the mortality from penetrating neck injuries was 4% to 7%. The current mortality rate in civilians is approximately 2% to 6%. Patients with zone I injuries (**Fig. 77.1**) at the base of the neck are at highest risk. Currently, spinal cord injuries and thrombosis of the common and internal carotid arteries account for 50% of all deaths from penetrating neck injury.

## PATHOPHYSIOLOGY

Unstable cervical spine fractures and spinal cord injuries are extremely unlikely in the presence of low-risk National Emergency X-radiography Utilization Study I (NEXUS I) criteria—that is, the patient:

1. Is alert and awake
2. Is not intoxicated
3. Has no signs or symptoms of neurologic injury
4. Has no spinous process tenderness

## ANATOMY

The neck consists of three anatomic zones (see Fig. 77.1):

- Zone I—base of the neck to the cricoid cartilage (**Fig. 77.2**)
- Zone II—cricoid cartilage to the angle of the mandible
- Zone III—above the angle of the mandible (**Fig. 77.3**)

The major muscles of the neck are the platysma muscles, which extend from the lower jaw to the clavicle (**Fig. 77.4**). Other critical structures are shown in **Figures 77.5 through 77.7**.

## PRESENTING SIGNS AND SYMPTOMS

### AIRWAY INJURY

Symptoms of airway injury include dyspnea, hemoptysis, subcutaneous air, stridor, hoarseness, and dysphonia (**Fig. 77.8**).

### VASCULAR INJURY

"Hard signs" that indicate severe vascular injury include the following:

- Bruit or thrill suggestive of a traumatic arteriovenous fistula
- Expanding or pulsatile hematoma
- Pulsatile or severe hemorrhage
- Pulse deficit—pulses may be normal in patients with nonocclusive injuries that require surgical repair, such as intimal flaps or pseudoaneurysms

**Table 77.1 Incidence of Neck Injuries**

| VASCULAR | % | AERODIGESTIVE | % | NEUROLOGIC | % |
|---|---|---|---|---|---|
| Subclavian artery | 2.6 | Trachea | 6.0 | Spinal cord | 1.9 |
| External carotid artery | 2.5 | Pharynx | 5.0 | Brachial plexus | 2.1 |
| Internal carotid artery | 1.3 | Esophagus | 5.0 | Cranial nerves VII, X, XI, XII | 1.9 |
| Common carotid artery | 0.6 | Larynx | 2.4 | Sympathetic chain | 0.2 |

From Carducci B, Lowe RA, Dalsey W. Penetrating neck trauma: consensus and controversies. Ann Emerg Med 1986;15:208-15.

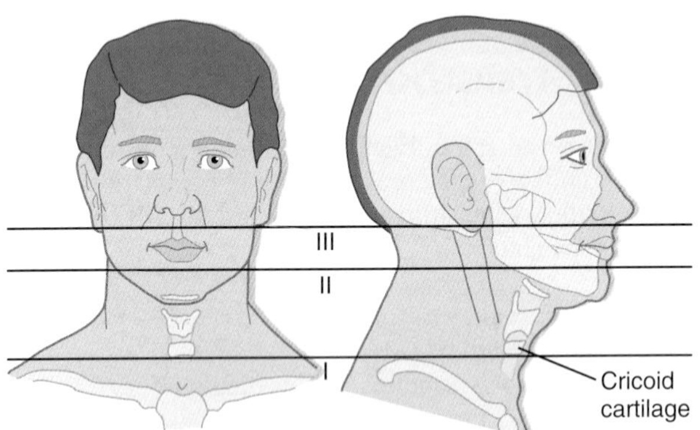


**Fig. 77.1 Zones of the neck.**

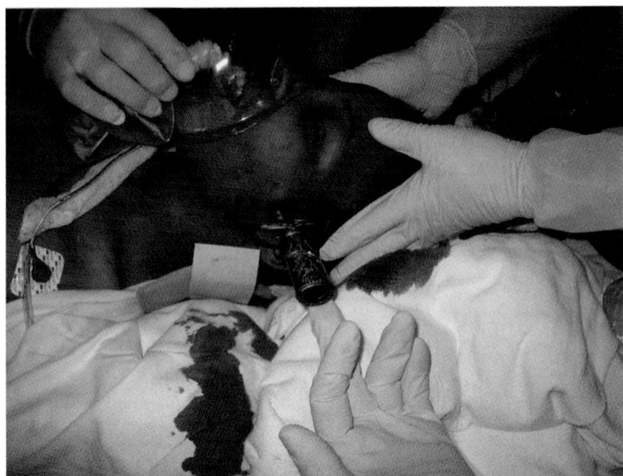

**Fig. 77.3 Injury in zone III of the neck.**

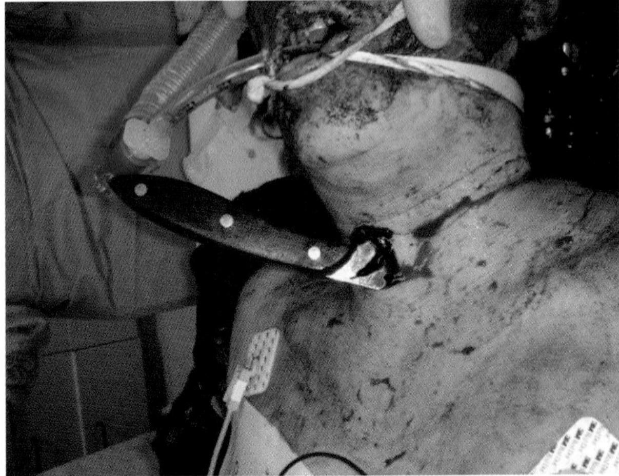

**Fig. 77.2 Stab wound in zone I of the neck.**

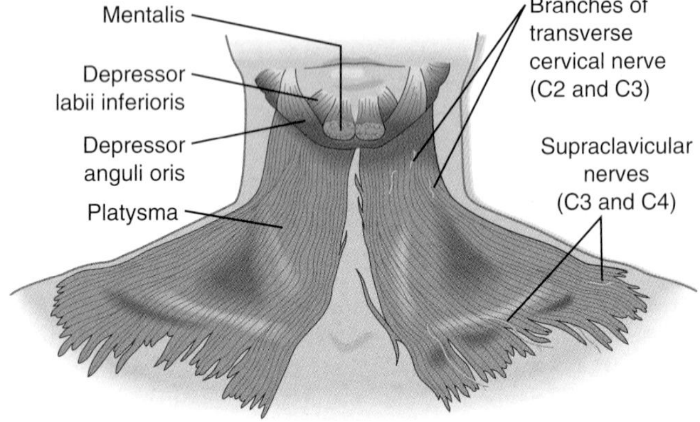


**Fig. 77.4 Surface anatomy: the platysma.** (From Agur AMR, Dalley AF, editors. Grant's atlas of anatomy. 9th ed. Baltimore: Williams & Wilkins; 1991.)

"Soft signs," which are less predictive of severe vascular injury, include the following:

- Hypotension and shock
- Stable, nonpulsatile hematoma
- Central nervous system ischemia—a neurologic deficit that develops over the course of 1 to 2 hours after injury is consistent with ischemic neurologic injury; an immediate deficit is more likely to be due to a primary neurologic injury
- Proximity to a major vascular structure is not considered a high-risk feature in the absence of the preceding criteria (**Fig. 77.9**)

## DIGESTIVE TRACT

The pharynx must be examined by visual inspection. Under normal conditions, the esophagus is mobile and collapsed. Symptoms and signs of esophageal injury include

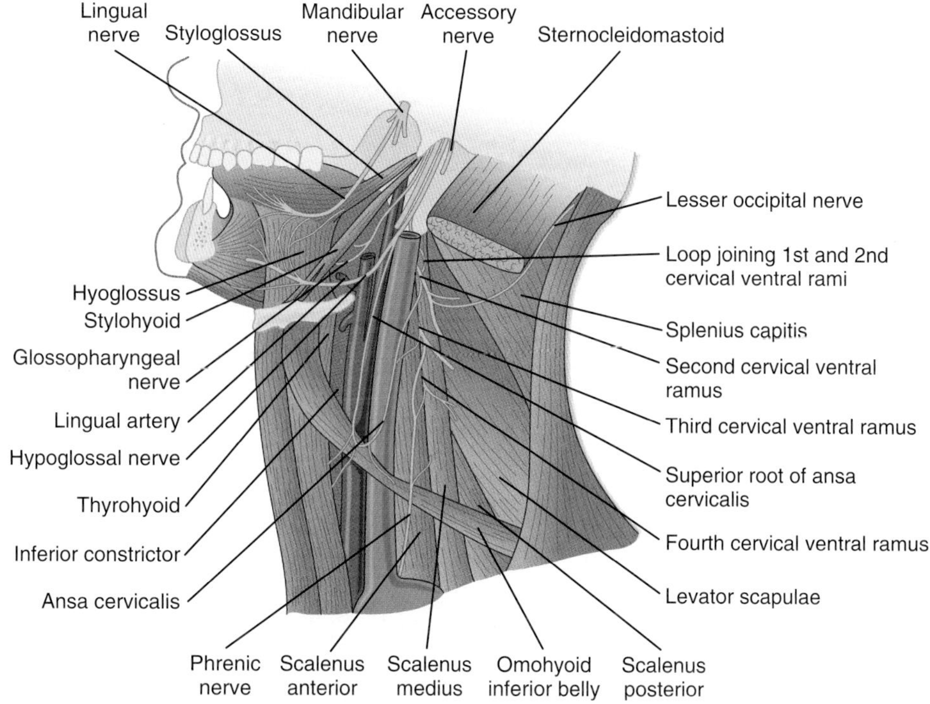


**Fig. 77.5 Anterior triangle—anterior border of the sternocleidomastoid muscle to the midline.** (From Agur AMR, Dalley AF, editors. Grant's atlas of anatomy. 9th ed. Baltimore: Williams & Wilkins; 1991.)

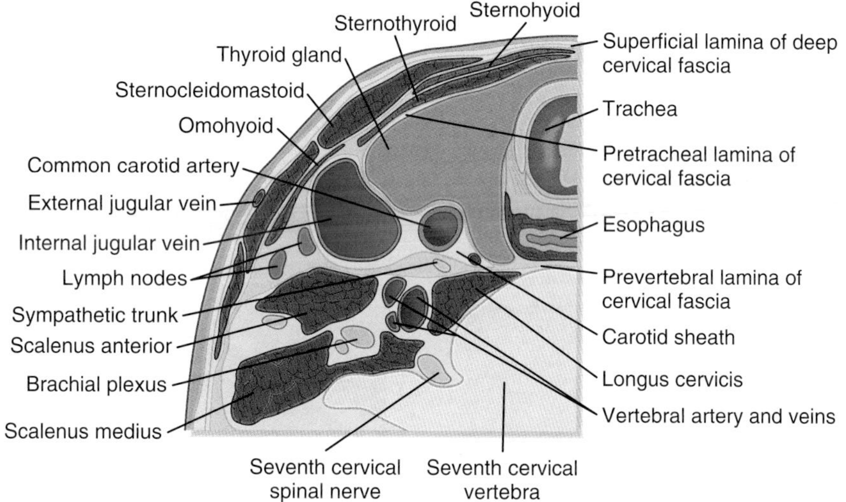


**Fig. 77.6 Transverse section of the neck at the level of C7.** (From Agur AMR, Dalley AF, editors. Grant's atlas of anatomy. 9th ed. Baltimore: Williams & Wilkins; 1991.)

subcutaneous air, crepitus, dysphagia, odynophagia, drooling, and hematemesis.

## DIAGNOSTIC TESTING

### VASCULAR INJURY

#### *Conventional Angiography*

The "gold standard" of diagnostic modalities is four-vessel angiography with venous-phase imaging (sensitivity > 99%) (**Fig. 77.10**). Very rarely do injuries missed by angiography require repair. A normal study is highly predictive of survival from vessel injury.[2]

#### *Duplex Ultrasonography*

Duplex ultrasonography is noninvasive, convenient, and relatively inexpensive, but its sensitivity in detecting vascular injury is highly operator dependent. However, its sensitivity in comparison with conventional angiography is 90% to 100% for injuries requiring intervention.[3] Duplex ultrasonography can miss nonocclusive injuries with preserved flow, such as intimal flaps and pseudoaneurysms.

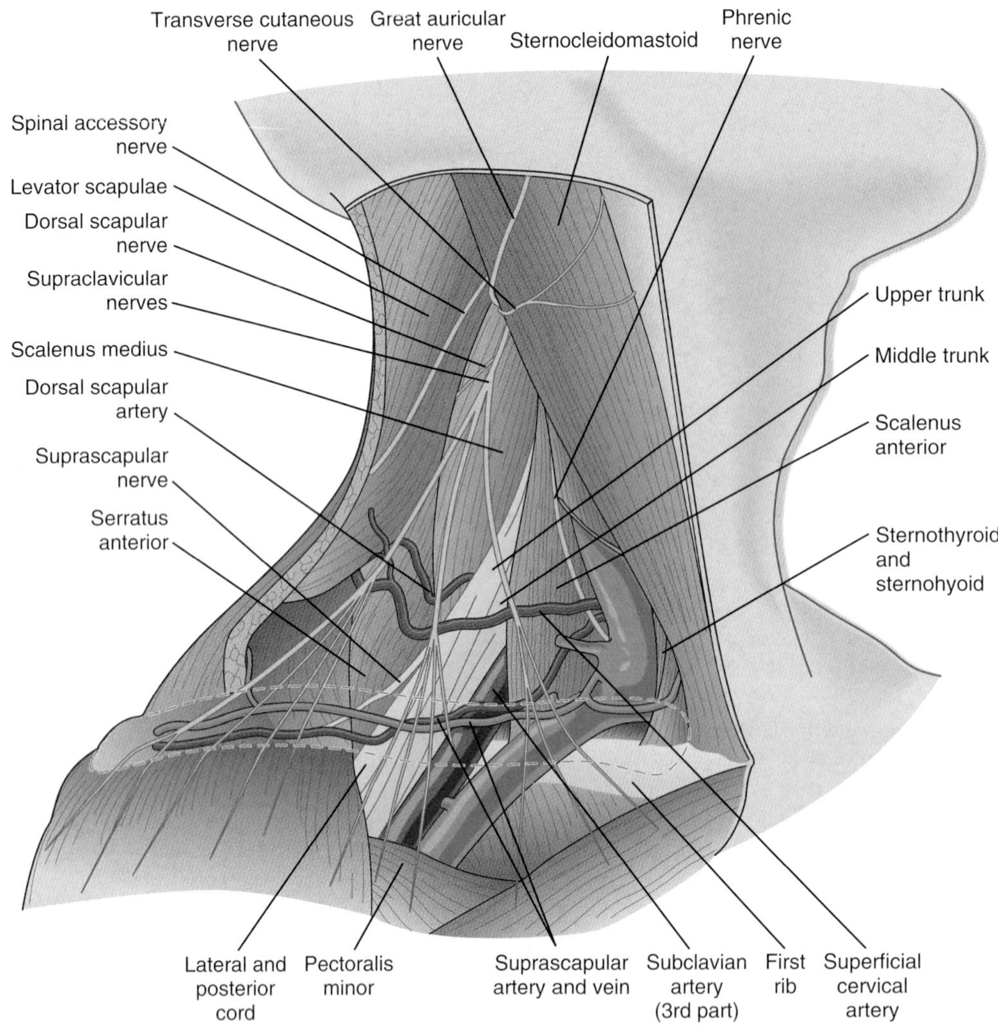


**Fig. 77.7 Posterior triangle—posterior border of the sternocleidomastoid muscle to the trapezius muscle.** (From Agur AMR, Dalley AF, editors. Grant's atlas of anatomy. 9th ed. Baltimore: Williams & Wilkins; 1991.)

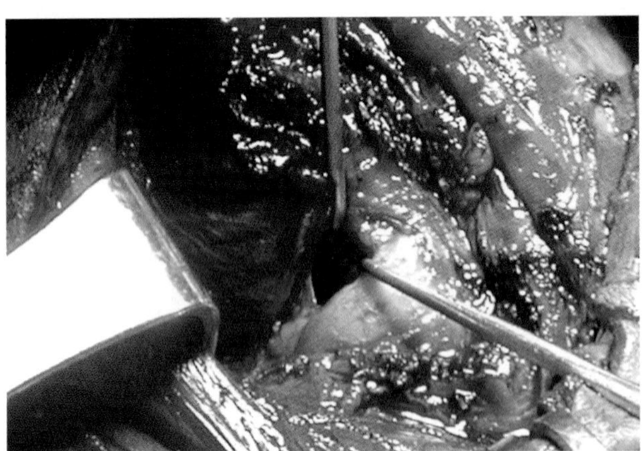

**Fig. 77.8 Tracheal injury.**

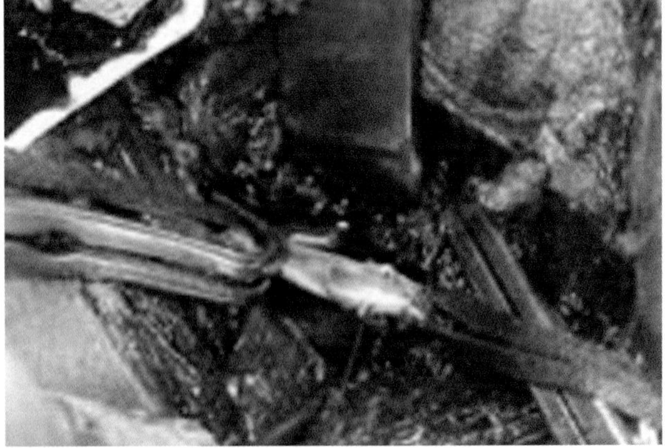

**Fig. 77.9 Injury to the common carotid artery.**

## *Multidetector Helical Computed Tomographic Angiography*

This diagnostic modality has largely supplanted duplex ultrasonography in patients without obvious indications for immediate operative intervention (**Fig. 77.11**). The sensitivity of multidetector computed tomographic (MDCT) angiography is 90% to 100% with respect to conventional angiography and surgical exploration.[4,5]

Sensitivity is further improved with high-resolution computed tomography scanning, such as 64-row technology, and with increased technical experience using this modality. When compared with conventional angiography, MDCT angiography is faster, less expensive, and noninvasive and does not involve interventional radiology.

## PHARYNGEAL INJURY

Hypopharyngeal injuries may be difficult to visualize on radiographic contrast swallow studies, especially if patients are intubated. Videolaryngoscopy is an alternative diagnostic modality that is effective in detecting these injuries.[6]

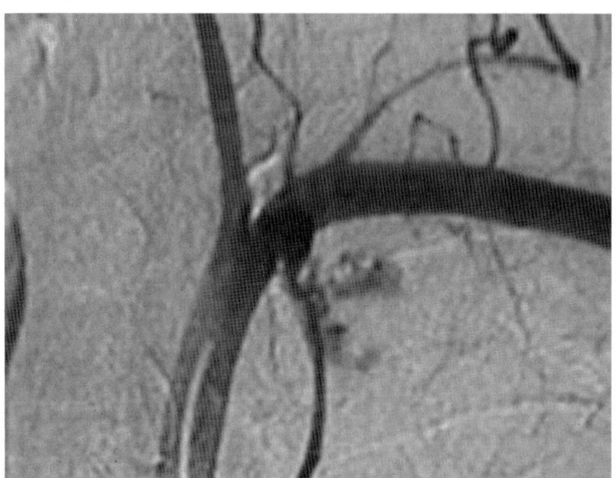

**Fig. 77.10 Angiogram revealing extravasation of contrast agent caused by a stab wound in the subclavian artery.**

## ESOPHAGEAL INJURY

Esophageal injuries may be clinically silent initially. Radiographs do not exclude esophageal injury. Contrast-enhanced studies have a sensitivity of 50% to 90%. Esophagoscopy has a sensitivity of 43% to 100% (**Table 77.2**).

Rigid endoscopy has higher diagnostic yield than flexible endoscopy does; however, it is associated with a higher incidence of complications, including iatrogenic rupture. A combined approach that includes both contrast-enhanced studies and esophagoscopy has a sensitivity of 100%.[7,8]

**Table 77.2 Sensitivities of Diagnostic Modalities for Esophageal Injury**

| DIAGNOSTIC TEST | SENSITIVITY (%) |
|---|---|
| Physical examination | 80 |
| Contrast-enhanced study | 89 |
| Rigid esophagoscopy | 89 |
| Contrast-enhanced study plus esophagoscopy | 100 |

From Weigelt JA, Thal ER, Snyder 3rd WH, et al. Diagnosis of penetrating cervical esophageal injuries. Am J Surg 1987;154:619-22.

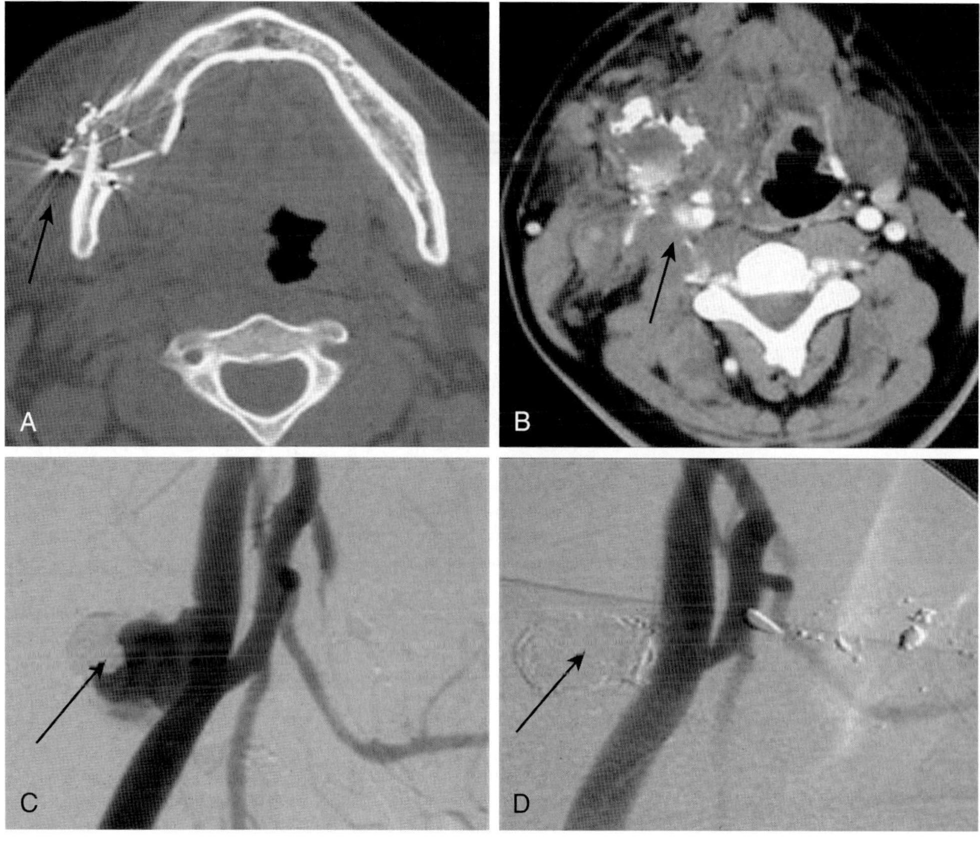


**Fig. 77.11 Gunshot wound to the mandible. A** and **B,** Helical computed tomographic angiography reveals diminished flow through the right common carotid artery *(arrow)*. **C** and **D,** Conventional angiography demonstrates a pseudoaneurysm *(arrow)* of the vessel proximal to its bifurcation.

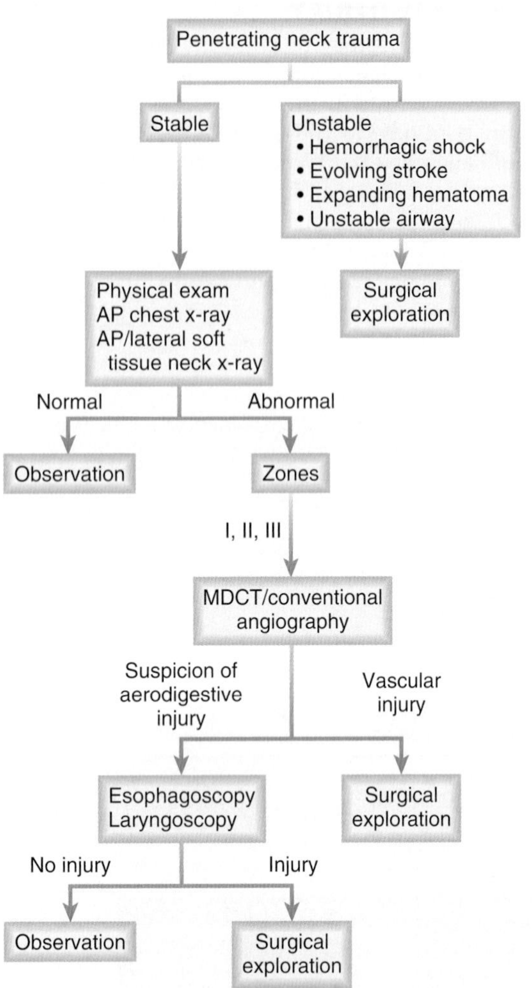


**Fig. 77.12 Algorithm for the diagnosis of penetrating neck injuries.** *AP*, Anteroposterior; *MDCT*, multidetector computed tomography.

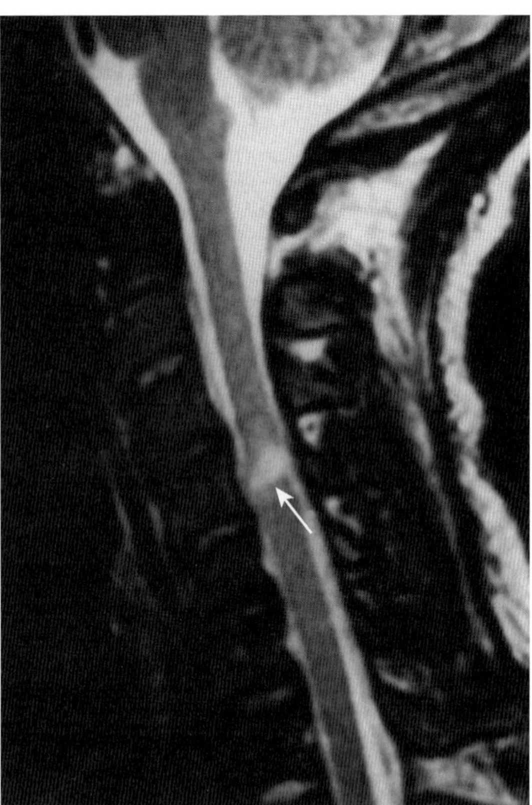

**Fig. 77.13 Magnetic resonance image showing hemisection of the spinal cord at C4 *(arrow)* as a result of a zone III stab wound.** (From Firlik AD, Welch WC. Images in clinical medicine: Brown-Séquard syndrome. N Engl J Med 1999;340:285.)

## SELECTIVE EVALUATION

Selective surgical exploration is recommended for patients without obvious indications for surgical repair.[9-13] Nonoperative techniques (**Fig. 77.12**) are sufficiently sensitive to safely rule out injuries that require an operation. Esophageal and arterial injuries have reportedly been missed during exploration. A selective approach is more cost-effective than mandatory exploration.

## NEUROLOGIC INJURY

Fortunately, injuries to the brain, spinal cord, and peripheral nerves are uncommon (**Fig. 77.13**; see Table 77.1). Patients with primary neurologic injuries are seen initially with focal deficits or alteration in mental status.

# TREATMENT

## PREHOSPITAL MANAGEMENT

Prehospital care should focus on maintenance of an open airway. Establishment of a definite airway should be performed only when absolutely necessary because of the complexity of the procedure in these patients. Partial airway injuries may lead to complete airway obstruction during endotracheal intubation. Hemorrhage should be controlled with direct pressure only. Spine immobilization is secondary to airway maintenance and control of bleeding in patients who are neurologically intact and awake.

## AIRWAY INTERVENTIONS

Direct visualization of the airway is optimal, and orotracheal intubation is the initial method of choice because the procedure is frequently performed and rarely associated with complications.[14,15] Ideally, intubation is accomplished with topical anesthesia while the patient is awake.[16] If not possible, rapid-sequence induction should be performed. Fiberoptic intubation is reserved for semielective airway management unless an experienced operator and the necessary equipment are immediately available. Visualization may be impaired because of extensive hemorrhage and secretions.

Cricothyrotomy or tracheostomy is necessary if orotracheal or fiberoptic intubation is unsuccessful. A surgical airway should not be delayed because an expanding hematoma can quickly distort the anatomy and result in complications. Intubation through an accessible neck wound has a very high success rate (**Fig. 77.14**). In this instance, care must be taken to control the proximal end of the trachea so that it does not retract into the thorax.

Nasotracheal intubation is *not* a preferred airway technique. Its success rate varies from 0% to 75%. It is potentially associated with complications because of the "blind" nature of the procedure. A more direct, visualized approach is suggested (**Fig. 77.15**).

When diagnosed, injuries to the larynx or trachea are treated by primary surgical repair in the operating room. Immediate surgical exploration should also be performed in patients with progressive subcutaneous or mediastinal emphysema, pneumothorax, severe dyspnea, or associated esophageal trauma. This is followed by a mid or low tracheostomy, depending on the site of the injury.

## WOUND CARE AND EVALUATION

The emergency physician (EP) may gently spread the wound edges without probing. The patient should be placed in the Trendelenburg position if there is any concern about internal jugular vein injury and possible air embolism. Wounds should be closed only if the depth is clearly visualized; caution is urged because assessment of depth is difficult. The EP must suspect deep penetration and ensure complete diagnostic evaluation.

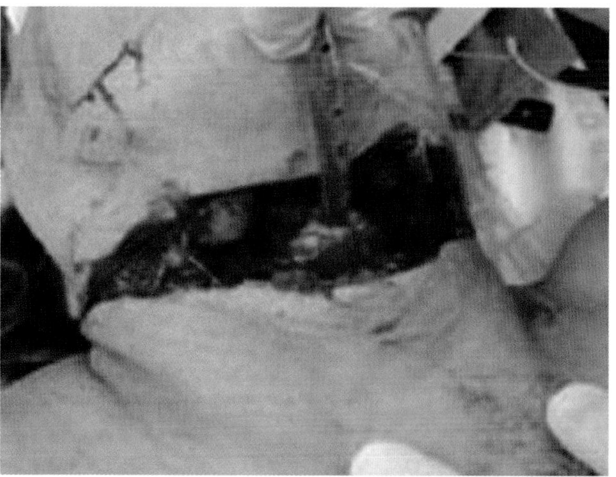

**Fig. 77.14 Emergency airway through an accessible wound.**

### *Vascular Injury*

Direct pressure should be used; blindly clamping structures with poor visualization should be avoided. Pharyngeal packing for severe oral bleeding may be necessary. Subclavian vein injury should be suspected in patients with zone I injuries. Intravenous access should be established on the side opposite the injury to avoid potential extravasation of fluids.

Emergency department thoracotomy is indicated for patients with zone I injuries and refractory shock. Subclavian artery injury should be suspected in these cases. Treatment is determined by angiographic grading of the vascular injuries. Primary repair is preferred over graft placement when possible.

Surgical repair of carotid and vertebral artery injuries is preferred over ligation except in the following cases:

- Coma without antegrade flow because of the high risk of converting an ischemic to a hemorrhagic brain injury
- Uncontrollable hemorrhage
- Inability to place a temporary shunt

### *Esophageal Injury*

Delay in diagnosis and repair of esophageal injuries is associated with increased morbidity and mortality because of the potential for mediastinitis. When surgery is performed less than 24 hours after the injury, the survival rate is greater than 90%; when surgery is performed more than 24 hours after the injury, it is just 65%.

### *Cervical Spine Injury*

Rigorous spinal precautions should not be maintained at the expense of managing life-threatening airway or vascular injuries in patients who are awake and neurologically intact without focal deficits.[17,18] Unstable spine fractures are almost

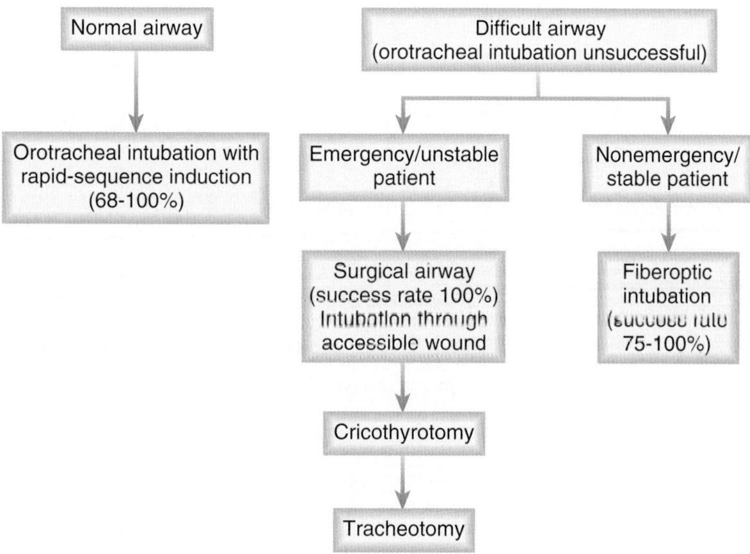


**Fig. 77.15 Algorithm for emergency airway management.**

invariably associated with focal neurologic deficits or altered mental status. Early fracture stabilization and fixation are mandatory. Corticosteroids have no role in spinal cord injury caused by penetrating trauma.

## ADMISSION AND DISCHARGE

Admission criteria include (1) any signs or symptoms of organ damage and (2) penetration of the platysma, which is only 2 to 3 mm in depth.

## REFERENCES

***References can be found on Expert Consult @ www.expertconsult.com.***

# Thoracic Trauma 78

*John Bailitz and Tarlan Hedayati*

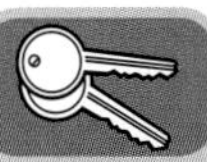

**KEY POINTS**

- Emergency life-threatening conditions that need to be detected during the primary survey include airway obstruction, tension pneumothorax, open pneumothorax, massive hemothorax, flail chest, and pericardial tamponade (**Table 78.1**).
- Urgent life-threatening conditions to detect during the secondary survey include simple pneumothorax, hemothorax, pulmonary contusion, tracheobronchial injury, blunt cardiac injury, traumatic aortic injury, diaphragmatic injury, and esophageal injury.
- Common thoracic cage injuries are not always associated with serious injury, but some individuals, especially pediatric and elderly patients, may require admission for associated injuries and respiratory therapy.

## EPIDEMIOLOGY

Head and thoracic injuries from moving vehicle collisions (MVCs) and firearms account for the majority of the more than 160,000 injury-related deaths in the United States each year. Most fatalities occur immediately as a result of massive cardiac or vascular injury. Rib fractures are the most common thoracic cage injury following blunt thoracic trauma. Isolated first and second rib, sternum, and scapula fractures are no longer considered markers of traumatic aortic injury.[1] However, rib fractures must still be considered markers of significant injury. Most patients seen in trauma centers with rib fractures will have hemothorax, pneumothorax, or a pulmonary contusion. Three or more rib fractures at any anatomic site dramatically increases the risk for spleen and liver injury. Likewise, scapula fractures are uncommon yet signify a high-energy mechanism of injury, almost always with important associated injuries.

Seat belts have increased the incidence of sternum fractures while reducing the number of lives lost in MVCs. Isolated nondisplaced sternum fractures are no longer considered markers of blunt cardiac injury.[2] More complicated fracture patterns predict associated injuries. Fractures of the manubrium, manubrium-sternum synchondrosis, and proximal part of the sternum and severely displaced sternum fractures are associated with an increased incidence of spinal fractures. Displaced fractures of the body of the sternum are associated with a higher incidence of intrapulmonary and cardiac injuries.[3]

## PATHOPHYSIOLOGY

The most common mechanism of blunt thoracic trauma is an MVC, followed by falls, assaults, and crush injuries. Compressive forces directly injure the thoracic cage and underlying viscera and result in rib fractures and pulmonary contusion. Deceleration produces traction on fixed structures such as the isthmus of the aorta and the carina and results in traumatic aortic and tracheobronchial injuries. Blunt thoracic trauma causes penetrating thoracic trauma when rib or clavicle fractures impale thoracic or abdominal viscera.

Gunshot wounds and stab wounds are the most common mechanisms of penetrating thoracic trauma. Low-velocity stab wounds disrupt only the structures penetrated. Medium-velocity handguns and high-velocity military assault rifles produce temporary and permanent cavities of tissue damage. Missile injuries to the thorax often involve multiple anatomic regions, including the neck, diaphragm, abdomen, and retroperitoneum.

## THORACIC CAGE INJURIES: RIB, STERNUM, AND SCAPULA FRACTURES

MVCs are the most common cause of rib and sternum fractures. Other mechanisms include pedestrian injury by a moving vehicle, falls, contact sports, and altercations. Fractures occur at the site of direct blows or at their posterior weak point as a result of compressive forces. Ribs 4 to 9 are the most commonly fractured.

All thoracic cage injuries result in significant pain, splinting, atelectasis, and increased risk for pneumonia. Multiple rib fractures interfere directly with the mechanics of ventilation. Fracture fragments may penetrate the pleura and lungs and result in pneumothorax and hemothorax. Traditionally, fractures of the 6th to 12th rib on the right suggest liver injury and on the left suggest splenic injury. However, any fracture, especially multiple fractures, increases the risk for liver and splenic injuries.[4]

**Table 78.1 Life-Threatening Emergencies in the Primary Survey**

| EMERGENCY | CLASSIC FINDINGS | INITIAL TESTING | FURTHER MANAGEMENT |
|---|---|---|---|
| Airway obstruction as a result of retrosternal clavicular dislocation | Deformity over the clavicle and stridor; depressed medial clavicle on a chest radiograph | Clinical Dx | Immediate reduction if unable to intubate |
| Tension pneumothorax | JVD, tracheal deviation, and unilaterally absent breath sounds | Clinical Dx | Needle decompression followed immediately by tube thoracostomy |
| Open pneumothorax | Respiratory distress as a result of a sucking chest wound | Clinical Dx | Three-sided tape over the wound and tube thoracostomy |
| Flail chest | Respiratory distress, tenderness, crepitus, and paradoxic movement | Three or more ribs fractured in two or more places on a chest radiograph | Early CPAP and close attention to pain control and fluid status |
| Cardiac tamponade | Hypotension and tachycardia, JVD, and the Beck triad late | Ultrasound confirms the diagnosis; chest radiograph; ECG insensitive | Intravenous fluids, pericardiocentesis, and thoracotomy |
| Massive hemothorax | Respiratory distress, chest wall injury, diminished breath sounds, and dullness to percussion | Ultrasound confirms the diagnosis; chest radiograph with fluid collection | Initial chest tube output of 1.5-2 L is an indication for surgical intervention |

*CPAP*, Continuous positive airway pressure; *Dx*, diagnostic testing; *ECG*, electrocardiogram; *JVD*, jugular venous distention.

Because children have more elastic chest walls, more energy is transmitted to the underlying lung, and greater force is required for fractures. Excluding other major trauma, 71% of rib fractures in children younger than 2 years result from abuse.[5]

## PRESENTING SIGNS AND SYMPTOMS

Classically, rib fractures are accompanied by localized tenderness and pleuritic chest pain, as well as splinting, crepitus, and ecchymosis. Patients with a classic sternum fracture have localized pain and tenderness along with ventral compression, ecchymosis, and deformity. Pain at the site of thoracic cage injuries increases with cough and deep inspiration. Patients with scapular fractures typically have rib and extremity fractures that often mask the diagnosis of scapula fracture.

## DIFFERENTIAL DIAGNOSIS AND MEDICAL DECISION MAKING

The initial portable anteroposterior (AP) chest radiograph should be inspected to confirm the diagnosis of rib fracture and underlying pleura or lung injury. Upright posteroanterior (PA) and lateral radiographs should be obtained if a high clinical index of suspicion remains for fracture or underlying injury. The presence of an occult "clinical rib fracture" with tenderness over the rib should be assumed even in the absence of radiographic findings. Rib radiographs seldom add to the clinical evaluation and are not routinely indicated.

Sternum fractures are best detected on the lateral chest radiograph. Associated rib fractures and mediastinal abnormalities may be evident on the PA view. In experienced hands, bedside ultrasound may be more sensitive than radiographs for detection of both rib and sternum fractures, as well as associated hemothorax or pneumothorax.[6,7] The electrocardiogram (ECG) should be examined for evidence of cardiac injury. Scapula fractures are often missed on the initial chest radiograph unless the scapular outline is specifically inspected. Shoulder radiographs can confirm suspected fractures (**Fig. 78.1**).

Helical computed tomographic (CT) angiography should be performed on hemodynamically stable patients when clinically significant underlying injury is suspected. An abdominal CT scan can rule out intraabdominal injury in patients with tenderness or fracture of the sixth rib or below, three or more rib fractures, hypotension noted in the field or emergency department (ED), abdominal or flank tenderness, pelvic or femoral fractures, or gross hematuria.[8]

## TREATMENT

Adequate pain control should be provided to prevent atelectasis in patients with simple acute rib fractures. Patients should be instructed to perform incentive spirometry or take 10 deep breaths every hour. Binders and belts are not recommended because such devices promote hypoventilation, which results in atelectasis and pneumonia. Shoulder slings and pendular exercise should be prescribed for most scapular fractures. Displaced fractures, especially those involving the scapular spine and neck, often require consultation with an orthopedic surgeon for repair.

## FOLLOW-UP, NEXT STEPS IN CARE, AND PATIENT EDUCATION

Otherwise healthy patients with isolated rib fractures or sternum or scapula fractures may be discharged home. Elderly

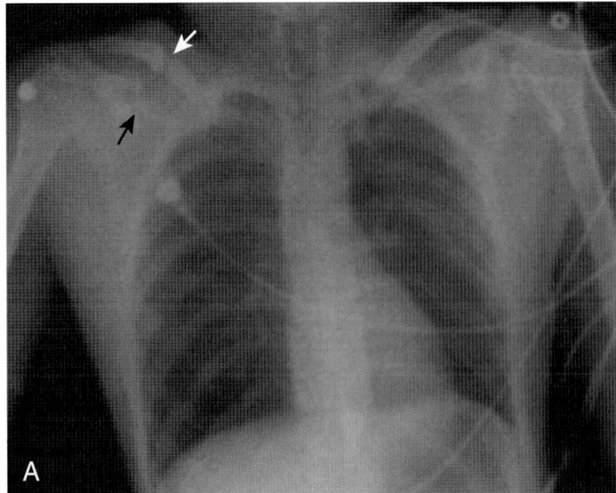


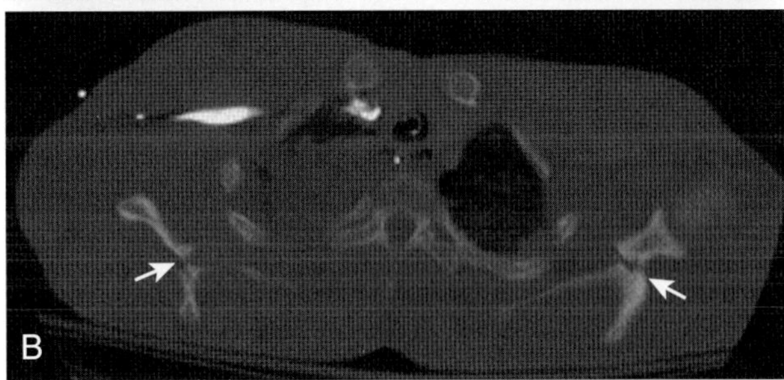


**Fig. 78.1** **A,** Chest radiograph showing fractures of the clavicle *(white arrow))* and scapula *(black arrow)*. **B,** Lateral scapula fractures *(arrows)* visible on a computed tomography scan. (From Westra SJ, Wallace EC. Imaging of pediatric chest trauma. Radiol Clin North Am 2005;43:267-81.)

patients and those with multiple comorbid conditions may require admission for pain control and pulmonary therapy. An intercostal nerve block can be of marked benefit. Discharged patients should be informed that the pain will diminish after 2 weeks but may persist for up to 6 weeks. Follow-up with a trauma surgeon should be scheduled if pain persists beyond 4 weeks to detect delayed rib fracture complications.

## FLAIL CHEST

Flail chest occurs when three or more ribs are fractured in two or more places and a discontinuous segment of the thoracic wall is produced and moves paradoxically with respiration. Flail chest is diagnosed in approximately 5% of thoracic trauma patients seen in level I trauma centers, typically in the setting of multisystem trauma. Mechanisms include MVCs, crush injuries, assault, falls, and even minimal trauma in elderly patients. Respiratory insufficiency results primarily from the underlying pulmonary contusion. Pneumothorax occurs in 50% of cases and pulmonary contusion in 75%.[9]

### PRESENTING SIGNS AND SYMPTOMS

Patients may have the classic signs and symptoms of respiratory distress, tenderness, crepitus, deformity, and paradoxic motion of the affected thoracic wall. Affected segments will move inward during inspiration and outward during expiration. More commonly, splinting secondary to severe pain or mechanical ventilation masks the diagnosis. Forced expiration and coughing accent the paradox.

### DIFFERENTIAL DIAGNOSIS AND MEDICAL DECISION MAKING

A chest radiograph can confirm the diagnosis and detect complications such as pneumothorax and hemothorax. A chest CT scan can further evaluate the underlying pulmonary contusion and assess for other underlying injuries such as traumatic aortic injury.

### TREATMENT

Immediate chest tube placement is required for assessment and management of other injuries, including pneumothorax and hemothorax. Continuous positive airway pressure is the first-line treatment in awake and cooperative patients with worsening oxygenation or ventilation.[10] Criteria for intubation include airway obstruction, respiratory distress, shock, closed head injury, and need for surgery. Endotracheal intubation should be performed only when necessary to avoid the increased mortality associated with nosocomial pneumonia.

Fluid replacement should be managed carefully to avoid overhydration and worsening of lung injury. Analgesia is titrated so that patients are more willing to make sufficient inspiratory effort, but excessive sedation should be avoided. Intercostal nerve blocks, epidural anesthesia, or even surgical fixation of the flail segment may be beneficial.[11] Stabilization of the flail segment in the ED or prehospital setting has not been shown to be helpful, and aggressive stabilizing efforts impede overall thoracic mechanics.

### FOLLOW-UP, NEXT STEPS IN CARE, AND PATIENT EDUCATION

Consultation and admission for trauma or cardiothoracic surgery is advised when flail chest is suspected. Overall mortality from flail chest, though dependent on other injuries, ranges up to 35%. All patients with flail chest should be admitted to the intensive care unit, preferably at a level I trauma center for close observation of respiratory mechanics and worsening of pulmonary contusion.

## PNEUMOTHORAX AND HEMOTHORAX

A simple pneumothorax occurs when air accumulates in the pleural space without shifting the mediastinum or communicating with the atmosphere. Mechanisms include laceration of the pleura or lung by a fractured rib, alveolar rupture from compression of the chest against a closed glottis, or a penetrating wound in the thorax.

Tension pneumothorax occurs when injury to the chest wall acts as a one-way valve. Outside air enters the pleural space during inspiration but cannot exit during expiration. Accumulating air increases intrapleural pressure, which eventually shifts the mediastinum, compresses the vena cava, reduces venous return, and ultimately decreases cardiac output. Open or communicating pneumothorax occurs when a significant thoracic wall defect causes the lung to collapse on inspiration and expand on expiration, with air being "sucked" into and out of the chest and thus preventing effective ventilation. Mechanisms include high-velocity assault rifle injuries and shotgun wounds.

Hemothorax occurs when blood accumulates in the pleural space, typically from minor lacerations in the lung parenchyma. Massive hemothorax is defined as greater than 1.5 L of blood in the initial chest tube drainage and is an indication for immediate surgery. Hemopneumothorax occurs when both air and blood fill the pleural space and commonly results from rib fractures or penetrating trauma.

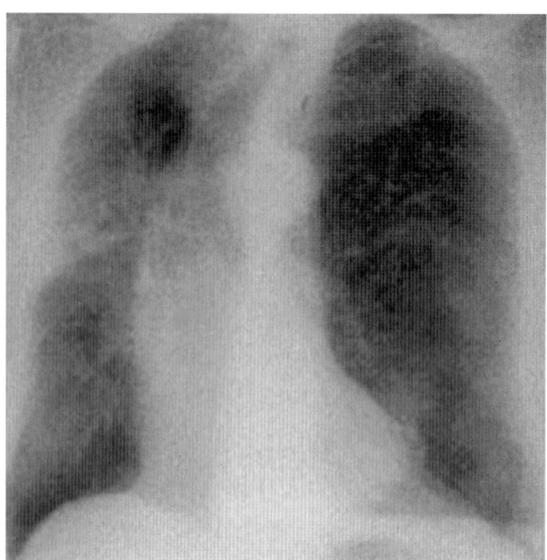

**Fig. 78.2 Chest radiograph showing obvious left-sided tension pneumothorax with mediastinal shift.** (From Ullman EA, Donley LP, Brady WJ. Pulmonary trauma emergency department evaluation and management. Emerg Med Clin North Am 2003; 21:291-313.)

## PRESENTING SIGNS AND SYMPTOMS

Patients with a simple pneumothorax classically have chest pain, diminished breath sounds, crepitus, hyperresonance, and mild to moderate respiratory distress. Patients with tension pneumothorax are classically seen in extremis and exhibit jugular venous distention, tracheal deviation, unilaterally absent breath sounds, or tachycardia followed by hypotension immediately before death (or any combination thereof).[12] Patients with open pneumothorax have chest wall wounds that produce sonorous sounds and are in severe respiratory distress. Typical symptoms of hemothorax are respiratory distress, chest pain, and diminished breath sounds with dullness to percussion.

Atypical manifestations are more common than classic ones. Respiratory distress may occur as a result of multiple other causes. Patients can have severe pain from distracting injuries. Breath sounds may be difficult to hear in a noisy environment. Physical examination in patients with penetrating thoracic trauma is unreliable for the detection of pneumothorax or hemothorax.[13] Patients with simple pneumothorax may be minimally symptomatic or may be cyanotic and in severe respiratory distress. Tension pneumothorax most commonly occurs in intubated patients as a result of positive pressure ventilation, sometimes after overzealous bagging.

Clinical reassessment of ventilated patients with decreasing oxygen saturation and hypotension may allow faster detection and treatment, even before chest radiographic diagnosis. Open pneumothorax may be missed if the patient is not completely exposed and rolled during the primary survey.

## DIFFERENTIAL DIAGNOSIS AND MEDICAL DECISION MAKING

The differential diagnosis for tension pneumothorax includes cardiac tamponade, massive hemothorax, and right mainstem intubation with left lung collapse. All will produce respiratory distress, hypotension, and tachycardia. Cardiac tamponade results in diminished heart sounds with normal breath sounds and a midline trachea. Massive hemothorax produces decreased or absent unilateral breath sounds and dullness to percussion. Chest tube insertion confirms the diagnosis. Right mainstem intubation results in jugular venous distention, tracheal deviation to the left, normal resonance, and diminished breath sounds on the left versus the right. In an intubated patient, the endotracheal tube should be checked and pulled back. In the field or resuscitation bay, bilateral needle thoracostomy should be performed when the patient is in distress, even if the diagnosis is uncertain. A rush of air confirms the diagnosis of tension pneumothorax. Chest tubes must be placed after needle decompression.

A chest radiograph can confirm the diagnosis of simple pneumothorax and hemothorax. A distance of 1 cm or one fingerbreadth between the chest wall and visceral pleural line correlates with a small, 10% to 15% pneumothorax. Anything larger requires immediate chest tube insertion. On a supine portable AP chest radiograph, a deep sulcus sign suggests pneumothorax. The affected costophrenic angle appears clearer and deep with depression of the hemidiaphragm as a result of localized air collection in a supine patient. In patients with a high index of clinical suspicion based on symptoms or penetrating injuries, some authorities advocate expiratory upright PA and lateral chest radiographs to make the lung volume smaller and the pneumothorax volume relatively larger and easier to visualize. Clinically significant pneumothorax should be evident on standard chest radiographs. The chest CT scan is more sensitive in visualizing pneumothorax; it often detects small occult pneumothoraces, which require close monitoring.

In an upright patient, a hemothorax appears as a fluid layer in the affected hemithorax. Early collections are noted to blunt the costophrenic angles on the AP and lateral radiographic views. Hemothorax often appears as only a diffuse hazy infiltrate in a supine trauma patient. Hemopneumothorax has a fluid layer with a flat superior border, in contrast to the round meniscus of an isolated hemothorax (**Figs. 78.2 and 78.3**). Decubitus views better demonstrate a small hemothorax.

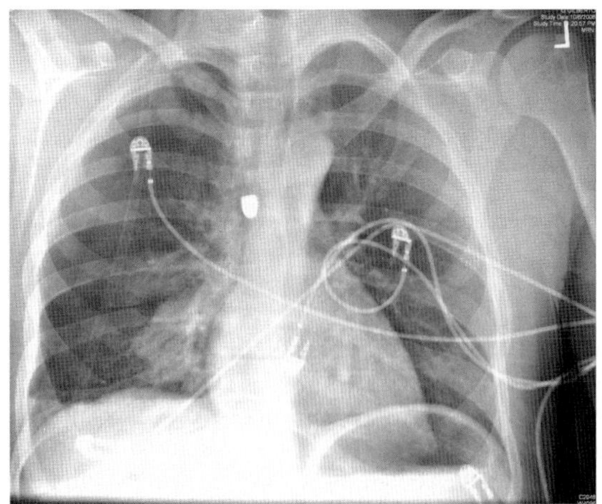

**Fig. 78.3 Chest radiograph showing right hemopneumothorax along with a bullet.** (Image courtesy Dave Andreski, MD.)

An extended focused assessment with sonography for trauma (FAST) scan can diagnose pneumothorax and hemothorax with higher sensitivity than portable chest radiography can in experienced hands. An extended FAST scan is especially helpful when chest radiography is not immediately available and in mass casualty situations.[14]

## TREATMENT

Tension pneumothorax and open pneumothorax are both clinical diagnoses that require immediate treatment with needle thoracostomy followed by tube thoracostomy, even when based on clinical evaluation, before radiographic confirmation. All suspicious open chest wounds should be covered with petrolatum gauze secured on three sides to prevent the entry of air during inspiration and allow the exit of air during expiration. Postprocedure radiographs should be obtained to confirm placement, drainage of air and blood, and reexpansion of lung. Prophylactic antibiotics with chest tube insertion do not reduce the risk for empyema or pneumonia.[15]

Operating room thoracotomy is indicated for patients with massive hemothorax (initial drainage of 1.5 to 2 L of blood), persistent bleeding of more than 200 mL/hr for 4 hours, and persistent hypotension or instability despite blood replacement. Autotransfusion should be performed in patients with massive hemothorax or persistent significant bleeding. It is prudent to prepare for autotransfusion early because most blood loss occurs at the time of initial chest tube insertion.

## FOLLOW-UP, NEXT STEPS IN CARE, AND PATIENT EDUCATION

Traumatic pneumothorax and hemothorax generally require tube thoracostomy. The exception is a small stable pneumothorax in an otherwise healthy and symptom-free patient, which may be managed with observation.

Occult traumatic pneumothorax detected on a CT scan requires only close observation for respiratory distress, progression, and the development of complications. Tube thoracostomy must be immediately available but is not required even with positive pressure ventilation.[16] Any prolonged surgery, diagnostic testing, or transport preventing immediate tube thoracostomy requires prophylactic placement.

In patients with penetrating injuries and a negative initial chest radiograph, upright PA and lateral chest radiographs should be repeated in 3 to 4 hours.[17] Patients with normal findings on repeated radiographs and no significant associated injuries are discharged with wound care and follow-up instructions. Patients with asymptomatic blunt chest trauma and normal findings on the initial chest radiographs do not require repeated films before discharge. All patients with chest tubes are admitted to the trauma, cardiothoracic, or general surgery service in the care of personnel experienced in managing chest tube equipment.

## PULMONARY CONTUSION

Pulmonary contusion is the most common parenchymal lung injury in victims of blunt chest trauma. Though typically described in the setting of flail chest, pulmonary contusion can occur with less significant chest wall fractures and occasionally even in the absence of overlying injury.

Pulmonary contusion occurs with blunt, blast, or high-energy penetrating injuries. MVCs and falls are the most commonly reported mechanisms. Injury to the lung-parenchyma causes hemorrhage and edema of the alveoli and interstitium, which results in ventilation-perfusion mismatching and ultimately hypoxia and hypercapnia. Hemorrhage worsens over the first 24 to 48 hours and then typically resolves over the next 7 days. Acute respiratory distress syndrome and pneumonia are the most frequent complications, both with significant morbidity and mortality.

## PRESENTING SIGNS AND SYMPTOMS

Patients with pulmonary contusion typically have significant chest wall injury accompanied by dyspnea and tachypnea and progressing to hemoptysis, cyanosis, and hypotension. Inspection often reveals an obvious flail chest or ecchymosis overlying rib fractures. Auscultation reveals rhonchi, wheezes, rales, or minimal breath sounds. Blast injuries may result in significant pulmonary contusion with minimal chest wall injury. Delayed manifestations of pulmonary contusion can occur in initially well-appearing patients. Because the hemorrhage and edema will worsen, patients with even mild initial symptoms must be observed closely with continuous monitoring. The clinical findings usually progress over the initial hours through the first 2 days.

## DIFFERENTIAL DIAGNOSIS AND MEDICAL DECISION MAKING

The differential diagnosis in a trauma patient with respiratory distress and infiltrates on initial chest radiographs includes pulmonary contusion, congestive heart failure, aspiration pneumonia, and acute respiratory distress syndrome. Symptomatic congestive heart failure may predispose patients to blunt trauma, result from blunt myocardial injury, or develop during fluid resuscitation. Aspiration pneumonia leads to

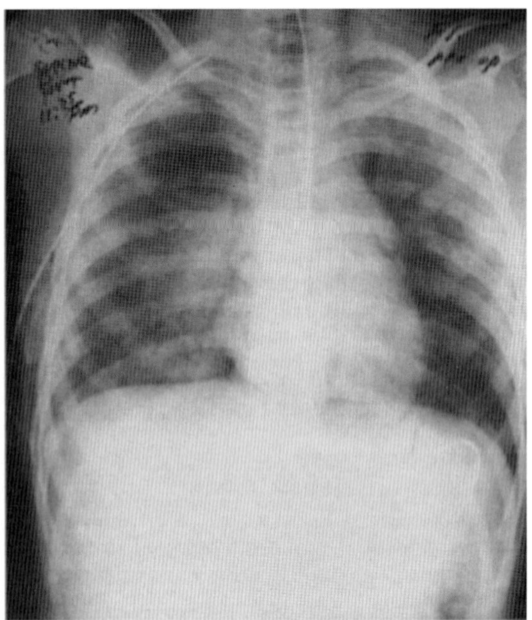

**Fig. 78.4 Chest radiograph showing right pulmonary contusion with pneumomediastinum and pneumopericardium.** (From Marx J, Hockberger R, Walls R, editors. Rosen's emergency medicine: concepts and clinical practice. 6th ed. St. Louis: Mosby; 2006.)

lobar opacification. Acute respiratory distress syndrome typically occurs 24 to 48 hours after the injury, often with diffuse bilateral infiltrates and a normal heart size.

The patchy or diffuse air space opacification above the site of injury with pulmonary contusion is often present on the initial chest radiograph and typically progresses over the first 6 hours (**Fig. 78.4**). Initial CT scanning is more sensitive than chest radiography but seldom changes the initial management of pulmonary contusion. Pulse oximetry is essential to detect early clinical deterioration.

## TREATMENT

Prophylactic intubation is not recommended for patients with minimal symptoms. Indications for intubation in adult patients with pulmonary contusion include airway compromise, moderate to severe respiratory distress, hypoxia, hypercapnia, and the need for general anesthesia, as well as to facilitate the care of other injuries.

## FOLLOW-UP, NEXT STEPS IN CARE, AND PATIENT EDUCATION

Patients with pulmonary contusion require admission to the intensive care unit for oxygen administration, chest physical therapy, incentive spirometry, suctioning, analgesia, and close monitoring. Overhydration must be avoided to prevent iatrogenic worsening of capillary leak and lung function. Prophylactic steroids and antibiotics are not recommended.[18] Isolated pulmonary contusions typically resolve within 14 days without long-term complications. Disability and mortality rates are higher in patients with larger areas of contusion, flail chest, acute respiratory distress syndrome, and pneumonia.

## TRACHEOBRONCHIAL INJURY

Tracheobronchial injuries are infrequent but present unique challenges to the emergency physician (EP). Emergency airway management is often both required and complicated by these devastating injuries.

Penetrating tracheobronchial injuries are more common than blunt injuries. Penetrating injuries to the relatively exposed cervical trachea occur more frequently than injuries to the protected thoracic trachea. Gunshot wounds involving the thoracic trachea occur more often than stab wounds. Blunt injuries to the cervical trachea occur with rapid deceleration and result in shear stress at the junction of the larynx and trachea; examples of these types of injury include hyperextension injury, direct dashboard strikes, and "clothesline" injuries in snowmobile and motorcycle accidents.

Blunt injuries to the thoracic trachea are typically caused by high-energy MVCs, crush injuries, and falls. Rapid deceleration produces a shearing force with injury typically within 2 cm of the fixed carina. Injuries to the esophagus and spine are the most common associated injuries. Head, vascular, nerve, and intrathoracic injuries also occur frequently with both blunt and penetrating tracheobronchial injuries (**Box 78.1**).

## PRESENTING SIGNS AND SYMPTOMS

Patients with tracheobronchial injuries typically have dramatic but nonspecific symptoms, including hoarseness, dysphagia, hemoptysis, and dyspnea. Careful inspection for penetrating wounds should be made, and the trajectory and proximity of the injury to the trachea should be estimated. Findings on physical examination include escape of air from wounds, subcutaneous emphysema in the neck and supraclavicular region, hypoxia, stridor, pneumothorax, and pneumomediastinum. Patients with blunt trauma often have few signs of external injury. Persistent air leaks despite a functioning chest tube suggest tracheobronchial injury. Rarely, patients with tracheobronchial injuries without communication with the pleural space maintain respiration with minimal symptoms until granulation tissue obstructs the airway and results in delayed lobar atelectasis.

## DIFFERENTIAL DIAGNOSIS AND MEDICAL DECISION MAKING

Chest radiographs may have subtle evidence of tracheobronchial injuries such as high rib fractures, the fallen lung sign, pneumomediastinum, deep cervical emphysema, peribronchial air, abnormal location of the endotracheal tube, and a spherical shape of the normally oval endotracheal tube balloon. The fallen lung sign occurs when the apical segments of the lung have collapsed and fallen to the level of the hilum. Flexible fiberoptic bronchoscopy usually confirms the injury. Helical CT angiography is particularly effective in diagnosing blunt laryngeal injury and often provides additional informa-

**BOX 78.1 Approach to Thoracic Trauma***

**Blunt Trauma**

High-energy mechanisms: Falls greater than 3 m or motor vehicle collisions at more than 30 mph

All injuries: CXR and pulse oximetry. If pneumothorax or hemothorax, insert a chest tube

Traumatic aortic injury: A mechanism with chest wall tenderness or abnormal CXR evidence requires helical CT angiography; if negative, evaluate for traumatic aortic injury; if findings indeterminate, obtain an aortogram; if positive, transfer the patient to the operating room

Blunt cardiac injury: With abnormal ECG, hypotension, or dysrhythmia, cardiac monitoring and hospitalization for 24 hours with repeated ECGs every 8 hours; with hypotension or symptomatic dysrhythmia, formal echocardiography

**Penetrating Injuries**

All injuries: Continuous pulse oximetry and PA and lateral CXR at 0 and 6 hours

Anterior cardiac box: FAST examination to evaluate for pericardial fluid

Posterior box and transmediastinal gunshot wounds: Angiography for great-vessel injury; with signs and symptoms of injury, esophagography or esophagoscopy and bronchoscopy

Posterior box stab wounds: If abnormal mediastinum on CXR, angiography for great-vessel injury; with signs and symptoms of injury, esophagography or esophagoscopy and bronchoscopy

Thoracoabdominal: DPL with a red blood cell count of 10,000 cells/μL, laparoscopy/thoracoscopy or laparotomy to evaluate for diaphragmatic injury

*CT*, Computed tomography; *CXR*, chest radiograph; *DPL*, diagnostic peritoneal lavage; *ECG*, electrocardiogram; *FAST*, focused assessment with sonography for trauma; *PA*, posteroanterior.

*Protocols and approach may vary depending on institutional experience and availability.

tion in the evaluation of penetrating thoracic and tracheobronchial injuries.

## TREATMENT

Patients with tracheobronchial injuries who are in respiratory distress require immediate intubation and mechanical ventilation. Fiberoptic bronchoscopy is the best diagnostic and management option for patients with cervical and intrathoracic tracheal injuries. When not available and immediate airway intervention is required, some authorities recommend orotracheal intubation without paralysis to prevent loss of paratracheal muscle support of the injured trachea. The benefits must be weighed against the suboptimal intubating conditions in a nonparalyzed patient. If paralysis is required, prior preparation for a surgical airway and right-sided thoracotomy is necessary.

During orotracheal intubation, a smaller-size endotracheal tube should be inserted and placed past the injury if possible. To prevent worsening of the injury, force should be avoided during placement of the endotracheal tube. When orotracheal intubation is not possible, the endotracheal tube should be placed through the anterior neck wound into the trachea. The EP must be careful to avoid pushing a transected trachea deeper into the thorax. In patients with complete transection and retraction of the trachea, major intervention is required. A right-sided thoracotomy should be performed (to avoid the aortic arch on the left), and the EP should attempt to visualize the injured trachea, support it, and establish an airway. Extension to a left-sided thoracotomy may be needed for complex distal injuries.[19] Tube thoracostomy is required, often with multiple tubes to drain the resulting pneumothorax and reexpand the affected lung.

## FOLLOW-UP, NEXT STEPS IN CARE, AND PATIENT EDUCATION

Stable patients with tracheobronchial injuries and a maintained airway are best transported to the operating room immediately for fiberoptic bronchoscopy, intubation, and possible thoracotomy. Definitive surgical repair is necessary to prevent acute and late complications. Acute complications include persistent air leak, pneumothorax, empyema, and mediastinitis. Delayed complications include granulation of partial injuries with resultant atelectasis and significant loss of pulmonary function. Penetrating and blunt injuries are typically managed early by exploration and repair.

## BLUNT CARDIAC INJURY

The pathologic spectrum of blunt cardiac injury begins with cardiac concussion; includes myocardial contusion, coronary artery injury, and valve and septal injury; and ends with myocardial rupture. Myocardial contusion remains the most common clinical challenge to the EP. A definitive diagnosis can be made only at autopsy, and complications are rare but life-threatening.

Blunt cardiac injury typically results from MVCs but may occur after falls, crush injuries, blast injuries, direct blows, and chest compression. Low-speed deceleration injuries occasionally result in significant injury. Proposed mechanisms include compression of the heart between the sternum and vertebral bodies and sudden striking of the heart against the sternum in deceleration injuries.

Cardiac concussion, or commotio cordis, occurs when a blow to the chest briefly "stuns" the heart; it results in dysrhythmia, hypotension, syncope, and often sudden death but without permanent cellular damage. Commotio cordis may result from an anterior chest wall impact at a moment when the myocardium is refractory to depolarization and can result in fatal arrhythmia, also known as the R-on-T phenomenon.[20]

Myocardial contusion occurs when injury to the anterior wall, formed by the right ventricle, results in well-defined areas of red blood cell extravasation and eventually in subendocardial and transmural necrosis. Infrequent delayed complications include mural thrombus, pericardial effusions, constrictive pericarditis, and ventricular aneurysms. Direct injury to already atherosclerotic coronary arteries or severely contused myocardium can result in myocardial infarction. The rare blunt cardiac rupture is typically immediately fatal except when limited to the low-pressure right side of the heart or to small, self-sealing ventricular injuries.

## PRESENTING SIGNS AND SYMPTOMS

Blunt cardiac injury typically occurs in patients with multiple blunt trauma injuries. Patients with commotio cordis generally experience immediate dysrhythmia and loss of consciousness. Though usually fatal, the survival rate is increasing as a result of increased public awareness, immediate cardiopulmonary resuscitation, and increased availability of automatic external defibrillators.[21]

Patients with myocardial contusion typically complain of angina-type chest pain unrelieved by nitroglycerin, pleuritic pain, or pain from associated injuries. Evidence of external trauma is usually but not always present. Information about the scene of the injury often provides the only evidence of blunt cardiac injury.

Initial and vital sign trends should be carefully noted, including mental status, color, jugular venous distention, and the presence of chest wall ecchymosis or tenderness, gallop rhythms, and friction rubs. Persistent unexplained tachycardia, hypotension, or dysrhythmia suggests blunt cardiac injury. Patients with valve dysfunction typically have a loud murmur, acute heart failure, and jugular venous distention. The rare patient with cardiac rupture who survives to arrive at the ED generally exhibits signs of cardiac tamponade or overt cardiogenic shock.

## DIFFERENTIAL DIAGNOSIS AND MEDICAL DECISION MAKING

An ECG should be recorded in all patients with suspected blunt cardiac injury. Traditionally, stable patients with normal results on the initial ECG were considered to be at low risk for complications and safe for discharge. However, more recent literature suggests that patents may still be at risk for complications of blunt cardiac injury, including lethal dysrhythmias up to 12 hours after trauma and non–life-threatening dysrhythmias up to 72 hours later.[22] New findings on the ECG suggestive of myocardial contusion include unexplained tachycardia, ST- and T-wave changes, conduction abnormalities, and dysrhythmias.

Evaluation of cardiac markers is not routinely indicated in patients with blunt cardiac injury. The exception is serial troponin I measurement in patients with an ischemic pattern on the initial ECG and in patients in whom cardiac ischemia may have precipitated the trauma. However, a recent metaanalysis supports the use of troponin I as a sensitive test for myocardial contusion when determined at admission and 4 to 6 hours later.[23]

Emergency bedside echocardiography is recommended for unstable patients with suspected blunt cardiac injury or with evidence of myocardial infarction on the ECG. Pericardial effusions are easily identified on the initial subxiphoid view of the FAST scan. Formal echocardiography with parasternal and apical views will better identify small effusions, valve dysfunction, and wall motion abnormalities. Transesophageal echocardiography is more sensitive than transthoracic echocardiography and provides additional imaging of the aorta in unstable patients. Routine echocardiography does not predict complications in stable patients with suspected blunt cardiac injury.

## TREATMENT

Unstable patients with blunt cardiac injury require definitive airway control to ensure optimal oxygenation and ventilation. A large-bore internal jugular catheter should be inserted for fluid resuscitation, monitoring of central venous pressure, and placement of a Swan-Ganz catheter. Cardiogenic shock secondary to myocardial contusion or cardiac rupture typically requires careful fluid replacement and inotropic support. Refractory cases may require temporary stabilization with an aortic balloon pump after an aortic injury has been ruled out. Cardiac catheterization is necessary in patients with myocardial infarction because antithrombotic therapy is contraindicated after trauma.

## FOLLOW-UP, NEXT STEPS IN CARE, AND PATIENT EDUCATION

Stable patients with a normal initial ECG and without significant associated injuries can be safely discharged from the ED. Stable patients with changes on the ECG suggestive of myocardial contusion require observation with continuous monitoring for 24 hours and electrocardiography repeated every 8 hours for 24 hours. Brief dysrhythmias seldom require treatment, and prophylactic antidysrhythmic therapy is not indicated.

Unstable patients with ventricular dysrhythmias, atrial fibrillation, sinus bradycardia, and bundle branch block require intensive care unit admission. In patients with abnormal findings on the initial ECG, the complication rate is low, with complications predominantly occurring in older patients with multiple injuries. Wall motion abnormalities and rhythm disturbances typically resolve within hours. Most patients with myocardial contusion require only supportive care and aggressive management of complicating injuries. Morbidity and mortality are directly related to the presence of other injuries.

# PENETRATING CARDIAC INJURY, CARDIAC TAMPONADE, AND EMERGENCY DEPARTMENT THORACOTOMY

Penetrating cardiac injuries most commonly result from gunshot wounds, followed by stab wounds. Any gunshot wound involving the torso can result in penetrating cardiac injury. Survival is better in patients with stab wounds, single-chamber involvement, and low-pressure right heart injuries.

Cardiac tamponade most commonly results from stab wounds to the chest or upper part of the abdomen, followed by gunshot wounds and infrequently by blunt chest trauma.

Penetrating injuries to the heart result in either death at the scene or tamponade, which allows transport to the ED. Tamponade is more likely to occur with smaller injuries from stab wounds. The tough fibrous sac surrounding the heart prevents immediate exsanguination. As blood accumulates, cardiac filling and eventually output are impaired, which often results in rapid decompensation after arrival at the ED. Acutely accumulated pericardial blood may be difficult to visualize on cardiac ultrasonography. The right ventricle is the most commonly injured structure, followed by the left ventricle. Approximately three of four patients will die of the injury.

## PRESENTING SIGNS AND SYMPTOMS

Patients with pericardial tamponade classically but uncommonly exhibit the Beck triad of hypotension, jugular venous distention, and muffled heart sounds. Most patients will have at least one of these signs, with all three appearing only briefly before cardiac arrest. More frequently, patients either appear relatively stable or are in extremis. Stable-appearing patients have small wounds in the pericardium that allow intermittent decompression of the accumulated blood. Patients with more rapid accumulation are panic-stricken, appear to be in severe respiratory distress, and often have needle thoracostomy performed for presumed tension pneumothorax. In these patients, agitation, tachycardia, and hypotension predominate before progressing to obtundation, bradycardia, and pulseless electrical activity.

## DIFFERENTIAL DIAGNOSIS AND MEDICAL DECISION MAKING

An ultrasonographic subxiphoid view (**Fig. 78.5**) may detect pericardial fluid in patients with suspected cardiac injury. Pericardial fluid with diastolic collapse of the right atrium and ventricle is diagnostic of pericardial tamponade. Any pericardial effusion in unstable trauma patients with equal bilateral breath sounds signals tamponade requiring immediate operative intervention. Although the sensitivity of FAST scans approaches 100% for hemopericardium, false-negative results may occur when blood drains rapidly into the thorax. The possibility should be considered in patients with small anterior stab wounds and persistent left hemothorax despite tube thoracostomy.[24]

An initial ECG should be obtained to evaluate for findings suggestive of pericardial tamponade and other cardiac injury. Electrical alternans, low voltage, and PR-segment depression are specific but not sensitive for the diagnosis of pericardial effusion. A chronic pericardial effusion is more likely to reveal such findings. Acute traumatic pericardial effusion resulting in tamponade does not change the size of the heart on the chest radiograph. However, a chest radiograph can be useful in identifying other injuries and the presence of retained foreign bodies. It is important to remember that normal findings on the ECG and chest radiograph do not rule out traumatic pericardial effusion or tamponade.

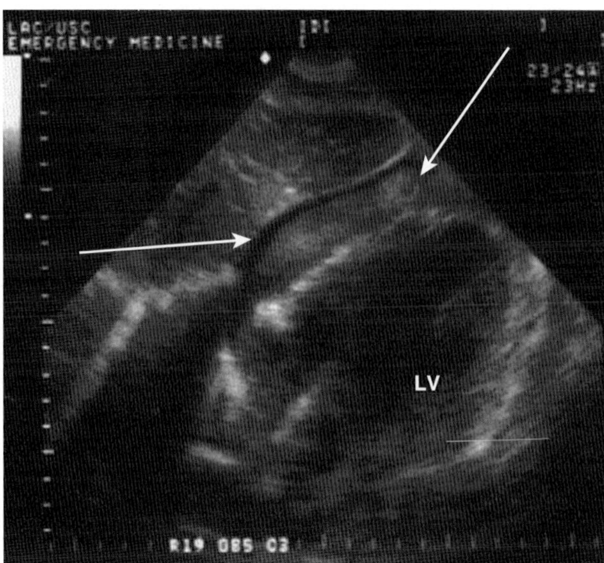


**Fig. 78.5 Subxiphoid view of a focused assessment with sonography for trauma scan showing traumatic hemopericardium *(arrows)*.** *LV*, Left ventricle. (From Mandavia DP, Joseph A. Bedside echo in chest trauma. Emerg Med Clin North Am 2004;22:601-19.)

## TREATMENT

A central venous line should be placed for volume infusion and monitoring of central venous pressure. The injured hemithorax is preferred for central line placement to avoid iatrogenic complications in the uninjured side. The exception is a patient with obvious injury to the clavicle and suspected injury to the subclavian vein.

Aggressive fluid resuscitation is mandatory for patients with suspected pericardial tamponade to maximize cardiac filling pressure and cardiac output. Elevated central venous pressure in persistently hypotensive and tachycardic trauma patients suggests impending tamponade. Pericardiocentesis with catheter placement should be performed in patients with deteriorating vital signs. Pericardiocentesis may serve as a diagnostic and temporizing measure but is never a replacement for thoracotomy and definitive repair of the injury. Ultrasonography or ECG-guided pericardiocentesis is preferred, if available. Nonclotting blood traditionally signifies pericardial blood, but aspiration may be unsuccessful because of needle placement, continuous brisk pericardial bleeding, or other reasons. However, removal of even a small amount of pericardial blood can restore vital signs and aid survival until surgical intervention is available.

Thoracotomy is reserved for patients with cardiac tamponade who are in cardiac arrest or impending arrest. The likelihood of functional survival after ED thoracotomy is greatest for victims of stab wounds with isolated cardiac injury who have signs of life on ED arrival. At the trauma center, thoracotomy is performed on victims of penetrating trauma who experienced cardiac arrest in the ED or within 10 minutes of arrival at the ED and on blunt trauma patients who experienced cardiac arrest in the ED. In the ED without surgical support, thoracotomy is best performed by a skilled EP only on patients with thoracic stab wounds or isolated gunshot

**Table 78.2** Indications for ED Thoracotomy

| SETTING | PENETRATING INJURIES | BLUNT TRAUMA |
|---|---|---|
| Trauma center | Cardiac arrest in the ED or within 10 min of ED arrival | Cardiac arrest in the ED |
| Community ED without emergency surgical backup | Patients with thoracic stab wounds or isolated gunshot wounds who lose signs of life in the ED or within 10 min of ED arrival | All other ED thoracotomies should be performed only when a surgeon is available within 10 min |

*ED*, Emergency department.

wounds who lost signs of life in the ED or within 10 minutes of arrival in the ED. In all other cases, ED thoracotomy should be performed only if a qualified surgeon is present or immediately available (**Table 78.2**).[25-28]

## FOLLOW-UP, NEXT STEPS IN CARE, AND PATIENT EDUCATION

Immediate operative repair is indicated for all penetrating injuries of the heart to relieve tamponade and repair the initial injury. Identification and initial management of all associated injuries ensure optimal outcomes, but operative intervention must not be delayed. Diagnostic peritoneal lavage should be performed in the operating room to identify intraperitoneal bleeding and assess the need for laparotomy.

# GREAT VESSEL INJURY

Great vessel injury is a significant cause of morbidity and mortality with both blunt and penetrating thoracic trauma. Traumatic aortic injury is the second most common cause of blunt traumatic death. Eighty percent of victims of traumatic aortic injury die immediately. The majority of survivors can be saved with prompt ED diagnosis, blood pressure control, and operative repair. Five percent of patients will be unstable on arrival and have a mortality rate of up to 98%. The remaining 15% will be hemodynamically stable, which often contributes to a delay in diagnosis and a mortality rate as high as 25%.[29]

The descending aorta is fixed within the thorax by the ligamentum arteriosum and the intercostal arteries. Sudden deceleration causes the aortic arch to swing forward and produces a shearing force with resultant injury just distal to the takeoff of the left subclavian artery. Traditionally, traumatic aortic injuries have been considered only in patients with "major mechanisms of injury," including high-speed MVCs with frontal or side impact and motorcycle crashes. However, the injury has been reported with less impressive mechanisms such as pedestrian-versus-auto collisions, falls, and crush injuries. Use of restraint systems does not protect persons from traumatic aortic injuries.[30,31] Penetrating injuries to the great vessels typically result from both gunshot penetration and stabbing.

## PRESENTING SIGNS AND SYMPTOMS

Signs and symptoms of traumatic aortic injury are often not present or are masked by other injuries. Up to one half of all patients have no signs of chest wall injury. Common signs and symptoms include interscapular or retrosternal pain, decreased blood pressure in the left arm, upper extremity hypertension with absent femoral pulses, bruit, and a harsh systolic murmur heard over the precordium or interscapular area. Uncommon findings include extremity pain from distal ischemia, dysphagia from concomitant esophageal injury, and hoarseness as a result of compression of the laryngeal nerve.

Evidence of penetrating injury to the great vessels depends on the mechanism and location of the injury. High-energy proximal arterial injury typically results in immediate exsanguination or hemorrhagic shock with massive hemothorax. Contained mediastinal hematoma can occasionally impair superior vena cava return and produce engorgement of the soft tissues of the neck, face, and airway. Distal injuries may result in diminished pulses, expanding hematomas, and limb ischemia. Careful palpation for pulse symmetry and measurement of blood pressure in both arms are advisable.

Stab wounds should be inspected carefully to help determine the general trajectory. Deep probing of wounds should be avoided to prevent iatrogenic worsening of the initial injury, dislodgment of clot and massive hemorrhage, and infection. Chest tube output should be closely monitored. The chest tube should be clamped when the patient is being transported to the operating room; when massive hemothorax and heavy, continuous bleeding are present, temporary tamponade within the pleural cavity may be required for this short time.

## DIFFERENTIAL DIAGNOSIS AND MEDICAL DECISION MAKING

The initial chest radiograph should show evidence of traumatic aortic injury (**Fig. 78.6, *A***). The most sensitive criterion is mediastinal widening, usually larger than 8 cm on an AP view; however, a subjective interpretation of mediastinal widening is more reliable. Other mediastinal abnormalities suggesting mediastinal hematoma secondary to traumatic aortic injury are an obscured aortic knob, loss of the AP window, a displaced nasogastric tube, widened paratracheal stripe, widened paraspinal interface, depression of the left mainstem bronchus, left hemothorax, left apical pleural cap, deviation of the trachea to the right, and multiple rib fractures. The more abnormalities seen on the chest radiograph, the higher the sensitivity in identifying an aortic injury. A normal chest radiograph, however, does not rule out a traumatic aortic injury.

With sensitivity near 100%, a normal CT scan rules out traumatic aortic injury.[32] If the results are indeterminate, aortography should be performed. Rarely, a positive helical CT angiogram in a stable patient is followed by aortography for further localization of the injury and identification of other injuries, such as a pseudoaneurysm (see Fig. 78.6, *B*). Advantages of helical CT angiography over aortography are that it is faster, is noninvasive, requires a smaller volume of contrast agent, and provides information about other thoracic injuries. A high index of suspicion and low threshold for performing screening helical CT angiography are required

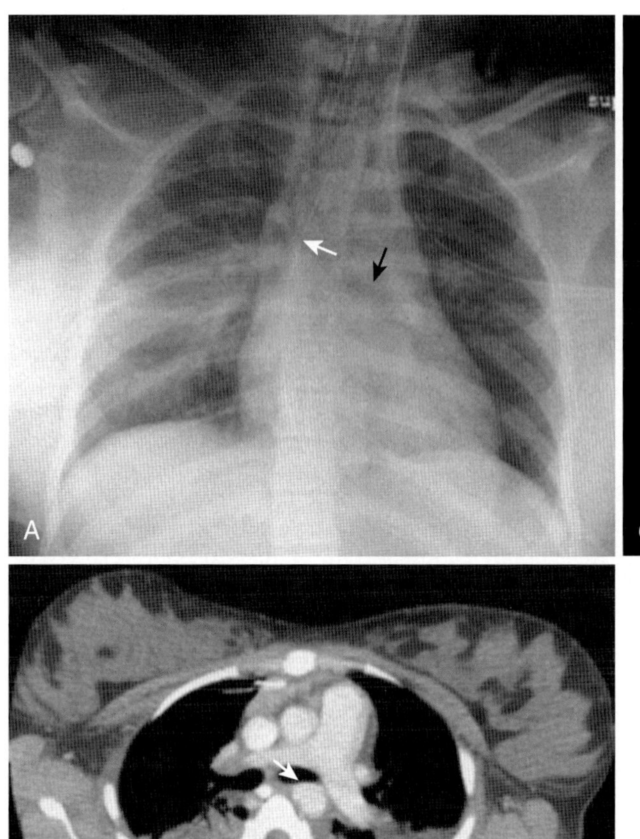


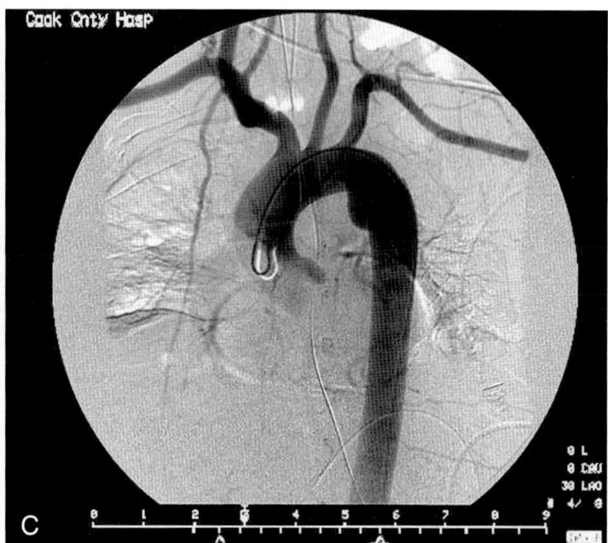


**Fig. 78.6 Chest radiographs showing traumatic aortic injury. A,** Widened mediastinum, loss of mediastinal contours, depression of the left mainstem bronchus *(black arrow)*, and deviation of the nasogastric tube *(white arrow)*. **B,** Traumatic pseudoaneurysm in the proximal descending aorta *(arrow)*. **C,** Traumatic pseudoaneurysm seen on an aortogram. (**B,** From Westra SJ, Wallace EC. Imaging of pediatric chest trauma. Radiol Clin North Am 2005;43:267-81; **C,** image courtesy Scott Sherman, MD.)

to save patients with traumatic aortic injury who survive to arrive at the ED.

Transesophageal echocardiography should be performed in unstable patients with suspected traumatic aortic injury but is contraindicated in patients with esophageal injuries. Very high sensitivity and specificity approaching 100% have been reported, but it varies widely depending on operator experience.

Aortography remains the "gold standard" for the diagnosis of traumatic aortic injury. False-positive and false-negative results are rare but do occur. Better sensitivity with helical CT angiography has been reported. Aortography offers improved localization of injury before surgical repair. Newer techniques such as intravenous digital subtraction angiography have improved the speed while reducing the cost of aortography (see Fig. 78.6, *C*).

A chest radiograph should be obtained in all patients with suspected penetrating great vessel injury, and all wounds should be noted and marked. The examination should be focused specifically on evidence of mediastinal hematoma, hemothorax, foreign bodies near vessels or in the trajectory of a missile, "fuzzy" missiles created by arterial pulsations, and the absence of a missile in patients with a gunshot wound to the chest, which suggests distal embolization. An angiogram should be obtained to further assess the injuries and plan an operative approach in the rare stable patient. With the added benefit of evaluating nearby structures, helical CT angiography will probably replace aortography in the evaluation of stable patients with transmediastinal penetrating injury.[33]

## TREATMENT

Early orotracheal intubation is required because hematoma expansion can make both orotracheal intubation and creation of a surgical airway impossible. Tracheostomy is contraindicated in patients with great vessel injury involving the upper mediastinum or zone I of the neck because major bleeding can result.

Patients with penetrating great vessel injuries often require ED thoracotomy or immediate thoracotomy in the operating room. In patients with penetrating wounds involving the subclavian vessels, traditional left lateral thoracotomy will often not provide adequate exposure.

Before operative repair of traumatic aortic injury, blood pressure must be controlled, with systolic pressure maintained at 100 to 120 mm Hg to decrease shear stress and progression of the injury. Patients with isolated aortic injuries may be hypertensive and will require short acting titratable agents such as nitroprusside and esmolol.

## FOLLOW-UP, NEXT STEPS IN CARE, AND PATIENT EDUCATION

Surgical repair of traumatic aortic injury is performed after stabilization of other life-threatening intracranial or intraabdominal injuries. Delayed surgical repair is frequently indicated in elderly patients with multiple comorbid conditions. The mortality rate during surgery is approximately 10%, and such mortality is primarily related to the extent of the injury and condition of the patient.

## ESOPHAGEAL INJURY

Esophageal injuries occur infrequently with both blunt and penetrating trauma. More immediate life-threatening injuries often mask the clinical findings, and esophageal leakage can progress to fatal mediastinitis. Esophageal evaluation is indicated in patients with a significant penetrating injury to the neck. The majority of esophageal perforations result from medical endoscopic procedures, not from traumatic injuries.

Penetrating esophageal injury must be considered in any patient with injury near or trajectory through the esophagus. Common mechanisms of penetrating injury include laceration, missile penetration, iatrogenic perforation, and ingested foreign body. Stab wounds to the neck often directly injure the esophagus. High-velocity gunshots result in direct esophageal perforation, as well as delayed necrosis. The majority of penetrating injuries occur at the proximal or distal end of the esophagus during routine endoscopy.

Blunt esophageal injuries are much less common than penetrating injuries. Common mechanisms include crush injuries to the cervical esophagus and barotrauma. Blunt laryngotracheal trauma and cervical spine fractures are associated with injuries to the upper part of the esophagus. Blunt injuries to the lower third of the esophagus occur with sudden increases in intraabdominal pressure against a closed upper esophageal sphincter, analogous to Boerhaave syndrome. The initial rupture typically originates from an inherent weakness in the left posterior aspect of the distal end of the esophagus.

Both cardiopulmonary resuscitation and the Heimlich maneuver have been associated with perforation of the thoracic esophagus. Blast injury can result in primary esophageal injury as a result of the pressure wave, in secondary injury from impact of the patient against fixed structures, and in tertiary injury from blast projectiles.

### PRESENTING SIGNS AND SYMPTOMS

Typical symptoms of esophageal injury include pleuritic chest pain anywhere along the course of the esophagus, dyspnea, odynophagia, dysphagia, hoarseness, and pain with flexion or extension of the neck. The physical examination should include palpation for subcutaneous emphysema and auscultation for a systolic Hamman crunch produced by mediastinal air.

Commonly, patients have emergency life-threatening injuries that obscure the clinical findings, which can lead to delayed recognition and management. Fever, tachycardia, hypotension, and progressive dyspnea are noted as mediastinitis develops.

### DIFFERENTIAL DIAGNOSIS AND MEDICAL DECISION MAKING

AP or PA chest radiographs should be examined for evidence of mediastinal air, subcutaneous emphysema, left-sided pleural effusion, pneumothorax, and a widened mediastinum. A lateral neck radiograph may reveal prevertebral air displacing the tracheal air column forward. Early in the course of a perforation, radiographic evidence is often minimal. Later CT scans of the chest may demonstrate collections of air or fluid as infection develops, but CT scans are not usually performed for esophageal injury.

Esophagography and esophagoscopy should be performed in all patients with suspected esophageal injury, although neither modality alone is sensitive enough to rule out esophageal injury. The initial esophagography is done with Gastrografin to avoid mediastinal irritation from leakage of barium. Incidentally, a CT scan after barium ingestion may detect small esophageal perforations and small metallic foreign bodies better than plain radiographs can. Negative findings on an esophagogram with Gastrografin enhancement should be followed by the more sensitive barium-enhanced esophagography. Neither contrast agent prevents the use of endoscopy. If findings on both esophagograms are negative, flexible endoscopy can be used to exclude subtle injuries.

### TREATMENT

Chest tube drainage is often necessary for associated pneumothorax. Persistent air leak is suggestive of esophageal injury. Food particles in the chest tube confirm major injury. Patients should be kept on nothing-by-mouth status. Fluid resuscitation is mandatory. Broad-spectrum antibiotics that cover oral anaerobes should be administered. Placement of a nasogastric tube is controversial because of the risk for mediastinitis and should be done in consultation with trauma or general surgery services.

### FOLLOW-UP, NEXT STEPS IN CARE, AND PATIENT EDUCATION

Management can be operative or nonoperative. Small, minimally symptomatic or chronic perforations, particularly those involving the cervical esophagus secondary to instrumentation, are most amenable to a nonsurgical approach.[34] Consultation with trauma or general surgery specialists for primary surgical repair dramatically improves outcomes.

## DIAPHRAGMATIC INJURIES

Diaphragmatic injuries are a diagnostic challenge and are associated with significant delayed complications. Complications often develop weeks to years after the initial trauma and consist of symptoms of visceral herniation. Both blunt and penetrating trauma can cause diaphragmatic injuries, but with very different injury patterns. The most common mechanisms for blunt diaphragmatic injuries are MVCs and falls, followed by pedestrian-versus-vehicle collisions, motorcycle accidents, and crush injuries. Penetrating injuries result from gunshot or stab wounds. When detected initially, diaphragmatic injury signals that other severe injuries are probably present.

Gunshot and stab wounds result in injuries to the diaphragm with nearly equal incidence. Stab wounds with a trajectory reaching the 4th intercostal space superiorly or the 12th intercostal space inferiorly must be considered to have perforated the diaphragm and require prudent evaluation. Stab wounds outside this area may also penetrate the diaphragm, depending on the length and angle of the blade. Gunshot wounds anywhere in the neck, chest, abdomen, or pelvis can penetrate the diaphragm. Blunt force to the chest or abdomen often results in large tears in the diaphragm. Left-sided injuries are more common in survivors, whereas an equal incidence of right- and left-sided injuries is noted at autopsy. The negative pressure of inspiration prevents closure and promotes herniation through the wound into the chest cavity. If not detected initially, diaphragm injuries frequently result in visceral herniation months to years later.

## PRESENTING SIGNS AND SYMPTOMS

Three phases of injury have been described. The acute phase begins with the injury and ends with the initial recovery. A patient with acute diaphragmatic rupture will typically complain of chest pain, abdominal pain, and dyspnea. Findings on physical examination include diminished breath sounds in the lung bases, respiratory distress, bowel sounds in the chest, peritoneal signs, and palpation of viscera during chest tube placement. Large left-sided blunt injuries are more obvious than smaller penetrating and right-sided injuries. Acute diaphragmatic injuries are often overshadowed by other injuries. Frequently, no abdominal tenderness is noted.

In the second, or latent, phase, intermittent herniation of abdominal viscera results in mild and vague symptoms suggesting biliary, gastric, coronary artery, or pulmonary disease. Patients with latent manifestations often appear to have other gastrointestinal or cardiovascular diseases and complain of vague abdominal pain relieved when upright or cough and vague chest pain.

In the last, or obstructive, phase, incarceration, strangulation, and ischemia develop.[35] Additionally, the compressive effects of the intrathoracic bowel on the heart and lung can result in tension enterothorax or viscerothorax.[36] In this phase, symptoms of visceral obstruction, ischemia, and ultimately visceral infarction develop. Rarely, tension viscerothorax also develops. Herniation should be considered in any patient with vague complaints of chest or abdominal pain and a history of thoracoabdominal trauma.

## DIFFERENTIAL DIAGNOSIS AND MEDICAL DECISION MAKING

The initial chest radiograph should be inspected for the classic diagnostic finding, which is a nasogastric tube or viscera in the left hemithorax. Other important but more subtle signs include an indistinct or elevated left hemidiaphragm and left lower lobe atelectasis. Hemopneumothorax is present in 50% of patients with penetrating injury. Up to 25% of patients with penetrating diaphragmatic injuries have normal chest radiographic findings and no abdominal tenderness. CT scanning is 100% specific but only 66% sensitive for the diagnosis of blunt diaphragmatic injury.[37]

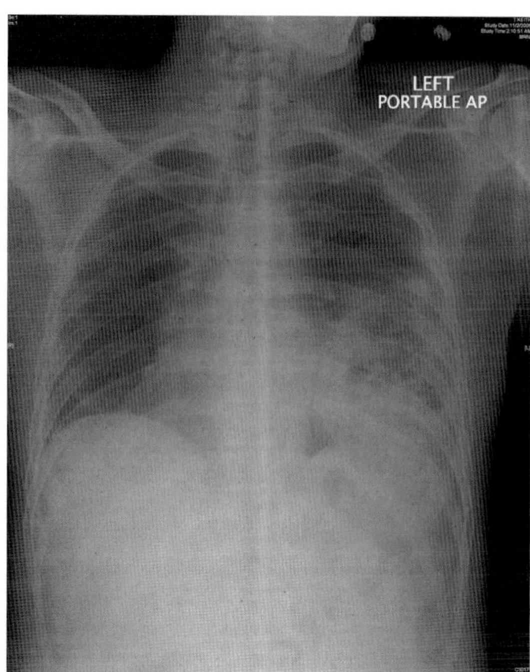


**Fig. 78.7 Chest radiograph showing obvious left-sided viscerothorax secondary to a stab wound in the diaphragm 3 years earlier.** (Image courtesy Dave Andreski, MD.)

In the latent phase of injury, the chest radiograph is typically abnormal. Findings can be subtle, such as a unilaterally elevated hemidiaphragm, unilateral pleural thickening, or basilar atelectasis, or can be significant, such as a shift of the mediastinum or viscera evident above the diaphragm. In cases of delayed herniation, upper or lower gastrointestinal contrast-enhanced studies may be needed to demonstrate herniation (**Fig. 78.7**).

FAST can also be used in the diagnosis of diaphragmatic rupture. The sonographic features of a ruptured diaphragm include nonvisualization of the spleen or heart, poor diaphragmatic movement, elevated diaphragm, liver sliding sign, pleural effusion, subphrenic effusion, or viscera visualized in the thorax.[38,39] Traditionally, a diagnostic peritoneal lavage count of less than 10,000 red blood cells/μL is used to rule out a diaphragmatic injury in patients with penetrating thoracoabdominal trauma. Lavage fluid draining from the chest tube is diagnostic. However, diagnostic peritoneal lavage misses up to 25% of diaphragmatic injuries because of bleeding into the chest. Laparoscopy or thoracoscopy is the diagnostic study of choice in patients with high clinical suspicion for diaphragmatic injury not otherwise needing surgery.

## TREATMENT

A nasogastric tube should be placed carefully in obstructed patients to avoid further trauma to a herniated gastroesophageal junction. In cases of tension viscerothorax, a chest tube should be placed into the thoracic cavity while taking care to avoid the viscera. The EP should palpate for viscera and diaphragmatic injuries before insertion of a chest tube.

## FOLLOW-UP, NEXT STEPS IN CARE, AND PATIENT EDUCATION

Consultation and admission to trauma or general surgery services is recommended for early surgical repair to prevent delayed complications. Patients with suspected diaphragmatic injuries typically have multiple injuries requiring treatment and hospitalization. An asymptomatic patient with a mechanism for diaphragmatic injury but a negative work-up should be instructed about the need for immediate evaluation if signs of delayed herniation and obstruction develop, such as abdominal discomfort, chest discomfort, shortness of breath, or vomiting.

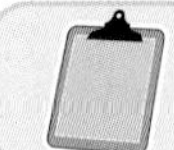

### DOCUMENTATION

Careful documentation helps ensure identification and evaluation of all significant injuries. The documentation chart should reflect the following thought processes and actions:

- Primary survey assessment and management
- Secondary survey findings: Use a figure or drawing of the patient to describe the injuries
- *Ample* history
- Initial laboratory and imaging findings
- Definitive testing
- Results of consultations
- Main assessment and plan: Patient, mechanism, and list of injuries with a plan for each.
- Tertiary survey or reassessment before discharge:
  - Follow-up provided
  - Patient education provided

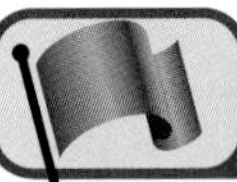

### RED FLAGS

**Subtle Life-Threatening Emergencies in the Secondary Survey**

**Traumatic Aortic Injury**

Patients may have no external sign of trauma. Never say "She looks too good to have a traumatic aortic injury," "It was only a lateral impact," or "He was wearing a belt and the airbag went off." The patient will look good until the aorta ruptures; with lateral impact in a moving vehicle collision, there may be increased risk for traumatic aortic injury, and restraints alone do not reduce the risk for traumatic aortic injury.

**Esophageal Injury**

For any injury near the esophagus, esophagography and esophagoscopy should be performed. Injuries are often subtle until fatal mediastinitis develops.

**Diaphragmatic Injury**

Penetrating injury anywhere near the diaphragm requires chest radiography, computed tomography, and in some cases, diagnostic peritoneal lavage.

**Tracheobronchial Injury**

Persistent air leaks despite a functioning chest tube indicate a tracheobronchial injury until proved otherwise. Bronchoscopy must be performed to prevent delayed infection, atelectasis, and loss of lung function.

**Liver and Splenic Injuries**

Three or more rib fractures or any fracture or tenderness of the sixth rib or below is an indication for abdominal computed tomography to rule out liver and splenic injury.

## SUGGESTED READINGS

EAST management of pulmonary contusion and flail chest practice guidelines 2006. Available at http://www.east.org/.

Eroglu A, Turkyilmaz A, Aydin Y, et al. Current management of esophageal perforation: 20 years experience. Dis Esophagus 2009;22:374-80.

Holmes JF, Ngyuen H, Jacoby RC, et al. Do all patients with left costal margin injuries require radiographic evaluation for intraabdominal injury? Ann Emerg Med 2005;46:232-6.

Practice management guidelines for emergency department thoracotomy: Working Group, Ad Hoc Subcommittee on Outcomes, American College of Surgeons–Committee on Trauma. J Am Coll Surg 2001;193:303-9.

Soreide E, Deakin CD. Pre–hospital fluid therapy in the critically injured patient—a clinical update. Injury 2005;36:1001-10.

## REFERENCES

***References can be found on Expert Consult @ www.expertconsult.com.***

# 79 Blunt Abdominal Trauma

*Carlo L. Rosen, Eric L. Legome, and Richard E. Wolfe*

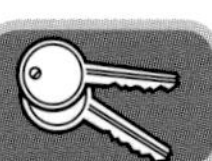

**KEY POINTS**

- Intraperitoneal bleeding is an immediately life-threatening injury after blunt trauma.
- Management of intraperitoneal bleeding takes priority over injuries to many other systems (**Box 79.1**).
- Physical examination is unreliable for predicting the presence or absence of injury except for certain high-risk findings such as the seat belt and Kehr signs.
- Bedside ultrasonography is an excellent initial screening tool that facilitates early triage of patients for either laparotomy or transfer to the radiology suite for computed tomography (CT).
- Helical CT provides excellent, accurate detail of intraperitoneal injuries. CT is highly sensitive for solid organ injuries but has lower sensitivity for detecting pancreatic, small bowel, and diaphragmatic injuries.
- Detailed CT images allow grading of organ injuries and nonoperative management of solid organ trauma in stable patients and the use of angiographic embolization in patients with liver, spleen, and renal injuries.
- Early detection of intraperitoneal injuries after blunt trauma and a team approach to management of these injuries significantly improve mortality rates.

## EPIDEMIOLOGY

In the United States, trauma is a serious health problem, both as a cause of mortality and as a significant financial burden.[1] In recent years, management of blunt abdominal trauma has started to change because of the high success rates of more conservative, nonoperative treatment. Such management is a safer, successful, and more cost-effective way to care for these patients and consequently has led to an increasingly selective approach to performing explorative laparotomy.

Abdominal injuries occur in approximately 1% of all trauma patients.[2] Blunt trauma is far more common than penetrating trauma in the United States and is associated with greater mortality because of multiple related injuries and greater diagnostic and therapeutic challenges. The mechanism of blunt trauma may range from high-speed injuries to minor falls or direct blows to the abdomen. Motor vehicle collisions are responsible for approximately 75%, blows to the abdomen for approximately 15%, and falls for approximately 9% of injuries.[3] Evaluation is further complicated by extraabdominal injuries, as well as by altered mental status from head trauma, alcohol intoxication, or recreational drugs.

## PATHOPHYSIOLOGY

Blunt trauma leads to injury when the elastic limit or breaking point of an organ is exceeded by the impact force applied. Impact force is defined by the amount of energy involved (e.g., the speed of a vehicle, the height of a fall), the location and surface of the blow to the body, and the duration of the impact. Understanding the mechanism of injury is imperative for assessing the initial risk and subsequent evaluation.

The risk for injury may vary slightly according to predisposing factors such as age and gender. Because men are more commonly engaged in dangerous activities, they are more frequently injured than women. A gravid uterus in a pregnant woman may offer some degree of protection to the intraperitoneal structures but adds the unique threat of placental abruption or uterine rupture.

A child's abdomen is less well protected than an adult's because of the thinner musculature, and it is far easier to injure abdominal organs such as the duodenum via compression against the posterior vertebrae. The elastic pediatric rib cage also provides less protection to the spleen and liver.

The risk for specific organ injury is linked to its structure and size. In particular, injuries to the spleen are far more common than injuries to other abdominal organs because of its poor elasticity. This is particularly true of abnormal spleens (e.g., patients with mononucleosis); such spleens are injured with far less force because of their larger size, which favors a greater mass effect, and because of their thinner capsule, which lacerates more easily. A spleen can be injured by a minor mechanism such as falling over a chair.

Blunt trauma can lead to injury to any abdominal structure. Direct, focused blows to the epigastrium may result in contusions and even perforation of the duodenum, as well as pancreatic injuries. Deceleration injuries may cause vascular sheering and subsequent thrombosis or tears of the renal artery (grade IV renal injury).

**BOX 79.1 Management of Intraperitoneal Injuries**

Intraperitoneal bleeding is an immediately life-threatening injury after blunt trauma, and management of intraperitoneal bleeding takes priority over injuries to other systems.

Physical examination is unreliable in predicting the presence or absence of injury except for certain high-risk findings such as the seat belt and Kehr signs.

Bedside ultrasonography is an excellent initial screening tool that facilitates early triage of patients to either laparotomy or the radiology suite for computed tomography (CT).

CT is highly sensitive for detecting solid organ injuries but has lower sensitivity for detecting pancreatic, small bowel, and diaphragmatic injuries.

Detailed CT allows grading of organ injuries and nonoperative management of solid organ trauma in stable patients and the use of angiographic embolization in patients with liver, spleen, and renal injuries.

## ANATOMY

The abdominal compartment is bounded by the diaphragm, pelvis, and abdominal wall. The boundaries include the vertebral column and the muscles of the abdomen, the most important being the external oblique and rectus. The rib cage below the fourth intercostal space is considered part of the abdominal wall, and thus the abdominal compartment extends up into the chest.

The abdominal compartment is subdivided by the peritoneum into an anterior intraperitoneal cavity and the retroperitoneum. The lack of skeletal protection of the muscular anterior abdominal wall leads to a greater risk for injury to the intraperitoneal organs, notably the spleen, liver, and small bowel. Injured organs in the intraperitoneal cavity may bleed freely because of the substantial fluid capacity of this cavity, whereas brisk bleeding will be contained more by the limited space in the retroperitoneum.

## PRESENTING SIGNS AND SYMPTOMS

Certain signs and symptoms suggest the presence of intraperitoneal injury. Blood pressure and heart rate are the most important vital signs when assessing for significant intraabdominal injury. Isolated prehospital hypotension has been shown to be a predictor of mortality and of chest or abdominal injury requiring operative intervention. Prehospital abnormal vital signs should not be discounted even if the patient arrives with "stable" vital signs. Normal vital signs do not rule out intraperitoneal injury.

Patients in shock usually demonstrate tachycardia. However, up to 44% of trauma patients in shock may have relative bradycardia, defined as a heart rate of less than 90 beats per minute and a systolic blood pressure lower than 90 mm Hg. Relative bradycardia has been identified as an independent risk factor for mortality.[4]

Significant complaints and findings include abdominal pain or tenderness, ecchymoses and abrasions on the abdominal wall, and hematemesis. Increasing abdominal distention may be a marker of ongoing intraperitoneal bleeding. Peritonitis, even in the absence of hypotension, is a strong predictor of intraabdominal injury, although it does not necessarily predict the need for laparotomy in a stable patient.

Physical examination is limited in its ability to identify the presence or absence of intraabdominal injury. Therefore, further diagnostic testing should be performed, despite minimal clinical findings, if the abdomen sustained significant direct trauma such as a baseball bat or handlebar injury or if the patient is difficult to evaluate because of concomitant injuries or altered mental status for any reason. Other significant mechanisms, such as a rollover motor vehicle collision, a motor vehicle collision with ejection or significant intrusion, or a substantial fall, should be evaluated in light of the patient's clinical picture. A motor vehicle collision with steering wheel deformity is associated with serious abdominal injury in front seat passengers but not in drivers; direct impact from a bicycle handlebar suggests an increased likelihood of abdominal injury requiring laparotomy. Intraperitoneal injury can also result from minor mechanisms, such as a fall from the standing position onto the abdomen.

Several insensitive clinical signs suggest specific injuries in a blunt trauma patient. The Kehr sign, which is left shoulder pain, suggests splenic rupture. The Cullen sign is ecchymosis around the umbilicus, and the Turner sign is ecchymosis in the flank area. These signs suggest retroperitoneal hemorrhage but are very rarely found in acute trauma patients. They occur only hours after injury and thus are of little use in the initial assessment of patients who have sustained blunt abdominal trauma.

The presence of the seat belt sign (erythema, ecchymosis, or abrasions in the pattern of a seat belt) is associated with intraperitoneal injuries—specifically, pancreatic, hollow viscus, and mesenteric injuries. Multiple studies have shown a significantly higher incidence of intraabdominal operative pathology in patients with the seat belt sign than in those lacking this sign after motor vehicle trauma. The seat belt sign usually results from incorrect use or improper placement of a seat belt restraint. It should be used as a predictor of intraperitoneal injury and therefore as an indication to perform diagnostic imaging in patients with blunt abdominal trauma. Negative findings on computed tomography (CT) in a patient with abdominal tenderness and the seat belt sign should be followed by observation, diagnostic peritoneal lavage (DPL), or laparotomy, depending on the findings and clinical suspicion. Although evisceration and clear-cut peritonitis are diagnostic of intraabdominal pathology, neither is a common finding.

Abdominal tenderness is often absent in patients with intraperitoneal injury. Drugs, alcohol, hypotension, and the presence of head injury reduce the patient's ability to sense pain or tenderness. Additionally, other significant injuries such as fractures or large lacerations may distract the patient from feeling the pain associated with abdominal injury. In a large prospective study, 19% of patients with positive findings on CT for intraabdominal injury did not have abdominal tenderness.[3] Other studies have reported abdominal tenderness in only 42% to 75% of patients with small bowel or mesenteric injury.[5,6] The sensitivity, specificity, and negative and positive predictive values of abdominal pain or tenderness in predicting intraabdominal injury are reported to be 82%, 45%, 93%, and 21%, respectively.[7] Furthermore, patients with chest wall injuries and pneumothorax are at risk for injury and may not exhibit abdominal pain or tenderness. Thus, it is important to avoid relying solely on the physical examination, especially in a multitrauma patient or one with altered mental status, when deciding whether to perform diagnostic testing on a patient after blunt abdominal trauma.

## EVALUATION

Physical examination of the abdomen following trauma consists of observation and palpation. The abdomen should be observed for signs of disruption, evisceration, ecchymoses, abrasions, and distention. Although it is important to perform a rectal examination to assess rectal tone and the prostate for possible urethral injury, a positive stool guaiac test is not predictive of injury. If gross blood is present on rectal examination, large bowel or rectal injury should be suspected.

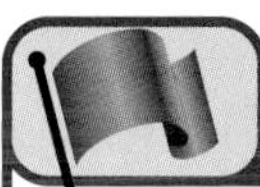

**RED FLAGS**

Prehospital hypotension indicates the need for diagnostic imaging of the abdomen.
Abdominal ecchymosis is predictive of intraperitoneal injury.
The presence of a Chance fracture is predictive of intraperitoneal injury.
Left shoulder pain suggests splenic injury.
Low rib fractures are associated with liver and spleen injuries.

The initial physical examination includes assessment of the pelvis for stability and the urethral meatus for blood as an indicator of associated urethral injury. These aspects of the examination will help the emergency physician (EP) plan the subsequent evaluation. Patients with pelvic instability may need stabilization of a pelvic fracture and embolization, whereas those with a urethral injury may need retrograde urethrography and suprapubic placement of a Foley catheter.

## DIFFERENTIAL DIAGNOSIS

The specific injuries to be concerned with after blunt abdominal trauma can be broken down into several categories: solid organ (liver and spleen), hollow viscus, mesenteric, vascular (inferior vena cava and aorta), diaphragmatic, and retroperitoneal (renal, bladder, pelvic fractures, and vascular). Other less common injuries are gallbladder, pancreas, and rectus sheath hematomas.

### CHANCE FRACTURES

A single lap belt restraint can result in Chance fractures of the lumbar spine. In a recent report, 33% of patients with Chance fractures had associated intraabdominal injury, and of these patients, 22% had hollow viscus injuries.[8] In other studies, up to 89% of patients with Chance fractures had small bowel injuries.[5,9] Some centers consider the presence of Chance fractures and the seat belt sign to be an indication for exploratory laparotomy.

### UPPER ABDOMINAL INJURIES

Low rib injuries may be associated with spleen or liver trauma, as well as kidney injuries. The incidence of splenic injury in patients with "isolated" low rib pain or tenderness (no abdominal tenderness) was 3% in a recent report. Although the only prospective study on the subject is not definitive, it suggests that patients with pleuritic pain and isolated low left rib pain or tenderness, regardless of whether abdominal tenderness is present, should undergo imaging.[10] In addition, patients with abdominal tenderness following low chest trauma should undergo diagnostic imaging (e.g., CT).

### LOWER ABDOMINAL INJURIES

Blunt abdominal trauma may result in retroperitoneal injury to the kidneys or ureters. Intraperitoneal or extraperitoneal bladder rupture may also occur. Major pelvic fractures are associated with abdominal injuries in 30% of patients.[11] Injury to the abdominal aorta is rare after blunt abdominal trauma. Other less serious injuries are abdominal wall hematomas, which do not usually require operative intervention but can result in significant blood loss.

### INJURIES WITH DELAYED PRESENTATION

Several injuries are notoriously seen in delayed fashion or have subtle clinical findings. Pancreatic injuries may be manifested as abdominal pain and tenderness several hours after the trauma. Duodenal hematomas typically become evident 5 to 7 days after the trauma as vague abdominal pain and vomiting. This is in contrast to patients with duodenal perforations, who usually have acute pain and tenderness immediately after the trauma.

Traumatic diaphragmatic hernia can also occur in delayed fashion. These injuries are frequently missed because the sensitivity of CT for diaphragmatic injuries is low and the majority of patients have associated injuries.[12] Most of these injuries result from a vehicular collision. Because the right hemidiaphragm is protected by the liver, the left hemidiaphragm is more commonly involved.

Diaphragmatic injuries occur in three phases. In the acute phase, immediately after injury, patients may have decreased or absent breath signs on one side of the chest or bowel sounds in the chest. If the injury is not detected, patients may go through a latent phase consisting of intermittent visceral herniation into the chest through the diaphragmatic rupture. These patients may have vague postprandial abdominal pain (which improves with standing because the herniated bowel is reduced), nausea, vomiting, and belching. During this phase the injury can go undetected for months to years. With time, patients will eventually enter the obstructive phase, which is associated with herniation and incarceration of bowel, intestinal obstruction, and ischemia. These patients exhibit abdominal pain, distention, and vomiting.

In the acute setting, patients with a diaphragmatic injury can also have tension viscerothorax–herniation of bowel into the chest, which results in increased intrathoracic pressure and mediastinal shift with compression of the superior vena cava. These patients have hypotension and decreased breath sounds on the affected side of the chest.

## SOLID ORGAN INJURIES

The most common type of injury is solid organ injury. More than 90% of the injuries sustained in blunt trauma are isolated to the liver and spleen. Patients with hypotension as a result of blunt trauma usually have free rupture of a solid organ. Delayed onset of symptoms or pain without hypotension should raise concern about encapsulated hepatic or splenic trauma or hollow viscus injury. Although most intraperitoneal injuries today are managed nonoperatively, delayed diagnosis in some cases can lead to severe morbidity or mortality. Free intraperitoneal bleeding is the most urgent diagnosis in patients with blunt abdominal trauma. This immediately life-threatening condition may require interventions, including transfusion, exploratory laparotomy, and angiography with embolization.

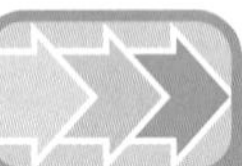

**PRIORITY ACTIONS**

1. Follow the advanced trauma life support protocols for initial resuscitation.
2. Determine the stability of the patient.
3. Perform chest and pelvic radiography on all unstable trauma patients.
4. Perform ultrasound examination on all major trauma patients.
5. Arrange transfer immediately for all patients with multi-system trauma or with the potential for intraperitoneal injury if a trauma surgeon is not available.
6. Triage the patient to either computed tomography scanning, laparotomy, the angiography suite (pelvic fractures or for embolization of abdominal injuries), intensive care unit, admission for observation, or discharge.

# THE UNSTABLE PATIENT

## INITIAL MANAGEMENT

The initial therapeutic intervention in patients with presumed intraperitoneal injury is to address the ABCs of trauma (airway, breathing, and circulation). Initially, all patients should receive high-flow oxygen. Intubation should be performed on unstable or severely injured multitrauma patients or those with the potential for rapid decline. After breathing is attended to, circulatory status is addressed. Antecubital venous or central line access should be obtained.

## IMMEDIATE OPERATIVE INTERVENTION

There are several indications to proceed immediately to the operating room without further diagnostic testing, including evisceration, gross blood per rectum, blood per nasogastric tube or hematemesis, evidence of diaphragmatic injury, and hemodynamic instability with evidence of intraperitoneal injury (e.g., positive ultrasound findings).

### *Focused Abdominal Sonography for Trauma*

Bedside ultrasonography has many advantages as an initial triage tool in an unstable trauma patient. It is readily accessible at most level I trauma centers and, in the hands of trained EPs, is accurate in detecting hemoperitoneum.[13] Focused abdominal sonography for trauma (FAST) can be performed in less than 2 minutes and can triage patients to the operating room or further diagnostic testing, depending on the patient's stability. In trauma patients, the incidence of an indeterminate sonographic result is low (less than 7%),[14] and the reported sensitivity and negative predictive value in unstable patients approach 100%.[15,16] The presence of hemoperitoneum in an unstable patient is an indication for operative intervention. The only caveat is that in patients with major pelvic trauma who may have bladder rupture with uroperitoneum, diagnostic peritoneal aspiration may be indicated to distinguish blood from urine. If the sonographic findings are negative, other sources of bleeding should be addressed, such as pelvic fractures and retroperitoneal bleeding.

### *Diagnostic Peritoneal Lavage*

Some authors take a conservative approach and recommend confirming the results of negative ultrasonography with DPL in hypotensive patients. If ultrasonography is unavailable or if the results are indeterminate, DPL is required to determine the presence of intraperitoneal bleeding as an indication for immediate laparotomy. Before performing DPL, the EP should place a nasogastric tube and Foley catheter to decompress the stomach and drain the bladder.

DPL involves placement of a catheter into the peritoneal space and aspiration with a 10-mL syringe to see whether blood is present. In an unstable patient, an initial aspirate of 10 mL of blood is an indication for laparotomy. The presence of bile, food particles, or other gastrointestinal contents is also considered an indication for laparotomy. If the aspirate is negative, other sources of bleeding should be addressed (e.g., pelvic fractures). One liter of normal saline should be instilled into the abdomen if the initial aspirate is negative and then drained from the abdomen and sent to the laboratory for analysis.

# THE STABLE PATIENT

## LABORATORY TESTING

Laboratory tests are rarely helpful in the initial resuscitation of patients after blunt abdominal trauma. The utility of ordering individual laboratory tests when a specific clinical need is present versus routinely ordering a standard "trauma panel" has been studied. A significant cost savings, without adverse events, occurs if this practice is followed.[17,18]

Several laboratory tests are useful in the initial evaluation of blunt trauma patients. The hematocrit should be measured for use as a baseline value and may be helpful as an indicator of bleeding if it is very low. Patients with a high likelihood of requiring an operation should have their blood typed and cross-matched in the event that a transfusion is required. A bedside glucose test should be performed on patients involved in a single-car accident and in patients with altered mental status after trauma.

All women of childbearing age should undergo a pregnancy test and be questioned about whether they are pregnant. Serial ultrasonography can be used as the initial and often definitive modality, and CT should be used sparingly in the first 20 weeks of gestation to avoid unnecessary exposure to radiation.[19]

Coagulation profiles should be performed in patients with a significant mechanism of trauma and in those who will probably require an operation. In addition, any patient receiving warfarin (Coumadin) therapy should have a coagulation profile performed.

Lactate levels and base excess are two laboratory tests that have been shown to predict bleeding.[20] In one recent study of stable trauma patients, an increased lactate level (>2.5 mmol/L in ethanol-negative patients and >3 mmol/L in ethanol-positive patients) and an increased base deficit (>0.0 in ethanol-negative patients and >3.0 in ethanol-positive patients) were associated with a significant risk for torso injury, whereas patients with a normal base deficit were unlikely to have injury.[21] Other authors consider a base deficit cutoff value of 6 or less to be predictive of intraabdominal injury and an indication for diagnostic imaging or DPL.[22]

Urinalysis should be performed in all blunt trauma patients with a significant mechanism of injury. The presence of gross hematuria is an indication for evaluation of the genitourinary tract. Microscopic hematuria is a sign of mild renal injury that does not require treatment; its presence in a stable patient without a significant deceleration injury (associated with renal pedicle injury) is not an indication for additional diagnostic imaging. Some evidence also suggests that microscopic hematuria consisting of 25 or more red blood cells per high-power field may be one of the predictors of intraperitoneal injury.[23]

Amylase and lipase levels do not predict pancreatic injury in the acute setting. However, they may be helpful for detecting traumatic pancreatitis in patients initially evaluated hours after trauma.

## PLAIN RADIOGRAPHS

Plain radiographs cannot rule out intraperitoneal injury after blunt trauma. Chest radiography may be used to diagnose a diaphragmatic rupture (**Fig. 79.1**). However, plain radiographs of the chest are diagnostic of diaphragmatic rupture in only 50% of patients with left-sided rupture and in only 17% of those with right-sided rupture.[24,25] Free air is a rare finding on an upright chest radiograph that indicates hollow viscus rupture (stomach or colon), but upright chest radiography is not usually feasible after blunt trauma. Thus, plain radiographs should not be used to rule out intraperitoneal injury.

Radiography is also useful for detecting pelvic fractures as a cause of hypotension after blunt trauma and can help guide evaluation for the management of associated genitourinary injuries. Although pelvic radiography is not necessary in patients with normal mental status and no pain or tenderness, it should be performed in unstable or seriously injured patients with an appropriate mechanism of injury.

## ULTRASONOGRAPHY

FAST is recommended for all blunt trauma patients with any significant mechanism of injury as an initial screening test regardless of patient stability. Ultrasonography is now listed in the advanced trauma life support algorithm for abdominal trauma and is used in the majority of level I trauma centers.[26] In the blunt trauma setting, ultrasonography has become part of the secondary survey to detect hemoperitoneum as an indicator of intraperitoneal injury.

If the sonogram shows free fluid and the patient is hemodynamically unstable, exploratory laparotomy is indicated. A stable patient with free fluid should undergo CT immediately to identify the type of injury and determine the need for laparotomy. A clinical algorithm that incorporates FAST is presented in **Figure 79.2**.

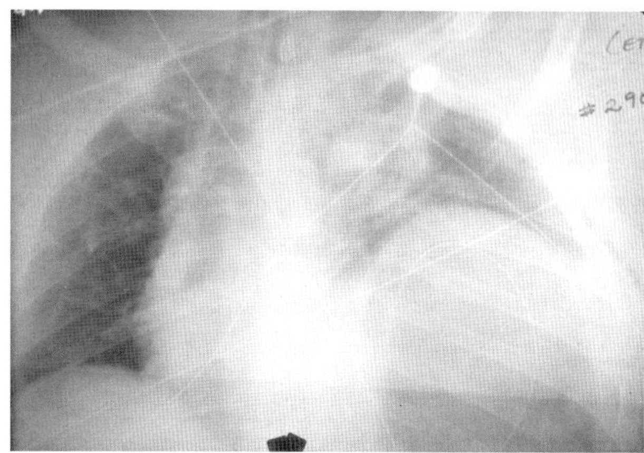

**Fig. 79.1 Chest radiograph of a patient with left diaphragmatic rupture.**

FAST is also used for the rapid detection of pericardial fluid, hemothorax, and pneumothorax. It does not replace chest radiography for hemothorax and pneumothorax but may be obtained faster and can be used to expedite thoracostomy tube placement.

The major limitation of ultrasonography is its inability to identify or grade solid organ injury. Its sensitivity for detecting hemoperitoneum as an indicator of intraperitoneal injury ranges from 76% to 90%, and its specificity ranges from 95% to 100%.[13] However, its sensitivity is as low as 33% with splenic injuries and 12% with hepatic injuries for identifying encapsulated solid organ bleeding.[13,27] Ultrasonography is also limited in assessing injuries that are not associated with a large amount of hemoperitoneum, such as retroperitoneal bleeding and injuries to the small bowel or diaphragm. Up to one third of patients with intraperitoneal injury will have negative findings on FAST, including as many as 10% of patients who require surgery.[28] Thus, FAST does not replace more definitive tests such as CT, but it can be a triage tool to expedite the evaluation and management of patients with blunt abdominal trauma. The amount of intraperitoneal fluid that must be present to have abnormal FAST findings is at least 150 mL and may be as much as 1 L.[29,30]

The technique of bedside ultrasonography in trauma patients consists of four standard views (**Fig. 79.3**): right upper quadrant (Morison pouch), subxiphoid, left upper quadrant, and suprapubic (pouch of Douglas). Although this examination has no standard sequence, the suprapubic view takes advantage of the full bladder as a sonographic window and should therefore be obtained before placement of a Foley catheter. Most operators start with the Morison pouch view because it is technically the easiest.

Obtaining all the views rather than one single view increases the sensitivity of the test.[31] Performing serial examinations every 30 minutes into the resuscitation—or if a change in clinical status occurs—increases the sensitivity further. Trendelenburg positioning may improve the sensitivity by causing the hemoperitoneum to pool in dependent spaces. The differential diagnosis for fluid seen on ultrasonography includes

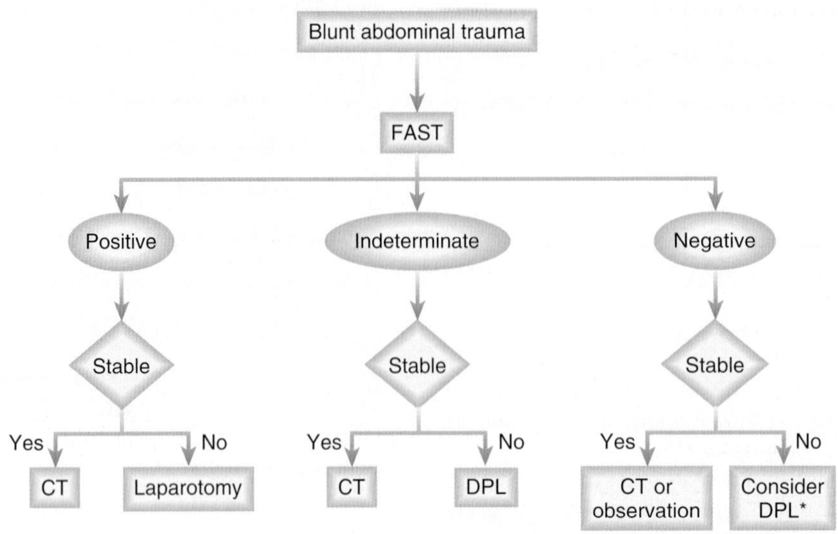


**Fig. 79.2 Algorithm for the management of blunt abdominal trauma.** *CT*, Computed tomography; *DPL*, diagnostic peritoneal lavage; *FAST*, focused abdominal sonography for trauma. (From Rosen CL, Promes SB. Use of ultrasound in emergency medicine. Clinical bulletin: State of the Art Emergency Medicine 2003;7[2]:1. Reprinted with permission from Sterling Healthcare. All rights reserved.)

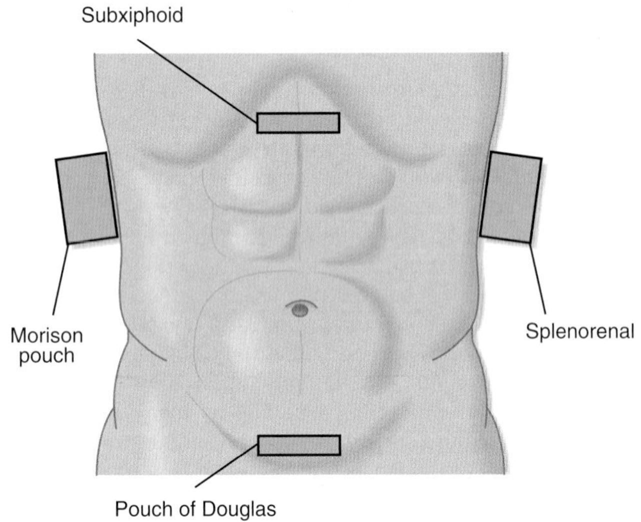


**Fig. 79.3 Focused abdominal sonography for trauma: four views.**

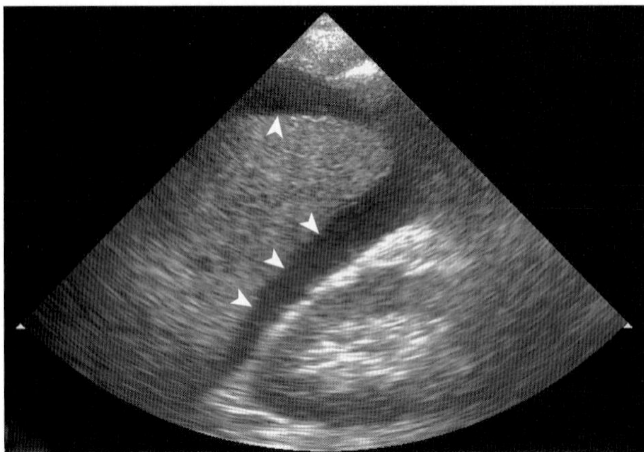

**Fig. 79.4 Morison pouch showing fluid *(arrowheads)* in the space between the liver and the right kidney.**

ascites, as well as urine from intraperitoneal bladder rupture. All fluid will result in the same black stripe seen on the sonogram.

The finding suggestive of injury is hemoperitoneum, which appears as a black (anechoic) stripe between the kidney and the liver (**Fig. 79.4**), between the kidney and the spleen, or posterior to the bladder. Because ultrasonography is insensitive in detecting actual parenchymal injury, the operator should not waste time evaluating the spleen and liver for evidence of injury.

## DIAGNOSTIC PERITONEAL LAVAGE

DPL was formerly the primary method for evaluating unstable patients after blunt abdominal trauma, but its use has markedly decreased with the widespread application of bedside ultrasonography. Currently, DPL is indicated when ultrasonography is unavailable or if the results are indeterminate in an unstable patient. Some authors recommend DPL to confirm the absence of hemoperitoneum in unstable patients with negative results on ultrasonography.[32]

DPL is very sensitive in detecting intraperitoneal bleeding, can be performed rapidly, and is inexpensive. It can detect small amounts of intraperitoneal blood (as little as 20 mL).[33] The accuracy of DPL for predicting or ruling out intraperitoneal bleeding is close to 98%.[34,35] DPL has, however, been shown to be less accurate in patients with major pelvic fractures. The false-positive rate may be higher in this group of patients because of the presence of uroperitoneum as a result of bladder injury. Consequently, in the presence of a pelvic fracture, diagnostic peritoneal aspiration may be indicated to determine whether a positive FAST result is due to blood or urine.[36]

The disadvantages of DPL are that it is invasive, does not identify the specific organ that is injured, and does not sample the retroperitoneal space. It will also detect small amounts of bleeding associated with injuries that do not require operative intervention. The nontherapeutic laparotomy rate for patients with a positive DPL finding is reported to be as high as 35%.[37] Thus, in stable patients, a positive DPL result is not an indication for laparotomy.

The only absolute contraindication to DPL is a clear need for emergency laparotomy. Relative contraindications include morbid obesity, previous abdominal surgery (because of the presence of adhesions), and late-term pregnancy.

DPL findings that predict the presence of intraperitoneal injury after blunt trauma are a red blood cell count greater than 100,000/mm$^3$, a white blood cell count greater than 500/mm$^3$, amylase level greater than 10 IU/L, and alkaline phosphatase level of 3 IU/L or greater. The complication rate for DPL is less than 1%. The most serious complication is bowel perforation; other complications include wound infection and bleeding.

## COMPUTED TOMOGRAPHY

Abdominal and pelvic CT is the standard diagnostic imaging modality for a stable patient with possible intraabdominal injury. CT provides excellent detail of solid organ and retroperitoneal injuries. Its performance in diagnosing hollow viscus injuries continues to improve. Because of the accuracy and detail of CT images, nonoperative management of solid organ injury can now be performed safely. With the use of three-dimensional reconstruction, radiologists can also image the lumbar spine and pelvis to evaluate for fractures.

The disadvantages of CT are the difficulty in monitoring and resuscitating a patient in the radiology suite and the risk for contrast allergy and renal failure from administration of the dye. The complication rate is 3%, which includes aspiration of oral contrast material.

CT is indicated in stable patients when intraabdominal injury is clinically of concern because of abdominal wall findings, traumatic distracting injuries, and a significant mechanism of injury. The presence of distracting injury and the need for operative intervention for other injuries (e.g., orthopedic injuries) are also indications for performing CT. In awake patients who have a reliable abdominal examination and no abdominal tenderness, the yield of performing abdominal CT scanning because they are undergoing extraabdominal surgery is very low. Less than 2% of patients undergoing abdominal CT scanning only because of the need for general anesthesia for urgent extraabdominal surgery actually had an abdominal injury, and less than 0.5% required laparotomy.[38,39]

Recent studies have looked at determining clinical predictors for identifying patients at low risk for intraperitoneal injury after blunt trauma who may not need CT. One such clinical prediction rule consists of a Glasgow Coma Scale score of less than 14, costal margin tenderness, abdominal tenderness, femoral fracture, hematuria consisting of greater than 25 red blood cells per high-power field, hematocrit of less than 30%, and abnormal chest radiograph findings (pneumothorax or rib fracture). In the absence of any of these clinical variables, patients are at very low risk of having intraperitoneal injury (96% sensitivity and 99% negative predictive value).[23]

Many trauma centers in the United States and Europe are using a newer technique, the "pan scan," for obtaining a rapid CT scan of the head, neck, and torso in patients with a high mechanism of trauma who are at higher risk for traumatic injuries. The advantage of this technique is that it is faster than performing segmental, sequential CT scans and may detect injuries that would otherwise be missed or diagnosed in delayed fashion, such as spine and chest injuries. The biggest risk, however, is that this technique will be overused and expose patients to unnecessary radiation and cancer risk. The exact indications for performing a pan scan are controversial. However, a conservative approach would be to obtain a pan scan in patients with a major traumatic mechanism who are also not evaluable because of head injury, intubation, or depressed mental status from alcohol. A pan scan is also recommended for elderly trauma patients who may sustain significant injuries with lesser mechanisms and for patients with prehospital hypotension who are stable in the emergency department because they are also at risk for torso trauma.[40,41]

Determining when a patient is stable enough to undergo CT remains a point of controversy. An unstable patient should not be sent to the radiography suite, where it is difficult to monitor and resuscitate a sick patient. Most centers use the response to fluid resuscitation and transfusion as an indicator of whether the patient is stable enough to be transferred to the radiography suite for CT. This decision may also be influenced by the proximity and type of CT scanner.

CT is very accurate in diagnosing intraperitoneal injury, especially for detecting solid organ injury, as stated previously. Another advantage of CT is its higher accuracy and sensitivity than plain radiographs for detecting fractures of the thoracolumbar spine (TLS). In one prospective study, the accuracy of CT of the torso for detecting TLS fractures was 99% versus 87% for plain radiographs, with the "gold standard" for fracture being the discharge diagnosis of acute fractures confirmed by thin-cut CT or clinical examination of the patient when alert (or both). It is also much faster to obtain a torso CT scan than it is to obtain multiple plain radiographic spine images.[42]

The limitations of CT lie in its low sensitivity for diaphragm, mesenteric, hollow viscus, and pancreatic injuries. Although the newer-generation multidetector CT scanners appear to have better resolution and sensitivity for these rare injuries, they are still not highly accurate. The sensitivity for diaphragmatic injury is between 67% and 84%, with specificities reported to be between 77% and 100%.[12,43-46]

The sensitivity of CT for detecting hollow viscus injury is reported to range from 83% to 94%.[10,12,46-50] Multidetector CT without oral contrast enhancement was 82% sensitive and 99% specific for detecting bowel and mesenteric injuries.[51] The reported sensitivity of CT for detecting pancreatic injuries after blunt trauma ranges from 50% to 68%, even with spiral CT technology.[52,53] The use of oral contrast is not associated with an increase in sensitivity for detecting pancreatic injury.[53] In a recent multicenter study, the sensitivity of CT was 76% for pancreatic injuries and 70% for duodenal injuries.[54]

### *Oral Contrast or No Oral Contrast?*

An ongoing controversy on the use of CT scanning for blunt abdominal trauma is the utility of oral contrast versus intravenous contrast alone. Oral contrast is associated with increased time and the potential for vomiting, aspiration, and other complications, as well as discomfort if a nasogastric tube is placed. Several studies have documented that oral contrast enhancement is not essential for identifying solid organ, mesenteric, or bowel injuries.[55-58] Because use remains controversial and local customs often prevail, oral contrast agents are still commonly used in many trauma centers.

### *Findings in Patients with Blunt Abdominal Trauma*

CT findings suggesting solid organ injury are disruption of the parenchyma, extravasation of contrast material, and hemoperitoneum. Patients with blunt intestinal or mesenteric injuries may have more subtle findings such as free fluid without obvious organ injury, mesenteric stranding or edema, and bowel wall hematoma. Other indicators of bowel and mesenteric injury are pneumoperitoneum, tears in the bowel wall, and wall thickening.

Isolated intraperitoneal fluid in patients without solid organ injury is associated with a high incidence of bowel or mesenteric injury. In patients without solid organ injury and with more than trace amounts of free fluid, the therapeutic laparotomy rate is 54% to 94%.[59] At surgery, small bowel, mesenteric, and diaphragm injuries are usually found.

### ANGIOGRAPHY

When combined with embolization, angiography is both a diagnostic and therapeutic modality. Though classically used in blunt trauma for the treatment of pelvic fractures, it has been found to be especially helpful in the nonoperative treatment of active bleeding from solid organ injuries. High-grade spleen and liver injuries, as well as renal lacerations, are amenable to this technique. Patients selected for this procedure must be stable and have solid organ injuries with active extravasation (contrast blush) on abdominopelvic CT.

## TREATMENT

The initial treatment of patients with blunt abdominal trauma includes fluid resuscitation, transfusion, and simultaneous consultation with the trauma surgery facility for operative intervention, angiography, or admission for observation.

Intravenous fluid resuscitation with normal saline or lactated Ringer solution is indicated for patients who are hemodynamically unstable (tachycardia or hypotension). The optimal amount and goal of resuscitation are controversial. Although the standard has been to immediately infuse 2 L of crystalloid followed by blood transfusion in patients with continued instability, many institutions move rapidly to blood transfusion and limit resuscitation so that patients are kept "underresuscitated" with a systolic blood pressure of approximately 90 mm Hg.[32,60] This can usually be accomplished with type O-negative blood in women of childbearing age and type O-positive in all others. Once the bleeding lesion is identified and definitively controlled, full resuscitation is instituted. However, this practice is not typically recommended for patients with possible traumatic brain injury.

The presence of an unstable pelvis on physical examination or on the initial pelvic radiograph is another indication for early blood transfusion because patients with this condition will bleed profusely. EPs should place a pelvic stabilization binder or simply wrap a sheet tightly around the pelvis to stabilize the fractures as an early intervention.

For patients requiring large amounts of blood products, new evidence suggests that early administration of plasma and a higher ratio of plasma to packed red blood cells (PRBCs) transfused will result in lower mortality rates. In patients who require massive transfusion (defined as 10 or more units of PRBCs in 24 hours), it is recommended that they receive plasma, platelets, and PRBCs in a ratio close to 1:1:1.[61,62]

Indications for operative intervention include hemodynamic instability, diaphragmatic injury, and hollow viscus injury. Although high-grade spleen and liver injuries once routinely underwent surgery, the use of angiography with embolization has become more common. Other CT findings that trauma surgeons may consider indications for operative intervention include the presence of intraperitoneal fluid without obvious organ injury and evidence of active extravasation. Because of the high incidence of associated small bowel injury, many institutions consider the presence of a Chance fracture in conjunction with abdominal wall ecchymosis an indication for laparotomy.

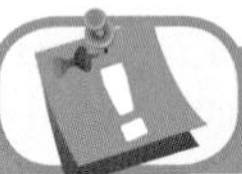

**TIPS AND TRICKS**

- Do not underestimate the mechanism of injury. A significant mechanism of injury requires evaluation for intraperitoneal injury even if the patient is stable and the findings on physical examination are normal.
- The presence or absence of abdominal tenderness does not predict intraperitoneal injury.
- Alcohol and distracting injuries can make the findings on physical examination unreliable.
- All blunt abdominal trauma patients should undergo FAST.
- Before performing DPL, place a nasogastric tube and Foley catheter and obtain a pelvic radiograph.
- Positive FAST findings or DPL aspirate in an unstable patient is an indication for laparotomy.
- Unstable patients should not be transferred to the radiology suite for CT.
- Significant intraperitoneal fluid without solid organ injury on a CT scan suggests the presence of small bowel injury.
- CT can fail to identify injuries of the pancreas, diaphragm, small bowel, and mesenterium.

*CT*, Computed tomography; *DPL*, diagnostic peritoneal lavage; *FAST*, focused abdominal sonography for trauma.

### PRIORITIZING MANAGEMENT OF INJURIES

Emergency department management of unstable patients with blunt abdominal trauma becomes challenging when associated injuries are present. In general, intraperitoneal bleeding trumps other injuries in terms of the immediate need for operative management. An unstable patient with known intraperitoneal hemorrhage and associated pelvic trauma should undergo laparotomy first, followed by management of pelvic injuries (e.g., angiographic embolization of pelvic vessels). In unstable patients with evidence of associated traumatic brain injury, neurosurgical consultation should be obtained for intracranial bolt placement in the operating room while the intraperitoneal injuries are being addressed. Suspicion of aortic injury presents an added challenge in management. The aortic injury is not usually the cause of hemodynamic instability, and intraperitoneal bleeding should be the presumed source of the hypotension. Thus, in patients with concomitant aortic and abdominal injuries, laparotomy should be performed first. Abdominal bleeding takes priority over orthopedic injuries; frequently, however, the trauma surgeon can perform laparotomy at the same time that the orthopedic surgeon is repairing an open fracture.

## NONOPERATIVE TREATMENT

Many reports in the surgical literature document success with nonoperative management of patients with spleen and liver lacerations.[63] Most centers, however, consider the presence of hemodynamic instability or transfusion requirements as indications to operate on patients with solid organ injuries. Age may also be used as an indicator for surgery; children do well with nonoperative management, whereas elderly patients may have lower success rates with nonoperative care. Nonoperative salvage rates in patients with lacerations of the spleen are 94%, and up to 80% of grade 4 and 5 splenic injuries can be managed successfully without operative intervention.[64]

In one prospective study, the failure rate of nonoperative treatment of kidney, liver, and splenic lacerations was 22%; the failure rate was higher for splenic injury than for liver or kidney injuries.[65] Independent predictors of failure of nonoperative management were fluid identified on screening ultrasonography, significant blood on CT (>300 mL), and the need for blood transfusion.[65]

## INTERVENTIONAL RADIOLOGY

In major trauma centers, interventional radiologists in conjunction with trauma surgeons are performing angiography with embolization instead of operative management. The nonoperative salvage rate in patients with splenic lacerations who undergo embolization is 90%.[64] Angiography with embolization may be performed in patients who are hemodynamically stable and do not have associated hollow viscus or other injuries requiring operative intervention.[66,67]

For splenic injuries, arterial embolization may be indicated for patients with active extravasation of contrast material, pseudoaneurysm or arteriovenous fistula, large hemoperitoneum, and a higher grade of injury (III to V), assuming that no indications for operative intervention are present. The combination of contrast blush and significant hemoperitoneum may also predict a high failure rate for nonoperative management and may be an indication for arterial embolization or laparotomy with splenectomy.[68]

## FOLLOW-UP, NEXT STEPS IN CARE, AND PATIENT EDUCATION (ADMISSION AND DISCHARGE)

If the patient is initially transported to a hospital that is not a designated trauma center, the EP must decide when to transfer the patient to the trauma center and what tests to perform before transfer. If the trauma is isolated to the abdomen and a general surgeon is available to admit the patient or perform therapeutic laparotomy, transfer may not be necessary. Patients with multisystem trauma or hemodynamic instability require transfer to a trauma center.

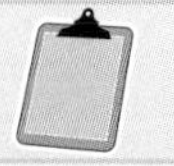

### DOCUMENTATION

Mechanism and timing of the injury
Findings on physical examination
Timing and ordering of tests and consultations
Emergency department procedures
Changes in clinical status

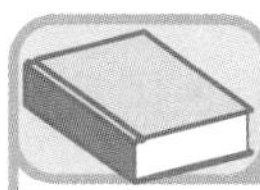

### PATIENT TEACHING TIPS

For patients with nonoperative splenic injuries, avoid contact sports until follow-up and for several weeks.

Return to the emergency department if experiencing abdominal pain, light-headedness, vomiting, or blood per rectum.

## SUGGESTED READINGS


ACEP Clinical Policies Committee, Clinical Policies Subcommittee on Acute Blunt Abdominal Trauma: clinical policy: critical issues in the evaluation of adult patients presenting to the emergency department with acute blunt abdominal trauma. Ann Emerg Med 2004;43:278-90.

Borgman MA, Spinella PC, Perkins JG, et al. The ratio of blood products transfused affects mortality in patients receiving massive transfusion at a combat support hospital. J Trauma 2007;63:805-13.

Farahmand N, Sirlin CB, Brown MA. Hypotensive patients with blunt abdominal trauma: performance of screening US. Emerg Radiol 2005;235:436-43.

Haan JM, Bochicchio GV, Kramer N, et al. Non-operative management of blunt splenic injury: a 5-year experience. J Trauma 2005;58:492-8.

Hauser CJ, Visvikis G, Hinrichs C, et al. Prospective validation of computed tomographic screening of the thoracolumbar spine in trauma. J Trauma 2003;55:228-35.

Holmes JF, Schauer BA, Nguyen H, et al. Is definitive abdominal evaluation required in blunt trauma victims undergoing urgent extra-abdominal surgery? Acad Emerg Med 2005;12:707-11.

Holmes JF, Wisner DH, McGahan JP, et al. Clinical prediction rules for identifying adults at very low risk for intra-abdominal injuries after blunt trauma. Ann Emerg Med 2009;54:575-84.

Jayal V, Neilsen A, Jones A, et al. Accuracy of trauma ultrasound in major pelvic injury. J Trauma 2006;61:1453-7.

Velmahos GC, Toutouzas KG, Radin R, et al. Non-operative treatment of blunt injury to solid abdominal organs: a prospective study. Arch Surg 2003;138:844-51.

Zink KA, Sambasivan CN, Holcomb JB, et al. A high ratio of plasma and platelets to packed red blood cells in the first 6 hours of massive transfusion improves outcomes in a large multicenter study. Am J Surg 2009;197:565-70.


## REFERENCES

***References can be found on Expert Consult @ www.expertconsult.com.***

# 80 Penetrating Abdominal Trauma

*Eric L. Legome and Carlo L. Rosen*

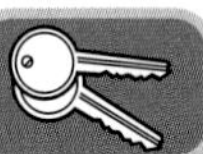

**KEY POINTS**

- Patients with diffuse peritonitis or hypotension after penetrating abdominal trauma require immediate operative intervention.
- Conversely, mandatory laparotomy for *all* wounds that penetrate the anterior abdominal fascia is no longer the sole approach.
- Evaluation of patients with *stable* penetrating trauma depends on the anatomic site of injury, the weapon used, serial examinations, and local diagnostic and surgical resources.

## EPIDEMIOLOGY

Since the 1960s, U.S. mortality rates of 9.5% to 12.7% for civilian gunshot wounds and up to 3.6% for stab wounds have been reported. Most deaths caused by penetrating trauma take place in the first 24 hours; about 70% occur in the first 6 hours of the patient's course, most commonly in the emergency department (ED), followed by the operating room. Most of these patients tend to have vascular injuries and succumb to exsanguination or refractory hemorrhagic shock.[1] If patients survive the first 24 hours, later deaths tend to cluster after 72 hours and are related mainly to acute systemic complications such as multiple system organ failure, acute respiratory distress syndrome, pulmonary embolism, and pneumonia.[2,3]

Management of penetrating abdominal trauma has undergone many changes over the last 20 years. Major transformations include rapid transport to trauma centers, "scoop and run" protocols in the field, damage control surgery, increased use of interventional radiologic techniques, and recognition and treatment of abdominal compartment syndrome. Better diagnostic studies, including rational use of computed tomography (CT) and ultrasonography, as well as expanded use of laparoscopy, have also improved morbidity rates, but no marked change in mortality has occurred.[1] Although management of patients with obvious peritonitis or hypovolemic shock remains essentially unchanged from the perspective of the emergency physician (EP), a patient without obvious intraperitoneal injury still presents a diagnostic dilemma. The benefits of nonoperative management, when performed appropriately, include lower hospital costs, less morbidity, and shorter hospital stays.[4,5]

## PATHOPHYSIOLOGY

Physiologic evaluation of patients with penetrating abdominal trauma concentrates on two major findings related to the pathophysiologic basis of the injury—peritonitis and hemodynamic instability. Peritonitis develops when the peritoneal envelope and the posterior aspect of the anterior abdominal wall are inflamed by enteric contents. Intraperitoneal or retroperitoneal blood and organ contents inflame the deeper nerve endings (visceral afferent pain fibers), thereby resulting in poorly defined and localized pain. Direct contact of the parietal peritoneum with blood or bowel contents can cause inflammation, which may be manifested as tenderness on palpation of the abdomen, as well as involuntary guarding of the abdominal wall musculature. Patients may also have referred pain. Because of the afferent, embryologically related pain fibers that ascend during development, a back or shoulder distribution of pain may provide a clue to the damaged organ (e.g., left shoulder pain from splenic rupture with subphrenic blood). Even though penetrating trauma is associated with multiple specific mechanisms, for most purposes it is divided into low- and high-energy injury; in general, these categories correlate with stab wounds or gunshot wounds. Gunshot wounds may be further divided into low- and high-velocity injuries, although both have the ability to cause secondary injury by energy transfer, fragmentation, and secondary missiles such as bone fragments. Handguns and lower-caliber rifles such as .22 gauge tend to have lower energy transfer than do military rifles and hunting rifles. Shotgun injuries, despite having lower velocity, often cause massive tissue damage if the wound is sustained at close range (i.e., less than 3 feet).

## PRESENTING SIGNS AND SYMPTOMS

The *anterior part of the abdomen* is the region between the anterior axillary lines from the anterior costal margins to the groin. The thoracoabdominal area is the region in which an injury can enter the chest, abdomen, or both. In addition to the anterior abdominal boundaries, it includes the lower part of the chest bordered by the nipple line or the fourth intercostal space anteriorly, the sixth intercostal space laterally, and the inferior scapular tip posteriorly because the diaphragm may extend to this level with expiration. The flank is the area between the anterior and posterior axillary lines bilaterally and ranges from the sixth intercostal space to the iliac crest. The back is bordered by the posterior axillary lines, with the inferior scapular

**BOX 80.1 Approximate Percentage of Organs Injured with Penetrating Trauma**

| Stab Wounds | Gunshot Wounds |
|---|---|
| Liver (40%) | Small bowel (50%) |
| Small bowel (30%) | Colon (40%) |
| Diaphragm (20%) | Liver (30%) |
| Colon (15%) | Abdominal vasculature (25%) |

tip located superiorly and the iliac crest inferiorly. In addition, depending on the type of penetrating object, simultaneous abdominal and thoracic penetration may be present. Within the abdominal cavity, both the intraperitoneal and retroperitoneal organs may be injured. The intraperitoneal organs include the liver, spleen, small bowel, transverse colon, gallbladder, and bladder. The retroperitoneal structures include the duodenum, pancreas, kidneys, ureters, bladder, ascending and descending colon, aorta and branching vessels, and rectum.[6]

Classic teaching is that the majority (about 90%) of gunshot wounds to the abdomen penetrate the peritoneum.[7] However, recent studies looking at nonoperative management show that a larger number of nontangential wounds do not penetrate. If a patient is initially stable and peritoneal signs are absent, the rate is probably closer to about 40%; however, abdominal gunshot wounds associated with peritonitis or instability have penetrated the peritoneum.[8,9] The majority of wounds that penetrate the peritoneum require laparotomy for repair. The most commonly injured organs are the small bowel, colon, and liver, followed by vascular structures, the stomach, and the kidneys (**Box 80.1**).

Stab wounds, as opposed to gunshot wounds, tend to follow the track of the wound and have more predictability. Approximately one fourth to one third of anterior abdominal stab wounds penetrate the peritoneum. Of those that do penetrate, about one third cause intraabdominal injury that requires operative repair. In addition to wounds involving the abdominal cavity, injuries to the thoracic cavity must also be considered in patients with thoracoabdominal stab wounds or any gunshot wound.

Physical examination often plays a major role in the management of patients with penetrating abdominal trauma, especially those who are hemodynamically stable. Serial examinations are a common and time-tested management strategy for low-velocity wounds. Studies show that it is an effective approach and that delay in diagnosis, if less than 24 hours, does not lead to a significant increase in complications. Furthermore, the decrease in morbidity and cost of nontherapeutic laparotomy is considerable.[10-12] In fact, in some centers, even patients with evisceration (especially omentum alone) without peritonitis are observed successfully after replacement of the eviscerated peritoneal contents, although such management remains controversial.[13-15]

## DIFFERENTIAL DIAGNOSIS AND MEDICAL DECISION MAKING

Examination may be used as a sole modality or in conjunction with other modalities. In patients with an anterior stab wound, local wound exploration can be a valuable diagnostic aid and should shorten a prolonged evaluation or observation if the results are negative. Its utility is dependent on the wound's mechanism and location. Stab wounds involving the anterior aspect of the abdomen are well suited for local wound exploration because many do not penetrate the fascia and can easily be visualized. Back, flank, and thoracoabdominal wounds do not allow clear delineation of the wound track and extent and are not candidates for this procedure. Likewise, this is a poor option for gunshot wounds or wounds from a sharp pinpoint instrument (e.g., ice pick).

Over the last decade, patients with gunshot wounds have also been managed by serial observation, though generally in conjunction with some other modality, usually CT. The length of observation varies by institution. Standard practice is usually a 24-hour observation period, but recent data suggest that all important injuries will become apparent within a 12-hour period.[16] Until more data are available or a clear institutional protocol has been established, approximately 24 hours of observation seems appropriate.

## DIAGNOSTIC MODALITIES

### PLAIN RADIOGRAPHY

Although plain abdominal radiography rarely adds to the evaluation of patients with blunt abdominal trauma, in cases of penetrating trauma with projectiles or retained foreign bodies it allows one to account for bullets, shrapnel, and foreign bodies. If all foreign bodies are not accounted for, one must consider the possibility that the foreign body is intraluminal or intravascular and a potential source of emboli. In patients with stab wounds or injuries without a foreign body, radiography's utility lies in ruling out a broken instrument in the abdomen or in evaluating a large amount of free air consistent with a hollow viscus injury.

In thoracoabdominal trauma, chest radiography can identify the presence of hemothorax, pneumothorax, and possibly diaphragmatic injury. Unfortunately, its sensitivity for pneumothorax is variable, and at least two separate radiographs 4 to 6 hours apart must be taken to exclude clinically significant pneumothorax. Diaphragmatic injuries are seen clearly on plain radiographs only about 30% of the time. They cannot be excluded on the basis of normal radiographic findings.

### ULTRASONOGRAPHY

Focused abdominal sonography for trauma (FAST) is a useful test if positive (i.e., free fluid is found during the examination). Several authors have shown specificity and positive predictive values in the low 90th percentile for therapeutic laparotomy if ultrasound reveals free fluid. A positive ultrasound finding after penetrating abdominal trauma should lead to exploration by either laparotomy or laparoscopy. Unfortunately, although its specificity is very high, its sensitivity ranges from 21% to 70%, which is not acceptable to rule out an injury requiring laparotomy.[17-21] Therefore, FAST findings negative for free fluid should be considered indeterminate, and further observation or testing is required. FAST should be able, in trained hands, to rule out significant pericardial effusion after thoracoabdominal trauma.

## COMPUTED TOMOGRAPHY

The expanded use of CT is a major change in the initial evaluation of patients with penetrating trauma in the past decade. In the past, use of CT had been limited in patients with penetrating abdominal trauma because of the high incidence of bowel injury and its lack of sensitivity in diagnosing bowel and mesenteric injuries, as well as rents in the diaphragm. The newest-generation CT scanners (i.e., multidetector scanners), as well as increased familiarity with their use, have markedly improved resolution and diagnostic capabilities. It is generally agreed that CT scanning of stab wounds in stable patients without the need for immediate laparotomy is a useful approach and can obviate admission when the wound is found to be superficial. In addition, it may reveal the path of a knife, identify or rule out peritoneal violation, and show with increasing sensitivity signs of hollow viscus perforation (free intraperitoneal air, unexplained free fluid, or bowel edema). These signs remain excellent in diagnosing solid organ injury. In addition, CT may show a "contrast blush," a sign of active bleeding or false aneurysms in patients with solid organ injuries, and may establish whether early laparotomy or angiographic intervention is warranted.[22] Although the negative predictive value of the need for operative intervention is high, patients with peritoneal penetration and no other clear operative requirements still merit an overnight observation period. In the case of gunshot wounds the literature is a bit less clear, but it generally shows that for tangential wounds in a stable patient, CT is excellent for ruling out abdominal penetration.

Even though it has not been shown to have high enough sensitivity to rule out diaphragmatic injuries, CT has improved and may one day be useful for this role.[21] CT is now accepted for use in stable patients with penetrating flank trauma. "Triple-contrast" (intravenous, oral, rectal) CT has been found to be highly sensitive in diagnosing injuries to retroperitoneal structures, including bowel and renal injuries. At this time, however, its sensitivity is too low to fully exclude a bowel injury, and a negative CT scan should be followed by a period of observation, usually 24 hours. The one caveat is that it should be clear on CT that the wound track is superficial and that no intraperitoneal or retroperitoneal penetration has occurred.

## DIAGNOSTIC PERITONEAL LAVAGE

Though not practiced as commonly as in the past, diagnostic peritoneal lavage (DPL) is still a useful and acceptable screening tool for penetrating abdominal trauma. In unstable patients with blunt trauma, it has been supplanted by ultrasonography. With penetrating trauma, its major benefit is its high sensitivity in screening for intraabdominal penetration and injury to abdominal structures. The main drawback, in addition to a small but real number of complications, is its lack of specificity. That is, DPL tends to diagnose injuries that may be treated by observation alone. For this reason, DPL is sometimes used in patients with penetrating trauma in conjunction with less invasive (in comparison with laparotomy) procedures such as laparoscopy. It is still not entirely clear where it best fits in the overall algorithm and is probably best reserved for patients with equivocal findings on examination or concern for diaphragmatic injuries. One recent multicenter study looking at the various diagnostic options for penetrating abdominal trauma found that in stable patients, DPL did not perform markedly better than admission and serial examination.[17] In patients with penetrating trauma who are hemodynamically unstable, it is not usually required to confirm what is already a high pretest probability that surgery is required. It may be of use, however, in patients with other possible causes of instability, especially in those with thoracoabdominal trauma, although it does not screen for retroperitoneal injuries.

A grossly bloody lavage effluent (10 mL of blood on initial aspiration) is always considered positive, although even with this finding, some surgeons will not operate immediately. If the effluent is not bloody on initial aspiration, 1 L of normal saline is instilled and then drained, and the effluent is sent to the laboratory for analysis. In patients with penetrating anterior abdominal wounds, lavage is always considered positive if the aspirate contains food particles, bile, or urine.

Cell counts tend to be a bit more controversial in that no cell count value is universally accepted to be indicative of a positive lavage result. If one is looking for penetration only, which may be useful when assessing gunshot wounds or diaphragm injuries, some institutions use as little as $1000/mm^3$; a more common and specific value, however, is $10,000/mm^3$. Although some centers use the cell count as an indication for laparotomy, others consider it complementary to observation or use CT or laparoscopy, depending on the wound. When assessing anterior abdominal wounds for injury and not just penetration, many institutions consider a cell count between $50,000/mm^3$ and $100,000/mm^3$ to be positive; a white blood cell count greater than $500/mm^3$ has also been used. However, these values do not seem to be particularly sensitive or specific.[23] Alkaline phosphatase and amylase lavage effluent levels have been advocated, but it is not clear that they add much to the standard criteria.[24]

## LAPAROSCOPY

Minimally invasive laparoscopic surgery has gained general acceptance as a diagnostic and therapeutic modality in several circumstances. Although the specific injury may not always be identified, laparoscopy appears to be highly specific in identifying the need for therapeutic laparotomy. More important, in many instances it can rule out the need for laparotomy completely with a high degree of sensitivity. Its most accepted use is for low-velocity wounds when diaphragmatic injury (i.e., wounds involving the left thoracoabdominal area) is a possibility. It is also a reasonable tool to use in stable patients with anterior abdominal wounds to screen for peritoneal penetration and the need for laparotomy. The overall benefit, however, in this group of patient, over less invasive approaches such as serial examination, has not been well proven. It may be used in the operating room as an initial intervention in a stable patient with penetrating abdominal trauma and equivocal findings on physical examination. It allows a survey of the abdominal contents, repair of minor injuries, and possible avoidance of laparotomy with its associated complications. Its major drawbacks are its relative invasiveness, need for general anesthesia, and cost, as well as some literature showing suboptimal sensitivity for hollow viscus injury.[25-27]

## DIAGNOSTIC TESTING FOR SPECIFIC INJURIES

### *Anterior Stab Wounds*

In patients with anterior stab wounds, the first step is to decide whether peritoneal penetration has occurred. This may be accomplished by local wound exploration, DPL, or CT. If lavage or local exploration is clearly negative, no further management other than local wound care is indicated. If lavage or CT shows peritoneal penetration but no indication for emergency surgery, options include laparoscopy, laparotomy, and serial observation. Depending on the center, all may be appropriate, although laparoscopy or serial observation provides the best risk-benefit balance. For observation to be successful, patients must be able to cooperate with serial examinations and have evidence of continued hemodynamic stability, and peritonitis should not develop. Prolonged observation is rarely possible in the ED, and these patients are generally admitted to a surgical service where serial examinations are possible.

### Flank Wounds

Flank wounds require triple-contrast CT scanning. If the results are negative, a period of observation is standard. In patients with a left-sided thoracoabdominal wound, a negative ED work-up is often followed by laparoscopy to exclude an occult diaphragmatic injury. Patients who have stab wounds in the flank or back and are stable without obvious signs of bowel injury (peritonitis, hypotension) should undergo triple-contrast CT scanning of the abdomen and pelvis. If the results are negative, such patients should be admitted for 24-hour observation, as previously described.

### Gunshot Wounds

It is common and acceptable to explore all gunshot wounds that penetrate the peritoneum. If it is unclear whether penetration has taken place, a plain film radiograph may show an intraperitoneal bullet. Alternatively, DPL with appropriate cell counts is sensitive for intraperitoneal penetration. A positive FAST finding with free fluid in the abdomen should prompt operative exploration. Although serial physical examinations have been advocated, this is usually performed in conjunction with an intravenous or oral contrast-enhanced (or both) CT scan of the abdomen and pelvis. CT has been shown to be effective in stable patients with tangential gunshot wounds to rule out intraperitoneal penetration. If it is clear that penetration of the peritoneum did not occur, the patient may be discharged. If penetration occurred, the patient may remain under observation or may undergo laparotomy or possibly laparoscopy or angiography, depending on the injury complex.

### Other Injuries

ISOLATED BOWEL INJURIES Patients with bowel injury alone or injury to the liver or spleen without significant bleeding may have minimal symptoms initially. Given that hollow viscus injury is much more common with penetrating trauma than with blunt trauma, the EP must search for these sometimes subtle or delayed findings. Tenderness at the wound site is normal, but peritoneal findings such as diffuse tenderness and muscular rigidity, regardless of stability, are generally indicative of the need for operative intervention.[28] These findings may become apparent several hours into a patient's course if the injury involves rupture of a hollow viscus. Over time, intraperitoneal inflammation increases, stimulates somatic pain fibers, and becomes evident clinically.

DIAPHRAGMATIC INJURIES Diaphragmatic injuries may have dramatic findings but can also be occult and be accompanied by symptoms or even fatal complications years after the initial injury. Any patient with a thoracoabdominal injury may have a diaphragmatic injury. The rate of diaphragmatic injury varies from 7% to 42% in patients with penetrating thoracoabdominal trauma. The diagnostic rate varies with the aggressiveness of evaluation; if it is not looked for, many diaphragmatic injuries will be missed. It tends to be highest in patients with left costal penetration.[25,26,29] Most left-sided tears can be repaired surgically. A small right-sided tear may not need to be repaired because herniation is much less likely on this side as a result of protection by the liver. In cases of potential left diaphragmatic injury, laparoscopy or DPL is a reasonable addition to the diagnostic approach.

## TREATMENT

Most interventions and procedures in patients with penetrating trauma (**Table 80.1**) are aimed at first determining whether intraabdominal penetration occurred and, if so, deciding

**Table 80.1** Options for Evaluation

| DIAGNOSTIC MODALITIES | ADVANTAGES | DISADVANTAGES |
|---|---|---|
| Local wound exploration | Inexpensive bedside test; if negative, can discharge the patient | Operator dependent; may be inconclusive; not good for gunshot wounds or impalement |
| Ultrasonography | Inexpensive bedside test; high positive predictive value (90%) for therapeutic laparotomy | Operator dependent; poor sensitivity for bowel injury; if negative, cannot exclude injury |
| Diagnostic peritoneal lavage | Highly sensitive, inexpensive; can diagnose small bowel and diaphragm injuries | Poor specificity; up to 25% negative laparotomies when using lower limits of red blood cell counts |
| Computed tomography | Excellent for solid organ injuries; can often show lack of peritoneal penetration and obviate the need for observation; test of choice for flank and back injuries because it shows the retroperitoneal structures | Expensive; requires radiation; variable sensitivity for bowel and diaphragm injuries; unless penetration of the peritoneum is clearly excluded, observation is required afterward |
| Laparoscopy | Test of choice for left-sided thoracoabdominal wounds; can exclude peritoneal penetration and also screen for more serious injury; can be used for repair in selected cases | Expensive; associated complications; requires operating room |

whether the patient can avoid a nontherapeutic laparotomy. The options are varied and may be performed alone or in series depending on the test, findings, and local custom. Although mandatory exploration was once the paradigm for penetrating injuries, knowledge of significant morbidity from negative laparotomy has pushed surgeons toward a much more conservative approach to management.[22,30,31]

Exploration requires aseptic technique, good overhead lighting, and local lidocaine and epinephrine anesthesia. Inserting a digit or cotton swab into the wound is not an acceptable alternative. Obese or noncooperative patients and those with abdominal scarring from previous operations are not optimal candidates. Paralleling the natural skin lines, the wound is enlarged as necessary so that the posterior fascia may be evaluated. If penetration of the anterior fascia has occurred or if the wound exploration is inconclusive, the wound is considered intraperitoneal and must be evaluated further by more invasive methods or by observation and serial examinations. A recent multicenter observational study suggested that serial examinations are a safe option. Operative evaluation based solely on penetration would lead to a high number of nontherapeutic laparotomies (57%).[17] If the fascia is clearly intact, the wound can be irrigated and closed by primary intention if clean and the patient discharged. Alternatively, the initial wound can be closed by secondary intention or delayed primary closure.[23]

## FLUID RESUSCITATION

Resuscitation of hypotensive patients remains a widely discussed and controversial area of treatment. The advanced trauma life support standard treatment is to administer 2 L of intravenous fluid followed by transfusion of blood; however, some EPs and surgeons prefer to limit resuscitation until definitive control is obtained[32,33] because of concerns that elevation in blood pressure through aggressive administration of fluids may disrupt clots and clotting factors, as well as evidence in multiple animal studies that less aggressive resuscitation or "permissive hypotension" leads to improved outcomes.

Two well-done large prospective trials have been carried out in humans, a study of penetrating torso injuries by Bickell et al. and a study of a combination of blunt and penetrating injuries by Dutton et al.[32,34] The Bickell trial enrolled 598 patients with penetrating trauma and a systolic blood pressure of 90 mm Hg or lower. The authors found a trend toward lower mortality and morbidity in the minimally resuscitated patients, although the "appropriately resuscitated" patients—or those with standard high fluid volume—had blood pressure values that were significantly higher after resuscitation but before surgery. The Dutton study[32] of approximately 100 patients compared the outcomes of actively bleeding patients treated via the standard resuscitation protocol with the outcomes of patients treated with a "hypotensive resuscitation" protocol consisting of a target systolic blood pressure of 70 mm Hg. Neither the standard group nor the hypotensive group showed improvements in mortality or worse outcomes; however, there was difficulty reaching the target blood pressures. In the authors' judgment, limiting resuscitation with normal saline and blood to reach a target systolic blood pressure of around 90 mm Hg appears to be reasonable. Moving more rapidly to blood replacement rather than excessive saline is probably a reasonable approach also. In patients with massive blood loss, the current literature suggests blood replacement protocols with increased use of platelets and clotting factors, although the exact ratios remain unclear and somewhat controversial.[35,36] It may not be feasible, appropriate, or beneficial to allow the blood pressure to decrease much lower.

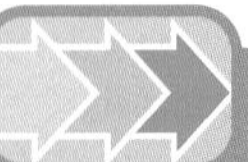

**PRIORITY ACTIONS**

- Immediate attention to the ABCs (airway, breathing, and circulation)
- Immediate transport to the operating room for diffuse peritonitis or hemodynamic stability
- Evaluation of stable patients with local wound exploration when possible to exclude peritoneal penetration
- Admission if penetration has occurred or evaluation is unclear
- Antibiotics if surgery is planned
- Documentation of the location and appearance of all wounds
- Consultation with a trauma practitioner or general surgeon
- Exclusion of pulmonary, diaphragm, or cardiac injury

## ANTIBIOTICS

Despite the dearth of high-quality prospective research to support the practice, most expert opinion and guidelines recommend that antibiotics be administered to any patient with a penetrating injury who will undergo operative intervention. The antibiotics are generally continued for 24 hours postoperatively. Perioperative antimicrobial coverage directed against skin and enteric flora will decrease postoperative wound infections. A single agent with broad-spectrum aerobic and anaerobic coverage is recommended. Alternatively, combination therapy with clindamycin or cefazolin and an aminoglycoside is appropriate. Patients allergic to cephalosporin or penicillin may receive vancomycin instead for gram-positive coverage.[37]

No clear guidelines have been established for patients with wounds that have not penetrated the peritoneum and who will not undergo surgery. Essential to decreasing wound infection is high-pressure irrigation. It may be reasonable to offer a 5-day course of prophylactic antibiotics to patients who have significant devitalized tissue or irretrievable foreign bodies. It is more judicious to allow closure of these wounds by secondary or delayed primary intention.

## TETANUS PROPHYLAXIS

Because of the rarity of the disease and successful public health measures, clinical tetanus is exceedingly rare in the United States. Only one case of a traumatic gunshot wound was reported to cause tetanus in the United States between 1998 and 2000. Penetrating trauma may carry *Clostridium tetani* into the wound, but most patients born in the United States are properly immunized. A prospective observational case series in 2004 found a 90.2% seroprevalence of tetanus immunity in 1988 patients with acute wounds seen in five U.S. urban EDs. Elderly patients and those from outside North America or western Europe are at higher risk. Mexican Americans between 20 and 44 years of age who were born outside the United States appear to be at higher risk. Most cases worldwide are due to neonatal tetanus.[38]

If they have not received a tetanus shot within the previous 10 years, patients with stab or gunshot wounds should be treated with tetanus toxoid. All patients not previously fully immunized or with unclear status should be given both tetanus toxoid and tetanus immunoglobulin. It is not always necessary to give the booster in the ED because it may be administered up to several days after the injury. However, it is often preferable because tetanus immunization may not be part of the usual care in the hospital or outpatient setting.

## PAIN CONTROL

Although pain control is generally thought to be appropriate and safe in patients with nontraumatic abdominal pain, little scientific literature is available to guide the treatment of patients with traumatic injury when observation is planned.

It seems clear that in a patient who will require operative intervention, withholding pain control offers no diagnostic benefit. Care should be taken, however, before giving large doses of pain medication that may decrease the blood pressure or when treating patients with preexisting shock. Fentanyl, titrated appropriately, may be a better choice than morphine sulfate in these patients because of its better hemodynamic profile.

# FOLLOW-UP, NEXT STEPS IN CARE, AND PATIENT EDUCATION

Final disposition is usually based on the location of the injury, the implement used, the patient's hemodynamic status, and the EP's and surgeon's preferred evaluation methods. As discussed previously, several different approaches can be taken, from conservative observation to aggressive operative approaches. As is true with all trauma, the ABCs (airway, breathing, and circulation) are the first line in management. In general, patients with evidence of signs of shock or diffuse peritoneal findings should be taken to the operating room. The one final caveat is that patients who may have concomitant cardiac or pulmonary injuries should have them ruled out as a source of the hypotension.

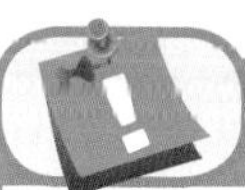

### TIPS AND TRICKS

- Always undress the patient fully and examine the back, axilla, and groin areas for occult penetrating trauma.
- Always account for all bullets in cases of penetrating trauma (e.g., if only one wound is present, the bullet should still be inside the body).
- In general, the number of bullets and the number of entrance and exit wounds should add to an even number. For example, a single wound would suggest that a bullet is still in the body (1 bullet + 1 wound = 2). Three wounds suggest either one or three bullets in the body (2 entrance wounds + 1 exit wound + 1 bullet = 4; 3 entrance wounds + 3 bullets = 6).
- Ultrasonography can always be used to rapidly distinguish hypovolemic shock from distributive shock by looking for collapse of the inferior vena cava with inspiration.
- Penetrating trauma is a reportable injury in most of the United States. Make sure that your emergency department is in compliance with local laws.
- A single chest radiograph cannot exclude pneumothorax with a thoracoabdominal wound.
- Negative results on ultrasonography have little predictive value with penetrating abdominal trauma; however, positive findings on ultrasonography have high predictive value for therapeutic laparotomy.

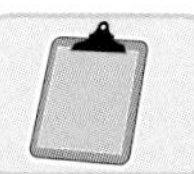

### DOCUMENTATION

**History**

- Record the time of injury, number of assailants, gunshots, and so on, if known.
- List all field interventions.

**Physical Examination**

- Document all wounds. Do not document as "entrance and exit" but as specific areas. Draw simple picture of the wounds.
- Consider having police or security in the hospital take photographs of the injuries.
- Document that the patient was completely examined, including the groin, back, and perineal and axillary regions.

**Treatment**

- Document all interventions and response to treatment. If the patient is to be transferred, document reasons for the decision, as well as the name of the accepting physician. Document whether the surgical service is involved and the time of call and arrival.
- Document all radiologic tests and results.
- Document procedure notes for all significant interventions (e.g., wound exploration, chest thoracostomy, diagnostic peritoneal lavage).
- Save and bag all clothing removed from the patient.

# SUGGESTED READINGS

Bickell WH, Wall Jr MJ, Pepe PE, et al. Immediate versus delayed fluid resuscitation for hypotensive patients with penetrating torso injuries. N Engl J Med 1994;331:1105-9.

Biffl W, Kaups K, Cothren CC. Management of patients with anterior abdominal stab wounds: a Western Trauma Association Multicenter Trial. J Trauma 2009;66:1294-301.

Como J, Bokhari F, Chiu W, et al. Practice management guidelines for selective nonoperative management of penetrating abdominal trauma. J Trauma 2010;68:721-33.

Quinn AC, Sinert R. What is the utility of the Focused Assessment with Sonography in trauma (FAST) exam in penetrating torso trauma? Injury 2011;42:482-7.

Udobi KF, Rodriguez A, Chiu WC, et al. Role of ultrasonography in penetrating abdominal trauma: a prospective clinical study. J Trauma 2001;50:475-9.

# REFERENCES

***References can be found on Expert Consult @ www.expertconsult.com.***

# 81 Pelvic Fractures

*Leigh A. Patterson*

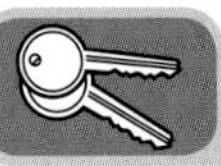

**KEY POINTS**

- Approximately 70% of patients with a traumatically disrupted pelvic ring will have a major associated injury.
- If a patient has displacement of 0.5 cm at any fracture site in the pelvis or has an "open book" pelvic fracture, massive transfusion may be needed.
- Blood loss from open book pelvic fractures and vertical shear injuries can be life-threatening.
- Emergency binding of the pelvis can help reduce pelvic volume and tamponade the bleeding. Binding the fractured pelvis too tightly should be avoided.
- Interventional radiology can embolize the vessels.

## EPIDEMIOLOGY

Fractures of the bony pelvis account for 3% of all fractures; however, the overall mortality from pelvic ring injuries is 10% to 15%. Motor vehicle collisions (MVCs) involving cars or cars and pedestrians cause approximately 60% of pelvic fractures.[1] Side-impact car collisions more commonly cause pelvic fractures than do head-on car collisions.[2] Falls and motorcycle accidents are also significant causes of pelvic ring injuries.

The blood supply and innervation of the pelvic organs and lower extremities are intimately linked to the pelvic architecture. Major disruptions lead to life-threatening blood loss, damage to urogenital organs, and neurologic deficits. The emergency physician (EP) must identify patients at risk for pelvic ring disruption and aggressively work to control bleeding.

## PATHOPHYSIOLOGY

The pelvis provides support for upright mobility by connecting the spine to the lower extremities. When viewed as a whole, the pelvis contains a major ring and two inferior rings. The triangular sacrum and two innominate bones form the major pelvic ring (**Fig. 81.1**). The sacrum is a fusion of the five sacral vertebrae and distributes the weight of the upper part of the body to the innominate bones. The sacrum also conducts the sacral nerve roots to the pelvic organs. Each innominate bone is a fusion of the ilium, ischium, and pubic bones. The intersection of the fusion forms the acetabulum, which articulates with the femur. Posteriorly, the innominate bones are anchored to the sacrum by the anterior and posterior iliac ligaments, two of the body's strongest ligaments. The sacrotuberous and sacrospinous ligaments attach the sacrum to the ischial tuberosity and the ischial spines bilaterally, thus further reinforcing the posterior arch of the pelvic ring.

Anteriorly, the innominate bones are anchored to each other at the cartilaginous pubic symphysis. Because the innominates and sacrum are dense bone anchored together with equally dense connective tissue, disruption of the architecture of the major pelvic ring requires tremendous force and usually results in bony fractures or ligamentous disruptions at two or more sites in the ring. The inferior rings are formed by the pubic and ischial rami. They serve as attachments for muscles of the thighs and do not bear weight from the upper part of the body. Low-force mechanisms such as straddle injuries and falls onto the buttocks can fracture the rings, usually an isolated pubic ramus.

The left and right internal iliac arteries course in the region of the sacroiliac joints; they branch and form a network of vessels in the posterior pelvic arch. Posteriorly, the superior gluteal artery is commonly injured. Throughout the pelvis, arteries and veins are easily injured during the impact that causes the pelvic fracture, and blood collects in the retroperitoneal space.

*Lateral compression*, caused by injuries involving the side, crushes the pelvis inward; therefore, massive pelvic bleeding is uncommon with these types of injury. Sacral crush fractures and horizontal pubic ramus fractures can be diagnosed radiographically. Sacroiliac diastasis may also occur.

*Anteroposterior compression* forces cause the iliac wings to rotate outward, as when a pedestrian is struck directly anteriorly or posteriorly by a car. The fractures are unstable and pelvic volume increases, which allows massive retroperitoneal venous or arterial pelvic bleeding to occur. Diastasis of the anterior pelvic ring may be evident and is often termed an open book pelvic fracture. The posterior ligaments (as a guiding principle) can withstand about 2.5 cm of symphyseal diastasis before the sacral ligaments are disrupted. Associated acetabular fractures are commonly present in about half of cases.

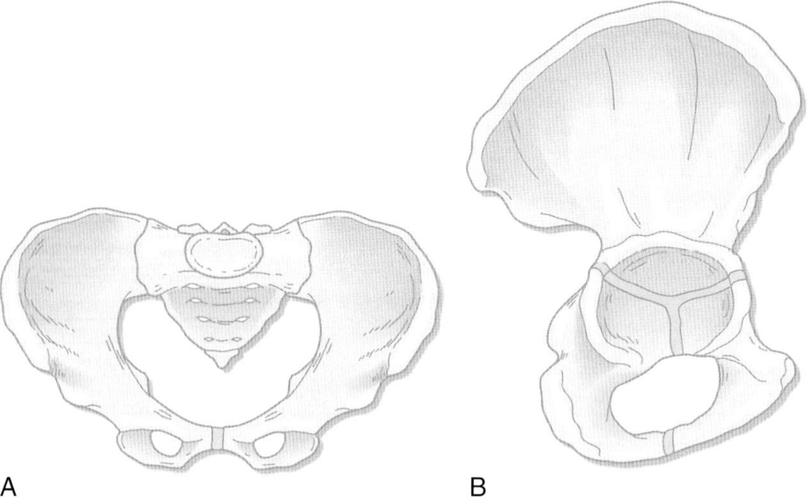


**Fig. 81.1 Bony pelvis. A,** Anteroposterior view. **B,** Innominate bone (lateral view).

**BOX 81.1 Most Common and Most Threatening Pelvic Fractures***

**Most Common**
Inferior pubic ramus fractures (type A)
Avulsion fractures (type A)
Lateral compression fractures (type B)

**Most Threatening**
Open book pelvic fractures (type B)
Type C fractures

*See "Tile Classification of Pelvic Fractures" in text for discussion of types of fractures.

*Vertical shear* injuries are less common and result from axial force through the legs or spine to the pelvis. The anterior and posterior rings are both disrupted. As the hemipelvis is forcibly sheared, pelvic volume increases, which results in massive bleeding.

Several classification schemes involving the direction of force applied to the pelvis, the bones injured, the degree of instability of the ring, and any associated injuries are used for pelvic ring disruptions. Fracture stability and increases in pelvic volume determine the magnitude of blood loss and potential mortality. See **Box 81.1**.

## TILE CLASSIFICATION OF PELVIC FRACTURES

The Tile classification adopted by the Orthopedic Trauma Association[3] describes pelvic fractures by the degree of stability. The type and degree of stability predict outcome and associated injuries (see Box 81.1). Type A fractures are stable and include avulsion fractures and isolated fractures of an inferior pubic ramus, iliac wing, or distal sacrum. These fractures cause local pain but do involve the major pelvic ring.

Type B and C fractures are unstable fractures resulting from high-energy force. In both types the pelvic ring is disrupted in two or more places. These disruptions can consist of any combination of fractures and ligament tears. Disruptions may be unilateral, with involvement of only one hemipelvis, or bilateral, with one or more disruptions in both hemipelves.

Type B fractures are vertically stable but rotationally unstable. These ring disruptions usually involve anterior structures, the superior pubic rami and pubic symphysis and the anterior iliac ligaments. The sacrum and the posterior iliac ligaments are spared. Lateral trauma from a side-impact MVC or anteroposterior trauma from a frontal-impact MVC can cause fractures in this class. The axis of a bony fracture is determined by the orientation of the force applied to the pelvis.

Type C fractures are both vertically and rotationally unstable because the posterior elements of the major pelvic ring are disrupted by a fracture through the sacroiliac joint, which is a complete tear. In addition to lateral and anteroposterior forces, vertical shear mechanisms, including falls, can cause type C fractures.

Avulsion fractures of the pelvis at muscle insertion sites are caused by forced contraction of the thigh muscles when moving the hip.[4] The apophyses at the anterior superior iliac spine, the anterior inferior iliac spine, and the ischial tuberosity fuse between the ages of 16 and 25. Adolescent athletes involved in strenuous sports are vulnerable to these injuries. EPs should suspect these injuries based on the mechanism of injury (**Table 81.1**).

## PRESENTING SIGNS AND SYMPTOMS

The classic findings in patients with a major pelvic ring disruption include a chief complaint of pelvic pain or pain with movement at the hips.[5] However, nearly 70% of patients with disruption of the major pelvic ring have associated injuries, such as closed head trauma, blunt chest and abdominal trauma, and long-bone fractures,[1] that may mask the symptoms of pelvic pain.

The EP should first suspect a pelvic fracture based on the mechanism of injury and then search for additional signs of

**Table 81.1 Avulsion Pelvic Fractures**

| FRACTURE SITE | MUSCLE INVOLVED | TYPE OF SPORT | HIP MOVEMENT | INITIAL TREATMENT | HEALING TIME |
|---|---|---|---|---|---|
| ASIS | Sartorius | Soccer | Flexion, abduction | Limit weight bearing with crutches | 10 wk |
| AIIS | Rectus femoris | Sprint runner<br>Kicking | Forced flexion in the starting block<br>Hyperextension of the hip with knee flexion | Bed rest with the rectus femoris relaxed (hip and knee flexed) | 6 wk |
| Ischial tuberosity | Hamstring | Hurdler, long jumper, gymnast | Forced extension at the hip | Bed rest | 12 wk |

*AIIS*, Anterior inferior iliac spine; *ASIS*, anterior superior iliac spine.

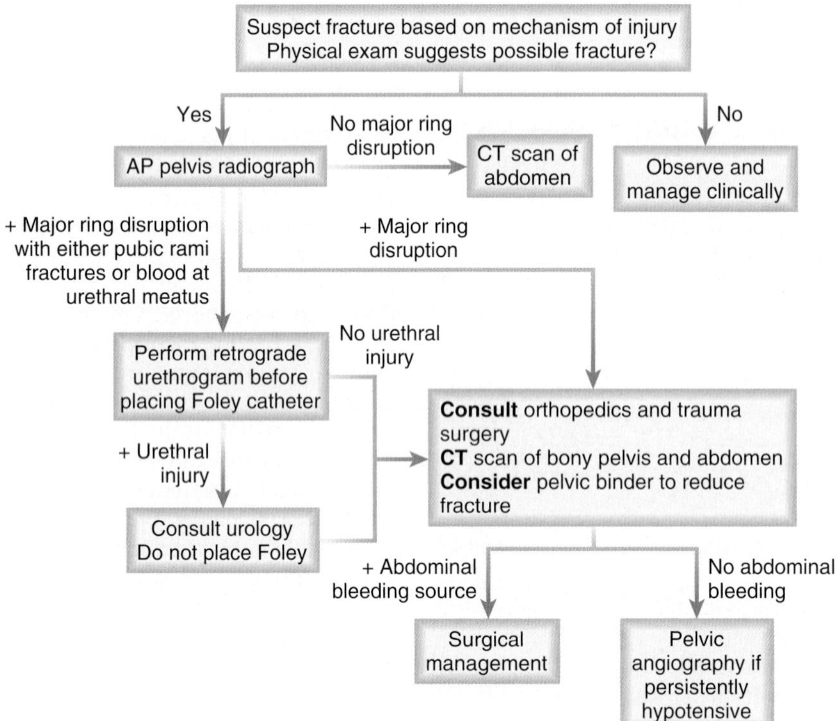


**Fig. 81.2 Diagnostic and treatment approach to a patient with suspected disruption of the major pelvic ring.** *AP*, Anteroposterior; *CT*, computed tomography.

fracture during the physical examination. Uneven leg length or asymmetry of the iliac wings may indicate a pelvic fracture. The perineum is carefully exposed to visualize any flank ecchymoses, scrotal or labial hematomas, and blood at the urethral meatus. When examining the pelvis, the EP should assume that it is fractured and avoid actions that may distract or displace a fracture. The iliac wings are gently palpated and compressed medially. The pubic symphysis is palpated anteriorly, and the sacrum and sacroiliac joints are palpated posteriorly. The rectum is examined for tone; in females, a manual vaginal examination is performed to check for bone protruding into the vagina.

If no obvious fractures of the lower extremities are found, the femurs are rotated at the hips to assess for pain in the acetabula. Pain elicited by physical examination is 98% sensitive and 94% specific for predicting fracture of the posterior aspect of the pelvic ring.[6]

## DIFFERENTIAL DIAGNOSIS AND MEDICAL DECISION MAKING

**Figure 81.2** outlines a diagnostic and treatment approach to patients with suspected pelvic ring disruption.

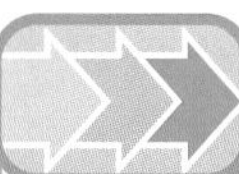

PRIORITY ACTIONS

**RESCUE Pelvis Mnemonic for the Treatment of Patients with Pelvic Fractures**

**Resuscitate the Patient**
ATLS protocols, IV fluids, pain control

**Examine and Obtain Radiographs of the Pelvis and Perineum**
Signs of pelvic fracture or instability, urethral injury, neurologic injury

**Stabilize the Pelvic Ring**
Circumferential sheet, commercial pelvic binder

**Consult Trauma, Orthopedics, and Urology**
Consult early

**Evaluate for Nonpelvic Sources of Bleeding**
FAST, DPL, CT of the abdomen

**Pelvis Angiography**
Persistent hypotension despite stabilization efforts

*ATLS*, Advanced trauma life support; *CT*, computed tomography; *DPL*, diagnostic peritoneal lavage; *FAST*, focused assessment with sonography for trauma.

## TREATMENT

Pelvic fractures need to be reduced rapidly and fixated to prevent ongoing blood loss and promote healing. Reduction of a major pelvic ring disruption should increase interstitial pressure in the pelvis and at the bony surfaces of a fracture to tamponade any venous bleeding. Pelvic volume is also directly related to diastasis at the sites of ligamentous disruption, namely, the pubic symphysis and sacroiliac joints. A 1-cm widening of the pubic symphysis allows pelvic volume to expand 4.6%. A combined 8-cm widening of the pubic symphysis and sacroiliac joints would allow potentially 500 mL of blood to accumulate in the pelvis before the soft tissues even begin to tamponade the bleeding.[7]

Prehospital providers should obtain large-bore intravenous access and immobilize the patient on a long spine board.

Initially, the EP can reduce the fracture by applying a sheet circumferentially around the pelvis and tying it so that pelvic volume is reduced (**Figs. 81.3 to 81.5**). Commercial binders can be applied in the same manner. Such reduction works best for fractures with external rotation of one or both hemipelves, such as an open book pelvic fracture.[8] The EP should be careful to not overcorrect the external rotation by binding the pelvis too tightly. Overcorrection could force sharp bony fragments into the pelvic vasculature and organs.

Orthopedic surgery should be consulted early for reduction of pelvic ring disruptions. Circumferential binding is a temporary reduction and will not stabilize a vertically unstable fracture. Patients with ongoing blood loss may need external fixators to stabilize the ring.

Bleeding can be life-threatening, and the posterior pelvic venous plexus accounts for more than 80% of hemorrhages.[9]

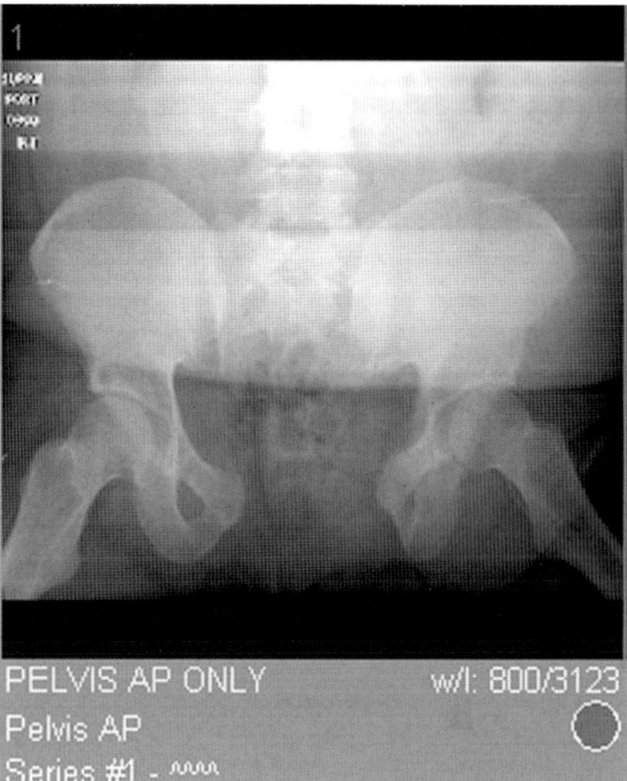


**Fig. 81.3** Open book pelvic fracture.

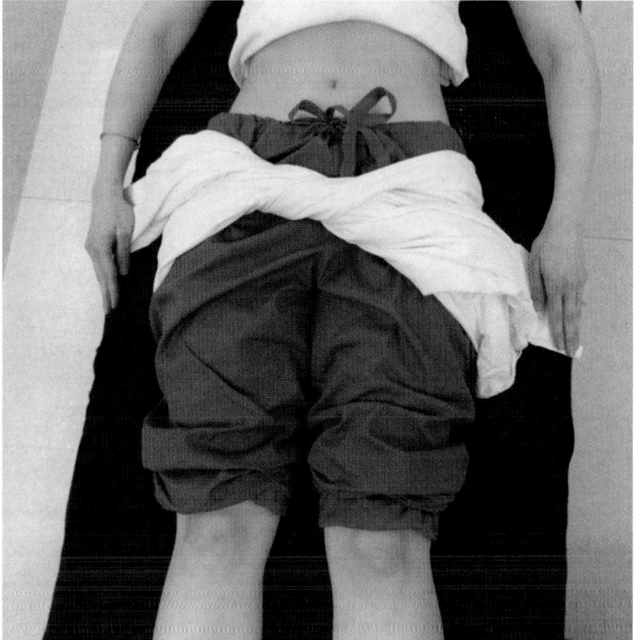

**Fig. 81.4** Sheet binder application.

Early transfusion is indicated, particularly for patients with vertical shear or anteroposterior compression fractures. If a patient has 0.5-cm displacement at any fracture site in the pelvis or an open book pelvic fracture, massive transfusion will probably be needed. Patients who are persistently

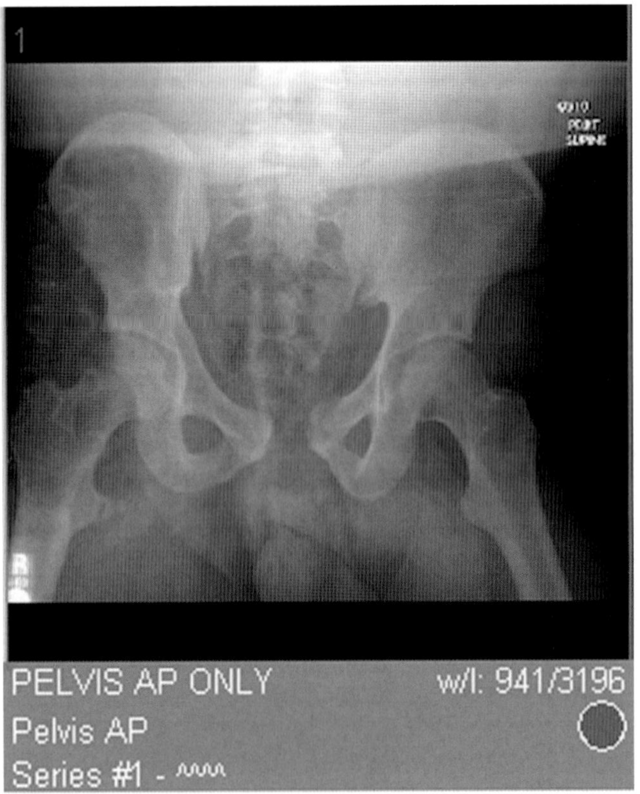


**Fig. 81.5** Binder reduction of an open book pelvic fracture.

hypotensive despite fixation and transfusion may have an arterial bleeding source. Interventional radiology for embolization of the bleeding vessels can be lifesaving.[9]

For avulsion fractures, initial treatment is supportive, and physical activity is resumed slowly over a period of weeks to prevent repeated avulsion.[5] After pain control has been achieved, these patients can be discharged home with follow-up by their primary care physician.

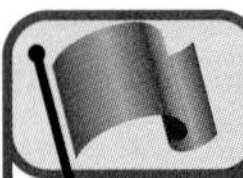

**RED FLAGS**

Mortality in patients with hemorrhagic shock from a pelvic fracture is about 50%.

Patients who undergo repair of major pelvic ring injuries may have chronic pelvic pain and typical operative complications, including infection and bleeding.

Concomitant head, chest, and abdominal injuries will contribute to the overall complication rate of pelvic fractures.

## FOLLOW-UP, NEXT STEPS IN CARE, AND PATIENT EDUCATION

Patients with unstable pelvic fractures will need to be admitted to a surgical intensive care unit for close hemodynamic and neurologic monitoring. Because many of these patients will have additional head, chest, abdomen, and limb injuries, they are best managed primarily by a trauma surgeon in consultation with orthopedists, vascular surgeons, urologists, and interventional radiologists. If multidisciplinary trauma services are not available at the initial facility, the EP must stabilize the patient and arrange emergency critical care transport for these patients to a designated trauma center.

Patients with single ring disruptions who are able to bear weight and ambulate with minimal assistance may be discharged home with pain control and referral to physical therapy. If they are unable to bear weight, they may need admission to a primary care service for physical and occupational therapy consultation.

Follow-up should also be scheduled with a sports medicine specialist or orthopedic surgeon who will monitor healing and guide the patient's return to athletic activity.

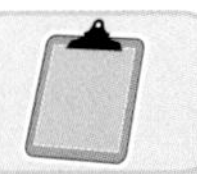

**DOCUMENTATION**

**History**

Mechanism of injury

Prehospital treatment and transport time

**Physical Examination**

Complete undressing and logrolling of the patient with special attention to the pelvis and perineum

Neurologic examination

Hemodynamic examination and any evidence of vascular injury

**Treatment**

Imaging modalities selected, plain films, computed tomography, and other modalities

Consideration of binder application if open book injury

Specialists consulted

If transfer to a trauma facility is indicated, documentation of indications for transfer, efforts to stabilize, and neurovascular status at the time of transfer

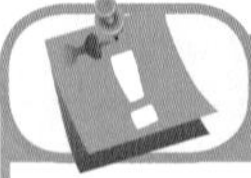

**TIPS AND TRICKS**

**Pelvic Binder Application**

To reduce the volume of an open book pelvic fracture, a bedsheet can be used in place of a commercial binder (see Fig. 81.4).

Fold the sheet lengthwise into thirds. Logroll the patient to place the sheet or binder posterior to the pelvis.

The superior edge of the sheet should be just inferior to both iliac crests. The umbilicus or natural waist should not be covered by the sheet. The inferior edge should not extend below the lesser trochanter.

The sheet should be knotted anterior to the patient with enough torque to reduce the symphysis diastasis to *nearly* normal: 1 to 3 cm for many patients.

## SUGGESTED READINGS

Gonzalez RP, Fried PQ, Bukhalo M. The utility of clinical examination in screening for pelvic fractures in blunt trauma. J Am Coll Surg 2002;194:121-5.
Krieg JC, Mohr M, Ellis TJ, et al. Emergent stabilization of pelvic ring injuries by controlled circumferential compression: a clinical trial. J Trauma 2005;59:659-64.
McCormick JP, Morgan SJ, Smith WR. Clinical effectiveness of the physical examination in diagnosis of posterior pelvic ring injuries. J Orthop Trauma 2003;17:257-61.
Scopp JM, Moorman CT. Acute athletic trauma to the hip and pelvis. Orthop Clin North Am 2002;33:555-63.

## REFERENCES

***References can be found on Expert Consult @ www.expertconsult.com.***

# 82 Genitourinary Trauma

*Michael S. Runyon and Michael A. Gibbs*

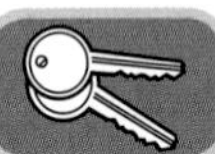

**KEY POINTS**

- Evaluate suspected genitourinary tract injuries in retrograde fashion; check for urethral disruption before bladder rupture and bladder rupture before ureteral or kidney injury.
- Suspect urethral injury in blunt trauma patients with a significant pelvic fracture, blood at the urethral meatus, gross hematuria, absent or abnormally positioned prostate on digital rectal examination, and ecchymosis or hematoma involving the penis, scrotum, or perineum.
- Evaluate urethral integrity by retrograde urethrography when urethral injury is suspected and a urinary catheter cannot easily be placed with a single gentle attempt.
- Suspect bladder rupture in blunt trauma patients with pelvic trauma and gross hematuria and in those sustaining a significant pelvic fracture.
- Suspect upper tract (kidney or ureter) injury in blunt trauma patients with gross hematuria or with microscopic hematuria when the patient has sustained a significant decelerating mechanism or exhibits hypotension.
- Suspect genitourinary involvement when any penetrating injury is inflicted in proximity to the genitourinary system.

## EPIDEMIOLOGY

Approximately 10% of trauma patients sustain injury to the genitourinary system. The majority of these injuries (approximately 80%) are the result of a blunt trauma mechanism. Timely identification and management of genitourinary injuries can minimize the associated morbidity, which may include impairment of urinary continence and sexual function. Identification of injury depends on a stepwise evaluation with consideration of the mechanism of injury, pertinent findings on physical examination, urinalysis, and appropriate diagnostic imaging performed in the correct sequence.

## PATHOPHYSIOLOGY

Anatomically, the genitourinary system is divided into lower and upper tracts. This division is clinically important because specific mechanisms tend to injure different parts of the genitourinary system. The lower genitourinary tract consists of the external genitalia, urethra, and bladder (**Figs. 82.1 and 82.2**). The upper genitourinary tract consists of the ureters and kidneys.

### EXTERNAL GENITALIA

The male external genitalia consist of the penis, scrotum, testicles, and ejaculatory complex. The female external genitalia consist of the vagina and vulva; the latter includes the labia majora, labia minora, and clitoris.

Injuries to the external genitalia may occur by blunt or penetrating mechanisms or by circulatory compromise induced by constricting devices applied either accidentally (as in the case of a hair tourniquet) or intentionally (e.g., to enhance sexual performance and pleasure). Additionally, the skin of the penis, scrotum, or labia may become ensnared by a metal zipper. Blunt trauma mechanisms include a kick or other direct blow to the genitals, falls, and straddle injuries. Penile fracture is a blunt injury that occurs when an erect penis is bent suddenly and forcefully, with rupture of the tunica albuginea of one or both of the corpora cavernosa. This injury occurs most commonly during sexual intercourse when the penis slips out of the vagina and strikes the partner's pubis or perineum, but it may also occur during masturbation. Significant injury to the external genitalia may accompany pelvic fractures. Penetrating injuries may be inflicted by gunshot wounds, knives, or other sharp objects.

### URETHRA

The male urethra is divided into anterior (bulbous and pendulous) and posterior (prostatic and membranous) portions. Traditionally, this division has been described at the level of the urogenital diaphragm; however, recent work has questioned the existence of this structure, as classically taught.[1-3] Regardless, the weakest point of the posterior urethra is the bulbomembranous junction, and it is the area where the majority of posterior urethral disruptions occur.[1]

Injuries to the anterior urethra occur from direct blows, straddle injuries, or instrumentation or in conjunction with a penile fracture (**Fig. 82.3**). By contrast, posterior urethral injuries usually occur in the setting of significant pelvic fractures, often caused by motor vehicle collisions (**Fig. 82.4**). Penetrating injuries may be inflicted by gunshot wounds, knives, or other sharp objects. Urethral injuries are much less common in women because the female urethra is short and relatively mobile and lacks significant attachment to the pubis.

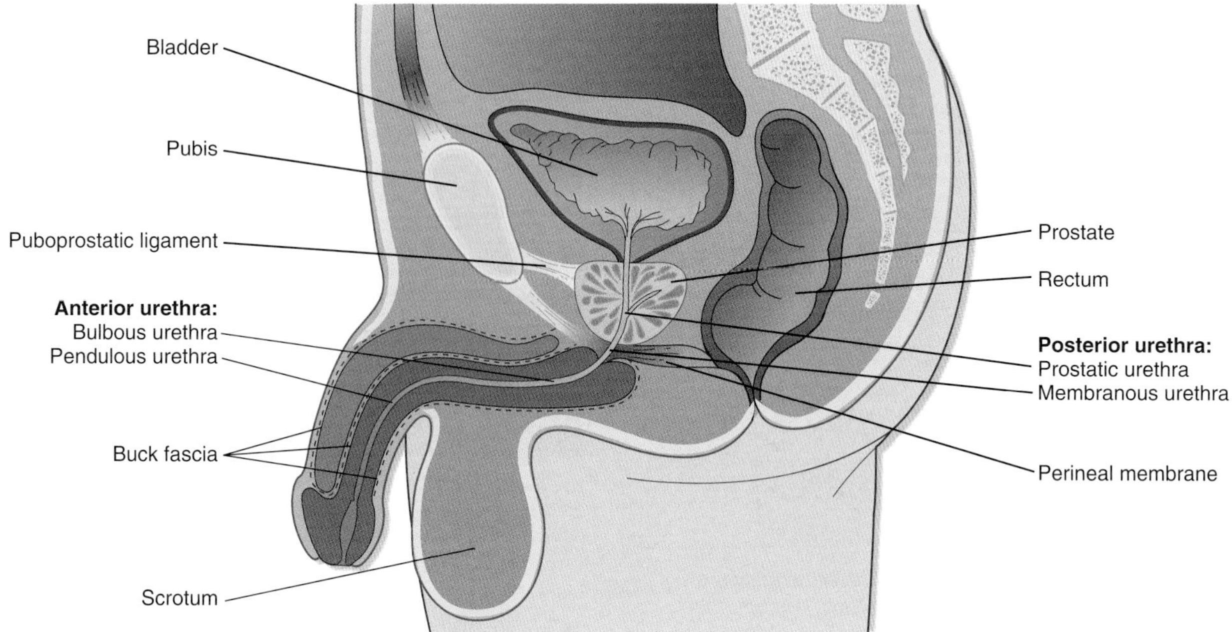


**Fig. 82.1** Sagittal view of the normal male pelvis.

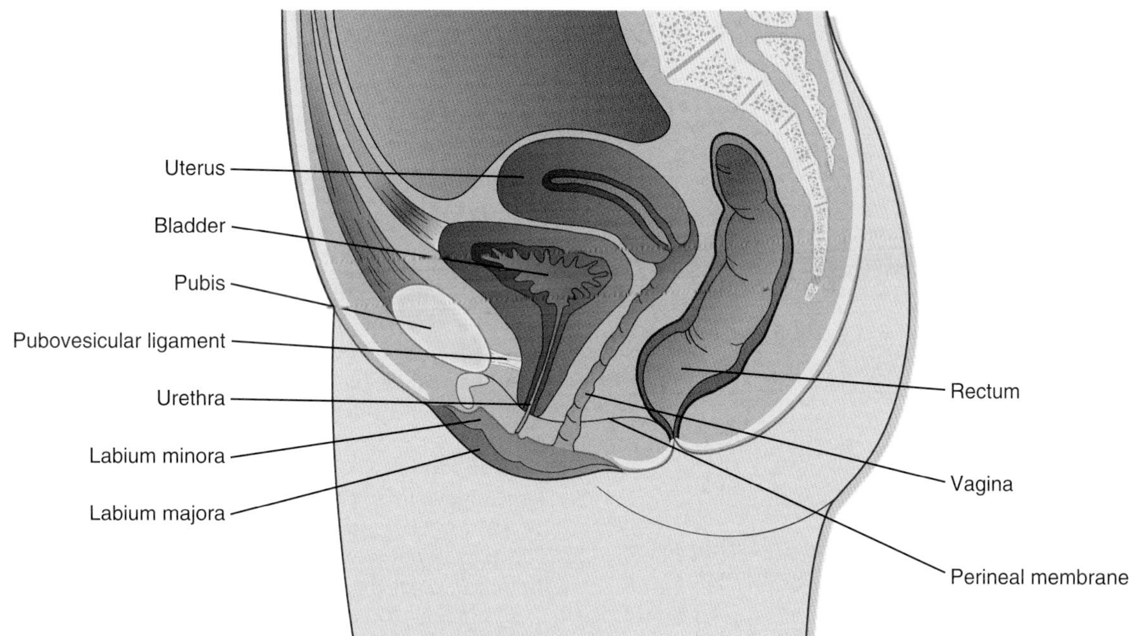


**Fig. 82.2** Sagittal view of the normal female pelvis.

Overall, urethral disruption accompanies pelvic fracture in approximately 5% of cases in women and up to 25% of cases in men.[1,4] However, the risk for urethral injury varies with the type of pelvic fracture. High-risk fractures include concomitant fractures of all four pubic rami (straddle fractures; **Fig. 82.5**) or fractures of both ipsilateral rami accompanied by massive posterior disruption through the sacrum, sacroiliac joint, or ilium. Low-risk injuries include single ramus fractures and ipsilateral ramus fractures without disruption of the posterior ring. The risk for urethral injury approaches zero with isolated fractures of the acetabulum, ilium, and sacrum.[1]

Posterior urethral disruption occurs when a significant pelvic fracture causes upward displacement of the bladder and prostate. Avulsion of the puboprostatic ligament is followed by stretching of the membranous urethra and subsequent partial or complete disruption at the anatomic weak point, the bulbomembranous junction.[1]

## BLADDER

When empty, the bladder lies along the floor of the pelvis, where it is relatively protected unless the force of an injury fractures the bony pelvis. When distended by urine, the

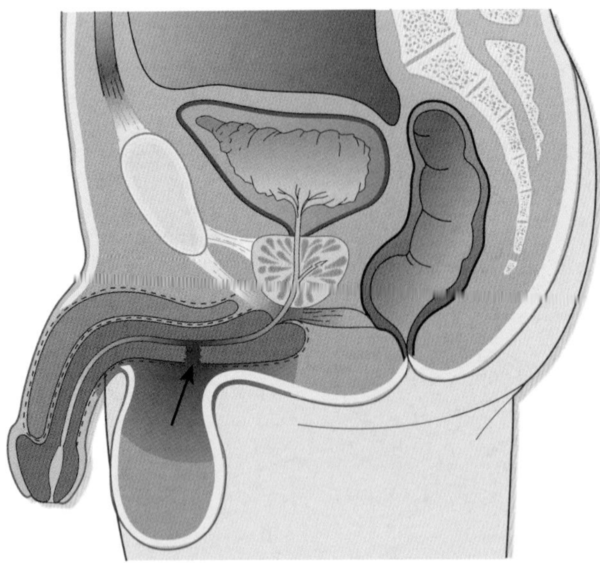

**Fig. 82.3 Anterior urethral injury.** Note the extravasation of blood at the injury site *(arrow)* with dissection into tissues of the scrotum and perineum.

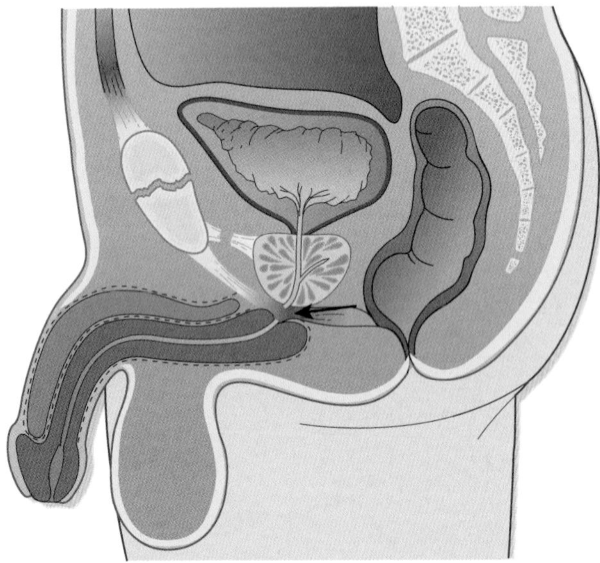

**Fig. 82.4 Posterior urethral injury.** Note the displacement of the prostate by the hematoma at the site of injury *(arrow)*.

bladder may extend up to the level of the umbilicus, where it is vulnerable to blunt force trauma inflicted on the lower part of the abdomen. The weakest and most mobile area of the bladder is at the peritoneal surface of the dome.

Blunt force bladder injuries are seen with lower abdominal trauma and in conjunction with pelvic fractures, often resulting from a motor vehicle collision. They are classified as contusions, intraperitoneal rupture, or extraperitoneal rupture. Contusions are partial-thickness injuries to the bladder wall without rupture. Intraperitoneal rupture is caused by a blunt force injury to the lower part of the abdomen in a patient with a full bladder, which results in rupture at the bladder dome followed by extravasation of urine into the peritoneal cavity. Extraperitoneal rupture occurs most often in association with

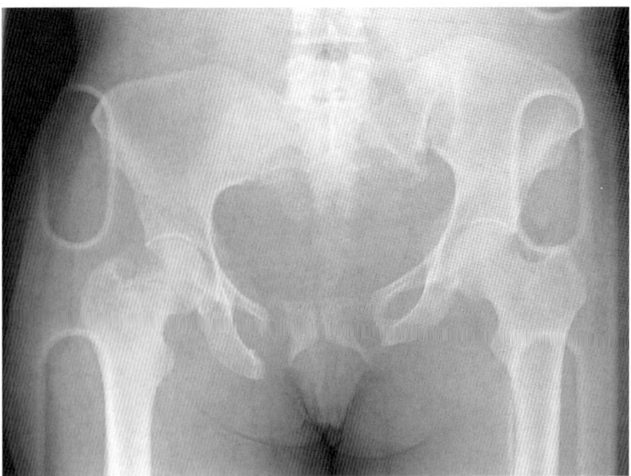

**Fig. 82.5 Straddle pelvic fracture.** Note the concomitant fractures of all four pubic rami. This injury confers a high risk for urethral disruption.

a pelvic fracture, and the injuring force causes rupture at the anterior or anterolateral wall. In other cases, bony fragments from the pelvic fracture impale the bladder and result in extraperitoneal rupture. Penetrating injuries may be inflicted by gunshot wounds, knives, or other sharp objects.

### URETERS

The ureters course distally along the psoas muscles and enter the bladder posteriorly and inferiorly at the trigone.

Ureteral injury is rare and occurs in less than 1% of all genitourinary injuries.[5] In adults, penetrating injuries account for approximately 90% of cases, most commonly inflicted by gunshot wounds.[6] In children, the most common mechanism is blunt avulsion at the ureteropelvic junction as a result of a motor vehicle collision or a fall from a height. This injury pattern is thought to be due to the increased mobility of the pediatric vertebral column, which allows extreme hyperextension that results in upward displacement of the kidney and separates it from the relatively immobile ureter.

### KIDNEYS

The kidneys lie in the retroperitoneal space and are protected by the lower ribs, the back musculature, and perinephric fat. The right kidney extends lower than the left one because of the presence of the liver.

Significant force is required to injure the kidney. Motor vehicle collisions, falls, direct blows, and lower rib fractures are common mechanisms. Significant decelerating force may cause avulsion of the renal pedicle. In children, bicycle accidents represent a prominent mechanism of renal injury.[7] Penetrating injuries may be inflicted by gunshot wounds, knives, or other sharp objects.

## PRESENTING SIGNS AND SYMPTOMS

### EXTERNAL GENITALIA INJURIES

Blunt scrotal trauma may result in superficial ecchymosis and swelling or testicular rupture, torsion, or displacement. In testicular rupture, the tunica albuginea is disrupted. Even in the absence of testicular rupture, blood or fluid may accumulate between the tunica albuginea and tunica vaginalis and result in a hematocele or hydrocele, respectively. Testicular torsion disrupts the vascular supply and causes ischemia. Testicular displacement occurs when the testicle is forced from the scrotum, usually into the peritoneal cavity. Physical examination may be limited because of pain and swelling.

Penile fracture is often accompanied by an audible snapping sound and is followed immediately by severe pain, detumescence, swelling, and ecchymosis. The corpus spongiosum is involved in 20% to 30% of cases, and urethral injury occurs in 10% to 20%. If the Buck fascia remains intact, the swelling and ecchymosis are confined to the penile shaft. If not, blood and urine may dissect into the scrotum, perineum, and suprapubic spaces.[8,9]

In patients with penetrating mechanisms, a careful and complete physical examination should be conducted to search for associated or additional occult injuries. In one series, gunshot wounds involving the penis were associated with injury to other organ structures in 80% of cases.[10] Violation of the corpora cavernosa requires operative intervention and is heralded by an expanding penile hematoma, significant bleeding from a wound to the penile shaft, or a palpable corporal defect.

Injuries to the female genitalia are often associated with pelvic fractures. Important mechanisms include physical or sexual assault, consensual intercourse, and penetrating injuries. In the presence of a pelvic fracture or blood at the introitus, meticulous vaginal examination is mandated. Complications of missed vaginal injuries include infection, fistula formation, and significant hemorrhage.[11,12] In one series, 25% of women sustaining injury to the external genitalia required red blood cell transfusion because of blood loss from the genital injury alone.[11]

## URETHRAL INJURIES

In blunt trauma, the signs and symptoms of urethral injury include blood at the urethral meatus, gross hematuria, inability to void, absent or abnormally positioned prostate on digital rectal examination, or ecchymosis or hematoma involving the penis, scrotum, or perineum. In penetrating trauma, urethral disruption should be suspected when the injury trajectory lies in proximity to the course of the urethra.

## BLADDER INJURIES

The vast majority of blunt bladder injuries are accompanied by gross hematuria, significant pelvic fracture, or both. In general, the diagnosis may be excluded clinically when both are absent. Bladder injury may occur with any pelvic fracture but is more likely with fractures of the anterior arch or when all four pubic rami are fractured. A minority of patients will have a pelvic fracture with microscopic hematuria. Additional signs and symptoms include lower abdominal pain or tenderness and inability to void. In patients with penetrating trauma, bladder rupture should be evaluated when the injury trajectory lies in proximity to the bladder.

## URETERAL INJURIES

Hematuria (gross or microscopic) is not a reliable predictor of ureteral injury because the findings on urinalysis are normal approximately 25% of the time.[7,13] The diagnosis is frequently missed on the initial evaluation because the signs and symptoms are minimal and nonspecific. Delayed findings include fever, flank pain, and a palpable flank mass (urinoma). Ureteral injury should be considered in patients with any penetrating injury that has a trajectory in proximity to the ureter.

## KIDNEY INJURIES

Clinical clues to a potential renal injury include bruising, pain, or tenderness in the flank or abdomen; rib or spine fractures; and hematuria, injury to other organs, and shock. In patients with penetrating trauma, renal involvement should be suspected when the injury trajectory is in proximity to the kidney.

## DIGITAL RECTAL EXAMINATION

Classic teaching has held that digital rectal examination provides useful clinical information in the evaluation of a blunt trauma patient who has sustained a pelvic fracture or in whom a urethral injury is suspected. The technique described includes evaluation for an absent or high-riding prostate, the presence of which may be associated with posterior urethral disruption and the need for prompt investigation for urethral integrity. However, multiple studies have now demonstrated a relative lack of utility of digital rectal examination for the detection of urethral injuries.[14-16] Accordingly, the decision to evaluate for urethral injury should not rely solely on the findings of digital rectal examination but instead should consider additional clinical features, including the mechanism of injury, physical examination findings such as a scrotal or perineal hematoma or blood at the urethral meatus, and the presence and type of any associated pelvic fracture.

## VAGINAL EXAMINATION

Although most multiply injured patients receive a digital rectal examination, the vaginal examination is often omitted in error. To avoid missing occult injuries that may result in significant and potentially life-threatening hemorrhage and infection, a careful vaginal examination should be performed to identify any lacerations or bone fragments in all women with pelvic fractures. This is especially critical in patients with fractures of the anterior pelvic ring.

## HEMATURIA

Hematuria is a marker of potential injury to the genitourinary tract. It is important to inspect the initial urine output to avoid missing transient hematuria that may clear with ongoing fluid resuscitation. A spontaneously voided specimen is ideal but is frequently impractical in a multiply injured patient.

Gross hematuria is defined as urine that is any color other than clear or yellow. This is a necessarily conservative definition because the degree of gross hematuria does not correlate with the severity of the injury; a relatively minor urethral injury may result in impressive hemorrhage, whereas major vascular disruption may be accompanied by only slightly discolored urine. False-positive results may be due to many factors, including ingestion of certain food products or dyes, various medications, or the presence of free myoglobin because of rhabdomyolysis.

Microscopic hematuria is defined as more than five red blood cells per high-power field (RBCs/HPF) or a positive dipstick evaluation. The significance of gross versus microscopic hematuria varies with the mechanism of injury (blunt versus penetrating) and is discussed in more detail later in the chapter.

## DIFFERENTIAL DIAGNOSIS AND MEDICAL DECISION MAKING

Ideally, investigation for genitourinary injury is conducted in a retrograde fashion beginning with evaluation of the external genitalia and urethra before the bladder. The ureters and kidneys are evaluated after lower tract injury is excluded or after appropriate emergency management of an identified lower tract injury is initiated.

### EXTERNAL GENITALIA

Diagnosis of injuries to the external genitalia is based largely on the mechanism of injury and physical examination. Unexplained penile or clitoral swelling necessitates a careful search for a hair tourniquet, especially in infants and young children. Concomitant urethral injury should be considered and a retrograde urethrogram performed to assess urethral integrity in any patient with a penile fracture, blood at the urethral meatus, or penetrating trauma that violates the Buck fascia. Plain radiographs revealing a significant pelvic fracture should prompt a careful examination for occult rectal or vaginal injury.

Ultrasonography is used to evaluate testicular blood flow in cases of suspected torsion and to supplement the physical examination in cases of testicular trauma. However, this modality has only modest sensitivity and specificity in detecting testicular rupture and is quite operator dependent.[9,17]

### URETHRA

After the initial history and physical examination, an anteroposterior (AP) pelvic radiograph should be obtained to assess for fracture. In cases of suspected urethral injury, classic teaching has held that it is imperative to evaluate the integrity of the urethra with a retrograde urethrogram before attempting to place a urinary catheter to avoid worsening a partial urethral disruption. Although the literature on this topic is sparse, one small retrospective review of 13 cases of urethral injury demonstrated no evidence that a blind attempt to insert a urinary catheter worsened the initial injury.[18] Consequently, in the presence of gross hematuria without other signs of urethral injury, it is reasonable to make one attempt at passing a Foley catheter. If resistance is encountered, the attempt should be aborted and urethral integrity evaluated by retrograde urethrography. This procedure should be deferred if pelvic angiography is indicated because extravasation of contrast material from a urethral injury may obscure computed tomography (CT) and angiography images and complicate attempts to control significant pelvic hemorrhage by vascular embolization.[19]

#### *Retrograde Urethrography Procedure*

The patient should be kept supine to avoid potentially disrupting a stable pelvic hematoma. Obtain a baseline kidneys, ureter, and bladder (KUB) radiograph and ensure that the film captures the entire course of the urethra and bladder. Retract the foreskin, if present, and control the shaft of the penis with a 4 × 4-inch gauze pad to prevent slippage. Stretch the penis obliquely over the thigh to promote unfolding and visualization of the entire urethra. Fill a 60-mL syringe with 10% water-soluble contrast material (diluted in sterile saline) and attach a Christmas tree adaptor. Insert the adaptor snugly into the urethral meatus and ensure a tight fit because leaking contrast material will result in spurious findings.

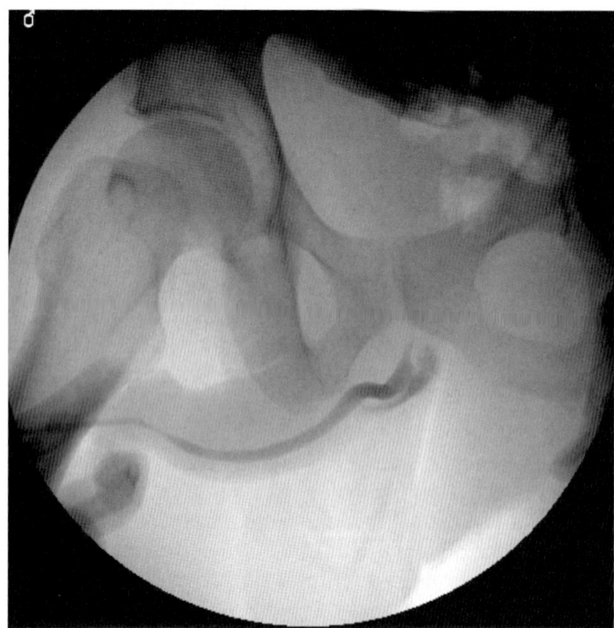

**Fig. 82.6 Retrograde urethrogram showing complete urethral rupture at the level of the membranous urethra.** Note that no contrast agent reaches the bladder.

Alternatively, a Foley catheter can be inserted a few centimeters into the urethra and the balloon inflated to ensure a snug fit within the fossa navicularis; next, attach a catheter-tip syringe filled with contrast material as described previously. Inject 50 to 60 mL (0.6 mL/kg in children) of contrast agent and obtain a KUB radiograph simultaneously with infusion of the final 10 mL. Lack of urethral extravasation with filling of the bladder indicates a normal study. Partial disruption is indicated by urethral extravasation accompanied by partial filling of the bladder. Complete disruption results in urethral extravasation with no filling of the bladder (**Fig. 82.6**).

If urethral injury is suspected, obtain a retrograde urethrogram first to ensure urethral integrity before placement of a Foley catheter. Once urethral injury is excluded and a Foley catheter has been placed, evaluate for bladder rupture in all patients with gross hematuria and in those who have sustained a significant pelvic fracture. This is accomplished by retrograde cystography or retrograde CT cystography. Additional relative indications for bladder imaging include gross hematuria without pelvic fracture and microscopic hematuria with pelvic fracture.[20]

#### *Retrograde Cystography Procedure*

As with the procedure for retrograde urethrography, the patient should be kept supine to avoid potentially disrupting a stable pelvic hematoma and care taken to avoid spillage of the contrast agent, which will result in a spurious study. Obtain a baseline KUB radiograph. Remove the central piston from a 60-mL catheter-tip syringe and attach it to the Foley catheter. Hold the syringe upright above the level of the bladder and instill 400 mL of 10% water-soluble contrast agent (diluted in sterile saline) by gravity. In patients younger

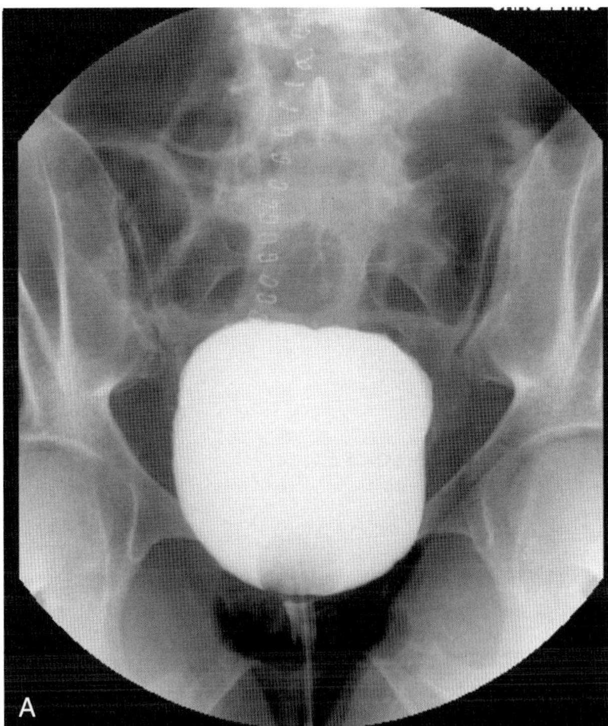


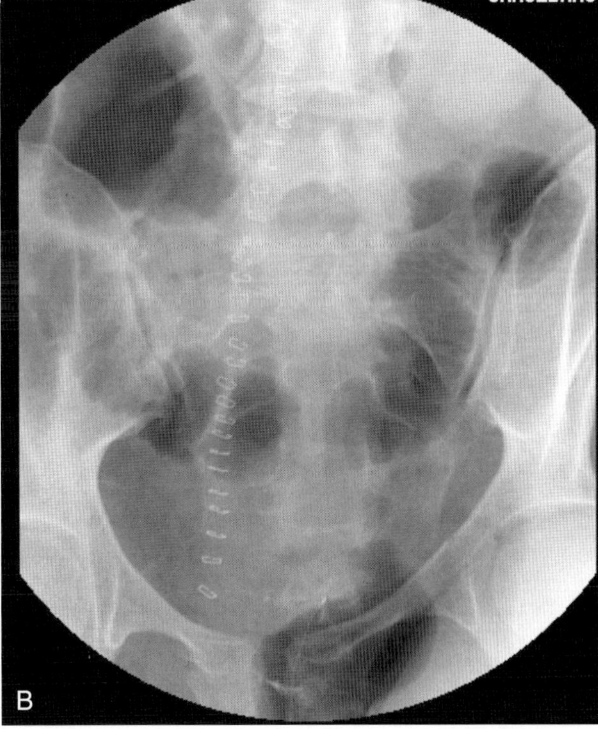


**Fig. 82.7** **A,** Normal retrograde cystogram. Note the complete retrograde filling of the bladder via a Foley catheter. **B,** Normal retrograde cystogram. Note the complete evacuation of contrast material on the postvoid film.

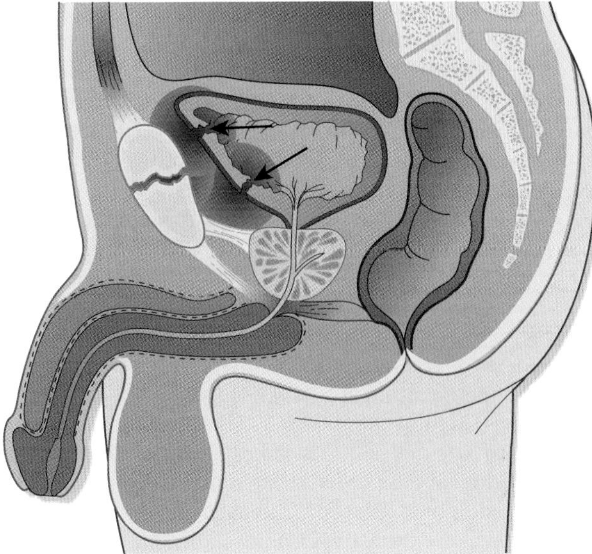

**Fig. 82.8** Extraperitoneal rupture *(arrows)*.

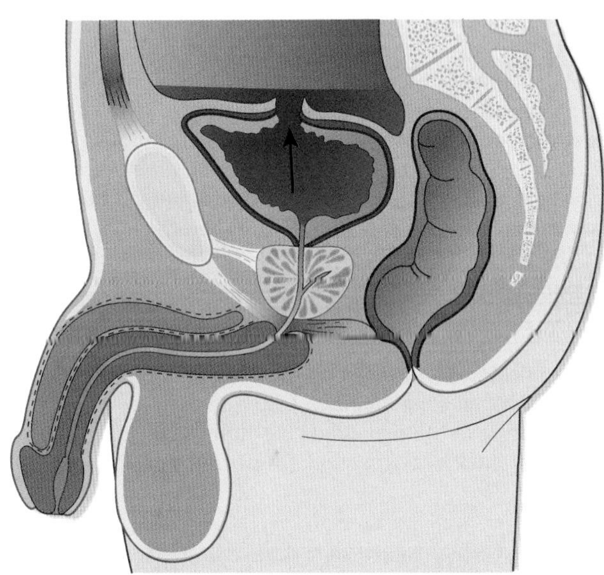

**Fig. 82.9** Intraperitoneal rupture *(arrow)*.

than 11 years, calculate the appropriate amount of contrast agent in milliliters with the following formula: (age in years/2) × 30. If a bladder contraction occurs before the instillation of 400 mL of contrast material (as evidenced by the contrast level rising in the syringe), wait for the contraction to pass, refill the bladder to the point of contraction, and then forcefully inject another 50 mL of contrast agent. The goal is to adequately distend the bladder to avoid missing injuries.

The most common reason for false-negative cystographic results is failure to instill enough contrast material. Once the bladder is filled, clamp the catheter and obtain a KUB radiograph (**Fig. 82.7**). After ensuring adequacy of the contrast film, unclamp the catheter, allow the bladder to drain, and obtain a postevacuation film. Extraperitoneal rupture appears as a flamelike area of contrast material confined to the pelvis, often extending lateral to the bladder (**Fig. 82.8**). In cases of intraperitoneal rupture, contrast material outlines the bowel and other structures in the peritoneal cavity (**Fig. 82.9**). Using the baseline film for comparison, carefully scrutinize the postevacuation film for any subtle areas of extravasation not seen on the contrast-distended view.

For retrograde CT cystography, the bladder is filled in an identical manner. Do not simply clamp the Foley catheter and rely on passive filling of the bladder by intravenously administered contrast material for CT cystography. Multiple studies have demonstrated missed injuries with this approach.[21-24] A postevacuation film is not necessary with retrograde CT cystography.

## URETER

The diagnosis of ureteral injury is elusive. Intravenous pyelography has long been the test of choice, although its reported sensitivity is highly variable.[6,13,25] CT imaging has gained popularity of late and is often indicated for identification of related injuries. In cases of suspected ureteral or renal pelvis disruption, additional delayed CT images (obtained 10 minutes after injection of contrast agent) are indicated to allow time for the intravenous contrast material to be excreted by the kidneys (**Fig. 82.10**). If operative exploration is indicated, the ureters may be directly evaluated in the surgical suite. When the diagnosis remains in doubt, retrograde pyelography may be useful.

## KIDNEY

Renal imaging is indicated in all patients with penetrating trauma proximate to the kidneys and in those with blunt injuries and gross hematuria or microscopic hematuria with shock (defined as systolic blood pressure lower than 90 mm Hg). Additional relative indications include a significant decelerating mechanism, such as a high-speed motor vehicle collision or a fall from a height.[26,27] The imaging study of choice is CT scanning with intravenous contrast enhancement. If injury to the collecting system is suspected, additional cuts should be obtained 10 minutes after injection of the contrast agent. Intravenous pyelography has been used extensively in the past but has largely been supplanted by CT.

In an unstable patient requiring immediate laparotomy, a "one-shot" intravenous pyelogram obtained in the operating room has some utility. Although this limited study does not provide sufficient sensitivity to exclude all clinically important renal injuries, it will demonstrate major renal disruption and confirm the presence of a functioning contralateral kidney. This study is accomplished by obtaining a KUB radiograph 10 minutes after rapid intravenous bolus injection of contrast material (2 mL/kg).[27,28] Angiography performed on an emergency basis can be both diagnostic and therapeutic, but it is time-consuming and impractical in many centers. Ultrasonography lacks sensitivity in visualizing renal trauma and should not be relied on to exclude significant injury.

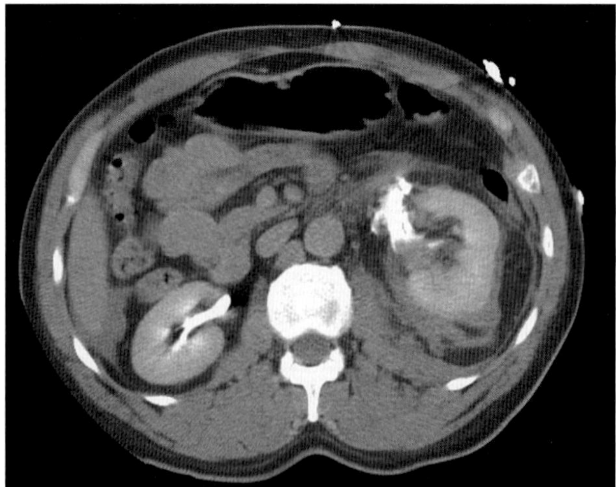

**Fig. 82.10 Injury to the collecting system of the left kidney.** This delayed image demonstrates extravasation of contrast material from the renal pelvis.

### DOCUMENTATION

Note the presence or absence of any abnormalities that suggest genitourinary injury. In blunt trauma patients, such abnormalities include the following:

- Flank tenderness, bruising, or swelling
- The presence (and type) of a pelvic fracture
- Blood at the urethral meatus
- Ecchymosis or hematoma involving the penis, scrotum, or perineum

In patients with penetrating trauma, note whether the injury trajectory occurs in proximity to the genitourinary tract.

Document the presence or absence of hematuria in the initial urine specimen.

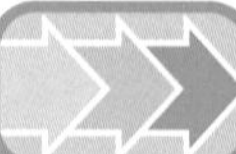

### PRIORITY ACTIONS

Because genitourinary injuries are rarely life-threatening, initial assessment of a multiply injured patient is focused on rapid identification of potentially life-threatening injuries with prompt intervention to preserve life.

During the initial resuscitation, note any findings, such as gross hematuria or an unstable pelvic fracture, that may herald genitourinary injury so that the appropriate investigation may be undertaken once the patient has been stabilized.

# TREATMENT

Except in the rare instance of a shattered kidney or major renal vascular laceration with significant hemorrhage, genitourinary injuries seldom pose a threat to life. Therefore, in a multiply injured patient, evaluation for genitourinary injury is deferred until other, potentially life-threatening injuries are excluded and the patient's condition is stabilized. During the initial evaluation and stabilization, the emergency physician should note any findings that may herald genitourinary injury so that the appropriate investigation can be undertaken once the immediately life-threatening conditions have been addressed. The patient should not receive any oral fluids until the need for operative intervention has been excluded. Intravenous fluids and analgesics may be administered as needed.

## EXTERNAL GENITALIA INJURIES

Bleeding should be controlled with direct pressure. An amputated penis should be wrapped in saline-moistened gauze and placed in a sealed plastic bag, which is then placed on ice in a second plastic bag until reimplantation.

Any constricting devices should be removed promptly. This may be accomplished by unwinding a hair tourniquet, cutting a tight-fitting constricting ring or band, or wrapping a string or Penrose drain around the penis distal to the object to decrease swelling and facilitate removal. Liberal use of a water-based lubricant may be beneficial. After significant underlying injury has been excluded, copiously irrigate any superficial lacerations of the scrotum or penis and close with absorbable suture.

Zipper entrapment injuries are managed by infiltrating the affected area with 1% plain lidocaine followed by the application of mineral oil and carefully "unzipping" the zipper. If this fails, cut the slide bar of the zipper with an orthopedic pin cutter and gently pull the teeth apart.

Traumatic testicular torsion and displacement are treated surgically. All but the most superficial penetrating injuries to the external genitalia require operative exploration, especially those that violate the corpora cavernosa. Prompt surgical exploration plus repair of penile fractures minimizes the late complications of penile curvature, erectile dysfunction, and dyspareunia.[8,9] Likewise, in patients with testicular rupture, early operative intervention maximizes the rate of testicular salvage.[9] Reimplantation of an amputated penis should be performed as expeditiously as possible but has been successful after 16 hours of cold ischemia.[17] The majority of women with vaginal injuries will require operative repair or washout to prevent significant morbidity and mortality.[11]

## URETHRAL INJURIES

In patients with a low-risk pelvic fracture (as defined previously) and no evidence of urethral injury on physical examination, it is reasonable to make a gentle attempt at passage of a Foley catheter. If any significant resistance is met, remove the catheter and obtain a retrograde urethrogram. If the retrograde urethrogram is normal, insert the catheter and inspect the initial output for evidence of hematuria.

If a urethral injury is suspected subsequent to successful placement of a Foley catheter, do not remove the catheter. A retrograde urethrogram may be obtained by inserting a small feeding tube alongside the catheter and proceeding as described previously. A urologist should be consulted for management of patients with abnormal retrograde urethrogram results or in cases of suspected urethral injury when a retrograde urethrogram cannot be obtained. In female patients, suspected urethral injury mandates urologic consultation; retrograde urethrography is not indicated in the emergency department (ED).

Optimal definitive management of urethral injuries depends on several factors, including the location (anterior or posterior) and severity (partial or complete) of the injury and the preference and expertise of the consulting urologist. Options vary from simple placement of a Foley catheter to allow a partial anterior urethral injury to heal by secondary intention to early endoscopic realignment or delayed urethroplasty of posterior urethral injuries. Frequently, placement of a suprapubic cystostomy tube is required to promote decompression of the bladder and divert urine from the healing urethral injury or anastomosis. Regardless of the approach, the ultimate goal is maintenance of urinary continence and sexual function.

## BLADDER INJURIES

The Foley catheter should be irrigated as needed to clear any clots and ensure adequate drainage; the primary goal is to keep the bladder completely decompressed. Because bladder injuries are often associated with intraabdominal trauma, a diligent search for the latter should be undertaken in all patients with positive cystography results.

Operative repair is the rule for most intraperitoneal bladder ruptures. By contrast, the majority of extraperitoneal ruptures can be managed nonoperatively with catheter drainage alone. Exceptions include injuries involving the bladder neck, associated rectal or vaginal injuries, and patients requiring laparotomy for other indications.

## URETERAL INJURIES

Identification and urologic consultation are the main priorities in the emergency management of ureteral injuries. Depending on the degree and location of the ureteral disruption, management options include cystoscopic stent placement or surgical repair over a stent. Urinary diversion may be required.

## KIDNEY INJURIES

The need for operative intervention correlates with the severity of injury as classified by the American Association for the Surgery of Trauma organ injury severity scale for the kidney (**Fig. 82.11** and **Table 82.1**). Most grade I and II injuries can

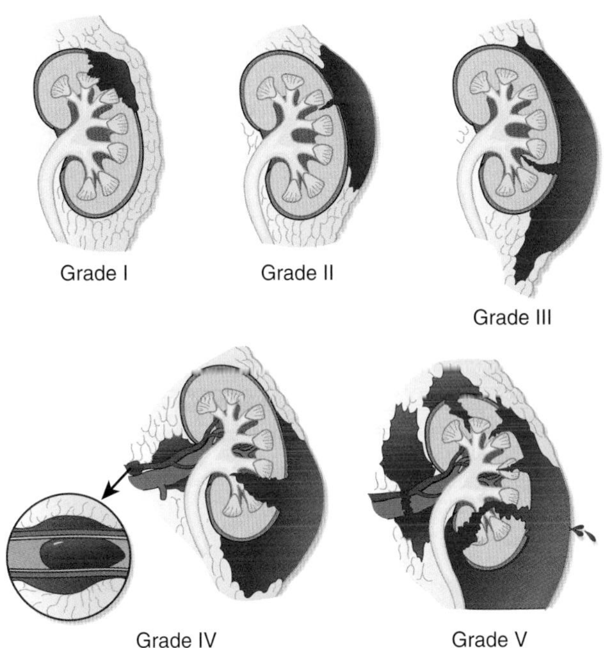


**Fig. 82.11 American Association for the Surgery of Trauma organ injury severity scale for the kidney.**

**Table 82.1 AAST Organ Injury Severity Scale for the Kidney***

| GRADE† | TYPE | DESCRIPTION |
|---|---|---|
| I | Contusion | Microscopic gross hematuria, urologic studies normal |
| | Hematoma | Subcapsular, nonexpanding hematoma without parenchymal laceration |
| II | Hematoma | Nonexpanding perirenal hematoma confined to the renal retroperitoneum |
| | Laceration | <1-cm parenchymal depth of the renal cortex without urinary extravasation |
| III | Laceration | >1-cm parenchymal depth of the renal cortex without collecting system rupture or urinary extravasation |
| IV | Laceration | Parenchymal laceration extending through the renal cortex, medulla, and collecting system |
| | Vascular | Main renal artery or vein injury with contained hemorrhage |
| V | Laceration | Completely shattered kidney |
| | Vascular | Avulsion of the renal hilum with devascularization of the kidney |

*AAST*, American Association for the Surgery of Trauma.
*Appears online at http://www.aast.org/injury/injury.html.
†Advance one grade for bilateral injuries up to grade III.

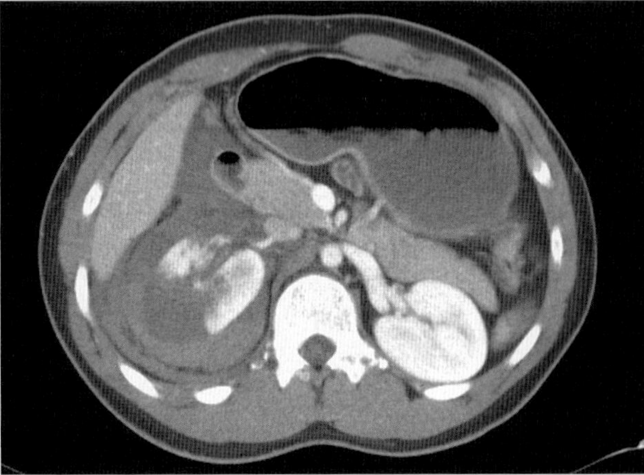

**Fig. 82.12 American Association for the Surgery of Trauma grade V renal laceration *(right)* with significant perinephric hematoma secondary to renal artery disruption with devascularization of the lower pole of the kidney.**

be managed nonoperatively, and nearly all grade V injuries (**Fig. 82.12**) require nephrectomy, which may be lifesaving in the rare case of exsanguinating hemorrhage from a renal vascular injury. Delayed nephrectomy may be indicated in the small subset of patients in whom hypertension or symptomatic renal infarction develops.[27]

## PEDIATRIC CONSIDERATIONS

It is somewhat controversial whether the criteria used to determine the need for renal imaging after blunt trauma in adults may be applied to children. One issue is whether the presence of microscopic hematuria in children warrants imaging even in the absence of shock. Some authors have recommended imaging in children when urine microscopy reveals more than 50 RBCs/HPF.[29,30]

Certainly, the criterion of shock as defined by a systolic blood pressure lower than 90 mm Hg is unhelpful in the pediatric population. Even age-specific definitions of hypotension are of little utility because children manifest shock differently than do adults. A recent study reviewing 720 consecutive pediatric patients with suspected renal trauma concluded that using the criteria of gross hematuria, shock, and significant deceleration injury can identify all cases of renal injury.[31] However, like the definition of shock, "significant deceleration injury" was not well defined in this study.

For now, consensus guidelines recommend that hemodynamically stable children with blunt trauma undergo imaging if they have gross hematuria (i.e., more than 50 RBCs/HPF) on urine microscopy.[31] All children with penetrating trauma in proximity to the kidneys warrant imaging.

## FOLLOW-UP, NEXT STEPS IN CARE, AND PATIENT EDUCATION

Most patients with significant genitourinary injuries require urgent or emergency urologic consultation in the ED. Additionally, many patients will have associated, nonurologic injuries that mandate trauma surgery or general surgery consultation. In the event that the appropriate specialists are unavailable, expeditious transfer to an appropriate referral center is indicated after the initial evaluation and stabilization.

A minority of hemodynamically stable patients with no other indications for admission may be considered for discharge from the ED after telephone consultation with the urologist who will see the patient for follow-up care. Such cases include minor lacerations, zipper injuries, and isolated partial anterior urethral injuries in the presence of a functioning Foley catheter. These patients should be counseled on the signs and symptoms of infection and Foley catheter dysfunction and be asked to return to the ED if these or any other concerning symptoms develop. Finally, make sure that they understand the importance of complying with the scheduled follow-up plan.

$SI = \frac{SV}{BSA}$ **FACTS AND FORMULAS**

**Pediatric Contrast Agent Dosage**

The pediatric dose of a contrast agent for a retrograde urethrogram is 0.6 mL/kg to a maximum of 60 mL.

In patients younger than 11 years, calculate the appropriate amount of contrast agent in milliliters for retrograde cystography by using the formula (age in years + 2) × 30 to a maximum of 400 mL.

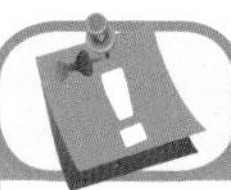

### TIPS AND TRICKS

If a urethral injury is suspected subsequent to successful placement of a Foley catheter, a retrograde urethrogram may be obtained by injecting the contrast agent through a small feeding tube inserted alongside the catheter.

Cautions for the emergency physician:

- To avoid the risk of completing a partial urethral disruption, defer Foley catheter placement in a patient with a suspected urethral injury until urethral integrity is ensured by the retrograde urethrogram.
- Perform a careful rectal examination in all patients and a vaginal examination in women with a pelvic fracture to evaluate for rectal or vaginal lacerations.
- For computed tomographic cystography, do not simply clamp the Foley catheter and rely on passive filling of the bladder by intravenously administered contrast material. Multiple studies have demonstrated missed injuries with this approach.[21-24]
- In the setting of penetrating trauma, significant renal vascular injury may exist in the absence of hematuria.

## SUGGESTED READINGS

Ball CG, Jafri M, Kirkpatrick AW, et al. Traumatic urethral injuries: does the digital rectal examination really help us? Injury 2009;40:984-6.

Netto FACS, Hamilton P, Kodama R, et al. Retrograde urethrocystography impairs computed tomography diagnosis of pelvic arterial hemorrhage in the presence of a lower urologic tract injury. J Am Coll Surg 2008;206:322-7.

Santucci RA, Langenburg SE, Zachareas MJ. Traumatic hematuria in children can be evaluated as in adults. J Urol 2004;171:822-5.

Santucci RA, Wessells H, Bartsch G, et al. Evaluation and management of renal injuries: consensus statement of the renal trauma subcommittee. BJU Int 2004; 93:937-54.

Shlamovitz GZ, McCullough L. Blind urethral catheterization in trauma patients suffering from lower urinary tract injuries. J Trauma 2007;62:330-5.

## REFERENCES

***References can be found on Expert Consult @ www.expertconsult.com.***

# 83 Hip and Femur Injuries

*Philip Bossart*

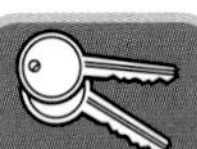

**KEY POINTS**

- Most hip fractures result from ground-level falls in patients with osteoporosis.
- Patients with intertrochanteric fractures can experience significant blood loss into the thigh and may require fluid or blood resuscitation.
- Hip dislocations and femoral fractures are often caused by high-energy trauma such as motor vehicle collisions and falls from heights; associated injuries are therefore common and should always be looked for.
- Computed tomography is more sensitive than radiography in detecting fractures and can be considered when radiographs appear to be negative and clinical suspicion for fracture is present.
- Emergency physicians may relocate hip dislocations in the emergency department; however, most hip and femoral fractures require orthopedic consultation and operative repair.

## EPIDEMIOLOGY

Approximately 300,000 hip fractures occur each year in the United States,[1] and this number is projected to increase significantly as the population ages. The major cause of hip fractures is ground-level falls in elderly patients with osteoporosis. Hip injuries are a major cause of morbidity and mortality, especially in the elderly, in whom 1-year mortality after a hip fracture is approximately 25%. Femoral shaft and distal femoral fractures are usually the result of high-energy trauma such as motor vehicle collisions and falls from heights, and thus open wounds and associated traumatic injuries are common.

## PATHOPHYSIOLOGY

The leading cause of hip fractures is falls in elderly people with underlying osteoporosis. Osteoporosis is a common condition in the elderly, and its incidence increases with advancing age. After about the age of 30, bone resorption slowly begins to exceed bone formation, and as a result bone mass and bone strength lessen. The lifetime risk of fracturing a hip is about 17% in white women and 5% in white men.[2]

The major cause of hip dislocations is motor vehicle collisions. A great deal of force is required to dislocate a hip, and thus associated injuries are common. Up to 88% of hip dislocations will be accompanied by an associated fracture.[3] Patients with hip dislocations have about a 25% risk for osteoarthritis and a 20% risk for avascular necrosis. In addition, sciatic nerve injuries occur in approximately 10% to 14% of patients with posterior hip dislocations.[4] These risks may be decreased by prompt diagnosis and treatment in the emergency department (ED).

Osteonecrosis (also known as aseptic necrosis, ischemic necrosis, or avascular necrosis) may be caused by acute disruption of the blood supply to the femoral head as a result of a hip fracture or dislocation. Fractures of the femoral neck can also disrupt the blood supply and result in osteonecrosis. Other causes are sickle cell disease, barotrauma, radiation therapy, chemotherapy, atherosclerosis, and Gaucher disease. Associated conditions include steroid use, excessive alcohol consumption, smoking, connective tissue diseases, pancreatitis, and chronic liver and renal diseases.[5] The incidence of osteonecrosis after hip dislocation depends on the degree of trauma involved and the duration of the dislocation. Some data suggest that reduction of the hip within 6 hours after dislocation decreases the incidence of osteonecrosis.[6] Therefore, every effort must be made to relocate dislocated hips as soon as possible. Femoral neck fractures are also associated with a high incidence of osteonecrosis. It is thought that the synovial fluid around the fracture site interferes with normal bone healing. Intertrochanteric fractures and other more distal fractures of the femur are rarely complicated by osteonecrosis.

## ANATOMY

The hip joint is a ball-and-socket articulation located between the femoral head and the acetabulum. The ligamentum teres, the capsular ligaments, and the proximal muscles of the leg make the hip a stable joint that requires very strong force to dislocate it. The femur is the largest and strongest bone in the body. The femoral neck is about 8 to 10 cm in length. The intertrochanteric line is an oblique line that connects the greater trochanter and the lesser trochanter and marks the junction of the femoral neck and the shaft.

The muscles of abduction (gluteus medius and gluteus minimus) insert on the laterally located greater trochanter, and the muscles of flexion (iliopsoas) insert on the medially located lesser trochanter. The major blood supply to the head and neck of the femur is the medial and lateral circumflex arteries, which are branches of the femoral artery.

The hip region has approximately 18 bursae. The most common source of hip pain and inflammation is the deep trochanteric bursa, which lies between the gluteus maximus and the greater trochanter.

## PRESENTING SIGNS AND SYMPTOMS

Pain is the most common complaint in patients with hip problems.[7] The location and character of the pain are very helpful in making a diagnosis. Increased pain during and after weight bearing and improvement with rest suggest a structural joint problem such as osteoarthritis. Constant pain, unrelated to use, suggests an infectious, inflammatory, or neoplastic process.

Lateral hip pain, especially with tenderness over the greater trochanter, suggests trochanteric bursitis. Lateral hip pain with paresthesias suggests meralgia paresthetica—lateral femoral cutaneous nerve entrapment. This condition is characterized by a local area of pain (often burning or dysesthesia) that is not influenced by direct pressure on the hip or back movement.

Anterior hip or groin pain made worse by joint motion suggests a problem with the hip joint, such as osteonecrosis, occult fracture, synovitis, or a septic joint. Anterior hip pain that is not made worse by hip motion or weight bearing suggests an inguinal hernia, lower abdominal pathology, or referred lumbar nerve root pain. Posterior hip pain suggests sacroiliac joint inflammation, lumbar radiculopathy, or herpes zoster. Anterior thigh pain may be secondary to injury to the hip joint or femur, stress fracture of the femoral neck, or lumbar radiculopathy.

## DIFFERENTIAL DIAGNOSIS AND MEDICAL DECISION MAKING

See **Box 83.1**.

## DIAGNOSTIC TESTING

Anteroposterior (AP) and lateral radiographs of the hip are usually sufficient to diagnose hip dislocations and fractures.

**BOX 83.1 Differential Diagnosis of Hip Pain**

- Bursitis
- Osteoarthritis
- Hip dislocation
- Hip fracture
- Meralgia paresthetica
- Lumbar radiculopathy
- Osteonecrosis
- Acute synovitis
- Septic arthritis
- Herpes zoster
- Stress fracture of the femoral neck
- Aortoiliac occlusive disease
- Sacroiliac joint disease

For the AP view, the patient is placed supine with about 15 degrees of internal rotation of the feet. For the lateral view, the patient is placed supine with the uninvolved hip flexed and abducted. The radiograph cassette is placed against the lateral aspect of the affected leg, and the x-ray beam is directed horizontally toward the groin with 20 degrees of cephalic tilt.

Frog-leg views of the pelvis should not be ordered if hip fracture or dislocation is a possibility.

## HIP FRACTURES

Hip fractures are classified as intracapsular or extracapsular. Intracapsular fractures include femoral head and femoral neck fractures (**Fig. 83.1**). These fractures are further categorized as either displaced or nondisplaced. Extracapsular fractures include intertrochanteric and subtrochanteric fractures, as well as the less common greater and lesser trochanteric fractures. These fractures can be further categorized by the degree of comminution.

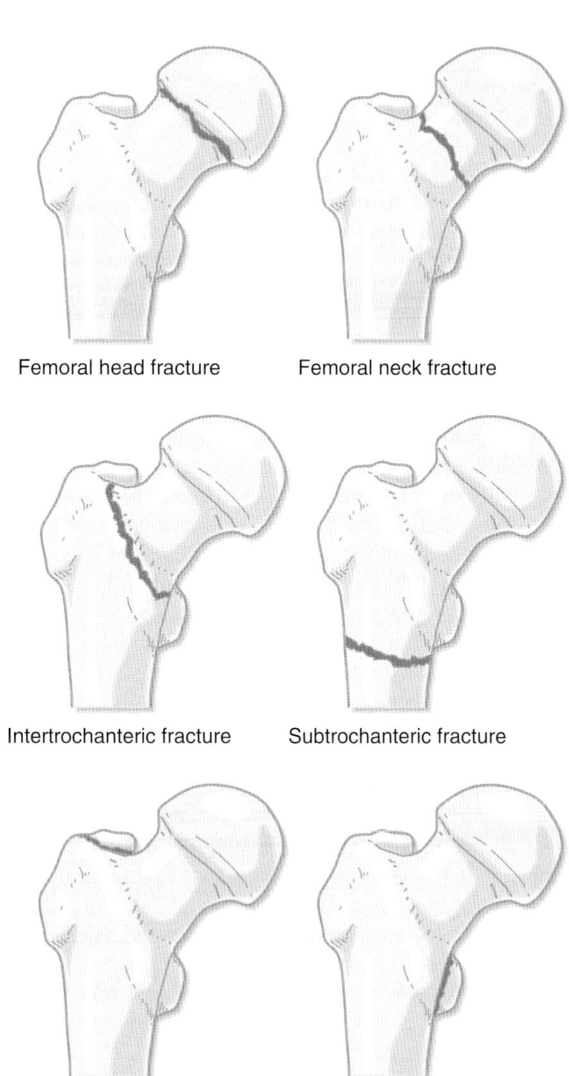


**Fig. 83.1 Types of hip fractures.**

## FEMORAL HEAD FRACTURES

These relatively uncommon fractures usually occur in conjunction with hip dislocations in young people involved in motor vehicle collisions. Because these fractures may not be visualized on plain radiographs, computed tomography or magnetic resonance imaging may be necessary for diagnosis.

## FEMORAL NECK FRACTURES

Fractures of the femoral neck, which is located between the femoral head and the trochanters, occur within the joint capsule and include subcapital fractures (fractures through the fused epiphyseal plate). These fractures are common and usually occur secondary to ground-level falls in older patients with osteoporosis and in young people involved in motor vehicle collisions.

This area of the femur has relatively little cancellous bone and very thin or absent periosteum; in addition, blood supply to the femoral head may be disrupted. As a result, degenerative changes involving the femoral head and frank avascular necrosis are common after these fractures.[8]

Because patients may be able to bear weight with some of these fractures, radiologic examination is important even if the patient is able to walk. Most femoral neck fractures can be treated by open reduction and internal fixation. Early surgical correction, usually within 12 hours, reduces the incidence of aseptic necrosis.

## INTERTROCHANTERIC FRACTURES

Intertrochanteric fractures are extracapsular injuries and are the most common type of hip fracture. The majority occur in elderly patients with osteoporosis as a result of ground-level falls. About 80% are comminuted fractures. Because patients cannot bear weight, the diagnosis is probably evident clinically and usually easily confirmed with an AP radiographic view of the hip.

Patients with intertrochanteric fractures may lose as much as 1 to 2 L of blood, and therefore intravenous crystalloid infusion or blood transfusion may be necessary. Affected patients are typically elderly and frail; ED evaluation includes determining the reason for the fall (e.g., syncope, near-syncope, transient ischemic attack), as well as evaluation for other significant medical problems. The treatment of choice is surgical repair; however, because avascular necrosis is uncommon, surgery does not have to be performed immediately. Medical and postoperative complications are common, and about one third of these patient die within 1 year of the injury.

## GREATER TROCHANTERIC FRACTURES

Fractures of the greater trochanter are uncommon. In adults they are generally the result of direct trauma; in children they are usually secondary to muscle avulsion. These fractures may be difficult to visualize on radiographs. Fractures caused by direct trauma are generally comminuted but not displaced; those caused by avulsion are usually displaced but not comminuted.

If displacement is greater than 1 cm, open reduction with internal fixation is often recommended. However, most of these fractures are generally minimally displaced and do not need surgery. If plain radiographs are uninformative, computed tomography or magnetic resonance imaging may be needed to make the diagnosis.

## LESSER TROCHANTERIC FRACTURES

Fractures of the lesser trochanter typically occur in people younger than 20 years. If they occur in adults, a pathologic fracture should be suspected. The usual mechanism is forceful contraction of the iliopsoas muscle during strenuous activity. Patients are unable to lift the affected leg when in the sitting position. Treatment is usually bed rest.

## SUBTROCHANTERIC FRACTURES

Subtrochanteric fractures are defined as fractures between the lesser trochanter and a point 5 cm distally. They are associated with severe trauma in young people or mild trauma in people with pathologic bone disease. Like intertrochanteric and midshaft femoral fractures, these fractures can be associated with significant blood loss. In addition, associated injury to the profunda femoris artery, branches of the lateral circumflex artery, the lateral femoral cutaneous nerve, and the femoral nerve is possible. If the patient has severe swelling in the proximal part of the thigh, angiography or duplex scanning should be performed to look for a vascular injury.

Treatment consists of open reduction and internal fixation. Because of the large stress forces in this area, nonunion is a relatively common complication.

## FEMORAL SHAFT FRACTURES

The diagnosis of femoral shaft fractures is usually obvious on physical examination because of marked deformity and tenderness. These fractures most commonly occur after high-energy injuries such as motor vehicle collisions and falls, and thus associated injuries are common and must be carefully searched for.

If the fracture is associated with an open wound, the wound should be irrigated and covered with moist sterile dressings. Treatment of small, relatively clean wounds includes administration of a first-generation cephalosporin. An aminoglycoside should be given if more extensive soft tissue injury is present.

Because associated fractures in the hip and knee are common, radiographs should be obtained. Blood loss can be significant, but associated neurovascular injuries are rare. On average, these patients lose about 2 to 3 units of blood, and about 50% will require blood transfusions.

Traction devices should be removed when patients arrive at the ED, but limb immobilization should be maintained.

Treatment includes internal fixation with intramedullary rods. Severely comminuted fractures may be treated by closed reduction. In general, patients do better if the fractures are stabilized within 24 hours of injury. Early stabilization is associated with early patient mobilization and therefore less risk for the development of deep vein thrombosis, pressure ulcers, and pneumonia. Fat embolism syndrome is a possible complication. This condition is manifested by signs of pulmonary or central nervous system dysfunction, fever, and rash starting about 12 to 72 hours following the injury. In almost all cases, the fractures will have healed and the patients will be functional in 6 months. Nonunion is rare.

## DISTAL FEMORAL FRACTURES

Fractures of the distal end of the femur tend to occur in older patients with severe osteoporosis or in young people with multiple trauma. Supracondylar and intercondylar fractures of the femur are difficult to treat. They are generally unstable and often comminuted. Most are treated operatively.

However, malunion, nonunion, and infections are relatively common.

### STRESS FRACTURES

Stress fractures occur when normal bone is subjected to repeated stress. The bone fails because osteoblasts are unable to lay down new bone fast enough. Symptoms of a femoral neck stress fracture can be very mild pain only. Consequently, the injury may be mistaken for a muscle strain or arthritis. Pain is typically felt in the groin and medial aspect of the thigh, is worse with use, and may make weight bearing very painful or impossible.

Findings on physical examination are usually normal, except perhaps some pain at the extremes of hip flexion and internal rotation. Because plain films are generally unrevealing until 14 days after the injury, computed tomography or magnetic resonance imaging may be needed to make the diagnosis. This condition is often bilateral, so any pain in the other hip needs evaluation as well.

## HIP DISLOCATIONS

In approximately 90% of hip dislocations, the femoral head is posterior to the acetabulum. Typically, posterior hip dislocations occur when the knee hits the dashboard during a motor vehicle collision. In posterior hip dislocations the limb is adducted, internally rotated, and shortened. In anterior dislocations the limb is abducted, externally rotated, and shortened.

### POSTERIOR HIP DISLOCATIONS

Several techniques for reducing posterior hip dislocations have been described in the literature. All these methods require adequate sedation and analgesia. The Stimson method requires the patient to lie with the legs hanging over the edge of the bed. This position is seldom practical in a trauma patient, however.[4]

The Allis technique involves keeping the patient supine on the bed. The hip is then flexed to 90 degrees and upward traction is applied with some gentle internal and external rotation. It is usually necessary to stand on the bed over the patient to perform this technique. An assistant stabilizes the pelvis and may apply some lateral force to the leg.

The Whistler technique involves lying the patient supine on the bed with the knees flexed about 130 degrees.[9] An assistant stabilizes the pelvis while the operator stands on the side of the bed near the affected hip. The operator places an arm under the knee on the leg with the dislocation and then grips the top of the other knee. The other hand stabilizes the patient's ankle. The operator then raises up the arm by using the patient's knee as a lever in an attempt to relocate the hip. After reduction, the legs are immobilized in slight abduction with a pillow between the knees, and the patient should be sent for radiographs and hospital admission.

### ANTERIOR HIP DISLOCATIONS

A modification of the Allis maneuver can be used to relocate anterior hip dislocations. The patient is placed supine and an assistant stabilizes the pelvis and applies lateral force to the affected thigh. Traction is then applied along the long axis of the femur with the hip slightly flexed. Gentle leg adduction and internal rotation may facilitate the reduction.

Postreduction care is the same as for posterior hip dislocations.

### PROSTHETIC HIP DISLOCATIONS

A patient with a hip arthroplasty may dislocate the hip with minimal force. Frequently, a minor twisting motion is all that it takes. As with native hips, the majority of these dislocations are posterior. The reduction methods are the same as with a native hip. Orthopedic consultation should be considered. Because aseptic necrosis is not an issue, there is no urgency to reduce the hip. Unlike patients without artificial hips, these patients will often not require hospitalization after reduction.

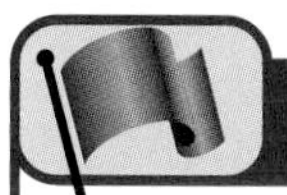

**RED FLAGS**

- It is important to look for acetabular fractures before performing closed reduction of a hip dislocation.
- On average, patients with femoral shaft fractures lose about 2 to 3 units of blood at the fracture site, and about half of these patients will require blood transfusions.
- Hip dislocation or fracture in a young person is strong evidence of serious multisystem trauma.

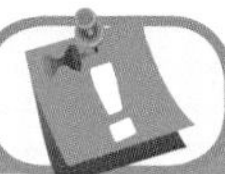

**TIPS AND TRICKS**

- Consider avascular necrosis in patients with nontraumatic hip, thigh, or knee pain.
- If hip pain prevents weight bearing and plain films do not reveal a fracture, perform computed tomography or magnetic resonance imaging to rule out a fracture.

## ULTRASOUND-GUIDED FEMORAL NERVE BLOCK

Pain relief for hip fractures and femoral shaft fractures can be achieved with ultrasound-guided femoral nerve blocks.[10] Contraindications to this procedure include hypersensitivity to the local anesthetic and infections near the injection site. In addition, patients with neurologic deficits in the affected leg or those at risk for compartment syndrome should not have a femoral nerve block performed because it may make it difficult to detect new or worsening neurologic changes. A femoral nerve block is also relatively contraindicated in patients taking anticoagulants or with a bleeding diathesis.

Because high energy is generally required to dislocate a hip, associated injuries are common.[11] Ligamentous knee injuries, acetabular and femoral fractures, and sciatic nerve palsies should be considered. If an associated fracture is not clearly seen on plain films, a computed tomography scan should be ordered.

Posterior dislocations are likely to cause a fracture of the inferior aspect of the femoral head and may cause injury to the sciatic nerve.[12] Anterior dislocations are associated with fractures of the anterior femoral head and also with vascular injuries.

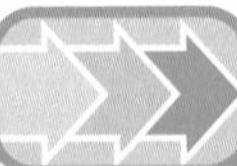

**PRIORITY ACTIONS**

Hip dislocations are true orthopedic emergencies. Reduction should be done as soon as possible. Reduction within 6 hours reduces the incidence of avascular necrosis.

Significant blood loss is common with hip and femoral fractures, especially fractures in young people, which usually involve a high-energy force. Good intravenous access, fluid resuscitation, and monitoring for blood loss are mandatory.

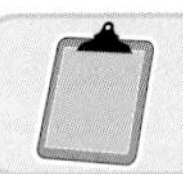

**DOCUMENTATION**

Always carefully record the findings on neurovascular examination in patients with fracture involving an extremity.

If hip reduction is delayed, record the reason for delay.

Hip dislocations are orthopedic emergencies. Reduction should be performed as soon as possible because the incidence of avascular necrosis, traumatic arthritis, and joint instability increases with the length of time that the hip is dislocated. In addition, orthopedic consultation should be obtained.

Hip relocations require procedural sedation in the ED or general anesthesia in the operating room.

## SUGGESTED READINGS

Christos S, Chiampas G, Offman R, et al. Ultrasound guided three-in-one nerve block for femur fractures. West J Emerg Med 2010;11:310-3.

Fracture dislocations of the hip. In: Wheeless' textbook of orthopedics (online). Available at www.wheelessonline.com/ostho/fracture_dislocations_of_the_hip.

LaVelle DG. Fractures of hip. In: Canale ST, editor. Campbell's operative orthopaedics. 10th ed. St. Louis: Mosby; 2003. pp. 2874-8.

## REFERENCES

***References can be found on Expert Consult @ www.expertconsult.com.***

# Knee and Lower Leg Injuries 84

Christy Hopkins

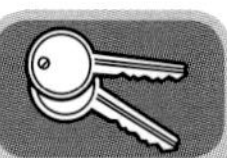

**KEY POINTS**

- Knee dislocations are associated with a high risk for neurovascular injury and constitute an orthopedic emergency.
- A grossly unstable knee should be assumed to have been dislocated.
- Patients with fractures or dislocations of the knee and lower extremity and neurovascular compromise should undergo emergency reduction or realignment before any radiographic evaluation.
- Patients discharged home in knee immobilizers with stable injuries should be instructed to remove the device several times a day and perform range-of-motion and quadriceps-strengthening exercises.
- The cast or splint should be removed from any patient with increasing pain after a lower leg fracture to allow careful assessment of neurovascular status and evaluation of the lower leg compartments.

## EPIDEMIOLOGY

Knee and lower leg injuries are common orthopedic problems seen in the emergency department (ED). This chapter divides such injuries into discussions of traumatic injuries (soft tissue and cartilaginous injuries, dislocations, and fractures), overuse injuries, and other disorders of the knee and lower part of the leg.

## PATHOPHYSIOLOGY

### KNEE

#### *Anatomy*

The knee is the largest and most complex joint in the body. Injuries to this joint are common, so a clear understanding of the anatomy and pathophysiology of the knee is essential for appropriate evaluation, diagnosis, and treatment of disorders in this area.

The knee has a wide range of motion, including flexion, extension, abduction, adduction, and internal and external rotation. Three different articulations are present in the knee: the patellofemoral articulation (anterior) and articulations between the lateral and medial tibial and femoral condyles. In full extension, the stabilizing ligaments of the knee are tight and prevent rotary motion of the knee. Beyond 20 degrees of flexion, the ligaments are relaxed and allow axial rotation of the joint.

Knee stability is provided solely by ligaments and tendons in and around the joint (**Fig. 84.1**). The knee joint is encapsulated by fibrous connective tissue lined by a synovial membrane. The knee capsule is continuous with the suprapatellar bursa, which expands when a joint effusion is present.

The popliteal fossa contains the popliteal artery and vein and the peroneal and tibial nerves. The popliteal fossa is delineated laterally by the biceps femoris muscle, medially by the semimembranosus and semitendinosus muscles, and inferiorly by the gastrocnemius muscle.

The popliteal artery is a continuation of the femoral artery after it leaves the adductor hiatus. It gives rise to the geniculate arteries, which form a rich vascular anastomosis around the knee, and divides to form the anterior and posterior tibial arteries at the level of the tibial tubercle. The popliteal artery is immobilized proximally and distally within the popliteal fossa, which predisposes it to vascular injury in the setting of traumatic knee injuries.

The tibial nerve and common peroneal nerve (a branch of the tibial nerve) innervate the knee. Because the tibial nerve is not immobilized proximally, it is less likely than the popliteal artery to be injured in the setting of joint disruption. The common peroneal nerve travels around the head of the fibula and divides into the deep and superficial peroneal nerves.

#### *Evaluation*

Key aspects of evaluation of knee are listed in **Box 84.1**. In general, evaluation of knee complaints should also include an examination of the hip and back to prevent overlooking a source of pain referred to the lower extremity.

During evaluation, the point of maximal tenderness should be assessed last. Specific tests for evaluating ligamentous and meniscal injuries are detailed in **Table 84.1**. Comparison with the uninjured or normal knee is helpful, especially for assessment of ligamentous laxity.

Joint pain or swelling may limit full evaluation of the knee in the acute setting. Patients with limited evaluations should

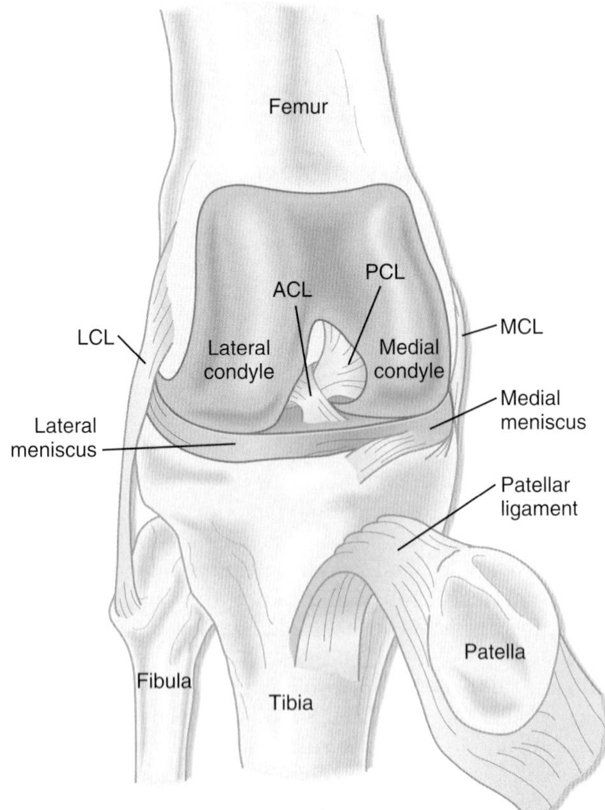


**Fig. 84.1 Knee anatomy.** *ACL*, Anterior cruciate ligament; *LCL*, lateral collateral ligament; *MCL*, medial collateral ligament; *PCL*, posterior cruciate ligament. (From Brown JR, Trojian TH. Anterior and posterior cruciate ligament injuries. Prim Care 2004;31: 925-56.)

**BOX 84.1 Evaluation of the Knee**

**History**

Mechanism of injury:

- Direction and type of force (high or low energy)
- Position of the extremity at the time of injury

Nature and duration of symptoms
Previous injuries
Previous surgical procedures
Associated complaints
Joint effusion
Locking of the joint
Ability to ambulate
Associated injuries

**Physical Examination**

Inspection of the entire limb with the patient sitting or lying and walking (if possible):

- Deformity, ecchymosis, edema, cutaneous lesions
- Joint effusions
- Previous scars
- Gait and functional range of motion
- Neurovascular status

Palpation:

- Extensor mechanism: quadriceps tendon, patella, patellar tendon, tibial tubercle (tendinitis, prepatellar bursitis, knee effusion, Osgood-Schlatter disease)
- Femoral or tibial epiphysis in adolescents (physeal fractures)
- Joint line (meniscal and/or collateral ligament injuries)
- Posterior aspect of the knee (popliteal cyst or pseudoaneurysm)
- Neurovascular status

Range of motion:

- Flexion or extension
- Internal or external rotation
- Active straight leg raise

Stability testing:

- Anterior or posterior stability (cruciate ligaments)
- Medial or lateral stability (collateral ligaments)

undergo immobilization and follow-up examination within 7 days. Key physical findings are listed in discussions of specific disorders later in the chapter.

### *Diagnostic Testing*

Because acute injuries to the knee commonly involve soft tissue, plain radiographic examination is not always indicated. The Ottawa Knee Rules[1] (**Box 84.2**) and the Pittsburgh Knee Rules[2] (**Box 84.3**) are useful guides to aid in the decision of whether to order plain radiographs. Both criteria are sensitive for fractures, but the Pittsburgh criteria are more specific and can be applied to both children and adults.

If plain radiographs are indicated, a minimum of an anteroposterior (AP) and a lateral view should be obtained. Oblique radiographs are helpful for detecting subtle tibial plateau fractures. The intercondylar or tunnel view is helpful in evaluating for tibial spine fractures and osteochondral defects (**Fig. 84.2**). Assessment of the patellofemoral joint and evaluation for the presence of patellar tilt (increased propensity for patellar subluxation or dislocation) can be done with the Merchant or sunrise view (**Fig. 84.3**). Comparison radiographs of the unaffected extremity are helpful in discerning problems in skeletally immature patients.

When describing the knee radiograph, the examiner should note the alignment and joint spacing of the femoral condyles in relation to the tibial plateau. Narrowing of the joint space (particularly in weight-bearing views) indicates articular cartilaginous and meniscal degeneration. The patella should be examined for possible fractures (in the event of a direct blow to the anterior aspect of the knee) and the presence of a bipartite or tripartite patella. Significant joint effusions are evident as a water-density radiolucency on the lateral view, anterior to the distal end of the femur.[3] Effusions seen shortly after injury are suggestive of anterior cruciate ligament (ACL) or posterior cruciate ligament (PCL) tears, tibial plateau fractures, femoral condyle fractures, or patellar fractures.[4]

In the setting of acute injuries, radiographs should be examined for the presence of fractures involving the tibial plateau (depression fracture) or tibial spine (suggesting rupture of the ACL). Segond fractures are avulsion fractures of the lateral tibial plateau at the site of attachment of the lateral capsular ligament. These fractures are associated with ACL and meniscal injuries. The presence of posterior opaque bodies should

**Table 84.1** Stability Testing

| TEST | HOW PERFORMED | DEFINITION OF A POSITIVE RESULT | COMMENTS |
|---|---|---|---|
| **Anterior Cruciate Ligament** | | | |
| Lachman (see Fig. 84.13) | Hold the knee in 15-30 degrees of flexion<br>Attempt to pull the tibia forward with one hand while holding the femur stationary with the other hand | Anterior laxity in conjunction with the lack of a firm end point (displacement > 5 mm in comparison with the opposite side) | Most sensitive test for ACL injury |
| Anterior drawer (see Fig. 84.14) | Flex the hip to 45 degrees and the knee to 90 degrees<br>Stabilize the foot with pressure directed toward the examination table<br>Grasp the proximal end of the tibia and pull forward<br>Perform with the knee in neutral and internal and external rotation | Increased laxity in a neutral position suggests ACL injury (displacement > 6 mm with respect to the opposite side)<br>Increased displacement with external rotation suggests injury to the posteromedial capsule<br>Increased displacement with internal rotation suggests injury to the posterolateral capsule | Not a reliable test for acute ACL injuries |
| Pivotal shift (see Fig. 84.15) | Flex the hip to 45 degrees and fully extend the knee while holding the heel<br>The second hand holds the knee with the thumb behind the fibular head<br>Internally rotate the ankle and knee<br>Apply valgus stress to the knee and then flex the knee while maintaining internal and valgus stress | If anterior subluxation of the knee is present, reduction of the subluxation will occur at 20-40 degrees of flexion | May be painful<br>Highest positive predictive value for ACL rupture |
| **Posterior Cruciate Ligament** | | | |
| Posterior drawer (see Fig. 84.16) | Flex the hip to 45 degrees and the knee to 90 degrees<br>Stabilize the foot with pressure directed toward the examination table<br>Apply backward force to the tibia | >5-mm posterior displacement of the tibia or a soft end point | Best test for evaluation of a PCL injury |
| Posterior sag | Put a pillow under the patient's thigh so that the knee is flexed to 45-90 degrees<br>The patient's heel should be resting on the examination table | Posterior tibial sag with regard to the femur<br>The tibia usually sits 10 mm anterior to the femoral condyles in this position | Assess before performing the posterior drawer test to avoid misinterpreting it |
| **Lateral and Medial Collateral Ligaments** | | | |
| Collateral ligament | Apply varus and valgus stress to the knee in full extension and at 30 degrees<br>Assess the joint line opening between the tibia and femur | Laxity in full extension suggests a complete collateral ligament tear in addition to injury to the secondary stabilizers (ACL, PCL)<br>Laxity at 30 degrees (but not in full extension) isolates injury to the collateral ligament undergoing testing | |
| **Meniscal Tears** | | | |
| McMurray | Hyperflex the knee<br>Hold the lower part of the leg and flex/extend the knee while simultaneously internally and externally rotating the tibia in relation to the femur | Clicking sensation felt along the joint line with internal/external rotation or the patient experiences pain<br>Internal rotation tests the lateral meniscus<br>External rotation tests the medial meniscus | Hyperflexion may not be possible in an acutely injured knee<br>Poor sensitivity |
| Apley | Place the patient in the prone position<br>Flex the knee to 90 degrees<br>Internally and externally rotate the leg with pressure on the heel | Pain while applying downward pressure suggests meniscal injury | |

*ACL*, Anterior cruciate ligament; *PCL*, posterior cruciate ligament.

**BOX 84.2 Ottawa Knee Rules**

Radiographs indicated if any *one* of the following is present:

- Age 55 years or older
- Tenderness at the head of the fibula
- Isolated tenderness of the patella
- Inability to flex the knee to 90 degrees
- Inability to bear weight for four steps both immediately after the injury and in the emergency department

Data from Stiell IG, Wells GA, McDowell I, et al. Use of radiography in acute knee injuries: need for clinical decision rules. Acad Emerg Med 1995;2:966-73.

**BOX 84.3 Pittsburgh Knee Rules**

Radiographs are indicated if the patient sustained a fall or a blunt trauma mechanism and one of the following two conditions is present:

- The patient is younger than 12 or older than 50 years.
- The patient is unable to walk four weight-bearing steps in the emergency department.

Data from Seaberg DC, Yealy DM, Lukens T, et al. Multicenter comparison of two clinical decision rules for the use of radiography in acute, high-risk knee injuries. Ann Emerg Med 1998;32:8-13.

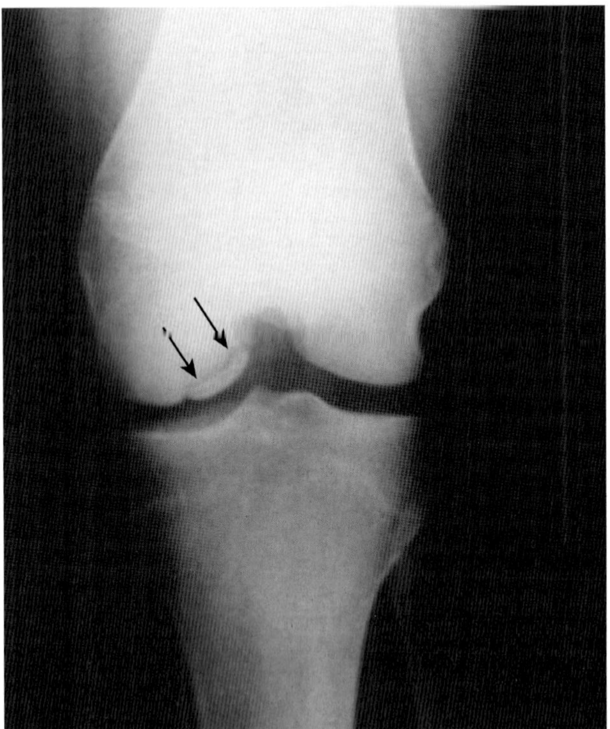

**Fig. 84.2 Knee radiograph, tunnel or intercondylar view, showing an osteochondritis dissecans lesion *(arrows)*.**

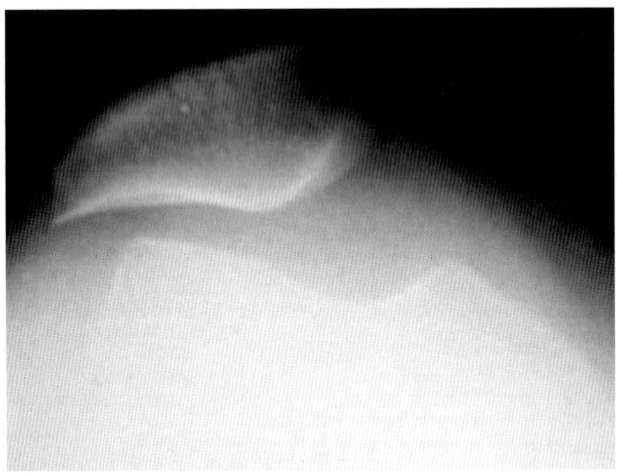

**Fig. 84.3 Merchant view of the knee showing patellar tilt and subluxation.**

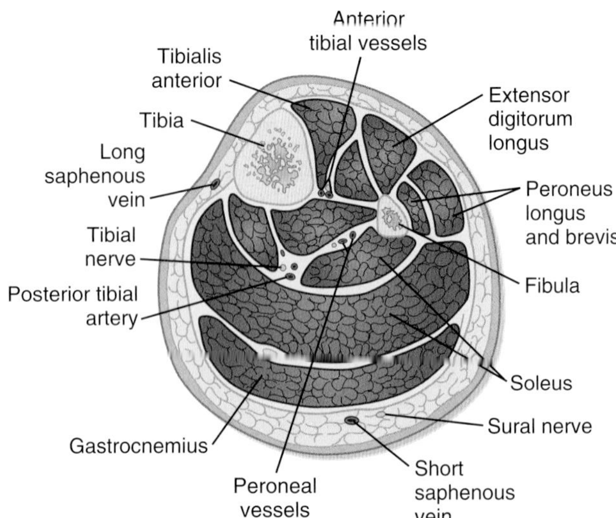


**Fig. 84.4 Cross section of the lower extremity at the level of the calf.** (From Khatri VP, Asensio JA. Operative surgery manual. Philadelphia: Saunders; 2003.)

also be noted. These may be fabellae (congenital sesamoid) or loose bodies. More than 75% of loose bodies originate from osteochondral lesions.[3] Occult fractures that are commonly missed on plain radiographs include patellar, tibial plateau, fibular head, and Segond fractures.[5]

Musculoskeletal ultrasound techniques can be used to diagnose ACL and PCL tears and may be helpful in the diagnosis of meniscal injuries.[4] Magnetic resonance imaging (MRI) can be used to confirm suspected meniscal injuries, ligamentous disruptions, osteochondral lesions, and occult fractures; however, it is rarely indicated in the acute setting. Computed tomography (CT) is helpful for establishing the extent of certain fractures (e.g., tibial plateau fractures) and is often more readily available than MRI.

## LOWER LEG

### *Anatomy*

The lower part of the leg contains the tibia and fibula. The tibia is the only weight-bearing bone in this part of the leg and is the most commonly fractured long bone in the body. Its superficial course predisposes it to a higher incidence of open fractures. The two bones are bound together by the superior and inferior tibiofibular joint along with an interosseous membrane. The interosseous membrane aids in stability of the ankle mortise.

The thigh muscles attach to the upper part of the tibia and lend stability to the knee joint. The muscles of the lower part of the leg, which are enclosed by fascia, can be divided into four compartments: anterior, posterior, deep posterior, and lateral (**Fig. 84.4**). Specific motor and sensory nerve distributions are listed by compartment in **Table 84.2**.

### *Evaluation*

A directed history of the traumatic events, duration of symptoms, and exacerbating events or activities is necessary to assess lower leg injuries. Examination of lower leg complaints should include an evaluation of the back, hips, knee, and ankle to assess for pain referred to the lower part of the leg or associated injuries.

Thorough assessment of skin integrity, neurovascular status, and the leg compartments is essential in the evaluation of any traumatic lower leg injury. The point of maximal tenderness should be evaluated last.

### *Diagnostic Testing*

Imaging of the lower part of the leg should include the joint above and the joint below the injury. Oblique views are useful for detecting tibial plateau fractures, which may not be seen on routine views.

**Table 84.2 Peripheral Nerve Assessment of the Leg**

| COMPARTMENT | NERVE | MOTOR FUNCTION | SENSORY FUNCTION |
|---|---|---|---|
| Anterior | Deep peroneal | Toe dorsiflexion | Dorsal I-II web space |
| Lateral | Superficial peroneal | Foot eversion | Lateral dorsum of the foot |
| Deep posterior | Tibial | Toe plantar function | Sole of the foot |
| Superficial posterior | Sural | Gastrocsoleus | Lateral aspect of the heel |

## DISLOCATIONS AND FRACTURES

### DISLOCATIONS

#### *Knee Dislocations*

Knee dislocations are relatively uncommon and represent, at most, 0.2% of all orthopedic injuries. They require disruption of at least three of the four major ligaments of the knee. Common mechanisms include traffic accidents, sporting injuries, or simple mechanical falls. Dislocations are classified on the basis of the direction of tibial movement in relation to the femur. Anterior and posterior dislocations account for approximately 70% of all knee dislocations. Knee dislocations may also have associated intraarticular fractures involving the tibial plateau or femoral condyles.[6]

Knee dislocations are associated with a high risk for neurovascular injury and should be considered an orthopedic emergency. The neurovascular bundle runs posterior to the bony and ligamentous structures in the popliteal fossa. The popliteal artery and nerve are fixed in the fibrous tunnel of the adductor magnus muscle proximally and traverse the fibrous arch of the soleus muscle and interosseous membrane distally. The relative immobility of the neurovascular bundle makes it susceptible to injury. The popliteal artery may be injured in up to 14% of all knee dislocations (**Fig. 84.5**). Traction injuries to the common peroneal and, less commonly, to the tibial nerve may also be present.[6]

A grossly unstable knee after a traumatic injury should be assumed to be a reduced dislocation until proved otherwise. Any patient suspected of having sustained a knee dislocation should undergo a careful neurovascular examination. Anterior and posterior dislocations have a higher incidence of vascular injury. Vascular compromise in a dislocated knee requires immediate reduction.

Neurovascular status should be documented before and after reduction. All patients with a suspected or confirmed knee dislocation should have the ankle-brachial index (ABI) calculated. An ABI of less than 0.9 has high predictive value for a vascular injury, and such patients should undergo either CT or traditional angiography. Patients with normal findings on vascular examination and an ABI lower than 0.9 should be observed for at least 24 hours with neurovascular checks every 2 to 3 hours.[4] Prompt diagnosis of vascular injury is essential given the chance of development of progressive distal ischemia. When injury to the popliteal artery has occurred, patient outcome is directly related to the duration of ischemia.

Standard AP and lateral radiographs are adequate for initial evaluation of knee dislocations. After appropriate analgesia and sedation, emergency reduction of the dislocated knee should be attempted. Longitudinal traction on the tibia (to free it from the femur) should be followed with a force in the opposite direction of the dislocation. The rotary components should also be corrected to restore normal leg alignment. After reduction, the knee should be immobilized in 15 to 20 degrees of flexion.[4] Orthopedic consultation in the ED is mandatory for all suspected and confirmed knee dislocations.

#### *Patellar Dislocation*

The patella normally articulates in the groove between the femoral condyles. The vastus medialis, medial and lateral patellofemoral, and patellotibial ligaments and the medial retinaculum all stabilize the patella (**Fig. 84.6**).

The overall incidence of patellar dislocations is estimated to be 7 per 100,000 per year and as high as 31 per 100,000 per year in patients between the age of 10 and 19 years.[7] Patellar dislocations most commonly occur when a varus force is applied to a flexed knee or after forced contraction of a flexed quadriceps. Dislocations may be associated with meniscal tears, disruption of the medial collateral ligament, and osteochondral fractures.[4]

The patient may report that the knee "gave out," followed by pain and swelling. Patients may not be able to bear weight on or flex the knee. An acute hemarthrosis is most commonly seen if an associated osteochondral fracture is present. A patellar apprehension test may be useful in a patient who reports a dislocation that resolved spontaneously. This test is performed by moving a nondisplaced patella laterally. The result is positive if the patient shows apprehension, senses pain, or feels a sensation of impending dislocation when the patella is moved laterally (**Fig. 84.7**). AP, lateral, and sunrise radiographs are adequate to evaluate for acute dislocations and associated fractures.

After proper sedation, the emergency physician (EP) should reduce a lateral patellar dislocation by flexing the hip and pushing medially on the patella while extending the knee. Postreduction radiographs are mandatory to rule out osteochondral fractures. Intraarticular, horizontal, and superior dislocations typically require open reduction. Dislocations associated with osteochondral fractures are generally treated surgically.

After reduction, the patient should be told to use conservative therapeutic measures, such as ice, elevation, and pain control. The knee should be placed in a straight leg immobilizer, and the patient can start progressive weight bearing when comfortable. Follow-up should be arranged within 1 to

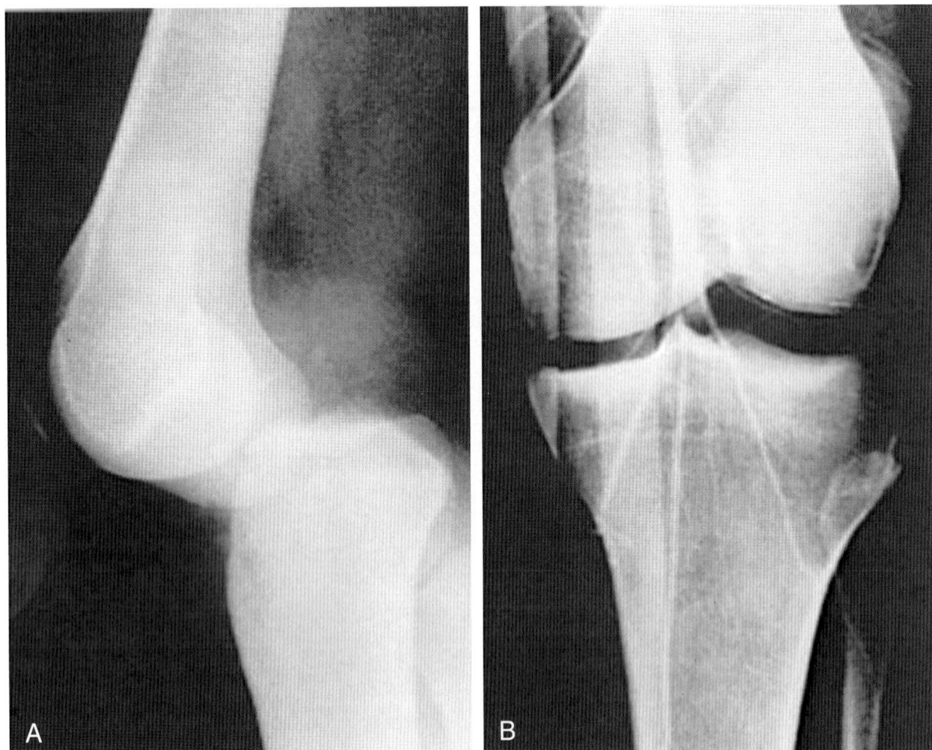


**Fig. 84.5 A,** Radiograph demonstrating posterior knee dislocation from a dashboard injury. **B,** Arteriogram showing an injury to the popliteal artery. (From Browner BD, Jupiter JB, Levine AM, et al. Skeletal trauma; basic science, management, and reconstruction. 3rd ed. Philadelphia: Saunders; 2003.)

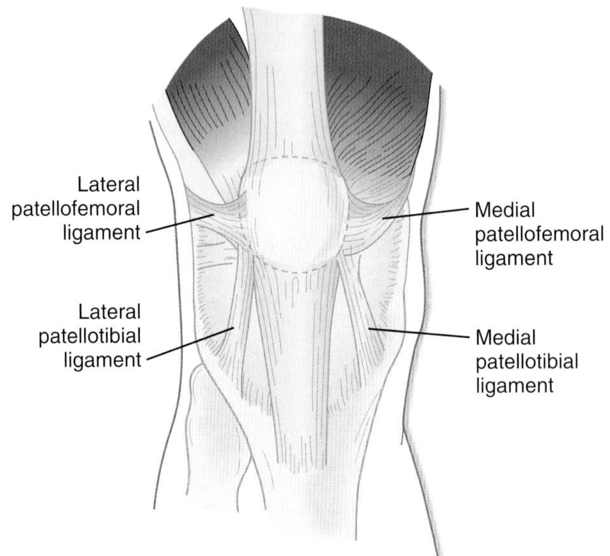


**Fig. 84.6 Patellofemoral and patellotibial ligaments.** These structures act as static stabilizers of the patella. (From DeLee JC, Drez Jr D, Miller MD. DeLee & Drez's orthopaedic sports medicine: principles and practice. 2nd ed. Philadelphia: Saunders; 2003.)

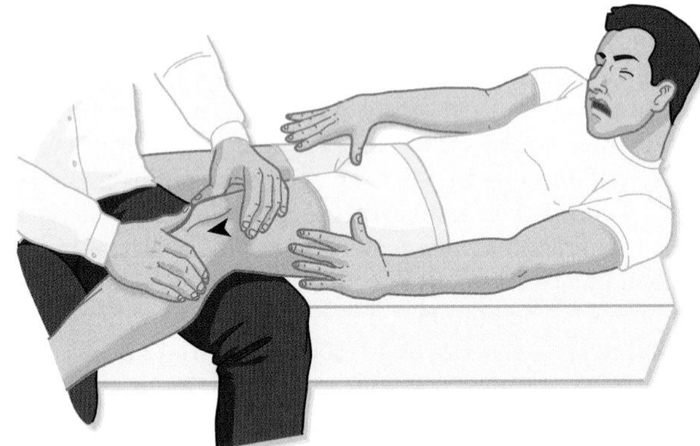

**Fig. 84.7 Positive apprehension test.** As the patella is displaced laterally over the lateral femoral condyle, the patient experiences apprehension and discomfort. (From DeLee JC, Drez Jr D, Miller MD. DeLee & Drez's orthopaedic sports medicine: principles and practice. 2nd ed. Philadelphia: Saunders; 2003.)

2 weeks. Complications include persistent instability, subluxation, repeated dislocation, and osteoarthritis.[4]

### Proximal Tibiofibular Joint Dislocations

The proximal tibiofibular joint is a small joint between the head of the fibula and the inferior aspect of the lateral tibial condyle. Dislocations can be anterior (most common), posterior, or superior. This rare injury is seen more in adolescents and young adults. It is typically associated with motor vehicle crashes and sports such as skydiving and hang gliding.

Pain and tenderness are felt over the proximal tibiofibular joint. On physical examination the patient has worsening pain with inversion and eversion of the foot or flexion and extension of the ankle. Instability may be present when anterior or posterior pressure is applied to the fibular head. Peroneal nerve injury occurs in approximately 5% of these dislocations.

AP and lateral radiographs are indicated. A comparison view may be helpful to make the diagnosis. Radiographs may demonstrate lateral displacement of the fibular head or diastasis of the proximal ends of the tibia and fibula.

Tibiofibular dislocations are reduced by flexing the knee to 90 degrees and everting and dorsiflexing the ankle while applying direct pressure to the head of the fibula. General anesthesia may be necessary. After reduction, the knee should be immobilized in extension or partial flexion. Posterior dislocations may be unstable, and recurrent subluxation may be seen. Degenerative joint disease and arthritis can develop after injury to this joint.[8]

## FRACTURES

### *Patellar Fracture*

The patella, the largest sesamoid bone in the body, is enveloped within the quadriceps tendon and articulates with the trochlear groove of the distal end of the femur. The superficial location of the patella makes it more susceptible to injury.

Patellar fractures account for approximately 1% of skeletal injuries and are the result of either a direct injury (dashboard injury) or an indirect injury (violent flexion). Indirect injuries result in an avulsion injury of the patella as a result of pull of the quadriceps muscle against resistance. Transverse patellar fractures are the most common type of fracture and are more likely to be displaced and be manifested as a disrupted extensor mechanism.

The patient usually has a swollen, painful knee. Patellar evaluation includes palpation for pain and bony disruption and assessment for extensor weakness. AP, lateral, and sunrise views of the knee should be obtained. A bipartite patella may be difficult to distinguish from a patellar fracture and is most often seen in the superolateral part of the patella. A high-riding patella, or a patella alta position, may signify disruption of the distal extensor mechanism; this is best visualized on AP and lateral views.[8]

Acute treatment of patellar fractures consists of ice, elevation, pain control, and a straight leg knee immobilizer. Nonoperative intervention is considered for nondisplaced fractures (<3 to 4 mm) when the extensor mechanism is intact. Patients with a disrupted extensor mechanism should have immediate orthopedic consultation because these injuries are often repaired within 24 hours.[4]

### *Proximal Tibial Fractures*

Proximal tibial fractures include fractures above the tibial tuberosity.

TIBIAL PLATEAU FRACTURES The proximal end of the tibia comprises the medial and lateral condyles, which make up approximately three fourths of the proximal tibial surface. The condyles ensure appropriate knee alignment, stability, and motion. Tibial plateau fractures account for about 1% of all proximal tibial fractures.[9]

Tibial plateau fractures are caused by side loading secondary to either a varus or a valgus force combined with axial compression, which results in the femoral condyle impacting on the tibia. Common mechanisms are motor vehicle crashes, falls, and athletic activities such as skiing (**Fig. 84.8**). A Segond fracture is bony avulsion of the lateral tibial plateau at the site of attachment of the lateral capsular ligament. This fracture is an important marker for ACL disruption and anterolateral rotary instability. Associated soft tissue injuries to the collateral ligaments, menisci, and neurovascular structures are common, although low-energy injuries (from athletic activities) usually result in less soft tissue damage.[9]

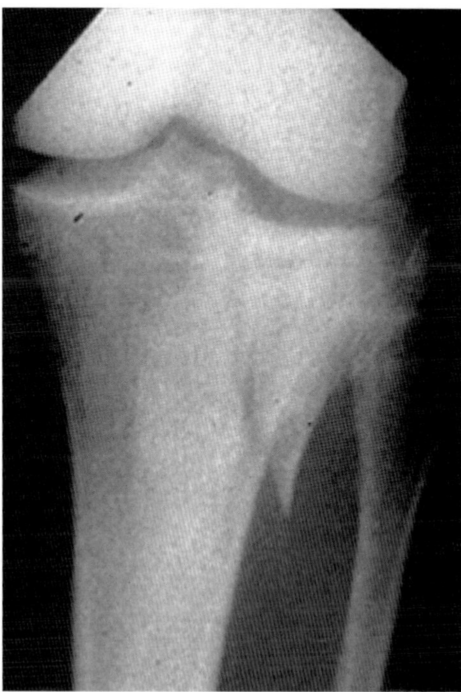

**Fig. 84.8 Lateral tibial plateau fracture.** (From Browner BD, Jupiter JB, Levine AM, et al. Skeletal trauma: basic science, management, and reconstruction. 3rd ed. Philadelphia: Saunders; 2003.)

Patients with tibial plateau fractures exhibit pain and swelling of the knee and hold their knee in a slightly flexed position. A valgus or varus deformity of the knee generally indicates a depressed fracture. Careful assessment of associated ipsilateral bony, soft tissue, and neurovascular status is essential given the high rate of association of such injuries with tibial plateau fractures.[9]

AP, lateral, and oblique radiographs are necessary to evaluate tibial plateau fractures. In addition, a tibial plateau view is helpful in assessing the amount of depression present. CT with 2-mm cuts and three-dimensional reconstruction is useful to further investigate indeterminate plain films, evaluate fracture patterns, show the precise extent of articular depression, and assist in planning for optimal operative treatment.[4]

Nonoperative treatment is indicated for minimal or nondisplaced fractures (<2 to 3 mm of articular incongruity), peripheral (submeniscal) fractures, and fractures in elderly, low-demand, or osteoporotic patients. Patients should not bear weight on the affected leg for 4 to 6 weeks.

Absolute indications for surgery are open fractures, arterial injuries, and compartment syndrome. Relative indications for surgery are displaced fractures leading to joint instability and depression of the plateau. The amount of depression that requires operative intervention is controversial and ranges from 3 to 10 mm; however, 3 mm is the usual cutoff in athletic patients.[9]

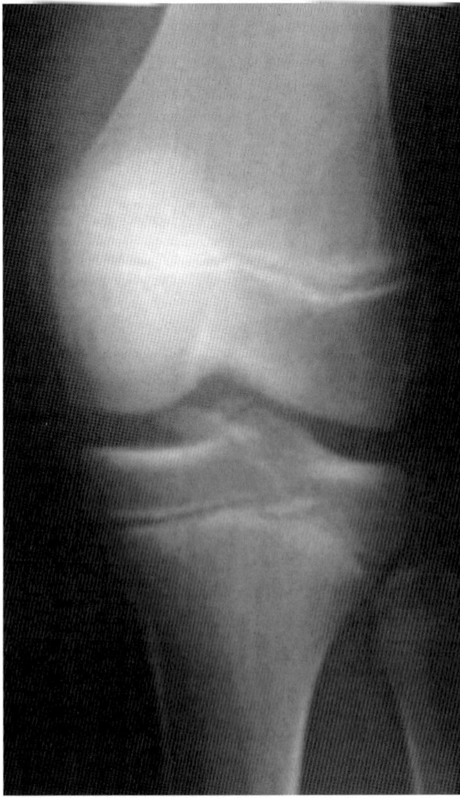

**Fig. 84.9 Type III eminence fracture.** Note the complete displacement of the avulsed fragment.

TIBIAL SPINE FRACTURES Tibial eminence avulsion fractures occur most often in children 8 to 14 years of age but can be seen in skeletally mature patients as well. A fracture of the anterior tibial spine in children is equivalent to an ACL rupture in adults.

The intercondylar eminence, or tibial spine, is the central portion of the proximal tibial surface. Tibial spine injuries usually result from a hyperextension force with or without a valgus or rotational moment about the knee. The fracture may also occur after a direct blow to the distal end of the femur while the knee is flexed (**Fig. 84.9**).

Affected patients have a suggestive history and a painful, swollen knee. In most cases, patients are unable to fully extend the knee and exhibit an effusion, and findings on stability tests (Lachman, anterior drawer) are abnormal. The examiner should carefully evaluate such patients for associated ligamentous injuries.

Routine AP and lateral radiographs are adequate to define these fractures. CT is helpful for evaluating displacement, whereas MRI is superior in assessing any accompanying soft tissue injuries.

Fractures with little or no displacement should be immobilized in a long leg splint with the knee flexed at approximately 10 to 20 degrees. Displaced fractures necessitate orthopedic consultation because they may require closed reduction (if no ligamentous damage is present) or open or arthroscopic reduction with fixation of the fragments.[10]

SUBCONDYLAR FRACTURES Subcondylar fractures involve the proximal tibial metaphysis and are usually transverse or oblique. Isolated subcondylar fractures are rare, and such fractures are generally associated with tibial plateau fractures.

Routine AP and lateral radiographs are adequate for evaluation of subcondylar fractures. Acute management of these injuries involves ice, elevation, and immobilization in a long leg splint. Stable extraarticular nondisplaced transverse fractures are treated with a long leg cast for 8 weeks. Fractures that are comminuted or associated with a condylar component require open reduction and internal fixation.[8]

### *Tibial Shaft Fractures*

Tibial shaft fractures are the most common long-bone fractures, as well as the most common open long-bone fracture. They are commonly associated with a fibular fracture or ligamentous injury. The fibula remains intact in only 15% to 25% of tibial shaft fractures. These fractures are associated with a high incidence of infection, delayed union, nonunion, and malunion.

Tibial shaft fractures result from either direct (motor vehicle accidents) or indirect (rotary or compressive forces) trauma. High-energy direct injuries usually cause transverse or comminuted fractures (most common). Indirect trauma commonly results in spiral or oblique fractures (**Fig. 84.10**).

A good neurovascular examination is essential. Skin integrity should be noted, and documentation of the integrity of the peroneal nerve is mandatory, as is a thorough examination of the knee and ankle.

AP and lateral radiographs should be obtained and must include the knee and ankle in both views. Closed tibial shaft fractures are immobilized in a long leg posterior splint with 10 to 20 degrees of knee flexion. Closed tibial and fibula shaft fractures, especially if displaced, are at risk for the development of compartment syndrome. Such injuries may necessitate observation in the hospital. It is estimated that compartment syndrome may develop in approximately 8% of tibial diaphyseal fractures. Any patient discharged home from the ED with a closed tibial fracture should be educated about the signs of compartment syndrome.

Open fractures should be gently cleaned, dressed with sterile dressings, and placed in a splint while awaiting orthopedic consultation. Patients should receive prophylactic antibiotics and tetanus prophylaxis. Emergency reduction is necessary for injuries accompanied by neurovascular compromise. Nonunion or delayed union is more likely with fractures that are open, severely displaced, or comminuted or with fractures associated with severe soft tissue injuries or infections.[11]

### *Proximal Fibular Fractures*

Proximal fibular fractures are often seen in conjunction with tibial fractures. Isolated proximal fibular fractures are rare given that the fibula runs parallel to the tibia and is bound to the tibia via ligaments. These fractures may be associated with significant knee injuries.

Isolated proximal fibular fractures are treated with protected weight bearing. The EP must rule out other associated injuries, such as lateral collateral ligament injury, common peroneal nerve injury, arterial injuries, and Maisonneuve fractures.[11]

### *Tibial Tuberosity Fractures*

The tibial tubercle is a bony prominence that is found approximately 3 cm distal to the proximal articular surface of

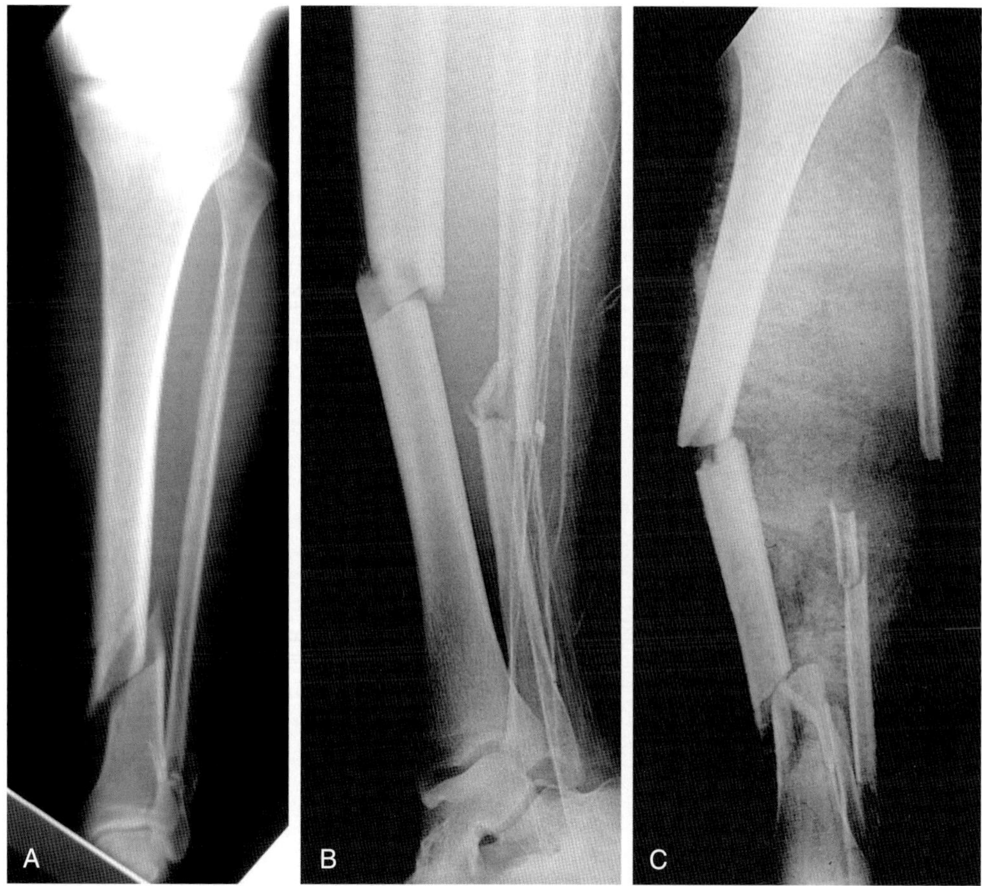


**Fig. 84.10 Radiographic examples of the three grades of severity of tibial fractures. A,** Minor: spiral fracture caused by a simple slip and fall. **B,** Moderate: fracture in a pedestrian struck by a slowly moving vehicle. **C,** Major: fracture caused by a high-velocity motorcycle crash. (From Browner BD, Jupiter JB, Levine AM, et al. Skeletal trauma: basic science, management, and reconstruction. 3rd ed. Philadelphia: Saunders; 2003.)

the tibia and in line with the medial half of the patella. It is the insertion point of the extensor mechanism, and thus accurate reduction and healing of this structure are essential.

Tibial tubercle avulsion fractures are rare injuries. Although they can occur in adults, these fractures are more commonly seen in adolescents undergoing a growth spurt. Most fractures are the result of an indirect force delivered by an eccentric load.[12] A sudden flexion force is applied while the knee is in flexion and the quadriceps is tightly contracted. The quadriceps resists the force, which causes avulsion of the tibial tubercle.

The physical findings depend on the extent of the injury. Swelling and tenderness are present over the anterior aspect of the tibia. A joint effusion may result from associated intraarticular injuries. The injured knee is usually held in 20 to 40 degrees of flexion secondary to hamstring spasm. In addition, the patient may not be able to extend the knee because of either pain or loss of the extensor mechanism.[13]

Routine AP and lateral radiographs are useful for ruling out associated fractures (**Fig. 84.11**). Initial treatment is similar to that for both quadriceps and patellar tendon injuries. Minimally displaced fractures are treated conservatively. Displaced fractures frequently require open reduction and internal fixation.[12]

## SOFT TISSUE AND CARTILAGINOUS INJURIES

### EXTENSOR MECHANISM INJURIES

The extensor mechanism of the knee is composed of the quadriceps muscles and tendon, the patella, the patellar tendon, and the tibial tubercle. Injuries can result from direct trauma (direct blow or laceration) or an indirect force (forced flexion of the knee). Rupture of the extensor mechanism is relatively uncommon in comparison with other injuries involving the knee joint.[12]

### QUADRICEPS AND PATELLAR TENDON INJURIES

The quadriceps tendon represents the convergence of the rectus femoris, vastus intermedius, vastus lateralis, and vastus medialis muscles. It inserts on the superior pole of the patella. The patellar tendon travels from the inferior pole of the patella to the tibial tubercle.

Quadriceps ruptures typically occur in patients older than 40 years. Rupture is usually the result of forced quadriceps contraction with a flexed knee, which loads the tendon. Direct blows and lacerations can also cause disruption of the tendon.

The most common site of rupture is at or near its insertion on the patella. Predisposing factors are listed in **Box 84.4**.

Patellar tendon ruptures are less common. Risk factors for patellar tendon rupture are similar to those for quadriceps rupture, with the exception that they generally occur in patients younger than 40 years. Most patellar tendon ruptures occur along the inferior pole of the patella.

Pain, swelling, and ecchymosis are usually localized to the superior pole (quadriceps tendon) or inferior pole (patellar tendon) of the patella. A defect in the patella or quadriceps tendon may be palpable on physical examination. Other physical findings include a low-riding patella (patella baja) with inferior retraction of the patella (quadriceps tendon rupture) or a high-riding patella (patella alta) with superior retraction of the patella (patellar tendon rupture). The integrity of the extensor mechanism should always be evaluated.

AP and lateral radiographs help define the patellar position (alta or baja) and rule out associated fractures. Ultrasound has also been shown to be useful in diagnosing quadriceps tears. MRI is helpful in the diagnosis of partial tears.

Orthopedic consultation in the ED is indicated for suspected injuries and complete ruptures. Initial treatment consists of ice, elevation, and a straight leg immobilizer. Partial tears are treated by immobilization for 4 to 6 weeks, whereas complete tears are treated surgically. Diagnosis is essential given the better outcomes with prompt referral and repair.

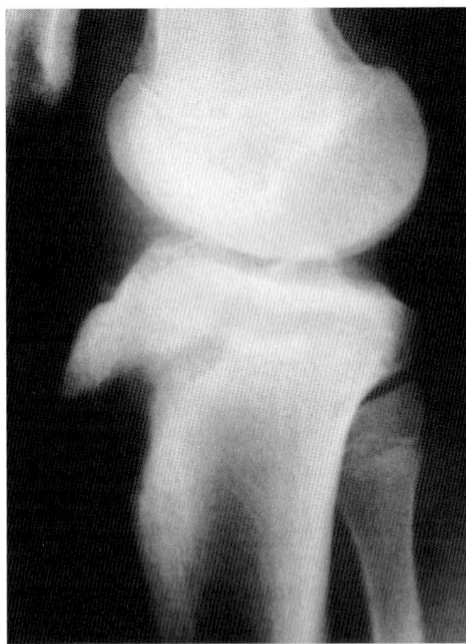

**Fig. 84.11 Lateral knee radiograph in a 14-year-old boy with a displaced fracture of the tibial tubercle.** (From Green NE, Swiontkowski MF. Skeletal trauma in children, vol 3. 3rd ed. Philadelphia: Saunders; 2003.)

## LIGAMENTOUS AND MENISCAL INJURIES

Knee stability depends on the static stability of the ligaments and the dynamic stability of the muscles. Injuries to the knee involve the following six common mechanisms: (1) valgus stress (laterally directed), (2) varus stress (medially directed), (3) hyperextension, (4) rotational stress, (5) direct anterior stress, and (6) direct posterior stress. These stressors, working in isolation or combination, may result in myriad of ligamentous, meniscal, or chondral injuries.[12]

Common mechanisms of ligamentous knee injuries are shown in **Figure 84.12**. Diagnosis is based on clinical

**BOX 84.4 Risk Factors for Quadriceps Tendon Rupture**

Age > 40 years
Steroid use
Insertional tendinopathy
Chronic metabolic disorders
Chronic systemic conditions (rheumatoid arthritis, systemic lupus erythematosus, gout)

Data from Perryman JR, Hershman EB. The acute management of soft tissue injuries of the knee. Orthop Clin North Am 2002;33:575-85.

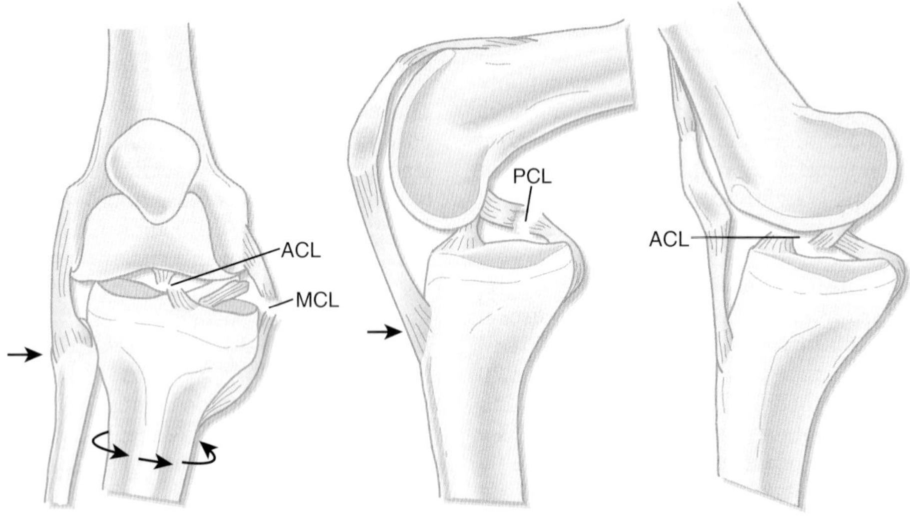


**Fig. 84.12 Common mechanisms of knee injuries.** *ACL*, Anterior cruciate ligament; *LCL*, lateral collateral ligament; *MCL*, medial collateral ligament; *PCL*, posterior cruciate ligament. (From Browner BD, Jupiter JB, Levine AM, et al. Skeletal trauma: basic science, management, and reconstruction. 3rd ed. Philadelphia: Saunders; 2003.)

examination; plain radiographs are indicated if a fracture is suspected. MRI offers a direct, noninvasive view of the knee ligaments, menisci, and other soft tissue structures; however, it is rarely indicated in the ED setting.

Stability testing for ligamentous and meniscal injuries is outlined in Table 84.1 and **Figures 84.13 to 84.16**. Ligament function, mechanism of injury, diagnosis, and treatment are outlined in **Table 84.3**. Most ligamentous and meniscal injuries should be reevaluated by an orthopedist in 3 to 5 days.[4]

## MUSCLE STRAINS

### *Gastrocnemius Muscle Strain*

The gastrocnemius, soleus, and plantaris muscles form the posterior muscles of the calf. The tendon of the gastrocnemius muscle has two heads that arise from the posterior surfaces of the medial and lateral femoral condyles. The tendons of the gastrocnemius and soleus muscles form the Achilles tendon, which inserts on the posterior tubercle of the calcaneus. The gastrocnemius muscle acts primarily as a plantar flexor but also provides some passive support to the

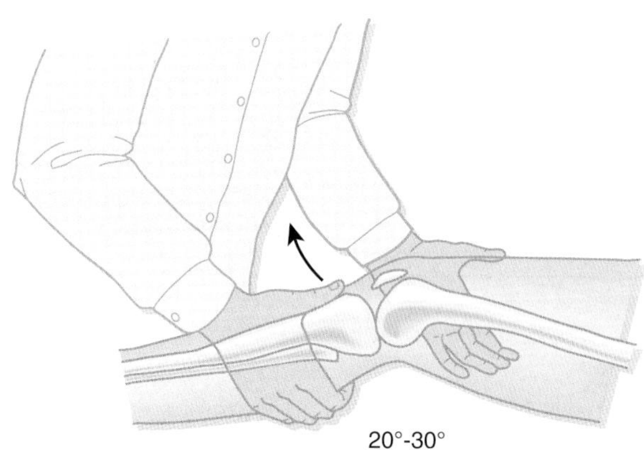


**Fig. 84.13 Lachman test for anterior drawer instability.** The test is done at 20 to 30 degrees of flexion. The examiner stabilizes the femur with one hand and draws the tibia anteriorly with the other hand. (From Browner BD, Jupiter JB, Levine AM, et al. Skeletal trauma: basic science, management, and reconstruction. 3rd ed. Philadelphia: Saunders; 2003.)

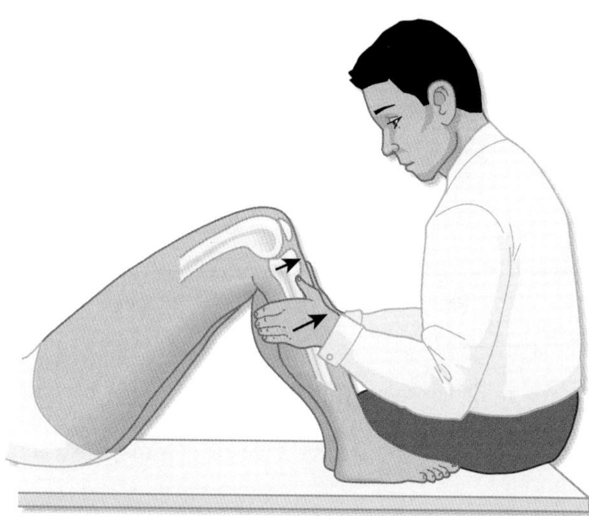

**Fig. 84.14 Anterior drawer test.** The knee is placed in 90 degrees of flexion, the foot is stabilized with pressure toward the examination table, and the proximal end of the tibia is grasped and pulled forward. (From Brown JR, Trojian TH. Anterior and posterior cruciate ligament injuries. Prim Care 2004;31:925-56.)

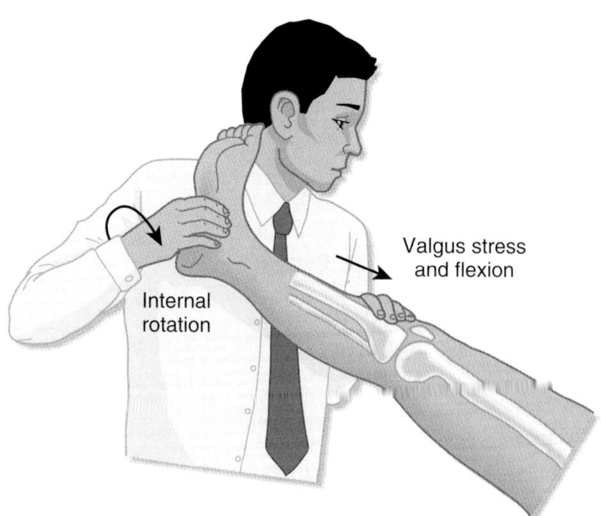


**Fig. 84.15 Pivot shift test.** With one hand the examiner flexes the hip to 45 degrees, extends the knee, and holds the heel. With the other hand the examiner holds the knee with the thumb behind the fibular head. The examiner then internally rotates the leg at the heel and applies valgus stress and flexion at the knee. (From Brown JR, Trojian TH. Anterior and posterior cruciate ligament injuries. Prim Care 2004;31:925-56.)

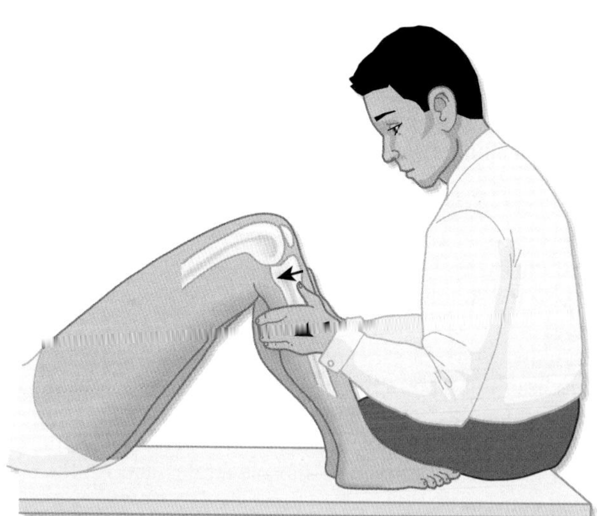

**Fig. 84.16 Posterior drawer test.** The knee is placed in 90 degrees of flexion and the foot is stabilized with pressure toward the examination table. The proximal end of the tibia is then grasped and a posterior force applied to it. (From Brown JR, Trojian TH. Anterior and posterior cruciate ligament injuries. Prim Care 2004;31:925-56.)

**Table 84.3 Static Knee Stabilizers: Function, Mechanism of Injury, and Treatment**

| STRUCTURE | FUNCTION | MECHANISM OF INJURY | TEST | INITIAL TREATMENT |
|---|---|---|---|---|
| Anterior cruciate ligament | Prevents forward displacement of the tibia on the femur | Deceleration, hyperextension, or twisting | Lachman, anterior drawer, pivot shift (see Figs. 84.13 to 84.15) | Ice, elevation, pain control, hinged knee brace (unlocked) |
| Posterior cruciate ligament | Primary restraint against posterior tibial displacement | Forced hyperflexion, direct blow to the proximal end of the tibia | Posterior drawer (see Fig. 84-16), posterior sag | Ice, elevation, pain control, hinged knee brace (unlocked) |
| Lateral collateral ligament | Lateral joint stability | Direct force to the anteromedial aspect of the knee when extended | Varus stress testing in extension and 30 degrees of flexion | Ice, elevation, pain control, hinged knee brace (unlocked) |
| Medial collateral ligament | Medial joint stability | Direct force to the lateral aspect of a partially flexed knee | Valgus stress testing in extension and 30 degrees of flexion | Ice, elevation, pain control, hinged knee brace (unlocked) |
| Meniscal injuries | Load-share and reduce contact stress across the joint | Cutting, deceleration, landing from a jump | McMurray test, Apley test | Partial weight bearing or hinged knee brace (unlocked). A "locked" knee requires attempted reduction and orthopedic consultation |

posterior joint capsule. The most common mechanism of injury to this muscle is hyperextension of the knee. Posterior dislocation of the tibia during knee flexion may also injure this muscle.

Patients may describe sudden calf pain while running or making a sudden stop or cut. Pain and swelling of the calf develop over the next day, and tenderness is typically found at the musculotendinous junction of the medial (more common) or lateral head of the gastrocnemius muscle. Complete rupture of the head of the gastrocnemius muscle is associated with retraction of the muscle belly. Acute posterior compartment syndrome has been associated with rupture of the medial head of the gastrocnemius muscle.[14]

Plain radiographs are not indicated. MRI may be helpful if a soft tissue injury is in doubt. Acute strains of the gastrocnemius muscle are treated conservatively with ice, compression wraps, and antiinflammatory medications. Gentle passive and active stretching exercises are begun early.

### *Strain or Rupture of the Plantaris Muscle*

The plantaris is a pencil-shaped muscle that originates at the lateral condyle of the femur and passes below the soleus to attach to the Achilles tendon. Strain of the proximal plantaris muscle may occur with an injury to the ACL.

Patients with plantaris muscle rupture may experience a deep, disabling pain in the calf followed by a dull, deep ache. On examination, tenderness is greatest just lateral to the midline of the posterior aspect of the calf. No diagnostic testing is indicated. Plantaris muscle strains and ruptures are treated conservatively.

### *Shin Splints*

Shin splints are also known as the medial tibial stress syndrome, which is characterized by diffuse tenderness over the posteromedial aspect of the distal third of the tibia. It is believed to represent a periostalgia or tendinopathy along the tibial attachment of the tibialis posterior or soleus muscle. It may be confused with a stress fracture.

Common contributing factors are improper shoe wear, rapid transition in training, inadequate warm-up, running on uneven or hard surfaces, running in cold weather, and anatomic considerations. Patients with mild cases of shin splints have pain during exercise, whereas those with more severe cases have pain at rest.

Diagnostic tests are not indicated for shin splints unless a tibial stress fracture is a consideration. Treatment of shin splints involves relative rest, training adjustment, and antiinflammatory medications. Runners should be instructed to avoid running on hills and uneven surfaces.[15]

## OVERUSE INJURIES

Common tendinopathies and bursitis of the knee are described in Chapter 86.

### OSGOOD-SCHLATTER DISEASE

Osgood-Schlatter disease is an overuse injury that involves traction apophysis at the tibial tubercle. It is often seen in adolescents during a growth spurt, when the apophysis in this region becomes weaker than the surrounding bony and tendinous tissues. The condition is bilateral in 20% to 30% of cases. Its cause is unknown.

Patients with Osgood-Schlatter disease complain of pain and swelling over the tibial tuberosity. They may describe worsening of the pain with jumping, squatting, or kneeling. The pain may be intermittent and is rarely severe enough to interrupt daily activity. Physical examination demonstrates localized pain and swelling over the tibial tuberosity.

A lateral knee radiograph is the most useful view and may show separation of the apophysis or fragmentation of a portion of the tibial tubercle. The appearance of tibial tubercle fragmentation may represent a normal variant in ossification of the tibial tubercle. Radiographic findings without associated clinical symptoms should be interpreted with caution.

Osgood-Schlatter disease is generally a self-limited condition. In most cases, treatment is nonoperative and consists of modification of activity, nonsteroidal antiinflammatory drugs (NSAIDs), and physical therapy. The family of an adolescent with this disorder should be counseled that the symptoms may take up to 12 to 18 months to resolve.[13]

### STRESS FRACTURES

A stress fracture is a partial or complete bone fracture that results from repeated stress. Stress fractures are most common in the lower extremities (tibia, fibula, and metatarsal bones). They occur as a result of a repetitive use injury that exceeds the intrinsic ability of the bone to repair itself. Tibial stress fractures are commonly seen in military recruits, as well as in track and long-distance runners.

Patients have localized dull pain in the lower extremity that is not related to trauma. The pain typically worsens during exercise or weight bearing. Stress fractures can be manifested in a similar fashion as shin splints but are associated with more focal bony tenderness.

Evidence of a stress fracture may not appear on plain radiographs for up to 2 to 10 weeks after the onset of symptoms. The presence of a transverse fracture line across the entire anterior shaft of the tibia on a plain radiograph is considered a poor prognostic sign and is associated with a greater likelihood of nonunion.[8] Radionuclide scintigraphy can confirm the diagnosis as early as 2 to 8 days after the onset of symptoms.

Initial treatment consists of conservative therapy: ice, antiinflammatory pain medication, and rest for several weeks or until the extremity is free of pain. Tibial fractures that do not improve with conservative management may require splinting in a walking boot or air splint. A midshaft tibial fracture is splinted until the extremity is pain free with radiographic evidence of healing.[15]

## OTHER DISORDERS

### OSTEOCHONDRITIS DISSECANS

Osteochondritis dissecans is a potentially reversible idiopathic lesion of subchondral bone. It is seen more often in children and adolescents. Osteochondritis dissecans of the knee occurs most commonly on the posterolateral aspect of the medial femoral condyle (70% to 80%) (**Fig. 84.17**). Inflammation, genetics, ischemia, ossification, and repetitive trauma have all been hypothesized as possible causes.

Most children and adolescents with this disorder have a stable lesion and nonspecific complaints, such as aches or activity-related knee pain localized to the anterior aspect of the knee. Both knees should be examined because the condition is bilateral in 20% to 25% of cases. Initial plain radiographs should include AP, lateral, and tunnel views of the knee.

Stable osteochondritis dissecans lesions have a favorable healing rate with conservative management alone (modified activity, NSAIDs, rehabilitative exercises). Patients and their

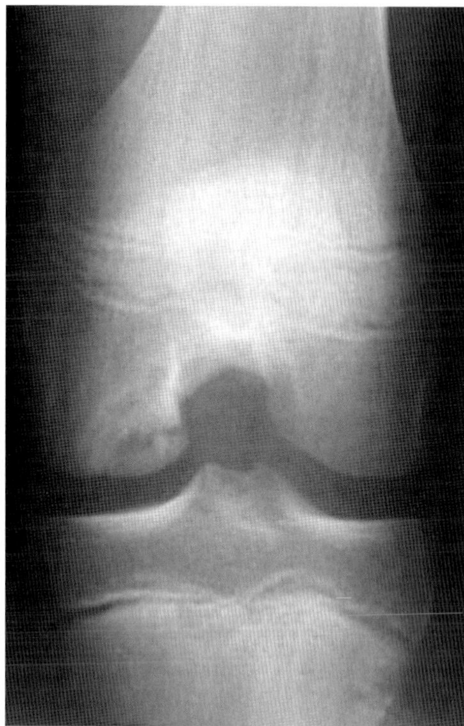

**Fig. 84.17 Tunnel radiograph of a juvenile osteochondritis dissecans lesion of the medial femoral condyle.** The lesion can be difficult to see on an anteroposterior radiograph and is often more apparent on the notch view, which images the posterior aspect of the femoral condyle with knee flexion.

parents should be instructed that it takes up to 12 to 18 months for healing to be complete.[16]

### OSTEONECROSIS

Osteonecrosis of the knee is usually idiopathic and is most commonly located on the medial femoral condyle. It may be associated with steroids, irradiation, and systemic diseases such as sickle cell anemia and rheumatologic disorders. Osteonecrosis occurs when the blood supply to the bone is disrupted, which results in bone infarction.

The patient has a sudden onset of pain over the anteromedial (most common) aspect of the knee. The pain may become worse at night or increase with activity. Idiopathic osteonecrosis is typically seen in women older than 60 years. The patient may have a joint effusion or decreased range of motion of the knee joint.

Radionuclide scintigraphy or CT may be required to detect the disease in its early stages. Plain radiographic findings in patients with early disease are usually normal.

Patients with early stages of osteonecrosis are treated conservatively with partial weight bearing and antiinflammatory medications. Patients with advanced disease may require surgery to restore the articular surface. Total knee arthroplasty is reserved for disease that has expanded to the lateral compartment.[17]

### PATELLOFEMORAL PAIN SYNDROME

Patellofemoral pain syndrome refers to the clinical manifestation of anterior knee pain related to changes in the patellofemoral articulation. Patients are generally between the ages of 10 and 20 years and usually have complaints of nonspecific anterior knee pain that is not related to trauma. Athletes may experience symptoms after periods of overactivity. Elderly patients may exhibit symptoms if they have arthritis that affects the patellofemoral joint. The most important risk factors are overuse, quadriceps weakness, and soft tissue tightness. In most cases the etiology is multifactorial.[18]

The patient has a history of mild to moderate anterior knee pain. The knee may be more painful with prolonged flexion, stair climbing, or kneeling. Physical examination may show a slight effusion, along with patellar crepitus on range of motion. Applying direct pressure to the anterior aspect of the patella may reproduce the patient's pain.[5]

Plain radiographs are not indicated. CT or MRI can detect abnormalities in the articular surface of the patella. In most cases, a physical therapy program that strengthens the quadriceps muscle can successfully reduce the symptoms. Surgery may be required for the minority of patients who do not respond to conservative management.[18]

## POPLITEAL CYST

A popliteal cyst, or Baker cyst, is an inflammation of the semimembranosus or medial gastrocnemius bursa. A Baker cyst is produced by herniation of the synovial membrane through the posterior knee capsule. It is usually the result of synovitis, arthritis, or an internal derangement of the knee that results in excess synovial fluid in the bursa.

Intermittent swelling can develop behind the knee. If the bursa ruptures, the patient may complain of calf pain, and the findings may be similar to those in patients with thrombophlebitis.

Ultrasonography is helpful to distinguish Baker cysts from other disorders, such as popliteal artery aneurysms, neoplasms, and thrombophlebitis. Treatment is based on the underlying cause. Asymptomatic cysts found incidentally need no further treatment.[19]

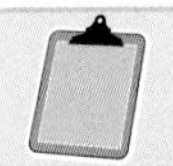

### DOCUMENTATION

The following issues should be clearly documented in a patient with knee or lower leg injury:

- History: Mechanism of injury; duration and location of symptoms; associated symptoms; exacerbating or alleviating factors; complaints of weakness, numbness, or instability; complicating medical factors; and previous interventions, imaging, or evaluations
- Physical examination: Neurovascular status (before and after splint placement or reduction), compartment assessment, skin integrity, stability assessment, and associated injuries
- Radiography: Anteroposterior or lateral films of the joint above and below the injury; prereduction and postreduction films indicated for most reductions
- Medical decision making: Any emergency reduction secondary to neurovascular compromise and reasons for emergency or nonemergency consultation or follow-up
- Procedures: Neurovascular status both before and after reduction or splint placement, skin integrity, and postreduction fracture alignment
- Patient instructions: Discussion with the patient regarding splint care, appropriate crutch use, importance of range-of-motion exercises, weight-bearing status, warning signs for neurovascular impairment and compartment syndromes, and arrangements for follow-up or return to the emergency department

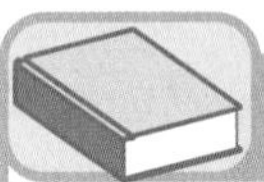

### PATIENT TEACHING TIPS

A patient in whom a strain, sprain or stable injury of the knee is diagnosed should be discharged home in a hinged brace (fully unlocked). If discharged in a knee immobilizer, the patient should be instructed to perform gentle range-of-motion exercises multiple times per day to prevent joint stiffness.

A patient with a tibia fracture who is sent home should be educated about compartment syndrome and told to return to the emergency department if either severe pain or numbness in the foot or leg develops within the first 48 hours.

A patient with an acute injury should be instructed to:

- Elevate the injured area above the level of the heart for the first 48 hours after the injury.
- Apply ice to the injured area while avoiding direct contact of ice with bare skin and getting the splint moist.

In a patient discharged from the emergency department on crutches:

- Crutch training should be given.
- The ability of the patient to safely use crutches should be observed before discharge.

## SUGGESTED READINGS

Davenport M. Knee and leg injuries. Emerg Med Clin North Am 2010;28:861-84.

Howells NR, Brunton LR, Robinson J, et al. Acute knee dislocation: an evidence based approach to the management of the multiligament injured knee. Injury 2010. Available at http://www.ncbi.nlm.nih.gov/pubmed/21156317.

Seaberg DC, Yealy DM, Lukens T, et al. Multicenter comparison of two clinical decision rules for the use of radiography in acute, high-risk knee injuries. Ann Emerg Med 1998;32:8-13.

Stiell IG, Wells GA, McDowell I, et al. Use of radiography in acute knee injuries: need for clinical decision rules. Acad Emerg Med 1995;2:966-73.

## REFERENCES

*References can be found on Expert Consult @ www.expertconsult.com.*

# Foot and Ankle Injuries 85

Jorge del Castillo

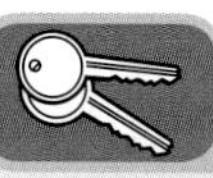

**KEY POINTS**

- Most ankle sprains are due to inversion during plantar flexion of the ankle, and 85% involve the lateral ligaments.
- Isolated injury to the medial (deltoid) ligament is uncommon; such injury is usually associated with a medial malleolar fracture.
- Examination techniques that cause pain make complete examination less feasible; do not start the examination at the point of maximal swelling and tenderness.
- Because magnetic resonance imaging is better at detecting ligamentous injuries involving the ankle, stress testing is less commonly performed in the acute phase of injury.
- Do not mistake subluxating peroneal tendons for an ankle sprain because the treatment and prognosis are different.
- The Thompson test to assess Achilles tendon rupture can be misleading, especially with partial tears.
- Dislocations at the level of the tibiotalar joint require prompt anatomic reduction to minimize cutaneous and neurovascular injury.
- Talar dome fractures are often missed; further evaluation is required in patients with swelling or locking of the ankle 4 to 5 weeks after injury.

## PERSPECTIVE

Injuries to the ankle and foot are the most common orthopedic injuries and the most frequently seen athletic injuries in the emergency department (ED). The lateral ligaments are most often involved because of the anatomy of the tibiotalar joint.

The frequency of these injuries often leads physicians to minimize their seriousness and morbidity. It is important to avoid this pitfall and adhere to a methodic physical and radiographic examination. Additionally, one must avoid undertreatment of these injuries, maintain a guarded prognosis, and ensure proper follow-up when necessary.

## EPIDEMIOLOGY

Inversion injuries occur at a rate of 1 per 10,000 people per day, which equates to about 28,000 injuries per day in the United States. Injury to the dominant ankle is more likely than injury to the nondominant ankle. These injuries are common during recreational sports involving running, such as basketball, soccer, baseball, and volleyball.

Inversion injuries may at first glance appear to be common and minor. A large percentage of these injuries continue to be symptomatic for a year or longer after the injury. Chronic instability eventually develops in some individuals and requires surgical repair.[1]

## PATHOPHYSIOLOGY

### ANATOMY

The ankle is composed of two joints: the talar mortise and the subtalar joint. The talar joint is a modified hinge joint similar to a "mortise and tenon," as referred to in carpentry. It is composed of three bones: the tibia, the mortise, and the talus of the fibula, which form the tenon (**Fig. 85.1**). The plafond or "ceiling" of this joint is formed by the tibia with its medial malleolus and articulation with the fibula.

The dome of the talus has a trapezoidal shape—wider anteriorly and narrower posteriorly. This anatomic shape confers greater stability in dorsiflexion. However, when the ankle moves into plantar flexion, the narrow part of the talus sits in the mortise, which results in ankle instability and predisposes it to injury.[2,3]

#### *Ligaments of the Ankle*

The medial side of the ankle is supported by the deltoid ligament (**Fig. 85.2**). The deltoid ligament has five components: one deep and four superficial. The deep ligament attaches to the tibia and the undersurface of the talus. The superficial ligaments are the tibionavicular, anterior talotibial, calcaneotibial, and posterior talotibial.

The lateral aspect of the ankle has three supporting ligaments: the anterior talofibular, calcaneofibular, and posterior talofibular (**Fig. 85.3**). The tibiofibular ligaments include the anterior and posterior inferior ligaments, which bind the distal ends of the tibia and fibula, and the superior ligaments of the

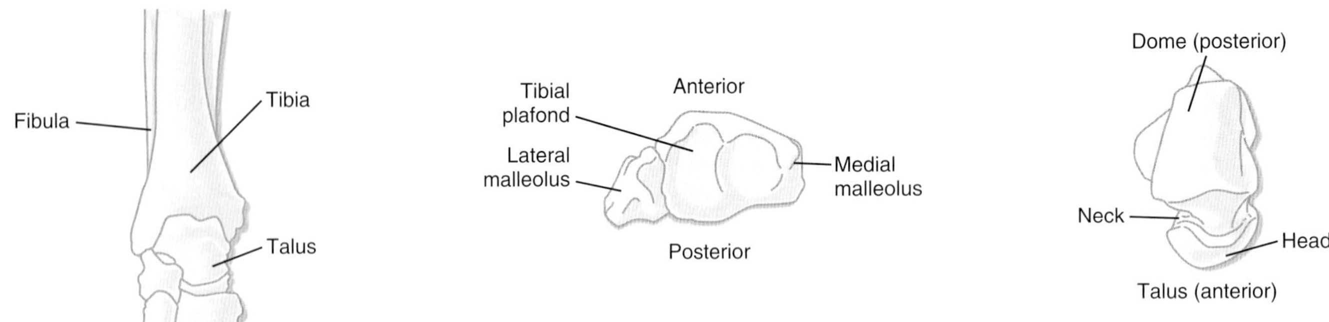


**Fig. 85.1** Bony anatomy of the ankle.

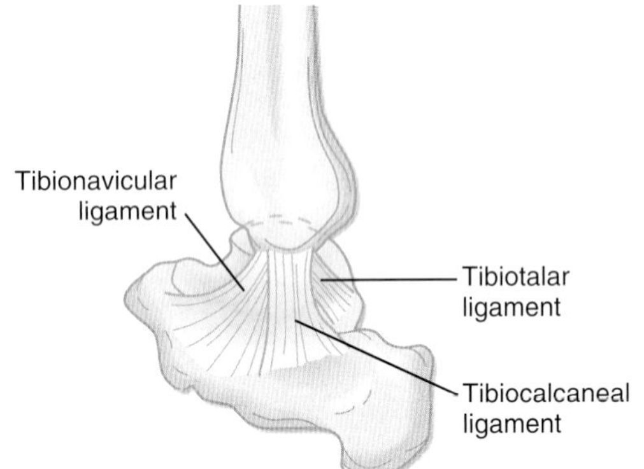


**Fig. 85.2** Medial ligaments of the ankle.

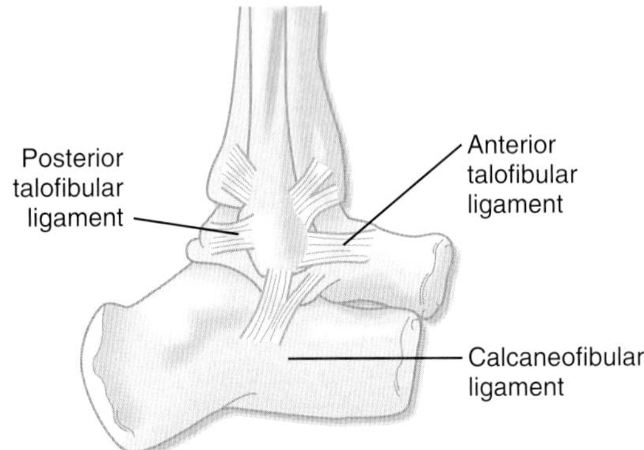


**Fig. 85.3** Lateral ligaments of the ankle.

same name, which bind the tibia and fibula at the proximal articulation. Other supporting structures are the inferior transverse ligament and the interosseous ligament. The latter is not part of the ankle but nevertheless provides a strong bond between the tibia and fibula.[2,3]

## PRESENTING SIGNS AND SYMPTOMS

As noted previously, the ankle is a modified hinge joint; its motion is predominantly executed in a sagittal plane.

Most ankle sprains are due to inversion during plantar flexion of the ankle. Thus approximately 85% of injuries involve the lateral ligaments: the anterior talofibular ligament, the calcaneofibular ligament, and the posterior talofibular ligament. Of sprains caused by inversion, 65% are isolated to the anterior talofibular ligament. In some patients the subtalar complex may also be injured. The calcaneofibular ligament is rarely injured in isolation. Classification of these injuries and examination findings are presented in **Table 85.1**.

**Table 85.1** Classification of Ankle Sprains

| TYPE OF INJURY | EXTENT OF INJURY | PHYSICAL FINDINGS |
|---|---|---|
| Grade I | Stretch of the ligament with microscopic but not macroscopic tearing | Minor swelling but no joint instability |
| Grade II | Involves partial tearing of the particular ligament | Minor to moderate swelling and some instability of the affected ankle |
| Grade III | Involves complete rupture of the ligament | Significant swelling, tenderness, and ecchymosis; instability of the joint and inability to bear weight |

Isolated injury to the medial (deltoid) ligament is uncommon, and such injury is usually accompanied by a medial malleolar fracture. Distal tibiofibular syndesmotic rupture is very rare and is associated with forceful dorsiflexion and external rotation.[2,4]

## HISTORY AND PHYSICAL EXAMINATION

A methodic approach to elicitation of the history of the injury and examination of the ankle joint is of paramount importance. Frequently, the mechanism is unknown because of the sudden and rapid occurrence of the injury. Specific questions about the mechanism, time of the injury, ability to bear weight, and previous history of injury involving the affected joint are helpful in arriving at an accurate diagnosis (**Box 85.1**).

The physical examination (**Box 85.2**) should be thorough and orderly with the intent of assessing joint stability and possible neurovascular compromise. The emergency physician (EP) should make sure that the patient is in a comfortable

**BOX 85.1 Suggested Questions During the History in Patients with Ankle Injuries**

Has the same ankle been injured before?
Is there any other relevant medical history?
What was the mechanism of the injury?
Where is the point of maximal tenderness?
Was a popping or snapping sound heard?
Did the swelling occur immediately?
Were you able to bear weight?
Was any emergency treatment performed?

**BOX 85.2 Sequential Examination of the Injured Ankle**

1. Visual inspection
2. Neurovascular assessment
3. Proximal fibula
4. Midshaft tibia and interosseous membrane
5. Medial malleolus and deltoid ligament
6. Lateral malleolus and ligaments
7. Syndesmosis
8. Anterior talofibular ligament
9. Calcaneofibular ligament
10. Posterior talofibular ligament
11. Peroneal tendons
12. Achilles tendon
13. Navicular and bifurcated ligament
14. Base of the fifth metatarsal
15. Range of motion
16. Other manouvers (anterior drawer, tilt, side-to-side tests)

position for the examination. Many times patients are examined in hallways while sitting in chairs with their feet resting on the floor or a wheelchair footrest. Uncomfortable approaches to examination of the ankle—or any joint for that matter—are detrimental to the welfare of both the patient and physician. All that is derived from this approach is an incomplete examination and an uncomfortable patient and physician.

The EP should make sure that the patient is seated at a level higher than the examiner (e.g., seated on a gurney with the affected limb dependent, seated on the examining table with both extremities on the table). Never begin the examination at the point of maximal swelling and tenderness. The examination should begin with visual inspection to assess the degree of swelling and the presence of any deformity and discoloration. The neurovascular status of the extremity is evaluated by testing sensation, capillary refilling, and presence of pulses. Once a preliminary assessment is done, the EP should proceed in detail from distal to proximal in an orderly fashion as noted in Box 85.2.[5]

## OTHER MANEUVERS

Other maneuvers sometimes used in the evaluation of an injured ankle are worth mentioning. The *anterior drawer test* (**Fig. 85.4**) is used to determine the integrity of the anterior talofibular ligament. It is, unfortunately, not very reliable, especially in acute injuries with significant swelling and pain. It is performed by holding the foot at the calcaneus with one hand while the other hand stabilizes the extremity at its middle third. The foot is moved forward while one observes or feels (or both) for displacement of the foot and ankle anteriorly.

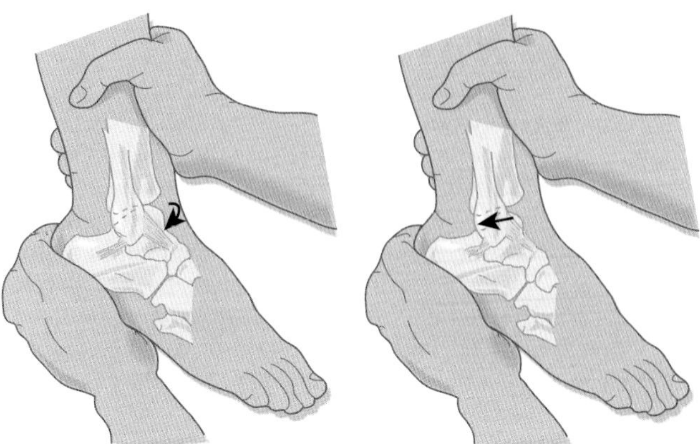

**Fig. 85.4** Anterior drawer test.

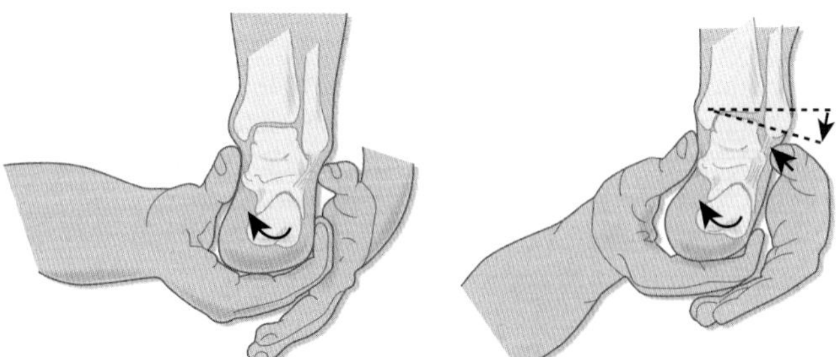

**Fig. 85.5** Talar tilt test.

The *side-to-side test* (clunk test) evaluates the integrity of the tibiofibular ligament. The foot is held in a neutral position and then moved from side to side. A "clunk" is heard or felt if the ligament is ruptured.

The *talar tilt test* can be used to assess the deltoid ligament and the calcaneofibular ligament by applying eversion and inversion stress, respectively. The calcaneus is held in one hand while the examiner moves the ankle into inversion or eversion (**Fig. 85.5**). Frequently, it is accompanied by simultaneous radiographic evaluation to determine the amount of tilt at the level of the talus.[2]

Stress testing is not generally performed in the acute phase of an injury because of its inaccuracy and the pain that it inflicts on the patient. Since the advent of magnetic resonance imaging (MRI), which can reveal soft tissue injuries of varying degrees, stress testing is rarely used at all.[2]

## DIFFERENTIAL DIAGNOSIS AND MEDICAL DECISION MAKING

Ankle sprains result from traumatic rotational forces applied to the ankle and usually occur in individuals who are involved in sports activities. They have been classified to better understand treatment modalities, as well as prognosis.

## CLASSIFICATION OF ANKLE SPRAINS

### *Subluxation of the Peroneal Tendons*

The peroneus longus and brevis tendons lie in a shallow groove immediately posterior to the distal end of the fibula. Rupture of the superior peroneal retinaculum results in subluxation or dislocation of the peroneal tendons. This injury is often mistaken for a common sprain in the emergency department (ED). However, it differs in that the pain and swelling are located along the posterior border of the lateral malleolus. It results from forced dorsiflexion with reflex contraction of the peroneal muscles. Patients complain of pain and a snapping sensation over the posterolateral aspect of the ankle with weakness of eversion.[6]

During physical examination, pain is elicited on palpation of the area, and swelling is also noted. The subluxation can be reproduced with dorsiflexion and eversion of the foot.

Do *not* mistake subluxation of the peroneal tendons for an ankle sprain because the treatment and prognosis are different.

Treatment is directed at stabilization of the subluxed tendon. A U-shaped felt pad is placed over the lateral aspect of the ankle with the tip of the fibula lying inside the "U." The ankle is then taped to ensure that the U-shaped pad stays in place. Refer to an orthopedic surgeon for further evaluation in the event that corrective surgery is warranted.

### *Achilles Tendon Injuries*

The most common conditions affecting the Achilles tendon in patients seen in the ED range from tendonitis to rupture. Rupture of the Achilles tendon is missed in more than 20% of patients with this injury. The rupture may be partial or complete. Occasionally, because of significant swelling and a hematoma over the area, a discernible defect in the tendon may be difficult to identify.

The history usually includes some form of violent motion around the ankle; the injury is often seen in basketball and tennis players. Weekend athletes in their third or fourth decade are most commonly affected.

Physical examination reveals swelling and tenderness, as well as a partial or complete defect in the tendon. A positive Thompson test is diagnostic. It is performed by having the patient lie prone on a gurney or stand with the knee of the affected leg resting on a chair (**Fig. 85.6**). The examiner then squeezes the calf muscles. Individuals with normal Achilles tendons will plantar flex as the maneuver is performed.[3]

Note that the Thompson test can be misleading, especially with partial tears, because the accessory ankle flexors are often squeezed together with the contents of the superficial leg compartment.

Treatment consists of either a compression wrap or a short leg plaster splint with the foot positioned in equinus (plantar flexion). Crutches, non–weight bearing, and analgesics are also indicated. Prompt orthopedic consultation to determine the necessity for surgical repair is advised.

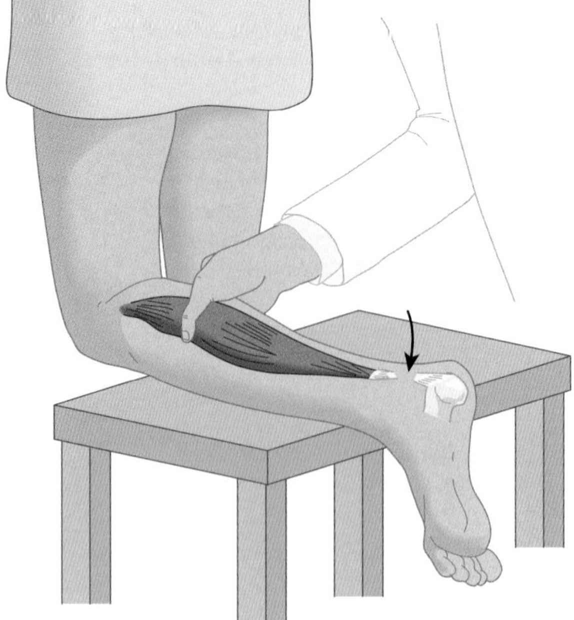

**Fig. 85.6** Thompson test.

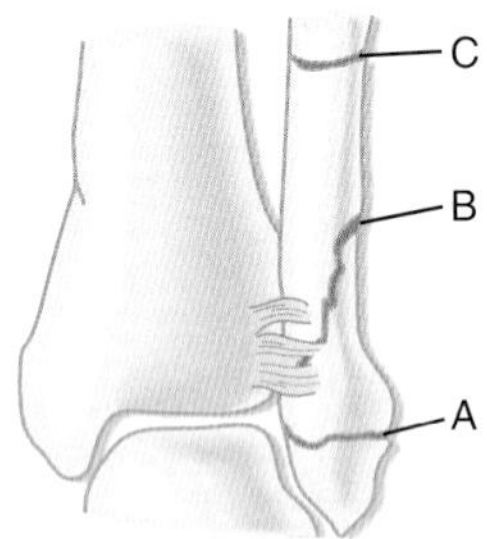


**Fig. 85.7** Danis-Weber classification (see text).

## CLASSIFICATION OF FRACTURES

Several classifications of ankle fractures have been published over the years in an effort to facilitate accurate description and subsequent treatment. The most comprehensive classification, still in use, was proposed by Lauge-Hansen in 1950 and was based on cadaver experiments involving the use of foot position (supination or pronation) and direction of the force exerted on the joint (external rotation, adduction, or abduction) at the time of the injury. The Danis-Weber Arbeitsgemeinschaft für Osteosynthesefragen (AO) classification proposes a simpler description based on the location and appearance of the fibular fracture. The fracture lines are designated A, below the syndesmosis; B, at the level of the syndesmosis; and C, above the syndesmosis (**Fig. 85.7**).

The Orthopedic Trauma Association has since expanded the Danis-Weber classification by keeping the three types (A, B, and C) and adding nine groups (1, 2, and 3 for each type) and 27 subgroups.[3]

In 1987, Tile recommended another classification that identifies ankle fractures by their stability. Because *unstable* fractures require a different treatment approach than *stable* fractures do, such distinction is clinically important. For example, identification of a medial injury will generally determine the stability of the ankle joint. *Therefore, always suspect an unstable fracture of the ankle when the medial structures are identified as injured clinically or radiographically.*[4,7]

### *Danis-Weber Classification System*

This classification system has four injury patterns: (1) supination adduction (SA or Weber A), (2) supination external rotation (SE or Weber B), (3) pronation abduction (PA or Weber

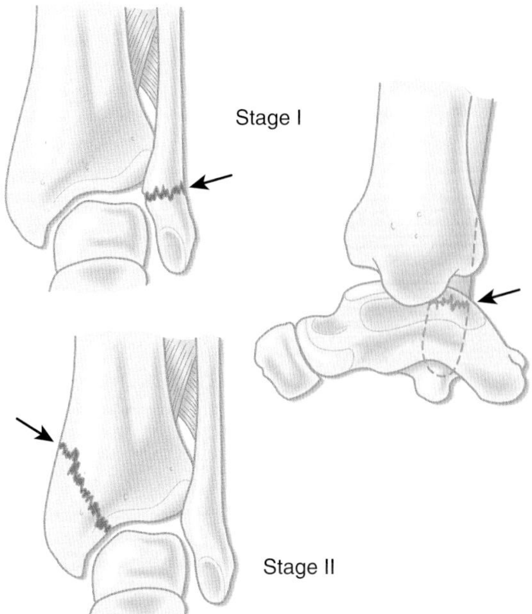


**Fig. 85.8** Supination adduction (SA, Weber A).

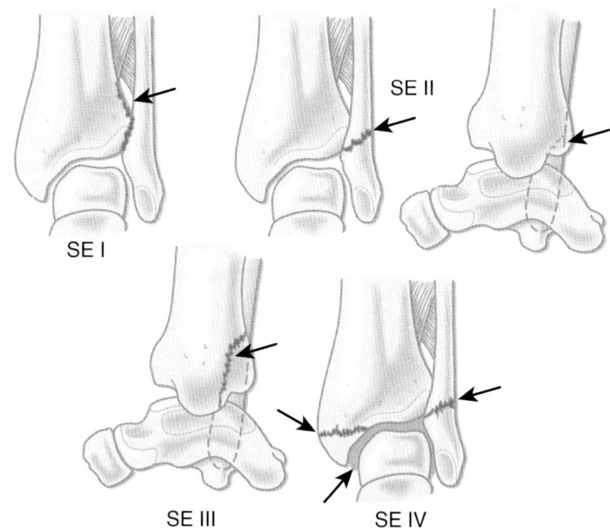


**Fig. 85.9** Supination external rotation (SE, Weber B).

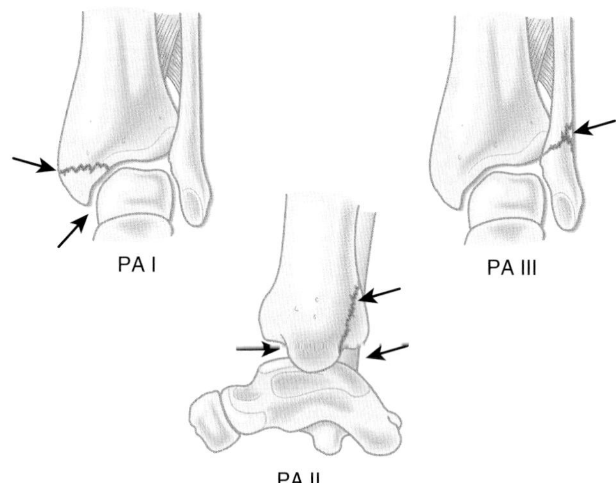


**Fig. 85.10** Pronation (eversion) of the foot and application of an abducting force on the talus can result in up to three sequential injuries.

C1), and (4) pronation external rotation (PE or Weber C2). The names of these injury patterns can be thought of in simple terms as indicating the initial position of the foot (supination or pronation) and the direction of the injuring force acting through the talus (adduction, abduction, external rotation). The location and type of fibula fracture are the key to understanding the classification.[2]

SUPINATION ADDUCTION (SA, WEBER A) Supination (inversion) of the foot and application of an adducting force on the talus result in two sequential injuries: transverse fracture of the lateral malleolus below or up to the level of the tibiofibular joint and a ligament tear (SA I). As the force progresses, the talus impacts the medial malleolus and causes an oblique medial malleolar fracture (SA II) (**Fig. 85.8**).

SUPINATION EXTERNAL ROTATION (SE, WEBER B) This is the most common mechanism of a "twisted ankle" injury. Supination of the foot and application of an external rotation force on the talus result in up to four sequential injuries (**Fig. 85-9**): tear of the anterior inferior tibiofibular ligament (SE I); short oblique fracture of the fibula (SE II), which is best seen on a lateral radiograph; fracture of the posterior malleolus (SE III); and transverse fracture of the medial malleolus (SE IV) or a tear of the deltoid ligament (or both).

PRONATION ABDUCTION (PA, WEBER C1) In this injury, pronation (eversion) of the foot and application of an abducting force on the talus result in up to three sequential injuries (**Fig. 85.10**). First, a transverse fracture of the medial malleolus occurs (PA I), and then as the forces progress, the anterior inferior tibiofibular ligament tears (PA II). Finally, further abduction of the talus results in an oblique fracture of the distal end of the fibula (PA III). This fibula fracture ends just above the level of the joint line and is best seen on an anteroposterior (AP) or mortise view.

PRONATION EXTERNAL ROTATION (PE, WEBER C2) In pronation external rotation, pronation (eversion) of the foot and application of an external rotation force through the talus result in up to four sequential injuries (**Fig. 85.11**). Similar to the pronation abduction mechanism, the first two injuries are the same: transverse fracture of the medial malleolus (PE I), followed by a tear of the anterior inferior tibiofibular ligament (PE II). The third injury is a short spiral or oblique fracture, usually 6 to 8 cm above the syndesmosis but possibly as high as the midshaft level (PE III). The fourth injury is fracture of the posterior malleolus (PE IV).

### *Maisonneuve Fracture (Weber C3)*

The exact mechanism leading to a Maisonneuve fracture is not clear. It appears to combine different forces and possibly shifting foot positions. Patients have isolated medial ankle tenderness and swelling. On further examination, tenderness at the level of the proximal end of the fibula is also identified. *This fracture is unstable and warrants clinical and radiographic evaluation of the entire lower extremity below the*

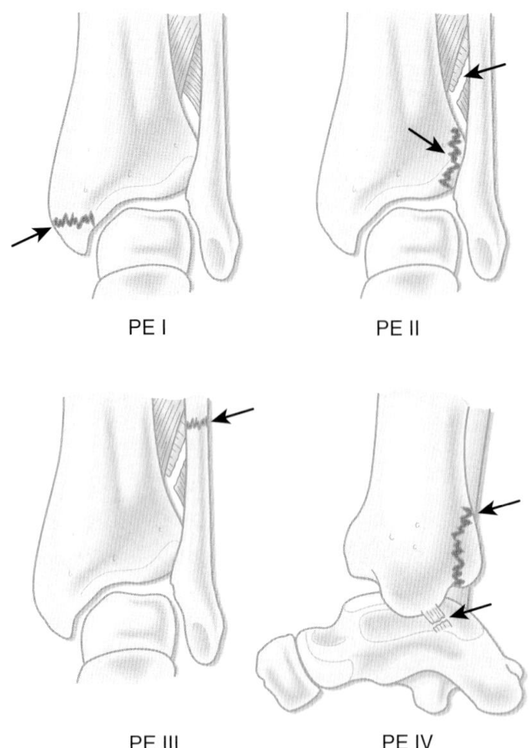


**Fig. 85.11 Pronation external rotation (PE, Weber C2).** Pronation (eversion) of the foot and application of an external rotation force through the talus can result in up to four sequential injuries.

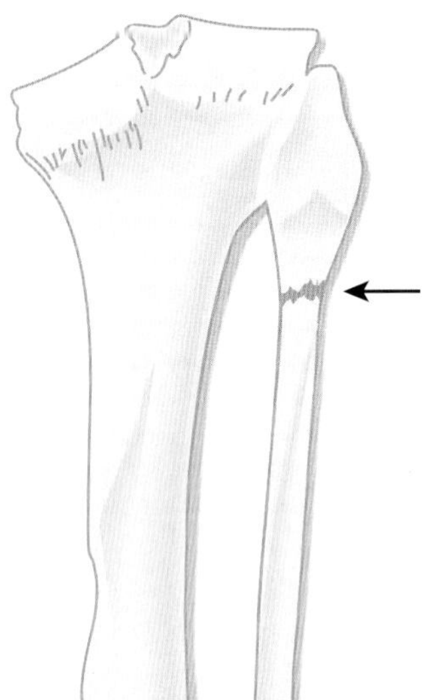

**Fig. 85.12 Maisonneuve fracture.**

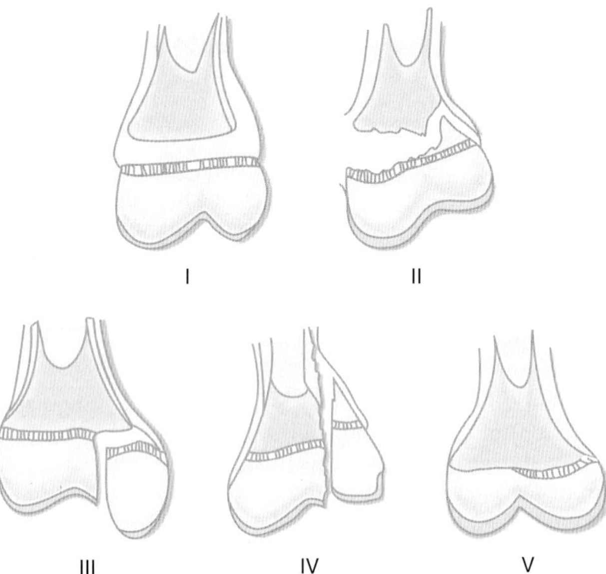


**Fig. 85.13 Salter-Harris fractures are generally broken down into five categories.**

*knee.* It often goes unrecognized and is identified merely as "just another ankle sprain." *Therefore, vigilance must be exercised when a medial ankle injury is identified in any patient.* These medial ankle injuries could be limited to the deltoid ligament, an isolated fracture of the posterior tibial tubercle, or a medial malleolar fracture in the absence of a lateral malleolar fracture. The classic appearance of the injury is a fracture of the neck of the fibula—either linear or comminuted (**Fig. 85.12**). Emergency orthopedic consultation is necessary.[4]

### Salter-Harris Classification System

The Salter-Harris classification system describes injuries that occur only around growth plates. Hence, just children have Salter-Harris fractures.

Injuries to the ankle in the pediatric population generally occur at the level of the bone physis. The Salter-Harris classification system enables definition of the type and severity of the fracture. Salter-Harris fractures are generally broken down into five categories as shown in **Figure 85.13** and **Table 85.2**.[5]

### Triplane Fractures

This type of fracture is generally seen in older children with partially closed epiphyses and resembles a Salter-Harris type IV fracture. The mechanism is usually external rotation. Even with proper care and reduction, this fracture can result in epiphyseal growth arrest and deformity. If unsure of the fracture lines on plain film radiographs, computed tomography (CT) is recommended to ascertain the position of the fracture fragments (**Fig. 85.14**).

Treatment consists of reduction and immobilization in a long leg cast for 4 weeks followed by a short leg cast for an additional 2 weeks. Displaced fractures that cannot be easily or anatomically reduced will require open reduction and internal fixation.

## DISLOCATIONS

Dislocations can occur at multiple sites in the foot and ankle. An in-depth description of these dislocations is beyond the scope of this chapter. Nevertheless, two of these types of dislocations are worth mentioning.

Dislocations at the level of the tibiotalar joint, or *tibial dislocations*, are generally associated with fractures. On occasion, a pure tibial dislocation will occur. They require prompt anatomic reduction in an effort to diminish cutaneous and neurovascular injury. If orthopedic consultation is not readily available, reduction under conscious sedation should be performed by the EP.

**Table 85.2 Salter-Harris Classification of Fractures**

| TYPE | DESCRIPTION | RADIOGRAPHIC FINDINGS | TREATMENT |
|---|---|---|---|
| I | Separation of the two portions of bone, with the growth plate being the area of weakest link | No changes seen on radiographs, although the growth plate may look wider than that in the other limb | Immobilization for a short period |
| II | Most common fracture; occurs partially through the growth plate, with the rest of the fracture extending back into the shaft of the bone; that fragment of bone is known as the Thurston-Holland sign | Separation of the physis and metaphyseal fragment with varying degrees of displacement | Immobilization in a short leg splint or cast and orthopedic follow-up |
| III | Fracture occurring partially across the growth plate and then extending out through the epiphysis and into the joint space | The fracture fragment is epiphyseal, with varying degrees of displacement | Because these fractures may affect the joint, the prognosis is more guarded; immobilization as described previously for type II fractures and orthopedic follow-up |
| IV | Fracture extending from the metaphysis, across the growth plate, and into the joint through the epiphysis; premature arrest of normal growth is common | Combination of types II and III, with varying degrees of displacement | Immobilization and prompt orthopedic follow-up; surgical repair usually needed to restore proper anatomic alignment |
| V | Fracture involving compression of the growth plate; the prognosis is variable, with premature arrest of normal growth being the biggest risk | Radiography is generally of little help in diagnosing this fracture; however, obliteration of the physis is an indication of severity | Immobilization and emergency orthopedic consultation; surgical repair usually needed to restore proper anatomic alignment |

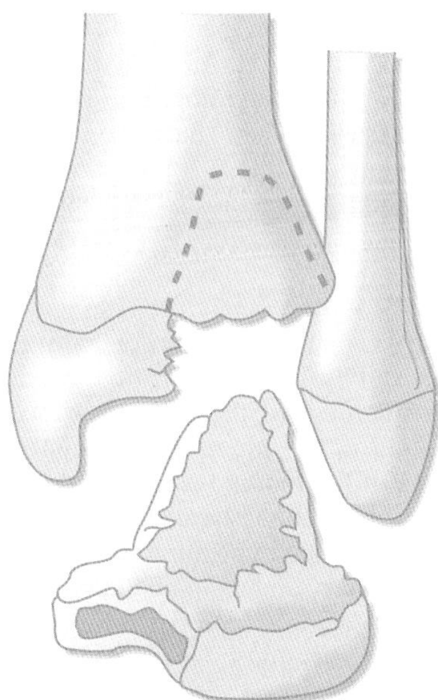

**Fig. 85.14** Triplane fracture.

The second type is *subtalar dislocation*. This injury occurs at the level of the talocalcaneal and talonavicular joints. Subtalar dislocations can be medial or lateral, depending on the direction of the foot and the effecting forces. These high-energy injuries result from sports (basketball and baseball), as well as from motor vehicle accidents and falls from heights.[6]

Clinical examination of patients with subtalar dislocations shows significant and obvious deformity. Skin tenting and neurovascular compromise should be promptly assessed and remediated by reduction. Standard lateral radiographs are sometimes not diagnostic, and an AP projection of the foot may be the only view that depicts the actual talonavicular dislocation. CT is recommended to further assess for associated fractures and the integrity of the reduction. Open subtalar dislocations carry significant morbidity and require emergency orthopedic intervention.

## FOOT INJURIES

### Talar Fractures

Injuries to the talus result from high-energy trauma such as falls from heights or motor vehicle accidents. These injuries may occur at the neck or the body of the talus. Avascular necrosis is common when the injury involves the neck of the talus because of the limited blood supply to this area of the bone. Most of these injuries are significant and all warrant orthopedic consultation. For complete classification details, see Fracture and dislocation compendium. Orthopaedic Trauma Association Committee for Coding and Classification. J Orthop Trauma 1996;10(Suppl 1):104-8.

### Osteochondritis Dissecans (Osteochondral Fracture)

These fractures result from a mechanism similar to that of ankle sprains. When the ankle is forcibly inverted while in plantar flexion or dorsiflexion, the dome of the talus is compressed against the fibula or the tibial plafond. This results in several degrees or "stages" of lesions (**Fig. 85.15**). More often than not, the initial radiographs are negative, and diagnosis will require CT or MRI. The diagnosis is missed in 40% to 50% of patients seen in the ED with an ankle injury. Therefore, a high index of suspicion is warranted with these injuries, especially if the patient has experienced reinjury, chronic swelling, or locking of the ankle 4 to 5 weeks after the injury.[2]

## Calcaneal Injuries

The calcaneus is the most frequently fractured tarsal bone and accounts for more than 60% of tarsal fractures. These fractures are frequently work-related injuries in roofers or other individuals working at heights. The majority are intraarticular, with the remainder being classified as extraarticular.

The most common extraarticular fracture is a calcaneal body fracture. In decreasing frequency, other locations of calcaneal fractures are at the anterior process, the superior tuberosity, and the area of the sustentaculum tali; isolated injuries are rarely seen at these sites. Calcaneal fractures are infrequently encountered as open fractures. Open injuries are reported to occur in only 2% of cases. As a result of the accompanying mechanisms and forces related to calcaneal fractures, other pathology such as spinal injuries and extremity fractures are usually associated with injuries to the os calcis. Multiple complications such as gait abnormalities, arthritis, and leg length discrepancy are generally the sequelae of calcaneal fractures.[8]

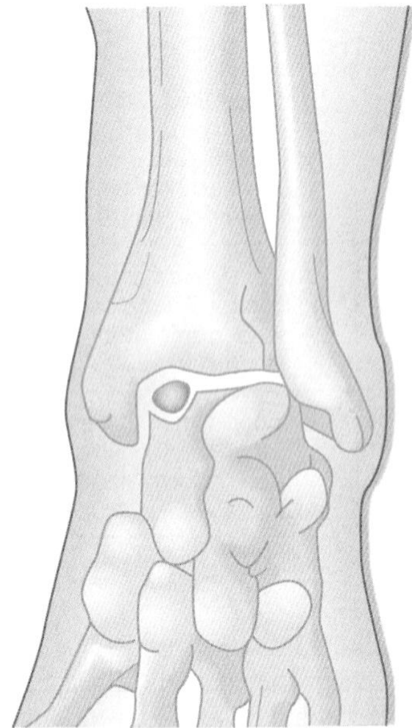

**Fig. 85.15** Osteochondritis dissecans (osteochondral fracture).

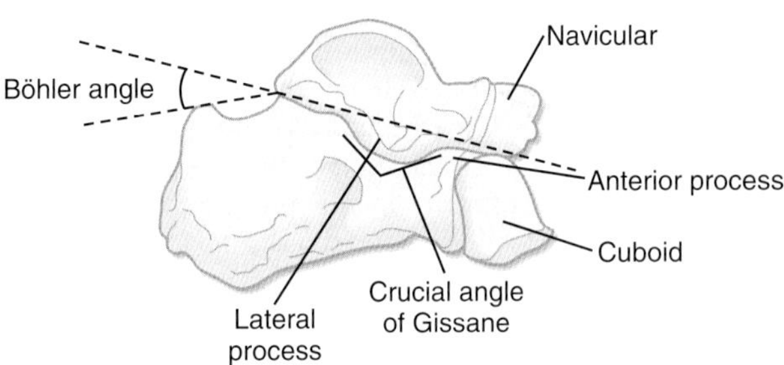


**Fig. 85.16** Critical angles for evaluating calcaneal fractures.

Plain films, including AP, lateral, and axial views of the hindfoot, provide a good initial assessment. CT is generally used to ascertain the true extent of these complex fractures.

One method of assessing the integrity of the calcaneus is measurement of the Böhler angle. This angle is normally 30 to 35 degrees and is determined by tracing two lines on a lateral view of a radiograph of the foot (**Fig. 85.16**). One line is drawn from the posterior tuberosity to the apex of the posterior facet. A second line connects the apex of the posterior facet to the anterior (beak) process. An angle of 20 degrees or less should raise suspicion for a compression fracture of the calcaneus.[3]

Another less frequently used angle measurement is the crucial angle of Gissane. This angle is formed by the downward portion of the posterior facet where it connects to the upward portion. This angle normally measures 100 degrees.[3]

## Other Tarsal Conditions

Avascular necrosis occurs in many areas of the skeleton. The foot is not spared, with the tarsal navicular experiencing the greatest frequency of this condition. Stress fractures can result in avascular necrosis when they go unrecognized and untreated.[8] Examples of these injuries, with a description of the clinical findings, diagnosis, and treatment, appear in **Table 85.3**.

## Lisfranc Injury

A Lisfranc injury is uncommon and generally associated with significant force. Physical examination reveals significant swelling and tenderness of the midfoot area commensurate with the magnitude of the injury. On occasion, ecchymoses of the midarch area of the foot are present and are diagnostic of this injury. The vasculature should be scrutinized carefully, especially if the intercommunicating arterial branch between the dorsalis pedis artery and the plantar arterial arch has been disrupted. It can lead to a compartment syndrome, which requires prompt intervention by an orthopedic surgeon.[8]

**Table 85.3** Other Tarsal Conditions

| | ETIOLOGY | HISTORY/PHYSICAL | DIAGNOSIS | TREATMENT |
|---|---|---|---|---|
| Kohler disease | Self-limited from repetitive trauma; occurs in children aged 3 to 7 | Limp and tenderness over the navicular | Radiography of the foot | Simple orthotic device; short leg cast for 4-6 wk in recalcitrant cases |
| Tarsal navicular stress fracture | Occurs in track athletes | Pain in the midfoot relieved by rest | Magnetic resonance imaging best; plain film radiography 33% accurate | Immobilization in a cast; no weight bearing for 6 wk |

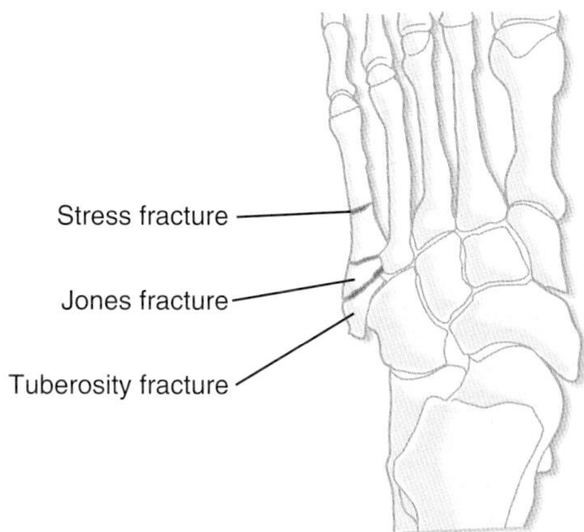


**Fig. 85.17** **Metatarsal fracture.**

### *Metatarsal Injuries*

METATARSAL FRACTURES Three types of fractures commonly occur in the proximal fifth metatarsal (proximal to distal): tuberosity avulsion fracture, Jones fracture, and proximal diaphysial stress fracture. Each has distinct characteristics, and the approach to treatment is often controversial. Nevertheless, most of these fractures heal with immobilization over a period of 3 to 8 weeks, depending on location. Treatment of displaced intraarticular fractures, delayed union, and nonunion usually requires operative methods. A Jones fracture has a high rate of nonunion and may require surgical intervention. Patients must be warned of this potential problem. Tuberosity fractures and Jones fractures must not be confused despite their proximity on the fifth metatarsal (**Fig. 85.17**).[3,9]

FREIBERG DISEASE Freiberg disease is caused by repetitive trauma to the head of the second metatarsal, which deprives the epiphysis of adequate circulation, with consequent necrosis of the metatarsal head and pain in the area of the second metatarsal in the forefoot. Radiography shows flattening of the metatarsal head with a fragmented epiphysis.

Freiberg disease is most common in adolescent girls and is associated with the wearing of high-heeled shoes.

Treatment is directed at prevention of trauma by rest and diminishing sports activities, as well as by wearing flat shoes instead of high heels. Nonsteroidal antiinflammatory drugs (NSAIDs) may be used as necessary to decrease inflammation.[10]

### *Sesamoid Bone Fractures*

The foot has many sesamoid bones. However, those most commonly injured are in the area of the great toe and occasionally in the os trigonum located posterior to the posterior tubercle of the talus. These fractures are infrequent and often go unrecognized. They can occur as a result of direct and indirect trauma. Direct traumatic injuries result from crush-type mechanisms such as falling from a height or direct impact with an external object. Indirectly, the great toe suffers a hyperdorsiflexion-type injury that results in the fracture. In the case of the os trigonum, plantar flexion is the mechanism. Ballet dancers suffering from these injuries may at some time require removal of the bone because of chronic pain.[3]

Examination reveals localized tenderness over the sesamoid and reproducible pain on dorsiflexion of the great toe. In the case of the os trigonum, physical examination almost always reveals tenderness anterior to the Achilles tendon and posterior to the tibia, as well as decreased plantar flexion. Pain is reproduced by plantar flexion or resisted plantar flexion of the great toe.

Radiographically, sesamoid fractures appear to have irregular margins, as opposed to the smooth contours of a bipartite sesamoid bone. Nonunion is frequent because of their poor vascular supply. This can result in chronic pain and swelling, as well as disability. It is therefore important to stress the need for orthopedic follow-up.

Treatment is directed at protection and immobilization of the affected area in either a walking cast or boot for 4 to 6 weeks.[3]

### *Toe Fractures*

Toe fractures are generally the result of direct trauma such as a heavy object falling on the foot. Occasionally, walking or kicking an immobile object will result in a displaced fracture. The eponym "nightwalker" fractures has been given to injuries that occur at night while navigating in a dark room.

Treatment is directed at anatomic integrity and immobilization. Therefore, reduction of displaced fractures with "buddy tape" immobilization is the standard. All other fractures that are not displaced warrant immobilization in the same fashion; a hard-soled cast shoe is recommended until the pain resolves, at which time an athletic shoe can be worn. In the event of a large intraarticular fracture fragment or significant displacement of the fragments, emergency orthopedic consultation is required.[8]

### *Plantar Fasciitis*

Plantar fasciitis is a fairly common condition in runners and long-distance walkers. It can have an acute cause from sudden excessive loading of the foot; more commonly, however, it becomes symptomatic in a gradual manner from excessive pronation of the foot. These chronic insults result in microtears of the plantar fascia.

Individuals with a high-arched foot are more prone to this injury. The patient reports pain in the plantar area of the foot, especially in the morning. Occasionally, the pain can be sharp and lancinating and resemble neuropathic pain.

Physical examination reveals tenderness along the plantar area of the hindfoot, near the origin of the plantar fascia. Swelling may be noted occasionally, as well as reproduction of the pain with dorsiflexion of the foot.

Treatment consists of ice massage and gentle stretching of the fascia. The latter is accomplished by stretching of the Achilles tendon, as well by rolling the foot back and forth over an object such as a can of soup. An orthotic device is helpful for individuals with excessive pronation on ambulation. Physical therapy in the form of massage and ultrasonography is sometimes necessary. Steroid injections can occasionally be used but should be done judiciously.[5]

### *Tarsal Tunnel Syndrome*

Compression of the posterior tibial nerve as it courses through the tarsal tunnel is known as tarsal tunnel syndrome. The tarsal canal is covered by the flexor retinaculum, which extends posteriorly and distally to the medial malleolus. The

**BOX 85.3 Causes of Tarsal Tunnel Syndrome**

Trauma
Medications
Heavy metals or solvents
Flat feet (pes planus)
Tendonitis in the posterior tibialis
Varices
Space-occupying mass
Medical conditions: diabetes, hypothyroidism
Alcoholism
Transition from a raised heel to a flat shoe

floor is formed by the calcaneus, tibia, and talus. Tendons of the flexor hallucis longus, flexor digitorum longus, and tibialis posterior muscles, the posterior tibial nerve, and the posterior tibial artery and vein pass through the tarsal tunnel.

Patients complain of shooting or radiating pain to the forefoot or the plantar arch. Numbness or a burning or tingling sensation may also be present in the ankle, heel, arch, or toes. Activity will often aggravate the symptoms.

Shooting pain distally may be elicited when the entrapped nerve is percussed (Tinel sign). Nerve conduction velocity studies are helpful in obtaining a definitive diagnosis. The multiple causes of tarsal tunnel syndrome are listed in **Box 85.3**.

Several treatment options are available, depending on the cause. Conservatively, the area can be put at rest with the use of night splints. Orthotics can be used to correct hyperpronation of the foot. Women should stop wearing high-heeled shoes.

NSAIDs and occasionally physical therapy may be of benefit. Steroid injections may also be of some help. Ultimately, tarsal tunnel release can be performed to alleviate the condition.

## DIAGNOSTIC TESTING

### IMAGING

Views of the ankle should include AP, lateral, and mortise views. The mortise view allows a fairly good image of both the mortise and the talar dome.

Stress views are sometimes helpful but are not presently used as much as in the past. A posteroanterior or mortise view is obtained while stressing the affected ligaments (lateral ligaments) to ascertain the degree of instability as identified by talar tilt. Comparison with the uninjured ankle is necessary, and joint stability is defined as less than 5 degrees of difference between the injured and uninjured sides. A tilt angle greater than 15 degrees with respect to the uninjured side often signifies rupture of the anterior talofibular and calcaneofibular ligaments.[2]

Another radiographic method of assessing ankle joint stability is identification of the medial clear space. This is the distance, as measured on a mortise view, between the lateral border of the medial malleolus and the medial border of the talus. Any value greater than 4 mm is considered abnormal and is a sign of instability (**Fig. 85.18**).[3]

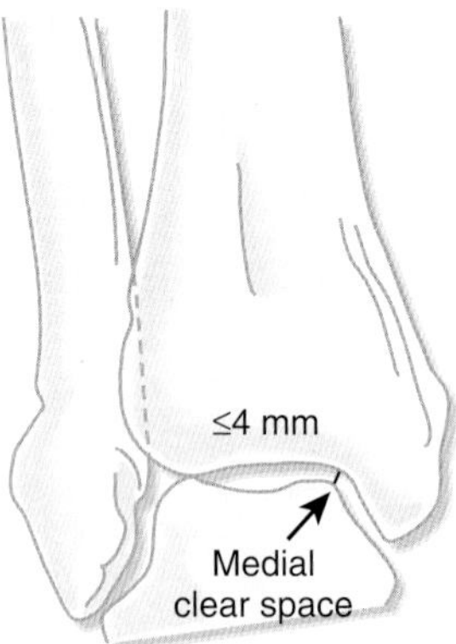


**Fig. 85.18 Distance between the tibial surface and the medial wall of the fibula.** Any measurement greater than 4 mm is considered abnormal and a sign of instability.

**BOX 85.4 Ottawa Ankle Rules**

Age 55 years or older
Inability to bear weight immediately and in the emergency department
Bone tenderness at the posterior edge or tip of either malleolus

Finally, CT and MRI have become very popular in the diagnosis of these injuries but are still not in common use in the ED.

#### *Ottawa Ankle Rules*

In an effort to decrease the number of ankle radiographs used in the diagnosis of acute ankle injuries, Stiell et al. from the Ottawa Civic and the Ottawa General Hospitals in Canada conducted a prospective study that included more than 750 patients seen in the ED with acute blunt ankle injuries. They determined that ankle films were necessary only when patients with pain near the malleoli exhibited one or more of the findings shown in **Box 85.4**.

Likewise, for injuries to the foot, radiographs would be necessary only with pain in the midfoot area *and* with bone tenderness at the navicular, the cuboid, or the base of the fifth metatarsal.[11]

## TREATMENT

In general, the approach to treatment of foot and ankle injuries is directed at protecting the affected limb from further injury at the same time that other modalities, including early mobilization, are used. **Box 85.5** outlines a brief summary of the standard and basic treatment of these injuries.

An ankle stirrup will protect the joint by preventing lateral motion of the ankle. At the same time it allows plantar flexion and dorsiflexion, which contribute to early motion and rehabilitation of the affected joint. These devices can be inflated and deflated by the patient to allow a tolerable degree of compression, as well as stability.

**BOX 85.5 ICEMM Mnemonic for Treatment of Fractures of the Foot and Ankle**

***I*CE:** Every 2 hours or as needed for the first 24 to 48 hours
***C*OMPRESSION:** Compression dressing (Webril or Ace) to decrease swelling; ankle stirrup to lend stability, if indicated
***E*LEVATION:** To reduce swelling
***M*OBILIZATION:** Early, as soon as patient is pain free
***M*EDICATION:** Nonsteroidal antiinflammatory drugs or narcotics when applicable

## FOLLOW-UP, NEXT STEPS IN CARE, AND PATIENT EDUCATION

The patient can begin exercises when the pain subsides (do not use heat) and can return to full activity when full pain-free motion and equal strength are attained in both ankles.

For weekend and other athletes, depending on age and conditioning, **Box 85.6** outlines some guidelines when sports activities can be resumed safely.

**BOX 85.6 Guidelines for When Sports Activities Can Be Resumed Safely**

**Type I injury** (ligament stretch or minor tear): Return to play in 1 to 10 days
**Type II injury** (partial ligament tear): Return to play in 2 to 4 weeks
**Type III injury** (complete ligament tear): Return to play in 5 to 8 weeks

## SUGGESTED READINGS

Anderson RB, Hunt KJ, McCormick JJ. Management of common sports-related injuries about the foot and ankle. J Am Acad Orthop Surg 2010;18:546-56.
Davis KW. Imaging of pediatric sports injuries: lower extremity. Radiol Clin North Am 2010;48:1213-35.
Hanlon DP. Leg, ankle and foot injuries. Emerg Med Clin North Am 2010;28: 885-905.
Khan W, Oragui E, Akagha E. Common fractures and injuries of the ankle and foot: functional anatomy, imaging, classification and management. J Perioper Pract 2010;20:249-58.
Scott AM. Diagnosis and treatment of ankle fractures. Radiol Technol 2010;81: 457-75.

## REFERENCES

*References can be found on Expert Consult @ www.expertconsult.com.*

# 86 Tendinitis and Bursitis

*Erin M. Lareau*

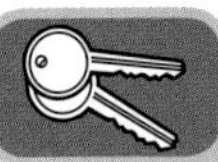

**KEY POINTS**

- Emergency department treatment of tendinopathy and aseptic bursitis should be initiated conservatively with rest, immobilization of the involved tendon, compression of superficial bursae, and oral analgesia.
- Nonsteroidal antiinflammatory drugs may be useful in providing pain relief for patients with tendinopathy and bursitis but are no longer preferred over other analgesic regimens.
- Other emergency medical conditions such as septic arthritis, suppurative tenosynovitis, septic bursitis, fractures, and rheumatologic conditions should be excluded in the differential diagnosis.

## PERSPECTIVE

Tendinopathy and bursitis are two of the most common joint complaints affecting adults seen in the emergency department (ED). Tendinopathy refers to pain, swelling, microscopic tearing, or degeneration of a tendon at its bony insertion. Bursitis refers to pain, swelling, or inflammation of the fluid-filled sac covering a joint. Both may be caused by overuse injuries or arthritis or may be symptoms of underlying systemic disease.

## EPIDEMIOLOGY

The incidence of tendinitis increases with age as muscles and tendons lose some of their elasticity, and it is highest in the age group 25 to 54 years. Bursitis affects approximately 1 in 31 (3.2%) or 8.7 million people in the United States. According to the Centers for Disease Control and Prevention, in 2001 tendinitis was responsible for a median of 10 days away from work as compared with 6 days for all cases of nonfatal injury and illness.[1] Most cases of tendinitis involved white, non-Hispanic women whose occupations had a highly repetitive component.

## PATHOPHYSIOLOGY

Most often, tendon injury is caused by chronic overuse resulting in degenerative changes.[2,3] The classic inflammatory signs of pain, warmth, erythema, and swelling may sometimes be experienced acutely, although tendinitis is no longer thought to be an inflammatory disorder.[4] Bursae may become inflamed for many reasons: chronic friction, trauma, crystal deposition, infection, and systemic diseases (rheumatoid arthritis, ankylosing spondylitis, psoriatic arthritis, tuberculosis, and gout). Because tendons frequently cross over bursae, it is not uncommon for bursitis to be secondary to overlying tendonitis (e.g., supraspinatus tendinitis, subacromial bursitis).

### TENDONITIS

The signs and symptoms of tendinitis can be quite variable. Pain is the most common complaint of patients with joint problems seen in the ED. Particular attention should be paid to the location of the pain; it can be articular (within the joint capsule), as in septic arthritis, or periarticular (outside the joint capsule), as in tendinitis or bursitis (**Table 86.1**).

### BURSITIS

Inflammation of a bursa may be infectious or traumatic, degenerative, or due to underlying systemic disease.[5] Risk factors for the development of bursitis are acute trauma, repetitive injury to the painful area, infections, tuberculosis, gout, pseudogout, uremia, and rheumatoid arthritis. The diagnosis is made clinically based on tenderness at a bursal site, swelling of a superficial bursa, and localized pain with motion and at rest. Regional loss of active motion may occur as a result of swelling; however, range of motion should not be affected in patients with aseptic bursitis (see the Red Flags box on tendinopathy and bursitis).

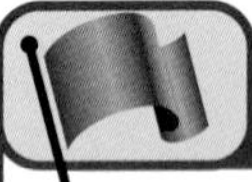

**RED FLAGS**

**Tendinopathy and Bursitis**

Any joint effusion with systemic symptoms is septic arthritis until proved otherwise.

Any injury in a patient with a history of trauma is considered a fracture until proved otherwise.

Pain with passive motion indicates joint involvement; further investigation for an inflammatory or infectious cause is needed.

A history of steroid injection into a large tendon greatly increases the risk for rupture.

Steroid injections or systemic steroids increase the risk for infection.

Fluoroquinolone use increases the risk for tendonitis and tendon rupture.

**Table 86.1** Clinical Features of Articular versus Periarticular Joint Pain

| CLINICAL FEATURE | ARTICULAR | PERIARTICULAR |
|---|---|---|
| Associated conditions | Septic or other arthropathies | Tendinitis and bursitis |
| Range of motion | Decreased | Preserved |
| Pain | With passive and active motion | Only with certain active movements |
| Fever | Yes | No* |
| Trauma | Fractures | Repetitive use or stress |
| Risk factors | Rheumatoid and psoriatic arthritis, osteoarthritis, crystal arthropathy | Corticosteroid or fluoroquinolone use, connective tissue disease |
| Association with rest | Morning stiffness improves throughout the day | Night pain prevents sleep |

*Exceptions are septic bursitis and suppurative tenosynovitis.

**Table 86.2** Shoulder Tendinopathies

| CONDITION | CHARACTERISTICS | SYMPTOMS | TESTS | TREATMENT |
|---|---|---|---|---|
| Adhesive capsulitis (frozen shoulder) | Fibrosis of the joint capsule secondary to immobilization | Diffuse pain, atrophy, stiffness | Pain when forcing limits of motion (not palpation) | Analgesia, orthopedic referral |
| Biceps tendinitis | Inflammation of the long head of the biceps | Acute, intense, localized pain | Tenderness along the biceps groove | Analgesia, sling if subluxating, orthopedic referral |
| Calcific tendinitis | Calcium hydroxyapatite deposition | Acute attacks last 1-2 wk, pain at rest | Radiograph confirms deposits, pain and "catching" with abduction | Analgesia, orthopedic referral |
| Biceps rupture | Secondary to contracting against resistance | Snap or pop, anterior shoulder pain | Swelling, crepitus over the biceps groove, "Popeye" deformity | Analgesics, rest with a sling, orthopedic referral for surgical repair |

## PRESENTING SIGNS AND SYMPTOMS

### SHOULDER

#### *Supraspinatus Tendinitis/ Impingement Syndrome*

Because of its complex structure and extensive range of motion, the shoulder is a joint predisposed to overuse injuries. The muscles of the rotator cuff (supraspinatus, infraspinatus, teres minor, subscapularis) and the glenohumeral ligaments serve to stabilize the joint. Impingement of these tendons occurs because of their position between the humeral head and acromion, which predisposes to chronic tendinosis[6,7] (**Table 86.2**). Impingement syndrome is the number one cause of shoulder pain. It occurs in three progressive stages that worsen over time. Testing and staging of impingement syndrome are reviewed in **Table 86.3**.

In addition to the classic tests for impingement, the examiner should isolate and test individual muscles of the rotator cuff. The empty beer can position tests the supraspinatus by applying downward resistance to an arm in 90 degrees of abduction and 30 degrees of flexion with the thumb pointed downward. Applying resistance to external rotation when the elbow is against the patient's body and bent at 90 degrees tests the infraspinatus and teres minor. The subscapularis is tested with the arm in the same position and applying resistance to internal rotation.

#### *Subacromial Bursitis*

The subacromial bursa lies under the acromion and coracoacromial ligament, to which it is attached. This bursa separates the ligament from the supraspinatus muscle and rotator cuff. Subacromial bursitis is thus thought to be an extension of supraspinatus tendinitis and typically follows this disorder's stages of impingement. Pain and tenderness are localized to the lateral aspect of the shoulder, and signs of impingement are noted on physical examination (see Table 86.3).

### ELBOW

#### *Lateral and Medial Epicondylitis*

The lateral and medial epicondyles are commonly injured as a result of repetitive use (**Table 86.4**). Pain often begins as a dull ache that increases with the inciting activity. Approximately 50% of tennis players will experience lateral

**Table 86.3 Impingement Syndrome of the Supraspinatus Tendon**

| GRADE | CHARACTERISTICS | TESTS | TREATMENT |
|---|---|---|---|
| Stage 1: days to weeks | Dull achy, diffuse pain; reversible; no limits of motion | *Painful arc*: flexion, abduction to 70-130 degrees | Analgesics, activity modification |
| Stage 2: weeks to months | Night pain, localizes to lateral acromion and humeral head, active motion limited | *Neer test*: straight arm forcibly forward-flexed while preventing scapular rotation | As above, orthopedic referral for subacromial steroids (controversial) |
| Stage 3: chronic | Rotator cuff tears, muscular atrophy, weakness | *Drop arm test*: cannot hold arm extended at 90 degrees | Analgesia, orthopedic referral for surgical decompression |

**Table 86.4 Elbow Tendinopathies**

| CONDITION | CHARACTERISTICS | TESTS | TREATMENT |
|---|---|---|---|
| Lateral epicondylitis (tennis elbow) | Overuse microtrauma of the wrist extensors, supinators | Pain with grasp or resisted wrist dorsiflexion, tender lateral epicondyle | Analgesia, compression banding over the elbow, rest with a splint if severe |
| Medial epicondylitis (golfer's, bowler's, pitcher's elbow) | Overuse microtrauma of the flexor carpi radialis | Pain with resisted wrist flexion, tender medial epicondyle | Analgesia, circumferential compression banding to the proximal end of the forearm |

epicondylitis, although less than 5% of those with the syndrome play tennis. Radiographs may be helpful in atypical or prolonged cases to exclude rare pathologic conditions such as tumors.[8]

### *Olecranon Bursitis*

Because of its superficial location at the posterior tip of the elbow, the olecranon bursa is vulnerable to injury. When traumatized, the resulting bursal hematoma causes pain and swelling mimicking acute bursitis. Infection is frequent and most often occurs locally as a result of puncture wounds or lacerations. If fever is present, septic bursitis must be considered and septic arthritis excluded.

## WRIST AND HAND

The wrist and hand are composed of several tendons that pass through thick, fibrous retinacular tunnels. Overuse syndromes are thought to result from degenerative changes in the synovial lining between these tendons and the retinaculum (**Table 86.5**).

The differential diagnosis of wrist and hand tendinopathy also includes osteoarthritis of the carpometacarpal joint, rheumatoid or psoriatic arthritis of the flexor or extensor tendons, gonococcal tenosynovitis, and suppurative tenosynovitis. It is therefore important to review the clinical history for trauma, systemic symptoms, fever, penile or vaginal discharge, or rash (see the Red Flags box on suppurative tenosynovitis).

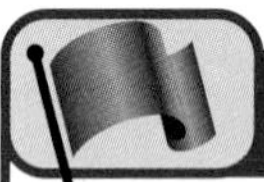

**RED FLAGS**

**Suppurative Tenosynovitis**

Infection of the closed synovial sheaths of the flexors (rarely extensors), often of the fingers and hand

Usually caused by trauma, with the type of bacteria depending on the traumatic exposure (bite wound, puncture, skin flora)

Kanavel signs: tenderness over the flexor sheath, symmetric swelling of the digit, slightly flexed finger at rest, pain with passive extension of the finger

Additional signs: local erythema, edema, lymphangitic streaking, fever, leukocytosis

Treatment with broad-spectrum antibiotics, admission to the hospital, emergency surgical evaluation for incision and drainage

Prophylaxis of all bite wounds recommended to prevent flexor tenosynovitis

## HIP

### *Trochanteric Bursitis*

Patients with trochanteric bursitis are generally middle-aged or older women who complain of acute or chronic pain over the bursal area and lateral aspect of the thigh. The pain is increased when lying on the hip or walking down or climbing stairs and is classically worse at night. The pain associated with superficial bursitis can be reproduced by adduction and that of deep trochanteric bursitis by abduction. Approximately 50% of patients have pain with sequential flexion, abduction, external rotation, and extension of the hip while the contralateral knee is held in flexion (Patrick-Fabere test). Internal rotation does not usually provoke symptoms. The hip joint itself appears normal on examination, and no pain is elicited with flexion or extension.

**Table 86.5 Wrist and Hand Tendinopathies**

| CONDITION | CHARACTERISTICS | TESTS | TREATMENT | PEARLS |
|---|---|---|---|---|
| de Quervain tendinitis | Overuse inflammation (repetitive motion) of the abductor pollicis longus and extensor pollicis brevis synovia causes radial wrist pain | Thumb held in the palm with ulnar deviation of the wrist (Finkelstein test) causes pain | Rest, splinting, NSAIDs, referral to an orthopedist for cortisone injections; refractory cases require orthopedic consultation for tendon release | Carrying heavy objects (grocery bags) over the wrists can cause symptoms; pregnancy precipitates a flare; the differential diagnosis includes SLE, rheumatoid arthritis, CMC joint osteoarthritis, scaphoid fracture or nonunion |
| Gonococcal tenosynovitis | Hematogenous seeding of the CMC joint | Fluid culture, sensitivity | Antibiotics, rest, NSAIDs | Fever, penile or vaginal discharge, skin findings, polyarticular arthritis; the differential diagnosis includes Reiter syndrome and de Quervain tendinitis |
| Trigger finger | Overuse tenosynovitis or congenital sheath narrowing causes nodules and A-1 palmar pulley stenosis; "catching" sensation with flexion | Symptoms vary from pain to complete locking of the finger in flexion, palpable "pop" during extension | Rest, NSAIDs, splinting; refer to an orthopedist for cortisone injections | The differential diagnosis includes infectious flexor tenosynovitis, trisomy 13, rheumatoid arthritis, diabetes mellitus |
| Dupuytren contracture | Proliferative disorder of the subcutaneous palmar fascia; autosomal dominant with variable penetrance | Place the palm down on a flat surface; the digits cannot simultaneously lie flat because of contractures (Hueston tabletop test) | No effective treatment; observation; refer to an orthopedist for fasciotomy | Commonly occurs in older men and patients with alcohol abuse, epilepsy, diabetes, COPD; not symmetric; some patients have Dupuytren diathesis, involvement of the hands and feet (Letterhose disease) or penis (Peyronie disease) |

*CMC*, Carpometacarpal; *COPD*, chronic obstructive pulmonary disease; *NSAIDs*, nonsteroidal antiinflammatory drugs; *SLE*, systemic lupus erythematosus.

### *Ischial Bursitis*

Ischial bursitis develops secondary to trauma or sitting on a hard surface (weaver's bottom). Sometimes the pain radiates down the back of the thigh and mimics sciatic nerve inflammation. The pain can be reproduced by applying pressure over the ischial tuberosity by sitting, standing on tiptoes, or bending forward.

## KNEE

### *Iliotibial Band Syndrome*

Iliotibial band syndrome, or "runner's knee," is a common tendinopathy that occurs in long-distance runners. Patients report pain in the lateral portion of the knee as the distal iliotibial tract becomes injured, and they may state that the pain resolves after an initial warm-up phase, may return at the end of running, and is always prominent the next morning on awakening. Examination reveals point tenderness to palpation, and crepitus may be appreciated.

### *Biceps Femoris and Popliteal Tendinopathy*

These two disorders are grouped together because of their common anatomic location. The biceps femoris (hamstring) is a large muscle that inserts on the proximal end of the fibula. The popliteal muscle inserts on the lateral aspect of the distal end of the femur. Both tendons cross the knee joint and are subject to acute and overuse injuries, especially in athletes. In acute injuries, radiography should be performed to exclude an avulsion fracture. The diagnosis is made clinically. Patients report that the symptoms occur while running or playing sports. Tenderness to palpation at the insertions of these muscles is noted. Knee tendinopathies are treated conservatively with rest, ice, and referral for physical therapy. Surgery is rarely indicated.

### *Prepatellar Bursitis*

Prepatellar bursitis (housemaid's knee, nun's knee) causes visual swelling over the lower pole of the patella. Range of motion may increase the pain as the bursa is placed under tension. Findings on examination of the joint are usually normal. Pyogenic prepatellar bursitis is an infection of this bursa and is common in children. This condition requires aspiration, immobilization, and antibiotic coverage. If acute episodes are not resolved within 2 days, incision and drainage should be considered.[9]

### *Infrapatellar Bursitis*

The infrapatellar bursa is divided into two parts. Between the patellar ligament and the superior anterior surface of the tibia lies the deep part. The superficial aspect lies between the skin and patellar ligament. Deep infrapatellar bursitis is associated with tenderness on both sides of the tendon that increases with extreme flexion.[10]

If signs of infection such as loss of full extension of the knee or resistance to full flexion are present, aspiration of the infrapatellar bursa should be performed along with antibiotic therapy. If infection exists, evaluation for surrounding osteomyelitis is advisable.

### *Anserine Bursitis*

Anserine bursitis most commonly occurs in obese older women with osteoarthritis and in endurance athletes. Pain characteristically occurs in the medial knee region over the proximal end of the tibia, increases on climbing stairs and with extremes of range of motion, and can radiate to the inner part of the thigh and midcalf region. The area of tenderness is localized to the medial aspect of the knee 2 inches below the joint margin, where the medial hamstrings (sartorius, gracilis, and semitendinosus) attach. The area is usually neither swollen nor warm.

## ANKLE

### *Achilles Tendinitis*

The Achilles tendon can be injured as a result of direct trauma, overuse, and medications such as steroids or fluoroquinolones[11] (**Table 86.6**; also see the Red Flags box on fluoroquinolones and tendinopathy). It can also become inflamed as part of a systemic disease (ankylosing spondylitis, Reiter syndrome, gout, pseudogout). However, most causes of Achilles tendinitis are thought to be multifactorial. Additionally, the vascular supply creates a watershed area approximately 2 to 6 cm above the calcaneal insertion and is thought to be responsible for the clinical symptoms and pathologic disruption at this site. Tendon rupture must be ruled out. Diagnosis and treatment of Achilles tendon rupture are discussed further in Chapter 85.

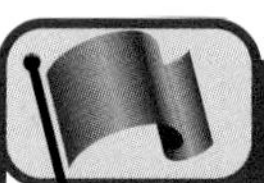

**RED FLAGS**

**Fluoroquinolones and Tendinopathy**

The Food and Drug Administration has issued a black box warning for all fluoroquinolone antibiotics because of the increased risk for tendinopathy and tendon rupture.

Risks are increased in patients older than 60 years, those taking corticosteroids, and transplant recipients.

Patients prescribed fluoroquinolones should be advised to stop the medication at the first sign of pain, swelling, or inflammation in a tendon area and to avoid exercise and use of the area.

Signs of tendon rupture include an audible snap or pop, immediate bruising, and loss of motor function or inability to bear weight in the area.

Initial conservative treatment includes pain control, splinting in plantar flexion, and referral to orthopedics for stretching, eccentric load strength training, and correction of limb misalignment with orthotics. Surgical referral is urgent if there is any concern for tendon rupture.[12]

## CALCANEAL BURSITIS

Two bursae are found at the insertion of the Achilles tendon. The superficial bursa lies between the skin and the tendon. It may become inflamed secondary to Achilles tendinitis or from repetitive friction or overuse. The deep bursa lies between the tendon and calcaneus and is rarely affected. Pain with range of motion and tenderness anterior to the Achilles tendon will be noted.

## DIFFERENTIAL DIAGNOSIS

The differential diagnosis of tendonitis and aseptic bursitis is related to the clinical features accompanying the patient's joint pain (see Table 86.1). Febrile patients need evaluation for septic bursitis and septic joints. Additional differential diagnostic considerations include inflammatory arthritis and gout.

**Table 86.6** Ankle Tendinopathies

| CONDITION | CHARACTERISTICS | TESTS | TREATMENT |
|---|---|---|---|
| Achilles tendinopathy | Pain, morning stiffness | Posterior calf, ankle tenderness | Analgesia, splint in plantar flexion |
| Achilles tendon rupture | Pop or snap after forced dorsiflexion, distal calf swelling at the watershed area | Thompson test, weakness of plantar flexion, palpable defect | Analgesia, splint as above, no weight bearing, orthopedic referral for surgery |
| Peroneal tendon subluxation | Subluxation of tendons over the lateral malleolus, clicking sensation | Tenderness, ecchymosis, anterior subluxation with forced dorsiflexion | Radiographs for avulsion fractures (50%), analgesia, dorsal splint |
| Plantar fasciitis | Tender facia at the plantar calcaneal insertion, heel pain on first morning steps | Pain with passive dorsiflexion of the toes, tenderness in the anteromedial part of the heel | Analgesia, arch supports |

If multiple joints are involved and the swelling is symmetric, viral infection, drug-induced reaction, and osteoarthritis should be considered. If the joint swelling is asymmetric, rheumatoid arthritis, lupus, and serum sickness should be considered. If a characteristic rash is present, rheumatologic diseases, Reiter syndrome, Lyme disease, and dermatomyositis should be considered. If the pain is migratory, one should consider gonococcal disease and rubella. If the pain occurred after trauma and a joint effusion is present, hemarthrosis is a possibility. If an audible "pop" is heard, tendon rupture should be considered. If no joint effusion is present, one should look for radiographic evidence of fracture.

## DIAGNOSTIC TESTING

Patients with bursitis who have local signs of inflammation or any systemic symptoms should be evaluated for septic bursitis (see the Red Flags box on septic bursitis). Some distinguishing characteristics of septic bursitis are rapid onset, marked warmth, erythema, and extremely tense and painful bursae. The most commonly infected bursae are those most superficial: the olecranon and the prepatellar and superficial infrapatellar bursae. Bursae are most often directly inoculated with *Staphylococcus aureus* as a result of subcutaneous trauma. Hematogenous spread of infection is rare. If a deep bursa becomes infected, it is probably due to contiguous cellulitis or septic arthritis.[5]

Gram stain, culture, crystal analysis, and a bursal white blood cell (WBC) count should be obtained. Because systemic leukocytosis is neither sensitive nor specific, a routine complete blood count can be omitted. A bursal fluid WBC count higher than 5000/mm$^3$ suggests bursal fluid infection; however, this may not be clear-cut because of overlap in the WBC count of bursa fluid in septic versus aseptic cases (synovial fluid analysis is discussed in more detail in Chapter 107). Therefore, if infection is suspected, regardless of the Gram stain results, treatment with antistaphylococcal antibiotics should be instituted pending culture results.

### IMAGING STUDIES

A diagnosis of tendinitis or bursitis is generally made on clinical grounds, but radiologic studies are sometimes required to confirm the diagnosis by ruling out other causes of pain. Plain radiographs help distinguish extraarticular from articular sources of pain.[13] In acute injury, radiographs are essential to exclude an avulsion fracture. Ultrasonography is useful in the evaluation of joint effusions and lesions involving tendons, ligaments, and skeletal muscles. It can be very helpful in guiding difficult joint aspirations in the ED and is particularly useful in imaging of the shoulder region.[14] Ultrasound has been shown to be more sensitive than magnetic resonance imaging and is now considered the "gold standard" for evaluating tendon involvement with concomitant trauma or rheumatic diseases.

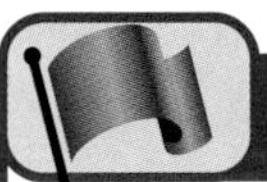

**RED FLAGS**

**Septic Bursitis**

Erythema, edema, pain, or adjacent cellulitis over a bursa is a possible indication of septic bursitis.

Patients with septic bursitis may have fever, leukocytosis, an elevated erythrocyte sedimentation rate, or neutrophilic bandemia, although systemic findings are not universal and are more common with deep bursa infection.

Joint mobility may be preserved if no direct joint involvement is present.

Any swollen bursa with signs of infection should be aspirated and sent for culture and Gram stain.

Eighty percent of cases of bacterial septic bursitis are due to *Staphylococcus aureus*; the rest are due mostly to β-hemolytic streptococci.

Antibiotic coverage should cover staphylococcal and streptococcal species, preferably guided by Gram stain results.

Empiric choices for outpatients include dicloxacillin and clindamycin (with or without trimethoprim-sulfamethoxazole for patients at risk for methicillin-resistant *S. aureus*.

Empiric intravenous antibiotic choices include cefazolin or vancomycin.

The duration of therapy is between 1 and 4 weeks, depending on culture results and response to treatment.

Any patient with severe inflammation, systemic signs, diabetes, or immunosuppression should be admitted for intravenous antibiotics and consultation with orthopedics for incision and drainage.

## TREATMENT

Most patients seen in the ED with tendinopathy can be managed conservatively by resting the affected region, administering adequate pain medication, and referral to orthopedics or physical therapy for biomechanical rehabilitation and gradual eccentric load exercises (**Box 86.1**). Aseptic bursitis can be managed conservatively with joint protection, modification of activity, and pain control. Exceptions are olecranon bursitis and prepatellar bursitis, which have a moderate risk of being infected, most likely with *S. aureus*. These bursae require needle aspiration and treatment with antibiotics until culture results are negative. Documentation should support the clinical suspicion of infection (see the Documentation box).

**BOX 86.1 Treatment of Tendinopathy and Aseptic Bursitis**

Rest
Ice for 24 to 48 hours after trauma
Immobilization of the involved tendon
Aspiration of the swollen bursa
Circumferential compression band for the swollen bursa
Oral analgesics tailored to the patient

**DOCUMENTATION**

**History**

Acute or chronic pain? Treatments attempted? Occupation, frequent activities, aggravating factors, or history of trauma? Diffuse articular pain or focal periarticular pain? Monoarticular or polyarticular? Migratory pain? Any systemic complaints?

**Physical Examination**

Does the patient look ill? Any abnormal vital signs? Fever?

**Studies**

Radiography: soft tissue swelling, erosions, calcification, osteoporosis, deformity, joint narrowing or separation, fractures

Synovial or bursal fluid analysis: cell count, Gram stain, crystals, culture results

**Medical Decision Making**

Concerns for infection, reasons for starting or not starting antibiotics, alternative diagnoses entertained

**Procedures**

Fluid aspiration: indication, approach used, analgesia, results

**Patient Instruction**

Discussion regarding diagnosis, warming signs and what to do if they occur, follow-up, when to return

Patients should rest the involved joint. Many patients with tendinopathy benefit from splinting followed by graduated range-of-motion exercises. Shoulders should not be immobilized for more than a few days because of the risk for adhesive capsulitis. Patients with superficial bursitis should have a compression dressing with an elastic bandage applied to prevent recurrent swelling after drainage of the bursa.

Nonsteroidal antiinflammatory drugs (NSAIDs) provide pain relief when compared with placebo and are well ingrained in the literature as treatment of both tendinopathy and bursitis. Because tendinopathies are now thought to be due to degenerative changes and abnormal healing responses, NSAIDs may not provide any additional benefit over other oral analgesics such as acetaminophen.[15] NSAIDs have not been found to improve healing in patients with chronic tendinopathy and probably should not be used long-term for the management of recurrent pain.[4] Further research is needed in this area. Oral analgesia should therefore be tailored to the patient. Regardless of the medication chosen, a short (1- to 2-week) course of oral analgesia should be administered as first-line treatment along with rest and modification of activity.

Glucocorticoid injections are often used in treating refractory rotator cuff tendonitis, de Quervain tendonitis, trigger finger, subacromial bursitis, trochanteric bursitis, and olecranon bursitis, although good-quality research to support their use is lacking.[4,16] Complications of intrabursal injections are infection, local subcutaneous atrophy, bleeding, postinjection flare as a result of the release of microcrystals, and tendon rupture. Steroid injections are best managed by the follow-up physician after conservative measures have failed and culture results have definitively ruled out infection.

Multiple alternative treatments of chronic tendinopathy exist as well, including massage, stretching, cryotherapy, heat, therapeutic ultrasound, laser, orthotics, and various types of tendon injections. Evidence to support the use of these treatments is lacking.[4,17,18] Some evidence supports eccentric load rehabilitation exercises for the treatment of chronic tendinopathy.[4]

## ADMISSION AND DISCHARGE

Most patients can be managed conservatively as outpatients as long as close follow-up is ensured (see the Patient Teaching Tips box). Referral to the primary medical physician, orthopedic surgery, and physical therapy is appropriate. Patients who undergo fluid aspiration of bursitis should follow up within 48 hours for culture results. Otherwise, patients may schedule follow-up within 1 to 2 weeks so that further treatment can be initiated if conservative measures fail. Patients with suppurative tenosynovitis or septic bursitis require admission for intravenous antibiotics and consultation with orthopedic surgery for incision and drainage.[5]

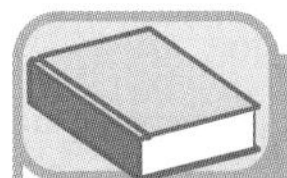

**PATIENT TEACHING TIPS**

Instructions should be given regarding proper rest, analgesia, and immobilization.

If a joint or bursa is aspirated, prompt follow-up must be obtained for culture results.

Septic bursitis requires antistaphylococcal antibiotics and immediate orthopedic consultation. Patients with systemic symptoms require admission for intravenous antibiotics and operative washout.

Patients should call their primary provider or return to the emergency department for the following:

- Increased pain, swelling, or redness around the area
- Fever
- Inability to move a joint because of pain

## SUGGESTED READINGS

Khaliq Y, Zhanel GG. Fluoroquinolone-associated tendinopathy: a critical review of the literature. Clin Infect Dis 2003;36:1404-10.

Rees JD, Wilson AM, Wolman RL. Current concepts in the management of tendon disorders. Rheumatology 2006;45:508-21.

Small LN, Ross JJ. Suppurative tenosynovitis and septic bursitis. Infect Dis Clin North Am 2005;19:991-1005.

## REFERENCES

*References can be found on Expert Consult @ www.expertconsult.com.*

# Injuries to the Shoulder Girdle and Humerus 87

M. Scott Linscott

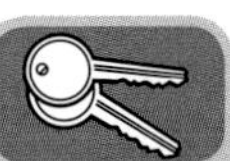

**KEY POINTS**

- Scapular fractures require high force and are therefore associated with a high percentage of injuries to the ipsilateral chest wall and lung.
- Posterior dislocation of the sternoclavicular joint may damage vital structures within the superior mediastinum and thorax.
- Proximal and middle third clavicle fractures and type I and type III distal third clavicle fractures should be treated by placement of an arm sling.
- Open clavicle fractures require urgent open reduction and internal fixation.
- The degree of acromioclavicular separation can be diagnosed from an acromioclavicular view radiograph taken with the patient in the sitting or standing position.
- Axillary nerve function, both sensory and motor, should be tested in all patients with glenohumeral dislocation.
- Most proximal humerus fractures, especially in older individuals, can be treated conservatively.
- Injuries to the radial nerve should always be considered in patients with midshaft humerus fractures.
- Supracondylar fractures in children, especially those with significant displacement, may be associated with injuries to the brachial artery and the median and radial nerves.

## EPIDEMIOLOGY

### FRACTURES

The most commonly injured bone in the shoulder girdle in adults is the proximal end of the humerus (114 per 100,000 population), followed by the clavicle (30 to 50 per 100,000 population), with middle third fractures making up the majority (80%), followed by the lateral third (15%) and middle third (5%). The next most common fractures in adults involve the humeral shaft. Scapular fractures are uncommon (10 to 12 per 100,000 population) and result from significant force (e.g., high speed motor vehicle crashes, falls from heights). Supracondylar distal humeral fractures rarely occur after the age of 15 years.

### DISLOCATIONS

The most common dislocations are glenohumeral (85% being anterior), followed by acromioclavicular, sternoclavicular, and the very rare dislocation of the entire shoulder girdle from the thorax.

### SOFT TISSUE INJURIES

The most common soft tissue injuries are the shoulder impingement syndromes, including subacromial tendinitis and bursitis with rotator cuff tears (95% are chronic and 5% acute), as well as tendinitis and rupture of the long head of the biceps tendon.

## PATHOPHYSIOLOGY

The shoulder girdle connects the upper extremity to the thorax and axial skeleton. It consists of three bones (scapula, clavicle, and humerus), three joints (sternoclavicular, acromioclavicular, and glenohumeral), and one articulation (scapulothoracic). Injuries to the shoulder girdle include disarticulation (rare), fractures, ligament sprains, joint dislocations, musculotendinous strains, and contusions, as well as injuries to the nerves and vascular structures of the shoulder girdle and humerus.

The scapula and clavicle are attached to the axial skeleton by ligaments at the sternoclavicular joint and by muscles from the blade or body of the scapula to the thorax. The clavicle is attached to scapula by the coracoclavicular and acromioclavicular ligaments. The coracoacromial ligament serves as the roof of the coracoacromial arch, beneath which the neurovascular bundle traverses (**Figs. 87.1 and 87.2**).

## PRESENTING SIGNS AND SYMPTOMS

### STERNOCLAVICULAR JOINT SPRAINS AND DISLOCATIONS

These injuries are graded as type I, a simple sprain of the joint; type II, subluxation of the joint, either anterior or posterior; and type III, complete dislocation of the joint. Dislocation usually results from a lateral force applied to the shoulder and an indirect force applied to either a rolled-back shoulder

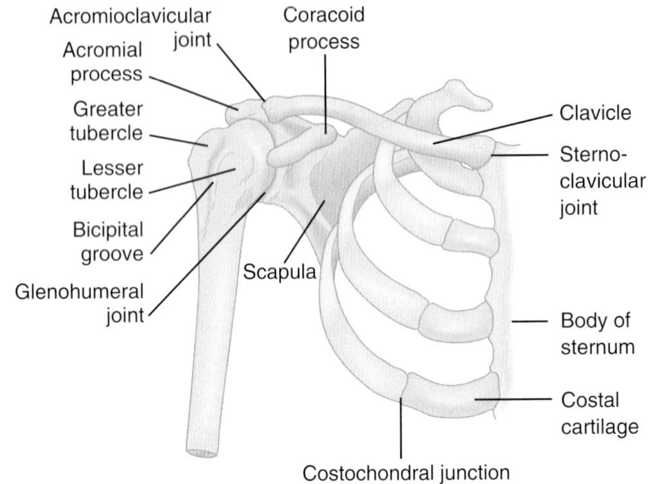


**Fig. 87.1 Anatomy of the shoulder girdle.**

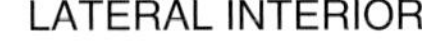


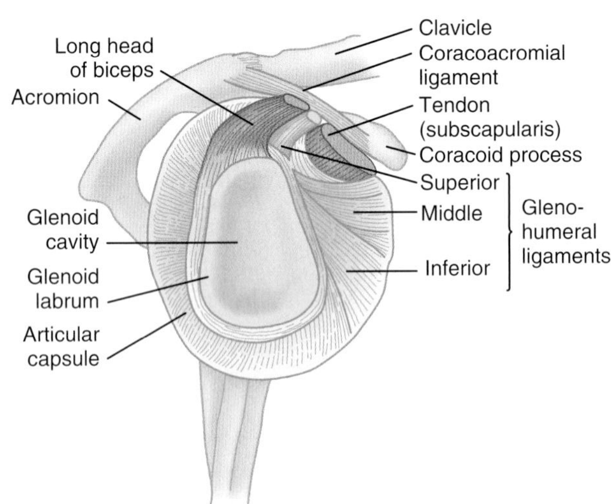


(anterior dislocation) or a rolled-in shoulder (posterior dislocation). Posterior dislocations are potentially life-threatening because the dislocated medial head of the clavicle may cause pneumothorax or injuries to the great vessels, esophagus, or trachea (all structures in the superior mediastinum).[1]

The patient complains of severe pain in the affected sternoclavicular joint. In anterior dislocations, the protruding medial end of the clavicle is visible, easily palpable, and tender. In posterior dislocations, there is often a cavity where the medial end of the clavicle would normally lie, which is especially noticeable when compared with the uninjured side. Patients with posterior dislocations may also have signs and symptoms of pneumothorax, vascular occlusion, and esophageal or tracheal injury.[2] Routine radiographs may not be diagnostic, and computed tomography (CT) is usually required to make the diagnosis. This should always be performed with intravenous (IV) contrast media when a posterior sternoclavicular dislocation is suspected to rule out injuries to the superior mediastinal vascular structures[3] (**Fig. 87.3**).

## ACROMIOCLAVICULAR JOINT DISLOCATION OR SEPARATION

Acromioclavicular separations are generally caused by a fall onto the point of the shoulder or acromioclavicular joint with the arm adducted (thus the lay term *shoulder pointer* to describe this injury). It is caused less frequently by a fall onto the outstretched arm in extreme abduction, which drives the acromion below the clavicle. Acromioclavicular separations are classified as six types, although only the first three (I to III) are commonly seen. Types IV to VI are very uncommon and usually require surgical repair.[1] In type I acromioclavicular separations, the acromioclavicular ligaments are partially torn and the coracoclavicular ligaments are intact, which results in less than 50% superior dislocation or separation of the clavicle from the acromion (**Fig. 87.4, *A* to *C***). In type II injuries, the acromioclavicular ligaments are completely torn and the coracoclavicular ligaments are stretched or partially torn, which results in at least 50% superior dislocation or separation of the clavicle from the acromion. In type III injuries, both the acromioclavicular and coracoclavicular ligaments are completely torn, with complete superior dislocation or separation of the clavicle from the acromion.

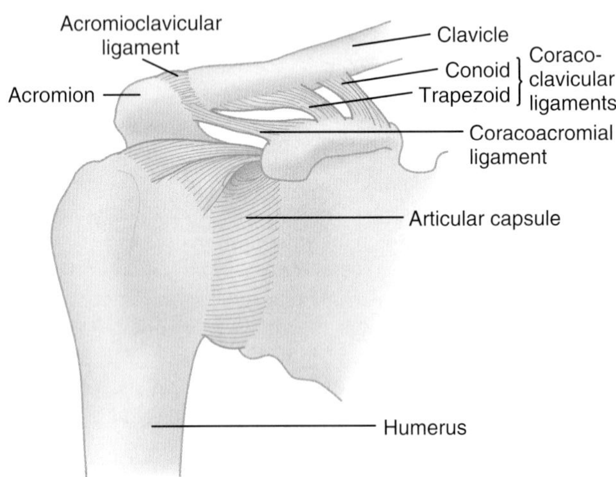


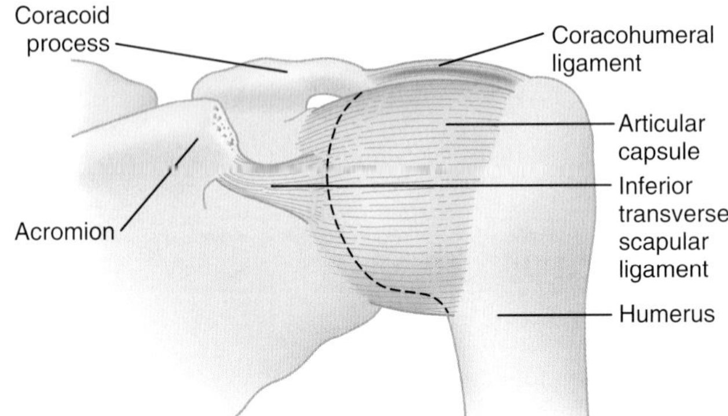


**Fig. 87.2 Anatomy of the glenohumeral joint.**

The patient complains of severe pain in the acromioclavicular joint. Type I dislocations are characterized by tenderness and some swelling over the acromioclavicular joint, with little or no tenderness over the distal end of the clavicle and coracoid process. With type II dislocations, patients have tenderness and more swelling over the acromioclavicular joint and some tenderness over the coracoid process. In type III dislocations, the clavicle is obviously dislocated superiorly when the patient is sitting or standing, with less deformity noted when the patient is supine. Shoulder radiographs may miss an acromioclavicular separation if the radiograph is taken with the patient supine. Acromioclavicular views (a single radiograph that includes both acromioclavicular joints) should be taken with patients in the sitting or standing position and the arms unsupported. In type I injuries there is less than 50% cephalad dislocation of the clavicle on the acromion of the affected shoulder. Type II injuries are marked by greater than 50% cephalad displacement of the clavicle on the acromion on the affected side. In type III dislocations, complete dislocation is seen on sitting or standing films. Use of weight-bearing films (the patient holds weights with the affected arm) is of no benefit.[4]

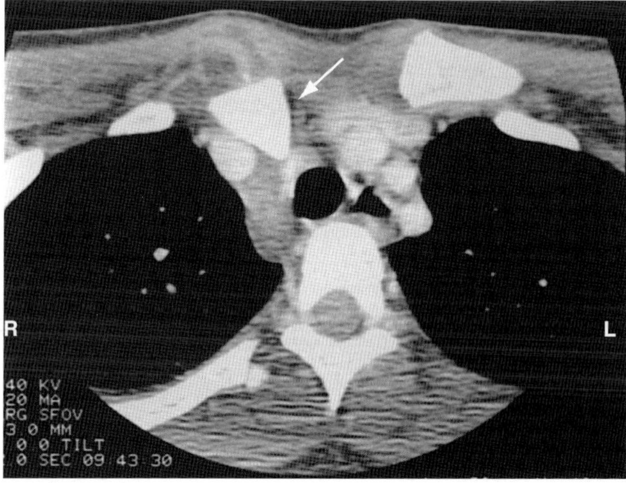


**Fig. 87.3 Computed tomography scan of the right sternoclavicular joint revealing posterior dislocation of the right proximal aspect of the clavicle into the posterior mediastinum.** (Courtesy Donald Sauser, MD.)

## CLAVICLE FRACTURES

The most common mechanism of injury is a medially directed blow to the shoulder, usually from a ground-level fall. Children frequently have a bowing deforming or a greenstick fracture, whereas in adults the fracture fragments are often significantly displaced. Clavicle fractures are divided into proximal third, middle third, and lateral third. Lateral third fractures are divided into types I, II, and III (**Fig. 87.5**). Type II lateral third fractures are relatively unstable because the coracoclavicular ligament has been disrupted.

Patients complain of severe pain at the site of the fracture. They may support the adducted arm on the injured side with the other hand. A deformity is usually obvious, and the fracture site is tender. The diagnosis is made by radiography of the injured clavicle. If a type II distal third clavicle fracture is suspected, both supine and upright films will reveal the degree of instability of the fracture.

## SCAPULA FRACTURES

Scapular fractures are typically associated with high-energy force and are thus often associated with significant life-threatening injuries, especially injuries to the ipsilateral ribs, pleura, and lungs. Most scapular fractures are caused by a direct blow, although fractures of the glenoid and scapular neck may occur as a result of a fall on an outstretched arm.[5]

The patient complains of pain at the site of the fracture. Any movement of the ipsilateral arm will exacerbate the pain, especially with fractures of the glenoid. Fractures of the scapular spine are usually seen clearly on plain films. However, fractures of the neck and the glenoid may not be seen, and if suspected, a CT scan of the scapula should be obtained.

## GLENOHUMERAL DISLOCATIONS

Dislocations of the glenohumeral joint are divided into anterior, posterior, and inferior (luxatio erecta). Most glenohumeral dislocations are anterior and are caused by an indirect

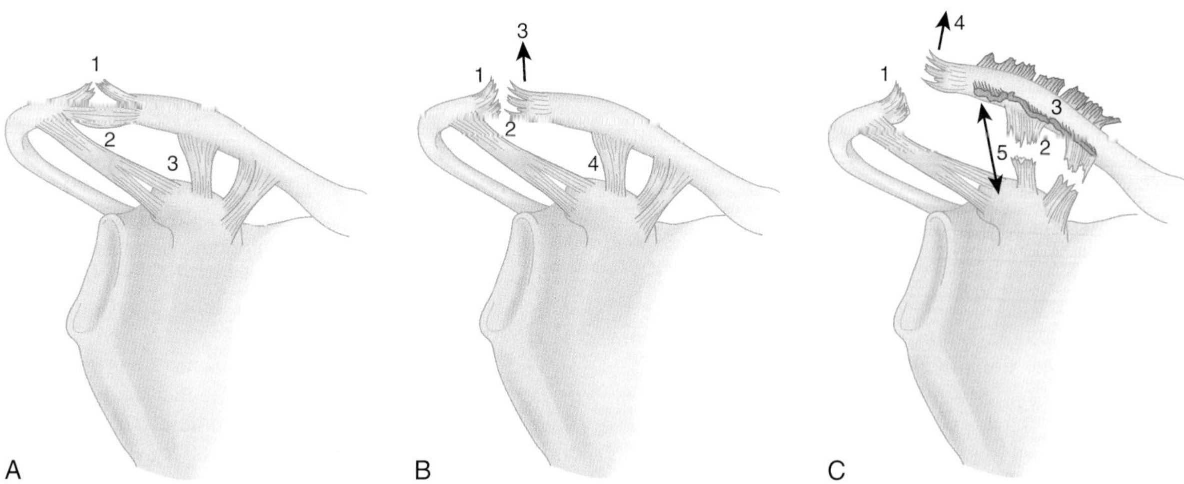


**Fig. 87.4 A,** First-degree acromioclavicular (AC) sprain. **B,** Second-degree AC sprain. **C,** Third-degree AC sprain.

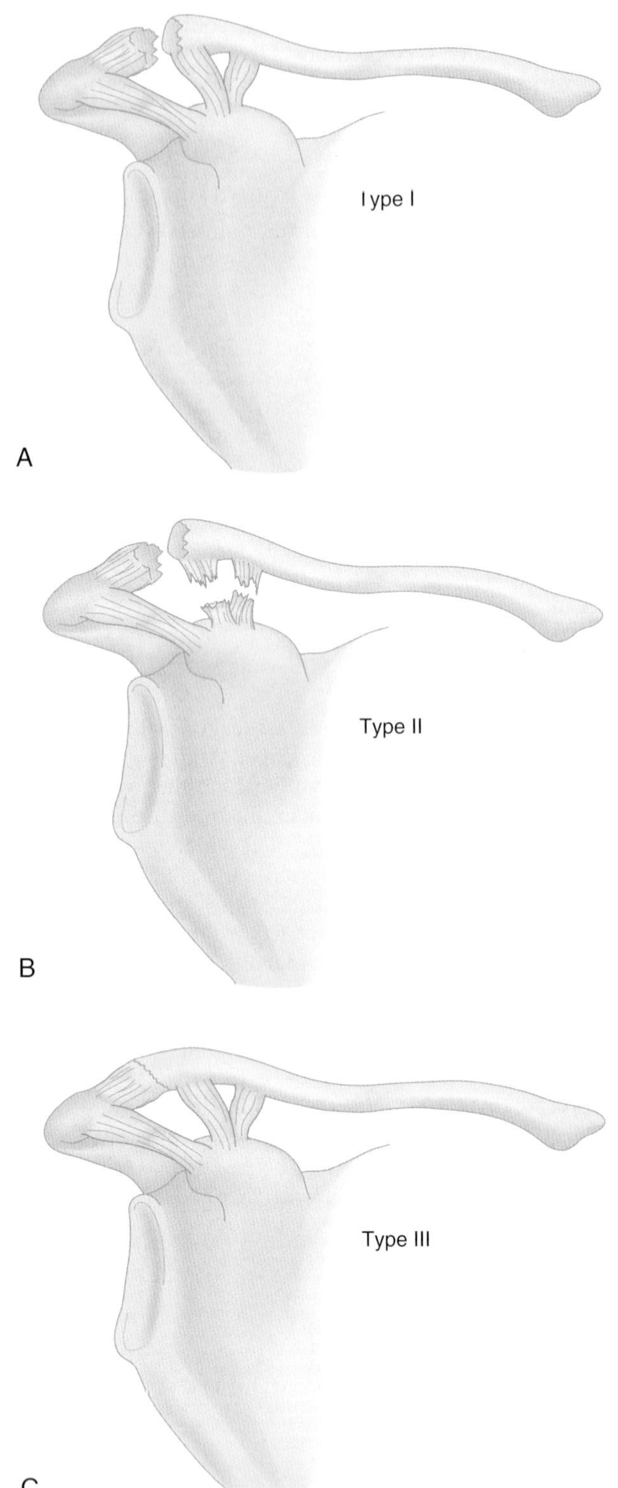


Fig. 87.5 A-C, Three types of lateral third clavicle fractures.

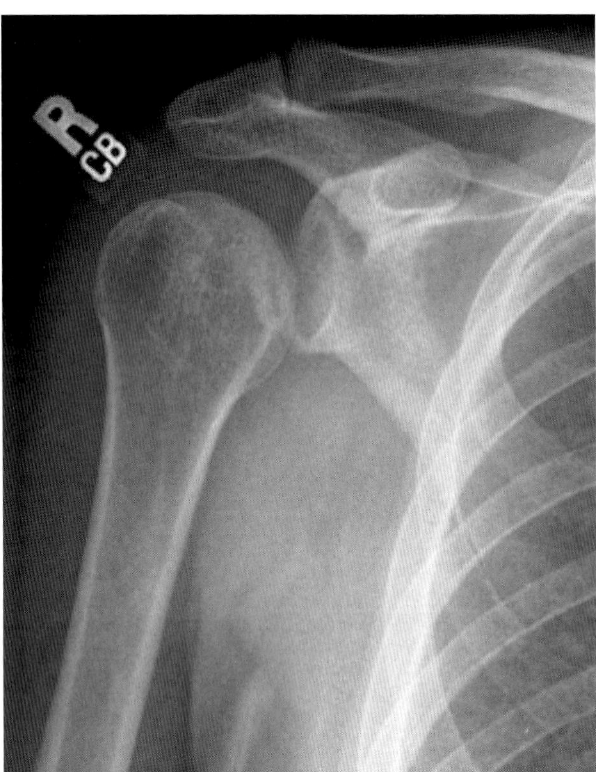


**Fig. 87.6 Anteroposterior shoulder radiograph of a patient with a posterior glenohumeral dislocation.**

force such as abduction, extension, and external rotation; however, they are occasionally caused by a direct blow to the proximal end of the humerus.

Patients generally have severe pain in the glenohumeral joint and hold the affected arm in adduction and internal rotation. There is lack of the normal contour, with a depression where the humeral head would normally reside. Patients report extreme pain in the joint with any attempted movement of the arm. Anteroposterior (AP) and axillary or transthoracic lateral radiographic views should be obtained in all patients with suspected dislocations, even if the patient has a history of multiple dislocations, because occasionally an associated fracture of the proximal end of the humerus or a posterior dislocation will be present.[6,7] If displaced fractures of the glenoid or proximal end of the humerus are suggested on plain radiographs, CT scans of the shoulder should be obtained. Although the AP film usually shows the "light bulb" appearance of the humeral head, it is not always present (**Fig. 87.6**). Though rare, with luxatio the patient has the classic picture of holding the arm in marked adduction and over the head (**Fig. 87.7**). The radiograph reveals the humeral head to lie inferior to the glenoid and the humeral shaft adducted superiorly (**Fig. 87.8**).

## PROXIMAL HUMERUS FRACTURES

The two mechanisms that most commonly cause fractures of the proximal end of the humerus are (1) a direct blow to the lateral aspect of the upper part of the arm and (2) indirect forces generated by a fall on an outstretched arm. The position of the humeral shaft in relation to the proximal fragments depends on whether the fall is onto an abducted or adducted arm.

The Neer fracture classification is most commonly used and is based on the position of the articular segment, the greater and lesser tuberosities, and the humeral shaft. According to the Neer classification, a fracture is considered displaced if any major fracture fragment is displaced 1 cm or more or is angulated greater than 45 degrees.[8] Fractures are classified as

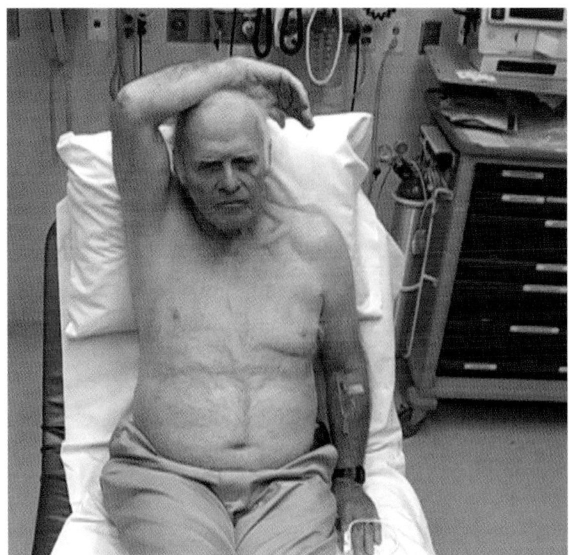

**Fig. 87.7 Photograph of a patient with luxatio erecta.** (From Thomsen T, Setnick G, editors. Procedures consult—emergency medicine module. Copyright 2008 Elsevier Inc. All rights reserved.)

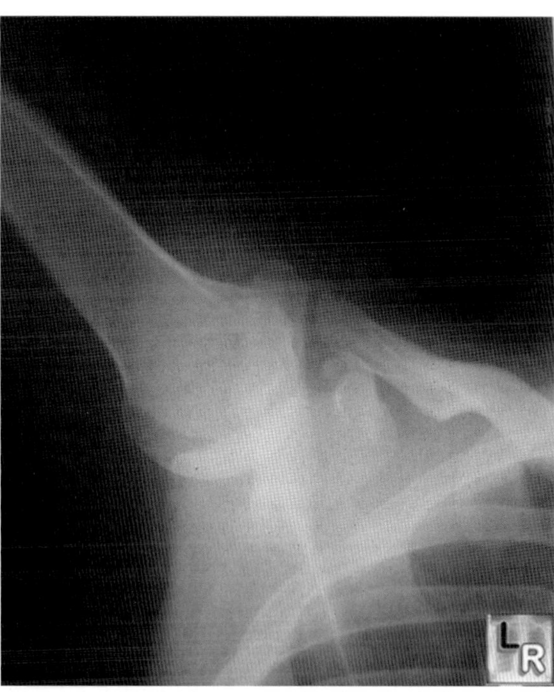


**Fig. 87.8 Radiograph of the shoulder of a patient with luxatio erecta.** (From Thomsen T, Setnick G, editors. Procedures consult—emergency medicine module. Copyright 2008 Elsevier Inc. All rights reserved.)

one-, two-, three-, or four-part fractures and are usually differentiated along the classic epiphyseal lines (anatomic neck, surgical neck, greater tuberosity, and lesser tuberosity) (**Fig. 87.9**).

The patient has severe pain in the proximal end of the humerus. An obvious deformity may be present, as well as swelling and extreme tenderness over the proximal end of the humerus. The trauma radiographic series recommended by Neer,[8] as well as an AP internal rotation view and an axillary lateral view, provides the most complete diagnostic information. A CT scan of the shoulder may be necessary to better define the extent of injury.

## HUMERAL SHAFT FRACTURES

Humeral shaft fractures are almost always caused by a direct blow to the bone, and this mechanism usually results in a transverse fracture. Occasionally, a fall onto an outstretched hand or a severe twisting force brought about by supination or pronation or by twisting of the entire arm may result in spiral fractures.

Symptoms include pain and deformity at the fracture site. In addition, the fracture is usually very unstable. If the radial nerve is injured, the patient will not be able to extend the wrist or fingers and generally has decreased sensation on the dorsum of the hand. The diagnosis is based on radiographs of the humerus. As with all long-bone fractures, the joints above and below the fracture—in this case the shoulder and elbow—should also be radiographed.

## DISTAL HUMERUS (SUPRACONDYLAR) FRACTURES

Supracondylar fractures are classified as either flexion or extension fractures and occur almost exclusively in children, usually between the age of 4 and 10 years. More than 95% of these fractures are the extension type and occur when the child falls onto an outstretched arm with the elbow in full extension or hyperextension. In the flexion-type fracture, the child falls onto the arm with the elbow flexed.

The patient is generally seen holding the injured arm in extension with the unaffected hand. Swelling, as well as tenderness to palpation over the distal end of the humerus, is typical. An S-shaped deformity may be present if significant displacement of the fracture fragments has occurred. The patient resists any attempt to flex or extend the elbow. Elbow radiographs (AP and lateral views) should be obtained. The fracture will often be visible only on the lateral view unless fracture fragments are significantly displaced. Normally, the anterior humeral line should pass through the capitellum (**Fig. 87.10, *A* and *B***). If the capitellum is anterior to the anterior humeral line, it is diagnostic of a flexion-type supracondylar fracture in a child. If the capitellum is posterior to the anterior humeral line, it is diagnostic of an extension-type supracondylar fracture. Based on radiographic findings, extension fractures are often classified into three types: type I has minimal or no displacement; type II is a displaced fracture with the posterior cortex intact; and type III is a completely displaced fracture, with both the anterior and posterior cortices disrupted.

## ROTATOR CUFF TENDINITIS/SUBACROMIAL BURSITIS, ROTATOR CUFF TEARS, AND IMPINGEMENT SYNDROMES

These three disorders have much in common; rotator cuff tears are the end result of rotator cuff tendinitis and subacromial bursitis. Most rotator cuff tears occur in patients older than 40 years and result from long-term degeneration and entrapment of the rotator cuff tendons as they pass between the humeral head and the acromion (impingement syndrome). The injury occurs with a sudden, powerful elevation of the arm (as when grabbing a tree limb during a fall). Occasionally, the injury occurs in weight lifters and in patients who fall onto

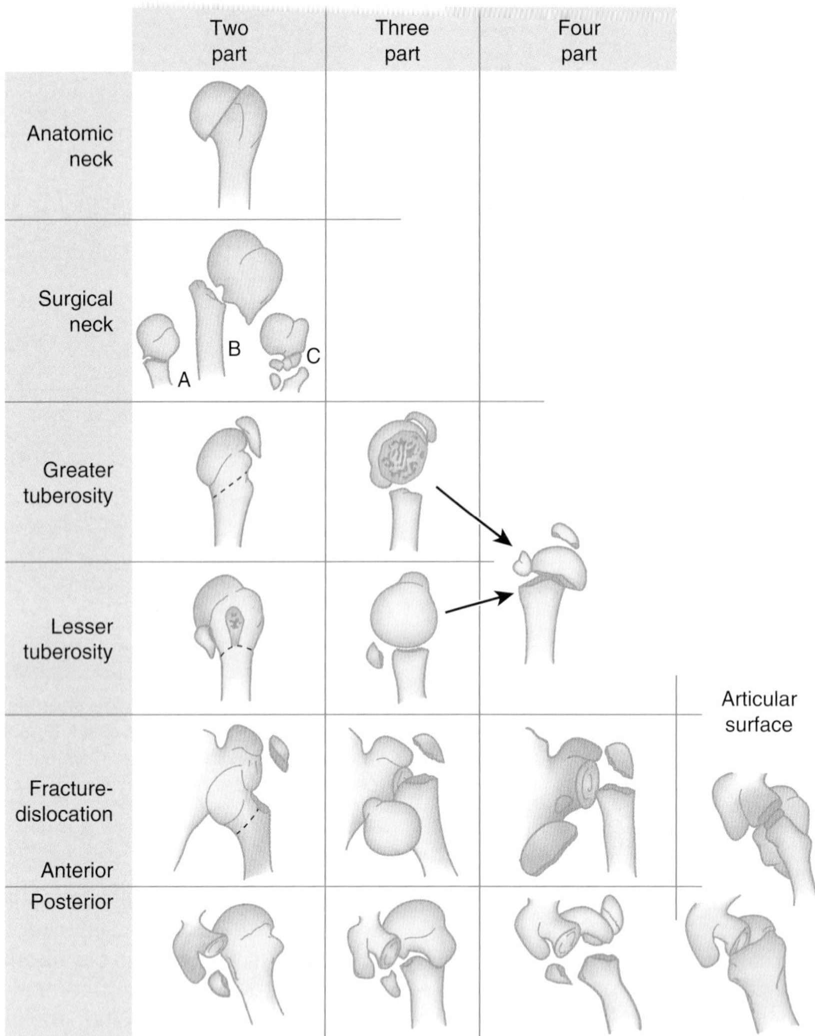


**Fig. 87.9 Neer classification of proximal humerus fractures.**

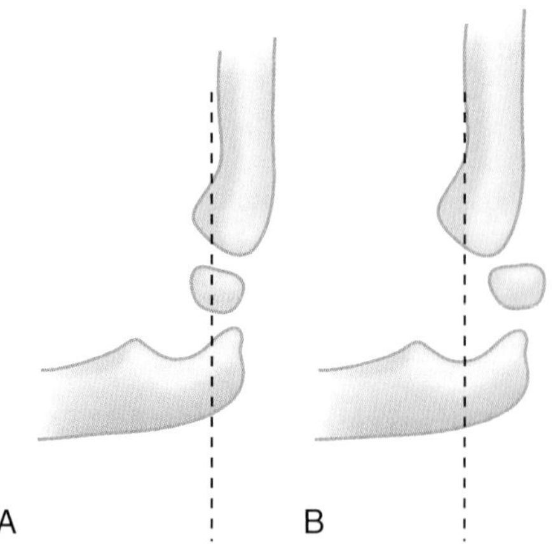


**Fig. 87.10 A,** Normal anterior humeral line alignment. **B,** Supracondylar fractures. (From Simon R, Koenigsknecht S. Emergency orthopaedics: the extremities. 2nd ed. Norwalk, Conn.: Appleton & Lange; 1987.)

the shoulder. In younger patients, these injuries frequently result in avulsion of bone because their tendons are normal.

The patient complains of pain over the proximal end of the humerus, where the rotator cuff tendons attach to the greater tuberosity. Significant pain is felt with both active and passive abduction of the shoulder. In other impingement syndromes (supraspinatus tendinitis and subacromial bursitis), the symptoms are similar, but with less tenderness over the rotator cuff and greater tenderness proximally.[9] The drop arm test is positive if a significant rotator cuff tear has occurred. The patient extends the injured arm to 90 degrees and the operator lightly taps the wrist or forearm. In a positive test, the patient suddenly drops the arm. In addition, the patient cannot slowly lower the arm from the abducted position—rather, it drops suddenly to the side. In patients with rotator cuff tendinitis or subacromial bursitis, significant pain occurs with abduction, but the drop arm test is negative.[9]

## TENOSYNOVITIS AND RUPTURE OF THE LONG HEAD OF THE BICEPS TENDON

The long head of the biceps tendon inserts into the glenoid rim and traverses the bicipital groove between the greater and lesser tuberosities. The tendon is irritated by multiple shoulder

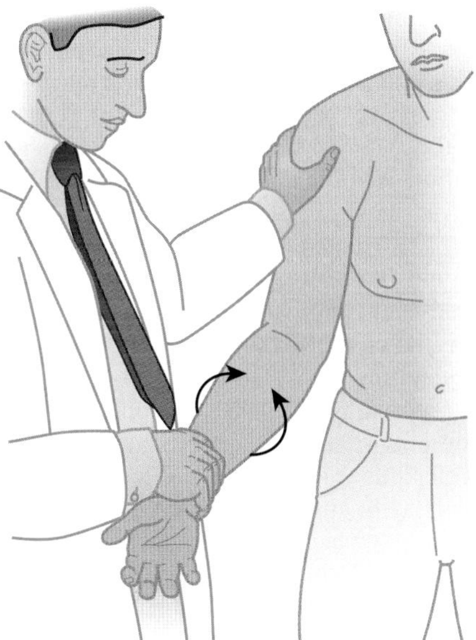

**Fig. 87.11** Yergason test.

movements and becomes inflamed. Eventually, the tendon becomes weakened and may rupture completely.

Pain in the anterior aspect of the shoulder may radiate to the elbow. The pain is made worse with abduction and external rotation. There is tenderness over the biceps tendon in the bicipital groove. The Yergason test is a reliable method for confirming the diagnosis of tenosynovitis of the long head of the biceps tendon. The patient's elbow is flexed to 90 degrees and the patient tries to supinate the forearm against resistance. If this action causes increased pain in the bicipital groove, the test is positive[10] (**Fig. 87.11**).

### ADHESIVE CAPSULITIS

Adhesive capsulitis is caused by inflammation within the glenohumeral joint capsule, which leads to the formation of adhesions within the joint capsule and marked limitation of range of motion of the shoulder. The exact mechanism is unclear; however, this disease usually results from prolonged immobilization of the shoulder joint, particularly when associated with inflammation, such as in subacromial bursitis.

In most cases the nondominant arm is affected and the patient experiences pain with minimal activity. The pain is generally worse at night. There is tenderness in the subacromial area and marked limitation of glenohumeral motion in all ranges, especially abduction and rotation.[9] The diagnosis is made primarily on the basis of the symptoms and signs described previously. Radiographs are typically normal. Arthroscopy or arthrography may be diagnostic, but these modalities are invasive and should be avoided if possible. Adhesive capsulitis is usually due to prolonged immobilization of the shoulder in patients with subacromial bursitis or rotator cuff tendinitis.

## TREATMENT

### STERNOCLAVICULAR DISLOCATION

Closed reduction of an anterior dislocation is accomplished with the patient in the supine position and rolled blankets

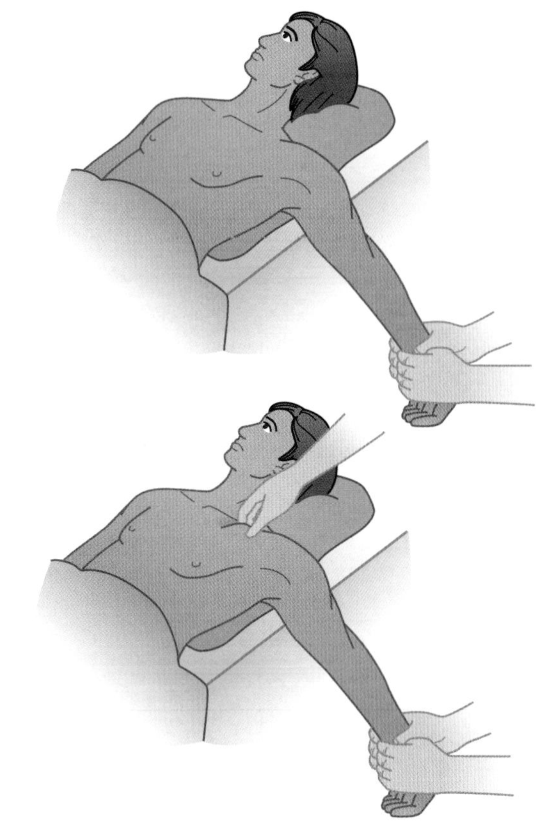

**Fig. 87.12** Closed reduction of anterior sternoclavicular dislocation.

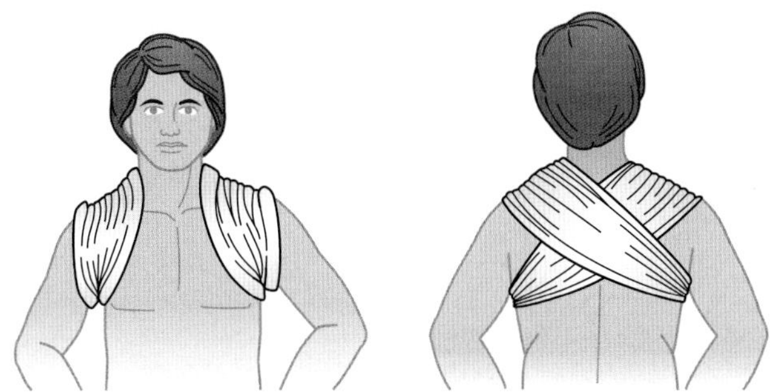

**Fig. 87.13** Clavicular (figure-of-eight) splint.

placed between the shoulder blades. Significant downward pressure on the distal and proximal ends of the clavicle with elevation of the proximal end usually reduces the dislocation (**Fig. 87.12**). If reduction is accomplished, the patient should be placed immediately in a clavicle or figure-of-eight splint to maintain the reduction (**Fig. 87.13**), as well as an arm sling and swath (**Figs. 87.14 and 87.15**). Patients with posterior sternoclavicular dislocations require immediate orthopedic consultation; open reduction is usually necessary. Most reductions should be performed in the operating room with thoracic surgery backup in the event of injury to the superior mediastinal structures. Complications include pneumothorax and vascular, esophageal, and tracheal injuries. Although nonoperative attempts at reduction are occasionally successful, most patients with posterior sternoclavicular dislocations require

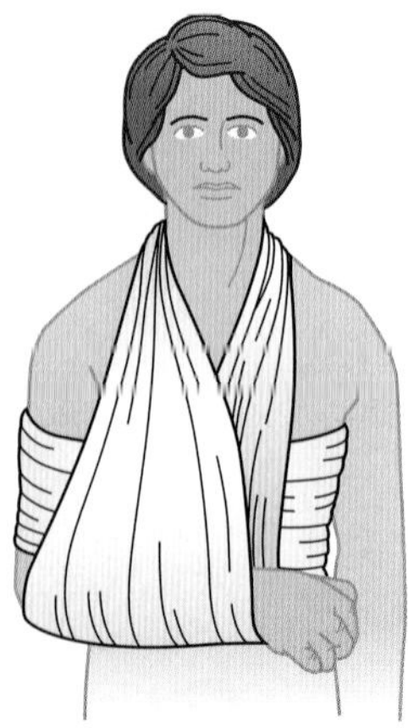

**Fig. 87.14** **Sling and swath shoulder immobilization.**

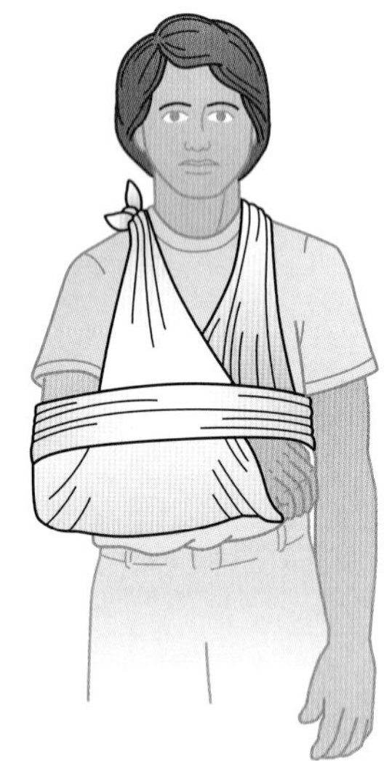

**Fig. 87.15** **Velpeau sling immobilization.**

reduction in the operating room, especially to check for damage to the vital superior mediastinal structures.

## ACROMIOCLAVICULAR DISLOCATION OR SEPARATION

Types I, II, and III acromioclavicular separation should initially be treated conservatively. In the emergency department (ED), the patient should be given adequate analgesia and have ice applied to the area of injury. Following diagnosis, the patient should wear a shoulder immobilizer, be instructed to apply ice to the injured area for 20 to 30 minutes every hour, and be given adequate oral analgesia. The more superiorly the clavicle is displaced in type II dislocations, the more likely patients are to benefit from surgical repair.[11] Type IV, V, and VI injuries are generally severe, and these patients should be referred to an orthopedic surgeon for consultation because most will require open reduction with internal fixation (ORIF).

## CLAVICLE FRACTURES

Almost all proximal third, middle third, and type I and III distal third fractures heal with conservative treatment (a sling or a sling and swath for the ipsilateral arm). Even markedly displaced fractures generally heal without surgical intervention. Some attempts at closed reduction may be appropriate if these fractures are markedly displaced or if significant skin tenting is noted. Many orthopedic surgeons believe that surgical intervention is indicated only if the fracture is open, if there is marked diastasis between the two fracture fragments that cannot be corrected with closed reduction, or in some cases of a type II distal clavicle fracture.[12,13] Recently, one study showed that surgical repair of middle third clavicle fractures may be cost-effective after 9 years when compared with nonsurgical therapy.[14] However, even type II distal third clavicle fractures may do well with nonoperative therapy,[15] although nonunion occurs frequently and surgical therapy is probably preferred.

For patients with middle and proximal third fractures, a figure-of-eight clavicle splint may decrease the pain and, in occasional patients, help keep the fracture reduced. However, such splints are primarily for the patient's comfort and should not be used if their application increases pain from the fracture, which it often does, especially with lateral third clavicle fractures. No evidence has shown any difference in healing time, severity, duration of pain, or any other parameter with an arm sling versus a figure-of-eight clavicle splint or both.[16]

## SCAPULA FRACTURES

Most scapular fractures are treated nonsurgically with a sling, ice, analgesics, and range-of-motion exercises. Displaced fractures of the glenoid, neck, and coracoid and some acromial fractures may need ORIF; patients with such fractures should be referred for consultation with an orthopedic surgeon.[2]

## GLENOHUMERAL DISLOCATIONS

### *Anterior Dislocations*

Multiple techniques for closed reduction of anterior glenohumeral dislocations have been recommended. The three main categories are scapular manipulation, traction, and leverage.[17] The hippocratic method (foot in the axilla with traction on the extended arm) and the Kocher maneuver (traction, adduction, internal rotation) should not be used because of the increased incidence of brachial plexus injuries with the hippocratic method and the increased incidence of proximal humerus fractures with the Kocher maneuver. For almost all reduction techniques to be successful, adequate sedation/analgesia or anesthesia must be obtained. Conscious sedation with IV fentanyl (50 to 100 mcg) and IV midazolam (1 to 3 mg) is adequate for most reductions. However, some patients require deep sedation with propofol or etomidate, and occasionally a patient may require general anesthesia to accomplish the reduction. Frequently, injecting 10 to 20 mL of 1% lidocaine or 0.25% bupivacaine into the vacated glenohumeral joint will significantly facilitate reduction of the dislocation.[18]

Several methods commonly used to reduce anterior glenohumeral dislocations are described in the following sections.

SCAPULAR MANIPULATION Ideally, the patient is in the prone position with the dislocated arm hanging over the edge of the stretcher. Traction is applied to the arm, and the operator pushes the tip of the scapula medially while stabilizing the

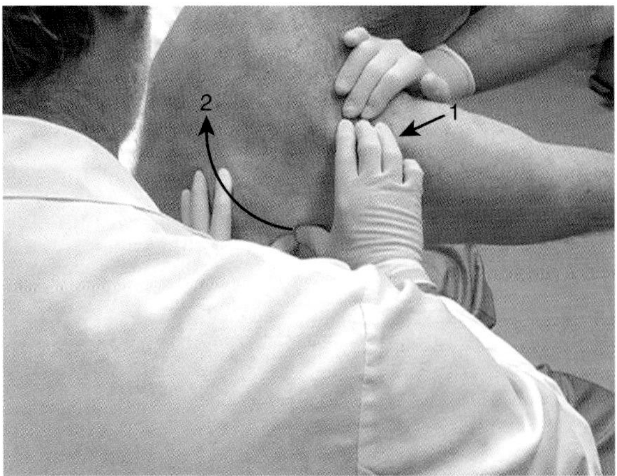


**Fig. 87.16 Scapular manipulation technique for reduction of anterior glenohumeral dislocation.** (From Thomsen T, Setnick G, editors. Procedures consult—emergency medicine module. Copyright 2008 Elsevier Inc. All rights reserved.)

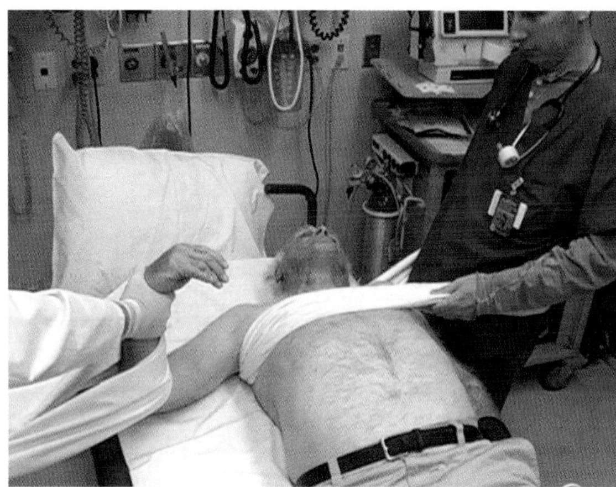

**Fig. 87.18 Traction-countertraction technique for reduction of anterior glenohumeral dislocation.**

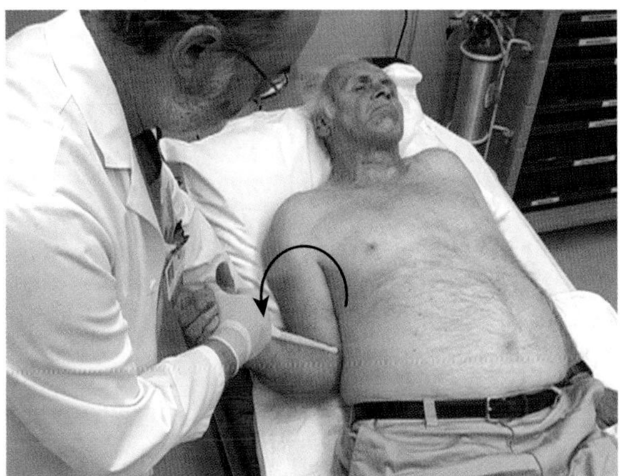

**Fig. 87.17 External rotation technique for reduction of anterior glenohumeral dislocation.** (From Thomsen T, Setnick G, editors. Procedures consult—emergency medicine module. Copyright 2008 Elsevier Inc. All rights reserved.)

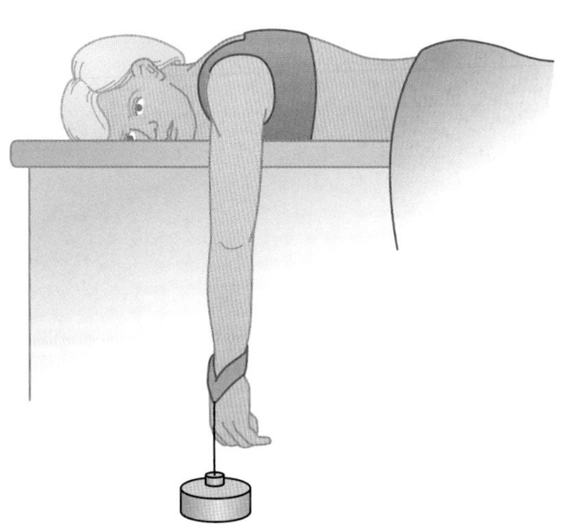

**Fig. 87.19 Stimson method for reduction of anterior glenohumeral dislocation.**

upper part of the scapula (**Fig. 87.16**). If the patient insists on sitting up, this same technique can be combined with a modified hippocratic method in which one operator applies countertraction superiorly with a sheet sling in the axilla, another operator places traction on the arm, and a third operator manipulates the scapula. This is the technique of choice for the author. It requires relatively little sedation or analgesia and is successful in more than 90% of cases.[19]

EXTERNAL ROTATION With the patient supine, the affected arm is adducted close to the thorax. The elbow is flexed to 90 degrees and the operator very slowly externally rotates the arm without applying longitudinal traction. This method is safe, easily learned, and relatively atraumatic for the patient[20] (**Fig. 87.17**).

MODIFIED HIPPOCRATIC (TRACTION-COUNTERTRACTION) METHOD With the patient supine, the elbow is slightly abducted and flexed to 90 degrees. The operator ties a sheet around his or her waist and to the proximal end of the patient's forearm. An assistant slings another sheet around the thorax and under the affected armpit and ties it around his or her own waist. The operator and the assistant pull in opposite directions with their arms and bodies (**Fig. 87.18**).

STIMSON METHOD With the patient prone, the affected arm is dangled over the edge of the stretcher and a 10- to 20-lb weight is attached to the wrist to produce constant, gentle traction. This method is one of the oldest and has the advantage of not requiring the physician to be present for the reduction and probably being the least traumatic for the patient. The disadvantage is that it often takes 20 or more minutes to complete the reduction and ties up a nurse for this period if the patient has been consciously sedated (**Fig. 87.19**). Several other techniques have also been proposed for reduction of anterior glenohumeral dislocations.[21-25]

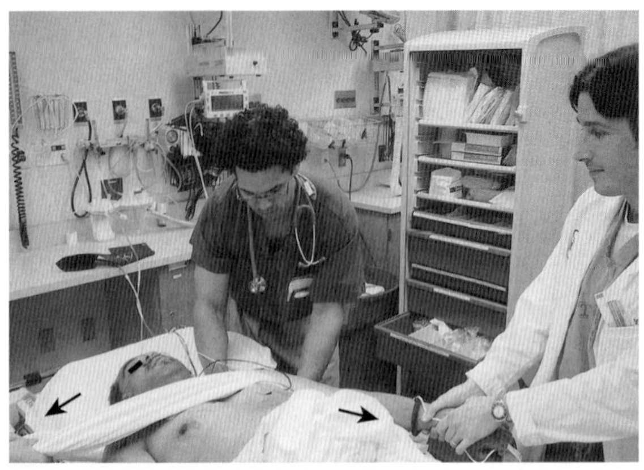

Fig. 87.20 Technique for reduction of posterior glenohumeral dislocation.

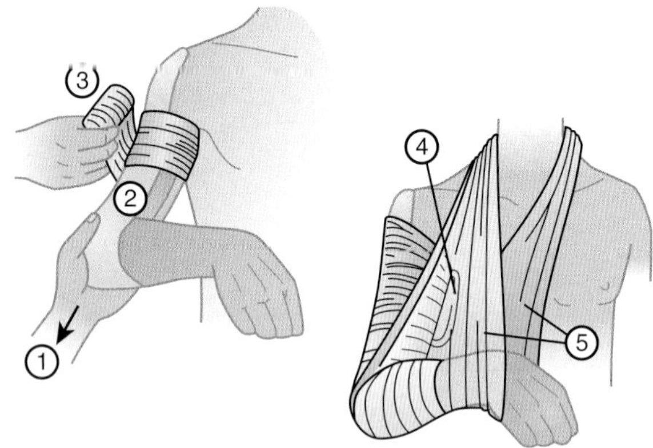


Fig. 87.22 Sugar-tong splint for humeral shaft fractures.

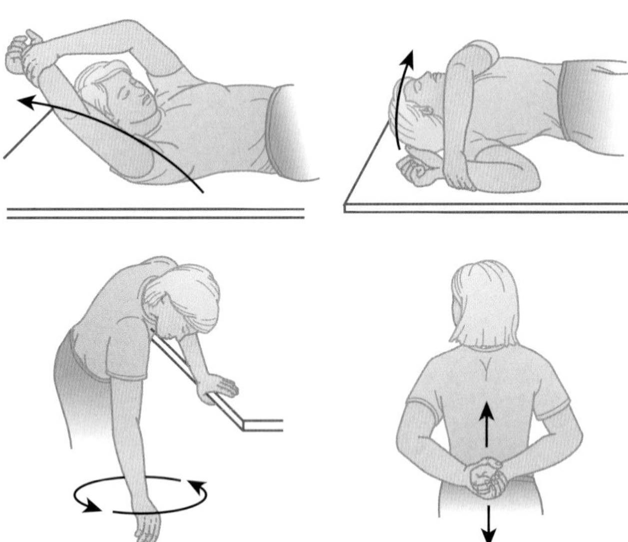

Fig. 87.21 Passive and active shoulder range-of-motion exercises to prevent adhesive capsulitis.

### *Posterior Dislocations*

The most common technique for reduction of a posterior dislocation is to apply axial traction in line with the humerus while an assistant applies countertraction with a sheet slung under the axilla of the affected arm. Gentle pressure is applied by the operator, who also applies slow external rotation to the affected humerus (**Fig. 87.20**).

### *Luxatio Erecta (Inferior Dislocations)*

If possible, orthopedic consultation should be obtained before reduction. The traction-countertraction method is most effective in reducing this dislocation, although deep sedation or general anesthesia may be required. Recently, a technique by which the luxatio erecta is converted to an anterior-inferior dislocation and then relocated in a separate step has been shown to be more successful and requires less analgesia and sedation.[26]

## PROXIMAL HUMERUS FRACTURES

With a glenohumeral dislocation, the patient will usually need ORIF to reduce the dislocation and repair the proximal humeral fracture. If the fractures are not displaced (<1 cm of displacement), wearing a sling or a sling and swath may be all the treatment that is required. If significant displacement remains after closed reduction, ORIF will be necessary.[8] Orthopedic consultation should be obtained in almost all cases.

Successful treatment is most dependent on early mobility. Prolonged immobilization without range-of-motion exercises often results in adhesive capsulitis or a marked reduction in mobility of the glenohumeral joint. Patients should be encouraged to perform circumduction range-of-motion exercises after a few days of immobilization, especially elderly patients (**Fig. 87.21**).

## HUMERAL SHAFT FRACTURES

Most humeral shaft fractures can be treated conservatively. If the fracture fragments are minimally displaced, no reduction is necessary. If the fragments are widely separated, reduction may be carried out before splinting.[27] If the fracture fragments are in reasonable apposition (within 1 to 2 inches) following the reduction, the most commonly used splinting technique is the coaptation or sugar-tong splint, whereby a 5-inch plaster or Orthoglass splint is applied over the shoulder, down the lateral side of the upper part of the arm, around the elbow, and up the medial side of the upper part of the arm near the axilla. The arm is then placed in a sling with the sling around the wrist so that the weight of the splint will bring the fracture fragments together (**Fig. 87.22**). If the fracture fragments are separated more than 2 inches after reduction or if a spiral fracture is present, the hanging cast technique may be used. A lightweight cast is applied 1 to 2 inches proximal to the fracture site up to the palmar crease of the hand. The elbow is flexed to 90 degrees and a loop is placed at the wrist either on the dorsal side to reduce lateral angulation or on the volar side to reduce medial angulation (**Fig. 87.23**). The hanging cast has the disadvantage of needing gravity for traction; therefore, patients must remain upright at all times, even during sleep. Many patients cannot tolerate this.

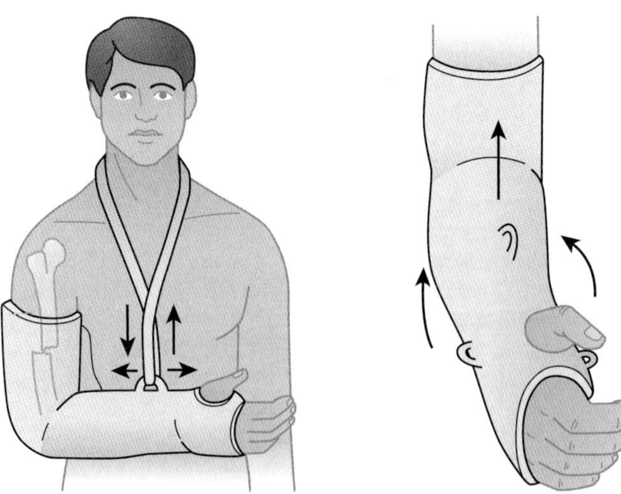

**Fig. 87.23** Hanging cast technique on the dorsal side to reduce lateral angulation or on the volar side to reduce medial angulation.

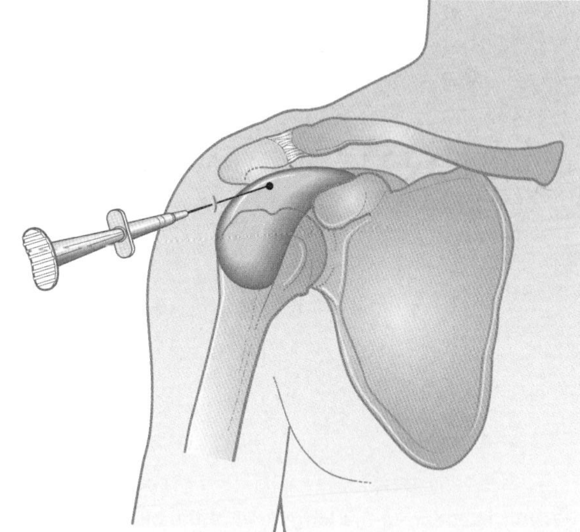

**Fig. 87.24** Subacromial injection for subacromial bursitis or tendinitis and adhesive capsulitis.

The most common and most feared complication of humeral shaft fractures is radial nerve injury. If nerve function is lost before reduction, most authorities treat it expectantly. Most of the time nerve function returns because the nerve has been either contused or stretched. After reduction, function of the radial nerve should again be tested.[28] If radial nerve function is compromised but was normal before reduction, most authorities recommend ORIF because the probability is high that the radial nerve is entrapped within the fracture.[29]

## SUPRACONDYLAR FRACTURES

Type I supracondylar fractures are treated with a long arm splint and the elbow flexed to 90 degrees. The arm is placed in a sling. Protected active range-of-motion exercises are begun in 3 to 4 weeks.

Type II fractures require reduction even though they are minimally displaced. Following reduction, a long arm splint is applied with the elbow flexed to 100 to 120 degrees. Flexion greater than 90 degrees places tension on the intact posterior periosteum to maintain the reduction. Because this degree of hyperextension may compromise neurovascular structures volar to the elbow, careful attention should be paid to ensure that this complication does not arise, especially in the first 2 to 3 days after the fracture.[30,31] Orthopedic consultation should be obtained in all cases.

Type III injuries are problematic because they may increase the chance for a varus deformity and are more likely to cause injury to the neurovascular structures passing through the elbow. Rarely should an attempt be made to reduce these fractures in the ED. The only exception might be the unavailability of immediate orthopedic consultation for a patient who has an obviously occluded brachial artery. The vast majority of these patients should be taken to the operating room immediately and undergo either closed or open reduction.[32] Orthopedic consultation is mandatory in all cases.

The most common complication is loss of the normal carrying angle, which results in a cubitus varus deformity. This complication has decreased in incidence as the practice of percutaneous pinning of the fracture has evolved. More serious complications of supracondylar fractures include brachial artery injury and injuries to the radial, median, and ulnar nerves. Most often these injuries are due to contusion or stretching of the nerves, and full recovery is the rule.[30]

## ROTATOR CUFF TENDINITIS/SUBACROMIAL BURSITIS, ROTATOR CUFF TEARS, AND IMPINGEMENT SYNDROMES

Treatment depends on the degree of disability (incomplete versus complete tear), the patient's age, and the patient's activity level. In patients with tendinitis or subacromial bursitis, an injection into the subacromial bursa usually results in relief of pain (**Fig. 87.24**). In young, active patients with significant rotator cuff tears, arthroscopic repair is indicated. In older patients with a sedentary lifestyle, repair should rarely be attempted because the outcome is often worse than that with conservative therapy. For evaluation, patients should be referred for consultation with an orthopedist who specializes in shoulder injuries.[33]

## TENOSYNOVITIS AND RUPTURE OF THE LONG HEAD OF THE BICEPS TENDON

Conservative treatment consists of a sling and nonsteroidal antiinflammatory drugs (NSAIDs). If after a week of immobilization the patient continues to have pain, the bicipital canal can be injected with a combined local anesthetic and steroid (**Fig. 87.25**). Range-of-motion exercises should be performed daily to prevent adhesive tenosynovitis.

## ADHESIVE CAPSULITIS

The most important form of therapy should be directed at prevention of this problem. All patients with shoulder injuries or inflammation should be encouraged to perform circumduction range-of-motion exercises daily to prevent adhesive capsulitis. Conservative treatment consists of a gentle exercise program, NSAIDs, and corticosteroid injections.[33] Such treaent results in significant improvement in many patients;

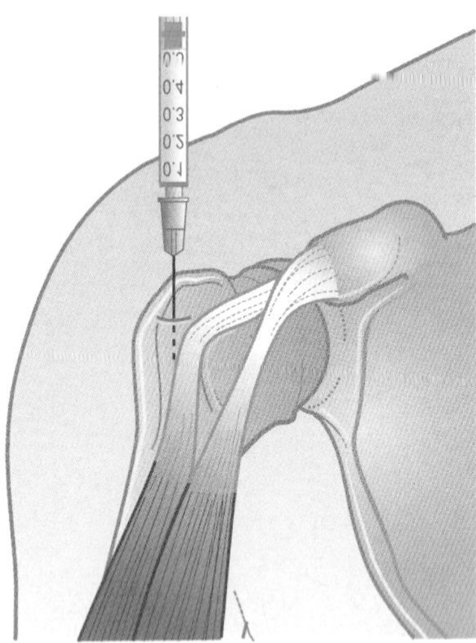

**Fig. 87.25 Injection of the long head of the biceps tendon in the bicipital groove.**

however, many others require the adhesions to be broken up by putting the shoulder through full range of motion under general anesthesia.

## FOLLOW-UP, NEXT STEPS IN CARE, AND PATIENT EDUCATION

### STERNOCLAVICULAR STRAINS, SUBLUXATIONS, AND DISLOCATIONS

Anterior dislocations can be reduced in the ED. The patient should be placed in a sling and swath and be told to wear it for 2 to 3 weeks and follow up with an orthopedic surgeon. If an anterior dislocation cannot be reduced in the ED, the patient should be placed in a sling and figure-of-eight clavicle splint and be referred to an orthopedic surgeon. A patient with a posterior dislocation should undergo CT of the sternoclavicular joint and be seen urgently by an orthopedic surgeon. The patient must also be seen by a cardiothoracic surgeon if injury to a superior mediastinal structure is suspected.

### ACROMIOCLAVICULAR SEPARATION OR DISLOCATION

Patients with a type I or II separation should be put in a sling or a sling and swath for their comfort. They should be treated with ice and analgesics and be told to follow up with their primary care physician. Patients with type III separations should be put into a sling, be told to apply ice to the injury, and be referred for follow-up consultation with an orthopedic surgeon within 1 to 2 weeks. Most type III fractures should be treated conservatively. Although some orthopedic surgeons may elect to perform open reduction of these injuries in an athlete who uses the injured arm in overhead activities (e.g., baseball pitcher, football quarterback), no good evidence has shown a difference in outcome with surgical versus nonsurgical therapy, even in these patients. Type IV, V, and VI injuries are usually severe, and these patients should be referred to an orthopedic surgeon for consultation because most will require ORIF.

### CLAVICLE FRACTURES

The only indication for immediate surgery is an open fracture or fractures with neurovascular compromise. Some orthopedic surgeons would consider a significantly displaced type II distal third clavicle fracture, any fracture with skin tenting, or any widely displaced middle or proximal third clavicle fracture as an orthopedic urgency. All such patients should be referred immediately to an orthopedic surgeon. If patients are to be discharged, they should be put in a sling, be told to put ice on their injured clavicle, and be prescribed potent opioid analgesics. Patients should leave their arm in a sling (with a figure-of-eight bandage if it provides additional comfort). Patients should be told to perform circumduction range-of-motion exercises at least once daily to prevent adhesive capsulitis. The sling should be left on for 2 to 4 weeks in children younger than 14 years and for 4 to 8 weeks in adolescents and adults. Referral to an orthopedic surgeon is necessary only for patients with severely displaced fractures (>20 mm of shortening), open fractures, fractures associated with neurovascular injury or skin tenting, and type II distal third clavicle fractures. Complications are uncommon and consist of osteoarthritis of the acromioclavicular joint (in type II and III distal third clavicle fractures) and nonunion in type II distal third clavicle fractures (primarily a cosmetic issue).

### SCAPULA FRACTURES

Most scapular fractures heal without surgery, and patients should be discharged with a sling, instructions to apply ice, and analgesics, as well as arrangements for follow-up with an orthopedic surgeon. Patients with fractures of the scapular neck and glenoid that are widely displaced or angulated may need ORIF and should be referred immediately to an orthopedic surgeon. These fractures are associated with internal injuries, which should be ruled out before discharge.

### GLENOHUMERAL DISLOCATIONS

Most dislocations can be reduced with some type of conscious sedation in the ED. In some cases the relocation will be unsuccessful and the patient must be taken to the operating room for relocation. Following relocation, the patient may be discharged with a sling or a sling and swath. The sling should be kept on for 3 to 5 weeks, and the patient should perform circumduction range-of-motion exercises until the sling is removed. Complications include fracturing of the humerus during reduction and injury to the axillary nerve, which should be checked before and after reduction. Prereduction radiographs are recommended. However, routinely obtaining postreduction radiographs is controversial, especially if the patient is asymptomatic.[34] The sling should be left on for approximately 4 weeks.

### PROXIMAL HUMERAL FRACTURES

Most patients with these fractures do not require admission unless it is needed for pain control. Successful treatment is most dependent on early mobility. Prolonged immobilization without range-of-motion exercises often results in adhesive capsulitis or a marked reduction in mobility of the glenohumeral joint. Patients should be encouraged to perform circumduction range-of-motion exercises after a few days of immobilization, especially elderly patients.

## HUMERAL SHAFT FRACTURES

Unless the fracture is open, most patients can be discharged home. The coaptation splint or hanging cast should remain in place until the patient sees the orthopedic surgeon 2 to 3 days following the injury. The patient should be given potent oral analgesics for pain.

## SUPRACONDYLAR HUMERAL FRACTURES

Patients with type I fractures are usually discharged with a long arm splint in 90 degrees of flexion at the elbow and orthopedic follow-up scheduled within 2 weeks. Patients with type II and III fractures are generally admitted to the hospital and undergo ORIF. The most common complication is loss of the normal carrying angle, which results in a cubitus varus deformity. This complication has decreased in incidence as the practice of percutaneous pinning of the fracture has evolved. More serious complications of supracondylar fractures include brachial artery injury and injuries to the radial, median, and ulnar nerves. Most often these injuries are due to contusion or stretching of the nerves, and full recovery is the rule.

## ROTATOR CUFF TENDINITIS/SUBACROMIAL BURSITIS, ROTATOR CUFF TEARS, AND IMPINGEMENT SYNDROMES

Conservative therapy for rotator cuff tears consists of improving the patient's ability to abduct the arm. Having the patient "crawl up the wall" with the affected hand until the pain is unbearable and repeat this exercise daily is beneficial. In addition, subacromial injection of a local anesthetic and steroid mixture reduces pain and allows greater range of motion. This should probably be limited to two or three times per year because of the tendency for steroids to cause tendon rupture. Treatment of subacromial bursitis and supraspinatus tendinitis is similar to that for conservative therapy for rotator cuff tears, with initial treatment consisting of the application of ice and NSAIDs and, in refractory cases, subacromial steroid or local anesthetic injections.

## SUGGESTED READINGS

Baratz M, Micucci C, Sangimino M. Pediatric supracondylar humerus fractures. Hand Clin 2006;22:69-75.

Dodson CC, Cordasco FA. Anterior glenohumeral joint dislocations. Orthop Clin North Am 2008;39:507-18.

Klein SM, Badman BL, Keating CJ, et al. Results of surgical treatment for unstable distal clavicular fractures. J Shoulder Elbow Surg 2010;19:1049-55.

Lenza M, Belloti JC, Andriolo RB, et al. Conservative interventions for treating middle third clavicle fractures in adolescents and adults. Cochrane Database Syst Rev 2009;2:CD007121.

Macdonald PB, Lapointe P. Acromioclavicular and sternoclavicular joint injuries. Orthop Clin North Am 2008;39:535-45.

Malik S, Chiampas G, Leonard H. Emergent evaluation of injuries to the shoulder, clavicle and humerus. Emerg Med Clin North Am 2010;28:739-63.

## REFERENCES

***References can be found on Expert Consult @ www.expertconsult.com.***

# 88 Forearm Fractures

*Trevor J. Mills*

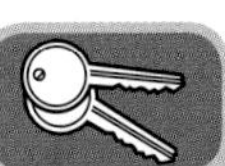

**KEY POINTS**

- The goal of treatment of forearm fractures is to restore length, correct angulation, and ideally, achieve normal function.
- Radiographs of the proximal and distal joints of patients with a forearm fracture should always be considered to rule out concurrent dislocations (i.e., Monteggia fracture).

## EPIDEMIOLOGY

Injury is a leading cause of mortality, morbidity, and lost days of work. The annual health care cost of injuries exceeds $9.2 billion. Traumatic injuries result in more than 34 million emergency department (ED) visits each year.[1] The highest rate of injuries occurs in persons between the ages of 15 and 24 years. Likewise, forearm fractures are commonly seen in young adults but have a bimodal distribution, with a second increased incidence in the elderly.[2]

### PATHOPHYSIOLOGY

The bones of the forearm consist of the radius and ulna. These two bones lie in parallel and are connected by joint capsules at the elbow and at the wrist, whereas the shafts are interlocked by a fibrous interosseus membrane.[3] Most forearm fractures are caused by a sudden force, such as a fall on an outstretched arm. Because of the interlocking joint capsules, interosseus membrane, and contraction of the forearm muscles, multiple fractures, displaced fragments, and concurrent dislocations may be present. Alternatively, forearm fractures may be due to smaller repetitive injuries, which result in a stress fracture over time. Any pathophysiologic process that reduces the integrity of the bone, such as osteopenia, osteomyelitis, and bone metastasis, increases the likelihood of fracture, even with normal external stress.[4]

## PRESENTING SIGNS AND SYMPTOMS

Symptoms of forearm fractures include pain, forearm edema, forearm ecchymosis, abnormal or reduced mobility from the wrist through the elbow, and complaints of neurovascular compromise. Findings on physical examination can include obvious bony deformity; shortening of the forearm; crepitus; tenderness to palpation of the forearm; joint effusions; abnormal mobility of the wrist, forearm, or elbow; and neurologic and vascular deficits of the forearm, wrist, or hand.

**BOX 88.1 Signs and Symptoms of Fractures and Complications That Suggest Serious Injury**

**Open Fracture**

Open wounds in proximity to the fracture, bone fragments protruding from the skin

Skin tenting may indicate a high potential for progression to an open fracture

**Fracture-Dislocation**

In patients with intraarticular fractures and displaced fractures, additional radiographs above and below the injury may reveal concurrent dislocations

Physical examination should include the joints above and below the fracture site

**Vascular Compromise**

Loss or reduction of pulses distal to the injury

Reduced capillary refill

Skin pallor; patient complaints of a "cold" extremity or pain out of proportion to the injury

**Neurologic Compromise**

Loss of strength, sensation, reflexes, or two-point discrimination distal to the injury

Complaints of paresthesias or pain distal to the injury

**Compartment Syndrome**

Tense forearm

Neurologic or vascular compromise distal to the injury

**Box 88.1** lists the signs and symptoms of fractures and complications that indicate serious injury.

In general, forearm fractures are classified by the bone (or bones) involved, anatomic location, trajectory of the fracture and alignment of the fracture fragments, and the presence of angulation, rotation, comminution, and concurrent dislocations. All fractures should be further described as open or closed, and the presence (or absence) of distal neurologic and vascular function should be noted (**Fig. 88.1**).

Types of forearm fractures that are frequently mentioned in the medical literature are described in **Table 88.1**.

## PEDIATRIC FRACTURES

Forearm fractures in the pediatric population include several additional entities because children have a plastic bone matrix and active growth plates, both of which contribute to unique fractures (**Table 88.2**). In children, when an external force bends a long bone, one side of the cortex may be disrupted while the other side remains intact (greenstick fracture).

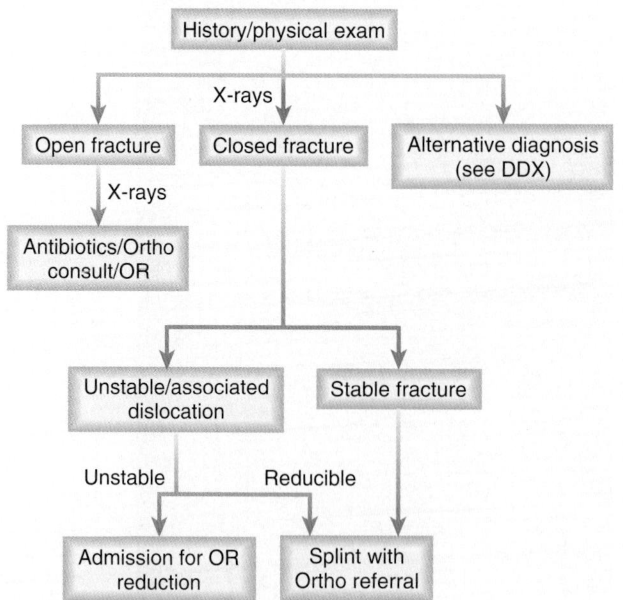


**Fig. 88.1 Approach to patients with a suspected forearm fracture.** *DDX*, Differential diagnosis; *OR*, operating room; *Ortho*, orthopedics.

**Table 88.1 Types of Forearm Fractures**

| NAME | DESCRIPTION |
|---|---|
| Colles | Distal radial extension fracture (may also include the ulna) with dorsal displacement of the distal fragments |
| Smith | Distal radial flexion fracture with volar displacement of the distal fragments |
| Barton | Intraarticular fracture of the dorsal rim of the distal end of the radius, often associated with carpal dislocation. Treatment is typically operative |
| Hutchinson | Radial styloid fracture associated with carpal dislocation |
| Galeazzi | Distal radial shaft fracture with concurrent distal radioulnar dislocation |
| Monteggia | Ulnar shaft fracture with dislocation of the radial head |

**Table 88.2 Types of Pediatric Fractures**

| NAME | DESCRIPTION |
|---|---|
| Torus | Fracture involving compression buckling of one or both sides of the cortex |
| Greenstick | Fracture involving distraction of one side of the cortex without apparent disruption of the other |
| Plastic deformity | Bowing of the radius or ulna without obvious fracture lines (multiple microfractures) |
| Salter-Harris | Fracture involving the growth plates |

**BOX 88.2 Differential Diagnosis of Forearm Fractures**

**Traumatic**
Wrist sprain, elbow sprain
Ligamentous injuries, forearm contusions, hematomas
Dislocations of the elbow or wrist (including nursemaid's elbow)

**Infectious**
Cellulitis of the forearm, abscesses
Necrotizing fasciitis

**Vascular**
Acute arterial occlusion
Venous thrombosis

**Neurologic**
Neurapraxias, carpal tunnel syndrome
Systemic neurologic syndromes involving the nerves of the upper extremities

**Arthritis**
Septic joint, gonococcal arthritis, rheumatoid arthritis, osteoarthritis
Pseudogout, gout
Systemic lupus erythematosus, rheumatic fever, viral syndrome
Reiter syndrome, Lyme disease, serum sickness

**Other**
Olecranon bursitis, soft tissue masses
Normal growth plates, nutrient vessels

Alternatively, a deformity of the bone may occur without an obvious fracture line (plastic deformity). With compression, buckling of the cortex may be seen (torus fracture). Depending on the age of the child, fractures through the various growth plates of the elbow and wrist may also occur (Salter-Harris fractures).[5]

## DIFFERENTIAL DIAGNOSIS AND MEDICAL DECISION MAKING

The differential diagnosis for forearm fractures includes any soft tissue injury to the forearm, in addition to acute skin, soft tissue, and joint infections (**Box 88.2**). Some clinical aspects of acute arterial occlusion, as well as venous thrombosis, may mimic forearm fractures. Any acute neurologic change, including paresthesias, weakness, and functional loss, should be considered along with forearm fractures. Two normal variants sometimes mistaken for forearm fractures on radiographs are normal growth plates in children and nutrient vessels.

The orthopedic literature often recommends radiographs of a suspected fracture and additional films of the joints above and below the injury (**Fig. 88.2; Table 88.3**). This is true for forearm fractures if they are close to the joint (either elbow or wrist) or are suspected of having a concurrent dislocation (**Fig. 88.3**).

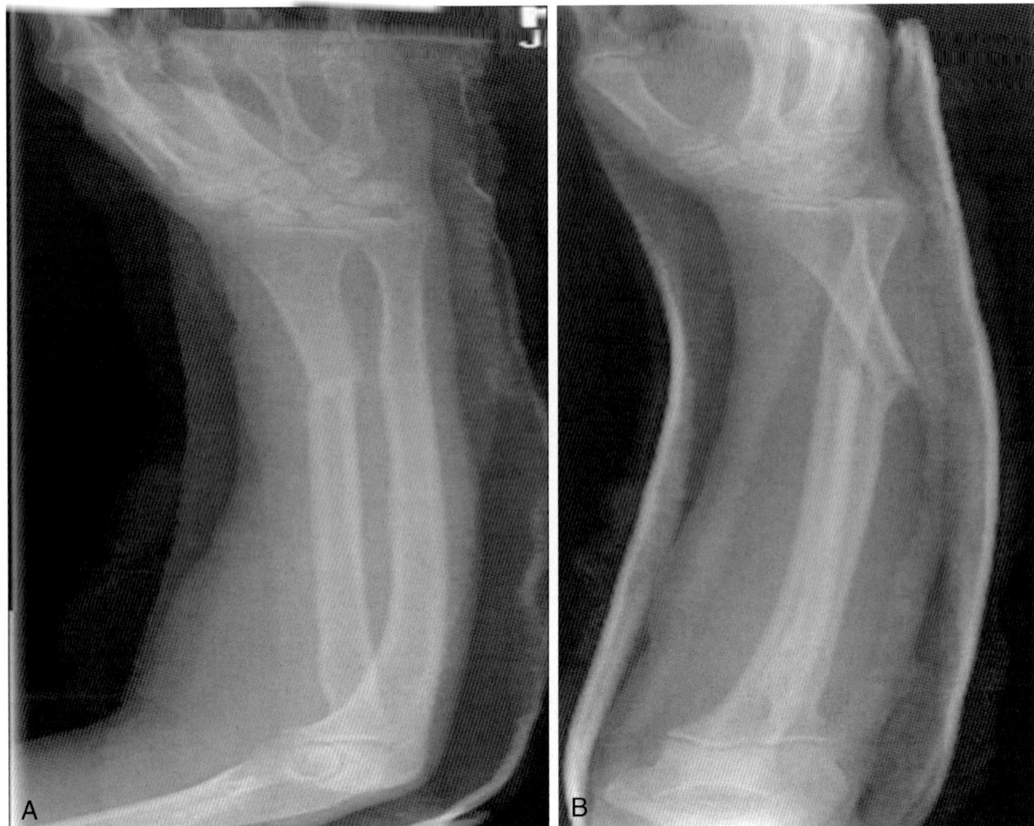


**Fig. 88.2 Radiographs demonstrating the need for at least two views of a fracture.** In **A** (anteroposterior view), there appears to be good alignment; in **B** (lateral view), a large amount of displacement is obvious.

**Table 88.3 Radiographs Useful in the Differential Diagnosis of Forearm Fractures**

| SUSPECTED INJURY | VIEWS |
|---|---|
| Proximal forearm fracture | Elbow series (AP and lateral) and forearm series (AP and lateral forearm) |
| Shaft fracture | Forearm series |
| Distal forearm fracture | Wrist series (AP and lateral wrist) and forearm series |

*AP*, Anteroposterior.

Because isolated proximal ulnar fractures are unusual, a Monteggia fracture must be suspected and specific attention paid to the radial head to assess for dislocation. Specific radiographs of the radioulnar joint should be obtained if dislocation is suspected because the overall forearm radiograph may not reveal subtle injury. A longitudinal line through the radial shaft and head must transverse the capitellum in all views. Open reduction with internal fixation (ORIF) will probably be required, although children may be treated with casting.

Galeazzi fractures are two to three times more common than Monteggia fractures and have the potential for higher morbidity as a result of disruption of the distal radioulnar joint accompanying fracture of the distal end of the radius. Disruption of the radioulnar joint must be suspected in patients with a fracture of the ulnar styloid, shortening of the radius (5 mm), or widening of the radioulnar joint (2 mm). ORIF will probably be required.

Additional films are not usually necessary with uncomplicated shaft fractures (one bone, nondisplaced). If the fracture is intraarticular, additional radiographic views or computed tomography or magnetic resonance imaging may be suggested (**Table 88.4**).

A Colles fracture is probably unstable if the fracture is comminuted and exhibits ulnar styloid displacement, loss of radial height of 2 mm or greater, intraarticular displacement of more than 1 mm, or dorsal angulation greater than 20 degrees.

Although most forearm fractures are evident on plain radiographs, occult fractures of the elbow may be difficult to interpret. One indication of an elbow fracture is the fat pad or sail sign, which indicates hemarthrosis of the elbow joint and thus a fracture.[6]

The fracture is probably unstable if it is comminuted

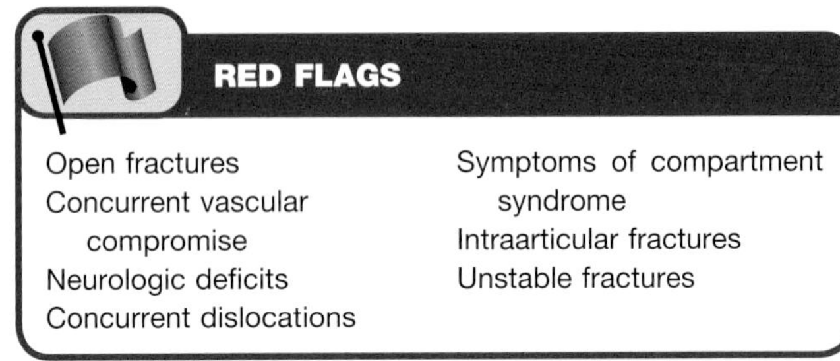

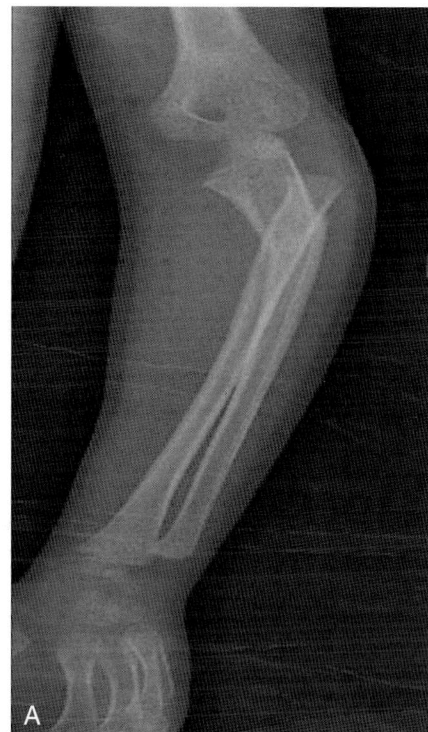


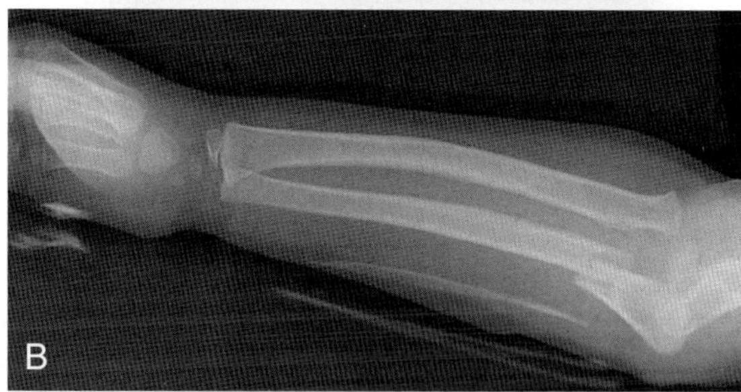


**Fig. 88.3 Anteroposterior (A) and lateral (B) radiographs of a Monteggia (fracture of the ulna and dislocation of the radial head).** (Courtesy Dr. Alan Nemeth, Brookhaven Memorial Hospital Medical Center, East Patchogue, New York.)

**Table 88.4 Special Circumstances in the Differential Diagnosis of Forearm Fractures**

| SUSPECTED INJURY | ADDITIONAL RADIOLOGY |
|---|---|
| Proximal forearm fracture—olecranon | Elbow series (AP and lateral) with the elbow in 90 degrees of flexion; forearm series (AP and lateral) |
| Proximal forearm fracture—radial head and neck | Elbow series, including oblique views, if the coronoid process is involved; forearm series |
| Fracture of the distal end of the forearm | If the radiocarpal or radioulnar joint is involved, CT or MRI to define subluxation or dislocation |

*AP*, Anteroposterior; *CT*, computed tomography; *MRI*, magnetic resonance imaging.

**Table 88.5 Immobilization of Forearm Fractures**

| FRACTURE | IMMOBILIZATION |
|---|---|
| Proximal forearm fracture (olecranon and radial head and neck) | Long arm posterior splint |
| Shaft fracture without displacement | Long arm posterior splint |
| Shaft fracture with displacement | Long arm posterior splint with urgent orthopedic referral for surgical reduction |
| Shaft fracture with concurrent dislocations | Reduction and long arm posterior splint |
| Distal fracture—Colles, Smith, shaft | Reduction in the emergency department and sugar-tong splint |
| Hutchinson | Short dorsal forearm splint (reduction) |
| Barton | Short volar forearm splint (reduction) |

## TREATMENT

Prehospital treatment includes immobilization to reduce the development of further injury and help control pain. The mainstays of ED treatment include pain control, reduction of further injury, immobilization, and appropriate disposition.[7] Pain control should include elevation of the arm and cooling via ice packs. Oral or parenteral pain medications are usually indicated, depending on the age and size of the patient and the amount of pain.

Reduction of further injury depends on the fracture. Patients with open fractures and suspected open fractures should be given early parenteral antibiotic therapy and tetanus prophylaxis (if indicated). Displaced fractures and fractures with associated dislocations require early relocation, either by the emergency physician in consultation with an orthopedic surgeon or, if the patient's condition is unstable, by an orthopedic surgeon in the ED.[8]

The preferred method of fracture immobilization in the ED is splinting rather than casting because fracture edema will tend to increase in size over the first 24 hours. Specific splints for particular fractures are listed in **Table 88.5**.

## FOLLOW-UP, NEXT STEPS IN CARE, AND PATIENT EDUCATION

Patients with forearm fractures can be classified into three categories: those who need immobilization with routine orthopedic follow-up, those who need interventions in the ED with very close follow-up, and those who should be admitted to the hospital.[9]

Admission criteria include all open fractures, fractures with suspected compartment syndrome or neurovascular compromise, and fractures (or fracture-dislocations) that cannot be adequately reduced in the ED. Patients who have difficulty with pain control or social issues that reduce their ability to take care of their injuries may also require admission. Any suspicion of child abuse, interpersonal violence, or elder abuse may also necessitate admission.

Forearm injuries that require urgent orthopedic referral include unstable fractures, fractures that can be reduced and splinted but need further internal fixation, and dislocations that are reduced.

Forearm fractures that can be evaluated by an orthopedist in a 1-week range include stable nondisplaced fractures that show no evidence of neurovascular compromise.

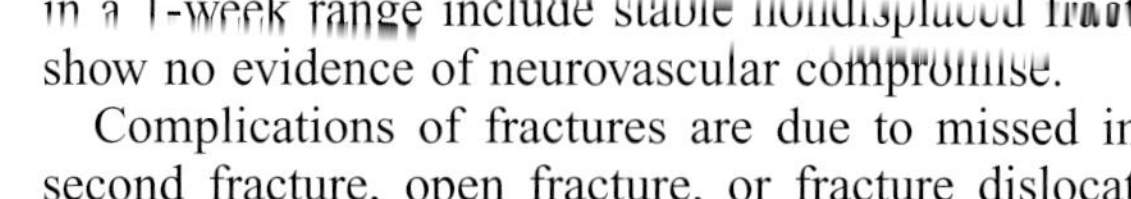

Complications of fractures are due to missed injuries (a second fracture, open fracture, or fracture dislocation) and include early signs of neurovascular compromise or impending compartment syndrome. For most forearm injuries, return to full function can be anticipated.

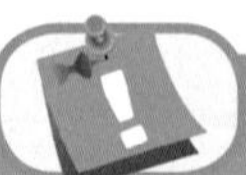

### TIPS AND TRICKS

**Splinting Procedure**

Use extra padding on the elbow and wrist.

Cast padding should be smooth to avoid pressure points.

To avoid irregularities, use constant pressure (palms, not fingers) to shape the splint.

Always repeat the distal neurovascular examination after the splint dries.

If in doubt, splint joints in the position of use and avoid flexion contractures.

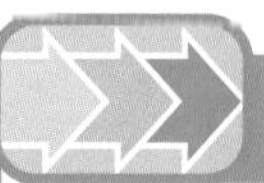

### PRIORITY ACTIONS

History: Elucidate mechanisms with a high potential for open fractures.

Physical examination: Check the joints above and below the injury, examine the skin for open wounds, and evaluate and reevaluate neurovascular status distal to the injury.

Radiography: Always look for a second fracture or associated dislocation.

Treatment: Antibiotic therapy is needed for patients with open fractures; early reduction of dislocations and displaced fractures is essential.

### DOCUMENTATION

**History**

Details of the mechanism and circumstances (fall, penetrating trauma, motor vehicle collision)

Timing of the event; time elapsed before arrival at the emergency department

Concurrent medications, drugs, or alcohol use; allergies; last meal; immunizations

Past orthopedic injuries or surgeries; other surgeries

**Physical Examination**

Initial examination, including evaluation of motor, neurologic, and vascular function

Reexamination over time, including after any intervention (e.g., splinting)

**Diagnostic Studies**

Emergency department interpretation of radiographs, computed tomography scans, magnetic resonance images, and angiograms

**Medical Decision Making**

Indications for studies and choice of consultant

Discussion with the consultant and mutual care plan decisions

**Procedures**

Details of each procedure, including the type of splint or immobilization device used

**Patient Instructions**

Discussion of injuries and potential outcomes with the patient, family, or both

Discussion of splint care with the patient, family, or both

Documentation of pain medications prescribed or the recommended plan for breakthrough pain

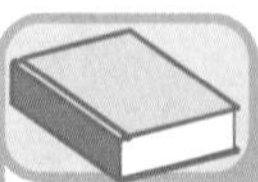

### PATIENT TEACHING TIPS

Recovery from orthopedic injuries takes time and often involves extensive rehabilitation.

Provide a cast or splint care instruction sheet; for example, "Don't get it wet."

Inform the patient about the side effects of pain control medication.

Educate the patient about warning signs for which to seek immediate care—for example, increased pain, cold fingers, or loss of mobility.

## SUGGESTED READINGS

Blakeney WG. Stabilization and treatment of Colles' fractures in elderly patients. Clin Interv Aging 2010;5:337-44.

Cheng JC, Shen WY. Limb fracture pattern in different pediatric age groups: a study of 3,350 children. J Orthop Trauma 1993;7:15-22.

Handoll HH, Madhok R. Closed reduction methods for treating distal radial fractures in adults. Cochrane Database Syst Rev 2003;1:CD003763.

Morgan WJ, Breen TF. Complex fractures of the forearm. Hand Clin 1994;10:375-90.

Simon R, Koenigsknecht S. Fractures of the radius and ulna. In: Emergency orthopedics: the extremities. 4th ed. New York: McGraw-Hill; 2001. pp. 195-230.

## REFERENCES

*References can be found on Expert Consult @ www.expertconsult.com.*

# Hand and Wrist Injuries 89

*Sara W. Nelson and Michael A. Gibbs*

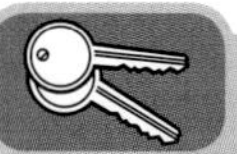

**KEY POINTS**

- Irrigation is the greatest ally in preventing wound infections.
- The final step in the management of almost all hand and wrist injuries is effective splinting.
- All but the most minor hand and wrist injuries merit scheduled follow-up.

## PERSPECTIVE

Effective use of the hand is such a fundamental human skill that none of us can imagine living without it. Injuries that threaten this vital function have an impact on patients of all ages and walks of life but tend to cluster in productive young adults who use their hands to make a living. It goes without saying that the stakes are high for both the patient and physician. Emergency physicians (EPs) must develop a sophisticated understanding of hand anatomy and function, as well as injury patterns and optimal management strategies.

## EPIDEMIOLOGY

Annually, more than 16 million people suffer some form of hand injury, and more than 4.8 million will seek treatment of these injuries at the emergency department (ED).[1] Traumatic injuries may include lacerations, fractures, and tendon or ligamentous injuries. Most injuries are readily identified in the ED, provided that the assessment is effective.[2] Because the morbidity associated with undiagnosed, misdiagnosed, or mistreated hand injuries is significant, a high level of expertise is required of the EP.

## PATHOPHYSIOLOGY

This chapter assumes that the reader is familiar with the basic structures of the hand. The back of the hand is referred to as the dorsal surface; the palm is called either the palmar or volar surface. The lateral borders of the hand are referred to as radial or ulnar. Movement may occur in any of these planes. Additionally, fingers may abduct away from or adduct toward an imaginary plane bisecting the third finger. The thumb has further planes of movement. In general, we refer to the digits by their numerical designations, but the common names are also acceptable—first (thumb), second (index finger), third (middle finger), fourth (ring finger), and fifth (little finger).

## PRESENTING SIGNS AND SYMPTOMS

When assessing hand injuries, the history should focus on the mechanism of the injury, hand position at the time of the insult, perceived resultant functional impairment, and the time elapsed since the injury. Some mechanisms yield classic injury patterns, such as the jersey finger and mallet finger. Other injury patterns are known for their poor outcomes, such as fight bites or high-pressure injection injuries, and require specific managements. Some wounds are more prone to infection, such as crush injuries and grossly contaminated wounds.

During the history the patient's hand dominance and career should also be ascertained and documented. Factors that may compromise wound healing, such as smoking, drug use, or an immunocompromised state, are important to document.[2] Tetanus status should be verified.

Despite its complicated nature, the hand can be examined adequately in a short period. Developing a rapid, reproducible hand examination strategy and performing it regularly will decrease the chance of missing subtle injuries. Even when a specific injury is obvious, it is important to examine the entire hand to avoid overlooking less obvious, coincident injuries. **Box 89.1** lists one approach to comprehensive assessment of the hand.

Assuming that no active bleeding is occurring and requires immediate attention, examination of the hand begins with inspection. All rings, watches, and other potentially constricting devices should be removed immediately.[3] Lacerations and other disruptions in skin integrity are usually recognized easily; erythema, soft tissue swelling, and ecchymoses should also be noted. It is important to compare the general position of the hand with that of the unaffected side inasmuch as many fractures or tendon disruptions will cause characteristic deformities that are recognizable on inspection.

Vascular integrity should be determined by comparing skin temperature with that of the opposite hand, feeling for ulnar and radial pulses, and documenting intact and symmetric distal capillary refill.

**BOX 89.1 Two-Minute Hand Examination**

**General**
General appearance
Obvious deformity

**Vascular**
Hemorrhage control
Ulnar and radial pulses
Capillary refill less than 2 seconds

**Neurologic**
Ulnar
- Sensation: light touch distal, volar fifth digit
- Motor: interosseous—abduction of the second digit

Median
- Sensation: light touch distal, volar second digit
- Motor: thenar eminence—adduction of the first digit toward the ceiling

Radial
- Sensation: light touch to the dorsal web space between the second and third digits
- Motor: wrist extension, otherwise sensation only in the hand

Digital
- Two-point discrimination—2 to 5 mm at the fingertip

**Musculoskeletal**
Bony palpation of all digits and joints
Active range of motion: make a fist; fully extend all digits
Passive range of motion: passively take all digits and joints through all ranges
Resistance: test all joints, all ranges with resistance to diagnose partial ligament injuries

**Ligamentous**
Flexor digitorum profundus tendon—hold the proximal interphalangeal joint in extension; flex the distal interphalangeal joint against resistance
Flexor digitorum sublimis tendon—hold the metacarpophalangeal joint in extension; flex the proximal interphalangeal joint against resistance
Extensor tendons—place the hand palm down; extend the digit with resistance at the nail bed
Ulnar collateral ligament—adduct the thumb against resistance

Neurologic testing should be performed before local or regional anesthesia. Radial, median, and ulnar nerve function should be individually assessed and the digital nerves interrogated via both light touch and two-point discrimination. Comparison with the unaffected side can be useful. To evaluate for radial neuropathy, the dorsal aspect of the second and third web space is tested for decreased sensation. Proximal limb radial nerve lesions will cause wristdrop. However, the superficial radial nerve, as it courses through the hand, is sensory only. To test for median neuropathy, the distal, palmar surface of the second digit is assessed for decreased sensation. Placing the hand dorsal side down and abducting the fifth digit toward the ceiling tests motor function. Resistance is applied to the thenar eminence, followed by palpation, to test for contraction of the abductor pollicis brevis muscle. To test for ulnar neuropathy, the distal, palmar surface of the fifth digit is assessed for decreased sensation. Challenging the interosseous muscles best tests ulnar motor function. One method is to ask the patient to place the injured hand on a surface with the fifth digit down and the thumb pointing at the ceiling. The patient then abducts the second finger (spreads the fingers) against resistance; weakness of the first interosseous muscle verifies contraction.

Musculoskeletal assessment is targeted at identifying injuries to bones, joints, and ligaments. Bone structures should be palpated thoroughly, as should all joints, to look for signs of pain, laxity, and limited range of motion. Every digit and joint should be put through complete active and passive range of motion. All extensor and flexor tendons should be tested individually. Specific tendon function is evaluated by ranging every joint individually. Extensor tendon function is tested by extending all interphalangeal and metacarpophalangeal (MCP) joints against resistance. Flexor digitorum profundus tendon injury limits flexion at the distal interphalangeal (DIP) joint; its presence is confirmed by holding the proximal interphalangeal (PIP) and MCP joints in extension and flexing the DIP joint against resistance. Flexor digitorum sublimis tendon injury limits flexion at the PIP joint. This injury is confirmed by holding the MCP joint in extension and flexing the PIP joint against resistance. False-negative results occur if all the other digits are not held in complete extension. The uninjured thumb will have complete active range of motion without pain and should be able to oppose the fifth digit. Full flexion to a fist and full extension should be normal.

## DIFFERENTIAL DIAGNOSIS AND MEDICAL DECISION MAKING

### FRACTURES OF THE HAND

#### *Metacarpal Bone Fractures*

Metacarpal bone fractures cannot be discussed simply as a single group because of the vast differences in inherent mobility and function among them. For each, the tolerance for unreduced angulation varies. The first metacarpal is very mobile and fractures are relatively uncommon. Management includes proper reduction, placement of a thumb spica splint, and follow-up with hand surgery. The second and third metacarpals are the fixed center of the hand, and proper reduction of fractures is important for full return of function. The fourth and fifth metacarpals are more mobile and have greater ability to compensate for angular deformities. Hand surgery consultation is necessary for all metacarpal fractures; for unstable reductions; for irreducible, open, or intraarticular fractures; and for any fracture with rotational malalignment.

Metacarpal base fractures are uncommon and usually of little significance.[2] The exception is at the base of the fifth metacarpal bone, where there can be associated subluxation of the metacarpal-hamate joint. The injured hand should be immobilized in an ulnar gutter splint and scheduled for referral to hand surgery.

#### *Bennett/Reverse Bennett and Rolando Fractures*

A Bennett fracture is a fracture of the proximal first metacarpal bone (**Fig. 89.1**). The classic mechanism is an axial load onto a flexed and adducted thumb. For example, a

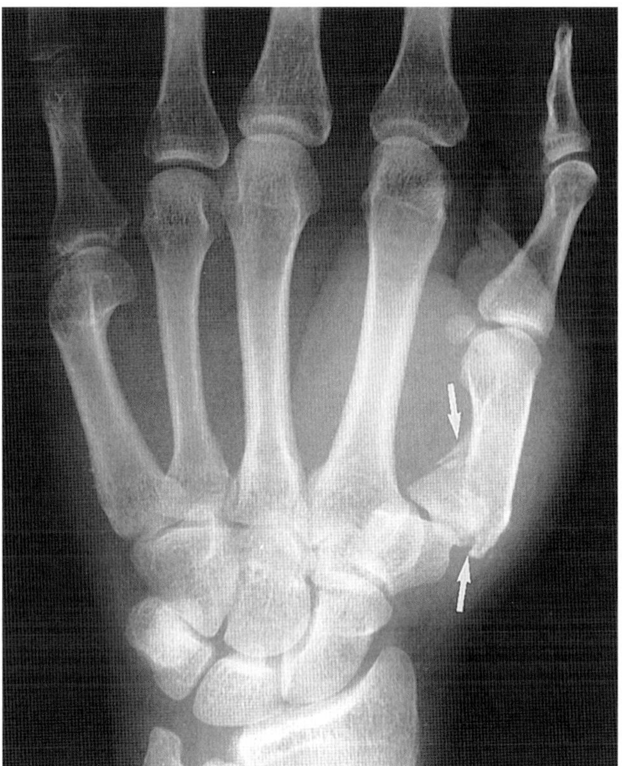

**Fig. 89.1 Bennett fracture *(arrows).*** (From Mettler Jr FA. Essentials of radiology. 2nd ed. Philadelphia: Saunders; 2004.)

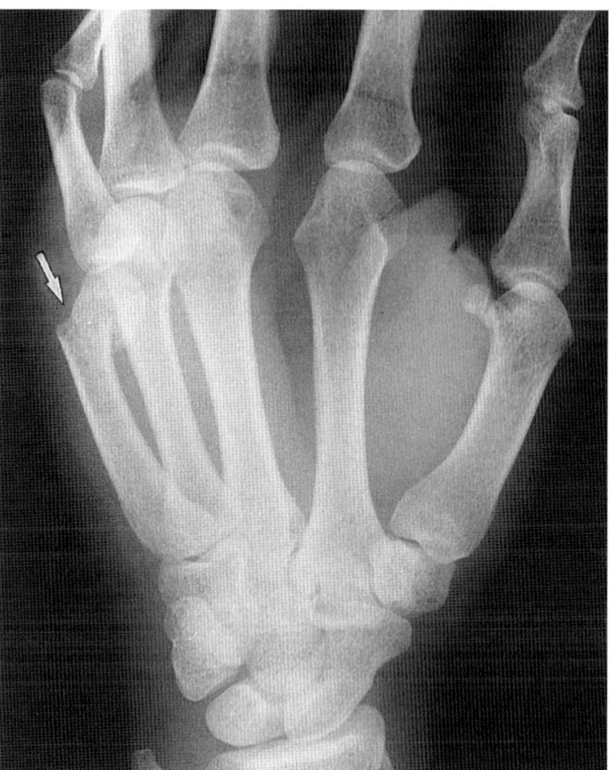

**Fig. 89.2 Boxer's fracture *(arrow).*** (From Mettler Jr FA. Essentials of radiology. 2nd ed. Philadelphia: Saunders; 2004.)

football quarterback strikes the helmet of an opposing player after releasing a throw. In this avulsion injury, the strong abductor pollicis longus muscle fractures the bone at the point of its insertion at the ulnar aspect of the first metacarpal bone. This causes displacement of a bony fragment, which can be seen on a plain film radiograph. It is usually an unstable fracture, and ED management should consist of referral to a hand surgeon and immobilization in a thumb spica splint. Potential long-term morbidity includes malunion, decreased function, and significant arthritis.

The same injury pattern and mechanism of injury can also occur in the fifth metacarpal bone and is called a reverse Bennett fracture, which is as unstable as a Bennett fracture because of the traction exerted by the extensor carpi ulnaris muscle on the distal aspect of the fifth metacarpal. Traction tends to pull the distal segment ulnarly. Closed reduction with ulnar gutter splinting may be attempted, but any articular incongruity must be recognized and referred on an emergency basis to a hand surgeon for potential immediate operative repair.

A Rolando fracture is similar to a Bennett fracture; however, it is comminuted and by definition extends into the joint space. ED management is identical to that for a Bennett fracture.

### Boxer's Fracture

Although many people refer to any fracture of the fifth metacarpal as a boxer's fracture, the specific injury is a fracture through the neck of the bone (**Fig. 89.2**). This injury is most frequently seen when a solid object is forcefully struck with a closed fist. True boxer's fractures may carry significant morbidity because in addition to being an unstable fracture, the injury often has a rotational component. If allowed to heal in this position, the hand will be deformed and weakened.

ED management consists of an attempt at closed reduction and placement of a dorsal-volar splint. Regardless of the type of splint used, at a minimum the fourth and fifth MCP joints should be splinted at 90 degrees of flexion. Because of the instability of this fracture, all patients should be referred to a hand surgeon and warned of the significant likelihood that the injury will require operative management.

### Proximal and Middle Phalanx Fractures

Proximal and middle phalanx fractures are managed similarly. The degree of instability depends on the nature of the fracture. Transverse and spiral fractures have greater instability than simple fractures do and are therefore more likely to require percutaneous fixation. It is important to keep in mind that rotational deformity cannot be tolerated. When the hand is held in a relaxed fist, the fingers should all point to the scaphoid region. Visible deviation from this plane suggests a rotational deformity of greater than 10%. All nondisplaced proximal and middle phalanx fractures should be splinted in the ED and referred for outpatient follow-up. Rotated, transverse, displaced, or intraarticular fractures should be reduced and splinted, and contemporaneous hand surgery consultation should be obtained.

### *Distal Phalanx Fractures*

The most common distal phalanx fracture is a tuft fracture, and nail bed injuries are the most common complication of this fracture.[2] There is some controversy regarding the need to repair nail bed injuries; however, most authors recommend performing trephination only for nail bed hematomas involving 30% to 50% or greater of the nail bed surface. When the nail bed is involved, tuft fractures are considered open fractures. Although some physicians prescribe antibiotics empirically, evidence suggests that prophylactic antibiotics are not indicated.[4] Proximal distal phalanx fractures are often unstable and require hand surgeon referral for percutaneous wire placement. An attempt to reduce any rotational deformity or angulation should be made before splinting. Splinting should isolate the DIP joint alone.

## LIGAMENTOUS INJURIES OF THE HAND

### *de Quervain Tenosynovitis*

de Quervain tenosynovitis is an overuse injury of the thumb. The classic example of the mechanism is a fly fisherman who repetitively collects the line after each cast by using the thumb and index finger to grasp the line, thereby resulting in inflammation of the abductor pollicis longus and extensor pollicis brevis tendons. The diagnosis is made clinically, and a positive Finkelstein test is said to be pathognomonic. The Finkelstein test is considered positive when pain is elicited with passive ulnar deviation of a closed fist.

It is important to note that patients with this condition may complain of pain on palpation of the anatomic snuffbox because the aforementioned tendons form the radial border of that structure. If the history is suggestive of a possible scaphoid injury, radiography should be performed and a thumb spica splint applied. Treatment of simple de Quervain tenosynovitis consists of rest, application of ice, and nonsteroidal antiinflammatory drugs (NSAIDs); more severe cases may require splinting to rest the injured joint.

### *Gamekeeper's/Skier's Thumb*

Gamekeeper's thumb is also called skier's thumb. The mechanism is hyperextension of an abducted thumb causing injury to the ulnar collateral ligament, and it is often associated with an avulsion fracture (**Fig. 89.3**). Historically, old-world gamekeepers sustained this injury while dispatching wounded birds during hunts. Today, this injury often occurs when a skier falls while grasping the ski pole.

Physical examination will be remarkable for tenderness at the ulnar collateral ligament, laxity at the MCP joint, and inability to actively oppose the thumb (**Fig. 89.4**). Most ulnar collateral ligament ruptures occur at the distal attachment. If the injured joint demonstrates 40 degrees of radial angulation during stressing, complete ligament rupture should be assumed. An associated avulsion fracture may be present. Treatment consists of immobilization in a thumb spica splint, NSAIDs, and referral to a hand surgeon for open reduction with internal fixation.

The initial examination may be compromised secondary to pain and spasm. In these cases, the most prudent course of action is immobilization in a thumb spica splint and referral for reevaluation.

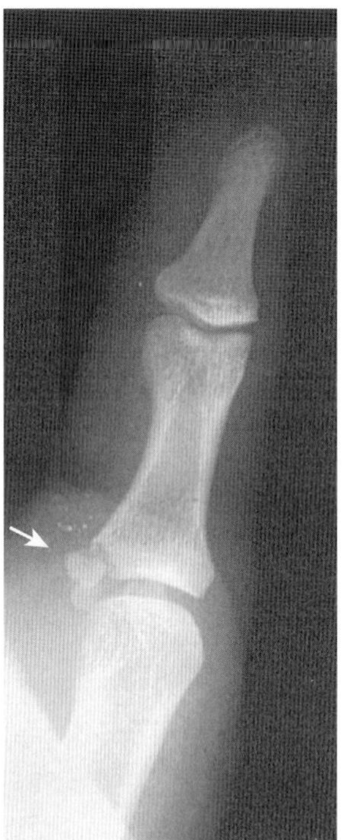

**Fig. 89.3 Gamekeeper's thumb *(arrow).*** (From Perron AD, Brady WJ. Evaluation and management of the high-risk orthopedic emergency. Emerg Med Clin North Am 2003;21:159-204.)

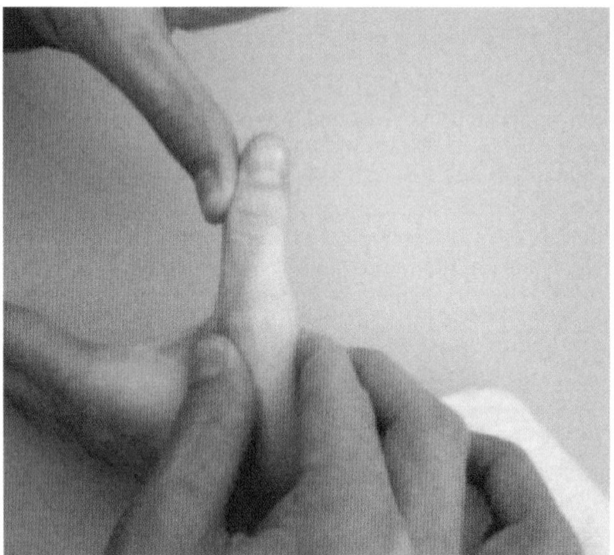

**Fig. 89.4 Testing for ulnar collateral ligament integrity.** (From Patel D, Dean C, Baker R. The hand in sports: update on clinical anatomy and physical examination. Prim Care 2005;32:71-89.)

### *Jersey Finger*

Jersey finger is an injury often associated with tackling sports (**Fig. 89.5**). The injury itself consists of disruption of the flexor digitorum profundus joint, which is responsible for flexion of the digit at the DIP joint. It occurs when a digit (often the second digit) is forced into extension while actively being flexed, as might occur when grabbing an opponent's jersey during a tackle.

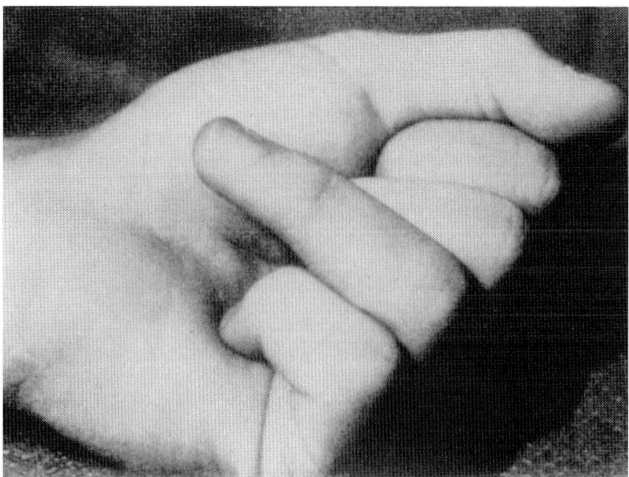

**Fig. 89.5 Jersey finger.** (From Perron AD, Brady WJ. Evaluation and management of the high-risk orthopedic emergency. Emerg Med Clin North Am 2003;21:159-204.)

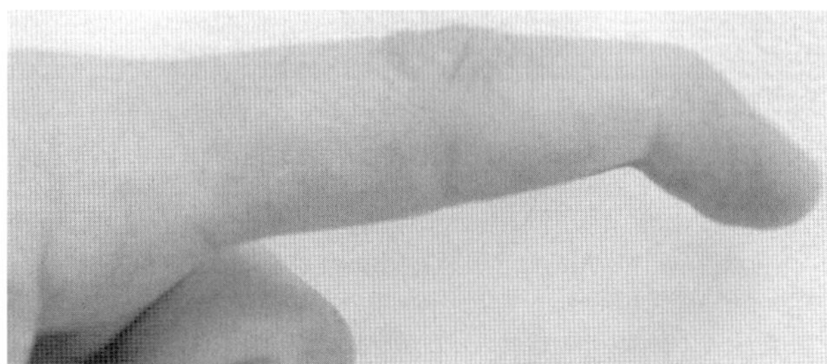

**Fig. 89.6 Mallet finger.** (From Perron AD, Brady WJ. Evaluation and management of the high-risk orthopedic emergency. Emerg Med Clin North Am 2003;21:159-204.)

On physical examination an injured patient will not be able to flex the digit at the DIP joint when the PIP joint is held (by the examiner) in extension. Examining the DIP joint without holding the PIP joint may result in a false-negative test result because of contribution from the lateral bands. The patient may complain of pain more proximally along the flexor tendon sheath or even in the palm because the ruptured flexor digitorum profundus tendon will retract. It is therefore imperative to challenge the distal joint despite only proximal pain. With full disruption the best outcomes depend on early surgical repair, and all patients should be scheduled for hand surgeon referral.

### Mallet Finger

Mallet finger is in many ways the functional opposite of jersey finger. In mallet finger the distal extensor tendon is ruptured (**Fig. 89.6**). It often occurs when the distal phalanx of a finger (or thumb) is forced into flexion while being actively extended. In sports the middle finger is most often affected because of its length, and it occurs when the finger is jammed, as when attempting to catch a ball.

Because this injury is often painless, it is not always manifested immediately. Physical examination is remarkable for the inability to extend the finger at the affected DIP joint. Radiographs may demonstrate an avulsion fracture. Treatment consists of immobilization by splinting the DIP in full extension, which allows full range of motion at the PIP joint. The patient should be referred to a hand surgeon for follow-up. Most mallet fingers are treated nonoperatively; however, those with large avulsion fracture fragments may require operative management.

### Digital Dislocations

Dislocation of the DIP joint is a rare injury, but when it does occur, it most commonly dislocates in the dorsal direction after direct force on the finger pad. Relocation is best accomplished after a digital block with traction longitudinally and pressure directing the proximal aspect of the distal phalanx back to correct alignment. After relocation, the entire digit is splinted in extension. Some injuries are nonreducible and require operative repair because the volar plate or profundus tendon (or both) may occupy the joint space. Any indication of joint involvement should prompt referral to a hand surgeon.

PIP joint dislocations result in more complications than do DIP joint dislocations. The complex biomechanics of the joint adds a degree of intricacy that often results in the need for operative repair. The volar plate may be injured with dorsal dislocations, and the lateral collateral ligaments may be injured with ulnar or radial dislocations. It is important to assess any relocated joint for stability to better rule out the potential for ligament or volar plate injury. Patients with an irreducible or unstable joint should be referred to a hand surgeon for operative repair. If stable, the joint should be splinted in 30 degrees of flexion for 2 to 4 weeks.

MCP joint dislocations are seen less commonly than PIP dislocations but have a similar rate of complications. Dislocations may be partial or complete and may involve the volar plate. Care should be taken during the examination to not convert a partial dislocation to a complete dislocation. Injury most commonly occurs as a hyperextension mechanism. With complete dislocations and volar plate involvement, relocation is often impossible because the volar plate may become entrapped in the joint space. For the best chance of relocation, the wrist should be placed in full flexion to relieve all flexor tendon tension and exert longitudinal and volar force. The MCP joint should be splinted in full flexion.

### Extensor Tendon Injuries

Open wounds on the dorsum of the hand and digits should trigger suspicion for extensor tendon injury. The Verdan extensor tendon injury classification system uses eight anatomic zones to direct treatment (**Table 89.1**).

Treatment of extensor tendon injuries should usually be coordinated with a hand surgeon. Data on suture repair of partial tendon lacerations are lacking, and current treatment is based on flexor tendon treatment. Conservative treatment of injuries involving less than 50% of a cross-sectional area has been proposed.

Injuries to zones I and II occur with axial loading onto a fully extended DIP joint, which forces the DIP joint into flexion and disrupts the distal aspect of the extensor tendon. This creates a mallet injury, as described previously.

Zone III injuries are caused either by axial loading and forced flexion of the PIP joint or by direct trauma to the PIP joint. These injuries should be splinted with the joint in extension, and the patient should be referred to a hand surgeon. With complete disruption of the central slip, the lateral bands slide toward the volar surface of the digit, which causes the extensor tendons to act as flexors. Untreated injuries lead to

**Table 89.1 Verdan Classification of Extensor Tendon Injuries with Appropriate Disposition**

| ZONE | ANATOMIC LOCATION | DISPOSITION |
|---|---|---|
| I | Distal phalanx to distal interphalangeal joint | Splint, hand surgeon referral |
| II | Middle phalanx | Splint, hand surgeon referral |
| III | Proximal interphalangeal joint | Splint, hand surgeon referral |
| IV | Proximal phalanx | ED primary repair, splint |
| V | Metacarpophalangeal joint | Splint, hand surgeon referral |
| VI | Dorsum of the hand/ metacarpals | ED primary repair, splint |
| VII | Dorsum of the wrist, carpals | Hand surgeon primary repair |
| VIII | Distal forearm, proximal wrist | Hand surgeon primary repair |

Data from Verdan CE. Primary and secondary repair of flexor and extensor tendon injuries. In: Flynn JE, editor. Hand surgery. 2nd ed. Baltimore: Williams & Wilkins; 1975.

*ED*, Emergency department.

**Table 89.2 Verdan Classification of Flexor Tendon Injuries with Appropriate Disposition**

| ZONE | ANATOMIC LOCATION | DISPOSITION |
|---|---|---|
| I | Distal to insertion of the flexor digitorum sublimis tendon | Hand surgeon primary repair |
| II | Area of the flexor sheath with both the flexor digitorum sublimis and flexor digitorum profundus tendons | Hand surgeon primary repair |
| III | Carpal tunnel to the proximal aspect of the flexor sheath | Hand surgeon primary repair |
| IV | Carpal tunnel | Hand surgeon primary repair |
| V | Forearm proximal to the carpal tunnel | Hand surgeon primary repair |

Data from Verdan CE. Primary and secondary repair of flexor and extensor tendon injuries. In: Flynn JE, editor. Hand surgery. 2nd ed. Baltimore: Williams & Wilkins; 1975.

a boutonnière deformity in which the PIP is flexed and the DIP is hyperextended.

Most zone IV injuries are caused by direct trauma. Open injuries may be treated primarily as in zone IV; by definition, no joint involvement is present. Closed injuries should be splinted with extension of the PIP joint. The extensor tendons of the phalanx are broad and flat, which allows easier primary repair.

"Fight bite" must be considered in all patients with zone V ligament injuries. Patients with open injuries should be referred to a hand surgeon for primary repair. Closed injuries can be treated by splinting the MCP joint in extension while allowing free range of motion of the PIP joint.

Zone VI injuries are usually superficial and easily repaired by the EP. Suture material should be strong, such as braided nylon, and the lacerated tendon completely apposed. After closure, the wrist should be splinted in 30 degrees of extension and the MCP joint in 15 degrees of flexion, and the PIP joint should be free. The patient should be referred to a specialist for dynamic splinting.

Zone VII and VIII injuries often involve the extensor retinaculum, and the patient should be scheduled for referral to a hand surgeon for primary closure. The affected tendon often retracts into the forearm, thus complicating the repair. Because of the density of associated anatomic structures, operative survey of the injury to identify additional injuries is indicated.

### *Flexor Tendon Injuries*

All patients with open flexor tendon injuries should be referred to a hand surgeon for emergency evaluation (**Table 89.2**). However, some knowledge of the nomenclature and prognoses associated with flexor tendon injuries will aid the EP in conversations with both the consultant and the patient.

Repair of complete lacerations within 24 hours is most commonly recommended. Operative repair is usually limited to injuries involving greater than 50% of a cross-sectional area. Injuries involving less than 50% are frequently treated conservatively with splinting. Newer data suggest that conservative management is adequate for injuries occupying less than 75% of a cross-sectional area; however, this decision should be deferred to the consulting hand surgeon.[1] When splinting flexor tendon injuries, the wrist should be placed in 30 degrees of flexion, MCP joint injuries in 70 degrees of flexion, and DIP or PIP joint injuries in 10 degrees of flexion. Classification of flexor tendon injuries is based on anatomic location, treatment, and prognosis. All patients with flexor tendon injuries should be referred to a hand surgeon for operative exploration and repair.

## FRACTURES OF THE WRIST

Carpal bone fractures can result in significant long-term morbidity and are easily missed during the physical examination. The two most common carpal fractures are fractures of the scaphoid and triquetrum. Scapholunate, perilunate, and lunate dislocations are the most common dislocations.

### *Scaphoid Fractures*

The scaphoid is the most commonly injured carpal bone. A high index of suspicion is needed when considering this injury because plain film findings are often subtle or even absent (a dedicated scaphoid view will increase plain film sensitivity). The mechanism of injury is most often a fall onto an outstretched hand.

Morbidity is high with this injury because the bone is anatomically predisposed to avascular necrosis and nonunion. The blood supply to the scaphoid originates from the radial and palmar arteries and flows from distal to proximal. The

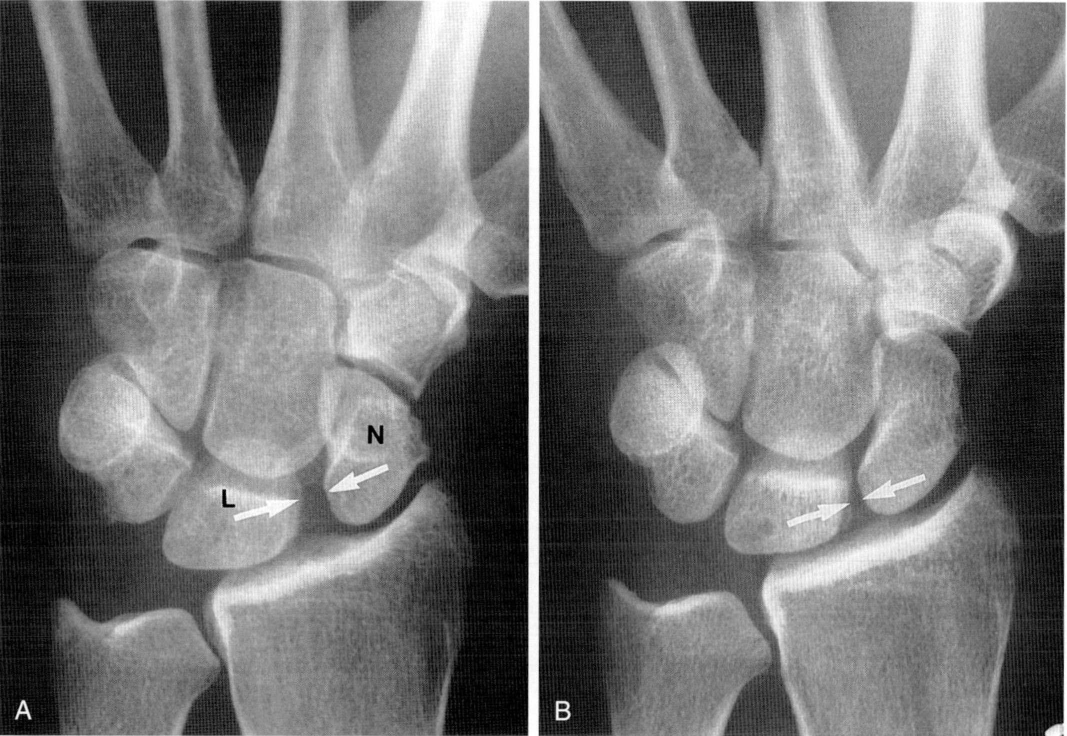


**Fig. 89.7 Scapholunate dislocation. A,** Terry-Thomas sign *(arrows).* **B,** Normal wrist. *L,* Lunate; *N,* navicular. (From Mettler Jr FA. Essentials of radiology. 2nd ed. Philadelphia: Saunders; 2004.)

most proximal aspect of the scaphoid receives blood only from this distal to proximal flow, and if this flow is interrupted by a fracture, the risk for avascular necrosis and nonunion is high. For this reason all patients with a traumatic mechanism and scaphoid tenderness, as assessed by palpation of the anatomic snuffbox or pain with axial loading of the thumb, should be treated with a thumb spica splint and referred for follow-up. Roughly 15% of these patients will have a scaphoid fracture despite unrevealing plain films.[5]

### Triquetrum Fractures

Triquetrum fractures are less common than scaphoid fractures but frequently have a similar mechanism of hyperextension. Most often the fracture is secondary to avulsion with an avulsion fragment noted at the dorsal aspect of the triquetrum. This is best seen on a lateral plain film projection. The prognosis is better than with scaphoid fractures because avascular necrosis is not a common occurrence with these injuries.

Occasionally, triquetrum body fractures can be seen; in this case the EP should look for associated lunate or perilunate dislocations. The wrist should be splinted and the patient referred to a hand surgeon for follow-up.

## DISLOCATIONS OF THE WRIST

Scapholunate, perilunate, and lunate dislocations are varying degrees of the same disease process. The mechanism is one of hyperextension. In cadaver work it was shown that progressive force applied to the wrist in a hyperextension mechanism will reliably re-create these injuries in a persistent pattern.[6] The reason is anatomically based and the result of progressive ligament injuries.

### Scapholunate Dislocation

Scapholunate dislocation is the most common of these injuries and occurs with the least amount of force. It can be diagnosed on plain film radiography. Scapholunate dislocation results in a classic radiologic finding—the Terry-Thomas sign (**Fig 89.7**). Terry-Thomas was a 20th-century British comedian who possessed a noticeable gap between his two front teeth, reminiscent of the wide space (2 mm when measured on an anteroposterior view) seen between the scaphoid and lunate bones when they are dislocated.[3] Stress views accentuate this finding. Additionally, the scaphoid may twist on its axis and cause a ringlike shadow known as the signet ring sign. This artifact is caused by the x-rays traveling longitudinally down the twisted scaphoid, unlike the normal crosswise orientation. Mayfield et al. classified this injury as a stage I injury.[6]

### Perilunate Dislocation

Stage II injury is associated with progressively more force (e.g., an automobile accident versus a slip and fall) and results in perilunate dislocation (**Fig. 89.8**). Perilunate dislocations may be a difficult concept because there is no "perilunate" bone. Perilunate dislocation is a disruption of the ligamentous structures around ("peri") the lunate bone. One of these structures is the capitate, which most often dislocates dorsally. Perilunate dislocation may perhaps better be called capitate dislocation; however, perilunate dislocation is actually a more accurate description of the stepwise disease process as outlined by Mayfield et al.[6] Dislocation of the capitate can be associated with a scaphoid fracture. The EP should be diligent in assessing for one in the setting of the other. Perilunate dislocation is frequently overlooked despite the classic plain

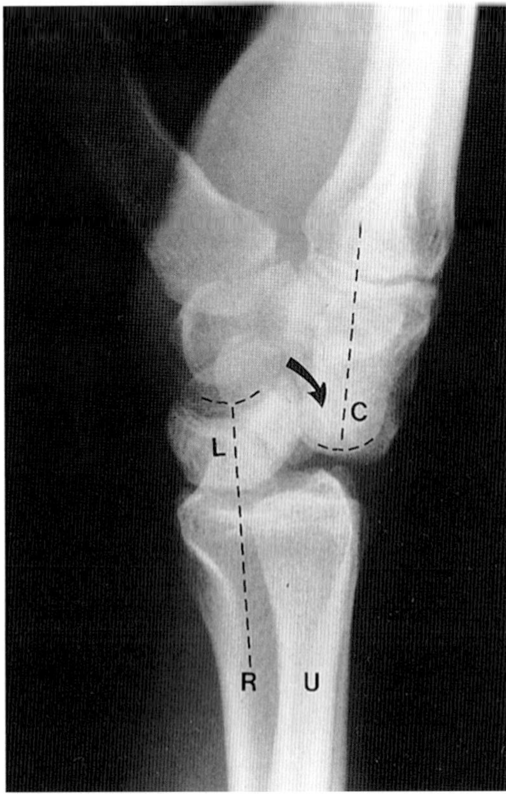


**Fig. 89.8 Perilunate dislocation.** *C*, Capitate; *L*, lunate; *R*, radius; *U*, ulna. (From Mettler Jr FA. Essentials of radiology. 2nd ed. Philadelphia: Saunders; 2004.)

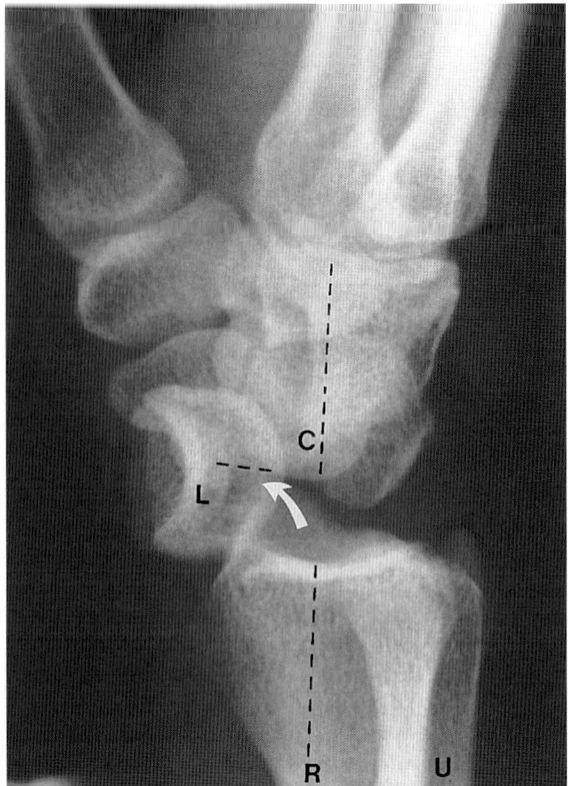


**Fig. 89.9 Lunate dislocation: spilled teacup sign.** *C*, Capitate; *L*, lunate; *R*, radius; *U*, ulna. (From Mettler Jr FA. Essentials of radiology. 2nd ed. Philadelphia: Saunders; 2004.)

film finding of the capitate and the remainder of the distal part of the hand lying dorsal to the lunate on the lateral projection.

### *Triquetrum Dislocation*

Stage III injury involves dislocation of the triquetrum but is difficult to differentiate radiographically from stage II perilunate dislocation.

### *Lunate Dislocation*

Stage IV injury is defined by the presence of a lunate dislocation. It is a complete disruption of the ligamentous structures of the wrist. In stage I the scaphoid dislocates from the lunate, in stages II and III the capitate and triquetrum dislocate from the lunate, and in stage IV the lunate dislocates from its articulation with the distal end of the radius. The dislocated capitate, which lies dorsal to the lunate, will often collapse onto the distal end of the radius as a result of muscular spasm because the lunate is no longer present to prevent such spasm.

The result is a distal radius and capitate pseudoarticulation, with the lunate lying palmar to the "new" wrist articulation. This is best viewed on a lateral plain film projection and causes the "spilled teacup" sign (**Fig. 89.9**). When teaching this concept, the author has asked students to imagine a watermelon seed being squeezed between two fingers and then popping forward with force. This is essentially what happens to the lunate as it is "squeezed" by the radius and distal wrist structures, including the capitate, in an extreme hyperextension mechanism. Lunate dislocation often compresses the carpal tunnel and can cause median neuropathy.

Plain film radiography is in general adequate to diagnose carpal bone dislocations, although computed tomography can be helpful in ambiguous cases. The EP may attempt closed reduction; however, many of these injuries are unstable. All injuries should be splinted in a long arm splint and patients should be referred to a hand surgeon. Many of these injuries will require internal fixation.

## BITES TO THE HAND

Because of the potential for injury and morbidity, all open injuries of the MCP joint should be treated as closed-fist bite wounds, or "fight bites," until proved otherwise. These often minor-appearing injuries are by definition caused by a clenched fist versus human teeth and are well known for poor outcomes. Potential complications include violation of the joint capsule, extensor tendon injury, and contamination of the deep fascial space.[7] The potential for infection is great because of the poor vascular supply of the extensor tendon and joint capsule. Treatment of these injuries is threefold: surgical decontamination, antibiotics, and dynamic splinting.[8] These injuries are not limited to fist fights and also commonly occur during sporting events.

Delayed manifestations most commonly occur 2 to 3 days after the inciting event and consist of signs and symptoms of local or significantly advanced infection. Any indication of infection or joint space or tendon sheath involvement should prompt referral to a hand surgeon for irrigation and débridement. The timing of initiation of intravenous antibiotics should be determined in consultation with the hand surgeon, who may wish to delay antibiotic treatment until after tissue for culture has been obtained intraoperatively. Antimicrobial therapy should cover common pathogens found in the human oral and skin flora, including aerobic and anaerobic pathogens. *Staphylococcus aureus* is the most common pathogen, followed by *Streptococcus* species, *Corynebacterium* species, and *Eikenella corrodens*.[9]

If the signs and symptoms are acute with no indication of fracture, joint space involvement, or extensor tendon injury, antibiotic therapy and local wound care are sufficient. In this nonoperative patient group, wounds should be treated with high-volume irrigation, and they should be left open to heal by secondary intention. The injured hand should be splinted in the position of function, and the patient should be instructed to elevate the affected limb and to return if any evidence of infection is seen.

Prophylactic antibiotics for clenched-fist bite wounds should be initiated for all but the most superficial injuries. Recommended regimens include amoxicillin–clavulanic acid, a combination of penicillin and dicloxacillin, and a combination of penicillin and a first-generation cephalosporin.[9]

### HIGH-PRESSURE INJECTION INJURIES

High-pressure injection injuries occur when substances such as paint, oil, grease, solvents, and water are sprayed under high pressure. These substances can penetrate deeply into the soft tissues of the hand and cause inflammation, infection, fibrosis, and severe disability. In one series the rate of amputation approximated 50%, and when patients are initially seen more than 6 hours after the injury, amputations are the rule rather than the exception.[10,11] Even a small puncture wound with a history of high-pressure injection should be considered a high-priority emergency.

Historical information, including time since the injury, the material injected, the amount injected, the temperature of the material, and the velocity and pressure of the injection may be helpful in determining the prognosis. For example, the amputation rate is considerably lower with grease injection than with injection of paint or solvent-based material. Thinner and less viscous material is more apt to lead to amputation because of easier spread and a subsequently larger extent of injury.

Plain film radiographs should be obtained to look for subcutaneous air and radiopaque material. The hand should be elevated and maintained in a position of comfort. Parenteral analgesics are often required. Infiltration of anesthetics directly into the area of injury may worsen local inflammation and is therefore contraindicated. All these injuries require immediate consultation with a hand surgeon. Even though several authors recommend prophylactic antibiotics and some suggest systemic corticosteroids to decrease inflammation, few data support either recommendation.

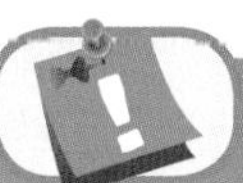

**TIPS AND TRICKS**

Regional anesthesia of the median, radial, and ulnar nerves can easily be mastered. These techniques improve the patient's comfort and the physician's ability to assess and manage injury.

Use plain radiography to assess for air or radiopaque material in patients suffering high-pressure injection injuries.

## TREATMENT

Although individual hand and wrist injuries require specific treatment, several generalizable steps should be taken to optimize management in the ED.

### ANESTHESIA AND ANALGESIA

The hand is densely innervated to increase tactile discrimination and complex function. Accordingly, hand injuries can be very painful. The decision to manage an injury by infiltration of a local anesthetic, a regional anesthetic technique, oral or parenteral analgesics, or a combination of these approaches will vary. It is worth noting that the hand is highly amenable to regional anesthetic techniques that can be mastered quickly by EPs with a bit of practice. Local and regional anesthesia is discussed in Chapter 10. A number of instructional websites also provide detailed information on these techniques, including a site developed at our institution (see www.mmc.org/em_body.cfm?id=3235).

### TREATMENT OF OPEN WOUNDS

Unless a plan for intraoperative washout is in place, all open hand and wrist injuries should undergo meticulous irrigation. When performing irrigation, a 60-mL syringe and an 18-gauge angiocatheter or splashguard device will generate the proper irrigation pressure. No study has shown any benefit of wound soaking or the use of antiseptic solution during irrigation. Tap water irrigation has proved to be as safe as irrigation with sterile solutions.[6] As a rule, patients with all but the most minor hand injuries should receive prophylactic antibiotics.

### SPLINTING

For almost every hand and wrist injury, the most important last step is effective splinting. Splinting decreases pain, speeds healing, and reduces the likelihood of fracture displacement.

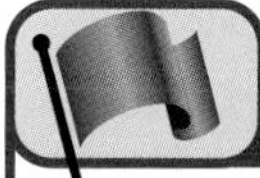

**RED FLAGS**

**Cautions for Physicians**

Do not cut corners during physical examination of the hand. This will invariably lead to misdiagnosis, mistreatment, and loss of function.

All lacerations involving the extensor surface of the hand are "fight bites" until proved otherwise. Never accept the history at face value when the injury pattern is suspicious.

In patients with a history of high-pressure injection injuries, do not be fooled by a seemingly innocuous skin puncture wound.

Failure to immobilize, failure to consult, and failure to arrange timely follow-up are common avoidable pitfalls in the management of hand and wrist injuries.

Digital injuries can usually be managed with a simple aluminum finger splint. When the injuries are unstable, more complete immobilization of the hand and wrist is recommended. Splinting of the hand should preserve the "position of function"—that is, extension at the wrist, flexion at the MCP joint, and nearly complete extension of the PIP and DIP joints. The objective is to maintain an appropriate amount of tension on ligaments that may shorten over time if relaxed. The position of function can be achieved by asking the patient to hold the hand as though holding a tennis ball and facing it forward.

## FOLLOW-UP, NEXT STEPS IN CARE, AND PATIENT EDUCATION

The vast majority of hand injuries are amenable to outpatient follow-up. Care pathways should be established between the ED and hand surgeons to ensure that patients are not lost to follow-up when follow-up is vital. A relatively small subset of acute hand injuries will require immediate operative repair (e.g., vascular injuries with compromised perfusion, major crush injuries, amputations) or washout in the operating room (e.g., open fractures and joint injuries, grossly contaminated soft tissue injuries, high-pressure injection injuries, bite wounds at high risk for infection). When in doubt, the EP should not hesitate to obtain phone consultation or call a colleague to the bedside.

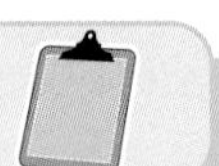

### DOCUMENTATION

Hand dominance, the profession of the patient, and the timing and mechanism of injury are essential elements of the history in patients with hand and wrist injuries.

"Neurovascular intact" is not enough for a hand injury! Documentation should carefully reflect assessment of the pulses and capillary refill. Motor and sensory function of the median, radial, and ulnar nerves should be individually tested and documented.

Because follow-up is such a crucial element in the management of hand and wrist injuries, documentation of phone consultation and agreed-on decisions for definitive management should be explicitly documented.

## SUGGESTED READINGS

Amadio P. What's new in hand surgery. J Bone Joint Surg Am 2005;87:468-73.
Harrison B, Holland P. Diagnosis and management of hand injuries in the emergency department. Emerg Med Pract 2005;7:1-28.
Hogan CJ, Ruland RT. High-pressure injection injuries of the upper extremity: a review of the literature. J Orthop Trauma 2006;20:503-11.
Perron AD, Miller MD, Brady WJ. Orthopedic pitfalls in the ED: fight bite. Am J Emerg Med 2002;20:114-7.
Southall JC, Sanders SP. Adult hand trauma. Trauma Rep 2006;7(5):1-12.

## REFERENCES

*References can be found on Expert Consult @ www.expertconsult.com.*

# Arterial and Venous Trauma and Great Vessel Injuries 90

*Stephen J. Wolf and Margaret M. DiGeronimo*

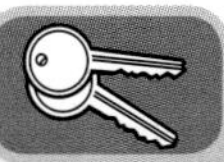

**KEY POINTS**

- Thirty percent of patients with great vessel injury (GVI) die within 6 hours of hospital arrival.
- Thirty percent to 50% of patients with blunt aortic injury have no signs of trauma.
- A normal chest radiograph does not exclude GVI.
- Computed tomographic angiography is the diagnostic test of choice to rule out traumatic aortic injury in hemodynamically stable patients.
- For patients too large for a computed tomography scanner, transesophageal echocardiographic evaluation of the aorta should be considered.
- Medical management of GVI is typically used as a bridge to more definitive operative care.
- β-Adrenergic blockade is instituted before nitroprusside in the medical management of GVI to avoid possible reflex tachycardia.

## EPIDEMIOLOGY

Few traumatic injuries are more devastating than great vessel injury (GVI). With an average circulating volume of 5 L and a flow rate of up to 4.8 L/min in the circulatory system, it is easy to see why GVI can result in catastrophic outcomes quickly. The true incidence of traumatic aortic injury may never be known; however, according to the National Trauma Data Bank, blunt thoracic aortic injury occurred in 0.3% of trauma patients admitted to the hospital during a 5-year period.[1] When patients survive an initial injury to their great vessels, rapid diagnosis and treatment are imperative to prevent subsequent exsanguination within the next minutes to hours. This highlights the ever-emphasized "golden hour" of trauma resuscitation.

Several contributing factors are important when evaluating potential GVI (**Fig. 90.1**). Although the mechanism and specific vessel injured are the most important of these factors, significant attention must be paid to the role of concomitant injuries and comorbid conditions on patients' morbidity and mortality. Unfortunately, on initial evaluation the emergency physician is often lucky to be privy to one, let alone all, of these factors.

The most important branch point for both the likelihood and the type of GVI is a penetrating versus blunt mechanism. Penetrating mechanisms are associated with greater than 90% of great vessel trauma, and any thoracic vascular structure is at risk.[2] Patients who survive to arrive at the emergency department, particularly if they are not in hemorrhagic shock, have a survival rate that approaches 50%.[3]

In contrast, blunt traumatic injuries to the great vessels most often affect the aorta, although the innominate artery, pulmonary hilar vessels, and vena cava are also susceptible. Blunt aortic rupture carries an immediate mortality rate of greater than 80% and is responsible for 10% to 15% of motor vehicle accident fatalities.[4] Because of the high association of blunt ascending aortic injury with fatal cardiac injury, the vast majority of those who survive to hospital evaluation have descending injuries. Of patients who survive until medical evaluation, 30% die within 6 hours and 40% within 24 hours.[4] Because most of these injuries occur in young healthy males, the overall survival rate is much better than expected given the severity of injury.

Though incompletely understood, it is proposed that blunt aortic injury can result from any combination of shearing forces, rotational forces, increased intraluminal aortic pressure, or a pinching mechanism between the sternum and vertebral column. Given these forces, it is not a surprise that motor vehicle collisions cause the majority of blunt aortic injuries. This association increases with the speed of the accident.[5,6] Shearing forces were originally thought to be the highest in frontal-impact accidents, where deceleration forces are the greatest. More recent studies, however, have shown that side-impact accidents are associated with a higher risk for blunt aortic injury. A review of 119 cases of known blunt aortic injury as a result of car accidents in the United Kingdom found that lateral impact direction to the same side was highly associated with aortic injury.[7] A review of accident data from the United Kingdom and United States in 2004 mirrored these results and found that side impact involving the patient's side of the vehicle carried a significantly higher risk for aortic injury than did frontal impact.[8] Although motor vehicle accidents account for the majority of blunt GVI, falls from a height and crushing forces have also been known to cause the disease process.[5]

In part because of difficulty isolating the hilum, injuries to the pulmonary arteries, veins, and thoracic vena cava are associated with mortality rates greater than 60%, regardless of whether they are caused by blunt or penetrating force, although the latter is much more common.[9]

Concomitant injuries clearly play a role in the epidemiology, morbidity, and mortality of GVI. One study on blunt thoracic trauma showed that patient with traumatic aortic injury carried a mean injury severity score (ISS) of 40

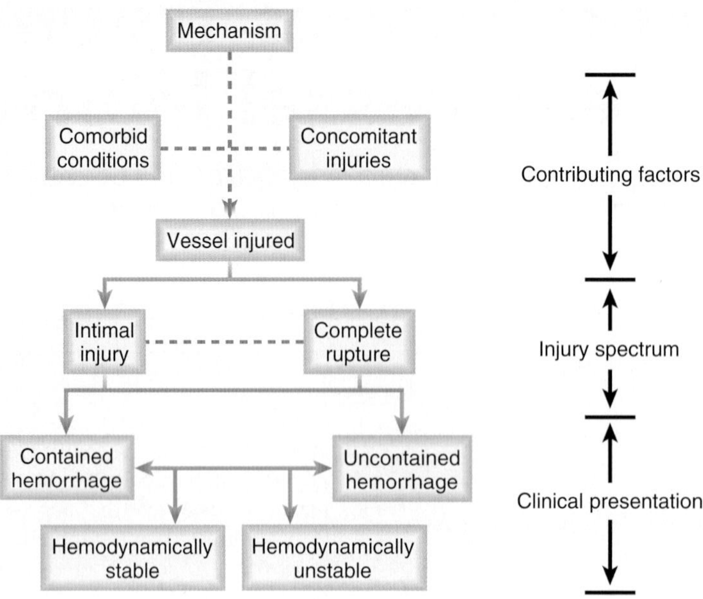


**Fig. 90.1 Great vessel injury paradigm of disease, including associated contributing factors, injury spectrum, and variable clinical findings.**

whereas patients without vascular injury had a mean ISS of just 16.[5] Another showed that closed head injury was diagnosed in more than half of patients with GVI, with one quarter having intracranial hemorrhage.[3]

Comorbid conditions such as underlying vascular disease, cardiopulmonary disease, and renal insufficiency contribute to the morbidity and mortality associated with GVI. Many disease processes affect a patient's ability to tolerate the initial and delayed physiologic insults accompanying severe GVI.

## PATHOPHYSIOLOGY

Knowledge of the vascular anatomy of the great vessels and the particular branch points of the more distal vasculature is important in identifying and potentially preventing morbidity and mortality in the setting of injury. This anatomy can be broken down into arterial, venous, and pulmonary components.

### ARTERIAL SYSTEM

The systemic arterial great vessels include the ascending aorta, arch, and descending thoracic aorta. The innominate artery is the first branch of the aortic arch and gives rise to the right subclavian and common carotid arteries. The left carotid and then the left subclavian artery are the next two branches. These structures course in close approximation to the clavicle, the first and second ribs, and the brachial plexus. Just distal to the left subclavian takeoff, the descending aorta becomes a more fixed structure in comparison with the arch. The ligamentum arteriosum, a remnant of the ductus arteriosus, and the intercostal arteries tether it to other thoracic structures. This junction, often called the isthmus region, proves to be the most susceptible site for blunt aortic injury as the arch moves in relation to the relatively fixed descending aorta. The spinal arteries branching off the descending aorta are of particular importance because they supply the spinal column. Compromised flow to these small branches as a result of direct injury or vascular clamping plays a significant role in patients' risk for paraplegia.

The microanatomy of the artery wall, with its intimal, medial, and adventitial layers, is integral in the spectrum of disease. Injuries range from isolated thrombogenic intimal flaps to full-thickness tears with free hemorrhage (**Fig. 90.2**).

### VENOUS SYSTEM

The venous components of the great vessel system include the confluence of the subclavian and internal jugular veins, which ultimately combine to form the superior vena cava. The inferior vena cava receives blood from the portal system through the hepatic vein in the retrohepatic region. As a whole, this system is characterized by low pressure and resistance and high flow and compliance, unless tamponade or heart failure is present, which results in increased right-sided pressure. These factors make control of hemorrhage difficult.

### PULMONARY CIRCULATION

The final component of the great vessel system is the pulmonary circulation. As mentioned earlier, the structures of this system reside in the hilum and are deep in the thorax, thus making them difficult to access. The pulmonary arteries and veins possess mediastinal and intrathoracic portions, which can result in different clinical findings, including mediastinal hematoma or hemothorax.

## PRESENTING SIGNS AND SYMPTOMS
(Box 90.1)

Traditionally, aortic dissection as a result of nontraumatic causes is believed to be manifested as tearing pain radiating

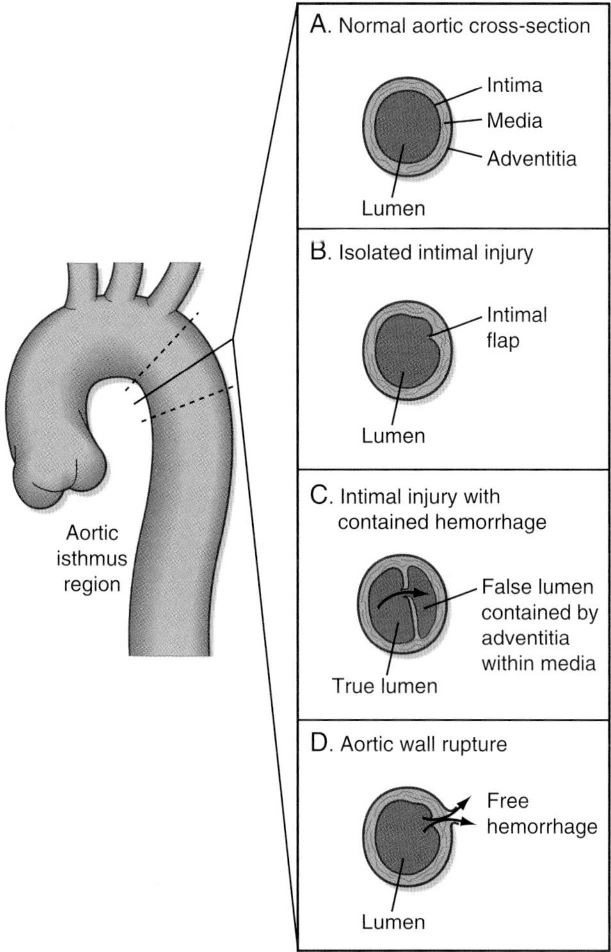


**Fig. 90.2 Continuum of aortic vessel injury. A,** Normal aortic cross section. **B,** Isolated intimal injury. **C,** Intimal injury with contained hemorrhage. **D,** Complete aortic wall rupture.

through the chest to the interscapular region of the back. This pain can be accompanied by various degrees of associated symptoms, including shortness of breath or vagal complaints. In patients with traumatic injury, this symptom pattern is seen less than 25% of the time; these patients most frequently either have vague chest-related complaints or no complaints at all because of distracting injuries. A remarkable 30% to 50% of patients with a blunt aortic injury may have no external signs of trauma.[10]

The signs and symptoms of GVI often result from its effect on blood flow, which can be secondary to direct vessel injury, traumatic thrombus formation, or vascular compression from surrounding hematoma. Of great concern are clinical signs of hemorrhagic shock such as hypotension, tachycardia, altered mental status, pallor, or diaphoresis. Frequently, hypertension occurs as a result of increased stimulation of sympathetic nerve fibers in close proximity to the aortic arch.[11] Additionally, many of the other signs can be subtle. Dyspnea may result for any number of reasons, such as associated pulmonary injury, hemothorax, hypovolemia with poor tissue oxygenation, or tamponade. Neurologic symptoms can be found in patients with arterial injury involving the carotids or spinal arteries.

Extremity findings of altered transmission or diminished intensity of the pulse pressure wave suggest intravascular

**BOX 90.1 Signs and Symptoms of Great Vessel Injury**

**Signs**
Hemorrhagic shock
- Hypotension
- Tachycardia
- Altered mental status
- Pallor
- Diaphoresis

Hypertension
Dyspnea
Asymmetric pulse pressure
Vascular bruits
Focal neurologic findings

**Symptoms**
Tearing pain
Pain radiating to the back
Difficulty breathing
Vagal complaints
Vague chest-related complaints
Asymptomatic
Neurologic complaints

volume depletion or, if asymmetric, direct vascular injury. Femoral pulses are important to note, particularly with respect to upper extremity pulses, because change can indicate vascular injury in the descending aorta resulting in a pseudocoarctation syndrome. Vascular bruits, which result from turbulent blood flow in the arterial system, either over the precordium or in the interscapular region, are heard in up to 30% of patients with aortic injury.

Unfortunately, none of the aforementioned signs and symptoms are sensitive or specific for making the diagnosis of GVI.[10]

## DIFFERENTIAL DIAGNOSIS AND MEDICAL DECISION MAKING

GVI should be considered in the differential diagnosis of all patients with thoracoabdominal trauma and an appropriate mechanism of injury. Care must be taken to not exclude the diagnosis solely on the basis of identification of other injuries that might also be contributing to the patient's clinical findings.

GVI is easily misdiagnosed in hemodynamically stable patients, particularly those without external signs of trauma, because of the nonspecific nature of the initial signs and symptoms of GVI. Penetrating injury in proximity to any of the great vessels mandates consideration of GVI. However, a diagnosis of blunt injury requires assessment of the severity of the causative mechanism (e.g., speed, forces), in combination with the patient's complaints and findings on physical examination. This pretest probability will ultimately be used by the clinician to guide further diagnostic evaluation for GVI (**Box 90.2**).

GVI is often associated with either significant multisystem trauma or distinct penetrating injury. In the first situation, the signs and symptoms of GVI are frequently obscured by other distracting injuries, altered mental status, or intubation, thereby necessitating a high level of suspicion and a low threshold for diagnostic testing. In the second situation, diagnostic testing is driven mainly by the pretest probability of GVI (i.e., the location and mechanism of the injury). **Figure 90.3** depicts a diagnostic management algorithm for suspected traumatic aortic injury.

**BOX 90.2 Pros and Cons of Imaging Modalities for Great Vessel Injury**

**Chest Radiography**

Pros

- Inexpensive
- Performed at the bedside
- Easy to interpret

Cons

- Nonspecific
- False-negative rate of 7% to 10% for traumatic aortic injury

**Computed Tomographic Angiography**

Pros

- Identifies mediastinal hematoma and differentiates its causes
- Identifies aortic injury, including intimal tears
- Sensitivity and specificity approaching 100% for traumatic aortic injury

Cons

- Poor delineation of nonaortic vascular injuries
- Requires relative hemodynamic stability to obtain

**Aortography**

Pros

- Traditional "gold standard"
- Beneficial in the diagnosis of branch vessel injuries
- Delineates equivocal computed tomographic angiographic findings

Cons

- Difficult to obtain on an emergency basis
- Requires relative hemodynamic stability

**Transesophageal Echocardiography**

Pros

- May be performed at the bedside
- Not limited by body habitus

Cons

- Poor availability on an emergency basis
- Contraindicated in patients with an unstable cervical spine or suspected esophageal trauma

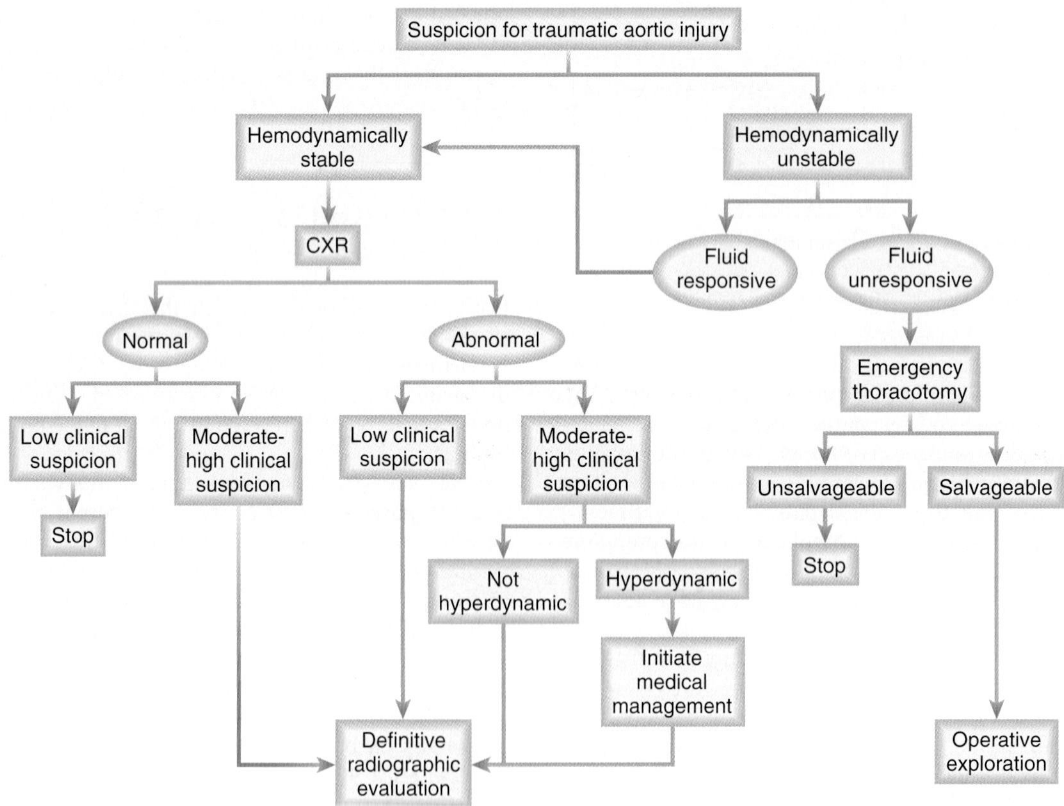


**Fig. 90.3 Diagnostic management algorithm for suspected traumatic aortic injury.** *CXR*, Chest radiograph.

The chest radiograph is the initial diagnostic screening tool in patients with history of chest trauma. An upright, posteroanterior view provides the best evaluation of the mediastinum. In patients with concern for spinal injury, a portable supine, anteroposterior view is commonly performed. Note that in the recumbent position the mediastinum may appear artificially widened and hemothorax can be obscured.

Chest radiography is not diagnostic of GVI; rather, it is used to identify any of the multiple findings suggestive of aortic injury. **Box 90.3** reviews the classic findings on chest

**BOX 90.3 Radiographic Findings Associated with Great Vessel Injury**

Superior mediastinal widening
Indistinct aortic knob
Left pleural effusion or hemothorax
Left apical cap
Deviation of the trachea
Deviation of the nasogastric tube to the right
Depressed left mainstem bronchus
Narrowing of the carinal angle
Opacification of the aortopulmonary window
Widening of the left or right paraspinous stripe
Sternal or rib fractures

Data from references 3, 5, and 12.

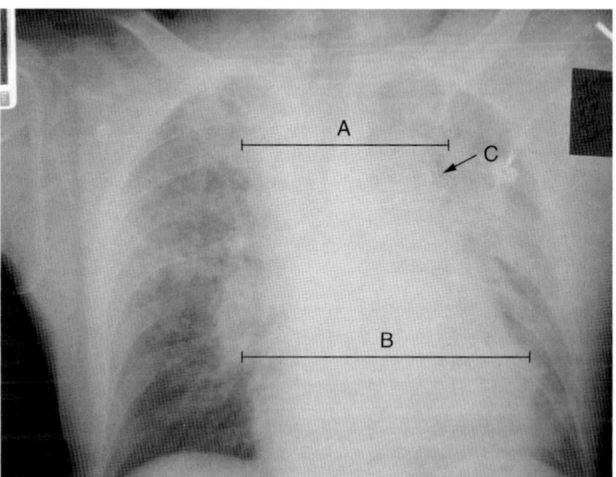


**Fig. 90.4 Chest radiograph demonstrating the three most common findings of traumatic aortic injury: widened superior mediastinum *(A)*, increased mediastinal width *(B)*, and obscured aortic knob *(C)*.**

radiography associated with GVI; a widened superior mediastinum (50% to 92%), increased mediastinal width (67% to 85%), and indistinct aortic knob (21% to 24%) occur with the greatest frequencies.[3,12] **Figure 90.4** is a chest radiograph demonstrating these three findings.

No individual radiographic finding is sensitive enough to rule out GVI. A normal radiograph is found in 7% to 10% of injured patients; such a finding should not dissuade one from further testing if the patient's initial complaint, physical examination, or mechanism of injury generates a significant pretest probability.

When GVI is a persistent concern following or despite the chest radiograph, computed tomographic angiography (CTA) of the chest should be carried out. This test provides significant information on patients with thoracic trauma, including identification of mediastinal hematoma and differentiation of the various causes. Recent advances in technology of helical computed tomography (CT) have improved its sensitivity and specificity for aortic injury, including isolated intimal tears, such that it approaches 100%.[13,14] More recent studies focusing on the use of 64-slice multidetector CT have added to the evidence that sensitivity and specificity approaching 100% make this the preferred imaging modality.[15] An additional benefit is its ability to identify concomitant or alternative injuries. Limitations of CTA of the chest for GVI include poor delineation of nonaortic vascular injuries and the need for relative hemodynamic stability in the patient.[5,13]

Because of the ease and accuracy of CTA, use of the traditional "gold standard" for traumatic aortic injury, aortography, has markedly diminished over the past decade. In fact, newer studies are questioning the role of aortography even in the setting of equivocal CT findings. Several studies have shown that catheter angiography following equivocal findings on CTA is unlikely to reveal GVI, which has led some authors to suggest that patients be monitored clinically with or without repeated cross-sectional imaging, thus obviating the need for aortography.[16]

Transesophageal echocardiography (TEE) is another modality that can be used to evaluate aortic injury. Availability reduces its usefulness in the emergency setting, but it should be considered for patients who are too unstable to leave the department or when body habitus prohibits the use of a CT scanner. Its use is contraindicated in patients with unstable cervical spine injuries or suspected esophageal trauma. TEE has similar sensitivity as CTA of the chest in the evaluation of traumatic aortic injury.[14]

## TREATMENT

### INITIAL INTERVENTIONS AND PROCEDURES

When great vessel trauma is suspected, adequate vascular access should be obtained immediately. Although two large-bore peripheral intravenous lines are frequently cited as being sufficient for trauma patients, the benefits of central venous pressure monitoring and rapid large-volume resuscitation may necessitate central access. Ideally, the suspected vascular injury should not be affected by the site chosen for central venipuncture. For example, with penetrating injury involving the descending aorta, concomitant vena cava injury is possible; solely femoral or lower extremity access would therefore not be optimal. Unfortunately, in the setting of undifferentiated thoracic trauma, the options may be limited.

Many of the initial emergency resuscitative efforts needed in patients with great vessel trauma are dictated by hemodynamic instability. Patients with traumatic cardiac arrest or extreme hemodynamic compromise unresponsive to crystalloid and packed red blood cell transfusions are candidates for emergency department resuscitative thoracotomy. This procedure is usually performed without knowledge of the exact injury. Consequently, it must be executed methodically such that all potential lifesaving interventions are performed. Injuries to the ascending aorta or aortic arch mandate manual pressure for control of hemorrhage, whereas injuries to the descending aorta require cross-clamping above the site of injury until stability and repair can be achieved. Injuries to aortic arch branch vessels may be tempered by packing the apex of the injured hemithorax. Suspected injury to the right hemithorax requires extension of the thoracotomy into the right side of the chest. Right-sided thoracotomy could be considered in the rare incidence of an isolated transthoracic right-sided penetrating injury.

Identification of pulmonary hilar injury or excessive bleeding from deep in the thorax, despite aortic cross-clamping, suggests the need to clamp the affected pulmonary hilum. This is achieved either through manual compression or with a vascular clamp. The goal of emergency department thoracotomy is to achieve enough clinical stabilization to allow definitive operative repair.

## DEFINITIVE TREATMENT

Definitive treatment of GVI is usually surgical or endovascular repair. With mortality rates associated with these injuries increasing at an estimated rate of 1% per hour over the 48 hours after arrival at the hospital, expediting time to intervention is imperative.[4] Surgical techniques usually include clamping and aortic reconstruction with or without vascular bypass. In part because of the need for vascular clamping, paraplegia can be a complication of repair in up to 4% to 20% of patients.[3,17] Although cross-clamp times are not thought to directly correlate with the incidence of paraplegia, keeping times under 30 minutes is believed to be beneficial.[3,17]

More recently, endovascular stenting has become an alternative to open surgical repair.[18,19] Potential benefits of endovascular repair include a less invasive approach and avoidance of aortic cross-clamping (which may lead to lower rates of paraplegia), cardiopulmonary bypass, and systemic heparinization. Endovascular stenting can be performed in less time and in patients too unstable for operative intervention. A metaanalysis of endovascular versus open repair published in 2008 showed lower mortality rates and lower risk for paraplegia with endovascular repair. It is thought that the mortality benefit relates to the less invasive approach and lack of systemic heparinization given that the majority of these patients have concomitant intraabdominal, intracerebral, or intrapulmonary injuries at high risk for bleeding complications.[20]

Before surgical or endovascular intervention, medical management is critical and should include pharmacologic reduction of wall tension and shearing forces to prevent propagation of intimal tears and minimize the risk for subsequent in-hospital catastrophic rupture of a contained hemorrhage. One study demonstrated that by starting pharmacologic management as soon as possible, even before a confirmative diagnostic test when suspicion is high enough, morbidity and mortality were reduced significantly.[13]

Beta-blockers are the first-line medication for reducing wall stress and controlling the heart rate. Esmolol is ideal because of its rapid onset of action and short half-life, which makes it easy to titrate in a continuous infusion. When further blood pressure control is desired, vasodilators such as nitroprusside can be added after beta-blockade has been established. Because of the potential for reflex tachycardia, which increases shearing forces, caution should be exercised when using nitroprusside alone.[21,22] **Table 90.1** lists drug dosages for esmolol and nitroprusside.

A second but controversial intervention is permissive hypovolemia, in which blood pressure is controlled by limiting fluid administration. Lower systolic pressures of 60 to 90 mm Hg are thought to decrease the risk for clot rupture and minimize the shear force on traumatized vessels. Patients often have associated pulmonary contusions, which strengthens the rationale for limiting fluid administration before operative intervention.[23,24] Animal studies using permissive hypovolemia have shown consistent benefit, whereas human trials have been few and the results conflicting.

**Table 90.1** Medical Management of Great Vessel Injury

| DRUG | DOSE |
|---|---|
| Esmolol* | |
| Bolus | 0.5 mg/kg over 1-min period |
| Continuous infusion | 50-200 mcg/kg/min |
| Nitroprusside | 0.3-10 mcg/kg/min |

*A beta-blocker is first-line treatment; nitroprusside should be added if blood pressure control is not achieved. The goal is systolic blood pressure between 100 and 120 mm Hg.

Two other interventions that are often used during global resuscitation require special consideration in the setting of GVI. Central line access provides important information during resuscitative efforts; however, caution must be taken to avoid further vessel damage by choosing a site farthest from the suspected vessel injury. Similar caution must be undertaken when considering chest tube placement to resolve hemothorax. This action may disrupt the containment of a great vessel hemorrhage with the catastrophic result of exsanguination of the patient.

Ideally, immediate surgical or endovascular repair of GVI has been recommended. However, recent studies have looked at delayed repair, particularly in patients with significant associated injuries or hemodynamic instability. Repair of great vessels has been delayed as long at 6 to 8 months.[25] One prospective multicenter study in 2009 examined delayed repair of blunt traumatic aortic injury in stable patients and found significant survival benefits in all patient groups, particularly striking in those with associated injuries.[26] Delayed repair is not routinely performed yet but may become more prevalent as further studies focus on this approach.

If a patient survives the first 24 hours without rupture, a stable pseudoaneurysm may develop. In such cases nonoperative management, including close monitoring and pharmacologic control of blood pressure, may be considered.

## SUGGESTED READINGS

Fitzharris M, Franklyn M, Frampton R, et al. Thoracic aortic injury in motor vehicle crashes: the effect of impact direction, side of body struck, and seat belt use. J Trauma 2004;57:582-90.

Lee WA, Matsumura JS, Mitchell RS, et al. Endovascular repair of traumatic thoracic aortic injury: clinical practice guidelines of the Society for Vascular Surgery. J Vasc Surg 2011;53:187-92.

Xenos E, Abedi N, Davenport D, et al. Meta-analysis of endovascular versus open repair for traumatic descending thoracic aortic rupture. J Vasc Surg 2008;48:1343-51.

## REFERENCES

*References can be found on Expert Consult @ www.expertconsult.com.*

# Acute Compartment Syndromes 91

*David A. Peak*

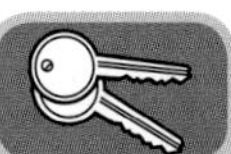

**KEY POINTS**

- Severe pain out of proportion to the clinical situation is the main feature of acute compartment syndrome and often the only early finding.
- Early diagnosis, consultation, and treatment are the keys to a good outcome.

## EPIDEMIOLOGY

The true incidence of acute compartment syndrome (CS) varies with the inciting event. Almost half of all cases of CS are related to tibia fractures. The incidence of CS with tibia fractures is 1.2% with closed fractures, 6% with open fractures, and as high as 19% with concomitant vascular injury.[1,2] The forearm is the second leading site. CS can occur in any contained compartment.

## PATHOPHYSIOLOGY

CS is a condition of impaired microcirculatory perfusion related to increased interstitial pressure within a closed compartment. CS begins when increased pressure as a result of increased volume within or external pressure compromises microcirculatory perfusion within that space. Once autoregulatory reductions in the arteriovenous gradient are overwhelmed, interstitial pressure will rise above capillary perfusion pressure (normally between 20 and 30 mm Hg in a normotensive patient for most compartments), and tissue ischemia will occur.[3] CS is characterized by a self-propagating cycle of impaired perfusion resulting in ischemia, release of osmotically active particles, and edema, which further increase interstitial pressure and diminished perfusion (**Fig. 91.1**).

## PRESENTING SIGNS AND SYMPTOMS

CS should be on the working list of "worst-case" diagnoses for every patient with musculoskeletal pain. CS may result from either externally applied compressive force or internally expanding force, and a suggestive history should be elicited (**Box 91.1**). Myofascial causes include long-bone fracture, vascular injury, reperfusion after ischemia, burns, prolonged positioning from a drug overdose or operating procedures, compression from tight casts and dressings (including military antishock trousers), overexertion, hemorrhage, injection of fluid into the compartment, massive intravenous fluid infusions, envenomations, hypothyroidism, and rhabdomyolysis. CS has also been reported with deep vein thrombosis and ruptured Baker cysts (see Box 91.1). High-risk patients with an altered sensorium may be unable to provide an appropriate history. CS usually develops hours after the inciting event and rarely more than 48 hours after the inciting event.

Clinicians must remain vigilant and retain a high index of suspicion to avoid missing the diagnosis. Patients with a high mechanism of trauma and an altered sensorium should be examined carefully. The physical examination should focus on evidence of trauma and gross deformity, as well as assessment of neurovascular abnormalities. Comparing one extremity with the unaffected side is often very useful.

Serial examinations are often required.

Acute CS is a clinical diagnosis. The essential clinical feature in a conscious patient is severe pain out of proportion to the injury that is aggravated by active or passive stretching of the muscles of the affected compartment or by palpation of the affected compartment. In early cases, pain is the *only* abnormality. Increasing pain or pain refractory to analgesics suggests the diagnosis. Severe pain while at rest or without any movement should raise suspicion for acute CS. Increasing need for analgesia or increased analgesic dosing is common. The diagnosis is far more challenging in patients who cannot communicate (i.e., altered mental status).

The natural progression of untreated acute CS is severe pain, decreased sensation, decreased strength, and eventual paralysis of the affected limb. With the exception of pain and paresthesia, the traditional five P's (pain, paresthesia, pallor, pulselessness, poikilothermia) are misleading and more relevant for arterial injury or occlusion. Patients with severe CS, even those with extensive myonecrosis, may have palpable pulses and preserved capillary refill until late in the course. Pulse deficits should raise suspicion for a vascular injury alone or coexisting with acute CS. Decreased two-point discrimination is consistently the earliest physical abnormality and can help differentiate which compartments are affected. Correlation has also been reported between decreasing vibratory sense (256 cycles per second) and increasing compartment pressure.

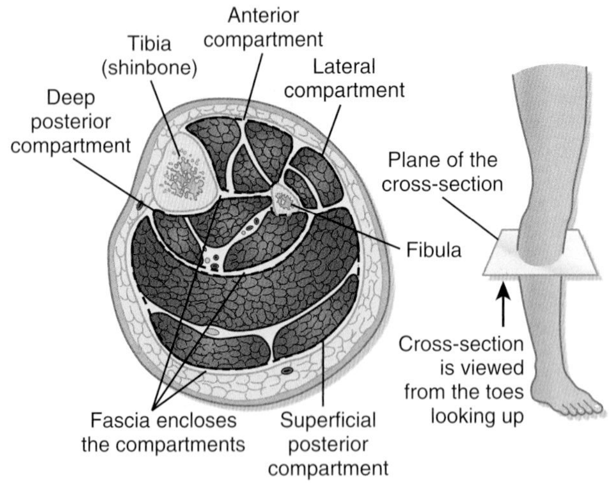


**Fig. 91.1 Compartments of the leg.**

**BOX 91.1 Causes of Acute Compartment Syndrome**

**Internally Applied Force, Increased Content Within the Compartment**

Long-bone fractures
Vascular injury
Overexertion (including seizures)
Hemorrhage, coagulopathy
Injection of fluid into the compartment
Massive intravenous infusions
Envenomations
Deep vein thrombosis, ruptured Baker cyst
Reperfusion after ischemia

**Externally Applied Force, Decreased Volume of the Compartment**

Burns
Tight casts, dressings, military antishock trousers
Prolonged awkward positioning
Closure of fascial defects

## DIFFERENTIAL DIAGNOSIS AND MEDICAL DECISION MAKING

The differential diagnosis includes any disorder that can cause musculoskeletal pain, including fracture, contusions, and hematomas; however, pain from other causes generally diminishes after the inciting event, whereas in acute CS, the pain generally increases even while the patient is at rest. Arterial injury will be manifested as abnormal pulses at the onset. Crush injury shares some overlapping features with CS, but the primary pathophysiology is thought to be direct tissue injury, and fasciotomy is rarely indicated.

The diagnosis cannot be made with radiographic imaging. However, because the differential diagnosis for acute CS includes fracture or dislocation and because the risk for CS increases with fracture, radiographic imaging may be useful. Computed tomography or ultrasound is rarely indicated but may be helpful in establishing the cause of the CS (i.e., fracture, hematoma).

## TREATMENT

### PREHOSPITAL MANAGEMENT

The affected limb should be placed at the level of the heart. Elevation is contraindicated because it decreases arterial flow, which narrows the arteriovenous pressure gradient and thus worsens ischemia.[4] Circumferential bandages should be removed, and casts should be removed or split.[5] Because hypotension potentiates CS, it should be corrected with crystalloid or blood products. Supplemental oxygen should be administered routinely to improve tissue oxygenation.[6]

### HOSPITAL MANAGEMENT

Surgical speciality evaluation is mandatory in suspected cases because the therapy for CS is usually surgical decompression. Full trauma evaluation and correction of hypotension, anemia, and coagulopathy, as well as preoperative assessment, are expected. CS can cause rhabdomyolysis, acute renal failure, and death, and these complications should be anticipated and treated accordingly.

Measurement of intracompartmental pressure is not necessary if the diagnosis of acute CS is clinically apparent.[7] Equivocal cases may require further evaluation. Multiple methods and devices for measuring compartmental pressure are available. Devices that use a side-ported needle or slit catheter are recommended rather than those using a simple needle.

Normal intracompartmental pressure is in the range of 0 to 10 mm Hg. Pain and paresthesias are common at 20 to 30 mm Hg, and ischemia generally ensues at pressures greater than 30 mm Hg. Many surgeons traditionally consider a measured compartment pressure of 30 mm Hg or higher as an indication for fasciotomy,[8] although higher values have been used, especially for the thigh. More recently, some authors have recommended the use of a ΔP value (diastolic blood pressure minus the measured intracompartmental pressure) of less than 30 to 50 mm Hg as an indication for fasciotomy and have found it to be more reliable than an absolute compartment pressure (**Box 91.2**).

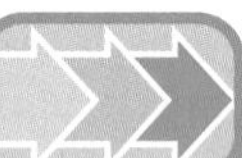

**PRIORITY ACTIONS**

Suspect acute compartment syndrome when a patient has severe pain, especially with passive movement, but few other objective physical findings.
Measure compartment pressures when indicated.
Consult the orthopedic or general surgery department.
Treat hypotension and anemia, provide oxygen, and reverse coagulopathy if present.[6]
The affected compartment should be positioned at the level of the heart.[7]

## FOLLOW-UP, NEXT STEPS IN CARE, AND PATIENT EDUCATION

All patients with acute CS must be admitted to the hospital. Most will be transferred to the operating room for emergency fasciotomy or surgical decompression. Patients with abnormal

**BOX 91.2 Management of Acute Compartment Syndrome**

Consult surgery.
Maintain the affected area at the level of the heart.
Reverse hypoperfusion/hypotension.
Maximize oxygenation/administer supplemental oxygen.
Correct coagulopathy if present.
Correct anemia if present.
Modify the cast, splint, or dressing if this is the precipitant of the syndrome.
Order antivenom if envenomation is the cause of the syndrome.

compartment measurements that do not reach the threshold for emergency surgical decompression should be admitted for observation. Patients with suspected impending acute CS should be admitted for serial examinations and observation.

The prognosis depends on early diagnosis and treatment. Severe disability, amputation, and even death may occur when the diagnosis is delayed or missed. Pitfalls include failure to make the diagnosis or consult surgery when indicated.

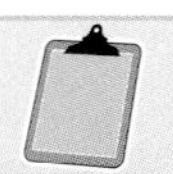

**DOCUMENTATION**

*History*: A careful history will include the mechanism, timing, history of paresthesia or weakness, medical conditions that may impair oxygenation or perfusion, coagulopathy or anticoagulation therapy, intravenous drug use, increasing pain, and pain with active or passive movement

*Physical examination*: Including neurovascular signs, compartment palpation, discoloration, masses, range of motion

*Medical decision making*: Reasons to pursue or not pursue work-up or consultation

*Patient teaching*: Patients with significant extremity pain but who do not have clinical evidence of acute compartment syndrome should be counseled to avoid activity, maintain the extremity at the level of the heart, and return if any increase in pain occurs

## SPECIAL CIRCUMSTANCES

### ACUTE ORBITAL COMPARTMENT SYNDROME

Acute orbital CS is considered a rare complication of facial trauma (usually blunt) or surgery. The globe and retrobulbar contents are encased in a continuous cone-shaped fascial envelope that is bound on all sides by seven rigid bony walls, except anteriorly, where the orbital septum and eyelids form another, fairly inflexible boundary. The medial and lateral canthal tendons attach the eyelids to the orbital rim and limit forward movement of the globe.

**BOX 91.3 Primary Indications for Lateral Canthotomy/Cantholysis**

Suspected orbital compartment syndrome with one or both of the following:

- Decreasing vision
- Increasing intraocular pressure

When vision cannot be assessed and clinical suspicion is high (e.g., a comatose patient)

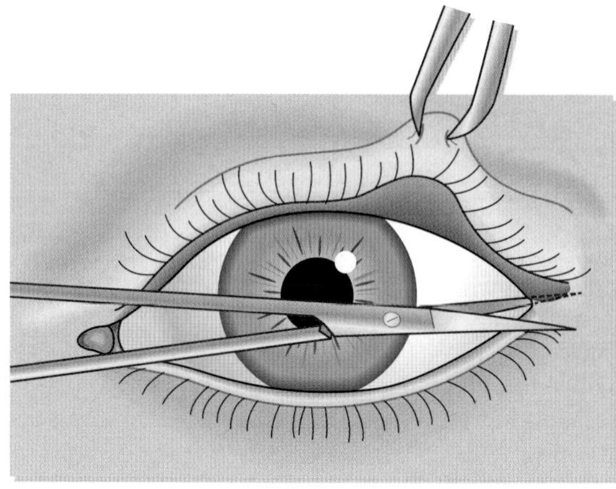

**Fig. 91.2** Lateral canthotomy.

The orbit may compensate for small increases in orbital volume by forward movement of the globe and prolapse of fat, followed immediately by a rapid rise in orbital tissue pressure. The orbit therefore follows pressure-volume dynamics with a pathophysiology akin to that with CS in other compartments: increased tissue pressure in an enclosed space is associated with decreased perfusion. Ischemia ensues when orbital pressure exceeds central retinal artery pressure.

Symptoms and signs include eye pain, visual loss, proptosis, reduction of ocular mobility, diplopia, increased intraocular pressure, chemosis, and (late) afferent pupillary defect. Diagnosis requires high clinical suspicion and may require serial examinations, including visual acuity tests.

Suspected acute orbital CS with a decrease in vision, loss of vision with increasing intraocular pressure, or high suspicion in a comatose patient requires treatment to prevent permanent blindness. Computed tomography or magnetic resonance imaging is not necessary to make the diagnosis. Irreversible optic nerve pathology may occur with as little as 2 hours of ischemia.

Medical therapy and ophthalmologic consultation should proceed promptly, before the diagnosis is established. Osmotic agents and carbonic anhydrase inhibitors are part of established protocols at many centers. Most experts also recommend high-dose steroid therapy. Less agreement exists about the use of topical beta-blockers and multiple osmotic agents.

The emergency procedure of choice for loss of visual acuity associated with acute orbital CS is lateral canthotomy and cantholysis of the canthal ligaments (**Box 91.3; Figs. 91.2 and 91.3**; also see the Tips and Tricks box). Primary indications for lateral canthotomy and cantholysis include intraocular pressure greater than 40 mm Hg with visual loss

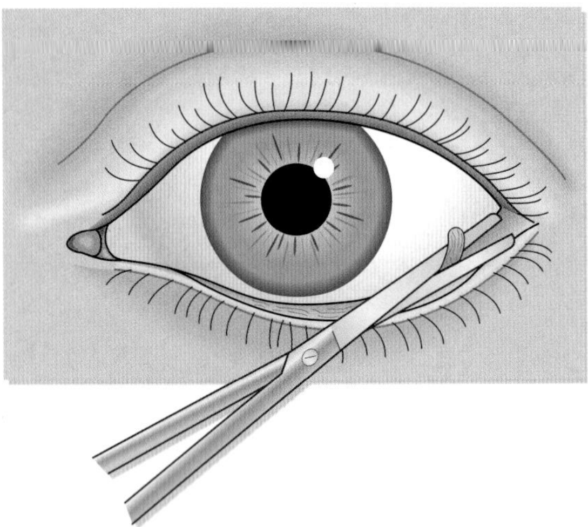

**Fig. 91.3 Canthal ligament cantholysis.**

and proptosis, which may be used as a criterion for an unconscious patients whose visual acuity cannot be determined. Secondary criteria include an afferent pupillary defect, ophthalmoplegia, cherry-red macula, optic nerve head pallor, and severe pain, but these signs are all considered less sensitive or very late.

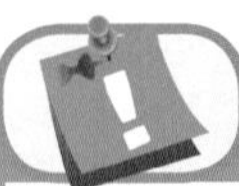

**TIPS AND TRICKS**

**Lateral Canthotomy and Canthal Ligament Cantholysis Procedures**

**Lateral Canthotomy**

Stabilize the patient's head and lids.

Anesthetize the lateral canthus with lidocaine with or without epinephrine.

Crush the canthus with a hemostat for 30 to 60 seconds.

Incise the canthus with straight sharp-edged scissors, make a horizontal incision over the crushed canthus, and continue to the bony orbital rim (see Fig. 91.2).

Avoid the orbit during the incision.

**Cantholysis Sweep Technique**

Starting lateral to the midline, carefully sweep the lateral edge of the open-faced straight or curved blunt-edged scissors along the palpebral conjunctiva toward the canthotomy incision, with care taken to avoid the orbit and orbital conjunctiva.

The canthal ligament will be identified as the structure along the orbital rim that prevents a completely smooth sweep to the canthotomy incision.

Identify and isolate the ligament with the open scissor blade (see Fig. 91.3).

Carefully maneuver the opposing scissor blade into place while avoiding the globe.

Cut the canthal ligament.

The lid will now be freely mobile with distraction.

A contraindication to lateral canthotomy is a suspected ruptured globe. In an experimental model, lateral canthotomy/cantholysis produced a mean decrease in intraocular pressure of 30.4 mm Hg.[9] Emergency department personnel should be familiar with and able to perform this procedure in the event that emergency ophthalmology consultation is delayed.

## ABDOMINAL COMPARTMENT SYNDROME

Abdominal CS is a sudden increase in intraabdominal pressure that results in dysfunction of the respiratory, cardiovascular, and renal systems.[10] Normal intraabdominal pressure is 0 to 5 mm Hg. Acute abdominal CS was defined by the 2004 International Abdominal Compartment Syndrome Consensus Definitions Conference Committee as sustained intra-abdominal pressure greater than 20 mm Hg that is associated with new organ dysfunction or failure. It is most common after abdominal surgical procedures but can also occur with peritonitis, intraabdominal abscesses, intestinal obstructions, ruptured abdominal aneurysms, acute pancreatitis, intraperitoneal or retroperitoneal hemorrhage, ascites, ovarian tumors, and massive edema following resuscitation.

The diagnosis depends on high clinical suspicion combined with the presence of clinical parameters, including intra-abdominal pressure elevated to greater than 20 to 25 mm Hg (most commonly assessed with a device used to measure bladder pressure), a distended abdomen, elevated peak airway pressure, large intravenous fluid requirements, elevated central venous pressure, oliguria or anuria not responding to volume repletion, decreased cardiac output, hypoxemia, hypercapnia, acidosis, and a wide pulse pressure.

Treatment consists of rapid surgical decompression, as well as restoration of intravascular volume, maximization of oxygen delivery, and correction of acidosis and coagulopathies. Mortality associated with abdominal CS can exceed 50%.

## CHRONIC COMPARTMENT SYNDROME

Chronic CS was first described in 1956 and initially thought to be a form of shin splints (anterior tibial enthesitis). Chronic CS (also known as exertional or recurrent CS) is not a surgical emergency. It is commonly reproducible with a certain specific exercise or exercise distance. Symptoms subside with termination of the exercise and are minimal with normal daily exercise. When suspected, patients should be advised to rest and be referred to an orthopedic or sports medicine specialist.

## SUGGESTED READINGS

Matsen III FA. Compartment syndrome. A unified concept. Clin Orthop Relat Res 1975;113:8-14.

Wall CJ, Lynch J, Harris IA, et al. Clinical practice guidelines for the management of acute limb compartment syndrome following trauma. Aust N Z J Surg 2010;80:151-6.

## REFERENCES

*References can be found on Expert Consult @ www.expertconsult.com.*

# Low Back Pain 92

*Gerard S. Doyle*

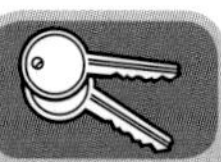

**KEY POINTS**

- Nonspecific low back pain is usually self-limited and of short duration: about 60% of cases will resolve within 1 week and 90% within 2 to 6 weeks.
- Clues pointing to inflammatory, infectious, and oncologic disorders as possible causes of low back pain may be subtle and easily missed.
- Testing should be directed toward specific diagnostic concerns rather than screening studies.
- The primary treatment option for back pain is nonsteroidal antiinflammatory drugs along with judicious opioid use.
- Skeletal muscle relaxants and steroids have not been shown to improve outcomes and have significant side effects, although some patients do report relief.
- Patients who have pain longer than 2 weeks or in whom leg weakness, bowel or bladder dysfunction, fever, or new adverse symptoms develop at any time should be reevaluated.

## PERSPECTIVE

Low back pain (LBP) is associated with large economic costs, both direct and indirect. Estimates vary depending on the types of care included (i.e., allopathic medicine versus chiropractic or complementary-alternative medicine), with direct costs being estimated at anywhere from $12 to $91 billion per year in the United States. Lost productivity is thought to be the major indirect costs of LBP; one study puts this annual U.S. cost at $24 billion for workers with LBP versus $7 billion for those without LBP.

## EPIDEMIOLOGY

Most adults will experience LBP at some point in their lifetime, and about one in five adults experience LBP within a single year. LBP costs billions of dollars per year. About 85% to 90% of patients with LBP in a variety of outpatient settings are considered to have nonspecific LBP.[1] This may lead to physician complacence in the evaluation of a presumably benign disorder.

Conversely, LBP can be incapacitating, and the patient may perceive the problem as a harbinger of death or disability, regardless of the cause. Patient expectations of a specific diagnosis of the pain source and a complete cure are rarely met and are probably unrealistic. Psychologic, social, and economic factors play a role in the natural history of many pain-related conditions, including progression of LBP from an acute to a chronic condition. LBP often becomes a chronic condition subject to exacerbations, akin to asthma and diabetes mellitus.[2] These issues combine to make LBP a source of frustration for patients and physicians alike.

## PATHOPHYSIOLOGY

LBP is a symptom complex caused by a variety of diseases and anatomic abnormalities. Multiple potential sources of pain intrinsic to the spinal column (joints between vertebrae, sacroiliac joint, intervertebral disks, vertebral bones, periosteum, ligaments, meninges, paraspinous muscles, fascia, blood vessels, and nerves) have been implicated. Additionally, a number of visceral structures may be a source of pain referred to the low back region.

LBP is often classified as specific or nonspecific, mechanical or nonmechanical, or primary or secondary or is classified on the basis of presumed etiology (structural, neoplastic, referred pain or visceral, infectious, inflammatory, or metabolic). All these classification systems recognize that in the majority of cases a specific pathoanatomic diagnosis cannot be assigned. Indeed, clear correlation between a specific anatomic abnormality and pain is rarely established in patients, and proposed mechanisms of pain in the medical literature have been fraught with controversy. For example, many asymptomatic subjects have evidence of bulging, prolapsed, or herniated intervertebral disks.[3]

## PRESENTING SIGNS AND SYMPTOMS

### CLASSIC SYMPTOMS

In general, patients complain of pain described as a dull ache that is mild to moderate in intensity. Its onset is frequently attributed by patients to lifting, bending, or twisting activities and may be abrupt. Movement tends to exacerbate the pain, whereas rest, especially recumbency, minimizes or relieves it. The pain can be midline, unilateral, or bilateral and may radiate to the buttocks or thighs. Because of the recurrent nature of LBP, many patients have experienced similar pain in the past.

### TYPICAL VARIATIONS

Pain that is not relieved or worsens when the patient lies down or pain that awakens the patient from sleep is concerning because it may portend a systemic source of the pain. Pain that is unremitting for more than 4 to 6 weeks or that continues despite rest and adequate analgesia often has a specific cause.

LBP can occur alone or as one of a constellation of associated symptoms that are frequently more important than the pain itself in determining an accurate diagnosis and treatment plan. Certain symptoms, comorbid diseases, medication use, and signs are "red flags" in that they point to specific, often serious diagnoses.

## DIFFERENTIAL DIAGNOSIS AND MEDICAL DECISION MAKING

Nonmechanical causes must be distinguished from mechanical causes of LBP. The key to such distinction rests on eliminating systemic (infectious, neoplastic, metabolic, or inflammatory) and visceral causes. **Figure 92.1** shows one diagnostic approach, and **Box 92.1** lists the differential diagnosis for LBP.

Specific causes of LBP are shown in **Table 92.1**, together with red flag signs or symptoms suggesting these diagnoses. When the history and physical examination suggest a nonmechanical cause of LBP, appropriate diagnostic testing or specialty consultation (or both) is necessary to confirm or rule out the suspected specific cause or causes.

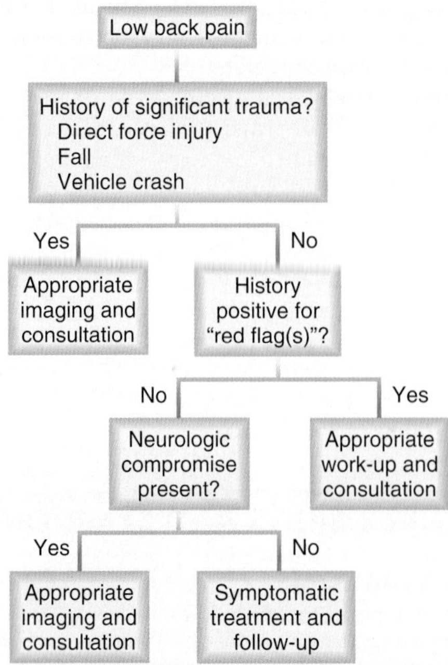


**Fig. 92.1 Diagnostic approach to low back pain.**

Visceral and systemic causes of LBP, though rarely found in most ambulatory care settings, must be addressed. Visceral sources of referred pain that cause LBP can result from a variety of vascular, pelvic, renal, and gastrointestinal pathology. Pain from aortic dissection, for example, can be referred to the back. Similarly, retroperitoneal pathology of any source, including hematomas and metastatic disease, can cause LBP. Patients with pain from these sources may or may not have other clues to the source of their pain. Clues to the diagnosis of aortic dissection may include a diminished femoral pulse or mottling of a leg. Because testicular cancer metastasizes to the retroperitoneum, genitourinary examination might identify the pathology.

A retroperitoneal hematoma may be heralded only by tachycardia or, rarely, by hypotension from blood loss. More commonly, warfarin or an antiplatelet agent may be a contributing factor. Any of these clues may be subtle but may also be the only evidence of an important diagnosis.

Systemic causes of LBP are disease processes that involve the structures of the spinal column, including cancer, infection, inflammation, and degenerative processes. Cancer (with metastatic or primary tumor invasion of the spinal column) typically occurs in those older than 50 years. Weight loss, pain with bed rest, and failure of therapy (with pain lasting a month or longer) are frequent symptoms. Back pain in any patient with a history of cancer should be considered to be due to a cancerous lesion of the spine until ruled out.[4]

Infections involving the spine (spinal epidural abscess [SEA], osteomyelitis, and diskitis) are rare. Prudent suspicion, deliberate consideration, and attention to patient risks are the most important ways to facilitate successful diagnosis. Patients with sickle cell disease are predisposed to *Salmonella* osteomyelitis. Patients with immunosuppression, chronic corticosteroid therapy, injection drug use, and recent bacterial infections (cellulitis, pneumonia, urinary tract infection) are at increased risk for SEA, osteomyelitis, and diskitis. Patients with SEA may have isolated back pain, spotty neurologic changes that do not fit a discrete distribution, or pain that mimics sciatica.

Inflammatory arthritides such as ankylosing spondylitis can cause LBP but are frequently associated with other arthritic and systemic symptoms. Patients with these diseases usually report pain that worsens with lying down, as well as morning stiffness that gradually improves with activity. The pain is usually chronic, with a duration of 3 or more months, and is of gradual onset. Ankylosing spondylitis is most common in young men, with symptoms usually appearing before the age of 40.

Once possible visceral and systemic causes of the patient's symptoms have been excluded, the focus should be shifted to determine whether neurologic compromise has occurred. Additionally, diagnoses that may lead to spinal instability (fracture and spondylolisthesis) should be considered.

LBP can be associated with leg pain secondary to radiating pain, but other causes include sciatica (or lumbosacral radiculopathy) with pain radiating from the back to the buttock and posterior or lateral aspect of the leg. Sciatica is frequently caused by lumbar degenerative disk disease. True sciatica usually causes pain below the knee; at least 95% of degenerative disks in the lumbar spine occur at the L4-L5 and L5-S1 vertebral levels. For this reason, the neurologic examination should be focused on both sensory and motor testing of the lumbosacral nerve roots. **Table 92.2** details the motor, sensory, and reflex test components of the neurologic examination of patients with LBP. Note that functional strength testing is more likely than simple motor testing to detect subtle muscle weakness.

Passive straight leg raise (SLR) testing appears to help in the diagnosis of sciatica by stretching the sciatic nerve. A positive ipsilateral SLR test (which results in pain below the knee when the leg to which LBP radiates is raised higher than 30 to 60 degrees with the patient supine) is sensitive but not specific for sciatica, whereas a positive crossed SLR test (in which pain in the affected leg is provoked or worsened when the contralateral leg is raised) is specific but insensitive.[5] A negative SLR test may be of greater value because patients with this finding generally have good long-term outcomes.

Spinal stenosis can result from a variety of processes that impinge on the spinal cord (usually hypertrophy of the ligamentum flavum) and cause pseudoclaudication—back and leg pain with walking and extension of the spine that improves with sitting and lumbar flexion. Most cases occur in patients 55 years or older; they usually report an insidious onset of symptoms.

Cauda equina syndrome (CES) results from compression of the conus medullaris of the spinal cord or the nerve roots that make up the cauda equina. It is typically caused by a large central disk herniation but can also be due to other space-occupying lesions such as spinal stenosis, tumor, SEA, and hematoma.[2] The most consistent findings in patients with CES are LBP, urinary symptoms, and sacral and perineal ("saddle") paresthesias.[6] Bilateral sciatica is also a concerning symptom. Central disk herniations may not cause sciatica, and back pain may be a minor component of the patient's symptoms. The presence of urinary retention has good sensitivity and specificity for CES.[7] Magnetic resonance imaging (MRI) is diagnostic and usually shows severe spinal canal impingement by a disk.

Expeditious diagnosis and therapy may help maximize the long-term outcome (in terms of pain and disordered bladder, bowel, and sexual function) in these patients. Despite some controversy regarding the role of impairments already present at diagnosis, there appears to be some improvement in the

**BOX 92.1 Differential Diagnosis of Low Back Pain***

**Mechanical Lower Back or Leg Pain (97%)†**
Lumbar strain, sprain (70%)‡
Degeneration of disks and facets, usually age related (10%)
*Herniated disk* (4%)
*Spinal stenosis* (3%)
Osteoporotic compression fracture (4%)
Spondylolisthesis (2%)
Traumatic fracture (<1%)
Congenital disease (<1%)
Severe kyphosis
Severe scoliosis
Transitional vertebrae
Spondylolysis§
Internal disk disruption, diskogenic low back pain¶
Presumed instability¶

**Nonmechanical Spine Conditions (≈1%)****
Neoplasia (0.7%)
Multiple myeloma
Metastatic carcinoma
Lymphoma and leukemia
Spinal cord tumors
Retroperitoneal tumors
Primary vertebral tumors
Infection (0.01%)
Osteomyelitis
Septic diskitis
Paraspinous abscess
*Shingles*
Inflammatory arthritis (often associated with HLA-B27) (0.3%)
Ankylosing spondylitis
Psoriatic spondylitis
Reiter syndrome
Inflammatory bowel disease
Scheuermann disease (osteochondrosis)
Paget disease of bone

**Visceral Disease (2%)**
Disease of pelvic organs
Prostatitis
Endometriosis
Chronic pelvic inflammatory disease
Renal disease
Nephrolithiasis
Pyelonephritis
Perinephric abscess
Aortic aneurysm
Gastrointestinal disease
Pancreatitis
Cholecystitis
Penetrating ulcer

From Jarvik JG, Deyo RA. Diagnostic evaluation of low back pain with emphasis on imaging. Ann Intern Med 2002;137:586-97.
*HLA-B27*, Human leukocyte antigen B27.
*Figures in parentheses indicate the estimated percentages of patients with these conditions among all adult patients with low back pain in primary care. Diagnoses shown in italics are often associated with neurogenic leg pain. Percentages may vary substantially according to demographic characteristics or referral patterns in a practice. For example, spinal stenosis and osteoporosis are more common in geriatric patients, spinal infection in injection drug users, and so forth.
†The term *mechanical* is used here to designate an anatomic or functional abnormality without underlying malignant, neoplastic, or inflammatory disease. Approximately 2% of cases of mechanical low back or leg pain are accounted for by spondylolysis, internal disk disruption, or discogenic low back pain and presumed instability.
‡*Strain* and *sprain* are nonspecific terms with no pathoanatomic confirmation. *Nonspecific low back pain* or *idiopathic low back pain* may be a preferable term.
§Spondylolysis is as common in asymptomatic persons as in those with low back pain; thus its role in causing low back pain remains ambiguous.
¶Internal disk disruption is diagnosed by provocative diskography (injection of contrast material into a degenerated disk with assessment of pain at the time of injection). However, diskography often causes pain in asymptomatic adults, and the condition in many patients with positive diskogram findings improves spontaneously. Thus the clinical importance and appropriate management of this condition remain unclear. The term *diskogenic lower back pain* is used more or less synonymously with the term *internal disk disruption*.
¶Presumed instability is loosely defined as greater than 10 degrees of angulation or 4 mm of vertebral displacement on lateral flexion and extension radiographs. However, the diagnostic criteria, natural history, and surgical indications remain controversial.
**Scheuermann disease and Paget disease of bone probably account for less than 0.01% of nonmechanical spinal conditions.

outcome of CES if decompression is performed within 48 hours of arrival in the emergency department (ED).[8]

LBP without a systemic or visceral cause and without neurologic compromise may nevertheless occur as a result of a specific mechanical cause, usually involving the spinal column itself. Lumbar fractures generally result from significant trauma (e.g., falls from heights, external trauma) but can be caused by minor trauma in older patients, in patients receiving chronic corticosteroid therapy, and in persons at risk for pathologic fractures (e.g., because of bony metastases or osteoporosis of the spine).

A history of trauma and bone tenderness (to palpation or percussion) suggests fracture as a possible cause of LBP. Stress fractures of the sacrum and lumbar spine and insufficiency fractures of the sacrum are other causes of LBP to which athletes (especially young athletes) and older patients (especially women), respectively, are predisposed.

Spondylolisthesis, or slippage of one vertebral body relative to an adjacent vertebral body, is a specific mechanical cause of LBP that can lead to progressive instability. It occurs as a result of a defect in the pars interarticularis from either a fracture or spondylolysis, which can be congenital or degenerative in etiology. Spondylolisthesis can also lead to degenerative disk disease and osteophyte development. Instability causes symptoms similar to those of spinal stenosis.

**Table 92.1 "Red Flags" in the History and Physical Examination of Patients with Low Back Pain**

| DISORDER | HISTORY | PHYSICAL EXAMINATION |
|---|---|---|
| All | Duration of pain > 1 mo<br>Bed rest with no relief<br>Age < 20 or >50 yr* | |
| Cancer | Age ≥ 50 yr<br>Previous cancer history<br>Unexplained weight loss† | Neurologic findings‡<br>Lymphadenopathy |
| Compression fracture | Age ≥ 50 years (≥60 yr more specific)<br>Significant trauma§<br>History of osteoporosis<br>Corticosteroid use<br>Substance abuse‖ | Fever (>100° F [38° C])<br>Tenderness of spinous processes |
| Infection | Fever or chills<br>Recent skin or urinary infection<br>Immunosuppression<br>Injection drug use | |
| Inflammatory arthritis | Insidiously causing pain for >3 mo<br>Bed rest with no relief<br>Morning stiffness improved with activity | |

Adapted from Atlas SJ, Deyo RA. Evaluating and managing acute low back pain in the primary care setting. J Gen Intern Med 2001;16:120-31.

*Age younger than 20 years is associated with increased risk for spondylolysis, spondylolisthesis, and stress fractures; age older than 50 years suggests increased risk for cancer and compression fractures.

†Unexplained weight loss is defined as more than 10 lb over the preceding 6 months.

‡Most commonly caused by a herniated lumbar disk or lumbar spinal stenosis rather than malignancy.

§Significant trauma is a fall from a height or external trauma such as a motor vehicle accident.

‖Substance abuse can increase the risk for fracture through higher rates of trauma. Alcohol abuse can also increase the risk for fracture as a result of decreasing bone density.

**Table 92.2 Neurologic Examination Components in Patients with Low Back Pain**

| NERVE ROOT | MOTOR EXAMINATION | FUNCTIONAL TEST | SENSATION* | REFLEX |
|---|---|---|---|---|
| L3 | Extend the quadriceps | Squat down and return to standing | Lateral thigh/medial femoral condyle | Patellar tendon |
| L4 | Dorsiflex the ankle | Heel walking | Medial leg/medial ankle | Patellar tendon |
| L5 | Dorsiflex the great toe | Heel walking | Medial leg/medial ankle | NA |
| S1 | Stand on toes for ≥5 repetitions | Walk on toes | Plantar foot/lateral ankle | Achilles tendon |

*NA*, Not applicable.
*Sharp/dull or pinprick.

Children have back pain at higher rates than previously appreciated and are at higher risk for spondylolysis and spondylolisthesis, especially adolescent and teenage athletes. A one-legged hyperextension test may help diagnose these conditions. Bone scans using single-photon emission computed tomography may be the most appropriate initial test, assuming that the findings on plain radiography are normal.[9]

Finally, nonspecific mechanical causes of LBP may be the root of patients' symptoms when possible systemic and visceral sources have been ruled out and no signs of instability or neurologic compromise are present. Nonspecific LBP syndromes have been called lumbago, lumbar sprain or strain, idiopathic LBP, myofascial strain, and a variety of other names. These patients tend to be most comfortable at rest, and their symptoms worsen with activity and movement. They do not have red flags (that suggest specific musculoskeletal, systemic, or visceral sources of their pain) in their history and physical examination, nor do they have signs or symptoms of neurologic compromise.

The Waddell signs have been promoted as tools to help demonstrate a "nonorganic" cause of patients' symptoms, but they are mainly useful for predicting patients at risk for prolonged recovery from LBP.[10] Waddell signs may also point to a diagnosis of depression or another psychoneurosis.

## DIAGNOSTIC TESTING

Plain films of the lumbosacral spine, rectal examination, postvoid residual bladder volume, the erythrocyte sedimentation rate, and MRI are useful diagnostic adjuncts in the ED (**Table 92.3**). Other studies such as myelography (plain or computed tomographic [CT]), electromyography, and diskography should be obtained at the discretion of consultants.

**Table 92.3 Diagnostic Adjuncts for Low Back Pain**

| TEST | COMMENTS |
|---|---|
| Plain radiography | Reserve for <15 *OR* >50 yr old *OR* significant trauma* |
| Rectal examination | To check for neurologic compromise *OR* a prostate mass |
| Erythrocyte sedimentation rate | >20 mm/hr is concerning in patients with possible infection or cancer† |
| Postvoid residual bladder volume | >100-200 mL implies possible CES; bladder scan accurate to ±25 mL‡ |
| Magnetic resonance imaging | Reserve for suspected CES, SEA, or spinal cord compression§ |

CES, Cauda equina syndrome; *SEA*, spinal epidural abscess.

*Deyo RA, Weinstein JN. Low back pain. N Engl J Med 2001;344:363-70.

†Henschke N, Maher CG, Refshauge KM. Screening for malignancy in low back pain patients: a systematic review. Eur Spine J 2007;16:1673-9.

‡Small SA, Perron AD, Brady WJ. Orthopedic pitfalls: cauda equina syndrome. Am J Emerg Med 2005;23:159-63.

§Gilbert FJ, Grant AM, Gillan MG, et al. Low back pain: influence of early MR imaging or CT on treatment and outcome—multicenter randomized trial. Radiology 2004;231:343-51.

If an abdominal aortic aneurysm or dissection is a consideration in the diagnosis, it must be ruled out by an appropriate imaging study, either ultrasound or CT scanning. Urinalysis (and culture as indicated) is recommended for patients in whom urinary tract infection or renal disease is likely. Other specific conditions causing LBP may be diagnosed with appropriate tests as indicated by their differential diagnosis.

## TREATMENT

### PREHOSPITAL MANAGEMENT

Prehospital treatment of LBP consists of immobilization of patients who may have spinal instability or a neurologic deficit, resuscitation of those with systemic or visceral causes of their symptoms, and analgesia.

### HOSPITAL MANAGEMENT

ED diagnostic and treatment priorities are shown in the Priority Actions box. Early institution of intravenous corticosteroids such as dexamethasone (for tumors or disks causing cord or conus medullaris compression) or intravenous antibiotics (for osteomyelitis, SEA, and other infectious processes) should be considered if these diagnoses are likely.

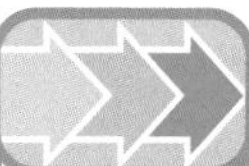

**PRIORITY ACTIONS**

**Diagnosis and Treatment of Low Back Pain**

Establish the absence of a systemic or visceral source of the pain.

Rule out fracture and orthopedic instability.

Check for neurologic compromise, especially cauda equina syndrome.

Treat specific systemic, visceral, and orthopedic diseases as indicated.

Use conservative therapy for nonspecific back pain.

Manage patient expectations regarding nonspecific back pain.

Counsel patients regarding concerning symptoms accompanying the pain.

Placement of a Foley catheter may provide improved comfort and convenience in nonambulatory patients, and decompression of the distended bladder in patients with neurogenic bladder may improve later voiding function.

Nonspecific LBP is usually self-limited and of short duration: about 60% of cases will resolve within 1 week and 90% within 2 to 6 weeks. Treatment is conservative. Acetaminophen and nonsteroidal antiinflammatory drugs (NSAIDs) are first-line analgesics; they are usually prescribed for all patients who do not have contraindications.[11] Patients should be instructed to use NSAIDs routinely because administration only as needed does not seem to be as effective. Narcotic administration is restricted to patients with severe pain and only for short courses. Narcotics are not more beneficial than

**Table 92.4 Treatment of Nonspecific Low Back Pain and Sciatica**

| TREATMENT | EVIDENCE-INFORMED CONSIDERATIONS |
|---|---|
| **Medications** | |
| Acetaminophen | As effective as NSAIDs for short-term pain relief[*] |
| NSAIDs | Offer modest short-term pain relief[*] |
| Skeletal muscle relaxants | No improvement in outcomes; have significant side effects[†] |
| Corticosteroids | No improvement in outcomes; have significant side effects[‡] |
| Narcotic analgesics | Not recommended by guidelines; may foster chronic pain[§] |
| **Nonpharmacologic Modalities** | |
| Symptom-limited activities of daily living | Equal or superior to bed rest or specific therapeutic exercise[‖] |
| Self-paced walking | Seems to reduce recurrence and speed recovery[¶] |
| Superficial heat | Good evidence for moderate relief of low back pain[**] |

*NSAIDs,* Nonsteroidal antiinflammatory drugs.

*Roelofs PD, Deyo RA, Koes BW, et al. Nonsteroidal anti-inflammatory drugs for low back pain: an updated Cochrane review. Spine 2008;33:1766-74.

†Turrurro MA, Frater CR, D'Amico FJ. Cyclobenzaprine with ibuprofen versus ibuprofen alone in acute myofascial strain: a randomized, double-blind clinical trial. Ann Emerg Med 2003;41:818-26.

‡Holve RL, Barkan H. Oral steroids in initial treatment of acute sciatica. J Am Board Fam Med 2008;21:469-74.

§Wevster BS, Verma SK, Gatchel RJ. Relationship between early opioid prescribing for acute occupational low back pain and disability duration, medical costs, subsequent surgery and late opioid use. Spine 2007;32:2127-32.

‖Dahm KT, Brurberg KG, Jamtvedt G, et al. Advice to rest in bed versus advice to stay active for acute low-lack pain and sciatica. Cochrane Database Syst Rev 2020;6:CD007612.

¶Sculco AD, Paup DC, Fernhall B, et al. Effects of aerobic exercise on low back pain patients in treatment. Spine J 2001;1:95-101.

**Ghou R, Huffman LH. Nonpharmacologic therapies for acute and chronic low back pain: a review of the evidence for an American Pain Society/American College of Physicians clinical practice guideline. Ann Intern Med 2007;147:492-504.

other medications for acute or subacute LBP and may lead to higher rates of chronic pain.[12] See **Table 92.4** for other treatment modalities.

Patients frequently prefer "alternative" modes of therapy (e.g., chiropractic or osteopathic spinal manipulation, acupuncture, massage, magnets) over traditional allopathic approaches. In most cases there are neither proven benefits nor drawbacks to these therapies[13]; however, patients will often use them regardless of physician recommendations. Risk for CES may be increased following manipulation in patients with disk disease, tumors, or other specific diseases of the spinal column.

## ADMISSION AND DISCHARGE

Admission to the hospital may be required for further evaluation, testing, and treatment, including further diagnostic testing and consultation, as well as relief of symptoms.

Patients with nonspecific LBP can be discharged home in almost all circumstances; there appears to be limited need or utility in admitting patients for pain control. All patients with LBP who are discharged from the ED should be warned about the risk for CES and be told to return if they experience neurologic or bowel or bladder symptoms.[14]

Counseling patients with nonspecific LBP that the ED work-up has not found any concerning pathology, that they can expect their pain to get better, and that pain does not necessarily mean danger will help manage their expectations. They should be told to continue their normal activities of daily living as limited by their symptoms. Finally, they should be advised to arrange follow-up with a primary care provider because LBP can recur frequently and may better be managed with continuity of care.

Patients with specific systemic or visceral sources of their LBP require specialist consultation.

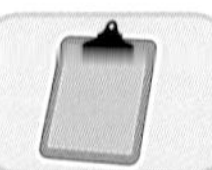

**DOCUMENTATION**

Presence or absence of "red flags" suggesting specific, systemic, or visceral sources of the patient's complaints

Findings from a systematic neurologic examination of the lower extremities, including sacral nerve function

Discussion of findings requiring urgent work-up, including consultations (because of a possible specific cause, neurologic compromise, or spinal instability)

Discussions with patients and their families or friends (specific instructions about follow-up and warning signs suggesting cauda equina syndrome requiring immediate evaluation)

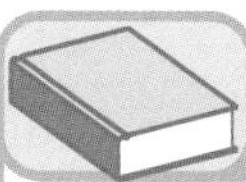

### PATIENT TEACHING TIPS

Low back pain is a common problem, with four of every five adults having back pain at some time in their lifetime.

The most common causes of low back pain are:

- *Muscle strains and spasm*: Poor posture and improper or excessive lifting or twisting may cause strains or spasms of the muscles that support the back.
- *Degenerative processes*: As people age, the disks between the spine's bones that provide cushioning and lubrication dry and harden, and the spine stiffens, which leads to pain and discomfort.
- *Sciatica*: Compression or "pinching" of nerves (perhaps from a disk that bulges out from between the backbones) causes pain from the back to travel down the leg.

Treatment of low back pain (what doctors call "conservative therapy") includes:

1. Over-the-counter pain relievers such as ibuprofen (Advil, Motrin, Nuprin), naproxen sodium (Aleve), and aspirin:
   - Aspirin and other nonsteroidal antiinflammatory drugs (NSAIDs) can cause stomach problems and should be taken with food or milk.
   - If you are taking blood thinners, ask your doctor or pharmacist whether it is safe to take NSAIDs or aspirin.
   - Acetaminophen (Tylenol) is less likely than aspirin and other NSAIDs to bother your stomach.
2. Application of ice in the first 24 hours of symptoms, with moist heat on the following days.
3. Gradual return to normal activities, including walking, without the need for special exercises.
   - "Bed rest" does not help and may actually slow the recovery process.

Follow up with your primary care provider to make sure that you are getting better and to help minimize recurrence of your symptoms. If you have back pain plus *any* of the following signs or symptoms, call your doctor:

- Fever above 100.5° F (38° C)
- Past use of steroids, such as prednisone, for more than 1 week
- Unexplainad weight loss
- Pain that gets worse or does not get better when you stop moving and rest or lie flat in bed
- Pain that awakens you from sleep
- An injury to your back from a fall, a car crash, or an assault
- Bladder or bowel problems
- Weakness in your legs, as opposed to pain
- Severe pain despite the use of medications prescribed by your doctor
- A personal history of cancer

## REFERENCES

*References can be found on Expert Consult @ www.expertconsult.com.*

# 93 Intimate Partner Violence

*Abigail D. Hankin and Debra E. Houry*

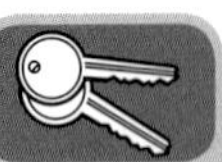

**KEY POINTS**

- The estimated prevalence of intimate partner violence victimization in women accessing emergency departments is as high as 36% in some populations.
- Interpersonal violence occurs across all populations regardless of social, economic, religious, cultural, or sexual orientation factors.
- More than 40% of women murdered by an intimate partner had visited an emergency department within 2 years of the homicide, and more than 90% had at least one visit for an injury.
- The emergency department serves a critical role to screen for, identify, and provide help to victims of intimate partner violence.

## EPIDEMIOLOGY

The Centers for Disease Control and Prevention defines intimate partner violence (IPV) as threatened or current physical, sexual, or verbal abuse inflicted by a spouse, former spouse, or current or former boyfriend, girlfriend, or dating partner. Among women alone, IPV is estimated to result in 2 million injuries and 1300 deaths annually. Costs associated with IPV are estimated to be $5.8 million in the United States each year.[1] It is estimated that 40% to 60% of homicides of women in the United States occur as a result of IPV.[2]

Although IPV is commonly thought to affect women and be perpetrated by men, studies suggest that women may be perpetrators of IPV as often as men, but male victims may be less likely to sustain physical injuries and seek medical care.[3] Additionally, counter to these perceptions, a recent emergency department (ED)-based study performed in an urban ED found that 31% of men who had been in a relationship during the previous year had experienced some form of IPV victimization.[4] In same-sex partners, IPV appears to occur at rates similar to that in heterosexual couples and with similar patterns, types of violence, and inciting factors.[5]

## PATHOPHYSIOLOGY

The etiologic factors and mechanisms mediating IPV are both complex and the subject of ongoing dispute by researchers in the field. Known factors associated with increased risk for IPV include poverty, societal and individual views of gender relationships, relationship conflict, alcohol use, and societal views about the use of violence in conflict.[6] The sequelae of IPV range from mental health issues and minor injuries to multisystem trauma and death.[7]

## PRESENTING SIGNS AND SYMPTOMS

### HISTORY

Victims of IPV often do not disclose their abuse to health providers, and studies have shown that some victims will even deny abuse when directly asked.[8] Surveys of IPV victims suggest that women fail to disclose victimization when physicians do not ask about abuse, when patients perceive that the provider lacks time or interest in their disclosure, or when they have concerns about police involvement or loss of confidentiality.[9] The probability of IPV disclosure may be increased if clinicians provide a reason for inquiring about abuse, create an atmosphere of concern and support, and provide informational resources about IPV regardless of patient disclosure.[8]

In addition to direct inquiry by a clinician, recent ED-based studies have found that patient disclosure of abuse is increased when the ED uses an automated system of IPV screening, such as a computer-based screening questionnaire.[10]

### PHYSICAL FINDINGS

Most commonly, IPV victims seek treatment in health care settings for complaints not directly related to their abuse or with obvious physical trauma.[11] When IPV victims are seen in the ED with evidence of physical trauma, women who are victims of IPV are more likely to have trauma involving the head, face, neck, thorax, breasts, and abdomen than are women with trauma attributable to other causes.[12] In addition, injuries in various stages of healing or defensive injuries may be noted.

Although any pattern or mechanism of injury may be the result of IPV, clinicians should have a low threshold for suspecting IPV when seeing women with blunt trauma to the head, neck, and face (particularly as a result of punching or

**BOX 93.1 Common Acute Patterns of Injury Associated with Intimate Partner Violence Victimization**

**Mechanisms**
Blunt trauma with a hand (slapping, punching)
Blunt trauma with a household object used as a weapon
Penetrating trauma with a sharp object or knife
Strangulation with hands or a ligature
Sexual assault

**Locations of Injuries**
Face
Head
Neck
Chest
Genitals

From Sheridan DJ, Nash KR. Acute injury patterns of intimate partner violence victims. Trauma Violence Abuse 2007;8:281.

slapping). Across all injuries, women who are victims of IPV are more likely to have blunt trauma injuries caused by being struck or kicked or by objects used as weapons than to have an injury caused by a knife or gun. Two other common injury patterns are strangulation and sexual assault, both of which may leave scant or no physical evidence and thus may be missed by a clinician who does not suspect abuse.[7]

Persistent health problems resulting from IPV include chronic headaches; chronic back pain; neurologic symptoms, including fainting and seizures; gastrointestinal complaints, including poor appetite, eating disorders, and irritable bowel syndrome; and cardiac symptoms, including recurrent chest pain and hypertension.[11] IPV victimization is also significantly correlated with an increased risk for mental health problems, including depression, suicidality, and posttraumatic stress disorder.[13] Long after the abuse has ended, IPV victimization has long-term consequences on health status, quality of life, and use of health care resources[11] (**Box 93.1**).

## DIFFERENTIAL DIAGNOSIS AND MEDICAL DECISION MAKING

The differential diagnosis of injuries attributable to IPV include injuries related to unintentional causes, such as household injuries or motor vehicle collisions, as well as self-inflicted injuries. The cause of the injury may be distinguished by the physical patterns of injury and the history provided by patients, although no approach can entirely rule out the possibility that an injury was caused by IPV. Additionally, IPV victimization should be considered in the differential diagnosis of many patients seen in the ED with complaints unrelated to injury, including depression, abdominal pain, headaches, and chest pain, among others.

If IPV victimization is suspected, the physician should perform a thorough social history, including living situation and perceived safety at home, relationships, and access to social, familial, and financial support. Even though no diagnostic test can confirm or refute an abuse history, in some cases obtaining radiographic or photographic documentation (or both) of injuries may be useful for subsequent prosecution of the perpetrator (see the Red Flags box).

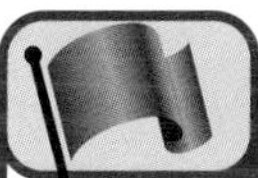

**RED FLAGS**

**Symptoms and History Suggestive of Interpersonal Violence**
Blunt trauma to the head, face, and neck
Frequent headaches
Sexually transmitted diseases
Chronic pelvic pain
Abdominal pain, indigestion, or frequent diarrhea or constipation
Vague history of injury or a history inconsistent with injuries
Injuries in multiple stages of healing
Partner will not leave patient's side

From Coker AL, Smith PH, Bethea L, et al. Physical health consequences of physical and psychological intimate partner violence. Arch Fam Med 2000;9:451.

## TREATMENT

Interventions for patients who are known or suspected to be victims of IPV focus on (1) treating any acute injury resulting from the violent incident, (2) ensuring the patient's physical safety after discharge, and (3) providing referrals and resources to at-risk patients.

In the prehospital and hospital setting, priority should be placed on identifying and stabilizing physical injuries. A complete physical examination and detailed history are a priority because the patient may have prior, incompletely healed injuries that are unrelated to the trauma prompting the present visit.

History taking should focus on the mechanism of injury, as well as inquiries into the patient's safety at home. A majority of states have laws mandating physicians to report injuries resulting from IPV; clinicians should be aware of laws pertaining to mandatory reporting in the locations where they practice. In addition to facilitating contact with law enforcement agencies, the treating clinician should ensure that the patient and any children will have a safe place to stay after discharge and should facilitate referrals to social services or local support agencies if the patient does not have a safe home setting.

If a clinician suspects that a patient may be at risk for IPV but there is no clear history of recent or current victimization, providing the patient with educational material about the warning signs of at-risk relationships and information about local support organizations and shelters may be appropriate (see the Priority Actions box).

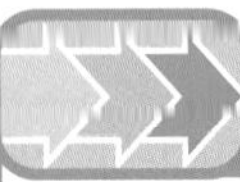

### PRIORITY ACTIONS

Stabilize and manage any physical injuries caused by interpersonal violence (IPV).

Identify and treat any secondary or partially healed injuries.

Contact law enforcement if reporting is locally mandated or desired by the patient.

Ensure that the patient has a safe place to stay and that any children are in a safe location.

Provide the patient with referral to social services or local resources for victims of IPV (or to both).

Educate patients who may be at risk for IPV about the danger signs and local resources.

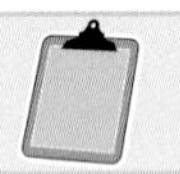

### DOCUMENTATION

**History of Present Illness**

Mechanism of injury

Name and relationship of assailant

Other recent injuries

Any threats of further violence by the assailant

**Physical Examination**

Locations of injuries, as well as any evidence of old injuries (e.g., bruises in various stages of healing)

Physical evidence of the mechanism of injury (e.g., hand or bite marks)

**Social History**

Home situation:

- Children present and safe?
- Other occupants of the home?
- Does the victim live with the assailant?
- Temporary housing options?
- Does the victim believe that he or she will be safe if discharged?

Other:

- Symptoms of depression?
- Any homicidal or suicidal ideation?
- Substance abuse?

**Plan of Care**

Document any reports to law enforcement or refusal by the patient of an offer to contact local law enforcement.

Document contact with social services and plan for ensuring the patient's safety on discharge.

If the social history revealed coexisting mental health problems, document referrals or consultation with psychiatry service.

## FOLLOW-UP, NEXT STEPS IN CARE, AND PATIENT EDUCATION

The decision to admit patients victimized by IPV should be dictated by the severity of the injuries or non trauma related complaints, as well as the patient's safety at home. If the patient has minor injuries but no safe place to stay, admission may be indicated to allow time for the patient to work with social services staff to ensure safe discharge.

In addition to thorough documentation of the patient's history of the present illness and findings on physical examination, it is essential that the treating clinician document details about the patient's home situation, including (1) whether the patient lives with the assailant, (2) whether children are living in the home and plans for ensuring the safety of the children, (3) temporary alternative housing options available to the patient, and (4) whether the patient believes that she will be safe if discharged. In addition, given the high correlation between IPV and depression, the social history should also include inquiries into the patient's substance use, as well as symptoms of depression or any suicidal or homicidal ideation (see the Documentation box).

## SUGGESTED READINGS

Houry D, Kaslow N, Kemball R, et al. Does screening in the emergency department hurt or help victims of intimate partner violence? Ann Emerg Med 2008;51:433-42.e7.

Jewkes R. Intimate partner violence: causes and prevention. Lancet 2002;359:1423-9.

Rodríguez MA, Sheldon WR, Bauer HM, et al. The factors associated with disclosure of intimate partner abuse to clinicians. J Fam Pract 2001;50:338-44.

Wu V. Pattern of physical injury associated with IPV in women presenting to the ED: a systematic review and meta-analysis. Trauma Violence Abuse 2010;11:71-82.

## REFERENCES

*References can be found on Expert Consult @ www.expertconsult.com.*

# Altered Mental Status and Coma 94

Benjamin S. Bassin, Jeremy L. Cooke, and William G. Barsan

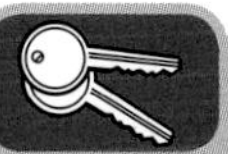

**KEY POINTS**

- Because the differential diagnosis of coma is broad, a systematic approach to patient evaluation and diagnostic testing is required.
- Patients with altered mental status may have subtle neurologic dysfunction, so careful neurologic examination is necessary.
- Quickly reversible causes should be sought before the initiation of a more lengthy diagnostic work-up. Naloxone, dextrose, and thiamine administration should be considered initially in patients with undifferentiated coma.
- Structural brain lesions that may require operative intervention dictate immediate consultation with a neurosurgical service.

## PERSPECTIVE

Altered mental status is a spectrum of disease ranging from sleepiness and confusion to frank coma. Approximately 3% of patients arrive at the emergency department (ED) in a altered state.

## EPIDEMIOLOGY

Roughly 85% of cases of altered mental status are caused by metabolic or systemic derangements, whereas 15% are caused by structural lesions. Once the ABCs (airway, breathing, and circulation) have been controlled and the patient stabilized, it is the role of the emergency physician (EP) to quickly distinguish structural from metabolic and systemic causes.

## PATHOPHYSIOLOGY

Consciousness is collectively made up of arousal and cognition. Arousal is defined as the awareness of self and the surroundings. The neuroanatomic structure primarily responsible for arousal is the ascending reticular activating system, which is located in the dorsal part of the brainstem. It controls the input of somatic and sensory stimuli to the cerebral cortex and functions to initiate arousal from sleep. Cognition is the combination of *orientation* (accurate perception of what is experienced), *judgment* (the ability to process input data to generate more meaningful information), and *memory* (the ability to store and retrieve information). The brain's cognition centers are located primarily in the cerebral cortex.

Coma can be caused by damage to the brainstem (**Fig. 94.1**), the cerebral cortex, or both. These structures are vulnerable to toxins, metabolic derangements, and mechanical injury. Localized, unilateral lesions in the cerebral cortex do not usually induce altered mental status or coma, even with other cognitive functions being impaired. However, if both cerebral hemispheres are affected, altered mental status or coma can occur, depending on the size of the insult and its speed of progression. The ascending reticular activating system can also be vulnerable to small, focal lesions in the brainstem, which can result in coma.[1,2]

## PRESENTING SIGNS AND SYMPTOMS

The chief complaints of patients and their family members are highly variable along the spectrum of altered mental status. Patients may report increased sleepiness or periods of confusion and disorientation. They may have trouble concentrating or maintaining focus on tasks that were previously performed without difficulty. Family members may describe the patient as being less interactive or more difficult to arouse from sleep.

Regardless of the circumstance, the EP will frequently need to use alternative sources of information to answer key historical questions that may alter the breadth and speed of the diagnostic work-up undertaken. Common sources of information include family members, neighbors, prehospital personnel, law enforcement, and nursing home staff.[3] They may know of preceding symptoms such as headache, nausea, vomiting, or fever. It is important to determine the rate of symptom onset and whether the patient had any history of trauma, exposure to drugs or toxins, or new medications or change in dosage. Family members usually have some knowledge regarding the patient's past medical history. Additionally, previous medical records should be reviewed whenever possible to confirm or augment the information provided. If the patient's historical baseline mental status cannot be established, the current findings must be assumed to be an acute change.[4]

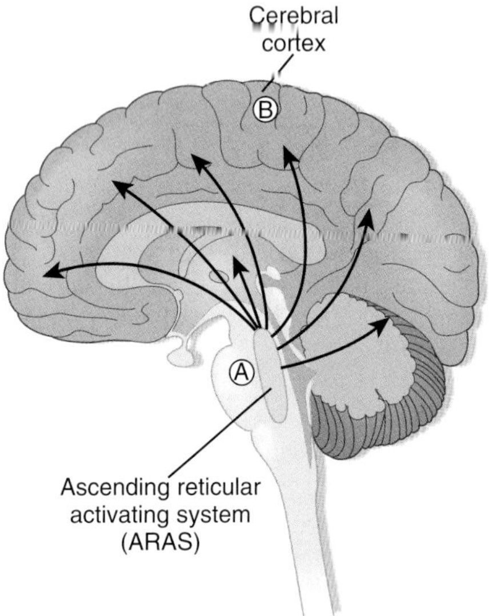


**Fig. 94.1 Cerebral insults leading to a depressed level of consciousness.** *A*, Ascending reticular activating system; *B*, bilateral cerebral cortex.

**BOX 94.1 Common Age-Related Causes of Altered Mental Status and Coma**

**Infant**
Infection
Trauma, abuse
Metabolic

**Child**
Toxic ingestion

**Adolescent, Young Adult**
Toxic ingestion
Recreational drug use
Trauma

**Elderly**
Medication changes
Over-the-counter medications
Infection
Alterations in living environment
Stroke
Trauma

The age of the patient can be a key historical tool that may focus the physician on the most probable cause of the patient's symptoms (**Box 94.1**).

In infants, infectious causes of altered mental status are most common; however, nonaccidental trauma and metabolic derangements from inborn errors of metabolism are also possible causes.[5] Toxic ingestions are commonly seen in young children. Adolescents and young adults are often seen in the ED after recreational drug use. The elderly are particularly susceptible to infectious causes and to disorders related to changes in medications or drug doses, use of over-the-counter medications, and alterations in their living environment. Psychiatric illness should be considered in the adolescent through elderly population and must be distinguished from medical illness as a cause of the patient's symptoms.

**BOX 94.2 Structural Causes of Altered Mental Status and Coma**

Trauma
- Subdural hematoma
- Epidural hematoma
- Cerebral concussion, contusion

Stroke syndromes
- Embolism
  - Cardiac (atrial fibrillation, endocarditis)
  - Paradoxic (fat embolus)
- Thrombosis
  - Basilar artery occlusion
  - Cerebral venous sinus thrombosis

Hemorrhage
- Subarachnoid hemorrhage
- Pontine hemorrhage
- Cerebellar hemorrhage
- Intracerebral hemorrhage

Tumor
- Brainstem tumors
- Metastatic disease
- Angiomas

Pituitary apoplexy
Acute hydrocephalus
Infection
- Subdural empyema, abscess

As with all patients, specific attention should first be paid to assessment of the ABCs and specific vital signs. Alterations in respiratory patterns such as hyperventilation, Kussmaul or Cheyne-Stokes breathing, agonal breathing, or apnea should be noted and may suggest toxic or metabolic derangements or primary central nervous system abnormalities. Marked hypotension or hypertension should be addressed immediately even if the underlying cause is unknown. Bradycardia may be the result of increased intracranial pressure as seen in the Cushing response and suggests a state of hypoperfusion. Tachycardia may also result in hypoperfusion and can be the result of toxic, metabolic, or primary cardiac causes. Assessment of temperature is crucial because both hypothermia and hyperthermia can cause altered mental status from infectious, structural (**Box 94.2**), environmental exposure, or toxic or metabolic causes (**Box 94.3**).

Any signs of trauma should be sought immediately. Scalp lacerations or hematomas, depressed skull fractures, hemotympanum, raccoon eyes, Battle sign, cerebrospinal fluid oto-rhinorrhea, cervical spine step-offs, and crepitus all suggest a traumatic cause. Other signs of trauma include lesions on the chest, abdomen, or pelvis; long-bone deformities; and gross blood in the rectum or vagina or at the urethral meatus.

In the absence of trauma, breath odors may be helpful, including the smell of alcohol, ketones (diabetic or alcoholic ketoacidosis), and bitter almonds (cyanide toxicity). Abdominal findings include ascites, hepatosplenomegaly, ecchymosis, and striae. Lesions on the skin such as rashes, signs of drug use (needle tracks, medication patches), and embolic phenomena can be telling.

**BOX 94.3 Metabolic and Systemic Causes of Altered Mental Status and Coma**

**Hypoxia, Hypercapnia**
Severe pulmonary disease (hypoventilation)
Severe anemia
Environmental, toxic
Methemoglobinemia
Cyanide
Carbon monoxide
Decreased atmospheric oxygen (high altitude)
Near-drowning

**Glucose Disorders**
Hypoglycemia
- Chronic alcohol abuse and liver disease
- Excessive dosage of insulin or other hypoglycemic agents
- Insulinoma

Hyperglycemia
- Diabetic ketoacidosis
- Nonketotic hyperosmolar coma

**Decreased Cerebral Blood Flow**
Hypovolemic shock
Cardiac
- Vasovagal syncope
- Arrhythmias
- Myocardial infarction
- Valvular disorders
- Congestive heart failure
- Pericardial effusion, tamponade
- Myocarditis

Infectious
- Septic shock
- Bacterial meningitis

Vascular, hematologic
- Hypertensive encephalopathy
- Pseudotumor cerebri
- Hyperviscosity (sickle cell, polycythemia)
- Hyperventilation
- Cerebral vasculitis as a manifestation of systemic lupus erythematosus
- Thrombotic thrombocytopenic purpura
- Disseminated intravascular coagulation

**Metabolic Cofactor Deficiency**
Thiamine (Wernicke-Korsakoff syndrome)
Pyridoxine (isoniazid overdose)
Folic acid (chronic alcohol abuse)
Cyanocobalamin
Niacin

**Electrolyte, pH Disturbances**
Acidosis, alkalosis
Hypernatremia, hyponatremia*
Hypercalcemia, hypocalcemia
Hypophosphatemia
Hypermagnesemia, hypomagnesemia

**Endocrine Disorders**
Myxedema coma, thyrotoxicosis
Hypopituitarism
Addison disease (primary or secondary)
Cushing disease
Pheochromocytoma
Hyperparathyroidism, hypoparathyroidism

**Endogenous Toxins**
Hyperammonemia (liver failure)
Uremia (renal disease)
Carbon dioxide narcosis (pulmonary disease)
Porphyria

**Exogenous Toxins**
Alcohols
- Ethanol, isopropyl alcohol, methanol, ethylene glycol

Acid poisons
- Salicylates
- Paraldehyde
- Ammonium chloride

Antidepressant medications
- Lithium
- Tricyclic antidepressants
- Selective serotonin reuptake inhibitors
- Monoamine oxidase inhibitors

Stimulants
- Amphetamines, methamphetamines
- Cocaine
- Over-the-counter sympathomimetics

Narcotics, opiates
- Morphine
- Heroin
- Codeine, oxycodone, meperidine, hydrocodone
- Methadone
- Fentanyl
- Propoxyphene

Sedative-hypnotics
- Benzodiazepines
- Barbiturates
- Rohypnol
- Bromide

Hallucinogens
- Lysergic acid diethylamide
- Marijuana
- Mescaline, peyote
- Mushrooms
- Phencyclidine

Herbs, plants
- Aconite
- Jimsonweed
- Morning glory

Volatile substances
- Hydrocarbons (gasoline, butane, toluene, benzene, chloroform)
- Nitrites
- Anesthetic agents (nitrous oxide, ether)

Other
- γ-Hydroxybutyrate
- Ketamine
- Penicillin
- Cardiac glycosides

Continued

**BOX 94.3 Metabolic and Systemic Causes of Altered Mental Status and Coma—cont'd**

- Anticonvulsants
- Steroids
- Heavy metals
- Cimetidine
- Organophosphates

**Disorders of Temperature Regulation, Environmental**
Hypothermia
Heat stroke
Malignant hyperthermia
Neuroleptic malignant syndrome
High-altitude cerebral edema
Dysbarism

**Primary Glial or Neuronal Disorders**
Adrenoleukodystrophy
Creutzfeldt-Jakob disease
Progressive multifocal leukoencephalopathy
Marchiafava-Bignami disease
Gliomatosis cerebri
Central pontine myelinolysis

**Other Disorders with Unknown Etiology**
Seizures
Postictal states
Reye syndrome†
Intussusception†

*Can be associated with dilution of formula in infant feeding.
†Prominent in the pediatric population.

## NEUROLOGIC EVALUATION

A systematic neurologic examination is a key tool in determining whether the cause is structural, systemic, or metabolic. The basic examination includes evaluation of the patient's level of alertness, cranial nerves, strength, sensation, reflexes, gait, and cerebellar function.

The Glasgow Coma Scale (GCS) can be used to assess the patient's level of consciousness. The GCS does not differentiate between causes of altered mental status or coma or assess cognition. However, it is useful in monitoring changes in mental status when serial examinations are performed and serves as an objective reference when communicating with consultants (**Table 94.1**).[6]

A focal neurologic deficit usually suggests a structural cause. Pupillary findings such as unilateral dilation or a "blown pupil" and loss of reactivity indicate uncal herniation, which is a neurosurgical emergency. Funduscopic examination can demonstrate hemorrhage in the setting of trauma or papilledema, which suggests increased intracranial pressure.[2]

Testing of eye movements is a hallmark in the neurologic examination of patients with altered mental status or coma. Eye movements are coordinated by ocular centers in the cerebral cortex and the medial longitudinal fasciculus located in the brainstem. The extraocular muscles are innervated primarily by cranial nerves III, IV, and VI. Disconjugate gaze in the horizontal plane is common and can be associated with sedated or drowsy states or alcohol intoxication. Disconjugate gaze in the vertical plane is more ominous and points to pontine or cerebellar lesions. A persistently *adducted* eye is caused by cranial nerve VI paresis, whereas a persistently *abducted* eye is caused by cranial nerve III paresis. These are nonlocalizing lesions; however, elevated intracranial pressure or mass effects from trauma, for example, can compromise cranial nerve functions via extrinsic compression. In the absence of contraindications, oculocephalic (doll's eyes) or oculovestibular reflex testing can be very helpful. If intact, these reflexes demonstrate functional integrity of a significant

**Table 94.1 Glasgow Coma Scale**

| | | SCORE |
|---|---|---|
| Eye opening | Spontaneous | 4 |
| | To voice | 3 |
| | To pain | 2 |
| | None | 1 |
| Verbal response | | |
| Adult | Oriented | 5 |
| | Confused | 4 |
| | Inappropriate words | 3 |
| | Incomprehensible words | 2 |
| | None | 1 |
| Pediatric | Appropriate | 5 |
| | Cries, consolable | 4 |
| | Persistently irritable | 3 |
| | Restless, agitated | 2 |
| | None | 1 |
| Motor response | Obeys commands | 6 |
| | Localizes pain | 5 |
| | Withdraws to pain | 4 |
| | Flexion to pain | 3 |
| | Extension to pain | 2 |
| | None | 1 |
| Maximum score | | 15 |

majority of the brainstem, thus making it exceedingly unlikely as the anatomic location for the cause of the patient's altered mental status.[1,2,5,7]

## DIFFERENTIAL DIAGNOSIS AND MEDICAL DECISION MAKING

The differential diagnosis of altered mental status and coma is extensive and can be daunting for the busy EP (see Boxes 94.1 to 94.3). Fortunately, there are many distinguishing features in the physical examination that, when combined with information gleaned from the patient's history of the present illness, past medical history, and response to therapy (i.e., dextrose, naloxone), point to a particular cause and are frequently of greater diagnostic value than imaging, electrocardiograms (ECGs), and laboratory tests.[1] However, a systematic approach is best and reduces the likelihood of missing an important clue.[1,2,8]

## DIAGNOSTIC TESTING

Diagnostic testing in patients with altered mental status or coma is based on information gathered from the history and physical examination, which in most cases will point toward a structural versus systemic or metabolic cause. Extensive metabolic work-ups should not precede neuroimaging studies in patients with altered mental status or coma that may be due to structural causes. Similarly, treatment of suspected narcotic overdose or hypoglycemia should not be delayed in favor of imaging studies. However, in undifferentiated patients, diagnostic tests should be performed in parallel whenever possible to avoid unnecessary delays in initiating treatment. A general approach to the diagnostic work-up of patients with altered mental status or coma is shown in **Figure 94.2**.

### LABORATORY EVALUATION

Basic laboratory studies are useful in determining the most common metabolic causes of altered mental status. Capillary blood glucose measurement, both prehospital and on arrival at the ED, can often avoid further extensive work-ups, especially in patients with diabetes or alcohol intoxication. Serum electrolytes and renal function studies may demonstrate an anion gap acidosis or significant sodium or potassium imbalance or uremia. Serum calcium may be a marker for metastatic disease, and severe hypercalcemia can be associated with altered mental status.

A complete blood cell count may demonstrate profound anemia from witnessed or occult blood loss. A low white blood cell count raises concern for an immunocompromised state, but an elevated white blood cell count is less helpful in making the diagnosis as a nonspecific marker for infection, inflammation, or stress. Low platelet levels may indicate sepsis, disseminated intravascular coagulation, or intracranial bleeding. Serum coagulation studies may be performed to look for bleeding dyscrasias or supratherapeutic levels of anticoagulants (warfarin) or, when combined with other liver function studies, may provide evidence of liver dysfunction. Both platelet counts and coagulation studies should be performed before obtaining central venous access and performing lumbar puncture or other invasive procedures if time or the patient's condition allows. Checking the serum ammonia level is controversial; it has not been shown to be a reliable marker for the cause of altered mental status because it can be normal in patients with hepatic encephalopathy but can also be elevated in those with acute hepatic failure from other causes, as well as valproic acid toxicity and inborn errors of metabolism.[9]

Thyroid function studies are useful in patients with suspected myxedema coma secondary to hypothyroidism. Arterial blood gas (ABG) analysis can demonstrate hypercapnia or hypoxia and aid in the classification of acid-base disturbances. Cooximetry can be added to ABG analysis to determine carbon monoxide levels or methemoglobinemia. In the absence of contraindications, cerebrospinal fluid analysis is mandatory when considering a central nervous system infectious cause or to rule out subarachnoid hemorrhage after a negative, non–contrast-enhanced computed tomography (CT) scan of the brain.

Urinalysis is a useful tool that provides information about volume status (specific gravity), spilling of glucose as in hyperosmolar coma, and evidence of infection, which is a common cause of altered mental status in the elderly. Urine drug screening for illicit drug use as a cause of altered mental status is often less helpful unless other causes are not forthcoming, but it may help confirm a suspected diagnosis. Microscopic analysis of urine can reveal calcium oxalate crystals in the setting of ethylene glycol ingestion.

### IMAGING

The mainstay of diagnostic imaging in the setting of altered mental status is non–contrast-enhanced CT of the brain. It is fast and readily available in most ED settings and can reveal the vast majority of intracranial hemorrhages large enough to induce coma. Hydrocephalus is also readily detected on non–contrast-enhanced CT. If subarachnoid hemorrhage is suspected, negative CT findings should be followed by lumbar puncture. When tumor or infection is suspected, contrast-enhanced CT may be indicated.

A limitation of brain CT scanning is the potential poor view of the posterior fossa as a result of linear artifacts created by the thick skull base. Magnetic resonance imaging (MRI) of the brain is more helpful in identifying structural lesions in this area; however, its cost and limited availability, as well as the inability to monitor unstable patients, make this imaging modality less feasible in some ED settings.[4] CT angiography or venography may be available for the diagnosis or treatment (or both) of vertebral or basilar artery stenosis or occlusion, intracerebral aneurysms, cerebral venous sinus thrombosis, or arteriovenous malformations. If brain abscess or metastatic lesions are a concern, contrast-enhanced head CT can be useful in making the diagnosis.

Other diagnostic tools include plain radiography, which can reveal serious pneumonia, acute respiratory distress syndrome, ingested illicit substances seen in "body packers," or specific types of ingestions such as mercury, iron, and lead. This can be particularly helpful in the pediatric population when the history is not reliable. ECGs are useful for diagnosing certain ingestions (e.g., tricyclic antidepressants), electrolyte abnormalities (e.g., potassium, calcium), and hypothermia. Though not commonly used in the ED, electroencephalographic monitoring is mandatory for comatose patients with suspected status epilepticus.

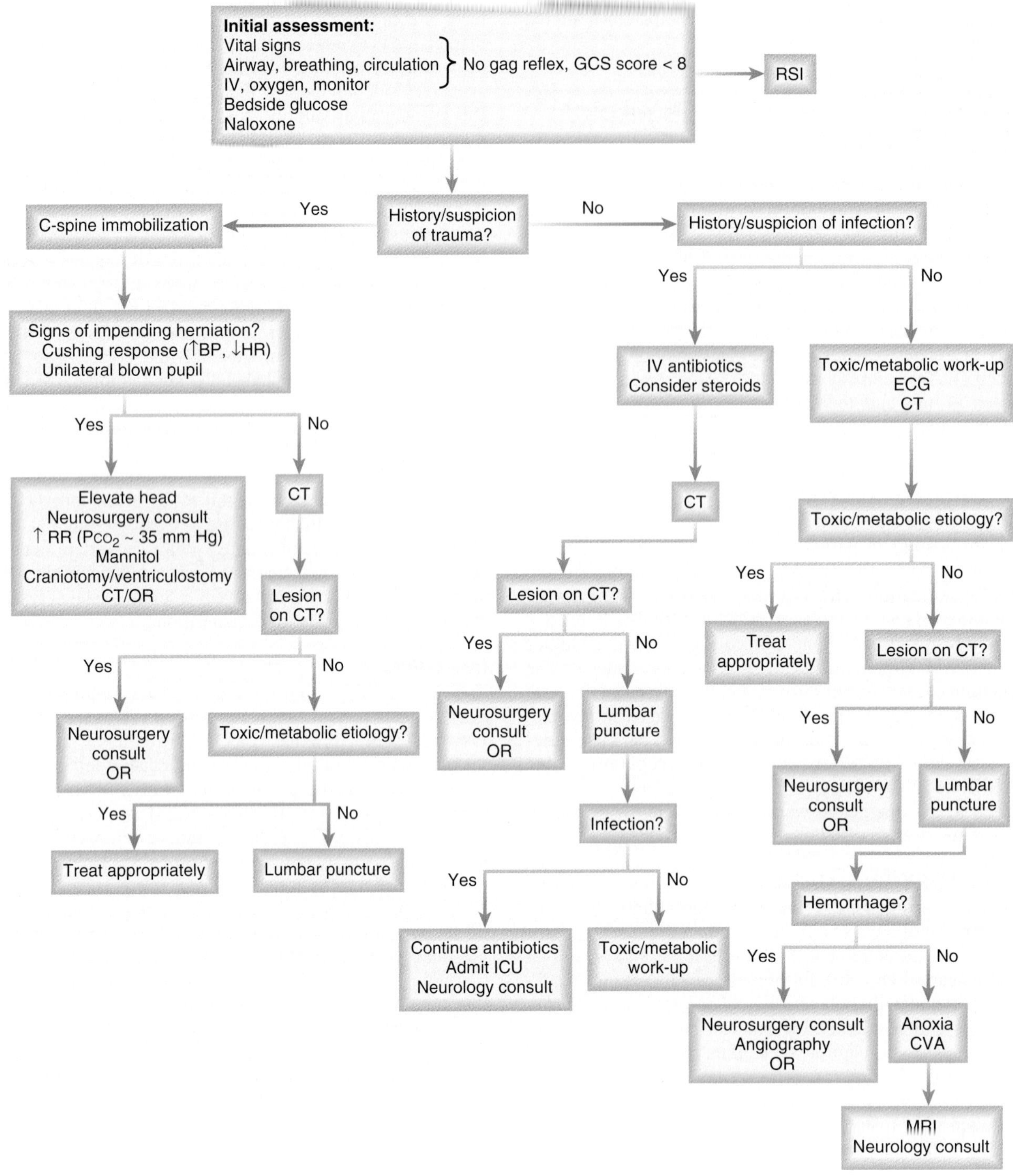


**Fig. 94.2 Diagnostic approach to altered mental status and coma.** *BP*, Blood pressure; *CT*, computed tomography; *CVA*, cerebrovascular accident; *ECG*, electrocardiography; *GCS*, Glasgow Coma Scale; *HR*, heart rate; *ICU*, intensive care unit; *MRI*, magnetic resonance imaging; *OR*, operating room; *RR*, respiratory rate; *RSI*, rapid-sequence intubation.

## TREATMENT

Initial stabilization and quick control of the ABCs are paramount in patients with altered mental status. Patients should be placed immediately on telemetry with concomitant administration of oxygen and initiation of intravenous access. Definitive airway control with endotracheal intubation is critical in patients without a gag reflex or with a GCS score lower than 8. Lidocaine premedication should be used for rapid-sequence intubation in patients with suspected elevated intracranial pressure. In the setting of trauma, maintaining spinal precautions with a backboard in addition to initiation of intravenous fluid therapy is mandatory.

Once initial stabilization has been addressed, reversible causes must be sought. A bedside ECG and capillary blood glucose test should be obtained immediately. Blood and urine should be sent to the laboratory for studies early after the patient's arrival, and the patient should be scheduled for emergency head CT. Empiric administration of a "coma cocktail" consisting of dextrose, thiamine, and naloxone is controversial but may bring immediate results and significantly narrow the differential diagnosis.

Physical examination with specific attention to brainstem function dictates further work-up and therapy. Patients whose brainstem function is compromised with evidence of brain herniation require immediate evaluation by neurosurgery. Empiric therapy with mannitol may be indicated in this setting. Elevating the head of bed to 30 degrees (if not contraindicated) and hyperventilation to a $P_{CO_2}$ of 35 mm Hg are additional temporizing measures. Evidence of brain herniation secondary to a traumatic cause may necessitate the use of burr holes on the side of the dilated pupil as a last resort. Ventriculostomy and monitoring of intracranial pressure are often performed by a neurosurgeon in the ED.

Patients with compromised brainstem function but no evidence of herniation should have immediate consideration for basilar artery or bilateral vertebral artery occlusion and undergo CT or magnetic resonance angiography while receiving supportive care with a concomitant toxic and metabolic work-up. Patients are considered to have unsalvageable brain tissue if they have no brainstem reflexes, have not received neuroactive medications, and are normothermic.

In patients whose brainstem function is intact, supportive care is provided while the work-up proceeds. Lesions discovered on brain CT require immediate evaluation by neurosurgery. In general, patients with operable lesions are transferred immediately to the operating room; patients with inoperable lesions continue to receive supportive care. In cases in which an infectious cause is suspected, empiric antibiotic coverage should not be delayed for lumbar puncture or other diagnostic modalities.

In the setting of suspected toxic ingestion, activated charcoal with or without sorbitol is indicated. Gastric lavage has been used in patients with recent (less than 60 minutes since ingestion), potentially lethal toxic ingestion (e.g., tricyclic antidepressants, beta-blockers); however, this intervention is somewhat controversial and associated with potential complications, including aspiration and esophageal damage. Specific antidotes, if applicable based on the history and physical examination, should be initiated early. Finally, early hemodialysis should be considered in patients who have ingested substances amenable to this therapeutic modality.[10]

## ADMISSION AND DISCHARGE

The majority of patients who have significant alterations in mental status require admission for further work-up and treatment. The exception is patients with an easily reversible cause, such as opiate overdose or hypoglycemia, who may be discharged after a period of observation during which there is a return to baseline mental status. In addition, patients with alcohol intoxication and no other cause of altered mental status may be discharged once they are deemed clinically sober. Placement in an intensive care unit setting is usually appropriate for patients whose mental status is persistently altered.

Immediate consultation with the neurosurgical service is paramount for patients with potentially operable lesions. After definitive airway control and stabilization of vital signs, rapid transfer to a center with neurosurgical diagnostic and therapeutic capabilities should be sought if the necessary resources are not available locally.

## SUGGESTED READINGS

American College of Emergency Physicians. Clinical policy for the initial approach to patients presenting with altered mental status. Ann Emerg Med 1999;33:251-81.

Feske SK. Coma and confusional states: emergency diagnosis and management. Neurol Clin 1998;16:237-56.

Hoffman R, Goldfrank L. The poisoned patient with altered consciousness. JAMA 1995;274:562-9.

Kanich W, Brady WJ, Huff JS, et al. Altered mental status: evaluation and etiology in the ED. Am J Emerg Med 2002;20:613-17.

Koita J, Riggio S, Jagoda A. The mental status examination in emergency practice. Emerg Med Clin North Am 2010;28:439-51.

## REFERENCES

***References can be found on Expert Consult @ www.expertconsult.com.***

# 95 Cranial Nerve Disorders

*Ernest E. Wang*

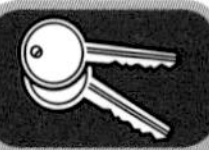

**KEY POINTS**

- The 12 cranial nerves supply motor and sensory innervation to the head and neck.
- Cranial nerve disorders generally cause visual disturbances, facial weakness, or facial pain or paresthesias, depending on the nerve or nerves involved.
- Trigeminal neuralgia and Bell palsy are common cranial nerve disorders.
- A thorough history and physical examination should focus on assessing the potential for trauma (skull fracture), tumor, cerebrovascular accidents, vascular derangements (aneurysm, dissection, thrombosis), and infection (meningitis, abscess).
- The presence of concomitant focal neurologic or systemic signs should heighten suspicion for a central rather than a peripheral cause of the neurologic dysfunction.

## PERSPECTIVE

The 12 cranial nerves provide motor and sensory innervation to the head and neck. Some nerves serve purely motor functions (cranial nerves III, IV, VI, XI, and XII), some serve purely sensory functions (cranial nerves I, II, and VIII), and the remainder serve mixed motor and sensory functions (cranial nerves V, VII, IX, and X).

In addition to somatic and visceral sensory components, the cranial nerves provide the special sensory functions of sight, smell, hearing, taste, and balance. Understanding the functions of individual cranial nerves aids in recognition of patterns of the clinical syndromes classically associated with disorders of specific cranial nerves.

## EPIDEMIOLOGY

Cranial neuropathies are a heterogeneous group of disorders with a variety of causes. Trauma is a common cause, and diabetes and hypertension are common comorbid conditions. Cranial nerves I, VI, and VII are the most frequently affected after minor head trauma.[1] Trigeminal neuralgia is a common cause of facial pain that affects approximately 4.5 per 100,000 individuals; women are affected twice as often as men, and it is more common in those older than 60 years.[2] Trigeminal neuralgia can be severely debilitating and has been termed the "suicide disease."[3] Bell palsy is the most common cause of acute facial paralysis worldwide. The peak age at incidence has been reported to be between 15 and 45 years,[4] but other investigators have noted an increased incidence in individuals older than 70.[5,6] Pregnant women and patients with diabetes have an associated increased incidence of the disease. A familial association of Bell palsy is noted in 4% of cases,[4] and it can cause both significant psychologic and physical morbidity.

## PATHOPHYSIOLOGY

### CRANIAL NERVE I (OLFACTORY NERVE)

#### *Anatomy*

Cranial nerve I is a special sensory nerve that provides the sense of smell. Inhaled scents are detected by the olfactory epithelium lining the nasal cavity and transmitted to the olfactory bulb, which lies adjacent to the cribriform plate of the ethmoid bone. Olfactory sensations are relayed from the olfactory bulb to the brain via the olfactory tract.

#### *Presenting Signs and Symptoms*

The patient should be questioned about a history of head trauma. An anteroposterior skull fracture parallel to the sagittal suture or an anteroposterior shearing injury can tear the olfactory fibers traversing the cribriform plate and lead to disruption of the synapses from the olfactory epithelium to the olfactory bulb.

A frontal lobe mass such as a tumor, meningioma, or abscess can compress the olfactory bulb as well, but the signs and symptoms associated with such masses tend to be more subacute.

#### *Treatment*

Treatment depends on the presence of concomitant injury. Basilar skull fracture and cerebrospinal fluid rhinorrhea associated with trauma require immediate neurosurgical consultation. A subacute mass or abscess should be managed in consultation with neurosurgery, depending on the acuity of the findings. Patients with anosmia secondary to trauma and normal findings on head computed tomography (CT) can referred to neurology or neurosurgery for outpatient follow-up.

## CRANIAL NERVE II (OPTIC NERVE)

### *Anatomy*

Visual stimuli are transmitted from the retina to the optic nerve through the optic chiasm to the lateral geniculate nucleus in the thalamus, where they synapse. From there, impulses are transmitted along the optic radiations (geniculocalcarine tracts, including the Meyer loop) to the primary visual cortex in the occipital lobes.

### *Presenting Signs and Symptoms*

Unilateral loss of vision is most common with injuries to the optic nerve. Patients with bilateral visual loss may not be aware of any such injury until an examination is performed. Acute visual loss is often of vascular origin, including central retinal arterial or venous occlusion and cerebrovascular disease. Neurologic causes, such as multiple sclerosis, may be suggested by progression of the visual loss over a period of hours or days, pain, and a history of additional neurologic complaints with a recurrent waxing and waning pattern. Inflammatory processes such as optic neuritis may be the initial symptom of multiple sclerosis.

Neuropathy from temporal arteritis usually occurs in elderly patients and is associated with progressive loss of vision (unilaterally or bilaterally), constitutional symptoms, jaw claudication, and headache.

Idiopathic intracranial hypertension should be considered in patients with a history of headache, visual scotomata, and visual changes. The typical patient is a young, heavy-set woman who is taking oral contraceptives. The headache and visual changes are typically worsened by coughing, bending over, or performing techniques such as the Valsalva maneuver.

Orbital compressive tumors or aneurysms cause mass effects that compromise optic nerve function.

### *Differential Diagnosis*

The differential patterns of visual loss are described in **Box 95.1**.

**BOX 95.1 Differential Patterns of Visual Loss**

A central retinal etiology of the fovea or optic disk compromises visual acuity or causes central loss of vision in the affected eye only.

Unilateral blindness is usually associated with an optic nerve lesion, and only the affected eye has complete visual field loss.

Unilateral nasal visual field loss can be caused by an internal carotid artery aneurysm compressing the lateral optic chiasm.

Bitemporal hemianopia can be caused by a midchiasmatic lesion.

Homonymous hemianopia from an optic tract lesion causes full contralateral visual field loss in both eyes.

Homonymous quadrantanopia secondary to a Meyer loop lesion causes contralateral one-quarter visual field loss in both eyes.

### *Treatment*

Treatment depends on the cause. Emergency ophthalmologic consultation is essential for vascular causes. Treatment of central retinal artery occlusion should focus on lowering intraocular pressure. Inpatient evaluation for neurologic causes is warranted depending on the clinical findings. Temporal arteritis requires high-dose steroid therapy. Idiopathic intracranial hypertension requires urgent diagnostic and therapeutic lumbar puncture.

## CRANIAL NERVE III (OCULOMOTOR NERVE)

### *Anatomy*

The oculomotor nerve is a pure motor nerve that works in conjunction with cranial nerves IV and VI to coordinate extraocular movements. The oculomotor nerve controls the superior rectus (globe elevator), medial rectus (globe adductor), inferior rectus (globe depressor), and inferior oblique (globe elevator) muscles. It also controls the levator palpebrae superioris muscle (upper eyelid elevator) and the intrinsic visceral motor function of the sphincter pupillae muscles and the ciliary muscles, which perform pupillary constriction and accommodation, respectively.

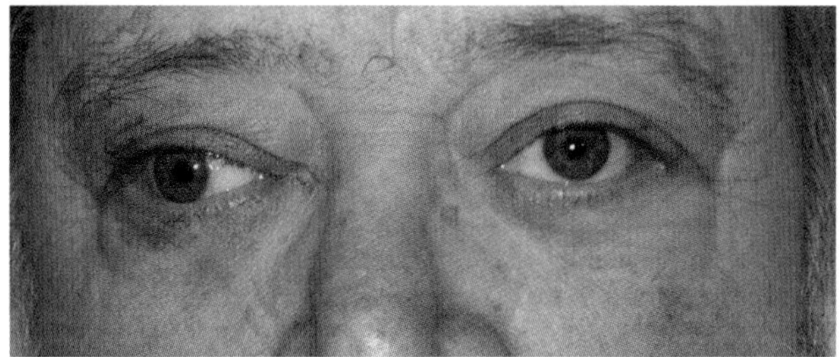

**Fig. 95.1** This 60-year-old man had diabetes mellitus, hypertension, coronary artery disease, chronic renal failure, and multiple myeloma. He sought medical care because of double vision (he described the images as "a little side by side but mostly up and down"), diplopia, ptosis, and papillary sparing. Findings on laboratory tests, magnetic resonance imaging, and magnetic resonance angiography were negative. The patient was evaluated by a neurologist and an ophthalmologist, and diabetic cranial nerve palsy was ultimately diagnosed. He was given an eye patch and scheduled for ophthalmologic follow-up.

### *Presenting Signs and Symptoms*

The patient typically complains of double vision or difficulty seeing out of the affected eye. There may be mild photophobia in bright light. The patient may also complain of an inability to raise the eyelid (ptosis).

Cranial nerve III palsy is more common in patients older than 60 years and in those with diabetes or hypertension (**Fig. 95.1**).

Patients with herniation syndromes will have a history of trauma (**Fig. 95.2**), tumor, or other neurologic findings.[7]

Pain associated with unilateral mydriasis should alert the emergency physician (EP) to look for an aneurysm involving the terminal internal carotid artery. Computed tomographic angiography is more sensitive than magnetic resonance angiography.[8]

Patients with an abscess or cavernous sinus thrombosis may have headaches, altered mental status, and seizures. This diagnosis should be considered in patients with signs and symptoms in the contralateral eye, previous sinus or midface infection, fever, chemosis, eyelid or periorbital edema, and exophthalmos. Extension of internal carotid artery dissection intracranially into the cavernous sinus can result in third, fourth, and sixth cranial nerve palsies.[9]

### Treatment

Treatment is dependent on the cause. CT should be performed to exclude a herniating mass. Admission for magnetic resonance imaging (MRI) and neurology or neurosurgical consultation is indicated for acute-onset deficits.

## CRANIAL NERVE IV (TROCHLEAR NERVE)

### Anatomy

The trochlear nerve innervates the superior oblique muscle of the eye and causes inward rotation and downward and lateral movement of the globe. It is the smallest cranial nerve but has the longest intracranial course.

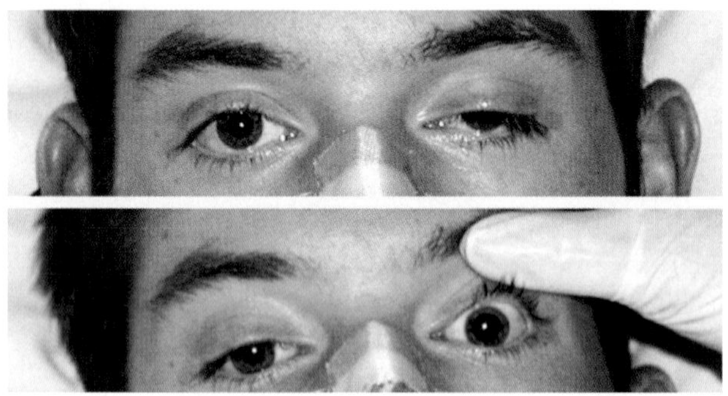

**Fig. 95.2 Ptosis and mydriasis suggest a cranial nerve III palsy.** The appearance of these signs after a crush injury indicates that a skull fracture is impinging on the nerve canal. (Reproduced with permission from Baker C, Cannon J. Images in clinical medicine. Traumatic cranial nerve palsy. N Engl J Med 2005;353:1955.)

### Presenting Signs and Symptoms

Patients with a fourth cranial nerve palsy have double vision exacerbated by looking downward. The classic complaint is difficulty going down stairs. Most commonly, a history of trauma is reported. On physical examination the patient may unconsciously tilt the head away from the affected side (**Fig. 95.3**). Etiologic mechanisms are similar to those for the third cranial nerve and include inflammatory processes, trauma, and vascular causes.[10]

### Treatment

Treatment of isolated fourth nerve palsy is generally conservative, and the patient should be referred to neurology or neurosurgery as appropriate.[10] CT, MRI, and neurology consultation are warranted if multiple cranial nerves are involved.

## CRANIAL NERVE V (TRIGEMINAL NERVE)

### Anatomy

The trigeminal nerve is a mixed motor and sensory nerve. It provides motor innervation to the muscles of mastication, as well as sensation from the face, scalp, conjunctiva, globe, mucous membranes of the sinuses, tongue, teeth, and part of the external tympanic membrane.

The trigeminal sensory ganglion is located in the middle cranial fossa and branches into three divisions: the ophthalmic nerve (V1), the maxillary nerve (V2), and the mandibular nerve (V3).

### Presenting Signs and Symptoms

Patients with trigeminal nerve dysfunction have either sensory or motor deficits. Sensory dysfunctions include paroxysmal pain, paresthesias (abnormal sensations such as burning, pricking, tickling, or tingling), dysesthesias (disagreeable, unpleasant, or painful sensations produced by ordinary stimuli), and anesthesia (loss of sensation). The motor dysfunction is usually described as difficulty chewing and difficulty swallowing.

Peripheral lesions cause loss of sensation or pain in only one division. Positive findings in two or more divisions (e.g., loss of light touch in one division and loss of sensitivity to pain, temperature, or pinprick in another division) should raise suspicion for a central cause.

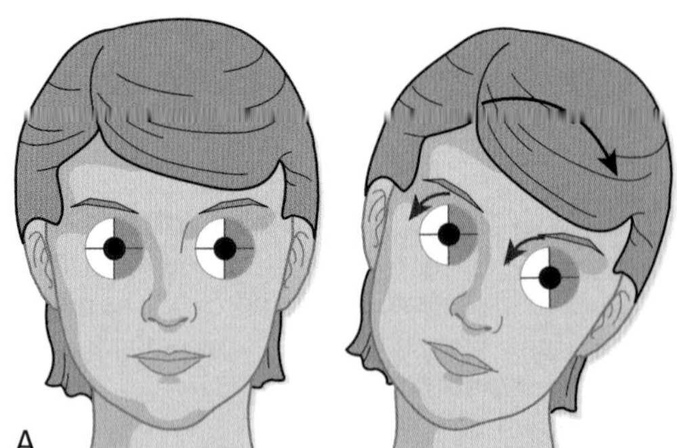


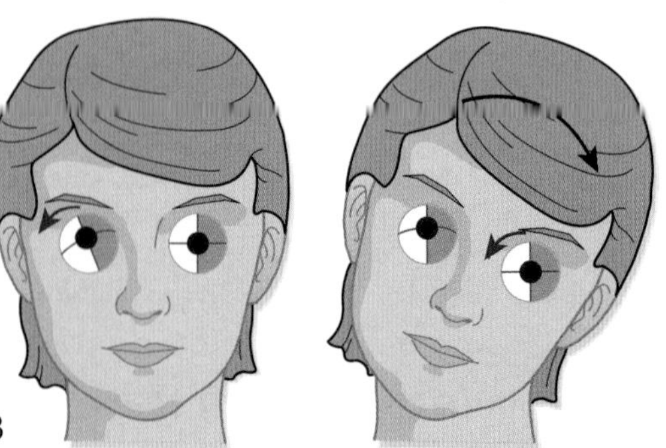


**Fig. 95.3 A,** Normal eye rotation. When the head tilts, both eyes rotate in the opposite direction. **B,** Cranial nerve IV palsy (right eye). The right eye is extorted and slightly elevated, which is causing double vision. The patient compensates by tilting the head to the left.

The presence of associated cranial nerve deficits (III, IV, IV, or any combination of these nerves) suggests cavernous sinus involvement. In the setting of trauma, if a bruit over the orbit can be detected, a carotid–cavernous sinus fistula may be present. Associated involvement of cranial nerve VII or VIII or gait ataxia should raise suspicion for a cerebellopontine angle or lateral pontine tumor (**Table 95.1**).

Associated Horner syndrome may indicate a cervical or lateral brainstem lesion.

The main categories of trigeminal nerve dysfunction are trigeminal neuralgia and trigeminal neuropathy. A sudden onset of symptoms should raise suspicion for a vascular, traumatic, or demyelinating cause, whereas a more indolent course suggests tumor or inflammation (**Table 95.2**).

TRIGEMINAL NEUROPATHY Causes include compression by an extrinsic mass, trauma, and vascular, inflammatory, or demyelinating disorders.

Symptoms include neuralgia or paresthesia (or both) involving half of the face. Unlike trigeminal neuralgia, the pain with trigeminal neuropathy is more constant. Loss of the corneal reflex is evident. The patient's mouth may become more oval

**Table 95.1 Clinicoanatomic Correlation of Localization of Lesions of Cranial Nerve V**

| ANATOMIC SITE OF DAMAGE | CLINICAL FINDINGS | OTHER NEUROLOGIC AND MEDICAL FINDINGS | COMMON CAUSES |
|---|---|---|---|
| **Supranuclear** | | | |
| Sensory cortex | Facial numbness, paresthesias | Neglect, apraxia, aphasia | Stroke, tumor, hemorrhage |
| Internal capsule | Hemifacial sensory loss | Hemiparesis of the arm | Stroke, tumor, hemorrhage, MS |
| Corona radiata | | Central seventh cranial nerve paresis | |
| VPM thalamus | Facial numbness, paresthesias, pain; cheirooral syndrome | Anosmia, hemisensory deficit | Stroke, tumor, hemorrhage |
| Midbrain | Facial numbness, paresthesias, pain | Ophthalmoparesis | Stroke, MS, tumor, aneurysm |
| **Nuclear** | | | |
| Pons | Facial numbness and weakness, paresthesias, pain; trigeminal neuralgia | Ophthalmoparesis; CN VI, CN VII, CN VIII palsies; Horner syndrome | Stroke, tumor, hemorrhage; MS, syringobulbia, abscess, trauma |
| Medulla | Facial numbness, paresthesias, pain; trigeminal neuralgia | Ataxia, CN X palsy, ophthalmoparesis, nystagmus, Horner syndrome, Wallenberg syndrome | Stroke, MS, tumor, aneurysm, abscess, vasculopathy |
| **Preganglionic** | | | |
| Cerebellopontine angle | Facial numbness | CN VII, CN VIII palsies; headache, cerebellar dysergia | Neuroma, meningioma, meningitis (bacterial, TB, cancer), aneurysm, trauma |
| Middle cranial fossa | | | |
| Gasserian ganglion | Facial numbness and weakness | Gradenigo syndrome; CN VI, CN VII palsies | Tumor, infection, trauma |
| Skull base | Facial numbness and weakness | Headache, meningismus | Meningitis (bacterial, TB, cancer, sarcoid) |
| **Trigeminal Nerve Branches** | | | |
| V1: Cavernous sinus | Facial numbness, pain | Headache, ophthalmoparesis; Horner syndrome | Tumor, thrombosis, infection, trauma |
| V1: Carotid-cavernous fistula | Facial numbness | Proptosis, bruit, ophthalmoparesis | Trauma |
| V2: Maxillary region | Facial numbness; numb cheek syndrome | | Tumor, infarct, vasculopathy, trauma |
| V3: Mandibular region | Weakness of mastication; numb chin syndrome | | Tumor, trauma, infarct |

*CN*, Cranial nerve; *MS*, multiple sclerosis; *TB*, tuberculosis; *VPM*, ventroposteromedial.

**Table 95.2 Selected Specific Causes Associated with Trigeminal Nerve Disorders**

| ETIOLOGIC CATEGORY | SELECTED SPECIFIC CAUSES |
|---|---|
| **Structural Disorders** | |
| Developmental | Brainstem vascular loop, syringobulbia |
| Degenerative and compressive | Paget disease |
| **Hereditary and Degenerative Disorders** | |
| Chromosomal abnormalities, neurocutaneous disorders | Hereditary sensorimotor neuropathy type I, neurofibromatosis (schwannoma) |
| Degenerative motor, sensory, and autonomic disorders | Amyotrophic lateral sclerosis |
| **Acquired Metabolic and Nutritional Disorders** | |
| Endogenous metabolic disorders | Diabetes |
| Exogenous disorders (toxins, illicit drugs) | Trichloroethylene, trichloroacetic acid |
| Nutritional deficiencies, syndromes associated with alcoholism | Thiamine, folate, vitamin $B_{12}$, pyridoxine, pantothenic acid, vitamin A deficiencies |
| **Infectious Disorders** | |
| Viral infections | Herpes zoster, unknown |
| Nonviral infections | Bacteria, tuberculous meningitis, brain abscess, Gradenigo syndrome, leprosy, cavernous sinus thrombosis |
| HIV infection, AIDS | Opportunistic infection; abscess, herpes zoster<br>Stroke, hemorrhage, aneurysm |
| **Neurovascular Disorders** | |
| **Neoplastic Disorders** | |
| Primary neurologic tumors | Glial tumors, meningioma, schwannoma |
| Metastatic neoplasms, paraneoplastic syndromes | Lung, breast; lymphoma, carcinomatous meningitis |
| **Demyelinating Disorders** | |
| Central nervous system disorders | Multiple sclerosis, acute demyelinating encephalomyelitis |
| Peripheral nervous system disorders | Guillain-Barré syndrome, chronic inflammatory demyelinating polyneuropathy<br>Tolosa-Hunt syndrome, sarcoidosis, lupus, orbital pseudotumor |
| **Autoimmune and Inflammatory Disorders** | |
| **Traumatic Disorders** | Carotid-cavernous fistula, cavernous sinus thrombosis, maxillary/mandibular injury |
| **Epilepsy** | Focal seizures |
| **Headache and Facial Pain** | Raeder neuralgia, cluster headache |
| **Drug-Induced and Iatrogenic Neurologic Disorders** | Orbital, facial, dental surgery |

From Goetz CG, editor. Textbook of clinical neurology. 2nd ed. Philadelphia: Saunders; 2003.
*AIDS*, Acquired immunodeficiency syndrome; *HIV*, human immunodeficiency virus.

and oblique in appearance, and because of loss of masseter muscle strength, the chin may be deviated toward the affected side.

Until proved otherwise, neuropathies of cranial nerve V, the chin (numb chin; V3), and the suborbital region (numb cheek) should be presumed to be due to malignancies.[11]

TIC DOULOUREUX The term *tic douloureux* was coined by Nicolaus André, a French surgeon, in 1756. Its mechanism is probably compression of the trigeminal nerve root within millimeters of entry into the pons.[12] The maxillary and mandibular divisions are most commonly affected, either alone or in combination. In one longitudinal case series, no cases of trigeminal neuralgia affecting both the ophthalmic and mandibular divisions were reported.[2] Causes of tic douloureux are listed in **Box 95.2**.

The International Association for the Study of Pain defines tic douloureux as "a sudden usually unilateral, severe, brief, stabbing, recurrent pain in the distribution of one or more branches of the fifth cranial nerve." The pain is classically precipitated by normal activities such as eating, talking, washing the face, or cleaning the teeth.

### *Diagnostic Testing*

The presence or absence of a corneal reflex should be checked. An intact reflex indicates normal function of the afferent V1 division, as well as normal cranial nerve VII motor efferent function. Absence of a corneal reflex can be caused by tumors in the posterior fossa or cerebellopontine angle, multiple sclerosis, brainstem strokes (Wallenberg or lateral medullary syndrome), and Parkinson disease.

Motor function is evaluated by having the patient open and close the mouth and laterally deviate the jaw against resistance. Loss of muscle bulk or the presence of fasciculations in the temporalis or masseter musculature indicates a lower motor neuron lesion.

The jaw jerk reflex test determines the integrity of the V3 division. The examiner places a thumb on the patient's chin, after which the patient is instructed to relax the jaw completely with the mouth closed, and the examiner then taps the chin to elicit the jaw jerk reflex. The reflex will be diminished in patients with a lower motor neuron lesion and accentuated in patients with a supranuclear lesion.

### *Treatment*

A trial of carbamazepine can be therapeutic as well as diagnostic because failure to improve with carbamazepine suggests some other cause. Treatment options are listed in **Box 95.3**.[3] Surgical approaches are considered when medication cannot control the pain or pain medication is not tolerated.[13]

## CRANIAL NERVE VI (ABDUCENS NERVE)

### *Anatomy*

The abducens nerve is a pure motor nerve that supplies the ipsilateral lateral rectus muscle of the eye and controls globe abduction.

## PRESENTING SIGNS AND SYMPTOMS

Patients with an abducens nerve palsy usually complain of double vision. The head may be turned away from the affected side to maintain binocularity. Diabetes and hypertension are common risk factors. Another common sign is "crossed eyes" (esotropia or strabismus) (**Fig. 95.4**).[14]

### *Differential Diagnosis*

Children are more likely to have a tumor as the principal cause, and older individuals are more likely to have an ischemic cause such as temporal arteritis.

An abducens nerve palsy occurring in isolation is rare. Usually, the seventh and eighth cranial nerves are also involved, which signals a central cause. Causes of abducens nerve palsy are listed in **Box 95.4**.

**BOX 95.2 Causes of Tic Douloureux**

Vascular compression by an artery or vein
Saccular aneurysm
Arteriovenous malformation
Vestibular schwannomas
Meningioma
Epidermoid cyst
Tumor
Primary demyelinating disorders
- Multiple sclerosis
- Charcot-Marie-Tooth disease (rare)

Infiltrative disorders
- Trigeminal amyloidoma

Nondemyelinating lesions
- Small infarct or angioma in the brainstem

Familial

**BOX 95.3 Treatment of Trigeminal Neuralgia**

**First-Line Agent**

Carbamazepine (Tegretol)—Start at 150 mg daily and increase by 100 mg every 3 days as needed to a total daily dose of 800 to 1600 mg divided into three doses.

**Second-Line Agents**

Oxcarbazepine (Trileptal)—Start at 300 mg daily and increase by 300 mg every 3 days as needed to a total daily dose of 1200 to 1800 mg divided into two doses.

Gabapentin (Neurontin)—Start at 300 mg three times daily and increase as needed to a total daily dose of 3600 mg divided into three doses. Also commonly used as first-line therapy.

Phenytoin (Dilantin)—Start at 300 mg daily and increase as needed, divided into two or three doses.

**Third-Line Agents (Add-On Therapy or Monotherapy)**

Lamotrigine (Lamictal)—Start at 25 mg daily and increase by 25 mg every 7 days as needed to a total daily dose of 200 to 400 mg divided into two doses.

Baclofen (Lioresal)—Start at 15 mg daily and increase by 5 mg every 3 days as needed to a total daily dose of 60 to 80 mg divided into three doses.

Reprinted with permission from Prasad S, Galetta S. Trigeminal neuralgia: historical notes and current concepts. Neurologist 2009;15:87-94.

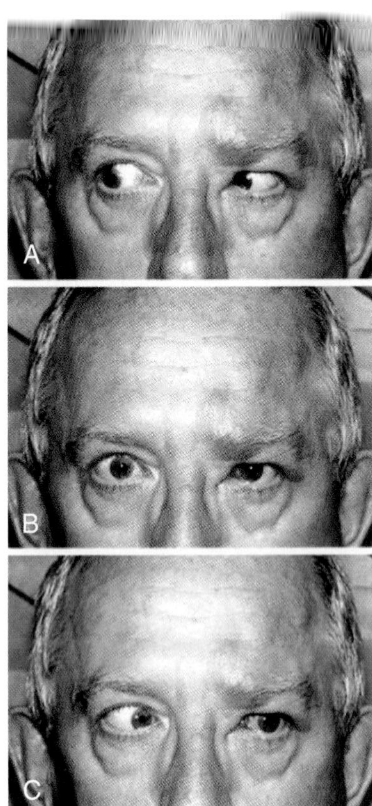


**Fig. 95.4** This 62-year-old man reported acute left retroorbital pain of 1 week's duration. Double vision developed, a rash appeared on his forehead, and he had restricted abduction in his left eye; this finding is diagnostic of a left sixth cranial nerve palsy (right, center, and left gaze seen in panels **A, B,** and **C,** respectively) and binocular horizontal diplopia. A diagnosis of herpes zoster ophthalmicus was made. The patient was treated with gabapentin and acyclovir for 1 week. Six weeks later, he had minimal residual diplopia with no postherpetic neuralgia. (Reproduced with permission from Jude E, Chakraborty A. Images in clinical medicine. Left sixth cranial nerve palsy with herpes zoster ophthalmicus. N Engl J Med 2005;353:e14.)

**BOX [illegible] Causes of Abducens Nerve Palsy**

Trauma—a blowout fracture of the orbit may result in a trapped medial rectus muscle and mimic a sixth nerve palsy
Subarachnoid disorders—hemorrhage, infection (meningitis), tumor
Vascular—intracavernous aneurysms; sixth nerve palsies are almost always the first clinical feature because of this nerve's close relationship to the carotid artery and the fact that it is unsupported by a fibrous covering
Giant cell arteritis
Pontine glioma (in children)
Pseudotumor cerebri—may be manifested as an isolated abducens nerve palsy in 30% of cases
Inflammatory (postviral or demyelinating) leptomeningeal involvement secondary to carcinomatous meningitis; inflammatory or infiltrating lesions of the cavernous sinus
Metabolic—vitamin B deficiency, Wernicke-Korsakoff syndrome
Congenital absence of cranial nerve VI (Duane syndrome)

### *Treatment*

Truly isolated sixth nerve palsies are often caused by microvascular ischemia secondary to hypertension or diabetes. A thorough work-up must be performed to rule out a central, inflammatory, infectious, or neoplastic cause. Close follow-up by a neurologist over a 6-month period is indicated; most cases resolve within 3 to 6 months.

## CRANIAL NERVE VII (FACIAL NERVE)—BELL PALSY

### *Mechanisms*

The pathophysiology of Bell palsy has not been clearly established. Several theories have been proposed, including infectious or ischemic inflammation leading to nerve compression within the narrow canal as the nerve exits the stylomastoid foramen. Because the nerve is encased in a tight dural sheath within the temporal bone, this edema then causes additional compression of the vascular supply to the nerve.[15]

The cause of Bell palsy is most commonly idiopathic (66%).[4] Numerous observed associations have been described in the literature. The palsy is often preceded by a viral syndrome, and a correlation has been noted with herpes simplex virus (HSV). Its association with shingles and the characteristic blistering (from varicella-zoster virus [VZV]) is given the designation Ramsay Hunt syndrome. Reactivation of VZV has also been theorized as a cause. In addition, Bell palsy may be seen in patients with Lyme disease in places where the disease is endemic.

Diabetes, hypertension, human immunodeficiency virus infection, sarcoidosis, Sjögren syndrome, parotid nerve tumors, eclampsia, amyloidosis, and the intranasal influenza vaccine have been associated with the development of Bell palsy.[5,16] Other common triggers include stress, trauma, fever, tooth extraction, and a chilling episode from exposure to drafts and cold.

Complete facial weakness, severe non–ear-related pain (e.g., retroauricular, cheek), late onset of recovery or no recovery by 3 weeks, diabetes, pregnancy, age older than 60 years, hypertension, and Ramsay Hunt syndrome are risk factors for incomplete recovery.[17,18]

Electroneurographic studies demonstrate a steady decline in electrical activity on days 4 to 10. When excitability is retained, 90% of patients recover fully, but when excitability diminishes to absence, only 20% of patients recover completely.[5]

### *Anatomy*

Cranial nerve VII is a mixed motor and sensory cranial nerve, which accounts for the varied symptoms. It travels adjacent to cranial nerves V, VI, and VIII as it traverses the cerebellopontine angle, the internal auditory meatus, and the temporal bone.

Motor function involves the muscles of facial expression, the posterior digastric muscle, the stylohyoid muscle, and the stapedius muscle of the inner ear.

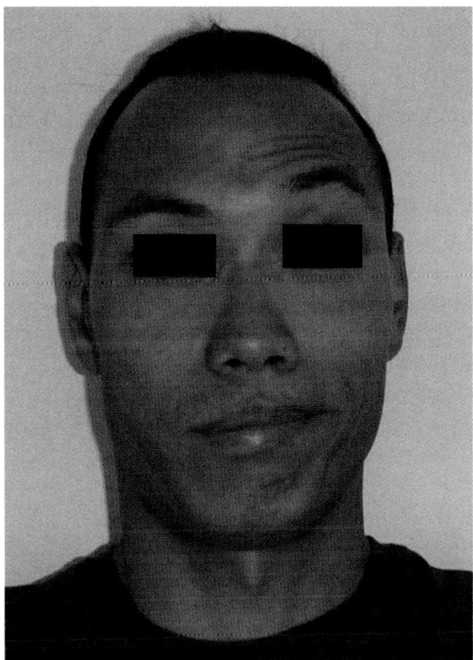

**Fig. 95.5 "Raise your eyebrows."** A patient with a peripheral seventh nerve palsy (i.e., Bell palsy) will have loss of forehead wrinkles at rest and an inability to wrinkle the forehead and raise the eyebrow on the affected side (right side in this patient).

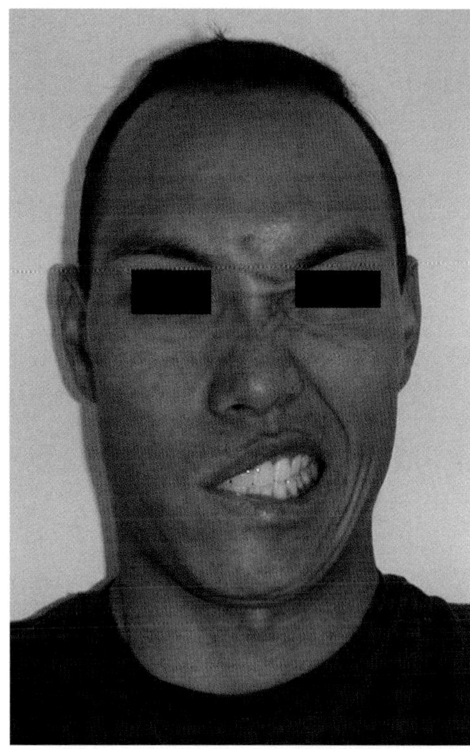

**Fig. 95.6 "Show me your teeth"; "wrinkle your nose."** The risorius and orbicularis oris muscles are denervated. Notice the inability to corrugate the nose on the affected right side because of loss of function of the nasal and buccal musculature.

Parasympathetic innervation includes the lacrimal glands, the mucous membranes of the nose, the hard and soft palate, and the submandibular and sublingual glands.

The geniculate ganglion contains the nerve cell bodies of the sensory taste fibers of the anterior two thirds of the tongue.[19]

### *Presenting Signs and Symptoms*

To the patient, the most alarming symptom of Bell palsy is the abrupt onset of unilateral facial paralysis. Approximately 50% of patients believe that they have suffered a stroke, 25% think that they have an intracranial tumor, and the remaining 25% have no clear conception of what is wrong but are extremely anxious.[4]

The EP may note drooping of the eyebrow or the corner of the mouth (or both) and loss of wrinkles on the forehead or the nasolabial folds (or both). Inability to raise the eyebrow and furrow the forehead is a cardinal sign of Bell palsy (**Fig. 95.5**). Preservation of forehead motor neuron innervation should raise suspicion for a central cause.[17] Because the forehead receives bilateral upper motor neuron innervation, a central stroke will spare the forehead and allow the patient to raise the eyebrow. If the patient can do this, it is not Bell palsy.

Loss of nasolabial fold and nasal flaring is common. Loss of buccinator strength causes an inability to blow out the cheeks. An inability to close the eye on the affected side is a hallmark of Bell palsy. Speech is affected and may sound slurred or garbled, similar to dysarthria from a stroke. An asymmetric smile is often noted on examination (**Fig. 95.6**).

The signs and symptoms vary depending on the site of the affected nerve. They are listed in **Box 95.5**.

**BOX 95.5 Signs and Symptoms of Bell Palsy**

- Ipsilateral tongue numbness
- Loss of taste or a dull taste
- Overt paralysis preceded by a sensation of subjective numbness or weakness on the affected side
- Ear pain in the external auditory canal
- Retroauricular pain
- Occipital headache
- Hyperacusis
- Fullness or snapping sound in the affected ear
- Tinnitus
- Drooling
- Inability to keep liquids in the mouth or chew
- Noticeable dryness of the oral and nasal mucous membranes on the affected side
- Anxiety

### *Diagnostic Testing and Differential Diagnosis*

The "blow out your cheeks" test (**Fig. 95.7**) demonstrates loss of buccinator function. A sensitive variation of this test is to ask patients to hold water in their mouth and contract the buccal muscles. The water will either dribble out of the corner of the mouth or shoot across the room.

On testing of hearing, hyperacusis may be observed on the affected side because of denervation of the stapedius. The patient should have no hearing loss.

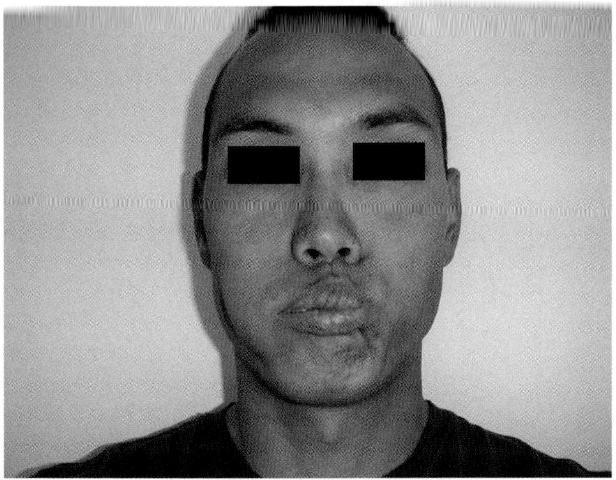

**Fig. 95.7 "Blow out your cheeks."** Loss of buccinator function prevents pursing of the lips and allows air (and food and liquids) to escape.

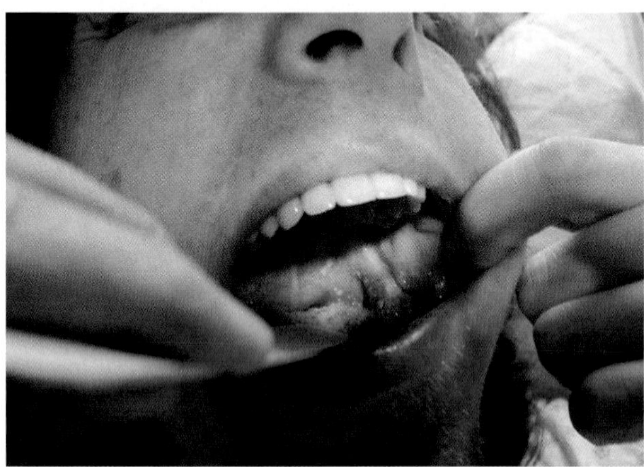

**Fig. 95.8 Buccal herpetic lesions in an individual with Ramsay Hunt syndrome.**

To evaluate taste sensation, a few granules of sugar are placed on the tip of the patient's tongue on the affected side. Decreased taste sensation may be noted.

Other cranial nerves should be normal. The abducens nucleus lies at the level of the genu of cranial nerve VII; infarction in the area can cause concomitant palsy of cranial nerve VI, which signals an upper motor neuron lesion rather than Bell palsy. No evidence of expressive or receptive aphasia should be present.

The presence of vesicles on the tympanic membrane or in the oropharynx (**Fig. 95.8**) or the presence of grouped vesicular lesions on the face or around the ear (**Fig. 95.9**) suggests a diagnosis of Ramsay Hunt syndrome.

Residual synkinesis can result from abnormal regeneration of nerve fibers. This can be manifested as abnormal motor function (e.g., blinking causes involuntary contracture of the risorius); as abnormal parasympathetic function, which is classically accompanied by "crocodile tears"—lacrimation after a salivary stimulus; or as hemifacial spasm, which can be bothersome, especially when the patient is tired.

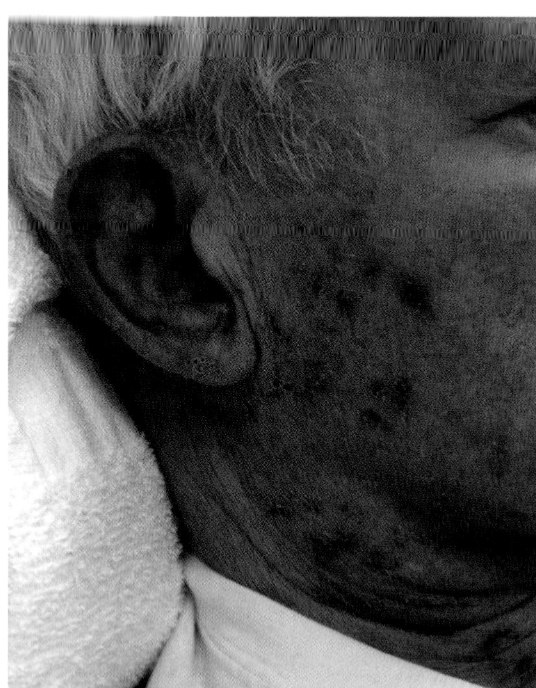

**Fig. 95.9 Characteristic auricular rash of Ramsay Hunt syndrome.**

## *Treatment*

The algorithm shown in **Figure 95.10** outlines the treatment of patients with Bell palsy.

Patients can be discharged home with oral medication, instructions for eye care, and expedited follow-up with a neurologist. Additional investigation for Lyme disease may be indicated for patients at risk.

The evidence available indicates that steroids are safe and effective in shortening the course of the neurologic deficit and improving facial function.[5,20-24] Patients receiving steroid therapy are up to 1.2 times more likely to attain good functional outcomes than untreated patients are.[25] Corticosteroids reduce the risk for unsatisfactory recovery by 9%, with the number needed to benefit (NNTB) being 11.[21] Corticosteroids were also associated with a 14% absolute reduction in risk for synkinesis and autonomic dysfunction, with an NNTB of 7.[22]

No studies have demonstrated significantly worse facial functional outcomes in patients treated with steroids.[21,22,25]

The most commonly reported treatment regimen is oral prednisone, 1 mg/kg up to 70 mg/day for a 10-day course. Dosing can be once daily or split into twice daily. The starting dose is continued for 6 days and tapered over the next 4 days.[22,25] Alternatively, prednisone, 1 mg/kg/day, may be given for 7 days without a taper.[4]

Recent studies and metaanalyses have questioned the benefit of using antivirals for the treatment of Bell palsy.[20-24,26] Antiviral agents used alone did not provide any benefit over placebo, and their use as the sole therapeutic agent is not recommended.[20] When combined with corticosteroid therapy, antiviral therapy may have incremental benefit,[21] but this remains to be shown conclusively. Therefore, until definitive studies are performed, clinical judgment will probably guide the use of antiviral therapy in cases in which a viral cause is strongly suspected (i.e., patients in whom HSV or VZV is

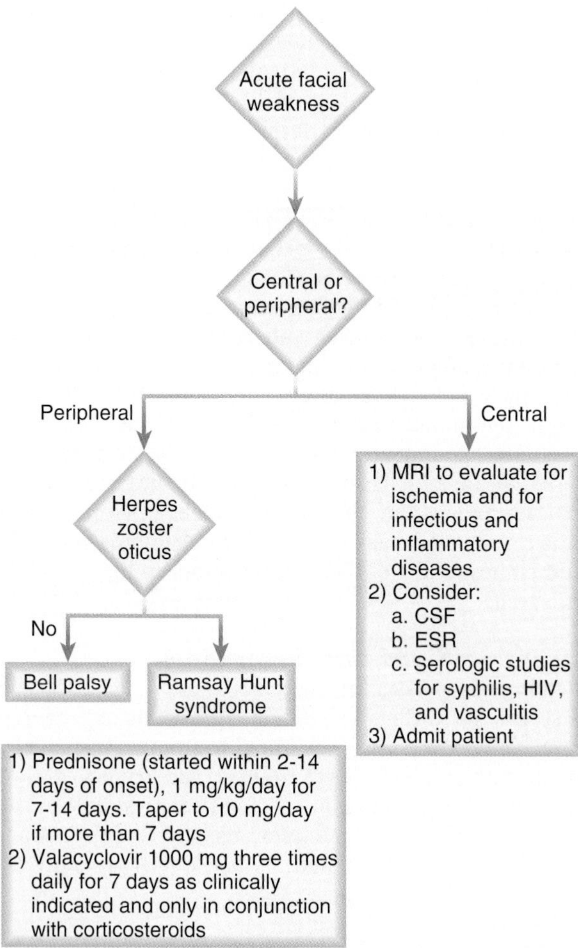


**Fig. 95.10 Algorithm outlining the treatment of patients with Bell palsy.** *CSF*, Cerebrospinal fluid; *ESR*, erythrocyte sedimentation rate; *HIV*, human immunodeficiency virus; *MRI*, magnetic resonance imaging.

contributory). Valacyclovir, 1 g three times daily for 7 days, can be prescribed in conjunction with corticosteroids.

An eye shield or an eye patch should be worn during the night to prevent drying of the cornea. Liberal use of artificial tears during the day and an ophthalmic ointment such as Lacri-Lube at night should be prescribed to prevent drying of the cornea. Pain medication should be prescribed because the otalgia and cephalgia can be debilitatingly painful.

### Prognosis

In a prospective study describing the spontaneous untreated course of idiopathic peripheral nerve palsy in patients with diabetes, 38% of patients had complete palsies, and only 25% regained normal facial muscle function.[4] This is significantly worse than the observed rate of spontaneous full recovery in nondiabetic patients.[27] Recurrence is rare (6.3%[28]) and should prompt a work-up for other causes such as myasthenia gravis, lymphoma, sarcoidosis, Lyme disease, and rarely, Guillain-Barré syndrome.[5,29,30]

Although the prognosis for recovery is good, the psychologic consequences can be long-lasting and are perhaps more significant than the physical disability. Patients report self-consciousness about the facial disfigurement, fear of permanent disfigurement, loss of self-esteem, and social ostracism.

## CRANIAL NERVE VIII (VESTIBULOCOCHLEAR NERVE)

### Anatomy

The vestibulocochlear nerve is a special sensory nerve that transmits auditory signals from the cochlea (hearing) and signals from the semicircular canals (balance). The vestibular apparatus also sits in the petrous temporal bone and is composed of a body consisting of the saccule and utricle and three semicircular canals aligned in three different planes. Hair cells within the endolymph of the canals detect angular movement and transmit the impulses to the vestibular nuclear complex in the floor of the fourth ventricle. The hair cells collectively combine to form the vestibular ganglion.

### Presenting Signs and Symptoms

Patients with vestibulocochlear nerve dysfunction usually exhibit various degrees of hearing loss, tinnitus, vertigo, falling, and imbalance. The mechanism is asymmetric integration of vestibular input to the central nervous system or asymmetric disruption of sensory input from the vestibular organs.[31] If the vertigo is severe, nausea and vomiting also occur. Symptoms may be constant or episodic. Vestibular neuronitis causes vertigo that lasts for weeks, and central vertigo may persist for years.[32]

Patients should be asked about triggers, particularly positional triggers because this may indicate benign paroxysmal positional vertigo. Recent viral and upper respiratory tract infections may be significant because they predispose to vestibular neuronitis. The history should also include the use of medications such as anticonvulsants, antihypertensives, sedatives, and ototoxic drugs.

The examination should be focused on determining reproducibility of the symptoms, gait, balance, and ataxia; on evaluation of possible acute stroke symptoms; and on the character of the nystagmus and severity of the ataxia. The presence or absence of associated cerebellar signs such as lateralizing dysmetria, motor weakness, sensory loss, and abnormal reflexes should be noted, as well as the Babinski reflex and cranial nerve abnormalities such as ophthalmoplegia, dysarthria, and Horner syndrome.[31] Abnormalities in cerebellar function should prompt consideration of a central cause. Patients should also be examined for vertical and rotatory nystagmus, which are not typically present in patients with peripheral vertigo; their presence warrants imaging and neurologic evaluation.

### Diagnostic Testing and Differential Diagnosis

The Dix-Hallpike maneuver is commonly used to elicit positional nystagmus (see Fig. 96.1), which is associated with benign paroxysmal positional vertigo and usually lasts 5 to 60 seconds. Prolonged nystagmus is unlikely to be a result of this disorder. Gait and balance can be assessed with tandem walking and the Romberg test. Ataxia and lateralizing dysmetria can be assessed with finger-to-nose and heel-knee-shin testing. Hearing can be evaluated with the finger rub or finger snap, the Weber test, and the Rinne test. The ear and external auditory canal should be examined for evidence of cerumen, otitis media, perforation of the tympanic membrane, and mass lesions.

CT lacks sensitivity in the evaluation of cranial nerve VIII disorders but may be useful in evaluating the bony temporal region. MRI with gadolinium enhancement is useful in identifying acoustic neuroma.

When a central cause is suspected because of abnormalities on cerebellar testing or clinical suspicion, MRI or magnetic resonance angiography (or both) should be performed to rule out a posterior circulation stroke as a central cause of the vertigo.

The differential diagnosis should include other cranial nerve deficits that are not typically present in benign causes of cranial nerve VIII dysfunction. Acoustic neuromas may compress the trigeminal nerve when they attain a size of 3 cm or greater; patients with complaints of facial numbness should therefore be evaluated for trigeminal neuropathy, as well for a mass lesion. Because large tumors can affect cranial nerves IX, X, and XI, these nerves should also be tested.

### *Treatment*

Some patients who come to the emergency department with sudden or severe symptoms may not be able to comply with testing because the severity of the symptoms limits the ability to open their eyes and turn their head without experiencing nausea and vomiting or exacerbating the symptoms. In these cases it is appropriate to treat the patient symptomatically, initiate a work-up, and reassess clinically for improvement before attempting to move the patient or perform provocative testing.

## CRANIAL NERVE IX (GLOSSOPHARYNGEAL NERVE)

### *Anatomy*

The glossopharyngeal nerve provides branchial motor function to the stylopharyngeus muscle; visceral motor function to the otic ganglion and parotid gland; visceral sensory function from the carotid body; somatic sensory function to the posterior third of the tongue, the skin of the external ear, and the internal surface of the tympanic membrane; and the special sensory function of taste sensation from the posterior third of the tongue.

### *Presenting Signs and Symptoms*

Patients with glossopharyngeal nerve palsy usually have associated symptoms involving other cranial nerves, most commonly cranial nerves X and XI. The most common symptoms are dysphagia and choking. If the vagus nerve is involved, the patient complains of hoarseness and demonstrates ipsilateral paralysis of the soft palate. Head, neck, and oral trauma or surgery can cause acute dysfunction of cranial nerve IX. Glossopharyngeal nerve palsy is a known complication of tonsillectomy surgery.[33]

Glossopharyngeal neuralgia is a rare disorder consisting of paroxysms of pain in the back of the throat and tongue. The pain is similar to that of trigeminal neuralgia in that the attacks are brief, lasting seconds to minutes. It is unilateral and usually triggered by chewing, swallowing, coughing, or sneezing.

### *Treatment*

CT scanning is warranted to evaluate for a cerebrovascular event or tumor. Rarely, vasovagal syncope can result from bradycardia or asystole caused by vagus nerve cardioinhibitory input. Medical management is similar to that for trigeminal neuralgia. If involvement of other [illegible] is evident on examination, the patient should be admitted for further evaluation and neurologic consultation.

## CRANIAL NERVE X (VAGUS NERVE)

### *Anatomy*

The vagus nerve is a mixed motor and sensory nerve that provides motor function to striated muscle of the pharynx, tongue, larynx, and tensor veli palatini, as well as motor function to smooth muscle and glands of the pharynx, larynx, and thoracic and abdominal viscera. Cranial nerve X provides general sensation from the skin at the back of the ear, the external auditory meatus, the pharynx, and part of the external surface of the tympanic membrane, as well as visceral sensation from the larynx, trachea, esophagus, and thoracic and abdominal viscera; from chemoreceptors in the aortic bodies; and from stretch receptors in the walls of the aortic arch.

### *Presenting Signs and Symptoms*

Patients with palsies of the vagus nerve generally have hoarseness or difficulty swallowing. A history of recent carotid or thyroid surgery should prompt suspicion for a recurrent laryngeal nerve injury. The patient may also complain of regurgitation of food and liquid into the nose. Oropharyngeal examination usually reveals a drooped arch of the soft palate and uvular deviation away from the affected side.

### *Treatment*

A CT scan of the head without contrast enhancement should be performed to evaluate for a cerebrovascular accident (hemorrhagic or ischemic) or skull-based lesions. Further inpatient evaluation may include MRI of the head and neck and work-ups for metabolic, infectious, or inflammatory disorders as warranted.

## CRANIAL NERVE XI (ACCESSORY NERVE)

### *Anatomy*

The accessory nerve provides motor function to the sternocleidomastoid and trapezius muscles.

### *Presenting Signs and Symptoms*

Patients with accessory nerve palsies have neck and shoulder weakness on the affected side. Inspection may reveal a "dropped" shoulder—that is, the affected shoulder lying downward and in lateral rotation. Testing of the sternocleidomastoid reveals weakness when turning the head against resistance to the contralateral side. Because of the proximity of cranial nerves IX and X, particular attention should be paid to these nerve functions on examination. The most common causes are postoperative trauma (e.g., from cervical lymph node dissection) and a cerebrovascular accident.

### *Treatment*

Treatment and disposition are similar to that for cranial nerves IX and X.

## CRANIAL NERVE XII (HYPOGLOSSAL NERVE)

### Anatomy

The hypoglossal nerve provides motor function to all the intrinsic tongue muscles and three of the four extrinsic tongue muscles: the genioglossus, styloglossus, and hypoglossus.

### Presenting Signs and Symptoms

Patients with hypoglossal nerve palsies usually have unilateral tongue weakness.

### Differential Diagnosis

The primary diagnostic consideration is distinguishing an upper from a lower motor neuron lesion. An upper motor neuron lesion causes contralateral tongue deviation and fasciculations, and tongue atrophy is absent. A lower motor neuron lesion causes ipsilateral tongue deviation and fasciculations, and tongue atrophy is present. A 26-year review of 100 cases of hypoglossal nerve palsy revealed that tumors, predominantly malignant ones, produced nearly half of the palsies. Only 15% of patients made a complete or nearly complete recovery.[34] External lesions that cause compression or stretching of the nerve include internal carotid artery dissection or aneurysm, intracranial tumor, abscess, and other pharyngeal space tumors.

### Treatment

Treatment and disposition are similar to that for cranial nerves IX, X, and XI. If there is concern for a cerebrovascular accident or space-occupying lesion, the patient should be admitted for evaluation.

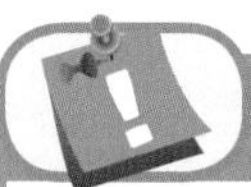

**TIPS AND TRICKS**

- Patients with palsies of any of the 12 cranial nerves have heterogeneous symptoms reflecting the intrinsic function of each nerve.
- Patients with cranial nerve disorders generally have visual disturbances, facial weakness or pain, or paresthesias, depending on the nerve or nerves involved.
- Knowledge of the function of each of the cranial nerves helps the emergency physician recognize the classic signs and symptoms of cranial nerve palsies.
- Trigeminal neuralgia and Bell palsy are common cranial nerve disorders encountered in the emergency department.
- Corticosteroids are beneficial in the treatment of Bell palsy. Additional benefit of antiviral therapy is unclear.
- The majority of patients with an acute onset of facial weakness are concerned about a stroke.
- A thorough history and physical examination should be focused on assessing the potential for trauma (skull fracture), tumor, cerebrovascular accident, vascular derangements (aneurysm, dissection, thrombosis), and infection (meningitis, abscess). Morbidity primary results from these entities.
- The diagnostic work-up and disposition depend on the clinical findings.
- The presence of concomitant focal neurologic or systemic signs should heighten suspicion for a central rather than a peripheral cause of the neurologic dysfunction.

## SUGGESTED READINGS

de Almeida JR, Al Khabori M, Guyatt GH, et al. Combined corticosteroid and antiviral treatment for Bell palsy: a systematic review and meta-analysis. JAMA 2009;302:985-93.

Engström M, Berg T, Stjernquist-Desatnik A, et al. Prednisolone and valaciclovir in Bell's palsy: a randomised, double-blind, placebo-controlled, multicentre trial. Lancet Neurol 2008;7:993-1000.

Gilden DH. Clinical practice. Bell's palsy. N Engl J Med 2004;351:1323-31.

Gilden D. Treatment of Bell's palsy—the pendulum has swung back to steroids alone. Lancet Neurol 2008;7:976–7.

Salinas RA, Alvarez G, Daly F, et al. Corticosteroids for Bell's palsy (idiopathic facial paralysis). Cochrane Database Syst Rev 2010;3:CD001942.

Sherbino J. Evidence-based emergency medicine: clinical synopsis. Do antiviral medications improve recovery in patients with Bell's palsy? Ann Emerg Med 2010;55:475-6.

Worster A, Keim SM, Sahsi R, et al; Best Evidence in Emergency Medicine (BEEM) Group. Do either corticosteroids or antiviral agents reduce the risk of long-term facial paresis in patients with new-onset Bell's palsy? J Emerg Med 2010;38:518-23.

## REFERENCES

***References can be found on Expert Consult @ www.expertconsult.com.***

# 96 Vertigo

Andrew K. Chang

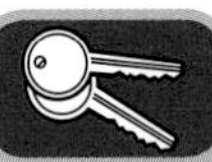

**KEY POINTS**

- The majority of cases of vertigo arise from a peripheral source (e.g., cranial nerve VIII, vestibular structures) rather than a central source.
- The Dix-Hallpike test (also called the Nylan-Bárány test) can help confirm the diagnosis of benign paroxysmal positional vertigo.
- Other causes should always be considered because the signs and symptoms of central vertigo can mimic those of peripheral vertigo.
- Central vertigo should be suspected in patients with any abnormal neurologic findings.

## PERIPHERAL VERTIGO

## EPIDEMIOLOGY

### GENERAL

Vertigo is diagnosed in roughly half of patients reporting dizziness. It is defined as the sensation of movement when none exists. About 80% of cases of vertigo are due to a peripheral lesion (pathology of the vestibular structures or cranial nerve VIII). Although peripheral vertigo is benign and not life-threatening, it may cause significant disability.

### BENIGN PAROXYSMAL POSITIONAL VERTIGO

The most common type of vertigo is benign paroxysmal positional vertigo (BPPV).[1] It occurs in all age groups but becomes more common with aging. Women are affected twice as often as men.

### VESTIBULAR NEURITIS AND LABYRINTHITIS

These disorders most commonly occur in patients in the third to fifth decades of life. Peripheral vestibulopathies typically follow viral gastrointestinal or upper respiratory infections.

## PATHOPHYSIOLOGY

Peripheral vertigo results from pathology involving the vestibular system or the eighth cranial nerve. The vestibular organs are responsible for equilibrium. The two main components—the three semicircular canals and the two otolith organs (utricle and saccule)—are interconnected and contain endolymph. The three semicircular canals—posterior (inferior), horizontal (lateral), and anterior (superior, vertical, dorsal)—are arranged at right angles to each other and allow detection of rotation via movement of endolymph. Otoliths (also known as otoconia), which are calcium carbonate particles, are found in the saclike utricle and provide information on head tilt.

When there is no disease and the head is held motionless, the bilateral vestibular systems fire at a tonic resting frequency. When the head rotates, there is increased firing from one semicircular canal and decreased firing from the others. The cerebral cortex interprets this information, synthesizes it with signals from the visual and proprioceptive systems, and translates it into the consciousness of movement. Vertigo results when the end-organs fire inappropriately at different frequencies, which causes unequal input to the brainstem and cerebral cortex.

Nystagmus is an involuntary rhythmic movement of the eyes to and fro that is often seen in patients with vertigo. Nystagmus is defined in terms of the direction of the fast-phase component. The factors listed in **Table 96.1** should be noted in all patients with nystagmus. It should be kept in mind that on extremes of lateral gaze, several-beat nystagmus is a normal finding in 60% of patients.

### BENIGN PAROXYSMAL POSITIONAL VERTIGO

BPPV results from a mechanical defect in the inner ear. Canalolithiasis is the most accepted hypothesis. According to this premise, the culprits are free-floating otoliths that have become displaced from the utricle and inappropriately enter and activate the end-organs of the semicircular canals.[2] With certain head movements, a clump of otoliths moves, causes the endolymph to move with resultant inappropriate displacement of the cupula. Movement of the cupula triggers neural firing, with consequential vertigo and nystagmus. Less commonly, otoliths can adhere to the cupula and result in vertigo. This mechanism is called cupulolithiasis.

Although any semicircular canal can be affected, the posterior (inferior) canal is involved approximately 95% of the time because the otoliths, when displaced from the utricle, fall into the most dependent part of the system—the long arm of the posterior semicircular canal. BPPV is generally unilateral.

**Table 96.1 Characteristics of Nystagmus**

| | |
|---|---|
| Direction | Left or right |
| Axis | Upbeat or downbeat |
| Nature | Rotary/torsional or vertical |
| Duration | Seconds, minutes, or persistent |
| Associated Factors | Spontaneous or positional<br>Effect of visual fixation |

**Table 96.2 Pathophysiology of Various Causes of Peripheral Vertigo**

| CAUSE | PATHOPHYSIOLOGY |
|---|---|
| BPPV | Otoliths inappropriately displaced into the semicircular canals |
| VN/L | Inflammation of the vestibular nerve |
| Meniere disease | Excessive endolymph in the vestibule |
| Posttraumatic vertigo | Trauma to the occiput or temporal area |
| Perilymph fistula | Abnormal opening between the middle and inner ear |
| Acoustic neuroma | Slowly expanding tumor compressing cranial nerve VIII |

*BPPV,* Benign paroxysmal positional vertigo; *VN/L,* vestibular neuritis/labyrinthitis.

## VESTIBULAR NEURITIS AND LABYRINTHITIS

Sometimes referred to as vestibular neuronitis, vestibular neuritis occurs as a result of viral inflammation of the vestibular nerve. Unlike labyrinthitis, no auditory symptoms are present.

Labyrinthitis is caused by an infectious inflammation of the labyrinth. Viral causes are most common, although labyrinthitis may also occur as a result of Lyme neuroborreliosis or otosyphilis infections. Disruption of the round window by otitis media or cholesteatoma gives pathogens access to the labyrinth. Tumors, fistulas, meningitis, or mastoiditis may also create a portal of entry. Unilateral hearing loss and tinnitus are the distinguishing factors of labyrinthitis.

See **Table 96.2** for the pathophysiology of other causes of peripheral vertigo.

**BOX 96.1 Evaluation of Vertiginous Patients**

Consider the following factors when questioning patients during emergency department evaluation:

**General**
Sensation
Length of each episode of vertigo
Frequency of episodes
Intermittent or constant
Whether symptoms are mild, moderate, or severe

**Precipitating Factors**
Noise
Stress
Head position
Ameliorating circumstances
Head or neck trauma
Barotrauma (airplane flight, scuba diving)
Ototoxic drugs (aspirin, aminoglycoside, loop diuretic)

**Symptoms**
Do you tend to fall? Which side do you fall to?
Any nausea or vomiting?
Sensation of linear movement?

***Symptoms Associated with Central Vertigo***
Diplopia
Blurred vision
Weakness of the arms or legs
Numbness in the face or extremities
Confusion or decreased consciousness
Slurring of speech
Clumsiness of the arms or legs
Difficulty swallowing
Associated headache
Gait ataxia

***Symptoms Associated with Migraine***
Photophobia
Phonophobia
Preceding aura

***Associated Auditory Symptoms***
Hearing impaired in one or both ears
Pressure in the ears
History of ear infections
Ear drainage
Recent viral illness
Tinnitus (constant or pulsatile)

***Associated Cardiac Symptoms***
Chest pain
Shortness of breath
Palpitations

## PRESENTING SIGNS AND SYMPTOMS

Most patients describe vertigo as a spinning sensation (usually of the room or surrounding environment). In general, the emergency physician should ask open-ended questions when interviewing vertiginous patients because patients with dizziness are often very suggestible and will usually answer affirmatively to descriptions given to them. One should thus ask, "What do you mean by dizzy?" and not "Does the room spin?"

Diagnosis of peripheral vertigo is often based on the quality of the accompanying nystagmus. Peripheral nystagmus may be spontaneous or positional. In general, nystagmus is often provoked by having the patient lie with the affected ear dependent. With peripheral vertigo the nystagmus is generally fatigable—the symptoms and nystagmus decrease with repeated testing.

Details of the patient's history, as well as findings on physical examination, can help narrow the differential diagnosis (**Box 96.1**).

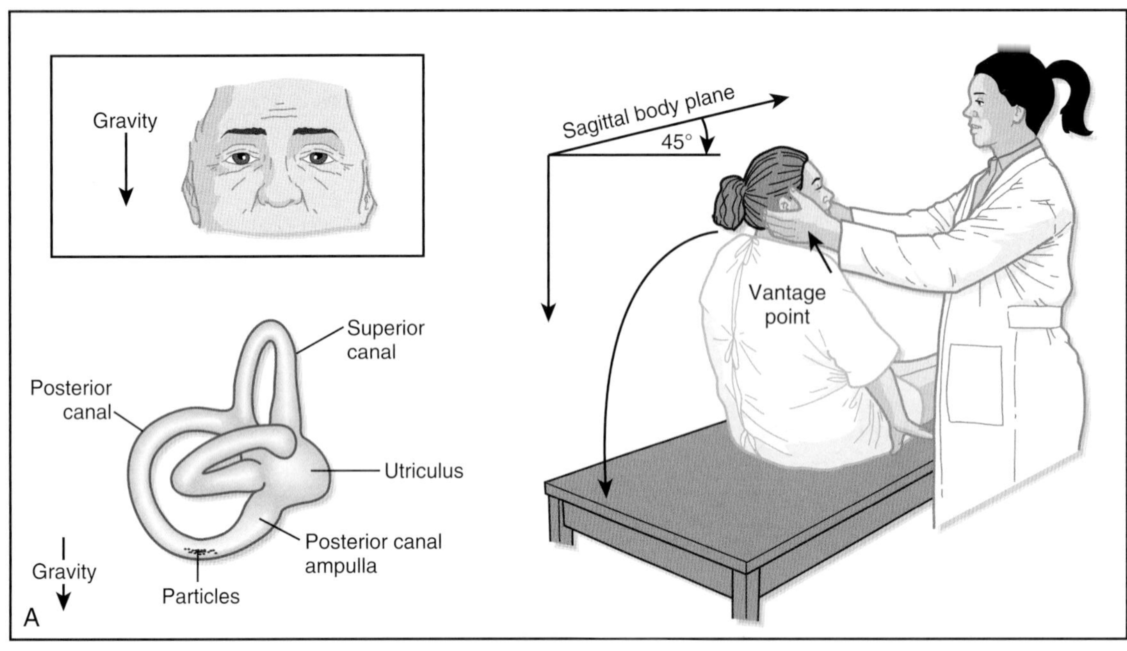


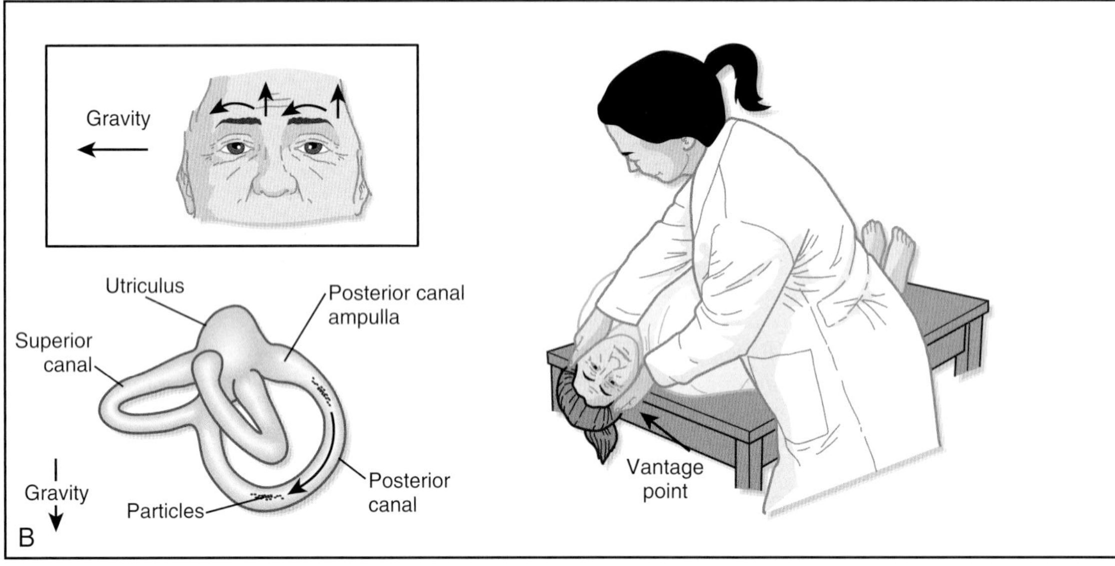


**Fig. 96.1 The Dix-Hallpike test of a patient with benign paroxysmal positional vertigo affecting the right ear.** In **A,** the examiner stands at the patient's right side and rotates the patient's head 45 degrees to the right to align the right posterior semicircular canal with the sagittal plane of the body. In **B,** the examiner moves the patient, whose eyes are open, from the seated to the supine right ear–down position with the head extended past the edge of the examination table. The latency, duration, and direction of nystagmus, if present, and the latency and duration of vertigo, if present, should be noted. The *arrows* in the inset depict the direction of nystagmus in patients with typical benign paroxysmal positional vertigo. The presumed location in the labyrinth of the free-floating otoliths thought to cause the disorder is also shown. (From Furman JM, Cass SP. Benign paroxysmal positional vertigo. N Engl J Med 1999;341:1590-6.)

## BENIGN PAROXYSMAL POSITIONAL VERTIGO

In BPPV, sudden transient vertigo is brought on by a change in head position. After head movement there is a delay of a few seconds, and then the room starts to spin and the patient experiences nausea or vomiting, or both. If the head is kept motionless, these symptoms typically resolve within 10 to 30 seconds. The symptoms are generally worse in the morning, probably because the otoliths have clumped together during sleep and exert a greater mass effect when the patient rolls over on awakening in the morning. The vertigo will tend to lessen as the day goes on because the otoliths become more dispersed and exert less of a mass effect.

The diagnosis of BPPV is confirmed with the Dix-Hallpike test,[3] also called the Nylan-Bárány test (**Fig. 96.1; Box 96.2**).

The patient should sit on one end of the examination table so that the head hangs over the edge when lying down. Because visualization of the direction of nystagmus is important, the patient should be instructed to keep the eyes open during the test. The purpose of the Dix-Hallpike test is to determine whether otoliths are inappropriately placed in the

**BOX 96.2 Findings on the Dix-Hallpike Test in Patients with Benign Paroxysmal Positional Vertigo**

Latency is approximately 3 to 10 seconds.
Significant subjective vertigo is present.
The intensity of vertigo escalates and then slowly resolves.
Vertigo and nystagmus last for approximately 5 to 30 seconds.
The nystagmus is upbeat (toward the forehead) and torsional toward the abnormal ear.
The nystagmus often reverses direction when the patient returns to the seated position.
Fatigability—the vertigo and nystagmus decrease and eventually subside with repeated positioning.

posterior semicircular canal. Thus the goal is to try to move potential otoliths that are located in the posterior semicircular canal, which will elicit symptoms and nystagmus. The most provocative way to get otoliths to move is to first align the posterior canal in the same plane as the upcoming movement (lying supine). This is why the patient's head, while sitting up, is first turned 45 degrees to the side being tested. The patient then lies back down so that the head overhangs the edge of the examination table. A positive test results in transient reproduction of the patient's symptoms and transient torsional nystagmus in which the fast phase is upbeat (toward the forehead). The patient then sits up and the test is repeated with the head rotated 45 degrees to the opposite side. In general, the test should be positive with the head turned only to one side, and this becomes the starting side for the potentially curative Epley maneuver (to be discussed later).

Occasionally, the horizontal semicircular canal is affected, and this is diagnosed with the roll test. The patient lies supine (unlike the Hallpike test, the head does not need to extend off the edge of the examination table). The head is then turned to each side approximately 90 degrees. Reproduction of the symptoms and nystagmus should occur, with the fast phase of the nystagmus beating downward toward the dependent ear. The side that is involved is the one that has the more acute symptoms and more severe nystagmus.

### VESTIBULAR NEURITIS AND LABYRINTHITIS

Spontaneous vertigo develops over a period of hours. Nausea and vomiting may occur. Symptoms that accompany a viral illness may also be present. The vertigo is initially severe, may require 1 or 2 days of bed rest, and then gradually resolves over a few weeks.

Spontaneous nystagmus with peripheral features may be seen on examination. Postural imbalance with a tendency to fall toward the side with the lesion is also seen. Middle ear infection or serous fluid may be present. Patients have a positive head-thrust test,[4] also known as the head impulse test.

The head-thrust test begins by directing the patient to look straight ahead. The examiner then places both hands on the patient's head and rapidly thrusts the patient's head to one side approximately 10 degrees. Normally, the patient's eyes will remain focused straight ahead when the head is turned rapidly. In patients with unilateral peripheral vestibular loss, such as occurs with vestibular neuritis and labyrinthitis, the eyes will move with the head but then a corrective saccade will bring the eyes back to the midline. Visualization of a corrective saccade (a positive test) confirms the diagnosis. Both sides should be tested.

**Table 96.3** Characteristics Differentiating Peripheral from Central Vertigo

| SYMPTOMS | PERIPHERAL | CENTRAL |
|---|---|---|
| Latency | 3-10 sec | None |
| Intensity of vertigo | Marked | Mild |
| Duration | <1 min | >1 min |
| Reproducibility | Variable | Present |
| Fatigability | Yes | No |
| Habituation | Yes | No |
| Nausea/vomiting | Moderate to severe | Variable |
| Nystagmus | Rotatory | Vertical or downbeat |
| Associated neurologic findings | Absent | Present |

## DIFFERENTIAL DIAGNOSIS AND MEDICAL DECISION MAKING

**Table 96.3** presents characteristics that differentiate peripheral from central vertigo.

## DIAGNOSTIC TESTING

### COMPUTED TOMOGRAPHY

Because skull-related artifacts are common with computed tomography, it has limited utility for evaluating the posterior fossa. If a patient has a focal neurologic finding and normal results on computed tomography, further imaging is necessary.

### MAGNETIC RESONANCE IMAGING AND MAGNETIC RESONANCE ANGIOGRAPHY

For assessment of pathologic causes of vertigo, magnetic resonance imaging (MRI) is the modality of choice. Magnetic resonance angiography is a noninvasive technique that can be used to visualize the vessels of the posterior circulation. It can detect aneurysms, atherosclerosis, dissections, vasculitis, thrombosis, and other processes.

### LABORATORY TESTING

Laboratory testing is rarely useful in the initial evaluation of a vertiginous patient. Screening tests include hematocrit, glucose, and electrolyte levels.

**Table 96.4 Medications for Treating Vertigo**

| CATEGORY | DRUG | DOSAGE |
|---|---|---|
| Anticholinergic | Scopolamine | 0.5-1.5 mg transdermally q3-4d |
| Antihistamine | Diphenhydramine | 25-50 mg IM, IV, or PO q4-6h |
| | Meclizine | 25-50 mg PO q6-12h |
| | Promethazine | 12.5-25 mg IM, PO, or PR q6-8h |
| Antiemetic | Hydroxyzine | 25-50 mg PO q6h |
| | Promethazine | 12.5-25 mg IM, IV, or PO q6-12h |
| | Prochlorperazine | 5-10 mg PO q6-8h; 10-25 mg PR q6-12h |
| | Ondansetron | 4 mg IM, IV |
| Benzodiazepine | Diazepam | 2-5 mg PO qd-tid |
| | Clonazepam | 0.25-0.5 mg PO bid-tid |

## ELECTROCARDIOGRAPHY

An electrocardiogram is useful to evaluate for signs of cardiac ischemia or dysrhythmia.

# TREATMENT

Short-term treatment with vestibular suppressants is useful in the management of peripheral vertigo (**Table 96.4**). The sensory conflict theory states that a mismatch of information from vestibular, visual, or proprioceptive input will temporarily result in nausea and vertigo but will resolve as habituation occurs. This mechanism occurs via γ-aminobutyric acid, acetylcholine, serotonin, and histamine receptors. In the emergency department (ED) setting, parenteral antiemetics such as benzodiazepines (e.g., valium, 2 to 5 mg intravenously), promethazine, and ondansetron are generally most helpful. Note that the Food and Drug Administration recently recommended that promethazine be administered only via the intramuscular route when given parenterally.

Vestibular exercises such as Brandt-Daroff exercises may be helpful for BPPV, poorly compensated vestibular neuritis, end-stage Meniere disease, and chronic and psychiatric vertigo.[5] These exercises, which can be performed in the physical therapy unit or at home, are based on the concept of fatigue and facilitation of central compensatory mechanisms.

## BENIGN PAROXYSMAL POSITIONAL VERTIGO

The Epley maneuver takes approximately 3 minutes and has been shown to be safe and effective in treating posterior canal BPPV.[6] It is also easily performed in the ED setting. Gravity is used to move the otoliths out of the posterior semicircular canal into the utricle, where they will no longer cause vertigo.

The starting position of the Epley maneuver is determined by the diagnostic Hallpike test (recall that only one side should be positive). As in the Hallpike test, the patient sits upright with the head turned 45 degrees to the affected side and then lies down with the head overhanging the edge of the examination table. This maneuver should cause reproduction of the symptoms and torsional nystagmus.

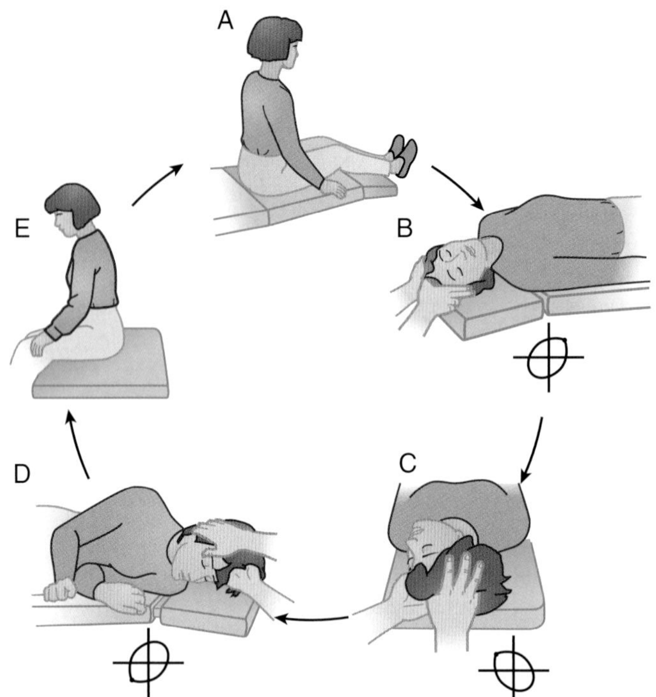


**Fig. 96.2 Epley maneuver.** (Adapted from Timothy C. Hain, MD. Available at http://www.dizziness-and-balance.com/disorders/bppv/bppv.html.)

Next, the head is rotated 90 degrees to the opposite side while it remains overhanging the edge of the examination table. The patient now rolls over onto the side and turns the head toward the ground. The patient is instructed to not lift the head up while turning onto the side. The patient is then brought up to the sitting position (the legs can hang over the side of the examination table or return to the original starting position), and the head is brought forward slightly.

Each position is held for approximately 30 seconds or until the symptoms and nystagmus resolve. It is currently recommended that the patient remain upright at least 20 minutes after the maneuver, which may be sufficient time for the otoliths to reattach to hair cells in the utricle (**Fig. 96.2**).

The Semont liberatory maneuver can also be used to treat BPPV. The patient sits upright in the middle of the examining table with his legs overhanging the edge of the gurney. The head is turned 45 degrees to the side opposite the involved canal. The patient is then rapidly laid down sideways to the side opposite of the direction his head is turned. Then the patient is rapidly laid down sideways to the other side, such that the patient's face is now directed toward the gurney. The patient then returns to the sitting position. The author does not recommend the use of this maneuver because the rapid movements are not likely to be tolerated, especially by elderly patients.

Patients with a positive roll test (indicating horizontal semicircular canal involvement) can be treated with the barbeque roll maneuver in which the patient is placed in the supine position with the head turned 90 degrees to the affected side as determined by the roll test. The head is then turned in 90-degree intervals in the opposite direction back to the original starting position. This requires the patient to eventually turn onto the abdomen. Each position is held for 30 seconds or until resolution of the vertigo and nystagmus. Anterior canal BPPV is diagnosed by a characteristic history, as well as by downbeat torsional nystagmus during the Dix-Hallpike test. Because downbeat (fast phase beating toward the feet) nystagmus can also indicate a central cause of vertigo and anterior canal involvement is extremely rare,[7] the author cautions against making this diagnosis and recommends consideration of a central cause of vertigo.

### VESTIBULAR NEURITIS AND LABYRINTHITIS

A recent multicenter trial sought to treat vestibular neuritis in a manner similar to Bell palsy. The study found that a 22-day taper of methylprednisolone was beneficial but that valacyclovir was not.[8]

## FOLLOW-UP, NEXT STEPS IN CARE, AND PATIENT EDUCATION

Once the symptoms are controlled, patients with peripheral vertigo can be discharged from the ED with meclizine as needed. Arrangements for follow-up should be made with the primary care physician and, if needed, a specialist. Peripheral vertigo is typically self-limited, although its duration is variable. Fixed unilateral lesions may produce steady symptoms that eventually diminish as a result of habituation and compensatory mechanisms by the central nervous system (CNS), although this process can take several weeks or months.

### BENIGN PAROXYSMAL POSITIONAL VERTIGO

BPPV is generally self-limited but recurs up to 50% of the time.[7] Persistent or recurrent vertigo is managed with the maneuvers described previously. Vestibular suppressants may also be prescribed.

Patients who work at heights (builders, roofers) should curtail activities until their symptoms have resolved. All patients can benefit from specialist referral. Outpatient contrast-enhanced MRI may be used to look for an acoustic neuroma or other pathology that can mimic BPPV.

In some intractable incapacitating cases, patients may benefit from neurectomy or nonampullary plugging of the semicircular canal.[9]

## CENTRAL VERTIGO

Central vertigo occurs as a result of disorders of the CNS. Major causes of central vertigo are listed in **Box 96.3**. Migraine and stroke are emphasized in the rest of this section.

**BOX 96.3 Major Causes of Central Vertigo**

Demyelination
- Acquired
- Leukodystrophies
- Multiple sclerosis

Familial disorders
- Friedreich ataxia
- Spinocerebellar ataxia
- Familial episodic ataxia (type 1 and type 2)
- Olivopontocerebellar atrophy

Central nervous system infections
- Lyme neuroborreliosis
- Meningitis
- Tuberculosis

Intrinsic brainstem lesion
- Tumor
- Arteriovenous malformation
- Trauma

Migraine
- Basilar
- Benign paroxysmal positional vertigo of childhood

Toxins
- Drugs, alcohol
- Analgesics
- Anticonvulsants
- Antihypertensives
- Hypnotics
- Tranquilizers

Metabolic and endocrine disorders
- Hyperinsulinism
- Impaired glucose tolerance
- Diabetes mellitus
- Hypertriglyceridemia
- Hypothyroidism

Systemic conditions
- Paget disease

Stroke/ischemia
- Vertebrobasilar
- Cerebellar
- Posterior inferior cerebellar artery syndrome
- Lateral medullary syndrome
- Medial medullary infarct
- Basilar artery syndrome
- Anterior inferior cerebellar artery

Other causes of posterior ischemia
- Subclavian steal syndrome
- Rotational vertebral artery occlusion syndrome
- Vertebral artery dissection
- Vertebral or basilar artery dolichoectasia
- Neoplasm of the fourth ventricle
- Chiari malformation

Superficial siderosis of the central nervous system

Vestibular epilepsy

## EPIDEMIOLOGY

### MIGRAINE

The lifetime prevalence of migraine (16%) and vertigo (7%) leads to an expected comorbidity of the two conditions in 1.1% of the general population.[10] A recent German survey, however, found a prevalence of 3.2%.[11] Vestibular migraines are the most common cause of central vertigo and occur in 25% of patients suffering from migraines. Vestibular migraines tend to occur in women between the third and fifth decades of life.

### STROKE

Each year 795,000 people suffer a new or repeated stroke, and stroke remains the third leading cause of death in the United States. Twenty percent of strokes involve the posterior circulation, which can affect the vestibular structures or pathways leading to vertigo.

## PATHOPHYSIOLOGY

Central vertigo is caused by disorders of the CNS. The visual, proprioceptive, and vestibular systems inform the brain about movement and location of the body. Input from these systems is integrated by the CNS, and any mismatch in information leads to vertigo. Overlapping of these systems allows two of them to compensate when one is deficient.

### MIGRAINE

It has been theorized that the increased sensitivity to vestibular input in patients with vestibular migraine is analogous to the increased sensitivity causing photophobia and phonophobia in patients with typical migraines.

### STROKE

The CNS obtains its blood supply from the carotid and vertebral arteries. The carotid arteries are referred to as the anterior circulation and the vertebral arteries as the posterior circulation. These two arterial systems join at the base of the brain in the vascular circle of Willis. Smaller arteries branch off from this anastomosis to supply specific areas of the brain. Blockage of one of these arteries results in a recognizable pattern of signs and symptoms consistent with the brain territory affected. A stroke is caused by thrombosis, hemorrhage, or embolism in one of the cerebral arteries. Vertigo secondary to stroke generally indicates involvement of the posterior circulation.

### OTHER

The pathophysiology of selected other causes of central vertigo are listed in **Box 96.4**.

## PRESENTING SIGNS AND SYMPTOMS

The most important clue to the diagnosis of central vertigo is the presence of associated neurologic signs and symptoms. Symptoms may occur insidiously with a slow growing lesion such as a tumor or rapidly from stroke, intracranial hemorrhage, or trauma. In general, central vertigo is not positional, its intensity is mild, and there is no associated diaphoresis, nausea, vomiting, tinnitus, or hearing abnormality. It is important to note that these clues are generalizations with many published exceptions.

### MIGRAINE

If a preceding aura occurs, the migraine will usually develop over a period of minutes and subside within an hour. This is followed by the acute onset of vertigo. Patients usually have an associated headache; however, vertigo may be the headache equivalent.[12] Fluctuating low-frequency hearing loss and tinnitus can also occur (**Box 96.5**).

**BOX 96.4 Pathophysiology of Other Causes of Central Vertigo**

Lateral medullary syndrome (Wallenberg syndrome): ipsilateral ischemia (usually from the posterior inferior cerebellar artery or one of its branches) or rarely demyelination of the lower brainstem. Cranial nerves IX and X are most commonly affected.

Subclavian steal syndrome: occurs when blood is siphoned away from the central circulation to the left upper extremity, which leads to ischemia of the posterior circulation.

Rotational vertebral artery occlusion syndrome: turning of the head may cause occlusion of the vertebral artery at the C1-C2 level.

Vertebral artery dissection: sudden strain of the neck and even trivial injuries can cause dissection, which leads to ischemia of the posterior circulation. Blood penetrates the arterial wall and compresses the lumen or forms an aneurysmal dilation. Small emboli and subarachnoid hemorrhages may also occur.

**BOX 96.5 Findings Associated with a Migrainous Etiology of Vertigo**

Onset early in life
Female gender
Occurring during menses
Episodic vertigo
Spontaneous or positional vertigo
Episodes lasting no more than a few days
Frequent recurrences within a year
Interferes with daily activities
History of motion sickness as a child
Hearing loss
Symptoms associated with the vertigo
- Migrainous headache
- Photophobia
- Aura (visual, vertiginous)
- Phonophobia

Migraine history according to International Headache Society criteria
Migraine-specific precipitants of vertigo
Personal history of migraines
Atypical positional nystagmus
Migraine medications terminating the symptoms
Other causes of vertigo ruled out
At least two attacks

### STROKE

Twenty percent of strokes involve the posterior circulation, which can affect the vestibular structures or pathways leading to vertigo. Symptoms of stroke vary depending on the affected anatomy and vasculature but often involve one or more of the "five D's": dizziness, diplopia, dysarthria, dysphagia, and dystaxia. The vascular structures most commonly affected by stroke and other lesions can be divided into anatomic territories, including the vertebrobasilar territory, the

**Table 96.5 Symptoms of Stroke and Central Nervous System Lesions Based on the Affected Anatomy and Vasculature**

| SYMPTOM | PICA | AICA | SCA | MMI | VBAT |
|---|---|---|---|---|---|
| Vertigo | + | + | + | | + |
| Nystagmus | + | | | + (upbeat) | + |
| Dysarthria | + | | + | | + |
| Dysphagia | + | | | | + |
| Nausea and vomiting | + | | + | | + |
| Slurred speech | | | + | | |
| Paresis | – | C body | – | C body | U/B |
| Sensory loss | I—face; C—body | C | – | C | B |
| Horner syndrome | I | | I | | U |
| Dysmetria | + | | | | + |
| Hearing loss | | I, U | + | | + |
| Ataxia | I, U | + | I | | + |
| Facial weakness | | I | – | – | + |
| Pain and temperature loss | I—face; C—body | | C | | |
| Respiratory failure | | | | | + |
| Headache | + | | + | | + |
| Diplopia | + | | | | + |
| Visual loss | – | | | | + |
| Hoarseness | + | | | | |
| Babinski sign | | | | | + |
| Position and vibration loss | | | | C | |
| Altered consciousness | | | | | + |
| Crossed findings | + | + | + | + | + |
| Tinnitus | | + | + | | + |
| Autonomic instability | + | | | | + |
| Other | Hiccups, facial pain | | | I—tongue weakness | Locked-in syndrome |

*AICA*, Anterior inferior cerebellar artery territory; *B*, bilateral; *C*, contralateral; *I*, ipsilateral; *MMI*, medial medullary infarction; *PICA*, posterior inferior cerebellar artery territory (Wallenberg, lateral medullary); *SCA*, superior cerebellar artery territory; *U*, unilateral, *VBAT*, vertebral basilar artery thrombosis; *VBI*, vertebrobasilar insufficiency.

superior cerebellar artery territory, and the posterior inferior cerebellar artery territory (see **Table 96.5**).

The hallmark of many brainstem strokes is crossed signs (e.g., contralateral sensory and motor findings). Vertigo and nystagmus occur early in the progression of ischemia. Dysarthria and oculomotor deficits develop later in the course and portend major neurologic catastrophe.

## DIFFERENTIAL DIAGNOSIS AND MEDICAL DECISION MAKING

### MIGRAINE

MRI may be performed to evaluate for a cerebellar or brainstem lesion if suspected.

### STROKE

Although computed tomography may show large bleeding, MRI is best for imaging the posterior fossa.

Acute posterior circulation infarcts are best seen on diffusion-weighted MRI. Magnetic resonance angiography is used to additionally assess the vertebral arteries. Patients with contraindications to MRI should undergo computed tomography and computed tomographic angiography. Carotid ultrasound scanning is not helpful in patients with posterior ischemia. Electrocardiography, echocardiography, and rhythm monitoring are important in evaluating cardiac and aortic sources of embolism.

## TREATMENT

Causes of central vertigo are serious and appropriate consultation should be obtained. Although compensation may occur with peripheral lesions, the CNS has relatively less plasticity and diminished capacity for compensation over time.

### MIGRAINE

Information on specific treatment of vertiginous migraines is limited (e.g., patients should avoid migraine triggers) and is not based on controlled studies. Patients should be referred to a neurologist for follow-up.

### STROKE

Although intravenous tissue plasminogen activator (t-PA) may enhance recovery if given within 3 hours of the onset of ischemic stroke, mixed results are found when t-PA is used for vertebrobasilar disease.[13]

### OTHER

Ventriculostomy and occipital craniotomy are often performed to relieve pressure within the posterior fossa associated with hemorrhage or a mass effect. Administration of mannitol should be considered for patients with signs of herniation.

Hypotension should be corrected because it worsens symptoms and outcome. Intravenous fluids, blood, and pressors should be administered as needed. Neurologic consultation may be useful to guide treatment.

## SUGGESTED READINGS

Baloh RW. Neurotology of migraine. Headache 1997;37:615-21.

Hilton M, Pinder D. The Epley (canalith repositioning) maneuver for benign paroxysmal positional vertigo. Cochrane Database Syst Rev 2002;1:CD003162.

Hoston JR, Baloh RW. Acute vestibular syndrome. N Engl J Med 1998;339:680-5.

Lempert T, Von Brevern M. Episodic vertigo. Curr Opin Neurol 2005;18:5-9.

Savitz S, Caplan L. Current concepts in vertebrobasilar disease. N Engl J Med 2005;352:2618-26.

## REFERENCES

***References can be found on Expert Consult @ www.expertconsult.com.***

# Peripheral Nerve Disorders 97

*Phillip Andrus and Swathi Nadindla*

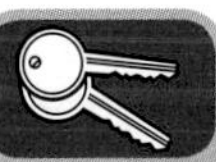

**KEY POINTS**

- Nerve compression is the most common cause of radiculopathy and mononeuropathy.
- Radiculopathy and radicular pain are typically associated with symptoms within a dermatome or myotome.
- Patients with mononeuropathy have symptoms limited to a single peripheral nerve.
- Guillain-Barré syndrome is an autoimmune demyelinating disease that results in primarily motor symptoms, with severe disease leading to respiratory compromise.
- Myasthenia gravis and Lambert-Eaton myasthenic syndrome are both autoimmune disorders of the neuromuscular junction; myasthenia gravis affects the postsynaptic membrane, whereas Lambert-Eaton syndrome affects the presynaptic membrane.
- Botulism is a toxin-mediated disorder of the neuromuscular junction.
- Systemic diseases such as diabetes mellitus and human immunodeficiency virus infection can result in several peripheral nerve disorders.

## PERSPECTIVE

Peripheral nerve disorders can result in varied findings, including proximal or distal weakness, symmetric or asymmetric symptoms, and acute or chronic manifestations. Motor symptoms range from weakness to paralysis, whereas sensory symptoms range from numbness to pain.

Evaluation of peripheral nerve disorders requires an understanding of the anatomy of the spinal cord and the peripheral nervous system (**Fig. 97.1**). The peripheral nervous system is composed of 12 cranial nerves and 31 spinal nerves. Spinal nerves are formed from motor fibers whose cell bodies reside in the ventral horn of the spinal cord and from sensory fibers whose cell bodies are found in the dorsal root ganglion. The motor and sensory fibers join to form one nerve as it exits the spinal canal. Spinal nerves from several spinal levels merge at the cervical, brachial, lumbar, and sacral plexuses. Peripheral nerves originate either at these plexuses or, if they are formed from nerves of only one spinal level, as they exit the vertebral foramina.

Peripheral nerves consist of mixed fibers with variable amounts of motor, sensory, and autonomic fibers; small and large fibers; and myelinated and unmyelinated fibers. These fibers, which are surrounded by endoneurial fluid and covered in perineurium, form fascicles that are bundled together by the epineurial sheath. This sheath forms a protective barrier akin to the blood-brain barrier in the central nervous system.

In patients with symptoms concerning for a peripheral nerve disorder, the history and physical examination are important in localizing the lesion. Spinal nerve, or nerve root, lesions are called radiculopathies and result in myotomal weakness or dermatomal sensory loss. Plexus lesions can be variable, with symptoms that cross myotomes and dermatomes or involve multiple peripheral nerves. Symptoms depend on which trunk or cord is involved. Peripheral nerve lesions cause weakness and sensory loss that is limited to a specific peripheral nerve.

Systemic diseases affect the peripheral nervous system as well, and multiple peripheral nerves may be involved. Examples include disorders of the neuromuscular junction (NMJ), demyelinating disorders, diabetes, and toxic effects of drugs or chemicals (**Box 97.1**).

# Radiculopathies

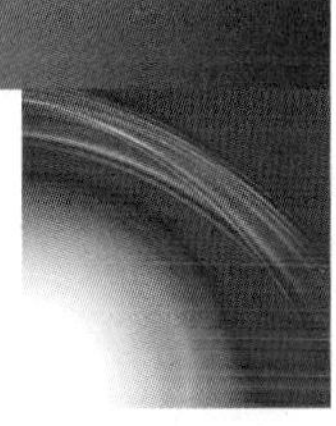

## PATHOPHYSIOLOGY

Spinal nerve compression results in radiculopathy, radicular pain, or both. Radiculopathy is due to blocked conduction along a spinal nerve and results in a neurologic deficit: dermatomal sensory loss or myotomal weakness. Radicular pain is due to irritation or inflammation of the spinal nerve, neurologic deficits are absent, and patients have purely painful symptoms that may not be isolated to a dermatome.

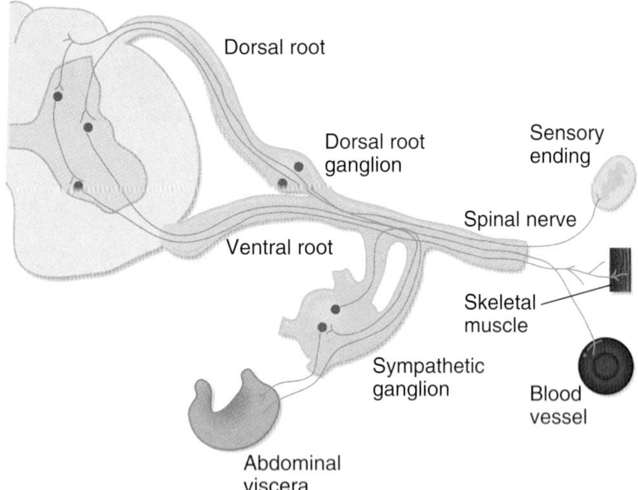


**Fig. 97.1 Cross section of the spine showing the relationship among the ventral and dorsal roots, dorsal root ganglion, spinal cord, vertebrae, and peripheral nerve.**

**BOX 97.1 Differential Diagnosis of Suspected Peripheral Nerve Disorders**

**Central Nervous System**
Cerebrovascular accident (stroke)
Spinal cord compression
Brown-Sequard syndrome
Amyotrophic lateral sclerosis

**Autoimmune**
Myasthenia gravis
Lambert-Eaton myasthenic syndrome
Guillain-Barré syndrome

**Demyelination**
Multifocal motor neuropathy
Critical illness polyneuropathy

**Drug and Toxin Related**
Medications: amiodarone, isoniazid
Metals: gold, arsenic, lead
Diphtheria
Botulism
Tick paralysis

**Hereditary**
Charcot-Marie-Tooth disease
Acute intermittent porphyria

**Infections**
Human immunodeficiency virus–related neuropathy
Chronic hepatitis
Acute infectious mononucleosis (Epstein-Barr virus)

**Inflammatory**
POEMS (polyneuropathy, endocrinopathy, M-protein production, skin changes)

**Metabolic**
Alcoholic neuropathy
Vitamin $B_{12}$ deficiency
Hypokalemia

**Table 97.1 Nerve Root and Associated Reflex**

| NERVE ROOT | REFLEX |
|---|---|
| C5-6 | Brachioradialis |
| C7 8 | Triceps |
| L3-4 | Patellar |
| S1 | Achilles |

Causes of spinal nerve compression are varied; if a patient is younger than 50 years, the symptoms are more likely to be caused by disk herniation, and if older than 50 years, by degenerative changes.

## PRESENTING SIGNS AND SYMPTOMS

As noted, sensory loss and weakness follow a dermatomal or myotomal distribution. Diminished reflexes may also assist in determining the nerve root that is involved (**Table 97.1**).

In the cervical region, C6 and C7 are the most commonly affected, with higher roots less frequently involved. This is true for the lumbosacral spinal nerves as well, with more patients having signs in the L5-S1 distribution. Sciatica is a particularly common syndrome of radicular pain and involves more than one of the L2-S1 spinal nerves.

## DIAGNOSTIC TESTING

A careful history and physical examination will help localize the symptoms of a radiculopathy. The straight leg raise should be used to test for lumbosacral involvement. While the patient is lying supine, the leg is raised with the knee in extension. The test is considered positive for spinal nerve involvement when symptoms are reproduced within 60 degrees of elevation.

If a patient has solely radicular pain, imaging may not be necessary because the symptoms resolve in 60% to 80% of patients within 6 to 12 weeks with conservative treatment. In patients whose symptoms fail to resolve, progress, or involve sensory loss or weakness, either computed tomography or magnetic resonance imaging (MRI) is indicated. Patients should also undergo imaging if they have a history of malignancy, long-term steroid use, intravenous drug abuse, human immunodeficiency virus (HIV) infection, diabetes, acute loss of neurologic function, or known trauma. In general, MRI is preferred because it has higher soft tissue resolution. For disk disease, it is important to note that the size of a disk herniation does not always correlate with clinical symptoms: patients without evidence of herniation may have significant symptoms, whereas patients with an incidental finding of disk herniation may have no symptoms.

## TREATMENT

In the acute phase of injury, painful symptoms are typically treated conservatively with nonsteroidal antiinflammatory drugs (NSAIDs) and physical therapy. Low-quality evidence suggests that there is no difference between bed rest and activity for patients with sciatica.[1] However, a randomized controlled trial showed that the addition of physical therapy is more effective than counseling and pain medications alone, although it may not be as cost-effective.[2] Persistent or severe symptoms may require more invasive measures, from local corticosteroid injections to neurosurgical intervention.[3] For the cervical spinal nerves, some evidence has shown that conservative therapy consisting of pain control has favorable short-term outcomes when compared with surgical intervention, although long-term outcomes appear to be similar.[4] Surgical outcomes can be dependent on the mechanism of injury; for example, with spinal stenosis, 70% of patients will still have persistent loss of function. Chronic pain symptoms may be treated with medications used for neuropathic pain, such as antidepressants or anticonvulsants.

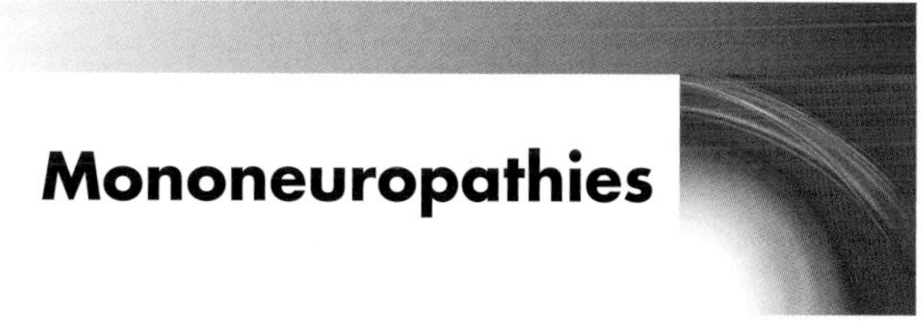

# Mononeuropathies

## EPIDEMIOLOGY

As with radiculopathy, compression of peripheral nerves is the most common cause of peripheral mononeuropathy, the most frequent being median mononeuropathy (**Fig. 97.2**). Women older than 55 years are most commonly affected, with a 4.6% prevalence in women and 2.8% in men.[5] The second most frequent cause is ulnar mononeuropathy; specifically, cubital tunnel syndrome. Other common peripheral mononeuropathies include involvement of the radial nerve in the upper extremity and the peroneal and lateral cutaneous femoral nerves in the lower extremity.

## PATHOPHYSIOLOGY, PRESENTING SIGNS AND SYMPTOMS, AND DIAGNOSTIC TESTING

For mononeuropathies, the history and physical examination largely lead to the appropriate diagnosis. Findings in patients with common mononeuropathies and diagnostic maneuvers are presented in **Table 97.2**.[6-12] In patients with a history of trauma or acute symptoms, plain films may be necessary to rule out fracture or dislocation. Patients with subacute or chronic symptoms should be asked about chronic conditions. Mononeuropathies can occur with several systemic diseases, including diabetes mellitus, amyloidosis, HIV, and states that cause edema, such as pregnancy.[13] Outpatient testing may be more appropriate for individuals with chronic symptoms. MRI or electrodiagnostic testing such as electromyography or nerve conduction studies may be necessary, and the patient should be referred to a neurologist. MRI may demonstrate chronic nerve injury, whereas electrodiagnostic testing may show slowing of nerve conduction. These studies may aid in deciding whether surgical repair or decompression is necessary for certain syndromes.

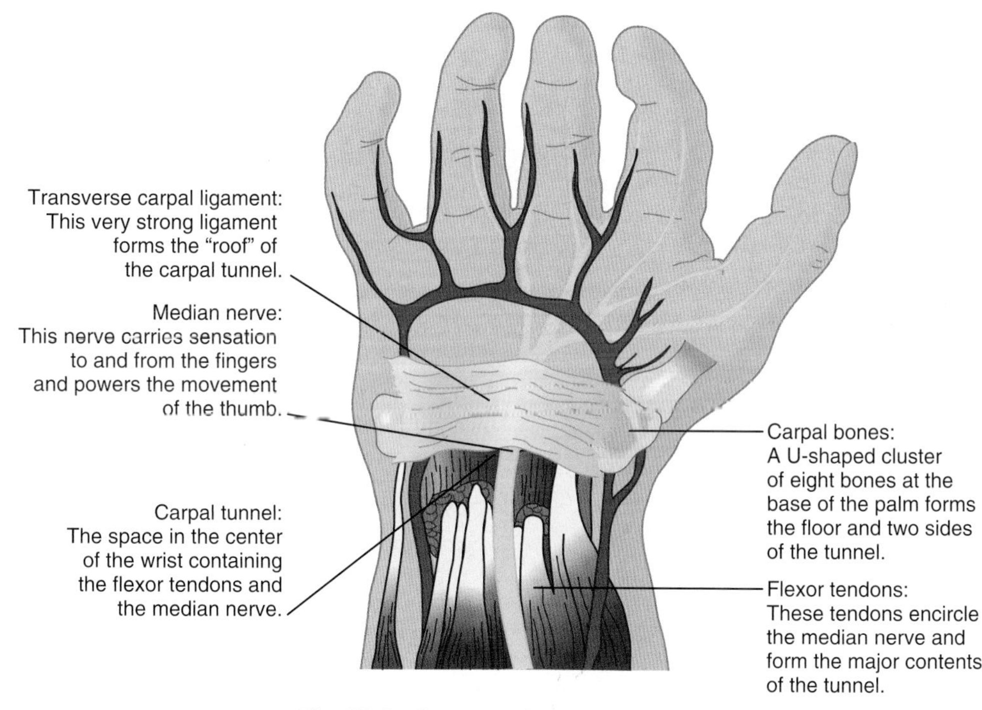


**Fig. 97.2 Anatomy of the carpal tunnel.**

**Table 97.2 Specific Peripheral Mononeuropathies**

| PERIPHERAL NERVE | SYNDROME | COMPRESSION SITE | CAUSES | SIGNS AND SYMPTOMS | TESTING |
|---|---|---|---|---|---|
| Median | Carpal tunnel | Carpal tunnel: by carpal bones and the flexor retinaculum (see Fig. 97.2) | Repetitive use, trauma | Burning, numbness, pain in the palmar aspect of the 1st, 2nd, 3rd, and radial aspect of the 4th finger | Tinel sign: symptoms with tapping on the palmar aspect of the wrist<br>Phalen sign: symptoms when the wrists is held in flexion for 60 seconds[6] |
| Ulnar | Cubital tunnel | Cubital tunnel: behind the medial epicondyle[7] | Repetitive use, trauma | Tingling of the 5th and lateral aspect of the 4th fingers; weakness of intrinsic muscles of the hand | Tinel sign: symptoms with tapping on the elbow at the cubital tunnel<br>Elbow flexion sign: symptoms when the elbow is flexed and the wrist is extended for 3 min<br>Froment sign: the thumb interphalangeal joint flexes when attempting to hold a card between the 1st and 2nd digits |
| | Guyon's canal, handlebar palsy | At the Guyon canal at the wrist, bounded by the pisiform and hamate bones | Repetitive use, trauma | Weakness of the intrinsic muscles of the hand | Unable to abduct the fingers |
| Radial | Saturday night palsy | Upper part of the arm at the spiral groove | Compression injury or midshaft humeral fracture | Wristdrop, dorsal sensory loss in the hand[8,9] | |
| | Radial tunnel syndrome | Sensory branch at the elbow | Repetitive motion | Forearm pain | |
| | — | Motor branch at the elbow | Radial fracture, elbow fracture or dislocation | Extensor muscles of the hand more than the wrist | |
| Peroneal | — | Below the fibular head | Compression (crossing the legs, rapid weight loss, casting, any source of direct pressure on the fibular head, fracture, knee dislocation[10,11]) | Footdrop, steppage gait | |
| Lateral cutaneous femoral | Meralgia paresthetica | | Compression (inguinal ligament, seat belt, tight pants, pregnancy[12]) | Anterolateral thigh pain, paresthesias, numbness; no motor component | Worsening pain with hip extension, pain with palpation of the inguinal ligament |

## TREATMENT

Primary treatment should be aimed at the precipitating event for both acute and chronic mononeuropathy.

With acute mononeuropathy, the primary cause of injury is generally trauma. Fractures and dislocations should be reduced appropriately and immobilized with the guidance of surgical consultation.

Initial treatment of chronic mononeuropathy is typically conservative and supportive. Modification of behavior is a key component of treatment and prevention of further injury. For carpal tunnel syndrome, behavior modification includes weight loss and avoidance of caffeine, nicotine, and alcohol. Patients should be instructed to decrease any possible trauma related to repetitive use by making changes in workplace ergonomics, reducing repetitive use, and changing posture. Some neuropathies may require supportive devices; for example, the carpal tunnel may benefit from wearing a wrist splint, the ulnar nerve from wearing a sling or a long arm posterior splint, the radial nerve from wearing a volar splint, and the peroneal nerve from wearing a posterior splint.[8,9] NSAIDs are typically prescribed for relief of symptoms, although they may be ineffective without appropriate behavioral modification. In patients with a systemic disease, the primary process should be treated. Diuretics may be given if edema is believed to be contributing significantly to the patient's symptoms. More invasive procedures, such as local nerve block for meralgia paresthetica or surgical decompression for carpal tunnel syndrome, are reserved for severe cases.

# Autoimmune Disorders

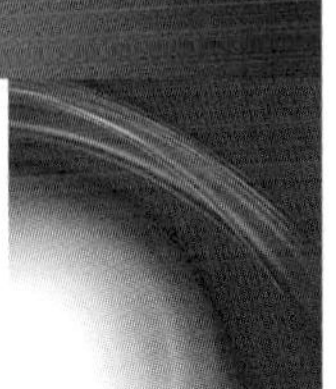

## GUILLAIN-BARRÉ SYNDROME

### EPIDEMIOLOGY

Guillain-Barré syndrome (GBS) is also known as acute inflammatory demyelinating polyradiculopathy or Landry-Guillain-Barré syndrome. Its worldwide incidence is 0.6 to 4 per 100,000 individuals annually.[14]

### PATHOPHYSIOLOGY

GBS is characterized by immune-mediated destruction of the myelin sheath of peripheral nerves. Biopsy frequently reveals a mononuclear inflammatory infiltrate. Although its exact etiology remains unknown, two thirds of cases are preceded by an infection. Associations have been made with viral or febrile illness, *Campylobacter jejuni* infection, vaccinations, and even surgery or trauma.

GBS is a monophasic illness with progressive symptoms that reach a nadir in 2 to 4 weeks. Recovery can vary from weeks to a year. Mortality has been reported in 4% to 15% of patients, whereas another 10% to 20% have significant residual motor dysfunction.

### PRESENTING SIGNS AND SYMPTOMS

#### CLASSIC GUILLAIN-BARRÉ SYNDROME

Classic GBS is preceded by a viral prodrome and followed by acute or subacute ascending symmetric weakness or paralysis and loss of the deep tendon reflexes. Paralysis may ascend to the diaphragm and compromise respiratory function to the extent that mechanical ventilation is required. One third of patients will require intubation and 15% will experience dysautonomia. Specific findings are strongly suggestive of this diagnosis (**Box 97.2**).

**BOX 97.2 Findings Suggesting Guillain-Barré Syndrome**

Relative symmetry of symptoms
Mild sensory signs and symptoms
Cranial nerve involvement
Autonomic dysfunction
Absence of fever at onset
Cytoalbuminologic dissociation of cerebrospinal fluid
Typical electrodiagnostic findings
Progression over days to weeks
Recovery beginning 2 to 4 weeks after cessation of progression

#### VARIANTS OF GUILLAIN-BARRÉ SYNDROME

##### *Acute Motor Axonal Neuropathy*

This purely motor form of GBS is associated with *C. jejuni* infection and is more often preceded by diarrhea than by a viral prodrome. It results in axonal injury rather than demyelination.

##### *Acute Motor and Sensory Axonal Neuropathy*

This variant involves loss of both motor and sensory function. As with acute motor axonal neuropathy, electrodiagnostic testing reveals axonal degeneration.

##### *Miller-Fisher Syndrome*

Identified in 1956, Miller-Fisher syndrome is characterized by ophthalmoplegia, ataxia, and decreased or absent reflexes. Patients have significantly less weakness and a milder course than do those with classic GBS.

### DIAGNOSTIC TESTING

It is critical that respiratory function be assessed early and often because maintenance of airway protection well in advance of respiratory compromise decreases the incidence of aspiration and other complications of emergency intubation (**Box 97.3**). The most studied monitoring parameter is vital capacity (VC), with normal values ranging from 60 to 70 mL/kg. However, a simple bedside assessment of respiratory status can be obtained by having the patient count from 1 to 25 with a single breath and trending the values over time.

**BOX 97.3 Indications for Intubation in Patients with Guillain-Barré Syndrome**

Rapid progression of respiratory compromise
Vital capacity less than 20 mL/kg
Negative inspiratory force less than –30 cm $H_2O$
Greater than a 30% decrease in either vital capacity or negative inspiratory force in the first 24 hours
Autonomic instability

If the patient's condition does not initially meet the criteria for intubation, VC should be monitored closely—every hour for the first 4 hours and then every 4 hours.[15]

Lumbar puncture often reveals the classic "albuminocytologic dissociation" in which cerebrospinal fluid (CSF) protein is high without pleocytosis. The protein level is greater than 45 mg/dL. Cell counts are typically below 10/mL and usually

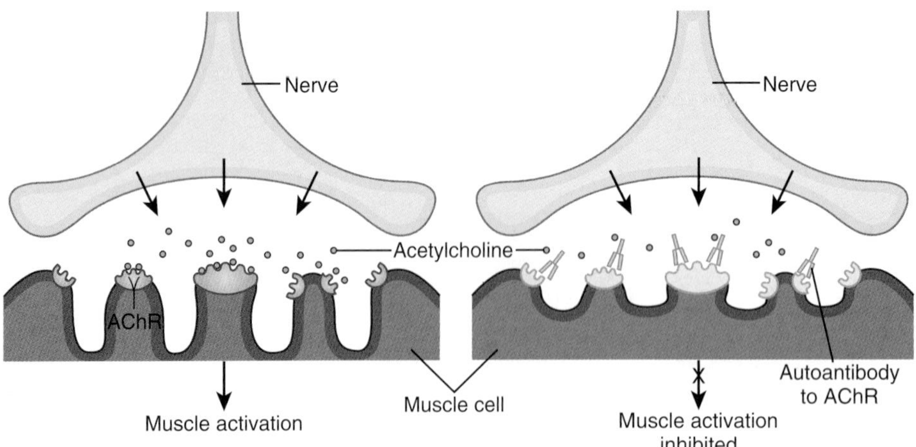


**Fig. 97.3** Diagram of the motor end plate illustrating blocking of autoantibodies to acetylcholine receptors (AChRs).

consist predominantly of mononuclear cells. Up to 80% of patients demonstrate this classic pattern. Of note, CSF studies are more likely to be negative in the first week of illness. With counts higher than 100 cells/mL, other causes should be considered, including HIV infection, Lyme disease, syphilis, sarcoid, tuberculosis, bacterial meningitis, leukemic infiltration, and central nervous system vasculitis.

Electrodiagnostic testing confirms the demyelination typical of GBS. In patients with the acute motor axonal neuropathy or acute motor and sensory axonal neuropathy variants, electromyography and nerve conduction studies reveal axonal injury rather than demyelination.

## TREATMENT

The first priority in the treatment of patients with GBS is airway management. Along with frequent assessment of the need for intubation, early consultation with neurology or critical care specialists (or both) will ensure a coordinated management strategy.

Corticosteroids have shown no benefit in the management of GBS and may be harmful. The two modalities that have clearly proved to be beneficial are intravenous immunoglobulin (IVIG) and plasmapheresis. Both provide an equal, but not additive reduction in the duration of symptoms if given within 2 weeks of onset to ambulatory patients and within 4 weeks to nonambulatory patients. Plasmapheresis has been associated with more treatment complications and adverse events, including hemodynamic instability, which has resulted in a higher rate of discontinuation. However, it is also associated with a lower relapse rate. Overall, fewer complications occur with IVIG, although thromboembolism and aseptic meningitis have been reported.[16]

The decision to admit the patient to the hospital should be made in consultation with a neurologist and may be based on clinical criteria alone or confirmation by CSF analysis and nerve conduction studies. Patients who require or may require intubation, are unable to ambulate, or are being considered for plasmapheresis should be admitted to the intensive care unit.

# MYASTHENIA GRAVIS

## EPIDEMIOLOGY

Myasthenia gravis has a prevalence of 50 to 125 individuals per million. The age at onset is bimodal: the first peak involves persons in their 20s to 30s, with women being affected more than men, and the second peak occurs during the sixth and seventh decades, with men being affected more than women.

## PATHOPHYSIOLOGY

Myasthenia gravis has many causes, but they all lead to the formation of autoantibodies directed against nicotinic acetylcholine receptors (AChRs) at the NMJ (**Fig. 97.3**). This results in autoimmune destruction of AChRs through complement-mediated destruction, as well as increased endocytosis by muscle cells. The autoantibodies further compete with acetylcholine (ACh) for binding at the remaining receptors. Thus with repeated stimulation of the same muscle, fewer and fewer sites are available and fatigue develops.

## PRESENTING SIGNS AND SYMPTOMS

### NEW ONSET

Muscular weakness and fatigability are the hallmarks of myasthenia gravis. When patients are seen in the emergency department (ED) with an initial manifestation of the disease, the symptoms usually consist of mononeuropathy involving the ocular or bulbar muscles. The typical finding is ptosis, diplopia, or blurred vision. Ocular muscle weakness may be the first sign in up to 40% of patients, although it will develop in 85% in due course. When present, ptosis is often worse toward the end of the day. When the bulbar muscles are involved, dysarthria or dysphagia occurs. Respiratory failure is a rare initial sign. Nevertheless, up to 17% of patients may have weakness of the muscles of respiration.

**BOX 97.4 Drugs That May Exacerbate Myasthenia Gravis**

| Cardiovascular Drugs | Other Drugs |
|---|---|
| Calcium channel blockers | Phenytoin |
| Quinidine | Neuromuscular blockers |
| Lidocaine | Corticosteroids |
| Procainamide | Thyroid replacement drugs |
| **Antibiotics** | |
| Aminoglycosides | |
| Tetracycline | |
| Clindamycin | |
| Lincomycin | |
| Polymyxin B | |
| Colistin | |

### ACUTE MYASTHENIC CRISIS

Acute myasthenic crisis is defined as respiratory failure eventually requiring mechanical ventilation. It occurs in 15% to 20% of patients, generally within the first 2 years of the disease. With the use of better and more aggressive techniques in the intensive care unit, mortality has declined tremendously.

Underlying infection, aspiration, and changes in medications most often trigger myasthenic crisis, but the precipitant may not be found in up to 30% of cases (**Box 97.4**).

Some patients experience an increase in weakness when starting chronic steroid therapy. Other precipitants include surgery and pregnancy.

As with GBS, the initial step in managing patients in myasthenic crisis is assessing respiratory status and securing the airway, if necessary. A patient who is complaining of shortness of breath or difficulty breathing should have VC measured frequently. In contrast to the steady deterioration associated with GBS, patients in myasthenic crisis may have fluctuating weakness. In these patients a lower VC of 15 mL/kg is considered an indication for intubation, but the trend of their respiratory function is more useful than a single measurement.

### CONGENITAL MYASTHENIA GRAVIS

Approximately 12% of pregnant women with myasthenia gravis will give birth to symptomatic infants because of placental transfer of autoantibodies. An infant's symptoms develop within 2 days of life and include impaired sucking, weak cry, limp limbs, and rarely, respiratory insufficiency. The symptoms disappear within days or weeks as antibody titers in the infant decline. In severe cases of respiratory failure, intubation is necessary, and exchange transfusion should be considered.

## DIAGNOSTIC TESTING

The diagnosis is based on clinical findings, bedside testing, and serologic studies.

### BEDSIDE TESTING

The edrophonium test is a pharmacologic test involving the use of a short-acting acetylcholinesterase (AChE)-blocking agent that can be done at the patient's bedside.[17] The test confirms the diagnosis of myasthenia if the ptosis improves after the intravenous administration of edrophonium. An initial dose of 1 mg is given and the patient is observed for an adverse reaction or improvement in the symptoms of ptosis, medial rectus weakness, or dysphonia. If unimproved in 30 to 90 seconds, a second dose of 3 mg is given. Another 3-mg dose of edrophonium is administered if no response is seen after 30 to 60 seconds. If there is still no response, a final dose of 3 mg is given, for a total maximum dosage of 10 mg. Edrophonium may result in a severe anticholinergic reaction, especially in the elderly, cardiac disease patients, those with chronic obstructive pulmonary disease, or asthmatics. Symptoms include salivation and gastrointestinal cramping but may be more severe, such as bradycardia, bronchorrhea, bronchospasm, and worsening weakness. Because of the potential for bradycardia, atropine should be at the bedside during edrophonium testing.

The ice test is another bedside test that can be used to quickly confirm the diagnosis. Cooling decreases the symptoms of myasthenia gravis, whereas heat exacerbates them. In this test the distance between the upper and lower lids is measured before the application of an ice pack for 2 to 3 minutes to the most severely affected eye.[18]

### SEROLOGIC TESTING

Receptor antibody testing is positive in 80% to 90% of patients. Many patients found to be seronegative nonetheless respond to traditional therapy aimed at lowering levels of circulating antibodies, thus suggesting that antibodies are present but not detected.

## TREATMENT

### ACETYLCHOLINESTERASE INHIBITORS

AChE inhibitors such as pyridostigmine and neostigmine are the backbone of outpatient chronic therapy and provide symptomatic improvement.[2] This class of drugs inhibits the hydrolysis of ACh, which leads to an increased circulating concentration of ACh to compete with the antibody for AChR binding sites. The most common side effects are those of excessive cholinergic stimulation as mentioned earlier. These drugs are not directed at the underlying immunologic basis of the disease and are often used as adjunctive therapy to control symptoms while allowing time for other therapy to take effect, after which they are discontinued.[19]

The use of intravenous pyridostigmine in the setting of acute exacerbation of myasthenia gravis is controversial. Some evidence indicates that its use may complicate ventilation by worsening pulmonary secretions.[20] Consequently, cholinergic drug therapy should be discontinued during a myasthenic crisis. In addition, a cholinergic crisis characterized by acute decompensation and excessive muscarinic stimulation may be caused by excessive medication with AChE inhibitors. Cholinergic crisis should be distinguished from an exacerbation of the disease by muscarinic findings on physical examination: excessive sweating, salivation, lacrimation, miosis, tachycardia, and gastrointestinal hyperactivity.

### IMMUNOSUPPRESSION

Immunosuppressant drugs are often used for chronic control of the symptoms of myasthenia gravis. They have no role in the acute management of myasthenic crisis, although they may be started before extubation of patients recovering from a crisis. Corticosteroids, azathioprine, and cyclosporine have all been used.

### THYMECTOMY

Thymectomy in otherwise well patients between adolescence and 60 years of age results in remission or improvement in up to 50% of cases. However, the onset of improvement after thymectomy is often delayed for 2 to 3 years.

### IMMUNOMODULATORY THERAPY

Plasmapheresis and IVIG are reserved for patients with severe exacerbations or are administered preoperatively to patients with stable myasthenia gravis. Of patients treated with IVIG, 50% to 90% have some improvement following infusion. These treatment modalities should be administered in conjuction with a neurologist.

## LAMBERT-EATON MYASTHENIC SYNDROME

### EPIDEMIOLOGY

Lambert-Eaton myasthenic syndrome (LEMS) is relatively uncommon, with a prevalence of 1 in 100,000 individuals. The disease occurs predominantly in those older than 50 years, with both genders affected equally.[22]

### PATHOPHYSIOLOGY

In healthy presynaptic neurons, depolarization opens channels that allow calcium to enter. This results in ACh-filled vesicles fusing with the presynaptic membrane and release of ACh into the synapse. ACh then stimulates the postsynaptic neuron, which results in transmission of the impulse from one neuron to the next.

LEMS is an autoimmune presynaptic disorder of the NMJ. IgG autoantibodies bind to the presynaptic calcium channels, thereby inhibiting entry of calcium into the cell during depolarization. The net effect is decreased release of ACh and absent or diminished transduction of signal to the postsynaptic membrane. This disease affects not only the NMJ but also muscarinic receptors and results in autonomic dysfunction.

Frequently, this disease is associated with other pathology. Malignancies are often seen with LEMS, with upward of 70% of cases having a concomitant malignancy. The most common association is with small cell lung cancer: 62% of cases have this link.[19] Diagnosis of the malignancy may come after the diagnosis of LEMS. Because LEMS is an autoimmune disorder, it is also associated with other autoimmune disorders, including hypothyroidism, pernicious anemia, and celiac disease.[23]

### PRESENTING SIGNS AND SYMPTOMS

The typical symptoms involve weakness of the proximal muscles, with the lower extremities being affected more than the upper ones, and decreased or absent reflexes. Bulbar symptoms may be present, though with significantly less frequency and severity than in myasthenia gravis. Autonomic symptoms are reported in 75% of patients; symptoms include dry eyes and mouth, impotence, constipation, and orthostatic hypotension.

Patients often have symptoms of weakness with minimal associated disability; the symptoms frequently improve with repetitive use because calcium is able to accumulate in the presynaptic neuron. This is demonstrated with the Lambert sign, in which there is a progressive increase in grip when maintained over a few seconds. It can also be seen in reflexes, which improve after exercising the muscle.

### DIAGNOSTIC TESTING

Testing specific to this disease is typically not conducted in the ED, and a neurologist should be consulted for evaluation. Antibody testing is positive in 85% of patients. LEMS may develop up to 2 years before the diagnosis of a malignancy, and therefore patients should be evaluated for malignancy.

### TREATMENT

The most effective treatment of LEMS involves treatment of the primary malignancy if present. Other treatments have been used over the years, including immunosuppressants such as prednisone, pyridostigmine (AChE inhibitor), plasma exchange, IVIG, and 3,4-diaminopyridine (3,4-DAP). 3,4-DAP is an oral medication that blocks potassium channels and prevents repolarization and removal of calcium from the cell. Evidence for the efficacy of these therapies is limited because the disease itself is uncommon, although randomized controlled trials have found improvement with IVIG and 3,4-DAP.[24]

# Systemic Disorders

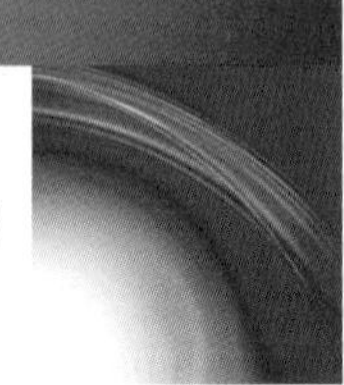

## BOTULISM

### EPIDEMIOLOGY

Botulism is a toxin-mediated illness that can cause acute weakness leading to respiratory failure. In 2009, the Centers for Disease Control and Prevention reported 121 cases of botulism: 69% were categorized as infantile, 19% as wound, and 9% as food-borne botulism. In 2009, of the 23 cases of wound botulism, 21 resulted from injection drug use.[25]

### PATHOPHYSIOLOGY

*Clostridium botulinum*, the causative organism, is an anaerobic spore-forming bacterium. Three of eight known toxins produced by *C. botulinum* cause human disease: toxin types A, B, and E. Most cases of botulism are isolated events associated with improperly preserved canned foods, although the incidence of botulism from wound infections has recently increased. Toxin type E is associated with preserved or fermented fish and marine mammals. These are the most important sources of botulism in Alaska, Japan, Russia, and Scandinavia.[26]

The botulinum toxin binds irreversibly to the presynaptic membrane of peripheral and cranial nerves and inhibits release of ACh at the peripheral nerve synapse. As new receptors are generated, patients improve.

## PRESENTING SIGNS AND SYMPTOMS

### CLASSIC BOTULISM

The disorder occurs at the NMJ, so neither sensory deficit nor pain occurs. Symptoms begin 6 to 48 hours after ingestion of the tainted food. The classic finding is a descending, symmetric paralysis. The nerves and muscles often affected first are the cranial nerves and bulbar muscles, which results in diplopia, dysarthria, dysphagia, and blurry vision. The deep tendon reflexes are normal or diminished. Signs and symptoms consistent with gastroenteritis may develop: nausea, vomiting, abdominal cramps, diarrhea, and constipation.

Because the toxins cause decreased cholinergic output, anticholinergic signs may be seen in the form of constipation, urinary retention, dry skin and eyes, and increased temperature. Pupils are often dilated and not reactive to light—an important point of differentiation from myasthenia gravis.

### INFANTILE BOTULISM

Infantile botulism occurs as a result of the ingestion of *C. botulinum* spores that are able to germinate and produce toxin in the high pH of the gastrointestinal tract of infants (the same spores are not active in the gut of adults because of the lower pH). It occurs in infants between the age of 1 week and 11 months and has been implicated as a cause of sudden infant death syndrome. Clinical findings include constipation, poor feeding, lethargy, and weak cry; consequently, this diagnosis must be included in the differential diagnosis of a "floppy" infant.

## DIAGNOSTIC TESTING

The diagnosis is based on clinical findings and exclusion of other processes. The toxin can be identified in both serum and stool, but the assay is not commonly available in most hospitals and thus requires a prolonged turnaround time. If the suspected food source is available, it should also be tested for the toxin.

## TREATMENT

Treatment is initially focused on evaluating respiratory effort and securing the airway if respiratory compromise has occurred. The course of the disease can be shortened by administering botulinum antitoxin. A trivalent equine antitoxin is available from the Centers for Disease Control and Prevention, as well as from local poison control centers. Skin testing to assess for horse serum sensitivity should be carried out before administration.

# DIABETIC PERIPHERAL NEUROPATHY

## EPIDEMIOLOGY

A common complication of diabetes, diabetic peripheral neuropathy has a varied prevalence ranging from 34% to 60%, although higher rates often include asymptomatic neuropathies. It is a highly variable entity that is composed of several subsets. Of the various subsets of diabetic neuropathy, distal symmetric polyneuropathy is the most common, with up to 54% of patients with diabetic neuropathy having this variant. It is seen in patients with type 1 diabetes after 5 years and early in the course of type 2 diabetes.[27,28]

## PATHOPHYSIOLOGY

Diabetic peripheral neuropathy encompasses any neuropathy in a diabetic patient not attributable to other causes. Although the most common form is distal symmetric polyneuropathy, diabetes also leads to focal and autonomic neuropathies. It is accompanied by significant morbidity: the most common cause of nontraumatic amputation is injury resulting from the impaired sensation associated with diabetic peripheral neuropathy that fails to heal because of the impaired blood flow in patients with diabetic vasculopathy.

Hyperglycemia affects the peripheral nerves by several proposed mechanisms:

1. Oxidative stress
2. Glycosylation of nerve proteins
3. Changes in the diabetic vasculature resulting in increased resistance and decreased flow to the peripheral nerves

Motor, sensory, and small and large fibers can all be involved. Diabetic peripheral neuropathy is an example of a distal axonopathy resulting in length-dependent "dying back" of the affected nerves. This dying-back phenomenon produces the typical stocking-and-glove distribution of diabetic neuropathy.[29]

## PRESENTING SIGNS AND SYMPTOMS

Several neuropathic syndromes can be found in diabetic patients and are often present concurrently (**Table 97.3**). For example, patients may have a sensorimotor polyneuropathy with subsequent development of a mononeuropathy of the upper extremity.[30]

## TREATMENT

Disease modification has the greatest effect on the progression of diabetic neuropathy; although the cause is multifactorial, a clear relationship between glycemic control and neuropathy exists. The Diabetes Control and Complications Trial showed

**Table 97.3 Syndromes of Diabetic Neuropathy**

| SYNDROME | TIME COURSE | HALLMARKS | NERVES INVOLVED |
|---|---|---|---|
| Diabetic sensorimotor polyneuropathy | Chronic and progressive | Stocking glove distribution | Sensory: pain, paresthesias, numbness, cramping<br>Motor: weakness, atrophy, imbalance, ataxia |
| Diabetic autonomic neuropathy | Chronic and progressive | | Autonomic: dysmotility, gastroparesis, orthostatic hypotension, erectile dysfunction, incontinence |
| Acute painful diabetic neuropathy | Duration < 6 mo | Intermittent, worse at night or when attentive | Sensory: pins and needles, throbbing, burning, aching, cramping, cold sensation |
| Chronic painful diabetic neuropathy | Duration > 6 mo | Same as above | Same as above |
| Insulin neuritis | | Associated with insulin therapy, may resolve with time or cessation | Sensory: pain, paresthesias |
| Diabetic neuropathic cachexia | Monophasic, unrelated to duration of the disease | Rare syndrome | Initial weight loss<br>Sensory: pain in the limbs and trunk |
| Hyperglycemic neuropathy | Newly diagnosed diabetes | Resolves with glycemic control | |
| Asymmetric proximal diabetic neuropathy | Duration of several months | Usually asymmetric, may be bilateral | Sensory: low back, hip, anterior thigh; with or without weakness, weight loss |
| Diabetic radiculopathy | Chronic | | See Table 97.2 |
| Diabetic mononeuropathy | Chronic | Higher incidence of mononeuropathy in diabetics | See Table 97.2 |

a 60% reduction in risk for the development of neuropathy with tight glycemic control.[31]

Foot care should be stressed to the patient because neuropathy-associated anesthesia may result in inadvertent trauma. These injuries, coupled with impaired healing from diabetic vasculopathy, can result in ulcers, cellulitis, and even amputation.

Management of symptoms is the patient's most immediate concern. NSAIDs may alleviate discomfort but are relatively contraindicated in diabetic patients. Narcotics carry addictive potential. Off-label use of tricyclics, antidepressants, anticonvulsants, and topical capsaicin have all proved beneficial (**Table 97.4**).[32,33]

**Table 97.4 Initial Therapy for Diabetic Peripheral Neuropathy (Based on a 70-kg Adult)**

| | |
|---|---|
| Tricyclic antidepressants | Amitriptyline, 25-100 mg PO daily<br>Nortriptyline, 10-25 mg PO daily |
| Anticonvulsants | Gabapentin, 900 mg PO daily or divided TID<br>Valproate, 500-1200 mg PO daily or divided BID |
| Topical | Capsaicin 0.075%, up to 4 times daily<br>Lidocaine 5% patch, 1 patch daily |

## HUMAN IMMUNODEFICIENCY VIRUS–ASSOCIATED PERIPHERAL NEUROPATHY

### EPIDEMIOLOGY

Peripheral nervous system disease associated with HIV infection most commonly takes the form of a distal sensory polyneuropathy. The prevalence of symptomatic patients is 35%, although an additional 20% of asymptomatic patients have electrophysiologic evidence of disease.[34]

### PATHOPHYSIOLOGY

The distal peripheral neuropathy associated with HIV disease has two causes. There does not appear to be direct nervous invasion by HIV, although proteins produced by the virus may have associated neurotoxicity. The resultant inflammatory mediators, including macrophages and cytokines, probably play a role as well. Since the introduction of highly active antiretroviral therapy (HAART), a second proposed mechanism has implicated mitochondrial toxicity because of the medications themselves. Both causes primarily affect small unmyelinated fibers and may progress to involve larger myelinated fibers. The neuropathy demonstrates a dying-back axonal pattern with distal axonal degeneration.[35]

## PRESENTING SIGNS AND SYMPTOMS

The initial signs and symptoms may be similar to those found with diabetic peripheral neuropathy, thus making it difficult to distinguish between them. Patients typically have the symptom of painful feet, usually without associated weakness. Physical examination will probably demonstrate decreased sensation distally, as well as diminished deep tendon reflexes.

## DIAGNOSTIC TESTING

Before HIV-associated peripheral neuropathy is diagnosed, other causes such as diabetes, vitamin $B_{12}$ deficiency, or other neurotoxic drugs must be ruled out. The history and physical examination largely drive the diagnosis of HIV-associated peripheral neuropathy. HAART-associated and non–HAART-associated neuropathy can be very difficult to distinguish clinically. Some patients with antiretroviral toxicity may have a more rapidly progressive course, at times temporally linked to the initiation of medication. The most effective diagnostic strategy is cessation of the suspected medication, which may result in improvement or resolution of the symptoms over a period of several weeks.

## TREATMENT

The goals of treatment are similar to those for diabetic peripheral neuropathy: control of the primary disease process is important. Potential toxic drugs should be discontinued if appropriate. Painful neuropathy may be managed with NSAIDs, topical analgesics such as lidocaine patches, anticonvulsants, antidepressants, or narcotic analgesics.[36] Randomized controlled trials have demonstrated the effectiveness of pain control over placebo along with the use of specific antiepileptics such as gabapentin and lamotrigine.[35,37]

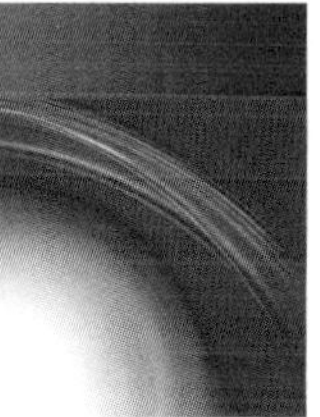

# Follow-up, Next Steps in Care, and Patient Education

Most patients with peripheral nerve disease can be treated on an outpatient basis. For patients with radiculopathy, compression mononeuropathy, or plexopathy, conservative treatment with analgesics and physical therapy is appropriate initially. This conservative treatment may take several weeks to reach maximal effect, which is important to convey to patients to improve compliance. Diabetics in particular may also benefit from referral to podiatry to prevent the complications of diabetic peripheral neuropathy. Patients with persistent symptoms despite a trial of conservative care may require referral for diagnostic testing with MRI or electrodiagnostics, pain management, or surgical evaluation.[38] Patients with acute injury, such as fracture or dislocation, will require either immediate consultation by or follow-up with an orthopedist or hand specialist.

For patients with GBS, myasthenia gravis, LEMS, or botulism in whom respiratory compromise or aspiration is a concern, close monitoring as an inpatient is required, usually in an intensive care setting. If these patients are being discharged, the effect of changing or initiating pharmacologic therapy should be considered because a number of medications can exacerbate the underlying disease (notably aminoglycosides and immunosuppressants, including prednisone).

## SUGGESTED READINGS

Dahm KT, Brurberg KG, Jamtvedt G, et al. Advice to rest in bed versus advice to stay active for acute low back pain and sciatica. Cochrane Database Syst Rev 2010;6:CD007612.

Lawn ND, Fletcher DD, Henderson RD, et al. Anticipating mechanical ventilation in Guillain-Barré syndrome. Arch Neurol 2001;58:893-8.

Pascuzzi RM. The edrophonium test. Semin Neurol 2003;23:83-8.

The effect of intensive treatment of diabetes on the development and progression of long-term complications in insulin-dependent diabetes mellitus: the Diabetes Control and Complications Trial Research Group. N Engl J Med 1993;329:977-86.

## REFERENCES

*References can be found on Expert Consult @ www.expertconsult.com.*

# 98 Demyelinating Disorders

*Scott E. Rudkin*

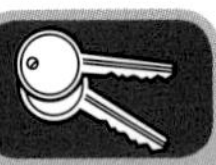

**KEY POINTS**

- Monocular vision loss from optic neuritis is a characteristic manifestation of multiple sclerosis (MS).
- Elevated body temperature worsens the symptoms of MS.
- Treatment of MS typically requires steroids to decrease autoimmune, inflammatory myelin damage.
- Transverse myelitis usually causes flaccid paraparesis initially, but it becomes spastic later.
- Back pain may precede neurologic symptoms in patients with MS and Guillain-Barré syndrome (GBS).
- Patients with GBS can initially have paresthesias followed by ascending weakness.
- Respiratory evaluation of forced vital capacity should be performed in patients with GBS.
- Succinylcholine should be avoided in patients with GBS because it can cause hyperkalemia.
- Treatment of acute optic neuritis requires admission for intravenous steroids.

## PERSPECTIVE

Second only to trauma, demyelinating diseases are a major cause of neurologic disability. Nerve conduction relies on the insulation that myelin provides the axon for transmission of impulses; demyelination disrupts this insulation, thereby resulting in abnormal signal propagation. This disruption results in sensory abnormalities, visual dysfunction, and muscle weakness.

Of the demyelinating conditions encountered by emergency physicians (EPs), multiple sclerosis (MS) is the most common. Other demyelinating conditions include optic neuritis, transverse myelitis, and acute inflammatory polyneuropathy (Guillain-Barré syndrome [GBS]).

## EPIDEMIOLOGY

Approximately 250,000 to 350,000 people in the United States have MS. It is more than twice as common in women as in men and more frequently afflicts Caucasian patients, but all races can be affected. Onset of disease usually occurs in people between 20 and 50 years of age, with a peak occurring in those 30 years of age. The prevalence of MS varies widely with location; the highest prevalence is found at higher latitudes. This geographic variation suggests that MS may in part be caused by the action of some environmental factor.

GBS has an incidence of 3 per 100,000 individuals, which makes it the most common cause of flaccid paralysis. It has a slight male preponderance. The age at onset is bimodal, with the elderly and young adults most commonly being afflicted. There does not appear to be a geographic effect.

## PATHOPHYSIOLOGY

The exact cause of demyelinating conditions is unknown, but an autoimmune or immune-mediated etiology is most likely. A molecular mimicry model postulates that an autoimmune attack on myelin is precipitated by an infectious organism that contains a protein similar to a myelin protein. The infection elicits an immune response by lymphocytes that recognize the cross-reactive protein; the activated lymphocytes then damage the myelin. The majority of the demyelinating disorders cause demyelination of the myelin sheath with relative sparing of the axon.

MS, transverse myelitis, and optic neuritis all affect the central nervous system. GBS, which primarily afflicts the peripheral nervous system, is now believed to cause both demyelination of the myelin sheath and axonal loss. Inflammatory lesions in peripheral nerve fibers cause focal demyelination with resultant slowing of conduction. Cranial nerves can also be affected.

## PRESENTING SIGNS AND SYMPTOMS

In general, all the demyelinating disorders are characterized by an abrupt episode of loss of function. Depending on the area of the brain or nervous system affected, the patient may have sensory, motor, or autonomic symptoms.

### MULTIPLE SCLEROSIS

In MS, the initial attack occurs abruptly (minutes to hours) from a single lesion. These attacks last between 6 and 8 weeks. Recovery between bouts of demyelination can be incomplete or complete, depending on the amount of remyelination. Any part of the central nervous system can be affected. In decreasing order of frequency, the patient may exhibit optic neuritis, paresthesias in a limb, diplopia, trigeminal neuralgia, urinary retention, vertigo, or transverse myelitis. Depending on the spinal cord level, transverse myelitis can also cause loss of bladder or bowel function.

Ocular findings are the most common initial symptom. Optic neuritis is manifested as subacute monocular vision loss, although it can affect both eyes, and pain exacerbated with eye movement. It is the initial symptom in 25% and ultimately affects 50% of patients.[1] The course usually progresses over a period of 2 weeks and may be include headache, retroorbital or periocular pain, and alterations in color vision and visual fields. Slit-lamp examination may demonstrate cell and flare in the anterior chamber. The optic disk is frequently swollen on initial evaluation. In addition to optic neuritis, the patient may have an afferent pupillary defect (Marcus Gunn pupil, or decreased pupillary constriction on direct light confrontation but a normal consensual response) or intranuclear ophthalmoplegia, which is characterized by dysconjugate gaze with limited adduction of one eye and nystagmus in the abducting eye on lateral gaze as a result of a lesion involving the medial longitudinal fasciculus.

Sensory symptoms in patients with MS usually include numbness, tingling, pins and needles sensation, and tightness and coldness of the limbs and trunk. Radicular pain and itching may also occur. Symptoms result from involvement of the spinothalamic, posterior column, and dorsal nerve roots. The loss of vibration sense is often most prominent. Ataxia is uncommon at the onset of MS, but it occurs to some degree in most patients. Exacerbation of sensory symptoms can occur frequently and in different patterns with a patchy distribution. Patients may note either paresthesias or loss of sensation.

Sensitivity to heat is a characteristic complaint. Exercise, fever, a hot bath, or other activities that raise body temperature may result in the appearance of new symptoms or the recurrence of old symptoms. These events occur as a result of a temperature-induced conduction block across partially demyelinated fibers. Symptoms resolve when body temperature returns to normal.

In addition to loss of sensation, patients may also report "positive" symptoms. In addition to causing a slowing of conduction, demyelination may result in ectopic impulses with resultant abnormal signal transmission and abnormal mechanical sensitivity. These aberrant signals can produce the Lhermitte sign—an electric-like tingling or vibrating sensation in the torso or extremities with neck flexion. The patient may also report flashes of light (phosphenes) and paroxysmal symptom, including trigeminal neuralgia, ataxia, and dysarthria or painful tetanic posturing of the limbs triggered by touch or movement.

Motor weakness may occur in any pattern, including paraparesis, hemiparesis, and monoparesis; the lower extremities are usually affected more than the upper ones. Upper motor neuron dysfunction accompanied by spasticity and increased reflexes may also be present. Transverse myelitis with ascending weakness and numbness below the level of the lesion can occur as an initial symptom.

Autonomic symptoms are a frequent finding. Patients have difficulty with bladder function, including frequency and urgency, and may experience urge incontinence from bladder spasticity or hesitancy, retention, and overflow incontinence from poor signal conduction. Constipation is the most common bowel complaint. This autonomic dysfunction is frequently very embarrassing and distressful.

Normal disease progression is variable: MS may remain indolent or occur in a progressive manner, with steady accumulation of neurologic deficits in the absence of clearly defined exacerbations. Typically, acute exacerbations are followed by partial or complete resolution. New neurologic deficits develop over the course of several hours or days, remain stable for a few days to a few weeks, and then gradually improve.

With repeated exacerbations, permanent neurologic deficits tend to develop. Patients usually have symptom-free intervals of months or years between attacks. Patients who initially have relapsing-remitting disease (two or more episodes lasting more than 24 hours separated by more than 1 month) and who then enter a progressive phase are said to have *secondary progressive disease* (initial exacerbations and remissions followed by slow progression over at least a period of 6 months), whereas those whose symptoms are progressive from the onset are said to have *primary progressive disease* (slow or stepwise progression over a period of at least 6 months). About 15% of patients have primary progressive disease; of those who initially have relapsing-remitting disease, 30% to 50% will experience progressive symptoms during the first 10 years.

## OPTIC NEURITIS

Optic neuritis may occur by itself or be the initial symptom of MS. The relationship of optic neuritis to MS is controversial. Some regard optic neuritis as a distinct entity, but others consider it part of the clinical continuum of MS. More than half of all patients with MS have optic neuritis at some time during the disease. Patients with completely normal results on magnetic resonance imaging (MRI) and comprehensive cerebrospinal fluid (CSF) evaluation seldom progress to MS. Optic neurits is usually manifested initially as unilateral vision loss and retrobulbar pain with eye movement.

## TRANSVERSE MYELITIS

Like optic neuritis, transverse myelitis may occur in isolation or be part of the symptomatology of MS. It is usually manifested as paraparesis, which is initially flaccid and then spastic; as loss of sensation at a sensory level on the trunk; and as bowel and bladder dysfunction. Back pain precedes the neurologic symptoms, and the sensory symptoms may begin distally and ascend. The thoracic cord is most often affected.

## GUILLAIN-BARRÉ SYNDROME

Patients with GBS have weakness, paresthesias, and decreased or absent deep tendon reflexes. The distribution typically includes distal involvement with symmetric paresthesias (pins and needles). It spreads proximally, with weakness occurring a few days later; weakness also progresses to involve the upper extremities. Weakness is most prominent in the lower extremities and tends to involve the proximal muscles. It is usually first manifested as difficulty rising from a chair. The disease progresses from a few days to 3 to 4 weeks *(progressive phase)*, followed by a *plateau phase* (days to weeks) and then by a *recovery phase* lasting from weeks to months. Weakness is varied but can be profound and involve the face and respiratory muscles. A loss or decrease in deep tendon reflexes is frequently the initial finding, and these reflexes should be tested if GBS is suspected. Variants include the acute axonal form, which has a poor prognosis, and the Miller-Fisher syndrome, which is characterized by ataxia, ophthalmoplegia, and areflexia.

## DIFFERENTIAL DIAGNOSIS AND MEDICAL DECISION MAKING

The differential diagnosis of demyelinating diseases includes conditions that cause progressive weakness. In due course the diagnosis of a demyelinating disorder becomes clear because few disorders relapse and remit over time. The role of the EP is to exclude other diseases that need immediate treatment.

Clinical factors that suggest a diagnosis other than MS (**Table 98.1**) include normal findings on neurologic examination, aphasia, predominance of pain, abrupt hemiparesis, quick (seconds or minutes) resolution of symptoms, and age younger than 10 or older than 50 years.

The diagnosis is usually made from the clinical signs and symptoms; MRI and other laboratory tests play a supporting role. Diagnosis requires evidence of *dissemination of lesions in time and space* and careful exclusion of other causes. The patient should have had more than one episode of neurologic dysfunction and evidence of white matter lesions in more than one part of the central nervous system or a change in a previous lesion. Although it is possible for a neurologist to diagnoses MS during an initial attack, provided that two clinical lesions are present and with corroborating laboratory testing, it is prudent for the EP to use a more conservative approach that requires two distinct attacks.

The EP should consider the diagnosis in a young adult with a history of two or more clinically distinct episodes of central nervous system dysfunction or the presence of highly suggestive symptoms (optic neuritis or intranuclear ophthalmoplegia). In 2005, the McDonald criteria revised the 2001 guidelines of the International Panel on MS[2] to incorporate specific MRI findings and reaffirm the need for separation of clinical events and lesions in space and time. Diagnostic confidence is based on whether the criteria are fully met (diagnosis of MS), partially met (possible MS), or not met (not MS). **Table 98.2** lists characteristic factors differentiating demyelinating disorders.

Differential diagnoses for optic neuritis include anterior ischemic optic neuropathy, which is usually painless and found in patients older than 50 years; hereditary diseases such as Leber hereditary optic neuropathy; and toxic or nutritional optic neuropathies.

Transverse myelitis may superficially resemble GBS, but its asymmetric involvement, definite sensory level, lack of upper extremity involvement, urinary incontinence symptoms, and CSF pleocytosis make the diagnosis of GBS less likely. The differential diagnosis includes other causes of acute myelopathy such as compression of the cord by an extradural structural lesion, spinal cord neoplasms, ischemia, and systemic lupus erythematosus.

Heavy metal poisoning can also mimic GBS, but it is usually preceded by a gastrointestinal phase with vomiting and diarrhea. As discussed previously, transverse myelitis can superficially resemble this syndrome.

**Table 98.1 Differential Diagnosis of Multiple Sclerosis**

| DISEASE/SYSTEM | IMPORTANT FACTORS |
|---|---|
| Seizures, syncope, or dementia | Present diffusely or globally; MS is usually focal; consider Todd paralysis in seizure patients |
| SLE | Neurologic findings normally occur in patient with a known diagnosis of SLE |
| Sarcoid | CNS and pulmonary involvement normally occurs in patients with known disease |
| Lyme disease | Can mimic MS; look for tick exposure, travel history, and Lyme disease titers |
| CNS infection | Intracranial abscess, meningitis/encephalitis, or epidural abscess can produce focal findings |
| Bleeding (CNS) | Subdural, subarachnoid, intraparenchymal, or epidural hemorrhage can produce focal findings |
| Neoplasm | Usually progressive course with a more insidious onset |
| Vascular | Patients with thrombosis, embolism, or vasculitic conditions do not usually have resolution of symptoms |
| Metabolic | Vitamin $B_{12}$ deficiency, hypoglycemia, hyperglycemia (hyperosmolar) |
| Neurologic | Migraine headache, postictal state, Bell palsy |
| Psychiatric | Diagnosis of exclusion; includes conversion reaction |

*CNS*, Central nervous system; *MS*, multiple sclerosis; *SLE*, systemic lupus erythematosus.

## DIAGNOSTIC TESTING

Findings on routine laboratory tests are usually normal in patients with myelinating disorders, including MS, transverse myelitis, and GBS. Because the respiratory muscles are frequently affected in GBS, measurement of forced vital capacity (FVC) is essential to determine disposition.

Most cases of optic neuritis are diagnosed clinically. In questionable cases of optic neuritis, serum testing (erythrocyte sedimentation rate, angiotensin-converting enzyme, rapid plasma reagin, thyroid function testing, and antinuclear antibody studies) can be ordered to exclude other causes of optic neuropathy.

### CEREBROSPINAL FLUID ANALYSIS

With MS, CSF analysis (with electrophoresis) frequently demonstrates albuminocytologic dissociation with increased protein (usually less than 100 mg/dL) and a normal cell count.

**Table 98.2 Differentiating Between the Demyelinating Disorders**

| | MULTIPLE SCLEROSIS | OPTIC NEURITIS | TRANSVERSE MYELITIS | GUILLAIN-BARRÉ SYNDROME |
|---|---|---|---|---|
| Epidemiology | 2:1 female-to-male ratio; usually northern European descent; peaks at 30 yr of age | Patients usually 15 to 45 yr of age; generally idiopathic | Peak incidence between 10 and 19 yr and 30 to 39 yr of age | Annual incidence of 1 to 2 per 100,000; equal male and female incidence |
| Onset | Abrupt (minutes to hours); lasts 6-8 wk | Visual loss over days (rarely over hours) | Hours to weeks; 45% within 24 hr | 3 days to 3 wk; usually 1-3 wk after respiratory infection |
| Duration | 6-8 wk | 4-12 wk | 1-3 mo | Weeks to months |
| Symptoms | Motor weakness; paresthesias; ocular symptoms common (optic neuritis, intranuclear ophthalmoplegia) | Unilateral vision loss and retrobulbar pain with eye movement; loss of light, color, and depth perception more pronounced; bilateral vision loss possible; more common in children | Flaccid, then spastic paresis; loss of sensation and motor function at a specific cord level; bowel and bladder dysfunction common | Rapidly ascending, symmetric paralysis with paresthesias and decreased deep tendon reflexes; autonomic dysfunction common |
| Diagnosis, testing | MRI (white matter lesions); lumbar puncture (oligoclonal bands); diagnosis largely clinical | MRI with gadolinium may show enhancement of optic nerves; visual field testing; diagnosis largely clinical | MRI (intramedullary lesion at level of symptoms); hyperintense on T2-weighted imaging; CSF may show elevated protein and leukocytes | CSF analysis (albuminocytologic dissociation); MRI with gadolinium may show abnormal enhancement of nerve roots in region of conus medullaris and cauda equina; electrodiagnostic testing shows abnormal motor and sensory conduction |
| Treatment | High-dose, pulsed steroid therapy for exacerbations; interferon and glatiramer acetate for prevention of relapse; treat fevers aggressively | IV methylprednisolone (1 g/day for 3 days), followed by oral taper for 11 days | Largely supportive; test FVC to determine respiratory function (intubate if FVC < 20 mL/kg) with high cord lesions; steroids may be helpful to reduce inflammation, and plasmapheresis can be attempted for refractory cases | Largely supportive; test FVC to determine disposition (intubate if FVC < 15 mL/kg; admit to ICU if FVC < 20 mL/kg); plasmapheresis or intravenous immunoglobulin |
| Disposition | Acute exacerbations require IV therapy and admission; oral, high-dose outpatient steroid therapy possible | Admit for IV methylprednisolone therapy if known flare; outpatient therapy possible if unilateral vision loss and good follow-up arranged | Admit for respiratory function testing and observation; early mobility therapy for paralyzed limbs can help reduce risk for muscle atrophy and pressure sores | Admit for respiratory function testing and observation |

*CSF*, Cerebrospinal fluid; *FVC*, forced vital capacity; *ICU*, intensive care unit; *IV*, intravenous; *MRI*, magnetic resonance imaging.

However, 10% of patients have a normal CSF protein level. Mild mononuclear cell pleocytosis can be found during acute MS relapses, but total cell counts greater than 50/mm$^3$ are uncommon. During acute attacks of MS, especially those involving the spinal cord and brainstem, CSF may contain measurable amounts of myelin basic protein. Oligoclonal bands or abnormal immunoglobulin synthesis is found in about 90% of patients with a diagnosis of MS. Though not specific to MS, these findings support the diagnosis of MS in equivocal cases.

CSF studies may demonstrate elevated protein levels and leukocytes in patients with transverse myelitis; such studies are not generally required for optic neuritis but are usually obtained to help in the diagnosis of MS.

## NERVE CONDUCTION STUDIES

Electrodiagnostic testing may demonstrate conduction blocks, differential slowing, or focal slowing. Slowing of conduction over demyelinated segments of axons or over incompletely remyelinated pathways provides a useful marker for identifying additional subclinical lesions in the sensory pathways. Conduction can be measured along the visual, auditory, and somatosensory pathways with the use of summated cortical evoked responses. In these tests, a time-locked recording of the electroencephalogram over the afferent cortex of interest is obtained after repeated visual, auditory, or sensory stimulation. If the demyelination is significant, conduction is delayed.

Electrodiagnostic testing may demonstrate abnormal motor and sensory conduction, but these signs can take a few weeks to develop.

### MAGNETIC RESONANCE IMAGING

MRI permits the exclusion of many diseases that mimic MS and identifies certain lesions that are hyperintense on T2-weighted or proton density imaging and hypointense or isointense on T1-weighted imaging. Typical lesions are ovoid and periventricular, with the long axis perpendicular to the ventricle, but lesions may appear anywhere in the white matter. Although MRI is extremely sensitive in detecting white matter lesions in patients with MS, it is not very specific because many other diseases produce multiple white matter lesions. Useful features for increasing the predictive value of MRI for the diagnosis of MS include the presence of three or more white matter lesions, lesions that abut the body of the lateral ventricles, infratentorial lesions, lesions larger than 5 mm in diameter, and lesions that demonstrate gadolinium enhancement.

MRI is extremely useful for confirming the presence of an intramedullary lesion at the level in the spinal cord commensurate with the symptoms of transverse myelitis. The lesions are typically hyperintense on T2-weighted imaging; they involve the majority of the cross-sectional area of the cord over several segments and may be enhanced with contrast agents. The lesions may cause swelling of the spinal cord. Gadolinium-enhanced MRI may show abnormal enhancement of the nerve roots in the region of the conus medullaris and cauda equina.[3]

MRI is also useful for diagnosing optic neuritis and evaluating for concomitant MS. Gadolinium enhancement may demonstrate optic nerve involvement. In questionable cases, visually evoked potentials may demonstrate prolonged latency.

## TREATMENT

For all demyelinating conditions, the EP's goal is to reduce the current demyelinating episode while ensuring that the ABCs (airway, breathing, and circulation) are maintained. Because inflammation is a central component of demyelination, corticosteroids are frequently used; their effectiveness in patients with GBS and optic neuritis is questionable. Preventing and aggressively treating fever are important because an increased core temperature can worsen the demyelination.

### MULTIPLE SCLEROSIS

Treatment of MS can be discussed in terms of the management of acute relapses, prevention of relapses as a modification of the disease process, and management of symptoms and fixed neurologic deficits. High-dose pulsed corticosteroid therapy is indicated for exacerbations of acute relapses that adversely affect the patient's function. Intravenous (IV) methylprednisolone at doses of 0.5 to 1 g daily for 5 days reduces the maximal neurologic signs and hastens the resolution of associated fatigue. A controversial study by Sellebjerg et al. supports the use of oral methylprednisolone (500 mg daily for 5 days with a 10-day tapering period).[4]

In patients with relapsing-remitting MS, disease-modulating drugs reduce the frequency of attacks, the rate of increase in lesions seen on MRI, and the accumulation of disability. In patients with relapsing disease of mild to moderate severity, interferon beta-1b, given subcutaneously every other day, reduced the year-on-year relapse rate by one third and severe attacks by one half. The effect was maintained for up to 5 years.[5,6] In another study, interferon β1b reduced MRI contrast-enhanced lesions by 1.6%, as opposed to a 15% increase in those receiving placebo. The number of enlarging or new lesions was also significantly reduced.[7] Antibodies developed in 35% of patients taking interferon β1b, but there is a lack of consistent effect of antibodies on clinical outcome. Additionally, these antibody levels were found to have disappeared in the majority of patients after 8 years of treatment.[8,9]

Interferon β1a produced similar benefits when given intramuscularly three times per week, with a 17% reduction in the relapse rate. When compared with weekly, low-dose interferon β1a, high-dose interferon β1a given three times per week demonstrated a 32% relative reduction in steroid use to treat relapses.[10]

Glatiramer, a synthetic random compound composed of four amino acids, is found in myelin. Its exact mechanism is unknown, but it is believed that glatiramer acetate binds to the major histocompatibility complex class II antigen and induces organ-specific T helper type 2 cell responses, thus converting proinflammatory T cells to antiinflammatory agents.[11] Treatment with glatiramer reduces the relapse rate by 30% and may delay disease progression.[12]

Natalizumab, a monoclonal antibody against $\alpha_4$ integrins, is effective for relapsing-remitting MS. The reduction in annualized relapse rates with natalizumab is similar to that with glatiramer or interferon β.[13] However, it is not a first-line agent because it can cause progressive multifocal leukoencephalopathy in 0.1% of cases.[14]

Mitoxantrone is an anthracenedione, antineoplastic agent approved for the relapsing-remitting and progressive forms of MS. Cardiotoxicity, acute leukemia, and questionable efficacy limit it to treatment failures or cases of rapidly progressive MS.

Fingolimod, the first oral treatment option for MS approved by the Food and Drug Administration, is a sphingosine analogue that blocks lymphocyte release from lymph nodes through interaction with the sphingosine 1-phosphate receptor. Fingolimod can significantly reduce relapse rates when compared with interferon β1a. However, fingolimod is associated with life-threatening infections, bradycardia, atrioventricular block, tumor development, and macular edema.[15]

Specific therapies for relief of symptoms are provided in **Table 98.3**.

### TRANSVERSE MYELITIS

Corticosteroids and plasma exchange may be beneficial in the treatment of transverse myelitis.[16] In a small case series, patients treated with steroids were able to walk after a median time of 23 days versus 97 days for historical controls.[17] Plasma exchange is often used for those with more severe disease (e.g., unable to walk) who fail to improve with IV steroid therapy.[18] The prognosis for transverse myelitis is variable.

**Table 98.3 Symptomatic Treatment of Multiple Sclerosis**

| SYMPTOM | TREATMENT OPTIONS |
|---|---|
| Fatigue | Amantadine, pemoline, methylphenidate, modafinil, or selective serotonin reuptake inhibitor |
| Weakness | Steroids, potassium channel blocker |
| Loss of balance or coordination, tremor, ataxia | Clonazepam for tremor, steroids for balance |
| Sexual dysfunction | Sildenafil, intracavernosal prostaglandins (for erectile dysfunction) |
| Vertigo | Meclizine, prochlorperazine, diazepam, metoclopramide |
| Paroxysmal symptoms (itching, burning, twitching, Lhermitte sign) | Carbamazepine, phenytoin, tricyclic antidepressants, low-dose antipsychotics, gabapentin |
| Bladder urgency | Oxybutynin, tolterodine, imipramine, hyoscyamine, propantheline |
| Bladder dyssynergia | Phenoxybenzamine, clonidine, terazosin |
| Bladder retention | Intermittent catheterization, bethanechol |
| Spasticity (commonly increased tone in the lower extremities) | Baclofen, diazepam, tizanidine, clonazepam, clonidine (adjunctive to baclofen), dantrolene |
| Paresthesias | Amitriptyline, carbamazepine, gabapentin, corticosteroids if disabling |
| Optic atrophy, blurred vision, central scotomata | Intravenous methylprednisolone for acute optic neuritis |
| Intranuclear ophthalmoplegia | Corticosteroids |
| Ataxia | Clonazepam, gabapentin |
| Paroxysmal pain | Carbamazepine, phenytoin, misoprostol (trigeminal neuralgia) |
| Dysesthetic pain | Amitriptyline, phenytoin, gabapentin, valproic acid, carbamazepine, baclofen |

## OPTIC NEURITIS

IV methylprednisolone (1 g/day for 3 days) followed by oral prednisone (1 mg/kg/day for 11 days with a 4-day taper) and interferon β1a (30 mcg intramuscularly once a week) for patients at high risk for MS based on MRI has been shown to hasten recovery of vision in patients with optic neuritis.[19] However, this therapy shows little residual benefit at 1 year. Additionally, oral prednisone therapy alone was found to actually increase the recurrence rate.[20] Regardless of therapy, most patients recover their vision within a month.

## GUILLAIN-BARRÉ SYNDROME

Therapy is largely supportive. Most patients recover function if they survive the acute phase. The key therapeutic measure is ventilatory support. FVC should be measured in all patients in whom GBS is suspected. Patients with an FVC of less than 20 mL/kg should be admitted to the intensive care unit because of their high risk for ventilatory insufficiency. For those with FVC lower than 15 mL/kg, intubation is indicated. If intubation is necessary, succinylcholine should be avoided because it can cause hyperkalemia with resultant arrhythmia and hypotension. Dysautonomia can result in severe paroxysmal hypertension, orthostatic hypotension, and arrhythmias. Cardiovascular function should be monitored carefully. Plasmapheresis and IV gamma globulin therapy have both been shown to reduce recovery time by 50%. IV gamma globulin is less expensive and easier to administer, but the risk for viral transmission is greater. IV steroids are frequently administered, but their actual benefit is questionable.

# FOLLOW-UP, NEXT STEPS IN CARE, AND PATIENT EDUCATION

All patients with a first episode of a demyelination disorder merit neurology consultation. Although outpatient therapy is possible for a subset of these patients, this decision is best left to the neurologist. As discussed previously, the typical course of MS is a relapsing-remitting pattern. During an acute exacerbation, the patient is frequently admitted for IV steroid therapy, but oral treatment is possible.

Hospital admission is required for GBS, and FVC measurement typically guides selection of the appropriate level of care. The majority of patients are hospitalized for a month or

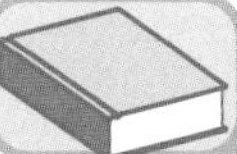

**PATIENT TEACHING TIPS**

- The National Multiple Sclerosis Society (http://www.nmss.org), Guillain-Barré Foundation (http://www.gbsfi.com/), and Transverse Myelitis Foundation (http://www.myelitis.org/) provide excellent patient resources and offer support groups for both patients and family.
- Patients are at risk for exacerbation of symptoms and progression of disease from an elevated core temperature. Aggressive fever control and determination of its cause are important.
- There is no cure for demyelinating disorders, but current therapies can reduce their frequency and severity.
- Patients with optic neuritis have a worse prognosis with *oral* steroid therapy. If steroids are used, they must be given intravenously.
- Patients with symptoms of progressive weakness and sensory symptoms must be assessed rapidly for Guillain-Barré syndrome. With aggressive therapy, respiratory failure can be avoided.

longer, and with careful attention to respiratory function, mortality is now less than 5%.

Patients should undergo ophthalmology and neurology evaluation for manifestations of optic neuritis. If steroid therapy is needed, hospital admission is necessary because steroids may worsen the clinical outcome.

## SUGGESTED READINGS

Balcer LJ. Clinical practice. Optic neuritis. N Engl J Med 2006;354:1273-80.

Panitch H, Goodin D, Francis G, et al. EVIDENCE (Evidence of Interferon Dose-response: European North American Comparative Efficacy) Study Group and the University of British Columbia MS/MRI Research Group. Benefits of high-dose, high-frequency interferon beta-1a in relapsing-remitting multiple sclerosis are sustained to 16 months: final comparative results of the EVIDENCE trial. J Neurol Sci 2005;239:67-74.

Polman CH, Reingold SC, Edan G, et al. Diagnostic criteria for multiple sclerosis: 2005 revisions to the "McDonald criteria." Ann Neurol 2005;58:840-6.

Ropper AG. Selective treatment of multiple sclerosis. N Engl J Med 2006;354:965-7.

## REFERENCES

***References can be found on Expert Consult @ www.expertconsult.com.***

# Seizures 99

*Asim F. Tarabar, Andrew S. Ulrich, and Gail D'Onofrio*

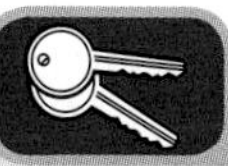

**KEY POINTS**

- Seizures are classified by the clinical finding of abnormal electrical impulses within the cerebral cortex.
- Direct morbidity and mortality are the result of inadequate cerebral perfusion of oxygen and glucose to the brain, as well as secondary trauma.
- Serum glucose levels should be checked in all seizure patients immediately.
- Emergency department treatment is directed at urgent cessation of seizures, prevention of further activity, and diagnosis and correction of the underlying cause.
- Intravenous benzodiazepines are the initial treatment of most seizures.
- Isoniazid can cause intractable seizures with an overdose; the antidote is pyridoxine.
- Eclamptic seizures, most common in the third trimester, can also occur postpartum; the antidote is intravenous magnesium sulfate.
- One third of eclamptic woman do not have the classic triad of hypertension, proteinuria, and edema.
- Most chronic seizure patients can be discharged home safely after emergency department evaluation and correction of anticonvulsant levels if needed.
- Patients with seizure disorders should have adequate control and close follow-up with a neurologist before driving vehicles or operating machinery.

## EPIDEMIOLOGY

Seizures are a common complaint of patients seeking care in emergency departments (EDs). By some estimates, seizures account for 1% to 2% of all ED visits.[1,2] Epilepsy, a condition resulting in recurrent, unprovoked seizures, affects upward of 4 million people; however, as much as 10% of the population will have at least one seizure during their lifetime.[3,4]

The natural history of untreated epilepsy is essentially unknown. Based on retrospective data, it was found that 32% of patients with a first epileptic seizure will experience a second attack within 1 month, 51% within 3 months, and 87% within the first year. Some strong predictors for recurrence of seizures include a history of previous neurologic insult, abnormal findings on neurologic examination, or an electroencephalogram (EEG) with epileptiform abnormalities and circadian timing. Approximately 50% patients in whom epilepsy is diagnosed will become seizure free with only single-drug treatment. The addition of a second or third drug will control another 20%, and intractable seizures that are poorly responsive to standard medical treatment will develop in about 30%.

## PATHOPHYSIOLOGY

Seizures are the result of inappropriate electrical activity in the brain, whereas syncope is caused primarily by transient hypoperfusion within the brain. Uncontrollable electrical discharges can originate from a single area as a result of an underlying structural condition (e.g., tumor, scar, bleeding), or it can be caused by an imbalance in inhibitory (γ-aminobutyric acid [GABA]) and excitatory (*N*-methyl-D-aspartate) receptor activities. The latter is usually due to toxic or metabolic causes.

The specific seizure activity is determined by the area in the brain involved (**Box 99.1**). Some of these abnormal electrical discharges may remain localized, whereas others may involve larger areas of the brain. Subsequently, the resultant clinical spectrum includes isolated focal motor activity, as well as generalized motor and sensory abnormalities, including altered mental status and behavioral changes.

## PRESENTING SIGNS AND SYMPTOMS

If available, the previous medical history may reveal risk factors (**Box 99.2**) associated with the development of seizures. The history can be obtained from the patient (after normalization of mental status), family, primary care physicians, old medical records, or emergency medical service (EMS) personnel.

## DIFFERENTIAL DIAGNOSIS AND MEDICAL DECISION MAKING

The most common serious condition that can be misinterpreted as a seizure is syncope.[5] There may be important

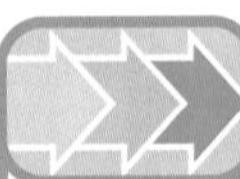

PRIORITY ACTIONS

### Signs and Symptoms of Seizures

**Central Nervous System**
Behavioral manifestations
Focal deficits (Todd paralysis or cerebrovascular accident/transient ischemic attack)
Hyperreflexia
Loss of consciousness (generalized or complex seizures)
Sensory abnormalities (visual, olfactory)
Thought disturbances

**Constitutional**
Hypertension, hypotension (late)
Hyperthermia

**Metabolic**
Lactic acidosis
Rhabdomyolysis, disseminated intravascular coagulation

**Musculoskeletal**
Any trauma caused by a fall or motor activity
Involuntary minor physical activity
Head or neck injury
Shoulder dislocation (posterior)
Physical convulsions

**Obstetric/Gynecologic**
Pregnancy or recent delivery

**Pulmonary**
Hypoxia
Hypercapnia
Cyanosis
Pulmonary edema

### BOX 99.1 Seizure Classification

**Partial (Focal) Seizures (One Area or Brain Hemisphere Involved)**
Simple (awareness retained)
Motor
Somatosensory
Autonomic
Psychogenic
Complex (altered awareness and behavior)
**Secondary Generalized Seizures (Spreading from One Area to the Whole Brain)**
**Generalized Seizures (Seizures Involving the Whole Brain with Alteration of Consciousness)**
Tonic-clonic
Grand mal, convulsions
Positive loss of consciousness, stiffening of the body with the jerking movements of the limbs
**Secondary Seizures**
Toxin induced
Substance withdrawal
Metabolic
**Absence**
Petit mal: staring fit or trancelike state
Tonic or atonic
- Drop attack: abrupt fall, either with stiffening (tonic) or with loss of muscle tone (atonic)

Myoclonic
- Sudden muscle jerks

### BOX 99.2 Differential Diagnosis of Conditions Resulting in Seizurelike Symptoms

Breath-holding spells
Episodic dyscontrol syndrome, rage attacks
Fugue states
Heat stroke, exhaustion
Hyperventilation
Migraine narcolepsy, cataplexy
Movement disorders
Night terrors
Nonepileptic seizures
Panic attacks
Paroxysmal vertigo
Psychogenic seizures
Syncope
Transient global amnesia
Transient ischemic attack, stroke (ischemic, hemorrhagic)

clinical signs or preceding events that can help differentiate these two entities (**Table 99.1**). In many circumstances patients will be unable to provide critical information, so it is important to try to obtain an accurate description from anyone who witnessed the event (e.g., family, coworkers, EMS personnel). Aside from syncope, several other medical conditions need to be included in the differential diagnosis of seizures (**Boxes 99.3 and 99-4; Table 99.2**).

Though rare, various disturbances in electrolytes may precipitate seizures, including hyponatremia, uremia, and hypocalcemia. A serum electrolyte assay is recommended for patients with new-onset seizures. Between 2.4% and 8% of patients with seizures will have electrolyte abnormalities. Despite the fact that the majority of these abnormalities will be clinically insignificant, they should be evaluated and can often be easily corrected in the ED.

If an overdose is suspected, both blood and urine toxicologic screens should be performed.

Measuring the serum prolactin level has no clinical utility in the ED because the results cannot be obtained in a timely manner. However, it may be useful for the consulting service that will conduct further work-up to help differentiate between epileptic (generalized tonic-clonic or complex partial seizures) and psychogenic nonepileptic seizures. It should be performed within 10 to 20 minutes after a suspected event. Prolactin levels of at least twice baseline are considered abnormal (positive). Prudent clinicians may decide to have prolactin levels measured, especially in patients with the symptoms suggestive of nonepileptic or psychogenic seizures.[6]

An electrocardiogram (ECG) should be obtained in every patient with a first onset of seizures or with suspicion of a

**Table 99.1 Seizure Disorder versus Syncope**

| SEIZURES (SPECIFIC) | NONSPECIFIC (CAN OCCUR IN BOTH) SYMPTOMS | SYNCOPE (SPECIFIC) |
|---|---|---|
| Prodromal symptoms | Incontinence | Lightheadedness |
| Déjà vu | Loss of consciousness | Sweating |
| Rising abdominal or epigastric sensation | | Prolonged standing |
| Stereotyped tastes or smells | | Precipitants: |
| Postictal confusion | | Micturition |
| Tongue biting | | Painful stimuli |
| | | Chest pain |
| | | Palpitations |
| | | Bradycardia |
| | | Neck turning (carotid sinus) |
| | | Rapid recovery of awareness |
| | | Myoclonus |
| | | Pallor |
| | | Sweating |

**BOX 99.3 Differential Diagnoses of Secondary Seizures**

Central nervous system infections (encephalitis, meningitis)
Eclampsia
Metabolic
- Hypoglycemia
- Hyponatremia
- Hypothyroidism
- Hyperammonemia

Trauma (subarachnoid hemorrhage)
Toxic
- Anticholinergics
- Baclofen overdose, withdrawal
- Cyclic antidepressants
- Carbon monoxide
- Isoniazid
- Sedative-hypnotic drug withdrawal

**BOX 99.4 Factors Precipitating Seizures**

Flashing lights (strobe light, Pokémon seizures)
Menstrual period (catamenial seizures)
Recent head trauma
Metabolic
- Hypoglycemia, hyperglycemia
- Hypomagnesemia
- Hyponatremia, hypernatremia

New medications (interfering with the metabolism of anticonvulsants)
Sleep deprivation
Toxins, drugs of abuse
- Alcohol use, withdrawal
- Baclofen pump malfunction; overdose, withdrawal
- Cocaine, sympathomimetics

Medication noncompliance
- Lack of insurance, unable to refill medications
- Substance abuse
- Change in dose or generic versus brand medications

cardiac cause of decreased central nervous system (CNS) perfusion. In addition to ischemia, the most important disorders that have to be excluded are related to conduction abnormalities and consequent dysrhythmias. ECGs are used to evaluate widening of the QRS complex because of sodium channel blockade after an overdose of certain medications, particularly cyclic antidepressants. More specific changes on the ECG, such as a terminal 400-msec R wave in the aVR lead, can also assist in identifying toxicity from cyclic antidepressants. A prolonged QTc interval can be found with overdose of citalopram (a selective serotonin reuptake inhibitor with proconvulsive properties). Tachyarrhythmias are often seen in the setting of cocaine and methylxanthine toxicity (theophylline, caffeine) (**Box 99.5**).

Patients at high risk for meningitis or encephalitis should be treated with ceftriaxone (2 g intravenously [IV]), vancomycin (1 g IV), and acyclovir (500 mg IV), even before the results of a spinal tap are available. In addition, patients should be placed in an isolation room with droplet precautions.

**BOX 99.5 Conduction Disorders That Should Be Considered as a Cause of Seizurelike Activity**

Brugada syndrome: right bundle branch block with ST-segment elevation in leads $V_1$ to $V_3$
Short QTc interval
Long QTc interval
Wolff-Parkinson-White syndrome
Torsades de pointes
Widening of the QRS complex
Sodium channel blockade: cyclic antidepressants, lidocaine, anticholinergics

Neurocysticercosis (NCC) is the most common parasitic CNS infection in the world and has been increasing in the United States since 1980.[7] In endemic areas (Latin America, Asia, Africa), NCC is considered to be main cause of late-onset epilepsy, and seizures are reported to be the most

**Table 99.2 Seizure Work-up**

| DIAGNOSTIC TEST | COMMENT |
|---|---|
| Complete blood count | May reveal anemia or an infectious process |
| Electrolytes (including Ca and Mg) | Hypocalcemia and hypomagnesemia can be associated with seizures and should be corrected |
| Anticonvulsants—serum levels | For patients currently taking anticonvulsants, see Table 99.5 |
| Pregnancy test (women of childbearing age) | Rule out eclamptic seizures |
| Serum glucose | Should be determined immediately and corrected before further management |
| Computed tomography of the brain | Indications:<br>First-onset seizures<br>Persistent altered mental status<br>Change in seizure character or pattern:<br>New focal neurologic deficit<br>History of trauma or blood thinner use<br>AIDS, fever |
| Spinal tap | In the event of suspected CNS infection or HIV/AIDS population |
| Electroencephalography | Only if intubated in the emergency department or in a patient with persistent unconsciousness with an identifiable cause (rule out non–tonic-clonic status) |
| Magnetic resonance imaging | May reveal additional CNS diagnosis and identify smaller CNS lesions |
| Electrocardiography | Rule out dysrhythmias or drug toxicity (anticholinergics, sodium channel blockade, cyclic antidepressants)<br>Rule out a prolonged QTc or widened QRS interval |

*AIDS*, Acquired immunodeficiency syndrome; *CNS*, central nervous system; *HIV*, human immunodeficiency virus.

common symptom and occur in 70% to 90% of patients. The majority of patients will respond to treatment with phenytoin or carbamazepine.

Albendazole is the mainstay antiparasitic drug for the treatment of NCC (15 mg/kg/day divided into two doses twice daily for 8 to 30 days). Patients in whom NCC is diagnosed may require treatment with steroids to control the inflammation and treat meningitis, cysticercal encephalitis, and angiitis. Treatment is usually started with dexamethasone (4 to 12 mg/day), and it can be replaced with prednisone (1 mg/kg/day) for long-term treatment.

Computed tomography (CT) of the brain should be performed in *every patient with a first onset of seizures* and in those with persistent change in mental status, focal neurologic deficit, or suspicion of an organic intracerebral lesion. Early CT scanning is essential for identifying surgically correctable causes. If there is a concern that trauma occurred, CT can be used to rule out cervical spine and intracerebral injury (**Box 99.6**).

Magnetic resonance imaging (MRI) is more sensitive than CT and can be effective in diagnosing additional lesions; namely, temporal sclerosis, cortical dysplasia, vascular malformations (e.g., arteriovenous aneurysms), and some tumors. Its use will depend on availability and time constraints, but MRI is not typically done on an emergency basis. The majority of patients will be able to undergo MRI as an outpatient.

The EEG records brain electrical activity and is used for definitive diagnosis of epilepsy and related conditions. The need for EEG in the emergency setting is limited, usually to patients whose seizure activity is uncontrollable despite aggressive treatment or to patients whose seizure activity is more difficult to diagnose.

**BOX 99.6 Indications for Computed Tomography Scanning of the Brain**

Advanced age
Human immunodeficiency virus, acquired immunodeficiency syndrome
Suspicion of parasitic central nervous system infection (neurocysticercosis)
Persistent change in mental status
New focal neurologic deficit
History or evidence of trauma

Intubated patients who are paralyzed or have undergone induction of phenobarbital coma and general anesthesia should be monitored continuously with an EEG to exclude seizure activity because in these situations obvious seizure activity may not be apparent as a result of neuromuscular paralysis. Another indication may be patients who have unexplained altered consciousness that can be due to persistent non–tonic-clonic seizure activity.

If patient is transported by EMS, multiple steps in the treatment (**Fig. 99.1**) protocol can be initiated and completed by

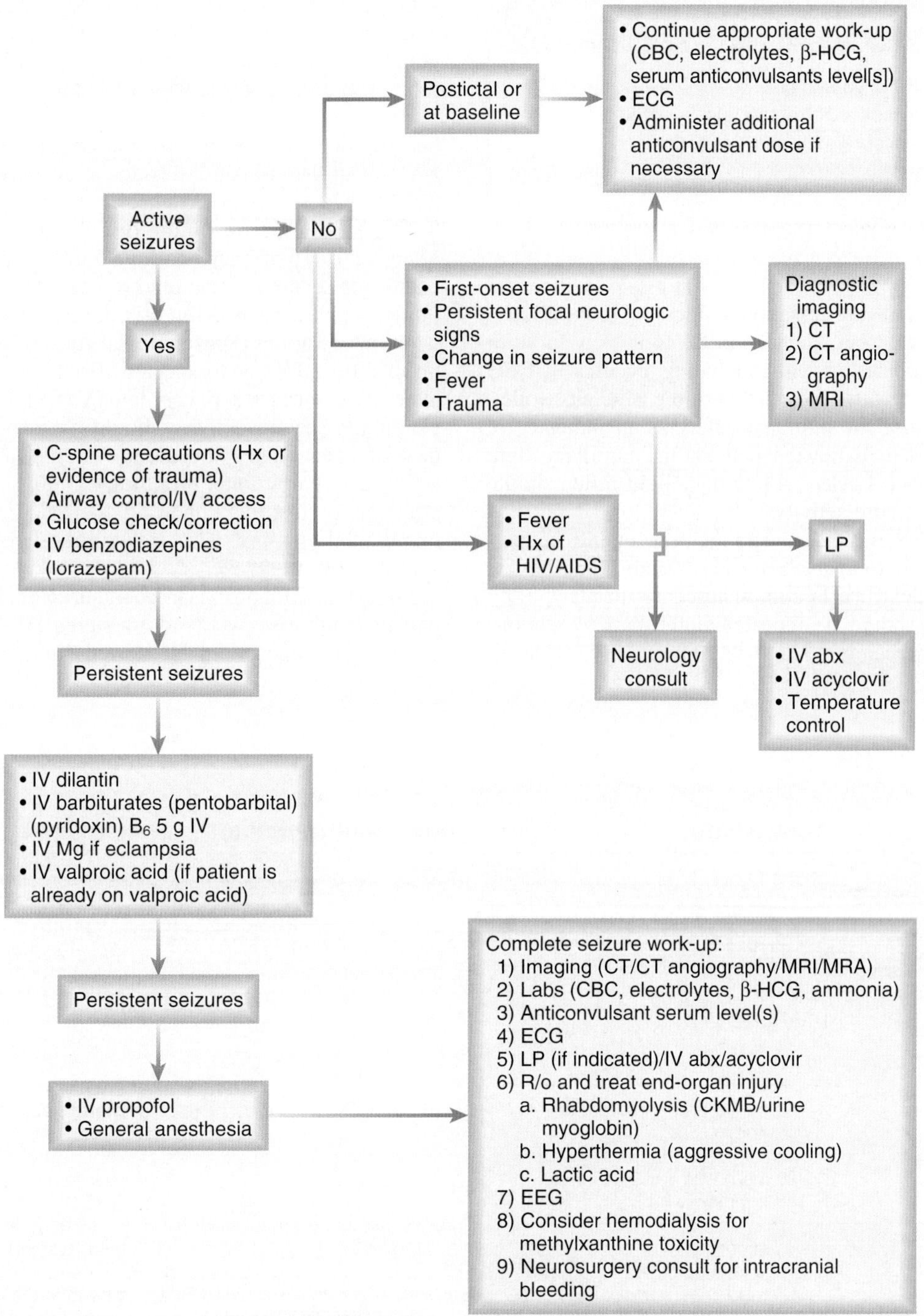


**Fig. 99.1 Steps in treatment.** *abx*, Antibiotics; *AIDS*, acquired immunodeficiency syndrome; *CBC*, complete blood count; *C-spine*, cervical spine; *CT*, computed tomography; *ECG*, electrocardiogram; *EEG*, electroencephalogram; *β-HCG*, β-human chorionic gonadotropin; *HIV*, human immunodeficiency virus; *Hx*, history; *IV*, intravenous; *LP*, lumbar puncture; *MRA*, magnetic resonance angiography; *MRI*, magnetic resonance imaging; *r/o*, rule out.

EMS personnel, including administration of anticonvulsants, airway protection, correction of glucose, and elicitation of the initial history, including drug exposure. It is essential that an attempt be made to control seizure activity immediately on arrival at the ED, so discussion of treatment will occur simultaneously with discussion of the diagnostic approach. Maintenance of adequate cerebral perfusion and consequent oxygen and glucose supply to the brain is the goal of treatment.

Most seizures will stop spontaneously or soon after the initiation of appropriate treatment. One of the primary goals during the evaluation and treatment of patients with seizures is to preserve a patent airway and oxygenation, as well as prevent aspiration in patients who are in the postictal phase. Despite very dramatic signs and symptoms, including cyanosis, very few patients who are actively experiencing seizures will require endotracheal intubation.

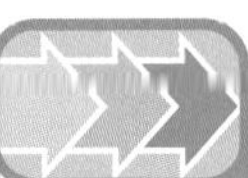

**PRIORITY ACTIONS**

Airway control and oxygenation
Cervical spine protection if trauma is suspected
Serum glucose measurement and correction
Intravenous administration of benzodiazepines and other anticonvulsants

Cessation of motor seizure activity as a result of chemical paralysis does not indicate cessation of neuronal seizure activity. It is essential that clinicians continue to closely monitor for seizures in intubated patients, including, eventually, EEG monitoring. While awaiting placement of the EEG electrodes, clinicians should use the pupillary reflex as an indicator of seizure activity. In a paralyzed patient, the pupillary light reflex remains intact. Lack of a pupillary light reflex should suggest ongoing seizure activity.

A rapid bedside or field fingerstick test should be performed immediately to evaluate for low serum glucose. One ampule of 50% dextrose is administered IV to a hypoglycemic patient. It should be repeated if the patient remains hypoglycemic. Glucagon, 1 mg intramuscularly (IM) or subcutaneously, should be given to hypoglycemic patients without intravenous access as a temporizing measure. Glucagon, however, can cause vomiting, thus increasing the risk for aspiration in an unresponsive or seizing patient.

Benzodiazepines should be administered immediately because they have been shown to control the majority of seizures regardless of cause through an increase in GABA activity. Studies have shown that lorazepam (Ativan, 0.05 to 0.1 mg/kg up to a maximum of a 4-mg initial dose) is more effective than diazepam (Valium, 5 to 15 mg IV) for the initial control of seizures, although both agents are acceptable.[2,4] If intravenous access is difficult, intramuscular or rectal administration of valium (Diastat, rectal form of valium, 0.2 mg/kg up to 20 mg PR) or lorazepam (0.1 to 0.2 mg/kg IM) is an alternative. Intranasal midazolam (Versed) has also been used. Continued seizure activity should be treated with a second dose of a benzodiazepine, along with the addition of a second agent (e.g., barbiturate, propofol, pyridoxine/vitamin $B_6$) and attention to disorders inciting the seizure (e.g., increased intracranial pressure, CNS infection, eclampsia, drug-related seizures) (**Table 99.3**).

Phenytoin (Dilantin) is a second drug of choice but requires patient monitoring when administered IV. A loading dose of 15 to 20 mg/kg should be started simultaneously with the

**Table 99.3 Treatment of Acute Seizures: Medication Summary**

| MEDICATION | DOSE (LOAD) | DOSE (MAINTENANCE) | COMMENTS |
|---|---|---|---|
| Diazepam | 10 mg IV over 2 min | Repeat q5-10min | Respiratory depression, hypotension |
| Lorazepam | 2-8 mg IV | Repeat once in 10-15 min if seizure persists | Respiratory depression, hypotension |
| Midazolam | 0.1-0.2 mg/kg or 2.25-15 mg IV | | Respiratory depression, hypotension |
| Phenytoin | 15-20 mg/kg IV at max rate of 50 mg/min | 100 mg IV/PO q6-8h | Hypotension, ataxia |
| Fosphenytoin | 15-20 mg/kg IM at max rate of 150 mg/min | | Faster loading time, needs to be metabolized to be effective |
| Pentobarbital | 1.5-20 mg/kg<br>5 mg/kg is effective for induction of anesthesia in most cases | 2.5 mg/kg/hr | Severe respiratory depression<br>Faster effect than with phenobarbital |
| Phenobarbital | 15-20 mg/kg at max rate of 50 mg/min | 120-240 mg q20min | Severe respiratory depression, hypotension |
| Propofol | 1-2 mg/kg IV | 2-4 mg/kg/hr | Severe respiratory depression, acidosis (children) |
| Valproic acid (VA) | 20 mg/kg IV at 20 mg/min | Repeat if needed | Only if everything else fails; may be beneficial for patients already taking VA but the level is subtherapeutic |
| Isoflurane | Up to 1.5% volume | | Severe respiratory depression |
| Magnesium sulfate (eclampsia) | 4 gr IV over 15 min | 2 mg/hr | Respiratory depression with rapid administration, monitor deep tendon reflexes |

administration of benzodiazepines. This should be done for patients with elevated intracranial pressure (e.g., tumor, bleeding, hydrocephalus), as well as for those who are not compliant with the phenytoin prescribed. Phenytoin has poor water solubility and has to be formulated with propylene glycol, so intravenous delivery is rate-limited (no faster than 50 mg/min) to prevent hypotension.

If the emergency physician suspects drug-induced seizures, including withdrawal (alcohol, sedative-hypnotics, baclofen), phenytoin should not be used as a second drug of choice because it has disadvantageous properties (negative inotropic and proarrhythmogenic properties). For drug-related seizures resistant to benzodiazepines, barbiturates, propofol, and pyridoxine should be considered.

Fosphenytoin (Cerebyx) is less irritating to veins, less toxic to tissues, and less likely to induce dysrhythmias and can be administered either IV or IM, but it is more expensive. Fosphenytoin is a prodrug of phenytoin. Plasma phosphatase enzymes cleave phenytoin from fosphenytoin, which takes 8 to 15 minutes when administered IV. With intramuscular dosing, approximately 30 minutes is needed for therapeutic levels to be achieved. The loading dose is 15 to 20 mg/kg (phenytoin equivalent) IV or IM. Fosphenytoin is water soluble and associated with far less tissue toxicity at the infusion site; however, it is just as cardiotoxic as phenytoin. Fosphenytoin is typically reserved for short-term parental administration.

Barbiturates are potent respiratory depressants, much more so than benzodiazepines, so clinicians should be concerned about the potential for intubation. Traditionally, phenobarbital (10 to 20 mg/kg IV administered at a rate of 25 to 50 mg/min) has been used as a drug of choice, but because of rate-limited administration, pentobarbital (100 mg IV administered at a rate of 25 mg/min), a shorter-acting barbiturate, should be considered for resistant seizures.

Patients whose seizure activity has ceased before arrival at the ED might be candidates for oral loading of antiepileptic medications. The oral loading regimen for patients who have no detectable serum level of phenytoin (Dilantin) is 20 mg/kg in divided doses administered over a day, with a maximum dose of 400 mg every 2 hours. A suspension formulation is preferred over tablets because of better absorption and higher serum levels. Adverse reactions to phenytoin, such as ataxia, somnolence, and confusion, are decreased with a slower loading rate.

The usual typical outpatient oral dose is 100 mg three times per day. Because the half-life of phenytoin is about 24 hours, some patients take 300 mg once a day. The therapeutic serum level is 10 to 20 mg/L. Even at this level, some patients will experience mild sedation and cognitive effects. With long term use, gum and skin thickening can occur and may not be reversible. One in 10,000 will experience Steven-Johnson syndrome. Phenytoin can cause folate deficiency, which leads to anemia and bone problems, so daily use of multivitamins is recommended.

Patients with chronic seizures who have a typical event may require only evaluation of the antiepileptic level and triggering factors. However, new organic pathology that may lower the seizure threshold (e.g., infection, electrolyte abnormality, trauma) should be excluded. Any precipitating factors that may unmask a chronic seizure disorder or explain an increase in seizure reoccurrence in patients with therapeutic levels of anticonvulsants should be identified (see Box 99.4). In the absence of concomitant pathology, the majority of patients with chronic seizures can be discharged home if they return to baseline.

In addition to the classic or traditional anticonvulsants (phenytoin, carbamazepine, phenobarbital), the emergency physician may encounter many new anticonvulsants. The majority of new drugs do not have timely measurable serum levels.

Patients who are undergoing chronic anticonvulsant treatment should receive an additional oral dose before discharge if the level is found to be subtherapeutic. It is also reasonable to give a dose of one of the newer anticonvulsants in the ED to patients who are noncompliant with treatment (**Table 99.4**).

Neurology consultation should be considered for patients in status epilepticus (SE) or for breakthrough seizures. Trauma and neurosurgery consultation should be obtained for patients with intracranial bleeding and complex trauma. Finally, an infectious disease consultation could be considered for some patients with infectious pathology and acquired immunodeficiency syndrome (AIDS).

## SPECIAL CIRCUMSTANCES

### STATUS EPILEPTICUS

SE is defined as continuous seizure activity in excess of 5 minutes or consequent seizure activity without return to consciousness. Diagnostic assessment of patients in SE should be performed in parallel with treatment, and most of the time the diagnosis can be based on clinical findings.

Early aggressive administration of intravenous anticonvulsants is the keystone for successful treatment of SE. Benzodiazepines and barbiturates will control seizure activity through the increased action of GABA. With longer durations of SE, there may be loss of responsiveness to GABAergic medications because of a theoretically time-dependent loss of synaptic $GABA_A$ receptors.

For patients who fail to respond to first-line anticonvulsant therapy, especially if exposure to isoniazid (INH) is suspected because of tuberculosis, 5 g of vitamin $B_6$ should be administered IV.

### PREGNANCY

Pregnancy can precipitate seizure episodes in patients with underlying seizure disorders. Women with epilepsy can also experience seizures during and after abortions. Sometimes during cervical dilation, woman can experience cervical shock, which is a type of vasovagal syncope resulting in bradycardia, relative CNS hypoperfusion, and occasional tonic-clonic activity that is much shorter in duration and lacks any postictal phase.

The incidence of eclampsia in the western world ranges from 1 in 2000 to 3000 pregnancies. The incidence of seizures in woman with preeclampsia is approximately 1 in 300. Eclamptic seizures can occur from the 20th week of gestation up to 7 days after delivery. Seizures up to 26 days after delivery have been reported. During this period every new-onset seizure should initially be treated as eclamptic until proved otherwise. Clinician should be aware that up to 30% of eclamptic woman do not necessarily have the "classic symptoms"—hypertension, proteinuria, and

**Table 99.4 Miscellaneous Treatment of Active Seizures**

| MEDICATION | INDICATION | DOSE | COMMENT |
|---|---|---|---|
| Calcium gluconate, calcium chloride | Hypocalcemia | 10 mL of 10% calcium gluconate solution<br>Repeat as needed | Watch for hypercalcemia<br>Calcium chloride has 3 times more calcium and is more caustic (requires administration through a central line) |
| Magnesium sulfate | Hypomagnesemia | 2-4 g of 50% magnesium sulfate diluted in saline or dextrose IV over 30-60 min<br>IV push if symptoms severe | Watch for respiratory arrest and hyporeflexia |
| 3% Normal saline solution | Hyponatremia with persistent seizures and neurologic findings | 300-500 mL of 3% NaCl solution over 1-2 hr until resolution of seizures | Calculate total sodium deficit<br>Avoid too rapid correction |
| Baclofen | Baclofen withdrawal | Same dose that the patient was already taking (PO or IV)<br>Consult toxicologist before administration | May require restoration of intrathecal pump |
| Pyridoxine | Persistent status epilepticus; isoniazid overdose | 5 g empirically | Requires 50 ampules of 100 mg vitamin $B_6$ |

edema. Other than early detection of preeclampsia, no tests are reliable in predicting the development of eclampsia. All female patients of childbearing age who are seen following seizure activity should be tested for pregnancy. Pregnant women who have hypertension, proteinuria, headache, visual disturbances, abdominal pain with nausea, or edema should be presumed to have eclampsia until proved otherwise. The cerebral abnormalities with eclampsia (mostly vasogenic edema) are similar to those found with hypertensive encephalopathy.

The treatment of choice is magnesium and concomitant delivery of the fetus. Magnesium sulfate is administered at a dose of 4 to 6 g IV over a 15-minute period, followed by a maintenance infusion of 2 g/hr. Magnesium sulfate is not an anticonvulsant, and its mechanism of activity remains unclear. After administration, deep tendon reflexes should be monitored closely because hyporeflexia will precede respiratory insufficiency, a complication of hypermagnesemia. Hydralazine is usually indicated in conjunction to manage blood pressure. Benzodiazepines and phenytoin, though not typically first-line agents for the treatment of eclamptic seizures, may also have some short-term benefit.

## HUMAN IMMUNODEFICIENCY VIRUS

People infected with human immunodeficiency virus (HIV) may have a CNS mass or infection as a cause of the seizure. This can be the first manifestation of AIDS. HIV-positive patients who have a seizure require a CT scan and, if negative, a lumbar puncture. HIV encephalopathy or meningitis must be considered (**Box 99.7**).

**BOX 99.7 Causes of Seizures in the Human Immunodeficiency Virus–Infected Population**

Focal central nervous system lesions
- Cerebral toxoplasmosis
- Primary central nervous system lymphoma
- Progressive multifocal leukoencephalopathy

Focal viral encephalitis
- Cytomegalovirus
- Varicella-zoster virus
- Herpes simplex virus

Bacterial abscess
Cryptococcoma
Tuberculous abscess
Mass lesion
- Toxoplasmosis
- Lymphoma

Meningitis, encephalitis
- Cryptococcal
- Bacterial, aseptic
- Herpes zoster
- Cytomegalovirus

Human immunodeficiency virus–associated encephalopathy, acquired immunodeficiency syndrome–dementia complex
Progressive multifocal leukoencephalopathy
Central nervous system tuberculosis
Neurosyphilis

## CENTRAL NERVOUS SYSTEM PATHOLOGY

Patients with underlying intracranial hemorrhage who are taking anticoagulants or have an elevated international normalized ratio may require the administration of fresh frozen plasma and vitamin K to prevent further bleeding. Patients with brain tumors, evidence of increased intracranial pressure, or hydrocephalus require immediate neurosurgical consultation.

## DRUG- AND TOXIN-INDUCED SEIZURES

Any drug that decreases GABA activity in the CNS can cause seizures. Drug-related seizures are a result of either overstimulation (glutamate) or lack of inhibition (GABA withdrawal) of electrical brain activity. Treatment is generally directed at increasing GABA activity with benzodiazepines. However, certain drugs are associated with particular types of toxicities that may require specific treatments or antidotes (**Tables 99.5 and 99.6**).

Removal of the toxin or drug plus secondary decontamination is the hallmark of treatment of drug- and toxin-induced seizures.

### *Cocaine*

The most commonly abused substance that causes seizures is cocaine. Benzodiazepines will help control seizures, agitation, and hyperthermia. In patients with prolonged seizures, focal neurologic findings, or persistent changes in mental status, CT of the brain should be used to exclude intracerebral bleeding. Fluid resuscitation is important to protect against renal damage from potential rhabdomyolysis. If the patient is hyperthermic, cooling measures with intravenous fluids, ice packs, and even ice baths for refractory hyperthermia should be applied to avoid multiorgan failure and death.

### *Alcohol*

Alcohol-related seizures (ARSs) are defined as adult-onset seizures, generally after the age of 25, that occur in the setting of chronic alcohol dependence or withdrawal. Preexisting epilepsy, structural brain lesions, use of illicit drugs, or other metabolic disorders can also increase the frequency of seizures in patients who drink heavily. They are typically brief, generalized tonic-clonic seizures that occur 6 to 48 hours after the last drink. Without treatment, 60% of patients will experience multiple seizures over a period of approximately 6 hours.

The diagnosis of ARSs is made only after exclusion of other potential causes. New-onset seizures in an alcohol-dependent patient should prompt a thorough evaluation similar to that described for any person with a new-onset seizure.

In majority of the patients, lorazepam (Ativan), 2 mg IV, has been shown to prevent subsequent seizures after the first one. In a randomized controlled trial of patients with ARSs, only 3% had a subsequent seizure during a 6-hour observation period as compared with 24% in the placebo group ($P < .001$).

All patients should be offered referral to a specialized alcohol treatment facility (when possible) where they can be treated with longer-acting benzodiazepines. If patients are unwilling to be referred, they should be observed for at least 3 hours.

### *Opioids*

Despite the fact that opioids are not generally associated with the seizures, it is worth mentioning several exceptions, including meperidine (Demerol), propoxyphene (Darvon), and tramadol (Ultram). Administration of naloxone can actually precipitate and worsen meperidine-associated seizures.

### *MDMA; 3,4-Methylenedioxymethamphetamine ("Ecstasy")*

MDMA is an amphetamine-related drug that is associated with seizure activity. Typically, patients who are ingesting MDMA during "rave parties" experience brief tonic-clonic seizures as a result of hyponatremia. MDMA can cause a transient syndrome of inappropriate antidiuretic hormone secretion, in addition to the dilutional hyponatremia secondary to excessive free water consumption. Most patients can be treated by fluid restriction and observation.

## OTHER MEDICATIONS TYPICALLY ASSOCIATED WITH SEIZURES (Table 99.7)

### *Cyclic Antidepressants*

Cyclic antidepressants are notorious for their propensity to cause seizures as a result of GABA inhibition. Seizures are typically a manifestation of severe toxicity, so airway protection, complete gastrointestinal decontamination (charcoal, lavage if indicated), and intravenous benzodiazepines should be initiated immediately. Sodium bicarbonate, a primary treatment of cyclic antidepressant overdose, is effective in treating cardiac conduction abnormalities but does not affect seizure activity.

### *Isoniazid*

The typical manifestation of INH-induced seizures is SE that does not respond to conventional treatment with GABAergic drugs or phenytoin. INH prevents GABA synthesis, and the treatment is vitamin $B_6$ (pyridoxine). If the dose of ingested INH is known, the antidote treatment is 1 g of vitamin $B_6$ for each gram of INH. However, if the dose is not known, empiric administration of 5 g is recommended. Pyridoxine should be diluted to a concentration of 50 mL/g and administered IV over a period of 5 to 10 minutes. The dose should be repeated if seizures continue or if the patient remains lethargic.

### *Methylxanthines (Caffeine, Theophylline)*

Overdoses of caffeine and theophylline are notorious for causing seizures through the antagonism of adenosine, an inhibitory neurotransmitter. Usually, the seizures are short acting and can be controlled with benzodiazepines. However, in severely toxic patients, hemodialysis may be necessary.

## FOLLOW-UP, NEXT STEPS IN CARE, AND PATIENT EDUCATION

Every patient with persistent seizures, change in mental status, or underlying medical condition that requires hospital treatment (e.g., sepsis, overdose, trauma) should be admitted. Patients in SE should be admitted to an intensive care setting (**Box 99.8**).

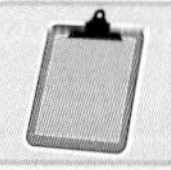

**DOCUMENTATION**

Subtherapeutic levels should be documented in addition to the planned strategy to achieve therapeutic serum levels in a reasonable time frame.

If computed tomography and laboratory work are deemed unnecessary, adequate documentation should support the medical reasoning and clinical findings.

Discussion with the neurology service should be documented with respect to diagnosis, treatment, and close follow-up.

**Table 99.5 Anticonvulsants**

| NAME | INDICATIONS | SIDE EFFECTS | ADULT DOSING | LEVELS | SERUM TURNAROUND TIME |
|---|---|---|---|---|---|
| Carbamazepine (Carbatrol, Tegretol, Tegretol XR) | Partial seizures and epilepsy | Anemia<br>Neutropenia<br>Ataxia<br>Drowsiness<br>Nausea | 200 mg bid, can titrate to maximum of 500 mg bid | Therapeutic concentration: 2.0-10.0 mcg/mL<br>Toxic concentration: ≥12.0 mcg/mL | 2 hr |
| Clobazam (Frisium, Canada) | Adjunctive therapy for tonic-clonic, complex partial, and myoclonic seizures | Ataxia<br>Diplopia<br>Dysarthria<br>Lethargy | 5-15 mg/day; may increase up to 80 mg/day | 50-300 ng/mL | N/A |
| Clonazepam (Klonopin, Epitril, Rivotril) | Single or adjunctive therapy for treatment of Lennox-Gastaut (petit mal variant), akinetic, and myoclonic seizures | Ataxia<br>Confusion<br>Lethargy | 0.5 mg tid; can increase up to 20 mg/day | 20-80 ng/mL<br>Toxic > 80 ng/mL | N/A |
| Diazepam (Diastat) | Tonic-clonic seizures | Ataxia<br>Confusion<br>Lethargy | Mainly used IV for acute seizures | 200-600 ng/mL | N/A |
| Ethosuximide (Zarontin) | Absence (petit mal) seizures | Ataxia<br>Euphoria<br>Hyperactivity<br>Lethargy | 500 mg/day, up to 1500 mg/day | Therapeutic concentration: 40-100 mcg/mL<br>Toxic concentration: ≥100 mcg/mL | 2-3 days |
| Felbamate (Felbatol, Taloxa) | For patients who have failed alternative therapies<br>Consultation needed | Aplastic anemia<br>Hepatic failure | 1200 mg/day divided into 3-4 doses, up to 3600 mg/day | 30.0-60.0 mcg/mL | 3-5 days |
| Gabapentin (Neurontin) | Adjunctive therapy for partial seizures | Fatigue<br>Dizziness<br>Imbalance | 300-600 mg tid | 2.0-20.0 mcg/mL | N/A |
| Lacosamide (Vimpat) | Adjunctive therapy for partial seizures | Mood or behavior changes<br>Depression<br>Anxiety | 50-100 mg bid PO IV up to 400 mg/day | Expected values: up to 15.0 mcg/mL | N/A |
| Lamotrigine (Lamictal) | Adjunctive therapy for partial seizures | Headache, nausea, dizziness, potentially life-threatening skin rash (with valproate) | 50-250 mg bid | 2.5-15.0 mcg/mL | 2-5 days |
| Levetiracetam (Keppra, Keppra XR) | Adjunctive therapy for partial seizures | Fatigue, imbalance, behavioral changes | 500-2000 mg bid | 12.0-46.0 mcg/mL | 2-5 days |
| Lorazepam (Adivan) | Active partial and grand mal seizures | Ataxia<br>Lethargy<br>Respiratory depression | IV medication for acute seizures | 30-100 ng/mL | N/A |
| Oxcarbazepine (Trileptal) | Monotherapy, adjunctive therapy for partial seizures with and without secondary generalized seizures in adults<br>Adjunctive therapy for partial seizures in children | Abdominal pain, nausea, vomiting, dizziness, diplopia, drowsiness, fatigue, loss of coordination | 300-600 mg bid | Assessment of compliance and potential toxicity<br>Oxcarbazepine metabolite: 3-35 mcg/mL | 2-5 days |

**Table 99.5 Anticonvulsants—cont'd**

| NAME | INDICATIONS | SIDE EFFECTS | ADULT DOSING | LEVELS | SERUM TURNAROUND TIME |
|---|---|---|---|---|---|
| Phenobarbital (Luminal) | Monotherapy for epilepsy | Respiratory depression, constipation | 60-200 mg daily divided bid-tid | Therapeutic concentration: Infants and children, 15.0-30.0 mcg/mL Adults, 20.0-40.0 mcg/mL Toxic concentration: ≥60.0 mcg/mL | 2 hr |
| Phenytoin (Dilantin) | Monotherapy for epilepsy | Anemia<br>Ataxia<br>Gingival hyperplasia | 100-200 mg tid | 10-20 mcg/mL | 2 hr |
| Pregabalin (Lyrica) | Adjunctive therapy for partial-onset seizures | Blurred vision<br>Difficulty concentrating<br>Dizziness<br>Dry mouth<br>Peripheral edema<br>Somnolence | 100 mg bid-tid | Up to 9.5 mcg/mL | 3-5 days |
| Primidone (Mysoline) | Refractory grand mal seizures and partial seizures | Blurred vision<br>Fatigue<br>Incoordination<br>Nausea, vomiting<br>Erectile dysfunction<br>Vertigo<br>Weight loss | Day 1-3: 100-125 mg qhs<br>Day 4-6: 100-125 mg bid<br>Day 7-9: 100-125 mg tid<br>Day 10 and maintenance: 250 mg tid | Therapeutic concentration: Children (<5 yr), 7.0-10.0 mcg/mL Adults, 9.0-12.5 mcg/mL<br>Toxic concentration: ≥15.0 mcg/mL | N/A |
| Rufinamide (Banzel, Inovelon) | Children 4 yr and older with Lennox-Gastaut syndrome | Fatigue<br>Headaches<br>Nausea | 200-400 mg bid, up to 3600 mg/day | Not established | N/A |
| Tiagabine (Gabitril) | Adjunctive therapy for partial seizures | Dizziness<br>Somnolence | 4-8 mg qid (start at 4 mg/day, titrate up to 32 mg/day bid-qid) | Peak: 110-520 ng/mL<br>Trough: 5-35 ng/mL | 7-10 days |
| Topiramate (Topamax) | Treatment of partial and generalized tonic-clonic seizures | Drowsiness, nausea, dizziness, coordination problems<br>Caveat: acute glaucoma | 12.5-25 mg bid, up to 100-200 mg bid | Assessment of compliance and potential toxicity<br>2-20 mcg/mL | 2-5 days |
| Valproic acid (Depakene, Depakote, Depakote ER) | Monotherapy or adjunctive therapy for complex partial seizures | Hepatotoxicity, hyperammonemia, nausea, weight gain, alopecia, tremor | Start at 10-15 mg/kg/day, can titrate up to 60 mg/kg/day (max dose of 4000 mg/day) | 40-100 mcg/mL | 2 hr |
| Vigabatrin (Sabril) | Epilepsy<br>Infantile spasms | Dizziness<br>Lethargy<br>Memory impairment<br>Hyperactivity in children | 500 mg bid, up to 3 g/day | Therapeutic and toxic doses not established<br>Expected levels of 20-160 mcg/mL | N/A |
| Zonisamide (Zonegran) | Adjunctive therapy for treatment of partial seizures in adults | Dizziness, imbalance, fatigue<br>Cross-allergy with sulfonamides | 25/50/100mg (qd-bid), max of 400 mg/day (100-600 mg qd) | 10-40 mcg/mL | 2-5 days |

*N/A*, Not available.

**Table 99.6 Most Common Drugs Associated with Seizures**

| MEDICATION/DRUG | COMMENT |
|---|---|
| Camphor | Brief, tonic-clonic seizures, usually self-limited |
| Cocaine<br>Amphetamines<br>Phencyclidine | Control agitation and hyperthermia aggressively<br>Treatment of choice: benzodiazepines |
| Cyclic antidepressants | Can be excluded with electrocardiogram<br>Severe toxicity can cause cardiac dysrhythmias<br>Treatment with bicarbonate will control electrocardiographic changes, but not the seizures<br>Benzodiazepines are the drug of choice |
| Isoniazid | Suspect isoniazid in patients with intractable seizures not responsive to benzodiazepines<br>Treat with intravenous vitamin $B_6$ |
| Lindane | Usually ingestion of topical preparation |
| MDMA (Ecstasy) | Usually associated with hyponatremia<br>Morning after "rave" party<br>Fluid restriction is usually sufficient therapy |
| Strychnine | Consciousness preserved<br>Pseudoseizures |
| Theophylline | Adenosine antagonism<br>Wide pulse pressure<br>Tachycardia<br>Hypokalemia<br>Hyperglycemia<br>Possible hemodialysis for intractable seizures |

*MDMA*, 3,4-Methylenedioxymethamphetamine.

**BOX 99.8 Admission Criteria for Patients with Seizures**

Change in mental status
- Drowsiness, coma

Neurologic deficit
- Underlying structural condition
- Tumor, bleeding

Underlying treatable medical condition
- Central nervous system infection

Unable to follow up
Elderly
Inability to ambulate
Lack of social support
Need for the placement in a facility with a higher level of care

**BOX 99.9 Discharge Criteria**

Normal findings on neurologic examination
- Syncope or cardiogenic cause of loss of consciousness ruled out
- Trauma ruled out
- Central nervous system infectious pathology ruled out
- Toxic and metabolic etiology ruled out

Patients with chronic seizures
- Correction of subtherapeutic serum levels

Reasonable plan for follow-up with neurology service or consultant established

Patients with a chronic seizure disorder can be discharged if they return to their normal baseline neurologic level (**Box 99.9**). If the drug level is found to be subtherapeutic, an additional dose of antiepileptics should be given prior to discharge. Before discharge, patients may inquire about their prognosis. In the absence of precipitating factors, secondary seizures may be avoidable in the future, but there will always be some risk, depending on the underlying condition and lifestyle. Patients should avoid sleeplessness, heavy alcohol use, and other physiologic stressors that can alter seizure thresholds.

**Table 99.7 Different Drug Classes Associated with Seizures**

| CLASS | REPRESENTATIVE AGENTS |
|---|---|
| Analgesics | Tramadol |
| | Propoxyphene |
| | Meperidine |
| Anesthetics | General: enflurane |
| | Local: lidocaine, bupivacaine |
| Anthelmintics | Albendazole |
| Antiasthmatics | Terbutaline |
| | Theophylline |
| Antibacterials | Erythromycin |
| | Fluoroquinolones |
| Anticholinergics | Scopolamine |
| Anticholinesterases | Physostigmine |
| Antidepressants | Cyclic antidepressants |
| | Citalopram |
| | Wellbutrin |
| Antifungals | Amphotericin B |
| Antihistamines | Diphenhydramine |
| Antimalarials | Quinine |
| Antipsychotics | Haloperidol |
| Antivirals | Amantadine |
| Contrast agents | Iohexol |
| Hypoglycemics | Chlorpropamide |
| Immunosuppressives | Azathioprine |
| Miscellaneous | Baclofen |
| | Flumazenil |
| | Nicotine |
| NSAIDs | Mefenamic acid |
| Sympathomimetics | Amphetamines |
| | Ephedrine |
| Vaccines | DTP |

*DTP*, Diphtheria and tetanus toxoids and pertussis vaccine; *NSAIDs*, nonsteroidal antiinflammatory drugs.

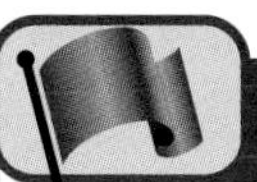

**RED FLAGS**

Patients with status epilepticus should be treated aggressively with the administration of multiple medications at once. Clinician should be aware that administration of phenytoin and phenobarbital is rate dependent and that patients may continue to have seizures for 30 minutes before effective serum levels are achieved.

Patients with cocaine abuse, persistent seizures, and a recent history of travel abroad should be evaluated for body packing and decontaminated by whole-bowel irrigation.

Not recognizing that a patient is pregnant (or postpartum) may lead to delayed treatment and obstetrics consultation.

Patients with seizures should be counseled to not drive and should be accompanied because a recurrent seizure is possible.

Timely administration of antibiotics and antiviral medication in patients with central nervous system infection can improve survival and reduce morbidity.

## REFERENCES

***References can be found on Expert Consult @ www.expertconsult.com.***

# 100 Transient Ischemic Attack and Acute Ischemic Stroke

*Holly K. Ledyard*

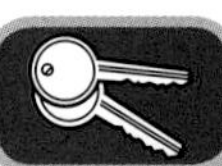

**KEY POINTS**

- Transient ischemic attack (TIA) is a high-risk warning sign for stroke within 90 days, with the highest risk occurring in the first 2 days.
- Patients with TIA can be accurately risk-stratified for recurrent stroke.
- Large artery atherosclerosis, cardioembolism, and small vessel disease are the leading causes of TIA and acute ischemic stroke.
- Magnetic resonance imaging is valuable in differentiating TIA from acute ischemic stroke.
- The goal of management of patients with TIA is to prevent recurrent stroke with antiplatelet, anticoagulation, or surgical therapy.
- The best outcomes for strokes treated with thrombolytic therapy are found with early delivery of recombinant tissue plasminogen activator (rt-PA) within established guidelines.
- Recent evidence supports extending the time window for treatment of ischemic stroke with rt-PA to 4.5 hours for specific patient populations.
- Stroke units and stroke teams provide comprehensive stroke care that improves patient outcomes.

## PERSPECTIVE

Transient ischemic events and acute ischemic strokes are separate points on a continuum of cerebral vascular disease and share a relationship similar to that of unstable angina and acute myocardial ischemia.[1] The most common causes are large artery atherosclerosis, cardioembolism, or small vessel (lacunae) disease. Patients with transient ischemic attacks (TIAs) have a significant short-term risk for recurrent stroke, myocardial infarction, and death. Although TIA is typically a reversible process, ischemic stroke is a pathologic process that permanently injures the brain. Ischemic stroke is defined as a permanent cerebral injury secondary to prolonged disruption of cerebral blood flow (typically <10 mL/100 g brain/min).[2]

Acknowledgment and thanks to Scott Jolley and Todd L. Allen for contributions from the first edition.

## EPIDEMIOLOGY

The yearly incidence of TIA in the United States has been estimated to be approximately 200,000 to 500,000 but may be higher because of the high frequency of underreporting of these events by medical professionals.[3-6] The annual incidence of TIA may be less and the annual incidence of stroke may be higher if the tissue-based definition were applied to all patients evaluated for TIA.[4] It has been estimated that the overall incidence rate of TIA is 1.1 per 1000 U.S. population.[7] This incidence increases with age from 0.1 per 1000 for patients younger than 50 years to 11.7 per 1000 for patients older than 80 years.[3] The incidence of TIA also varies with race and gender: it is significantly greater in blacks and men than in whites and women. The greatest incidence of TIA occurred in black men older than 85 years, who had an incidence of 16 events per 1000.[3]

TIAs account for 0.3% of all emergency department (ED) visits, and it is estimated that 8.7% to 30% of patients will have a TIA before stroke.[8,9] Only 28% of TIA patients arrive via ambulance, and 36% of patients arrive during daylight hours. Emergency physicians (EPs) obtain computed tomography (CT) scans on 56% to 70% of all TIA patients and magnetic resonance imaging (MRI) scans on 7% of TIA patients. Nearly half of all patients with TIA are admitted to the hospital, although there is geographic variability in this practice; another 20% of patients are referred for follow-up. Finally, patients seen in the ED with TIA receive preventive aspirin therapy in 18% of cases, other antiplatelet therapy in 7%, and no preventive therapy in an estimated 42%.[7]

Clearly defined risk factors for stroke and adverse events following a TIA are now well described in the literature, and several groups of investigators have independently developed short-term risk stratification methods applicable to TIA patients in the ED.[10-13] These investigators reported a 10% rate of stroke in the 90 days following the TIA, with 50% of these strokes occurring in the immediate 48 hours after the TIA.

Recently, the ABCD2 score, which combines elements from existing risk stratification systems, was devised to create a robust prediction standard for determining high-risk populations that will benefit from emergency investigation and therapy to prevent short-term adverse events (**Table 100.1**).[12] Patients with the following characteristics were at high risk for having a stroke in the next 2 to 90 days: age older than 60 years, blood pressure higher than 140 mm Hg systolic or 90 mm Hg diastolic, clinical features such as unilateral weakness or speech disturbance, longer duration of symptoms of TIA, and diabetes.

Ischemic stroke accounts for 80% to 88% of the total strokes occurring annually.[14] Each year approximately 795,000 people experience a new or recurrent stroke. It is an important cause of death in the United States and ranks third behind heart disease and cancer.[15]

Approximately 8% to 12% of all patients suffering an ischemic stroke die within 30 days of the initial stroke. Ischemic stroke disproportionately affects the elderly, with a mean age at onset of 70.5 years. Ischemic stroke affects black and Hispanic populations more frequently than white populations. The age-adjusted incidence of first ischemic stroke per 100,000 population is 88 in whites, 149 in Hispanics, and 191 in blacks.[16] Ischemic stroke is an enormous economic burden, with an average 30-day cost of $20,346 for a severe stroke and mean lifetime cost of $140,048.[15,17] The United States spends approximately $73.7 billion yearly on the direct and indirect cost of stroke care.[15]

$SI = \frac{SV}{BSA}$ **FACTS AND FORMULAS**

8.7% to 30% of stroke patients suffer a TIA before the stroke.

10% of TIA patients have a stroke in the next 90 days, 25% to 50% of whom will have their stroke within the first 2 days.

33% of TIA patients with symptoms lasting less than 1 hour will have an infarct shown on diffusion-weighted magnetic resonance imaging.

50% of TIA patients never report symptoms to a physician.

19.2% of patients with untreated symptomatic carotid stenosis of greater than 70% will have a stroke in the next 90 days.

For each minute that reperfusion is delayed, 1.9 million neurons die.

*TIA*, Transient ischemic attack.

**Table 100.1 Two-Day Risk for Stroke Stratified According to the ABCD2 Score**

| RISK FACTOR | NUMBER OF POINTS |
|---|---|
| Age > 60 yr | 1 |
| Initial blood pressure > 140/90 mm Hg | 1 |
| Symptoms of focal motor weakness | 2 |
| Symptoms of speech impairment without weakness | 1 |
| Duration > 60 min | 2 |
| Duration 10-59 min | 1 |
| Diabetes mellitus | 1 |
| **ABCD2 SCORE** | **2-DAY RISK FOR STROKE** |
| 0-1 | 0% |
| 2-3 | 1.3% |
| 4-5 | 4.1% |
| 6-7 | 8.1% |

Adapted from Johnston SC, Rothwell PM, Nguyen-Huynh MN, et al. Validation and refinement of scores to predict very early stroke risk after transient ischaemic attack. Lancet 2007;369:283-92.

## PATHOPHYSIOLOGY

An ischemic injury involving the central nervous system disrupts normal cerebral blood flow to the brain (40 to 60 mL/100 g brain/min). The extent of injury is based on three principles: the duration of disrupted flow, the flow rate, and collateral circulation. Loss of consciousness occurs within 10 seconds and cell death within minutes of disrupted cerebral circulation.

Cerebral tissues with blood flow between 12 and 20 mL/100 g brain/min are termed the ischemic penumbra. These cells are at risk for permanent injury but have the ability to recover if flow is reestablished. When cerebral blood flow falls below 10 mL/100 g brain/min, electrical activity ceases and cell death occurs. Many areas of the brain may be protected by collateral circulation between the anterior and posterior circulation through vessels that make up the circle of Willis.

Classification of TIAs is important because the pathophysiology and risk for recurrent stroke differ among the subtypes. The five mechanisms described are large artery atherosclerosis, cardioembolism, small vessel disease, other rare determined cause, and undetermined cause.[9,18]

Large artery atherosclerosis is defined as greater than 50% narrowing of vessel caliber. It accounts for 15% of all ischemic strokes and is the most common cause of low-flow TIA. Symptoms are the result of thrombus formation in a ruptured atherosclerotic plaque. The most commonly affected vascular territories are the origin of the internal carotid and intracranial portion of the internal carotid (siphon), the middle cerebral artery stem, and the junction of the vertebral and basilar arteries. It is found more commonly in men and has a greater incidence in African and Hispanic populations. Patients with large artery atherosclerosis have a higher recurrence rate than do patients with other stroke subtypes: 4%, 12.6%, and 19.2% at 7, 30, and 90 days, respectively.[19] These patients have transient or stuttering symptoms in the same vascular territory. Symptoms and disability may be less severe than those in patients with cardioembolic stroke.[14]

Cardioembolic disease represents 20% to 25% of ischemic cerebrovascular events. The most common sources are abnormal cardiac rhythm, abnormal left ventricular wall motion, and aortic and mitral valve disease.[20] The clinical features are abrupt in onset, with nonprogressive symptoms that may occur in multiple vascular territories. Cardioemboli affect the anterior circulation in 70% of patients. These patients tend to have more severe symptoms and higher mortality rates; disability is more severe in survivors.[14] Patients with embolic TIA have a lower recurrence rate of 2.5%, 4.6%, 11.9% at 7, 30, and 90 days, respectively.[19]

Lacunar strokes represent 20% of all ischemic strokes and are caused by small vessel disease—obstruction of the small vessels that penetrate the brain parenchyma at right angles to major parent arteries and supply the basal ganglia, internal capsule, thalamus, and pons.[21,22] The vessels most commonly involved are small branches of the middle cerebral and basilar arteries.[21] The most common causes of small vessel disease are microatheroma and lipohyalinosis, which are increased in the setting of older age, hypertension, diabetes, and smoking. Small embolic events rarely cause ischemia in these vessels.[21,22] Patients with lacunar TIA and stroke commonly have hypertension and diabetes. Black populations are affected more than white populations, and there does not seem to be a gender preference in patients with lacunar infarcts. These patients have a favorable prognosis with low, short-term recurrence rates of 0%, 2%, and 3.4% at 7, 30, and 90 days, respectively.[19,21,22]

Rare causes of stroke account for approximately 2% to 3% of annual cases. Common causes are nonatherosclerotic vasculopathies (acute arterial dissection, vasculitis, polyarteritis, giant cell arteritis, infectious arteritis), hypercoagulable conditions (deficiencies in proteins C and S and antithrombin III, antiphospholipid antibody syndrome/systemic lupus erythematosus, pregnancy, postmenopausal hormone replacement), hematologic disorders (sickle cell disease, polycythemia, myeloproliferative disorders), and other causes of emboli (patent foramen ovale, endocarditis, air).[23]

Cryptogenic stroke is the designation used for stroke without a well-defined etiology despite extensive evaluation. It accounts for 30% to 40% of all strokes in some stroke databases. Patients with cryptogenic stroke have a better 1-year prognosis than do those with other subtypes; the 2-year risk for recurrence is 14% to 20%.[14]

Systemic hypoperfusion is an uncommon cause of cerebral ischemia that represents a global decrease in cerebral blood flow. Causes include cardiac arrest and reduced cardiac output as a result of cardiac ischemia, pericardial effusion, arrhythmias, pulmonary emboli, hemorrhage, and medications. Symptoms consist of diffuse brain dysfunction in the setting of unstable vital signs.[14,23]

## PRESENTING SIGNS AND SYMPTOMS

Patients who have suffered a TIA often have no physical findings but a variety of historical clinical symptoms. Several studies have demonstrated that interobserver disagreement is high when making the diagnosis of TIA.[24,25]

A few basic principles can guide accurate diagnosis of TIA. The symptoms are sudden in onset and vascular in nature. TIAs are commonly brief, lasting less than 1 to 2 hours with many lasting less than 10 to 15 minutes. Symptoms are associated with loss of function such as hemiparesis, hemiparesthesia, dysarthria, aphasia, monocular vision loss, diplopia, and gait and balance disturbances. Symptoms such as shaking, scotomata, and marching of symptoms to other body parts are more consistent with migraine or seizure.[26]

Approximately 80% of ischemic strokes occur in the distribution of the anterior circulation and give rise to deficits in behavior, sensation, movement, and speech, as well as some elements of visual awareness. The minority of strokes occur in the distribution of the posterior circulation. Common posterior circulation symptoms are limb weakness, gait and limb ataxia, oculomotor palsy, and oropharyngeal dysfunction. In addition, patients often exhibit nausea and vomiting because of brainstem involvement, as well as vertigo and balance disorders related to cerebellar and brainstem injury.

### OPTHALMIC ARTERY

Transient monocular blindness, known as amaurosis fugax, is caused by transient occlusion of the ophthalmic artery. It is commonly associated with internal carotid artery stenosis and carries a better prognosis than does carotid disease associated with hemispheric TIA.[27]

### MIDDLE CEREBRAL ARTERY

Patients with middle cerebral artery occlusion typically exhibit sensory loss hemiplegia, contralateral sensory loss, and contralateral homonymous hemianopia. Patients with dominant hemispheric lesions have aphasia; those with nondominant hemispheric lesions demonstrate contralateral hemisensory neglect. Subtle findings include gaze preference toward the side of the lesion and contralateral gaze weakness.

### ANTERIOR CEREBRAL ARTERY

Occlusion of branches of the anterior cerebellar artery is more common than stem lesions and is associated with well-recognized clinical findings: contralateral motor weakness and sensory deficit in the lower extremity. Other symptoms include urinary incontinence because of contralateral weakness of the pelvic floor muscles, memory loss or apathy secondary to occlusion of the orbital or frontopolar branch, dysarthria secondary to compromise of the medial striate artery, and ideomotor apraxia (inability to perform skilled movements) as a result of occlusion of the pericallosal branch.

### SMALL VESSEL DISEASE (LACUNAE)

Patients with lacunar ischemia are commonly hypertensive, diabetic, or both, and they do not have associated cortical dysfunction (speech, calculation, and spatial orientation deficits). Lacunar infarcts result from ischemic events involving small penetrating branches of the middle cerebral, anterior cerebral, posterior cerebral, and basilar and anterior choroidal arteries. These lesions affect the basal ganglia, internal capsule, thalamus, putamen, and internal capsule. Five major lacunar syndromes are recognized: pure motor hemiparesis, ataxic hemiparesis, pure sensory syndrome, mixed sensorimotor syndrome, and dysarthria–clumsy hand syndrome.

Pure motor hemiparesis is the most common lacunar syndrome and occurs in 50% of patients with lacunar strokes. Patients have stuttering symptoms that develop over hours, as well as contralateral facial and arm weakness, but do not have sensory or higher cortical dysfunction. The injury involves the corona radiata or internal capsule.[22]

Ataxic hemiparesis syndrome is characterized by weakness and dysmetria (inability to fix the range of movement) on the same side. The lower extremity is more often affected and the face is least affected. The injury involves the internal capsule, basis pontis, or corona radiata.[22]

Patients with pure sensory syndrome have contralateral sensory loss in the face, arm, and leg. Symptoms include sensory ataxia, a movement disorder secondary to sensory impairment; a wide-stance gait with gaze directed to the feet; and a walking pattern characterized by a stamping action that maximizes any remaining proprioception. The injury involves the ventral posterior nucleus of the thalamus.[22]

In mixed sensorimotor syndrome, patients have hemiparesis or hemiplegia associated with sensory loss on the same side. This syndrome is distinguished from the other syndromes by the lack of associated cortical symptoms. The posterolateral thalamus and the posterior limb of the internal capsule are the sites of injury.[22]

Dysarthria–clumsy hand syndrome is the least common of the lacunar syndromes and affects 6% of patients with lacunar stroke. Patients are typically dysarthric secondary to paresis of the lip, tongue, and jaw musculature and report clumsiness of hand movement. The injury involves fibers descending through the genu of the internal capsule.[22]

### VERTIBROBASILAR ARTERIES

Twenty percent of ischemic events affect brain tissue supplied by the posterior circulation. Patients with posterior circulation ischemia rarely have a single initial sign or symptom. Typical symptoms are dizziness, vertigo, headache, vomiting, double vision, loss of vision, transient interruption of consciousness, numbness, weakness, and ataxia. These patients often have crossed signs that include ipsilateral cranial nerve deficits associated with contralateral motor deficits. The most common signs include contralateral limb weakness, gait and limb ataxia, oculomotor palsy, and oropharyngeal dysfunction.

### POSTERIOR CEREBRAL ARTERY

Occlusion of the posterior cerebral artery and its branches leads to a variety of defects in the cerebral cortex, midbrain, thalamus, subthalamic nuclei, and corpus callosum. Stem lesions in the posterior cerebral artery cause isolated contralateral homonymous hemianopia. Midbrain lesions result in crossed symptoms with ipsilateral third nerve palsy accompanied by contralateral motor hemiplegia. Thalamic branch lesions cause contralateral sensory loss accompanied by hemianopia. Injury to the subthalamic nuclei results in ballism of the contralateral arm. Finally, corpus callosum injury results in an inability to transfer written information from right to left, as well as alexia (inability to read written material).[23]

### CEREBELLAR INFARCT

The most common cause of an ischemic injury involving the cerebellum is an embolic infarct in the upper part of the cerebellum. Symptoms include dizziness, vertigo, vomiting, blurred vision, and difficulty walking. Patients may report that they veer to a specific side or are unable to sit upright without assistance. Cerebellar infarcts are distinguished from infarcts in other anatomic locations by the lack of hemiparesis or hemisensory deficits.[23,28] Hypotonia may be present in the arm on the affected side. This sign is best elicited by having patients hold their arms straight out at 90 degrees from the trunk, quickly lower them, and then abruptly stop the lowering motion. The affected side is detected because the hypotonic arm will overshoot the rapid descent.

### LATERAL MEDULLARY SYNDROME (WALLENBERG SYNDROME)

Occlusion or narrowing of the intracranial vertebral artery causes signs and symptoms related to ischemic injury to the lateral medullary tegmentum. Symptoms include ipsilateral facial sensory loss, ataxia, and nystagmus. Patients may also have Horner syndrome, hoarseness, difficulty swallowing, and contralateral hemisensory loss of pain and temperature sense.

## DIFFERENTIAL DIAGNOSIS AND MEDICAL DECISION MAKING

Evaluation of patients with suspected ischemic injury is summarized in **Box 100.1**. The results of these fundamental tests combined with risk stratification can guide the EP in determining whether cerebral injury has occurred, as well as the cause of the ischemia.

Patients with TIA and ischemic stroke require rapid and accurate diagnosis to determine the cause and location of the event and the extent of damage. This knowledge allows the EP to estimate the risks and benefits associated with therapies that will reestablish cerebral blood flow and preserve viable brain tissue.

Rapid diagnosis of acute ischemic stroke begins with public education about recognition of the major warning signs of stroke. Prehospital personnel also play a crucial role in early diagnosis and rapid transport of stroke patients to treatment facilities. Tools such as the Cincinnati Prehospital Stroke Scale and the Los Angeles Prehospital Stroke Screen (LAPSS) are used to evaluate facial droop, arm weakness, and speech abnormalities in patients with suspected stroke. In addition, the LAPSS screens for mimics of stroke such as hypoglycemia, hyperglycemia, and seizure and has high sensitivity (93%) and specificity (97%) for the diagnosis of acute stroke.[29,30]

EPs caring for patients with acute ischemic stroke are often under enormous time constraints. A systematic method is necessary to distinguish patients with stroke from those with conditions that mimic stroke.[31] In addition, the EP must combine historical and physical data with the results of

**BOX 100.1 Diagnostic Evaluation for Transient Ischemic Attack and Stroke**

- History
- Physical examination—blood pressure; cardiac, vascular, and neurologic evaluation; National Institutes of Health Stroke Scale score
- Laboratory tests—chemistry, coagulation, complete blood count, fasting lipid panel
- Electrocardiogram
- Cerebral imaging—computed tomography and magnetic resonance imaging if available
- Vascular and cardiac imaging

neurologic imaging to exclude hemorrhage and determine the extent of injury. These elements, coupled with basic laboratory tests and an electrocardiogram (ECG), as recommended by the American Heart Association (AHA), are the foundation for accurate diagnosis of an acute ischemic stroke.

The history is the cornerstone of accurate stroke diagnosis. Historical evidence that has been identified as being predictive of a patient having a stroke includes persistent focal neurologic deficits, acute onset during the previous week, and no history of head trauma.[31] Clinical symptoms such as arm and leg weakness and speech impairment are more reliable indicators than subjective isolated sensory symptoms are. The single most important piece of historical information is the time of onset of the symptoms. This is considered to be the last time that the patient was at the previous baseline or symptom-free state. For patients unable to provide this information or awaken with stroke symptoms, onset is defined as time when the patient was last seen to be normal.[32] Other key historical factors include contraindications to thrombolytic therapy, medications being taken by the patient, heart disease, previous stroke, TIA, seizures, vomiting, or headache occurring at the beginning of the patient's acute symptoms.

EPs must use a reproducible standardized physical examination to assess the severity of injury in stroke patients. Three key physical findings—facial paresis, arm drift, and abnormal speech—are highly predictive of an acute stroke. The National Institutes of Health Stroke Scale (NIHSS) (see the Documentation box) is a valid, standardized tool that records clinical findings and provides information that is helpful in determining the prognosis and therapeutic options. This 42-point scale evaluates level of consciousness, cranial nerves, motor function, ataxia, sensation, speech, and neglect. It can be used for serial examinations and is a predictor of patient outcome and risk associated with therapy, which can be useful when discussing treatment options with specialists, patients, and family members.

### DOCUMENTATION

- Time of onset of symptoms or the last time that patient was seen to be normal
- Initial National Institutes of Health Stroke Scale (NIHSS) score
- Resolution of symptoms and NIHSS score of 0 for patients with a transient ischemic attack (TIA)
- Single or multiple events
- History of stroke risk factors
- Current medications, including antiplatelet drugs and anticoagulants
- Results of cerebral imaging
- ABCD2 score for patients with TIA
- Suspected cause and initiation of preventive or thrombolytic therapy
- Specialist consultation and early (within 48 hours) follow-up for low-risk patients with TIA discharged from the emergency department
- Specialist consultation and admission to a stroke unit for patients with stroke

Patients with an NIHSS score lower than 6 have a predicted excellent outcome at 6 months, and 81% are discharged home. Nearly half the patients with an NIHSS score higher than 15 will require transfer to a nursing facility. Patients with an NIHSS score higher than 20 have a 17% risk for intracerebral hemorrhage when treated with recombinant tissue plasminogen activator (rt-PA). Finally, each additional point on the NIHSS decreases the likelihood of an excellent outcome by 17%.[33-35]

Although the history and physical examination are important elements in making an accurate diagnosis of patients with acute neurovascular events, neuroimaging is the key diagnostic tool. The goals of modern neuroimaging evaluation are to (1) obtain evidence of a vascular origin of the symptoms; (2) exclude an alternative nonischemic origin; (3) ascertain the underlying vascular mechanism of the event, which helps guide therapy; (4) identify prognostic outcome categories; and (5) improve selection of patients to be treated with reperfusion therapies by identifying those with regions of salvageable brain tissue, low risk for hemorrhagic transformation, or occlusion of large arteries that might be amenable to therapy.[1,32] Currently, EPs have a multitude of imaging options that are based on availability of the imaging modality and local expertise in interpretation of the images.

Non–contrast-enhanced CT remains the standard imaging technique for evaluating patients with acute stroke. It can be performed in the majority of hospitals, images are acquired rapidly, and it is sensitive in detecting acute hemorrhage. For patients with TIA, CT has been shown to provide an alternative diagnosis in 1% of all cases, and a new infarct has been found within 48 hours in 4% of patients with TIA. Of these patients, 38% eventually experienced a new ischemic stroke in the next 90 days.[26] CT findings not associated with an increased short-term risk for stroke include old infarction, periventricular white matter disease, cerebral atrophy, and vascular calcification.[36] Unfortunately, CT scans are frequently negative in the first hours after an ischemic stroke, are limited in defining posterior fossa structures and discriminating between infarct and viable at-risk tissue (penumbra), and provide no information on the presence or location of vascular pathology.[32]

Subtle clues found on CT scanning are cortical hypodensity, hyperdense middle cerebral artery, middle cerebral artery dot sign, sulcal effacement, hypoattenuation of the insular ribbon, and obscuration of the lentiform nucleus. The Alberta Stroke Program Early CT Score (ASPECTS) organized these early subtle clues into a semiquantitative 10-point grading system for early ischemic changes in the middle cerebral artery territory found on CT scans. Patients with an ASPECTS higher than 7 were found to have a much higher incidence of parenchymal hematoma after receiving rt-PA therapy.[37]

Perfusion CT is an advanced neuroimaging technique that uses intravenous (IV) contrast material to provide semiquantitative information on cerebral blood flow and cerebral blood volume. Other useful calculations include the mean transit time of the contrast agent from the arterial to the venous circulation and time to peak, which measures the time between the first arrival of contrast agent in the artery and the peak of the bolus within the brain tissue.[38] Studies suggest that a CT battery that includes non–contrast-enhanced CT, CT angiography, and CT perfusion can be performed quickly in patients with acute stroke and can provide comprehensive information.[1,39] Benefits include more rapid identification of the location of ischemia and the presence of viable tissue. Disadvantages include the need for IV contrast material and normal renal function, which limits imaging of the posterior fossa, and lack of local expertise in interpretation of the images.

MRI with diffusion-weighted imaging (DWI) is very accurate in early detection of hyperacute stroke and determination of the stroke subtype.[40] It is more sensitive than standard CT in identifying both new and preexisting ischemic lesions in patients with TIA.[1] Multimodal MRI provides physiologic data and distinction between cytotoxic edema (diffusion-weighted MRI), reduced cerebral blood flow (perfusion MRI), and increased water content, which is a marker of permanent brain injury (T2 imaging). On average, 42% of TIA patients will have abnormalities on diffusion-weighted MRI, and in up to one third of cases the results of diffusion-weighted MRI change the clinically suspected vascular location and cause of the TIA.[41] Clinical predictors of positive findings on diffusion-weighted MRI include a duration of symptoms longer than 1 hour, motor deficits, and aphasia, as well as large vessel occlusion on magnetic resonance angiography (MRA).[1,24] Additionally, patients with TIA who exhibit abnormalities on DWI have a higher risk for recurrent ischemic events than do those without such abnormalities.[42] DWI positivity also correlates with the ABCD2 score for predicting stroke risk.[43]

MRI coupled with perfusion-weighted imaging and MRA increases diagnostic certainty and allows detection of ischemic injury, determination of tissue viability, and localization of vascular clot, stenosis, and dissection. MRI provides better imaging of the brainstem and posterior fossa than CT does. Furthermore, MRI is as accurate as CT in detecting acute hemorrhagic transformation and is more accurate in distinguishing acute from chronic hemorrhage.[44] Limitations include cost, availability, incompatibility with implantable devices, and requirement for patient tolerance and stability. However, if available, MRI is a first-line imaging modality for patients whose neurologic symptoms are transient.

Diagnostic testing is completed with laboratory and ancillary tests. Laboratory tests recommended by the AHA include a complete blood count with platelets, prothrombin time, partial thromboplastin time, international normalized ratio (INR), chemistry panel including renal function and glucose, and cardiac enzymes. Other laboratory tests to consider in selected patients include liver function tests, pregnancy testing, arterial blood gas analysis (if hypoxia is suspected), drug toxicology, and urinalysis. An ECG should be obtained to look for atrial fibrillation, acute myocardial infarction, or other disturbances in rhythm. Ancillary testing includes a chest radiograph if pulmonary pathology, aspiration, or congestive heart failure is suspected.[1] Echocardiography and carotid Doppler ultrasonography also play limited roles in the diagnostic evaluation and are generally part of a complete inpatient work-up.[32]

## TREATMENT

The goal of management of patients with TIA is the introduction of therapy that will prevent stroke and thus avoid permanent disability and untimely death. Three types of medical therapy to achieve this goal are available: antiplatelet therapy, anticoagulation therapy, and surgical or endovascular therapy. In addition, patients should be instructed about measures that modify risk factors for stroke.

ED management of patients with acute ischemic stroke requires a team approach that is organized, time sensitive, and goal directed. The goal of ED care is to ensure medical stability, identify the cause of the ischemic event, determine the extent of injury, and create a therapeutic plan that reestablishes cerebral function and prevents or limits further injury.[45] Four time goals for therapy have been established (see the Priority Actions box).

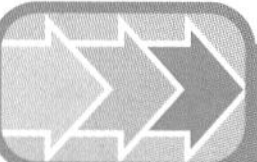

**PRIORITY ACTIONS**

**10 Minutes from Time of Arrival**

Secure the ABCs, obtain vital signs, and check a fingerstick blood glucose level.
Establish an IV line, administer $O_2$, and place the patient on a cardiac monitor.
Calculate the NIHSS score.
Consult the stroke team or neurology.
Send the patient for a CT scan.

**25 Minutes from Time of Arrival**

CT scan is completed.
Establish an accurate time of onset with the patient, family, or EMS personnel.
Review the history with the stroke team or neurologist.

**45 Minutes from Time of Arrival**

CT scan is reviewed and interpreted.
Review contraindications to thrombolysis (see Box 100.5).
Repeat the neurologic examination to assess for worsening clinical status.
Treat hypertension (SBP > 185 mm Hg, DBP > 110 mm Hg), hyperglycemia (glucose > 120 mg/dL), and fever (temperature > 38° C).

**60 Minutes from Time of Arrival**

Establish a plan of care.
Review the risks and benefits of the plan of care with the patient and family.
Initiate thrombolytic therapy for patients who are candidates.
Screen for aspiration in patients who are not candidates for thrombolysis and administer aspirin orally or rectally.
Admit for further monitoring and therapy.

*ABCs*, Airway, breathing, and circulation; *CT*, computed tomography; *DBP*, diastolic blood pressure; *EMS*, emergency medical service; *IV*, intravenous; *NIHSS*, National Institutes of Health Stroke Scale; *SBP*, systolic blood pressure.

### ANTIPLATELET THERAPY

The use of antiplatelet agents rather than oral anticoagulation is the treatment of choice for the prevention of stroke in patients with TIA secondary to atherothrombotic disease (**Box 100.2**).[46,47] Aspirin is the most widely used and the most economical drug available for prevention of stroke. Currently,

**BOX 100.2 Antiplatelet Recommendations**

Acceptable options for initial therapy are aspirin monotherapy, 50 to 325 mg/day; the combination of aspirin, 25 mg, and extended-release dipyridamole, 200 mg twice daily; and clopidogrel monotherapy, 75 mg.

The addition of aspirin to clopidogrel increases the risk for hemorrhage and is not recommended for routine secondary prevention after a transient ischemic attack.

Clopidogrel is a reasonable option for patients allergic to aspirin.

For patients who have an ischemic stroke while taking aspirin, no evidence has indicated that increasing the dose of aspirin provides additional benefit; the addition of alternative antiplatelet agents in this scenario has not been studied.

From Furie KL, Kasner SE, Adams RJ, et al. Guidelines for the prevention of stroke in patients with stroke or transient ischemic attack: a guideline for healthcare professionals from the American Heart Association/American Stroke Association. Stroke 2011;42:227-76.

clopidogrel, ticlopidine, and combined dipyridamole-aspirin (DPA) are antiplatelet agents that are effective alternatives to aspirin. Unfortunately, despite being the standard of care in the AHA guidelines, these agents are often underused, with only 18% of TIA patients encountered in the ED receiving aspirin, 7% receiving other antiplatelet agents, and 42% receiving no treatment.[7]

Aspirin is a mainstay of antiplatelet therapy for prevention of atherothrombotic stroke in TIA patients. It achieves this benefit though irreversible block of the enzyme cyclooxygenase, which in turn prevents the metabolism of arachidonic acid to the potent vasoconstrictor and platelet aggregator thromboxane $A_2$. The effective dose of aspirin is 50 to 325 mg. It is associated with an overall reduction of 15% to 18% in the combined end points of stroke, myocardial infarction, and death.[47] It is well tolerated and inexpensive; however, gastrointestinal bleeding is a documented major side effect.

Clopidogrel (75 mg daily) and ticlopidine (250 mg twice daily) are adenosine diphosphate receptor antagonists that prevent platelet aggregation. Clopidogrel has the advantages of once-daily dosing, less neutropenia, and fewer gastrointestinal side effects. It must be noted that clopidogrel has been reported to induce thrombotic thrombocytopenic purpura in a very small percentage of patients.[48] In addition, clopidogrel has not been compared with placebo for secondary stroke prevention.[46]

Large, multicenter randomized controlled trials have compared clopidogrel with aspirin[49] and combined clopidogrel-aspirin with clopidogrel alone in the prevention of stroke, myocardial infarction, and death.[50] Subgroup analysis failed to find a statistically significant reduction in ischemic stroke in favor of clopidogrel or the combined drugs. In addition, no increase in reduction of the risk for stroke was achieved by giving aspirin to symptomatic patients currently taking clopidogrel; in fact, major bleeding increased with the combination of the two drugs.[51] Clopidogrel remains a viable option for patients who are aspirin sensitive, and it has been shown to be beneficial in patients who have concomitant cerebral vascular and coronary disease or recent stent placement.

Dipyridamole is a cyclic nucleotide phosphodiesterase inhibitor that inhibits platelet aggregation by increasing levels of cyclic adenosine monophosphate. Extended-release dipyridamole in combination with aspirin has been shown to reduce the risk for stroke by 37% when compared with placebo and to reduce risk by 23% when compared with aspirin alone.[36] Studies comparing extended-release DPA and clopidogrel have demonstrated that they are not different in their efficacy.[52] Common side effects include headache and gastrointestinal disturbances.

## ANTICOAGULATION

Atrial fibrillation (AF) is responsible for 50% of all cardiogenic embolic events. Patients with a TIA or ischemic stroke and paroxysmal or sustained AF should receive warfarin as the therapy of choice for the prevention of stroke.[46,53] These patients have a target INR of 2.5 (range, 2.0 to 3.0). Risk factors for stroke in patients with AF include congestive heart failure, hypertension, age older than 75 years, diabetes, and previous stroke or TIA.[54] For these high-risk patients who require temporary interruption of oral anticoagulation, bridging therapy with low-molecular-weight heparin administered subcutaneously is reasonable.[46]

Other cardiac risk factors include left ventricular thrombus in the setting of acute myocardial infarction, native valvular heart disease, and prosthetic heart valves. Warfarin is a reasonable option for all these conditions with slight variations. With a left ventricular thrombus, oral anticoagulation with a target INR of 2.5 (range, 2.0 to 3.0) should be continued for at least 3 months. In the setting of rheumatic mitral valve disease, oral anticoagulation with a similar target is also reasonable. Because of the increased risk for stroke in patients with mechanical prosthetic heart valves, the target range for anticoagulation is increased and the target INR should be 3.0 (range, 2.5 to 3.5). Patients with bioprosthetic valves can be maintained at an INR of 2.5 (range, 2.0 to 3.0). In general, to avoid additional bleeding risk, antiplatelet agents should not be routinely added to warfarin unless a patient with a prosthetic heart valve has an ischemic stroke or systemic embolism despite adequate therapy with oral anticoagulants and is not at high risk for bleeding.[46] Warfarin has not been shown to be superior to aspirin in the prevention of noncardioembolic forms of stroke.[55]

## SURGICAL MANAGMENT

Carotid endarterectomy (CEA) performed in patients with symptomatic severe carotid stenosis greater than 70% to 99% results in a long-term benefit in preventing strokes.[56-58] Patients with symptomatic stenosis of 50% to 69% may also benefit from CEA, depending on age, sex, and comorbid conditions, if their perioperative risk for morbidity and mortality is estimated to be less than 6%.[46] Finally, CEA is not beneficial or is harmful in symptomatic patients with stenosis of less than 50% (**Box 100.3**).[59-61] When performed within 2 weeks, surgery is reasonable in patients with no contraindications to early revascularization.[46]

Recently, carotid angioplasty plus stenting (CAS) has been deemed a possible alternative to surgical carotid therapy and has been shown to have outcomes comparable with those achieved with CEA.[62-64] The AHA now recommends CAS as

**BOX 100.3 Carotid Endarterectomy (CEA)/Carotid Angioplasty and Stenting (CAS) Recommendations***

CEA is recommended for symptomatic stenosis of 70% to 99%.
CEA may be recommended for symptomatic stenosis of 50% to 69%, depending on patient-specific factors such as age, sex, and comorbid conditions.
CEA is best performed within 2 weeks of symptomatic events.
No benefit is achieved with performance of CEA for stenosis of less than 50%.
CAS is an alternative to CEA in patients at low to average risk for complications when the luminal diameter of the internal carotid artery is found to be reduced more than 70% by noninvasive imaging or more than 50% by catheter angiography.
CAS may be considered in patients with greater than 70% stenosis if the stenosis is difficult to access surgically or if they are deemed to be poor surgical candidates.

From Furie KL, Kasner SE, Adams RJ, et al. Guidelines for the prevention of stroke in patients with stroke or transient ischemic attack: a guideline for healthcare professionals from the American Heart Association/American Stroke Association. Stroke 2011;42:227-76.
*Assumes that the perioperative or periprocedural risk for stroke or death is less than 6% for surgeon, interventionalist, or center.

an alternative to CEA for symptomatic patients at average or low risk for complications associated with endovascular intervention when the diameter of the lumen of the internal carotid artery is found to be reduced by more than 70% by noninvasive imaging or by more than 50% by catheter angiography, and CAS can be used in patients with greater than 70% stenosis if they are deemed to be poor surgical candidates.[46]

## RISK FACTOR REDUCTION

Several factors portend an increased risk for stroke in patients who have experienced a TIA. Modifiable risk factors include hypertension, diabetes, hyperlipidemia, cigarette smoking, and heavy alcohol consumption. The AHA recommends that blood pressure be reduced in all patients with TIA beyond the first 24 hours of symptoms, with an average reduction of approximately 10/5 mm Hg and an ultimate goal of less than 120/80 mm Hg. Reduction of blood pressure can be attained through lifestyle modification and antihypertensive therapy.[46] In diabetic patients, diet, exercise, oral hypoglycemic drugs, and insulin are recommended to gain glycemic control.

Elevations in total cholesterol or low-density lipoprotein cholesterol (LDL-C) and low levels of high-density lipoprotein cholesterol (HDL-C) are modest risk factors for stroke. A metaanalysis of statin trials showed that the larger the reduction in LDL-C, the greater the reduction in risk for stroke.[65] Therefore, the AHA recommends statin therapy with intensive lipid-lowering effects in patients with TIA who have evidence of atherosclerosis and an LDL-C level higher than 100 mg/dL. It is reasonable to target a reduction of at least 50% or levels of less than 70 mg/dL. For patients with TIA and low HDL-C, treatment with niacin or gemfibrozil can be considered.[46]

Additional lifestyle risk factor reduction includes providing TIA patients with smoking cessation counseling and advising patients to avoid environmental (passive) tobacco smoke. Patients who are heavy drinkers should eliminate or reduce their consumption of alcohol to no more than two drinks per day for men and one drink per day for women who are not pregnant.[46]

## THROMBOLYSIS

The only treatment of acute ischemic stroke approved by the Food and Drug Administration (FDA) is IV rt-PA therapy, which has traditionally been recommended for carefully selected patients older than 18 years who are seen within 3 hours of the onset of an acute ischemic stroke.There have been some recent updates to recommendations for the use of IV rt-PA outside the traditional 3-hour time window, as well as the use of intraarterial thrombolysis for patients initially seen between 3 and 6 hours after the onset of symptoms.[32,66]

Adjuncts to intraarterial thrombolysis include angioplasty, stenting, and clot retrieval devices. Other therapies include prevention of hypoxemia and dehydration, administration of antiplatelet and anticoagulation agents, normalization of glucose, and temperature control.[32]

The era of emergency intravenous thrombolysis for acute ischemic stroke began in 1995 with the National Institute of Neurological Disorders and Stroke (NINDS) rt-PA trial.[67] This study was a single randomized controlled trial that compared patients with ischemic stroke treated with IV rt-PA versus placebo (given at 0 to 90, 90 to 180, and 0 to 180 minutes). Despite no difference in the NIHSS score at 24 hours, the main outcome of the trial was a 30% decrease in disability at 3 months in patients treated with IV rt-PA versus 20% in those treated with placebo. This benefit was similar 1 year after stroke.[68] Adverse events included a 10-fold increase in the rate of intracerebral hemorrhage 36 hours after treatment with rt-PA (6% versus 0.6%); however, the death rate in the two treatment groups was similar at 3 months (17% versus 20%) and at 1 year (24% versus 28%).[67]

Concern over data that support the use of thrombolytics for acute ischemic stroke and external validity in community hospitals has been raised by some EPs.[69] Some community hospital groups have reported high rates of intracranial hemorrhage and fewer favorable outcomes. In these studies the risk for hemorrhage is proportional to the degree to which the NINDS protocol is not followed.[70-72] Critics also observed that the relative predominance of mild strokes (NIHSS score < 5) with a probably good outcome in the rt-PA group may explain the entire benefit reported in patients treated between 91 and 180 minutes. Neither reanalysis of the data by the NINDS study group nor a separate analysis by an independent group could demonstrate that the effect of the imbalance in severity influenced the overall result that rt-PA therapy positively influenced outcome.[73,74] Several recent studies also demonstrated improved neurologic outcomes and similar hemorrhage rates as the original NINDS data.[75-79]

The effectiveness of thrombolysis is determined by several variables. Time until treatment is extremely important: 75% of patients in one pooled analysis who were treated within 60 minutes of the onset of stroke in the initial pooled analysis had the best chance of achieving complete or partial reopening of the occluded artery.[78] Patients with mild to moderate strokes (NIHSS score < 20) and patients younger than 75 years had the greatest potential for a favorable response to treatment.[80] Predictors of a poor postthrombolysis prognosis include older patient age, higher stroke severity (NIHSS score > 22), systemic hypertension or hypotension, hyperglycemia, and fever.

Despite its effectiveness in improving neurologic outcomes, the majority of patients with ischemic stroke are not treated with rt-PA, largely because they arrive after the 3-hour window for treatment. One potential solution would be to designate a longer time window for treatment. A pooled analysis of previous large trials suggested that the upper limit of the treatment window may be as late as 5 to 6 hours.[78] The ECASS-3 trial enrolled patients to either rt-PA or placebo by using the current guideline protocols of between 3 and 4.5 hours after the onset of symptoms. It excluded patients older than 80 years, those taking oral anticoagulants, those with a history of both previous stroke and diabetes, and patients with a baseline NIHSS score higher than 25. The rate of symptomatic intracranial hemorrhage (as defined by NINDS criteria) was 7.9% for the treatment group and 3.5% for the placebo group, neurologic improvement was significantly higher in the rt-PA group than in the placebo group, and mortality in the two treatment groups did not differ significantly.[66] These findings are consistent with the results in this time window from pooled analyses of previous trials.[78] Subsequently, the AHA made recommendations regarding expansion of the time window for the treatment of ischemic stroke with IV rt-PA (**Box 100.4**).[81]

Centers that care for stroke patients must develop guidelines for the appropriate selection of patients and develop systems to rapidly deliver thrombolysis therapy to these patients. Candidates for IV thrombolysis must have a clearly defined time of symptom onset of less than 270 minutes, must be older than 18 years, and must have no contraindications to thrombolytic therapy (**Box 100.5**).[32] The dosing regimen is 0.9 mg/kg (maximum of 90 mg) of rt-PA, with 10% (maximum of 9 mg) given as a bolus over a 1- to 2-minute period, followed by the remaining dose (maximum of 81 mg) infused by pump over a 1-hour period. Any indwelling catheters should be placed before the administration of thrombolytics. The patient should be admitted to an intensive care or stroke unit for frequent neurologic examination and blood pressure checks, with the goal of maintaining blood pressure lower than 180/105 mm Hg. If severe headache, acute hypertension, nausea, or vomiting develops, the infusion should be discontinued and an emergency non–contrast-enhanced head CT scan should be obtained. The institution must have a protocol for the management of thrombolytic-induced intracerebral hemorrhage. The patient should not receive aspirin or heparin during the first 24 hours after thrombolytic therapy. A follow-up non–contrast-enhanced head CT scan should be done at 24 hours and before starting anticoagulant or antiplatelet therapy.[32]

## ENDOVASCULAR PROCEDURES

Procedures such as intraarterial thrombolysis with or without mechanical embolectomy, angioplasty, and carotid stenting are considered experimental therapies that may benefit

**BOX 100.4 Recommendations of the American Heart Association Regarding Extension of the Time Window for Administration of Recombinant Tissue Plasminogen Activator in Patients with Ischemic Stroke**

Recombinant tissue plasminogen activator should be administered to eligible patients who can be treated in the 3- to 4.5-hour period after the onset of stroke.

Exclusion criteria for the extended treatment window include:

- Patients older than 80 years
- Baseline National Institutes of Health Stroke Scale score higher than 25
- Patients with a history of both stroke and diabetes
- All patients receiving oral anticoagulants regardless of their international normalized ratio

Delays in evaluation and initiation of therapy should be avoided because of the opportunity for greater neurologic improvement with earlier treatment.

From del Zoppo GJ, Saver JL, Jauch EC, et al. Expansion of the time window for treatment of acute ischemic stroke with intravenous tissue plasminogen activator: a science advisory from the American Heart Association/American Stroke Association. Stroke 2009;40:2945-8.

**BOX 100.5 Contraindications to Administration of Recombinant Tissue Plasminogen Activator**

Head trauma or stroke in the previous 3 months
Myocardial infarction in the previous 3 months
Gastrointestinal or urinary tract hemorrhage in the previous 3 weeks
Major surgery in the past 2 weeks
Arterial puncture at a noncompressible site in the previous 7 days
History of previous intracranial hemorrhage
Systolic blood pressure higher than 185 mm Hg, diastolic blood pressure higher than 110 mm Hg
Evidence of active bleeding or acute trauma (fracture) on examination
Oral anticoagulation with an international normalized ratio higher than 1.7
Receiving heparin in the previous 48 hours with an abnormal activated partial thromboplastin time
Platelet count lower than 100,000/mm$^3$
Blood glucose level lower than 50 mg/dL
Seizure with postictal residual neurologic impairments
Computed tomography scan demonstrating multilobar infarction (hypodensity in more than a third of the cerebral hemisphere)

Adapted from Adams HA, del Zoppo G, Alberts MJ, et al. Guidelines for the early management of adults with ischemic stroke. Stroke 2007;38:1655-711.

specific patient groups who are seen outside the 3-hour window or have contraindications to IV thrombolysis, such as recent surgery.[82] Benefits of this therapy include a lower dose of thrombolytic, direct visualization of the occluded vessel, and higher recanalization rates. The FDA has approved use of the MERCI (Mechanical Embolus Removal in Cerebral Embolism) devise. Treatment requires the patient to be at an experienced stroke center with immediate access to cerebral angiography and qualified interventionalists.[32]

## ADJUVANT THERAPIES

### *Blood Pressure Management*

Management of blood pressure in an acute stroke patient is controversial. In an ED study of patients with acute ischemic stroke, systolic blood pressure outside the range of 155 to 220 mm Hg and diastolic blood pressure outside the range of 71 to 105 mm Hg were associated with increased 90-day mortality. These findings demonstrate the harmful effects of both hypertension and hypotension and indicate that there is an optimal range of blood pressure required to perfuse at-risk tissue in these patients.[83]

Current American Stroke Association and European Stroke Initiative guidelines recommend withholding antihypertensive therapy in patients with acute ischemic stroke unless they are thrombolysis candidates or show evidence of end-organ dysfunction (acute myocardial infarction, aortic dissection, pulmonary edema, and renal failure). Short-acting IV medications with reliable dose response and safety profiles should be used. Medications that meet these requirements include labetalol, nicardipine, and esmolol.[32,84] Despite concern that lowering blood pressure in the acute stroke setting might be harmful, pilot data from the CHHIPS trial demonstrated that labetalol and lisinopril are effective antihypertensive drugs for patients with acute stroke and do not increase serious adverse events. Early lowering of blood pressure also resulted in a reduction in mortality. However, in view of the small sample size, care must be taken when these results are interpreted, and further evaluation in larger trials is needed.[85] Conversely, small clinical studies suggest that drug-induced hypertension could be used in the management of some patients with acute ischemic stroke to improve cerebral blood flow, but data from large clinical trials are lacking. The AHA recommends using this method only in exceptional cases or within the setting of clinical trials.[32]

### *Glucose Management*

Hyperglycemia (glucose > 185 mg/dL) and hypoglycemia (glucose < 60 mg/dL) are associated with worsening of clinical and tissue outcome in patients with acute ischemic stroke. Hyperglycemia can accelerate the course of ischemic injury, actively convert penumbra to infarcted tissue, and increase the risk for hemorrhagic events and poor outcome in patients receiving rt-PA therapy.[86,87] Glycemic control with rapidly acting insulin should be instituted to maintain blood glucose between the suggested levels of 140 to 185 mg/dL while taking care to avoid hypoglycemia.[32]

### *Temperature Management*

Hyperpyrexia (temperature > 38.0° C) is associated with increased morbidity and mortality. The pathologic effects stem from increased neurotransmitter and free radical production and adverse effects on the blood-brain barrier, which seem to be most pronounced at the border zone or penumbra of the infarct and lead to loss of potentially viable tissue. Therefore, the source of the fever should be actively sought and treated with acetaminophen.[88]

### *Anticoagulation*

Currently, early administration of heparin is not recommended for any type of acute ischemic stroke because of the increased risk for secondary hemorrhagic conversion; furthermore, clinical trial data have shown no reduction in stroke recurrence or improvement in patient outcome.[89-93] Additionally, initiation of anticoagulant therapy within 24 hours of treatment with IV rt-PA is not recommended.[32]

### *Antiplatelet Therapy*

The goals of antiplatelet therapy in patients with stroke are a reduction in stroke recurrence and stroke-related morbidity and mortality. Aspirin (50 to 325 mg/day) therapy resulted in a significant reduction in death and disability when given within 48 hours of ischemic stroke.[89,94] It reduced the risk for early recurrent stroke in all stroke subtypes. Therefore, patients who are not aspirin sensitive or at risk for aspiration and are not being administered t-PA should receive aspirin within 48 hours of ischemic stroke.

Other oral antiplatelet agents, including clopidogrel, ticlopidine, and combination drugs such as DPA, have not been proved to be safer or more cost-effective than aspirin alone. Clopidogrel is recommended for aspirin-sensitive patients who require emergency antiplatelet therapy in the ED. The use of IV antiplatelet agents such as glycoprotein IIb/IIIa inhibitors is still investigational and is not recommended for use outside the setting of clinical trials.[32]

## FOLLOW-UP, NEXT STEPS IN CARE, AND PATIENT EDUCATION

The areas that should be emphasized when making decisions regarding admission or discharge are the completeness of the evaluation, the source of the event, and resolution of the symptoms. These issues, coupled with proper risk stratification and cerebral vascular imaging, represent a logical approach to achieving safe and proper disposition of the patient.

A thorough diagnostic evaluation that determines the cause of the TIA plays a crucial role in the decision to hospitalize or discharge patients from the ED. Patients who are at high risk for recurrent events and are unable to undergo appropriate cerebral and vascular imaging should be hospitalized to expedite the evaluation and allow observation for recurrent events in the period of vulnerability (hours or days) after the event.[8] Diagnostic benefits of hospital admission include rapid evaluation, monitoring for acute neurologic deterioration, and cardiac telemetry monitoring. Therapeutic benefits include the ability to deliver thrombolytic therapy, rapid institution of antiplatelet and anticoagulation therapy, and early consideration for carotid surgery.[95]

The AHA has recently recommended hospital admission for patients initially seen with TIA within 72 hours of the event and when any of the following criteria are present: (1) ABCD2 score higher than 3, (2) ABCD2 score of 0 to 2 and uncertainty that diagnostic work-up can be completed within 2 days as an outpatient, and (3) ABCD2 score of 0 to 2 and other evidence indicating that the patient's event was caused by focal ischemia.[1]

Patients deemed to be at low risk after a complete evaluation and those who have a clear cause and are receiving preventive therapy can be discharged after appropriate consultation with a neurologist, cardiologist, or vascular surgeon. It should be emphasized to all patients that a TIA is a high-risk event and that the risk for stroke is highest in the next 2 to 90 days (see the Patient Teaching Tips box). All patients discharged from the ED should be scheduled for follow-up during the next 2 days, which is the most critical period for recurrent events. Preventive therapy, especially antiplatelet therapy, should be initiated before discharge.[1]

with physical and occupation therapy. Stroke units have been found to be effective for patients with large artery–associated stroke and more costly but equally efficacious as medical ward care for patients with small vessel–associated stroke.[97] Hospitals without stroke units should have comprehensive protocols and quality assurance programs that actively manage the variables shown to affect outcome and ensure optimal care for all patients.

Patients who require intensive care unit admission are those with severe stroke and the potential for decompensation. High-risk populations include patients treated with IV or intraarterial thrombolysis or catheter-based therapies, patients with an NIHSS score higher than 17, and patients with large strokes in the cerebellar or middle cerebral artery distribution who are at risk for the development of cerebral edema.

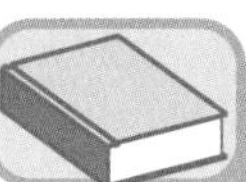

**PATIENT TEACHING TIPS**

A transient ischemic attack is a serious warning sign for stroke, myocardial infarction, and death in the next 2 to 90 days.

Patients should understand the warning signs of stroke and be instructed to return to the emergency department if symptoms recur.

Patients with significant carotid disease should be evaluated promptly for surgery within the next 2 weeks and should be treated with antiplatelet agents.

Patients who are discharged should have early outpatient follow-up and evaluation in the following 2 to 7 days.

Patients should control modifiable risk factors and adhere to antiplatelet, anticoagulation, and antihypertensive therapy.

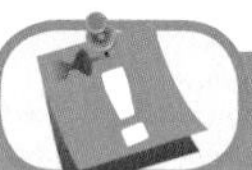

**TIPS AND TRICKS**

Use diffusion-weighted magnetic resonance imaging to differentiate a true transient ischemic attack from ischemic stroke.

Use risk stratification criteria to determine the need for hospitalization.

Patients with motor and speech deficits and prolonged symptoms are more likely to have positive findings on diffusion-weighted imaging.

An antiplatelet agent should be prescribed for patients with transient ischemic attacks to minimize the risk for stroke.

A stroke team or neurologist should be consulted early for patients who may be candidates for thrombolytic therapy.

Patients with acute stroke should be admitted to a stroke unit for further care.

Unlike TIA, all patients with acute ischemic stroke require admission to the hospital to be observed for changes in their condition, facilitate medical or surgical procedures, receive preventive therapy, and recover neurologic function with rehabilitative services. Optimal disposition is dependent on local hospital expertise, severity of the stroke, and intensity of therapy. Following early therapy initiated at a community hospital, patients may be transferred to a stroke center for more comprehensive care, which is often coordinated by stroke teams in hospitals throughout the United States. Patients undergoing thrombolysis should have access to the intensive care unit, neurology and neurosurgery consultation, and blood bank services.

Admission to a stroke unit has been validated in clinical trials as being statistically significant in decreasing disability and mortality while increasing the probability that the patient will return home and resume daily living activities.[96] These effects are independent of age, sex, and severity of stroke and are reproducible in a community setting.

Intensive monitoring in a stroke unit allows early detection and treatment of fever, hypoxemia, hyperglycemia, and cardiac rhythm disturbances and permits early mobilization coupled

## SUGGESTED READINGS


Adams HA, del Zoppo G, Alberts MJ, et al. Guidelines for the early management of adults with ischemic stroke. Stroke 2007;38:1655-711.

del Zoppo GJ, Saver JL, Jauch EC, et al. Expansion of the time window for treatment of acute ischemic stroke with intravenous tissue plasminogen activator: a science advisory from the American Heart Association/American Stroke Association. Stroke 2009;40;2945-8.

Easton JD, Saver JL, Albers GW, et al. Definition and evaluation of transient ischemic attack: a scientific statement for healthcare professionals from the American Heart Association/American Stroke Association Stroke Council; Council on Cardiovascular Surgery and Anesthesia; Council on Cardiovascular Radiology and Intervention; Council on Cardiovascular Nursing; and the Interdisciplinary Council on Peripheral Vascular Disease. Stroke 2009;40:2276-93.

Furie KL, Kasner SE, Adams RJ, et al. Guidelines for the prevention of stroke in patients with stroke or transient ischemic attack: a guideline for healthcare professionals from the American Heart Association/American Stroke Association. Stroke 2011;42:227-76.


## REFERENCES

*References can be found on Expert Consult @ www.expertconsult.com.*

# Headache 101

*Joshua N. Goldstein and Jonathan A. Edlow*

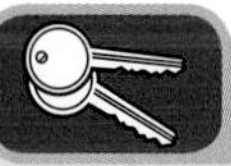

**KEY POINTS**

- Inquire about the onset, quality, severity, associated symptoms, and past history of the headache; a new headache that is due to a serious "cannot miss" cause will usually have unique features.
- The most frequently missed components of the neurologic examination are visual fields and gait; they are helpful in the diagnosis of subtle disorders.
- New abnormal neurologic findings must be evaluated and explained.
- Patients whose headaches are abrupt, with maximal intensity at or close to onset ("thunderclap" headaches), should be evaluated for subarachnoid hemorrhage even if the findings on neurologic examination are entirely normal.
- When evaluating for a nontraumatic subarachnoid hemorrhage, a negative computed tomography scan should be followed by a lumbar puncture.

## PERSPECTIVE

Headache is a high-risk symptom because it is very common and a small percentage of patients with headache will have serious treatable life-, brain-, or eye-threatening causes. Emergency physicians (EPs) must use the history and physical examination to decide which patients need diagnostic testing beyond the history and physical examination because a delayed or missed diagnosis of disorders such as meningitis or subarachnoid hemorrhage can lead to catastrophic outcomes.

## EPIDEMIOLOGY

Approximately 2% to 4% of all emergency department (ED) visits are for headache. Only a small proportion (as low as 2%) of patients seen in the ED with a headache suffer a life-, limb-, or vision-threatening illnesses.

## PATHOPHYSIOLOGY

The sensation of headache is rarely due to injury to the brain parenchyma itself. Rather, head pain results from tension, traction, distention, dilation, or inflammation of pain-sensitive structures external to the skull, portions of the dura mater, and blood vessels. Each of these mechanisms is probably mediated by a final common biochemical pathway that results in pain; therefore, a favorable response to analgesics should not be used to judge the cause of an individual headache.[1]

## PRESENTING SIGNS AND SYMPTOMS

EPs should develop a logical, practical, and accurate approach to identification of patients with serious pathology. A comprehensive organizational scheme developed by the International Headache Society has recently been updated (**Table 101.1**); however, this scheme is cumbersome in emergency practice. For practical purposes, headaches can be divided into "benign" and "cannot miss" categories (**Table 101.2**).

Treatment of pain should occur in parallel with the history and physical examination. Appropriate analgesia is all that most patients require, and comfortable patients are more willing to undergo tests and procedures (e.g., lumbar puncture [LP]). Immediate pain control results in greater patient satisfaction and more rapid disposition. That said, a given patient's response to analgesics should not alter the diagnostic strategy, so there is no reason to withhold treatment.

Evaluation should focus on signs and symptoms that can differentiate a benign headache from one requiring emergency work-up and treatment. For example, although location of the headache is often considered significant, unilateral headache is a hallmark of both primary (migraine, cluster) and secondary (intracerebral hemorrhage, glaucoma) headaches, thus limiting its usefulness in diagnosis. In contrast, fever and neck stiffness are uncommon with primary headache and are therefore very useful.

### TIMING AND DURATION

Identifying the timing and duration of the headache is useful. Questions such as "What brings you here today rather than any other day?" can help focus patients on the timing of their symptoms. Worrisome features include a new acute headache

**Table 101.1 International Headache Society Classification of Headaches**

| HEADACHE ASSOCIATED WITH | COMMENTS |
|---|---|
| Migraine | Requires 5 or more attacks of a specific nature lasting 4-72 hr. Can be unilateral, pulsating, moderate, or severe in intensity; aggravated by physical activity; or associated with nausea, vomiting, or photophobia |
| Tension type | Requires 10 or more attacks of a specific nature lasting 30 min to 7 days; absence of nausea, vomiting, and photophobia |
| Cluster type | Requires 5 or more attacks of a specific nature lasting 15-180 min; always unilateral; associated with eye, nose, or face symptoms |
| Other primary headaches | Includes a variety of brief (idiopathic stabbing headache) and situational (cough, exertional, coital) headache syndromes |
| Head trauma | Includes minor postinjury headaches |
| Vascular disorders | Includes cerebral ischemia and infarction, all forms of intracranial hemorrhage, venous sinus thrombosis, giant cell arteritis, arterial dissections |
| Nonvascular intracranial disorders | Includes idiopathic intracranial hypertension, post–lumbar puncture headache, tumor |
| Substance abuse or withdrawal | Includes drugs and food additives (e.g., monosodium glutamate headache, or Chinese restaurant syndrome); also includes headache from carbon monoxide poisoning |
| Infections | Includes headaches secondary to intracranial (meningitis, abscess) or extracranial infection |
| Disorders of homeostasis | Includes headaches secondary to hypercapnia, high-altitude illness, hypertensive encephalopathy, preeclampsia |
| HEENT (head, eyes, ears, nose, and throat) disorders (includes dental) | Includes narrow angle-closure glaucoma, sinusitis, temporomandibular joint disorder |
| Cranial neuralgias, nerve trunk and deafferentation pain | Most of these are cranial neuropathies or associated with herpes zoster |

From Olesen J. International Classification of Headache Disorders, Second Edition (ICHD-2): current status and future revisions. Cephalalgia 2006;26:1409-10.

or a subacute headache that is increasing in severity. An abrupt or "thunderclap" onset suggests intracranial hemorrhage or cerebral venous sinus thrombosis. If the maximum intensity of the pain occurred at the onset, aneurysmal bleeding should be considered. Very fleeting headaches, termed "jabs and jolts," that last seconds are typically benign. In abrupt-onset headaches, the activity at the onset sometimes suggests the cause, such as with coital headache or benign exertional headache. However, even though a history of these activities can be a sensitive indicator of the corresponding diagnoses, specificity is poor. Therefore, subarachnoid hemorrhage cannot be excluded on the basis of activity before the headache.

## LOCATION

Location of the pain is not very helpful in diagnosing headaches because of the significant overlap between benign and serious causes. Some recommend work-up of patients whose headaches always occur on the same side.

## SEVERITY

Severity of the pain also has limitations in differentiating benign from serious headaches. Although the "worst-of-my-life" headache suggests a more serious problem, most severe headaches seen in the ED have benign causes. Patients without a previous history of similar, severe headaches should be evaluated for a secondary cause of the headache. In patients with a history of previous headaches, ask about details and consider evaluating those whose headaches are clearly increased in severity or different in quality.

## QUALITY

The quality of the patient's pain is critical. Most secondary headaches are qualitatively unique, unusual, or distinctly different from prior headaches. Diagnostic work-up of patients with chronic headaches that have new or unusual features should be strongly considered.

## ASSOCIATED SYMPTOMS

Specific associated symptoms can provide important clues to a dangerous cause of the headache. Fever and neck stiffness suggest meningitis. Syncope, seizure, or any focal neurologic symptoms or new signs associated with a headache should prompt an evaluation. Diplopia suggests a mass, cerebral aneurysm, or elevated intracranial pressure (ICP).

Unfortunately, migraine headaches can produce an array of associated symptoms traditionally associated with secondary

**Table 101.2 "Cannot Miss" Diagnoses**

| DIAGNOSIS | SUGGESTIVE HISTORY AND PHYSICAL FINDINGS | DIAGNOSTIC TESTING |
|---|---|---|
| Meningitis and encephalitis | Fever, stiff neck, accentuation by jolts, altered mental status, seizure | LP; if preceded by CT, administer antibiotics before CT |
| Subarachnoid hemorrhage* | Abrupt onset of severe headache, stiff neck, third nerve palsy | CT scan; LP if CT is not diagnostic |
| Stroke (ischemic or hemorrhagic) | Abrupt onset and focal neurologic deficit conforming to an arterial territory | CT scan; if available, MRI will give more information (should not delay thrombolytic therapy) |
| Dissection of craniocervical arteries | Neck pain, abrupt onset, variable presence of neurologic deficit | CT angiography, MRA, or conventional angiography |
| Hypertensive encephalopathy | Severe (usually chronic) hypertension; often papilledema and other signs of end-organ damage | Careful, titratable lowering of blood pressure by ≈25% of the peak level will decrease the headache |
| Idiopathic intracranial hypertension | Obese, female patient; papilledema; often sixth nerve palsy | LP (following an imaging study, which by definition will be normal) |
| Giant cell arteritis | Nearly always age > 50 yr, symptoms of polymyalgia rheumatica, abnormal scalp vessels | ESR, temporal artery biopsy |
| Acute angle–closure glaucoma | Painful red eye with midposition pupil and corneal edema | Tonometry |
| Intracranial mass (tumor, abscess, hematoma)† | Any focal or generalized neurologic finding | CT scan; if available, MRI will provide more information |
| Cerebral venous sinus thrombosis | Hypercoagulable state of any type | MRI and MRA with venous phase, CT with venous phase |
| Carbon monoxide poisoning | Cluster of cases, winter season | COHb level |
| Pituitary apoplexy | Visual acuity or field abnormalities<br>Known pituitary tumor | MRI |

*COHb*, Carboxyhemoglobin; *CT*, computed tomography; *LP*, lumbar puncture; *MRA*, magnetic resonance angiography; *MRI*, magnetic resonance imaging.
*See Figure 101.1.
†See Figure 101.2.

headaches. Although nausea, vomiting, and photophobia can occur with increased ICP or infection, they are also associated with migraines. A helpful differentiating factor in migraineurs is whether these symptoms accompanied previous migraines or whether the finding is new. Visual abnormalities are associated with migraine headaches but also with idiopathic intracranial hypertension, temporal arteritis, and pituitary apoplexy.

### EXACERBATING AND ALLEVIATING FACTORS

Determining exacerbating and alleviating factors is occasionally helpful. Post LP headache tends to worsen on standing upright, and headache from sinusitis often worsens on bending forward with the head dependent. In contrast, the classic history of a headache caused by a brain tumor—worse on awakening—is neither specific nor sensitive because it is also seen in patients with hypercapnic chronic lung disease (in which the headache worsens during sleep). In terms of alleviating factors, diagnostic significance should not be ascribed to pain relief, even with over-the-counter medications.

### OTHER FACTORS

Age is useful as a consideration because new-onset headache at older ages suggests a secondary cause such as giant cell arteritis, tumors, subdural hematoma, and side effects of medications. Environmental considerations include winter season and common-source clusters, which can indicate carbon monoxide poisoning.

## PAST AND FAMILY HISTORY

Predisposing factors for a secondary cause of headache should be determined. For example, poorly treated hypertension may lead to hypertensive encephalopathy, vascular risk factors can result in stroke, and a past or family history of cerebral aneurysm increases the likelihood of subarachnoid hemorrhage (**Box 101.1**).

A history of thromboembolic events should raise the possibility of cerebral venous sinus thrombosis. In contrast,

**BOX 101.1 Critical Features of the History in the Emergency Department**

**Timing**
Abrupt onset, "thunderclap" (pain rapidly reaches maximal intensity)

**Location**
Nonspecific with regard to the differential diagnosis

**Severity**
Worst of my life, most severe; have never been to an emergency department before for headache

**Quality**
New type, qualitatively different from previous headaches

**Associated Symptoms**
Fever, neck stiffness
Seizure, syncope
Focal neurologic complaints
Visual abnormalities (diplopia, decreased or altered vision)

**Exacerbating or Alleviating Factors**
Worse with cough or lying down suggests increased intracranial pressure (but is not specific)

**Past Medical History**
Stroke, vascular disease, cancer
Immunocompromised status
Hypercoaguable states or bleeding diathesis

**Family History**
Hypercoaguable states, bleeding diathesis, cerebral aneurysm

patients with hemophilia are at higher risk for bleeding. Obesity suggests idiopathic intracranial hypertension (pseudotumor cerebri), especially in women. A history of cancer can raise suspicion for brain metastasis, and patients infected with human immunodeficiency virus or taking immunosuppressive medicines are at higher risk for infection.

## PHYSICAL EXAMINATION

The physical examination (**Box 101.2**) is critical in guiding the differential diagnosis and appropriate work-up.

**BOX 101.2 Critical Features (Potential Diagnoses) of the Physical Examination**

**Vital Signs**
Fever (meningitis, encephalitis, abscess)
Elevated blood pressure (stroke or problems associated with elevated intracranial pressure)

**Head**
Vesicles on the scalp (herpes zoster of the upper two cervical roots or the root of the fifth trigeminal nerve)
Tender temporal artery (giant cell arteritis)
Tender sinuses (sinusitis)

**Eyes**
Red, edematous (acute angle–closure glaucoma)
Proptosis (cavernous sinus thrombosis)
Papilledema (increased intracranial pressure)

**Ears**
Vesicles in the external ear canal (Ramsay Hunt syndrome)

**Nose**
Vesicles on the tip of the nose (herpes zoster of the root of the fifth trigeminal nerve)

**Neck**
Meningismus with positive jolt accentuation, Kernig or Brudzinski sign (infection, subarachnoid hemorrhage)

**Neurologic Examination**
Change in mental status (increased intracranial pressure, infection, carbon monoxide poisoning)
Decreased visual acuity (giant cell arteritis, acute angle–closure glaucoma)
Visual field cut (mass lesion, pituitary apoplexy)
Third nerve palsy (subarachnoid hemorrhage, cavernous sinus thrombosis)
Sixth nerve palsy (increased or decreased intracranial pressure, basilar meningitis)
Direction-changing nystagmus (cerebellar or brainstem stroke)
Lower motor neuron seventh nerve palsy (Bell palsy, Ramsay Hunt syndrome)
Eighth nerve palsy (diminished hearing or vertigo, Ramsay Hunt syndrome)
Gait ataxia (cerebellar stroke)
Any focal sensory or motor deficit (mass lesion, stroke)

### GENERAL APPEARANCE AND VITAL SIGNS

General appearance can be deceiving. For example, shielding one's eyes from the light is seen with both migraine and meningeal irritation. Fever is not a symptom of migraine and suggests infection or a several-day-old subarachnoid hemorrhage. Hypertension suggests hypertensive encephalopathy, stroke, or other secondary causes but also can be due to pain or stress. The EP should have a low threshold for brain imaging (and possibly LP) in patients with headache and persistent hypertension. However, it should be remembered that patients with secondary headaches can appear well and neurologically intact.

### HEAD AND NECK

The head, eye, ear, nose, and throat examination may reveal the cause of the headache. Vesicles on the scalp, nose, or external ear canal suggest herpes zoster. Temporal artery tenderness, nodularity, or thickening suggests giant cell arteritis. A red eye with an edematous cornea and midposition pupil suggests narrow angle–closure glaucoma. A proptotic eye or chemosis is suggestive of cavernous sinus thrombosis. Papilledema is specific but poorly sensitive for increased ICP, whereas venous pulsations in the retina indicate normal ICP.

Examination of the neck should be directed at signs of meningeal irritation. Meningismus (stiffness on passive flexion of the neck) may be seen in patients with infections (meningitis) or irritation (subarachnoid hemorrhage). However, this finding is not reliably present, and its absence does not exclude these diagnoses. One physical finding that is more reliable in diagnosing meningitis is "jolt accentuation"; when the patient is asked to turn the head

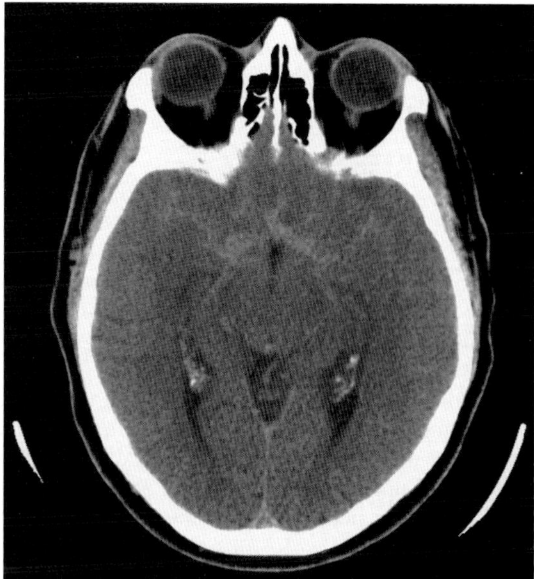

**Fig. 101.1** Subarachnoid hemorrhage.

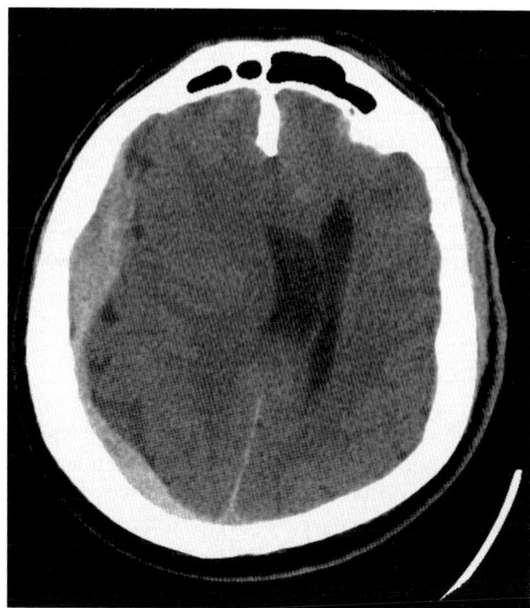

**Fig. 101.2** Subdural hematoma.

horizontally in alternate directions (as though rapidly shaking one's head "no") two to three times per second, the baseline headache increases in intensity.

## NEUROLOGIC EXAMINATION

A complete neurologic examination of all patients with the chief complaint of headache should be performed and documented. Although some patients with migraine headaches may have neurologic deficits, the presence of new neurologic abnormities should trigger a work-up beyond the history and physical examination. Abnormalities may suggest a diagnosis and the location of a mass lesion or cerebrovascular accident. Abnormal mental status with a new headache suggests increased ICP, a diffuse process such as meningitis, or carbon monoxide poisoning.

## DIFFERENTIAL DIAGNOSIS AND MEDICAL DECISION MAKING

Following the history and physical examination, the EP must determine whether further diagnostic testing is necessary. Patients with new abnormal findings on physical examination clearly need further evaluation. Similarly, patients with a reassuring history and normal physical examination findings may require only appropriate analgesia and follow-up arrangements. Diagnostic dilemmas usually arise with patients who have normal findings on physical examination but some worrisome aspect of the history. No well-studied and validated decision rules have been published; for the most part, experience, judgment, and careful attention to the clinical examination and differential diagnosis guide further testing.

### COMPUTED TOMOGRAPHY

Computed tomography (CT) is often the first neuroimaging test because it is both rapid and widely available. A non–contrast-enhanced CT scan is extremely sensitive for acute intraparenchymal bleeding and very sensitive for subarachnoid bleeding (**Fig. 101.1**), but small or less acute subarachnoid bleeding may not be visible. Although some small tumors and abscesses are not visible on a non–contrast-enhanced scan, some abnormal finding will usually be seen on such scans in patients with masses large enough to cause a significant headache or focal neurologic findings (**Fig. 101.2**). Any focal neurologic signs or symptoms should be conveyed to the radiologist reading the CT scan so that appropriate attention can be directed to the anatomic site in question.

**BOX 101.3 Indications for Computed Tomography**

**History**

New or qualitatively different type of headache, thunderclap headache
Hemophilia or other coagulopathy
Blunt trauma (especially in the elderly)
Immunocompromised status (human immunodeficiency virus infection, chemotherapy)
Elderly
Fever with neurologic findings

**Physical Examination**

Glasgow Coma Scale score less than 15 with no clear explanation
Any new focal neurologic finding
Signs of increased intracranial pressure

Which patients require CT scanning is a matter of some debate. Hard and fast rules do not exist, but in general, high-risk factors indicate the need for CT (**Box 101.3**). The American College of Emergency Physicians has a clinical policy about the use of CT in some situations.[2]

The type of CT to perform depends on the specific differential diagnosis under consideration. Imaging of a mass or an abscess can be improved with intravenous infusion of a contrast agent. CT angiography (CTA) can be performed with multidetector scanners. Depending on the number of detectors, the software, and the skill of the neuroradiologist, CTA can approach conventional angiography in direct visualization of the cerebral vasculature. For patients in whom an arteriovenous malformation or aneurysm is suspected, CTA is a useful modality, although the standard diagnostic algorithm is still CT followed by LP.[2-4] CT venography can be useful in the diagnosis of cerebral venous sinus thrombosis.

### MAGNETIC RESONANCE IMAGING

In general, magnetic resonance imaging (MRI) is superior to CT, especially in evaluating vascular and neoplastic lesions and infections and pathology at the cervicomedullary junction and in the posterior fossa. Brain tumors, abscesses, ischemia, and pituitary apoplexy are easily visible. Recent studies suggest that MRI may even identify small cerebral hemorrhages that are not detected by CT scanning. Arterial and venous blood vessels can be evaluated by magnetic resonance angiography. Carotid and vertebral artery dissections, cerebral aneurysms, and cerebral venous sinus thrombosis can be diagnosed with magnetic resonance angiography and magnetic resonance venography.

Given the expense and scarcity of this resource, it is important that the EP carefully evaluate its necessity. For example, a headache patient with known thrombophilia or signs of cerebellar ischemia may require MRI evaluation for venous sinus thrombosis or a cerebellar stroke. Similarly, any newly documented neurologic deficit must be explained, and if contrast-enhanced CT scanning is not sufficient to find the cause, the EP should consider arranging for MRI, with the urgency depending on the clinical situation.

### LUMBAR PUNCTURE

LP remains an important diagnostic tool for headache patients. In patients with subarachnoid hemorrhage, the EP must be aware that CT scanning may be nondiagnostic and that LP is the next step necessary.[2]

LP can establish the diagnosis of suspected meningitis with nearly 100% sensitivity. Elevated opening pressure suggests idiopathic intracranial hypertension or cerebral venous sinus thrombosis. However, as with all tests in medicine, even LP has limitations. In particular, patients taking prednisone, who are otherwise immunocompromised, may not have the elevated cerebrospinal fluid white blood cell count expected. LP to rule out subarachnoid hemorrhage can be traumatic as well, thus making interpretation difficult. In such cases, an elevated opening pressure may help identify pathology such as subarachnoid hemorrhage.

### LABORATORY STUDIES

Routine laboratory studies are rarely helpful and not recommended in the work-up of patients with headache. In a few very specific circumstances, targeted laboratory tests can be helpful. Such tests include an erythrocyte sedimentation rate if giant cell arteritis is suspected, a toxicology screen for cocaine or other sympathomimetics in cases of intracranial hemorrhage in which they might play a role, and a carboxyhemoglobin level in patients with suspected carbon monoxide poisoning.

### TONOMETRY

Tonometry is a critical test in the ED for patients with headache, eye complaints, and findings that suggest acute narrow angle–closure glaucoma.

### TEMPORAL ARTERY BIOPSY

Temporal artery biopsy helps diagnose giant cell arteritis. When this diagnosis is suspected, high-dose oral steroid therapy should be started and arrangements made for the patient to see a surgeon for biopsy within the next week or so.

### NEUROLOGY CONSULTATON

One final issue to be considered is neurology consultation. The timing of consultation can vary, depending on the differential diagnosis and the duration of the headache. In patients with a new, definite neurologic finding on physical examination and normal results on brain imaging, the physician should consider neurologic consultation on an urgent or emergency basis.

## TREATMENT

Airway protection is always paramount in a critically ill patient. Patients with impending herniation from a mass lesion or intracranial bleeding may require intubation. Although neurologic examination is important in the acute phase of the patient's hospitalization, short-term paralysis for rapid-sequence intubation can and should be used to achieve the optimal intubation conditions. Lidocaine and fentanyl are sometimes advocated to blunt the transient rise in ICP that accompanies tracheal intubation. If feasible, a quick neurologic examination should be performed first.

Once the airway is secure, sedation should be adequate (to avoid elevations in ICP), but oversedation should be avoided to provide the best possible serial neurologic examination (propofol is a short-acting sedative that is useful for this purpose). If airway management precedes imaging, emergency neuroimaging should rapidly follow intubation.

For patients with signs or symptoms of acute bacterial meningitis, a critical early decision is whether to perform a CT scan or proceed directly to LP (**Box 101.4**). Administration of antibiotics should not be delayed in patients who have signs of acute meningitis. Performing LP directly in an alert, neurologically intact patient with no medical history is usually safe, especially in those with normal venous pulsations on funduscopy.

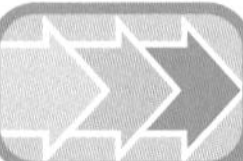

**PRIORITY ACTIONS**

Treat pain early and adequately. The response to pain should not affect the work-up, so there is no reason to withhold appropriate analgesia.

Patients with hemophilia and headache require coagulation factor repletion on an emergency basis, sometimes even before head computed tomography, given their high risk for intracranial hemorrhage.

Patients with signs and symptoms of acute bacterial meningitis require early antibiotics, even if the diagnosis is not yet established.

**BOX 101.4 Patient Features Suggesting That Computed Tomography Be Performed Before Lumbar Puncture**

**History**
Age older than 60 years
Immunocompromised status
History of central nervous system disease (e.g., tumor)
Recent seizure

**Physical Examination**
Altered mental status
Any new focal neurologic finding
Papilledema

## BLOOD PRESSURE

The three major indications for reduction of blood pressure (BP) are hypertensive encephalopathy, ruptured cerebral aneurysm, and intraparenchymal hemorrhage.

### *Hypertensive Encephalopathy*

Reduction of mean arterial pressure (MAP) by 25% should improve the headache and other signs of end-organ damage.

### *Ruptured Cerebral Aneurysm*

Although high-quality evidence is lacking, it is generally considered prudent to lower systolic BP to less than 140 or even 120 mm Hg with labetalol, nitroprusside, or nicardipine. This is in contrast to an ischemic stroke, in which higher BP levels (up to 220/120 mm Hg) are acceptable or even desired.

### *Intraparenchymal Hemorrhage*

Data to guide BP management in patients with intraparenchymal hemorrhage are limited, and no trial has demonstrated improved outcomes with reduction in BP. The American Heart Association published updated guidelines in 2010.[5] There has been a trend away from nitroprusside and toward nicardipine and labetalol.

The 2010 guidelines state the following:

1. If systolic BP is higher than 200 mm Hg (MAP > 150), aggressive reduction with continuous intravenous medication and monitoring of BP every 5 minutes should be considered.

2a. If systolic BP is higher than 180 mm Hg (MAP > 130) *AND* ICP is possibly increased, monitoring ICP and reducing BP to maintain cerebral perfusion pressure higher than 60 should be considered.

2b. If systolic BP is higher than 180 mm Hg (MAP > 130) with *NO* increased ICP, modest reduction (target of 160/90 or MAP of 110) and monitoring every 15 minutes should be considered.

3. In patients with a systolic BP of 150 to 220 mm Hg, acute lowering to 140 systolic is "probably safe."

## GIANT CELL ARTERITIS (TEMPORAL ARTERITIS)

Giant cell arteritis is classically manifested as a sudden, severe temporal headache in patients older than 50 years. A major differentiating feature of this disease is the presence of ischemic symptoms such as jaw claudication, scalp tenderness, or visual loss. In the ED, giant cell arteritis is a clinical presumptive diagnosis; therefore, high-dose prednisone should be administered empirically immediately. Temporal artery biopsy should be scheduled within a week or so to establish a definitive diagnosis, although even a negative biopsy result does not definitively exclude this disorder. The decision whether to continue steroid therapy following negative biopsy findings should be made by the primary care physician in consultation with appropriate specialists.

## ACUTE ANGLE–CLOSURE GLAUCOMA

Patients with acute angle-closure glaucoma typically have a recurrent unilateral headache behind the eye associated with blurred vision and erythema; there will often be a prolonged course of symptoms before appropriate diagnosis. Although the diagnosis is usually based on clinical findings, tonometry can establish the condition. Intraocular pressure in the affected eye will be elevated up to 40 to 80 mm Hg. In addition to appropriate pain control, any or all of the following therapies may be considered:

1. Acetazolamide, 500 mg intravenously followed by 500 mg orally
2. Timolol, 0.25% to 0.5% applied topically
3. Prednisolone, 1 to 2 drops onto the affected eye
4. Pilocarpine, 2% applied topically
5. Isosorbide, 1.5 g/kg orally, or glycerin, 1 to 2 g/kg orally
6. Mannitol, 1.5 to 2 g/kg intravenously
7. Antiemetics and analgesia as needed
8. Anterior chamber paracentesis

An ophthalmologist should be consulted on an emergency basis for definitive peripheral iridectomy or laser iridotomy.

## SINUSITIS-RELATED HEADACHE

A diagnosis of sinus-related headache should be made with caution because paranasal sinus mucosal thickening is a common incidental finding on CT and does not imply causality. Pain control is the cornerstone of treatment. Nonsteroidal agents and decongestants can be provided. Oxymetazoline nasal spray should be used for no more than several days. The Centers for Disease Control and Prevention recommends that the diagnosis of bacterial sinusitis be made only after 7 days of symptoms and that amoxicillin should be a first-line agent for mild sinusitis in patients with no previous antibiotic use.

## MIGRAINE HEADACHE

Migraine headache is classically defined as a throbbing unilateral headache with associated symptoms, including photophobia, phonophobia, nausea, and vomiting. The headache can be preceded by an aura, such as scintillating scotomata, jagged lines, or other visual abnormalities. Neurologic signs, including hemiparesis, paresthesias, ophthalmoplegia, and aphasia, can complicate migraine. Patients will usually have a history of similar headaches and frequently a family history of migraines.

Migraine is most confidently diagnosed by a history of at least five similar headaches with several specific criteria. New-onset headaches or those of a different or unusual quality often require further work-up. One cannot definitively

**BOX 101.5 Management of Moderate to Severe Acute Migraine Headaches**

Antiemetics (first-line agents)—often combined with diphenhydramine; consider using both to prevent akathisia
- Metoclopramide, 10 mg IV—supported by multiple clinical trials
- Prochlorperazine, 10 mg IV—supported by multiple clinical trials
- Promethazine, 25 mg IV
- Ondansetron, 1-4 mg IV

Nonsteroidal antiinflammatory drugs (first-line agents)—use in combination with antiemetics
- Naproxen, 500 mg PO
- Ibuprofen, 200-800 mg PO
- Diclofenac, 50 mg PO
- Ketorolac, 15-30 mg IV

Analgesics (first-line agents)—use in combination with antiemetics
- Aspirin, 81-325 mg
- Acetaminophen, 325-1000 mg
- Paracetamol—available outside the United States

5-$HT_1$ receptor agonists—use in combination with antiemetics, analgesics
- Sumatriptan, 6 mg SC—also available as a nasal spray
- Zolmitriptan, 2.5-5 mg PO
- Frovatriptan, 2.5 mg PO
- Eletriptan, 20-40 mg PO
- Almotriptan, 6.25-12.5 mg PO
- Rizatriptan, 5-10 mg PO

Ergotamines
- Dihydroergotamine, 0.5-1 mg IV—may be second line with respect to triptans or antiemetics
- Ergotamine

Steroids—no clear benefit acutely but may decrease recurrence
- Dexamethasone, 10 mg IV

diagnose migraine or tension headache at the initial onset of a new headache.

**Box 101.5** summarizes the various agents that are useful in the management of acute migraine. Although opiates are used frequently in the ED, they should not be first-line treatment and should be reserved for rescue therapy in patients who do not respond to the initial medications—and even in this situation they should be used sparingly.

## CLUSTER HEADACHE

Cluster headache is typically a severe unilateral headache that can be accompanied by conjunctival injection, lacrimation, ptosis, miosis, rhinorrhea, and nasal congestion. Attacks can occur up to eight times a day and are severe but short-lived; the autonomic symptoms are typically unilateral and ipsilateral to the pain. Recognition is important because this headache subtype is uniquely sensitive to oxygen. Mainstays of emergency management include administration of oxygen and subcutaneous sumatriptan (**Box 101.6**).

**BOX 101.6 Acute Management of Cluster Headache**

Oxygen, 7 L/min for 15 minutes by face mask
Sumatriptan, 6 mg subcutaneously or 20 mg by nasal spray
Dihydroergotamine nasal spray (*Note*: Do not combine ergotamines with sumatriptan)
Lidocaine intranasally, 1 mL of a 4% solution ipsilaterally

**BOX 101.7 Acute Management of Tension Headache**

Nonsteroidal antiinflammatory drugs
Antihistamines
- Diphenhydramine (Benadryl)
- Promethazine (Phenergan)

Antiemetics
- Metoclopramide (Reglan)
- Prochlorperazine (Compazine)

Butalbital-containing agents
- Acetaminophen + caffeine + butalbital
- Aspirin + caffeine + butalbital

## TENSION HEADACHE

Tension headache is usually characterized by throbbing pain that radiates bilaterally from front to back and to the neck muscles. As with migraine headaches, one cannot firmly diagnose tension headache after a single episode, and this diagnosis requires more than nine previous episodes. Pain control consists of nonsteroidal antiinflammatory drugs, antiemetics, and perhaps caffeine (**Box 101.7**). Butalbital-containing agents (as with migraine headaches) may be used with caution, given the risk for dependency and rebound headache.

# FOLLOW-UP, NEXT STEPS IN CARE, AND PATIENT EDUCATION

Disposition is entirely a function of the cause of the headache and the need for further treatment or, in some cases, pain control.

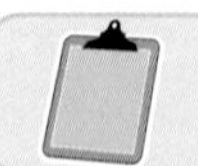

**DOCUMENTATION**

The history in every headache patient should include the onset, timing, severity, comparison with previous headaches, and any new neurologic complaints.

The physical examination should include a complete neurologic and head, eye, ear, nose, and throat examination. Any new neurologic findings must be explained.

Visual fields and gait assessment cover a wide range of neuroanatomic territory and are often either inadequately tested or inadequately documented.

Be very careful assigning the diagnosis of migraine headache to patients if they do not already have this diagnosis or if the current headache is different from their usual migraines.

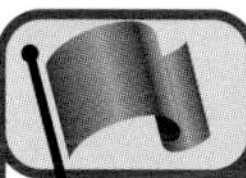

**RED FLAGS**

**Complications and Pitfalls**

Just because a patient states that he or she has had "migraine" (or "tension" or "sinus") headaches does not mean that the headaches ever formally met these criteria or have ever been evaluated or that this headache is the same as the previous headaches. This is especially true for recent-onset headaches.

If head computed tomography is performed to evaluate for subarachnoid hemorrhage, it should always be followed by lumbar puncture to evaluate for xanthochromia and the presence of blood.

Visualization of mucosal thickening in the paranasal sinuses on computed tomography is a common incidental finding and should not be used to diagnose acute sinusitis.

A favorable response to analgesics has little or no diagnostic significance and should not be used to exclude a secondary cause of headache.

## REFERENCES AND SUGGESTED READINGS

***References and suggested readings can be found on Expert Consult @ www.expertconsult.com.***

Derby Teaching Hospitals
NHS Foundation Trust
Library and Knowledge Centre

# 102 Intracranial and Other Central Nervous System Lesions

*Steven M. Zahn*

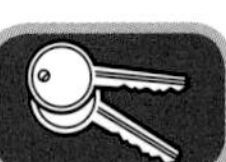

**KEY POINTS**

- A comprehensive patient history is imperative to narrow the differential diagnosis when a new mass lesion is discovered on radiographic imaging.
- A complaint of dizziness requires cerebellar testing, including finger-nose, heel-shin, dysdiadochokinesia, and gait evaluation.
- Fever in the setting of a neurologic complaint requires both a neurologic examination and consideration of neuroimaging.
- Any patient with a first-time seizure warrants a non–contrast-enhanced computed tomography (CT) scan of the head regardless of age (**Box 102.1**).
- CT scans reliably demonstrate lesions 1.0 cm or larger.
- Magnetic resonance imaging should be performed if there is significant concern for a central nervous system lesion in patients with negat ive CT findings.

**BOX 102.1 Indications for Computed Tomography of the Brain in Patients with First-Time Seizures**

New focal deficit
Persistently altered mental status
Fever
Recent trauma
Persistent headache
History of cancer
Anticoagulant use
Suspicion or known history of acquired immunodeficiency syndrome
Age older than 40 years
Partial complex seizure

Adapted from guidelines developed by the U.S. Headache Consortium, American College of Emergency Physicians, and the American College of Radiology. American College of Emergency Physicians. Clinical policy: critical issues in the evaluation and management of patients presenting to the emergency department with acute headache. Ann Emerg Med 2002;39:108.

## EPIDEMIOLOGY

Patients with intracranial lesions typically have headaches, seizures, focal neurologic changes, weakness, fatigue, or any combination of these findings. Headaches occur in approximately 50% of patients with central nervous system (CNS) tumors; however, brain tumors are uncommon in patients with a headache and normal findings on neurologic examination (<1% of the time).[1] Thus emergency physicians should always consider the presence of a brain tumor in the differential diagnosis but should use neuroimaging judiciously (**Table 102.1**).[2,3] Focal neurologic changes always warrant further investigation, including laboratory tests, radiographic imaging, and neurologic or neurosurgical consultation (or both).

## PATHOPHYSIOLOGY

Small intracranial lesions can drastically affect important neural pathways within the CNS. Frequently, a non-CNS malignancy is first identified by a neurologic manifestation of a metastatic lesion. Lesions located near or within the ventricular system can be manifested as changes in intracranial pressure (ICP) and thus affect the clinical findings. However, slow-growing lesions of a primary CNS origin located in clinically silent regions of the brain such as the frontal lobe may be present for years before detection.

Autopsy diagnosis reveals that nearly 25% of patients who die of cancer had intracranial metastasis (**Fig. 102.1**). The lung is the most common origin of brain metastases. Breast cancer (especially ductal carcinoma) has a propensity to metastasize to the cerebellum and the posterior pituitary gland; however, breast cancer that metastasizes to bone tends to not metastasize to the brain.

Other common origins of brain metastases are gastrointestinal malignancies (most commonly colon and rectum), renal carcinoma, and melanoma. In contrast, prostate, esophageal, and ovarian cancer and Hodgkin disease rarely metastasize to the brain.

Although metastatic disease is a common form of intracranial mass lesion, other mass lesion considerations include lymphoma (**Fig. 102.2**), glioblastoma multiforme (**Fig. 102.3**), astrocytoma, ependymoma, meningioma, oligodendroglioma,

**Table 102.1 Guidelines for Neuroimaging in Patients with a Headache**

| CLINICAL FINDING | RECOMMENDATION |
|---|---|
| "Thunderclap" headache with abnormal neurologic findings | Emergency neuroimaging recommended |
| Signs of increased intracranial pressure; fever and nuchal rigidity | Safe performance of lumbar puncture recommended |
| "Thunderclap" headache<br>Headache radiating to the neck<br>Temporal headache in an older individual<br>New-onset headache in a patient who:<br>Is HIV positive<br>Has a previous diagnosis of cancer<br>Is in a population at high risk for intracranial disease<br>Accompanied by an abnormal neurologic findings, including but not limited to papilledema, unilateral loss of sensation, weakness, and hyperreflexia | Neuroimaging should be considered |
| Migraine and normal neurologic findings | Neuroimaging not usually warranted |
| Headache worsened by the Valsalva maneuver, wakes the patient from sleep, or is progressively worsening | No recommendation (some data revealing increased risk for intracranial abnormality, not sufficient for recommendation) |
| Tension headache with normal neurologic findings | No recommendation (insufficient data) |

Adapted from guidelines developed by the U.S. Headache Consortium, American College of Emergency Physicians, and American College of Radiology. American College of Emergency Physicians. Clinical policy: critical issues in the evaluation and management of patients presenting to the emergency department with acute headache. Ann Emerg Med 2002;39:108.

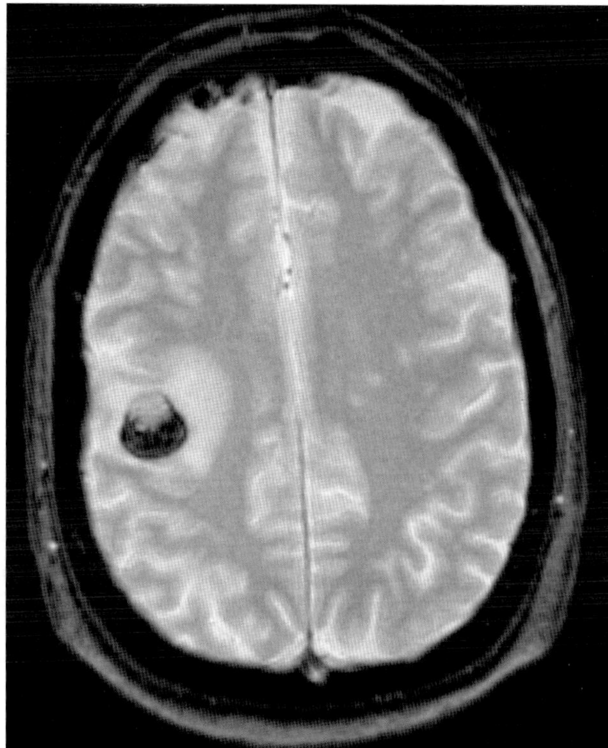

**Fig. 102.1** Axial magnetic resonance image demonstrating a metastatic lesion present at the gray-white matter junction with significant surrounding edema. The hyperdense focus within the lesion probably represents calcification or blood.

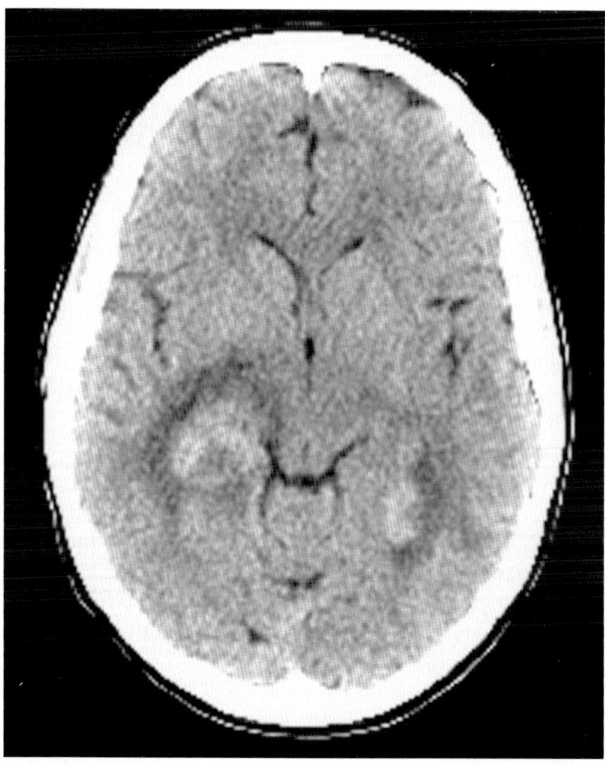

**Fig. 102.2** This computed tomography scan demonstrates the classic periventricular homogeneous lesion of a central nervous system lymphoma; it has a ring-enhancing appearance when viewed with contrast enhancement.

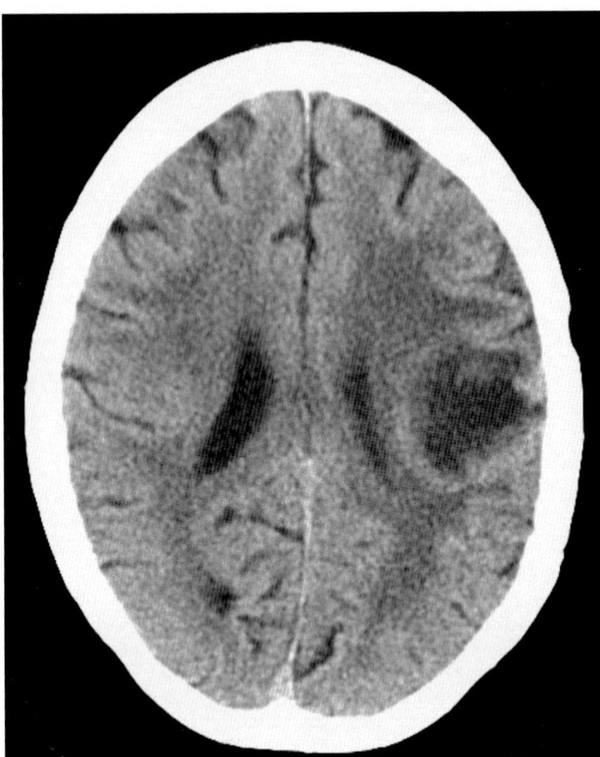

**Fig. 102.3** The lesion in this computed tomography scan illustrates the characteristic features of glioblastoma multiforme: heterogeneous irregular ring of enhancement, hypointense core, and significant surrounding edema.

**BOX 102.2 Differential Diagnosis of a Brain Mass**

Metastatic brain tumor
Primary brain tumor
- Meningioma
- Glioma
- Pituitary adenoma
- Vestibular schwannoma
- Primary or secondary central nervous system lymphoma

Infections
- Abscess
- Toxoplasmosis
- Neurocysticercosis
- Tuberculoma
- Progressive multifocal leukoencephalopathy

Vascular disease
Hemorrhage
- Anomalies (arteriovenous malformation)
- Intratumoral
- Hypertensive

Infarct
- Embolism
- Thrombosis (sinus venous)

Inflammatory
- Multiple sclerosis
- Encephalomyelitis

medulloblastoma, hemangioblastoma, neurocysticercosis, toxoplasmosis, tuberculoma, tuberous sclerosis, and arteriovenous malformations.

## PRESENTING SIGNS AND SYMPTOMS

CNS mass lesions are usually manifested as one of three syndromes: (1) subacute progression of a focal neurologic deficit; (2) seizure; or (3) a nonfocal neurologic disorder such as headache (especially with nocturnal features or occurrence on awakening), dementia, changes in personality, or gait disorder. The presence of systemic symptoms (malaise, fever, weight loss) suggests a metastatic rather than a primary brain tumor or an infectious process such as toxoplasmosis or tuberculoma.[4]

The initial complaint related to a CNS lesion may be attributable to an increase in ICP. Nausea, vomiting, lethargy, and morning headaches are common symptoms that are mistaken for other organ system involvement but are classic findings in patients demonstrating a rise in ICP. Hydrocephalus arising from a strategic location of a CNS lesion can lead to dizziness, ataxia, and vomiting as a result of obstruction to flow of cerebrospinal fluid.

## DIFFERENTIAL DIAGNOSIS AND MEDICAL DECISION MAKING

The initial diagnostic modality in a patient with a new neurologic complaint is a non–contrast-enhanced computed tomography (CT) scan. Most brain tumors causing clinical symptoms are visible on CT scans, and all are visible with the various contrast-enhanced techniques of CT and magnetic resonance imaging (MRI). On nonenhanced CT, brain tumors are visualized by mass effect and altered attenuation. Masses may be hypodense, isodense, or hyperdense with respect to surrounding structures and can be associated with vasogenic edema, which is visualized by low attenuation of the white matter (**Box 102.2**). Extraaxial lesions can best be appreciated with bone window settings because bone erosion or hyperostosis may be present.

Calcification can be useful in isolating brain tumors. Oligodendrogliomas contain calcification in 90% of cases. Other tumors with calcification include choroid plexus tumors, ependymoma, central neurocytoma, meningioma (**Fig. 102.4**), craniopharyngioma, teratoma, and chordoma. Nonmalignant lesions such as neurocysticercosis, toxoplasmosis, and tuberous sclerosis exhibit calcific changes on radiographic imaging as well (**Table 102.2**).

Ring enhancement on contrast-enhanced imaging modalities may expand the differential diagnosis to toxoplasmosis, neurocysticercosis, or even multiple sclerosis. Multiple lesions in various stages of development are characteristic of neurocysticercosis. Multiple sclerosis is a common misdiagnosis in the setting of primary CNS lymphoma because both have features of white matter lesions on MRI.

Hemorrhage within a defined lesion on a CT scan should suggest the possibility of an arteriovenous malformation or hemangioblastoma (**Fig. 102.5**). Contrast-enhanced CT or MRI may identify more than 95% of arteriovenous malformations. Lesions appear as a heterogeneous, hypodense mass

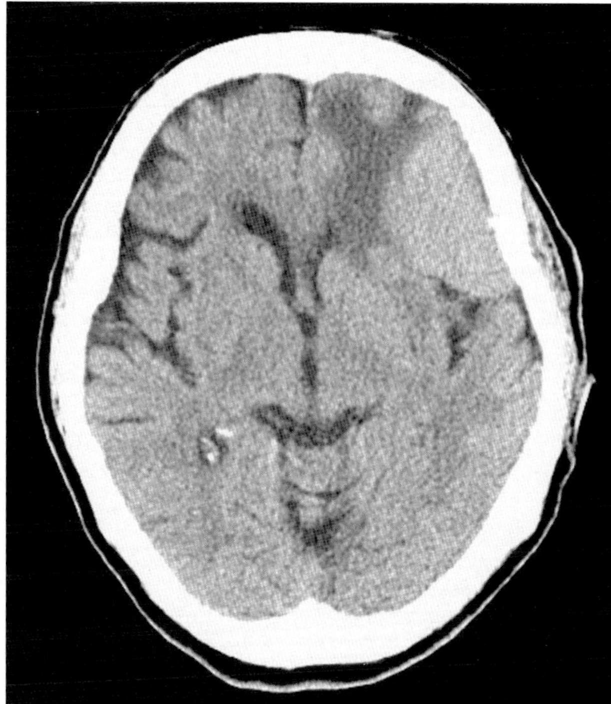

**Fig. 102.4** The meningioma seen on this computed tomography scan has the classic extraaxial appearance of this lesion. Meningiomas are often hyperdense and may demonstrate calcification.

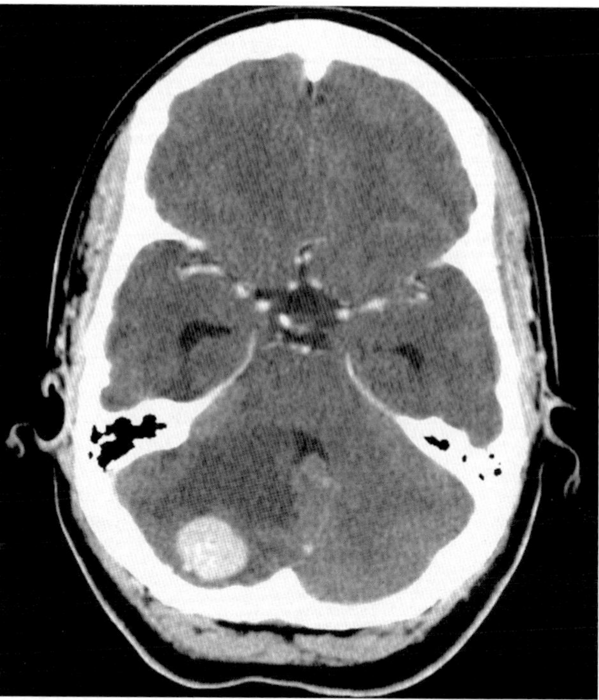

**Fig. 102.5** Computed tomography scan with contrast enhancement demonstrating the typical cystic appearance of a cerebellar hemangioblastoma. A nodular lesion is visible within the wall of the cerebellar cyst.

with hyperdense regions within the mass; an enhancing rim may also be visible (**Fig. 102.6**). In patients with negative CT findings but a high index of clinical suspicion, lumbar puncture with cerebrospinal fluid analysis is necessary. If the index of clinical suspicion is high and the diagnosis is suggested by findings on CT, angiography is required to better define the lesion and develop a management strategy. Laboratory analysis of coagulation, including the prothrombin time, partial thromboplastin time, and international normalized ratio, should also be undertaken.

Constitutional symptoms should be accounted for when interpreting CNS lesions on radiographic images. Fever or laboratory findings such as leukocytosis or an unusual differential feature (elevated lymphocyte or eosinophil count) may raise suspicion for an infectious cause such as tuberculoma or toxoplasmosis instead of a primary brain tumor or a metastatic lesion.

## TREATMENT

Prehospital evaluation for possible intracranial lesions involves basic emergency medicine principles for airway support and monitoring of breathing. Seizure may be a manifestation that should require standard antiepileptics and airway management. Mass lesions near the pons and medulla, as well as those leading to hemorrhage and a mass effect, will require emergency airway support.

A variety of treatment options are available for the myriad of intracranial lesions possible. Most, if not all modalities should

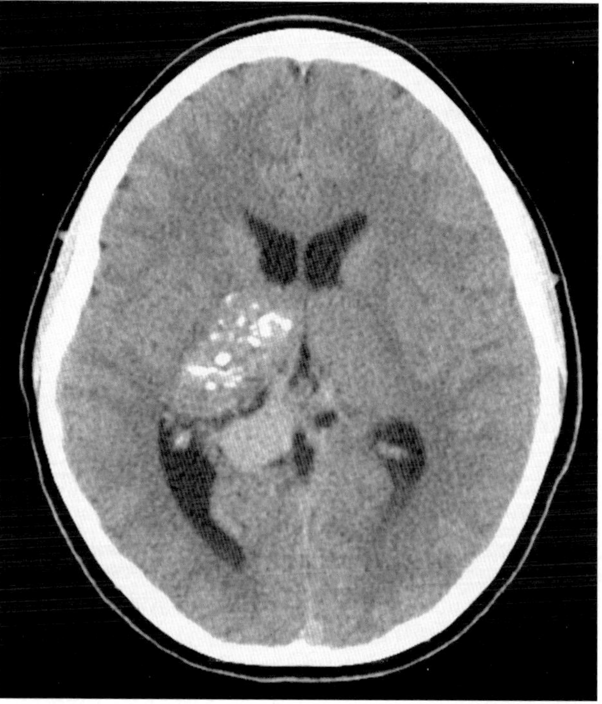

**Fig. 102.6** Arteriovenous malformations, as demonstrated in this non–contrast-enhanced computed tomography scan, are heterogeneous, with hyperdense regions throughout the mass signifying the presence of blood.

**Table 102.2 Characteristic Appearance of Intracranial and Central Nervous System Lesions**

| TYPE OF LESION | EDEMA | BORDER | CALCIFICATION | CHARACTERISTICS |
|---|---|---|---|---|
| Metastatic brain lesion | + | Irregular | ± | Present at the gray-white matter junction following cerebral blood flow |
| Central nervous system lymphoma | ± | Irregular | – | Dense, homogeneous enhancing periventricular mass; white matter, ring-enhancing mass |
| Low-grade astrocytoma | + | Irregular | ± | Isodensity or hypodensity with minimal enhancement |
| High-grade astrocytoma, glioblastoma multiforme | + | Irregular | ± | Heterogeneous, hypointense enhancing mass with surrounding edema; can involve both cerebral hemispheres |
| Ependymoma | ± | ± | + | Uniformly enhancing mass; well demarcated from adjacent tissue |
| Meningioma | ± | Irregular | + | Extraaxial, uniformly enhancing mass |
| Oligodendroglioma | ± | ± | + | Well-demarcated frontal-temporal mass with calcific streaks |
| Medulloblastoma | ± | Irregular | ± | Contrast-enhancing heterogeneous mass near or involving the fourth ventricle |
| Hemangioblastoma (von Hippel-Lindau disease) | ± | Irregular | – (Blood may mimic) | Enhancing cerebellar cyst with a nodule on the wall of the cyst; angiography important |
| Schwannoma | ± | Irregular | – | Dense hyperdense mass around the eighth cranial nerve; can have a mass effect on the pons/posterior fossa |
| Neurocysticercosis | + | Regular | + | Ring-enhancing, low-density lesions; often multiple |
| Toxoplasmosis | + | Regular | + | Ring-enhancing, low-density lesions; often multiple |
| Tuberculoma | – | Irregular | ± | Isodense or hypodense lesions that mimic malignancy with contrast enhancement |
| Tuberous sclerosis | – | Irregular | + | Periventricular mass; often multiple |
| Arteriovenous malformation | – | Irregular | – (Blood may mimic) | Heterogeneous hypodense mass with a contrast-enhancing rim; lumbar puncture for diagnosis of subarachnoid hemorrhage; angiography required for diagnosis |

+, Present; –, not present; ±, may or may not be present.

be performed in consultation with neurology and neurosurgery. The majority of lesions require additional specialized diagnostic testing such as serologic analysis and biopsy, which makes the final diagnosis a responsibility of the consultants.

Primary and metastatic brain lesions may require a multifaceted approach to medical care. In the emergency department setting, glucocorticoids and prophylactic antiepileptics (phenytoin, fosphenytoin, phenobarbital) may be given before admission. Surgery, radiation therapy, and chemotherapy are options for further long-term treatment plans, but they are usually tailored to the specific tissue diagnosis when it pertains to a solid mass lesion.[5]

Infectious lesions such as abscesses (**Fig. 102.7**), neurocysticercosis, toxoplasmosis, and tuberculomas usually require consultation with infectious disease specialists. Serologic examination may prove useful for determining a diagnosis and treatment approach. Antibiotic and antiparasitic medications may be administered under the guidance of these consultants; regimens including clindamycin, albendazole, praziquantel, sulfadiazine, and pyrimethamine may be instituted with or without glucocorticoids.

Special situations include hemorrhaging lesions, such as metastatic lesions or arteriovenous malformations, which may necessitate the use of coagulation factors such as fresh frozen plasma, platelets, or factor VII given the location, mass effect, and patient-specific comorbid conditions.

## FOLLOW-UP, NEXT STEPS IN CARE, AND PATIENT EDUCATION

Most lesions that are discovered on CT or are due to a neurologic abnormality require further inpatient diagnosis and treatment as stated in the previous section. Patients with

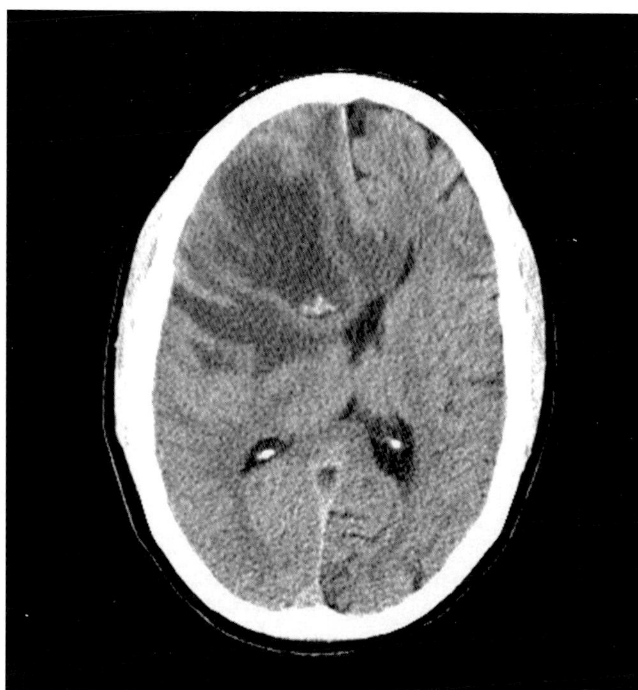

**Fig. 102.7** This irregularly shaped mass may ultimately reveal edema surrounding a large intrinsic brain tumor on subsequent imaging, but this lesion is a result of a central nervous system abscess.

meningiomas or those with a known diagnosis of a chronic condition such as tuberous sclerosis may be discharged and close follow-up with primary and specialty physicians arranged. Any new lesion (except for a solitary meningioma, for example) or signs of a mass effect require emergency consultation with a specialty service.

## SUGGESTED READINGS

American College of Emergency Physicians. Clinical policy: critical issues in the evaluation and management of adult patients presenting to the emergency department with seizures. Ann Emerg Med 2004;43:605-25.

Cavaliere R, Farace E, Schiff D. Clinical implications of status epilepticus in patients with neoplasms. Arch Neurol 2006;63:1746.

Engstrom JW. Tumors of the nervous system. In: Braunwald E, Fauci AS, Kasper DL, et al, editors. Harrison's manual of medicine. 15th ed. New York: McGraw-Hill; 2001. p. 842-4.

Evans RW. Diagnostic testing for the evaluation of headaches. Neurol Clin 1996;14:1-26.

Schaefer PW, Miller JC, Singhal AB, et al. Headache: when is neuroimaging indicated? J Am Coll Radiol 2007;4:566-9.

## REFERENCES

*References can be found on Expert Consult @ www.expertconsult.com.*

# 103 Intracranial Hemorrhages

J. Stephen Huff, Max Wintermark, and Chris A. Ghaemmaghami

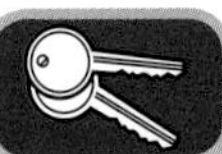

**KEY POINTS**

- "Head bleed" is an oversimplified term for intracranial hemorrhage because different types of hemorrhages have different causes, signs and symptoms, diagnostic strategies, and therapies.
- Descriptions of intracranial hemorrhage should include the anatomic location, estimation of size, presence of midline shift, and whether the hemorrhage is thought to be spontaneous or secondary to another process.
- Treatment recommendations regarding blood pressure management and anticonvulsant therapy remain controversial and lack strong evidence-based support.

## PERSPECTIVE

Intracranial hemorrhages have different clinical manifestations ranging from subtle to catastrophic. The efforts of the emergency physician (EP) are directed toward identifying the correct diagnosis, confirming the diagnosis by cranial computed tomography (CT) or other diagnostic tests, and providing supportive care. Liberal consultation plus collaboration with specialists is required. Strong evidence of the best course of action regarding basic treatment issues such as blood pressure management and the use of anticonvulsants is lacking. Definitive therapy is most often in the hands of consulting and admitting physicians.

It is tempting to place any intracranial hemorrhage in the diagnostic category head bleed. Different types of intracranial hemorrhage may have different causes, different natural histories, different diagnostic strategies, different treatments, and frequently different prognoses. It is important to delineate the various types of intracranial hemorrhage so that correct diagnostic steps and therapeutic interventions can be performed.

## EPIDEMIOLOGY

Estimates of the incidence of intracranial hemorrhage in patients seen in the emergency department (ED) are difficult because the findings include isolated headache, stroke syndromes, and head trauma, but a few generalities may be made. It is estimated that approximately 800,000 strokes occur each year in the United States, with intracranial hemorrhages accounting for 20% of the strokes. About 1% to 2% of patients seek treatment in EDs with a primary complaint of headache, and it is thought that 1% of these patients may have subarachnoid hemorrhage (SAH). If a filter of "worst headache of my life" is used, that estimate increases to up to 12% of patients with SAH. Approximately 500,000 moderate and severe traumatic head injuries occur each year in the United States. One percent to 2% of these patients have epidural hematomas, with estimates of an additional 5% to 25% having acute subdural hematomas.

## PATHOPHYSIOLOGY

Intracranial hemorrhage is the umbrella term used to encompass the many types of bleeding within the cranial vault (**Figs. 103.1 to 103.5** and **Table 103.1**). Intraparenchymal hemorrhage implies blood within the substance of the brain. When the hemorrhage is not clearly secondary to a detectable cause, it is deemed a spontaneous hemorrhage. This term is often used synonymously with the terms *hypertensive hemorrhage* and, when anatomically appropriate, *intracerebral hemorrhage*. Intraparenchymal hemorrhages may also occur in the brainstem or cerebellum. SAH literally describes blood in the subarachnoid space, and if nontraumatic, a vascular lesion such as an aneurysm is the implied cause of the bleeding. SAH and intraparenchymal hemorrhage may coexist. Intraventricular hemorrhage means that blood is visualized within the ventricles by cranial CT, and it is most often present with other types of intracranial hemorrhage. Intracranial hemorrhages outside the brain substance are referred to as extraaxial hemorrhages and include both subdural hemorrhages and epidural hemorrhages. Although uncommon exceptions exist, extraaxial hemorrhages almost always have a traumatic etiology. The term *hemorrhagic stroke* might literally describe abrupt symptoms with any of the previously mentioned hemorrhages, but it is sometimes used in a more restrictive sense to describe hemorrhagic changes in an area of ischemic stroke to the point of being visible on cranial CT; this is termed hemorrhagic transformation of ischemic stroke.

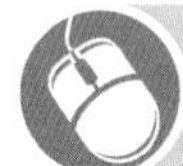

See Table 103.1, Types of Intracranial Hemorrhage, online at www.expertconsult.com

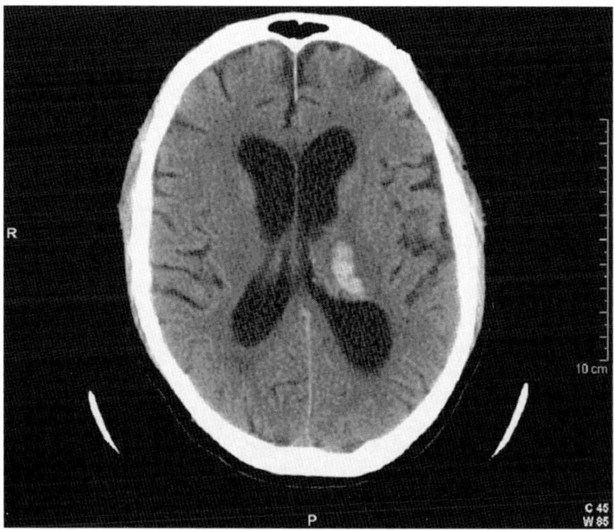


**Fig. 103.1 Computed tomography scan: supratentorial intracerebral hematoma.** Note the bright white appearance consistent with an acute hemorrhage. The anatomic location is thalamic.

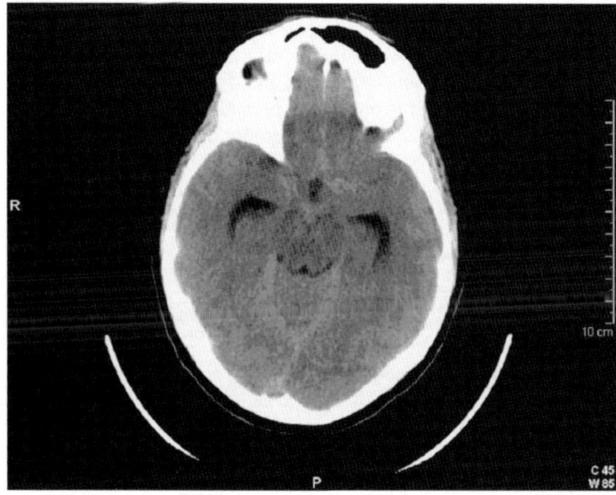


**Fig. 103.2 Computed tomography scan: acute subarachnoid hemorrhage.** Blood density is not as dramatic as in Figure 103.13. Hydrocephalus with enlarged temporal horns of the lateral ventricle is present.

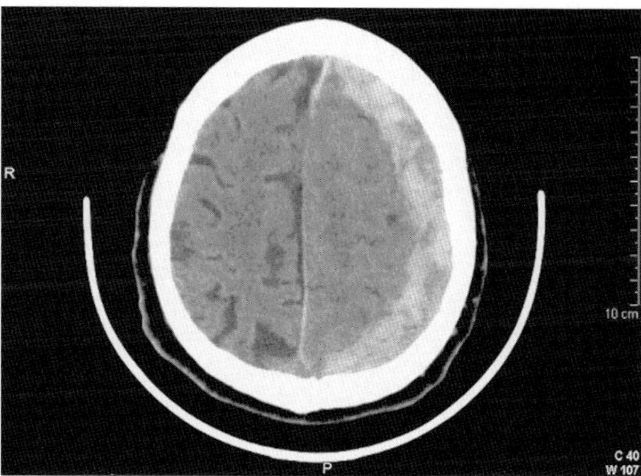


**Fig. 103.3 Computed tomography scan: acute subdural hematoma.** Note the crescent-shaped hemorrhage extending the length of the left hemisphere. The mottled appearance is consistent with ongoing bleeding.

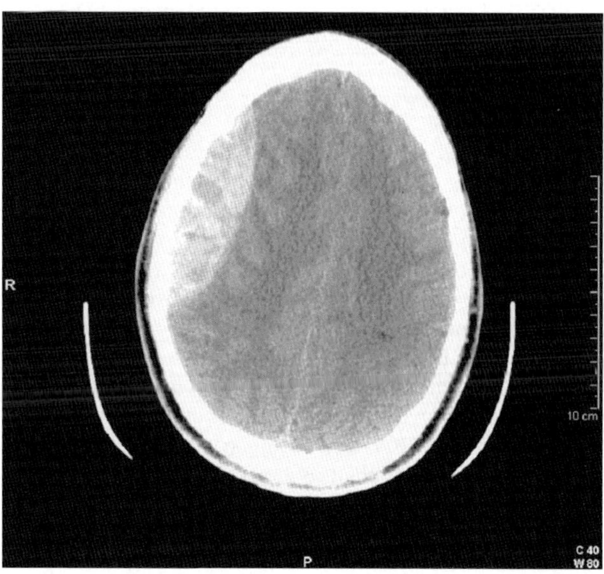


**Fig. 103.4 Computed tomography (CT) scan: acute epidural hematoma with the "swirl" sign.** This is a slice from a repeated CT scan of the patient in Figure 103.10 taken approximately 1 hour later. The marbled density of the clot is consistent with ongoing hemorrhage. Note the lens shape of the hematoma.

Intracranial bleeding may be of either arterial or venous origin. Because of the closed nature of the cranial vault, any increase in intracranial volume from bleeding may result in increased intracranial pressure (ICP) and decreased cerebral perfusion pressure (CPP). As a mass expands, some initial compensation occurs in the form of diminished intracranial vascular and cerebrospinal fluid volume. However, at some point the compensatory mechanisms fail and ICP will dramatically rise with a further increase in size of the mass. A key concept is CPP, the effective blood pressure exerted on the intracranial contents. CPP is equal to mean arterial pressure (MAP) minus ICP:

$$CPP = MAP - ICP$$

If ICP increases abruptly or if MAP falls, CPP decreases and central nervous system ischemia may follow and exacerbate the neuronal injury.

Hemorrhages also cause injury by direct tissue destruction or compression of adjacent structures. Edema formation around a hematoma may further increase the mass effect. For example, with cerebellar hemorrhages, tissue damage may cause the initial symptoms, but increased ICP and rapid progression to coma result from compression of the adjacent brainstem.

Spontaneous intraparenchymal hemorrhages (e.g., intracerebral hemorrhages, lobar hemorrhages, hypertensive hemorrhages) are most often associated with chronic hypertension. Cerebral amyloid angiopathy is increasingly being recognized

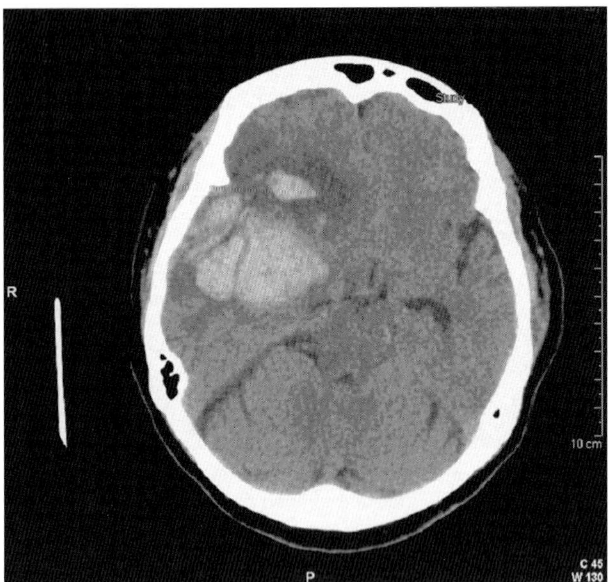


**Fig. 103.5 Computed tomography scan: hemorrhagic transformation of ischemic stroke.**

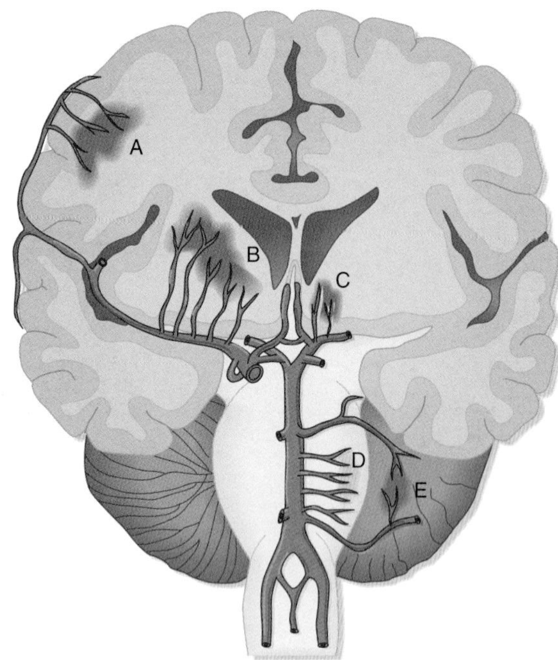


**Fig. 103.6 Common sites and sources of intracerebral hemorrhage.** Intracerebral hemorrhages most commonly involve the cerebral lobes, with origin from penetrating cortical branches of the anterior, middle, or posterior cerebral arteries (*A*); the basal ganglia, with origin from ascending lenticulostriate branches of the middle cerebral artery (*B*); the thalamus, with origin from ascending thalamogeniculate branches of the posterior cerebral artery (*C*); the pons, with origin from paramedian branches of the basilar artery (*D*); and the cerebellum, with origin from penetrating branches of the posterior inferior, anterior inferior, or superior cerebellar arteries (*E*).

as a contributing process in the elderly. Chronic excessive alcohol use is also a risk factor. Hemorrhage usually originates from rupture of small penetrating branch arteries of the vessels at the base of the brain[1] (**Fig. 103.6**).

Serial cranial CT demonstrates that many intracerebral hemorrhages expand over the course of several hours.[2] The initial hemorrhage may infiltrate the white matter with little direct destruction, but continued hematoma expansion, white matter edema, additional hemorrhage from surrounding vessels, and the development of hydrocephalus may all contribute to increased ICP and secondary neuronal injury. The frequency of anticoagulant-associated intracerebral hemorrhage is increasing.[3] Warfarin therapy does not appear to increase hematoma volume initially, but it does increase the risk for later hematoma expansion.[4]

SAH literally means "blood in the subarachnoid space." Trauma is the most common cause. Spontaneous, or nontraumatic, SAH has an entirely different differential diagnosis. About 80% of spontaneous SAHs are caused by rupture of saccular (berry) aneurysms of the intracranial vessels, which are commonly located near intracranial arterial bifurcations of the circle of Willis[5,6] (**Fig. 103.7**). Aneurysms are often named after the vascular site of origin, such as the anterior communicating artery or middle cerebral artery. Aneurysms that develop following vascular infection from endocarditis are termed mycotic aneurysms. Some aneurysms also cause symptoms without rupture from a mass effect or from emboli originating within the aneurysm. Rupture of an intracranial aneurysm abruptly raises ICP and leads to the onset of symptoms. The bleeding may be confined to the subarachnoid space, or a hematoma may extend into the brain substance and create an intraparenchymal hemorrhage, which in turn may rupture into the ventricles. Vasospasm of the vascular tree related to the aneurysm typically takes hours to develop and may worsen regional ischemia.

Arteriovenous malformations are another cause of intracranial hemorrhage of both the subarachnoid and intraparenchymal anatomic subtypes. These arteriovenous shunts vary in their anatomy, and many patients have saccular aneurysms as well. Lesions with deep venous drainage and high pressure in the feeding vessels are at increased risk for bleeding.[7] Cavernous angiomas are low-pressure vascular lesions associated with small hemorrhages.

Closed head injury may cause diffuse or localized subarachnoid bleeding. Cerebral contusion is a loosely defined term that describes the CT appearance of low density consistent with edema and often with some hemorrhage within that region.

An epidural hematoma usually reflects arterial bleeding into the epidural space following injury to a meningeal artery. A common mechanism is a skull fracture in the temporal area with associated laceration of the middle meningeal artery. The arterial pressure hematoma may increase in size until tamponade occurs as a result of resistance of distorted intracranial structures and increased ICP (at the expense of CPP).

Subdural hematomas reflect bleeding from small vessel sources and from diffuse brain injury with hemorrhage accumulating over the surface of the brain. Again, distortion of the cranial contents may occur, as well as increased ICP. The cortical atrophy that occurs with aging is thought to make the bridging vessels from the cortex to the dura increasingly susceptible to rupture from even trivial trauma in the elderly.

Less common causes of intracranial hemorrhage include dural sinus thrombosis with venous infarction and

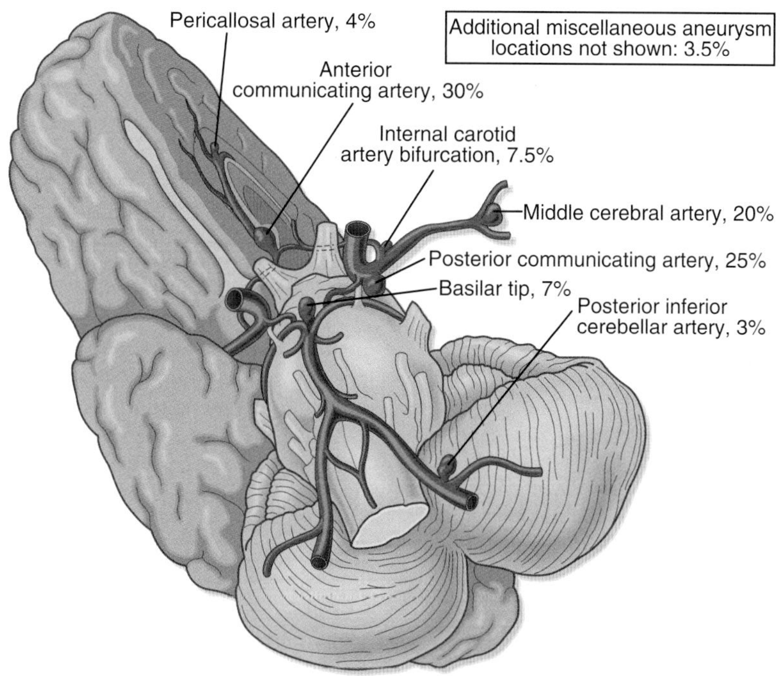


**Fig. 103.7 The intracranial vasculature showing the most frequent locations of intracranial aneurysms.**

hemorrhage, intracranial neoplasms, brain abscesses, coagulopathies, vasculitides, and toxins. Cocaine and other sympathomimetic agents are believed to cause transient severe hypertension with resultant hemorrhage.

The anatomic terminology regarding intracranial hemorrhage historically comes from postmortem neuropathology descriptions. In the ED, intracranial hemorrhages are most often diagnosed by cranial CT, which remains the initial diagnostic modality of choice. The appearance of acute hemorrhage usually contrasts vividly with that of the other intracranial contents. The types of intracranial hemorrhage are anatomically classified primarily by their relationship to the substance of the brain and the meninges.[8] Simplistically, hemorrhages may be thought to be located in the brain substance (intraparenchymal, intracerebral), within the ventricles (intraventricular), in the subarachnoid space between the meninges and the brain, or outside the brain and meninges (subdural, epidural) (**Figs. 103.8 and 103.9**).

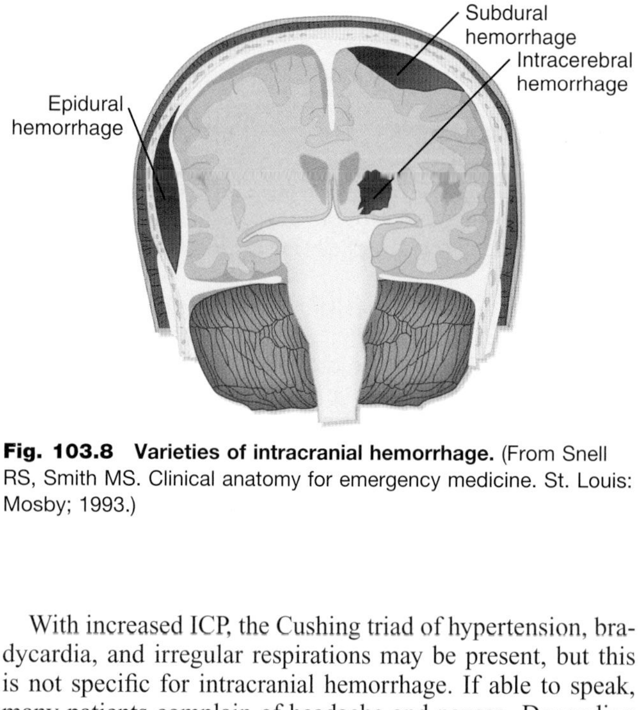

Subdural hemorrhage
Intracerebral hemorrhage
Epidural hemorrhage

**Fig. 103.8 Varieties of intracranial hemorrhage.** (From Snell RS, Smith MS. Clinical anatomy for emergency medicine. St. Louis: Mosby; 1993.)

## PRESENTING SIGNS AND SYMPTOMS

Intracranial hemorrhages of any type may be associated with a continuum of changes in mental status ranging from mild headache to agitation, confusion, and coma. Seizures and stroke symptoms are also common findings.

Patients with a large intracranial hemorrhage typically have a diminished level of consciousness with or without a focal neurologic deficit. Intracerebral hemorrhages are responsible for about 20% of acute strokes. It is not possible at the bedside to reliably distinguish between an ischemic stroke and an intracerebral hemorrhage.[9] Patients with a diminished level of consciousness often have a larger hemorrhage and increased ICP or distortion of the thalamic and brainstem reticular activating system.[1]

With increased ICP, the Cushing triad of hypertension, bradycardia, and irregular respirations may be present, but this is not specific for intracranial hemorrhage. If able to speak, many patients complain of headache and nausea. Depending on the region of brain injured, the examiner will often find corresponding neurologic deficits. With hemispheric lesions, the picture may be similar to ischemic stroke—that is, patients with a large left cerebral hemorrhage may have right-sided hemiparesis and aphasia. Other stroke syndromes of neglect, visual field defects, and cortical sensory abnormalities may be present. With frontal lesions, conjugate eye deviation toward the side of the lesion is common. Large hematomas with mass effects may present the clinical picture of uncal herniation with diminished consciousness and third nerve dysfunction,

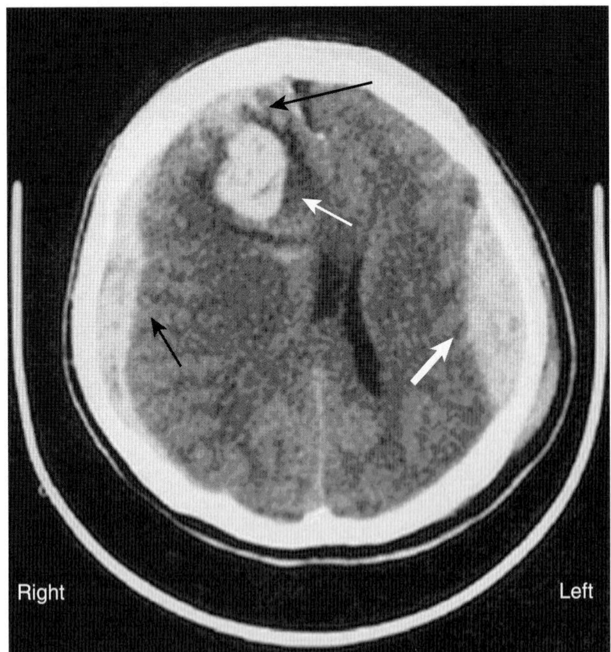


**Fig. 103.9** An axial section of a non–contrast-enhanced computed tomography scan of the head reveals four types of acute posttraumatic intracranial hemorrhage: an epidural hematoma *(thin white arrow)* on the left side, a laminated subdural hematoma *(short black arrow)* on the right side, right-sided periventricular and frontal lobe contusions containing an intraparenchymal hematoma *(thick white arrow)*, and a subarachnoid hemorrhage *(long black arrow)* in the right frontal region.

including a large, nonreactive pupil. Third nerve dysfunction usually occurs on the side of the mass lesion but in about 10% of cases is on the opposite side (falsely localizing third nerve palsy).

Patients with brainstem and posterior fossa hematomas may show brainstem dysfunction, including alteration in consciousness, abnormalities in extraocular motion, other cranial nerve abnormalities, and the so-called crossed signs, with cranial nerve dysfunction on one side and long-tract findings of weakness on the opposite side. One pathognomonic finding on physical examination occurs in patients with pontine hemorrhage, in whom truly pinpoint pupils (not just small) may be present.

Patients with cerebellar hemorrhages may have profound vegetative signs of diaphoresis and vomiting. A common finding is acute headache and inability to ambulate. Smaller cerebellar hemorrhages may demonstrate nystagmus, ataxia, dysmetria, or abnormalities in extraocular motion. If brainstem compression develops, consciousness may deteriorate abruptly.

SAH is typically manifested as the "worst headache of my life." Abrupt onset of a severe headache that quickly attains maximal intensity is the classic finding. This manifestation—abrupt severe headache reaching maximal intensity within seconds or moments of onset, perhaps occurring with exertion—often leads to the diagnosis. Syncope may be present at the onset of a hemorrhage. Meningismus may also be present. However, initial misdiagnosis of SAH occurs in up to 50% of cases.[10,11] The high-risk clinical characteristics of SAH have led to the derivation of preliminary decision rules, which remain under study.[12]

It is important to identify the diagnosis at the time of an initial or "sentinel" hemorrhage or warning leak. The sentinel hemorrhage may be manifested as a transient headache or confusional episode. If the patient complains of headache of abrupt onset or that the headache is different from the kind that the patient usually experiences, the possibility of SAH exists. Patients in whom the diagnosis is made at subsequent visits often have worse outcomes.

An expanding unruptured aneurysm may be accompanied by cranial nerve abnormalities. Typically, this is a third nerve paresis with asymmetric pupils and impairment of extraocular movement. The pupillary reflex may or may not be impaired.

With SAH and increased ICP, cardiac arrhythmias and changes on the electrocardiogram (ECG) consistent with myocardial ischemia may at times confound the diagnosis.[10] Usually, these patients have severe neurologic symptoms, but cases in which the arrhythmia overshadows the clinical findings are reported as well.

Intracerebral hemorrhage is the most common manifestation of arteriovenous malformations and accounts for roughly half the presentations. Other manifestations include seizures and focal neurologic deficits.[7]

A history of trauma suggests the possibility of an extraaxial hematoma. Progression of symptoms or deterioration in level of consciousness mandates investigation for an expanding mass lesion. With epidural hematoma, the classic description (present in only a minority of patients) is a transient loss of consciousness followed by an alert or lucid interval and later by progressively decreased level of consciousness. Headache out of proportion to the head blow or the presence of persistent vegetative symptoms such as nausea and vomiting is the more common manifestation. As the mass progresses, the neurologic findings may progress. Altered mental status following trauma is the typical clinical scenario.

Chronic large subdural hematomas may be found during evaluation of patients for altered mental status or headaches. Occult manifestations of intracranial injury are more common in the elderly.

## DIFFERENTIAL DIAGNOSIS AND MEDICAL DECISION MAKING

The major differential diagnosis of intracranial hemorrhage with focal neurologic signs or symptoms is ischemic stroke. Both processes may be associated with an abrupt onset of symptoms and focal neurologic deficits. Intracranial neoplasms are also in the differential diagnosis. However, the spectrum of findings in patients with intracranial hemorrhage is wide. Seizures are not a frequent initial complaint of patients with intracranial hemorrhage, although they do occur with enough frequency to include intracerebral hemorrhage and SAH in the differential diagnosis of seizures. Abnormal decerebrate posturing, which may occur with intracranial hemorrhage, is sometimes mistaken as seizure activity, particularly if it is brief and repetitive. Though counterintuitive, infectious processes such as encephalitis and meningitis may at times also have an abrupt onset of symptoms.

If altered mental status is the initial finding, all the causes of altered mental status should be included in the differential

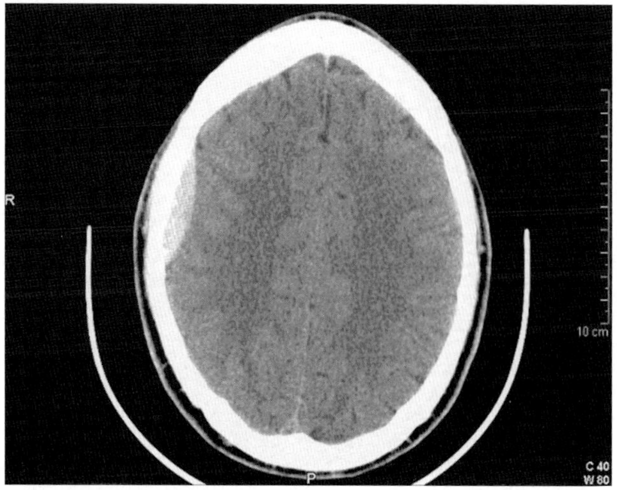

**Fig. 103.10 Computed tomography scan: acute epidural hematoma.** Note the high density of the hemorrhage and the lens-shaped clot.

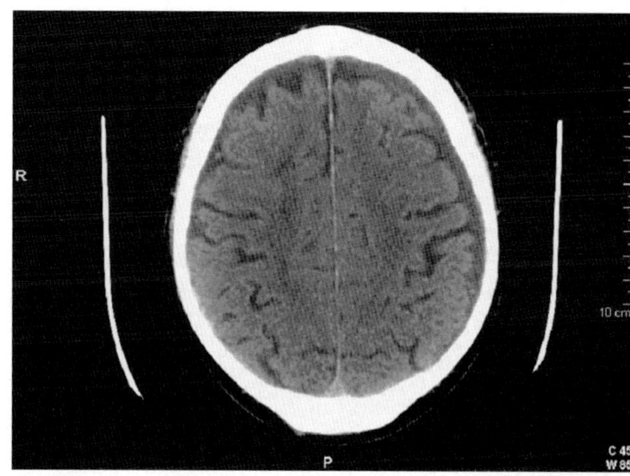

**Fig. 103.11 Computed tomography scan: chronic subdural hematoma (left hemispheric and bifrontal section).** Low density is consistent with the presence of hemorrhage for some days to weeks.

diagnosis (see Chapter 104). The expanded differential diagnosis for hemorrhages without focal lesions or altered mental status includes the universe of headache types. Functional headaches or thunderclap headaches are at times related to different types of exertion; however, they must be part of a diagnosis of exclusion for the EP.

Cranial CT is the current initial imaging test of choice for evaluation of intracranial hemorrhage because of the ability of non–contrast-enhanced cranial CT to demonstrate the presence of acute hemorrhage. Cranial CT is readily available in most U.S. EDs. Expert interpretation of cranial CT scans is sometimes not as readily obtainable, however, and EPs should be familiar with the basics of CT interpretation as it applies to immediate patient care.

In patients with suspected SAH, CT is very sensitive in detecting acute hemorrhage, with estimates of 95% or better.[11,13] Sensitivity starts to diminish as time from the hemorrhage increases, and CT sensitivity is estimated to be less than 50% 7 days after the event.

A suggested approach to analyzing CT scans (see Chapter 74) and a useful structure for communicating with consultants can be determined by asking the following series of simple questions:

1. Is blood present?
2. Where is the hemorrhage?
3. How much blood is present, and what is the effect?
4. What is causing the bleeding?

## QUESTION 1—IS BLOOD PRESENT?

Acute blood appears white or hyperdense on non–contrast-enhanced CT scans (**Fig. 103.10**). Some intracranial structures such as the dura or choroid plexus may calcify and at times simulate hemorrhage. As blood ages, it becomes increasingly low density or dark (**Fig. 103.11**). There is a time during this evolution when blood is nearly the same CT density as brain parenchyma and is therefore termed isodense. Rarely, the existence of an isodense hematoma must be inferred from cortical sulcus markings that do not reach the cranium. Clinically, the terms *acute, subacute,* and *chronic* are used to reflect the change in appearance on the CT scan, from hyperdense to isodense and finally hypodense. Nonhomogeneous density may be observed in some cases and is an indication of acute or acute on chronic bleeding. The possibility of hyperacute bleeding should always be kept in mind, with the areas of rapid bleeding appearing relatively hypodense within a larger, more dense area on CT (see Fig. 103.4).

## QUESTION 2—WHERE IS THE HEMORRHAGE?

If hemorrhage is present, it is then described as external to the brain substance (extraaxial), within the substance of the brain (intraaxial or intraparenchymal), or visible in the intraventricular and subarachnoid or cisternal spaces. Extraaxial hematomas have two basic types of appearance. Subdural hematomas are most often crescentic (see Fig. 103.3), whereas epidural hematomas have a typical lens-shaped pattern (see Fig. 103.4). An intraparenchymal hemorrhage may be located in the cerebrum (intracerebral hemorrhage) or in subcortical or brainstem structures. Intracerebral hemorrhages of hypertensive origin tend to be situated in deep white matter or the basal ganglia or are confined to one lobe of the brain (lobar) (see Fig. 103.1). These hemorrhages tend to have a stereotypic pattern, and deviation from these patterns may suggest an uncommon cause of the hemorrhage.

Cerebellar hemorrhages may be midline or hemispheric (**Fig. 103.12**) and may cause brainstem compression. SAH may be detected by high density in the suprasellar or perimesencephalic cistern or by blood in the cortical sulci, where ordinarily there should be low-density images from the cerebrospinal fluid signal. Depending on the degree of hemorrhage, SAH may be obvious (**Fig. 103.13**) or relatively subtle (see Fig. 103.2). Intraventricular hemorrhage (literally "blood within the ventricles") may result from rupture of an intracerebral hemorrhage into the ventricular system, from trauma, or from SAH (**Fig. 103.14**).

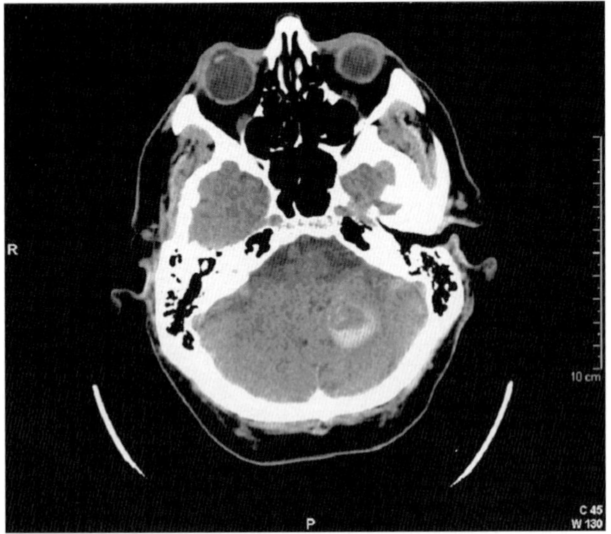


**Fig. 103.12 Computed tomography scan: acute hemispheric cerebellar hemorrhage.** The expanding mass in the posterior fossa places the brainstem at risk for compression.

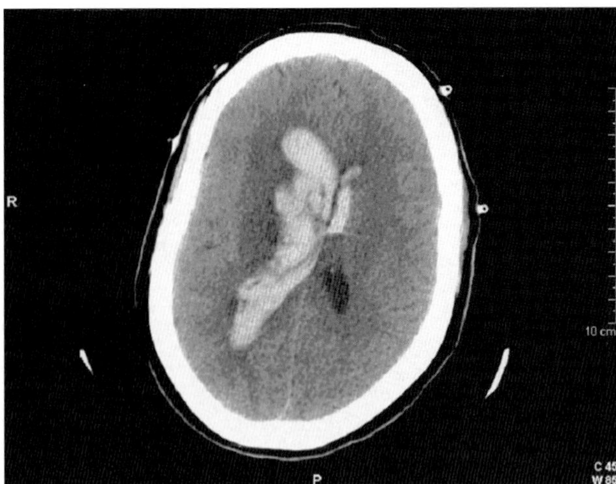


**Fig. 103.14 Computed tomography scan: intraventricular blood from extension of deep intracerebral hemorrhage.** The right lateral and third ventricles are filled with blood casts.

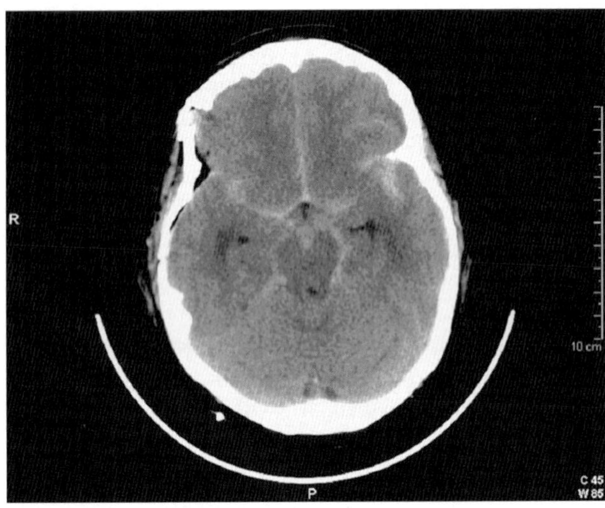


**Fig. 103.13 Computed tomography scan: acute subarachnoid hemorrhage.** Blood is present in the suprasellar cistern and over the hemispheres.

## QUESTION 3—HOW MUCH BLOOD IS PRESENT, AND WHAT IS THE EFFECT?

Some quantification of the hemorrhage should follow. For extraaxial hemorrhage, the greatest thickness of the hematoma is easily estimated from the ruler on the CT scan. Volumetric estimation of intraparenchymal hematomas may be estimated from information present on the cranial CT scan, although this is not usually done frequently by EPs. Because most hemorrhages are ellipsoid, the formula ABC/2 may be used to estimate the volume, where *A* is the greatest hemorrhage diameter on CT, *B* is the diameter 90 degrees to *A*, and *C* is the approximate number of CT slices with hemorrhage multiplied by slice thickness.[14] Of more importance is any effect that the hematoma is having on adjacent structures. This may be estimated qualitatively by noting any compression on the ventricular system and the amount of shift of midline structure, as well as by CT signs of herniation (subfalcine, uncal, tonsillar herniations).

## QUESTION 4—WHAT IS CAUSING THE BLEEDING?

Some cranial CT scan patterns of intracranial hemorrhage are sufficiently typical that an etiologic diagnosis may be suspected. For example, in a middle-aged or elderly patient with a spontaneous intracerebral hemorrhage in the deep white matter, the term *hypertensive hemorrhage* may be used. The same hemorrhage in a much younger patient might suggest a vascular lesion such as an arteriovenous malformation as the cause. One must remember that the specific cause of a hemorrhage seen on a CT scan is garnered from pattern recognition and is speculative to some degree.

Conventional angiography with selective injection of contrast material has traditionally been used when vascular lesions such as aneurysms or arteriovenous malformations are suspected. CT angiography with intravenously administered radiographic contrast material is increasingly being used instead of conventional angiography. Selection of direct vascular imaging is determined by a radiologist, neurologist, or neurosurgeon. (Discussion of this modality is outside the scope of this chapter.)

The role of magnetic resonance imaging (MRI) in current emergency medicine practice is evolving. In some centers, magnetic resonance angiography or venography is used, although again this is done in consultation with the admitting physicians or services. The traditional view is that MRI is inferior to CT when acute intracranial hemorrhage is suspected; however, recent literature suggests that with some technical adaptations, MRI may readily detect hemorrhages.

Lumbar puncture can increase the sensitivity for the detection of SAH in patients with negative or equivocal results on CT scanning. The common procedure is to collect cerebrospinal fluid in four tubes and obtain a cell count in tubes 1 and 4. Findings consistent with SAH include the presence of xanthochromia and a red blood cell count that does not diminish from tube 1 to tube 4. Xanthochromia from the breakdown of red blood cells may take more than 12 hours to develop and may not be present when lumbar puncture is performed soon after the onset of symptoms. The most common method of determining xanthochromia in the clinical laboratory is visual inspection, although some studies show that spectrophotometry is superior. Lumbar puncture performed to exclude SAH sometimes reveals unexpected diagnoses such as meningitis. Basic laboratory work should include coagulation studies and platelet counts if hemorrhage is suspected.

## TREATMENT

Supportive care including appropriate management of the ABCs—airway, breathing, and circulation—is of course important. The decision to perform endotracheal intubation is based on the judgment of the physician who assesses the patient's ability to protect the airway. It is recommended that certain steps be taken for rapid-sequence induction in patients with intracranial hemorrhage or other conditions with suspected increased ICP, including the use of lidocaine and a defasciculating dose of a paralytic agent, although rigorous proof of efficacy is lacking. In the past, hyperventilation was recommended with the goal of reducing abnormally increased ICP. Again, evidence is lacking, but the consensus is that hyperventilation beyond that needed to reduce $PaCO_2$ to only a small degree ($PaCO_2$ of 30 to 35 mm Hg) is not indicated.[15]

Blood pressure management in the setting of intracranial hemorrhage is controversial. In multiple-trauma patients with central nervous system injury, hypotension is associated with a poor outcome. In patients with intracerebral hemorrhage, the risk of expanding a hematoma associated with sustained hypertension must be weighed against the risk of impairing cerebral perfusion if blood pressure is reduced. A 2010 study suggested a trend toward more favorable outcomes in patients with aggressive blood pressure reduction but admitted that the study was underpowered and called for further investigation.[16] In patients with established intracerebral hematoma and hypertension, consensus at this time is to use intravenous agents that can be titrated, such as nitroprusside, labetalol, esmolol, or carvedilol, if needed, to maintain blood pressure with an MAP of less than 130 mm Hg. Systolic blood pressure greater than 180 mm Hg or diastolic blood pressure higher than 105 mm Hg on two readings taken 5 minutes apart are the criteria recommended for intervention.[15]

In patients with SAH, there is also no clear evidence-supported management strategy. Hypertension should be avoided in patients with a ruptured aneurysm by administering intravenous titratable agents, as described previously. Some experts argue that relative hypotension should be induced based on the theory that a ruptured aneurysm is at risk for rebleeding in the presence of hypertension. Once the aneurysm is secured by interventional techniques, blood pressure is allowed to return to normal levels. The calcium channel antagonist nimodipine is recommended to reduce the chance of ischemia from vasospasm.[5,6]

Management of increased ICP is conjectural if its existence is unknown. However, basic steps such as elevating the head of the bed, keeping the head midline, and avoiding painful stimulation are clearly indicated. Hyperventilation with the goal of reducing ICP is currently out of favor. Steroids have no proven benefit in patients with intracranial hemorrhage. Use of osmotic agents such as mannitol in cases in which a herniation syndrome is present may be useful as a temporizing measure when decompressive neurosurgical therapy is planned.

ICP monitoring may be useful in the ED but should be performed under the direction of a neurosurgeon or neurointensivist. Ventriculostomy may be performed in the ED by a neurosurgeon.

If a patient with intracranial hemorrhage has a seizure, the use of anticonvulsants is clearly indicated. Phenytoin and fosphenytoin are the current drugs of choice. Increasingly, levetiracetam seems to be used in these settings, though rigorous evidence for superiority is lacking. Use of anticonvulsants is common in patients with intracerebral hematomas who have not had seizures, although their efficacy is not based on evidence. Likewise, use of anticonvulsants in patients with SAH who have not had seizures is controversial.

Hyperglycemia and hyperthermia are associated with neuronal injury and should be avoided if possible and treated if present. No specific guidelines exist for the clinician at this time. If a coagulopathy is detected, appropriate treatment should be initiated (see the following discussion on warfarin coagulopathy).

In patients with intracranial hemorrhage, most activity in the ED is directed at diagnosis. Treatment is governed by the type of hemorrhage, its cause, and any associated medical and surgical conditions. Definitive treatment is under the direction of the consulting and admitting physicians, and the EP should work in concert with them. In most institutions, SAH and traumatic hemorrhage will be managed by neurosurgeons. Intracerebral hemorrhage is also often managed by neurosurgeons, but institutional management patterns vary. Intensive care and monitoring are necessary in many cases.

For deeply comatose patients, intensive supportive care is indicated in the short term. Evidence of the development of hydrocephalus on CT should lead to consideration of ventriculostomy. Drainage of cerebrospinal fluid and other supportive measures may be guided by continuous measurement of ICP by a variety of invasive techniques.

Cerebellar hemorrhage is an emergency requiring removal of the hematoma and relief of brainstem compression, which offers the possibility of good recovery in selected cases.[1] Surgery for removal of supratentorial intracerebral hematomas is controversial and not generally recommended.[17] Other inpatient supportive measures for intracerebral hemorrhage might include prophylaxis for thromboembolic events.

Patients with an acute intracerebral hematoma who are taking warfarin should receive fresh frozen plasma (FFP) and vitamin K as soon as possible to correct the coagulopathy. The best dosing regimens are not known, but for patients with a prolonged international normalized ratio, a reasonable recommendation is 5-10 mg of vitamin K (administered intravenously over a 10-minute period) plus 10 mL/kg of FFP administered as soon as possible. Type AB FFP is available in some blood banks and can speed administration time by eliminating the time needed for cross-matching. Institutional recommendation many vary. Time to treatment of warfarin-associated coagulopathy in patients with intracerebral hemorrhage has been found to be the most important determinant of 14-hour reversal of anticoagulation.[18]

Antiplatelet therapy has been noted to be associated with clinical deterioration.

Acute administration of recombinant activated factor VII limits expansion of hematomas, but it has limited use for thromboembolic complications.[19,20] Other procoagulant pharmaceutical preparations are under study.

In recent years the trend has continued for early surgical intervention for SAH—that is, intervention to isolate the aneurysm or occlude it within 1 to 2 days of bleeding.[5,6] Until the aneurysm is secured, the consensus is that blood pressure should be lowered with parenteral medications if necessary. A recent study reported that interventional endovascular coiling may lead to better outcomes in selected patients with ruptured aneurysms.[21]

Treatment of arteriovenous malformations is complex, controversial, and outside the practice of EPs other than providing supportive care as outlined previously. The risk for rebleeding is less than that with saccular aneurysms. Should seizures occur, anticonvulsant medication should be administered. Additional diagnostic vascular studies besides cranial CT are required and may include angiography, CT angiography, and MRI. Treatment may include radiotherapy, embolization of the arteriovenous malformation, resection, or any combination of these modalities.

All but the smallest epidural hematomas must be treated by craniotomy and surgical evacuation plus investigation of the bleeding site to secure hemostasis. Treatment of subdural hematomas depends on the size and chronicity of the hematoma, the general medical condition of the patient, and signs and symptoms referable to the hematoma. In some patients, chronic subdural hematomas may be of large size with seemingly minimal or no effect on the patient; the problem is underlying atrophy, with the subdural hematoma filling the void. Acute subdural hematomas are generally evacuated if they are causing any mass effect, but at times this may be difficult to assess because the underlying brain is usually injured and edematous.

In hemorrhages complicating abscesses, tumors, or other conditions, treatment is generally directed at the underlying lesion.

## FOLLOW-UP, NEXT STEPS IN CARE, AND PATIENT EDUCATION

If the facility does not have the necessary specialty care, the patient should be transferred after stabilization to an appropriate facility. The urgency of transport corresponds roughly with the clinical condition of the patient; for example, patients with a headache, a chronic subdural hematoma, and no other findings may probably be transferred electively. The necessity for transfer of stable alert patients with minimal symptoms and minute traumatic hemorrhages detected on CT has not been studied. The notable exceptions in which emergency transport is indicated include acute SAH, cerebellar hemorrhage, and epidural hematoma when the natural history includes early clinical deterioration.

## SUGGESTED READINGS

Brisman JL, Song JK, Newell DW. Cerebral aneurysms. N Engl J Med 2006;355:928-39.

Broderick JP, Connolly S, Feldman E, et al. Guidelines for the management of spontaneous intracerebral hemorrhage in adults. Stroke 2007;38:2001-23.

Edlow JA, Caplan LR. Avoiding pitfalls in the diagnosis of subarachnoid hemorrhage. N Engl J Med 2000;342:29-36.

Kothari RU, Brott T, Broderick JP, et al. The ABC's of measuring intracerebral hemorrhage volumes. Stroke 1996;27:1304-5.

Runchey S, McGee S. Does this patient have a hemorrhagic stroke? Clinical findings distinguishing hemorrhagic stroke from ischemic stroke. JAMA 2010;308:2280-6.

## REFERENCES

***References can be found on Expert Consult @ www.expertconsult.com.***

# Delirium and Dementia 104

Andy Jagoda and Haru Okuda

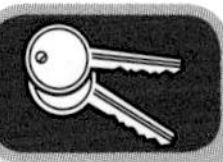

**KEY POINTS**

- Delirium is a medical emergency (not a psychiatric emergency) that can be superimposed on a chronic condition such as dementia.
- Because delirium is associated with high mortality, especially in the elderly, early recognition and treatment are essential.
- A systematic, detailed evaluation, including cognitive assessment, is critical to the diagnosis of delirium and differentiation of delirium from dementia.
- Hypoglycemia and hypoxia are easily identified and reversible causes of delirium.
- Infections and medication effects are common causes of delirium, and the management plan must focus on identifying and treating these processes.

## EPIDEMIOLOGY

Altered mental status affects 5% to 10% of patients seen in the emergency department (ED) and in up to 30% of the older population.[1] Delirium and dementia account for a significant proportion of the altered mental status. Hustey and Meldon reported that of 78 ED patients with changes in mental status, 62% had cognitive impairment without delirium and the remaining 38% had delirium.[2] In a study at a single tertiary care center, it was found that emergency physicians (EPs) missed the diagnosis of delirium in up to 75% of patients older than 65 years; either the condition was misdiagnosed or the patients were discharged home.[3] Some studies suggest a mortality rate as high as 9% in patients who are admitted to the hospital because of altered mental status. One study found that patients who were discharged home with unrecognized delirium had a mortality of 30.8% at 6 months.[4] The challenge for the EP, who has not generally seen the patient previously, is recognizing delirium—an acute process—when it is superimposed on dementia—a chronic process. Therefore, a systematic approach to ED evaluation is necessary.

Alzheimer dementia is the most common form of dementia in adults (occurring in 50% to 60% of patients), followed by vascular dementia (15% to 25%), Lewy body dementia (5%), and Parkinson dementia (5%).[5,6]

## DELIRIUM

### PATHOPHYSIOLOGY

The exact mechanism of delirium is not known, but it is believed to arise from an imbalance of neurotransmitters at the cortical and subcortical levels. The principal neurotransmitters implicated in causing delirium include dopamine, an excitatory neurotransmitter, and acetylcholine and γ-aminobutyric acid, inhibiting neurotransmitters.[7] Physiologic stressors such as infection, medications, and metabolic disturbances can alter the balance of the levels of neurotransmitters and lead to changes in cognition and attention. Inflammatory mediators such as cytokines and histamines are thought to be involved as well.

### PRESENTING SIGNS AND SYMPTOMS

Delirium is a syndrome and not a specific disease; therefore, identifying the underlying cause requires a comprehensive approach that includes a medical and family history, physical examination, bedside cognitive assessment, and diagnostic testing. The confusion assessment method is a useful tool to screen for delirium in the medical setting.[8] In an uncooperative or severely confused patient, information obtained from emergency medical service personnel and the patient's family, personal items brought in with the patient, and a detailed physical examination with close attention to vital signs are important. **Figure 104.1** provides a structured approach to assessing cognition at the bedside; patients who are oriented with immediate recall and the ability to sustain attention and recite months or digits in reverse but no delayed recall are unlikely to have delirium and should be suspected of having dementia.[8] The EP should consider all possible reversible medical causes of delirium so that treatment can be initiated as soon as possible (**Box 104.1**).

#### *Infection*

One of the most common causes of delirium in the elderly is infection. A simple urinary tract infection or pneumonia, which is easily handled by the immune system of a healthy adult, can have deleterious effects on the mental balance of an elderly patient who has little physiologic reserve. Progression to sepsis often worsens the delirium and can lead to

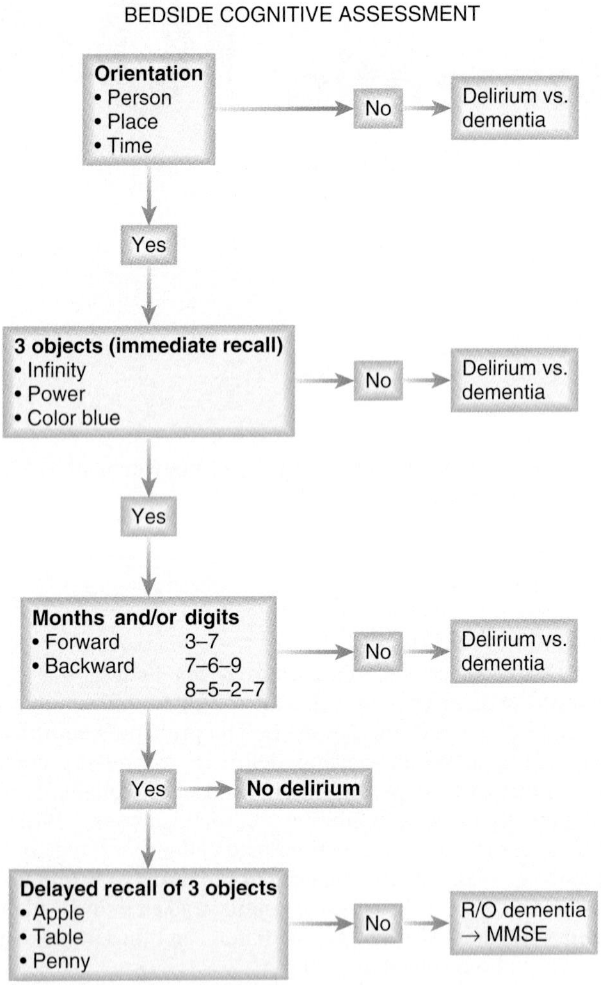

BEDSIDE COGNITIVE ASSESSMENT

**Orientation**
- Person
- Place
- Time

→ No → Delirium vs. dementia

↓ Yes

**3 objects (immediate recall)**
- Infinity
- Power
- Color blue

→ No → Delirium vs. dementia

↓ Yes

**Months and/or digits**
- Forward 3–7
- Backward 7–6–9, 8–5–2–7

→ No → Delirium vs. dementia

↓ Yes → **No delirium**

**Delayed recall of 3 objects**
- Apple
- Table
- Penny

→ No → R/O dementia → MMSE

**Fig. 104.1 Bedside assessment of cognition.** *MMSE*, Mini-Mental State Examination; *R/O*, rule out.

**BOX 104.1 Causes of Delirium**

**Infections**

Systemic
- Urinary tract infection, pneumonia

Central nervous system
- Meningitis, seizures, encephalitis, abscess, mass

Human immunodeficiency virus
- Toxoplasmosis, cytomegalovirus, *Cryptococcus*

**Metabolic and Fluid Disorders**

Electrolyte
- Hypoglycemia, hyperglycemia, hyponatremia, hypercalcemia

Hypovolemia
- Dehydration, bleeding

Other
- Uremia, hepatic encephalopathy

**Drugs**

Withdrawal
- Alcohol, benzodiazepines

Illicit and abuse
- Sympathomimetics, hallucinogens, alcohol

Prescription medications (see Box 104.2)

**Cerebrovascular**

Medical
- Hypertensive emergency, stroke

Traumatic

**Hypoxia and Hypercapnia**

Pulmonary
- Asthma, chronic obstructive pulmonary disease, pulmonary embolism

Hematologic
- Carbon monoxide, methemoglobinemia

Endocrine
- Hyperthyroidism, hypothyroidism, Cushing syndrome, hyperparathyroidism

**Environment and Toxicity**

Toxic exposure
- Pesticides, cyanide, carbon monoxide, methemoglobinemia, lead, mercury

Temperature
- Heat stroke, hypothermia

Other
- Bites, stings, plants (see Box 104.4)

**Vitamin Deficiency**
- Vitamin $B_1$, vitamin $B_{12}$

coma. A history of recent coughing, fever, or urinary symptoms can help establish the diagnosis of delirium in elderly patients. Central nervous system infections range from localized abscess, meningitis, and encephalitis to late manifestations of syphilis. All these disease forms may be accompanied by symptoms of delirium ranging from minimal changes in mental status to severe confusion.

## *Metabolic, Fluid, and Electrolyte Disturbances*

Hypoglycemia is a common cause of delirium seen in the ED and one that is readily treatable. Patients can have symptoms ranging from mild agitation to coma. As a note of caution, delirium from hypoglycemia may not be suspected in patients with a hypoglycemia-induced focal neurologic deficit or seizure. A history of diabetes, medications, and the time of the last meal are important; documentation of the administration of dextrose and other medications by the emergency medical service should be obtained.

Diabetic ketoacidosis and hyperosmolar hyperglycemic nonketotic coma can both be manifested as an acute confusional state. Hyperosmolar hyperglycemic nonketotic coma is seen more commonly in elderly patients with no history of diabetes or in patients with adult-onset diabetes and an underlying stressor such as infection.

Hyponatremia can cause delirium, but it is related to the rate of sodium reduction and not the absolute quantity. A patient with a slight, sudden decrease in serum sodium can have delirium, whereas a larger, more gradual reduction (over days) is well tolerated by many patients. Hyponatremia has many causes, from underlying medical conditions such as the syndrome of inappropriate secretion of antidiuretic hormone to intentional and unintentional water ingestion.

Hypercalcemia may be associated with delirium. The normal range of total serum calcium is between 8.5 and 10.5 mg/dL. Patients with calcium elevated above this range can exhibit confusion, depending on the rate of increase.

Patients with end-stage kidney and liver disease can also have delirium. The patient's medical history or family members may document dialysis or a history of encephalopathy. The underlying process causing the encephalopathy, such as infection or lack of compliance with treatment, should be investigated.

### *Drug Withdrawal*

Alcohol withdrawal in its severe form can cause delirium, which is known as delirium tremens. These patients will be seen in the ED with agitation and possible confusion. Visual or auditory hallucinations (or both) and delusions can also be part of the clinical findings and can contribute to misdiagnosis in these patients with a primary psychiatric disorder. Diagnosis of delirium tremens is based on a history of chronic alcohol abuse and symptoms of acute confusion and sympathetic hyperactivity. Typically, the last drink of alcohol was more than 48 hours before arrival at the ED. Vital signs may show severe hypertension, hyperthermia, and tachycardia. On physical examination, the patient often exhibits postural tremor and hyperreflexia.

Withdrawal from chronic benzodiazepine abuse can have a similar manifestation, although the onset of the symptoms varies, depending on the time of the last dose and the half-life of the drug.

### *Drug Toxicity*

Alcohol intoxication is a common finding in the ED. The patient is often agitated, confused, and combative. This patient population is more susceptible to other causes of delirium, including infection, trauma, and concomitant ingestion of drugs; a thorough, unbiased evaluation is therefore important.

Common classes of abused drugs causing delirium include sympathomimetics such as cocaine and amphetamine and hallucinogens such as lysergic acid diethylamide (LSD) and ketamine. Close attention to vital signs and identification of a toxic syndrome (toxidrome) are essential in making the diagnosis. Patients with sympathomimetic toxicity may have significant increases in heart rate, blood pressure, and temperature with associated hyperactivity, agitation, and diaphoresis. Clinical findings associated with ketamine abuse include vertical and rotatory nystagmus, midpositioned pupils, hallucinations, labile affect, hyperthermia, and muscle rigidity. Mild tachycardia and hypertension may be seen. Investigation of personal belongings for pills and interview with family members may augment the diagnosis. Anticholinergic medications are also commonly used in the ED and outpatient settings. Delirium associated with mydriasis, hyperthermia, anhydrosis, and hyperemia is seen in this toxidrome.

Many commonly prescribed medications can cause delirium as a result of improper dosing, change in metabolism, intentional overdose, and drug-drug interactions (**Box 104.2**).[9] Family members or the patient's personal physician may be able to provide valuable information about recent changes in medication dosages or the addition of new medications.

**BOX 104.2 Medications Associated with Delirium**

**Anticholinergics**
$H_1$ receptor blockers (diphenhydramine, meclizine, hydroxyzine)
Antiparkinson drugs (benztropine)
Phenothiazine (promethazine)

**Antidepressants**
Tricyclics (amitriptyline, nortriptyline)
Selective serotonin reuptake inhibitors (fluoxetine, sertraline)

**Sedatives**
Benzodiazepine (alprazolam, diazepam)

**Analgesics**
Opioids (codeine, morphine)

**Antiinflammatory Agents**
Nonsteroidal antiinflammatory drugs (aspirin, ibuprofen)
Corticosteroids (hydrocortisone, prednisone)

**Antihypertensives and Antiarrhythmics**
Beta-blockers (metoprolol, propranolol)
Angiotensin-converting enzyme inhibitors (lisinopril, captopril)
Calcium channel blockers (amlodipine, nifedipine)
Other (digoxin)

**Antibiotics**
Quinolones (levofloxacin, ciprofloxacin)
Macrolides (azithromycin, clarithromycin)

**Anticonvulsive Agents**
Barbiturates (phenobarbital)

### *Cerebrovascular Disorders*

Delirium is a common complication after an acute stroke and is reported in up to 48% of patients.[10] Despite case reports of delirium being the primary manifestation of an acute stroke,[11] it is more frequently reported as a sequela of the event. Delirium has been associated with left-sided infarcts and thalamic and caudate nucleus strokes. Delirium after stroke has been linked to longer hospital stay and increased mortality.

Hypertensive emergency is associated with delirium if target organ damage affects the brain and causes hypertensive encephalopathy. Blood pressure is typically elevated significantly. Other signs of end-organ damage include heart failure and renal failure.

Delirium can develop as a result of a primary traumatic brain injury or the consequent secondary injury. Aggressive systematic evaluation of the reversible secondary causes of acute confusion after a traumatic brain injury is necessary while maintaining optimal cerebral perfusion and oxygenation. Intracerebral bleeding or edema, or both, must be suspected in patients in whom a change in mental status develops after a traumatic brain injury.

### *Hypoxemia and Hypercapnia*

Acute elevations in $P_{CO_2}$ and low $P_{O_2}$ can cause alterations in cognition and awareness. Pulmonary disorders such as pneumonia, pulmonary embolism, asthma, and pneumothorax can cause hypoxia. Abnormal chest excursion and rate, depth, and effort of breathing are significant findings on the physical examination. Symptoms important in the history include dyspnea, fever, cough, and pleuritic chest pain, as well as recent travel and a family history of connective tissue disease.

Hypercapnia is a normal finding in many patients with chronic obstructive pulmonary disease, but an acute rise in $P_{CO_2}$ can lead to an alteration in consciousness. Oxygenation is not an adequate measurement of ventilation, and therefore serial monitoring of the patient's mental status should be initiated in the absence of bedside capnography.

### Endocrine Disorders

Patients with endocrine disorders such as hyperthyroidism, hypothyroidism, Cushing syndrome, and hyperparathyroidism may have altered mental status when seen initially in the ED.[12] Delirium is more common with severe manifestations of these diseases, as in the case of thyroid storm and myxedema coma. Abnormalities in vital signs, such as tachycardia and fever in thyroid storm and bradycardia and hypotension in myxedema coma, may be the only initial clues to the diagnosis.

### Chemical Exposure

Delirium may be the initial symptom in patients exposed to a chemical weapon or contaminated environment. History of the exposure is important, but the patient often displays confusion and no history is available. If chemical exposure is suspected, the patient must be brought to the proper decontamination area immediately. Universal precautions should be practiced, as well as use of a proper-level hazmat suit. The patient should be stabilized and evaluated for findings on examination and vital signs suggesting the cause of the contamination and thus the antidote (**Box 104.3**).

**BOX 104.3 Chemical Agents Associated with Delirium**

**Organophosphates**
Sarin (isopropyl methylphosphonofluoridate)
Diethyl parathion
VX (*O*-ethyl *S*-2-[diisopropylamino]ethyl-methylphosphonothioate)

**Carbamates**
Aldicarb (Tres Pasitos)
Propoxur (Baygon)

**Organochlorines**
DDT (dichlorodiphenyltrichloroethane)
Lindane

**Other**
DEET (diethyltoluamide)
Pyrethrins

### Environmental Agents

Stroke from heat exposure occurs in the very young and the elderly, but exertional heatstroke can occur acutely in persons of all age. Heatstroke can be manifested as confusion, hyperthermia (temperature typically higher than 40° C), tachycardia, tachypnea, and hypotension. Delirium may be the initial finding because the central nervous system is often the first organ system to be affected by the elevation in temperature.

In contrast to heat illnesses, patients suffering from cold exposure can exhibit acute confusion. Patients with temperatures below 35° C can demonstrate apathy, slurred speech, confusion, forgetfulness, and shivering. As the temperature drops further, the symptoms progress from delirium to coma.

Exposure to plants, insect stings, and animal bites may all result in delirium related to the toxin or chemical involved in the exposure. The initial finding may be related to the cause of the injury or rash, but progression to systemic complications can ensue rapidly.

### Central Nervous System Disease

Depending on the location of the mass, intracerebral tumors can be manifested as delirium without focal motor deficits. Frontal lobe tumors are more commonly associated with acute changes in personality or behavior.

Absence seizures, seen primarily in children 5 to 10 years of age, are characterized by acute-onset altered mental status without motor activity. The seizure episodes typically last for seconds and resolve without a postictal state. Complex partial seizures can also be accompanied by an acute change in mental status. Patients with nonconvulsive status epilepticus (absence or complex partial) may have a change in mental status that can vary in intensity and duration.[13] Nonconvulsive status can occur in patients of all ages and without any previous history of a seizure disorder. Clinical findings vary from a minor change in mental status to full-blown psychotic or comatose states. The hallmark of nonconvulsive status epilepticus is a change in mental status that occurs in the absence of motor activity and is associated with characteristic electroencephalographic changes. Motor activity, when present, is subtle and in the form of mild twitching of the lips or the upper or lower extremities, but no clear tonic-clonic activity is present.

### Vitamin Deficiency

Deficiency in certain vitamins can cause altered mental status. Patients with Wernicke encephalopathy, which is caused by a deficiency of thiamine (vitamin $B_1$), can exhibit delirium, ataxia, and ophthalmoplegia. Advanced cases of vitamin $B_{12}$ deficiency can also cause altered mental status, along with a history of paresthesias, weakness, diarrhea, and loss of appetite.

## DIFFERENTIAL DIAGNOSIS AND MEDICAL DECISION MAKING

If delirium is excluded after a thorough work-up of a patient with confusion, other causes of altered cognition should be considered. An elderly patient with newly recognized or worsening dementia may arrive at the ED with an acute decline in consciousness. Family members may recall changes in memory and function over a longer period, thus suggesting dementia rather than delirium (**Table 104.1**).

First-time manifestations of psychiatric disorders or exacerbation of underlying psychiatric disease can often be confused with delirium as a result of their similar characteristics. Because patients with psychiatric illness can exhibit delirium, medical and reversible causes of the confusion must be excluded before transfer of care to a psychiatrist[14] (see the

**Table 104.1 Clinical Characteristics of Delirium versus Dementia**

| CHARACTERISTIC | DELIRIUM | DEMENTIA |
|---|---|---|
| Onset | Acute | Insidious |
| Course | Fluctuating | Progressive |
| Orientation | No | Yes |
| Attention | Impaired | Intact |
| Cognitive function | Impaired* | Impaired |
| Speech | Pressured or unintelligible | Normal |

*Some of the cognitive impairments reported in patients with delirium may actually be due to inattention.

Priority Actions box "Tests Useful in the Diagnosis of Delirium").

## TREATMENT

Once the cause of the delirium is discovered, appropriate treatment should be initiated immediately. Antibiotic therapy should be started in patients with suspected meningitis, hypoglycemia should be corrected with dextrose, and patients with hypoxia should receive oxygen supplementation. Delay in diagnosis and treatment can increase overall morbidity and mortality.

Pharmacologic management of agitation is sometimes necessary when a patient with delirium is a danger to self or others or if the agitation is impeding medical evaluation and management. Current pharmacologic options include typical and atypical antipsychotic agents and benzodiazepines.[15] Both droperidol and haloperidol are generally safe and effective and cause less respiratory depression than benzodiazepines do. However, the benzodiazepines, midazolam or lorazepam, may be preferable in particular clinical scenarios such as drug withdrawal or overdose. It is important to remember to reduce dosing in elderly patients because they have altered pharmacodynamics and pharmacokinetics. There is currently no good literature to support the use of atypical antipsychotics in the acute management of delirium.

# DEMENTIA

## PATHOPHYSIOLOGY

At the anatomic level, Alzheimer dementia is characterized by atrophy of both cortical and subcortical structures, which is seen most prominently in the hippocampus and temporal cortex. Histologic examination reveals an accumulation of extracellular amyloid plaques and neurofibrillary tangles that attract inflammatory mediators and impede delivery of neurotransmitters along the axons, respectively. Deficiencies in the neurotransmitters acetylcholine and norepinephrine are also thought to be responsible for the dementia in Alzheimer disease. Pathophysiologic and clinical characteristics of the types of dementia are presented in **Table 104.2**.[16]

**PRIORITY ACTIONS**

### Tests Useful in the Diagnosis of Delirium

**Infections**

Pneumonia—Chest radiography, blood culture
Urinary tract infection—Urinalysis, urine culture
Human immunodeficiency virus—Head contrast-enhanced CT, lumbar puncture

**Metabolic Disorders**

Hypoglycemia, hyperglycemia—Glucose fingerstick test, serum chemistry panel
Electrolyte abnormalities—Serum chemistry panel, ECG
Hypovolemia—Vital signs, hematocrit
Uremic encephalopathy—Blood urea nitrogen, serum chemistry panel

**Drugs**

Withdrawal—History and vital signs
Illicit and abuse—History and vital signs

**Cerebrovascular Disorders**

Hypertensive emergency—ECG, serum chemistry panel
Stroke—Head CT and/or head MRI, ECG, radiography
Intracerebral bleeding, axonal injury—Head CT

**Hypoxia and Hypercapnia**

Asthma and chronic obstructive pulmonary disease—Pulse oximetry, capnography
Pulmonary embolism—$\dot{V}/\dot{Q}$ scan or CT angiography of the chest, D-dimer
Carbon monoxide—Carboxyhemoglobin level, CO-oximetry
Methemoglobinemia—Serum methemoglobin level, CO-oximetry

**Endocrine Disorders**

Thyroid storm—Vital signs
Myxedema coma—ECG, serum chemistry panel, glucose fingerstick test
Acute adrenal failure—Serum chemistry panel (K ↑, Na ↓, glucose ↓)

**Toxic Exposure**

Pesticides—Toxidrome

**Thermal Disorders**

Heat stroke—Temperature, ECG, liver function test, serum chemistry panel
Hypothermia—Temperature, ECG

**Central Nervous System Disorders**

Meningitis and encephalitis—Lumbar puncture
Abscess—Head contrast-enhanced CT or MRI
Mass—Head CT
Seizure—Head CT

**Vitamin Deficiency**

Vitamins $B_1$ and $B_{12}$—Serum vitamin assays

*CT*, Computed tomography; *ECG*, electrocardiogram; *MRI*, magnetic resonance imaging; $\dot{V}/\dot{Q}$, ventilation-perfusion.

## PRESENTING SIGNS AND SYMPTOMS

Alzheimer disease is characterized by a gradual onset of dementia, as defined by the *Diagnostic and Statistical Manual of Mental Disorders*, fourth edition (**Box 104.4**), with continuous functional decline. The cognitive impairment seen in Alzheimer disease is not explained by other causes of dementia. Most patients in the ED with Alzheimer disease will already carry the diagnosis and probably have an associated complication such as infection or exacerbation of the dementia.

Because the clinical manifestation of dementia is subtle and gradual, it is important to maintain a high index of suspicion in the evaluation of elderly patients in the ED. Initial symptoms, such as depression, fatigue, insomnia, and irritability, can be nonspecific. Inquiring about missing appointments and increased forgetfulness can be helpful, but patients often avoid discussing difficulties in cognitive abilities by changing the subject. Family members or caregivers may bring patients to the ED because they are unable to care for them or because the patients are no longer able to care for themselves. It is important to recognize early dementia (mild cognitive impairment) in the ED setting to prevent secondary complications such as injuries from falls and fires, noncompliance with medications, and malnutrition and dehydration. Evaluation for a reversible cause of dementia and delirium must be initiated.

Although dementia has a reversible cause in less than 5% of these patients, a thorough history and physical examination must be undertaken to identify this subcategory (see the Priority Actions box "Tests Useful in the Diagnosis of Reversible Causes of Dementia"). Normal-pressure hydrocephalus is characterized by ataxia, urinary incontinence, and dementia, all of which are reversible. Diagnosis is made by CT scan of the head and the finding of elevated opening pressure on lumbar puncture. Treatment is surgical insertion of a shunt.

### BOX 104.4 DSM-IV Criteria for Dementia

1. Memory impairment (inability to learn new information or to recall previously learned information)
2. At least one of the following:
   a. Aphasia (language disturbance)
   b. Apraxia (problems with motor activities despite intact motor function)
   c. Agnosia (problems recognizing or identifying objects despite intact sensory function)
   d. Disturbance in executive functioning (planning, organizing, sequencing, abstracting)
3. The deficits listed above significantly impair social or occupational functioning and are a significant decline from a previous level of functioning.
4. The deficits do not occur exclusively during the course of an episode of delirium.
5. The deficits are not better accounted for by another disorder.

*DSM-IV, Diagnostic and Statistical Manual of Mental Disorders*, fourth edition.

## DIFFERENTIAL DIAGNOSIS AND MEDICAL DECISION MAKING

*Pseudodementia* is a term used to describe patients who appear to be demented but are actually severely depressed. Differences from genuine dementia can be subtle; patients with pseudodementia usually have a preexisting history of depression with acute onset (often after a specific event), emphasize and appear more distressed about the cognitive deficits, and have preserved attention. If the diagnosis of depression is suspected, patients should be asked about thoughts of suicidality and their social support structure. Appropriate consultation and follow-up with a psychiatrist or social worker or hospitalization may be necessary to ensure the patient's safety.

**Table 104.2** Clinical and Pathophysiologic Symptoms and Signs in Types of Dementia

| | SYMPTOMS AND SIGNS | |
|---|---|---|
| DISORDER | CLINICAL | PATHOPHYSIOLOGIC |
| Alzheimer disease | Gradual and continuing functional decline not explained by another cause of dementia | Amyloid plaques, neurofibrillary tangles, hippocampal and temporal atrophy |
| Vascular dementia | Sudden onset, focal neurologic findings, stepwise deterioration | Multiple infarcts |
| Lewy body dementia | Visual hallucinations, fluctuating cognition, mild parkinsonism seen less than 1 yr before dementia | Lewy bodies, Lewy neuritis |
| Parkinson dementia | Extrapyramidal signs, visual hallucinations, fluctuating cognition | Lewy bodies, Lewy neuritis |
| Frontotemporal dementia (Pick disease) | Personality changes, restlessness, disinhibition, impulsiveness, ataxia, parkinsonism | Pick bodies, frontal and temporal atrophy |
| Infectious dementia (Creutzfeldt-Jakob) | Visual disturbances, ataxia, myoclonus, progressive dementia | Prion protein accumulation, spongiform change of brain |

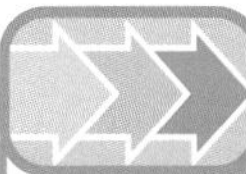

**PRIORITY ACTIONS**

**Tests Useful in the Diagnosis of Reversible Causes of Dementia**

**Central Nervous System Disorders**
Normal-pressure hydrocephalus—Head CT, lumbar puncture
Subdural hematoma—Head CT

**Infections**
Neurosyphilis—VDRL and RPR tests, lumbar puncture
AIDS—HIV titers

**Heavy Metal Toxicity**
Lead—Blood lead assay
Mercury—Urine mercury assay

**Endocrine Abnormalities**
Hypothyroidism—Serum assay for thyroid-stimulating hormone

**Vitamin Deficiency**
- Vitamins $B_1$ and $B_{12}$—Serum vitamin assay

*AIDS*, Acquired immunodeficiency syndrome; *CT*, computed tomography; *HIV*, human immunodeficiency virus; *RPR*, rapid plasmin reagin; *VDRL*, Venereal Disease Research Laboratory.

### TREATMENT

As with the treatment of delirium, reversible causes of dementia should be addressed and treatment initiated immediately. Frequently, the dementia will have no reversible cause; the patient has a new diagnosis of dementia or worsening of an underlying condition. In such cases, disposition is based on the patient's ability to function independently at home or on the family's capacity to care for the patient. If the family is unable to further care for the patient, admission to the hospital for evaluation for nursing home placement or assisted home care is necessary. If there is adequate support by family and patient safety can be ensured, the work-up of patients with new-onset dementia can be done in an outpatient setting with appropriate coordinated care by the primary physician.

Cholinesterase inhibitors are often used in the treatment of mild to moderate Alzheimer-type dementia; vitamin E has also been recommended to slow the progression of Alzheimer dementia.[17] Cholinesterase inhibitors have been recommended to improve quality of life and cognitive function. However, despite the frequent use of these medications, the literature on the benefit of cholinesterase inhibitors remains controversial.[18]

## FOLLOW-UP, NEXT STEPS IN CARE, AND PATIENT EDUCATION

Disposition depends on the cause of the delirium or dementia and the patient's response to treatment. If the patient does not improve or the cause is not found, the patient should be transferred to the appropriate inpatient facility. In some cases, with improvement in baseline values the patient can be discharged home.

## SUGGESTED READINGS

American Academy of Neurology. Detection, diagnosis and management of dementia: AAN guideline summary. Available at http://www.aan.com/professionals/practice/pdfs/dementia_guideline.pdf. Downloaded January 2, 2011.

American College of Emergency Physicians. Clinical policy for the initial approach to patients with altered mental status. Ann Emerg Med 1999;33:251-81.

Han J, Wilson A, Ely EW. Delirium in the older emergency department patient: a quiet epidemic. Emerg Med Clin North Am 2010:28:611-31.

Han JH, Zimmerman EE, Cutler N, et al. Delirium in older emergency department patients: recognition, risk factors, and psychomotor subtypes. Acad Emerg Med 2009;16:193-200.

Koita J, Riggio S, Jagoda A. The mental status examination in emergency practice. Emerg Med Clin North Am 2010; 28:439-51.

## REFERENCES

***References can be found on Expert Consult @ www.expertconsult.com.***

# 105 Neurologic Procedures

*Brian A. Stettler and Edward C. Jauch*

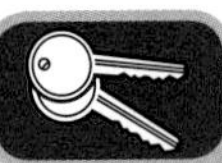

**KEY POINTS**

- Topical anesthetics (especially in children), liberal use of subcutaneous lidocaine, and small doses of anxiolytic agents can expedite performance of lumbar puncture in an anxious patient.
- To obtain an accurate opening pressure, patients should lie on their side with the head supported by a pillow and the legs straight. Cerebrospinal fluid should be allowed to equilibrate in the manometer before reading.
- A smaller-gauge needle with the bevel of the needle angled parallel to the dural fibers or use of a small-diameter blunt-tipped needle will decrease the frequency of post–dural puncture headache.

## EPIDEMIOLOGY

Lumbar puncture (LP), the most common invasive neurologic procedure, is performed daily by emergency physicians (EPs) to evaluate a wide range of chief complaints in the emergency department (ED), including headache, altered mental status, and fever. To optimize patient care, it is important for the EP to be knowledgeable about the indications for this procedure, as well as be proficient in its performance.

Other emergency neurologic procedures, including ventriculostomy for drainage of cerebrospinal fluid (CSF), intracranial pressure (ICP) monitoring, and aspiration of an indwelling ventriculoperitoneal (VP) shunt, are performed less frequently and usually only in consultation with a neurosurgeon.

## LUMBAR PUNCTURE

EPs perform LP to diagnose and treat a variety of neurologic complaints. Currently, this procedure is used mainly in the ED for assessment of headache or altered mental status. CSF analysis and opening pressure (OP) measurements obtained from the LP can make or exclude the diagnosis of meningitis, subarachnoid hemorrhage (SAH), pseudotumor cerebri, and other diseases with high morbidity. Although performance of LP is considered relatively safe, patients with a suspected mass lesion or ventricular obstruction may have a theoretic risk for herniation; in such cases neuroimaging may be warranted before LP.[1]

### PROCEDURE

After explaining the procedure to the patient and obtaining informed consent, the patient is placed on the side on a flat stretcher with a pillow under the head. The procedure is typically started with the patient placed in the fetal position and the person performing the procedure seated facing the patient's back. Administration of a small dose of an anxiolytic, such as midazolam, is helpful in anxious patients. Depending on the response to the medication, pulse oximetry may be appropriate.

The iliac crest is located and the thumbs used to palpate and identify the spinous processes in the midline of the back. This is roughly the L4-L5 interspace and is an appropriate interspace to use. In adults, the L3-L4 interspace can also be used because both lie below the termination of the spinal cord within the spinal canal. An absorbent towel is placed under the patient, and the patient's back is cleansed with the skin preparation solution (povidone-iodine or chlorhexidine) by making circular motions to scrub the back in gradually expanding circles, starting at the midline of the L4-L5 interspace and out to the iliac crests and lower thoracic spine; the skin should be allowed to dry between wipes (**Figs. 105-1 and 105-2**). The procedure may be facilitated by having the patient sit and lean over a bedside table while being stabilized by a helper, but this prevents measurement of OP. In anatomically challenging patients, ultrasonography and fluoroscopic guidance may aid in the identification of landmarks.

Once the patient and physician are in positions of comfort, the landmarks are reassessed and lidocaine is injected subcutaneously with a 27- or 25-gauge needle at the identified interspace to anesthetize the skin (**Fig. 105.3**). In children, topical application of anesthetic before injection may reduce the initial discomfort. After 1 to 2 minutes the deeper tissues are anesthetized by advancing a longer, 22-gauge needle slowly and injecting lidocaine. Achieving sufficient anesthesia is critical to success of the procedure.

Once anesthesia is achieved, the landmarks are checked yet again. A 22-gauge spinal needle is used to advance into the previously identified space (**Fig. 105.4**). The bevel of the needle is kept parallel to the dural fibers, which run cephalad

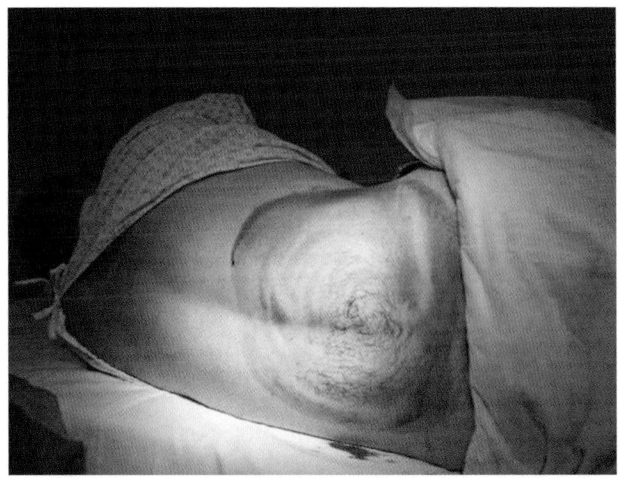

**Fig. 105.1** Lumbar puncture procedure showing patient preparation.

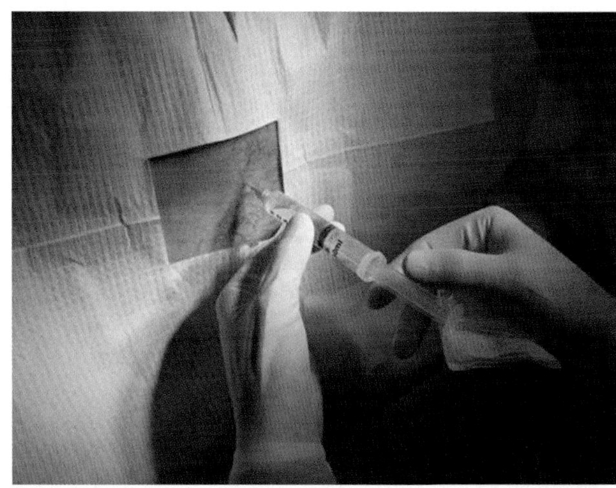

**Fig. 105.3** Lumbar puncture procedure showing placement of local anesthetic.

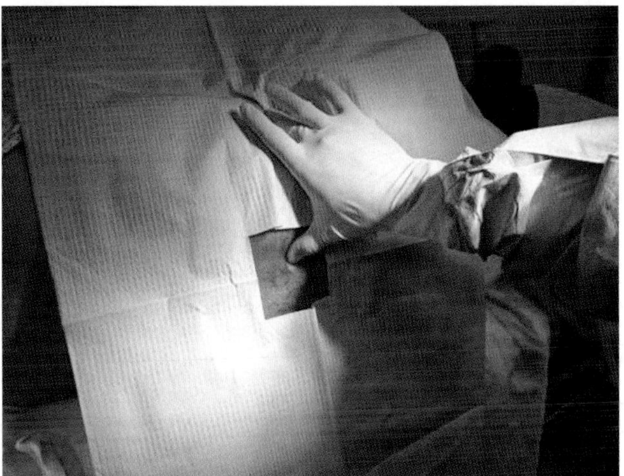

**Fig. 105.2** Lumbar puncture procedure showing identification of the interspace.

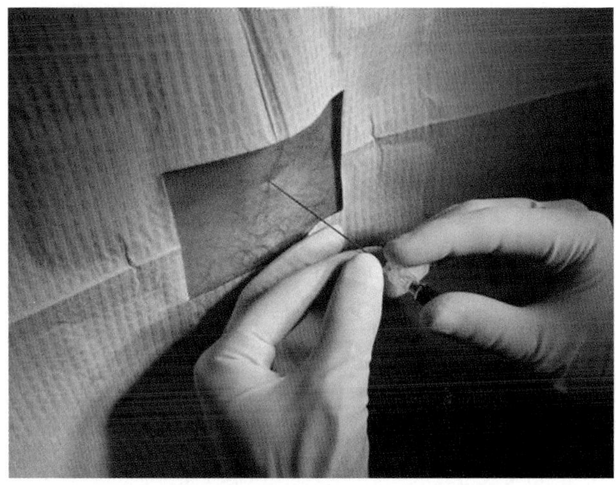

**Fig. 105.4** Lumbar puncture procedure showing insertion of the needle.

to caudad, to minimize the incidence of post–dural puncture headache (PDPH). The needle is advanced slowly while controlling it at the skin with the nondominant hand. Angling the needle slightly cephalad may be required because of the orientation of the spinous processes. The widely discussed "pop" of the needle penetrating the dura is not always felt; after traversing the ligamentum flavum, removal of the introducer every few millimeters of advancement may identify CSF. It is important to keep the orientation of the needle in the midline to avoid nerve roots as they exit the spinal canal.

Once CSF is observed, the manometer is attached to measure OP (**Fig. 105.5**). The patient's legs are straightened while the patient is lying on the side, and the EP waits for CSF to equilibrate in the manometer column (slight respiratory variation will be noted) (**Fig. 105.6**). The fluid meniscus is the OP, which in the absence of obstructive hydrocephalus is equivalent to ICP.

One to 2 mL of CSF is placed into each of four tubes, the introducer stylet is replaced in the needle, the needle is

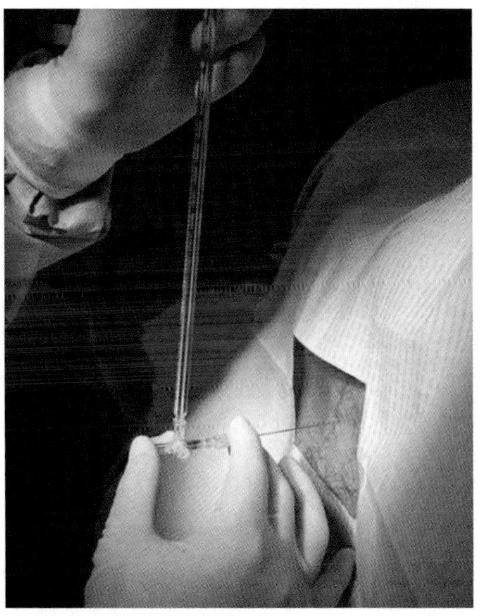

**Fig. 105.5** Lumbar puncture procedure showing measurement of intracranial pressure.

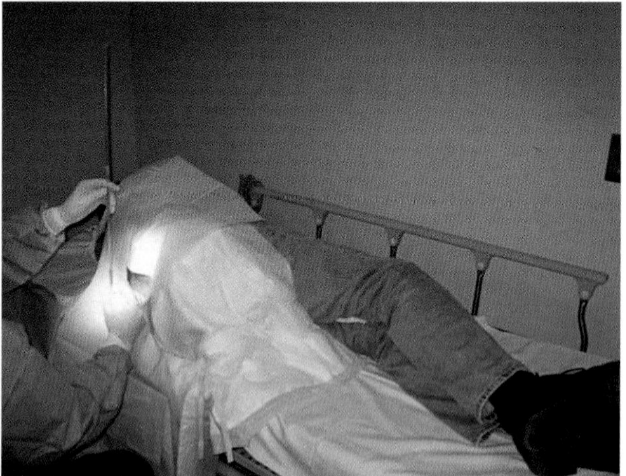

**Fig. 105.6 Lumbar puncture procedure showing measurement of intracranial pressure.**

removed from the patient's back, and pressure is briefly applied over the puncture site with a piece of gauze. Residual skin preparation solution is washed off and a bandage applied over the puncture site. At this point the patient may be returned to any position of comfort.

### COMPLICATIONS

PDPH is the most common complication associated with LP, with a rough incidence of 5% to 40%. Factors associated with PDPH include the technique and the type and gauge of needle used.[2] PDPH develops about 2 days after the performance of a dural puncture, is worse with standing, and is partially relieved by lying down. The exact cause of this complication is uncertain, but it possibly due to continued leakage of CSF through the dural rent created by the needle. The headache is typically self-limited but can last up to a week and be fairly debilitating.

Several strategies can be used to reduce the incidence of PDPH, including orientation of the bevel of sharp-tipped needles parallel to the dural fibers to avoid cross-cutting of the fibers, the use of atraumatic blunt-tipped spinal needles (Pajunk, Sprotte) with a noncutting tip and side port, and reinsertion of the introducer into the noncutting needle before removal of the needle.[3-5] The patient's position following dural puncture or the periprocedural use of intravenous (IV) fluids is not associated with the development or prevention of PDPH. PDPH can be treated by reassurance and administration of IV fluids, analgesics, and IV caffeine. Severe headaches may require the placement of a blood patch, which is curative in 80% to 90% of cases.

Other complications of LP are less common, but potentially more serious. Development of a spinal epidural hematoma is more common in the setting of anticoagulation, platelet disorders, thrombocytopenia, and hypocoagulable conditions and may represent a surgical emergency. As with all invasive procedures, infections such as vertebral osteomyelitis, meningitis, or abscess can be minimized by observing strict sterile technique. In procedures performed at the proper level (i.e., L3-L4 or lower in an adult and L4-L5 or lower in a child), cauda equina or nerve root injury is not a common complication.

## CEREBROSPINAL FLUID ANALYSIS

CSF testing varies depending on the indication for LP. If central nervous system (CNS) infection is suspected, a Gram stain and bacterial culture should be obtained. This may be performed on any CSF sample because all fluid should be sterile. CSF cultures, assays, or tests for other organisms should be ordered as indicated, including viral and fungal cultures, assay for cryptococcal antigen, India ink, testing for acid-fast bacilli, and other specific pathogens. Some of these assays may require more than 1 to 2 mL of CSF, so extra fluid should be obtained from immunocompromised patients or when unusual pathogens are suspected.

In the setting of infection, CSF protein concentrations may be elevated and absolute CSF glucose concentrations and CSF-serum glucose ratios are often depressed. In general, when CSF analysis reveals high protein and low glucose concentrations relative to serum glucose, the EP should maintain a high index of suspicion for infection.

CSF cell counts must be determined in the setting of infection, primarily to assess the number and type of leukocytes present in the CSF.[6] If the CSF obtained during LP is obviously bloody or blood-tinged, cell counts should be performed on multiple tubes and the number of leukocytes corrected for the number of erythrocytes present.[7] The typical anecdotal correction applied in the past is 1 leukocyte for every 500 erythrocytes in a traumatic tap. More than 5 leukocytes per high-power field in CSF is considered abnormal, although CNS infections typically yield higher values. Lower leukocyte counts still above the cutoff may also signify CNS vasculitis, viral infection, or malignancy, depending on the cell type present.

When concern for SAH exists, cell counts obtained from tubes 1 and 4 should be used for comparison. A specific value has not been established to determine the number of erythrocytes that differentiate a traumatic tap from SAH; however, the number of cells in the last tube collected should be substantially less than those in the first sample collected in the setting of a traumatic tap. CSF should also be analyzed for the presence of xanthochromia (yellow discoloration) when SAH is suspected, preferably by spectrophotometry for maximum sensitivity and specificity. Xanthochromia from erythrocyte lysis and enzymatic degradation of hemoglobin in CSF develops 12 hours after the initial hemorrhage. The presence of xanthochromia suggests SAH versus traumatic LP; its absence immediately after the onset of symptoms does not rule out SAH, however. Xanthochromia persists for at least 1 week, and its presence thereafter suggests repeated bleeding or an alternative explanation.

## INTRACRANIAL PRESSURE MONITORING

Placement of an invasive ICP monitor is typically performed in the setting of traumatic brain injury (TBI).[8] Patients with suspected TBI and an associated Glasgow Coma Scale score of 7 to 8 or less often require ICP monitoring because an adequate neurologic examination may be difficult to perform in these patients. Sustained elevations in ICP, greater than 15 to 20 mm Hg, are associated with worse clinical outcomes. To assess ICP in patients with an unreliable neurologic examination, a monitor can be placed directly overlying the dura or into the ventricles.[9] When performed on an emergency basis in the ED, these devices are typically placed by neurosurgeons in sterile fashion at the bedside. Furthermore, placement of an invasive monitor should be reserved for patients with some chance for meaningful recovery from their injuries.[10]

## VENTRICULOPERITONEAL SHUNT ASPIRATION

VP shunts are placed for persistent hydrocephalus caused by congenital malformations, previous SAH, obstructive processes such as neoplasms, and normal-pressure hydrocephalus. Aspiration of a VP shunt is typically performed when CNS infection is suspected in patients seen in the ED with headache, fever, or altered mental status. The reservoir can also be used to aspirate larger volumes of CSF in the setting of a malfunctioning shunt and acute hydrocephalus. A standard shunt assembly consists of a catheter tip located in the ventricle, shunt tubing traversing the cerebrum and exiting the skull, and a CSF reservoir and check valve placed subcutaneously under the scalp. The shunt is tunneled down the neck and empties into the peritoneum. Aspiration of a VP shunt should be done only in consultation with a neurosurgeon; the EP performing the procedure should have some experience in the procedure. Only shunts that have a reservoir are amenable to aspiration.

### PROCEDURE

Shunt aspiration is a relatively simple procedure that involves palpation of the reservoir under the scalp as a landmark. Once the landmark is identified, the skin is prepared in sterile fashion. Absolute sterility is imperative because the procedure violates the sterile space of the CNS through a retained foreign body (i.e., the shunt) and infection can result.

The location of the reservoir is subcutaneous, so its depth below the skin and therefore the depth of needle penetration should be only the thickness of the scalp. Once sterility is ensured, a 23- or 25-gauge butterfly needle is introduced into the reservoir, with the bevel of the needle contained within the reservoir. If desired, a manometer can be connected to the butterfly needle so that pressure within the CNS can be assessed. If so, a larger-gauge needle such as a 23 gauge may be needed to produce more accurate results. CSF is then aspirated for standard CSF analysis as discussed previously.

### COMPLICATIONS

The most common complication of VP shunt aspiration is infection, which can potentially result in meningitis or encephalitis. Other complications include subdural hemorrhage from overly aggressive CSF decompression, bleeding or persistent CSF leakage from the site of aspiration, and disruption of the valve by a misplaced attempt at aspiration.

## SUGGESTED READINGS

Arendt K, Demaerschalk BM, Wingerchuk DM, et al. Atraumatic lumbar puncture needles: after all these years, are we still missing the point? Neurologist 2009;15:17-20.

Ellenby MS, Tegtmeyer K, Lai S, et al. Videos in clinical medicine. Lumbar puncture. N Engl J Med 2006;355(13):e12.

Straus SE, Thorpe KE, Holroyd-Leduc J. How do I perform a lumbar puncture and analyze the results to diagnose bacterial meningitis? JAMA 2006;296:2012-22.

## REFERENCES

***References can be found on Expert Consult @ www.expertconsult.com.***

# Allergic Disorders

*Aaron N. Barksdale and T. Paul Tran*

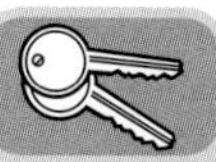

**KEY POINTS**

- Allergy refers to inappropriate responses (hypersensitivity) by the host's immune system.
- Anaphylaxis is an acute, potentially fatal, systemic allergic reaction. Deaths in patients with anaphylaxis are caused by acute respiratory failure.
- Foods, medications, and insect stings are the most common agents causing anaphylaxis.
- Epinephrine is the first-choice medication in the treatment of anaphylaxis, with $H_1$ and $H_2$ antihistamines and steroids being helpful adjuncts.
- Most cases of angioedema are mediated by IgE and respond to allergic therapy. Certain forms of angioedema, however, are mediated by bradykinin and may respond to new classes of medications, the kallikrein inhibitor (ecallantide) and C1 esterase inhibitor concentrates (Cinryze, Berinert).

## ALLERGIC DISEASE: ALLERGIC RHINITS, INSECT STINGS, DRUG ALLERGY

## EPIDEMIOLOGY

The prevalence of allergic disorders, including the incidence of anaphylaxis, has been increasing worldwide in the last few decades and is a topic of intensive study.[1,2] Features of Western lifestyles, such as changes in infant diets, widespread use of antibiotics, smaller family size, and cleaner child care, are believed to reduce stimulatory antigenic exposure in an individual's early years. This has led to an environment in which the immune system is dominated by a persistent allergy-prone system.[3]

### ALLERGIC RHINITIS

It is estimated that up to 42% of Americans suffer from some form of allergic rhinitis at any one time,[4] and it has been shown to have a strong correlation with asthma. In recent studies, nearly 40% of adults with allergic rhinitis were also found to have asthma, and 80% of asthmatics demonstrated signs of rhinitis.

### INSECT STINGS

Serious systemic reactions to insect stings are rare and occur in 1% of children and 3% of adults. Anaphylactic reactions account for approximately 50 deaths annually in the United States. There is a 2 : 1 male-to-female distribution, and adult male agricultural workers are considered the most vulnerable population. Individuals who experience large local reactions are less likely to have a systemic reaction (5% to 10%).[5]

### DRUG ALLERGY

A drug allergy is defined as an immune-mediated adverse response to a drug. An adverse drug reaction is defined as a noxious, unintended, or undesired response to a drug taken at a normal dose for the prevention, diagnosis, or treatment of a disease,[6] and a drug side effect is an expected and known (adverse) effect of taking the drug that is not the intended therapeutic outcome. Although the true frequency is unknown, drug allergy is thought to account for approximately one third of adverse drug reactions.[7] Adverse drug reactions affect 10% to 20% of hospitalized patients and more than 7% of the general population.

## PATHOPHYSIOLOGY

The immune system protects the host by distinguishing self from nonself; it tolerates the former but attacks the latter.[8,9] Allergy, allergic diseases, and hypersensitivity reactions arise when our immune system reacts inappropriately to allergens with resultant harm to the host.[1,2,10,11] For allergic diseases to occur, predisposed individuals need to first be exposed to an allergen through a process called sensitization.

The term *atopy* is used to describe the propensity in affected patients to produce IgE in response to otherwise innocuous environmental allergens. Atopic patients have higher serum levels of IgE antibody and a propensity for the development of one or more atopic diseases (e.g., allergic asthma, allergic rhinoconjunctivitis, atopic dermatitis, urticaria, angioedema).

Hypersensitivity reactions are mechanistically divided into four types of reactions according to the Gell and Combs classification system (**Box 106.1**). The immediate hypersensitivity reaction (type I), which is mediated by IgE, serves as the classic model of the immune response to allergen. On initial exposure to allergen, T helper 2 ($T_H2$) cells are activated, which results in the production of an array of cytokines that exert their effects on the T cells themselves, B cells, and antigen-presenting cells. IgE is elaborated and attached to the high-affinity Fc receptor on the surface of mast cells and basophils. Fixation of allergen-specific IgE leads to a series of cellular and molecular changes that prime these cells for future exposure. On reexposure, allergen cross-links the cell-bound IgE on the surface of mast cells and basophils, thereby setting in motion a complex cascade of events that lead to the release of preformed mediators such as histamine, lipid mediators, and cytokines and subsequent activation of various inflammatory pathways. These mediators and products of secondary inflammatory pathways cause adherence and chemotaxis of inflammatory cells, increased capillary permeability, vasodilation, smooth muscle contraction, and sensory nerve stimulation. A few allergen molecules can thus cause the release of a large number of mediator molecules in a designed amplification response. Examples of type I hypersensitivity reactions include allergic rhinitis, allergic asthma, urticaria, angioedema, and anaphylaxis.

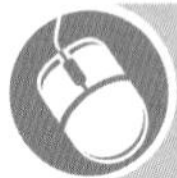

See Box 106.1, Types of Hypersensitivity, online at www.expertconsult.com.

Allergens are typically carbohydrate or protein molecules (or parts of a larger molecule) that elicit an immune response.[10]

The inflammation that occurs in allergy is divided into three temporal phases.[10] Early-phase reactions occur within minutes of exposure and are considered immediate type I hypersensitivity reactions. Late-phase reactions typically occur within 2 to 6 hours and peak 6 to 9 hours after exposure. This response is thought to be due to newly synthesized cytokines, growth factors, and chemokines, which were released more slowly than the preformed mediators primarily responsible for the early-phase reaction. This reaction often involves airway narrowing and hypersecretion of mucus in the lungs, in addition to the erythema, warmth, and pain experienced in the skin. In some individuals there is no clinical distinction between the early and late phases. Chronic allergic inflammation is the final phase in the inflammatory process. It occurs after persistent or repetitive exposure to specific allergens and results in tissue remodeling and structural changes in affected cells. Chronic allergic inflammation can further increase epithelial injury, mucus production, and thickening of airway walls.

The majority of serious sting-related reactions are caused by insects belonging to the order Hymenoptera (yellow jackets, hornets, honeybees, wasps, and fire ants).[5] Their venom contains histamine, dopamine, various peptides, and protein enzymes that are either vasoactive or can elicit significant allergic reactions (IgE mediated).

## PRESENTING SIGNS AND SYMPTOMS

### ALLERGIC RHINITIS

A detailed history is important in making the diagnosis of allergic rhinitis. Patients often acknowledge a history of seasonal allergies (hay fever). Patients with allergic rhinitis frequently suffer from symptoms such as eye itching, swelling, and discharge (clear or can resemble strings of cheese); nasal congestion; itching of the nose; sneezing; rhinorrhea; and mild cough. Patients may report a temporal association with exposure to certain environment allergens (seasonal allergy, pollen, mold, animal dander). On physical examination, the nasal membranes are swollen with enlarged, pale turbinates and a clear nasal discharge. The maxillary sinuses may feel full and tender on palpation.

### INSECT STINGS (HYMENOPTERA VENOM ALLERGY)

Patients with systemic allergic reactions from stings may exhibit generalized urticaria, angioedema, wheezing, stridor, anxiety, or other signs of respiratory and circulatory insufficiency. Most stings, however, cause self-limited local reactions consisting of redness, pain, and itching at the site of the sting. These reactions typically develop within minutes and usually last for a few hours. Local reactions rarely put patients at risk for future systemic reactions.[5] Fire ant stings tend to produce pustulelike lesions. Local stings that result in subsequent swelling near the oropharynx (either cutaneous or deep) can cause airway compromise, and affected patients should be observed in the emergency department (ED) until the symptoms have resolved.

### DRUG ALLERGY

Most allergic reactions occur within 1 hour of taking the medication, and symptoms typically include urticaria, morbilliform rash, itching (lips, tongue, face), or sensitivity to light. Symptoms of anaphylaxis may also occur (see later in chapter). Late symptoms (1 to 2 weeks) include fever, muscle and joint aches, and swollen lymph nodes.

## DIFFERENTIAL DIAGNOSIS AND MEDICAL DECISION MAKING

### ALLERGIC RHINITIS

**Box 106.2** lists other diagnostic considerations in patients with symptoms that may mimic allergic rhinitis.[12] Patients older than 20 years should be investigated for nonallergic causes (e.g., polyps). Atopic patients with severely inflamed conjunctivae, lids, and periorbital structures should raise the possibility of atopic keratoconjunctivitis (**Fig. 106.1**) and vernal keratoconjunctivitis (**Fig. 106.2**). These two types of chronic allergic conjunctivitis have the potential to cause corneal erosions and ulcers leading to vision loss and should be managed in consultation with an ophthalmologist.

Typically, no diagnostic tests need to be performed in the ED. Specific IgE serum assays such as the radioallergosorbent test (RAST), enzyme-linked immunosorbent assay (ELISA), skin prick test, and nasal smears are usually performed by allergists.

### INSECT STINGS (HYMENOPTERA VENOM ALLERGY)

Considerations include secondary bacterial infection, cellulitis, abscess, urticaria, angioedema, and anaphylactic reaction. Screening laboratory examinations for infection (complete blood count, wound culture) should be done if signs of infection are noted on physical examination.

**BOX 106.2 Causes of Rhinorrhea and Nasal Obstruction**

**Nonallergic Rhinitis with Eosinophilia Syndrome**
Nasal smears negative for allergens but with an abundance of eosinophils

**Mechanical Obstruction**
Foreign body
Previous trauma involving the septum
Polyps
Adenoid disease

**Infectious Rhinosinusitis**
Primary or secondary bacterial, viral, or fungal infections

**Vasomotor Rhinitis**
Profuse, clear rhinorrhea and nasal congestion—may be triggered by environmental conditions such as cold air, odors, or changes in atmospheric pressure or by the ingestion of hot or spicy foods

**Drug Induced**
Includes entities such as rhinitis medicamentosa (rebound from prolonged use of topical decongestants)
May be triggered by aspirin, nonsteroidal antiinflammatory drugs, or oral contraceptive use

**Systemic Disease**
Wegener disease, sarcoidosis
Head trauma

Modified from Greiner AN. Allergic rhinitis: impact of the disease and considerations for management. Med Clin North Am 2006;90:17-38.

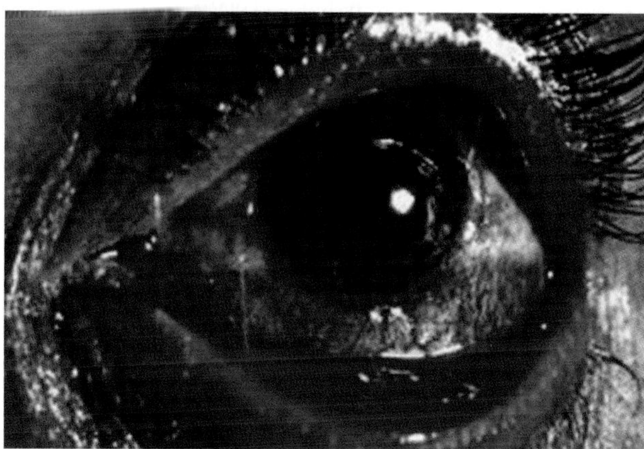

**Fig. 106.1** **Atopic keratoconjunctivitis.** (From Baba I. Red eye—first aid at the primary level. Community Eye Health 2005;18:70-72.)

## DRUG ALLERGY

Understanding the involvement of an immunologic mechanism in drug allergy may help physicians in determining whether a reaction represents an adverse drug reaction or a true drug allergy. For example, the stomach discomfort that may result from taking nonsteroidal antiinflammatory drugs (NSAIDs) is an adverse drug event and not a drug allergy. Factors that favor a drug allergy include a history of previous

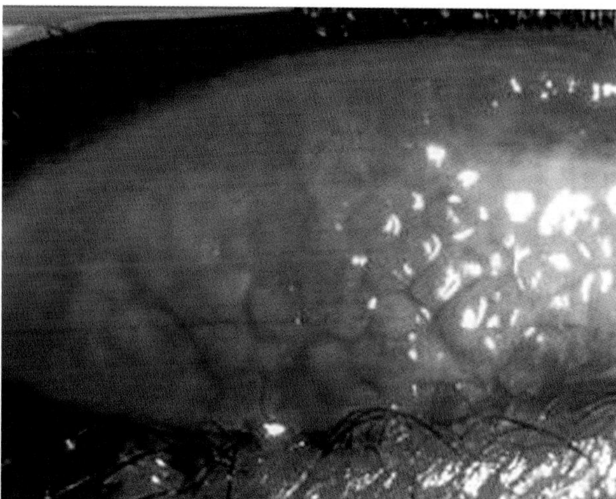

**Fig. 106.2** **Vernal keratoconjunctivitis.** Notice the lumpy appearance on the conjunctivae. (From Yorston D, Zondervan M. Red eye picture quiz. Community Eye Health 2005;18:72-78.)

sensitization (the drug was taken before) and typical allergic symptoms (urticaria, angioedema, wheezing).

Common entities to consider are infection (viral exanthem, mononucleosis, Rocky Mountain spotted fever, syphilis, cellulitis, sepsis), insect bite, pityriasis rosea, serum sickness, vasculitides, contact dermatitis, fixed drug eruption, and drug hypersensitivity syndrome.

Diagnosis of an adverse drug reaction relies on a careful history and thorough skin examination. A complete blood count, chemistry panel, and erythrocyte sedimentation rate may be ordered to evaluate possible infections or vasculitis. Skin testing is of limited value. RAST and ELISA for serum IgE require known immunogenic epitopes for the drugs, information that is usually unavailable. In cases of hemolytic anemia, the indirect Coombs test can be used to diagnose immune-mediated destruction of red blood cells.

Studies show that 4.4% of patients whose penicillin allergy history was confirmed by a positive skin test experienced an allergic reaction to cephalosporins.[13] Only 10% to 20% of patients who report a history of penicillin allergy are truly allergic when assessed by skin testing.[14] Although the overall risk for a cross-allergic reaction to cephalosporins in patients with a history of a penicillin allergy is low, the use of cephalosporins requires weighing the risks versus benefits based on an informed discussion between the patient and treating physician. **Table 106.1** shows the incidence of allergic reactions to penicillin.[15] Some factors can transiently cause T cells to falsely identify the penicillin epitope as being allergic. For example, in up to half (50%) of patients with mononucleosis, a maculopapular rash develops after taking amoxicillin. These same patients often have no adverse drug reaction on subsequent challenge with amoxicillin at a later time. Penicillin allergy should not be diagnosed in such patients.

# TREATMENT

## ALLERGIC RHINITIS

Oral second-generation $H_1$ blockers (loratadine, fexofenadine), oral decongestants (pseudoephedrine), and nasal

**Table 106.1 Estimated Incidence of Allergic Reactions to Penicillin**

| TYPE OF REACTION | MANIFESTATION | TIME OF OCCURRENCE AFTER FIRST DOSE | PERCENTAGE OF PATIENTS SHOWING REACTION |
|---|---|---|---|
| Late | Rash | ≥72 hr | 1.4 |
| Accelerated | Urticaria | 1-72 hr | 0.3 |
| Immediate | Generalized urticaria | 2-30 min | 0.3 |
| | Anaphylaxis | 2-30 min | 0.04 |
| | Death from anaphylaxis | | 0.001 |

From Asthma and the other allergic diseases. NIAID Task Force Report, NIH Publ No. 79-387. Bethesda, MD: National Institutes of Health; 1979.

decongestants (oxymetazoline, phenylephrine) can be used for mild, intermittent symptoms.[16] Moderate to severe and persistent nasal symptoms may require the addition of intranasal steroid (fluticasone, triamcinolone, budesonide), or chromone derivative such as cromoglycate and nedocromil. An intraocular antihistamine (olopatadine), intraocular chromone, or intraocular ketorolac can be used for ocular allergies, including conjunctivitis.[17]

### INSECT STINGS (HYMENOPTERA VENOM ALLERGY)

The stinger should be removed if present. For minor local reactions, antihistamines and NSAIDs such as ibuprofen should be sufficient. Ice can be used to decrease the inflammation, and elevation will decrease the swelling. The pseudopustules caused by fire ant stings contain mostly necrotic material and should not be unroofed. These lesions should be managed similar to second-degree burns, with the therapeutic goal being pain control and minimization of the risk for secondary bacterial infection.

Treatment of large local reactions includes cold compresses, NSAIDs, $H_1$ antihistamines, and high-potency topical steroids. Prednisone (1 mg/kg or 60 mg orally) as a single dose or for 5 days might decrease local swelling. The swelling typically resolves in 7 to 10 days. Antibiotics should be prescribed only if signs of secondary bacterial infection are present. Coverage for methicillin-resistant *Staphylococcus aureus* should be considered. Management of systemic reactions to stings is similar to that for anaphylaxis.

### DRUG ALLERGY

The most prudent approach in managing possible drug allergy–related complaints in the ED is to discontinue use of the suspect medication or medications, treat the allergic symptoms, and prescribe a suitable alternative drug or drugs. Severe symptoms should be treated in the same way as anaphylaxis (see Box 106.8). Patients with Stevens-Johnson syndrome and toxic epidermal necrolysis require a multidisciplinary approach that includes an intensivist, burn surgeon, and endocrinologist or allergist. For minor allergic drug reactions, $H_1$ antihistamines can be prescribed for itching, flushing, and rash. Steroids are reserved for serious or extensive drug reactions.

## FOLLOW-UP, NEXT STEPS IN CARE, AND PATIENT EDUCATION

### ALLERGIC RHINITIS

Patients are advised to avoid allergens when practically feasible. Those who are sensitive to pollen should minimize time spent outdoors during periods of high pollen counts and lessen the allergen load indoors by keeping windows closed. Use of HEPA (high-efficiency particulate air) filters, infestation control (cockroach), and impermeable covers for mattresses and pillows may also decrease the severity of symptoms.

### INSECT STINGS (HYMENOPTERA VENOM ALLERGY)

Patients with systemic reactions to stings warrant overnight observation in the hospital. Patients with limited or large local reactions can be managed as outpatients.

Patients with urticaria or angioedema reactions should be referred to an allergist for possible skin testing and v enom immunotherapy. These patients should wear a Med-Alert bracelet. Before discharge it is important that patients be educated about prevention of stings (always wearing shoes when outdoors and not wearing brightly colored clothes or fragrances in high-risk areas), the early signs of a systemic reaction, and how to self-administer an Epi-Pen. At least two Epi-Pens should be prescribed for emergency self-injection.

### DRUG ALLERGY

The majority of patients with late (>1 hour to days) reactions to medications who have a mild to moderate rash can be safely discharged home. Those with immediate drug reactions (<1 hour) need to be observed in the ED. Patients with a systemic reaction whose symptoms resolve after a 4- to 6-hour observation period in the ED can be discharged home in the company of a family member. They should be prescribed two Epi-Pens, $H_1$ antihistamines, a short course of steroids, and a Med-Alert bracelet. Patients at risk for a recurrent systemic drug reaction who have poor social support, comorbid conditions, and moderate to severe allergic syndromes warrant a hospital stay. At the end of the ED visit, patients should be educated about the nature of a drug allergy versus an adverse drug reaction.

# URTICARIA

## EPIDEMIOLOGY

Urticaria (hives) is a fairly common reaction that affects approximately 20% of the population at some point in their lifetime.[18] It has numerous different underlying causes and consists of several different types and subtypes. Spontaneous urticaria is broadly divided into acute (<6 weeks) and chronic (≥6 weeks) forms, with the latter representing approximately 10% to 20% of cases.

## PATHOPHYSIOLOGY

The classic wheal lesions associated with urticaria are the result of edema within the mid and upper dermal layers of the skin. Dilation of lymphatic vessels and capillary venules allows extravasation of protein-rich fluid into the surrounding tissue. This complex inflammatory process involves a variable mixture of macrophages, T cells, neutrophils, eosinophils, and mast cells.[19]

## PRESENTING SIGNS AND SYMPTOMS

Patients with urticaria usually have hives of variable duration and location.[20,21] Urticarial lesions are pruritic, erythematous, raised rashes that blanch on palpation. The lesions are typically round or oval with serpiginous borders, but they may vary in color, size, and shape (**Fig. 106.3**). They may be localized or appear throughout the body, but there is a slight predilection for the trunk, hands, feet, lips, tongue, and ears. Urticaria usually starts with erythema (flare) as a result of capillary vasodilation in the superficial layer of the dermis. As the protein-rich fluid extravasates into surrounding tissue, it evolves into raised wheals and may change from red to white. A history of pruritic red rash that changes in size and shape, with extension and regression over a period of hours or days, favors the diagnosis of urticaria.

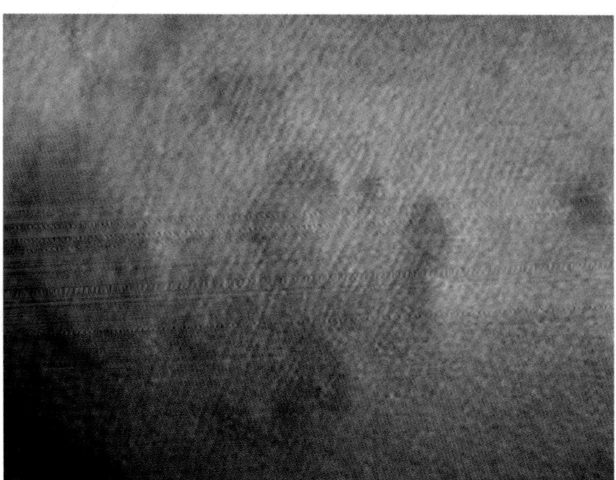

**Fig. 106.3 Acute urticaria.** (Copyright 2001–03, Johns Hopkins University School of Medicine. Shahbaz Janjua: Dermatlas. Available at http://www.dermatlas.org. With permission.)

## DIFFERENTIAL DIAGNOSIS AND MEDICAL DECISION MAKING

The first step in narrowing the differential diagnosis of urticaria is to determine whether the urticaria is acute (<6 weeks of symptoms) or chronic (≥6 weeks of symptoms).[20,21] The differential diagnosis of urticaria is outlined in **Box 106.3** and illustrated in **Figure 106.4**.

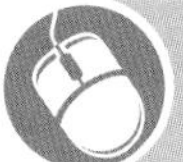

See Box 106.3, Differential Diagnosis of Urticaria, online at www.expertconsult.com

Evaluation of acute urticaria and angioedema is based on a careful history and skin examination; little additional laboratory testing should be needed. The work-up for chronic urticaria is usually performed by an allergist in the office.

## TREATMENT

Therapy for acute urticaria includes avoidance of the suspected causative agent and administration of $H_1$ antihistamines (see Fig. 106.4). The second-generation $H_1$ antihistamines (cetirizine, loratadine, fexofenadine, desloratadine) are currently recommended as the first-line drugs.[18,20]

For urticaria judged difficult to control with antihistamines alone, prednisone can be added.[20] If the urticarial rash is extensive and pruritus is severe, epinephrine can be administered (0.3 to 0.5 mL of a 1 : 1000 dilution intramuscularly). It may be repeated every 1 to 2 hours as needed. Caution is advised when administering epinephrine to patients at risk for coronary heart disease (>35 years of age, other risk factors for coronary artery disease). Patients with chronic urticaria can be prescribed a nonsedating $H_1$ antihistamine (in higher dosages) as a temporizing measure and be referred to an allergist for further care.

## FOLLOW-UP, NEXT STEPS IN CARE, AND PATIENT EDUCATION

Most patients with urticaria (acute and chronic) can be managed as outpatients. Usually, a 7-day course of a second-generation $H_1$ antihistamine is sufficient, although a corticosteroid (prednisone) in a tapering course is sometimes added for moderate to severe cases.

# ANGIOEDEMA

## EPIDEMIOLOGY

Angioedema (not including hereditary angioedema [HAE]) may affect 10% to 20% of the population at some time in

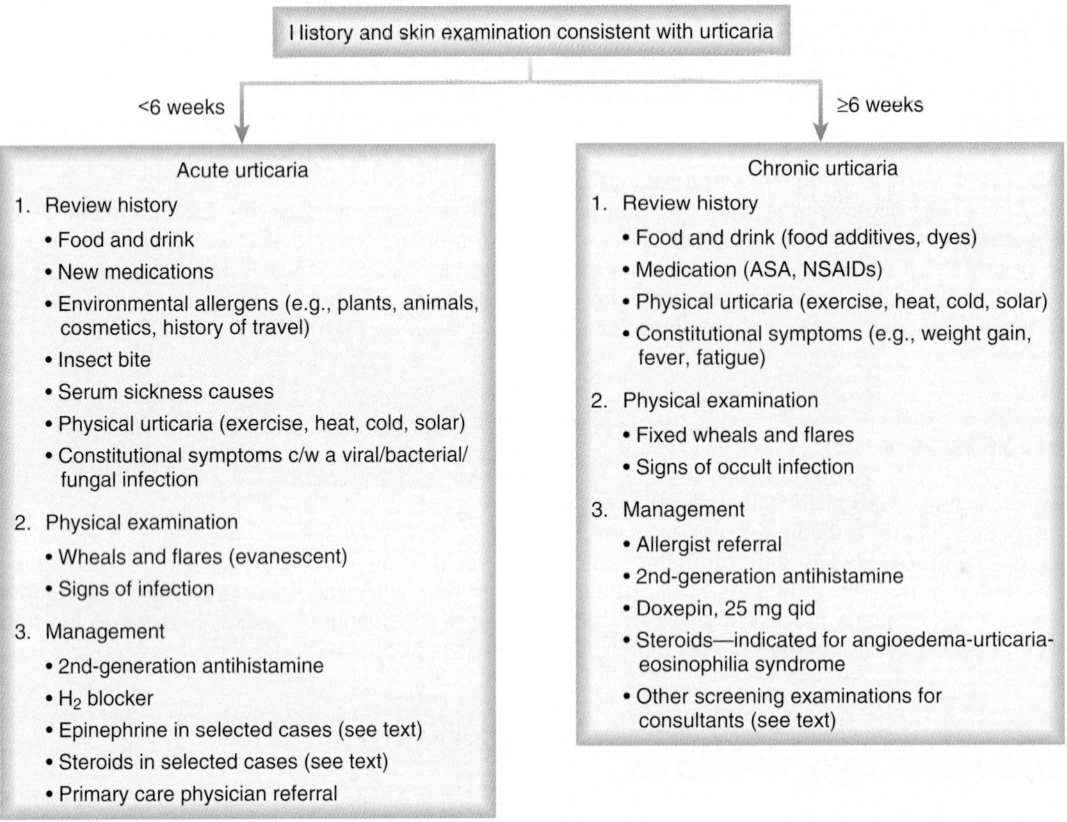


**Fig. 106.4 Algorithm for the diagnosis and treatment of urticaria.** *ASA*, Acetylsalicylic acid; *c/w*, consistent with; *NSAIDs*, nonsteroidal antiinflammatory drugs.

their lives; most chronic angioedema is idiopathic. HAE is an autosomal dominant genetic disorder with an estimated prevalence of 1 per 10,000 to 150,000 persons. The incidence of angiotensin-converting enzyme inhibitor (ACEI)-associated angioedema is approximately 0.2% to 0.7% and slightly higher in the African American population. Episodes have been reported to occur within days of initiating ACEI therapy and up to 8 years later, with an average onset of approximately 10 months. Ten percent to 25% of cases of angioedema encountered in the ED are considered to be life-threatening. African Americans are more susceptible to angioedema induced by ACEIs. Other forms of angioedema have no clear association between race and the frequency or severity of the disease. In HAE, affected women tend to have more frequent attacks and a more severe clinical course. Chronic idiopathic angioedema is more common in females than in males.

Angioedema can affect patient of all ages. For patients with HAE, the onset of symptoms is often around puberty. Idiopathic angioedema is more common in those aged 30 to 50 years than in other age groups. Patients typically experience minor swelling in childhood that may go unnoticed, with increased severity noted around puberty. However, type III HAE is found in the second decade of life or later and occurs only rarely before puberty. Five percent of adult HAE carriers are asymptomatic and identified only after their children are found to be symptomatic.

Urticaria-associated angioedema occurs in nearly 50% of children with urticaria. Because urticaria occurs in 2% to 3% of children, urticaria-associated angioedema is estimated to occur in 1% to 2% of the general population.

## PATHOPHYSIOLOGY

Angioedema (swelling) refers to vasodilation and edema in the lower dermis and subcutaneous layers of the skin.[22] In the majority of cases angioedema shares a similar allergic mechanism, but in selected cases it is the result of a reaction mediated by bradykinin. Both forms of angioedema can appear similar clinically, with bradykinin-mediated angioedema typically being manifested as angioedema without urticaria. They both commonly affect the eyelids, face, lips, and tongue and can potentially cause life-threatening respiratory compromise. It is important to distinguish the two forms because bradykinin-mediated angioedema may respond better to the new classes of medications, including recombinant C1 factor, kallikrein inhibitor, or a bradykinin receptor antagonist.

Bradykinin-mediated angioedema typically falls into one of two groups, HAE or acquired angioedema (AAE). HAE was first described by William Osler in 1888. It is a rare autosomal dominant disorder with an overall incidence of 1 in 50,000.[23] Approximately 25% of cases are the result of a spontaneous mutation. HAE has three subtypes. Type I (85%) is characterized by low levels of C1 esterase inhibitor (C1 INH), type II (<15%) consists of normal but poor functioning levels of C1 INH, and type III (rare) has normal C1 INH levels and activity but probably involves another unidentified defect or gene mutation at the receptor level. Currently, bradykinin is thought to be the primary molecule responsible for angioedema in patients with HAE. Documented triggers include infection, stress, trauma, oral contraceptives, pregnancy, and menstruation.[23]

AAE comprises a heterogeneous group that includes drug-induced, idiopathic, and environmental agent–related angioedema and acquired C1 INH deficiency (ACID). ACID is characterized by a lack of inheritance and low-level or nonfunctional C1 INH. Drug-induced angioedema is most commonly caused by ACEIs.[24] Up to 50% of those who still take an ACEI after an episode of angioedema will experience recurrent episodes. Discontinuation of the medication results in resolution of the symptoms in the majority of patients (within 24 to 48 hours). ACEIs block the degradation of kinins and thereby lead to elevated levels of bradykinin and other peptides. This results in vasodilation and tissue edema of the deeper layers of the skin, which is clinically manifested as angioedema.[24]

**BOX 106.4 Differential Diagnosis of Angioedema**

Cellulitis, erysipelas
Acute contact dermatitis
Crohn disease (of the mouth and lips)
Dermatomyositis
Venous obstructive disease (superior vena cava syndrome)
Heart failure
Photodermatitis
Tumid discoid lupus erythematosus
Melkersson-Rosenthal syndrome
Ascher syndrome
Facial lymphedema
Renal disease

From Kaplan AP, Greaves MW. Angioedema. J Am Acad Dermatol 2005;53:373-88.

## PRESENTING SIGNS AND SYMPTOMS

Angioedema has a brawny appearance and occurs when extravasation of fluid occurs at the subcutaneous and deep dermal layers of the skin. Patients with angioedema experience less pruritus than urticaria and often complain of a pain or burning sensation at affected sites. Angioedema also tends to involve the face, tongue, lips, and larynx but can occur in the mucosal layer of the gastrointestinal tract and genitalia in men. Involvement of the gastrointestinal tract can cause nausea, vomiting, diarrhea, and abdominal pain.

HAE is usually manifested in the second decade of life and appears either alone or with urticaria. Recurrent angioedema without urticaria later in life (e.g., middle age) may suggest some form of AAE, including ACID- and ACEI-induced angioedema (if undergoing ACEI therapy). Both HAE and ACEI-induced angioedema tend to have a predilection for the face, tongue, lips, oropharynx, and larynx. Patients with HAE may complain of a lump or tightness in the throat and progressive dyspnea. Physical examination may reveal hoarseness, inspiratory stridor, and rarely, urticaria. Prompt attention to airway management can be lifesaving. After stabilization, these patients need to be identified and referred to an allergist for further work-up and treatment.

## DIFFERENTIAL DIAGNOSIS AND MEDICAL DECISION MAKING

When angioedema is suggested by the history and physical examination, it is important to determine whether it is associated with other allergic findings, urticaria, a family history, or other medications (ACEIs). The differential diagnosis of angioedema is outlined in **Box 106.4**.

Patients suspected of having HAE should first have their complement 4 (C4) and complement 2 (C2) levels checked. As recommended by the consulting allergist or internist, other tests can include a $CH_{50}$ (total complement activity) test, C1 INH test, or C1 functional assay. Additional screening tests may be considered to help rule out occult infection, hematologic or oncologic pathology, and rheumatologic or inflammatory disorders, which may aid the consultant in subsequent evaluation of these patients.

## TREATMENT

The first priority in the management of patients with acute angioedema is to secure a patent airway if needed.[22,23] Endotracheal intubation should be considered early in patients with progressive laryngeal edema. As soon as the patient is situated, intravenous access should be established, oxygen administered, and the patient placed on a monitor.

The majority of cases of angioedema are type I hypersensitivity reactions. If signs of airway compromise or hypoxia are present, epinephrine should be administered (0.3 to 0.5 mL of a 1:1000 dilution intramuscularly) and repeated every 5 minutes as needed. Nebulized racemic (or regular) epinephrine (0.5 mL of a 2.25% racepinephrine solution; multiple doses are acceptable in patients without intravenous access) can be a temporizing measure for pharyngeal and laryngeal edema before or in addition to parenteral administration of epinephrine. In patients with mild symptoms and no airway involvement, $H_1$ and $H_2$ antihistamines should be used first. Parenteral steroids (methylprednisolone, 125 mg intravenously) should be administered for moderate to severe attacks.

Epinephrine, antihistamines, and corticosteroids are generally ineffective in the treatment of HAE and ACEI induced angioedema, although they are commonly given in the acute setting. The use of new drugs for acute HAE attacks and ACEI-induced angioedema is still in the formative stage. Plasma-derived C1 INH concentrate (Berinert, 20 U/kg intravenously, Cinryze, 1000 units intravenously) is currently available in the United States.[15] Ecallantide, a kallikrein inhibitor (30 mg subcutaneously in adults), is another recent agent approved by the Food and Drug Administration for the treatment of acute HAE. Aminocaproic acid, tranexamic acid, and anabolic androgens (danazol, stanozolol) are often prescribed for HAE prophylaxis but may be considered for the treatment of acute episodes. Additional treatment alternatives include solvent detergent–treated plasma or fresh frozen plasma, although these therapies are considered less safe.[23]

## FOLLOW-UP, NEXT STEPS IN CARE, AND PATIENT EDUCATION

Patients with mild symptoms who improved clinically after treatment and were observed for 4 to 6 hours in the ED can be discharged home with $H_1$ antihistamines and a short course of steroids. If the patient was taking an ACEI, its use should be stopped. Replacement candidates include calcium channel blockers and thiazides. Angiotensin receptor blockers are deemed acceptable by some authorities because the risk for angioedema from these agents is considered acceptably low.[24,25] Beta-blockers are not advised in the initial setting because of the theoretic risk of exacerbating the angioedema and potential antagonistic effects with epinephrine.

Inpatient admission is warranted for those with moderate to severe symptoms who fail to display signs of resolution after 4 to 6 hours in the ED. In particular, patients with HAE should be managed in consultation with their primary physician or allergist. Most of these patients, especially those with face and laryngeal involvement, warrant observation overnight in the hospital.

# ANAPHYLAXIS

## EPIDEMIOLOGY

Anaphylaxis is a life-threatening systemic hypersensitivity reaction that is rapid in onset and usually precipitated within minutes of exposure to an allergen. Because of lack of data the true incidence of anaphylaxis is unknown, but recent evidence suggests that it is increasing and its incidence may be as high as 2%.[26,27] Risk factors for anaphylaxis include atopy, higher socioeconomic status, northern locations, female sex (adults), and route of allergen exposure. An individual with a history of asthma is more likely to experience a severe or fatal reaction.[27]

### TRIGGERS

Foods, predominantly peanuts, tree nuts, shellfish, fish, eggs, soy, and cow milk, are the most common cause of anaphylaxis and are responsible for up to 30% of all fatal cases. Insect stings, primarily by those belonging to the order Hymenoptera, are the second most common cause of anaphylaxis. They account for approximately 18.5% of anaphylactic cases. Medications are the third most common cause of anaphylaxis (13.7%). Although the β-lactams (penicillin) are commonly involved, several other drugs are known to cause anaphylaxis, including NSAIDs, aspirin, protamine, vancomycin, neuromuscular blocking agents, and newer biologic modifiers such as omalizumab, infliximab, and cetuximab.[27,28]

Although the three groups just mentioned (foods, stings, and drugs) are responsible for the majority of anaphylactic reactions, other prominent triggers of anaphylaxis include latex, seminal fluid, transfusion products, allergen immunotherapy, contrast dye, methylmethacrylate (bone cement), and physical activity (exercise). Exercise-induced anaphylaxis is noteworthy because its pathophysiology is unknown. Some authorities suspect co-triggers, such as a specific food, drug, or recent high pollen exposure as the actual culprit.[29] In approximately 20% of anaphylactic cases, no identifiable triggers are found, and the reaction is termed idiopathic anaphylaxis.[30]

## PATHOPHYSIOLOGY

Anaphylaxis is commonly an IgE-mediated type I hypersensitivity reaction, but it can also occur through other immunologic mechanisms or direct mast cell activation (formerly known as an anaphylactoid reaction). The resultant degranulation of mast cells and basophils causes the release of preformed mediators such as histamine, tryptase, carboxypeptidase $A_3$, chymase, and tumor necrosis factor-α, as well as newly generated mediators such as leukotrienes, prostaglandins, cytokines, and platelet-activating factor. These vasoactive molecules together are believed to be responsible for the pathophysiology of anaphylaxis. Of these mediators, histamine is probably the most important. It mediates systemic vasodilation and increases vascular permeability, cardiac contractility, and glandular secretion. The leukotrienes, together with platelet-activating factor, contribute to vascular permeability and, in combination with prostaglandins ($D_2$), cause bronchoconstriction.

## PRESENTING SIGNS AND SYMPTOMS

Anaphylaxis is a systemic reaction of rapid onset that involves multiple organ systems, principally the cutaneous, respiratory, cardiovascular, gastrointestinal, and central nervous systems (**Box 106.5**).[31] Patients may initially experience warmth and tingling of the face, mouth, and chest, followed by nasal congestion, sneezing, and ocular itching and tearing. Urticaria, pruritus, and angioedema occur roughly 90% of the time.

The majority of anaphylactic reactions become clinically evident within minutes after parenteral exposure (average of 5 to 30 minutes), with a longer latent time (2 hours) after the ingestion of a triggering agent. In general, the sooner the clinical syndrome is manifested after exposure to the allergen, the more severe the reaction. Most fatalities occur within the first 30 minutes after exposure. In the setting of shock, cutaneous symptoms may be absent as a result of compensatory vasoconstriction. Anaphylaxis may precipitate an acute coronary syndrome in what is known as cardiac anaphylaxis.[32] More commonly in the elderly, the initial complaint may be abdominal pain and cramping.

In approximately 20% of patients, anaphylaxis may recur 1 to 72 hours after apparent clinical resolution of all signs and symptoms in what is called a biphasic reaction.[33] There is currently no evidence or expert consensus on clinical predictors of the occurrence of a biphasic anaphylactic reaction, although it has been suggested that a biphasic reaction is rare in patients without hypotension and airway obstruction during the initial evaluation.[34] Most authorities recommend an observation period (8 to 24 hours) after the initial manifestation to minimize the untoward effects of the biphasic reaction.[33]

**BOX 106.5 Common Clinical Findings in Patients with Anaphylaxis**

**Cutaneous, Subcutaneous, Mucosal Tissue**
Urticaria (hives), angioedema, flushing, pruritus, morbilliform rash, pilar erection
Conjunctival erythema, tearing
Pruritus and swelling of the lips, tongue, uvula/palate
Pruritus of the genitalia, palms, soles

**Respiratory**
Nasal congestion, rhinorrhea, sneezing
Throat tightness and soreness, dysphonia and hoarseness, dry staccato cough, stridor, dysphagia
Dyspnea, chest tightness, deep cough, wheezing, bronchospasm

**Gastrointestinal**
Nausea, vomiting (stringy mucus), dysphagia, cramping abdominal pain, diarrhea

**Cardiovascular**
Chest pain, palpitations, tachycardia, bradycardia, or other dysrhythmia
Dizziness, altered mental status, hypotension, shock

**Central Nervous System**
Aura of impending doom, uneasiness, throbbing headache, dizziness, confusion, tunnel vision
Infants and children: sudden behavioral changes, such as irritability, cessation of play, and clinging to parent

**Other**
Metallic taste in the mouth
Uterine contractions in postpubertal female patients

Modified from Simons FE. Anaphylaxis. J Allergy Clin Immunol 2010; 125(Suppl 2):S161-81 (with permission).

**BOX 106.6 Differential Diagnosis of Anaphylaxis**

**Flush Syndromes**
Hereditary angioedema
Urticaria vasculitis
Carcinoid syndrome
Systemic mastocytosis
Urticaria pigmentosa
Vasoactive intestinal polypeptide–secreting tumors
Medullary carcinoma of the thyroid
Pheochromocytoma
Acute alcohol syndrome
Monosodium glutamate toxicity
Sulfites
Scombroidosis

**Infections, Respiratory Syndrome**
Epiglottitis, supraglottitis
Retropharyngeal, peritonsillar abscess
Laryngeal spasm, foreign body aspiration, tumor
Acute asthma exacerbation, chronic obstructive pulmonary disease

**Shock Syndromes**
Hemorrhagic
Cardiogenic
Septic
Spinal shock

**Somatoform, Psychogenic**
Panic attacks
Munchausen, factitious disorder
Somatoform idiopathic anaphylaxis

**Miscellaneous**
Idiopathic
Vasodepressor (vasovagal) reactions
Progesterone anaphylaxis
Red man syndrome (vancomycin)
Capillary leak syndrome

## DIFFERENTIAL DIAGNOSIS AND MEDICAL DECISION MAKING

The clinical spectrum of anaphylaxis overlaps that of several other syndromes, especially those involving the skin and cardiorespiratory system (**Box 106.6**). Vasovagal reactions may mimic early anaphylaxis, although these patients usually have bradycardia, hypotension, diaphoresis, and pallor, as opposed to the tachycardia, hypotension, diaphoresis, and urticaria usually associated with anaphylaxis. Anaphylactic shock may also appear clinically indistinguishable from other forms of shock (distributive, septic, or cardiogenic). The acute onset and characteristic angioedematous urticarial rash favor the diagnosis of anaphylactic shock. Flushing syndromes also frequently mimic anaphylactic reactions. They may be associated with dry skin or diaphoresis and are the result of numerous different drugs, ingestants, and other physiologic syndromes.

Anaphylaxis is diagnosed clinically. The diagnosis is considered highly likely when any of three clinical criteria in **Box 106.7** are met.[35]

Currently, histamine and tryptase are the only measurable markers of anaphylaxis in clinical laboratories.[31] Histamine plasma levels become elevated approximately 10 minutes after the onset of symptoms and remain so for up to an hour. Peak levels of serum tryptase occur between 60 and 90 minutes and persist for as long as 6 hours. These markers must be determined within the time frames mentioned and may be helpful when it is uncertain whether anaphylaxis has occurred. It should be noted that food-induced anaphylaxis may not be accompanied by elevated levels of tryptase. Additional laboratory tests and imaging may be necessary to help rule out other disease processes.

## TREATMENT

Early administration of epinephrine is the mainstay of treatment of anaphylaxis (**Box 106.8**). It should be administered quickly and preferably intramuscularly in the lateral aspect of the thigh (vastus lateralis). Epinephrine should be considered if anaphylaxis is suspected even when only one system (e.g., skin) is involved. Doses can be repeated every 5 to 10 minutes or more frequently as indicated clinically.[27,31] Caution should be exercised in patients with risk factors for ischemic heart disease, although there are no absolute contraindications to epinephrine in those initially seen in anaphylactic shock.

**BOX 106.7 Clinical Diagnosis of Anaphylaxis**

Anaphylaxis is highly likely when any of the following three criteria are fulfilled:

1. Acute onset (minutes to hours) of an illness with cutaneous or mucosal involvement *AND* at least one of the following:
   a. Respiratory compromise (e.g., dyspnea, wheezing/bronchospasm, stridor, hypoxia)
   b. Reduced blood pressure or symptoms of end-organ dysfunction
2. Two or more of the following occurring rapidly after exposure to a probable allergen (minutes to several hours):
   a. Involvement of skin or mucosal tissue
   b. Respiratory compromise
   c. Persistent gastrointestinal symptoms (e.g., crampy abdominal pain, vomiting)
3. Reduced blood pressure after exposure to a known allergen for that patient (age specific, less than 90 mm Hg, or 30% decline from baseline)

Reproduced from Sampson HA, Munoz-Furlong A, Campbell RL, et al. Second symposium on the definition and management of anaphylaxis: summary report—Second National Institute of Allergy and Infectious Disease/Food Allergy and Anaphylaxis Network symposium. Ann Emerg Med 2006;47:373-80.

Intravenous infusion should be used only in patients who remain hypotensive and have failed to respond to multiple intramuscular injections.[27,31] Inhaled epinephrine may be used as adjunctive therapy for laryngeal edema but should never replace the intramuscular or intravenous route (**Fig. 106.5**).

In conjunction with the administration of epinephrine, the patient should be placed in the supine position with the lower extremities elevated. Intravenous access should be established, supplemental oxygen administered, and the patient placed on a monitor. Patients with rapidly progressive respiratory insufficiency will benefit from early endotracheal intubation. Use of rapid-sequence intubation should be approached with great caution because of the potential for rapid deterioration of the oral and laryngeal edema. Plans for backup airway support and rescue airway devices, including a surgical airway, may be prudent.

Hypotension is treated aggressively with crystalloid infusion and colloid as indicated clinically. Caution should be taken in patients with a history of congestive heart failure. Patients with persistent hypotension despite appropriate doses of epinephrine and intravenous fluid resuscitation should be administered vasopressors drips (see Box 106.8).

$H_1$ antihistamine (diphenhydramine) should be given to improve the itching and hives in patients with anaphylaxis. $H_2$ antihistamines (ranitidine, cimetidine) have a synergistic effect with $H_1$ antihistamines and should be given because

**BOX 106.8 Treatment Options for Anaphylaxis**

**General**

Two large-bore intravenous lines (intraosseous if unable to acquire intravenous access)

Placement of the patient on a monitor

Supplement oxygen (nasal canula, non-rebreather mask)

Consideration of a tourniquet—if anaphylaxis is due to an insect sting at the distal end of an extremity (blood pressure cuff inflated to approximately 20 mm Hg greater than systolic blood pressure), release every 10 minutes for 1 minute or when the symptoms resolve

**Epinephrine**

Intramuscular (subcutaneous acceptable)—1:1000; adult: 0.3 to 0.5 mL every 5 minutes as necessary, titrated to effect; pediatric: 0.01 mL/kg every 5 minutes as necessary, titrated to effect)

Alternatively, EpiPen (0.3 mL) or EpiPen Jr (0.15 mL) can be administered into the anterolateral aspect of the thigh; removal of clothing unnecessary

Intravenous infusion—1:100,000; 0.1 mL of a 1:1000 dilution in 10 mL of normal saline (NS), 100 mcg, over a 10-minute period; equivalent to 10 mcg/min for a 10-min period, titrated to effect; repeat as necessary; continuous hemodynamic monitoring required

Continuous infusion—1 mL of a 1:1000 dilution of epinephrine in 250 mL of 5% dextrose in water ($D_5W$) results in a concentration of 4 mcg/mL; can be started at 1 mcg/min and increased to 4 mcg/min if needed

Pediatric continuous infusion—rate of 0.1 mcg/kg/min (up to 30 kg) advised, with increasing increments of 0.1 mcg/kg/min to a maximum of 1.5 mcg/kg/min

**Second-Line Medications**

***Antihistamines***

Diphenhydramine (IV or PO)—adult: 50 to 100 mg, up to 400 mg/24 hr, titrated to effect; pediatric: 0.02 mg/kg, up to 300 mg/24 hr, titrated to effect

Ranitidine or other $H_2$ blocker (IV or PO)—adult: 50 mg IV, 300 mg PO (4 mg/kg); pediatric: 1 mg/kg

***Aerosolized Beta-Agonists and Others***

Albuterol—adult: 2.5 mg; pediatric: 0.02 mL/kg up to 2.5 mg in 3 mL of NS; may be given continuously

Ipratropium—adult: 0.5 mg; pediatric: 0.25 mg in 3 mL of NS; repeat as necessary

***Prednisone***

Adult: 40 to 60 mg PO; pediatric: 1 to 2 mg/kg PO

***Methylprednisolone***

Intravenous infusion—adult: 125 to 250 mg; pediatric: 40 to 80 mg

***Glucagon***

Intravenous infusion—adult: 1 to 5 mg over a 5-minute period; pediatric: 0.5 mg, followed by 5 to 15 mcg/min as drops (gtt); for refractory hypotension or patients receiving beta-blockers

***Dopamine***

Intravenous infusion—5 to 20 mcg/kg/min gtt, and/or dobutamine, 5 to 20 mcg/kg/min gtt

***Norepinephrine***

Intravenous infusion—8 to 12 mcg/min gtt (2 to 3 mL/min; 4 mg added to 1000 mL of $D_5W$ provides a concentration of 4 mcg/mL)

they improve vascular permeability, flushing, gastric secretion, and mucus production in the airway. Antihistamines, however, should be considered second-line agents after epinephrine. Inhaled β-agonists (albuterol) can be administered for bronchospasm refractory to appropriate doses of epinephrine. Glucocorticosteroid provides no immediate benefit in the acute treatment of anaphylaxis, although it may be helpful in preventing biphasic reactions.

## SPECIAL CONSIDERATIONS

### PATIENTS TAKING BETA-BLOCKERS

Patients currently taking beta-blockers may not respond adequately to epinephrine and intravenous fluids. A glucagon

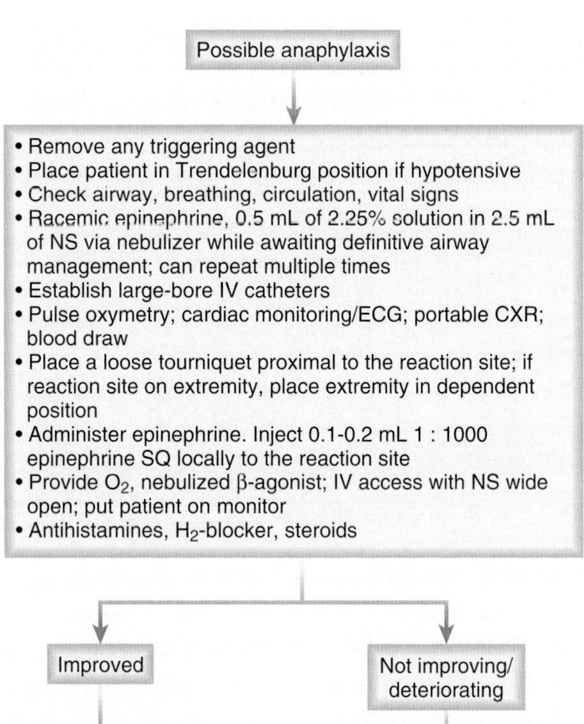


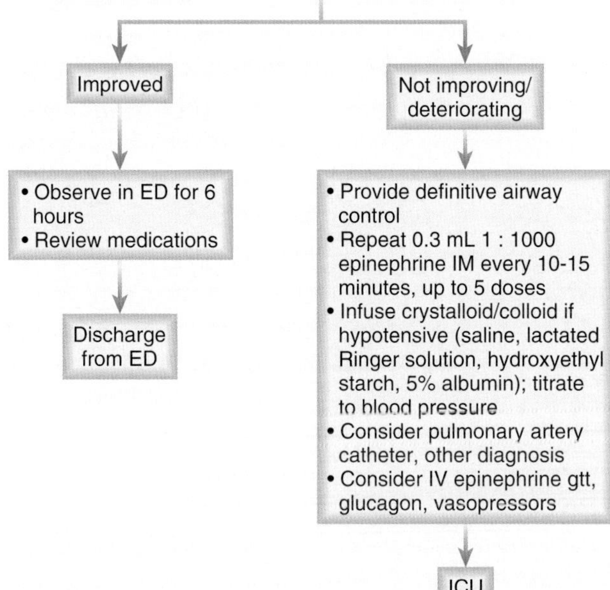


**Fig. 106.5 Treatment algorithm for possible anaphylaxis (see Box 106.8 for drug dosages and indications).** *CXR*, Chest radiograph; *ECG*, electrocardiogram; *ED*, emergency department; *gtt*, drops; *ICU*, intensive care unit; *IM*, intramuscularly; *IV*, intravenous; *NS*, normal saline; *SQ*, subcutaneously.

**BOX 106.9 Standard Pharmacologic Treatment Protocol for Patients with a History of Radiocontrast-Induced Anaphylaxis**

Prednisone, 50 mg PO given 13 hours, 7 hours, and 1 hour before the procedure
Diphenhydramine, 50 mg IM given 1 hour before the procedure
Consider giving an $H_2$ antagonist, such as ranitidine, 300 mg PO as drops 3 hours before the procedure

Modified from Lieberman P. Anaphylaxis. Med Clin North Am 2006; 90:77-95.

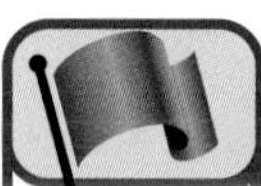

**RED FLAGS**

**Management of Anaphylaxis**

Failure to diagnose anaphylaxis early or to recognize the need to secure the airway early
Delayed administration of epinephrine
Incorrect administration of intravenous epinephrine (e.g., not diluting it, wrong concentration)

infusion should be strongly considered in these cases (see Box 106.8).[27,31] Conversely, these patients may also demonstrate unopposed α-adrenergic effects after epinephrine administration and may require an alpha-blocker such as phentolamine.

### PATIENTS WITH ALLERGY TO INTRAVENOUS CONTRAST MEDIA

Pretreatment with antihistamines and steroids significantly decreases the frequency and severity of anaphylactoid reactions in patients who have sustained a previous reaction to intravenous radiocontrast media. Each hospital has its own pretreatment protocols for clinical procedures; **Box 106.9** reproduces one such protocol.[36]

## FOLLOW-UP, NEXT STEPS IN CARE, AND PATIENT EDUCATION

Patients who experience complete resolution of symptoms and were never hypotensive can potentially be discharged home. Although the time frame for biphasic reactions varies significantly, limited literature suggests that patients be observed in the ED for up to 8 hours.[33] Oral $H_1$ antihistamines such as diphenhydramine (50 mg every 6 hours for 72 hours) and $H_2$ blockers such as ranitidine (150 mg every 12 hours for 72 hours) along with oral prednisone may prevent possible relapse.[37] These patients should be instructed to return to the ED if they experience any recurrent symptoms consistent with their previous anaphylactic reaction.

All patients who have experienced an anaphylactic or significant allergic reaction should be prescribed at least two

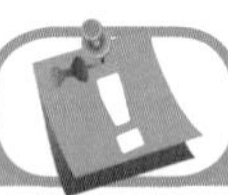

TIPS AND TRICKS

**Prevention of Anaphylaxis and Anaphylactic Death**

Obtain a thorough drug allergy and atopic history.
Check all drugs for proper labeling.
Give drugs orally rather than parenterally when possible.
Give drugs in distal end of the extremity if possible when a parenteral route is necessary.
Always have resuscitation equipment available when administering antigenic compounds.
Ensure that patients remain in the emergency department for at least 30 minutes after drug administration.
Use unrelated drugs when feasible in susceptible patients.
Encourage patients to carry warning identification (Medic-Alert, wallet ID).
Educate patients on the technique of self-injection of epinephrine and urge them to carry the treatment kit at all times.
Instruct patients to avoid known antigens (stinging insects, foods, antibiotics).
Refer patients to an allergist for a skin test and possible immunotherapy.

Epi-Pens, one kept at the common residence and another in the purse or briefcase. In addition, patients should be taught how to self-administer it. Predisposed patients should be encouraged to wear a Medic-Alert bracelet or carry a wallet card identifying their hypersensitivity. Patients should also be referred to an allergist for possible skin testing and hyposensitization immunotherapy.

Hospital admission should be considered for patients who show slow clinical improvement, were hypotensive, and had upper airway involvement or persistent bronchospasm. Patients at risk for a biphasic reaction, such as those maintained on chronic beta-blocker therapy, may also be candidates for extended observation in the hospital.

## REFERENCES

*References can be found on Expert Consult @ www.expertconsult.com.*

# Joint Disorders 107

*Kathleen S. Schrank*

**KEY POINTS**

- A white blood cell count higher than 50,000/mm$^3$ is suggestive of a septic joint; however, lower counts do not rule out this diagnosis. If the index of clinical suspicion for a septic joint is high but the test results are nondiagnostic, the disorder should be treated as an infection.
- Severely painful acute monarticular arthritis, with or without fever, is highly likely to be a septic joint; it is an emergency requiring parenteral antibiotics and possible surgical intervention.
- Joint prostheses, diabetes, rheumatoid arthritis, concurrent infection, and age older than 80 years are significant risk factors for bacterial joint infections. Acute problems in a prosthetic joint merit immediate discussion with an orthopedic surgeon.
- A sexually active young adult with an inflamed, painful joint is considered to have gonococcal arthritis until proved otherwise and should be treated accordingly.
- Gout and pseudogout are crystal-induced arthritides that although benign, may cause significant pain and morbidity. The patient's pain can be significantly improved by anesthetic and steroid injection after arthrocentesis.
- Overlying soft tissue infection may preclude arthrocentesis or warrant a different approach.
- Syncope may be a warning of high risk for sudden cardiac death in patients with systemic inflammatory arthritides.
- Cervical spine disease is common with rheumatoid arthritis and osteoarthritis and must be considered before any attempt at endotracheal intubation that involves forced flexion.
- Serious complications of arthritides are rare but may be life- or limb-threatening.

## ARTHRITIS

### EPIDEMIOLOGY

An estimated 20 million people in the United States have osteoarthritis (OA), and 2 to 3 million have rheumatoid arthritis (RA). The total cost of medical care, lost work time, and disability for OA alone is estimated to run 2% of the gross national product. The most common cause of joint pain is OA, but the most crucial challenge is identification of a septic joint. Septic arthritis occurs in all age groups but is more common in children than in adults, and about 10% of patients with an acutely painful joint will be found to have infection.[1]

### PATHOPHYSIOLOGY

The structure of diarthrodial joints (the most common type) includes the synovium, synovial fluid, articular cartilage, intraarticular ligaments, joint capsule, and juxtaarticular subchondral bone. The delicate synovium provides oxygen and nutrients to cartilage and produces lubricants. Articular cartilage deforms under mechanical load to minimize stress and provides a smooth surface for joint motion with minimal friction. Causes of joint disorders (**Box 107.1**) often overlap. Cumulative microdamage and remodeling occur with use and aging. Mechanical or metabolic disturbances may lead to a secondary inflammatory response, or an inflamed structure (e.g., a tendon) may rupture. Arthrosis is due to a mechanical insult, whereas arthritis is due to inflammation of the synovium. With inflammation comes white blood cell (WBC) infiltration, release of cytokines (e.g., tumor necrosis factor-α [TNF-α], interleukins) and other inflammatory mediators, and proliferation of cells or tissue. Edema collects around the joint, which causes stiffness. With prolonged inflammation, erosion of bone and destruction of the joint eventually occur and can produce deformity and chronic disability.

In addition to bone, muscles, and joints, "joint" pain may derive from nerves, skin, or periarticular structures (ligaments, tendons, bursae, bone). The enthesis is the structural insertion of tendon or ligament into bone. Inflammatory enthesitis is prominent in the spondyloarthropathies, such as reactive arthritis.

### PRESENTING SIGNS AND SYMPTOMS

The clinical findings can narrow the potential cause of a patient's symptoms (**Table 107.1**). Initial assessment must determine whether the anatomic site of the problem is the joint and then a general category of the disease, either inflammatory (septic versus aseptic) or noninflammatory (mechanical). A red, hot, swollen, painful joint is the classic finding with septic and other inflammatory arthritides. Arthritis patients may also have serious nonarticular complications of their disease or its treatment.

The onset and pattern of pain are important to determine (**Box 107.2**). Mechanical pain is worse with use, rapidly relieved with rest, and often least in the morning. If present, morning stiffness resolves quickly. Rapid onset over a period of minutes suggests trauma, internal derangement, or a loose fragment in the joint. Inflammatory pain is often worse with use as well, but not so quickly relieved with rest, and is commonly associated with morning stiffness (short duration with OA, prolonged with RA). "Gelling" (stiffness and immobility) after sitting in one position occurs with either type. Widespread pain with stiffness is typically due to inflammatory arthritis or fibromyalgia. Subjective pain without joint findings on examination is termed arthralgia. If the patient has tried medications without relief, the dosage should be determined because inadequate dosing is common.

**BOX 107.1 Initial Causes of Joint Disorders**

**Mechanical**
Loss of articular surface
Trauma
Microfractures, remodeling, arthrosis
Congenital dysplasias

**Metabolic**
Crystal deposition
Osteoporosis
Inherited storage diseases (e.g., Gaucher disease)
Endocrinopathies (e.g., acromegaly, hyperparathyroidism)
Other metabolic bone disease (e.g., Paget disease)

**Inflammatory**
Infection
Immunologic response

Although pain is usually the main concern of patients with joint disease, it is important to determine whether other associated symptoms (e.g., fever, rash, eye symptoms) or findings are present that can aid in the diagnosis. For example, examination of the skin may reveal the malar or butterfly facial rash associated with lupus, the pustular lesions of gonococcemia, or the subcutaneous nodules of RA and gout.

The musculoskeletal examination attempts to identify the exact site of the problem—joint versus bone, muscle, periarticular, or superficial skin pain. Particular joint involvement may aid in making the diagnosis (**Box 107.3**). True joint pain is usually diffuse on palpation and increases with active and passive motion. Periarticular inflammation (tendonitis, bursitis, cellulitis) is generally more focal, with pain reproduced only by certain movements—most often resisted active

**Table 107.1 Clinical Features of the Arthritides**

| | PAIN | MONOARTICULAR vs. POLYARTICULAR | EFFUSION | SKIN | FEVER | OTHER |
|---|---|---|---|---|---|---|
| Osteoarthritis | Long onset | Usually mono at first; often DIP or first CMC<br>Later lumbosacral spine | Possibly | Possible swelling, minimal redness | No | Presence of osteophytes, morning stiffness (<1 hr) |
| Rheumatoid arthritis | Long onset (weeks to months) | Mono or poly; symmetric; often MCP, PIP, or wrist; later cervical spine | Often | Mild swelling, minimal to mild redness | May be low grade | Rheumatoid nodules, morning stiffness (>1 hr); systemic symptoms, heart and lung involvement |
| Reactive arthritis | Short onset | Asymmetric mono or oligo, smaller joints<br>Enthesitis | Often | Swelling and redness<br>Rashes common | Common | GU, eye, systemic symptoms; follows GU or GI infection |
| Septic joint | Quick onset | 80% mono; often knee | Yes | Swelling and redness | Yes; may be high | May be toxic appearing, systemic sepsis possible |
| Gout | Quick onset | Mono or oligo; often first MTP (podagra), knee | Often | Swelling and redness<br>May appear cellulitic | May be low grade | Tophi |
| SLE | Variable onset | Poly | Often | Swelling ± redness<br>Butterfly, malar rash | Possibly | Oral lesions, systemic symptoms, multiple organ involvement |
| Gonococcal arthritis | Short onset<br>Often migratory | Mono in 25%, poly in >60%; arthritis and arthralgias<br>Localized septic joint in 40%<br>Usually wrists, hands, knees, elbows, or shoulders | Often | Swelling ± redness<br>Pustular lesions | May be low grade | May have cervicitis, urethritis |

*CMC*, Carpometacarpal; *DIP*, distal interphalangeal joint; *mono*, monarticular; *MTP*, metatarsophalangeal joint; *oligo*, oligoarticular; *PIP*, proximal interphalangeal joint; *poly*, polyarticular; *SLE*, systemic lupus erythematosus.

contraction or passive stretching of the involved muscles or tendons and usually only toward one side.

## DIFFERENTIAL DIAGNOSIS AND MEDICAL DECISION MAKING

Mechanical, inflammatory, or metabolic causes of arthritis may be present, and the whole picture must be considered in narrowing the lengthy differential diagnosis (**Box 107.4**). A new diagnosis of a specific type of inflammatory arthritis may not be possible in one visit, but recognition that the case is inflammatory is important for interim care. The severity of a patient's discomfort will determine the urgency of analgesia, which may be initiated well before refining the list of possible diagnoses.

Early identification of septic arthritis is a top priority. An infected joint is especially likely to be present in patients with inflammatory, acute monarticular arthritis, with or without fever. The presence of another site of infection (skin, lungs, urine, heart) or a joint prosthesis increases the likelihood considerably. Moderate fever is typical with a septic joint, whereas low-grade fever may be present with any inflammatory arthritis. Treatment (antibiotics and drainage) must be initiated empirically while awaiting culture results. Infections in nearby sites (bursae, skin, periosteum) should be distinguishable by careful examination and radiologic studies; ultrasonography may be very helpful in looking for joint effusions. High fever, chills, and signs of sepsis should prompt fluid resuscitation as needed and studies to identify any additional site of infection.

Although patients usually have a history of trauma or very sudden monarticular pain, fractures may occasionally be surprises, especially in those with severe osteopenia or altered mentation (e.g., alcohol abuse, seizures), in whom trauma might not have been noticed.

Signs and symptoms may overlap, but crystals found on arthrocentesis are diagnostic of crystal-induced arthritis. The recent addition of a medication that can cause hyperuricemia may be a clue, but serum uric acid levels alone do not make or rule out the diagnosis of gout. Frequently, the patient has had multiple bouts of gout in the same joint, most commonly the great toe.

### DIAGNOSTIC STUDIES

Blood tests are rarely diagnostic in patients with synovial disorders but may be ordered sparingly to assist in management decisions. A complete blood count (CBC) and basic chemistry profile will identify anemia, an elevated WBC count, and renal dysfunction (which affects selection of

**BOX 107.2 Key Historical Points**

What is the source and type of pain?
- Muscle, nerve, skin, periarticular or articular structures, or joint?
- Acute, chronic, or chronic with acute complication?
- Monarticular, oligoarticular (2 or 3 joints) or polyarticular (>3 joints)?
- If polyarticular, is there a symmetric or migratory pattern?

What is the OPQRST (onset, palliation/aggravation, quality, radiation, severity, timing)?

Associated symptoms?
- Brief or prolonged morning stiffness?
- Evidence of inflammation?
- Fever, chills, fatigue, weight loss?
- Rash, eye complaints, mucosal lesions?

Personal history
- Previous diagnosis of arthritis or other diseases? How does this compare?
- Trauma?
- Recent infection?
- Joint surgery? Prosthesis?
- Joint instability or locking?
- Repetitive use?
- Intravenous drug use?

Family history of arthritis?

Medications, especially thiazides (can increase serum uric acid), isoniazid, procainamide, and hydralazine (can precipitate lupus)?

Current and previous treatments? Nontraditional remedies? Results?

**BOX 107.3 Articular Diseases Associated with Joint Location**

**Monarticular**
Osteoarthritis (OA, often oligoarticular)
Septic arthritis
Gout
Pseudogout
Trauma
Hemarthrosis

**Polyarticular**
Rheumatoid arthritis (RA)
Systemic lupus erythematosus
Viral arthritis
Rheumatic fever
Reiter syndrome
Lyme disease
Serum sickness
Drug induced

**Periarticular**
Bursitis
Tendinitis
Cellulitis

**By Specific Joint or Joints**
First metatarsophalangeal (MTP): Gout
Knee: Septic arthritis, pseudogout, gout, OA
Metacarpophalangeal, MTP, proximal interphalangeal, tarsometatarsal, and cervical spine: RA
Distal and proximal interphalangeal, first carpometacarpal, knee, hip, cervical and lumbosacral spine: OA
Sternoclavicular: Injection drug abusers with septic joints
Axial: Seronegative spondyloarthropathies

**BOX 107.4 Differential Diagnoses for Acute Arthritis**

**Monarticular Disorders**
Abscess
Bone tumor
Bursitis
Cellulitis
Compartment syndrome
Fibromyalgia, myofascial pain syndromes
Inflammatory myopathies
Myalgia, myositis
Neuropathic pain
Osteomyelitis
Polychondritis
Polymyalgia rheumatica
Reflex sympathetic dystrophy
Shoulder capsulitis
Temporal arteritis
Tendinitis, tenosynovitis
Trauma (ligament, tendon, muscle, bone)

**Noninflammatory Joint Disorder**
Avascular necrosis of the hip (including Legg-Calvé-Perthes disease*)
Charcot (neuropathic) arthropathy
Congenital hip dysplasia
Decompression sickness, bends
Hemarthrosis, hemophilic arthropathy
Hemoglobinopathies
Hypertrophic pulmonary osteoarthropathy
Inherited storage diseases (e.g., Gaucher)
Liquid lipid microsphere disease
Malignancy
Osteoarthrosis
Osteochondritis desiccans
Osteochondroma
Osteonecrosis
Pigmented villonodular synovitis
Slipped capital femoral epiphysis
Trauma

**Inflammatory Joint Disorder**
Amyloidosis
Connective tissue diseases: systemic lupus erythematosus, scleroderma, Sjögren syndrome, mixed connective tissue disease
Crystal deposition: gout, pseudogout
Drug reaction (serum sickness)
Erythema nodosum
Familial Mediterranean fever
Foreign body reaction
Infection related
Juvenile idiopathic arthritis and subtypes*
Multicentric histiocytosis
Osteoarthritis, degenerative joint disease
Palindromic rheumatism
Polymyalgia rheumatica with joint involvement
Rheumatoid arthritis
Sarcoidosis
Seronegative spondyloarthropathies*
Vasculitides

*Additional information is provided in the online appendix to this chapter.

medications). The erythrocyte sedimentation rate (ESR) and C-reactive protein (CRP) are nonspecific but useful markers of inflammation. Coagulation studies are needed only if a patient is taking anticoagulants or a bleeding disorder is suspected. Creatine phosphokinase is helpful if muscle pain or weakness is detected. If clinical assessment raises concern for other autoimmune or systemic diseases, additional screening for multiorgan involvement with urinalysis, liver enzymes, electrocardiogram, and chest films may help. Serologic testing (e.g., rheumatoid factor [RF], antinuclear antibody, and Lyme serology, depending on the clinical impression) is generally done in follow-up settings.[2]

Plain radiographs are ordered if a fracture, foreign body, septic joint, or tumor is suspected. If the initial films show no fracture but suspicion remains, films repeated in 1 to 2 weeks may show callus formation or abnormal alignment. Radiographic findings may also assist in diagnosing the type of arthritis (**Box 107.5**),[3] although they may remain normal early in the course. The presence of degenerative changes in a painful joint supports the clinical suspicion of OA as the cause, but such changes also become common with age, even in asymptomatic joints; conversely, a normal film does not rule out OA. Similarly, calcified fibrocartilage is often found in patients with calcium pyrophosphate deposition (CPPD) disease but is common in asymptomatic patients as well. Ultrasonography is useful in confirming joint effusion, especially in joints that are difficult to assess, such as the hip. Other modalities are rarely indicated in the emergency department (ED). Although magnetic resonance imaging (MRI) can distinguish synovitis from effusion and identify rotator cuff tears or be used to evaluate ligament trauma, emergency MRI or computed tomography (CT) is indicated only if a severe joint complication is strongly suspected or if axial skeletal pain merits evaluation for stenosis or metastatic disease.

Arthrocentesis with synovial fluid analysis is an important diagnostic and therapeutic procedure for joint disease (see the Tips and Tricks box and **Box 107.6**). It is the only reliable means to rule out a septic joint, and it is essential in acute monarthritis to look for joint infection, crystals, or hemarthrosis. Possible complications of arthrocentesis include introduction of infection into the joint space, hemarthrosis, and adverse reactions to medications. Arthrocentesis of prosthetic joints is best done with orthopedic consultation.

Normal synovial fluid is clear and yellow in appearance. In degenerative joint disease the fluid itself is normal and thus remains clear. Bloody fluid suggests hemarthrosis. Fat droplets may confirm a fracture. Turbid fluid is observed in

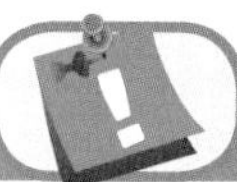

**TIPS AND TRICKS**

**Joint Fluid Collection**

Identify and mark landmarks before infiltration with an anesthetic.

Preprocedure use of an ice pack will decrease pain.

Support the joint in a position of comfort during and after the procedure.

Contact the laboratory technicians before collecting the fluid to verify the following:

- Quantity of fluid required for the studies desired
- Correct tubes required and their availability (e.g., a liquid heparin tube is optimal for specimen for crystal analysis because inflamed fluid may clot)
- Where the fluid is to be sent (e.g., cell count to the hematology laboratory, Gram stain to the microbiology laboratory)

Use sonographic localization of joint fluid.

Prepare the area thoroughly with the antiseptic of choice. Use sterile gloves and equipment.

Use an 18- to 22-gauge needle depending on the size of the joint; smaller needles may not be sufficient to collect joint fluid.

Attachment of extension tubing between the needle hub and the syringe helps decrease movement of the needle in the joint space and makes changing syringes with large-volume arthrocentesis and injection of medications into the joint space easier. Tubing must be flushed when injecting corticosteroids so that the full dose actually enters the joint space.

Collect enough fluid for appropriate testing (this is not an easily repeated procedure).

Send fluid for a cell count and differential, Gram stain and culture, crystals, glucose, and viscosity.

Seeding the fluid into blood culture flasks immediately after aspiration may increase the yield.

Have the patient rest the joint for 12 to 24 hours after the injection of corticosteroids.

inflammatory conditions: gout, pseudogout, and septic, rheumatoid and seronegative arthritides (**Table 107.2**).

Crystal analysis is performed under compensated polarizing microscopy. In patients with acute gout, monosodium urate crystals are present inside neutrophils in fluid from the affected joint. The crystals are typically needle shaped and appear yellow when parallel to the compensator; this is negative birefringence. Sensitivity is at least 85%, and specificity for gout is 100%.[4] In pseudogout, the crystals are positively birefringent (blue when parallel to the compensator), usually rhomboid shaped, and also phagocytized by neutrophils. Acute gouty arthritis may occasionally coexist with septic arthritis or pseudogout.

Glucose may be decreased relative to serum glucose in severe inflammatory disorders: down to less than 50% of the serum glucose level in septic arthritis and 50% to 75% in rheumatoid and seronegative arthritides. However, evidence suggests that chemistry studies on joint fluid should be discouraged because their results may be misleading or redundant.[5]

**BOX 107.5 "Seconds" Mnemonic for Radiographic Evaluation of Arthritis**

**S**oft tissue swelling—Nonspecific, often seen with acute arthritides such as gout, pseudogout, and septic arthritis, as well as with tuberculous arthritis; also present in trauma

**E**rosions—May be present in late rheumatoid arthritis as a result of the pannus eroding into articular cartilage and bone

**C**alcification—In late pseudogout, there may be linear calcification in cartilage

**O**steoporosis—Sometimes present in late septic arthritis as a result of joint destruction (about 8 to 10 days of disease before changes are evident on plain films). Osteoporosis or periarticular bone may be seen with late rheumatoid arthritis but *not* with pseudogout or osteoarthritis

**N**arrowing of the joint space—Present in late septic arthritis; asymmetric narrowing is consistent with late pseudogout and osteoarthritis; symmetric narrowing is consistent with late rheumatoid arthritis. Joint space is typically preserved with tuberculous arthritis

**D**eformity—In late septic arthritis, subchondral bone destruction and periosteal new bone may be visualized; in late pseudogout and osteoarthritis, changes may include sclerosis, osteophyte formation, and subchondral cyst formation

**S**eparation from fracture

Adapted from Beachley MC, Franklin JW, Ostlund W, et al. Radiology of arthritis. Prim Care 1993;20:771-94.

**BOX 107.6 Arthrocentesis**

**Indications**

Suspected septic arthritis

Diagnosis of nontraumatic joint disease by synovial fluid analysis

Diagnosis of ligamentous or bony injury by confirmation of blood in the joint

Establishment of the existence of an intraarticular fracture by the presence of blood with fat globules in the joint

Relief of pain accompanying acute hemarthrosis or a tense effusion

Local instillation of medications

Obtaining fluid for analysis (culture, cell count, crystal studies)

**Contraindications (Relative)**

Infection in tissue overlying the site to be punctured

Presence of bacteremia

Coagulopathy

Joint prosthesis (contact an orthopedic consultant)

Uncooperative patient

Viscosity can be measured grossly in the laboratory and ED. Inflammation decreases the hyaluronate portion of synovial fluid, and thus viscosity decreases. When dropped from a syringe, normal synovial fluid makes a 5- to 10-cm string of fluid before dropping. With inflammation, the string of fluid will be shorter or the fluid may simply form droplets.

**Table 107.2 Joint Fluid Analysis of the Various Arthritides**

| DIAGNOSIS | APPEARANCE | WBCs/MM³ | PMN LEUKOCYTES | GLUCOSE (% BLOOD LEVEL) | CRYSTALS UNDER POLARIZED LIGHT | CULTURE |
|---|---|---|---|---|---|---|
| Normal | Clear | <200 | <25% | 95-100 | None | Negative |
| Osteoarthritis | Clear | <4000 | <25% | 95-100 | None | Negative |
| Traumatic | Straw colored, bloody, xanthochromic, occasionally with fat droplets | <4000 | <25% | 95-100 | None | Negative |
| Acute gout | Turbid | 2000-50,000 | >75% | 80-100 | Negative birefringence; needlelike | Negative |
| Pseudogout | Turbid | 2000-50,000 | >75% | 80-100 | Positive birefringence; rhomboid | Negative |
| Septic arthritis | Turbid, purulent | 5000 to >50,000 | >75% | <50 | None | Usually positive |
| Rheumatoid arthritis | Turbid | 2000-50,000 | 50-75% | ≈75 | None | Negative |

*PMN*, Polymorphonuclear; *WBCs*, white blood cells.

Although a joint WBC count higher than 50,000/mm³ is generally said to be positive for infection, septic arthritis can occur with lower joint WBC counts, especially early in infection (36% of patients with septic arthritis had joint WBC counts lower than 50,000/mm³).[6] In addition, patients with inflammatory arthritides such as RA, gout, and pseudogout may have very high joint WBC counts. Thus fluid must also be sent for Gram stain and culture. The yield is increased by immediate plating in the laboratory and perhaps by inoculating blood culture bottles with joint fluid in the ED. The serum WBC count, ESR, and joint WBC count are extremely variable in adults with septic arthritis.[7] In the absence of a positive Gram stain, the ED clinician must consider the whole picture when determining the probability of septic arthritis.

## TREATMENT

ED care focuses on early relief of pain, typically with nonsteroidal antiinflammatory drugs (NSAIDs) such as ibuprofen (800 mg orally) or acetaminophen (1 g orally) (or both), ice, and limb support in a position of comfort (usually partial flexion). If the pain is severe or unrelieved by initial analgesia, tramadol or narcotic analgesics are used, and the joint may be immobilized with an elastic bandage, splint, or brace. "Buddy taping" to the adjacent digit helps relieve the pain in finger joints.

Removal of fluid from a joint effusion provides considerable relief. Intraarticular corticosteroids (e.g., triamcinolone hexacetonide, ranging from 5 mg in a finger joint to 40 mg in a large joint, or methylprednisolone, 2 to 5 mg in small joints and 10 to 25 mg in large joints) are recommended for effusions unless infection is suspected. The patient should be informed that the pain relief with corticosteroids typically begins in 1 to 2 days, peaks at about 1 week, and lasts for 1 week to a few months, during which time compliance with adjunctive measures helps prevent recurrence. Although minimal evidence supports the concern, repeated steroid use traditionally raises concern over cartilage damage, so use in the same joint is limited to every 3 to 4 months. Long-acting local anesthetic may be added to the injection for same-day short-term relief.[8,9]

If suspicion for an infected joint is high, intravenous antibiotics are administered after appropriate material is sent for culture (see discussion later under "Septic Arthritis").

## FOLLOW-UP, NEXT STEPS IN CARE, AND PATIENT EDUCATION

Serious situations may warrant admission (**Box 107.7**). Patients with joint infections require admission and early consultation with an orthopedic surgeon or rheumatologist.

Most other patients will be discharged home with an analgesic and general treatment measures to relieve pain. Full-dose acetaminophen (650 to 1000 mg four times daily) may be adequate (especially if a history such as gastrointestinal [GI] bleeding, heart failure, or renal failure makes use of an NSAID risky), or an NSAID may be selected based on low cost and safety profile (e.g., celecoxib may be safer for the stomach). The NSAID is begun at a high dose (e.g., ibuprofen, 600 to 800 mg three times daily), continued for at least 2 to 3 days (or with inflammatory arthritis, for at least a few days after the pain stops), and then may be continued as needed. The patient is advised to take NSAIDs with food, especially with a history of stomach upset, and cotreatment with a stomach-protective drug ($H_2$ blocker, proton pump inhibitor, or sucralfate [Carafate]) should be considered. Nonresponders

**BOX 107.7 Emergency Department Disposition Decisions**

**When to Admit**
Septic joint
Inability to control pain without parenteral analgesics
Acute inability to ambulate despite treatment in the emergency department (ED)
Inability to care for self at home (physical and occupational therapy; social, placement issues)
Need for urgent operative intervention
Need for parenteral medications
Possible infection in a prosthetic joint
High-risk complications (e.g., acute renal failure, systemic vasculitis, cardiac involvement, hypoxic lung disease)

**Indications for Rheumatology or Orthopedic Outpatient Follow-up**
Diagnostic uncertainty in inflammatory arthritis
Failure of adequate treatment regimens
Increasing disability or deformity
Disease complications
Management dilemmas
Consideration of immunosuppressive therapy
Proposed surgical intervention
Complication of a complex treatment regimen
Concern regarding a prosthetic joint
Patient request for a specialist's opinion

**Time Line for Follow-up**
**In 2 to 3 days**: Significant inflammation, serious risk if diagnostic delay, culture results to be checked (if timely outpatient visit not possible, schedule return to the ED)
**Within 1 week**: Lupus flare (no central nervous system or renal involvement; laboratory results not seriously altered); consultation with a rheumatologist for a possible increase in steroids
**In 1 to 2 weeks**: Patient with rheumatologic disease sick enough to merit an ED visit but not severely ill; intraarticular corticosteroids administered in the ED; most inflammatory arthritides (not septic)
**In 2 to 4 weeks**: Chronic, mild, or noninflammatory complaints

may be switched to a different NSAID, often with good relief, or may be given concomitant acetaminophen or tramadol. Judicious short-term use of narcotic analgesics is also helpful.

Topical analgesics may help, especially if only a single joint is problematic. Topical NSAIDs (diclofenac or ketoprofen, but not salicylates) and capsaicin (thin film of 0.025% cream applied four times per day) have been shown in trials to be beneficial, but maximal relief may take 3 to 4 weeks. Topical NSAIDs avoid the GI and renal complications of oral agents.[10,11] Lidocaine patches are another option, although unstudied.

General treatment measures should be recommended, including ice packs or heat (or both), temporary support (elastic wrap; brace, cane, or walker) and joint rest, but unnecessary or prolonged immobilization should be avoided. Patient education should include simple measures to avoid repetitive injury (e.g., patients with shoulder pain often ignore the obvious trigger of carrying a heavy shoulder bag). Simple splinting or ergonomic advice may assist patients with pain related to repetitive motions when the activity is unavoidable.

Appropriate lifestyle recommendations for patients with chronic arthritis are to stay as active as possible with daily activities and reasonable exercise programs. Physical and occupational therapy[12] may contribute greatly to improved quality of life and ability to maintain independence in self-care but are usually arranged by the continuity physician. Initial range-of-motion (ROM) and later strengthening and aerobic exercise regimens are recommended; swimming pool exercise programs are quite helpful. Obese patients with lower extremity arthritis should be educated about the importance of weight reduction.

Follow-up care includes referral to a primary care physician for most patients. Rheumatology referral is recommended for patients with clinical suspicion of new inflammatory or autoimmune arthritides such as RA or for patients not improving despite adequate general care. Chronic severe pain with significant disability merits orthopedic referral. Patient education is vital for achieving an optimal outcome (see the Patient Teaching Tips box).

# RHEUMATOID ARTHRITIS

## EPIDEMIOLOGY

RA is the most common inflammatory arthritis, with about 0.8% of the world's population afflicted, and it has a 3 : 1 female preponderance. It begins most commonly in the 40s. Overall, life expectancy is only modestly reduced, but quality of life may be significantly impaired. The majority of patients experience chronic remitting but overall progressive disease, including about 10% with an aggressive, severely destructive pattern and 15% to 30% with intermittent remissions lasting up to 1 year; about 15% experience a long-lasting remission with excellent function.[13]

## PATHOPHYSIOLOGY

RA is a systemic inflammatory autoimmune disease that primarily targets the synovium and transforms it into hyperplastic inflamed and thickened tissue that proliferates into a pannus. The pannus is unique to RA, where it grows over the articular cartilage, erodes into bone, and causes destruction and deformity. Synovial fluid contains abundant neutrophils, cytokines, proteolytic enzymes, prostaglandins, and leukotrienes. The etiology of RA remains unknown, but it is probably caused by a combination of environmental factors and genetic susceptibility, with several contributing genes, particularly the class II major histocompatibility complex. An ongoing and uncontrollable immune response is elicited, perhaps against an autoantigen. RFs are IgM or IgG antibodies synthesized in the synovium that form immune complexes with IgG in the blood or joints.

## PRESENTING SIGNS AND SYMPTOMS

RA is characterized by symmetric polyarthritis persisting for more than 6 weeks, prolonged morning stiffness (>30 minutes),

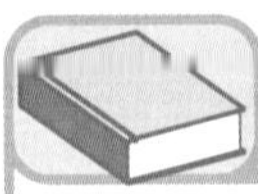

**PATIENT TEACHING TIPS**

**At Discharge**

Instruct patients to return to the emergency department (ED) for temperatures higher than 101° F or if the redness or swelling spreads; also state specific problems to watch out for—for example, patients given nonsteroidal antiinflammatory drugs should "stop the medicine and come to the ED if you have black or bloody stools."

Educate patients about their specific condition. Examples of teaching points include the following:

- Osteoarthritis is a chronic condition that often requires medications, general support measures, physical and occupational therapy, and in some cases surgical intervention (joint replacement).
- Gout may recur, so it is important to stay well hydrated; avoid excessive meat, seafood, and alcohol and certain medications. Discuss preventive medication with your primary doctor.
- Gonococcal infections spread through sexual contact, so all sexual partners must be treated. Protected sex can prevent transmission. The patient requires further testing for other sexually transmitted diseases, including human immunodeficiency virus, hepatitis B and C, and syphilis.

Understanding plus compliance with the recommended medication dose and directions is important for a good outcome. Patients with inflammatory arthritis may benefit from continuing the antiinflammatory medications even after the pain improves.

Follow-up visits are important for a good outcome:

- The results of the ED visit and treatment need to be reviewed with a primary physician.
- Many rheumatologic diseases are chronic, cannot be diagnosed in a single ED visit, or need specialized care or treatments not normally done in the ED.
- Patients must inform their caregivers about *all* the medications that they are taking, including over-the-counter and herbal and alternative preparations.

Preprinted discharge instructions and disease education pamphlets are helpful, especially if notes are added to adapt them to the specific needs of individual patients. Additional information is available at sites such as www.arthritisfoundation.org.

and systemic symptoms of fatigue, malaise, and weight loss. Diagnostic criteria are listed in **Table 107.3**.[14] Arthritis typically starts in the small joints (metacarpophalangeal [MCP], metatarsophalangeal [MTP], and proximal interphalangeal [PIP] joints of the hands and feet but not the distal interphalangeal [DIP] joints) and later affects larger extremity joints. Migratory polyarthralgia occurs, and the symptoms may wax and wane. The onset of RA is typically insidious but can be abrupt. Cervical spine involvement is prevalent, although the rest of the spine is usually spared. RA increases the risk for a septic joint or tendon rupture, and temporomandibular joint (TMF) problems are common.

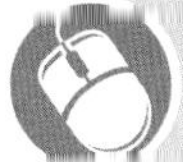

See Table 107.3, 2010 American College of Rheumatology Revised Criteria for the Classification of Rheumatoid Arthritis, online at www.expertconsult.com

Examination in the early stages usually finds tenderness, swelling, and limited ROM in at least three joints, especially in the hands and feet.[15] Warmth and erythema are uncommon. Palpation may reveal loss of the normal contour across joints (especially the MCP joints) because of pannus. Rheumatoid nodules are found in 20% of patients and can appear anywhere but especially over bony prominences, pressure points, and tendon sheaths. These nodules may be fixed or mobile with a rubbery or granular texture and are sometimes indistinguishable from gouty tophi. They are not a serious problem unless they occur in the vocal cords or cardiac conduction tissue. Typical later joint deformities are radial deviation at the wrist (usually the earliest deformity), ulnar deviation at the MCP joints (the most characteristic deformity of RA), swan neck or boutonnière deformities of the fingers, cock-up toes, loss of arches, and hallux valgus.

Extraarticular manifestations are common. Acutely life-threatening complications are rare but disastrous. Patients may also have serious complications of chronic treatment, particularly with infections from immunosuppression.

## DIFFERENTIAL DIAGNOSIS AND MEDICAL DECISION MAKING

Identification of septic arthritis is the top priority given its risk for rapid joint destruction or systemic infection. Patients with known RA are at significantly increased risk, and clinical findings may be more subtle because of their drug regimens. Joint fluid analysis is essential. Systemic infections may seed a joint or induce an immunologic arthritis; mild systemic symptoms may be difficult to distinguish from those of exacerbation of RA.

OA is the most common consideration in the differential diagnosis, but its pattern of joint involvement (especially in the hands) and minimal to absent systemic symptoms distinguish it from RA. Self-limited arthritic syndromes (e.g., viral infections, Lyme disease) can be difficult to distinguish clinically from the initial findings in patients with RA, and thus the RA criteria require persistence of the joint symptoms for longer than 6 weeks. The usual time from onset to diagnosis of RA is 6 to 12 months, but joint damage occurs early, with 30% of patients exhibiting bone erosion at time of diagnosis.

Studies may assist in the differential diagnosis. RA typically produces a mild normochromic normocytic anemia and thrombocytosis but normal WBC count (unless infected or Felty syndrome is present), an ESR of 30 to 60 mm/hr, and an elevated CRP level. On plain films, RA is characteristically associated with joint space narrowing (especially in the MCP, PIP, and wrist joints), marginal bony erosions, periarticular osteopenia, and soft tissue swelling (**Fig. 107.1**). Joint destruction (e.g., femoral head protruding through the acetabulum) occurs late.

Serologic testing (RF IgM or anti–citrullinated protein antibody [ACPA]) for a new diagnosis is generally best done in

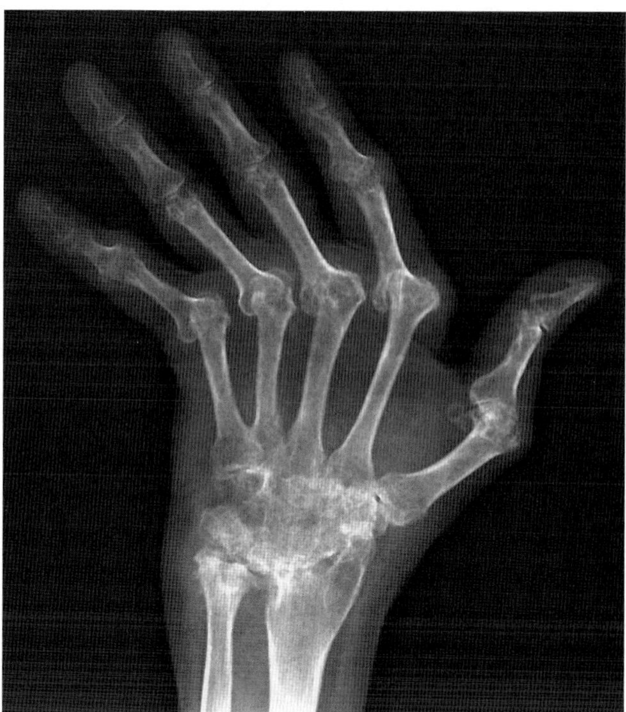

**Fig. 107.1 Ulnar deviation in a patient with rheumatoid arthritis.** Severe ulnar deviation with extensive erosions is present at the metacarpophalangeal joints. Pancompartmental bony ankylosis and erosion are also seen in the wrist. (From Harris E, editor. Kelley's textbook of rheumatology. 7th ed. Philadelphia: Saunders; 2005.)

the follow-up setting. False positives and negatives occur, so the results must always be interpreted in the clinical context. Although a positive RF titer (>1 : 80) develops in 85% of patients with RA in the first year of the disease, unfortunately half are negative for the first 6 months, just when early intervention is most effective. RF is frequently positive in other settings, such as subacute bacterial endocarditis and rheumatic fever, and is present in low titer in 20% of elderly patients without disease. ACPA testing is newer, becomes positive earlier, but is not as widely available as RF.[16]

## TREATMENT

General measures (analgesics, ice, rest, joint support) are needed for relief of pain. NSAIDs are the mainstay of initial symptomatic treatment, although these drugs do not modify the overall course. Unless contraindicated, the maximal dose of an NSAID is administered for a minimum 2-week trial. Concomitant use of an additional analgesic is often helpful.

Low-dose corticosteroids (prednisone, 5 to 10 mg daily) are often tremendously helpful for rapid relief of symptoms but are generally initiated after failure of general measures and an adequate NSAID trial. In RA, corticosteroids are usually superimposed on other treatment regimens. If the patient has only one or two very problematic joints that are clearly *not* infected, intraarticular corticosteroids can produce rapid improvement lasting for several weeks to months.

## FOLLOW-UP, NEXT STEPS IN CARE, AND PATIENT EDUCATION

The majority of RA patients will be discharged (see Box 107.7). Immunosuppressed patients warrant high suspicion for infection and a low threshold for admission. Follow-up visits with either a primary care physician or rheumatologist (if a new diagnosis or not responding to treatment) are essential. Chronic severe joint dysfunction merits orthopedic referral for potential surgical intervention (joint replacement, arthrodesis, synovectomy).

Disease-modifying antirheumatic drugs (DMARDS) are essential for all RA patients to prevent joint damage[17,18] and are now initiated as early as possible after diagnosis (but not in the ED). The mainstay remains methotrexate, alone or in combination.[19] Leflunomide (an immunomodulatory drug) and sulfasalazine are alternatives.[20] Exciting new and effective biologic agents include anticytokine therapies such as etanercept, anakinra, abatacept, and rituximab.[21]

# OSTEOARTHRITIS

## EPIDEMIOLOGY

OA is the most common cause of joint pain and frequently leads to chronic pain and disability. In the United States, symptomatic knee OA occurs in 6% of persons older than 30 years and hip OA in 3%. About one third of adults aged 25 to 74 years have radiographic evidence of OA in at least one joint group, most commonly the hands and then the feet and knees. Prevalence increases considerably with age, and OA is a major cause of disability, lost work time, and early retirement. Before the age of 50, prevalence in most joints is higher in men, but at older ages women are more often affected in the hands, feet, and knees.[22]

Other risk factors include obesity, trauma, family history, and occupations involving repetitive knee or hip bending and lifting (e.g., farmers, dockworkers). The role of aggressive exercise remains unclear, although moderate running appears to be low risk. High-intensity contact sports and those involving repetitive joint impact and twisting are higher-risk categories.

## PATHOPHYSIOLOGY

OA is a disease of articular cartilage and subchondral bone that is characterized by patchy loss of cartilage, overgrowth of bone at the joint margins (osteophytes are hallmarks of OA), hypertrophy of subchondral bone, fibrosis in the joint capsule, loss of joint space, and mild inflammation of the synovium. Loss of cartilage allows the underlying bones to rub together, which produces pain, swelling, and limited ROM. The primary process is mechanical, not inflammatory, but past views of OA as being entirely mechanical (hence names used in the past such as degenerative joint disease and osteoarthrosis) are inaccurate because recent evidence shows considerably more synovial inflammation than was previously considered. Its pathogenesis involves chronic mechanical microdamage, disturbed chondrocyte regulation of the synthesis and degradation of cartilage matrix, genetic factors, and inflammatory pathways. Local mechanical factors (malalignment, laxity, proprioception) contribute in specific joints.

Most cases are classified as idiopathic or primary. Secondary osteoarthritis may result from congenital or developmental diseases, trauma, deposition diseases (calcium, hemochromatosis), neuropathic arthropathy, or endocrinopathies (e.g., acromegaly, hyperparathyroidism).

## PRESENTING SIGNS AND SYMPTOMS

OA most commonly affects the knees, hips, spine, fingers (especially the DIP joints and first carpometacarpal joint), and toes (especially the MTP joints). ED visits are usually prompted by significant pain in a large joint (knees or hips) that is often associated with an acute but minor injury. Neck or back pain is also common. Patients typically report a gradual onset of pain and stiffness in one or a few joints with limited ROM. Locking or instability of the knee is common, as is joint effusion. Baseline pain is mild to moderate, worse with use, and rapidly better with rest, and the symptoms are worse in damp, cool weather.

On examination, disease is found to be limited to the symptomatic joints. Joint tenderness, bone enlargement, and crepitus on joint motion are common findings. Heberden nodes (hard nodules on the dorsal aspect of the DIP joints) are commonly seen in older women with OA. Malalignment is found in about half of knees with OA, typically with a varus (bowleg) deformity and often with instability on excess ROM. Joints may be mildly warm, especially if an effusion is present, but not dramatically inflamed. Late in the disease course, significant joint disability is evident (**Fig. 107.2**).

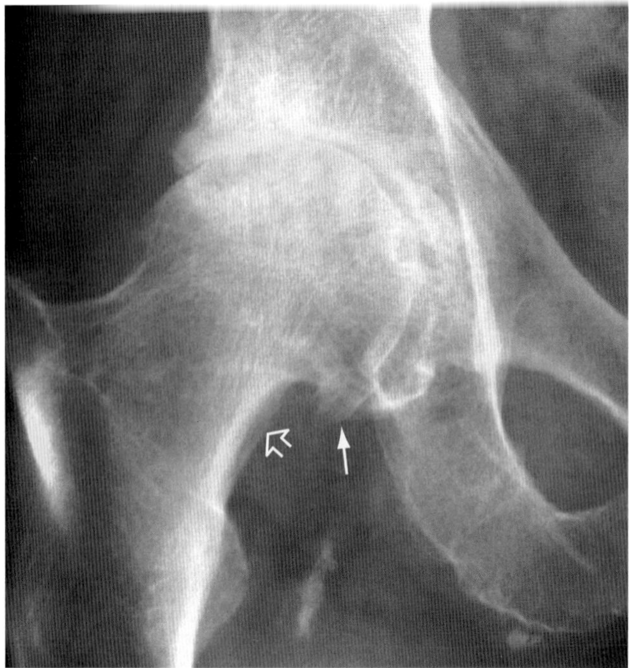

**Fig. 107.2 Osteoarthritis of the hip.** This anteroposterior view of the hip shows complete loss of cartilage space superiorly. There is osteophytic lipping from the femoral head, especially medially *(arrow)*, and buttressing bone *(open arrow)* is present along the femoral neck. (From Harris E, editor. Kelley's textbook of rheumatology. 7th ed. Philadelphia: Saunders; 2005.)

## DIFFERENTIAL DIAGNOSIS AND MEDICAL DECISION MAKING

Although OA is a polyarthritis, it most commonly affects just a few joints in each patient. Prominent general systemic symptoms point to another diagnosis, such as RA or fibromyalgia, whereas active involvement of other organs suggests other autoimmune arthritides. Patients are prone to coexisting pseudogout in the knee, or gout may develop. A red, hot swollen joint is probably infected or acute crystal-induced arthritis.

If ordered, laboratory results are generally normal. Joint fluid is usually noninflammatory, with a WBC count lower than $2000/mm^3$; inflammatory fluid may occur in OA but more often suggests gout or infection. Radiologic results must be correlated with the clinical picture. In asymptomatic patients older than 40 years, radiographic studies often show degenerative joint changes, but a label of OA would be incorrect. The classic changes with OA are degenerative with marginal osteophyte formation, subchondral bony sclerosis, and asymmetric joint space narrowing. Later, subchondral cysts with sclerotic walls form, and bone remodeling distorts the ends of bones. Bone demineralization and marginal erosions suggest an inflammatory arthritis such as RA.

## TREATMENT

Initial attempts at pain relief in the ED include analgesics, ice, and support in a position of comfort. Acetaminophen or ibuprofen may be adequate. If a patient has already adequately tried and failed to obtain relief with these medications, tramadol or narcotic analgesics should be considered. If a significant effusion is causing pain and disability, removal of fluid provides considerable relief. Intraarticular corticosteroids are also effective, especially in the knee or MCP joints, with pain relief lasting weeks to months. Intraarticular hyaluronic acid injections have been used in the knee, but their efficacy is limited.[23]

## FOLLOW-UP, NEXT STEPS IN CARE, AND ADMISSION

As with other arthritides, the vast majority of patients with OA are discharged home with recommendations for primary care follow-up, whereas those with known or strongly suspected joint infection are treated and admitted to the hospital. Several options are available for discharge analgesia.[24,25] Patients with mild symptoms may need only general care measures. Acetaminophen and NSAIDs are the first-line choices. In studies both have been shown to be effective in reducing pain, although NSAIDs or celecoxib is modestly better. However, acetaminophen has less risk for side effects and thus remains a good first choice. Effective additions or alternatives include tramadol or short-term use of narcotics.

Topical NSAIDs (not salicylates) are considered core treatment of OA of the knee or hands, and topical capsaicin is considered adjunctive to core treatment of these joints; strong evidence supports their benefits.[10,11] Glucosamine sulfate (1500 mg/day) and chondroitin sulfate (1200 mg/day) may shift cartilage metabolism toward a positive balance and are widely popular among patients, but the overall evidence to date shows limited efficacy[26,27]; these over-the-counter preparations may vary considerably in composition.

General care measures and patient education are also important (see the Patient Teaching Tips box presented earlier and **Box 107.8**).[28] Evidence supports the benefit of exercise regimens and weight loss in patients with knee arthritis. Correction of knee malalignment with a neoprene sleeve, valgus brace, orthotics, or a combination of such devices is beneficial.[29] Evidence on the benefit of acupuncture is mixed.[30] Surgical interventions are useful in selected situations; knee arthroscopy is beneficial if cartilage flaps, loose bodies, or meniscal disruption is causing mechanical locking or instability. Total joint replacement for knee or hip OA often dramatically improves severe refractory pain and disability, particularly if the patient has a relatively low body mass index. Chondrocyte transplantation is an exciting intervention for future care.

**BOX 107.8 General Treatment Measures for Chronic Arthritis**

**Patient Education**
Nature and usual course of the disease
Exacerbating and relieving factors
Avoidance of repetitive injuries, impacts
Arthritis self-help course available from the Arthritis Foundation (www.arthritis.org)

**Painful Joint**
Analgesics (take a bedtime dose if early morning pain), oral and/or topical
Acute exacerbations:
- Rest, ice, compression, elevation
- Temporary limitation of range of motion and forceful use

Correction of misalignment—joint sleeve or brace, orthotics
Chronic pain—trials with ice, heat, in-water therapy
Unloading joint stress with a cane or crutch (contralateral to the affected leg)

**Physical Therapy**
Relief of pain and muscle spasm (massage, heat, ultrasonography, electrical stimulation therapy, physical maneuvers)
Improvement in and preservation of range of motion
Strengthening (general or surrounding a specific joint)
Progressive individualized exercise regimen
General conditioning

**Occupational Therapy**
Improved activities of daily living
Assist devices
Temporary splinting
Protective techniques
Energy conservation skills

**Lifestyle**
Weight loss program
Adequate nutrition and calcium intake
Range-of-motion preservation
Exercise program with low-impact aerobic conditioning
Evaluation of the home for fall prevention, improved functionality
Well-cushioned shoes or orthotics

**Acupuncture**
Role unclear; efficacy not well supported by available evidence; appears beneficial for knee pain

**Glucosamine and Chondroitin**
Role unclear; efficacy not well supported by available evidence

# REACTIVE ARTHRITIS

## EPIDEMIOLOGY

Reactive arthritides are seronegative spondyloarthropathies that are much less common than OA and RA; however, identification is important to guide management. Most are self-limited illnesses, but persistent and severe disease develops in a minority of patients (particularly those with acquired immunodeficiency syndrome). Prevalence parallels that of the human leukocyte antigen (HLA) B27 genes in different populations. In the United States, 6% to 14% of Caucasians have HLA-B27, as do 2% to 3% of African Americans. The peak onset is during the third decade of life. Reactive arthritis has a 5 : 1 to 6 : 1 male preponderance, but cases in women may be underdiagnosed—women tend to have milder symptoms, and their genitourinary (GU) manifestations may be occult. The incidence of reactive arthritis is estimated to be 3 to 6 cases per year per 100,000 males younger than 50 years.

## PATHOPHYSIOLOGY

In reactive arthritides, a sterile inflammatory arthropathy arises, commonly after a primary infection elsewhere in the body. Onset typically occurs 1 to 4 weeks after a diarrheal or GU infection, once the triggering infectious illness is over. Enteric pathogens include *Shigella, Yersinia, Salmonella, Campylobacter*, and *Clostridium difficile*. Sexually transmitted pathogens include *Chlamydia* (mainly *Chlamydia trachomatis*), *Ureaplasma urealyticum*, and human immunodeficiency virus (HIV). Presumably, microbial material or products are disseminated to the joints and extraarticular structures and trigger an inflammatory response consisting of mononuclear infiltration into the joints and entheses, synovial effusions, and inflammatory mediators. Most patients carry HLA-B27 genes. In many, the inciting infection is not identifiable.

Inflammation of the entheses, eyes, and mucosal surfaces is a distinctive feature of reactive arthritis. The illness tends to be self-limited over several months, but relapses occur in about one third of patients. HIV-associated disease is often severe and disabling.

**BOX 107.9 Classic Signs of Reactive Arthritis (Formerly Known as Reiter Syndrome)**

Enthesitis—periarticular, classically Achilles or plantar tendinitis
Peripheral arthritis pattern—may be a hot erythematous joint for which active infection must be ruled out; often asymmetric oligoarthritis
Dactylitis—"sausage digits"
Conjunctivitis—bilateral or unilateral, usually painful
Urethritis, cervicitis
Circinate balanitis on the shaft or glans of the penis; vulvitis in women—ranging from vesicles to ulcerations
Keratoderma blenorrhagicum—painless papulosquamous rash on the palms and soles, similar to pustular psoriasis
Oral ulcerations—painless

## PRESENTING SIGNS AND SYMPTOMS

Cases of reactive arthritis seen in the ED are likely to be a new diagnoses. Typically, the patient reports one or a few sites of acute joint pain, often asymmetric and with sequential onset. Common sites include large joints (one or both ankles, wrists, knees) and small joints in the feet; the upper extremities may be involved later. Fever (up to 102.2° F [39° C]), constitutional symptoms (fatigue, malaise, weight loss), and mucosal problems are common findings (**Box 107.9**). Low back pain, back stiffness, or sacroiliitis occurs in half the patients.[31] The involved joints are often inflamed. The classic triad that was formerly named Reiter syndrome includes acute peripheral arthritis (asymmetric, oligoarticular, additive), conjunctivitis (mild, usually several days before the appearance of joint pain), and nongonococcal urethritis or cervicitis (generally mild, precedes the joint pain).

Most patients do not manifest the full triad. Some may not volunteer information about other symptoms before their joint pain or about recent diarrheal or GU infections.

Later complications can include ankylosing spondylitis, uveitis, and cardiac involvement (in about 10% of patients) with conduction blocks, nonspecific ST-segment changes, Q waves, or aortic regurgitation.

## DIFFERENTIAL DIAGNOSIS AND MEDICAL DECISION MAKING

With an acute hot joint, infection (especially gonococcal) must be ruled out. Active infection elsewhere (especially the GI and GU tracts) must also be considered. Reactive arthritis should be distinguished from seronegative RA, crystal-induced arthritis, sarcoidosis, acute rheumatic fever, psoriatic arthritis, and erythema nodosum. A carefully constructed clinical picture will usually distinguish reactive arthritis, but this may not easily be done in the ED.

Given the frequent finding of fever, acute arthritis, and involvement of mucosal surfaces in patients with reactive arthritis, laboratory studies are appropriate (CBC, chemistries, liver enzymes, urinalysis, ESR, arthrocentesis, joint fluid cultures, and usually blood cultures). In reactive arthritis, a modest increase in WBCs, platelets, and ESR is expected, and mild anemia is common. Active urethral or GI infection should be considered, and tests for *Chlamydia* and gonorrhea are appropriate if the patient has had any recent GU symptoms. If the precipitating infection was dysenteric, stool should be sent for culture. Serologic and HLA studies are not done in the ED.

## TREATMENT

Full-dose NSAIDs are the mainstay of therapy for reactive arthritis—a good response is typical.[32] General care measures are also appropriate (see earlier), especially encouragement of continuing exercise. Systemic corticosteroid therapy is not generally indicated, but intraarticular glucocorticoids may help in alleviating persistently problematic joints after ruling out infection. Second-line medications for nonresponders include sulfasalazine or methotrexate. Experience with anti-TNF agents is limited but promising.

Antibiotic treatment of *Chlamydia* is appropriate if the initial infection was untreated or is found on testing. Empiric administration of an antibiotic to patients with a previous history of GI infection is not useful unless current stool cultures show persistence of a pathogenic trigger.

## FOLLOW-UP, NEXT STEPS IN CARE, AND PATIENT EDUCATION

Most patients with reactive arthritis can be discharged home with primary care follow-up, but admission is indicated if the patient is febrile or if active joint infection is likely. Referral to ophthalmology is advised if uveitis is suspected.

# SEPTIC ARTHRITIS

## EPIDEMIOLOGY

The incidence (expressed per 100,000 per year) of septic arthritis varies between 2 and 5 in the general population, 5 and 12 in children, 28 and 38 in patients with RA, and 40 and 68 in patients with joint prostheses. Males are usually affected more commonly than females, although with underlying RA, females are affected more often. About 10% of patients with acutely painful joints will have septic arthritis.[1]

The organisms causing bacterial arthritis depend on the epidemiologic circumstances (**Table 107.4**). For example, monarthritis of a prosthetic joint is probably due to *Staphylococcus* species, whereas a migratory arthritis in a sexually active woman is probably due to disseminated gonococcal infection. Rarely, the cause may be fungal, protozoal, or mycobacterial, particularly in immunosuppressed patients. Viral joint infections are not considered part of the "septic" category.

Major risk factors for septic arthritis in adults include age older than 80 years, diabetes mellitus, RA, prosthetic joint or recent joint surgery, skin infection or ulceration, alcoholism,

**Table 107.4 Most Common Organisms and Suggested Antibiotics for Various Patient Groups with Arthritis**

| AGE/GROUP | MOST COMMON ORGANISMS | SUGGESTED EMPIRIC ANTIBIOTICS |
|---|---|---|
| Overall | *Staphylococcus aureus* most common; also streptococci, gram-negative organisms, anaerobes, *Neisseria gonorrhoeae* | At risk for STD—ceftriaxone; not at risk for STD—oxacillin/nafcillin + ceftriaxone |
| Infants (<6 mo) | *Escherichia coli*, group B streptococci | Oxacillin/nafcillin + cefotaxime/ceftriaxone |
| Children 6-24 mo | Staphylococci, *Kingella kingae* (no longer *Haemophilus influenzae*) | Oxacillin/nafcillin + cefotaxime/ceftriaxone |
| Pediatric (>24 mo) | *N. gonorrhoeae*, pneumococci | Oxacillin/nafcillin + cefotaxime/ceftriaxone |
| Intravenous drug abusers | *S. aureus*, gram-negative organisms | Oxacillin/nafcillin + ceftriaxone |
| Prosthetic joint | MSSA/MRSA, MSSE/MRSE, Enterobacteriaceae, *Pseudomonas* | Vancomycin + ciprofloxacin |

*MSSA/MRSA*, Methicillin-sensitive/resistant *Staphylococcus aureus; MSSE/MRSE*, methicillin-sensitive/resistant *Staphylococcus epidermidis; STD*, sexually transmitted disease.

intravenous drug use, and prior intraarticular corticosteroid injection.[1] Previous joint damage from any cause also appears to increase risk.

## PATHOPHYSIOLOGY

Bacteria can infect the joint via hematogenous spread, direct inoculation (arthrocentesis, trauma, surgery), or contiguous contact (cellulitis, bursitis, tenosynovitis). Any microorganisms, including bacteria, fungi, and protozoa, may invade joints; however, the overwhelming majority of cases (90%) are caused by the pyogenic bacteria *Staphylococcus* and *Streptococcus*.[33] Once the pathogen penetrates the joint space, it initiates a series of inflammatory reactions that may lead to joint destruction and permanent damage. Microorganisms or their products (or both) activate the release of proinflammatory cytokines, such TNF-$\alpha$ and interleukin-1, and proteolytic enzymes, such as metalloproteinases and other collagen-degrading enzymes. These proteins induce synovial membrane proliferation, granulation tissue, neovascularization, and infiltration by polymorphonuclear cells and may result, if untreated, in cartilage and bone destruction. The articular damage may progress even after eradication of microorganisms because persistence of bacterial antigens and metalloproteinases within the joint will continue to promote an inflammatory response.

## PRESENTING SIGNS AND SYMPTOMS

Septic arthritis is generally manifested acutely as a "hot joint"—with joint pain, swelling, erythema, limited and painful ROM, and tenderness. Septic arthritis is usually monarticular, but about 10% of patients have polyarticular involvement (of those, >50% have underlying RA). The knee is the most common site, followed by the hip, wrist, ankle, and shoulder. Fever is common, though often absent in the elderly, and patients frequently have another site of recent infection.

## DIFFERENTIAL DIAGNOSIS AND MEDICAL DECISION MAKING

The differential diagnosis for septic arthritis is focused on other inflammatory diagnoses.[39] Although low-grade fever is common with many types of inflammatory arthritis, higher fevers are more commonly associated with a septic joint, and the physician must rule out a septic joint with joint fluid analysis (see Table 107.2).

A history of gout makes a recurrent gout attack more likely. However, patients with gout are more susceptible to septic arthritis. Gouty arthritis is more likely than septic arthritis to be manifested in a polyarticular fashion. In general, a septic joint will be redder and warmer, whereas a gouty joint will have more fluid.

Unfortunately, laboratory tests, including synovial fluid analysis, do not diagnose or rule out septic arthritis with accuracy. Therefore, if suspicion for septic arthritis is high in the setting of negative testing, the emergency physician should not hesitate to treat for infection while awaiting the results of bacterial culture.[35] Imaging studies are indicated when trauma, bone infection, malignancy, or a foreign body is suspected and are recommended before arthrocentesis. Ultrasonography may assist in identification of joint effusion.

## TREATMENT

Pain management should be initiated early. After appropriate material for culture is obtained, parenteral antibiotics should be selected to treat the most likely pathogens (see Table 107.4). Another reasonable approach is to treat according to Gram stain results (for gram-positive cocci, start vancomycin; for gram-negative organisms, start ceftriaxone or cefotaxime). If the Gram stain is negative, vancomycin is reasonable for an immunocompetent host and vancomycin plus ceftriaxone (or cefotaxime) for an immunosuppressed individual, injection drug user, or traumatic bacterial arthritis.

## FOLLOW-UP, NEXT STEPS IN CARE, AND PATIENT EDUCATION

Hospital admission is needed, along with orthopedic consultation and repeated arthrocentesis if fluid reaccumulates. The patient should be advised about the probable diagnosis and plan of care.

## GOUT AND PSEUDOGOUT

### EPIDEMIOLOGY

The incidence of gout ranges from 1% to 15% in the general population and increases with age and with elevations in serum urate. In adults, serum urate levels correlate strongly with serum creatinine levels, body weight, height, age, blood pressure, and alcohol intake. Acute gout is much more common in men (peak age at onset between the fourth and sixth decades) but tends to occur at older ages in women (sixth to eighth decades). Radiography and autopsy studies have found the incidence of pseudogout to be 15% at age 65 and 50% at age 85.

### PATHOPHYSIOLOGY

Gout and pseudogout are characterized by crystal deposition in joints with recurring attacks of acute inflammatory arthritis, as well as chronic arthropathy.

Although acute gout never develops in most hyperuricemic individuals, all patients with gouty arthritis have hyperuricemia at some point. Microscopic tophaceous deposits of urate crystals develop in synovial membranes, but deposits alone are asymptomatic. Abrupt increases and decreases in serum urate levels may promote the release of free urate crystals from deposits, which have considerable proinflammatory potential because of their ability to activate synovial epithelial cells and promote the ingress of leukocytes into the joint, which triggers multiple inflammatory cascades. Precipitants include initiation of diuretics and other drugs that inhibit the excretion of uric acid (including aspirin), alcohol use, initiation of urate-lowering drugs, starvation, and tumor lysis. Repetitive joint microtrauma may produce locally increased urate concentrations, which perhaps explains the predilection for the first MTP joint.

An acute gouty attack is spontaneously self-limited (usually lasting 7 to 10 days) and probably mediated by an altered balance between proinflammatory and antiinflammatory mediators in the joint. Low-grade synovitis may persist in affected joints. Inflammation, especially with untreated disease, can lead to chronic synovial proliferation, cartilage loss, and bone erosion. Tophi commonly develop in osteoarthritic interphalangeal joints, thus suggesting a role of connective tissue matrix structure and turnover in urate crystal deposition.

Calcium-containing crystals in the pericellular matrix of cartilage are often deposited in the form of CPPD and therefore lead to a disorder termed chondrocalcinosis, pyrophosphate arthropathy, CPPD crystal deposition disease, or when associated with acute arthritis, pseudogout.[36] Precipitation of CPPD crystals in connective tissue is most often asymptomatic. Acute attacks are generally self-limited and often triggered by trauma, surgery, or severe medical illness.

### PRESENTING SIGNS AND SYMPTOMS

Acute inflammatory joint pain, swelling, erythema, and tenderness with painful limited ROM are typical. Inflammatory signs often extend beyond the involved joint and resemble cellulitis. Classically, acute gout affects the first MTP joint, but more than 50% of pseudogout attacks affect the knee. Eighty percent of first gouty attacks are monarticular. Low-grade fever is common in both diagnoses, and a previous history of the joint disease is common.[37]

### DIFFERENTIAL DIAGNOSIS AND MEDICAL DECISION MAKING

A known history of gout, typical precipitants, or location in the great toe suggests gout. Chondrocalcinosis (radiographic evidence of calcification in hyaline cartilage, fibrocartilage, or both) is common in pseudogout; though highly suggestive of the diagnosis, it is neither absolutely specific nor universal. Leukocytosis with a left shift and an elevated ESR may be present but are more common in pseudogout than gout. An elevated uric acid level may or may not be found in acute gout and is nondiagnostic by itself. Normal to low levels are reported in 12% to 43% of patients with acute gout attacks.[38,39] The pattern of symptoms in chronic pseudogout is often similar to OA and may sometimes mimic RA. A significant minority of patients have coexisting arthritides.

Evaluation for septic arthritis is the diagnostic priority in the ED. Joint aspiration with evaluation of synovial fluid for acute inflammation, crystals, or evidence of infection is necessary, and fluid must be sent for Gram stain and culture. Urate crystals inside neutrophils diagnose gout; phagocytosed CPPD crystals are seen in pseudogout. Some patients have concurrent gout and pseudogout, with both types of crystals being found. Coexistence of crystalline and infectious arthritis in the same joint is well reported. If joint fluid analysis cannot be done, a clinical diagnosis may be made from historical and clinical data,[40] but specificity is reduced (**Table 107.5**).

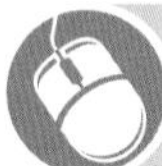

See Table 107.5, Clinical Diagnostic Rule for Acute Monarticular Gout, online at www.expertconsult.com

### TREATMENT

Although acute attacks will resolve spontaneously, antiinflammatory medications are essential for more rapid relief of pain. Even though colchicine has traditionally been used for the acute treatment of gout, rheumatologists prefer NSAIDs (other than aspirin), oral prednisone (30 to 50 mg/day for 5 to 7 days), or intraarticular corticosteroids. Low-dose oral colchicine (1.2 mg and then 0.6 mg in 1 hour or 0.5 mg every 8 hours for 1 day) is safe and effective and avoids the diarrhea and vomiting that were common with higher-dose regimens.[41,42] Pseudogout is treated with NSAIDs or intraarticular cortisone (or both); effective prevention is often achieved with low-dose colchicines or NSAIDs.

### FOLLOW-UP, NEXT STEPS IN CARE, AND PATIENT EDUCATION

Drugs that lower uric acid production (e.g., allopurinol, febuxostat) or enhance excretion (e.g., probenecid) may be

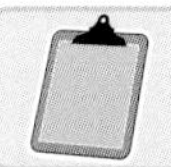

## DOCUMENTATION

**Arthritis**

Presence or absence of the following:

- Cardinal signs of inflammation (pain, tenderness, heat, erythema, swelling)
- Functional impairment and ability to bear weight
- Constitutional and systemic symptoms
- Traumatic injury
- Risk factors for joint space infection
- Risk factors for adverse effects of the planned treatment regimen

Clearly identify the specific anatomic sites of tenderness, swelling, and erythema

Assess and document the following:

- Characteristics of pain (PQRST mnemonic)
- Full set of vital signs
- Approximate range of motion of the affected joints; level of activity
- Witnessed functional impairment, weight bearing, and gait
- Distal neurovascular status
- Patient consent, procedure note, results of a tap if arthrocentesis is performed

Document specific discharge instructions:

- Medications and potential serious side effects and drug interactions
- Adjunctive measures as indicated (splinting, rest, ice, elevation)
- Follow-up plan for any pending test results
- Recommended follow-up visits
- Need to bring all medications to follow-up visits
- Potential reasons to return to the ED for reassessment

*PQRST*, Palliation/aggravation, quality, radiation, severity, and timing.

used as preventive therapy but can be started at follow-up visits.[43] Adjunctive measures include a diet low in uric acid (decreased meat and seafood) plus lifestyle modification. Unless an infected joint is suspected, these patients are discharged home with primary care follow-up.

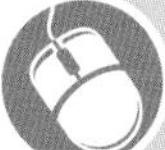

A discussion of Legg-Calvé-Perthes disease, juvenile idiopathic (rheumatoid) arthritis, and psoriatic arthritis can be found online at www.expertconsult.com

## SUGGESTED READINGS

Carter JD, Hudson AP. Reactive arthritis: clinical aspects and medical management. Rheum Dis Clin North Am 2009;35:21-44.

Lavelle ED, Lavelle L. Intra-articular injections. Med Clin North Am 2007;91:241-50.

Margaretten ME, Kohlwes J, Moore D, et al. Does this adult patient have septic arthritis? JAMA 2007;297:1478-88.

Rott K, Agudelo C. Gout. JAMA 2003;289:2857-60.

Saag KG, Teng GG, Patkar NM, et al. American College of Rheumatology 2008 recommendations for the use of nonbiologic and biologic disease-modifying antirheumatic drugs. Ann Rheum Dis 2010;69:762-84.

Salzman BE, Nevin JE, Newman JH. A primary care approach to the use and interpretation of common rheumatologic tests. Clin Fam Pract 2005;7:335-58.

## REFERENCES

***References can be found on Expert Consult @ www.expertconsult.com.***

# 108 Systemic Lupus Erythematosus

James G. Adams

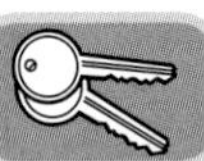

**KEY POINTS**

- Systemic lupus erythematosus is an autoimmune disease that damages the skin, kidneys, bones, lungs, brain, and nearly every other organ in the body.
- The damage is due to inflammation as a result of a direct antibody reaction to body tissues, deposits of immune complexes, and secondary thrombosis.
- A characteristic finding is fever, malar rash, and joint pain in a young, premenopausal woman.
- Sunlight and certain viruses and drugs can induce an autoimmune response in a genetically susceptible host.
- Basic treatment of pain is with nonsteroidal antiinflammatory medications or steroids. Many patients additionally require immunosuppressants, antimalarial drugs, and other therapies prescribed by a rheumatologist.
- Patients with systemic lupus erythematosus have increased risk for serious infection, often because of the steroids and immunosuppressants required to treat the disease.
- Morbidity is due to organ failure, primarily of the kidney and brain.

## PERSPECTIVE

Systemic lupus erythematosus (SLE) is a chronic autoimmune disease with widespread physical effects caused by the production of autoantibodies to components of cellular nuclei.[1] The term *lupus* (Latin for "wolf") is attributed to the 13th-century physician Rogerius, who used it to describe the characteristic facial lesions that were reminiscent of a wolf's bite.

In some patients the illness is mild. Other patients suffer early, catastrophic organ damage. Early deaths are frequently due to injury to the kidney and brain. Later deaths often occur as a result of acute myocardial infarction, stroke, or infection. Steroids used for treatment may cause or worsen complications.

Acknowledgment and thanks to Clare Sercombe for contributions to the first and second editions of this chapter.

## EPIDEMIOLOGY

SLE is more common by a ratio of 12:1 in women aged 15 to 45 years and by a ratio of 2:1 in younger and older women. The overall prevalence of this disease is about 1 in 1000. In most studies of SLE, about 90% of enrollees are women. In the United States, the disease is three times more common in black women than in white women. In addition to genetic factors, age, sex, race, and socioeconomic status have an impact on disease expression and prognosis. With optimal management, the 20-year survival rate approaches 70% and the 1-year survival rate is about 90%.[2]

## PATHOPHYSIOLOGY

SLE is a prototypic autoimmune disease characterized by tissue damage from excessive antibody production and immune complex deposition. The chronic inflammation characteristic of the disease originates from overproduction of autoantibodies and failure of the body to suppress them.

Nearly every tissue in the body can be affected. Autoantibodies directly react to human antigens, immune complexes are deposited in tissue and blood vessels, and the complement cascade is activated, which results in inflammation and organ damage.

The exact cause is unknown, but genetic predisposition, viruses, ultraviolet light (including sunlight), and medications such as hydralazine, isoniazid, and procainamide are known to be involved in certain patients. There is a relationship to specific human leukocyte antigen genotypes.

Autoantibodies to lupus erythematosus are found in laboratory workers who handle lupus sera. Exposure to certain drugs can produce a SLE-like syndrome. Hormonal factors include an association with estrogens, which may explain the higher prevalence in women.

## PRESENTING SIGNS AND SYMPTOMS

The triad of fever, joint pain, and rash in a woman of childbearing age suggests SLE. The most well-recognized cutaneous finding is the red, raised butterfly rash (**Fig. 108.1**), but malaise, fatigue, aches, fever, and weight loss are the most common symptoms. The rash, which does not cross the

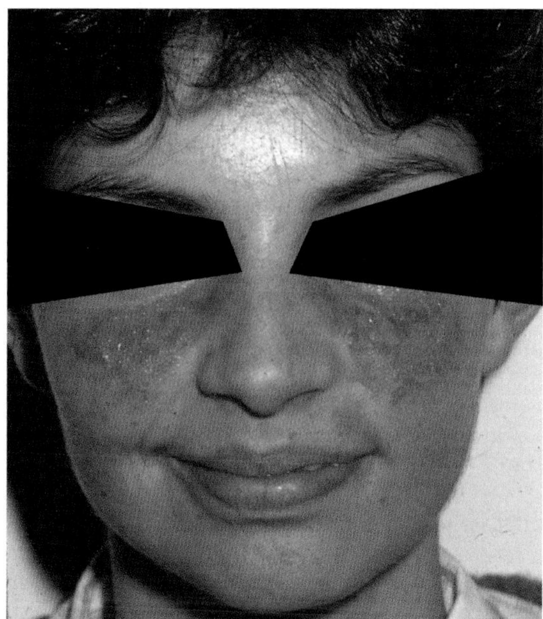

**Fig. 108.1 Erythematous malar rash of systemic lupus erythematosus.** Note that the rash does not cross the nasolabial fold. (From Gladman DD, Urowitz MB. Clinical features. In: Hochberg MC, Silman AJ, Smolen JS, editors. Rheumatology. Philadelphia:, Mosby; 2003. pp. 1359-79.)

nasolabial fold, may be painful or pruritic. It may be precipitated by sunlight and can last from days to weeks.

More than two thirds of patients have vague constitutional symptoms. A thorough evaluation is required before attributing such symptoms to lupus alone. Patients can have kidney failure, infections, adrenal failure, and other complications with similar symptoms (**Box 108.1**).

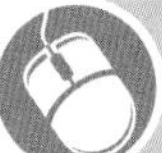

See Box 108.1, Criteria for the Classification of Systemic Lupus Erythematosus, online at www.expertconsult.com

Clinical manifestations range widely from mild to life-threatening. About half of patients have severe disease, defined as complications that threaten life or organ function.

Some rash or arthritis (or both) develops in a substantial majority of patients. At least half of patients have the Reynaud phenomenon, mucous membrane involvement, and renal or central nervous system involvement. About half of patients report photosensitivity. Pleurisy, vasculitis, or gastrointestinal involvement will develop in a quarter to a third of patients. Less common but important manifestations include pancreatitis, myositis, and myocarditis.

## DIFFERENTIAL DIAGNOSIS AND MEDICAL DECISION MAKING

### ARTHRITIS, ARTHRALGIA, MYALGIA, AND OSTEONECROSIS

Almost all patients occasionally have arthralgias and myalgias. The hand inflammation is symmetric, as in rheumatoid arthritis, but joint deformities are less common. "Hitchhiker's thumb" (hyperextension of the interphalangeal joint of the thumb) develops in 30% of patients. Tenosynovitis and tendon rupture may also occur, especially in patients taking corticosteroids. In addition, vascular necrosis of the large joints, especially the femoral heads, may be present as a result of ischemia caused by the vasculitis or as a complication of corticosteroid therapy.

### SKIN

The characteristic facial eruption, seen in up to 40% of patients, may be the first sign or may accompany flares of the disease. It can be exacerbated by exposure to ultraviolet light.

### KIDNEYS

Clinical nephritis, defined as persistent proteinuria, develops in approximately 50% of patients with SLE, although mesangial and glomerular immunoglobulin deposition occurs in almost all patients. Usually, the nephritis does not cause any symptoms until it progresses to an advanced stage. Serum creatinine is an important but insensitive indicator of early renal disease because many nephrons must be damaged before the creatinine level is elevated. Renal complications are recognized by hematuria, proteinuria, and red blood cell casts. Active urine sediment with excretion of red blood cell casts and increasing proteinuria is cause for concern.

Patients with active urine sediment may benefit from aggressive steroid or other immunosuppressive therapy. Indications for treatment include worsening renal failure, decreasing serum complement levels, increasing anti–double-stranded DNA levels, and nephritic urinary sediment, especially when accompanied by increasing or nephrotic-range proteinuria.[3]

### CENTRAL NERVOUS SYSTEM

Seizures, stroke, migraines, peripheral neuropathies, and psychosis are common. These symptoms may appear early but are rarely the initial sign of SLE. Central nervous system involvement develops in approximately 50% of patients with SLE. Full recovery from the neuropsychiatric manifestations occurs in approximately 70% to 85% of patients, although mortality from such events is 10% to 15%.

Seizures are the most frequent central nervous system manifestation. Strokes as a result of vascular inflammation and thrombosis are also common, especially in association with antiphospholipid syndrome.

Cerebritis should be considered when a patient with SLE exhibits a change in behavior or altered mental status. Infection should also be considered, particularly in patients receiving immunosuppressive therapy. These patients are at risk for bacterial, fungal, and tuberculous infections, in addition to brain abscesses. A head computed tomography scan and lumbar puncture are generally required to clarify the diagnosis. Symptoms may range from subtle changes in behavior to frank psychosis. Steroids are an important therapy for patients who have lupus-associated cerebritis.

### CARDIOVASCULAR SYSTEM

#### *Pericarditis*

Pericarditis is the most common heart-related problem and is reported to occur in 20% to 30% of patients, but it is present in up to 60% at autopsy. Electrocardiographic (ECG) findings alone may lead to the diagnosis because the pericarditis can be clinically inapparent. Alternatively, some patients will have fever, tachycardia, chest pain, and a cardiac rub. The pericarditis is usually fairly benign and responds well to ibuprofen or, in severe cases, to corticosteroids. Pericardial effusion, typically a transudative serous fluid, occurs in about 20% of patients. Tamponade is rare but has been noted. An uncommon but dangerous complication is purulent pericarditis, which should be suspected in patients who appear especially ill. Typical causes are *Staphylococcus aureus* and *Mycobacterium tuberculosis*. Purulent pericarditis is exudative with a high C-reactive protein level and elevated white blood cell count.

### Myocarditis

Myocarditis is rarely diagnosed clinically but is found on autopsy in about 40% of patients. The 10% of patients in whom the diagnosis is made typically have symptoms that resemble those of cardiomyopathy, including congestive heart failure, ventricular dysrhythmia, tachycardia, and nonspecific ECG changes. Severe myocarditis should be treated with high-dose systemic corticosteroids, control of hypertension, and correction of volume overload.

### Endocarditis

Libman-Sachs vegetations, present in up to 10% of patients with SLE, are growths on heart valves that usually cause no symptoms. Occasionally, these vegetations may be complicated by infection, valvular dysfunction, and rarely thromboembolism. The mitral valve is most commonly involved, although all four valves may have vegetations.

### Coronary Artery Disease and Coronary Vasculitis

Accelerated atherosclerosis as a result of corticosteroid use may cause coronary ischemia. Mortality from coronary artery disease is seen in up to 30% of patients with SLE despite improved survival of patients with renal and cerebral SLE. Hypertension, smoking, and hypercholesterolemia significantly increase the risk for mortality in these patients. Patients with acute cardiac ischemia should be treated with standard interventions.

Coronary vasculitis is rare and best treated with steroids. Differences in treatment make the distinction between coronary vasculitis and coronary artery disease important. The diagnosis can be made by coronary angiography. Evidence of aneurysmal dilation of the coronary arteries is seen in patients with coronary vasculitis.

### Hypertension

Between 25% and 50% of patients with SLE often have systemic hypertension as a result of lupus nephritis and steroid use.

## PULMONARY SYSTEM[4]

### Pleuritis

Pleurisy and pleural effusions occur in more than half of patients with SLE.[5] The pleural effusions are usually small and bilateral but can occasionally be very large. Pleural fluid is generally exudative, with glucose levels similar to serum glucose levels. In contrast, the pleural fluid of patients with rheumatoid arthritis has very low glucose levels.

### Pneumonitis

Pneumonitis in patients with SLE causes diffuse interstitial infiltrates, although patients have usually had the disease for several years before they suffer from pneumonitis. Bacterial, fungal, and opportunistic infections must be considered before confirming the diagnosis, especially in patients taking immunosuppressive agents. Patients with SLE are particularly at risk for pneumococcal disease, in part because of autosplenectomy or splenic dysfunction.

### Pulmonary Fibrosis

Chronic interstitial infiltrates leading to pulmonary fibrosis may also develop in patients with SLE. These patients need inpatient treatment, and their condition may progress to chronic hypoxia, pulmonary hypertension, and right-sided heart failure.

### Shrinking Lung Syndrome

When a patient has shortness of breath, low lung volumes seen on a chest radiograph, and no other identifiable cause, shrinking lung syndrome is signaled. An elevated diaphragm but clear lung fields is characteristic. This syndrome may be chronic as a result of impaired respiratory mechanics, weak muscles, and poor diaphragmatic function. If the findings are acute, the patient may have a good response to steroids.

## GASTROINTESTINAL SYSTEM

Mucous membrane lesions (small, shallow ulcerations in the mouth) occur in up to 19% of patients. Oral ulcerations usually accompany disease flares. Esophageal dysmotility is occasionally seen; however, it is much less common in patients with SLE than in patients with scleroderma.

Patients with intestinal pseudoobstruction may have crampy abdominal pain and a clinical and radiographic picture consistent with obstruction. They should be observed for resolution.

Mesenteric vasculitis is the most serious gastrointestinal complication. Patients have abdominal pain and, typically, bloody diarrhea along with evidence of vasculitis elsewhere. Bowel vasculitis may progress to perforation, gangrene, and peritonitis.

## HEMATOLOGIC DISORDERS

Anemia, which affects up to 40% of patients with SLE, may result from hemolysis, drugs, renal disease, blood loss, or chronic disease. The most important cause is autoimmune hemolytic anemia. The Coombs test, which detects hemolysis caused by antibodies directed against red blood cell antigens, is usually positive.

Thrombocytopenia occurs in 25% of patients. Antiplatelet antibodies may be the cause of the low platelet count seen in patients with active SLE. Treatment of severe lupus-related thrombocytopenia is controversial; some authors advocate the use of vinca alkaloids and intravenous gamma globulin.

An important cause of thrombocytopenia is thrombotic thrombocytopenic purpura, which may be difficult to distinguish from acute autoimmune hemolysis. Patients with thrombotic thrombocytopenic purpura typically have low platelets, hemolytic anemia, central nervous system dysfunction, renal insufficiency, and fever. Symptoms can appear similar to those of a lupus flare. Treatment requires plasma exchange, so it is

**Table 108.1 Drugs Implicated in Lupuslike Syndromes**

| SYSTEM | DRUG | RISK |
|---|---|---|
| Cardiovascular | Procainamide, quinidine, practolol* | High |
| Antihypertensive | Hydralazine, methyldopa, reserpine | High |
| Antimicrobial | Isoniazid, nitrofurantoin, penicillin, sulfonamides, streptomycin, tetracycline | Moderate |
| Anticonvulsant | Ethosuximide, mephenytoin, phenytoin, primidone | Moderate |
| Antithyroid | Methylthiouracil, propylthiouracil | Low |
| Psychotropic | Chlorpromazine, lithium carbonate | Low |
| Miscellaneous | Allopurinol<br>Aminoglutethimide, gold salts, D-penicillamine, phenylbutazone, methysergide | High<br>Low |

Adapted from Marx J. Rosen's emergency medicine: concepts and clinical practice. 5th ed. St. Louis: Mosby; 2001.
*Removed from the market because of lupuslike syndrome.

important to either clinically distinguish or empirically initiate plasma exchange. Thrombotic thrombocytopenic purpura should be considered when a patient has a combination of microangiopathy, seizures, coma or altered mental status, and renal failure.

### DRUG-INDUCED LUPUS ERYTHEMATOSUS

Procainamide has been known for more than 40 years to induce a lupus reaction. Since then, a large number of agents have been implicated, with hydralazine and procainamide being the most common (**Table 108.1**). The clinical manifestations vary, with most patients experiencing arthralgias and occasional pleuropericardial pain. The full manifestations are present in less than 1% of patients taking high-risk drugs, although a positive antinuclear antibody titer can be found in more than 50%. Patients are generally women, middle-aged or older, and rarely African American, but this may be representative of the group of patients. The condition is usually reversible when drug therapy is stopped, with resolution occurring within days or weeks. Manifestations lasting for years have been reported. In patients with significant pleuropericardial disease, a short course of tapered steroids has been used successfully once use of the implicated medication has been discontinued.

## TREATMENT

Medical therapy attempts to reduce inflammation, suppress the immune system, and control pain. Nonsteroidal antiinflammatory drugs (NSAIDs), corticosteroids, and immunosuppressive agents are the mainstays of treatment. Aspirin and other NSAIDs are the primary treatment of arthralgias, pleurisy, and pericarditis. The maximum standard recommended doses of these agents are usually needed. These agents should be avoided in patients with severe gastrointestinal complications, renal insufficiency, nephritis, or thrombocytopenia. Treatment with NSAIDs can worsen lupus nephritis, either by causing interstitial nephritis or by inhibiting prostaglandins.[5]

Topical corticosteroids control most rashes. Although antiinflammatory and antimalarial drugs are often advocated for patients with minor symptoms to avoid the long-term complications of corticosteroid therapy, symptoms such as arthralgias, fatigue, pleurisy, and others may require lower-dose steroids, such as prednisone (0.5 mg/kg or less).

High-dose steroids (e.g., 1 mg/kg/day of prednisone or 1 g of methylprednisolone intravenously [IV]) are used when major organs are involved and also for hemolytic anemia and severe thrombocytopenia. For example, in patients with lupus-related cerebritis or acute worsening of lupus nephritis, 1 g/day of methylprednisolone IV may be given for several days.

Corticosteroids are associated with well-known complications, including steroid-induced diabetes, osteoporosis, weight gain, pancreatitis, osteonecrosis, accelerated atherosclerosis, and immunosuppression. Patients receiving chronic steroid therapy should be evaluated promptly for any episode of fever or potential infection. When patients who are taking corticosteroids have an acute serious illness or other physiologic stress (e.g., surgery, childbirth), they should also be given hydrocortisone (100 mg IV every 8 hours). Patients with overwhelming sepsis or shock should be given stress-dose steroids (e.g., 100 mg of hydrocortisone IV), in addition to the usual treatment with broad-spectrum antibiotics and intravenous resuscitation fluid.

Antimalarial drugs are effective for the cutaneous and musculoskeletal manifestations of SLE. Hydroxychloroquine and chloroquine are given on an outpatient basis in a loading dose for 4 weeks, followed by maintenance dosing once the symptoms are under control. Withdrawal of the drug may result in flare of the disease.

Immunosuppressive agents (azathioprine, methotrexate, cyclophosphamide) are reserved for patients with severe renal or cerebral disease in whom other therapies have failed and for patients who cannot tolerate corticosteroids. Studies of the use of immunosuppressants have shown decreased chronic renal scarring and a reduced likelihood of end-stage renal disease without an increase in mortality. The toxic effects of such drugs are numerous and include myelosuppression, risk for neoplasms, and infections,[6] especially with gram-negative organisms, encapsulated gram-positive organisms, herpes zoster, and opportunistic organisms. Febrile patients who are taking azathioprine, methotrexate, or cyclophosphamide should be admitted regardless of whether a source is evident because gram-negative or streptococcal sepsis occurs in this population. Immunosuppressed patients with localized herpes zoster should be admitted for intravenous acyclovir treatment to prevent viral dissemination.

## FOLLOW-UP, NEXT STEPS IN CARE, AND PATIENT EDUCATION

Patients with known disease and increasing arthritic pain or with a mild flare and no fever may be treated with NSAIDs or corticosteroids as an outpatient. Pleuritis and arthralgias can be treated on an outpatient basis. It may be prudent to perform urinalysis to ensure that there is no evidence of renal involvement, which might signal significant disease activity. In the absence of major organ involvement, the patient can be scheduled for prompt follow-up with a rheumatologist.

Patients with a new diagnosis of pericarditis, myocarditis, pleural effusion, or infiltrates or with evidence of vasculitis or renal insufficiency should almost always be admitted to the hospital. If there is uncertainty regarding diagnosis or severity of any circumstance, patients should be admitted for observation, testing, and treatment. Patients with worsening disease who are taking large doses of steroids or immunosuppressive agents should be admitted for aggressive treatment.

Patients with evidence of lupus nephritis and worsening renal failure should be admitted for therapy with steroids and, frequently, immunosuppressive agents.[6] The serum creatinine level may be elevated, but serious disease may be present even with normal creatinine levels. Proteinuria may be present, or red blood cell casts in urine may be the only sign of severe renal involvement.

Patients with SLE have a higher risk for coronary artery disease, so a complaint of chest pain should prompt evaluation for cardiac ischemia. If pericarditis is suspected, evaluation for pericardial effusion may be necessary, although tamponade is rare. Patients with myocarditis should be observed for evidence of congestive heart failure and dysrhythmias.

Shortness of breath suggests lung infection from typical or atypical organisms. Opportunistic infection, tuberculosis, and lupus pneumonitis need to be considered. In a hypoxic patient, it is prudent to consider the possibility of pulmonary embolism secondary to antiphospholipid antibody with thrombosis. Patients with significant pleural effusions should be admitted for consideration of diagnostic thoracentesis and treatment. Pleural effusions may be complicated by infection, tuberculosis, or malignancy.

SLE predisposes patients to anemia and thrombocytopenia. Patients should be admitted if there is evidence of active hemolysis with decreased hematocrit levels or hemolysis that is evident on the blood smear. Patients with thrombocytopenia should be admitted if evidence of bleeding is seen or if platelet counts are severely decreased (<50,000/mm$^3$). If the patient is actively bleeding, platelet transfusion is appropriate; however, rapid destruction of the platelets may occur. Simultaneous administration of intravenous corticosteroids and gamma globulin will aid in increasing the platelet count and decreasing the amount of platelet destruction.

Patients with evidence of arterial or venous thrombosis should be admitted for anticoagulation and possible embolectomy. Anticoagulation can be achieved acutely with heparin, although large doses are occasionally needed to overcome the antibody effect. The partial thromboplastin time (PTT), if not elevated, can be monitored to assess for evidence of adequate anticoagulation, with careful observation for bleeding in patients who are also thrombocytopenic. Otherwise, patients with a prolonged PTT and evidence of lupus anticoagulant can be monitored with thrombin times if necessary. Patients with an international normalized ratio of less than 2.5 should nevertheless be considered to have a possible thrombus if they have a history of antiphospholipid syndrome.

Pregnant patients should undergo early follow-up with a high-risk obstetrician. Emergency delivery for a pregnant patient with SLE should include stress-dose steroid administration and close observation of the neonate for congenital complete heart block (i.e., neonatal lupus). Emergency cardiac pacing may be necessary for the infant.

## REFERENCES

*References can be found on Expert Consult @ www.expertconsult.com.*

# Connective Tissue and Inflammatory Disorders 109

*Raveendra S. Morchi*

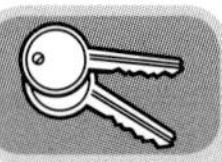

**KEY POINTS**

- Dry eyes and dry mouth unrelated to a medication side effect suggest primary Sjögren syndrome.
- Loss of sensation, paresthesias, and pain in the digits on exposure to cold or emotional stress are characteristics of Raynaud phenomenon.
- Many patients in whom systemic sclerosis eventually develops are initially found to have symptoms of Raynaud phenomenon and symmetric, nonpitting digital edema (without any fibrosis).
- Gastrointestinal symptoms in the presence of symmetric, digital edema or fibrosis suggest systemic sclerosis.
- Symptoms of edema and fibrosis proximal to the elbows or knees can represent an aggressive, diffuse form of systemic sclerosis with a high likelihood of internal organ involvement.
- An angiotensin-converting enzyme inhibitor should be considered for hypertensive patients with a presumed or definite diagnosis of systemic sclerosis.
- The diagnosis of sarcoidosis should be suspected in patients with only bilateral hilar lymphadenopathy on chest radiography, especially if they either have long-standing pulmonary complaints or are entirely asymptomatic.
- Early, vague subjective symptoms of fatigue, joint pain, or muscle discomfort may herald autoimmune disease.

## SJÖGREN SYNDROME

### EPIDEMIOLOGY

Sjögren syndrome is a slowly progressive dysfunction of the lacrimal and salivary glands. The resulting exocrinopathy produces the characteristic symptoms of dry eyes and dry mouth. An incidence of 4 per 100,000 per year has been noted. Ninety percent of cases occur in women, and the incidence increases with age. Patients may be anywhere in age from the fourth to the eighth decades.

### PATHOPHYSIOLOGY

Activation of the innate immune system, possibly in response to environmental or as yet unrecognized infectious triggers, results in elevated levels of type 1 interferon and characteristic cytokine profiles, including increased B-cell–activating factor. The ensuing infiltration of the salivary or lacrimal glands by periductal and periacinar foci of aggressive T lymphocytes marks the adaptive immune response. What follows is destruction and eventual loss of exocrine function.[1] In addition to T cells, polyclonal activation of B cells within and at the border of foci can result in hypergammaglobulinemia.

More recently, animal models suggest that lacrimal and salivary gland dysfunction need not always rely on innate and adaptive inflammation as a prerequisite. Rather, they may be related to abnormalities in water and ion channels as a result of genetic, hormonal, or autonomic imbalances antecedent to the inflammatory response.[2] Other exocrine glands in the body (lining the respiratory tree, integument, and vagina) can also be affected in Sjögren syndrome and produce a dry cough, dry skin, dysuria, or dyspareunia.

Regardless of whether the lacrimal and salivary gland dysfunction is bound to an inflammatory infiltrate, it is known that the hallmark of Sjögren syndrome is eventual systemic lymphocyte activation, which means that organs other than glandular tissue can be affected. Such a level of immune activation could be responsible for the increased risk for lymphoproliferative disorders and autoimmune endocrinopathies that have been noted in patients with Sjögren syndrome.

### PRESENTING SIGNS AND SYMPTOMS

#### GLANDULAR

Dry eyes, foreign body sensation, ocular grittiness, fatigue, and easy irritation are common complaints related to the lacrimal system. The patient may also have blurred vision, trouble with bright lights, or red eye. Signs include keratitis, conjunctivitis, mucous filaments at the inner canthus, blepharitis from meibomian gland dysfunction, and lacrimal enlargement.

Dry mouth and lips, an unpleasant taste in the mouth, difficulty chewing and swallowing dry food, and possibly a clicking quality of speech from the tongue sticking to the hard palate are all symptoms of diminished saliva production. Signs of poor salivary flow include secondary dental caries, gingivitis, irritation of oral mucosa, oral candidiasis, parotid gland enlargement, and diminished pooling of sublingual saliva on direct inspection.

### EXTRAGLANDULAR

The T- and B-lymphocyte activity that infiltrates exocrine glands can also affect other nonglandular organs. These extraglandular manifestations portend a worse prognosis. Fatigue, myalgias, arthralgias, arthritis, and subjective fever are nonspecific and will not help distinguish Sjögren syndrome. Most renal disease will be tubular in origin and related to invading lymphocytes. Signs can be minimal, but urinary sediment consisting of small amounts of protein or evidence of tubular malabsorption, with or without systemic acidosis (renal tubular acidosis), may be seen.

Patients may have abdominal pain or nausea and vomiting consistent with gastritis or hepatitis. In some instances there is an association between Sjögren syndrome and hepatitis C or celiac disease, another condition characterized by aggressive lymphocyte activity.

Patients may have symptoms of Raynaud phenomenon because of abnormal regulation of vascular caliber. Purpuric, maculopapular, or urticarial rash results from hypergammaglobulinemia or cryoglobulinemia secondary to polyclonal B-cell activation.

Peripheral (median or peroneal) and cranial (V, VII, VIII) neuropathies are secondary to autoimmune-mediated vasculitis. Central nervous system involvement is less common and consists of focal lesions mimicking multiple sclerosis, diffuse encephalopathy, or aseptic meningitis.

## DIFFERENTIAL DIAGNOSIS AND MEDICAL DECISION MAKING

If dry eyes and dry mouth dominate the clinical picture, the patient may have primary Sjögren syndrome. However, these symptoms can be associated with a number of other autoimmune disorders that more accurately characterize the clinical findings (rheumatoid arthritis, systemic lupus erythematosus, scleroderma), in which case such patients probably have secondary Sjögren syndrome (**Box 109.1**).

The cracker test, in which the patient tries to chew and swallow a dry cracker, is probably the most useful bedside diagnostic maneuver. Patients with Sjögren syndrome will have a difficult time completing this task, with adherence of food to the buccal mucosa. Slit-lamp testing with fluorescein may show epithelial defects over the cornea consistent with keratitis secondary to dryness. Rose bengal staining (**Fig. 109.1**) is generally regarded as a more sensitive means of depicting these defects but is usually performed by an ophthalmologist. The Schirmer test involves placing standardized tear testing strips between the unanesthetized eyeball and the lateral margin of the lower lid and noting advancement of a tear film over a period of 5 minutes. Anything less than 5 mm is considered abnormal.

## TREATMENT

Treatment of Sjögren syndrome has two objectives: improve the symptoms of exocrine gland dysfunction and attempt to control the underlying autoimmune lymphocyte activity. The former has had more success than the latter.

### XEROPHTHALMIA

Artificial tears with or without preservatives may be used throughout the day, and lubricating ointments can be used at night. Oral pilocarpine, 5 mg four times per day, will stimulate muscarinic gland receptors, increase lacrimal flow, and provide subjective improvement.[3,4] More severely affected patients with keratoconjunctivitis sicca who are taking cevimeline, 30 mg three times per day, have reported a reduction in the severity of symptoms.[5,6] Topical ocular nonsteroidal and steroidal preparations or topical 0.05% cyclosporine can be prescribed by an ophthalmologist for a short term.[5] Occlusion of the nasolacrimal duct temporarily with plugs or permanently by surgical intervention is last-line therapy.

**BOX 109.1 Differential Diagnosis of Sjögren Syndrome**

**Most Common**

- Medication effects (antihypertensives, antipsychotics, antihistamines, antidepressants)
- Viral sialadenitis, human immunodeficiency virus, human T-cell lymphotropic virus type I
- Lacrimal gland infiltration in sarcoidosis or amyloidosis
- Chronic sialadenitis, conjunctivitis, blepharitis
- Previous radiation treatment
- Malnutrition (alcoholism, bulimia)
- Diabetes

**Most Threatening**

- Bacterial sialadenitis or parotitis
- Lymphoproliferative disorders
- Graft-versus-host disease
- Salivary gland tumor

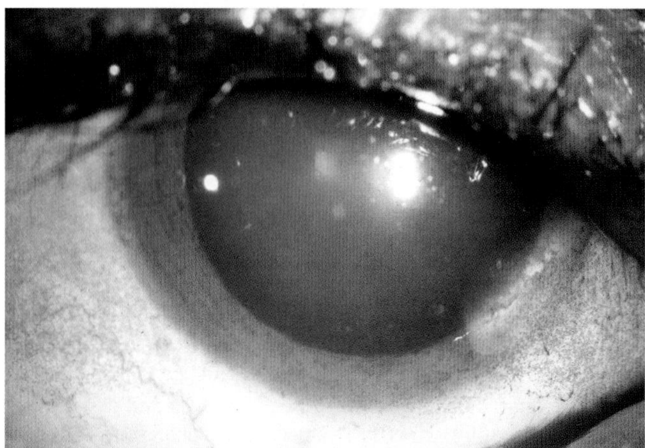

**Fig. 109.1 Keratitis seen with rose bengal stain.** (From Yanoff M, Duker JS, editors. Ophthalmology. 2nd ed. St. Louis: Mosby; 2004.)

### XEROSTOMIA

Though available, artificial saliva tends to be short-lived and less well accepted by patients. Meticulous oral hygiene is necessary to prevent dental caries, gingivitis, or periodontitis secondary to dryness. Sugarless sialogogues (lemon drops) stimulate flow. Lifestyle modifications such as the use of a humidifier or avoidance of dry environments and excessive air conditioning can help retain moisture. Mycostatin oral suspension, Mycostatin vaginal tablets (also dissolve orally), or clotrimazole troches should be considered for the treatment of oral candidiasis in patients with Sjögren syndrome. Oral pilocarpine, 5 mg four times per day, or cevimeline, 30 to 60 mg three times per day, can stimulate muscarinic receptors and improve salivary flow in those with more significant symptoms.[5,7-9] One must beware of side effects related to systemic muscarinic activation, including bradycardia, bronchospasm, gastrointestinal symptoms, or impaired mydriasis and trouble with night vision.

### OTHER TYPES OF XEROSIS

Humidified air and guaifenesin are useful for a dry respiratory tree. Avoidance of tight or restrictive clothing and the use of moisturizing creams, lotions, and bathing products can help with dry skin. Mild corticosteroid cream may be added for pruritus. Propionic acid gel is an effective vaginal lubricant.

### AUTOIMMUNE LYMPHOCYTE ACTIVITY

Nonsteroidal antiinflammatory drugs (NSAIDs) can be prescribed from the emergency department (ED) for symptomatic control of minor rheumatic complaints. Hydroxychloroquine has no clear benefit in ameliorating these symptoms.[5] The rheumatologist may prescribe prednisone, methylprednisolone, cyclophosphamide, methotrexate, or azathioprine to control lymphocyte activity. Newer therapies include monoclonal antibodies (rituximab) that target B cells.[5] Future investigations are directed at blocking type 1 interferon, B-cell–activating factor, and other cytokines that link the initial innate immune response to the subsequent adaptive response composed of activated lymphocytes.

## PATIENT DISPOSITION AND NEXT STEPS IN CARE

Patients with suspected primary or secondary Sjögren syndrome should undergo outpatient primary care and rheumatology follow-up within 2 to 4 weeks. Outpatient ophthalmology or dental evaluation is also advisable. Patients should be told to return to the ED for significant ocular pain or visual disturbance, which may signify keratitis and can be complicated by globe perforation.

# SYSTEMIC SCLEROSIS (SCLERODERMA)

## EPIDEMIOLOGY

Systemic sclerosis is a generalized thickening and fibrosis of the skin and internal organs that affects 1 in 4000 adults in the United States.[10] Its incidence ranges from 2 to 23 cases per million per year.[11] Women are more likely to be affected than men, with the onset of disease peaking between 30 and 50 years of age.

## PATHOPHYSIOLOGY

Patients can have localized patches of skin fibrosis, or the disorder may progress to diffuse skin involvement with fibrosis and dysfunction of internal organs. Although the precise trigger is not known, an underlying functional and microstructural vascular abnormality is believed to play a central role. In association with oxygen radical species, findings include endothelial cell dysfunction and apoptosis, an imbalance favoring endothelin over prostacyclin, vascular smooth muscle hyperplasia, and pericyte proliferation in the perivascular space. Concomitantly, an adjacent inflammatory response occurs and is composed of lymphocytes, macrophages, and fibroblasts that lay down increasing amounts of extracellular matrix, including collagen.[12] Cytokines and growth factors such as transforming growth factor-β and platelet-derived growth factor are involved in the amplification of this response, which includes activation and differentiation of fibroblasts.[10] The types of systemic sclerosis are listed in **Box 109.2**.

## PRESENTING SIGNS AND SYMPTOMS

Raynaud phenomenon is the initial complaint in the majority of patients and precedes clinically detectable skin fibrosis, probably because vascular malfunction antedates the edema and collagen deposition in patients with systemic sclerosis. The skin blanching associated with Raynaud phenomenon may not be present, but paresthesias or sensory deficits followed by throbbing pain in the fingers, toes, and sometimes the cheeks, nose, or tongue on exposure to cold are more

**BOX 109.2 Types of Systemic Sclerosis**

*Localized scleroderma* consists of fibrosis in scattered, circular patches of skin (morphea), linear streaks (linear scleroderma), or nodules and is seen primarily in children. There is no systemic or internal organ involvement, and sequelae are cosmetic and sometimes functional.

*Limited systemic sclerosis* implies that fibrosis occurs distal to the elbows or knees and above the clavicles only. It is generally slowly progressive.

*CREST syndrome* previously referred to a fibrotic process that involved the skin, digits, and esophageal wall. Patients have calcinosis cutis, Raynaud phenomenon, esophageal dysmotility with symptoms of reflux and dysphagia, sclerodactyly, and telangiectasia. This particular classification is no longer commonly used.

*Diffuse systemic sclerosis* is characterized by fibrosis extending proximal to the elbows and knees. It may be rapidly progressive and can be associated with significant internal organ fibrosis.

consistent findings. It should be noted, however, that systemic sclerosis never develops in most patients with Raynaud phenomenon.

Musculoskeletal complaints consisting of arthralgias, myalgias, and generalized weakness are nearly universal in patients with systemic sclerosis and other connective tissue disorders. Sometimes patients will have palpable or audible tendon friction rubs. Musculoskeletal problems are often some of the first symptoms and may be refractory to standard therapy with NSAIDs.

Skin findings are the most useful in the ED. Edema is a hallmark of early scleroderma, as well as rheumatoid arthritis, systemic lupus erythematosus, and other connective tissue disorders. Painless swelling of the fingers and hands is common (**Fig. 109.2**). Erythema and pruritus are associated findings caused by an early inflammatory response and deposition of components of the extracellular matrix. Nonpitting edema need not be limited to the distal end of extremities but may spread proximally or to the face and neck over the course of weeks.

Fibrosis can ensue in weeks or months. Gradually, collagen is deposited and the edematous areas are replaced by firm, thick, taut skin that may become bound to underlying tissue. In the fingers, tight skin can produce joint flexion contractures plus breaks or ulcerations as it is stretched over bony prominences (knuckles) in the condition termed sclerodactyly (see Fig. 109.2). Digital ulcerations, pitting scars, and loss of the finger pad can result from poor distal perfusion through intervening fibrotic tissue. This may be followed by calcium deposition (calcinosis).

A masklike appearance of the face (**Fig. 109.3**) with loss of the natural skin creases and diminished hair growth is characteristic. "Salt and pepper" alterations in pigmentation may be present. Disorganized arrays of blood vessels (telangiectases) scattered over the extremities, face, and mucous membranes are sequelae of deranged angiogenesis after the initial vascular obliteration and fibrotic inflammatory response.

Gastrointestinal symptoms are very common and related to intestinal wall edema and fibrosis, which can occur anywhere from the esophagus to the rectum. Reflux esophagitis, strictures, and even Barrett esophagus can occur. Throughout the rest of the bowel, complications include smooth muscle dysfunction with dysmotility and ileus, pulsion diverticula as a result of uncoordinated peristaltic activity, bacterial overgrowth, and malabsorption. Nausea, anorexia, bloating, constipation, and diarrhea are potential complaints.

Pulmonary symptoms generally include dyspnea on exertion and a nonproductive cough. Interstitial fibrosis is more common in the diffuse form of scleroderma, and scattered rales may be heard. As with other fibrotic conditions, systemic sclerosis produces a restrictive lung disease. Pulmonary hypertension from obliteration of pulmonary vasculature associated with changes in the intimal and medial vessel walls can occur in the absence of significant interstitial fibrosis and is seen in a subset of patients with the limited form of systemic sclerosis.

Renal vascular involvement parallels that of other organs. The main difference is that when flow through the arcuate and interlobular renal arterioles is diminished secondary to the microvasculopathy and spasm characteristic of systemic sclerosis, the distal glomerulus and juxtaglomerular apparatus will respond to this decrease in perfusion by producing renin and beginning a cycle of fluid retention and vascular constriction via angiotensin II and aldosterone. The result is hypertension with systemic vasoconstriction, which can cause further damage to blood vessels and even hemolysis of red cells as they pass through the injured vasculature. In this sense, patients with renal involvement can seen be anywhere along a spectrum between asymptomatic hypertension and a

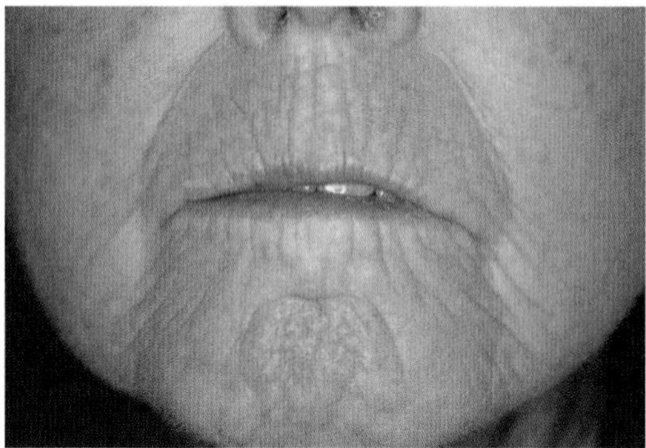

**Fig. 109.3 Facial features in scleroderma.** Note the vertical lines or furrowing around the mouth in this patient with diffuse scleroderma. (From Goldman L, Ausiello D, editors. Cecil textbook of medicine. 22nd ed. Philadelphia: Saunders; 2004.)

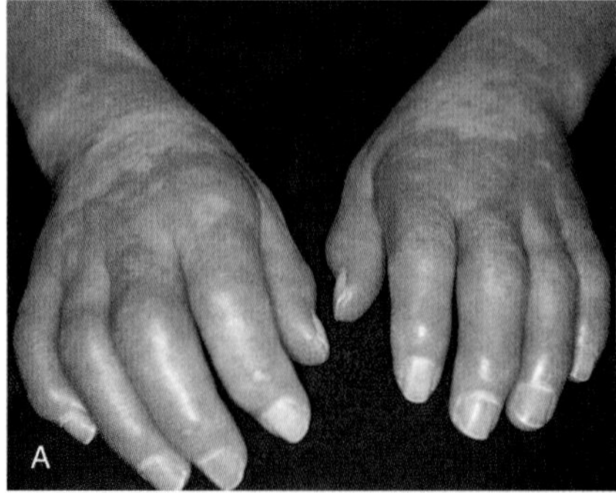


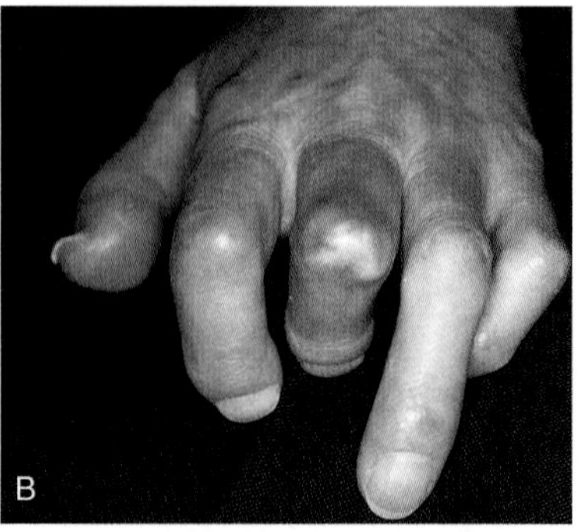


**Fig. 109.2 Changes in the hands associated with connective tissue diseases. A,** Edematous phase. **B,** Atrophic phase with contractures and skin thickening (sclerodactyly). (From Goldman L, Ausiello D, editors. Cecil textbook of medicine. 22nd ed. Philadelphia: Saunders; 2004.)

hypertensive emergency or malignant hypertension with characteristic funduscopic changes.

Cardiac inflammation results in pericarditis with effusion. In the myocardium, patchy areas of fibrosis can physically impair cardiac conduction or provide scar tissue that serves as points of electrical reentry. Secondary conduction deficits and supraventricular or ventricular arrhythmias will follow. Myocardial involvement and arrhythmias are asymptomatic in most, but dyspnea on exertion, congestive heart failure, syncope, or sudden death can occur. Additionally, coronary artery vasospasm may be associated with the underlying vasculopathy of systemic sclerosis.

Other features include thyroid, salivary, and lacrimal gland dysfunction secondary to fibrosis. Fibrosis in soft tissue can result in an entrapment neuropathy of susceptible peripheral nerves, including the median, lateral femoral cutaneous, trigeminal, and facial nerves. Men may have erectile dysfunction from impaired blood flow secondary to vasculopathy and fibrosis.

## DIFFERENTIAL DIAGNOSIS AND MEDICAL DECISION MAKING

The differential diagnosis for systemic sclerosis includes several other connective tissue diseases (**Box 109.3**).

Skin examination is the most important diagnostic tool for the emergency physician (EP). Nail fold capillary examination may be useful for patients with Raynaud phenomenon who do not yet have skin changes indicative of sclerosis. Using an ophthalmoscope and immersion oil applied to the skin, dilated and tortuous capillaries mixed with areas of capillary loss can be seen as evidence of a burgeoning connective tissue disease in patients with secondary Raynaud phenomenon.

Serum electrolyte levels should be measured and urinalysis performed to evaluate renal function. Because the disease does not usually involve the glomerulus or nephron tubular cells directly, but rather the arterioles upstream, findings on urinalysis are frequently normal or limited to mild proteinuria with few cells or casts. Therefore, elevations in serum creatinine alone in a patient with other clinical evidence of systemic sclerosis would raise the possibility of scleroderma renal disease.

A complete blood count and smear should be obtained for patients with suspected microangiopathic hemolysis from malignant hypertension. An electrocardiogram and rhythm strip can be evaluated for suspected conduction deficits or arrhythmia secondary to myocardial fibrosis.

Nonemergency work-up includes specific autoantibody profiling, gastrointestinal contrast studies for dysmotility, pulmonary function testing, echocardiography to evaluate myocardial contractile function or pulmonary hypertension, and biopsy to reveal the characteristic fibrotic skin or gland changes.

**BOX 109.3 Differential Diagnosis of Systemic Sclerosis**

**Most Common**
Primary Raynaud phenomenon
Localized scleroderma (linear or morphea)
Other connective tissue disorders
Scleredema and scleromyxedema
Eosinophilic fasciitis and eosinophilia-myalgia
Amyloidosis
Reflex sympathetic dystrophy
Diabetic sclerodactyly
Myxedema

**Most Threatening**
Chronic graft-versus-host disease
Bleomycin toxicity
Mycosis fungoides

## TREATMENT

Because the mechanics and primary inciting events of systemic sclerosis are not yet well understood, therapy is generally aimed at improving symptoms and curbing end-organ dysfunction. Treatment of Raynaud phenomenon includes lifestyle changes, calcium channel blockers, alpha-blockers, antiplatelet agents, and sympathectomy.

Musculoskeletal symptoms may respond to ibuprofen or another NSAID in standard doses combined with physical and occupational therapy.

Skin therapy includes moisturizers, topical glucocorticoid or antihistamine cream for pruritus, and local wound care with topical antibiotics for ulceration. High- or low-dose D-penicillamine cannot be recommended as an effective treatment at this time.[13]

Gastroesophageal reflux responds to standard changes in dietary habits and daily oral administration of omeprazole, 10 to 20 mg. Refractory cases may require surgical intervention, and reflux esophagitis–induced strictures may need periodic dilation.

Pulmonary hypertension is managed with endothelin receptor antagonists, phosphodiesterase inhibitors, and prostacyclin analogues.[10,14] Control of interstitial fibrosis has proved more difficult. Aggressive treatment with methotrexate, cyclophosphamide, or other immunosuppressives should be left to a specialist because their benefit is unclear.

Asymptomatic hypertension in a patient with known or suspected systemic sclerosis is presumed to be hyperreninemic in origin secondary to renal arteriolar disease and should be treated as such with an angiotensin-converting enzyme inhibitor. Oral administration of captopril, 6.25 to 12.5 mg three times per day, is a recommended starting point.[15,16] These patients require close outpatient monitoring of renal function. Patients with a hypertensive emergency or malignant hypertension may require intravenous enalaprilat or tighter control of systemic vascular resistance and heart rate via short-acting agents. Dialysis and renal transplantation remain last-line treatments for patients whose condition progresses to end-stage renal disease despite medical management.

Current emerging therapies include intravenous immune globulin, mycophenolate mofetil, B-cell antibodies (rituximab), and autologous or allogeneic hematopoietic stem cell transplantation to curb the role of immune cells in the pathogenesis of systemic sclerosis. Interferon therapy, downstream tyrosine kinase inhibition, and other novel antifibrotic approaches may be used to limit fibroblast proliferation and collagen production in the future.[17]

## SARCOIDOSIS

### EPIDEMIOLOGY

Because granulomatous inflammation can be due to many causes, the exact worldwide prevalence and incidence of sarcoidosis are not known. Most patients with the disease are younger than 50 years, and the peak age seems to be 20 to 39 years. Women are affected slightly more often than men. Worldwide, the majority of cases occur in white persons in northern European countries, but in the United States the disease is more frequent in African Americans.[18]

### PATHOPHYSIOLOGY

Sarcoidosis is characterized by the presence of noncaseating granulomas in multiple organs. Granulomas are composed of macrophages and other antigen-presenting cells, as well as T lymphocytes helping organize the response. They represent the immunologic reaction to organisms or antigens that cannot be properly disposed of and instead are simply contained and walled off. Sometimes the contents of the granuloma undergo what is described pathologically as caseous necrosis (i.e., the granulomatous response to tuberculosis). At other times necrosis is absent, and the granulomas are termed noncaseating. In sarcoidosis, noncaseating granulomas can be found anywhere in the body but are primarily situated in the mediastinal and hilar lymphatic tissue, airways, and pulmonary parenchyma. Respiratory or not, nearly every clinical manifestation of sarcoidosis can be traced to the physical presence of granulomas within the organ.

Although the exact cause of sarcoidosis is unknown, some evidence indicates that an environmental, chemical, or infectious agent provides the antigenic stimulus to macrophages. Once processed and presented, these antigens trigger a $CD4^+$ T-cell–mediated reaction that subsequently incites increasing numbers of macrophages and neighboring epithelial cells to partake in the formation of noncaseating granulomas and thereby produce the clinical signs and symptoms of sarcoidosis.

In addition to the environmental trigger, a genetic component mediating T-cell hypersensitivity may be required. In this way, clinical sarcoidosis may develop in only a genetically susceptible individual exposed to the unidentified antigen.

### PRESENTING SIGNS AND SYMPTOMS

Pulmonary disease is the hallmark of sarcoidosis. Granulomas occur throughout the mediastinal and hilar lymph nodes, in the lining of bronchi, and within the pulmonary parenchyma. Dyspnea on exertion, nonproductive cough, and nonspecific retrosternal chest pain are common complaints. Depending on the location and extent of the granulomatous tissue, patients may have primarily wheezing and a prolonged expiratory phase from endobronchial lesions or rales from parenchymal involvement. Alternatively, many patients have no symptoms and clear lung findings despite radiographic evidence of disease.

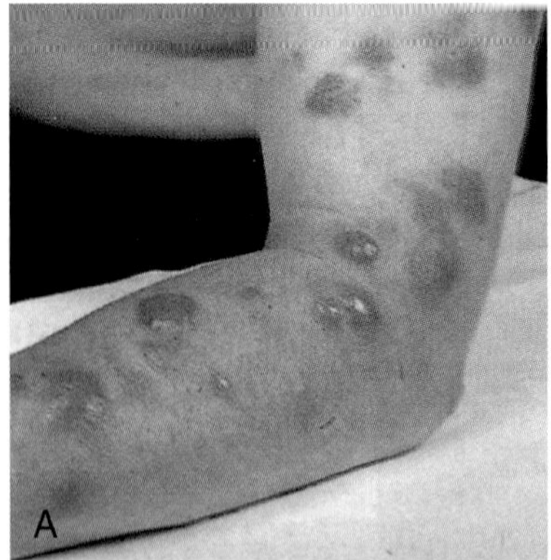

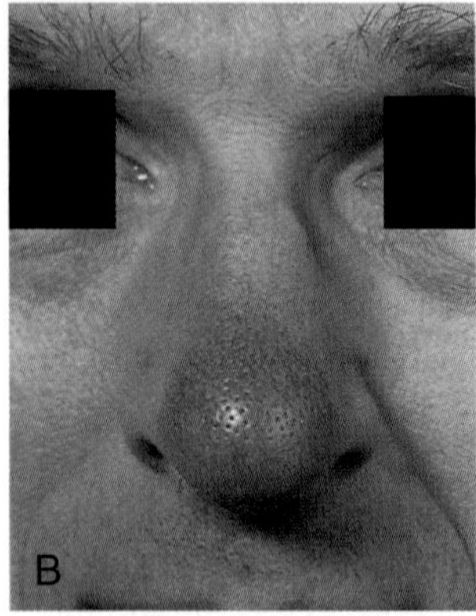

**Fig. 109.4 Skin lesions of sarcoidosis. A,** Sarcoid lesions may occur at any site, and they may take a nodular, papular, or plaque form. Biopsy is often necessary for diagnosis. **B,** *Lupus pernio* is the term used to describe a dusky-purple infiltration of the skin of the nose, cheeks, or ears in chronic sarcoidosis. (From Goldman L, Ausiello D, editors. Cecil textbook of medicine. 22nd ed. Philadelphia: Saunders; 2004.)

Skin lesions are present in up to 25% of patients (**Fig. 109.4**). Most are chronic and due to direct granulomatous involvement of the dermis. Unfortunately, they may take the form of papules, plaques, nodules, keloids at the site of surgical scars, or even lupus pernio (a violaceous discoloration over the nose, cheeks, chin, and ears). Thus it is difficult for the EP to make the diagnosis of sarcoidosis based on the presence of skin lesions alone.

Erythema nodosum may be one exception. Unlike other lesions, it is acute in onset and does not consist of granulomas but instead cellular inflammation and edema involving the dermis and subcutaneous tissue; it produces the characteristic raised, red, tender, nodular lesions most often seen on the anterior tibial surface. Erythema nodosum can be used to confirm the diagnosis of sarcoidosis in patients found to have bilateral hilar lymphadenopathy on chest radiography.

This combination of findings describes a subset of sarcoidosis patients said to have Löfgren syndrome. Note that erythema nodosum without bilateral hilar adenopathy may be present in a number of other infectious or neoplastic conditions and should not be considered diagnostic of sarcoidosis.

**Table 109.1 Summary of Connective Tissue Diseases**

| SYNDROME | TESTING | TREATMENT | TIPS |
|---|---|---|---|
| Sjögren syndrome | Cracker test<br>Slit-lamp examination<br>Schirmer test | Artificial tears<br>Sialogogues<br>Pilocarpine<br>Nasolacrimal duct occlusion | Use humidifier and moisturizers<br>Avoid dry environments |
| Systemic sclerosis and Raynaud phenomenon | Skin examination<br>Serum creatinine<br>Urinalysis | Omeprazole<br>Captopril | GERD precautions<br>Regular BP checks<br>Patients should be advised of the chronic and progressive nature of systemic sclerosis |
| Sarcoidosis | Chest radiograph<br>ECG<br>Slit-lamp examination | Prednisone<br>NSAIDs<br>Cycloplegics | Most cases abate within 2 yr |
| Raynaud phenomenon | Normal nail fold capillary examination | Nifedipine | Avoid cold<br>Avoid tobacco<br>Wear warm clothing |

*BP*, Blood pressure; *ECG*, electrocardiogram; *GERD*, gastroesophageal reflux disease; *NSAIDs*, nonsteroidal anti-inflammatory drugs.

Ocular sarcoidosis most frequently takes the form of anterior uveitis with symptoms of eye pain, irritation, and visual disturbances, including red eye and photophobia. Cell and flare or even hypopyon may be seen on slit-lamp examination. Posterior uveal tissue can also be involved, with signs of chorioretinitis noted on funduscopy. Keratitis and globe perforation are sequelae of corneal involvement, and nodules representative of granulomatous tissue can be seen on the conjunctiva of affected patients.

Cardiac disease, though less common, can be life-threatening. Appropriately placed septal granulomas can block the normal conduction system, with complete heart block being the most common manifestation. They may also serve as foci for electrical reentry and thereby predispose to arrhythmias. Within papillary tissue, granulomas can result in muscle dysfunction and secondary atrioventricular valve incompetence. Extensive ventricular muscle involvement or valvular insufficiency can result in congestive heart failure.

Musculoskeletal manifestations consist of symmetric arthralgias or inflammatory arthritis of the ankles, knees, wrists, and elbows. Most patients do not have a chronic destructive arthritis, however. Although lytic or sclerotic bony lesions can be noted in the hands and feet, many patients will be asymptomatic. Granulomatous muscle involvement is also often subclinical.

Neurologic complications develop in up to 10% of patients and can involve any part of the central or peripheral nervous system. Aseptic (predominantly basal) meningitis, encephalopathy, seizures, hypothalamic and pituitary disturbances (with diabetes insipidus or secondary thyroid or adrenal dysfunction), cranial neuropathies (especially unilateral or bilateral cranial nerve VII palsies), and communicating or noncommunicating hydrocephalus from granulomatous impairment of ventricular drainage are all potential intracranial manifestations. Peripheral neuropathies and spinal cord dysfunction are secondary to extracranial granulomatous inflammation.

Glandular exocrine insufficiency from granulomatous involvement can produce swollen lacrimal, parotid, and salivary glands, with resultant symptoms of dry eyes and mouth. Other signs and symptoms related to systemic T-cell activation and granuloma formation include nonthoracic lymphadenopathy, splenomegaly, fever, and malaise. Increased granulomatous calcitriol production with long-standing hypercalcemia and hypercalciuria may result in renal calcium deposition.

## DIFFERENTIAL DIAGNOSIS AND MEDICAL DECISION MAKING

Pulmonary symptoms and typical radiographic signs in a young or middle-aged patient with erythema nodosum, iritis, or nonspecific, symmetric musculoskeletal complaints can help the EP distinguish sarcoidosis from other infectious or autoimmune processes (**Table 109.1**). Even then, a definitive bedside diagnosis may be difficult to make, and the EP may need to consider tuberculosis, histoplasmosis, community-acquired pneumonia, and lymphoma before diagnosing sarcoidosis (**Box 109.4**). Some of these patients will have to be admitted or treated empirically for an infectious process before a diagnosis can be secured via a more extensive workup. Given the array of organ systems affected and the lack of pulmonary symptoms in many patients, sarcoidosis may go unrecognized in the ED.

A chest radiograph is the most useful tool for patients with cough, dyspnea, or chest pain. Patients in whom the diagnosis of sarcoidosis is being considered because of erythema nodosum, iritis, or cranial neuropathy should also undergo chest radiography, even in the absence of pulmonary signs or symptoms. The four stages of pulmonary sarcoidosis are described in **Table 109.2**. Patients normally do not progress from one stage to the next. A higher stage indicates a lower likelihood of spontaneous resolution.

An electrocardiogram should be obtained for any patient with syncope, dyspnea, or rhythm abnormalities. Cardiac granulomas can produce first- through third-degree atrioventricular block, fascicular block, or bundle branch block.

Patients should undergo a slit-lamp examination for evaluation of the red eye. Consensual photophobia, pain at a given distance of accommodation, and cell and flare are indicative of iritis. Funduscopic examination may provide evidence of posterior uveitis (vitreous, retinal, or choroid disease). Corneal staining and the Seidel test are useful for the diagnosis of keratitis and corneal perforation.

Findings on arthrocentesis will be consistent with nonseptic, inflammatory arthritis. A computed tomography scan of the brain or a lumbar puncture should be performed in patients with suspected focal intracranial or diffuse meningeal neurologic involvement. Two thirds of patients will have elevated cerebrospinal fluid protein, and half may have a predominantly mononuclear pleocytosis. These findings in some patients with extraneural sarcoid features may suggest the diagnosis of neurosarcoidosis.

Laboratory work will probably not help the EP make a diagnosis, but findings may include anemia of chronic disease, thrombocytopenia from splenomegaly, elevated serum calcium levels from granuloma-related abnormalities in calcitriol production, and nonspecific transaminitis as a result of asymptomatic hepatic granulomas.

Further work-up consisting of a tuberculin skin test, chest computed tomography scan, pulmonary function tests, echocardiography, angiotensin-converting enzyme levels, radionuclide imaging, endomyocardial biopsy for myocardial involvement, bronchoalveolar lavage, or endobronchial, transbronchial, mediastinal, or thoracoscopic biopsy may be considered for patients on an inpatient or outpatient basis with specialist consultation.

**Table 109.2 Stages of Pulmonary Sarcoidosis**

| | |
|---|---|
| Stage I | Bilateral hilar lymphadenopathy (**Fig. 109.5**) |
| Stage II | Bilateral hilar lymphadenopathy plus parenchymal infiltrate |
| Stage III | Parenchymal infiltrate without hilar adenopathy (see Fig. 109.5) |
| Stage IV | Parenchymal fibrosis |

**BOX 109.4 Differential Diagnosis of Sarcoidosis**

**Most Common**

Other granulomatous disease (tuberculosis, fungal, spirochetes, viral, parasitic)
Environmental antigens
Chemical antigens (silica, beryllium)
Other autoimmune conditions (Sjögren syndrome)
Human immunodeficiency virus

**Most Threatening**

Primary cardiac arrhythmia, conduction deficit, cardiomyopathy
Neoplasm (pulmonary or lymphoma)
Globe perforation
Bacterial or aseptic meningitis

## TREATMENT

Two thirds of cases of sarcoidosis will resolve spontaneously within 2 years, and many patients can be managed by observation alone. Treatment focuses on suppression of granuloma formation with glucocorticoids and is reserved for individuals with functional impairment or chronic disease.

Many patients with pulmonary involvement will not require ED treatment. Simple observation by a primary care physician

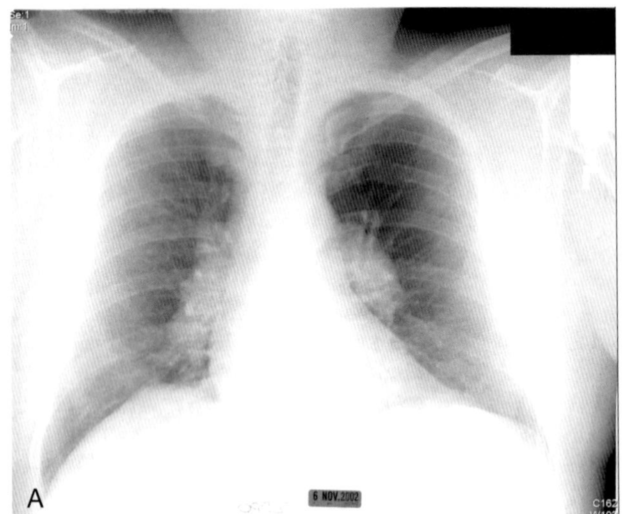


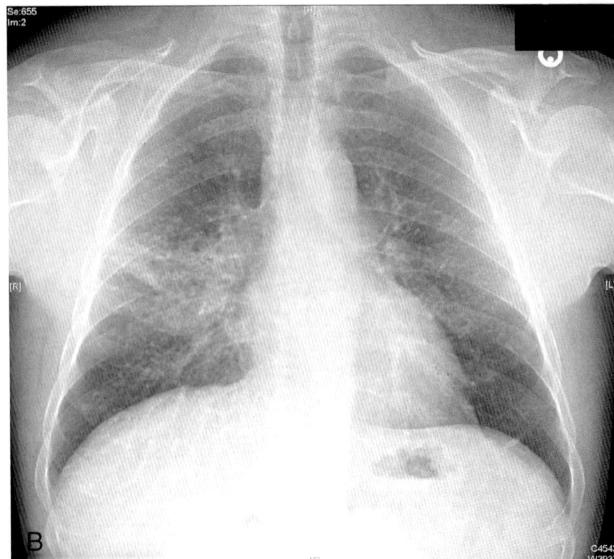


**Fig. 109.5 A,** Stage I sarcoidosis: prominent hilar lymphadenopathy and normal lungs. **B,** Stage III sarcoidosis: interstitial infiltrate without hilar lymphadenopathy. (From Mason RJ, Broaddus VC, Murray JF, et al. Murray and Nadel's textbook of respiratory medicine. 4th ed. Philadelphia: Saunders; 2004.)

on an outpatient basis for the development of treatable symptoms or abnormal findings on pulmonary function tests will suffice. Patients seen in the ED with significant dyspnea, functional impairment, and parenchymal disease noted on radiography are candidates for therapy with prednisone, 0.5 to 1 mg/kg/day, if bacterial, mycobacterial, fungal, and neoplastic processes can be excluded. Patients may need specialist consultation, hospital admission, or (at the very least) close outpatient follow-up. Depending on symptomatic response, doses can be tapered over a 6- to 12-month period by the patient's primary physician.

Musculoskeletal complaints and erythema nodosum are best treated with NSAIDs. Patients with cardiac or neurologic involvement should first undergo standard ED management, with subsequent specialist consultation and consideration given to systemic treatment with glucocorticoids. Invasive interventions such as transvenous cardiac pacing or an intraventricular drain for obstructive hydrocephalus may be required. Ocular manifestations can be treated with topical cycloplegics and, after consultation with an ophthalmologist, topical corticosteroids. Suspected globe perforation as a result of severe keratitis warrants an ophthalmologic evaluation in the ED.

Weekly methotrexate and daily azathioprine are corticosteroid-sparing agents that can be prescribed by a pulmonologist or rheumatologist for steroid-dependent patients. Anti–tumor necrosis factor medication may be a future option in severe cases.[18,19] Tetracyclines are occasionally used for the treatment of skin lesions.[18,20] Radiation therapy and surgical intervention have been used for focal intracranial disease refractory to multiple agents. Lung, heart, or liver transplantation are last-line treatments.

## PATIENT DISPOSITION AND NEXT STEPS IN CARE

The EP should give first consideration to bacterial, mycobacterial, or fungal causes of the patient's signs and symptoms. Lymphoma and other neoplastic processes are also potential diagnoses. If these entities can be excluded or if patients are known to have sarcoidosis, they may be discharged provided that they are minimally symptomatic. Oral prednisone can be prescribed if needed for control of symptoms. However, close outpatient primary care or rheumatology follow-up is mandatory in all cases.

Most patients with functional impairment and no known history of sarcoidosis will need to be admitted for evaluation of other infectious and neoplastic processes before a definitive diagnosis can be made and treatment started.

# PRIMARY RAYNAUD PHENOMENON

## EPIDEMIOLOGY

Raynaud phenomenon is a vasospastic disorder marked by minute- to hour-long episodes of digital ischemia on exposure to cold or emotional stress. Up to 20% of the population may suffer from Raynaud phenomenon. Cases commonly involve women and occur in cooler environments.

## PATHOPHYSIOLOGY

In primary Raynaud phenomenon, the microstructure of distal vessels is entirely normal and symptoms are due to intrinsic hyperreactivity of these vessels when exposed to a trigger. In secondary Raynaud phenomenon, symptoms result from arterial luminal occlusion or stasis of flow, external compression, fibrosis, or abnormal neural innervation.

## PRESENTING SIGNS AND SYMPTOMS

Intense vasoconstriction results in decreased perfusion, well-demarcated pallor, and loss of sensation in the fingers and toes and rarely the nose and ears. With the return of sluggish flow, the extremity turns from white to blue. Paresthesias may be present. Subsequently, with increased flow, the digits become bright red in a phase termed reactive hyperemia. It is during this time of reperfusion that patients will have throbbing pain. Although the triphasic color changes are not always present, it is the predictable response to cold or stress that defines Raynaud phenomenon.

In primary Raynaud phenomenon, the appearance of the vasculature and the patient's digits is normal between attacks.

In secondary Raynaud phenomenon, the symptoms are not always symmetric. Over time, there may be structural changes in distal vessels and permanent changes in the appearance of the patient's digits.

## DIFFERENTIAL DIAGNOSIS AND MEDICAL DECISION MAKING

The cardinal stigmata of autoimmune diseases (sclerodermatous skin changes, muscle weakness, rash) may not be present at the time that a patient has symptoms of Raynaud phenomenon (**Box 109.5**). A diagnosis of primary Raynaud phenomenon is sometimes made on the initial visit when in actuality the patient later turns out to have secondary Raynaud phenomenon caused by an underlying autoimmunity yet to be manifested.

**BOX 109.5 Differential Diagnosis of Raynaud Phenomenon**

**Most Common**
Scleroderma
Systemic lupus erythematosus
Other connective tissue diseases
Occupational arterial injury (hypothenar hammer syndrome)
Medications (beta-blockers, ergotamines)
Thoracic outlet syndrome
Carpal tunnel syndrome
Cryoglobulinemia

**Most Threatening**
Arterial occlusion
Thromboangiitis obliterans

A well-demarcated symmetric change in color occurs during an attack or can be precipitated by placement of the extremity in ice water. Fibrosis, pitting, or ulceration of the fingertips is indicative of the structural vascular and dermal changes in secondary Raynaud phenomenon. In the nail fold capillary examination, immersion oil is placed over the skin at the proximal end of the nail and an ophthalmoscope is used to denote normal-appearing capillaries. Abnormally tortuous, enlarged capillaries or a heterogeneous appearance may be indicative of Raynaud phenomenon secondary to scleroderma, idiopathic inflammatory myopathy, or another vascular disease.

Autoantibodies, cryoglobulins, and serum or urine protein electrophoresis to determine secondary causes of Raynaud phenomenon are not standard parts of the ED work-up.

## TREATMENT

Patients should be instructed to avoid cold and stress, cease tobacco consumption, and wear warm clothing. Oral administration of nifedipine, 10 to 20 mg taken 30 minutes before exposure to cold, can minimize attacks.[21] Alternatively, patients may take up to 60 mg/day divided into three doses. Once-a-day extended-release tablets are also available. Caution should be used in the elderly and those with cardiac and vascular disease. One study suggested that the angiotensin receptor blocker losartan (50 mg/day) outperforms nifedipine.[22] Prazosin (1 to 2 mg three times daily) and topical nitrates are second-line agents for primary Raynaud phenomenon.[23] Endothelin antagonists, phosphodiesterase inhibitors, and intravenous infusions of prostacyclin analogues are newer therapies for severe or secondary Raynaud phenomenon.[22,24] Temporary relief of symptoms can be achieved by chemical sympathectomy via local or regional infiltration of an anesthetic. Surgical treatments, including palmar sympathectomy, thoracoscopic cervical sympathectomy, or arteriolysis (release of fibrotic adventitia), are last-line therapy.

## PATIENT DISPOSITION AND NEXT STEPS IN CARE

Most patients with primary or secondary Raynaud phenomenon may be discharged home for primary care follow-up in the following 2 to 4 weeks.

Admission is occasionally required. In addition to prolonged arteriolar constriction and the occasional limb threat, chest pain can occur as a result of coronary artery vasospasm.

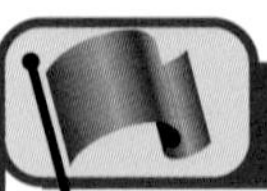

**RED FLAGS**

Many connective tissue diseases have associated severe keratitis that may be complicated by globe perforation.

Sarcoid granulomas can block the normal conduction system, with complete heart block being the most common manifestation.

Consider sarcoidosis in patients with only bilateral hilar lymphadenopathy shown on a chest radiograph, especially if they are asymptomatic or have insidious pulmonary complaints.

Before diagnosing sarcoidosis, consider tuberculosis, histoplasmosis, community-acquired pneumonia, and lymphoma. Some of these patients will have to be admitted or treated empirically for an infectious process before a diagnosis can be secured via more extensive work-up.

Patients who have functional impairment and no known history of sarcoidosis will need to be admitted for evaluation of other infectious and neoplastic processes before a definitive diagnosis can be made and treatment started.

## REFERENCES

*References can be found on Expert Consult @ www.expertconsult.com.*

# Vasculitis Syndromes 110

*Paul J. Allegretti and Keri Robertson*

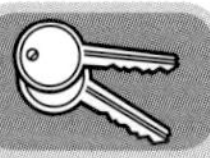

**KEY POINTS**

- A patient's combined genetic predisposition and regulatory mechanisms control expression of the immune response to antigens.
- Negative test results for antineutrophil cytoplasmic antibodies do not exclude disease, nor do positive results indicate a specific syndrome.
- The combination of clinical, laboratory, biopsy, and radiographic findings usually points to a specific vasculitis syndrome.
- Definitive diagnosis of a vasculitic syndrome depends on demonstration of vascular involvement and may be accomplished by biopsy or angiography.
- Differentiation of primary and secondary vasculitis is essential because their pathophysiologic, prognostic, and therapeutic aspects differ.
- The diagnosis of vasculitis should be considered in any patient with febrile illness and organ ischemia without other explanation.

## EPIDEMIOLOGY

In 1994, the Chapel Hill Consensus Conference named and defined the 10 most common forms of vasculitis according to vessel size (**Box 110.1**). This system is based on the fact that different forms of vasculitis attack different vessels.[1,2] These criteria were established to differentiate specific types of vasculitis, but they are often used as diagnostic criteria. The vasculitic syndromes feature a great deal of heterogeneity and overlap, which leads to difficulty with regard to categorization.[3] In addition, many patients display incomplete manifestations, thereby adding to the confusion. Emergency physicians should keep in mind the fact that nature does not always follow the patterns and artificial boundaries drawn by classification systems.[4]

### TEMPORAL (GIANT CELL) ARTERITIS

Temporal, or cranial or giant cell, arteritis is a granulomatous large vessel vasculitis that affects the extracranial branches of the carotid artery, particularly the temporal artery. Females are affected two to four times more often than males, and the disorder usually occurs in patients older than 55 years. Its incidence is estimated to be 1 per 3000 individuals older than 50. Up to 59% of the time it is associated with polymyalgia rheumatica, which is characterized by pain and stiffness in the shoulders, neck, and pelvis, along with an elevated erythrocyte sedimentation rate (ESR).

### TAKAYASU ARTERITIS

Takayasu arteritis (also referred to as aortic arch syndrome) is a granulomatous large vessel vasculitis that primarily affects the aorta, its branches, and the pulmonary and coronary arteries.[1] This rare disease predominantly affects women in the 20- to 30-year-old age group and is more common in Asian and South American women. Mortality ranges from 10% to 75%.

### POLYARTERITIS NODOSA

Polyarteritis nodosa is a multisystem necrotizing vasculitis of small- and medium-sized muscular arteries. Visceral and renal artery involvement is characteristic.[3] The mean age at onset is 50 years, although it can occur at any age. Men, women, and racial groups are all affected equally. This rare disease affects fewer than 10 per 1 million persons worldwide.

### KAWASAKI DISEASE

Kawasaki disease, also referred to as mucocutaneous lymph node syndrome, primarily affects children younger than 5 years. This acute systemic vasculitis is a febrile multisystem disease that is the leading cause of acquired heart disease in children in the United States.[1] The disease occurs worldwide but predominates in Japan, Asia, and the United States.

### WEGENER GRANULOMATOSIS

Wegener granulomatosis is a vasculitis of the upper and lower respiratory tract and kidneys. A systemic small vessel vasculitis is also involved. It may occur at any age but has a mean onset at 40 years of age. Wegener granulomatosis affects men and women equally and involves whites more commonly than blacks.

### CHURG-STRAUSS SYNDROME

Churg-Strauss syndrome is a rare small vessel vasculitis manifested by fever, asthma, and hypereosinophilia.[1] This disease is also referred to as allergic angiitis and granulomatosis,

**BOX 110.1 Chapel Hill Consensus Conference Classification of Primary Vasculitides**

**Large Vessel**
Giant cell (temporal) arteritis
Takayasu arteritis

**Medium Vessel**
Polyarteritis nodosa
Kawasaki disease

**Small Vessel**
Wegener granulomatosis
Churg-Strauss syndrome
Microscopic polyangiitis
Henoch-Schönlein purpura
Cryoglobulinemic vasculitis
Cutaneous leukocytoclastic vasculitis

From Kallenberg CG. Vasculitis: clinical approach, pathophysiology, and treatment. Wien Klin Wochenschr 2000;112:656-9.

**BOX 110.2 Three Potential Mechanisms of Blood Vessel Damage in Vasculitis with Corresponding Diseases**

**Pathogenic Immune Complex Formation**
Henoch-Schönlein purpura
Vasculitis associated with collagen vascular diseases
Serum sickness
Cutaneous vasculitic syndromes
Hepatitis C, cryoglobulinemia
Hepatitis B, polyarteritis nodosa

**Antineutrophilic Cytoplasmic Antibodies**
Wegener granulomatosis
Churg-Strauss syndrome
Microscopic polyangiitis

**Pathogenic T-Lymphocyte Responses and Granuloma Formation**
Temporal arteritis
Takayasu arteritis
Wegener granulomatosis
Churg-Strauss syndrome
Kawasaki disease

From Fauci AS, Sneller MC. Pathogenesis of vasculitis syndromes. Med Clin North Am 1997;81:221-42.

particularly when it affects the lungs. It is estimated that about 3 million people are affected worldwide, with an equal incidence between sexes. It is seen at all ages with a mean onset at 44 years of age.

## HENOCH-SCHÖNLEIN PURPURA

Henoch-Schönlein purpura (anaphylactoid purpura) is a small vessel vasculitis that predominantly affects children and is characterized by palpable purpura, arthralgia, glomerulonephritis, and gastrointestinal symptoms.[3] Though also seen in adults, 75% of cases occur in children younger than 8 years. It is more common than other vasculitides and affects males more frequently than females in a 2:1 ratio. It has a peak incidence in winter and spring and usually follows an upper respiratory tract infection.

## CUTANEOUS LEUKOCYTOCLASTIC VASCULITIS

This disorder, also called hypersensitivity vasculitis or predominantly cutaneous vasculitis, involves small vessels of the skin and is the most common vasculitic manifestation seen in clinical practice.[1] It has an incidence of 15 per million.[4] In about 70% of cases, cutaneous vasculitis occurs along with an underlying process such as infection, malignancy, medication exposure, and connective tissue disease or as a secondary manifestation of a primary systemic vasculitis.

## BEHÇET SYNDROME

Behçet syndrome is a multisystem inflammatory disease that affects vessels of all size.[1] It is manifested as recurrent aphthous oral and genital ulcerations along with ocular involvement. Behçet syndrome is most prevalent at ages 20 to 35 years, with males suffering more severe disease.

# PATHOPHYSIOLOGY

Vasculitis, also known as the vasculitides or the vasculitis syndromes, is a clinicopathologic process that results in inflammation and damage to blood vessels.[3] Cell infiltration with inflammatory modulators causes swelling and changes in function of the vessel walls. This compromises vessel patency and integrity and leads to tissue ischemia, necrosis, and bleeding. Because most forms of vasculitis are not restricted to a certain vessel type or organ, the syndromes are broad and heterogeneous. Vasculitis is a systemic multiorgan disease, so the findings may be dominated by a single or a few clinical organ manifestations.[4]

Vasculitis can be separated into two broad categories. It may develop de novo as a primary manifestation of vessel inflammation without a known cause. Alternatively, it may be a secondary manifestation of an underlying disease or exposure to a drug. Distinction between primary and secondary vasculitis is essential because their pathophysiologic, prognostic, and therapeutic aspects differ.

Management of patients with the secondary forms of vasculitis needs to be directed toward the underlying disease process. The primary vasculitides, once thought to be uncommon, have proved to be much less rare than previously estimated, and awareness of the incidence and prevalence of all forms of vasculitis has recently increased.[5] This chapter focuses on the primary or de novo vasculitides.

The pathophysiology of the vasculitis syndromes remains poorly understood, with variation between disease states contributing to the difficulty. It is also not clear why vasculitis develops in certain patients in response to antigenic stimuli and not in others; however, in each disease state, immunologic mechanisms play an active role in mediating blood vessel inflammation.[1] Blood vessels can be damaged by three potential mechanisms (**Box 110.2**).[6]

Immune complex deposition in vessel walls is the most well-known pathogenic mechanism of vasculitis and results in tissue damage from such deposition. Complement components are then activated and infiltrate the vessel walls. The immune complexes are phagocytosed and release damaging enzymes. As the condition progresses and becomes subacute, the vessel lumen may become compromised with subsequent tissue ischemia.

Antineutrophil cytoplasmic antibodies (ANCAs) develop in a large number of patients with systemic vasculitis, especially Wegener granulomatosis. These antibodies attack proteins in the cytoplasm of neutrophils. Two main types of ANCA are differentiated by the different targets of the antibodies: perinuclear ANCA (p-ANCA) attacks the enzyme myeloperoxidase, whereas cytoplasmic ANCA (c-ANCA) attacks the proteinase-3 enzyme.

The exact role of ANCAs in the pathogenesis of vasculitis is unclear. Although a number of mechanisms have been proposed, confusion remains because vasculitis develops in many patients without ANCAs, there is a lack of correlation with the quantitative value of ANCAs and disease activity, and many patients in remission continue to exhibit high ANCA titers.

Pathogenic T-lymphocyte responses and granuloma formation may also be involved in damaging blood vessels. Delayed hypersensitivity and cell-mediated immune injury are the most common mechanisms in this category. Direct cellular toxicity or antibody-dependent cellular toxicity may also occur.

Two main factors are involved in the expression of a vasculitic syndrome: genetic predisposition and regulatory mechanisms associated with the immune response to antigens. Only certain types of immune complexes cause vasculitis, and the process may be selective for only certain vessel types. Other factors are also involved—for example, the reticuloendothelial system's ability to clear the immune complex, the size and properties of the complex, blood flow turbulence, intravascular hydrostatic pressure, and the preexisting integrity of the vessel endothelium.[3]

## TEMPORAL (GIANT CELL) ARTERITIS

Giant cell arteritis is a panarteritis characterized by inflammatory mononuclear cell infiltrates and giant cell formation in vessel walls. The intima proliferates and the internal elastic lamina fragments. Organ pathology results from ischemia related to the involved vessel derangement.[3]

## TAKAYASU ARTERITIS

The inflammation in Takayasu arteritis involves all vessel wall layers of medium- and large-sized vessels, especially the aorta and its branches. Panarteritis with inflammatory mononuclear cell infiltrates and giant cells predominates. This results in scarring and fibrosis with disruption and degeneration of the elastic lamina. Narrowing of the vessel lumen (**Fig. 110.1**) follows with frequent thrombosis.[3] Vessel dilation and the formation of aneurysms may also occur. Organ pathology results from ischemia.

## POLYARTERITIS NODOSA

The inflammatory lesions associated with polyarteritis nodosa are segmental and involve the bifurcations and branches of arteries. Polymorphonuclear neutrophils infiltrate all layers of the vessel wall. The resultant intimal proliferation and degeneration of the vessel wall lead to vascular necrosis, which in turn results in thrombosis, compromised blood flow, and infarction of the involved tissues and organs. Characteristic aneurysmal dilations of up to 1 cm are common. Multiple organ systems are involved.[3]

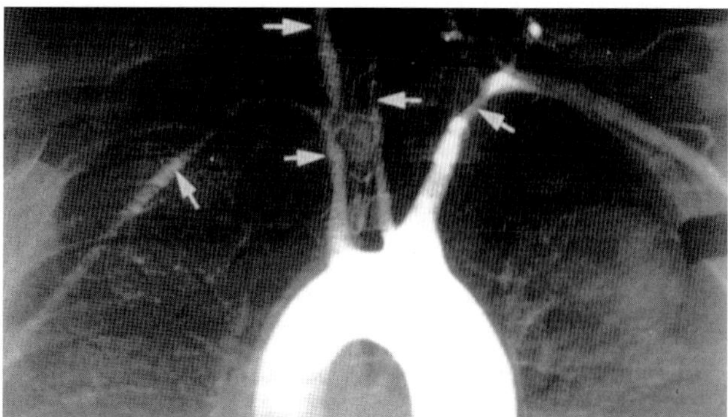

**Fig. 110.1 Aortic arch angiogram showing narrowing of the brachiocephalic, carotid, and subclavian arteries *(arrows)*.** (From Kumar V, editor. Robbins and Cotran pathologic basis of disease. 7th ed. Philadelphia: Saunders; 2005.)

## KAWASAKI DISEASE

The etiology of Kawasaki disease is unknown, but increasing evidence supports an infectious cause; however, whether the inflammatory response results from a conventional antigen or a superantigen continues to be debated. Although a strong predilection for the coronary arteries is seen, this vasculitis is systemic and may involve medium-sized arteries with corresponding manifestations. Initially, neutrophils are present in great numbers, but the infiltrate rapidly switches to mononuclear cells, T lymphocytes, and immunoglobulin A (IgA)-producing plasma cells. Inflammation involves all three layers of vessels. As in other vasculitides, there is typical intimal proliferation and infiltration of the vessel wall with mononuclear cells, which leads to beadlike aneurysms and thrombosis. Cardiomegaly, pericarditis, myocarditis, myocardial ischemia, and infarction may result.[3]

## WEGENER GRANULOMATOSIS

The pathology of Wegener granulomatosis involves a necrotizing vasculitis of small vessels with granuloma formation. The typical necrotizing granulomatous vasculitis in the lungs commonly leads to scarring, atelectasis, and obstruction. The upper airways also become inflamed, with necrosis and granuloma formation. Renal involvement takes the form of a focal and segmental glomerulonephritis that may become rapidly progressive. Few or no immune complexes are found on biopsy; the involvement of immunopathology is unclear. c-ANCAs develop in a large number of these patients, but this correlation is not clear.[3] Besides the typical sinus, lung, and kidney involvement, other organs may be affected because Wegener granulomatosis is a systemic small vessel vasculitis.

## CHURG-STRAUSS SYNDROME

The characteristic histopathologic features of Churg-Strauss syndrome include tissue infiltration by eosinophils, necrotizing small vessel vasculitis, and extravascular "allergic" granulomas.[1] The process can occur in any organ, but lung involvement predominates, and its association with asthma is strong. The combination of asthma, eosinophilia, granulomas, and vasculitis strongly suggests a hypersensitivity reaction as the triggering factor.[3]

### HENOCH-SCHÖNLEIN PURPURA

Henoch-Schönlein purpura is an immune complex disease characterized by deposition of IgA-containing complexes. Suggested but unproved inciting antigens include upper respiratory infections, foods, drugs, insect bites, and vaccinations.[3] All aspects of the disease are more serious when an adult is affected.

### CUTANEOUS LEUKOCYTOCLASTIC VASCULITIS

The pathology predominantly involves small vessels, especially postcapillary venules. Acutely, neutrophils infiltrate the vessels, cause destruction, and result in nuclear debris—thus the term *leukocytoclastic*. As the process becomes more chronic, mononuclear cells and eosinophils become involved. Erythrocytes frequently extravasate and cause a classic palpable purpura, which is a hallmark of the disease.[3]

### BEHÇET SYNDROME

The main pathology in Behçet syndrome is vasculitis with a tendency to form venous thrombi.

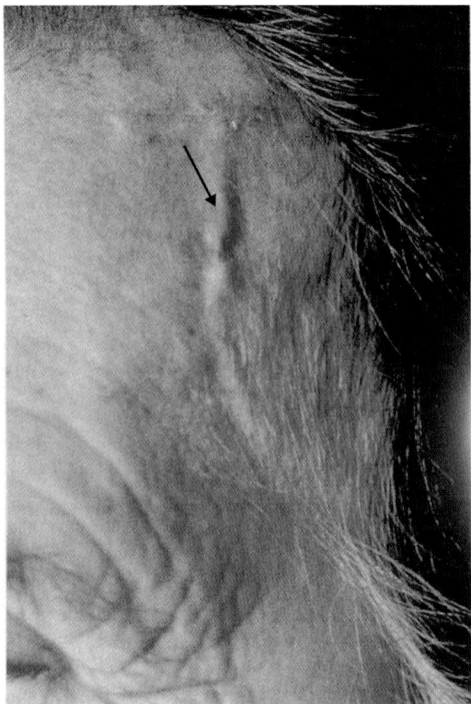

**Fig. 110.2 Temporal artery inflammation.** (From Kumar V, editor. Robbins and Cotran pathologic basis of disease. 7th ed. Philadelphia: Saunders; 2005.)

## PRESENTING SIGNS AND SYMPTOMS

The diagnosis of many vasculitic syndromes is based more on the clinical findings than on laboratory results; therefore, a detailed history plus physical examination is an essential first step in the diagnosis.[7] A high index of suspicion is necessary. The diagnosis should be considered in any patient with systemic febrile illness and signs of organ ischemia without a direct explanation. Nonspecific symptoms such as weight loss, night sweats, and malaise are common. The vessels involved may correlate with the specific symptoms displayed.[8]

### TEMPORAL (GIANT CELL) ARTERITIS

Patients with temporal arteritis have local symptoms related to the arteries involved. Headache, scalp tenderness associated with the inflamed temporal artery (**Fig. 110.2**), jaw claudication, and visual disturbances are typical. Symptoms associated with polymyalgia rheumatica are frequently displayed. Constitutional symptoms such as fever, malaise, fatigue, anorexia, weight loss, arthralgias, and night sweats are also common. The most serious complication is ocular involvement as a result of ischemic optic neuropathy, which may lead to blindness; however, loss of vision is usually avoided with proper treatment. A later complication may be an aortic aneurysm.[9-11]

### TAKAYASU ARTERITIS

Patients with Takayasu arteritis have ischemic symptoms of the involved vessels; such symptoms include visual problems, faint or absent pulses in the upper extremities, and myocardial, abdominal, and lower extremity ischemia. Differences in extremity blood pressure and bruits may also be present. Up to 40% of patients may experience systemic symptoms such as fever, malaise, night sweats, arthralgias, myalgias, weight loss, and anorexia. Death usually occurs from congestive heart failure or stoke. The course may be progressive and unremitting and become fulminant or may stabilize into remission.[3]

### POLYARTERITIS NODOSA

The most common symptoms of polyarteritis nodosa are fever, hypertension, myalgias, arthralgias, weight loss, malaise, and headache. Renal involvement evolves as flank pain, hematuria, renovascular hypertension, and renal failure. Skin lesions range from subcutaneous nodules to distal ischemia. Gastrointestinal manifestations include pain, malabsorption, bleeding, and perforation. Congestive heart failure secondary to coronary artery vasculitis may occur. A classic symptom is orchitis, which may occur in one third of male patients.[4]

### KAWASAKI DISEASE

The characteristic clinical features of Kawasaki disease are fever for at least 5 days, conjunctivitis, changes in the oral mucosa, a generalized rash, red palms and soles, indurative edema with subsequent skin desquamation, and cervical lymphadenopathy.[4] The presence of five of these symptoms confirms the diagnosis. Of course, atypical cases with fewer symptoms occur.

### WEGENER GRANULOMATOSIS

The characteristic manifestation of Wegener granulomatosis involves symptoms in the upper or lower airways (or both) for a prolonged period before the disease becomes systemic. Up to 90% of patients have sought medical attention for sinus or pulmonary problems earlier.[1] Upper respiratory symptoms include pain, purulent or bloody drainage, ulcerations, hoarseness, stridor, and deafness. Pulmonary findings are manifested as cough, dyspnea, chest pain, and hemoptysis, which may become severe. Pulmonary nodules, infiltrates, or cavitations may be seen on chest radiographs. Hypoxemia ensues when the lungs become affected.

Other manifestations include ocular inflammation ranging from conjunctivitis, episcleritis, and scleritis to retinal vasculitis and retroorbital masses. Skin lesions may appear as ulcerations, subcutaneous nodules, or purpura with necrosis. Central nervous system symptoms stem from infarction, cranial nerve neuropathy, and mononeuritis multiplex. Bowel perforation and bleeding may be symptoms of gastrointestinal involvement; pericarditis, coronary ischemia, and cardiomegaly may signal cardiac involvement.[3] Vague symptoms such as malaise, weakness, arthralgia, fever, and anorexia are common.

Glomerulonephritis is present in 20% of patients at the time of diagnosis and develops in 80% at some point as the disease progresses. If not treated properly, renal involvement accounts for most mortality.

## CHURG-STRAUSS SYNDROME

Symptoms such as fever, anorexia, malaise, and weight loss suggest a multisystem disease. Churg-Strauss syndrome has three identifiable phases. It begins with a prodrome of allergic rhinitis, nasal polyps, and asthma. The next phase includes peripheral eosinophilia and eosinophilic tissue infiltrates, especially in the lungs. The third phase is marked by a systemic vasculitis involving the lungs, heart, kidneys, central nervous system, and gastrointestinal tract. These phases may not occur in sequence and may not be seen in all patients.

The disease is best known for its severe and frequent exacerbations of asthma and relapsing vasculitis.[1] The asthma associated with Churg-Strauss syndrome is not a classic allergic asthma that begins early in life; rather, it begins later in life around 35 years of age. It is severe, and patients frequently become steroid dependent.[4]

## HENOCH-SCHÖNLEIN PURPURA

The classic clinical picture of Henoch-Schönlein purpura includes four cardinal manifestations—palpable purpura, arthralgias, gastrointestinal involvement, and glomerulonephritis. The palpable purpura develops in nearly all cases and occurs most commonly over the buttocks and legs (**Fig. 110.3**). Polyarthralgia also develops in most patients. Gastrointestinal symptoms include abdominal pain with nausea, vomiting, diarrhea, constipation, and occasional gastrointestinal bleeding.

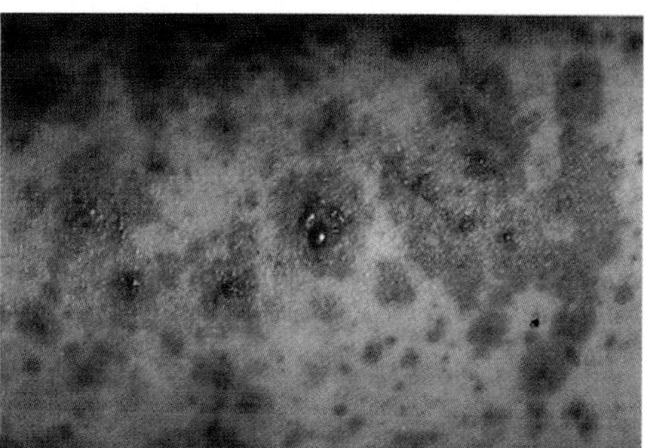

**Fig. 110.3 Palpable purpura in a patient with Henoch-Schönlein purpura.** (From Hoffman R, Benz Jr EJ, Shatttil SJ, et al, editors. Hematology: basic principles and practice. 4th ed. Philadelphia: Saunders; 2005.)

Renal disease is characterized by a mild glomerulonephritis with hematuria and proteinuria. Glomerulonephritis is seen in 20% to 50% of patients, with 2% to 5% progressing to end-stage renal disease.[1]

## CUTANEOUS LEUKOCYTOCLASTIC VASCULITIS

Clinically, besides purpura, patients may exhibit macules, papules, vesicles, bullae, subcutaneous nodules, or urticaria. The skin usually becomes pruritic and painful, and the lesions may progress to ulcers. Although the skin is predominantly involved, patients may exhibit systemic symptoms such as myalgias, fever, anorexia, and malaise.[3] The course of the disease ranges from a brief single episode to multiple prolonged recurrences with infrequent progression to systemic vasculitis.

## BEHÇET SYNDROME

Patients with Behçet syndrome have painful ulcers that occur as one ulcer or multiple ulcers; the ulcers last for 1 to 2 weeks and resolve without scarring. Besides oral ulcers, patients with Behçet syndrome may exhibit two or more of the following signs or symptoms: recurrent genital ulcers, skin lesions, eye lesions, and a positive pathergy test.[1]

The genital ulcers resemble the oral ulcers. Skin lesions range from erythema nodosum and folliculitis to a general inflammatory exanthem. The ocular manifestations usually arise at onset of the disease but may develop later in the first few years. Iritis, posterior uveitis, retinal artery and vein occlusion, and optic neuritis may be seen. Hypopyon uveitis is rare but is pathognomonic of the disease. The ocular involvement may lead to blindness.

Other symptoms include mild arthritis of the lower extremity joints, gastrointestinal inflammation, and ulcerations. Central nervous system manifestations include meningoencephalitis, benign intracranial hypertension, multiple sclerosis–like symptoms, and psychiatric disturbances. Large venous or arterial thrombi or occlusions occur in 25% to 38% of patients.[1,3] Pulmonary emboli are possible.

# DIFFERENTIAL DIAGNOSIS AND MEDICAL DECISION MAKING

## LABORATORY TESTS

The complete blood count may reveal leukocytosis, normocytic normochromic anemia, and thrombocytosis. C-reactive protein (CRP) levels and the ESR may be elevated. Complement levels may be low. Because of renal involvement, urinalysis may reveal proteinuria or active sediment. Cerebrospinal fluid findings in patients with central nervous system vasculitis reveal elevated protein.

The ANCA associated with Wegener granulomatosis, first reported in 1985, is now an established entity in the evaluation of patients with suspected vasculitis. As with any diagnostic test, the predictive value of ANCA depends on the pretest probability of the disease. A negative test result does not exclude the disease, nor should the diagnosis of a vasculitic syndrome be made or treatment initiated based on a positive ANCA titer alone. There have been reports of positive ANCA titers in patients with chronic infections and clinical features similar to systemic vasculitis. Therefore, caution is advised and testing for c-ANCA should not replace tissue biopsy.

## BIOPSY AND ANGIOGRAPHY

Definitive diagnosis is dependent on demonstration of vascular involvement and may be accomplished by biopsy or angiography. Biopsy is preferred and should be directed toward tissue showing evidence of clinical involvement. Biopsy provides the distinct advantage of differentiating active from chronic disease. Such differentiation allows appropriate treatment.

Angiography is an excellent diagnostic modality when medium and large vessels are involved and visceral organ involvement is likely. This modality is the "gold standard" in the work-up of Takayasu arteritis, for which a full evaluation of the aorta is recommended. Angiography demonstrates luminal patency but provides no information about cellular or tissue status. Early vessel inflammation may still be present in a fully patent vessel. Conversely, vessel narrowing may also be due to fibrosis, not active disease.[8] Therefore, clinical correlation is advised with each angiographic finding.

## NONINVASIVE IMAGING

Noninvasive imaging modalities are useful in evaluating changes in the vessel wall not evident on angiography. They are associated with less morbidity than angiography and biopsy and have recently gained popularity in the serial evaluation and detection of early disease in patients with vasculitis.

High-resolution ultrasonography is an efficient, noninvasive, and inexpensive method of monitoring known cases of vasculitis. An example of clinical application is the evaluation of stenotic segments of the carotid arteries. Progression—and hopefully resolution—with treatment of this pathology can also be monitored with ultrasonography. The fact that it cannot detect disease in all vessels, particularly the pulmonary, thoracic, and abdominal visceral vessels, limits this modality.

Computed tomography (CT) can be useful to detect vessel wall thickening, especially in early Takayasu arteritis. CT angiography, high-resolution CT, and electron beam CT have all improved diagnostic outcomes. CT may also be used to evaluate sinus pathology or pulmonary lesions in patients with Wegener granulomatosis. To exclude infection, sarcoidosis, and malignancy, biopsy should follow CT when evaluating these lesions.

Magnetic resonance imaging (MRI) can be used to assess vessel wall thickening and has the advantage of axial, sagittal, and coronal plane views. Magnetic resonance angiography (MRA) correlates well with findings on CT angiography when evaluating the aorta or renal arteries. Further studies are needed before MRI or MRA can be considered first-choice diagnostic tools.

Positron emission tomography measures glucose metabolism in tissues. Increased glycolysis is seen in inactivated leukocytes and macrophages and is a hallmark of inflammation in certain vasculitides, especially giant cell arteritis.

Single-photon emission computed tomography (SPECT) uses multiplanar nuclear imaging to investigate abnormalities in perfusion, especially when evaluating central nervous system vasculitis. Clinical correlation is necessary because perfusion defects may not distinguish vasculitis from entities such as vasospasm, thromboembolism, atherosclerosis, and malignant hypertension. SPECT may also be useful in evaluating the coronary arteries in patients with Kawasaki disease.[8]

## DIAGNOSIS OF SPECIFIC VASCULITIC SYNDROMES

### *Temporal (Giant Cell) Arteritis*

Classic laboratory manifestations include an elevated ESR and CRP. Normochromic anemia and thrombocytosis secondary to the chronic inflammation are common. Liver function abnormalities, particularly an elevated alkaline phosphatase level, are common.

The diagnosis can be determined clinically because of the classic scenario of headache, fever, anemia, and an elevated ESR. Temporal artery biopsy is confirmatory. Because involvement of the vessel may not be contiguous, several separate biopsies may be needed. Color duplex ultrasonography, angiography, or MRI may play a role in making the diagnosis. A rapid clinical response to treatment also confirms the diagnosis.

### *Takayasu Arteritis*

Laboratory findings during active disease include an elevated ESR and increased CRP levels.[4] Angiography demonstrates stenosis, occlusion, dilation, and aneurysms of the aorta and its branches. The entire aorta should be visualized to fully appreciate the spectrum of this disease.[3] Spiral CT angiography and MRA have been shown to be useful.

The diagnosis should be suspected in any young woman with the systemic signs and symptoms previously described and with any blood pressure or pulse discrepancies or bruits. Establishment of the diagnosis must then be achieved by radiologic procedures.

### *Polyarteritis Nodosa*

No diagnostic serologic tests are available for polyarteritis nodosa, and laboratory findings are nonspecific; the ESR, CRP, and leukocytes are elevated. Normochromic anemia is present and is indicative of chronic disease. The diagnosis may be achieved by biopsy demonstrating histologic necrotizing inflammation in the arteries. If biopsy is not possible, angiography demonstrating microaneurysms, stenosis, or sequential narrowing and dilation suggests the diagnosis.

### *Kawasaki Disease*

Echocardiography and angiography confirm the cardiac complications and vasculitis. Laboratory findings include elevated leukocytes, platelets, ESR, and CRP.

Although the disease is generally benign and self-limited, coronary artery aneurysms occur in 20% to 30% of patients, usually during the third or fourth week as convalescence ensues. The presence of four symptoms along with coronary artery aneurysms is diagnostic. The case fatality rate secondary to coronary artery aneurysm is 0.5% to 2.8%.

### *Wegener Granulomatosis*

Laboratory findings include an elevated ESR and CRP, anemia with leukocytosis, thrombocytosis, and positive tests for ANCA, which is seen especially when the kidneys are affected.

The diagnosis is made by biopsy demonstrating necrotizing granulomatous vasculitis with an aggregation of neutrophils in nonrenal tissue. Renal biopsy reveals focal, segmental, necrotizing, crescentic glomerulonephritis.[4] Biopsy findings coincide with the characteristic clinical findings of sinus, pulmonary, and renal symptoms. Although the use of ANCA testing is only adjunctive, its specificity is 90% for Wegener granulomatosis if active glomerulonephritis is present.

### *Churg-Strauss Syndrome*

Classic laboratory findings include leukocytosis with notable eosinophilia, anemia, and elevated ESR and CRP. The diagnosis is confirmed via biopsy in a patient with the characteristic clinical manifestations.

### *Henoch-Schönlein Purpura*

Laboratory studies are nonspecific and may reveal a mild leukocytosis and occasional eosinophilia. Serum IgA levels are elevated in 50% of patients.[3] The diagnosis remains a clinical diagnosis based on the characteristic findings. A skin biopsy is occasionally necessary for confirmation and reveals leukocytoclastic vasculitis with IgA immune deposition. Renal biopsy better serves as a prognostic indicator.[1]

### *Cutaneous Leukocytoclastic Vasculitis*

Laboratory values are usually within normal limits, including ESR and CRP levels. Mild leukocytosis and eosinophilia may be present. Laboratory studies should be used primarily to rule out the presence of systemic vasculitis. Minimal to no signs of inflammation should be found.[4] The diagnosis is made by skin biopsy and by carefully ruling out systemic disease or exogenous reasons for the vasculitis.

The clinical and histopathologic appearance of the lesions is indistinguishable from the cutaneous manifestations of the systemic vasculitides; therefore, the diagnosis should be one of exclusion after other causes have been ruled out.[2] Only then can the disorder be called true cutaneous leukocytoclastic vasculitis or idiopathic cutaneous vasculitis.

### *Behçet Syndrome*

Laboratory findings indicate nonspecific inflammation such as leukocytosis and elevated ESR and CRP levels. Half of patients are found to have autoantibodies to human oral mucous membranes. The diagnosis is based on the clinical findings of recurrent aphthous oral ulcerations.

## TREATMENT

The combination of clinical, laboratory, biopsy, and radiographic findings usually points to a specific syndrome (**Table 110.1**). Therapy should then be initiated as appropriate. If the vasculitis is associated with a specific disease such as neoplasm, infection, or connective tissue disease, the underlying disease should be treated. If the syndrome resolves, no further treatment is needed. If the syndrome persists, treatment of vasculitis should be initiated. Likewise, if an offending antigen is recognized, it should be removed if possible. No further treatment is needed if the syndrome resolves; however, if the syndrome continues, treatment must be initiated. Treatment initiated for a primary vasculitis syndrome should focus on using the most effective and least toxic options based on published experience.[12]

### TEMPORAL (GIANT CELL) ARTERITIS

Treatment should commence immediately and not be delayed by diagnostic procedures. Administration of 40 to 60 mg of prednisone daily for 1 month is followed by a taper to 7.5 to 10 mg daily. This should be continued for 1 to 2 years to prevent relapse. Aspirin, 81 mg daily, has been shown to reduce cranial ischemic complications and should be given to patients without contraindications.[13] Clinical symptoms and the ESR are used to monitor disease activity.

### TAKAYASU ARTERITIS

Treatment consists of the combination of 40 to 60 mg/day of prednisone and aggressive surgical or angiographic procedures directed toward stenotic vessels. This approach corrects hypertension caused by renal artery stenosis, improves blood flow in ischemic vessels, and decreases risk for stroke,[3] thereby resulting in decreased morbidity and improved survival.

### POLYARTERITIS NODOSA

Combination therapy consisting of prednisone (1 mg/kg/day) and cyclophosphamide (2 mg/kg/day) has resulted in a long-term remission rate of 90% after therapy has been discontinued. Glucocorticoids may be used alone in mild cases.

### KAWASAKI DISEASE

Treatment consists of high-dose intravenous gamma globulin (2 g/kg infused over a 10-hour period) administered concurrently with aspirin (80 to 100 mg/kg/day for 2 weeks followed by 3 to 5 mg/kg/day for several more weeks). Early therapy has proved beneficial in reducing coronary artery abnormalities.

### WEGENER GRANULOMATOSIS

Administration of cyclophosphamide (2 mg/kg/day) combined with prednisone (1 mg/kg/day) has proved to be the most successful therapy. Reported results are complete remission in 75%, a survival rate of 80%, and marked improvement in 91%.[1] Though very effective, cyclophosphamide may be associated with severe bone marrow toxicity. Leukocytes must be monitored closely and kept at a level above 3000 mcg.

Full-dose cyclophosphamide therapy should be continued for 1 year after remission and then tapered off. Prednisone therapy may be changed to alternate-day administration after 1 month and then tapered off by 6 months.[3] Methotrexate has shown some success in patients who cannot tolerate cyclophosphamide.

### CHURG-STRAUSS SYNDROME

The most effective therapy is prednisone (1 mg/kg/day). The vasculitis usually remits more readily than the asthma, which may remain moderate to severe and thus make discontinuation of prednisone therapy difficult.[1] Cyclophosphamide at 2 mg/kg/day may be added to the prednisone in patients not responsive to prednisone alone.

### HENOCH-SCHÖNLEIN PURPURA

Although renal failure is the most common cause of death, Henoch-Schönlein purpura usually resolves without therapy. In general, the disease is self-limited with an excellent prognosis for full recovery in as little as a few weeks.

**Table 110.1 Comparing the Vasculitides**

| DISEASE | PATHOPHYSIOLOGY | CLASSIC FEATURES | TESTING | TREATMENT |
|---|---|---|---|---|
| Temporal arteritis | Mononuclear cell infiltration and giant cell formation | Headache<br>Scalp tenderness<br>Visual disturbance | ESR<br>CRP<br>Biopsy | Prednisone |
| Takayasu arteritis | Mononuclear cell infiltration and giant cell formation | Visual disturbance, chest pain, abdominal pain, differences in extremity blood pressure and pulses | Angiography | Prednisone<br>Surgical or angiographic intervention |
| Polyarteritis nodosa | Polymorphonuclear infiltration | Fever, hypertension, myalgias, abdominal pain, hematuria, CHF, GI bleeding, orchitis | ESR, CRP<br>Biopsy<br>Angiography | Prednisone plus cyclophosphamide |
| Kawasaki disease | Polymorphonuclear infiltration | 5-day fever, conjunctivitis, oral lesions, rash, red palms and soles, edema, cervical lymphadenopathy | ESR, CRP<br>Leukocytosis<br>Thrombocytosis<br>Echocardiography | Aspirin plus IV gamma globulin |
| Wegener granulomatosis | Granuloma formation secondary to aggregating neutrophils | Upper and lower respiratory symptoms, renal insufficiency, skin lesions, visual disturbance | ESR<br>CRP<br>c-ANCA | Cyclophosphamide plus prednisone |
| Churg-Strauss syndrome | Eosinophilic infiltration<br>Allergic granulomas | Allergic rhinitis<br>Nasal polyps<br>Asthma | Leukocytosis<br>Eosinophilia<br>ESR, CRP<br>Biopsy | Prednisone with or without cyclophosphamide |
| Henoch-Schönlein purpura | IgA complex deposition | Palpable purpura, arthralgias, GI disturbances, glomerulonephritis | Leukocytosis<br>Eosinophilia<br>IgA elevation<br>Skin biopsy | Usually self-limited<br>Prednisone if necessary |
| Cryoglobulinemic vasculitis | Cold precipitable monoclonal or polyclonal immunoglobulins | Palpable purpura, glomerulonephritis, myalgias, weakness, peripheral neuropathy | Low complement levels<br>Hepatitis C<br>Renal biopsy | Interferon alfa plus ribavirin |
| Cutaneous leukocytoclastic vasculitis | Neutrophilic infiltration<br>Mononuclear and eosinophilic infiltration | Palpable purpura, macules, vesicles, bullae, urticaria | Skin biopsy | Prednisone |
| Behçet syndrome | Polymorphonuclear infiltration | Recurrent oral aphthous ulcers, genital ulcers, skin lesions, visual disturbance | ESR, CRP<br>Leukocytosis<br>Oral mucosa autoantibodies | Topical glucocorticoids<br>Prednisone |

*c-ANCA*, Cytoplasmic antineutrophil cytoplasmic antibody; *CHF*, congestive heart failure; *CRP*, C-reactive protein; *ESR*, erythrocyte sedimentation rate; *GI*, gastrointestinal; *IgA*, immunoglobulin A; *IV*, intravenous.

However, when required, prednisone at 1 mg/kg/day is effective in lessening tissue edema, arthralgias, and abdominal pain. The dose should be tapered as the symptoms abate. Glucocorticoids have no proven benefit on skin and renal involvement and have not been shown to shorten the course of the disease or prevent relapse.[3]

## CUTANEOUS LEUKOCYTOCLASTIC VASCULITIS

If an underlying process is discovered to be the cause of the cutaneous symptoms, treatment should be aimed at the underlying process. If an exogenous agent is the culprit, removal of it usually results in remission of the skin process. If true cutaneous leukocytoclastic vasculitis is determined to be the etiology, glucocorticoids administered at a dosage of 1 mg/kg/day have proved effective.[3]

Frequently, the disease is self-limited; otherwise, it generally responds very rapidly to steroid therapy. Some symptomatic agents may be used on occasion, such as antihistamines, nonsteroidal antiinflammatory drugs, and colchicine. In the rare scenario in which glucocorticoids are not effective, cytotoxic agents such as methotrexate, azathioprine, and cyclophosphamide may be used, but these drugs should be reserved for severe cases.

### BEHÇET SYNDROME

Treatment is based on disease manifestations. Oral and skin lesions respond well to topical glucocorticoids, dapsone, or colchicine. Thrombophlebitis is treated with aspirin. Ocular and central nervous system manifestations require aggressive treatment with immunosuppressive agents such as glucocorticoids, azathioprine, or cyclosporine.[1]

## FOLLOW-UP, NEXT STEPS IN CARE, AND PATIENT EDUCATION

### TEMPORAL (GIANT CELL) ARTERITIS

The prognosis is good; the majority of patients go into remission and remain in remission after discontinuation of steroids. Patients with severe disease or impending vision loss should be hospitalized and given high-dose intravenous steroids.

### TAKAYASU ARTERITIS

Hospital admission for diagnostic testing and treatment should be considered for suspected cases. It is the best practice but not always possible to control the vascular inflammation with prednisone before any surgical procedures.

### POLYARTERITIS NODOSA

Discharge home with follow-up is appropriate except in patients with evidence of end-organ failure.

### KAWASAKI DISEASE

Except for rare fatal cardiac complications, the prognosis is good, typically with full recovery.[3] Children in whom aneurysms develop require close follow-up after discharge, and some patients with severe disease may need long-term anticoagulation.

### WEGENER GRANULOMATOSIS

Outpatient management is appropriate except in patients with advanced end-organ involvement. On achievement of remission, long-term follow-up is essential. Up to 50% of patients have one or more relapses. With close follow-up and immediate reinstitution of therapy, induction of remission is almost always a success. In many patients, especially those with multiple relapses, some degree of long-term morbidity develops, such as renal insufficiency, tracheal stenosis, hearing loss, or sinus impairment.[3] Aggressive prompt therapy during the initial manifestation of the disease, as well as during relapses, helps diminish the degree of chronic morbidity.

### CHURG-STRAUSS SYNDROME

Outpatient management is appropriate except in patients with advanced end-organ involvement. The prognosis of untreated patients is a 25% 5-year survival rate, which improves to 50% with proper treatment.[1]

### HENOCH-SCHÖNLEIN PURPURA

Patients with Henoch-Schönlein purpura who have severe abdominal pain, significant gastrointestinal bleeding, or marked renal insufficiency may require hospitalization.

### CUTANEOUS LEUKOCYTOCLASTIC VASCULITIS

This disorder may be managed on an outpatient basis.

### BEHÇET SYNDROME

Treatment may be managed on an outpatient basis unless ocular or central nervous system manifestations are evident.

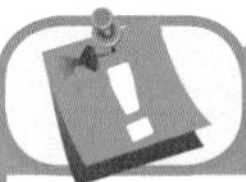

**TIPS AND TRICKS**

- Although antineutrophil cytoplasmic antibodies (ANCAs) are quite common in patients with vasculitis, their role is not clear. ANCA testing may actually confuse the diagnostic picture when results are negative in a patient with clinical vasculitis, when there is a lack of quantitative correlation with disease activity, and when high titers are found in patients whose disease has fallen into remission.
- Vision loss associated with temporal arteritis may be prevented with immediate and proper treatment. In patients with any signs of this complication, treatment must not be delayed because permanent vision loss may ensue.
- Patients with Wegener granulomatosis often have prolonged signs and symptoms of upper or lower airway dysfunction, or both. Ninety percent of these patients have previously been evaluated for sinus problems that became chronic. A high index of suspicion is required.
- The asthma associated with Churg-Strauss syndrome is a severe condition that usually begins when the patient is about 35 years of age. With treatment, the vasculitis commonly subsides much more readily than the asthma.

## REFERENCES

*References can be found on Expert Consult @ www.expertconsult.com.*

# Male Genitourinary Emergencies 111

*Jonathan E. Davis*

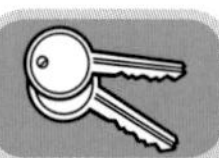

**KEY POINTS**

- The five major male genitourinary emergencies are testicular torsion, Fournier gangrene (necrotizing fasciitis of the perineum), priapism, paraphimosis, and genitourinary tract trauma. An associated emergent condition is an incarcerated or strangulated inguinal hernia.
- Ultrasound examination is the primary diagnostic tool for differentiation of causes of acute scrotal pain.
- Urology services should be consulted immediately after initial patient evaluation when testicular torsion is suspected.
- Pain out of proportion to the findings on physical examination is the hallmark of early Fournier gangrene.
- In the setting of severe scrotal pain, a necrotic or ischemic cause should be suspected. Testicular torsion, Fournier gangrene, and an incarcerated or strangulated inguinal hernia are surgical emergencies.
- A trial of oral terbutaline, a β-adrenergic agonist, is the least invasive initial treatment of priapism. Corporal blood aspiration with or without irrigation or injection of an α-adrenergic receptor agonist (e.g., phenylephrine) may be necessary if the condition is not reversed rapidly.
- Successful reduction of paraphimosis can often be performed at the bedside without specialty consultation.
- A urologist should be engaged in the care of all but the most minor cases of genitourinary trauma.

## ANATOMY AND PATHOPHYSIOLOGY

The male genitalia is composed of the penis, with paired erectile bodies and the penile urethra, and the scrotum, which encases the testis, epididymis, and spermatic cord bilaterally. Beneath the scrotal skin is the superficial scrotal (dartos) fascia (which is contiguous with the fascia of the abdomen, known as the fascia of Scarpa), the perineal (Colles) fascia, and the penile (dartos) fascia. The spermatic fascia lies beneath the dartos fascia; it has three layers, with the middle layer forming the cremaster muscle. These anatomic layers may provide a conduit for the rapid spread of infection.

The fibrous capsule of the tunica albuginea surrounds each testis. A break in the integrity of the tunica albuginea represents a "ruptured" testicle, which can be caused by blunt trauma. External to the testicular parenchyma and tunica albuginea is the tunica vaginalis, which envelops each testicle and fastens it to the posterior scrotal wall.

The gubernaculum, or scrotal ligament, anchors each testis inferiorly and provides additional stability. The tunica vaginalis consists of both visceral (contiguous with the tunica albuginea) and parietal (contiguous with the deep spermatic fascia) layers, with an interposed potential space. A lack of firm attachment of the testicle to the posterior scrotal wall makes the testis prone to rotation in a horizontal plane about the spermatic cord, a condition termed testicular torsion.

The testicular artery originates from the aorta just below or directly from the renal artery. The spermatic cord contains both the blood supply to each testicle via the gonadal vessels and the vas deferens. Interruption of blood flow to the testis by twisting of the spermatic cord can lead to rapid ischemia and subsequent infarction of the affected testicle in cases of testicular torsion.

The appendix testes are embryologic remnants with no known physiologic function. These appendages are prone to torsion as well, which can lead to localized, self-limited necrosis. It results in clinical findings that may be confused with testicular torsion.

The epididymis adheres closely to the posterolateral aspect of each testis. It is involved in promoting sperm maturation and motility. The appendix epididymis is an embryologic remnant typically attached to each epididymis. These too are prone to torsion.

The vas deferens is a tubular structure involved in sperm transit; it extends from the epididymis distally to the prostatic portion of the urethra proximally.

The penis consists of the corpora cavernosa (erectile bodies) and the corpus spongiosum, which surrounds the urethra. In uncircumcised males, the retractile penile foreskin covers the glans. The potential constricting effect of proximally retracted foreskin may lead to paraphimosis. In paraphimosis, venous engorgement of the glans and edema resulting from constriction can potentially progress to arterial compromise and necrosis of the distal end of the penis. Each corpus cavernosum is surrounded by the tunica albuginea as well.

Priapism is a pathologic condition defined as the presence of a persistent erection lasting longer than 4 hours in the

**BOX 111.1 Selected Causes of Low-Flow Priapism**

**Medications**

Impotence agents

- Intracavernosal therapies (prostaglandin $E_1$, papaverine, phentolamine)
- Oral agents (e.g., sildenafil)

Antihypertensives

- Hydralazine, prazosin, doxazosin

Antidepressants

- Trazodone, fluoxetine, sertraline, citalopram

Antipsychotics

- Phenothiazines, atypical antipsychotics

Illicit substances

- Cocaine, marijuana, alcohol

General anesthetics

Miscellaneous

- Hydroxyzine, metoclopramide, omeprazole, total parenteral nutrition, anticoagulant hormones

**Hematologic Disorders**

Sickle cell disease

Leukemia

Myeloma

Other malignancies

**Central Nervous System**

Brain

- Cerebrovascular accident

Spinal cord

- Spinal stenosis, spinal cord injury, lumbar disk herniation

**Others**

Infections

- Malaria, rabies

Toxins

- Black widow, scorpion

Carbon monoxide

Trauma

Hypertriglyceridemia

Idiopathic

absence of sexual desire or stimulation. It most frequently results from engorgement of the corpora cavernosa with stagnant blood (termed low-flow priapism). **Box 111.1** lists several causes of low-flow priapism.

High-flow priapism is rare and is caused by the development of traumatic arterial-cavernosal fistulas, which results in the accumulation of oxygen-rich blood in the corpora.

## PRESENTING SIGNS AND SYMPTOMS

Genitourinary complaints are often influenced by patient embarrassment and apprehension, especially in children and adolescents. Complaints of abdominal pain, fever, or nausea may be offered by the patient, but information about scrotal or penile issues may be withheld. It is important to speak with the patient alone to maximize patient disclosure, privacy, and confidentiality.

### ACUTE SCROTAL PAIN

One of the most challenging aspects of male genitourinary complaints is that a wide variety of clinical conditions may all be manifested as acute, unilateral (or bilateral) pain and swelling of the scrotum. Although the differential diagnosis for such symptoms is extensive, threats to life and fertility need to be excluded. Testicular torsion, Fournier gangrene, and an incarcerated or strangulated inguinal hernia are surgical emergencies. The vast majority of acute testicular pain, however, can be attributed to one of three diagnostic entities: testicular torsion, epididymitis, or appendage torsion (**Table 111.1**).[1]

### HISTORY

Pain may be due to structures within or adjoining a particular region or may be referred from other areas. Delineation of the source of the pathology is essential. For example, pain from abdominal aortic aneurysms, renal colic, and pyelonephritis can radiate to the testicles.

### ONSET OF SYMPTOMS

Pain that begins abruptly and is severe suggests testicular torsion.[2] Intermittent severe pain can signal intermittent torsion. Twisting of the spermatic cord leads to rapid diminution of blood supply to the affected testicle and resultant ischemic pain. This is in contrast to the more indolent pain of epididymitis, a gradually progressive inflammatory process. Patients with long-standing inguinal hernias often complain of isolated genital pain of prolonged duration. However, patients with an incarcerated (cannot be reduced) or strangulated hernia (with ischemic or infarcted, herniated bowel) may experience more acute pain.

Testicular torsion may accompany a report of minor scrotal trauma.[3] Testicular torsion can also take place in the absence of such events and may even occur during sleep.

### CHARACTER OF SYMPTOMS

The distinction between constant progressive and intermittent colicky pain is potentially useful in the diagnosis of acute scrotal pain. Constant and progressive pain typically results from progressive inflammatory processes such as epididymitis. Patients may exhibit pain with ambulation and other movements as a result of the inflammation. Intermittent and colicky pain is more consistent with rapid onset and offset conditions, as occurs with twisting of the spermatic cord, either suddenly or intermittently.

Patients with testicular torsion often complain of severe pain as a consequence of ongoing testicular ischemia. Pain resulting from inflammatory processes (epididymitis) may be relieved temporarily by rest and scrotal elevation with a supportive undergarment such as a jockstrap. Similarly, the inflammatory pain is often exacerbated by movement, thus leading a patient to remain still. Alternatively, patients exhibiting the colicky symptoms of testicular torsion may writhe in pain as they try (and often fail) to find a position of comfort. These symptoms are generalizations and, when considered alone, lack high sensitivity or specificity.

### ASSOCIATED SYMPTOMS

Patients with nausea or emesis are less likely to have torsion of an appendage or simple, uncomplicated epididymitis. It is more likely that substantial pathology is present. Patients

**Table 111.1 Differentiation of Testicular Torsion, Epididymitis, and Appendage Torsion**

| | TESTICULAR TORSION | EPIDIDYMITIS* | APPENDAGE TORSION |
|---|---|---|---|
| **Historical Features** | | | |
| Age | Peak incidence in neonatal and adolescent groups but may occur at any age | Primarily adolescents and adults but may occur at any age | Typically prepubertal boys |
| Risk factors | Undescended testicle (neonate), rapid increase in testicular size (adolescent), failure of previous orchiopexy | Sexual activity or promiscuity, GU anomalies, GU instrumentation | Presence of appendages |
| Pain onset | Sudden | Gradual | Gradual or sudden |
| Previous episodes of similar pain | Possible (spontaneous detorsion) | Unlikely | Occasional |
| History of trauma | Possible | Possible | Possible |
| Nausea, vomiting | More likely | Less likely | Less likely |
| Dysuria | Less likely | More likely | Less likely |
| **Physical Findings** | | | |
| Fever | Less likely | More likely, particularly with advanced disease (epididymoorchitis) | Less likely |
| Location of swelling and tenderness | Testicle, progressing to diffuse hemiscrotal involvement | Epididymis, progressing to diffuse hemiscrotal involvement | Localized to head of affected testicle or epididymis |
| Cremasteric reflex | Testicular torsion less likely if present | May be present or absent | May be present or absent |
| Testicle position | High-riding testicle, transverse alignment | Normal position, vertical alignment | Normal position, vertical alignment |
| Pyuria | Less likely | More likely | Less likely |

*GU*, Genitourinary.
*Including epididymoorchitis.

with abdominal pain, nausea, or constitutional symptoms may have testicular torsion, an incarcerated hernia, or another process.[2,4,5] Patients with epididymitis may have a low-grade fever, nausea, and malaise; those with advanced infection (e.g., epididymoorchitis) may demonstrate more pronounced constitutional symptoms.[6]

Urinary symptoms such as dysuria and urgency may accompany epididymitis. Inability to void spontaneously may indicate either urethral obstruction or severe volume depletion. A yellow-green penile discharge may provide clues to the diagnosis of urethritis or epididymitis, often caused by gonorrhea or *Chlamydia* infection in sexually active males.

## PHYSICAL EXAMINATION

### ABDOMINAL EXAMINATION

Because many intraabdominal conditions may be associated with genitourinary pain, abdominal, flank, and back evaluation is useful. It is important to assess for lower abdominal tenderness or a mass, which potentially signals acute appendicitis, inguinal hernia, genitourinary malignancy, abdominal trauma, or an advanced perineal infection such as Fournier gangrene. Tenderness at the costovertebral angle may be present with retroperitoneal processes such as pyelonephritis, renal colic, and an expanding or ruptured abdominal aortic aneurysm.

### GENITAL EXAMINATION

The genitalia should be examined while the patient is both standing and lying supine. Caution should be used when examining a standing patient because some males experience a strong vagal response to scrotal (or prostate) stimulation that can lead to presyncope or syncope. In addition, examination of the testicles and epididymis may cause significant discomfort, even in the absence of pathology. Because many patients have unilateral pain, the unaffected side should be examined first. This serves as a control and helps gain the trust of the patient.

Visual examination of the genitals may reveal cutaneous rashes or lesions, abnormal testicular symmetry or position, edema evident by loss of the scrotal skin folds, and masses. Key visual features of testicular torsion include a high-riding and transverse lie of the affected testicle.[2,4,7]

It is important to look for evidence of scrotal and perineal erythema or ecchymoses, particularly in older patients with scrotal pain. This may be the only clue to the presence of Fournier gangrene, which often affects diabetics and other immunocompromised individuals. However, a prominent feature of necrotizing fasciitis is significant pain in the absence of pronounced physical findings.

A digital rectal examination provides information regarding the prostate and the prostatic portion of the urethra. Exquisite prostate tenderness may indicate acute prostatitis. Firmness and enlargement of the prostate are typically signs of benign prostatic hypertrophy; nodularity is concerning for prostatic carcinoma. These conditions may be accompanied by variable genitourinary symptoms.

## ACUTE PENILE PAIN

Patients with low-flow priapism often complain of an exquisitely painful and prolonged erection. Stagnant, oxygen-poor, acidic blood accumulates in the corpora and results in ischemic pain. Ischemia may lead to irreversible cellular damage, permanent fibrosis, and impotence if the duration of the pathologic erection is prolonged. Of note, the use of oral erectile dysfunction treatments such as sildenafil (Viagra) have only rarely been associated with priapism.[8] Patients with high-flow priapism often complain of a persistent, yet painless erection that is caused by continuous inflow of well-oxygenated blood through traumatic arterial-cavernosal fistulas.

Paraphimosis classically develops in uncircumcised males when the proximally retracted foreskin acts as a constricting band on the mid to distal portion of the penile shaft. Disruption of venous drainage by the constricting foreskin leads to a vicious cycle of progressive glans edema. Progressive glans edema will eventually cause arterial compromise, ischemic pain, glans necrosis, and gangrene. Penile foreskin should always be replaced after retraction during examination or placement of a urethral catheter to avoid the development of iatrogenic paraphimosis.

Penile constriction analogous to paraphimosis can also occur. Objects constricting the penile shaft lead to the same pathophysiologic derangements seen with paraphimosis. These objects may be placed intentionally (e.g., string, metal, rubber rings), or the constriction may occur sporadically, as in the case of a hair tourniquet in infants. Hair tourniquets may be very difficult to diagnose because the offending hair is nearly invisible within an edematous coronal sulcus. An occult hair tourniquet should be considered along with testicular torsion in a male infant with inconsolable crying. Removal of the offending hair from the coronal sulcus can be difficult. It has been reported that over-the-counter hair removal products, including depilatories such as Nair, have been used successfully for the removal of digital (finger, toe) hair tourniquets, thus suggesting its utility for penile hair tourniquets as well.[9]

## GENITOURINARY TRAUMA

Trauma to the testicle and its associated structures (epididymis and spermatic cord) occurs infrequently because of testicular mobility and the protective cremasteric reflex. In addition, each testicle is encapsulated by the tunica albuginea, which may protect the testicular parenchyma from injury. Blunt force injury may cause a testicular contusion or, less frequently, rupture of the tunica albuginea. In addition, traumatic dislocation of the testicle to a location outside the scrotal confines is possible with significant blunt force injury.

All but the most superficial penetrating scrotal injuries require specialty consultation for possible exploration.[10]

Blunt or penetrating genitourinary trauma may cause a hematocele, which is a painful, tender ecchymotic scrotal mass resulting from accumulation of blood in the tunica vaginalis.

Trauma to the penis is often accompanied by distressing pain. A penile fracture is an acute tear or rupture of the tunica albuginea of the corpus cavernosum. Patients often relate a history of a sudden "snapping" sound during intercourse or other sexual activity or as a result of blunt trauma to an erect penis. Physical examination reveals a swollen, ecchymotic, detumescent penis that is tender to palpation at the site of injury.

A penile contusion results from less severe direct blunt force trauma to the penis. In a penile contusion, the tunica albuginea remains intact and the patient has localized bruising and tenderness at the trauma site. It may result from a toilet seat injury sustained while "potty training" in the toddler age group or be caused by a "straddle" mechanism at any age.

Penetrating penile injuries require specialty consultation in virtually all cases.

## SEXUALLY TRANSMITTED DISEASES

Genital infections that are likely to cause acute symptoms can generally be divided into diseases characterized by genital ulceration (e.g., genital herpes) and diseases causing penile discharge (urethritis).

Among the many infections that can cause genital ulceration, genital herpes, syphilis, and chancroid are the most common in the United States; genital herpes is the most prevalent.[11]

Primary or recurrent genital herpes may be manifested as severe pain, pruritus, or burning localized to the penis, scrotum, rectum, or elsewhere in the perineum. The typical pattern of multiple grouped vesicular or ulcerative lesions may be absent entirely in many acutely infected persons, however, thus rendering the diagnosis elusive.

Syphilis is a systemic disease caused by *Treponema pallidum*. Patients with syphilis may seek treatment for signs or symptoms of primary infection, which is often a painless ulcer (chancre) at the infection site, typically on the head or distal shaft of the penis.

Chancroid is caused by *Haemophilus ducreyi* and is classically manifested by the combination of a painful ulcer and tender inguinal adenopathy.

Diagnosis of any of these ulcerative infections is frequently inaccurate when based on the history and physical examination alone.[11] Therefore, evaluation of all patients with genital ulcers should include a serologic test for syphilis and a diagnostic evaluation for genital herpes. Testing for *H. ducreyi* should be performed in settings where chancroid is prevalent.

Findings on urinalysis suggestive of a urinary tract infection may be present in cases of urethritis or epididymitis. Urethritis is typically characterized by discharge of mucopurulent or purulent material, with or without accompanying dysuria or urethral pruritus. The principal bacterial pathogens of proven clinical importance in men who have urethritis are *Neisseria gonorrhoeae* and *Chlamydia trachomatis*. Asymptomatic infections are common as well.

## SPECIAL SIGNS AND TECHNIQUES

Several adjuncts to the traditional examination are commonly used when assessing the male genitourinary tract.

An intact ipsilateral cremasteric reflex is frequently used, though imperfect, for excluding the diagnosis of testicular torsion.[12-14] This reflex is elicited by stroking the ipsilateral inner aspect of the thigh, which results in a reflexive elevation of the testicle through contraction of the cremaster muscle. Absence of this reflex is nonspecific in that healthy individuals may lack the reflex altogether, particularly boys in the first few years of life.[15] Of note, there have been several published reports of testicular torsion with an intact cremasteric reflex.[16-18]

The Prehn sign, or relief of pain with scrotal elevation, was previously thought to help in differentiating epididymitis from testicular torsion (the latter condition having no improvement in symptoms with elevation). However, this sign has been found to be unreliable in distinguishing these two disorders, and its use for this purpose should be abandoned.

In appendage torsion, the "blue dot sign" is pathognomonic. Appendage torsion is most common in the prepubescent age group, and the infarcted appendage (the blue dot) is seen through thin, non–hormonally stimulated prepubertal skin.

Scrotal transillumination may be performed in cases of suspected hydrocele. The scrotal contents should become transilluminated when filled with light-transmitting fluid, as is the case with a hydrocele. However, transillumination is neither sensitive nor specific for the diagnosis of hydrocele, and the results should be interpreted with caution.

## DIFFERENTIAL DIAGNOSIS AND MEDICAL DECISION MAKING

Most routine diagnostic aids, such as blood work or urinalysis, add little to distinguish the emergency causes of acute scrotal pain. Rather, they may actually worsen the outcome of patients by causing delays in consultation and therapeutic action. If the history and physical examination suggest the diagnosis of testicular torsion, urology (or general surgery) services should be consulted and plans made for immediate surgical exploration without delay. A patient of appropriate age with the classic history and examination findings of testicular torsion does not require any diagnostic tests. In low-risk or unclear circumstances, a confirmatory imaging study is indicated, and ultrasonography is typically used for this purpose.

In cases of Fournier disease, a delay in recognition and surgical débridement can be life-threatening. Early consultation plus administration of broad-spectrum antibiotics is indicated in all suspected cases. However, prompt surgical débridement remains the definitive treatment.[19,20]

### LABORATORY TESTING

Any patient encountered in the emergency department (ED) with penile discharge should be assumed to have infectious urethritis. Centers for Disease Control and Prevention (CDC) guidelines recommend testing to determine the specific cause.[11] Urine polymerase chain reaction testing for *N. gonorrhea* and *Chlamydia* infection is available at most institutions. Urine samples to test for urethritis should be collected at the initiation of the urine stream without cleansing of the glans; midstream collection and glans cleansing are necessary for urine culture in patients with suspected cystitis or pyelonephritis. If polymerase chain reaction testing is unavailable, swabs of the lining of the distal 1 to 2 cm of the penile urethra are necessary for testing.

An elevated systemic white blood cell count may be present in cases of inflammation, as well as infection, but does little to narrow the differential diagnosis—awaiting results could delay definitive management. Patients with advanced infections (e.g., scrotal abscess, epididymoorchitis, Fournier gangrene) may have a markedly elevated white blood cell count or granulocyte predominance, but the test lacks sufficient sensitivity and specificity.

### ULTRASONOGRAPHY

Ultrasound visualization is the most useful diagnostic modality for the evaluation of genitourinary complaints. Color flow duplex Doppler ultrasound is generally helpful in distinguishing potential causes of acute scrotal pain. The classic finding suggestive of testicular torsion is diminished intratesticular blood flow. In addition, examination of the spermatic cord with high-resolution gray-scale sonography may reveal kinking of the spermatic cord.[21] In epididymitis, perfusion is normal or increased because of the effects of inflammatory mediators on local vascular beds.

Ultrasonography may also identify an infarcted appendage, hydroceles, hematoceles, varicoceles, hernias, tumors, abscesses, and gonadal vasculitis, among other conditions. In patients with testicular trauma, ultrasonography may identify disruption of the tunica albuginea, which signals testicular rupture. Doppler blood flow studies can measure the adequacy of blood flow. Absent blood flow means that traumatic torsion or vascular injury has occurred.

Ultrasound evaluation of acute scrotal problems has its limitations. Surgical scrotal exploration remains the only definitive diagnostic modality in assessing for testicular torsion. When is the risk low enough to safely send a patient home following "normal" ultrasound findings? Even though some series have found ultrasound to be unreliable, other larger series have reported a negative predictive value approaching 97%.[22] However, if ultrasound is nondiagnostic of testicular torsion and the clinical picture is still concerning, emergency surgical consultation is prudent.

### COMPUTED TOMOGRAPHY

Computed tomography may be helpful in assessing the extension or depth of a genitourinary abscess or Fournier disease and may aid in the search for coexisting injuries or foreign bodies in the evaluation of a trauma patient.

## TREATMENT

### ANALGESIA

Analgesia should be administered parenterally in most cases because of the significant pain associated with the majority of the aforementioned conditions. Analgesia should not be withheld pending consultation. If the likelihood of surgical intervention is low or if the pain is mild on arrival, a trial of oral medications can be offered. The agents used most frequently are narcotic analgesics, nonsteroidal antiinflammatory drugs, and acetaminophen.

### MANUAL TESTICULAR DETORSION

In the case of prolonged time until definitive treatment, manual testicular repositioning may be attempted. Because testicular torsion usually occurs in a lateral to medial fashion, detorsion is often accomplished by rotation of the affected testicle from medial to lateral. However, medial to lateral torsion occurs up to a third of the time.[23] The end point of the detorsion procedure is relief of pain.

#### *Emergency Surgery for Testicular Torsion*

Testicular salvage rates are time dependent; more than 90% of testicles are salvaged if detorsion occurs within 6 hours after the onset of symptoms, whereas the salvage rate is less than 20% when treatment is delayed by more than 24 hours.[24] Immediate surgical consultation is important when testicular torsion is likely.

### SCROTAL ELEVATION

Elevation of the scrotum may be beneficial in patients with inflammatory conditions such as epididymitis. It is easily accomplished with the use of a towel roll or supportive undergarments, such as a jockstrap. In addition, ice may reduce edema and provide mild symptomatic relief.

**Table 111.2** Medication Dosages for Sexually Transmitted Diseases

| | RECOMMENDED TREATMENT | ALTERNATIVE |
|---|---|---|
| **Ulcerative Disease** | | |
| Genital herpes | | |
| Primary | Acyclovir, 400 mg tid × 7-10 days | Valacyclovir, 1 g bid × 7-10 days |
| Recurrent | Acyclovir, 400 mg tid × 5 days | Valacyclovir, 1 g once daily × 5 days |
| Syphilis | Benzathine penicillin G, 2.4 million units IM × 1 dose | Doxycycline, 100 mg bid × 14 days |
| Chancroid | Azithromycin, 1 g PO × 1 dose | Ceftriaxone, 250 mg IM × 1 dose |
| **Urethritis** | | |
| Gonorrhea | Ceftriaxone, 250 mg IM × 1 dose | Cefixime, 400 mg PO × 1 dose |
| *Chlamydia* | Azithromycin, 1 g PO × 1 dose | Doxycycline, 100 PO bid × 7 days |

Data from Centers for Disease Control and Prevention (CDC). Sexually transmitted disease treatment guidelines, 2010. MMWR Recomm Rep 2010;59(RR-12):18-55.

### ANTIBIOTIC THERAPY

Antimicrobial agents are indicated in cases of suspected or proven infection. Early broad-spectrum antibiotic therapy is imperative in any patient with suspected Fournier disease. Recommended empiric intravenous antimicrobials include ampicillin-sulbactam plus clindamycin and ciprofloxacin or clindamycin plus an aminoglycoside in individuals with known penicillin hypersensitivity.[25] The addition of vancomycin to either regimen for expanded gram-positive coverage is reasonable.

### SEXUALLY TRANSMITTED DISEASES

Because timely follow-up counseling and treatment of patients with abnormal test results are impractical in the ED setting, empiric antimicrobial treatment of the probable pathogens should be initiated (**Table 111.2**), and counseling regarding notification of the patient's sexual contacts should be underscored. Patients should wear a condom during intercourse following treatment for at least 1 week after the symptoms have resolved, although the CDC recommends consistent use of latex condoms to reduce the risk for many sexually transmitted diseases, including human immunodeficiency virus.[26]

Antibiotics are the cornerstone of therapy for epididymitis. Antimicrobial selection is guided by patient demographics: sexually active males younger than 35 years are treated presumptively for *N. gonorrhoeae* and *C. trachomatis* with intramuscular ceftriaxone and oral doxycycline, respectively. Broader coverage should be considered for coliform and fungal species in males who engage in anal insertive intercourse (with presumed gonorrhea and *Chlamydia* coinfection).

Patients older than 35 years are treated with agents that cover the common urinary pathogens. This age distinction, however, is arbitrary and variability exists.

Distinction between urethritis with or without accompanying epididymitis is important in patients with a penile discharge. When accompanying epididymal pain or tenderness is present, the duration of antimicrobial treatment is lengthened because epididymitis represents a more advanced stage of reproductive tract disease. The typical treatment regimen for isolated urethritis is a single dose of ceftriaxone, 250 mg intramuscularly (IM), for gonorrhea, plus a single dose of azithromycin, 1 g orally, for *Chlamydia*; typical treatment of epididymitis is a single dose of ceftriaxone, 250 mg IM, plus doxycycline, 100 mg orally given twice a day for 10 days.

Epididymitis may also occur in prepubescent boys as a result of reflux of sterile urine into the epididymis; it often results from minor congenital genitourinary anomalies that need diagnostic evaluation. Treatment typically includes prophylactic antimicrobials to cover the common urinary pathogens.[27]

## PRIAPISM

A urologist usually manages the treatment of priapism; however, in certain circumstances the emergency physician may have to initiate treatment of low-flow priapism. The classic teaching is that the initial treatment—oral (or subcutaneous) terbutaline—is the same regardless of the inciting etiology, although its utility is debated.[28-30] It is thought that terbutaline, a $\beta_2$-adrenergic agonist, increases venous outflow from the engorged corpora by way of relaxation of venous sinusoidal smooth muscle. Terbutaline is of unproved benefit; however, given its limited propensity for adverse effects, a trial is reasonable in selected circumstances while awaiting urology consultation.[31]

If terbutaline fails to work rapidly, the next step in the treatment of priapism is corporal blood aspiration with or without irrigation and injection of an $\alpha$-adrenergic receptor agonist such as dilute phenylephrine. Phenylephrine should be diluted in normal saline to a concentration of 0.1 to 0.5 mg/mL and 1-mL injections made intermittently for upward of 1 hour. Lower concentrations in smaller volumes should be used in children and patients with severe cardiovascular disease.[30]

The goal of treatment for patients with sickle cell disease and priapism is reduction of red blood cell sickling, thereby reducing vascular sludging and vasoocclusion. Treatments in this setting include oxygen, intravenous hydration, and simple or exchange transfusions.

Regardless of the precipitating cause of priapism, surgical shunt procedures are used as a last resort in patients with low-flow priapism unresponsive to the aforementioned treatments.

## PARAPHIMOSIS

Paraphimosis can frequently be managed in the ED without the need for emergency specialty consultation. Many methods for successful reduction of paraphimosis have been reported; however, the most commonly used initial maneuver involves manual compression of the distal glans penis to decrease edema, followed by reduction of the glans penis back through the proximal constricting band of foreskin.[32]

## TESTICULAR TRAUMA

Patients with penetrating injury to the scrotum generally undergo exploration in the operating room. Patients with blunt testicular trauma and ultrasonographic evidence of significant testicular injury also generally undergo surgical exploration for débridement of devitalized tissue, treatment of an acute hematocele larger than 5 cm, or repair of the tunica albuginea.[33] Documented testicular injury requires early repair to minimize the potential for infection, infarction, necrosis, abscess, infertility, atrophy, and testicular loss.

### PRIORITY ACTIONS

**Testicular Torsion**

Emergency urology consultation in all moderate- to high-probability cases

Consider ultrasound imaging only if the diagnosis is equivocal based on the history and findings on physical examination

**Fournier Disease**

Emergency surgical consultation for débridement

Broad-spectrum antibiotics (covering gram-positive, gram-negative, and anaerobic species)

Intravenous fluids and supportive measures as dictated by the clinical picture

**Priapism**

Urology consultation

Consider treatment with terbutaline

Corporal aspiration, saline irrigation, or injection of an $\alpha$-adrenergic receptor agonist may be necessary at the bedside

**Paraphimosis**

Attempt reduction in the emergency department; urology consultation if unsuccessful

**Genitourinary Trauma**

Maintain a very low threshold for urology consultation and ultrasound imaging

Search meticulously for other coexisting injuries

## SUGGESTED READINGS

Beni-Israel T, Goldman M, Bar Chaim S. Clinical predictors of testicular torsion as seen in the pediatric ED. Am J Emerg Med 2010;28:786-9.

Centers for Disease Control and Prevention (CDC). Sexually transmitted disease treatment guidelines, 2010. MMWR Recomm Rep 2010;59(RR-12):67-9.

Choe JM. Paraphimosis: current treatment options. Am Fam Physician 2000;62:2623-6.

Erectile Dysfunction Guideline Update Panel. The management of priapism. Baltimore: American Urological Association; 2003 [Reaffirmed September 28, 2009]. Available at http://guidelines.gov/content.aspx?id=3741. Accessed January 29, 2012.

Roberts JR, Price C, Mazzeo T. Intracavernous epinephrine: a minimally invasive treatment for priapism in the emergency department. J Emerg Med. 2009;36:3:285-9.

Van Der Horst C, Martinez Portillo FJ, Seif C, et al. Male genital injury: diagnostics and treatment. BJU Int 2004;93:927-30.

## REFERENCES

*References can be found on Expert Consult @ www.expertconsult.com.*

# 112 Nephrolithiasis

Carl R. Menckhoff

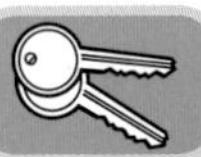

**KEY POINTS**

- Ureteral calculi smaller than 5 mm in diameter spontaneously pass through the urinary tract in 90% of cases, whereas stones larger than 8 mm in diameter cause impaction in 95% of instances.
- Impaction most commonly occurs at the ureterovesical junction, the ureteropelvic junction, or the pelvic brim.
- Abdominal aortic aneurysms are commonly misdiagnosed as renal colic.
- Hematuria is absent in 15% of patients with symptomatic nephrolithiasis.

## SCOPE AND OUTLINE

Renal colic is defined as severe, spasmodic pain caused by the impaction or passage of a calculus in the renal pelvis or ureter. Symptomatic nephrolithiasis will develop in approximately 15% of the U.S. population during their lives[1]; the majority of these patients seek treatment in the emergency department (ED).

## EPIDEMIOLOGY

Most cases of renal colic occur in men between 20 and 50 years of age. The incidence of first-time ureteral stones in men is 0.3% per year, with recurrence rates of 37% and 50% at 1 and 5 years, respectively.[2,3] The most significant risk factors for renal stone disease are listed in **Box 112.1**.

## PATHOPHYSIOLOGY

Renal stones form when the urine becomes supersaturated with calcium, oxalate, cystine, uric acid, or struvite. Hypercalciuria accounts for the development of 60% of calculi and results from increased intestinal absorption, decreased renal tubular reabsorption, or excessive bone resorption of calcium. Decreased urine output can further promote calculus formation as a result of reductions in citrate, magnesium pyrophosphate, and other inhibitors of urine crystallization. **Table 112.1** describes features of the five main types of renal calculi.

**BOX 112.1 Risk Factors for Renal Calculus Formation**

Family history of nephrolithiasis
Age (third to sixth decade of life)
Male gender
Living in a hot, dry climate
Low water intake
Primary hyperparathyroidism
Type 1 renal tubular acidosis
Crohn disease
Laxative abuse
Sarcoidosis
Recurrent urinary tract infections
Milk-alkali syndrome
Sedentary lifestyle
Diet high in animal protein

Stone impaction may occur anywhere along the path of the genitourinary tract. The resultant ureteral obstruction can shift hydrostatic pressure and cause blood flow to be redistributed to the opposite renal artery. The overall rate of glomerular filtration decreases as renal excretion becomes a task of the unaffected kidney. A transient increase in serum creatinine may follow this decrease in the glomerular filtration rate.

Although an initial rise in creatinine may quickly resolve, irreversible kidney damage can begin to occur after 7 days of complete obstruction.[3,4] Prolonged obstruction impairs recoverable kidney function over time,[4,5] but case reports show that some recovery may be possible for up to 150 days.[5,6]

Ureteral obstruction is primarily determined by calculus size. Most stones smaller than 5 mm in diameter will pass spontaneously (90%), whereas passage of stones larger than 8 mm is unlikely (5%). **Table 112.2** compares ureteral stone size with the percent likelihood of spontaneous passage.

## ANATOMY

Stone impaction most commonly occurs at the ureterovesical junction, the narrowest part of the genitourinary tract. Other common areas of impaction include the ureteropelvic junction (where the renal pelvis narrows from 1 cm down to 3 mm)

**Table 112.1 The Five Main Types of Renal Calculi**

| MINERAL TYPE | FREQUENCY (%) | CAUSES | PEARLS |
|---|---|---|---|
| Calcium oxalate | 70 | Hypercalciuria<br>High calcium intake (cheese, milk, antacids)<br>Jejunal hyperabsorption<br>Hyperparathyroidism<br>Hyperoxaluria<br>Dietary (tea, coffee, sodas, plums, rhubarb, cranberries, citrus fruit, green leafy vegetables)<br>Inflammatory bowel disease | Most common |
| Calcium phosphate | 10 | Type 1 renal tubular acidosis | Most dense |
| Struvite (magnesium-ammonium-phosphate) | 10 | Urinary tract infections with urea-splitting bacteria such as *Klebsiella, Serratia, Enterobacter, Pseudomonas, Proteus, Staphylococcus* | Alkaline urine (pH > 7.6), staghorn calculi |
| Uric acid | 10 | Hyperuricosuria (dietary: meat, fish, poultry) | Radiolucent<br>Least dense |
| Cystine | 1 | Inborn error of metabolism causing increased cystine secretion | Rare, radiolucent, staghorn calculi |

**Table 112.2 Renal Calculus Size and Likelihood of Spontaneous Passage**

| STONE SIZE (DIAMETER) | PERCENT LIKELIHOOD OF SPONTANEOUS PASSAGE |
|---|---|
| <5 mm | 90 |
| 5-8 mm | 15 |
| >8 mm | 5 |

and the pelvic brim (where the ureter arches anteriorly across the iliac vessels) (**Fig. 112.1**).

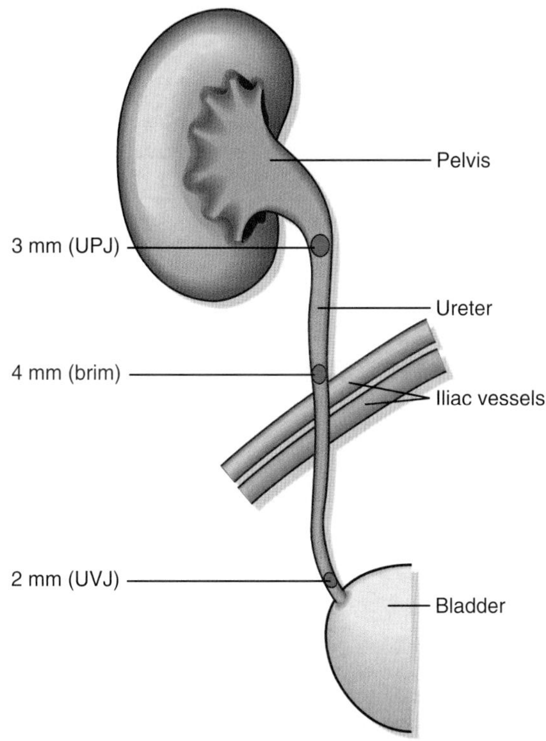


**Fig. 112.1 Common sites of renal calculus impaction.**

## CLINICAL PRESENTATION

### HISTORY

Renal colic is classically manifested as a sudden onset of excruciating, intermittent flank pain that radiates to the groin. This swift onset of pain is often accompanied by a deeper flank ache, nausea, and vomiting. The severe, spasmodic pain of renal colic is thought to be caused by hyperperistalsis of smooth muscle from the calices to the ureter. The dull, deep, aching pain reflects ureteral obstruction and distention of the renal capsule.

The location of the ureteral calculus determines the symptoms, as outlined in **Table 112.3**.

### PHYSICAL EXAMINATION

Patients with renal colic typically appear uncomfortable and are commonly described as "writhing" on the gurney. Findings on the abdominal examination are generally unremarkable, although thin patients with distal ureteral stones and obstruction may exhibit some tenderness. Tenderness at the costovertebral angle can develop as a result of worsening hydronephrosis; this sign is mild or absent early in the course of the disease. Abnormal findings on physical examination should raise suspicion for alternative diagnoses, as reviewed in **Table 112.4**.

## DIFFERENTIAL DIAGNOSIS

Many disease processes can mimic symptomatic nephrolithiasis. Abdominal aortic aneurysm, aortic dissection, renal artery

**Table 112.3 Ureteral Calculus Location and Associated Symptoms**

| LOCATION OF CALCULUS | SYMPTOMS |
|---|---|
| Renal pelvis or calyx | Deep flank ache |
| Proximal or middle part of the ureter | Severe flank pain radiating to the groin |
| Distal end of the ureter | Flank discomfort and/or low abdominal pain |
| Bladder | Dysuria, frequency, urgency, retention, suprapubic discomfort |

**Table 112.4 Physical Examination Findings and Potential Alternative Diagnoses**

| FINDING | CONSIDERATION |
|---|---|
| **Vital Signs** | |
| Fever | Infected stone, pyelonephritis, perinephric abscess |
| Hypotension | Sepsis, abdominal aortic aneurysm |
| **Abdomen** | |
| Bruit | Abdominal aortic aneurysm, renal artery stenosis |
| Pulsatile mass | Abdominal aortic aneurysm |
| Pronounced costovertebral angle tenderness | Pyelonephritis |
| Lower abdominal or pelvic tenderness | Ectopic pregnancy, appendicitis, pelvic inflammatory disease, tuboovarian abscess, ovarian torsion |
| **Genitourinary** | |
| Testicular tenderness | Torsion, epididymitis, orchitis |
| Mass | Hernia, cancer |
| **Pulmonary** | |
| Focal findings | Lobar pneumonia |
| **Cardiovascular** | |
| Asymmetric lower extremity pulses | Abdominal aortic aneurysm |
| **Skin** | |
| Vesicular rash | Herpes zoster |

dissection, and renal infarction are the most lethal conditions that may manifest similar to renal colic. In one study, abdominal aortic aneurysms were initially misdiagnosed as kidney stones in approximately 20% of patients older than 60 years.[7] **Box 112.2** lists the differential diagnosis for renal colic.

**BOX 112.2 Differential Diagnoses of Renal Colic**

**Vascular**
Abdominal aortic aneurysm
Aortic dissection
Renal artery dissection
Renal artery stenosis
Renal vein thrombosis
Renal infarct
Mesenteric ischemia
Retroperitoneal hemorrhage

**Gastrointestinal**
Incarcerated hernia
Appendicitis
Cholecystitis
Biliary colic
Pancreatitis
Bowel obstruction
Diverticulitis

**Gynecologic**
Ectopic pregnancy
Ovarian torsion
Tuboovarian abscess
Pelvic inflammatory disease
Endometriosis

**Genitourinary**
Testicular torsion
Pyelonephritis
Perinephric abscess
Urinary tract tumor
Renal papillary necrosis
Upper urinary tract hemorrhage

**Musculoskeletal**
Lumbar strain
Radiculopathy
Disk herniation
Vertebral compression fracture

**Dermatologic**
Herpes zoster

**Miscellaneous**
Factitious

## DIAGNOSTIC TESTING

### LABORATORY TESTS

#### *Urinalysis*

A bedside urine dipstick test or urinalysis should be performed in all patients with suspected renal colic to evaluate for hematuria and infection. Urine culture should be ordered if leukocytes, nitrites, or bacteria are identified.

Hematuria is a common but inconsistent finding in patients with ureteral stones. The amount of gross or microscopic hematuria does not correlate with stone impaction or the degree of obstruction; rather, hematuria results from direct ureteral trauma caused by the passing stone.[8] Hematuria is absent in 15% of patients with ureteral stones.[9,10]

Alkaline urine (pH > 7.6) may indicate infection with a urea-splitting organism, a common finding in patients with struvite stones. Urine pH lower than 5.0 suggests the presence of a uric acid stone.

Uric acid or oxalate crystals may be detectable in urine in a variety of conditions; this finding does not imply the presence of nephrolithiasis, however, and should be interpreted with caution.

#### *Urine Pregnancy Test*

Urine human chorionic gonadotropin levels should be checked in female patients of childbearing age. Although pregnant patients may have renal colic, a newly positive result should raise suspicion for ectopic pregnancy in the differential diagnosis.

#### *Blood Tests*

Blood urea nitrogen and creatinine can be measured if the symptoms have been prolonged or renal impairment is a concern, but these tests are not routinely indicated.

**Table 112.5 Imaging Modalities for Detection of Nephrolithiasis**

| TEST | SENSITIVITY (%) | SPECIFICITY (%) | PROS AND CONS |
|---|---|---|---|
| Computed tomography | 94-100 | 96-100 | Pros: no contrast agent used, rapid, identifies alternative diagnoses |
| | | | Cons: radiation exposure, cost |
| Intravenous pyelography | 52-85 | 97-100 | Pro: functional study |
| | | | Cons: need for contrast agent, radiation exposure, duration of imaging |
| Ultrasonography | 66-93 | 83-100 | Pros: no contrast agent used, no radiation |
| | | | Con: false-negative results in patients with small, nonobstructing stones |
| Kidney-ureter-bladder radiography | 58-62 | 67-69 | Pros: quick, readily available |
| | | | Cons: lower sensitivity and specificity |

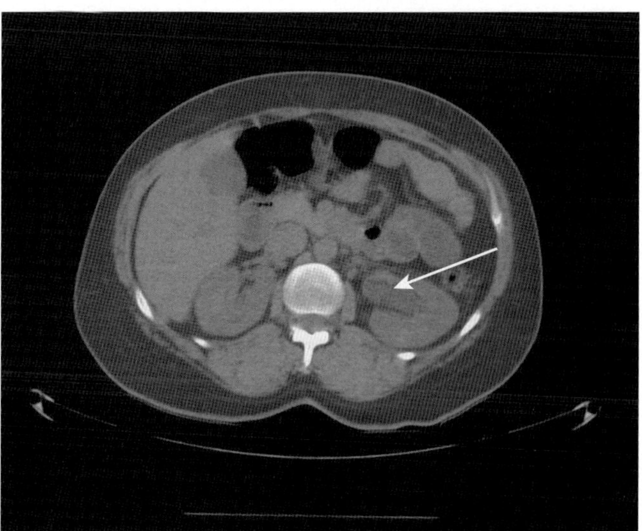

**Fig. 112.2 Noncontrast renal protocol computed tomography scan showing moderate hydronephrosis of the left renal pelvis *(arrow)*.**

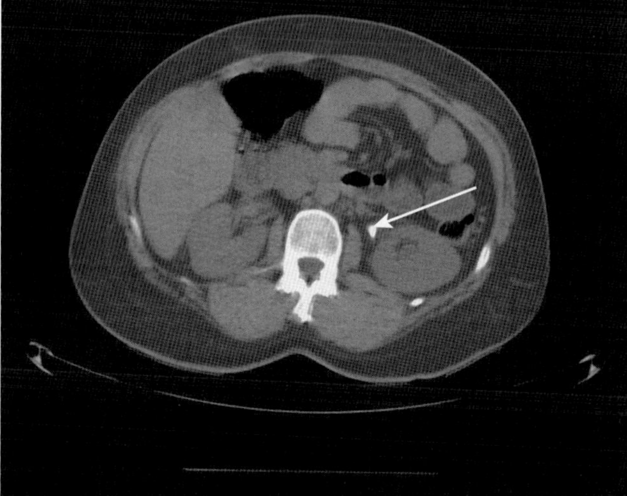

**Fig. 112.3 Noncontrast renal protocol computed tomography scan showing a stone at the left ureteropelvic junction *(arrow)*.**

If a complete blood count is obtained, increased leukocytosis should be interpreted with caution because it can indicate either pain-induced demargination or infection.

A baseline hemoglobin level should be considered in the evaluation of patients with persistent gross hematuria or hemodynamic compromise.

## IMAGING

ED imaging (**Table 112.5**) is used to confirm the diagnosis of nephrolithiasis, evaluate stone size, identify obstruction, and exclude alternative diagnoses. Patients with decreased renal reserve (solitary kidney, uncontrolled diabetes mellitus, uncontrolled hypertension), concurrent infection, first occurrence of stone disease, advanced age, and prolonged or unrelenting symptoms should undergo imaging during their initial evaluation. Indications for emergency imaging in cases of suspected renal colic are summarized in **Table 112.6**.

### *Helical Computed Tomography*

Noncontrast helical computed tomography (CT) of the abdomen and pelvis is the preferred imaging modality for the evaluation of patients with suspected nephrolithiasis. CT imaging for renal stones can be performed without contrast material, demonstrates both high sensitivity (94% to 100%) and specificity (96% to 100%),[11-15] and allows alternative diagnoses to be simultaneously identified.[15,16] Sagittal images are obtained at 5-mm intervals from the top of the kidney to the bottom of the bladder (**Figs. 112.2 and 112.3**).

### *Intravenous Pyelography*

Intravenous pyelography (**Fig. 112.4**) has a sensitivity of 52% to 85% and specificity of 97% to 100% for detection of ureteral calculi.[11,17,18] It provides a visual interpretation of renal function, as well as genitourinary anatomy. The earliest sign of ureteral obstruction on an intravenous pyelogram

**Table 11[illegible] Indications for Diagnostic Imaging of Patients with Suspected Renal Colic**

| FINDING | INDICATION FOR DIAGNOSTIC IMAGING |
|---|---|
| Solitary kidney, uncontrolled diabetes,* uncontrolled hypertension* | To exclude obstruction in a patient with decreased renal reserve |
| Advanced age | To exclude alternative diagnoses, especially vascular disease |
| Concurrent infection | If concurrent with obstruction, a urologist should be involved to evaluate the need for intervention |
| Prolonged symptoms | To evaluate for prolonged obstruction, which may cause renal impairment |
| Refractory symptoms, first occurrence* | To exclude alternative diagnoses, especially ischemia or infarction |

*Relative indication.

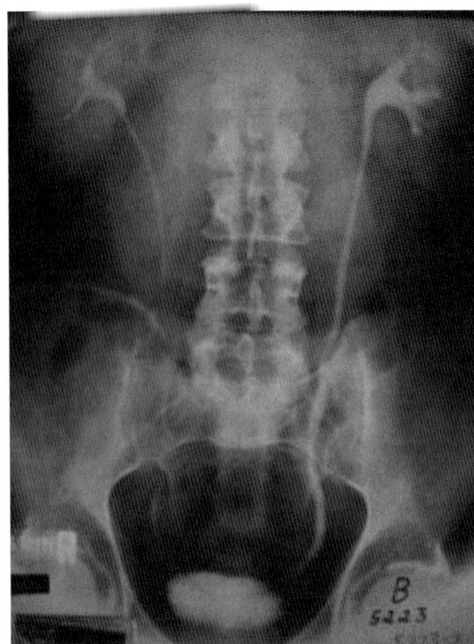

**Fig. 112.5 Intravenous pyelogram showing the entire left ureter in one view.** This is known as a standing column and is caused by lack of ureteral peristalsis because of a ureteral stone.

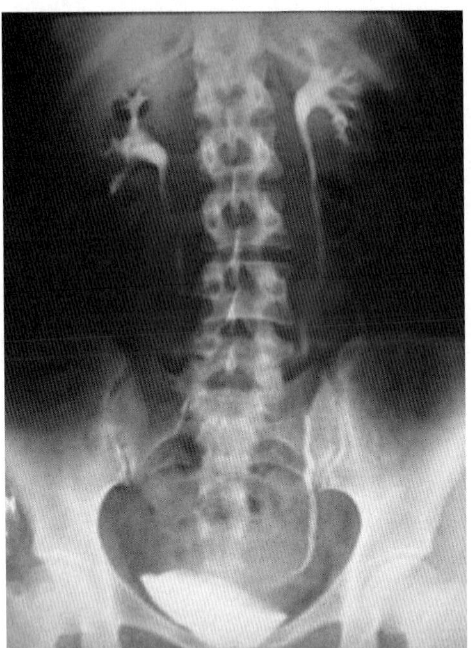

**Fig. 112.4 Normal findings on an intravenous pyelogram.**

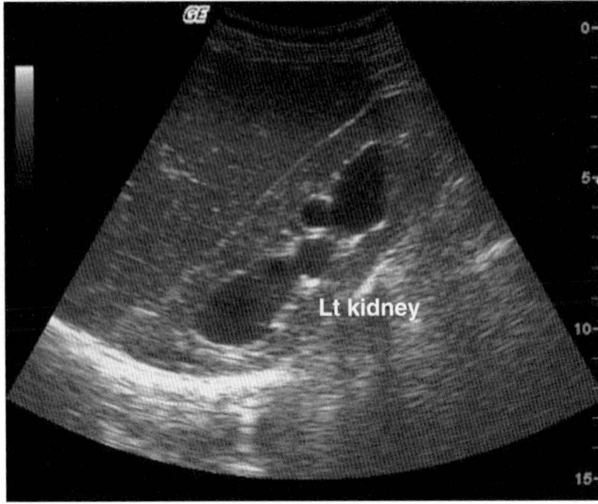


**Fig. 112.6 Renal ultrasound showing moderate hydronephrosis.**

is a delayed nephrogram; other abnormal findings include a "standing column" (the entire ureter seen on one image; **Fig. 112.5**), hydroureter, hydronephrosis, contrast cutoff at the point of impaction, and extravasation of contrast material. The use of intravenous pyelography is limited by the need for contrast material, decreased sensitivity in comparison with helical CT, and the length of time required to obtain multiple delayed images.

### *Sonography*

Ultrasonography is a useful modality for identifying hydronephrosis caused by ureteral obstruction (**Fig. 112.6**). Advantages include its ease of use and rapid acquisition of diagnostic images at the bedside without the need for contrast agents or radiation. It is the imaging technique of choice for the evaluation of suspected renal colic in pregnancy. Ultrasonography is limited by false-negative results, which occur in patients with small calculi that do not cause significant obstruction or hydronephrosis. The sensitivity and specificity of ultrasonography for the diagnosis of urologic stone disease is 66% to 93% and 83% to 100%, respectively.[18-20]

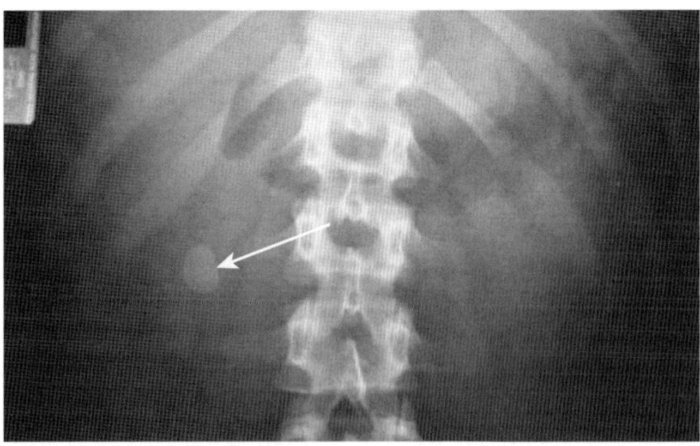

**Fig. 112.7 Kidney-ureter-bladder radiograph showing a large kidney stone on the right *(arrow)*.**

### *Plain Radiography*

The utility of plain radiography (kidney-ureter-bladder [KUB] projection performed in the supine position) is dependent on the radiodensity of the suspected kidney stone. Although 90% of stones are radiopaque (**Fig. 112.7**), uric acid and cystine calculi are radiolucent. KUB imaging is limited technically by overlying soft tissue, air, and bone; low sensitivity (58% to 62%) and specificity (67% to 69%) are observed in clinical practice.[21,22] The combination of ultrasonography and KUB radiography improves the usefulness of these imaging modalities. Studies that used both ultrasound and plain radiography for the detection of nephrolithiasis demonstrated a sensitivity and specificity of 89% and 100%, respectively, when both tests were positive[20] and a sensitivity and specificity of 95% and 67%, respectively, when either test was positive.[23]

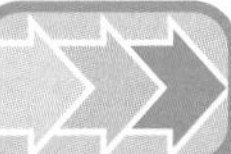

**PRIORITY ACTIONS**

Institute symptom management (nonsteroidal antiinflammatory drugs, opiates, antiemetics).

Evaluate the need for imaging:

- Advanced age
- Signs of infection—treat with antibiotics if present
- Symptoms for longer than 7 days
- Symptoms refractory to treatment
- Known renal impairment

Determine the need for urgent urology consultation and intervention.

## TREATMENT

### PHARMACOLOGIC MANAGEMENT

Patients with renal colic will probably require immediate pain control. Several options are available for rapid analgesia.

### *Nonsteroidal Antiinflammatory Drugs*

Nonsteroidal antiinflammatory drugs (NSAIDs) decrease ureteral spasm by inhibiting prostaglandin synthesis. Renal blood flow may be reduced when NSAIDs are administered in the setting of ureteral obstruction,[24] thereby improving symptoms through a decrease in urine production and ureteric pressure. Ketorolac (Toradol) (30 mg intravenously or 60 mg intramuscularly) has efficacy equivalent to the oral administration of 800 mg of ibuprofen, although the latter may be less well tolerated in patients with concomitant nausea.

Some urologists debate the routine use of NSAIDs for the treatment of nephrolithiasis because these medications may promote bleeding after the placement of a ureteral stent. Data to support such observations are inconclusive.

### *Opiates*

Intravenous narcotics provide adequate relief of symptoms for most patients with renal colic. Opiates have similar analgesic effects at equivalent dosing. Although meperidine (Demerol) demonstrates smooth muscle relaxation when tested in vitro,[25] this spasmolytic effect does not appear to improve its clinical utility in therapy for renal colic.[26] Given the potential for drug interactions with meperidine, preferred opiates for ED use include hydromorphone (0.015 mg/kg) and morphine (0.1 mg/kg starting dose).

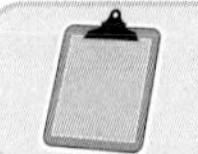

**DOCUMENTATION**

Patient's age
Onset, location, and duration of pain
Urinalysis results
Medical decision making for imaging
Medical decision making for disposition
Discharge instructions and return precautions
Follow-up within 7 days

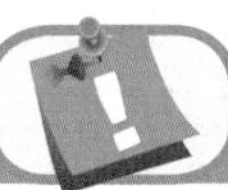

**TIPS AND TRICKS**

A young, healthy patient with the typical findings of renal colic, a history of previous nephrolithiasis, no signs of infection, and easily managed symptoms may be discharged with analgesics, antiemetics, and a urine strainer for follow-up within 7 days.

All other patients require evaluation of the need for imaging and possible urology consultation.

Multiple studies have shown that both NSAIDs and opiates are effective and appropriate treatments of renal colic.[24-31] One metaanalysis of 19 studies showed that NSAIDs and opiates are equally effective in the acute management of renal colic symptoms.[28] Many experts recommend the use of NSAIDs followed by opiates for continued pain.

### MANAGEMENT OF OTHER SYMPTOMS

Tamsulosin (Flomax), an α-adrenergic blocker, reduces ureteral spasm. Early studies suggested that oral tamsulosin (0.4 mg/day) helps promote ureteral passage of juxtavesical stones.[32] There continue to be more studies supporting such treatment,[33-35] as well as studies now indicating that tamsulosin may be useful for more proximal stones as well.[36] Calcium channel blockers have been studied for their smooth muscle relaxant effects, and some studies suggest that they also promote stone expulsion.[34,37,38]

Antiemetics should be administered to patients experiencing concomitant nausea or vomiting. Intravenous crystalloid administration was once thought to promote stone migration by stimulating ureteral peristalsis; however, no supporting evidence has shown that hydration consistently improves symptoms by this mechanism.[39]

**RED FLAGS**

Patients older than 60 years: Consider a vascular cause of their pain.
Signs of infection: Exclude concurrent obstruction.
Large calculi: 5-mm stones have a 50% chance of passing; stones larger than 8 mm have a 5% chance of passing.

## DISPOSITION

Patients with uncomplicated renal colic whose symptoms are easily controlled should be discharged with analgesics, a urine strainer, antiemetics, and follow-up within 7 days. Stones captured by urine straining should be brought to the urologist for pathologic evaluation. Return precautions include uncontrolled pain, protracted vomiting, and fever (**Fig. 112.8**).

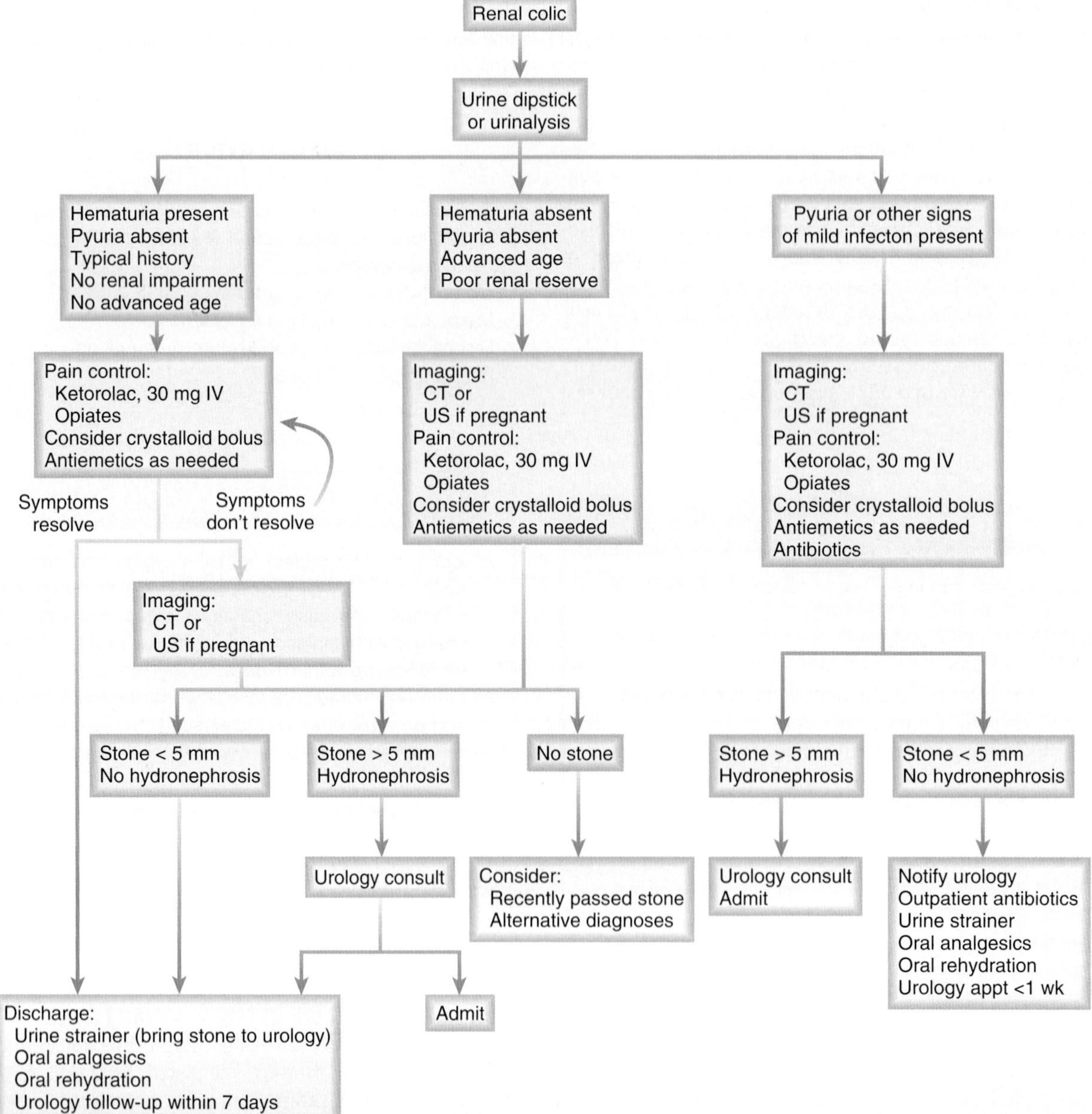


**Fig. 112.8 Guideline algorithm for the evaluation, treatment, and disposition of patients with presumed renal colic.** *CT*, Computed tomography; *IV*, intravenously; *US*, ultrasonography.

A urologist should be consulted if patients have uncontrollable pain or evidence of infection. The presence of white blood cells in urine may indicate an infection and, in the presence of obstruction, warrants urology consultation for urgent stone removal or stenting.

**BOX 112.3 Indications for Admission or Consultation with a Urologist**

**Indications for Admission**

Obstruction with significant infection

Solitary kidney with obstruction or a stone unlikely to pass spontaneously

Refractory pain

Refractory emesis

**Indications for Consultation with a Urologist**

Infection

Stone unlikely to pass spontaneously

Moderate to severe hydronephrosis

Solitary kidney

Intrinsic renal disease

Some patients will have a few white blood cells in their urine (e.g., <10) but no clinical signs of infection. These patients will be otherwise asymptomatic following medication for pain (i.e., afebrile). In the absence of concomitant obstruction, urgent stone removal in such cases is not routine. Patients with coexisting, complicating diseases may be treated with antibiotics and observed in the hospital. Patients without underlying disease may be treated with antibiotics as an outpatient and monitored carefully. A urine culture should be performed for patients with white blood cells in their urine.

**Box 112.3** summarizes common indications for admission or urology consultation.

## REFERENCES

***References can be found on Expert Consult @ www.expertconsult.com.***

# 113 Hematuria

M. Kit Delgado and Eva M. Delgado

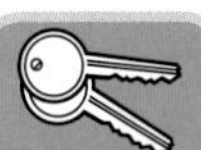

**KEY POINTS**

- Hematuria can be a transient and incidental finding, or it can be caused by underlying and otherwise silent life-threatening disease.
- Infection is the most common cause of symptomatic hematuria in all age groups. Crystalluria and glomerulonephritis are more common in children; malignancy and nephrolithiasis are more common in adults.
- Patients with microscopic hematuria should have urinalysis repeated with their primary care provider about 1 week after discharge from the emergency department.
- All patients with gross hematuria warrant careful evaluation to ensure adequate urinary drainage. Those with difficulty passing clots, evidence of retention, or poor mobility should have a three-way Foley catheter placed in the emergency department.
- Although hematuria alone is rarely grounds for admission, emergency associated disease processes should be considered and excluded. Such processes include urosepsis, obstructing ureteral stone, renal parenchymal disease, coagulopathy, symptomatic anemia, intraabdominal injury in the setting of trauma, renal vein thrombosis, and aortic abdominal aneurysm.

## SCOPE AND DEFINITIONS

Hematuria is the abnormal excretion of red blood cells (RBCs) in urine. Regardless of whether it is a chief complaint or an unexpected discovery, the emergency provider must be able to distinguish between serious and nonserious causes of hematuria. Evaluation begins with classification into four broad categories: (1) gross (macroscopic); (2) microscopic, symptomatic; (3) microscopic, asymptomatic; and (4) pigmenturia (pseudohematuria).

Gross (macroscopic) hematuria, visualized as red-colored urine, is disconcerting to most patients, but it does not always imply significant blood loss: as little as 1 mL of blood may turn 1 L of urine red. Dysuria is common in patients with gross hematuria, and urinary retention may develop if high-volume bleeding leads to clots that obstruct urethral outflow.[1]

Microscopic hematuria refers to the detection of more than three RBCs per high-power field (HPF) in a spun sample of urine sediment not visible to the naked eye.[1,2] Screening of asymptomatic individuals suggests that up to 10% of adults and 6% of children may have some degree of microscopic hematuria at any given time.[2-4] Typically an incidental and transient discovery, it can be associated with dysuria or pain. Because microscopic hematuria may be the only clue to previously undiagnosed structural, neoplastic, or inflammatory conditions, follow-up is essential.[2-5]

Pigmenturia (pseudohematuria) refers to urine that appears red or dark without RBCs detected by urine microscopy. A urine dipstick may register a positive test result for blood if hemoglobin, myoglobin, or bilirubin is present in the urine, as in the case of hemolysis, rhabdomyolysis, or jaundice. Pigmented urine with a negative dipstick test result may be caused by certain foods or medications (**Table 113.1**).

## PATHOPHYSIOLOGY

Hematuria results from the admixture of blood and urine as a result of infection, inflammation, or injury at any point along the genitourinary tract. Causes of hematuria can be divided into glomerular and nonglomerular (see Table 113.1). Glomerular causes, such as glomerulonephritis, are more common in children than in adults and are frequently associated with systemic medical illness. Nonglomerular causes of hematuria can be further classified as renal (e.g., papillary necrosis), extrarenal (e.g., bladder cancer), traumatic (e.g., renal contusion), coagulopathy related (e.g., patient taking warfarin), and factitious (e.g., Munchausen syndrome).

Minor trauma caused by high-impact exercise, such as long-distance running, can produce transient microscopic hematuria.[5,6] Persistent or high-volume bleeding is generally pathologic and mandates further evaluation.

## CLINICAL PRESENTATION

The signs and symptoms in patients with hematuria vary greatly, depending on the underlying cause and degree of hematuria. Incidental discovery of microscopic hematuria is generally noted when providers have urinalysis performed for another reason (e.g., suspected urinary tract infection). Increasing concentrations of blood in urine and persistent

**Table 113.1 Differential Diagnosis of Hematuria**

| DIAGNOSTIC CLUES | POSSIBLE DIAGNOSIS (NONGLOMULAR CAUSES) | POSSIBLE DIAGNOSIS (GLOMULAR CAUSES) |
|---|---|---|
| **Hematuria in the Adult and Pediatric Patient** | | |
| Trauma (blunt or penetrating) | Renal or bladder injury, at risk for other intraabdominal injuries | |
| Suprapubic pain or lower tract symptoms (dysuria, urgency, frequency, suprapubic pain) | UTI | |
| Flank pain | Stones, pyelonephritis, renal vein thrombosis, renal cyst, renal arteriovenous malformation | IgA nephropathy, glomerulonephritis |
| Hypercoagulable state and acute-onset flank pain | Renal vein thrombosis | |
| Elevated blood pressure | | Glomerulonephritis |
| Risk factors for muscle injury; viremia, exertion, crush injury, sympathomimetic drug use | Rhabdomyolysis | |
| Cough, hemoptysis | | Vasculitis |
| Sickle cell disease | Papillary necrosis | Glomerulonephritis |
| Cancer treatment | Radiation- or cyclophosphamide-associated cystitis | |
| Travel history | Schistosomiasis, tuberculosis | |
| Coagulopathy (hemophilia, idiopathic thrombocytopenic purpura) or anticoagulation | Bleeding diathesis | |
| Pregnancy | | Preeclampsia |
| Diet: beets, berries, rhubarb<br>Medications: quinine sulfate, phenazopyridine, rifampin, phenytoin | Pseudohematuria (pigmenturia) | |
| Nail or patellar abnormalities | | Nail-patella syndrome |
| **Hematuria in the Pediatric Patient** | | |
| Recent illness (pharyngitis, impetigo, viral illness) | | Postinfectious glomerulonephritis |
| Abdominal pain | UTI, hypercalciuria, stone | HSP |
| Concurrent illness | | IgA nephropathy |
| Arthralgias | | HSP, SLE |
| Diarrhea (± bloody) | | HUS |
| Hearing loss | | Alport syndrome |
| Family history of hematuria or kidney disease | Polycystic kidney disease, hypercalciuria | Benign familial hematuria, thin basement disease, Alport syndrome |
| Rash (purpura, petechiae) | Bleeding dyscrasia, abuse | HSP, SLE, HUS |
| Edema | | Glomerulonephritis, nephrotic syndrome |
| Abdominal mass | Wilms tumor, hydronephrosis, polycystic kidney disease | |
| Conjunctivitis, pharyngitis | Adenovirus (hemorrhagic cystitis) | |
| Meatal erythema or stenosis | Masturbation, infection, trauma | |

Continued

**Table 113.1 Differential Diagnosis of Hematuria—cont'd**

| DIAGNOSTIC CLUES | POSSIBLE DIAGNOSIS (NONGLOMULAR CAUSES) | POSSIBLE DIAGNOSIS (GLOMULAR CAUSES) |
|---|---|---|
| **Hematuria in the Adult Patient** | | |
| Age > 40, smoking history, analgesic abuse, *Schistosoma* exposure, pelvic irradiation, exposure to chemicals | Urogenital tract cancer | |
| Flank pain | Angiomyolipoma, AAA | |
| Pulsatile abdominal mass | AAA | |
| Atrial fibrillation | Anticoagulation (warfarin), renal emboli | |
| New heart murmur, fever | Renal emboli from endocarditis | |
| Dribbling with urination, urinary retention | Benign prostatic hypertrophy | |
| Dysuria, discharge | Urethritis, sexually transmitted disease | |
| Dysuria, frequency, perineal pain | Prostatitis | |
| Scrotal pain | Epididymitis | |
| Cyclic hematuria during menstrual pain | Endometriosis | |
| NSAID use, diabetes, sickle cell disease | Papillary necrosis | |

*AAA*, Abdominal aortic aneurysm; *HSP*, Henoch-Schönlein purpura; *HUS*, hemolytic-uremic syndrome; *NSAID*, nonsteroidal antiinflammatory drug; *SLE*, systemic lupus erythematosus; *UTI*, urinary tract infection.

bleeding will result in dysuria, clot formation, and eventually bladder outlet obstruction. If left untreated, urinary retention, suprapubic pain, flank pain, and renal failure may ensue.

## DIFFERENTIAL DIAGNOSIS

Hematuria may be a sign of a large number of diseases (see Table 113.1).[1-9] Infection at any location in the genitourinary tract can cause hematuria and is the most common cause of hematuria in both adults and children.

Nephrolithiasis is the second most common cause of hematuria in adults (see Chapter 112). Microscopic hematuria is a common finding in patients with suspected ureteral colic and is caused by abrasion of mucosal tissue by the stone; however, hematuria may be absent in patients with complete ureteral obstruction.[6] Thus, exclusion of the diagnosis of a ureteral stone should not be based solely on negative findings on urinalysis. Although nephrolithiasis is not as common in children, it must remain part of the differential diagnosis. Hypercalciuria is often associated with recurrent asymptomatic microscopic hematuria, and affected children may face higher risk than their peers for the development of nephrolithiasis.[2,7]

Glomerulonephritis, responsible for 10% of cases of gross pediatric hematuria, is usually accompanied by systemic symptoms such as hypertension.[8] Systemic lupus erythematosus and other chronic inflammatory disorders can also cause hematuria by similar mechanisms.[2,5,6,8]

The family history may provide a clue to glomerulonephritis and other disorders associated with hematuria that are due to rare genetic causes (see Table 113.1).[2,5,6,8]

A particularly common cause of pigmenturia in newborns is urate crystals, which result from poor oral intake and decreased urine output (**Fig. 113.1**).[2,8] Discovery of these crystals in the diaper should prompt evaluation for dehydration with no further work-up for hematuria. Pigmenturia can also be due to a medication side effect and usually has no clinical significance (see Table 113.1).

Anticoagulant use may be associated with varying degrees of hematuria, yet serious underlying causes such as malignancy should not be excluded without further investigation or close follow-up.[1,6,9] It is important to understand that painless hematuria, whether transient or persistent, may be the only symptom of a malignancy, which accounts for 10% to 20% of underlying causes of hematuria in adults.[3,9]

## DIAGNOSTIC TESTING

The point-of-care urine dipstick test can detect the equivalent of 1 to 2 RBCs/HPF. False-positive results can occur with

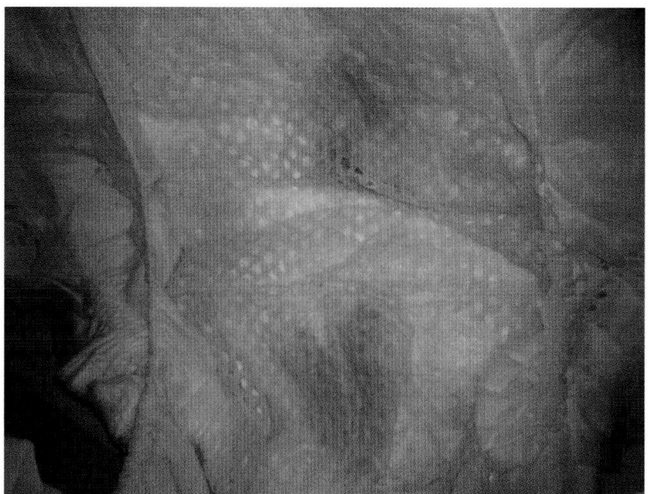

**Fig. 113.1 Urate crystals, a common finding in the diaper of a newborn.** These crystals form as a result of poor oral intake and decreased urine output. Further laboratory investigation of hematuria is not indicated. (Courtesy Janelle Aby, MD, Newborn Nursery, Lucile Packard Children's Hospital, Stanford University.)

**Table 113.2 Glomerular versus Nonglomerular Hematuria**

| FACTOR | GLOMERULAR | NONGLOMERULAR |
|---|---|---|
| Color | Smoky, tea or cola colored, red | Red or pink |
| RBC morphology | Dysmorphic | Normal |
| Casts | RBC, WBC | None |
| Clots | Absent | Present (±) |
| Proteinuria | ≥2+ | <2+ |

Reproduced from Massengill S. Hematuria. Pediatr Rev 2008;29:342-7.
*RBC*, Red blood cell; *WBC*, white blood cell

myoglobinuria and hemoglobinuria.[5,6] If a urine dipstick test is positive for the detection of blood, standard urinalysis should be performed. Urinalysis is highly sensitive and specific; however, it is more expensive and time intensive than the urine dipstick test. Urinalysis quantifies the amount of blood present and can differentiate the presence of myoglobin or hemoglobin.[5] Thus in the appropriate context, patients with a urine dipstick positive for blood and negative findings on urinalysis should be evaluated for rhabdomyolysis, hemolysis, or hyperbilirubinemia.

The presence of casts, dysmorphic RBCs, and proteinuria is associated with glomerular causes of hematuria (**Table 113.2**).

Incidental microscopic hematuria without associated symptoms or hemodynamic instability mandates confirmation of normal blood pressure in pediatric patients as a screen for glomerulonephritis, obstructive uropathy, or other systemic disease.[2,8] Normotensive patients require no further testing in the emergency department (ED), but all patients will need follow-up evaluation as an outpatient.[2,5,6,8]

Urine culture should be considered in the setting of suspected infection, especially in pediatric patients or those with indwelling Foley catheters. Urine calcium and creatinine determination is useful in a child with hematuria who does not have a urinary tract infection or a glomerular cause to confirm the diagnosis of hypercalciuria (urine calcium-creatinine ratio > 0.2).[2,7,8] Urine cytology for malignancy has poor sensitivity in the ED setting and should not be ordered as part of the ED evaluation.[1]

In patients with gross hematuria or symptomatic microscopic hematuria, blood should be sent for a complete blood cell count and renal function testing (blood urea nitrogen, creatinine). A coagulation panel should be ordered for patients who are taking anticoagulants or have a suspected or known coagulopathy.[1] Patients with unstable vital signs, heavy bleeding, and symptomatic anemia should have blood typed and screened for a potential transfusion.

Although hematuria associated with flank pain may suggest a ureteral stone, a rupturing abdominal aortic aneurysm or renal vein thrombosis should be considered in the differential diagnosis (see Table 113.1).[6] For this reason, imaging can be used to exclude these emergency diagnoses when clinically indicated (**Fig. 113.2**).[1,6] Ultrasonography is useful for the evaluation of microscopic hematuria in children and as a screen for obstruction, hydronephrosis, and abdominal aortic aneursym.[1,2,6] It less expensive than computed tomography (CT) and is safer because of lack of radiation and intravenous contrast agents. Non–contrast-enhanced CT may be used to indentify the size and location of renal stones. Contrast-enhanced CT is more sensitive than ultrasound for the detection of small renal masses. Contrast-enhanced CT is necessary to elucidate the integrity of intraabdominal and retroperitoneal structures in the setting of significant trauma associated with hematuria.[3,4,10-12]

In pediatric victims of significant blunt thoracoabdominal trauma, microscopic hematuria consisting of more than 5 RBCs/HPF indicates the need for further evaluation with abdominal and pelvic CT.[10] For pediatric trauma patients who are not toilet-trained, bag urine collection may be preferred over catheterization as a screen for hematuria because the trauma from catheterization can lead to false-positive urine specimens.

In adults with blunt trauma, a higher cutoff (>50 RBCs/HPF) for microscopic hematuria is associated with increased risk for intraabdominal injury worthwhile of abdominal and pelvic CT.[11] As a screen for bladder injury, gross hematuria has greater sensitivity and specificity than microscopic hematuria does.[12]

## TREATMENT AND DISPOSITION

Treatment varies depending on the underlying diagnosis and degree of hematuria (see Fig. 113.2). Intravenous fluids, analgesics, and antiemetics may be needed in patients with gross hematuria.

Patients with gross hematuria who are able to void should be asked about the presence of clots in their urinary flow and the ease with which they are passed. Foley catheterization may

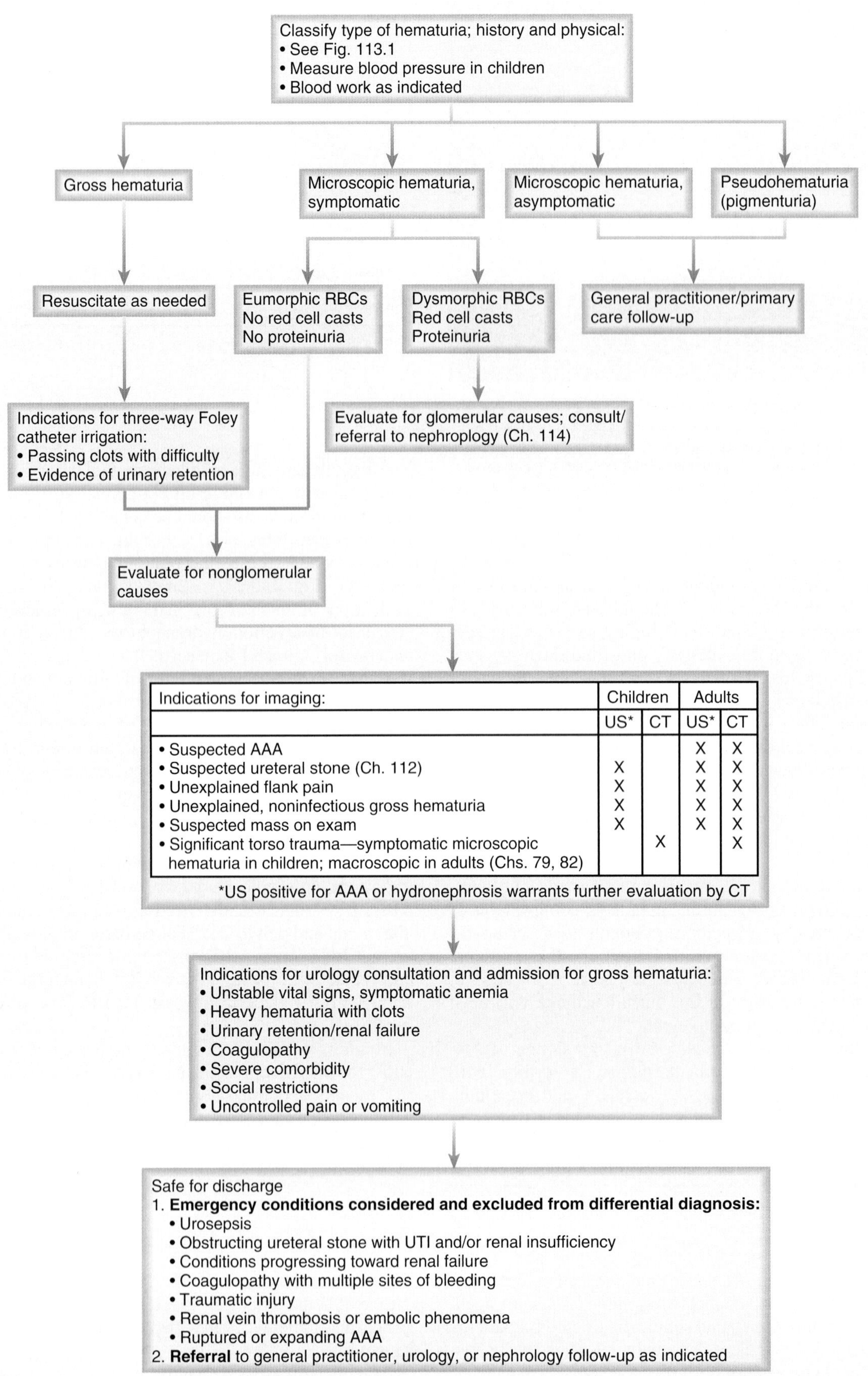


| Indications for imaging: | Children | | Adults | |
|---|---|---|---|---|
| | US* | CT | US* | CT |
| • Suspected AAA | | | X | X |
| • Suspected ureteral stone (Ch. 112) | X | | X | X |
| • Unexplained flank pain | X | | X | X |
| • Unexplained, noninfectious gross hematuria | X | | X | X |
| • Suspected mass on exam | X | | X | X |
| • Significant torso trauma—symptomatic microscopic hematuria in children; macroscopic in adults (Chs. 79, 82) | | X | | X |

*US positive for AAA or hydronephrosis warrants further evaluation by CT

**Fig. 113.2 Management algorithm for hematuria.** *AAA*, Abdominal aortic aneurysm; *CT*, computed tomography; *RBCs*, red blood cells; *US*, ultrasound; *UTI*, urinary tract infection.

be avoided in stable, sensible, and mobile patients who are able to void easily and who have a few small clots that pass with ease. If clot retention or significant dysuria is present, the treatment of choice is insertion of a three-way Foley catheter to facilitate irrigation of the bladder to dislodge clots and allow bladder decompression.[1] Saline should be irrigated continuously through the third port until the urine turns pink to clear and is free of clots. In the setting of trauma, urethral injury should be excluded before catheter placement (see Chapter 82). Stable patients with improved symptoms may be discharged with a leg bag and instructions for urology follow-up in 3 to 5 days.

Consultation with a nephrologist may be helpful in cases of suspected glomerular disease or obstructive uropathy in a child. Urology consultation should be obtained for patients with malignancies and for patients with high-volume, noninfectious gross hematuria. Hematuria alone is rarely an indication for admission, except as noted in Figure 113.2.[1,6]

The vast majority of patients with hematuria are discharged with further care as an outpatient. Incidental cases require repeated urinalysis in 1 week.[1,4,6] Patients treated for gross hematuria should be instructed to drink plenty of fluids and return if they have an inability to void, fever, pain, worsening dysuria, and gross hematuria that fails to clear.

## SUGGESTED READINGS

Hicks D, Li C. Management of macroscopic hematuria in the emergency department. Emerg Med J 2007;24:385-90.

Massengill S. Hematuria. Pediatr Rev 2008;29:342-7.

Sokolosky M. Hematuria. Emerg Med Clin North Am 2001;19:621-32.

## REFERENCES

***References can be found on Expert Consult @ www.expertconsult.com.***

# 114 Renal Failure

*William J. Brady and Amita Sudhir*

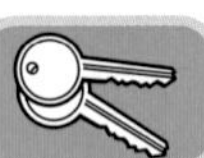

**KEY POINTS**

- Management of renal failure in the emergency department should be aimed at identifying and treating life-threatening abnormalities associated with the disorder, identifying reversible causes of renal failure, and preventing further injury to the kidneys.
- Acute pulmonary edema and hyperkalemia are potentially life-threatening complications of renal failure.
- Severe hyperkalemia should be suspected as the cause of cardiac arrest in patients with a possible history of renal failure.
- An electrocardiogram should be obtained for all patients with renal failure on arrival at the emergency department to screen for hyperkalemia.

## DEFINITIONS

Renal failure can be the result of a wide variety of conditions that cause injury to the kidneys. Recently, there has been a change in terminology with respect to kidney disease: the entities previously known as acute renal failure and chronic renal failure are now known as acute kidney injury and chronic kidney disease, respectively.

The Acute Kidney Injury Network (AKIN) provides the following criteria for the diagnosis of acute kidney injury: an abrupt (within 48 hours) reduction in kidney function currently defined as an absolute increase in serum creatinine of 0.3 mg/dL or greater (≥26.4 μmol/L), a 50% or greater increase in serum creatinine of (1.5-fold higher than baseline), *or* a reduction in urine output (documented oliguria of less than 0.5 mL/kg/hr for more than 6 hours).[1]

Two classification systems describe the stage of renal disease. The first, created by the Acute Dialysis Quality Initiative, is the RIFLE (risk, injury, failure, loss, and end-stage kidney disease) classification system, which bases severity on the degree of change in serum creatinine or urine output from a baseline measurement (**Table 114.1**).[2] The second was created by AKIN. Although it is modeled on the RIFLE classification, it does not require the physician to know the patient's baseline creatinine level. Its ease of use in the emergency department (ED) is improved by the fact that it does not use the glomerular filtration rate (GFR) as one of the criteria for staging kidney injury. The AKIN criteria are to be applied after adequate fluid resuscitation has taken place, and the authors of the criteria also recommend excluding easily reversible causes of kidney failure, such as urinary outflow obstruction (**Table 114.2**).[1]

The National Kidney Foundation's clinical practice guidelines define patients with chronic kidney disease as meeting one of the following criteria: (1) kidney damage for 3 or more months, defined as structural or functional abnormalities of the kidney, with or without an increased GFR, and demonstrated by either pathologic abnormalities or markers of kidney damage, including abnormalities in blood or urine or abnormal findings on imaging tests; *or* (2) a GFR lower than 60 mL/min/1.73 $m^2$ for 3 or more months, with or without kidney damage.[3] The complicated definition of chronic kidney disease plus the need to monitor kidney function over an extended period means that it is unlikely that chronic kidney disease will be convincingly diagnosed in the ED. However, it is useful for the emergency physician (EP) to understand what it means when a patient has preexisting chronic kidney disease, as well as to be vigilant for suspected, but previously undiagnosed chronic kidney disease in a patient with the appropriate signs and symptoms.

## EPIDEMIOLOGY

The prevalence and incidence of kidney failure in the United States are rising. The prevalence of chronic kidney disease is estimated to be greater than 10%.[4] The annual incidence of acute kidney injury is 100 per 1 million population. The incidence of acute kidney injury in the community varies widely depending on the population, but hospital-acquired rates can be quite high, with as many as 30% of critical care patients in some studies developing acute kidney injury.[5]

## PATHOPHYSIOLOGY

The kidneys are located in the retroperitoneal space and are composed of three basic structures: vasculature, parenchyma,

**Table 114.1 RIFLE Classification System**

| | GFR CRITERIA | URINE OUTPUT CRITERIA |
|---|---|---|
| *R*isk | Increased Cr × 1.5<br>*or*<br>GFR decreased >25% | UO < 0.5 mL/kg/hr × 6 hr |
| *I*njury | Increased Cr × 2<br>*or*<br>GFR decreased >50% | UO < 0.5 mL/kg/hr × 12 hr |
| *F*ailure | Increased Cr × 3<br>*or*<br>GFR decreased >75% | UO < 0.5 mL/kg/hr × 12 hr<br>*or*<br>anuria × 12 hr |
| *L*oss | Persistent ARF = complete loss of renal function for >4 wk | None |
| *E*nd-stage kidney disease | End-stage kidney disease > 4 mo | None |

*Cr*, Creatinine; *GFR*, glomerular filtration rate; *UO*, urine output.

**Table 114.2 AKIN Criteria for Staging Acute Kidney Injury**

| | CREATININE CRITERIA | URINE OUTPUT CRITERIA |
|---|---|---|
| Stage 1 | Increased Cr × 1.5<br>*or*<br>Increased ≥0.3 mg/dL | UO < 0.5 mL/kg/hr > 6 hr |
| Stage 2 | Increased Cr × 2 | UO < 0.5 mL/kg/hr > 12 hr |
| Stage 3 | Increased Cr × 3<br>*or*<br>≥4 mg/dL with acute increase of 0.5 mg/dL<br>*or*<br>Patient receiving renal replacement therapy | UO < 0.5 mL/kg/hr > 24 hr or anuria for 12 hr |

*AKIN*, Acute Kidney Injury Network, *Cr*, creatinine; *UO*, urine output.

and the collecting system. The kidneys receive about a quarter of the body's total cardiac output through the renal arterial system and an extensive network of arteries, arterioles, and capillaries that eventually drain into the renal vein. The renal parenchyma is composed of the medulla and cortex, which houses the functional unit of the kidney, the nephron. A single nephron consists of a glomerulus, proximal tubule, thin limbs of Henle, and a distal tubule. The connecting tubule joins the nephron to the collecting system, including the renal pelvis, minor and major calyces, and the ureter, bladder, and urethra (**Fig. 114.1**).

The kidney is responsible for maintaining the volume and ionic composition of body fluids, excreting metabolic waste products such as urea, and eliminating exogenous drugs, hormones, and toxins. The kidneys also serve as a major endocrine organ through the production of renin, erythropoietin, 1,25-dihydroxycholecalciferol, prostaglandins, and kinins. Metabolic functions of the kidney include catabolism of small-molecular-weight proteins and anabolic roles in ammoniagenesis and gluconeogenesis.

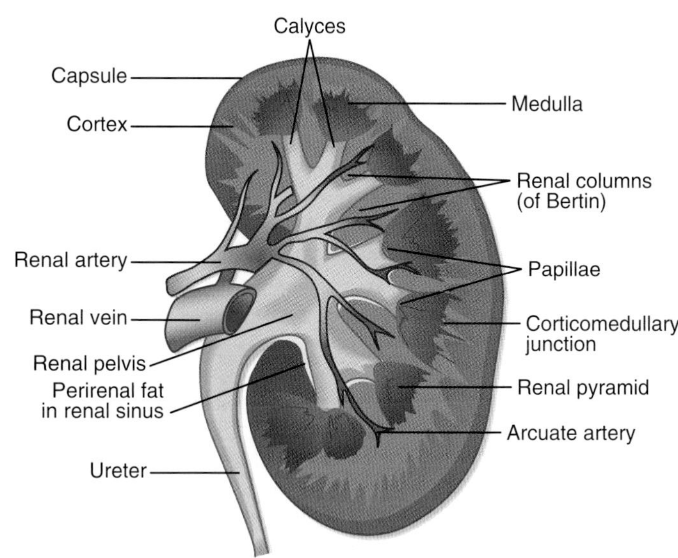


**Fig. 114.1 Gross anatomy of the kidney.**

In a person weighing 70 kg, the kidney forms approximately 180 L of glomerular filtrate each day. Cardiac output in combination with effective intravascular volume generates hydraulic pressure that drives fluid from the capillaries into the urinary space, which represents the main mechanism of urine formation. The final urinary filtrate is determined by a complex interaction between hydraulic and oncotic pressure, molecular size and charge, absorption, reabsorption, and secretion under hormonal control.

Renal failure can be the result of dysfunction in any part of this system. It is helpful to understand the pathophysiology of renal disease as a set of three etiologic categories: prerenal, intrinsic renal, and postrenal causes.

1. Prerenal failure results from the kidneys not receiving enough blood via a cause external to the kidneys themselves; it results in a reduced GFR, buildup of toxic waste products, and damage to the kidneys persisting after the underlying cause has been corrected. Causes of prerenal failure include hypovolemia, decreased cardiac output, and septic shock.
2. Renal failure may be caused by diseases intrinsic to the kidneys, including genetic syndromes such as polycystic kidney disease, infections, vascular diseases, and toxins or drugs.
3. Postrenal failure may result from obstruction to urinary flow external to the kidneys themselves. The obstruction causes increased fluid pressure within the nephron, which ultimately leads to loss of function. Ureteral stones, prostatic hypertrophy, tumors, and anticholinergic medications are some possible causes of postrenal kidney failure.

Renal failure can be divided into two categories: primary disturbances and secondary disturbances. Primary disturbances reflect a direct failure of the kidneys to perform critical functions, such as failure to excrete sodium (leading to volume overload) or a decrease in erythropoietin production (leading to anemia). Secondary disturbances result from an accumulation of metabolic products in other organ systems, as when hyperphosphatemia causes hyperparathyroidism or when nitrogenous waste products promote platelet dysfunction. The combination of primary and secondary disturbances disrupts the homeostatic balance of almost every organ system.

## PRIMARY DISTURBANCES

When the kidney can no longer perform excretory functions, the result is volume overload, hyperkalemia, and hyperphosphatemia. As renal endocrine function declines, hypocalcemia and anemia develop. Renal failure can cause an increased circulating concentration of insulin and lower insulin requirements in diabetics. Loss of ammoniagenesis and the ability to excrete phosphate impairs clearance of the metabolic acid load by the kidneys and may lead to acidosis. Adverse drug reactions at normal dosages can occur when drugs that are metabolized or excreted by the kidneys are administered.

## SECONDARY DISTURBANCES

Accumulation of nitrogenous waste products, generically referred to as uremia, is a characteristic of not only renal excretory failure but also a host of metabolic and endocrine disease states. Derangements in protein, carbohydrate, and lipid metabolism will ensue and are associated with anemia, malnutrition, and metabolic bone disease. Loss of renal catabolism and an increase in endocrine secretion affect many hormones, including insulin, glucagon, luteinizing hormone, and prolactin. A normal platelet count may be maintained, although platelet function and bleeding time will probably become abnormal. Poorly understood immune system interactions can lead to immunosuppression, overwhelming infection, septic shock, and death.

# PRESENTING SIGNS AND SYMPTOMS

Manifestations may vary greatly depending on the cause of the renal failure, but patients may describe a history of volume overload or decreased urine output. They may also have one or many of a long list of end-organ effects (**Table 114.3**). Renal failure is not a diagnosis that is necessarily obvious on initial encounter and is often made only after screening laboratory data are obtained.

Once the laboratory diagnosis of renal failure is made, the EP should go back through the patient's history to look for signs and symptoms and findings on physical examination that suggest the cause of the renal failure, as well as signs of any complications that must be dealt with urgently. Pulmonary edema, cardiac arrhythmias, and altered mental status are particularly concerning findings.

**Table 114.3 Organ System Effects of Renal Failure**

| ABNORMALITY CAUSED BY RENAL FAILURE | PHYSICAL FINDINGS, END-ORGAN EFFECT |
|---|---|
| **Cardiovascular** | |
| Pulmonary edema | Crackles |
| Hypertension | |
| Pericardial effusion | |
| **Metabolic** | |
| Hyperkalemia | Peaked T waves, arrhythmias, bradycardia, cardiac arrest |
| Hypocalcemia | Tetany, cardiac arrhythmias |
| Hypermagnesemia | Nausea and vomiting, arrhythmias |
| **Neurologic** | |
| Uremia | Seizures |
| Acute and chronic neurologic changes | Hyperreflexia<br>Encephalopathy, including asterixis<br>Sensory neuropathy |
| Hyponatremia or hypernatremia | Altered mental status, seizures |
| Dialysis-associated dementia | Loss of cognitive function |
| **Immunologic** | |
| Immunosuppression | Recurrent infections |
| **Pulmonary** | |
| Fluid overload: pleural effusions, pulmonary edema | Shortness of breath, hypoxia, crackles, dullness to percussion, peripheral edema |
| **Gastrointestinal** | |
| Gastritis | Abdominal pain |
| Bleeding | Melena |
| Malnutrition | Cachexia, anemia |
| **Endocrine** | |
| Glucose intolerance | Hyperglycemia |
| Renal osteodystrophy<br>Myopathy<br>Amyloid arthropathy<br>Secondary hyperparathyroidism | Bone and joint pain, myalgias |
| **Skin** | |
| Uremia | Pruritus, uremic frost (urea crystals from sweat on skin) |

**Table 114.3** Organ System Effects of Renal Failure—cont'd

| ABNORMALITY CAUSED BY RENAL FAILURE | PHYSICAL FINDINGS, END-ORGAN EFFECT |
|---|---|
| **Cardiovascular** | |
| Uremic pericarditis | Pericardial friction rub, chest pain worse with lying down, ECG changes: ST elevation and PR depression (only some or none of these may be seen) |
| Myocardial infarction | ST elevation in anatomic distribution or elevated enzymes |
| Acidosis | Hypotension |
| **Hematologic** | |
| Uremic platelets | Bleeding |
| **Musculoskeletal** | |
| Arthritis | |
| Spontaneous tendon rupture | |
| Carpal tunnel syndrome | |

*ECG*, Electrocardiographic.

**BOX 114.1 Diagnostic Criteria for Acute Kidney Injury**

An abrupt (within 48 hours) reduction in kidney function as defined by the following:

- An absolute increase in serum creatinine of 0.3 mg/dL or greater

*or*

- A 50% or greater increase in serum creatinine (1.5-fold higher than baseline)

*or*

- A reduction in urine output (documented oliguria of less than 0.5 mL/kg/hr for more than 6 hours)

**BOX 114.2 Causes of Renal Failure Secondary to Vessel Injury**

| Small and Medium Vessel | Large Vessel |
|---|---|
| Scleroderma | Renal artery thrombosis or stenosis |
| Malignant hypertension | Renal vein thrombosis |
| Hemolytic-uremic syndrome | Atheroembolic disease |
| Thrombotic thrombocytopenic purpura | Aortic dissection |
| Sickle cell nephropathy | Angiography |
| Preeclampsia | |
| Trauma | |

## DIFFERENTIAL DIAGNOSIS AND MEDICAL DECISION MAKING

Although the classic teaching has been that fractional excretion of sodium and urea be used to determine the source of the renal dysfunction—prerenal, intrinsic renal, or postrenal—these calculated values are often unreliable indicators of the cause of renal failure, especially in the setting of diuretic use and underlying chronic renal disease. Their diagnostic value or usefulness in guiding therapy in the ED is questionable. Physical examination findings and the clinical history are more useful in determining the cause of the renal failure. Fractional excretion of sodium and urea can be used to support a conclusion or help eliminate alternative diagnoses.

Once a diagnosis of renal failure is made through creatinine screening or the presence oliguria or anuria (**Box 114.1**), a differential diagnosis of underlying conditions and complications should be generated by considering potential diseases of the vasculature, parenchyma, and collecting system, as well as conditions external to the kidneys that lead to decreased blood flow or obstruction to the flow of urine.

### INTRINSIC RENAL FAILURE: VASCULAR CAUSES

Vascular diseases of the kidney are manifested differently according to the size of the artery involved (**Box 114.2**). Sudden back or flank pain suggests large vessel aneurysm, dissection, embolism, or trauma. Poorly controlled hypertension and chronic renal insufficiency suggest renal artery stenosis. Systemic manifestations such as rash and fever suggest vasculitis in the smaller vessels of the kidney.

### INTRINSIC RENAL FAILURE: PARENCHYMAL CAUSES

The working unit of the kidney is the nephron, which is composed of a variety of cell types that are susceptible to many disease processes (**Box 114.3**). The medical history is invaluable in identifying the root cause within this category of kidney failure.

### OBSTRUCTIVE RENAL FAILURE

The collecting system of the kidneys is composed of the calyces, renal pelvis, ureter, bladder, and urethra—obstruction may occur at any level (**Box 114.4**). Obstruction to urinary flow is generally a reversible cause of renal failure. Alert patients may have symptoms of urinary retention or nephrolithiasis that are dramatic and obvious. Occult, potentially reversible renal obstruction should be considered in patients with altered mental status and acute renal failure.

### URINE FORMATION PROBLEMS RESULTING IN RENAL FAILURE

Also known as prerenal kidney failure, problems with urine formation should be suspected in patients with volume depletion, decreased cardiac output, or third spacing of fluid as a result of any cause. The various causes of prerenal kidney failure are summarized in **Box 114.5**.

## TREATMENT

### PREHOSPITAL MANAGEMENT

If the patient's history suggests a possible diagnosis of renal failure, the prehospital provider should consider hyperkalemia

**BOX 114.3 Causes of Renal Failure Secondary to Parenchymal Injury**

Systemic disease
- Systemic lupus erythematosus
- Infective endocarditis
- Systemic vasculitis
- Henoch-Schönlein purpura
- Essential mixed cryoglobulinemia
- Goodpasture syndrome

Primary renal disease
- Poststreptococcal glomerulonephritis
- Rapidly progressive glomerulonephritis

Ischemia
- Shock
- Severe volume depletion

Nephrotoxins
- Antibiotics
- Contrast agents
- Pigment induced (rhabdomyolysis)
- Drugs (nonsteroidal antiinflammatory drugs)
- Toxins
- Multiple myeloma

Hereditary
- Polycystic kidney disease
- Alport syndrome
- Medullary cystic disease

Infections
Severe liver disease
Allergic reactions

**BOX 114.4 Causes of Renal Failure Secondary to Collecting System Obstruction**

**Intrarenal and Ureteral**
Kidney stone
Sloughed papilla
Malignancy (obstructive)
Crystal precipitation
Retroperitoneal fibrosis

**Bladder**
Kidney stone
Blood clot
Prostatic hypertrophy
Bladder carcinoma

**Anticholinergic Medications**
Neurogenic bladder

**Urethra**
Phimosis
Stricture
Reflux nephropathy

as a cause of any electrocardiographic (ECG) changes and treat the patient accordingly. Fluid should be administered judiciously to patients with renal failure, with awareness of the patient's impaired ability to excrete fluid and the possibility of subsequent volume overload.

## HOSPITAL MANAGEMENT

ED management of patients with renal failure should be aimed at (1) identifying any easily reversible causes of renal failure, (2) preventing and treating life-threatening abnormalities caused by renal failure, and (3) supportive therapy to prevent further injury to the kidneys. Patients receiving renal

**BOX 114.5 Prerenal Causes of Renal Failure**

**Volume Loss**
Vomiting and diarrhea
Diuresis
Blood loss
Insensible losses
Third spacing
Peritonitis
Trauma and burns

**Oncotic Pressure**
Hypoalbuminemia
Nephrotic syndrome
Liver disease

**Decreased Perfusion**
Congestive heart failure
Valvular disease
Septic shock
Anaphylaxis
Antihypertensive medications
Neurogenic shock

replacement therapy (dialysis of any kind) and those with known renal abnormalities who exhibit worsening of their renal function ("acute on chronic failure") should be treated the same as patients without a history of renal insufficiency.

### *Treating Reversible Causes of Renal Failure*

Hypovolemic patients should be given appropriate fluid resuscitation while taking precautions to avoid volume overload. Appropriate fluid resuscitation may result in return of renal function.

Patients with known or suspected urinary outflow obstruction in or distal to the bladder should be treated with a Foley catheter.

In cases of parenchymal injury, any obvious toxic exposures (drugs, antibiotics, toxins) should be stopped, proper hydration should be provided, and infections or severe shock states should be treated.

The use of specific antidotes and pharmacologic treatments (e.g., bicarbonate and mannitol for patients with rhabdomyolysis) and the use of diuretics to improve urine flow are controversial; consultation should be obtained before initiating any therapy (beyond fluid replacement) aimed at maintaining adequate urine output.[6]

Treatment of vascular compromise in large vessels (embolization, thrombosis, dissection) should focus on return of normal blood flow. Consultation with urology, vascular surgery, or interventional radiology may be required. Treatment of small vessel disease should be focused on therapy for the underlying illness.

### *Other Treatment Considerations*

Particular care should also be taken with the administration of renally cleared drugs, such as morphine or insulin, which could be harmful or even fatal if blood concentrations rise.

Intravenously administered contrast material may cause additional kidney injury. If patients are receiving renal replacement therapy, contrast material may be administered in consultation with a nephrologist if dialysis is to take place in a timely manner (**Box 114.6**).

### *Life-Threatening Complications of Renal Failure*

Volume Overload Extracellular fluid volume is determined by the balance between sodium and water. Renal failure may promote sodium retention or result in failure to excrete

**BOX 114.6 Management Considerations for Patients with Renal Failure**

**Intravenous Access**
Avoid the side of grafts and fistulas.
In life-threatening emergencies, grafts and fistulas may be accessed.

**External Blood Pressure Measurements**
Avoid the side of grafts and fistulas.

**Volume and Electrolyte Replacement**
Careful titration of fluid administration is necessary to avoid volume overload and pulmonary edema.
Avoid aggressive electrolyte replacement.

**Medications**
Adjust dosages according to creatinine clearance.
Avoid nephrotoxic antibiotics.
Anticoagulants may need to be adjusted (low-molecular-weight heparin).

**Radiographic Contrast Agents**
If no renal function remains, contrast dye should be tolerated.
Avoid intravenous contrast agents in patients with remaining renal function.

**Procedures**
Increased risk for bleeding is possible.

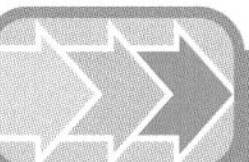

**PRIORITY ACTIONS**

**Volume Overload and Pulmonary Edema**

Assess the airway and ventilation
- Intubation, CPAP, or BiPAP as necessary

Provide supplemental $O_2$
- 100% non-rebreather mask if the above measures are not used

Position the patient upright
Apply a cardiac monitor
- Look for contributing dysrhythmias

Obtain intravenous access
Obtain an ECG
- Screen for hyperkalemic changes

Venodilating agents
- Nitroglycerin: SL or intravenous drip
- Nitroprusside
- ACEI if hypertensive

Diuretics
Inotropes or vasopressors as necessary
Urgent consultation for dialysis

*ACEI*, Angiotensin-converting enzyme inhibitor; *BiPAP*, bilevel positive airway pressure; *CPAP*, continuous positive airway pressure; *ECG*, electrocardiogram; *SL*, sublingual.

excessive sodium intake, thereby leading to a positive sodium balance and extracellular fluid volume expansion. The most concerning clinical manifestation of volume overload is pulmonary edema with respiratory distress. The presence or lack of previous renal replacement therapy should not alter the management of acute pulmonary edema. Volume overload remains one of the most common reasons for emergency dialysis—dialysis should be considered as early as possible in patients with renal failure and severe pulmonary edema.

**Hyperkalemia** One of the most lethal complications of renal failure is hyperkalemia. Any patient suspected of having renal failure or hyperkalemia should undergo a screening ECG study on arrival at the ED. Peaked T waves are pathognomonic for hyperkalemia. Later changes include bradycardia, widening of the QRS complex, and degeneration into a sine wave pattern. These changes can all occur without preceding peaked T waves. Patients with ECG changes consistent with hyperkalemia should receive treatment immediately—do not wait for serum confirmation. However, because normal ECG findings do not exclude hyperkalemia, serum confirmation should be made when suspicion for hyperkalemia remains high, as it should in all patients with known or suspected renal failure. In patients with previous chronic kidney disease, significant dietary changes, new medications, and noncompliance with dialysis can precipitate hyperkalemia.

All patients with known renal failure who are initially seen in cardiac arrest should be treated for the hyperkalemia along with the usual resuscitative measures. The extremities and upper part of the chest should be checked for dialysis access devices when patients are in cardiac arrest, and their presence should be assumed to be diagnostic of preexisting renal failure.

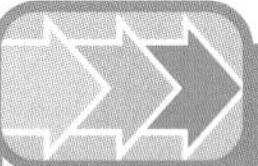

**PRIORITY ACTIONS**

**Treatment of Hyperkalemia**

Stabilize the myocardium against the effects of potassium
- Calcium gluconate or calcium chloride, 1 g IV

Induce an intracellular shift of potassium
- Insulin, 10 units IV, plus glucose, 1 ampule of $D_{50}$ IV
- Sodium bicarbonate, 1 ampule IV
- Inhaled albuterol: continuous nebulization
- Magnesium sulfate, 2 g IV

Reduce total-body potassium
- Oral polystyrene sulfonate (Kayexalate)
- Dialysis

*$D_{50}$*, 50% dextrose; *IV*, intravenously.

**Other Electrolyte and Acid-Base Disturbances** Additional metabolic derangements seen in cases of renal failure include hypermagnesemia, hypernatremia, hyponatremia, hypercalcemia, hypocalcemia, hyperglycemia, hypoglycemia, and metabolic acidosis (refer to specific treatment strategies in corresponding chapters of this text). In many instances, severe electrolyte disturbances mandate urgent dialysis.

**Chest Pain** The leading cause of death in patients with renal failure is acute coronary syndrome. Preceding illnesses (diabetes, hypertension) compounded with complications of renal failure (dyslipidemia, chronic volume overload, hyperphosphatemia, anemia, hyperparathyroidism) present a host of risk factors for cardiovascular disease. Renal failure does not change the treatment of acute myocardial infarction.

Other causes of life-threatening chest pain should be considered. Patients with renal failure have abnormalities in platelet adhesion that make pulmonary embolism more likely.

**Uremic Pericarditis** Uremic pericarditis may occur in patients with a high blood urea nitrogen level. Classic findings of chest pain, pericardial friction rub, worsening of pain when supine, and ECG changes may or may not be present. The presence of any of these signs should trigger a differential diagnosis that includes uremic pericarditis. If no signs of pericardial tamponade are present, pain control and hospital admission are appropriate. Uremic pericarditis traditionally prompts the initiation of dialysis in patients not already receiving renal replacement therapy.

Dialysis-associated pericarditis can also occur. It is not well understood, but large effusions may be present and require either increased dialysis or surgical correction.[7]

**Pericardial Tamponade** Many patients with long-standing renal failure have preexisting pericardial effusions and volume overload that complicate the diagnosis of pericardial tamponade. Chest radiography may not reveal classic abnormalities in heart shape because many patients may have coincident cardiomegaly. Echocardiographic findings may also be altered.[8]

**Hemorrhage** Prolongation of the bleeding time, decreased activity of platelet factor 3, abnormal platelet aggregation, and impaired prothrombin consumption contribute to the abnormal hemostasis in patients with renal failure. Patients may have abnormal bleeding as a result of minor wounds or surgery, epistaxis, spontaneous gastrointestinal bleeding, or hemorrhage in the liver, pericardial sac, or brain. Gastrointestinal bleeding is both more common and more severe in patients being maintained on renal replacement therapy.[7] Patients with renal failure may have preexisting anemia, and therefore small drops in hemoglobin may be detrimental. Blood transfusions that maintain the hematocrit above 30% have been shown to improve platelet dysfunction. Desmopressin, erythropoietin, cryoprecipitate, and conjugated estrogens may all be of benefit (**Box 114.7**).

**BOX 114.7 Interventions to Reduce Bleeding in Patients with Renal Failure**

Packed red blood cell transfusions
Conjugated estrogens
- 0.6 mg/kg/day intravenously for 5 consecutive days or 25 mg orally or 50 to 100 mcg/24 hr transdermally every three days

Intensification of the dialysis regimen
Recombinant erythropoietin
Desmopressin (DDAVP)
- 0.3 mcg/kg (intravenously, subcutaneously, or intranasally)

Cryoprecipitate

Data from Dember LM. Critical care issues in the patient with chronic renal failure. Crit Care Clin 2002;18:421-40.

**Infection** Both immunomodulators and cellular components of the immune system are altered in patients with renal failure and lead to a greater risk for infections. Vascular grafts, recurrent needlesticks, and peritoneal ports break the skin's protective barrier down and offer more opportunities for bacteria to enter the circulation. Patients undergoing peritoneal dialysis are at risk for peritonitis. Most infections are bacterial. Patients often need to be treated with coverage for hospital-acquired pathogens; pneumonia in a dialysis patient is treated as a health care–associated pneumonia with broad empiric antibiotic coverage. Fever in a dialysis patient with an indwelling line should be assumed to be bacteremia until proved otherwise, and empiric antibiotic coverage for line-associated infections should be initiated. The catheter may also need to be removed. *Pseudomonas*, methicillin-resistant *Staphylococcus aureus*, and vancomycin-resistant *Enterococcus* should all be treated with appropriate antibiotics until cultures allow more specific treatment.

## COMPLICATIONS OF RENAL REPLACEMENT THERAPY

Renal replacement therapy produces its own unique set of complications. Patients with grafts and fistulas may have infections, bleeding, or thrombosis of their access sites. Port malfunction, infection, or peritonitis may develop in peritoneal dialysis patients. Dialysis-related complications include hypotension and disequilibrium syndrome (refer to Chapter 116 for a detailed discussion of dialysis-related emergencies).

## CONSULTATION

Urgent nephrology consultation should be obtained for patients with volume overload or significant electrolyte abnormalities requiring dialysis. Indications for dialysis are summarized in **Boxes 114.8 and 114.9**.

**BOX 114.8 Indications for Dialysis in Patients with Chronic Renal Failure**

Pericarditis or pleuritis
Uremic encephalopathy or seizures
Significant bleeding secondary to uremic platelets
Fluid overload refractory to diuretics
Hypertension poorly responsive to antihypertensive medications
Metabolic disturbances refractory to medical therapy
Persistent nausea and vomiting
Evidence of malnutrition

**BOX 114.9 Indications for Dialysis in Patients with Acute Kidney Disease**

Acute volume overload in patients with pulmonary edema and significantly compromised pulmonary function
Hyperkalemia with compromising dysrhythmia, widened QRS complex, or other worrisome electrocardiographic finding
Symptomatic uremia (encephalopathy, emesis)
Severe metabolic acidosis
Severe hyponatremia
Uremic myopericarditis

A urology consultation should be initiated if the cause of the renal failure is thought to be obstruction. In cases of easily reversible outflow obstruction, the consultation can be delayed and deferred to the admitting physician's discretion. If renal function improves and the patient is able to urinate independently without a catheter in place, outpatient follow-up with a urologist may be all that is required.

A pharmacist may also be consulted to determine renal dosing of drugs based on the patient's creatinine clearance. In general, a single dose of antibiotics given in the ED does not need to be adjusted; subsequent doses can be adjusted by a pharmacist based on blood levels and the patient's renal function. However, if the patient is to be sent home on medication, doses may need to be adjusted with the help of a pharmacist.

## NEXT STEPS IN CARE

### ADMISSION VERSUS DISCHARGE

A small subset of patients may be discharged home safely. Those undergoing chronic dialysis who are stable, have no life-threatening electrolyte abnormalities, and otherwise have no indications for admission may be discharged to follow-up with their regularly scheduled dialysis appointment.

The majority of patients with acute or acute on chronic kidney injury will require admission to the hospital. Stable patients may be admitted to non–critical care units; patients with significant volume overload or ECG changes, patients in respiratory distress, those with altered mental status, or patients who have experienced a life-threatening arrhythmia should be admitted to an intensive care unit. All dialysis patients with an indwelling catheter and a fever should be admitted to the hospital for intravenous antibiotics because of the high risk for line infection.

Patients undergoing peritoneal dialysis in whom peritonitis is suspected should be managed in conjunction with a nephrologist; if well appearing with normal vital signs, discharge with intraperitoneal antibiotics and close follow-up is a reasonable option.

### PITFALLS

EPs should be vigilant for volume overload, iatrogenic overdosing of renally cleared drugs, and failure to identify hyperkalemia. Normal ECG findings do not exclude hyperkalemia. Hyperkalemia should always be investigated as the cause of arrhythmias or bradycardia in a patient with known renal failure.

### PROGNOSIS

The prognosis of an individual patient with renal failure depends on a multitude of factors—the underlying cause of the renal failure, the patient's preexisting renal function, and comorbid conditions. In patients with chronic kidney disease, the mortality rate, especially from cardiovascular causes, is much higher than in the general population and worsens as kidney function decreases.[3]

## SUGGESTED READINGS

Albright R. Acute renal failure: a practical update. Mayo Clin Proc 2001;76:67-74.

Dember LM. Critical care issues in the patient with chronic renal failure. Crit Care Clin 2002;18:421-40.

Minnaganti V, Cunha B. Infections associated with uremia and dialysis. Infect Dis Clin North Am 2001;15:385-406.

## REFERENCES

***References can be found on Expert Consult @ www.expertconsult.com.***

Derby Teaching Hospitals
NHS Foundation Trust
Library and Knowle... Centre

# 115 Emergency Renal Ultrasonography

*Mark W. Byrne, Heidi H. Kimberly, and Vicki E. Noble*

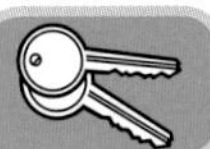

**KEY POINTS**

- The presence of unilateral hydronephrosis in the correct clinical context is used as an indirect finding for the diagnosis of renal colic. Obstructing stones are not typically visualized directly during bedside sonography.
- Identification of hydronephrosis in one kidney should prompt evaluation of the contralateral side to rule out bilateral hydronephrosis as a result of bladder outlet obstruction.
- Ultrasound measurements of the urinary bladder can be used to estimate bladder volume and identify a distended bladder in patients with suspected urinary retention.
- Abdominal aortic aneurysm should always be included in the differential diagnosis of renal colic. Emergency practitioners should maintain a low threshold for performing screening ultrasound of the aorta in patients with risk factors for an aneurysm.

## INTRODUCTION

Acute flank pain is a common complaint in the emergency department. The presence of unilateral flank or groin pain, especially in the setting of gross or microscopic hematuria, raises clinical suspicion for renal colic secondary to an obstructing ureteral stone. Bedside renal ultrasonography is a rapid and safe imaging modality for evaluation of renal colic. The presence of unilateral hydronephrosis in the correct clinical context is often sufficient to make the diagnosis. Because pain from a rapidly expanding or leaking abdominal aortic aneurysm (AAA) can masquerade as renal colic, additional evaluation of the aorta should be considered, especially in patients with risk factors for AAA.

Acute urinary retention is a common cause of abdominal pain. Bedside ultrasound is a rapid, noninvasive diagnostic tool for the evaluation of suspected urinary retention. Sonographic estimation of urinary bladder volume provides an accurate quantitative assessment of retention in the emergency setting. Additionally, screening ultrasound for the presence of adequate urine volume has been shown to decrease the number of unsuccessful attempts at catheterization in the pediatric population.

## EVIDENCE-BASED REVIEW

Computed tomography (CT) currently has the greatest sensitivity and specificity of imaging modalities used for the diagnosis of renal colic. When compared with ultrasound, non–contrast-enhanced CT is more sensitive in identifying obstructing ureteral stones[1-4] and more accurate in measuring stone size.[4,5] CT also more consistently locates the specific site of obstruction along the course of the ureter and can identify other causes of abdominal pain that may mimic acute renal colic.

However, routine use of CT for suspected renal colic has significant limitations. Patients are exposed to significant amounts of ionizing radiation when they undergo CT of the abdomen and pelvis,[6,7] which makes CT inadvisable during pregnancy and less appealing in the pediatric population. Because renal colic is a recurrent diagnosis, patients may eventually receive multiple CT scans over time, and cumulative radiation doses may rise to concerning levels[8] and place patients at risk for cancer later in life. Additionally, radiologic imaging has been shown to be the largest contributor to the cost of hospitalization in patients with renal colic, with CT being the most expensive imaging modality.[9,10]

Ultrasound offers a safe, noninvasive means of assessing for renal colic that does not subject the patient to any ionizing radiation. Traditionally, ultrasound has been thought to have only fair sensitivity (37% to 64%) for detecting stones and better sensitivity (74% to 85%) for the diagnosis of acute obstruction,[1] whereas CT has consistently shown sensitivity greater than 90% for the diagnosis of ureteral stones.[1-4] Recent studies using modern ultrasound equipment in the hands of skilled operators have demonstrated comparable sensitivity (76% to 98%) of ultrasound for the detection of ureteral stones.[11-14] Although specific stone location and size cannot always be determined with ultrasound, surrogate findings may have prognostic value in guiding patient management. One study showed that normal renal ultrasound findings in the setting of suspected renal colic predicted a very low risk (0.6%) for subsequent urologic intervention.[15]

The goal of bedside ultrasound is to identify unilateral hydronephrosis as an indirect sign of obstructing ureteral

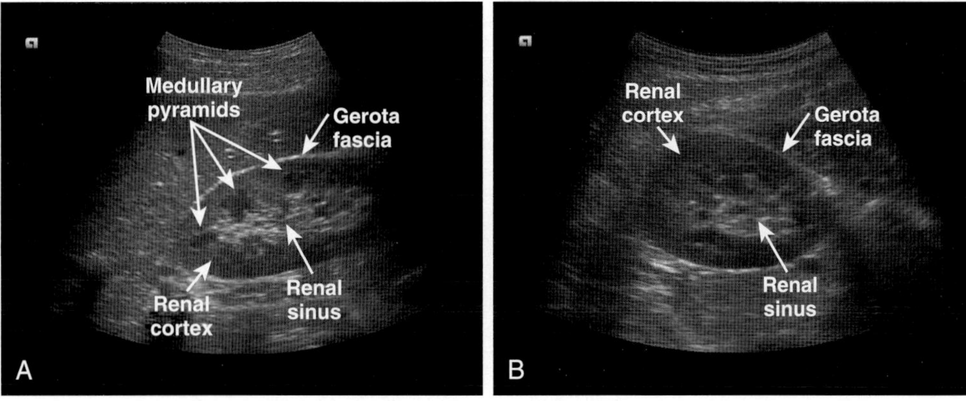


**Fig. 115.1** Longitudinal (A) and transverse (B) images of the kidney.

stones. In the emergency department setting, Rosen et al. demonstrated a sensitivity of 72% and specificity of 73% for the detection of hydronephrosis with bedside ultrasound.[16] More recently, Gaspari and Horst reported a sensitivity of 87% and specificity of 85% for the diagnosis of hydronephrosis.[17] These results are comparable to a sensitivity of 81% and specificity of 92% for bedside ultrasound performed by on-call urologists; however, this study evaluated other renal findings in addition to hydronephrosis.[18] Although the specific size of the obstructing stone is not typically demonstrated on bedside ultrasound, the degree of hydronephrosis may correlate with the size of the obstructing stone. A 2010 study showed that no or mild hydronephrosis predicted smaller stone size (<5 mm) as opposed to moderate or severe hydronephrosis.[19]

Bedside ultrasound for the measurement of urinary bladder volume has been well described in the literature. Bedside ultrasound provides a quantitative assessment of bladder volume when evaluating for urinary retention in the emergency department setting and can guide the need for emergency catheterization.[20,21] Many studies have shown good correlation between sonographic bladder volume calculations and urine volumes obtained via catheterization.[22-24] In the pediatric population, ultrasound has been shown to predict patients with volumes sufficient for successful catheterization of urine samples (>3 mL).[25-28] This may help avoid multiple attempts at urinary catheterization, which can result in unnecessary patient discomfort and the potential for iatrogenic infection. Additionally, bedside ultrasound has demonstrated increased success rates during attempts at suprapubic aspiration when compared with traditional, landmark-based techniques.[29-31]

## HOW TO SCAN

Emergency renal ultrasonography is performed with a 2- to 5-MHz curvilinear transducer. When rib shadows limit adequate sonographic windows for the kidneys, switching to a phased-array probe may be helpful. In general, patients can be positioned supine for renal ultrasound. The right lateral recumbent position may be necessary when imaging the left kidney because this kidney tends to be located more posteriorly and the spleen is not as large an acoustic window as the liver.

For the right kidney, the probe is initially placed along the lower portion of the rib cage in the midaxillary line with the probe marker directed toward the patient's head. The resulting coronal view is the traditional right upper quadrant view of the focused assessment with sonography for trauma (FAST) examination. The kidney lies in a plane oblique to the long axis of the body, and the probe usually needs to be rotated slightly counterclockwise to obtain a maximally longitudinal view of the kidney (**Fig. 115.1,** *A*). This orientation also helps the ultrasound transducer align the image in between the ribs, thus minimizing rib shadows. The transducer should then be angled anterior to posterior so that it fans through the entire kidney. To obtain a transverse view of the kidney, the probe is rotated 90 degrees in a counterclockwise direction (Fig. 115.1, *B*). The transducer should then be fanned superior to inferior to image the entire kidney in the transverse plane.

For the left kidney, the probe is initially placed along the lower part of the rib cage in the posterior axillary line with the probe marker directed toward the patient's head. The resulting coronal view is the traditional left upper quadrant view of the FAST examination. The transducer often needs to be moved relatively posterior and superior with respect to the right side to obtain adequate views of the left kidney. The spleen is not as large an acoustic window as the liver, and bowel gas from the stomach and colon may interfere with images of the left kidney. When a satisfactory sonographic window is located, the probe should be rotated slightly clockwise to maximize the longitudinal view of the kidney and align the transducer in between the ribs. The transducer should then be angled anterior to posterior to fan through the entire kidney. To obtain a transverse view of the kidney, the probe is rotated 90 degrees in a counterclockwise direction. The transducer should then be fanned superior to inferior to image the entire kidney in the transverse plane.

To image the urinary bladder, the transducer is placed in the midline above the symphysis pubis with the probe marker directed toward the patient's head. The resulting sagittal view is the traditional pelvic view of the FAST examination. The transducer should then be moved or angled to the right and left to image the entire bladder. To obtain a transverse view

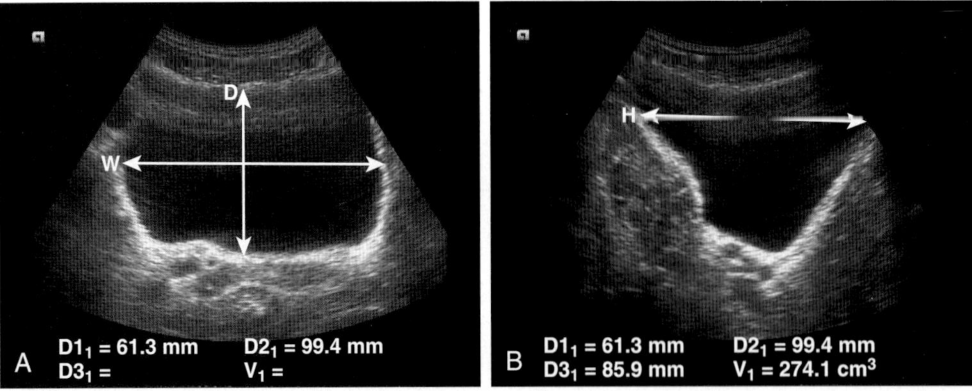


**Fig. 115.2 Transverse (A) and sagittal (B) images of the urinary bladder with bladder dimension measurements.** *D*, Depth; *H*, height; *V*, volume; *W*, width.

of the bladder, the probe is rotated 90 degrees counterclockwise so that the probe points toward the patient's right. The transducer should then be moved or angled superior and inferior to image the entire bladder.

When measuring urinary bladder volume, the bladder should first be imaged in the transverse plane at the level where the largest view of the bladder is obtained. The image is frozen, and bladder depth and width are measured (**Fig. 115.2,** *A*). The bladder is then imaged in the sagittal plane, again at the level where the largest view of the bladder is obtained. The image is frozen, and bladder height is measured (Fig. 115.2, *B*). Bladder volume can be estimated with the simplified formula 0.75 × depth × width × height.[20-22] On many ultrasound machines, software will automatically calculate bladder volume by using measurements obtained by the sonographer.

## IMAGES—NORMAL AND ABNORMAL

The kidneys are paired, bean-shaped retroperitoneal structures that lie slightly oblique to the long axis of the body. A normal kidney measures 9 to 12 cm in length and is between 4 and 5 cm in width. A difference of up to 2 cm in measurements between the right and left kidney is considered within the normal range. On longitudinal images, the kidney will appear oval in shape (see Fig. 115.1, *A*); on transverse images, the kidney will appear circular (see Fig. 115.1, *B*).

The kidneys consist of a renal cortex, medullary pyramids, and renal sinus (see Fig. 115.1). The renal cortex has a homogeneous sonographic appearance and is slightly less echogenic than normal liver and spleen. The medullary pyramids may or may not be well visualized on bedside sonography. They appear as multiple hypoechoic cone-shaped structures between the renal sinus and cortex, with their apices directed toward the renal sinus. The renal sinus appears hyperechoic because of its fibrous and fatty tissue content. The renal collecting system, which consists of the renal pelvis and multiple calices, resides within the renal sinus. The kidney is surrounded by a hyperechoic fibrous capsule (Gerota fascia), as well as perinephric fat.

Hydronephrosis is manifested as varying degrees of dilation of the collecting system as a result of distal obstruction. It is best visualized on longitudinal images of the kidney. Hydronephrosis may be graded as mild, moderate, or severe. Mild hydronephrosis is defined as dilation of the renal pelvis and blunting of the normally concave renal calices. Anechoic areas will appear in the normally hyperechoic renal sinus as fluid fills and distends the renal pelvis (**Fig. 115.3,** *A*). Mild hydronephrosis may be difficult to appreciate on bedside ultrasound. Careful comparison with the contralateral kidney can help reveal more subtle cases of unilateral hydronephrosis. Prominent renal vessels within the renal sinus may be mistaken for mild hydronephrosis. Application of color flow or power Doppler can help differentiate whether an anechoic space within the renal sinus is due to blood vessels or actual dilation of the renal pelvis. Moderate hydronephrosis is defined as more prominent dilation of the renal pelvis and rounding of the renal calices (Fig. 115.3, *B*). Severe hydronephrosis is defined as extreme calyceal distention causing thinning of the renal cortex (Fig. 115.3, *C*). When chronic, hydronephrosis can result in a marked degree of cortical atrophy. In the setting of acute obstruction, calyceal rupture may occur and result in a urinoma. A urinoma appears as a stripe of anechoic free fluid surrounding a portion of the kidney.

Kidney stones appear as brightly echogenic structures and will exhibit posterior acoustic shadowing when sufficient size has been attained.[3,5] Obstructing ureteral stones are not typically visualized directly during bedside ultrasonography. Nonobstructing stones within the renal pelvis are more frequently visualized, although they may be hard to distinguish from adjacent hyperechoic fibrofatty tissue within the renal sinus. Obstructing stones may occasionally be visualized at the ureteropelvic or ureterovesical junction. Obstructing stones within the remainder of the ureter are more challenging to identify because of overlying bowel gas. The ureters themselves are not discernible during bedside ultrasonography unless significantly dilated.

Renal cysts appear as rounded anechoic structures with thin, smooth walls and exhibit posterior acoustic enhancement (**Fig. 115.4**). Though not a primary indication for performing emergency renal sonography, renal cysts are not an uncommon finding and occur in roughly 50% of patients 50 years or older.[32] When internal echoes, septations, or thick walls are visualized, other diagnoses, such as a hemorrhagic cyst, renal

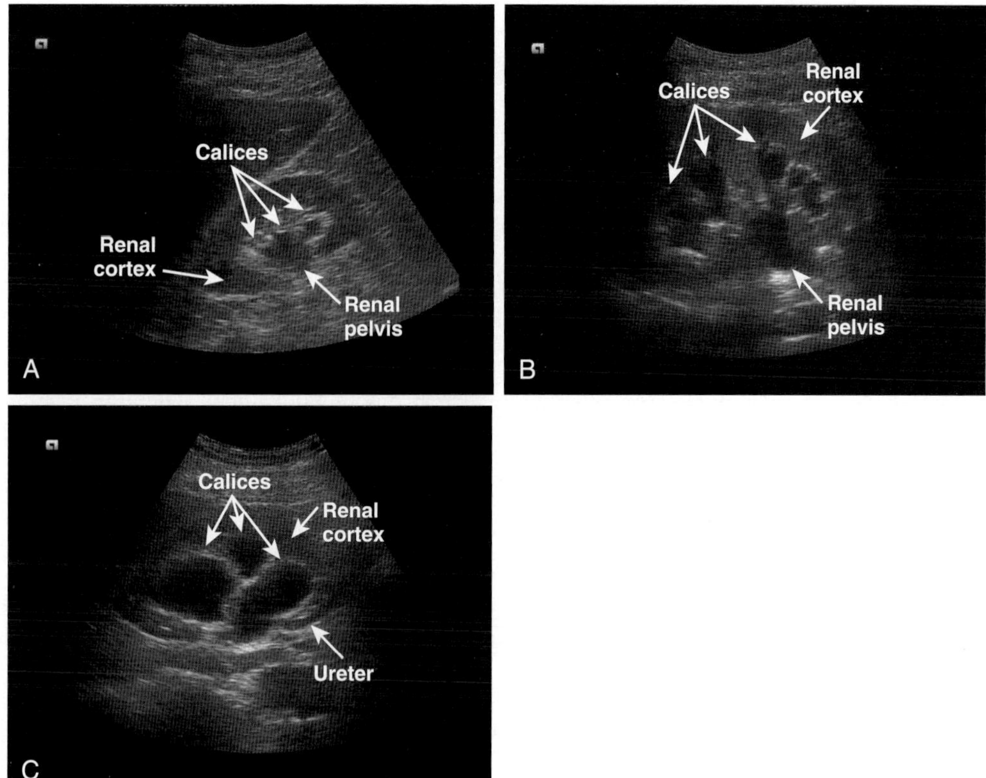


**Fig. 115.3** Longitudinal images of the kidney demonstrating mild (A), moderate (B), and severe (C) hydronephrosis.

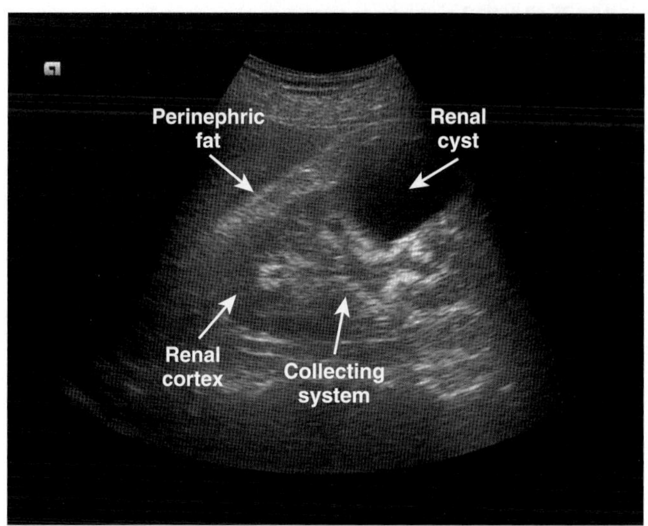


**Fig. 115.4** Longitudinal image of the kidney demonstrating a simple renal cyst.

abscess, or carcinoma, are more likely. Making these diagnoses is outside the scope of bedside ultrasonography, and such findings should prompt comprehensive radiologic imaging. Additionally, any structure that distorts the normal renal architecture is concerning for malignancy. Renal cancers and pseudoaneurysms may have an appearance similar to simple renal cysts,[33] and it is recommended that color flow or power Doppler be applied to evaluate for internal blood flow within any cystic structure seen in the kidneys.

## HOW TO INCORPORATE INTO PRACTICE

Ultrasound serves as a valuable initial screening examination in patients suspected of having renal colic. It can be performed directly at the bedside by the emergency physician to rapidly categorize the likelihood of an obstructing ureteral stone. Though not specifically studied in the setting of renal colic, bedside ultrasound has been shown to expedite patient care and decrease length of stay in the emergency department when performing other focused studies.[34,35] Bedside ultrasound may also speed the identification of life-threatening conditions such as a leaking AAA when being considered in the differential diagnosis.[36]

In patients with clinical findings suggestive of renal colic, especially in those with microscopic or gross hematuria, the presence of unilateral hydronephrosis may be adequate evidence of a ureteral stone. If findings on the initial bedside ultrasound are normal, it may be repeated after a period of hydration, which can subsequently reveal hydronephrosis. When mild to moderate hydronephrosis is identified as a surrogate for an obstructing ureteral stone, the patient may undergo standard treatment of renal colic. When severe hydronephrosis is seen as a new finding, comprehensive imaging by radiology and urgent urologic consultation are advised.[20,21]

Ultrasound may be especially helpful in patients with known renal colic who have recurrent or worsening pain. In these patients, in whom the diagnosis of renal colic has already been established, ultrasound is an excellent tool to screen for significant obstruction and assess for complications of obstructing stones, such as calyceal rupture and resultant urinoma. In comparison, patients with complicating comorbid conditions such as a solitary kidney, known abdominal or pelvic tumor, or recent instrumentation should not be assessed solely with bedside ultrasound. These patients are more likely to have ureteral obstruction unrelated to renal colic, and the presence of unilateral hydronephrosis should not be interpreted as a surrogate for ureteral stones. Of note, mild unilateral (commonly on the right) or bilateral hydronephrosis may be a normal finding during pregnancy because the enlarging uterus exerts a mass effect on the ureter.

Bilateral hydronephrosis carries a completely distinct differential diagnosis and is rarely due to kidney stones. Identification of unilateral hydronephrosis should always prompt an evaluation of the contralateral kidney to rule out the presence of bilateral hydronephrosis. Bilateral hydronephrosis is typically caused by bladder outlet obstruction. In men, bladder outlet obstruction most commonly results from prostate enlargement. Neurogenic bladder, obstructing bladder clot, and prolonged urinary retention of any origin also may lead to bilateral hydronephrosis. Ultrasound evaluation of the bladder should always follow when bilateral hydronephrosis is identified.

Bedside ultrasound serves as a straightforward examination for the presence of a distended bladder when urinary retention is clinically suspected. A grossly enlarged bladder after the patient attempts to void indicates the need for urinary catheterization. In contrast, a collapsed bladder in the setting of suspected urinary retention should prompt a search for alternative diagnoses. Intermediate bladder sizes necessitate calculation of bladder volume with sonographic measurements. Although threshold values for what constitutes an elevated postvoid residual urine volume are poorly defined,[37] a volume greater than 100 mL in the setting of symptoms of obstruction (urgency, frequency, hesitancy, decreased flow) is generally used as the lower threshold for acute urinary retention.[38] It is important to remember that urinary retention, especially when prolonged, may lead to bilateral hydronephrosis, and ultrasound evaluation of the kidneys should reflexively follow identification of a distended bladder.

In the pediatric population, bedside ultrasound may guide the timing of urinary catheterization. Attempts at catheterization are unsuccessful in obtaining urine from pediatric patients approximately 25% of the time.[25-27] A brief ultrasound evaluation of the bladder identifies patients with urine volumes adequate for collecting a urine sample via catheterization. A transverse bladder dimension larger than 2 cm and a sonographic bladder volume calculation of greater than 3 mL both predict successful urinary catheterization.[25-27] In cases in which suprapubic bladder aspiration is indicated to obtain a urine sample, ultrasound provides procedural guidance and increases the rate of successful bladder taps.[29-31]

In summary, bedside ultrasound is a rapid, noninvasive imaging modality useful for the evaluation of flank pain. It may identify hydronephrosis as a surrogate finding in patients with renal colic and can be used to exclude AAA from the differential diagnosis. Ultrasound can also assist in the diagnosis of urinary obstruction and provide guidance for the timing of urinary catheterization in children. Emergency renal sonography is a focused application that must be interpreted within the clinical context of the patient's signs and symptoms. Patients with findings outside the scope of the bedside ultrasound examination should be referred for consultative radiologic imaging.

## REFERENCES

***References can be found on Expert Consult @ www.expertconsult.com.***

# Dialysis-Related Emergencies 116

*Yi-Mei Chng and Gregory H. Gilbert*

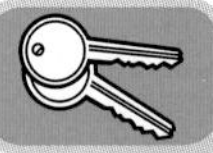

**KEY POINTS**

- Infection is a common cause of morbidity and mortality in dialysis patients. Tunneled lines and temporary dialysis catheters are more likely to become infected than grafts and native arteriovenous fistulas.
- The differential diagnosis of hemodynamic instability in a hemodialysis patient is dependent on the associated signs or symptoms (e.g., fever, chest pain), as well as the duration and speed of onset of the instability.
- Early vascular surgery consultation is necessary for patients with clotted hemodialysis access.
- Peritonitis is a common infection associated with peritoneal dialysis. Turbidity is one of the earliest signs of infection.
- Empiric treatment of peritoneal dialysis–associated peritonitis should include intraperitoneal antibiotics with both gram-positive and gram-negative coverage.

## SCOPE

In the United States, in excess of 380,000 patients with renal failure rely on some form of dialysis as life-sustaining renal replacement therapy. More than 90% of these patients are managed with hemodialysis, whereas about 7% use peritoneal dialysis (PD).[1] The most common complication associated with either dialysis modality is infection, although many access site malfunctions and dialysis-related emergencies prompt visits to the emergency department (ED) by this population.

## HEMODIALYSIS

## STRUCTURE AND FUNCTION

Hemodialysis can be performed through native arteriovenous (AV) fistulas, prosthetic AV grafts composed of polytetrafluoroethylene, tunneled (PermCath) central venous catheters, and nontunneled (temporary) central venous catheters. Different modalities offer different advantages.

Connecting an artery (usually in the forearm) directly to a vein via surgery creates a native AV fistula (**Fig. 116.1**). Over months, the increased blood flow creates a larger, stronger vein with adequate blood flow for dialysis. Native AV fistulas are less likely than other forms of hemodialysis access to become infected or form clots.

Synthetic AV grafts (**Fig. 116.2**) are used when forearm veins are unsuitable for native grafts. Synthetic grafts can be used within weeks of placement; however, they have higher infection and clotting rates than native AV fistulas do.

Central venous catheters (**Fig. 116.3**) are used when dialysis access is needed before permanent AV grafts have had time to mature or when fistula or graft surgery fails. Approximately 25% of the hemodialysis patients in the United States use central venous catheters as their primary vascular access. Tunneled, cuffed catheters have a lower infection rate than nontunneled catheters do. All these catheters have a double lumen and are at higher risk for infection and clotting than AV fistulas or grafts are.

## COMPLICATIONS

### INFECTION

Infectious complications are among the foremost causes of morbidity and mortality in hemodialysis patients. The risk for infection results from both impaired immune function related to the renal failure (e.g., altered granulocyte function in uremia) and repetitive access of the vasculature across the protective skin barrier. Vascular access is the source of bacteremia in 48% to 73% of infected hemodialysis patients.[2]

Clinical findings may include fever, hypotension, altered mental status, skin infection at the access site, and severe sepsis. Patients with diabetes may have ketoacidosis. The differential diagnosis of the various clinical findings in hemodialysis patients is described in **Table 116.1**.

Antimicrobial therapy for potential infections related to hemodialysis access (whether catheter or graft) should cover gram-positive species, including methicillin-resistant *Staphylococcus aureus* (MRSA) and gram-negative species. Gram-positive species account for up to two thirds of cases of hemodialysis access–related bacteremia. *Enterococcus* and gram-negative rods are also frequently implicated. Broad-spectrum antibiotic coverage should be initiated empirically until the results of culture are available, especially in patients

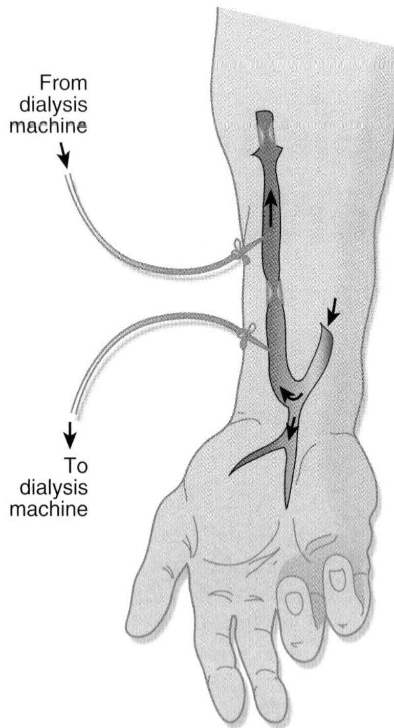


Fig. 116.1 Native arteriovenous graft.

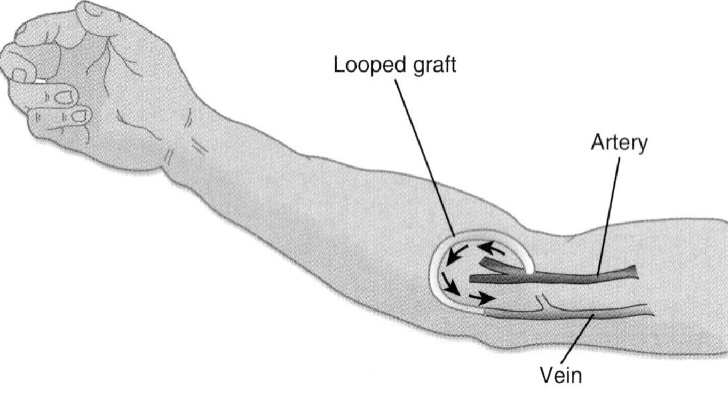


Fig. 116.2 Arteriovenous graft.

**Table 116.1 Differential Diagnosis of Various Clinical Findings in Hemodialysis Patients**

| CLINICAL FINDING | DIFFERENTIAL DIAGNOSIS AND CRITICAL ACTIONS |
|---|---|
| Hypotension | If accompanied by fever, consider sepsis.<br>If sudden onset during dialysis, consider hypovolemia secondary to excessive ultrafiltration, anaphylaxis or anaphylactoid reaction, or air embolism.<br>If accompanied by chest pain, consider tamponade, arrhythmia, or acute coronary syndrome. |
| Altered mental status | If onset immediately after first hemodialysis session, consider dialysis disequilibrium syndrome.<br>If the onset is gradual, consider dialysis dementia.<br>Infection is a common cause of altered mental status (delirium) in hemodialysis patients, and the presence of a fever should prompt antibiotic administration and a search for the source.<br>Also consider stroke, hypotension, drug effect, seizure, and metabolic derangement (acidosis, hyperkalemia). |
| Chest pain | Consider acute coronary syndrome, pulmonary embolism, air embolism, uremic pericarditis, and arrhythmias caused by electrolyte imbalance. |
| Shortness of breath | Consider fluid overload, cardiac tamponade, acute coronary syndrome, air embolism, and anaphylactoid reactions. |
| Bleeding | Bleeding can be due to excessive anticoagulation during dialysis or uremic coagulopathy. |
| Fever | Consider line infection in patients with warmth or erythema of the skin overlying the dialysis access site.<br>Consider sepsis if the patient is hypotensive or in shock; obtain blood for culture and administer antibiotics.<br>Fever is almost always due to infection, but overheated dialysate is a potential cause. |

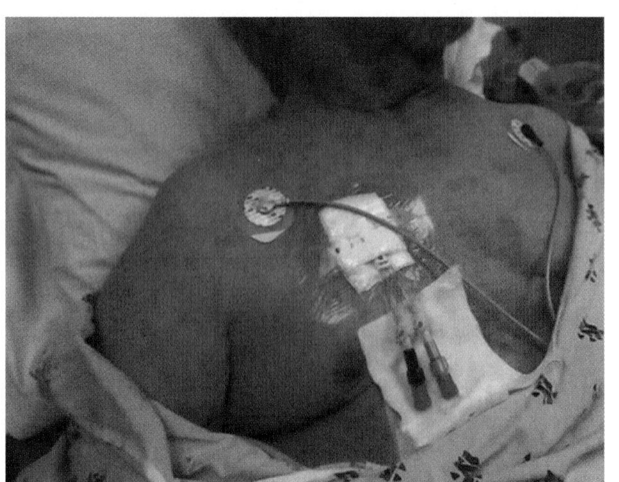

Fig. 116.3 Tunneled central venous catheter.

who have a history of gram-negative bacteremia or who may be septic from a secondary source. The recommended regimen is 1 g of vancomycin intravenously (with sequential doses according to the level of the drug at dialysis) plus gram-negative coverage with either an aminoglycoside or a third-generation cephalosporin.

Removal or exchange of an infected catheter is advisable because a bacterial biofilm can form rapidly in the lumens of most indwelling central venous catheters and serve as a source of continued infection. Systemic antibiotics given alone are relatively ineffective in eradicating infection if the catheter is not removed. There are occasional protocols that have demonstrated catheter salvation, but none have done so reliably. Catheter removal with delayed replacement is required in patients who are clinically unstable, who have metastatic infectious complications, or who have tunnel infections.[3] Tunneled catheters can be replaced with temporary nontunneled catheters or can be changed over a guidewire, thus avoiding disruption of the patient's dialysis schedule.

## THROMBOSIS

Thrombosis of hemodialysis access grafts and catheters is a significant cause of morbidity. Failure of hemodialysis grafts is mainly due to progressive intimal hyperplasia at the venous anastomosis and resultant decreased flow and graft thrombosis.[4]

Signs and symptoms of impending graft thrombosis include loss of the thrill or bruit, increased water-hammer pulses, increased venous pressure, and poor flow rates.

Success of treatment decreases with time. A vascular surgeon should be consulted immediately for definitive treatment with thrombectomy (percutaneous or surgical) or surgical revision. To avoid rupture or distal embolization, the access site should not be forcibly irrigated or manipulated.

Thrombolytic agents can be initiated in consultation with a vascular surgeon. Several different thrombolytic regimens can be used. One protocol involves the use of 2 to 4 mg of alteplase infused through an 18- to 22-gauge intravenous line while waiting for the availability of angiography. If the wait time exceeds 30 minutes, an additional 2 mg is given.[5] Care must be taken to confirm that the intravenous tubing has actually been inserted into the graft pointing toward the occlusion and not into surrounding tissue or another vessel before infusion of the thrombolytic agent. The arterial limb of the graft should also be occluded while the thrombolytic agent is being infused.

## BLEEDING

Bleeding from dialysis puncture sites or around tunneled catheters can occur hours after hemodialysis is complete. Bleeding from needle hole punctures can usually can be controlled with firm (but nonocclusive) direct pressure on the site. A thrill should be documented after the bleeding stops in peripheral hemodialysis grafts. Surgicel may be placed around the entry port of a tunneled catheter to promote hemostasis. Patients should be evaluated for significant blood loss and observed in the ED to ensure that rebleeding does not occur. If the bleeding cannot be controlled or if skin erosion has occurred, a vascular surgeon should be consulted.

Hemodialysis patients are at risk for hemorrhage from other sites because of anticoagulation during dialysis. Platelet dysfunction secondary to uremia also contributes to hemorrhage in patients with renal failure, and it is only partially corrected by hemodialysis. Administration of desmopressin (DDAVP) (0.3 mcg/kg intravenously with 50 mL saline over a 3-minute period, 0.3 mcg/kg subcutaneously, or 2 mcg/kg intranasally) improves the hemostatic function of platelets and is useful in treating hemorrhage in hemodialysis patients. The maximal effect of DDAVP occurs after 1 hour, and if immediate hemostasis is needed, 10 units of cryoprecipitate can be infused over a 30-minute period.[4]

## PSEUDOANEURYSM

Pseudoaneurysms are more likely to occur with prosthetic grafts, but they can also develop with autogenous access. Duplex ultrasound can be used to distinguish between pseudoaneurysms and other perigraft fluid collections. Small puncture site pseudoaneurysms can sometimes be monitored, but pseudoaneurysms at the anastomosis of the graft require surgical or endovascular revision and are often associated with infection. Vascular surgery consultation is necessary for suspected pseudoaneurysms.[4]

## DIALYZER REACTIONS

Patients undergoing their first hemodialysis session or those switching to a new dialyzer may experience anaphylaxis or an anaphylactoid reaction to a component of the dialyzer or dialysate. Anaphylactoid reactions have been observed with dialyzers made of cuprophane and with polyacrylonitrile dialysis membranes (particularly in patients taking angiotensin-converting enzyme inhibitors). Treatment consists of epinephrine, antihistamines, and steroids.[6]

## AIR EMBOLISM

Venous air embolism is a rare complication of hemodialysis that can occur during a session or during insertion of (or more

**TIPS AND TRICKS**

**Use of Hemodialysis Graft or Catheter for Emergency Vascular Access**

Peripheral hemodialysis access sites may be used for placement of an intravenous catheter in an emergency when no other access is available:

- Do not use a tourniquet.
- Avoid puncturing the back wall of the vessel.
- Use a small intravenous catheter if possible.
- Secure all sources of intravenous access tightly. Infusions may need to be given under pressure because of the relatively high pressure within the peripheral graft.
- Apply firm but nonocclusive pressure for 10 to 15 minutes after removing the intravenous catheter. Ask a nurse experienced in hemodialysis for assistance with removal if available.
- Document the presence or absence of a thrill before and after the procedure.

Central venous hemodialysis access may also be used in an emergency when no other access is available:

- Either the red or blue port may be used because both lead to the vein (even though one is used to withdraw blood during hemodialysis and the other to return it). The "arterial" (red) port is proximal to the "venous" (blue) port to avoid recirculation during dialysis.
- Aspirate at least 2 mL from the port being used because it usually contains heparin between hemodialysis sessions.
- After use, contact a nurse experienced in hemodialysis to clear and prepare the catheter according to standard protocols.

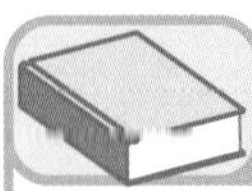

PATIENT TEACHING TIPS

**Hemodialysis**

Keep your access site clean and allow it to be used only for dialysis or emergency access.
Do not allow placement of a blood pressure cuff on your access arm.
Do not lift heavy objects or put pressure on your access arm.
Check the pulse (thrill) in your forearm access graft daily.

rarely during removal of) a tunneled venous catheter. Air enters the systemic venous system and is transported to the right heart and pulmonary arteries, thereby potentially leading to changes in gas exchange, cardiac arrhythmias, and death.

When air embolism is suspected, 100% oxygen is administered and the patient is intubated if necessary. The patient is placed in the Trendelenburg and left lateral decubitus positions in an attempt to trap air in the apex of the right ventricle and prevent migration to the pulmonary arterial system. Transfer to a hyperbaric chamber should be considered if the patient is stable. If the patient is unstable or suffering arrest, chest compressions may break up the air bubbles—aspiration of intracardiac air should be considered.

### CARDIAC TAMPONADE

Many dialysis patients have small pericardial effusions that are not clinically significant. Symptomatic cardiac tamponade can occur in these patients either as a result of an acute pericardial hemorrhage (possibly after heparin administration during hemodialysis) or as an exacerbation of volume overload in the setting of a preexisting effusion. Hemodynamically compromised patients with significant pericardial effusions confirmed by ultrasonography (particularly if right ventricular collapse in diastole is noted) may be treated with emergency pericardiocentesis if they are not sufficiently stable to be transferred for a pericardial window. Providers should be prepared for complications of hemorrhage in renal failure patients requiring pericardiocentesis.

### DIALYSIS DISEQUILIBRIUM SYNDROME

Dialysis disequilibrium syndrome is characterized by nausea, headache, malaise, vomiting, fatigue, and muscle cramps that occur during or immediately after hemodialysis. In severe cases, patients may exhibit altered mental status, seizures, or coma (although other probable causes of these altered mentation states should be excluded first before attributing such symptoms to dialysis disequilibrium syndrome).

The exact pathogenesis of the syndrome is unclear; it is believed to result from cerebral edema caused by shifts in osmolarity and pH during dialysis. Removal of small solutes such as urea from serum causes a rapid drop in serum osmolarity in the brain. This leads to the rapid ingress of free water, which results in cerebral edema.

The mainstay of treatment is prevention by avoiding rapid shifts in serum osmolarity during dialysis. Symptoms are usually self-limited and resolve within a few hours; severe cases can be treated by raising serum osmolarity with infusions of hyperosmolar solutions such as hypertonic saline or mannitol, in consultation with a nephrologist.[7,8]

### DIALYSIS DEMENTIA

Dialysis dementia is a form of dialysis-related encephalopathy that is associated with dyspraxia and multifocal seizures. Unlike dialysis disequilibrium syndrome, dialysis dementia is slowly progressive in onset and generally occurs in patients who have been undergoing hemodialysis for at least 2 years. There are three forms of dialysis dementia:

1. An epidemic form believed to be due to contamination of dialysate with aluminum, which is usually excreted by the kidneys (the use of deionized water in dialysis has decreased the incidence of this form)
2. A sporadic endemic form whose cause remains unclear
3. A pediatric form that occurs in children with renal failure even when they have not yet undergone dialysis (this may be related to exposure to aluminum-containing medications)

Seizures in the ED should be treated with benzodiazepines; a serum aluminum level should be obtained in addition to performance of other standard laboratory tests if dialysis dementia is suspected (see Table 116.1).

## PERITONEAL DIALYSIS

### STRUCTURE AND FUNCTION

PD can be performed in a number of different ways; however, the complications associated with the various methods are similar. Typically, PD is performed with a Tenckhoff catheter (it can be straight or curved, single or dual cuffed) inserted in a median or paramedian line with or without omentectomy. Omentectomy is associated with fewer complications. The dialysate is infused into the abdomen via either a pump or gravity. It remains in the abdomen for a period, known as the dwell time, long enough to allow osmosis and diffusion. The effluent (or dialysate after dwelling in the abdomen) is then drained (**Fig. 116.4**).[9]

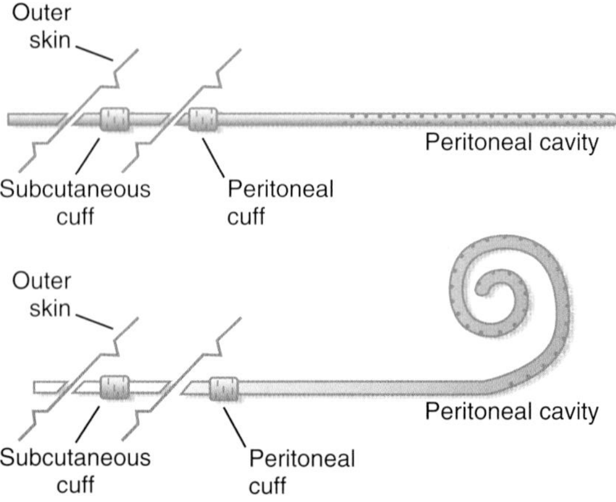


**Fig. 116.4 Peritoneal dialysis catheters.**

**BOX 116.1 Complications of Peritoneal Dialysis (In Order of Frequency)**

**Mechanical**
Catheter dislodgment
Catheter malfunction
Leakage, hernias, effusions

**Infectious**
Peritonitis
Cellulitis, tunnel infection
Abscess

**Medical**
Malnutrition, hypoalbuminemia
Bowel obstruction
Hyperglycemia

Data from U.S. Renal Data System, USRDS 2005 Annual Data Report. Atlas of end-stage renal disease in the United States. Bethesda, MD: National Institutes of Health, National Institute of Diabetes and Digestive and Kidney Diseases; 2005.

## COMPLICATIONS

Complications of PD are organized into three groups: mechanical, infectious, and medical (**Box 116.1**).

The most common and life-threatening complication is peritonitis, which causes the effluent to be turbid and cloudier than usual. This symptom should not be ignored. Patients are typically afebrile and otherwise well appearing. They do not have a rigid abdomen—instead, findings on physical examination are usually unimpressive, and the patient may at most complain of mild abdominal pain.

Peritonitis is usually the most common finding in patients with PD catheter malfunction, but other problems can arise.[1] Blood in the effluent suggests solid organ damage (especially if the catheter was placed recently), ruptured or leaking abdominal aortic aneurysm, or coagulopathy.

### MECHANICAL COMPLICATIONS

Mechanical complications are related to the process of dialysis and include pump malfunction (for patients maintained on continuous cyclic or intermittent dialysis); inability to instill the dialysate or failure of the effluent to drain because of catheter malfunction or dislodgment; or leakage of fluid into the groin, across the diaphragm, or out of the abdominal wall.

### INFECTIOUS COMPLICATIONS

Infectious complications include peritonitis, cellulitis at the catheter site, infection in the tunnel site itself, or intraabdominal abscesses.

### MEDICAL COMPLICATIONS

Most frequently, medical complications are related to nutrition. Hypoalbuminemia results from poor dietary intake and daily loss of 15 g of protein, which promotes infection by impairing normal immune function. Hyperglycemia occurs as a result of a large glucose load in the dialysate. Bowel obstruction can occur secondary to abdominal surgery.[10]

## DIFFERENTIAL DIAGNOSIS

Although peritonitis is the most common cause of fever and abdominal pain or tenderness in a PD patient, patients with other intraabdominal infections may also have these symptoms. Swelling in the groin or shortness of breath suggests leakage of the dialysate because of the high intraabdominal pressure associated with instilling 2 L of fluid. Common abdominal infections in patients undergoing PD reflect those in the general population: appendicitis, cholecystitis, pancreatitis, and small bowel obstruction.

## DIAGNOSTIC TESTING

### MECHANICAL COMPLICATIONS

Abdominal radiography is the most important modality. Radiographs confirm that the tube is placed correctly in the true pelvis, that no kinks are present, and that the tube has not broken into multiple pieces. Chest radiographs can reveal evidence of pleural effusion, and bowel obstruction is apparent on upright and lateral decubitus abdominal views. For suspected leaks, intraperitoneal water-soluble contrast material can be instilled to demonstrate communication with noted areas of swelling.

### INFECTIOUS COMPLICATIONS

Culture is critical when testing for infectious complications. PD-associated peritonitis is defined as two of the following three: (1) signs and symptoms; (2) white blood cell (WBC) count higher than 100/mL in the PD effluent, with more than 50% neutrophils after a dwell time of at least 2 hours; and (3) positive culture of an organism from the PD effluent.[11] For patients undergoing automated PD who are being evaluated during their nighttime treatment, the dwell time will not be 2 hours, so the percentage of neutrophils should be used for diagnostic purposes even if the absolute WBC count is not higher than 100/mL. Bacteria in the peritoneal cavity have been diluted significantly by the dialysate, which can lead to negative cultures at standard volumes. To improve diagnostic results, 50 mL of effluent should be centrifuged down and the sediment resuspended in 3 to 5 mL of sterile saline before inoculation into both solid and liquid blood culture media. Alternatively, a minimum of 10 mL of effluent per blood culture bottle can be used. Blood cultures are not helpful unless the patient appears septic.[12]

### MEDICAL COMPLICATIONS

A comprehensive metabolic panel and serum lipase level should be obtained. Liver function tests and serum lipase levels can differentiate other causes of abdominal pain. Albumin levels are useful markers of malnutrition, which is present in 40% of these patients (25% of whom are severely malnourished). Hypoalbuminemia significantly increases the incidence of morbidity and mortality, especially in patients with peritonitis and those with a serum albumin concentration lower than 35 g/L. Hypokalemia causes decreased gut motility and constipation, which is associated with peritonitis; both conditions should be treated. Hyperglycemia, inadequate dialysis, and volume depletion or overload can be evaluated by physical examination and standard laboratory testing.[10]

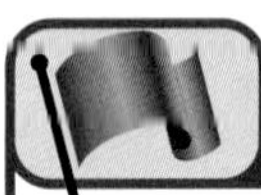

RED FLAGS

**Complications of Peritoneal Dialysis**
Fever
Vomiting
Severe abdominal tenderness
Known or suspected fungal infection
Cloudy or turbid effluent

## TREATMENT

### MECHANICAL COMPLICATIONS

Most complications require removal of the peritoneal catheter or some type of surgical repair; patients need to be switched to hemodialysis until the catheter malfunction is resolved.

For a clogged catheter, attempts to empty the bladder and then the bowel (with laxatives) may improve function. If the catheter is clogged with fibrin or clot, heparin (500 U/L) can be added to the dialysate. If this fails, urokinase can be used as a last resort (5000 IU diluted in saline), which has a success rate of 10% to 15%.[9]

For catheter leakage, the amount of dialysate infused is decreased to lower intraabdominal pressure; the patient will probably still need surgical repair for correction.

In patients with catheter migration, kinking, dislodgment, and cuff extrusion, a one-time 2-g intravenous dose of ampicillin should be given for prophylaxis in the setting of tube manipulation.[9]

### INFECTIOUS COMPLICATIONS

Gram-positive organisms account for three fourths of PD-associated infections, half of which are due to *Staphylococcus epidermidis*. Concerning organisms observed in infections are *Pseudomonas*, *S. aureus* (including MRSA), and fungal species.[11]

If the patient has had culture-positive results in the past, these results can help guide antibiotic therapy. Otherwise, empiric antibiotic therapy should cover gram-positive and gram-negative organisms based on local hospital sensitivities.

Intermittent or continuous antibiotic therapy can be used with continuous ambulatory peritoneal dialysis (**Table 116.2**). Dosing regimens are different for patients undergoing automated PD. For intermittent treatment, antibiotics are added to only one of the four daily exchanges. For continuous therapy, a loading dose is given in the first exchange and then a

**Table 116.2** Intraperitoneal Antibiotic Dosing Recommendations for Patients Undergoing Continuous Ambulatory Peritoneal Dialysis*

| ANTIBIOTIC | INTERMITTENT | CONTINUOUS† |
|---|---|---|
| **Aminoglycosides** | | |
| Amikacin | 2 mg/kg | LD 25, MD 12 |
| Gentamicin, netilmicin, or tobramycin | 0.6 mg/kg | LD 8, MD 4 |
| **Cephalosporins** | | |
| Cefazolin, cephalothin, or cephradine | 15 mg/kg | LD 500, MD 125 |
| Cefepime | 1000 mg | LD 500, MD 125 |
| Ceftazidime | 1000-1500 mg | LD 500, MD 125 |
| Ceftizoxime | 1000 mg | LD 250, MD 125 |
| **Penicillins** | | |
| Amoxicillin | ND | LD 250-500, MD 50 |
| Ampicillin, oxacillin, or nafcillin | ND | MD 125 |
| Azlocillin | ND | LD 500, MD 250 |
| Penicillin G | ND | LD 50,000 units, MD 25,000 units |
| **Quinolones** | | |
| Ciprofloxacin | ND | LD 50, MD 25 |
| **Others** | | |
| Aztreonam | ND | LD 1000, MD 250 |

maintenance dose is given in each exchange for the remainder of the course of treatment.[12]

One suggested regimen is cefazolin (15 mg/kg/day intraperitoneally [IP]) for intermittent treatment, or for continuous therapy administer a 500-mg loading dose with 125-mg maintenance doses. For gram-negative coverage, an antibiotic that also treats *Pseudomonas* infection should be given, such as ceftazidime (1000 to 1500 mg/day IP), or for continuous therapy use a 500-mg loading dose and 125-mg maintenance doses. If MRSA infection is suspected, vancomycin (15 to 30 mg/kg) can be added to the dialysate and should be used in place of cefazolin.[12] Of note, vancomycin and ceftazidime must be mixed in a dialysate solution of greater than 1 L to be compatible. Aminoglycosides should not be mixed with penicillins in an intraperitoneal infusion.[11]

Doses for renally excreted drugs should be increased by 25% if the patient produces more than 100 mL of urine per day.[12]

Fungal infections may occur after antibiotic treatment. They require early removal of the catheter and are associated with a mortality of 25%.[12]

Exit site infections should be treated with oral antibiotics except in some cases of MRSA.[11] Therapy is guided by Gram stain of the purulent drainage and by previous treatment regimens, although *S. aureus, S. epidermidis*, and *Pseudomonas aeruginosa* are responsible for the majority of infections. For first-time infections, immediate empiric antibiotic treatment of gram-positive organisms should be initiated (cephalexin, 500 mg orally two to three times daily). Suspected MRSA infections should be treated with vancomycin, clindamycin, Bactrim, or rifampin (do not use rifampin as monotherapy). Patients with MRSA infections may also be given intranasal and local mupirocin (cream, not ointment, because the polyethylene glycol in the ointment can damage the polyurethane in some PD catheters) twice a day for 5 to 7 days. Suspected pseudomonal infections should be treated with quinolones, although double therapy in accordance with local susceptibility patterns is recommended because of the rapid rise of resistance.[11] The duration of treatment is at least 2 weeks for gram-positive organisms and 3 weeks for pseudomonal organisms.

### MEDICAL COMPLICATIONS

Management of most medical complications in PD patients is similar to that in the general population. Hyperglycemia can be treated with intraperitoneal insulin, but at higher doses.[11] Hypokalemia should be treated aggressively because it leads to constipation and risk for peritonitis. Hypoalbuminemia should be managed with protein supplements and education of the patient. In severe cases, total parenteral nutrition or intravenous albumin (or both) may be necessary.[10]

## DISPOSITION

### MECHANICAL COMPLICATIONS

Patients can be safely discharged home if dialysate goes in, effluent comes out, and no signs of infection are present. If a patient is unable to use the PD catheter, hospital admission

**Table 116.2 Intraperitoneal Antibiotic Dosing Recommendations for Patients Undergoing Continuous Ambulatory Peritoneal Dialysis—cont'd**

| ANTIBIOTIC | INTERMITTENT | CONTINUOUS† |
|---|---|---|
| Daptomycin | ND | LD 100, MD 20 |
| Linezolid | 200-300 mg/day orally | |
| Teicoplanin | 15 mg/kg | LD 400, MD 20 |
| Vancomycin | 15-30 mg/kg every 5-7 days | LD 1000, MD 25 |
| **Antifungals** | | |
| Amphotericin | NA | 1.5 mg/L |
| Fluconazole | 200 mg IP every 24-48 hr | |
| **Combinations** | | |
| Ampicillin-sulbactam | 2 g every 12 hr | LD 1000, MD 100 |
| Imipenem-cilastin | 1 g bid | LD 250, MD 50 |
| Quinupristin-dalfopristin | 25 mg/L in alternate bags‡ | |
| Trimethoprim-sulfamethoxazole | 960 mg orally bid | |

*bid*, Two times per day; *IP*, intraperitoneally; *LD*, loading dose; *MD*, maintenance dose; *NA*, not applicable; *ND*, no data.

*For dosing of drugs with renal clearance in patients with residual renal function (defined as >100 mL/day of urine output), the dose should be empirically increased by 25%.

†Per exchange, once daily (mg/L; all exchanges).

‡Given in conjunction with 500 mg intravenously twice daily.

and scheduling for hemodialysis in consultation with a nephrologist are necessary.

## INFECTIOUS COMPLICATIONS

The majority of patients with peritonitis are stable and can be treated at home. Those with fever, vomiting, intractable pain, fungal infection, or concomitant catheter site infection and those refractory to outpatient treatment require hospital admission. Discharge and urgent follow-up should be arranged with the team that placed the catheter and with the patient's nephrologist.[1]

## MEDICAL COMPLICATIONS

The disposition of patients with medical complications depends on the severity of the specific disease process. Nutritional problems can usually be managed with patient education and close outpatient follow-up.

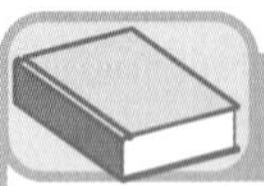

### PATIENT TEACHING TIPS

**Peritoneal Dialysis**

Wear loose clothing.

Do not submerge yourself in unchlorinated water (baths, rivers, lakes).

Avoid heavy lifting and abdominal exercise.

Wash your hands and peritoneal dialysis site with antibacterial soap.

## SUGGESTED READINGS

Himmelfarb J. Hemodialysis complications. Am J Kidney Dis 2005;45:1122-31.

Nassar GM, Ayus JC. Infectious complications of the hemodialysis access. Kidney Int 2001;60:1-13.

Padberg FT, Calligaro KD, Sidawy AN. Complications of arteriovenous hemodialysis access: recognition and management. J Vasc Surg 2008;48:55S-80S.

## REFERENCES

***References can be found on Expert Consult @ www.expertconsult.com.***

# Renal Transplant Complications 117

*Gerald Maloney*

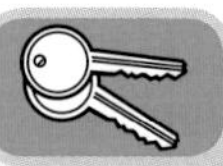

**KEY POINTS**

- Renal transplantation is highly successful. With appropriate immunosuppressive therapy, the rate of acute rejection during the first posttransplant year is less than 25%; 1-year survival rates approach 100%.
- Surgical complications that may be seen in the emergency department include hematoma formation, ureteral anastomotic leak, and ureteral obstruction. Computed tomography is the diagnostic imaging modality of choice for these surgical emergencies.
- Surgical infections that are common in the first posttransplant month include pneumonia, line sepsis, and wound infection. Opportunistic infections reach their peak incidence during the remainder of the first posttransplant year. After the first year, community-acquired infections predominate.
- Renal transplant patients have a high risk for atherosclerotic disease. Cardiovascular conditions account for 30% to 50% of deaths during the first posttransplant year.
- Fluoroquinolones and macrolides may increase levels of cyclosporine and tacrolimus; these antibiotic classes should not be used as first-line agents for the treatment of patients with posttransplant pneumonia.
- Fever and tenderness over the graft site may indicate acute rejection.
- Transplant recipients treated with corticosteroid therapy have functional adrenal insufficiency and require pulse doses of corticosteroids when they encounter physiologic stress.

## EPIDEMIOLOGY

The kidney is the most commonly transplanted solid organ. According to the U.S. Organ Procurement and Transplantation Network, more than 298,260 kidney transplants have been performed to date.[1] It is important that providers have a general understanding of the expected surgical and medical complications commonly observed in posttransplant patients.

## DEVELOPMENTS IN RENAL TRANSPLANTATIONS

The primary indication for renal transplantation is stage V chronic kidney disease (formerly called end-stage renal disease). Transplantation is recognized as the most effective form of renal replacement therapy for these patients.

Specific disease entities that causing chronic kidney disease are outlined in **Box 117.1**. Diabetic nephropathy is the most common single disease process leading to renal transplantation.[1]

Most renal grafts now function for longer than 10 years. The 1-year survival rate of renal transplant recipients is 95% to 98%. Renal transplants are more effective than hemodialysis at prolonging the life of patients with chronic kidney disease.[2]

Previously, the highest surgical success rates were achieved with histologically matched donor kidneys from a living recipient. Advances in immunosuppressive medication regimens have improved the success rate of cadaveric kidney transplantation, which now approaches that seen with living donors.

Preoperative clearance for renal transplantation is extensive. For patients with cancer, the suggested disease-free interval before transplantation is 5 years. Infection with human immunodeficiency virus is considered a contraindication to renal transplantation in many institutions, although transplantation has been successful in many patients with well-maintained CD4+ T-cell counts.

Cholecystectomy was previously performed in all patients undergoing renal transplantation. Currently, cholecystectomy is performed only in patients with evidence of cholelithiasis or cholecystitis.

The surgical approach to renal transplantation varies with the age of the patient, as well as with the location of the kidney and the anastomosis. The recipient's native kidneys and collecting system are generally left in place unless there is another indication for nephrectomy. The donor kidney is placed in one of the lower abdominal quadrants (more commonly the right), and the ureter is anastomosed to the bladder; arterial and venous anastomoses generally arise from the iliac vessels, aorta, or inferior vena cava. The transplanted kidney is usually palpable on abdominal examination.

Immunosuppression is initiated after transplantation and is divided into two phases: induction and maintenance.[3] Agents such as tacrolimus and monoclonal and polyclonal antibodies are often included in the induction and maintenance phases of treatment (**Box 117.2**). With the use of immunosuppressive medications, the 1-year incidence of acute rejection is 15% to 25%.

## COMPLICATIONS

Complications of renal transplantation can be categorized by cause as either surgical or medical and further divided by time of occurrence as either early or delayed.

**BOX 117.1 Diseases Leading to Renal Transplantation**

Chronic kidney disease
Polycystic kidney disease
Trauma
Rapidly progressive glomerulonephritis
Toxic nephropathies

**BOX 117.2 Common Immunosuppressive Drugs Used in Renal Transplant Recipients**

Cyclosporine (Sandimmune, Neoral)
Tacrolimus (Prograf)
Azathioprine (Imuran)
Mycophenolate mofetil (CellCept)
Sirolimus (Rapamune)
Prednisone, methylprednisolone
Polyclonal antithymocyte globulin
Rituximab
Daclizumab

**BOX 117.3 Infections in Posttransplant Patients**

**First Month After Transplantation**

Typical postsurgical infections (pneumonia, urinary tract infection, line sepsis, wound infection)
Opportunistic infections uncommon

**Infections in the First Posttransplant Year**

Opportunistic infections (*Pneumocystis pneumoniae*, *Cryptococcus*, fungal infections, viral infections; highest incidence in months 2 to 6)
Cytomegalovirus (most common)
Tuberculosis

**Infections More Than 1 Year After Transplantation**

Community-acquired more common than opportunistic infections
Typical organisms causing cellulitis, pneumonia, urinary tract infections

## SURGICAL COMPLICATIONS

Surgical complications include graft malfunction, thrombosis, aneurysms of the graft vessels, and stricture or obstruction of the ureter. Some of these complications will be evident shortly after surgery; others may occur years after the procedure and cause symptoms that will probably prompt emergency department (ED) evaluation.

Graft function may be delayed in up to 30% of cadaveric transplants, probably as a result of prolonged cold ischemia of the kidney during the period between harvesting and transplantation.[4] Delayed graft function is a rare complication with living donor transplants. Patients may require continued dialysis until adequate posttransplant function is demonstrated.

Acute thrombosis of the arterial or venous anastomoses is usually seen within the first posttransplant week.[3,4] Treatment is surgical exploration in an attempt to salvage the donor kidney.

Renal artery stenosis has been reported in allografts and can cause hypertension in posttransplant patients. This is generally a delayed complication. Aneurysms of the graft vessels are uncommon, delayed events.

Hematomas may develop around the transplanted kidney. Hematoma formation may be an early postoperative complication or rarely may result from acute rejection with spontaneous rupture of the kidney.[4] Acute hematomas are surgical emergencies.

Ureteral complications include anastomotic leakage (generally within the first posttransplant month), acute ureteral obstruction, and lymphocele. These complications will occur within the first 3 months following transplantation. Computed tomography of the abdomen is the preferred imaging modality for ureteral complications. Ureteral obstruction often requires emergency surgical intervention.

## MEDICAL COMPLICATIONS

Medical complications are numerous and often subtle. Posttransplant patients are at risk for atypical infections, cardiovascular death, renal failure, and rejection. Adverse reactions from immunosuppressive medications account for many delayed medical complications in transplant patients.

### *Fever*

Management of fever in posttransplant patients should be approached similar to that of fever in other immunocompromised patients.[5] Because of suppressed immunologic and inflammatory responses, posttransplant patients may not exhibit the common findings of acute infection. Fever may or may not be associated with clinically significant infection.

Acute rejection is one cause of fever that may develop at any time. Decisions regarding appropriate diagnostic testing and disposition of a posttransplant patient with fever should be made in consultation with a transplant service.

### *Infections*

The incidence of infection in the first posttransplant year has been reported to be as high as 25% to 80%. Expected infections vary according to posttransplant time (**Box 117.3**). Infections in the first posttransplant month are typical postoperative infections—pneumonia, sepsis from central lines or urinary catheters, and wound infections.[3,5] Atypical or opportunistic infections are uncommon.

After the first month through the end of the first posttransplant year, opportunistic infections reach their peak incidence. A variety of atypical bacterial, viral, fungal, protozoal, and parasitic infections may occur. Individual transplant services maintain current information on the opportunistic infections seen in their institution. Cytomegalovirus is one of the most common opportunistic infections and occurs in up to 25% of renal transplant recipients.[5] It can cause systemic or invasive disease and is associated with acute rejection.

After the first year, the incidence of opportunistic infections decreases and typical community-acquired pathogens predominate.

Leukocytosis is a poorly sensitive and inconsistent indicator of the source of the fever, and therefore a normal white blood cell count should not be used to exclude a potential infectious illness in a transplant patient. Peritoneal findings

**BOX 117.4 Drug Interactions in Patients Taking Immunosuppressive Medications**

**Cyclosporine**

Levels increased (potential nephrotoxicity) by diltiazem, verapamil, azole antifungals, macrolides

Levels decreased (potential subtherapeutic levels and risk for rejection) by phenobarbital, phenytoin, carbamazepine, isonicotinic hydrazine (INH), rifampin, nafcillin

Aminoglycosides—can exacerbate nephrotoxicity

Statins—may predispose to hepatotoxicity or rhabdomyolysis; cyclosporine may increase statin levels

**Azathioprine**

Allopurinol—levels of azathioprine increased, which results in an increased risk for myelosuppression

may be minimal or absent in the presence of an acute intraabdominal catastrophe. As a result of the degree of immunosuppression, infections may follow a fulminant course.

## *Cardiovascular Emergencies*

Because the majority of renal transplant recipients in the United States have diabetes or hypertension (or both), the risk for concomitant cardiovascular disease is high. Furthermore, the combination of cyclosporine and corticosteroids worsens dyslipidemias and atherogenesis.[6] Cardiovascular disease accounts for 30% to 50% of deaths in the first posttransplant year, and the incidence of atherosclerotic vascular disease is up to five times greater in transplant recipients than in other hospitalized patients.[7]

The approach to diagnosis and management of suspected cardiac ischemia in the posttransplant population is similar that in the general population; however, higher-risk stratification for these patients is critical.

Varying degrees of hypertensive urgencies or emergencies may be seen in posttransplant patients. Likewise, patients may have acute or chronic dysrhythmias (e.g., chronic atrial fibrillation) unrelated to the transplant. Although no single antihypertensive or antidysrhythmic agent is contraindicated, care should be taken to avoid drug interactions (**Box 117.4**).

## *Pulmonary Emergencies*

Pneumonia remains the most common pulmonary emergency in transplant recipients.[8] The causative organisms vary depending on the timing after transplantation. Chest radiograph findings may be nonspecific; immunosuppressive medications blunt the appearance of infiltrates.[3,8] Additionally, sirolimus has been noted to cause interstitial pneumonitis.[9] Chest computed tomography may be required to help delineate the cause of abnormal findings on chest radiography.

The threshold for hospital admission of posttransplant patients with pneumonia is lower given the potential for rapidly progressive disease and opportunistic infections. Appropriate effort should be made to obtain sputum for Gram stain and culture because of the potential for unusual organisms. Antimicrobial choices need to be tailored to the most likely organisms based on the clinical findings, time after transplantation, and history of recent hospitalization.

Fluoroquinolones and macrolides may increase levels of cyclosporine and tacrolimus; these antibiotic classes should not be used as first-line agents for the treatment of patients with posttransplant pneumonia. Discussion with the transplant service may be beneficial in determining the preferred choice of antibiotic.

## *Gastrointestinal Emergencies*

Abdominal pain in renal transplant recipients may be due to a variety of causes. Diagnostic imaging studies should be used liberally given the potential for patients with serious intraabdominal processes to have relatively minimal findings on physical examination.[3,10]

Mortality from cholecystitis is high in renal posttransplant patients. Diverticulitis is the most common bacterial gastrointestinal infectious process.[10] Diarrhea may be due to any number of infectious organisms, including *Salmonella, Listeria*, cytomegalovirus, and *Cryptosporidium*.

Abdominal pain in the area of the allograft should prompt consideration of acute rejection.

Opportunistic infections may affect any area of the gastrointestinal tract, from the mouth to the anus. Common opportunistic infections include candidiasis, cytomegalovirus, and herpes simplex.[10,11] Cytomegalovirus and Epstein-Barr virus can cause acute hepatitis.

Various immunosuppressive drugs can cause stomatitis, ulcerations, or acute hepatitis.[10] Renal transplant recipients have an increased incidence of acute pancreatitis that may be related to immunosuppressive agents.[10]

## *Genitourinary and Renal Emergencies*

Renal transplant recipients are prone to the same genitourinary and renal disorders as the general population. The one truly unique renal emergency in this population is rejection.

Urinary tract infections are more severe in transplant recipients.[12] Pyelonephritis may follow a fulminant course and necessitate inpatient management. These patients often require two broad-spectrum antibiotics for adequate treatment. Aminoglycosides are nephrotoxic and should be avoided if possible.

Hematuria in renal transplant recipients may be due to infection or obstruction in the allograft or in the native kidneys; imaging studies are recommended. Hemolytic-uremic syndrome is a cause of hematuria and acute renal failure in posttransplant patients that may be related to infection (cytomegalovirus), rejection, or medication toxicity (cyclosporine and tacrolimus).[13]

Common causes of renal insufficiency normally observed in nontransplant patients should be considered when evaluating acute renal failure in posttransplant patients; rejection is a later consideration, after other, more likely causes have been excluded.

If hydronephrosis is present, ultrasound studies should be ordered to look for ureteral obstruction. Arterial Doppler imaging may be needed to evaluate the adequacy of blood flow to a graft. Obstruction of an allograft is a true surgical emergency that generally requires placement of a percutaneous nephrostomy tube.

Rejection can be acute, chronic, or acute on chronic. Acute rejection occurs in the early posttransplant period. Chronic rejection is the most common cause of renal allograft dysfunction after the first posttransplant year.

A common cause of acute renal failure in renal transplant patients is nephrotoxicity from cyclosporine or tacrolimus.[3,14] Rejection may not be able to be distinguished from nephrotoxicity without a biopsy. Fever and tenderness over the graft site suggest the presence of rejection, whereas elevated trough levels of cyclosporine or tacrolimus suggest drug-induced nephrotoxicity.

If acute rejection is the most likely diagnosis, the transplant service should be consulted for inpatient management and high-dose methylprednisolone therapy begun at 500 to 1000 mg daily.

### Endocrine and Metabolic Emergencies

Transplant recipients receiving corticosteroid therapy have functional adrenal insufficiency and require pulse doses of corticosteroids when they encounter physiologic stress. Stress-dose hydrocortisone should be administered to transplant patients with unexplained or refractory hypotension unless they have not been taking corticosteroids for more than 6 months.

Electrolyte disorders, especially hyperkalemia, are common in posttransplant patients as a result of cyclosporine- or tacrolimus-induced impairment of potassium excretion.[15] This impairment may be exacerbated by the use of potassium-sparing diuretics and angiotensin-converting enzyme inhibitors.

Cyclosporine and corticosteroids both contribute to an increased incidence of new-onset diabetes in transplant recipients.[16]

### Neurologic Emergencies

Cryptococcal meningitis and central nervous system lymphoma are seen with greater frequency in posttransplant patients because of the immunosuppression.[17] Patients with fever of unknown origin, headache, or altered mental status should undergo intracranial imaging and lumbar puncture as appropriate. Computed tomography scanning of the brain with and without contrast enhancement is preferable in this population to more readily identify space-occupying lesions. The risk for contrast-induced nephrotoxicity must be weighed against the benefit of diagnostic accuracy when brain lesions are suspected. Similarly, use of gadolinium-enhanced magnetic resonance imaging may be contraindicated given the risk for nephrogenic systemic fibrosis in patients with abnormal creatinine clearance.[18]

### Adverse Drug Reactions

Immunosuppressive medications cause illness through the direct toxic effects of these drugs or through interaction with other common medications. Medication reconciliation is critical as new drug regimens become more complex.

Initial posttransplant regimens typically consist of three agents: a corticosteroid, a calcineurin inhibitor (cyclosporine, tacrolimus, sirolimus), and a purine synthesis inhibitor (azathioprine, mycophenolate mofetil).[19] Most patients are weaned off corticosteroids in 6 months, and maintenance is continued with only two drugs.

During the initial induction phase of immunosuppression, other agents such as antithymocyte monoclonal and polyclonal antibodies are used. Because these medications are generally reserved for inpatient use, it is unusual for patients to be seen in the ED with an acute complication from these agents.

Corticosteroid therapy has many well-recognized complications. In addition to functional adrenal suppression, corticosteroids can induce diabetes, steroid psychosis, gastric ulceration, pancreatitis, changes in body habitus, and avascular necrosis.

Azathioprine is one of the oldest agents used to treat rejection. It is an alkylating agent similar to other chemotherapeutic drugs, and thus its primary toxicity is bone marrow suppression (particularly leukopenia). When given with allopurinol, increased levels of azathioprine may result in myelosuppression. Azathioprine and mycophenolate mofetil demonstrate an additive risk for myelosuppression. The hepatotoxicity from azathioprine is less than that with other agents.

Cyclosporine interacts with multiple other medications and demonstrates significant nephrotoxicity. Increased serum creatinine levels are observed in up to one third of patients taking cyclosporine.[15] As these levels rise, cyclosporine excretion decreases and renal failure worsens. Trough measurements of cyclosporine (3 hours before the next scheduled dose) differentiate drug-induced nephrotoxicity from other causes of renal insufficiency.

Tacrolimus and sirolimus both carry a risk for multiple drug interactions and worsening nephrotoxicity. Drugs that increase the metabolism of these agents may decrease their effective serum levels and thus result in acute rejection because of inadequate immunosuppression.

## DISPOSITION

Concerns about chronic immunosuppression, graft rejection, and multiple drug interactions make management of transplant patients among the most difficult challenges encountered in the ED. As a rule, these patients require extensive laboratory and imaging studies; there are no data to predict which of these patients can safely forgo such testing in an emergency setting.[20] Consultation with an experienced transplant team will improve outcomes. The majority of transplant patients with serious chief complaints require hospital admission for observation and further management.

## SUGGESTED READINGS

Abou-Saif A, Lewis JH. Gastrointestinal and hepatic disorders in end-stage renal disease and renal transplant recipients. Adv Renal Replace Ther 2000;7:220-30.

Djamali A, Kendziorski C, Brazy PC, et al. Disease progression and outcomes in chronic kidney disease and renal transplantation. Kidney Int 2003;64:1800-7.

Kendrick E. Cardiovascular disease and the renal transplant recipient. Am J Kidney Dis 2001;38:36-43.

Unterman S. A descriptive analysis of 1251 solid organ transplant visits to the emergency department. West J Emerg Med 2009;10:46-54.

Venkat KK, Venkat A. Care of renal transplant recipients in the emergency department. Ann Emerg Med 2004;44:330-41.

## REFERENCES

*References can be found on Expert Consult @ www.expertconsult.com.*

# The Healthy Pregnancy 118

*Jacqueline Khorasanee and Matthew Kippenhan*

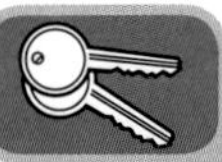

**KEY POINTS**

- The incidence of venous thromboembolism increases by a factor of 5 during pregnancy; pulmonary embolism is a leading cause of maternal mortality in the United States.
- Approximately 2% to 10% of gravid and nongravid patients have asymptomatic bacteriuria, which will eventually progress to acute pyelonephritis in as many as 40% of gravid patients.
- Acute pyelonephritis during pregnancy increases the risk for preterm labor; these patients should be admitted for intravenous antibiotic therapy.
- One third of patients will have improvement in their asthma symptoms during pregnancy, one third will remain the same, and one third will have worsening symptoms.
- As many as one third of patients with epilepsy will experience an increase in seizure activity during pregnancy.
- Treatment of human immunodeficiency virus infection during pregnancy with zidovudine can reduce the incidence of perinatal transmission from mother to infant by 70%.

## EPIDEMIOLOGY

Each year, 4.1 million live births in the United States result from approximately 6.5 million pregnancies.[1,2] These women routinely go to the emergency department (ED) for general medical complaints, as well as for pregnancy-specific issues. In addition, more patients with complex medical problems are becoming pregnant because of advances in fertility treatments. Pregnancy can be an emotionally stressful condition that requires special attention from caregivers. Because diagnostic and management strategies are altered in pregnancy, a thorough understanding of the physiologic changes that accompany pregnancy is mandatory (**Box 118.1**).

## PATHOPHYSIOLOGY

Gravidity refers to the total number of pregnancies conceived, including the current pregnancy. Parity characterizes the outcome of the pregnancy, and it is further subdivided into four categories described by the mnemonic TPAL (number of term infants, preterm infants, abortions, and living children; **Box 118.2**).

A term pregnancy lasts from 37 to 42 weeks and is divided into trimesters. The first trimester begins at conception and lasts until the 14th week. The second trimester encompasses weeks 14 to 28, and the third trimester lasts from the 28th to the 42nd week. Infants delivered before 37 weeks are considered premature, whereas those delivered after 42 weeks are considered postterm. The due date can be estimated with the Naegele rule, which is applied by subtracting 3 months from the first day of the patient's last menstrual period and adding 7 days to that date. First trimester ultrasound scans provide more reliable estimates of gestational age.

## PRESENTING SIGNS AND SYMPTOMS

Emergency physicians (EPs) should consider the possibility of pregnancy in every female patient of childbearing age regardless of the chief complaint or symptoms. One study documented pregnancy in 7% of ED respondents who indicated that their last menstrual period was on time and normal and that there was "no chance" that they were pregnant.[3] Early signs of pregnancy include missed menses, vaginal bleeding, nausea, vomiting, breast tenderness, urinary frequency, fatigue, near-syncope, and abdominal pain or bloating. Some patients may not have these symptoms or may ignore them and later go to the ED with an obviously enlarged uterus or in labor.

### RESPIRATORY SYSTEM

The physiology of breathing in pregnancy is altered by both anatomic and hormonal changes. Anatomic changes include an increase in chest diameter and circumference, as well as a rise in the level of the diaphragm. The result is a reduction in total lung capacity by 5% and functional residual capacity by 20%. In contrast, vital capacity does not change.[4] The

**BOX 118.1 Physiologic Changes in Pregnancy**

**Respiratory System**
Reduction of total lung capacity
Reduction of functional residual capacity
Increased tidal volume
Increased minute ventilation
Decreased $Pa{CO_2}$

**Hematologic and Immunologic Systems**
Increased blood volume
Increased plasma volume
Decreased hemoglobin (dilutional)
Increased procoagulation factors
Increased white blood cell count

**Cardiovascular System**
Increased cardiac output
Increased heart rate
Increased stroke volume
Decreased systemic vascular resistance
Decreased blood pressure

**Gastrointestinal System**
Decreased stomach motility and tone
Increase in gastroesophageal reflux

**Dermatologic System**
Striae gravidarum
Linea nigra
Chloasma or melasma
Spider angioma

**Urinary System**
Increased glomerular filtration rate
Dilation of the ureters, renal pelvis, and renal calices
Decrease in creatinine and blood urea nitrogen

**Musculoskeletal System**
Increased spinal lordosis
Increased pubic ligament laxity
Breast enlargement and tenderness

**Endocrine System**
Increased pituitary gland size
Glucose intolerance

**BOX 118.2 Gestation and Parity Notation**

**Gestatation (G):** Total number of pregnancies
**Parity (P):** Subdivided into four categories described by the mnemonic *TPAL*—number of term infants, preterm infants, abortions, and living children
**Example:** G4P3 describes a woman who has had four pregnancies and three deliveries; G4P3 (2-1-1-3), also written as G4P2113, describes a woman who has had two term deliveries, one preterm delivery, and one abortion (spontaneous or induced) and has three living children.

respiratory rate also remains constant, but because of a progesterone-mediated increase in both tidal volume and minute ventilation, $Pa{CO_2}$ decreases to an average of 30 mm Hg. The sensation of dyspnea is increased during pregnancy.

## HEMATOLOGIC AND IMMUNOLOGIC SYSTEMS

Blood volume increases during pregnancy by an average of 40% to 50% secondary to both plasma volume expansion and increased erythrocyte mass. Plasma volume increases approximately 50%, with a plateau reached at 30 weeks of gestation. Erythrocyte mass increases 20% to 30% over prepregnancy levels and peaks near term, with greater increases associated with iron supplementation. Asymmetric expansion of the plasma and erythrocyte mass results in a relative anemia, referred to as the physiologic anemia of pregnancy. Plasma expansion begins earlier than erythropoiesis but then stabilizes, with the nadir in hemoglobin concentration occurring between weeks 16 and 28.[5] Hemoglobin levels normally do not drop below 10.5 g/dL during the nadir period and should measure 11 g/dL or higher during the remaining pregnancy.

Procoagulation factors are increased during pregnancy, whereas inhibitors of coagulation are reduced or unchanged. These changes in the coagulation cascade may serve to protect the mother against peripartum hemorrhage, but when combined with venous stasis and vessel wall injury, they predispose a patient to thromboembolic disease.[6]

Pregnancy has been described as a state of immunodeficiency but is more accurately described as a period of modified immune response.[7] The peripheral white blood cell count is elevated during pregnancy; it ranges from 5110/$mm^3$ to 12,200/$mm^3$ during gestation and rises even higher during labor. Additionally, changes in both chemotaxis and adherence of neutrophils occur during pregnancy, as well as a shift by the immune system away from the cell-mediated immune response toward antibody-mediated immunity. This altered immune focus allows tolerance of the maternal immune system to paternal antigens but increases susceptibility to pathogens and variation in the activity of autoimmune diseases.[8]

## CARDIOVASCULAR SYSTEM

Changes in diaphragm position and rib cage dimension cause the heart to be displaced to the left and upward and rotated on its long axis. On radiographic studies these changes are manifested as an increase in heart silhouette in the absence of actual cardiomegaly. Likewise, this change in position is responsible for apparent left axis deviation on an electrocardiogram.

Cardiac output consistently and dramatically increases during pregnancy, with a 37% to 53% increase over prepregnancy values.[9] This change is driven by increases in both heart rate and stroke volume. The heart rate increases 15 to 20 beats/min over pregravid rates, and stroke volume increases by 20% to 30%. In the later stages of pregnancy, decreased venous return as a result of compression of the inferior vena cava leads to decreased cardiac output. The highest levels of cardiac output occur in the right and left lateral positions; the lowest levels occur in the supine, sitting, and standing positions. Supine hypotension with symptoms such as dizziness, nausea, and syncope develop in a small number of pregnant patients (5% to 10%).[6] Despite the increase in cardiac output, the pregnancy-associated reduction in systemic vascular resistance causes an overall reduction in maternal blood pressure. Blood pressure, like cardiac output, is dependent on position, highest when sitting and lowest in the lateral recumbent position.

### DERMATOLOGIC SYSTEM

Striae gravidarum ("stretch marks") occur in 50% to 90% of pregnancies during the late second or third trimester. Mechanical stretching of the skin along with hormonal changes affecting the dermis are implicated. Hormonal stimulation of melanocyte activity is responsible for the hyperpigmentation seen in as many as 90% of pregnancies.

### GENITOURINARY SYSTEM

Changes in the urinary system during normal pregnancy include increases in kidney size, glomerular filtration rate, and renal blood flow. Additionally, dilation of the ureters, renal pelvis, and renal calices occurs as a result of mechanical compression by the expanding uterus and ovarian structures, as well as progesterone-mediated smooth muscle relaxation. The right ureter is more commonly affected than the left one, probably secondary to anatomic susceptibility. The glomerular filtration rate increases 50% over nongravid values by the end of the first trimester and is maintained throughout pregnancy. This increase and the subsequent increase in filtration fraction leads to decreases in both creatinine and blood urea nitrogen levels. The dependent edema accumulated during the day is mobilized at night, which results in increased nocturia during pregnancy. An increased incidence of glycosuria is common during pregnancy and may be unrelated to blood glucose levels or kidney dysfunction, but hematuria or proteinuria before labor should be considered pathologic.

The weight of the uterus increases from 70 to 1100 g, and intrauterine volume increases from 10 to 5000 mL. The gradual change in color of the vaginal walls to dark blue or black (Chadwick sign) is secondary to venous congestion.

### GASTROINTESTINAL SYSTEM

Changes in the gastrointestinal system during pregnancy include an overall decrease in gastric tone and motility. There is also a decrease in lower esophageal sphincter tone caused by altered hormone levels. This muscle relaxation, coupled with compression of the stomach by the expanding uterus, leads to an increase in gastroesophageal reflux disease. Paradoxically, a concurrent decrease in peptic ulcer disease takes place.

Liver anatomy and function are essentially unchanged. However, serum alkaline phosphatase levels are elevated during the third trimester secondary to placental production of the isoenzyme. Gallbladder emptying is slower and less efficient during pregnancy. In addition to stasis, changes in the chemical composition of bile lead to increased formation of cholesterol crystals. The result is an increase in symptomatic cholelithiasis.

### MUSCULOSKELETAL SYSTEM

To counterbalance the expanding uterus and prevent an anterior shift in the center of gravity, the degree of lordosis of the lumbar spine increases throughout pregnancy, which often results in low back pain. Increased laxity of the ligament of the pubic symphysis and sacroiliac joints can also cause pain. Increasing tenderness of the breasts is common in pregnancy.

### ENDOCRINE SYSTEM

Enlargement of the breasts and nipples is normal, and discharge of colostrum from the nipples during the later stages of pregnancy is not uncommon. Despite histologic changes, women remain euthyroid during pregnancy, and the slight increase in thyroid size that does occur is not clinically detectable. A palpable increase in the thyroid during pregnancy is pathologic and must be further evaluated. The results of laboratory tests commonly used to evaluate thyroid function should be within normal limits. Significant hypothyroidism during pregnancy is associated with fetal neurologic defects such as mental retardation and lower IQ scores.[10,11]

The pituitary gland increases 136% in comparison with its prepregnancy size. This increase in size makes the gland more susceptible to infarction with hemorrhage (Sheehan syndrome) but does not impair the optic chiasm.

Some level of glucose intolerance is associated with pregnancy. Normal pregnancy is marked by hyperglycemia after eating, followed by hypoglycemia when fasting. Postprandial hyperglycemia ensures adequate delivery of nutrients to the fetus.

## COMMON MEDICAL DISEASES AND PREGNANCY

### DIABETES

Diabetes occurs in approximately 3% to 5% of all gestations.[12] Three types of diabetes affect pregnancy: type 1, type 2, and gestational diabetes. Gestational diabetes accounts for 90% of cases. Fetal risks during pregnancy in women with diabetes include congenital malformation, intrauterine growth retardation, macrosomia, fetal hypoglycemia, fetal respiratory distress syndrome, neonatal hypocalcemia, hyperbilirubinemia, polycythemia, intrauterine demise, and neonatal jaundice.[13] These risks are greatest for women with type 1 diabetes, although type 2 and gestational diabetes are also associated with a significant increase in fetal mortality.

With tight glucose control, the perinatal mortality rate of diabetic pregnancies can approach that of uncomplicated pregnancies. However, maintaining normal blood sugar levels is extremely difficult because of the changing degree of insulin resistance throughout pregnancy.

Patients who are unable to achieve glucose control with diet and exercise require insulin therapy. The side effects of oral hypoglycemic agents in pregnant patients have not been studied extensively. Some agents may be associated with an increased rate of congenital malformation, and frequently they do not provide adequate glucose control.

Diabetic ketoacidosis occurs in as many as 10% of patients with type 1 diabetes. Treatment during pregnancy is the same as for nongravid patients but should include assessment of fetal status and supportive measures such as oxygen and use of the left lateral decubitus position to maximize fetal blood flow.

### URINARY TRACT INFECTIONS

The incidence of acute cystitis or acute pyelonephritis is approximately 1% during pregnancy. Asymptomatic bacteriuria is a related condition in which urine culture is positive in an asymptomatic patient. The incidence of asymptomatic bacteriuria is similar in both gravid and nongravid populations, with 2% to 10% of the population being affected.[14,15] However, gravid patients have a much higher rate of progression to symptomatic infection, and as many as 40% of cases eventually progress to acute pyelonephritis. Chronic cystitis and chronic and acute pyelonephritis are associated with negative outcomes, and patients should receive antibiotic therapy. Patients with recurrent asymptomatic bacteriuria or urinary tract infection may require daily suppressive therapy or postcoital prophylaxis.

Treatment of asymptomatic bacteriuria and acute cystitis can be accomplished with 3 to 7 days of oral therapy consisting of amoxicillin, a cephalosporin, or nitrofurantoin. Unless sensitivities are known, nitrofurantoin is the preferred agent because of higher levels of resistance to the other agents. Acute pyelonephritis during pregnancy increases the risk for preterm labor and should be managed aggressively. Patients require admission and intravenous antibiotic therapy until clinical improvement is demonstrated.

## ASTHMA

Approximately 4% of pregnancies are complicated by asthma,[16,17] roughly mirroring its incidence in women of childbearing age. The course of asthma during pregnancy is not uniformly predictable. One third of patients will have improvement in their symptoms during pregnancy, one third will experience stable disease, and another third will have worsening of their symptoms.[18] Though somewhat controversial, patients with asthma have been reported to have increased rates of preeclampsia, cesarean delivery, and preterm rupture of membranes. Fetal risks include increased mortality, prematurity, intrauterine growth retardation, and low birth weight.

Monitoring and treatment of asthma in pregnant patients are much the same as for nonpregnant patients. Commonly used measures include the peak expiratory flow rate and forced expiratory flow in 1 second. Beta-agonists are the initial medication of choice both for acute exacerbation and for maintenance. Inhaled corticosteroids are safe and effective, but intravenous corticosteroids may be required during acute exacerbations.

## SEIZURE DISORDERS

Epilepsy is associated with an increased incidence of obstetric and fetal complications. However, more than 90% of pregnant women with epilepsy have a normal pregnancy with a good outcome.[19] Seizure disorders affect approximately 1% of the general population and affect a similar percentage of gestations. As many as one third of women with epilepsy experience an increase in seizure activity during pregnancy. Patients with a higher pregravid incidence of seizures are at greater risk for increased seizure frequency during pregnancy. Increased seizure activity may result from decreased compliance with medical therapy, altered pharmacologic distribution, increased elimination of medications, or a combination of factors.

Status epilepticus during pregnancy is a grave danger for both the mother and fetus and should be treated aggressively with early intubation, pharmacologic therapy, and evaluation for eclampsia. Benzodiazepines, phenytoin, and fosphenytoin are all effective in the treatment of status epilepticus. New seizure activity during pregnancy merits investigation to determine its cause; eclampsia should be suspected in the third trimester.

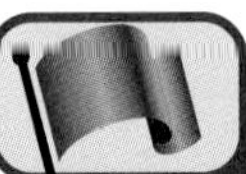

**RED FLAGS**

- New seizure activity during pregnancy merits investigation; eclampsia must always be suspected in the third trimester.
- Hemoglobin levels do not normally drop below 10.5 g/dL during pregnancy and should usually measure 11 g/dL. More significant anemia should be investigated.
- Pregnancy is a state of modified immune response, and pregnant women have increased susceptibility to pathogens.

## MIGRAINE

Migraine symptoms are reduced or resolved in 60% to 80% of women during pregnancy.[20] Acceptable pharmacologic agents to treat symptoms include acetaminophen, narcotics, and antiemetics such as prochlorperazine, promethazine, and metoclopramide. Caffeine is sometimes effective and may be used in moderation. Propranolol is generally considered safe for migraine prophylaxis but may carry a risk for intrauterine growth retardation.

Other commonly used agents should be avoided. Ergotamines may cause birth defects secondary to vascular alteration. Triptans may cause vasospasm resulting in an increased incidence of preterm birth and intrauterine growth retardation. As is the case in other conditions, nonsteroidal antiinflammatory drugs (NSAIDs) should be avoided.

## THROMBOEMBOLIC DISEASE

Thromboembolic disease is a major source of maternal morbidity and mortality during pregnancy. The incidence of venous thromboembolism increases by a factor of 5 during pregnancy, and pulmonary embolism is a leading cause of maternal mortality in the United States.[21] Factors believed to contribute to the increased incidence of venous thromboembolism include alteration of normal clotting factor levels, increased stasis, and vessel damage. These factors may be aggravated by advanced maternal age and inherited or acquired thrombophilias.

Ultrasonography safely and reliably detects lower extremity deep vein thrombosis. If pelvic or iliac thrombosis is suspected, venography may be required for diagnosis, but magnetic resonance imaging is increasingly being used. Ventilation-perfusion scans are useful in assessing for pulmonary embolism; however, spiral computed tomography, available at most institutions, is associated with lower fetal radiation exposure than ventilation-perfusion scans are. Both heparin and low-molecular-weight heparin are commonly used for the treatment of acute thromboembolism. Warfarin is contraindicated in pregnant patients because of its association with fetal malformation and fetal demise.

## HYPERTENSION

Pregnant women with elevated blood pressure may have preexisting hypertension, gestational hypertension, preeclampsia, or eclampsia.[22]

No consensus regarding initiation of antihypertensive therapy during pregnancy has currently been established.

Most authorities prescribe treatment for patients with a blood pressure of 160/105 or higher; others argue that a lower threshold of 150/100 should be the criteria for treatment. In one review of pregnant patients experiencing stroke secondary to preeclampsia, systolic blood pressures recorded before the event were 159 to 198 mm Hg, and diastolic blood pressures were 81 to 113 mm Hg[23]; arterial hemorrhage was the cause of stroke in 93% of patients who underwent intracranial imaging. Of note, evidence is not sufficient to recommend bed rest as an effective or practical treatment of hypertension during pregnancy.[24]

## ALCOHOL AND OTHER RECREATIONAL DRUGS

Alcohol use is reported in 10% to 15% of pregnancies; no safe level of intake has been determined. Alcohol abuse is associated with fetal alcohol syndrome. Common features of this syndrome include low IQ, microcephaly, short palpebral fissures, smooth filtrum, thin upper lip, and ventricular septal defects.

Cigarette smoking increases the risk for spontaneous abortion, prematurity, small-for-gestational-age births, placental abruption, placenta previa, and premature rupture of membranes. The adverse effects of smoking are dose related and reduced by cessation of smoking, even after a pregnancy is diagnosed.

Opiates, cocaine, and methamphetamine are all associated with obstetric complications. Cocaine use during pregnancy is believed to cause increased rates of placental abruption, preterm labor, and small-for-gestational-age infants. However, these studies are limited in that many of the mothers using cocaine have polysubstance abuse.

EPs should be aware of the reporting requirements of drug abuse in the states in which they practice.

## HUMAN IMMUNODEFICIENCY VIRUS AND ACQUIRED IMMUNODEFICIENCY SYNDROME

Treatment of human immunodeficiency virus (HIV) infection during pregnancy with antivirals can reduce the incidence of perinatal transmission from mother to infant by 70%. The combination of antiviral therapy and elective cesarean delivery may reduce perinatal HIV transmission by as much as 85%. In the United States, where safe breast milk replacement is readily available, breastfeeding is discouraged because of the risk for transmission from mother to child. Referral to infectious disease and high-risk obstetric services is mandatory for pregnant women found to be HIV positive.

# MEDICATION USE DURING PREGNANCY

Medication use during pregnancy can be a source of apprehension for both patients and physicians because of the paucity of data on safety. Pharmaceutical companies have excluded pregnant patients from testing of new agents for decades, thus resulting in little knowledge about the teratogenicity of products in humans. Additionally, animal models may not be representative of human risk. EPs prescribing medication for pregnant or lactating women should use the resources available in both electronic and text format.

Fetal toxicity is affected by the dose, duration of exposure, and gestational age when the exposure occurs. During the 31-day period following the last menstrual period, teratogens have essentially a binary (all-or-nothing) effect—the conceptus is either aborted or survives without harm. The next stage of development is the crucial period of organogenesis and lasts from 31 to 71 days after the last menstrual period. The effect of exposure to a teratogen depends on the time during this period that the fetus was exposed. Early exposure may affect the cardiovascular or central nervous systems (or both), whereas later exposure may affect the musculoskeletal system, such as palate and ears.

The U.S. Food and Drug Administration classifies medications into five categories according to potential fetal risk based on animal and human studies (**Table 118.1**).[25] Medications commonly used in the ED and generally considered safe are listed in **Box 118.3**; often-used medications considered unsafe for use during pregnancy are listed in **Table 118.2**.

**Table 118.1** U.S. FDA Pharmaceutical Pregnancy Categories

| PREGNANCY CATEGORY | DESCRIPTION |
|---|---|
| A | Adequate well-controlled studies in pregnant women have not shown an increased risk for fetal abnormalities. |
| B | Animal studies have revealed no evidence of harm to the fetus; however, there are no adequate and well-controlled studies in pregnant women.<br>*or*<br>Animal studies have shown an adverse effect, but adequate and well-controlled studies in pregnant women have failed to demonstrate a risk to the fetus. |
| C | Animal studies have shown an adverse effect, and there are no adequate well-controlled studies in pregnant women.<br>*or*<br>No animal studies have been conducted, and no adequate well-controlled studies have been performed in pregnant women. |
| D | Adequate well-controlled or observational studies in pregnant women have demonstrated a risk to the fetus. However, the benefits of therapy may outweigh the potential risks. |
| X | Adequate well-controlled or observational studies in animals or pregnant women have demonstrated positive evidence of fetal abnormalities. Use of the product is contraindicated in women who are or may become pregnant. |

Modified from Meadows M. Pregnancy and the drug dilemma. FDA Consum 2001;35:16-20. Available at http://www.fda.gov/fdac/features/2001/301_preg.html.
*FDA*, Food and Drug Administration.

**BOX 118.3 Medications Considered Safe During Pregnancy**

**Analgesics**
Acetaminophen
Opiates*

**Antiemetics**
Dopamine agonists (phenothiazines, promethazine, chlorpromazine, perphenazine, metoclopramide)
Serotonin 5-$HT_3$ receptor antagonist (ondansetron)
Other (vitamin $B_6$, ginger)

**Antihypertensives**
$\alpha$-Methyldopa
Hydralazine
Beta-blockers (labetalol, metoprolol, propranolol)
Calcium channel blockers (nifedipine, diltiazem, verapamil)
Diuretics

**Antimicrobials**
Penicillin and derivatives (ampicillin, nafcillin, ticarcillin, piperacillin)
Cephalosporins (first, second, third, fourth generation)
Macrolides (erythromycin,† azithromycin, clarithromycin)
Benzodiazepines‡
Others (clindamycin, nitrofurantoin)

**Anticoagulants**
Heparin
Low-molecular-weight heparin

**Antiepileptics**
Benzodiazepines‡

**Asthma Medications**
Beta-agonists
Corticosteroids

**Diabetes Medications**
Insulin (lispro, aspart, regular, glargine)

**Prophylaxis**
Tetanus toxoid
Influenza vaccine

*Avoid chronic use of opiates during pregnancy. Also use caution when giving opiates near the time of delivery because of the risk for respiratory and central nervous system depression.
†Do not give the estolate salt of erythromycin because of the risk for maternal hepatic toxicity.
‡Use caution when giving benzodiazepines near the time of delivery because of the risk for respiratory depression. Early studies showed teratogenicity, which was unconfirmed in later studies; however, the drug is still class D and should be used with caution in the first trimester.

## ANALGESIC AGENTS

No evidence has implicated acetaminophen as a teratogen, and thus it is the preferred agent when a mild analgesic or antipyretic is indicated. The use of NSAIDs such as ibuprofen and naproxen is generally discouraged during pregnancy, although the risk appears to be mostly in the third trimester. Indomethacin has been reported to be associated with oligohydramnios, pulmonary hypertension, and constriction of the ductus arteriosus.

Despite the lack of conclusive human data indicating that aspirin is a teratogen, its other ill effects limit its use during pregnancy. Aspirin has been linked to delayed onset of labor, protracted labor, and increased risk for prolonged pregnancy. It inhibits prostaglandin synthesis, which leads to premature closure of the ductus arteriosus, as well as increases the incidence of hemorrhage because of a decrease in platelet aggregation.

The use of opiates is considered safe throughout pregnancy. However, opiate use shortly before delivery can result in respiratory and central nervous system depression in the newborn. Because long-term opiate use during pregnancy can cause newborn addiction and withdrawal, patients using opiates chronically should be monitored carefully by their physician during pregnancy.

## ANTICOAGULANTS

Warfarin is a known human teratogen associated with nasal bone hypoplasia, bone stippling, ophthalmologic abnormalities, and mental retardation; therefore, it is contraindicated in pregnancy. Heparin and low-molecular-weight heparin are thought to be safe during pregnancy and can be used when anticoagulation is indicated.

## ANTIEMETICS

Multiple antiemetic agents are commonly prescribed during early pregnancy. Dopamine agonists such as the phenothiazines, promethazine, chlorpromazine, perphenazine, and metoclopramide are all well tolerated and appear to be safe in pregnancy. The serotonin 5-$HT_3$ receptor antagonist ondansetron also appears to be both safe and effective for nausea and vomiting during pregnancy, although fewer data are available about this agent. Vitamin $B_6$ has been reported to be an effective treatment of nausea and vomiting in several randomized, double-blind, placebo-controlled trials.

## ANTIMICROBIAL AGENTS

All antibiotics have been shown to cross the placenta and enter the fetal circulation to some degree.[26,27] Penicillin and its derivative compounds, including nafcillin, dicloxacillin, amoxicillin, and ampicillin, have been used extensively in pregnant patients without any ill effects on fetal development being reported. Newer derivatives, such as piperacillin and ticarcillin, have not been used as extensively but are believed to be safe in pregnancy. Cephalosporins are prescribed routinely, although there is less experience with the use of cephalosporins than with penicillin and ticarcillin.

**Table 118.2 Common Emergency Department Pharmaceutical Agents Contraindicated in Pregnancy**

| AGENT | CONTRAINDICATION |
|---|---|
| **Analgesics** | |
| Aspirin | Premature closure of the ductus arteriosus, increased incidence of hemorrhage |
| NSAIDs (ibuprofen, indomethacin, naproxen) | Oligohydramnios, pulmonary hypertension, constriction of the ductus arteriosus |
| **Antimicrobials** | |
| Tetracyclines | Discolored teeth, inhibition of bone growth |
| Fluoroquinolones | Arthropathy in immature animals |
| Aminoglycosides | Ototoxicity, nephrotoxicity |
| **Anticoagulants** | |
| Warfarin | Nasal bone hypoplasia, bone stippling, ophthalmologic abnormalities, mental retardation |
| **Antiepileptics** | |
| Phenytoin | Fetal hydantoin syndrome (ossification abnormalities, cleft lip and palate, impaired growth, cardiac abnormalities) |
| Carbamazepine, valproic acid | Dysmorphic syndrome, similar to fetal hydantoin syndrome |
| **Antihypertensives** | |
| ACE inhibitors | Renal malformation, oligohydramnios, craniofacial malformations, lung malformations |
| Angiotensin II receptor blockers | Linked to malformations similar to those from ACE inhibitors |
| **Other** | |
| Isotretinoin | Craniofacial, cardiac, thymic, and CNS malformations |

*ACE*, Angiotensin-converting enzyme; *CNS*, central nervous system; *NSAIDs*, nonsteroidal antiinflammatory drugs.

The macrolides (erythromycin, azithromycin, clarithromycin) are considered safe during pregnancy with the exception of erythromycin estolate, which is contraindicated because of the risk for maternal hepatotoxicity. Clindamycin and nitrofurantoin, both commonly used during pregnancy, are considered safe.

Metronidazole has not been shown to be a human teratogen. However, its use is somewhat controversial because of potential mutagenesis and carcinogenicity. Trimethoprim-sulfamethoxazole has two contraindications, one related to each of its constituents—trimethoprim should be avoided during the first trimester because it is a folate antagonist and its use may lead to an increased incidence of neural tube defects; use of sulfamethoxazole is discouraged near term because of competitive binding of albumin with bilirubin, which leads to concern for an increased risk for kernicterus. Although this concern exists for all sulfonamides, no cases of kernicterus resulting from prenatal use have been reported.[27]

Tetracyclines are contraindicated during pregnancy as a result of calcium binding, which causes staining of deciduous teeth, poor development of tooth enamel, and inhibition of skeletal growth in the fetus. Fluoroquinolones have not been shown to increase the rate of fetal malformation in humans but are contraindicated because of the development of arthropathy in immature animals exposed to quinolones.[28,29]

The aminoglycosides streptomycin and kanamycin are associated with ototoxicity and are potentially nephrotoxic. Gentamicin is potentially ototoxic and nephrotoxic; dosing must be adjusted for renal function, and it should be used with caution.

## ANTIVIRAL AGENTS

Women with disseminated herpes infection or a first genital herpesvirus infection occurring during pregnancy should be treated with acyclovir. No cases of fetal abnormalities caused by acyclovir have been reported. A genital herpes outbreak at term necessitates cesarean delivery.

## ANTIEPILEPTIC DRUGS

Management of epilepsy during pregnancy is difficult and requires a multidisciplinary approach. The risk for maternal death during pregnancy can be up to 10 times higher than that for patients without epilepsy.[30] In addition, rates of intrauterine fetal demise and malformation are also increased.[31] Many commonly available anticonvulsive medications are known or suspected teratogens, which can make management decisions difficult for both caregivers and patients.

Phenytoin, carbamazepine, valproate, and lamotrigine are associated with an increased incidence of congenital abnormalities. A recent review of data from 25 epilepsy centers recorded the following rates of serious adverse outcomes: valproate, 20.3%; phenytoin, 10.7%; carbamazepine, 8.2%; and lamotrigine, 1.0%.[32] Newer antiepileptic drugs, including levetiracetam, felbamate, gabapentin, oxcarbazepine, tiagabine, and topiramate, seem to be safe for use in pregnancy, although fewer data are available for these agents.[33]

Despite these risks, most physicians agree that patients with a well-established diagnosis of epilepsy should continue taking their medications during pregnancy. Women taking antiepileptic drugs during pregnancy should receive folic acid supplementation and undergo frequent monitoring. Seizures occurring during pregnancy or labor may be treated with benzodiazepines on an as-needed basis. Early studies demonstrated a risk for teratogenesis (mostly cleft abnormalities), but these findings have not been reproduced in more recent studies. Lorazepam does not cross the placenta at as fast a rate as other benzodiazepines do and, except during the first trimester, is considered safe. Sedation of the fetus around delivery is a minor concern and should not be considered a contraindication if needed for maternal seizures.

## ANTIHYPERTENSIVE MEDICATIONS

Several agents for the treatment of hypertension during pregnancy have favorable safety profiles. Commonly used medications include α-methyldopa and hydralazine. Hydralazine has been used extensively in pregnancy and is available in both intravenous and oral formulations.[34-36] Beta-blockers are believed to be safe in pregnancy, although some association with lower placental and fetal weight has been reported with atenolol.[37] Labetalol is the preferred agent because it does not carry this risk. The combined alpha- and beta-blocking characteristics of labetalol may act to preserve uteroplacental blood flow.

Although fewer data are available on calcium channel blockers, they also appear to be safe and effective for use during pregnancy. Short-acting sublingual formulations of nifedipine should be avoided because they may cause maternal hypotension and fetal distress. Diuretics are safe but are not often used during pregnancy because preeclampsia may arise from a fluid-depleted state.

Two classes of antihypertensive agents, angiotensin-converting enzyme inhibitors and angiotensin II receptor blockers, are contraindicated during pregnancy. Angiotensin-converting enzyme inhibitors have been associated with fetal renal malformation, oligohydramnios, craniofacial malformations, and lung malformations. Angiotensin II receptor blockers are associated with a similar set of malformations, probably caused by a similar mechanism.

## ANTIHYPERGLYCEMIC AGENTS

Insulin is the primary medication for the treatment of diabetes during pregnancy and has been proven to be safe and effective. A regimen that includes multiple daily doses of both short- and long-acting insulin is often required. Data regarding the use of oral hypoglycemic agents in pregnancy are still limited. Glyburide and metformin have been used and appear to be safe, but there is little indication for initiating these agents in the ED setting. Patients are at increased risk for hypoglycemic episodes associated with oral hypoglycemic use and thus should be monitored closely.

## IMMUNIZATIONS

Indications for vaccines composed of toxoid or inactivated virus are similar to those for nongravid females. In general, the protection gained by vaccination during pregnancy usually outweighs the risks.[38] Live virus or attenuated vaccines (measles, mumps, poliomyelitis, rubella, yellow fever, and varicella) may cause infection or malformation (or both) in the fetus and are therefore contraindicated. Patients planning to became pregnant should ideally have their vaccines updated several months before conceiving.

Influenza is indicated for all women who will be pregnant during the flu season (October to March) and for all women at high risk for pulmonary complications.[39] Tetanus–diphtheria toxoid vaccine should be administered as usual for tetanus-prone wounds.

## OVER-THE-COUNTER MEDICATIONS

Most over-the-counter cold medications contain a combination of compounds. Little information is available regarding the effects of these agents alone and even less when they are used in combination. Decongestants act via vasoconstriction, and this mechanism also serves, at least theoretically, to decrease placental blood flow; their use during pregnancy should be avoided. Antihistamines such as diphenhydramine have been used during pregnancy and are considered safe. However, it should be noted that over-the-counter cold remedies are effective for relief of symptoms only and do not modify the course of disease; rest, hydration, and time are still the best treatment of the common cold.

## ACKNOWLEDGMENT

Thanks to Dr. Jon D. Van Roo for his work on the first edition.

## SUGGESTED READINGS

ACOG educational bulletin. Antimicrobial therapy for obstetric patients. Number 245, March 1998 (replaces no. 117, June 1988). American College of Obstetricians and Gynecologists. Int J Gynaecol Obstet 1998;6:299-308.

Barton JR. Hypertension in pregnancy. Ann Emerg Med 2008;51(2 Suppl):S16-7.

Hodder R, Lougheed MD, Rowe BH, et al. Management of acute asthma in adults in the emergency department: nonventilatory management. CMAJ 2010;182(2):E55-67.

Stead LG. Seizures in pregnancy/eclampsia. Emerg Med Clin North Am 2011;29:109-16.

## REFERENCES

*References can be found on Expert Consult @ www.expertconsult.com.*

# Disorders of Early Pregnancy 119

*Matthew Kippenhan*

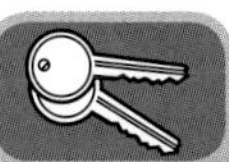

**KEY POINTS**

- Spontaneous abortion (before 12 weeks) will progress to completion with few complications, and incomplete or missed abortion (without shock, fever, or significant bleeding) can be managed expectantly.
- $Rh_0$ immune globulin is effective for up to 12 weeks; no repeated dose is required if bleeding recurs in that time.
- Ectopic pregnancy is responsible for the greatest morbidity and mortality in early pregnancy; ruptured ectopic pregnancy remains responsible for 10% of pregnancy-related deaths.
- Women with a previous ectopic pregnancy have a 15% recurrence rate.
- Serum human chorionic gonadotropin (HCG) levels can vary by as much as 15% between laboratories, and an HCG level should be ordered when suspicion is high despite a negative urine HCG.
- Gestational trophoblastic disease (up to 75% of malignant cases) may develop after a nonmolar pregnancy (spontaneous and elective abortion, ectopic pregnancy, and term gestation); these patients have prolonged bleeding after delivery or miscarriage, with subsequent HCG levels that fail to return to undetectable values.

## SPONTANEOUS ABORTION

## EPIDEMIOLOGY

Spontaneous abortion, also known as miscarriage, occurs when a pregnancy ends before the fetus has reached viability. Viability correlates to a fetus larger than 500 g—or approximately the size at 20 to 22 weeks of gestation. Miscarriage is common and occurs in 25% to 30% of all pregnancies. Eighty percent of miscarriages occur before the 12th week of gestation, and up to 25% occur in pregnancies that are not even recognized clinically; in such cases human chorionic gonadotropin (HCG) can be detected in urine but the patient has no missed menses.[1]

Approximately 25% of patients will experience some bleeding in the first trimester of pregnancy, with half of these patients proceeding to miscarriage. Risks for spontaneous abortion include advanced maternal age, previous spontaneous abortion, and prolonged time from ovulation to implantation. Other risk factors are smoking, alcohol, cocaine, caffeine, and use of nonsteroidal antiinflammatory drugs.

### PATHOPHYSIOLOGY

The etiology of miscarriage can be classified as either intrinsic or extrinsic to the embryo. Intrinsic factors include genetic abnormalities and congenital conditions. Most cases of spontaneous abortion are due to genetic factors, either anembryonic gestations or chromosomal abnormalities. The majority of these defects arise de novo during fertilization and are not inherited. Genetic factors tend to lead to miscarriage early because of abnormal growth and development.[2] In contrast, later miscarriage is more often a result of extrinsic factors.

Extrinsic causes of miscarriage include host factors such as such as fibroids, intrauterine adhesions, septate uterus, maternal infections, hypercoagulable states, endocrine abnormalities, and teratogen exposure. Although blunt trauma to the abdomen is an unlikely cause of miscarriage because of the well-protected placement of the uterus in the pelvis, traumatic procedures such as chorionic villus sampling and amniocentesis may induce miscarriage.

## PRESENTING SIGNS AND SYMPTOMS

Spontaneous abortion is classified as threatened, inevitable, incomplete, complete, missed, or septic. **Table 119.1** lists characteristics of these categories. Symptoms of spontaneous abortion include vaginal bleeding, suprapubic cramping or pain, and passage of tissue. Bleeding can vary from minor spotting to severe hemorrhage.

Threatened abortion is defined by vaginal bleeding with or without mild suprapubic cramping or pain. It is the most common manifestation of spontaneous abortion seen in the emergency department (ED). Examination shows a closed cervix, uterine size that correlates to gestational age, and bleeding varying from scant to heavy. Ultrasound imaging confirms an intrauterine pregnancy and fetal heart tones in appropriate gestational ages. Threatened abortion may resolve with progression to normal pregnancy, or it may progress to other forms of miscarriage.

**Table 119.1 Classification of Spontaneous Abortion**

| CATEGORY | DEFINITION, CLINICAL CHARACTERISTICS | ULTRASONOGRAPHIC FINDINGS |
|---|---|---|
| Threatened | Bleeding and/or cramping with no passage of tissue, closed os, uterine size appropriate for dates, pregnancy viable | Intrauterine pregnancy (IUP), fetal heart tones (if age appropriate) |
| Inevitable | Open os without passage of products, pregnancy nonviable | IUP or products in the cervical canal |
| Incomplete | Partial passage of products; open os, uterus not well contracted; variable bleeding; pregnancy nonviable | Persistent gestational tissue in the uterus |
| Complete | Products of pregnancy completely passed, closed os, minimal bleeding, uterus well contracted | Empty uterus |
| Missed | Intrauterine demise with no spontaneous passage of products, closed os | Absent fetal cardiac activity or anembryonic gestation, absent heart tones with a crown rump length > 5 mm, absent fetal pole with >18-mm mean sac diameter |
| Septic | Infection complicating any of the previously described categories | Persistent products of conception or hemorrhage within the uterine cavity |

Before the 12th week of gestation, most spontaneous abortions will progress to completion with few complications. After this time, patients are more likely to have an incomplete abortion and require medical or operative intervention.

A septic abortion occurs when infection develops during any stage of the abortion process. Implicated agents include *Staphylococcus aureus*, gram-negative rods, gram-positive cocci, and anaerobes. Risk factors include elective abortion, cytomegalovirus infection, amniocentesis, and incomplete abortion.

## DIFFERENTIAL DIAGNOSIS AND MEDICAL DECISION MAKING

As mentioned previously, bleeding in early pregnancy is common. It may represent benign bleeding from implantation or marginal separation of the placenta. Many cases are idiopathic. Pathologic processes in the differential diagnosis include ectopic pregnancy, gestational trophoblastic disease, cervicitis, subchorionic hemorrhage, and cervical or vaginal malignancy. Vaginal lacerations from intercourse or trauma may be to blame. Occasionally, nongynecologic sources such as rectal bleeding or hematuria are mistaken for vaginal bleeding.

Pregnancy should be confirmed by a positive urine HCG test. A speculum examination should be performed to assess the degree of bleeding and cervical dilation, as well as to inspect for expelled products of conception. Bimanual examination can assess uterine size, cervical opening, and any abnormal masses or tenderness.

Laboratory studies include a complete blood count, quantitative HCG, and blood type with Rh status. With significant bleeding or other medical disease, coagulation parameters and typing and crossmatching for blood products should be ordered. Ultrasonography is essential for a full diagnosis and for guiding further management (**Fig. 119.1**). Even if it appears that the patient has passed the embryo, she should undergo ultrasound imaging to evaluate for any retained products.

## TREATMENT

Many patients with spontaneous abortion often need little or no intervention following accurate diagnosis and exclusion of other pathology. Expectant management is the only option for threatened abortion; education and ensuring adequate follow-up care are essential. The presence of fetal heart tones in women with symptoms of threatened abortion is reassuring; less than 5% of women younger than 36 years will miscarry, but this risk rises to 29% in those older than 40.[3]

Inevitable abortions may be managed either expectantly or by dilation and curettage. Both methods are generally acceptable. If products of conception are visible in the cervical os, gentle removal with ring forceps may allow the cervix to close and may control the bleeding. A complete abortion requires no further treatment as long as ultrasound scanning confirms that no retained products are present. Any retrieved tissue should be examined for villi, which will have a frondlike appearance.

Incomplete or missed abortions can be managed expectantly as long as shock, fever, or significant ongoing bleeding are absent. The time course for completion of a spontaneous abortion is highly variable, and patients will need education and routine gynecologic care to plan for dilation and curettage if tissue does not pass spontaneously or if the bleeding becomes heavy. Patients should attempt to collect the products of conception for examination and should undergo subsequent ultrasonography to assess whether all products of conception have passed. Studies have proved the safety of this practice.[4] Approximately 90% of patients with incomplete and 76% of those with missed abortions require no surgical treatment when managed expectantly for 4 weeks. Complications occur in 1%, less than in those managed medically.[5]

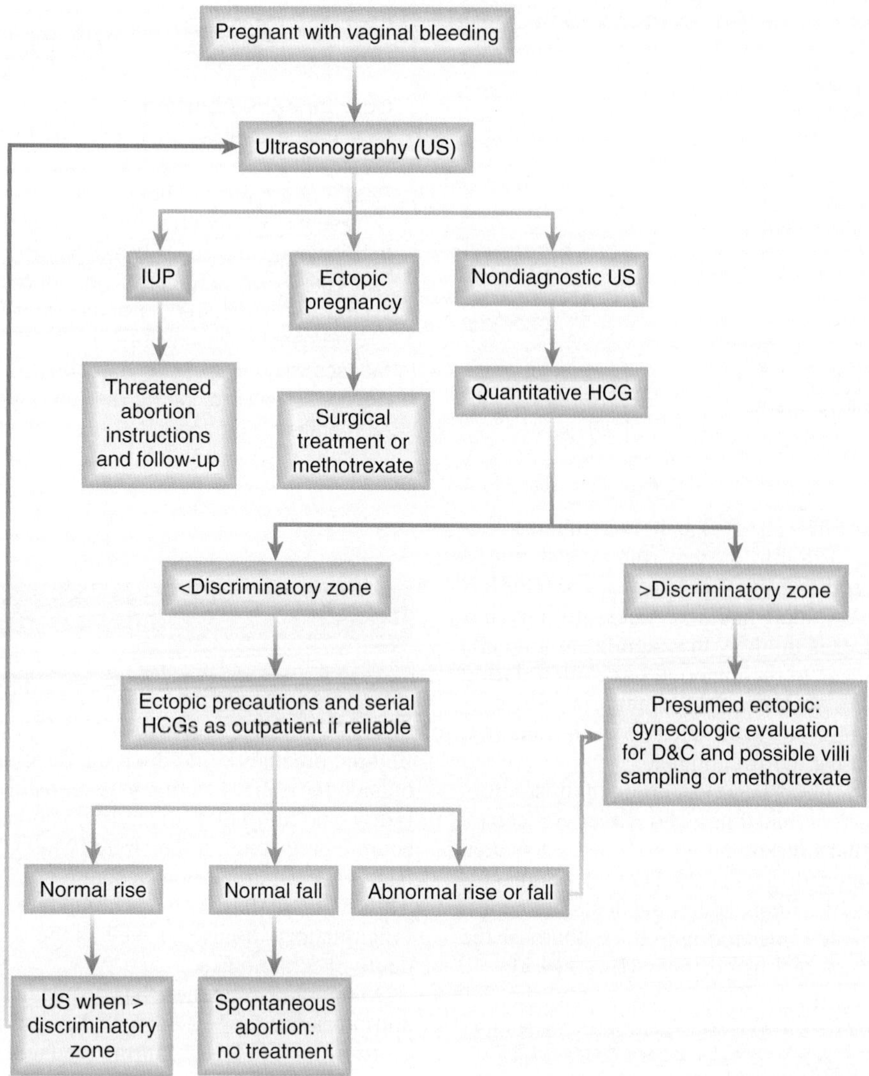


**Fig. 119.1 Algorithm for evaluation of vaginal bleeding in a pregnant patient.** *D&C*, Dilation and curettage; *HCG*, human chorionic gonadotropin; *IUP*, intrauterine pregnancy.

Prostaglandins such as misoprostol can effectively induce abortion for pregnancy failure of longer than 12 weeks and may help control bleeding in patients with inevitable or incomplete abortions. The dose of misoprostol is 800 mcg administered vaginally or rectally, but this drug should be given only after consultation with a gynecologist. One large study showed an 84% success rate.[6] Misoprostol induces spontaneous abortion, so any possibility of a desired viable pregnancy must be excluded.

Surgical management includes dilation and curettage or dilation and evacuation. Indications are listed in **Box 119.1**. Risks associated with surgical management are small and include uterine perforation, infection, adhesions, and anesthetic complications.

Women with significant hemorrhage or hemodynamic instability should first receive crystalloid volume replacement. If no response is seen or if the bleeding persists, either type-specific or type O-negative blood should be administered. Patients with septic abortions should be given broad-spectrum antibiotics in addition to dilation and curettage.

**BOX 119.1 Indications for Dilation and Curettage in Patients with Spontaneous Abortion**

Incomplete abortion
Significant hemorrhage
Signs of septic abortion
Documented fetal demise or blighted ovum with no spontaneous passage (after a period of observation)
Patient unwilling or unable to comply with expectant management

## $RH_0$ IMMUNE GLOBULIN

$Rh_0$ immune globulin ($Rh_0$ IG) should be administered to any Rh-negative woman with signs of spontaneous abortion unless the father is also known to be Rh negative. It is administered in a dose of 50 mcg before the twelfth week of gestation and

**BOX 119.2 Indications for $Rh_0$ Immunization**

Spontaneous abortion (any phase)
Elective pregnancy termination
Ectopic pregnancy
Amniocentesis
Chorionic villus sampling
Gestational trophoblastic disease
Blunt abdominal trauma
Placenta previa
Placental abruption
Immune thrombocytopenic purpura
Routinely at 28 weeks of gestation
Postpartum (if Rh-positive infant)

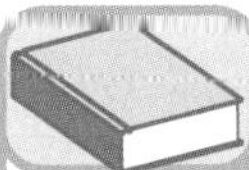

**PATIENT TEACHING TIPS**

**Spontaneous Abortion**

Miscarriage affects up to one third of pregnancies. Most patients will subsequently have normal pregnancies.

Reassure the patient that in most cases genetic factors are responsible—not patient behavior.

In threatened abortion with a detectable fetal heartbeat, 95% of cases will progress to normal pregnancy.

Women with recurrent miscarriage should receive fertility and genetic evaluation.

Menses will usually resume in about 6 weeks.

Advise 2 weeks of pelvic rest and suggest waiting 2 to 3 months before trying to get pregnant again (although no studies have confirmed either recommendation).

in a dose of 300 mcg after 12 weeks. It is estimated that 50 mcg will neutralize 2.5 mL of fetal blood and that a 300-mcg dose will neutralize 15 mL. A 12-week-old fetus has approximately 4.8 mL of blood, and a 16-week-old fetus has about 30 mL of blood. It is unlikely that significant amounts of fetal blood will transfer to the maternal circulation during a first-term miscarriage, so the single, appropriate dose of immune globulin will be fully sufficient to prevent maternal antibody formation against the Rh antigen.

$Rh_0$ IG is effective for up to 12 weeks after administration, so patients with recurrent bleeding who already received immunization within that time frame do not need a repeated dose. If significant hemorrhage occurs later in pregnancy, especially in the setting of trauma, additional doses are necessary. Ideally, $Rh_0$ IG is administered within 72 hours of the event leading to fetal-maternal hemorrhage (**Box 119.2**).

## NEXT STEPS IN CARE AND FOLLOW-UP

Emergency gynecologic consultation is needed for patients with significant hemorrhage or signs of infection. Others may be managed expectantly or with close follow-up as long as adequate outpatient care is ensured. Patients with missed abortions may ultimately need surgical management if they do not spontaneously pass tissue.

Patients should be instructed to contact their physician or return to the ED if heavy bleeding, severe pain, or fever develops. Bleeding should resolve over the course of a few weeks, and menses will generally resume within 6 weeks. Pelvic rest (no vaginal intercourse, tampons, or douching) for 2 weeks is often recommended because of the theoretic risk for infection, although no studies support this risk. Patients are often advised to not become pregnant for 2 to 3 months, but again no studies show worse outcomes if another pregnancy is achieved during this interval.

Psychosocial issues surrounding miscarriage are common, including feelings of guilt and sadness. Reassuring women that most miscarriages are due to genetic abnormalities and are not the result of their actions is essential. Women with substance abuse leading to abortion should be counseled appropriately. Referral for grief counseling may be appropriate. Patients with recurrent miscarriages should be offered referral for fertility treatment and genetics counseling.

# ECTOPIC PREGNANCY

## EPIDEMIOLOGY

Ectopic pregnancy, in which the developing embryo implants outside the uterine cavity, is responsible for the greatest morbidity and mortality in early pregnancy. The incidence of ectopic pregnancy in the United States has increased over the past 30 years, and it now accounts for 2% of all pregnancies.[7] This increase has been attributed to rising rates of pelvic inflammatory disease, as well as the advent of assisted reproductive technologies.

At the same time there has been a decrease in the morbidity and mortality associated with ectopic pregnancy because of more widespread use of ultrasound and methotrexate. Despite advances in diagnosis and management, ruptured ectopic pregnancy remains responsible for 10% of pregnancy-related deaths.

## PATHOPHYSIOLOGY

Risk factors for ectopic pregnancy are outlined in **Box 119.3**. Tubal pathology, the most significant risk factor, leads to abnormal transport and implantation of the embryo. The majority of cases arise in women with a history of pelvic inflammatory disease, and women with a previous ectopic pregnancy have a 15% recurrence rate. However, up to 50% of patients with an ectopic pregnancy have no identifiable risk factor.[8]

Genetic abnormalities in the embryo have not been found to be a risk factor for abnormal implantation. Although women using an intrauterine device or those who have undergone a sterilization procedure are at decreased overall risk for pregnancy, the incidence of ectopic pregnancy is increased in those who do become pregnant. For example, the pregnancy rate after tubal ligation is 0.1% to 0.8%, but as many as one third of these pregnancies are ectopic.

The most common location for ectopic implantation is the fallopian tube, which accounts for 95% of all ectopic pregnancies. The growing blastocyst leads to tubal distention and bleeding into the peritoneal cavity. If the pregnancy continues and is undetected, it can lead to rupture of the tube with subsequent hemorrhage. Less commonly, ectopic pregnancies implant on the ovary, abdominal viscera, or cervix. In these cases, significant hemorrhage or perforation of abdominal structures may occur. See **Figure 119.2** for sites of ectopic implantation.

## PRESENTING SIGNS AND SYMPTOMS

Most ectopic pregnancies are detected 6 to 8 weeks after missed menses, and significant tubal distention and bleeding have usually occurred by that point. Symptoms may mimic the signs of spontaneous abortion. The classic triad consists of abdominal pain, vaginal bleeding, and a missed menstrual period, although these symptoms vary with the stage of the pregnancy. Patients with early ectopic pregnancies may have no abdominal tenderness or vaginal bleeding, and the ectopic implantation may be found only incidentally on ultrasonography.

In contrast, a woman with tubal rupture may display hemodynamic instability and signs of a surgical abdomen. Approximately one half of patients are asymptomatic before tubal rupture. Of those with rupture, 99% have abdominal pain, 74% have amenorrhea, and 56% have vaginal bleeding.

An interstitial, or cornual, pregnancy occurs when the embryo is implanted in the proximal portion of the tube that is embedded in the muscle of the uterus. The tube at this location is more distensible, so the embryo may grow undetected for a longer period. It may not be discovered until 12 weeks or later. Ultrasonography demonstrates an asymmetric uterine thickness surrounding the gestational sac. However, a skilled ultrasonographer is required, and in the early stages it may be mistaken for a normal intrauterine pregnancy. Cornual pregnancy is associated with a 2% to 2.5% maternal mortality rate and is more likely than other tubal pregnancies to require hysterectomy.

A heterotopic pregnancy occurs when an intrauterine pregnancy is present simultaneously with an ectopic gestation. Its incidence was at one time estimated to be 1 in 30,000, but the true incidence is unknown. Thus an ectopic gestation can essentially be excluded if an intrauterine pregnancy is demonstrated by ultrasonography. Patients using assisted reproductive techniques have up to a 1% incidence of ectopic pregnancy, highest in patients with transfer of multiple embryos. In these patients, an ectopic gestation should not be excluded solely on the basis of the presence of an intrauterine pregnancy.[9]

**BOX 119.3 Risk Factors for Ectopic Pregnancy**

**High Risk**
History of pelvic inflammatory disease
Tubal surgery
Previous ectopic pregnancy
Tumor or congenital tubal abnormality
In utero diethylstilbestrol exposure

**Moderate Risk**
Previous genital infection, especially if recurrent
Infertility
More than one lifetime sexual partner

**Low Risk**
Smoking
Douching
First intercourse when younger than 18 years
Age older than 35 years
In vitro fertilization
Tubal ligation

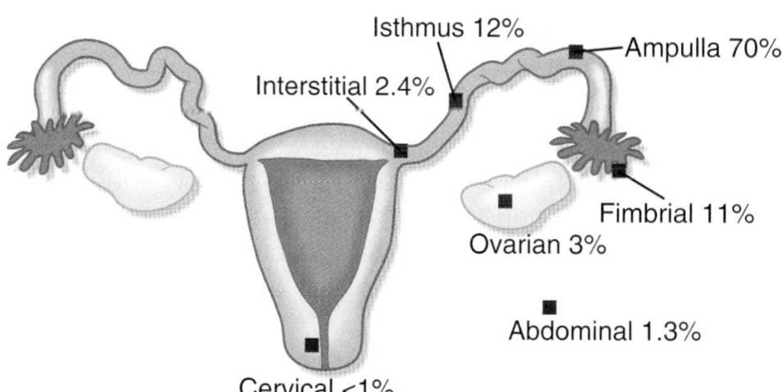


**Fig. 119.2 Sites and rate of occurrence at each site of ectopic implantation.**

## DIFFERENTIAL DIAGNOSIS AND MEDICAL DECISION MAKING

The differential diagnosis of ectopic pregnancy is listed in **Box 119.4**. Because of the high potential for morbidity, any patient with abnormal vaginal bleeding or abdominal or pelvic pain should be considered to have an ectopic pregnancy until proved otherwise (see Fig. 119.1).

### QUANTITATIVE HUMAN CHORIONIC GONADOTROPIN TESTING

Urinary HCG testing is essential for any woman of childbearing age with abdominal pain. Commercially available kits detect as low as 20 mIU/mL, although there have been case reports of ectopic pregnancy with an undetectable urine HCG

**BOX 119.4 Differential Diagnosis of Ectopic Pregnancy**

Spontaneous abortion
Benign bleeding from implantation
Hemorrhage, rupture, or torsion of a corpus luteum cyst
Molar pregnancy
Pelvic inflammatory disease
Endometriosis
Appendicitis
Diverticulitis
Urinary tract infection
Nephrolithiasis

level.[10] If high clinical suspicion still exists despite negative urinary HCG, a serum HCG test should be ordered.

In normal pregnancy, HCG production begins shortly after fertilization with a peak of about 100,000 mIU/mL at approximately 41 days' gestational age. In the early weeks of normal pregnancy, HCG levels are expected to double roughly every 48 hours, with a range of 1.4 to 2.1 days. In contrast, HCG levels generally rise more slowly with ectopic and nonviable intrauterine pregnancies. However, in some normal pregnancies, HCG levels may increase as little as 66% over a 48-hour period,[11] and up to 17% of ectopic pregnancies have normal doubling times. Patients should have serial measurements done by the same laboratory because interassay variability may be as high as 15%.

### ULTRASONOGRAPHY

Transvaginal ultrasonography is essential for making the diagnosis. A visible extrauterine gestational sac with a yolk sac or embryo confirms the diagnosis of ectopic pregnancy, but this is seen in less than half of cases. Highly suggestive findings include a complex adnexal mass or free fluid in the pelvis in conjunction with an empty uterus.

#### *Ultrasonographic Findings Plus Human Chorionic Gonadotropin*

To obtain the full benefit of transvaginal ultrasonography, serum HCG levels must be taken into consideration.

The earliest ultrasonographic confirmation of intrauterine pregnancy is a true gestational sac seen within the uterine cavity. The sac is routinely visualized when HCG levels reach 1500 to 2000 mIU/mL, but it can be detected with levels as low as 800 mIU/mL. The discriminatory zone refers to the level of HCG at which a true gestational sac can be seen. Lack of an intrauterine pregnancy with an HCG level above the discriminatory zone raises concern for ectopic pregnancy or a failed intrauterine gestation. The discriminatory zone is generally accepted to be in the range of 1500 mIU/mL but is dependent on equipment quality and operator skill.

Transvaginal sonograms are more likely to be nondiagnostic in women with very low HCG levels, but they may still be useful. Given its safety, transvaginal ultrasonography should be performed on all women with a suspected ectopic pregnancy, even those with HCG levels below the discriminatory zone.[12] In a study by Kaplan et al., 19% of patients with HCG levels higher than 1000 mIU/mL at the time of evaluation had transvaginal sonograms diagnostic of an ectopic pregnancy.[12] The specificity of the ultrasonography findings was 100%.

As discussed previously, ectopic pregnancy is visualized by ultrasonography only half of the time; therefore, women with serum HCG levels below the discriminatory zone and nondiagnostic ultrasonographic findings present a clinical challenge. These findings may represent an ectopic pregnancy or a nonviable early intrauterine pregnancy. In these cases, HCG testing and ultrasonography should be repeated at 48 to 72 hours. HCG levels increasing normally at 48 to 72 hours should be monitored until the intrauterine pregnancy can be seen on the sonogram. A decreasing HCG level is most consistent with a failed pregnancy or spontaneously resolving ectopic pregnancy. In these cases, serial measurements should be monitored until HCG reaches nondetectable levels.

Patients with HCG levels that plateau or rise by less than double in 72 hours are likely to have either a nonviable intrauterine or an ectopic pregnancy. Repeated transvaginal ultrasonography may be helpful to distinguish the two. Failure to visualize an intrauterine gestation with HCG levels higher than 2000 mIU/mL excludes the possibility of a viable pregnancy. These patients have a high likelihood of having an ectopic gestation and should be treated accordingly.[13]

Patients with HCG levels higher than 1500 mIU/mL may undergo dilation and curettage to obtain tissue for examination. Confirmation of villi in the curettage specimen confirms the diagnosis of a failed intrauterine pregnancy, whereas their absence suggests an ectopic pregnancy. Laparoscopy may then be used to provide a definitive diagnosis and guide treatment.

## TREATMENT

Ruptured ectopic pregnancy may have dramatic findings, with the patient in hemorrhagic shock. Rapid stabilization with intravenous fluids and packed red blood cells is essential. Unstable patients may require O-negative blood until a full crossmatch is performed. Laboratory studies include a complete blood count, quantitative HCG, and coagulation studies. The gynecology department should be consulted for operative management. Rh-negative patients should receive $Rh_0$ IG.

In stable patients, treatment of confirmed unruptured ectopic pregnancy may be medical, surgical, or expectant.

### METHOTREXATE THERAPY

The medical treatment of choice is methotrexate, a folate antagonist that inhibits DNA synthesis in rapidly dividing cells such as embryonic tissue. This action leads to medically induced abortion of the embryo. Despite limitations, use of methotrexate allows noninvasive management and has proved successful in properly selected patients. Methotrexate protocols vary by institution, but single-dose treatment consisting of an intramuscular injection of 50 mg/m$^2$ of body surface area is widely used.

The ideal candidate for methotrexate therapy is relatively asymptomatic with no significant pain or bleeding. A minority of patients will fail treatment or progress to rupture, and the patient must be made aware of these possibilities. Criteria predicting success include diameter less than 3.5 cm, absence of cardiac activity on ultrasonography, and HCG level lower than 5000 mIU/mL. Patients with lower HCG levels tend to have fewer treatment failures.[14]

Patients should be counseled on the risks and benefits of methotrexate therapy. They must be willing to comply with follow-up visits and have ready access to care. The patient should be aware of the possibility of treatment failure.

Relative contraindications include a high HCG level (>6000 mIU/mL), visible cardiac activity, and a large ectopic mass. Although visible cardiac activity is generally considered a contraindication, one study showed good results despite this finding.[15] Absolute contraindications to the use of methotrexate include hemodynamic instability, as well as the factors listed in **Box 119.5**.

Side effects of methotrexate include stomatitis, conjunctivitis, enteritis, pleuritis, bone marrow suppression, and elevated liver function test results. Thirty percent of patients are affected, but most symptoms are mild and self-limited. The

**BOX 119.5 Contraindications to Methotrexate Therapy**

Hypersensitivity to methotrexate
Breastfeeding
Immunodeficiency
Alcoholic or other liver disease
Blood dyscrasias
Active pulmonary disease
Peptic ulcer disease
Renal dysfunction

majority of patients will experience some abdominal pain, usually 2 to 3 days after methotrexate administration, because of tubal abortion with subsequent hematoma formation. In contrast to the pain from rupture, this pain is milder, and patients do not have hemodynamic instability or signs of a surgical abdomen. Although only 20% of patients with abdominal pain following methotrexate administration will ultimately need laparoscopy to evaluate for rupture, this subset can be difficult to identify. Transvaginal ultrasonography should be performed in these patients to evaluate for rupture.[16]

It is normal for HCG levels to increase for as long as 4 days following methotrexate administration. Patients typically have HCG testing repeated between days 4 and 7. By day 7, if the serum HCG level has not decreased by 25%, a second dose of methotrexate is given (required in 15% to 20% of patients), and HCG values are monitored weekly until levels decrease to less than 10 to 15 mIU/mL. Success rates with methotrexate range from 86% to 94%.

**TIPS AND TRICKS**

**Methotrexate**

Relative contraindications to methotrexate include an HCG level higher than 6000 mIU/mL, visible cardiac activity, and a large ectopic mass because of a high rate of treatment failure.
It is normal for HCG to increase for as long as 4 days after treatment.
On day 7, if HCG has not decreased by 25%, a second dose is needed (15% to 25% of patients).
Most patients will have some abdominal pain 2 to 3 days after administration; this pain is milder than that with rupture. Twenty percent of these patients will need laparoscopy to exclude rupture, however.

### SURGICAL TREATMENT

Surgical treatment is the only option for unstable patients with ectopic pregnancy. It is also indicated for patients with large ectopic masses, patients unable or unwilling to comply with the monitoring associated with methotrexate therapy, and patients with poor access to emergency care.

Resection of the ectopic mass with preservation of normal anatomy is ideal. Consequently, salpingostomy is preferred over salpingectomy. Laparoscopic resection is the standard approach, although laparotomy is occasionally required. After surgery, patients should be monitored with weekly HCG testing given the slight possibility of persistent ectopic tissue following resection.

A recent review showed the highest success rates with salpingostomy, although single-dose methotrexate therapy had the lowest financial cost and the least impact on quality of life.[17] Methotrexate therapy was less costly in patients with HCG levels lower than 1500 mIU/mL. The cost of medical therapy increases in patients with higher HCG levels because of the increased risk for failure, the requirement for multiple doses, and the need for extended monitoring.

Stable patients with nondiagnostic HCG and ultrasound findings are designated as having a pregnancy of unknown location. Expectant management relies on the fact that the spontaneous resolution rate of pregnancies of unknown location is 70%.[18] These patients are monitored with serial HCG levels and ultrasonography until a definitive diagnosis can be made. Expectant management is most successful in patients with HCG levels lower than 200 mIU/mL; increased complications occur in those with HCG levels higher than 1500 mIU/mL. However, the complication of tubal rupture can develop in as many as 30%, and it may occur even with decreasing HCG levels, so patients must be aware that treatment failures do occur.

## NEXT STEPS IN CARE AND FOLLOW-UP

In consultation with the patient's gynecologist, patients with a confirmed ectopic pregnancy should receive methotrexate or be transferred for operative management. Low-risk patients with an indeterminate work-up who are clinically stable may be discharged with appropriate follow-up in 48 to 72 hours for repeated HCG testing and ultrasonography. Patients without access to follow-up may be admitted for observation. Patients with a pregnancy of unknown location should be counseled about the possibility of an ectopic pregnancy.

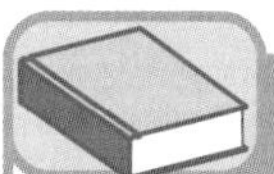

**PATIENT TEACHING TIPS**

**Instructions After Receiving Methotrexate**

Use acetaminophen for pain instead of nonsteroidal antiinflammatory drugs (methotrexate interacts with them).
No intercourse or pelvic examination for 7 days or as advised by the gynecologist (theoretically could rupture the ectopic mass).
No pregnancy for at least one cycle.
Return to the emergency department if the pain increases, especially if it has an acute onset.

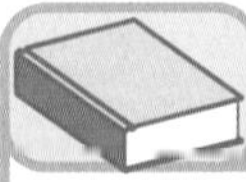

PATIENT TEACHING TIPS

**Ectopic Pregnancy**

Patients should understand that they *must* obtain follow-up in 2 days for evaluation and repeated HCG measurements because of the potential dangers associated with ectopic pregnancy. (Many patients fail to return for scheduled follow-up.)

Patients should return to the emergency department immediately if any of the following symptoms occur:

- Increased or continuous abdominal pain
- Heavy vaginal bleeding
- Weakness, dizziness, or lightheadedness

The patient should have ready access to emergency care and should avoid distant travel or rural locations.

Patients undergoing fertility treatment with gonadotropins or multiple embryo transfers should be educated about the possibility of recurrence of ectopic pregnancy (e.g., 15% recurrence rate after one ectopic pregnancy, 30% recurrence rate after two ectopic pregnancies).

**Table 119.2 Characteristics of Molar Pregnancies**

| CHARACTERISTIC | COMPLETE MOLE | PARTIAL MOLE |
|---|---|---|
| Genetics | Paternal DNA only; 90% 46XX, 10% 46XY | Paternal and maternal DNA; 69XXX, 69XXY, or tetraploid |
| HCG level | Increased | High normal |
| Uterine size | Greater than expected at gestation dates | Normal |
| Fetal tissue | Absent | Present |
| Malignant transformation | 15%-20% | 5% |

*HCG*, Human chorionic gonadotropin.

# GESTATIONAL TROPHOBLASTIC DISEASE

## EPIDEMIOLOGY

The incidence of gestational trophoblastic disease (GTD) varies from 1 per 1000 pregnancies in the United States to 2 per 1000 pregnancies in Japan.[19] Well-established risk factors include nulliparity, personal history of GTD, and maternal age younger than 20 or older than 35 years. Heavy smoking, oral contraceptive use, infertility, and maternal blood types AB or B are also risk factors. Although the disease carried significant morbidity in the past, earlier diagnosis with ultrasonography and more sensitive HCG measurements have led to more successful treatment in recent years.

## PATHOPHYSIOLOGY

GTD is a disorder of abnormal proliferation of trophoblastic tissue. The benign form is a hydatidiform mole, whereas the malignant forms are grouped as gestational trophoblastic neoplasia, which includes choriocarcinoma, placental site trophoblastic tumor, and persistent or invasive GTD. Although GTD is classically associated with molar pregnancy, it may result from any gestational event, such as spontaneous abortion or term pregnancy.

The most common form of GTD is a hydatidiform mole, either partial or complete. A partial mole contains fetal tissue and arises from fertilization of a haploid ovum by two sperm or by a single sperm that then duplicates. In contrast, a complete mole has no fetal tissue or maternal DNA and results from fertilization of an enucleate egg. Up to 15% of complete moles result in malignancy, whereas malignant transformation of a partial mole is less common. **Table 119.2** lists the typical characteristics of molar pregnancies.

The abnormal trophoblastic tissue in GTD secretes HCG, thereby resulting in quantitative serum levels much higher than predicted in normal pregnancy. Patients with GTD have an increased incidence of hyperemesis gravidarum and early preeclampsia. Hyperthyroidism may result because of the structural similarity of HCG and thyroid-stimulating hormone. Theca lutein cysts seen in patients with GTD are bilateral, multiloculated ovarian cysts that are present in 15% to 25% of patients with complete moles.

Trophoblastic hyperplasia causes uterine enlargement abnormal for the stage of pregnancy. Deeper uterine invasion may result and lead to severe hemorrhage from destruction of the myometrium or uterine vasculature. Malignant forms of GTD may spread into the pelvis or be manifested as distant metastases, most commonly to the liver, lungs, vagina, and brain.

## PRESENTING SIGNS AND SYMPTOMS

The most common complaint with molar pregnancy is first trimester vaginal bleeding. Patients may also complain of pelvic pain or pressure, and there may be passage of hydropic vesicles from the vagina.

Complete moles have a more striking clinical manifestation, with uterine size larger than expected at the stage of pregnancy, absent fetal heart tones, and markedly elevated HCG levels. Vaginal bleeding may be heavy. Medical complications include pregnancy-induced hypertension, early preeclampsia, hyperthyroidism, anemia, and hyperemesis gravidarum.[20]

In contrast, the manifestation of a partial mole is subtle. Symptoms are similar to those of spontaneous abortion, with mild to moderate bleeding and cramping. Patients typically do not have significant uterine enlargement, and the diagnosis is made only when the abnormal placental tissue is visualized on ultrasonography. Patients with partial moles are less likely to have the medical complications associated with complete moles because HCG levels are lower.

As mentioned earlier, GTD may also develop after a nonmolar pregnancy, such as spontaneous and elective abortion, ectopic pregnancy, and term gestation. These patients have prolonged bleeding after delivery or miscarriage, with subsequent HCG levels that fail to return to undetectable measurements. Up to 75% of cases of malignant GTD occur after nonmolar pregnancies. Because placental site trophoblastic tumors may occur years after pregnancy, GTD should be considered in a woman with metastatic disease from an unknown primary site.[21]

## DIFFERENTIAL DIAGNOSIS AND MEDICAL DECISION MAKING

Molar pregnancy should be included in the differential diagnosis of any patient with first trimester bleeding (see Box 119.4). Abnormally elevated quantitative HCG levels suggest the diagnosis, although there is no absolute level that identifies molar pregnancy. Pelvic ultrasonography is diagnostic in almost all cases. Tissue obtained from uterine evacuation provides histologic confirmation.

Ultrasonographic findings in a patient with a complete mole include diffuse hydatidiform swelling of chorionic villi ("snowstorm pattern"), bilateral theca lutein cysts, and absence of fetal tissue or amniotic fluid. The ultrasonographic appearance of a partial mole is not as striking and may be misinterpreted by an inexperienced ultrasonographer. There is only focal hydatiform swelling with absence of theca lutein cysts. Growth-restricted embryonic tissue or amniotic fluid may also be seen.

Laboratory tests should include a complete blood count, blood typing and antibody screen, clotting function analysis, renal and liver studies, and measurement of the serum HCG level. For patients with malignant disease, additional work-up includes chest radiography to search for metastases. Other appropriate studies include computed tomography of the chest and magnetic resonance imaging of the abdomen, pelvis, and brain.

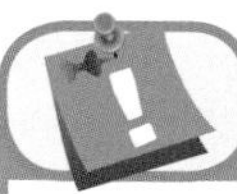

**TIPS AND TRICKS**

**Gestational Trophoblastic Disease**

Molar pregnancy should be in the differential diagnosis of patients with exaggerated symptoms of pregnancy such as hyperemesis and early preeclampsia.

In patients with spontaneous abortion, the products of conception should be sent for pathologic evaluation because of the possibility of incidental molar pregnancy.

The clinician should consider gestational trophoblastic disease in patients with prolonged or abnormal bleeding after delivery or miscarriage.

## TREATMENT

GTD is likely to be diagnosed only incidentally in the ED during evaluation for spontaneous abortion or ectopic pregnancy. Most patients have few or mild symptoms. Initial ED management includes supportive care for significant hemorrhage, including intravenous fluids and blood products. $Rh_0$ IG should be administered to Rh-negative women. Patients with rupture or torsion of theca lutein cysts may require operative management, although rupture is rare.[22]

## NEXT STEPS IN CARE AND FOLLOW-UP

Any woman with suspected or diagnosed GTD should be referred to a gynecologic oncologist urgently because the disease may progress quickly. Definitive management of molar pregnancy includes dilation and curettage. As long as serial HCG levels decline appropriately, no further treatment is needed. Persistent local disease is usually treated with chemotherapy, although hysterectomy may be performed in women with locally invasive disease who no longer desire fertility.

Posttreatment monitoring for malignant or persistent disease consists of serial HCG measurements. Patients should have frequent pelvic examinations to monitor for local recurrence or vaginal metastases. Patients should be instructed to use contraceptive methods for 12 months because an increase in HCG levels as a result of pregnancy would obscure the monitoring results. Affected patients have an approximately 1% chance for a recurrent mole in future pregnancies, although this risk increases to as high as 28% after two molar pregnancies.[23]

# HYPEREMESIS GRAVIDARUM

## EPIDEMIOLOGY

Estimates of the incidence of hyperemesis gravidarum range from 0.3% to 2% of all pregnancies. Risk factors include multiple gestations, GTD, personal or family history of hyperemesis, and female sex of the fetus. Protective factors include advanced maternal age, cigarette smoking, and anosmia. Hyperemesis gravidum is responsible for the highest percentage of hospital admissions during the first half of pregnancy.[24,25]

## PATHOPHYSIOLOGY

Up to 85% of pregnant patients experience nausea and vomiting to some degree. Hyperemesis gravidarum has no strict diagnostic criteria, but it is generally defined as nausea and vomiting that results in loss of 5% or more of prepregnancy weight, as well as ketonuria. In addition, the symptoms must not be attributable to another medical condition.

Hormonal factors are believed to be the pathogenesis. Studies have shown that women with higher HCG and estradiol concentrations have an increased incidence of hyperemesis, but the mechanism is unknown.[26] In contrast, no correlation of progesterone levels and symptoms has been shown. Other potential causes such as vitamin deficiencies, gastric motility, and *Helicobacter pylori* infection have not been consistently linked to the disease. The belief in the past that psychologic issues were causative has no supporting data.

## PRESENTING SIGNS AND SYMPTOMS

Hyperemesis classically begins early in the first trimester, with symptoms peaking at 9 to 10 weeks and generally resolving by 16 to 18 weeks. Most patients report more severe symptoms in the morning hours, often made worse by noxious smells. Frequently, multiple ED visits or interactions with a primary care provider occur because of the persistence of symptoms.

Symptoms of abdominal pain and tenderness are usually minimal; such findings suggest another pathology. The physical examination confirms varying levels of dehydration.

Complications include dehydration, weight loss, and vitamin deficiencies. Esophagitis, Mallory-Weiss tears, and Wernicke encephalopathy have been reported in patients with persistent vomiting and malnutrition. Anxiety, as well as depressive symptoms, may occur in response to the illness.

## DIFFERENTIAL DIAGNOSIS AND MEDICAL DECISION MAKING

The diagnosis of hyperemesis gravidarum is one of exclusion given the lack of confirmatory testing available. A careful history should confirm that the symptoms began in the first trimester, with review of systems negative for symptoms consistent with coexistent pathology. Physical examination is aimed at identifying these other conditions. **Box 119.6** outlines the differential diagnosis of hyperemesis.

Serum HCG measurements and ultrasonography can determine the time of gestation and rule out a hydatidiform mole. Urinalysis can rule out infection and may reveal ketonuria and high specific gravity. Laboratory evaluation can be helpful in excluding other pathology. Initial testing includes a complete blood count; basic chemistry panel; and liver, amylase, lipase, and thyroid function assays, including thyroid-stimulating hormone and free thyroxin levels.

As many as half of patients with hyperemesis will have mild elevations in transaminases; levels are usually in the low hundreds, with alanine transaminase levels being higher than aspartate transaminase levels. Amylase and lipase may be elevated, but much less so than with pancreatitis. Typical laboratory test results include hemoconcentration, electrolyte abnormalities, and mildly elevated hepatic and pancreatic function via urinalysis. The laboratory test abnormalities generally resolve by the 20th week of gestation, and no treatment is necessary.

## TREATMENT

After coexistent pathology has been ruled out, treatment consists of rehydration, correction of electrolyte abnormalities, control of nausea, and reinstitution of nutrition. Volume resuscitation is accomplished with normal saline or lactated Ringer solution. Dextrose-containing solutions can then be used for maintenance fluids. Potassium, magnesium, and phosphorus supplements should be added to fluids as needed. Patients with prolonged vomiting should be given thiamine (100 mg/day) and multivitamins intravenously.

Pharmacotherapy is appropriate significant nausea, although patients may have reservations about using these medications. The combination of pyridoxine (10 mg) and doxylamine (12.5 mg) three to four times a day is considered safe; randomized, placebo-controlled studies have shown a 70% reduction in nausea and vomiting. This combination should be considered first-line therapy.[27,28]

Various antiemetics (**Table 119.3**) have been used for hyperemesis with good results and reasonable safety data. Antihistamines have the best safety profile, but phenothiazines, metoclopramide, and ondansetron are considered safe as well. Gynecologists may prescribe oral corticosteroids for patients with refractory nausea and vomiting. Studies have shown conflicting results of effectiveness, and the incidence of cleft palate appears to be slightly increased in infants whose mothers received methylprednisolone in the first trimester of pregnancy. Steroids should thus be reserved as a last resort.[29,30]

**BOX 119.6 Differential Diagnosis of Hyperemesis Gravidarum**

**Gastrointestinal**
Gastroenteritis, pancreatitis, cholelithiasis, hepatitis, peptic ulcer disease, bowel obstruction, gastroparesis

**Metabolic**
Hyperthyroidism, hyperparathyroidism, diabetic ketoacidosis, toxic ingestions, porphyria

**Central Nervous System**
Intracranial mass, migraine headache, vestibular dysfunction, pseudotumor cerebri

**Other**
Pyelonephritis, nephrolithiasis, ovarian torsion, acute fatty liver of pregnancy, psychogenic disorders

**Table 119.3 Antiemetics for Hyperemesis Gravidarum**

| MEDICATION | SAFETY CLASSIFICATION | DOSAGE |
|---|---|---|
| Doxylamine | A | 12.5 mg PO |
| Dimenhydrinate | B | 50-100 mg PO, PR; 50 mg IV |
| Metoclopramide | B | 5-10 mg PO, IV, IM |
| Ondansetron | B | 4-8 mg PO, IV, IM |
| Promethazine | C | 12.5-25 mg IV, IM, PO, PR |
| Prochlorperazine | C | 5-10 mg IV, IM, PO; 25 mg PR |

*IM*, Intramuscularly; *IV*, intravenously; *PO*, orally; *PR*, parenterally.

Many patients are reluctant to use pharmacotherapy because of a perceived fear of birth defects. These patients may be agreeable to adjunctive therapies such as acupuncture, hypnosis, and powdered ginger. Studies of acupuncture and acupressure have yielded conflicting results,[31] whereas hypnosis has been shown to decrease vomiting in patients with hyperemesis. Powdered ginger (250 mg to 1 g/day) is as effective as pyridoxine, but its safety is not well established.[32]

The ultimate goal of treatment is restoration of nutrition. Many patients are able to tolerate feeding after a short course of rehydration along with gut rest. The Patient Teaching Tips box outlines dietary suggestions.

Patients who cannot maintain their weight despite rehydration and antiemetics are candidates for enteral nutrition. Those who cannot tolerate enteral feedings should be given total parenteral nutrition. This regimen carries the usual risks of infectious and metabolic complications.

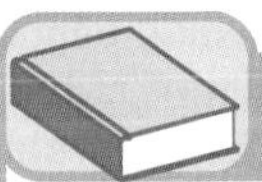

### PATIENT TEACHING TIPS

**Hyperemesis**

Daily multivitamin use at the time of conception may decrease the severity of nausea and vomiting.

Avoid triggers such as noxious odors, brushing teeth after eating, and iron supplements.

Eat small, frequent meals rich in protein and carbohydrates and low in fat. Avoid spicy foods.

Eat as soon as you feel hungry.

Drink small amounts of liquids often. Cold, clear, carbonated, and sour liquids are best tolerated.

Aromatic mint tea and teas with lemon or orange flavoring may be helpful.

## NEXT STEPS IN CARE AND FOLLOW-UP

Patients with mild dehydration may be discharged home after fluid and electrolyte repletion. Antiemetics can be prescribed for home use after appropriate discussion with the patient and primary physician. Many patients come to the ED before they have established prenatal care; ensuring adequate outpatient care is essential. Patients with severe dehydration, significant electrolyte abnormalities, progressive weight loss, and intractable vomiting despite antiemetics should be admitted to the hospital.

Patients should be instructed to return to the ED if vomiting persists or if they experience new symptoms such as abdominal pain and fever. Patients with only mild nausea and vomiting are not at increased risk for low-birth-weight infants or birth defects. Although patients with true hyperemesis do have a higher incidence of low-birth-weight infants, appropriate weight gain later in pregnancy reduces this risk.[33]

## SUGGESTED READINGS

ACEP Clinical Policies Committee and Clinical Policies Subcommittee on Early Pregnancy. American College of Emergency Physicians. Clinical policy; critical issues in the initial management of patients presenting to the emergency department in early pregnancy. Ann Emerg Med 2003;41:123-33.

Adhikari S, Blavias M, Lyon M. Diagnosis and management of ectopic pregnancy using bedside transvaginal ultrasonography in the ED: a 2-year experience. Am J Emerg Med 2007;25:591-6.

Kohn MA, Kerr K, Malkevich D, et al. Beta-human chorionic gonadotropin levels and the likelihood of ectopic pregnancy in emergency department patients with abdominal pain or vaginal bleeding. Acad Emerg Med 2003;10:119-26.

Stein JC, Wang R, et al. Emergency physician ultrasonography for evaluating patients at risk for ectopic pregnancy: a meta-analysis. Ann Emerg Med 2010;56:674-83.

## REFERENCES

*References can be found on Expert Consult @ www.expertconsult.com.*

# 120 First Trimester Ultrasonography

*Cindy W. Chan, Michael Lambert, and Vicki E. Noble*

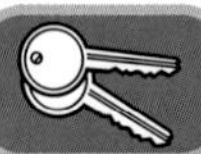

**KEY POINTS**

- Patients with ectopic pregnancy have highly variable and often unhelpful findings on physical examination.
- Ultrasound is the initial imaging modality of choice to locate a pregnancy in the first trimester.
- Emergency physicians proficient in ultrasound are capable of rapidly diagnosing ectopic pregnancy and expediting definitive care.
- Most first trimester pregnancies can be localized within the uterus on initial ultrasound in the emergency department.
- All patients discharged from the emergency department without a confirmed intrauterine pregnancy by ultrasound should thoroughly understand the "ectopic precautions," have close outpatient follow-up arranged with their obstetrician, and have the means to return immediately to the emergency department if complications arise.

## INTRODUCTION

All female patients of reproductive age seen in the emergency department (ED) with vaginal bleeding or abdominal or back pain should have a urine or serum pregnancy test performed. Ectopic pregnancy is the number one cause of death in patients in the first trimester.[1] Emergency physicians (EPs) caring for these patients understand that no historical clues or physical findings can effectively affirm or refute an ectopic pregnancy.[2] The rate-limiting step is finding the location of the pregnancy. Ultrasound imaging and interpretation play a crucial role in this decision-making process. The faster this information is available, the quicker management can be implemented. In the late 1980s, a few EP pioneers invested the time and effort to learn the technical and interpretive skills necessary to bring ultrasound to the bedside.[3] The ability to locate a first trimester pregnancy saves valuable time in the search for an ectopic pregnancy.[4] Ultrasound performed at the patient's bedside quickly classifies patients by ultrasound criteria.[5] Based on this ultrasound classification, management strategies can be implemented. The following sections describe the ultrasound techniques and management skills used in symptomatic patients in the first trimester of pregnancy.

## EVIDENCE-BASED REVIEW

In most EDs, when "formal" ultrasound is traditionally ordered, it is actually performed in the department of radiology. This requires (1) time to transport the patient out of the ED, (2) a sonographer available to obtain the images, and (3) a radiologist to interpret the study. Ultimately, the combination of these factors postpones the diagnosis, delays definitive care, and increase the patient's length of stay.[4] As an alternative to formal ultrasound, many EPs have learned how to perform and interpret ultrasound images at the patient's bedside. As early as 1989, a number of small studies suggested that EPs were able to perform ultrasound for ectopic pregnancies with high sensitivity.[3] When previous studies from multiple institutions are compiled to increase the sample size ($N = 2057$), it is estimated that EPs have a pooled sensitivity of 99.3% when diagnosing ectopic pregnancies at the bedside. Sensitivity is defined as the proportion of bedside ultrasound images demonstrating a true absence of definitive intrauterine pregnancy (IUP) in patients with ectopic pregnancies.[4]

Multiple retrospective and prospective studies from the late 1990s and early 2000s have reported that when compared with formal imaging, the use of bedside ultrasound to evaluate first trimester bleeding reduced length of stay in the ED by a mean time of 48 to 169 minutes. Time of day, day of the week, and whether ultrasound technicians were in house 24 hours a day were some of the factors that had an impact on the length of stay.[5] Finally, based on two separate studies from the early 2000s, bedside ultrasound performed by EPs saved an estimated $229 to $1244 per ED visit when compared with patients who underwent radiology-performed ultrasound. In some cases this was a 40% savings in billed charges.[5] Literature from the past 20 years has and continues to demonstrate that ultrasound performed by an EP to evaluate for ectopic pregnancies is feasible, fast, and accurate. Bedside ultrasound in symptomatic first trimester pregnant patients has high sensitivity in ruling out ectopic pregnancy, speeds time to diagnosis, and decreases true costs.

## HOW TO SCAN

The pelvic organs may be evaluated with one of two different sonographic methods of interrogation: the transabdominal or the endovaginal technique. In the transabdominal approach, the probe is positioned over the lower portion of the abdomen, just superior to the pubic symphysis, and directed inferiorly into the pelvis because the uterus typically remains a pelvic organ until approximately the 12th week of pregnancy. In the endovaginal approach, the probe is inserted into the vaginal vault, directly in touch with the cervix. These "windows" into the pelvis are illustrated and discussed in the following sections.

## TRANSABDOMINAL TECHNIQUE

The transabdominal technique has long been used to evaluate first trimester pregnant patients and is best done with a curvilinear probe. Before the ultrasound examination, a Foley catheter can be inserted to fill the bladder. The practice of filling the bladder accomplishes two things. First, a full bladder displaces bowel out of the anterior cul-de-sac and acts as an acoustic window to the pelvic organs. Second, a full bladder generally aligns the uterus such that its long axis parallels the abdominal wall. This allows the transmitted sound waves to strike the uterus at a nearly perpendicular angle, which produces better reflections when the returning echoes are received by the transducer and plotted on the monitor. Although this optimizes image quality, adequate images can often be achieved without this maneuver.

In the sagittal view, in which the uterus is seen in its long axis, the probe is placed just superior to the pubic symphysis with the indicator pointed toward the patient's head. The anterior-most organ on screen is the fluid-filled, triangular-shaped bladder. Just posterior to the bladder is the pear-shaped uterus. The uterus more commonly lies in an anteverted position, with the fundus pointed toward the anterior abdominal wall, but it may also be seen in a retroverted lie with the fundus pointing posteriorly toward the spine. The endometrial stripe serves as the landmark for identifying the longitudinal uterus in the midline. The endometrial stripe is a result of the endometrial mucosal lining coming together to form a hyperechoic, curvilinear line that continues as the cervical stripe more inferiorly (**Fig. 120.1,** *A* and *B*). After the midline of the longitudinal uterus is identified, the probe is panned from side to side to evaluate the entire width of the uterus. Much of the hyperechoic area surrounding the uterus is the bowel and rectum, which are poorly defined because of their solid and gas contents.

In the transverse view, the probe is rotated 90 degrees counterclockwise so that the indicator is pointed toward the patient's right. With the probe angled inferiorly to visualize into the pelvis, the anterior-most organ is the fluid-filled, rectangular-shaped bladder. Posterior to the bladder is an ovular-shaped cut of the uterus in the transverse view with the hyperechoic endometrial stripe in the center. The rectum and bowel are hyperechoic areas surrounding the bladder and uterus posteriorly and laterally. The uterus should be evaluated from the top of the fundus inferiorly through to the cervix. Though not always visualized, the ovaries may be seen lateral to the fundus of the uterus in either the sagittal or transverse view.

Advantages of the transabdominal technique include (1) an overall view of the true pelvis and (2) a faster examination. The lower-frequency curvilinear probe will penetrate deeper into the pelvis, and although the images might be a little fuzzy, a "full" view of the pelvis is provided. Second, in patients who are farther along in the first trimester or whose bladder is not completely empty, adequate transabdominal views can be obtained without filling the bladder. Less preparation time is needed to scan these patients, and enlisting the assistance of a coworker to chaperone is unnecessary.

The main disadvantage of the transabdominal technique results from the use of a lower-frequency probe. The lower frequency (2- to 5-MHz curvilinear probe) means less resolution and thus the pregnancy must be farther along (usually 7 to 8 weeks' gestational age) to be visualized. The transvaginal probe is a higher-frequency probe (5 to 9 MHz) with increased resolution, which means that pregnancies as early as 5 to 6 weeks can be visualized.

## ENDOVAGINAL TECHNIQUE

The arrival of endovaginal transducers in the 1980s significantly improved the quality of ultrasound imaging in female patients. Simplified, the engineering design placed an ultrasound transducer on the end of a stick that could be inserted

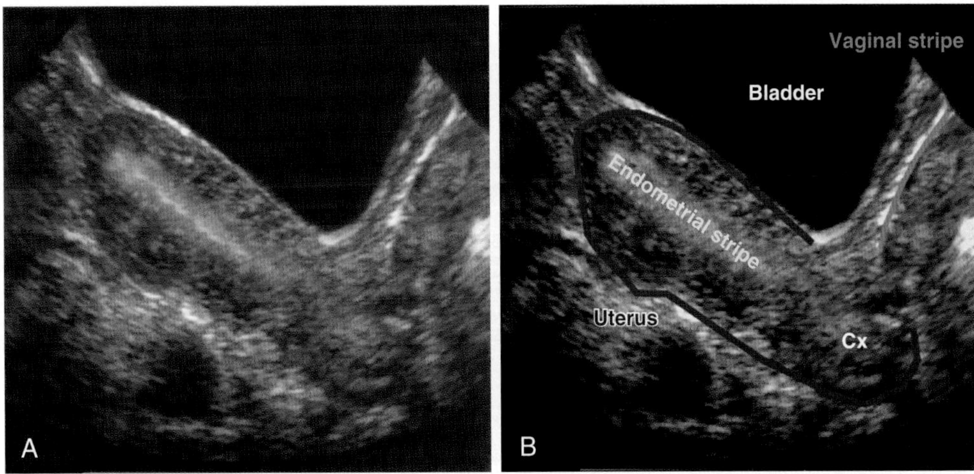


**Fig. 120.1** **A** and **B,** Transabdominal views of the sagittal plane of the uterus revealing the typical landmarks of the uterus, endometrial stripe, cervix, bladder, and vaginal stripe.

into the vaginal vault. This permits the transducer scanning head to be in close proximity to the pelvic organs, which has several important implications in ultrasound imaging. First, there is a clearer path to transmit and receive echoes, and second, the shorter distance between the transducer and the pelvic organs allows higher transducer frequencies to be used.[6] In contrast to the transabdominal approach, the quality of images from an endovaginal approach is enhanced with an empty bladder because of less distortion of the pelvic anatomy.

The high-frequency endocavitary probe is prepared by directly placing ultrasound gel on the transducer head, sheathing the probe with a sterile cover, and then adding more sterile gel over the sheathed transducer head. If it is not possible to place the patient in the lithotomy position on a gynecology examination table, it is important to adequately prop up the patient's pelvis for any modified positioning. It is often necessary to manipulate the handle of the probe below the level of the pelvis for better visualization. The covered probe is then inserted into the vaginal vault to begin scanning. Some patients and practitioners have found it more comfortable for patients to insert the probe.

For the sagittal view, the transducer is inserted so that the indicator is straight up and down, with the body sliced into left and right halves. Even after voiding, the bladder usually retains a small amount of fluid, which enables this anechoic structure to be used as a landmark in endovaginal imaging. After initially placing the probe into the vaginal vault, the bladder or uterus (or both) may not initially be visible. To look for these structures, the handle of the probe should be brought down and the footprint of the probe tilted more anteriorly and angled up to get the uterus in its full, longitudinal (sagittal) plane. In this plane, the anterior-most structure is a sliver of bladder, the pear-shaped uterus is posterior to the bladder, and the more hyperechoic bowel and rectum surround the uterus (**Fig. 120.2,** *A* to *C*). As in transabdominal imaging, the endometrial stripe serves as the landmark for identifying the longitudinal uterus in its midline. Once it is identified, the uterus should be interrogated along its entire width by fanning from side to side.

For the coronal view the probe is rotated 90 degrees counterclockwise, with the body cut into anterior and posterior components. As in the sagittal view, the probe is tilted anteriorly by moving the handle of the probe downward to obtain transverse cuts of the uterus. Depending on the depth of probe insertion, some part of the bladder may be seen. Deep to the bladder lies the ovular uterus, which is surrounded by the rectum and bowel.

Advantages of the endovaginal technique include (1) superior resolution and (2) a wider field of view. The shorter pathway from the transducer to the pelvic structures permits the use of higher frequencies. Sound attenuation is limited, and waves reflected from nearby objects are maximized. These higher-frequency probes, with their inherent enhanced resolution, provide the EP with more clinical confidence when interpreting images. In addition, most endovaginal transducers incorporate a beam angle that provides a 120- to 180-degree field of view.

Disadvantages of the endovaginal technique include (1) increased invasiveness, (2) more time to prepare and perform the scan, and (3) decreased depth of view. As the endovaginal probe is inserted into vaginal vault, there is a small risk of transmitting disease through an improperly sanitized probe. Second, the taboo of having an unknown physician insert a probe into the vaginal vault may require greater explanation of the procedure. Optimal examination is performed with a gynecology table, which may be a limited resource. More time commitment is involved in preparation for the endovaginal study and obtaining a chaperone. Third, the higher-frequency probes used for endovaginal scanning limit the range of the transmitted echo. Generally, a full view of the pelvis is not achieved with transvaginal scanning.

## IDENTIFICATION AND LOCALIZATION OF THE PREGNANCY

First trimester pregnancies can be categorized into three groups according to location: intrauterine, extrauterine, or indeterminate (**Box 120.1**). Within these three categories, further subdivisions into one of five diagnostic possibilities based on specific criteria (**Box 120.2**) are possible. The significance of this unambiguous classification scheme is that it corresponds with EP management strategies for first trimester symptomatic patients.

### INTRAUTERINE PREGNANCY

To define a pregnancy as intrauterine, it is imperative to have a clear understanding of the criteria necessary to support the

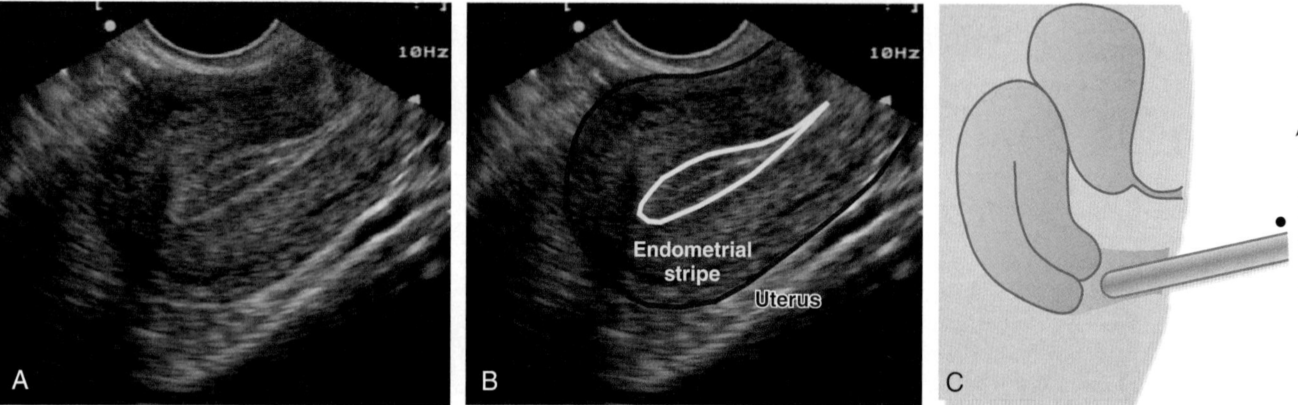


**Fig. 120.2** **A** and **B,** Transvaginal views of the sagittal plane of the uterus revealing the typical landmarks of the uterus and endometrial stripe. **C,** Illustration depicting positioning of the probe.

diagnosis by ultrasound (**Box 120.3**). The first component of the criteria is to visualize a gestational sac with a mean sac diameter (height, width, and length) larger than 5 mm and an echogenic ring. Second, this gestational sac must be clearly visualized within the endometrial lining of the uterus and many times may demonstrate a "double decidual sac sign." Finally, this gestational sac, which lies within the endometrial echo of the uterus, must contain a yolk sac or a fetal pole. Although this may be excessive for a radiologist who uses the double decidual sac sign as the earliest criteria for an IUP, it is a conservative safety measure that has served EPs well to avoid confusing the pseudogestational sac of an ectopic pregnancy with a true IUP. Because ectopic pregnancies secrete hormones that stimulate the endometrial lining, occasionally there may be changes in the endometrial lining that can approximate the appearance of a gestational sac. This pseudosac will never have an inner yolk sac or fetal pole. Use of these two additional findings for defining an IUP helps ensure that the EP will not be confused. Whether scanning from a transabdominal or an endovaginal approach, all these criteria should be visualized and documented on every sonogram. The safest way to ensure that these criteria are present is a systematic approach to documenting these landmarks. In the endovaginal approach, documentation is best achieved by obtaining a single sagittal view of the gestational and yolk sacs clearly within the endometrial echo of the uterus, along with the inferiorly positioned endometrial stripe as it passes through the corpus and cervical region of the uterus (**Fig. 120.3,** *A* and *B*). In the transabdominal approach, documentation is best achieved by obtaining a single sagittal view of the gestational and yolk sacs clearly within the endometrial echo of the uterus, along with the anteriorly positioned bladder and the inferiorly positioned vaginal stripe (**Fig. 120.4,** *A* and *B*). By identifying pregnancies as intrauterine, ectopic pregnancy has effectively been excluded with reasonable certainty. There is a theoretic risk for a heterotopic pregnancy of approximately 1 in 30,000 pregnancies.[7] When assisted reproduction is involved, the heterotopic rate is 1 in 7000 overall and as high as 1 in 900 with induction of ovulation.[8] Even when a live IUP is identified in an assisted reproduction patient, close follow-up with the fertility specialist is recommended.

**BOX 120.1 Ultrasound Categorization of First Trimester Pregnancies by Location**

Intrauterine
Extrauterine
Indeterminate

**BOX 120.2 First Trimester Ultrasound Diagnosis**

| Intrauterine | Extrauterine |
|---|---|
| Intrauterine pregnancy | Extrauterine gestation: ectopic |
| Live intrauterine pregnancy | **Indeterminate** |
| Abnormal intrauterine pregnancy | No definitive pregnancy |

**BOX 120.3 Diagnostic Criteria**

*Intrauterine pregnancy*—Gestational sac with a concentric echogenic ring lying within the endometrial echo of the uterus that is greater than 5 mm in mean sac diameter (height, width, and length) and contains a yolk sac with or without a fetal pole

*Live intrauterine pregnancy*—Gestational sac with a concentric echogenic ring lying within the endometrial echo of the uterus that is greater than 5 mm in mean sac diameter (height, width, and length) and contains a yolk sac plus a fetal pole and cardiac activity

*Abnormal intrauterine pregnancy*—Gestational sac with a concentric echogenic ring lying within the endometrial echo of the uterus that is greater than 13 mm in mean sac diameter (height, width, and length) without a yolk sac or greater than 18 mm in mean sac diameter (height, width, and length) without a fetal pole or with an obvious fetal pole without cardiac activity

*No definitive pregnancy*—No definite gestational sac is apparent within the endometrial echo of the uterus, or if a gestational sac is visualized, it is less than 5 mm in mean sac diameter (height, width, and length)

*Extrauterine gestation: ectopic*—Gestational sac with a concentric echogenic ring lying outside the endometrial echo of the uterus that is greater than 5 mm in mean sac diameter (height, width, and length) and contains a yolk sac with or without a fetal pole and cardiac activity

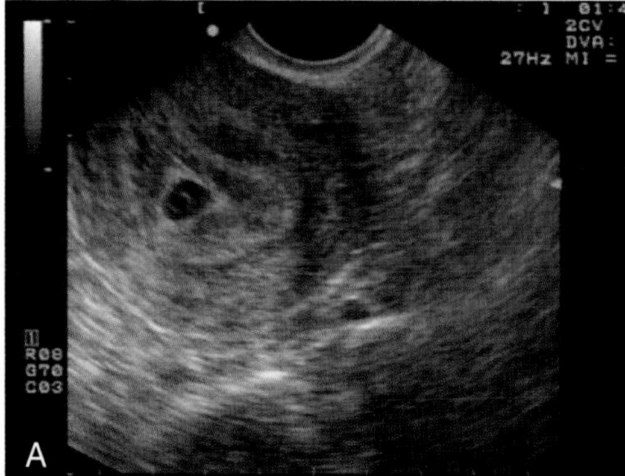


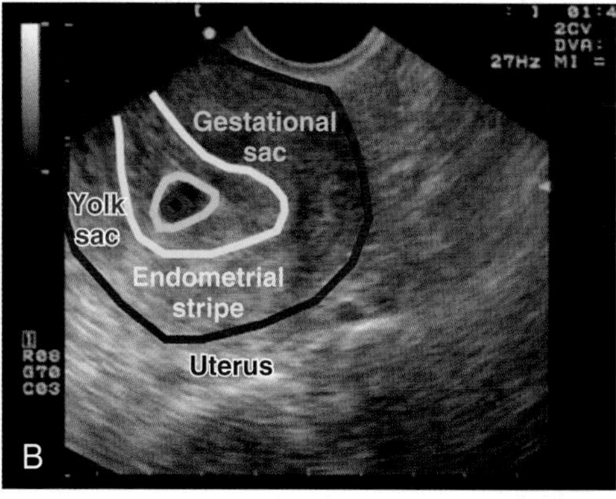


**Fig. 120.3** **A** and **B,** Endovaginal views of the sagittal plane showing an intrauterine pregnancy. The gestational sac is located within the endometrial echo of the uterus and contains a yolk sac.

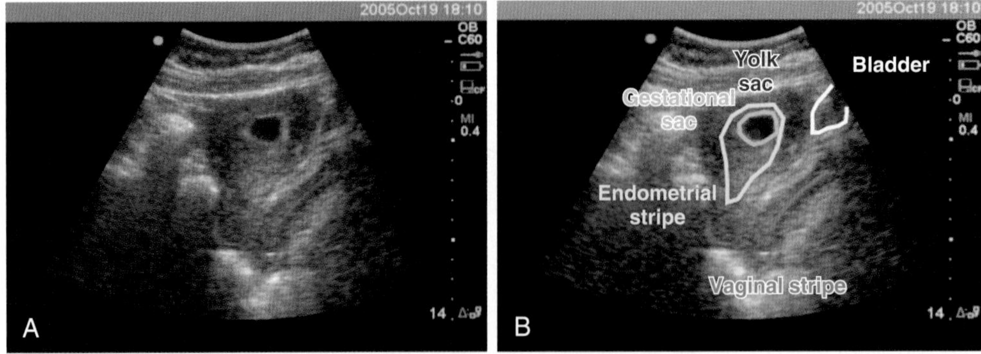


**Fig. 120.4** **A** and **B,** Transabdominal view of the sagittal plane showing an intrauterine pregnancy. The gestational sac is located within the endometrial echo of the uterus and contains a yolk sac. The landmarks of the vaginal stripe and bladder help confirm the proper location.

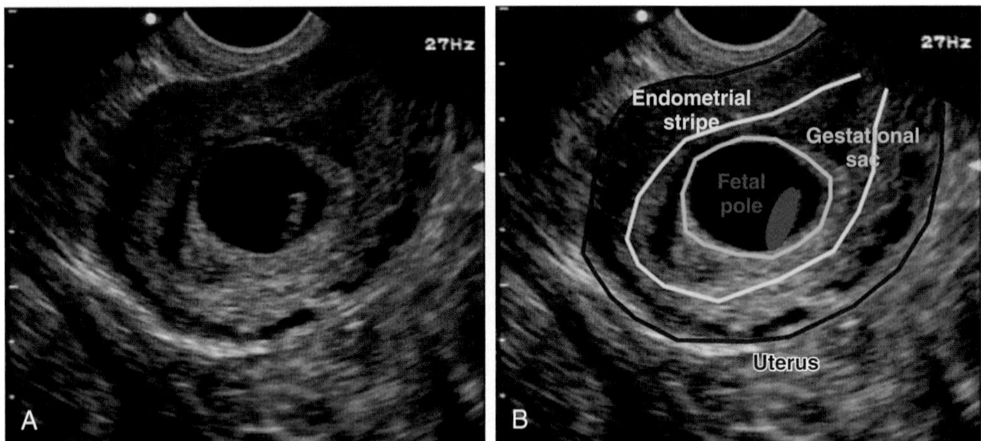


**Fig. 120.5** **A** and **B,** Endovaginal views of the sagittal plane showing an intrauterine pregnancy. The gestational sac is located within the endometrial echo of the uterus and contains a fetal pole.

## LIVE INTRAUTERINE PREGNANCY

Once the pregnancy is determined to be intrauterine, the next designation is viability. This involves real-time documentation of the cardiac activity normally present at 6 weeks' gestational age when using the endovaginal technique and at 7 to 8 weeks' gestation when using the transabdominal technique. The criteria for documentation of a live IUP is detailed below (see Box 120.3). Simply having a fetal pole within the endometrial echo of the uterus will not suffice (**Fig. 120.5,** *A* and *B*). For our purposes, an IUP is not live until cardiac activity is documented. The flickering of cardiac activity is an unmistakable sign of life that can be identified by the novice sonographer and the patient as well. Documentation can be confirmed by video in B mode or by identifying the fetal heart rate by M mode (**Fig. 120.6**). Pulsed wave Doppler should never be used to document fetal heart rates because of the theoretic risk to the fetus of the increased heat generated by this form of ultrasound. Novice sonographers will occasionally use the zoom feature and record or print an image of a pregnancy without any definite landmarks confirming the pregnancy as intrauterine (**Fig. 120.7**). The problem is that ectopic pregnancies can be indistinguishable with this particular example of a cone-down view, which does not allow visualization of the landmarks that support the criteria for an IUP.

## ABNORMAL INTRAUTERINE PREGNANCY

A pregnancy can be categorized as abnormal when the gestational sac is disproportionate to its contents. For example, by the time that a gestational sac measures 13 mm in diameter, a yolk sac should clearly be visualized. Likewise, by 18 mm, all intrauterine gestational sacs containing live embryos should have cardiac activity. When using conservative criteria, it is safe to conclude that any sac larger than 13 mm without a yolk sac or larger than 18 mm without evidence of cardiac activity is termed abnormal (**Fig. 120.8,** *A* and *B*). It has been shown in the obstetric ultrasound literature that gestational sacs reaching 13 mm in size with no yolk sac or fetal pole have virtually no viability and ultimately result in miscarriage. In most cases in which viability is equivocal, there is no rush to make a specific diagnosis (IUP versus abnormal IUP). Because these pregnancies have only a gestational sac visualized on ultrasound, obstetric consultation and close follow-up in 48 hours, repeated ultrasound, and quantitative measurement of β-human chorionic gonadotropin will be required.

## EXTRAUTERINE PREGNANCY

Ectopic pregnancies represent approximately 2% of reported pregnancies, and ectopic pregnancy–related deaths account for 9% of all pregnancy-related deaths.[9] The most common

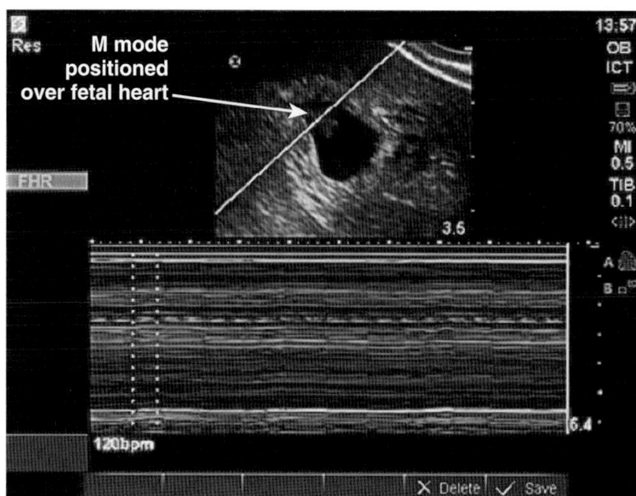


**Fig. 120.6 M-mode documentation of the fetal heart rate confirming that an intrauterine pregnancy is a live intrauterine pregnancy.**

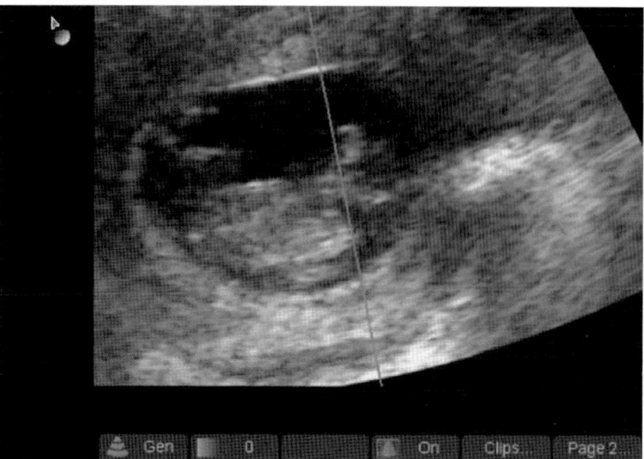

**Fig. 120.7 Transabdominal technique in an unknown plane of a live pregnancy.** This image demonstrates that with the zoom function, proper identification of landmarks (bladder, vaginal stripe, uterine fundus) is lost such that proper documentation of intrauterine location is not possible.

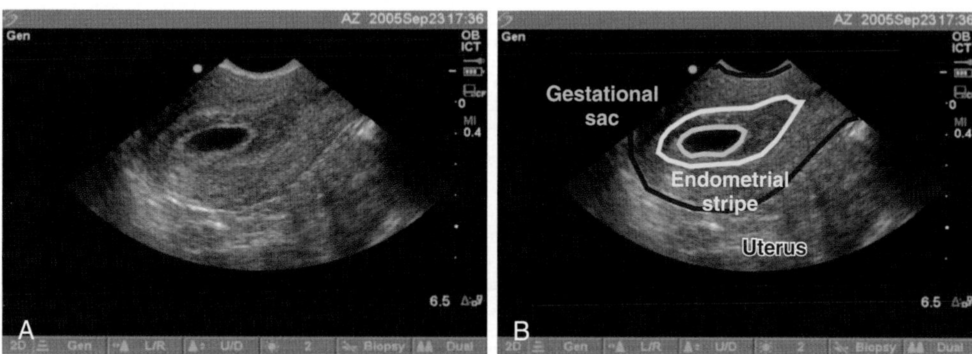


**Fig. 120.8** **A** and **B,** Endovaginal coronal plane views of an abnormal intrauterine pregnancy. The gestational sac is located within the endometrial echo of the uterus but is larger than 10 mm and does not have a fetal pole.

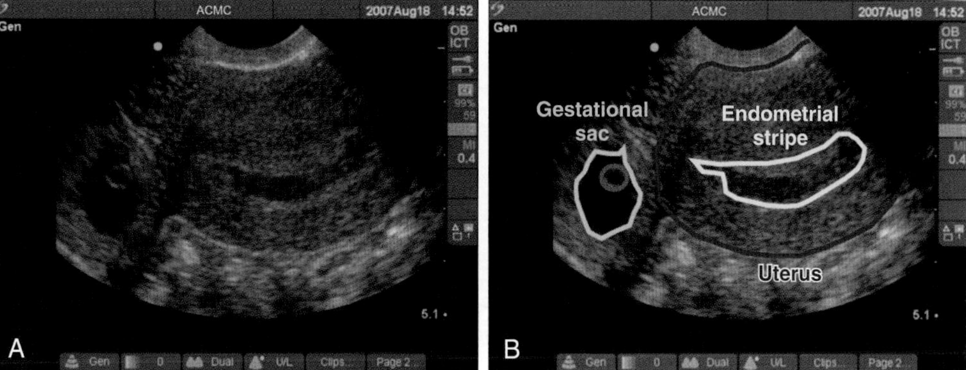


**Fig. 120.9** **A** and **B,** Endovaginal coronal plane views of an extrauterine gestation. The gestational sac is located outside the endometrial echo of the uterus and has a yolk sac.

implantation site is within the fallopian tube (95.5%). Sites of tubal implantation in descending order of frequency are ampullary (73.3%), isthmus (12.5%), fimbrial (11.6%), and interstitial (2.6%). The remaining sites are ovarian (3.2%) and abdominal (1.3%).[10] Visualization of an ectopic pregnancy on ultrasound, even for experienced sonographers, is frequently difficult. As opposed to an IUP, for which ultrasound confirms the diagnosis, an extrauterine pregnancy is often not substantiated by ultrasound and is just presumed because of the absence of an IUP or other findings of a normal pregnancy. The criteria for diagnosis of an extrauterine gestation is a gestational sac outside the endometrial echo of the uterus with evidence of a yolk sac or fetal pole (**Fig. 120.9,** *A* and *B*). In patients who do not have this definitive finding, the diagnosis can be made either intraoperatively or by serial ultrasound in patients who are being monitored very closely. A "ruptured"

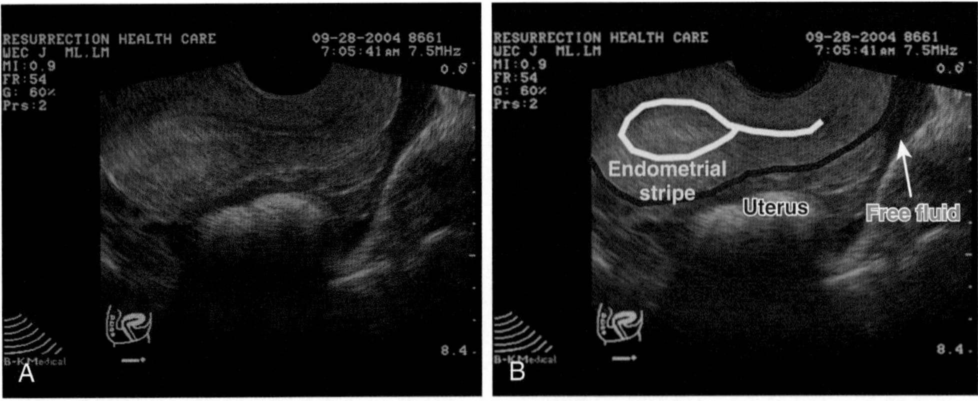


**Fig. 120.10** **A** and **B,** Endovaginal sagittal plane views of a uterus with no definitive pregnancy identified. There is no gestational sac in the uterus. In addition, free fluid is seen in the pouch of Douglas.

ectopic pregnancy is frequently suspected on clinical grounds. Supportive sonographic findings of an intraperitoneal fluid collection or an adnexal mass (or both) further strengthen this suspicion.[11] Recent literature suggests that a transabdominal approach in which a large intraperitoneal fluid collection is revealed will decrease the time to diagnosis and treatment.[14] A pregnant female with free fluid visualized in the right upper quadrant should have these findings communicated immediately to obstetric consultants to help facilitate a shorter time to the operating room.

## NO DEFINITIVE PREGNANCY

The diagnosis of no definitive pregnancy is established when a technically adept emergency ultrasound examination fails to diagnose an intrauterine or extrauterine gestation (**Fig. 120.10,** *A* and *B*). When this is encountered, three possible diagnoses exist. First, it is possible that an early IUP is present but no definitive signs are visualized within the uterus by ultrasound. Second, the products of conception my have been aborted and the empty uterus is a result of a miscarriage. Finally, a concealed ectopic pregnancy is not identified by emergency ultrasound.

Absence of proof is not proof of absence. It should be borne in mind that patients in whom no definitive pregnancy is diagnosed are at high risk for an ectopic pregnancy. The presence of free fluid in the pouch of Douglas or elsewhere in the pelvis should increase suspicion for an ectopic pregnancy substantially. The literature varies widely in defining ectopic pregnancy rates in patients with indeterminate or no definitive pregnancy. This may be due to variation in the specific criteria used to define this category. Many researchers have added subgroups such as probable ectopic pregnancy and probable IUP.[11,12] The take-home message is that all patients in whom no definitive IUP is diagnosed should be managed closely with our obstetric colleagues regardless of the β-human chorionic gonadotropin level. An interdepartmental policy addressing this issue would clearly be advantageous to each specialty and the patient.

## HOW TO INCORPORATE INTO PRACTICE

Use of bedside ultrasound for the evaluation of first trimester pregnancy is a skill that can grow with the experience and practice of the EP. Obtaining the basic skills necessary to safely and consistently identify a live IUP is an excellent foundation. This skill alone will enable EPs to discharge home more than half the pregnant patients seen in the ED by identification of an IUP. The important caveat is to pay attention to detail. Identification of an IUP means finding a gestational sac within the endometrial echo of the uterus *and* a yolk sac or fetal pole within the gestational sac. A systematic approach should be undertaken each and every time to document the location by ultrasound landmarks (uterus, bladder, and endometrial stripe). With time, the ability to recognize abnormal IUPs and adnexal masses will grow, but the goal of EP-performed first trimester ultrasound should be to identify IUPs and refer all others for consultation and further imaging as necessary per local practice standards.

After years of providing ultrasound education, a pattern of learning is so consistent that it is worth printing to help others forgo the same mistakes. First, there is the "puzzled stage" in which everything looks like shades of gray and seems uninterpretable. The second phase is the "eureka phase" in which things start to make sense. The third phase is the most dangerous—also known as the "who's the man (or woman)!" phase in which overconfidence should be closely monitored and the scope of practice closely followed to prevent mistakes. Finally, in the "safe again" phase, limitations are recognized and confident practice is achieved. To achieve the "safe again" phase, a few tips on scanning practice are helpful. Strive to approach every patient systematically. Attempt to define the boundary of each organ that is being evaluated. Document the landmarks pertinent to each ultrasound image obtained. Discipline yourself to systematically save images that provide a clear "story" that other sonographers can follow and interpret. Always obtain confirmatory studies in cases in which the diagnosis is unclear or the images are inadequate. Finally, develop a quality assurance process to share interesting cases, provide technical and interpretative teaching points, and help avoid common errors.

## REFERENCES

***References can be found on Expert Consult @ www.expertconsult.com.***

# Third Trimester Pregnancy Emergencies 121

*Sally A. Santen and Robin R. Hemphill*

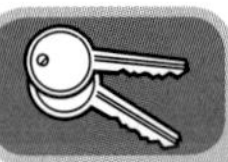

**KEY POINTS**

- Preeclampsia, a disease of the third trimester of pregnancy, is characterized by a sustained elevation in blood pressure and proteinuria. Edema is common in patients with preeclampsia but is no longer considered to be necessary for the diagnosis.
- HELLP syndrome is a particularly severe form of preeclampsia associated with high maternal morbidity and characterized by hemolysis, elevated liver enzymes, and low platelet counts.
- Eclampsia is defined by seizures, usually in the setting of preeclampsia.
- In patients with severe preeclampsia and eclampsia, basic management involves support of maternal vital signs, control of hypertension, prevention and treatment of seizure activity, and close consultation with obstetrics colleagues to determine the appropriate disposition.
- Placental abruption and placenta previa are the most serious causes of vaginal bleeding in late pregnancy.
- Painful bleeding in late pregnancy is probably due to placental abruption. In contrast, when the vaginal bleeding is painless, the cause is more likely to be placenta previa.
- Ultrasound evaluation of third trimester bleeding is diagnostic for placenta previa, but placental abruption is diagnosed clinically because ultrasound detects only 25% to 50% of abruptions.
- Treatment of third trimester bleeding includes stabilization of the patient, assessment of fetal status with ultrasound and fetal monitoring, and consultation with obstetrics colleagues to determine the need for delivery.

## PREECLAMPSIA AND ECLAMPSIA

Preeclampsia is a disease of pregnancy characterized by a sustained elevation in blood pressure (sitting blood pressure of ≥140 mm Hg systolic or ≥90 mm Hg diastolic) and proteinuria (≥1+ in a random urine sample or 300 mg in a 24-hour urine sample) occurring after the 20th week of gestation. Edema is common in patients with preeclampsia but is not necessary for the diagnosis. Eclampsia is defined by seizures, usually in the setting of preeclampsia. Seizures are rare without underlying preeclampsia. Although preeclampsia develops most commonly after the 20th week of pregnancy, it may occur in the postpartum period, usually within the first 24 to 48 hours, but delayed manifestations of 2 weeks or longer have been reported.

### EPIDEMIOLOGY

Preeclampsia complicates 5% to 11% of pregnancies in the United States. The rate is higher in developing nations. This disease accounts for a significant percentage of both maternal and fetal mortality. Fetal complications such as prematurity and low birth weight are common, with death occurring in 129 of every 1000 cases. Maternal complications are common in both eclampsia and severe preeclampsia, including HELLP syndrome (hemolysis, elevated liver enzymes, and low platelet count) (11%), placental abruption (10%), disseminated intravascular coagulation (DIC) (6%), neurologic deficits (6%), aspiration pneumonia (6%), pulmonary edema (5%), renal failure (4%), and death (1%).

First pregnancies are at greatest risk. Other risk factors include extremes of reproductive age, more than 10 years between pregnancies, multiple gestations, molar pregnancies, previous or family history of preeclampsia, underlying diseases (hypertension, diabetes, autoimmune or renal diseases, obesity), and thrombophilia (e.g., antiphospholipid syndrome, factor V Leiden deficiency, activated protein C resistance).[1]

### PATHOPHYSIOLOGY

Preeclampsia is a multisystem disorder of gestation. Its exact cause is unclear, and several mechanisms have been implicated. The disease is thought to originate within the placenta, which for reasons that remain obscure, has inappropriately decreased perfusion. Hypoperfusion and multiorgan effects ensue in some patients as a result of decreased intravascular volume and endothelial vascular leakage causing increased interstitial volume, interstitial protein leakage, and vasoconstriction.[2] Preeclampsia affects nearly every organ system.

Severe preeclampsia is characterized by hypertension secondary to increased peripheral resistance. However, the profound elevation in blood pressure is the result rather than the cause of the underlying pathophysiology. Effects on the liver include edema, hepatocellular necrosis, and periportal and subcapsular hematomas. Decreased renal flow with high perfusion pressure can cause glomerular and tubular injury resulting in proteinuria or, worse, renal failure. Cerebral vasospasm leads to edema, microinfarction, and hemorrhage. Patients experience a variant of chronic DIC with thrombocytopenia and hemolysis that can worsen the already present organ system dysfunction.

HELLP syndrome is a particularly severe form of preeclampsia associated with severe maternal morbidity.

Preeclampsia has long-term implications for the health of these patients. After delivery, women with preeclampsia are at increased risk for the development of chronic hypertension, cardiovascular diseases, and psychosomatic disorders.[3]

**BOX 121.1 Clinical Manifestations of Severe Preeclampsia**

**Cardiovascular**

Increased cardiac output, systemic vasoconstriction, systemic hypertension, increased hydrostatic pressure, generalized edema

**Obstetric**

Uteroplacental insufficiency, fetal growth retardation, fetal hypoxemia and distress, decidual ischemia or thrombosis, placental abruption, placental infarcts

**Renal**

Decreased renal blood flow and glomerular filtration rate, endothelial damage, proteinuria, elevated creatinine levels and decreased creatinine clearance, oliguria, elevated uric acid levels, renal tubular necrosis, renal failure

**Hematologic**

Intravascular hemolysis (schistocytes, burr cells, elevated free hemoglobin and iron, decreased haptoglobin levels), thrombocytopenia, disseminated intravascular coagulation (increased fibrin split products, decreased fibrinogen)

**Cerebrovascular**

Ischemia, generalized grand mal seizures (eclampsia), high cerebral perfusion pressure with regional ischemia, cerebral hemorrhage, cerebral edema, coma, central blindness, loss of speech

**Hepatic**

Ischemia, hepatic cellular injury, elevated liver enzymes, mitochondrial injury, intracellular fatty deposits

## PRESENTING SIGNS AND SYMPTOMS

Classic clinical findings in patients with preeclampsia include proteinuria and an associated elevation in blood pressure; when these signs develop late in the pregnancy of a previously healthy woman, the diagnosis of preeclampsia is clear. However, preeclampsia does not always occur in such a straightforward manner. For instance, a patient with chronic hypertension complicated by chronic renal disease can be difficult to differentiate from one who has preeclampsia. Likewise, seizures in pregnant patients do not always herald eclampsia, and other structural, toxic, and metabolic causes have to be considered.

Patients may have the classic symptoms of severe preeclampsia, such as seizures superimposed on hypertension and proteinuria, or may have incidentally noted hypertension and proteinuria with or without edema.

Persistent elevation in blood pressure is the hallmark of preeclampsia. Hypertension is defined as a sitting blood pressure of 140 mm Hg systolic or 90 mm Hg diastolic or greater. Blood pressure readings should ideally be taken more than 6 hours apart; however, for most patients in the emergency department (ED), if concern is high, therapy should not be delayed. Early in pregnancy, diastolic blood pressure decreases but returns to normal toward the 28th week of gestation. Therefore, a sustained diastolic blood pressure of greater than 90 mm Hg at the midpoint of pregnancy should be considered elevated unless the patient has a clearly documented history of hypertension.

If the patient's blood pressure before pregnancy is known, an increase in systolic blood pressure of 30 mm Hg or greater and an increase in diastolic blood pressure of 15 mm Hg or greater are diagnostic of preeclampsia. In addition to hypertension, the patient will have proteinuria of 1+ or greater on urinalysis.

Patients with severe preeclampsia may have additional symptoms of organ involvement (**Box 121.1**),[4] including significant edema, especially facial edema, and documented weight gain of more than 5 pounds per week. Findings ominous for severe preeclampsia include a blood pressure of 160 mm Hg systolic and 110 mm Hg diastolic or greater, visual disturbances (blurred vision or scotomata), severe headache, altered mental status, seizures (which defines eclampsia), hyperreflexia with clonus, severe epigastric or right upper quadrant pain on examination, retinal hemorrhage with exudates and papilledema (which is rare and more commonly indicates underlying chronic hypertension), bibasilar rales and evidence of frank pulmonary edema, oliguria, and petechiae and bleeding from puncture sites.

Fetal growth retardation and oligohydramnios may be seen in cases of severe preeclampsia, but this information is not usually available. Sudden onset of abdominal pain with a firm painful uterus suggests placental abruption, which complicates up to 10% of preeclamptic pregnancies.

## DIFFERENTIAL DIAGNOSIS AND MEDICAL DECISION MAKING

The current classification of hypertension in pregnancy is divided into four categories: preeclampsia, gestational or transient hypertension, chronic hypertension, and preeclampsia superimposed on chronic hypertension (**Box 121.2**).[5] In addition, occult renal disease can be manifested as proteinuria and associated hypertension.

The differential diagnosis of severe preeclampsia is broad and distinction may be difficult, particularly with concomitant HELLP syndrome.[6] Thrombotic thrombocytopenic purpura (TTP) and preeclampsia can have identical findings

**BOX 121.2 Classification of Hypertension in Pregnancy**

**Preeclampsia and Eclampsia**
Hypertension and proteinuria detected for the first time after the 20th week of gestation
Eclampsia is the occurrence of seizures in a patient with preeclampsia

**Gestational or Transient Hypertension**
Hypertension without proteinuria after the 20th week of gestation (resolves within 3 months of delivery)

**Chronic Hypertension**
Hypertension diagnosed before the 20th week of gestation or before the pregnancy

**Preeclampsia Superimposed on Chronic Hypertension**
Development of accelerated hypertension or proteinuria after the 20th week of gestation in a patient with hypertension diagnosed before the 20th week or before the pregnancy

of thrombocytopenia, hemolytic anemia, renal disease, and neurologic abnormalities. In patients with preeclampsia, the hypertension, proteinuria, and edema tend to precede the hematologic findings. In patients with TTP, they generally follow and are a result of the hematologic abnormalities. However, by the time that the patient arrives in the ED, these subtle distinctions may be almost impossible to delineate.

Laboratory tests may help clarify the diagnosis and determine the severity of the preeclampsia. If proteinuria is 1+ or greater on urinalysis, a hypertensive pregnant woman should be considered to have preeclampsia unless proved otherwise. A 24-hour urine collection is more sensitive for this purpose, but its use is not realistic in the ED.

A complete blood count should be performed with a manual differential and haptoglobin assay to evaluate for hemolysis. Decreased platelet counts (<100,000/mm$^3$) are associated with severe disease. Fibrinogen levels, fibrin split products, and a prothrombin time (PT) and partial thromboplastin time (PTT) should be ordered to evaluate for DIC, which may complicate severe preeclampsia.

A comprehensive metabolic profile should be obtained because elevated serum creatinine, especially when associated with oliguria, and elevated liver transaminases suggest severe preeclampsia. Uric acid levels should be assayed; the degree of elevation of uric acid has been shown to correlate with the severity of the preeclampsia. Elevated lactate dehydrogenase (LDH) levels indicate hemolysis but can also be a result of liver involvement. Typing plus crossmatching of blood is necessary in cases of severe preeclampsia or anticipated delivery.

HELLP syndrome is characterized by peripheral smears showing schistocytes and burr cells, elevated LDH levels (>600 U/L), elevated liver enzymes (bilirubin > 1.2 and aspartate transaminase > 70 U/L), and low platelet count (<100,000).[7] In addition, the abnormal laboratory test results in patients with HELLP syndrome can be seen in the other diseases noted in **Box 121.3**.

**Table 121.1** shows the frequency of certain signs and laboratory values that may help distinguish between several of the key conditions that mimic severe preeclampsia with HELLP syndrome.[6]

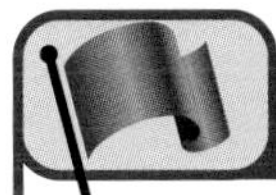

**RED FLAGS**

**Preeclampsia and Eclampsia**
Pain with a firm painful uterus suggests placental abruption, which is a complication in up to 10% of preeclamptic pregnancies.
Diagnosing preeclampsia may be difficult in patients with chronic hypertension complicated by chronic renal disease.
Seizures in pregnant patients do not always herald eclampsia, and other structural, toxic, and metabolic causes should be considered.
Both thrombotic thrombocytopenic purpura and preeclampsia can have the identical findings of thrombocytopenia, hemolytic anemia, renal disease, and neurologic abnormalities. In patients with preeclampsia, the hypertension, proteinuria, and edema tend to precede the hematologic findings, and in patients with thrombotic thrombocytopenic purpura, they generally follow and are a result of the hematologic abnormalities.

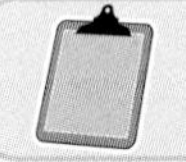

**DOCUMENTATION**

**Preeclampsia and Eclampsia**
Pregnant women being evaluated should have their blood pressure documented; any elevation needs to be addressed. A complete history should include symptomatic clues (e.g., headache, vision changes, abdominal pain) identifying causes of the elevation.
Review of records may indicate that the elevation is chronic and that the patient is being monitored for this finding.
If the blood pressure is not dangerously high and no other evidence of preeclampsia is present, it may be addressed by making arrangements for close outpatient follow-up.
Documentation should include completion of appropriate laboratory testing.
Patients with severe preeclampsia and eclampsia require documentation of all actions taken, interventions given, consultations requested, and the time at which all were ordered.

## TREATMENT

It is important to differentiate between mild and severe preeclampsia[8] (**Table 121.2**) when discussing the patient with the obstetrics consultant because acute management depends on the severity of disease, as well as fetal maturity. Recent research favors delivery over observation for gestational age older than 36 weeks.[9]

In patients with severe preeclampsia and eclampsia, basic management involves the following measures: (1) support of

**Table 121.1 Differentiating HELLP Syndrome from Other Critical Conditions**

| FINDINGS | HELLP SYNDROME | AFLP | TTP | HUS |
|---|---|---|---|---|
| Jaundice (%) | 5-10 | 40-90 | Rare | Rare |
| Urine findings | Proteinuria and evidence of hemolysis | Occasional proteinuria with conjugated bilirubin | Proteinuria with blood | Proteinuria |
| Thrombocytopenia | Present | Present | Present | Present |
| Hemolysis (%) | 50-100 | 15-20 | 100 | 100 |
| Anemia | Sometimes | No | Yes | Yes |
| DIC (%) | <20 | 50-100 | Uncommon | Uncommon |
| Hypoglycemia | No | Common | No | No |
| Elevated ammonia | Rare | Sometimes | No | No |
| Elevated transaminases | High | High | Usually mild | Usually mild |
| Elevated bilirubin | Sometimes | Always | Always | Always |
| Impaired renal function (%) | 50 | 90-100 | 30 | 100 |

Adapted from Sibai BM. Imitators of severe preeclampsia. Obstet Gynecol 2007;109:956-66.

*AFLP*, Acute fatty liver of pregnancy; *DIC*, disseminated intravascular coagulation; *HELLP*, hemolysis, elevated liver enzymes, and low platelets; *HUS*, hemolytic-uremic syndrome; *TTP*, thrombotic thrombocytopenic purpura.

**BOX 121.3 Differential Diagnosis of Severe Preeclampsia with HELLP Syndrome**

Hemolytic-uremic syndrome
Acute fatty liver of pregnancy
Thrombotic thrombocytopenic purpura
Immune thrombocytopenic purpura
Systemic lupus erythematosus
Antiphospholipid antibody syndrome
Cholecystitis
Fulminant viral hepatitis
Acute pancreatitis
Disseminated herpes simplex
Hemorrhagic or septic shock

*HELLP*, Hemolysis, elevated liver enzymes, and low platelets.

**Table 121.2 Comparison of Symptoms of Severe and Mild Preeclampsia**

| | MILD | SEVERE |
|---|---|---|
| Hypertension | 140-150/90-100 mm Hg | >160/110 mm Hg |
| Proteinuria | 1+ | >3+ |
| Oliguria | Absent | Present |
| Visual disturbances, particularly scotomata | Absent | Present |
| Epigastric pain | Absent | Present |
| Headache | Absent | Present |
| Pulmonary edema or cyanosis | Absent | Present |
| Seizures (eclampsia) | Absent | Present |
| Laboratory test abnormalities (elevated creatinine and liver enzymes; thrombocytopenia) | Absent | Present |

maternal vital functions and initiation of laboratory test evaluation, (2) control of severe hypertension, (3) prevention and treatment of seizures, and (4) early consultation for determination of final treatment (capability of the hospital to deliver material and fetal care, decision regarding immediate delivery).[10]

The patient should be placed in the left lateral decubitus position with large-bore intravenous (IV) access; however, large fluid boluses should be avoided. Patients should receive supplemental oxygen and, if the airway is in danger of compromise, should be intubated, with attempts to minimize elevations in intracranial pressure. Vital signs should be monitored continuously. Fever may indicate infection, may mean that the patient has a disorder other than preeclampsia (e.g., acute fatty liver of pregnancy, TTP), or may be the result of prolonged seizures. As the maternal condition is stabilized, fetal heart rate monitoring should begin.

In preeclamptic patients, the mainstay of treatment is administration of magnesium for seizure prophylaxis when diastolic

**Table 121.3 Priority Medications for Preeclampsia: Antihypertensive Agents**

| DRUG | DOSAGE | COMMENTS |
|---|---|---|
| Hydralazine | 5-10 mg IV q20min; consider another drug after a total of 20 mg; can be given as infusion | Side effects include tachycardia, nausea, vomiting, headache, epigastric pain |
| Labetalol | 20-40 mg IV q20min; continue up to 220 mg; followed by 1-2 mg/min as an infusion or repeat IV doses q3h | Side effects include flushing, orthostatic hypotension, tremulousness; do not use in patients with asthma or heart failure |
| Nifedipine | 10 mg sublingually; repeat in 30 min; if no response after 20 mg, consider alternatives | Third-line treatment; avoid in older patients or those with a family or personal history of coronary disease, especially if smokers; may cause a precipitous decrease in blood pressure, especially when used with magnesium |
| Clonidine | 0.1 mg PO, may repeat in 30 min, then 0.1 mg every hour | Third-line treatment; no parenteral form; not good for initial management |

blood pressure exceeds 100 mm Hg. Magnesium is superior to phenytoin (Dilantin) or diazepam for prevention of eclamptic seizures.[11] The recommended dosage is 4 to 6 g of magnesium administered intravenously over a 15-minute period, followed by a maintenance infusion of 1 to 2 g/hr, with a goal of serum levels of 4 to 6 mEq/L. The maintenance dosing should be started only if the patient still has patellar reflexes and an adequate respiratory rate. Magnesium should be used cautiously in patients with renal insufficiency or oliguria.

When systolic blood pressure reaches 160 mm Hg or diastolic pressure reaches 105 mm Hg, most experts recommend the use of an antihypertensive agent. The ideal antihypertensive agent for preeclampsia is one that reduces blood pressure in a controlled manner and has minimal side effects (**Table 121.3**).[12,13] The exact degree of reduction is controversial, but it is reasonable to maintain diastolic blood pressure between 90 and 110 mm Hg.

Hydralazine hydrochloride (Apresoline) has been commonly used as an antihypertensive agent for patients with severe preeclampsia. Its mechanism of action is through direct relaxation of arteriolar smooth muscle. This drug can be given as 5- to 10-mg boluses every 15 to 20 minutes until a response in blood pressure is seen. Side effects include tachycardia, nausea, vomiting, headache, and epigastric pain.

Labetalol, a combination α- and β-adrenergic blocking agent, is another commonly used medication, and some authors prefer this agent over hydralazine.[14] The dose is 20 to 40 mg administered as a slow IV push every 20 minutes. This can be followed by 1 to 2 mg/min given by continuous infusion or by IV dosing every 3 hours after the blood pressure has been controlled. Side effects include flushing, orthostatic hypotension, and tremulousness. Labetalol should not be used in patients with asthma or evidence of heart failure.

Antihypertensive agents to use with caution, if at all, include nifedipine and nitroglycerin. Calcium channel blockers such as nifedipine (10 mg orally every 30 minutes) have been used for refractory cases of hypertension. However, there is concern about a precipitous decrease in blood pressure when magnesium and nifedipine are used together. Nitroglycerin, a venous (predominantly) and arterial vasodilator, has also been used for refractory cases of hypertension, particularly if the patient has evidence of congestive heart failure resulting from the hypertension. However, when high doses are used, the patient should be monitored for the development of methemoglobinemia.

Other antihypertensive agents to avoid include sodium nitroprusside and angiotensin-converting enzyme inhibitors. Sodium nitroprusside should be used only as a last resort because fetal cyanide poisoning has been reported in animal studies.[15] However, if the blood pressure is not responding to other agents, use of this medication is appropriate. Angiotensin-converting enzyme inhibitors have been shown to cause fetal death in animals and possibly renal failure in neonates and thus should not be used in pregnancy. Clonidine and α-methyldopa are not administered parenterally and are therefore rarely used in initial management of preeclampsia.

The treatment of eclampsia and severe preeclampsia is delivery. The method of delivery (cesarean or vaginal) depends on gestational age, cervical maturation, and clinical status. In patients with less than 32 weeks' gestation and mild preeclampsia, care is controversial and detailed discussion with an obstetrician is needed. If a decision is made to observe the patient, low-dose aspirin is sometimes recommended. Blood typing and crossmatching should be ordered if the severity of illness indicates the need for delivery.

Treatment of specific complications of preeclampsia includes dexamethasone, which may be useful in patients with HELLP syndrome. However, this is therapy is not yet universally accepted and consultation is recommended. Betamethasone, which will accelerate fetal lung maturity after 24 hours, may also be considered. DIC should be treated with replacement of blood products and coagulation factors as indicated clinically; however, heparin is not usually recommended. Epidural anesthesia in the setting of DIC or thrombocytopenia may be contraindicated because of the risk for epidural hematoma.

## FOLLOW-UP, NEXT STEPS IN CARE, AND PATIENT EDUCATION

In pregnant women evaluated in the ED for any complaint, blood pressure should be considered carefully. Mild preeclampsia may progress rapidly to severe preeclampsia with

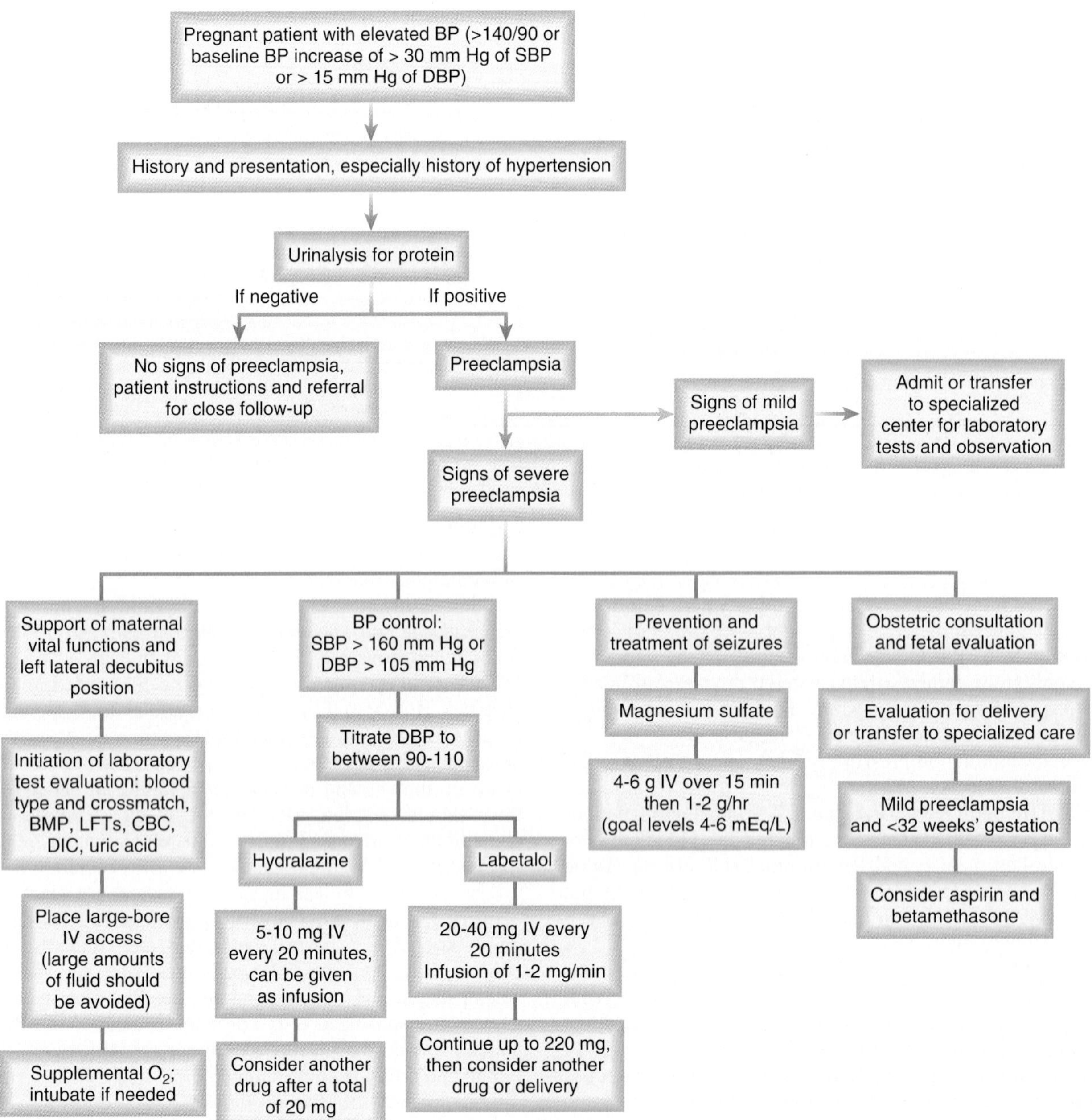


**Fig. 121.1 Algorithm for the approach to a patient with suspected preeclampsia.** *BMP*, Basic metabolic profile; *BP*, blood pressure; *CBC*, complete blood count; *DBP*, diastolic blood pressure; *DIC*, disseminated intravascular coagulation; *LFTs*, liver function tests; *IV*, intravenous; *SBP*, systolic blood pressure.

little warning. If a pregnant patient is found to have elevated blood pressure, the initial assessment should include a complete history and physical examination with attempts to determine whether the elevated blood pressure is new or old and whether other evidence of preeclampsia is present (**Fig. 121.1**). If there is concern that the elevated blood pressure indicates preeclampsia, the patient will usually need admission for close monitoring and therapy.

Patients with preeclampsia and eclampsia will need emergency obstetrics consultation to assist in management and admission versus transfer decisions.

# THIRD TRIMESTER BLEEDING

## EPIDEMIOLOGY

Vaginal bleeding occurs in about 3% to 4% of second and third trimester pregnancies. It can herald catastrophic problems for both the mother and fetus.[16] Placental abruption and placenta previa are the most serious causes of vaginal bleeding in late pregnancy. In 20% of women the bleeding is due to placenta previa, and in 33% it is due to placental abruption.

Placental abruption is estimated to occur in about 1% of all pregnancies. Of these pregnancies, 20% to 40% will be associated with perinatal morbidity or mortality involving the mother or fetus. Maternal death, though diminishing in incidence (0.03% of pregnant women), remains significant.[17] Additionally, women who sustain trauma in pregnancy are at risk for abruption, even when the trauma appears to be minimal.

Ultrasound studies estimate that the incidence of placenta previa is higher (about 5%) in the second trimester. The incidence decreases to about 0.5% of pregnancies at delivery as the uterus enlarges and pulls the placenta away from the cervical os.

Vaginal bleeding in late pregnancy has causes other than placenta previa or placental abruption (e.g., cervical and vaginal abrasions or polyps) in about 50% of patients; nonetheless, these women need close follow-up. The risk for second trimester miscarriage or perinatal morbidity is as high as 30% in this group. Investigation of other causes of vaginal bleeding should be delayed until the diagnosis of placenta previa or placental abruption is ruled out. Vaginal bleeding in all patients should receive serious consideration, even if the bleeding appears to be self-limited.

## PATHOPHYSIOLOGY

### PLACENTAL ABRUPTION

Placental abruption, or abruptio placentae in Latin (meaning "rending asunder of the placenta"), is premature separation of the normally implanted placenta from the uterine decidual lining. Initially, there is bleeding into the placental decidua basalis, a thin layer adherent to the myometrium, and then bleeding into the abrupted placental tissue. The pathophysiology causing the initial bleeding is not clearly understood in many cases. The blood creates a potential space and can track to the cervix and cause vaginal bleeding. The margin, part, or all of the placenta may separate and result in minimal to a large amount of bleeding. Women will bleed vaginally with revealed abruption, or the blood may be contained behind the placenta with concealed abruption. It can also disrupt the placenta and result in bloody amniotic fluid.

The vascular placental bed can bleed significantly and cause maternal hypotension. Loss of the placental circulation may cause fetal distress or death because the hematoma between the layers prevents that area of placenta from exchanging nutrients and oxygen. In addition, significant uterine spasm is typically present. The combination of spasm and decreased perfusion causes the fetus to become hypoxic. Fetal bleeding can occur but is more likely with traumatic placental abruption. The hallmark of placental abruption is vaginal bleeding and uterine tenderness.

Risk factors for placental abruption include previous placental abruption, cocaine use, smoking, hypertension in pregnancy (preeclampsia, gestational or chronic hypertension), trauma, advanced maternal age, multiparity, and multiple gestation. Other risk factors are fetal malformation, premature rupture of membranes, uterine leiomyomas, previous cesarean section, and malnutrition.[17]

Hypertension increases not only the risk for placental abruption but also the risk for more severe placental abruption and increased fetal mortality. Elevations in blood pressure may predispose the placenta to bleeding, but the exact initiating event is still elusive.

Major trauma, as well as seemingly insignificant trauma, is an important cause of placental abruption. Because pregnant trauma patients are initially managed in the ED, the emergency physician should be vigilant for signs of placental abruption. Abruption may be seen in up to 30% of patients with severe abdominal trauma and in up to 3% with minor trauma in late pregnancy.[18,19]

Additional complications of placental abruption include maternal morbidity, massive blood loss, renal failure, fetal mortality, preterm birth, and low birth weight. Coagulopathy and progression to DIC may develop, and the cause is multifactorial. The larger the abruption, the more likely DIC is to develop because clot serves as a nidus for activation of the intrinsic and extrinsic pathways of coagulation. Another mechanism for the development of DIC is the loss of endothelial integrity; exposure of thromboplastin stimulates the coagulation cascade.

### PLACENTA PREVIA

Painful bleeding in late pregnancy is probably due to placental abruption; however, when the vaginal bleeding is painless, the cause is more likely to be placenta previa, with the placenta being located either partially or completely over the cervical os.[16,20] In preparation for labor, softening of the lower uterine segment and effacement of the cervix tear the implanted placenta previa, which results in painless vaginal bleeding. Only 10% of women have contractions or uterine tenderness coincident with the initial vaginal bleeding. Many women have brief painless bleeding initially, which is a warning that placenta previa is present. As the cervix dilates further, the bleeding can become rapid and life-threatening.

Placenta previa can be total, partial, marginal, or low lying. The exact cause of placenta previa is unclear, but it is thought that factors that decrease the richness of the vascular bed of the uterus (defective decidual vascularization) or "scar" the uterus predispose to placental implantation in the lower uterine segment and cervix. The risk for placenta previa is increased with previous cesarean section and advanced maternal age. Other risk factors include previous placenta previa, assisted reproduction, cocaine use, and smoking. The presence of multiple implantation sites in multiparous women and multiple gestations also increases the risk. In addition, the placenta often preferentially implants near the scar of a previous cesarean section but then expands to cover the cervix as well. It is uncertain whether the lower uterine scar prevents the normal elongation of the lower uterine segment that would normally pull the placenta away from the cervix or whether the uterus is not rich enough to support the placenta, which causes it to enlarge and cover the cervix. Whatever the cause, the eventual vaginal bleeding is caused by softening of the lower uterine segment and subsequent disruption of the placental attachment.

Although placenta previa may be diagnosed in the second trimester, in many women, as the uterus enlarges, it pulls the placenta away from the cervix, thereby eliminating the previa; in this manner 90% of cases of placenta previa diagnosed before the 20th week of gestation resolve. Therefore, definitive diagnosis of placenta previa is made after the 24th week of gestation.

## PRESENTING SIGNS AND SYMPTOMS

In women with late pregnancy bleeding, there are three key historical points: painful or painless bleeding, volume of bleeding, and presence of fetal movement. The classic manifestation of placental abruption is painful vaginal bleeding associated with fetal distress. However, the clinical findings of abruption vary from asymptomatic to significant painful bleeding to catastrophic maternal or fetal death. Most women have uterine contractions, and about one third have uterine hypertonus. Symptoms may also include back pain when the placental location is posterior. Fetal distress may be noted from lack of movement and fetal heart rate patterns that include fetal decelerations, reduced variability, and bradycardia. In the majority of cases the abruption is not due to trauma; however, in the ED population, trauma is an important cause. The shearing force of minor trauma such as a fall or motor vehicle crash might initiate abruption.

In contrast to placental abruption, the classic finding in patients with placenta previa is painless bleeding.[16] The bleeding varies from mild to massive and from intermittent to continuous. Bleeding usually occurs after the 28th week of gestation.

Vaginal bleeding past the first trimester of pregnancy is abnormal and should be taken seriously. The patient's obstetric history, as well as social and medical history, may contribute to the diagnosis and alert the physician to complicating factors. The onset, duration, and quantity of vaginal bleeding are relevant to determine the patient's stability; trauma and sexual activity may stimulate bleeding. Bleeding after trauma is more likely to be due to placental abruption, whereas intercourse may provoke bleeding from placenta previa.

The duration of bleeding, estimated volume of blood lost, and number of pads used can help determine the volume of blood loss. A typical saturated pad holds about 30 mL of blood. Because several liters of blood can remain concealed in the uterus, it is easy to underestimate the volume of blood lost.

During the initial evaluation, women should be asked whether they felt any fetal movements in the past few hours. Lack of movement may indicate fetal death or compromise.

The physical examination should not include speculum or manual pelvic examination as part of the evaluation of patients with third trimester bleeding. In the presence of placenta previa, cervical manipulation may cause torrential vaginal bleeding. If the patient has had second trimester ultrasound performed with no placenta previa documented, internal examination may be performed.

The evaluation should include fundal height measurement and evidence of uterine tenderness, contractions, or a hypertonic uterus. Severe placental abruption causes uterine irritability manifested as frequent contractions with increased baseline tone (high-frequency contractions). In patients with placenta previa, the uterus should be soft, although 10% of these patients may be in labor and have contractions that should not be confused with the uterine irritability of placental abruption. Fetal descent into the pelvis should be noted, and the presenting part may be determined with Leopold maneuvers.

In cases of vaginal bleeding caused by trauma, placental abruption is highest on the list of differential diagnoses. However, if the pain is caused by trauma to other organs, the bleeding might be due to placenta previa. In about 10% of cases, abdominal pain occurs with placenta previa. The pain may be due to the bleeding or the onset of labor.

Although vaginal bleeding occurs in 80% of cases of placental abruption, some abruptions are concealed without any evidence of overt bleeding, thereby making diagnosis difficult. It is thus important to realize that abruption may be accompanied by symptoms that can be either minor or severe (shock, fetal demise, tetanic contractions).

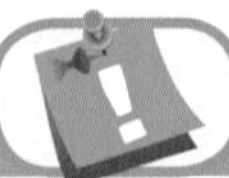

### TIPS AND TRICKS

**Third Trimester Bleeding**

Do not perform a speculum examination in patients with third trimester bleeding.

Major trauma, as well as seemingly insignificant trauma, is an important cause of placental abruption.

All vaginal bleeding during the third trimester should be considered serious; investigation for other causes of the vaginal bleeding should be delayed until the diagnosis of placenta previa or placental abruption is ruled out.

Focus on maternal stabilization—when mom does well, the fetus has a better chance to do well.

Diagnosis of placental abruption is based on clinical signs; the diagnosis should always be considered in pregnant women seen in the ED with significant uterine contractions and fetal distress.

**Placental Abruption**

Painful vaginal bleeding
Concealed abruption is difficult to diagnose
Uterine contractions
More likely after trauma

**Placenta Previa**

Painless vaginal bleeding
Usually occurs after the 28th week of gestation
Uterine irritation not present
Bleeding more likely to start after sexual intercourse

## DIFFERENTIAL DIAGNOSIS AND MEDICAL DECISION MAKING

Uterine rupture is a rare but catastrophic event that should be considered in the differential diagnosis of placental abruption. It is most commonly seen in women with previous cesarean section or after severe trauma. Fetal mortality is close to 100%, and maternal mortality is significant. Bleeding may or may not be present, but there is usually severe abdominal pain and a rigid gravid abdomen. The diagnosis is made operatively or by ultrasonography. With trauma, other injuries such as liver or splenic lacerations need to be considered and ruled out.

The maternal response to volume depletion is to decrease blood flow to nonvital organs, including the uterus, with resultant fetal hypoxia manifested as bradycardia with a fetal heart rate lower than 100 beats/min. Bradycardia and fetal distress may have a variety of causes and may be present in placental abruption without maternal compromise. In addition, it should

**BOX 121.4 Differential Diagnosis of Third Trimester Bleeding**

Placental abruption
Placenta previa
Bloody show (extrusion of cervical mucus)
Vasa previa
Disseminated intravascular coagulopathy
Uterine rupture
Cervicitis, cervical cancer, or other cervical abnormality
Vaginal laceration

be noted that up to 20% of cases of placental abruption are initially manifested as fetal demise.

Following clinical examination, ultrasound imaging may be performed, which may result in another diagnosis in 25% to 50% of cases (**Box 121.4**). About 10% of pregnant patients with abdominal pain and bleeding may have preterm labor, heavy bloody show with the onset of labor, or marginal placental or subchorionic bleeding. These patients should be admitted for monitoring. Other causes of vaginal bleeding are vaginal or cervical polyps, cervical lacerations or erosions, cervical carcinoma, and vulvar injury.

Patients in the second half of pregnancy with abdominal or back pain but without vaginal bleeding should first be considered to have placental abruption because concealed hemorrhage is present in 10% of placental abruptions. Other causes of abdominal pain should also be considered, such as pyelonephritis, nephrolithiasis, appendicitis, ovarian torsion, and other abdominal processes. Abnormal laboratory findings such as blood in the urine and an elevated white blood cell count may help in the differential diagnosis.

## DIAGNOSTIC TESTING

In patients with third trimester bleeding, ultrasonography may be performed to rule out placenta previa, to determine fetal age and viability, and to look for placental abruption. However, only 25% to 50% of placental abruptions are identified on ultrasound, and the appearance may be unimpressive because the clot looks similar to the placenta. When abruption is seen on ultrasound, its specificity is 95%.[21] The diagnosis of placental abruption is clinical, and the emergency physician should suspect placental abruption in a pregnant woman with significant uterine contractions and fetal distress. Monitoring of the fetal heart rate and uterine contraction (tocography) should be initiated early. The diagnosis is confirmed by examination of the placenta after delivery.

In trauma patients with abdominal pain in late pregnancy, other injuries must be considered and are best managed by a multispecialty team consisting of emergency medicine, trauma, and obstetrics. Early evaluation with focused assessment with sonography for trauma (FAST), as well as assessment of fetal size (for dates) and fetal heart rate, is key. Chest and pelvis radiographs, as well as computed tomography (CT) scans, may be necessary. Though not the test of choice for abruption, abdominal CT scans have a sensitivity of 50% to 100%, depending on the expertise of the radiologist.[22] During the evaluation it is important that the fetus be monitored continuously as early as possible. Resuscitation of the mother is the best treatment for the fetus. If the mother has loss of vital signs, perimortem cesarean section should be considered. See Chapter 11, Resuscitation in Pregnancy; Chapter 79, Blunt Abdominal Trauma; and Chapter 122, Emergency Delivery and Peripartum Emergencies, for further details.

Laboratory evaluation includes a complete blood count, comprehensive metabolic profile, PT and PTT, DIC panel (fibrinogen, fibrin split products), urinalysis, and blood type and crossmatch. Anemia is a concern with both placental abruption and placenta previa. Because DIC can complicate placental abruption, it is important to perform the relevant tests. The Kleihauer-Betke test, which confirms the presence of fetal blood cells in the maternal circulation, may be performed if fetal-maternal transfusion is suspected. It is neither sensitive nor specific for abruption but quantifies that volume of fetal-to-maternal transfusion if positive.[17-19]

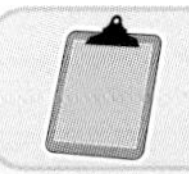

**DOCUMENTATION**

**Third Trimester Bleeding**

Vital signs of the patient, as well as fetal monitoring
Size of the gravid uterus and the degree of uterine spasm as determined during the physical examination
Presence or absence of vaginal bleeding and its onset, quantity, and duration
Events before the onset of bleeding
Type and time of interventions, as well the time when consultation was requested
Personal and family history with a focus on risk for placental abruption
Medical (including obstetric) history, especially in regard to cesarean section

## TREATMENT

Basic management of vaginal bleeding in third trimester pregnancy includes determination of the hemodynamic status of the mother and resuscitation as needed, assessment of fetal condition and age by fetal monitoring and ultrasonography, and decision making about the optimal timing of delivery. Early consultation with obstetrics colleagues is critical.

The patient should be placed on her left side to increase venous return. Initial management of significant vaginal bleeding is volume resuscitation and transfusion as needed. Although normal vital signs are optimal, they may be falsely reassuring because of the physiologic increase in maternal volume. After stabilization of the mother is ensured, the status of the fetus is assessed with continuous monitoring and ultrasound imaging to determine viability and age. The fetal heart rate may be a good indicator of maternal status; however, it is not specific.

Ultrasonography will diagnose placenta previa, which is managed by delaying delivery if the patient is stable and the fetus is premature. If there is heavy bleeding or the pregnancy is near term, delivery should be undertaken by cesarean section, regardless of fetal viability.

Management of placental abruption is contingent on the viability or distress of the fetus. In cases of mild placental abruption without fetal distress and severe placental abruption with fetal mortality, infants are delivered vaginally. In cases of moderate placental abruption with fetal distress, cesarean section is preferred.

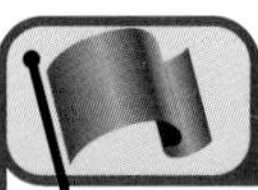

**RED FLAGS**

**Third Trimester Bleeding**

Hypertension not only increases the risk for placental abruption but also predisposes to more severe placental abruption and increased fetal mortality.

Although vaginal bleeding occurs in 80% of cases of placental abruption, some abruptions are concealed, with no evidence of overt bleeding.

Placental abruption in patients seen in the emergency department may be the result of abuse.

Many women with vaginal bleeding will have brief painless bleeding initially; this is a sign of placenta previa.

Rh-negative women should be given 300 units of RhoGAM. This dose is adequate to prevent maternal sensitization to up to 15 mL of fetal blood. A larger dose may be necessary if fetal-to-maternal transfusion is greater as determined by the Kleihauer-Betke test.

## FOLLOW-UP, NEXT STEPS IN CARE, AND PATIENT EDUCATION

Women with vaginal bleeding late in pregnancy need to be admitted. If the hospital does not have critical obstetrics and neonatal care facilities, transfer to a tertiary hospital is required.

## SUGGESTED READINGS

Oxford CM, Ludmir J. Trauma in pregnancy. Clin Obstet Gynecol 2009;52:611-29.

Shah DM. Preeclampsia: new insights. Curr Opin Nephrol Hypertens 2007;16:213-20.

Sibai BM. Imitators of severe preeclampsia. Obstet Gynecol 2007;109:956-66.

Sinha P, Kuruba N. Ante-partum haemorrhage: an update. J Obstet Gynecol 2008;28:377-81.

Vidaeff AC, Carroll MA, Ramin SM. Acute hypertensive emergencies in pregnancy. Crit Care Med 2005;33(10 Suppl):S307-12.

## REFERENCES

***References can be found on Expert Consult @ www.expertconsult.com.***

# Emergency Delivery and Peripartum Emergencies 122

*Jeremy B. Branzetti*

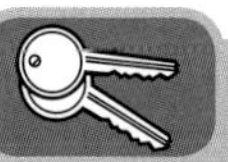

**KEY POINTS**

- If shoulder dystocia is encountered, attempt the McRoberts maneuver with suprapubic pressure while simultaneously calling for obstetric assistance.
- Practitioners underestimate blood loss in postpartum hemorrhage by as much as 50%.
- Uterine inversion is relatively uncommon but is associated with significant morbidity if not recognized and treated promptly.
- Up to 87% of patients with uterine rupture have no pain, and up to 89% have no vaginal bleeding.
- Perimortem cesarean delivery is indicated in gravid patients if more than 24 weeks pregnant and if arrest continues after 4 to 5 minutes of cardiopulmonary resuscitation.
- The clinical examination of a term pregnant patient is notoriously unreliable.
- Treatment of anaphylactoid syndrome of pregnancy is similar to that for sepsis and disseminated intravascular coagulation and should begin immediately; the diagnosis is one of exclusion, and patients must be treated promptly to survive.

## EMERGENCY DELIVERY

### PATHOPHYSIOLOGY

During labor the fetus follows a series of stereotypic movements known as the cardinal movements of labor. Although the specifics have little bearing on the emergency physician's approach to labor, the final movement typically leaves the baby with the occiput anterior (relative to the maternal pelvis) and the head sharply flexed. This position offers the smallest fetal head diameter and is therefore optimal for passage through the pelvis. Any deviation from this position is by definition a malpresentation, and these different presentations are all associated with increasing morbidity and mortality. The overwhelming majority of births, however, will require little physician intervention beyond timely encouragement and vigilance for complications.

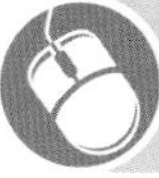

For a description of potential malpresentation, along with management recommendations, see www.expertconsult.com

### PRESENTING SIGNS AND SYMPTOMS

Labor is classically heralded by shedding of the mucous plug that was occluding the cervix (the "bloody show"), passage of clear fluid from the vagina from ruptured membranes (the "water breaking"), and contractions. True contractions are organized and detectable by tocometry; tend to increase in pain, frequency, and strength with time; and have associated cervical changes. Braxton-Hicks contractions, commonly called false labor, are characterized by unorganized myometrial activity without cervical changes. Other common symptoms at labor onset include abdominal pain and back pain.

In the emergency department (ED), the majority of patients seen in labor are in the latter part of stage I or stage II.[1] Precipitous delivery is a common occurrence because most patients whose labor progresses more slowly will have time to get to their designated obstetric facility.

### DIFFERENTIAL DIAGNOSIS AND MEDICAL DECISION MAKING

For any woman encountered after 20 weeks of pregnancy, labor must be in the differential diagnosis. Although the ultimate differentiation of false labor, or Braxton-Hicks contractions, is made by continuous tocometry, a good history can often make the diagnosis.

For patients with a chief complaint of vaginal bleeding, placental abruption and placenta previa should be considered. When the only complaint is passage of clear fluid from the vagina, premature rupture of membranes (PROM) and preterm premature rupture of membranes (PPROM) should be assumed until proved otherwise.

For an uncomplicated delivery, no diagnostic testing is needed. In those without any prenatal care, a complete blood count and Rh status should be obtained.

For patients complaining of vaginal bleeding, placenta previa or abruption should be assumed. Ultrasound is required to evaluate for previa. It is essential that placenta previa be diagnosed early because vaginal delivery is absolutely contraindicated with this condition. Ultrasound is not useful in ruling out the diagnosis of placental abruption because tococardiographic monitoring in an obstetric suite is required.

### TREATMENT

The major point of triage is during stage I of labor. If care is available in-house, transfer can be accomplished at any point before crowning. If care requires out-of-hospital transfer, it is imperative to establish early and reliable contact with the treating obstetrician to facilitate a safe plan of care.

Even though multiple physical interventions may be necessary with an abnormal delivery, an uncomplicated one typically only requires measures that support smooth fetal passage. Resuscitation equipment should be available immediately. Episiotomies are no longer recommended during routine pregnancies. They should be used sparingly and typically only with complicated deliveries. If shoulder dystocia is encountered, hyperflexion of the maternal hips and knees (McRoberts maneuver) and suprapubic pressure are first-line interventions that resolve most instances of dystocia.

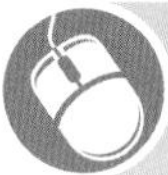

For more information on the management of difficult labor, see www.expertconsult.com

After determination of hemodynamic stability, the next priorities are to determine whether true labor is occurring and the appropriate disposition to achieve optimal medical care. For any patient with a complaint of passage of clear fluid from the vagina without other signs and symptoms of labor (bloody show and regular, progressing, often painful contractions), a sterile speculum examination should be performed before a gloved digital examination to evaluate for PROM.

Once labor is confirmed, the goal is to evaluate the positioning (orientation in space relative to the maternal pelvis) and presentation (body part palpable at the cervix) of the fetus, along with the degree of change in the uterine cervix. This includes assessment of station (level of decent into the pelvis relative to the maternal ischial spines), effacement (degree of cervical thinning), and dilation of the cervical aperture. For the emergency physician, determination of dilation and effacement is the most important part of the examination—a fetus that is still contained within a closed and minimally effaced cervix will probably be transferred to obstetrics whether or not it is vertex (fetal head as the presenting part).

If delivery is imminent, the patient will have to remain in the ED. A gynecologic bed with lithotomy position capability is ideal, and a resuscitation bay with greater accessibility and equipment is recommended. A radiant warmer and appropriate airway equipment should be available. Positioning of the mother may require an approximate 10-degree tilt to the left to prevent uterine pressure on the inferior vena cava and associated hypotension. When crowning occurs, the mother should be instructed to push along with the contractions, with the physician positioned in front of the introitus ready to accept the fetus. As soon as the head is accessible, continuous gentle countertraction should be administered to maintain it in a flexed position. This technique provides control of an explosive delivery, as well as avoidance of the high morbidity associated with fetal neck hyperextension. Though once recommended, the modified Ritgen maneuver has recently been shown to be associated with an increased rate of third-degree lacerations and episiotomy in comparison with a "hands-off" approach.[2] Similar rates of perineal tears were found for each modality.

When the head is clear, the fetus rotates 90 degrees. Suction of the fetal mouth and nose should be performed as soon as possible in the setting of meconium staining. Typically, the shoulders will then be delivered, anterior first, without assistance. Mild downward traction on the torso (not lateral flexion of the neck) may be required to assist passage of the anterior shoulder. Once clear, the posterior shoulder is typically delivered spontaneously or with upward traction in a similar manner as just described. At this point the largest fetal diameter has passed, and labor is generally smooth. The cord may be clamped once it is accessible after passage of the fetus. If the cord is tightly wound around the fetus, knotted, or abnormal in any way, it is clamped (typically at 7 and 10 cm) and cut once accessible. When free, the neonate is dried and warmed and its resuscitation needs evaluated. If available, a neonatologist should be present at any ED delivery.

Three classic signs indicate delivery of the placenta: sudden lengthening of the cord, a gush of blood, and a change in the shape of the uterine fundus. Once the fetus is clear, gentle traction on the cord should continue until these signs are seen. After the placenta is delivered, typically within 20 minutes, it is inspected for irregularities that may suggest retained tissue. Manual abdominal massage of the uterine fundus will often assist in uterine contraction. An infusion of oxytocin, typically 20 units in a 1000-mL bag of normal saline infused at about 200 mL/hr, can be administered to hasten separation and assist in contraction of the uterus back into the pelvis.

## FOLLOW-UP, NEXT STEPS IN CARE, AND PATIENT EDUCATION

After the placenta is delivered and the neonate is stabilized, the mother should be evaluated for bleeding—the causes and treatment of which are covered next. If hemodynamically stable after the first postpartum hour, the mother may be transferred to the postpartum floor.

# POSTPARTUM HEMORRHAGE

## EPIDEMIOLOGY

Hemorrhage is a significant cause of maternal morbidity and is the second most common cause of peripartum deaths (following amniotic fluid embolism). Hemorrhage was a direct cause of more than 18% of 3201 pregnancy-related maternal deaths in the United States from 1991 to 1997.[3] Worldwide, hemorrhage has been identified as the single most important cause of maternal death and is responsible for almost half of all postpartum deaths in developing countries.[4]

*Postpartum hemorrhage* is the term used to describe excessive blood loss after delivery. Classically, it is defined as more than 500 mL of blood loss in a vaginal delivery or more than 1000 mL of blood loss in a cesarean delivery; however, careful quantitative measures reveal that blood loss in the range of 500 to 1000 mL is actually average for both types of delivery. Of note, practitioners often underestimate blood loss by as much as 50%.[5] For the ED physician, the most important causes of hemorrhage in the postpartum period are birth trauma, uterine atony, uterine rupture, and uterine inversion.

## PATHOPHYSIOLOGY

Separation and delivery of the placenta constitute the third stage of labor. With separation of the placenta, there is also severance of the numerous uterine arteries and veins that carry 600 mL/min of blood through the intervillous space. The most important factor for hemostasis is contraction and retraction of the myometrium to compress and obliterate the open lumens of the vessels.

Uterine atony, the most common cause of postpartum hemorrhage, is the result of a hypotonic uterus after delivery. Factors that lead to uterine overdistention or that interfere with uterine contractility can cause uterine atony and are associated with postpartum hemorrhage. Although it is important to keep these associations in mind, most cases of postpartum hemorrhage occur without any known predisposing factors.

Trauma to the genital tract during labor and delivery (lacerations of the perineum, vagina, vulva, or cervix) is the second most common cause of postpartum hemorrhage. Abnormal placentation (placenta accreta, increta, or percreta) can contribute to postpartum hemorrhage in different ways: (1) an adherent placenta or large blood clots prevent effective contraction of the myometrium, thereby impairing hemostasis at the implantation site, and (2) significant bleeding from the implantation site is more likely with placental separation of abnormally adherent tissue.

Uterine inversion is prolapse of the uterine corpus to or through the cervix. Uterine inversion may be incomplete (inverted but does not go through the cervix) or complete (the fundus protrudes through the cervix). In the more extreme cases, the entire uterus may prolapse out of the vagina. Most cases are acute and occur immediately after delivery and before the cervical ring constricts. If inversion occurs (or is noted) after cervical contraction, the inversion is termed subacute. Chronic inversion takes place weeks after delivery. The majority of cases of uterine inversion occur as a result of traction on the umbilical cord during removal of the placenta. Acute, significant hypotension is common.

Uterine rupture is classified by the degree (complete or incomplete) and cause (spontaneous or traumatic) of the defect. A complete uterine rupture is defined as a full-thickness tear of the uterine wall and overlying serosa; it is associated with life-threatening maternal and fetal compromise. After complete rupture, the uterine contents may escape or partially extrude from the uterus and into the peritoneal cavity. An incomplete uterine rupture is defined as uterine muscle separation with an intact visceral peritoneum (often from uterine scar dehiscence). In an incomplete rupture, hemorrhage frequently extends into the broad ligament, which has a tamponading effect.

## PRESENTING SIGNS AND SYMPTOMS

Peripartum patients may lose a substantial amount of blood before becoming hypotensive or feeling symptomatic. Immediate postpartum hemorrhage should be recognized as a potential complication of a precipitous delivery. The classic clinical manifestation is a woman with sudden massive vaginal bleeding who is tachycardic, pale, and possibly diaphoretic or hypotensive. However, three factors make this classic manifestation flawed. First, an elevated pulse and decreased blood pressure are insensitive indicators until large amounts of blood have been lost. Second, many patients will have steady bleeding that, although moderate in appearance, may escape notice until serious hypovolemia develops. Third, intrauterine, intravaginal, intraperitoneal, and retroperitoneal accumulation of blood can be overlooked.

In a reported case series on uterine inversion, the most common signs were shock and hemorrhage.[6] With a complete inversion, the prolapsed uterus may be visible as a large, dark red polypoid mass within the vagina or protruding through the introitus. If the fundus remains within the vagina, the diagnosis may be suspected because of dimpling, indentation, or absence of the uterine fundus on abdominal examination or because a mass is palpated in the cervix on bimanual examination. Establishing the diagnosis of incomplete inversion can be quite difficult; severe hypotension, postpartum hemorrhage, and subtle abnormalities on abdominal examination may be the only clues.

Uterine rupture is also a difficult clinical diagnosis and should be considered in any patient with unexplained peripartum hemorrhage or hypotension. The classic findings of uterine rupture are "ripping" or "tearing," suprapubic pain and tenderness, absence of fetal heart sounds, recession of the presenting parts, and vaginal hemorrhage. Signs and symptoms of hypovolemic shock and hemoperitoneum may follow. This classic manifestation is actually rare; 87% of patients with uterine rupture have no pain and 89% have no vaginal bleeding. Pain is also an unreliable finding because of the altered response to noxious intraperitoneal stimuli by a stretched abdominal wall. Fetal distress is the most consistent finding (80% to 100%), with fetal bradycardia being the most common sign.[7] Most reports of uterine rupture describe patients with normal blood pressure or even elevated blood pressure without tachycardia. Abnormal maternal vital signs are late indicators of severe hemorrhage. The most important risk factor for uterine rupture is a previous uterine scar; other factors are listed in **Box 122.1**.

**BOX 122.1 Risks for Uterine Rupture**

**Surgery or Procedure**
Previous cesarean delivery (most common by far—1 in 125 subsequent pregnancies)
Previous uterine rupture
Previous myomectomy incision (1 in 40 subsequent pregnancies)
External or internal version
Breach extraction
Forceful uterine pressure during delivery

**Trauma or Environmental**
Trauma
Cocaine use

**Structural Anomaly**
Congenital fetal or uterine anomaly
Previous invasive molar pregnancy
Uteroplacental abnormalities: adenomyosis or placenta increta or percreta

**Pregnancy Related**
Silent rupture in a previous pregnancy
Persistent, intense contractions (spontaneous or iatrogenic)
High parity (1 in 100 subsequent pregnancies); grand multiparity (>7) increases the risk for rupture 20-fold[8]
In vitro fertilization

## DIFFERENTIAL DIAGNOSIS AND MEDICAL DECISION MAKING

Postpartum hemorrhage is a sign, not a diagnosis; it is important to consider the cause of the postpartum hemorrhage because it will often direct the treatment. The key to identifying the cause of postpartum hemorrhage is the physical examination. Because uterine atony is the most common cause of postpartum hemorrhage, accurate assessment of uterine tone is essential. To assess uterine tone, a hand is placed on the anterior wall of the uterus (over the fundus) to palpate it. If a soft, boggy, or very large uterus is felt, the diagnosis of uterine atony is established. At this point, management of uterine atony should be a priority over inspection for secondary causes of bleeding. If a firm, contracted uterus is felt, a search for other causes should be initiated promptly.

Without palpation or visualization of a frankly prolapsed uterus, it may be difficult to differentiate uterine inversion from severe atony. Heavy bleeding may make visualization of the cervix impractical. In addition, accurate abdominal palpation for a uterine fundus may be impossible in an obese patient. Depending on factors such as patient stability, resources, and diagnostic uncertainty, ultrasonography or laparotomy may be necessary. In stable patients in whom the diagnosis is uncertain and resources are available, prompt ultrasound scanning may be helpful.[9] Ultrasonography may be able to identify retained products or clot in the uterus, but manual exploration is still needed. Ultrasound can also help detect peritoneal free fluid suggestive of uterine rupture. In selected circumstances in stable patients, a computed tomography scan can be useful in making the diagnosis in those with postpartum hemorrhage (retroperitoneal hematoma). If the accompanying hemorrhage or shock is sufficiently alarming to require immediate exploration, the correct diagnosis may be established only at laparotomy.

Although congenital coagulation defects may be relatively rare, consumptive, dilutional, and disseminated intravascular coagulopathies are important considerations. Depletion of platelets and soluble clotting factors after blood loss and subsequent crystalloid and packed red blood cell replacement is difficult to distinguish clinically from disseminated intravascular coagulopathy. Placental abruption, amniotic fluid embolism, HELLP syndrome (hemolysis, elevated liver enzymes, and low platelet count), and intrauterine demise are pregnancy-related risk factors for disseminated intravascular coagulation. Initial laboratory studies include a complete blood count, coagulation studies, disseminated intravascular coagulation panel, liver function tests, and basic metabolic panel.

## TREATMENT

The most important aspects of managing postpartum hemorrhage are obtaining hemostasis and treating shock, including supplemental oxygen, placement of two large-bore intravenous (IV) lines, hemodynamic monitoring, and volume replacement. In addition, blood should be typed and crossmatched and 4 to 6 units of packed red blood cells should be available. Consultation with the obstetrics service should be arranged. Along with the initial resuscitation, bimanual massage and IV oxytocin should be initiated (**Fig. 122.1** and **Table 122.1**). A Foley catheter should be placed.

If the placenta has been delivered, manual uterine exploration may reveal uterine rupture or retained products or clots (which should be removed manually to improve uterine contraction). If the placenta is still in place and bleeding is ongoing, the placenta should be removed if a distinct cleavage plane is palpated on exploration. If an indistinct cleavage plane is revealed, the diagnosis of placenta accreta is likely. In this case the placenta should not be removed in the ED. Bimanual uterine compression should continue, with the goal being to stabilize patients until they can be taken to the operating room.

Trauma to the genital tract can be diagnosed by careful inspection of the labia, vagina, and cervix for laceration or hematoma. Noncomplex (first or second degree), easily accessible lacerations can be repaired with absorbable suture. Cervical lacerations and third- and fourth-degree lacerations should be repaired by an obstetrician. Temporary hemostasis may be achieved by direct pressure or, in the case of cervical lacerations, by gentle application of ring forceps to the bleeding point.

Retroperitoneal hematoma is a potentially life-threatening condition that may be manifested as hypotension, cardiovascular shock, or flank pain. Once a diagnosis is made, treatment should be supportive until the obstetrician, interventional radiology, or the operating room is available.

First-line interventions for atony are part of the initial management of postpartum hemorrhage—namely, initiation of bimanual uterine compression, IV oxytocin, and clearing of products of conception and clots from the uterus. If bleeding persists after the initial interventions, additional uterotonic medications should be given (see Table 122.1). The choice of agent may be influenced by the side effect profile, but the best drug is probably the agent that is the most quickly available in the ED. Interventional radiology may be beneficial because embolization may control the bleeding. In any case, temporizing measures may be required until definitive intervention (**Table 122.2**).

Uterine tamponade with sterile gauze and balloon tamponade are commonly used temporizing measures. Uterine balloon tamponade has been described with large Foley catheters, Sengstaken-Blakemore tubes, condom catheters, sterile gloves, and Rusch urologic catheters, as well as with catheters specifically designed to be used for uterine tamponade in patients with postpartum hemorrhage (SOS Bakri tamponade balloon).[10]

### UTERINE INVERSION

Management of uterine inversion has two important components: treatment of hemorrhagic shock and immediate repositioning of the uterus (**Fig. 122.2**). Resuscitation should be initiated immediately and continued while attempts are made to reposition the uterus manually. If oxytocin is being infused, it should be stopped once uterine inversion is suspected.

The success of nonsurgical replacement depends on completion before the myometrium regains its tone. The reported rate of successful immediate reduction is between 40% and 80%.[11] If initial measures are delayed or fail to relieve the condition, the inversion may progress to the point at which operative treatment or even hysterectomy is necessary.

The most common nonsurgical replacement method is a variation of the Johnson maneuver.[12] The prolapsed uterus is

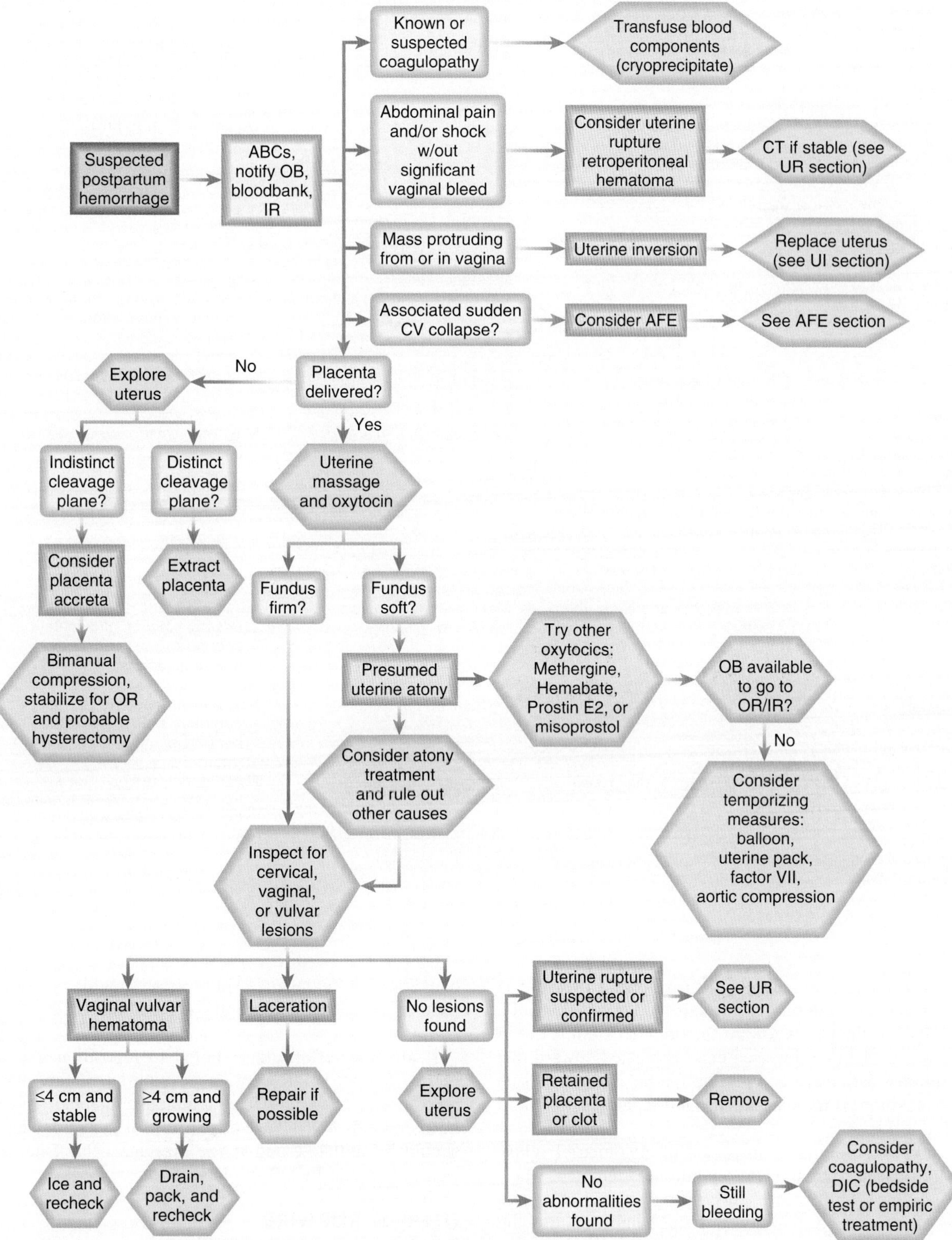


**Fig. 122.1 Algorithm for postpartum hemorrhage management strategies.** *ABCs*, Airway, breathing, and circulation; *AFE*, amniotic fluid embolism; *CT*, computed tomography; *CV*, cardiovascular; *DIC*, disseminated intravascular coagulation; *IR*, interventional radiology; *OB*, obstetrics; *OR*, operating room; *UI*, uterine inversion; *UR*, uterine rupture.

Table 122.1 Medications

| DRUG | DOSAGE | CLASS | COMMENTS |
|---|---|---|---|
| **Uterotonic** | | | |
| Oxytocin (Pitocin) | 20-40 U/L by wide-open IV infusion at 10 mL/min or 10-20 units IM | | Do not give an IV push; IV infusion first-line choice, IM second choice |
| Methylergonovine (Methergine, Ergonovine) | 0.2 mg IM, may repeat q2h (max 5 doses) | Ergot | Contraindicated in those with preeclampsia or hypertension |
| Carboprost tromethamine (Hemabate) | 0.25 mg (250 mcg) IM, may repeat q15-90min (max 8 doses) | Prostaglandin (15-methyl prostaglandin $F_{2\alpha}$ analogue) | May cause transient $O_2$ desaturation; contraindicated in those with active cardiac, renal, pulmonary, or hepatic disease |
| Misoprostol (Cytotec) | 600-1000 mcg SL or PR; single dose | Prostaglandin (prostaglandin $E_1$ analogue) | May cause bronchospasm |
| Prostaglandin $E_2$ (Dinoprostone or Prostin E2) | 20-mg uterine suppository, may repeat q2h | Prostaglandin | May transiently decrease blood pressure |
| Factor VIIa (NovoSeven) | 35-200 mcg/kg, may repeat q2h until hemostasis achieved | Human recombinant factor VIIa | |
| **Tocolytic** | | | |
| Magnesium sulfate | 4 g IV over 20-min period, then 2- to 3-g/hr infusion | Magnesium enzymes cofactor | Monitor for side effects; has prolonged effects; calcium gluconate may be needed to reverse tocolysis when the uterus in place |
| Terbutaline | 0.25 mg SC, may repeat q20min | Terbutaline beta-agonist | May cause hypotension; tachycardia common; hold if heart rate >120 beats/min |
| Nitroglycerin | 50 to 100 mcg IV, may repeat as needed | Nitroglycerin nitrate | Rapid onset and half-life; transient hypotension; have ephedrine (10 mg IV) available as remedy |

*IM*, Intramuscular/intramuscularly; *IV*, intravenous/intravenously; *PR*, per rectum; *SL*, sublingually.

cupped in the operator's palm, and firm upward pressure is applied to move the uterus up through the cervix along the natural curve of the pelvis toward the umbilicus until it is in place. Usually when the inverted mass is pushed upward, the uterus automatically reverts, with the fundus returning to its anatomic position. If the placenta has not separated, it should not be removed.

If initial repositioning is unsuccessful, myometrial relaxation with pharmacologic agents should be attempted. Magnesium sulfate, terbutaline, and nitroglycerin (attractive because of its easy availability and short half-life) are the agents most commonly used (see Table 122.1).[13] Attempts at manual repositioning of the uterus should continue.

After successful reduction, the uterus should be supported for several minutes to allow the ligaments to return to their original state while uterotonics are administered. If magnesium sulfate was administered as a tocolytic, calcium gluconate can be given to reverse the tocolytic effect. Fluid and blood replacement and manual uterine massage should be maintained until the uterus is well contracted and the bleeding has stopped. Antibiotics should be started as soon as practical. Uterotonics are continued for at least 24 hours.

If all other efforts have failed to reposition the inverted uterus, operative intervention is required. If the uterus was repositioned with the placenta attached, manual removal can be attempted once the use of relaxants is stopped. Uterotonics should be initiated, and if the placenta cannot be removed easily, it should be left in place.

## UTERINE RUPTURE

Initial management of uterine rupture differs and is based on the stability of the patient and fetus. Because the results of examination are normal in most patients with uterine rupture and because fetal distress is the most common finding, initial management will probably be the same as that for other causes of acute fetal distress—urgent delivery.

The physician should consult obstetrics on an emergency basis, ensure adequate IV access, notify the blood bank, and alert the neonatal team to be ready for intensive care newborn

**Table 122.2 Temporizing Measures for Hemostasis of Postpartum Hemorrhage**

| METHOD | PROCEDURE | COMMENTS |
|---|---|---|
| Uterine packing | Layer sterile gauze within the uterus, with the distal end going out through the os | May adhere to the uterine wall and removal required; does not allow monitoring of ongoing bleeding; start prophylactic antibiotics |
| Balloon tamponade | | If available and time allows, use bedside ultrasonography to confirm that the balloon is beyond the internal os before inflation to avoid damage to the cervical canal; give prophylactic antibiotics and continue oxytocin infusion |
| Foley catheter | Insert a large bulb catheter (24 French) into the uterus<br>Instill with 80-100 mL of saline<br>Pack the vagina to avoid expulsion of the catheter | Multiple catheters may be needed (in a sterile overbag), which makes the inner lumen difficult to monitor |
| SOS Bakri balloon | Insert into the uterus<br>Instill 300-500 mL of saline through the stopcock<br>Pack the vagina | Best option if available; allows direct measurement of ongoing bleeding via the open inner lumen; developed for postpartum hemorrhage; balloon conforms to the shape of the uterine cavity |
| Sengstaken-Blakemore tube | Cut off the distal ("stomach") end of the tube<br>Insert inside the uterine cavity<br>Infuse 75-300 mL of saline<br>Pack the vagina to avoid expulsion of the tube | Does not conform to the shape of the uterine cavity; with the end cut off, proximal bleeding can be monitored through the lumen; may be available from the gastrointestinal department laboratory if not available in the emergency department |
| Rusch catheter | Using a 60-mL bladder syringe, inflate the balloon via the drainage port with 150-500 mL of saline<br>Pack the vagina to avoid expulsion of the tube | Urologic catheter used for bladder stretching; may be available in the urology department |
| Condom catheter | Slide the condom over the end of the Foley catheter and tie it off with string to close the end<br>Inflate with 250-500 mL of saline and clamp the end<br>Pack the vagina to avoid expulsion of the tube | A sterile rubber catheter is fitted with a condom |
| Vaginal packing | Pack the vagina with a blood pressure cuff placed inside a sterile glove<br>Increase pressure to 10 mm Hg above systolic blood pressure | Various techniques have been described; concern for bleeding proximal to the vaginal pack |
| Noninflatable antishock garment | Begin application at the ankles and progress sequentially up to the abdomen | Adjust the panels if any discomfort or dyspnea; contraindicated in women with heart failure or mitral stenosis |

resuscitation. If these resources are not available in the hospital, arrangements should be made for immediate transfer.

For unstable patients, prompt, aggressive resuscitation is an important temporizing measure until definitive surgical repair is performed. Fetal morbidity almost invariably occurs because of catastrophic hemorrhage, fetal anoxia, or both. In a study of 99 cases of uterine rupture, the best fetal outcomes were noted when surgical delivery was accomplished within 17 minutes from the onset of fetal distress.[7]

If the patient is stable, no signs of fetal distress are present, or the diagnosis is unclear, ultrasonography can be useful. Ultrasound findings include lack of normal orientation, uncertain placental location, fetal demise, and absence of amniotic fluid.

## FOLLOW-UP, NEXT STEPS IN CARE, AND PATIENT EDUCATION

Obstetric consultation should be obtained on an emergency basis to assist in the delivery and postpartum care of the mother, as well as pediatric or neonatal services for the newborn. All patients who deliver in the ED should be admitted to an obstetric floor after delivery or stabilization of the acute complication.

# PERIMORTEM CESAREAN DELIVERY

## EPIDEMIOLOGY

Maternal arrest is estimated to occur in 1 in 4000 to 6500 pregnancies in the United States.[14-16] In any maternal arrest that occurs beyond 24 weeks' gestation, perimortem cesarean delivery should be considered as a potentially lifesaving intervention for both the mother and the fetus.[17]

When comparing causes of death in the cohort of women undergoing perimortem cesarean delivery with all maternal deaths, trauma accounts for a larger proportion in the former group.[18] Perimortem cesarean delivery is one of the oldest

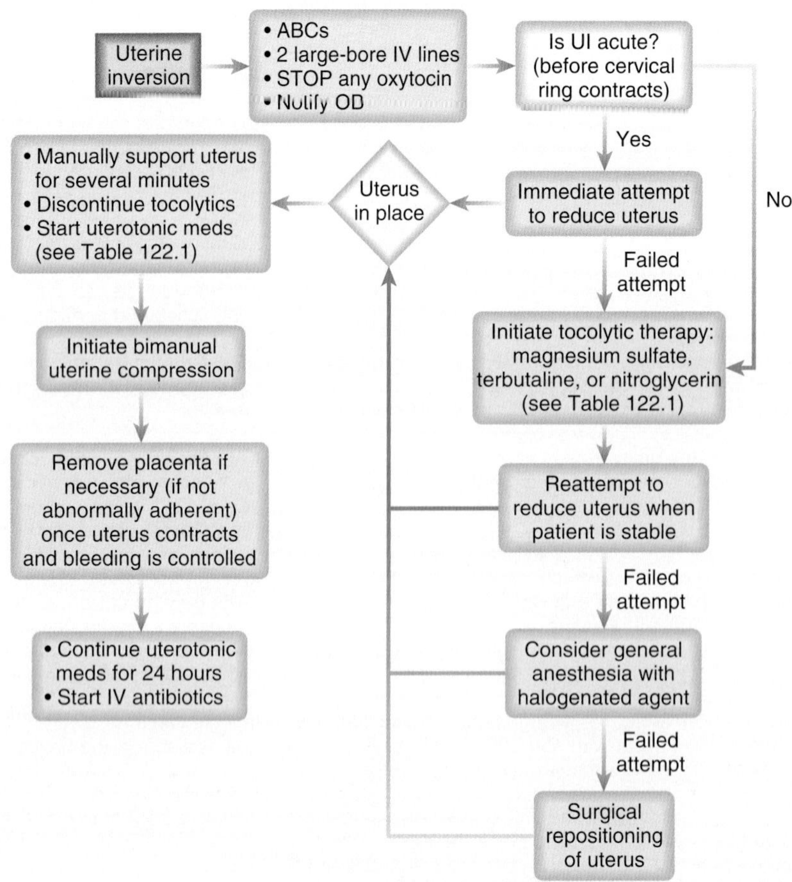


**Fig. 122.2 Algorithm for uterine inversion management strategies.** *ABCs*, Airway, breathing, and circulation; *IV*, intravenous; *OB*, obstetrics; *UI*, uterine inversion.

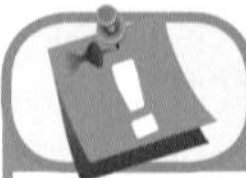

**TIPS AND TRICKS**

**Peripartum Hemorrhage**

Use an endotracheal tube 0.5 to 1 mm smaller than you would normally use because the airway may be narrowed from edema.

Compensate for reduced ventilation volumes (because of an elevated diaphragm) with a higher respiratory rate.

The left lateral position, manual uterine displacement, and perimortem cesarean delivery may improve the maternal circulation.

Do not use a femoral vein for a central line.

Follow the standard advanced cardiac life support guidelines for resuscitation, medications, and defibrillation doses (remove any fetal or uterine monitors before defibrillation).

Administer calcium gluconate (1 ampule or 1 g) for arrest from suspected magnesium toxicity.

surgical procedures in history, with the first reference to a successful postmortem cesarean section recorded in 237 BCE.[19] Under the emperors of Rome, the Caesars, a law decreeing that a child be excised from the womb of any woman who died late in pregnancy became known as the "lex caesare"—consequently the name *cesarean operation*. The first documented maternal survival after cesarean delivery was a Swiss woman sectioned by her husband in 1500.

## PATHOPHYSIOLOGY

Even under ideal conditions, cardiac output from chest compressions in a gravid patient is about 10% of normal. Cardiac output can be improved by displacing the uterus or tilting the patient (left lateral decubitus position); however, a decrease in effective chest compressions occurs with an increase in the patient's body tilt.[20]

Fetal outcomes are most directly related to the time from maternal arrest to delivery. Other important variables are the maturity of the fetus, the performance and effectiveness of maternal cardiopulmonary resuscitation, the cause of the maternal arrest, and the availability of a neonatal intensive care unit (NICU).

## DIFFERENTIAL DIAGNOSIS AND MEDICAL DECISION MAKING

Perimortem cesarean delivery is indicated for gravid patients more than 24 weeks pregnant (or the uterine fundus is four

**BOX 122.2 Procedure for Perimortem Cesarean Delivery**

Using a No. 10 blade, make a midline vertical incision that goes through all abdominal layers to the peritoneal cavity, which extends from the umbilicus to the pubic symphysis.

Separate the rectus muscles in the midline and enter the peritoneum. If available, retractors can be used to expose the anterior surface of the uterus. If the bladder is full, it may be seen inferior to the uterus. A Foley catheter is optimal, but under pressing conditions the bladder can be drained with a small scalpel incision and applied pressure.

To enter the uterus, start with a vertical incision through the lower uterine segment until amniotic fluid is obtained or the uterine cavity is clearly entered. Next, lift the uterine wall away from the fetus with two fingers and use blunt scissors to extend the incision vertically to the fundus; allow generous exposure. The membranes should be ruptured and the baby delivered.

Suction the infant's mouth and nose, and clamp and cut the cord. If the mother regains stable vital signs, remove the placenta and repair the uterus, abdomen, and bladder.

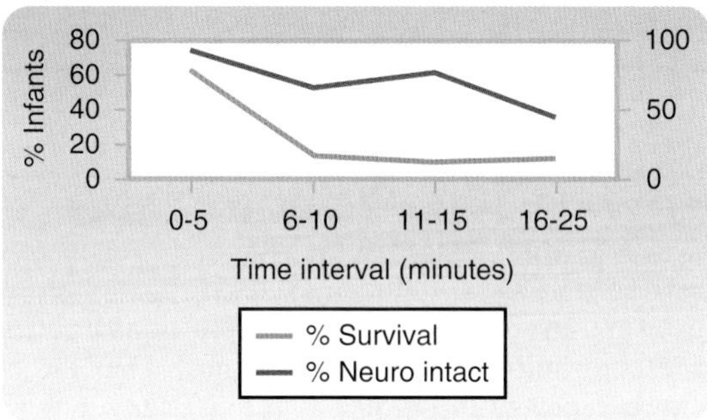


**Fig. 122.3 Perimortem cesarean delivery: fetal outcomes in relation to time interval from maternal arrest to delivery.**

fingerwidths above the umbilicus if the gestational age is unknown) if arrest continues after 4 to 5 minutes of cardiopulmonary resuscitation. In a study by Katz et al.,[17] among the cases with available data on maternal hemodynamics during resuscitation, more than half the women had a "sudden and often profound improvement, including return of pulse and blood pressure at the time the uterus was emptied." The study concluded that perimortem delivery should be performed within 4 minutes of maternal arrest if resuscitation was ineffective. An update published in 2005 strongly supported this conclusion,[17] and the 2010 American Heart Association guidelines for cardiac arrest associated with pregnancy agree with this window (even sooner if it is clear that the mother has a grave or nonsurvivable injury).[21]

## TREATMENT

See **Box 122.2**, "Procedure for Perimortem Cesarean Delivery," and **Fig. 122.3**.

# AMNIOTIC FLUID EMBOLISM

## EPIDEMIOLOGY

Amniotic fluid embolism and the resulting anaphylactoid syndrome of pregnancy occur in late pregnancy or immediately postpartum. Though rare (roughly 1 in 8000 to 80,000 pregnancies), it is responsible for about 10% of all maternal deaths in the United States and is the most common cause of peripartum death.[22]

## PATHOPHYSIOLOGY

Despite knowledge of this deadly syndrome for more than 80 years, its cause and pathophysiology are not fully understood. The criteria to make the diagnosis are still controversial, and no management interventions have been proved to improve outcomes or prevent the syndrome.[23] The term *anaphylactoid syndrome of pregnancy* is considered more appropriate than the term *amniotic fluid embolism* because of lack of evidence supporting a causative embolic event.[24]

Anaphylactoid syndrome of pregnancy, from a clinical, hemodynamic, and hematologic standpoint, is similar to anaphylaxis and septic shock and suggests the possibility of a shared pathophysiologic mechanism.[25] The syndrome appears to be initiated after maternal intravascular exposure to fetal tissue. Fetal-maternal tissue transfer is common and probably normal. It is proposed that when fetal antigens breach a maternal immunologic barrier in some women, release of endogenous mediators is triggered, and an anaphylactoid syndrome can occur.[24]

Neurologic damage is seen in as many as 85% of survivors of anaphylactoid syndrome.[25] The mechanism of neurologic injury is thought to be severe hypoxia leading to encephalopathy and seizures. The increased metabolic demand concurrent with seizures (seen in 50%) may worsen the brain injury, especially in the setting of hypoxia.[3] Disseminated intravascular coagulation developed within 4 hours of initial evaluation in more than 80% of patients.[25] If diffuse bleeding occurs, hemorrhagic shock can contribute to the hypotension.

## PRESENTING SIGNS AND SYMPTOMS

The classic manifestation of anaphylactoid syndrome of pregnancy is acute hypoxia or respiratory arrest with associated cardiovascular failure, altered mental status, seizures, and coagulopathy in the immediate peripartum period. It typically occurs abruptly and with catastrophic outcomes, but less severe forms of this syndrome have been described. In about 10% of patients the diagnosis is made postpartum, and it has been diagnosed as late as 48 hours postpartum.

## DIFFERENTIAL DIAGNOSIS AND MEDICAL DECISION MAKING

The National Registry's criteria for the diagnosis of amniotic fluid embolism are included in **Box 122.3**. The diagnosis of

**BOX 122.3 National Registry Criteria for the Diagnosis of Amniotic Fluid Embolism**

Acute hypotension or cardiac arrest
Acute hypoxia (defined as dyspnea, cyanosis, or respiratory arrest)
Coagulopathy (defined as laboratory evidence of intravascular consumption or fibrinolysis or severe clinical hemorrhage in the absence of other explanations)
Onset during dilation and evacuation, labor, cesarean delivery, or within 30 minutes postpartum
Absence of other significant, confounding conditions or explanation of the symptoms and signs listed here

Modified from Clark SL, Hankins GD, Dudley DA, et al. Amniotic fluid embolism: analysis of the national registry. Am J Obstet Gyrecol 1995;172:1158-69.

**BOX 122.4 Differential Diagnosis of Anaphylactoid Syndrome of Pregnancy (Amniotic Fluid Embolism)**

**Cardiovascular Collapse, Hypotension**
Acute coronary syndromes, myocardial infarction
Cardiomyopathy
Pulmonary embolism
Anesthesia complications, transfusion reaction
Sepsis, systemic inflammatory response syndrome

**Respiratory Arrest**
Pulmonary embolism, air embolism
Anesthesia complications, transfusion reaction
Aspiration

**Altered Mental Status, Seizure**
Eclampsia
Cerebrovascular accident
Hypoglycemia

**Coagulopathy**
Disseminated intravascular coagulation
Consumptive coagulopathy from hemorrhage

anaphylactoid syndrome of pregnancy is one of exclusion. Its dramatic and rapid onset should prompt immediate action; death has been reported in 30 minutes to 7 hours after onset, with most deaths occurring within the first 2 hours. The initial signs and symptoms can be difficult to differentiate from those seen with other serious causes, but management, with a focus on cardiopulmonary stabilization, is similar (**Box 122.4**).

## TREATMENT

No studies have shown that targeted intervention improves maternal prognosis. Management includes early definitive airway control with endotracheal intubation, IV fluids, vasopressors, and inotropes as needed. The blood bank should be notified and packed red blood cells, platelets, fresh frozen plasma, cryoprecipitate, and factor replacement should all be used as needed to treat disseminated intravascular coagulation. If the fetus is still not delivered at the time of arrest, perimortem cesarean delivery should be initiated within 4 to 5 minutes of resuscitation.

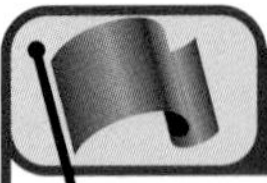

**RED FLAGS**

Underestimating the degree of blood loss in patients with peripartum hemorrhage or not appreciating moderate-appearing bleeding
Delaying uterine inversion replacement, which increases mortality (increases the risk and degree of hemorrhage and shock) and decreases the likelihood of successful nonsurgical repositioning because of cervical constriction
Not performing emergency cesarean delivery in maternal (>24 weeks of gestation) cardiac arrest not immediately reversed by cardiopulmonary resuscitation
Overlooking intrauterine, intravaginal, intraperitoneal, or retroperitoneal accumulation of blood in a hemodynamically unstable peripartum patient
Presuming that patients with active bleeding are stable because they have normal vital signs

## FOLLOW-UP, NEXT STEPS IN CARE, AND PATIENT EDUCATION

Patients who survive long enough to be transferred to the intensive care unit have a better prognosis, but the overall mortality is reported to be 60%.[25] In one study, only 8% of patients who had cardiac arrest as part of the initial findings survived neurologically intact. The infant survival rate was reported to be 70%, but almost half of the survivors had neurologic damage. If arrest occurs, a short arrest-to-delivery interval is associated with improved neonatal outcomes.[25]

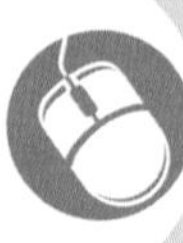

For expanded content on nonvertex presentation in delivery, cord-related complications, shoulder dystocia, premature rupture of membranes and preterm premature rupture of membranes, and multiple gestations, see www.expertconsult.com.

## REFERENCES

*References can be found on Expert Consult @ www.expertconsult.com.*

# Postpartum Emergencies 123

*Fiona E. Gallahue*

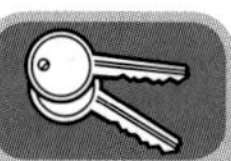

**KEY POINTS**

- The most common infection after childbirth is a genital tract infection.
- Because lochia will contaminate a clean-catch specimen in the first 4 to 8 weeks postpartum, urine should be obtained by catheterization in the immediate postpartum period to rule out a urinary tract infection.
- In the immediate postpartum period, an acute abdomen may not be manifested as abdominal rigidity on examination because of laxity of the abdominal wall tissue at this time.
- Leukocytosis cannot be used to help differentiate an infection in the first 2 weeks postpartum because of the physiologic leukocytosis that occurs during pregnancy and delivery.
- Fever is the most important criterion for the diagnosis of postpartum metritis.

## EPIDEMIOLOGY

Despite the fact that the first postpartum visit is generally scheduled at 6 weeks, most life-threatening complications arise within the first 3 weeks following delivery and are thus likely to be seen in the emergency department (ED). These complications are primarily related to infection, hemorrhage, pregnancy-induced hypertension, and embolic events.[1,2] Infection is one of the top five causes of mortality, with approximately 13% of pregnancy-related deaths between 1991 and 1999 being due to infection.[2] In the general population, the incidence of pregnancy-induced venous thromboembolism (VTE) is approximately 0.49 to 1.72 per 1000 deliveries.[3] The risk for VTE is five times higher in a pregnant than in a nonpregnant patient. When compared with pregnancy, the risk for VTE is even higher postpartum: a postpartum woman's risk for VTE is 20- to 80-fold higher in the first 6 weeks, and in the first postpartum week the risk is 100-fold higher.[3,4] The majority of deaths from VTE occur during the first 2 weeks of the puerperium, but a significant number of nonfatal events occur 2 to 6 weeks after delivery.[4] Approximately 75% of cases of pregnancy-associated VTE are deep vein thrombosis (DVT) and approximately 25% are pulmonary embolism (PE).[3]

Additionally, there is a high frequency of late maternal morbidity from a variety of causes; up to 87% of women note problems in the first 6 weeks postpartum, and as many as 76% of these patients continue to have these problems for as long as 18 months following delivery.

## PATHOPHYSIOLOGY: THE PUERPERIUM

Originally, the puerperium was defined as the period of confinement during and just after birth; it is now generally accepted to mean the 6 weeks after delivery. The puerperium has also been referred to as "the fourth trimester." This period is marked by multiple physiologic changes (**Table 123.1**) as the woman returns to the prepregnant state, including healing physically from any trauma during delivery, and adjusts to the many physiologic and psychologic demands involved in caring for a newborn. Just as in pregnancy, when there are so many physiologic changes, the potential exists for the normal healing process to go awry and emergencies to occur.

Certain significant changes in the physiology of the coagulation system during pregnancy persist past delivery and into the puerperium, including major changes in the coagulation and fibrinolytic system, as well as a reduction in venous blood flow in the deep venous system. Combined, these alterations increase the thrombotic potential in near-term and immediate postpartum patients.

A pregnant patient around term and immediately postpartum has significant increases in factors I, V, VII, IX, X, and XII; von Willebrand factor antigen; and ristocetin cofactor activity. The endogenous anticoagulants protein C and antithrombin remain unchanged throughout pregnancy, but levels of protein S are reduced. Fibrinolytic activity is impaired during pregnancy as a result of placentally derived plasminogen activator inhibitor type II and pregnancy-induced increases (approximately threefold) in endothelial and hepatic-derived inhibitor of plasminogen activator type I. These changes rapidly return to normal following delivery.

During normal pregnancy there is a significant reduction in blood flow to the deep venous system, as well as an increase in diameter of the major leg veins. These changes do not occur evenly in both legs. Studies of patients in the puerperium have reported greater diameter and slower blood flow in the left common femoral vein than in the right. These differences are manifested clinically; in nonpregnant patients, the left leg was affected in 55% of cases of DVT, whereas in pregnancy the

**Table 123.1 Physiologic Changes in the Puerperium**

| IMMEDIATELY FOLLOWING DELIVERY | BY POSTPARTUM TIME* |
|---|---|
| Uterus palpable at the umbilicus | By the 2nd wk, the uterus has shrunk back into the pelvis; complete involution takes 6-8 wk |
| Uterine blood flow via the uterine artery = 500-600 mL/min | By the 2nd wk, uterine blood flow = 30-45 mL/min |
| Cardiac output and blood volume increased by 30% to 50% | By the 2nd week, values are normalized to baseline |
| Breasts produce colostrum | By day 5, mature breast milk produced |
| Thyroid size and function increase | In 3 mo, the size of thyroid decreases; by the 4th wk, biochemical changes resolve ($T_3$,$T_4$, TSH are normalized) |
| Bladder has enlarged capacity and insensitivity to increased intravesicular pressure; renal pelvis and ureters dilated | 2-3 mo to return to normal |
| GFR increased | 8 wk to return to prepregnant GFR |
| Rectus abdominis muscles lengthened | 3-4 wk minimum to shorten; may be altered by exercise and overall baseline tone of the mother |
| Leukocytosis | 2 wk to return to baseline |
| Fibrinogen level elevated | Increases on days 2-4; returns to normal levels by the end of the first week |
| Stretch marks | 6-12 mo; depigmentation occurs but never fully resolves |
| Thicker and fuller hair | 3-4 mo; delayed alopecia |
| Lower mean velocity of blood flow in the common femoral vein after cesarean section | 6 wk to return to baseline |

*GFR*, Glomerular filtration rate; $T_3$, triiodothyronine; $T_4$, thyroxine; *TSH*, thyroid-stimulating hormone;
*Approximate time.

rate was 85%. The mode of delivery also affects the deep venous system. Women who delivered by cesarean section had a lower mean velocity of blood flow in the common femoral vein during the puerperium than did those who had delivered vaginally. These changes in flow velocity and diameter take approximately 6 weeks to return to baseline. Another significant clinical difference observed in pregnant and immediate postpartum patients is that the majority of DVT events seen during this time occur in the iliofemoral segments rather than in the calf veins and are therefore more likely to result in PE. Additional underlying risk factors that increase the likelihood for thrombotic complications are age older than 35 years, delivery by cesarean section, weight greater than 175 lb, and a family or personal history of thrombosis and thrombophilia (protein C or S deficiency, factor V Leiden).

## PRESENTING SIGNS AND SYMPTOMS

The most common complaints in the postpartum period are fatigue (56%), breast problems (20%), backache (20%), depression (17%), hemorrhoids (15%), and headache (15%).[5]

The signs and symptoms of metritis are fever, uterine tenderness, abdominal pain, and either purulent lochia or a positive culture of endometrial fluid or tissue usually between the second and seventh days postpartum. Fever (>38° C [100.4° F]) is the most important criterion for the diagnosis of metritis. Lochia may be foul smelling or have no odor.

Peritonitis is manifested as severe abdominal pain but may be misdiagnosed because abdominal rigidity, guarding, or rebound tenderness are often not present on physical examination as a result of laxity of the rectus abdominus muscles. Commonly, an adynamic ileus is the first sign.

Symptoms of toxic shock syndrome (TSS) include fever with a temperature of 39° C (102.2° F) or higher; erythematous diffuse rash; headache, photophobia, myalgias, and altered sensorium; gastrointestinal complaints, including nausea, vomiting, and watery diarrhea; and rapid progression to renal failure, hepatic failure, disseminated intravascular coagulation, and circulatory collapse.

Clinical signs and symptoms associated with cardiopulmonary complications may include fatigue, dyspnea, cough, orthopnea, hemoptysis, chest pain, palpitations, abdominal pain, tachycardia, elevated blood pressure, pulmonary rales, third heart sound, mitral regurgitant murmur, and peripheral edema.

Symptoms of postpartum mood disturbance include mild depression, irritability, confusion, mood instability, anxiety, headache, fatigue, and forgetfulness. Usually, the postpartum blues appear in the first 2 weeks after delivery and last from a few hours to a few days. More severe symptoms may include delusions, hallucinations, rapid mood swings, sleep disturbances, and obsessive thoughts about the baby.

## DIFFERENTIAL DIAGNOSIS AND MEDICAL DECISION MAKING

### INFECTIONS

Puerperal fever is defined as a temperature of 38° C (100.4° F) or higher that occurs on any 2 of the first 10 days postpartum, exclusive of the first 24 hours; the temperature should be taken orally by a standard technique at least four times daily.[6] The usual cause is a genital tract infection, which can lead to significant morbidity and mortality.

In a small proportion of women, postpartum fever will develop as a result of breast engorgement, but the fever rarely exceeds 39° C (102.2° F) in the first few postpartum days and usually lasts less than 24 hours.

The most common infection in the postpartum period is a genital tract infection, but other sources must be eliminated, especially urinary tract infection and pneumonia. The puerperal bladder is prone to urine retention, especially after instrumental delivery and epidural analgesia; in addition, dilation of the ureters and renal pelvis makes them potential sites of infection.

Mild hypoventilation after delivery as a result of pain or limited ambulation, or both, predisposes some women to pneumonia. Additionally, minor elevations in temperature are occasionally caused by thrombosis of the superficial or deep veins of the lower extremities (**Box 123.1**).[1,6]

### GENITOURINARY

#### *Metritis and Pelvic Infections*

In the past, uterine infections had different names based on the assumed location of the infection; however, the accepted terminology is now metritis or metritis with cellulitis because uterine infection often involves multiple tissue layers, usually the decidua and myometrial and parametrial tissue.

The single most significant risk factor for the development of metritis is the route of delivery. Women who deliver by cesarean section have a 6% to 18% incidence of metritis versus 0.9% to 3.9% with vaginal deliveries.[7,8] Other recognized risk factors for the development of metritis are chorioamnionitis, anal sphincter laceration, prolonged rupture of membranes, and weight on admission of more than 200 lb.

**BOX 123.1 Differential Diagnosis of Postpartum Fever**

| Most Common | Most Threatening |
|---|---|
| Metritis | Toxic shock syndrome |
| Urinary tract infection | Necrotizing fasciitis |
| Pneumonia | Pelvic phlegmon |
| Wound infection | Pelvic abscess |
| Mastitis | Peritonitis |
| Superficial or deep vein thrombosis | Septic pelvic thrombosis |
| | Breast abscess |

Rates of metritis are lower now than in the past 2 decades because of the routine use of prophylactic antibiotics for cesarean deliveries.[6,7]

Leukocytosis is often present but the white blood count is frequently elevated during the first 2 weeks postpartum. Chills may indicate bacteremia, which occurs in 10% to 20% of women with pelvic infection. Blood for culture is best obtained during the peak temperature elevations and chills that are associated with bacteremia.[9] Complications of pelvic infections can be quite severe. If a patient with metritis does not respond to antibiotics after 48 to 72 hours, suspicion for complications should be high.

Wound infections are the most common cause of antimicrobial failure in women treated for metritis and are usually associated with fever around the fourth postoperative day in patients who deliver by cesarean section. Wound dehiscence, or separation of the fascial layer, is a complication of incisional infections and is associated with fascial infection and tissue necrosis.

One of the most severe complications of a pelvic infection is necrotizing fasciitis. It has a devastatingly high mortality of approximately 50%, even with appropriate treatment, and may be a complication of a cesarean incision, episiotomy, or perineal laceration. Risk factors for necrotizing fasciitis are diabetes, obesity, and hypertension.

Other complications include pelvic phlegmon, which is cellulitis that has extended to the broad ligament. These infections can extend into any blood collections that develop after a cesarean delivery, such as under the bladder flap, and cause an infected hematoma. If left untreated, a phlegmon can suppurate into an abscess. Pelvic abscesses can develop in the broad ligament, ovaries, rectovaginal septum, or psoas muscle.

Infections can extend into the veins and cause septic pelvic thrombosis, which usually involves one or both ovarian venous plexuses and occurs more predominantly on the right because of the slightly longer vein on the right and dextrotorsion of the puerperal enlarged uterus. In 25% of patients, these clots extend into the inferior vena cava and occasionally into the renal veins.

#### *Toxic Shock Syndrome*

TSS is a rare but worrisome postpartum infection with a mortality of 10% to 15%. Group A streptococci and *Staphylococcus aureus* are the predominant causes of TSS. These bacteria colonize the mucosa of the vaginal tract and infect the postpartum uterus, cervix, and vagina, all of which are susceptible as a result of the trauma that accompanies delivery. Most cases of TSS occur in the first 8 weeks postpartum, but TSS can be seen up to week 10.

#### *Perineal Pain*

Although some discomfort is to be expected after delivery because of disruption and distention of the soft tissues of the birth canal, painful perineal tissue is a significant issue for many women. In fact, perineal pain was noted by 42% of recently delivered women to be a significant problem in the first 2 weeks following delivery, and as might be expected, the percentage was higher in patients with assisted vaginal deliveries (84%). By 8 weeks postpartum the percentage was down to 22% and by 12 weeks down to approximately 7%.[5]

Careful examination is required for these patients, especially those with persistent and significant discomfort, to look for evidence of hematoma formation, abscess, or genital tract infections such as cellulitis and necrotizing fasciitis.

### Urinary Tract Dysfunction

The puerperal bladder is predisposed to some urinary retention, as well as urinary tract infections, especially in patients who had instrumentation or prolonged labor in delivery, as well as epidural or spinal analgesia. In the immediate postpartum period, the bladder has increased capacity and relative insensitivity to increased intravesical pressure. The ureteral and renal pelvic dilation seen in late pregnancy takes approximately 2 to 3 months to resolve. These factors, combined with stasis of urine, create an excellent environment for development of a urinary tract infection. Any patient with a complaint of urinary retention should have catheterized urinalysis performed and urine sent the laboratory for culture to rule out urinary tract infection.

## LACTATION AND BREAST DYSFUNCTION

Milk leakage, breast engorgement, and breast pain peak at 3 to 5 days postpartum.

A milk duct can be clogged by inspissated secretions or milk forming a galactocele. It may form a fluctuant mass and resultant pain.

### Mastitis

In women who breastfeed, mastitis is a common problem that usually peaks between the second and sixth postpartum weeks. Most often the mastitis is unilateral and is caused by infant oral bacterial flora and relative obstruction of a milk duct. The most commonly isolated organism is *S. aureus*.

The affected breast appears hard and reddened, and the patient complains of severe pain. An abscess develops in 10% of women with mastitis. Patients with breast abscesses may have constitutional symptoms of fevers, chills, or rigor along with fluctuance of the area. Ultrasonography can be useful in detecting an abscess.

## GASTROINTESTINAL

Abdominal pain is a common complaint in the puerperium. In fact, one questionnaire given to women 48 hours after vaginal delivery noted that 50% of primiparous and 86% of multiparous women complained of lower abdominal pain.[10]

Abdominal pain can be a difficult complaint to evaluate in postpartum patients and requires a higher level of suspicion for a surgical emergency or infectious or thrombotic complications. Because patients expect to experience a certain amount of pain and discomfort after delivery, they often come late to the ED with these symptoms. During the preliminary ED evaluation it may be difficult for the emergency physician to adequately assess these patients without imaging, and the proper diagnosis may be further delayed.

### Appendicitis

In puerperal patients with appendicitis, peritoneal tenderness may not be present as a result of laxity of the rectus abdominis muscles following pregnancy. The uterus is still enlarged for much of the puerperium, and because the appendix is displaced upward toward the right upper quadrant and the abdominal wall is lifted away from the inflamed appendix, clinically apparent signs of peritoneal irritation are minimized. The psoas, obturator, and Rovsing signs are not predictive of appendicitis in pregnant and postpartum women. Other tests have been suggested such as the Bryan sign (pain elicited by movement of the enlarged uterus to the right) for appendicitis and the Alder test (maintaining constant pressure at the area of maximum tenderness while the patient rolls from a supine position to the left side) to differentiate pain of intrauterine origin (which diminishes as the uterus falls away with the maneuver) from pain of extrauterine origin. The sensitivity and specificity of these tests are unknown.

The incidence of appendicitis is not increased during the puerperium, although outcome is poorer because of delayed diagnosis. The incidence of certain pathologies such as obstruction, ileus, acute cholecystitis and perihepatitis, and Fitz-Hugh-Curtis syndrome (often misdiagnosed as acute cholecystitis) is increased during this period. Postpartum ileus is usually associated with cesarean section; other obstructions may occur more frequently as a result of compression of the enlarged uterus. Perihepatitis is often a sequela of latent or asymptomatic infection. Ovarian cysts and torsion need to be ruled out in the differential diagnosis, as well as complications of metritis and urinary tract infections.

Evaluation tools include a careful pelvic examination with appropriate cultures to rule out infection of the genital tract, a catheterized urine specimen to avoid contamination with lochia for urinalysis and culture, and standardized laboratory values such as electrolytes, liver function tests, serum amylase, and a complete blood count. In puerperal patients with appendicitis, urinalysis may show a sterile pyuria of more than five white blood cells per high-power field, and 15% to 30% of these patients have hematuria as a result of the proximity of the inflamed appendix to the ureter. The white blood cell count is difficult to interpret in puerperal patients because of the leukocytosis that normally occurs during the first 2 weeks of the puerperium.

Radiographs are typically nonspecific. Ultrasonography is useful to identify uterine, adnexal, ovarian, pelvic, or hepatobiliary abnormalities and may diagnose appendicitis. Contrast-enhanced computed tomography (CT) is better for identifying appendicitis and complications of metritis such as septic pelvic thrombophlebitis.[11,12]

## HEMATOLOGIC

### Hemorrhage

Severe bleeding complications usually occur early in the puerperium. The most common cause of early postpartum hemorrhage is uterine atony. Because this complication usually occurs immediately after delivery of the placenta, it is not likely to be seen in the ED unless the mother delivered at home or at a birth center without medical backup.

The second most common cause of early postpartum bleeding is vaginal or cervical laceration of the reproductive tract. Sometimes these areas of bleeding can be concealed, especially if the source is above the pelvic diaphragm; they can be very uncomfortable and not obvious on examination.

Delayed bleeding is the hemorrhagic complication most likely to be evaluated in the ED. Most cases of delayed postpartum hemorrhage are associated with infected retained placental fragments or membranes. A persistently patent cervix, particularly if associated with bright red bleeding, should suggest retained products of conception.

A rare cause of hemorrhage (0.2 to 1 case per million) is an acquired hemophilia that usually occurs within the first

4 months after delivery, occasionally as early as the first postpartum day. The mortality from such hemorrhage is 12% to 22%. Of these patients, 54% have other previously diagnosed immune system diseases such as rheumatoid arthritis, systemic lupus erythematosus, and inflammatory bowel disease. A prolonged partial thromboplastin time with a normal prothrombin time localizes the coagulation defect to the intrinsic pathway of the coagulation cascade and thus suggests hemophilia as the cause of the hemorrhage.

### *Thromboembolic Complications*

The index of suspicion for VTE should remain high because although complaints of dyspnea, tachypnea, leg swelling, and leg discomfort are common at term, they may also indicate PE or DVT. One study found that approximately 24% of women in whom DVT developed during pregnancy or the puerperium were asymptomatic and 55% complained of isolated leg swelling.[4]

DVT is best diagnosed by duplex ultrasonography because no radiation is involved; if the diagnosis is still uncertain, ultrasonography can be repeated or venography can be performed. To confirm the diagnosis of PE, ventilation-perfusion lung scanning or spiral CT could be performed safely in patients in the puerperium.

Neurologic embolic events such as cerebral embolism and cerebral venous thrombosis can also occur in the puerperium. Cerebral embolism generally involves the middle cerebral artery and is commonly associated with a cardiac arrhythmia, especially atrial fibrillation associated with rheumatic heart disease. However, these emboli may also be associated with rheumatic heart disease without arrhythmia, mitral valve prolapse, and infective endocarditis.

Central venous thrombosis is a rare but serious postpartum embolic complication with a frequency of 8.9 to 11.6 cases per 100,000 deliveries. The clinical findings are extremely variable and range from isolated headache to focal deficits to encephalopathy to psychiatric manifestations to coma.[13] The diagnosis is made by brain imaging, commonly magnetic resonance imaging with gadolinium enhancement, magnetic resonance venography, magnetic resonance angiography, CT four-vessel angiography, CT angiography, or any combination of these modalities.

## CARDIAC

Peripartum cardiomyopathy is a rare disorder that occurs in 1 of every 15,000 pregnancies in the United States, but it is a potentially fatal complication in the puerperium. Diagnostic criteria include onset of heart failure in the last month of pregnancy or in the first 5 months postpartum, absence of a determinable cause of the cardiac failure, absence of demonstrable heart disease before the last month of pregnancy, and impairment of left ventricular systolic function as demonstrated by echocardiography. The cause of peripartum cardiomyopathy is not known. Multiparity, multiple gestations, advanced maternal age (>30 years), preeclampsia, hypertension, and African descent are documented risk factors. The mortality associated with peripartum cardiomyopathy ranges from 18% to 56%.[14] Survival is largely dependent on recovery of left ventricular function. Most who recover significant left ventricular function show improvement by 2 months after diagnosis.

Patients who fail to recover within 6 months may require cardiac transplantation. Those who undergo transplantation have a 30% higher rate of early rejection than do patients with idiopathic cardiomyopathy, but the survival rate at 2 years is 86%.[15] Without transplantation, patients with persistent or progressive cardiomyopathy have a 5-year mortality rate approaching 50%.

Initial diagnostic evaluation includes electrocardiography, plain chest radiography, serum tests (electrolytes, liver function panel, complete blood count), and urinalysis. The electrocardiogram may be normal or tachycardic and may show nonspecific ST-segment or T-wave changes, atrial or ventricular dysrhythmias, left ventricular hypertrophy, PR or QRS prolongation, and conduction disturbances. Plain chest radiography usually shows cardiomegaly with pulmonary venous congestion and occasionally pleural effusion.

The diagnostic study of choice is echocardiography because it can be performed at the bedside, presents no radiation risk to pregnant patients, can differentiate between PE and amniotic embolism, and can provide prognostic information based on the degree of left ventricular dysfunction. The biggest drawback is often lack of availability in the ED.

Patients with peripartum cardiomyopathy are at especially high risk for thromboembolic events because of blood stasis from the severe left ventricular dysfunction, which may lead to left ventricular thrombi and subsequent emboli.

## ENDOCRINE

### *Sheehan Syndrome*

This syndrome of pituitary ischemia and necrosis associated with obstetric blood loss, first described in 1937, is an extremely rare occurrence in the developed world now that hemorrhage and shock are managed aggressively.

### *Thyroiditis*

Postpartum thyroiditis is usually a self-limited autoimmune disorder marked by the development of postpartum thyroid dysfunction that occurs up to 9 months following delivery. Classically, a period of transient hyperthyroidism occurs between postpartum months 2 and 6, followed by a transient hypothyroid stage, with return to the euthyroid state by 1 year postpartum. Its incidence ranges from 1.1% to 16.7%.

Risk factors include the presence of thyroid antibodies, a previous episode of postpartum thyroiditis, type 1 diabetes mellitus, and a family history positive for thyroid disease. These patients have an increased risk for the development of permanent hypothyroidism in the following 5 to 10 years. The diagnosis is based on thyroid-stimulating hormone (TSH) levels and free triiodothyronine ($T_3$) and thyroxine ($T_4$) levels.

During the hyperthyroid state of postpartum thyroiditis, TSH is suppressed and free $T_3$ and $T_4$ levels are elevated. Symptoms include fatigue, palpitations, irritability, heat intolerance, and nervousness. Many of these symptoms are often attributed to the stress of motherhood, and the diagnosis is frequently missed. During the hypothyroid state, TSH is elevated with suppressed levels of free $T_3$ and $T_4$. Symptoms include impaired concentration, carelessness, lack of energy, poor memory, dry skin, cold intolerance, and aches and pains.

## NEUROLOGIC

Headache is a common complaint in postpartum patients; it has been noted by about 15% of patients to occur in the first 2 weeks after delivery. The differential diagnosis of the cause of headache is extensive, and certain life-threatening complications need to be excluded, such as central venous thrombosis, stroke, meningitis, and intracranial bleeding from an undiagnosed aneurysm or arteriovenous malformation. The patient's personal and medical history is of the greatest importance to aid in diagnosis because it may suggest a cause such as migraine, post–dural puncture headache, or pneumocephalus.

The pain from pneumocephalus associated with epidural anesthesia is a result of direct injection of air into the subarachnoid space and is immediately felt as back pain at the level of needle insertion that spreads to the posterior aspect of the neck and then to the occipital and frontal areas. Generally, this complication, which occurs when the patient is in labor, resolves with supportive care, and the patient has no neurologic deficits.[16]

Post–dural puncture headache is also associated with epidural anesthesia. It is a "nonthrobbing" headache that is worsened on change of posture from a horizontal to an upright position. These headaches are postulated to be caused by persistent loss of cerebrospinal fluid at a dural puncture site. Most of these headaches begin within 5 days of the procedure. Auditory and ocular symptoms may occur with prolonged or severe manifestations.

Other less common causes of headache in postpartum patients include central venous thrombosis (see the earlier section "Thromboembolic Complications") and late postpartum preeclampsia, which may be manifested as hypertension with blood pressure greater than 140 mm Hg systolic and 90 mm Hg diastolic, proteinuria, and a headache not responsive to analgesics. Late postpartum eclampsia occurs in 3% to 26% of eclamptic patients. Late postpartum preeclampsia or eclampsia is defined as the development of signs and symptoms after 48 hours and before 4 weeks following delivery. Most patients with postpartum preeclampsia or eclampsia do not have a preceding history of gestational preeclampsia or eclampsia. A postpartum woman with a new history of convulsions occurring more than 48 hours after delivery plus proteinuria and hypertension should be considered eclamptic while other causes are being ruled out. Neuroimaging generally demonstrates a posterior reversible encephalopathy syndrome.[17]

## PSYCHIATRIC

Fatigue is one of the most common complaints during the puerperium. Some fatigue is normal given the demands of taking care of a newborn infant after the physical rigors of labor and delivery; however, this complaint should be taken seriously because it can be the first symptom of anemia, new-onset diabetes, hypothyroidism, or a psychiatric disorder.

The most common postpartum mood disturbance is the postpartum blues, which affects 50% to 80% of new mothers. Physicians must evaluate the patient to differentiate postpartum blues from the more severe symptoms associated with postpartum depression. Up to 20% of women with postpartum blues will have a major depressive episode in the first postnatal year. Multiple risk factors for postpartum depression have been identified: personal or family history of depression, previous episode of postpartum depression, depression or anxiety during pregnancy, an unplanned or unwanted pregnancy, recent stressful life events, poor social support, and marital discord. Neonatal medical problems or the occurrence of postpartum blues also increases the risk for postpartum depression.

Usually beginning within the first 4 weeks after delivery, postpartum depression is highly variable in severity and duration. It occurs in 5% to 20% of new mothers and is especially prevalent in adolescent mothers. The diagnosis of depression is difficult to make in a postpartum mother because the typical signs and symptoms have significant overlap with normal issues of the puerperium, such as disturbances in sleep, weight, and energy.

The most severe form of psychiatric disease in the postpartum period is postpartum psychosis. Fortunately, this condition is rare and occurs in fewer than 2 of every 1000 deliveries. The onset of postpartum psychosis is usually within the first 3 weeks after delivery and occasionally within a few days after delivery. Many of these patients have a history of schizophrenia or bipolar disorder. Symptoms include delusions, hallucinations, rapid mood swings, sleep disturbances, and obsessive thoughts about the baby.

# TREATMENT AND FOLLOW-UP

## GENITOURINARY

### *Metritis and Pelvic Infections*

Low-risk patients in whom mild metritis develops after being sent home following vaginal delivery can be treated with an oral microbial agent such as doxycycline or azithromycin. Patients with moderate to severe metritis, as well as those who have delivered by cesarean section, should be treated with broad-spectrum intravenous antibiotics to cover mixed flora and should be observed in the hospital.

Most patients should improve with antibiotics within 48 to 72 hours, and failure to improve suggests a complication of metritis such as parametrial phlegmon, pelvic or incisional abscess, infected hematoma, septic pelvic thrombi, retention of fetal parts, or bacteria resistant to the treatment regimen.

Treatment of pelvic abscesses includes intravenous antibiotics and possible percutaneous drainage. In cases of septic pelvic thrombi, intravenous antibiotics are currently the mainstay of therapy because studies indicate that the use of heparin does not alter the outcome.

Empiric treatment of necrotizing fasciitis varies widely. Treatment typically consists of a four-antibiotic regimen that includes gram-positive coverage with a penicillin or extended-spectrum penicillin; gram-negative coverage with aminoglycosides, cephalosporins, or carbapenems; anaerobic coverage with clindamycin; empiric coverage for methicillin-resistant *S. aureus* (MRSA) such as vancomycin; and emergency operative débridement of the area.[18]

### *Toxic Shock Syndrome*

Treatment of TSS includes aggressive fluid management with crystalloids, supportive care, and pressors as needed. Antibiotics do not alter the course of TSS, but they decrease the recurrence rate by 50%. An agent to cover gram-positive organisms plus coverage for MRSA, such as vancomycin combined with an aminoglycoside such as gentamicin, is appropriate.[19]

### *Perineal Pain*

Early application of cold compresses or ice packs to soft tissue trauma reduces swelling and discomfort. Sitz baths are also recommended to alleviate discomfort. Acetaminophen or nonsteroidal antiinflammatory drugs (generally considered safe in breastfeeding patients) are the initial medications of choice for pain.

### Urinary Tract Dysfunction

Most patients with urinary retention will note incomplete voiding and will not require catheterization, but they should be referred to the urology or urogynecology department for urodynamic testing.

Stress urinary incontinence is another complaint that occurs in the postpartum period. The ED usually lacks the facilities to address this complaint, but these patients should be referred to the urology or urogynecology department for work-up and management.

## LACTATION AND BREAST DYSFUNCTION

### Breast Engorgement

During the state of engorgement, breast pain can be partially alleviated by a supportive brassiere or breast binder, avoidance of nipple stimulation, ice packs, and oral analgesics.[1,6]

### Galactocele

Warm compresses may help the situation resolve spontaneously, but in patients with a large amount of pain and fluctuance, needle aspiration may be required.

### Mastitis

First-line agents for the treatment of mastitis are penicillin, cephalosporin, clindamycin, and erythromycin (for penicillin-sensitive patients); all are considered safe in lactating women. The infection should show improvement within 48 hours. Lack of improvement over this period suggests an abscess or resistant organism. Abscesses require incision and drainage with packing or ultrasound-guided needle aspiration, which has a success rate of 80% to 90%.

If resistant organisms are suspected, milk from the affected breast should be sent on a swab for culture, and an antimicrobial agent effective against MRSA should be started. Continued breastfeeding on the affected side is important to help clear the infection. If the baby is having difficulty latching on because of surrounding erythema or induration, the affected breast can be pumped gently. Patients should be referred for a follow-up visit within 72 hours to their primary care physician or gynecologist to ensure that they are responding to the medication prescribed.

## HEMATOLOGIC

### Postpartum Bleeding

Treatment consists of broad-spectrum antibiotics and emergency obstetric consultation for dilation and curettage. Disseminated intravascular coagulation can occur in these cases and may require aggressive management with platelets, fresh frozen plasma, and packed red blood cells.[1]

Hemorrhage from acquired hemophilia should prompt a hematology consultation. Management of the hemorrhage consists of the administration of blood products to replace the blood loss, coagulation factor, and immunosuppressants. Selection of a product for control of acute bleeding depends on the clinical severity and on coagulation factor VIII inhibitor titers. Immunosuppressive therapy with corticosteroids and cytotoxic drugs, alone or in combination, has been the mainstay of therapy in stable patients. In most of these cases, the acquired hemophilia spontaneously remits within months of delivery.[20]

### Deep Vein Thrombosis

Treatment of postpartum patients with DVT consists of unfractionated or low-molecular-weight heparin and transition to warfarin (Coumadin), which is safe in lactating patients because it does not significantly cross over into breast milk.[4,21]

### Central Venous Thrombosis

Management includes anticonvulsants to control seizures, emergency neurology consultation, and antimicrobials if septic thrombosis is suspected. Heparin therapy is controversial because of the bleeding complications that may develop.[6]

## CARDIAC

Treatment of postpartum cardiomyopathy is the same as that for nonischemic dilated cardiomyopathy. Management should be supportive with restriction of sodium (no more than 4 g daily of salt) and fluid (no more than 2 L of daily fluid intake). Preload- and afterload-reducing agents plus positive inotropic agents, if the patient is acutely ill, are the cornerstones of treatment. For antepartum patients, afterload reduction can be accomplished with hydralazine; positive inotropy with digoxin; and preload reduction with diuretics, nitroglycerine, and beta-blockers. Postpartum patients should receive angiotensin-converting enzyme inhibitor therapy, which has been shown to improve survival in patients with dilated cardiomyopathy.[14] Breastfeeding mothers should curtail breastfeeding because angiotensin-converting enzyme inhibitors are excreted in breast milk and their safety is unproved.[21]

## ENDOCRINE DISORDERS

### Thyroiditis

Most women in the hyperthyroid stage need no treatment or intervention. Symptomatic patients in this stage can usually be managed with beta-blockers and referral to an endocrinologist. The hypothyroid stage is multifactorial, and management is more difficult; these patients should also be referred to an endocrinologist for long-term follow-up. Patients with a TSH level greater than 10 mU/L or who are symptomatic with a TSH level between 4 and 10 mU/L should be treated with levothyroxine. Women who are planning to become pregnant again should be cautioned to wait until they have discussed the issue with an endocrinologist because even subclinical hypothyroidism can cause an increased miscarriage rate and may result in impaired cognitive performance in the child.[22]

## NEUROLOGIC

Headaches that result from the pneumocephalus associated with epidural anesthesia generally occur when the patient is in labor and resolve with supportive care.[15]

Treatment of post–dural puncture headaches includes hydration and analgesic agents initially. If these measures fail, an anesthesia consultation to consider an epidural blood patch is recommended.[16,23]

Postpartum preeclampsia or eclampsia can develop as late as 2 or more weeks postpartum. Magnesium sulfate therapy should be initiated with a loading dose of 4 g administered over a 30-minute period, followed by a maintenance dose of 2 g/hr for at least 24 hours after the last seizure, along with close monitoring and observation. More detail about the diagnosis and management of these patients can be found in Chapter 121.

## PSYCHIATRIC

Postpartum blues is generally a self-limited and benign condition, but patients should be evaluated for a personal or family history of depression, as well as the strength of their social support structure. Patients with postpartum blues should be referred to their primary care physicians for follow-up. Those with risk factors for a major depressive episode should be educated about the signs and symptoms of major depression and be encouraged to seek help if they experience these symptoms. Patients who show signs of psychosis or major depression require psychiatric evaluation and follow-up before they can be discharged. Patients with postpartum psychosis require emergency hospitalization because 5% of these patients commit suicide and 4% commit infanticide.[24]

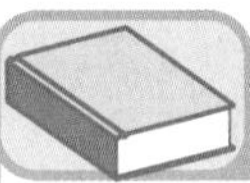

### PATIENT TEACHING TIPS

After starting antibiotics for mastitis, improvement should be seen by 48 to 72 hours; if the condition does not improve or worsens, an abscess or resistant organism may be the cause of the infection, and reevaluation is necessary.

Patients with mastitis should be instructed to continue breastfeeding on the affected side to help clear the infection.

To avoid complications in a second pregnancy, patients with hypothyroidism should not become pregnant again until management of the disorder is successful and cleared by an endocrinologist.

Patients with abdominal pain should be counseled on the difficulty of making intraabdominal diagnoses in the puerperium and should have clear follow-up and return visit instructions.

Patients with postpartum blues should be reassured that this is normal and usually resolves within a few days. If no improvement in symptoms is seen by the end of a week, patients should be reevaluated either in the emergency department or by a psychiatrist.

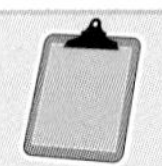

### DOCUMENTATION

The mode of delivery is an important factor in puerperium complications; delivery by cesarean section is associated with higher rates of infection, as well as other disorders. Note the method of delivery, pregnancy and delivery complications, and associated risk factors.

Document social support for the patient and infant.

Give and record instructions about potential complications.

Patients with abdominal pain are at increased risk for complications; provide clear instructions on where and when follow-up should be carried out, list reasons to return to the emergency department, and discuss potential causes of abdominal pain.

In patients with headache in the first 3 postpartum weeks, document the timing of the headache, worsening with change of position, and quality of the headache.

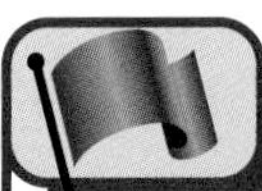

### RED FLAGS

Metritis should improve within 48 to 72 hours with antibiotics; failure to improve suggests complications such as parametrial phlegmon, pelvic or incisional abscess, infected hematoma, septic pelvic thrombi, retained products of conception, or bacterial resistance.

Initial diagnosis of peripartum cardiomyopathy (PPCM) may be difficult to make, and it is often manifested by symptoms similar to amniotic fluid or pulmonary thromboembolism. Patients with PPCM are at high risk for thromboembolic events. Severe left ventricular dysfunction from PPCM results in blood stasis and may lead to left ventricular thrombi and subsequent emboli.

Postpartum thyroiditis is associated with a period of transient hyperthyroidism occurring 2 to 6 months postpartum; symptoms include fatigue, palpitations, irritability, heat intolerance, and nervousness. These symptoms are often attributed to the stress of motherhood, and the correct diagnosis may be missed.

Sterile pyuria and hematuria may be seen in patients with appendicitis. The uterus is still enlarged for much of the puerperium, with the appendix displaced upward toward the right upper quadrant and the abdominal wall lifted away from the inflamed appendix, which minimizes clinically apparent signs of peritoneal irritation.

Patients with postpartum psychosis may have symptoms such as delusions, hallucinations, rapid mood swings, sleep disturbances, and obsessive thoughts about the baby. These patients require emergency hospitalization because approximately 5% commit suicide and 4% commit infanticide.

### TIPS AND TRICKS

Because lochia will contaminate a clean-catch urine specimen during the first 30 to 60 days postpartum, a catheterized urine specimen should be obtained and sent to the laboratory to rule out urinary tract infection.

The second most common cause of early postpartum bleeding is laceration of the reproductive tract. In some of these cases, areas of bleeding may be concealed, especially if the source is above the pelvic diaphragm; this condition is very uncomfortable and not always obvious on examination.

Although 75% of deep vein thrombosis events occur antepartum, 66% of pulmonary thromboembolism events occur postpartum.

The psoas, obturator, and Rovsing signs are not predictive of appendicitis in pregnant and postpartum patients.

## REFERENCES

*References can be found on Expert Consult @ www.expertconsult.com.*

# Gynecologic Pain and Vaginal Bleeding 124

*Jamie L. Collings and Nicholas A. Borm*

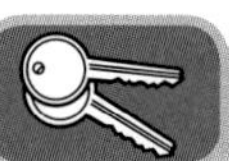

**KEY POINTS**

- The possibility of pregnancy should be considered in every patient with a chief complaint of vaginal bleeding or pelvic pain.
- Ectopic pregnancy, acute appendicitis, and ovarian torsion must be considered in female patients with acute pelvic pain.
- Up to 50% of patients with ovarian torsion have normal findings on ultrasound.
- Malignancy should be considered in postmenopausal women with new-onset vaginal bleeding.
- With the exception of physiologic withdrawal bleeding in the neonate, vaginal bleeding in a prepubescent girl is always abnormal.

## VAGINAL BLEEDING

This section of the chapter addresses common causes of vaginal bleeding, including dysfunctional uterine bleeding (DUB), uterine leiomyomas (fibroids), vaginal foreign body, endometrial cancer, and cervical cancer.

## EPIDEMIOLOGY

### DYSFUNCTIONAL UTERINE BLEEDING

DUB affects an estimated 30% of women in the United States, is most common at the extremes of the reproductive years, and has no predilection for race. DUB rarely causes mortality but is accountable for two thirds of all hysterectomies and the majority of endoscopic endometrial destructive surgery.[1]

### UTERINE LEIOMYOMAS (FIBROIDS)

Uterine leiomyomas (fibroids) are the most common pelvic tumor in women and have been noted on pathologic examination in approximately 80% of surgically excised uteri.[2] Risk factors include African American race, early menarche (<10 years of age), nulliparity, and family history. Several studies have shown more subtle correlations with obesity and diet.[3,4]

### VAGINAL FOREIGN BODY

The epidemiology of vaginal foreign bodies is largely unknown, but one study theorizes that approximately 20% of preteenage girls with vaginal bleeding with or without discharge and 50% of those with bleeding and no discharge will prove to have vaginal foreign bodies.

### ENDOMETRIAL CANCER

Endometrial cancer is the fourth most common cancer in women and occurs in approximately 25 per 100,000 women.[5,6] This malignant disease develops during the reproductive and menopausal years, with most patients being 50 to 59 years of age. About 5% of women younger than 40 have adenocarcinoma, and it is diagnosed in a quarter of patients before menopause. Many cases of endometrial cancer go undetected given that Papanicolaou smears detect only 50% of cases and the diagnosis is rarely considered in perimenopausal women despite the aforementioned statistics.

### CERVICAL CANCER

Cervical cancer is the second most common malignancy in women worldwide. Approximately 11,000 new cases are diagnosed annually in the United States, and it accounts for around 4000 deaths per year. Minority populations are more commonly affected. The peak incidence of cervical cancer occurs in women 45 to 54 years of age; however, there is a surge in prevalence in women in their 20s and 30s as human papillomavirus (HPV) rates have increased.[5,6]

## PATHOPHYSIOLOGY

Common terminology and definitions for vaginal bleeding are listed in **Box 124.1**. An understanding of the normal female reproductive cycle is useful when caring for patients with vaginal bleeding and pelvic pain. The normal reproductive cycle is 28 days, with a range of 21 to 35 days, and the average age at menarche is approximately 12.5 years. The complex hormonal feedback mechanism that governs the female reproductive cycle is controlled by the hypothalamic-pituitary-ovarian (HPO) axis. Days 1 to 14 are known as the follicular or proliferative phase and are dominated by the release of gonadotropin-releasing hormone (GnRH) from the hypothalamus; GnRH in turn stimulates pituitary release of follicle-stimulating hormone (FSH). During this phase a dominant ovarian follicle matures and produces estrogen, which causes

**BOX 124.1 Differential Diagnosis of Vaginal Bleeding in Nonpregnant Females**

**Trauma**
Blunt force
Penetrating force
Foreign bodies

**Infectious**
Vaginitis
Cervicitis
Endometritis

**Dysfunctional Uterine Bleeding**
Ovulatory
Anovulatory
Adenomyosis

**Benign Growths**
Uterine leiomyomas
Cervical polyps

**Malignancy**
Vulvar
Cervical
Uterine
Ovarian

**Systemic Disease**
See Table 124.2

**Medications**
Anticoagulation (warfarin [Coumadin], low-molecular-weight heparin, clopidogrel [Plavix])
Antipsychotics
Corticosteroids
Tamoxifen
Selective serotonin reuptake inhibitors
Contraceptives (oral, intrauterine devices, intramuscular)

the endometrium to thicken and prepare for possible embryo implantation. Positive feedback of estrogen to the pituitary gland induces a surge in luteinizing hormone (LH) on day 14 of the cycle, which results in ovulation. Days 14 to 28 are known as the luteal or secretory phase; this phase is predominated by progesterone production from the corpus luteum, which induces maturation of the endometrium. If conception and implantation do not occur, the corpus luteum involutes, estrogen and progesterone levels fall, and menstruation occurs.

Changes in the endometrium occur at each step of the reproductive cycle. During the proliferative phase the endometrium grows and thickens in response to estrogen as it prepares for implantation of an embryo. During the secretory phase the endometrium matures under the influence of progesterone and glands and secretory vacuoles develop. As progesterone levels drop at the end of the secretory (luteal) phase, prostaglandins are released and cause vasospasm within the endometrial vasculature. This leads to sloughing of the outer layers of the endometrium, and thus menstruation occurs.

Disruption at any point in this feedback loop may cause pelvic pain or abnormal vaginal bleeding.

## DYSFUNCTIONAL UTERINE BLEEDING

DUB is the most common cause of menorrhagia in menstruating females and is defined as abnormal uterine bleeding in the absence of organic disease. DUB can be ovulatory or anovulatory. Ovulatory DUB is hallmarked by regular intervals of increased menstrual flow. The root cause is an abnormality in uterine hemostasis secondary to cytokine and prostaglandin production. More commonly (accounting for 90% of cases of DUB), anovulatory DUB is hallmarked by irregular intervals of alternating heavy and light flow. This can be caused by primary ovarian disorders or a disruption in the HPO axis.[7]

Polycystic ovarian disease is classically associated with anovulatory uterine bleeding. It is defined by ovulatory failure, which leads to the absence of a corpus luteum and thus the lack of progesterone production and therefore unopposed action of estrogen on the endometrium. The uterine lining persists in the proliferative phase until it outgrows its vascular supply and degenerates, thereby leading to irregular menses with alternation between heavy and light flow. Women often have signs of hyperandrogenism, including hirsutism, obesity, acne, palpable enlarged ovaries, and acanthosis nigricans (hyperpigmentation typically in the folds of the skin of the neck, groin, or axilla).

Anovulatory DUB is most commonly seen in postpubescent girls secondary to immaturity of hypothalamic function. In general, it is failure to mount an LH surge that causes this dysfunction. As the central nervous system matures, the menses are ultimately regulated. In addition, systemic disease such as thyroid disorders, extreme fluctuations in weight, excessive exercise, or stress can all disrupt the HPO axis and lead to anovulation.

## UTERINE LEIOMYOMAS (FIBROIDS)

Uterine leiomyomas are benign tumors arising from the myometrium that ultimately disrupt the normal contour of the endometrium. Abnormal uterine bleeding is the most common symptom and is usually manifested as chronic heavy and prolonged menses, or menometrorrhagia. The location of the myomas seems to determine the majority of the symptomatology, whereas size is of secondary importance.

The disease process just described generally occurs in the fourth decade of life and usually abates after menopause. Approximately 10% to 40% of fibroids will regress over a period of 6 months to 3 years, and almost all symptomatology will abate at the time of menopause because these uterine tumors are estrogen sensitive. With the use of postmenopausal hormone replacement therapy, however, symptoms may continue past the cessation of menses.[8,9]

## VAGINAL FOREIGN BODY

Vaginal foreign bodies can lead to vaginal bleeding secondary to direct trauma, local irritation, superimposed infection, or any combination of these causes. The two most common foreign bodies are toilet tissue (minors) and tampons, although a wide range of vaginal foreign bodies have been reported.

## ENDOMETRIAL CANCER

Risk factors for the development of endometrial cancer include age older than 35 years, history of anovulatory cycles, nulliparity, obesity, tamoxifen therapy, exogenous estrogen use without progestins, and diabetes mellitus. Almost all these risk factors are associated with elevated levels of estrogen or prolonged exposure to estrogen.

### CERVICAL CANCER

Risk factors for cervical cancer are strongly correlated with sexual activity and include multiple sexual partners, early age at first coitus, early pregnancy, and previous history of sexually transmitted diseases. All these risk factors increase exposure to HPVs, which have been implicated as a major risk factor for the development of cervical cancer and high-risk lesions.[10]

## PRESENTING SIGNS AND SYMPTOMS

Vaginal bleeding can vary greatly in amount and severity. A thorough history and physical examination should be performed to evaluate the onset, duration, amount, and timing within the menstrual cycle of the bleeding. Assessment of severity includes determining the number of tampons or pads changed over a 12- to 24-hour period, whether they were saturated, and whether any clots were associated with the bleeding. Associated symptoms such as orthostatic complaints, fatigue, and dyspnea on exertion should point to underlying anemia from chronic blood loss or hypovolemia from acute blood loss. Vaginal bleeding may not be the primary disorder, and thus a thorough search for causes of secondary vaginal bleeding is prudent. The age of the patient, medical and surgical history, and medication profiles will also provide clues to the cause of the bleeding.

### DYSFUNCTIONAL UTERINE BLEEDING

The typical finding of DUB is irregular menses with alternation between heavy and light flow. Women often have signs of hyperandrogenism, including hirsutism, obesity, acne, palpable enlarged ovaries, and acanthosis nigricans (hyperpigmentation typically in the folds of the skin of the neck, groin, or axilla).

### UTERINE LEIOMYOMAS (FIBROIDS)

The symptoms that arise from uterine myomas can be classified into abnormal uterine bleeding, pelvic pressure and pain, and reproductive dysfunction. The number, size, and location of these tumors dictate the severity of symptoms. Abnormal uterine bleeding is the most common symptom and is usually manifested as chronic heavy and prolonged menses, or menometrorrhagia. Bulk-related symptoms of fibroids include urinary frequency, difficulty voiding, urinary obstruction, constipation, and occasionally back pain. In addition, leiomyomas have the propensity to degenerate or twist on their stalk and cause torsion. In this setting, pelvic pain may be accompanied by low-grade fevers, uterine tenderness, leukocytosis, or even peritoneal signs. Distortion of the uterine cavity secondary to leiomyomas may result in difficulty conceiving and has been associated with an increased risk for miscarriage, placental abruption, fetal growth restriction, and preterm labor.

### VAGINAL FOREIGN BODY

Mild vaginal bleeding may be the initial sign in a patient with a retained vaginal foreign body. If associated with infection, the patient may also have a purulent discharge or vaginal irritation.

### ENDOMETRIAL CANCER

Symptoms include painless postmenopausal vaginal bleeding. In perimenopausal patients, the menses typically lighten and become farther apart. Heavy or frequent menstrual periods or intermenstrual bleeding in this patient population should be evaluated.

### CERVICAL CANCER

The typical manifestation of cervical cancer is painless, abnormal vaginal bleeding, often postcoital secondary to localized inflammation.

## DIFFERENTIAL DIAGNOSIS AND MEDICAL DECISION MAKING

The first step in evaluating any woman with vaginal bleeding should be to determine whether the patient is pregnant because this will drastically alter the diagnostic and therapeutic approach.

The most common causes of abnormal vaginal bleeding in nonpregnant patients are DUB and uterine leiomyomas. **Tables 124.1** and **124.2** list the differential diagnosis of vaginal bleeding in nonpregnant females. **Figure 124.1** details an approach to patients seen in the emergency department (ED) with the complaint of vaginal bleeding.

### DYSFUNCTIONAL UTERINE BLEEDING

The majority of the work-up for DUB, including laboratory analysis and diagnostic imaging, is completed in the outpatient setting. However, several critical actions should be done by an emergency physician (EP) when these patients are encountered in the ED. Initial screening in appropriate patients includes human chorionic gonadotropin because the most common cause of abnormal uterine bleeding during the

**Table 124.1 Common Terminology and Definitions**

| TERMINOLOGY | DEFINITION |
|---|---|
| Amenorrhea | Cessation of menses for >6 mo |
| Dysmenorrhea | Pain associated with menses |
| Hypomenorrhea | Menstrual volumes < 20 mL/cycle |
| Menorrhagia | Menses > 80 mL/cycle or occurring for >7 days |
| Metrorrhagia | Vaginal bleeding between menstrual cycles or irregular cycles |
| Menometrorrhagia | Prolonged or heavy bleeding at irregular intervals |
| Oligomenorrhea | Decreased frequency of cycles (>35 days per cycle) |
| Polymenorrhea | Increased frequency of cycles (<21 days per cycle) |
| Postmenopausal bleeding | Bleeding 6-12 mo after menopause |

**Table 124.2 Systemic Causes of Abnormal Vaginal Bleeding**

| CAUSE | MECHANISM |
|---|---|
| Weight loss<br>Stress<br>Excessive exercise | Hypothalamic suppression of GnRH |
| Polycystic ovarian disease | Excessive estrogen effects on the endometrium<br>Anovulatory cycles |
| Hypothyroidism | Anovulatory cycles |
| Hyperthyroidism | Changes in androgen and estrogen production |
| Hyperprolactinemia (prolactinoma) | Mass effect on the pituitary stalk reduces GnRH secretion |
| Liver failure | Decreased production of vitamin K–dependent clotting factors<br>Increased estrogen levels secondary to decreased metabolism |
| Renal failure | Inherent platelet dysfunction |
| Primary coagulopathies:<br>Immune thrombocytopenia<br>von Willebrand disease<br>Myeloproliferative disorders | Platelet dysfunction |
| Cushing disease | Mass effect on the pituitary stalk reduces GnRH secretion<br>Decreased LH, FSH function |

*FSH*, Follicle-stimulating hormone; *GnRH*, gonadotropin-releasing hormone; *LH*, luteinizing hormone.

reproductive years is an abnormal pregnancy. Once pregnancy is ruled out, further laboratory testing and diagnostic imaging can be tailored to each particular patient.

Complete blood count analysis is prudent in most patients with abnormal vaginal bleeding and can both provide analysis for anemia and establish a baseline hemoglobin and hematocrit level for the patient. Further laboratory analysis could include thyroid function tests and prolactin levels because these abnormalities are associated with ovulatory dysfunction. If significant bleeding is a concern, liver function tests and coagulation factor assay should be performed because hepatic disease and inborn errors of coagulation can complicate abnormal vaginal bleeding.

The mainstay of imaging for patients with abnormal vaginal bleeding is pelvic ultrasonography. Ultrasound imaging can be helpful in evaluating the status of the endometrium to look for hyperplasia, carcinoma, polyps, and uterine fibroids and, if available, can direct treatment and follow-up care for the EP.

## UTERINE LEIOMYOMAS (FIBROIDS)

The diagnosis of fibroids is based on the physical examination finding of an enlarged, mobile uterus with irregular contours in combination with pelvic ultrasound imaging. It is important that the physician keep a broad differential diagnosis when identifying a new uterine mass because both benign and malignant lesions may be manifested similarly. Other conditions characterized by an enlarged uterus include pregnancy, adenomyosis, hematometra, uterine sarcoma, uterine carcinosarcoma, endometrial carcinoma, and metastatic disease.

Transvaginal ultrasound remains the primary imaging modality in this patient population. This study has high sensitivity (95% to 100%) for detecting myomas in mild to moderate cases of uterine enlargement. Other imaging modalities include diagnostic hysteroscopy, magnetic resonance imaging (MRI), and hysterosalpingography.[11]

## VAGINAL FOREIGN BODY

Once a vaginal foreign body is suspected, a thorough gynecologic examination, including a speculum and bimanual examination, should be completed. The physician should make every attempt to identify secondary injury from the foreign body and intervene as necessary.

If secondary systemic infection is a concern, urgent laboratory testing and diagnostic imaging should take place to evaluate for end-organ injury. Testing may include laboratory tests such as a complete blood count, chemistry panel, lactate analysis, and blood cultures. Diagnostic tools such as plain film radiographs or computed tomography (CT) scans of the abdomen and pelvis may be indicated depending on the severity of the symptoms.

## ENDOMETRIAL CANCER

No specific laboratory testing is necessary in the ED setting to evaluate for endometrial adenocarcinoma. As with all vaginal bleeding, assessment of the patient and the need for a complete blood count analysis and other laboratory testing founded on a differential diagnosis is done on a case-by-case basis.

## CERVICAL CANCER

Again, no specific laboratory testing is necessary in the ED setting to evaluate for cervical cancer. The patient may need a complete blood count analysis and other laboratory testing

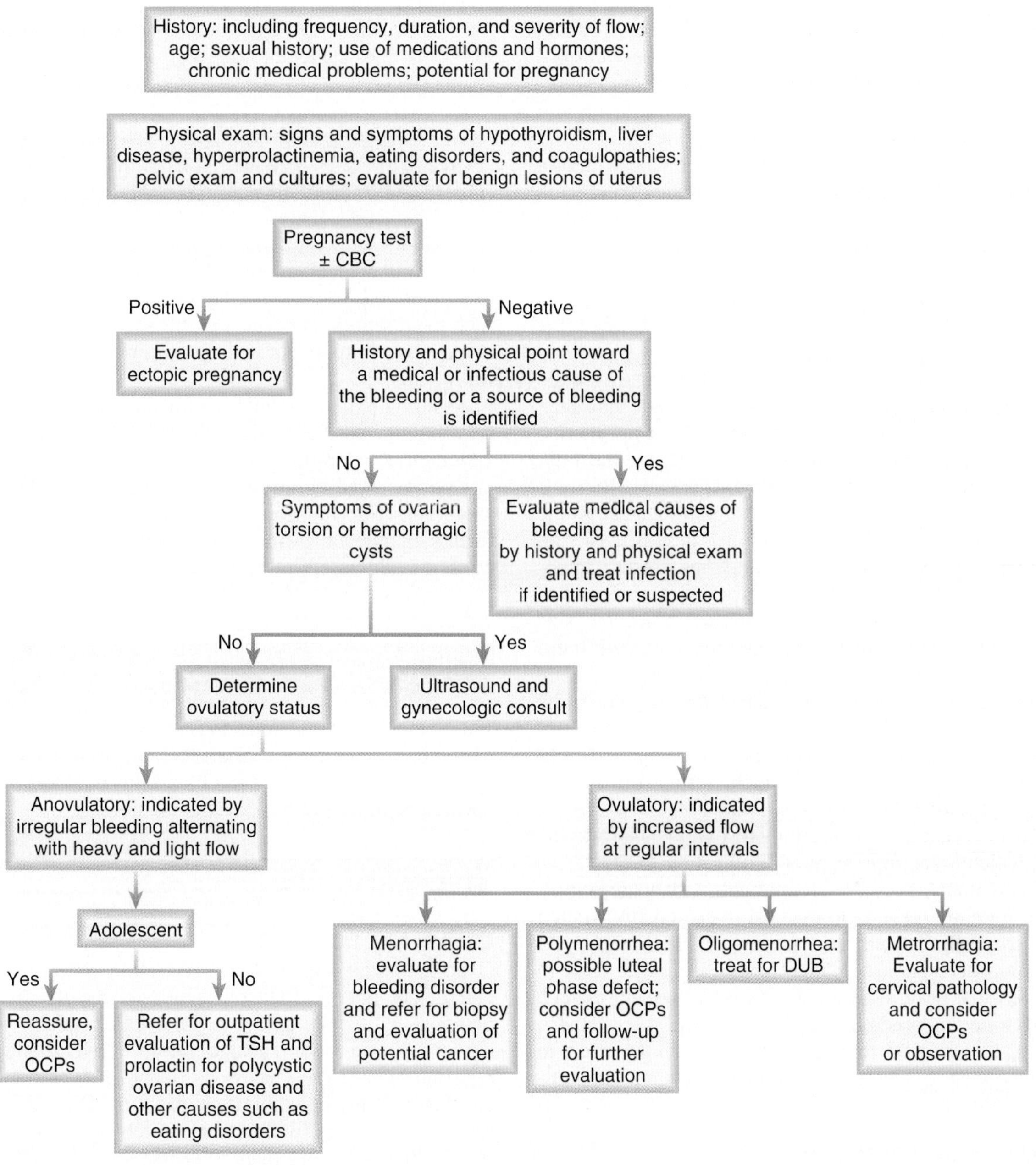


**Fig. 124.1 Algorithm outlining an approach to patients with abnormal vaginal bleeding.** *CBC*, Complete blood count; *OCPs*, oral contraceptive pills; *TSH*, thyroid-stimulating hormone.

on a case-by-case basis, depending on the degree of bleeding and other factors associated with the findings and evaluation for malignant spread. Further diagnostic imaging is generally performed for staging purposes and may include chest radiography, CT, or positron emission tomography.

## TREATMENT

### DYSFUNCTIONAL UTERINE BLEEDING

Oral contraceptive pills (OCPs) remain first-line therapy for DUB. OCPs suppress endometrial development, reestablish predictable bleeding patterns, decrease menstrual flow, and lower the risk for iron deficiency anemia. Treatment can be effective in either a cyclic or continuous regimen, and many gynecologists recommend tapering of OCPs over 1-week period to control acute blood loss in patients with DUB. The typical regimen includes low-dose OCPs two to three times daily for 7 days, 7 days off for withdrawal bleeding, followed by once-daily OCP use for 3 months. Single-agent therapy with estrogen or progesterone alone is used in selected cases and is best prescribed with gynecologic consultation.

If significant hemorrhage from a uterine source is leading to hemodynamic instability, the physician must consider a primary bleeding disorder. In this case, laboratory analysis should focus on identification of disseminated intravascular coagulation, thrombocytopenia, or inherited coagulopathies with a focus on repletion of blood products as necessary and prompt gynecologic consultation. In certain cases, desmopressin has been shown to be effective in controlling hemorrhage because it rapidly increases von Willebrand factor and factor VIII with duration of action lasting about 6 hours.

In these extreme cases or in patients with medical failure, surgical intervention may be necessary, including dilation and curettage or endometrial ablation; if all else fails, abdominal or vaginal hysterectomy may be indicated.

### UTERINE LEIOMYOMAS (FIBROIDS)

Treatment of leiomyomas is generally initiated when the tumors become symptomatic and is dependent on size, location, severity, age, and reproductive plans. OCPs again are the first-line treatment for medical management; however, although they may work well in regulating abnormal uterine bleeding, they are not very effective in reducing the bulk symptoms. More effective at medical management of fibroids are GnRH agonists. They work by causing an increase in the release of gonadotropins, which in turn desensitizes and downregulates the reproductive tissue and thus causes a hypogonadal state.[12,13] Most women will experience amenorrhea and a significant reduction (35% to 60%) in uterine size within 3 months of initiation of therapy. Even though these medications are quite effective, initiation of therapy should be guided by a gynecologist, and they are rarely started in the ED setting. The addition of nonsteroidal antiinflammatory drugs (NSAIDs) is useful in this population to regulate painful menses, but they do not have much action on uterine bleeding.

Surgical intervention is the definitive treatment of uterine myomas, which is the most common indication for hysterectomy. Hysterectomy is reserved for patients with acute hemorrhage that does not respond to medical management, women with increased risk for malignancy, those in whom minimally invasive procedures fail, or patients who no longer wish to preserve fertility. Several minimally invasive procedures such as myomectomy, endometrial ablation, or uterine artery embolization have increased in popularity and can be used in patients who wish to retain their uterus or have not yet completed childbearing.

### VAGINAL FOREIGN BODY

Generally, prompt removal of the foreign body will result in resolution of the patient's symptoms and is often the only intervention necessary. If toxin-mediated disease such as toxic shock syndrome is suspected, urgent administration of antibiotics is paramount and lifesaving. An antibiotic regimen targeted against staphylococcal and streptococcal species is prudent and should be augmented with clindamycin because it is a potent suppressor of the synthesis of bacterial toxin.

### ENDOMETRIAL CANCER

Depending on the histopathology noted on endometrial biopsy and staging of the cancer, surgical or chemotherapeutic interventions may be initiated.

### CERVICAL CANCER

As with other gynecologic malignancies, the primary role for the EP is timely recognition and referral to a gynecologic specialist who can arrange for a Papanicolaou test, colposcopy, directed biopsies, and endocervical curettage. Surgical, radiation, or chemotherapeutic interventions are tailored to the stage of cervical cancer and directed by specialty care.

## FOLLOW-UP, NEXT STEPS IN CARE, AND PATIENT EDUCATION

Any patient with vaginal bleeding and evidence of symptomatic anemia or hypovolemia should be admitted for definitive treatment and observation. However, the majority of patients with the diseases mentioned in this section can be treated and managed as outpatients with strong emphasis on gynecologic follow-up.

As an outpatient, a patient with abnormal vaginal bleeding may undergo further testing, including a Papanicolaou smear, endometrial sampling, hormonal assays, or hysteroscopy, and can be managed by a practicing gynecologist. Most patients should be referred for follow-up, continued treatment, or further diagnostic evaluation, depending on the findings or concerns addressed in the ED.

# PELVIC PAIN

This section of the chapter focuses on gynecologic causes of pelvic pain, including ovarian torsion, ovarian cysts, ovarian tumors, and endometriosis. Other causes of pelvic pain are covered in other sections of this textbook.

## EPIDEMIOLOGY

### OVARIAN TORSION

Ovarian torsion is the fifth most common gynecologic surgical emergency, and because of vague, nonspecific findings, the diagnosis is usually delayed, which can result in necrosis of the ovary and poor salvage rates.[14] Several studies have reported salvage rates as low as 10% to 25%. Adnexal torsion can occur at any age, but the highest incidence is in the early reproductive years, with approximately 80% of cases occurring in those younger than 50 years.

### OVARIAN CYSTS

Ovarian cysts are estimated to affect 7% to 10% of premenopausal and postmenopausal woman. Up to 4% of women will be admitted to the hospital with a primary diagnosis of ovarian cysts. Approximately 3% of theca lutein cysts are complicated by torsion or hemorrhage, and approximately 30% of these cysts can cause maternal androgen excess. Ovarian cysts affect all age ranges of females, from those in utero to postmenopausal women.

### OVARIAN TUMORS

Ovarian cancer is the most common cause of death from gynecologic tumors in the United States. Worldwide, the reported lifetime risk for the development of ovarian malignancy is 1 in 70, and it accounts for 100,000 deaths annually.[15] Ovarian cancer affects white women more than black women, and the incidence increases with age. The mean age of females with ovarian carcinoma is 56. The overall prognosis for ovarian cancer is poor, with reported 5-year mortality rates reaching 46%, but it is closely related to staging. In girls younger than 9 years, 80% of ovarian masses are malignant, with the majority being germ cell tumors. These tumors are generally localized to the ovary and have cure rates of 90% after chemotherapy.

### ENDOMETRIOSIS

Endometriosis is commonly a disease of reproductive-age women, with the highest incidence of disease in those 25 to 35 years of age. It is uncommon in prepuberal girls and postmenopausal women who are not receiving estrogen replacement therapy. The disease is reported to occur in approximately 7% to 10% of the general population of women and is found in 20% to 50% of infertile women and 80% of women with chronic pelvic pain. There is a strong familial relationship, with the incidence in women who have an affected first-degree relative being significantly increased.[16,17]

## PATHOPHYSIOLOGY

Causes of gynecologic pelvic pain in nonpregnant females can be divided into infectious, ovarian, cervical, uterine, or extrauterine. As with vaginal bleeding, an understanding of the female reproductive cycle is paramount in understanding the pathophysiology of disease.

### OVARIAN TORSION

Ovarian torsion is caused by mechanical obstruction of the vascular supply to the ovary, and progressive edema and eventually necrosis ensue if the torsion is untreated.

Classically, ovarian torsion occurs unilaterally in a pathologically enlarged ovary, almost always secondary to a cyst or neoplasm. Approximately 80% of cases of torsion occur in ovaries that are 5 cm or larger, and it occurs on the right more than on the left. In young children, ovarian torsion may develop in a normal ovary secondary to developmental abnormalities such as a long fallopian tube or absent mesosalpinx. Pregnancy is a strong risk factor for ovarian torsion because of the corpus luteum increasing the ovarian mass, and it is responsible for approximately 20% of cases. Ovarian tumors and pelvic surgery also increase the risk for torsion, and it has even occurred in patients following laparoscopic hysterectomy.

### OVARIAN CYSTS

Different kinds of functional ovarian cysts can form during the menstrual cycle. Follicular cysts may result from lack of physiologic release of the ovum because of excessive FSH stimulation or from lack of the normal LH surge at midcycle just before ovulation. Hormonal stimulation causes these cysts to continue to grow. Follicular cysts are typically larger than 2.5 cm in diameter.

In the absence of pregnancy, the life span of the corpus luteum is 14 days. If the ovum is fertilized, the corpus luteum continues to secrete progesterone for 5 to 9 weeks until its eventual dissolution in 14 weeks, when the cyst undergoes central hemorrhage. Failure of dissolution to occur may result in a corpus luteal cyst, which is arbitrarily defined as a corpus luteum that grows to 3 cm in diameter.

Theca lutein cysts are caused by luteinization and hypertrophy of the theca interna cell layer in response to excessive stimulation of β-human chorionic gonadotropin. This type of cyst can occur in the setting of gestational trophoblastic disease, multiple gestation, or exogenous ovarian hyperstimulation. Theca lutein cysts are usually bilateral and result in massive ovarian enlargement.

### OVARIAN TUMORS

The peak incidence of ovarian tumors occurs at 55 to 65 years of age; however, the majority of ovarian masses in children are malignant. Consequently, a palpable ovary in a postmenopausal woman or prepubescent girl should be considered a malignancy until proved otherwise. Risk factors include frequent ovulation, nulliparity, late menopause, family history, and late childbearing age. Oral contraceptives are believed to decrease risk for the development of ovarian malignancies.

Epithelial tumors represent the most common histologic type (90%), with other causes including sex cord stromal tumors, germ cell tumors, and metastatic disease. These tumors appear as partially cystic lesions with solid components.[18] Metastatic disease is often found on the peritoneal surfaces but can be found in the liver, small bowel, uterus, lymphatic system, and lungs. In the prepubescent population, germ cell tumors are the most common histologic type, and the risk for teratomas increases into adolescence.

### ENDOMETRIOSIS

Endometriosis is defined as the presence of endometrial tissue in a location outside the uterine cavity and can be definitively diagnosed only by direct visualization via laparoscopy. There is no clear-cut explanation for the pathogenesis of endometriosis; however, several hypotheses have been proposed, including retrograde menstruation, surgical transplantation, lymphatic or hematogenous spread, cellular metaplasia, altered immunity, or genetic disposition.

The most common sites are ovarian and dependent portions of the pelvis, including the ovaries, broad ligament, fallopian tubes, sigmoid colon, and appendix. Endometriosis can sometimes be found outside the pelvis and has been reported in the breast, pancreas, liver, kidney, vertebrae, and lung.

## PRESENTING SIGNS AND SYMPTOMS

Pelvic pain may be acute or chronic. Acute pain should raise concern for a life-threatening or organ-threatening process that may warrant urgent treatment or intervention. Chronic pain is more likely to represent an indolent process such as scarring or malignancy. A good history and complete physical examination focusing on the abdomen and genitourinary system will provide great insight into possible causes of the pain. Paying close attention to age, past medical and surgical history, sexual history, and timing in the reproductive cycle will further narrow the differential diagnosis.

### OVARIAN TORSION

The typical finding is an acute onset of unilateral pelvic pain that can be intermittent and associated with nausea and vomiting. Approximately 25% of patients experience bilateral lower quadrant pain, and as many as 70% of patients have an element of nausea and vomiting that can often mimic a gastrointestinal cause. Fever is evidence that necrosis of the tissue has occurred.

Findings on physical examination are traditionally nonspecific and variable. Bimanual examination will reveal a tender adnexal mass or fullness in between 50% and 90% of patients. However, absence of this finding should not exclude this diagnosis. Peritonitis usually occurs late in the disease process.

### OVARIAN CYST

Ruptured cysts may cause an acute onset of unilateral pelvic pain and can mimic ovarian torsion or acute appendicitis. They usually occur in the second half of the menstrual cycle and begin during strenuous physical activity. Though rare, other associated symptoms may be present, including vaginal bleeding, nausea and vomiting, syncope, orthostatic changes, shoulder pain, and circulatory collapse.

### OVARIAN TUMORS

Ovarian tumors may be accompanied by abnormal vaginal bleeding secondary to hormone secretion; however, they generally cause signs and symptoms related to a mass effect. Patients are often asymptomatic, and ovarian tumors are commonly found during evaluation or imaging for an unrelated issue. Adults generally have typical bulk-related complaints, including urinary frequency, constipation, rectal fullness, pelvic pressure, and bloating. Conversely, the pediatric population will generally have pelvic pain initially.

### ENDOMETRIOSIS

The sometimes diffuse pelvic pain caused by endometriosis is cyclic and estrogen responsive. Pain is the most common initial symptom and can be manifested as chronic pelvic pain, dysmenorrhea, dyspareunia, back pain, or dyschezia. Bleeding can be an initial sign and may be manifested as abnormal menstrual bleeding, as rectal bleeding, or if located under the skin, as abdominal ecchymosis. Unfortunately, physical findings in patients with endometriosis are nonspecific and highly related to the location and size of the implants.

**BOX 124.2 Differential Diagnosis of Pelvic Pain in Nonpregnant Females**

**Gynecologic Diagnoses**

***Infectious***
Vaginitis
Cervicitis
Endometritis
Tuboovarian abscess
Pelvic inflammatory disease

***Ovarian***
Ovarian torsion
Ruptured ovarian cyst
Ovarian tumor
Degenerating ovarian tumor
Mittelschmerz

***Cervical***
Cervical polyps
Cervical stenosis
Cervical cancer

***Uterine***
Uterine fibroids
Degenerating uterine fibroids
Adenomyosis
Endometrial carcinoma

***Extrauterine***
Endometriosis
Adhesions
Residual accessory ovary

**Nongynecologic Diagnoses**

***Gastrointestinal***
Acute appendicitis
Mesenteric lymphadenitis
Diverticulitis
Inflammatory bowel disease
Irritable bowel syndrome
Bowel obstruction
Intraabdominal abscess
Colorectal carcinoma

***Urinary***
Cystitis
Renal colic
Bladder cancer

***Musculoskeletal***
Abdominal wall pain
Lumbar back pain
Fibromyalgia
Muscular strain
Piriformis syndrome

***Neurologic***
Lumbar radiculopathy
Shingles
Spondylosis

***Psychologic***
Personality disorders
Major depressive disorder

## DIFFERENTIAL DIAGNOSIS AND MEDICAL DECISION MAKING

The differential diagnosis of pelvic pain in women is quite extensive and includes disease processes in the gastrointestinal, urinary, and reproductive systems (**Box 124.2**). Careful consideration should always be given to the possibility of acute appendicitis and ovarian torsion in a nonpregnant female with pelvic pain.

### OVARIAN TORSION

The clinical diagnosis of ovarian torsion is based on findings on physical examination and clinical suspicion, in coordination with pelvic imaging; however, definitive diagnosis is based on surgical findings.[19,20] Pelvic ultrasound is the first-line diagnostic imaging modality used to aid in identification of ovarian torsion. Doppler ultrasound can be used to identify the physical anatomy of the pelvic organs, as well as to detect ovarian vessel flow. Data on the sensitivity of Doppler ultrasound in detecting ovarian torsion are controversial, especially with regard to vessel flow. Sensitivities as low as 43% and as high as 100% have been reported. In contrast, Doppler ultrasound is quite specific for diagnosing torsion, with sensitivities found to be anywhere from 92% to 97%.[21] It has been reported that up to 50% of patients with torsion may have normal findings on pelvic ultrasound. Therefore, despite negative findings on imaging, if the EP has high enough suspicion for ovarian torsion, prompt gynecologic consultation is warranted. CT and MRI have also been shown to aid in the diagnosis, but their cost and the time required for imaging are prohibitive to regular use of these imaging modalities as long as ultrasound is readily available.

Laboratory testing is generally performed in the setting of acute abdominal pain. Changes in the white blood cell count, hematocrit, and electrolytes have been seen with torsion but are quite nonspecific. Research to identify serum markers is promising, with several studies reporting that increased levels of interleukin-6 are associated with ovarian torsion; however, further investigation is warranted.[22,23]

### OVARIAN CYSTS

Routine laboratory studies will generally be ordered in patients with acute abdominal pain, especially with hemodynamic changes, as the physician attempts to rule out a ruptured ectopic pregnancy or acute appendicitis. Laboratory tests specifically helpful in the setting of hemorrhagic cysts are a hemoglobin level, coagulation profile, and blood type and screen or crossmatch. Again, these tests are nonspecific but aid in monitoring and treatment of patients if they become unstable.

Pelvic ultrasonography is the best imaging modality because it can identify the location and size of a cyst, as well as detect free pelvic fluid, but it is not specific. The physician may also apply the concept of focused assessment with sonography for trauma (FAST) to evaluate for free intraperitoneal fluid, which if positive would raise suspicion for significant hemorrhage. If the diagnosis is unclear after pelvic ultrasound, CT of the abdomen and pelvis may be necessary, especially because it may help evaluate for nongynecologic causes.

### OVARIAN TUMORS

Many laboratory tests and serum markers can be used to evaluate an ovarian mass; however, much of the work-up is done on an outpatient basis and is guided by a gynecologist. The laboratory testing done by an EP is usually limited to evaluation of pelvic pain in conjunction with vomiting. Further laboratory testing will probably include serum markers such as CA 125, which can be elevated in 80% of women with ovarian malignancy and is 90% sensitive in women with advanced disease. However, given that it has low sensitivity in women with early disease and can be associated with several other gynecologic and nongynecologic illnesses, routine testing in the regular population is discouraged.[24,25] Promising studies of human epididymal secretory protein E4 have been shown to be more specific for ovarian carcinoma, but further investigation is warranted.

If the EP suspects or finds an ovarian mass on examination, pelvic ultrasound should be performed. Several characteristics of ovarian tumors should raise the EP's suspicion for malignancy, such as having a complex internal structure, including complex cysts with solid components; masses in prepubescent or postmenopausal women; or persistence beyond the length of a normal menstrual cycle.

If the findings on ultrasound are equivocal or limited, further diagnostic imaging could include CT scanning of the abdomen and pelvis or MRI. CT scanning is often helpful to the EP who may be trying to evaluate or rule out other causes of pelvic pain or symptoms of a mass effect in these specific patients.

### ENDOMETRIOSIS

As noted earlier, the diagnosis of endometriosis is made by direct visualization of the implants by surgical methods such as laparoscopy or laparotomy. Laboratory analysis is rarely conducted by the EP aside from evaluating abdominal pain in an undifferentiated patient. Serum CA 125 has been shown to correlate with endometriosis but is not a sensitive marker because it can be elevated in other gynecologic and nongynecologic disease, most notably ovarian carcinoma.

Transvaginal ultrasound is the initial diagnostic imaging test for endometriosis. The classic finding on ultrasound is an ovarian cyst containing low-level homogeneous internal echoes consistent with old blood that correlates with the chocolate cyst found on laparoscopy. MRI has been reported to be useful in cases that require identification of peripheral implant spread, but it is rarely used for this purpose in the ED setting.

## TREATMENT

Both acute and chronic pelvic pain can be debilitating, and thus early pain management is essential. In a patient with acute pelvic pain a diligent search for the cause in concert with pain management is the best course of action. Oral and intravenous narcotic medications are often needed in this patient population. Unfortunately, in patients with chronic pelvic pain, acute control of pain may be the only intervention that EPs can offer. Disease-specific diagnostic testing and treatment options are described in the following sections.

### OVARIAN TORSION

Management of ovarian torsion is emergency operative intervention in an attempt at detorsion of the affected adnexal structures and restoration of blood flow and venous drainage. In the past the adnexal structures were surgically resected; however, recent studies and practice have shown that mechanical detorsion is effective and safe. The most important factor in preservation of ovarian function is early recognition and treatment. Several studies have reported high salvage rates when treatment is initiated within the first 24 hours of the onset of symptoms.[20,26]

### OVARIAN CYSTS

The mainstay of treatment in the majority of patients with ovarian cysts is pain control. Cyst ruptures are typically self-limited and treated with pain control and expectant management in an outpatient setting. However, significant rupture and intraperitoneal hemorrhage occasionally occur and cause hemodynamic instability. In these cases, urgent gynecologic evaluation and performance of diagnostic laparoscopy or laparotomy are indicated. An unstable patient may require aggressive fluid resuscitation and, in extreme cases, blood products and more aggressive hemodynamic stabilization with pressors or intubation.

### OVARIAN TUMORS

When the EP finds a highly suspicious ovarian mass, prompt gynecologic referral or consultation must be arranged so that further diagnostic work-up and possible medical or surgical therapy can be initiated. Symptomatic control of bulk-related or pain-related symptoms can include urinary catheter insertion, disimpaction, or narcotic pain medications.

### ENDOMETRIOSIS

Although optimal treatment of this chronic disease is unclear, options are focused on three main categories—pelvic pain, infertility, and pelvic mass—and tailored to each specific patient. The EP will primarily focus on the treatment of pelvic pain with NSAIDs and combined estrogen-progestin contraceptives. NSAIDs are thought to control pain, as well as affect prostaglandin production, thus altering growth and secretion of the endometrial implants. In a similar manner, OCPs induce decidualization and atrophy of the endometrial tissue and ectopic implants, which may control the cyclic pain and limit progression of the disease. The EP can initiate this therapeutic regimen in the ED setting, but it should be done with close gynecologic consultation or follow-up.

If a conservative medical approach fails, further treatment with GnRH agonists, danazol, aromatase inhibitors, or

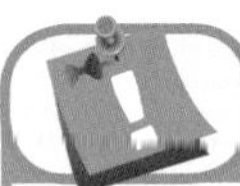

### TIPS AND TRICKS

Assume that all women of childbearing age are pregnant until proved otherwise.

In patients with strong suspicion for ovarian torsion despite negative ultrasound findings, prompt gynecologic evaluation is warranted.

About 20% to 25% of cases of endometrial cancer occur before menopause; any patient without a definitive cause of the vaginal bleeding should be referred to a gynecologist for endometrial evaluation.

### DOCUMENTATION

Age of the patient
Gravid and parous status
Bedside pregnancy test results
Onset and duration of symptoms
Recent trauma
Duration and frequency of past menstrual cycles
Complete sexual history, including contraception methods, number of partners, history of sexually transmitted diseases
History of previous abnormal Papanicolaou smears
Associated symptoms, including fever, breast changes, anorexia, weight changes, hirsutism, bowel or bladder changes
Past medical history
Current medications

conservative surgery may be indicated. All these treatments are coordinated by a gynecologist on an outpatient or inpatient basis, depending on severity of the symptoms.

## FOLLOW-UP, NEXT STEPS IN CARE, AND PATIENT EDUCATION

Most patients with pelvic pain can also be managed on an outpatient basis with directed therapy and gynecologic follow-up. However, acute gynecologic pain, such as ovarian torsion, necessitates admission to the gynecologic service for definitive management.

## SUGGESTED READINGS

Berger K. Ovarian cyst/torsion. In: Rosen & Barkin's 5-minute emergency medicine consult. Philadelphia: Lippincott Williams & Wilkins; 2007.

Schorge J, Schaffer J, Halvorson L, et al, editors. Williams gynecology. New York: McGraw-Hill; 2008.

Valentine C. Vaginal bleeding. In: Rosen & Barkin's 5-minute emergency medicine consult. Philadelphia: Lippincott Williams & Wilkins; 2007.

## REFERENCES

*References can be found on Expert Consult @ www.expertconsult.com.*

# Complications of Gynecologic Procedures, Abortion, and Assisted Reproductive Technology

# 125

*Christine Yang-Kauh*

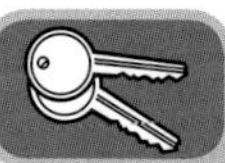

**KEY POINTS**

- Complications with the highest morbidity and mortality are severe hemorrhage, serious infection, damage to intraabdominal structures, and pulmonary embolism.
- Complications seen in the emergency department are usually delayed in presentation, and often difficult to diagnose due to insidious onset, resulting in increased morbidity and mortality and a higher risk for litigation (i.e., ureteral injuries) High suspicion must be maintained.
- Emergency department bedside ultrasonography can provide rapid, early imaging for the evaluation of postprocedural patients, particularly unstable ones.
- Abortion is one of the most common procedures in the United States and overall has very low serious complication rates.
- Ovarian hyperstimulation syndrome is a potentially fatal complication of assisted reproduction in a generally healthy young woman. With no cure, early recognition, aggressive intervention, and close monitoring are key.

This chapter is divided into three main sections—complications of gynecologic procedures, complications following medical and surgical abortion, and complications of assisted reproductive technology (ART).

Gynecologic procedures run the gamut from minor office procedures to major invasive surgery. They can be diagnostic or therapeutic and may initiate pregnancy or terminate it. They represent some of the most common surgical procedures performed in the United States today.

More than 146,000 cycles of ART were reported to the Centers for Disease Control and Prevention from 441 sites in the year 2009. In addition, approximately 600,000 hysterectomies are performed annually, which ranks it behind cesarean section as the most common major surgery in women of reproductive age.[2]

Shortened hospital stays and minimally invasive or outpatient surgery have led to the delayed diagnosis of complications in the emergency department rather than during the postoperatve hospitalization period.

## COMPLICATIONS OF GYNECOLOGIC PROCEDURES

This section focuses on complications particular to gynecologic procedures that one might encounter in the ED setting and their evaluation and management (**Fig. 125.1**). Many complications of gynecologic procedures may go unrecognized before discharge, only to be seen later in the ED (**Box 125.1**). **Box 125.2** lists the typical timing of these complications.

## DIFFERENTIAL DIAGNOSIS AND MEDICAL DECISION MAKING

During the evaluation of postoperative patients it is essential to avoid narrowing the differential diagnosis to postoperative complications alone. Other conditions, particularly preexisting ones that may have served as the original indication for surgery (e.g., malignancy, anemia) must be taken into consideration. Laboratory testing and imaging studies should be guided by the differential diagnoses under consideration (see the Priority Actions box).

For patients with complications after a gynecologic procedure, bedside ultrasonography (US) in the hands of a skillful operator can provide rapid recognition of intraabdominal and intrapelvic pathology. Possible ultrasonographic findings include free fluid heralding leakage from a perforated vessel, urinary tract, or viscus (**Fig. 125.2**); hydronephrosis as a result of ureteral obstruction; a full bladder secondary to urinary retention; fluid collections; and intrauterine contents. US can also be used to guide paracentesis for definitive fluid diagnosis or for the drainage of subcutaneous abscesses. It is important to remember that sensitivity and accuracy are very dependent on the user and interpreter and that anatomy, habitus, and elements such as bowel gas can greatly interfere with adequate imaging. US is a poor modality for evaluating the bowel or retroperitoneal space.

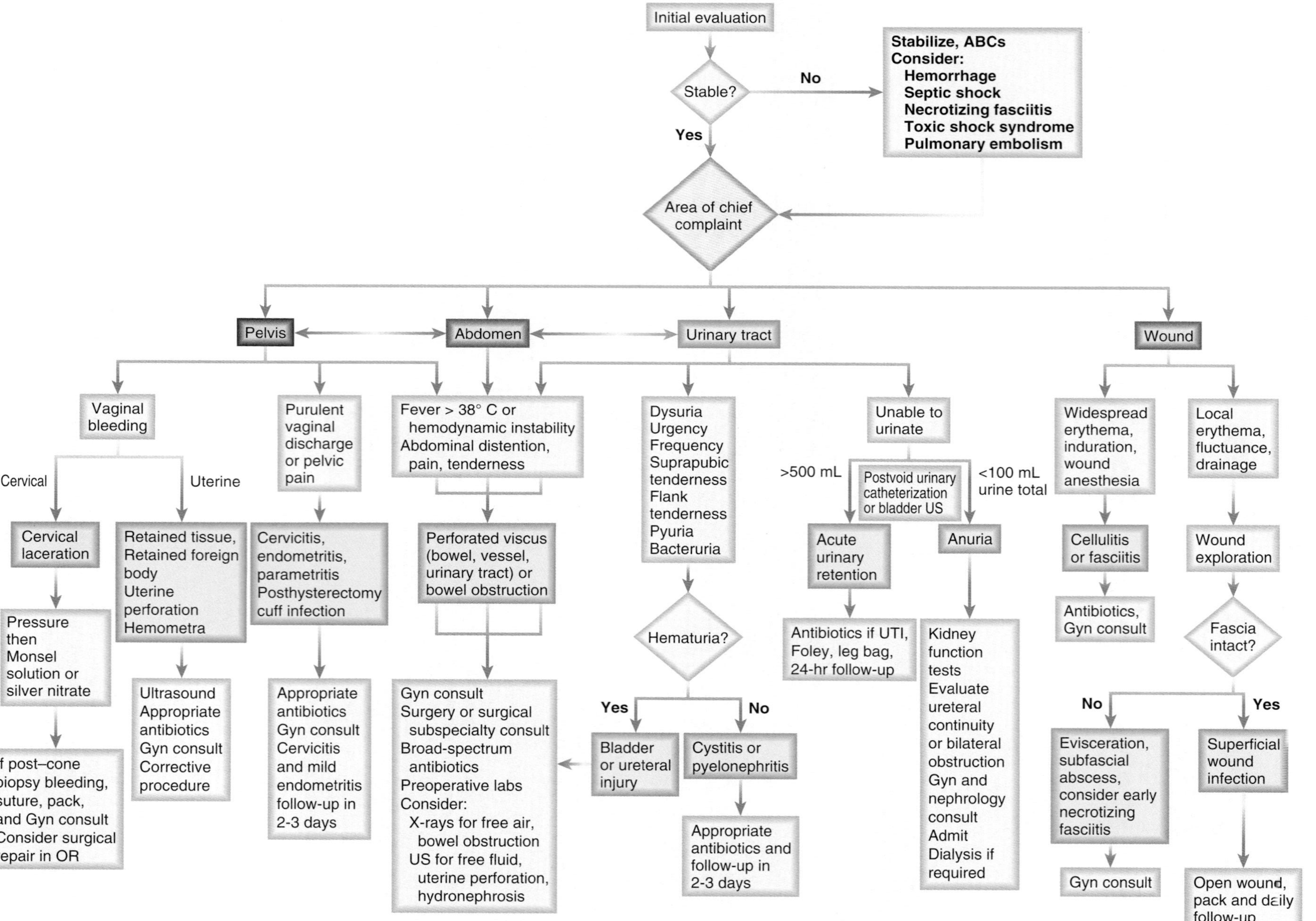


**Fig. 125.1 Suggested algorithm for the evaluation and treatment of postoperative gynecologic patients.** *ABCs*, Airway, breathing, and circulation; *Gyn consult*, gynecology consultation; *OR*, operating room; *US*, ultrasonography; *UTI*, urinary tract infection.

**BOX 125.1 Most Threatening and Most Common Complications of Gynecologic Procedures**

**Most Threatening**
Vascular injury—consider both intraperitoneal and retroperitoneal
Bowel injury
Urinary tract injury—bladder more likely than ureteral
Sepsis, severe infection
Pulmonary embolism

**Most Common**
Pain
Bleeding
Fever
Wound concerns
Nausea and vomiting

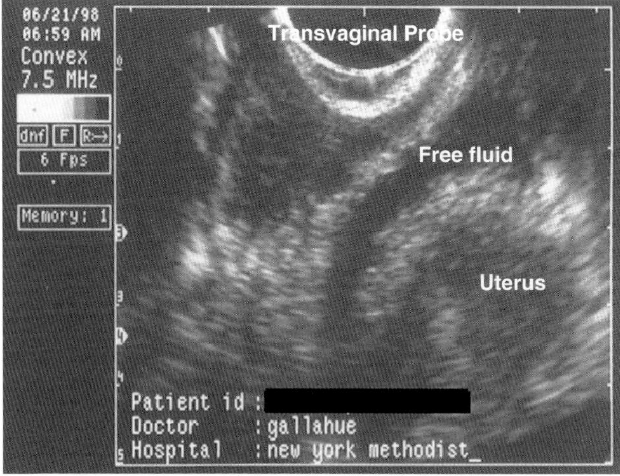


**Fig. 125.2 Transvaginal ultrasound image showing free fluid in the cul-de-sac consistent with hemorrhage.**

**BOX 125.2 Complications of Gynecologic Procedures by Estimated Time Line**

**Immediate (<24 Hours)**
Complications of anesthesia
- Emesis
  - Postoperative ileus
  - Medication reaction

Fever
- Atelectasis
- Hematoma
- Pyogenic reaction to tissue trauma

Bleeding
- Vaginal or cervical laceration
- Uterine perforation
- Visceral perforation
- Vascular injury
- Retained tissue
- Retained foreign body

Laparoscopic
- Visceral injuries
- Fluid overload
- Gas embolization
- Pneumothorax
- Pneumomediastinum

**Early (1 Day to 1 Week)**
Bleeding
- Laceration
- Perforation
- Injury to vasculature
- Infection
- Retained tissue
- Retained foreign body

Infection
- Superficial wound infection
- Clostridial infections
- Pelvic cellulitis, abscess
- Septic pelvic thrombophlebitis
- Necrotizing fasciitis
- Septic shock
- Toxic shock syndrome

Postoperative ileus
Constipation
Urinary retention
Thrombosis
- Venous thrombosis
- Pulmonary embolism

Retained foreign body

**Delayed (1 Week to 1 Year)**
Wound dehiscence
Suture sinuses
Postoperative small bowel obstruction
Incisional hernia
Vaginal evisceration
Fistula formation
Amenorrhea

**Late (Years)**
Postoperative small bowel obstruction
Fistula formation
Incisional hernia
Vaginal eversion
Vaginal evisceration
Decreased fertility
- Amenorrhea
- Uterine synechiae
- Cervical stenosis

When a patient with postprocedural complications is seen in the ED, the physician who performed the procedure should be contacted; definitive management often requires gynecologic or other surgical intervention.

## URINARY TRACT INJURY

The incidence of urinary tract injury in gynecologic surgery is between 0.33% and 4.8%. The great majority (80%) of these injuries involve the bladder. Ureteral injuries occur in just 0.3% to 1.0% of cases, but unilateral injury is discovered postoperatively in the majority of cases.[3] This delayed recognition leads to increased morbidity. As a result, ureteral injury has become the leading cause of legal action against gynecologic surgeons.

Typical symptoms are fever, flank pain, prolonged ileus, and prolonged abdominal distention. Unexplained hematuria or watery vaginal discharge may be present as well. The most common causes of these symptoms are cystitis and pyelonephritis secondary to perioperative bladder catheterization.

Inability to urinate may represent anuria or urinary retention, which are differentiated by postvoid urinary catheterization or US. No output at all indicates anuria as a result of bilateral compromise or renal failure. Urine residual volume greater than 500 mL suggests urinary retention instead. Bedside US can also detect intraabdominal fluid or hydronephrosis.

Laboratory testing includes a complete blood count and differential, electrolytes, kidney function tests, preoperative blood assays, urinalysis, and urine culture. If ascites or other fluid is obtained, fluid creatinine levels should be measured to determine whether it is urinary in origin. Imaging to evaluate the urinary system is indicated, such as intravenous urography, abdominal/pelvic computed tomography with contrast enhancement, or renal US with retrograde ureteropyelography.

Complications of ureteral obstruction (secondary to ligation, stricture, or external compression by another structure) include hydronephrosis and progressive kidney damage, which ultimately leads to failure of the ipsilateral kidney if

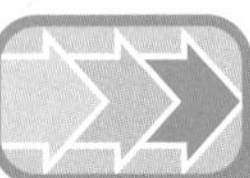

**PRIORITY ACTIONS**

**Differential Diagnosis: Complications of Gynecologic Procedures**

**Abnormal Symptoms or Vital Signs?**

Anemia, bleeding

- Hemorrhage may be internal or exsanguinating; emergency resuscitation and exploratory laparotomy are required if unstable. Bedside US for detection of free intraabdominal fluid. For emergency transfusion, use O-negative blood in women with childbearing potential; otherwise, use O positive blood.

Fever

- Consider septic shock, toxic shock syndrome, and necrotizing fasciitis; administer broad-spectrum antibiotics and search for the source of infection. Emergency surgical débridement is required for necrotizing fasciitis.

Abdominal distention

- Consider bowel obstruction or injury to the vasculature, bowel, or urinary tract; bedside US to evaluate for free fluid; upright chest and abdominal radiographs; antibiotics; abdominal/pelvic CT with contrast enhancement if stable; and early surgical evaluation.

Shortness of breath

- Consider pulmonary embolism, fluid overload, and aspiration pneumonia.
- If occurring after laparoscopy, also consider pneumothorax.

**Vaginal Bleeding—Is It Cervical or Uterine in Origin?**

Cervical or vaginal lacerations: Controlled by simple measures in the ED?

- If yes, discharge with close follow-up with gynecology.
- If not or if after conization, pack and gynecology consultation for management in the operating suite.

Uterine bleeding: Is retained tissue or hemometra noted on ultrasound imaging?

- If yes, gynecology consultation for definitive care.
- If not, consider uterine perforation, and if uterine perforation is present, maintain high suspicion for a perforated viscus and obtain abdominal/pelvic CT. Consider other specific evaluation of nearby structures (i.e., cystoscopy).

**Abdominal Pain with Distention?**

Ileus or small bowel obstruction on radiography? Nasogastric tube if excessive vomiting; surgical consultation required.

If not, consider intestinal, urinary, or vascular injury. Abdominal/pelvic CT imaging.

**Unable to Urinate?**

Postvoid catheterization or bedside US:

- >500 mL of urine noted? Maintain the urinary catheter and check for a UTI. Substitute a leg bag and treat the UTI if present; discharge to follow-up with urology.
- <200 mL, consider renal failure from medications or bilateral ureteral obstruction. Renal function tests, US to evaluate for hydronephrosis or free fluid. Admit for further evaluation.

**Dysuria?**

Hematuria and abdominal pain? Persistent or recurrent UTI? Suspect urinary tract injury; obtain imaging to evaluate for ureteral or bladder compromise.

If not, treat the UTI with antibiotics, urine culture, and close follow-up.

**Wound Redness and Drainage?**

Localized? If so, check the fascia; if it is intact, treat as a superficial wound infection with packing and close follow-up. If the fascia is not intact, consider a subfascial abscess, early necrotizing fasciitis, or hernia or evisceration; make sure that it is not an incarcerated hernia; gynecology consultation and possible surgical evaluation are required.

Widespread? Consider cellulitis or fasciitis; administer antibiotics and hospitalize the patient. If only mild cellulitis is present, oral antibiotics, very close follow-up, and explicit return instructions are required (consider priming with first dose of intravenous antibiotics).

*CT*, Computed tomography; *ED*, emergency department; *US*, ultrasound; *UTI*, urinary tract infection.

treatment is delayed. Bilateral injury (or unilateral injury to a solitary functioning kidney) may simply manifest as anuria and subsequent total renal failure. Urinary leakage from ureteral disruption can cause urinary ascites or an enclosed urinoma.

Months to years after the procedure, watery drainage from the vagina heralds an ureterovaginal or vesicovaginal fistula, whereas watery wound drainage suggests a ureterocutaneous or vesicocutaneous fistula (**Table 125.1**).

## TREATMENT

Antibiotics covering urinary and gastrointestinal pathogens should be initiated early. Gynecology and urology services should be consulted for definitive repair once the diagnosis is made. Ureteral injury can be repaired urgently on the day of diagnosis, or if the patient is unstable, percutaneous nephrostomy can be performed to decompress the kidney while awaiting surgical repair.

If urinary tract injury is ruled out and the diagnosis is simple infection, the patient can be discharged with oral antibiotics.

## VAGINAL BLEEDING

Bleeding from the vagina must be evaluated in the context of the procedure performed. A careful history and speculum examination are key to determining the source, quantity, and persistence of the bleeding.

Blood flowing from the cervical os implies a uterine cause. It may be a result of hemometra (intrauterine hematoma), retained tissue, retained foreign bodies, infection, or uterine

**Table 125.1 Clinical Findings and Bedside Diagnosis of Pelvic Fistulas**

| TYPE OF FISTULA | FINDINGS | BEDSIDE DIAGNOSIS |
|---|---|---|
| Ureterovaginal | Copious, watery vaginal discharge; multiple urinary tract infections | To confirm and differentiate these fistulas:<br>1. Place a tampon in the vagina.<br>2. Administer phenazopyridine, 200 mg orally.<br>3. Instill normal saline tinted with methylene blue into the bladder.<br>Results:<br>Orange tampon = a ureterovaginal fistula.<br>Blue tampon = a vesicovaginal fistula.<br>Note that *both* types may be present concurrently and that blue may overpower orange. |
| Vesicovaginal | Copious, watery vaginal discharge; multiple urinary tract infections | |
| Enterovaginal | Vaginal discharge may contain intestinal contents; severe vaginovulvar irritation may be present because of the pH | Acidity can be tested with litmus paper or the pH portion of a urine dipstick.<br>Place a tampon in the vagina and administer oral activated charcoal. A stained tampon is diagnostic. |
| Colovaginal | Brown, feculent vaginal discharge | Place a tampon in the vagina and instill normal saline tinted with methylene blue into the rectum. A stained tampon is diagnostic of a rectovaginal fistula.<br>Higher colonic lesions may be diagnosed by oral administration of activated charcoal. |
| Vesicocutaneous | Copious watery suprapubic wound discharge | Place a clean wound dressing and administer saline tinted with methylene blue into the bladder. A blue-stained dressing is diagnostic.<br>To differentiate from ureterocutaneous fistulas, insert a urinary catheter, instill methylene blue via the catheter and clamp it off, wait ½ hour, and then drain the bladder until clear and perform the test described below. |
| Ureterocutaneous | Copious, watery wound drainage | Place a clean dressing and then administer methylene blue intravenously. A blue-stained dressing is diagnostic. |

injury. Bimanual examination helps ascertain the size and tenderness of the uterus. A pelvic US scan must be performed to assess the uterine contents. It can be done at the bedside if the patient is unstable. An acute abdominal radiographic series (flat and upright abdominal views with an upright chest radiograph) to look for signs of perforation may be obtained, but it must be kept in mind that residual pneumoperitoneum from laparotomy or laparoscopy often persists for at least 24 hours and may be present for up to 72 hours.

Uterine perforation is manifested as pelvic cramping and vaginal bleeding. It is of serious concern because of risk for associated injury to adjacent bowel, pelvic vessels, bladder, or other structures. Rapid bedside US by the emergency physician (EP) can be useful to assess for free pelvic fluid suggesting hemorrhage or bladder leakage.

Symptoms of acute hemometra include severe, progressive, cramping pelvic pain. Vaginal bleeding may be minimal if the os is obstructed by the enlarging hematoma. The total blood loss is usually insufficient to cause hypotension or anemia. An extremely distended and tender uterus on bimanual pelvic examination is diagnostic, and bedside US can be used to further support the diagnosis.

In rare cases of persistent bleeding without explanation, an unrecognized bleeding diathesis must be considered. von Willebrand disease is the most common bleeding disorder in women of childbearing age.

## TREATMENT

Minor vaginal or cervical lacerations can be managed in the ED with direct pressure followed by the application of Monsel solution or silver nitrate. Persistent bleeding despite these measures may require sutures or electrocautery. Bleeding following cold knife conization is often profuse and frequently requires surgical management.

Minor cases of uterine perforation in which the damage was inflicted by a small blunt instrument (e.g., dilator) may be managed conservatively with close observation and consideration of antibiotics if the bleeding is minimal and the patient is otherwise stable. All cases of perforation with a sharp instrument—or significant damage with a blunt instrument—require definitive management with laparoscopy or laparotomy to evaluate the extent of the damage and to stop the bleeding. Cystoscopy may also be necessary if the bladder lies in the path of the perforation. Broad-spectrum antibiotic coverage is indicated.

Definitive treatment of an intrauterine hematoma is suction evacuation of the uterus. This provides prompt relief and can typically be performed without anesthesia or cervical dilation. Afterward, methylergonovine maleate (0.2 mg intramuscularly [IM]) should be administered to induce uterine contraction unless contraindicated by hypertension, in which case a 1000-mcg rectal suppository of misoprostol can be given instead.

## ENDOMETRITIS

Patients with endometritis are typically initially seen 3 to 7 days after instrumentation with fever and pelvic or lower abdominal pain and tenderness. Vaginal bleeding is frequently present. Potential pathogens are those of pelvic inflammatory disease, in addition to organisms that may have been introduced during the procedure. Risk factors include retained tissue, as well as pelvic inflammatory disease and insufficiently aseptic operating conditions.

Evaluation consists of pelvic US to assess for retained products and laboratory tests, including a complete blood count and assay for the β subunit of human chorionic gonadotropin (β-hCG).

### TREATMENT

Mild endometritis without retained products can be managed on an outpatient basis. Many antibiotic regimens can be used, including a single shot of ceftriaxone, 250 mg IM, plus doxycycline, 100 mg orally twice per day for 14 days, or amoxicillin-clavulanate, 875 mg twice daily, along with the doxycycline. Anaerobic coverage such as metronidazole, 500 mg every 8 hours, may be required as well.

For severe endometritis, inpatient admission is necessary for intravenous (IV) administration of clindamycin, 900 mg every 8 hours, and gentamicin, 1.5 mg/kg every 8 hours. Alternatives are triple IV therapy consisting of ampicillin, 2 g every 6 hours, plus gentamicin, 1.5 mg/kg every 8 hours, and metronidazole, 500 mg every 6 hours, or IV ampicillin-sulbactam, 3.0 g every 8 hours as monotherapy. Doxycycline, 100 mg twice per day for 14 days, should be added if *Chlamydia* is a possible pathogen.

## WOUND AND ABDOMINAL WALL INFECTIONS

Superficial wound infections occur in up to 10% of patients who have undergone gynecologic surgery without perioperative antibiotics. The most common causes are *Staphylococcus aureus* and vaginal or enteric flora. The great majority of these infections are minor, although systemic toxicity or extensive infection may occur if the initial infection is neglected or in patients who are immunosuppressed, have diabetes, or are obese.

Thorough evaluation requires opening the wound for drainage and examination for deep fascial or muscular involvement. Superficial wound infections can be managed without antibiotics by meticulous wound care, irrigation with diluted hydrogen peroxide or Dakin solution four times per day, and dry gauze packing. Delayed wound closure can be performed if necessary. **Table 125.2** details the clinical findings, evaluation, and treatment of wound infections, dehiscence, and necrotizing fasciitis.

## VAGINAL EVISCERATION

Vaginal evisceration (bowel and organs protruding from the vagina) is rare, yet dramatic and has a mortality of up to 10% because of associated intestinal necrosis, peritonitis, or other underlying or global illness. It occurs as a result of increased intraperitoneal pressure in the setting of a ruptured vaginal enterocele or unrecognized uterine perforation. The diagnosis is based on findings on physical examination.

**BOX 125.3 Most Threatening and Most Common Complications of Laparoscopy Seen Postoperatively**

| Most Threatening | Most Common |
|---|---|
| Vascular injury | Ileus |
| Thermal bowel injury | Wound concerns |
| Traumatic bowel injury | Urinary tract infection |
| Urinary tract injury | |
| Sepsis | |

### TREATMENT

A moist covering must be placed immediately to protect the viscera. Bed rest in the supine or Trendelenburg position is recommended to prevent further outward pressure. Broad-spectrum antibiotics should be administered, and gynecology consultation should be obtained immediately for surgical repair.

## COMPLICATIONS SPECIFIC TO LAPAROSCOPY

Laparoscopic procedures are characterized by more rapid recovery and lower complication rates than seen with open surgical procedures. However, unique complications are associated with needle or trocar insertion, induced pneumoperitoneum, and extensive use of electrocautery[4,5] (**Box 125.3**). Most catastrophic complications are recognized intraoperatively. Management in the ED in the first month postoperatively is usually for wound complaints or symptoms caused by injury to the bowel, bladder, or ureters. Remote complications include hernias.

### BLEEDING

Abdominal wall hematomas may occur as a result of damage to superficial vessels at laparoscopic sites. If the injury is extensive or if the size cannot be estimated because of habitus, a complete blood count can be obtained to estimate and track the blood loss, although the blood lost is not usually sufficient to require transfusion.

Injury to the inferior epigastric vessels can cause intraperitoneal and retroperitoneal bleeding. Patients with slow retroperitoneal bleeding may possibly be seen in the ED if the postoperative observation time was short. Bedside US is of limited utility for evaluating the retroperitoneal space. Worsening flank or back pain soon after the procedure must raise concern for retroperitoneal bleeding. Work-up includes laboratory tests to evaluate for anemia and computed tomography with intravenous contrast enhancement to identify the bleeding.

**Table 125.2 Wound and Abdominal Wall Infections**

| | FINDINGS | EVALUATION | TREATMENT |
|---|---|---|---|
| Superficial wound infections<br>*Incidence*: ≈10% in surgeries without antibiotic prophylaxis<br>*Risk factors*: diabetes, obesity, immunosuppression<br>Low mortality and morbidity if recognized and treated | *Staphylococcus aureus*, vaginal or enteric flora—presents 5-7 days postoperatively with serosanguineous or seropurulent drainage<br>With or without fever and leukocytosis | Open incision to drain and rule out deep fascial or muscular involvement<br>Cultures not helpful | Wound care—irrigate with diluted hydrogen peroxide or Dakin solution four times a day, dry gauze wound packing<br>No antibiotics if no surrounding cellulitis<br>Delayed wound closure if desired |
| | Group A β-hemolytic streptococci—presents 1-2 days postoperatively with rapidly advancing erythema, lymphangitis, lymphadenopathy, and scant, watery drainage | External examination<br>If little drainage, leave wound intact<br>Cultures not helpful | Wound care as above<br>Amoxicillin-clavulanate, 875 mg orally q12h for 7-10 days, or a first-generation cephalosporin. Initial IV dose of nafcillin or oxacillin, 2 g for more severe cases<br>If suspected, add coverage for community-acquired MRSA |
| Wound dehiscence (complete fascial disruption)<br>*Incidence*: 0.5% of gynecologic surgical cases<br>*Mortality*:10-35%<br>*Risk factors*: obesity, poor nutrition, cancer, previous radiation exposure, previous incision, infection, distended abdomen, bronchopulmonary disease, corticosteroid use, absorbable sutures, layered closure | Lump, bloody drainage, pain, or wound opening after a sudden movement or abrupt increase in intraperitoneal pressure, such as a violent cough<br>Evisceration (herniation of abdominal contents through the wall) in extreme cases<br>Complications include sepsis, death, hernias, and poor cosmetic outcome | Diagnosis based on interruption of fascia. Skin may still be closed<br>If open, gently probe with a sterile gloved finger or sterile cotton swab to evaluate the integrity of the fascial layer<br>Ultrasound may be useful if skin is intact to reveal subcutaneous herniated bowel loops<br>Laboratory tests, wound cultures<br>CT scan if deeper infection suspected | Cover exposed viscera with a wet sterile dressing<br>Decompress the stomach and bladder with a nasogastric tube and Foley catheter<br>IV antibiotics<br>Resuscitation and repletion of fluid, electrolyte, and nutritional deficits<br>Once stabilized, operative management with removal of old suture material, abscess drainage, wound débridement, and peritoneal cavity lavage before closure of abdominal wall<br>Skin closure often by secondary intention |

*Continued*

**Table 125.2 Wound and Abdominal Wall Infections—cont'd**

| | FINDINGS | EVALUATION | TREATMENT |
|---|---|---|---|
| Necrotizing fasciitis<br>Necrosis of superficial fascia and connective tissue, undermining skin but sparing muscle<br>*Incidence*: about 50% of these cases associated with surgical incisions<br>High morbidity and mortality (70-80%)<br>*Risk factors*: immunosuppression, diabetes, elderly, peripheral vascular disease, poor nutrition, obesity, hypertension, malignancy, radiation exposure, renal insufficiency | Mixed aerobic-anaerobic, group A streptococci, *Clostridium perfringens*, community-acquired MRSA, *Vibrio vulnificus*<br>Early findings nonspecific—pain, edema, and firm induration with erythema<br>Duskiness of skin, anesthesia of the area, or pain out of proportion to findings on examination may be the keys to early recognition<br>Fever and leukocytosis<br>Superficial bullae and altered mental status may develop<br>May present already in septic shock<br>Progression over hours to a few days<br>Complications: limb loss, organ failure, death | Lack of fascial resistance to probing in the wound of a toxic-appearing patient is highly suspicious<br>Laboratory testing includes a complete blood count with differential, electrolytes, renal and liver function tests, lactate, preoperative tests and cultures of the wound and blood<br>Chest radiograph and urine cultures to rule out other sources of infection<br>If stable, CT may help assess extent of involvement (should not delay surgical evaluation)<br>ABGs and lactate if septic shock | Immediate IV antibiotics—assume polymicrobial infection from recent hospitalization: ampicillin-sulbactam, 3.0 g q6-8h, or piperacillin-tazobactam, 3.375 g q6-8h<br>*Plus* clindamycin, 600-900 mg q8h<br>*Plus* ciprofloxacin, 400 mg q12h<br>*Or* imipenem-cilastin, 1 g q6h, or meropenem, 1 g q8h<br>Community-acquired infection: assume group A streptococci (penicillin G, 18 million units daily in 3-4 divided doses; clindamycin, 900 mg q8h for streptococcal or clostridial infection; with or without vancomycin, 30 mg/kg/day divided q12h for *Staphylococcus* infection)<br>Aggressive IV repletion of fluids, colloids, and calcium<br>Immediate surgical consultation for emergent wide surgical débridement<br>Central venous monitoring and admission to intensive care unit<br>Hyperbaric therapy can be considered postoperatively<br>If toxic shock, IV immunoglobulin, 1 g/kg on day 1 followed by 0.5 g/kg for 2 more days, decreases sepsis-related organ failure |

*ABGs*, Arterial blood gases; *CT*, computed tomography; *IV*, intravenous; *MRSA*, methicillin-resistant *Staphylococcus aureus*.

### TREATMENT

Treatment depends on the site and degree of bleeding. The EP should be prepared for blood transfusion and involve the gynecologic surgeon early.

## BOWEL INJURY

The incidence of bowel injury from laparoscopic surgery is estimated to be 0.06% to 0.5%, with higher rates for therapeutic procedures than for diagnostic ones, and about 50% to 70% of the time it is diagnosed postoperatively.[5]

Most of these bowel injuries are caused by the initial needle insertion or thermal injury with electrocautery. Major injuries are typically discovered intraoperatively because of excessive bleeding or spillage of intestinal contents, but some are less obvious.

Thermal bowel injuries are serious and typically manifested days or even weeks after laparoscopy. Symptoms include abdominal distention, severe lower abdominal pain and tenderness, and fever, often accompanied by nausea, vomiting, and peritoneal signs. Blood tests reveal leukocytosis. Abdominal radiographs may show free air or ileus. Although residual induced pneumoperitoneum may persist for up to 72 hours, in a symptomatic patient the EP should not assume that the free air is benign if it persists longer than 24 hours after laparoscopy.

### TREATMENT

Early gynecology consultation should be obtained if thermal injury is suspected. The EP should also consider early empiric antibiotics effective against gastrointestinal pathogens if perforation is suspected or confirmed.

## COMPLICATIONS OF UTERINE FIBROID EMBOLIZATION

Uterine fibroid embolization is typically performed by an interventional radiologist to treat bleeding fibroids in patients who are poor candidates for major surgery, are not interested in reproduction, or wish to preserve their menses for personal or for ethnic or religious reasons. The procedure consists of the injection of a mass of microspheres (tris-acryl gelatin) or polyvinyl alcohol directly into the uterine artery to occlude it. The goal is to cut off the blood supply to the fibroids so that they will shrink and degenerate.

A relatively new procedure, uterine fibroid embolization has been rapidly gaining in popularity in the United States, from 50 cases performed in 1996 to now more than 100,000 worldwide. Early results show a success rate of about 90% and a complication rate of about 5% by American College of Gynecology criteria.[6] Patients have a shorter hospitalization and return to activities sooner but have a higher rate of treatment failure and delayed rehospitalization than patients undergoing surgery.

Postembolization syndrome (low-grade fever, malaise, pelvic pain, nausea, and vomiting) affects most of these patients to some degree. Only symptomatic treatment is warranted as long as other causes have been ruled out.

These patients are at risk for angiographic complications such as femoral hematoma, site infection, pseudoaneurysm, arteriovenous fistula, thromboembolism, and contrast agent–induced nephropathy.

**BOX 125.4 Most Threatening and Most Common Complications of Uterine Fibroid Embolization**

| Most Threatening | Most Common |
|---|---|
| Sepsis | Postembolization syndrome |
| Nontarget embolization | Severe pain |
| Uterine ischemia, rupture | Vaginal bleeding |
| Endometritis, pyometrium | Allergic reaction |
| Contrast agent–induced renal failure | Groin hematoma |
| Thromboembolic disease | Retained tissue |
| | Embolization failure |
| | Iatrogenic menopause* |

*The incidence is 1% to 5% in all women but up to 43% in women older than 45 years.

Occasionally, the embolization goes awry ("nontarget embolization"), and severe tissue ischemia and necrosis occur in undesirable areas such as the buttock, labia, and vaginal vault. **Box 125.4** lists the most common and most life-threatening complications.

### TREATMENT

Severe pain from degenerating fibroids can be treated with nonsteroidal antiinflammatory drugs and oral opioids (e.g., acetaminophen with hydrocodone). Infected necrotic tissue or intractable pain may require hysterectomy. Severe bleeding or a sloughed fibroid that is not spontaneously expulsed vaginally requires evacuation.

## BLEEDING AFTER CERVICAL PROCEDURES

Cervical cancer used to be the top cancer killer of women in the United States. Even though numbers have declined over the past few decades because of the emphasis on regular Papanicolaou tests, in 2007 cervical cancer was diagnosed in 12,280 women, and 4021 died of the disease.[7] Cervical procedures such as cervical conization (laser conization, cold knife conization, loop electrosurgical excision), colposcopy, and cryotherapy are used for the diagnosis and treatment of early cervical neoplasia.

Cold knife conization (surgical excision with a scalpel) is always performed in the operating room, usually with general or spinal anesthesia. Because intraoperative and postprocedural bleeding can be profuse, cerclage is often performed prophylactically before the procedure as a tourniquet. Postconization bleeding is usually manifested 1 to 2 weeks after the procedure.

Laser conization has only slightly lower rates of bleeding. Cervical cryotherapy and loop electrosurgical excision cause just minor bleeding and thus are performed in the outpatient setting.

### TREATMENT

Vaginal packing may be attempted, but the patient often needs to return to the operating room for control of hemorrhage.

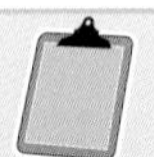

**DOCUMENTATION**

**Patients with Complications of Gynecologic Procedures**

**History**

Gravida, para, aborta, current pregnancy status
Last normal menstrual period or onset of menopause
Procedure performed, including any previous associated complications
Time lapsed since the procedure
If bleeding, quantify the rate and whether symptoms of anemia are present

**Physical Examination**

Are the vital signs stable?
Does the patient look ill? pale? febrile? uncomfortable?
Abdominal examination—Distention, soft, tender, peritoneal signs
Speculum examination—Vaginal discharge, bleeding, color, quantity
Bimanual examination—Uterine and ovarian size and texture, tenderness
Wound evaluation—Is there discharge? Erythema? Tenderness? Is it intact at all layers?

**Diagnostic Studies**

Bedside ultrasound imaging results, if performed, to evaluate for free fluid, bladder fullness, hydronephrosis, or uterine contents
Other imaging or blood and urine laboratory study results

**Medical Decision Making**

Time and person contacted for gynecology consultation

**Patient Instructions**

Documentation of discussion with the patient regarding diagnosis, anticipated course, recognition of warning signs, what to do if they occur, follow-up, and reasons to return to the emergency department

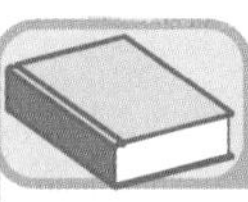

**PATIENT TEACHING TIPS**

**After a Gynecologic Procedure**

Explain the normal postoperative course to the patient.
If the patient is not being admitted, schedule follow-up with the patient's physician in the next 1 to 3 days.
If antibiotics are prescribed, instruct the patient to complete the entire course of therapy as indicated.
Tell the patient to call her physician or return to the emergency department if she has:

- Worsening abdominal or pelvic pain or abdominal distention
- Intractable vomiting
- Any evidence of wound infection or discharge
- Vaginal bleeding soaking more than 1 maxi-pad an hour for at least 4 hours (instruct her that there may be an initial gush in the morning or on standing after lying down)
- Foul-smelling, milky, green, or other abnormal vaginal discharge
- Fever with a temperature higher than 100.3° F
- Any other concerning symptoms

# POSTABORTION COMPLICATIONS

## EPIDEMIOLOGY

Since becoming legalized nationwide in 1973, termination of pregnancy has become among the most frequently performed operative procedures in the United States, with more than 1 million performed yearly. A total of 1.2 million cases were reported in 2008.[8] An estimated half of all pregnancies are unplanned, and 40% of unintended pregnancies are terminated. In fact, each year approximately 3% of all women of childbearing age have abortions, thus accounting for almost one fourth of all pregnancies. Most abortions are performed during the first trimester—62% within the first 8 weeks and 95% within the first 16 weeks.[9] Overall complication rates are low, ranging from 1% to 5% of cases, and associated maternal mortality is extremely rare. Death is infrequent, with seven occurring after the almost 1 million legal abortions reported in the United States in 2005.[8] In fact, for every gestational age, mortality is lower with abortion than with pregnancy and childbirth.[10]

Medical abortion has a success rate of 80% to 97% (higher for gestations <50 days); 2% to 5% of patients with failed abortions require subsequent surgical abortion, with a 5% to 10% rate of incomplete evacuation of products of conception.[11,12]

## PATHOPHYSIOLOGY

### MEDICAL ABORTION

The three most commonly used abortion medications are mifepristone (an antiprogestin), misoprostol (a prostaglandin), both of which trigger uterine contraction, and methotrexate, an antimetabolite that interrupts embryonic development. Methotrexate and misoprostol are also teratogenic. Thus once used, termination must be completed, even if surgical means are ultimately necessary.

Medical abortion of both live and deceased fetuses between 13 and 28 weeks of gestation is uncommon but can be achieved with prostaglandin $E_2$ suppositories, carboprost tromethamine, misoprostol, or high-dose oxytocin (80% to 90% effective).

### SURGICAL ABORTION

Dilation plus curettage is the most frequently used abortion method in the United States (>90% of abortions).[8] The cervix is dilated and the uterine contents scraped out with a curette or aspirated via vacuum extraction. In the first trimester the overall risk profile is very low (0.1% to 0.3%) and even lower with regional anesthesia. However, the complication rate does increase with increasing gestational age.

Dilation plus evacuation is performed to terminate pregnancies more than 16 weeks of gestation. Dilation is achieved via osmotic dilators (i.e., laminaria) or vaginally administered prostaglandins, as opposed to instrumentation, and the uterine contents are removed with forceps or vacuum. This technique is also used for the management of spontaneous abortion, retained products of conception, intrauterine fetal demise, and gestational trophoblastic neoplasia. Its application

**Table 125.3** Postabortion Complications

| ABORTION METHOD | GESTATIONAL AGE | COMPLICATIONS: IMMEDIATE (<24 HR) | EARLY (1 DAY-4 WK) | DELAYED | LATE |
|---|---|---|---|---|---|
| **Medical** | | | | | |
| Mifepristone (single 200-mg dose)<br>Methotrexate with or without misoprostol | <8 wk | Nausea<br>Bleeding<br>Pain, cramping<br>Ruptured ectopic pregnancy<br>Rh isoimmunization | Bleeding<br>Retained pregnancy<br>Retained products<br>Infection:<br>Endometritis<br>Sepsis<br>Toxic shock syndrome<br>Rh isoimmunization | Psychologic trauma<br>Rh isoimmunization | Psychologic trauma<br>Rh isoimmunization |
| Misoprostol, vaginal or buccal prostaglandins | Up to 23 wk | | | | |
| **Surgical** | | | | | |
| Curettage (suction or sharp): without dilation | <7 wk | Pain<br>Bleeding<br>Cervical laceration<br>Uterine perforation<br>Inability to complete procedure<br>Heterotopic pregnancy<br>Rh isoimmunization<br>Disseminated intravascular coagulation (rare) | Bleeding<br>Retained products<br>Infection:<br>Endometritis<br>Sepsis<br>Toxic shock syndrome<br>Rh isoimmunization | Postabortive amenorrhea<br>Psychologic trauma<br>Rh isoimmunization | Postabortive amenorrhea<br>Psychologic trauma<br>Rh isoimmunization |
| Curettage (suction or sharp): with dilation | 7-13 wk | | | | |
| Dilation and evacuation | >13 wk | | | | |

depends on uterine volume, age of gestation, and operator experience.[13]

## DIFFERENTIAL DIAGNOSIS AND MEDICAL DECISION MAKING

Abortion is a commonly performed procedure and, when performed under medical supervision, rarely has severe complications. The vast majority of terminations are procedural (including vacuum aspiration, sharp curettage, and dilation and evacuation). Medical abortion can be used earlier in the pregnancy and avoids the risks and stigma of procedural termination, but it has a higher incidence of incomplete abortion and failed termination and can be accompanied by severe side effects of the medication and physical discomfort.

General complications of abortion include retained pregnancy, hemorrhage, infection, and incomplete evacuation (**Table 125.3**); the most threatening and most common complications of abortion are listed in **Box 125.5**.

In the long term there is a risk for decreased fertility and amenorrhea. Postabortion infection seems to be the only predictor of decreased fertility. For instance, the risk for ectopic pregnancy increases only in cases of postabortion infection. Because ovulation can resume as early as 2 weeks after abortion, contraception should be initiated soon after abortion.

**BOX 125.5 Most Threatening and Most Common Complications of Induced Abortion**

**Most Threatening**
- Vascular injury
- Bowel injury
- Urinary tract injury
- Sepsis
- Uterine perforation or rupture

**Most Common**
- Bleeding
- Pain, cramping
- Medication intolerance (medical abortion)
- Cervical laceration (surgical abortion)
- Retained products of conception
- Retained pregnancy
- Infection, endometritis

### COMPLICATIONS OF MEDICAL ABORTION

The most feared complication is uterine rupture with intraabdominal expulsion of the fetus, especially in women with a scarred uterus (e.g., from a previous cesarean delivery), grand multiparity, and nulliparity with an insufficiently ripened cervix. Common side effects include nausea, vomiting, diarrhea, headache, dizziness, back pain, and fatigue, but it is the severe cramping and heavy bleeding that occur with medical induction that are most likely to bring patients to the ED. Treatment is symptomatic, and regardless of whether the

**BOX 125.6 Complications of Surgical Abortion**

**Immediate Complications (<24 Hours)**

***Minor***

Mild infection
Incomplete abortion
Hematometra (uterine distention syndrome)

***Major***

Hemorrhage secondary to:

- Incomplete abortion (retained products of conception)
- Uterine perforation with or without injury to adjacent structures
- Cervical laceration

Severe infection and sepsis
Injury to adjacent structures
Missed heterotopic pregnancy

**Delayed Complications (1 Day to 4 Weeks)**

Infection (e.g., endometritis)
Hemorrhage
Retained foreign body or products of conception
Cervical stenosis

**Long-Term Complications**

Future fertility problems
Postabortion amenorrhea
Adhesions
Uterine synechiae
Ectopic pregnancy
Premature labor
Very-low-birth-weight infants

**Table 125.4 Findings in Patients with Uterine Perforation**

| SITE | SIGNS AND SYMPTOMS |
|---|---|
| Any site | Unexpected pain<br>Vaginal bleeding<br>Symptoms of anemia |
| Any site with bowel injury | Abdominal pain with or without distention or peritoneal signs<br>Fever |
| Fundal | Unexpected pain |
| Lateral | Diffuse lower abdominal pain<br>Pelvic mass<br>Fever |
| Anterior | Hematuria |

bleeding is heavy, transfusions are rarely required. It is important to distinguish the natural course of medical termination from incomplete abortion or uterine rupture.

## COMPLICATIONS OF SURGICAL ABORTION

Surgical abortion carries the risks associated with anesthesia, in addition to those related to the procedure. Complications categorized as immediate, delayed, and long term are listed in **Box 125.6**.

Complications include uterine perforation, cervical laceration, hemorrhage, incomplete removal of the fetus and placenta, and infection. Very rarely, curettage performed in advanced pregnancy results in a severe, fatal consumptive coagulopathy.

The most common postprocedural complaints are bleeding and pain. Uterine bleeding may be due to retained products of conception, uterine atony, infection, uterine arteriovenous malformation, placenta accreta, coagulopathy (secondary to high levels of tissue thromboplastin released during the procedure), or uterine perforation.

## HEMORRHAGE

Posttermination vaginal bleeding in the natural course of abortion must be differentiated from pathologic causes. Determination of the abortion method, rate of bleeding, and accompanying symptoms such as fever, abdominal pain, and symptoms of acute anemia is essential.

Diagnostic testing includes a complete blood count, coagulation studies, basic metabolic profile, type and screen (or crossmatch if the bleeding is brisk and uncontrolled), and US to evaluate for intrauterine contents. Bedside US revealing free fluid or an upright chest radiograph revealing free air is sufficient evidence of perforation and the need for emergency exploratory laparotomy. Heavy bleeding or a nonfundal perforation requires evaluation of the adjacent intraabdominal organs for collateral damage. In a stable patient, US is required to evaluate the pelvic structures, followed by a computed tomography scan if the US image is equivocal. Incomplete abortion is one of the most common causes of ongoing bleeding, and US is extremely useful for making the diagnosis.

Uterine atony is a diagnosis of exclusion and can be treated medically after the findings on US and hemoglobin levels are within normal limits.

Uterine perforation carries a high risk for concomitant damage to the intraperitoneal structures and severe hemorrhage. Delayed manifestation is not uncommon because fundal perforations (accounting for two thirds of all perforations) have scant bleeding. Lateral perforations may have heavy bleeding hidden in the broad ligament, and a lacerated uterine artery may initially spasm. The signs and symptoms depend on the site of perforation (**Table 125.4**). Uterine perforation related to surgical abortion or uterine rupture from medical abortion must be considered in patients with vaginal bleeding and abdominal pain.

# TREATMENT

The EP must first establish that the patient is stable, resuscitate if necessary, and then determine whether the source of bleeding is vaginal, cervical, or uterine. Resuscitation of unstable patients is paramount. Management includes rapid diagnosis, large-bore IV access, fluid resuscitation or transfusion (or both), and gynecologic consultation.

Uterine perforation related to surgical abortion and uterine rupture from medical abortion are surgical emergencies, so gynecology must be involved early. Laparotomy or laparoscopy to examine the abdominal contents is usually indicated, although small perforations may be managed expectantly with consideration of antibiotic treatment. In the presence of rapid bleeding, insertion of a Foley catheter into the uterus and inflation of the balloon with 60 mL of saline can serve as a temporizing tamponade (**Table 125.5**).

Definitive treatment of incomplete abortion with retained products of conception is dilation and curettage. Gynecology should be consulted and antibiotics should be considered because retained products place patients at risk for infection.

**Table 125.5 Treatment of Postabortion Hemorrhage Without Perforation**

| CAUSE OF HEMORRHAGE | TREATMENT |
|---|---|
| Uterine atony | Methylergonovine maleate (Methergine), 0.2 mg IM<br>Carboprost tromethamine (Hemabate), 250 mcg IM q15-90 min (maximum total dose, 2 mg)<br>Misoprostol, 1000-mcg suppository per rectum<br>Oxytocin (Pitocin), 40 units in 1 L of 5% dextrose in NS by IV drip, with the rate titrated to bleeding control |
| Retained products of conception | Dilation and curettage<br>Antibiotics if endometritis is suspected |
| Placenta accreta | Uterine artery embolization |
| Severe continued bleeding | Temporizing measure: intrauterine tamponade via uterine packing or transcervical placement of a Foley catheter and inflation of the balloon with 30 mL of sterile NS (or 100 mL of NS for a 30-mL balloon) |

*IM*, Intramuscularly; *IV*, intravenous; *NS*, normal saline.

Lacerations of the vagina or cervix are treated with direct pressure, followed by the application of Monsel solution or silver nitrite if needed.

Treatment options for uterine atony are methylergonovine maleate (Methergine), 0.2 mg IM, carboprost tromethamine (Hemabate), 250 mcg IM every 15 to 90 minutes with a maximum total dose of 2 mg, misoprostol, 1000-mcg suppository per rectum, or oxytocin (Pitocin), 40 units in 1 L of 5% dextrose in normal saline (D5NS) IV, with the drip rate titrated to control the bleeding.

Heavy ongoing hemorrhage without an obvious source and with symptomatic or profound anemia requires temporizing packing and exploration in the operating room or uterine artery embolization.

## POSTABORTION INFECTION

Postabortion infection is infrequent, but when it does occur, it is usually a result of retained products of conception or unrecognized preexisting infection.

Patients with endometritis usually have fever, prolonged vaginal bleeding, and pelvic pain. A midline boggy mass may be noted on examination. Laboratory tests include a complete blood count, coagulation profile, β-hCG level, and cervical cultures. Transvaginal pelvic US should be performed to evaluate for retained tissue.

Though extremely rare and seen mostly following illegal abortions, severe and fatal infections are possible. Other major complications include severe hemorrhage, septic shock, disseminated intravascular coagulation, and acute renal failure. Uterine infection is most common, but parametritis, endocarditis, peritonitis, and septicemia may occur and are typically due to anaerobic coliforms.

Diffuse abdominal tenderness with guarding, fever, tachycardia, and hypotension suggests severe sepsis. Laboratory tests should include a complete blood count with differential, electrolytes, kidney and liver function, coagulation profile, lactate studies, β-hCG, a blood bank sample, urinalysis, and cervical and urine cultures.

### TREATMENT

Postabortion infections require antibiotics, as well as suction curettage. The antibiotic regimens recommended are usually based on guidelines of the Centers for Disease Control and Prevention for treating pelvic inflammatory disease and include IV clindamycin, 900 mg every 8 hours, plus gentamicin, 1.5 mg/kg every 8 hours; triple coverage with ampicillin, gentamicin, and metronidazole is indicated for sicker patients; and ampicillin-sulbactam is used as monotherapy in less severe cases. Treatment of sepsis begins with rapid stabilization and aggressive IV fluid resuscitation. Broad-spectrum intravenous antimicrobials and gynecology consultation for definitive evacuation of the products of conception should not be delayed.

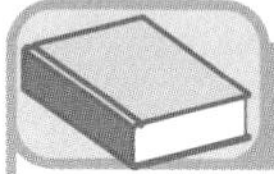

**PATIENT TEACHING TIPS**

**Postabortion Instructions**

Instruct the patient about the natural course of recovery, in particular how much bleeding and pain can be anticipated and when to be concerned.

If antibiotics are prescribed, the patient should complete the entire course as indicated.

Inquire whether the patient wishes to use contraception. Also clarify that only barrier contraception protects against sexually transmitted diseases as well.

Tell the patient to call her physician or return to the emergency department if she has
- Vaginal bleeding soaking more than 1 maxi-pad per hour for at least 4 hours
- Foul-smelling, milky, or green vaginal discharge
- Increasing abdominal or pelvic pain
- Fever with a temperature higher than 38° C
- Any other concerning symptoms

## COMPLICATIONS OF ASSISTED REPRODUCTIVE TECHNOLOGY

### EPIDEMIOLOGY

On July 25, 1978, Louise Brown, the original "test tube baby," was born in England. Conceived by in vitro fertilization, her birth was a landmark in the history of ART. Four years later, the first child conceived by ART in the United States was born. In 2009, 146,244 ART procedures were reported by 441 sites in the United States, resulting in more than 60,000 babies.[1] and it is estimated that more than 1% of children conceived worldwide can be attributed to ART each year.

Despite the growing frequency of ART, however, published data on complications are limited. What does exist focuses primarily on outcomes of the pregnancy (multiple-birth gestations, low-birth-weight babies, cesarean sections, and preterm delivery), as well as long-term effects on women and the resultant children.[14] These complications are dealt with only indirectly in the ED.

## PATHOPHYSIOLOGY

The subfertility of a couple can be attributed to male factor, female factor, or incompatibility issues. Male factor infertility includes dysfunctional sperm, inadequate sperm concentration, and obstruction. Female factor infertility can be due to ovulatory dysfunction, poor egg quality, anatomic abnormalities, or hormonal imbalance. Compatibility factors include a hostile environment.

Many techniques are used in the course of assisted reproduction, and rapid advances have been made over the last 2 decades. ART incorporates techniques of controlled ovarian hyperstimulation, egg or sperm retrieval, insemination, and embryo transfer. Selection of the ART methods used depends on the specific fertility issues identified. During the course of evaluation and preparation, each party may undergo diagnostic and corrective procedures before the initiation of assisted reproduction.

The five basic stages of ART for women are ovulation (natural or induced), egg harvesting, implantation of the egg and sperm or fertilized zygote, pregnancy, and delivery. Each stage has its own risks. For men, the risks are limited mostly to procedures for the acquisition of sperm.

## DIFFERENTIAL DIAGNOSIS AND MEDICAL DECISION MAKING

When dealing with these patients, the EP must keep in mind that infertility specialists are typically very involved in the management of their patients and would prefer to have close communications regarding the patient's status while being able to provide close monitoring and follow-up.

Major complications of ART likely to be encountered in the ED include ovarian hyperstimulation syndrome (OHSS), ectopic or heterotopic pregnancy, miscarriage, ovarian torsion, ovarian rupture, thromboembolism, and postprocedural complications (**Table 125.6** and **Box 125.7**).

**Table 125.6 Complications of Assisted Reproductive Technology**

| | *Time of Onset* | | | |
|---|---|---|---|---|
| **PHASE OF ART** | **IMMEDIATE** | **EARLY** | **DELAYED** | **LATE** |
| Controlled ovarian hyperstimulation: clomiphene citrate, gonadotropins (FSH/LH, GnRH, hMG) | Medication side effects | OHSS,* ovarian torsion, ovarian cyst, cyst rupture | Multifetal pregnancy, thromboembolic disease* | Ovarian cancer is *not* supported by trials |
| Oocyte retrieval | Risks of anesthesia, bleeding from the vaginal puncture site, intraperitoneal bleeding | Bleeding from the vaginal puncture site, intraperitoneal bleeding, ovarian torsion, infection | Bowel endometriosis | |
| Embryo transfer | Contractions expelling the embryos | Infection, OHSS* | Multifetal pregnancy | |
| Pregnancy | Early pregnancy, bleeding, placenta previa | OHSS,* ectopic or heterotopic pregnancy,* spontaneous abortion, thromboembolic disease* | Multifetal pregnancy, preeclampsia or eclampsia,* thromboembolic disease,* placental abruption | Multifetal pregnancy, preeclampsia or eclampsia,* thromboembolic disease* |
| Delivery | Preterm labor or PROM, preeclampsia or eclampsia,* primary inadequate contractions, secondary uterine inertia; increased risk for cesarean section, multifetal delivery; EVLBW, VLBW, LBW infants | Thromboembolic complications,* retained placenta, bleeding associated with vaginal delivery, preeclampsia or eclampsia* | | |

*Major complication.

*ART*, Assisted reproductive technology; *EVLBW*, extremely very low birth weight; *FSH/LH*, follicle-stimulating hormone/luteinizing hormone; *GnRH*, gonadotropin-releasing hormone; *hMG*, human menopausal gonadotropin; *LBW*, low birth weight; *OHSS*, ovarian hyperstimulation syndrome; *PROM*, premature rupture of membrane; *VLBW*, very low birth weight.

**BOX 125.7 Most Threatening and Most Common Complications of Assisted Reproductive Technology**

**Most Threatening**
Ovarian hyperstimulation syndrome
Ectopic or heterotopic pregnancy
Ovarian torsion
Pulmonary embolism, deep vein thrombosis

**Most Common**
Medication side effects
Multiple-gestation pregnancies
Preterm labor
Bleeding
Infection
Miscarriage
Pain

## OVARIAN TORSION

Ovarian enlargement predisposes to torsion. ART patients are at particular risk because they are actively seeking to attain hyperovulation and pregnancy. In addition, patients with elevated risk because of preexisting conditions such as polycystic ovarian syndrome are overrepresented in the ART population.

Severe unilateral adnexal or pelvic pain may initially be intermittent as the ovary twists and untwists; the pain then becomes sustained when the torsion persists and the ovary becomes ischemic. Immediate pelvic Doppler US of the ovarian vessels is the key to diagnosis and differentiation from benign causes of pelvic pain. Emergency surgical intervention is indicated to avoid permanent damage to the ovary.

## THROMBOEMBOLIC DISEASE

ART patients are at increased risk for thromboembolism because of the elevated levels of hormones. A high index of suspicion must be maintained, but evaluation should take into consideration the ongoing attempts at pregnancy.

Before any type of imaging is performed, pregnancy status should be established. Chest computed tomography with intravenous contrast enhancement to evaluate for pulmonary embolism can be performed with shielding. The patient should first be informed of the risks and benefits of the procedure and provide written consent. Echocardiography can be used to evaluate for signs of critical pulmonary embolism such as right heart strain when the patient refuses a radioactive study, although this is not the preferred method of evaluation.

Lower extremity vascular studies can be performed, but their sensitivity is low if no leg symptoms are present. Nevertheless, confirmed deep vein thrombosis must be treated and may save the patient and her early pregnancy from further exposure to radiation.

Bedside US by an EP trained in echocardiography and lower extremity Doppler studies can speed the diagnosis of thromboembolic disease.

## OOCYTE HARVESTING

Transvaginal US–guided oocyte aspiration is typically an ambulatory procedure involving intravenous analgesia and sedation. Risks include vascular injury with bleeding from the vaginal puncture site, hemoperitoneum, rupture of ovarian cysts, bowel perforation, injury to pelvic organs, and infection.

Bleeding from the vaginal mucosa because of the harvesting punctures typically resolves spontaneously by the end of the procedure or with direct pressure. Topical hemostatic agents may be used if compression fails. Persistent or significant bleeding despite these measures requires suturing.

Intraabdominal bleeding should be suspected in patients with postprocedural symptoms of anemia even before peritoneal signs become evident.

If vital signs remain stable and the patient is minimally symptomatic, conservative management is possible; however, hemodynamic instability unresponsive to basic fluid resuscitation or a falling hemoglobin level in a symptomatic patient requires emergency exploratory laparotomy for definitive diagnosis and correction. Typed and crossmatched blood should be used for transfusion if the patient is sufficiently stable. Uncrossmatched O-negative blood can be used for immediate transfusion if necessary.

## EMBRYO TRANSFER

Pelvic infection, ectopic or heterotopic pregnancy, spontaneous expulsion of the embryo, and multiple-gestation pregnancy may complicate embryo transfer.

## ECTOPIC AND HETEROTOPIC PREGNANCIES

Despite careful placement of embryos in the uterus, approximately 4% of in vitro fertilization pregnancies are ectopic. This incidence is slightly reduced with US guidance of embryo placement; however, migration of the embryo may occur occasionally. Ectopic pregnancies as a result of ART are usually diagnosed very early because of close monitoring by the fertility specialist.

Heterotopic pregnancies (multigestational pregnancies with at least one ectopic and one intrauterine pregnancy) are very rare with spontaneous conception (1 in 30,000) but occur in up to 1% of assisted conception cycles. This number is expected to decrease as technology continues to improve and the use of single-embryo transfer increases. In patients with symptoms consistent with a possible ectopic pregnancy, the presence of an intrauterine pregnancy does not rule out a heterotopic ectopic pregnancy, and a full work-up should be performed.

Management of patients who have undergone the psychologic, physical, and financial burden of using ART and have a heterotopic pregnancy should be focused on maintaining the intrauterine pregnancy while eliminating the ectopic pregnancy and avoiding excessive risk to the mother.

## MULTIPLE-GESTATION PREGNANCIES

In 2009, 31% of infants born as a result of ART were multiple-gestation births, in contrast to approximately 3% of births in the general population.[13]

Multiple embryos are often placed in the uterus because of the low implantation rate per embryo (10% to 25%). Although this can be welcome news to the expectant parents, these multifetal pregnancies are associated with an increased risk for mortality and morbidity in both the mother and fetuses.

Maternal complications include preterm labor, placental abruption and placenta previa, cesarean section, postpartum hemorrhage, gestational diabetes, and preeclampsia. Fetuses are at risk for the secondary effects of maternal complications, as well as premature birth, low birth weight, intrauterine demise, and congenital conditions such as cerebral palsy. As new technologic developments increase the success of implantation, however, protocols are changing to dictate the transfer of only one or two embryos.

## OVARIAN HYPERSTIMULATION SYNDROME

### Epidemiology

OHSS is the most feared complication of ovulatory stimulation. Severe OHSS is life-threatening and occurs in an estimated 0.5% to 5% of ART cycles. It also occurs occasionally in spontaneous pregnancy. The estimated mortality rate is 1 in 400,000 to 500,000 patients.[15]

### Pathophysiology

OHSS is characterized by increased capillary permeability with third spacing of protein-rich fluid. This results in hemoconcentration with severe intravascular hypovolemia manifested as edema, ascites, and pleural and pericardial effusions. Multisystem organ failure, renal failure, immunosuppression, pulmonary failure, thromboembolism, and death may result.

Through an unclear mechanism, hCG appears to be a trigger for OHSS. The syndrome is usually manifested within a week of exogenous hCG administration and oocyte retrieval and has a second peak of incidence after implantation as a result of the rise in endogenous hCG.

Risk factors include young age, low body mass index, use of gonadotropin-releasing hormone analogues and exogenous hCG, elevated estradiol levels, increased number of stimulated follicles during controlled ovarian hyperstimulation ("necklace sign" or "string of pearls" appearance on US images), polycystic ovarian disease, and previous OHSS (**Box 125.8**).

### Presenting Signs and Symptoms

Patients have abdominal pain and distention, nausea, and vomiting and may complain of constipation or diarrhea. Chest discomfort, dyspnea, concentrated oliguria, rapid weight gain, and peripheral edema are symptoms of more severe cases.

Physical examination reveals abdominal distention with tenderness in the bilateral lower quadrants and tender, enlarged ovaries. Increasing evidence of third spacing such as peripheral edema, ascites, dull lung fields consistent with pleural effusion, and distant heart sounds are evident in patients with severe disease.

**BOX 125.8 Risk Factors for Ovarian Hyperstimulation Syndrome**

- Younger than 35 years
- Low body mass index
- Use of gonadotropin-releasing hormone analogues and gonadotropins
- Elevated estradiol levels
- Increased number of stimulated follicles during controlled ovarian hyperstimulation
- Polycystic ovarian disease
- Previous episode of ovarian hyperstimulation syndrome

### Differential Diagnosis and Medical Decision Making

Laboratory testing reveals serum estradiol levels elevated to higher than 3000 pg/mL, hemoconcentration with hyponatremia and hyperkalemia, and decreased renal function. Pelvic US with Doppler is essential to evaluate for the presence of ascites (**Fig. 125.3**) and the extent of follicular recruitment (**Fig. 125.4**) while ruling out alternative diagnoses such as ovarian torsion.

### Treatment

No specific cure is available for OHSS; treatment is empiric and focused on supportive care until spontaneous resolution occurs (**Table 125.7**). The syndrome is usually self-limited.

Early detection and prevention are key. Individuals at risk should receive only low-dose gonadotropins and be monitored closely by the fertility specialist. The development of symptoms, elevated estradiol levels (>3000 pg/mL), or excessive follicular recruitment (>20) calls for the initiation of preventive treatment strategies such as decreasing hormone dosages, freezing the embryos rather than waiting for fresh embryo transfer, administering albumin during oocyte harvesting, and

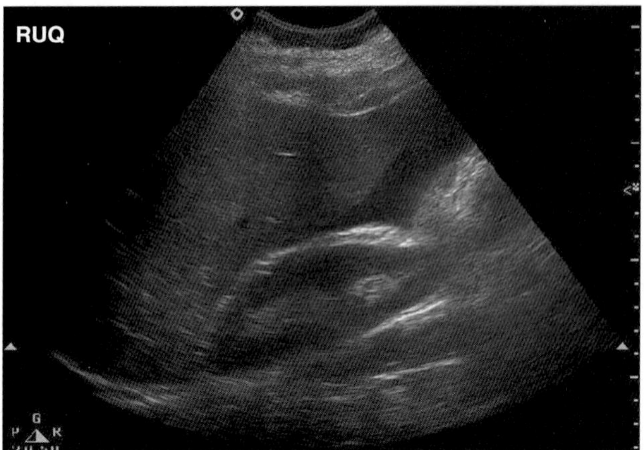


**Fig. 125.3** Ascites and pleural effusion in a patient with ovarian hyperstimulation syndrome.

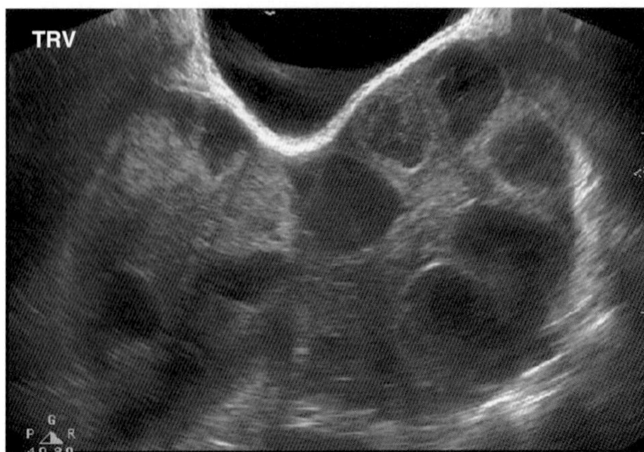


**Fig. 125.4** Polycystic ovarian syndrome affecting both ovaries in a patient with ovarian hyperstimulation syndrome.

**Table 125.7 Management of Patients with Ovarian Hyperstimulation Syndrome**

| SEVERITY | SIGNS AND SYMPTOMS | MANAGEMENT |
|---|---|---|
| Mild | Abdominal discomfort, distention, pain<br>Enlarged ovaries (up to 5 cm)<br>Minimal ascites<br>Weight gain of <10 lb | Outpatient management<br>Analgesia<br>Increased oral fluid intake (high-salt solutions)<br>Close follow-up with regular visits<br>Report if symptoms worsen |
| Moderate | **AS ABOVE, PLUS:**<br>Enlarged ovaries (5-12 cm)<br>Nausea, vomiting, diarrhea<br>Ultrasonographic evidence of ascites<br>Hemoconcentration (Hct < 45%) | Admit to the hospital<br>Daily assessment<br>Thromboembolic prophylaxis<br>Monitor laboratory tests—CBC, electrolytes, blood urea nitrogen, creatinine, liver function tests, coagulation profile |
| Severe | **AS ABOVE, PLUS:**<br>Clinical evidence of ascites<br>Palpable ovaries<br>Hepatic dysfunction<br>Hydrothorax, dyspnea<br>Peripheral edema, anasarca<br>Oliguria<br>Hemoconcentration (Hct > 45%, Hg > 15 g)<br>Hypotension<br>Renal insufficiency (Cr=1.0-1.5 mg/dL) | Admit to the intensive care unit<br>Strict fluid balance with input of 3 L or more<br>2 large-bore IV catheters (18 gauge or larger)<br>Consider central venous pressure line<br>Consider IV albumin<br>Thoracentesis or paracentesis as needed<br>Thromboembolic prophylaxis<br>Terminate the ART cycle |
| Critical | **AS ABOVE, PLUS:**<br>Severely contracted blood volume (Hct > 55%, WBC count > 25,000)<br>Renal failure (Cr > 1.6 mg/dL)<br>Thromboembolism<br>Acute respiratory distress syndrome | Admit to the intensive care unit<br>Strict fluid balance with input of 3 L or more<br>2 large-bore IV catheters, central venous pressure line<br>IV albumin<br>Intubation and ventilation<br>Thoracentesis or paracentesis as needed<br>Hemodialysis as needed<br>Anticoagulation or IVC filter as required<br>Terminate the ART cycle |

*ART*, Assisted reproductive technology; *CBC*, complete blood count; *Cr*, creatinine; *Hct*, hematocrit; *Hg*, hemoglobin; *IV*, intravenous; *IVC*, inferior vena cava; *WBC*, white blood cell.

"coasting" (withholding further gonadotropin administration until estradiol levels decrease, which allows fresh embryo retrieval and transfer). In extreme circumstances, the stimulation protocol should be terminated.

MILD CASES Mild cases can be managed on an outpatient basis with very close follow-up and daily monitoring of weight, abdominal girth, and urine output. Conservative management focuses on treating pain and maintaining hydration, although some treatment strategies include high-protein diets and high-sodium drinks (e.g., exercise rehydration drinks). Progressive symptoms or weight gain of more than 2 lb should prompt hospital admission. In the absence of pregnancy, the symptoms are expected to resolve about 2 weeks after hCG was administered.

MODERATE CASES Patients with moderate disease require a complete work-up, including laboratory tests and US, and hospitalization is recommended for close observation and serial examinations, as well as for symptomatic care if the patient has disabling nausea, intractable abdominal pain, tense ascites, abnormal laboratory values, or other indications of a downward trajectory. Pelvic examination is *not* recommended in moderate or severe cases because of the risk for cyst rupture with hemorrhage.[16] There should be a low threshold for admission to the hospital for monitoring, but typically these patients are being very closely followed by their fertility specialist; if the symptoms are controlled adequately, the patient can be discharged to follow-up in the next 1 to 3 days. She should be instructed to maintain a record of fluid balance and avoid physical activity.

SEVERE CASES Severe OHSS requires inpatient care in the intensive care unit.[17] Strict monitoring of fluid balance and hemodynamics is critical. Large-bore IV access must be established for fluid resuscitation, and a subclavian line for central venous pressure is advised.

Aggressive repletion of the intravascular space starts with at least 2 to 3 L of normal saline. If urine output remains inadequate (<50 mL/hr), salt-poor IV albumin (or hydroxyethyl starch) is the next step. Lactated Ringer solution should be avoided because of elevated potassium levels.

Ongoing oliguria and renal failure in the face of aggressive volume repletion may be due to abdominal compartment syndrome with elevated intraperitoneal pressure compressing the renal vasculature. This can be relieved with therapeutic paracentesis. Bedside US guidance is recommended to avoid puncturing the enlarged ovaries.

Diuretics are not suggested as first-line care because they may deplete the intravascular space and increase the risk for thromboembolism; however, once hemodilution has been achieved, following each 100 mg of albumin with 10 to 20 mg of furosemide may be of benefit in patients with recalcitrant prerenal azotemia.

Prophylaxis for deep vein thrombosis is essential given the high risk for thromboembolic disease.

Syndrome-associated hypoglobulinemia results in a relative immunosuppression. Antibiotic choice should target specific suspected infectious causes.

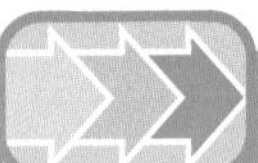

**PRIORITY ACTIONS**

**Complications of Assisted Reproductive Technologies**

**Induction Phase**

Abdominal pain, distention or ascites? Initiate a work-up and symptomatic treatment of OHSS. Obtain a US scan and estradiol levels.

Difficulty breathing and unstable? If signs of third spacing are present, suspect severe OHSS; start aggressive symptomatic and supportive treatment. Admit to the ICU.

Dyspnea with only leg edema or without any evidence of third spacing? Consider PE; obtain a chest radiograph. Anticoagulation and lower extremity vascular Doppler US are required to evaluate for DVT. If still equivocal, obtain a helical CT scan of the chest with IV contrast enhancement

Pelvic pain? Consider early OHSS.

**Any Time During ART**

Pelvic pain? Perform Doppler US to evaluate for ovarian torsion versus ovarian cyst rupture.

**After Oocyte Harvesting**

Fever? Consider infection; administer antibiotics and evaluate whether stable for discharge.

Vaginal bleeding from a puncture site? Place pressure. If the bleeding does not stop, consider Monsel solution or silver nitrate.

Abdominal pain or peritoneal signs? Consider intraperitoneal hemorrhage; cardiovascular stabilization and definitive exploratory laparotomy are required.

**After Implantation or Embryo Transfer**

Pelvic pain or vaginal bleeding? Perform or obtain a pelvic US and check quantitative β-hCG to evaluate for ectopic or heterotopic pregnancy or threatened spontaneous miscarriage.

*ART*, Assisted reproductive technology; *DVT*, deep vein thrombosis; *hCG*, human chorionic gonadotropin; *ICU*, intensive care unit; *IV*, intravenous; *OHSS*, ovarian hyperstimulation syndrome; *PE*, pulmonary embolism; *US*, ultrasonography.

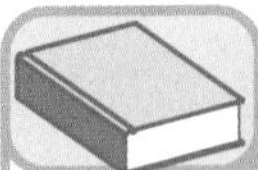

**PATIENT TEACHING TIPS**

**Ovarian Hyperstimulation Syndrome**

Clarify the details of the anticipated therapeutic course.

Schedule follow-up with the patient's physician in 1 to 3 days.

Instruct her to call her physician or return to the emergency department immediately if progressive symptoms of ovarian hyperstimulation syndrome develop, including:

- Chest discomfort
- Difficulty breathing
- Abdominal pain
- Bloating and swelling, rapid weight gain
- Decreased urination
- Severe or persistent vomiting

Warn the patient that there can be a second peak in symptoms *after* implantation triggered by her own hormonal surge.

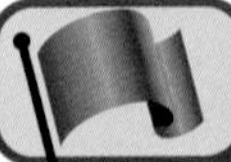

**RED FLAGS**

**Complications of Assisted Reproductive Technology**

Increased abdominal girth, abdominal pain, edema, and dyspnea during induction of ovulation or early after implantation are suspicious for ovarian hyperstimulation syndrome.

Unilateral pelvic pain is suspicious for ectopic pregnancy or ovarian torsion.

Severe pain, fever, brisk bleeding, and peritoneal signs are suspicious for perforation.

Shortness of breath, possibly with pleuritic chest pain, should prompt evaluation for pulmonary embolism, although pleural effusions as a result of ovarian hyperstimulation syndrome are also possible.

Selection of medication must take into careful consideration the possible presence of early pregnancy.

CRITICAL CASES Critical cases with complications such as renal failure, thromboembolism, or acute respiratory distress syndrome require all of the previously described measures and termination of the pregnancy.

## REFERENCES

*References can be found on Expert Consult @ www.expertconsult.com.*

# Gynecologic Infections 126

*Jamil D. Bayram and Mamta Malik*

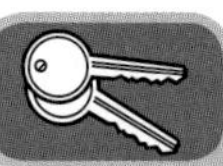

**KEY POINTS**

- Not all gynecologic infections, including pelvic inflammatory disease, are sexually transmitted, although many are. They are often asymptomatic in women and their sex partners.
- Sexually transmitted diseases are common, particularly in young, sexually active women with multiple sex partners.
- A careful history, physical examination, and diagnostic tests are important to differentiate gynecologic infections because modalities of treatments vary.
- Microscopic diagnosis of yeast infections has a sensitivity of only 50% and fails to diagnosis the disorder in a large percentage of patients with symptomatic vulvovaginal candidiasis.
- Most young, sexually active patients with genital ulcers have a genital herpes infection; syphilis or chancroid disease should be considered as well.
- Treatment should be instituted for most gynecologic infections based on the presumed diagnosis because many patients with genital infections will not have a laboratory-confirmed diagnosis.
- Gonorrhea is becoming increasingly resistant to antibiotics; the clinician should check local susceptibilities before treatment.

## EPIDEMIOLOGY

Gynecologic infections are often asymptomatic in women, and the majority of these infections are transmitted sexually. In 2009, the Centers for Disease Control and Prevention (CDC) reported approximately 19 million new sexually transmitted infections with an estimated cost of $16.4 billion annually.[1] Many cases of sexually transmitted diseases in the United States, such as human papillomavirus (HPV) and genital herpes, are not reported to the CDC.

## Diseases Characterized by Genital Ulcers

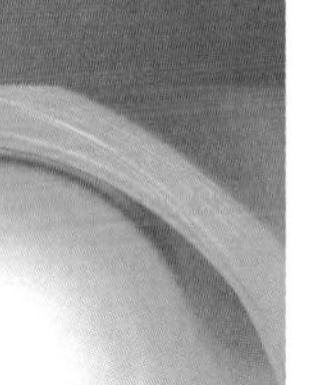

Genital ulcers may also be caused by chancroid, granuloma inguinale, herpes simplex virus (HSV), lymphogranuloma venereum (LGV), and syphilis.

## CHANCROID

### EPIDEMIOLOGY

The number of reported cases of chancroid in the United States has varied for the past 10 years but remains very low. Only 28 cases were reported domestically in 2009.[1]

### PATHOPHYSIOLOGY

Chancroid, a sexually transmitted disease caused by the short gram-negative bacillus *Haemophilus ducreyi*, is characterized by painful genital ulcers and painful lymphadenopathy.[2] The incubation period is 4 to 7 days.

*H. ducreyi* infection occurs through loss of integrity of the epithelial layer of the skin, most commonly following minor trauma such as sexual intercourse. Once the bacteria have breached the integument, secretion of a cytologically lethal toxin causes apoptosis and necrosis of cells, which results in the characteristic ulcer formation seen with chancroid.

### PRESENTING SIGNS AND SYMPTOMS

*H. ducreyi* forms a vesicopustule that progresses to a painful ulcer with a necrotic base and surrounding erythema. Because of autoinoculation, multiple lesions may develop.

The adenitis is generally unilateral and tender with overlying erythema. The lesions may become fluctuant and rupture spontaneously. Fever, chills, and malaise may accompany the lymphadenitis. Women may have adenitis without external ulcerative lesions.

## DIFFERENTIAL DIAGNOSIS AND MEDICAL DECISION MAKING

Chancroid must be differentiated from other genital ulcers based on clinical findings. The chancre of syphilis, for example, is clean and painless with a hard base. The diagnosis of chancroid is established by culturing a swab of the lesion onto a specific medium.

The presence of more than one sexually transmitted disease is very common (including syphilis, HSV infection, and human immunodeficiency virus [HIV] infection), as is infection of the ulcer with fusiforms, spirochetes, and other organisms.

## TREATMENT

Several treatment regimens have been recommended and are listed in **Box 126.1**.[3,4]

## FOLLOW-UP, NEXT STEPS IN CARE, AND PATIENT EDUCATION

Follow-up within 1 week to reevaluate the ulceration is recommended. Safe sex practices, such as condom use, as well as regular genital self-examination, should be discussed. Sexual partners should be informed.

# GRANULOMA INGUINALE (DONOVANOSIS)

## EPIDEMIOLOGY

The incidence of granuloma inguinale is low, with less than 100 cases reported in the United States per year. The peak demographic of occurrence is in people between the ages of 20 and 40 years who are sexually active.

**BOX 126.1 Recommended Treatment Regimens for Chancroid**

Azithromycin, 1 g orally once
*or*
Ceftriaxone, 250 mg intramuscularly once
*or*
Ciprofloxacin, 500 mg orally twice per day for 3 days*
*or*
Erythromycin base, 500 mg orally three times per day for 7 days

*Ciprofloxacin is contraindicated in pregnant and lactating women.

## PATHOPHYSIOLOGY

Granuloma inguinale is a chronic granulomatous anogenital infection caused by *Calymmatobacterium granulomatis*. Granuloma inguinale is primarily a sexually transmitted disease, but gastrointestinal transmission is possible. Its onset is insidious, with a median incubation period of about 50 days.

## PRESENTING SIGNS AND SYMPTOMS

The lesions, which can occur on the skin and mucous membranes of the genitalia or perineal area, are relatively painless nodules that transform into shallow, sharply demarcated ulcers with a red base. The lesions spread by contiguity, and the ulcer then becomes purulent, painful, and foul smelling.

## DIFFERENTIAL DIAGNOSIS AND MEDICAL DECISION MAKING

*C. granulomatis* is difficult to culture because it is an intracellular parasite. Identification is usually made from scraped material or a biopsy specimen obtained from the periphery of the lesion. Bipolar-staining bacteria are best identified within mononuclear cells (Donovan bodies) by Wright or Giemsa staining. Note that genital ulcers are also caused by syphilis, chancroid, and LGV.

## TREATMENT

See **Box 126.2** for treatment.

## FOLLOW-UP, NEXT STEPS IN CARE, AND PATIENT EDUCATION

Risk for relapse remains a concern for up to 18 months after treatment. Carcinoma (squamous and basal cell variants) is

**BOX 126.2 Treatment Regimens for Donovanosis**

A. **Recommended regimen:**
- Doxycycline, 100 mg orally twice per day for at least 3 weeks and until all lesions have healed completely*

B. **Alternative regimens** (all given orally for a duration of at least 3 weeks and until all lesions have healed completely):
- Azithromycin, 1 g/wk
  *or*
- Ciprofloxacin, 750 mg twice per day*
  *or*
- Erythromycin base, 500 mg four times per day
  *or*
- Trimethoprim-sulfamethoxazole, 160 mg/800 mg (1 tablet) twice per day*

*Doxycycline and ciprofloxacin are contraindicated in pregnant and lactating women. Sulfonamides are relatively contraindicated.

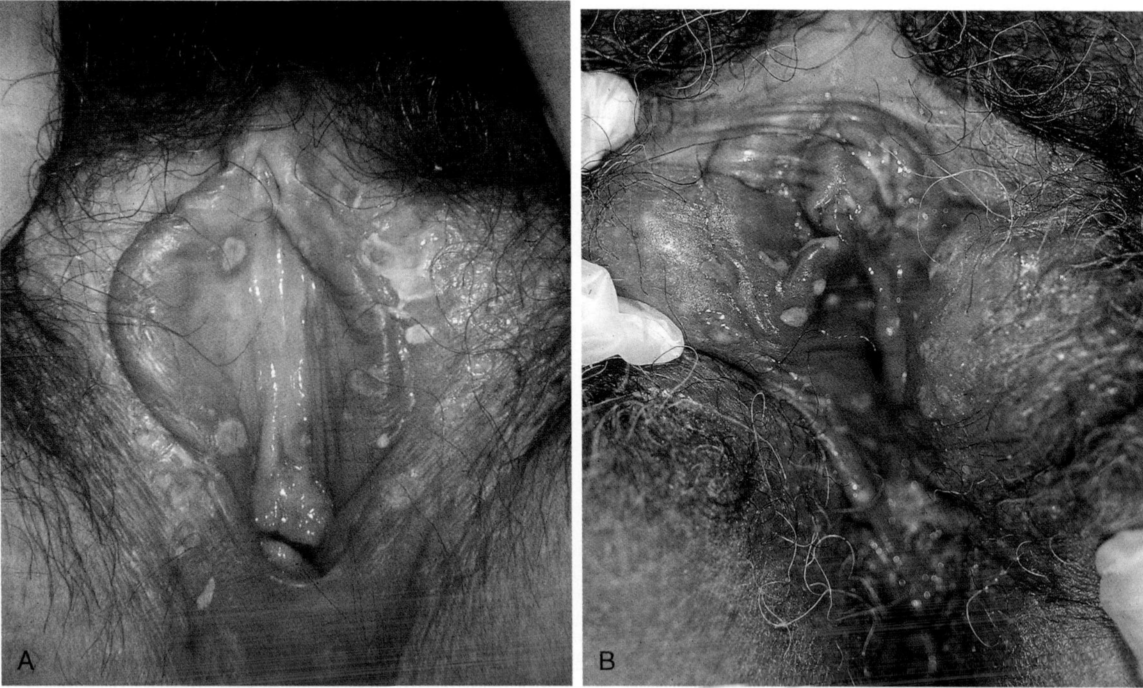

**Fig. 126.1** **Primary herpes simplex. A,** Scattered erosions covered with exudate. **B,** Numerous erosions appeared 4 days after contact with an asymptomatic carrier. (From Habif TP. Clinical dermatology. 4th ed. Philadelphia: Mosby; 2004.)

the most concerning sequela of granuloma inguinale and occurs in 0.25% of patients. Lymphatic destruction may result in elephantiasis of the genitals. Increased risk of acquiring HIV infection exists when granuloma inguinale is present.

## HERPES SIMPLEX VIRUS

### EPIDEMIOLOGY

HSV is widespread in the United States, with approximately 50 million people infected,[5] and it is the most common cause of genital ulcers. The overall domestic seroprevalence of subtype 2 (HSV-2) is 16.2%, but infection rates are considerably higher (39.2%) in African Americans.[1] HSV-2 is the most common variant causing genital infections, but subtype 1 (HSV-1) is the causative agent in up to 10% to 15% of all cases.[1]

### PATHOPHYSIOLOGY

Two types of HSV may cause genital herpes: HSV-1 and HSV-2. Once acquired, genital herpes becomes a lifelong infection. Herpes simplex is a DNA virus with an incubation period ranging from 2 to 7 days.[5] Transmission occurs through exposure to infectious secretions of mucosal surfaces or through skin microabrasions during sexual contact.

### PRESENTING SIGNS AND SYMPTOMS

Of all HSV-2 infections studied, 81.1% were reported to be asymptomatic or were not recognized.[5] Symptoms usually begin with painful lesions that are often described as burning (**Fig. 126.1**). These lesions begin as vesicles and then rupture to expose an ulcerated base that persists for 1 to 2 weeks before crusting over and healing without scars. The vesicles and ulcers contain many highly infectious virus particles, and viral shedding occurs until the lesions disappear. Vulvar lesions may last for 3 or more weeks before complete healing. The cervix and vagina may also be involved, with a gray, necrotic cervix and profuse leukorrhea. External dysuria is common, and bilateral inguinal lymphadenopathy is usual.

The primary episode, defined as genital herpes without antibodies to HSV-1 and HSV-2, is typically associated with systemic symptoms, including headache, fever, malaise, and other flulike symptoms in about two thirds of the cases.

Following primary infection, latent HSV usually localizes in the sacral ganglion and perhaps the dermis. Recurrent attacks tend to be more subtle and are the most frequently seen outbreaks in the emergency department (ED). Recurrence can be precipitated by immunodeficiency, trauma, fever, or sexual intercourse.

### DIFFERENTIAL DIAGNOSIS AND MEDICAL DECISION MAKING

A significant number of patients with the typical signs and symptoms of herpesvirus infection are later found to have syphilis; therefore, screening for treponemal antibodies is an important part of the ED evaluation. The diagnosis of HSV infection can be made clinically if the typical, painful, shallow multiple vulvar ulcers are present. Laboratory confirmation is best attained by polymerase chain reaction (PCR) testing.

**BOX 126.3 Treatment Regimens for Herpes Simplex Virus**

A. **Initial infection** (first episode): Recommended regimens for initial infection should be given orally for 7 to 10 days (may be extended if healing is incomplete).
- Acyclovir, 400 mg three times per day or 200 mg five times per day
  *or*
- Famciclovir, 250 mg three times per day
  *or*
- Valacyclovir, 1 g twice per day

B. **Recurrent infection** (episodic treatment): Recommended regimens are given orally.
- Acyclovir, 400 mg three times per day for 5 days, 800 mg twice per day for 5 days, or 800 mg three times per day for 2 days
  *or*
- Famciclovir, 125 mg twice per day for 5 days, 1 g twice per day for 1 day, or 500 mg once followed by 250 mg twice daily for 1 day
  *or*
- Valacyclovir, 500 mg twice per day for 3 days or 1 g once per day for 5 days

C. **Suppressive therapy**: Given for frequent recurrent infections and includes several recommended oral regimens.
- Acyclovir, 400 mg twice per day
  *or*
- Famciclovir, 250 mg twice daily
  *or*
- Valacyclovir, 1 g once per day

From Centers for Disease Control and Prevention. Sexually transmitted diseases treatment guidelines, 2010. Atlanta: U.S. Department of Health and Human Services; 2010. Available at http://www.cdc.gov/mmwr/preview/mmwrhtml/rr5912a1.htm. Accessed May 30, 2012.

## TREATMENT

Treatment of HSV infection is dependent on the onset of clinical symptoms (acute versus recurrent) and their frequency, which determines the need for suppressive therapy (**Box 126.3**).

## FOLLOW-UP, NEXT STEPS IN CARE, AND PATIENT EDUCATION

Timely outpatient referral to gynecology should be made. Patients should be informed of the potential for recurrent episodes, as well as the potential for transmission of HSV even when symptoms are not present. Sexual activity should be avoided when active genital lesions or prodromal symptoms are present. In pregnant patients, immediate referral to obstetrics for potential cesarean section to avoid transmission of the virus from mother to fetus should be made if rupture of membranes has occurred. HSV serves as a cofactor in the transmission of HIV.

# LYMPHOGRANULOMA VENEREUM

## EPIDEMIOLOGY

LGV is rarely reported in developed countries—perhaps in part because of the lack of a standardized diagnostic test or surveillance requirements. However, outbreaks have been reported in populations of homosexual men in Western Europe and North America since 2003, with the largest cluster of case reports occurring in the United Kingdom and New York City.[6]

## PATHOPHYSIOLOGY

LGV is an acute or chronic sexually transmitted disease caused by *Chlamydia trachomatis* types L1, L2, and L3. The disease is acquired during intercourse or through contact with contaminated exudates from active lesions. *C. trachomatis* enters the system through loss of skin integrity (breaks and abrasions) or by crossing the epithelial cells of mucous membranes and multiplies in regional lymph nodes after lymphatic dissemination. The primary mode of transmission is sexual; however, spread by fomites, nonsexual personal contact, and laboratory accidents has been documented.

## PRESENTING SIGNS AND SYMPTOMS

The most common clinical manifestation of LGV in heterosexuals is tender inguinal or femoral lymphadenopathy (or both), which is typically unilateral. The initial vesicular or ulcerative lesion is transient and often goes unnoticed. Inguinal buboes appear 1 to 4 weeks after exposure and have a tendency to fuse, soften, and break down to form multiple draining sinuses with extensive scarring. In women, genital lymph drainage is to the perirectal glands. Early anorectal manifestations include proctitis with tenesmus and bloody purulent discharge; late manifestations are chronic inflammation of rectal and perirectal tissue. These changes can lead to obstipation, rectal stricture, and occasionally, rectovaginal and perianal fistulas.

## DIFFERENTIAL DIAGNOSIS AND MEDICAL DECISION MAKING

The early lesion of LGV must be differentiated from the lesions of syphilis, genital herpes simplex, chancroid, and granuloma inguinale; lymph node involvement must be distinguished from that caused by tularemia, tuberculosis, plague, neoplasm, or pyogenic infection; and rectal stricture must be distinguished from that secondary to neoplasm and ulcerative colitis.

The complement fixation test may be positive, but cross-reaction with other chlamydiae occurs. Although a positive reaction may reflect remote infection, high titers usually indicate active disease. Specific immunofluorescence tests for immunoglobulin M are more specific for acute infection.

**BOX 126.4 Treatment Regimens for Lymphogranuloma Venereum**

A. **Recommended regimen**: It is the preferred treatment.
   - Doxycycline, 100 mg orally twice per day for 21 days*
B. **Alternative regimen**: Recommended regimens are given orally.
   Erythromycin, 500 mg four times per day for 21 days

From Centers for Disease Control and Prevention. Sexually transmitted diseases treatment guidelines, 2010. Atlanta: U.S. Department of Health and Human Services; 2010. Available at http://www.cdc.gov/mmwr/preview/mmwrhtml/rr5912a1.htm. Accessed May 30, 2012.
*Doxycycline is contraindicated in pregnant women.

## TREATMENT

**Box 126.4** details the treatment regimen for LGV.

## FOLLOW-UP, NEXT STEPS IN CARE, AND PATIENT EDUCATION

Appropriate treatment should resolve all symptoms and result in no significant sequelae. Patients should be advised to notify sexual contacts to be evaluated for possible infection. Complications of LGV include cervicitis, perimetritis, salpingitis, fistula development, and rectal stricture.

# SYPHILIS

## EPIDEMIOLOGY

Rates in women increased from 0.8 case per 100,000 in 2004 to 1.4 cases per 100,000 in 2009 despite a previously decreasing incidence.[1]

## PATHOPHYSIOLOGY

Syphilis is a systemic, sexually transmitted disease caused by the spirochete *Treponema pallidum*. It can also be acquired congenitally. The risk for transmission following sexual exposure depends on many factors and is estimated to be about 30%.[7] *T. pallidum* causes infection after traversing mucous membrane surfaces or denuded skin and then extending systemically through hematogenous and lymphatic routes.

## PRESENTING SIGNS AND SYMPTOMS

Syphilis can be seen in the ED in any of the four stages through which untreated syphilis can pass. Primary infection is manifested as a single, painless ulcer, usually within 3 weeks but sometimes 2 to 3 months after infection. The labia and vaginal walls are most often affected; however, lesions can also occur on the cervix (**Fig. 126.2**). Secondary syphilis is associated with a characteristic maculopapular generalized rash on the palms and soles and may include components of arthralgia, pharyngitis, and lymphadenopathy. This stage is typically seen 4 to 10 weeks after the initial appearance of a chancre. Infectivity can occur in the first two stages (up to 2 to 4 years following infection).

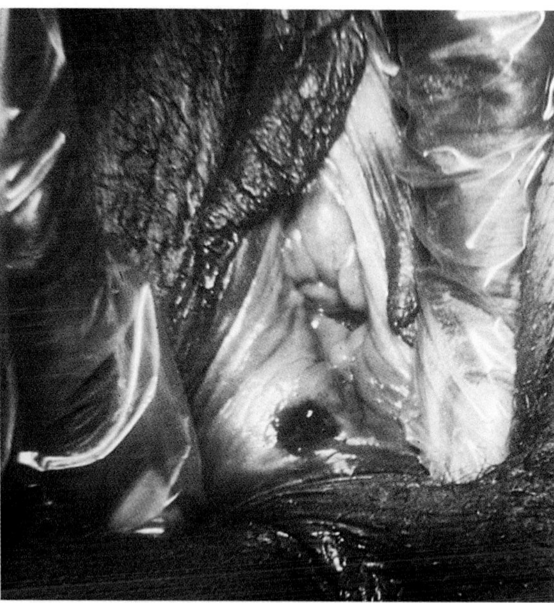

**Fig. 126.2 Primary syphilis with a chancre in the vagina.** The lesions are painless and may never be detected.

The third stage—the asymptomatic latent phase—may last many years. It is defined as syphilis characterized by seroreactivity without other evidence of disease.

The fourth stage—tertiary syphilis—has numerous neurologic, cardiovascular, and other systemic effects and develops in about 25% of untreated patients.[6]

## DIFFERENTIAL DIAGNOSIS AND MEDICAL DECISION MAKING

The diagnosis of syphilis should be considered in any patient with an ulcerative lesion in the genital area, as well as in patients with unexplained rashes, arthralgia, and neurologic or systemic complaints.

Screening includes the rapid plasma reagin and Venereal Disease Research Laboratory tests, which must be followed by confirmatory testing when positive. If the serologic results are nonreactive and spirochetes cannot be demonstrated by darkfield examination, the serologic tests should be repeated in 1 month.

## TREATMENT

Penicillin remains the mainstay of treatment across the board (**Box 126.5**). According to the CDC guidelines, parenteral penicillin is considered to be the only treatment documented to be efficacious in pregnancy.[3] Treatment with penicillin is the same as for the corresponding stage of syphilis in nonpregnant women. For pregnant patients who are allergic to penicillin, tetracycline and doxycycline are contraindicated. Pregnant patients who are allergic to penicillin should be skin-tested and desensitized.

**BOX 126.5 Treatment Regimens for Syphilis**

A. **Primary and secondary infections**:
- Benzathine penicillin G, 2.4 million units intramuscularly [IM]
- For penicillin-allergic nonpregnant patients:
  - Doxycycline, 100 mg orally twice daily for 14 days

  *or*
  - Tetracycline, 500 mg orally four times daily for 14 days
- For children and infants:
  - Benzathine penicillin G, 50,000 U/kg IM up to the adult dose of 2.4 million units

B. **Latent syphilis**:
- Benzathine penicillin G, 7.2 million units total administered as 3 doses of 2.4 million units IM each at 1-week intervals
- For penicillin-allergic nonpregnant patients:
  - Doxycycline, 100 mg orally twice daily for 28 days

  *or*
  - Tetracycline, 500 mg orally four times daily for 28 days
- For children and infants:
  - Benzathine penicillin G, 50,000 U/kg IM up to the adult dose of 2.4 million units administered as 3 doses at 1-week intervals (total of 150,000 U/kg up to the adult total dose of 7.2 million units)

C. **Tertiary syphilis** (with no evidence of neurosyphilis): For example, patients with gumma and cardiovascular syphilis.
- Benzathine penicillin G, 7.2 million units total administered as 3 doses of 2.4 million units IM each at 1-week intervals
- Consult infectious disease specialists for penicillin-allergic patients

D. **Neurosyphilis**:
- Recommended regimen: Aqueous crystalline penicillin G, 18 to 24 million U/day administered as 3 to 4 million units intravenously (IV) every 4 hours or as a continuous infusion for 10 to 14 days
- Alternative regimen: Procaine penicillin, 2.4 million units IM once daily, plus probenecid, 500 mg orally four times per day, both for 10 to 14 days
- Limited data suggest that ceftriaxone, 2 g daily either IM or IV for 10 to 14 days, may be effective for patients with neurosyphilis

From Centers for Disease Control and Prevention. Sexually transmitted diseases treatment guidelines, 2010. Atlanta: U.S. Department of Health and Human Services; 2010. Available at http://www.cdc.gov/mmwr/preview/mmwrhtml/rr5912a1.htm. Accessed May 30, 2012.

The Jarisch-Herxheimer reaction, caused by massive release of treponemal antigens and manifested by fever, headache, and myalgias, can occur in any patient in the first 24 hours following initiation of therapy and is observed most often in patients with early syphilis (frequently in those with secondary syphilis). Because this reaction in pregnant women may precipitate early labor or cause fetal distress, these patients should be hospitalized for monitoring. Concern for this reaction should not prevent or delay therapy. Systemic glucocorticoids administered 12 hours before or concurrent with antibiotics may minimize the effects, and antipyretics have been used for supportive care.

## FOLLOW-UP, NEXT STEPS IN CARE, AND PATIENT EDUCATION

Quantitative serologic tests should be performed in patients with syphilis to monitor the results of treatment. Sexual contacts must be notified and evaluated for possible infection. All patients with syphilis should be tested for HIV to assess for possible coinfection. Delay in diagnosis during pregnancy past 20 weeks' gestation should prompt fetal ultrasound to rule out congenital syphilis.

# Diseases Characterized by Vaginal Discharge

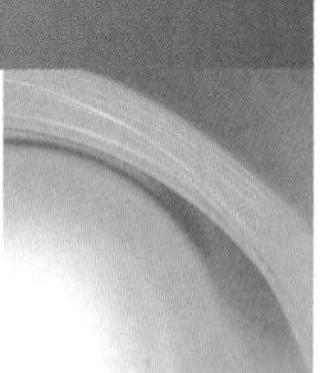

## BACTERIAL VAGINOSIS

### EPIDEMIOLOGY

Although the range is wide, depending on the population, prevalence rates for bacterial vaginosis (BV) have been estimated to be 4% to 40%. However, because *Gardnerella vaginalis* is present in 50% to 70% of asymptomatic women, the exact incidence of BV is difficult to estimate.[8]

### PATHOPHYSIOLOGY

BV is a polymicrobial infection that results from replacement of the normal *Lactobacillus* species in the vagina by high concentrations of the anaerobic *G. vaginalis, Mycoplasma hominis*, and *Mobiluncus curtisii*. It can be a precursor infection to upper genital tract extension, including cervicitis and pelvic inflammatory disease (PID). Infection is related to the *Lactobacillus* concentration and changes in pH within the vaginal vault but remains primarily multifactorial.

### PRESENTING SIGNS AND SYMPTOMS

Clinical signs include a thick, homogeneous, milky vaginal discharge sometimes with a fishy odor. Usually, no other symptoms are present.

### DIFFERENTIAL DIAGNOSIS AND MEDICAL DECISION MAKING

BV can be diagnosed with the use of clinical criteria (see Amsel's diagnostic criteria below) or Gram stain, with the latter considered to be the "gold standard" laboratory method for diagnosis.

Clinical diagnosis requires three of the following four criteria:

- Homogeneous, thin vaginal fluid that adheres to the vaginal walls
- Presence of vaginal epithelial cells with borders obscured by adherent small bacteria (clue cells)
- Vaginal fluid pH higher than 4.5
- Release of an amine "fishy" odor with alkalinization (adding 10% KOH) of the vaginal fluid ("whiff test")

## TREATMENT

Only women with symptoms require treatment (**Box 126.6**).

## FOLLOW-UP, NEXT STEPS IN CARE, AND PATIENT EDUCATION

Recurrence rates for BV have not been shown to be affected by treatment of males; therefore, sex partners do not need to be referred for evaluation. Follow-up is recommended only if symptoms persist after treatment.

# TRICHOMONIASIS

## EPIDEMIOLOGY

Trichomoniasis affects 2 to 3 million women in the United States per year. A total of 216,000 visits to physician offices were reported in women 15 to 44 years of age for this issue in 2009 alone.[1]

### BOX 126.6 Treatment Regimens for Bacterial Vaginosis

A. **Recommended regimens**:
- Metronidazole, 500 mg orally twice per day for 7 days
  *or*
- Metronidazole gel 0.75%, one full applicator (5 g) intravaginally once per day for 5 days
  *or*
- Clindamycin cream 2%, one full applicator (5 g) intravaginally at bedtime for 7 days

B. **Alternative regimens**:
- Tinidazole, 2 g orally once daily for 2 days or 1 g orally once daily for 5 days
  *or*
- Clindamycin, 300 mg orally twice daily for 7 days
  *or*
- Clindamycin ovules, 100 mg intravaginally once at bedtime for 3 days

From Centers for Disease Control and Prevention. Sexually transmitted diseases treatment guidelines, 2010. Atlanta: U.S. Department of Health and Human Services; 2010. Available at http://www.cdc.gov/mmwr/preview/mmwrhtml/rr5912a1.htm. Accessed May 30, 2012.

## PATHOPHYSIOLOGY

Trichomoniasis is caused by *Trichomonas vaginalis*, an anaerobic protozoan that is transmitted primarily through sexual activity. *T. vaginalis* measures 10 μm in diameter and structurally has a flagellum that allows it to move around vaginal and urethral tissues. The incubation period for infection ranges from 4 to 28 days.

## PRESENTING SIGNS AND SYMPTOMS

Many women infected with *T. vaginalis* are asymptomatic. Typical symptoms, if present, include vulvar irritation, dyspareunia, dysuria, urinary frequency, and a malodorous, profuse, purulent vaginal discharge. Physical examination may reveal an erythematous vaginal mucosa or punctate hemorrhages on the cervix.

## DIFFERENTIAL DIAGNOSIS AND MEDICAL DECISION MAKING

Although candidiasis and BV are included in the differential diagnosis of vaginitis, trichomonal infections are less typically associated with pruritus or malodor.[1] The diagnosis is made by identification of motile trichomonads on a saline wet preparation but are seen in only 60% to 70% of confirmed cases when cultures are performed.

## TREATMENT

Treatment regimens are listed in **Box 126.7**. Patients with allergy to a nitroimidazole may undergo metronidazole desensitization. Because of adverse pregnancy outcomes with *Trichomonas* infection, such as premature rupture of membranes, preterm delivery, and low birth weight, women can be treated with 2 g metronidazole in a single dose at any stage of pregnancy.

### BOX 126.7 Treatment Regimens for Trichomoniasis

**Recommended Regimens**
- Metronidazole, 2 g orally in a single dose
  *or*
- Tinidazole, 2 g orally in a single dose

**Alternative Regimen**
- Metronidazole, 500 mg orally twice per day for 7 days

From Centers for Disease Control and Prevention. Sexually transmitted diseases treatment guidelines, 2010. Atlanta: U.S. Department of Health and Human Services; 2010. Available at http://www.cdc.gov/mmwr/preview/mmwrhtml/rr5912a1.htm. Accessed May 30, 2012.

## FOLLOW-UP, NEXT STEPS IN CARE, AND PATIENT EDUCATION

Patients in whom trichomoniasis is diagnosed should be advised to notify sex partners to seek treatment because of the known exposure. Investigation for persistent trichomoniasis versus an alternative diagnosis such as candidiasis or gonorrhoea should be pursued on follow-up via repeated examination if vaginal discharge is still present.

# VULVOVAGINAL CANDIDIASIS

## EPIDEMIOLOGY

Vulvovaginal candidiasis (VVC) is exceedingly common, with 75% of women expected to have at least one episode during their lifetime. However, only 10% to 20% of women will have symptoms to the extent that diagnostic and therapeutic considerations are warranted.[2]

## PATHOPHYSIOLOGY

*Candida albicans* is a normal vaginal flora that is the primary cause of 25% of cases of vaginitis and approximately 90% of vaginal yeast infections (noncandidal species cause the remaining infections). These saprophytic fungi are isolated from the vagina in 20% to 40% of asymptomatic women. Infection should especially be suspected in women who have recently been taking antibiotics or high-dose estrogen oral contraceptives and in women who are immunosuppressed (e.g., due to diabetes or corticosteroid therapy). The pH of vaginal secretions is maintained by the normal vaginal flora (lactobacilli, diphtheroids, and *Staphylococcus epidermidis*) and should be 4.0 to 4.5. Several factors such as age, phase of the menstrual cycle, hormonal contraception, and sexual activity may change the vaginal milieu by causing an increase in vaginal pH and hence may result in vulvovaginitis.

## PRESENTING SIGNS AND SYMPTOMS

Common symptoms include vulvovaginal pruritus, dyspareunia, external dysuria, and a white, thick, curdlike vaginal discharge. Physical examination typically reveals erythematous or edematous mucosa in addition to the classic discharge described previously.

## DIFFERENTIAL DIAGNOSIS AND MEDICAL DECISION MAKING

Several infections may mimic VVC; however, the diagnosis is based on the characteristic clinical findings along with microscopy. Microscopic evaluation reveals a normal pH (4 to 4.5) with hyphae, pseudohyphae, or budding yeast on a saline wet preparation or 10% potassium hydroxide preparation. Fifty percent of women with candidiasis have a negative wet mount but a positive *Candida* culture. Recurrent VVC, defined as four or more episodes of symptomatic VVC in 1 year, affects 5% of women. Vaginal cultures should be performed for patients with recurrent VVC to confirm the clinical diagnosis and to identify unusual species (including non-*albicans* species), particularly *Candida glabrata*.[9]

## TREATMENT

Treatment regimens are listed in **Box 126.8**. For recurrent VVC caused by *C. albicans*, some specialists recommend a longer duration of initial therapy (e.g., 7 to 14 days of topical therapy or a 100-mg, 150-mg, or 200-mg oral dose of fluconazole every third day for a total of three doses [days 1, 4, and 7]) before initiating a maintenance antifungal regimen. Maintenance regimens include oral fluconazole (i.e., 100-mg, 150-mg, or 200-mg dose) weekly for 6 months, which is the first line of treatment. If this regimen is not feasible, topical treatments used intermittently as a maintenance regimen can be considered. For severe VVC (i.e., extensive vulvar erythema, edema, excoriation, and fissure formation), either 7 to 14 days of topical azole or 150 mg of fluconazole in two

**BOX 126.8 Treatment Regimens for Uncomplicated Vulvovaginal Candidiasis**

**Over-the-Counter Intravaginal Agents**

- Butoconazole 2% cream, 5 g intravaginally for 3 days
  *or*
- Clotrimazole 1% cream, 5 g intravaginally for 7 to 14 days, or 2% cream, 5 g intravaginally for 3 days
  *or*
- Miconazole 2% cream, 5 g intravaginally for 7 days, or 4% cream, 5 g intravaginally for 3 days, or 100-mg vaginal suppository for 7 days, or 200-mg vaginal suppository for 3 days, or 1200-mg vaginal suppository for 1 day
  *or*
- Tioconazole 6.5% ointment, 5 g intravaginally in a single application

**Prescription Intravaginal Agents**

- Butoconazole 2% cream (single-dose bioadhesive product), 5 g intravaginally for 1 day
  *or*
- Nystatin 100,000-unit vaginal tablet, one tablet for 14 days
  *or*
- Terconazole 0.4% cream, 5 g intravaginally for 7 days, or 0.8% cream, 5 g intravaginally for 3 days, or 80-mg vaginal suppository, one suppository for 3 days

**Oral Agent**

- Fluconazole, 150-mg oral tablet, one tablet in a single dose

From Centers for Disease Control and Prevention. Sexually transmitted diseases treatment guidelines, 2010. Atlanta: U.S. Department of Health and Human Services; 2010. Available at http://www.cdc.gov/mmwr/preview/mmwrhtml/rr5912a1.htm. Accessed May 30, 2012.

sequential doses (second dose 72 hours after the initial dose) should be used.[3]

Options for the treatment of non-*albicans* VVC include a longer duration of therapy (7 to 14 days) with an azole drug other than fluconazole (oral or topical) as first-line therapy. If VVC recurs, 600 mg of boric acid in a gelatin capsule administered vaginally once daily for 2 weeks is recommended.[2]

Azole drugs are not absorbed to any degree from the vagina, and these local regimens applied for 7 days are the only ones recommended to be used safely in pregnancy.

## FOLLOW-UP, NEXT STEPS IN CARE, AND PATIENT EDUCATION

Patients in whom VVC is diagnosed should be advised to have their sex partners evaluated as well given that males with symptomatic balanitis should be identified and treated to prevent recurrent female infection. Avoidance of vaginal douching is encouraged to minimize disruption of the normal vaginal milieu.

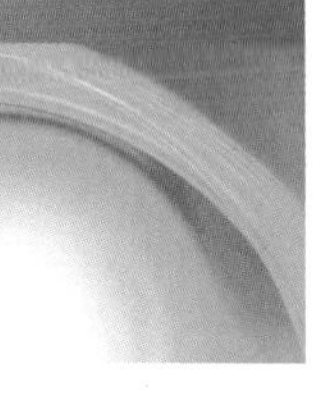

# Diseases Characterized by Cervicitis and Urethritis

## CHLAMYDIA

### EPIDEMIOLOGY

*C. trachomatis* infection is the most commonly reported notifiable disease in the United States. *C. trachomatis* and *Neisseria gonorrhoeae* are isolated in combination in about 20% to 40% of women with purulent cervicitis,[10] but accurate disease rates are limited by the fact that 80% of women infected with these pathogens are asymptomatic. During the period 2005 to 2009, the chlamydial infection rate in women increased by 20.3% (from 492.2 to 592.2 cases per 100,000 females).[1]

### PATHOPHYSIOLOGY

*C. trachomatis* is an obligate intracellular bacterium that is transmitted sexually. Chlamydial infections in women are usually asymptomatic and may lead to PID, which is a major cause of infertility and ectopic pregnancy. Women are most commonly seen with infection of the genital tract, typically 1 to 3 weeks after exposure.

### PRESENTING SIGNS AND SYMPTOMS

Chlamydial infection is usually asymptomatic and frequently not identified until overt infection develops. It causes a variety of clinical signs and symptoms, including intermenstrual or postcoital bleeding, lower abdominal pain, and even fever. *Chlamydia* can cause cervicitis, PID, and Fitz-Hugh–Curtis syndrome (FHCS).

### DIFFERENTIAL DIAGNOSIS AND MEDICAL DECISION MAKING

Chlamydial infections can be diagnosed by culture. However, newer DNA methods using ligase chain reaction or PCR offer both sensitivity and specificity not achieved with the older tests. For DNA tests, samples should be taken from the cervix or from urine.

### TREATMENT

Treatment regimens are listed in **Box 126.9**. In pregnant women, treatment with doxycycline, ofloxacin, and levofloxacin are contraindicated. Therefore, the recommended regimen is azithromycin, 1 g orally in a single dose, or amoxicillin, 500 mg orally three times per day for 7 days, with erythromycins being the alternative regimen.

### FOLLOW-UP, NEXT STEPS IN CARE, AND PATIENT EDUCATION

Repeated testing 3 to 4 weeks after completion of therapy (test of cure) is recommended only in pregnant women, patients with persistent symptoms, and those with suspected reinfection. Testing for coinfection with HIV or syphilis (or both) should be performed. Patients should be advised to notify sex partners to undergo evaluation, testing, and treatment.

**BOX 126.9 Treatment Regimens for Uncomplicated Genital Chlamydia Infections**

**Recommended Regimens**

- Azithromycin, 1 g orally in a single dose
  *or*
- Doxycycline, 100 mg orally twice per day for 7 days

**Alternative Regimens**

- Erythromycin base, 500 mg orally four times per day for 7 days
  *or*
- Erythromycin ethylsuccinate, 800 mg orally four times per day for 7 days
  *or*
- Levofloxacin, 500 mg orally once daily for 7 days
  *or*
- Ofloxacin, 300 mg orally twice per day for 7 days

From Centers for Disease Control and Prevention. Sexually transmitted diseases treatment guidelines, 2010. Atlanta: U.S. Department of Health and Human Services; 2010. Available at http://www.cdc.gov/mmwr/preview/mmwrhtml/rr5912a1.htm. Accessed May 30, 2012.

# GONORRHEA

## EPIDEMIOLOGY

The highest incidence of infection is found in the 15- to 24-year-old age group, and transmission occurs via sexual contact. In 2009, the gonorrhea rate was 105.5 cases per 100,000 population in women.[1]

## PATHOPHYSIOLOGY

*N. gonorrhoeae*, a gram-negative diplococcus typically found inside polymorphonuclear cells, is the causative agent in gonorrhea infections. Incubation times for gonorrhea range from 3 to 5 days. Infection is usually asymptomatic, but if present, the most common clinical sign is endocervicitis. The virulence and pathophysiology of *N. gonorrhoeae* subtypes depend on the antigenic characteristics of the organism.

## PRESENTING SIGNS AND SYMPTOMS

As mentioned in the previous section, infection is often asymptomatic, but if manifestations do develop, they often occur during menses and have a clinical picture similar to that of *Chlamydia* infection. Patients may have dysuria, urinary frequency, and urgency with a purulent urethral discharge. Vaginitis and cervicitis with inflammation of the Bartholin glands are common findings. Infection may be asymptomatic with only slightly increased vaginal discharge and moderate cervicitis on physical examination. Infection may remain as a chronic cervicitis—an important reservoir of gonococci. Systemic complications follow dissemination of gonococci from the primary site via the bloodstream and include meningitis, endocarditis, and arthritis.

## DIFFERENTIAL DIAGNOSIS AND MEDICAL DECISION MAKING

Gonococcal urethritis or cervicitis must be differentiated from nongonococcal urethritis; from cervicitis or vaginitis secondary to *C. trachomatis, G. vaginalis, T. vaginalis,* or *C. albicans*; and from many other pathogens associated with sexually transmitted disease. Gram stains are often negative.

In the past, culture has been the gold standard for diagnosis; however, nucleic acid amplification tests that detect both *N. gonorrhoeae* and *C. trachomatis* in cervical and urethral swab specimens and urine have become more widely used.

## TREATMENT

Therapy is typically administered before antimicrobial susceptibilities are known (**Box 126.10**). The decision to treat can be based on laboratory confirmation; however, in patients with high clinical suspicion for the disease or in those likely to be lost to follow-up, empiric therapy should not be delayed. Specific antibiotic regimens are recommended for patients with complicated gonococcal infections such as bacteremia, endocarditis, arthritis, meningitis, and conjunctivitis. Because antibiotic resistance is becoming an increasing problem, the physician should check local sensitivities before treating.

**BOX 126.10 Treatment Regimens for Uncomplicated Genital Gonorrhea Infections***

**Recommended Regimens**

- Ceftriaxone, 250 mg intramuscularly (IM) in a single dose (treatment of choice)
  *or*
- Cefixime, 400 mg orally in a single dose
  *or*
- Ceftizoxime, 500 mg IM
  *and*
  Azithromycin 1 gm orally in a single dose
  *or*
  Doxycycline 100 mg orally twice daily for 7 days

**Alternative Regimens (less desirable)**

- Cefpodoxime, 400 mg orally
  *or*
- Cefuroxime axetil, 1 g orally
  *or*
- Azithromycin, 2 g orally (use in limited circumstances)

From Centers for Disease Control and Prevention. Sexually transmitted diseases treatment guidelines, 2010. Atlanta: U.S. Department of Health and Human Services; 2010. Available at http://www.cdc.gov/mmwr/preview/mmwrhtml/rr5912a1.htm. Accessed May 30, 2012.

*Because coexistent chlamydial infection is common, it is recommended that doxycycline (100 mg twice daily orally for 7 days) be added if Chlamydia trachomatis has not been excluded.

## FOLLOW-UP, NEXT STEPS IN CARE, AND PATIENT EDUCATION

Patients should be advised to notify sex partners to be treated based on exposure regardless of the presence or absence of symptoms. Unprotected sexual intercourse should be avoided until 7 days after completion of the treatment regimen. Uncomplicated cases should be referred to follow-up with a primary care or public health provider within 72 hours for reevaluation. Use of condoms should be recommended with the understanding that they offer partial protection. Serologic testing for syphilis should be performed in all patients with gonorrhea.

# URETHRITIS

## EPIDEMIOLOGY

Causative agents of nongonococcal urethritis include *Ureaplasma urealyticum* (40% to 60% of cases), *C. trachomatis*

(15% to 55% of cases), *M. hominis* (5% to 10% of cases), and *T. vaginalis* (<5% of cases).[1]

## PATHOPHYSIOLOGY

Urethritis can result from infectious and noninfectious conditions. Infectious urethritis is usually transmitted sexually and is categorized as gonococcal urethritis *(N. gonorrhoeae)* or nongonococcal urethritis (i.e., *C. trachomatis, U. urealyticum, M. hominis, Mycoplasma genitalium, T. vaginalis*). Asymptomatic infections are common. Rare infectious causes of urethritis most commonly include LGV, herpes genitalis, syphilis, and adenovirus.

## PRESENTING SIGNS AND SYMPTOMS

Symptoms, if present, include discharge of mucopurulent or purulent material, dysuria, and urethral pruritus.

## DIFFERENTIAL DIAGNOSIS AND MEDICAL DECISION MAKING

Gram stain is the preferred rapid diagnostic test for evaluating urethritis. The presence of gram-negative intracellular diplococci on a urethral smear is indicative of gonorrhea infection, which is frequently accompanied by chlamydial infection. If Gram stain microscopy is not available, patients should be treated with drug regimens effective against both gonorrhea and chlamydia.

Urethritis can be documented on the basis of any of the following signs or laboratory tests:

- Mucopurulent or purulent discharge on examination
- Microscopy of urethral secretions demonstrating five or more white blood cells (WBCs) per oil immersion field
- Positive leukocyte esterase test on first-void urine or microscopic examination of first-void urine sediment demonstrating 10 or more WBCs per high-power field

## TREATMENT

For gonococcal urethritis, refer to the treatment of uncomplicated gonorrhea infections. Because of possibility of concomitant infection, *Chlamydia* infection should be presumed and also treated unless it is ruled out. See **Box 126.11** for the treatment of nongonococcal urethritis.

## FOLLOW-UP, NEXT STEPS IN CARE, AND PATIENT EDUCATION

Reevaluation is recommended if the symptoms persist or recur following completion of therapy. Alternative causes (*T. vaginalis*, HSV, adenovirus, *Mycoplasma*, and *Ureaplasma* species) should be pursued when nongonococcal urethritis does not improve with the recommended treatment.

**BOX 126.11 Treatment Regimens for Nongonococcal Urethritis**

**Recommended Regimens**

- Azithromycin, 1 g orally in a single dose
  *or*
- Doxycycline, 100 mg orally twice per day for 7 days

**Alternative Regimens**

- Erythromycin base, 500 mg orally four times per day for 7 days
  *or*
- Erythromycin ethylsuccinate, 800 mg orally four times per day for 7 days
  *or*
- Levofloxacin, 500 mg orally once daily for 7 days
  *or*
- Ofloxacin, 300 mg orally twice per day for 7 days

**Recurrent or Persistent Urethritis**

- Metronidazole, 2 g orally in a single dose
  *or*
- Tinidazole, 2 g orally in a single dose, plus azithromycin, 1 g orally in a single dose (if not used for the initial episode)

From Centers for Disease Control and Prevention. Sexually transmitted diseases treatment guidelines, 2010. Atlanta: U.S. Department of Health and Human Services; 2010. Available at http://www.cdc.gov/mmwr/preview/mmwrhtml/rr5912a1.htm. Accessed May 30, 2012.

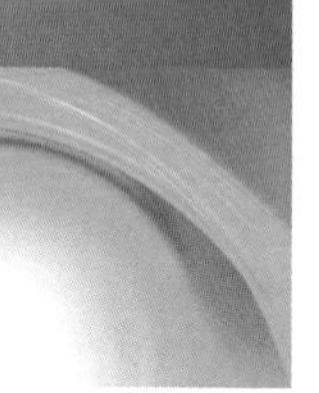

# Diseases Characterized by Abdominal or Pelvic Pain

## PELVIC INFLAMMATORY DISEASE

### EPIDEMIOLOGY

PID is diagnosed in more than 1 million women each year.[1] Infertility as a result of tubal involvement after PID is the second most common cause of female infertility in the United States. Following PID, infertility occurs in 12% of women; the risk for ectopic pregnancy increases 7- to 10-fold, and chronic pelvic pain develops in approximately 20% of women.[11]

### PATHOPHYSIOLOGY

PID is a polymicrobial infection of the upper genital tract (endometrium, fallopian tubes, ovaries) that is associated most commonly with *N. gonorrhoeae* and *C. trachomatis* and, to a lesser extent, with some endogenous organisms, including anaerobes, *Haemophilus influenzae*, and enteric gram-negative rods. Retrograde spread of the organisms occurs in as many as 20% of women with cervicitis and often results in PID with salpingitis, endometritis, or tuboovarian abscess (TOA). PID is most common in young, nulliparous, sexually active women with multiple sex partners.

The specific mechanism of infection in PID is unknown. However, numerous risk factors have been identified, including previous sexually transmitted disease, high number of sexual partners, inconsistent or no regular use of condoms, sexual intercourse at an early age, and intrauterine devices. Pregnancy can be a protective factor because of the mucous plug, which helps prevent upward transmission of infection.

## PRESENTING SIGNS AND SYMPTOMS

Symptoms suggesting PID include bilateral lower abdominal pain, dyspareunia, vaginal discharge (75% of patients), abnormal vaginal bleeding, low back pain, nausea and vomiting, and fever. Mucopurulent discharge or leukorrhea in the vaginal vault has good sensitivity but low specificity for PID.

## DIFFERENTIAL DIAGNOSIS AND MEDICAL DECISION MAKING

Diagnosis of PID is usually based on the clinical findings of lower abdominal tenderness, cervical motion tenderness, or adnexal tenderness for which another cause is not likely (**Box 126.12**). Women with PID may have subtle or mild symptoms, thus complicating the diagnosis.

The differential diagnosis includes appendicitis, ectopic pregnancy, septic abortion, hemorrhagic or ruptured ovarian cysts or tumors, degeneration of a myoma, and acute enteritis (**Fig. 126.3**).

## TREATMENT

Antimicrobial coverage should include *N. gonorrhoeae, C. trachomatis*, gram-negative facultative bacteria, anaerobes, and streptococci. No single therapeutic regimen has been established (**Box 126.13**). Outpatient management is appropriate for most patients with mild to moderate PID who do not meet the criteria for admission.

As a result of the emergence of quinolone-resistant *N. gonorrhoeae*, regimens that include a quinolone agent are no longer recommended for the treatment of PID.[13]

Parenteral therapy may be discontinued 24 hours after the patient improves clinically, and oral therapy with doxycycline, 100 mg orally twice daily, should be continued for a total of 14 days.

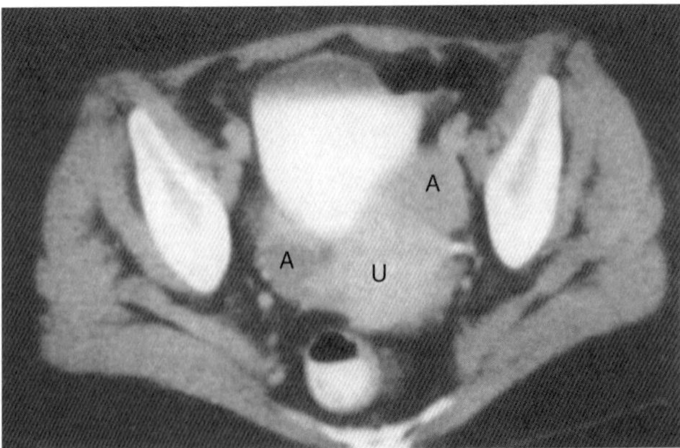


**Fig. 126.3 Computed tomography scan of a patient with pelvic inflammatory disease showing bilateral adnexal masses.** *A*, Tuboovarian abscesses; *U*, uterus.

**BOX 126.12 CDC Suggested Criteria for Diagnosis, Empiric Treatment, and Hospitalization for Patients with PID**

A. **Minimum diagnostic criteria** (for diagnosis and empiric treatment of PID in sexually active young women experiencing pelvic or lower abdominal pain if no other cause is identified):
- Cervical motion tenderness
  *or*
- Adnexal tenderness
  *or*
- Uterine tenderness

B. **Additional diagnostic criteria** (used to enhance specificity of the diagnosis of PID once any of the minimum criteria listed above is met):
- Oral temperature higher than 101° F (>38.3° C)
- Abnormal cervical or vaginal mucopurulent discharge
- Presence of abundant numbers of WBCs on saline microscopy of vaginal fluid
- Elevated erythrocyte sedimentation rate
- Elevated C-reactive protein
- Laboratory documentation of cervical infection with *Neisseria gonorrhoeae* or *Chlamydia trachomatis*

C. **Additional diagnosis criteria** (most specific criteria for the diagnosis of PID):
- Histopathologic evidence of endometritis on an endometrial biopsy specimen
- Transvaginal ultrasonography, computed tomography[12] (see Fig. 126.3), or magnetic resonance imaging showing thickened, fluid-filled tubes with or without free pelvic fluid and a tuboovarian complex
- Laparoscopic abnormalities consistent with PID

D. **Criteria for hospitalization** (recommended criteria for hospitalization of patients with PID):
- Unable to exclude surgical emergencies such as appendicitis in the diagnosis
- Pregnancy
- Presence of tuboovarian abscess
- Severe illness such as intractable nausea and vomiting, high fever, or leukocytosis
- Inability to follow or tolerate an outpatient oral regimen
- Failure to respond clinically to oral antimicrobial therapy

From Centers for Disease Control and Prevention. Sexually transmitted diseases treatment guidelines, 2010. Atlanta: U.S. Department of Health and Human Services; 2010. Available at http://www.cdc.gov/mmwr/preview/mmwrhtml/rr5912a1.htm. Accessed May 30, 2012.
*CDC*, Centers for Disease Control and Prevention; *PID*, pelvic inflammatory disease; *WBCs*, white blood cells.

**BOX 126.13 Treatment Regimens for Pelvic Inflammatory Disease**

**Outpatient Treatment Regimens**

Recommended regimens:

- Ceftriaxone, 250 mg intramuscularly (IM) once, plus doxycycline, 100 mg orally (PO) twice daily for 14 days, with or without metronidazole, 500 mg PO twice daily for 14 days

  *or*
- Cefoxitin, 2 g IM in a single dose, and probenecid, 1 g PO, administered concurrently in a single dose, plus doxycycline, 100 mg PO twice daily for 14 days, with or without metronidazole, 500 mg PO twice daily for 14 days

  *or*
- Cefotaxime, 500 mg (or ceftizoxime, 500 mg) IM once, plus doxycycline, 100 mg PO twice daily for 14 days, with or without metronidazole, 500 mg PO twice daily for 14 days

Alternative regimen:

- If parenteral cephalosporin therapy is not available: Fluoroquinolones (levofloxacin, 500 mg PO once daily, or ofloxacin, 400 mg twice daily for 14 days) with or without metronidazole (500 mg PO twice daily for 14 days)

**Inpatient Treatment Regimens (Parenteral)**

Recommended regimen:

- Cefotetan 2, g intravenously (IV) every 12 hours (or cefoxitin, 2 g IV every 6 hours), plus doxycycline, 100 mg PO or IV every 12 hours

  *or*
- Clindamycin, 900 mg IV every 8 hours, plus a gentamicin loading dose IV or IM (2 mg/kg of body weight), followed by a maintenance dose (1.5 mg/kg) every 8 hours. Single daily dosing (3 to 5 mg/kg) can be substituted

Alternative regimen:

- Ampicillin-sulbactam, 3 g IV every 6 hours, plus doxycycline, 100 mg PO or IV every 12 hours

From Centers for Disease Control and Prevention. Sexually transmitted diseases treatment guidelines, 2010. Atlanta: U.S. Department of Health and Human Services; 2010. Available at http://www.cdc.gov/mmwr/preview/mmwrhtml/rr5912a1.htm. Accessed May 30, 2012.

## FOLLOW-UP, NEXT STEPS IN CARE, AND PATIENT EDUCATION

Compliance with the full 2-week course of oral antibiotic therapy should be encouraged. Advise against sexual activity pending resolution of the disease process. Patients should be referred for follow-up in 72 hours for reevaluation. Patients should be advised to notify any sex partners who were active with the patient during the 60 days before the onset of symptom to receive treatment as per CDC recommendations.

# TUBOOVARIAN ABSCESS

## EPIDEMIOLOGY

TOA is the most common intraabdominal abscess in premenopausal women and develops in up to one third of patients hospitalized with PID. Rupture is categorized as a surgical emergency with rates of occurrence as high as 15%.

## PATHOPHYSIOLOGY

TOA is usually a complication of PID, although cases can infrequently occur without the preexisting presence of PID. TOAs typically result from salpingitis that progresses to oophoritis.[14] Ovarian infection occurs after contamination with purulent material from the fallopian tube. Adherence of tubal fimbriae to the ovary forms a large, cylinder-shaped TOA. Most TOAs consist of polymicrobic anaerobic bacteria.

## PRESENTING SIGNS AND SYMPTOMS

Patients with TOA typically have abdominal pain and severe, asymmetric tenderness, often with peritoneal signs on palpation. Fever and leukocytosis are usually but not always present as well. TOA can be bilateral, although unilateral disease is more common and accounts for 60% of such abscesses.

## DIFFERENTIAL DIAGNOSIS AND MEDICAL DECISION MAKING

Definitive diagnosis is made by direct visualization or use of an imaging study. Pelvic ultrasonography has a reported sensitivity of 93% and specificity of 98%. Computed tomography may be used to define the abscess better or may be appropriate if the ultrasound evaluation is inconclusive. Appendicitis, PID, and ovarian torsion are common entities in the differential diagnosis.

## TREATMENT

All patients with suspected TOA should be hospitalized. Initial parenteral therapy options are the same as those listed for PID, but continued oral therapy should include clindamycin (or metronidazole) for 14 days in addition to doxycycline.

TOAs may require transcutaneous or transvaginal aspiration. Surgical excision is also an option. Unless rupture is suspected, high-dose antibiotic therapy should be instituted, and the efficacy of therapy should be monitored with ultrasonography. Ruptured TOA is a life-threatening condition that requires immediate medical therapy associated with surgery.

Unilateral adnexectomy is acceptable for unilateral abscesses. Hysterectomy and bilateral salpingo-oophorectomy may be necessary for overwhelming infection or in cases of chronic disease with intractable pelvic pain.

## FOLLOW-UP, NEXT STEPS IN CARE, AND PATIENT EDUCATION

Compliance with the full 2-week course of oral antibiotics should be encouraged. Patients should be referred for follow-up in 72 hours for reevaluation. Advise against sexual activity pending resolution of the disease process.

# FITZ-HUGH–CURTIS SYNDROME

## EPIDEMIOLOGY

The incidence of FHCS is lower in adult women (4% to 14%) than in adolescent girls (27%).[15]

## PATHOPHYSIOLOGY

FHCS is described as inflammation of the liver capsule (perihepatitis) without damage to the liver parenchyma. A purulent or fibrinous exudate appears on the capsular surface, and swelling of the liver capsule produces pleuritic right upper quadrant pain. This syndrome is an extrapelvic manifestation of PID.

## PRESENTING SIGNS AND SYMPTOMS

Illness consists of two phases. The acute phase is characterized by sharp, right upper quadrant, pleuritic abdominal pain that can radiate to the shoulder; the chronic phase results from the formation of peritoneal adhesions, which cause persistent, typically right upper quadrant abdominal pain. Tubal infections may or may not be present concurrently.

## DIFFERENTIAL DIAGNOSIS AND MEDICAL DECISION MAKING

Perihepatitis was formerly believed to be caused solely by *N. gonorrhoeae*, but *C. trachomatis* is now known to more often be the causative agent. Salpingitis is invariably the source, but the syndrome occasionally follows appendicitis and other causes of peritonitis. FHCS is frequently misdiagnosed as cholecystitis, pneumonia, perforated peptic ulcer, or renal colic. Liver enzyme levels may be mildly elevated.

Diagnosis is difficult and based on clinical features. A high index of suspicion should be maintained in women seen in the ED with upper abdominal pain and normal routine results on gallbladder and liver function tests. FHCS is a more likely cause of upper quadrant pleuritic pain than cholecystitis is and should be suspected in any woman with pleuritic upper quadrant pain and physical signs of salpingitis. Associated signs and symptoms of fever, leukocytosis, abdominal pain, cervicitis, or PID may be present, but their absence does not exclude the diagnosis.

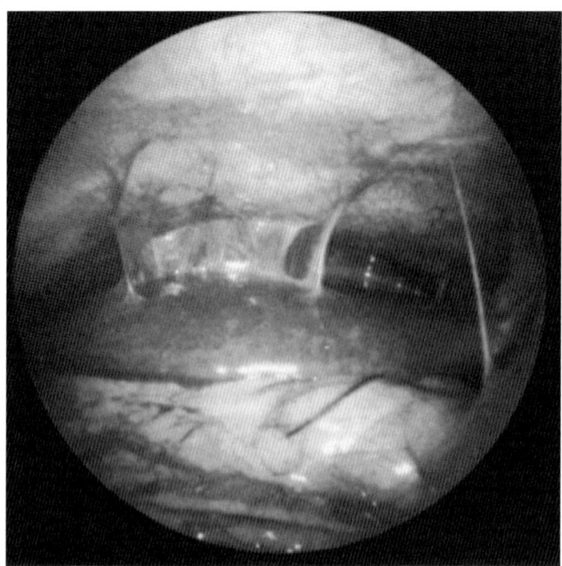

**Fig. 126.4** "Violin string" adhesions are visualized in this scan of a patient with Fitz-Hugh–Curtis syndrome. (From Ferri FF. Ferri's clinical advisor 2007: instant diagnosis and treatment. 9th ed. Philadelphia: Mosby; 2007.)

Laparoscopy is useful to identify unclear cases and, in conjunction with positive cervical or abdominal cultures, represents the standard criterion for diagnosis. Negative cervical cultures alone, however, do not rule out the diagnosis. "Violin string" adhesions may be seen on ultrasound or computed tomography scans (**Fig. 126.4**).

## TREATMENT

The goal of treatment is bacterial eradication with antibiotics to prevent chronic abdominal pain and adhesions. Complications are uncommon but can include subdiaphragmatic abscess and small bowel obstruction.

Although no formal antibiotic recommendations exist, patients with FHCS usually require admission for observation and parenteral antibiotic therapy. Initial options are the same as those listed for inpatient treatment of PID. Like TOA, continued outpatient oral therapy should include clindamycin (or metronidazole) for 14 days in addition to doxycycline.[2]

## FOLLOW-UP, NEXT STEPS IN CARE, AND PATIENT EDUCATION

Compliance with the full 2-week course of oral antibiotic therapy should be encouraged. Advise against sexual activity pending resolution of the disease process. Patients should be referred for follow-up in 72 hours for reevaluation. Patients should be advised to notify any sex partners who were active with the patient during the 60 days before the onset of symptom to receive treatment as per CDC recommendations.

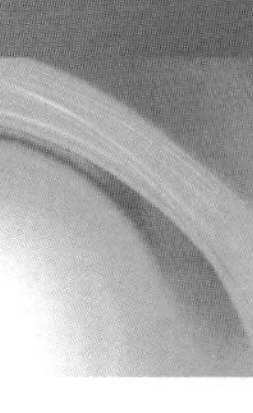

# Diseases Characterized by Genital Warts or Mucosal Abscess

## HUMAN PAPILLOMAVIRUS

### EPIDEMIOLOGY

HPV is the most common sexually transmitted virus in the United States. Its prevalence corresponds inversely with age (highest in younger age groups, 50% in females 20 to 24 years of age) and declines substantially after the age of 24 years.[16] However, the gross clinical prevalence of HPV is less than 1%.[11]

### PATHOPHYSIOLOGY

HPV is a double-stranded DNA virus that infects the epithelial cells of skin and mucosa and can cause cellular changes leading to formation of warts. HPV infection is a sexually transmitted illness that is most commonly asymptomatic but has been associated with various disease processes such as benign anogenital warts, as well as with invasive cancer. Of the greater than 100 types of HPV, more than 40 can infect the genital area. A quadrivalent HPV vaccine that provides protection against types 6, 11, 16, and 18 was licensed for use in the United States in June 2006. HPV subtypes 6 and 11 most commonly cause genital warts (condylomata acuminata),[3] which can occur on the vulva, perianal area, urethra, vaginal walls, or cervix. These subtypes have also been identified as the causative agent of laryngeal or respiratory papillomatosis in infants and children, but the route of transmission is not completely understood.

### PRESENTING SIGNS AND SYMPTOMS

The average incubation period for visible warts is about 3 months. Genital warts may be asymptomatic but can be pruritic. On clinical examination the lesions are generally papillary, verrucous (wartlike), or macular in character (**Fig. 126.5**).

Lesions usually first appear individually, but large confluent growths can develop.

Vaginal and cervical warts are more common than labial warts, although most of them are flat lesions visible only with colposcopy.

### DIFFERENTIAL DIAGNOSIS AND MEDICAL DECISION MAKING

Several laboratory methods such as PCR have been developed for confirmation of genital HPV infection, but the ED diagnosis remains primarily clinical.

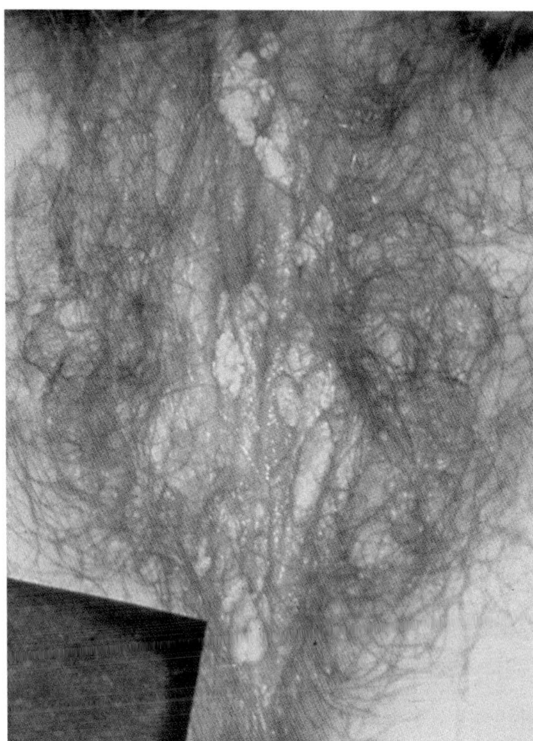

**Fig. 126.5 Vulvovaginal human papillomavirus infection.** (From Cohen J, Powderly WG. Infectious diseases. 2nd ed. Philadelphia: Mosby; 2004.)

Vulvar warts must be differentiated from the less verrucous, flatter growths of syphilitic condyloma latum and from carcinoma in situ of the vulva. Darkfield examination or punch biopsies may be required to differentiate these lesions.

Vulvar lesions may be obviously wartlike or may be diagnosed with colposcopy following the application of 4% acetic acid (vinegar), after which they appear whitish with prominent papillae.

### TREATMENT

Subclinical genital HPV infection usually clears spontaneously. Treatment is indicated for those with genital warts or precancerous lesions and not for subclinical HPV infection (**Box 126.14**).

Extensive warts may require $CO_2$ laser treatment under local or general anesthesia. Intralesional interferon, photodynamic therapy, and topical cidofovir are associated with more side effects and are no more effective than other therapies.

In women who have exophytic cervical warts, biopsy evaluation to exclude high-grade squamous intraepithelial lesions must be performed before treatment is initiated. Management of exophytic cervical warts should include consultation with a specialist.

### FOLLOW-UP, NEXT STEPS IN CARE, AND PATIENT EDUCATION

Curative measures to prevent transmission once infected are not available, and therefore routine examination of sex

**BOX 126.14 Treatment Regimens Recommended for External Genital Warts Caused by Human Papillomavirus**

**Patient Applied**

- Podofilox 0.5% solution or gel, twice per day for 3 days, followed by 4 days of no therapy. This cycle can be repeated, as necessary, for up to four cycles
  *or*
- Imiquimod 5% cream, once daily at bedtime three times per week for up to 16 weeks
  *or*
- Sinecatechin 15% ointment, three times daily for up to 16 weeks

**Provider Administered**

- Cryotherapy with liquid nitrogen or cryoprobe. Applications repeated every 1 to 2 weeks
  *or*
- Podophyllin resin, 10% to 25% in a compound tincture of benzoin
  *or*
- Trichloroacetic acid or dichloroacetic acid, 80% to 90%
  *or*
- Surgical removal by either tangential scissors excision, tangential shave excision, curettage, or electrosurgery

From Centers for Disease Control and Prevention. Sexually transmitted diseases treatment guidelines, 2010. Atlanta: U.S. Department of Health and Human Services; 2010. Available at http://www.cdc.gov/mmwr/preview/mmwrhtml/rr5912a1.htm. Accessed May 30, 2012.

partners is not emphasized as part of the management plan. Patients should still be encouraged to notify partners to facilitate their decision making regarding further evaluation. Imiquimod, podophyllin, and podofilox should not be used for treatment during pregnancy because of the risk for systemic absorption and their ability to cross the placenta.

# BARTHOLIN GLAND ABSCESS

## EPIDEMIOLOGY

Swelling of the Bartholin glands occurs in 2% of women of reproductive age, most commonly between the ages of 20 and 30. Development of this disease process in patients older than 40 years is atypical and should lead to assessment for possible malignancy as part of the diagnostic and treatment plan.

## PATHOPHYSIOLOGY

The Bartholin glands are bilateral vulvovaginal secretory structures located in the labia minora on the posterolateral aspect of the vestibule. Normally pea sized, these glands drain fluid through a 2.5-cm duct into a fold between the hymeneal ring and the labium that serves to maintain moisture of the vaginal mucosa. Duct occlusion can result in cyst and subsequently abscess formation. Isolates from cultures of abscesses are most commonly anaerobic organisms *(Bacteroides fragilis, Peptostreptococcus),* aerobic *N. gonorrhoeae* is the causative agent in approximately 10% to 15% of cases, and *C. trachomatis* is found even less frequently.

## PRESENTING SIGNS AND SYMPTOMS

Onset of disease can occur rapidly over a period of several hours or may progress more gradually over several days. The initial symptoms are pain, dyspareunia, and sometimes fever. Findings on physical examination are a unilateral labial mass with tenderness, redness, and swelling in the Bartholin gland area. Elevated temperature is observed in approximately one third of patients.

Microscopically, acute inflammation is present within the Bartholin duct, as well as within the gland stroma about the duct. The abscess, when fully developed, contains purulent exudate.

## DIFFERENTIAL DIAGNOSIS AND MEDICAL DECISION MAKING

Cultures and Gram staining of material expressed from the duct may identify gonococci. Cervical gonococcal and chlamydial cultures should be performed and the organisms treated if present.

## TREATMENT

Management of the abscess consists of simple incision and drainage. After sterile preparation of the area, a scalpel stab incision, ideally no longer than 1.5 cm (longer incisions will make it difficult to keep the Word catheter in place), should be made deep into the abscess from the inside of the labium. An outside incision can cause permanent fistula formation.[17] Loculations should be broken manually followed by placement of a Word catheter with its balloon tip inserted into the abscess before inflation with water or lubricating gel (**Fig. 126.6**). Simple incision and drainage without Word catheter placement may be inadequate and result in recurrence.

After successful drainage, routine antibiotic therapy is not recommended for uncomplicated Bartholin gland abscesses in otherwise healthy women. Treatment of *N. gonorrhoeae* and *C. trachomatis* should be initiated only in patients with confirmed disease.

## FOLLOW-UP, NEXT STEPS IN CARE, AND PATIENT EDUCATION

Follow-up in 72 hours for reevaluation should be arranged. Refer the patient to gynecology for removal of the catheter in 2 to 4 weeks.

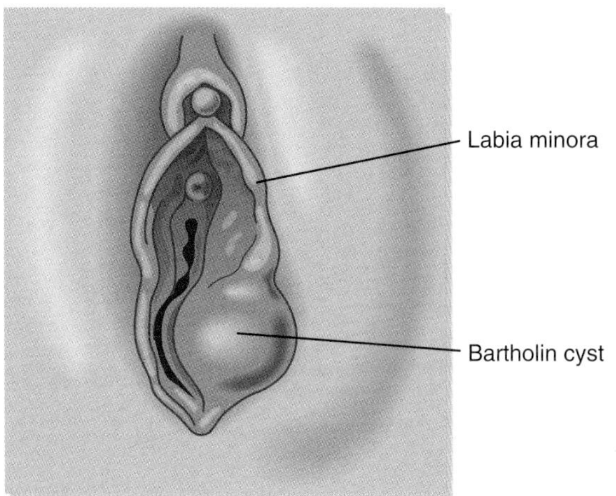


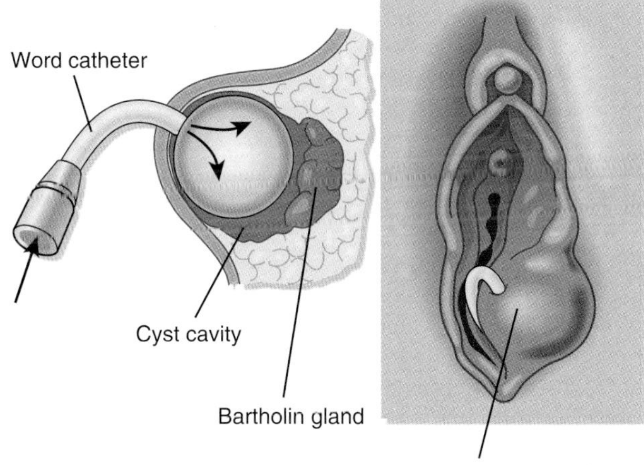


**Fig. 126.6** **A,** Scalpel incision of a Bartholin duct cyst. **B,** Placement of a Word catheter in the cyst.

## SUGGESTED READINGS


Centers for Disease Control and Prevention. Sexually Transmitted Disease Surveillance 2009. Atlanta: U.S. Department of Health and Human Services; 2010. Available at http://www.cdc.gov/STD/stats09/surv2009-Complete.pdf. Accessed January 18, 2011.

Centers for Disease Control and Prevention. Sexually Transmitted Diseases Treatment Guidelines, 2010. Atlanta: U.S. Department of Health and Human Services; 2010. Available at http://www.cdc.gov/mmwr/preview/mmwrhtml/rr5912a1.htm. Accessed January 18, 2011.

Ramin SM, Wendell JD, Hemsell DL. Sexually transmitted diseases and pelvic infections. In: DeCherney AH, Pernoll ML, editors. Current obstetric and gynecologic diagnosis and treatment. 10th ed. New York: McGraw-Hill; 2007.


## REFERENCES

*References can be found on Expert Consult @ www.expertconsult.com.*

# 127 Breast Disorders

*Robert Lockwood and Jamie L. Collings*

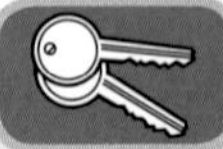

**KEY POINTS**

- There are very few true breast emergencies, and immediately life-threatening causes such as traumatic breast rupture or necrotizing fasciitis are exceedingly rare.
- Breast pain, particularly if cyclic, is common, and benign causes predominate.
- Breast cancer is a possible diagnosis in any patient with a chief complaint related to the breast, including breast pain or a mass, nipple discharge, or skin lesions.
- Most patients in whom breast cancer is diagnosed have no risk factors except age older than 50 years and female sex, and eight of nine patients have no family history of breast cancer.
- The emergency physician can play a role in reduction of the risk for lymphedema by early and aggressive treatment of even very minor infections and burns.
- Most medications are safe for use while breastfeeding, and the benefits of continuing breastfeeding generally outweigh the potential for harm.
- Few maternal infections, other than human immunodeficiency virus, present a significant risk to the breastfeeding infant.

## EPIDEMIOLOGY

Approximately one half of visits to physicians for breast complaints are for pain. New, palpable masses represent another common breast-related complaint. Although a benign condition will be diagnosed in 9 of 10 premenopausal women with a palpable breast mass, a new mass in a 75-year-old woman is malignant up to 70% of the time. Breast cancer is the most common cause of cancer-related mortality in women worldwide and second only to lung cancer in women in the United States. In 2006, it accounted for one third of all cancer diagnoses in women in the United States.[1]

Although there are few true breast-related emergencies, perioperative issues represent a second significant group of emergency department (ED) visits. Breast surgery is relatively common in the United States. In addition to the 90,000 mastectomies performed annually, approximately 100,000 cosmetic augmentations and 100,000 reduction mammoplasties take place each year.[2] Many patients undergoing breast augmentation, either for reconstruction or cosmesis, experience significant complications and require additional surgery.

## PATHOPHYSIOLOGY

The unique anatomic structure of the breast contributes to the wide variety of pathologic conditions that may occur. Each breast contains approximately 20 glandular units (lobes) composed of glands and adipose tissue (**Fig. 127.1**). Each lobe drains into a lactiferous duct, which fuses with other ducts to form lactiferous sinuses just below the skin. The lactiferous sinuses store milk during lactation. Disruption (obstruction, infection, inflammation) of the glandular system may occur at any time during a female's lifetime but predominates between menarche and menopause. The breast's diffuse vascular network predisposes it to hematogenous spread of malignancy, as well as infection.

Virtually all breast conditions that occur in women are seen in men as well, including benign conditions such as fat necrosis, allergic and irritant dermatitis, mastitis and abscess, and mammary tuberculosis. Malignant entities such as adenocarcinoma of the breast, Paget disease of the nipple, and lymphoma occur less frequently in men than in women. Breast cancer in men accounts for less than 1% of the total number of breast malignancies diagnosed in the United States. However, in other areas in the world (e.g., central Africa), male breast cancer is significantly more common. Men are at higher risk for the development of malignant melanoma and basal cell carcinoma of the breast. One condition, gynecomastia, occurs exclusively in men.

## PRESENTING SIGNS AND SYMPTOMS

Similar to other sensitive or visible areas, ED visits for breast complaints are often precipitated by a change in appearance of the tissue. Discoloration, erythema, and engorgement are some of the more notable changes that may occur. It is very important to determine the context within which these changes are taking place. Patients with breast pain while lactating are clearly quite different from those whose pain is a result of an automobile accident. Patients can typically be segregated into

Acknowledgment and thanks to Dr. Karen Jubanyik for her contribution to the first edition.

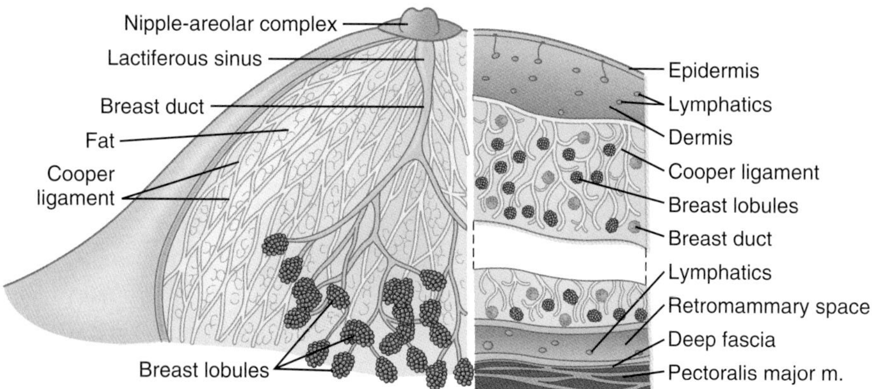


**Fig. 127.1** The breast contains approximately 20 glandular units (lobes), each composed of a tubuloalveolar gland and adipose tissue. (From Iglehart JD, Kaelin CM. Diseases of the breast. In: Townsend CM, Beauchamp RD, Evers BM, et al, editors. Sabiston's textbook of surgery. 17th ed. Philadelphia: Saunders; 2004.)

**BOX 127.1 Differential Diagnosis of Breast-Related Complaints**

**Mastalgia**
Cyclic mastalgia
Noncyclic mastalgia
Extramammary pain

**Dermatologic Conditions**
Dermatitis
Infection
Inflammation
Malignancy
Skin necrosis
Partner violence

**Masses and Malignancy**
Malignancy
Fibrocystic changes
Infection
Benign tumors
Treatment effects

**Trauma**
Partner violence
Blunt trauma
Penetrating trauma
Posttraumatic complications

**Perioperative Conditions**
Pain
Seroma
Hematoma
Infection
Failure of patency

**Lactation-Related Complaints**
Mastitis
Abscess
Special conditions

subgroups, each of which has a distinct set of concerns. Patients may have atraumatic complaints (pain, dermatologic changes, masses or discharge) perioperatively, following trauma, or while lactating. This initial categorization facilitates narrowing of the differential diagnosis. Special consideration should be reserved for victims of domestic abuse. All patients with isolated breast complaints should be screened to ensure their safety.

## DIFFERENTIAL DIAGNOSIS AND MEDICAL DECISION MAKING

See **Box 127.1** for an overview of causes of breast-related complaints.

### MASTALGIA

Breast pain, especially as an isolated symptom, can be thought of as originating from one of three broad categories: cyclic mastalgia, noncyclic mastalgia, or extramammary.

Cyclic mastalgia occurs in premenopausal women, is associated with worsening symptoms in the late luteal phase of the menstrual cycle, and accounts for two thirds of patients with mastalgia. The typical pain of cyclic mastalgia is "achy" or "heavy" and bilateral. Resolution with the onset of menses is very reassuring.

Findings on physical examination may be normal, or tender nodularities may be detected. Fibrocystic breast conditions (the term *fibrocystic breast disease* has been replaced by the term *fibrocystic breast condition* to emphasize that it represents a spectrum of histologic entities) are not associated with axillary lymphadenopathy, skin thickening, edema or discoloration, or nipple abnormalities such as retraction or discharge. The presence of any of these findings raises the probability that the patient has another condition instead of or in addition to cyclic mastalgia.

Noncyclic mastalgia may be caused by a variety of conditions[3] (**Box 127.2**). It may be constant or intermittent, but it is not associated with the menstrual cycle. Noncyclic mastalgia tends to be unilateral and localized to a discrete area. Women with noncyclic breast pain are generally older than 40 years, and the cause is likely to be related to an anatomic lesion in the breast. It is rare for breast cancer to have pain as the sole initial symptom.[4]

Extramammary breast pain can arise from the chest wall or from other sources. Although most of the conditions that cause isolated breast pain are not immediately life-threatening, some emergency conditions, including acute coronary syndrome and pulmonary embolism, can be accompanied by pain that appears to be originating from the breast.

Mondor disease (**Fig. 127.2**) is a superficial phlebitis of the lateral thoracic, thoracoepigastric, or superior epigastric vein. It typically occurs in middle-aged women. The condition can be unilateral or bilateral. It is often idiopathic but may be associated with other conditions.[5] The classic Mondor cord is 2 to 3 mm in diameter and typically red and tender, tracks from the lateral margin of the breast across the costal margin, and extends from 2 to 30 cm. Any tenderness should resolve within weeks, but the cord may remain palpable for up to 6 months. There is no risk for systemic embolization.

### DERMATOLOGIC CHANGES AND DISCHARGE

A wide variety of skin conditions can affect the breast, nipple, or both; the most threatening and most common

**BOX 127.2 Causes of Noncyclic Mastalgia and Extramammary Pain**

**Breast-Related Mastalgia**
Mastitis
Breast trauma
Mondor disease
Breast cancer
Benign breast mass
Breast cyst
Duct ectasia
Postoperative pain
Diabetic mastopathy
Medication side effects

**Extramammary Pain**
Costochondritis
Chest wall trauma
Acute coronary syndrome or angina
Pericarditis
Pulmonary embolism
Pleurisy
Biliary disease
Peptic ulcer disease
Arthritis
Phantom pain (after mastectomy)

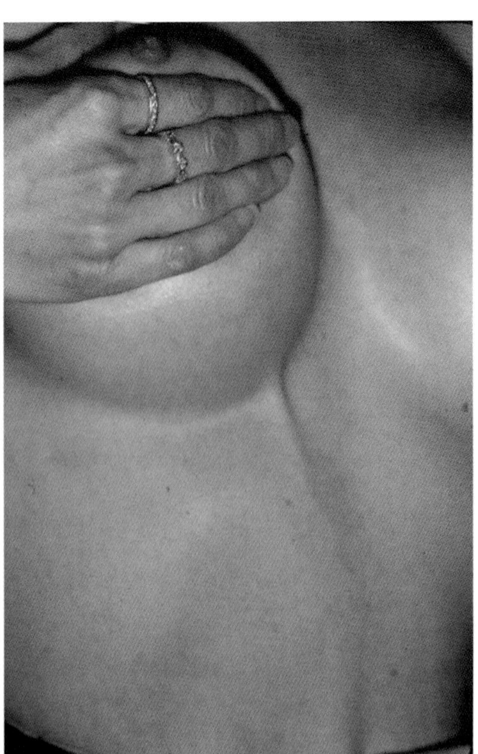

**Fig. 127.2 Mondor disease.** (Photo courtesy Edward Pechter, MD.)

are listed in **Box 127.3** and are discussed in the following sections.

### *Inflammatory Breast Cancer*

Inflammatory breast cancer is the breast malignancy most likely to be manifested with acute changes. It accounts for 4% of invasive breast cancers and typically develops from invasive ductal carcinoma. It is associated with particularly high mortality. Patients may have rapid, unilateral breast enlargement because infiltration of the dermal and intramammary lymphatics by tumor causes an inflammatory response. The breast typically exhibits tenderness, erythema, warmth, and the classic peau d'orange appearance. Nipple retraction or flattening is common. In one half of cases an underlying mass is detectable.

### *Necrotizing Fasciitis*

Although patients with necrotizing fasciitis are usually found to be quite ill systemically on initial evaluation, examination of the breast may show only mild changes suggesting the location of the disease. Signs of inflammation with changes in skin color from red to dusky blue along with severe pain disproportionate to the findings on examination, particularly in a patient with significant systemic toxicity, should increase suspicion for necrotizing fasciitis.

Risk factors include advanced age, diabetes mellitus, peripheral vascular disease, acquired immunodeficiency syndrome (AIDS), and use of immunosuppressive medications, including steroids, cytotoxic agents, and antirejection medications.

### *Dermatitis*

Dermatitis of the breast and nipple-areola complex is common and may be caused by a number of benign and malignant conditions. Frequently, the clinical history and physical examination will yield the probable diagnosis.

**BOX 127.3 Skin Conditions Involving the Breast, Nipple, or Both**

**Most Threatening**
Inflammatory breast carcinoma
Necrotizing fasciitis
Direct spread of invasive carcinoma
Mammary Paget disease
Metastatic disease
Malignant melanoma
Lymphomas, sarcomas
Systemic infections
Skin necrosis, warfarin (Coumadin) induced

**Most Common**
Contact dermatitis (irritant, allergic)
Atopic dermatitis (nipple eczema)
Candidiasis
Lactational mastitis or abscess
Periductal mastitis
Psoriasis
Hidradenitis suppurativa
Herpes zoster
Papillary adenoma of the nipple

Nipple eczema is the most common manifestation of atopic dermatitis involving the breast. The patient typically complains of burning and itching. Examination of the breast may reveal erythema, erosions, weeping, crusting, fissures, or lichenification. The condition is often bilateral. In breastfeeding women, nipple dermatitis tends to develop after initiating supplemental foods, probably as a result of an allergy to food residue in the infant's mouth.

The signs and symptoms of allergic contact dermatitis of the breast are similar to those of atopic dermatitis. Triggers include soaps, shampoos, detergents, or body lotions. Most ointments available for use in lactation contain ingredients that can induce allergic contact dermatitis.

Irritant dermatitis of the nipple—"jogger's nipple"—is common in long-distance runners; during a marathon, up to 15% of runners will experience this problem. The repetitive friction between the runner's shirt and nipple can cause painful, erythematous, crusted erosions of the nipple and areola.

### Candidal Breast Infections

*Candida albicans* intertrigo is a common skin condition, especially in the inframammary area. The nipple-areola complex may be involved as well, particularly in lactating women. The rash is often beefy red with typical satellite lesions. Pruritus and maceration are common.

### Nonpuerperal Mastitis and Abscess

Recent evidence suggests that ductal ectasia and periductal mastitis are really two distinct inflammatory entities. Ductal ectasia is minimally inflammatory, generally asymptomatic, and characterized by normal aging and dilation of the subareolar ducts. Occasionally, a mass may be palpated. In contrast, periductal mastitis is a symptomatic inflammatory condition seen especially in middle-aged female smokers and has the following characteristics: fistular or erosive lesions in the periareolar area, erythema and peau d'orange appearance, axillary adenopathy, and nipple discharge.

Periductal mastitis may be confused with cellulitis, abscesses, or inflammatory breast cancer. Approximately 90% of nonpuerperal breast abscesses are subareolar.[6]

### Piercing-Related Infections

Infection within the first year following nipple piercing is common (incidence as high as 20%) and is of special concern in patients who are immunosuppressed. Other high-risk patients are those who have previously undergone breast augmentation or surgery for congenital heart defects. Nipple piercing, especially in these high-risk patients, can lead to endocarditis or sepsis.

### Nipple Discharge

Discharge from the nipple is a common complaint. Nipple discharge is often categorized according to the following factors: color, unilateral versus bilateral, number of ducts involved, and whether the fluid requires pressure for expression. In the absence of a mass, most physiologic discharge is yellow, milky, or green; occurs bilaterally from multiple ducts; and is seen only with compression. Other types of physiologic discharge include persistent lactation in women for up to 3 months postpartum or for as long as 2 years after discontinuation of lactation.

Galactorrhea may be caused by hyperprolactinemia secondary to medications, medical conditions, or a pituitary adenoma. Nipple discharge that is spontaneous, unilateral, localized to a single duct, and either clear or bloody is pathologic and requires outpatient follow-up. The most common cause of bloody discharge from a single duct is a benign intraductal papilloma.

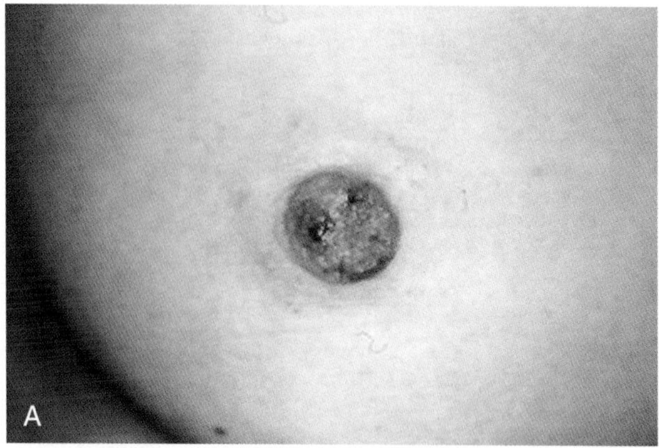

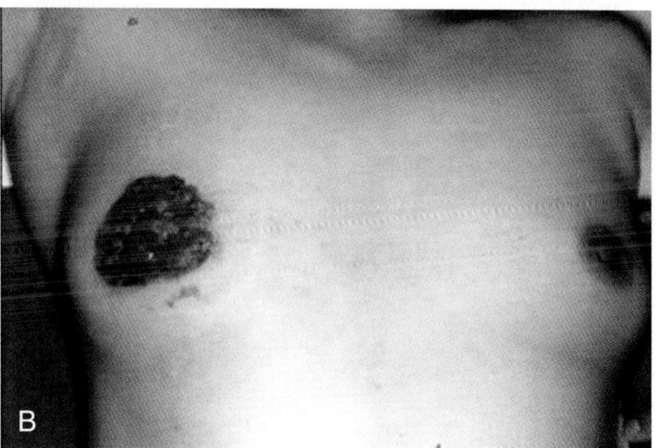

**Fig. 127.3** **A** and **B**, Paget disease of the nipple. (Courtesy Sehwan Han, MD.)

### Mammary Paget Disease

Paget disease of the nipple (**Fig. 127.3, *A* and *B***), first described by James Paget in 1874, is a neoplastic condition that accounts for 2% to 4% of breast malignancies. The lesion involves the nipple-areola complex and may spread to the surrounding skin. Patients with early disease may have only a burning and itching sensation around the nipple area. A central palpable breast mass is present in 60% of cases.[7] Patients with mammary Paget disease usually undergo mastectomy with either lymph node dissection or sentinal node biopsy.

### Skin Necrosis

Warfarin-induced skin necrosis is a rare complication of oral anticoagulant therapy that affects only 0.01% to 0.1% of patients who take the medication.[8] The typical patient is a middle-aged, obese woman who recently initiated Coumadin therapy, although cases have been reported occurring well into a year of therapy.

The lesions can be single or multiple and are accompanied by intense pain.

## MASSES

Although breast pain is the most common symptom causing women to seek medical care related to their breasts, a palpable breast mass is associated with significant anxiety and

**Table 127.1 Benign Breast Tumors**

| TUMOR | TISSUE | AGE | SIZE | CHARACTERISTICS | DIAGNOSTIC FINDINGS | FOLLOW-UP |
|---|---|---|---|---|---|---|
| Fibroadenoma | Both glandular and stromal tissue elements; typically solitary | Common in women < 40 yr; uncommon in those >50 yr | From microscopic to 5 cm | Tender premenstrually, often asymptomatic; complex fibroadenomas increase risk for malignancy | MF: poor (look the same as surrounding parenchyma); USF: well-circumscribed, homogeneous, hypoechoic lesions with edge shadowing; diagnosis depends on fine-needle, core, or surgical biopsy | Specialist evaluation and follow-up |
| Cyst | Lobular lesions; obstruction, involution, and aging of ducts produce loculations that enlarge as cysts | Common in women 40-50 yr but rare in postmenopausal women | Microscopic to several cm | Usually round, mobile; can be tender premenstrually | MF: poor; USF: typical simple cyst (well-defined round or oval anechoic lesions) | Ultrasonography for benign cysts; biopsy for atypical cases |
| Phyllodes tumor | Glandular tissue and stromal tissue (mostly stromal) | Any age; median of 50-60 yr | 5 cm average size; up to 30 cm seen | Rare; painless, rapidly growing; 5% are malignant | MF and USF similar to findings for fibroadenoma; definitive diagnosis depends on tissue sampling and biopsy | All tumors, including benign growths, are resected; high mortality at 3 yr |
| Intraductal papilloma | Wartlike growths of glandular and fibrovascular tissue within ducts | Typically 45-50 yr | Usually <1 cm | Single tumors involving large ducts near the nipple; clear or bloody discharge; may be felt as a small lump behind or adjacent to the nipple | Ductography is particularly helpful | Surgical treatment generally recommended; involves removal of papilloma and portion of the duct |

*MF*, Mammography findings; *USF*, ultrasound findings.

frequently prompts a visit to a physician. For patients with a chief complaint of a breast mass, evaluation and treatment will probably be based on findings on physical examination, the patient's age, and other risk factors.

Breast cancer is exceedingly rare in women younger than 20 years and accounts for only a small fraction of a percent of breast disease in women younger than 30 years. Most women younger than 35 years with a solitary painless breast mass will have a fibroadenoma (see **Table 127.1** for a comparison of benign breast tumors). Common benign breast masses include fibroadenomas, cysts, phyllodes tumors (malignant 5% of the time), and intraductal papillomas. Other benign tumors found in breast tissue, but not limited to the breasts, include lipomas, hamartomas, hemangiomas, neurofibromas, granular cell tumors, and fat necrosis. None of these conditions appear to increase the risk for subsequent development of breast cancer.

### *Breast Cancer*

Emergency physicians (EPs) are in a unique position to provide education about breast cancer and screening (**Box 127.4**) to many women who do not have other contact with the health care system,[9-11] in particular, minority and lower socioeconomic groups, who have both higher mortality rates and decreased access to preventive services. A female born in the United States today has a 13% probability of breast cancer developing during her lifetime. Most women in whom breast cancer develops have only two risk factors (being female and age older than 50 years).

COMPLICATIONS OF BREAST CANCER Patients undergoing treatment of breast cancer frequently visit the ED because of complications related to their disease or treatment. Breast cancer metastasis commonly includes local, regional, and distant sites: lung, pleura, pericardium, bone, and brain.

**BOX 127.4 American Cancer Society Recommendations for Breast Cancer Screening, 2010**

Women 40 years and older should have a screening mammogram every year and should continue to do so for as long as they are in good health.

Breast self-examination (BSE) is an option for women starting in their 20s. Women should be told about the benefits and limitations of BSE. Women should report any changes in their breasts to their health professional right away.

Women in their 20s and 30s should have a clinical breast examination (CBE) as part of a periodic (regular) health examination by a health professional at least every 3 years. After 40 years of age, women should undergo CBE by a health professional every year.

Women at high risk (greater than 20% lifetime risk) should undergo magnetic resonance imaging (MRI) and mammography every year. Women at moderately increased risk (15% to 20% lifetime risk) should talk with their doctors about the benefits and limitations of adding MRI screening to their yearly mammogram. Yearly MRI screening is not recommended for women whose lifetime risk for breast cancer is less than 15%.

From American Cancer Society guidelines for breast cancer screening. Available at www.cancer.org. Revised 2/9/11.

Because breast cancer is the most common extrathoracic primary neoplasm that causes metastases to the heart and pericardium, the EP should facilitate emergency echocardiography when managing a patient with breast cancer and symptoms consistent with pericardial effusion.

The development of back pain in a woman with a history of breast cancer should prompt initiation of diagnostic studies and treatment of cord compression. The most sensitive imaging study is magnetic resonance imaging, and it should be performed for back pain even when no associated neurologic finding is present (waiting for symptoms to appear may be too late).

Most patients who are treated for breast cancer undergo surgery that includes some degree of lymph node dissection. Lymphedema affects 10% to 30% of women who undergo axillary lymph node dissection; radiation and infection increase the risk. Lymphedema may range from mild to severe and can develop even years after treatment. Those at risk for the development of lymphedema are encouraged to have blood drawn and intravenous lines placed in the unaffected arm. It is usually permanent, although a few institutions have reported success with autologous lymph node transplantation.[12]

Women who choose lumpectomy or partial mastectomy usually undergo 6 weeks of external beam radiation therapy. Radiotherapy may also be given in the form of radioactive seeds placed at the tumor site. In another method, a saline-filled balloon is placed in the lumpectomy site and radioactive material is instilled and drained twice daily for 5 days. Regardless of the radiation method, the most common complications are radiation-induced dermatitis[13] (90% of patients), which can progress to dry desquamation (50% of patients) in the first few weeks, and moist desquamation (<10% of patients), which appears within 3 to 6 weeks. A corticosteroid cream such as mometasone furoate can be used as prophylaxis or treatment of dry desquamation, preferably in consultation with a medical or radiation oncologist. Wet desquamation, a partial-thickness injury, is best treated with hydrocolloid dressings and should be managed in consultation with a plastic surgeon or radiation oncologist.

Late effects of radiation may develop months or years after therapy. Pneumonitis is typically manifested as cough, fever, and shortness of breath 1 to 10 months after completion of radiation therapy. Radiographic changes, which can start as diffuse haziness and progress to patchy consolidations, are generally confined to the field of radiation. Dermal necrosis is a complication that may develop years after treatment. Radiation-induced brachial plexopathy,[14] which may develop up to 30 years after breast cancer therapy, is a permanent debilitating condition that can progress to complete sensory and motor impairment of the ipsilateral upper extremity and chronic neuropathic pain.

Adverse reactions to chemotherapy are beyond the scope of this chapter. However, the EP should be aware of all drugs being used by the patient. In addition, the EP should always query patients about their use of complementary and alternative medicine.

## TRAUMA

Trauma to the breast can be divided into the traditional divisions of blunt and penetrating. All but the most minimal trauma to the breast will require additional consideration of disruption of the underlying structures. The breast tissue itself may diminish the utility of physical examination in accurately identifying pathology.

Blunt trauma to the breast rarely appears in isolation. Multiple thoracic injuries are typical. Mandatory three-point lap-shoulder restraint laws have been effective in decreasing overall mortality from motor vehicle crashes; however, there has been a concurrent increase in the incidence of soft tissue injury to the chest wall. The chest restraint belt produces both shearing and compressive force. Simple hematomas are the most common problem after trauma. Although these hematomas typically resolve spontaneously, they may recur and become infected, even months after an injury.

Crush injuries from seat belts that involve the breast have, in rare cases, caused subcutaneous transection of the breast. A permanent furrow deformity may result. Because the breast is mobile over the pectoral fascia, sudden forceful movement of the breast can also cause complete avulsion of the breast from the chest wall and potentially rupture the perforating arteries to the breast. A transected artery may bleed massively immediately or may retract into the pectoral musculature and result in life-threatening hemorrhage after the vascular spasm resolves.

### *Fat Necrosis*

The most common long-term complication after trauma to the breast is fat necrosis.[15] Fat necrosis is an inflammatory condition that is typically a sequela of trauma, but it may also develop following surgery, infection, or radiation therapy. Women with pendulous breasts seem to be at higher risk for fat necrosis. The pathophysiology is multifactorial but primarily involves the breakdown of fat cells by blood and tissue lipases. Clinically, mammographically, and sonographically, the condition may mimic carcinoma of the breast. Usually, a firm, poorly mobile, nontender mass is present in the superficial subcutaneous tissues. The overlying skin may be erythematous, ecchymotic, or indurated. Axillary lymphadenopathy and nipple retraction may be present. Fat necrosis typically resolves spontaneously but requires biopsy to reliably differentiate it from malignancy.

## PERIOPERATIVE COMPLAINTS

More than 2 million women in the United States have undergone breast augmentation. Although 80% of augmentations are performed purely for cosmetic reasons, the 20% representing reconstruction following mastectomy account for a disproportionate percentage of local complications. Roughly 30% will require additional surgeries within 5 years.[16]

Postoperative pain can be prolonged; 30% to 40% of patients report significant pain 1 year after reduction or augmentation mammoplasty, and the number is higher after mastectomy with reconstruction. Phantom breast pain after mastectomy occurs in up to 12% of patients 1 year after surgery.[17]

### *Seroma or Hematoma*

The most common perioperative complication after any type of breast surgery is a seroma, or collection of serous fluid. On physical examination, the accumulation is manifested as a soft, movable mass with no evidence of infection and a "water bed" consistency when depressed and released. Seromas typically appear 7 to 10 days after surgery or 1 to 2 days after removal of a drain; in most cases they will resolve independently as the fluid is absorbed into surrounding tissues. A persistent, untreated seroma can lead to infection or skin flap necrosis. Hematomas may also occur after surgery, and management depends on multiple factors, including size and when they develop in relation to surgery.

### *Galactorrhea*

In the first days of recovery from surgery, 1% of women will experience galactorrhea (inappropriate lactation). This figure is slightly higher in women who have previously breastfed.

### *Capsular Contracture*

In capsular contracture, tightly woven collagen fibers form about an implant; they represent the body's attempt to isolate the implant from endogenous tissue. In 15% of women, this capsule becomes hard and resistant, contracts around the implant, and causes pain, deformation, and rupture. The risk is greater in women who experienced perioperative seroma, hematoma, or infection and in those who opt for silicone implants or subglandular placement.

### *Rupture*

The median life span of an implant is approximately 16 and 10 years for silicone gel and saline prosthetics, respectively. Although most ruptures do not result from ascertainable trauma, they have been reported following mammography, motor vehicle collisions, gunshots, falls, and surgical procedures in the chest, including central venous catheter insertion and thoracostomy. Clinical examination alone is unsatisfactory to identify most ruptures and should be supplemented with magnetic resonance imaging (90% accurate) or computed tomography (80% accurate).

### *Infection*

Many surgeons advocate perioperative antibiotic prophylaxis. This precaution has decreased the rate of postoperative infections, which otherwise ranges from 2% to 4% within the first month. The highest risk for infection occurs in patients who choose reconstruction at the time of mastectomy. The most common pathogen is *Staphylococcus aureus* (75%), followed by *Staphylococcus epidermidis* (10%). Toxic shock syndrome has been reported in some patients after augmentation or explantation; patients exhibit sudden pyrexia (>102° F), swelling of the infected breast, vomiting, diarrhea, dizziness, and often a sunburnlike rash.

## LACTATION AND PUERPERAL CHANGES

### *Puerperal Mastitis*

Puerperal mastitis, or mastitis that develops while breastfeeding, is a common cause of premature cessation of lactation and results in voluntary discontinuation of breastfeeding in up to 25% of patients.[18] It develops in about one third of nursing mothers. Eighty percent of cases occur in the first 3 months of lactation. Mastitis can rarely progress to abscess formation; this is significantly more common in the first 6 weeks after birth. Risk factors for puerperal mastitis include older age, primiparity, nipple damage, employment outside the home, ineffective nursing technique, and milk stasis.

Symptoms of puerperal mastitis include a painful, erythematous area or mass on the breast and systemic symptoms of fever, chills, malaise, and myalgia. The most common causative organism is *S. aureus*, although other organisms have been identified and infections may be polymicrobial. Fungal infection in the lactating breast is more common than was previously thought. *C. albicans* is the most frequently identified organism.

Differentiating between mastitis and abscess is important, and it is possible that the two conditions exist on a continuum. However, making the appropriate distinction is significant because the treatment for each is markedly different. Although an abscess is usually associated with significant fluctuance, it may appear as only a focal induration. Ultrasonography of the affected area should be performed to identify a subcutaneous fluid collection.

### *Risks Associated with Lactation in Special Circumstances*

Breastfeeding is superior to manufactured infant formula for its nutritional, cognitive, emotional, and immunologic benefits. Not all medications contraindicated during pregnancy are similarly dangerous to the nursing infant. Inappropriate cross-referencing of drug information in pregnancy to lactation may result in early cessation of lactation. Similarly, not all maternal infections necessitate cessation of lactation[19] (**Table 127.2**).

On average, 1% to 2% of a maternal dose of a drug is delivered to the infant, although the amount varies depending on the drug. Because the milk compartment is bidirectional, a drug that peaks in milk after 30 minutes may leave the milk compartment before the next feeding. It is therefore recommended that when possible, a nursing mother take medications immediately after a feeding to decrease the amount delivered to the infant in the next feeding. Little evidence-based data are available to determine which drugs are safe to use in lactation. EPs concerned about the safety of a particular

**Table 127.2 Breastfeeding Recommendations with Selected Maternal Infections**

| INFECTION | CLINICAL SIGNIFICANCE AND IMPACT ON BREASTFEEDING |
|---|---|
| CMV | Rarely causes illness in full-term infants because of placentally acquired antibodies |
| Hepatitis A | Found in breast milk but is an unusual mode of transmission; give immunoglobulin to the infant and continue breastfeeding |
| Hepatitis B | Give the infant routine hepatitis B vaccine and immunoglobulin and continue breastfeeding |
| Hepatitis C | Not proved to be transmitted by breastfeeding; continue breastfeeding. |
| VZV | Close contact with a person with acute VZV infection requires VZV immunoglobulin; the infant must avoid an infected person until the lesions crust over; expressed breast milk may be given unless lesions are present on the nipple-areola complex |
| HSV-1 and HSV-2 | Breastfeeding can be continued unless lesions are present on the breast |
| Lyme disease | If organism can be detected in breast milk by PCR but the infant has no signs of clinical illness, continue breastfeeding |
| Syphilis | Delay breastfeeding and express breast milk until maternal therapy has been given for 24 hr; treat the infant empirically |
| TB | Transmission via breast milk is seen only with TB mastitis; if no breast lesions are present, stop breastfeeding for 14 days and give isoniazid to the infant; expressed breast milk may be used |
| Gonorrhea | If the mother is treated with ceftriaxone, continue breastfeeding; if other medications are used, delay breastfeeding for 24 hr |

Data from Lawrence RM, Lawrence RA. Breast milk and infection. Clin Perinatol 2004;31:501-28.

*CMV*, Cytomegalovirus; *HSV*, herpes simplex virus; *PCR*, polymerase chain reaction; *TB*, tuberculosis; *VZV*, varicella-zoster virus.

**Table 127.3 Radioactive Drugs That Require Temporary Cessation of Breastfeeding**

| DRUG | TIME OF CESSATION |
|---|---|
| Gallium 67 | 14 days |
| Iodine 125 | 12 days |
| Iodine 131 | 2-14 days, depending on the study |
| Radioactive sodium | 4 days |
| Copper 64 | 50 hr |
| Technetium 99m | 15-36 hr |
| Iodine 123 | 36 hr |
| Indium 111 | 20 hr |

Data from American Academy of Pediatrics Committee on Drugs. Transfer of drugs and other chemicals into human milk. Pediatrics 2001;108:776-89.

medication in a lactating woman can consult the American Academy of Pediatrics Committee on Drugs.[20]

Administration of radioactive compounds to a lactating mother may require temporary cessation of breastfeeding (**Table 127.3**). Expression and discarding of milk for the duration of five half-lives are recommended. When ordering a nuclear medicine study for a lactating woman, the EP should speak directly to the nuclear medicine radiologist to determine whether a radionuclide with a shorter half-life could be used.

## TREATMENT

### MASTALGIA

Most patients require only mild analgesics, such as acetaminophen or ibuprofen. Discomfort from Mondor disease can also be managed with warm compresses. A number of alternative potential treatment modalities are available to women with cyclic mastalgia[21] (**Box 127.5**). Women with severe cyclic mastalgia, despite treatment with conservative measures, should be referred to an endocrinologist or reproductive specialist. All patients with mastalgia should receive follow-up care.

### DERMATOLOGIC CHANGES AND DISCHARGE

All patients with new onset of a dermatologic breast condition require outpatient follow-up regardless of their ED course. In particular, patients who fail to respond to traditional therapy should receive prompt evaluation and work-up for possible inflammatory breast cancer.

Local infections such as mastitis may be managed with oral broad-spectrum antibiotics; amoxicillin–clavulanic acid or levofloxacin with metronidazole is an appropriate regimen. All but the simplest abscesses require the consultation of a breast surgeon, admission for parenteral antibiotics (appropriate choices include cephalexin, doxycycline, gentamicin, and trimethoprim-sulfamethoxazole), and definitive surgical care.

**BOX 127.5 Adjuvant Treatment of Cyclic Mastalgia**

Improvement in mechanical support with a properly fitting bra and use of a sports bra during exercise
Application of warm compresses or ice packs
Decreasing dietary fat to less than 20% of energy intake
Eliminating caffeine in the diet
Smoking cessation
Oral contraceptive pills with low estrogen content
Parenteral medroxyprogesterone acetate (Depo-Provera)
Micronized progesterone vaginal cream applied to the breast
Vitamin E
Acupuncture

Patients with any findings suggestive of necrotizing fasciitis or skin necrosis require prompt surgical consultation. Broad-spectrum antibiotics and early, aggressive surgical débridement are necessary to minimize mortality in patients with necrotizing fasciitis. Emergency management of skin necrosis includes cessation of warfarin therapy, administration of vitamin K along with fresh frozen plasma, and initiation of heparin if anticoagulation is necessary.

Patients with dermatitis can typically be discharged safely. Management includes topical steroids, lubricants, friction-reducing agents, and avoidance of atopic triggers. Close outpatient follow-up of all patients is mandatory and may include short-term reevaluation of the response to treatment.

## MASSES

A physical examination that demonstrates any of the following necessitates prompt surgical referral: axillary or supraclavicular lymphadenopathy, rash, ulceration or dimpling, and nipple changes or discharge. Women without these worrisome findings still need referral for outpatient evaluation and follow-up, although many can be managed in a primary care setting. All women older than 35 years with masses require triple testing in the outpatient setting, including clinical evaluation, mammography with or without ultrasonography, and biopsy.

## TRAUMA

Simple hematomas can be managed conservatively with analgesics and instructions to wear a tight-fitting bra. Caution must be exercised in patients with an acute injury and an expanding hematoma, particularly those who have coagulopathies or are taking anticoagulant medication. Prompt reversal of anticoagulation should be considered. Patients initially seen more than 48 hours after sustaining an injury seldom have bleeding from a discrete vessel and only rarely are amenable to surgery.

Findings consistent with avulsion or transection require immediate surgical consultation. Further studies should be expedited to ascertain the true extent of the injuries. Patients will require admission for definitive care.

Hematomas occasionally occur spontaneously or in the setting of very minor trauma in women with breast cancer, and they may be the first symptom of occult malignancy. Breast trauma normally heals within 4 to 6 weeks. Symptoms that persist require evaluation for possible malignancy.

Penetrating trauma to the breast warrants careful scrutiny, and all but the most superficial injuries require consideration of intrathoracic penetration. Most wounds that penetrate the full dermis and all that affect the nipple should receive the attention of a breast surgeon.

Management strategies in patients with an infected hematoma include antibiotics and drainage (either open or guided by ultrasound). Appropriate antibiotics include first-generation cephalosporins or an antistaphylococcal penicillin.

## PERIOPERATIVE COMPLAINTS

Local infections may be treated with first-generation cephalosporins. Toxic shock is clearly a more significant progression of the infection and requires immediate surgical removal of the prosthesis, surgical débridement of surrounding tissue, parenteral antibiotics, and admission to an intensive care unit.

Seromas, hematomas, contractures, and ruptured implants all require consultation with a breast surgeon for definitive treatment and assurance of appropriate follow-up care.

Persistent or painful seromas or those that compromise surrounding tissue may require fine-needle aspiration. Because drainage may result in rupture of the prosthesis, aspiration is best performed by a plastic surgeon.

Hematomas seen within 48 hours of breast surgery may require additional surgery or drainage. Hematomas initially seen later than 48 hours after surgery are best managed conservatively with a cold compress or a compressive bra. Patients should avoid aspirin and ibuprofen because these medications can exacerbate the bleeding. As with seromas, there is a possibility of associated infection, and draining of the hematoma should be left to the discretion of the surgeon.

Galactorrhea is a benign symptom that should resolve spontaneously after a few days. Bromocriptine can be administered if the symptoms are persistent and bothersome.

In cases of capsular contracture in which notable breast hardness and distortion are present, surgery may be required to remove the implant via open capsulotomy. The patient should be counseled that manual manipulation of the breast to sever resistant fibrous capsules is not advised because it can lead to rupture.

Saline implant rupture rarely requires emergency intervention because the saline is quickly absorbed into surrounding tissue. Patients should be referred to a plastic surgeon for removal of the silicone lumen and cosmetic correction of breast deflation. Following rupture of a silicone gel–filled implant, however, extruded silicone may cause localized inflammation or silicone granulomas (siliconomas) that can migrate as far as the lower part of the back, groin, abdomen, and upper extremities.

## PUERPERAL MASTITIS

If mastitis is suspected, a 10-day course of oral therapy with dicloxacillin (500 mg four times daily) or cephalexin (500 mg four times daily) is indicated; either may be given as 1 g twice daily for increased compliance. Penicillin-allergic patients can be treated with clindamycin (300 mg four times daily) for 10 days. The patient should be instructed to continue breastfeeding, even on the affected side. If breastfeeding is painful, she should pump the affected breast frequently.

If an abscess is identified or suspected, oral or parenteral antibiotics may be prescribed, depending on the extent of tissue involvement, degree of systemic toxicity, and host factors. Parenteral choices include nafcillin (2 g intravenously [IV] every 6 hours), cefazolin (1 g IV every 8 hours), and vancomycin (1 g IV every 8 hours). Patients should pump and discard all milk until the abscess has healed to prevent transmission of the infection to the infant. Although aspiration with a 16-gauge needle may be performed, surgical consultation is required for definitive care.

Patients must have close follow-up and should be instructed to return to the ED if the symptoms worsen at any time or fail to improve within 48 hours. Additional management may include referral to a lactation specialist, if available.

Indications for possible inpatient admission include failure of outpatient therapy, infections in immunocompromised patients (AIDS, diabetes, therapy with cytotoxic agents or glucocorticoids), and patients with significant signs of systemic toxicity. Rarely, sepsis, gangrene, or necrotizing soft tissue infections can develop.

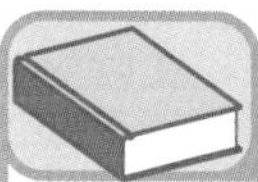

**PATIENT TEACHING TIPS**

Any new breast symptom requires evaluation by a physician; the patient should seek prompt reevaluation if initial treatment of a diagnosed condition is not effective.

Although most causes of breast lumps, skin changes, breast pain, and nipple discharge are benign, many conditions (including malignancy) appear similar on physical examination and even on imaging studies.

Making a definitive diagnosis of any breast condition may require several follow-up outpatient visits and tests.

Patients should be familiar with the American Cancer Society's recommendations for breast cancer screening for their age group.

Most patients fail to appreciate the significance of the false-negative rate of mammography. Mammograms fail to diagnose breast cancer in up to 15% of cases; therefore, a recent "normal" screening mammogram should not falsely reassure a patient with a suspicious complaint. Tissue sampling is indicated in these situations.

Patients who have undergone surgery or radiation therapy (or both) for breast cancer are at high risk for the development of lymphedema. They should be instructed to avoid compression of the ipsilateral arm and should seek immediate medical care for the treatment of insect bites, burns, lacerations, and infections, all of which increase the risk for lymphedema.

## SUGGESTED READINGS

Hartmann LC, Sellers TA, Frost MH, et al. Benign breast disease and the risk of breast cancer. N Engl J Med 2005;353:229-37.

Michie C, Lockie F, Lynn W. The challenge of mastitis. Arch Dis Child 2003;88:818-21.

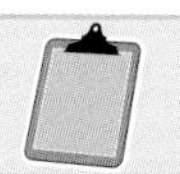

**DOCUMENTATION**

Meticulous documentation of the physical examination, as well as all results, when evaluating a patient with a complaint related to the breast or when an abnormality is discovered incidentally is a necessity.

Documentation of the physical examination should include the appearance of the breasts, including the nipple-areola complex, with the patient sitting, with the arms raised, and supine. Results of palpating the breast with the patient supine and the ipsilateral hand under the head should be recorded, as well as the results of gentle nipple squeezing.

All abnormalities should be diagrammed and described. Size, mobility, consistency, and symmetry in comparison with the opposite breast are important to document. Lymph nodes should be noted in terms of number, size, consistency, and mobility.

Impeccable documentation is required in cases of suspected intimate partner violence or sexual assault.

When treating a lactating patient, all discussions about the advisability and possible risks associated with continuing breastfeeding should be documented, especially when diagnosing infectious conditions, prescribing medications, and ordering radionuclide imaging.

The history should include attention to current medications, as well as past hormonal therapy, menopausal status, reproductive and breastfeeding history, family history of cancer, radiation exposure, and previous breast problems.

An inclusive differential diagnosis should be documented, specifically listing cancer if it is a possibility. In these cases, documented discussions with the patient should include mention of the physician's concerns and need for prompt follow-up.

Written discharge instructions should include follow-up plans and phone numbers for referral physicians. Special arrangements may be necessary to ensure timely specialist care. All such efforts should be documented.

Smith RL, Pruthi S, Fitzpatrick L. Evaluation and management of breast pain. Mayo Clin Proc 2004;79:353-72.

Whitaker-Worth DL, Carlone V, Susser WS, et al. Dermatologic diseases of the breast and nipple. J Am Acad Dermatol 2000;43:733-51.

## REFERENCES

*References can be found on Expert Consult @ www.expertconsult.com.*

# 128 Sexual Assault

*Monique Iris Sellas*

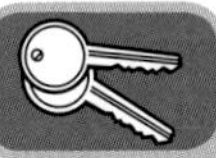

**KEY POINTS**

- Sexual assault requires the emergency physician to competently and comprehensively evaluate and treat the physical, emotional, and legal needs of the patient.
- Management includes medical stabilization, treatment of physical injuries, emergency contraception, prophylaxis for sexually transmitted diseases, assessment of risk for nonoccupational postexposure prophylaxis, forensic evaluation and evidence collection, crisis intervention, arrangement for follow-up medical care, and referral to social support and legal services.

## EPIDEMIOLOGY

Sexual assault is sexual contact of one person with another without appropriate legal consent. The precise definition varies slightly from state to state, and health care providers should familiarize themselves with the definition in their jurisdiction. It is a widespread occurrence that permeates every facet of our society and can affect anyone regardless of gender, age, race, or socioeconomic status. In 2009, 88,097 forcible rapes were reported to law enforcement in the United States.[1] This number is estimated to represent only 40% of the total sexual assaults because the majority of cases go unreported.[2] The National Violence Against Women Survey found that 18% of surveyed women (1 in 6) and 3% of surveyed men (1 in 33) had experienced an attempted or completed rape at some time in their lives.[3] The majority of females are assaulted by acquaintances or intimate partners and 32% by a stranger. Young females between the ages of 16 and 24 are disproportionately affected.[4] For affected males, underreporting of their victimization is the norm. During the last decade, an alarming increase has been observed in reports of drug-facilitated sexual assault (DFSA).[5]

## PRESENTING SIGNS AND SYMPTOMS

A sexual assault patient will most often walk into the emergency department (ED) alone or in the company of a friend or family member. Alternatively, she or he may be accompanied by law enforcement officers or be transported by emergency medical services. The individual may be seen immediately after or long after the assault. A sexual assault patient initially evaluated within 120 hours (5 days) of the assault should be considered a high-priority patient and be brought to a designated treatment area as soon as possible. The reason for this is manifold and includes providing crisis intervention, treating injuries, administering time-sensitive medications, and expediting the evidentiary examination to minimize loss or deterioration of forensic evidence. It is prudent for EDs to have a systematic management plan in place for these patients from triage to discharge.

## DIFFERENTIAL DIAGNOSIS AND MEDICAL DECISION MAKING

### MULTIDISCIPLINARY APPROACH

Emergency physicians (EPs) are responsible for managing both the medical and forensic needs of patients with a report of sexual assault. This is best accomplished in an organized manner, such as with a sexual assault response team (SART). Members include a sexual assault forensic examiner (SAFE), victim advocates, law enforcement officers, crime laboratory personnel, and prosecutors. A SAFE has specialized knowledge and training to perform the forensic evaluation with a standardized sexual assault evidence collection kit (SAECK). Research has shown that use of a SART/SAFE program improves the quality of forensic evidence with an increase in prosecution rates over time.[6] In jurisdictions in which such teams are unavailable, ED providers are responsible for the forensic examination, and it is therefore prudent that EPs familiarize themselves with their state-specific SAECK.

### CONSENT FOR FORENSIC EVALUATION AND EVIDENCE COLLECTION

Patients should be informed of all of the options available to them, including forensic evaluation and evidence collection, depending on timing of examination. Before proceeding with any part of this evaluation, written informed consent for all aspects of the evaluation must be obtained as listed in **Box 128.1**. The patient has the right to refuse all or some parts of a forensic examination, and consent can be withdrawn at any time during the examination.

**BOX 128.1 Forensic Evaluation Tasks That Require Written Informed Consent**

Medical evaluation and treatment
History and documentation of the testimonial
Physical examination of the body and genitals with documentation of injuries
Evidence collection, including clothing, hair, blood samples, body fluid samples, and fingernail scrapings
Forensic photography

## ONE PATIENT, TWO MEDICAL RECORDS

The clinical encounter with a sexual assault patient is unique in that two medical records are generated for one patient. One is the usual ED medical record and the other is the forensic legal record. These records serve very different purposes, and consequently what is documented in each will differ.

## HISTORY

For the ED medical record, the history of the assault should be focused on details that affect medical management of the patient in the ED, including information that will help determine the risk for injuries and what treatment of sexually transmitted diseases (STDs) should be offered. In contrast, the forensic record is driven by strict policies and procedures and should include only medical information that has a direct bearing on evaluation of the reported crime. Material that is generally considered to constitute useful background in a therapeutic context may have a prejudicial effect in a forensic context and should not be included in the forensic record. Examples include the number of previous pregnancies, past mental health treatment, and remote substance abuse. Documentation should be concise and directly relevant to the assault, including any information that is necessary to properly interpret the current physical findings. Many SAECKs contain preprinted forms that help the examiner with the history-taking process to facilitate proper documentation. Salient features of the history that should be obtained for documentation in the forensic medical record are listed in **Box 128.2**.[7,8]

**BOX 128.2 Pertinent Historical Features of a Sexual Assault for Forensic Documentation**

Date, time, location, and physical surroundings of the assault
Date and time of hospital examination
Loss of memory or periods of unconsciousness
Patient's narrative of events as they pertain to sexual acts or the trauma sustained
Total number of assailants and relationship to the patient
Weapons, restraints, or force used
Specific sexual acts, including:

- Vaginal, anal, or oral penetration by the assailant's penis, finger, tongue, or an object
- Ejaculation inside or outside a body cavity
- Condom or lubricant use
- Any injuries to the victim or assailant resulting in bleeding

Physical trauma sustained
Pertinent health history

- Recent medical or gynecologic procedures or treatment that may affect the physical findings or evidence collection
- Presence of menstruation at the time of the assault
- Consensual intercourse in the past 120 hours (5 days)
- Use of any type of contraception in the past 24 hours

Hygiene events after the assault

- Has the patient changed clothes, bathed or showered, washed off, brushed teeth, taken anything by mouth, vomited, urinated, douched, defecated, or used an enema since the assault?

## PHYSICAL EXAMINATION

Physical examination is necessary to evaluate for signs of any trauma sustained during the sexual assault. The reported incidence of nongenital physical injuries ranges from 23% to 85%.[8-15] When injuries are sustained, those most commonly seen are soft tissue injuries involving the head, face, neck, and extremities. Blunt force trauma, including penetrative blunt mechanisms, may produce contusions, which are associated with swelling, pain, tenderness, and discoloration, and lacerations from tearing of the tissues. A friction mechanism may cause abrasions. Sharp-force trauma may produce incised wounds. Bites may involve multiple mechanisms of injury. Patterned injuries suggest the specific object, weapon, or mechanism used to produce its characteristic shape.

The physical examination should be dictated by the history of the events. Close attention should be paid to the skin for signs of victim resistance, applied restraints, or defensive wounds. The oral cavity should be inspected for a torn lingual or labial frenulum or contusions to the palate with report of an oral assault. With a report of strangulation, the examination should focus on assessing for and documenting abrasions or contusions of the neck, facial petechiae, and subconjunctival hemorrhage.

Published rates of female genitoanal injury vary widely from 6% to 65%, with most investigators reporting a range of 10% to 30%.[8-18] Risk factors for injuries included examination within 24 hours of the assault, presence of nongenital injury, threats of violence, and age younger than 20 and older than 40 years.[8-18] The genital structures most frequently injured as a result of a penetrative mechanism are the fossa navicularis and posterior fourchette, followed by the labia minora and hymen. It is paramount that these areas be inspected carefully during the examination.

Physical examination consists largely of gross visual inspection, which may readily miss documentable injuries. Adjuncts to assist in detecting subtle injuries include anoscopy, colposcopy, Wood lamp, and application of toluidine blue.

A large number of sexual assault patients do not sustain obvious injuries. It is important that the EP understand that the absence of objective physical or genital injury does not preclude the possibility of sexual assault. The presence of such injuries is dependent on many assault-specific and patient-specific factors, including the age of the victim, the state of the tissues such as lubrication and elasticity, the degree of force involved, and the use of objects or implements.

In addition, detection of subtle injuries is largely dependent on examiner training and experience.

For the forensic record, documentation of the physical findings should include thorough, precise written descriptions in standard anatomic position, including injury location, measured size, shape, colors, contours, and depth. In addition, the use of anatomic body maps and forensic photography is encouraged, both of which can be invaluable in court proceedings. Many SAECK preprinted forms include body maps on which to note injuries.

## FORENSIC EVALUATION: EVIDENCE COLLECTION AND CHAIN OF CUSTODY

The premise of evidence collection in sexual assault cases is to link the victim and assailant, relate both to the crime scene, identify the assailant via a DNA profile, and establish some features of the crime. The SAECK, also known as a "rape kit," is stocked in most hospitals and is state specific. It is used to guide the process of evidence collection within 96 to 120 hours (4 to 5 days) of an assault. EPs should familiarize themselves with the SAECK used in their jurisdiction.

Once a patient consents to evidence collection, the steps delineated in the kit should be followed. Evidence collection should be guided by the history of the assault. **Box 128.3** lists potential specimens to be gathered for forensic evidence collection.[19,20]

Evidence is lost in an exponential manner over time. As a result, evidence collection may have to be augmented based on time of evaluation after the assault. Oral and anal swabs should be collected only if the patient is initially evaluated within 24 hours of the assault because the yield thereafter is 0%. In addition, cervical sampling should be considered for evaluations between 96 and 120 hours after the assault to increase the chance of detecting spermatozoa. Seminal fluid, as evidenced by spermatozoa, high levels of acid phosphatase, or p30 prostate-specific antigen, is recovered from 38% to 48% of sexual assault patients.[9]

Chain of custody, also referred to as the chain of evidence, refers to detailed documentation of the trail of the evidence from the time that it is collected until it is exhibited during a legal trial. To comply with the chain of custody, the kit must be accounted for at all times without failure, and all transfers must be documented, including the police officer who assumes responsibility for the kit. If police are unavailable to collect the kit at that point, it should be locked in a secure area reserved for such instances so that the data are not invalidated. If there are any gaps in the chain of custody, the evidence may not be admissible in court. It is prudent for EDs to develop protocols for these encounters.

**BOX 128.3 Potential Specimens to Be Gathered for Forensic Evidence Collection**

Clothing
- Each article of clothing should be packaged in separate paper bags to avoid cross-contamination
- If the patient has changed her clothing, only underwear should be collected

Known blood sample
- Crime laboratory assesses for the secretor status and blood type of the patient

Toxicology testing (urine and blood)
- For use in cases in which drug-facilitated sexual assault is suspected
- Collect for evaluation less than 72 to 96 hours after the assault (the time varies by crime laboratory)

Oral swabs and smears
- Collect for evaluation up to 24 hours after the assault

Head hair combings

Fingernail scrapings

Foreign material collection

Swabs of bite marks or areas where the assailant's mouth touched the patient

Pubic hair combings

External genital swabs

Vaginal swabs and smears
- Cervical sampling should be considered for evaluation between 96 and 120 hours after the assault

Perianal swabs

Anorectal swabs and smears
- Collect for evaluation up to 24 hours after the assault

Forensic photography
- Three views per injury, one with a ruler for scale

**TIPS AND TRICKS**

**Forensic Evaluation**

SART/SAFE programs coordinate patient care and improve evidence collection and prosecutions.

Emergency physicians should familiarize themselves with the SAECK used in their jurisdiction.

If the patient wants something to drink before the forensic evaluation has started and she consents, collect the oral swabs first and be sure to maintain chain of custody.

If the patient wants to urinate before the forensic evaluation has started, give her a collection cup for the urine pregnancy test and toxicology screen, and inform her not to wipe the genital area afterward. Be sure to maintain chain of custody of this sample.

*SAECK*, Sexual assault evidence collection kit; *SAFE*, sexual assault forensic examiner; *SART*, sexual assault response team.

## DIAGNOSTIC TESTING

Although selection of the initial laboratory studies and radiographic imaging is guided by the trauma assessment, certain tests should be ordered for all sexual assault patients. All female sexual assault victims should undergo urine pregnancy testing because a positive result will alter the choices for prophylaxis. If nonoccupational postexposure prophylaxis (nPEP) will be administered, a baseline complete blood count, liver function tests, and blood urea nitrogen and creatinine levels should be ordered before initiation. If the patient is initially seen many days after the assault and has symptoms and signs suggestive of active infection with an STD, culture for gonorrhea and *Chlamydia* should be obtained in addition to a vaginal wet mount and culture for *Trichomonas* and bacterial vaginosis (BV). Further testing should be reserved for an outpatient follow-up appointment, including human immunodeficiency virus (HIV) antibody testing, syphilis testing, hepatitis B and C serology, and gonorrhea and *Chlamydia* screening.

The influence of drugs must be considered in each sexual assault case. Samples for hospital toxicology screening should be drawn only if they affect medical management of the patient. During the forensic examination, if the patient is amnestic and DFSA is suspected, urine and blood should be collected with the victim's consent for a forensic drug screen for assaults occurring less than 72 to 96 hours before the evaluation. These samples are considered forensic evidence, and the chain of custody should be maintained at all times for analysis in the crime laboratory, not in the hospital laboratory.

## MANDATORY REPORTING

Laws regarding mandatory reporting of adult sexual assault victims vary from state to state and can be broken down into laws that specifically require providers to report treatment of a rape victim to law enforcement, laws that require reporting of injuries that may include rape, laws relating to other crimes or injuries that may have an impact on rape and sexual assault victims, and laws regarding sexual assault forensic examinations that may affect rape and sexual assault reporting.[21,22] It is prudent for EPs to be well informed of the local reporting regulations in their jurisdictions.

## CONSULTATION

A multidisciplinary approach to the care of sexual assault patients is prudent to optimize medical care and forensic and legal considerations. In patients with significant physical or genital trauma, consultation with trauma surgery and gynecology should be considered. The local victim advocacy group and hospital social worker should be consulted for patient support. A SAFE should be consulted for forensic evaluation and evidence collection once the patient consents to this course of action. For patients who are at high risk for HIV, consultation with an infectious disease (ID) specialist is important to facilitate the best nPEP regimen based on the characteristics of the assault.

## TREATMENT

### PREHOSPITAL MANAGEMENT

Prehospital care should proceed as usual with medical stabilization and treatment of injuries. In clinically stable victims without significant injury, it is best practice for the prehospital providers to minimize touching the patient so that potential forensic evidence is not altered. If the sheet that the patient is transported on contains foreign material, it should be folded up and given to the responsible clinical staff member in the ED for possible inclusion in the evidence collection kit while maintaining the protocol for chain of custody.

### HOSPITAL MANAGEMENT

A patient with a report of sexual assault may go to the ED immediately after or long after the assault. The time since the assault determines how these patients are managed, including what interventions and treatments are recommended. **Figure 128.1** outlines the scope of evaluation and treatment of sexual assault based on the timing of initial evaluation.

Sexual assault is a disempowering experience, and giving patients options about their management and treatment is important in supporting the process of recovery. If conducted in a sensitive and supportive way, the ED encounter may be the first step toward healing. The local victim advocacy group should be notified, with patient permission, so that an advocate can come to the ED to provide support, crisis intervention, and information to the patient.

#### *Medical Stabilization and Management of Physical Injuries*

Injuries related to the assault, such as soft tissue injuries and fractures, should be treated appropriately. The advanced trauma life support protocol should be followed when assessing a trauma patient. Nearly 20% of sexual assault victims require medical procedures or interventions.[10,23] Tetanus prophylaxis should be considered in patients with violation of skin integrity who have not had a booster within 10 years. After treatment of the physical injuries, the focus should transition to emergency contraception, STD prophylaxis, and risk assessment for nPEP. **Table 128.1** lists the recommended prophylaxis regimen for sexual assault patients. Forensic evaluation and evidence collection follow suit.[24-27]

#### *Emergency Contraception*

Overall, the risk for pregnancy following sexual assault is 5%.[28] The risk varies throughout the menstrual cycle, as shown in Table 128.1. Regardless of where she is in her cycle, following a negative pregnancy test, all females of childbearing age with a report of sexual assault should be offered emergency contraception (see Chapter 129 for further details).[29-31]

#### *Sexually Transmitted Disease Prophylaxis*

The risk of acquiring an STD following a sexual assault is significant, with reported rates of 4% to 56%, depending on the circumstances of the assault.[32] Given the difficulty in accurately assessing risk, as well as poor compliance with follow-up visits in this patient population, which has been estimated to be 10% to 35%, empiric prophylaxis should be offered routinely to these patients.[24,33,34] STD prophylaxis should be guided by the 2010 Centers for Disease Control and Prevention (CDC) guidelines and includes dispensation of medication for prophylaxis against *Neisseria gonorrhea, Chlamydia trachomatis, Trichomonas vaginalis*, BV, hepatitis B, and HIV in high-risk cases.[24]

Table 128.1 includes the 2010 CDC-recommended regimen for STD prophylaxis after a sexual assault. Although the efficacy of these medications in preventing infections after sexual assault has not been evaluated, administration is still considered standard of care given the high single-exposure transmission rate in the case of a disease-positive assailant.[24,25]

Screening for STDs in asymptomatic sexual assault patients is very controversial. Those in favor of not testing argue that a positive test represents preassault disease and could be used against a victim in court. Laws exist in every state that protect

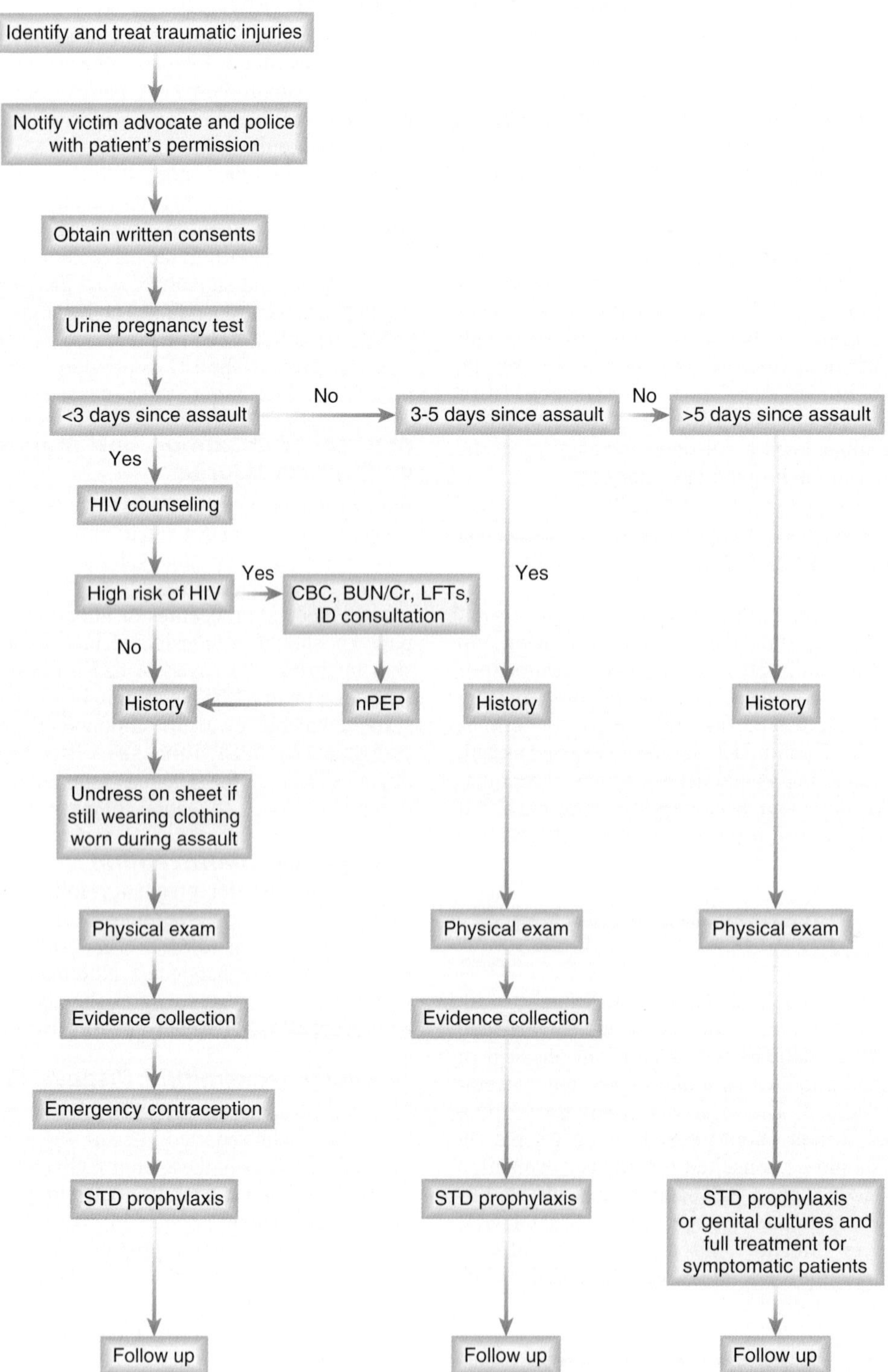


**Fig. 128.1 Emergency department management of patients after sexual assault.** *BUN*, Blood urea nitrogen; *CBC*, complete blood count; *Cr*, creatinine; *HIV*, human immunodeficiency virus; *LFTs*, liver function tests; *nPEP*, nonoccupational postexposure prophylaxis; *STD*, sexually transmitted disease.

the victim's previous sexual history, but if medical records are subpoenaed, the STD diagnoses may be discovered. As a result, the patient and clinician might opt to defer testing. The American College of Emergency Physicians states that in cases in which prophylaxis will be given, acute cultures are not necessary unless obvious signs of an STD are present.[24,35]

If the patient is seen in the ED days after the sexual assault with symptoms of active infection, including vaginal discharge or pelvic pain, a pelvic examination must be performed to assess for cervicitis and pelvic inflammatory disease. Cervical and vaginal cultures should be obtained and full treatment administered for symptomatic disease.

**Table 128.1** Recommended Prophylaxis Regimen and Treatment of Sexual Assault Patients

| RISK | MEDICATION | SINGLE-EXPOSURE TRANSMISSION RATE | INDICATION AND CAVEATS |
|---|---|---|---|
| Pregnancy | Levonorgestrel (Plan B), 1.5 g PO × 1 | Risk varies throughout the menstrual cycle:<br>15% 3 days before ovulation<br>30% 1-2 days before ovulation<br>12% on the day of ovulation<br>Approaches 0% 1-2 days after ovulation | Offer to all victims at risk seen <72 hr after assault.<br>Pregnancy should be ruled out with urine β-hCG. |
| Gonorrhea | Ceftriaxone, 250 mg IM × 1 (also covers incubating syphilis)<br>*or*<br>Cefixime, 400 mg PO × 1 | 20-78% | Offer to all victims at risk |
| *Chlamydia* | Azithromycin, 1 g PO × 1<br>*or*<br>Doxycycline, 100 mg PO bid × 7 days | 20-70% | Offer to all victims at risk.<br>Doxycycline is FDA pregnancy class C. |
| Trichomonas *and* bacterial vaginosis | Flagyl, 2 g PO × 1 | High | Offer to all victims at risk.<br>Do not administer within 48 hr of alcohol use. |
| Hepatitis B | Hepatitis B vaccine × 1<br>2nd and 3rd vaccines of the series are given at 4 wk and 6 mo | 1-30% | Offer to all victims at risk who are unimmunized or unsure of immunization status. |
| Tetanus | Td toxoid, 0.5 mL IM × 1 | | Offer to all victims with violation of skin who have not had a booster within 10 yr.<br>FDA pregnancy class C. |
| HIV | NNRTI-based therapy: efavirenz plus lamivudine or emtricitabine plus zidovudine or tenofovir<br>*or*<br>Protease inhibitor–based therapy: Kaletra plus lamivudine | Receptive vaginal: 0.1-0.2%<br>Receptive anal: 0.5-3% | Offer to high-risk victims seen <72 hr after the assault.<br>Consult with a specialist in HIV treatment.<br>Adjustments to the regimen will have to be made in pregnant women and women of childbearing potential. |
| | × 28 days or until the source patient is proved to be HIV negative<br>*Note:* Many alternative regimens are available.<br>Administration of an antiemetic is highly suggested because the combination of medications listed in concert with the traumatic event may induce nausea and vomiting. | | |

Data from Centers for Disease Control and Prevention (CDC). Sexually transmitted diseases treatment guidelines, 2010. MMWR Recomm Rep 2010;59(RR-12):1-110; National Institute of Allergy and Infectious Diseases, National Institutes of Health, Department of Health and Human Services. Scientific evidence on condom effectiveness for sexually transmitted disease (STD) prevention. July 20, 2001. Retrieved January 2011 from http://www.niaid.nih.gov/about/organization/dmid/documents/condomreport.pdf; Varghese B, Maher JE, Peterman TA, et al. Reducing the risk of sexual HIV transmission: quantifying the per-act risk for HIV on the basis of choice of partner, sex act, and condom use. Sex Transm Dis 2002;29:38-43; and Centers for Disease Control and Prevention (CDC). Antiretroviral postexposure prophylaxis after sexual, injection-drug use, or other non-occupational exposure to HIV in the United States: recommendations from the U.S. Department of Health and Human Services. MMWR Recomm Rep 2005;54(RR-2):1-20.

*FDA*, Food and Drug Administration; *β-hCG*, β subtype human chorionic gonadotropin; *HIV*, human immunodeficiency virus; *IM*, intramuscularly; *NNRTI*, nonnucleoside reverse transcriptase inhibitor; *PO*, orally; *Td*, tetanus-diphtheria toxoid.

### *Nonoccupational Postexposure Prophylaxis for Human Immunodeficiency Virus Infection*

The frequency of HIV seroconversion as a result of sexual assault is difficult to estimate but probably low. In consensual sex, the risk for HIV transmission from receptive penile-vaginal intercourse is 0.1% to 0.2% and for receptive penile-rectal intercourse is 0.5% to 3%.[26] Various factors increase risk for HIV transmission, including trauma with resultant bleeding, site of exposure to the ejaculate, high viral load in the ejaculate, multiple assailants, and the presence of an STD or genital lesion in either party.[24,27]

nPEP has not been proved to be effective in decreasing transmission of HIV in cases of sexual assault but, instead, is extrapolated from health care workers with occupational exposure. As a result, a risk-benefit analysis must be performed to determine whether this therapy should be offered.

nPEP should be considered only if the exposure occurred less than 72 hours previously, and its efficacy is maximal when administered soonest after exposure.[27] Absolute indications for starting nPEP include initial evaluation less than 72 hours after exposure to a known HIV-positive assailant with an exposure that carries substantial risk for transmission. This will rarely be the case because the majority of sexual assault patients do not know the HIV status of their assailant. Consequently, the clinician will have to make a case-by-case determination for starting nPEP based on the characteristics of the assault. The EP should consult with an ID specialist to decide whether therapy is indicated and which regimen would be most appropriate given the assault-specific details. If one is not readily available, assistance with nPEP-related decisions can be obtained by calling the National Clinician's Post-Exposure Prophylaxis Hotline (PEP line) at (888) 448-4911.[24] When the decision is made to administer nPEP, the first dose should be given as soon as possible and prophylaxis continued for 28 days. nPEP is not recommended for patients initially evaluated more than 72 hours after exposure because the risks associated with the medications outweigh the benefits by this time.[27] Table 128.1 includes the CDC-recommended regimen for nPEP after a sexual assault.

### *Prescriptions*

As illustrated in Table 128.1, sexual assault patients may be administered multiple medications during the ED visit, the majority of which require only one dose. The exceptions are doxycycline and nPEP. If doxycycline is chosen for *Chlamydia* prophylaxis, a prescription for a 7-day course should be given. For nPEP, the CDC recommends a 3- to 5-day starter pack to last until the follow-up visit, at which time an additional prescription can be given if appropriate.[24,27] If the patient has consumed alcohol in the last 48 hours, she should not be administered metronidazole (Flagyl) in the ED. She should be sent home with the dose or given a prescription so that she can take it when outside the window of a disulfiram-type reaction.

## FOLLOW-UP, NEXT STEPS IN CARE, AND PATIENT EDUCATION

After all medical treatment and forensic evaluation are complete, the patient's environment should be assessed for safety. The SAFE or hospital social worker can help the patient identify resources if she feels unsafe returning home. If deemed safe for discharge, a hospital aftercare packet should be given to the patient because victims of traumatic events frequently cannot remember the events immediately following a crisis. She should be given contact information for the rape crisis center or hospital counseling services because the mental health morbidity associated with sexual assault is profound.[32]

Within 1 to 5 days of the ED visit, the patient should follow up with an ID specialist for testing for HIV, hepatitis B and C, and syphilis. Additional counseling and support can be offered in addition to assessing for medication adherence and side effects if nPEP was started in the ED. The rest of the 28-day course of medication should then be prescribed or an altered regimen recommended if indicated by side effects. Two weeks after the ED visit the patient should follow up for STD screening. Four weeks after the ED visit the patient should follow up for pregnancy testing and receive the second dose of the hepatitis B vaccine if applicable.[24,36]

Note that management of pediatric sexual abuse varies significantly from the management of adult sexual assault outlined in this chapter.

## SUGGESTED READINGS

Centers for Disease Control and Prevention (CDC). Antiretroviral postexposure prophylaxis after sexual, injection-drug use, or other non-occupational exposure to HIV in the United States: recommendations from the U.S. Department of Health and Human Services. MMWR Recomm Rep 2005;54(RR-2):1-20.

Centers for Disease Control and Prevention (CDC). Sexually transmitted diseases treatment guidelines, 2010. MMWR Recomm Rep 2010;59(RR-12):1-110.

Green WM. Sexual assault. In: Riviello RJ, editor. Manual of forensic emergency medicine: a guide for clinicians. Boston: Jones & Bartlett; 2010. p. 107.

Scalzo TP. Rape and sexual assault reporting requirements for competent adult victims. Retrieved January 2011 from http://www.usmc-mccs.org/famadv/restrictedreporting/National%20Rape%20Reporting%20Requirements%206.15.06.pdf.

Tjaden P, Thoennes N. Extent, nature, and consequences of rape victimization: findings from the National Violence Against Women Survey. Washington, DC: U.S. Department of Justice, Office of Justice Programs; 2006. NCJ 210346. Retrieved January 2011 from http://www.ncjrs.gov/pdffiles1/nij/210346.pdf.

## REFERENCES

***References can be found on Expert Consult @ www.expertconsult.com.***

# Emergency Contraception 129

*Tomer Begaz*

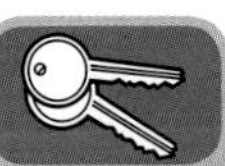

**KEY POINTS**

- Emergency contraception (EC) is more effective the sooner it is administered, and its effectiveness decreases with time. It can be administered up to 120 hours after intercourse with reasonable effectiveness.
- EC is not effective in pregnancy, but it is also not harmful.
- Progestin-only EC (levonorgestrel, "Plan B") is more effective than combined estrogen-progestin EC and has fewer side effects.
- In the United States, levonorgestrel EC ("Plan B") is available to women older than 17 years without a prescription.
- Both levonorgestrel doses (1.5 mg total) can be administered as a single, one-time dose.
- Hormonal EC can cause nausea. Antiemetics can help if administered 30 to 60 minutes before taking contraceptive pills.
- Because patients can still become pregnant for the remainder of the cycle after the use of EC, alternative methods of contraception must still be used, and patients should immediately resume taking their regular oral contraceptive pills.
- A pelvic examination is not a prerequisite to providing EC.
- Many pharmacies do not have Plan B available in timely fashion; therefore, it is prudent to give the pills directly to the patient.

**Table 129.1** Failure Rates of Selected Contraceptive Methods Within 1 Year (%)

| METHOD | PERFECT USE | TYPICAL USE |
|---|---|---|
| Chance | 85 | 85 |
| Combination pill | 0.1 | 5.0 |
| Progestin-only pill | 0.5 | 5.0 |
| Male condom | 3.0 | 14.0 |
| Diaphragm | 6.0 | 20 |
| Spermicide | 6.0 | 26 |
| Periodic abstinence—calendar method | 9.0 | NA |
| Hormonal emergency contraception | 0.1 | 3.0 |
| Copper IUD | 0.1 | NA |

From Kafrissen M, Adashi E. Fertility control: current approaches and global aspects. In: Larsen PR, Kronenberg HM, Melmed S, et al, editors. Williams textbook of endocrinology. 10th ed. Philadelphia: Saunders; 2003. pp. 665-708.

*IUD*, Intrauterine device; *NA*, not available.

## EPIDEMIOLOGY

Emergency contraception (EC) refers to methods of preventing pregnancy that are used after sexual intercourse. Circumstances making visits to the emergency department (ED) necessary include rape, contraceptive failure (e.g., condom breakage), and failure to use a contraceptive.

Approximately 50% of women between the ages of 15 and 44 years have had at least one unwanted pregnancy, which amounts to more than 3 million unwanted pregnancies annually in the United States.[1] No contraceptive method is 100% effective, and the failure rates of contraceptives are surprisingly high (**Table 129.1**).[2] Because contraceptive failure is so common, most emergency physicians (EPs) will deal with this issue on a regular basis, and they should be aware of the indications and complications of this treatment.

## PATHOPHYSIOLOGY

The primary mechanism of action of estrogen-progestin EC is inhibition of ovulation. Additional possible contributing mechanisms include thickening of cervical mucus, altered sperm transport, and changes in the endometrial lining.[3] Progestin-only methods (levonorgestrel) do not appear to have an effect on the endometrium. Ulipristal is a progesterone receptor modulator, similar to mifepristone. The primary mechanism of these drugs at the EC dose is inhibition of ovulation, although the possibility of an additional affect on uterine implantation cannot be entirely excluded. Once an embryo is implanted in the endometrium, hormonal EC has no effect on a pregnancy and does not cause abortion.[4]

It is important for the EP to understand the mechanism of action of EC to accurately address the concerns of individual patients. According to the definition of the American College of Obstetrics and Gynecology, pregnancy is established at the time of implantation of the embryo in the uterus.[5] By this definition, hormonal EC drugs are *not* abortifacients because these medications do not interfere with already established (implanted) pregnancies. However, individual patients may have a different understanding of terms such as *conception* and *abortion* than the medical community does. The known facts should be presented to patients simply and clearly so that they will be informed participants in their health care (**Table 129.2** and **Boxes 129.1 and 129.2**).[6,7]

## PRESENTING SIGNS AND SYMPTOMS

Patients seen immediately afterward in the ED should have no symptoms. If pregnancy or any symptoms such as abdominal pain are of concern, further evaluation is indicated. See the Red Flags box.

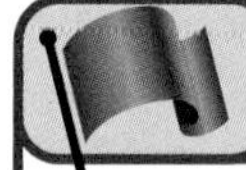

**RED FLAGS**

Patients seen immediately after coitus should have no symptoms.

Patients requesting emergency contraception (EC) who are having medical symptoms (abdominal pain) should be evaluated for the cause of their symptoms.

If signs or symptoms consistent with pregnancy are present, a pregnancy test should be performed because EC is not effective in pregnant patients.

Patients requesting EC may be at risk for sexually transmitted diseases and should be counseled and either tested or referred for outpatient follow-up or testing.

**Table 129.2 Myths and Facts About Emergency Contraception**

| MYTH | FACT |
|---|---|
| EC causes a "medical abortion." | EC has no effect on an established pregnancy, and EC agents are not teratogenic. |
| | The primary mechanism of action of EC is inhibition of ovulation. |
| | Estrogen-progestin combination EC may inhibit implantation of a fertilized egg. |
| If EC is too easily available, women will "abuse" it and use EC instead of regular forms of birth control. | Women who receive advance prescriptions for EC agents are not less likely to use regular forms of birth control. |
| EC agents contain high doses of hormones and are dangerous to use. | The small dose of hormones in EC agents is extremely safe and can be used by virtually any woman. |
| EC is readily available in the United States. | Although FDA approval for over-the-counter EC medications is an improvement, availability in EDs, as well as pharmacies, is variable. The emergency physician must be a patient advocate and ensure that the patient is able to obtain the medication that has been prescribed. |

*EC*, Emergency contraception; *FDA*, U.S. Food and Drug Administration.

## DIFFERENTIAL DIAGNOSIS AND MEDICAL DECISION MAKING

EC may be indicated in several circumstances, as listed in Box 129.1.

## TREATMENT

Four regimens for EC are commonly used in the United States: combined estrogen-progesterone ("Yuzpe method"), progestin only (levonorgestrel), progesterone agonist-antagonist (ulipristal), and the copper intrauterine device (IUD). A combined regimen of estrogen and progesterone

**BOX 129.1 Sample Indications for Using Emergency Contraception**

Failure to use a contraceptive method

Dislodged, broken, or improperly used condom, diaphragm, or cervical cap

Unprotected intercourse within 7 days of starting oral contraceptives

Two or more missed estrogen-progestin birth control pills

One or more missed progestin-only birth control pills

Removal of a contraceptive skin patch or ring

Unprotected intercourse within 14 days of first depot medroxyprogesterone (Depo-Provera) injection

Ejaculation on the external genitalia without reliable contraception

Sexual assault when the woman is not using reliable contraception

Miscalculation of the periodic abstinence method

Data from Conard LA, Gold MA. Emergency contraception. Adolesc Med Clin 2005;16:585-602; and WHO Fact Sheet. Levonorgestrel for emergency contraception. October 2005. Available at http://www.who.int/reproductive-health/family_planning/docs/ec_factsheet.pdf.

pills for EC was first reported and popularized in the 1970s by Yuzpe et al.[8] and is often referred to as the Yuzpe method. The standard dosing in this regimen is two 100-mcg doses of ethinyl estradiol and 1 mg of norgestrel taken 12 hours apart. When taken within 72 hours of unprotected intercourse, this regimen will prevent approximately 75% of pregnancies.[9] This method of EC has been effectively supplanted by progestin-only methods, which are more effective and have fewer side effects. The Yuzpe method is thus primarily a historical regimen.

A preferred, progestin-only method of EC has become popular and is marketed in the United States under the brand name Plan B, which consists of two 0.75-mg doses of levonorgestrel taken 12 hours apart. The recommended approach is to take the two doses simultaneously, which increases compliance, decreases side effects, and is equally effective. The EP should instruct the patient on this method because the packaging lists only the two-dose method (**Table 129.3**).

Ulipristal acetate (brand name Ella) is a progesterone agonist-antagonist that became available for use in the United States late in 2010. It is available by prescription only. Its effectiveness is similar to that of levonorgestrel, and ulipristal has been found to not be inferior to levonorgestrel in two well-conducted studies.[10,11] It is administered as a single 30-mg dose taken within 120 hours of intercourse. The side effect profile of Ulipristal is remarkably similar to that of levonorgestrel, with about 20% of women experiencing headache and 10% to 15% experiencing nausea or dysmenorrhea (or both).[11] Unlike levonorgestrel, which tends to bring about the next menses sooner than expected, thus relieving the patient of the fear of being pregnant, ulipristal is associated with a delay in subsequent menses by a mean of 2 days.

Of the hormonal EC methods, levonorgestrel and ulipristal are more effective and are recommended over the Yuzpe method. The difference in effectiveness varies with the timing of treatment (**Fig. 129.1**).[9] Both levonorgestrel and ulipristal are less likely to cause nausea and vomiting than combined estrogen-progestin formulations are. Other hormonal methods have been used for EC but are less popular either because of questionable efficacy (danazol) or because of a higher incidence of side effects (high-dose estrogens).

The IUD is the most effective postcoital contraceptive and prevents more than 99% of pregnancies if inserted within 5 days of intercourse.[12] This can be an ideal form of EC in patients who prefer to continue using an IUD as their contraceptive device for an extended period. IUDs should be avoided in patients with a history of sexually transmitted disease and in those with multiple sexual partners because IUD use increases the likelihood of pelvic inflammatory disease. This drawback makes an IUD unsuitable for patients seen after rape and for adolescent patients. Other contraindications to copper IUD insertion are cervical or endometrial cancer, unexplained vaginal bleeding, and copper allergy. Patients should be informed of its marked superiority in effectiveness over other methods of EC and be referred for IUD insertion if they choose this method.

Mifepristone (RU-486) is a progesterone antagonist that is effective in EC. It functions by inhibiting ovulation, as

**BOX 129.2 Contraindications to and Complications of Emergency Contraception (EC)**

There are no absolute contraindications to hormonal EC.

EC agents are not abortifacients, and EC is not effective in pregnancy. A urine pregnancy test should be performed before administering EC if the patient might be pregnant.

Relative contraindications to estrogen-containing EC include smokers older than 35 years and patients with a history of thrombophilia, stroke, heart attack, malignancy, deep vein thrombosis, and migraine with neurologic symptoms. In these cases, a progestin-only form of EC is recommended.

An intrauterine device should not be used by patients with multiple sexual partners or those at risk for sexually transmitted diseases.

**Table 129.3 Common Hormonal Methods of Emergency Contraception**

| METHOD | CONTAINS | DOSING |
|---|---|---|
| Combination oral (Yuzpe method) | 0.1 mg ethinyl estradiol and 0.5 mg levonorgestrel | Two doses 12 hr apart |
| Progestin-only oral (Plan B) | 0.75 mg levonorgestrel | Two doses 12 hr apart |
| Progestin-only oral, single-dose regimen* | 1.5 mg levonorgestrel | One dose |
| Progesterone agonist-antagonist | 30 mg ulipristal acetate | One dose |

*Recommended.

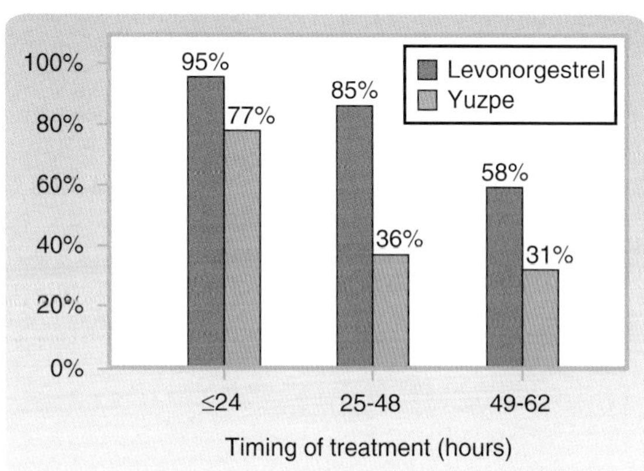


**Fig. 129.1 Proportion of pregnancies prevented by levonorgestrel versus the Yupze method by timing of treatment.** (Adapted from Task Force on Postovulatory Methods of Fertility Regulation. Randomised controlled trial of levonorgestrel versus the Yuzpe regimen of combined oral contraceptives for emergency contraception. Lancet 1998;352:428-433. With permission.)

well as endometrial maturation. In the United States, a 600-mg dose of mifepristone is approved as an abortifacient for pregnancies up to 49 days. Lower doses of mifepristone, from 10 to 50 mg, are at least as effective as and probably more effective than levonorgestrel for EC and have a very good side effect profile.[13] Mifepristone is administered as a single dose within 120 days of intercourse. The 10-mg dose is currently used routinely in several countries as EC. Mifepristone causes a 1-week delay in subsequent menses in about 20% of women who use it for EC, which understandably can cause patients anxiety. Currently, administration of mifepristone is limited to registered providers who contract with the patient to schedule three office visits. This restriction makes prescribing mifepristone in the ED impractical. Additionally, its use as an abortifacient has given the drug some notoriety that may make universal implementation a challenge in the future.[14]

## TIMING OF ADMINISTRATION OF EMERGENCY CONTRACEPTION

Hormonal EC is effective when administered up to 120 hours after intercourse. There is an inverse linear relationship between the time of administration of EC after unprotected intercourse and its effectiveness—the sooner that EC is started, the more effective it is.[15] For this reason, it is of the utmost importance to begin EC as soon as possible. Many EDs stock levonorgestrel; if it is available through the hospital pharmacy, it can be given directly to the patient by the EP. If this is not possible, in addition to a prescription (if necessary) and instructions, the patient should be provided with a list of local 24-hour pharmacies that provide EC. It is advisable to call the pharmacies to confirm availability and expedite the preparation because as many as half of the pharmacies will not stock many forms of EC.[16]

## SIDE EFFECTS

The adverse effects of estrogen-progestin contraceptive drugs are primarily related to the estrogen component. The most common side effect is nausea, which affects half of women taking this regimen. Approximately 20% of women vomit as a result. Nausea and vomiting are significantly less common with progestin-only regimens (nausea in 18% and vomiting in 4%).[17] The incidence and severity of nausea and vomiting can be decreased with the administration of an antiemetic 30 to 60 minutes before taking the EC agent. Meclizine (50 mg) has been used with success,[18] but any antiemetic can be administered. If a patient vomits more than 1 hour after taking an EC drug, the dosage does not need to be repeated.[19]

A common side effect of all regimens is vaginal spotting; between 10% and 20% of patients report this symptom. Spotting should resolve without intervention and does not indicate failure of this method. Breast tenderness is another side effect of EC, particularly of estrogen-progestin methods, and can be troublesome because it is also an early sign of pregnancy. Patients should be advised to have a pregnancy test if their next period is not normal and they have signs of pregnancy.

## FOLLOW-UP, NEXT STEPS IN CARE, AND PATIENT EDUCATION

### ACCESS TO EMERGENCY CONTRACEPTION

On April 22, 2009, the U.S. Food and Drug Administration approved over-the-counter sales of levonorgestrel, packaged as Plan B, for women 17 years or older. Men with proof of age could also buy Plan B for a partner. Women younger than 17 years can still purchase EC with a prescription. Because over-the-counter availability is unlikely to change the reluctance of many pharmacies to stock Plan B and provide it in timely fashion, administration of EC in the ED is recommended to ensure patient access. Increased knowledge about the availability of EC methods is likely to increase the number of adolescents younger than 17 years who access the ED for Plan B.

Patients should be advised of the common side effects of EC. More serious symptoms such as fever, severe abdominal pain, and heavy bleeding should *not* be attributed to EC, and patients should be advised to be reevaluated for serious symptoms.

Patients should be told to use barrier protection or resume taking oral contraceptive pills (or both). If they have not been tested for sexually transmitted diseases in the ED, patients should follow up with a primary care provider for counseling and testing. For the majority of women, their next menstrual period should fall within 1 week of the time that the menstrual period is regularly due. The patient should be instructed to have a pregnancy test if the menstrual cycle is delayed by more than 1 week.

Patients should be advised that the actual effectiveness of EC depends on the timing of administration so that they understand that EC is not 100% effective even when taken as directed (see Table 129.2).

## REFERENCES

***References can be found on Expert Consult @ www.expertconsult.com.***

# Heat-Related Emergencies 130

Virgil Davis

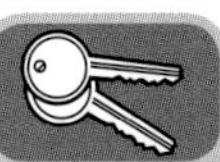

**KEY POINTS**

- Heat stroke is a life-threatening hyperthermic syndrome characterized by central nervous system dysfunction and associated multisystem organ failure.
- The main goal of therapy is rapid reduction of the patient's core temperature to about 39° C with one of two methods—evaporative cooling or cold water immersion.

## PERSPECTIVE

Heat-related injury spans a wide spectrum from the unpleasant and transient conditions of heat cramps or prickly heat to the life-threatening multisystem organ failure of heat stroke. The most important risk factors for heat illness are listed in **Box 130.1**. Mechanisms of acclimatization are listed in **Table 130.1**.

## EPIDEMIOLOGY

Roughly 688 people die yearly of heat-related causes, Arizona has the highest incidence at 1.7 per 100,000, followed by Nevada (0.8 per 100,000) and Missouri (0.6 per 100,000).[1] An estimated half of the deaths are weather related, and 5% result from being enclosed in motor vehicles, boiler rooms, or kitchens; in the remaining cases, the causes are unspecified.[2] Mortality from heat stroke with appropriate treatment is reported to be between 0% and 28%.[3-5]

## PATHOPHYSIOLOGY OF HEAT STROKE

Severe heat illness is thought to result from three main mechanisms: physiologic alterations in response to hyperthermia, direct cytotoxic effects of heat, and inflammatory and coagulation responses of the host, which interact to create a spiraling deterioration resulting in circulatory collapse and multisystem organ failure.

Failure of thermoregulation occurs when fluid and electrolyte replacement is inadequate; it results in diminished cardiac output, hypotension and acute renal failure, and shunting of blood away from the splanchnic circulation, which leads to intestinal ischemia. Increased gut permeability and the entrance of endotoxins stimulate additional inflammatory mediators.

Heat itself has a direct cytotoxic effect and causes cell death over a period of 45 minutes to 8 hours at body temperatures of 41.6° C to 42° C[6]; below these temperatures, cell death can still occur through apoptosis.[7]

Heat induces higher production of numerous inflammatory cytokines that contribute to the neuronal injury and hypotension seen in patients with heat stroke, and it results in coagulation and endothelial cell injury, which can lead to disseminated intravascular coagulation and greater vascular permeability.

**Figure 130.1** diagrams the current understanding of the pathophysiology of heat stroke.

## MINOR HEAT-RELATED SYNDROMES

## PRESENTING SIGNS AND SYMPTOMS

As stated earlier, heat-related illness is a continuum. **Table 130.2** summarizes the various types of heat illness.

### HEAT EDEMA

Heat edema is a self-limited illness characterized by mild swelling of the hands and feet as a result of increased interstitial fluid after heat exposure.

### PRICKLY HEAT

Clogging of the sweat glands leads to an erythematous, maculopapular, and pruritic rash commonly called prickly heat.

### HEAT SYNCOPE

Heat syncope results from heat-induced volume depletion and peripheral vasodilation, which often occur in people with decreased vasomotor tone, such as the elderly, and in people poorly acclimated to the heat. It is important to regard heat syncope as a diagnosis of exclusion and to evaluate for other plausible causes of syncope. In addition, the emergency physician (EP) should remember to evaluate for any injuries sustained during a fall as a result of syncope. The patient should have a rapid response to hydration. Electrolytes should be evaluated in patients with signs of volume depletion.

### HEAT CRAMPS

Heat cramps are involuntary muscle spasms, most commonly of the calves, thighs, or shoulders, that occur either during or after vigorous physical activity. Cellular hyponatremia and hypokalemia are thought to cause this problem. Rhabdomyolysis is a very rare complication that can result from prolonged muscle spasm.

## TREATMENT

Most minor heat-related syndromes are mild and require simple or no treatment. Treatment is summarized in Table 130.2 for these conditions.

**BOX 130.1 Risk Factors for Severe Heat Illness**

Extremes of age (children and people 65 and older)
Alcohol and drug intoxication
Impaired cardiac function
- Illness (e.g., heart failure)
- Drug therapy (e.g., beta-blockers)

Dehydration
Exertion
Anhydrosis from the use of anticholinergic agents or phenothiazines
Intercurrent illness
Psychiatric Illness
Stimulants
Lack of air conditioning
Lower socioeconomic status.

## FOLLOW-UP, NEXT STEPS IN CARE, AND PATIENT EDUCATION

Minor heat-related illnesses rarely require admission. Patients with heat syncope and significant electrolyte abnormalities should be admitted for correction. Patients with heat cramps who show evidence of impending rhabdomyolysis require

**Table 130.1 Acclimatization Mechanisms**

| | |
|---|---|
| Cardiac | Increased cardiac performance: higher cardiac output |
| Vascular | Increases in:<br>Plasma volume<br>Renal flow<br>Shunting of blood away from the visceral circulation |
| Endocrine | An enhanced renin-angiotensin-aldosterone system and improved salt retention by the kidneys and sweat glands result in better fluid retention |
| Renal | Increased glomerular filtration rate |
| Sweat glands | The increased volume of sweat produced and the more dilute sweat reduce salt loss and indirectly diminish dehydration |
| Muscle | Improved ability to resist rhabdomyolysis from exertion |
| Cellular | Upregulated transcription of heat shock proteins |

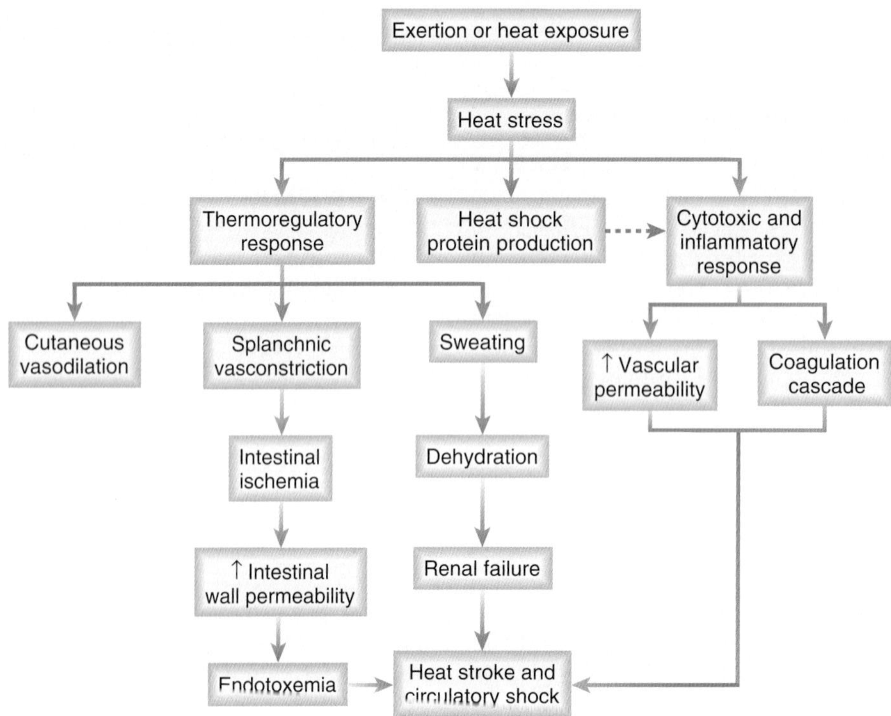


**Fig. 130.1** Algorithm of the pathophysiology of heat stroke.

**Table 130.2 Heat-Related Illnesses and Treatment**

| DIAGNOSIS | KEY FEATURES | TREATMENT |
|---|---|---|
| **Mild** | | |
| Heat edema | Mild edema of the hands and feet as a result of interstitial edema | Elevation, compression<br>Self limited<br>Diuretics not indicated |
| Prickly heat | Erythematous, maculopapular rash | Antihistamines<br>Antibiotics effective against staphylococci if secondary cellulitis present |
| Heat cramps | Severe muscle spasms during or after vigorous exercise | Intravenous or oral rehydration |
| **Severe** | | |
| Heat exhaustion | Dehydration, weakness, fatigue<br>Normal or mildly elevated temperature (<40° C)<br>Normal mental status | Remove clothing<br>Remove from heat<br>Intravenous or oral fluids<br>Check electrolytes and creatinine<br>Generally discharge<br>Drink fluids and rest for 1-2 days |
| Heat stroke | Abnormal mental status<br>Multisystem organ failure<br>Hyperthermia<br>Often temperature >40° C<br>Often anhydrosis | Rapid cooling with immersion or evaporative methods to core temperature <39° C<br>Supportive care<br>Hospital admission |

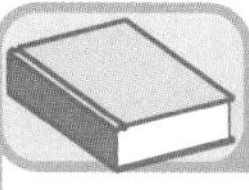

## PATIENT TEACHING TIPS

### Heat Illness

The three main types of heat illness are heat cramps, heat exhaustion, and heat stroke.

Heat cramps are painful muscle spasms and a mild form of heat illness that occur when you sweat too much or do not drink enough fluids.

Heat exhaustion is due to dehydration and is more serious.

Heat stroke is marked by severe dehydration and confusion secondary to overheating; it is life-threatening.

### Prevention

During hot weather:

- Reschedule strenuous activities to cooler times of the day.
- Reduce your overall level of physical activity.
- Drink additional water or electrolyte solution (sports drink).
- Wear lightweight and light-colored clothing.
- Increase time spent in air-conditioned environments.
- Frequently check the elderly, homebound, or disabled people, all of whom are at greater risk for heat illness.

### Children

Never leave children enclosed in motor vehicles. Yearly, 30 to 40 children die of heat stroke after being left in cars.

### Athletics and Strenuous Labor

Drink 500 mL of water or sports drink 2 hours before vigorous exercise or work.

Continue to replace 250 mL of fluid for every 20 minutes of exertion and replace 150% of weight loss with fluid after exertion.

Acclimatization takes at least 2 weeks, and a gradual increase in activity is recommended to safely adjust to hotter environments.

### Treatment of Heat Illness

If you have serious heat illness, you may feel lightheaded, nauseated, tired, anxious, and confused.

Get out of the heat into a cool, shaded place or air-conditioned building, and take off some clothing.

Put cold water or cold wet towels on your skin, and drink cold liquids.

If you are confused or lethargic or have a fever, seek medical attention immediately.

hospital admission for aggressive hydration and monitoring of renal function. Informing patients about how to avoid severe heat illness when they have mild heat illness may prevent future recurrence or more serious injury. The Patient Teaching Tips box lists information that can be given in the form of an educational handout to patients with heat illness.

## SEVERE HEAT-RELATED SYNDROMES

## PRESENTING SIGNS AND SYMPTOMS

### HEAT EXHAUSTION

Heat exhaustion is a systemic illness that develops as a result of heat stress and depletion of water or salt. Common symptoms are extreme thirst, dizziness, lightheadedness, fatigue, weakness, syncope, headache, malaise, and vomiting. Usually, core body temperature is normal or slightly elevated (but often lower than 40° C). Signs include tachycardia, orthostatic hypotension, tachypnea, and diaphoresis.

All patients with presumed heat exhaustion should undergo neurologic assessment to distinguish heat exhaustion from heat stroke. Heat exhaustion does not cause signs of central nervous system (CNS) dysfunction, such as delirium, ataxia, and seizures.

### HEAT STROKE

The classic definition of heat stroke was a core body temperature higher than 40° C, CNS dysfunction, and anhydrosis. However, many cases of heat stroke have been reported in which sweating was present and the core temperature was not higher than 40° C. Therefore, the definition has been amended to a form of hyperthermia associated with a systemic inflammatory response leading to a syndrome of multiorgan dysfunction in which encephalopathy predominates.[8]

Heat stroke resulting from failure to stay normothermic in high environmental temperatures is usually termed classic or nonexertional heat stroke, as opposed to exertional heat stroke, in which a significant component of the heat is generated by the body's muscle tissue through strenuous work or exercise. Although both types of heat stroke are very similar, acute renal failure, rhabdomyolysis, and disseminated intravascular coagulation are more common in patients with exertional heat stroke.

The signs and symptoms of heat stroke are similar to those of heat exhaustion, except for the addition of CNS dysfunction in the form of delirium, hallucinations, ataxia, convulsions, or coma.

## DIFFERENTIAL DIAGNOSIS AND DECISION MAKING

Many other conditions are associated with elevated core body temperature and altered mental status. **Box 130.2** contains an extensive list. The EP should regard infection as a strong possibility in patients with these signs. Toxicologic, neurologic (e.g., hemorrhage, seizures), and endocrinologic (e.g., thyroid storm) causes should also be kept in mind and appropriate neuroimaging and laboratory workup ordered. Many cases of heat stroke involve victims with concomitant substance abuse, overdose, or psychiatric illnesses. Evaluation for common overdoses, medication toxicities and substances of abuse should be performed. Additionally, heat stroke often occurs in patients who have significant comorbid conditions, such as cardiac or respiratory diseases, or have another concomitant acute illness, such as infection. Therefore, it is reasonable to assess cardiac function, perform a sepsis evaluation, and evaluate for any additional conditions that the EP suspects.

**BOX 130.2 Differential Diagnosis of Heat Stroke**

Sepsis
Encephalitis
Meningitis
Brain abscess
Malaria (cerebral falciparum)
Typhoid fever
Tetanus
Alcohol withdrawal syndrome
Neuroleptic malignant syndrome (see Tips and Tricks box)
Anticholinergic toxicity
Salicylate toxicity
Phencyclidine hydrochloride (PCP), cocaine, or amphetamine toxicity
Status epilepticus
Cerebral hemorrhage
Diabetic ketoacidosis
Thyroid storm

**TIPS AND TRICKS**

- Both neuroleptic malignant syndrome and heat stroke cause altered mental status and hyperthermia; unlike patients with heat stroke, however, all patients with neuroleptic malignant syndrome also have extrapyramidal rigidity.
- Hospital maintenance often has large fans used to dry hospital floors, which can be used to enhance evaporative cooling of a patient with heat illness.

## DIAGNOSTIC TESTING

Heat stroke is a clinical diagnosis, but associated multiorgan dysfunction may be present. Therefore, the EP must assess the patient for the severity of dysfunction to provide appropriate supportive management. Examples of multiorgan dysfunction seen in patients with heat stroke are listed in **Box 130.3**.

## TREATMENT

### PREHOSPITAL MANAGEMENT

Morbidity and mortality are correlated with the duration and intensity of elevation in core body temperature. Therefore,

**BOX 130.3 Organ Dysfunction Seen in Patients with Heat Stroke**

Encephalopathy
Rhabdomyolysis
Acute renal failure
Acute respiratory distress syndrome
Myocardial injury
Hepatocellular injury
Intestinal ischemia and infarction
Pancreatic injury
Hemorrhagic complication (e.g., disseminated intravascular coagulation)

field management in which patients with possible heat stroke are identified quickly and cooling measures initiated immediately should have a significant positive effect on outcome. Measures include placing the patient in a cool, shaded environment and removing clothing. Next is either immersion in iced water (immersion) or wetting the skin with water and using a fan to aid evaporation (evaporative cooling).

Continuous monitoring and assessment of core body temperature every 5 to 10 minutes are also recommended. The ability and resources to execute these measures will vary significantly according to the setting (wilderness versus an Ironman triathlon medical tent), but even simple measures such as those recommended by the Israeli defense forces—splashing 20 to 40 mL of water on the skin and fanning the person or driving the person in an open car—effectively cool the core body temperature at a rate of 0.14° C/min.[9]

## HOSPITAL MANAGEMENT

Some experts liken the treatment of heat stroke to that of trauma, for which there is a "golden hour" for effective intervention and stabilization of the patient. Frequently after this time, aggressive measures cannot overcome the circulatory collapse and organ failure.

The EP's main goal is to cool the core body temperature to 38.5° C or 39° C as quickly as possible. Active cooling is not continued to normothermic temperatures to avoid the risk of overshooting and causing hypothermia. Usually, significant improvement is noted in the patient's cardiovascular stability and mental status immediately after cooling. Methods of body cooling are defined in **Table 130.3**.

Debate and research continue about which cooling method is most effective and safest in treating heat stroke. Current research does not definitively answer the question of whether water immersion or evaporative cooling is significantly more effective. However, most evidence indicates that cold water immersion is superior for exertional heat stroke and that the cooler the immersion water bath, the faster the cooling,[5,10,11] whereas for classic heat stroke both methods are thought to be equally effective. Additionally, if temperature can be reduced within 30 to 60 minutes, the risk for mortality is decreased.[11] The choice often depends on which method can be instituted more quickly and effectively. Cold water immersion may be most useful when planned in advance for event medicine and other field applications. Evaporative cooling with the application of ice packs is a practical and effective method that can be instituted with equipment normally available in the emergency department (ED). Ice packs, wet sheets, and a fan will provide rapid cooling. **Table 130.4** lists the advantages, disadvantages, and efficacy of various cooling methods.

**Table 130.3 Methods of Core Temperature Cooling**

| | |
|---|---|
| Immersion | Placement of the body into a bath of cold or iced water |
| Immersion of extremities | Putting only the hands and forearms in iced water |
| Evaporative cooling | Spraying tepid water or placing a wet sheet on the skin with a fan to facilitate evaporation |
| Ice packing | Application of ice or cold packs to the groin, axilla, and neck |
| Invasive measures | |
| Gastric lavage | Lavage with iced water via a nasogastric tube |
| Peritoneal lavage | Lavage with sterile cold water |
| Dantrolene, 2-4 mg/kg | Decreases muscle contraction and, in theory, reduces heat production |
| Benzodiazepines | Theoretically, control shivering and heat production |

### Shivering and Vasoconstriction

Experts differ about whether shivering and vasoconstriction hinder cooling measures. Some believe that shivering and vasoconstriction require intervention, such as massage or a benzodiazepine, to prevent their negative effects on cooling. Others believe that shivering and vasoconstriction do not significantly slow the rate of cooling and may help prevent hypotension.

### Hypotension

Hypotension is a common problem in patients with heat stroke and should be treated aggressively with fluid boluses, which are generally adequate. Central venous pressure of 3 to 8 mm Hg is targeted.[5] If the patient's blood pressure remains unresponsive, vasopressors are indicated. One study used isoproterenol (β-adrenergic agonist) to increase peripheral blood flow and cutaneous circulation, but this agent is used infrequently and is unlikely to result in a significant rise in blood pressure.[12] An α-adrenergic agent (e.g., dopamine, which is commonly used) may be more effective in raising blood pressure but has the theoretic disadvantage of causing peripheral vasoconstriction and hence diminishing cutaneous perfusion when given in higher doses.

## ADDITIONAL MANAGEMENT

Initial treatment of heat stroke is identical to that for all patients in critical condition: assessment of the ABCs (airway, breathing, circulation), cardiac monitoring, establishment of

**Table 130.4 Advantages, Disadvantages, and Efficacy of Various Cooling Methods**

| COOLING METHOD | ADVANTAGES | DISADVANTAGES | EFFECTIVENESS |
|---|---|---|---|
| Antipyretics | | Can worsen liver or renal injury | Not effective (the temperature set-point is not elevated in hyperthermia)<br>Not effective in controlling pathologic inflammation |
| Evaporative cooling | Noninvasive, easy to monitor, readily available | Labor-intensive—requires constant moistening of skin | Comparison studies show the cooling rate on average to be slower than immersion<br>Published rate range: 0.05-0.31° C/min |
| Immersion | Noninvasive, rapid | Cumbersome, poorly tolerated, safety questionable if comorbid conditions present, monitoring difficult, shivering and vasoconstriction | Comparison studies show the cooling rate on average to be faster than evaporation<br>Published rate range: 0.04-0.35° C/min |
| Immersion of the hands and forearms | Noninvasive, easy to perform in the field | Shivering and vasoconstriction | Slower cooling but appropriate for mildly ill patients such as those with heat exhaustion |
| Ice packing | Noninvasive, readily available | Shivering and vasoconstriction, poorly tolerated | Less effective than immersion or evaporation<br>Some authorities recommend using both evaporation and ice |
| Cold gastric or peritoneal lavage | Very rapid | Invasive, cumbersome (cold sterile saline needed for peritoneal lavage) | In canine studies, questionably faster than evaporation or immersion |
| Dantrolene | In theory, decreases heat production by inhibiting muscle contraction | | No clear efficacy; it may be more effective for exertional than for classic heat stroke |
| Benzodiazepines | Treatment of shivering to decrease heat production and heat-induced seizures | Sedation | Whether treatment increases cooling is unknown but may make cooling treatments tolerable<br>Also effective for heat-related seizures |

intravenous access and administration of normal saline or lactated Ringer solution, and liberal oxygen supplementation. Placement of a Foley catheter with temperature monitoring capability will help guide management and determine whether the cooling measures are working. Liberal use of diagnostic studies to assess organ dysfunction and other potential diagnoses is important. However, these tests must not delay the initiation of cooling measures. Empiric antibiotic treatment is appropriate when sepsis remains in the differential diagnosis.

### CONSULTATIONS AND EXPECTATIONS

Admitting services consulted should include a medical or surgical intensive care unit physician. In patients with acute renal failure, a nephrologist should be involved to determine the need for dialysis. Patients with drug ingestions should be discussed with a toxicologist. Other specialty services may need to be involved depending on the individual situation, such as neurosurgery for cerebral edema and infectious diseases for suspected sepsis. Generally, the admitting service can coordinate these consultations.

## FOLLOW-UP, NEXT STEPS IN CARE, AND PATIENT EDUCATION

All patients with heat stroke require hospital admission. The majority will require admission to an intensive care unit or step-down unit, depending on the resources of the hospital and the severity of the illness.

Selected patients with heat stroke who respond well to ED cooling may be suitable for ward admission. Prudence would dictate consultation with an intensivist before admission to the general medical floor. Usually, these will be patients in whom heat stroke was suspected but, based on further evaluation and response to treatment, heat exhaustion seems to be a more appropriate diagnosis.

Patients with heat exhaustion who respond well to fluids, have no serious electrolyte derangements, have no evidence of mental status changes, and who are reliable with good follow-up can generally be managed as outpatients. If in doubt, overnight admission to a medical ward or an observation unit for continued hydration and reevaluation may be appropriate.

## DOCUMENTATION

Because mental status changes and evidence of end-organ dysfunction are key components of the diagnosis and treatment of heat stroke, careful documentation of these features is important. Additionally, most patients will require documentation of bedside critical care. Patients with heat exhaustion who are able to be discharged need careful documentation of the lack of mental status changes and end-organ dysfunction, normal electrolytes, and follow-up plans and precautions. This will help justify the decision to not admit a patient with potentially serious heat-related illness.

## PATIENT TEACHING

Patients with heat stroke will require admission. Patients with heat exhaustion who are able to be discharged will benefit from the information noted in the Patient Teaching Tips box.

## PROGNOSIS

The prognosis of patients with heat exhaustion and more mild forms of heat illness is good, and no long-term morbidity is anticipated. The prognosis of patients with heat stroke depends on the severity, underlying comorbid conditions, and time elapsed until appropriate cooling. Mortality between 0% and 28% with appropriate treatment is reported. Survivors of exertional heatstroke that is treated aggressively rarely have long-term sequelae, whereas up to one third of survivors of classic heat stroke will have moderate to severe neurologic sequelae.[1] Independent risk factors for mortality include hypotension (systolic blood pressure < 90 mm Hg), temperature higher than 42° C, and a Glasgow Coma Scale score lower than 12.4.

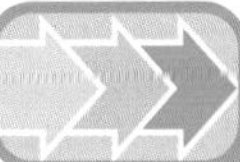

**PRIORITY ACTIONS**

- Use advanced cardiac life support principles to assess and monitor cardiac and respiratory stability.
- Obtain intravenous access, as well as cardiac and core temperature monitoring, and place a Foley catheter for monitoring urine output and core temperature continuously.
- Start cooling measures immediately, preferably in the field if possible with either immersion or evaporative cooling.
- Actively cool the patient as quickly and safely as possible to a core temperature of 38.5° C to 39° C.
- Continue monitoring for rebound hyperthermia.
- Assess for other organ dysfunction and intercurrent illness.
- Admit to the intensive care unit.

## PITFALLS

The primary pitfall to avoid is delaying rapid cooling in any patient with suspected heat stroke. Further diagnostic and therapeutic modalities should not delay institution of cooling. Priority stabilizing actions such as airway management, vascular access, and circulatory support should occur simultaneously with cooling measures.

Avoid failure to recognize that mental status abnormalities and end-organ dysfunction in a patient with heat-related illness represent heat stroke and mandate more aggressive treatment than needed for heat exhaustion.

## SUGGESTED READINGS

Bouchama A, Dehbi M, Chaves-Carballo E. Cooling and hemodynamic management in heatstroke: practical recommendations. Crit Care 2007;11:R54.

Lugo-Amador NM, Rauthenhaus T, Moyer P. Heat-related illness. Emerg Med Clin North Am 2004;22:305-27.

Smith JE. Cooling methods used in the treatment of exertional heat illness. Br J Sports Med 2005;39:503-7.

## REFERENCES

***References can be found on Expert Consult @ www.expertconsult.com.***

# 131 Hypothermia and Frostbite

*Robert L. Stephen*

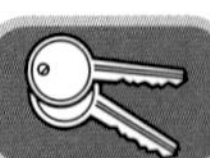

**KEY POINTS**

- Accidental (primary) hypothermia occurs when the ambient temperature outstrips a person's ability to thermoregulate.
- Secondary hypothermia is due to an underlying medical problem that alters thermoregulation.
- Mild hypothermia is treated by passive external rewarming, moderate hypothermia by a combination of passive and active external and active internal rewarming, and severe hypothermia by active external and active internal rewarming techniques.
- For patients without a pulse or blood pressure, aggressive, invasive measures should be pursued.
- One should hesitate to declare death in a hypothermic patient. Consider rewarming to a temperature of 32° C to 35° C.
- Frostbite remains a clinical diagnosis and needs to be distinguished from nonfreezing injuries (frostnip, pernio, and trench foot).
- The cornerstone of therapy is rapid rewarming in a circulating bath of heated water.
- In all aspects of care a subsequent "freeze-thaw-freeze" cycle must be avoided.
- Additional therapies involve the use of antiprostaglandins, both topical and systemic, and possibly thrombolytics.
- The full extent of frostbite injury can take weeks to become evident.

## PERSPECTIVE

Accidental hypothermia is responsible for approximately 700 deaths per year in the United States.[1] It primarily affects those least able to ward off the effects of cold weather: the very young, the very old, and the poor, disabled, pharmacologically inquisitive, environmentally adventurous, and mentally ill. Urban people are common victims. Hypothermia can occur in many latitudes, with episodes reported even in Florida.[2] It occurs when a person's ability to generate heat and remain warm is outstripped by the ambient temperature.

In the United States, frostbite is often a disease of the indigent, the intoxicated, the mentally ill, and winter outdoor recreation enthusiasts. For both frostbite and hypothermia the literature consists of primarily case reports, case series, and reviews.

## EPIDEMIOLOGY

Accidental hypothermia is generally manifested as progression from an initial state of catecholamine release and stimulation (mild hypothermia) to one marked by a predictable slowing of metabolism and all critical body functions to the extent that patients may appear dead. The profound physiologic changes and metabolic slowing all reverse with rapid rewarming, and reports of remarkable neurologically intact survival despite hours of pulselessness and resuscitation are not infrequent. This has given rise to the adage "No one is dead until they are warm and dead." Not surprisingly, there is little strong scientific evidence for treatment recommendations because trials cannot be conducted. The medical literature is composed mostly of animal experiments, case reports and series, and retrospective reviews. Still, rational approaches can be inferred from the extant literature for this uncommon but serious problem (**Table 131.1**).

Frostbite is a freezing injury to soft tissues secondary to cold exposure and results in loss of circulation to and therefore viability of the affected area. The extremities, nose, ears, and male genitalia are the most commonly affected areas.

# HYPOTHERMIA

## PATHOPHYSIOLOGY

### MECHANISMS OF HEAT LOSS

The mechanisms of heat loss are as follows:

- *Radiation* of heat occurs when the ambient temperature is less than body temperature and heat is lost directly to the environment via electromagnetic radiation.
- *Conduction* is heat transfer from one (warmer) solid to another (cooler) when they are in contact.

- *Convection* is loss of heat from a surface to a (usually moving) gas or fluid, typically air or water. It can be considered an adjunct to conduction.
- *Evaporation* causes heat loss through the energy required to vaporize water (i.e., sweat).

As a person cools, a fairly predictable procession of pathophysiologic changes occurs, as seen in **Table 131.2** and **Figure 131 .1**.

## PRESENTING SIGNS AND SYMPTOMS

Patients with mild hypothermia are awake, occasionally drowsy, uncomfortable, and shivering. They simply need insulation (blanket), dry clothes, and food. They will recover completely and can be discharged when normothermic and feeling better.

Patients with moderate hypothermia are generally confused and lethargic, often have slurred speech, and are typically not shivering. They require more energetic rewarming measures, including heated blankets, resistive and hot air blankets (Bair Hugger), and close monitoring, including core temperature. Though strictly considered active internal rewarming, the use of heated, humidified oxygen and warmed intravenous (IV) fluids is reasonable in this situation. Patients whose hypothermia responds to these measures may be discharged when normothermic, awake, alert, and ambulatory. Patients with severe hypothermia require prompt intervention, close monitoring, and potentially aggressive, invasive rewarming therapies.

It is of the utmost importance to learn the circumstances that led to the patient becoming hypothermic. The possibility of a verify drug overdose, trauma, infection, drowning, or decompensated comorbid conditions—to name but a few examples—must be considered, sought, and treated along with the hypothermia.

The critical element of the diagnosis of hypothermia is accurate measurement of core temperature. Several methods exist, all of which have potential drawbacks (**Table 131.3**). Laboratory and physiologic changes are correlated with the temperature. For example, a normal hematocrit value in a

**Table 131.1** Definitions of Hypothermia

| LEVEL OF HYPOTHERMIA | CORE TEMPERATURE (° C) |
|---|---|
| General | >35 |
| Mild | 32-35 |
| Moderate | 28-32 |
| Severe | <28 |

**Table 131.2** Pathologic Changes Seen with Hypothermia

| | LEVEL OF HYPOTHERMIA | | |
|---|---|---|---|
| **SYSTEM** | **MILD** | **MODERATE** | **SEVERE** |
| Cardiovascular | ↑ HR<br>↑ CO<br>↑ PVR | Progressive ↓ HR, ↓ CO, ↑ PVR<br>Osborn waves possible on electrocardiogram | Profound ↓ HR, ↓ CO, ↓ PVR<br>Ectopy (especially atrial fibrillation)<br>Ventricular fibrillation<br>Asystole |
| Central nervous system | Drowsiness, shivering | Confusion<br>Lethargy<br>Dysarthria<br>Shivering cessation at <30°-32° C | Coma<br>Muscular rigidity<br>Pupils fixed and dilated<br>Electroencephalogram flat at –20° C |
| Hematologic | In general, hematocrit ↑ ≈2% for every 1° C ↓ in temperature | Continuum | Coagulopathy<br>Thrombocytopenia |
| Renal | Diuresis secondary to ↑ PVR with ↑ renal blood flow | Progressive loss of distal tubular resorption<br>Resistance to antidiuretic hormone | Continued diuresis<br>Limitation of clearance of electrolytes and glucose<br>Acute renal failure |
| Respiratory | Tachypnea | Progressive bradypnea<br>Loss of protective reflexes<br>Bronchorrhea | Profound bradypnea<br>Apnea<br>Pulmonary edema (rare) |
| Gastrointestinal | Clinically silent | Progressive hepatic impairment | Decreased lactate clearance and detoxification and metabolism of drugs<br>Pancreatitis in 20-30% of cases |
| Acid-base | | Can be either alkalotic or acidotic | |
| Endocrine | | Patient usually hyperglycemic<br>Thyroid, adrenal glands usually normal | Preexisting hypothyroidism or hypoadrenalism can impair rewarming |

*CO*, Cardiac output; *HR*, heart rate; *PVR*, peripheral vascular resistance.

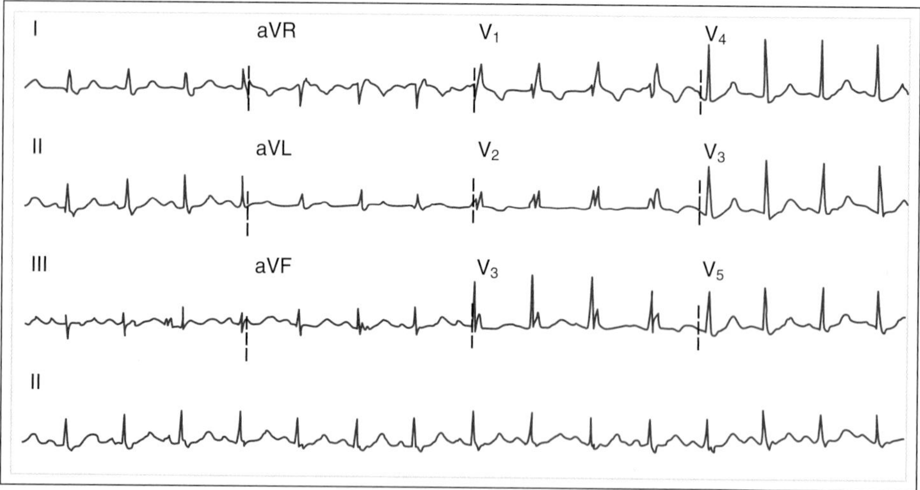


**Fig. 131.1 Osborn wave seen on the electrocardiogram of a patient with hypothermia.** The wave is usually seen at body temperatures lower than 30° C; however, it is neither diagnostic nor prognostic of hypothermia and is thus of academic interest only.

**Table 131.3 Methods of Measuring Core Temperature**

| METHOD | COMMENTS |
|---|---|
| Esophageal probe | Easy to insert<br>Falsely high temperature readings possible with warmed oxygen via an endotracheal tube |
| Rectal probe | Insert to 15-20 cm<br>If the probe is in or surrounded by cold stool, temperature recordings will lag behind true changes |
| Temperature-recording Foley catheter | Inflowing cold urine may falsely lower temperature recordings |
| Pulmonary artery catheter | Most accurate and most invasive method<br>Higher potential for iatrogenic injury, especially ventricular fibrillation in cold, irritable myocardium |

severely hypothermic patient should prompt concern for hemorrhage because the hematocrit should rise in a predictable fashion with ever-lowering temperature. Alternatively, arterial blood gas values should be interpreted as though the patient is normothermic (the alpha-stat method) and not corrected for the actual core temperature (the pH-stat method). Evaluation for infection, metabolic derangement, and cardiac, neurologic, renal, and other organ system abnormalities is important because comorbid conditions are common as a cause, a consequence, or coincidence of hypothermia.

## TREATMENT

### MILD HYPOTHERMIA

Patients with mild hypothermia may be treated with passive external rewarming. Such treatment, which consists of the use of blankets, dry clothes, ambient warmth, oral hydration, and energy substrate (food), produces a rewarming rate of about 0.5° C to 1° C per hour. The approach uses the patient's inherent ability to keep warm, primarily through shivering, and insulation.

### MODERATE HYPOTHERMIA

Patients with moderate hypothermia should undergo active external rewarming. Heat is actively supplied to the body via electric blankets, forced-air blankets, and space heaters. This method achieves rewarming rates of about 1° C to 2° C per hour.

### SEVERE HYPOTHERMIA

Active internal rewarming is needed for patients with moderate and severe hypothermia. Actions are directed toward heating the core preferentially over the periphery. This goal is accomplished via methods of variable invasiveness and complexity, as follows:

- Heated, humidified oxygen (40° C to 45° C) administered via face mask or endotracheal tube; it primarily serves to prevent additional heat loss.
- Administration of heated IV fluids (40° C to 42° C) adds negligible heat overall but does aid in preventing further heat loss.
- Gastric or bladder lavage (or both) via nasogastric tube and Foley catheter is relatively easily accomplished; however, the small volume of these cavities limits the effectiveness of these modalities.
- Peritoneal lavage with prepackaged dialysate or standard crystalloid fluids heated to about 45° C. This method is quicker if two catheters, one for afferent flow and one for efferent flow, are used. Rewarming rates average 2° C to 3° C per hour.[3,4]
- Closed thoracic cavity lavage (pleural lavage) of the left hemithorax is done with two 36-French thoracostomy tubes and isotonic fluid heated to about 42° C. Large volumes are required. The afferent tube is placed in the second intercostal space (ICS) in the midclavicular line. The efferent tube is placed in the usual location, the fourth or fifth ICS in the

midaxillary line. Fluid is literally poured in by hand, infused with a large (60-mL) syringe, or administered directly with a rapid infuser (the hub of the rapid infuser fits snugly into the bore of a 36-French chest tube). Rewarming rates average about 3° C per hour.[5,6]

- Left thoracotomy with mediastinal irrigation and internal cardiac massage is quite invasive with high attendant morbidity. It is very effective and self-explanatory and has rewarming rates as high as 5° C to 6° C per hour.[7,8]
- Cardiopulmonary bypass (CPB) is the definitive method for rewarming. It is rapid, with rewarming rates of 9° C per hour or higher achieved, and supports blood pressure; however, CPB also requires specialized equipment and personnel that are not readily available in most hospitals.[9,10]

The use of medications, particularly cardioactive medications and vasopressors, is theoretically unappealing and thought to be potentially dangerous in a patient with a core temperature lower than 30° C, primarily because of decreased metabolism, which can lead to toxic levels. Similarly, defibrillation is less likely to be effective at temperatures lower than 30° C. However, citing the solely theoretic basis of these concerns, the 2010 American Heart Association guidelines now state that in patients with persistent ventricular fibrillation or tachycardia after a single shock it may be "reasonable to perform further defibrillation attempts according to the standard BLS [basic life support] algorithm concurrent with rewarming strategies." Furthermore, regarding medication administration "it may be reasonable to consider administration of a vasopressor during cardiac arrest according to the standard ACLS [advanced cardiac life support] algorithm concurrent with rewarming strategies."[11] It is clear that very little is known about the utility of defibrillation and administration of vasoactive medications in patients with hypothermic cardiac arrest. Providers will have to decide each case on an individual basis and be guided by any response to the therapy used.

The phenomenon of core temperature afterdrop refers to the observation that a patient's temperature can fall after rewarming efforts have begun. It is believed to be due to a combination of temperature equilibration and return of cold blood from the periphery to the patient's core as perfusion is restored and strengthened. The clinical importance of core temperature afterdrop is keenly contested, and no consistent recommendations can be made regarding it. Certainly, attempts to rapidly rewarm a patient should not be delayed for fear of this consequence.

## NEXT STEPS IN CARE

Patients with mild hypothermia and (most) patients with moderate hypothermia can be treated in the emergency department and released when normothermic. This statement relies on the assumption that no other complicating social or medical problems are present that must be addressed. All patients with severe hypothermia should be admitted to the hospital, usually to an intensive care unit. Successful revival of these patients will require considerable time and resources.

Clear, universally accepted criteria on declaration of death in hypothermic patients are lacking, beyond the obvious recommendations regarding terminal injuries, rigidity that precludes chest compressions, and physical blockage of the mouth or nose by ice.

Numerous case reports have described neurologically intact survival after prolonged, severe hypothermia with cardiac arrest.[7,12] A serum potassium level higher than 10 mmol/L has been postulated to be a marker of irreversible cell and therefore patient death[13]; however, another case report has called this approach into question.[14] Pronouncement of death in a severely hypothermic patient should be made with reluctance until the patient's core temperature has been warmed to higher than 30° C to 32° C and signs of life remain absent.

A reasonable approach to the hypothermic patient is presented in **Figure 131.2.**

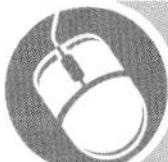

See Figure 131.2, Algorithmic Approach to Patiens with Hypothermia, online at www.expertconsult.com

# FROSTBITE

## PATHOPHYSIOLOGY

Frostbite is a freezing injury to tissues. During this process it is believed that deposits of ice crystals causing interstitial, cellular, and vascular endothelial cell damage are one part of the pathophysiologic process.[15] The vascular endothelial damage results in activation of the clotting cascade with resulting thrombosis, which leads to hypoperfusion, ischemia, and eventually tissue necrosis. The prominence of the clotting that can cause vascular occlusion can be seen on angiography and is the basis for the concept of treating selected patients with thrombolysis.

## PRESENTING SIGNS AND SYMPTOMS

The classic victim of frostbite has either a dusky or a white affected area that is brawny to solid in texture, insensate, and without capillary refill. Variations are time dependent, and patients seen in delayed fashion may have blisters that are either hemorrhagic or clear and even some tissue loss or frank necrosis already evident. Classification systems exist for frostbite, but they are controversial and are also problematic for the emergency physician because the initial clinical appearance can be misleading and it takes time for the full extent of the damage to become clear. It is simpler and more realistic to start to treat the affected part and consult surgeons for ongoing wound care and treatment (**Fig. 131.3**).

## TREATMENT

Frostbite is a clinical diagnosis. Other cold-related tissue injuries to be considered are frostnip, pernio (chilblains), and trench foot. These injuries, however, are nonfreezing ones, in contrast to frostbite.

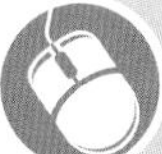

For a concise summation of nonfreezing injuries, see www.expertconsult.com

## PREHOSPITAL MANAGEMENT

Treatment of frostbite in the field consists of the application of dry sterile dressings to separate the involved digits and elevation of the affected extremity. Avoid rewarming with dry heat, such as with fires or heaters, and also assiduously prevent further cold injury. Rubbing the affected part with snow is soundly condemned. It is paramount to avoid a freeze-thaw-freeze cycle, which worsens the tissue damage.

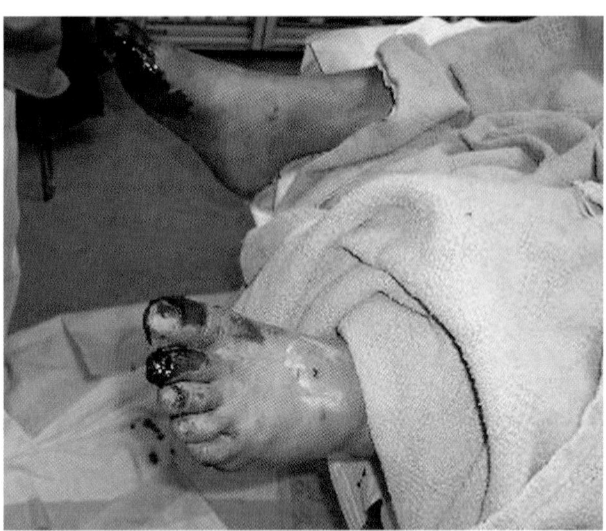

**Fig. 131.3 Frostbitten feet of a young man who had been running barefoot all night in winter secondary to drug-induced paranoia.**

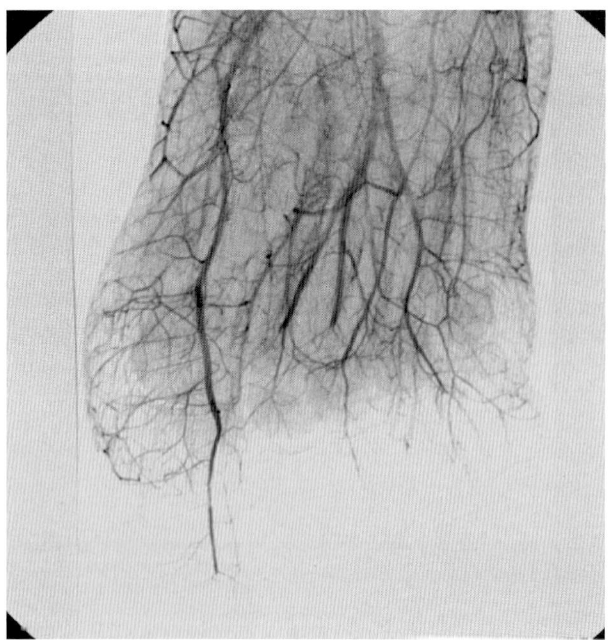

**Fig. 131.4 Angiogram of the left foot of a young female with frostbite after she wandered in the desert all night under the influence of illicit drugs.**

## HOSPITAL MANAGEMENT

Once the patient is in the hospital, the mainstay of treatment is rapid rewarming with a circulating bath of water heated to 40° C to 42° C for 10 to 30 minutes until the involved area is erythematous and pliable. Because rewarming is extraordinarily painful, liberal use of parenteral analgesics is usually necessary. Clear, large blisters should generally be débrided, but hemorrhagic ones should be left intact (their presence implies much deeper damage, and desiccation of the area is a concern). Débridement removes fluid that is rich in thromboxanes and prostaglandins, which are thought to be destructive to tissue. Aloe vera may be applied topically every 6 hours and the wounds bandaged.

Prophylactic antibiotics are controversial. Penicillin G has been advocated. Additionally, ibuprofen, 400 mg by mouth twice daily, is recommended in an attempt to interrupt the arachidonic acid cascade.[15,16] Both catheter-directed intraarterial and systemic thrombolytic therapies have been used with impressive success in preventing amputations (**Figs. 131.4 and 131.5**). This novel therapy holds considerable promise but does have several limitations, including restriction to patients initially seen within 24 hours of the injury and risk for bleeding.[17,18]

Most recently, a small, randomized trial of frostbite therapies showed remarkable success with intravenous iloprost, a prostacyclin (no digit amputations), over an IV nonsteroidal antiinflammatory drug (≈40% digit amputation rate) or recombinant tissue plasminogen activator plus iloprost (≈3% digit amputation rate).[19] Whether this promising success can be repeated and confirmed elsewhere remains to be seen.

Early surgical management is not indicated for frostbite because of the difficulty of ascertaining the full extent of the

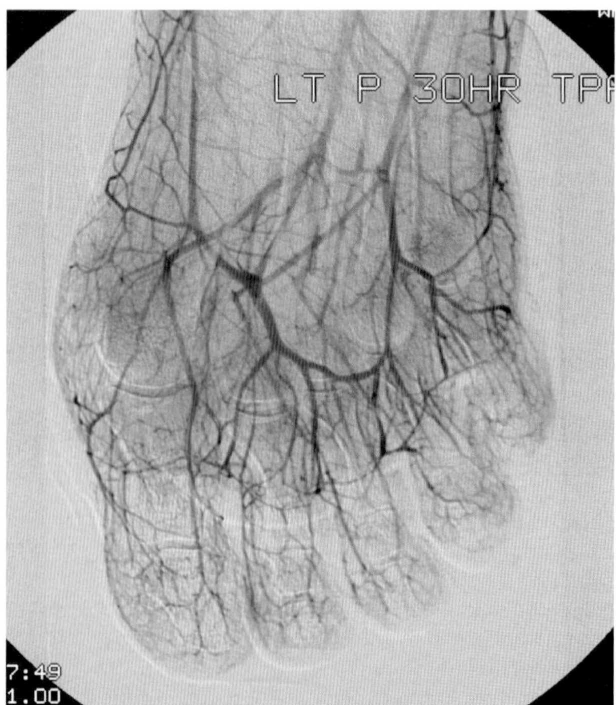


**Fig. 131.5 Angiogram of the foot shown in Figure. 131.3 after approximately 30 hours of tissue plasminogen activator infusion showing restoration of perfusion.** An amputation was averted with this therapy.

tissue damage initially. Typically, the affected area is left to mummify and essentially autoamputate before the formal procedure is carried out. Some newer imaging modalities, such as nuclear scanning and magnetic resonance angiography, may be able to shorten the time to definitive surgery by delineating viable tissue earlier than possible with simple observation.

## NEXT STEPS IN CARE

Because of the severity of frostbite, the need for daily hydrotherapy and wound care, and the often tenuous social circumstance of those afflicted, most patients with frostbite should be admitted to the hospital under the care of a physician skilled in treating this illness. In many cases, burn centers are an excellent option.

## SUGGESTED READINGS

Bruen KJ, Ballard JR, Morris SE, et al. Reduction of the incidence of amputation in frostbite injury with thrombolytic therapy. Arch Surg 2007;142:546-51; discussion 551-553.

Danzl DF, Pozos RS, Auerbach PS, et al. Multicenter hypothermia survey. Ann Emerg Med 1987;16:1042-55.

Mulcahy A, Watts M. Accidental hypothermia: an evidence-based approach. Emerg Med Pract 2009;11:1-24.

Murphy JV, Banwell PE, Roberts AH, et al. Frostbite: pathogenesis and treatment. J Trauma 2000;48:171-8.

Walpoth BH, Walpoth-Aslan BN, Mattle HP, et al. Outcome of survivors of accidental deep hypothermia and circulatory arrest treated with extracorporeal blood warming. N Engl J Med 1997;337:1500-5.

## REFERENCES

***References can be found on Expert Consult @ www.expertconsult.com.***

# 132 Lightning and Electrical Injuries

Christopher B. Colwell

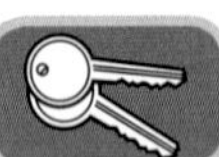

**KEY POINTS**

- In high-voltage electrical injuries, the internal damage that the victim has suffered can be significantly greater than the external damage or surface injury indicates.
- Fixed, dilated pupils are not a reliable indicator of brain death in the victim of a lightning strike.
- Oral burns in children can represent electrical injury from chewing on electrical wires.
- Victims in cardiac arrest may respond quite well to defibrillation, so these patients should receive highest priority for treatment at the scene.
- Victims of electrical injuries who have any symptoms are at high risk for compartment syndrome.
- Blunt trauma can occur in up to one third of victims of lightning or high-voltage electrical injuries.

## EPIDEMIOLOGY

A strike of lightning is one of the most common environmental causes of sudden cardiac death and is responsible for between 50 and 300 deaths annually in the United States.[1,2] Cloud-to-ground lighting strikes, the most destructive form of lightning, occur approximately 30 million times each year,[3] most often in Florida and along the southeastern coast of the Gulf of Mexico.[4] Lightning has struck more than 10 miles away from the rain of a thunderstorm, so the danger may not always be obvious or apparent.[3] Electrical injuries can be equally devastating. The spectrum of injuries from both can range dramatically from minor, localized injuries to death.

Although lightning injury may be one of the most common injuries caused by natural phenomena, its incidence has not been tracked accurately. The incidence is higher in males and in people between 20 and 44 years of age, three of every four occurred in the South or Midwest, and one in four was work related.[5] Sport-, wilderness-, and travel-related activities also place people at higher risk for lightning injuries.

Electrical injuries tend to occur in patients in three distinct age groups. The first group is toddlers who encounter household electrical sockets, cords, and appliances. The second is adolescents who engage in risky behavior. The third group comprises adults who work with electricity. Electrical burns account for between 3% and 7% of admissions to burn centers in the United States each year, many of which are occupational injuries. The annual occupational death rate from electrocution is 1 per 100,000; this type of death occurs more frequently in utility workers, miners, and construction workers.[6]

## PATHOPHYSIOLOGY

Definitions that should be familiar to those caring for patients with electrical injuries are listed in **Box 132.1**. Electrical current is the movement of electrical charge from one location to another. Current strength is expressed in amperes. Materials that allow electrical current to flow easily (low resistance) are referred to as conductors. Materials that do not allow flow of electrical current are called insulators.

All body tissues conduct electricity to some extent. Tissues with high fluid content conduct better than those with lower fluid content. Nerves tend to offer the least resistance, whereas bones offer the most. **Table 132.1** lists body tissues according to level of resistance. Skin resistance can vary substantially, with wet skin having the lowest resistance. Factors determining the severity of the injury caused by the electrical current are listed in **Box 132.2**.

Any electrical charge greater than 1000 V is generally considered high voltage, although some authorities have argued that the risk for significant injury increases with charges exceeding 600 V. Typical household circuits in the United States are 110 V, with bigger appliances operating on 220-V circuits. Power lines in residential areas can have more than 7000 V.

Electricity causes injury in several ways, as listed in **Box 132.3**. As current passes through the body, the tissues through which it passes are heated, and significant damage can occur. The emergency physician (EP) must be aware of the potential for internal damage when caring for a victim of electrical injury; not all patients with significant internal injuries display significant external damage. Arc burns result from an electrical source through the air and can cause significant damage. Temperatures can reach 2500° C, which can ignite clothes or nearby material and cause thermal injuries. Flash burns occur when current strikes the body but does not penetrate the skin.

**BOX 132.1 Definitions of Electrical Injuries**

Alternating current (AC): Electrical source with changing direction of current flow
Current: Flow of electrons per second (measured in amperes)
Direct current (DC): Electrical source with unchanging direction of current flow
Frequency: Number of transitions from positive to negative per second in AC
Resistance: Tendency of a material to resist the flow of electrical current (measured in ohms)
Volt: Unit of electrical force

**BOX 132.2 Factors Determining the Severity of Electrical Injury**

Type of circuit
Whether the current was alternating or direct
Duration of contact
Voltage (electrical potential)
Resistance of tissues
Amperage (current intensity)
Environmental circumstances
Pathway of the current

From Arrowsmith J, Usgaocar RP, Dickson WA. Electrical injury and the frequency of cardiac complications. Burns 1997;23:576-8.

**Table 132.1 Level of Resistance of Body Tissues to Electricity**

| LEVEL OF RESISTANCE | TISSUE |
|---|---|
| Low | Nerves<br>Blood vessels<br>Mucous membranes<br>Muscle |
| Intermediate | Skin |
| High | Tendon<br>Fat<br>Bone |

**BOX 132.3 Mechanisms of Electrical Injury**

Direct tissue damage (entry and exit sites)
Internal thermal heating
Induced muscle contraction
Flash burns
Arc burns
Blunt trauma

**BOX 132.4 Mechanisms of Injury from Lightning Strikes**

Direct strike
Contact strike: Lightning strikes an object that the victim is touching
Side flash: Lightning strikes a nearby object, and electrical current then traverses the air to strike the victim (can involve multiple victims)
Ground strike: Lightning hits the ground and is transferred to a person standing near the site of the strike. If there is a difference in potential between the legs of the victim, lightning can enter one leg and exit the other and thereby result in temporarily paretic, cold, insensate, and pulseless legs (keraunoparalysis)

Lightning delivers high-voltage direct current that tends to flow over the body rather than enter it. This event, often referred to as flashover, is one explanation for how people are able to sometimes survive exposure to such high voltage. Lightning current can also enter the victim and cause significant damage, particularly to the cardiac, respiratory, and neurologic systems. Blunt injury has been reported in up to one third of lightning victims[7] as a result of both the direct force of the strike and rapid expansion of the surrounding air, which often causes the victim to fall or be struck by flying debris. Lightning can also cause thermal injury (burns) by hot steam produced from surrounding moisture or by metal objects heated by the electricity. **Box 132.4** lists the mechanisms of injury from lightning strikes.

## ANATOMY

Cardiac arrest is the primary cause of immediate death after both electrical and lightning injuries. Electrical injuries can result in virtually any type of dysrhythmia, although rhythm disturbances are unlikely if the exposure is to less than 120 V and water is not involved.[8] Lighting also causes a variety of cardiac rhythm disturbances. Acute myocardial infarction is uncommon with both electrical and lightning injuries. Other cardiac sequelae of lightning injuries have been described and include cardiogenic shock[2] and Takotsubo cardiomyopathy.[1]

The head is a common point of contact for high-voltage injuries, and skull and cervical spine injuries occur as a result of blunt trauma from lightning and electrical injuries. Eye and ear injuries can both occur with electrical or lightning injuries, although they are more commonly associated with lightning.

The skin is commonly affected by electrical or lightning injuries, primarily in the form of burns. Injury to the extremities occurs with both lightning and electrical injuries, but high-voltage electrical injuries are far more likely to result in compartment syndromes.

Kidney damage or even acute renal failure can develop as a result of myoglobinemia, although this condition often responds well to fluid resuscitation. Gastrointestinal tract dysfunction, including bleeding and ulcer formation, has been described as well.

## PRESENTING SIGNS AND SYMPTOMS

Victims of high-voltage electrical injury typically have significant burns with a very dramatic appearance. Victims of low-voltage electrical injury or lightning injury may appear quite well. The most severe injuries are generally those affecting the cardiovascular and neurologic systems, and cardiac arrest is the most common cause of immediate death and is generally manifested as asystole (direct current) or ventricular fibrillation (alternating current).

Other than cardiac arrest, the most significant obvious injuries caused by exposure to electricity are usually burns, which are frequently most severe at the source of the electricity, as well as at the exit point, which is commonly a ground contact point (usually the heel). The EP should assume significant underlying damage in all patients with electrical or lightning injuries. Lightning contact is generally instantaneous and leads to flashover burns that are more often superficial and minor. Extensive burns and deeper injury are more common with high-voltage electrical injuries, frequently because of more prolonged contact.

The neurologic effects of electrical and lightning injuries can be immediate (which are often transient) or delayed (which last for a longer period and are more likely to be progressive). The prognosis is usually better for patients with more immediate symptoms than for those with delayed manifestations.[9] Initial findings include altered mental status, which is frequently transient but can range from slightly agitated to comatose. As current passes through the skull, heat-induced coagulation can occur and result in subdural and epidural hematomas, as well as intraventricular hemorrhage. Weakness and paresthesias of the extremities also occur and are more common in the lower than the upper extremities. Seizures have likewise been described.

Up to two thirds of victims of lightning strikes experience keraunoparalysis, a temporary paralysis specific to lightning injuries that is characterized by blue, mottled, and pulseless extremities (lower more commonly than upper).[10] Permanent paresthesias can result but are unusual.

Blood is a good conductor of electricity, and vascular damage from electrical and lightning injuries has been well described. Thrombosis, hemorrhage, and ischemia can occur as a result of direct damage to vessel walls, vasospasm, or burns. Small arteries to muscle are at particular risk.[11]

Skin findings include feathering burns, flash burns, contact burns, punctate burns, blistering, and linear streaking. A specific type of burn associated with electrical injury is referred to as a "kissing burn," which occurs at the flexor creases of the knees, elbows, and axilla. Kissing burns indicate extensive underlying damage, so EPs must be sure to look at the flexor surfaces for lightning or electrical injury when evaluating patients who are victims.

Contact with electrical current tends to produce burns that result in discolored (often gray or yellow), painless, depressed, punctate areas of the skin. It is important to recognize that tissue damage under these burns can be massive.

Feathering burns (also known as Lichtenberg figures) are specific to lightning injuries and result from electron showers induced by the lightning that make a fern pattern on the skin. No permanent damage to the skin occurs, and no specific therapy is required. Punctate burns are full-thickness burns that look like multiple small burns from a cigarette. Deep burns are rare with lightning injuries.

Oral burns in children often represent electrical injury from chewing or sucking on electrical wires. These injuries are particularly worrisome because of the possibility of delayed bleeding, which can be massive from the labial artery when the eschar separates, sometimes 5 days or more after the injury.

High-voltage electrical injuries and lightning injuries can both result in damage to the eyes and ears. Electrical injury is more likely to injure the eye if the exposure involves the head or neck, and such injuries include corneal burns, retinal detachment, and intraocular hemorrhage. Delayed cataract formation has been described in up to 6% of patients.[12] Lightning injuries can also cause uveitis, iridocyclitis, mydriasis, anisocoria, or Horner syndrome. It is for this reason that fixed, dilated pupils are not a reliable indicator of brain death in lightning strike victims. Damage to the ear is common with lightning injuries; rupture of the tympanic membrane is the most common finding, and the symptoms are generally transient hearing loss and vertigo.

Blunt trauma is common in the setting of electrical and lightning injuries, either from being thrown back from the source or from incidents resulting from the exposure, such as falls. Long-bone fractures, dislocations, and solid internal organ injury have been associated with both electrical and lightning injuries.

## DIFFERENTIAL DIAGNOSIS AND MEDICAL DECISION MAKING

Electrical injuries are generally more obvious than lightning injuries. With the exception of bathtub electrical injuries, where burns may not be apparent, a good history and thorough physical examination usually reveal the cause of the electrical injuries, ideally including the type of current, voltage, duration of contact, and symptoms immediately after the attack. Lightning injuries are not always as evident (lightning can strike when no rain or snow is present and even on mostly sunny days) and may be manifested as cardiac arrest, altered mental status, or paralysis. Recognition of classic patterns of lightning injury, such as feathering, may be the only way to initially distinguish these injuries from other causes of cardiac arrest, altered mentation, or acute neurologic injury. Differential diagnoses in which a history of lightning injury or high-voltage electrical injury is not obvious are listed in **Box 132.5**.

$SI = \frac{SV}{BSA}$ **FACTS AND FORMULAS**

Ohm's law: V = I × R

where V = potential (in volts); R = resistance (in ohms); I = current (an amperes)

P = I2Rt

where P = heat (in joules); I = current (in amperes); R = resistance (in ohms); t = time (in seconds)

**BOX 132.5 Differential Diagnosis of Lightning Injury**

Intracranial disease:
- Cerebrovascular accident
- Intracranial hemorrhage

Seizure disorder
Closed head injury
Spinal trauma
Encephalopathy
Primary cardiac dysrhythmia
Toxic ingestion

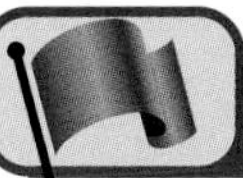

**RED FLAGS**

Do not underestimate the potential for significant underlying tissue damage, particularly with high-voltage electrical injury, even when the skin findings appear minor.
Traditional rules of triage do not apply to lightning victims. In this situation, care should be focused on rather than withheld from those in cardiopulmonary arrest.
Do not miss compartment syndrome, particularly with high-voltage electrical injury.
Consider the potential for rhabdomyolysis in all victims of high-voltage electrical injury, and provide adequate hydration. Beware of overaggressive hydration in lightning victims.
Admit patients for cardiac monitoring who have lost consciousness, have any evidence of cardiac instability or dysrhythmia, or have a transthoracic injury pattern.
Ensure good follow-up and provide careful instructions for the parents of children with oral burns, who are at risk for both cosmetic defects and delayed labial artery bleeding.
Remember the risk for blunt trauma in victims of high-voltage electricity and lightning.
Patients with neurologic complaints or deficits are at risk for permanent neurologic sequelae, particularly when the symptoms are delayed.
Remember to evaluate for tetanus immunization status and update as needed.

## DIAGNOSTIC TESTING

Cardiac monitoring and electrocardiography are indicated for all but the most benign electrical injuries and for virtually all lightning injuries. QT prolongation is a common finding. Complete blood counts are usually recommended, but their results should be normal. Abnormalities are more likely to be found when checking electrolyte, blood urea nitrogen, and creatinine values. Urinalysis should be performed to look for evidence of myoglobinuria, the presence of which indicates rhabdomyolysis. The serum creatine kinase value may also point to rhabdomyolysis. Acute myocardial infarction is rare with either lightning or electrical injuries. Computed tomography of the head should be performed in anyone with altered mental status or a significant headache given the risk for intracranial bleeding from either direct contact (particularly lightning) or the resulting head trauma. Cervical spine films should be obtained for patients with altered mental status or significant cranial injuries, including burns. A pregnancy test should be performed on all women of childbearing age.

## TREATMENT

Prehospital providers must be particularly vigilant about scene safety. With electrical injuries involving a discrete electrical source other than intact electrical outlets, the power must be turned off before the victim is approached. Any provider at the scene of a lightning injury must remember that lightning can strike in the same place twice. In addition, both electrical injuries and lightning injuries should be considered to pose a high risk for concomitant blunt trauma, and spinal immobilization should be initiated unless clearly not indicated.

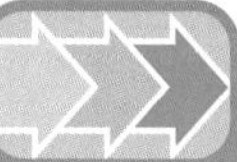

**PRIORITY ACTIONS**

Ensuring scene safety
Intravenous access; aggressive fluid resuscitation
Cardiac monitoring
Electrocardiography in all victims of lightning or high-voltage electrical injuries
Aggressive resuscitation of victims in cardiac arrest
Fasciotomy:
- May be needed early with high-voltage electrical injuries
- Rarely, if ever, needed with lightning injuries

Lightning injuries are an exception to the general rule that in mass casualty and disaster situations, people in cardiac arrest should be categorized or tagged as “black” (expectant or dead) and receive the lowest priority for treatment on the scene. Unlike the situation in most other mass casualty situations, cardiac arrest in the setting of lighting or electrical injury may be quickly reversed with defibrillation. Triage for multiple victims of lightning injuries at one scene should concentrate on those in cardiorespiratory arrest, and immediate treatment of those who are breathing can be reasonably delayed when necessary. Regardless of whether there are multiple casualties, victims of lightning injuries who are in cardiac arrest should be aggressively resuscitated whenever possible because evidence suggests that success rates are higher than in patients in cardiac arrest from other causes, even when the interval before resuscitation is prolonged.[2]

Rhabdomyolysis can be treated effectively by aggressive fluid administration, with the goal of urine output greater than 1 mL/kg/hr. Formulas used to determine fluid resuscitation in burn victims cannot be used for electrical injuries. Fluid resuscitation in patients with lightning-related injuries does not have to be very aggressive unless they are hemodynamically compromised. Fluid overload is a common iatrogenic complication in patients with lightning injuries.

Fasciotomy must be considered in patients with extremity burns from high-voltage electrical injuries in which compartment syndrome is a concern. Circumferential burns are more likely to result in compartment syndrome.

Tetanus boosters should be administered to patients whose immunization status is not up to date and even to those whose immunization status is current if they have significant muscle damage or contamination of the wounds because electrical wounds are especially prone to tetanus.

## FOLLOW-UP, NEXT STEPS IN CARE, AND PATIENT EDUCATION

Asymptomatic patients with normal physical findings who were victims of low-voltage electrical injury can be discharged safely without significant evaluation or observation. Patients with low-voltage injuries for whom risks are higher include those whose skin was wet during the injury, those with tetany, and those in whom the current traversed the thorax. Patients with mild symptoms, normal electrocardiographic findings, and no evidence of myoglobinuria can be discharged after a period of observation (generally 4 to 6 hours, although no research has confirmed this interval) and with recommendation for outpatient follow-up.

Any patient who experienced cardiac or respiratory arrest or clear loss of consciousness or has abnormal or changed electrocardiographic findings, hypoxia, chest pain, dysrhythmia observed by a medical care provider, or serious concomitant injury should be admitted.

### DOCUMENTATION

A large percentage of electrical injuries involve legal claims of some sort (e.g., worker's compensation, manufacturers), so the medical record should be complete with particular emphasis on the available history, physical findings, and treatment rendered. The record should include the following:

- Whether loss of consciousness was involved
- Voltage of the exposure if known
- Initial symptoms
- Skin findings
- Electrocardiographic findings
- Condition and symptoms at discharge

## SUGGESTED READINGS

Cooper MA, Andrews CJ, Holle RL. Lightning injuries. In: Auerbach P, editor. Wilderness medicine: management of wilderness and environmental emergencies. 5th ed. St. Louis: Mosby; 2005.

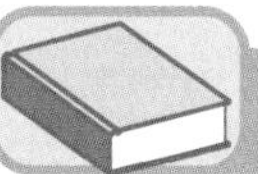

### PATIENT TEACHING TIPS

**For Parents**

Hazards of unused sockets

Hazards of extension cords

Dangers of oral burns; in particular, delayed labial artery bleeding and cosmetic defect

**For Electrical Injuries**

Never work with electrical equipment alone.

Sweaty or otherwise wet skin can decrease resistance significantly and turn a low-risk exposure into a higher-risk one.

Insulation of electrical lines is meant to protect the lines from environmental challenges, *not* to protect humans from contact with the line.

**For Lightning Injuries**

Seek shelter indoors or in a vehicle if lightning is anticipated.

If shelter is not available, seek dense woods or a ditch to lie in.

Lightning can strike even when the sun is out.

Stay clear of metallic objects in a storm, particularly those that would elevate your height from the ground, because the highest object is generally struck by lightning.

Get out of water and off small boats.

Discard metallic objects such as golf clubs, umbrellas, and jewelry.

A lightning strike is imminent when an individual's hair stands on end.

Lightning *can* strike in the same place twice.

Do not resume activity in the area of a storm until more than 30 minutes has elapsed after the last flash of lighting or sound of thunder.

**For Patients with an Electrical or Lightning Injury**

Delayed neurologic symptoms can be serious and should prompt a return to the emergency department.

Up to 74% of victims of lightning injuries suffer some sort of permanent sequela, such as sleep disturbance or chronic pain syndrome.

Koumbourlis AC. Electrical injuries. Crit Care Med 2002;30:S424-30.

Price TG, Cooper MA. Electrical and lightning injuries. In: Marx JA, editor. Rosen's emergency medicine: concepts and clinical practice. 7th ed. Philadelphia: Mosby; 2010.

## REFERENCES

***References can be found on Expert Consult @ www.expertconsult.com.***

# Dysbarisms, Dive Injuries, and Decompression Illness 133

*Heather Murphy-Lavoie and Tracy Leigh LeGros*

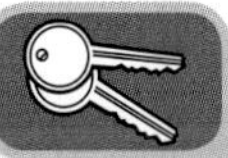

**KEY POINTS**

- Decompression illness describes diving-related injuries, including decompression sickness and arterial gas embolism.
- Any neurologic symptoms that occur in a diver immediately or soon after resurfacing are highly suspicious for arterial gas embolism and require urgent medical attention.
- A thorough neurologic examination is crucial with any suspicion of decompression illness.
- Dive injuries are best differentiated into the following categories: disorders of descent, disorders at depth, disorders of ascent, and disorders that occur after resurfacing.
- Decompression illness is treated on the scene by rapid implementation of high-flow oxygen and intravenous hydration; definitive treatment is recompression with hyperbaric oxygen therapy.
- One should delay flying after diving for at least 12 hours following a single no-decompression dive and at least 24 hours for dives involving decompression stops.
- Consultation with a diving physician or the Divers Alert Network (or both) is needed for a patient with any symptoms associated with recent diving.

## EPIDEMIOLOGY

Dysbarisms refer to the pathophysiologic effects of changes in ambient (surrounding) pressure on the body. Decompression illness (DCI) includes decompression sickness (DCS or "the bends") and arterial gas embolism (AGE). DCI occurs during or after ascent (decompression) when dissolved gases come out of solution, form bubbles, and then become lodged in various tissues (instead of being filtered by the lungs). Diagnosis of DCI in the emergency department (ED) is vital because delayed treatment or missed cases can have permanent sequelae (**Box 133.1**).

With the advent of "extreme sports" that involve water contact, sport diving, and the increasing number of people engaging in breath-hold diving, a sharp increase in diving injuries has been seen in EDs (**Box 133.2**). Deaths from breath-hold diving alone have almost doubled in the last 5 years, thus illustrating the potential for injury associated with this form of diving.[1] With acute DCI, rapid assessment and treatment are the foundation of management. Three keys to successful ED treatment are having a high index of suspicion (DCI may have nonspecific findings), performing a thorough neurologic examination, and obtaining hyperbaric medicine consultation when DCI is suspected.

## PATHOPHYSIOLOGY

Dysbarism refers to the effects of variations in ambient (surrounding) pressure on the body. Hypobaric (low-pressure) exposure, such as that experienced by climbers, pilots, and astronauts, can result in symptoms and injuries similar to those found in divers with DCI who are exposed to high pressure while at depth. Decompression injuries during high-pressure (hyperbaric) exposure are far more common.

### DIVING PHYSIOLOGY

Evaluation of a diver with a water-associated injury requires a basic understanding of diving physiology and the physics of pressure and gases. Different gases have different properties at different depths, which allows gases to be used alone or in combination for different types of diving. The gases of most interest are air, oxygen, nitrogen, helium, and occasionally argon. Deep diving (past 180 feet of sea water [fsw]) often requires helium-oxygen combinations (heliox) to mitigate the effects of nitrogen narcosis (discussed later). Moreover, enriched nitrogen-oxygen combinations (nitrox) may be used to reduce obligations for decompression stops, which is the time spent at more shallow depths to help divers offload the nitrogen built up in the body before exiting a dive.

In general, most recreational divers breathe compressed air and use a self-contained underwater breathing apparatus (SCUBA) when diving to depths of less than 135 fsw. Nitrogen represents about 78% of the gas inhaled with compressed air diving. During diving, hydrostatic pressure "pushes" nitrogen into tissues; nitrogen (an inert gas) then becomes dissolved in plasma and permeates tissues. While at depth, gases remain in solution, and most divers experience minimal difficulty. The deeper that divers travel and the longer that they remain at depth, the more saturated the blood and tissues

**BOX 133.1 Typical Signs and Symptoms of Decompression Illness**

| Symptoms | Signs |
|---|---|
| Pain | Sensory deficits |
| Numbness | Weakness |
| Dizziness | Paralysis |
| Extreme fatigue | Ataxia |
| Headache | Rash |
| Itching | Urinary retention |
| Vertigo | |
| Nausea | |
| Changes in personality | |
| Loss of consciousness | |

**BOX 133.2 Fatality Statistics for Diving**

Deaths: 120 diving fatalities in the United States and Canada (2007)

Death analyses: men (85%); median age 50 years (men) and 43 years (women)

Obesity: 76% of deaths involved overweight or obese divers

Causes of death: drowning (86%); acute heart condition (9%); arterial gas embolism (3%); decompression sickness (1%)

Activities: 66% of deaths during pleasure of sight-seeing diving

Data from Divers Alert Network. DAN report on decompression illness, diving fatalities and project dive exploration, 2008. Available at www.diversalertnetwork.org/.

become with nitrogen (or other inspired inert gases). One of the tenets of diving is to ascend slowly when resurfacing. Doing so allows the dissolved (inert) gases to escape the tissues slowly and be cleared via normal respiration. If a person ascends to the surface too quickly, the dissolved gases come out of solution and form bubbles in tissues or within the vasculature. When these bubbles are not cleared by the lungs ("blown off") they can embolize and cause downstream injury or they can cause local damage at the site of formation (autochthonous bubbles). When bubbles cause symptoms, the disorder is called DCI. Depending on the size, number, and location of the bubbles, DCI has a wide range of manifestations, from pain (most common symptom), numbness, and fatigue to severe neurologic symptoms such as seizure, paralysis, and loss of consciousness (LOC).

## BUBBLE PHYSIOLOGY

Knowledge of bubble mechanics and the effects of bubbles in various tissues is critical to understanding the pathophysiology and treatment of DCI. Venous bubbles are not usually problematic because the lungs can filter large gas loads. Bubbles have damaging effects when they remain within tissues or embolize. Bubbles can pass from the venous circulation to the arterial circulation via a right-to-left shunt (patent foramen ovale or arteriovenous malformation). Bubbles can grow from "nucleation sites" within body tissues, such as the joint spaces, tendon sheaths, periarticular sheaths, and peripheral nerves.[2] Once inside these areas, bubbles can act as emboli and block perfusion of distal tissues or act as foreign bodies with resultant vascular damage through activation of the inflammatory and clotting cascades. Interestingly, scientists are now evaluating a possible biologic marker of DCI. As gas emboli within the circulation induce decompression stress, endothelial cells release microparticles in response to cellular activation or cell death. These microparticles may, in the future, reflect a biologic marker of decompression stress that can be used to gauge the extent of disease, efficacy of treatment, or prophylaxis.[3]

## PRINCIPLES OF GAS LAWS AND DYSBARISM

An understanding of the pertinent diving gas laws, units of measurement, abbreviations, and mathematic conversions helps facilitate the treatment and disposition of dive-injured patients. At sea level, the pressure of the atmosphere on the body (ambient pressure) is 760 mm Hg, which equals 1 atm. The term for the absolute pressure on a diver at sea level is called *atmospheres absolute* (ATA), and it represents the total sum of the pressure on a diver. Therefore, at sea level, a dive computer gauge reads zero, but sea level also represents one surrounding atmosphere of pressure (1 ATA). This knowledge helps the physician better comprehend the circumstances surrounding a dive injury. Although there are a large number of gas laws, the two that are the most important in diving medicine are Boyle's law and Dalton's law.

### *Boyle's Law*

Boyle's law aids in understanding why a diver needs to exhale while ascending from depth. According to Boyle's law, the volume of a quantity of gas *(V)* varies inversely with the pressure on that gas *(P)* if it is kept at a constant temperature. It is often represented by the following formula:

$$P_1V_1 = P_2V_2$$

where the subscripts *1* and *2* indicate two different combinations of pressure and volume; in other words, the product of pressure and volume will always remain a constant.

Usually, as a diver descends deeper, the surrounding pressure increases in linear fashion. Water pressure at the surface is referenced as 1 ATA. In general, for every 33 fsw that the diver descends, there is an increase in pressure of 1 ATA. Therefore, a descent to 33 fsw would equal 2 ATA, a descent to 66 fsw would equal 3 ATA, and so on. Furthermore, for the first 33 fsw descended, the volume of gas present is reduced by half the original amount of gas at the surface. At 66 fsw, the volume is one third the original volume. The greatest changes in volume occur closest to the water surface and represent a significant vulnerability to injury (**Fig. 133.1**).

### *Dalton's Law*

Dalton's law of partial pressures is critical to understanding the mechanisms for DCS, nitrogen narcosis, and oxygen toxicity. It is represented by the formula

$$P_{total} = P_1 + P_2 + P_3$$

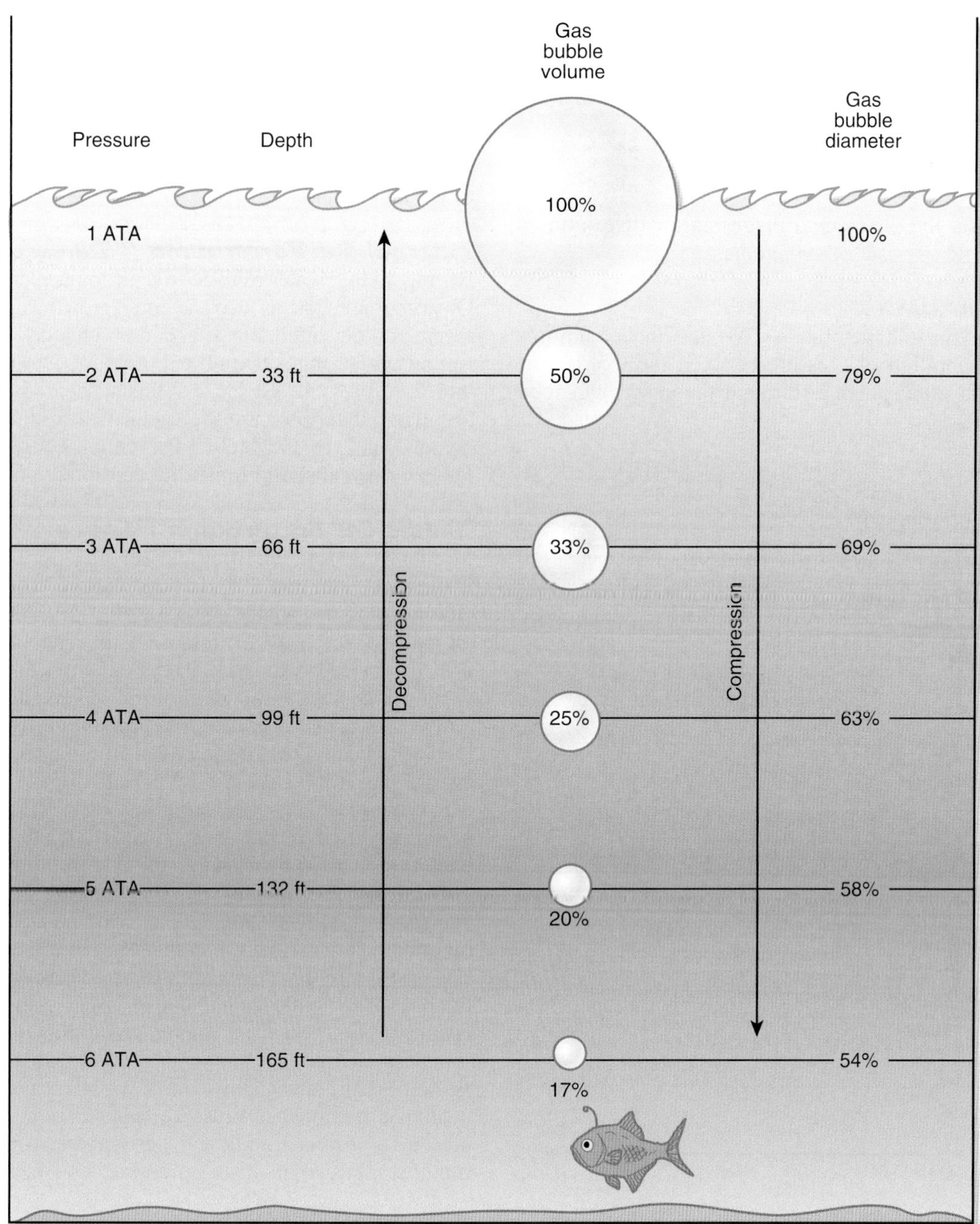


**Fig. 133.1 Boyle's law.** *ATA*, Atmospheres absolute.

where $P_{total}$ is the total pressure of the gases that a diver breathes and the subscripts *1, 2,* and *3* indicate the partial pressure of each individual gas. This law explains why the effects of the individual gases increase as a diver travels deeper during a dive. Put simply, as a diver descends, the amount of each gas inhaled increases proportionally with increasing depth. When diving with air tanks, divers are exposed to higher partial pressures of both oxygen and nitrogen the farther down that they travel. Importantly, nitrogen at high concentrations has a narcotic effect (nitrogen narcosis), and oxygen at high concentrations can be toxic (oxygen toxicity). Both problems are described in further detail later in the chapter.

## PRESENTING SIGNS AND SYMPTOMS

### BAROTRAUMA

Barotrauma is sustained from failure to equalize the pressure of an air-containing space with that of the surrounding environment. The most common examples of barotrauma occur during air travel and scuba diving.[1,4] Barotrauma occurs only in gas-containing (compressible) body spaces. More than 95% of the body is composed of water (incompressible). Typical gas-filled spaces include the sinuses, middle and inner ears, air-filled areas within carious or filled teeth, and hollow viscous organs such as the intestines and lungs. Barotrauma incurred during descent is called a "squeeze." Barotrauma incurred during ascent is called a "reverse squeeze," "reverse block," or expansion injury.

## DIFFERENTIAL DIAGNOSIS AND MEDICAL DECISION MAKING

**Table 133.1** lists the differential diagnosis for dive injuries based on the time of onset of symptoms.

### EAR BAROTRAUMA

With an intact tympanic membrane (TM), the only communication for equilibration of pressure between the middle ear and the ambient atmosphere is through the eustachian tube (ET).[5] Divers typically perform Valsalva maneuvers during decent to equalize pressure in the middle ear. Failure to equalize leads to pain and damage from injury to the middle or inner ear and results in TM edema, rupture, or hemorrhage, as well as rupture of the oval or round window (may lead to a perilymphatic fistula).[5] **Table 133.2** summarizes the types of ear barotrauma.

**Table 133.1 Differential Diagnosis of Dive Injuries Based on the Onset of Symptoms**

| SYMPTOM ONSET | INJURIES TO CONSIDER |
|---|---|
| Descent | Ear or sinus barotrauma<br>Inner ear barotrauma |
| Bottom | Nitrogen narcosis<br>Oxygen toxicity<br>Trauma |
| Ascent | Arterial gas embolism<br>Pneumothorax<br>Pneumomediastinum<br>Subcutaneous emphysema<br>Severe decompression sickness<br>Ear or sinus barotrauma<br>Barodontalgia<br>Gastrointestinal barotrauma<br>Trauma<br>Alternobaric vertigo<br>Alternobaric facial palsy |
| 15 min after resurfacing | Arterial gas embolism |
| 15 min to 24 hr after resurfacing | Decompression sickness |

#### *External Ear Barotrauma ("Squeeze")*

During diving, water replaces the air in the external ear canal. Obstructions such as wax, a bony growth, or earplugs can create an unvented air space that changes in volume in response to changes in ambient pressure. During descent, the increased pressure "squeezes" this space and causes the TM to bulge outward toward the canal with resultant pain, small hemorrhages, or TM blebs.[4] Prevention consists of cleaning the external canal and removing any foreign bodies.

#### *Middle Ear Barotrauma ("Squeeze")*

Middle ear barotrauma (middle ear squeeze, barotitis media) is the most common disorder in divers and hyperbaric medicine patients. It usually occurs during descent as a result of an inability to equalize pressure across the TM. It occurs in 30% of novice divers and 10% of experienced divers.[6] When water exerts pressure on the external TM and pushes it inward, a diver can usually equalize the pressure in the ears by swallowing, yawning, performing a Valsalva maneuver, or blowing against closed nostrils. Divers are often unable to clear their ears because of anatomic variability of the ET, inflammation, a viral infection, or upper aerodigestive dysfunction. Without equalization of the pressure, the TM ruptures. As little as 100 mm Hg (5 fsw) can create a pressure differential large enough to rupture the TM.[7] Symptoms of middle ear barotrauma are ear pain, pressure, and muffled hearing. If the TM is ruptured, vertigo may occur because of the effects of cold water on the middle ear or TM. Treatment consists of decongestants, rest from diving, and follow-up with an otorhinolaryngologist (refractory cases). In general, these injuries are self-limited. However, if a patient needs hyperbaric medicine treatments, pressure equalization tubes may be placed to prevent middle ear barotrauma. Any form of TM rupture, placement of a pressure equalization tube, or

**Table 133.2 Barotrauma of the Ear**

| | MIDDLE EAR BAROTRAUMA | INNER EAR BAROTRAUMA | ALTERNOBARIC VERTIGO |
|---|---|---|---|
| Symptoms | Ear pain on descent<br>Hearing loss<br>Possible transient vertigo | Ear pain on descent<br>Hearing loss<br>Severe vertigo and nausea | Ear pain on ascent<br>Transient hearing loss<br>Nausea |
| Signs | Conductive hearing loss<br>TM injury<br>Unilateral facial paralysis (rare) | Nystagmus<br>Vomiting<br>Ataxia<br>Romberg sign<br>Neural hearing loss | Nystagmus<br>Vomiting<br>TM injury<br>Abrupt relief with descent |
| Treatment | Decongestants | Referral to an otorhinolaryngologist | None if resolved |

Modified from Shockley L. Scuba diving and dysbarism. In: Hockberger RM, Walls JA, Marx RS, editors. Rosen's emergency medicine. 6th ed. St. Louis: Mosby; 2006.
*TM*, Tympanic membrane.

myringotomy would be a contraindication to wet water diving because water comes in direct contact with the middle ear.

ALTERNOBARIC FACIAL PALSY Alternobaric facial palsy, a complication of middle ear barotrauma after diving, is a syndrome consisting of unilateral facial nerve palsy, ataxia, vertigo, nausea, and vomiting. The symptoms can be confused with those of AGE or DCS; however, the mechanism is elevated middle ear pressure pressing against the facial nerve and causing ischemic neurapraxia.[7] Alternobaric palsy is also observed in those who fly after diving, fly at high altitude in unpressurized airplanes, and experience explosive decompression in flight.[7] Though uncomfortable, the symptoms usually resolve within minutes once middle ear pressures equilibrate.

REVERSE MIDDLE EAR BAROTRAUMA Reverse middle ear barotrauma, or reverse squeeze, is similar to middle ear squeeze but involves increased pressure in the middle ear pushing outward on the TM. It is often due to ET obstruction and occurs on ascent. The symptoms are similar to those of middle ear squeeze; however, reverse squeeze can rupture the round window as well.

### Inner Ear Barotrauma

The inner ear is a complicated and delicate organ, and any diver complaining of hearing loss, vertigo, or ear pain might have inner ear barotrauma (IEBT). Though less common than middle ear squeeze, IEBT is associated with significantly higher morbidity because it often involves damage to the cochleovestibular organs. Separating the middle and inner ear are the thin membranes of the round and oval windows. Damage to these structures may cause leakage of fluid from the inner to the middle ear. IEBT can result from difficulty equalizing pressure during a dive. Performing a vigorous Valsalva maneuver or forcefully attempting to clear the ears can cause damage to the round window. The symptoms can be quite significant and include extreme dizziness, vertigo, nausea, and vomiting. The patient might also have nystagmus, ataxia, and hearing loss. IEBT is considered an emergency and mandates immediate evaluation by an otolaryngologist.

### Alternobaric Vertigo

Alternobaric vertigo occurs on ascent as a result of differences in pressure between the two middle ear spaces. This difference causes asymmetric stimulation of each vestibular organ, which leads to vertigo. Symptoms include severe nausea and vomiting, as well as transient hearing loss. The patient will report abrupt relief with clearing of the ears or return to pressure.

### Sinus Barotrauma

Sinus barotrauma ("sinus squeeze") is the second most common disorder in divers, but it is significantly less common than middle ear barotrauma, with only 1% of divers affected.[5] Symptoms include sinus pain on descent and bloody nasal discharge on ascent.[4] Treatment consists of decongestants, antiinflammatory agents, and rest from diving.

### Pulmonary Barotrauma and Pulmonary Overpressurization Syndromes

Pulmonary overpressurization syndromes can occur during rapid ascent with breath-holding in which the pulmonary parenchyma is ruptured. Ascending too fast without exhaling allows the rapidly expanding gases in the lungs to enlarge and stretch the lung parenchyma, followed by overdistention and ultimately parenchymal rupture. Gas then enters the perilung spaces, which creates a pathway for bubbles to embolize to the brain. As little as an 80–mm Hg pressure differential is sufficient to rupture the alveolar lining. It can occur with breath-holding during the last 3 to 4 fsw of ascent.

PNEUMOMEDIASTINUM AND MEDIASTINAL EMPHYSEMA Pneumomediastinum occurs when alveolar rupture allows gas to enter the mediastinum through the perivascular sheath; it causes chest pain and sometimes crepitus that is appreciated with auscultation (Hamman sign). Treatment consists of supplemental oxygen and observation; the diagnosis is made by chest radiographic evaluation and physical examination. Recompression is usually unnecessary, although a thorough neurologic examination to screen for AGE is recommended. Approximately 30% of divers with AGE will be found to have pneumomediastinum on a chest radiograph.

SUBCUTANEOUS EMPHYSEMA Similar to pneumomediastinum, subcutaneous emphysema is due to alveolar rupture causing release of gas into tissues that can track up into the neck and under the skin. Symptoms include palpable crepitus, a sensation of fullness in the chest, possible alteration of voice, and occasionally dysphagia. Treatment is similar to that for pneumomediastinum; recompression is not generally necessary for isolated subcutaneous emphysema.

PNEUMOTHORAX Pneumothorax is a severe, potentially life-threatening pulmonary overpressure syndrome. Rupture allows bubbles and gas to enter the pleural space, which can place pressure on the lung itself. Symptoms vary greatly, depending the volume of air entering the pleural space and the patient's baseline lung function. Patients may have simple dyspnea or exhibit shock or life-threatening cardiac arrest (tension pneumothorax). The most common symptoms are sharp chest pain, shortness of breath, and occasionally a sudden, dry, hacking cough. Pain may also be felt in the shoulder, neck, or abdomen. Treatment is immediate administration of high-flow oxygen and possible needle decompression or tube thoracostomy (or both). If pneumothorax occurs during hyperbaric treatment or surface decompression table treatment, immediate venting of the pneumothorax (Heimlich valve) may be necessary to prevent the development of tension pneumothorax.

ARTERIAL GAS EMBOLISM AGE, the most lethal result of pulmonary barotrauma, is a common cause of death in recreational divers.[8] Its incidence is underestimated because many in-water deaths are classified as drowning. When rupture of the lung parenchyma leads to intravascular bubbles, these bubbles can embolize and cause end-organ damage. Sadly, this disorder is often seen in inexperienced divers who panic at depth and shoot to the surface without exhaling slowly. The symptoms are dramatic, usually LOC immediately or within minutes of the diver reaching the surface. Death is common. The arterial emboli are most deadly when they travel to the coronary or cerebral circulation. Cerebral AGE is manifested very much like a stroke and results in headache, confusion, agitation, hemiplegia, or sudden LOC. Air embolism can also block blood flow through the coronary circulation and lead to cardiac ischemia, dysrhythmias, shock, and death.

Definitive treatment of AGE consists of high-flow oxygen on site and immediate hyperbaric recompression. The sooner patients are recompressed, the less likely they are to have permanent neurologic injury. Full recovery is common when recompression is available immediately. It is important to remember that AGE can occur in shallow water while breathing compressed gas or during breath-hold diving. This is in contrast to DCS, which usually occurs following a deep or prolonged dive when high nitrogen partial pressure develops.[9] AGE also occurs in the hospital setting as a result of iatrogenic errors (central line manipulation, hemodialysis), but it can occur with any procedure or trauma that can entrain gas into the bloodstream.

### Gastrointestinal Barotrauma

The stomach and intestine are both air-filled organs and, though rarely affected, are susceptible to barotrauma. Specifically, gas expansion occurring on ascent can cause nausea, belching, flatulence, mild stomach pain, and reflux. These symptoms resolve fairly quickly after the diver resurfaces because these spaces are typically easily vented.

### Tooth Barotrauma

The small air pockets that exist in teeth and under fillings are susceptible to barotrauma (barodontalgia). Most people experience pain only on ascent, but tooth fractures have occurred (odontocrixis). Decompressions as mild as those experienced during commercial air flight pressurization (8000 feet or 0.75 ATA) are sufficient to cause barodontalgia. Such patients should be referred for dental evaluation, and divers should make their dentists aware of their diving hobby so that air pockets can be avoided.

## DECOMPRESSION SICKNESS

DCS, or "the bends," is a type of DCI that usually occurs after diving at deeper depths. In accordance with Dalton's law, tissues become highly permeated with inspired inert gases with increasing depth. DCS can also occur after long shallow dives if significant tissue saturation has occurred. It can cause a spectrum of symptoms. Diagnosis can be difficult because divers may complain of only mild to moderate symptoms, which they tend to ignore or attribute to other causes. Frequently, a diver complains, "I just don't feel right," or has limb pain without trauma that is assumed to be muscular in origin. DCS symptoms rarely develop while the diver is in the water. The key to diagnosing dive-related injuries is to (1) elicit the timing of the onset of symptoms (before, during, or after a dive), (2) determine the presence of any dive-related DCS risk factors (dehydration, alcohol use, inexperience, failure to follow the decompression tables, flying after diving, reverse-profile diving, multiple dives per day, decompression diving, smoking, advanced age, cold water, patent foramen ovale, and obesity), and (3) have a low threshold for suspicion of DCS when symptoms develop. DCS is classically divided into three types according to the severity of illness and the location of symptoms. In reality, DCS symptoms overlap and the basic treatment is usually the same for all types—recompression with hyperbaric oxygen.

### *Type I ("Mild" Symptoms)*

Type I DCS describes mild symptoms such as joint pain (most common), dermatologic manifestations, and lymphatic-associated swelling and edema as a result of the effects of gas bubbles in the tissues (**Box 133.3**). Bubble formation in joints is due to the greater negative pressure that exists in the joint spaces.[10] Pain is most often felt in the shoulders or knees but can appear in any joint. The pain is gradual and aching and varies in intensity, usually worsening with time. Limb pain in divers affects the upper extremities three times more often than the lower extremities, and its distribution is often asymmetric.[11] Caisson workers, however, are affected more often in their lower limbs.[8] Merritt makes the point that type I DCS usually involves pain in the extremities whereas type II DCS usually involves central structures.[7]

Dermatologic DCI ("skin bends") can have several manifestations. A diver can experience itching alone (without a rash) in localized or generalized areas of the arms, legs, face, or trunk ("fleas"). This form is commonly thought to follow dry dives, appears shortly after resurfacing, and lasts only a few minutes to a few hours.[12] Other dermatologic manifestations of DCS are mottling (cutis marmorata) and rindlike skin (peau d'orange).

### *Type II ("Severe" Symptoms)*

Type II DCS causes more severe symptoms that have a high risk of leading to major disability or death. Cardiopulmonary,

**BOX 133.3 Type I Decompression Sickness**

**Musculoskeletal Pain ("Limb Bends")**
- Most common manifestation of DCS
- Dull, aching pain often in the shoulder or knee
- Pain occurring both at rest and with movement
- No evidence of joint inflammation on examination
- Occurs within 24 hours of resurfacing but almost never at depth and rarely within the first few minutes after surfacing

**Cutaneous DCS ("Skin Bends")**
- Itching and pruritus most common symptoms (self-resolving)
- Cutis marmorata (mottled appearance of the skin)
- Peau d'orange (rindlike skin seen in the truncal area)
- "Fleas" (formication-like symptoms of insects on the skin)

**Lymphatic Effects and Edema**
- Swelling in the soft tissues or in areas of lymph nodes
- Usually localized
- Very uncommon

**Definitive Treatment**
- Definitive treatment is recompression
- All patients require oxygen. Remember to consult a hyperbaric medicine specialist early if the patient is being brought from a dive accident

Adapted from Bove AA, Davis J. Bove and Davis' diving medicine. 4th ed. Philadelphia: Saunders; 2004; and U.S. Department of Commerce: NOAA Navy diving manual. 5th ed. Flagstaff, Ariz: Best Publishing; 2005.
*DCS*, Decompression sickness.

neurologic, and inner ear manifestations predominate (**Box 133.4**). All patients with type II DCS symptoms require emergency recompression in a hyperbaric chamber. The sooner they are recompressed, the more likely they are to have a full recovery. However, even if treatment is delayed several days, recompression can still be helpful. Multiple treatments may be necessary to maximize recovery.

### *Type III Decompression Sickness*

Type III includes both type II symptoms and AGE.

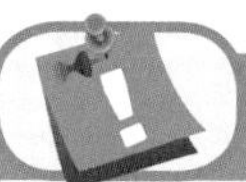

**TIPS AND TRICKS**

Limb pain as a result of DCS usually persists even at rest, whereas the pain of a traumatic injury often improves with rest or nonuse.

Resolution of the pain at a joint when a blood pressure cuff is inflated is a strong indicator of joint DCS.

Neurologic examination of an injured diver is best performed with the patient out of the stretcher or bed to unmask any neurologic deficits.

Serious diving injuries are much more common in recreational divers than in commercial or military divers.

Abdominal pain may be an early signal of spinal cord injury in divers with DCS.

*DCS*, Decompression sickness.

**BOX 133.4 Type II Decompression Sickness**

Type II is associated with a higher risk for permanent disability or death than type I.

**Pulmonary DCS ("Chokes")**

Persistent, dry, nonproductive cough
Substernal, pleuritic chest pain
Seen more with high-altitude DCS and in tunnel and caisson workers

**Neurologic DCS**

Represents 60% to 70% of DCS injuries
Spinal cord affected three times more often than the cerebrum
Seen more often in recreational divers.
Symptoms usually occur hours after ascent:

- Tingling in the trunk
- Progressive numbness and paresthesias
- Ascending motor weakness
- Bowel, bladder incontinence
- Paralysis
- Memory impairment, aphasias, visual disturbances, personality changes

**Vestibular DCS ("Staggers")**

Dizziness, nausea, vomiting, nystagmus, hearing loss, tinnitus
Uncommon in recreational divers
Can be confused with middle ear barotrauma

**Definitive Treatment**

Recompression

*DCS*, Decompression sickness.

## NEUROLOGIC EXAMINATION

The importance of performing a thorough neurologic examination cannot be understated. Unless an obvious neurologic deficit is noted, many dive-injured patients do not realize that they have an injury. However, if "hard" neurologic symptoms are observed, the patient requires immediate recompression with hyperbaric oxygen therapy without delay (**Box 133.5**). The neurologic examination should include a diver's mental status, cranial nerves, balance, coordination, sensory testing, deep tendon reflexes, pathologic reflexes, and both fine and gross motor skills. Preprinted neurologic examination forms enable the physician to maximize diagnosis and treatment, as well as to standardize findings.

**BOX 133.5 Definitive Treatment of Dive-Injured Patients**

**Recompression with Hyperbaric Oxygen in a Chamber**

Counteracts new bubble formation
Reduces existing bubble size
Creates a strong gradient for nitrogen washout
Improves oxygenation of ischemic tissues
Reduces edema
Inhibits leukocyte-mediated reperfusion injuries

**Other Therapies**

***Prostaglandins and Platelet Inhibitors***

Nonsteroid antiinflammatory drugs, aspirin
Inhibit inflammation and platelet formation
Not routinely used, no proven benefit

***Lidocaine***

May be beneficial for arterial gas embolism
Shown to be helpful in animal studies
Decreases neuronal irritability

## TREATMENT

### PREHOSPITAL MANAGEMENT AND AIR EVACUATION FROM THE SITE

Prehospital treatment of a dive injury is similar to that given in the ED. However, the hyperbaric team should be notified early that the patient is incoming to minimize delays (**Box 133.6**).

### EMERGENCY DEPARTMENT EVALUATION AND TREATMENT

ED treatment of dive-injured patients must follow a standard approach. In addition to ordering routine laboratory tests, oxygen, and intravenous fluids, obtaining a thorough history is critical to treatment (**Boxes 133.7 and 133.8**).

**BOX 133.6 Prehospital Treatment and Air Evacuation Instructions for Dive-Injured Patients**

1. Maintain the ABCs of resuscitation and evaluate the patient's serum glucose level.
2. Use ACLS protocols to stabilize the patient.
3. Administer high-flow oxygen, establish intravenous lines, and begin fluid administration.
4. Keep the patient flat; avoid the Trendelenburg position. If aspiration is a risk, lay the patient on the left side or in the right lateral position.
6. If air evacuation is being performed, ensure that the cabin of the airplane is pressurized or have the pilot fly at altitudes below 1000 feet.
7. Transport the patient along with all gear (it will have to be examined later).
8. Remember that the other members of the diving party might also need transport and evaluation for decompression sickness; they should accompany the patient to the ED.
9. Alert the consultant dive physician and hyperbaric center ahead of time that a dive injury has occurred and the patient is being brought to the ED.

*ABCs*, Airway, breathing, and circulation; *ACLS*, advanced cardiac life support; *ED*, emergency department.

**BOX 133.7 Emergency Department Diagnostic Work-up for Dive-Injured Patients**

**Laboratory Tests**
Complete blood count
Measurement of serum electrolytes
Consider markers of injury LDH, CPK
Oxygen saturation measurement
Add these tests for altered mental status:

- Urine and blood toxicologic tests with acetylsalicylic acid or acetaminophen and ethanol levels
- Arterial blood gas measurements, including a carboxyhemoglobin level

**Imaging**
Consider the following evaluations for suspicion of pulmonary barotrauma:

- Chest radiograph
- Computed tomography of the chest (evaluation for blebs, small pneumothoraces, and other pulmonary problems)

**BOX 133.8 Dive History Interview: Questions to Ask Dive-Injured Patients**

1. Where did the dive occur (e.g., ocean, river, pool)?
2. When was the onset of the patient's symptoms (on resurfacing, during descent or ascent, at the bottom)?
3. How deep did the patient go? Was a dive computer being used?
4. Was the patient intoxicated or dehydrated?
5. What type of diving equipment was used? What type of gas was used (compressed air, mixed gas, enriched air)? What was the source of the gas?
6. Did the patient perform heavy exertion or work during the dive?
7. Did the dive approach or exceed decompression limits?
8. How many dives did the patient perform and what were the depths, bottom times, total times, and resurface intervals for all dives in the previous days preceding symptoms (the dive "profiles")?
9. Were decompression stops missed? Was in-water recompression attempted?
10. What was the time delay from the last dive to the time of air travel or travel to altitude such as a mountain range?
11. Did the patient experience ear or sinus problems on this dive or in the past?
12. Does the patient have any other medical problems? What medications does the patient take?
13. Was oxygen given at the scene?

## FOLLOW-UP, NEXT STEPS IN CARE, AND PATIENT EDUCATION

Although each patient is unique, many patients with DCI can be safely discharged from the hospital. However, any diver with serious DCS symptoms should be admitted. All patients who have experienced DCS or embolic dive injuries should be transferred immediately to the closest emergency hyperbaric facility. The physician should err on the side of caution; any patient with concerning symptoms should not be discharged until a hyperbaric physician has been consulted (**Boxes 133.9 and 133.10**).

## FLYING AFTER DIVING

One of the most important factors in the disposition of divers is how long the diver should wait to fly after diving or a diving-related injury. Forgetting to counsel a patient about

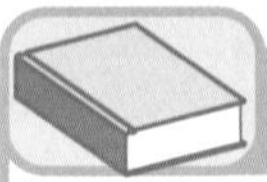

**PATIENT TEACHING TIPS**

Avoid diving when you have any symptoms of upper respiratory infection.
Do not drink alcohol and dive.
Never dive alone.
Do not dive and fly within the same 24 hours.
Do not "push" dive tables or dive profiles.
Do not perform heavy exercise after diving.
Drink plenty of fluids and get plenty of rest.
Plan deeper dives at the beginning of a dive trip.

**BOX 133.9 Indications for Immediate Hyperbaric or Dive Medicine Consultation**

A hyperbaric or dive medicine consultation should be sought immediately for divers exhibiting the following:

- ANY alteration in mental status
- ANY neurologic deficit
- ANY loss of consciousness
- ANY worsening of symptoms during evaluation
- ANY worrisome sign, symptom, or behavior
- ANY limb pain after ascent from depth

**BOX 133.10 Using the Divers Alert Network (DAN) Emergency Hotline**

(919) 684-8111 or (919) 684-4DAN (collect)

DAN handles all diving emergencies, including decompression sickness, arterial gas embolism, pulmonary barotrauma, and other diving-related injuries. DAN's medical staff is on call 24/7/365.

flying limitations has the potential for serious injury. A number of guidelines are available. For the most part, it is unwise to fly within 12 to 24 hours after diving. A diver should delay flying for at least 12 hours after a single no–decompression obligation dive. A diver who participates in multiple-day, unlimited diving should delay flying for at least 24 hours after the last dive. A diver who has experienced DCS should be advised to not fly for 3 to 7 days after treatment of type I DCS or for 4 weeks after recompression therapy for type II DCS.

## SUGGESTED READINGS

Barratt M, Harch P, Van Meter K. Decompression illness in divers: a review of the literature. Neurologist 2002;8:186-202.

Bove AA, Davis J. Bove and Davis' diving medicine. 4th ed. Philadelphia: Saunders; 2004.

U.S. Department of Commerce. NOAA navy diving manual. 5th ed. Flagstaff, Ariz: Best Publishing; 2005.

## REFERENCES

*References can be found on Expert Consult @ www.expertconsult.com.*

# 134 Submersion Injuries

*Mohammed A. Abu Aish and Naranjan Kisson*

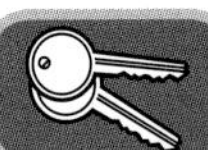

**KEY POINTS**

- Drowning is the second leading cause of death in children.
- Inadequate supervision is the main risk factor for drowning in children.
- Some patients with relatively mild symptoms initially can deteriorate.
- Cardiopulmonary resuscitation at the scene is the most important factor in improving survival.
- Most drowning victims should be transferred to the emergency department regardless of the initial appearance at the scene.
- The degree of hypoxia determines the outcome.
- Cervical spine immobilization is unnecessary unless trauma is suspected.
- Asymptomatic patients should be observed for at least 4 to 6 hours before being discharged.

## EPIDEMIOLOGY

Submersion simply means going under water. To avoid confusion, especially in reporting, the International Liaison Committee on Resuscitation recommends that the following previously used terms no longer be used: dry and wet drowning, active and passive drowning, silent drowning, secondary drowning, and drowned versus near-drowned.[1] In 2002, the World Congress on Drowning adopted a uniform definition of drowning: "the process resulting in primary respiratory impairment from submersion/immersion in a liquid medium."[2]

Drowning is an important cause of childhood morbidity and is among the top 10 causes of mortality (**Fig. 134.1**). Drowning is estimated to kill 500,000 people every year worldwide. Eighty percent of these episodes take place in low-income countries and low-income groups. About 80% of drowning episodes are deemed preventable.[3,4]

Overall rates of drowning have dropped in all age groups, probably as a result of improved awareness, use of preventive measures, and other factors (**Box 134.1**). Inadequate supervision is the main risk factor for drowning in children. Most toddlers who drown do so in their own home pools, most infants drown in bathtubs, and adults and older children drown in fresh water. Fencing of private pools reduces the risk for drowning.[5]

## PATHOPHYSIOLOGY

Injuries from drowning result mainly from asphyxia and subsequent hypoxic-ischemic damage to vital organs. The event starts with panic because of air hunger and, eventually, aspiration of fluid into the hypopharynx. Reflex laryngospasm occurs but is usually brief before the victim aspirates large amounts of fluid into the lungs. Further aspiration can occur if the victim vomits and aspirates gastric contents. Aspiration is the end result of all drowning, and the old terminology of dry and wet drowning should not be used.[6,7] Changes in intravascular volume, hematocrit, and electrolyte concentration as a result of aspiration are usually mild and not clinically significant. Both salt water and fresh water cause lung injury. The effect of tonicity on the intravascular compartment is minimal.[8,9]

The diving reflex is one of the unique phenomena described in children. Caused by vagal stimulation when the face is exposed to cold water (<10° C), this reflex is characterized by apnea, bradycardia, and intense vasoconstriction. It is presumed that this reflex can play a neuroprotective role in cold water submersion. Hypothermia slows cerebral metabolism when the body has had time to cool before aspiration or with submersion in extremely cold water and may also contribute to neuroprotection.

### RESPIRATORY

Aspiration of fluid causes loss of surfactant, noncardiogenic pulmonary edema, and acute respiratory distress syndrome. Some patients have mild respiratory symptoms and then deteriorate rapidly because of gradual leakage and influx of proteins and fluid into the alveoli as a result of loss of surfactant and the effect of acidosis and hypoxia on the respiratory membranes.

### CENTRAL NERVOUS SYSTEM

Hypoxia and acidosis lead to neuronal injury, which results in diffuse brain edema and eventually increased intracranial pressure. Brain injury is the major cause of death and disability from drowning.

| | Age groups | | | | | | | | | | |
|---|---|---|---|---|---|---|---|---|---|---|---|
| **Rank** | **<1** | **1-4** | **5-9** | **10-14** | **15-24** | **25-34** | **35-44** | **45-54** | **55-64** | **65+** | **Total** |
| 1 | Unintentional suffocation **959** | Unintentional drowning **458** | Unintentional MV traffic **456** | Unintentional MV traffic **696** | Unintentional MV traffic **10,272** | Unintentional MV traffic **6,842** | Unintentional poisoning **7,575** | Unintentional poisoning **9,006** | Unintentional MV traffic **4,177** | Unintentional fall **18,334** | Unintentional MV traffic **42,031** |
| 2 | Homicide unspecified **174** | Unintentional MV traffic **428** | Unintentional fire/burn **136** | Homicide firearm **154** | Homicide firearm **4,669** | Unintentional poisoning **5,700** | Unintentional MV traffic **6,135** | Unintentional MV traffic **6,262** | Unintentional poisoning **3,120** | Unintentional MV traffic **6,632** | Unintentional poisoning **29,846** |
| 3 | Unintentional MV traffic **122** | Unintentional fire/burn **204** | Unintentional drowning **122** | Suicide suffocation **119** | Unintentional poisoning **3,159** | Homicide firearm **3,751** | Suicide firearm **2,879** | Suicide firearm **3,531** | Suicide firearm **2,786** | Unintentional unspecified **4,855** | Unintentional fall **22,631** |
| 4 | Homicide other spec., classifiable **85** | Homicide unspecified **174** | Homicide firearm **47** | Unintentional drowning **102** | Suicide firearm **1,900** | Suicide firearm **2,306** | Homicide firearm **2,038** | Suicide poisoning **2,015** | Unintentional fall **1,739** | Suicide firearm **3,895** | Suicide firearm **17,352** |
| 5 | Unintentional drowning **57** | Unintentional suffocation **149** | Unintentional suffocation **42** | Unintentional other land transport **80** | Suicide suffocation **1,533** | Suicide suffocation **1,770** | Suicide suffocation **1,839** | Suicide suffocation **1,589** | Suicide poisoning **1,147** | Unintentional suffocation **3,209** | Homicide firearm **12,632** |
| 6 | Unintentional fire/burn **39** | Unintentional pedestrian, other **124** | Unintentional other land transport **40** | Unintentional fire/burn **78** | Unintentional drowning **630** | Suicide poisoning **802** | Suicide poisoning **1,419** | Unintentional fall **1,304** | Suicide suffocation **725** | Adverse effects **1,631** | Suicide suffocation **8,161** |
| 7 | Undetermined suffocation **34** | Homicide, other spec., classifiable **61** | Unintentional pedestrian, other **32** | Unintentional poisoning **69** | Homicide cut/pierce **444** | Undetermined poisoning **687** | Undetermined poisoning **1,020** | Homicide firearm **1,159** | Unintentional fire/burn **505** | Unintentional fire/burn **1,179** | Suicide poisoning **6,358** |
| 8 | Homicide suffocation **30** | Homicide firearm **48** | Homicide suffocation **21** | Unintentional suffocation **60** | Undetermined poisoning **365** | Homicide cut/pierce **466** | Unintentional fall **593** | Undetermined poisoning **1,155** | Unintentional suffocation **484** | Unintentional poisoning **1,149** | Unintentional unspecified **6,019** |
| 9 | Undetermined unspecified **28** | Unintentional struck by or against **44** | Unintentional firearm **20** | Suicide firearm **53** | Suicide poisoning **362** | Unintentional drowning **381** | Unintentional drowning **417** | Unintentional fire/burn **496** | Homicide firearm **446** | Suicide poisoning **604** | Unintentional suffocation **5,997** |
| 10 | Unintentional fall **24** | Unintentional fall **36** | Unintentional struck by or against **20** | Unintentional firearm **26** | Unintentional other land transport **310** | Unintentional fall **334** | Homicide cut/pierce **409** | Unintentional drowning **481** | Adverse effects **398** | Suicide suffocation **583** | Undetermined poisoning **3,770** |

**Fig. 134.1 Ten leading causes of injury deaths by age group highlighting unintentional injury deaths, United States—2007.** *MV*, Motor vehicle. (Adapted from National Center for Injury Prevention and Control, Centers for Disease Control and Prevention. Web-based Injury Statistics Query and Reporting System [database]. Available at http://www.cdc.gov/ncipc/wisgars/.)

**BOX 134.1 Risk Factors for Drowning**

Inability to swim
Hyperventilation
Trauma
Use of alcohol and illicit drugs
Intoxications
Hypoglycemia
Seizures
Arrhythmias (long QT syndromes)
Child abuse and neglect
Vascular events (cerebrovascular accident, myocardial infarction)

## CARDIOVASCULAR SYSTEM

Arrhythmias secondary to hypoxia and hypothermia are common. Sinus bradycardia, atrial fibrillation, and less commonly, asystole and ventricular fibrillation are reported to occur in patients who drown.

## OTHER ORGANS

Acute tubular necrosis can develop but is uncommon. Significant electrolyte abnormalities are not seen unless drowning occurs in exceptionally concentrated media. Coagulopathy can occur with hypoxia but is uncommon.

# PRESENTING SIGNS AND SYMPTOMS

Manifestations vary from no symptoms to death and depend on the severity of hypoxemia. Cervical spine injuries are uncommon with drowning unless trauma is suspected (e.g., diving and boating accidents, falls, crashes).

Respiratory signs and symptoms can vary in severity and may be delayed. They result from aspiration of fluid and loss of surfactant and include shortness of breath, wheezing (rhonchi, crepitations), pulmonary edema, and acute respiratory distress syndrome. Symptoms of aspiration pneumonia may develop later from aspiration of infected material.

Neurologic symptoms also vary. Patients may be asymptomatic, irritable, or confused; have seizures; or be comatose at initial evaluation. Deterioration can occur in asymptomatic patients and those with mild symptoms. Symptoms and signs of increased intracranial pressure appear late and are due to hypoxic brain injury.

Arrhythmias can also develop early or late and further compromise cardiorespiratory status. Hypoxia, acidosis, and hypothermia can lead to bradycardia, tachycardia, hypotension, hypertension, arrhythmias, and asystole.

## DIFFERENTIAL DIAGNOSIS

Although the diagnosis of drowning is obvious, it is important to rule out medical conditions that may predispose a person to submersion, as well as the possibility of child abuse.

### DIAGNOSTIC INVESTIGATIONS

Investigations are not as important on initial evaluation as clinical assessment and emergency therapy. Chest radiographic findings may be normal initially, even in symptomatic patients. However, pulmonary edema (localized or diffuse) and various degrees of atelectasis may be noted on examination. The initial chest radiograph will also help check endotracheal and gastric tube position. Measurement of arterial blood gas concentrations may be useful in guiding resuscitation efforts and in adjusting ventilator settings but should not be used as the sole predictor of outcome. Neuroimaging has no role in acute management but becomes important later to rule out unrecognized brain disease or to confirm hypoxic changes in the brain. When major trauma is suspected, the need for further imaging (e.g., head and cervical spine computed tomography [CT], abdominal CT) is determined by the severity of suspected injuries.

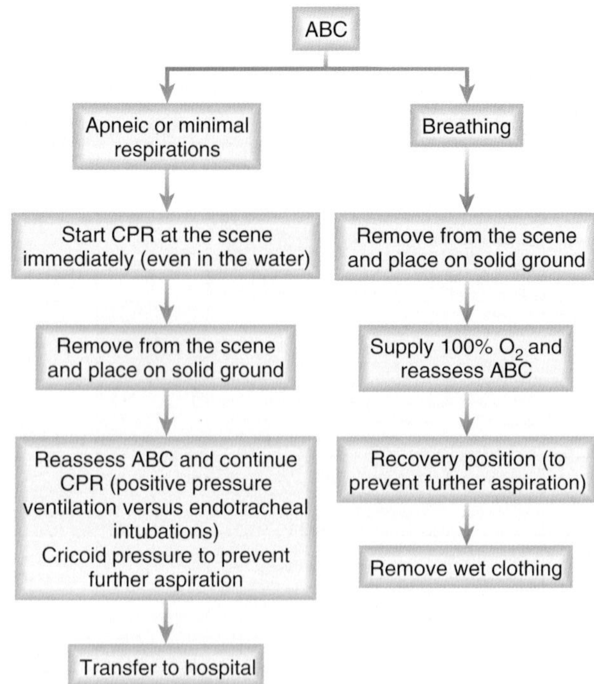


**Fig. 134.2 Algorithm for prehospital treatment of drowning victims.** *ABC*, Airway, breathing, and circulation (ABCs of resuscitation); *CPR*, cardiopulmonary resuscitation.

## PROGNOSTIC FACTORS

### AT THE SCENE

Performance of cardiopulmonary resuscitation (CPR) at the scene has been documented to improve survival in some cases, especially after cold water submersion. Generally, hypothermia is a poor prognostic sign unless the victim has fallen into extremely cold water (<10° C) or has undergone rapid cooling. Several case reports of survival of victims in such circumstances were attributed to a protective effect of cooling on the brain, which has led some authorities to recommend continuing CPR in hypothermic victims while actively rewarming them before declaring them dead.[10]

### IN THE EMERGENCY DEPARTMENT

Many factors have been suggested as predictors of a bad outcome, but none alone were consistently reliable across studies. Prognostic factors such as a low Glasgow Coma Scale (GCS) score and ineffective respiratory efforts become more predictive after resuscitation and stabilization and hence may be more useful in the intensive care unit. Because no single prognostic factor is reliable in the immediate period after submersion, it is recommended that CPR be performed on most submersion victims until their condition is fully assessed.

## TREATMENT

### PREHOSPITAL MANAGEMENT

CPR at the scene is the most important initial step. It can be started even if the victim is still in the water. After the airway is secured and oxygenation and ventilation are ensured, the patient should be transferred to the nearest hospital. Further management at the scene depends on the availability of personnel experienced in advanced life support (**Fig. 134.2**). Most drowning victims should be transferred to an emergency department (ED) regardless of the initial appearance at the scene. Exceptions are those with obvious rigor mortis, lividity, and decay.

Emergency personnel dealing with a drowning victim should avoid the following:

- Maneuvers to expel water out of the lungs (i.e., abdominal thrusts)
- Cervical spine immobilization if no trauma is suspected
- Rough handling of a hypothermic patient (may induce arrhythmias)
- Delay in transport to the hospital after optimizing respirations

### EMERGENCY DEPARTMENT MANAGEMENT

The main aims of treatment of a drowning victim in the ED are to avoid further hypoxia and restore effective ventilation and circulation (**Table 134.1**). ED personnel should assume the triad of hypoxia, acidosis, and hypothermia to be present in every drowning victim until proved otherwise. The need for cervical spine immobilization should be assessed, but in atraumatic drowning, immobilization is not mandatory. Vomiting occurs frequently, so early airway protection should be considered in distressed patients.

#### *Airway*

- For breathing patients, the $FiO_2$ value should be kept at 1.0.
- For patients in respiratory distress, emergency personnel should have a low threshold for intubation. Treatment may start with positive pressure and positive end-expiratory pressure (PEEP) ventilation with a nasal cannula or mask.

**Table 134.1 Summary of Emergency Department Management of Drowning**

| ASPECT | INTERVENTION |
|---|---|
| Airway | 100% $O_2$ (mask)<br>Bag-valve-mask ventilation<br>Positive end-expiratory pressure ventilation<br>Endotracheal intubation |
| Breathing | Respiratory status<br>$O_2$ status<br>Signs of trauma |
| Circulation | Cardiac status (pulses, perfusion, blood pressure)<br>Intravenous access (intraosseous if the intravenous route is difficult)<br>Monitor<br>Blood work<br>Glucometer<br>Fluid management (crystalloid boluses of 20 mL/kg as needed) to correct hypovolemia and acidosis<br>Management of arrhythmias<br>Inotropic agents (e.g., dobutamine for cardiogenic shock) |
| Disability | Glasgow Coma Scale score<br>Focal signs<br>Management of seizures |
| Exposure | Temperature<br>External injuries<br>Active rewarming if temperature <30° C<br>Passive rewarming if temperature >30° C with a goal of 30° to 33° C |

- Indications for intubation are as follows: unconsciousness, respiratory insufficiency, and high $O_2$ requirements to keep the oxygen saturation value higher than 90% or $PO_2$ higher than 60 to 90 mm Hg (or both).

### *Breathing*

- The oxygen saturation value and respiratory status should be checked. The onset of respiratory distress may be delayed and progressive.
- In cases of trauma, life-threatening disorders (e.g., hemothorax, pneumothorax) should be ruled out.

### *Circulation*

- Vascular access, either intravenous or intraosseous, should be established.
- Arrhythmia, which can be the inciting event or a complication of hypoxia and hypothermia, should be ruled out.
- Fluid and electrolyte management and inotropic support are important to reverse depressed myocardial function, shock, and acidosis.

### *Disability*

- The GCS score should be documented at baseline; it can be used to monitor the patient's status over time because all drowning victims are at risk for worsening brain edema.
- Seizures can occur in patients with hypoxia, focal lesions, and worsening edema.

### *Exposure*

- The patient's whole body should be exposed to check for injuries that might suggest trauma, abuse, suicide, and other causes.
- Rectal temperatures should be recorded.

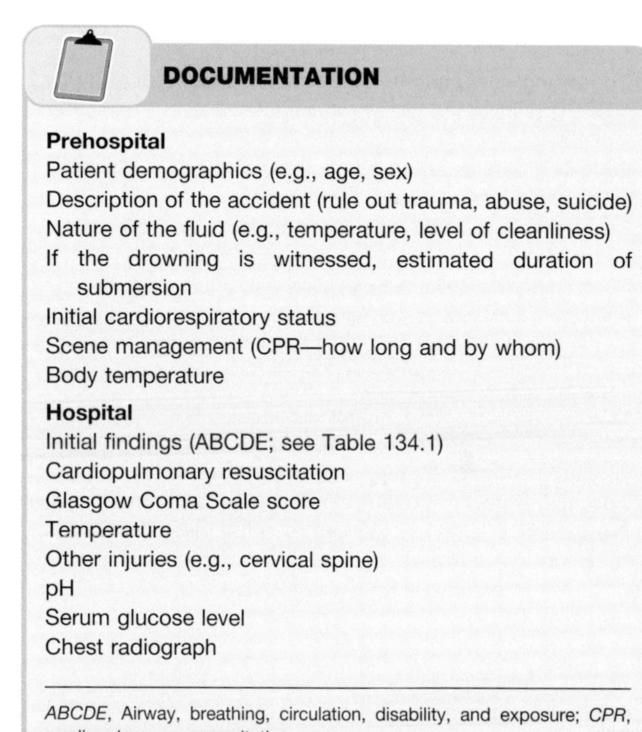

**DOCUMENTATION**

**Prehospital**

Patient demographics (e.g., age, sex)
Description of the accident (rule out trauma, abuse, suicide)
Nature of the fluid (e.g., temperature, level of cleanliness)
If the drowning is witnessed, estimated duration of submersion
Initial cardiorespiratory status
Scene management (CPR—how long and by whom)
Body temperature

**Hospital**

Initial findings (ABCDE; see Table 134.1)
Cardiopulmonary resuscitation
Glasgow Coma Scale score
Temperature
Other injuries (e.g., cervical spine)
pH
Serum glucose level
Chest radiograph

*ABCDE*, Airway, breathing, circulation, disability, and exposure; *CPR*, cardiopulmonary resuscitation.

## MANAGEMENT OF HYPOTHERMIA

For a detailed discussion of hypothermia, refer to Chapter 131. Hypothermia is defined as a core body temperature lower than 35° C. Depending on the temperature, hypothermia may be mild, moderate, or severe. This condition should be anticipated and treated in drowning victims. Notably, standard thermometers may not accurately measure low temperatures. Rewarming techniques are discussed in Chapter 131.

## NEXT STEPS IN CARE AND PATIENT EDUCATION

Because of lung injury, loss of surfactant, and pulmonary edema, some patients will need higher end-expiratory pressure for optimal oxygenation. As PEEP is increased, blood pressure and cardiac output should be monitored because they can be compromised by high end-expiratory pressure. Intensive monitoring of cardiac, respiratory, and neurologic status and for complications such as aspiration pneumonia is indicated.

Some reports suggest that therapeutic hypothermia can improve neurologic outcome after out-of-hospital cardiac arrest and therefore recommend induction of hypothermia in drowning victims after restoration of spontaneous circulation

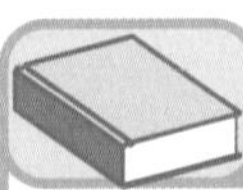

**PATIENT TEACHING TIPS**

**Prevention of Drowning**

Fencing private pools

Using personal flotation devices

Minimizing alcohol and substance abuse at beaches and around water

Counseling new parents about the importance of supervision, as well as the safety of bathtubs, buckets, and other vessels

Educating parents about safe bathing of babies: a child can drown in just a few inches of water

Recommending cardiopulmonary resuscitation courses for the public

Recommending swimming lessons with adult supervision

Identifying risk factors to help prevent a second incident if the victim survived

as a neuroprotective therapy. Further studies of this approach are needed, especially regarding its use in children.[11,12]

No evidence supports the use of prophylactic antibiotics, corticosteroids, barbiturate therapy, or intracranial pressure monitoring in patients who have drowned.

Patients who are completely asymptomatic in the ED and whose arterial blood gas levels in room air, electrolytes, and chest radiographic findings are normal can be discharged after being observed for 6 hours. All others should be admitted to the hospital.

## SUGGESTED READINGS

Bierens JJ, editor. Handbook on drowning: prevention, rescue, treatment. Amsterdam: Springer; 2004.

Bierens JJ, Knape JT, Gelissen HP. Drowning. Curr Opin Crit Care 2002;8:578-86.

Ibsen L, Koch T. Submersion and asphyxial injury. Crit Care Med 2002;11(Suppl):S402-8.

National Center for Injury Prevention and Control, Centers for Disease Control and Prevention. Web-based Injury Statistics Query and Reporting System (database). Available at http://www.cdc.gov/ncipc/wisqars/.

Olshaker J. Submersion. Emerg Med Clin North Am 2004;22:357-67, viii.

Zuckerbraun N, Saladino R. Pediatric drowning: current management strategies for immediate care. Clin Pediatr Emerg Med 2005;6:49-56.

## REFERENCES

***References can be found on Expert Consult @ www.expertconsult.com.***

# Acute Radiation Emergencies 135

*Bradley A. Dreifuss*

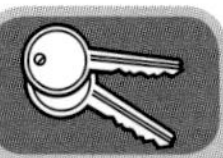

**KEY POINTS**

- The nature and extent of an acute radiologic emergency should be identified to determine whether hospital disaster plans should be activated.
- Large-scale radiologic emergencies require triage of multiple patients based on the estimated radiation dose, presence of traumatic injuries, and availability of local resources.
- An emergency physician can use the symptoms and findings on physical examination to estimate the whole-body radiation dose (rad or gray) for predicting a patient's course and subsequent need for treatment.
- A complete blood count with differential at triage and 24 to 48 hours later can be used to guide the diagnosis, treatment, and prognosis of acute radiation syndrome.
- Decontamination is an important aspect of acute radiation emergencies but should *not* supersede stabilization of unstable patients.
- Recognition of patients who have been exposed to moderate to high doses of radiation and triage to early treatment of acute radiation syndrome can significantly decrease mortality.

## EPIDEMIOLOGY

Acute radiologic emergencies are a rare occurrence, yet with increasing use of radioisotopes in medicine, research, and industry, as well as ongoing use in national defense and electrical power generation, it is imperative that emergency physicians (EPs) be versed in acute medical management after radiologic emergencies. The relative magnitude of the situation and the resources needed to address an emergency vary depending on the scale of the exposure event. Small-scale events include contained exposure in hospitals or research facilities or contained breaches at nuclear power plants in which small amounts of material may lead to exposure or contamination of a limited number of individuals. Large-scale events involve relatively large quantities of radioactive material or potential widespread exposure or contamination of a significant population. Examples of large-scale events include nuclear reactor meltdowns (e.g., Fukushima Daiichi, Japan, in March 2011; the Chernobyl meltdown in April 1986), detonation of nuclear weapons, or terrorist attacks with a radiologic dispersal device—otherwise known as a "dirty bomb."[1,2] Hospitals are required by The Joint Commission to have disaster plans in place for mass casualty events, including radiologic emergencies, and EPs and emergency medical service personnel will be at the forefront of decision making and patient care when a radiologic event occurs.

The first priority during an acute radiation emergency is to *establish the reality and type of radiologic event.* Information received from the field is essential in mounting an effective response in the emergency department (ED) and the hospital. Important information to obtain from the field, if possible, is listed in the Documentation box. With large events, EDs should anticipate patients arriving from multiple field triage and stabilization sites, as well as individuals who arrive on their own accord without first being triaged or evaluated for injury or radiation exposure or contamination.

Communication between the field triage team and the ED must be clear because no federal or internationally agreed-upon medical triage systems have been established

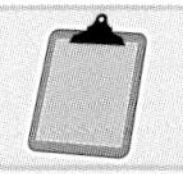

**DOCUMENTATION**

**Important Information to Obtain from the Field After Acute Radiologic Emergencies**

Type of radioactive material involved. Different types of radioactive material can expose patients in different ways. Important specifics include the type of radioisotope or source (α-, β-, γ-emitters, or neutrino), the form that it was in when the exposure occurred, and whether those exposed were also contaminated via inhaled dust or ingestion

Types of traumatic injuries occurring with the radiation exposure (blast or burn)

Type of decontamination procedures taking place at the scene or in field triage

Number of patients expected to require triage, evaluation, and treatment

What local, regional, or federal resources have been activated and notified of the acute radiologic emergency specifically for radiation mass casualty incidents, and thus existing mass casualty emergency triage algorithms should be used with modifications for the impact of the radiation exposure or contamination.[1,3-5] The Scarce Resources for a Nuclear Detonation Project has published new triage recommendations for the first 4 days following a possible nuclear detonation, and formal guidelines will probably be recommended in the near future.[5-7]

The disaster response coordinator should prepare the ED to receive patients triaged at all levels with blast, thermal, and radiation injuries. Importantly, *standard personal protective equipment sufficient to protect the emergency personnel treating these patients in the decontamination area and in the ED must be used.*[1,8-11] Those triaging and caring for patients with possible contamination should be using strict isolation precautions.

In any acute radiation emergency, initial mass casualty field triage should not be confused with the subsequent clinical triage used by EPs and other providers for more definitive medical management. It is essential that those involved in triage and provision of emergency care for radiologic emergencies understand that *lifesaving medical stabilization takes precedence over other concerns*, including external radiation decontamination.[1,4,10-12]

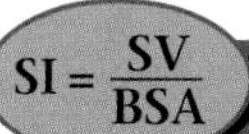

### FACTS AND FORMULAS

**Radiation Absorbed Dose**

Amount of energy deposited in tissue by ionizing radiation

Measured in both U.S. and SI units:

- U.S. unit = rad (1 rad = 100 ergs [$10^{-7}$ J] of energy deposited into 1 g of tissue)
- SI unit = gray (1 Gy = 1 J of energy deposited into 1 kg of tissue)
- Therefore, 1 Gy = 100 rad

**Dose Equivalent or Equivalent Dose (SI Terms)**

Difference in future risk (i.e., risk for induction of cancer) with different types of radiation and calculated by applying a constant that is unique for each type of radiation: quality factor (U.S.) and radiation weighting factor (SI)

- U.S. unit = rem
- SI unit = sievert (Sv)

For example, the constant for x-radiation or γ-radiation = 1

100 rad × 1 = 100 rem; 1 Gy × 1 = 1 Sv

**Triage Formula for Irradiated Patients When CBC with Differential Is Available (Adapted from AFRRI, 2010; REAC/TS, 2011)**

In otherwise healthy adult patients who have been exposed to external irradiation without trauma or burn, a clinically detrimental radiation dose can be distinguished from a dose lower than 1 Gy 4 hours after exposure by using a triage score involving two criteria: the N/L ratio and whether emesis has occurred in the 4 hours since exposure

The triage score T is assigned as follows:

$$T = N/L + E$$

Given: N = WBC × (% neutrophils); L = WBC × (% lymphocytes); E = 0 if no emesis is present by 4 hours; E = 2 if emesis is present by 4 hours

If T is higher than 3.7, the patient should be referred for further evaluation; otherwise can be discharged with follow-up if clinically stable

**Background**

In a normal, healthy human population, the N/L ratio from a CBC with differential has been found to be approximately 2.1. For time longer than 4 hours after the event, T is significantly elevated with doses higher than 1 Gy. Data from a REAC/TS Radiation Accident Registry was used in a case-control study ($n$ = 226 controls, $n$ = 36 radiation cases; median dose, 3 Gy) to show that this triage scoring tool has the ability to discriminate between patients with whole-body radiation doses lower than 1 Gy and those with higher, clinically significant doses (sensitivity of 89% and specificity of 93%).

*AFRRI*, Armed Forces Radiobiology Research Institute; *CBC*, complete blood count; *N/L*, neutrophil-lymphocyte ratio; *REAC/TS*, Radiation Emergency Assistance Center/Training Site; *WBC*, white blood cell.

## PATHOPHYSIOLOGY

Radioactivity refers to the loss of particles or energy from an unstable atom that is decaying. There are two distinct types of radiation: ionizing radiation (e.g., α and β particles from a decaying radioisotope and nonparticulate electromagnetic γ-rays and x-rays) and nonionizing radiation (e.g., all forms of the electromagnetic spectrum, except for γ-rays and x-rays). The main means of exposure to a dose of radiation are (1) from an external radiation source, (2) by loose radioactive material deposited on the skin or into wounds, and (3) by ingestion or inhalation of radioactive material.[1] Significant radiation injuries can occur from irradiation with or without contamination (contact of the substance directly with human tissue). A *contaminated patient* will have been exposed to radioactive material that could still be on or inside the patient's body. *Irradiated patients without contamination* have been exposed but do not have radioactive material on or in them. Irradiated patients are not "radioactive." Such differentiation in a radiologic emergency situation is important because it dictates whether decontamination is needed. A radioactivity meter (most commonly a Geiger counter is the initial screening tool) and the patient's history should be used to determine whether a patient has been contaminated.

To comprehend the physiologic effects of radiation, it is important to understand the units of measurement for types of doses (see the Facts and Formulas box). Radiation damage occurs within microseconds of exposure and most significantly affects rapidly reproducing types of cells (e.g., intestinal crypt cell, stem cells) or cells with a large nucleus, such as lymphocytes. The threshold of 2 Gy of whole-body irradiation is often used as the reference point for when cells have been irreparably damaged and symptoms of acute radiation syndrome (ARS) develop.[1,12]

## PRESENTING SIGNS AND SYMPTOMS

Depending on the cause of the radiologic emergency (spill or leak versus explosion), the emergency provider may be in the position of having to stabilize and treat traumatic injuries and burns before assessing patients for signs of ARS. In cases of blast and thermal injury, patients' traumatic injuries are of primary concern because poor outcomes after radiation injury are compounded by traumatic injury and thermal burns (e.g., combined injury).[12,13]

ARS is an acute illness that results from external exposure to radiation doses typically greater than 1 to 2 Gy (100 to 200 rad) delivered to a significant body surface area over a short period, and it occurs at an onset that varies from hours to weeks after exposure, depending on the dose. The severity and type of subsyndrome correspond to the amount and duration of exposure (dose).

ARS has four subsyndromes—hematopoietic, gastrointestinal, cutaneous, and neurovascular—and the time until onset and severity are related to the dose for all syndromes. The hematopoietic system is most vulnerable, with at least mild changes occurring at whole-body exposure to doses of less than 1 Gy, and acute treatment is typically considered at 2 Gy and higher.[4,11,14] The cutaneous, gastrointestinal, and cardiovascular subsyndromes generally occur with whole-body exposure to doses of greater than 4 Gy, greater than 6 Gy, and greater than 10 Gy, respectively.[11]

ARS and the subsyndromes typically follow four predictable phases. The first, or prodromal, phase can include the symptoms of nausea and vomiting, diarrhea, fatigue, fever, erythema, conjunctivitis, and respiratory difficulty. Altered mental status occurs in the cardiovascular subsyndrome in association with very high radiation doses (>10 Gy). This prodromal phase indicates that more serious manifestations may follow and provides important clues for triage.[5,9-12,14,15] Next is the latent phase, in which the symptoms subside; it lasts days to weeks, with patients exposed to higher doses typically having shorter latency. The latent phase is followed by the manifest illness phase, in which the four ARS subsyndromes are evident and patients require intensive medical management. The final phase is eventual recovery or death (**Fig. 135.1**; **Table 135.1**).

## DIFFERENTIAL DIAGNOSIS AND MEDICAL DECISION MAKING

Given that modern supportive care is effective in increasing $LD_{50/60}$ doses (lethal dose for 50% of the population surviving at 60 days) in nontrauma patients from 3.5 to 4 Gy (without medical care) to up to 6 to 8 Gy (treated with transfusions, antibiotics, colony-stimulating factors, and intensive care), it is of the utmost importance to triage and treat patients appropriately early in the postexposure period.[1,5,10,11] The goal is to provide the highest level of care possible to patients

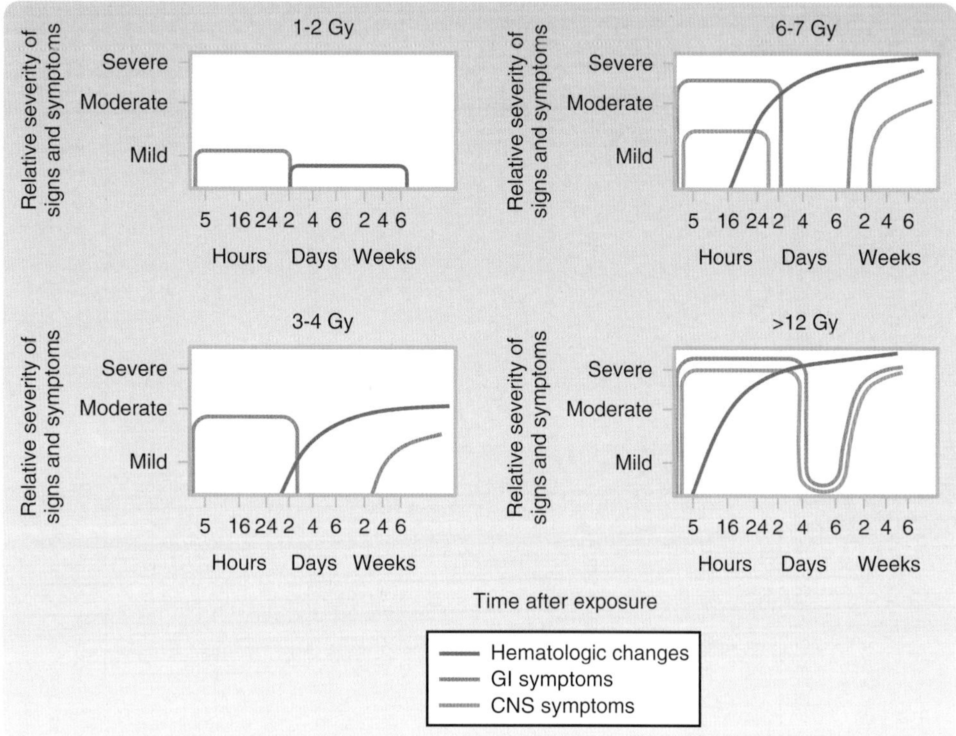


**Fig. 135.1 Nature and time course of symptoms based on radiation dose.** Approximate times are listed for hematopoietic, gastrointestinal (GI), and central nervous system (CNS) symptoms at different ranges of whole-body radiation doses for exposed living persons. Symptoms include lymphopenia, granulocytopenia, and thrombocytopenia (hematopoietic); nausea, vomiting, and diarrhea (GI); and headache, impaired cognition, disorientation, ataxia, seizures, prostration, and hypotension (cerebrovascular). Relative severity is measured on an arbitrary scale. (Adapted from Waselenko JK, MacVittie TJ, Blakely WF, et al. Medical management of the acute radiation syndrome: recommendations of the Strategic National Stockpile Radiation Working Group. Ann Intern Med 2004;40:1037-51.)

**Table 135.1** Phases, Symptoms, and Prognostication of Outcomes in Patients with Acute Radiation Syndrome (Whole-Body Irradiation from Acute Photon-Equivalent Doses)

| PHASE OF SYNDROME | SURVIVABILITY | HIGHLY SURVIVABLE | | SURVIVABLE TO LETHAL | | LETHAL | |
|---|---|---|---|---|---|---|---|
| | Degree of ARS | | Mild | Moderate to severe | Very severe | Lethal | |
| | Dose range (cGy) | 0-100 | 100-200 | 200-600 | 600-800 | 800-3000 | >3000 |
| Initial or prodromal | Vomiting | | 5-50% | 50-100% | 75-100% | 98-100% | 100% |
| | Time of onset | | 3-6 hr | 1-6 hr | <2 hr | <1 hr | <1 hr |
| | Duration | | <24 hr | <24 hr | <48 hr | <48 hr | <48 hr |
| | Lymphocyte count (cells/mm$^3$) | | <1400 at 4 days | <1400 at 48 hr | <1000 at 24 hr | <800 at 24 hr | |
| | CNS function | No impairment | No impairment | Routine task performance; cognitive impairment for 6-20 hr | Simple and routine task performance; cognitive impairment for >24 hr | Transient incapacitation | |
| Latent | Duration | N/A | 7-15 days | 0-21 days | 0-2 days | 0-20 days | |
| Manifest (obvious) illness | Signs and symptoms | None | Moderate leukopenia | Severe leukopenia, purpura, hemorrhage, pneumonia, hair loss after 300 rad (cGy) | | Severe diarrhea, fever, electrolyte disturbance | Convulsions, ataxia, tremor, lethargy |
| | Time of onset | | >2 wk | 2 days-2 wk | | 0-2 days | |
| | Critical period | | None | 4-6 wk | | 5-14 days | 1-48 hr |
| | Principal organ system | None | Hematopoietic | Hematopoietic and gastrointestinal | | Gastrointestinal(mucosal surfaces) | CNS |
| Hospitalization | % | 0 | <5% | 90% | 100% | 100% | 100% |
| | Duration | 0 | 45-60 days | 60-90 days | 90+ days | 2 wk | 2 days |
| Fatality | | 0% | 0% | 0-89% | 80-100% | 98-100% | |
| Time of death | | | | 3-12 wk | | 1-2 wk | 1-2 days |

Adapted from Armed Forces Radiobiology Research Institute. AFRRI pocket guide: emergency radiation medicine response. Bethesda, Md: Uniformed Services University of the Health Sciences; 2011.
*ARS*, Acute radiation syndrome; *CNS*, central nervous system; N/A, not applicable.

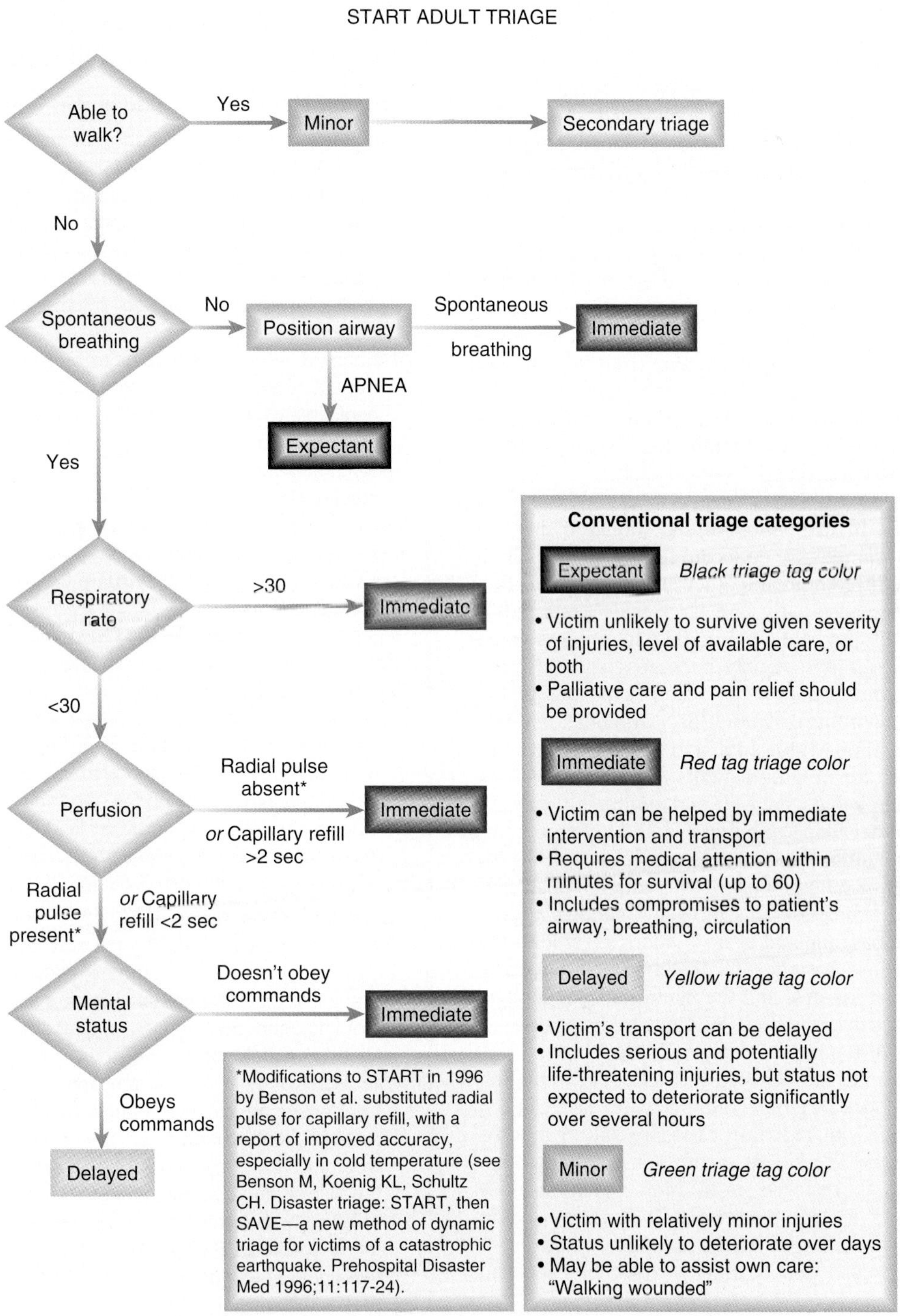

START ADULT TRIAGE

Able to walk? — Yes → Minor → Secondary triage

No ↓

Spontaneous breathing — No → Position airway — Spontaneous breathing → Immediate

Position airway — APNEA → Expectant

Yes ↓

Respiratory rate — >30 → Immediate

<30 ↓

Perfusion — Radial pulse absent* or Capillary refill >2 sec → Immediate

Radial pulse present* or Capillary refill <2 sec ↓

Mental status — Doesn't obey commands → Immediate

Obeys commands ↓

Delayed

*Modifications to START in 1996 by Benson et al. substituted radial pulse for capillary refill, with a report of improved accuracy, especially in cold temperature (see Benson M, Koenig KL, Schultz CH. Disaster triage: START, then SAVE—a new method of dynamic triage for victims of a catastrophic earthquake. Prehospital Disaster Med 1996;11:117-24).

**Conventional triage categories**

Expectant — *Black triage tag color*

- Victim unlikely to survive given severity of injuries, level of available care, or both
- Palliative care and pain relief should be provided

Immediate — *Red tag triage color*

- Victim can be helped by immediate intervention and transport
- Requires medical attention within minutes for survival (up to 60)
- Includes compromises to patient's airway, breathing, circulation

Delayed — *Yellow triage tag color*

- Victim's transport can be delayed
- Includes serious and potentially life-threatening injuries, but status not expected to deteriorate significantly over several hours

Minor — *Green triage tag color*

- Victim with relatively minor injuries
- Status unlikely to deteriorate over days
- May be able to assist own care: "Walking wounded"

**Fig. 135.2 START triage system used in mass casualty situations.** *START*, Simple triage and rapid treatment.

who may have had radiation exposure, are possibly contaminated, and may or may not have sustained concomitant trauma or burns.

Although several well-known mass casualty triage systems such START (**Figs. 135.2** and **135.3**) and JumpSTART have been devised, no federal or internationally agreed-up on medical triage systems have currently been established specifically for radiation mass casualty incidents.[4,6,14,] Existing mass casualty emergency triage algorithms are currently being used with modifications for the impact of radiation and need for decontamination.[5,8,14] However, large interorganizational efforts are currently being made at the federal level to further delineate triage protocols for different types of radiologic emergencies and for different levels of resource scarcity. See the Radiation Emergency Medical Management (REMM) website[9] for up-to-date triage recommendations.

A significant aspect of triage is determining the degree to which the patient may have been irradiated and whether external or internal contamination is present.[2,8-10,16] A Geiger counter and nasal swabs should be used at initial triage to determine whether a patient is externally (or potentially internally) contaminated. This should help dictate the amount and type of decontamination required to minimize the radiation dose. Removal of clothing alone is typically responsible for 70% to 90% of the external decontamination. In the setting of trauma and burn injury, additional wound decontamination and early wound care are necessary[1,2,8-11,16] (see the Tips and Tricks box).

Radiation injury and traumatic injury (blast and burn) interact synergistically. Patients with traumatic or burn injury who have been subjected to significant whole-body irradiation (>2 Gy) have a substantially worse prognosis because of effects on the hematopoietic syndrome and high risk for infection and poor healing. Consequently, they require a higher triage priority than do patients who are only irradiated (with or without contamination) and should be triaged and treated according to the Armed Forces Radiobiology Research Institute (AFRRI) treatment protocol[16] (**Fig. 135.4**).

Although the REMM website[9,17] has very useful biodosimetry tools to assist in estimation of the radiation dose, it requires that blood samples be collected for a complete blood count (CBC) with differential and other laboratory tests (**Box 135.1**). However, because early in a large-scale acute radiologic emergency it may not be possible to process large numbers of blood samples, it may be necessary to use the history and symptoms (mainly time from exposure to the onset of persistent vomiting) (**Table 135.2**) with other findings on physical examination (**Table 135.3**) to estimate the whole-body radiation dose for triaging patients to the four levels of care—expectant, immediate, delayed, and minimal. Ideally, all patients triaged higher than "minimal" should undergo additional work-up, including blood work and urine testing for more sensitive and specific biodosimetric radiation dose estimation. Current recommendations include obtaining a CBC with differential at baseline and every 6 hours for at least the first 48 hours because lymphocyte depletion follows dose-dependent first-order kinetics and the neutrophil-lymphocyte (N/L) ratio increases over the first 48 hours after exposure—a sensitive indicator of the radiation dose (**Table 135.4**).

The U.S. Department of Defense has used the Radiation Emergency Assistance Center/Training Site (REAC/TS) database of patients with radiation exposure and symptoms combined with the N/L ratio to create a triage score that differentiates patients exposed to a high radiation dose from those exposed to less than 1 Gy. It can be used in patients seen 4 or more hours after an exposure and has a sensitivity of 89% and specificity of 93%[1,2] (see the Facts and Formulas box).

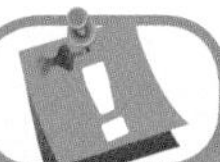

**TIPS AND TRICKS**

**Recommendations for Radiologic Decontamination**

**Principles of Radiologic Decontamination**

Ideally, decontamination takes place at field triage (area away from the emergency department [ED]), and patients arrive at the ED for evaluation and treatment already largely decontaminated. The exception should be when patients require medical stabilization and resources are available for the expected volume of severely injured patients.

The hazard of radiation exposure by health care providers from a radiologically contaminated patient is probably negligible when recommended personal protective equipment is used.

Decontamination begins *after* the patient is medically stabilized.

Patients with a risk for external or internal contamination should be evaluated with a Geiger counter and the nares swabbed and tested to evaluate the risk for inhalation of radioactive material.

Decontamination priorities are (1) wounds, (2) body orifices around the face, and (3) intact skin.

Patients should be reassessed with a Geiger counter after every attempt at decontamination (e.g., removal of clothing, washing, and wound cleansing). Decontamination procedures should be continued until less than two times the normal amount of background radiation is present.

All wound care material, irrigation fluid, and water used for washing or showering should be contained and disposed of properly as radioactive waste.

**Decontamination Techniques**

Clothing is removed by rolling the clothes off in an outward direction and away from the patient's skin and airway so that any radioactive contamination is trapped in the rolled clothing, and the clothing is placed in a sealed bag. Clothing should be cut, not torn.

Wound dressings are to be removed and the skin adjacent to the wound cleaned before cleaning the wound to prevent contamination of the wound. Areas around wounds should be draped to prevent contamination of the skin during copious wound irrigation.

Partial-thickness burns should be cleaned well with nonirritating solutions. Blisters should be left closed; open blisters should be irrigated well and treated as all other open partial-thickness burns.

Full-thickness burns with radioactive contaminants warrant typical care because of contamination sloughing with the eschar.

Data from references 1, 8 and 22.

## TREATMENT

The mainstay of acute medical treatment in a radiologic emergency is similar to the typical acute medical and trauma management in the ED, with attention paid to threats to life and limb first and symptomatic treatment as needed.

In ARS diagnosed by the onset of symptoms or biodosimetry assessment, treatment is based on the whole-body radiation dose. In general, treatment of ARS is not indicated for (1) a low exposure dose (<1 Gy) because the risk for complications is low and (2) a very high exposure dose (>10 Gy) because the prognosis is very poor in this population and palliative care is most appropriate.[1,11] With exposure to greater than 2 to 3 Gy, medical treatments are both supportive (appropriate use of intravenous fluids, antiemetics, and nutritional support) and preventive (prophylactic antibiotics, colony-stimulating factors, and transfusion of blood products)[2,10,11] (**Box 135.2**).

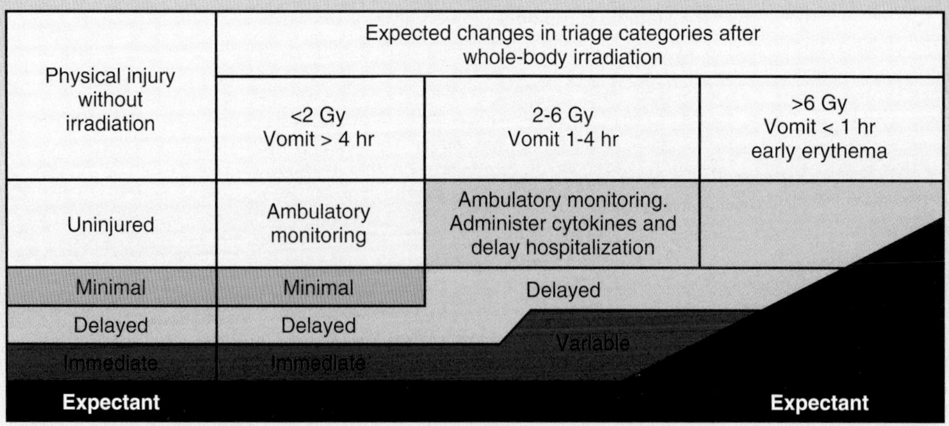


**Fig. 135.3 Alterations in triage categories because of a substantially worse prognosis with combined injury (radiation and traumatic or thermal burn injury).** (Adapted from Armed Forces Radiobiology Research Institute. Medical management of radiological casualties. Bethesda, Md: Uniformed Services University of the Health Sciences; 2010. p. 51.)

**BOX 135.1 Recommended Testing in Acute Radiation Emergencies**

Recommended initial laboratory tests (all patients with suspected irradiation):
- Complete blood count with differential and absolute lymphocyte count at baseline and at 48 hours
- Serum amylase at baseline and at 24 hours (if feasible); radiation dose–dependent increase expected after 24 hours
- Urine pregnancy test—advisable for women of child-bearing age

If the patient is vomiting less than 3 hours after exposure:
- CBC with differential and absolute lymphocyte count repeated every 6 to 12 hours
- Type and crossmatch for possible need for transfusion of blood products
- HLA subtyping for possible future need for stem cell transplantation
- Cytogenetic dosimetry—dicentric chromosome assay (if feasible)

If the history indicates internal contamination (inhalation or gastrointestinal):
- Twenty-four-hour urine sample (name of radioactive isotope)
- Stool sample (name of radioactive isotope)

Data from references 1, 2, 9, 12, and 17.

Hospital treatment of ARS is focused on supportive measures and management of the hematopoietic subsyndrome to minimize the complications of sepsis and bleeding. The goal is to reduce both the depth and duration of neutropenia and thrombocytopenia, as well as to prevent or manage neutropenic fever and sepsis.[2,10,11] Treatment recommendations for antibiotics (fluoroquinolone, acyclovir, and fluconazole) and cytokine therapy (hematopoietic colony-stimulating factors) vary depending on the estimated dose of radiation exposure, the presence of traumatic injury or burn, and the size of the

**Table 135.2** Radiation Dose Estimate by Time to Emesis After Irradiation

| TIME TO EMESIS | UPPER BOUND DOSE ESTIMATE |
|---|---|
| >2 hr | <9 Gy |
| >4 hr | <4 Gy |
| >10 hr | <2 Gy |

Adapted from Parker DD, Parker JC. Estimating radiation dose from time to emesis and lymphocyte depletion. Health Phys 2007;93:701-4.

**BOX 135.2 Recommended Medications and Treatments of Acute Radiation Emergency and Acute Radiation Syndrome**

**Supportive Care**
Antiemetics
Antidiarrheals
Fluids
Analgesia

**Preventive Care**
Antibiotics
Antivirals
Antifungals

**Preventive and Restorative**
Colony-stimulating factor
Transfusions

**Special Considerations**
Potassium iodide for pregnant women

Data from references 10, 11, and 21.

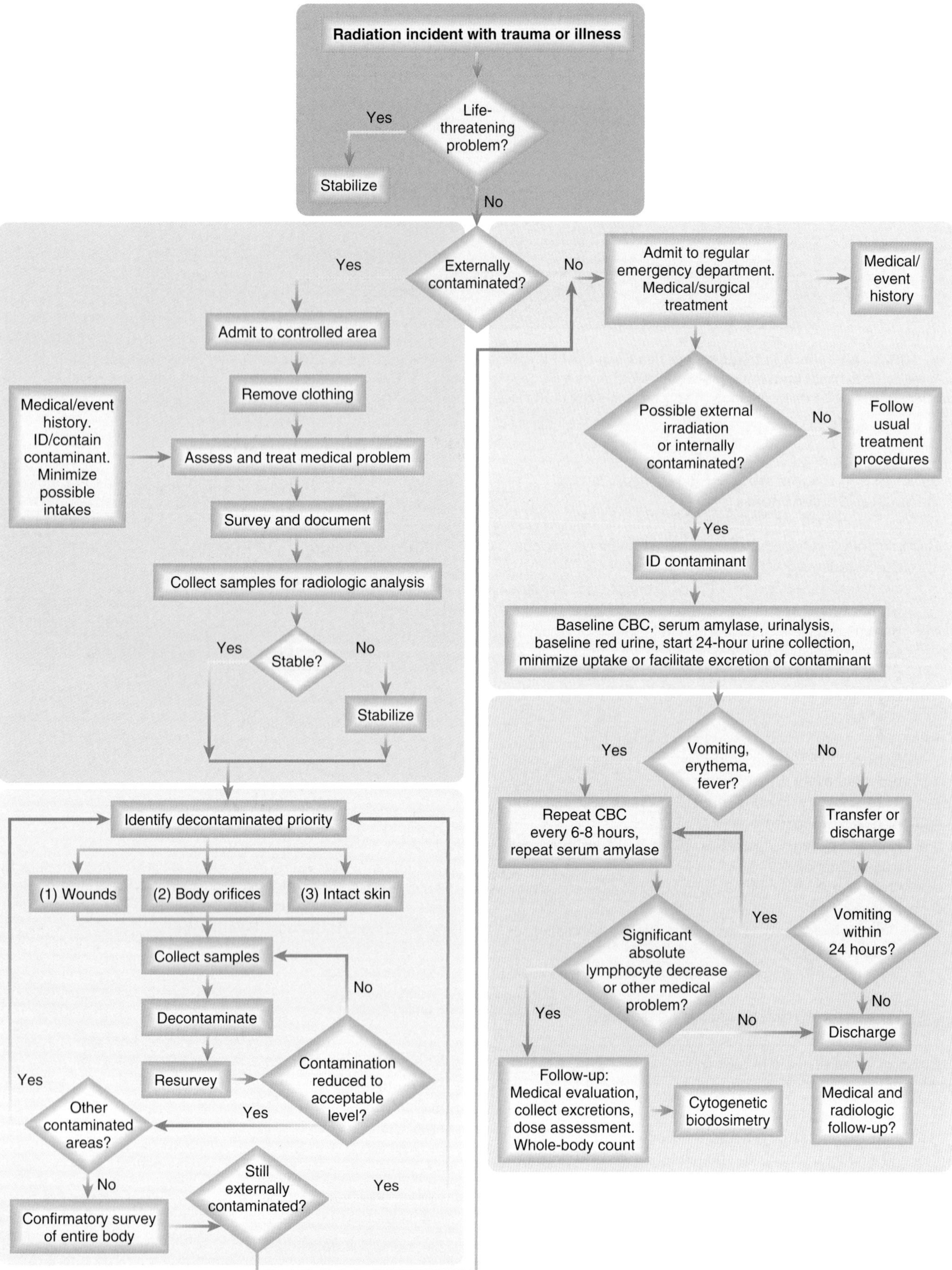


**Fig. 135.4 Treatment algorithm for patients with combined radiation and trauma or burn injury.** *CBC*, Complete blood count; *ID*, identify. (Adapted from Armed Forces Radiobiology Research Institute. AFRRI pocket guide: emergency radiation medicine response. Bethesda, Md: Uniformed Services University of the Health Sciences; 2011.)

**Table 135.3 Findings in Patients in the Prodromal Phase of Acute Radiation Syndrome for Dose Estimation Without Biodosimetry**

| SYMPTOMS AND MEDICAL RESPONSE | *ARS DEGREE AND APPROXIMATE DOSE OF ACUTE WBE* MILD (1-2 Gy) | MODERATE (2-4 Gy) | SEVERE (4-6 Gy) | VERY SEVERE (6-8 Gy) | LETHAL (>8 Gy)* |
|---|---|---|---|---|---|
| **Vomiting** | | | | | |
| Onset | 2 hr after exposure or later | 1-2 hr after exposure | Earlier than 1 hr after exposure | Earlier than 30 min after exposure | Earlier than 10 min after exposure |
| Incidence (%) | 10-50 | 70-90 | 100 | 100 | 100 |
| **Diarrhea** | None | None | Mild | Heavy | Heavy |
| Onset | | | 3-8 hr | 1-3 hr | Within minutes or 1 hr |
| Incidence (%) | | | <10 | >10 | Almost 100 |
| **Headache** | Slight | Mild | Moderate | Severe | Severe |
| Onset | | | 4-24 hr | 3-4 hr | 1-2 hr |
| Incidence (%) | | | 50 | 80 | 80-90 |
| **Consciousness** | Unaffected | Unaffected | Unaffected | May be altered | Unconsciousness (may last seconds to minutes) |
| Onset | | | | | Seconds to minutes |
| Incidence (%) | | | | | 100 (at >50 Gy) |
| **Body temperature** | Normal | Increased | Fever | High fever | High fever |
| Onset | | 1-3 hr | 1-2 hr | <1 hr | <1 hr |
| Incidence (%) | | 10-80 | 80-100 | 100 | 100 |
| **Medical response** | Outpatient observation | Observation in general hospital, treatment in specialized hospital if needed | Treatment in specialized hospital | Treatment in specialized hospital | Palliative treatment (symptomatic only) |

Adapted from Koenig KL, Goans RE, Hatchett RJ, et al. Medical treatment of radiological casualties: current concepts. Ann Emerg Med 2005;45:643-52.
*ARS*, Acute radiation syndrome; *WBE*, whole-body exposure.
*With appropriate supportive and marrow resuscitative therapy, individuals may survive for 6 to 12 months after whole-body doses as high as 12 Gy.

**Table 135.4 Expected Patient Outcome Based on Absolute Lymphocyte Count at 48 Hours**

| MINIMAL LYMPHOCYTE COUNT 48 HOURS AFTER EXPOSURE | APPROXIMATE ABSORBED RADIATION DOSE (GY) | PROGNOSIS |
|---|---|---|
| 1000-3000 | 0-0.5 | No significant injury |
| 1000-1500 | 1-2 | Significant but probably nonlethal, good prognosis |
| 500-1000 | 2-4 | Severe injury, fair prognosis |
| 100-500 | 4-8 | Very severe injury, poor prognosis |
| <100 | >8 | High lethality even with full treatment with CSFs |

Adapted from Goans RE, Halloway EC, Berger ME, et al. Early dose assessment in criticality accidents. Health Phys 2001;81:446-9.
*CSFs*, Colony-stimulating factors.

radiologic emergency, which is addressed in **Table 135.5**. Note that the current recommendations are based on healthy adults and that a lower threshold for treatment may be advisable for children younger than 12 years and the elderly, in whom few data are available for evidence-based recommendations.[5,11] When treatment is indicated, it should continue until the absolute neutrophil count is higher than $1.0 \times 10^9$ cells/L after recovery from the nadir.

For those with trauma and burns, there are caveats for decontamination of wounds (see the Tips and Tricks box). Because of the increased likelihood of infection and bleeding as a result of the hematopoietic effects of radiation exposure, any orthopedic reductions, splinting, casting, or surgery (orthopedic and otherwise) should be completed within the initial 48 hours of significant radiation exposure (>2 Gy).[1,2,9]

In addition to the aforementioned general recommendations for treatment of radiologic emergencies, specific approaches for treating internal contamination (ingestion or inhalation) have been established. Reduction of the internal radionuclide content is called radionuclide decorporation and can be helpful in reducing the absorbed radiation dose.[18] Approaches to decorporation include (1) reducing or inhibiting absorption in the gastrointestinal tract, (2) blocking uptake to the organ predisposed to injury (e.g., potassium iodide for blocking uptake by the thyroid), (3) diluting the isotope and

**Table 135.5 Guidelines for Treatment of Acute Radiation Syndrome***

| VARIABLE | PROPOSED RADIATION DOSE RANGE FOR TREATMENT WITH CYTOKINES (Gy) | PROPOSED RADIATION DOSE RANGE FOR TREATMENT WITH ANTIBIOTICS (Gy)† | PROPOSED RADIATION DOSE RANGE FOR REFERRAL FOR CONSIDERATION OF SCT (Gy) |
|---|---|---|---|
| **Small-Volume Scenario (≤100 Casualties)** | | | |
| Healthy person, no other injuries | 3-10‡ | 2-10§ | 7-10 for allogeneic SCT, 4-10 if previous autograft stored or syngeneic donor available |
| Multiple injuries or burns | 2-6‡ | 2-6§ | NA |
| **Mass Casualty Scenario (>100 Casualties)** | | | |
| Healthy person, no other injuries | 3-7‡ | 2-7§ | 7-10 for allogeneic SCT, 4-10 if previous autograft stored or syngeneic donor available |
| Multiple injuries or burns | 2-6¶ | 2-6§¶ | NA |

Adapted from Waselenko JK, MacVittie TJ, Blakely WF, et al. Medical management of the acute radiation syndrome: recommendations of the Strategic National Stockpile Radiation Working Group. Ann Intern Med 2004;140:1037-51.

*NA*, Not applicable; *SCT*, stem cell transplantation.

*Consensus guidance for treatment is based on threshold whole-body or significant partial-body exposure. Events caused by detonation of a radiologic dispersal device resulting in 100 or fewer casualties and those caused by detonation of an improvised nuclear device resulting in more than 100 casualties have been considered. These guidelines are intended to supplement (and not substitute for) clinical findings based on examination of the patient.

†Prophylactic antibiotics include a fluoroquinolone, acyclovir (if the patient is seropositive for herpes simplex virus or has a medical history of this virus), and fluconazole when the absolute neutrophil count is lower than $0.500 \times 10^9$ cells/L and the patient is not already receiving colony-stimulating factor.

‡Consider initiating therapy at a lower exposure dose in nonadolescent children and elderly persons. Initiate treatment with granulocyte colony-stimulating factor or granulocyte-macrophage colony-stimulating factor in victims with an absolute neutrophil count lower than $0.5000 \times 10^9$ cells/L who are not already receiving colony-stimulating factor.

§Absolute neutrophil count lower than $0.5000 \times 10^9$ cells/L. Antibiotic therapy should be continued until neutrophil recovery has taken place. Follow the Infectious Diseases Society of America guidelines for febrile neutropenia if fever develops while the patient is taking prophylactic medication.

¶If resources are available.

increasing elimination, (4) altering the chemistry of the substance, (5) displacing the isotope from receptors, (6) using chelation techniques to enhance elimination, (7) excising radionuclide from contaminated traumatic wounds early to minimize absorption, and (8) performing bronchoalveolar lavage for severe cases of insoluble inhaled particles.[1,2]

Treatment options are available if the radioactive contaminant is known and antidotes exist.[2,9,10,19,20] Poison control centers can provide help in identifying potential antidotes for the ingestion of known radionuclides. A limited selection of radionuclide-specific decorporation treatments are included in **Table 135.6**. In general, the risk versus benefit balance of using these decorporation agents depends on the estimated dose ingested and the time since the ingestion. Estimation of ingested radionuclide doses is typically beyond the scope of EPs and ED staff, and in many situations these treatments are not helpful early in the medical response following a large-scale radiologic disaster.[5] Therefore, guidance from poison control, the Centers for Disease Control and Prevention, or REMM (or any combination of these resources) is recommended before beginning treatment.[5,18,21]

Importantly, after a nuclear detonation or nuclear reactor incident, radioactive iodine is a significant concern, and specific treatment might include potassium iodide (KI).[2,8,19,22] The decision to treat with KI will probably involve multiple agencies, including the U.S. Centers for Disease Control and Prevention, the U.S. Food and Drug Administration, and the U.S. Department of Health and Human Services, and guidance should be sought before treating.[9,21] If indicated after a nuclear disaster, KI should be administered before or immediately coincident with passage of the radioactive cloud, although KI may still have a substantial protective effect even if taken 3 or 4 hours after exposure. Consult the REMM website or desktop application for prescribing details and note that pregnant women and children deserve special consideration for KI given their increased risk for malignancy and thyroid disease over time.[10,20]

The psychologic impact of a nuclear event can be overwhelming[22,23,24] and should not be underestimated. It has been suggested that if possible, educational material and counselors should be available at triage and receiving centers, as well as in the ED, and patients should be given instructions to see a health care provider if they are having signs of psychologic stress.[1,8,25]

## FOLLOW-UP, NEXT STEPS IN CARE, AND PATIENT EDUCATION

Disposition after a radiologic emergency depends on several factors, including the estimated radiation dose and associated trauma or burn. Patients who remain asymptomatic or only minimally symptomatic without persistent vomiting were probably triaged as “minimal” (radiation exposure < 1 Gy)

**Table 135.6 Specific Decorporation Treatments in Patients with Internal Radiation Contamination***

| RADIONUCLIDE | THERAPY† |
|---|---|
| Tritium | Dilution: force fluids |
| Iodine 125 or 131 | Blocking: saturated solution of potassium iodide<br>Mobilization: antithyroid drugs |
| Cesium 134 or 137 | Blocking: Prussian blue |
| Strontium 89 or 90 | Decrease absorption: aluminum phosphate gel antacids<br>Blocking: strontium lactate<br>Displacement: oral phosphate<br>Mobilization: ammonium chloride or parathyroid extract |
| Plutonium and other transuranic elements | Chelating: Zn or Ca-DTPA (investigational) |
| Unknown ingestion | Reduce absorption; consider emetics, gastric lavage, charcoal, whole-bowel irrigation |

Adapted from Koenig KL, Goans RE, Hatchett RJ, et al. Medical treatment of radiological casualties: current concepts. Ann Emerg Med 2005;45:643-52.

*Seek guidance from the Centers for Disease Control and Prevention or Radiation Emergency Medical Management (REMM) when administering any of these interventions because many have an unfavorable risk-to-benefit ratio in those with ingestion of a low to moderate dose. Treatment is strongly recommended for ingestion doses 10 times the annual limit of intake (REMM, 2011).

†Only potassium iodide, diethylenetriaminepentaacetic acid (DTPA), and Prussian blue are approved by the Food and Drug Administration for decorporation (REMM, 2011).

and can be discharged home safely from the triage area after decontamination, with follow-up by a primary care provider. Importantly, they should be registered with the designated governmental agency that is tracking patients and outcomes of acute radiation emergencies.[1,9] All patients not admitted to the hospital or transferred to a higher level of care should also receive (1) reassurance, (2) informative patient handouts on radiologic emergencies and symptoms that require additional care, (3) recommendations for follow-up, and (4) instruction on how to safely deal with possible contamination at home. Basic patient handouts are available from the REMM website.[25]

In mass casualty situations, mildly symptomatic patients typically receive acute first aid and symptomatic treatment of nausea and vomiting and are discharged with strict instructions to return in 24 to 48 hours for revaluation of their hematopoietic system and possible need for treatment of ARS. Patients are to return earlier if the symptoms worsen.[1,10,22]

Moderately symptomatic patients or those who have absorbed more than 2 Gy and are experiencing symptoms are hospitalized for observation and treatment of ARS and any injuries. Patients with moderate injury or burn (>10% body surface area) and moderate to severe ARS should taken to surgery (if needed) within 36 to 48 hours, as well as be treated for ARS in an inpatient setting.[2,10,12] Within these recommendations for disposition, it is specifically noted that any transfers to larger facilities for surgery or management of severe ARS should take place in the first 48 hours when possible to enable the greatest likelihood of a good outcome.

Severely symptomatic patients with gastrointestinal and cardiovascular syndromes (>10 Gy) of absorbed radiation are treated with as many resources as reasonable for the situation in recognition of the fact that the prognosis is very poor regardless of interventions. In the setting of a mass casualty, these patients are managed expectantly (i.e., with comfort measures for pain, nausea or vomiting, and anxiety). Similarly, patients with moderate to severe trauma or burns and more than 6 to 8 Gy of absorbed radiation dose will often be managed expectantly. In isolated cases, empiric antibiotic therapy, colony-stimulating factor therapy, transfusions, and a search for bone marrow donors might ensue in a heroic attempt to save the patient's life.[2,10,12] Unfortunately, data and experience in identifying the optimal disposition of children and the elderly who have experienced irradiation and trauma are limited, so clinicians will have to decide each case individually.[12]

## SUGGESTED READINGS


Armed Forces Radiobiology Research Institute. Medical management of radiological casualties. Bethesda, Md: Uniformed Services University of the Health Sciences; 2010. p. 51. Available at http://www.usuhs.mil/afrri/outreach/pdf/3edmmrchandbook.pdf.

Koenig KL, Goans RE, Hatchett RJ, et al. Medical treatment of radiological casualties: current concepts. Ann Emerg Med 2005;45:643-52.

Radiation Emergency Assistance Center/Training Site (REAC/TS) at Oak Ridge Institute for Science and Education (ORISE). Available at http://orise.orau.gov/reacts/default.aspx.

Radiation Emergency Assistance Center/Training Site (REAC/TS). The medical aspects of radiation incidents. Oak Ridge, Tenn: Department of Energy; 2011. p. 56. Available at http://orise.orau.gov/reacts/resources/radiation-accident-management.aspx.

U.S. Department of Health and Human Services Radiation Emergency Management. Available at http://www.remm.nlm.gov/.

Waselenko JK, MacVittie TJ, Blakely WF, et al. Medical management of the acute radiation syndrome: recommendations of the Strategic National Stockpile Radiation Working Group. Ann Intern Med 2004;140:1037-51.


## REFERENCES

***References can be found on Expert Consult @ www.expertconsult.com.***

# 136 Smoke Inhalation

*Thomas Kunisaki and Steven A. Godwin*

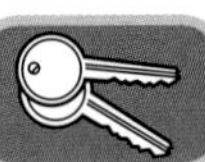

**KEY POINTS**

- The majority (50% to 80%) of deaths attributable to fire are caused by smoke inhalation rather than burns.
- Smoke is a combination of heated particles and gases (toxicants).
- Carbon monoxide has been implicated in more smoke inhalation deaths than any other single compound.
- In addition to inhalation of toxicants, smoke inhalation can cause upper airway burns that result in pulmonary parenchymal injury.
- The mainstay of treatment consists of ventilator support, early intubation, optimization of fluid resuscitation, pulmonary hygiene, and treatment of specific toxicants.

## EPIDEMIOLOGY

Fires are common events in the United States. It is estimated that fire departments respond to fire alarms every 20 seconds.[1] In 2007, more than 1 million fire incidents and nearly 3500 deaths were reported, with civilian fatalities occurring every 153 minutes on average.[1] An estimated 50% to 80% of fire-related deaths are the result of smoke inhalation. Incident after incident, most of the victims of fires in commercial buildings, such as clubs, escape burns but suffer from smoke inhalation

Smoke inhalation injuries related to fire result from the toxic gases generated. Deaths from smoke inhalation have increased in recent years because of the abundant use of newer synthetic material in building and furnishings.[2]

## PATHOPHYSIOLOGY

Deaths from fires are most often caused by smoke inhalation.[3,4] The injury from smoke inhalation is a result of direct thermal injury to the airway and lung parenchyma, as well as mucosal irritation, corrosive injuries, and asphyxiation from toxic gases. Toxic gases can be classified as irritant gases and asphyxiants. The danger from such toxic gases predominates in exposed fire victims. Smoke is composed of a complex mixture of suspended small particles, fumes, and gases. More than 400 toxic compounds have been demonstrated in the smoke of a typical house fire. Polyvinyl chloride, a component of many plastic goods, generates at least 75 different toxic products when burned. Of these toxic substances, carbon monoxide (CO) appears to be the most common fatal substance associated with fire victims.[5,6]

Thermal inhalation injuries are usually localized to the upper airway. Irritant gases, depending on their water solubility, affect either the upper or lower airway. Highly water-soluble agents such as ammonia, hydrogen chloride, and sulfur dioxide predominantly affect the upper airway. Their solubility directly correlates with rapid adverse upper airway symptoms. Agents with lower water solubility, such as phosgene and nitrogen dioxide, which do not produce immediate irritation, will be inhaled deeper in the pulmonary system and result in injury to the alveoli; victims typically have delayed noncardiogenic pulmonary edema.

Asphyxiants further compound the injury in smoke inhalation victims. Simple asphyxiants, such as carbon dioxide and methane, will produce an oxygen-deprived environment. Systemic asphyxiants, such as CO, cyanide, and hydrogen sulfide ($H_2S$), will prevent utilization of oxygen by cells. Either mechanism will promote an anaerobic state and the development of lactic acidosis.

CO is a colorless, odorless, nonirritating gas produced by the incomplete combustion of hydrocarbons and petroleum distillates, whether from a fire, fuel source, or automobile exhaust or from the metabolism of methylene chloride, a solvent commonly used as a paint stripper. One of the major mechanisms of CO toxicity is its affinity to bind hemoglobin, with an affinity estimated to be approximately 250 times greater than that of oxygen, which results in reduction in oxyhemoglobin. The impairment in delivery of oxygen is exacerbated by displacement of the oxygen dissociation curve to the left. Furthermore, CO interferes with cellular respiration by binding to mitochondrial cytochrome oxidase and is involved in the formation of oxygen free radicals and subsequent lipid peroxidation. All the aforementioned mechanisms produce oxidative stress on the brain, the main organ affected by CO; excitatory amino acids such as glutamate are activated, which results in neuronal injury and cell death. Areas of the brain that are highly sensitive to hypoxemia, such as the basal ganglia, appear to sustain the most injury. CO is known to bind to myoglobin as well, a feature that contributes to impairment in myocardial contractility. Fetal hemoglobin is more sensitive to the binding of CO; levels are reported to be approximately 10% higher than maternal levels, with a half-life five times longer. Over time, carboxyhemoglobin will dissociate, with its half-life on room air being approximately 4 to 6 hours. With 100% oxygen, the half-life decreases to approximately 90 minutes, and in the setting of hyperbaric oxygen therapy, it is about 20 minutes.

Cyanide is a highly toxic chemical. Hydrogen cyanide is a common by-product of the pyrolysis of wool, silk, and plastics. Cyanogenic compounds such as nitriles are used in industry as solvents and adhesives and are metabolized by the body to cyanide. Acetonitrile, which in the past was commercially available as an artificial nail glue remover, has resulted in fatality when accidentally ingested.[7] With increasing concern about terrorism, it is high on the potential lists of chemical agents. Its mechanism is binding of the cytochrome $aa_3$ site on the electron transport system of mitochondria. The result is an inability to use oxygen and subsequent cellular asphyxia.

$H_2S$ is the by-product of certain industries, such as paper factories, petroleum refineries, and dehairing of hides. It is produced naturally from decay of organic matter and from sulfur hot springs. These products have the characteristic "rotten egg" odor. Like cyanide, it is a potent inhibitor of the cytochrome oxidase system. The human nose is exquisitely sensitive to the odor of $H_2S$, and it is easily detected at levels as low as 0.13 parts per million (ppm). Irritation of mucous membranes occurs at levels of approximately 50 to 100 ppm, and such levels are also capable of causing bronchospasm, blepharospasm, and laryngeal edema. At levels greater than 500 ppm, a phenomenon classically described as a "rapid knockdown" effect occurs, which includes immediate loss of consciousness with the potential for cardiovascular collapse and respiratory arrest. Sulfhemoglobin may result from exposure to $H_2S$. Clinically, it may produce cyanosis. Unfortunately, it is an extremely stable compound and is eliminated only when the red blood cells are removed from the circulation. Recently, $H_2S$ was a popular means of suicide in Japan.[8] Bath sulfur, a product readily available, is added to water to mimic the water of natural sulfur hot springs. However, when the bath sulfur is combined with acid, such as toilet bowl cleaner, a lethal $H_2S$ gas is liberated. Any sulfur-containing substance, including laundry detergent, is a suitable substitute for bath sulfur. Reports of suicide in the United States with this method have been described in the media.

Methemoglobin is the oxidized form of hemoglobin and can result from exposure to oxidizing agents, such as nitrites and nitrates, as well as from smoke inhalation.[9] In this oxidized state, hemoglobin is no longer capable of carrying oxygen. Cyanosis is typically seen at levels approximately of 15% to 20%. Levels greater than 70% are usually lethal.

## PRESENTING SIGNS AND SYMPTOMS

Victims of smoke inhalation will typically be in various degrees of respiratory distress and altered mental status. Hoarseness, stridor, and aphonia may be early signs of impending respiratory arrest. Attention to vital signs is imperative. Hypoxemia despite supplemental oxygen is a poor prognostic sign and needs to be addressed immediately. Carboxyhemoglobinemia and methemoglobinemia will give false readings on pulse oximetry unless newer pulse oximetry instruments that can detect these hemoglobinopathies are used. In a normal patient, the pulse oximetry instrument is calibrated to measure the differences in light absorption between the red and infrared wavelengths. With oxyhemoglobin, the majority of light absorption is in the red wavelength region. With carboxyhemoglobinemia, the peak wavelength of light absorption is similar to that of oxyhemoglobin, and the instrument does not detect differences between the two. With methemoglobinemia, as its concentration increases, the pulse oximetry instrument interprets equal light absorption between the red and infrared wavelengths. As a result, the instrument interprets this ratio automatically as 85%.

Many of the toxicants associated with smoke inhalation can cause hypotension as result of either third spacing, peripheral vasodilation, or myocardial depression or arrhythmia. Seizure may be one of the early signs and results from either secondary hypoxemia, acidosis, or toxic gases and compounds.

## DIFFERENTIAL DIAGNOSIS AND MEDICAL DECISION MAKING

As a means of better understanding this complex problem, dividing smoke inhalation injury into toxidromes (toxic syndromes) may help identify clinically significant smoke inhalation. Aside from the potential concomitant thermal injuries associated with structural fires, these major toxidromes involve irritant gases, simple asphyxiants, systemic asphyxiants, and methemoglobinemia (**Table 136.1**).

Irritant gases can be divided into highly water-soluble and poorly water-soluble agents. Moderately water-soluble gases, such as chlorine, behave more like the highly water-soluble agents and are thus combined with the highly water-soluble agents. Highly water-soluble agents are very irritating to the mucous membranes, eyes, and upper airway, and affected individuals experience symptoms immediately. As with thermal injuries, early orotracheal intubation should be a priority in any individual with any degree of respiratory distress. These individuals can deteriorate rapidly. Generally, most individuals will be able to remove themselves from such an environment; however, if they are injured, incapacitated, or involuntarily confined, their outcome may be lethal. A prime example is the 1984 incident in Bhopal, India, where approximately 20,000 lb of isocyanate leaked from a nearby storage tank. By the time that the leak was discovered, the fumes covered nearly 5 square miles. It is estimated more than 200,000 individuals were victimized by the irritant gas and thousands of people died.

Poorly water-soluble gases have very poor warning properties, and thus they are inhaled deeper in the pulmonary system and affect the alveoli. Two examples of such agents are phosgene and nitrogen dioxide. The hallmark of these inhalation injuries is delayed pulmonary edema.

The asphyxiant toxidromes can be divided in simple and systemic. As asphyxiants, these agents affect the availability or utilization of oxygen by cells and therefore tissues and organs. Simple asphyxiants are generally inert gases, such as carbon dioxide, but they may be flammable, such as methane, and create an explosive hazard. Simple asphyxiants displace oxygen and thus create a hypoxic environment. Symptoms depend on the severity of the hypoxia and the duration of exposure. Because of the underlying mechanism, an excess

**Table 136.1 Major Toxidromes**

| | IRRITANT GASES (MODERATELY HIGHLY WATER SOLUBLE) | IRRITANT GASES (POORLY WATER SOLUBLE) | SIMPLE ASPHYXIANTS | SYSTEMIC ASPHYXIANTS | METHEMOGLOBINEMIA |
|---|---|---|---|---|---|
| Examples | Sulfur dioxide<br>Formaldehyde<br>Ammonia<br>Chloramine<br>Methylisocyanate<br>Hydrogen sulfide<br>Hydrogen chloride | Phosgene<br>Nitrogen dioxide | Methane<br>Butane<br>Carbon dioxide | Cyanide<br>Hydrogen sulfide<br>Hydrogen azide<br>Carbon monoxide | Nitrates, nitrites<br>Chlorates, chlorites<br>Aniline dyes<br>Nitric oxide<br>Hydrogen peroxide<br>Ozone<br>Iodine |
| Clinical findings | Immediate membrane irritation<br>Oral mucous burning<br>Excessive tearing<br>Laryngeal edema (hoarseness, stridor, aphonia)<br>Cough, bronchospasm, SOB | Gradual SOB<br>Delayed pulmonary edema | SOB<br>Altered mental status<br>Seizure, coma | SOB<br>Altered mental status<br>Seizure, coma<br>Metabolic acidosis<br>Cardiovascular collapse, shock | Cyanotic appearing<br>Asymptomatic in minority of cases<br>SOB<br>Altered mental status |
| Immediate treatment considerations | Removal from exposure environment<br>Resuscitation<br>ACLS<br>Oxygen<br>Intubation if necessary | Removal from exposure environment<br>Resuscitation<br>ACLS<br>Oxygen<br>Intubation if necessary | Removal from exposure environment<br>Resuscitation<br>ACLS<br>Oxygen<br>Intubation if necessary | Removal from exposure environment<br>Resuscitation<br>ACLS<br>Oxygen<br>Hydroxocobalamin if cyanide suspected<br>Hyperbaric oxygen for severe carbon monoxide toxicity | Removal from exposure environment<br>Resuscitation<br>ACLS<br>Oxygen<br>Methylene blue |

*ACLS*, Advanced cardiac life support; *SOB*, shortness of breath.

of deoxyhemoglobin, cyanosis is usually present. Systemic asphyxiates impair the body's ability to use oxygen by interfering with the transportation of oxygen, such as with methemoglobinemia, or by interfering with the utilization of oxygen at the cellular level, such as with cyanide. CO impairs both the transportation and utilization of oxygen.

The diagnosis of cyanide toxicity is generally based on a high index suspicion from the history. The victim will appear in a shocklike state. The classic bitter almond odor of cyanide is rarely detected. Hypoxia is a late finding because of its underlying pathophysiology. Oxygen is available, but the cells and tissues are unable to use it. Because cyanide assay is not immediately available in most institutions, indirect evaluation of the difference in the oxygen content of arterial and venous blood can provide valuable insight.[4] A small arterial ($PaO_2$)-venous ($PvO_2$) oxygen gap would support the diagnosis. Severe lactic acidosis should prompt further investigation of cyanide toxicity. A lactic acid level greater than 10 mmol/L has been correlated with a cyanide level of approximately 40 mmol/L, a level considered significant and warranting immediate action.

Methemoglobinemia is the result of oxidation of the iron in hemoglobin. Normal hemoglobin has iron in the 2+ state. When it is exposed to an oxidizing agent, the iron is converted to the 3+ state. In this oxidized state, it is unable to bind oxygen. A methemoglobin level of approximately 1.5 g/dL can produce cyanosis. The body normally reduces iron by various physiologic pathways, primarily via reduced nicotinamide adenine dinucleotide (NADH) methemoglobin reductase and by a minor pathway, reduced nicotinamide adenine dinucleotide phosphate (NADPH) methemoglobin reductase. This latter pathway is dependent on a functional glucose-6-phosphate dehydrogenase (G6PD) system. It is the pathway that is the target of administration of methylene blue, the treatment of methemoglobinemia.

## TREATMENT

The priority of treatment is supporting and stabilizing the primary survey—the ABCs (airway, breathing, and circulation). Aggressive airway management is essential, including high-flow supplemental oxygen and early orotracheal intubation and ventilator management if necessary.

Close monitoring is imperative to observe for the potential for rapid clinical deterioration. Good supportive care is vital and includes fluid resuscitation, anticonvulsant therapy, and correction of metabolic abnormalities, especially metabolic acidosis.

Hydroxocobalamin (Cyanokit) is a new cyanide antidote approved by the Food and Drug Administration in December 2006. It has essentially replaced the older antidote, which used sodium nitrite to generate a controlled methemoglobinemia, follow by the administration of sodium thiosulfate, a substrate required by the liver enzyme rhodanase to then detoxify the formation of cyanomethemoglobin. Use of hydroxocobalamin is indicated in any individual with cyanide toxicity or suspected cyanide toxicity. By mechanism, it binds to cyanide to form cyanocobalamin, which is vitamin $B_{12}$. It appears to be safe, with just a few clinically significant adverse effects, such as allergic reactions and transient hypertension. Generalized erythema and red chromaturia because of the dark red nature of the antidote once reconstituted are commonly reported. Unfortunately, laboratory studies that depend on colorimetric analysis are affected and will give false readings. Its clinical significance is unknown. Because of its safety profile, this antidote can be administered empirically at the scene of a fire to victims and fire rescuers who may be deemed at risk for toxic exposure to cyanide.[10] In at least one animal study evaluating the effect of hydroxocobalamin on mice poisoned with sodium sulfide (at a lethal dose for 90% of the population [$LD_{90}$]), the antidote resulted in improved survival following its administration.[11]

Methylene blue is the antidote for the treatment of methemoglobinemia. It is indicated in victims who are symptomatic and usually with methemoglobin levels greater than 20% to 30%. One contraindication to its use is G6PD deficiency. With multiple dosing, methylene blue may itself generate methemoglobinemia or cause hemolysis. Other therapeutic options for the treatment of methemoglobinemia are exchange transfusion or hyperbaric oxygen (HBO) therapy.

Treatment of CO toxicity is primarily supportive with 100% supplemental oxygen. HBO therapy has been studied clinically for years, but its role in treating CO toxicity remains controversial.[12,13] If considering HBO, generally accepted indications would include the following: loss of consciousness at the scene, comatose state, seizure, myocardial ischemia, and levels greater than 30% in adults and greater 15% in infants, children, or pregnant women.

## FOLLOW-UP, NEXT STEPS IN CARE, AND PATIENT EDUCATION

All smoke inhalation patients should be evaluated in an emergency department. If symptomatic, all will require admission. Depending on the severity of their exposure and injuries, they should be admitted to a monitor setting, including the intensive care unit if needed.

Patients with a brief exposure who are asymptomatic for a minimum of 6 hours can be discharged with good instructions to the patient and family member regarding the signs and symptoms of early respiratory distress, as long as they have the ability to access 911.

Patients in whom phosgene or nitrogen dioxide gases may be involved in the exposure should be admitted, despite being asymptomatic, and be observed for minimum of 24 hours with frequent assessment for signs and symptoms of delayed pulmonary edema.

## SUGGESTED READINGS


Borron SJ, Baud F, Barriot P, et al. Prospective study of hydroxocobalamin for acute cyanide poisoning in smoke inhalation. Ann Emerg Med 2007;49:794-801.

Cahalane M, Demling RH. Early respiratory abnormalities from smoke inhalation. JAMA 1984;251:771-3.

Clark WR, Nieman GF. Smoke Inhalation. Burns 1988;14:473-94.

Crapo RO. Smoke-inhalation injuries. JAMA 1981;246:1694-6.

Prien T. Toxic smoke compounds and inhalation injury—a review. Burns 1988;14:451-60.

Wolf SJ, Lavonas EJ, Sloan EP, et al. Clinical policy: critical issues in the management of adult patients presenting to the emergency department with acute carbon monoxide poisoning. Ann Emerg Med 2008;51:138-52.


## REFERENCES

*References can be found on Expert Consult @ www.expertconsult.com.*

# 137 Chemical and Nuclear Agents

*Christopher S. Kang and Ian S. Wedmore*

**KEY POINTS**

- Decontamination should take place immediately, before initial treatment and evacuation of exposed patients.
- For patients exposed to nerve agents, atropine and pralidoxime chloride should be administered rapidly.
- Treatment of blast injuries and emergency medical conditions should precede specific treatment of radiation exposure.

## EPIDEMIOLOGY

Tens of thousands of chemicals are manufactured, transported, and used every day. The 1984 Bhopal, India, disaster revealed the dangers posed by chemical agents. A 2008 U.S. Department of Health and Human Services database of 14 states reported more than 15,000 chemical-related events and over 4500 casualties.[1] Since World War I, chemical agents have also been used intentionally on civilian and military personnel, most recently in Japan in 1994-1995, in Russia in 2002 , and in Iraq in 2007. Of the 13 categories of chemical agents recognized by the U.S. Centers for Disease Control and Prevention, the four principal categories are nerve, vesicant, blood, and pulmonary agents[2] (**Box 137.1**).

Detonation of an atomic bomb over Hiroshima, Japan, in 1945 heralded the evolution of a new hazardous agent, radioactive material. Showcased by the 1987 accidental exposure of cesium 137 in Goiânia, Brazil, the threat from radiologic material has continued to increase with the proliferation of medical devices and radiation therapy. Though reduced by the end of the Cold War, the threat from nuclear agents continues to persist in light of the accidents at Chernobyl, Ukraine, in 1986 and Tokaimura, Japan, in 1997, as well as the acknowledgment that dozens of nuclear devices are missing.

Management of casualties from chemical and radioactive agents can be complicated by the types of agents and exposure, in addition to specialized logistic, safety, and security issues. Emergency physicians (EPs) must be familiar with the basic principles of managing contaminated patients and initial treatment of the principal chemical and radioactive agents.

## PERSPECTIVE

Casualties involving chemical and radiologic or nuclear agents have traditionally been associated with military armed conflicts. However, over the past 25 years, with the increased production and distribution of industrial chemicals, as well as the escalating threat of terrorist use of weapons of mass destruction, management of casualties from chemical, biologic, radiologic, nuclear, and high-yield explosive events has increasingly become the responsibility of the EP.[3]

Initially approved in 1999 and revised in 2006, the American College of Emergency Physicians (ACEP) issued a clinical policy statement that recognized the risk posed by accidental or intentional release of chemical and nuclear hazardous material (HAZMAT).[4] In another clinical policy statement, the ACEP also encouraged EPs to assume a primary role in the medical aspects of planning, management, and patient care during disasters, including those involving chemical, radiologic, and nuclear agents.[5]

## BASIC PRINCIPLES OF MANAGING CONTAMINATED PATIENTS

Management of casualties from chemical and radioactive agents can be complicated by one or more factors, such as the number of patients, type of agent or agents involved, severity of the exposure, and the availability of pharmaceutical and human resources. A current and accurate hazard vulnerability analysis is essential for an optimal response to a specific identified hazard. However, because no facility can prepare for every possible factor and scenario, adherence to several basic principles may facilitate effective management of contaminated patients.

### COMMUNICATION AND MOBILIZATION

Most events involving chemical or radioactive agents are rapidly identified by emergency services. Notification of health care facilities of a HAZMAT incident and casualties must also take place rapidly because 50% to 80% of the acute casualties will arrive at the closest health care facilities within 90 minutes following an event.[6] Some casualties may leave the scene under their own power and go to a nearby health care facility, even before other patients arrive via emergency medical services.[7,8]

**BOX 137.1 Categories of Chemical Agents**

| | |
|---|---|
| Biotoxins | Metals |
| Blister agents/vesicants | Nerve agents |
| Blood agents | Organic solvents |
| Caustics | Riot control agents |
| Choking/pulmonary agents | Toxic alcohols |
| Incapacitating agents | Vomiting agents |
| Long-acting anticoagulants | |

From U.S. Centers for Disease Control and Prevention. Chemical categories. Available at http://www.bt.cdc.gov/agent/agentlistchem-category.asp.

Concise and accurate communication of prehospital events is also crucial for an effective response. Collection of pertinent strategic details can guide mobilization of appropriate resources, including activation of an emergency management plan and the incident command system, consultation with material safety data sheets and HAZMAT experts, compilation of antidotes and medical equipment, and preparation of triage, decontamination, and personnel protection equipment.

### DECONTAMINATION

Decontamination should take place immediately, before initial treatment and evacuation of exposed patients. Although decontamination is usually completed at the scene before transportation, exposed and potentially contaminated patients may go on their own to nearby health care facilities.[9] In addition to requiring primary decontamination and triage, these patients may secondarily contaminate existing patients and medical personnel and thus create additional casualties and diminish the response by the affected facility.[7,9,10]

Removal of contaminated clothing can eliminate 70% to 90% of HAZMAT.[11,12] Once completed, patients should shower—or be showered if incapacitated—with copious amounts of tepid water. Several adjuncts, such as hypoallergenic liquid soap, may be helpful. Other adjuncts, including hard brushes and dilute additives such as bleach, are unlikely to provide additional benefit and, in some scenarios, could be harmful. Contaminated clothing and special items such as valuables and firearms should be labeled and securely contained to prevent accidental or continued secondary contamination, as well as for possible forensic analysis during a HAZMAT or criminal investigation.[12-16]

### SECURITY

Security personnel at health care facilities should be engaged promptly because their primary responsibility is to protect existing patients, staff, and the health care facility from contamination and distraction from avoidable crowds by controlling all access points to the facility. This responsibility may entail limiting visits from arriving friends, family, and other third parties, as well as sequestering contaminated patients.[17]

Security personnel should control traffic flow to and within the facility. Incoming patients should be directed to designated triage and decontamination sites, and the arrival of hospital personnel should be expedited. Patients awaiting further evaluation and disposition may be directed to secondary triage, holding, and treatment areas. Security personnel should coordinate with law enforcement and government agencies, safeguard valuables, and maintain the chain of custody of firearms and forensic evidence.[9,10,17]

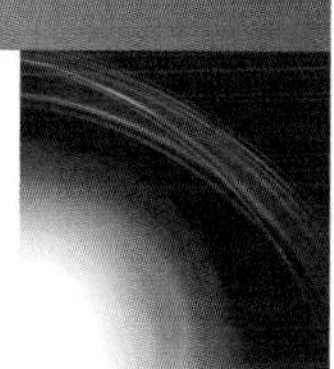

# Chemical Agents

## NERVE AGENTS

### PATHOPHYSIOLOGY

Nerve agents are potent anticholinesterases that can be divided into three categories: quaternary ammonium alcohols, carbamates, and organophosphates. Quaternary ammonium alcohols are used as disinfectants. Carbamates are found in household insecticides. Also in insecticides, some organophosphates have been designed for use as warfare agents. The G series consists of tabun (GA), sarin (GB), soman (GD), and cyclosarin (GF). The V series, which includes VE, VG, VM, and VX, was developed 20 years later and is more potent and persistent, which means that it is not removed as easily.

Absorbed through inhalation and skin contact, nerve agents irreversibly bind and inactivate acetylcholinesterase (AChE) receptors, thereby leading to excessive accumulation of acetylcholine and overstimulation of nicotinic and muscarinic receptors. Though dose dependent, the effects from inhalation begin within seconds and peak within minutes, whereas the effects from skin exposure may take minutes to hours to become evident.[18-20]

### PRESENTING SIGNS AND SYMPTOMS

The earliest symptoms from inhalation are rhinorrhea and dim vision secondary to miosis, and those from skin contact are anxiety and fasciculations. With greater exposure, the classic symptoms of a cholinergic crisis become apparent. Hyperactivity of muscarinic receptors leads to lacrimation and salivation, bronchoconstriction, and vomiting and diarrhea. Hyperactivity of nicotinic receptions produces diaphoresis, tachycardia, hypertension, and muscle weakness. With severe or prolonged exposure, end-organs fatigue and fail, and convulsions, incontinence, flaccid paralysis, and apnea ensue.

### TREATMENT

Atropine and pralidoxime chloride (2-PAM chloride) should be administered rapidly. When intubating patients, use of succinylcholine should be avoided. Atropine, a competitive cholinergic blocking agent, can mitigate muscarinic symptoms and should be administered every 5 to 10 minutes until

**Table 137.1 Initial Dosing of Medications After Exposure to Nerve Agents**

| POPULATION | ATROPINE | PRALIDOXIME | DIAZEPAM |
|---|---|---|---|
| Infants (<2 yr) | 0.05-0.1 mg/kg | 15-25 mg/kg | 0.2-0.5 mg/kg |
| Children (2-10 yr) | 1 mg | 15-50 mg/kg* | 0.2-0.5 mg/kg |
| Adolescents (11-17 yr) | 2-4 mg | 15-50 mg/kg* | 0.2-0.5 mg/kg |
| Adults | 2-4 mg | 600-1800 mg | 10 mg |
| Elderly | 1-4 mg | 10-25 mg/kg | 0.5 mg/kg |

From Davis D, Marcozzi D. Nerve agent attack. In: Ciottone GR, editor. Disaster medicine. 3rd ed. Philadelphia: Mosby; 2006; and Corvino TF, Nahata MC, Angelos MG, et al. Availability, stability, and sterility of pralidoxime for mass casualty use. Ann Emerg Med 2006;47:272-7.

*Maximum recommended dose of 2 g.

airway resistance is minimized and respiratory secretions have dried. Pediatric patients may receive 0.05 to 0.1 mg/kg, with a maximum dose of 1 mg. Adults can receive 2-mg doses, with total doses of 2 g having been reported anecdotally. 2-PAM chloride reactivates AChE. Pediatric patients may receive 15 mg/kg, whereas adults can receive 600-mg doses. With severe exposure, diazepam should be administered to reduce seizure activity and its sequelae[20-23] (**Table 137.1**).

# VESICANT AGENTS

## PATHOPHYSIOLOGY

Vesicating agents are highly penetrative oily substances that induce blister formation and include mustard agents and organic arsenicals. Mustard has a wide range of effects on the eyes, skin, lungs, nervous system, and bone marrow.[20] It has been produced and stockpiled by multiple countries.[24] Lewisite is an arsenical often combined with mustard, smells like geraniums, and is associated with renal failure and hepatic necrosis.

Absorbed through inhalation and topical contact, mustard agents are alkylating substances that damage DNA and nucleic acid synthesis. The mechanism of toxicity for lewisite is not known. Symptoms are dependent on the agent, as well as the severity and route of exposure. The effects of lewisite begin within seconds to minutes. DNA damage from mustard agents begins within minutes, but some symptoms may not be manifested for hours.

## PRESENTING SIGNS AND SYMPTOMS

For mustard agents, the earliest symptoms are irritation and burning of exposed areas, such as the eyes and upper airway. Subsequent symptoms include pruritus and erythema of the skin, especially warm, moist locations such as the axillae and groin. With higher doses or prolonged exposure, shortness of breath, bulla formation, and corneal damage develop. Vomiting, diarrhea, bone marrow suppression, and seizures are associated with severe exposure and imply a poor prognosis.[20,25,26]

Exposure to lewisite also produces eye, lung, and skin symptoms, which unlike those with mustard agents, begin immediately. With severe exposure, increased capillary permeability can lead to substantial loss of intravascular volume and end-organ damage.

## TREATMENT

Unless completed within minutes of exposure, decontamination will not prevent tissue and DNA damage. It can, however, reduce or prevent ongoing exposure and secondary contamination. Only lewisite has a specific antidote, the chelating agent British antilewisite (BAL). BAL can be toxic itself, may contain peanut oil, and thus should not be given to patients with peanut allergy.[20,27]

Additional treatment is primarily supportive. Eye injuries should be managed with lubrication and ophthalmologic antibiotics. Respiratory injuries may require oxygen, bronchodilators, and ventilatory support. Skin injuries should be treated similar to thermal burns, including wound care, tetanus prophylaxis, analgesia, and intravenous fluids. However, although fluid loss from mustard agents is less than that associated with thermal burns, lewisite casualties may require aggressive fluid replacement.

# BLOOD AGENTS

## PATHOPHYSIOLOGY

Blood agents include cyanide and arsenic-based chemicals. Absorbed through inhalation, ingestion, and topical exposure, blood agents disrupt the mitochondrial cytochrome oxidase complex, thereby inhibiting intracellular oxygen use and aerobic metabolism. Cyanide is the most well-known blood agent and is often associated with a pungent odor described as bitter almond. Cyanide is widely used in many industries, such as mining and plastic manufacturing, and can be released during the combustion of numerous natural and synthetic material. It has also been identified as a likely agent for use by terrorists.[20,28]

## PRESENTING SIGNS AND SYMPTOMS

The earliest symptoms begin within seconds to minutes and may include dyspnea, dizziness, nausea, and anxiety. With greater exposure, generalized weakness, diaphoresis, cyanosis, and hypotension may be observed, and with severe or prolonged exposure, dysrhythmias and seizures may progress rapidly to respiratory failure and death.

## TREATMENT

Treatment should be initiated immediately and presumptively based on prehospital information and clinical suspicion because diagnostic tests are not readily available. Traditionally, definitive treatment has been administration of the three components of the cyanide antidote kit: amyl nitrite, sodium nitrite, and sodium thiosulfate. Hydroxocobalamin, a precursor of vitamin $B_{12}$, has gained acceptance as another antidote because it can be used for prehospital management and has better safety and side effect profiles.[28-30]

# PULMONARY AGENTS

## PATHOPHYSIOLOGY

Pulmonary agents include phosgene and chlorine. Absorbed through inhalation and topical contact, pulmonary agents irritate and cause an inflammatory reaction of the peripheral and central airways. Phosgene is widely used in many industries, released during the combustion of foam plastics, and associated with the smell of newly cut grass. Chlorine is used widely in manufacturing and for purifying water and has its own distinctive odor. It was the first chemical warfare agent and has recently been involved in several large-scale disasters and terrorist attacks.[20,31]

## PRESENTING SIGNS AND SYMPTOMS

Symptoms begin within minutes and may start with eye irritation, rhinorrhea, coughing, and dyspnea. With greater exposure, skin irritation, vomiting, and shortness of breath may be observed, and with severe exposure, blistering and pulmonary edema may develop.[32]

## TREATMENT

Treatment is primarily supportive. Eye injuries should be managed with ophthalmologic antibiotics and follow-up. Skin injuries should be treated similar to thermal burns, including wound care, tetanus prophylaxis, and analgesia. Respiratory injuries may require oxygen, bronchodilators, and endotracheal intubation and ventilatory support. Corticosteroids are recommended, and nebulized lidocaine and sodium bicarbonate may be beneficial.[31]

# Radiologic and Nuclear Agents

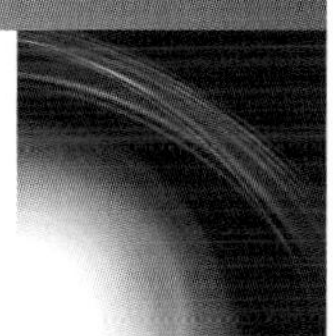

## PATHOPHYSIOLOGY

Radiation, regardless of type, causes injury through the production of charged water molecules and ionization of DNA. Because of its cellular effects, radiation can affect every organ, especially the hematopoietic, gastrointestinal, and central nervous systems.

Irradiation and external contamination by a radiologic agent may occur as a result of the surreptitious placement of a radiation emission device or detonation of a dirty bomb.[33,34] A dirty bomb involves the use of conventional explosives to disperse radioactive material, such as iodine 131. After decontamination, treatment of blast injuries should precede treatment of radiologic injuries because immediate death from the radiation is unlikely[35,36] (**Table 137.2**). If free of particulate matter and shrapnel, patients are unlikely to pose a significant threat to other patients and medical personnel.

**Table 137.2 Types of Blast Injuries**

| TYPE | MECHANISM | EXAMPLES/EFFECTS |
|---|---|---|
| Primary | Direct pressurization | Rupture of tympanic membranes, lungs, viscera |
| Secondary | Projectiles | Penetrating trauma from fragments |
| Tertiary | Secondary trauma | Structural collapse, being thrown by the blast wind |
| Quaternary | Other | Burns, radiation, hazardous materials |

From DePalma RG, Burris DG, Champion HR, et al. Blast injuries. N Engl J Med 2005;352:1335-42; and U.S. Department of Health and Human Services Radiation Emergency Medical Management. Available at http://www.remm.nlm.gov/nuclearexplosion.htm.

Irradiation and external contamination by a nuclear agent may occur during transportation of HAZMAT or a nuclear reactor accident. Though an unlikely scenario, detonation of a nuclear device would involve catastrophic levels of radiation.

## PRESENTING SIGNS AND SYMPTOMS

Within a few hours of exposure to greater than 1 Gy, three acute radiation syndromes may develop. Hematopoietic syndrome results in pancytopenia and a predisposition to infection, bleeding, and poor wound healing. Gastrointestinal syndrome results in abdominal cramping, vomiting, and diarrhea. Early intractable vomiting and bloody diarrhea imply a poor prognosis. Cerebrovascular syndrome results in confusion, ataxia, and seizures.[37]

## TREATMENT

After blast injuries and emergency medical conditions are treated, several radiation exposure–specific treatments should be discussed and initiated under the guidance of radiation safety, nuclear medicine, and hematology consultants. Any necessary surgeries should be performed within the first 24 to 36 hours before patients become immunologically incompetent. Cytokine therapy and the administration of chelating or blocking agents, such as potassium iodide and Prussian blue, should be considered.[37]

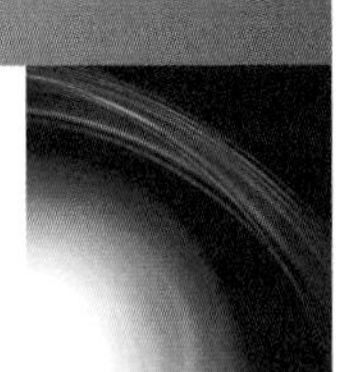

## Follow-Up, Next Steps in Care, and Patient Education

Patients with the mildest of exposure to a chemical or radiologic or nuclear agent may be eligible for discharge after confirmation of the agent and consultation with an appropriate HAZMAT expert. However, because the majority of chemical and radiologic or nuclear agents are associated with prolonged symptoms and delayed effects, most patients should be admitted. Patient disposition should also be coordinated with responding law enforcement and government agencies for possible interview during a HAZMAT or criminal investigation.

## SUGGESTED READINGS

Disaster Medical Services Clinical and Practice Management Policy Statement. American College of Emergency Physicians. October 2006. Available at http://www.acep.org/content.aspx?id=29176.

Koenig KL, Boatright CJ, Hancock JA, et al. Health care facility–based decontamination of victims exposed to chemical, biological, and radiological materials. Am J Emerg Med 2008;26:71-80.

Lawrence DG, Kirk MA. Chemical terrorism attacks: update on antidotes. Emerg Med Clin North Am 2007;25:567-95.

Wolbarst AB, Wiley Jr AL, Nemhauser JB, et al. Medical response to a major radiologic emergency: a primer for medical and public health practitioners. Radiology 2010;254:660-77.

## REFERENCES

***References can be found on Expert Consult @ www.expertconsult.com.***

# Mammalian Bites 138

*Ashley Booth Norse*

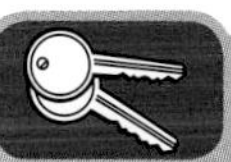

**KEY POINTS**

- Human bites, especially clenched-fist injuries (i.e., "fight bites") commonly cause septic joints, osteomyelitis, tenosynovitis, and fractures.
- Wound infections caused by human bites are usually polymicrobial.
- *Pasteurella* species are the most common organisms present in infected wounds from cat and dog bites.
- Injury to deeper structures should be suspected with all mammalian bites, and radiography should be considered to look for fractures, retained foreign bodies, gas in tissues, and osteomyelitis.

## EPIDEMIOLOGY

Two to 4 million cat, dog, and human bites are reported by the Centers for Disease Control and Prevention every year, as well as approximately 300,000 emergency department (ED) visits secondary to mammalian bites. The exact number of mammalian bites is difficult to determine because many cases are not reported. Although dog bites outnumber cat bites, 20% to 80% of cat bites become infected, whereas just 3% to 18% of dog bites will become infected.[1-4]

## PATHOPHYSIOLOGY

Wound infections from mammalian bites have a complicated microbiology profile. The majority of infections are polymicrobial with a mix of aerobic and anaerobic bacteria. Patients with acute cat bites (<24 hours from the time of the bite) most often have wound cultures that grow *Pasteurella* organisms, especially *Pasteurella multocida*. Patients with subacute cat bites (>24 hours) or who return to the ED more than 24 hours after initial treatment of an acute bite typically have cultures that grow mixed aerobic and anaerobic species, with *Pasteurella, Staphylococcus*, and *Streptococcus* species being the predominant pathogens. Other pathogens include the aerobe *Moraxella* and the anaerobes *Fusobacterium, Bacteroides*, and *Porphyromonas*.[2,3,5,6]

Dog bites are the most common mammalian bites seen in the ED. Dog bites tend to cause more damage, injure deeper structures, and crush tissues because of the animal's powerful jaws, which can exert a pressure of 200 to 450 psi when biting.[1] Damage to deeper structures is more common with police dogs.[2] Dogs trained specifically for guard duty or for fighting, such as pit bulls, rottweilers, German shepherds, and chows, tend to cause a disproportionate number of bites resulting in serious injury and death.[2]

Current research reveals that *Pasteurella* species are the most common organisms present in culture isolates from infected dog bite wounds, most frequently *Pasteurella canis*.[3] Other common aerobic pathogens in infected dog bite wounds include *Staphylococcus* and *Streptococcus* species.[2,3,5] Aerobes less frequently associated with cat and dog bite wound infections include *Moraxella* and *Neisseria*. Causative anaerobic organisms include *Fusobacterium, Bacteroides, Porphyromonas, Prevotella*, and *Capnocytophaga*. *Capnocytophaga canimorsus* causes an opportunistic infection that can result in severe infection and sepsis in immunocompromised patients. Mortality in patients with *C. canimorsus* infection approaches 30%.[3,6]

When compared with cat bite victims, patients with dog bites tend to be seen later after injury but have a lower infection rate. Conversely, patients whose injuries become infected secondary to cat bites tend to seek treatment earlier than those with infected dog bite wounds, at a mean time of 12 hours.[1] It is speculated that the infection rate is higher because wounds from cats are more likely to be punctures, involve the hand, and become infected with *Pasteurella* species.[1,2]

Human bites have long been associated with high rates of infection and complications such as septic joints, osteomyelitis, tenosynovitis, and fractures. However, recent studies show that human bites do not have a higher rate of infection than other bite wounds do.[1,2,5]

Human bites can be divided into two categories. The first category is referred to as occlusional bites, defined as intentional bites in which the teeth actually close down on the victim's skin. The second category is referred to as clenched-fist injuries (also called "fight bites"); these bites occur when the teeth hit or puncture the dorsum of the metacarpophalangeal region of a clenched hand. Clenched-fist injuries have a high propensity for causing injury to deep structures of the hand. Open fractures, joint involvement, and tendon injuries are common. Human bites to the hand, especially clenched-fist injuries, are at high risk for infection.[2,4,5]

**Table 138.1** Pathogens in Mammalian Bites

| MAMMALIAN BITE | <24 HOURS | >24 HOURS |
|---|---|---|
| Human | Polymicrobial: *Streptococcus* spp., 60-80% *Staphylococcus* spp., 37-46% Anaerobic spp., 44-60% (specifically *Eikenella corrodens*, 20-25%) | Mixed aerobic and anaerobic *Staphylococcus* spp., *Streptococcus* spp. |
| Cat | *Pasteurella* spp. | Mixed aerobic and anaerobic *Pasteurella* spp. *Staphylococcus* spp. *Streptococcus* spp. |
| Dog | *Pasteurella* spp. | Mixed aerobic and anaerobic *Pasteurella* spp. *Staphylococcus* spp. *Streptococcus* spp. |

Wound infections caused by human bites are usually polymicrobial. Streptococci are present in 60% to 80% of isolates. *Staphylococcus aureus* is found in 37% to 46% of isolates, and anaerobic species are present in 44% to 60% of isolates, specifically *Eikenella corrodens* (20% to 25%). Herpes simplex virus can also be transmitted through infected saliva and can cause herpetic whitlow, as well as wound infections (**Table 138.1**).[2]

## PRESENTING SIGNS AND SYMPTOMS

A thorough history should be obtained (**Fig. 138.1**), including the timing of the bite incident, the circumstances surrounding the bite, and whether a report was filed with animal control officials. If the victim knows the animal, it may be possible to ascertain the immunization status of the bite source and whether the animal is going to be quarantined to observe for signs of rabies. This information is especially important if the bite was unprovoked, if the animal was acting abnormally, or if the bite was caused by a wild animal. The patient's medical history (including a history of allergies, current medications, and immunization status) should also be obtained.

Patients with human bites, especially clenched-fist injuries, may not be forthcoming about how their injury occurred. If the wound is on the extensor surface of the metacarpophalangeal joint, the patient should be treated as though the wound is a human bite. In patients with human bites, it is important to ascertain the human immunodeficiency virus (HIV) and hepatitis status of both the patient and the attacker.

In major cases in which a patient suffers extensive injury, resuscitation from traumatic injury may be needed. Injury to deep structures, including major organs, and extensive blood loss are possible. It is usually apparent that a large animal has attacked the victim, but injuries from falls or other associated trauma can occasionally be occult. Disciplined, thorough evaluation of the patient's physical condition is warranted when associated injury may have occurred, especially since bite wounds draw the clinician's attention.

## DIFFERENTIAL DIAGNOSIS AND MEDICAL DECISION MAKING

Vital signs should be determined in all patients with bites because hypotension or tachycardia may be a sign of blood loss and fever may be a sign of infection. All bites mandate a full neurovascular examination, including a thorough motor and sensory examination distal to the bite, as well as evaluation of all the tendons and ligaments in the region of the bite. The physical examination should also include a thorough vascular examination and evaluation of any compartments involved.

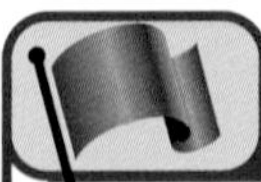

**RED FLAGS**

Emergency medical physicians must have a high level of suspicion with mammalian bites.

For clenched-fist injuries, a high index of suspicion should be maintained for tendon injuries, as well as for open fracture and open joints. The metacarpophalangeal joint and extensor tendons are covered by a thin layer of skin when the hand is clenched, and tendons can often retract proximally when the hand is unclenched and the fingers extended.

All bite wounds should undergo high-pressure irrigation of the wound with normal saline, dilute povidone-iodine solution, or poloxamer 188 (Shur-Clens).

Explore *all* wounds. Extend the margins of deep puncture wounds or small laceration so that all possible injured structures can be visualized if possible injury to deeper structures is suspected.

Radiography, angiography:

- If there is risk for a retained foreign body such as a tooth
- If there is risk for injury to deep structures such as a fracture
- If the patient has signs of infection (to look for retained foreign bodies, gas in tissues, and osteomyelitis)
- If a vascular injury is suspected, angiography may be needed to localize the injury or to determine the extent of the injury

## TREATMENT

All bite wounds should undergo high-pressure irrigation of the wound with normal saline, dilute (<1%) povidone-iodine solution, or poloxamer 188 (Shur-Clens) (**Table 138.2**). Recent studies have looked at the efficacy of tap water as an irrigation solution[2,7]; however, because no conclusive data exist at present for bite wounds, use of tap water as an irrigation solution for bite wounds cannot be supported at this time. Patients with larger or more complicated wounds may need to be anesthetized with lidocaine, bupivacaine, or another

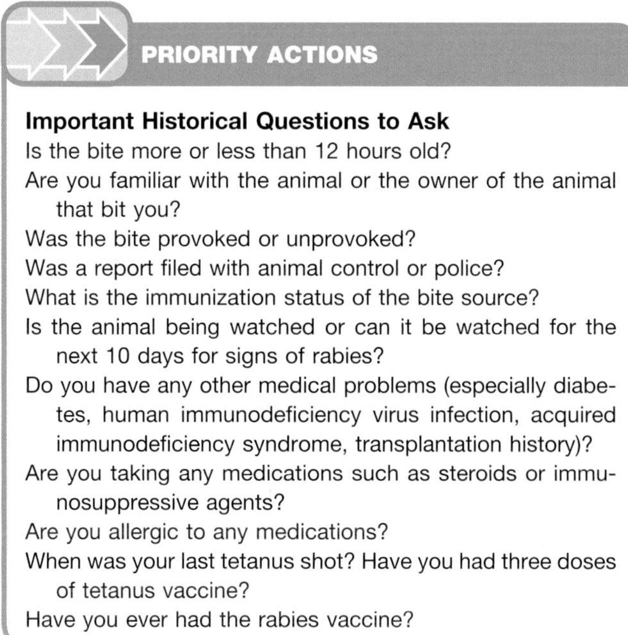
PRIORITY ACTIONS

**Important Historical Questions to Ask**

Is the bite more or less than 12 hours old?
Are you familiar with the animal or the owner of the animal that bit you?
Was the bite provoked or unprovoked?
Was a report filed with animal control or police?
What is the immunization status of the bite source?
Is the animal being watched or can it be watched for the next 10 days for signs of rabies?
Do you have any other medical problems (especially diabetes, human immunodeficiency virus infection, acquired immunodeficiency syndrome, transplantation history)?
Are you taking any medications such as steroids or immunosuppressive agents?
Are you allergic to any medications?
When was your last tetanus shot? Have you had three doses of tetanus vaccine?
Have you ever had the rabies vaccine?

anesthetic agent before irrigation and exploration of the wound. Epinephrine should be avoided if the bite involves the fingers, toes, nose, ears, or penis.[2]

All wounds should be explored for foreign bodies and injuries to deeper structures such as arteries, nerves, tendons, and ligaments. All tendons in the injured area should be isolated and tested through their full range of motion to assess for partial lacerations or tears, especially if the hands or feet are involved. Any devitalized tissue or ragged edges should be débrided.

There is no clear evidence whether suturing bite wounds increases the risk for infection, nor are there conclusive data on which wounds can safely be sutured. The safest course of action is to leave most bite wounds open and have the patient return for delayed primary closure if the wound does not become infected; however, primary closure may be necessary for cosmetic or functional reasons.

Recent studies show that the infection rate of sutured bite wounds may initially be lower in certain circumstances than historically predicted. Primary closure may be safe for simple bite wounds less than 6 hours old that involve the trunk and extremities (with the exception of the hands and feet) and for simple bite wounds involving the face and neck that are less than 12 hours old.[1,2]

The emergency physician should leave wounds open or consider closure by secondary intention for all infected wounds and all wounds at increased risk for infection, such as puncture wounds, hand and foot wounds, clenched-fist injuries, full-thickness wounds, wounds requiring débridement, wounds in patients older than 50 years or immunocompromised patients, wounds more than 12 hours old, and wounds involving damage to deep structures such as bones, joints, tendons, nerves, and blood vessels. Extremity wounds should be splinted and elevated.[2]

All patients sustaining mammalian (cat, dog, human, primate) bites should be given a dose of tetanus immune globulin and a dose of tetanus toxoid if they have never had

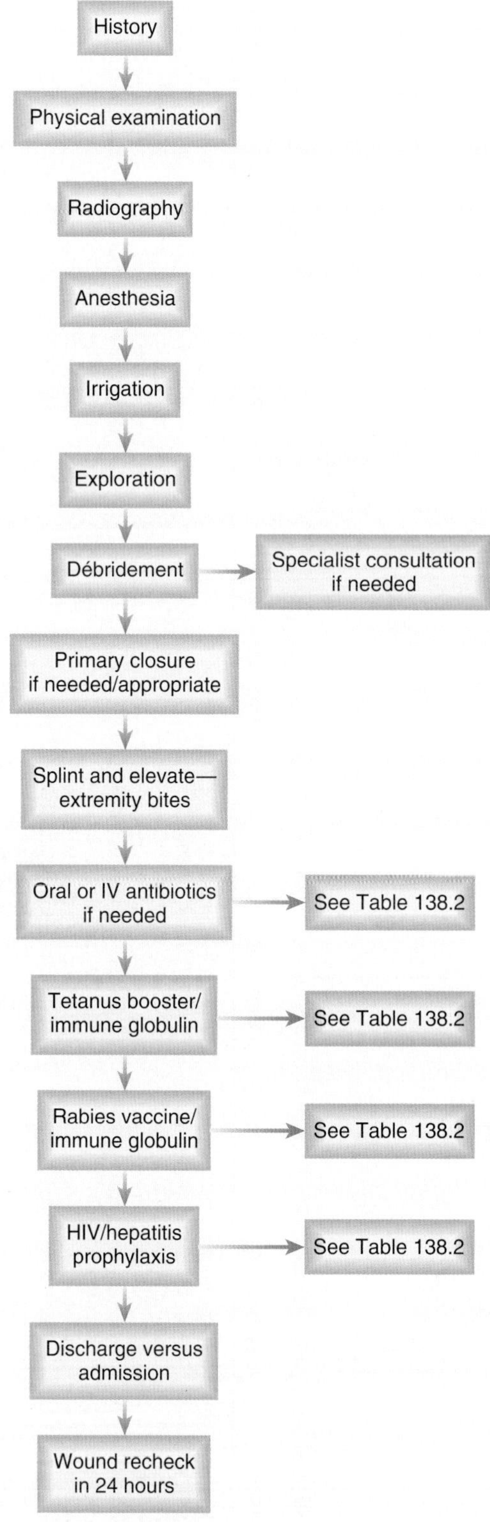


**Fig. 138.1 Algorithm for the management of human, cat, and dog bites.** *HIV*, Human immunodeficiency virus; *IV*, intravenous.

the tetanus vaccine series or if they have not had three doses of tetanus toxoid. Patients who have had a full course of the tetanus vaccine series should be given a tetanus toxoid booster of 0.5 mg intramuscularly if more than 5 years has elapsed since the previous tetanus booster.

**Table 138.2** Treatment of Mammalian Bites

| TYPE | WOUND CARE | ANTIBIOTIC PR. | TETANUS PR. | RABIES PR. | HIV PR. | HEPATITIS PR. |
|---|---|---|---|---|---|---|
| Human | High-pressure irrigation of the wound with normal saline or dilute (<1%) povidone-iodine solution; débride devitalized tissue or ragged edges | Amoxicillin-clavulanate, second-generation cephalosporin with anaerobic activity, penicillin plus dicloxacillin, clindamycin plus ciprofloxacin or trimethoprim-sulfamethoxazole | Tetanus immunoglobulin (250 units IM) and tetanus toxoid (0.5 mg IM) if never had a tetanus vaccine or have not had 3 doses of tetanus toxoid; tetanus toxoid (0.5 mg IM) if >5 yr since previous tetanus booster | None | HAART therapy started within the first 48-72 hr and continued for 28 days or bite source tested HIV negative; refer to the hospital for the specific drugs used in HAART therapy | HBIG (0.06 mL/kg IM); HBV given at separate site from HBIG |
| Cat | High-pressure irrigation of the wound with normal saline or dilute (<1%) povidone-iodine solution; débride devitalized tissue or ragged edges | Amoxicillin-clavulanate, second-generation cephalosporin with anaerobic activity, penicillin plus a first-generation cephalosporin, clindamycin plus a fluoroquinolone or trimethoprim-sulfamethoxazole | Tetanus immune globulin (250 units IM) and tetanus toxoid (0.5 mg IM) if never had a tetanus vaccine or have not had 3 doses of tetanus toxoid; tetanus toxoid (0.5 mg IM) if >5 yr since previous tetanus booster | HRIG (20 IU/kg) injected IM and/or around the bite site; rabies vaccine (1 mL IM) given in the deltoid in adults and in the thigh in children, on days 0, 3, 7, 14, and 28 | None | None |
| Dog | High-pressure irrigation of the wound with normal saline or dilute (<1%) povidone-iodine solution; débride devitalized tissue or ragged edges | Amoxicillin-clavulanate, second-generation cephalosporin with anaerobic activity, penicillin plus a first-generation cephalosporin, clindamycin plus a fluoroquinolone or trimethoprim-sulfamethoxazole | Tetanus immune globulin (250 units IM) and tetanus toxoid (0.5 mg IM) if never had a tetanus vaccine or have not had 3 doses of tetanus toxoid; tetanus toxoid (0.5 mg IM) if >5 yr since previous tetanus booster | HRIG (20 IU/kg) injected IM and/or around the bite site; rabies vaccine (1 mL IM) given in the deltoid in adults and in the thigh in children, on days 0, 3, 7, 14, and 28 | None | None |

*HAART*, Highly active antiretroviral therapy; *HBIG*, hepatitis B immune globulin; *HBV*, hepatitis B vaccine; *HIV*, human immunodeficiency virus; *HRIG*, human rabies immune globulin; *IM*, intramuscularly; *Pr.*, prophylaxis.

Patients who sustain dog, cat, or other animal bites should be evaluated for the potential need for rabies vaccination (see Chapter 179). Patients who sustain high-risk bites in which the animal cannot be quarantined should receive 20 IU/kg of human rabies immunoglobulin (HRIG) injected around the bite site or intramuscularly (or both) and 1 mL of rabies vaccine administered intramuscularly either in the deltoid in adults or in the thigh in children on days 0, 3, 7, 14, and 28. HRIG and rabies vaccine should be injected at separate sites if both are administered intramuscularly.[8]

Transmission of HIV and hepatitis B and C virus in human bites has been reported.[9] Patients who sustain human bites need to be evaluated and counseled about HIV and hepatitis B postexposure prophylaxis (PEP) (PEP for hepatitis C does not exist). HIV PEP should be started as soon as possible within the first 48 to 72 hours after a high-risk bite and continued for 28 days. High-risk bites are those in which the assailant is known to be HIV or hepatitis positive (or both) and bites in which blood exposure is involved. Hepatitis B PEP should include hepatitis B immune globulin (HBIG) and hepatitis B vaccine (HBV) if the patient has not previously been immunized. If the patient had previously received the hepatitis B vaccination series, a titer for anti-HBV should be drawn. If the patient has hepatitis B antibodies, no treatment is needed; if there are insufficient antibodies (anti-HBV < 10 mIU/mL), the patient needs HBIG and an HBV booster.[9]

Clinical evidence is limited on which cat and dog bites should receive prophylactic antibiotics. Cat bites—especially puncture wounds, wounds involving the hand and feet, wounds involving deeper structures, wounds in immunocompromised patients, and wounds closed primarily—are considered high-risk bites, and the patient should receive prophylactic antibiotics. Prophylactic antibiotics for cat and dog bites, specifically those seen within the first 24 hours, should cover *Pasteurella, Staphylococcus, Streptococcus*, and anaerobic species. Options include amoxicillin-clavulanate, a second-generation cephalosporin with anaerobic activity, and penicillin plus a first-generation cephalosporin. Clindamycin plus a fluoroquinolone or trimethoprim-sulfamethoxazole may be used in penicillin-allergic patients. Doxycycline plus metronidazole can also be used in penicillin-allergic patients.

Human bites are also considered high-risk bites. Prophylactic antibiotics should be considered for bites extending through the dermis, bites closed primarily, bites with significant crush injury or requiring considerable débridement, puncture wounds, bites in elderly or immunocompromised patients, and bites that involve the hands, feet, or deeper structures. Human bite prophylaxis should cover *Staphylococcus, Streptococcus*, and anaerobes, including *E. corrodens*. Amoxicillin-clavulanate or penicillin plus dicloxacillin may be used. Clindamycin plus ciprofloxacin or trimethoprim-sulfamethoxazole may be used in penicillin-allergic patients.

## FOLLOW-UP, NEXT STEPS IN CARE, AND PATIENT EDUCATION

Wounds with significant tissue loss may need plastic surgery or hand surgery consultation for skin grafting, depending on the location of the bite. Specialty consultation is also mandated for any hand or foot wound that involves a joint, tendon, artery, or nerve. Most patients can be discharged home safely with follow-up or recheck in the ED, or both.

## SUGGESTED READINGS

Broder J, Jerrard D, Olshaker J, et al. Low risk of infection in selected human bites treated without antibiotics. Am J Emerg Med 2004;22:10-3.

Eilbert W. Dog, cat and human bites: providing safe and cost-effective treatment in the ED. Emerg Med Pract 2003;5:1-20.

Griego R, Rosen T, Orengo IF, et al. Dog, cat and human bites: a review. J Am Acad Dermatol 1995;33:1019-29.

Oehler R, Velez A, Mizrachi M, et al. Bite-related and septic syndromes caused by cats and dogs. Lancet 2009;9:439-47.

## REFERENCES

***References can be found on Expert Consult @ www.expertconsult.com.***

# 139 Venomous Snakebites in North America

Robert L. Norris

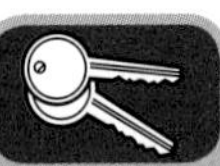

**KEY POINTS**

- Mortality following venomous snakebites in the United States is less than 1%, especially when patients are treated with antivenom.
- Permanent local sequelae following pit viper bites occur in at least 10% of patients.
- No field management (first aid) measure has been proved to be effective for pit viper bites other than expeditious transport to definitive medical care.
- The key to management of a venomous snakebite is judicious and timely use of antivenom.
- Hypotensive victims of snakebite are treated with antivenom and intravenous fluids; vasopressors are a last resort.
- All patients with a suspected venomous snakebite who have any signs or symptoms of envenomation are admitted to the hospital.
- Fasciotomy is rarely needed following pit viper bites and is performed only in the setting of objectively documented compartment syndrome.

## PERSPECTIVE

The two families of dangerously venomous snakes in North America are the pit vipers (family Crotalidae, subfamily Crotalinae) and the elapids (family Elapidae). Pit vipers found in the United States are the rattlesnakes (genera *Crotalus* and *Sistrurus*), cottonmouth water moccasins *(Agkistrodon piscivorus),* and copperheads *(Agkistrodon contortrix).* Mexico has a number of species of rattlesnakes and other genera of pit vipers (e.g., *Bothrops, Bothriechis, Porthidium*). The only indigenous elapids in North America are the coral snakes, which are found in the southern and southwestern part of the United States and Mexico. The coral snakes of the United States belong to two different genera—*Micrurus* (the eastern coral snake *Micrurus fulvius* and the Texas coral snake *Micrurus tener*) and *Micruroides* (the Sonoran coral snake *Micruroides euryxanthus*). Sixteen species of coral snakes are found in Mexico.[1]

## EPIDEMIOLOGY

Pit vipers inflict approximately 99% of the 7000 to 8000 venomous snakebites that occur in the United States each year.[2,3] The incidence of venomous snakebite is lower in Canada and higher in Mexico, although precise numbers are hard to determine.

## PATHOPHYSIOLOGY

Snake venom, particularly pit viper venom, is a complex mixture of enzymes, low-molecular-weight (nonenzymatic) proteins, metallic ions, and other constituents.[4,5] The venom is highly variable, depending on the species of snake; its geographic origin; its age, health, and diet; and the time of year.[6] Among the most important components found in pit viper venom are phospholipase $A_2$ enzymes, which cause cellular disruption and tissue damage; hyaluronidase, which facilitates the distribution of venom within tissues; and thrombin-like enzymes, which affect various aspects of the coagulation cascade and lead to coagulation abnormalities.

Also of major importance in pit viper venom–induced coagulopathy are metalloproteinases known as hemorrhagins, which increase vascular permeability and damage endothelial cells.[7,8] Some rattlesnakes, such as certain specimens of Mohave rattlesnakes *(Crotalus scutulatus),* possess neurotoxic components in their venom. These presynaptically acting toxins prevent the release of acetylcholine at neuromuscular junctions. Depending on their geographic location, Mohave rattlesnakes may possess this component and are termed venom A–producing rattlesnakes.[9,10]

Other rattlesnakes that may, based on their geographic origin, possess neurotoxic components closely related to Mohave toxin include the eastern diamondback rattlesnake *(Crotalus adamanteus)*, the timber rattlesnake *(Crotalus horridus),* the southern Pacific rattlesnake *(Crotalus oreganus helleri),* and the tiger rattlesnake *(Crotalus tigris).*[11-15]

Coral snake venom is less complex than pit viper venom but is among the most toxic venom in North America. The primary effects of coral snake venom are neurotoxic and are due to a component in the venom that blocks the postsynaptic end plates at neuromuscular junctions.[16,17]

## ANATOMY

Pit vipers get their name from the sensitive heat receptors (foveal organs) located on the anterior of their heads, slightly below and between the nostril and eye (**Fig. 139.1**). These organs aid the snake in finding prey, aiming its strike, and determining the volume of venom to be injected. Other characteristics typical of a pit viper include a triangular-shaped head (also found in many nonvenomous snakes), elliptical (catlike) pupils, and in the United States, the presence of a single row of scales that spans the underside of its tail (**Fig. 139.2**). Nonvenomous snakes in the United States generally have a double row of scales crossing the ventral aspect of the tail. Rattlesnakes can also usually be identified by the keratin plates that make up their unique caudal rattle.

Pit vipers range in size from the diminutive pygmy rattlesnake *(Sistrurus miliarius)*, typically 40 to 50 cm in length, to the massive eastern diamondback rattlesnake *(C. adamanteus)*, which can attain lengths of greater than 1.5 m (**Fig. 139.3**).[18]

Coral snakes are identified in the United States by their characteristic color pattern—red, yellow, and black bands that completely encircle the body, with the red and yellow bands

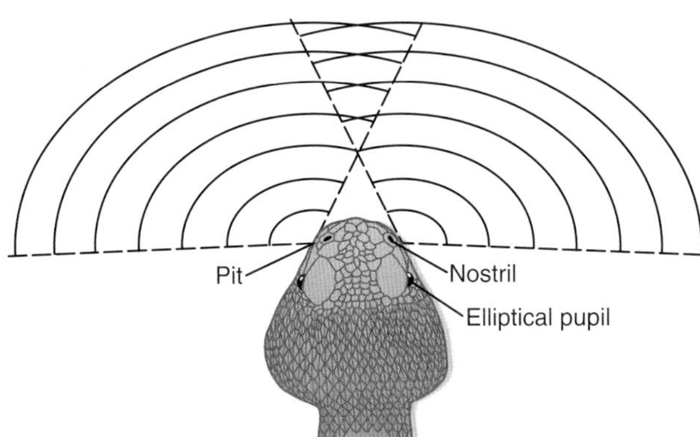


**Fig. 139.1 The heat-sensing pits or foveal organs of pit vipers.** (Adapted from original drawing by Marlin Sawyer. With permission.)

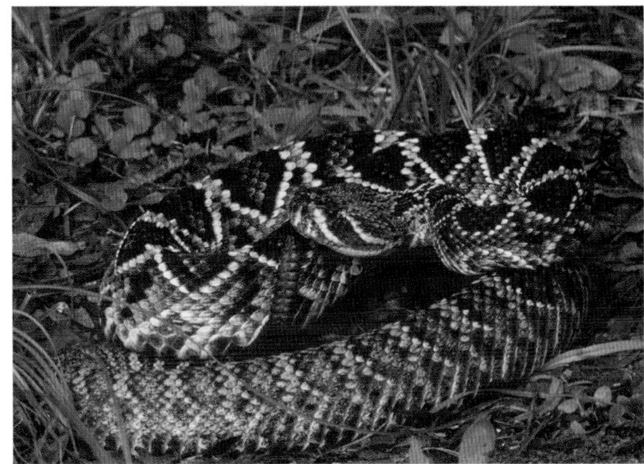

**Fig. 139.3** The eastern diamondback rattlesnake (*Crotalus adamanteus*), found in the southeastern United States, is the largest of the rattlesnakes in North America. (Courtesy Michael Cardwell, Extreme Wildlife Photography.)

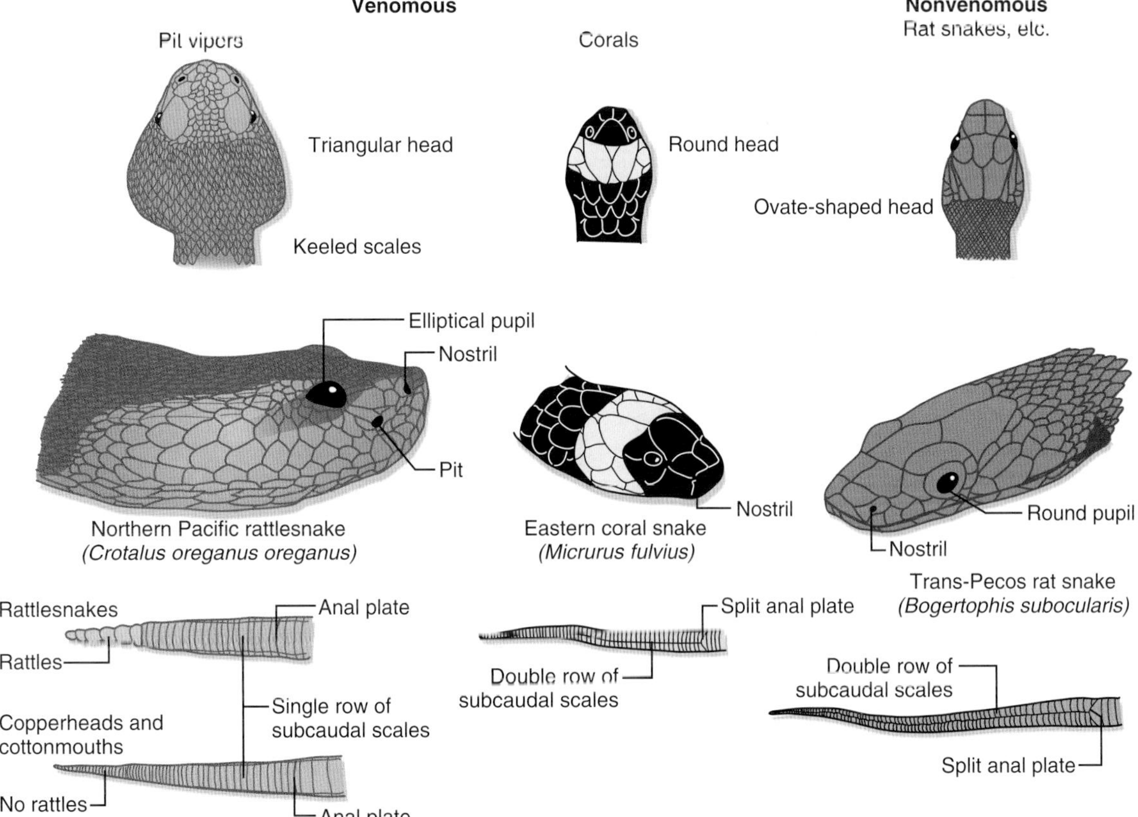


**Fig. 139.2 Anatomic comparison of pit vipers, coral snakes, and nonvenomous snakes of the United States.** Pit vipers have a triangular-shaped head, elliptical pupils, heat-sensing pits, and a single row of subcaudal scales on the ventral aspect of the tail. Coral snakes are identified by their color pattern (see Fig. 139.4) because they have round pupils and a single row of subcaudal scales, as do most harmless snakes in the United States. (Adapted from original drawing by Marlin Sawyer. With permission.)

being contiguous. In harmless coral snake mimics, such as milk snakes (*Lampropeltis* spp.), the red and yellow bands are separated by a band of black (**Fig. 139.4**). Color patterns cannot, however, be used outside the United States to reliably identify coral snakes.

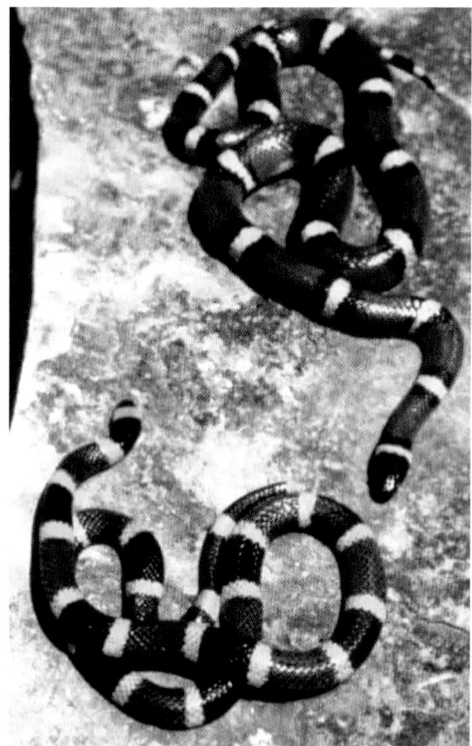

**Fig. 139.4** Venomous coral snakes in the United States can be identified by their color pattern, with the red and yellow bands being contiguous (*bottom,* the Texas coral snake, *Micrurus tener*). Harmless mimics such as the milk snake (*top,* the Mexican milk snake, *Lampropeltis triangulum annulata*) have red and yellow bands separated by black bands. (Courtesy Charles Alfaro.)

Venomous snakes possess venom-producing glands in the upper jaw, behind the eyes (**Fig. 139.5**). These glands produce the venom that at the time of a bite is passed via ducts to the hollow, needle-like fangs on the anterior maxillae. In pit vipers, these fangs range in length (proportional to the snake's overall length) from just a few millimeters to more than 2.5 cm.[18] The fangs are folded up against the roof of the snake's mouth when not in use. During a bite, the pit viper opens its mouth widely and swings its fangs into an upright position to drive them into the tissues of its target. Venom is then injected via a set of investing musculature. The speed of a pit viper's strike has been clocked at 8 feet per second[19]—faster than a human being can react.

The venom delivery apparatus of a coral snake is less sophisticated than that of a pit viper. Coral snakes have slightly enlarged, anterior, maxillary fangs fixed in an erect position, with which they inject venom (**Fig. 139.6**). For a coral snake to produce envenomation, it must chew on its victim for a few seconds. Bites by coral snakes frequently involve someone

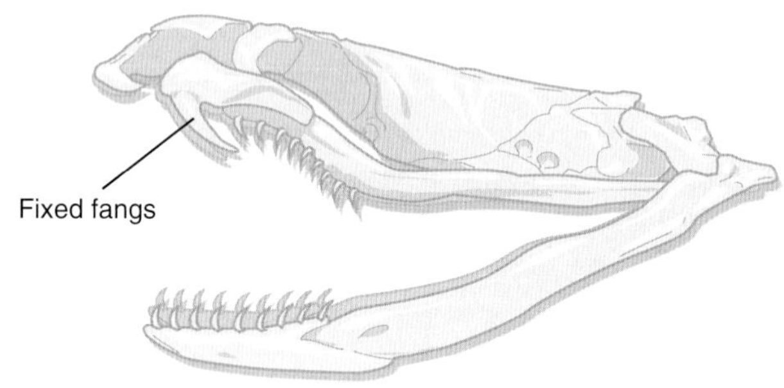


**Fig. 139.6 Coral snake skull demonstrating the smaller fixed anterior maxillary fangs of these reptiles.** (Adapted from original drawing by Marlin Sawyer. With permission.)

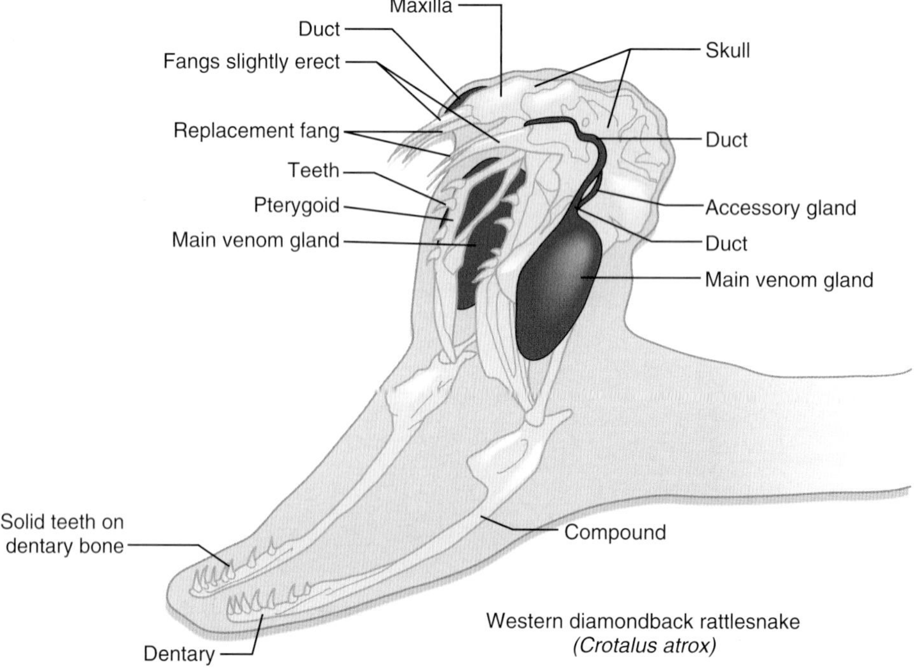


**Fig. 139.5 The venom apparatus of pit vipers.** (Adapted from original drawing by Marlin Sawyer. With permission.)

intentionally picking the snake up, often after misidentifying it as a harmless snake.[20]

## PRESENTING SIGNS AND SYMPTOMS

The signs and symptoms of pit viper envenomation are broken down into local and systemic findings. Locally, the victim will have puncture wounds, although the pattern may be misleading and cannot be used to reliably differentiate between a venomous bite and a bite by a harmless snake. Generally, severe, burning pain develops at the bite site within minutes, followed shortly by local swelling that can progress over time to involve the entire bitten extremity and even the trunk. There may be persistent bloody oozing from the fang marks, indicative of coagulopathy. Ecchymosis may be present at the site and, more remotely, as hemorrhagins induce vascular leaks and loss of red blood cells, in tissues (**Fig. 139.7**). Over several hours to days, blisters and blebs may form on the extremity, particularly at the bite site. These lesions are filled with clear serous fluid or bloody exudate.

Systemically, victims have a myriad of complaints, which can include nausea, vomiting, and dizziness; numbness of the mouth, tongue, or extremities; muscle fasciculations (myokymia); and shortness of breath. The victim's vital signs may be abnormal. Patients with severe bites may be tachycardic and hypotensive.

In the early stages, hypotension is due to systemic vasodilation. Later, the hypotension is compounded by third spacing of fluids into the bitten extremity and potentially hemolysis.[19] Some pit vipers, such as venom A–producing Mohave rattlesnakes, may produce few local signs and symptoms but may cause more systemic toxicity, particularly neurotoxic findings such as ptosis and difficulty swallowing and breathing.

Bites by a coral snake generally cause little in the way of local findings, and their fang marks may be difficult to see.[21] Swelling is usually slight and pain is variable (mild to more pronounced). Victims of significant bites by a coral snake may have a delay in the onset of systemic findings, sometimes for many hours.[22] Signs of neurotoxicity may then develop, with the earliest findings being altered mental status and cranial nerve dysfunction (e.g., ptosis). Neurotoxicity can progress to frank skeletal muscle paralysis and respiratory failure.

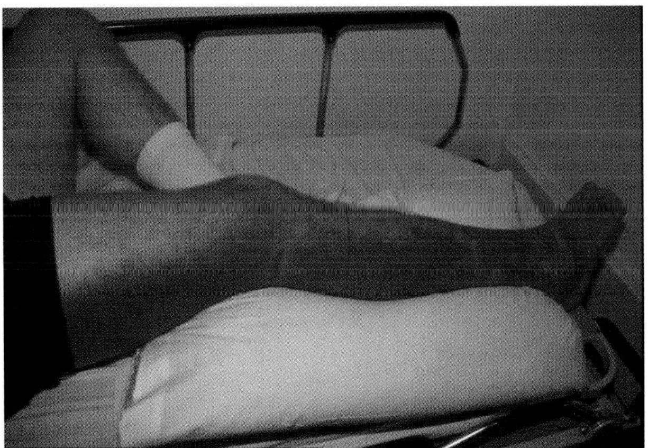

**Fig. 139.7 Extensive ecchymosis several days after a bite by a northern Pacific rattlesnake *(Crotalus oreganus oreganus)* on the victim's pretibial region.** (Photo © Dr. Robert L. Norris.)

## DIFFERENTIAL DIAGNOSIS AND MEDICAL DECISION MAKING

The differential diagnosis in a snakebite victim is generally limited. Most often the victim can recount being bitten by a snake. On rare occasion the victim may not have seen a snake, as when walking through high grass when bitten. In such cases, the presence of at least one puncture wound and progression of local and systemic findings are usually diagnostic. If the victim saw the snake but cannot adequately describe it, careful observation over time will reveal whether envenomation has occurred. Having color photographs on hand of the snakes found locally can aid in proper identification of the offending reptile.

Victims bitten by a coral snake almost always see the snake because of its need to actually chew on them to produce a significant bite. When a coral snake is implicated, the difficulty may be in differentiating the snake as a true coral snake versus a harmless coral snake mimic. Here again, color photos may help if the victim can recall the color pattern of the animal. All victims of a potential bite by a coral snake are observed carefully for at least 24 hours in the hospital because of the possible delay in onset of toxicity.

Young children have no innate fear of snakes and may be unable to describe precisely what bit them, particularly if they are preverbal. All children with possible venomous snakebites are admitted to the hospital for monitoring for at least 24 hours.

## DIAGNOSTIC TESTING

In the initial phase of evaluating a victim of a potential pit viper bite, a complete blood count and coagulation studies are repeated every 1 to 2 hours as long as the findings are normal (**Table 139.1**). If an abnormality appears (e.g., diminished platelets or fibrinogen), antivenom should be administered (see later) and laboratory tests rechecked every 6 hours thereafter until stable. This 6-hour period after antivenom administration is necessary for a healthy liver to replete coagulation factors.

## TREATMENT

### PREHOSPITAL MANAGEMENT

Field management focuses on providing reassurance and rapid transport to a facility equipped with antivenom. If possible to do so safely, the snake is identified. No attempt should be made to capture or kill the snake, although it may be possible to photograph the animal if a digital camera is available.

No first aid measures have ever been proved to be beneficial in victims of pit viper bites. For victims bitten by a coral snake, the Australian pressure-immobilization technique is applied quickly in the field to limit the spread of venom. This involves wrapping the entire bitten extremity snugly in an occlusive wrap followed by the application of a splint (**Fig. 139.8**). Victims must then be carried from the field for the

**Table 139.1 Diagnostic Testing in Victims of a Potential Venomous Snakebite in North America**

| DIAGNOSTIC STUDY | VENOM EFFECTS | COMMENTS |
|---|---|---|
| **Potential Pit Viper Bite** | | |
| Complete blood count | | |
| White blood cell count | May be elevated without evidence of infection | Caused by stress demargination |
| Hemoglobin/ hematocrit | Variable; may be normal, elevated, or decreased | May be elevated if dehydrated, may be low if bleeding or hemolysis is present |
| Platelets | May be low or very low | May see early profound thrombocytopenia |
| Metabolic panel | | |
| Renal function tests | Usually normal | May be abnormal if delayed renal dysfunction occurs |
| Hepatic function tests | Usually normal | May be abnormal with delayed hepatic dysfunction or underlying liver disease (e.g., alcohol abuse) |
| Coagulation studies | | |
| PT, APTT, INR | May be elevated | Abnormalities related to consumptive coagulopathy |
| Fibrinogen | May be reduced | |
| Fibrin degradation products | May be elevated | |
| D-dimer | May be elevated | |
| Type and screen | Venom effects and antivenom can interfere with this process[23] | Obtain on first available blood drawn; blood product replacement is rarely necessary, however |
| Blood gases (arterial or venous) | May demonstrate metabolic acidosis or hypoxia, depending on the clinical scenario | Consider in cases of severe envenomation (hypotension, shock, respiratory distress) or if significant underlying comorbidity; use caution in those with coagulopathy |
| Urinalysis | Hematuria, proteinuria | Test each voided sample until the patient is stable; positive blood on bedside testing in the absence of red blood cells on microscopic analysis may indicate myoglobinuria |
| Electrocardiogram | Variable; possible ischemia | Obtain in cases of severe envenomation or in patients with significant underlying comorbidity |
| Chest radiograph | Pulmonary edema, aspiration | Obtain in cases of severe envenomation or in patients with significant underlying comorbidity |
| Computed tomography | Variable | May be indicated if evidence of intracranial, intraabdominal, or retroperitoneal bleeding in patients with consumptive coagulopathy (based on clinical findings) |
| **Potential Coral Snake Bite** | | |
| Complete blood count | | |
| White blood cell count | May be elevated without evidence of infection | Caused by stress demargination |
| Hemoglobin/ hematocrit | Normal | |
| Platelets | Normal | |
| Metabolic panel | | |
| Renal function tests | Normal | |
| Hepatic function tests | Normal | May be abnormal if underlying liver disease (e.g., alcohol abuse) |

**Table 139.1 Diagnostic Testing in Victims of a Potential Venomous Snakebite in North America—cont'd**

| DIAGNOSTIC STUDY | VENOM EFFECTS | COMMENTS |
|---|---|---|
| **Potential Coral Snake Bite—cont'd** | | |
| Coagulation studies | All normal | |
| Type and screen | | Unnecessary (no need for blood products) |
| Blood gases (arterial or venous) | May demonstrate hypoxia and/or hypercapnia in the presence of respiratory insufficiency as a result of neurotoxicity | Consider in cases of severe envenomation (hypotension, shock, respiratory distress) or if significant underlying comorbidity is present |
| Urinalysis | Normal | |
| Electrocardiogram | Variable; possible ischemia | Obtain in cases of severe envenomation or in patients with significant underlying comorbidity |
| Chest radiograph | Usually normal; possible aspiration | Obtain in cases of severe envenomation or in patients requiring endotracheal intubation |
| Bedside pulmonary function testing | Variable; may reveal lowered peak flow in early respiratory embarrassment | May use to monitor respiratory status (at first sign of diminished flow, consider early airway control and assisted ventilation) |

*APTT*, Activated partial thromboplastin time; *INR*, international normalized ratio; *PT*, prothrombin time

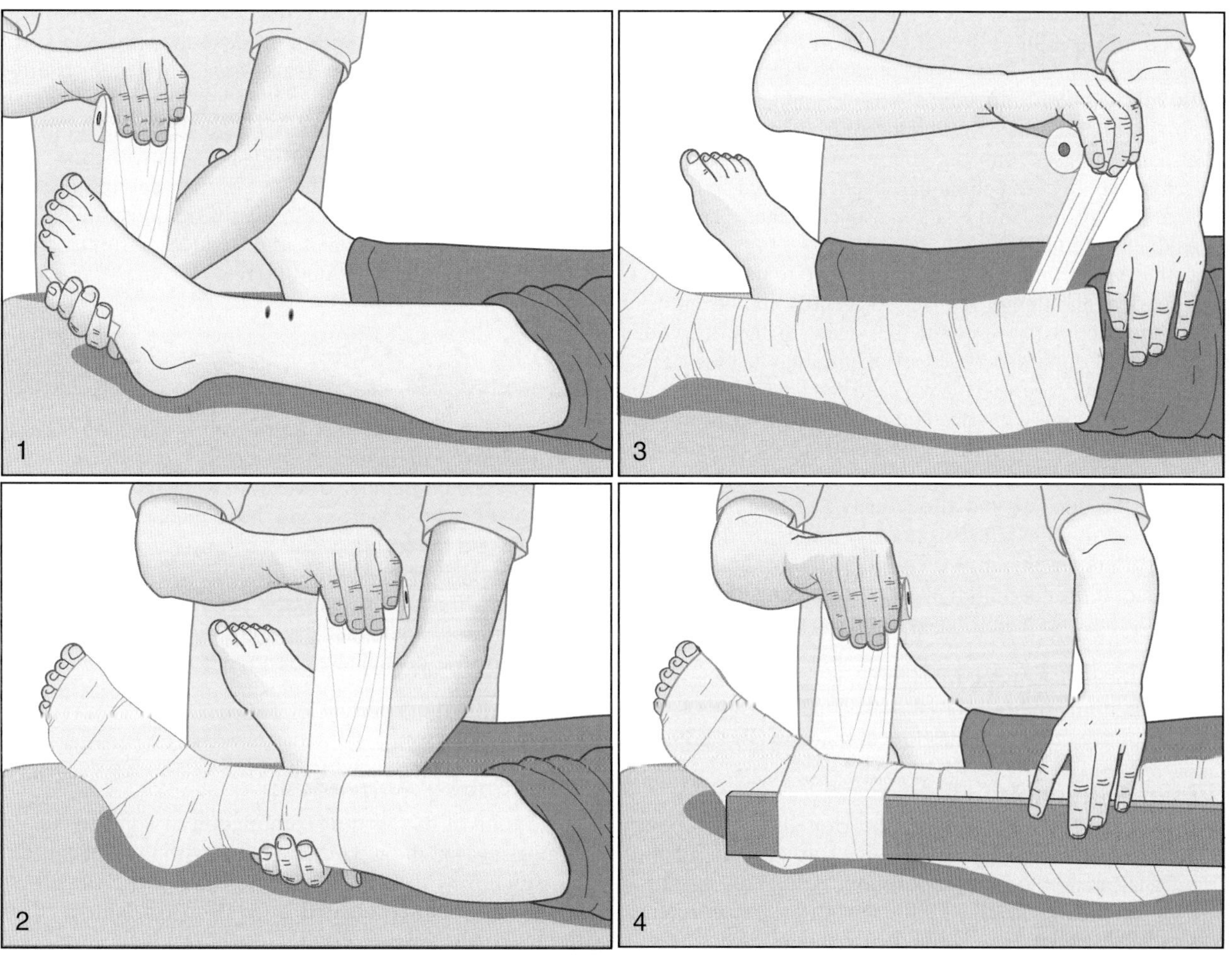


**Fig. 139.8 Australian pressure-immobilization technique for field management of nonnecrotizing elapid snakebites (e.g., coral snakes).** (Adapted from original drawing by Commonwealth Serum Laboratories. With permission.)

technique to be effective.[24] Rescuers may have difficulty applying the technique in correct fashion in that they tend to underestimate the degree of pressure that needs to be exerted under the wrap.[25] The pressure-immobilization technique has been shown to significantly limit the spread of venom after elapid snakebites[26] and was effective in one small animal study using eastern coral snake *(M. fulvius)* venom.[27] Although the pressure-immobilization technique may limit the spread of pit viper venom as well, it may actually exacerbate local tissue damage by restricting tissue-destroying venom to the bite site, and it should not be used for such bites.

## HOSPITAL MANAGEMENT

Hospital management of snakebite victims begins with assessment of respiratory and circulatory status. The patient is initially administered oxygen, and cardiac and pulse oximetry monitoring is begun while the emergency physician takes a directed history and performs a focused physical examination. It is uncommon for snakebite victims in North America to initially be seen with significant respiratory compromise. In patients bitten by coral snakes or rattlesnakes with neurotoxic venom, however, difficulty with airway patency and breathing can develop.

If signs of neurotoxicity are presence and any shortness of breath or difficulty speaking or swallowing develops, the airway should be promptly and definitively secured by endotracheal intubation to prevent aspiration. If the victim shows any signs of dehydration or shock, fluid resuscitation is begun with the administration of 1 to 2 L of normal saline (20 to 40 mL/kg for children). If the blood pressure does not respond promptly to crystalloid infusion, albumin is added because it may remain in the leaky vasculature for a longer period. Vasopressors are used only as a last resort after adequate intravascular volume repletion has been achieved.[28] Inadequately treated hypotension is a key aspect in many cases of fatal snake envenomation.[29,30]

Once the ABCs (airway, breathing, and circulation) have been addressed, an attempt is made to identify the offending snake. If the victim has brought the snake to the hospital, extreme caution should be used in examining it, even if it appears to be dead. A severed snake head can have a bite reflex for up to an hour following death and is capable of inflicting a serious bite.[31-33]

Circumferences of the bitten extremity are marked and measured at the bite site and at one or two sites more proximally every 15 minutes during the early stages of envenomation. This offers an objective measure of the progression of local swelling. If the circumferences are increasing, the envenomation is progressing and administration of antivenom is indicated.

The key to management of significant envenomation is antivenom administration. Initial decisions on antivenom administration are guided by the clinical findings (**Box 139.1**).

**BOX 139.1 Indications for Antivenom Administration for Venomous Snakebites in North America**

**Pit Viper Bite**

Progressive evidence of local envenomation (e.g., worsening local swelling)

*or*

Any evidence of systemic envenomation—i.e., systemic signs or symptoms (e.g., nausea or vomiting, abnormal taste, numbness or tingling, tachycardia, hypotension)

*or*

Laboratory abnormalities (e.g., low platelet count, evidence of coagulopathy)

**Coral Snake Bite**

Assuming that an appropriate antivenom can be located and obtained, administration should begin as soon as possible, including administration to an asymptomatic victim with a definite effective coral snake bite (see text)

### *Pit Viper Antivenom*

The current antivenom available in the United States for pit viper bites, Crotalidae polyvalent immune Fab, ovine (CroFab; BTG International, Inc., West Conshohocken, PA), is produced by immunizing sheep with the venom of four different pit vipers. The ovine IgG antibodies obtained are further refined by digestion with papain to yield Fc and Fab fragments. The Fc fragments—responsible for inducing many acute anaphylactoid reactions to antivenom—are discarded, and the protective Fab fragments are isolated with affinity column chromatography. CroFab is packaged in a lyophilized state and requires reconstitution before administration.

Antivenom administration is described in detail in **Box 139.2** and in the Tips and Tricks box. Antivenom is effective in reversing most systemic and laboratory derangements seen following snake envenomation. However, its ability to reverse thrombocytopenia, rhabdomyolysis, or myokymia is variable.[9,35,36] Antivenom's efficacy in preventing local tissue damage has never been definitively demonstrated. If given very early in the course, it may reduce or limit permanent local damage to some slight degree.

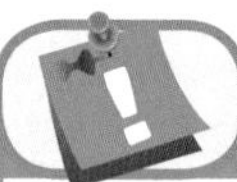

**TIPS AND TRICKS**

As soon as it is clear that antivenom is indicated, have the pharmacy or nursing staff begin reconstitution of the appropriate number of vials to be given. Reconstitution can be labor-intensive and, if the manufacturer's recommended procedure is used, can take almost 30 minutes to prepare each vial.

By using 25 mL of sterile water per vial (as opposed to the 10 mL recommended by the manufacturer) and hand mixing via continuous rolling and inverting of the vials, the reconstitution time can be reduced to less than 2 minutes per vial.[34]

### *Coral Snake Antivenom*

At the time of this writing, production of coral snake antivenom has ceased in the United States, with the current remaining stock set to expire October 31, 2012. Coral snake antivenom is still produced in Mexico (Coralmyn, Instituto Bioclon), but it is not commercially available in the United States. There is reportedly a plan in place for Pfizer to resume production of *Micrurus* antivenom in the United States.[37]

**BOX 139.2 Administration of Antivenom**

**Pit Viper Antivenom Administration**

Obtain informed consent if possible.

Expand the patient's intravascular volume with normal saline if safe to do so (e.g., no history of congestive heart failure).

Begin reconstitution of antivenom as soon as its need is evident because this process takes time (see the Tips and Tricks box).

Have epinephrine at the bedside, ready to administer immediately in the event of an acute reaction to the antivenom.

**CroFab**

Dilute the starting dose in 250 mL of normal saline.

Starting dose (children receive the same dose of antivenom as adults):

- Nonenvenomation (dry bite)—0 vials
- Progressive local findings only—4 vials
- Evidence of systemic toxicity—4 to 6 vials

Initially administer antivenom intravenously at a slow rate with the emergency physician at the bedside to intervene in the event of an acute (anaphylactoid) adverse reaction.

If tolerated, after 5 to 10 minutes increase the rate of infusion to allow the entire dose to be administered in 1 hour.

Observe the patient for 1 hour after administration—if findings of envenomation continue to worsen, repeat the starting dose (and continue this sequence until stable; generally no more than two initial doses are required).

Once the patient's condition is stabilized, admit the patient (to an intensive care unit if any evidence of instability, otherwise to a regular bed) for observation and further management (e.g., wound care; see text).

After stabilization, repeat the dosing of CroFab, 2 vials every 6 hours for 3 additional doses, to prevent recurrence of the effects of the venom.

**Coral Snake Antivenom Administration**

The basic principles (e.g., informed consent and presence of epinephrine at the bedside) are the same as for pit viper antivenom administration.

Use the manufacturer's product information to determine proper dosing.

Victims bitten by a coral snake should be admitted to a closely observed setting to allow early detection of any deterioration.

Even though the onset of neurotoxic findings following a bite by a coral snake may be delayed, once they start, they may be rapidly progressive and relatively unresponsive to antivenom administration. Management of a victim of a serious bite by a coral snake (definitively identified *Micrurus* specimen, particularly *M. fulvius*, and effective penetration of the fangs into the victim's skin) ideally includes prompt administration of antivenom before evidence of neurotoxicity begins. In the absence of appropriate coral snake antivenom, these victims must be managed conservatively, including securing the airway at the first sign of difficulty swallowing or breathing and providing mechanical ventilation (possibly for many days). If appropriate antivenom is available, it should be administered according to the manufacturer's guidelines, and all the precautions outlined for administration of pit viper antivenom should be taken (see Box 139.2). Pit viper antivenom is of no benefit to victims of bites by a coral snake.

No antivenom is available for Sonoran coral snake *(M. euryxanthus)* bites, but this species is quite small and inoffensive and has never caused a known fatality.[38] Management is purely supportive.

### *Other Treatment Considerations*

Blood products are rarely needed for victims of venomous snakebites, even with significant coagulopathy noted on laboratory tests.[39] Aggressive antivenom administration always precedes the administration of any blood products to avoid feeding further substrate to an ongoing venom-induced consumptive coagulopathy.

Wound management of pit viper bites includes placing the extremity in a well-padded splint and elevating it above heart level to reduce swelling. Tetanus prophylaxis is given if needed. Prophylactic antibiotics are not necessary unless misdirected first aid measures included incisions into the bite wound or mouth suction. In such cases, a broad-spectrum antibiotic (to cover both gram-positive and gram-negative bacteria) is administered in standard doses. Pit viper bites in the United States rarely become infected. When they do, however, antibiotic therapy is guided by wound culture testing. Tissue that is clearly necrotic is débrided after the patient is stabilized and once any attendant coagulopathy has been reversed. Intact blebs and blisters are left undisturbed, and those that rupture are conservatively unroofed. Physical therapy is started as early as possible to return the patient to an optimal level of functioning.

Indications for obtaining any consultations that may be needed are listed in **Box 139.3**.

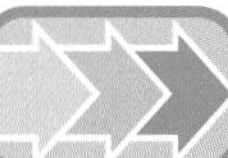

**PRIORITY ACTIONS**

Ensure that the airway, breathing, and circulation are adequate.

Begin intravenous crystalloid infusion in patients who are volume depleted or hypotensive.

Assess the severity of the envenomation and remain vigilant for signs of progression.

Measure and record the circumferences of the bitten extremity every 15 minutes during the early stages to assess for progression of local findings.

Send blood for appropriate screening laboratory tests, including blood typing and screening (see Table 139.1).

Begin the process of locating and obtaining appropriate antivenom as soon as possible.

To avoid delays in administration, begin reconstitution of antivenom as soon as it is clear that treatment is needed.

Seek consultation with an expert in snake envenomation as needed (see Box 139.3).

**BOX 139.3 When to Consider Consulting a Snakebite Expert***

The treating physician is uncomfortable evaluating or managing snakebite victims.
The envenomation is clearly severe (e.g., victim in respiratory distress, requiring intubation, or in shock).
The victim is pregnant.
The victim has significant underlying comorbid conditions (e.g., coronary artery disease, severe pulmonary disease).
No appropriate antivenom is available.
The victim has an acute adverse reaction to antivenom.
Recurrent coagulopathy is noted on follow-up evaluation.

*A regional poison control center can be reached in the United States at 1-800-222-1222.

**BOX 139.4 Management of Acute Reactions to Antivenom (Allergic or Nonallergic Anaphylaxis)**

Immediately stop the infusion.
Treat the signs and symptoms in standard fashion (airway management as needed, epinephrine, crystalloid infusion, antihistamines [$H_1$ and $H_2$ blockers], steroids, and vasopressors as needed).
In most cases the antivenom can be restarted (with the emergency physician at the bedside) once the reaction abates. If the reaction was severe and appears more life-threatening than the envenomation, a decision may be made to withhold further antivenom therapy. It is very helpful to consult an expert on snake envenomation in such cases.

## NEXT STEPS: ADMISSION AND DISCHARGE

All patients with any evidence of envenomation are admitted to the hospital for further observation and management. If the envenomation is severe, the victim is admitted to an intensive care unit. If it appears that the snake did not inject any venom (i.e., a dry bite—no signs or symptoms of envenomation, simple puncture wounds only), the victim is observed in the emergency department for a minimum of 8 hours. After 8 hours, victims who remain asymptomatic, with normal vital signs and laboratory results, are discharged in the care of a responsible adult and told to return if any evidence of envenomation occurs. Dry bites occur in as many as 20% of pit viper bites, although the precise reason for this remains unclear.[6,40] Any child with a possible venomous snakebite is admitted to the hospital regardless of the presence or absence of signs or symptoms of poisoning. Likewise, victims of a possible bite by a coral snake are admitted for observation because of the significant delay that can occur before any evidence of envenomation is apparent.

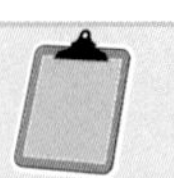

**DOCUMENTATION**

Record a careful history in the patient's own words, including a description of the snake.
Record the results of a thorough screening physical examination.
Have nursing staff measure and record the circumferences of the bitten extremity every 15 minutes until the swelling has stabilized and then every hour for 24 hours.
Note the specifics of any discussion with consultants (e.g., poison control specialists).
Measure and record intracompartmental pressures if concern arises about the development of compartment syndrome.
Document informed consent (for antivenom administration or fasciotomy) if possible.

## COMPLICATIONS

### ADVERSE REACTIONS TO ANTIVENOM

Adverse reactions to antivenom include early, acute reactions (which are probably anaphylactoid in nature [also known as nonallergic anaphylaxis]) and delayed serum sickness, an immunoglobulin (IgG and IgM) immune complex–mediated disease. Anaphylactoid reactions may be manifested as hives, wheezing, laryngeal edema, abdominal pain, vomiting, diarrhea, and hypotension. The incidence of anaphylactoid reactions to CroFab is approximately 15%,[41] with most reactions being minor and easily treated (**Box 139.4**).[42] Serum sickness occurs in approximately 3% of patients treated with CroFab[41] and may be manifested approximately 1 to 2 weeks after administration as fever, urticaria, myalgia, arthralgia, renal dysfunction, or neuropathy (or any combination of these signs). Serum sickness is easily treated with oral steroids (e.g., prednisone, 1 to 2 mg/kg orally per day) administered until the symptoms resolve, followed by a 2-week tapering of the dose. Oral antihistamines may provide additional symptomatic relief. Before discharge from the hospital, patients are warned to watch for signs and symptoms of serum sickness and told to return if they occur.

### COMPARTMENT SYNDROME

Some larger rattlesnakes have fangs long enough to penetrate deeply into muscle compartments. Because many significant pit viper bites result in swollen extremities that are discolored and painful on any attempted range of motion, it can be difficult to determine when a compartment syndrome is imminent. This complication is actually rare following pit viper bites, but if there is concern about rising intracompartmental pressure, it is objectively measured with any standard technique. If the pressure is elevated above 30 to 40 mm Hg, the limb is further elevated, more antivenom is administered, and mannitol is given (1.0 g/kg intravenously over a 30-minute period) if the patient is hemodynamically stable.[43] If the compartment pressure remains high 1 hour after these measures have been carried out, fasciotomy is considered. Although animal research has suggested an actual increase in myonecrosis following fasciotomy,[44] there is still a risk for ischemic

**BOX 139.5 Indications for Administering Further Antivenom to Patients with Delayed Coagulopathy**

Patients found on follow-up to have recurrent coagulopathy following a pit viper bite should receive further antivenom dosing in any of the following situations[48]:

- Evidence of clinically significant bleeding
- Platelet count < 25,000/mm$^3$
- Serum INR > 3 seconds
- Serum APTT > 50 seconds
- Serum fibrinogen < 50 mg/dL
- Multicomponent coagulopathy present
- Earlier, severe coagulopathy noted in the patient
- Patient at high risk for trauma (e.g., occupation risks) or with comorbid conditions such as systemic vasculitis, previous stroke, or seizures

*APTT*, Activated partial thromboplastin time; *INR*, international normalized ratio.

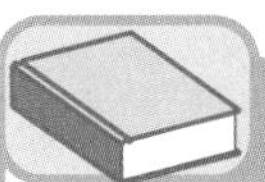

**PATIENT TEACHING TIPS**

Never approach, torment, or attempt to catch or kill a venomous or unidentified species of snake.

Do not keep any species of venomous snake as a "pet."

Never handle a venomous snake that you believe is dead. These snakes may still have a bite reflex and can inflict a serious or fatal bite.

If bitten by a venomous or unknown snake, proceed immediately to the nearest hospital for evaluation. No first aid measures are effective or necessary following bites by pit vipers.

If you have been treated for a venomous snakebite with antivenom, watch for signs of serum sickness (fever, muscle aches, joint aches, hives, or bleeding) in the first 2 weeks after you leave the hospital. If such signs occur, follow up immediately with your physician.

Avoid any elective surgery, contact sports, or high-risk activities for 2 to 3 weeks after a pit viper bite because your blood may not clot normally during this period.

$SI = \frac{SV}{BSA}$ **FACTS AND FORMULAS**

**Measurement of Intracompartmental Pressure**

If lower than 30 to 40 mm Hg, continue antivenom as indicated along with limb elevation and monitoring.

If higher than 30 to 40 mm Hg, give additional antivenom, keep the limb elevated, administer mannitol (1 g/kg intravenously if the patient's hemodynamic status allows), observe for 1 hour, and then recheck intracranial pressure.

If the pressure falls below 30 to 40 mm Hg, continue nonoperative treatment. If intracranial pressure remains elevated, consider fasciotomy (with informed patient consent).

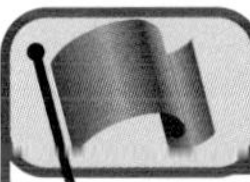

**RED FLAGS**

**Cautions for the Physician**

Remain vigilant for worsening severity of venom poisoning; it can progress rapidly and suddenly. Conversely, the onset of clinical findings may be delayed for hours.

Obtain consultation early from a clinician knowledgeable in snake envenomation (e.g., a regional poison control center specialist) whenever needed.

Obtain informed consent whenever possible before giving antivenom.

Give antivenom as soon as possible after its need is identified.

Remain at the patient's bedside during the initiation of antivenom therapy to intervene if an acute reaction occurs.

Have epinephrine available at the bedside before beginning antivenom infusion.

If a compartment syndrome is suspected, obtain objective measurements of intracompartmental pressure.

If fasciotomy is indicated, obtain and document informed consent.

Cases involving snake envenomation in the United States often end up in medicolegal litigation. Document carefully.

neuropathy following unabated rises in compartment pressure. It is important to obtain informed consent, if possible, before proceeding with fasciotomy.

## RECURRENT COAGULOPATHY

Patients in whom coagulopathy develops during the initial stages of pit viper envenomation may have delayed recurrence of abnormal coagulation studies for up to 2 weeks following the bite.[42,45] This is probably related to continued absorption of venom components from the depot site after all antivenom administered has been cleared from the body, particularly when a low-molecular-weight Fab antivenom (e.g., CroFab) is used. In most cases, delayed coagulopathy is benign, without evidence of clinically significant bleeding, but severe complications, including intracranial bleeding, have been reported.[46,47] Patients are warned of this possibility and instructed to avoid any elective surgery, contact sports, and other high-risk activities for a few weeks following the bite. Although administration of antivenom for delayed coagulopathy may be helpful, it is likely to be less effective than in the acute stages of envenomation. Reasonable indications for administering further antivenom in these cases are outlined in **Box 139.5**.

# PROGNOSIS

Deaths attributable to bites by endemic snakes are rare in the United States, with only 33 reported to the American Association of Poison Control Centers in the 26-year period from 1983 to 2008.[1] This is an underestimate of the total number of deaths because snakebite is not a reportable condition, but it does reflect the limited toll of snakebite in terms of loss of life in the United States. Deaths are even more infrequent in Canada, whereas in Mexico, as many as 150 people die each year of venomous snakebites.[43] The case fatality rate following venomous snakebite in the United States when antivenom is used is less than 1%.[49] However, long-term complications, such as loss of some degree of function in the bitten extremity, are more likely. Approximately 10% of victims will be left with some functional disability following pit viper bites, and this does not include permanent dysfunction directly related to surgical procedures.[43] The incidence of disability may actually be higher if careful, delayed evaluation of extremity function is performed (e.g., using goniometry and precise sensory testing).[50]

## SUGGESTED READINGS

Cannon R, Ruha AM, Kashani J. Acute hypersensitivity reactions associated with administration of Crotalidae polyvalent immune Fab antivenom. Ann Emerg Med 2008;51:407-11.

Kitchens C, Eskin T. Fatality in a case of envenomation by *Crotalus adamanteus* initially successfully treated with polyvalent ovine antivenom followed by recurrence of defibrinogenation syndrome. J Med Toxicol 2008;4:180-3.

Norris RL, Bush SP, Smith J. Bites by venomous reptiles in Canada, the U.S. and Mexico. In: Auerbach PS, editor. Wilderness medicine. 6th ed. Philadelphia: Saunders; 2012.

Seifert SA, Boyer LV, Benson BE, et al. AAPCC database characterization of native U.S. venomous snake exposures, 2001-2005. Clin Toxicol (Phila) 2009;47:327-35.

## REFERENCES

***References can be found on Expert Consult @ www.expertconsult.com.***

# Arthropod Bites and Stings 140

*Joshua N. Nogar and Richard F. Clark*

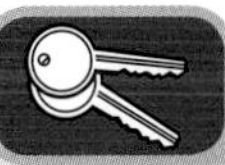

**KEY POINTS**

- Anaphylaxis, typically caused by Hymenoptera stings, is the most serious complication of all arthropod encounters and should be treated with steroids, epinephrine, and antihistamines when needed.
- Massive envenomations (>10 stings per kilogram or >100 stings per person) by Hymenoptera merit close monitoring for systemic effects of the venom.
- Latrodectism should be treated with adequate analgesia and benzodiazepines, but antivenom should be considered for severe cases.
- Dapsone, hyperbaric oxygen, colchicine, and electric shock therapy are no more effective than supportive care for the treatment of true dermonecrotic arachnidism.

## PERSPECTIVE

Arthropods are the most diverse, widespread, and numerous of all animal phyla inhabiting the planet. Not surprisingly, their contact with humans is a common occurrence. In 2009, 40,657 calls related to arthropods were made to poison centers in the United States, and although most do not require hospital attention, many patients will still come to the emergency department (ED) complaining of a bite or sting from an unknown or unidentified insect.[1] Fortunately, the vast majority of these patients can be treated with supportive care and medications for pruritus and pain; the challenge for the emergency physician (EP) is identifying more serious and rare complications of these encounters. The most clinically significant arthropods are summarized in **Table 140.1**.

Approaching this topic can be a daunting task because there are literally millions of arthropod species and hundreds of medical significance. This chapter focuses on the venomous and immunologic effects of these organisms. It is useful to divide arthropods into broad groups based on organism similarity and clinical findings: Hymenoptera (bees, wasps, hornets, yellow jackets, ants); arachnids (spiders, ticks, scorpions); centipedes, millipedes, and caterpillars; and scabies, fleas, and lice.

## EPIDEMIOLOGY

Arthropod venoms are complex mixtures of enzymes, proteins, histamines, and other bioamines that can either damage tissue directly or elicit an allergic response. The venoms of each family are unique, and cross-reactivity is rare with the exception of wasps, hornets, and yellow jackets (vespids). Local tissue reactions from dermal exposure to arthropod antigens result in the common pruritic, urticarial, and papular lesions seen after envenomation. The most immediately life-threatening complication of arthropod exposure is anaphylaxis either to the venom itself or to the antivenom administered in the ED. Treatment of anaphylaxis merits special discussion and is covered in the next section on Hymenoptera.

## HYMENOPTERA

### PATHOPHYSIOLOGY

Apidae (bees), Vespidae (wasps, yellow jackets, hornets), and Formicidae (ants) are the most clinically significant groups of arthropods for two reasons. First, the incidence of Hymenoptera venom allergy has been estimated to be 0.8% to 5% in the general population and is increasing, particularly in young people.[2] Second, because of their complex social organization, multiple stings are more likely to occur during Hymenoptera encounters than with arthropods that do not build nests or hives.

Recent research indicates that the major allergens in Hymenoptera venom are phospholipases and hyaluronidases, as well as mellitin, a peptide that causes degranulation of mast cells.[3] Hymenoptera venom is delivered via an ovipositor stinger and gland, although some anatomic variation does exist. Male bees have no stingers and are incapable of stinging when threatened. Females have barbed stingers that become lodged in human skin and eviscerate the bee after venom delivery. The retained stinger and venom sac can be removed with tweezers. Africanized "killer" bees deserve special mention in that (1) they are far more aggressive and territorial than the more docile domesticated varieties, (2) are known to pursue perceived threats for up to 1 km, and (3) do so in much larger swarms. Africanized bees are difficult to distinguish morphologically from domesticated bees, but fortunately, this distinction is of little clinical significance because of venom

**Table 140.1 Common Clinical Manifestations of Arthropod Envenomation**

| | |
|---|---|
| Bees and wasps | Urticarial eruptions, anaphylaxis, rhabdomyolysis, ARF, ARDS (after massive envenomations) |
| Widow spiders | Pain, muscle spasm, local diaphoresis, tachycardia, hypertension |
| Recluse spiders | Dermonecrosis; hemolysis, DIC, ARDS (rarely) |
| Scabies | Migratory pruritus, secondary infections |
| Ants | Urticarial and papular dermatitis, anaphylaxis risk |
| Scorpions | Pain, tingling, cranial neuropathy, ataxia, pancreatitis, DIC, ARDS (exotic species) |
| Caterpillars | Painful dermatitis, ocular and mucosal irritation |
| Mites | Papular urticarial dermatitis |
| Ticks | Local tissue reaction, tick paralysis, infectious complications |
| Reduviid bug | Bullous lesions, infectious complications |
| Lice and fleas | Papular urticarial dermatitis |
| Mosquitoes | Urticaria, pruritus, infectious complications |
| Tarantulas | Local pain (bite), urticarial dermatitis, ocular irritation (hairs) |
| Centipedes | Local pain |
| Millipedes | Skin discoloration from oily extractions |

*ARDS*, Acute respiratory distress syndrome; *ARF*, acute renal failure; *DIC*, disseminated intravascular coagulation.

homology between Hymenoptera Apidae. In contrast to bees, vespids (wasps, yellow jackets, and hornets) have the ability to withdraw their stinger from the victim and deliver multiple stings. Most severe allergic reactions to Hymenoptera are due to encounters with vespids, particularly wasps and yellow jackets.[3,4]

Ant venom is also delivered via a stinging apparatus, but ants are known to initially bite with their powerful jaws before stinging their victim and can do so en masse via a pheromone-coordinated attack. Multiple ant stings are most common with fire ants.

## PRESENTING SIGNS AND SYMPTOMS

Hymenoptera stings cause immediate pain with subsequent erythema, edema, and pruritus. Fire ants are known for their particularly painful sting, which can eventually develop into a sterile pustule. Delayed type IV reactions can occur with all Hymenoptera venoms and result in larger, albeit localized reactions.

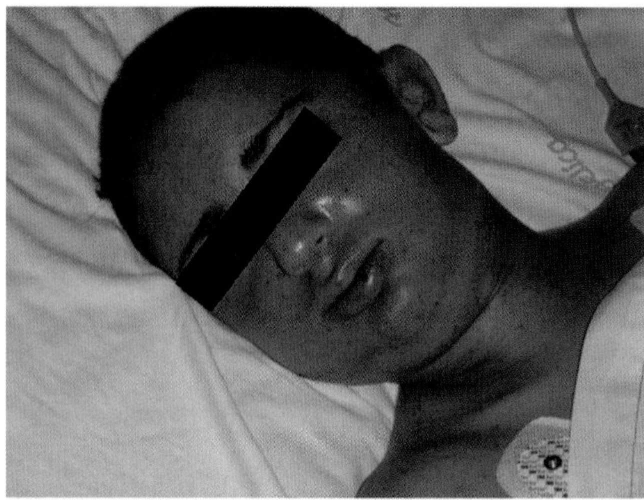

**Fig. 140.1 Massive Hymenoptera envenomation.** (Courtesy Richard Clark, MD.)

Massive envenomations are considered those in which the victim sustains more than 100 stings or more than 10 stings per kilogram (**Fig. 140.1**). Such cases merit special respect and victims should be considered for admission because of an increased risk for systemic symptoms, including nausea, vomiting, diarrhea, edema, dyspnea, hypotension, and rhabdomyolysis. Rarely, glomerulonephritis, acute renal failure, and acute respiratory distress syndrome can occur.[5-7]

## DIAGNOSTIC TESTING

No laboratory testing is necessary in cases limited to cutaneous symptoms from submassive envenomations. Massive envenomations or systemic reactions require investigation to evaluate for rhabdomyolysis, renal failure, or cardiac ischemia.[5,6,8] Appropriate testing should include a basic chemistry panel and creatine phosphokinase (CPK) level.

## ANAPHYLAXIS AND ALLERGIC REACTIONS

It has been estimated that 40 deaths occur per year in this country as a result of anaphylaxis from Hymenoptera stings.[4] Anaphylaxis is an IgE-mediated type I hypersensitivity reaction that leads to mast cell and basophil degranulation of vasoactive mediators, cytokines, prostaglandins, and platelet-activating factor. Some initial symptoms can be mild and include itchy eyes, urticaria, or cough. However, the symptoms can progress rapidly to shortness of breath, stridor, angioedema, and shock. Treatment should be initiated immediately and includes epinephrine, steroids, antihistamines, and bronchodilators (if bronchospasm is present). All available data suggest that failure or delay in the administration of epinephrine increases the chance for death from anaphylaxis. The risk for anaphylaxis with any event is dependent on the severity of the patient's previous reaction, and it seems to be proportional to the rate of symptom onset. Once the symptoms have been controlled, patients should be observed for at

**BOX 140.1 Treatment of Anaphylaxis Caused by Arthropod Venom or Antivenom Therapy**

Symptoms of allergy and anaphylaxis may be variable and include perioral or pharyngeal tingling, shortness of breath, tachypnea, bronchospasm and wheezing, stridor, chest pain, sudden tachycardia, hypotension, angioedema, and urticaria.

Bees and wasps are the most common sources of insect allergic reactions. Because animal-derived antibody products can also result in allergic reactions or anaphylaxis, each patient receiving antivenom must be monitored carefully. The antivenom infusion must be stopped immediately if allergic symptoms such as those listed develop.

Skin testing is a very imperfect (not sensitive, not specific) predictor of subsequent allergic reactions to antivenom.

Pretreatment includes antihistamines (e.g., diphenhydramine, 25 to 50 mg intravenously [IV], plus ranitidine, 50 mg IV) and antipyretics (acetaminophen, 500 mg or 15 mg/kg orally [PO]).

Treatment of any significant allergic reaction is prompt administration of epinephrine.

- The dose is 0.1 to 0.5 mg IV of a 1:10,000 concentration (0.1 mg/mL); repeat every 5 minutes as needed to titrate for symptoms.
- An infusion of 2 to 10 mcg/min may be used if continuous therapy is desired.
- For reference, the intramuscular dose is 0.5 mg of a 1:1000 concentration in a volume of 0.5 mL.
- The pediatric dose is 0.01 mg/kg IV of a 1:10,000 solution (equals 0.1 mL/kg per dose); continuous infusion is 0.1 to 1 mcg/kg/min.

Steroids are recommended to prevent delayed allergic effects.

- The typical dose is 125 mg of methylprednisolone IV, followed by a 5-day course of prednisone at a dose of 1 to 2 mg/kg PO.
- The pediatric dose of methylprednisolone is 2 mg/kg IV.

Pretreatment with steroids can be done in high-risk patients requiring antivenom.

Nebulized bronchodilators and supplemental oxygen can be used for bronchospasm.

Warn patients about the risk and signs of serum sickness, which occurs within 7 to 10 days of the envenomation or administration of antivenom. Serum sickness is characterized by a diffuse macular or urticarial rash, arthralgias, back pain, and sometimes hematuria. Therapy is a 10- to 14-day course of prednisone, 1 to 2 mg/kg/day PO, with tapering.

least 2 hours to ensure resolution of the symptoms. Patients with persistent cardiopulmonary symptoms should be admitted to the hospital. An outline of anaphylaxis treatment is found in **Box 140.1** and **Table 140.2**.[2-5]

## FOLLOW-UP, NEXT STEPS IN CARE, AND PATIENT EDUCATION

Patients treated for anaphylaxis should be educated on avoidance of the allergen and use of an epinephrine autoinjector. Wearing a medical bracelet is also advisable. Finally, patients should be referred to an allergist for sensitivity testing and possible venom immunotherapy.[3]

# Arachnids—Spiders, Scorpions, and Ticks

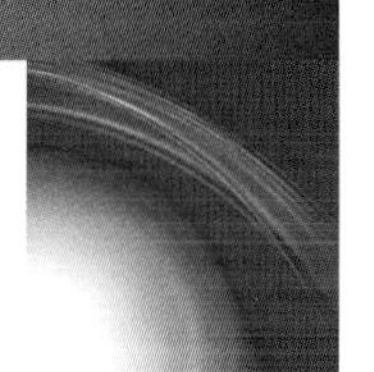

## SPIDERS (ARANEAE)

## PATHOPHYSIOLOGY

More than 40,000 species of spiders have been identified, but most of them lack venom or fangs large enough to deliver venom through human skin. In fact, fewer than 50 species are considered to be harmful to humans. The most clinically relevant spiders are widow spiders, recluse spiders, funnel-web spiders, and tarantulas.

## WIDOW SPIDERS (LATRODECTUS SPECIES)

With its distinct shiny black color, bulbous abdominal segment, and ventral orange-red markings, *Latrodectus* species are some of the most identifiable of all spiders. *Latrodectus mactans* (black widow) is perhaps the best known of the genus and possesses an hourglass-shaped ventral marking (**Fig. 140.2**). As is the case with many arthropods, females are the larger of the two sexes, and males do not have fangs capable of piercing human skin. *Latrodectus* venom contains a potent neurotoxin, α-latrotoxin, a well-characterized protein that induces massive release of neurotransmitters from presynaptic neurons. The resultant effect of these neurotransmitters is activation of the autonomic and somatic nervous systems.[9,10]

## PRESENTING SIGNS AND SYMPTOMS

The bite itself is typically painful, and this discomfort can spread throughout the affected extremity. Local erythema and diaphoresis occur early at the site with a resultant macule developing into a target lesion. The development of painful cramping in large muscle groups and autonomic instability is known as latrodectism. This systemic syndrome has been described as being so severe as to mimic an acute abdomen, even when the site of envenomation is remote from the center mass; the exact pathophysiology of this phenomenon is not well understood. Hypertension, tachycardia, headache, nausea,

**Table 140.2 Other Arthropod Rashes and Treatment**

| ARTHROPOD | SIGNS AND SYMPTOMS | TREATMENT |
|---|---|---|
| Fleas and mites | Pruritic, erythematous, red papules | Oral or topical antihistamines, topical steroid cream<br>Antimicrobials for secondary infections |
| Scabies | Significant nocturnal pruritus, intertriginous skin thickening, papules. The diagnosis can be made with microscopy of skin scrapings. Finger web spaces, wrists, elbows, and unscratched skin are the most productive sites for sampling | Topical and oral antihistamines<br>Topical scabicides: 5% permethrin cream applied once for 8-14 hr, then washed off. May be repeated in 1 wk; treatment failure typically results from incorrect application<br>Lindane cream no longer recommended<br>Ivermectin, 200 mcg/kg orally once, second dose recommended 14 days later. Only for topical treatment failure |
| Norwegian scabies | Severe scabies infection (thousands of organisms); typically indicates immunocompromised status | As above<br>Check for underlying immunodeficiency |
| Caterpillars | Stinging, pruritic lesions caused by contact with setae (spines) distributed in a pattern similar to those of the hairlike projections on the caterpillar. Mucosal and ophthalmic irritation, bronchospasm | Spine removal from the skin with tweezers, adhesive tape, or topical white school glue<br>Topical or oral steroid therapy for severe dermatitis<br>Ocular irrigation with 0.9% normal saline<br>Inhaled bronchodilators for bronchospasm<br>Antivenom for Brazilian *Lonomia* species |
| Centipedes | Carnivorous arthropod. Painful bite. Rare systemic reactions: nausea, vomiting, diaphoresis | Supportive care, analgesics, antihistamines |
| Millipedes | Herbivorous arthropod. Exoskeleton secretions can cause cutaneous irritation and discoloration | Wash the site copiously with soap and water, oral and/or topical antihistamines |

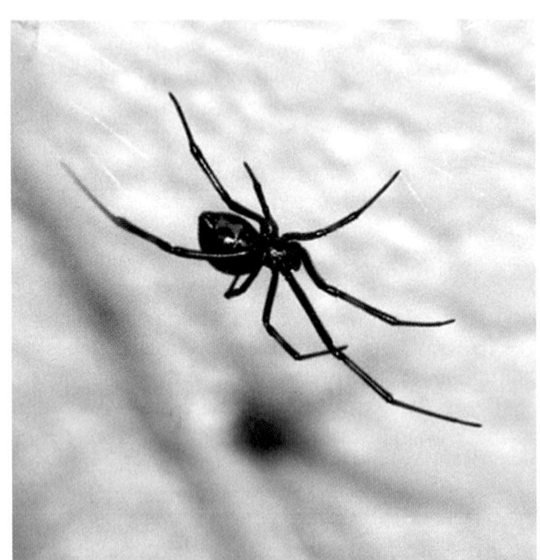

**Fig. 140.2** ***Latrodectus mactans.*** (Courtesy Richard Clark, MD.)

priapism, and dyspnea have also been described in association with *Latrodectus* bites.[9]

## TREATMENT

The mainstays of therapy for widow spider envenomation are adequate analgesia and muscle relaxants. The majority of patients respond to one or multiple doses of opioid analgesics and benzodiazepines, and these medications should be titrated according to patient symptoms.

IgG antivenom for *Latrodectus* envenomation is available in the United States, but this treatment is often reserved for the rare patients whose pain and muscle spasms are refractory to large doses of analgesics and relaxants. This antivenom is a whole-antibody horse-derived IgG preparation, and anaphylactoid reactions and serum sickness are potential consequences of its administration. Therefore, it should be administered slowly and with caution.[10]

One vial of antivenom is usually sufficient to relieve symptoms. This preparation should be infused slowly (over a 15- to 30-minute period). Premedication with antihistamines can be considered. The EP must be prepared to administer epinephrine if a severe allergic reaction to horse serum occurs. Additionally, patients must be informed that serum sickness (diffuse papular rash, glomerulonephritis, arthralgias) may occur 10 to 21 days following therapy, although this reaction will rarely be seen with administration of only one vial. *Latrodectus* antivenom is in very short supply and is not readily available in many facilities. A potentially safer, Fab fragment antivenom is currently being investigated and may be available for use in the United States in the near future.

## SPIDERS CAUSING DERMONECROTIC ARACHNIDISM

*Loxosceles*, or recluse, spiders cause the syndrome of dermonecrotic arachnidism. These spiders, as their name suggests, prefer dark and isolated spaces such as attics, basements, and closets. They bite only when threatened or disturbed. In contrast to *Latrodectus, Loxosceles reclusa* is more difficult to identify. Many possess a violin-shaped dorsal marking (hence in some regions they are called "fiddleback" spiders), but this is not a diagnostic feature of all *L. reclusa*. The only unifying feature of all *Latrodectus* spiders is that they possess only three pairs of eyes, as opposed to the four pairs found in most spiders. Hobo spiders in the Pacific Northwest and several other species are also theorized to cause necrotic complications following bites, but these associations are more controversial. The venom of recluse spiders is a complex mixture of hyaluronidase, ribonucleases, lipases, and sphingomyelinase D, the latter being thought to be responsible for the necrosis.[11,12]

## PRESENTING SIGNS AND SYMPTOMS

The most common clinical effect of true recluse spider bites is a progressively necrotic eschar. The lesion evolves from a nonspecific erythematous wheal into an eschar with surrounding rings of blanching and erythema ("red, white, and blue" sign) over a period of days to weeks. The slow destruction of skin structure occurs as a result of the effects of venom on the dermal microcirculation, and it can extend into adjacent tissues in a gravity-dependent manner. These lesions can be cosmetically disfiguring and stressful for patients because they expand and worsen over a period of many days to weeks. It is important to stress to patients that lesions from recluse spiders sometimes progress despite medical treatment.[11,12] It is also important to appreciate the rarity of these injuries in comparison with the frequency with which they are reportedly perpetrated; many cutaneous infections are mistaken for recluse bites. In one study, spider bites were confirmed in only 3.8% of all individuals with the chief complaint of a spider bite.[13] Rare cases of severe hematologic toxicity with hemolytic anemia, thrombocytopenia, and coagulopathy have been described in association with *Loxosceles* bites, particularly in Brazil.[14,15]

## TREATMENT

Therapies aimed at limiting or preventing the necrotic sequelae of recluse spider bites are controversial. The safest management regimen that can be recommended without reservation is gentle cleansing, tetanus prophylaxis, analgesia, antipruritic medications, and immobilization if needed. Disproved treatments include early wound excision, corticosteroids, cyproheptadine, and electric shocks delivered to the bite site to denature the venom components. Hyperbaric oxygen, dapsone, and colchicine have been tried as experimental therapies, but studies proving benefit are thus far lacking. Severely disfiguring or nonhealing bites may require delayed reconstructive procedures once the destructive effect of the venom has halted.

A *Loxosceles* antivenom has been developed for use in Brazil, but based on animal models, it must be given within 24 hours to be effective. Because most patients are seen 2 to 3 days after being bitten, this type of antivenom is not typically a useful adjunct in the treatment of *Loxosceles* spider bites.[15] Symptomatic and intensive supportive care is warranted in the rare case of disseminated intravascular coagulation, hemolytic anemia, renal failure, or acute respiratory distress syndrome following the bite of a recluse spider.

## TARANTULAS

Tarantulas are distributed worldwide and recognizable by their large size and prominent hairlike projections. Large or aggressive species can bite; the effects can range from relatively painless to deep throbbing pain with a febrile reaction that requires analgesics and antipyretics. By rubbing their hind legs against their abdominal wall, tarantulas can "flick" their hairs in the direction of perceived threats, and both dermal and ocular injuries have occurred from the highly irritating "urticating" hairs of tarantulas. The presence of urticaria, hives, intense pruritus, and mild erythema characterizes dermal lesions; ocular exposure to the urticating hairs has resulted in corneal abrasions, iritis, uveitis, and chronic granulomatous reactions (ophthalmia nodosum).[16]

## TREATMENT

Therapy is essentially supportive and consists of analgesics and antihistamines. Ophthalmic antibiotics or steroids in conjunction with close follow-up or emergency ophthalmology consultation may be necessary in cases of ocular exposure to tarantula hairs.

## SCORPIONS

Scorpions are easily recognized by the taillike abdominal segment that forms into a venom-filled bulb with a stinger (telson). In the United States, scorpions are commonly encountered hazards in the Southwest, where *Centruroides exilicauda* (formerly *Centruroides sculpturatus*), or the bark scorpion, is endemic. They commonly hide in dark spaces such as closets and shoes; the exoskeleton's ability to fluoresce under ultraviolet light is sometimes helpful in locating these creatures. Worldwide, species that represent significant hazards to human health include *Tityus* species in Trinidad and Brazil and *Buthus* and *Parabuthus* species in India, Africa, and the Middle East. Most scorpion stings occur when the creature feels threatened or alarmed.[17,18]

The venom of *C. exilicauda* is complex and targets excitable membranes. The result is abnormally prolonged opening of sodium channels at the neuromuscular junction and at both sympathetic and parasympathetic nerve endings. Dangerous varieties of scorpions from other countries can cause massive release of catecholamines from nerve terminals, particularly norepinephrine and acetylcholine, which can lead to diverse autonomic effects.

## PRESENTING SIGNS AND SYMPTOMS

Local effects of erythema and tingling may be present, but these findings may be quite subtle initially. Tapping the site of discomfort gently accentuates the reported symptoms, even in the absence of visible skin lesions. Systemic findings are often more dramatic than the local effects and peak around 5 hours after the sting; signs and symptoms commonly include hypertension, tachycardia, convulsions, cranial neuropathies, roving ophthalmoplegia (also known as oculogyric crisis), ataxia, abdominal cramps, and respiratory failure from neuromuscular dysfunction.[17,18]

The stings of other scorpion genera may produce unique syndromes. *Tityus* scorpions in Trinidad and South America can cause pancreatitis, and in India and Africa the *Buthus* and *Parabissesuthus* varieties can cause pulmonary hemorrhage, gastrointestinal bleeding, and disseminated intravascular coagulation, presumably because of the presence of phospholipase in the venom.

## DIAGNOSTIC TESTING

Testing of serum electrolytes, CPK, and cardiac isozymes, as well as chest radiography and electrocardiography, should be considered in patients at high risk for cardiac ischemia. Neurologic testing such as computed tomography of the head and lumbar puncture may be required in patients in whom other neurologic disease processes are suspected.

## TREATMENT

The majority of patients respond to supportive care and aggressive pain management with analgesics and muscle relaxants. Continuous infusion of benzodiazepines may be considered in well-monitored patients to decrease agitation and abnormal motor activity.[19] Short-acting antihypertensives such as esmolol or nitroprusside are also appropriate in the setting of severe hypertension and tachycardia.

Respiratory failure or fatigue warrant aggressive airway management and possibly intubation; this complication is especially concerning in the pediatric and elderly populations, which are most vulnerable to mortality from scorpion stings. Rarely, pancreatitis and coagulopathy require intensive supportive care with meticulous fluid management and transfusion of blood products.

Scorpion antivenom directed against different species has been produced for research or clinical use in more than 10 countries, and recommendations for their use are variable. In the United States, a recent study demonstrated improved outcome in critically ill children after treatment with *C. exilicauda* antivenom.[18]

## FOLLOW-UP, NEXT STEPS IN CARE, AND PATIENT EDUCATION

Patients with severe signs and symptoms require admission to the hospital, and intensive care may be necessary for pediatric and elderly patients. Patients who are comfortable and have normal vital signs and results of diagnostic testing can safely be discharged. Wounds from scorpion stings do not usually require specific therapy for infection.

# TICKS (*IXODES, DERMACENTOR,* OTHERS) AND TICK PARALYSIS

The overwhelming concern regarding ticks is their role as vectors for viral, bacterial, and protozoal infectious diseases. Ticks are arachnid bloodsucking parasites that painlessly attach to their host. In addition, several members of the *Dermacentor, Ixodes*, and *Amblyomma* genera of ticks can induce a rapidly progressive syndrome of ascending weakness and loss of deep tendon reflexes called tick paralysis. The condition is most common in the Rocky Mountain states and Pacific Northwestern region of the United States, but the true incidence is unknown because it is not a reportable entity. Girls seem to be affected more often because the pediatric population is more apt to harbor the tick for a longer period before being brought to medical attention and longer hair camouflages the offending tick.

Though not fully characterized, the neurotoxin is presumed to inhibit release of acetylcholine at the neuromuscular junction.

## PRESENTING SIGNS AND SYMPTOMS

The onset of lower extremity weakness is insidious, similar to Guillain-Barré syndrome, and reflexes tend to be diminished in both. Careful physical examination is the key to diagnosis because the paralytic neurotoxin is secreted by the tick as long as it remains attached to the skin. Although the tick can be found attached to the skin in any anatomic location, well-protected areas such as the clothing waistline and the occipital scalp in victims with long hair are common sites of injury. Respiratory failure is the most feared complication of a delayed diagnosis. In contrast to Guillain-Barré syndrome, the results of cerebrospinal fluid analysis are normal in patients with tick paralysis.

## DIFFERENTIAL DIAGNOSIS

The differential diagnosis for ascending paralysis is short and includes Guillain-Barré syndrome, cerebellar ataxia, spinal cord compression, hypokalemic periodic paralysis, and transverse myelitis. Work-up includes basic laboratory studies, lumbar puncture, and central nervous system imaging, all of which would be expected to show normal results in patients with tick paralysis.

## FOLLOW-UP, NEXT STEPS IN CARE, AND PATIENT EDUCATION

Removal of the offending tick rapidly leads to resolution of the symptoms and decreases the likelihood of tick-borne disease transmission. It can be achieved by grasping the tick near the skin with fine-point tweezers and pulling straight outward with steady, gentle traction. All patients with ascending paralysis should be admitted to the hospital, regardless of the cause. Once the tick has been removed and the neurologic symptoms are clearly improving, the patient can be safely discharged.[20,21]

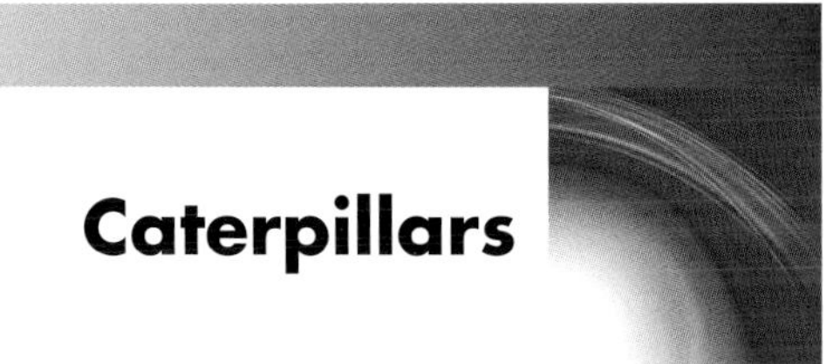

## Caterpillars

Caterpillars are the wormlike immature forms of butterflies and moths.[22] Of the 165,000 total species, only 12 families worldwide account for human injuries. In 2009, 1422 exposures were reported to poison centers in the United States. Most of these exposures occur in individuals younger than 18 years. The numerous hairlike projections of these organisms are called setae and, in some species, are actually hollow connections to venom glands capable of piercing the skin and result in envenomation on contact. These solid setae are highly irritating to the skin on contact and are light enough to be dispersed by the wind. In fact, dry weather and strong winds facilitated the dispersion of setae and resulted in an epidemic of dermatitis among Shanghai residents in 1972.[23]

Several illness syndromes caused by caterpillars or butterflies (order Lepidoptera) are recognized. The most common injuries are dermal lesions, sometimes referred to as erucism or cutaneous lepidopterism. In the United States, the most common form of lepidopterism is dermatitis caused by the puss caterpillar, also known as the woolly slug. This flat, fuzzy caterpillar is found in the southern United States from Maryland to Texas. The related flannel moth caterpillar is endemic to New England and the eastern U.S. seaboard. Other species that cause dermatitis include the *Automeris io, Megalopyge opercularis*, and saddleback caterpillars. All these species induce a stinging, itchy, or painful lesion on contact with the setae. Characteristic lesions are often teardrop shaped in a gridlike pattern and mimic the shape of the offending caterpillar.[24] The woolly slug induces a dull aching pain at the site of parallel papular eruptions. Caterpillar setae can occasionally irritate the eyes or respiratory passages on direct exposure to these surfaces. Distinguishing features and treatment of these lesions are summarized in Table 140.2.

## Centipedes and Millipedes

Centipedes and millipedes both possess multiple body segments. The front pair of legs in the centipede is modified into a hollow fanglike appendage called a maxillepede, which expresses venom from a muscular sac. This digestive aid is also capable of piercing human skin. These nocturnal creatures range from 3 to 250 mm in length and prefer moist, warm climates. Centipedes are carnivores and can cause painful bites. Rare systemic reactions include nausea, vomiting, and diaphoresis.[25] Solitary case reports have described more severe complications such as rhabdomyolysis and renal failure.[1]

In contrast to centipedes, millipedes are vegetarians but can induce dermal irritation injuries because they express a toxic substance onto the exoskeleton when threatened. This oily residue can cause ocular irritation and discoloration of the skin that can last for months.[26] Distinguishing features and treatment of these bites are summarized in Table 140.2.

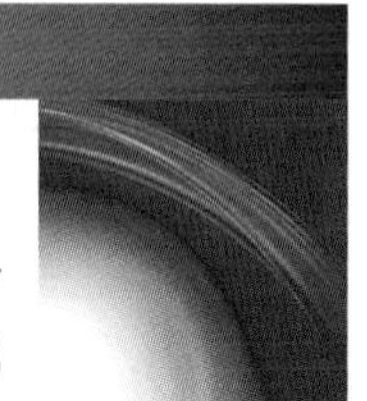

## Other Arthropods—Scabies, Fleas, Lice, and Bedbugs

Mites, fleas, lice, and bedbugs are small arthropods that reside in a wide variety of environments. Various mites thrive naturally in or on grains, pets, rodent pests, feathers, furniture, house floors, and straw. Fleas and lice are ectoparasites that feed on the skin surface, whereas the scabies mite is an arachnid endoparasite that burrows under the skin. Fleas and lice are probably more important from an infectious standpoint because of the zoonotic diseases that they can transmit, such as plague and typhus, respectively (**Box 140.2**). Bedbugs, in particular, have gained much publicity in recent years because of their increasing prevalence. Adults are oval shaped and resemble small (less than 5 mm) cockroaches. Bites from all four can produce self-limited pruritic papules at the feeding site, but scabies is more apt to cause a persistent dermatitis secondary to shedding and leaving fecal droppings embedded in the burrowed skin.[27]

The worldwide prevalence of scabies has been estimated to be approximately 300 million cases annually.[28] Most mites are transmitted via intimate interpersonal contact, but adult forms of the mite can survive remote from human tissue for 24 to 36 hours in bedding, clothing, and furniture. Dogs and cats can host other variants of the scabies mite that cannot complete their life cycle in humans but are able to survive up to

**BOX 140.2 Illnesses Transmitted by or Associated with Arthropods**

**Insects**

Lice: typhus, trench fever, relapsing fever

Fleas: plague, typhus, tungiasis

Bedbugs: possible hepatitis B transmission

Flies and mosquitoes: myiasis, malaria, yellow fever, dengue fever, viral encephalitis, West Nile fever

Reduviid (kissing) bugs: Chagas disease

**Arachnids**

Ticks: Lyme disease, Rocky Mountain spotted fever, Colorado tick fever, babesiosis, ehrlichiosis, Q fever, tularemia

96 hours in human skin. Contact with infected pets can cause self-limited illness, papules, and urticaria in humans.

Severe pruritus and erythematous papules are the most characteristic symptoms of all these bites. Distinguishing flea, lice, and mite bites from one another is very difficult without the offending arthropod present for microscopic examination. All clothing and linen must be laundered in hot water, and potential contacts (prolonged skin-to-skin contact) must be treated simultaneously to avoid reinfection. Scabies-affected pets should also be treated with a scabicide. Features and treatment of these bites are summarized in Table 140.2.

## SUGGESTED READINGS

Clark RF, Wethern-Kestner S, Vance MV, et al. Clinical presentation and treatment of black widow spider envenomations: a review of 163 cases. Ann Emerg Med 1992;21:782-7.

Edlow JA, McGillicuddy DC. Tick paralysis. Infect Dis Clin North Am 2008;22:397-413.

Gibly R, Williams M, Walter FG, et al. Continuous intravenous midazolam infusion for *Centruroides exilicauda* scorpion envenomation. Ann Emerg Med 1999;34:620-5.

Greeman TM. Hypersensitivity to hymenoptera stings. N Engl J Med 2004;351:1978-84.

Vetter RS. Spider research; brown recluse ID. 2009. Available at http://spiders.ucr.edu/recluseid.html.

## REFERENCES

***References can be found on Expert Consult @ www.expertconsult.com.***

# Non-Snake Reptile Bites 141

*Stephen C. Hartsell and Troy E. Madsen*

**KEY POINTS**

- Alligator and crocodile bites may inflict significant internal injury and should be managed as major trauma.
- Gila monster bites may leave teeth in the wound that are not visible by radiography.
- Patients with a Gila monster bite should be observed for 8 hours after the bite because of the risk for systemic toxicity.
- The Komodo dragon has joined the Gila monster and the beaded lizard as the only known venomous lizards of medical significance; its bites are known to cause hypotension and coagulopathy, in addition to infections.
- Green iguanas and snapping turtles may carry *Salmonella*.
- Delayed wound closure and prophylactic antibiotics should be considered in all patients with reptile bites.

## EPIDEMIOLOGY

Crocodilians account for more human injuries and fatalities worldwide than any other non-snake reptile. Three of the largest species are known for unprovoked attacks on humans: the American alligator *(Alligator mississippiensis),* the saltwater crocodile *(Crocodylus porosus),* and the Nile crocodile *(Crocodylus niloticus).* From 1928 through 2008, 567 reports of adverse encounters with American alligators resulted in 24 deaths in the United States. Most injuries were due to a single bite.[1,2] In Australia, 80% of unprovoked attacks by the saltwater crocodile involved people who were either swimming or wading in water. The Nile crocodile of Africa, though smaller and less territorial, probably accounts for more human fatalities than all other 23 species of crocodilians combined.[3]

Most Gila monster bites are nonaccidental and occur as a result of handling the reptile. Accidental bites have become exceedingly rare. No deaths from Gila monster bites have been reported in the United States in the past 50 years.[4,5] The Komodo dragon is now known to have a venom apparatus similar to that of the Gila monster, and deaths have been reported as a result of their bites.

## CROCODILIANS

### PATHOPHYSIOLOGY

Crocodilians survived the Ice Age and are the dominant predators in many of the world's tropical waterways. The American alligator may be found in the southeastern United States, from North Carolina to Louisiana. The saltwater crocodile is found in Southeast Asia and Australia, with males reaching lengths of up to 23 feet (7 m). Victims of crocodilian attacks sustain trauma from a combination of penetrating, blunt, and sheer force. The saltwater crocodile can generate 2000 psi when it bites. The sheer magnitude of the jaw muscle force sustained with extensive penetrating injuries devitalizes large areas of tissue, thereby making such injuries slow to heal and susceptible to infection. Bites must be considered to be heavily contaminated with multiple bacteria, including *Aeromonas hydrophila, Pseudomonas*, and *Proteus* (**Fig. 141.1**).

### PRESENTING SIGNS AND SYMPTOMS

Crocodilian bites are characterized by punctures and tears. Their teeth are conical and not designed for chewing but for grasping their prey. Among survivors, the extremities were the most commonly injured site, with less than 10% sustaining torso trauma.[3,6] Crocodilians may also roll their entire body (known as the "death roll") to disorient and drown the victim, as well as to tear pieces from the victim's body.[3] The force of the massive jaws may lead to extensive internal injury, but even when bite wounds are not present, the force of the animal's movement—or even blunt trauma from its tail—may also inflict significant internal trauma. Initial survivors of severe attacks may exhibit hypotension from massive hemorrhage, in addition to respiratory distress from submersion injury.

### DIFFERENTIAL DIAGNOSIS AND MEDICAL DECISION MAKING

Victims of crocodilian bites often have injuries comparable with those sustained in a severe motor vehicle collision. Prehospital care should start with movement of the patient to a safe environment well away from water's edge. The provider should make sure that airway control, breathing, and circulatory support are adequate with use of the advanced trauma life support (ATLS) protocols. External hemorrhage should be controlled with direct pressure or packing, and chest wounds should be dressed to prevent the development of tension physiology. Extremity fractures should be splinted and suspected major pelvic deformities bound or sheeted. Resuscitation in the hospital should continue according to ATLS protocols, including a focused assessment with sonography for trauma.

A secondary evaluation should be done to determine the extent of tendon, neurologic, and vascular injuries and possible internal organ damage. Underlying fractures and dislocations should be considered, particularly in light of the force and sheering mechanism of the animal's bite. Depending on

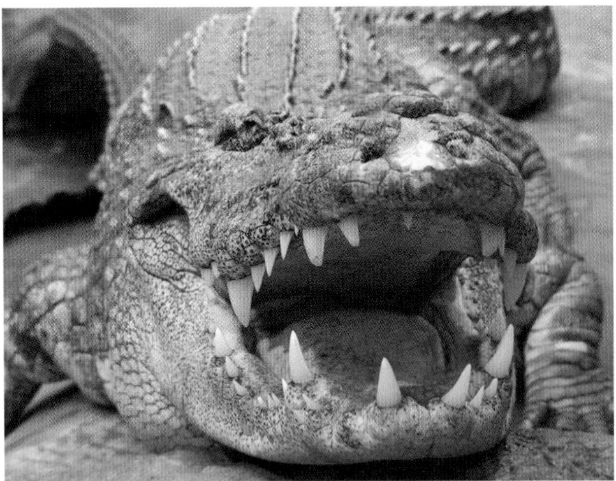

**Fig. 141.1 Crocodile.** (Courtesy Hogle Zoo, Salt Lake City, UT.)

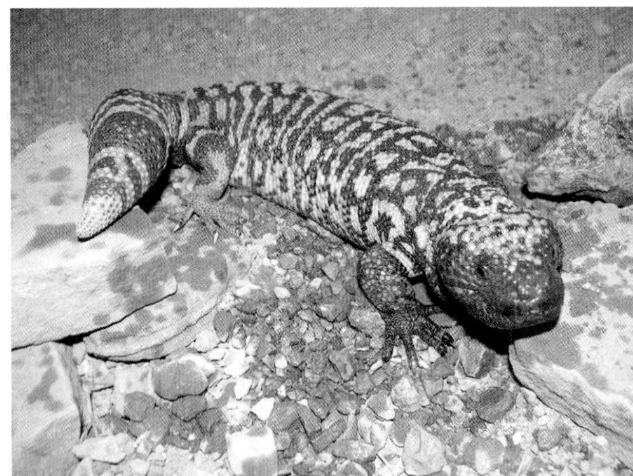

**Fig. 141.2 Gila monster.** (Courtesy Hogle Zoo, Salt Lake City, UT.)

the nature and location of the bite, radiographs can aid in evaluation for bony injury. Computed tomography may be useful to evaluate for internal injury.

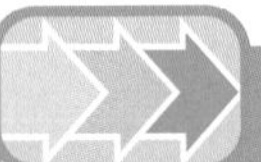

**PRIORITY ACTIONS**

**Reptile Bite Wounds**

Treat all victims of crocodilian bites as major trauma patients with the potential for massive internal injuries.

Extremity bites should be evaluated for underlying vascular, tendon, nerve, or bone injury.

Copiously irrigate and débride all wounds, especially crocodilian and Komodo dragon bites.

Facial wounds and others with significant cosmetic concern should be closed if the patient is seen early after the bite and does not show signs of infection.

Ensure tetanus prophylaxis.

Consider a 5-day course of prophylactic antibiotics with close outpatient follow-up to monitor for signs of infection.

## TREATMENT

Specialists should be consulted to evaluate and treat internal injuries, nerve and tendon damage, fractures, and major lacerations. Local wound care techniques are mandated to cleanse what are typically very contaminated wounds. Because of the high incidence of infection, all significant wounds need exploration, preferably in the operating room, where débridement of devitalized tissue and thorough decontamination can be accomplished. Prophylactic broad-spectrum antibiotic therapy may be necessary to prevent wound infection. The patient's tetanus status should be checked and brought up to date.

## FOLLOW-UP, NEXT STEPS IN CARE, AND PATIENT EDUCATION

Disposition is based on the extent of the injuries, but admission should be considered for all patients except those with minor cutaneous extremity trauma. If the patient is discharged, close follow-up is advisable for wound care and to evaluate for wound infection. Prolonged rehabilitation is frequently needed because of the extent of injuries. The public should be advised to contact local wildlife managers about crocodilian activity before recreating in crocodilian-inhabited environments. Care should be taken when swimming, wading in, or approaching water. If attacked, the best defense appears to be to "fight back" by gouging the crocodile's eyes with thumbs and fingers. If a hand or arm is within the reptile's mouth, reaching caudally may displace the palatal valve, causing the crocodile to aspirate water and open its mouth.

# GILA MONSTER AND BEADED LIZARD

## PATHOPHYSIOLOGY

The Gila monster *(Heloderma suspectum)* and the closely related beaded lizard *(Heloderma horridum)* are native to the southwestern United States and Mexico but may be found throughout the world in zoos and as illegal pets. They are characterized by black beadlike scales mixed with bandlike patterns of yellow, white, or pink scales (**Fig. 141.2**). These reptiles typically range in length from 9 to 32 inches (22 to 81 cm); the beaded lizard is the larger of the two species.

Unlike pit vipers, which inject their venom through fangs, *Heloderma* species have a very rudimentary venom delivery mechanism. The animal has individual vertical grooves in its lancet-shaped teeth to deliver venom by capillary-type action from anterior mandibular venom glands. The lizards tend to stay attached to their victims by using mastication to augment the delivery of venom.[5,6] Their venom is similar in some respects to rattlesnake venom and can stimulate the release of vasoactive kinin, which leads to hypotension.[5]

## PRESENTING SIGNS AND SYMPTOMS

Patients may arrive at the emergency department (ED) with the lizard still attached. Bite wounds are classically indurated and erythematous. Significant edema may develop at the site of the wound. Patients often describe excruciating pain associated with the bites. In envenomated patients, weakness, hypotension, and tachycardia are commonly seen as a result of systemic effects of the reptile's venom.[4,5]

## DIFFERENTIAL DIAGNOSIS AND MEDICAL DECISION MAKING

In addition to local pain and swelling, laboratory evaluation assists in determining the severity of envenomation. The most common reported laboratory abnormality in Gila monster bite envenomations is leukocytosis, although coagulopathy has also been reported. Minimum laboratory work-up should include a complete blood count with platelets, basic metabolic panel, and coagulation panel. An electrocardiogram and cardiacenzymes should be considered, especially in symptomatic patients with cardiac risk factors.

Radiographs may be obtained to rule out associated fractures. However, retained teeth do not show up radiographically, and local wound exploration should be performed to rule out this possibility.

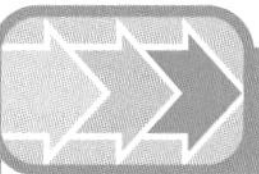

**PRIORITY ACTIONS**

**Envenomation by a Gila Monster or Beaded Lizard**

Observe all patients for 8 hours to watch for the development of signs of envenomation.
Initiate fluid therapy for hypotension and tachycardia.
Initiate vasopressor therapy for hypotension and tachycardia unresponsive to fluids.
Use adequate opiate analgesia to control pain.
Admit patients with systemic symptoms to the hospital for observation and resolution of symptoms.
Ensure tetanus prophylaxis if needed.

## TREATMENT

If still attached, the lizard must be removed from the patient. Increased time of mastication can increase the severity of envenomation. A flame placed under the animal's jaw will usually result in release within 3 to 5 seconds and decreases the possibility of leaving teeth in the wound. Other techniques, such as immersion in cold water, may also be used. Special care should always be taken to prevent reattachment of the animal to the victim or subsequent attachment to the person removing the reptile.

Envenomation may cause hypotension, tachycardia, and generalized weakness. These symptoms generally respond well to intravenous crystalloid administration. Refractory hypotension may require treatment with vasopressors such as dopamine. No antivenom is commercially available for Gila monster or beaded lizard envenomation.[4,6]

The most important aspect of evaluation of the wound is physical examination for evidence of vascular or tendon injury and local wound exploration for retained teeth from the animal. The pain typically requires large amounts of opiate

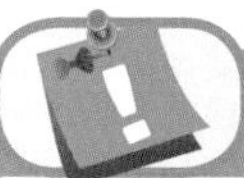

**TIPS AND TRICKS**

**Animal Removal**

Apply a flame under the animal's mandible.
Immerse the animal in cold water.
Use a large Kelly clamp or handheld cast spreader to manually disengage the animal's mouth from the victim.
Place a thin rod across the animal's mouth between the bite site and the jaw and push back on the jaw.
Avoid pulling the animal off, if possible; this may cause further tissue damage and detach teeth into the wound.

analgesics; the few patients who have experienced both rattlesnake and Gila monster bites report much greater pain associated with a Gila monster bite. The pain generally peaks between 15 and 45 minutes following the bite and may last for days.[4,7]

Although the use of prophylactic antibiotics for animal bites remains somewhat controversial, patients may benefit from treatment with broad-spectrum antibiotics, such as amoxicillin-clavulanate (Augmentin) for 3 to 5 days, with specific instructions to watch for signs of infection. Delayed or loose wound closure should be considered to prevent early infection, and the patient should be instructed about local wound care techniques.

## FOLLOW-UP, NEXT STEPS IN CARE, AND PATIENT EDUCATION

All symptomatic and potentially envenomated patients should be admitted for monitoring, supportive care, and pain management. Patients who remain asymptomatic and have normal laboratory values may be discharged after a period of 8 hours of observation. Tetanus prophylaxis is necessary if the patient's immunization status is not up to date. All patients should be reevaluated in 24 to 48 hours for evidence of the development of infection.

# KOMODO DRAGON

## PATHOPHYSIOLOGY

Native to the islands of Indonesia, the Komodo dragon *(Varanus komodoensis)* is the largest lizard in the world; it can reach lengths greater than 10 feet (3 m) and weigh as much as 300 lb (136 kg) (**Fig. 141.3**). These lizards can move as fast as 13 mph (20 km/hr) over short distances and take down prey as large as water buffalo. Komodo dragons' teeth are sharklike, with posterior serrations that create deep open wounds to facilitate envenomation. Its venom is known to cause coagulopathy, increased vascular permeability, and vasodilation.[8] Victims bleed profusely from large wounds. Hypotension and shock develop rapidly and lead to death. If the initial attack does not kill the victim, infections from multiple pathogenic bacteria in the Komodo's saliva can lead to sepsis and death.[9]

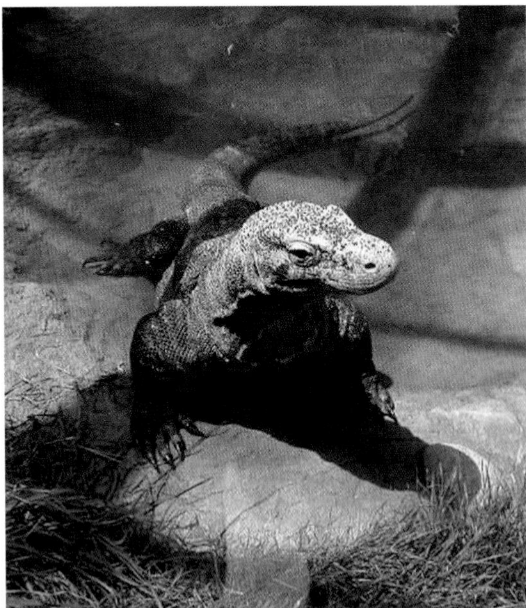

**Fig. 141.3 Komodo dragon.** (Courtesy Hogle Zoo, Salt Lake City, UT.)

## PRESENTING SIGNS AND SYMPTOMS

Most evaluations of Komodo dragon bites in the United States would expectedly come from exposure at zoos or zoologic parks. These bites typically occur on the extremities and produce puncture wounds and lacerations of the skin, along with the potential for local tendon, bone, and neurovascular damage. Bleeding from the wounds may be significant because of envenomation and subsequent coagulopathy. Patients who delay medical evaluation of their wounds will most likely show signs of local and/or systemic bacterial infection. Komodo dragon attacks in the wild may result in multiple large lacerations and areas of tissue loss, not unlike victims of shark attacks. The combination of extensive tissue loss and venom toxicity can lead to hypotension, exsanguination, and sudden death.[8]

## DIFFERENTIAL DIAGNOSIS AND MEDICAL DECISION MAKING

For victims of significant attacks, laboratory and radiologic studies should be ordered as directed by ATLS protocols for major penetrating trauma with associated coagulopathy. Blood and local wound cultures may be useful in the evaluation of hypotension and infection in patients whose arrival for initial medical care is delayed. Radiography can identify underlying damage to bony structures.

## TREATMENT

Victims of Komodo dragon attacks may experience trauma comparable with that sustained in a severe motor vehicle collision. Prehospital care should start with movement of the patient to a safe environment. The provider should make sure that airway control, breathing, and circulatory support are adequate with use of the ATLS protocols. External hemorrhage should be controlled with direct pressure or packing, and chest wounds should be dressed to prevent the development of tension physiology. Extremity fractures should be splinted. Resuscitation in the hospital should continue according to ATLS protocols, with immediate attention to large open wounds, control of hemorrhage, and potential coagulopathy. Because of possible significant blood loss, blood products, including packed red blood cells, platelets, and coagulation factors, should be started early. With the additional vasodilation from envenomation, vasopressors may be needed for refractory hypotension. A broad-spectrum intravenous antibiotic should also be started immediately. No antivenom is commercially available for treatment of komodo dragon enveromation.

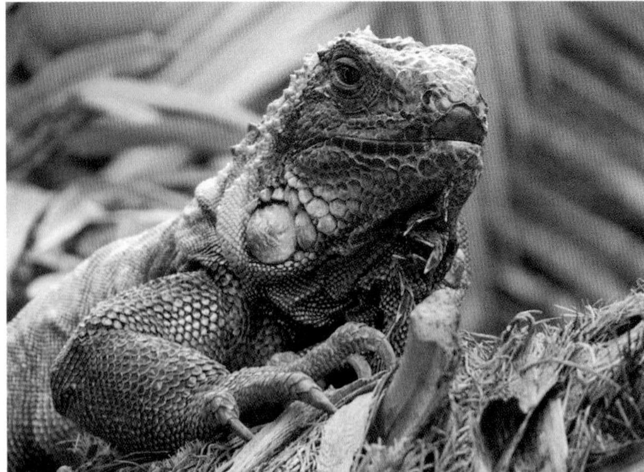

**Fig. 141.4 Iguana.** (Courtesy Hogle Zoo, Salt Lake City, UT.)

## FOLLOW-UP, NEXT STEPS IN CARE, AND PATIENT EDUCATION

Survivors of significant Komodo dragon attacks should be admitted to an intensive care unit. Victims of domestic attacks have required admission and speciality care as a result of underlying tendon and neurovascular injury from extremity wounds. As with all bite wounds, delayed closure of the wound may be required.

Outpatient treatment of simple lacerations or puncture wounds includes tetanus prophylaxis, broad-spectrum antibiotics, and close follow-up to monitor for signs of wound infection. Hospitalization for intravenous antibiotics should be considered because of the high risk for significant infection in these wounds.

# GREEN IGUANA

## PATHOPHYSIOLOGY

The green iguana *(Iguana iguana)* is native to Central and South America. It is the most common lizard sold as a pet in the United States (**Fig. 141.4**). Feral iguana populations can now be found in Florida, Hawaii, and southern Texas. Iguanas are usually docile but can cause injuries with their teeth, claws, and tail. They can also be a source of *Salmonella* infection.[10] No specific venom is associated with iguana bites.

## PRESENTING SIGNS AND SYMPTOMS

Most trauma from iguana bites is superficial soft tissue injury, although tendon injuries have been reported.[11] The majority of bites (80%) occur on the upper extremities, particularly the fingers, with 19% occurring on the face.[10] As with any bite, patients may have infectious complications, particularly those with delayed care or immunosuppression.

## DIFFERENTIAL DIAGNOSIS AND MEDICAL DECISION MAKING

Extensive diagnostic testing is not generally necessary in cases of iguana bites. Blood and local wound cultures may be useful for patients with established wound infections and systemic signs and symptoms. During physical examination the physician should look for underlying tendon and neurovascular injury. Associated bone damage is rare with iguana bites.[11]

## TREATMENT

As with any animal bite wounds, delayed closure should be considered and any underlying neurovascular or tendon injuries treated as appropriate. Prophylactic antibiotics remain somewhat controversial, but a 3- to 5-day course of ciprofloxacin should be considered in light of the *Salmonella* typically carried by the green iguana. In patients with wound infections, treatment with intravenous ceftriaxone may be beneficial. Tetanus prophylaxis is important.

# SNAPPING TURTLE

## PATHOPHYSIOLOGY

Both the common and the alligator snapping turtles have powerful beaklike jaws without teeth but with sharp occlusal surfaces adapted for cutting and holding prey. They are not aggressive but curious about activity occurring around them.

$SI = \frac{SV}{BSA}$ **FACTS AND FORMULAS**

**Antibiotic Therapy**

Crocodilian—multiple pathogens: Broad-spectrum coverage, such as with amoxicillin-clavulanate (Augmentin)

Gila monster—multiple pathogens: Broad-spectrum antibiotic coverage, such as with amoxicillin-clavulanate (Augmentin)

Komodo dragon—multiple pathogens, including *Escherichia coli* and *Staphylococcus* spp.: Consider hospitalization for intravenous broad-spectrum antibiotics, such as ampicillin-sulbactam (Unasyn), because of the high risk for infection

Green iguana—may carry *Salmonella* spp.: *Salmonella* coverage, such as with ciprofloxacin

Snapping turtle—may carry *Salmonella* spp.: *Salmonella* coverage, such as with ciprofloxacin

Snapping turtles will bite out of self-defense when cornered or cut off from their aquatic environment. Most bites tend to occur when victims put their fingers near the turtle's head. These turtles may be as long as 20 inches (50 cm) and have a long neck that may extend up to two thirds the length of their body. These freshwater turtles live in habitats ranging from southeastern Canada to Mexico and Ecuador.

## PRESENTING SIGNS AND SYMPTOMS

A snapping turtle's bite typically causes only soft tissue injury; however, the force of its bite may lead to digit amputation, fractures, or damage to underlying neurovascular structures. Patients with delayed arrival at the ED may show signs of infection.

## DIFFERENTIAL DIAGNOSIS AND MEDICAL DECISION MAKING

When performing the physical examination, the physician should be aware of the potential for damage to nerve, tendon, vascular, and bony structures because of the force of a snapping turtle's bite. Edema may be present and bleeding should be controlled with local wound pressure. Plain radiography may be helpful to evaluate for injury to bones.

## TREATMENT

Attempts to remove a turtle still attached to a patient will cause it to exert greater bite pressure and result in further injury. Although they rarely remain attached, they will typically release their bite if placed in water. The bite wound should be thoroughly irrigated and débrided. Management of tendon, neurovascular, and bony trauma may require specialty consultation. Delayed closure of wounds may be necessary. Because snapping turtles may carry *Salmonella*, antibiotic prophylaxis with ciprofloxacin is advisable; in patients with significant wound infections, treatment with intravenous ceftriaxone is recommended.

## FOLLOW-UP, NEXT STEPS IN CARE, AND PATIENT EDUCATION

All patients should be educated on the signs of infection and the need for elevation of any injured extremity. Reevaluation of the patient should be scheduled for 24 to 48 hours after discharge.

## SUGGESTED READINGS

Fry BJ, Wroe S, Teeuwisse W, et al. A central role for venom in predation by *Varanus komodoensis* (Komodo dragon) and the extinct giant *Varanus* (*Megalania*) *priscus*. Proc Natl Acad Sci U S A 2009;106;8969-74.

Gruen RL. Crocodile attacks in Australia: challenges in injury prevention and trauma care. World J Surg 2009;33;1554-61.

Hooker KR, Caravati EM, Hartsell SC. Gila monster envenomation. Ann Emerg Med 1994;24:731-5.

## REFERENCES

***References can be found on Expert Consult @ www.expertconsult.com.***

# 142 Marine Food-Borne Poisoning, Envenomation, and Traumatic Injuries

*Stephen Thornton and Richard F. Clark*

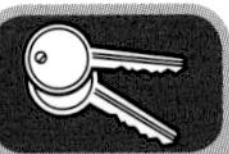

**KEY POINTS**

- Scombroid is thought to be caused by breakdown of histidine into histamine in dark-meat marine fish and can be managed with antihistamines.
- Ciguatera poisoning results from the consumption of large tropical predatory reef fish that have bioaccumulated ciguatoxin; it causes gastrointestinal distress and neurologic symptoms.
- Tetrodotoxin blocks sodium channels and can lead to ascending paralysis and respiratory failure.
- Box jellyfish (Cubozoa). Portuguese man-of-war (Hydrozoa), and other stinging marine invertebrates envenomate humans via nematocysts that contain a stinging barb and venom.
- The box jellyfish *(Chironex fleckeri)* and related species cause the most morbidity and mortality of all marine envenomations.
- Acetic acid immersion is recommended for the treatment of box jellyfish envenomation but may worsen man-o-war envenomation.
- Hot water immersion appears to be an effective treatment of almost all marine envenomations.
- Sea snake venom is neurotoxic and myotoxic. Treatment with antivenom is effective.
- Evaluation for a retained foreign body should be considered with stingray and spiny fish envenomation.
- Wound infection is a common complication of spiny fish and stingray envenomation, and prophylactic antibiotics effective against common pathogens such as *Vibrio* species should be considered.
- Direct marine injuries are usually abrasions and contusions, but fatal attacks by sharks and large predatory fish do occur.

## PERSPECTIVE

As human contact with the ocean and the organisms that live in it continues to increase, the impact of poisonings, envenomations, and direct trauma by these marine organisms will also grow. Marine food-borne poisonings can cause large outbreaks, and direct envenomation by the innumerable stinging organisms in the ocean cause significant morbidity. Less common but more dramatic, attacks by sharks and other large marine organisms cause deaths every year. Thus, it is important for physicians to be aware of the hazards posed by marine organisms and be familiar with appropriate treatment options.

## EPIDEMIOLOGY

Poisoning from the ingestion of marine animals such as shellfish and fish constitutes a small but consistent source of food poisoning outbreaks and illnesses.[1] Although mortality is low, morbidity can be significant, with many patients needing to seek medical care.[2] Tetrodotoxin poisoning is an exception, and significant mortality has been reported.[3]

Even though the vast majority of marine sea life is harmless to humans, a small but important percentage does cause human envenomation with resulting morbidity and mortality. It is difficult to quantify the annual number of marine envenomations because most victims will not seek medical care and reporting cases to health departments or poison centers is not mandatory. Some estimate the number of marine envenomations worldwide to be greater than 10 million per year, with the majority being caused by jellyfish.[4] Deaths are reported every year from envenomation by certain species of jellyfish, most commonly the box jellyfish.[5]

The true number of traumatic injuries caused by marine life is difficult to estimate. Most will consist of only minor abrasions and contusions, but occasional fatal traumatic injuries do occur. Attacks by sharks and large predatory fish cause human fatalities every year.[6] Stingray barbs can cause significant direct trauma and death.[7]

# MARINE FOOD-BORNE POISONINGS

## PATHOPHYSIOLOGY

The toxins responsible for the signs and symptoms of marine food-borne illnesses are primarily produced in microorganisms such as dinoflagellates, diatoms, and marine bacteria and are bioaccumulated by shellfish or fish, which are then ingested by humans and result in toxicity. Most of these toxins modulate neuronal and muscle sodium channels. Scombroid is not caused by a preformed toxin but rather by breakdown

**Table 142.1 Common Marine Food-Borne Poisonings**

| TYPE OF POISONING | TOXIN AND MECHANISM OF ACTION | SOURCE OF POISONING | TIME TO ONSET AND COMMON SYMPTOMS | TREATMENT |
|---|---|---|---|---|
| Scombroid | Histamine–histamine receptor agonist | Large, poorly refrigerated fish | Minutes<br>Flushing, pruritus urticaria<br>GI upset | Supportive<br>Antihistamines |
| Ciguatera | Ciguatoxin (from *Gambierdiscus toxicus*)—opens sodium channels | Large predatory reef fish | Hours<br>Cold allodynia<br>GI upset<br>Paresthesias | Supportive |
| Paralytic shellfish poisoning | Saxitoxin (from *Protogonyaulax* sp.)—blocks sodium channels | Mussels, clams, oysters | Minutes<br>Weakness<br>Paresthesias<br>GI upset<br>Rarely respiratory failure | Supportive<br>Respiratory support in severe cases |
| Neurotoxic shellfish poisoning | Brevetoxin (from *Ptychodiscus brevis*)—opens sodium channels | Mussels, clams, oysters | Minutes to hours<br>GI upset<br>Cold allodynia<br>Paresthesias | Supportive |
| Amnestic shellfish poisoning | Domoic acid (from *Pseudonitzschia* spp.)—activates glutamate receptors | Mussels | Minutes to hours<br>GI upset<br>Memory loss<br>Paresthesias<br>Seizures<br>Encephalopathy | Supportive |
| Tetrodotoxin poisoning | Tetrodotoxin (from marine bacteria species)—blocks sodium channels | Puffer fish, blue-ringed octopus, newt and frog species, horseshoe crabs | Minutes<br>Paresthesias<br>Muscle weakness<br>GI upset<br>Ataxia<br>Paralysis<br>Respiratory failure | Supportive<br>Respiratory support |

*GI*, Gastrointestinal.

of histidine into histamine in inadequately stored dark-meat fish. **Table 142.1** lists the common marine food-borne poisonings, causative toxins, and typical sources of such poisonings.[8]

## PRESENTING SIGNS AND SYMPTOMS

Table 142.1 lists the typical onset and common symptoms associated with marine food-borne poisonings. Typically, a history of seafood ingestion can be obtained. In most cases the symptoms are manifested within minutes to hours and include a mixture of gastroenteritis (nausea, vomiting, and diarrhea) and often dramatic neurologic findings.

## DIFFERENTIAL DIAGNOSIS AND MEDICAL DECISION MAKING

The differential diagnosis for marine food-borne poisoning includes disease processes that cause acute neurologic symptoms with or without gastrointestinal symptoms. Botulism, myasthenia gravis, poliomyelitis, and tick paralysis should be considered. In cases in which the neurologic symptoms are not as obvious, the more common bacterial causes of food-borne poisoning would also need to be considered. The diagnosis of marine food-borne poisoning must be made on a clinical basis because testing for the specific toxins is not readily available.

## TREATMENT

Treatment of marine food-borne poisoning is entirely supportive (see Table 142.1). Attention should be paid to fluid resuscitation and control of nausea and vomiting with antiemetics (ondansetron, 4 to 8 mg intravenously as needed). Although scombroid can be treated with antihistamine therapy, no antidotes are available for any other seafood toxin–mediated poisonings.

# MARINE ENVENOMATION

## PATHOPHYSIOLOGY

Envenomation can occur from both marine invertebrates and vertebrates. Members of the Cnidaria phylum, which includes the box jellyfish, true jellyfish, Portuguese man-o-war, and sea

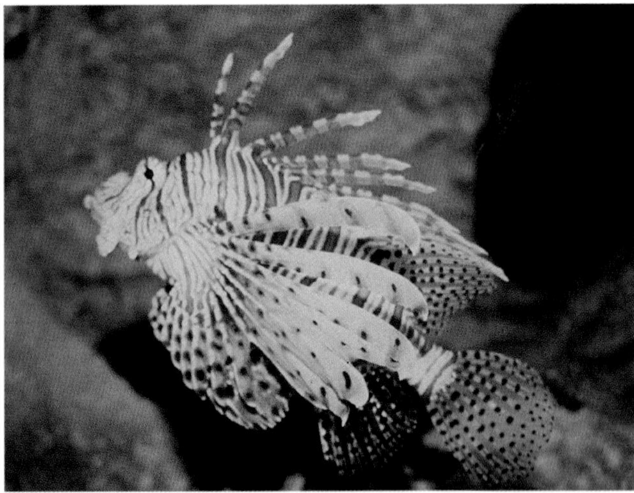

**Fig. 142.1** Lionfish—a member of the Scorpaenidae family of fish.

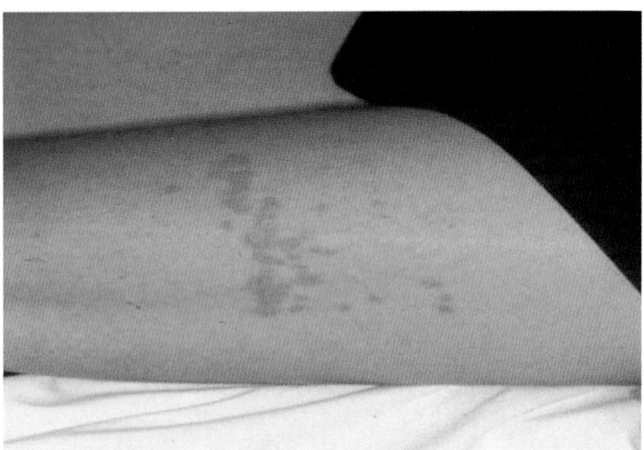

**Fig. 142.2** Skin lesions after envenomation by jellyfish species.

anemone, have nematocysts with hollow venomous barbs that deliver venom hypodermically. Stingrays have a serrated spine connected to a venom gland located on the tail that can be impaled into unsuspecting victims, whereas the Scorpaenidae family of fish (stonefish, lionfish, scorpion fish) have venomous spines on their fins (**Fig. 142.1**). **Table 142.2** lists the most medically important offending marine organisms and their toxicity.[5,9-15]

## PRESENTING SIGNS AND SYMPTOMS

The signs and symptoms of marine envenomation depend on the offending organism. Local pain and irritation are the most common symptoms, especially when nematocysts and spines are involved (**Fig. 142.2**). However, certain marine organisms can cause severe systemic symptoms and even death. The Australian box jellyfish *(Chironex fleckeri)* can cause sudden cardiopulmonary collapse.[5] The Irukandji jellyfish *(Carukia barnesi)* can cause Irukandji syndrome, a condition characterized by severe whole-body pain and spasms, tachycardia, and severe hypertension, and it has caused deaths.[12] The blue-ringed octopus has tetrodotoxin in its venom, which can cause paralysis and respiratory failure.[13] The cone snail's venom is a complex mixture of peptides that can lead to rapid paralysis and death.[14] Stonefish envenomation can result in cardiovascular instability and death, although severe local effects are more common.[10] Sea snake venom has both a neurotoxic component, which leads to ascending paralysis, and a myotoxic component, which causes muscle breakdown.[15] Table 142.2 summarizes the signs and symptoms of the more significant marine envenomations.

## DIFFERENTIAL DIAGNOSIS AND MEDICAL DECISION MAKING

Frequently, the identity of the offending marine organism will not be known. The geographic location can be a useful predictor, and physicians should be aware of the venomous marine organisms in their local area. It can be helpful to look for physical clues, such as retained jellyfish tentacles and puncture marks. The presence of severe local pain often indicates a Cnidaria or fish envenomation, whereas significant neurologic symptoms, such as weakness, should raise suspicion for cone snail or other neurotoxic organisms.

## TREATMENT

Treatment of marine envenomation begins with addressing the patient's airway, breathing, and circulation status. Typically, good supportive care and pain control are all that is needed. Hot water immersion is recommended to control the pain caused by Cnidaria, Scorpaenidae fish, and stingray envenomation and is efficacious because of the heat-labile properties of the neurotoxic component of the venom responsible for the pain. This is typically achieved by immersing the affected body part in water heated to approximately 42° C to 45° C for 20 minutes.[16,17] Acetic acid may have a role in inactivating the nematocysts of the box jellyfish and Irukandji jellyfish but should not be used on other types of jellyfish because it may worsen these envenomations.[18] Recently, topical lidocaine was shown to help in alleviating the pain and inactivating nematocysts from several different species of Cnidaria, including the Portuguese man-o-war.[19] Antivenom therapy is available to treat poisoning by the Australian box jellyfish, the stonefish, and the sea snake.[20] Evaluation for a retained foreign body should also be considered, especially with stingray and sea urchin envenomation[21,22] (**Fig. 142.3**). Table 142.2 summarizes the recommended treatments.

# MARINE TRAUMATIC INJURIES

## PATHOPHYSIOLOGY

Traumatic marine injuries are most often caused by the simple action of scraping against the rock-hard and sometimes razor-sharp exoskeletons of sponges, corals, and other sessile marine organisms. Bites from sharks and fish cause trauma directly related to the size of the animal, force of the bite, and

**Table 142.2 Signs and Symptoms of Significant Marine Envenomations**

| MARINE ORGANISM | METHOD OF VENOM DELIVERY | CLINICAL FINDINGS | TREATMENT |
|---|---|---|---|
| Australian box jellyfish *(Chironex fleckeri)* | Nematocysts | Linear rash, severe local and generalized pain, muscle spasms<br>Rare: rapid cardiopulmonary collapse, death | Supportive care<br>Pain management<br>Hot water immersion<br>Acetic acid irrigation<br>Antivenom |
| Irukandji jellyfish *(Carukia barnesi)* | Nematocysts | *Irukandji syndrome*: tachycardia, tachypnea, hypertension to hypotension, whole-body muscle spasms, pain<br>Rare: death | Supportive care<br>Pain management<br>Hot water immersion<br>Acetic acid irrigation<br>Vasodilators |
| Sea nettle *(Chyrsaora quinquecirrha)* | Nematocysts | Local pain and irritation | Supportive care<br>Pain management<br>Hot water immersion<br>Lidocaine spray |
| Portuguese man-o-war *(Physalia physalis)* | Nematocysts | Severe local pain, bullae, necrosis<br>Rare: hemolysis, shock, death | Supportive care<br>Pain management<br>Hot water immersion<br>Lidocaine spray<br>*Do not use* acetic acid |
| Thimble jelly *(Linuche unguiculata)* | Nematocysts | *Sea bather's eruption*: pruritic popular eruption on the skin covered by a bathing suit | Supportive care<br>Hot water immersion<br>Pain management |
| Fire coral *(Millepora alcicornis)* | Nematocysts | Local pain and irritation | Supportive care<br>Hot water immersion<br>Pain management |
| Sea anemones (class Anthozoa) | Nematocysts | Local pain and irritation, GI upset | Supportive care<br>Hot water immersion<br>Pain management |
| Blue-ringed octopus (*Hapalochlaena* sp.) | Beak | Flaccid paralysis, respiratory failure, death | Supportive care<br>Respiratory support |
| Cone snails (*Conus* spp.) | Modified radula | Rapid paralysis, respiratory failure, death | Supportive care<br>Respiratory support |
| Sea urchin (class Echinoidea) | Multiple spines | Local pain and irritation | Supportive care<br>Hot water immersion<br>Pain management<br>Wound care<br>Foreign body removal |
| Stonefish (*Synaceia* sp.) | Spines in dorsal, pelvic, anal fins | Severe local pain and edema, GI upset, cardiovascular instability, death | Supportive care<br>Hot water immersion<br>Pain management<br>Wound care<br>Antivenom |
| Other Scorpaenidae fish (*Pterois* sp. and *Scorpaena* sp.) | Spines in dorsal, pelvic, anal fins | Local pain and swelling, GI upset | Supportive care<br>Hot water immersion<br>Pain management<br>Wound care |
| Stingray (class Chondrichthyes) | Serrated tail barb | Severe local pain and edema | Supportive care<br>Hot water immersion<br>Pain management<br>Wound care |
| Sea snakes (genus *Hydrophiidae*) | Small, front fangs | Ascending paralysis, muscle pain and breakdown, respiratory failure, death | Supportive care<br>Respiratory support<br>Antivenom |

*GI*, Gastrointestinal.

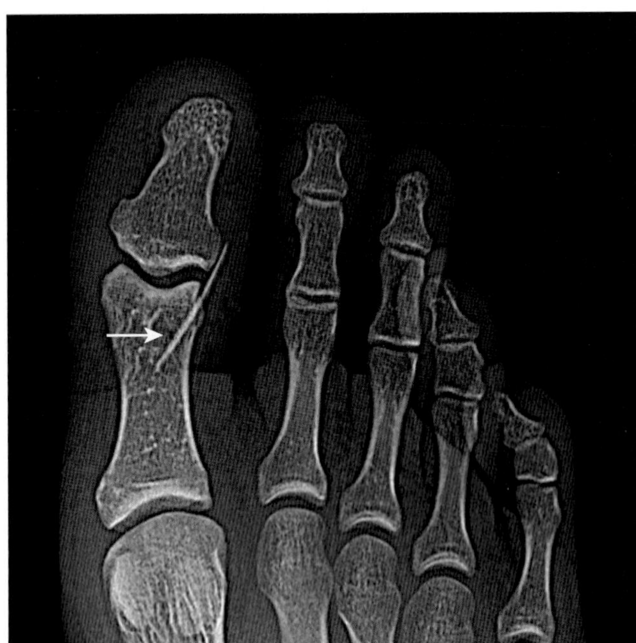

**Fig. 142.3 Retained stingray barb *(arrow)* in the foot.**

cutting nature of the teeth. The severity of direct injuries from stingray barbs depends on the location where the victim was impaled.

## DIFFERENTIAL DIAGNOSIS AND MEDICAL DECISION MAKING

The offending organisms may or may not be known to the victim, and concomitant envenomation should be considered. Radiographic evaluation may be needed. The most important medical decision to be made is whether the injury is severe enough to warrant specialist care by a trauma, vascular, or orthopedic surgeon.

## TREATMENT

After initially addressing the airway, breathing, and circulation, direct wound care is usually sufficient to treat most traumatic marine injuries. Control of bleeding and wound irrigation are important. Because infections can complicate these injuries, prophylactic antibiotics should be considered.[23] Injuries to tendons, ligaments, and other vital structures should be evaluated and addressed.

## FOLLOW-UP, NEXT STEPS IN CARE, AND PATIENT EDUCATION

All the marine food-borne illnesses are self-limited, although amnestic shellfish poisoning has been linked to long-term neurologic sequelae.[24] Patients with suspected tetrodotoxin poisoning should be admitted to the hospital for observation. Most other patients who are asymptomatic after treatment can be discharged. Those with ongoing or severe symptoms should be admitted. The local public health department should be informed of suspected cases of marine food-borne poisoning.

The vast majority of marine envenomations will be self-limited and resolve with simple supportive care. Infection from sea urchin spines, fish spines, and stingray barbs is well documented, and prophylactic treatment with antibiotics effective against pathogens such as *Vibrio* species should be considered.[21,22,25] Patients with persistent or severe pain may need to be admitted, as will any patient with envenomation by a potentially neurotoxic organism.

Serious injuries may need treatment by a trauma or orthopedic surgeon, either on an emergency basis or as an outpatient. Otherwise, good wound care measures should be explained to the patient and return precautions focusing on signs and symptoms of infection stressed.

## SUGGESTED READINGS

Atkinson PR, Boyle A, Hartin D, et al. Is hot water immersion an effective treatment for marine envenomation? Emerg Med J 2006;23:503-8.

Currie BJ. Marine antivenoms. J Toxicol Clin Toxicol 2003;41:301-8.

Fernandez I, Valladolid G, Varon J, et al. Encounters with venomous sea-life. J Emerg Med 2011;40:103-12.

Isbister GK, Kiernan MC. Neurotoxic marine poisoning. Lancet Neurol 2005;4:219-28.

Noonburg GE. Management of extremity trauma and related infections occurring in the aquatic environment. J Am Acad Orthop Surg 2005;13:243-53.

# General Approach to the Poisoned Patient 143

Amy E. Zosel

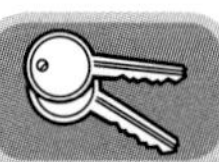

**KEY POINTS**

- The mainstay of treatment of a poisoned patient is good symptomatic and supportive care.
- Observation is one of the most critical aspects in the management of poisoned patients.
- The most common substance categories associated with fatalities are sedative-hypnotics, antipsychotics, cardiovascular medications, opioids, and acetaminophen combination products.
- All substances can be poisonous; toxicity usually depends on the dose and the duration of exposure.
- *Toxidromes* are symptom complexes that may provide clues to the identity of the offending agent on the basis of specific pharmacologic principles; they represent "physiologic fingerprints."
- In general, hypotension in the setting of poisoning is best treated with direct-acting pressors.
- In patients with an unknown ingestion, activated charcoal is the most efficacious decontamination method, but its use should be limited to those who are awake and alert *and/or* have a protected airway (self-protected or intubated).

## EPIDEMIOLOGY

Toxicology and poisons have always been of great interest to the public. *Toxicology* is the study of harmful interactions between chemical or physical agents and biologic systems.

It is believed that approximately 5.3 million poisoning exposures take place every year in the United States, but only about half are reported to poison control centers. The American Association of Poison Control Centers reported 2,479,355 cases of poisoning during 2009, with 93.8% occurring at a residence and just 1.5% at the workplace. Children younger than 3 years were involved in 46.0% of reported poisonings. About 82% of the poisonings were unintentional, and suicide attempts accounted for just 8.9% of cases.[1]

## PRESENTING SIGNS AND SYMPTOMS

A poisoned patient may have many different clinical symptoms, including cardiac dysrhythmias, altered mental status, seizures, nausea and vomiting, and respiratory depression. In many cases the offending agent is initially unknown. Vital signs, including pulse oximetry values, are important to obtain (**Table 143.1**) and should be measured often in a poisoned patient. Vital signs (temperature, pulse, respirations, blood pressure, pulse oximetry) are helpful because they can provide clues to the type of poisoning. Physical findings such as pupil size, odor, seizure activity, and dermatologic changes can also provide clues to the offending agent (**Tables 143.2 to 143.4**). Emergency physicians (EPs) should be sure to examine for diaphoresis under the axilla, which may be the only body part that exhibits this finding. It is essential to note that patients with mixed ingestions may not have the classic initial signs and symptoms.

Patients who have ingested poisons may not appear to be critically ill initially, but they all have the potential for clinical deterioration.

The history obtained from the patient may be unreliable.[2] It is crucial for emergency department (ED) personnel to also obtain additional history from family and friends. The paramedics who brought the patient can provide information about the scene where the overdose took place. What behavior did the patient have at the scene or before arrival? Were there seizures, emesis, changing vital signs? Were there any medicine bottles were found and, if so, were any pills were missing from the bottles? The patient's primary care physician or psychiatrist may provide important information. Frequently, the patient's pharmacy can be called to obtain lists of current medications and the last fill date. It is crucial to obtain an occupational history and to review past medical records for any poisoned patient. The initial work-up should determine whether a specific patient has been exposed to an agent for which an antidote (or other specific treatment) exists (**Box 143.1**).

## DIFFERENTIAL DIAGNOSIS AND MEDICAL DECISION MAKING

### TOXIDROMES

Several drugs and toxins are associated with specific toxidromes (**Table 143.5**). *Toxidromes* are symptom complexes that may provide clues to the identity of the offending agent. They are based on specific pharmacologic principles and represent the "physiologic fingerprints" of the associated substances. An anticholinergic toxidrome, for example, is caused by parasympatholytic substances such as antihistamines, jimsonweed, tricyclic antidepressants (TCAs), and phenothiazines. Affected patients may exhibit hypertension, tachycardia,

Acknowledgment and thanks to Victor Tuckler, MD, and Jorge Martinez, MD, for their work on the first edition.

**Table 143.1 Classic Examples of Ingested Substances Associated with Changes in Vital Signs***

| CHANGE IN VITAL SIGN | ASSOCIATED SUBSTANCES |
|---|---|
| Bradycardia | Anticholinesterase drugs<br>Beta-blockers<br>Calcium channel blockers<br>Clonidine<br>Digoxin<br>Ethanol, alcohols<br>Opioids |
| Tachycardia | Amphetamines<br>Anticholinergics<br>Cocaine<br>Sympathomimetics<br>Theophylline |
| Hypothermia | Ethanol<br>Insulin<br>Opioids<br>Oral hypoglycemics<br>Sedative-hypnotic agents |
| Hyperthermia | Anticholinergics<br>Antidepressants<br>Antihistamines<br>Salicylates<br>Sympathomimetics |
| Hypotension | Aminophylline, theophylline<br>Antidepressants<br>Antihypertensive agents<br>Opioids<br>Sedative-hypnotic agents, especially in combination with other depressants |
| Hypertension | Amphetamines<br>Anticholinergics<br>Caffeine<br>Cocaine<br>Sympathomimetics<br>Thyroid medications |
| Hypoventilation | Alcohols<br>Opioids<br>Sedative-hypnotic agents |
| Hyperventilation | Phencyclidine<br>Salicylates<br>Sympathomimetics (cocaine, amphetamines) |

*This is not an all-inclusive list. Victims of multiple substance exposure often do *not* have the classic signs and symptoms.

**Table 143.2 Specific Substances Associated with Pupillary Changes***

| PUPILLARY CHANGE | ASSOCIATED SUBSTANCES |
|---|---|
| Miosis | Carbamates<br>Cholinergics<br>Clonidine<br>Opioids<br>Organophosphates<br>Phenothiazine<br>Pilocarpine<br>Sedative-hypnotic agents |
| Mydriasis | Anticholinergics<br>Antidepressants<br>Antihistamines<br>Atropine |

*Patients with mixed ingestions often do not have the classic pupillary changes.

**Table 143.3 Specific Substances Associated with Skin Changes**

| SKIN CHANGE | ASSOCIATED SUBSTANCES |
|---|---|
| Diaphoresis | Organophosphates<br>Phencyclidine<br>Salicylates<br>Sympathomimetics |
| Red skin | Anticholinergics<br>Boric acid |
| Blue skin | Methemoglobin-forming agents (e.g., nitrates, nitrites, aniline dyes, dapsone, phenazopyridine) |
| Blisters | Barbiturates and other sedative-hypnotic agents<br>Carbon monoxide<br>Venom (snake bites, spider bites) |

fever, delirium, and mydriasis. Sympathomimetic toxidromes resemble anticholinergic toxidromes except that parasympatholytic agents produce silent bowel sounds and dry skin.

The following diagnostic studies should be performed in poisoned patients: serum acetaminophen and acetylsalicylic acid measurements, blood ethanol measurement, blood chemistry panel, electrocardiogram (ECG), pulse oximetry, and serum glucose measurement (**Box 143.2**). Toxicology screening may confirm exposure to a toxicant but does not usually change management (see later discussion). A blood chemistry profile can be extremely useful, especially in determining the anion gap.[3,4] The anion gap is calculated by the formula (mEq/L) = $Na^+ - [Cl^- + HCO_3^-]$; the normal range of anion gap varies from 3 to 12 mEq/L. An increase in the anion gap may indicate an intoxication, but EP must be aware that a normal anion gap does not rule out poisoning. Conditions such as hypoalbuminemia can alter the anion gap. Every 1-g/L decrease in plasma albumin leads in a drop in the anion gap of 2.5 mEq/L. Multiple conditions can cause metabolic acidosis with an elevated anion gap, and the mnemonic "A CAT MUD PILES" is an easy way to remember most of them (**Box 143.3**). It is important to note than any toxin that can cause seizures or other processes leading to lactic acidosis can also cause an anion gap. A decreased anion gap can be seen with bromide and lithium poisonings.

Measurement of serum osmolality may be useful for some toxin ingestions and should be ordered if toxic alcohols are suspected but results of toxic alcohol testing will be delayed (see Chapter 151).

A normal osmolar gap should be less than 10. An elevated osmolar gap suggests intoxication, although a low or no osmolar gap does not exclude intoxication. An elevated osmolar gap is seen early after the ingestion of methanol, ethylene glycol, diuretics (mannitol), ethanol, and isopropyl

**Table 143.4 Specific Substances Associated with Odors**

| ODOR | ASSOCIATED SUBSTANCE |
|---|---|
| Bitter almonds | Cyanide |
| Carrots | Water hemlock |
| Fruity | Ketones (from diabetic ketoacidosis), isopropanol (metabolized to acetone) |
| Garlic | Arsenic, organophosphates |
| Gasoline | Hydrocarbons |
| Mothballs | Camphor |
| Peanuts | Certain rodenticides |
| Pears | Chloral hydrate |
| Rotten eggs | Hydrogen sulfide, sulfur dioxide |
| Wintergreen | Methyl salicylates |

**BOX 143.1 Questions to Ask About a Poisoned Patient**

**Why?**
Was the poisoning unintentional or intentional?

**Where?**
Did the ingestion occur inside or outside? While the patient was alone, at a party, or at work?
What was the environment like?

**What?**
Question emergency medical services personnel and police, as well as family and friends of the patient, to learn what the substance is. What poisons or drugs were available?

**When?**
How long since the ingestion?
When was the person last seen in their general state of health (i.e., normal)?

**Who?**
Who was at the scene and knows what occurred?

alcohol and reflects the presence of the parent compound. Once the parent compound is metabolized to the toxic acid metabolite, in the case of methanol and ethylene glycol, the osmolar gap is low and the anion gap is high.

Patients with possible poisoning should undergo cardiac monitoring. In cases of unknown ingestion or ingestions for which cardiac abnormalities are a known side effect, a 12-lead ECG should be evaluated for QRS and QT intervals, morphology, and rhythm. A wide QRS interval may be seen with the ingestion of any agent that causes sodium channel blockade, such as TCAs and cocaine. A long QT interval may be seen with many ingestions, such as phenothiazine and methadone. Variable atrioventricular block is associated with digoxin overdose, and ischemic changes can be the result of hypoxemia secondary to carbon monoxide poisoning.

**BOX 143.2 Key Points for Ordering Diagnostic Studies in a Poisoned Patient**

Treat the patient, not the laboratory results.
Order laboratory tests according to the signs and symptoms.
The test results may not correlate with the toxidromes.
Drug screens lack clinical significance in some cases.
A test may not be rapidly available; check with the laboratory about turnaround times.
It is important to know what the specific laboratory drug panel covers.

**BOX 143.3 Mnemonic for Causes of Elevated Anion Gap Metabolic Acidosis: A CAT MUD PILES**

*A*lcoholic ketoacidosis
*C*yanide, *C*arbon monoxide
*A*lcohol
*T*oluene
*M*ethanol, *M*etformin, *M*assive acetaminophen
*U*remia
*D*iabetic ketoacidosis
*P*araldehyde
*I*ron, *I*soniazid
*L*actic acidosis
*E*thylene glycol
*S*alicylates, *S*trychnine

**BOX 143.4 Drug Detection on Routine Urinary Drug Screens**

**Drugs Detected**
Amphetamines, often misses MDMA, many false positives
Barbiturates
Benzodiazepines, often does *not* detect lorazepam or alprazolam
Cannabinoids
Cocaine metabolites
Ethanol
Opioids, naturally occurring (codeine, morphine, heroin) well detected, synthetics (fentanyl, oxycodone, meperidine, methadone) often *not* detected
Phencyclidine (PCP)
Propoxyphene

*MDMA*, Methylenedioxymethamphetamine.

## TOXICOLOGY SCREENS

Toxicology screens are of variable utility. Urine screens were specifically designed for the drugs of abuse but have high false-positive and false-negative rates (**Box 143.4**). Qualitative findings (i.e., yes/no tests) do not provide information about the exact time of ingestion or the severity of

**Table 143.5 Toxidromes and Their Causes**

| TOXIDROME | FEATURES | EXAMPLES OF CAUSES* |
|---|---|---|
| **Anticholinergic**: "Hot as a hare, dry as a bone, red as a beet, blind as a bat, mad as a hatter, full as a flask, tachy as a pink flamingo" | Delirium<br>Dry, flushed skin<br>Hyperthermia<br>Mydriasis<br>Tachycardia<br>Urinary retention | Amantadine<br>Antihistamines<br>Antiparkinsonian agents<br>Antipsychotics<br>Antispasmodics (dicyclomine)<br>Belladonna alkaloids (atropine)<br>Cyclic antidepressants<br>Glycopyrrolate<br>Phenothiazine<br>Plants (jimsonweed, nightshade, *Amanita muscaria*)<br>Scopolamine |
| **Cholinergic**: "SLUDGE syndrome and killer BBBs"[†] | *S*alivation<br>*L*acrimation<br>*U*rination<br>*D*iarrhea<br>*G*I hyperactivity<br>*E*mesis<br>*B*ronchorrhea<br>*B*ronchoconstriction<br>*B*radycardia | Acetylcholine<br>Carbamates<br>Mushrooms (some species)<br>Organophosphates<br>Physostigmine<br>Pilocarpine<br>Tobacco |
| **Extrapyramidal** | Ataxia<br>Choreoathetosis<br>Dystonic reactions<br>Hyperreflexia<br>Opisthotonos<br>Rigidity<br>Seizures<br>Torticollis<br>Tremor<br>Trismus | Haloperidol<br>Olanzapine<br>Phenothiazines<br>Risperidone |
| **Opioid** | Bradycardia<br>Coma<br>Decreased bowel sounds<br>Hypotension<br>Hypothermia<br>Hypoventilation<br>Miosis | Dextromethorphan<br>Opioids: codeine, diphenoxylate, fentanyl, heroin, hydrocodone, meperidine, methadone, morphine, oxycodone, pentazocine, propoxyphene[‡] |
| **Sedative-hypnotic** | Abnormal gait<br>Apnea<br>Coma<br>Confusion<br>Decreased level of consciousness<br>Hypoventilation<br>Pulse slow or normal<br>Sedation<br>Slurred speech<br>Stupor | Anticonvulsants<br>Antipsychotics<br>Barbiturates<br>Benzodiazepines<br>Ethanol<br>Meprobamate |
| **Serotonin** | Autonomic instability<br>Confusion<br>Diaphoresis<br>Fever<br>Flushing<br>Hyperreflexia<br>Irritability<br>Myoclonus<br>Tremor | Fluoxetine<br>MAOIs<br>Paroxetine<br>Sertraline<br>St. John's wort<br>Trazodone |
| **Sympathomimetic** | Agitation<br>Diaphoresis<br>Hypertension<br>Hyperthermia<br>Mydriasis<br>Seizures (CNS excitation)<br>Tachycardia | Aminophylline<br>Amphetamines<br>Caffeine<br>Cocaine<br>Ephedrine<br>Epinephrine<br>Fenfluramine<br>LSD<br>Methylphenidate<br>Phencyclidine<br>Phenylpropanolamine<br>Pseudoephedrine<br>Theophylline |
| **Delayed** | Patients may not have any initial symptoms | Acetaminophen<br>Extended-release cardiac medications<br>Oral hypoglycemic agents<br>Sustained-release or delayed-release formulations[§]<br>Warfarin |

*CNS*, Central nervous system; *GI*, gastrointestinal; *LSD*, lysergic acid diethylamide; *MAOIs*, monoamine oxidase inhibitors.

*This is by no means a comprehensive listing of causes of toxidromes.

†Killer BBBs are the true life threats of this toxidrome and indicate very severe poisoning.

‡Meperidine dilates the pupils; propoxyphene and pentazocine may not cause miosis.

§With transdermal patch–released medications, toxidromes may have a slower onset.

impairment (**Table 143.6**). Serum is useful for determining quantitative levels of a specific drug (**Box 143.5**). Treatment is best based on the signs and symptoms. When in doubt, talk to your laboratory manager regarding your particular laboratory assay's false-negative and false-positive rates, as well as which specific substances cross-react to cause a false-positive result. A comprehensive urine toxicology test, though not performed in most laboratories, can be helpful in cases in which the exact substance must be known. An example would be an intoxicated 3-year-old child whose parents deny any exposure.

When drug metabolites circulate in blood, they enter the scalp's blood vessels and are filtered through the hair. These metabolites remain in hair and may provide a permanent record of drug use when tested. Hair is constantly exposed to the extracorporal environment and can thus test positive for

**Table 143.6 Detection Periods for Toxic Substances in Urine***

| SUBSTANCE | DETECTION PERIOD† |
|---|---|
| Amphetamines | 2-4 days |
| Barbiturates: | |
| Short acting (e.g., secobarbital) | 1 day |
| Long acting (e.g., phenobarbital) | 2-4 wk |
| Benzodiazepines | 3-30 days |
| Cannabis: | |
| Single use | 24-72 hr |
| Habitual use | Up to 12 wk |
| Cocaine metabolite | 2-4 days |
| Codeine, morphine | 2-5 days |
| Ethanol | 6-24 hr |
| Euphorics (e.g., methylenedioxymethamphetamine) | 1-4 days |
| Heroin | 2-4 days |
| Lysergic acid diethylamide | 1-4 days |
| Methadone | 3-4 days |
| Methaqualone | 14 days |
| Opioids | 2-4 days |
| Phencyclidine | 2-7 days for casual use, several months for heavy use |
| Phenobarbital | 10-30 days |
| Propoxyphene | 6 hr-2 days |
| Steroids (anabolic), used as performance enhancers | |
| Oral | 1 mo |
| Parenteral | 14 days |

*These represent the approximate detection period. It may vary according to preparation and chronicity of use.

†Time after ingestion during which the substance can be detected.

substances that the patient has not ingested. Saliva testing is limited to detection of very recent drug use, so it will probably be confined to detecting current intoxication only.

If a sample tests positive on initial screening, a second method should be used to confirm the initial result. Positive results from two different methods operating on different chemical principles greatly decrease the possibility that a methodologic problem or a "cross-reacting" substance could have created the positive result. A confirmation assay should usually be carried out with a method that has comparable sensitivity and higher specificity (or selectivity) than a screening assay. Examples of confirmation methods are gas chromatography, gas chromatography with mass spectrometry, and high-performance liquid chromatography (**Table 143.7**).

**BOX 143.5 Drugs Commonly Quantified in Serum**

- Acetaminophen
- Carbon monoxide
- Digoxin
- Dilantin
- Ethanol
- Ethylene glycol
- Iron
- Lithium
- Methanol
- Methemoglobin
- Phenobarbital
- Salicylates
- Theophylline

**Table 143.7 False-Positive Results of Urine Drug Screening**

| SUBSTANCES FOR WHICH FALSE-POSITIVE RESULTS OCCUR | RESPONSIBLE DRUGS |
|---|---|
| Amphetamines | Asthma medications (Bronkaid tablets, Primatene tablets)<br>Ephedrine, pseudoephedrine, propyl ephedrine, phenylephrine (Nyquil-D, Contac, Sudafed, Allerest, Tavist-D, Dimetapp, Phenergan-D, Robitussin Cold and Flu)<br>Over-the-counter diet aids (Dexatrim, Acutrim)<br>Over-the-counter nasal sprays (Vicks inhaler, Afrin)<br>Prescription medications—many (e.g., Ritalin, Selegiline, Dexedrine) |
| Cocaine | Some antibiotics such as amoxicillin and ampicillin |
| Opiates | Cough suppressants with dextromethorphan (DXM or DM)<br>Most prescription pain medications<br>Nyquil-D<br>Poppy seeds<br>Quinine in tonic water<br>Some antidepressants, including amitriptyline, can cause false-positive opioid results for up to 3 days after use<br>Tylenol with codeine |
| Phencyclidine | Diazepam |
| Tetrahydrocannabinol | Dronabinol (Marinol)<br>Ibuprofen (Advil, Nuprin, Motrin, Excedrin)<br>Ketoprofen (Orudis)<br>Naproxen (Aleve)<br>Promethazine (Phenergan, Promethegan)<br>Riboflavin (vitamin $B_2$, hemp seed oil) |

Passive inhalation of marijuana smoke cannot lead to a positive urine test result for its metabolites. Inadvertent exposure to marijuana is commonly claimed as the basis for a positive urine drug screen result. Clinical studies have shown that it is unlikely that an individual who does not smoke marijuana could unknowingly inhale enough marijuana smoke

**Table 143.8 Radiographic Findings Associated with Toxic Ingestions**

| RADIOGRAPHIC FINDING | CAUSES |
|---|---|
| Concretions* | Barbiturates<br>Extended-release theophylline<br>Iron<br>Salicylates<br>Sedative-hypnotic agents |
| Noncardiogenic pulmonary edema | Meprobamate<br>Methadone<br>Opioids<br>Phenobarbital<br>Propoxyphene<br>Salicylates |
| Toxins appearing radiopaque on kidneys-ureters-bladder radiographs | Chloral hydrate<br>Illicit drug packets (well, densely packed)<br>Iron and other heavy metals (e.g., lead, arsenic, mercury)<br>Some neuroleptic agents<br>Sustained-release products and enteric-coated preparations |

*Should be suspected if the patient's clinical or laboratory status waxes and wanes.

passively for urine to contain a drug concentration detectable at the cutoff used in current urinalysis methods.

## RADIOGRAPHIC EVALUATION

**Table 143.8** summarizes the radiographic findings associated with toxic ingestions.

# TREATMENT

The primary treatment of a poisoned patient is to stabilize the airway, breathing, and circulation. Initial management includes attention to the ABCDs of resuscitation for a toxic ingestion:

*A*irway
*B*reathing, oxygen
*C*irculation
*D*extrose, naloxone

After initial stabilization of a critically ill patient, specific antidote therapy is administered if applicable (**Table 143.9**), a detailed history is elicited, and a physical examination is performed. Patients who are externally contaminated with a toxicant that may injure staff must be decontaminated immediately to avoid incapacitation of health care staff

**Table 143.9 Specific Toxins and Their Antidotes**

| TOXINS | ANTIDOTES* |
|---|---|
| Acetaminophen | *N*-acetylcysteine, 140 mg/kg PO, then 70 mg/kg q4h for up to 17 doses, *or* 150-mg/kg IV over 1-hr period with 50 mg/kg over 4 hr followed by 100 mg/kg over 16 hr |
| Anticholinergics | Physostigmine, 0.5-2 mg IV in adults or 0.2 mg/kg in children over 2-min period for anticholinergic delirium, seizures, or arrhythmias |
| Arsenic, lead, or mercury | Dimercaprol, 3-5 mg/kg IM only (followed by calcium EDTA for lead encephalopathy)<br>D-Penicillamine, 20-40 mg/kg/day divided tid or qid in adults for lead or mercury poisoning[†]<br>Oral succimer, 7.5 mg/kg PO q6h or 10 mg/kg q8h for lead, arsenic, or mercury |
| Benzodiazepines | Flumazenil, 0.2 mg, then 0.3 mg, then 0.5 mg, up to 3 mg; for nonchronic users only[‡] |
| Black widow spider bite | *Latrodectus* antivenin, 1 vial IV by slow infusion |
| Beta-blockers | Glucagon, 5-10 mg in adults, then infusion of the effective dose each hour |
| Calcium channel blockers | Calcium, as 1 g calcium chloride IV in adults or 20-30 mg/kg per dose in children delivered over a few minutes with continuous monitoring<br>When decreased myocardial activity is noted, a 1 U/kg regular insulin bolus can be initiated. If the blood sugar is less than 400 mg/dL, 0.5 g/kg of dextrose should be given with the insulin. After the insulin bolus, an insulin infusion of 0.5-1 U/kg/hour should be started along with a continuous dextrose drip of 0.5/kg/hour. The dextrose drip is titrated to maintain blood sugars between 100 and 250 mg/dL. Cardiac function should be monitored every 15-20 minutes, and blood glucose should be monitored every 15 sec initially and then can be spread out to every 30-60 min checks as blood glucose is consistently measured in the 100-250 mg/dL range. In addition, frequently monitor potassium concentration and judiciously replete as necessary. |
| Cyanide | Hydroxocobalamin, 5-g infusion IV over 30-min period in adults, 70 mg/kg in children. Each 5 g neutralizes about 40 μmol/L of cyanide in blood<br>Sodium thiosulfate, 50 mL of 25% solution (12.5 g; 1 ampule) in adults or 1.65 mL/kg IV in children<br>Sodium nitrate, 10 mL of 3% solution (300 mg; 1 ampule) in adults or 0.33 mL/kg slowly IV in children |
| Digitalis glycosides | Digoxin-specific Fab fragments, 10-20 vials if patient in ventricular fibrillation; otherwise dose based on serum digoxin concentration or amount ingested |

and the facility. Patients should undergo skin and eye decontamination, including removal of all clothing and washing of the skin with soap and water if indicated. Care should be taken to protect health care providers from exposure.

Establishing and maintaining an airway with adequate breathing should occur first. Supplemental oxygen should be administered through a nonrebreather mask. Death from intoxication can occur as a result of loss of the airway protective reflexes, and the patient should be intubated if the airway needs to be protected or the patient cannot be oxygenated or ventilated. Because it is hydrolyzed by plasma cholinesterase, succinylcholine can exacerbate cholinergic toxicity. Organophosphates can prolong the effects of succinylcholine. Electrical cardiac pacing may be effective in cases of mild to moderate drug-induced bradycardia. In patients with drug-induced cardiac arrest, electrical cardioversion or defibrillation per advanced cardiac life support guidelines is appropriate for those who are pulseless and have ventricular tachycardia or ventricular fibrillation. In extreme cases, cardiopulmonary bypass may be performed.

Circulation should be maintained and hypotension treated aggressively. Intravascular volume should be restored with crystalloid fluid, and if the hypotension has not resolved after fluid administration, direct-acting pressors, such as epinephrine or norepinephrine, are the preferred agents. In cases of symptomatic calcium channel blocker overdose, the antidote of choice is high-dose insulin-euglycemia therapy. The goal of this therapy is increased blood pressure leading to improved end-organ perfusion. The exact mechanism by which insulin-dextrose therapy improves ionotropy and increased peripheral vascular resistance is not well

**Table 143.9 Specific Toxins and Their Antidotes—cont'd**

| TOXINS | ANTIDOTES* |
|---|---|
| Ethylene glycol | Fomepizole, 15 mg/kg, then 10 mg/kg q12h for 4 doses, then increase dose to 15 mg/kg q12h until serum ethylene glycol level less than 20 mg/dL; dose should be adjusted during dialysis<br>Pyridoxine, 100 mg IV daily<br>Thiamine, 100 mg IV<br>Ethanol: loading dose, 10 mL/kg of 10% solution; maintenance dose, 0.15 mL/kg/hr of 10% solution; rate should be doubled during dialysis |
| Hydrofluoric acid | Calcium gluconate, calcium chloride |
| Iron | Deferoxamine, 15 mg/kg/hr IV |
| Isoniazid, hydrazine, and monomethylhydrazine | Pyridoxine, 5 g in adults, 1 g in children if ingested dose is unknown |
| Methanol toxicity | Folate or leucovorin, 50 mg IV q4h in adults<br>Ethanol: loading dose, 10 mL/kg of 10% solution; maintenance dose, 0.15 mL/kg/hr of 10% solution; rate should be adjusted during dialysis<br>Fomepizole, 15 mg/kg, then 10 mg/kg q12h for 4 doses, then increase to 15 mg/kg q12h until serum methanol level less than 20 mg/dL; dose should be adjusted during dialysis |
| Methemoglobin-forming agents | Methylene blue, 1-2 mg/kg IV (one 10-mL dose of 10% solution [100 mg]), may repeat in 30-60 min |
| Opioids | Naloxone, 0.4 mg IV titrated to 2 mg initially; higher doses may be needed for synthetic opioids<br>Nalmefene, 2 mg§ |
| Organophosphates and carbamates | Atropine, 1-2 mg IV in adults, 0.03 mg/kg in children; titrate to drying of pulmonary secretions<br>2-PAM (pralidoxime; loading dose, 1-2 g IV in adults, 25-50 mg/kg in children; adult maintenance, 500 mg/hr or 1-2 g q4-6h |
| Rattlesnake bite | CroFab antivenin injection, 4- to 6-vial loading dose by infusion in normal saline, then maintenance dosing of 2 vials q6h for 3 doses |
| Sulfonylureas | Octreotide, 50-100 mcg once or q 6-12h SC or IV as needed (most patients require 24 hr of therapy) |
| Tricyclic antidepressants | Sodium bicarbonate, 44-88 mEq in adults, 1-2 mEq/kg in children; best used with intravenous "push" rather than slow infusion |
| Valproic acid | Carnitine: loading dose, 100 mg/kg IV *or* PO; then 25 mg/kg q6h |

*EDTA*, Ethylenediaminetetraacetic acid; *IM*, intramuscularly; *IV*, intravenously; *PO*, orally; *SC*, subcutaneously.

*These are typical doses. Dosing may vary according to the patient and clinical picture. Consult with your medical toxicologist and pharmacist when in doubt. Your local poison center may be reached at 1-800-222-1222.

†May cross-react with penicillin in allergic patients.

‡Should not be used if the patient has signs of tricyclic antidepressant toxicity or a history of seizures.

§Has a much longer half-life than naloxone does.

understood. However, insulin seems to stimulate myocardial metabolism and improves glucose update by cardiac myocytes. Regular insulin, given as a 1 to 2 U/kg bolus followed by 0.5 to 2 U/kg while euglycemia is maintained (using 5% to 10% dextrose solution given as a bolus, then a drip), improves myocardial contractility, cardiac output, and blood pressure. Benzodiazepines are first-line agents for toxicant-induced hypertension. Beta-blockers are contraindicated because they may block the $\beta_2$ receptors, thereby leaving the $\alpha$-adrenergic stimulation unopposed and worsening the hypertension. In patients with a drug-induced hypertensive emergency refractory to benzodiazepines, short-acting antihypertensive agents, such as nitroprusside, should be administered. Labetalol is a third-line agent, effective at times for drug-induced hypertensive emergencies associated with sympathomimetic poisoning.

Treatment of drug-induced acute coronary syndromes is similar to that recommended for drug-induced hypertensive emergencies. Catheterization studies have shown that (1) nitroglycerin and phentolamine (an alpha-blocker) reverse cocaine-induced vasoconstriction, (2) labetalol has no significant effect, and (3) propranolol worsens it. Therefore, benzodiazepines and nitroglycerin are first-line agents, phentolamine is a second-line agent, and propranolol is contraindicated for drug-induced coronary syndromes.[5,6]

In cases of poisoning it is important to treat the patient, not the toxin. The EP should deal with the ABCDs of resuscitation, hypotension, seizures, and cardiac dysrhythmias aggressively. Such treatments can be started without knowledge of what the toxin is. Serial vital sign determination and physical examination are crucial. Progressive neurologic deterioration must be detected early and dealt with appropriately. Observation is one of the most critical aspects of the management of poisoned patients.

## "COMA COCKTAIL"

*Coma cocktail* is a slang term used to describe a combination of agents that have traditionally been given to poisoned patients with altered consciousness. It consists of **d**extrose, **o**xygen, **n**aloxone, and **t**hiamine. A mnemonic to remember this cocktail is DON'T forget. Use of a coma cocktail can be both therapeutic and diagnostic.

Hypoglycemia must be considered in all patients with altered mental status or active seizures. An overdosed patient can often be hypoglycemic because of the offending agent. An empiric therapy for coma, administer 50 to 100 mL (25 to 50 g) of 50% dextrose intravenously. Pediatric patients should receive 2 to 4 mL/kg of 25% dextrose IV. Neonates should receive 10% dextrose. Boluses should be given over several minutes and can be repeated, if necessary.

Naloxone reverses the coma and respiratory depression induced by opioids. It can also be used diagnostically. An initial dose of 0.2 to 0.4 mg is administered intravenously, and if no response is seen after 2 to 3 minutes, an additional 1 to 2 mg can be administered; doses can be repeated up to a total of 10 mg as needed. More than 10 mg may be required and may have to be given as an intravenous drip with higher grades of heroin, pentazocine, diphenoxylate, meperidine, propoxyphene, and methadone overdose.[7] Naloxone has a short half-life (20 to 30 minutes), and its effect does not last as long as the effects of most opioids. Therefore, if respiratory depression develops after an initial dose of naloxone, a naloxone drip should be started and the patient admitted to the intensive care unit. The naloxone is mixed with $D_5W$ and given at a rate that delivers two thirds of the initial reversal dose per hour.[8] Acute pulmonary edema, opioid withdrawal, and seizures have been reported with naloxone administration.[9-11]

Thiamine, 100 mg given intravenously or orally, should be reserved for alcoholic, malnourished patients. Despite traditional belief, giving thiamine to every comatose patient to prevent Wernicke-Korsakoff syndrome is not well supported by the literature. No evidence has shown that dextrose should be withheld until thiamine is administered.[12]

Flumazenil is a benzodiazepine reversal agent that can be used for a pure acute benzodiazepine overdose or when reversal of therapeutic conscious sedation is desired. It can potentially reverse the seizure-protecting properties of benzodiazepines in mixed drug ingestions (TCAs).[13] Because flumazenil can induce acute withdrawal symptoms in long-term benzodiazepine abusers, it is contraindicated in patients with a history of long-term benzodiazepine use, seizure disorder, and concomitant TCA ingestion. Flumazenil should not be used routinely to arouse an unconscious patient with overdose because it is often unknown whether a patient is a chronic benzodiazepine user. In a large prospective trial of unconscious patients suspected of benzodiazepine overdose, investigators did not observe any significant side effects with flumazenil.[14] However, serious complications of flumazenil have now been reported, including seizures, ventricular arrhythmias, and benzodiazepine withdrawal in patients who are chronic users.[15] If partial reversal of benzodiazepine intoxication is necessary, the smallest possible dose of flumazenil, 0.05 to 0.1 mg, should be diluted in 10 mL of saline or $D_5W$ and given slowly intravenously, over a period of several minutes. If there is no initial response, 0.3 mg may be given. If there is still no response, 0.5 mg can be given every 30 seconds for a maximum dose of 3 mg. Goals are respiratory sufficiency and verbal responsiveness, not complete arousal.

## DECONTAMINATION

Methods of decontamination include gastric emptying (administration of syrup of ipecac and gastric lavage), activated charcoal, and whole-bowel irrigation. There is some controversy about the roles of gastric lavage, activated charcoal, and cathartics in decontaminating a poisoned patient, as well as little support in the medical literature for such treatment. After a delay of 60 minutes or more after ingestion, very little of the ingested drug is likely to be removed by gastric lavage. In some circumstances, aggressive decontamination may be lifesaving, even more than 1 to 2 hours after ingestion. Examples are the ingestion of highly toxic drugs as calcium channel blockers, drugs not adsorbed by charcoal, and sustained-release or enteric-coated products.

Use of syrup of ipecac to induce emesis is no longer part of the treatment of any ingestion. Persistent vomiting after the use of ipecac is likely to delay the administration of activated charcoal. No evidence from clinical studies has shown that ipecac improves the outcome of poisoned patients, and its routine administration in the ED should be abandoned.[16] The only useful clinical situation would be a patient with a life-threatening ingestion many hours from medical care.with no other forms of decontamination available.

Gastric lavage is a time-consuming procedure that also poses a risk for aspiration and other injury. The concept is to try to wash out the stomach contents before absorption. It may still be useful when the toxin has not yet passed the pylorus. Gastric lavage should not be used routinely for the management of poisoned patients, however. In general, there is no advantage to gastric emptying more than 60 minutes after the ingestion. Gastric lavage is performed by inserting a 36- to 40-French tube into the patient's stomach and "washing out" the stomach with 300-mL aliquots of normal saline until clear. Unless a patient is intubated, gastric lavage is contraindicated if the airway protective reflexes are lost. It is also contraindicated if a hydrocarbon with high aspiration potential or a corrosive substance has been ingested. Gastric lavage should not be considered unless a patient has ingested a potentially life-threatening amount of a poison, no antidote exists, and the procedure can be undertaken within 60 minutes of the ingestion.[17] Multiple studies have shown no advantage of gastric emptying over activated charcoal in decreasing absorption.

In a patient with an unknown ingestion, administration of activated charcoal is the most efficacious decontamination method, with very few adverse side effects. Activated charcoal is produced by heating wood pulp, washing it, and then activating it with steam or acid. It has a large surface area for direct adsorption of agents in the gastrointestinal tract. It is usually safe and inexpensive, and it adsorbs most toxins (**Box 143.6**). This agent should be administered at a dose of 1 to 2 g/kg in overdose patients who are awake and alert or have a protected airway.

Charcoal does not adsorb all poisons. Infrequent complications include intestinal obstruction and aspiration pneumonitis. The effectiveness of activated charcoal has been found in volunteer studies to decrease with time; the greatest benefit occurs within 1 hour of ingestion, and single-dose activated charcoal should not be administered routinely for the management of poisoned patients. Administration of activated charcoal may be considered if a patient has ingested a potentially toxic amount of a poison (which is known to be adsorbed to charcoal) up to 1 hour previously; insufficient data support or exclude its use more than 1 hour after ingestion.[18]

Multiple-dose activated charcoal (every 4 hours) may be useful for the ingestion of some drugs with enterenteric enterohepatic circulation (see Box 143.6). Studies have shown decreases in the half-life of these drugs; however, clinical benefit of this approach has not been well established. Repetitive doses of charcoal, 0.25 to 1 g/kg, are given every 4 to 6 hours. Although many studies in animals and volunteers have demonstrated that multiple-dose activated charcoal increases drug elimination significantly, this therapy has not yet been shown in a controlled study to reduce morbidity and mortality. On the basis of experimental and clinical studies, therefore, administration of multiple-dose activated charcoal should be considered if a patient has ingested a life-threatening amount of carbamazepine, dapsone, phenobarbital, quinine, or theophylline.[19]

Not a single study has shown any benefit from the use of cathartics in poisoned patients. Cathartics include magnesium sulfate, sorbitol, and magnesium citrate. Drugs and toxins are usually absorbed within 30 to 90 minutes, and cathartics and laxatives take hours to work. Serious fluid and electrolyte shifts can occur as a result of the use of cathartics, and a few infant deaths have been reported. Complications of cathartics include electrolyte imbalance, dehydration, and hypermagnesemia. Administration of a cathartic alone has no role in the management of a poisoned patient and is not recommended as a method of gut decontamination.[20]

Whole-bowel irrigation should not be used routinely in the management of a poisoned patient. Although some volunteer studies have shown substantial decreases in the bioavailability of ingested drugs with this method, no controlled clinical trials have been performed, and there is no conclusive evidence that whole-bowel irrigation improves outcome in a poisoned patient.[21] Whole-bowel irrigation consists of the administration of a polyethylene glycol solution until the rectal effluent is clear. Whole-bowel irrigation should be reserved for life-threatening intoxications from sustained-release (CR, SR, LA, XL) beta-blockers, calcium channel blockers, lithium, iron, and lead. Most of the time, placement of a nasogastric tube is required for administration. Oral administration of charcoal followed by whole-bowel irrigation is the safest way to decontaminate people whose bodies have been stuffed with packets of illegal drugs. The dose is 20 mL/kg/hr, which translates to about 2 L/hr for adults and 0.5 L/hr for children. The end point is a clear rectal effluent, which usually requires 4 to 6 hours of treatment.

**BOX 143.6 Use of Activated Charcoal for Toxic Ingestions**

**Substances Poorly Adsorbed by Activated Charcoal**

*PHAILS* to bind charcoal

- *P*otassium
- *H*ydrocarbons, *H*eavy metals
- *A*lcohols, *A*lkali, *A*cidic
- *I*ron
- *L*axatives (sodium, magnesium, potassium based)
- *S*olvents

**Contraindications to Use of Activated Charcoal**

Unprotected airway
Altered mental status
Uncooperative patient
Intestinal obstruction
Poor gastrointestinal tract function
Decreased peristalsis
Ileus
Bowel obstruction
Aspiration

**Drugs with Enterohepatic Circulation**

Multiple-dose activated charcoal (every 4 hours) may be useful for some drugs with enterohepatic circulation, such as:

- Antidepressants: nortriptyline, amitriptyline
- Acetylsalicylic acid
- Aminophylline
- Carbamazepine
- Digitalis
- Dapsone
- Phenobarbital
- Phenylbutazone
- Phenytoin
- Quinine
- Theophylline

**DOCUMENTATION**

**History**

Name and concentration of the drug ingested

Time lapsed since the ingestion, if known

History of any other diseases that may complicate the ingestion

**Physical Examination**

Does the patient look ill? Pale? Febrile?

Mental status

Cardiac status (blood pressure, arrhythmias)

Respiratory and airway status

Physical examination should be repeated while the patient is in the emergency department

**Laboratory Studies**

Laboratory tests and time obtained

**Medical Decision Making**

Calculation of the amount (mg/kg) ingested if possible

Decision to begin treatment or delays

Consultations chosen and times of requests

If the patient is being discharged, documentation of medical reasons that the patient needs no further investigation or continuing care

**Treatment**

Availability of antidote, time antidote ordered, and any delays in treatment

**Patient Instructions**

Documentation of discussion with patient or parent regarding diagnosis, warning signs, what to do, follow-up, and when to return

With pediatric accidental ingestions, documentation of poison prevention counseling

Families should be given the phone number for their poison control center to address further concerns (1-800-222-1222)

Any time there is concern about the situation surrounding the ingestion or an ingestion has occurred in an infant younger than 12 months, social services should be contacted

## ENHANCEMENT OF ELIMINATION

Urine alkalinization should be considered first-line treatment in patients with moderately severe salicylate poisoning whose condition does not meet the criteria for hemodialysis. Alkalinization traps weak acids in an ionized state, thereby decreasing their reabsorption. Urine alkalinization increases ion trapping and thus urinary elimination of chlorpropamide, 2,4-dichlorophenoxyacetic acid, diflunisal, fluoride, mecoprop, methotrexate, phenobarbital, and salicylate. If the patient is acidemic, immediate correction with 1 to 2 mEq/kg of sodium bicarbonate can be performed immediately. Then a bicarbonate intravenous infusion of 100 to 150 mEq sodium dicarbonate in 1 L of $D_5W$ at 150 to 200 mg/hr. Sodium bicarbonate is administered as an intravenous drip at a rate of 0.5 to 2 mEq/kg/hr after a bolus of 1 to 2 mEq/kg. The dosage should be titrated to keep urine pH at 7.5 to 8.0. Urine pH should be tested every 30 minutes then once an hour to ensure adequate alkalinization. Check serum pH and potassium hourly. Urine alkalinization cannot be recommended as first-line treatment in cases of phenobarbital poisoning, for which multiple-dose activated charcoal is superior.[22]

In an unstable overdosed patient, consultation with a nephrologist for emergency hemodialysis may be indicated before the results of definitive diagnostic studies or drug level measurements are available. Toxins for which hemodialysis may be useful should have the following features: low molecular weight (<500 D), water solubility, low protein binding (<70% to 80%), and small volume of distribution (<1 L/kg). Toxins for which hemodialysis may be required include methanol, ethylene glycol, boric acid, salicylates, and lithium (**Box 143.7**).

**BOX 143.7 Examples of Agents Removed by Hemodialysis**

| | |
|---|---|
| Barbiturates | Lithium |
| Boric acid | Methanol |
| Ethylene glycol | Salicylates |
| Isopropanol | Theophylline |

## FOLLOW-UP, NEXT STEPS IN CARE, AND PATIENT EDUCATION

Patients who are cleared from a toxicology standpoint should be evaluated by psychiatric services if there is any question of an intentional overdose. Any patient with symptoms should be admitted for observation, and a sitter should be provided if the patient is suicidal. Typically, patients with unknown ingestions are observed for 6 hours; if asymptomatic, they can be released home or to psychiatric services as indicated. Patients should be observed until beyond the expected peak serum concentration or until asymptomatic (or both). Parents of children who have been evaluated for an ingestion or potential ingestion should be counseled about poisoning precautions and given contact information for the poison control center. Specific recommendations are provided in subsequent chapters related to the ingestion of specific toxins.

## REFERENCES

*References can be found on Expert Consult @ www.expertconsult.com.*

# Acetaminophen, Aspirin, and NSAIDs 144

*Heather Long*

## ACETAMINOPHEN

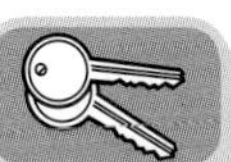

### KEY POINTS

- Acetaminophen (APAP) is available in numerous formulations, including cold, cough, and pain relief medications.
- ingestion of APAP is the most commonly reported exposure to a potentially toxic pharmacologic agent.
- APAP toxicity is clinically silent up to 24 hours after ingestion. If any abnormalities in vital signs or significant symptoms are present, a coingestant should be suspected.
- A blood specimen for serum APAP determination should be collected 4 hours after ingestion.
- The serum APAP result should be applied to the APAP nomogram for determination of the patient's risk for toxicity.
- *N*-Acetylcysteine (NAC) is the antidote for APAP poisoning, and the approach to treatment depends on the timing of the ingestion and the serum APAP level.
- Oral NAC dosing consists of a loading dose of 140 mg/kg and maintenance dose of 70 mg/kg every 4 hours for 17 doses. An intravenous formulation of NAC is now approved for use and should be given when oral administration is not feasible.
- The serum APAP level should be measured in any patient with clinical suspicion of an overdose or an attempt at suicide or if a patient with an overdose exhibits altered mental status.

## EPIDEMIOLOGY

Acetaminophen (APAP) is widely available in single-agent preparations, as well as in numerous cold, cough, and pain relief formulations. Though very safe at the recommended dosage, overdose and toxicity are common given its broad use. More than 100,000 calls are made to poison control centers in the United States each year regarding APAP exposure, and more hospitalizations take place for APAP overdose than for overdose of any other pharmacologic agent.

## PATHOPHYSIOLOGY

After therapeutic ingestion of APAP, more than 90% is metabolized in the liver to inactive and nontoxic glucuronide and sulfate conjugates that are subsequently excreted in urine. Less than 5% is metabolized by the cytochrome P-450 mixed-function oxidase system to form the highly reactive and toxic intermediate *N*-acetyl-*p*-benzoquinone imine (NAPQI). Glutathione quickly reduces NAPQI to a nontoxic metabolite that is eliminated in urine.

After an overdose of APAP, the normal nontoxic glucuronidation and sulfation pathways of metabolism become saturated, which allows more APAP to be metabolized by the cytochrome P-450 system to the toxic metabolite NAPQI. Once available stores of glutathione are diminished, the highly reactive NAPQI binds to intracellular proteins, thereby beginning the cascade of events that lead to cell death. Oxidative drug metabolism by the cytochrome P-450 system to NAPQI is concentrated in zone III (the centrilobular area of the hepatic lobule)—hence the characteristic centrilobular necrosis described with APAP toxicity.

## PRESENTING SIGNS AND SYMPTOMS

**Table 144.1** summarizes the four stages of APAP poisoning. The clinical manifestations of an APAP overdose arise from the hepatotoxicity and resultant complications. Patients, even those who eventually progress to fulminant hepatic failure, are initially asymptomatic. Significant abnormalities in vital signs or clinical findings that become evident soon after ingestion should not be attributed to APAP alone; the emergency physician (EP) should pursue diagnosis and treatment of a coingested agent.

## DIFFERENTIAL DIAGNOSIS AND MEDICAL DECISION MAKING

The differential diagnosis for APAP overdose includes other causes of liver damage such as shock liver, acute hepatitis A or B, mushroom exposure *(Amanita phalloides),* herbal preparations (cascara, chaparral, comfrey, kava, ma-huang), industrial chemicals (carbon tetrachloride, trichloroethylene, paraquat), angiotensin-converting enzyme inhibitors, anabolic steroids, aspirin, ibuprofen, isoniazid, calcium channel

**Table 144.1 Four Stages of Acetaminophen Poisoning**

| | | |
|---|---|---|
| Stage 1 (0-24 hr) | Asymptomatic | Patients are initially asymptomatic, with normal vital signs and no physical findings.<br>Laboratory results are normal.<br>Nonspecific complaints of nausea, vomiting, and malaise may start to develop near the end of this stage. |
| Stage 2 (24-72 hr) | Onset of hepatotoxicity | Right upper quadrant abdominal pain may develop.<br>Levels of AST, the most sensitive indicator of hepatotoxicity, and ALT begin to rise.<br>Later, INR values may begin to rise and renal function to deteriorate. |
| Stage 3 (72-96 hr) | Maximal hepatotoxicity | The patient exhibits clinical and laboratory manifestations of hepatic necrosis: varying degrees of hepatic encephalopathy, jaundice, renal failure, coagulation defects, and myocardial abnormalities.<br>AST and ALT levels peak, the INR value rises, blood urea nitrogen and creatinine levels rise, and pH drops.<br>Death may occur, typically 3-5 days after overdose.<br>Death from fulminant hepatic failure may be characterized by cerebral edema, sepsis, multisystem organ failure, hemorrhage, and adult respiratory distress syndrome. |
| Stage 4 (4 days to 2 wk) | Recovery phase | Patients who survive stage 3 undergo complete regeneration of the liver.<br>Laboratory abnormalities typically return to normal 5-7 days after overdose. |

*ALT*, Alanine transaminase; *AST*, aspartate transaminase; *INR*, international normalized ratio.

blockers, ketoconazole, methotrexate, phenytoin, statins, and valproic acid.

The objective of diagnostic testing after an overdose of APAP is to assist the clinician in determining which patients are at risk for hepatotoxicity and thus require further treatment. Laboratory evaluation is essential for all patients with potential risk because of the lack of reliable clinical manifestations early after APAP ingestion, when antidotal therapy is most effective. Risk is assessed through a thorough history and physical examination, as well as collection of a blood specimen for a serum APAP measurement 4 hours after ingestion—or as soon as possible in patients initially seen more than 4 hours after ingestion—and application of the result to the acetaminophen nomogram (**Fig. 144-1**). For patients who are seen late after ingestion and already exhibit signs and symptoms of hepatotoxicity or for whom the time of ingestion cannot be readily established, the serum aspartate transaminase (AST) level should also be measured. See **Figures 144.2** and **144.3** for guidelines to assess risk after acute and chronic APAP ingestion. Acute ingestion is defined as a single ingestion occurring over a single period shorter than 4 hours.

If there is any clinical suspicion of an overdose, even if the patient does not admit to APAP ingestion or if the patient with an overdose exhibits altered mental status, the serum APAP level should be measured.[1] Approximately 1 in 500 patients who have taken an overdose but do not admit to ingestion of APAP have a potentially hepatotoxic serum APAP concentration.

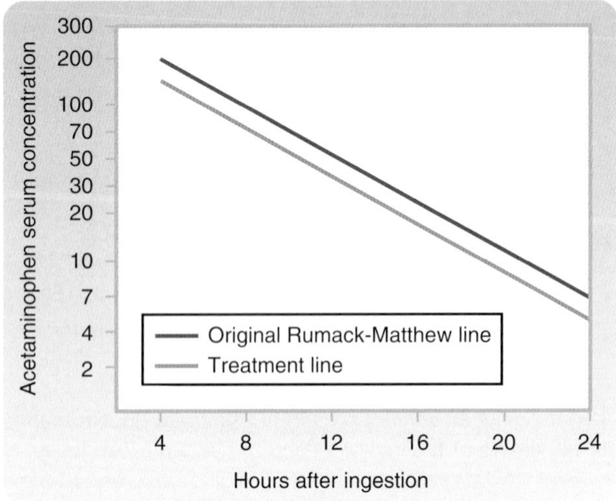


**Fig. 144.1 Treatment nomogram for acute acetaminophen overdose.** (From Marx JA, Hockberger RS, Walls RM, editors. Rosen's emergency medicine: concepts and clinical practice. 6th ed. Philadelphia: Mosby; 2006.)

## TREATMENT

Treatment with 50 g of activated charcoal should be considered in patients with large ingestions of APAP or coingestion of APAP and potentially toxic agents that bind to charcoal.[2] *N*-Acetylcysteine (NAC) is the antidote for APAP toxicity.[3] If given within 8 hours of ingestion, the risk for significant hepatotoxicity secondary to APAP toxicity is low. There does not appear to be a significant advantage to administering NAC within the first 2 or 3 hours after ingestion over giving it later as long as it is within the 8-hour window. See Figures 144.2 and 144.3 for guidelines in determining which patients should be given NAC after acute and chronic APAP ingestion and in managing patient care. NAC is available in both oral and intravenous formulations.[4] In general, both formulations are highly effective and well tolerated. Whether one formulation is superior remains controversial. See **Box 144.1** for a comparison of the two formulations and **Box 144.2** for dosing regimens.

Patients initially seen longer than 8 hours after ingestion should be treated with NAC on arrival at the emergency

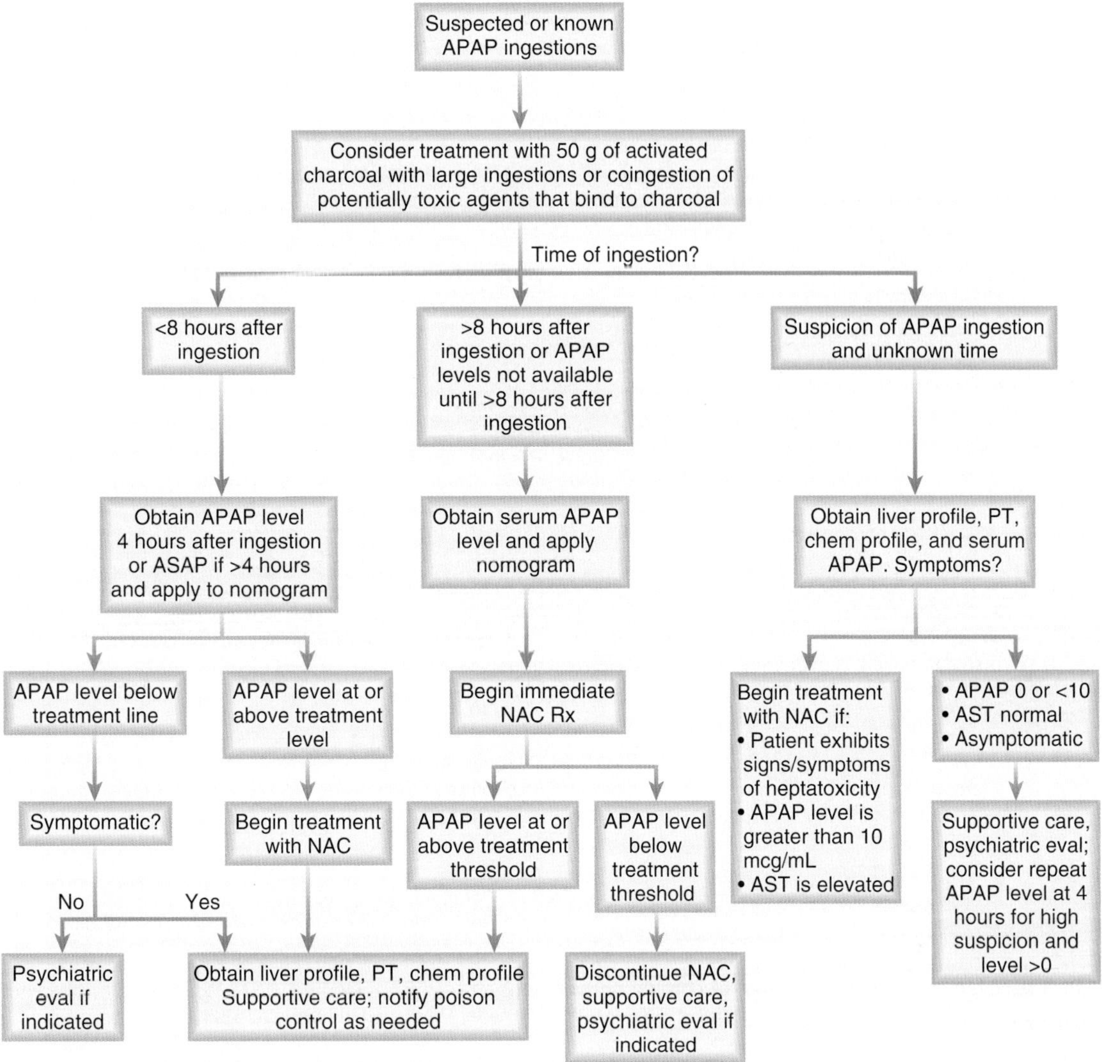


**Fig. 144.2 Risk assessment and management of acute acetaminophen (APAP) poisoning.** *AST*, Aspartate aminotransferase; *NAC*, *N*-acetylcysteine; *PT*, prothrombin time.

department and their serum APAP and AST levels measured. If the APAP level is above the treatment threshold on the nomogram (see Fig. 144.1), treatment with NAC should continue. If not and the patient has no signs or symptoms consistent with hepatotoxicity, NAC should be discontinued. NAC improves morbidity and mortality even if given late after ingestion and even if administered to patients in fulminant hepatic failure after APAP ingestion.[5] Rarely, patients with very high APAP levels or those seen late after ingestion may require a prolonged course of NAC. The EP should contact the regional poison control center for further assistance in managing patients with APAP overdose.

## PEDIATRIC CONSIDERATIONS

Children should be evaluated for potential risk for hepatotoxicity after both acute exposure and repeated excessive dosing. Serum APAP and AST levels should be measured in those

**BOX 144.1 Oral versus Intravenous Administration of *N*-Acetylcysteine**

**Oral**

Induces nausea or vomiting in more than 50% of patients
Inexpensive
Ease of dosing schedule
Safer than intravenous administration

**Intravenous**

Considered the preferred route in following settings:

- Fulminant hepatic failure
- Patient unable to tolerate oral administration

The preparation must be adjusted for children weighing less than 40 kg
Complicated dosing regimen
Risk for anaphylactoid reactions

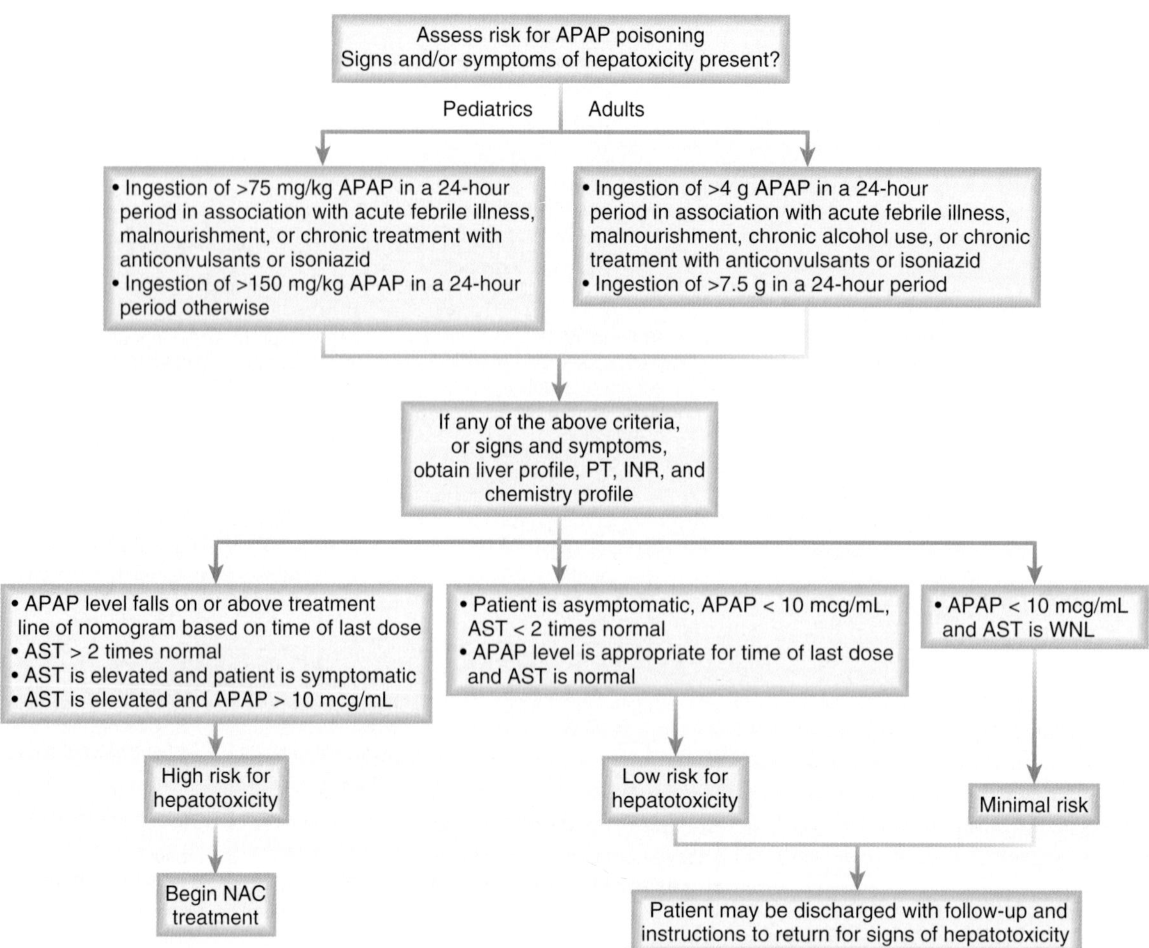


**Fig. 144.3 Risk assessment and management of chronic acetaminophen (APAP) poisoning.** *AST*, Aspartate aminotransferase; *INR*, international normalized ratio; *NAC*, *N*-acetylcysteine; *PT*, prothrombin time; *WNL*, within normal limits.

**BOX 144.2 Dosing Schedule for *N*-Acetylcysteine (NAC)**

**Oral (Adult and Pediatric)**

Loading dose (adult and pediatric): 140 mg/kg

Maintenance dose: 70 mg/kg every 4 hours for 17 doses (next 68 hours)

May be chilled or diluted with water, soda, or juice to ease administration

**Intravenous**

***Adult***

Loading dose: 150 mg/kg in 200 mL of 5% dextrose in water ($D_5W$) infused over a 60-minute period to reduce the risk for an anaphylactoid reaction

Second dose: 50 mg/kg in 500 mL $D_5W$ over a 4-hour period

Third dose: 100 mg/kg in 1 L $D_5W$ over a 16-hour period

***Pediatric (<40 kg)***

For patients weighing more than 10 kg, follow the package insert or regimen below

For infants less than 10 kg, dilute IV NAC to a 2% solution and then follow the dosing regimen below: Remove 50 mL from a 500-mL bag of $D_5W$, and add 50 mL IV NAC (20%) to 450 mL $D_5W$ to create a 2% solution

Loading dose: 7.5 mL/kg (150 mg/kg) of a 2% solution over a 1-hour period

Second dose: 2.5 mL/kg (50 mg/kg) of a 2% solution over a 4-hour period

Third dose: 5 mL/kg (100 mg/kg) of a 2% solution over a 16-hour period

with a large single ingestion or ingestion of more than 75 mg/kg of APAP in a 24-hour period, as well as in any child with signs or symptoms of hepatotoxicity (see Figs. 144.2 and 144.3). NAC should be administered if indicated according to the dosing guidelines (see Box 144.2).

## PREGNANT PATIENT

Oral NAC is routinely given to pregnant patients after potentially toxic APAP exposure and seems to be safe and effective. NAC appears to be safe for the fetus regardless of whether the mother receives the NAC orally or intravenously; however,

**BOX 144.3 Indications for Intensive Care Unit Admission or Transfer to a Liver Transplantation Center for a Patient with Hepatotoxicity**

Severe hepatotoxicity:

- Elevated aspartate transaminase and alanine tranaminase values
- Prolonged prothrombin time
- Elevated blood urea nitrogen or creatinine value
- Metabolic acidosis
- Hypoglycemia

Signs of hepatic encephalopathy

data are limited regarding the efficacy of NAC in the fetus, and whether there is an advantage with oral or intravenous administration remains unknown.

## FOLLOW-UP, NEXT STEPS IN CARE, AND PATIENT EDUCATION

Patients deemed to be at risk for hepatotoxicity should be treated with oral NAC within 8 hours of ingestion or as soon as possible thereafter and be admitted to the hospital for further medical and psychiatric evaluation as indicated. Patients with signs of severe hepatotoxicity, hepatic encephalopathy, or fulminant hepatic failure should be admitted to the intensive care unit (ICU), and early contact should be made with both the poison control center and a liver transplantation center (**Box 144.3**).

# ASPIRIN (SALICYLATES)

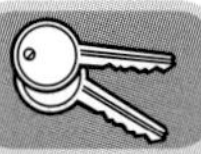

**KEY POINTS**

- Methyl salicylate is found in topical liniments and in oil of wintergreen.
- Aspirin toxicity in adults is characterized by a mixed respiratory alkalosis and metabolic acidosis.
- Acute toxicity is marked by tachypnea or hyperpnea, tachycardia, nausea, vomiting, and progressive central nervous system deterioration.
- Chronic aspirin toxicity is seen most commonly in the elderly and is frequently misdiagnosed as sepsis or dementia.[6]
- Aspirin toxicity is treated with multiple-dose activated charcoal, fluid resuscitation, urine alkalinization, and hemodialysis.

## EPIDEMIOLOGY

Aspirin (acetylsalicylic acid [ASA]) is found in single-agent preparations; in numerous cold, cough, and pain relief formulations; and in topical ointments and topical wart removal agents. Bismuth salicylate is included in the antidiarrheal medicine Pepto Bismol, and methyl salicylate is used in varying concentrations in liniments (30%) and oil of wintergreen (up to 100%). The incidence of unintentional salicylate poisoning has diminished with the growing use of APAP and nonsteroidal antiinflammatory drugs (NSAIDs) and with the increasing use of APAP rather than aspirin in children with viral illnesses to avoid Reye syndrome. In the United States, analgesics are the substances most frequently involved in human poison exposure for all age groups and the third most frequently involved substances in both pediatric (5 years and younger) and adult (>19 years) exposures. Aspirin alone caused 63 deaths in the United States in 2007 out of a total of 1597 fatalities from poisoning.

## PATHOPHYSIOLOGY

Salicylate toxicity in adults is characterized by a mixed respiratory alkalosis and metabolic acidosis. Salicylates stimulate the respiratory center in the brainstem, which causes hyperventilation and a primary respiratory alkalosis. In addition, salicylates cause an anion gap metabolic acidosis, probably through several mechanisms.[7] They uncouple oxidative phosphorylation, which leads to an accumulation of hydrogen ions, blocks the production of adenosine triphosphate, and favors the production of lactate. Salicylate toxicity interferes with the renal elimination of sulfuric and phosphoric acids and induces fatty acid metabolism, with the generation of $\alpha$-hydroxybutyric acid and acetoacetic acid.

In children, primary metabolic alkalosis is not commonly seen, either because they do not sustain the hyperventilation that adults do or because of a delay in medical care. In adults, the primary respiratory alkalosis may be blunted or absent as a result of salicylate-induced acute lung injury (noncardiogenic pulmonary edema), respiratory fatigue (a sign of severe toxicity), or concomitant ingestion of a central nervous system depressant.

Salicylate toxicity may induce acute lung injury, classically described as "noncardiogenic pulmonary edema." The mechanisms are unclear. Hypoxia is presumed to contribute to the pulmonary hypertension and release of vasoactive factors, which results in greater capillary permeability and more exudate in the interstitial and alveolar spaces.

The increased metabolic state associated with salicylate poisoning results in hypoglycemia and ketosis.

Ototoxicity, characterized by hearing loss and tinnitus, is a predictable manifestation of salicylate toxicity that occurs with serum ASA concentrations of 25 to 40 mg/dL. The cause is unknown, but it is postulated that salicylate has effects on glucose and protein metabolism that involve the endolymph and perilymph and thus alter nerve transmission.

## PRESENTING SIGNS AND SYMPTOMS

See **Box 144.4** for the clinical manifestations of salicylate toxicity and **Table 144.2** for comparison of acute and chronic salicylate toxicity.

**BOX 144.4 Clinical Manifestations of Salicylate Toxicity**

**Central Nervous System**
Tinnitus, decreased hearing
Confusion, agitation
Lethargy
Coma
Seizure
Syndrome of inappropriate antidiuretic hormone secretion

**Gastrointestinal**
Nausea, vomiting
Abdominal pain, gastritis
Decreased motility

**Cardiovascular**
Tachycardia (usually secondary to hypovolemia, hyperpyrexia)

**Pulmonary**
Tachypnea, hyperpnea
Acute lung injury

**Hematologic**
Prolongation of the prothrombin time
Platelet dysfunction

**Acid-Base, Electrolyte Abnormalities**
Respiratory alkalosis
Metabolic acidosis
Respiratory acidosis
Hypokalemia
Hyponatremia or hypernatremia

**Metabolic Changes**
Hyperthermia, diaphoresis
Hypoglycemia or hyperglycemia
Hypoglycorrhachia
Ketonemia, ketonuria

**Table 144.2** Comparison of Acute and Chronic Salicylate Toxicity

| ACUTE | CHRONIC |
|---|---|
| Seen in toddlers and suicidal adults | Seen primarily in the elderly |
| Typically caused by intentional overdose in suicidal adults or unintentional ingestion by children | Typically caused by unintentional overdose by the elderly for the treatment of chronic pain |
| Acute onset | Insidious onset |
| Gastrointestinal symptoms common | Gastrointestinal symptoms uncommon<br>Central nervous symptoms predominate<br>Typically misdiagnosed as altered mental status |
| Significant toxicity associated with high serum salicylate value | Significant toxicity associated with low to moderately elevated salicylate value |

**Table 144.3** Diagnostic Testing in Patients with Salicylate Toxicity

| TEST | FINDINGS AND SIGNIFICANCE |
|---|---|
| Serum acetylsalicylic acid measurement | Check every 2-4 hr<br>Therapeutic value: 15-30 mg/dL<br>>30 mg/dL: clinical manifestations evident<br>>90-100 mg/dL: severe toxicity (acute)<br>Chronic toxicity: patient may have significant toxicity with mild to moderately elevated acetylsalicylic acid value |
| Urinalysis | Ketonuria<br>Glucosuria<br>pH abnormality |
| Electrolytes | Elevated anion gap<br>Hyperglycemia or hypoglycemia<br>Hypokalemia |
| Arterial blood gas measurement | Initial respiratory alkalosis: pH > 7.4 (rarely seen in pediatric patients)<br>Metabolic acidosis: pH still >7.4; mixed metabolic acidosis and respiratory alkalosis<br>Worsening metabolic acidosis with acidemia: pH < 7.4; indicates severe toxicity |
| Chest radiograph | Acute lung injury |
| Electrocardiogram | Sinus tachycardia |

## DIFFERENTIAL DIAGNOSIS AND MEDICAL DECISION MAKING

The differential diagnosis for salicylate toxicity includes diabetic ketoacidosis, dementia, withdrawal syndromes, meningitis or encephalitis, acetaminophen overdose, toxic alcohol ingestion, lactic acidosis, and iron toxicity. See **Table 144.3** for laboratory and diagnostic tests useful in evaluating salicylate toxicity.

## TREATMENT

The mainstays of therapy after salicylate ingestion are multiple-dose activated charcoal, fluid and electrolyte replenishment, urine alkalinization, and in cases of severe toxicity, hemodialysis. **Table 144.4** lists guidelines for managing and treating patients with salicylate toxicity, instructions on urine alkalization, and indications for hemodialysis. The EP should contact the renal service early in cases of severe toxicity and consult with the regional poison control center for continued assistance soon after patient arrival.

**Table 144.4 Management and Treatment of Salicylate Toxicity**

| | |
|---|---|
| Gastric decontamination | Multidose activated charcoal: typically 1-2 g/kg every 4-6 hr up to 50 g for 2-3 doses<br>Do not administer with sorbitol more than once[8] |
| Fluid replacement | Patients often significantly dehydrated because of vomiting, hyperthermia, diaphoresis, and tachypnea or hyperpnea<br>Increasing fluids beyond resuscitation needs ("forced diuresis") not recommended |
| Urine alkalinization ("ion trapping")[9]<br>Goal is to alkalinize blood and urine to "trap" ionized salicylate, keep it out of the brain, and enhance urinary elimination<br>Acetazolamide administration is *not* recommended; it alkalinizes urine but acidifies blood and may increase the brain's salicylate concentration[9] | *Indications*:<br>Patient has signs or symptoms of salicylate toxicity<br>Serum acetylsalicylic acid level > 40 mg/dL<br>*Technique*:<br>1-2 mEq/kg sodium bicarbonate by IV bolus<br>Sodium bicarbonate infusion: 132 mEq sodium bicarbonate (3 ampules) + 40 mEq potassium chloride in 1 L of 5% dextrose in water to run at twice the maintenance fluid requirements<br>*Goals*:<br>Serum pH of 7.45-7.55<br>Urine pH of 7.5-8.0<br>Need to replenish or maintain serum potassium to achieve urine alkalinization<br>Monitor serum calcium and replenish as necessary during sodium bicarbonate therapy |
| Airway management | Avoid exacerbating the acidemia during endotracheal intubation<br>Important to maintain hyperventilation during mechanical ventilation |
| Hemodialysis | *Indications*:<br>Signs or symptoms of end-organ toxicity (altered mental status, acute lung injury, metabolic acidemia despite treatment)<br>Progressive clinical deterioration despite adequate supportive care<br>Renal failure<br>Serum acetylsalicylic acid level (acute) > 90-100 mg/dL |

## FOLLOW-UP, NEXT STEPS IN CARE, AND PATIENT EDUCATION

Patients with signs or symptoms of salicylate toxicity should be admitted to the hospital for continued monitoring of their clinical condition and serial laboratory evaluations. Patients with signs and symptoms of serious toxicity should be admitted to the ICU and evaluated early by the renal service for possible hemodialysis.

# NONSTEROIDAL ANTIINFLAMMATORY DRUGS

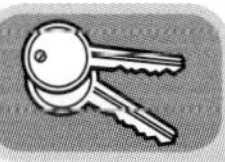

### KEY POINTS

- Nonsteroidal antiinflammatory drugs (NSAIDs) are a large class of drugs that include the over-the-counter drugs ibuprofen, naproxen, and ketoprofen.
- Nausea, vomiting, epigastric pain, and mild central nervous system depression are the most common clinical manifestations of NSAID poisoning.
- NSAID toxicity is usually mild and should be managed with gastrointestinal decontamination and supportive care.

## EPIDEMIOLOGY

NSAIDs are a large class of drugs, and exposure to and overdose of NSAIDs are common given their widespread use. Ibuprofen, naproxen, and ketoprofen are available over the counter. Ibuprofen accounts for 70% to 80% of all NSAID exposures reported to U.S. poison control centers. In 2007, calls to U.S. poison control centers (as documented by the National Poison Data System of the American Association of Poison Control Centers) included 307,590 cases involving NSAIDs (other than salicylates). Of these calls, 205,245 cases were found to be due to single exposures. More than 100,000 NSAID calls involved coingestants.

## PATHOPHYSIOLOGY

All NSAIDs competitively inhibit cyclooxygenase (COX), thereby preventing the formation of prostaglandins, prostacyclin, and thromboxane.[10] (Unlike salicylates, NSAIDs reversibly bind to COX.) There are two isoforms: COX-1 and COX-2. The analgesic and antiinflammatory properties are attributed to inhibition of COX-2. Most of the adverse effects and the acute toxicity of NSAIDs are attributed to inhibition of COX-1.

NSAIDs directly irritate the gastrointestinal mucosa; COX-1–mediated prostaglandin inhibition further contributes to gastrointestinal irritation, ulceration, and perforation.

Rarely, NSAID toxicity induces an anion gap metabolic acidosis associated with elevated serum lactate. This condition is attributed to NSAID metabolites, which are weak acids, rather than to COX inhibition and is favored by relative hypotension and hypoxia.

NSAID-induced renal toxicity is due to inhibition of prostaglandin and occurs in the setting of low intravascular volume such as seen with hypovolemia, congestive heart failure, cirrhosis, or intrinsic renal disease.

Via inhibition of thromboxane $A_2$, NSAIDs decrease platelet aggregation. Other idiosyncratic reactions associated with some NSAIDs are hemolytic anemia, aplastic anemia, agranulocytosis, and thrombocytopenia.

NSAID-induced COX inhibition is associated with anaphylactoid reactions. Acute bronchospasm may develop within minutes to hours of NSAID ingestion in adult patients with asthma and chronic urticaria or nasal polyps. Agents that block 5-lipoxygenase or leukotriene receptors may prevent adverse reactions.

## PRESENTING SIGNS AND SYMPTOMS

See **Box 144.5** for the signs and symptoms of NSAID toxicity. Gastrointestinal manifestations are the most common; rare findings after large ibuprofen ingestions include metabolic acidosis, coma, bradycardia, and hypotension.[11,12]

## DIFFERENTIAL DIAGNOSIS AND MEDICAL DECISION MAKING

The differential diagnosis for NSAID toxicity includes other ingestions such as APAP or salicylate, chronic anemia, anxiety, delirium or dementia, peptic ulcer disease, lactic acidosis, Stevens-Johnson syndrome, and toxic epidermal necrolysis.

Serum NSAID concentrations are not readily available from hospital laboratories and are not clinically useful. After a large overdose or in symptomatic patients, serum electrolyte, blood urea nitrogen or creatinine, serum bicarbonate, and arterial blood gas measurements should be obtained.

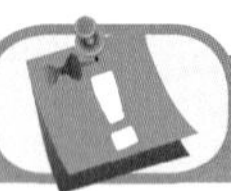

### TIPS AND TRICKS

- Measure serum acetaminophen in all patients with suspected overdose.
- Initiate treatment with *N*-acetylcysteine in patients seen late after an acetaminophen overdose.
- Initiate early contact with the poison control center and liver transplant center for patients with severe acetaminophen toxicity.
- Consider chronic salicylate poisoning in elderly patients with altered mental status.
- Initiate treatment with sodium bicarbonate and contact the renal service for potential hemodialysis in patients with salicylate poisoning.
- Beware of the risk of worsening the acidemia during intubation of patients with severe salicylate poisoning, and ensure adequate ventilation.

### BOX 144.5 Clinical Manifestations of Nonsteroidal Antiinflammatory Drug Toxicity

**Gastrointestinal**
Nausea, vomiting, abdominal pain
Gastritis, peptic ulcer disease
Gastrointestinal bleeding

**Renal**[12]
Sodium, potassium, water retention
Acute renal failure
Chronic interstitial nephritis
Papillary necrosis

**Central Nervous System**
Headache
Confusion, delirium, hallucinations (especially in the elderly)
Tinnitus, hearing loss
Coma

**Pulmonary**
Bronchospasm
Pneumonitis

**Hematologic**
Platelet dysfunction
Thrombocytopenia
Hemolytic anemia, immune mediated
Aplastic anemia

**Acid-Base Abnormality**
Metabolic acidosis (associated with large ibuprofen overdoses)

**Hepatic**
Elevated liver enzyme values

## TREATMENT

Life-threatening complications after an NSAID overdose are rare. Treatment consists of supportive care, fluid and electrolyte replacement, and gastric decontamination with activated charcoal. Asymptomatic patients should receive one dose of activated charcoal and be observed for 6 hours after ingestion.

## FOLLOW-UP, NEXT STEPS IN CARE, AND PATIENT EDUCATION

Patients who remain asymptomatic after 6 hours of observation may be further evaluated by the psychiatric service or may be discharged with arrangements for follow-up and instructions to return if gastrointestinal or central nervous system signs and symptoms develop. For symptomatic patients, the diagnostic tests already described should be performed, and the patients should be admitted to the hospital for further observation and evaluation.

## REFERENCES

*References can be found on Expert Consult @ www.expertconsult.com.*

# Anticholinergics 145

*Jessica A. Fulton and Lewis S. Nelson*

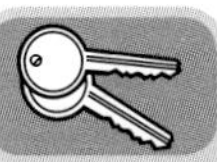

**KEY POINTS**

- Antimuscarinic poisoning syndrome is a more appropriate description than anticholinergic overdose because only the muscarinic receptors, not the nicotinic acetylcholine receptors, are involved. In this chapter the term *anticholinergic* will be used for consistency and is specifically meant to indicate *antimuscarinic*.
- Anticholinergic agents antagonize the neurotransmitter acetylcholine at both central and peripheral muscarinic acetylcholine receptors, which leads to altered mental status, mydriasis, tachycardia, urinary retention, ileus, and dry, flushed skin.
- The diagnosis of anticholinergic syndrome is largely clinical and should include physical examination, fingerstick serum glucose measurement, and an electrocardiogram.
- Anticholinergic syndrome is a key clinical finding leading to the diagnosis of poisoning by tricyclic antidepressants (a subset of antimuscarinic agents).
- Basic treatment involves supportive care of the vital signs, activated charcoal, benzodiazepines for agitation, sodium bicarbonate for a QRS complex longer than 100 msec or wide-complex tachycardia, and physostigmine for consequential central and peripheral anticholinergic (antimuscarinic) manifestations, if appropriate.

## EPIDEMIOLOGY

Because anticholinergic toxicologic syndrome (toxidrome) is common, recognition of its associated signs and symptoms is a necessary clinical skill. It occurs following exposure to many seemingly unrelated agents, many of which are available without prescription or used in patients with a propensity toward self-harm (**Box 145.1**). For example, according to data from the American Association of Poison Control Centers, 25,788 single exposures to diphenhydramine alone occurred in 2008, with 201 major outcomes and 3 deaths.[1]

## PATHOPHYSIOLOGY AND PHARMACOLOGY

Acetylcholine is the neurotransmitter released from cholinergic nerve endings in the central (brain and spinal cord) and peripheral (autonomic and somatic) nervous systems. In the autonomic (sympathetic and parasympathetic) nervous system, acetylcholine is released from all preganglionic neurons, as well as from postganglionic parasympathetic neurons. Degradation of acetylcholine by the enzyme acetylcholinesterase occurs in the synapse between the presynaptic and postsynaptic membranes.

There are two types of postsynaptic acetylcholine receptors: nicotinic and muscarinic. Nicotinic acetylcholine receptors are ion channels that open in response to stimulation. Found throughout the central nervous system (CNS) (most abundantly in the spinal cord), they are the postsynaptic receptors in the preganglionic sympathetic and parasympathetic neurons. Additionally, these receptors are found in the somatic nervous system at postganglionic skeletal neuromuscular junctions that mediate muscle contraction, as well as in postganglionic neurons of the adrenal medulla, which are subsequently responsible for the release of epinephrine and norepinephrine.

Muscarinic acetylcholine receptors are linked to G proteins to execute their postreceptor effects. They are found primarily in the CNS (most abundantly in the brain). They are also present at effector organs innervated by postganglionic parasympathetic neurons. Stimulation of these end-organs, either pharmacologically or through enhanced neuronal output, results in miosis, lacrimation, salivation, bronchospasm, bronchorrhea, bradydysrhythmia, urination, and increased gastrointestinal motility (**Table 145.1**). Finally, muscarinic receptors are located in sweat glands innervated by postsynaptic sympathetic neurons and cause diaphoresis when stimulated.

Muscarinic acetylcholine receptor antagonists competitively inhibit muscarinic acetylcholine receptors. These agents cause the classic anticholinergic poisoning syndrome, which perhaps may be more appropriately designated the antimuscarinic poisoning syndrome because nicotinic acetylcholine receptors are not affected. Muscarinic receptors in different organs are not equally sensitive to antimuscarinic agents.

Tricyclic antidepressants are a unique subset of antimuscarinic agents that deserve special attention. Their antidepressant effect is achieved pharmacologically through blockade of the reuptake of norepinephrine, dopamine, and serotonin in the CNS. Additionally, tricyclic antidepressants interact with other channels and receptors and cause considerably more profound clinical toxicity in overdose than occurs with most other agents that exhibit anticholinergic effects. Adverse effects of a tricyclic antidepressant overdose include competitive inhibition at both central and peripheral muscarinic acetylcholine receptors (antimuscarinic poisoning syndrome); histamine receptor antagonism (sedation); sodium channel blockade in the myocardium (widening of the QRS complex

**BOX 145.1 Agents That Produce Anticholinergic (Antimuscarinic) Poisoning Syndrome**

Anticholinergic syndrome can be caused by many agents, including atropine, diphenhydramine, and scopolamine.

**Plants**
*Atropa belladonna* (deadly nightshade)
*Datura stramonium* (jimsonweed)
*Mandragora officinarum* (mandrake)
*Hyoscyamus niger* (henbane)

**Belladonna Alkaloids (Natural) and Related Synthetic Compounds**
Atropine
Homatropine
Scopolamine
Glycopyrrolate (peripheral effects only)

**Antispasmodics**
Clidinium bromide (Librax)
Cyclobenzaprine (Flexeril)
Dicyclomine (Bentyl)
Propantheline bromide (Pro-Banthine)
Methantheline bromide (Banthine)
Orphenadrine (Norflex)
Flavoxate (Urispas)
Oxybutynin (Ditropan)

**Antiparkinsonian Medications**
Benztropine mesylate (Cogentin)
Biperiden (Akineton)
Trihexyphenidyl (Artane)

**Topical Mydriatics (Ocular)**
Cyclopentolate (Cyclogyl)
Homatropine (Isopto Homatropine)
Tropicamide (Mydriacyl)

**Antihistamines**
Brompheniramine (Dimetane)
Chlorpheniramine (Ornade, Chlor-Trimeton)
Cyclizine (Marezine)
Dimenhydrinate (Dramamine)
Diphenhydramine (Benadryl, Caladryl)
Hydroxyzine (Atarax, Vistaril)
Meclizine (Antivert)
Doxylamine (Unisom)
Promethazine (Phenergan)

**Antipsychotics**
Clozapine (Clozaril)
Chlorpromazine (Thorazine)
Prochlorperazine (Compazine)
Thiothixene (Navane)
Thioridazine (Mellaril)
Trifluoperazine (Stelazine)
Perphenazine (Trilafon)

**Others**
Amantadine (Symmetrel)
Disopyramide (Norpace)
Glutethimide (Doriden)
Procainamide (Pronestyl)
Quinidine (Quinidex)

**Table 145.1** Pathophysiology of Anticholinergic (Antimuscarinic Poisoning Syndrome) Symptoms

| ANTICHOLINERGIC EFFECT | SYMPTOMS |
|---|---|
| Central inhibition of muscarinic acetylcholine receptors | Confusion, disorientation, psychomotor agitation, ataxia, myoclonus, tremor, picking movements, abnormal speech, visual and auditory hallucinations, psychosis, seizures, cardiovascular collapse, coma |
| Inhibition of postsynaptic sympathetic muscarinic acetylcholine receptors in the sweat glands, as well as vasodilation of peripheral blood vessels | Dry, flushed skin |
| Inhibition of postsynaptic parasympathetic muscarinic acetylcholine receptors in the: | |
| Salivary glands | Dry mucous membranes |
| Eye | Paralysis of the sphincter muscle of the iris and the ciliary muscle of the lens resulting in mydriasis, cycloplegia, and blurred vision |
| Heart (vagus nerve) | Tachycardia |
| Bladder | Urinary retention and overflow incontinence |
| Bowel | Adynamic ileus |

or wide-complex dysrhythmias, atrioventricular block, QT prolongation, and rightward shift of the terminal 40-msec QRS axis on an electrocardiogram [ECG], as well as negative inotropy leading to hypotension); α-adrenergic receptor antagonism on vascular smooth muscle (vasodilation leading to hypotension); and although the mechanism of this effect is unclear, γ-aminobutyric acid (GABA) antagonism (seizures). In the right clinical setting, anticholinergic syndrome is a key clinical finding leading to the diagnosis of tricyclic antidepressant poisoning (**Table 145.2**).

## PRESENTING SIGNS AND SYMPTOMS

Central inhibition of muscarinic acetylcholine receptors results in confusion, disorientation, psychomotor agitation, ataxia, myoclonus, tremor, picking movements, abnormal speech, visual and auditory hallucinations, psychosis, seizures, cardiovascular collapse, and coma.

Inhibition of postsynaptic sympathetic muscarinic acetylcholine receptors in the sweat glands, as well as vasodilation of peripheral blood vessels, gives rise to dry, flushed skin. Inability to sweat, particularly in the presence of altered CNS regulation, may lead to hyperthermia. Inhibition of these receptors in the salivary glands results in dry mucous membranes, whereas inhibition of these receptors in the eye (which cause pupillary constriction when activated) leads to paralysis of the sphincter muscle of the iris and the ciliary muscle of the lens with subsequent mydriasis, cycloplegia, and blurred vision. Tachycardia is caused by inhibition of postsynaptic parasympathetic muscarinic acetylcholine receptors on the vagus nerve. Dysrhythmias may be caused by antimuscarinic agents that possess additional pharmacologic effects. For example, agents that produce sodium channel blockade in the myocardium (i.e., tricyclic antidepressants, diphenhydramine, pheniramine, orphenadrine, pyrilamine) cause widening of the QRS complex or wide-complex dysrhythmias, atrioventricular block, QT prolongation, and rightward shift of the terminal 40-msec QRS axis on the ECG, as well as negative inotropy leading to hypotension. Inhibition of postsynaptic parasympathetic muscarinic acetylcholine receptors in the bladder results in urinary retention and overflow incontinence, and in the bowel it causes adynamic ileus.

Frequently, patients with anticholinergic (antimuscarinic) poisoning do not have all the previously mentioned characteristics of the classic syndrome, especially the elderly and patients with organic brain syndrome, in whom central anticholinergic (antimuscarinic) poisoning syndrome is often more pronounced than or outlasts the peripheral syndrome.

See Tables 145.1 and 145.2, which detail the pathophysiology associated with the signs and symptoms of antimuscarinic poisoning syndrome and tricyclic antidepressants.

**Table 145.2 Pathophysiology of Tricyclic Antidepressants and Associated Symptoms**

| EFFECT | SYMPTOMS |
|---|---|
| Blockade of reuptake of norepinephrine, dopamine, and serotonin in the central nervous system | Mood elevation |
| Competitive inhibition at both central and peripheral muscarinic acetylcholine receptors | Antimuscarinic poisoning syndrome |
| Histamine receptor antagonism | Sedation |
| Sodium channel blockade in the myocardium | QRS complex widening or wide-complex dysrhythmias, atrioventricular block, QT prolongation and rightward shift of the terminal 40-msec QRS axis on the electrocardiogram, as well as negative inotropy leading to hypotension |
| α-Adrenergic receptor antagonism on vascular smooth muscle | Vasodilation leading to hypotension |
| γ-Aminobutyric acid antagonism | Seizures |

## DIFFERENTIAL DIAGNOSIS AND MEDICAL DECISION MAKING

### DIAGNOSTIC FEATURES

Patients who overdose with an anticholinergic (antimuscarinic) agent often have sufficient clinical findings to make the diagnosis apparent. However, the symptoms and signs in others may be less overt, and thus a substantially broader differential diagnosis is required.

Although patients with both adrenergic (sympathomimetic) and anticholinergic (antimuscarinic) poisoning may exhibit confusion, disorientation, psychomotor agitation, seizures, flushed skin, hyperthermia, mydriasis, and tachycardia, the two syndromes may be differentiated through examination of the skin and observation of the symptoms associated with the altered mental status. Patients with anticholinergic poisoning have dry skin and mucous membranes, and the alteration in mental status is characterized by mumbling speech, delirium, and tactile or visual hallucinations. In contrast, patients poisoned by sympathomimetic agents, such as cocaine toxicity, are typically, though not always, diaphoretic with agitated or violent behavior and hallucinations that are more commonly paranoid.

Multiple other toxicologic entities are associated with autonomic dysfunction (i.e., dysregulation of the heart rate, blood pressure, temperature, gastrointestinal secretion, metabolic and endocrine responses to stress). Acute withdrawal syndromes may be differentiated from anticholinergic (antimuscarinic) syndrome by a history of recent cessation of ethanol or another sedative-hypnotic agent, serotonin syndrome may be differentiated by a history of recent (minutes to hours) exposure to a serotonergic agent, and neuroleptic malignant syndrome may be differentiated by a history of exposure (within 3 to 9 days) to an agent capable of producing central dopamine blockade. Drug-induced psychosis mimicking central anticholinergic syndrome may be due to hallucinogens, phencyclidine, amphetamines, or corticosteroids.

Medical diseases that produce confusion, seizures, and tachycardia, such as hypoxia, hypoglycemia, and heat stroke, or those that cause hyperthermia, hypertension, tachycardia, and mydriasis, such as thyrotoxicosis and pheochromocytoma, may also be confused with anticholinergic toxicity.

Finally, diseases that may be manifested similar to central anticholinergic syndrome include schizophrenia and other psychotic disorders, cerebral vasculitis, CNS infection (e.g., encephalitis), sepsis, and psychiatric disease.

### DIAGNOSTIC TESTING

In the setting of anticholinergic (antimuscarinic) poisoning, results of the fingerstick serum glucose test and pulse oximetry analysis should be normal.

The ECG typically demonstrates sinus tachycardia. Some agents with anticholinergic (antimuscarinic) effects also have type IA antidysrhythmic effects that result in blockade of myocardial sodium channels. The blockade is seen on the ECG as prolongation of the QRS interval. Such agents include diphenhydramine, cyclobenzaprine, carbamazepine, and the tricyclic antidepressants.

With tricyclic antidepressant overdose in particular, the extent of prolongation of the QRS interval on an ECG is especially useful in predicting the severity of toxicity.

$SI = \frac{SV}{BSA}$ **FACTS AND FORMULAS**

A QRS duration shorter than 100 msec predicts that no serious clinical toxicity will occur, a QRS duration longer than 100 msec is associated with a 30% incidence of seizures, and a QRS duration longer than 160 msec is associated with a 50% likelihood of the development of ventricular dysrhythmia.[2] Additionally, an R wave in lead aVR measuring 3 mm or greater[3] or a terminal 40-msec right axis deviation between 130 and 270 degrees[4] is a predictor of tricyclic antidepressant–induced toxicity.

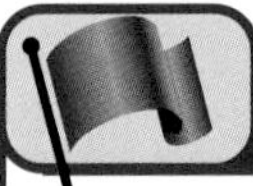

**RED FLAGS**

**Cautions for Physicians**

Physostigmine is contraindicated in patients after a tricyclic antidepressant overdose with a QRS interval longer than 100 msec because it may cause cardiac arrhythmias and profound hypotension.

Flumazenil should not generally be administered to patients with anticholinergic (antimuscarinic) toxicity because it may cause seizures or other complications.

Failure to become cholinergic (bradycardia, bronchorrhea, diaphoretic, drooling) after the administration of physostigmine is essentially diagnostic of anticholinergic toxicity.

Physostigmine will prolong the action of drugs metabolized by cholinesterases, such as succinylcholine. A nondepolarizing agent should be used instead.

Prolonged agitation and seizures can lead to the development of acidosis and rhabdomyolysis. Measurement of serum creatine phosphokinase and urine myoglobin aids in the recognition of patients at risk for the development of acute renal failure.

## TREATMENT

Most patients with anticholinergic (antimuscarinic) toxicity can be treated adequately with general supportive care of the airway, breathing, and circulation, followed by frequent reassessment and close observation (**Fig. 145.1**). To avoid the risk for aspiration, activated charcoal (1 g/kg) is recommended only for patients who are capable of spontaneously drinking and protecting their own airway. It may also be administered cautiously via a nasogastric tube to patients who are endotracheally intubated. Because anticholinergic (antimuscarinic) agents may slow gastrointestinal transit, activated charcoal may be useful several hours after ingestion.[5] The specific role of activated charcoal in most of these poisonings has not been studied.

The initial therapy for cardiovascular toxicity secondary to sodium channel blockade is hypertonic sodium bicarbonate in 1- to 2-mEq/kg boluses.[6] Treatment with sodium bicarbonate is indicated for patients with a QRS complex longer than 100 to 120 msec or a wide-complex or ventricular tachycardia until the abnormality is reversed or serum pH reaches 7.55. The ECG should be repeated within 60 seconds after a bolus of sodium bicarbonate to check for narrowing of the QRS complex. If narrowing has occurred, a continuous infusion at 1.5 times the maintenance intravenous fluid rate (three ampules [132 mEq] of sodium bicarbonate in 1 L of 5% dextrose in water [$D_5W$]) should be administered. Profound cardiovascular toxicity may require more aggressive interventions, such as the initiation of vasopressors or use of an intraaortic balloon pump.

Agitation should be addressed aggressively to prevent the development of more serious sequelae, such as hyperthermia, acidosis, and rhabdomyolysis. It is best controlled with benzodiazepines. The emergency physician should start with standard doses (i.e., diazepam, 5 to 10 mg intravenously) and repeat them until sedation (relief of agitation, myoclonus, tremor, picking movements, abnormal speech, and hallucinations) is achieved. Administration of physostigmine should also be considered for the treatment of agitation caused by an anticholinergic agent (see later).

Anticholinergic (antimuscarinic) agent–induced seizures should also be treated with standard doses of benzodiazepines (i.e., lorazepam, 2 mg intravenously) or with physostigmine. If this therapy fails, barbiturates or other GABAergic anticonvulsants should be administered. Phenytoin is rarely useful for toxin-induced seizures.

Patients with rhabdomyolysis should be administered saline intravenously at a rate sufficient to maintain brisk urine output (generally 3 to 5 mL/kg/hr after any lost intravascular volume has been replaced). If urinary pH is less than 6.0, urine alkalinization is necessary and is achieved with the use of a sodium bicarbonate infusion at 1.5 times the maintenance intravenous fluid rate (three ampules [132 mEq] of sodium bicarbonate in 1 L of $D_5W$). Serum pH must be monitored during the sodium bicarbonate infusion, which should be stopped if the pH reaches 7.55 or higher.

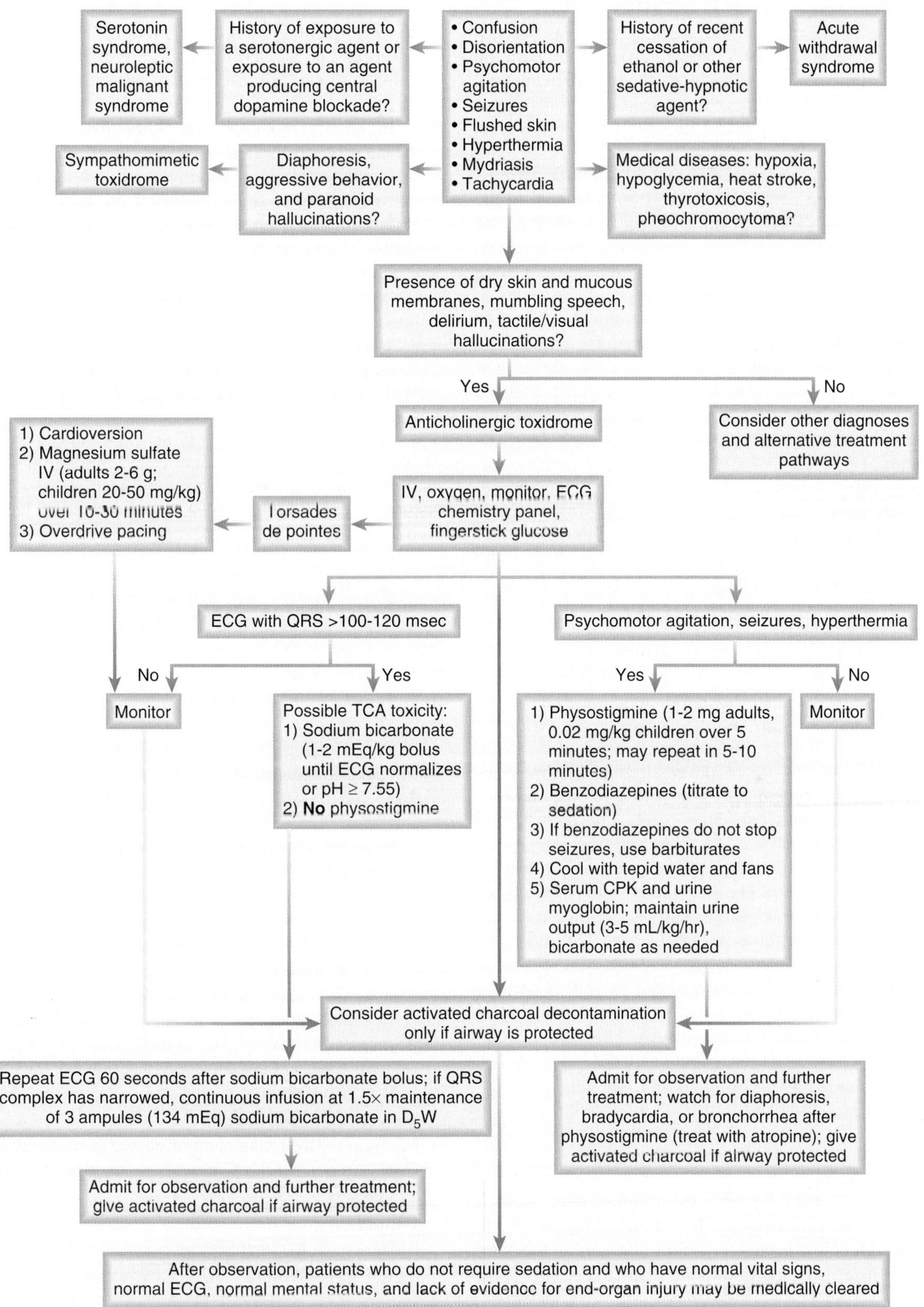


**Fig. 145.1 Algorithm for the recognition and treatment of anticholinergic toxicity.** *CPK*, Creatine phosphokinase; *$D_5W$*, 5% dextrose in water; *ECG*, electrocardiogram; *IV*, intravenous line; *TCA*, tricyclic antidepressant.

## ANTIDOTAL THERAPY PHYSOSTIGMINE

Physostigmine is a tertiary amine carbamate that penetrates into the CNS. It reversibly inhibits cholinesterases in both the central and peripheral nervous systems, thereby allowing acetylcholine to accumulate within the synapse. Accumulation of acetylcholine directly antagonizes the anticholinergic effects of antimuscarinic agents.

In the setting of a clear diagnosis of anticholinergic toxicity, physostigmine should be administered. It is beneficial in the treatment of agitation and delirium and also shortens the time to recovery after agitation. This agent should not be given once a benzodiazepine has been administered because the end point of clear mental status has been lost.[7]

During and immediately after the administration of physostigmine, patients must be monitored for early signs of cholinergic toxicity, such as diaphoresis and slowing of the heart rate. Atropine should be kept at the bedside and should be given in titrated doses if needed for cholinergic toxicity (development of bronchorrhea, hypoxia, bradycardia).

Physostigmine is indicated for patients with central (and perhaps peripheral) anticholinergic manifestations. It is contraindicated in patients with a QRS interval longer than 100 msec if the history suggests overdose of tricyclic antidepressant or other cardiotoxic agents. The latter contraindication is based on two case reports of patients with tricyclic antidepressant overdose in whom asystole developed after the administration of physostigmine. The cause of the asystole was theorized to be physostigmine-induced bradycardia that resulted in cardiac conduction defects and decreased cardiac output in the presence of tricyclic antidepressant–induced sodium channel blockade.[8] Other contraindications to the use of physostigmine are bronchospastic disease, peripheral vascular disease, intestinal or bladder obstruction, intraventricular conduction defects, and atrioventricular block.

Physostigmine is administered intravenously over a 5-minute period, 1 to 2 mg in adults and 0.02 mg/kg (maximum of 0.5 mg) in children. Its onset of action occurs within minutes.[9] This initial dose can be repeated in 5 to 10 minutes if an adequate response is not achieved and muscarinic effects are not noted. Failure of the patient to become cholinergic after the administration of physostigmine is essentially diagnostic of anticholinergic toxicity. Although the total effective dose of physostigmine depends on the individual, as well as the dose and duration of action of the anticholinergic (antimuscarinic) agent, 4 mg is usually a sufficient dose for most patients.[10] The half-life of physostigmine is 16 minutes, and its usual duration of action exceeds 1 hour.[11]

Adverse effects may occur if physostigmine is administered rapidly, in an excessive dose, or in the absence of an anticholinergic (antimuscarinic) agent. In all these instances, an excess of acetylcholine occurs at various sites within the body and has various effects, as follows:

- At nicotinic receptors: muscle fasciculations, weakness, and paralysis
- At muscarinic receptors: bronchospasm, bronchorrhea, bradycardia, salivation, lacrimation, urination, defecation, and emesis
- At CNS sites: anxiety, dizziness, tremors, confusion, ataxia, coma, and seizures

Accordingly, overdoses of physostigmine may require atropine to control the bronchial secretions, and mechanical ventilation may be needed for neuromuscular weakness because no specific antidote is available for the excess nicotinic activity.

Additionally, it is important to note that when other cholinergic agents are used concurrently with physostigmine, the effects may be additive. Examples of such agents are pilocarpine, carbamates, organophosphates, pyridostigmine, and depolarizing neuromuscular blocking agents. Because physostigmine is an acetylcholinesterase inhibitor, it also prolongs the action of drugs metabolized by plasma cholinesterases, such as cocaine, succinylcholine, and mivacurium.

## FOLLOW-UP, NEXT STEPS IN CARE, AND PATIENT EDUCATION

Patients in whom the anticholinergic toxicity resolves—who therefore do not require intervention for a period of 6 hours—and who have no evidence of complications of toxicity (e.g., aspiration pneumonia, rhabdomyolysis) may be medically

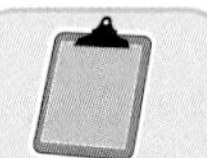

### DOCUMENTATION

**History**

Any history of psychiatric illness or previous suicidal ingestions?

Time since ingestion?

**Physical Examination**

Does the patient look ill? Febrile? What is the patient's mental status?

Cardiac (blood pressure, pulse, arrhythmias)?

Airway and respiratory status?

Urine output?

Repeated physical examinations while the patient is still in the emergency department

**Diagnostic Studies**

Electrocardiogram, blood chemistry panel with serum glucose, serum creatine phosphokinase, urine myoglobin measurements, pregnancy test?

Documentation of acetaminophen and aspirin levels if there is concern about coingestion

**Medical Decision Making**

Decision to begin treatment or delays in starting treatment

Consultations desired and times of calls to consulting services

**Treatment**

Response to treatment (especially for sodium bicarbonate, physostigmine)

**Patient Instructions**

Documentation of discussion with the patient regarding diagnosis, warning signs, what to do, follow-up, and when to return

With pediatric unintentional ingestions, documentation of poison prevention counseling and assessment of the home situation

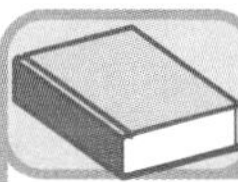

### PATIENT TEACHING TIPS

The regional poison control center can be contacted by telephone at 1-800-222-1222.

A dose of medication other than what was prescribed by the patient's physician should never be taken unless it has been approved by the ordering physician.

A second medication or herbal supplement should never be added to a previously taken medication without approval from the physician.

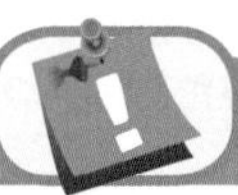

### TIPS AND TRICKS

Although patients with both adrenergic (sympathomimetic) and anticholinergic (antimuscarinic) poisoning may have similar clinical findings (altered mental status, tachycardia, mydriasis), the two syndromes may be differentiated by skin, type of alteration in mental status, and other clinical findings. Diaphoresis, agitation, paranoid hallucinations, and violent behavior are associated with sympathomimetic agents. Dry skin and mucous membranes, mumbling speech, delirium, and tactile or visual hallucinations are associated with anticholinergics.

cleared. All patients with suspected intentional overdose of any agent should be evaluated by a psychiatrist or otherwise appropriately cleared before hospital discharge according to local practice.

In patients with anticholinergic toxicity, admission to a critical care setting should be arranged for those with altered mental status, cardiac dysrhythmias or drug-related conduction abnormality, hyperthermia, or respiratory compromise requiring mechanical ventilation.

## SUGGESTED READINGS

Boehnert MT, Lovejoy FH. Value of the QRS duration versus the serum drug level in predicting seizures and ventricular arrhythmias after an overdose of tricyclic antidepressants. N Engl J Med 1985;313:474-9.

Niemann JT, Bessen HA, Rothstein RJ, et al. Electrocardiographic criteria for tricyclic antidepressant cardiotoxicity. Am J Cardiol 1986;57:1154-9.

Pentel P, Peterson CD. Asystole complicating physostigmine treatment of tricyclic antidepressant overdose. Ann Emerg Med 1980;9:588-90.

## REFERENCES

***References can be found on Expert Consult @ www.expertconsult.com.***

# 146 Insecticides, Herbicides, and Rodenticides

*Robert D. Cannon and Anne-Michelle Ruha*

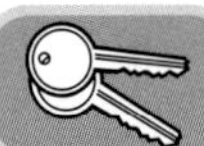

**KEY POINTS**

- Organophosphorus and carbamate poisonings cause excessive stimulation of muscarinic and nicotinic receptors by acetylcholine, which can potentially lead to life-threatening bronchorrhea and bronchospasm.
- Aggressive airway management and liberal use of atropine are important in the management of both organophosphorus and carbamate poisoning.
- Only a nondepolarizing neuromuscular blocker, such as vecuronium or rocuronium, should be used for intubation. Succinylcholine is metabolized by plasma cholinesterase, and prolonged paralysis may result if it is used in the setting of organophosphate poisoning.
- Timely administration of pralidoxime is key to the treatment of organophosphorus poisoning, but pralidoxime is not indicated for carbamate poisoning.
- Unintentional pediatric ingestion of 4-hydroxycoumarins (superwarfarins) accounts for the vast majority of rodenticide exposures and rarely results in toxicity.
- Ingestion of an anticoagulant rodenticide should be considered when a child younger than 6 years has an elevated prothrombin time or bleeding without another explanation.
- The prothrombin time should be measured at 24 and 48 hours after large ingestions of 4-hydroxycoumarins.
- Because no specific antidote or pharmacologic intervention has proved beneficial in treating paraquat or diquat poisoning, early decontamination is the most important step.

# Insecticides

## ORGANOPHOSPHORUS COMPOUNDS AND CARBAMATES

### EPIDEMIOLOGY

Organophosphate (OP) compounds and carbamates are used extensively worldwide for agricultural, industrial, and domestic pest control and, as a result, represent a significant public health issue in the developing world. An estimated 3 million poisonings and more than 200,000 deaths occur from OP compounds each year worldwide.[1] In the United States in 2008, 4642 exposures to OP compounds and 2644 exposures to carbamates were reported to the National Poison Data System of the American Association of Poison Control Centers.[2]

### PATHOPHYSIOLOGY

The clinical severity and toxicodynamics vary according to the agent, the route of absorption, and whether the exposure was intentional. Regardless of these factors, the toxicologic mechanism of acetylcholinesterase (AChE) inhibition remains consistent. The end result is an excess of the neurotransmitter acetylcholine (ACh), which results in overstimulation of muscarinic and nicotinic receptors and production of a cholinergic toxidrome.

Under normal circumstances, ACh is hydrolyzed by AChE to yield acetic acid and choline. In the presence of OP insecticides, AChE is phosphorylated, whereas in the presence of carbamate insecticides, the enzyme is carbamylated. As a result, the rate of regeneration of active AChE is slowed, and its function is inhibited. Within 24 to 72 hours of OP poisoning, an alkyl group may dissociate from the AChE-OP complex and thereby result in "aging" of the AChE. Once aging occurs, reactivation of AChE is no longer possible, and only synthesis of new enzyme can restore activity. In the case of carbamate poisoning, breakdown of the carbamate-AChE complex occurs much more rapidly and aging does not occur (**Box 146.1**).[3]

ACh accumulates in the autonomic nervous system at postganglionic muscarinic (parasympathetic and sympathetic) receptors and preganglionic nicotinic (sympathetic) receptors. It also accumulates at the neuromuscular junction and in the central nervous system (CNS). Overstimulation of these receptors is responsible for the cholinergic toxidrome seen with OP and carbamate insecticide poisoning (**Table 146.1**).

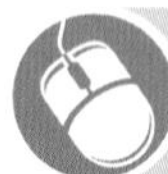

See Table 146.1, Effects of Organophosphorus and Carbamate Insecticides, at www.expertconsult.com

### PRESENTING SIGNS AND SYMPTOMS

The onset of symptoms can occur within minutes after massive exposure and intentional ingestions or be delayed up to 12 hours after accidental dermal, inhalational, or oral exposure in the occupational arena. Clinical effects may also be somewhat delayed because of the need for bioactivation of

**BOX 146.1 Effects of Organophosphate and Carbamate on Acetylcholinesterase (AChE)**

Organophosphate + AChE = phosphorylated AChE

Carbamate + AChE = carbamylated AChE

These complexes inactivate AChE and allow acetylcholine to sit on the nicotinic and muscarinic receptors and produce the symptoms of toxicity.

Three things can happen to the phosphorylated or carbamylated AChE:

- Breakdown of the complex (occurs more rapidly with carbamate) to release active AChE
- Complete binding and inactivation (aging), which occurs within 24 to 72 hours (with organophosphates) and requires that new AChE be produced
- Reactivation by a strong nucleophile such as pralidoxime

some OP insecticides after absorption (e.g., malathion). The mnemonic SLUDGE (salivation, lacrimation, urination, defecation, gastric secretions, emesis) has traditionally been used to describe the cholinergic toxidrome. However, the mnemonic DUMBBELS (defecation, urination, miosis, bronchorrhea, bradycardia, emesis, lacrimation, salivation) is probably more appropriate because it includes the life-threatening conditions bronchorrhea and bradyarrhythmias, as well as miosis, the distinguishing feature.

The clinical effects are summarized in Table 146.1; only caveats in the clinical findings are emphasized here. Bronchorrhea occurs commonly with moderate to severe poisonings[4] and can progress to pulmonary edema and respiratory failure. Miosis in the setting of cholinergic symptoms is fairly specific for OP and carbamate insecticide poisoning and may help make the diagnosis. Unfortunately, it is not consistently present.

Although the parasympathetic muscarinic effects are most often emphasized, certain sympathetic effects may predominate. Sinus tachycardia is more common than bradycardia,[4,5] and mydriasis may even be seen.[5] Nicotinic effects often predominate in mild cases and occur early in severe cases. Excessive nicotinic stimulation at the neuromuscular junction has effects that resemble the actions of a depolarizing neuromuscular blocking agent. Therefore, patients with OP or carbamate insecticide poisoning may exhibit muscle fasciculations and weakness. Paralysis occurs as the toxicity worsens, and the primary cause of death in acute poisonings is probably respiratory arrest secondary to paralysis and bronchorrhea.

One to 3 days after apparent resolution of the symptoms, patients may experience profound weakness and paralysis of the proximal muscles, neck flexor muscles, and cranial nerves. This development, termed the *intermediate syndrome*,[6] is probably explained by ongoing AChE inhibition (**Box 146.2**).

Finally, carbamates produce peripheral effects similar to those of OP compounds, but generally to a much lesser extent. A distinguishing clinical feature of carbamate toxicity is the paucity of central effects, which is secondary to their poor penetration of the CNS.

**BOX 146.2 Paralysis Seen After Organophosphate Poisoning**

**Type I**

Acute paralysis secondary to constant depolarization at the neuromuscular junction

**Type II (Intermediate Syndrome)**

- Develops 1 to 3 days after resolution of the acute organophosphate poisoning symptoms
- Manifested as paralysis and respiratory distress secondary to weakness of the proximal muscles, neck flexor muscles (with relative sparing of the distal muscle groups), and cranial nerve palsies
- Lasts for 4 to 18 days and may require mechanical ventilation
- Results from ongoing acetylcholinesterase inhibition or suboptimal treatment

**Type III (Organophosphate-Induced Delayed Polyneuropathy)**

Manifested 2 to 3 weeks after exposure

Results from inhibition of target esterase

Characterized by distal muscle weakness with relative sparing of the neck muscles, cranial nerves, and proximal muscle groups

Recovery can take up to 12 months

## DIFFERENTIAL DIAGNOSIS AND MEDICAL DECISION MAKING

A detailed history in a patient with signs and symptoms of cholinergic excess often elucidates exposure to OP or carbamate insecticides. The diagnosis of OP or carbamate insecticide poisoning is therefore usually straightforward; however, certain clinical aspects may be mimicked by other entities. **Table 146.2** is a partial list of other agents or diagnoses to consider.

All patients with potential OP poisoning should undergo erythrocyte (red blood cell [RBC], or true) cholinesterase and plasma (pseudo) cholinesterase measurement from specimens obtained after arrival at the emergency department (ED). Though not often useful or necessary for making a diagnosis in the ED, the results of this measurement may help guide continued therapy. RBC cholinesterase hydrolyzes ACh and correlates with toxicity, whereas plasma cholinesterase is the first to decline and may be a more sensitive marker of exposure.[7] Both substances should be measured because one may exhibit greater inhibition than the other, depending on the specific OP to which the patient was exposed. **Box 146.3** summarizes the tests that may be helpful in evaluating a patient with moderate to severe toxicity.

Cholinesterase values may prove useful in diagnosing OP toxicity if the history or findings on physical examination are unclear. The values must be interpreted with caution, however. There is great interindividual and intraindividual variation in baseline cholinesterase values. A patient may have a 50% depression in cholinesterase activity, yet the level still falls within the "normal" reference range. This makes cholinesterase measurements of limited value in the initial diagnosis of

**Table 146.2 Differential Diagnosis of Organophosphorus and Carbamate Poisoning**

| | |
|---|---|
| Other acetylcholinesterase inhibitors | Physostigmine, neostigmine, pyridostigmine |
| Other organophosphorus cholinesterase inhibitors (chemical weapon nerve agents) | Sarin, tabun, soman, VX |
| Cholinomimetics | Pilocarpine, carbachol, methacholine, bethanechol, muscarine-containing mushrooms |
| Nicotinic alkaloids | Nicotine, coniine, lobeline |
| Other (symptom based) | Coma, miosis, paralysis: Pontine hemorrhage<br>Salivation, fasciculations: Bark scorpion (*Centruroides* spp.)<br>Vomiting, diarrhea: Gastroenteritis<br>Respiratory failure: Any cause of pulmonary edema, status asthmaticus<br>Weakness: Myasthenic crisis, electrolyte disturbance, botulism |

**BOX 146.3 Ancillary Studies in the Management of Organophosphate or Carbamate Poisoning**

Laboratory tests:
- Red blood cell cholinesterase concentration
- Plasma cholinesterase concentration
- Complete blood count
- Electrolytes
- Blood urea nitrogen and creatinine levels
- Liver enzyme levels
- Arterial blood gas values

Electrocardiography
Chest radiograph

poisoning. The levels are helpful in confirming poisoning only if they are extremely low or undetectable at initial evaluation. The finding of "normal" levels does not necessarily rule out poisoning if the history and clinical picture are otherwise supportive.

## TREATMENT

Treatment focuses on aggressive airway management, liberal use of atropine for control of excessive airway secretions, and in the case of OP compounds, early administration of the antidote pralidoxime. Prompt recognition of toxicity and early intervention usually result in complete recovery.

The treatment algorithm for OP and carbamate insecticide poisoning is summarized in **Figure 146.1**. The first step is adequate decontamination of the patient by removal of wet clothing and washing of contaminated skin with soap and water. ED personnel should wear gowns, gloves, and masks to prevent exposure to contaminated body fluids.[8]

As the patient is being decontaminated, the emergency physician (EP) should focus on the ABCs (airway, breathing circulation), with particular attention paid to early airway, management for copious secretions, seizures, coma, severe weakness, and paralysis. If intubation is necessary, only a nondepolarizing neuromuscular blocking agent, such as vecuronium or rocuronium, should be used. Succinylcholine is metabolized by plasma cholinesterase, so prolonged paralysis may result if this agent is used a patient with OP poisoning.[9]

Treatment should next be directed at controlling muscarinic activity. Atropine is the drug of choice and should be administered intravenously at a dose of 2 to 5 mg (pediatric dose, 0.05 mg/kg) every 3 to 5 minutes, with the end point being control of respiratory secretions. Tachycardia is not a contraindication to atropine administration. Mild poisonings may resolve with just 1 to 2 mg of atropine, and severe poisonings may require more than 1000 mg.[10] Large doses of atropine may lead to antimuscarinic CNS toxicity. If such toxicity occurs, glycopyrrolate (1 to 2 mg; pediatric dose, 0.025 mg/kg) can be used in place of atropine.

Pralidoxime is the antidote for OP insecticide poisoning. Although its efficacy may vary according to the structure of the OP compound, it should be given to all OP-poisoned patients. It works by increasing the rate of AChE regeneration. It is a common belief that pralidoxime is not beneficial if given after 24 hours because of the "aging" of AChE. However, OP insecticides have been detected in blood weeks after exposure. Their presence may be secondary to redistribution from fat. Therefore, late pralidoxime therapy may still be of benefit. The adult dose is 1 to 2 g via the intravenous (IV) route delivered over a 15- to 30-minute period followed by a continuous infusion of 500 mg/hr. Pediatric dosing consists of a 25- to 50-mg/kg load followed by a 10- to 20-mg/kg/hr infusion. Pralidoxime is not indicated for carbamate poisoning, which is usually mild and self-limited.

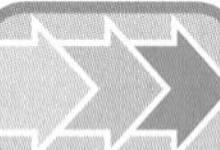

**PRIORITY ACTIONS**

**Organophosphates**

Protect the airway in patients with increased secretions from organophosphates or carbamates.
Administer atropine early and often to control airway secretions.
Give intravenous fluids to replace gastrointestinal losses.
Administer pralidoxime early in the course of organophosphate poisoning.
Treat seizures with benzodiazepines.

# ORGANOCHLORINES

## EPIDEMIOLOGY

Organochlorines are heavily chlorinated aromatic compounds that are nonvolatile and poorly water soluble. They are

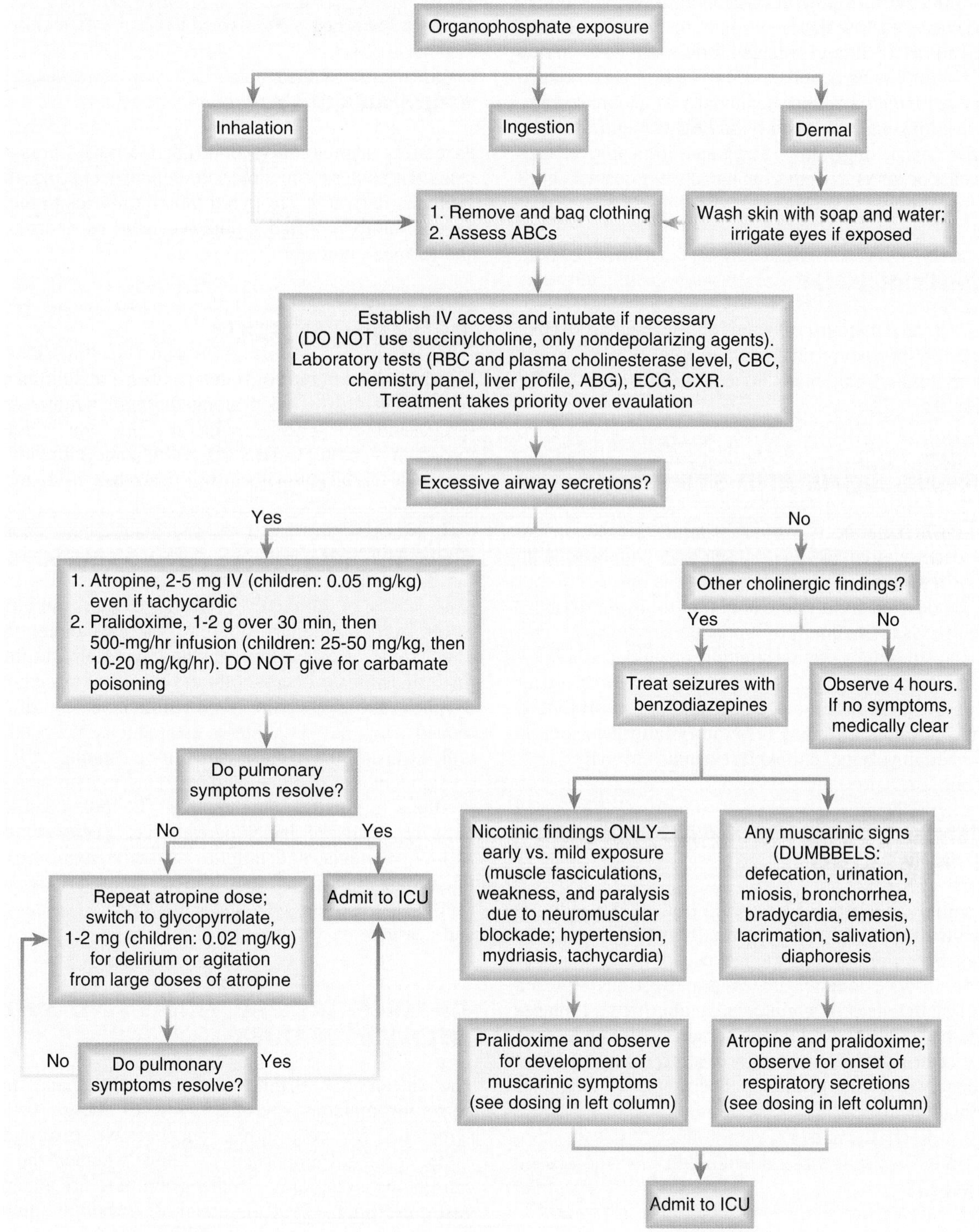

Organophosphate exposure

Inhalation

Ingestion

Dermal

1. Remove and bag clothing
2. Assess ABCs

Wash skin with soap and water; irrigate eyes if exposed

Establish IV access and intubate if necessary (DO NOT use succinylcholine, only nondepolarizing agents). Laboratory tests (RBC and plasma cholinesterase level, CBC, chemistry panel, liver profile, ABG), ECG, CXR. Treatment takes priority over evaulation

Excessive airway secretions?

Yes

1. Atropine, 2-5 mg IV (children: 0.05 mg/kg) even if tachycardic
2. Pralidoxime, 1-2 g over 30 min, then 500-mg/hr infusion (children: 25-50 mg/kg, then 10-20 mg/kg/hr). DO NOT give for carbamate poisoning

Do pulmonary symptoms resolve?

No

Repeat atropine dose; switch to glycopyrrolate, 1-2 mg (children: 0.02 mg/kg) for delirium or agitation from large doses of atropine

Do pulmonary symptoms resolve?

No

Yes

Yes

Admit to ICU

No

Other cholinergic findings?

Yes

Treat seizures with benzodiazepines

Nicotinic findings ONLY—early vs. mild exposure (muscle fasciculations, weakness, and paralysis due to neuromuscular blockade; hypertension, mydriasis, tachycardia)

Pralidoxime and observe for development of muscarinic symptoms (see dosing in left column)

Any muscarinic signs (DUMBBELS: defecation, urination, miosis, bronchorrhea, bradycardia, emesis, lacrimation, salivation), diaphoresis

Atropine and pralidoxime; observe for onset of respiratory secretions (see dosing in left column)

Admit to ICU

No

Observe 4 hours. If no symptoms, medically clear

**Fig. 146.1 Treatment algorithm for organophosphorus insecticide poisoning.** *ABCs*, Airway, breathing, and circulation; *ABG*, arterial blood gas determination; *CBC*, complete blood count; *CXR*, chest radiograph; *ECG*, electrocardiography; *ICU*, intensive care unit; *IV*, intravenous; *RBC*, red blood cell.

divided into four classes on the basis of their structural characteristics, and they vary tremendously with respect to dermal absorption, lipid solubility, and toxic doses. The clinical toxicity, which is similar for each of the classes, is summarized in (**Table 146.3**).

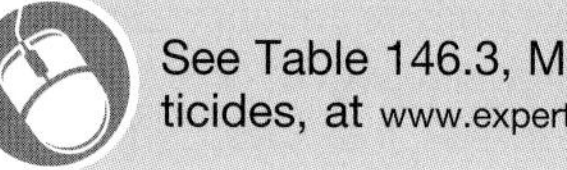

See Table 146.3, Major Organophosphorus Insecticides, at www.expertconsult.com

Most organochlorines have been banned in North America because of concern about their environmental persistence and bioconcentration. The only organochlorine still in common use in the United States is lindane (Kwell). It is used in agriculture as a seed treatment and medicinally as a topical scabicide in a 1% formulation. Toxicity from therapeutic lindane application is exceedingly rare, and most clinically relevant toxicity events occur as a result of inappropriate dermal application or ingestion.[11-13]

## PATHOPHYSIOLOGY

Lindane acts as an antagonist of γ-aminobutyric acid (GABA), the major inhibitory neurotransmitter in the CNS.[14] Toxicity results from loss of inhibitory tone and subsequent CNS hyperexcitability.

## PRESENTING SIGNS AND SYMPTOMS

Symptoms, which can occur within 30 minutes of the ingestion of lindane,[12] often include nausea and vomiting. With excessive or repeated topical applications, the onset of symptoms may be delayed from a few hours up to 4 to 5 days.[11,14] CNS excitation is the hallmark of lindane toxicity. It is manifested by paresthesias, agitation, tremor, myoclonus, hallucinations, and most important, seizures. Seizures may occur suddenly and without prodrome. Complications of prolonged seizures may develop, including respiratory failure, metabolic acidosis, rhabdomyolysis, and hyperthermia.

## DIFFERENTIAL DIAGNOSIS AND MEDICAL DECISION MAKING

The differential diagnosis for suspected lindane poisoning is extremely broad because it can potentially include any cause of seizures. Appropriate, therapeutic use of lindane is not expected to produce toxicity. Unless a patient has ingested lindane before the onset of symptoms, an alternative explanation should be sought to explain the seizures. Although some laboratories can measure lindane levels, the results will not be immediately available to the EP. Therefore, the diagnosis is primarily clinical.

## TREATMENT

No specific antidote is available for lindane toxicity. Although activated charcoal can be considered early after ingestion, it may be dangerous in a patient who may have seizures without warning. The mainstay of treatment is supportive. Benzodiazepines should be used to treat seizures. If that therapy is unsuccessful, barbiturates (phenobarbital) should be administered. As with other toxin-induced seizures, phenytoin is not indicated.

All symptomatic patients with lindane toxicity should be admitted to the hospital. Asymptomatic patients seen after the ingestion of lindane may be observed for 6 hours from the time of ingestion; if no symptoms develop, the patient can be medically cleared.

# PYRETHRINS AND PYRETHROIDS

## EPIDEMIOLOGY

Pyrethrins are naturally occurring esters of chrysanthemum resin that possess insecticidal activity, whereas pyrethroids are synthetic derivatives of pyrethrins. Exposures to these agents are commonly reported to poison centers. Most are accidental, and serious clinical effects are rare.[2]

## PATHOPHYSIOLOGY

Pyrethrins and pyrethroids delay closure of sodium channels. The delay results in prolonged depolarization, repetitive firing, and eventually conduction blockade.[15] Some pyrethroids may inhibit GABA chloride channels, but it is unlikely that such inhibition plays a significant role in toxicity.

## PRESENTING SIGNS AND SYMPTOMS

Most cases of clinically relevant toxicity from pyrethrins result from pulmonary allergic reactions rather than from direct toxic effects. The signs and symptoms are similar to those of asthma exacerbations and consist of wheezing, cough, dyspnea, and chest pain. Most reactions are mild and easily treated. However, fatal status asthmaticus has been reported with exposure to pyrethrin-containing shampoo.[16,17]

Accidental or occupational exposure to pyrethroids usually produces minimal, if any, toxicity. The most common symptoms reported are facial paresthesias, dizziness, headache, nausea, anorexia, and fatigue.[18] Massive exposures or large intentional ingestions may lead to more serious manifestations: seizures, altered mental status, coma, respiratory failure, and death.

## DIFFERENTIAL DIAGNOSIS AND MEDICAL DECISION MAKING

The differential diagnosis for pyrethrin and pyrethroid poisoning includes any other cause of allergic or asthmatic symptoms in most cases, but because treatment is the same, it is not important to know whether the exposure caused the symptoms. If the symptoms are neurologic or gastrointestinal, the differential diagnosis is quite broad; unfortunately, no laboratory or other test will help in differentiation.

## TREATMENT

Activated charcoal may be given to a patient initially seen within 1 hour of a large oral ingestion of pyrethrin or pyrethroid. Skin decontamination is accomplished with soap and water. Pyrethrin-induced bronchospasm is treated with oxygen, β-adrenergic agonists, and corticosteroids as needed. No specific antidote is available, and the symptoms resolve with supportive care.

## FIPRONIL

### EPIDEMIOLOGY

Fipronil is a relatively new insecticide that was first introduced in 1996, and over the past several years it has increasingly been used to control common household insects, in addition to being used in flea and tick treatment for pets. Until recently, limited human toxicity data existed. It is commonly found in Frontline and Maxforce products.

### PATHOPHYSIOLOGY

Fipronil acts as a GABA antagonist, which leads to excessive CNS excitation and death of the insect. It is more specific for the insect GABA receptor than it is for its mammalian counterpart.

### PRESENTING SIGNS AND SYMPTOMS

The majority of human exposures are unintentional and most commonly result in neurologic symptoms such as dizziness and headache. Ocular and upper respiratory irritation has been reported commonly in addition to nausea and vomiting.[19] More severe exposures or large intentional ingestions can cause CNS excitation and seizures.

### DIFFERENTIAL DIAGNOSIS AND MEDICAL DECISION MAKING

Again, depending on the neurologic or gastrointestinal symptoms, the differential diagnosis may be broad and cannot be narrowed with any laboratory or diagnostic test. A history of exposure or potential exposure remains the most important key.

### TREATMENT

Treatment of fipronil exposure remains primarily supportive and symptomatic. In patients with significant exposure who arrive at the ED in a state of CNS excitation or with seizures, the mainstay of treatment is airway protection and liberal use of benzodiazepines for sedation and control of the seizures.

**TIPS AND TRICKS**

**Insecticides**

Use glycopyrrolate in patients who need more atropine but show signs of central nervous system antimuscarinic toxicity, such as delirium and agitation.

Do not rely on the pupils to rule in or rule out the diagnosis.

The presence of tachycardia should not prevent administration of atropine to a patient with bronchorrhea or wheezing.

Base treatment on clinical signs and symptoms, not on acetylcholinesterase levels.

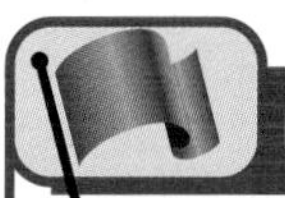

**RED FLAGS**

**Insecticides**

Miosis in the setting of cholinergic symptoms, though not consistently present, is fairly specific for organophosphate and carbamate insecticides and may help make the diagnosis.

Although the parasympathetic muscarinic effects are most often emphasized, certain sympathetic effects may predominate (sinus tachycardia is more common than bradycardia, and mydriasis may be seen).

Nicotinic effects often predominate in mild cases and occur early in severe cases.

"Normal" cholinesterase levels do not necessarily rule out poisoning if the history and clinical picture are otherwise indicative.

Symptoms can occur within 30 minutes of the ingestion of lindane, but with excessive or repeated topical applications, the onset of symptoms may be delayed from a few hours to 4 to 5 days.

# Herbicides

## PARAQUAT AND DIQUAT

### EPIDEMIOLOGY

Paraquat and diquat belong to the bipyridyl class of herbicides. They are both commonly used worldwide for weed control in the agricultural, horticultural, and forestry industries, and paraquat is marketed in more than 130 countries. Both compounds are available for home and commercial use in varying concentrations. Paraquat is commonly sold as a 0.2% solution for home use but can be found in 10% to 24% concentrated commercial solutions.

Paraquat and diquat account for only 4.9% of herbicide poisonings but are responsible for more than 50% of herbicide-related deaths.[20] This fact points to the extremely toxic nature of these compounds. Most serious toxicity events and deaths are secondary to intentional ingestion.[21]

### PATHOPHYSIOLOGY

Paraquat is rapidly absorbed after ingestion and is concentrated in type I and type II alveolar epithelial cells. It is subsequently reduced to a free radical, which then reacts with oxygen to form a superoxide anion ($O_2^-$). This anion then may form $H_2O_2$, which in the presence of $Fe^{2+}$, will generate highly reactive species such as the hydroxyl radical (OH). These reactive molecules cause lipid peroxidation and cellular destruction.[22] Initially, acute alveolitis may occur. Later, proliferative changes and pulmonary fibrosis are seen. Although paraquat concentrates mostly in the lungs, it is also distributed throughout the entire body and causes cellular destruction in multiple organs.

The pathophysiologic mechanism of diquat is similar to that of paraquat. Diquat does not concentrate in the lungs, however, and does not produce pulmonary fibrosis.[23]

## PRESENTING SIGNS AND SYMPTOMS

Paraquat poisoning can be classified as mild, moderate, or severe according to the amount ingested.[21] Physical examination findings are summarized in **Table 146.4**. Mild poisonings, which occur when small amounts of dilute preparations are ingested, are characterized by the development of gastrointestinal symptoms without other organ toxicity. As the amount of paraquat or diquat ion ingested rises, worsening gastrointestinal effects are seen, including severe oropharyngeal, esophageal, and gastric ulceration. Large ingestions produce renal and hepatic failure within a few days. Paraquat toxicity results in pulmonary fibrosis and refractory hypoxemia several days to weeks after ingestion, and death usually occurs within a few weeks. Massive ingestions cause multiorgan failure and death within a few days. Diquat toxicity does not produce pulmonary fibrosis. Diquat ingestion has been associated with brainstem infarction.[23] Effects from dermal exposure to paraquat and diquat are usually mild, but ulcers and blistering can occur with highly concentrated formulations.

## DIFFERENTIAL DIAGNOSIS AND MEDICAL DECISION MAKING

A qualitative urine test can be performed to aid in the diagnosis of paraquat or diquat poisoning. When alkaline sodium dithionate is added to urine, the color turns blue when paraquat is present and blue-green in the presence of diquat. Quantitative plasma measurements may also be obtained to confirm exposure and determine prognosis. Neither of these tests may be readily available in the emergency setting. Therefore, the diagnosis is often based on the history alone. The differential diagnosis of paraquat and diquat poisoning is wide and includes exposure to other caustic substances.

## TREATMENT

No specific antidote or pharmacologic intervention has been proven to affect outcome after paraquat or diquat poisoning. Early decontamination is the most important step in initial management and may be futile after large ingestions because of rapid absorption. There is little clinical or experimental evidence for the use of gastric lavage, and the procedure may even worsen the oral or esophageal ulceration. Therefore, activated charcoal (1 to 2 g/kg) is the agent of choice for gastric decontamination. Other agents, such as diatomaceous fuller's earth (1 to 2 g/kg in a 30% aqueous solution) and bentonite (1 to 2 g/kg of a 7% aqueous solution), have been used but are not as likely to be available to the EP, nor do they provide any advantage over charcoal. Gastric decontamination should be initiated as soon as possible.

Supportive care should be provided, with airway protection and ventilation being paramount. Supplemental oxygen may worsen the toxicity by accelerating the damage caused by oxygen radicals. It is generally accepted that supplemental oxygen be withheld until the $PaO_2$ value falls below 40 to 50 mm Hg. IV fluids should be given to ensure normal urine output and analgesics provided for the pain associated with mucosal ulcerations. Many other pharmacologic treatments of paraquat poisoning have been investigated, but none have proved useful.[22] Hemoperfusion and hemodialysis are effective in removing paraquat from the blood, but neither improves the prognosis.

# CHLORPHENOXY HERBICIDES

## EPIDEMIOLOGY

Chlorphenoxy herbicides are widely used to control the growth of broad-leaved weeds in pastures and crop fields and

**Table 146.4 Clinical Manifestations of Paraquat Poisoning**

| DEGREE | AMOUNT INGESTED | CLINICAL FEATURES |
|---|---|---|
| Mild | <20 mg/kg paraquat ion | Asymptomatic or gastrointestinal symptoms<br>Patients recover fully |
| Moderate to severe | 20-40 mg/kg | Oropharyngeal erythema and ulcerations may occur<br>Vomiting and diarrhea<br>Acute renal failure and hepatic dysfunction within 24 hr<br>Pulmonary fibrosis in all patients, but may be delayed days to weeks<br>Most die within 2-3 wk |
| Fulminant | >40 mg/kg | Definite ulceration of the oropharynx<br>Rapid development of multiorgan failure<br>Severe lung injury, cerebral edema, seizures, renal failure, hepatic necrosis, pancreatic necrosis, cardiovascular collapse<br>100% mortality<br>Death in 24 hr to a few days after the overdose |

along public streets. Poisoning is uncommon, and most ED encounters consist of accidental dermal or inhalational exposure, for which serious systemic toxicity is rare. However, intentional ingestion of these compounds carries high morbidity and mortality. From 1962 to 2004, 69 cases of ingestion of chlorphenoxy herbicides alone (excluding other pesticides as coingestants) were reported. One third of the patients in these reports died.[24]

## PATHOPHYSIOLOGY

The pathophysiology of chlorphenoxy herbicide toxicity involves three mechanisms. First, a dose-dependent disruption of cell membranes is thought to be responsible for mediation of CNS toxicity through disruption of the blood-brain barrier. Second, these compounds may form analogues of acetyl coenzyme A (CoA) and thereby disrupt its role in cellular metabolism. Because acetyl CoA is involved in formation of the neurotransmitter ACh, false cholinergic transmitters may be formed. A third mechanism of toxicity results from uncoupling of oxidative phosphorylation, which leads to depletion of cellular adenosine triphosphate.[25]

## PRESENTING SIGNS AND SYMPTOMS

Vomiting is common early after ingestion and may be accompanied by abdominal pain and diarrhea. Hypotension may occur secondary to volume loss, peripheral vasodilation, and direct myocardial toxicity. Severe ingestions are often associated with a rapid onset of coma. Other neurologic features that have been reported are hyperreflexia, hypertonia, seizures, hallucinations, clonus, and ataxia.[24,25] Peripheral neuromuscular effects include weakness, loss of deep tendon reflexes, and fasciculations. Common metabolic effects are acidosis, hyperthermia, and rhabdomyolysis.

## DIFFERENTIAL DIAGNOSIS AND MEDICAL DECISION MAKING

The diagnosis is made by obtaining a history of ingestion of or exposure to these agents. Plasma levels can be measured, but the results are not available in the emergency setting. When the history is lacking, the diagnosis is difficult to make because the differential diagnosis includes any potential cause of metabolic acidosis, myopathy, changes in mental status, and gastroenteritis.

## TREATMENT

Most patients can be managed with supportive care alone. Activated charcoal should be given if the patient is seen within 1 hour of a large ingestion. Other supportive measures are airway protection, IV fluids, and benzodiazepines for seizures, fasciculations, hyperreflexia, or clonus.

Alkaline diuresis has been reported to reduce the half-life of 2,4-dichlorophenoxyacetic acid (2,4-D).[26] Although hemodialysis and resin hemoperfusion enhance elimination of 2,4-D, no controlled trials have been conducted to assess whether these measures change the outcome. These modalities should be considered only for severe poisonings.

## GLYPHOSATE

Glyphosate is a widely used herbicide with formulations that range from a 1% household concentration to a 41% concentrate for commercial use. In addition, many of the commercial formulations are mixed with surfactants, which themselves produce toxicity by destroying mitochondrial cell walls and interfering with cellular energy production. The amine surfactants are also highly alkaline and corrosive and thus contribute to much of the toxicity of glyphosate.

Unintentional or small ingestions of glyphosate typically produce only mild gastrointestinal symptoms. An exception occurs with glyphosate-trimesium (Touchdown), which has produced rapid death after small ingestions.[27] Most cases of significant toxicity result from intentional ingestion of the concentrated formulation of Roundup (41% glyphosate and 15% polyoxyethyleneamine surfactant). Common features are corrosive effects, such as oropharyngeal ulcers, dysphagia, abdominal pain, and vomiting. Significant laryngeal injury may lead to aspiration and lung injury. Metabolic acidosis is common with large ingestions of concentrated formulations. Hypovolemia and hypoperfusion may lead to secondary hepatic and renal insufficiency.[28]

**TIPS AND TRICKS**

**Herbicides**

Withhold oxygen administration until a $PaO_2$ value of less than 40 mm Hg occurs in patients with paraquat poisoning because it may worsen toxicity through acceleration of damage by oxygen radicals.

Consider urinary alkalinization with severe chlorphenoxy herbicide poisoning.

Early decontamination with activated charcoal takes priority in paraquat and diquat ingestions.

Management is primarily supportive. Airway protection takes priority in patients with signs of oral and gastrointestinal corrosive effects. IV fluids should be given to normalize urine output. In the rare severe poisoning, acidosis and hypotension may be refractory to IV fluids and thus necessitate sodium bicarbonate and vasopressors, respectively.

## GLUFOSINATE

Glufosinate is a nonselective herbicide used worldwide and marketed under the trade names BASTA, Ignite, Challenge, and Harvest. A glutamic acid analogue, glufosinate is combined with surfactants. As with glyphosate, ingestion of these products can lead to symptoms attributable to surfactants, such as corrosive injury, gastrointestinal symptoms, and acidosis. However, glufosinate is unique in that it may cause delayed onset of CNS toxicity. Ataxia, depressed level of consciousness, coma, and central apnea may develop 4 to 12 hours after ingestion.[29,30] Delayed-onset seizures have been reported 29 hours after ingestion and may last for days.[29]

Treatment is supportive. Activated charcoal may be considered for patients seen within 1 hour after a large ingestion, but vomiting will probably limit its utility.

# Rodenticides

Rodenticides vary greatly with respect to pathophysiology, signs and symptoms, degree of toxicity, and management. Because these poisonings are rarely encountered by EPs, a detailed discussion on each one is beyond the scope of this text. Some of the characteristics can be found in **Table 146.5**. Instead, attention is directed to the anticoagulant rodenticides warfarin and superwarfarin and the compound strychnine, which can be found in some rodenticides today.

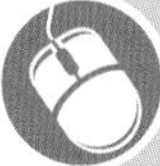

See Table 146.5, Characteristics of Some Rodenticides, at www.expertconsult.com

## ANTICOAGULANTS

### EPIDEMIOLOGY

Anticoagulant rodenticides can be categorized as warfarins or superwarfarins. The warfarins were the first anticoagulant rodenticides introduced, and their toxicity in rodents and humans depended on repeated ingestion. They are virtually nontoxic after a single small ingestion. This characteristic made them attractive from a safety standpoint but rendered them poor rodenticides.

In the 1980s, the 4-hydroxycoumarins and indanediones were developed (see **Table 146.6**). For a listing of brands and concentrations). These potent, long-acting superwarfarins are lethal to rodents and toxic to humans after a single acute ingestion. These compounds are now responsible for the majority of exposures to anticoagulant rodenticides. Of the 14,425 rodenticide exposures reported to poison control centers in 2008, 11,146 involved superwarfarins. Most were unintentional ingestions in children younger than 6 years.[2]

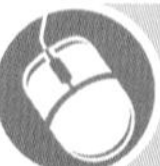

See Table 146.6, Anticoagulant Rodenticide (Superwarfarin) Brands and Concentrations, at www.expertconsult.com

### PATHOPHYSIOLOGY

The warfarins and superwarfarins inhibit the synthesis of vitamin $K_1$–dependent clotting factors (II, VII, IX, X) by blocking conversion of inactive vitamin K to the active form. Bleeding may occur when factor levels fall to 25% of baseline. Because factor VII has the shortest half-life (about 5 hours), a rise in the prothrombin time may be seen in three to four half-lives (15 to 20 hours after ingestion) and certainly will be present within 48 hours.[31]

### PRESENTING SIGNS AND SYMPTOMS

When a child is evaluated immediately after an unintentional ingestion, the child will be asymptomatic without signs of bleeding; 24 to 48 hours after a large ingestion, however, the child may have any manifestation of a coagulopathy, including, in order of decreasing frequency, ecchymosis, hematuria, uterine bleeding, gastrointestinal bleeding, epistaxis, spontaneous hematoma, gingival bleeding, hemoptysis, and hematemesis.[32]

### DIFFERENTIAL DIAGNOSIS AND MEDICAL DECISION MAKING

Ingestion of an anticoagulant rodenticide should be considered when a patient has an elevated prothrombin time or bleeding without other explanation. The differential diagnosis includes vitamin K deficiency, hemophilia or other factor deficiencies, and disseminated intravascular coagulation. The myriad causes of liver failure must also be considered, including viral hepatitis, alcoholic cirrhosis, hepatotoxic ingestions (e.g., acetaminophen, iron), and Wilson disease. A thorough laboratory evaluation aimed at sorting out these processes should be obtained, including a complete blood count, prothrombin and partial thromboplastin times, international normalized ratio, liver enzymes, fibrinogen and fibrin split products, measurements of coagulation factors (II, VII, VII, IX, X), and a 50:50 mixing test. Brodifacoum and difenacoum measurements may be performed, but their results will not be immediately available to the EP.

### TREATMENT

**Figure 146.2** summarizes the management of warfarin or superwarfarin poisoning, which depends on the timing, amount ingested, and symptomatology. Accidental ingestions of less than one box of 4-hydroxycoumarin are unlikely to result in clinically significant toxicity and may be managed without gastric decontamination or laboratory evaluation unless signs of bleeding occur.[33] Patients who ingest one or more boxes should be given activated charcoal if they are seen within 1 hour of ingestion. Acute hemorrhage is managed with oxygen and IV crystalloids to replace losses of volume. Fresh frozen plasma should be administered to patients with active bleeding and coagulopathy. Vitamin $K_1$ is given at doses of 1 to 5 mg in children and 10 mg in adults. It may be administered intravenously at no more than 1 mg/min to reduce the likelihood of anaphylactoid reactions. Oral or subcutaneous administration is also acceptable.

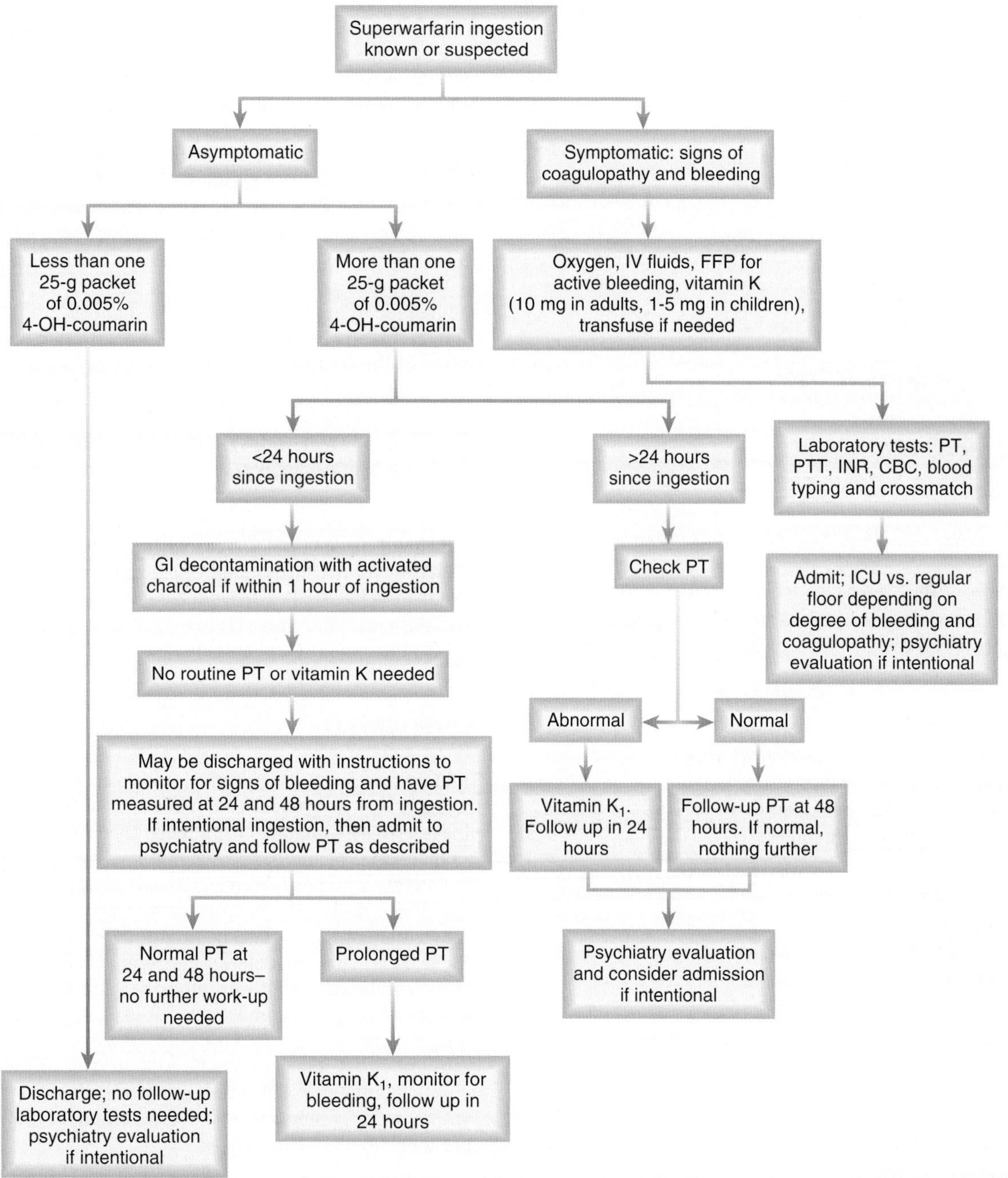


**Fig. 146.2 Algorithm for the management of superwarfarin ingestions.** *CBC*, Complete blood count; *FFP*, fresh frozen plasma; *GI*, gastrointestinal; *ICU*, intensive care unit; *INR*, international normalized ratio; *IV*, intravenous; *PT*, prothrombin time; *PPT*, partial thromboplastin time.

## FOLLOW-UP, NEXT STEPS IN CARE, AND PATIENT EDUCATION

All patients with signs and symptoms of bleeding should be admitted to the hospital for reversal of coagulopathy and control of bleeding. Those with severe or life-threatening hemorrhage warrant admission to the intensive care unit. Asymptomatic patients seen after ingestion can be discharged with arrangements to have blood specimens obtained for measurement of the prothrombin time on an outpatient basis in 24 and 48 hours.

## STRYCHNINE

### EPIDEMIOLOGY

Strychnine is a naturally occurring alkaloid derived from seeds of the tree *Strychnos nux-vomica*. Though rarely used as a rodenticide today, it is still available in some gopher, mouse, and rat poisons. It has also been found in certain traditional Cambodian home remedies. Strychnine is an odorless crystalline white powder with a bitter taste that is well absorbed in the gastrointestinal tract.

## PATHOPHYSIOLOGY

Strychnine blocks the postsynaptic binding of glycine in the spinal cord and brainstem. Because glycine is the major inhibitory neurotransmitter in these areas, disinhibition results in excessive stimulation of motor neurons.[34]

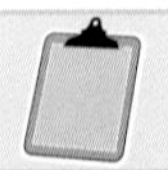

### DOCUMENTATION

**History**

Any history of psychiatric illness or previous suicide ingestions

Name, manufacturer, and concentration of the active ingredient

Amount ingested

Time elapsed since ingestion, if known

History of renal or cardiac disease or other illnesses that might exacerbate the complications of toxins

**Physical Examination**

Does the patient look ill? Pale? Febrile? What is the patient's mental status? Is bleeding present?

Cardiac status (blood pressure, arrhythmias)

Respiratory and airway status

Physical examinations should be repeated while the patient is in the emergency department

**Studies**

Laboratory tests and time that the specimens were obtained

**Medical Decision Making**

Decision to begin treatment or delays

Consultations and time of contact

**Treatment**

Availability of antidotes, time antidote ordered, and any delays in treatment

**Patient Instructions**

Document discussion with the patient regarding diagnosis, warning signs, what to do, follow-up, and when to return

With pediatric accidental ingestions, document poison prevention counseling for parents

For superwarfarin poisoning, instructions on where to return for measurements of the prothrombin time and who will monitor the results

## PRESENTING SIGNS AND SYMPTOMS

Symptoms usually begin within 15 to 30 minutes of ingestion. Initial symptoms include a heightened sense of awareness and muscle spasms. As the toxicity progresses, the muscular hyperexcitability worsens. Minimal stimuli can produce severe muscle spasms, opisthotonos, and trismus, which can be indistinguishable from seizures. Patients generally maintain a clear sensorium before and after these episodes, an effect unique to strychnine ingestion.[34] The complications of strychnine poisoning are secondary to muscle spasms and include hyperthermia, metabolic acidosis, and rhabdomyolysis. Death is usually the result of respiratory failure from spasm of the respiratory muscles.

## DIFFERENTIAL DIAGNOSIS AND MEDICAL DECISION MAKING

The diagnosis is based on a history of exposure in a patient with the aforementioned signs and symptoms. If the history is unknown, the differential diagnosis includes stimulant intoxication, alcohol or benzodiazepine withdrawal, neuroleptic malignant syndrome, serotonin syndrome, salicylate intoxication, encephalitis, meningitis, and tetanus.

## TREATMENT

Treatment is largely supportive, with a focus on airway protection and management of muscle spasms with benzodiazepines. Activated charcoal is unlikely to be of benefit given the rapid absorption and onset of symptoms. For mild symptoms, the patient should be administered diazepam or lorazepam and placed in a dark quiet environment to avoid stimuli. Airway and ventilatory status must be monitored closely and continually because sudden deterioration can occur. Patients with severe symptoms should be intubated and paralyzed with a nondepolarizing neuromuscular blocker. They should then be aggressively sedated with benzodiazepines, propofol, or barbiturates. If this approach fails to control the muscle activity, continuous neuromuscular paralysis is an option. All symptomatic patients should be admitted to the intensive care unit.

## REFERENCES

*References can be found on Expert Consult @ www.expertconsult.com.*

# Antidepressants and Antipsychotics 147

*Michael R. Christian and Sean M. Bryant*

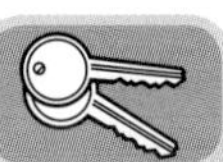

**KEY POINTS**

- Central nervous system depression is the most common sign of antidepressant or antipsychotic overdose.
- Tachycardia, hypotension, seizures, and ventricular dysrhythmias can also occur, especially after tricyclic antidepressant (TCA) overdose.
- Airway intervention, benzodiazepines, intravenous fluids, and cooling measures (especially for serotonin syndrome and/or neuroleptic malignant syndrome) are the mainstays of supportive care and treatment.
- Specific treatment options include sodium bicarbonate for TCA toxicity and crystalloid fluids or hemodialysis for lithium poisoning.
- Controversial treatment modalities include dantrolene for toxin-induced hyperthermia, cyproheptadine for serotonin syndrome, bromocriptine for neuroleptic malignant syndrome, and prophylactic magnesium for long QTc intervals without evidence of hypomagnesemia or torsades de pointes.

## EPIDEMIOLOGY

Data reported from United States poison control centers reveal that toxic exposures from antidepressants and antipsychotic agents continue to remain significant (**Figs. 147.1 and 147.2**). Tricyclic antidepressant (TCA) and monoamine oxidase inhibitor (MAOI) overdoses have historically resulted in the most significant morbidity and mortality. Currently, however, these agents are prescribed much less frequently than serotonin reuptake inhibitors (SRIs), atypical antipsychotics, and lithium. Atypical antipsychotic agents have largely replaced the older typical agents because these newer agents effectively reduce hallucinations, restructure thinking, and control agitation while assisting with the negative effects of psychotic disorders (flattened affect, avolition, social withdrawal). In addition, movement disorders such as dystonia, akathisia, tardive dyskinesia, and neuroleptic malignant syndrome occur less often with atypical antipsychotics than with the typical agents.

## PATHOPHYSIOLOGY

The prevailing theory of depression implicates an imbalance in various neurotransmitters and their receptors. Pharmacologic therapy has been engineered to neuromodulate these imbalances. Consequently, the signs and symptoms seen in a significant overdose of an antidepressant medication are the results of gross derangement of one or more neurotransmitters.

### TRICYCLIC ANTIDEPRESSANTS

TCAs have similar ring structures and, with only a few exceptions, result in a related toxicity. Examples are amitriptyline (Elavil), imipramine (Tofranil), and doxepin (Sinequan). The five major pharmacologic effects of TCAs are listed in **Table 147.1**.

### MONOAMINE OXIDASE INHIBITORS

Phenelzine (Nardil) and tranylcypromine (Parnate) are the two most commonly prescribed MAOIs in the United States, and they account for the majority of toxicity seen with this class of agents. The pharmacologic effects of MAOIs are listed in **Box 147.1**. These effects in overdose may result in a sympathomimetic toxidrome followed by profound hypotension. A therapeutic dose of an MAOI can interact with certain foods, drinks, and other pharmacologic agents and cause serious toxicity.

### SELECTIVE SEROTONIN REUPTAKE INHIBITORS

Selective SRI antidepressants commonly prescribed are sertraline (Zoloft), paroxetine (Paxil), fluoxetine (Prozac), citalopram (Celexa), and escitalopram (Lexapro). The clinically beneficial central nervous system (CNS) effects of SRIs are thought to result from blockade of presynaptic reuptake of serotonin at 5-hydroxytryptamine type 1 (5-$HT_1$) receptors. This blockade leads to higher synaptic serotonin levels and hence has positive effects on mood. Overdoses of these agents are much safer than overdoses of TCAs or MAOIs, although significant morbidity and mortality may occur with significant

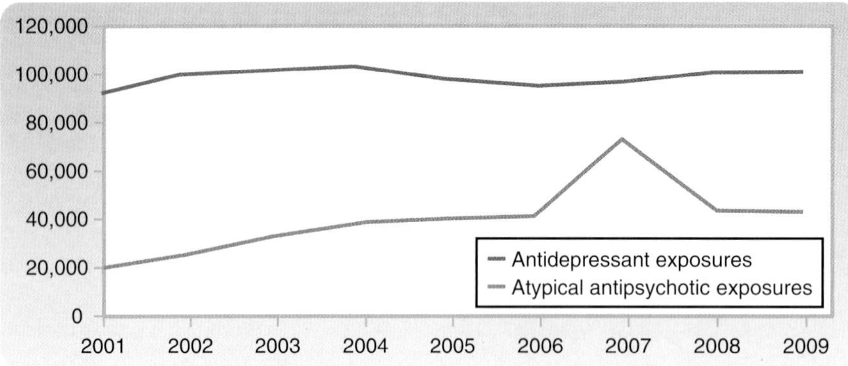


**Fig. 147.1 Trends in exposure to atypical antipsychotics and antidepressants.** (Compiled from the National Poison Data System, 2001 to 2009.)

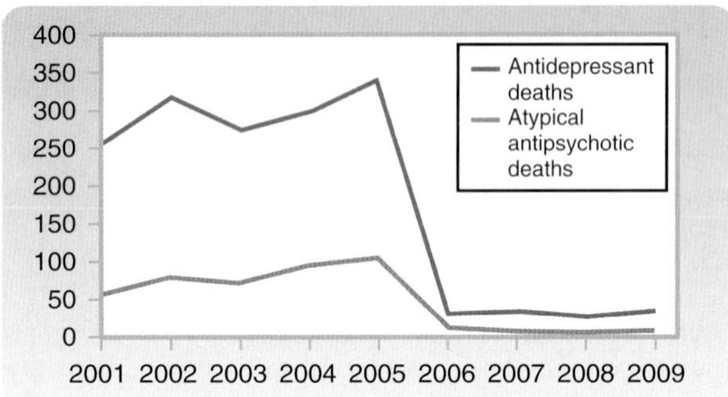


**Fig. 147.2 Trends in deaths related to atypical antipsychotics and antidepressants.** (Compiled from the National Poison Data System, 2001 to 2009.)

**Table 147.1 Five Major Pharmacologic Effects of Tricyclic Antidepressants**

| PHARMACOLOGIC EFFECT | SYMPTOMS |
|---|---|
| Blockade of sodium conductance through fast channels in the myocardium | Prolonged phase 0 of the cardiac action potential that results in a widened QRS complex on an electrocardiogram |
| Blockade of potassium efflux | Prolonged phase 3 of the cardiac action potential resulting in an increased QTc interval that lends itself to the development of torsades de pointes |
| Peripheral $\alpha_1$-receptor blockade | Vasodilation, decreased perfusion, and hypotension |
| Serotonin and norepinephrine reuptake inhibition | Agitation, delirium, or seizure activity |
| Anticholinergic activity | Range of physical findings (coma, delirium, urinary retention, mydriasis, seizures, tachycardia, flushing hyperthermia, dry skin)<br>"Hot as a hare, dry as a bone, red as a beet, blind as a bat, mad as a hatter, fast as a cat, full as a tick" |

**BOX 147.1 Pharmacologic Effects of Monoamine Oxidase Inhibitors**

Inhibition of monoamine oxidase isoenzymes that results in excessive activity of epinephrine, norepinephrine, serotonin, and tyramine
Effects on exogenous amphetamines and methamphetamine
Depletion of norepinephrine stores
Inhibition of pyridoxine-containing enzymes

**BOX 147.2 Examples of Atypical Antipsychotic Medications**

Clozapine (Clozaril)
Risperidone (Risperdal)
Quetiapine (Seroquel)
Ziprasidone (Geodon)
Aripiprazole (Abilify)
Paliperidone (Invega)
Olanzapine (Zyprexa; also Symbyax when combined with fluoxetine [Prozac])

overdose or, more commonly, with ingestion of an SRI in combination with ingestion of agents possessing proserotonergic activity.[1]

## ATYPICAL ANTIPSYCHOTICS

The pharmacologic mechanism of action of atypical agents includes blockade at dopamine ($D_2$) receptors and serotonin ($5\text{-}HT_{2A}$) receptors.[2] These agents can also cause repolarization abnormalities by blocking potassium efflux in the myocardium and thereby increasing the risk of torsades de pointes (**Box 147.2**).

## LITHIUM

The lightest metal known, lithium is in the same group of elements as sodium and potassium and therefore has similar chemical properties. Since the early 1970s, lithium has been

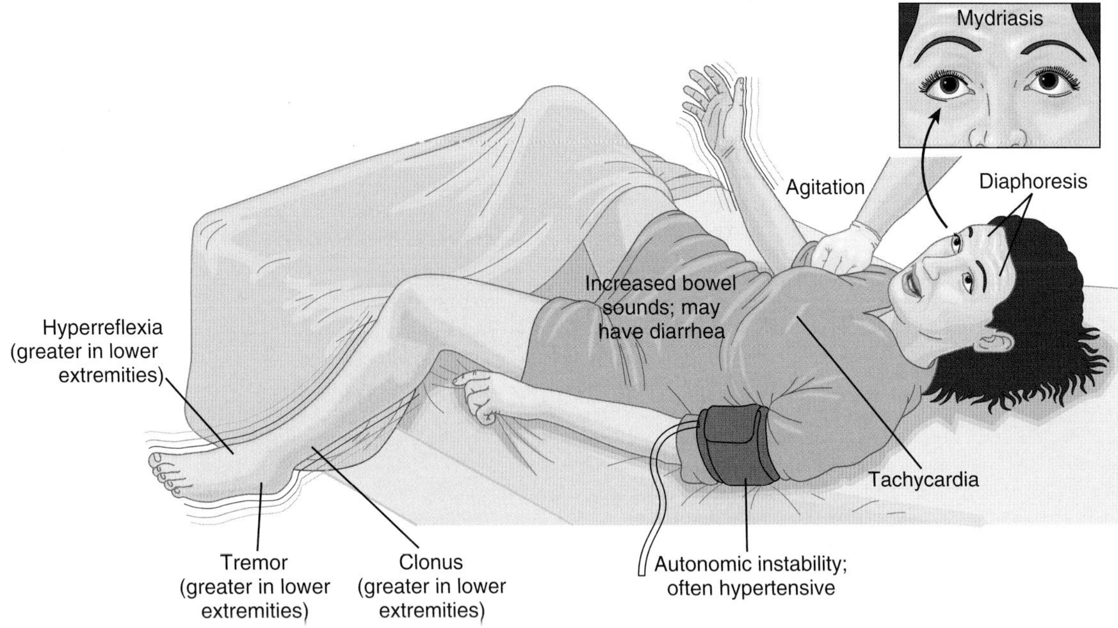


**Fig. 147.3 Signs and symptoms consistent with serotonin syndrome.** (From Boyer EW, Shannon M. The serotonin syndrome. N Engl J Med 2005;17:1112-20.)

a mainstay of treatment for bipolar disorder. Its mechanism of action, however, is still debated. Lithium may affect the synthesis and turnover of serotonin in the CNS. In addition, it may downregulate 5-$HT_{1A}$ receptors and α- and β-adrenergic receptors. Serving as a "false ion" and affecting second messenger systems (inositol triphosphate) in the CNS may also play parts in both the therapeutic and toxicologic manifestations of lithium ingestion.

## PRESENTING SIGNS AND SYMPTOMS

### TRICYCLIC ANTIDEPRESSANTS

Serious toxicity is usually seen within 6 hours of ingestion. Signs and symptoms include obtundation, seizures, hypertension (early), hypotension (late), tachycardia (supraventricular or ventricular), and respiratory depression. Patients can deteriorate rapidly and usually do so within an hour of ingestion of the drug.[3] Seizures and cardiovascular collapse can occur.[4-6] In addition, profound hemodynamic instability follows seizure activity in some patients who have been poisoned with TCAs. Seizures result in further acidemia, which contributes to cardiovascular poisoning.

### MONOAMINE OXIDASE INHIBITORS

Overdose of an MAOI results in sympathomimetic overdrive. Several phases have been described,[7,8] and they can be classified as follows:

1. Asymptomatic phase
2. Sympathetic hyperactivity
3. CNS depression and/or cardiovascular collapse (hypotension and bradycardia)
4. Subsequent complications

The onset of action occurs within 8 hours, but the effects may not manifest until 24 hours and may last for several days. Agitation, delirium, seizures, coma, and muscular rigidity predominate. Late in the clinical course of a significant poisoning, depletion of catecholamines can result in asystole. In the presence of increased sympathetic tone, rhabdomyolysis may occur.

MAOI interactions with foods or beverages (aged cheeses, fava beans, ales, wines) produce early onset of signs and symptoms within minutes to hours.[8] Because of tyramine's short-lived action on the adrenal medulla (to increase endogenous amines), these interactions last only several hours. Interactions of MAOIs with other drugs (sympathomimetics, methylxanthines, SRIs, meperidine) also lead to elevated sympathetic tone. This effect manifests within minutes to hours and can last several hours to days.

### SEROTONIN REUPTAKE INHIBITORS

Overdose of SRIs causes CNS abnormalities (sedation, agitation, delirium), peripheral alterations (tremor, hyperreflexia, rigidity), cardiovascular changes (tachycardia, bradycardia), nausea or vomiting, and lightheadedness.[9-11] The patient with citalopram or escitalopram overdose should be observed for seizures and QTc and/or QRS interval lengthening. Although isolated SRI ingestions frequently result in only mild toxicity, severe overdose or concomitant ingestion of proserotonergic medications can lead to serotonin excess and serotonin syndrome (**Fig. 147.3**). A history of ingestion of serotonergic agents, altered mental status, autonomic instability, and peripheral signs of rigidity or hyperreflexia are usually present.

### ATYPICAL ANTIPSYCHOTICS

Patients usually present within a few hours of atypical antipsychotic overdose with signs of CNS depression (sedation,

**Table 147.2 Comparison of the Manifestations of Serotonin Syndrome and Neuroleptic Malignant Syndrome**

| FEATURE | SEROTONIN SYNDROME | NEUROLEPTIC MALIGNANT SYNDROME |
|---|---|---|
| History | Drug(s) with serotonergic activity | Dopamine-blocking agents |
| Time of onset | Hours | Days |
| Mental status | Agitation to coma | Agitation to coma |
| Tone | Rigidity, greater in lower than in upper extremities | "Lead-pipe" rigidity |
| Vital signs | Hypertension, tachycardia, and hyperthermia | Hypertension, tachycardia, and hyperthermia |

confusion, coma). Hypotension and reflex tachycardia from peripheral vasodilation may also occur. Miosis may lead the examiner to consider opioid poisoning. QTc prolongation can be seen in therapeutic use, as well as in overdose. Other adverse effects, which are less commonly seen with the newer agents, are acute dystonias, akathisia, and tardive dyskinesia.

The most significant extrapyramidal effect is *neuroleptic malignant syndrome (NMS).*[12] NMS results when dopamine-blocking agents yield "dopamine-depleted" activity at $D_2$ receptors in the CNS. Although NMS can occur after an intentional overdose, it usually arises after an increase in dose or after the addition of agents with similar activity (e.g., lithium inhibition of dopamine secretion). Manifestations of NMS include CNS abnormalities (sedation, agitation, delirium), peripheral alterations (tremor, hyperreflexia, rigidity), and cardiovascular changes with autonomic instability (tachycardia, bradycardia, hyperthermia) much like those seen in serotonin syndrome. Unlike serotonin syndrome, in which onset of symptoms is normally rather quick, NMS occurs insidiously. Historical information and medication lists are often required to differentiate between the two conditions (**Table 147.2**).

### LITHIUM

The clinical effects of lithium overdose are gastrointestinal (nausea, vomiting, and diarrhea), neurologic (tremor, confusion, ataxia, weakness), and cardiovascular (QTc prolongation, bradycardia, T-wave flattening or inversion, bundle branch blocks). Adverse effects include nephrogenic diabetes insipidus, polyuria, psoriasis, alopecia, edema, and leukocytosis. Gastrointestinal distress is usually one of the first manifestations of lithium toxicity. Many presentations are chronic and result from continued lithium administration in the presence of dehydration (decreased fluid intake or vomiting and diarrhea). Physiologically, lithium cannot be differentiated from sodium and is retained by the kidney in patients with dehydration. The results are greater CNS levels and subsequent toxicity. Additionally, changes in a patient's renal function may decrease lithium clearance.

**BOX 147.3 Differential Diagnosis of Serotonin Syndrome**

**Medical Illnesses**
- Severe dystonic reaction
- Encephalitis
- Hyperthyroidism
- Malignant hyperthermia
- Tetanus
- Septicemia
- Meningitis

**Poisonings**
- Anticholinergics
- Amphetamines
- Cocaine
- Lithium
- Lysergic acid diethylamide (LSD)
- Phencyclidine (PCP)
- Salicylates
- Water hemlock

## DIFFERENTIAL DIAGNOSIS AND MEDICAL DECISION MAKING

Any sedating agent (e.g., opioids, ethanol, benzodiazepines) should be considered in the differential diagnosis of most antidepressant and antipsychotic overdoses. Serotonin syndrome (e.g., SRIs, ecstasy, meperidine, lithium, dextromethorphan, L-tryptophan), neuroleptic malignant syndrome (e.g., antipsychotics such as phenothiazines), malignant hyperthermia (e.g., volatile anesthetic agent use), sympathomimetic overdrive (e.g., cocaine, amphetamines), and MAOI overdose or drug-food interaction should also be considered (**Box 147.3**).

### TRICYCLIC ANTIDEPRESSANTS

The differential diagnosis of TCA overdose should be broader and should include anticholinergic and antihistamine products (e.g., diphenhydramine) and agents that can poison fast sodium channels, thereby lengthening the QRS interval (e.g., type I antidysrhythmics, cocaine, diphenhydramine, propoxyphene, carbamazepine, cyclobenzaprine, phenothiazines). Life-threatening features are hyperthermia associated with mental status changes, autonomic instability, and tremors, clonus, and rigidity. Life-threatening toxicity should be anticipated in an adult who has ingested TCA doses of 10 mg/kg or greater. Qualitative urine screens for TCAs are of no diagnostic benefit. Although quantitative serum levels of TCAs greater than 1000 ng/mL (therapeutic, 50 to 300 ng/mL) have been correlated with severe toxicity, quantitative testing may not be available in a timely fashion. In addition, depending on the time from ingestion, the type of TCA taken, and the chronicity of dosing, patients may be very ill with serum levels much lower than 1000 ng/mL. An electrocardiogram (ECG) is the diagnostic test of choice.[13] Normal ECG findings do not fully exclude TCA poisoning, but QRS prolongation greater than 120 msec should be a threshold for treatment (**Fig. 147.4**).[14] Cardiac monitoring helps discern the severity of

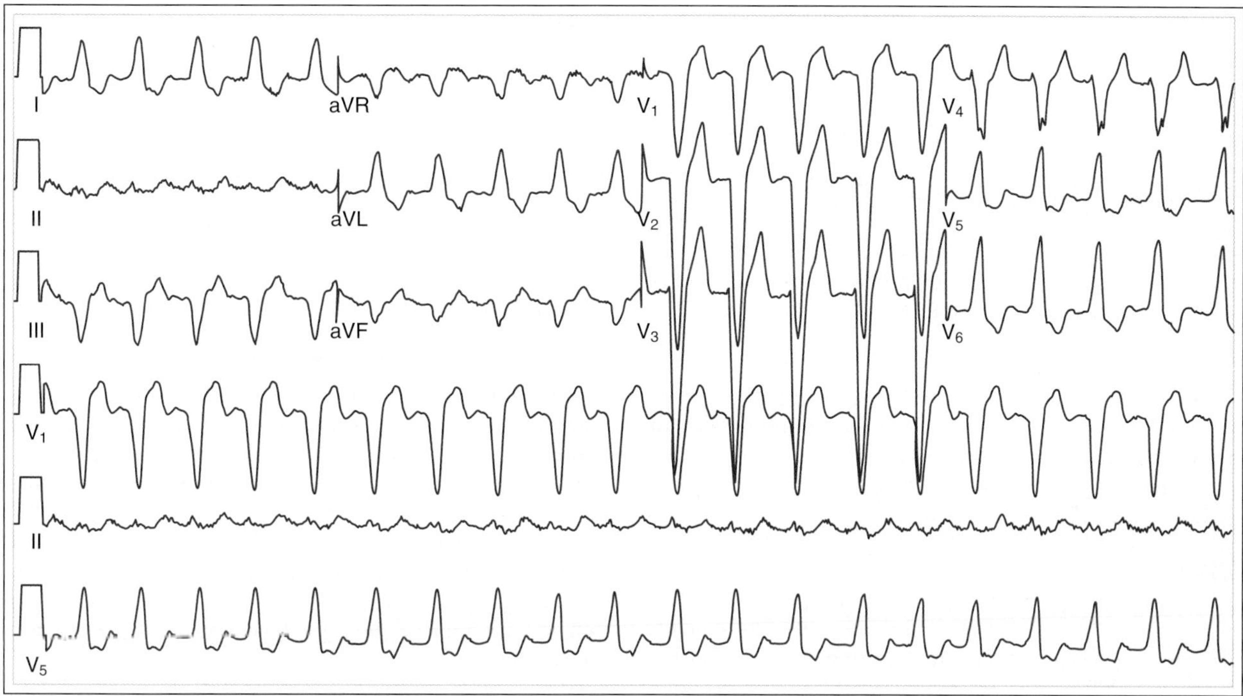


**Fig. 147.4 Electrocardiogram showing signs of poisoning by a tricyclic antidepressant.** Tachycardia and severe sodium channel poisoning are evidenced by a significantly widened QRS interval.

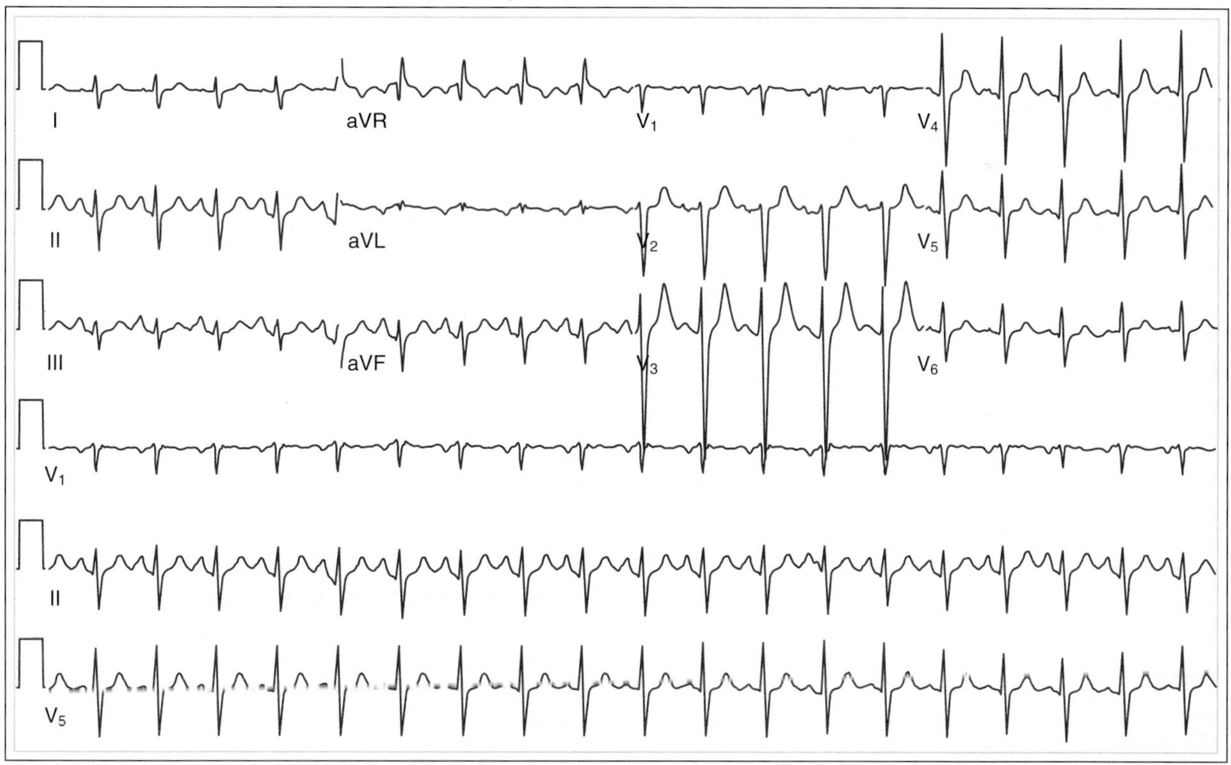


**Fig. 147.5 The electrocardiogram of a patient poisoned by a tricyclic antidepressant.** The tracing shows mild tachycardia and QRS interval lengthening in addition to a noticeable terminal R wave in lead aVR.

toxicity. Maximal limb-lead QRS interval duration is a sensitive indicator of illness.[15] Generally, QRS intervals longer than 100 msec are associated with a 33% incidence of seizure activity, and QRS intervals longer than 160 msec are associated with a 50% incidence of ventricular dysrhythmia. One study showed that the sensitivity of a QRS interval longer than 100 msec can be matched by two other parameters: the terminal 40 msec of lead aVR measuring longer than 3 mm (R wave in aVR > 3 mm), and a ratio of R-wave to S-wave amplitude in the aVR lead greater than 0.7[14] (**Fig. 147.5**).

### MONOAMINE OXIDASE INHIBITORS

A clinical diagnosis (largely based on historical facts) is required for MAOI overdose. No laboratory (urine or blood) test is readily available to make a diagnosis of MAOI poisoning.

### SEROTONIN REUPTAKE INHIBITORS

The diagnosis of SRI toxicity is purely clinical. The criteria for serotonin syndrome are met through focused elicitation of historical information and the finding of signs and symptoms consistent with the disorder (**Table 147.3**).[16]

### ATYPICAL ANTIPSYCHOTICS

Blood or urine testing plays no role in the diagnosis of atypical antipsychotic overdose. Although QTc prolongation can occur after both therapeutic and toxic ingestions, this finding is not specific for these agents. NMS is a clinical diagnosis coupled with diligent history taking.

### LITHIUM

Clinical suspicion, historical features, and serum lithium concentrations form the basis of the diagnosis of lithium poisoning. Serum concentrations must be interpreted in the context of chronicity and timing of ingestion. Because long-term users of this drug have higher CNS levels, ill effects occur at lower serum levels. Additionally, lithium has a long distribution time after absorption. In light of this feature, measurement of a serum lithium level less than 6 hours after the last dose may yield an excessively elevated concentration (therapeutic, 0.6 to 1.2 ng/mL). Generally, serum lithium levels greater than 4 ng/mL in acute ingestion and greater than 2.5 ng/mL in chronic poisoning are considered significant.

**Table 147.3 Criteria to Determine Serotonin Syndrome and Toxicity**

| | |
|---|---|
| Sternbach's diagnostic criteria for serotonin syndrome | 1. Recent addition or increase of proserotonergic medication<br>2. At least three of the following:<br>• Agitation<br>• Ataxia<br>• Diaphoresis<br>• Diarrhea<br>• Hyperreflexia<br>• Hyperthermia<br>• Mental status changes<br>• Myoclonus<br>• Shivering<br>• Tremor<br>3. Neuroleptic agent not added or dose increased before the onset of symptoms<br>4. Diagnosis of infections, withdrawal, and other poisoning or metabolic disruptions excluded |
| Hunter's criteria for serotonin toxicity (context of serotonergic medications) | 1. If patient has spontaneous clonus, serotonin toxicity present<br>2. If no spontaneous clonus, one of the following needed for a diagnosis of serotonin toxicity:<br>• Inducible clonus *and* agitation *or* diaphoresis<br>• Ocular clonus *and* agitation *or* diaphoresis<br>• Tremor *and* hyperreflexia<br>• Temperature > 38°C *and* ocular clonus *or* inducible clonus |

## TREATMENT

### TRICYCLIC ANTIDEPRESSANTS

The treatment of TCA overdose depends on symptoms and is most effectively judged from the ECG (**Fig. 147.6**). Decontamination is best done early after the overdose. Gastric lavage can be considered after life-threatening ingestion and early presentation (<1 hour). The mainstay of decontamination is activated charcoal. The risks of each technique should be weighed against the potential benefits. Unruly behavior, seizure activity, decreased mental status, and loss of airway reflexes are poor predictors of success and thus raise the risk of aspiration.

Focused therapy consists of serum alkalinization with intravenous sodium bicarbonate ($NaHCO_3$). Administration of boluses of 1 to 2 mEq/kg is accompanied by close examination of the QRS interval. Boluses should be repeated every 5 minutes until QRS widening resolves, dysrhythmias occur, or blood pH exceeds 7.55. Rarely, hypertonic saline solution can be considered for prolonged QRS intervals and severe alkalemia. $NaHCO_3$ drips—3 ampules added to 1 L of 5% dextrose in water ($D_5W$) and given at rates of 2 to 3 mL/kg/hour—and hyperventilation with ventilatory support are considered adjuncts to $NaHCO_3$ bolus therapy. Serum potassium levels should be monitored with this therapy, and potassium losses should be replaced as necessary.

Seizure activity should be managed with sedatives such as benzodiazepines and barbiturates. If muscle paralysis is necessary, continuous electroencephalographic techniques should be used to measure occult seizure activity. Lidocaine is an alternative to $NaHCO_3$ therapy for dysrhythmias. Class IA, IC, and III antidysrhythmics, beta-antagonists, and calcium channel blockers are contraindicated in the patient with TCA overdose. Flumazenil and physostigmine are also poor treatment strategies because they have been reported to cause seizure activity[4] and asystolic arrest,[17] respectively.

### MONOAMINE OXIDASE INHIBITORS

Decontamination techniques in patients with MAOI overdoses should include activated charcoal and, possibly, gastric lavage for significant ingestions without contraindication. No specific antidote is effective. Supportive care should be provided for hemodynamic compromise and/or hyperthermia. Beta-blockers and calcium channel blockers for treatment of tachycardia or hypertension should be avoided because of the theoretical concern of unopposed peripheral $\alpha_1$-adrenergic vasoconstriction and worsening hypertension or the development of hypotension and bradycardia, respectively. Rather, phentolamine (bolus of 5 mg in adults and 0.02 mg/kg to 0.1 mg/kg in children, repeated in 5 to 10 minutes as needed) or nitroprusside (0.3 mcg/kg/minute titrated to effect) should be considered for hypertensive emergencies. Ventricular

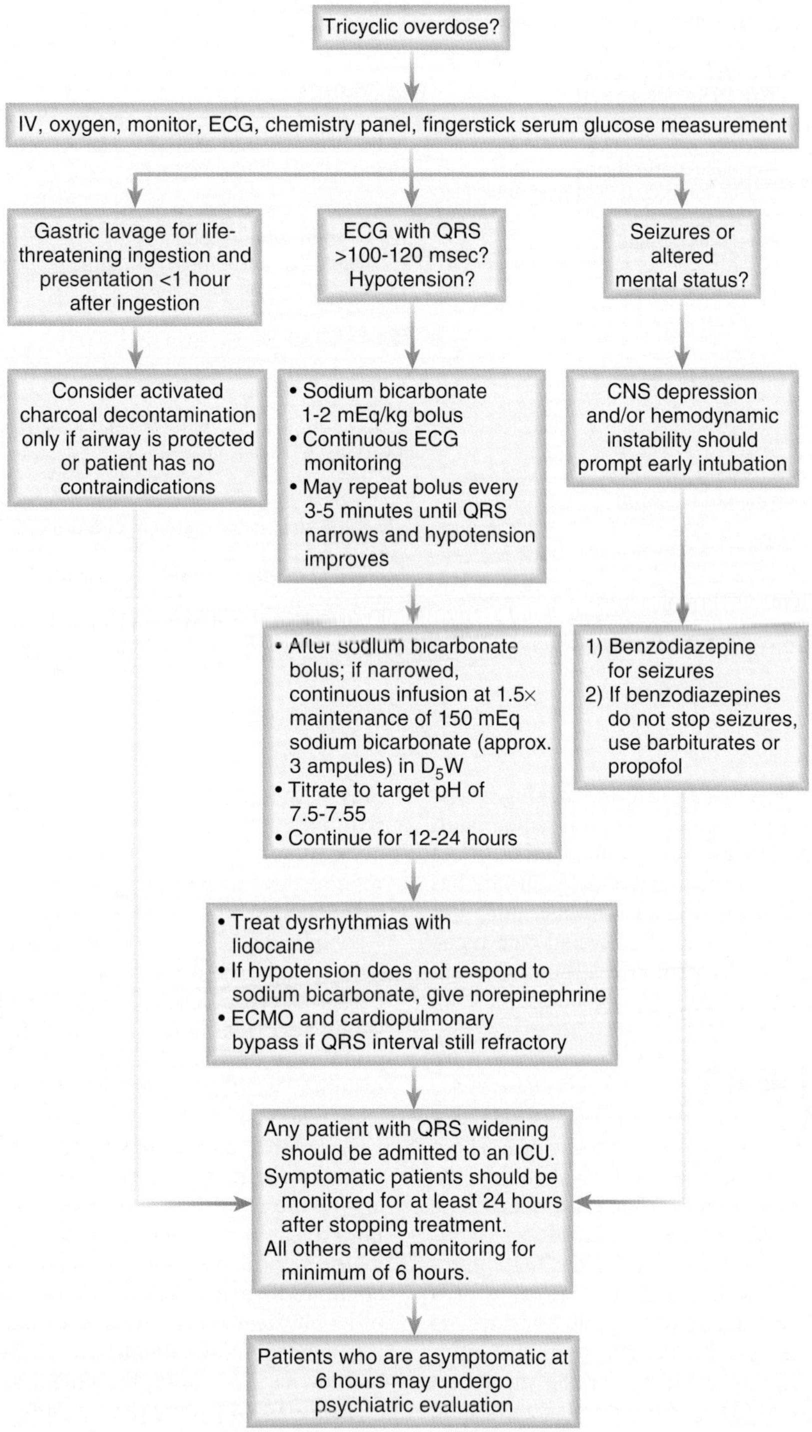


**Fig. 147.6 Algorithm for treatment of tricyclic antidepressant overdoses.** *CNS,* Central nervous system; *$D_5W$,* 5% dextrose in water; *ECG,* electrocardiogram; *ECMO,* extracorporeal membrane oxygenation; *ICU,* intensive care unit; *IV,* intravenous.

dysrhythmias should be treated with lidocaine. Controversy exists over the use of dantrolene for life-threatening hyperthermia in patients with MAOI overdose, and this agent should probably be reserved for patients with significant peripheral rigidity. Supportive cooling techniques (e.g., mist and fan) should be provided, as well as intravenous fluids and judicious use of benzodiazepines for agitation.

## SEROTONIN REUPTAKE INHIBITORS

Standard activated charcoal decontamination should be employed for SRI overdose. Supportive care of the airway, breathing, and circulation encompasses the majority of treatment. In cases of serotonin syndrome, aggressive cooling measures for hyperthermia, benzodiazepines for agitation, and intravenous fluids are usually the only interventions

**Table 147.4 Treatment of Non–Tricyclic Antidepressant Overdoses**

| DRUG | GASTROINTESTINAL DECONTAMINATION | TREATMENT |
|---|---|---|
| Lithium | Consider whole-bowel irrigation for sustained-release formulations (acute ingestions) | IV fluids at 1.5-2× maintenance levels<br>Hemodialysis in severe cases |
| Monoamine oxidase inhibitors | Activated charcoal<br>For significant ingestions, lavage before charcoal | For hypertension: IV phentolamine 2-5 mg infused over several minutes or nitroprusside 0.3 mcg/kg/min titrated to effect<br>For dysrhythmias: lidocaine<br>Cooling with mist and fan<br>Benzodiazepines for agitation |
| Selective serotonin reuptake inhibitors | Activated charcoal | Supportive care<br>Aggressive cooling<br>Benzodiazepines for cooling and/or agitation<br>For life-threatening hyperthermia: sedation, paralysis, and ventilation |
| Atypical antipsychotics | Activated charcoal | Supportive care<br>Benzodiazepines for agitation and/or rigidity<br>Aggressive cooling<br>Correction of electrolyte abnormalities |

*IV*, Intravenous.

required to decrease the risk of death. Life-threatening hyperthermia should be treated with sedation, neuromuscular paralysis, and ventilatory care. The use of cyproheptadine (8 mg by mouth; up to 24 mg per day) for serotonin syndrome has been described but remains controversial. Bromocriptine has been reported to worsen serotonin syndrome, and dantrolene (proven effective for malignant hyperthermia) should be considered only for life-threatening hyperthermia and significant rigidity.

## ATYPICAL ANTIPSYCHOTICS

Acute overdose of atypical antipsychotic agents is managed with supportive care because no specific antidote exists. These agents bind to activated charcoal, use of which should be the standard mode of decontamination. Correction of electrolyte (potassium, magnesium, and calcium) disturbances helps prevent widening or further lengthening of the QTc interval.[13,18] The prophylactic use of magnesium to prevent a widened QTc interval from degenerating into torsades de pointes has no proven benefit when magnesium concentrations are normal. Treatment of NMS is for the most part identical to that of serotonin syndrome (aggressive cooling, benzodiazepines for agitation, fluids, and ventilatory support as warranted). Bromocriptine, an antihistamine with dopamine agonist activity, has been used without consistent benefit. Dantrolene, which works peripherally to inhibit release of calcium from the sarcoplasmic reticulum, has never been proven to be of benefit in NMS but should be considered for the patient with significant rigidity and life-threatening hyperthermia.[19]

## LITHIUM

Treatment of lithium poisoning depends on the clinical context. Activated charcoal is contraindicated because lithium does not bind to it, and whole-bowel irrigation is considered only with ingestions of sustained-release products in patients with no contraindications. Sodium polystyrene sulfonate has been shown to bind to lithium in vitro, but in clinical use it requires excessive dosing at the risk of potentially causing hypokalemia.

Enhancing elimination through hemodialysis is a controversial topic in the setting of lithium poisoning.[16,20,21] The patient likely to benefit is the one with acute ingestion, mental status abnormalities, and/or significant renal dysfunction or pulmonary edema. Many patients experience lithium "redistribution" and an asymptomatic period after hemodialysis. This result often leads to further hemodialysis sessions, but whether this approach has an ultimate beneficial outcome remains controversial. The more common approach, barring any of the preceding abnormalities, is fluid hydration. Lithium's clearance depends on the glomerular filtration rate, which, in turn, depends on volume status. Dehydrated patients continue to reabsorb, rather than eliminate, lithium because of its physical characteristics. Crystalloids given at two times maintenance doses should suffice. Forced diuresis or diuretic therapy has no role in this situation.

**Table 147.4** summarizes treatment of overdoses involving antidepressant and antipsychotic agents other than TCAs.

# FOLLOW-UP, NEXT STEPS IN CARE, AND PATIENT EDUCATION

Any patient with a deliberate overdose of an antidepressant or antipsychotic medication or with clinical symptoms should be admitted to the hospital. Patients who are asymptomatic 6 hours after ingestion can be medically cleared for psychiatric evaluation. The exceptions are patients with elevated serum lithium values, who warrant further observation and subsequent lithium measurements, and patients with overdose of an

MAOI agent, which may not manifest for 24 hours. Patients should be admitted to the intensive care unit for any mental status changes that require close observation for loss of airway reflexes or seizure activity. In addition, patients with cardiovascular abnormalities, especially those requiring treatment in the emergency department with $NaHCO_3$, lidocaine, or other cardiovascular drugs, merit disposition to a critical care unit.

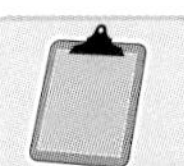

### DOCUMENTATION

**History**

- Any history of psychiatric illness or earlier suicide ingestions
- Time lapse since ingestion, if known
- History of renal or cardiac disease or other illnesses

**Physical Examination**

- Does the patient look ill? Febrile? What is his or her mental status?
- Cardiac status (blood pressure, arrhythmias)
- Respiratory and airway status
- Physical examination repeated while patient is in the emergency department

**Diagnostic Studies**

- Electrocardiogram, serum glucose measurement, blood chemistry panel
- Acetaminophen and aspirin concentration checked if concern exists about coingestion

**Medical Decision Making**

- Decision to begin specific treatment or delay it
- Consultations desired and times of phone calls to consulting services

**Treatment**

- Response to treatment (especially for sodium bicarbonate, cooling measures, and seizure treatment)

**Patient Instructions**

- Document the discussion with the patient regarding diagnosis, warning signs, what to do, follow-up, and when to return.
- With pediatric accidental ingestions, document poison prevention counseling and assessment of the home situation.
- The regional poison control center can be contacted by telephone at 1-800-222-1222. All poison emergencies should be reported by the patient to the local poison control center.
- A dose of medication other than what was prescribed by the patient's physician should never be taken or given unless it has been approved by the ordering physician.

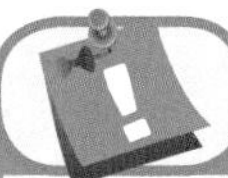

### TIPS AND TRICKS

- Although normal electrocardiographic findings do not fully exclude tricyclic antidepressant (TCA) poisoning, QRS prolongation to more than 100 to 120 msec should be a threshold for treatment.
- Generally, QRS duration longer than 100 msec is associated with a 33% incidence of seizure activity, and a QRS greater than 160 msec is associated with a 50% incidence of ventricular dysrhythmia. Cardiac monitoring is a valid way of discerning the severity of toxicity in TCA poisoning.
- Devastating hemodynamic instability follows seizure activity in 13% of patients with TCA poisoning.
- Rightward deviation of the terminal 40-msec QRS axis (R wave in aVR > 3 mm) should be a cause for concern in a patient with TCA overdose.
- Significant, late monoamine oxidase inhibitor poisoning results in asystole from depletion of catecholamines, so affected patients should be monitored for 24 hours.
- Atypical antipsychotic toxicity can be associated with sedation or coma and miosis and therefore can be confused with opiate intoxication.
- Lithium toxicity is often precipitated by dehydration or worsening renal function.
- A serum lithium value obtained less than 6 hours after the last dose may result in excessively elevated concentrations (therapeutic, 0.6-1.2 ng/mL).

## SUGGESTED READINGS

Boyer EW, Shannon M. The serotonin syndrome. N Engl J Med 2005;17:1112-20.

Burns MJ. The pharmacology and toxicology of atypical antipsychotic agents. J Toxicol Clin Toxicol 2001;39:1-14.

Ellison DW, Pentel PR. Clinical features and consequences of seizures due to cyclic antidepressant overdoses. Am J Emerg Med 1989;7:5-10.

McDaniel K. Clinical pharmacology of monoamine oxidase inhibitors. Clin Neuropharmacol 1986;9:207-34.

Rusyniak DE, Sprague JE. Toxin-induced hyperthermic syndromes. Med Clin North Am 2005;89:1277-96.

## REFERENCES

*References can be found on Expert Consult @ www.expertconsult.com.*

# 148 Cardiovascular Drugs

Kirk L. Cumpston

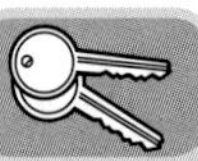

**KEY POINTS**

- Cardiovascular drugs are responsible for many fatalities.
- β-Receptor antagonists, calcium channel antagonists, and digoxin primarily cause toxicity by disruption of intracellular calcium homeostasis and lead to hypotension and dysrhythmias.
- With sustained-release forms of calcium channel antagonists and beta-receptor antagonists, toxicity has a delayed peak and longer duration, which can lead to cardiovascular collapse and arrest if treatment is delayed or there is insufficient cardiovascular moritoring.
- Diagnostic testing should include continuous cardiac monitoring; electrocardiogram; measurement of appropriate serum drug concentrations, electrolytes, and glucose; and investigation of coingestants.
- The call to the pharmacist to obtain the hyperinsulinemia-euglycemia infusion in calcium channel antagonist overdose should be made when the norepinephrine infusion is begun.

## EPIDEMIOLOGY

The pervasiveness of hypertension, congestive heart failure, and coronary artery disease in the United States has led to an immense number of prescriptions for β-receptor antagonists and calcium channel antagonists. The prevalence of digoxin as a therapy for atrial fibrillation and congestive heart failure has ostensibly diminished, but it is still prescribed.

The 2009 Annual Report of the American Association of Poison Control Centers National Poison Center Database System reported cardiovascular drugs as the second most common cause of fatalities overall (10%), and they were the second fastest in rate of exposure increase.[1] Cardiovascular drugs as a category were ranked as the fifth leading cause of death (44 total deaths: 5 from β-receptor antagonists, 16 from calcium channel antagonists, and 23 from cardiac glycosides). These specific cardiovascular drugs share the clinical effects of hypotension, bradycardia, and conduction disturbances. However, unique differences can help distinguish them in an unknown overdose (**Fig. 148.1**). Other pharmaceuticals included in the category of cardiovascular agents are angiotensin-converting enzyme inhibitors, antiarrhythmics, clonidine, and other antihypertensives; they are not discussed in this chapter.

## CALCIUM CHANNEL ANTAGONISTS

### PATHOPHYSIOLOGY

Calcium channel antagonists block the intracellular flow of calcium ions through L-type voltage-gated calcium channels in myocardial, smooth muscle, and pancreatic beta-islet cells. These mechanisms of action result in cardiovascular toxicity both directly and indirectly. Depending on the selectivity of the calcium channel antagonist, the direct cardiovascular toxicity is a combination of the effects on the cardiac conduction system, myocardial contractility, and vascular smooth muscle vasodilation. The dihydropyridine class (e.g., amlodipine, nifedipine) preferentially acts on the peripheral vasculature, thereby potentially leading to hypotension and reflex tachycardia. Verapamil operates on the sinoatrial and atrioventricular (AV) nodes and on the myocardium. Diltiazem acts to a lesser extent than verapamil on the cardiac tissue and nodes, and it also dilates peripheral vasculature (**Table 148.1**). The degree of contribution from each mechanism of cardiovascular toxicity can be difficult to predict. Despite the differences in therapeutic mechanisms, the distinctions among families of calcium channel antagonists are often blurred during an overdose, and the patient generally suffers from negative chronotropic, inotropic, and dromotropic effects.[2]

Calcium channel antagonist overdose also results in indirect toxicity from attenuation of the release of insulin from the pancreatic beta-islet cells. This inhibition leads to hyperglycemia and intracellular catabolism of fatty acids to create energy. The hypoinsulinemia contributes to impairment of cardiac function and shock by preventing the use of glucose as a metabolic substrate. Negative inotropy and diminished peripheral vascular resistance lead to shock and subsequently to metabolic acidosis; the result is a laboratory picture similar to that of diabetic ketoacidosis.

### PRESENTING SIGNS AND SYMPTOMS

Because the calcium channel antagonists were developed to affect the cardiovascular system, the presenting signs and symptoms of overdose with such agents are primarily related to a malfunction of this system. Hypotension is the hallmark of calcium channel antagonist toxicity.

Reflexive tachycardia can occur as a result of peripheral vasodilation after an overdose of a calcium channel antagonist in the dihydropyridine class, but this effect may be transient, and bradycardia usually develops in large overdoses. This

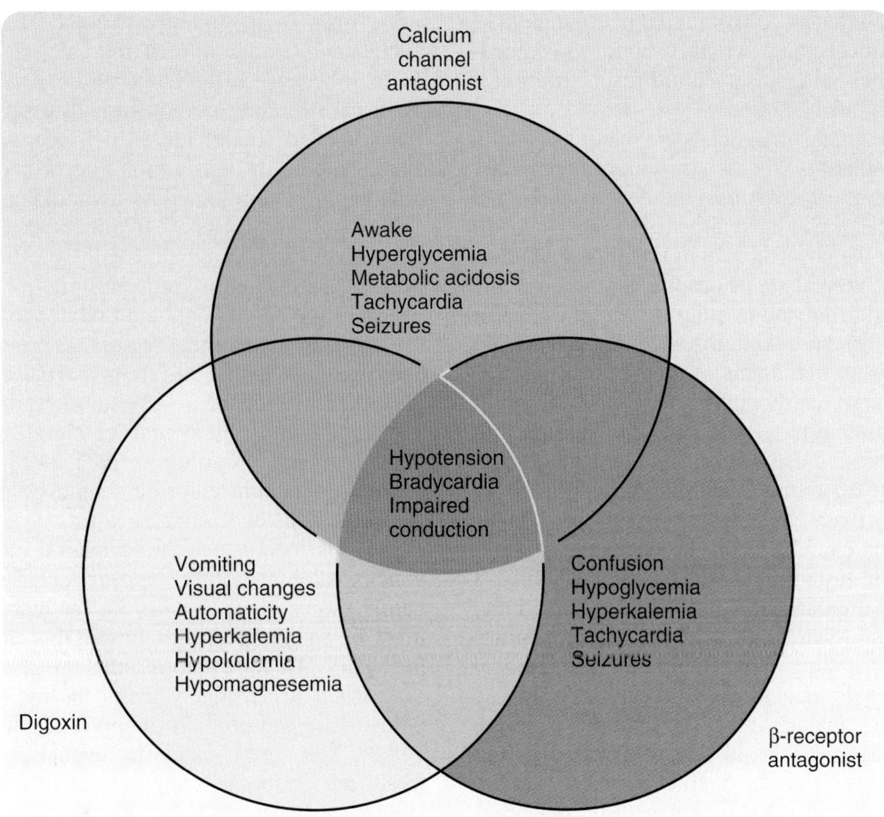


**Fig. 148.1 Differential diagnosis of cardiovascular drug overdoses.**

**Table 148.1 Classification of Calcium Channel Antagonists**

| CLASS | ACTION(S) | EXAMPLE(S) |
|---|---|---|
| Phenylalkylamines | Act on sinoatrial and atrioventricular nodes and the myocardium | Verapamil (Calan) |
| Benzothiazepines | Dilate peripheral vasculature and act to a lesser degree than verapamil on cardiac tissues and nodes | Diltiazem (Cardizem, Tiazac) |
| Dihydropyridines | Act on peripheral vasculature, leading to hypotension and reflex tachycardia | Nifedipine (Procardia)<br>Isradipine (DynaCirc)<br>Amlodipine (Norvasc)<br>Felodipine (Plendil)<br>Nimodipine (Nimotop)<br>Nisoldipine (Sular)<br>Nicardipine (Vascor) |

tachycardia may prove fortunate in maintaining organ perfusion by sustaining cardiac output when the stroke volume is depleted.

Verapamil and diltiazem overdoses cause bradycardia and numerous conduction abnormalities in and below the AV node. The decreased blood pressure results from vasodilation and decreased cardiac contractility from the negative inotropic and chronotropic effects.[2]

Patients often complain of chest pain, dyspnea, dizziness, syncope, and palpitations. Other clinical manifestations are confusion, agitation, seizures, pulmonary edema (cardiogenic and noncardiogenic), hyperglycemia, and metabolic acidosis.

## DIFFERENTIAL DIAGNOSIS AND MEDICAL DECISION MAKING

The differential diagnosis (see also Fig. 148.1) for overdose of calcium channel antagonists includes other cardiovascular drugs such as beta-blockers, clonidine, digitalis, and other antidysrhythmics. The emergency physician should also consider myocardial infarction and other causes of cardiogenic shock. The potency of the effect of calcium channel antagonists on the cardiovascular system is astounding. Significant cardiovascular toxicity can occur after supratherapeutic ingestion of calcium channel antagonists. Ingestion of double the therapeutic dose should instigate medical evaluation and treatment. Immediate-release calcium channel antagonists should have some clinical effect within 6 hours. Sustained-release calcium channel antagonists should result in clinical manifestations within 1 to 14 hours.[3]

Nearly all calcium channel antagonists are manufactured in modified-release formulation. This is convenient therapeutic dosing for the patient, but in overdose, the delayed peak and longer duration of toxicity can have disastrous consequences. The mistakes made by the physician are in finding reassurance in the patient's normal mental status despite hypotension and in not vigorously monitoring and treating the patient's hemodynamic condition. If close attention to hypotension is not maintained, the cardiovascular status of the patient will continue to deteriorate until cardiopulmonary arrest becomes imminent. This occurrence has no precise explanation, but investigators have suggested that cerebrovascular vasodilation may be cerebroprotective, acting much like nimodipine does in subarachnoid hemorrhage.

Diagnostic testing is contingent on the necessity of treatment for hemodynamic instability. Once the patient's airway, breathing, and cardiovascular status have been assessed and stabilized, testing should start with a 12-lead electrocardiogram (ECG) and chest radiography. Rapid determination of hyperglycemia and metabolic acidosis with capillary glucose and arterial blood gas analysis may demonstrate a severe calcium channel antagonist overdose. An elevated serum lactate concentration may be another marker of severe calcium channel antagonist overdose.[4] Testing for serum concentrations of calcium channel antagonists is not clinically useful or available to guide treatment. Otherwise, standard laboratory testing for a general overdose is a good comprehensive approach.

## TREATMENT

Because significant toxicity can occur after a small overdose of a cardiovascular drug, aggressive gastric decontamination is warranted, with activated charcoal as the primary agent. The general principle is that activated charcoal has the best efficacy if it is initiated within the first hour after ingestion. This is true but often not the circumstance, because most patients present beyond 1 hour from ingestion. If this is the case and the patient is still alert and hemodynamically stable, activated charcoal may prevent absorption, even if more than 1 hour because of sustained- or extended-redease formulation.

Whole-bowel irrigation has been suggested for overdose of calcium channel antagonists because many of these drugs are sustained-release preparations. Whole-bowel irrigation is not indicated for a patient with hemodynamic instability because a significant amount of the drug has already been absorbed,[5] and, therefore, the opportunity for prevention has passed. In addition, challenging a hypoperfused gastrointestinal system can have disastrous consequences, such as functional and physical obstruction by a calcium channel antagonist bezoar,[6-9] as well as perforation. Generally speaking, no evidence indicates that any gastric decontamination procedure improves outcome in the patient with an overdose, and the risks must be assessed against the benefits.

Enhanced elimination is the removal of the toxin at a greater rate than inherently done by the body. The modalities are multiple-dose activated charcoal, urinary alkalinization, and some form of hemodialysis. None of these techniques can adequately remove any of the calcium channel blockers or digoxin because of either too great a volume of distribution or protein binding or not enough enterohepatic circulation. Atenolol and sotalol are two β-receptor antagonists with a small volume of distribution and protein binding that could potentially be eliminated by hemodialysis.

The primary focus of treatment is the hypotension. The bradycardia and AV block usually improve as the hypotension improves. Atropine is frequently ineffective because the bradycardia and AV block are not related to increased vagal tone.

An antidotal treatment regimen is provided in **Figure 148.2**. This regimen emphasizes elemental calcium, either as calcium gluconate (30 mL of a 10% solution, or 3 g of calcium gluconate; 14 mEq elemental calcium) or calcium chloride (10 mL of a 10% solution, or 1 g; 13.5 mEq of elemental calcium). Calcium chloride should be administered through central venous access because it is an acidifying salt, which could cause necrosis of the peripheral vasculature. If the intravenous calcium boluses appear to have improved hemodynamic status, close monitoring for recrudescence of toxicity must be maintained, and further boluses must be given as necessary. An intravenous infusion of calcium is warranted only when it effectively treats the hypotension, and further boluses are required to support the blood pressure (**Table 148.2**). The serum calcium concentration should be monitored, but antidotal treatment rarely gives rise to clinically significant hypercalcemia.

Next, glucagon, in 5-mg intravenous boluses for two doses, may theoretically increase cardiac contractility by bypassing the antagonized calcium channels. When glucagon binds to its receptor, it activates cyclic adenosine monophosphate (cAMP). This may increase contractility by activating the phosphorylation cascade, which results in contraction of actin and myosin. Glucagon also stimulates release of endogenous insulin, a fortunate side effect explained later. Like a calcium infusion, a glucagon infusion is warranted only if a beneficial effect is seen after several boluses have been given. Glucagon can cause emesis because of relaxation of the lower esophageal sphincter.

Hyperinsulinemia euglycemia (HIE) therapy and catecholamines with inotropic and vasopressor activity are the next line of treatment for refractory hypotension in calcium channel antagonist overdose, but inotropics and vasopressors will be discussed first. A multicenter study compared dopamine and norepinephrine agents in all patients categorized as being in shock, regardless of cause. No difference was seen in the outcome (death at 28 days) for all patients in the study, but a predetermined subgroup analysis found greater mortality in patients with cardiogenic shock who were treated with dopamine.[10] Because calcium channel antagonists can cause cardiogenic shock, norepinephrine is probably a good first choice. If clinically significant hypotension persists, adding more agents may be necessary. Cardiovascular data from diagnostic modalities such as transthoracic echocardiogram, pulmonary artery catheter, arterial catheter, and central venous catheter should dictate which cardiovascular agent is the most appropriate choice. Vasopressin has been used in human cases when peripheral vasoconstriction is indicated.[11] Worsening of the cardiac index was demonstrated when vasopressin was used in an animal model to treat hypotension induced by calcium channel antagonist.[12]

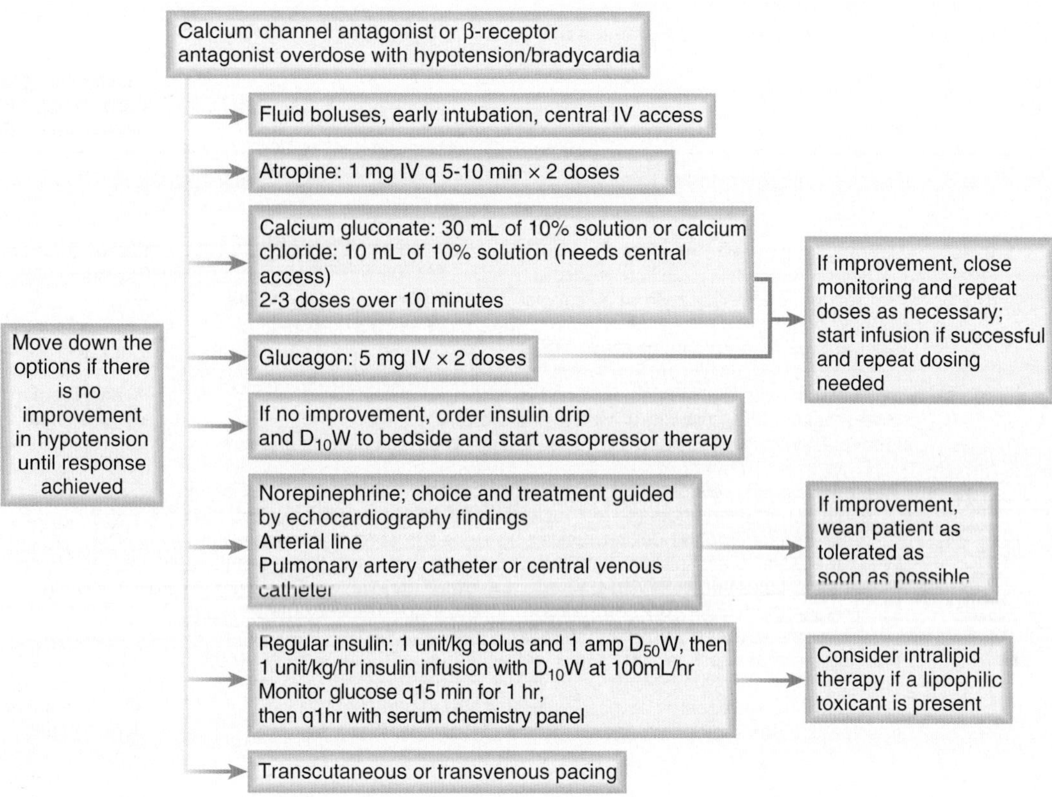


**Fig. 148.2 Treatment of overdose with calcium channel antagonist or β-receptor antagonist.** $D_{10}W$, 10% dextrose in water; $D_{50}W$, 50% dextrose in water; *IV*, intravenous(ly).

**Table 148.2 Antidotes, Treatments, Facts, and Formulas for Cardiovascular Drugs**

| ANTIDOTE OR TREATMENT | DOSING | ADVERSE EFFECTS AND SIGNS OF IMPROVING PERFUSION |
|---|---|---|
| Atropine | *Adult*: 1 mg IV bolus every 5 min as needed for symptomatic β-receptor antagonist bradycardia (maximum total dose: 0.04 mg/kg or 3 mg)<br>*Pediatric*: 0.02 mg/kg total dose, minimum of 0.1 mg | Anticholinergic toxicity |
| Glucagon | *Adult*: 5 mg IV bolus over 2 min (maximum total dose 10 mg)<br>*Adult infusion*: 1-5 mg/hr; titrate to MAP of 70 mm Hg<br>*Pediatric*: 0.05 mg/kg IV bolus over 2 min (maximum total dose 10 mg)<br>*Pediatric infusion:* 0.05 mg/kg/hr to 0.1 mg/kg/hr; titrate to MAP of 70 mm Hg and signs of improving perfusion | Emesis<br>Hyperglycemia |
| Calcium chloride (10 mL of 10% solution = 1 g = 13.5 mEq elemental calcium) | *Adult*: 1-3 g IV (central line) over 10 min as needed for hypotension<br>*Pediatric* (27.7 mg/mL of elemental calcium): 5-7 mg/kg of elemental calcium or 0.2-0.25 mL/kg IV (central line) over 10 min as needed for hypotension<br>*Infusion*: 20-50 mg/kg/hr | Sclerosis of veins<br>Hypercalcemia |
| Calcium gluconate (10 mL of 10% solution = 1 g = 4.65 mEq elemental calcium) | *Adult*: 3-9 g IV (central line) over 10 min as needed for hypotension<br>*Pediatric*: (9 mg/mL of elemental calcium) 5-7 mg/kg of elemental calcium or 0.6-0.8 mL/kg<br>*Infusion*: 20-50 mg/kg/hr | Hypercalcemia |
| Norepinephrine ($\alpha_1$ and $\beta_1$ agonist) | Start at 0.1 mcg/kg/min; titrate to MAP of 70 mm Hg and improvement in perfusion | Tachycardia<br>Hypertension<br>Arrhythmias<br>Extravasation<br>Anaphylaxis |
| Dopamine | For vasodilation of renal and splanchnic vasculature: 1-5 mcg/kg/min<br>For $\beta_1$ agonist: 5-10 mcg/kg/min<br>For $\alpha_1$ agonist 10-20 mcg/kg/min | Same as for norepinephrine |

*Continued*

**Table 148.2 Antidotes, Treatments, Facts, and Formulas for Cardiovascular Drugs—cont'd**

| ANTIDOTE OR TREATMENT | DOSING | ADVERSE EFFECTS AND SIGNS OF IMPROVING PERFUSION |
|---|---|---|
| Epinephrine ($\alpha_1$, $\beta_1$, and $\beta_2$ agonist) | Start at 1 mcg/min; titrate to effect | Same as for norepinephrine |
| Dobutamine ($\beta_1$ agonist) | 2.5 mcg/kg/min to 15 mcg/kg/min | Same as for norepinephrine |
| Isoproterenol ($\beta_1$, $\beta_2$ agonist) | Not recommended because of $\beta_2$ agonist vasodilation and dysrhythmias at high doses<br>Start at 0.02 mcg/kg/min; titrate to effect | — |
| Insulin (regular) | Consultation with a clinical toxicologist is recommended<br>Give a bolus of 1.0 units/kg IV with 1 ampule of $D_{50}W$<br>Immediately start an infusion of 1.0 units/kg/hr with a glucose infusion of $D_{10}W$ at 100 mL/hr<br>Titrate 0.5 units/kg every 30 min until desired effect; 1 ampule of $D_{50}W$ can be given during every increase in infusion; titrate to desired effect when blood pressure has reached desired value and signs of improving perfusion<br>When the blood pressure has reached the desired value with the insulin infusion, taper and wean pressor agent therapy<br>Monitor serum glucose concentration every 15 min for the first 60 min; when stable, monitor every 60 min thereafter<br>Monitor serum potassium and other electrolyte concentrations every 60 min | Hypoglycemia<br>Hypokalemia<br>Volume overload |
| Intralipid 20% | Bolus: 1.5 mL/kg repeated as needed for cardiovascular instability<br>Infusion: 0.25 mL/kg/min as needed for cardiovascular instability | Allergic reaction<br>Hyperthermia<br>Thrombocytopenia<br>Hypercoagulability<br>Antineutrophil activity<br>Pancreatitis<br>Elevated liver enzymes<br>Acute lung injury |
| Intravenous crystalloid | 20 mL/kg IV; repeat again if blood pressure has not improved | Pulmonary edema with severe cardiogenic shock |
| Vasopressin ($V_1$, $V_2$ receptor agonist) | 0.01-0.04 units/min; titrate to effect along with administration of 1-2 catecholamine vasopressors | Ischemia<br>Water intoxication |
| Phosphodiesterase inhibitor (Milrinone) | Give 50 mcg/kg IV bolus over 2 min; then 1.0 mcg/kg/min | — |
| Digoxin-specific Fab fragments | *For acute overdose (unknown amount in adult or child):* 5-10 vials IV as a bolus; repeat as needed every 30 min<br>*For chronic overdose in adult or child:* 1-2 vials IV as a bolus; repeat as needed every 30 min<br>*If amount ingested is known:* 1 vial binds 0.5 mg of digoxin<br>*Dosage calculated from serum digoxin concentration:*<br>$\text{Number of vials} = \frac{\text{Serum concentration (ng/mL)} \times \text{weight (kg)}}{100}$ | Anaphylaxis<br>Removal of therapeatic effect of digoxin on cardiovascular disease |
| Mechanical devices | Intraaortic balloon pump<br>Cutaneous or transvenous pacing<br>Extracorporeal membrane oxygenation<br>Cardiopulmonary bypass | — |

*$D_{10}W$,* 10% Dextrose in water; *$D_{50}W$,* 50% dextrose in water; *IV,* intravenous(ly); *MAP,* mean arterial pressure.

In 1999, Yuan et al.[13] described the first published use of high-dose insulin-euglycemia (HIE) therapy, in four patients with verapamil overdose and in one patient with amlodipine and atenolol overdose. HIE promotes inotropy by improving myocardial energy production. In addition, insulin has antiinflammatory attributes that protect against apoptosis and ischemic reperfusion injury.[2]

Subsequently, numerous case reports, reviews, and HIE regimens were published.[2,14-19] HIE therapy has successfully reversed cardiogenic shock from a polydrug overdose,[20] and historically it was used in multiple nontoxicologic conditions, such as acute myocardial infarction, post–cardiac surgery status, and septic shock.[21] The superiority of HIE therapy for cardiogenic shock resulting from calcium channel antagonist toxicity was also demonstrated dramatically in animal models.[22-25]

Failure of HIE therapy often occurs when it is started as rescue therapy and when the dose is inadequate.[26] A small prospective observational study of patients treated with HIE therapy supports it safety.[27] HIE therapy should be started when boluses of calcium, glucagon, atropine, and intravenous fluids have failed and the physician is considering a pressor agent to improve refractory hypotension. The call to the pharmacist to obtain the HIE infusion should be made when the norepinephrine infusion is begun.

HIE therapy should start with a 1.0 unit/kg bolus of regular insulin followed by an intravenous injection of 1 ampule of 50% dextrose in water ($D_{50}W$). Immediately thereafter, an infusion of 1.0 unit/kg/hour of regular insulin should begin, along with an infusion of $D_{10}W$ at 100 mL/hour. Serum glucose levels should be monitored every 15 minutes during the first hour and then, if stable, every hour. A serum electrolyte analysis must be performed every hour to monitor serum potassium, glucose, and other electrolyte values. Clinically significant hypoglycemia has not been described with HIE therapy. The amount of intravenous fluid administered must be taken into consideration and the patient closely monitored for signs and symptoms of pulmonary edema because the calcium channel antagonist overdose can result in cardiogenic or noncardiogenic pulmonary edema. The clinician must also be cognizant of the limitations of HIE therapy in patients with bradycardia, conduction abnormalities, and hypotension secondary to vasodilation.

When hemodynamic stability has been achieved, the vasopressor therapy should be tapered and stopped because of the potential detrimental effect on the myocardium from increased oxygen demand and metabolic acidosis. Consequently, HIE therapy can be gradually reduced when the patient becomes hemodynamically stable. After the insulin has been discontinued, the serum glucose concentration must be monitored continually for 4 to 6 hours after discontinuation of insulin.

A relatively new and novel antidote is increasingly being used to treat highly lipophilic toxicants, such as verapamil. Intralipid 20% was initially used for local anesthetic toxicity. In patients and animal models, dysrhythmias, hypotension, and even cardiac arrest from bupivacaine toxicity were reversed rapidly with intralipid bolus. Three theories on how this works have been proposed. One theory is the lipid forms a "sink" in the vascular compartment that pulls the toxicant from the tissues, where toxicity is occurring, and it becomes trapped and eliminated. The second is that bupivacaine inhibits transport of fatty acids into mitochondria required for energy production, and the exogenous lipids overcome this inhibition. The third is that fatty acids increase calcium in cardiac myocytes and therefore increase inotropy. Generally, boluses are used, but an infusion is sometimes necessary. Unfortunately, the safety of the boluses is unknown, but the complications of intralipid use are generally from prolonged total parenteral infusions.[28]

Young et al.[29] reported a case of a 32-year-old man who ingested 13.44 g of verapamil and bupropion, zolpidem, quetiapine, clonazepam, and benazepril. This patient had refractory hypotension after treatment with intravenous fluids, glucagon, calcium, and norepinephrine. He was then administered 100 mL of 20% intralipid over 20 minutes and then 0.5 mL/kg/hour for almost 24 hours. His blood pressure improved enough in 1 hour to begin weaning the norepinephrine, and the glucagon infusion was discontinued 2 hours after intralipid administration.[29] Consultation with a medical toxicologist can be very helpful when considering HIE or intralipid therapy.

Mechanical devices can also serve as adjunctive therapy in calcium channel antagonist poisoning. Transcutaneous or transvenous pacing is indicated when conduction is impaired beyond pharmacologic reversal. More invasive mechanical measures to support the cardiovascular system are an intraaortic balloon pump, extracorporeal membrane oxygenation, and cardiopulmonary bypass.

Often, the lack of mental status impairment coinciding with hypotension can beguile the physician into believing that the patient is not suffering severe clinical effects of a calcium channel antagonist overdose. At this point, elective intubation should be considered, before emergency intubation has to be performed during cardiopulmonary arrest.

## DISPOSITION

Asymptomatic patients who have ingested an immediate-release calcium channel antagonist can be monitored for 6 hours in the emergency department. After ingestion of a sustained-release calcium channel antagonist, the asymptomatic patient should undergo cardiovascular monitoring for 18 to 24 hours.[3] All symptomatic patients with cardiovascular instability after cardiovascular drug overdose should be admitted to the intensive care unit for cardiovascular monitoring, diagnostic studies, and treatment until the effects have resolved.

## SPECIAL CONSIDERATIONS: PEDIATRIC OVERDOSE

The 2009 National Poison Center Database System data noted one pediatric fatality of a suicidal 16-year-old girl, who ingested verapamil and an unknown drug.[1] The clinical consequences of accidental pediatric calcium channel antagonist ingestions depend on the dose.

One must consider that the major flaw of studies attempting to demonstrate a dose response of accidental pediatric drug ingestions is that many of the reports are nonexposures. The caretaker of the child may report the exposure to a poison center if a pill is missing and the child is implicated by his or her presence in the vicinity. If the child did not take the drug, the case may be referred to as having a good outcome, and the "dose" considered safe.[30]

A guideline for pediatric ingestions of calcium channel antagonists states that immediate referral to a health care center is necessary if the dose exceeded the usual therapeutic dose or was considered equal to or greater than the lowest toxic dose (whichever is lower).[3] At these doses, significant bradycardia or hypotension may occur. Accidental single ingestions of calcium channel antagonists in children are considered lethal enough to be fatal.[31]

Realistically, administration of activated charcoal is prudent if the patient has presented within 1 hour of the ingestion. Whole-bowel irrigation may be considered for ingestion of a modified-release product but is technically difficult. If the patient is near adult size, has ingested a potentially life-threatening amount of a calcium channel antagonist, and presents within 1 hour of the ingestion, gastric lavage may be helpful for gastrointestinal decontamination. However, many kits are not available, and the "act" of gastric lavage is labor intensive and does not change clinical outcome.

Cardiovascular monitoring for 6 to 8 hours for immediate-release medications and for at least 24 hours for sustained-release medications should reveal delayed toxicity. All symptomatic children should be admitted for cardiovascular monitoring and treated with standard therapy.[3]

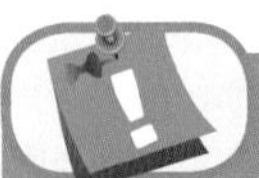

TIPS AND TRICKS

**Calcium Channel Antagonist Toxicity**

- The patient who presents with undifferentiated hypotension and bradycardia may paradoxically be relatively alert as a result of calcium channel antagonist toxicity, which may cause cerebrovascular vasodilation that is cerebroprotective.
- Insulin is an ideal inotropic agent because it can increase the contractility of the heart without raising oxygen demand.
- Monitor electrolyte concentrations and excess intravenous fluid closely.
- An echocardiogram, central venous pressure monitor, and pulmonary artery catheter can be helpful for diagnosing and treating the multiple components of the shock that occurs during calcium channel antagonist toxicity.
- Continue to monitor serum glucose concentrations after the insulin infusion is discontinued until consistent euglycemia is achieved.

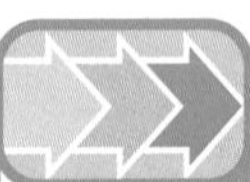

PRIORITY ACTIONS

**Treatment of Calcium Channel Antagonist Toxicity**

- Consult with a medical toxicologist.
- Intubate hemodynamically unstable patients electively, before emergency intubation is required because of cardiopulmonary arrest.
- Obtain central venous access for fluid resuscitation and administration of pharmaceutical infusions.
- Gastric decontamination is critical in the patient presenting with hemodynamic stability, but it should not be used if the patient is unstable.
- Use hyperinsulinemia/euglycemia (HIE) therapy early (in conjunction with medical toxicology consultation) after intravenous boluses of normal saline, atropine, calcium, and glucagon have failed.
- Titrate the HIE therapy in the same fashion as other standard inotropic medications to obtain a mean arterial pressure of 65 to 75 mm Hg and sings of improving perfusion. Tight glucose control is not the target of treatment.
- Maintain the insulin infusion and taper and stop vasopressor therapy when the mean arterial pressure has achieved 65 to 75 mm Hg and signs of organ perfusion are present.
- If hypoglycemic episodes occur in the setting of hemodynamic stability, decrease the rate of the insulin infusion. If hemodynamic instability occurs, increase the rate of the dextrose infusion.

# β-RECEPTOR ANTAGONISTS

## PATHOPHYSIOLOGY

As their name suggests, β-receptor antagonists antagonize the effects of beta agonists by competing for β-adrenergic receptors. The result within the cell is a decrease in cAMP, which inhibits the phosphorylation cascade, thus leading to decreased intracellular flow of calcium and actin-myosin contraction. The effects are bradycardia in the nodal cells and decreased contractility in the cardiac myocytes. Consequently, the attenuated stroke volume combined with a decreased heart rate elicits a decline in cardiac output and the promotion of cardiogenic shock.

β-Receptor antagonism is not the only pharmacologic mechanism of toxicity seen after β-receptor antagonist overdose. α-Receptor antagonism, sodium or potassium channel antagonism, central nervous system penetration leading to seizures with altered mental status, and sympathomimetic stimulation may also occur (**Table 148.3**).

Most of the actively prescribed β-receptor antagonists are first metabolized by hepatic enzymes and then processed by the kidney. One exception is atenolol, which is exclusively excreted in the urine. Atenolol also has a volume of distribution and protein-binding properties that permit hemodialysis as a method of enhancing elimination. Esmolol has the unique metabolic characteristic of rapid metabolism in the serum by red blood cell esterases.

## PRESENTING SIGNS AND SYMPTOMS

Immediate-release products should cause signs and symptoms within 6 hours. Unfortunately, most β-receptor antagonists are of modified-release formulation. They have some pharmacologic effect during the first 6 hours after ingestion, but the peak serum concentration is delayed, and the pharmacologic effect may last longer than with immediate-release formulations.[32]

Cardiovascular signs and symptoms are the predominant clinical manifestations of β-receptor antagonist toxicity. As with the calcium channel antagonists, cardiogenic shock results primarily from a decrease in cardiac output secondary to diminished stroke volume and heart rate. Patients may complain of chest pain, shortness of breath, palpitations, and dizziness in relation to their bradycardia and hypotension. The ECG may demonstrate sinus arrest, sinus bradycardia, junctional bradycardia, and all degrees of AV block.

If the β-receptor antagonist also possesses pharmacologic activity at other receptors, the clinical picture will be complicated. α-Receptor antagonism after ingestion of carvedilol or labetalol may contribute to hypotension by causing peripheral vasodilation. Propranolol can cause sodium channel antagonism (membrane-stabilizing effect). This pharmacologic activity is exhibited clinically as a prolonged QRS complex on the cardiac monitor and hypotension, much as in a tricyclic

**Table 148.3** Pharmacology of Selected β-Receptor Antagonists

| AGENT | RECEPTOR ACTIVITY | AGONIST ACTIVITY | MEMBRANE STABILIZING | VASODILATION? | LIPID SOLUBILITY | PROTEIN BINDING (%) | HALF-LIFE (HR) | METABOLISM | VOLUME OF DISTRIBUTION |
|---|---|---|---|---|---|---|---|---|---|
| Atenolol | $\beta_1$ | No | No | No | No | <5 | 5-9 | Renal | 1 |
| Carvedilol | $\alpha_1, \beta_1, \beta_2$ | No | No | Yes | Moderate | 98 | 6-10 | Hepatic | 115 |
| Esmolol | $\beta_1, \beta_2$ | No | No | No | Low | 50 | 8 min | Red blood cell esterases | 2 |
| Labetalol | $\alpha_1, \beta_1, \beta_2$ | No | Low | Yes | Moderate | 50 | 4-8 | Hepatic | 9 |
| Metoprolol | $\beta_1$ | No | Low | No | No | 10 | 3-4 | Hepatic | 4 |
| Pindolol | $\beta_1, \beta_2$ | Yes | Low | No | Moderate | 50 | 3-4 | Hepatic/renal | 2 |
| Propranolol | $\beta_1, \beta_2$ | No | Yes | No | High | 90 | 3-5 | Hepatic | 4 |
| Sotalol | $\beta_1, \beta_2$ | No | No | No | Low | 0 | 9-12 | Renal | 2 |

Data from Cave G, Harvey M. Intravenous lipid emulsion as antidote beyond local anesthetic toxicity: a systematic review. Acad Emerg Med 2009;16:815-24; and Brubacher JR. Beta adrenergic antagonists. In: Goldfrank L, Flomenbaum N, Lewin N, et al, editors. Goldfrank's toxicologic emergencies. 8th ed. New York: McGraw-Hill; 2006.

antidepressant overdose. The cardiac rhythm can potentially degenerate into ventricular tachycardia.

Sotalol is infamous for antagonizing the delayed rectifier potassium channels in the myocardium. The results are a prolonged QT interval and a higher risk of torsades de pointes (polymorphic tachycardia), monomorphic ventricular tachycardia, ventricular fibrillation, and asystole. These clinical effects can also be delayed and prolonged. In one case report, the onset of ventricular dysrhythmias occurred 4 to 9 hours after ingestion and did not normalize until 100 hours from the time of ingestion.[33]

Observation of sympathomimetic effects after β-receptor antagonist ingestion is rare because of the uncommon clinical use of β-receptor antagonists with intrinsic sympathomimetic activity, such as acebutolol, oxprenolol, penbutolol, and pindolol. Patients who have ingested these agents may have tachycardia, hypertension, tremor, and, possibly, some antidotal efficacy because some beta-antagonists can antagonize their own toxic effects.

Some of the β-receptor antagonists, such as propranolol, are more lipophilic and can cross the blood-brain barrier. Symptoms of delirium, coma, and seizures have been reported in patients with overdose of highly lipophilic β-receptor antagonists. Other less common clinical effects reported are respiratory depression, bronchospasm, hypoglycemia in children, and hyperkalemia.

**TIPS AND TRICKS**

**β-Receptor Antagonist Toxicity**

- Obtain a capillary blood glucose measurement to detect euglycemia or hypoglycemia.
- Identify the unique toxicity of each β-receptor antagonist.
- Do not start infusions of glucagon or calcium until multiple boluses have successfully reversed the toxicity.
- Avoid isoproterenol as an antidotal agent.
- Hyperinsulinemia/euglycemia therapy works to treat hypotension from β-receptor antagonist toxicity.
- Atenolol and sotalol have characteristics that allow the use of hemodialysis to enhance elimination.
- Monitor electrolyte concentrations and excess intravenous fluid closely.
- An echocardiogram, central venous pressure monitor, and pulmonary artery catheter can be helpful for diagnosing and treating the multiple components of the shock that occurs during β-receptor antagonist toxicity.
- If the beta-blocker is lipophilic (e.g., propranolol), intralipid therapy may be effective at reversing toxicity.

## DIFFERENTIAL DIAGNOSIS AND MEDICAL DECISION MAKING

The differential diagnosis (see also Fig. 148.1) of beta-blocker toxicity includes the following: congestive heart failure and pulmonary edema, cardiogenic or hemorrhagic shock, epidural hematoma, epidural and subdural infections, meningitis, other causes of electrolyte abnormalities, and overdoses of cardiac glycosides, calcium channel blockers, carbamazepine, carbon monoxide, cocaine, and antidepressants.

Measurements of serum concentrations of β-receptor antagonists are generally unavailable and unhelpful in the emergency department. No laboratory studies correlate beta-blocker concentrations with outcomes. Additional standard laboratory testing as for a general overdose is advisable, with particular focus on hypokalemia and hypoglycemia, along with other electrolytes. Cardiac enzymes should be obtained to evaluate for myocardial infarction. Therapeutic interventions and patient stabilization are the priorities. As resuscitation continues, a 12-lead ECG and cardiac monitoring may demonstrate bradycardia, AV conduction abnormalities, and prolonged QRS and QTc intervals. Monitoring for hypocalcemia, hypokalemia, and hypomagnesemia assists in treatment of coexisting causes of prolonged QTc intervals.

## TREATMENT

In a hemodynamically stable patient who has overdosed on a β-receptor antagonist, aggressive gastric decontamination is warranted. The limits of gastric decontamination use in calcium channel antagonist overdose apply to that in β-receptor antagonist overdose.

The end result of overdose of either β-receptor or calcium channel antagonists is shock, despite their different mechanisms of action. Because these agents have a final common pathway, antidotal therapy is analogous. Treatment follows the same algorithm as shown in Figure 148.2. Atropine can be used initially, followed by intravenous calcium, glucagon, HIE, and catecholamines with chronotropic and inotropic effects for refractory bradycardia and AV block. Unfortunately, severe bradycardia and AV block are often refractory to pharmaceutical efforts, and transcutaneous or transvenous pacing may be required.

Calcium reverses toxicity through circumvention of the β-receptor antagonist by entering open L-type calcium channels and increasing the cytoplasmic concentration of calcium, thus leading to contraction of the myosin-actin apparatus. Fear of hypercalcemia should not prohibit the use of elemental calcium as antidotal treatment of β-receptor antagonist toxicity.

Glucagon increases cardiac contractility by bypassing the antagonized β-receptors through activation of cAMP by agonism at the glucagon receptors. This activation increases contractility by activating the phosphorylation cascade, which leads to contraction of actin and myosin. Glucagon also stimulates release of endogenous insulin, a beneficial side effect. Unfortunately, glucagon is often ineffective at reversing β-receptor antagonist toxicity.[34]

Vasopressin was used in an experimental animal model poisoned by propranolol.[35] The investigators discovered equally dismal survival rates for treatment with glucagon and vasopressin.

HIE therapy is a therapeutic approach for β-receptor antagonist toxicity. Animal models demonstrated the superiority of HIE therapy over glucagon, epinephrine, and saline solution for the reversal of the toxic effects of propranolol.[36] Yuan et al.[13] reported effective reversal of the toxic effects of a β-receptor and calcium channel antagonist coingestion with this treatment. Despite the absence of the diabetic ketoacidosis metabolic state produced by calcium channel antagonist, HIE therapy is believed to be just as effective in β-receptor antagonist intoxication. Mechanistically, this antidote improves inotropy by promoting aerobic utilization of glucose by the myocardial myocytes, inhibition of fatty acid metabolism, decreased lactate production, and improvement of myocardial oxygen utilization without increasing oxygen demand. The mild hypokalemia that occurs also may beneficial.[17]

The evidence is convincing that HIE therapy is a remedy for a depressed inotropic state, but its reversal of the myriad other toxicologic effects mediated by β-receptor antagonists, such as bradycardia and conduction abnormalities, is unsubstantiated. The clinician must be aware of the limitations of HIE treatment and must treat other toxic effects appropriately. Vigilance in monitoring for the potential adverse effects of HIE therapy in this setting must be greater than for other uses of HIE therapy because of the lack of insulin resistance seen in most β-receptor antagonist intoxications.

A case of cardiac arrest induced by nebivolol, diazepam, and baclofen was reversed with a bolus of intralipid 20% and HIE therapy.[37] Intralipid therapy should be considered in lipophilic β receptor antagonist overdose.

## DISPOSITION

The asymptomatic patient who has no cardiovascular effects of overdose with an immediate-release or sustained-release β-receptor antagonist or sotalol can be discharged after 6, 8, or 12 hours of observation, respectively. All symptomatic patients should be admitted for intensive care monitoring of the hemodynamic effects.

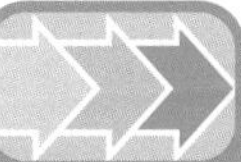

**PRIORITY ACTIONS**

**Treatment of β-Receptor Antagonist Toxicity**

- Supportive care of airway, breathing, and circulation is the first critical step.
- Gastric decontamination is critical in the patient presenting with hemodynamic stability.
- Administer doses of calcium and glucagon adequate to elicit a clinical response.
- Consider HIE therapy for cardiogenic shock.
- Consider norepinephrine as the first choice for vasopressor therapy.
- Electrical pacing is an option for symptomatic β-receptor antagonist bradycardia.

# DIGOXIN

## PATHOPHYSIOLOGY

Digoxin is a cardiac glycoside that was historically used for the treatment of congestive heart failure and for rate control in atrial fibrillation. Despite a reduction in popularity, digoxin is still clinically effective for many patients. Natural cardiac glycosides provide another possible exposure source (**Box 148.1**).

**BOX 148.1 Natural Cardiac Glycosides**

Oleander *(Nerium oleander)*, yellow oleander *(Thevetia peruviana)*
Lily of the valley *(Convallaria majalis)*
Foxglove (*Digitalis* spp.)
Red squill *(Urginea maritima)*
Dogbane *(Apocynum cannabinum)*
Skin secretions of *Bufo marinus* toad

Digoxin pharmacologically alters inotropy and conduction. This agent has the additive effect of increasing automaticity. The results of digoxin therapy are an increase in the intracellular concentration of calcium and higher efficiency of its use by the contractile apparatus. These effects are achieved largely by inhibition of the sodium, potassium adenosine triphosphatase ($Na^+,K^+$ ATP-ase) pump. This pump regulates the intracellular and extracellular concentrations of sodium and potassium by increasing the intracellular potassium concentration and decreasing the intracellular sodium concentration. Digoxin inhibits this function, with resulting serum hyperkalemia and increased intracellular sodium. This effect secondarily impairs the sodium, calcium ($Na^+,Ca^{++}$) exchange pump, which exchanges extracellular sodium for intracellular calcium. The consequence of this sequence of events is an elevated intracellular calcium concentration, which leads to a dysfunction of intracellular calcium homeostasis and a tetany-like state of the cardiac myocyte. Without myocardial relaxation, an increase in left end-diastolic pressure proceeds to decreased filling and decreased cardiac output, culminating in cardiac failure.

Several clinically important points must be remembered about the pharmacology of digoxin (**Table 148.4**). The drug is well absorbed, and the onset of action occurs within minutes to hours of administration. The serum digoxin concentration initially is supratherapeutic, until equilibrium between the serum and tissues has occurred. The optimum time for measurement of the serum digoxin concentration is at least 6 hours after ingestion. The volume of distribution is large and the enterohepatic circulation is small, thus rendering methods for enhancing elimination clinically ineffective. These properties effectively make the elimination half-life approximately 36 to 48 hours.[38,39] Most digoxin is eliminated as the parent compound in the urine. Consequently, a decrease in renal function often leads to acute-on-chronic digoxin toxicity in the geriatric patient. The clinician must keep in mind that these pharmacokinetic data are from controlled clinical situations. True toxicokinetic data are difficult to forecast in the patient with digoxin overdose because of inaccuracies about the timing and amount of the dose, comorbidities, drug interactions, and unpredictable variables in the human metabolism of digoxin.

## PRESENTING SIGNS AND SYMPTOMS

Patients may be asymptomatic from minutes to hours after ingestion of digoxin. Gastrointestinal symptoms are common, and patients have nausea and vomiting. Patients may complain of changes in vision, especially chromatopsia and xanthopsia.

**Table 148.4 Pharmacokinetics of Digoxin**

| | |
|---|---|
| Onset of action | Oral: 1.5-6 hr<br>Intravenous: 5-30 min |
| Maximal effect | Oral: 4-6 hr<br>Intravenous: 1.5-3 hr |
| Intestinal absorption (%) | 40-90<br>Mean: 75 |
| Metabolism | Small amount by bacteria in liver and gut |
| Plasma protein binding | 25% |
| Volume of distribution (L/kg) | Neonates: 10<br>Infants: 16<br>Adults: 6-7<br>Adults with renal failure: 4-5 |
| Routes of elimination | Renal: 50%-80% unchanged<br>Hepatic: limited metabolism<br>Enterohepatic circulation: 7% |
| Elimination half-life | Neonates:<br>Premature: 61-170 hr<br>Full-term: 35-40 hr<br>Infants: 18-25 hr<br>Children: 35 hr<br>Adults: 38-48 hr<br>Anephric patients: >4.5 days |

Data from Cave G, Harvey M. Intravenous lipid emulsion as antidote beyond local anesthetic toxicity: a systematic review. Acad Emerg Med 2009;16:815-24; And Wax PM, Erdman AR, Chyka PA, et al. Beta-blocker ingestion: an evidence-based consensus guideline for out-of-hospital management. Clin Toxicol (Phila) 2005;43:131-46.

**BOX 148.2 Dysrhythmias Associated with Digoxin Toxicity**

| | |
|---|---|
| Atrial fibrillation | Delayed afterdepolarizations |
| Atrial flutter | Bidirectional ventricular tachycardia (pathognomonic) |
| Atrial tachycardia with atrioventricular block | Bigeminy |
| Premature ventricular tachycardia | Junctional tachycardia |
| Ventricular tachycardia | Sinus arrest |
| Ventricular fibrillation | Sinus bradycardia |

Some mild confusion, weakness, and dizziness also can occur from the direct effect of the digoxin. The cardiac effects are usually represented by symptoms such as palpitations, chest pain, dizziness, and dyspnea. The cardiac signs in acute toxicity are a mixture of bradydysrhythmias, tachydysrhythmias with conductive blockade, and hypotension. Cardiac conduction can be impaired anywhere along the pathway from the sinus node to the AV node and the His-Purkinje fibers. Commonly reported dysrhythmias are listed in **Box 148.2**. Bidirectional ventricular tachycardia is considered pathognomonic for digoxin toxicity.

The patient with chronic digoxin toxicity is generally older and presents with nonspecific complaints that make diagnosis a challenge. Manifestations can be similar to those of patients with acute digoxin toxicity, but they differ in patients with more neuropsychiatric complaints, such as delirium, confusion, drowsiness, and hallucinations, and visual complaints. Ventricular tachydysrhythmias are more common in patients with chronic toxicity.

The patient with acute-on-chronic toxicity may have clinical manifestations of both the other types of toxicity. In general, acute-on-chronic toxicity is clinically more like acute digoxin toxicity.

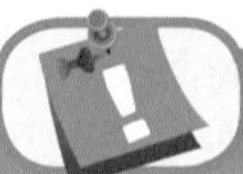

**TIPS AND TRICKS**

**Digoxin Toxicity**

- If the patient has life-threatening digoxin toxicity, treatment with the digoxin-specific Fab fragments is the first priority.
- Acute-on-chronic and acute digoxin toxicities have the same manifestations, but acute and chronic digoxin toxicities have distinct symptoms, dysrhythmias, and laboratory findings.
- The digoxin serum concentration may be only slightly elevated or normal in chronic digoxin toxicity.
- Digoxin toxicity can manifest as almost any dysrhythmia.
- The equilibrium concentration of serum digoxin occurs 6 hours after ingestion, and is inaccurate after administration of digoxin-specific Fab fragments.
- Recurrence of toxicity is typically related to underdosing of digoxin-specific Fab fragments.
- The indications and treatment of digoxin toxicity and concomitant renal impairment are the same.
- No method of enhancing elimination, including hemodialysis, is effective.

## DIFFERENTIAL DIAGNOSIS AND MEDICAL DECISION MAKING

Before considering digoxin toxicity, one must first define the different types of digoxin toxicity. They are as follows:

*Acute digoxin toxicity*: A patient who is naive to the medication is exposed to a single acute ingestion.

*Acute-on-chronic digoxin toxicity*: The serum digoxin concentration increases because of renal failure or an inadvertent or intentional increase in dose. The clinical presentations for this and acute toxicity are similar, so management is similar.

*Chronic digoxin toxicity*: A patient has clinical signs of digoxin toxicity with a mildly elevated or therapeutic serum digoxin concentration.

The differential diagnosis includes other cardiovascular drugs (see Fig. 148.1), acute renal failure, hypercalcemia, hyperkalemia and hypokalemia, hypernatremia and hyponatremia, and hypomagnesemia.

An ECG and continuous cardiac monitoring are crucial initial steps in determining cardiovascular instability in a patient with digoxin toxicity. These tests alert the clinician to dysrhythmias that require treatment with digoxin-specific Fab fragments and supportive care. A chest radiograph demonstrates any evidence of cardiac failure related to the digoxin overdose.

Laboratory testing should be performed expeditiously in any digoxin overdose, with the focus on serum potassium, magnesium, and digoxin concentrations. Rapid assessment of serum potassium concentration helps determine the severity of the toxicity. In acute digoxin poisoning, the serum potassium value is elevated. If this value is 5 mEq/L or greater, digoxin-specific Fab fragment therapy should be considered.[40] In chronic digoxin toxicity, the serum potassium concentration is often low, usually because of concomitant ingestion of a diuretic. The hypokalemia, in effect, worsens the inhibition of the $Na^+,K^+$ ATP-ase pump.

Obviously, assessment of the serum digoxin concentration is essential. The therapeutic range is 0.5 to 2.0 ng/mL. The steady-state serum concentration is most accurate 6 hours after ingestion. A serum digoxin concentration of 10 ng/mL at steady state or 15 ng/mL at any time is generally accepted as an indication for digoxin-specific Fab fragment therapy.

A serum digoxin concentration measured in blood collected after administration of digoxin-specific Fab fragments is clinically not useful and is uninterpretable. The assay often measures the antidote, the drug, and the combination of the two, and it interprets one or all of them as the serum digoxin concentration; the result may be higher than, lower than, or within the therapeutic range for serum digoxin.[41,42]

Screening for accompanying hypomagnesemia is important because this condition may lead to refractory hypokalemia, blockade of inward calcium channels and intracellular binding sites, blockade of extracellular movement of potassium, decrease in myocardial irritability, and a prolonged QT interval. Hypomagnesemia increases myocardial uptake of digoxin and worsens dysfunction of the $Na^+,K^+$-ATP-ase pump.[43]

## TREATMENT

A reasonable approach is to consider activated charcoal to minimize intestinal absorption in a person presenting within 1 hour of digoxin overdose. Gastrointestinal decontamination may be limited by emesis induced by the digoxin. Whole-bowel irrigation is also not indicated because of rapid absorption of digoxin and the availability of other, more practical options.

The successful use of digoxin-specific Fab fragments to treat digoxin intoxication was first described in 1976.[44] Since that time, multiple studies have demonstrated its safety and efficacy.[45,46] The best antidote to administer for digoxin toxicity is digoxin-specific Fab fragments, whether for hypotension, dysrhythmias, serum digoxin concentration, or hyperkalemia.

Two commercial formulations of digoxin-specific Fab fragments are available, Digibind and DigiFab. Literature for both products warns against anaphylaxis and administration of the agents to people with papain, chymopapain, or papaya allergies. Other adverse events associated with administration of digoxin-specific Fab fragments occur from removal of the therapeutic benefit of the digoxin—for example, recurrence of congestive heart failure[46] or atrial fibrillation with a rapid ventricular response.

**BOX 148.3 Indications for Administration of Digoxin-Specific Fab Fragments**

**Adult**

- Ingestion of 10 mg of digoxin
- Serum digoxin concentration of 15 ng/mL at any time
- Serum digoxin concentration of 10 ng/mL at 6 hr after ingestion
- Serum potassium value > 5 mEq/L
- Life-threatening dysrhythmia
- Hemodynamic instability

**Pediatric**

- Ingestion of 4 mg, or 0.3 mg/kg of digoxin
- Preexisting cardiac disease
- Serum potassium value > 5 mEq/L
- Serum digoxin concentration > 5 ng/mL
- Life-threatening dysrhythmia
- Hemodynamic instability

After an acute ingestion of digoxin, an empirical bolus of 5 to 10 vials (up to 10 to 20 vials) of digoxin-specific Fab fragments is indicated in the patient with life-threatening toxicity. When the clinical situation allows determination of a serum digoxin concentration, the simple dosing calculation is as follows:

$$\text{Dosage} = \frac{\text{Serum concentration (ng/mL)} \times \text{Patient weight (kg)}}{100}$$

The number obtained is the number of vials needed to treat the patient.

When the amount ingested is known, the digoxin-specific Fab fragment dose can be calculated by knowing that 1 vial will bind 0.5 mg, or multiply the amount ingested by 2 (see Table 148.4 for determining dose). In the noncritical patient, digoxin-specific Fab fragments should be reconstituted with 4 mL of saline, used immediately or within 4 hours if refrigerated, and infused over 30 minutes. Indications for digoxin-specific Fab fragments are listed in **Box 148.3**. A clinical response should be seen within 60 minutes.[46]

In patients with chronic digoxin toxicity, calculating the dosage of digoxin-specific Fab fragments with the serum digoxin concentration often overshoots the amount needed to reverse toxicity. The concern is precipitating an exacerbation of hypokalemia, congestive heart failure, or rapid atrial fibrillation. A prudent approach is to administer 1 or 2 vials initially. If toxicity has resolved or an adverse effect has occurred, no further vials should be given. If no adverse effect has arisen and toxicity has not resolved, 1 or 2 vials more are indicated.

Many patients presenting with acute-on-chronic digoxin toxicity have renal failure. Digoxin-specific Fab fragments should not be withheld in these patients because of concern about the inability of the kidney to remove the digoxin-Fab complex. This complex cannot be removed by dialysis either. Mild recrudescence of toxicity has been reported when the Fab fragments become unbound and are eliminated faster than digoxin.[47] However, multiple publications cite inadequate dosing as a much greater risk factor for recrudescence, and the transient rise in serum digoxin concentration has been within the therapeutic range and not clinically significant.[47,48] Simply administering another dose of digoxin-specific Fab fragments or giving conscientious supportive care may be the only additional therapy required. These patients typically have transient renal impairment, and once it has resolved, the digoxin, Fab fragments, and Fab-digoxin complex are removed. Finally, the use of digoxin-specific Fab fragments can be cost effective.[49]

Atropine may be effective in treating symptomatic bradycardia early in acute digoxin toxicity because it increases vagal tone. Treatment of bradycardia with atropine later in an acute presentation or in chronic digoxin toxicity is often unsuccessful because the bradycardia is may not be related to vaginal tone but to other toxic effects of the digoxin. The ultimate treatment of symptomatic bradycardia is administration of digoxin-specific Fab fragments.

Transcutaneous pacing and transvenous pacing have been used to treat symptomatic bradycardia, but transvenous pacing must be used with caution. One study reported a higher mortality rate in patients receiving transvenous pacing because of dysrhythmias.[50] In addition, iatrogenic complications (36%) were seen in patients receiving transvenous pacing.

This danger of transvenous pacing in the setting of digoxin toxicity has come into question, however. A retrospective review of 70 patients was divided into two groups. One group received transvenous pacing, and the other did not. No deaths occurred in the paced group, and 2 patients in the nonpaced group died of ventricular dysrhythmias, but no statistically significant difference was seen. Transvenous pacing was not an independent predictor of prognosis. The investigators reported no complications of venous thromboembolism, cardiac rupture, or infection. The investigators speculated that the previous study had poor outcomes from overdrive transvenous pacing, which can stimulate ventricular dysrhythmias. In their study, the heart rate was limited to 60 beats/minute.[51]

Unstable supraventricular or ventricular dysrhythmias can be treated by electrical cardioversion. Because of the hyperexcitability of the digoxin-poisoned myocyte and nodal tissue, however, low current is recommended. The concern is that high voltages may induce refractive lethal ventricular tachycardia.

The use of intravenous calcium in the treatment of hyperkalemia in the digoxin-poisoned patient was considered a contraindication during much of the twentieth century. The concern about calcium administration in digoxin toxicity is an additive toxic effect. During digoxin toxicity, patients already have a dysfunction in intracellular calcium regulation along with an elevated calcium concentration. If more calcium is added to this hypercontractile state, a condition referred to as "stone heart" could be produced. This concern was supported by an early human case series and two animal studies, all published before 1940.[52-54]

More recently, a case report and animal study found no synergistic effect of calcium and digoxin toxicity resulting dysrhythmia or death during treatment of hyperkalemia.[55,56] A retrospective review of 159 patients with digoxin toxicity over 17.5 years compared dysrhythmia in 1 hour from calcium or mortality in the patients treated with calcium versus no calcium. The investigators discovered no dysrhythmias and similar mortality in both groups and increased mortality in patients with higher serum potassium.[57]

An excellent review of the literature on this topic specified that the rate and amount of calcium administered is probably more contributory to dysrhythmias or the stone heart. The reviewers reasonably concluded that if the patient has signs of hyperkalemia toxicity, such as loss of P waves, peaked T waves, or a widened QRS complex, treatment with calcium should be undertaken. If the patient has manifestations of digoxin toxicity such as ectopic beats or ventricular tachycardia, then digoxin-specific Fab fragments should be the first-line treatment.[58] Ultimately, the anxiety created by calcium combined with digoxin toxicity is probably much greater than the true risk. This risk can be minimized even more by using other methods to decrease the serum potassium. If the patient is hemodynamically stable, administration of digoxin-specific Fab fragments should be the first choice to treat the hyperkalemia and all the other components of digoxin toxicity.

Treatment of hypotension should also include increasing the preload with intravenous fluids and pharmaceutical agents that have inotropic and vasopressor properties, such as norepinephrine. Little is known about the effectiveness of other antidotes, such as glucagon, to treat hypotension or bradycardia. Hypomagnesemia should be treated in standard fashion, with 2 g of intravenous magnesium given over 20 minutes.

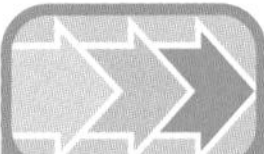

**PRIORITY ACTIONS**

**Treatment of Digoxin Toxicity**

- Supportive care of airway, breathing, and circulation is the first critical step.
- Gastric decontamination is critical in the patient presenting with hemodynamic stability, but refrain from challenging the gastrointestinal system of a patient with hemodynamic instability.
- Assess serum potassium and magnesium levels immediately.
- Digoxin-specific Fab fragments are the definitive treatment for all clinical manifestations of digoxin toxicity.
- Dosage of digoxin-specific Fab fragments can be (1) empirical (5-10 vials) in the hemodynamically unstable patient, (2) calculated according to the amount of digoxin bound by 1 vial, or (3) calculated from the serum digoxin concentration.
- Decrease the current for cardioversion in patients with digoxin toxicity.
- Use a small number of vials (1-2) to treat patients with chronic digoxin toxicity.

## DISPOSITION

If the patient is asymptomatic and has no clinical findings of acute digoxin toxicity, with a serum digoxin concentration at 6 hours in the therapeutic range, the physician is probably safe to reclassify this patient medically as no longer having digoxin toxicity. Of course, this decision depends on a reliable history. A 6-hour period of monitoring is adequate because the latest peak effect from oral digoxin is 6 hours, and that from intravenous digoxin is 3 hours. Clinical effects should appear before this time.

All symptomatic patients with clinical evidence of acute or chronic digoxin toxicity should be admitted to a monitored setting. The symptomatic patient who has life-threatening signs of toxicity and has been treated with digoxin-specific Fab fragments should be admitted to the intensive care unit. The symptomatic patient with relatively stable vital signs and cardiac rhythm should be admitted to a unit with cardiac monitoring capabilities with an adequate dose of digoxin-specific Fab fragments available at the bedside.

## REFERENCES

***References can be found on Expert Consult @ www.expertconsult.com.***

# 149 Sympathomimetics

*Mae F. De La Calzada-Jeanlouie and Gar Ming Chan*

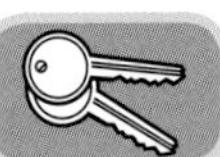

**KEY POINTS**

- Sympathomimetic agents comprise a large collection of over-the-counter, prescription, and illicit drugs.
- The sympathomimetic toxicologic syndrome (toxidrome) is a constellation of signs and symptoms: elevated mood, psychomotor agitation, diaphoresis, tremor, hypertension, tachycardia, and mydriasis.
- The toxidrome can mimic hypoglycemia, withdrawal syndromes, and the anticholinergic toxidrome.
- Treatment is generally symptomatic and supportive and includes control of the patient's psychomotor agitation. Occasionally, specific correction of the patient's vital signs is necessary.

## EPIDEMIOLOGY

A sympathomimetic agent is defined as any agent that may emulate the clinical effects of the endogenous sympathetic catecholamines epinephrine and norepinephrine. An exhaustive list of drugs falls into the class of sympathomimetics, ranging from over-the-counter and prescription agents to drugs of misuse and abuse (**Box 149.1**).

Clinically, sympathomimetics have been used as arousal agents in patients with barbiturate overdose, as weight loss preparations, and in the treatment of depression. Over-the-counter products are predominantly available as decongestants, and they also include weight loss and energy products. The U.S. Food and Drug Administration banned ephedrine and sibutramine, once popular dietary supplements for weight loss and arousal, but they can still be obtained illicitly.

Prescription and parenteral sympathomimetic agents are available for myriad medical illnesses, including hypersensitivity reactions, reactive airway disease, attention-deficit hyperactivity disorder, and cardiovascular compromise. Misused and abused licit and illicit agents comprise the remainder of sympathomimetics: cocaine, amphetamine derivatives (i.e., 3,4-methylenedioxymethamphetamine), and clenbuterol.

In 2010, data released by the University of Michigan in their Monitoring the Future Survey demonstrated that cocaine use among high school students had declined since 2007.[1] A difference in prevalence, which had decelerated, was noted. However, the year 2010 also saw a dramatic increase in the use of ecstasy, or 3,4-methylenedioxymethamphetamine (MDMA). Researchers believe that this shift may be the result of the adolescent population's perception of a lower risk associated with MDMA.

Prescription agents continue to be a source of misuse. The rate of misuse of combination sympathomimetic products rose from 2009 to 2010. Overall, sympathomimetics remain a public health concern. According to the Drug Abuse Warning Network, these drugs accounted for almost 30% of all emergency department (ED) substance-related visits in 2009.[2]

## PATHOPHYSIOLOGY

The biogenic amines (histamine, tyrosine, and serotonin) and the catecholamines (epinephrine, norepinephrine, and dopamine) are found within the central nervous system (CNS) and their synthesis, release, and metabolism are very similar. Tyrosine is converted into dopamine, and subsequently norepinephrine, whereas serotonin is derived from tryptophan and resides in separate vesicles. Despite differences in synthesis and packaging, calcium is the common stimulus for exocytosis. Once an amine is released into the synapse, reuptake can occur through transport proteins. Intracellularly, these products are either metabolized by the enzyme monoamine oxidase or repackaged and recycled. In the periphery, these amines may undergo extracellular metabolism by catechol-*O*-methyltransferase.

Sympathetic stimulation triggers the release of epinephrine and norepinephrine from the adrenal medulla. However, norepinephrine can also be released into the circulation, with effects consistent with α-adrenergic stimulation (i.e., vasoconstriction). Dopamine, found within nerve terminals in the CNS, is also present in the periphery. Excessive dopamine concentrations in the CNS can manifest as psychosis, which is clinically indistinguishable from primary psychosis. Similarly, serotonin found both centrally and peripherally can have a broad spectrum of effects modulating mood, appetite, sleep, and thermoregulation. In the CNS, an abundance of serotonin can induce euphoria, or an elevated mood.

Pharmacotherapeutics can mimic catecholamine release by stimulating release, inhibiting metabolism, and impairing reuptake. The specific clinical effects produced by a sympathomimetic agent are related to its pharmacology, whereas the relative effect on the two distinct adrenergic receptors, α and β, can be used to predict the clinical response. Generally, α-adrenergic receptor agonism results in vasoconstriction, whereas the inverse effect is appreciated with β-adrenergic receptor stimulation. The resultant vasodilatation produces hypotension and tachycardia. β-Adrenergic agonism can also lead to hypokalemia, hyperglycemia, tremor, and acidemia.

Sympathomimetics may act directly, indirectly, or in combination to produce sympathomimesis. Direct-acting sympathomimetics are the catecholamines epinephrine and norepinephrine, directly administered to the patient. Indirect-acting sympathomimetics are agents that either increase the release of endogenous catecholamines or impair their reuptake. In addition, indirect-acting sympathomimetics can trigger the release of other biogenic amines such as serotonin and dopamine. Finally, mixed-acting sympathomimetics exert their effect through direct and indirect-acting properties. Despite these underlying differences, the clinical presentation can be virtually indistinguishable. Clinical manifestations may also vary according to the location where the neurotransmitter predominance occurs.

## PRESENTING SIGNS AND SYMPTOMS

Tachycardia, hypertension, diaphoresis, mydriasis, hyperthermia, and psychomotor agitation characterize the sympathetic toxidrome, which can be further divided according to α- and β-adrenergic receptor effects. α-Adrenergic subtype 1, or $\alpha_1$, receptor agonism results in vasoconstriction, whereas postsynaptic $\alpha_2$ agonism results in hypotension and sedation. These effects are classically observed in the therapeutic use of clonidine. Like α receptors, β-adrenergic receptors have clinically distinct subtypes, 1 and 2. $\beta_1$ agonism increases cardiac output by improving chronotropy. $\beta_2$ agonism is specifically responsible for vasodilation, as well as secondary effects such as hypokalemia, hyperglycemia, acidemia, and tremor.

Methylxanthine exposure is virtually indistinguishable from β stimulation because of a shared final pathway, which increases intracellular cyclic adenosine monophosphate. Methylxanthines also result in increased circulating catecholamines and inhibit adenosine receptors. Potential clinical effects associated with sympathomimetics are listed in **Box 149.2**.

As a result of hypertension and tachycardia, vascular events can occur during exposure to a sympathomimetic. Cocaine use is associated with myocardial infarction, coronary artery dissection, aortic dissection, cardiomyopathy, splanchnic infarction, cerebrovascular accidents, and cerebrovascular hemorrhage. The vasoconstriction and resultant hypertension make β-adrenergic blockade a precarious pharmacologic intervention.

Similar to the cardiovascular effects, some of the CNS effects are secondary to hypertension and vasoconstriction, leading to CNS ischemia and hemorrhage. Animal studies suggested an association between extreme CNS stimulation and the development of seizures, hyperthermia, and increased mortality. Aggressive therapy should focus on inhibiting CNS hyperactivity, thus reducing morbidity and mortality. Other CNS effects associated with the cessation of amphetamines and cocaine use are termed withdrawal or "washout." The

**BOX 149.1 Common Sympathomimetic Agents**

**Over-the-Counter Agent or Dietary Supplement**

***Arousal Agents***
- Caffeine

***Weight Loss Products***
- Ephedrine*
- Synephrine
- Caffeine

***Nasal Decongestants***
- Pseudoephedrine
- Phenylpropanolamine (PPA)*
- Phenylephrine

**Prescription or Parenteral**

***For Hypersensitivity***
- Epinephrine (autoinjector)

***For Reactive Airway Disease***
- Albuterol
- Pirbuterol
- Salmeterol
- Levalbuterol
- Theophylline
- Ephedrine
- Epinephrine

***Vasopressors***
- Phenylephrine
- Epinephrine
- Norepinephrine
- Dopamine

***For Weight Loss***
- Dextroamphetamine
- Phentermine
- Sibutramine*

***For Attention-Deficit Hyperactivity Disorder***
- Methylphenidate
- Dextroamphetamine

***Inotropes***
- Dobutamine
- Isoproterenol
- Milrinone

**Illicit Misuse**
- Cocaine

***Amphetamine Derivatives***
- Methamphetamine
- 3,4-Methylenedioxymethamphetamine (MDMA)
- 3,4-Methylenedioxyethamphetamine (MDEA)
- Para-methoxymethamphetamine (PMA)
- Methcathinone

***For Sports Performance Enhancement***
- Clenbuterol
- Caffeine
- Ephedrine

*No longer available.

**BOX 149.2 Clinical Manifestations of Sympathomimetics**

**Cardiovascular**
- Hypertensive emergencies
  - Acute coronary syndrome
- Cerebrovascular accident
- Tachycardias, dysrhythmias
- Vasospasm and ischemia to end-organs

**Central Nervous System**
- Altered mentation
  - Anxiety
  - Mania
  - Psychosis
  - Agitated delirium
- Seizures
- Intracerebral hemorrhage

**Metabolic**
- Hypokalemia
- Hyperglycemia

**Other**
- Rhabdomyolysis
- Muscle rigidity
- Hyperthermia

**Unique**
- Syndrome of inappropriate antidiuretic hormone associated with 3,4-methylenedioxymethamphetamine

**BOX 149.3 Differential Diagnosis Sympathomimetic Toxidrome**

**Toxic and Metabolic**
- Hyponatremia
- Anticholinergics
- Withdrawal syndromes

**Endocrine**
- Hypoglycemia
- Hyperthyroidism and thyrotoxicosis
- Pheochromocytoma

**Pulmonary and Cardiovascular**
- Hypoxia
- Cerebrovascular accident
- Intracranial hemorrhage
- Subarachnoid hemorrhage, subdural hemorrhage, and epidural hemorrhage

**Infectious and Inflammatory**
- Sepsis
- Meningitis and encephalitis

**Environmental**
- Heat stroke

**Psychiatric**
- Psychosis not otherwise specified
- Schizophrenia
- Mania

resultant lethargy and depressed mood are secondary to catecholamine depletion.

Metabolic derangements during sympathomimetic exposure resemble the fight-or-flight response. The most common metabolic changes, hyperglycemia and hypokalemia, result from a surge in epinephrine. When the metabolic demands outstrip the supply of energy substrates, metabolic acidosis can develop. Because of the body's ability to achieve homeostasis, however, these metabolic effects usually do not require intervention.

Similarly, in combination with psychomotor agitation, this increased demand and activity can result in tremor, muscle rigidity, and rhabdomyolysis. Additionally, the syndrome of inappropriate antidiuretic hormone (SIADH) has been observed in association with MDMA use, as reflected by hyponatremia and inappropriately concentrated urine in the setting of euvolemia. Patients stereotypically develop symptoms the day after exposure, and they present with either altered mental status or seizures.

## DIFFERENTIAL DIAGNOSIS AND MEDICAL DECISION MAKING

The differential diagnosis of the patient with a sympathomimetic toxidrome is extensive (**Box 149.3**). It includes a spectrum of disease ranging from febrile illness to delirium.

Most individuals who misuse or abuse sympathomimetics do not present to the ED; those who do are usually symptomatic. While the physician is considering the extensive differential diagnosis and clinical effects, aggressive measures should be taken to evaluate and stabilize these individuals (**Fig. 149.1**). Urine screening for sympathomimetics, with the exception of cocaine, is fraught with error and misinterpretation. A negative result does not exclude an exposure, whereas a positive result does not confirm causation of the patient's clinical presentation. Therefore, this test is not recommended in the evaluation of a potentially poisoned adult patient.

If the patient is too agitated to allow a thorough evaluation, a bedside glucose measurement should be performed to exclude hypoglycemia. An intravenous line should be placed and secured, to allow parenteral administration of benzodiazepines to control the patient's behavior and thereby prevent further morbidity to the patient and hospital staff.

If the patient is well controlled or does not require sedation, a complete history and physical examination should be obtained while the physician pays close attention to the presence of a sympathomimetic toxidrome. The presence of this toxidrome supports the diagnosis of exposure but does not exclude other possibilities.

All patients with a potential exposure should have a 12-lead electrocardiogram (ECG) performed. Signs of ischemia, infarction, or electrolyte disturbance may be present despite the lack of patient endorsement. In the case of a suspected sympathomimetic toxidrome, patients should be resuscitated with isotonic fluid. Most of these individuals are volume depleted from agitation, diaphoresis, and increased metabolic demand. The only situation in which fluid resuscitation should not be initiated before laboratory evaluation is in the individual suspected of having SIADH from MDMA use.

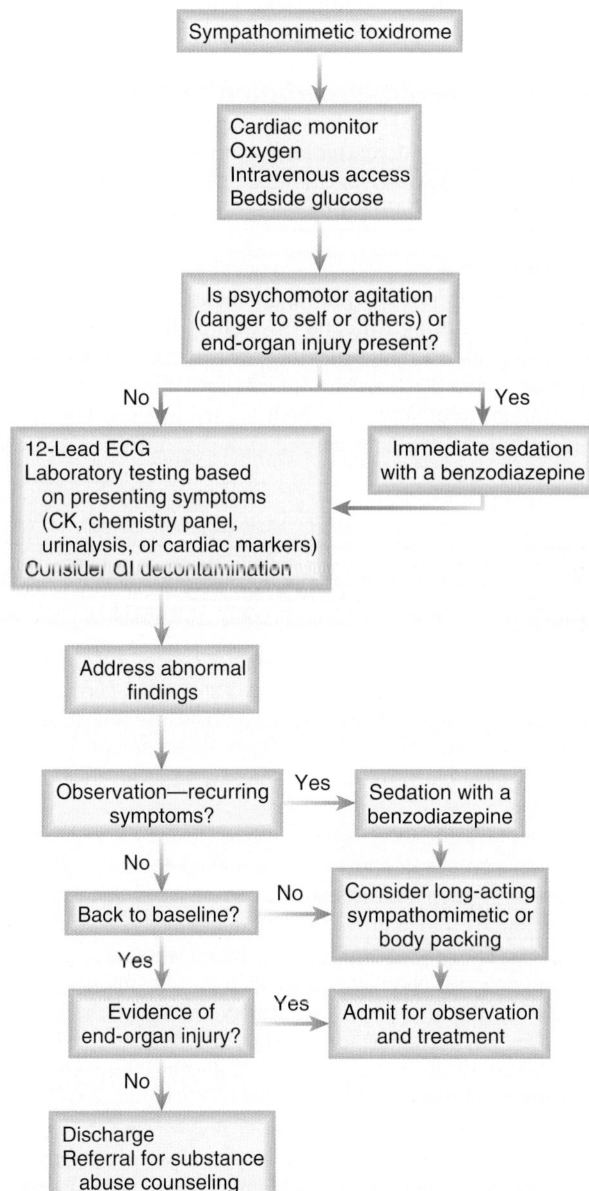


**Fig. 149.1 Treatment algorithm for sympathomimetic toxidrome.** *CK,* Creatine kinase; *ECG,* electrocardiogram; *GI,* gastrointestinal.

All patients should also undergo a chemistry panel to evaluate for the presence of metabolic acidosis, hypokalemia, rhabdomyolysis, renal insufficiency, glucose derangement, and hyponatremia. Individuals with suspected rhabdomyolysis should have serum myoglobin markers evaluated, as well as a urinalysis to check for myoglobinuria. Patients with symptoms of chest pain, an anginal equivalent, or an abnormal ECG should receive serial cardiac marker measurements and, in the appropriate setting, should undergo emergency cardiac catheterization. Individuals with headache, neurologic abnormalities, or persistent alteration in sensorium or cognition should have an emergency computed tomography (CT) scan of the brain to evaluate for injury, infarction, edema, or bleeding. If suspicion of a subarachnoid hemorrhage or an infectious origin persists, a subsequent lumbar puncture should be obtained in the setting of a normal-appearing CT scan of the brain.

## EVALUATION (SPECIAL CONSIDERATIONS)

### *Body Packers*

The concealment of illicit substances within the gastrointestinal tract in large quantities requires close and careful evaluation. Individuals who take part in this trafficking, also known as body packers or "mules," may be symptomatic or asymptomatic when they present to the ED. Those individuals with leaking or ruptured packets containing a sympathomimetic, often cocaine, need to be identified rapidly because they typically harbor enough drug to exceed multiple median lethal doses. Plain radiographs and oral contrast-enhanced CT scans of the abdomen have reasonable sensitivity in detecting packets; however, individuals already demonstrating signs and symptoms should receive an emergency surgical consultation with invasive removal of remaining packages.[3] Body packers, if asymptomatic, require the same consideration, but they may necessitate a prolonged treatment course and monitoring.[4]

### *Methylxanthines or Beta-Agonists*

Patients who present with signs and symptoms consistent with methylxanthine or beta-agonist exposure should have their serum theophylline levels tested. At-risk populations include individuals with a history of reactive airway disease and those with tachycardia, hypotension, widened pulse pressure, nausea, vomiting, tremor, hypokalemia, or hyperglycemia.

## TREATMENT

All patients should have vital signs recorded and continuously monitored, with close attention paid to core temperature. In addition, supplemental oxygen should be administered because of the increased metabolic demand.

Patients who have ingested sympathomimetics should receive activated charcoal if it can be safely administered. Individuals who overdose on theophylline should be considered for aggressive decontamination with multiple-dose activated charcoal because it has been shown to enhance elimination of theophylline from gastrointestinal circulation.

Because of the large drug burden and the risk of packet leakage or rupture in body packers or "mules," whole-bowel irrigation (WBI) can be used as first-line treatment in the asymptomatic patient. WBI can hasten the passage of packets through the gastrointestinal tract.[5] This decontamination modality requires stringent dosing, averaging 2 L/hour of polyethylene glycol orally for an adult patient, with dose adjustments for the pediatric population. Most patients are unable to maintain this rate voluntarily and therefore require nasogastric tube placement. WBI is not without complications.[6] Thus, consulting a toxicologist to discuss treatment is beneficial.

The focus of therapy should be reducing morbidity and mortality by controlling psychomotor agitation or seizures and correcting hyperthermia. Animal studies showed benzodiazepines to be the most effective treatment.

The psychomotor agitation and seizures can result in severe rhabdomyolysis, which, if unrecognized, may result in renal insufficiency or failure. A combination of hyperthermia, metabolic acidosis, and rhabdomyolysis can produce a vicious cycle, which should be recognized and treated immediately.

Mortality related to cocaine use has been associated with an elevation in core and ambient temperature.[7] An ice bath that covers the largest surface area can quickly and effectively reduce core temperature. Other common modalities employed include mist and fan, as well as strategic anatomic application of ice packs (i.e., axilla and groin).

Most patients present with hypovolemia secondary to increased metabolic demand, diaphoresis, and psychomotor agitation. Fluid resuscitation to the point of euvolemia is recommended.

## SPECIAL CONSIDERATIONS

### Beta-Agonists

For known beta-agonist exposures, it would seem logical to administer a β-adrenergic receptor antagonist. However, patients usually overdose on their own medications. In asthmatic patients, administration of a β-receptor antagonist is contraindicated and potentially dangerous. However, if no contraindication to beta-blocker use exists, careful administration and titration of an agent, such as esmolol and metoprolol, can be performed.

### Methylxanthines

Although they are not as common as in the past, theophylline overdoses can be treated aggressively with multiple-dose activated charcoal to enhance elimination, as well as hemoperfusion or hemodialysis. Tachydysrhythmias associated with theophylline overdose can be suppressed with $\beta_1$-selective antagonists. As mentioned previously, however, these patients usually overdose on their own medications, thus making the use of β-receptor antagonists precarious.

### Cocaine

Multiple agents are available to treat cocaine's unique properties of vasoconstriction and sodium channel blockade. The first-line agent for treatment of cocaine toxicity is a benzodiazepine; however, some patients do not respond to this therapy. Ongoing vasoconstriction or vasospasm can be treated with an α-adrenergic receptor antagonist, such as phentolamine. In the setting of cocaine-associated acute coronary syndrome, β-adrenergic blockade is contraindicated despite the mortality benefit observed in patients with acute coronary syndrome unassociated with cocaine.[8] The use of beta-blockers in cocaine toxicity is contraindicated because once the β-adrenergic receptor is blocked, these individuals suffer from unopposed α-adrenergic stimulation, thus worsening their clinical course. Even in the setting of suspected pure β-adrenergic agonist exposure, β-adrenergic blockade is rarely recommended because the underlying substrate usually depends on β- receptor agonism (i.e., asthmatic patients who overdose on albuterol).

A unique property of cocaine is its ability to block myocardial sodium channels. This manifests as wide complex tachydysrhythmia resulting from sodium channel blockade. These electrophysiologic effects are indistinguishable from those of other class I antidysrhythmics and require immediate attention and reversal with either sodium bicarbonate or lidocaine.

Symptomatic cocaine body packers require urgent surgical removal of residual packets. In some instances, body packers are not symptomatic, and WBI can be initiated. In the event that packets cause a mechanical obstruction, endoscopic removal is a successful treatment modality.[9]

### 3,4-Methylenedioxymethamphetamine

MDMA-associated SIADH usually responds to conservative fluid restriction. However, patients with severe CNS manifestations should receive hypertonic saline solution to correct a portion of the metabolic imbalance rapidly.

### Vasopressors

Epinephrine and norepinephrine can extravasate within tissue compartments during infusion, as well as from unintentional exposures related to autoinjectors. Warm compresses should be placed topically for mild cases, and nitroglycerin paste can be added topically to generate vasodilation. For severe cases, intradermal phentolamine may be introduced within the exposed tissue.

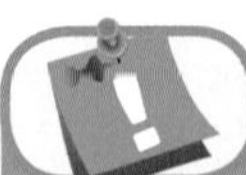

**TIPS AND TRICKS**

- The clinician should avoid neuroleptics (i.e., haloperidol) or antihistamines (i.e., diphenhydramine) to control the psychomotor agitation and psychosis associated with sympathomimetic overdose. Because neuroleptics have anticholinergic properties, decrease seizure thresholds, and increase QT intervals, these agents are a poor choice to achieve sedation. Anticholinergic toxicity is within the diagnostic consideration of the undifferentiated agitated delirium, such that administration of an anticholinergic agent may be additive to potential morbidity. Benzodiazepines are the preferred choice for sedation.
- The only situation in which fluid resuscitation should not be initiated before laboratory evaluation is in the individual suspected to have syndrome of inappropriate antidiuretic hormone from 3,4-methylenedioxymethamphetamine use.
- Because of persistent tachycardia and extrapolating data from acute coronary syndromes, emergency physicians often feel compelled to rate-control these patients with β-adrenergic receptor antagonists. Potential unopposed α-adrenergic agonism may lead to a hypertensive crisis, and these agents therefore should be avoided in the undifferentiated sympathomimetic toxidrome.
- Amiodarone is listed as a first-line agent in the treatment of wide complex tachycardia. Concern exists about the intrinsic β-adrenergic receptor antagonist properties of amiodarone, for the reasons stated. Amiodarone should not be used in the setting of cocaine toxicity because of this theoretical risk.

## DISPOSITION

The length of stay and disposition depend on the duration of action of the sympathomimetic, which is highly variable. Recreationally smoked or insufflated cocaine has a short duration of action, usually lasting no more than 4 hours, and patients can normally be discharged from the ED. Side effects such as rhabdomyolysis, heat stroke, or end-organ injury require ongoing monitoring and treatment. Prolonged effects may be seen in individuals who are body packers and in patients who use long-acting agents such as clenbuterol, a potent β-adrenergic receptor agonist. These individuals require admission and prolonged treatment.

The evaluation and treatment of cocaine-associated chest pain have evolved and have regional variation. A short observation period with serial ECGs and serial cardiac-specific markers performed 6 to 8 hours apart can be used to exclude cocaine-associated myocardial infarction.[10] Despite excluding the diagnosis of myocardial infarction, all patients should have urgent outpatient evaluation for coronary artery disease and drug abuse counseling.

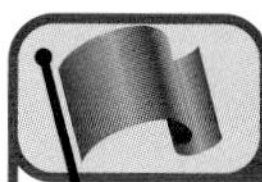

**RED FLAGS**

- Widened pulse pressure and hypokalemia, if present, may suggest exposure to either a methylxanthine or a β-adrenergic receptor agonist.
- A unique property of cocaine is its ability to block myocardial sodium channels, manifested as a widened QRS complex on the electrocardiogram. These electrophysiologic effects are indistinguishable from those of other class I antidysrhythmics and require immediate attention and reversal.
- Sympathomimetic stimulation of the central nervous system that results in psychomotor agitation and hyperthermia is associated with increased mortality and should be aggressively treated.
- Psychomotor agitation can result in rhabdomyolysis, tremor, and muscle rigidity. If left undetected, severe rhabdomyolysis may cause renal insufficiency or failure.
- The clinician should suspect a body packer when symptoms recur or are prolonged and when an individual develops signs and symptoms of sympathomimetic exposure associated with an international flight.
- Individuals already demonstrating signs and symptoms of packet leakage or rupture should receive an urgent surgical consultation and invasive removal of remaining packages because the lethality of the drug is high.

## SUGGESTED READINGS


de Prost N, Lefebvre A, Questel F, et al. Prognosis of cocaine body-packers. Intensive Care Med 2005;31:955-8.

Lange RA, Cigarroa RG, Flores ED, et al. Potentiation of cocaine-induced coronary vasoconstriction by beta-adrenergic blockade. Ann Intern Med 1990;112:897-903.

Marzuk PM, Tardiff K, Leon AC, et al. Ambient temperature and mortality from unintentional cocaine overdose. JAMA 1998;279:1795-800.

National Institute on Drug Abuse. Monitoring the future survey. Available at: http://www.nida.nih.gov/DrugPages/Stats.html. Accessed February 7, 2012.

Traub SJ, Hoffman RS, Nelson LS. Body packing: the internal concealment of illicit drugs. N Engl J Med 2003;349:2519-26.

Weber JE, Shofer FS, Larkin GL, et al. Validation of a brief observation period for patients with cocaine-associated chest pain. N Engl J Med 2003;348:510-7.


## REFERENCES

***References can be found on Expert Consult @ www.expertconsult.com.***

# 150 Hallucinogens and Drugs of Abuse

*Mark B. Mycyk*

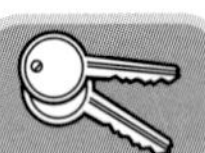

**KEY POINTS**

- The most common chief complaint when patients have hallucinogenic intoxication is altered mental status.
- Optimal treatment depends on *symptom-based* (rather than drug-based) diagnostic strategies and interventions.
- An elevated temperature is the most important prognostic sign of poor outcome.
- Most new drugs cannot be identified with hospital-based blood or urine tests, and results of urine drug screens should never be considered diagnostic.
- Treatment for drug-induced hypertension should involve generous doses of benzodiazepines before antihypertensive agents are considered.
- Substance abuse counseling and referral are required for all patients before discharge.

## EPIDEMIOLOGY

Recreational abuse of hallucinogens and other drugs is common among patients in the emergency department (ED) and is directly responsible for many ED visits. Although the exact prevalence of drug abuse in patients in the ED is unknown because so much drug abuse goes undetected, various surveillance studies all indicate that ED visits related to drug use continue to rise yearly.[1-3]

Patients who present to an ED immediately after using a drug do so for various reasons: an unfavorable or unanticipated reaction to the drug, an unintentional overdose, a traumatic injury, altered mental status, or suicidal and other dangerous behavior. In addition to the acute complications directly related to drug use, many cardiovascular, neurologic, infectious, psychiatric, and social health problems treated in the ED are linked to chronic drug abuse. Because drug abuse is often not declared by the patient at the time of arrival, recognition and optimal treatment require vigilance from the emergency physician, as well as attention to historical, clinical, and laboratory clues.

Recreational drug use today knows no demographic, age, or socioeconomic boundaries. Drug use is just as common (although perhaps less frequently suspected) in white, employed, and insured individuals as in patients who are nonwhite, unemployed, or homeless.[1,4] In the last 2 decades, first-time drug use has become more common among adolescents, and the variety of drugs used has exploded.[5,6] Drug use is no longer limited to what can be identified on a standard hospital toxicology screen, and many of the drugs people abuse to become high are not illegal, such as cough and cold products and prescription medications.[7-10] The rampant growth of drug use is likely linked to the proliferation of the Internet and the wide availability of unregulated partisan drug sites that enable potential users to learn about drugs, to order the raw ingredients and supplies to manufacture their own drugs, or simply to purchase drugs online in the safety of their own homes.[6]

## PATHOPHYSIOLOGY

The drugs available for recreational abuse are countless and are constantly evolving. In the past, recreational drugs were categorized, for the purposes of discussion, identification, and treatment, somewhat arbitrarily on the basis of structural class, predominant biochemical or neurotransmitter activity (e.g., dopaminergic versus serotonergic versus gamma-aminobutyric acid [GABA]–ergic), or expected clinical effect (e.g., hallucinogen versus stimulant versus entactogen). In reality, most drugs exhibit multiple biochemical effects of varying intensity that are not limited to a particular structural class, and clinical findings vary widely among different individuals even when these persons are exposed to the same drug. Physicians now recognize that clinical variability depends not only on the specific type of drug but also on the dose used, the form of drug (e.g., crystal versus powder versus liquid), the purity of the drug, the route of delivery (e.g., intranasal versus ingestion versus injection), the concomitant use of coingestants, individual genetic polymorphisms, and individual biochemical and physiologic adaptations from long-term exposure.

Most recreational drugs are highly lipophilic and easily cross the blood-brain barrier, so most result in some euphoria; otherwise, patients would have little reason to abuse them.[3] Although the exact mechanisms are still incompletely understood, modulation of central dopaminergic activity, which is responsible for pleasure seeking and reward reinforcement, is an important factor in the euphoric response and the development of drug addiction.[3] Recreational drugs also affect, to variable extents, peripheral and central norepinephrine, serotonin (5-HT), *N*-methyl-D aspartate (NMDA), and GABA activity.

## PRESENTING SIGNS AND SYMPTOMS

The most common presenting feature in all patients with recreational drug use is some degree of altered mental status. It may range from seemingly benign giddiness to life-threatening agitation or obtundation. Drug-associated altered mental status may be associated with any kind of vital sign abnormalities or evidence of end-organ damage. Cardiovascular, neurologic, infectious, and psychiatric complaints are also common (**Table 150.1**). Because the predominant drugs seen in a particular ED vary depending on local geographic preferences and because the types of drugs abused change far more quickly than published medical literature can keep up with, optimal treatment depends on *symptom-based* (rather than drug-based) diagnostic strategies and interventions.

The following paragraphs discuss some of the more common drugs of abuse historically prevalent in most EDs. Identifying previously undetected drug abuse requires some familiarity with these common drugs and the street slang associated with them (**Table 150.2**).

**Table 150.1 Signs and Symptoms of Recreational Drug Use**

| SIGN OR SYMPTOM | RESPONSIBLE DRUG(S) |
| --- | --- |
| Altered mental status | All |
| Agitation | Amphetamine<br>Cocaine<br>Dextromethorphan<br>Jimsonweed<br>MDMA<br>Mephedrone<br>Methamphetamine<br>PCP<br>Prescription medications |
| Obtundation | GHB<br>Opioids<br>Prescription medications |
| Hypothermia | Opiates<br>GHB |
| Hyperthermia | Amphetamine<br>Cocaine<br>Jimsonweed<br>MDMA<br>Mephedrone<br>Methamphetamine<br>PCP |
| Tachycardia | Amphetamines<br>Cocaine<br>Jimsonweed<br>Ketamine<br>LSD<br>Mephedrone<br>MDMA<br>Methamphetamine<br>PCP<br>Prescription medications |
| Bradycardia | GHB<br>Opioids<br>Prescription medications |
| Hypertension | Amphetamine<br>Cocaine<br>Jimsonweed<br>Ketamine<br>LSD<br>Methamphetamine<br>MDMA<br>PCP<br>Prescription medications |
| Hypotension | GHB<br>Opioids<br>Prescription medications |
| Seizures | Amphetamines<br>Cocaine<br>Dextromethorphan<br>GHB<br>Jimsonweed<br>MDMA<br>Methamphetamine<br>Prescription medications |

*GHB,* Gamma-hydroxybutyrate; *LSD,* D-lysergic acid diethylamide; *MDMA,* methylenedioxymethamphetamine; *PCP,* phencyclidine.

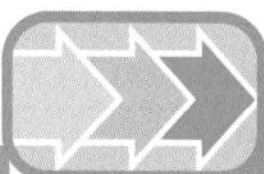

**PRIORITY ACTIONS**

**Altered Mental Status, Seizures, or Behavioral Changes?**

- Does the patient have a central nervous system infection, infarction, lesion, or mass?
- Consider brain imaging and lumber puncture if neurologic status is inconsistent with intoxication.

**Apnea or Depressed Respirations?**

- Consider treatment with naloxone to reverse potential narcosis or dextrose and thiamine for hypoglycemia.
- Intubation may be needed for persistent hypoxia or an inability to protect the airway.

**Chest Pain?**

- Evaluate the patient for myocardial ischemia with electrocardiography, telemetry, and cardiac enzyme measurements.

**Fever or Hyperthermia?**

- Does the patient have any history or evidence of intravenous drug use?
- Consider evaluation for endocarditis or epidural abscess.
- Consider active cooling and liberal benzodiazepine treatment if sympathomimetic intoxication is suspected.

### AMPHETAMINE

Commonly referred to as "crank" or "speed," amphetamine is a specific drug first synthesized in 1887 and initially marketed as a decongestant and appetite suppressant. Many other drugs with a similar chemical structure, such as methylenedioxymethamphetamine (MDMA) and methamphetamine, are collectively called *amphetamines,* even though their clinical effects vary. More precisely, these drugs are all derived from

**Table 150.2 New Drug Slang**

| | |
|---|---|
| Dextromethorphan | DXM<br>Red hots<br>Triple Cs |
| Gamma-hydroxybutyrate (GHB) | Georgia home boy<br>Easy lay<br>Liquid G |
| Ketamine | Special K<br>Kiddie Valium<br>Kitty Valium<br>Cat tranquilizer |
| Methylenedioxymethamphetamine (MDMA) | Ecstasy<br>XTC<br>X<br>ADAM<br>Hug drug |
| Mephedrone | Meow Meow<br>MCAT<br>Drone |
| Methamphetamine | Meth<br>Crystal<br>Chicken feed<br>Tweak<br>White man's crack |

a phenylethylamine core and should be collectively called *phenylethylamines* (MDMA and methamphetamine are discussed separately). Amphetamines are currently available as tablets in the form of a prescription (e.g., methylphenidate [Ritalin], proprietary mixture of amphetamine salts [Adderall]) or in a designer form produced in a clandestine laboratory.[11] The onset of symptoms occurs within 15 minutes of ingestion, and symptoms last 6 to 12 hours. The effects are primarily stimulant because of amphetamine's activity at peripheral and central norepinephrine and dopamine sites.[3] Varying levels of tachycardia, hypertension, hyperthermia, diaphoresis, and agitation are commonly seen in the ED in a patient who has ingested an amphetamine, and cardiac and central nervous system (CNS) complications have been frequently reported.

## COCAINE

Cocaine is also discussed in Chapter 149, Sympathomimetics. Derived from *Erythroxylon coca,* a shrub indigenous to South America, cocaine is well absorbed by any mucosal route and thus is abused when snorted, smoked (crack), or injected intravenously. Effects typically occur within 5 to 15 minutes and last 1 to 4 hours. The effects are primarily stimulant and are related to its effects on the sympathetic nervous system: increasing the release of norepinephrine and blocking its reuptake.[3,12] Concomitant use of cocaine with alcohol results in cocaethylene, a by-product with a clinical effect lasting longer than cocaine's and with direct myocardial depressant effects. After cocaine use, patients may present with chest pain, focal weakness, or altered mental status, and they typically exhibit tachycardia, hypertension, hyperthermia, diaphoresis, and agitation. Because of the intensity of the sympathomimetic stimulation, medical complications such as acute coronary syndrome, seizures, cerebral vascular accidents, intracranial hemorrhage, renal failure, and rhabdomyolysis are common.[12,13] *Cocaine washout syndrome* occurs after cocaine binging. Affected patients typically have a depressed mental status ranging from lethargy to obtundation that lasts up to 24 hours until depleted neurotransmitters are regenerated.

## DEXTROMETHORPHAN

Also known as DXM, dextromethorphan is a common antitussive agent found in over-the-counter and prescription medications in liquid or tablet form. It is a synthetic analogue of codeine but does not have the same analgesic effect because its activity is primarily at NMDA and 5-HT receptors.[7,10] Hallucinations are commonly reported, and in addition to some opioid features, patients may exhibit ataxia, slurred speech, nystagmus, tachycardia, hypertension, dystonia, and seizures.

## GAMMA-HYDROXYBUTYRATE

Gamma-hydroxybutyrate (GHB), also known as "Georgia Home Boy" and "Liquid G," has been variously used as an exercise supplement, for treatment of narcolepsy, for obtaining chemical submission of victims, and for euphoria. GHB works primarily at GABA receptors and the still poorly defined GHB receptor.[14,15] The analogues gamma-butyrolactone (GBL), 1.4-butanediol (1,4-BD), gamma-hydroxyvalerate methyl-GHB (GHV), and gamma-valerolactone 4-pentanolide (GVL) work similarly because they are all converted to GHB through various pathways after ingestion. GHB easily crosses the blood-brain barrier and produces loss of consciousness within 15 to 30 minutes of ingestion. Bradycardia, vomiting, myoclonic jerks, and hypothermia are commonly associated. Duration of unconsciousness lasts 2 to 6 hours in most cases.[16]

## JIMSONWEED

Jimsonweed is the common name of plants in the *Datura* genera. Intoxication with jimsonweed was first reported in 1676. The plants grow throughout the United States, and all parts of it—the fruit, flower, and seeds—can be abused for their hallucinogenic properties. Because these plants contains the alkaloids atropine, scopolamine, and hyoscyamine, clinical effects associated with jimsonweed hallucinations include anticholinergic findings such as dilated pupils, dry mouth, warm and flushed skin, diminished bowel sounds, and urinary retention. Cardiovascular instability, hyperthermia, and seizures have been reported after large ingestions.[17]

## KETAMINE

Also known as "Special K," "Kitty Valium," and "Kiddie Valium," ketamine is a structural and functional analogue of phencyclidine (PCP) and also works primarily at NMDA receptors.[18] Ketamine can be ingested or injected. Patients with ketamine abuse have symptoms similar to those of PCP intoxication, including rotatory nystagmus, excessive salivation, muscle rigidity, tachycardia, and hypertension, although the effects tend to last a shorter time.[5,18]

## LSD

D-Lysergic acid diethylamide (LSD) was first synthesized in 1938. It is available in tablets, liquid, powder, and gelatin squares, although the most commonly abused form of LSD is "blotter" acid (sheets of paper sprayed with LSD, dried, and then perforated into small squares). Effects occur within 30 minutes, can last for 16 to 24 hours, and cause powerful hallucinations from serotonergic (5-HT) and dopaminergic activity. Time is distorted, and visual hallucinations of bright colors are common. Tachycardia, hypertension, anxiety, and paranoia are frequently seen in patients who seek treatment in the ED as a result of LSD use. Significant medical complications are uncommon.[18]

## MARIJUANA

Also known as "grass," "weed," or "pot," marijuana is considered the most commonly used illegal substance in the United States. Marijuana is primarily smoked; its effects occur within 15 minutes and can last up to 4 hours. The psychoactive substance, delta-9-tetrahydrocannabinol, is derived from the plant *Cannabis sativa.*[3] Clinical effects are variable and seem to occur as a result of cannabinoid receptor activity in the brain. Inappropriate laughter, excessive hunger, anxiety, paranoia, ataxia, and tachycardia are commonly seen. Various synthetic cannabinoids (known by names such as Spice, K2, and Sky Incense) have become available to users in herb shops.[19] The duration of symptoms has reportedly been longer than for naturally growing marijuana. Medical complications associated with cannabinoid abuse alone are uncommon.

## METHYLENEDIOXYMETHAMPHETAMINE

MDMA is better known as "Ecstasy," "X," "XTC," and "ADAM" and is also discussed in Chapter 149, Sympathomimetics. It was first synthesized in 1914 but became wildly popular at rave parties and on college campuses in the 1980s and 1990s.[4,5] Although it is a phenylethylamine like amphetamine, MDMA's strong serotonergic activity has clinical effects that are primarily hallucinogenic and entactogenic.[3] Variable tachycardia and hypertension can also occur from some stimulant activity. Hyperthermia has been reported as a complication of excessive dancing in warm rave clubs without adequate hydration, although other individual variabilities and drug contaminants are also likely responsible.[5] Hyponatremia, another common occurrence with MDMA use, results from excessive ingestion of water or from MDMA-induced syndrome of inappropriate antidiuretic hormone secretion.

## METHAMPHETAMINE

Also known as "meth," "crystal," "chicken feed," and "white man's crank," methamphetamine has become one of the most popular drugs of abuse in the twenty-first century.[20,21] Its popularity is related to its multiple forms (crystal, powder, liquid, and tablet), its ease of manufacture from decongestants such as pseudoephedrine, and its low street cost (less than one third the cost of cocaine). Methamphetamine has strong norepinephrine activity and, of all the phenylethylamines, is the most quickly addictive because of its strong dopaminergic action.[3] It can be ingested, snorted, smoked, injected, or administered rectally. Clinical findings are similar to those associated with other stimulant intoxications, and acute coronary syndrome and cerebrovascular accident have been reported. Other hallmark features of methamphetamine are poor dentition, known as "meth mouth," from poor hygiene and bruxism and dermatologic lesions called "crank bugs" or "meth mites," from compulsive scratching that is likely delusional in origin.

## OPIOIDS

Naturally occurring or synthetic drugs with opium-like or morphine-like activity have always been popular. The poppy plant, *Papaver somniferum,* is the source of opium and contains the alkaloids morphine and codeine. Opioid effects are primarily modulated throughout the peripheral and CNS by interacting at three main opioid receptors: μ, κ, and δ.[3] The classic opioid toxidrome comprises CNS depression, respiratory depression, and miosis, although the intensity of each of those features varies among the different synthetic opioids. Prehospital deaths typically occur from untreated apnea.[22] Abuse of prescription opioids continues to rise, especially abuse of methadone and fentanyl patches. Data indicate that the abuse of combination acetaminophen-opioid analgesics is directly related to rising rates of acetaminophen-induced hepatic failure.[23]

## OTHER NATURAL PRODUCTS

Naturally found herbs, plants, and other related products have become especially popular during the Internet drug era. Adolescents and young adults have been reported to use morning glory seeds for LSD-like effects, nutmeg for myristicin-associated hallucinogenic effects, and the plant *Salvia divinorum* (known also as "Sally D" and "Diviner's mint") for κ-opioid–mediated hallucinogenic effects.[24] Naturally occurring recreational drugs are popular because they are considered "naturally" safe and can be used in various ways by users, including ingestion, insufflation, smoking, injection, and even tea consumption. Effects typically last 2 to 6 hours, and medical complications are uncommon, although long-term effects are still unknown.

## PRESCRIPTION MEDICATIONS

Nonmedical abuse of prescription drugs has been identified as a national epidemic. In 2005, nearly 15 million U.S. residents abused prescription drugs, including prescribed opioids, sedatives, antidepressants, and stimulants.[1] One of the reasons for the rapid rise of prescription drug abuse is the perception that these agents are safer than traditional street drugs. The growing rates of prescriptions written for analgesia, for mood disorders, and for attention-deficit hyperactivity disorder have resulted in experimentation with easily available tablets by the family members or friends of the person for whom the agents were prescribed.[9,11]

# DIFFERENTIAL DIAGNOSIS AND MEDICAL DECISION MAKING

Drug intoxication should always be considered in the differential diagnosis of any patient presenting to the ED with altered mental status. Infectious, metabolic, neurologic, endocrinologic, structural, and psychogenic causes should also be considered in the evaluation of the patient with suspected drug intoxication. The history of events immediately preceding onset of symptoms, if available to the clinician from the patient or witnesses, is most helpful in narrowing the diagnosis.

Asymptomatic patients with drug intoxication who have normal vital signs and normal physical findings do not require diagnostic testing. Patients with mild symptoms should undergo rapid blood glucose measurement because

**Table 150.3 Diagnostic Testing for Suspected Recreational Drug Use**

| TEST | INDICATION |
|---|---|
| Rapid blood glucose measurement | Altered mental status |
| Blood chemistry panel | Methylenedioxymethamphetamine intoxication or suspected rhabdomyolysis |
| Serum acetaminophen measurement | Prescription opioid ingestion |
| Blood alcohol evaluation | Suspected coingestant |
| Serum creatine phosphokinase (total) measurement | Agitation or suspected rhabdomyolysis |
| Urinalysis | Suspected rhabdomyolysis |
| Liver function tests | Prescription opioid ingestion |
| Electrocardiogram | Tachycardia, bradycardia, or dysrhythmia |
| Computed tomography of the head | Suspected trauma or mental status inconsistent with reported ingestion |

hypoglycemia or hyperglycemia may cause altered mental status. Ethanol measurement should be obtained if alcohol is suspected as a coingestant or to exclude alcohol ingestion as a cause of altered mental status. Patients who are agitated, hyperthermic, or seizing or were found after prolonged obtundation are all at risk for the development of rhabdomyolysis and should be evaluated with a basic metabolic profile, renal function tests, measurements of calcium, phosphorus, total creatine phosphokinase levels, and urinalysis.[25]

Electrocardiography should be performed in all patients with tachycardia or bradycardia, and telemetry monitoring should be instituted. Patients with altered mental status inconsistent with their reported drug use, new-onset seizure, or signs of traumatic injury or suspected trauma should be evaluated with computed tomography of the head (**Table 150.3**).

The toxicology drug screen has limited utility in the ED setting and should be used only for a patient in whom mental status is altered and the diagnosis is not clear. Several studies confirm that a careful patient history and attention to clinical signs make toxicology screens unnecessary in most cases of drug intoxication.[26,27] For example, a patient with depressed respirations, depressed mental status, and pinpoint pupils consistent with an opioid toxidrome who completely awakens after the administration of naloxone does not need a costly urine drug screen to confirm opioid toxicity. Furthermore, waiting for the results of a urine drug screen before administering lifesaving naloxone is impractical in cases of severe intoxication.

The drug screens available in most hospitals have a limited panel, and many of the nontraditional, emerging, and Web-based drugs (new drugs, including prescription medications and club drugs) cannot be detected by such hospital screens.[5] Toxicology screens are limited by what they cannot detect, and they can yield false-positive results related to contaminants. For example, over-the-counter decongestants used appropriately for an upper respiratory infection can yield a falsely positive amphetamine screen result, and quinolones can cause falsely positive opioid screen results.[28] Finally, urine drug screen results are not forensically defensible because most hospitals analyze urine with only one laboratory technique, and the chain of custody is not enforced from patient to laboratory (**Box 150.1**).

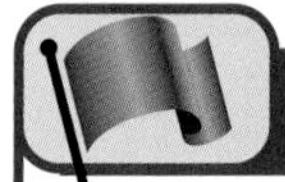

**RED FLAGS**

- An elevated temperature is prognostic of poor outcomes.
- Focal neurologic findings are indicative of seizure activity or intracranial lesion.
- Rhabdomyolysis can occur in cases of agitation or prolonged obtundation.
- Renal insufficiency or creatine phosphokinase elevation requires adequate fluid resuscitation to prevent renal failure.

**DOCUMENTATION**

- Amount ingested?
- Route of ingestion (oral, intravenous, subcutaneous dermal, sublingual, rectal)?
- Time of ingestion?
- Coingestants?
- History of trauma?
- Previous emergency department visits for drug abuse?
- Previous detoxification or other treatment programs?
- Referral for counseling, treatment program, or detoxification

## TREATMENT

Because the clinical presentation of drug intoxication varies widely, optimal treatment must be *symptom based.* Attempts to confirm identification of the drug should be postponed until the patient is stabilized. As with any patient in the ED,

**BOX 150.1 Hospital Urine Drug Screen**

It has limited utility and is never diagnostic.
Its primary use should be for altered mental status and unclear diagnosis.
It does not indicate time or dose of exposure because it identifies only the presence of drug metabolites from use within the last 72 to 96 hours.
It can result in false-positive results related to contaminants or cross-reactant medications.
It does not identify most new drugs used today.
It does not meet basic forensic standards.
Treatment decisions should be guided by clinical evaluation and never by a drug screen result.

attention to airway management is the top priority in all patients with drug intoxication. Obtunded patients with a poor respiratory effort should receive either naloxone, in an effort to reverse potential narcosis, or dextrose and thiamine for hypoglycemia. Intubation should be performed for persistent hypoxemia or the inability to protect a patient's airway. Intravenous fluids should be administered to treat hypotension. Dysrhythmias should be treated according to standard Advanced Cardiac Life Support guidelines. A thorough examination must be completed to exclude concomitant traumatic injuries that require emergency management.

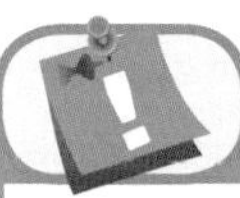

**TIPS AND TRICKS**

- Attempts to confirm or identify the drug should be postponed until the patient is stabilized.
- Attention to airway management is the top priority in all cases of drug intoxication.
- Close monitoring of the patient's core temperature is critical because an elevated temperature is the only vital sign abnormality consistently associated with poor outcomes in cases of drug intoxication.
- Physical restraints may be needed temporarily for patient and staff safety; chemical sedation with benzodiazepines must be given high priority, to minimize the duration of potentially harmful physical restraints.
- Drug-induced hypertension and tachycardia should also be treated first with benzodiazepines in very liberal doses.

Patients who are agitated or difficult to control should receive liberal benzodiazepine treatment for their own safety, as well as staff safety, and to ensure a complete examination. Butyrophenones, such as haloperidol, may be considered if benzodiazepines do not successfully control the difficult patient. Although physical restraints may be needed temporarily for patient and staff safety, chemical sedation with benzodiazepines must be given top priority, to minimize the duration of potentially harmful physical restraints.[29]

Drug-induced hypertension and tachycardia should also be treated first with benzodiazepines because these clinical findings primarily result from direct stimulant effects and are effectively managed in most cases with liberal benzodiazepine sedation. Short-acting antihypertensive agents with minimal beta-blocker activity may be considered only after sufficient doses of benzodiazepines have been administered.

Hyperthermia must be aggressively treated with external cooling measures and, if the patient is agitated, with liberal benzodiazepine therapy as well. Close monitoring of the patient's core temperature is critical because an elevated temperature is the only vital sign abnormality consistently associated with poor outcomes in cases of drug intoxication.[29]

Renal insufficiency or an elevated creatine phosphokinase value requires adequate fluid resuscitation. Drug-induced rhabdomyolysis results in renal failure and hemodialysis in 10% of patients hospitalized for drug intoxication and associated rhabdomyolysis.[25,29]

## FOLLOW-UP, NEXT STEPS OF CARE, AND PATIENT EDUCATION

Most patients with single-drug intoxication who have improved can be safely discharged after 4 to 6 hours of ED observation. In patients with multiple drug ingestion, prolonged clinical effects of long-acting agents such as methadone, or medical complications, admission to a monitored hospital bed is appropriate. Attention to signs of withdrawal is important before such a patient is discharged. Whether being discharged from the ED or from an inpatient bed, all patients with drug intoxication require substance abuse counseling and referral for support groups, detoxification, and other outpatient treatment.[30]

## SUGGESTED READINGS

Cami J, Farre M. Drug addiction. N Engl J Med 2003;349:975-86.
Cherpitel CJ, Ye Y. Trends in alcohol- and drug-related ED and primary care visits: data from three US National Surveys (1995-2005). Am J Drug Alcohol Abuse 2008;34:576-83.
Langdorf MI, Rudkin SE, Dellota K, et al. Decision rule and utility of routine urine toxicology screening of trauma patients. Eur J Emerg Med 2002;9:115-21.
Rockett IR, Putnam SL, Jia H, et al. Unmet substance abuse treatment need, health services utilization, and cost: a population-based emergency department study. Ann Emerg Med 2005;45:118-27.
Tominaga GT, Garcia G, Dzierba A, Wong J. Toll of methamphetamine on the trauma system. Arch Surg 2004;139:844-7.

## REFERENCES

*References can be found on Expert Consult @ www.expertconsult.com.*

# 151 Toxic Alcohols

*Mark B. Mycyk*

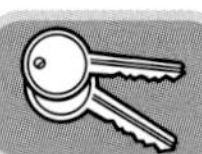

**KEY POINTS**

- Toxic alcohol poisoning may initially be mistaken for simple inebriation.
- Untreated ethylene glycol poisoning may result in renal failure.
- Untreated methanol poisoning may result in blindness.
- Acidosis from ethylene glycol or methanol may not be evident until several hours after exposure.
- An osmol gap may not be evident in patients whose presentation to the emergency department is delayed, and these patients benefit from early dialysis.
- An osmol gap measurement is only a screening test and is never diagnostic like a quantitative alcohol measurement.
- Isopropanol poisoning classically results in an elevated osmol gap without significant acidosis.
- Treatment with ethanol or fomepizole should be considered in cases of a witnessed ingestion of a toxic alcohol, when such an ingestion is highly suspected from the history, in the presence of an enlarged osmol gap alone with appropriate clinical suspicion, in the patient with both an enlarged osmol gap and anion gap acidosis, or when the serum concentration of a toxic alcohol exceeds 20 mg/dL.
- Early alcohol dehydrogenase inhibition minimizes metabolism of the toxic alcohol to organic toxic acids and reduces alcohol-specific complications.

## EPIDEMIOLOGY

Except for ethanol, no other alcohols are fit for human consumption, and they are properly termed *toxic alcohols*. Ethylene glycol, methanol, and isopropanol are the most common toxic alcohols associated with human poisoning.[1] Less commonly reported but still clinically important toxic alcohols are propylene glycol, diethylene glycol, and other glycol ethers. Unintentional ingestion from a mislabeled or contaminated container occurs commonly in children, whereas intentional ingestion of a toxic alcohol as an ethanol substitute or for self-harm occurs more commonly in adults. If untreated, toxic alcohol poisoning can result in metabolic acidosis, renal failure, blindness, central nervous system (CNS) injury, pulmonary edema, or death.

Ethylene glycol is present in antifreeze solutions, deicing solutions, foam stabilizers, and chemical solvents.[2] Methanol is a component of windshield-washing solutions, gas-line antifreeze solutions, solvents, and brake cleaners.[3] Isopropanol is found in rubbing alcohol, aerosols, and other cosmetic products. Propylene glycol is commonly found as a diluent in parenteral medications such as phenytoin, diazepam, and lorazepam.[4] The other toxic glycols can be found in various household and industrial cleaners, paints, resins, and solvents.

More than 35,000 toxic alcohol exposures are reported yearly to the American Association of Poison Control Centers.[1] Most cases are individual poisonings. However, contamination of beverages or pharmaceutical products has resulted in epidemic poisonings, including two significant outbreaks, in India and in Haiti in the 1990s, from diethylene glycol that affected hundreds of victims.[5]

Definitive laboratory confirmation of toxic alcohol poisoning is usually not immediately available to the emergency physician. However, early recognition of poisoning and emergency department (ED)–initiated interventions significantly improve patient outcomes and reduce the occurrence of alcohol-specific complications.[6]

## PATHOPHYSIOLOGY

Most toxic alcohol poisonings occur by oral ingestion. Significant methanol poisoning has also been reported to occur by inhalation of brake cleaning products, and isopropanol poisoning has occurred through transcutaneous absorption in children treated for fevers at home with rubbing alcohol baths.[7,8] Complete absorption is rapid by any route, each alcohol has a small volume of distribution (0.5 to 0.8 L/kg), and metabolism to toxic organic by-products occurs through hepatic alcohol dehydrogenase (ADH) (**Figs. 151.1 and 151.2**).

Toxicity from the parent products is limited to local mucous membrane irritation and CNS depression. The term *toxic* is specifically related to the production of different toxic by-products (oxalic acid and formic acid) by each of these alcohols. Ethylene glycol metabolism results in renal failure from deposition of oxalic acid in renal tubules.[2] Methanol

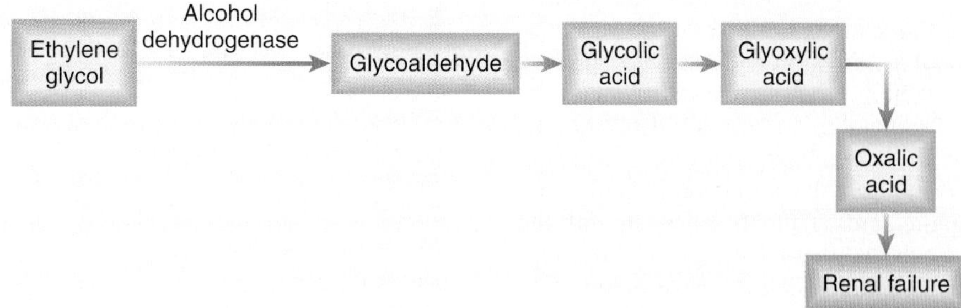


Fig. 151.1 Ethylene glycol metabolism pathway.

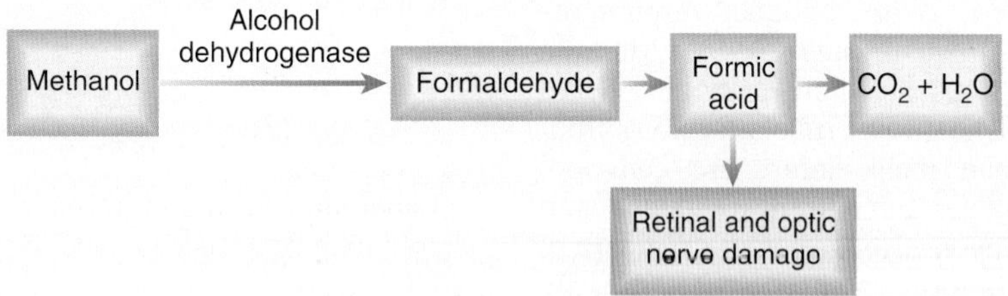


Fig. 151.2 Methanol metabolism pathway.

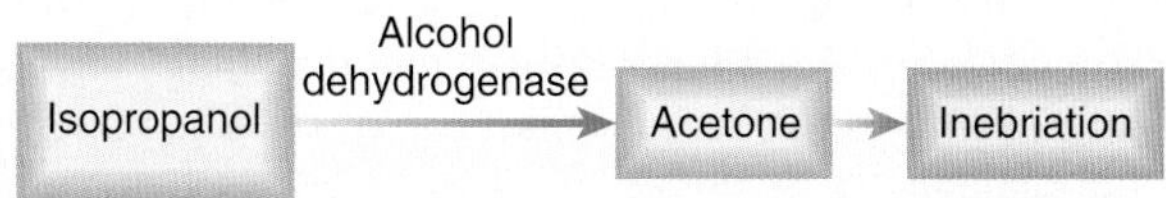


Fig. 151.3 Isopropanol metabolism pathway.

metabolism to formic acid results in blindness from direct injury to the retinal and optic nerves.[3]

Because the rate of metabolism through ADH varies by alcohol type and by individual variability in cytochrome P-450 genetic expression, clinical onset of worrisome symptoms can be delayed by 1 to 36 hours.[2,3] Furthermore, the concomitant presence of ethanol may delay metabolism to the toxic by-products because ethanol has a higher affinity for ADH than the toxic alcohols and competitively inhibits metabolism of these alcohols to toxic by-products until the serum ethanol concentration drops to less than 100 mg/dL.

Isopropanol is unlike ethylene glycol and methanol in that it is not metabolized to an organic acid. Instead, it is metabolized to acetone, an osmotically active CNS depressant, which leads to profound inebriation (**Fig. 151.3**).[8]

**Table 151.1 Symptoms and Signs of Toxic Alcohol Poisoning**

| | |
|---|---|
| Symptoms | Altered mental status<br>Headache<br>Nausea<br>Vomiting<br>Abdominal pain<br>Weakness<br>Unsteady gait<br>Visual blurring<br>Skin flushing |
| Signs | Hypotension<br>Tachycardia<br>Dysrhythmias<br>Hyperventilation<br>Hypoventilation<br>Hypothermia<br>Nystagmus<br>Sluggish pupils<br>Hyperemic optic disk<br>Seizures<br>Coma |

## PRESENTING SIGNS AND SYMPTOMS

### CLASSIC OR TYPICAL

Most patients poisoned with a toxic alcohol demonstrate some level of CNS depression consistent with inebriation (**Table 151.1**). Patients who arrive in the ED either shortly after a large ingestion or later after an ingestion, such that systemic accumulation of toxic metabolites has occurred, may be obtunded on presentation or may become obtunded during ED evaluation. The level of inebriation does not correlate with peak serum concentrations of the parent product or the accumulation of metabolic by-products.

Other clinical findings range from mild to life-threatening, depending on the type of alcohol and the dose consumed. Because the clinical toxicity from these alcohols results from the accumulation of specific toxic metabolites, some patients may appear relatively asymptomatic before the manifestation of significant symptoms. Hypotension with reflex tachycardia is common in significant ingestions because of the vasodilatory effects common to all alcohols. In patients with ethylene glycol or methanol poisoning, routine laboratory analysis classically shows anion gap metabolic acidosis and an enlarged osmol gap. Patients with isopropanol poisoning typically have only an enlarged osmol gap, because isopropanol is not metabolized to any organic acids. Patients poisoned with the other toxic alcohols, such as diethylene glycol or butyl ethers from household cleaning products, have acidosis of varying degrees and inconsistently demonstrate an enlarged osmol gap.

## TYPICAL VARIATIONS

Ethylene glycol poisoning that progresses to significant organic acid accumulation can cause Kussmaul respirations from severe acidosis, cerebral edema, and seizures. Multiple reports have described various self-limited cranial nerve palsies associated with ethylene glycol. Tubular necrosis from local oxalate deposition and renal failure are common. Because oxalic acid precipitates calcium, dysrhythmias and tetanic spasms secondary to hypocalcemia have been reported.

Metabolism of methanol to formic acid gives rise primarily to neurologic and ophthalmologic findings. Patients who are not obtunded may have severe headache, vomiting, dizziness, and amnesia. Cerebral edema, necrosis, and infarcts have been identified on intracranial imaging. Visual disturbances range from simple blurring to "snowstorm" vision to blindness. Worrisome eye findings include sluggish nonreactive pupils, papilledema, a hyperemic optic disk, and retinal edema.

Isopropanol ingestion is associated with a fruity breath odor from acetone accumulation and CNS depression that is reportedly two to four times more profound than would be expected from an equivalent dose of ethanol. Vomiting and hemorrhagic gastritis have also been reported in patients with isopropanol ingestion.

Propylene glycol is metabolized to lactic acid. This poisoning typically occurs iatrogenically from the diluent present in parenteral medications such as phenytoin and various benzodiazepines. Accumulated lactate in these cases has been associated with profound hypotension and cardiac dysrhythmias.

Diethylene glycol and the other butyl ethers have been associated with renal tubular necrosis, hepatitis, and pancreatitis.

## DIFFERENTIAL DIAGNOSIS AND MEDICAL DECISION MAKING

The differential diagnosis mnemonic "A CAT MUD PILES" should be used for any patient in whom ED evaluation demonstrates an anion gap acidosis (**Box 151.1**). Many of the possible conditions in the list can be easily excluded with a basic metabolic profile (e.g., uremia) and rapidly obtainable serum quantitative tests (e.g., salicylate). Although alcoholic ketoacidosis looks like toxic alcohol poisoning, it improves rapidly with only intravenous fluids and dextrose supplementation, whereas acidosis from a significant toxic alcohol exposure does not improve without antidotal treatment or enhanced elimination with hemodialysis, or both. In children, disorders of organic acid metabolism should be considered when poisoning is unlikely or has been excluded.

**BOX 151.1 Metabolic Acidosis with Elevated Anion Gap: "A CAT MUD PILES"**

**A**lcoholic ketoacidosis
**C**yanide, carbon monoxide
**A**lcohol
**T**oluene
**M**ethanol, metformin
**U**remia
**D**iabetic ketoacidosis
**P**araldehyde
**I**ron, isoniazid
**L**actic acidosis
**E**thylene glycol
**S**alicylates, strychnine

Laboratory testing in all patients with potential poisoning should include a basic metabolic profile to determine baseline renal function and acid-base status and to calculate the anion gap and osmol gap. In calculation of the osmol gap, the measured osmolality must be obtained *at the same time* as the basic metabolic panel (see "Facts and Formulas" box). The osmol gap value should be interpreted with caution because it is an imperfect screening test. The traditionally accepted normal value for an osmol gap is less than 10 mOsm/L. Unfortunately, an individual's normal gap may range between −14 and +10 mOsm/L, so the osmol gap by itself is imperfect and not diagnostic.[9-11]

$SI = \frac{SV}{BSA}$ **FACTS AND FORMULAS**

**Anion Gap**

- Anion gap = $Na^+ - (HCO_3 + Cl^-)$ [normal anion gap = 8-12 mEq/L]
- Osmol gap = measured osmols − calculated osmols
- Calculated osmols = ($2Na^+$ + BUN/2.8 + glucose/18 + ethanol/4.6) [normal osmol gap < 10 mEq/L]

*BUN,* Blood urea nitrogen; *$HCO_3$,* bicarbonate.

Additional serum tests include the following: (1) an ethanol measurement, to enable accurate calculation of the osmol gap and determine the need for additional ADH inhibition; and (2) measurement of the calcium level, which can be depressed in cases of ethylene glycol poisoning and may lead to prolonged QT, cardiac dysrhythmias, and tetany. Arterial blood gas measurements should also be obtained to determine the level of acidosis.

Urinalysis should be performed to look for crystals: monohydrate (spindle-like) or dihydrate (envelope-shaped) crystals are present in 50% to 60% of cases of ethylene glycol poisoning and suggest significant poisoning. However, the absence of these crystals does not reliably exclude poisoning. Some authorities have suggested examining the urine under a Wood

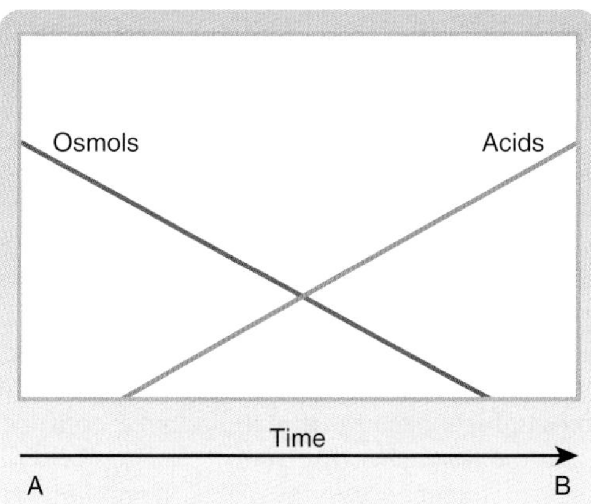


**Fig. 151.4 Mountain schematic.** Patients who present early may have elevated osmols without an anion gap *(A)*. Patients who present late may have an elevated anion gap without an elevation of osmol gap *(B)*.

lamp for fluorescence because antifreeze is commonly mixed with fluorescein. Unfortunately, urine may fluoresce in the presence or absence of ethylene glycol, so this maneuver has limited clinical utility.[12]

Although most clinicians are comfortable considering a diagnosis of ethylene glycol or methanol poisoning in patients with concomitant anion gap acidosis and an enlarged osmol gap, many patients do not arrive with those classic findings, and delays to definitive diagnosis and treatment are common.[6,11] Ethylene glycol and methanol are osmotically active and contribute to the enlarged osmol gap; the toxic metabolites are minimally osmotically active and primarily contribute to the anion gap. The Mountain schematic is useful in helping one understand the time course of acidosis and an osmol gap without needing to memorize the kinetics of each intermediate step (**Fig. 151.4**).[11]

### THE EARLY ARRIVAL

In a patient who arrives immediately after ingestion, as commonly occurs in children with an unintentional ingestion, anion gap acid acidosis is not present until enough time has elapsed for the parent product to be metabolized through ADH to produce laboratory evidence of acidosis. An enlarged osmol gap may be the only clue to potentially significant poisoning early after ingestion. In these cases, ADH inhibition with fomepizole or ethanol should be considered before acidosis develops (see Fig. 151.4, *A*).

### THE LATE ARRIVAL

In a patient who arrives with severe symptoms and significantly after ingestion, an abnormal osmol gap may no longer be present despite profound acidosis and other clinical findings suggestive of treatable toxic alcohol ingestion (e.g., visual disturbances in methanol ingestion, renal failure in ethylene glycol ingestion). In these cases, the parent product has already been metabolized to the toxic organic acids through ADH, so the osmotically active parent product no longer contributes significantly to the osmol gap. The benefit of an ADH inhibitor (fomepizole or ethanol) in these cases is less important than the benefit achieved from rapid hemodialysis and cofactor supplementation (see Fig. 151.4, *B*).

Although ED clinical decisions depend mostly on clinical suspicion and interpretation of imperfect laboratory data such as the anion gap, osmol gap, and urinalysis, cases of suspected toxic alcohol poisoning require that measurements of serum concentrations of ethylene glycol, methanol, and isopropanol be ordered as soon as possible. These measurements are the only definitive means of confirming the diagnosis and guiding duration of both antidotal therapy and hemodialysis. Unfortunately, most hospital laboratories are not equipped to run these tests and must send the specimens to an off-site reference laboratory.[11] Except when the patient arrives with the appropriately labeled product that was ingested in hand, a practical initial strategy is to order serum concentration measurements of all three of these alcohols because patients often do not know exactly what they ingested. Confirming the units of measure when these results are available is also important because different laboratories use different units, and management decisions may be significantly affected if test results are interpreted incorrectly. Serum concentration measurements for toxic alcohols other than ethylene glycol, methanol, and isopropanol are not routinely available; even if obtainable, test results do not guide management decisions.[13]

In cases of ethylene glycol poisoning, a baseline electrocardiogram should also be obtained because of the potential for dysrhythmias resulting from hypocalcemia.

## TREATMENT

Treatment decision making for the patient with toxic alcohol ingestion is easiest when the patient arrives with the ingested product in hand. Because this is an uncommon occurrence, definitive laboratory diagnosis is usually delayed by the need to send serum samples to off-site reference laboratories.[6,11] ED treatment in these cases should not be delayed and must be based on a presumptive clinical diagnosis. Attention to the airway in cases of CNS depression should be the first priority. Intravenous fluids should be administered to treat hypotension and maintain renal perfusion in all cases of toxic alcohol poisoning.

Because alcohols are so rapidly absorbed, gastric emptying procedures are not necessary in patients with toxic alcohol poisoning.

In cases of suspected ethylene glycol or methanol poisoning, immediate ADH inhibition should be considered to block continued metabolism of the ethylene glycol to toxic acids.[6] ADH inhibition is most effective when it is administered as early as possible after exposure and before significant acidosis develops.[11] This treatment should be considered in cases of a witnessed ingestion, when this agent is highly suspected from the history, in the presence of an elevated osmol gap alone with appropriate clinical suspicion, in the patient with both an elevated osmol gap and anion gap acidosis, or when the serum concentration of a toxic alcohol exceeds 20 mg/dL.

ADH inhibition can be achieved with either ethanol or fomepizole.[2,3,14] Until 1999, ethanol was the only clinically available antidote. Its affinity for ADH is higher than that of ethylene glycol and methanol, it is inexpensive, and it is readily available. An ethanol level of 100 mg/dL has been the accepted goal for ensuring complete ADH inhibition; after intravenous loading, ethanol levels must be checked regularly until the measured ethylene glycol or methanol concentration is lower than 20 mg/dL. An ethanol load may be administered orally or with an intravenous infusion (see "Facts and Formulas" box). Treatment difficulties associated with ethanol therapy include (1) iatrogenic inebriation of the patient and inability to monitor mental status, (2) potential occurrence of hypoglycemia in pediatric patients, and (3) difficulty maintaining a therapeutic level because of individual variability in ethanol metabolism and clearance.[14]

$SI = \frac{SV}{BSA}$ **FACTS AND FORMULAS**

**Antidotes for Toxic Alcohols**

**Fomepizole**

- Loading dose: 15 mg/kg IV (≤1 g)
- Maintenance therapy: 10 mg/kg IV every 12 hr for four doses, then 15 mg/kg every 12 hr (during hemodialysis, increase frequency to every 4 hr)

**Ethanol**

Goal: Maintain ethanol level of 100-150 mg/dL until ethylene glycol or methanol level is <20 mg/dL, pH normalizes, and patient is asymptomatic.

- 5% solution: 15 mL/kg IV load, then 2-4 mL/kg/hr
- 10% solution: 7.5 mL/kg IV load, then 1-2 mL/kg/hr
- 50% solution: 2 mL/kg oral load, then 0.2-0.4 mL/kg/hr

**Cofactor Supplementation**

- Folate: 50 mg IV every 6 hr until acidosis resolves (methanol only)
- Thiamine: 100 mg IV every 6 hr until acidosis resolves (ethylene glycol only)
- Pyridoxine: 50 mg IV every 6 hr until acidosis resolves (ethylene glycol only)

*IV*, Intravenously.

The use of fomepizole, which was approved by the U.S. Food and Drug Administration in 1999, is an easier form of ADH inhibition than the use of ethanol.[14-16] Dosing is weight based, and unlike ethanol, fomepizole does not require a constant infusion (see "Facts and Formulas" box). Fomepizole is given every 12 hours in patients not receiving hemodialysis or every 4 hours in patients undergoing hemodialysis, it does not cause inebriation, and it does not require monitoring of serum levels to ascertain therapeutic efficacy.[14] Fomepizole should not be given when ethanol concentrations are significantly elevated because ethanol works as an ADH inhibitor, and fomepizole's higher affinity for ADH will prolong the half-life and the clinical inebriation by the ethanol. Fomepizole is not available in all hospitals because of its high cost.[6]

In cases of poisoning with any of the toxic alcohols, the addition of a sodium bicarbonate infusion should be initiated when acidosis is severe. Alkalinization of serum is helpful in keeping acids in their ionic form. In patients with methanol poisoning, alkalinization of serum enhances the renal clearance of formate and may prevent formic acid from entering the CNS and affecting the optic nerves.

In cases of ethylene glycol poisoning, supplemental thiamine and pyridoxine should be administered to decrease the accumulation of oxalic acid (see "Facts and Formulas" box). In cases of methanol poisoning, supplemental folate should be given to enhance the elimination of formate by converting it to carbon dioxide and water. Although this approach is theoretically beneficial and has been found to be useful in some animal models, no human data demonstrate a clear benefit of cofactor administration.

Hemodialysis should be initiated in any patient with a significant ethylene glycol or methanol concentration and significant acidosis because it helps remove both the parent product and the resultant toxic acids.[17-19] When a serum concentration is not immediately available, hemodialysis should be initiated in patients with clinical indicators of significant toxicity, such as pH less than 7.30 despite aggressive intravenous fluid resuscitation, creatinine concentration indicative of renal failure, or other electrolyte abnormalities unresponsive to conventional therapy.[2,3,17] Hemodialysis should also be initiated soon after presentation in patients in whom ADH inhibition cannot be used because of antidote unavailability or a contraindication. Hemodialysis should also be considered to shorten the duration of antidote requirements and of hospitalization when acidosis has not occurred but the serum concentration of the toxic alcohol is extremely high.[17,18] For example, the half-life of methanol has been reported to be as long as 54 hours in patients receiving ADH inhibition, and these patients may require several days of hospitalization and antidotal therapy if hemodialysis is not performed as well (**Fig. 151.5**).

Management of the other toxic alcohol poisonings requires aggressive supportive therapy, attention to the medical complications of acidosis, and hemodialysis only in the presence of significant renal insufficiency or other electrolyte abnormalities.[13] Despite the similarity of its name to ethylene glycol, diethylene glycol does not produce oxalic acid, and any benefit from ADH inhibition in cases of diethylene glycol poisoning is uncertain.[20]

**TIPS AND TRICKS**

- Consult your local poison center: 800-222-1222.
- Refer to the Mountain schematic (see Fig. 151.4) to help interpret anion gap and osmol gap results.
- If long delays until definitive laboratory confirmation of the ingested substance are expected, consider repeating the basic metabolic profile or measure arterial blood gases.
- If alcohol dehydrogenase has not been blocked by fomepizole or ethanol, acidosis should worsen despite standard intravenous fluid resuscitation if ethylene glycol or methanol is present.
- Treatment difficulties associated with ethanol therapy are (1) iatrogenic inebriation and inability to monitor mental status, (2) potential occurrence of hypoglycemia in children, and (3) difficulty maintaining a therapeutic level because of individual variability in ethanol metabolism and clearance.

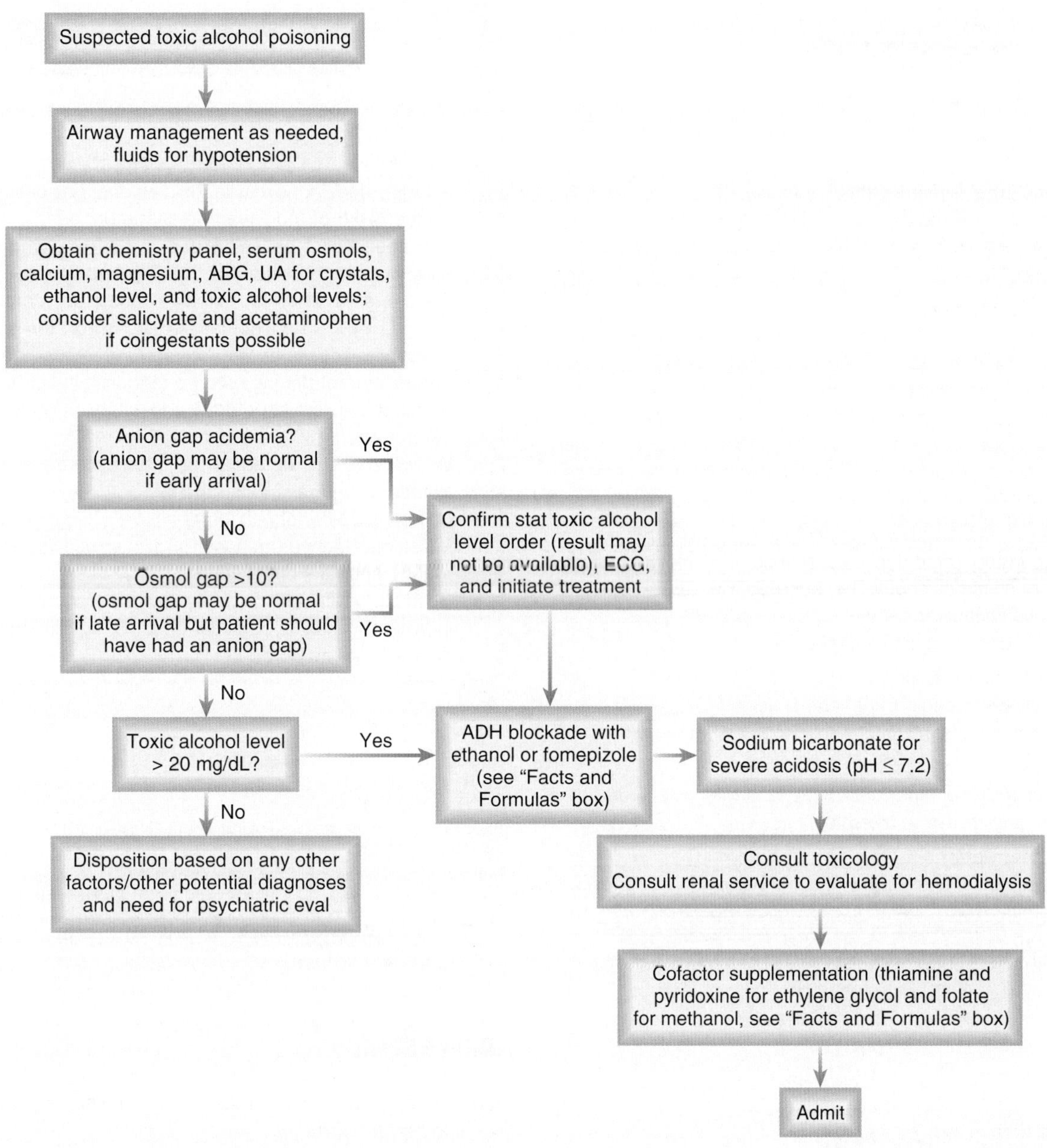


**Fig. 151.5 Treatment algorithm for toxic alcohol poisoning.** *ABG,* Arterial blood gas measurements; *ADH,* alcohol dehydrogenase; *ECG,* electrocardiography; *UA,* urinalysis.

## DISPOSITION

Patients without acidosis and with a toxic serum alcohol level less than 20 mg/dL may be discharged home if clinical findings and renal function are normal. Any patient receiving an ADH antidote must be admitted to the hospital until a definitive serum alcohol concentration is available. Patients with significant mental status depression or acidosis, patients who are receiving an intravenous ethanol infusion, or patients who need hemodialysis should be admitted to the intensive care unit because laboratory values must be checked frequently. Patients who arrive early after a significant ingestion may be considered for treatment in a setting other than the intensive care unit; these patients are given fomepizole therapy alone if no acidosis was detected before administration of the antidote.

In cases of intentional ingestion, appropriate psychiatric evaluation is warranted after the patient's medical issues are treated. In cases of unintentional poisoning, especially in children, appropriate poison prevention counseling for all caregivers is required before discharge.[21]

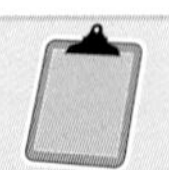

## DOCUMENTATION

**History**
- Any history of psychiatric illness or earlier suicidal ingestions
- Time lapse since ingestion if known
- History of renal or cardiac disease or other illnesses that will exacerbate the complications of toxic alcohols

**Physical Examination**
- Does the patient look ill? Pale? Febrile? Mental status? Cardiac status (blood pressure, arrhythmias)?
- Respiratory and airway status
- Visual acuity if concern exists for methanol poisoning
- Urine output
- Repeated examination while patient is in the emergency department

**Studies**
- Laboratory tests and time the samples were obtained (serum osmol should be done at the same time as blood chemistry panel)
- Availability of toxic alcohol levels

**Medical Decision Making**
- Decision to begin treatment or delays
- Consultations and times that contacts were made

**Treatment**
- Availability of antidotes, time antidote was ordered, and any delays to treatment

**Patient Instructions**
- Document discussion with patient regarding diagnosis, warning signs, what to do, follow-up, and when to return
- With accidental ingestions in children, document poison prevention counseling

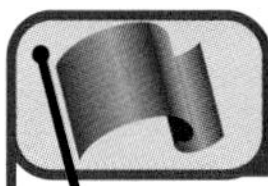

## RED FLAGS

- Urinalysis: The absence of crystals or fluorescence does *not* exclude poisoning.
- The absence of an osmol gap in patients with severe acidosis does *not* exclude toxic alcohol poisoning; it may be the result of a delayed presentation.
- The absence of an anion gap in patients who present early does *not* exclude toxic alcohol poisoning.
- Be prepared to have definitive laboratory confirmation delayed by 8 to 24 hours, depending on the individual hospital's access to an outside reference laboratory. Empirical treatment should be started if indicated.
- Renal specialists should be consulted early, to prevent complications.
- Be wary of the potential for hypoglycemia in patients treated with intravenous ethanol.
- *Do not* give ethanol with fomepizole. Both agents compete for alcohol dehydrogenase, and their use together may reduce antidotal effectiveness.
- Because metabolism varies by alcohol type and by individual variability, clinical onset of symptoms can be delayed by 1 to 36 hours.

## SUGGESTED READINGS

Barceloux DG, Krenzelok EP, Olson K, et al. American Academy of Clinical Toxicology practice guidelines on the treatment of ethylene glycol poisoning. Clin Toxicol 1999;37:537-60.

Barceloux DG, Bond GR, Krenzelok EP, et al. American Academy of Clinical Toxicology practice guidelines on the treatment of methanol poisoning. Clin Toxicol 2002;40:415-46.

Brent J Fomepizole for ethylene glycol and methanol poisoning. N Engl J Med 2009;360:2216-23.

Hoffman RS, Smilkstein MJ, Howland MA, Goldfrank LR. Osmol gaps revisited: normal values and limitations. Clin Toxicol 1993;31:81-93.

Mycyk MB, Aks SE. A visual schematic for clarifying the temporal relationship between the anion gap and the osmol gap in cases of toxic alcohol poisoning. Am J Emerg Med 2003;21:333-5.

## REFERENCES

*References can be found on Expert Consult @ www.expertconsult.com.*

# Hydrocarbons 152

*David D. Gummin*

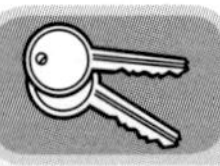

**KEY POINTS**

- Many hydrocarbons possess a characteristic odor similar to that of gasoline or lighter fluid. Solvents containing aldehyde or ketone groups smell sweet or fruity, and essential oils are characteristically pungent or aromatic. In acutely intoxicated patients, these odors are rarely missed.
- In assessing the patient with possible hydrocarbon exposure, important tasks are as follows:
  - Identification of the specific substance or substances
  - Quantification of the dose
  - Determination of the timing, duration, and course of exposure
  - Identification of the route or routes of exposure
  - Consultation or referral, or both, when indicated
- Many hydrocarbons are acutely cardiotoxic and have a propensity to induce tachyarrhythmias by sensitizing the myocardium to the arrhythmogenic effects of catecholamines.
- Gaseous or volatilized hydrocarbons are likely to cause toxicity through inhalation.
- Viscosity, surface tension, and volatility determine the aspiration potential and the risk of pulmonary toxicity.

## EPIDEMIOLOGY

Adolescents 12 to 17 years old comprise the most likely age group to abuse volatile substances; U.S. eighth grade students have a 15% lifetime prevalence of this abuse. Volatile substance use should be suspected in this population. The habitual abuser of volatile substances may have paint stains or other telltale findings on the clothing or skin (see "Presenting Signs and Symptoms").

Many hydrocarbons have a characteristic odor similar to that of gasoline or lighter fluid. Solvents containing aldehyde or ketone groups smell sweet or fruity. Essential oils are characteristically pungent or aromatic. In acutely intoxicated patients, these odors are rarely missed.

## PATHOPHYSIOLOGY

A hydrocarbon is an organic compound composed mainly of carbon and hydrogen atoms. In modern society, these compounds are virtually everywhere. Hydrocarbons are so common in our society that exposures—even illnesses related to exposures—are not usually documented. Hydrocarbons derive most commonly from distillation and processing of petroleum, but many derive from plants (pine oil, essential oils), animal fats, and natural gas. An example is gasoline, which is a mixture of alkanes, alkenes, naphthenes, and aromatic hydrocarbons. Commercial gasoline contains hundreds—up to 1500—individual chemical species.

The term *solvent* is often used to refer to an organic solvent—typically a hydrocarbon mixture—that is used to dissolve other substances. Occupational literature often uses the terms *solvent* and *hydrocarbon* interchangeably. Organic solvents are common in industry, and workers may suffer dermal or inhalational exposures. Children may suffer unintentional hydrocarbon exposures, often ingestions, with a risk of pulmonary hydrocarbon aspiration. More concerning is a trend toward greater intentional abuse of volatile hydrocarbon inhalants by adolescents and young adults. This form of substance abuse, often termed volatile substance abuse (VSA), is a growing problem worldwide.

One can predict many of the physical properties of hydrocarbons by knowing the molecular shape and size (number of carbon atoms in the molecule's chain). The nonpolar, covalent bonds between carbon-carbon and carbon-hydrogen atoms produce *dispersion forces,* which result in the attraction between hydrocarbon molecules. These same forces repel polar molecules (e.g., water) and make hydrocarbons generally hydrophobic. Once dissolved in aqueous solution, nonpolar hydrocarbons can transit rapidly through lipid membranes, including cell membranes and the blood-brain barrier. Small, light, aliphatic hydrocarbons with up to 4 carbons are gases at room temperature; those with 5 to 19 carbon molecules are liquids; and longer molecules form solids or *paraffins.* Branching in the molecule destabilizes intermolecular forces, so less energy is required to separate molecules. This makes it easier for a molecule to leave the liquid phase and enter the vapor phase (to *volatilize*). Therefore, for a given molecular size, more branching means a lower boiling point, and the compound is typically more volatile. Gaseous or volatilized hydrocarbons are likely to cause toxicity by inhalation.

**Table 152.1 Hydrocarbon Properties and Aspiration Risk**

| | DEFINITION | EXAMPLE | VALUE VS. RISK |
|---|---|---|---|
| Viscosity | Measure of a fluid's resistance to flow | Higher tendency for aspiration in animal models of low-viscosity substances (<60 SUS [e.g., turpentine, gasoline, naphtha]) | Lower value predicts higher risk |
| Surface tension | Indirect measure of dispersion forces between molecules; also the interaction with the surface that the fluid contacts | Adherence of the fluid along a surface ("the inability to creep") | Lower value predicts higher risk |
| Volatility | Tendency for a liquid to enter the gas phase | Tendency of highly volatile hydrocarbons, which have a high vapor pressure, to vaporize, enter the lungs, displace oxygen, and cause hypoxia | Higher value predicts higher risk |

*SUS,* Saybolt universal seconds.

Lipid-soluble solvents (aromatic, aliphatic, or halogenated hydrocarbons) are more likely than water-soluble hydrocarbons (alcohols, ketones, or esters) to cause acute central nervous system (CNS) effects. Clinicians are familiar with these effects from experience with inhaled anesthetic agents, which cause CNS sedation similar to that resulting from other hydrocarbons. The Meyer-Overton hypothesis suggests that inhaled anesthetics dissolve into some critical lipid compartment of the CNS and cause generalized inhibition of neuronal transmission. This mechanism is probably oversimplified, but it helps to explain partly the nonspecific inhibition of neuronal transmission that hydrocarbons produce in the CNS. Specific membrane interactions may also contribute to this process,[1] and several receptor-mediated interactions are known to occur.

Specific physical properties of ingested hydrocarbons help to predict the risk of pulmonary aspiration (**Table 152.1**). In particular, viscosity, surface tension, and volatility determine aspiration potential and the contribution to pulmonary toxicity.[2] *Viscosity* is a measure of a fluid's resistance to flow, commonly described in units of Saybolt universal seconds (SUS). This property is not the same as the fluid's density; in fact, these two properties correlate poorly.

Low-viscosity substances (less than 60 SUS), such as turpentine, gasoline, or naphtha, have higher tendency for aspiration in animal models. *A lower viscosity value predicts a higher risk.* The U.S. Consumer Products Safety Commission now requires child-resistant packaging for products that contain 10% or more hydrocarbons and have a measured viscosity less than 100 SUS.

*Surface tension* indirectly measures dispersion forces between molecules in a fluid, but it also characterizes the interaction with the surface that the fluid contacts. This property can be quantified on a modified Wilhelmy balance, which measures adherence of the fluid along a surface ("the inability to creep"). In theory, the lower the surface tension is, the higher is the aspiration risk.[2] *A lower surface tension value predicts a higher risk.*

*Volatility* is the tendency for a liquid to enter the gas phase. Hydrocarbons that are highly volatile have a high vapor pressure and so tend to vaporize, enter the lungs, displace oxygen, and cause hypoxia. *A higher volatility value predicts a higher risk.*

## MECHANISMS OF TOXICITY

Although organ-specific pathophysiology is often unique to individual agents, much of the toxicity of hydrocarbons results from their ability to dissolve fats or, similarly, to diffuse across hydrophobic barriers intended to protect anatomic structures (e.g., lipid bilayers, myelin). Hydrocarbon solvents cause irritation of skin and mucous membranes. Recurrent or prolonged contact results in "defatting" of skin, dissolving lipid components, and disrupting the normal architecture of the stratum corneum.[3]

Most hydrocarbons are flammable or combustible. Under appropriate conditions, most hydrocarbons can explode. The widespread availability of hydrocarbons and their use as organic solvents account for the frequent finding of stored quantities of these solvents in clandestine illicit drug laboratories and other places. Storage and use of these flammable agents appreciably contribute to the health hazards of these facilities.

### SKIN EFFECTS

The skin is a common site of contact and a potential portal of entry for hydrocarbons. Skin is composed of both hydrophilic and hydrophobic elements. Agents that contain both hydrophobic and hydrophilic regions (glycol ethers, dimethylformamide, dimethylsulfoxide) are highly absorbed. Dermal absorption usually constitutes a small fraction of the hydrocarbon dose absorbed by other routes (e.g., inhalation), however. The absorbed dose depends on the surface area exposed, the duration of contact, and skin's integrity (e.g., cut, abraded).[5]

## GASTROINTESTINAL EFFECTS

Ingested hydrocarbons typically cause local gastrointestinal (GI) irritation. Most hydrocarbons are poorly absorbed from the GI tract.

Chlorinated hydrocarbons are often hepatotoxic. Carbon tetrachloride is a prototype hepatotoxin that causes centrilobular necrosis through a reactive intermediate metabolite. Other halogenated and nonhalogenated hydrocarbons have been associated with hepatic insult, including trichloroethylene, tetrachloroethylene, benzene, and even petroleum distillates. Vinyl chloride is a well-known hepatic carcinogen.

## PULMONARY EFFECTS

Gaseous or volatilized hydrocarbons can be inhaled, thus displacing alveolar oxygen and causing hypoxia. Contact with lung tissue results in interstitial inflammation, polymorphonuclear infiltration and exudate, intraalveolar edema and hemorrhage, hyperemia, bronchial and bronchiolar necrosis, and vascular thrombosis. These results likely reflect both direct cytotoxicity and disruption of the surfactant layer that lead to poor oxygen exchange, atelectasis, and pneumonitis, with reductions in lung compliance and total lung capacity.

Severe hydrocarbon pneumonitis also results from intravenous injection of a hydrocarbon. In animals, intravascular hydrocarbons injure the first capillary bed encountered. The clinical course after intravenous hydrocarbon exposure mirrors that of aspiration injury.[5]

## CARDIAC EFFECTS

Many hydrocarbons are acutely cardiotoxic. Especially important is their propensity to induce tachyarrhythmias. The mechanism by which hydrocarbons cause malignant rhythms is poorly characterized, but some of these agents can precipitate ventricular tachycardia or fibrillation and can cause sudden death.

Endogenous or exogenous catecholamines (e.g., epinephrine) are proarrhythmic. Hydrocarbons enhance this potential and are said to sensitize the myocardium to the arrhythmogenic effects of catecholamines. Essentially every class of hydrocarbon compounds, including general anesthetic agents, can sensitize the heart. Some classes carry a high risk, however, and others sensitize the myocardium modestly, if at all. The ability of these substances to sensitize the heart constitutes an accepted system for grading halocarbon (e.g., Freon) toxicity. Unsaturated, aliphatic hydrocarbons (e.g., ethylene) and aliphatic ethers have been studied but do not appear to be sensitizers. Other unsaturated compounds (e.g., acetylene), are weak sensitizers. Aromatic hydrocarbons and, especially, halogenated hydrocarbons are often potent sensitizers.[6]

Sensitization appears to be mediated by slowed conduction velocity, possibly by chemical and functional changes in the membrane transport proteins at gap junctions. The major ventricular gap junction protein is composed of connexin 43. This protein is regulated by phosphorylation, such that the dephosphorylated state of the hexamers in the channel is associated with greater gap junction resistance. In the presence of epinephrine, halocarbons increase gap junction resistance in myocardial tissue and slow conduction velocity.[7]

## NERVOUS SYSTEM EFFECTS

The mechanism by which hydrocarbons depress consciousness is unknown. Diffusion across the blood-brain barrier with neuronal membrane stabilization provides the foundation of the Meyer-Overton hypothesis. To date, no specific receptor wholly explains this generalized effect. In cases of pulmonary toxicity, hypoxemia may contribute to depressed consciousness.[8]

Chronic solvent abuse leads to irreversible CNS toxicity, best described in the setting of toluene abuse. Volitional abusers demonstrate loss of cerebral white matter, with a characteristic syndrome of cognitive and motor deficits. Autopsied brains of long-term toluene abusers show profound atrophy and mottling of the white matter, as though the lipid-based myelin had been dissolved away. Microscopic examination shows a consistent pattern of demyelination, with relative preservation of axons. These pathologic features correlate with the clinical syndrome of subcortical dementia.[9] Mild cognitive deficits show improvement after 6 months of abstinence. In patients with advanced disease, regardless of the exposure history, full recovery is unlikely.[10]

Exposure to n-hexane or to methyl n-butyl ketone (MnBK) can cause peripheral neuropathy. This toxic axonopathy appears to result from 2,5-hexanedione, a metabolic intermediate common to both agents. The mechanism appears to involve decreased phosphorylation of neurofilament proteins, with disruption of the axonal cytoskeleton.[11]

Radiologically and histopathologically, prolonged and repeated exposures to toluene are associated with brain demyelination. Although the mechanism of this process is not fully understood, it is presumed to result from dissolution of myelin by the solvent. Toluene encephalopathy is characterized by a specific constellation of findings, alternatively described as "subcortical dementia," "white matter dementia," or "toxic leukoencephalopathy." Findings include the following: loss of cortical gray matter–white matter differentiation; atrophic changes in the basal ganglia, cerebellum, pons, and thalamus; and thinning of the corpus callosum. Changes noted on magnetic resonance imaging appear to progress in a lifetime dose–dependent fashion.[12] Unfortunately, toluene is an addictive substance, and progression of abnormalities is likely with persistent use. Resolution of neurologic abnormalities has not been documented once white matter loss becomes radiographically evident. Complete recovery from solvent encephalopathy is not considered likely, even with abstinence or removal from exposure.[10]

## RENAL EFFECTS

Halogenated hydrocarbons may be nephrotoxic. Examples include chloroform, carbon tetrachloride, and ethylene dichloride. Furthermore, recurrent or prolonged toluene exposure causes distal renal tubular acidosis. Sodium loss in the urine may transform the initial nongap metabolic acidosis into anion gap–positive metabolic acidosis. Toluene's principal metabolite, hippuric acid, contributes to the elevated anion gap. Renal potassium loss may be severe and can result in symptomatic hypokalemia. In one series, distal renal tubular acidosis was seen in 44% of hospitalized paint sniffers.[13]

## OTHER EFFECTS

Methylene chloride and other halomethanes are metabolized to carbon monoxide by CYP 2E1 (a member of the cytochrome P-450 enzyme system). Significant and prolonged carboxyhemoglobin levels can be measured after inhalational

**Table 152.2 Symptoms Associated with Hydrocarbon Exposure**

| SYMPTOM | NOTES |
|---|---|
| Coughing, choking, or vomiting | Heightens suspicion of pulmonary aspiration |
| Behavioral changes, impaired sense of smell, impaired concentration, and mildly unsteady movements or gait | Transient excitation initially possible after inhalation or ingestion, but early sedation more common |
| Elevated temperature | Initially noted in hydrocarbon aspiration<br>Often spiking at 8 to 12 hours and then declining over several days, unless bacterial superinfection occurs |
| Drying, cracking, pitting, or eczematous lesions | Contact dermatitis or frostbite injury with intentional abuse |
| Muscle weakness | Renal tubular acidosis associated with hypokalemia, with consequent muscle weakness or arrhythmia, possibly the presenting complaint |
| Seizures | Uncommon, probably because of overwhelming anesthetic effects, and should raise suspicion of a coingestant<br>Exceptions: (1) seizures that occur after large ingestion of pine oil or essential oils (e.g., oil of wormwood, fennel oil) and (2) anoxic seizures |
| Persistent hypoxia | Methemoglobinemia, carbon monoxide toxicity, and blood dyscrasias associated with specific ingestions |
| Peripheral neuropathy | Beginning in distal extremities and progressing proximally |

or dermal exposures. This metabolic toxicant appears to be exclusively generated by halomethanes.

Some hydrocarbon agents contain nitrogenous moieties, and mixtures may contain coloring additives (e.g., aniline) that can induce methemoglobinemia. Benzene is directly hematotoxic, and it is associated with hemolysis, aplastic anemia, and acute myelogenous leukemia. Because of benzene's cancer risk, toluene has largely replaced benzene in many commercial products worldwide.

## PRESENTING SIGNS AND SYMPTOMS

The route of exposure considerably influences the organs affected. The principal organ systems affected by hydrocarbons are the skin (from dermal contact), the GI system (when ingested), the CNS, and the lungs. Some classes of hydrocarbons are cardiotoxic. Certain agents may cause organ-specific toxicity to cranial or peripheral nerves, the liver, or the kidneys. Typical presenting symptoms can be found in **Table 152.2**.

The intentional inhalation in VSA can be challenging to diagnose because affected patients frequently withhold relevant history. Several common inhalational techniques have been identified. *Sniffing* involves inhaling vapor from an open container. *Huffing* involves placing a volatile hydrocarbon in a rag or cloth, then covering the nose and mouth with the cloth or rag and inhaling the agent through it. *Bagging* implies placing the substance inside a plastic (or other) bag and then putting the bag over the face to inhale hydrocarbon vapor.

Respiratory findings are uncommon after inhalation, but the patient may manifest tachypnea or cyanosis or may suffer sudden cardiac arrest. Classically, cardiac arrest occurs after a sudden fright or physical exertion (e.g., running to avoid an authority), with a sudden catecholamine surge and a sensitized heart. This phenomenon is termed the sudden sniffing death syndrome.

Cutaneous findings may be the chief complaints, with dermal exposure to solvents from work or hobbies. Drying, cracking, pitting, or eczematous lesions occur in up to 9% of workers who are repeatedly exposed. Allergic reactions are uncommon but may be seen with exposure to certain essential oils or to pine oil. Nonspecific skin irritation is the most common finding, and it may progress to blistering or contact dermatitis with recurrent, prolonged, or protracted VSA. With continued or recurring exposure, the skin changes may even progress to partial- or even full-thickness chemical burns.[4] When the dermatitis involves the skin surrounding the nose and mouth, it has been dubbed "huffer's rash" (**Fig. 152.1**). Abusers of volatile solvents may have telltale paint, shoeshine, or solvent stains on clothes or skin. Nonfreezing cold injury (frostbite) may occur on or about the face because of intentional release of liquid hydrocarbon propellant, which cools as it suddenly exits its container (**Fig. 152.2**).

Hydrocarbons cause CNS depression. Transient excitation may initially occur after inhalation or ingestion, but early sedation is more common. Initial findings include behavioral changes, impaired sense of smell, impaired concentration, and mildly unsteady movements or gait. As with alcohol or other sedatives, mild exposures produce euphoria, likely contributing to abuse potential. Further acute exposure leads to slurred speech and progressive incoordination. Physical signs are nystagmus, tremor, spasticity with hyperreflexia, abnormal plantar reflexes, hearing loss, impaired vision, and a broad-based, staggering gait. Pain inhibition explains why hydrocarbons were chosen as general anesthetic agents. Stupor, lethargy, or obtundation is seen in overdose. Coma and seizures occur in up to 3% of cases.[14]

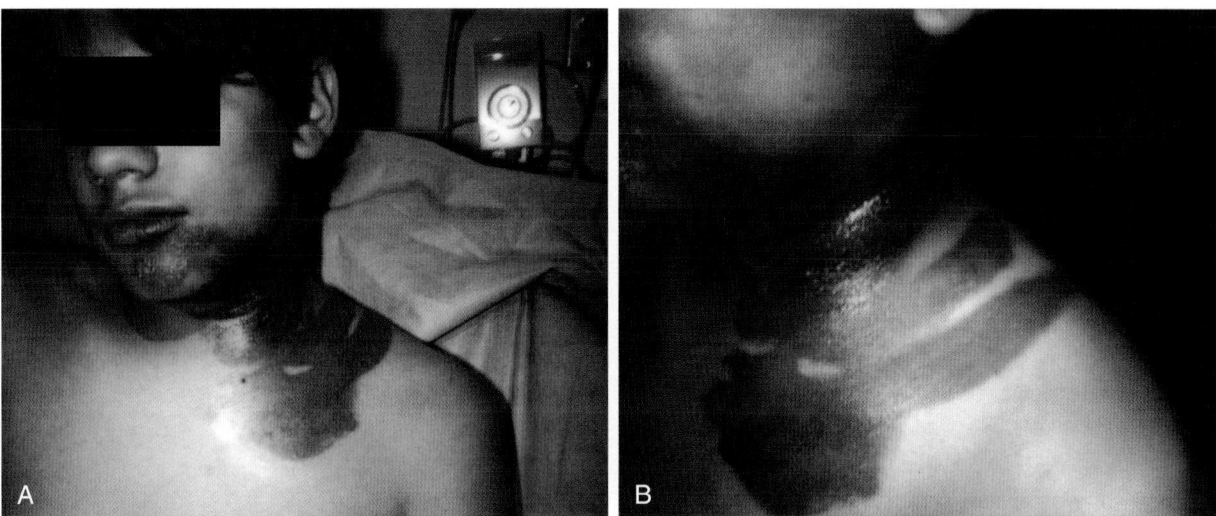


**Fig. 152.1 A and B, "Huffer's rash" resulting from repeated "sniffing" of liquid propane.** Both contact dermatitis and nonfreezing cold injury likely contribute to the skin findings in this characteristic distribution. (Courtesy of E. O'Connell, MD.)

Chronic CNS dysfunction occurs in recurrent abusers of volatile substances, and reports include optic neuropathy, sensorineural hearing loss, equilibrium disorders, ataxia, and cognitive deficits. Occupational solvent exposures are also associated with persistent CNS abnormalities, although the exposures and the clinical findings are typically less impressive than those in habitual VSA. Most published reports involve exposure to toluene, a very common workplace and household hydrocarbon solvent. Neurologic deficits are tremor, ataxia, impaired fine-motor skills, and mild cognitive defects. Long-term occupational exposures are associated with a clinical syndrome consisting of fatigue, poor short-term memory, attention difficulties, visuospatial abnormalities, personality changes, and mood disorder. Clinically, this presentation has been dubbed "the painter's syndrome."

Abdominal pain and vomiting are common, and diarrhea is likely after ingestion, particularly of insoluble hydrocarbons (mineral oil, paraffins). Vomiting increases the risk of pulmonary aspiration.

A typical case in the emergency department (ED) involves a young child who is suspected to have unintentionally ingested a hydrocarbon mixture. Infrequently, a parent may have witnessed the ingestion; more typically, the situation was discovered shortly thereafter. The caregiver often identifies the specific agent. A parent may report that the child was coughing, gagging, or vomiting, or that he or she noticed an odor of the suspected hydrocarbon. If the ingestion was unwitnessed, it may be difficult to quantify the amount ingested, but a "worst case scenario" can often be ascertained. A history of coughing, choking, or vomiting should heighten the ED's suspicion of pulmonary aspiration. Respiratory findings include coughing, choking, gagging, grunting, tachypnea, retractions, fever, cyanosis or poor coloration, and abnormal sounds on chest auscultation. Mental status depression is common in patients with larger ingestions but may not occur for 30 to 60 minutes after ingestion. In a prospective, multicenter study of 760 pediatric kerosene ingestions, no association was found between the age of the patient and the amount ingested. The risks of pulmonary toxicity and of CNS depression were significantly higher in children who ingested more than 30 mL of kerosene (according to history). The incidence of pulmonary aspiration was higher in children who vomited after ingestion.[15]

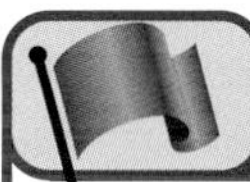

**RED FLAGS**

- History of coughing, choking, or vomiting should heighten the suspicion for pulmonary aspiration.
- Sudden sniffing death syndrome classically occurs after a sudden fright or physical exertion (e.g., running to avoid an authority), with a sudden catecholamine surge and a sensitized heart.
- Abusers of volatile solvents may have telltale paint, shoe-shine, or solvent stains on clothes or skin.
- Nonfreezing cold injury (frostbite) may occur on or about the face; it is caused by intentional release of liquid hydrocarbon propellant, which cools as it suddenly exits its container.
- Hypokalemia, with consequent muscle weakness or arrhythmia, may be the presenting complaint in abusers of volatile substances in whom renal tubular acidosis develops from recurrent toluene exposure.
- An adolescent or teen who presents to the emergency department with sudden death or a malignant tachyarrhythmia (especially ventricular tachycardia or ventricular fibrillation) must be considered to have been abusing hydrocarbons unless the emergency physician is able to demonstrate otherwise.
- Hydrocarbons do not generally affect systemic vascular resistance, so coingestants should be considered in the persistently hypotensive patient.
- Hypotension may relate to excessive positive end-expiration pressure (PEEP), and reducing PEEP may improve hemodynamics.

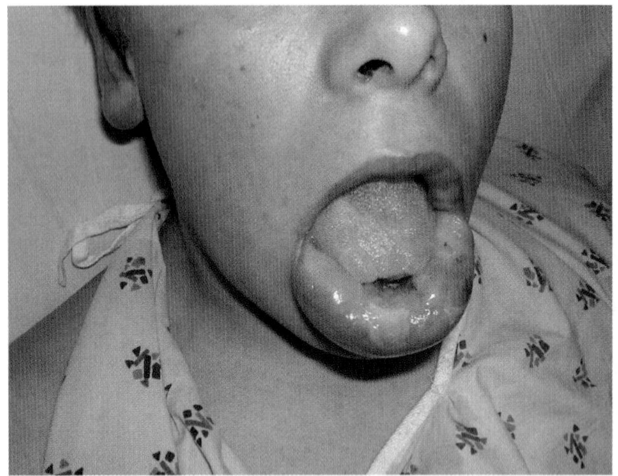

**Fig. 152.2 Nonfreezing cold injury resulting from intentional release and attempted inhalation of halocarbon propellant.**

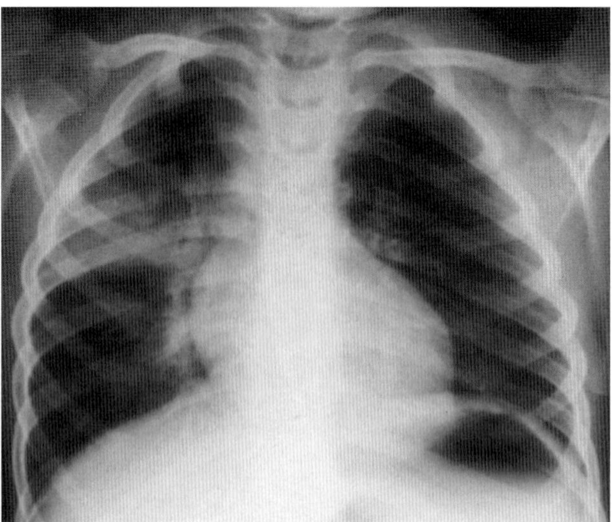

**Fig. 152.3 Aspiration pneumonitis in a child who ingested a hydrocarbon mixture.** Note the early consolidation in the right upper lobe. Although 75% of cases demonstrate right-sided findings, upper lobe involvement is not common.

## DIFFERENTIAL DIAGNOSIS AND MEDICAL DECISION MAKING

The differential diagnosis in hydrocarbon exposure is usually limited because the history often elucidates the exposure. Some possible differential diagnoses include adult respiratory distress syndrome, toxic alcohol exposure, barbiturate or benzodiazepine toxicity, and toluene exposure.

The diagnostic evaluation of a patient with hydrocarbon exposure depends heavily on the known patterns of toxicity associated with specific hydrocarbon agents and the route of exposure. It is more crucial to obtain and verify the history, with particular attention to identifying the specific type and composition of the agent or agents involved. The route of exposure should direct the clinician to the anticipated target organ or organs, which guide testing.

Renal function, serum electrolyte levels, and acid-base status should be evaluated in all patients with a history of chronic or recurrent toluene exposure. Liver transaminases and bilirubin should be assayed in patients with significant exposure to halocarbons or to benzene. Electrocardiographic monitoring and a formal 12-lead electrocardiogram are indicated when a patients has significant exposure to heart-sensitizing hydrocarbon agents. Head computed tomography and magnetic resonance imaging are valuable to assess the extent of brain involvement in chronic exposures. Pulse oximetry or arterial blood gas testing helps assess the severity of pulmonary injury. Carboxyhemoglobin or methemoglobin measurements are indicated for exposures involving specific agents (see "Other Effects").

Early chest radiography may be indicated for severely symptomatic patients, to gauge the extent of pulmonary injury and guide the inpatient placement decision. Radiographic evidence of pneumonitis may develop as early as 15 minutes or as late as 24 hours after hydrocarbon aspiration. Ninety percent of patients who have radiographic abnormalities do so within 4 hours.[16] After the initial episode of coughing, gagging, or choking, most patients with persistent respiratory signs and symptoms have pneumonitis and radiographic changes. Typical findings in hydrocarbon pneumonitis are audible abnormalities on chest auscultation, fever, leukocytosis, and abnormalities on chest radiograph (**Fig. 152.3**). These findings do not differ clinically from those of community-acquired pneumonia. Only the history differentiates the two entities. The elevated temperature initially noted in hydrocarbon aspiration often spikes at 8 to 12 hours, then declines over several days, unless bacterial superinfection intervenes. For an asymptomatic patient with hydrocarbon ingestion, however, early radiography does not help predict aspiration pneumonitis, and it is not cost-effective.

Results of bioassays and serum hydrocarbon levels are rarely available to the emergency physician and have little to no value in management of hydrocarbon exposure. These measurements are available through reference laboratories for occupational monitoring or to document exposure in forensic cases.

## TREATMENT

### DECONTAMINATION

An algorithm for the treatment of hydrocarbon exposure is shown in **Figure 152.4**. The first priority in managing toxicity is to protect rescuers. Personal protection is paramount at each level of health care delivery. Second, the exposure should be removed from the patient, and the patient should be removed from the exposure. Contaminated clothing and external contamination must be removed before the patient enters any patient care or trafficked area. For most hydrocarbons, soap and water are all that are required for decontamination. Most hydrocarbons are flammable and pose a fire risk to the hospital and staff. Personal protective equipment should be worn by anyone who will touch the patient or any articles brought with the patient. Once the patient is externally decontaminated, standard precautions generally suffice in the ED.

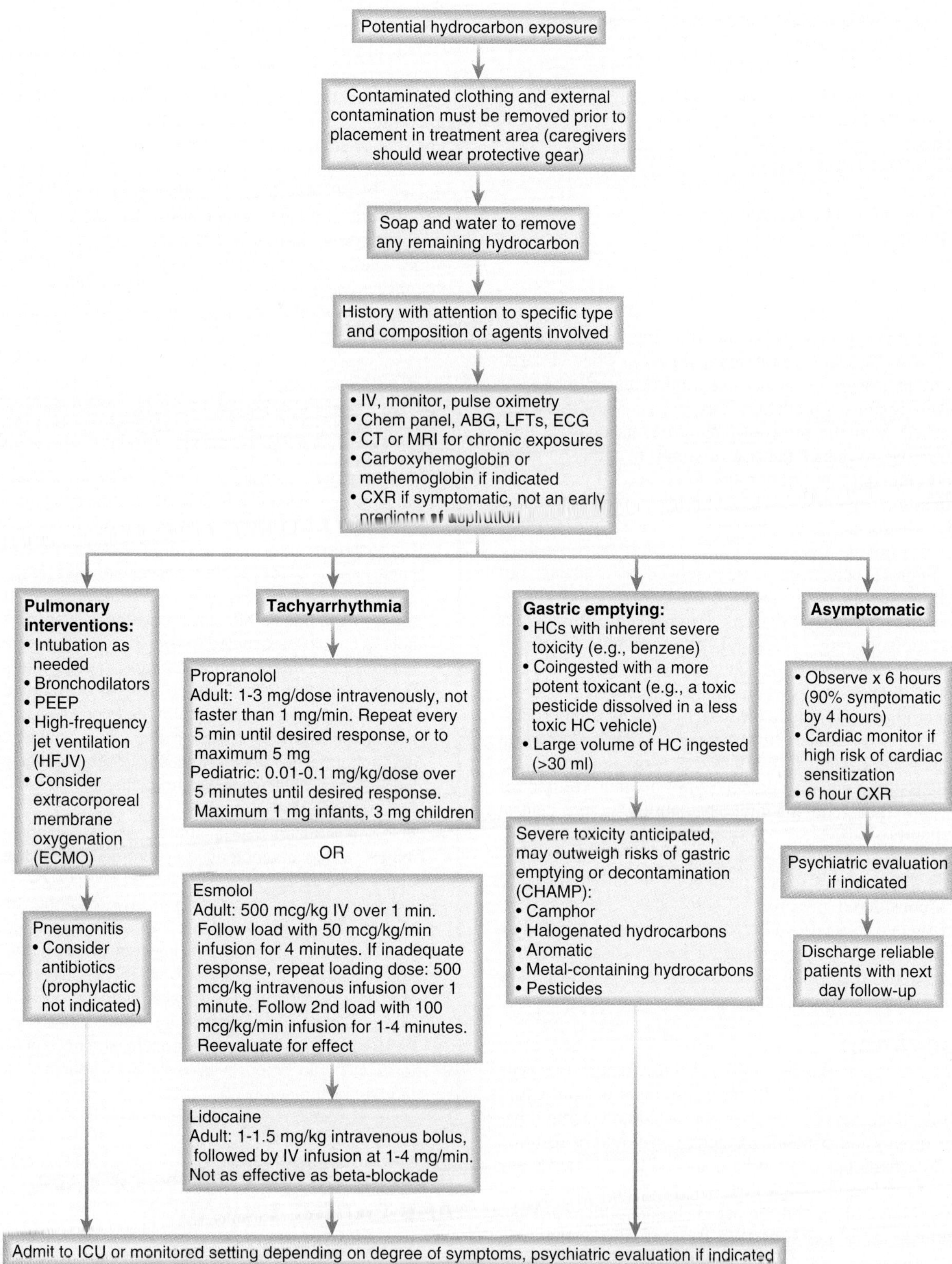


**Fig. 152.4 Treatment algorithm for hydrocarbon (HC) exposure.** *ABG,* Arterial blood gases; *Chem,* chemistry; *CT,* computed tomography; *CXR,* chest radiograph; *ECG,* electrocardiogram; *ICU,* intensive care unit; *IV,* intravenous; *LFTs,* liver function tests; *MRI,* magnetic resonance imaging; *PEEP,* positive end-expiratory pressure.

**BOX 152.1 Mnemonic for Potent Hydrocarbon Toxicants: "CHAMP"**

The clinician should consider decontamination/gastric emptying when these agents are ingested:

*C*amphor
*H*alogenated hydrocarbons
*A*romatic
*M*etal-containing hydrocarbons
*P*esticides

Gastric emptying may be useful when the hydrocarbon is extremely toxic (e.g., carbon tetrachloride), when a large volume of hydrocarbon is ingested (more than 30 mL), or when severe toxicity is predicted (**Box 152.1**). If gastric lavage is performed, a small-bore (not large-bore) nasogastric tube should be used, to reduce the risk of vomiting and aspiration. Activated charcoal has little ability to reduce GI absorption of hydrocarbons and may cause gastric distention and vomiting. Any role for activated charcoal in isolated hydrocarbon ingestion is limited, at best.

Most hydrocarbons cannot be removed by dialysis, but toxic agents that are water-soluble, small, highly polar molecules can be removed by dialysis. Examples are small alcohols and polyols (e.g., methanol, ethylene glycol). Small ketones (e.g., acetone) are also dialyzable. Chloral hydrate can be successfully removed by hemodialysis. Peritoneal dialysis has been employed to reduce the toxicity of both dichloroethane and trichloroethylene. Unfortunately, many hydrocarbon molecules are too large to be dialyzed. Most are lipophilic, so they dissolve into fat stores (with greater volume of distribution), thus reducing their availability in the central compartment.

Extracorporeal membrane oxygenation can successfully temporize the course of severe pulmonary toxicity. This technique is considered invasive, is not widely available, and requires special expertise. Use of extracorporeal membrane oxygenation is generally reserved for severe cases of hydrocarbon toxicity for which other available modalities have failed to achieve adequate oxygenation.

## RESUSCITATION

Priorities of resuscitation are similar to those in any other type of poisoning. Nuances include the requirement to limit exposure of the patient and caregivers by prioritizing decontamination. The airway and systemic oxygenation should be restored and secured first. This should be achieved by any necessary means and may require high-flow oxygenation, endotracheal intubation, ventilation, and the use of bronchodilators. Positive end-expiratory pressure (PEEP) ventilation may help oxygenate patients who are persistently hypoxemic. High-frequency jet ventilation may be required and has been used successfully in this situation.

Dysrhythmias in the setting of hydrocarbon toxicity should prompt investigations into electrolyte and acid-base status, hypoxemia, hypotension, and hypothermia. Ventricular fibrillation is especially concerning because resuscitation algorithms recommend epinephrine to treat this rhythm. If the dysrhythmia can be ascertained to emanate from myocardial sensitization by a solvent, catecholamines should be avoided. Exogenous catecholamines (e.g., epinephrine) should be avoided. In this setting, lidocaine has been used successfully, as have beta-blockers.[17,18]

Management of hypotension may be precarious. Hydrocarbons do not generally affect systemic vascular resistance, so coingestants should be considered in the persistently hypotensive patient. Hypotension may relate to excessive PEEP, and reducing PEEP may improve hemodynamics. Rarely, some hydrocarbons can cause myocardial depression; in a patient with this finding, an inotrope (but not isoproterenol or dobutamine) should be considered. Pressors such as dopamine, epinephrine, isoproterenol, and norepinephrine must be avoided, if possible, because of the risk of myocardial sensitization.[6]

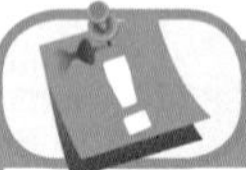

**TIPS AND TRICKS**

- The emergency physician should be aware of the intentional abuse of volatile hydrocarbon inhalants by adolescents and young adults, a growing problem worldwide.
- Hydrocarbons enhance the proarrhythmic potential of endogenous or exogenous catecholamines (e.g., epinephrine) and are said to sensitize the myocardium to the arrhythmogenic effects of catecholamines, so these agents should be avoided in hydrocarbon exposure.
- Mental status depression is common in larger ingestions but may not occur for 30 to 60 minutes after ingestion.
- Typical findings in hydrocarbon pneumonitis are audible abnormalities on chest auscultation, fever, leukocytosis, and abnormalities seen on chest radiograph; these findings do not differ clinically from those of community-acquired pneumonia.
- Volitional abusers demonstrate loss of cerebral white matter, with a characteristic syndrome of cognitive and motor deficits.
- Dysrhythmias in the setting of hydrocarbon toxicity should prompt investigations into electrolyte and acid-base status, hypoxemia, hypotension, and hypothermia.
- The possibility of methemoglobinemia should be evaluated in any patient who remains cyanotic once arterial oxygenation is normalized.
- Patients with hydrocarbon exposure who have no symptoms at home or on initial evaluation generally do not require gastric emptying.

## FOLLOW-UP, NEXT STEPS OF CARE, AND PATIENT EDUCATION

Patients who demonstrate clinical evidence of toxicity, and those who are suicidal or intend self-harm, should be hospitalized.

Patients who have been observed for 6 hours after an ingestion and who demonstrate no abnormal pulmonary findings, have adequate oxygenation, are not tachypneic, and have normal chest radiography findings have a good prognosis with a very low risk of subsequent deterioration.[19] These patients can be safely discharged. Care may be individualized for asymptomatic patients with radiographic abnormalities, as well as for patients who have initial respiratory symptoms but who quickly become asymptomatic during medical evaluation. Reliable patients may be considered for discharge with next-day follow-up.

Special care should be given to patients who ingest, or who otherwise have significant toxicity from, agents known to cause cardiac sensitization, including gasoline. The findings of mental status depression, seizures, or arrhythmias attributed to a known cardiac sensitizer (or to an unknown hydrocarbon ingestion) warrant at least 6 hours of continuous cardiac monitoring.

## REFERENCES

***References can be found on Expert Consult @ www.expertconsult.com.***

# 153 Inhaled Toxins

*Trevonne M. Thompson*

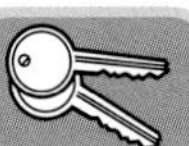

**KEY POINTS**

- Cyanide gas and hydrogen sulfide are rapid knockdown agents.
- The key characteristic of cyanide is profound metabolic acidosis with a wide anion gap and elevation of serum lactate.
- Clinical suspicion is paramount to the diagnosis of cyanide toxicity; treatment may be required before the diagnosis is confirmed.
- Hydroxycobalamin (Cyanokit) has fewer adverse events than the cyanide kit; it has one component instead of three.
- Rescuers must wear adequate personal protective equipment, including a self-contained breathing apparatus, to remove a victim from the source of exposure to hydrogen sulfide.
- Patients who present alert, without altered mental status and with normal respiratory effort after exposure to hydrogen sulfide, should have a good outcome.
- If administered shortly after severe hydrogen sulfide exposures, sodium nitrite may improve outcome.
- The mainstays of treatment for hydrogen sulfide toxicity are 100% oxygen and meticulous supportive care.

**BOX 153.1 Cyanogen-Containing Plants**

*Prunus* species (leaves, bark and seeds):
- Apricots
- Peaches
- Bitter almonds*
- Plums

Apple pits
Cassava beans and roots
Crab apple pits
Pear pits
Christmas berry
*Linum* species
Sorghum species

From Hall AH, Rumack BH. Clinical toxicology of cyanide. Ann Emerg Med 1986;15:1067-74.
*Bitter almonds are not the common almonds eaten in the United States.

**BOX 153.2 Combustion Sources of Cyanide**

Wool
Silk
Nylon
Synthetic rubber
Polyurethane
Nitrocellulose
Polystyrene

From Jones J, McMullen MJ, Dougherty J. Toxic smoke inhalation: cyanide poisoning in fire victims. Am J Emerg Med 1987;5:317-21.

## CYANIDE

### EPIDEMIOLOGY

Cyanide poisoning is uncommon. It is also potentially rapidly fatal. Cyanide is used in precious metal extraction, electroplating, metal hardening, photography, and various other industries. Cyanide has also been used as an agent of chemical warfare and in judicial executions.

Cyanide exists in several forms. The gaseous form is hydrogen cyanide (HCN); the salt forms are potassium cyanide and sodium cyanide. The inorganic salts release HCN gas when they are dissolved in water. *Cyanogens* are compounds that are metabolized to cyanide in vivo. The two clinically important cyanogens are amygdalin and acetonitrile. Amygdalin is a naturally occurring cyanogen found in the seeds of plants in the *Prunus* species and in the pits of other fruits (**Box 153.1**). Acetonitrile is found in some artificial nail removal products. Unlike other cyanide products, cyanogens may produce delayed cyanide toxicity because of the time required for their biotransformation. Cyanide gas is also released during combustion of certain natural and synthetic materials (**Box 153.2**). Consequently, cyanide poisoning can occur in victims of structure fires.

### PATHOPHYSIOLOGY

Cyanide is a potent cellular poison. The primary clinical effect occurs through the inhibition of oxidative phosphorylation. Cyanide binds to the ferric ($Fe^{3+}$) moiety of cytochrome oxidase $aa_3$, the last enzyme of the electron transport chain.[1] The net effects of cyanide poisoning are reduced oxygen consumption and conversion of aerobic to anaerobic metabolism;

**Table 153.1 Comparisons, Diagnosis, and Treatment of Various Gas Exposures**

| EXPOSURE | SYMPTOMS | DIAGNOSTIC TESTING | TREATMENT |
|---|---|---|---|
| Cyanide | Dependent on route of exposure and compound involved<br>Dyspnea, headache, weakness, nausea, vomiting, diarrhea, hypotension, and altered mental status early<br>Gas exposure a cause of rapid knock-down | Nonspecific:<br>ABGs (anion gap metabolic acidosis)<br>Serum lactate (elevated)<br>Electrocardiogram (arrhythmias) | Decontamination<br>Supportive care<br>Cyanide antidote kit or Cyanokit |
| Carbon monoxide | Generally, slow-onset alteration of mental status<br>Coma with severe poisoning<br>Nausea and vomiting, headache at low doses | Carbon monoxide level | Oxygen; hyperbaric in severe cases |
| Hydrogen sulfide | At high levels: rapid coma, collapse, seizures, respiratory arrest<br>At lower levels: headache, dizziness, nausea, dyspnea, chest pain, altered mental status | ABGs (hypoxia) and serum lactate (elevated) | Oxygen<br>Decontamination<br>Sodium nitrite component of cyanide antidote kit<br>Hyperbaric oxygen if readily available |
| Sodium azide | Similar to those in presentations of cyanide and hydrogen sulfide poisonings | None | Supportive care |
| Methane or butane | Alveolar hypoxia | None | Oxygen therapy with rapid improvement |

*ABGs,* Arterial blood gas measurements.

these effects lead to profound metabolic acidosis and an elevated serum lactate concentration.

## PRESENTING SIGNS AND SYMPTOMS

The clinical presentation of cyanide poisoning is protean and depends on the route of exposure and the cyanide compound involved. The early signs and symptoms are dyspnea, headache, weakness, nausea, vomiting, diaphoresis, hypotension, tachycardia, and altered mental status. The late signs and symptoms are bradycardia, atrioventricular heart block, ventricular dysrhythmias, asystole, seizures, and coma. Exposure to any form of cyanide can result in death.

Cyanide gas is a knockdown agent, causing those exposed to lose consciousness rapidly. Patients with exposure to 300 parts per million (ppm) of cyanide gas rapidly collapse and typically do not survive to admission to the emergency department. Exposure to 100 ppm for more than 30 minutes is considered life-threatening. An oral dose of 200 mg of potassium cyanide is considered a fatal ingestion. Features of cyanide poisoning typically develop 15 to 30 minutes after ingestion of cyanide salts. Exposure to cyanogens can result in delayed symptoms and signs because the parent compound must be metabolized before cyanide is produced.

## DIFFERENTIAL DIAGNOSIS AND MEDICAL DECISION MAKING

Without a history of cyanide exposure, the diagnosis is often difficult to make (**Table 153.1**). All medical causes of altered mental status, hypotension, and acidosis must be considered.

**BOX 153.3 Differential Diagnosis of Cyanide and Hydrogen Sulfide Poisoning**

| Medical Conditions Mimicking Cyanide and Hydrogen Sulfide Poisoning | Toxins Mimicking Cyanide and Hydrogen Sulfide Poisoning |
|---|---|
| Acute myocardial infarction | Arsine gas |
| Encephalitis and meningitis | Asphyxiant gases |
| Hyperglycemic coma | Carbon monoxide |
| Hypoglycemic coma | Cyclic antidepressants |
| Intracranial hemorrhage | Irritant gases |
| Pneumonia | Isoniazid |
| Pulmonary embolism | Phosphine gas |
| Shock | Salicylates |
| Stroke | Sodium azide |
| | Strychnine |
| | Toxic alcohols |

The differential diagnosis of cyanide poisoning is listed in **Box 153.3**.

Whole-blood cyanide measurement is not readily available in the emergency department. The hallmark findings in cyanide poisoning are profound metabolic acidosis with a wide anion gap and an elevation of serum lactate.

## TREATMENT

Aggressive supportive care and early administration of antidote therapy are the mainstays of treatment (**Fig. 153.1** and

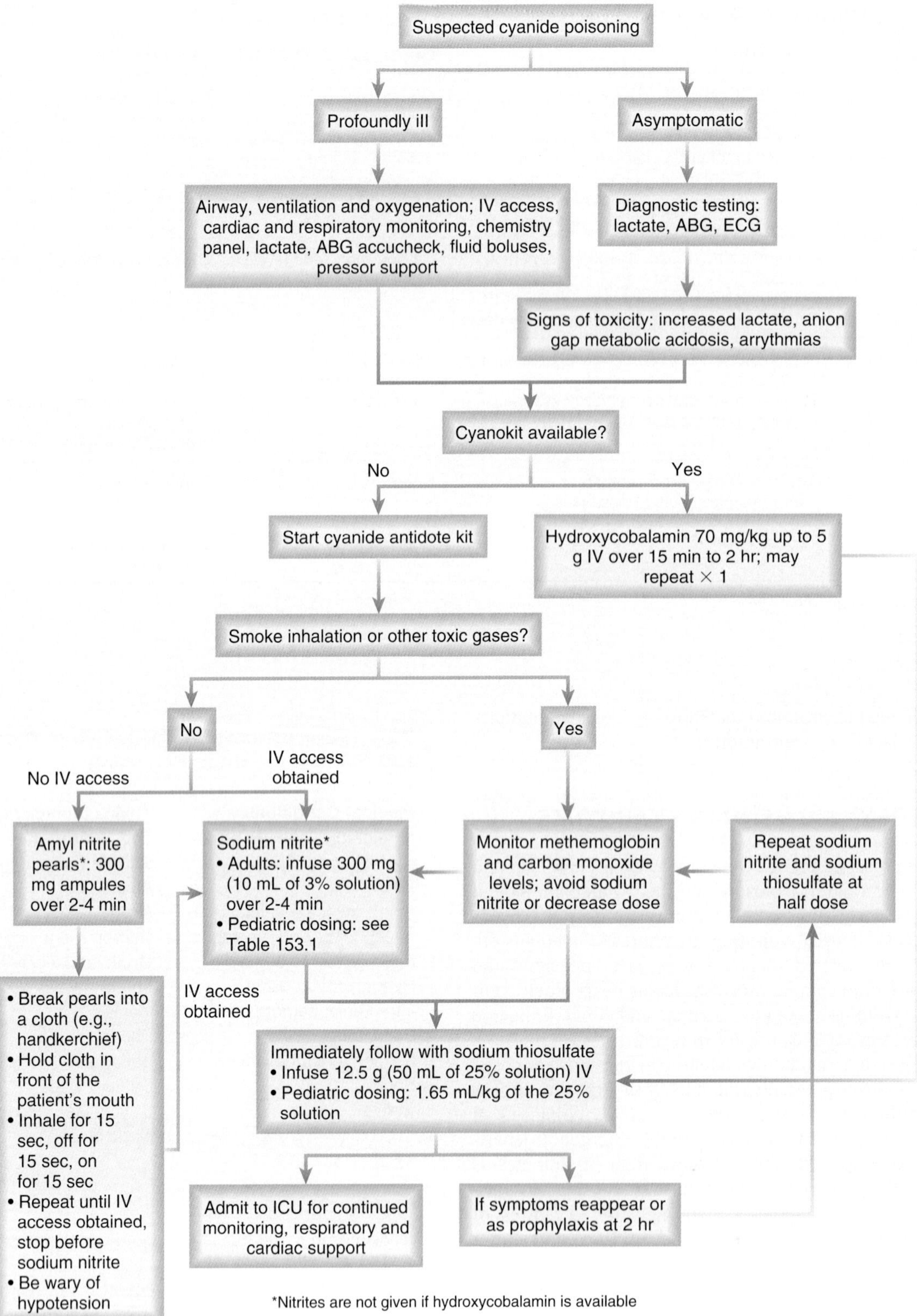


**Fig. 153.1 Diagnosis and treatment algorithm for cyanide poisoning.** *ABG,* Arterial blood gas measurement; *ECG,* electrocardiogram; *ICU,* intensive care unit; *IV,* intravenous(ly).

**BOX 153.4 Treatment Algorithm for Cyanide Poisoning**

**Suspected Cyanide Poisoning**

1. Immediate attention to supportive care
   - Airway, breathing, circulation, IV access, cardiac and respiratory monitoring
   - Initial laboratory evaluation: chemistry panel, complete blood count, lactate, ABGs
2. If signs of toxicity (hypotension, altered mental status, elevated lactate, wide anion gap, dysrhythmias):
   - Treatment with antidote: cyanide antidote kit or hydroxycobalamin
3. If smoke inhalation:
   - Use only of the sodium thiosulfate component of the cyanide antidote kit, *or*
   - Use of hydroxycobalamin alone, *or*
   - Use of sodium thiosulfate and hydroxycobalamin together (cannot use same IV site)
4. If no IV access immediately:
   - Use of amyl nitrite pearls
5. Readministration of antidotal therapy if necessary
6. Admission to the intensive care unit

*ABGs*, Arterial blood gases; *IV*, intravenous.

**Table 153.2** Pediatric Nitrite Dosing According to Hemoglobin Value*

| HEMOGLOBIN VALUE (G/dL) | 3% SODIUM NITRITE SOLUTION (mL/KG) |
|---|---|
| 7.0 | 0.19 |
| 8.0 | 0.22 |
| 9.0 | 0.25 |
| 10.0 | 0.27 |
| 11.0 | 0.30 |
| 12.0 | 0.33 |
| 13.0 | 0.36 |
| 14.0 | 0.39 |

Adapted from Berlin CMJ. The treatment of cyanide poisoning in children. Pediatrics 1970;46:793-6.

*If giving sodium nitrite empirically to a patient with no history of anemia, do not wait for hemoglobin results; assume that the hemoglobin level is 12 g/dL, and dose accordingly.

Box 153.4). Patients with cyanide exposure are often critically ill at presentation and may rapidly progress to respiratory and cardiovascular collapse. Antidote therapy options include the cyanide antidote kit (CAK) and hydroxycobalamin (Cyanokit).

The CAK contains three products: amyl nitrite, sodium nitrite, and sodium thiosulfate. The nitrates induce methemoglobinemia and thus allow cyanide to dissociate from cytochrome oxidase and preferentially bind to methemoglobin. This process sequesters cyanide in the serum and allows cellular metabolism to resume. The sodium thiosulfate component enhances the innate pathway of cyanide metabolism. The amyl nitrite component of the CAK is contained in pearls that are crushed to produce a vapor that is inhaled. This component is generally reserved for situations in which intravenous access is delayed or cannot be achieved. The sodium nitrite comes in 300-mg ampules, which are infused over 2 to 4 minutes in adult patients. The sodium thiosulfate dose is 12.5 g administered intravenously. The patient's blood pressure must be monitored carefully because the nitrites can induce hypotension. Methemoglobin levels must be monitored regularly during nitrite therapy because methemoglobin does not carry oxygen. The methemoglobin levels should be kept at less than 30%. Nitrites should not be administered to fire victims, who may have carbon monoxide poisoning, because carboxyhemoglobin also does not carry oxygen. Inducing methemoglobinemia in these patients may worsen oxygen delivery to tissues. In such cases, the physician should use the sodium thiosulfate alone, the hydroxycobalamin alone, or both the thiosulfate and hydroxycobalamin together. In the pediatric patient, the nitrite dose must be adjusted for the hemoglobin level. **Table 153.2** provides dosing guidelines for such a situation. Both the sodium nitrite and sodium thiosulfate components of the CAK may be readministered as clinically indicated.

Hydroxycobalamin (also hydroxocobalamin, vitamin $B_{12a}$) is the other antidote for cyanide poisoning and is much simpler and safer to use. Marketed as the Cyanokit, it has been approved in the United States for the treatment of cyanide poisoning. Hydroxycobalamin has a high affinity for cyanide and binds with cyanide to form cyanocobalamin (vitamin $B_{12}$), which is excreted in the urine. Transient hypertension and a self-limited reddish discoloration of the skin, mucous membranes, and urine are the only adverse effects of hydroxycobalamin. The adult dose is 5 g administered intravenously over 15 to 30 minutes; the pediatric dose is 70 mg/kg. The dose may be repeated as clinically indicated up to a maximum of 10 g.[2] Hydroxycobalamin can be used alone or in conjunction with the sodium thiosulfate component of the CAK. Hydroxycobalamin can be safely administered simultaneously with sodium thiosulfate, although the two agents cannot be administered through the same intravenous access site. Hydroxycobalamin and sodium thiosulfate may be synergistic in cyanide elimination.[3,4] Hydroxycobalamin does not induce methemoglobinemia.

## FOLLOW-UP, NEXT STEPS OF CARE, AND PATIENT EDUCATION

Cyanide-poisoned patients are critically ill. They should be admitted to an intensive care unit for continued respiratory and cardiovascular support and monitoring.

# HYDROGEN SULFIDE

## EPIDEMIOLOGY

Hydrogen sulfide is a known knockdown agent. It causes a patient to become rapidly comatose, with profound metabolic acidosis. Because of its rotten egg odor, it is commonly referred to as "sewer gas" or "stink damp."[5] In addition to being a well-known sewer hazard, hydrogen sulfide exposure can be seen in plumbing, mining, tanning, fisheries, drilling, and miscellaneous chemical manufacturing occupations. This agent can be produced by the decomposition of animal or organic material. It can also be produced by the addition of an acid to a metal sulfide. A clue to the presence of hydrogen sulfide is the blackening or tarnishing of silver coins, which results from the conversion of silver to silver sulfide on exposure to hydrogen sulfide.

## PATHOPHYSIOLOGY

Hydrogen sulfide is as potent as cyanide in binding to cytochrome $aa_3$, inhibiting oxidative phosphorylation, and leading to metabolic acidosis and impaired oxygen utilization.[5]

## PRESENTING SIGNS AND SYMPTOMS

Hydrogen sulfide is a rapid knockdown agent. An individual exposed to a large concentration of hydrogen sulfide may quickly lose consciousness. Exposure to low concentrations may cause headache, dizziness, and nausea; at higher concentrations, exposure can lead to dyspnea, chest pain, and a decreased level of consciousness. At the highest concentrations, exposures may quickly cause collapse, coma, seizures, respiratory arrest, and asphyxiation. **Table 153.3** illustrates the correlation of hydrogen sulfide air concentrations with clinical effect.[6]

**Table 153.3 Hydrogen Sulfide Air Concentrations and Clinical Effects**

| HYDROGEN SULFIDE CONCENTRATION (PPM) | CLINICAL EFFECTS |
|---|---|
| 30 | Local irritation<br>Sore throat<br>Eye irritation<br>"Rotten egg" odor |
| >30 | Over time, olfactory fatigue |
| 40-200 | Respiratory and mucous membrane irritation<br>Respiratory distress |
| >200 | Severe toxicity |
| >500 | Respiratory paralysis<br>Asphyxia<br>Death |

Adapted from the Agency for Toxic Substances and Disease Registry. Toxicological profile for hydrogen sulfide. Atlanta: Agency for Toxic Substances and Disease Registry, U.S Department of Health and Human Services, 2006.

## DIFFERENTIAL DIAGNOSIS AND MEDICAL DECISION MAKING

The differential diagnosis of hydrogen sulfide exposure includes the many medical and toxicologic causes of altered mental status, metabolic acidosis, and hypoxia. See Box 153.3 for an illustration of the differential diagnosis of hydrogen sulfide exposure.

No single diagnostic test establishes the diagnosis of hydrogen sulfide poisoning in the acute clinical setting. Blood gas measurement is useful to determine the degree of acidemia and hypoxemia present. An elevated serum lactate concentration suggests hydrogen sulfide exposure, but it is not specific to this toxin and does not distinguish it, for example, from other cellular poisons such as cyanide. Some emergency medical services and industrial hygienists have the capability to measure hydrogen sulfide air concentrations; this measurement could provide useful information at the scene and for clinical correlation.

## TREATMENT

The most important concept in hydrogen sulfide treatment is removal of the patient from the source of exposure (**Box 153.5**). Patients with significant signs and symptoms or a history of significant exposure should be given 100% oxygen. Comatose patients or those in severe respiratory distress should be intubated and given 100% oxygen. Principles of decontamination should be followed as indicated. The patient's clothes should be removed, and the skin should be decontaminated using water. Ocular examination with fluorescein and irrigation with saline solution are appropriate to address ocular exposures.

The sodium nitrite component of the CAK can be administered to patients presenting early after moderate to severe exposure to hydrogen sulfide. Animal evidence sup-

**BOX 153.5 Treatment of Hydrogen Sulfide Poisoning**

1. Remove the patient from the source of exposure by using a self-contained breathing apparatus.
2. Decontaminate the patient with water.
3. Administer 100% oxygen.
4. Intubate if the patient is comatose or has severe respiratory distress, and provide 100% oxygen.
5. If the patient is hypotensive, provide intravenous fluids and inotropes or pressors.
6. In moderate to severe cases in patients who present early, administer sodium nitrite: 300 mg (10 mL of 3% solution) over 2 to 4 minutes in adults. Measure methemoglobin levels 30 minutes after infusion.
7. Hyperbaric oxygen therapy may be tried in patients with moderate to severe cases if it is readily available at the treating institution.

ports the early administration of nitrites as antidote therapy for hydrogen sulfide toxicity.[7,8] Nitrates can be given intravenously in the same manner as described for cyanide poisoning.

Hyperbaric oxygen therapy (HBOT) has been used to treat hydrogen sulfide poisoning with anecdotal success.[9,10] Its use is based on a theoretical benefit, and the indications are controversial. Transfer of an unstable patient for HBOT is not justified by the current literature. HBOT may be considered if it is readily available at the treating institution.

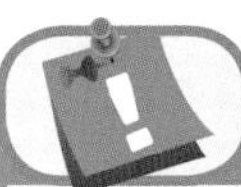

**TIPS AND TRICKS**

- Without a history of exposure, the diagnosis of cyanide poisoning is challenging.
- Hydrogen sulfide poisoning should be suspected whenever a person is found unconscious in an enclosed space, especially if an odor of rotten eggs is present.
- Hydroxycobalamin (Cyanokit) has fewer adverse effects compared with nitrites in treating cyanide poisoning and is preferred in the setting of smoke inhalation.
- Many patients with gas exposure respond rapidly to oxygen therapy; lack of response should raise suspicion of cyanide or hydrogen sulfide poisoning.
- Hyperbaric oxygen therapy for hydrogen sulfide toxicity is indicated only when it is readily available at the treating facility.
- Patients who do not survive cyanide poisoning are candidates for organ donation.

## FOLLOW-UP, NEXT STEPS OF CARE, AND PATIENT EDUCATION

Patients exposed to hydrogen sulfide who are asymptomatic at the scene can be monitored for a short observation period of approximately 4 hours and safely discharged. Patients with a history of significant exposure or those with moderate to severe symptoms should be admitted to an intensive care unit for close monitoring and meticulous supportive care.

## SUGGESTED READINGS

Hall AH, Saiers J, Baud F. Which cyanide antidote? Crit Rev Toxicol 2009;39:541-52.

Knight LD, Presnell SE. Death by sewer gas: case report of a double fatality and review of the literature. Am J Forensic Med Pathol 2005;26:181-5.

Morocco AP. Cyanides. Crit Care Clin 2005;21:691-705.

## REFERENCES

*References can be found on Expert Consult @ www.expertconsult.com.*

# 154 Ethanol and Opioid Intoxication and Withdrawal

*Patrick M. Lank and Shana Kusin*

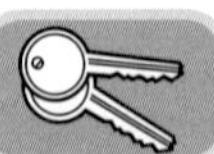

**KEY POINTS**

- Most organ systems in the body can be affected by ethanol consumption. Important associated disease states are electrolyte disturbances, traumatic injuries, infectious diseases, and primary central nervous system, gastrointestinal, and cardiovascular complications.
- Ethanol causes depressant effects, but abrupt cessation in long-term users causes hyperstimulation and dangerous withdrawal syndromes.
- Alcohol withdrawal is a spectrum of diseases ranging from minor signs and symptoms, such as anxiety and mild tremor, to severe withdrawal, including autonomic instability and delirium.
- Supportive care is the mainstay of treatment for acute ethanol intoxication and withdrawal. Benzodiazepines constitute the major form of pharmacotherapy for withdrawal syndromes.
- For admitted patients, underlying liver disease, need for intubation, hyperthermia, persistent tachycardia, and use of physical restraints are all associated with increased risk of death in alcohol withdrawal.
- Patients who have a history of major withdrawal and are currently in withdrawal or have significant associated disease states should be admitted for further treatment.
- Brief interventions in alcohol-dependent patients in the emergency department have been shown to have positive effects.
- Opioid intoxication is characterized by depressed central nervous system activity, respiratory depression, and miosis.
- Patients with opioid withdrawal syndrome can present with yawning, piloerection, and mydriasis.

## ETHANOL

## EPIDEMIOLOGY

Ethanol use is a common part of our society, as evidenced by the knowledge that approximately 80% of adults in the United States have consumed ethanol-containing beverages during their lifetimes.[1] Mild to moderate consumption (up to one drink/day for women and two drinks/day for men) has been shown to have beneficial cardiovascular effects, including a decreased risk of myocardial infarction and stroke, as well as overall decreased mortality (**Box 154.1**).[2-5]

Despite these possibly beneficial effects of alcohol, it has been found to be a top 10 cause of preventable deaths among all age groups in the United States.[6] Additionally, approximately 9% of adults meet the diagnostic criteria for alcohol abuse and alcoholism.[7] This maladaptive behavior can lead to numerous individual medical complications and societal problems, including motor vehicle collisions, assaults, homicide, suicide, and domestic violence. An estimated 7.6 million emergency department (ED) visits per year are for alcohol-related diseases and diagnoses.[8]

Alcohol withdrawal is seen in the ED in various forms and stages, including early withdrawal, hallucinosis, seizures, and fully developed delirium tremens (DT). DT, a severe withdrawal syndrome defined by the presence of tremors, seizures, and delirium, develops in 5% of patients who develop symptoms of alcohol withdrawal and itself carries a 5% to 15% risk of mortality.[9] Among patients admitted to the hospital with a diagnosis of alcohol withdrawal, the following clinical features have been found to be associated with an increased risk of death: underlying liver disease, the need for endotracheal intubation, hyperthermia, persistent tachycardia, and the use of physical restraints.[10,11]

## PATHOPHYSIOLOGY

### ALCOHOL INTOXICATION

Ethanol is readily absorbed from the gastrointestinal (GI) tract and is primarily metabolized by the liver through the alcohol dehydrogenase pathway (**Fig. 154.1**). Metabolism of ethanol differs in men and women. Although alcohol dehydrogenase is found in gastric mucosa and other tissues, women seem to have less ability to metabolize it by the gastric route.[12] Long-term ethanol users or those with high alcohol levels also use a second pathway, the microsomal ethanol-oxidizing system.[13]

Ethanol is a central nervous system (CNS) depressant involving multiple receptors and pathways. Likely its greatest effect is in enhancing gamma-aminobutyric acid (GABA) inhibitory action.[14] Ethanol is also known to block the excitatory *N*-methyl-D-aspartate (NMDA) glutamate receptor, thus leading to further CNS depression.[15]

The level of CNS depression depends on many factors affecting absorption and elimination, including age, weight, gender, the presence of food, gastric motility, the speed of consumption, and long-term alcohol use. Ethanol intoxication in most states is legally defined as a blood alcohol concentration (BAC) of 80 to 100 mg/dL (0.08 to 0.1% BAC). Elimination rates vary greatly, but a rate of 20 mg/dL/hour can be assumed for most intoxicated patients in the ED, regardless of initial alcohol level or chronic alcohol use.[16,17] Because alcohol follows zero-order kinetics, some sources advocate drawing two ethanol levels to determine the individual patient's exact rate of ethanol clearance, although this is most often medically unnecessary.

### ALCOHOL WITHDRAWAL

Alcohol withdrawal is best described as a pathologic excitation of the CNS and autonomic systems. GABA receptors are desensitized and downregulated in chronic ethanol use, with a resulting decrease in activity of the inhibitory effects of GABA when a patient reduces ethanol consumption. The excitatory glutamate neurotransmitter system is blocked by the NMDA receptor in the presence of ethanol, and this blockade leads to receptor upregulation in chronic alcoholism and excitation during withdrawal.[17] With repeated episodes of alcohol withdrawal, the patient will have more severe withdrawal, a phenomenon known as "kindling."[18] Cessation of alcohol consumption may be inadvertent, as in the patient who is unable to tolerate oral intake because of vomiting or in the hospitalized patient whose access to ethanol is restricted.

**BOX 154.1 Definition of One Standard Alcoholic Drink**

A standard alcoholic drink can be defined as one of the following:

- 12 fluid oz. regular beer
- 5 fluid oz. wine
- 1.5 fluid oz. 80-proof distilled spirits

Adapted from U.S. Department of Health and Human Services and the U.S. Department of Agriculture (USDA). Dietary guidelines for Americans 2005. 6th ed. Washington, D.C.: U.S. Government Printing Office; 2005.

## PRESENTING SIGNS AND SYMPTOMS

Ethanol use is associated with many disease states affecting many organ systems in the body. The Wernicke-Korsakoff syndrome bears special mention. This syndrome complex is composed of two disease processes, Wernicke encephalopathy and the Korsakoff amnestic state, which can manifest individually or concomitantly.

Classically, Wernicke encephalopathy consists of the following: ocular abnormalities such as nystagmus and motor palsies, seen in 29% of cases; ataxia, seen in 23% of cases; and mental status change, seen in 82% of cases. Presentations with this classic triad are rare, with only 10% of confirmed cases having all three symptom types.[19]

The Korsakoff amnestic state refers to the syndrome of memory deficits found in long-term alcohol abusers. Anterograde and retrograde amnesia is present, and confabulation is common. Thiamine deficiency is the cause, and ataxia and memory loss may persist despite treatment.

The CNS-depressive effects of ethanol range from diminished fine-motor control to coma and respiratory depression. Because of greater tolerance, patients with chronic alcoholism may exhibit a high level of functioning despite a high BAC. The intoxicated patient often presents with the smell of ethanol on the breath, slurred speech, emotional lability, and difficulty with coordination. Death can occur from respiratory depression or aspiration.

Alcohol is related to an estimated 35% of injury-associated ED visits.[20] In the setting of trauma, ethanol intoxication generally should not lower the Glasgow Coma Scale score dramatically; whenever a low score is found, further CNS evaluation is warranted.[21]

### ALCOHOL WITHDRAWAL

The patient in ethanol withdrawal usually presents to the ED approximately 24 hours after a significant decrease or cessation of ethanol consumption. The patient is anxious, tremulous, tachycardic, hypertensive, and hyperreflexic and may complain of sleep and GI disturbances.

Alcohol withdrawal syndrome represents a spectrum of disease, ranging from minor to major. An accompanying time frame within this spectrum of disease shows significant

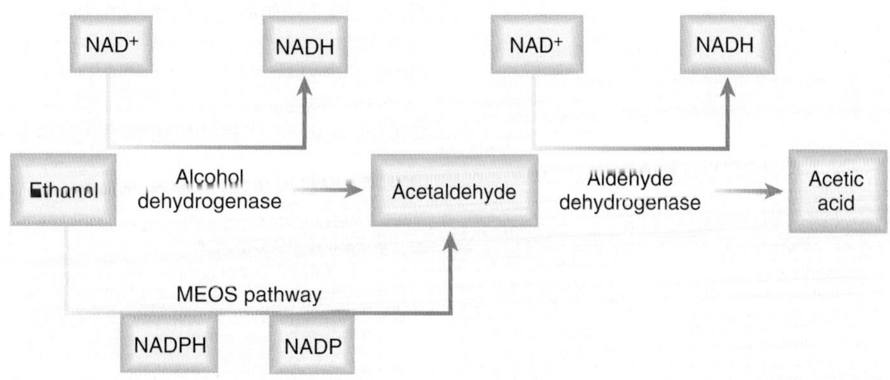


**Fig. 154.1 Alcohol dehydrogenase pathway, including the microsomal ethanol-oxidizing system (MEOS), the alternative metabolism seen in chronic alcoholics.** *NAD+*, nicotinamide adenine dinucleotide; *NADH*, reduced nicotinamide adenine dinucleotide; *NADP*, nicotinamide adenine dinucleotide phosphate; *NADPH*, reduced nicotinamide adenine dinucleotide phosphate.

overlap between timing and the signs and symptoms. Minor withdrawal begins within 6 to 24 hours and is characterized by hyperstimulation. Major withdrawal syndrome begins after 24 hours and peaks at approximately 48 to 72 hours. It may have any or all of the following features: progression of excitatory signs and symptoms, hyperpyrexia, seizures, altered mental status, hallucinations (visual, auditory, or tactile), and delirium.

True DT is rare and constitutes the most severe form of withdrawal, although patients may mistakenly equate it with generalized withdrawal syndrome. DT occupies the far end of the spectrum, and it consists of substantial tremor, autonomic hyperactivity, profound confusion, fever, and hallucinations (**Fig. 154.2**).[22]

## DIFFERENTIAL DIAGNOSIS AND MEDICAL DECISION MAKING

The diagnosis of ethanol intoxication is mainly one of exclusion, and a history consistent with ethanol consumption is important. The initial approach to the patient should be the same as for any patient with altered mental status. Traumatic injuries and coingestions (acetaminophen, illicit drugs, toxic alcohols) should be high on the differential diagnosis list (**Box 154.2**).

**BOX 154.2 Differential Diagnosis of Ethanol Intoxication and Withdrawal**

**Intoxication**
- Traumatic head injury
- Cerebrovascular accident
- Metabolic derangements (hypoglycemia)
- Hypoxia
- Drug ingestion
- Central nervous system infections

**Withdrawal**
- Infections (meningitis, encephalitis, sepsis)
- Toxidromes (sympathomimetic, anticholinergic)
- Thyrotoxicosis
- Neuroleptic malignant syndrome
- Heat stroke
- Acute psychosis
- Withdrawal from other sedative-hypnotic drugs (benzodiazepines, barbiturates) and from drugs used to treat spasticity (baclofen)

A history of previous ethanol withdrawal or of alcohol abuse with decreased intake or cessation of alcohol is the key to the diagnosis of ethanol withdrawal.

Diagnostic testing for the acutely intoxicated patient should be guided by suspicion of concomitant disease states and potential traumatic injury. A BAC measurement is necessary only to confirm a diagnosis or to guide treatment.

Patients presenting in withdrawal may mandate a comprehensive evaluation, but the same guidelines apply as for the intoxicated patient. The laboratory tests vary but may include a complete blood count, serum glucose measurement, blood chemistry panel with a full set of electrolyte measurements, urinalysis, toxicology screen, electrocardiogram, chest radiography, and head computed tomography. Lumbar puncture for cerebrospinal fluid analysis may be indicated if subarachnoid hemorrhage or CNS infection is in the differential diagnosis.

## TREATMENT

### ALCOHOL INTOXICATION

Supportive care is the mainstay of treatment for acute ethanol intoxication (**Fig. 154.3**). Airway and breathing must be assessed in the comatose patient, and endotracheal intubation, although rarely needed, should be used for airway protection if necessary. Circulation should be assessed, and isotonic intravenous fluids should be given initially for patients with hypotension or volume depletion.

In the comatose patient, naloxone (0.8 mg) should be considered, and glucose (25 to 50 g intravenously) should be given to a hypoglycemic patient. Thiamine (100 mg intravenously) can be given before glucose administration to prevent or treat Wernicke encephalopathy, but glucose administration need not be delayed.[23] Electrolyte and thiamine replacement can be achieved orally if the patient is tolerating oral intake, is not at risk of aspiration, and is not being treated for active Wernicke encephalopathy. Routine multivitamin replacement with vitamin $B_{12}$ and folate in patients presenting with alcohol intoxication is unnecessary.[24]

### ALCOHOL WITHDRAWAL

Patients who present to the ED with signs and symptoms of alcohol withdrawal should be evaluated using the Revised Clinical Institute Withdrawal Assessment for Alcohol (CIWA-Ar) scale to aid in determining the severity of withdrawal (**Box 154.3**). Initial treatment should focus on resuscitation with fluids, replacement of electrolyte deficiencies, and evaluation and treatment of concomitant diseases.

Benzodiazepines are the mainstays of treatment for withdrawal and are usually initiated when CIWA-Ar scores are

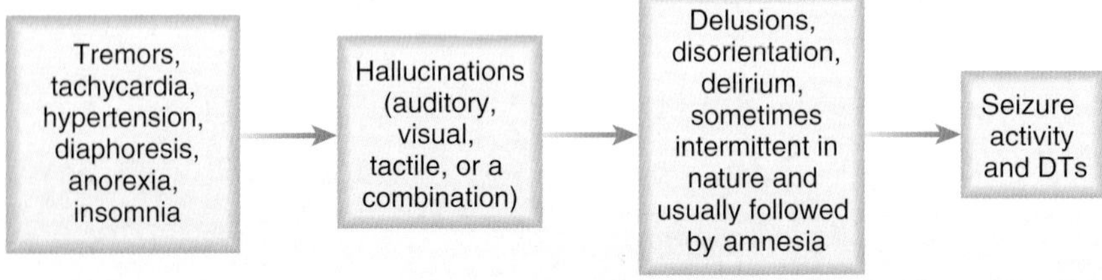


**Fig. 154.2 Progression of signs and symptoms of alcohol withdrawal.** Symptoms on the left predominate during the first 24 hours without alcohol and progress over the next 48 hours. *DTs,* Delirium tremens.

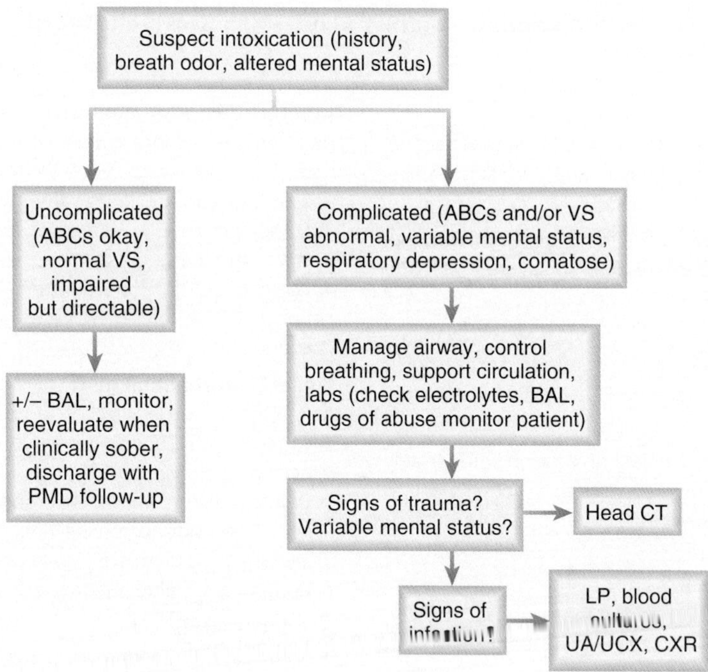


**Fig. 154.3 Treatment algorithm for ethanol intoxication.** *ABCs,* Airway, breathing, circulation; *BAL,* blood alcohol level; *CT,* computed tomography; *CXR,* chest radiograph; *LP,* lumbar puncture; *PMD,* primary care physician; *UA/UCX,* urinalysis/urine culture; *VS,* vital signs.

higher than 9. Lorazepam (1 to 4 mg) has an intermediate half-life and is easily used as either an oral, intramuscular, or intravenous agent. The dose can be repeated every 10 minutes as necessary. Other benzodiazepines, such as diazepam, chlordiazepoxide, and midazolam, can also be used. Massive amounts of benzodiazepines have been known to be given to patients in major withdrawal and may be necessary to control rapidly progressive symptoms, although a symptom-triggered approach has been shown to require less medication and shorter treatment.[25]

Propofol, butyrophenones (haloperidol), and barbiturates (phenobarbital, pentobarbital) are useful adjunct agents in patients not showing response to benzodiazepines. The airway must be closely monitored in these patients. Beta-blockers can also be used to decrease tachycardia in patients undergoing withdrawal from alcohol.

For patients being discharged from the ED and undergoing outpatient detoxification, a short course of benzodiazepines can be considered. Beta-blockers and clonidine may be useful additions to an outpatient treatment regimen for patients with minor withdrawal.

Alcohol-related seizures can result from withdrawal, precipitation of an underlying epileptic disorder, acute toxicity, metabolic causes such as hypoglycemia, trauma, or stroke. Benzodiazepines are first-line therapeutic agents for the treatment of acute seizure in the ED. Phenytoin is not recommended for treatment of an isolated, acute alcohol withdrawal seizure or as routine prophylaxis for patients with alcohol withdrawal and no history of seizures. Phenytoin can be continued in patients with alcohol withdrawal syndrome who are already taking the drug for seizures, and it can be given in the acute setting as deemed necessary for status epilepticus or for seizures resulting from other causes such as stroke or trauma.

## FOLLOW-UP, NEXT STEPS OF CARE, AND PATIENT EDUCATION

The patient with uncomplicated ethanol intoxication may be discharged home after an evaluation for associated disease states if the following criteria are met: (1) the patient is not at risk of airway or breathing complications; and (2) a responsible, sober adult is able to monitor the patient for the next 24 hours. Otherwise, the patient should be monitored in the ED until he or she is clinically and legally sober.

Patients with major ethanol withdrawal require admission and may need an intensive care unit setting. Patients with minor withdrawal may be discharged after observation for 4 to 6 hours if mental status, vital signs, and laboratory study results remain within normal limits. A short course of benzodiazepines can be considered for the patient undergoing outpatient detoxification.

Referral to an outpatient treatment program is appropriate for all patients being discharged who are recognized as having a substance abuse disorder. Options include the use of inpatient versus outpatient treatment programs and referral to Alcoholics Anonymous (AA). Because of the high incidence of underlying social and psychiatric problems, referral to the ED's social or psychiatric worker (if available) may also be helpful.

Patients presenting to the ED with alcohol-related issues should be screened for alcohol abuse and dependence. For patients thought to have or to be at risk for alcohol dependence, brief interventions have been shown to decrease at-risk drinking in the short term and provide an opportunity to provide information on long-term follow-up.[26] The brief intervention is described as a four-step conversation with the patient and consists of the following: (1) broach the subject,

**BOX 154.3 Alcohol Withdrawal Assessment Scoring Guidelines (Revised Clinical Institute Withdrawal Assessment for Alcohol Scale)**

**Nausea and Vomiting (0-7)**
0, none; 1, mild nausea with no vomiting; 4, intermittent nausea; 7, constant nausea, frequent dry heaves and vomiting

**Tremor (0-7)**
0, no tremor; 1, not visible, but can be felt fingertip to fingertip; 4, moderate, with patient's arms extended; 7, severe, even with arms not extended

**Paroxysmal Sweats (0-7)**
0, no sweats; 1, barely perceptible sweating, palms moist; 4, beads of sweat obvious on forehead; 7, drenching sweats

**Anxiety (0-7)**
0, no anxiety, patient at ease; 1, mildly anxious; 4, moderately anxious or guarded, so anxiety is inferred; 7, equivalent to acute panic states seen in severe delirium or acute schizophrenic reactions

**Agitation (0-7)**
0, normal activity; 1, somewhat more than normal activity; 4, moderately fidgety and restless; 7, pacing back and forth during, or constantly thrashing about

**Tactile Disturbances (0-7)**
Ask, "Have you experienced any itching, pins and needles sensation, burning or numbness, or a feeling of bugs crawling on or under your skin?"

0, none; 1, very mild itching, pins and needles, burning, or numbness; 2, mild itching, pins and needles, burning, or numbness; 3, moderate itching, pins and needles, burning, or numbness; 4, moderately severe tactile hallucinations; 5, severe hallucinations; 6, extremely severe hallucinations; 7, continuous hallucinations

**Auditory Disturbances (0-7)**
Ask, "Are you more aware of sounds around you? Are they harsh? Do they startle you? Do you hear anything that disturbs you or that you know isn't there?"

0, not present; 1, very mild harshness or ability to startle; 2, mild harshness or ability to startle; 3, moderate harshness or ability to startle; 4, moderate hallucinations; 5, severe hallucinations; 6, extremely severe hallucinations; 7, continuous hallucinations

**Visual Disturbances (0-7)**
Ask, "Does the light appear to be too bright? Is its color different than normal? Does it hurt your eyes? Are you seeing anything that disturbs you?"

0, not present; 1, very mild sensitivity to light; 2, mild sensitivity; 3, moderate sensitivity; 4, moderate hallucinations; 5, severe hallucinations; 6, extremely severe hallucinations; 7, continuous hallucinations

**Headache (0-7)**
0, not present; 1, very mild; 2, mild; 3, moderate; 4, moderately severe; 5, severe; 6, very severe; 7, extremely severe

**Orientation and Clouding of Sensorium (0-4)**
Ask, "What day is this? Where are you? Who am I?"

0, oriented; 1, cannot do serial additions or is uncertain about date; 2, disoriented to date by no more than 2 calendar days; 3, disoriented to date by more than 2 calendar days; 4, disoriented to place and/or person

**Total Score**
0-9: absent or minimal withdrawal
10-19: mild to moderate withdrawal
More than 20: severe withdrawal

From Sullivan JT, Sykora K, Schneiderman J, et al. Assessment of alcohol withdrawal: the revised clinical institute withdrawal assessment for alcohol scale (CIWA-Ar). Br J Addict 1989;84:1353-7.

(2) give feedback on current drinking patterns, (3) discuss readiness to change drinking habits, and (4) provide information. More information on ED-based brief alcohol interventions can be obtained at http://www.ed.bmc.org/sbirt/.

# OPIOIDS

## EPIDEMIOLOGY

Opioids are a class of drugs that comprise natural, semisynthetic, and synthetic substances that provide analgesic and anesthetic properties by acting at opioid receptors. **Box 154.4** gives the definition of terms associated with opioids. Opioids are most commonly used in the ED for the treatment of acute pain and for procedural sedation, although ED visits for patients with chronic opioid use for both medical and nonmedical reasons have steadily increased since 2000.[27] Between 2004 and 2008, the number of ED visits for nonmedical uses of prescription opioids increased by 111% and now is equivalent to the number of visits associated with illicit drugs.[28] This change parallels the marked increase in opioid prescription rates seen since 2000; approximately 4 million patients in the United States are receiving long-acting, long-term opioid therapy.[29]

Since 2002, opioids have become the leading cause of death from unintentional drug overdose in the United States, and they account for more deaths than heroin and cocaine combined. Opioid overdose can occur in several situations, including intentional self-injury, unintentional prescription, recreational or pediatric ingestion, and drug packing and stuffing.

## PATHOPHYSIOLOGY

Opioids as a medical class are defined by their agonist activity at opioid receptors, of which μ, κ and δ are the best described. Opioid receptor activity in the CNS, spinal cord, and GI system has widespread effects, including analgesia, anesthesia, euphoria, decreased GI motility, respiratory depression,

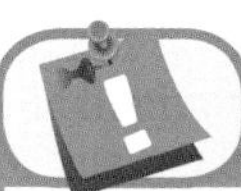

**TIPS AND TRICKS**

- Serum ethanol measurements are not needed in every patient. Obtain an ethanol measurement when needed for confirmation or to guide treatment.
- Remember to rule out any other disease process in the patient with complicated ethanol intoxication.
- Discharge time can be guided by the following: (1) a calculated sober time according to ethanol level; (2) an evaluation for clinical sobriety; or (3) whether the patient is awake and directable and will be in the care of a responsible, sober adult.
- Calculate sober time as follows: (1) subtract 80 to 100 (legal limit) from the blood ethanol level; (2) divide the remainder by 20 (mg/dL/hr); the resulting number is the time to sobriety in hours.
- Opioids may have a long half-life, so additional naloxone doses may be necessary if the patient seems to return to a depressed state after initially responding to naloxone.
- In patients with cancer or long-term pain medication use who present with symptoms of opioid withdrawal, treatment of nausea and vomiting and a dose of the prescribed opioid medications are appropriate.

**BOX 154.4 Definition of Terms Commonly Related to Opioids**

**Opium:** A resin from opium poppies (flowers) containing morphine, codeine, and thebaine

**Opiate:** Only the narcotic alkaloids directly found in opium (morphine, codeine, thebaine)

**Opioid:** Natural, semisynthetic, and synthetic opium derivatives that bind opioid receptors

**Narcotic:** Compounds with sedative properties, commonly including the opioids; in legal jargon, term referring to a controlled substance with illicit use

**Tolerance:** Physiologic adaptation to opioid use with escalating doses required for similar effects

**Dependence:** Continuous use despite negative impacts on life in addition to tolerance, withdrawal history, and compulsive use

**Withdrawal:** Physiologic response to decreased intake of opioids in dependent individuals with behavioral, cognitive, and physical changes

and miosis. Although the many opioids undergo varying types of initial conversion, all opioids undergo hepatic metabolism and renal elimination. These factors should be considered when caring for patients with hepatic and renal dysfunction.

Long-term opioid use can result in physiologic tolerance and dependency through changes in opioid receptor structure, receptor trafficking, and mechanism of action. Withdrawal can be precipitated in opioid-dependent individuals who decrease their intake or are given an opioid receptor antagonist such as naloxone. The timing of withdrawal symptoms depends on the variable half-life of the particular opioid.

Considered the opioid overdose antidote, naloxone is a competitive receptor antagonist that can reverse opioid activity and toxicity. Naloxone is used to reverse the dangerous consequence of respiratory depression in opioid overdose and can be given by various routes, including intravenous, subcutaneous, intramuscular, endotracheal, intranasal, and nebulized. Naloxone is not effective when given orally because of first-pass metabolism.

## PRESENTING SIGNS AND SYMPTOMS

Respiratory depression leading to apnea is the primary life-threatening presentation of opioid overdose. Because respiratory depression is reliably accompanied by altered mental status or coma, a history of opioid use is often not readily available and should be considered in patients who are found unconscious and who have a decreased respiratory rate or miosis. Patients with milder opioid intoxication may present with nausea, vomiting, constipation, miosis, depressed CNS level, and depressed respiratory status. **Table 154.1** contains a more extensive list of these symptoms.

The patient presenting with acute opioid overdose must be evaluated for additional emergency diagnoses, including trauma, infection (particularly in patients who inject opioids), coingestion, electrolyte abnormalities, and complications of prolonged immobility such as rhabdomyolysis, compartment syndrome, and mononeuropathies.

Certain opioids have unique toxicities that must be considered during ED evaluation (**Table 154.2**). Methadone, an agent used primarily for addiction therapy, is very long acting, with a half-life of more than 24 hours, and can cause prolongation of the QTc interval and torsades de pointes. Propoxyphene, tramadol, and meperidine may cause seizures, even in therapeutic doses. Propoxyphene was taken off the market because of its tricyclic antidepressant–like sodium channel activity and association with wide complex tachyarrhythmias and negative inotropy, even at therapeutic doses. Fentanyl, particularly when given as a rapid injection, can cause chest wall rigidity that can be difficult to manage, even with naloxone and endotracheal intubation.[30]

Noncardiogenic pulmonary edema is an uncommon complication of opioid overdose characterized by hypoxia despite resolution of altered mental status and bradypnea, production of frothy pink sputum, and chest radiograph evidence of diffuse pulmonary infiltrates.[31] Opioid-related pulmonary edema is short-lived and infrequently requires intubation, but it mandates admission to the hospital until resolution of symptoms and hypoxia. In the alert patient, noninvasive ventilation can be considered for improved oxygenation.

Patients with opioid withdrawal syndrome present with similarly varied symptoms, but as a rule they appear uncomfortable. Their symptoms may include yawning, rhinorrhea, mydriasis, piloerection, nausea, vomiting, diarrhea, myalgias, and abdominal pain. An acute withdrawal syndrome is seen after the administration of naloxone, particularly in patients with long-term opioid use with dependence.

Vital signs may include tachycardia, normal blood pressure to hypertension, and tachypnea. Another common picture of

**Table 154.1** Opioid Intoxication and Withdrawal Signs and Symptoms by Organ System

| | OPIOID INTOXICATION | OPIOID WITHDRAWAL |
|---|---|---|
| Central nervous system | Depression of activity<br>Respiratory depression<br>Increased parasympathetic activity | Excitation, restlessness, anxiety, seizures (rare)<br>Tachypnea<br>Adrenergic/sympathetic overdrive (lacrimation, piloerection, yawning, diaphoresis) |
| Head and neck | Miosis (pinpoint pupils)<br>Antitussive effect | Mydriasis<br>Rhinorrhea |
| Cardiovascular system | Hypotension to normal blood pressure<br>Bradycardia to normal heart rate | Normal blood pressure to hypertension<br>Normal heart rate to tachycardia |
| Gastrointestinal tract | Constipation<br>Nausea and vomiting | Diarrhea<br>Nausea and vomiting |
| Genitourinary tract | Sphincter constriction/spasm | Sphincter relaxation |
| Musculoskeletal system | Relaxation and flaccidity | Myalgias |
| Psychiatric manifestations | Euphoria or dysphoria | Drug craving |

**Table 154.2** Specific Opioid Toxicities

| COMPOUND | TOXICITY |
|---|---|
| Morphine | Acute lung injury |
| Meperidine | Seizures |
| Methadone | QTc prolongation, torsades de pointes |
| Fentanyl | Chest wall rigidity |
| Propoxyphene | QRS prolongation, seizures |
| Tramadol | Seizures |

Adapted from Gutstein HB, Akil H. Opioid analgesics. In: Brunton LL, editor. Goodman and Gilman's the pharmacological basis of therapeutics. 11th ed. New York: McGraw-Hill; 2006.

**BOX 154.5 Differential Diagnosis for Opioid Overdose**

**Opioid Overdose**

- All components of differential diagnosis for a patient who is unconscious or in a coma
- Alcohol (ethanol, isopropyl, ethylene glycol, methanol) intoxication or overdose
- Barbiturate overdose
- Benzodiazepine overdose
- Clonidine overdose
- Tricyclic antidepressant overdose
- Infection
- Head trauma
- Cerebrovascular accident

opioid withdrawal is seen in the patient who has cancer or uses an opioid for chronic pain and who misses a dose of medication. Such a patient presents to the ED with nausea, vomiting, and abdominal cramping. The history usually uncovers missed opioid doses.

## DIFFERENTIAL DIAGNOSIS AND MEDICAL DECISION MAKING

The differential diagnosis of mild opioid intoxication should include diagnoses that cause altered mental status and hypoventilation: hypoglycemia, head injury, and overdose of other medications (alcohols, benzodiazepines, barbiturates, tricyclic antidepressants). The differential diagnosis for the patient who is ill secondary to opioid overdose is similar to that for the patient in coma; infection, cerebrovascular accident, head trauma, and other overdoses should be considered (**Box 154.5**).

Diagnostic testing in opioid overdose usually does not guide treatment, given that the antidote is administered before test results are available. Tests are used to evaluate for complications of opioid toxicity including arrhythmias, acute lung injury, pulmonary edema, and comorbid diseases. Electrocardiograms and chest radiographs can be useful as adjuncts in these cases. Because intravenous drug abusers are prone to numerous and severe infections, the presence of fever or persistent altered mental status in this population should prompt a rapid and broad work-up.

Urine drug testing does not guide treatment in the acute setting of opioid overdose. Opioids can be detected for up to 36 hours in the urine, although false-positive results have been found after ingestion of poppy seeds. The urine drug screen is also poorly sensitive for detecting use of synthetic opioids, including methadone, fentanyl, hydromorphone, hydrocodone, and oxycodone. Acetaminophen, salicylate, and ethanol measurements should be included in the evaluation for unknown ingestions. A serum chemistry panel and complete blood count can be helpful in the broader evaluation of the sick opioid-toxic patient. The serum creatinine kinase level may be elevated in patients with prolonged immobility and rhabdomyolysis. Many patients awaken after treatment with naloxone, admit to opioid overdose, and may not require any further testing.

The diagnosis of opioid withdrawal can usually be obtained based on history and examination findings. However, because patients with opioid withdrawal can appear systemically ill, other emergency diagnoses such as infection, serotonin syndrome, and sympathomimetic or cholinergic toxicity should be considered.

Diagnostic testing in patients undergoing opioid withdrawal is guided by ruling out other causes of the presenting signs and symptoms. A comprehensive chemistry panel is useful when the patient has massive vomiting and diarrhea.

## TREATMENT

Treatment of opioid intoxication and overdose should begin with assessment of the airway, breathing, and circulatory status of the patient. Airway adjuncts such as an oral or nasal airway can be used to improve the viable airway. In patients with a decreased respiratory rate or apnea, bag-valve-mask ventilation may be necessary before intubation or naloxone administration.

Rapid administration of naloxone may preclude the need for intubation. If signs and symptoms are consistent with opioid intoxication, the antidote should be given immediately while preparations are being made for intubation. Naloxone should be administered intravenously in apneic patients, with starting doses of 0.4 to 1 mg and 2 mg in those with cardiopulmonary arrest. Naloxone can be repeated to reach the desired effect of increased respiratory rate. A higher dose of naloxone may be required for certain naloxone-resistant opioids (e.g., fentanyl, methadone, propoxyphene). Naloxone should take effect in minutes and has a duration of action between 20 and 90 minutes. Repeat dosing or continuous infusion may be necessary for patients who have ingested long-acting opioids such as methadone and extended-release formulations.

Hypotension should be treated with intravenous fluids according to resuscitation protocols. Blood glucose levels should be checked at the bedside, and patients with hypoglycemia should receive dextrose. Care should be taken to reevaluate the patient frequently and observe him or her for a return of respiratory depression.

Activated charcoal administration may be considered only in awake or intubated patients if they had a known recent oral ingestion and especially with coingestions. Opioid-induced seizures may respond to oxygen and naloxone administration. Seizures that do not respond to naloxone may be treated with benzodiazepines. Refractory seizures should prompt investigation of a complicating or additional process such as body packing, head trauma, or other ingestions. Hemodialysis is not indicated in opioid overdose because of the large and variable volume of distribution of these agents in the body.

Treatment of opioid withdrawal in the ED is aimed at stabilization of cardiopulmonary status and symptomatic therapy. Opioid replacement should be guided by the cause of the withdrawal: cessation of prescription medications, methadone

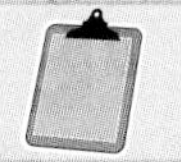

### DOCUMENTATION

**History**

- How much alcohol or opioid was ingested, by what route, and over what period?
- Other drugs ingested?
- History of delirium tremens or alcohol-related seizures?
- Was any trauma or loss of consciousness involved?
- Recent infections?
- Patterns of opioid use?
- Previous history of self-injury?

**Physical Examination**

- Stable or unstable vital signs (including repeat evaluation)?
- Does the patient look ill? Are signs of trauma present?
- Is the patient awake? Arousable? What is the Glasgow Coma Scale score?
- Cardiovascular status
- Respiratory and airway status
- Skin and musculoskeletal findings
- Eye examination: pinpoint pupils
- Findings of any repeat examinations made while the patient is in the emergency department
- Signs of intoxication at admission and discharge, especially if ethanol level was not measured

**Laboratory Studies**

- Levels of aspirin and acetaminophen; urine drug screen results if needed
- Ethanol level if measured
- Electrocardiogram and chest radiograph in patients with abnormal physical findings
- Tests for electrolyte levels, anion gap, complete blood count, serum creatinine, creatine kinase

**Medical Decision Making**

- Complex versus noncomplex alcohol intoxication
- Ruling out of concomitant diseases

**Treatment**

- Treatment strategy, including time monitored, fluid therapy, and any injuries addressed
- Decision to admit or discharge patient
- Time to administration of antidote, initial dose, redosing, or start of naloxone drip

**Patient Instructions**

- Discussion with patient regarding diagnosis, warning signs, what to do, follow-up, when to return
- Referral to outpatient primary medical follow-up and substance abuse centers
- For pediatric accidental ingestions: poison prevention counseling and child protective service notification if indicated

therapy for addiction, and decreased recreational intake. Administering missed doses of opioids and methadone replacement (20 mg orally or 10 mg intramuscularly) can be used to reverse withdrawal without overdose. Clonidine (0.1 to 0.3 mg orally every hour or in a sustained-release patch) can also help with high blood pressure and decrease withdrawal symptoms. Benzodiazepines can be used to aid in sedation and to temper withdrawal symptoms. Antiemetics can be given to the patient with persistent nausea and vomiting.

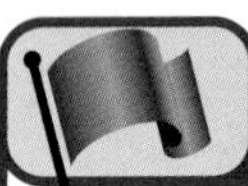

**RED FLAGS**

- Incorrectly assuming the patient is intoxicated
- Not suspecting ethanol abuse in an older patient
- Not recognizing concomitant head injury, intoxication, or associated diseases
- Not aggressively treating signs and symptoms of withdrawal
- Inappropriately discharging an acutely intoxicated patient
- Not managing the airway in a timely manner
- Not evaluating for other causes, including head trauma, infection, and cerebrovascular accident, after repeated doses of naloxone or continued altered consciousness in the patient with suspected intoxication or opioid overdose
- Not considering opioid withdrawal in patients with cancer and in other patients with long-term opioid use and treating appropriately

## FOLLOW-UP, NEXT STEPS OF CARE, AND PATIENT EDUCATION

Patients with opioid intoxication can probably be discharged from the ED after observation and evaluation of any active comorbid diseases at presentation. Patients with uncomplicated opioid overdose can be monitored in the ED for 2 to 4 hours after reversal because the half-life of most opioids is in this range. However, patients who present with overdose from opioids with long half-lives, such as methadone, should be admitted to the hospital for continued airway monitoring. Depending on the type of opioid, the route of administration, and the amount taken, additional doses of naloxone may be required to keep the patient from experiencing opioid reintoxication.

Any patient who requires a second dose of naloxone should be observed for an extended time, and intensive care unit admission should be considered. Patients with complicated opioid overdoses requiring respiratory assistance and those with severe toxicity must be admitted to the hospital's critical care unit.

Unlike alcohol withdrawal, opioid withdrawal is not life-threatening. Most patients may be discharged for outpatient treatment.

## SUGGESTED READINGS

Daeppen JB, Gache P, Landry U, et al. Symptom-triggered vs fixed-schedule doses of benzodiazepine for alcohol withdrawal: a randomized treatment trial. Arch Intern Med 2002;162:1117-21.

Holahan CJ, Schutte KK, Brennan PL, et al. Late-life alcohol consumption and 20-year mortality. Alcohol Clin Exp Res 2010;34:1961-71.

Monte R, Rabunal R, Casariego E, et al. Analysis of the factors determining survival of alcoholic withdrawal syndrome patients in a general hospital. Alcohol Alcohol 2010;45:151-8.

Okie S. A flood of opioids, a rising tide of deaths. N Engl J Med 2010;363:1981-5.

Pitzele HZ, Tolia VM. Twenty per hour: altered mental state due to ethanol abuse and withdrawal. Emerg Med Clin North Am 2010;28:683-705.

## REFERENCES

*References can be found on Expert Consult @ www.expertconsult.com.*

# Sedative-Hypnotic Agents 155

*James W. Rhee and Timothy P. Young*

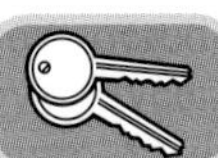

**KEY POINTS**

- Benzodiazepines account for the majority of overdoses with sedative-hypnotic drugs.
- Benzodiazepines can induce cardiovascular and pulmonary toxicity, but fatalities resulting from pure benzodiazepine overdoses are rare.
- Central nervous system depression is the primary symptom of sedative-hypnotic toxicity.
- Treatment should focus on supportive care, with particular attention to airway patency and respiratory function.
- Urinary alkalinization and multiple doses of activated charcoal can enhance the elimination of phenobarbital.
- Flumazenil is a reversal agent for benzodiazepine toxicity, but it should be used cautiously, to avoid the risk of seizures.
- Other possible causes of altered mental status should always be considered.

## EPIDEMIOLOGY

*Sedative-hypnotic agents* are a heterogeneous group of agents that have tranquilizing (sedative) or sleep induction (hypnotic) properties. Grouped with antipsychotics, they comprise the fourth leading class of substances reported to poison centers, and they are the leading cause of reported fatalities.[1] These drugs are widely used in clinical settings but are also used for suicide, illicit recreational activities, and facilitation of sexual assault ("date rape"). Several high-profile deaths have been attributed to sedative-hypnotic overdoses.

*Benzodiazepines* have largely supplanted older agents and have become the most widely used sedative-hypnotics in clinical settings. However, given their prevalence, benzodiazepines also account for the majority of sedative-hypnotic overdoses.[1] Flunitrazepam, sometimes referred to as "roofies,"[2] is a potent benzodiazepine that has been popularized as a street drug of abuse and has been implicated as a date-rape drug.[3]

*Barbiturates* were formerly the primary sedative-hypnotic agents used clinically. Currently, they are most often encountered as anticonvulsants, induction agents for anesthesia, and agents used for procedural sedation. Because the barbiturates have largely been replaced clinically by benzodiazepines due to safety concerns, their prevalence in overdoses has drastically decreased when compared with previous decades.[1] The reported use of barbiturates among high school seniors experienced a slow but steady surge throughout the 1990s and reached a peak in 2005, only to experience a decline since then.[4] Barbiturates accounted for only two single-substance deaths reported to poison centers in 2009.[1]

*Gamma-hydroxybutyrate (GHB)* was synthesized in 1960 as an anesthetic agent. Although it found limited use in this arena, GHB gained widespread acceptance in the body-building community in the 1990s as a purported anabolic agent. More recently, it has been used as a recreational drug for its euphoric and intoxicating effects.[5] It has also been implicated in date rape because of its "knockout" and amnestic properties.

Several *nonbenzodiazepine sedatives* have been introduced for sleep induction. Examples include zolpidem (Ambien), zaleplon (Sonata), and eszopiclone (Lunesta). Cases of abuse and dependence have been reported, albeit with much less frequency compared with benzodiazepines.[6] Nonbenzodiazepine sedatives have been implicated in cases of impaired driving.[7]

*Chloral hydrate* has been used as a sedative since the nineteenth century. In the early 1900s, chloral hydrate was used maliciously, added to alcoholic drinks consumed by unwary individuals to facilitate robberies. The drug-laced drink was referred to as a "Mickey Finn," named after the owner of a Chicago bar who used these drinks to rob unsuspecting patrons.[8] Currently, chloral hydrate is used primarily for procedural sedation.

*Propofol* is a short-acting sedative-hypnotic that has become widely used clinically for induction of anesthesia and procedural sedation. Despite its abuse potential, the literature is limited to case reports of toxicity from recreational use because of its limited availability to the general public.[9] Most reported cases involve self-administration by medical personnel.[10-12] Propofol is covered in greater detail elsewhere in this text.

**BOX 155.1 Benzodiazepines**

**Short Duration (A Few Hours)**
- Midazolam (Versed)
- Triazolam (Halcion)

**Intermediate Duration (Up to a Day)**
- Alprazolam (Xanax)
- Flunitrazepam (Rohypnol)
- Estazolam (ProSom)
- Lorazepam (Ativan)
- Oxazepam (Serax)
- Temazepam (Restoril)

**Long Duration (More Than a Day)**
- Chlordiazepoxide (Librium)
- Clonazepam (Klonopin)
- Clorazepate (Tranxene)
- Diazepam (Valium)
- Flurazepam (Dalmane)
- Halazepam (Paxipam)
- Prazepam (Centrax)
- Quazepam (Doral)

## PATHOPHYSIOLOGY

No strict criteria exist for defining this class of drugs other than possession of sedative-hypnotic properties. Consequently, this class has large numbers of substances with varying pharmacologic mechanisms. Given such a broad definition, many other substances, such as opioids, some antipsychotics, antihistamines, and alcohol, would also be considered part of this class, except that these substances have other unique properties that set them apart.

### BENZODIAZEPINES

Benzodiazepines vary in onset and duration of action according to their lipid solubility and the presence or absence of active metabolites (**Box 155.1**). The more lipid soluble the agent is, the more rapidly it crosses the blood-brain barrier, thus yielding a faster onset of action. The duration of action depends largely on the elimination half-life of specific agents, which can range from hours to days. The duration of action is also affected by the metabolism of certain benzodiazepines because their active metabolites extend the duration of symptoms.

The benzodiazepines produce central nervous system (CNS) depression through effects mediated by gamma-aminobutyric acid (GABA), a major inhibitory neurotransmitter. A specific benzodiazepine receptor exists on the $GABA_A$ receptor. When a benzodiazepine binds to this receptor, it subsequently promotes GABA binding to the $GABA_A$ receptor. Activation of the $GABA_A$ receptor results in influx of chloride into the neuronal cell and causes CNS inhibition. As such, benzodiazepines have anxiolytic, muscle relaxant, sedative, hypnotic, amnestic, and anticonvulsant properties.

Pure benzodiazepine overdoses cause mild to moderate CNS depression. Deep coma requiring assisted ventilation can occur, especially when a benzodiazepine is used with other sedating drugs. In severe overdoses, these agents can induce cardiovascular and pulmonary toxicity, but fatalities resulting from pure benzodiazepine overdoses are rare.

**BOX 155.2 Barbiturates**

**Ultra Short-Acting Barbiturates**
- Methohexital (Brevital)
- Thiamylal (Surital)
- Thiopental (Pentothal)

**Short-Acting and Intermediate-Acting Barbiturates**
- Pentobarbital (Nembutal)
- Amobarbital (Amytal)
- Secobarbital (Seconal)
- Tuinal (amobarbital and secobarbital combination)

**Long-Acting Barbiturates**
- Phenobarbital (Luminal)
- Mephobarbital (Mebaral)

### BARBITURATES

The barbiturates are often classified according to their therapeutic duration of action: ultrashort-acting, short-acting, intermediate-acting, and long-acting agents (**Box 155.2**). In overdoses, however, the duration of action varies with dose, rate of absorption, and rate of distribution and elimination. The ultrashort-acting and short-acting agents are highly lipid soluble and rapidly penetrate the CNS, so the onset of symptoms is also rapid. In addition, the ultrashort-acting barbiturates are more highly protein bound, have higher acid-dissociation constant ($pK_a$), values, and have larger volumes of distribution. Long-acting agents such as phenobarbital are metabolized more slowly in the liver, with a greater fraction of unchanged drug excreted in the kidney. These factors help explain why enhanced renal elimination through alkalinization may be more effective with phenobarbital, which also has a lower pKa than the other barbiturates, thus making it more sensitive to alkalinization. In addition, phenobarbital undergoes enterohepatic recirculation, which makes repeated use of activated charcoal potentially advantageous.

Barbiturates are primarily CNS depressants that mediate their effect through several mechanisms. The barbiturates promote GABA binding to the $GABA_A$ chloride channel complex. They can also bind directly to $GABA_A$ chloride ion channels in the CNS, and the influx of chloride into neuronal cells leads to greater CNS inhibition. Barbiturates may also reduce specific excitatory neurotransmission.

The reticular activating system and the cerebellum appear to be the most susceptible to the depressant effects of barbiturates. Toxicity can lead to suppression of skeletal, smooth, and cardiac muscles, with resulting depressed myocardial contractility, bradycardia, vasodilation, and hypotension (**Table 155.1**).

### GAMMA-HYDROXYBUTYRATE

GHB is a metabolite of GABA that occurs naturally in the human brain.[5] It is highly lipophilic and rapidly absorbed, and, unlike GABA, it readily crosses the blood-brain barrier. Presentation in a coma state and subsequent rapid recovery is characteristic of GHB overdose.

**Table 155.1 Classification of Barbiturates**

| DURATION OF ACTION | BARBITURATE | METABOLISM AND ACTIVITY | TREATMENT |
|---|---|---|---|
| Ultrashort-acting | Methohexital (Brevital)<br>Thiopental (Pentothal) | Highly lipid soluble with rapid CNS penetration | Supportive care<br>Airway protection<br>Activated charcoal |
| Short-acting | Pentobarbital (Nembutal)<br>Secobarbital (Seconal) | Highly lipid soluble with rapid CNS penetration | Supportive care<br>Airway protection<br>Activated charcoal |
| Intermediate-acting | Amobarbital (Amytal)<br>Aprobarbital (Alurate)<br>Butabarbital (Butisol)<br>Butalbital (Fiorinal) | Intermediate CNS penetration (30-60 min) | Supportive care<br>Airway protection<br>Activated charcoal |
| Long-acting | Barbital (Veronal)<br>Mephobarbital (Mebaral)<br>Phenobarbital (Solfoton, Luminal)<br>Primidone (Mysoline) | Metabolized slowly in liver; greater fraction excreted unchanged by kidney; undergoes enterohepatic recirculation | MDAC for phenobarbital<br>Urine alkalinization: use only if unable to give MDAC<br>Hemodialysis in severe cases |

*CNS,* Central nervous system; *MDAC,* multiple-dose activated charcoal.

## NONBENZODIAZEPINE SEDATIVES

This class can be divided into three general structural classes: imidazopyridines, pyrazolopyrimidines, and cyclopyrrolones. Their mechanisms of action are similar. They all act selectively at the benzodiazepine receptor to enhance $GABA_A$ receptor activity. Accordingly, their toxicity mimics that of the benzodiazepines.

## CHLORAL HYDRATE

Chloral hydrate is absorbed completely from the gastrointestinal tract and metabolized rapidly. One of its metabolites, trichloroethanol, is also pharmacologically active and produces sedation. In the presence of ethanol, the metabolism of trichloroethanol is inhibited, with resulting increase in sedation and prolongation of the sedative effects.

Although chloral hydrate has been used for more than a century to induce sedation, its mechanism of action is still largely unknown. It probably works through effects at the GABA receptor, similar to the other sedative-hypnotic agents discussed. Chloral hydrate can also induce cardiac dysrhythmias, most likely by increasing the sensitivity of the myocardium to catecholamines.[13]

## OTHER AGENTS

*Buspirone* is a nonbenzodiazepine used to treat generalized anxiety. Its mechanism of action involves serotonin, rather than GABA. Although buspirone is one of the more commonly reported miscellaneous sedative-hypnotic exposures, significant toxicity from overdose is extremely rare.[1] In one case report, overdose resulted in generalized seizure activity and subsequent full recovery.[14]

*Glutethimide, ethchlorvynol, meprobamate,* and *methaqualone* are older sedative-hypnotic agents that have fallen out of common use. Only meprobamate is still available in the United States. All these agents appear to act by enhancing the effects of GABA.

## PRESENTING SIGNS AND SYMPTOMS

The hallmark of sedative-hypnotic overdose is CNS depression. The degree of CNS depression depends on the dose, the specific agent, and the other agents ingested.

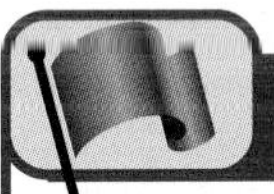

**RED FLAGS**

These signs, symptoms, and test results should prompt the clinician to search for other causes of central nervous system depression:

- Focal neurologic deficit
- Fever
- External evidence of trauma
- Seizure activity
- QRS prolongation on electrocardiogram (seen with agents that can block myocardial sodium channels, such as tricyclic antidepressants)
- Electrolyte abnormalities
- Metabolic acidosis
- Hypoglycemia
- Dysrhythmias (except with chloral hydrate)

Mild to moderate sedative-hypnotic overdoses may manifest with a reduced level of consciousness, slurred speech, and ataxia. At high doses, sedative-hypnotic agents can cause hypothermia, hypotension, bradycardia, flaccidity, hyporeflexia, coma, and apnea. These severe symptoms are more commonly encountered in barbiturate overdoses. Patients with severe overdoses may appear to be dead, with no electroencephalographic activity.

**TIPS AND TRICKS**

- Pear-like odor is associated with chloral hydrate.
- Chloral hydrate overdoses may manifest with cardiac toxicity as well as with central nervous system depression.
- Bullous lesions are sometimes associated with barbiturate overdoses.
- Consider rhabdomyolysis as a complication.
- A patient who appears brain dead after a severe sedative-hypnotic (barbiturate) overdose may not be brain dead.
- Use beta-blockers to treat chloral hydrate–induced cardiac dysrhythmias.
- Epinephrine and norepinephrine are relatively contraindicated in chloral hydrate overdose because the myocardium may have an increased sensitivity to these types of agents.
- The most common drug used to facilitate sexual assault is ethanol, not sedative-hypnotics.
- MDAC appears to be superior to urinary alkalinization in enhancing the elimination of phenobarbital, and performing both procedures concurrently has no apparent benefit.

*MDAC*, Multiple-dose activated charcoal.

## DIFFERENTIAL DIAGNOSIS AND MEDICAL DECISION MAKING

The differential diagnosis of sedative-hypnotic toxicity includes any condition or ingestion resulting in CNS depression. Many other substances are capable of producing profound CNS depression, including alcohol and opiates. However, care should be made not to miss other, nontoxicologic causes of CNS depression. Although sedative-hypnotic toxicity resolves with just supportive care, other mimickers of sedative-hypnotic overdose may need other acute interventions. Other diagnoses that should be considered include head trauma with intracranial hemorrhage, embolic and hemorrhagic stroke, electrolyte abnormalities, hypoglycemia, hyperglycemic crisis, hypoxemia, hypothyroidism, liver or renal failure, CNS infection, seizures, and significant alterations in temperature (**Table 155.2**).

Diagnostic testing should be used to help exclude other causes of altered mental status. A fingerstick blood glucose determination, pulse oximetry, and cardiac monitoring may help the clinician avoid missing hypoglycemia, hypoxemia, or dysrhythmia.

Further testing to help clarify the patient's presentation may include serum electrolytes, blood urea nitrogen, serum creatinine, serum ethanol, blood gas analysis, chest radiograph, computed tomography of the brain, cerebrospinal fluid analysis, serum transaminases, serum bilirubin, ammonia level, blood cultures, and urinalysis. If the patient is female, a urine pregnancy test is warranted. Directed quantitative serum levels of certain drugs may also be helpful; these may include acetaminophen, salicylate, lithium, and anticonvulsants.

Most institutions have a qualitative urine drug screen available, although this screen varies by institution. Most of the screens are immunoassays that detect the presence of certain drugs or metabolites in the urine. In the case of sedative-hypnotic agents, the commonly available screens usually test for benzodiazepines. The other sedative-hypnotic agents are typically not included in most urine drug screens. The typical benzodiazepine screen identifies metabolites of 1,4-benzodiazepines such as oxazepam or desmethyldiazepam. Benzodiazepines that are not metabolized or are metabolized to other compounds remain undetected. In addition, the detection cutoff may be set at a point at which the assay may not detect certain agents that can induce effects in very small amounts. A false-negative screen result may occur with

**Table 155.2** Differential Diagnosis of Sedative-Hypnotic Toxidromes and Priority Actions

| DIAGNOSTIC CONSIDERATION | PRIORITY ACTION(S) |
|---|---|
| Airway and respiratory status? | Provide airway protection and respiratory support as needed |
| Trauma? | If trauma is suspected, maintain spinal immobilization<br>Obtain computed tomography of the head |
| Cardiovascular status? | Start cardiac monitoring<br>Establish intravenous access<br>Administer vasopressors for refractory hypotension<br>Administer intravenous bolus(es) of isotonic crystalloid solution for hypotension<br>Avoid epinephrine and norepinephrine in known or suspected chloral hydrate overdose |
| Hypothermia or hyperthermia? | Actively rewarm severely hypothermic patients<br>Use active cooling for hyperthermia, and evaluate for infectious causes |
| Overdose or toxicity? | Consider administering activated charcoal to patients with a secure airway<br>Use MDAC in overdoses of long-acting barbiturates<br>Perform primary alkalinization for overdoses of long-acting barbiturates in which MDAC is not advised<br>Consider hemodialysis in severe cases |

*MDAC*, Multiple-dose activated charcoal.

certain benzodiazepines, including alprazolam, clonazepam, and flunitrazepam. The clinician must recognize the limitations of this screen.

Quantitative benzodiazepine concentrations correlate poorly with pharmacologic or toxicologic effects and are poor predictors of clinical outcome.

A quantitative serum phenobarbital level can be helpful to document toxicity, but it is not mandatory for definitive typically management. Therapeutic concentrations of phenobarbital range between 15 and 40 mg/L. Patients with levels higher than 50 mg/L exhibit mild toxicity, whereas patients with levels higher than 100 mg/L are typically unresponsive to pain and may suffer from respiratory and cardiac depression.

## TREATMENT

The mainstay of treatment for the patient with sedative-hypnotic overdose is supportive care, with particular attention to airway patency and respiratory status. When hypotension occurs, it should be managed with fluid resuscitation and vasopressors as needed.

Beta blockers have been successfully used to treat cardiac dysrhythmias resulting from chloral hydrate toxicity because myocardial catecholamine sensitivity is believed to induce the dysrhythmia.[15] Epinephrine and norepinephrine are relatively contraindicated because the myocardium may have increased sensitivity to these types of agents.

Patients who are stable after significant ingestions should receive activated charcoal as a means of preventing absorption of drugs still contained within the gastrointestinal tract. The efficacy of this procedure decays with time, so activated charcoal should be given expeditiously, ideally within the first hour after the ingestion occurred. The initial dose of activated charcoal is typically 1 g/kg. Ideally, at least a 10 : 1 ratio of charcoal to drug should be achieved. Given the CNS depression caused by sedative-hypnotics, careful attention should be directed to avoiding aspiration. If airway-protective reflexes are not intact, then administration of activated charcoal should be withheld unless the airway is protected by some other means.

Repeat dosing of activated charcoal has been recommended for increased clearance of certain drugs, one of which is phenobarbital.[16] This therapeutic procedure has been referred to as multiple-dose activated charcoal (MDAC). It is thought to be helpful for phenobarbital because this drug undergoes enterohepatic circulation and is excreted back into the gut, where activated charcoal present in the intestine may bind it before it is reabsorbed distally. Phenobarbital also has physical characteristics that allow it to diffuse from the blood into the intestinal lumen. With MDAC, activated charcoal avidly binds to the phenobarbital in the intestinal lumen, a process that creates a concentration gradient into the intestine and subsequently enhances the elimination of the phenobarbital.[17,18] Although MDAC has been shown to increase clearance phenobarbital, it has not been shown to improve overall clinical outcomes.

After the initial dose of activated charcoal, a reasonable dosing regimen for MDAC in adults can be accomplished by administering 25 g of activated charcoal without a cathartic every 2 hours. In pediatric patients, a dose of 0.25 g/kg every 2 hours may be used. The activated charcoal can be administered orally or through a nasogastric or orogastric tube. If a feeding pump is available, the activated charcoal can be administered continuously instead of at 2-hour intervals. Physicians must be aware that some charcoal preparations are premixed with a cathartic (usually sorbitol), and repeat doses are contraindicated because they may cause dehydration and electrolyte imbalances. A small dose of sorbitol (0.2 to 0.5 g/kg) may be given with the first dose of activated charcoal to prevent constipation. MDAC is contraindicated in patients who do not have protective airway reflexes or an otherwise secure airway. MDAC is also contraindicated in patients who have evidence of ileus or who are hemodynamically unstable.

Alkalinizing the urine with the intravenous administration of sodium bicarbonate can increase the elimination of phenobarbital. Urinary alkalinization with sodium bicarbonate to a pH of 7.5 to 8.0 can hasten the renal excretion of phenobarbital.[19] Urinary alkalinization can be accomplished with an initial sodium bicarbonate bolus of 1 mEq/kg, followed by a continuous infusion. This infusion is made by adding 100 to 150 mEq of sodium bicarbonate to 850 mL of dextrose 5% in water and titrating it to maintain a urine pH of greater than 7.5 with an arterial pH less than 7.5. The rate must be assessed hourly to avoid excessive administration of fluid or bicarbonate, which can cause pulmonary or cerebral edema or electrolyte imbalance. Although expediting the elimination of phenobarbital from the body has theoretical benefit, no difference in clinical outcome has been shown. Alkalinization does not increase excretion of short- and medium-acting agents, which are more lipid soluble.

MDAC appears to be superior to urinary alkalinization for enhancing the elimination of phenobarbital.[20] Performing both procedures concurrently appears to have no benefit.[21] Urinary alkalinization may still be useful in a patient who cannot undergo MDAC.

In patients who are not responsive to standard therapeutic measures, or in patients with renal failure, hemodialysis may help eliminate long-acting barbiturates.[22] These agents are less protein bound and less lipid soluble that the shorter-acting barbiturates, characteristics that enhance the role of hemodialysis. Fortunately, extracorporeal elimination is rarely indicated because most barbiturate overdoses resolve with supportive care alone.

Hemodialysis can enhance the elimination of chloral hydrate and its metabolites.[23] However, supportive measures are generally effective. Hemodialysis may have a role if a patient with chloral hydrate toxicity is not responding to conservative therapy.

Flumazenil is a specific antagonist for benzodiazepines (**Box 155.3**). It competitively binds at the benzodiazepine receptor, displaces benzodiazepines from the site, and inhibits GABA potentiation. Flumazenil is lipid soluble and readily crosses the blood-brain barrier to exert its effects quickly. Typically, benzodiazepine induced sedation is reversed within a couple of minutes.

In the setting of procedural sedation, flumazenil is an excellent rescue agent for inadvertent supratherapeutic administrations of a benzodiazepine agent.[24] Flumazenil may also be helpful in the setting of an isolated known benzodiazepine overdose. Unfortunately, this situation rarely occurs clinically. The use of flumazenil in the setting of a multiple drug overdose that includes a benzodiazepine is less clear.

Overall, for an unknown overdose, the administration of flumazenil is not indicated.[25] Flumazenil does not antagonize

**BOX 155.3 Flumazenil**

**Dose**
Adult: 0.2-3 mg IV, slowly titrate to response
Pediatric: 0.005-0.2 mg/kg IV, slowly titrate to response

**Indication**
Isolated benzodiazepine toxicity

**Contraindications**
Seizure disorder
Chronic benzodiazepine use
Suspected coingestion of a seizure-inducing substance

*IV*, intravenously.

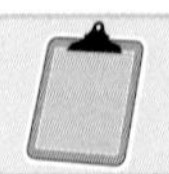

**DOCUMENTATION**

**History**
- Any history of psychiatric illness or prior suicide ingestions
- Time lapse since ingestion, if known
- History of renal or cardiac disease or other illnesses that will exacerbate the complications
- Drug taken, dose, and quantity

**Physical Examination**
- Does the patient look ill? Febrile? Mental status? Respiratory and airway status? Signs of trauma?
- Cardiac status (blood pressure, arrhythmias)?
- Should include repeat examinations while patient is in the emergency department

**Laboratory Studies**
For cases of alleged facilitated sexual assault, consult with local law enforcement regarding the handling of a patient's urine specimen because it may be tested at a forensic laboratory for the presence of "date-rape" drugs.

**Medical Decision Making**
- Decision to begin treatment or delays
- Consultations and time called

**Treatment**
- Interventions and timing

**Patient Instructions**
- Document discussion with the patient regarding diagnosis, warning signs, what to do, follow-up, and when to return.
- With pediatric accidental ingestions, document poison prevention counseling.
- Instruct the patient to avoid combination of these drugs with alcohol and antihistamines.

the CNS effects of alcohol, barbiturates, tricyclic antidepressants, or narcotics. Reports have noted precipitation of seizure activity in the setting of mixed overdose or benzodiazepine dependence.[26] Because supportive therapy is usually effective in benzodiazepine overdose, the benefit of flumazenil may not outweigh the risks of administration when circumstances surrounding the toxic ingestion are unclear. Flumazenil use has been described in the setting of overdose of the newer, non-benzodiazepine sedatives.[27] However, supportive care is usually effective in these cases as well.

## PARADOXICAL REACTIONS

Occasionally, patients who have been exposed to sedative-hypnotic agents experience a reaction that can be characterized by an increase in psychomotor activity. This has been most commonly described in benzodiazepines.[28] The reactions can range from increased talkativeness and excessive movement to rage and hostility. As a whole, these reactions have been termed paradoxical because they seem counter to the sedative properties of these agents.

The mechanism of these paradoxical reactions is unclear, but some characteristics seem to increase the risk of these reactions. These characteristics include the younger and older age groups, as well as underlying psychiatric disorders. A genetic predisposition to these reactions may also exist.[29]

The use of flumazenil,[30-32] haloperidol,[33] and other agents has been described for the treatment of these reactions, with variable success. However, the mainstay of treatment should focus on supportive care. This attention to supportive care should be all that is required.

## FOLLOW-UP, NEXT STEPS IN CARE, AND PATIENT EDUCATION

Patients who are symptom free from an isolated sedative-hypnotic overdose may be discharged home after a traditional 4- to 6-hour observation period. However, the events leading to the exposure may preclude discharge home. Psychiatry consultation is necessary for those patients with intentional overdoses.

Patients with prolonged sedation or other evidence of toxicity should be admitted for further observation and treatment.

Admission to a critical care setting is dictated by the severity of toxicity. Hemodynamic instability, respiratory failure, coma, severe hypothermia, and the need for hemodialysis are some indications for admission to an intensive care unit.

## SUGGESTED READINGS

Chudnofsky CR. Safety and efficacy of flumazenil in reversing conscious sedation in the emergency department: Emergency Medicine Conscious Sedation Study Group. Acad Emerg Med 1997;4:944-50.

Gueye PN, Hoffman JR, Taboulet P, et al. Empiric use of flumazenil in comatose patients: limited applicability of criteria to define low risk. Ann Emerg Med 1996;27:730-5.

Hall R, Zisook S. Paradoxical reactions to benzodiazepines. Br J Clin Pharmacol 1981;11(suppl 1):99S-104S.

Pond SM, Olson KR, Osterloh JD, Tong TG. Randomized study of the treatment of phenobarbital overdose with repeated doses of activated charcoal. JAMA 1984;251:3104-8.

## REFERENCES

*References can be found on Expert Consult @ www.expertconsult.com.*

# Hypoglycemic Agent Overdose 156

Mark Su

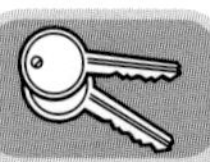

**KEY POINTS**

- Hypoglycemia is defined either by serum glucose level or on the basis of symptoms.
- Typically, an adult has enough glycogen to last approximately 6 to 8 hours.
- Insulin treatment is the most common cause of hypoglycemia in adults with diabetes.
- Extreme glucose values (either high or low) and hypoperfusion can cause a significant discrepancy in bedside glucose testing results.
- Sodium bicarbonate administered to alkalinize the urine has been shown to reduce the half-life of the sulfonylurea chlorpropamide.
- Patients with overdoses (intentional or unintentional) of insulin, sulfonylureas, and meglitinides should be admitted for inpatient observation because of the unpredictable kinetics of these agents.

## EPIDEMIOLOGY

For the purposes of this chapter, the term *hypoglycemia* refers to the condition of blood glucose concentration for which medical intervention is usually necessary. It is occasionally referred to in the literature as severe hypoglycemia.[1]

The exact incidence of hypoglycemia in nondiabetic persons is unknown. However, in patients with diabetes mellitus (DM), the occurrence of hypoglycemia depends on factors such as whether the patient has type 1 or type 2 DM and what type of pharmacologic therapy the patient is receiving (i.e., insulin, an oral antihyperglycemic agent). In patients with type 1 DM, hypoglycemia reportedly occurs at an approximate rate of 1.1 to 3.2 episodes per patient per year.[2]

The diagnosis is often made empirically by prehospital care providers before the patient's arrival in the emergency department (ED); however, death resulting from hypoglycemic coma may still occur if the condition is unrecognized.[3] A few patients intentionally overdose, and treating them can be extremely difficult. This chapter discusses important factors in the evaluation and treatment of patients with toxicity secondary to hypoglycemic agent overdose.

## PATHOPHYSIOLOGY

The primary metabolic substrate for the central nervous system (CNS) is glucose. Usual sources of glucose are diet, endogenous production (through gluconeogenesis), and storage (through glycogenolysis). Serum glucose concentrations are relatively tightly controlled by physiologic mechanisms. After dietary sources of glucose are completely used, glycogenolysis is the major physiologic mechanism for maintaining euglycemia. Typically, an adult has enough glycogen to last approximately 6 to 8 hours. When glycogen stores are depleted, gluconeogenesis, which is fueled by amino acids from muscle, takes over. The CNS cannot make or store glucose, and it relies on the previously mentioned mechanisms to maintain normal metabolic activity during fasting periods. As glucose use exceeds glucose production and serum glucose concentrations decrease, various counterregulatory pathways are activated. Counterregulatory pathways triggered at the glycemic threshold are increases in glucagon, epinephrine, growth hormone, and cortisol. Glycemic thresholds are fairly reproducible in research studies on healthy subjects, but these thresholds can vary significantly among patients with both type 1 and type 2 DM. These thresholds also depend on other factors, such as tightness of glucose regulation, the presence of chronic hyperglycemia, and recent episodes of hypoglycemia.[4]

Hypoglycemic agents induce hypoglycemia by various mechanisms. Insulins cause rapid transport of amino acids and glucose intracellularly. Sulfonylureas stimulate insulin secretion by binding to specific membrane receptors on the pancreatic beta-islet cell. These drugs also benefit glucose homeostasis by decreasing hepatic glucose production and improving insulin sensitivity at the receptor and postreceptor levels.[5] Other drugs may induce hypoglycemia by inhibition of gluconeogenesis, glycogenolysis, counterregulatory hormones, or other unknown mechanisms. Ethanol, a toxin commonly encountered in the ED, inhibits gluconeogenesis by depleting nicotinamide adenine dinucleotide and also inhibits the effects of cortisol, growth hormone, and epinephrine.[1]

## PRESENTING SIGNS AND SYMPTOMS

The symptoms of hypoglycemia can be divided into two basic groups: hyperadrenergic symptoms and neuroglycopenic

**BOX 156.1 Symptoms of Hypoglycemia**

**Hyperadrenergic Symptoms**

- Anxiety
- Nervousness
- Tremulousness
- Irritability
- Nausea and vomiting
- Palpitations and tachycardia
- Sweating
- Pallor
- Hypersalivation
- Pupillary changes

**Neuroglycopenic Symptoms**

- Decreased cognitive ability
- Agitation and emotional lability
- Sensations of warmth (despite cool, clammy skin)
- Blurred vision
- Slurred speech
- Lethargy
- Confusion
- Unresponsiveness
- Focal neurologic deficits
- Psychotic behavior
- Seizures

**Table 156.1** Three Categories of Hypoglycemia

| TYPE OF HYPOGLYCEMIA | CAUSES |
|---|---|
| Postprandial | Early diabetes<br>Alcohol intake<br>Postgastrectomy status<br>Renal failure<br>Drugs (e.g., salicylates, beta-blockers, pentamidine) |
| Fasting | Conditions of excess insulin, including insulinoma and self-administration of insulin or oral hypoglycemic agents (diabetic insulin overdose)<br>Alcohol abuse and liver disease (decreased gluconeogenesis)<br>Pituitary or adrenal insufficiency |
| Drug- or toxin-induced | Ethanol<br>Quinidine<br>Beta-blockers<br>Pentamidine<br>Monoamine oxidase inhibitors<br>Angiotensin-converting enzyme inhibitors<br>Salicylates<br>Haloperidol<br>Disopyramide<br>Ackee fruit<br>Trimethoprim-sulfamethoxazole |

symptoms (**Box 156.1**). Hyperadrenergic symptoms are more common with a rapid decrease in glucose and result from autonomic nervous system stimulation (both sympathetic and cholinergic). The other clinical features of hypoglycemia are mediated through altered brain activity; the resulting constellation of signs and symptoms of hypoglycemia is termed neuroglycopenia.[6] Three neuroglycopenic syndromes are described: acute, subacute, and chronic.[7] *Subacute neuroglycopenia* is characterized by episodic disorientation, somnolence, slurring of speech, personality changes, amnesia, and loss of consciousness. Precipitous loss of consciousness may occur as the sole manifestation of subacute neuroglycopenia. Both subacute and acute forms of neuroglycopenia may manifest as acute neurologic deficits (e.g., transient hemiplegia), strabismus, hypothermia, hyperthermia, seizures, and automatism. *Chronic neuroglycopenia* is a rare condition that usually occurs in patients with insulinoma and in patients with DM who are treated with excessive insulin and who demonstrate a gradual progressive mental illness similar to a chronic psychiatric disorder.[7]

## DIFFERENTIAL DIAGNOSIS AND MEDICAL DECISION MAKING

Hypoglycemia has numerous causes and may be classified into the following three categories: (1) postprandial, (2) fasting, and (3) drug- or toxin-induced (**Table 156.1**).[1] In healthy patients, fasting hypoglycemia is usually the result of unintentional or intentional drug ingestion and insulinoma. In patients who are severely ill or hospitalized, hypoglycemia may be a complication of the illness, drug interactions, or other iatrogenic factors.

Hypoglycemic agents can be divided according to their route of administration (i.e., parenteral or oral). Insulins and the newer agents, incretins (e.g., exenatide [Byetta], liraglutide [Victoza]), are the only medications for the treatment of DM that are given parenterally. Many antidiabetic medications are given orally, including the sulfonylureas (e.g., glyburide [Diabeta], glipizide [Glucotrol]), meglitinides (e.g., nateglinide [Starlix], repaglinide [Prandin]), biguanides (e.g., metformin), thiazolidinediones (e.g., rosiglitazone [Avandia], pioglitazone [Actos], and α-glucosidase inhibitors (e.g., acarbose [Precose]). Of all these antidiabetic drugs, only a few classes are commonly associated with hypoglycemia—the insulins, sulfonylureas, and meglitinides.

For adults with DM, insulin treatment is the most common cause of hypoglycemia. Factors associated with higher frequency of hypoglycemia in patients with type 1 DM include lower hemoglobin $A_{1c}$, higher daily insulin requirements, longer duration of DM, and a previous history of hypoglycemia. Approximately 25% of patients with DM are unable to recognize impending hypoglycemia because of a lack of autonomic warning symptoms; this characteristic is also an important predictor of hypoglycemia.[1] Patients with insulin-dependent type 2 DM are also susceptible to hypoglycemia, especially if their disease has been treated with insulin for a long time and if their DM is tightly controlled.[8]

For patients who are taking oral agents rather than insulin, sulfonylureas are a common cause of hypoglycemia. According to the 2010 annual report of the American Association of

Poison Control Centers' Toxic Surveillance System, 4109 reported sulfonylurea exposures, with 38 major outcomes and 1 death, occurred in 2009.[9] The incidence of hypoglycemia secondary to these agents rises in older patients and with long-acting agents (e.g., chlorpropamide).[10] Consequently, independent risk factors for hypoglycemia include recent hospitalization, advanced age, and polypharmacy. Other risk factors for sulfonylurea-induced hypoglycemia are hepatic and renal dysfunction because of decreased metabolism (e.g., glyburide, glibenclamide, glipizide) and decreased elimination (e.g., chlorpropamide, glyburide). The most commonly used sulfonylureas have a duration of effect of at least 24 hours, and hypoglycemia in a patient taking such an agent can be prolonged, especially in the setting of overdose. In one case report, sulfonylurea-induced hypoglycemia was reported to last up to 27 days.[11] Most other oral agents (e.g., thiazolidinediones, biguanides) used for the treatment of DM do not usually cause significant hypoglycemia.

Hypoglycemia is a simple diagnosis to make, provided it is considered early in a patient's presentation. In most cases, hypoglycemia is considered in a patient with altered sensorium or depressed mental status. Bedside blood glucose testing using a glucose meter in the patient with neuroglycopenic symptoms is generally the fastest technique, as well as a fairly reliable method, to determine hypoglycemia. In general, the correlation of capillary blood glucose levels (which are measured by a glucose meter) with venous or arterial glucose measurements seems to be good.[12,13] At extreme values (either high or low) and in cases of systemic hypoperfusion, however, a clinically significant discrepancy may be apparent. In the setting of suspected hypoglycemia, confirmatory laboratory testing of a serum specimen is therefore necessary. Furthermore, because symptoms of hypoglycemia vary among individuals, hypoglycemia is still a possible diagnosis even in a patient with a glucose level categorized as euglycemic.[14]

Additional diagnostic testing may be necessary, depending on the clinical situation. For most patients with DM who present with hypoglycemia, routine testing of liver and renal function is indicated. Ethanol (or other alcohol) ingestion may also result in hypoglycemia, and measurement of serum ethanol concentration may be useful in the setting of alcohol intoxication. Other tests that may be helpful are thyroid function tests and measurements of serum cortisol, insulin, and C peptide concentrations. Insulin and C peptide measurements are particularly useful in the setting of surreptitious exposure to insulin or sulfonylureas. Unlike endogenous insulin synthesized by the pancreas, exogenous insulin has no concomitant C peptide. In cases of intentional insulin poisoning, insulin concentrations are high, but C peptide concentrations are normal. On the contrary, sulfonylurea ingestions cause elevations in both insulin and C peptide, the same findings as in patients with insulinoma. Finally, in patients with intentional self-harm, testing of serum acetaminophen concentration is potentially useful.

**BOX 156.2 Treatment of Hypoglycemic Agent Overdose**

1. Basic support measures with attention to airway, breathing, circulation, and cardiopulmonary monitoring
2. Bedside glucose testing and an immediate bolus of glucose; hypoglycemia treated with IV glucose for severe episodes and when associated with obtundation: 0.5-1 g/kg of $D_{50}W$ for adults and of $D_{25}W$ for children
3. Consideration of thiamine and naloxone for obtunded patients
4. After initial euglycemia, continuous IV infusions of dextrose ($D_5W$ or $D_{10}W$) started and boluses repeated when indicated
5. Decontamination with activated charcoal, either a single dose or multiple doses, for agents such as glipizide (enterohepatic circulation)
6. Enhanced elimination with IV sodium bicarbonate to alkalinize urine and reduce the half-life for long-acting sulfonylureas (e.g., chlorpropamide)
7. Observation and admission for signs of neuroglycopenia and repeated serum glucose checks every 1 to 2 hr; monitoring of serum electrolyte levels every 4 hr
8. Octreotide, 50 mcg given subcutaneously every 6 to 8 hr, for at least 24 hr, in cases of prolonged hypoglycemia secondary to long-acting sulfonylurea overdose

*$D_5W$, $D_{10}W$, $D_{25}W$,* and *$D_{50}W$,* 5%, 10%, 25%, and 50% dextrose in water, respectively; *IV,* intravenous.

## TREATMENT

The emergency physician must institute basic supportive measures, with particular attention to airway, breathing, and circulation, along with cardiorespiratory monitoring on encountering the obtunded patient with hypoglycemia (**Box 156.2** has a treatment summary). Supplemental oxygen, intravenous (IV) thiamine, and naloxone are generally benign therapies that may be judiciously administered in a patient with depressed mental status of unknown origin.

After the primary survey has been performed and any needed measures taken, gastrointestinal decontamination should be considered for patients who have taken an intentional oral overdose of a hypoglycemic agent. The particular modality of decontamination implemented depends on the usual factors, such as time of ingestion, quantity of tablets, mental status of the patient, and potential harm to the patient. Activated charcoal has been shown to be very effective in binding to multiple sulfonylurea agents in vitro.[15] A single dose of activated charcoal may be beneficial in these ingestions. In theory, multiple-dose activated charcoal may enhance elimination of the sulfonylurea glipizide because glipizide undergoes enterohepatic circulation.[5] IV sodium bicarbonate administered to alkalinize the urine has been shown to reduce the half-life of the sulfonylurea agent chlorpropamide.[16] These and other forms of decontamination and enhanced elimination should be used on a case-by-case basis.

Patients who are documented to have hypoglycemia by rapid bedside glucose testing should be given glucose as soon as possible. If a patient is awake and is believed to have intact airway reflexes, oral carbohydrates in the form of flavored glucose tablets, juice, and soda may be given. The patient should show response within 10 to 15 minutes as he or she returns to a euglycemic state. After this initial therapy, the patient should be given additional nutrition in the form of a snack or meal for a sustained source of calories. If the patient does not show response to oral carbohydrates, parenteral therapy is required.

IV dextrose is the preferred treatment for severe hypoglycemia with obtundation and a patient's inability to take oral carbohydrates. The administration of 0.5 to 1 g/kg of IV dextrose rapidly reverses the clinical effects of hypoglycemia. Hypertonic dextrose solutions are commonly found in syringes containing 50 mL of 50% dextrose in water ($D_{50}W$), which is equivalent to 25 g of dextrose (4 calories/g of glucose or 100 calories). An average man weighing 70 kg would therefore require 35 to 70 g of dextrose. Administration of hypertonic dextrose is fairly safe, and only a few cases of significant adverse effects such as seizures, hyperosmolar coma, and death have been reported.[17] A much more common effect is phlebitis, which can be mitigated by injection of the dextrose into a large vein, followed by a saline flush.[1]

After initial euglycemia is achieved, patients should be given continuous IV infusions of dextrose. Dextrose-water solutions of 5% ($D_5W$) and 10% ($D_{10}W$) are usually used in this setting, and the dose is titrated along with other therapies to maintain euglycemia. For patients with repeated episodes of hypoglycemia, higher concentrations of dextrose and repeated boluses of $D_{50}W$ may be required. In this setting, hypertonic dextrose solutions should be administered by central line access because of the irritant venous effects of these solutions.

Treatment of overdose with a specific hypoglycemic agent depends on the agent. Some hypoglycemic agents, such as the meglitinides, are very short-acting drugs, and the resulting hypoglycemia is unlikely to be prolonged. For longer-acting insulins and the sulfonylureas, intensive therapy may be necessary for 1 or 2 days or even longer. The previously described approach to management is a general guideline to patients with hypoglycemia. Regardless of the cause of the hypoglycemia, patients should be frequently observed for signs of neuroglycopenia, bedside glucose checks should be performed every 1 to 2 hours at a minimum, and serum electrolyte levels should be monitored every 4 hours. Some patients may also require specific antidotal therapy, as described later.

Glucagon may also be administered by the subcutaneous, intramuscular, or IV route to stimulate hepatic glycogenolysis. Glucagon is most beneficial if it is given soon after the onset of hypoglycemic coma and to treat hypoglycemia in type 1 DM.[1,17] Glucagon is less effective in patients with type 2 DM because it causes the release of insulin.[18] These patients are also likely to already have depleted glycogen stores, thus limiting the efficacy of glucagon. Furthermore, glucagon administration may cause nausea and vomiting, which impair the ability to give oral carbohydrate therapy. Hypertonic IV dextrose is therefore the preferred initial therapy in the setting of acute hypoglycemia.

In patients with sulfonylurea-induced hypoglycemia, the same supportive measures as previously described are initially implemented. Occasionally, prolonged hypoglycemia may occur after a sulfonylurea overdose, especially with the long-acting agents. Antidotal therapy with octreotide should be considered in such refractory cases. A synthetic somatostatin analogue, octreotide inhibits the secretion of several neuropeptides, including insulin, and it is used clinically to suppress excessive growth hormone secretion, inhibit thyrotropin-secreting pituitary adenomas, and treat certain gastrointestinal and pancreatic neuroendocrine tumors (e.g., carcinoid insulinomas).[17]

Previously, the antihypertensive diazoxide was the recommended agent of choice for refractory hypoglycemia resulting from a sulfonylurea because of its ability to inhibit insulin secretion by opening adenosine triphosphate (ATP)–sensitive potassium ($K_{ATP}$) channels in pancreatic beta-islet cells.[19] Although the use of octreotide for sulfonylurea-induced hypoglycemia is "off label" (i.e., the agent has not been approved by the U.S. Food and Drug Administration for this purpose), multiple case reports and research document its efficacy and safety. On the contrary, diazoxide has been shown to be less effective and has several undesirable properties.[20] Diazoxide is usually administered by IV infusion, and its efficacy is limited in these situations because of associated hypotension, tachycardia, nausea, and vomiting. Adverse effects associated with octreotide are minimally significant; they include pain at the injection site, nausea, bloating, flatulence, diarrhea, and constipation. For these reasons, octreotide has supplanted diazoxide as the treatment of choice for sulfonylurea-induced hypoglycemia.

Octreotide has an IV half-life of 72 minutes, but when administered subcutaneously, it appears to be effective for approximately 6 hours.[19] Consequently, a reasonable dosing scheme for most sulfonylurea agents would be 50 mcg subcutaneously every 8 to 12 hours (one noted textbook recommends every 6 hours) for at least 24 hours.[19,21] After the octreotide is discontinued, an observation period for repetition of hypoglycemia is warranted for a minimum of 12 to 24 hours.

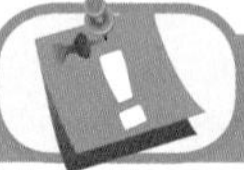

**TIPS AND TRICKS**

- Ill-appearing patients may have sepsis, chronic liver or renal failure, endocrinopathy resulting in deficiencies of cortisol or thyroid hormone, or acute-on-chronic alcohol abuse superimposed on chronic liver disease, with or without a state of chronic malnutrition.
- Hypoglycemia should be presumed to be present in *all* patients presenting to the emergency department with altered mental or psychiatric status, and hypoglycemia should be expeditiously excluded by rapid bedside glucose testing.
- For overdose with longer-acting insulins and the sulfonylureas, intensive therapy may be necessary for 1 or 2 days or even longer.
- Although the use of octreotide for sulfonylurea-induced hypoglycemia is "off label," multiple case reports and research document its efficacy and safety. On the contrary, diazoxide has been shown to be less effective and has several undesirable properties.

## FOLLOW-UP, NEXT STEPS IN CARE, AND PATIENT EDUCATION

The decision to admit patients after an episode of hypoglycemia is multifactorial and in all cases depends on the cause.

Patients with systemic conditions, such as sepsis, hepatic or renal failure, drug-induced hypoglycemia, hypoglycemia of unknown origin, and persistent neurologic signs and symptoms, usually require admission. Patients who present with overdoses (unintentional or intentional) of insulin, sulfonylureas, and meglitinides need inpatient observation because of the unpredictable kinetics of these agents in this setting. For patients with DM in whom hypoglycemia develops despite therapeutic dosing and without a history of an overdose, admission depends on the expected duration of effect of the drugs, the severity and recurrence of hypoglycemia, and other possible toxic effects. Because most commonly used sulfonylureas have a duration of effect of at least 24 hours, admission is warranted even for a single episode of hypoglycemia, even though in theory it may be possible to observe these patients closely at home. Discharge is possible for patients with hypoglycemia if the likelihood of recurrence is minimal or the patient has a simple explanation for the episode of hypoglycemia (e.g., a missed meal). In patients who do not require any treatment with glucose, observation for 8 hours may be considered. In all patients with hypoglycemia, the emergency physician should err on the side of caution and exercise good clinical judgment when deciding on disposition.

Patients who are discharged home from the ED must be educated on frequent home glucose monitoring, and they should be instructed to obtain rapid follow-up with their primary care physician. Educating patients on warning signs and symptoms of hypoglycemia is crucial to prevent severe episodes from recurring.

Complications associated with hypoglycemia may be severe and include death. Myocardial infarction, cardiac dysrhythmias (e.g., QT prolongation, increased QT dispersion, ectopy, sudden bradycardia) and seizures may all occur.[22] In the long term, neuroglycopenia may cause neurologic dysfunction and subsequent irreversible brain injury in patients with profound and prolonged hypoglycemia.[23] Even in mild cases of hypoglycemia, long-term neurologic dysfunction may occur.[23]

The prognosis of most patients with drug-induced hypoglycemia should be good, provided the diagnosis is promptly made and immediate therapy is instituted. The major pitfall in the treatment of hypoglycemia is usually the failure to make the diagnosis, by attributing the patient's symptoms to some other condition (e.g., stroke, acute psychosis). Other pitfalls include failure to perform frequent glucose checks and underestimation of the pharmacokinetics or toxicokinetics of the specific agent involved. Consultation with the regional poison control center or with a local medical toxicologist may be of assistance in the management of these cases.

## SUGGESTED READINGS

Carroll MJ, Burge MR, Schade DS. Severe hypoglycemia in adults. Rev Endocr Metab Disord 2003;4:149-57.

Choudhary P, Amiel SA. Hypoglycaemia: current management and controversies. Postgrad Med J 2011;87:298-306.

Dougherty PP, Klein-Schwatz W. Octreotide's role in the management of sulfonylurea-induced hypoglycemia. J Med Toxicol 2010;6:199-206.

Lacherade JC, Jacqueminet S, Preiser JC. An overview of hypoglycemia in the critically ill. J Diabetes Sci Technol 2009;3:1242-9.

Spiller HA, Sawyer TS. Toxicology of oral antidiabetic medications. Am J Health Syst Pharm 2006;63:929-38.

## REFERENCES

***References can be found on Expert Consult @ www.expertconsult.com.***

# 157 Over-the-Counter Medications

*Stephen Thornton and Binh T. Ly*

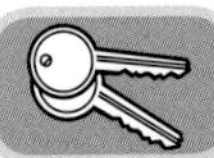

**KEY POINTS**

- Acetaminophen poisoning should be considered in patients presenting with over-the-counter medication misuse or overdose.
- Poisonings with antihistamine medications may manifest with antimuscarinic toxicity and sedation, but cardiac toxicity and seizures are also possible.
- Treatment for antihistamine poisoning is supportive care, but sodium bicarbonate and physostigmine may be helpful adjuncts.
- Dextromethorphan poisoning manifests as sedation, movement disturbances, and psychoactive dysphoria. Most of these effects are mediated by *N*-methyl-D-aspartate, rather than by opioid receptor activity.
- In overdose, poisoning with oral amphetamine-like decongestants may manifest as a sympathomimetic toxidrome.
- Imidazoline ocular and nasal decongestants such as oxymetazoline (Afrin) tetrahydrozoline (Visine), and naphazoline (Naphcon) may cause significant sedation when they are ingested orally.
- Diphenoxylate (Lomotil) can cause recurrent and delayed respiratory depression.
- Dietary supplements are mostly safe but are unregulated. Common conditions leading to poisoning include mislabeling, variations in concentration, contamination with unintended agents, and intentional adulteration.
- Vitamin A toxicity may cause increased intracranial pressure with associated symptoms.
- Vitamin D toxicity may cause significant hypercalcemia.

## ANTIHISTAMINES

### EPIDEMIOLOGY

Antihistamines are among the most frequently used medications in the United States.[1] Most of these drugs are available without a prescription. Although their efficacy is questionable, antihistamines are widely used for the symptomatic relief of cold and allergy symptoms. They are also found in nonprescription sleeping aids. Because of widespread access, these agents are commonly ingested intentionally, in suicide attempts, and unintentionally, particularly by children. Approximately 90,000 cases of antihistamine ingestions are reported to poison centers in the United States every year, and almost half of those involve children younger than 6 years.[2]

### PATHOPHYSIOLOGY

The antihistamines function as reversible competitive inhibitors of either $H_1$ or $H_2$ histamine receptors. Currently available antihistamines can be classified as first-generation, sedating $H_1$ receptor antagonists (e.g., diphenhydramine, hydroxyzine); second-generation, nonsedating $H_1$ receptor antagonists (e.g., loratadine, fexofenadine); or $H_2$ receptor antagonists. Antagonism of the $H_1$ receptors inhibits bronchoconstriction, vasoconstriction, and capillary permeability (the cause of edema and wheal), whereas $H_2$ receptor antagonism inhibits gastric acid secretion. In overdose, first-generation $H_1$ receptor antagonists may have some additional effects on other receptors and ion channels, particularly muscarinic-type cholinergic receptor inhibition, α-adrenergic receptor inhibition, and fast sodium channel blockade, whereas second-generation $H_1$ receptor blockers and $H_2$ receptor antagonists primarily cause sedation.

### PRESENTING SIGNS AND SYMPTOMS

Patients typically present with some degree of altered mental status or suicidality. A history of ingestion or coingestions should be sought. Emergency medical personnel and family members, if available, may need to be questioned. Pill bottles, if present, may help clarify the history.

Although sedation is common with larger ingestions, signs of antimuscarinic toxicity may also be present (**Box 157.1**). In addition, patients may have mild hypotension or more worrisome wide complex dysrhythmia resulting from sodium channel–blocking effects of some antihistamines (e.g., diphenhydramine). Cardiovascular toxicity associated with some antihistamines is indistinguishable from that associated with cyclic antidepressants (**Fig. 157.1**).

### DIFFERENTIAL DIAGNOSIS AND MEDICAL DECISION MAKING

The differential diagnosis of antihistamine toxicity is broad because many medications, street drugs, and disease processes can cause a presentation characterized by sedation or delirium, or both (**Box 157.2**). The emergency physician must consider nontoxicologic causes of altered mental status, such as infection and traumatic brain injury, and evaluate for these nontoxicologic conditions accordingly if the presence of the conditions cannot be excluded by other means. Computed tomography of the head and lumbar puncture may be warranted. In particular, patients presenting with antimuscarinic toxicity may be delirious, hyperthermic, and tachycardic, features that mimic infectious causes.

Bedside blood glucose measurements should be performed early in the course of management for individuals presenting with altered sensorium. An electrocardiogram should be obtained quickly to assess for conduction abnormalities, with particular attention paid to the QRS and QTc duration. Serum electrolyte concentrations should be measured to rule out metabolic abnormalities in patients who are confused or who exhibit evidence of cardiotoxicity. Laboratory evaluation of total creatinine kinase to evaluate for rhabdomyolysis may be indicated in acutely agitated patients. Serum acetaminophen levels should be measured in all patients with intentional overdose, because many cough and cold preparations combine antihistamines with antipyretics and analgesics. A urine

**BOX 157.1 Signs of Antimuscarinic Toxicity**

Delirium
Tachycardia
Anhidrosis
Mydriasis
Hyperthermia
Urinary retention
Ileus

**BOX 157.2 Drug Ingestions or Diseases That Manifest with Sedation or Delirium**

Ethanol
Benzodiazepines
Barbiturates
Opioids
Cyclic antidepressants
Antipsychotics
Anticonvulsants (carbamazepine)
Meningitis and encephalitis
Sepsis
Head injury
Metabolic derangements (hyponatremia)

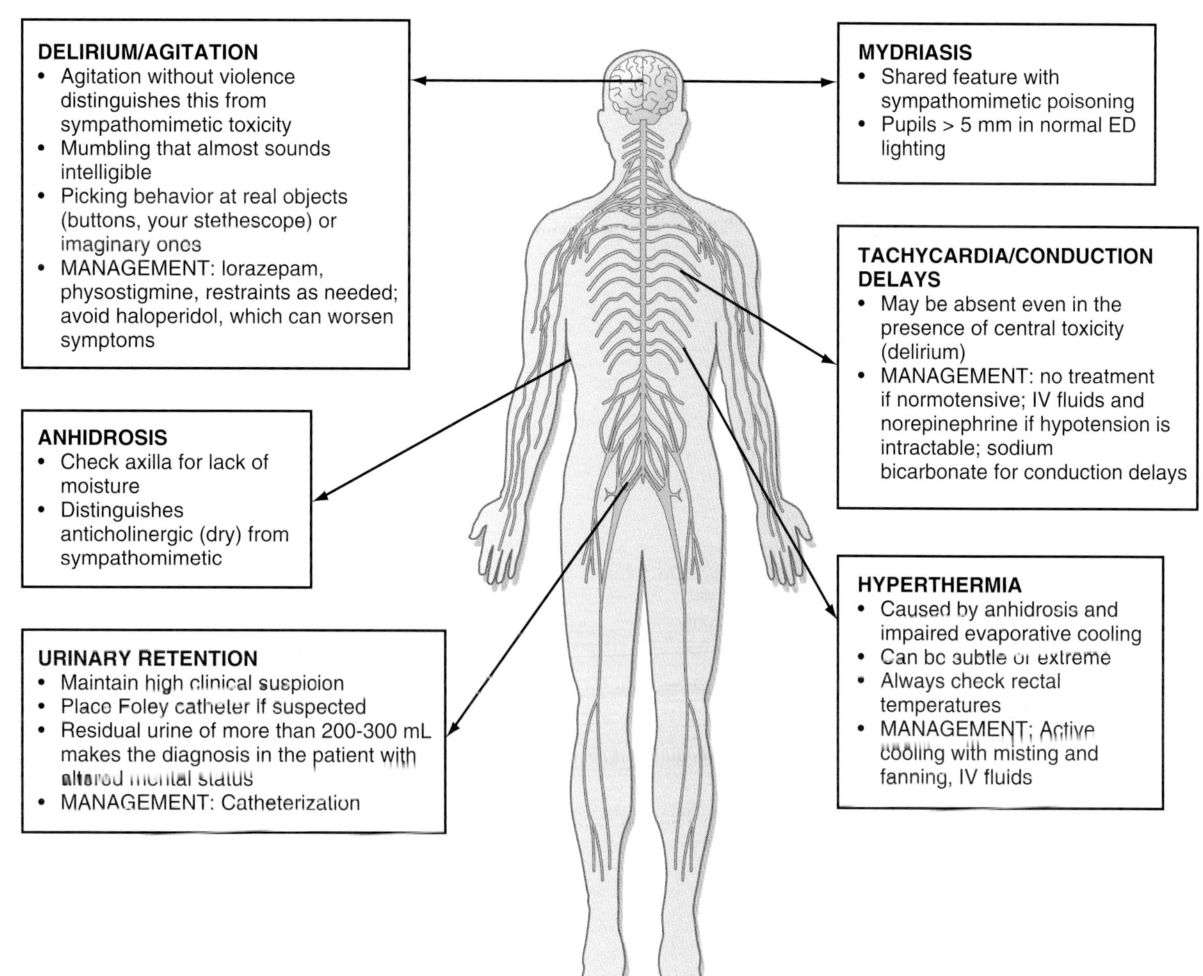


**Fig. 157.1 Recognizing the anticholinergic toxidrome.** *ED,* Emergency department; *IV,* intravenous.

immunoassay (standard urine drugs of abuse screen) may be considered to screen for recent exposure to opioids, benzodiazepines, or other drugs, although the clinical utility of this test is limited by frequent false-positive results. The emergency physician should recognize that a positive screening test result indicates only exposure to and not active toxicity of a compound. Qualitative testing for antihistamines is not useful and generally not readily available. Diphenhydramine may trigger a false-positive immunoassay result for tricyclic antidepressants or phencyclidine (PCP) on some urine drug immunoassays typically used in many hospitals.

## TREATMENT

Prehospital treatment of the acutely poisoned patient should be based on providing supportive care and preventing complications such as injury from agitation or aspiration from decreased mental status.

Hospital treatment should also be focused on supportive care with assessment of airway, breathing, and circulation. Particular attention should be paid to controlling agitation and hydration (**Table 157.1**). Agitation should be treated with benzodiazepines in doses titrated to desired effect (e.g., lorazepam, 1 to 2 mg by intravenous [IV] push to effect). In addition to chemical restraint, physical restraint for patient and staff safety may be needed. Hydration should be addressed with 1- to 2-L boluses of 0.9% saline solution to ensure adequate urine output.

In patients who present within 1 hour of drug ingestion and who are alert and cooperative, activated charcoal (50 g or 1 g/kg up to 50 g in children) should be considered. Data in humans are insufficient to support the use of activated charcoal beyond 1 hour.[3]

**Table 157.1 Toxicities of Over-the-Counter Medications**

| MEDICATION | TOXICITY | TREATMENT | DISPOSITION |
|---|---|---|---|
| **Antihistamines** | | | |
| First-generation $H_1$ antagonists<br>• Diphenhydramine<br>• Doxylamine | Sedation<br>Antimuscarinic toxidrome<br>• Tachycardia<br>• Delirium<br>• Anhidrosis<br>• Mydriasis<br>• Hyperthermia<br>Rhabdomyolysis<br>Hypotension<br>Dysrhythmia | Supportive care<br>Benzodiazepines<br>Physostigmine (for antimuscarinic delirium) | Observation<br>Admission for persistent symptoms |
| Second-generation $H_1$ antagonists<br>• Cetirizine<br>• Fexofenadine<br>• Loratadine | Sedation | Supportive care | Observation<br>Admission for persistent symptoms |
| **Antitussives** | | | |
| Dextromethorphan | Sedation<br>Agitation<br>Movement disorders<br>Serotonin syndrome | Supportive care<br>Benzodiazepines for agitation | Observation<br>Admission for persistent symptoms |
| **Decongestants** | | | |
| Amphetamine-like<br>• Ephedrine<br>• Pseudoephedrine<br>• Phenylephrine | Sympathomimetic toxidrome<br>• Tachycardia<br>• Agitated delirium<br>• Hypertension<br>• Mydriasis<br>Rhabdomyolysis | Supportive care<br>Benzodiazepines for agitation<br>Vasodilators for severe hypertension | Observation<br>Admission for persistent or severe symptoms |
| Imidazoline<br>• Tetrahydrozoline<br>• Oxymetazoline<br>• Naphazoline | Sedation<br>Hypotension or hypertension<br>Bradycardia | Supportive care | Observation<br>Admission for persistent or severe symptoms |
| **Antidiarrheals** | | | |
| Diphenoxylate | Opioid toxicity<br>• CNS depression<br>• [illegible]<br>• Respiratory depression | Supportive care<br>Naloxone | Admission<br>Awareness of recurrent or delayed symptoms |

Hyperthermia should be managed with sedation and active, evaporative cooling (misting with water and applying direct fanning). Rarely, endotracheal intubation with neuromuscular paralysis may be necessary if hyperthermia or agitation fails to improve with less aggressive measures.

Physostigmine is a reversible acetylcholinesterase inhibitor that crosses the blood-brain barrier; it increases synaptic acetylcholine and may temporarily reverse antimuscarinic delirium. Peripheral signs may also be reversed. It may also be used therapeutically to control agitation.[4] Physostigmine may have more value as a diagnostic tool by precluding the need for invasive tests (e.g., lumbar puncture) if complete reversal of delirium is achieved following administration.[5] Beyond diagnostic use, the role of physostigmine in the treatment of most antimuscarinic poisonings with minor symptoms is debatable, and caution should be used if a possibility of tricyclic antidepressant ingestion exists.

Severe cardiac conduction abnormalities as evidenced by QRS prolongation should be treated with sodium bicarbonate (1 to 2 mEq/kg IV push) to overcome impaired sodium conduction. Hypotension is usually mild and should be treated with IV fluids. Refractory hypotension may also be treated with sodium bicarbonate and direct-acting alpha agonists (norepinephrine, 2 to 12 mcg/min IV infusion).

As with all ingestions with significant toxicity, consultation with a medical toxicologist or a poison center should be considered.

## FOLLOW-UP, NEXT STEPS IN CARE, AND PATIENT EDUCATION

Patients with evidence of ongoing cardiovascular or neurologic toxicity should be admitted. Completely asymptomatic patients who have been observed for 6 hours after drug ingestion may be medically cleared for psychiatric evaluation or discharged, whichever is most appropriate.

# ANTITUSSIVES: DEXTROMETHORPHAN

## EPIDEMIOLOGY

Dextromethorphan was approved by the U.S. Food and Drug Administration (FDA) as an over-the-counter antitussive in 1958. It is a common component of cold preparations, and its nonmedical use (abuse) appears to be increasing, especially among adolescents.[6] Abuse of Coricidin (known on the streets as "Skittles") and Robitussin (known as "DXM" and "robo") has highlighted dextromethorphan's abusive potential.

## PATHOPHYSIOLOGY

Dextromethorphan is the structural analogue of the opioid analgesic levorphanol that is devoid of analgesic properties but has antitussive properties resulting from agonism of σ-opioid receptors. In addition, dextromethorphan inhibits *N*-methyl-D-aspartate (NMDA)–glutamate receptors and alters dopaminergic and serotonergic neurotransmission. Associated psychoactive effects are attributed to the active metabolite dextrorphan. At very high doses, typical opioid toxicity may be seen.

## PRESENTING SIGNS AND SYMPTOMS

Some degree of altered mental status (sedation or agitation) is the most common presenting manifestation. This feature may impair the ability to obtain a reliable history from the patient, and emergency medical personnel or family may need to be questioned.

Along with altered mental status, dextromethorphan may cause gait disturbances known as "robo-walking."[7] Serotonin syndrome, which consists of a triad of central nervous system (CNS) dysfunction, neuromuscular dysfunction (clonus, hyperreflexia), and autonomic instability (tachycardia, mild hyperthermia), may also be noted in patients with toxicity.[8]

## DIFFERENTIAL DIAGNOSIS AND MEDICAL DECISION MAKING

The initial approach to patients with altered mental status includes ruling out potential emergency conditions such as trauma, CNS infection, and metabolic derangements. Other common CNS depressants, such as benzodiazepines, opioids, and ethanol, may also cause sedation. Recreational drugs of abuse with similar actions at the NMDA receptor, such as PCP and ketamine, may also cause dysphoria and psychoactive features. Antimuscarinic poisoning does not result from dextromethorphan poisoning but can occur from coingested antihistamines such as chlorpheniramine (as found in Coricidin).

Although structurally considered an opioid, dextromethorphan does not trigger the opiate screen on a standard urine immunoassay, but it may result in a false-positive result for PCP. Dextromethorphan is often formulated as a hydrobromide salt; ingestions of such a formulation may cause false elevations of chloride on an autoanalyzer test, although true toxicity from bromide is rare.

Emergency physicians should be mindful of potential coingestants because many cough and cold preparations frequently contain aspirin, acetaminophen, decongestants, and antihistamines. Acetaminophen levels should be routinely checked in poisoned patients.

## TREATMENT

Prehospital treatment of the acutely poisoned patient should be based on providing supportive care and preventing complications such as injury from agitation or aspiration from decreased mental status.

Hospital treatment should be focused on supportive care with assessment of airway, breathing, and circulation. Attention should be paid to controlling agitation and hydration. Agitation should be treated with benzodiazepines in doses titrated to effect (IV lorazepam, 1 to 2 mg titrated to effect) (see Table 157.1). Reducing environmental stimuli may also be helpful. In addition to chemical restraint, physical restraint for patient and staff safety may be needed. Hydration should be addressed with 1- to 2-L boluses of 0.9% saline solution to ensure adequate urine output. Decontamination with activated charcoal may be considered in an alert, cooperative patient who presents within an hour of a possible ingestion. Supportive care is the treatment of choice. IV naloxone (1 to 2 mg) may be given for significant sedation, although reversal may not occur.[9]

## FOLLOW-UP, NEXT STEPS IN CARE, AND PATIENT EDUCATION

Patients with evidence of ongoing neurologic toxicity should be admitted. Completely asymptomatic patients who have been observed for 6 hours after drug ingestion should be evaluated by a psychiatrist to determine whether admission is indicated.

# DECONGESTANTS: PSEUDOEPHEDRINE, EPHEDRINE, PHENYLEPHRINE, OXYMETAZOLINE, AND TETRAHYDROZOLINE

## EPIDEMIOLOGY

Over-the-counter decongestants rank among the top five most commonly used medications.[1] They are frequently present in multiple ingredient cough and cold products. Some are abused for their stimulatory effects or diverted for the production of methamphetamines. As with other over-the-counter medications, children are frequent victims of unintentional poisonings or dosing errors, and decongestant exposure in this population has been linked to adverse outcomes.[2]

## PATHOPHYSIOLOGY

Over-the-counter decongestants have their therapeutic effects primarily by stimulating $\alpha_1$-adrenergic receptors and causing vasoconstriction and reducing edema in mucous membranes. They fall into two main classes. This first class is amphetamine-like substances (e.g., pseudoephedrine, ephedrine, phenylephrine), which cause release of catecholamines, and block their reuptake and breakdown and are taken orally. The other class is imidazoline decongestants (e.g., oxymetazoline, tetrahydrozoline, naphazoline), which directly stimulate α-adrenergic receptors on blood vessels and are applied topically.

## PRESENTING SIGNS AND SYMPTOMS

The presenting signs and symptoms from the ingestion of over-the-counter decongestants will vary depending on the agent ingested (see Table 157.1). Ingestion of an amphetamine-like decongestant typically presents signs and symptoms of sympathomimetic toxicity due to the increased stimulation of both α- and β-adrenergic receptors. This is typified by agitation, delirium, tachycardia, hypertension, hyperthermia and mydriasis. Ingestion of imidazolines, which are meant for topical use, usually presents with sedation, bradycardia and hypertension early with subsequent hypotension. Respiratory depression, sedation, and miosis, mimicking opioid toxicity, have been described.[10]

## DIFFERENTIAL DIAGNOSIS AND MEDICAL DECISION MAKING

If the history of ingestion is not clear then the differential diagnosis for decongestant ingestions can be broad, especially considering the disparate presentations of the amphetamine-like and the imidazoline classes (see Table 157.1). Coingestions and nontoxicologic processes must be considered. Rhabdomyolysis and cardiac ischemia should be evaluated for in patients with significant toxicity.

## TREATMENT

Standard prehospital care should be sufficient for decongestant-toxic patients, with particular attention paid to controlling agitation. Decontamination with activated charcoal is suitable for the alert patient with exposure in the previous hour. Agitation, tachycardia, and hypertension should be aggressively treated with benzodiazepines (IV lorazepam, 1 to 2 mg, or IV diazepam, 5 to 10 mg, titrated to effect). The physician must aggressively hydrate these patients to treat rhabdomyolysis. For refractory hypertension, an α-adrenergic antagonist (IV phentolamine, 5 mg) or a venous and arteriolar vasodilator (IV nitroprusside, 0.3 to 10 mcg/kg/min) should be given. In severe cases of CNS depression after imidazoline-type decongestant overdose, IV naloxone may be given (2 to 4 mg) but its effects are inconsistent, and endotracheal intubation may rarely be needed to support ventilation.[11]

## FOLLOW-UP, NEXT STEPS IN CARE, AND PATIENT EDUCATION

Symptoms of decongestant exposure, whether amphetamine-like or imidazoline, usually resolve within 8 hours or so. However, admission of symptomatic patients may be warranted. Depending on intent, psychiatry evaluation may be needed.

# ANTIDIARRHEALS: LOPERAMIDE AND DIPHENOXYLATE

## EPIDEMIOLOGY

Diarrhea remains an important and frequent health problem. Over-the-counter remedies are often sought by diarrhea sufferers, and many different over-the-counter agents are reported to be antidiarrheal. Loperamide (Imodium) is probably the best known of these agents. Diphenoxylate with atropine

(Lomotil) is a prescription medication and frequently used interchangeably with loperamide.

## PATHOPHYSIOLOGY

Loperamide and diphenoxylate are synthetic analogues of meperidine used to treat diarrhea. Loperamide's systemic absorption is restricted by its insolubility, and therapeutically only local μ-type opioid receptors in the gastrointestinal tract are affected, resulting in decreased intestinal motility. Diphenoxylate is combined with a small dose of atropine both to increase its antimotility effect and to discourage its abuse as an opioid (this combination is marketed as Lomotil). Diphenoxylate has a significantly worse adverse effect profile because it metabolizes to difenoxin, a compound with higher potency and a longer serum half-life.

## PRESENTING SIGNS AND SYMPTOMS

Loperamide is generally well tolerated even in large ingestions, and drowsiness is the most common effect.[12] Diphenoxylate is significantly more toxic, and overdoses commonly manifest with some degree of opioid toxicity (e.g., CNS depression, respiratory depression, miosis, decreased bowel motility), with or without the antimuscarinic effects of the atropine (see Table 157.1).

## DIFFERENTIAL DIAGNOSIS AND MEDICAL DECISION MAKING

The differential diagnosis includes conditions that cause altered mental status and respiratory depression. No specific tests are available to order in evaluating these patients. Common urine drug screens do not detect either drug. Any diagnostic tests ordered should be geared toward the standard evaluation of the poisoned or altered patient and not these agents in particular.

## TREATMENT AND DISPOSITION

Prehospital treatment should be oriented toward providing supportive care and preventing complications such as aspiration from decreased mental status. Prehospital administration of naloxone may be considered.

In general, loperamide has a high safety profile and has been associated with very few adverse events, even in overdose. However, diphenoxylate overdoses can cause significant symptoms, usually related to respiratory depression (see Table 157.1). Respiratory depression by can be recurrent or delayed, sometimes up to 24 hours after the ingestion, and children are particularly at risk.[13] Decontamination with activated charcoal in the cooperative patient may be useful even beyond the 1 hour, given the impairment of gastrointestinal motility with these agents. IV naloxone (0.4 to 2.0 mg) is effective in reversing the respiratory depression and other signs of opioid toxicity, but CNS and respiratory depression may recur, and an IV naloxone infusion may be needed.[13]

## FOLLOW-UP, NEXT STEPS IN CARE, AND PATIENT EDUCATION

Patients with loperamide ingestions can typically be observed for 6 hours and medically cleared for psychiatric evaluation if the ingestion was intentional or discharged if unintentional. Strong consideration should be given to admitting pediatric patients and patients with intentional and significant Lomotil ingestions because of the possibility of severe delayed or recurrent symptoms (e.g., respiratory depression).

# DIETARY SUPPLEMENTS

## EPIDEMIOLOGY

Any ingredient taken for the purpose of promoting health is considered a dietary supplement. Innumerable examples of dietary supplements exist, and a national surveyed showed that more than 15% of the U.S. population had used one or more in the previous week.[14] Ginkgo, St. John's wort, ginseng, echinacea, and synephrine are among the more commonly used dietary supplements (**Table 157.2**). Unlike with prescription drugs, proof of safety and proof of efficacy are not required for dietary supplements as long as the maker does not claim that the agent is a treatment for a particular disease. To be removed from the market, a dietary supplement must be proven unsafe. This situation occurred in 2006, when the FDA banned of ephedra over cardiovascular concerns.[15]

## PATHOPHYSIOLOGY

The exact mechanism of action of many of the dietary supplements is poorly understood. Severe toxicity from most supplements remains uncommon because of the low concentrations of specific agents in marketed products. Toxicity may arise not only from the product itself but also from unlisted active ingredients and from contaminants such as heavy metals. Supplements may also have interactions with certain drugs that affect metabolism and efficacy.

## PRESENTING SIGNS AND SYMPTOMS

Depending on the specific dietary supplement, presenting signs and symptoms vary. Table 157-2 lists some of the possible toxic manifestations of the more common dietary supplements.

## DIFFERENTIAL DIAGNOSIS AND MEDICAL DECISION MAKING

The differential diagnosis is driven by the particular supplement ingested. For example, ingestion of an ephedra-like supplement (bitter orange) suggests other causes of sympathomimetic toxicity such as cocaine and amphetamines. No diagnostic testing is specific to dietary supplements, and drug levels are of no value.

**Table 157.2 Toxicities of Dietary Supplements**

| DIETARY SUPPLEMENT | SIGNS AND SYMPTOMS OF TOXICITY |
|---|---|
| Synephrine (bitter orange) | Sympathomimetic toxidrome<br>Myocardial infarction<br>Stroke |
| Ephedra (Ma-Huang) | Sympathomimetic toxidrome<br>Myocardial infarction<br>Stroke |
| Ginkgo *(Ginkgo biloba)* | GI distress, headache, allergic reaction, bleeding, seizures |
| St. John's wort *(Hypericum perforatum)* | Photosensitization<br>Induction of CYP 3A4 that leads to decreased levels of certain drugs<br>Serotonin toxicity from weak MOAI properties |
| Ginseng *(Panax ginseng)* | Ginseng abuse syndrome (hypertension, sleepiness, nervousness, morning diarrhea) |
| Echinacea *(Echinacea purpurea)* | Normally none<br>Rarely hepatitis, asthma, anaphylaxis |
| Kava kava *(Piper methysticum)* | Mild euphoria, sedation, muscle weakness<br>Rarely hepatotoxicity |
| Nutmeg *(Myristica fragrans)* | GI upset, hallucinations |
| Hydroxycut (*Garcinia cambogia* extract, chromium polynicotinate, *Gymnema sylvestris* extract, and *Camellia sinensis*) | Hepatotoxicity, seizures |

*GI,* Gastrointestinal; *MAOI,* monoamine oxidase inhibitor.

## TREATMENT

Dietary supplement exposures pose unique challenges because of the lack of information on the toxicologic profiles, pharmacokinetics, and concentrations of their active ingredients. Most cases of toxicity stemming from therapeutic use can be managed with supportive care and symptom-based therapy.

## FOLLOW-UP, NEXT STEPS IN CARE, AND PATIENT EDUCATION

Symptomatic patients should be admitted for observation and symptomatic therapy. A psychiatric consultation should be obtained when warranted. Patients who are asymptomatic 4 to 6 hours after an acute accidental overdose of a known agent with known safety profiles can be discharged with appropriate follow-up.

# VITAMINS

## EPIDEMIOLOGY

Vitamins are frequently taken in supratherapeutic amounts. This is done typically under the premise of "more is better" or purportedly to treat or prevent conditions ranging from viral upper respiratory tract infections to Alzheimer dementia. Parents' concern about their children's eating patterns may result in vitamin oversupplementation.[16] All these factors, added to the ready availability of vitamins, make vitamins prime targets for potential toxic exposures.[17]

## PATHOPHYSIOLOGY

Vitamins can be grouped into two main categories: water soluble and fat soluble. Toxicity may be caused by either group, though in general toxicity from water-soluble vitamins are rarer and less severe as they do not accumulate as fat-soluble vitamins do. Vitamin A and D, which are both fat soluble, have well described toxicity. **Table 157.3** describes the normal function of the most common vitamins and their toxic effects.

## PRESENTING SIGNS AND SYMPTOMS

The presenting signs and symptoms of hypervitaminosis depend on the offending vitamin.[16-19] Table 157.3 lists the toxic effects of the most clinically relevant vitamins.

## DIFFERENTIAL DIAGNOSIS AND MEDICAL DECISION MAKING

Because of the relative infrequency of severe toxicity from hypervitaminosis, the more common causes of such conditions as sensory neuropathies, increased intracranial pressure,

**Table 157.3 Functions and Toxicities of Vitamins**

| VITAMIN | NORMAL FUNCTION(S) | TOXIC EFFECTS | TREATMENT |
|---|---|---|---|
| **Fat Soluble** | | | |
| Vitamin A | Vision<br>Gene transcription<br>Skin health | Increased intracranial pressure<br>Headaches<br>Vomiting<br>Lethargy<br>Hepatotoxicity<br>Alopecia | Cessation of exposure<br>Supportive care<br>Rarely: mannitol, steroids, hyperventilation for increased intracranial pressure |
| Vitamin D | Calcium homeostasis | Hypercalcemia<br>GI upset<br>Lethargy<br>Weakness<br>Hypertension<br>Renal injury | Cessation of exposure<br>Intravenous hydration<br>Loop diuretics<br>Glucocorticoids<br>Calcitonin |
| Vitamin E | Cell membrane antioxidation | Coagulopathy | Cessation of exposure<br>Rarely: FFP and platelet transfusion |
| Vitamin K | Coagulation | Rarely reported<br>Hepatotoxicity? | Cessation of exposure |
| **Water Soluble** | | | |
| Vitamin C (ascorbic acid) | Collagen synthesis<br>Carnitine synthesis<br>Neurotransmitter synthesis<br>Antioxidation | GI upset<br>Hematuria<br>Nephrolithiasis<br>Anemia | Cessation of exposure<br>Supportive care |
| Vitamin $B_6$ (pyridoxine) | Neurotransmitter metabolism | Neuropathy<br>Paresthesias<br>Weakness<br>Hyporeflexia | Cessation of exposure |
| Vitamin $B_3$ (niacin) | $NAD^+$/$NADP^+$ precursor status | Histamine release<br>Flushing (acute)<br>Hepatotoxicity<br>Gout | Cessation of exposure<br>Antihistamines<br>Aspirin |

*FFP*, Fresh frozen plasma; *GI*, gastrointestinal; *$NAD^+$/$NADP^+$*, oxidized nicotinamide adenine dinucleotide/oxidized nicotinamide adenine dinucleotide phosphate.

and hypercalcemia must be explored first. The diagnosis of a vitamin overdose is most often made from a history of ingestion. In patients with vitamin A toxicity, elevations of aminotransferase, alkaline phosphatase, and bilirubin concentrations, as well as prothrombin time, are indicators of hepatic toxicity. Computed tomography of the head or lumbar puncture with measurement of the opening pressure should be performed to confirm increased intracranial pressure. Vitamin D toxicity can be demonstrated with elevated calcium and vitamin D levels. Because many vitamin preparations contain iron or fluoride, these agents must be considered and evaluated as possible coingestants.

## TREATMENT

Typically, supportive care and cessation of the offending vitamin are sufficient to treat most vitamin toxicities. In the case of vitamin A toxicity, measures to reduce intracranial pressure may be warranted, and in the case of vitamin D

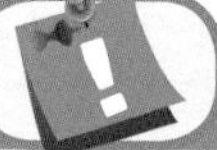

**TIPS AND TRICKS**

- Many vitamin preparations contain iron or fluoride, so it is imperative that these agents be considered and evaluated as possible coingestants.
- In patients with mixed ingestion, older patients, or very young patients, physical findings may be variable and the clinical picture unclear.
- Peripheral findings do not always accompany central findings in antihistamine overdose; therefore, a confused patient may not always have tachycardia or anhidrosis.
- In all cases of potential poisoning, nontoxicologic causes of altered mental status should also be considered.
- With dextromethorphan ingestions, genetic differences in speed of metabolism of the drug to dextrorphan can result in either predominance of sedation or dysphoria.

toxicity, standard treatment for hypercalcemia (IV hydration and loop diuretics) should be employed (see Table 157.3).

## FOLLOW-UP, NEXT STEPS IN CARE, AND PATIENT EDUCATION

Patients who are toxic from fat-soluble vitamin overdoses typically need admission because the effects of these agents may be prolonged. All patients should be educated on the risk of hypervitaminosis.

## SUGGESTED READINGS

Chyka PA, Erdman AR, Manoguerra AS, et al. Dextromethorphan poisoning: an evidence-based consensus guideline for out-of-hospital management. American Association of Poison Control Centers. Clin Toxicol (Phila) 2007;45:662-77.

Daggy A, Kaplan R, Roberge R, Akhtar J. Pediatric Visine (tetrahydrozoline) ingestion: case report and review of imidazoline toxicity. Vet Hum Toxicol 2003;45:210-12.

Haller C, Benowitz NL. Adverse cardiovascular and central nervous system events associated with dietary supplements containing ephedra alkaloids. N Engl J Med 2000;343:1833-8.

Tovar RT, Petzel RM. Herbal toxicity. Dis Mon 2009;55:592-641.

## REFERENCES

***References can be found on Expert Consult @ www.expertconsult.com.***

# Pediatric Overdoses 158

*Shana Kusin and Patrick M. Lank*

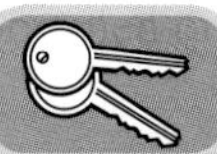

**KEY POINTS**

- Children less than 6 years old suffer the majority of toxic exposures seen annually in the United States.
- Many over-the-counter medications, household substances, and prescription medications can cause significant toxicity in young children when these substances are ingested in amounts as small as 1 to 2 pills or 1 to 2 teaspoons.
- As with adults, supportive care is the mainstay of treatment for pediatric overdoses. Specific antidotes and treatments are the same for pediatric patients as for adults.
- Salicylate overdose in the pediatric patient manifests similarly to overdose in adults, but the classic finding of a mixed metabolic acidosis and respiratory alkalosis may not be present. Methylsalicylate toxicity from oil of wintergreen ingestion can progress much more rapidly than toxicity from other salicylates, and treatment should not be delayed.
- When evaluating a child for potential caustic substance ingestion, the absence of burns in the mouth and oropharynx does not preclude burns in the esophagus and stomach.
- Sulfonylurea exposure in the pediatric patient warrants prolonged observation because of the risk of delayed hypoglycemia.

## EPIDEMIOLOGY

Pediatric exposures to toxic substances represent the majority of cases reported to poison centers in the United States. Children less than 5 years old accounted for 52%, or 1.29 million, of total reported exposures in 2009. In contrast, exposure-related fatalities in the same age group represented only 1.8%, or 21, of total fatalities in 2009, and 18 of these fatalities were classified as unintentional exposures.[1] This finding reflects the fact that toxic exposure in the child younger than 5 years old is generally the result of an inquisitive toddler exploring his or her environment.

The "One Pill Can Kill" list refers to a group of agents that are known to cause serious toxicity or death when they are ingested in very small quantities by a small child (**Box 158.1**). The emergency physician must be familiar with these agents to manage these patients appropriately and to anticipate the potential for poor outcomes. Many of these agents are covered in more detail in other chapters in this section.

## PATHOPHYSIOLOGY

### OVER-THE-COUNTER AGENTS

#### *Camphor*

Camphor is an aromatic terpene ketone, originally distilled from the bark of the camphor tree and now synthesized from turpentine oil. It is a common ingredient in some topical and vaporized medications intended to treat musculoskeletal pain or symptoms of common flu-like illnesses (**Table 158.1**). Camphor is marketed as an analgesic, an antipruritic, and an antitussive, and it is also found in older formulations of mothballs.

The exact mechanism by which camphor produces toxicity is unknown, although the cyclic ketone of its hydroaromatic terpene group is hypothesized to be a neurotoxin. Camphor is highly lipophilic, resulting in rapid movement across cell membranes and a large volume of distribution. Its metabolites are stored in fat deposits and are cleared over a prolonged period of time, which may be responsible for the delayed onset of seizures associated with camphor toxicity.[2] Camphor may also cause gastrointestinal toxicity from its direct effect on mucosal surfaces.

Doses between 750 and 1500 mg, and doses as low as 500 mg in some case reports, are associated with seizures and death.[2] For this reason, the U.S. Food and Drug Administration ruled in 1982 that products could not contain more than 11% camphor. However, some commercially available formulations contain 500 mg in 1 teaspoonful of product. In addition, a case series of pediatric seizures attributed to camphor toxicity highlights the role that camphor still plays in some ethnic and cultural practices. Illegally sold, high-concentration camphor products pose a risk in these populations.[3]

#### *Salicylates*

Salicylates are present in numerous over-the-counter products and are marketed as analgesics, antipyretics, and antiinflammatory agents (**Table 158.2**). Several Asian herbal remedies sold as topical treatments for musculoskeletal pain also contain salicylates.

Oil of wintergreen represents a specific concern in the pediatric population because of its extremely high concentration. One teaspoon of 98% oil of wintergreen contains 7000 mg of methylsalicylate, equivalent to 86 baby aspirin, a potentially lethal dose for children weighing less than 23 kg. This product has a pleasing aroma, thus rendering it

**BOX 158.1 Agents That Can Be Highly Toxic in Small Doses**

| | |
|---|---|
| Calcium channel blockers | Hydrofluoric acid |
| Camphor | Opioids |
| Caustic household agents | Salicylates |
| Clonidine and topical imidazolines | Sulfonylureas |
| Diphenoxylate-atropine (Lomotil) | Topical anesthetics (lidocaine, benzocaine) |
| Hydrocarbons | Toxic alcohols |
| | Tricyclic antidepressants |

**Table 158.1 Common Camphor-Containing Products**

| PRODUCT | CAMPHOR CONTENT (%) |
|---|---|
| Camphorated oil | 20.0 |
| Campho-Phenique | 10.8 |
| Camphor spirits | 10.0 |
| Vicks VapoRub | 4.8 |
| Heet | 3.60 |
| Tiger Balm | 11% |

**Table 158.2 Common Salicylate-Containing Products**

| PRODUCT | ACTIVE COMPONENT | CONTENT |
|---|---|---|
| Alka-Seltzer Plus | Acetylsalicylic acid | 325 mg/tablet |
| Ben Gay Arthritis Formula | Methylsalicylate | 30% |
| Clearasil Ultra Acne Scrub | Salicylic acid | 2% |
| Heet | Methylsalicylate | 18% |
| Oil of wintergreen | Methylsalicylate | 98% |
| Pepto-Bismol | Bismuth subsalicylate | 262 mg/ 15 mL |
| Sebulex Dandruff Shampoo | Salicylic acid | 2% |

**Table 158.3 Common Anesthetic-Containing Products**

| PRODUCT | CONTENT |
|---|---|
| Anbesol Maximum Strength | Benzocaine, 20.0% |
| Baby Orajel | Benzocaine, 7.5% |
| Baby Anbesol Gel | Benzocaine, 7.5% |
| EMLA Cream | 25 g each of lidocaine and prilocaine/1 g |
| Vagisil Cream | Benzocaine, 5% |

particularly vulnerable to accidental ingestion. A review of pediatric salicylate poisonings found that all published cases of life-threatening toxicity or death resulted from oil of wintergreen or Asian herbal oil ingestions.[4]

Salicylate toxicity is caused both by direct stimulation of the central nervous system (CNS) respiratory center, resulting in hyperventilation and respiratory alkalosis, and by uncoupling of oxidative phosphorylation, which results in anion gap metabolic acidosis. Pulmonary and cerebral edema is hypothesized to result from increased capillary permeability. Impaired glucose metabolism can lead to hyperglycemia or hypoglycemia. Doses greater than 150 mg/kg are potentially toxic in children, and serious toxicity is seen in the range of 300 to 500 mg/kg.

### *Topical Anesthetics*

Topical anesthetics are found in various pain-relieving products ranging from teething gels to hemorrhoid creams (**Table 158.3**). Amide anesthetics, which include lidocaine and dibucaine, work by blocking voltage-gated sodium channels and preventing action potential propagation. In toxic doses, these agents can cause CNS hyperstimulation secondary to central blocking of inhibitory pathways that can progress to seizures, respiratory depression, and coma. Amides can also cause cardiac toxicity because of their antiarrhythmic properties, but this is most frequently seen in intravenous, rather than oral, exposures.[5]

Benzocaine is an ester anesthetic whose metabolites can cause methemoglobinemia in toxic doses. Methemoglobin is formed by oxidation of iron from the ferrous ($Fe^{2+}$) to the ferric ($Fe^{3+}$) state within the hemoglobin molecule. This process causes a leftward shift in the hemoglobin-oxygen dissociation curve and decreased hemoglobin's oxygen carrying capacity. Patients less than 6 months old have a relative deficiency of methemoglobin reductase and may be more susceptible to toxicity.[5]

Prilocaine is an amide compound that has been shown to cause methemoglobinemia as its primary toxicity in overdose.[5] Both prilocaine and lidocaine are components in EMLA cream, so this particular cream can cause either CNS toxicity or methemoglobinemia in overdose.

A literature review found published cases of seizures resulting after single ingestions of 5 to 25 mL of viscous lidocaine by children 2 years of age or younger.[5] Although dibucaine is less commonly prescribed than lidocaine, it is 10 times more potent, and ingestion of 2 to 3 teaspoons has caused death secondary to cardiopulmonary arrest.[6] Published reports of benzocaine-induced toxicity vary; cyanosis secondary to methemoglobinemia may result from oral doses in the range of 15 to 40 mg/kg, although the development of methemoglobinemia may be idiosyncratic, rather than dose related.

## CAUSTICS

Many household products are caustic agents and can cause significant toxicity with small exposures. Caustic agents are classified as alkaline or acid corrosives, depending on their pH (**Table 158.4**). Passed in 1970, the Federal Hazardous Substances Act and the Poison Prevention Packaging Act stated that caustic agents with a concentration higher than 10% must be placed in child-resistant containers. By 1973, the household product concentration limit had been lowered to 2%.

**Table 158.4 Household Caustic Agents**

| PRODUCT | CAUSTIC INGREDIENT(S) |
|---|---|
| **Alkaline Corrosives** | |
| Drain cleaners | Sodium hydroxide (lye) |
| Oven cleaners | Sodium hydroxide |
| Hair relaxers | Sodium hydroxide |
| Automatic dishwasher detergents | Sodium tripolyphosphate<br>Sodium metasilicate |
| Household ammonia cleaning solutions (glass cleaners, antirust products, floor strippers, toilet bowl cleaners, wax removers) | Ammonium hydroxide |
| **Acidic Corrosives** | |
| Drain cleaners | Sulfuric acid |
| Rust removers | Hydrofluoric acid<br>Oxalic acid |
| Toilet bowl cleaners | Hydrochloric acid<br>Sulfuric acid<br>Phosphoric acid |
| Tire cleaning agent | Ammonium bifluoride |

Alkaline corrosives cause liquefaction necrosis, which is characterized by protein dissolution, collagen destruction, fat saponification, cell membrane emulsification, and cell death. Damage continues after surface exposure because of the ability of alkaline corrosives to penetrate tissue. In contrast, acids cause coagulation necrosis, which leads to desiccation of epithelial cells and produces eschar, with resulting edema, erythema, mucosal sloughing, ulceration, and necrosis of the surface tissues.

The dose of a caustic agent causing significant toxicity varies by product and concentration. Information on specific agents can be obtained from product packaging and from a poison control center.

## HYDROFLUORIC ACID

Hydrofluoric acid and related compounds, such as ammonium bifluoride, ammonium fluoride, potassium bifluoride, and sodium bifluoride, are found in rust removers, automobile wheel cleaners, toilet bowl cleaners, air conditioner coil cleaners, dentifrices, and insecticides. The bifluorides can form hydrofluoric acid in the presence of body water and can thus cause delayed presentation of symptoms.[7] The fluoride ion is directly toxic to numerous cellular enzymes and also forms complexes with calcium and magnesium. These complexes precipitate in tissues and cause significant pain and tissue destruction. At high enough levels of fluoride, these complexes can lead to systemic depletion of calcium and magnesium that can precipitate life-threatening arrhythmias.

The toxic ingested dose of hydrofluoric acid is between 5 and 10 mg/kg, and death occurs after a dose of 15 to 30 mg/kg. This translates into a lethal dose of 50 mg for a 10-kg child, a quantity contained in 5 mL of 10% hydrofluoric acid.

## CALCIUM CHANNEL BLOCKERS

Calcium channel blockers are widely prescribed for their chronotropic and antihypertensive effects. They exert their action through L-type voltage-gated channels present in cardiac myocytes, vascular smooth muscle, and the sinoatrial and atrioventricular nodes. The three main classes of calcium channel blockers are the phenylalkylamines, the benzothiaprines, and the dihydropyridines. The phenylalkylamines (verapamil) and the benzothiaprines (diltiazem) act predominantly on myocytes and cardiac tissue, and the dihydropyridines (nifedipine) work predominantly on vascular tissue. Bepridil, the sole agent representing a fourth class, is not in widespread use because of its poor side effect profile.

Calcium channel blocker overdose causes severe hypotension and bradycardia, although reflex tachycardia may also be seen in overdose of the vascular tone–predominant dihydropyridines. Calcium channel blockade is responsible for dysrhythmias ranging from heart block to idioventricular arrhythmias. Impaired insulin release and systemic insulin resistance lead to the classic finding of hyperglycemia. Pulmonary edema may occur; the mechanism is unknown, but the edema may be caused by selective precapillary vasodilation or aggressive fluid resuscitation.[8]

Data on the minimum dose required to produce significant toxicity in children are mixed, but published cases have reported that one to two pills caused significant morbidity or death in children less than 6 years of age.[9]

Calcium channel blocker overdose and beta-blocker overdose are commonly discussed together in the adult literature because of their similarity of presentation and the therapeutic coadministration of these medications. A review of the pediatric literature found no published cases of death in young children as a result of accidental ingestion of beta-blockers, so these agents do not appear on the "One Pill Can Kill" list.[10]

## CLONIDINE AND TOPICAL IMIDAZOLINES

Clonidine is a centrally acting α-receptor agonist that inhibits sympathetic pathways. It was developed in the 1960s as a nasal decongestant, but it is most commonly used as an antihypertensive and in the treatment of narcotic and alcohol withdrawal, of perimenopausal hot flashes, and, more recently, in the treatment of pediatric attention-deficit hyperactivity disorder and Tourette disorder. Topical imidazolines are found in over-the counter decongestants for the nose and eyes, including oxymetazoline (Afrin), naphazoline (Naphcon), xylometazoline (Otrivin Pediatric Nasal) and tetrahydrozoline (Visine).

The exact mechanism of clonidine toxicity is not fully understood. Because of functional overlap between $\alpha_2$ and μ receptors, symptoms of clonidine toxicity can mimic those of opioid toxicity. Peripheral $\alpha_1$-receptor stimulation may cause a transient period of hypertension before centrally mediated bradycardia and hypotension predominate. In contrast to clonidine, the topical imidazolines are specifically designed to induce local $\alpha_2$-mediated peripheral vasoconstriction for their desired clinical effect. Toxicity from these agents may manifest as agitation, tachycardia, and hypertension, although CNS and respiratory depression similar to that seen with clonidine toxicity have also been reported with these agents.[11,12]

A minimum toxic dose of imidazoline has not been established. A clonidine level as low as 0.01 mg/kg has been shown in case reports to cause altered mental status in children, which correlates with ingestion of a single 0.1-mg tablet by a 10-kg child. Larger doses have been associated with more severe symptoms.[12]

### DIPHENOXYLATE-ATROPINE (LOMOTIL)

Diphenoxylate-atropine, most commonly known as Lomotil, is an antidiarrheal agent consisting of a combination of opioid and anticholinergic medications. Diphenoxylate, a meperidine derivative, decreases smooth muscle action of the gut. Atropine is added to decrease the drug's abuse potential. Lomotil toxicity can be both prolonged and delayed, secondary to its combined opioid and anticholinergic effect on gut motility. Diphenoxylate's primary metabolite, difenoxine, is more active and has a longer half-life than diphenoxylate and thus exacerbates the phenomenon of delayed presentation.

Lomotil has classically been included on most "One Pill Can Kill" lists, but one review of the literature revealed a paucity of data demonstrating that significant morbidity is caused by small doses.[13] Most deaths are attributed to ingestion of multiple pills or repetitive, incorrect dosing over time. No established minimum toxic dose exists, but the review found no reports of significant toxicity with ingestions of fewer than six to eight tablets in small children.

### SULFONYLUREAS

Sulfonylureas are used for the treatment of non–insulin-dependent diabetes mellitus and can cause significant hypoglycemia after the ingestion of one or two pills by young children. Examples are chlorpropamide, glyburide, glimepiride, glipizide, tolazamide, and tolbutamide. Sulfonylureas lower blood glucose primarily by stimulating endogenous insulin secretion and secondarily by enhancing peripheral insulin receptor sensitivity and reducing glycogenolysis.

Death is rare with sulfonylurea exposure. Only one case was found in a literature review.[14] However, many children less than 6 years old become symptomatic from sulfonylurea ingestion, and numerous case reports have noted symptoms in children who ingested of one to two pills.

### TRICYCLIC ANTIDEPRESSANTS

Tricyclic antidepressants (TCAs) represent a diverse group of medications that have been historically responsible for many poisoning deaths. In addition to their use in the treatment of depression, TCAs have been used to treat migraines, chronic pain, and enuresis, and they have been administered as second-line therapy for several pediatric psychiatric disorders.

TCA toxicity manifests primarily with cardiovascular and CNS effects. Inhibition of the fast sodium channel causes cardiac conduction disturbances, resulting in a widened QRS complex. Blockade of catecholamine reuptake can cause tachycardia and mild hypertension, although these effects are usually offset by peripheral α-adrenergic blockade causing vasodilation and hypotension. CNS effects of delirium, seizure, and coma are likely caused by anticholinergic effects, as well as by central blockade of neurotransmitter uptake. Anticholinergic effects can also slow gastric emptying and produce delayed or unpredictable absorption.

Several case reports published since the 1970s demonstrated that one or two pills can kill a small child. Significant morbidity or mortality tends to occur at doses greater than 15 to 30 mg/kg; ingestion of one or two 150-mg pills by a 10-kg toddler can easily reach this level.[15]

## PRESENTING SIGNS AND SYMPTOMS

### CAMPHOR

Camphor toxicity most often develops 5 to 90 minutes from the time of ingestion, but some case reports have noted presentations as late as 9 hours after ingestion.[16] Clinical toxicity may first manifest with gastrointestinal complaints, from oral burning to nausea and vomiting. Initial CNS effects of hyperactivity such as irritability, hyperreflexia, and myoclonic jerking may progress to seizure, delirium, and coma. Seizures are common and may persist for up to 24 hours, although this does not seem to have prognostic implications.[2] When death occurs, it is usually the result of status epilepticus or respiratory failure.

### SALICYLATES

Patients may present with vomiting, hyperpnea, tinnitus, and a mixed metabolic picture of respiratory alkalosis and metabolic acidosis. In contrast to adults, children less than 2 years old tend to present with metabolic acidosis only, rather than the classic mixed picture, because respiratory alkalosis appears to be transient. Salicylate-induced hypoglycemia may also be more pronounced in children than in adults. More serious intoxications may progress to CNS symptoms, including lethargy, agitation, delirium, or seizures. Respiratory acidosis suggests pulmonary edema and fatigue. Hyperthermia reflects oxidative uncoupling and is often a preterminal finding.

Symptoms of oil of wintergreen ingestion may progress much faster than symptoms caused by other agents because of the high concentrations of salicylate. One review found that patients who progressed to life-threatening toxicity from oil of wintergreen ingestion almost uniformly experienced emesis within minutes to a few hours of ingestion, followed by signs of CNS toxicity.[4]

### TOPICAL ANESTHETICS

Lidocaine or dibucaine overdose manifests with signs and symptoms of CNS toxicity that progress from agitation, confusion, or ataxia to generalized seizures and coma. Cardiac toxicity, such as heart block or arrhythmia, is infrequently seen with ingestion other than dibucaine and usually occurs only after CNS toxicity has manifested. The onset of symptoms has been reported to occur any time from minutes to hours following exposure, with significantly faster onset if the exposure involves aspiration or the respiratory tract.[5]

Benzocaine exposures manifest with signs and symptoms that correlate with the percentage of methemoglobin present in the blood. At approximately 15%, patients may exhibit cyanosis unresponsive to supplemental oxygen; weakness, tachycardia, and nausea may occur at approximately 30%. Lethargy and stupor, seizure, coma, and dysrhythmia may occur when methemoglobin levels reach more than 55%; death related to methemoglobinemia, although never reported as a result of benzocaine ingestion, may occur at levels higher than 70%. The onset of symptoms following benzocaine ingestion is usually rapid, occurring within 30 to 60 minutes.

Pulse oximetry and arterial oxygen measurements are not accurate and may be falsely reassuring in these patients. If methemoglobinemia is suspected, methemoglobin must be measured on a cooximeter.

## CAUSTICS

Contact of caustic substances with mucosa generally causes severe pain, which often limits the quantity of substance ingested. However, even one mouthful of a sufficiently concentrated caustic substance may cause severe injury. Common signs include lip or tongue swelling and erythema or intraoral ulceration. The most common presenting features of a clinically significant exposure include drooling, vomiting, and refusal of oral intake. Substernal chest pain or abdominal pain should raise concern for esophageal or stomach perforation. In severe cases, progressive oropharyngeal edema may lead to drooling and rapid airway compromise.

The severity and rapidity of symptom development are related to the type of agent, concentration, volume, viscosity, duration of contact, and pH. The emergency physician must keep in mind that an absence of oropharyngeal burns does not exclude esophageal injury.[17]

## HYDROFLUORIC ACID

Local apparent injury may be minimal because of a paucity of free hydrogen ions, which are responsible for the caustic tissue injuries caused by other acids. A hallmark sign of dermal exposure to hydrofluoric acid is pain out of proportion to physical findings. Evidence of ingestion commonly manifests with gastrointestinal symptoms of nausea, vomiting, and abdominal pain. Respiratory symptoms ranging from dyspnea to acute respiratory distress syndrome can indicate direct inhalational injury, increased secretions caused by fluoride's effect on acetylcholinesterase, or muscle fatigue.[7]

CNS manifestations include lethargy, obtundation, weakness, and loss of deep tendon reflexes. Cardiac toxicity, in particular ventricular fibrillation and torsades de pointes, results from hypocalcemia and can develop precipitously. The QTc interval is often prolonged in these patients. The onset of severe systemic symptoms can be delayed, but cardiac toxicity generally occurs within 6 hours.

## CALCIUM CHANNEL BLOCKERS

Bradycardia and hypotension are the hallmarks of calcium channel blocker overdose. Patients may exhibit sequelae of hypoperfusion and shock, including mental status changes, lactic acidosis, renal or hepatic failure, and intestinal ischemia. Patients may have cardiac arrhythmias including second- and third-degree heart block. Seizures rarely occur in the absence of cardiovascular collapse because these agents, with the exception of nimodipine, do not cross the blood-brain barrier. CNS manifestations out of proportion to the cardiovascular effects should raise the suspicion of coingestions.[11] Hyperglycemia is a hallmark of calcium channel blocker toxicity.

Symptom onset usually occurs in 1 to 2 hours, but it may be delayed for up to 24 hours if an extended-release formulation is ingested.

## CLONIDINE AND TOPICAL IMIDAZOLINES

Clonidine toxicity often resembles opioid intoxication, with symptoms consisting of miosis, bradycardia, hypotension, and, in severe cases, respiratory depression and hypothermia. CNS depression is a common symptom. Unlike with opioid intoxication, patients are often rousable by stimulation, but they may quickly return to a depressed mental state.[12,18] Toxicity from topical imidazolines also manifests most commonly with altered mental status and respiratory depression.[12] Both topical imidazolines and clonidine may cause tachycardia or bradycardia and hypertension or hypotension.

Both clonidine and the topical imidazolines are rapidly absorbed. Symptoms usually appear in 30 to 90 minutes and may last for 1 to 3 days, depending on the dose ingested.

## DIPHENOXYLATE-ATROPINE (LOMOTIL)

The classic teaching regarding Lomotil toxicity is that it exhibits a biphasic course: an early, anticholinergic-predominant phase lasting 2 to 3 hours followed by a prolonged, opioid-predominant phase. This notion was challenged by a review in 1991 that suggested that most patients exhibited a prolonged opioid toxidrome, and only 11% presented with a biphasic course.[19] In serious intoxications, patients may exhibit CNS excitation, coma, or profound respiratory depression.

The onset of symptoms may occur as early as 2 hours or as late as 24 to 30 hours after ingestion. Respiratory or CNS depression may recur after 12 to 24 hours. The cause is thought to be an accumulation of the long-acting opioid metabolite of diphenoxylate.

## SULFONYLUREAS

The clinical presentation of sulfonylurea toxicity is that of hypoglycemia: lethargy, confusion, headache, seizures, tachycardia, and diaphoresis. If untreated, hypoglycemia can result in permanent neurologic sequelae or death. The onset of symptoms is usually seen within 8 hours of ingestion, but it can be delayed with ingestion of extended-release formulations. Chlorpropamide, glyburide, and the long-acting form of glipizide tend to have a longer clinical effect. Delayed presentation also seems to correlate with patients in whom a prophylactic dextrose drip is started; this practice may mask emerging hypoglycemia and create a false sense of security.[14]

## TRICYCLIC ANTIDEPRESSANTS

The TCA-poisoned pediatric patient presents similarly to the adult patient, with an anticholinergic syndrome of delirium, mydriasis, flushing, tachycardia, dry mucous membranes, or hyperthermia. Hypotension and a widened QRS complex are concerning findings. Pediatric patients exhibit electrocardiographic (ECG) changes similar to those seen adult patients, but no correlation between ECG findings and prognosis has been established.[15,18] As with adults, seizure is an ominous sign of potential impending circulatory collapse. When death occurs, it is usually the result of cardiac arrest.

# DIFFERENTIAL DIAGNOSIS AND MEDICAL DECISION MAKING

In the ideal situation, the differential diagnosis and medical decision making for a given exposure will be guided by knowledge of the ingested agent. Unfortunately, many children ingest toxic agents without direct observation by their caretakers, and the children come to medical care only when they exhibit signs of intoxication such as altered mental status, respiratory depression, and seizure.

In the patient with an undifferentiated condition who presents with any of these signs of systemic illness, the emergency physician must keep toxic exposure in the differential diagnosis while performing a broad work-up for infectious and metabolic causes of the patient's illness. A detailed history elicited from the child's parents and caregivers should include any possible household chemical, prescription, or over-the-counter medications with which the child may have come into contact. This history should include any visitors, such as grandparents, who may have transported their own medications into the home in a purse or suitcase.

The initial evaluation should include a complete blood count, basic chemistry panel with full electrolytes, and bedside glucose determination. An ECG study should be considered to evaluate for arrhythmia, heart block, and QRS widening. In general, serum drug levels are not helpful in guiding initial diagnosis and management because they may not provide clinically useful information other than confirming that a given exposure took place, and results may not be readily available. An exception is the salicylate level, which can be used to guide therapy and management. That said, treatment should not be delayed while awaiting this result when salicylate ingestion is strongly suspected or when the patient is symptomatic. Although acetaminophen is not included on the "One Pill Can Kill" list, an *N*-acetyl-*p*-aminophenol (APAP) level is often checked concurrently whenever undifferentiated ingestion is suspected.

During the history or physical examination, the astute physician may pick up a few agent-specific clues that will help guide the diagnosis of a particular toxic exposure in a child with altered mental status. The identification of a cluster of signs and symptoms suggestive of a toxidrome is helpful: anticholinergic symptoms should raise the suspicion of Lomotil or TCA exposure; an opioid toxidrome suggests possible imidazoline or Lomotil exposure. Salicylate overdose and camphor ingestion should be considered in the differential diagnosis of febrile seizure; in salicylate overdose, febrile seizure represents severe salicylate intoxication, whereas in camphor overdose, it reflects parents' use of camphor to treat symptoms of viral illness. A cyanotic child with symptoms out of proportion to pulse oximetry should raise suspicion of methemoglobinemia and should prompt cooximetry measurement. Significant hypotension should raise concern for TCA, clonidine, calcium channel blocker, or salicylate overdose. Hypoglycemia should raise the suspicion of sulfonylurea or salicylate exposure; hyperglycemia suggests calcium channel blocker ingestion.

In cases of suspected caustic exposure, pulse oximetry and a chest radiograph may be useful, but radiographic evidence of clinically significant aspiration may not be apparent for 6 hours or more. In a severe caustic ingestion accompanied by chest or abdominal pain, a radiograph should be obtained to evaluate for the presence of free air.

## TREATMENT

### PREHOSPITAL

Whenever possible, product or prescription containers should be transported to the hospital with the patient. Given the rapid onset of symptoms seen with many of the agents discussed in this chapter, patients should be transported by ambulance to a hospital facility.

The administration of syrup of ipecac at home is not recommended. A 2004 position paper from the American Academy of Clinical Toxicology (AACT) and the European Association of Poisons Centres and Clinical Toxicologists (EAPCCT) stated that data were insufficient to support or refute the use of syrup of ipecac in the prehospital setting.[20] In highly toxic ingestions by patients in remote locations (i.e., when hospital evaluation will be delayed by hours), ipecac may have a limited role in the prehospital setting if it is administered very early.[21]

Administration of a neutralizing agent, such as vinegar in the case of alkali ingestion, is not recommended because of concerns of inducing emesis or exacerbating injury by causing an exothermic reaction.

### HOSPITAL

Supportive care is the mainstay of treatment for toxic exposures. The ABCs (airway, breathing, and circulation) are of the utmost importance, and the airway is secured early in patients with compromised respiratory status, mental status depression, or risk of aspiration. Fluid resuscitation should be initiated early and aggressively in patients with hypotension. Seizures, regardless of causative agent, should generally be treated with benzodiazepines as first-line agents and with phenobarbital in refractory cases.

Gastric decontamination in toxic ingestions has historically been a controversial topic and poses unique problems in the pediatric patient. The AACT and EAPCCT's joint position on the routine use of gastric lavage states that the weight of evidence does not demonstrate a beneficial clinical effect and that the risk of adverse outcomes such as aspiration, laryngospasm, or perforation outweighs the questionable benefits.[22] An additional issue concerning lavage in the pediatric patient is that smaller children may not easily accommodate the 36 to 40 French catheter often needed to remove particulate material effectively.

Single-dose activated charcoal is similarly not recommended for routine use by the AACT and EAPCCT but may be considered in specific cases.[23] Risks associated with charcoal administration include vomiting and aspiration, decreased effectiveness of oral antidotes, and an obscured view of the oropharynx should intubation or endoscopy become necessary.[21] Data from volunteers implied that the reduction of toxin absorption may not be clinically significant if activated charcoal is administered more than 1 hour following ingestion, but a potential benefit after 1 hour cannot be excluded.[23] Charcoal use is contraindicated in a patient without an intact or protected airway. Convincing a toddler to drink a gritty slurry may prove extremely difficult, and the distress caused by forcibly administering this therapy must be weighed against the benefits on a case-by-case basis.

Whole-bowel irrigation is not routinely recommended but should be considered in a patients who has ingested sustained-release or enteric-coated tablets, particularly if the patient presents more than 2 hours following ingestion.[24] This procedure is contraindicated in cases of ileus, bowel obstruction or perforation, hemodynamic instability, or compromised airway.

Agents with specific treatment antidotes or guidelines are discussed next (**Table 158.5**).

**Table 158.5 Drugs That Are Highly Toxic in Small Doses**

| DRUG | TOXIC EXPOSURE* | MAJOR TOXIC EFFECTS | TREATMENT |
|---|---|---|---|
| Calcium channel blockers | Varied dose; one to pills | Bradycardia, hypotension | Atropine, glucagon, calcium, insulin |
| Clonidine | 0.01 mg/kg, or one 0.1 mg pill | Miosis, bradycardia, hypotension, respiratory depression, hypothermia | Supportive care; consider naloxone, atropine, dopamine |
| Diphenoxylate-atropine | Varies; six to eight pills | Bradycardia, hypotension, delayed gut motility, CNS excitation, coma, respiratory depression | Supportive care; consider bowel irrigation, naloxone |
| Sulfonylureas | One to two pills | Hypoglycemia | Supplemental glucose; consider octreotide |
| Tricyclic antidepressants | 15 mg/kg, or one 150-mg pill | Delirium, mydriasis, flushing, tachycardia, hyperthermia; seizures, hypotension (late) | Sodium bicarbonate, benzodiazepines, supportive care |

*CNS,* Central nervous system.
*For a 10-kg child.

### Salicylates

Depending on the clinical symptoms, blood salicylate concentration, and evidence of organ toxicity, urine and serum alkalinization or hemodialysis should be initiated following the same guidelines as for adult patients (see Chapter 144). Salicylate ingestion is a situation for which activated charcoal administration should be considered, given the high potential for significant morbidity.

When evaluating a suspected methylsalicylate exposure, the salicylate blood concentration should be obtained within 1 hour, as opposed to at the 2- to 4-hour mark. The Done nomogram should not be used because patients may progress far more rapidly than in other types of salicylate ingestion. Although the salicylate level is useful to guide management, treatment should never be delayed while awaiting laboratory results if a child's clinical presentation and metabolic status warrant intervention.

### Topical Anesthetics

Methylene blue is the antidote for benzocaine-induced methemoglobinemia. It works by reducing oxidized hemoglobin and increasing conversion of methemoglobin back to hemoglobin. Methylene blue should be given at a dose of 1 to 2 mg/kg intravenously in patients with serious symptoms or with methemoglobin concentrations greater than 30%. If treatment with methylene blue fails, exchange transfusion or hyperbaric oxygen may be considered. Methylene blue is contraindicated in patients with glucose-6-phosphate dehydrogenase deficiency.

### Caustics

Early intubation should be initiated for any patient with any symptom of airway compromise from caustic ingestion. Copious irrigation of the eyes and skin is indicated for dermal and eye exposures. Indications for endoscopy include vomiting, drooling, stridor, and dyspnea. Endoscopy should ideally be performed in the first 12 to 24 hours following exposure.

The administration of corticosteroids in the acute management of caustic ingestion is controversial, and the current evidence does not support use of these agents in preventing stricture formation.[25]

### Hydrofluoric Acid

For significant dermal exposures to hydrofluoric acid, topical use of calcium gel can be effective if it is applied immediately. Local injection of calcium gluconate or arterial calcium gluconate may be needed for significant hand exposures. Patients with severe systemic depletion of electrolytes require aggressive repletion and cardiac monitoring to avoid precipitous decline and progression to lethal arrhythmia.

### Calcium Channel Blockers

Calcium channel blocker overdoses in the pediatric patient should be managed aggressively following the same algorithm as for adult ingestions, with the use of atropine, calcium, glucagon, vasopressors, or hyperinsulinemia-euglycemic therapy, as warranted (see Chapter 148). Because of the danger of delayed and prolonged presentation, activated charcoal administration or whole-bowel irrigation should be considered in these patients if ingestion of extended-release formulations is suspected.

### Clonidine

Naloxone has been shown in some case reports to reverse both cardiovascular and respiratory depression caused by clonidine ingestion, but this is not well studied, and the use of naloxone is recommended only in severe cases or when intubation is imminent.[18] Atropine may be used to treat refractory bradycardia, and refractory hypotension may be treated with vasopressors; dopamine is the agent most commonly studied.

### Diphenoxylate-Atropine (Lomotil)

Because of the delayed and unpredictable gastric emptying associated with Lomotil, gastric decontamination should be considered in patients with significant Lomotil ingestions. Naloxone has been used in patients exhibiting significant opioid toxicity.

### *Sulfonylureas*

Management of sulfonylurea ingestion is controversial, with widely differing and contradictory recommendations published. Children suspected of ingesting a sulfonylurea should be monitored for a minimum of 8 hours, with blood glucose measurements performed every 1 to 2 hours. Patients should be managed expectantly unless they exhibit signs or symptoms of hypoglycemia. While under observation, patients may be allowed to eat, but they should not be given intravenous glucose infusion.

If a patient develops clinical symptoms or has a blood glucose level lower than 60 mg/dL, then a 1 g/kg bolus of glucose should be given, and the patient should be admitted for inpatient observation. A glucose infusion may be started at the physician's discretion. Giving exogenous glucose may stimulate an exaggerated endogenous insulin response and lead to rebound hypoglycemia.

For significant and persistent hypoglycemia, octreotide should be administered. Octreotide is a somatostatin analogue that inhibits the secretion of insulin and may obviate the need for exogenous glucose. The dose is 1 to 2 mcg/kg and can be administered subcutaneously or intravenously.

### *Tricyclic Antidepressants*

Pediatric TCA overdoses should be managed aggressively according to the same algorithm that is applied to adults: alkalinization with sodium bicarbonate, benzodiazepines for seizures, and supportive care (see Chapter 147). Given the lethality of a large enough dose and the concern for delayed gastric emptying secondary to anticholinergic effects, activated charcoal should be considered in the first 1 to 2 hours of a known exposure.

## FOLLOW-UP AND NEXT STEPS IN CARE

### OBSERVATION AND ADMISSION VERSUS DISCHARGE

Regardless of suspected agents, most pediatric patients with toxic exposures or suspected ingestions can be observed for 4 to 6 hours. Patients who remain asymptomatic may be safely discharged home. Exceptions and additional management information relevant to specific substances follow.

Children with suspected salicylate exposure who are found to have a positive blood level require hospital admission with levels rechecked every 2 hours until they are clinically improving, have a decreasing and nontoxic salicylate level, and have an alkalemic blood pH.[11]

With respect to calcium channel blocker ingestion, although a 6-hour period of observation is sufficient for ingestions of immediate-release formulations, a 12- to 24-hour observation period is recommended if concern exists about exposure to extended-release formulations.

The observation period for suspected Lomotil ingestion is not well described, especially if significant exposure is a concern. Because symptoms have been shown to be delayed by up to 24 hours, patients with concerning ingestions should be observed for at least this long.

Patients who have ingested sulfonylureas should be monitored for 8 hours because of the possibility of delayed presentation. Patients should be monitored for longer if the ingested medication is a sustained-release formulation.

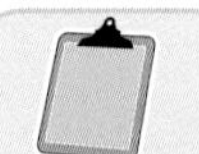

**DOCUMENTATION**

**History**
- Name and concentration of the drug ingestion
- Time lapse since ingestion, if known
- History of any other diseases that may complicate the ingestion

**Physical Examination**
- Does the patient look ill? Pale? Febrile?
- Mental status
- Cardiac status (blood pressure, arrhythmias)
- Respiratory and airway status
- Physical examination: repeated while patient is in the emergency department

**Laboratory Studies**
- Laboratory tests and time obtained

**Medical Decision Making**
- Calculation of the mg/kg dose ingested, if possible
- Decision to begin treatment or delays
- Consultation(s) chosen and time(s) of request(s)
- If patient being discharged, documentation of medical reasons that patient needs no further investigation or continuing care

**Treatment**
- Availability of antidote, time antidote ordered, and any delays of treatment

**Patient Instructions**
- Document a discussion with the patient or parent regarding the diagnosis, warning signs, what to do, follow-up, and when to return.
- With pediatric accidental ingestions, document poison prevention counseling.
- Families should be given the phone number for the poison control center to address further concerns (1-800-222-1222).
- Whenever concern exists about the situation surrounding the ingestion or when an ingestion has occurred in an infant younger than 12 months, social services should be contacted.

## SUGGESTED READINGS

Greene S, Harris C, Singer J. Gastrointestinal decontamination of the poisoned patient. Pediatr Emerg Care 2008;24:176-86.

Henry K, Harris CR. Deadly ingestions. Pediatr Clin North Am 2006;53:293-315.

Michael JB, Sztajnkrycer MD. Deadly pediatric poisons: nine common agents that kill at low doses. Emerg Med Clin North Am 2004;22:1019-50.

## REFERENCES

***References can be found on Expert Consult @ www.expertconsult.com.***

# Fluid Management 159

*Alan C. Heffner and Matthew T. Robinson*

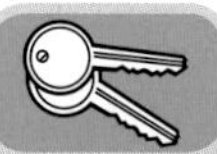

**KEY POINTS**

- Shock is defined by inadequate tissue perfusion and not by systemic blood pressure.
- The majority of emergency department patients who require resuscitation are in compensated shock with normal blood pressure.
- Volume expansion with isotonic fluid is the most important immediate therapy for most patients with circulatory insufficiency.
- Resuscitation and maintenance fluids should be tailored to an individual patient's acid-base and electrolyte status.
- The fluid dose titrated to appropriate end points is more important than the individual fluid class (i.e., crystalloid versus colloid) used for resuscitation.
- Normal vital signs do not guarantee adequate systemic perfusion and should not be the ultimate end point of resuscitation.
- Dynamic measures of fluid responsiveness should be used to assist in the management of patients who remain hypoperfused despite initial empiric volume therapy.

## PERSPECTIVE

Hypovolemia is a common crisis in acute care medicine. Loss of volume is often a direct consequence of acute fluid or blood loss, but relative hypovolemia complicates many clinical conditions. Its severity ranges from mild compensated hypovolemia to shock and hypotension that place end-organ perfusion and function at risk. Fluid therapy to optimize cardiac performance and restore fluid and electrolyte balance is a cornerstone of medical support. Timely and appropriate fluid therapy maintains macrocirculatory and microcirculatory support and reduces mortality.[1] In contrast, both underresuscitation and overly aggressive fluid therapy can have an adverse impact on organ function and outcome.[2,3] Inadequate resuscitation risks leaving a patient in compensated shock. Overly aggressive fluid administration results in volume overload without improving oxygen delivery and is associated with worse clinical outcomes.[4] In addition to sustaining circulating blood volume, intravenous (IV) fluids also correct and maintain normal acid-base and electrolyte balance. A thorough understanding of the appropriate selection, timing, and goals of fluid therapy is vital to optimize patient care.

## PATHOPHYSIOLOGY

### OXYGEN DELIVERY AND TISSUE PERFUSION

Oxygen is delivered to cells via the circulation as a function of red blood cell mass and cardiorespiratory function. Oxygen enables continuous production of energy by cells in the form of adenosine triphosphate. Poor oxygenation compromises cell energetics and function and results in the clinical manifestations of organ dysfunction and failure.

Cardiac output is the most important determinant of oxygen delivery, and it has sufficient flexibility to compensate for reduced oxygen-carrying capacity, as well as increased metabolic demands. The physiologic response to a decrease in cardiac output is catecholamine-induced tachycardia and enhanced cardiac contractility, which attempt to maintain oxygen delivery in the face of falling stroke volume. Concomitant venoconstriction maintains intrathoracic blood volume (preload), whereas arterial vasoconstriction shunts perfusion to vital organs and maintains critical organ perfusion pressure.

Cardiac output and organ perfusion vary dramatically under changing physiologic, pathologic, and pharmacologic stimuli. Organ blood flow is directly proportional to perfusion pressure in most vascular beds. In hypovolemia, protection of arterial (organ perfusion) pressure occurs via peripheral vasoconstriction at the expense of reduced flow to noncritical circulations (e.g., hepatosplanchnic, renal, cutaneous). Consequently, arterial pressure is maintained despite hypovolemia and organ hypoperfusion.

Effective circulating volume (ECV) conceptualizes the portion of intravascular volume contributing to organ perfusion. ECV decreases with hypovolemia but does not necessarily correlate with volume status because organ perfusion is also dependent on cardiac output, vasomotor tone, and circulatory distribution. As an example, ECV may be compromised by limited cardiac output despite optimized intravascular preload status.

Volume depletion describes a state of contracted extracellular fluid with clinical implications of compromised ECV, tissue perfusion, and function. This is distinguished from

**Table 159.1 Size and Composition of Body Fluid Compartments***

| COMPARTMENT | % BODY WEIGHT | VOLUME (L) | $H_2O$ (L) | NA (MMOL/L) | K (MMOL/L) | CL (MMOL/L) | $HCO_3$ (MMOL/L) |
|---|---|---|---|---|---|---|---|
| Total body | 60 | 45 | 42 | | | | |
| ICF | 40 | 30 | 28 (60%) | 16 | 150 | | 10 |
| ECF | 20 | 15 | 14 (40%) | 140 | 4 | 103 | 26 |
| Interstitial | 16 | 12 | | | | | |
| Plasma | 4 | 3 | | | | | |
| Blood | 7 | 5 | | | | | |

*ECF*, Extracellular fluid; *ICF*, intracellular fluid.
*Values based on a male weighing 70 kg (154 lb).

dehydration, which implies an intracellular water deficit characterized by plasma hypernatremia and hyperosmolarity.

## WATER

Water is the most abundant constituent of the body. An adult man weighing 70 kg (154 lb) contains approximately 45 L of water, which accounts for 60% of body mass (**Table 159.1**). Total body water (TBW) is proportional to lean body mass and affects maintenance fluid requirements. TBW is physiologically compartmentalized into intracellular and extracellular spaces. The extracellular compartment is anatomically and conceptually divided into vascular and interstitial spaces.

Water freely crosses cell membranes, and osmotic forces determine the distribution of water within the body. The intracellular and extracellular fluid environments remain isosmolar but physiochemically distinct via tight regulation of dissolved solutes and proteins. Membrane-bound sodium-potassium adenosine triphosphatase pumps compartmentalize sodium and potassium to the extracellular and intracellular spaces, respectively. Active restriction of sodium to the extracellular space is the foundation of isotonic sodium-based resuscitation solutions.

Starling's law describes the forces governing fluid flux across vascular endothelial membranes. In healthy persons, transcapillary hydrostatic force is nearly opposed by colloid oncotic pressure. Small net loss from the vascular space is ultimately returned to the systemic circulation via lymphatics. Albumin normally accounts for 80% of colloid oncotic pressure, whereas large cellular moieties such as red blood cells and platelets contribute little oncotic pressure effect. Positive hydrostatic pressure, hypoalbuminemia, and pathologic endothelial permeability are common clinical conditions that enhance extravasation of fluid from the vascular compartment. The clinical consequences include large and ongoing volume resuscitation requirements coupled with tissue (e.g., lung, gut, brain) edema, which may compromise function.

## PRESENTING SIGNS AND SYMPTOMS

*Absolute hypovolemia* occurs as a consequence of loss of water, electrolytes, or blood (or any combination of the three) (**Box 159.1**). Patients with hypovolemia most often have symptoms related to reduced cardiac output such as fatigue, dyspnea, postural dizziness, and near or true syncope. Tolerance is variable and depends on the acuity and severity of the hypovolemia, associated anemia, individual physiologic reserve, and primary cause. Organ dysfunction is often a heralding sign of hypovolemia and may occur in the absence of global hypoperfusion or frank hemodynamic instability.

**BOX 159.1 Anatomic Sites of Nonhemorrhagic Volume Loss**

**Gastrointestinal**
Vomiting
Diarrhea
Drainage (ostomy, fistula, nasogastric)

**Renal**
Diuresis (medication, osmotic)
Salt wasting
Diabetes insipidus

**Skin**
Burn
Wound
Exfoliative rash
Sweating

**Third-Space Sequestration**
Intestinal obstruction
Peritonitis
Crush injury
Pancreatitis
Ascites
Pleural effusion
Capillary leak

**Respiratory**
Respiratory distress

**Insensible Loss**
Fever

*Shock* is defined as a state of inadequate tissue perfusion in which oxygen delivery does not meet metabolic requirements. The term does not reflect perfusion pressure—shock may occur with low, normal, or elevated blood pressure. Unfortunately, clinical signs are unreliable indicators of oxygen delivery and blood volume.[5,6]

*Compensated shock* refers to inadequate perfusion in the setting of normal blood pressure. The majority of critically ill patients are in compensated shock. The difficulty in identifying these patients prompted the terms *occult* and *cryptic shock* to describe normotensive patients with alternative evidence of cardiovascular insufficiency. Hyperlactatemia (<3 mmol/L) is an important marker to aid in identification of these high-risk patients.[7] Left unresuscitated, these patients often progress to frank hypotension.

**BOX 159.2 Clinical Indicators of Hypoperfusion That Warrant Consideration for a Rapid Monitored Fluid Challenge**

Mean arterial pressure (MAP) < 65 mm Hg
Systolic blood pressure < 90 mm Hg
Decrease in MAP > 20 mm Hg from baseline
Shock index > 0.9
Sinus tachycardia > 100 beats/min
Serum lactate > 3 mmol/L
Base deficit ≤ 6
Oliguria (urine output < 0.5 mL/kg/hr)
Abnormal peripheral perfusion

Brief episodes of hypotension are important markers of hypoperfusion and herald progressive hemodynamic deterioration. These self-limited episodes of transient hypotension represent progressive exhaustion of cardiovascular compensation and are the first sign of uncompensated shock.[8] *Uncompensated shock* is characterized by hypotension that occurs when physiologic attempts to maintain normal perfusion pressure are overwhelmed or exhausted. Sustained hypotension signifies a late stage of shock.

Volume status and perfusion should be evaluated during every emergency department (ED) examination (**Box 159.2**). Delayed capillary refill, dry axillae and mucous membranes, abnormal skin turgor, sunken eyes, and a depressed fontanelle are classic but imperfect hallmarks of hypovolemia.[9,10] Peripheral cyanosis, cool extremities, and cutaneous mottling (cutis marmorata) characterize classic hypodynamic shock but are not a primary indication of hypovolemia. In contrast, early hyperdynamic septic shock may be manifested as peripheral vasodilation with warm extremities and brisk capillary refill.

Generalized tissue edema reflects total body sodium and fluid excess but does not quantify intravascular status and may be accompanied by hypovolemia, especially in acute illness. Acute weight change implies loss of fluid rather than lean body mass and is helpful in patients with a reliable comparison weight.

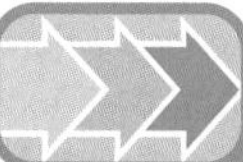

**PRIORITY ACTIONS**

**Prioritized End Points of Fluid Resuscitation**

Adequate intravenous access
Mean arterial pressure > 65 mm Hg
Systemic perfusion
- Central venous oxygen saturation ($Scvo_2$) > 70%
- Serum lactate clearance (>5%/hr) and normalization (<2 mmol/L)

Regional perfusion
- Urine output (>0.5 mL/kg/hr)
- Normalized peripheral perfusion

## TREATMENT

Circulatory failure is the final common pathway of many diseases. Inadequate circulating volume is the most common and immediately reversible factor in patients with acute circulatory insufficiency. Accordingly, fluid therapy is the initial management of undifferentiated shock. Pathologic vasodilation compounds the fluid deficit in common conditions such as sepsis, anaphylaxis, adrenal failure, neurogenic shock, and toxin-induced shock. Acute cardiac decompensation and pulmonary embolism are two exceptional situations in which limited volume resuscitation takes secondary priority to catecholamine and mechanical support.

**BOX 159.3 Conditions Warranting a Strategy of Limited-Volume Resuscitation Pending Surgical Control of Hemorrhage**

| | |
|---|---|
| Penetrating thoracoabdominal trauma | Traumatic aortic injury |
| Ruptured abdominal aortic aneurysm | Severe pelvic fracture |
| Major hemothorax | Gastrointestinal bleeding |
| Major hemoperitoneum | Ectopic pregnancy |
| | Postpartum hemorrhage |

Early recognition of hypovolemia and shock must be coupled with aggressive resuscitation to have an effect on patients. Timely resuscitation is important because the window to reverse critical organ hypoperfusion and affect clinical outcome is measured in hours and often transpires in the ED.[11] Equivalent but delayed resuscitation yields greater morbidity and mortality.[12-15] The immediate goal of fluid resuscitation is intravascular expansion to optimize stroke volume and oxygen delivery.

## FLUID RESUSCITATION

### *Resuscitation Targets (End Points)*

The target end point of resuscitation guides the dose and selection of interventions, including fluid therapy. In high-risk patients, fluid selection appears to be less important than volume dosage titrated to an appropriate therapeutic end point.[1,16] Rapid restoration of systemic pressure (mean arterial pressure > 65 mm Hg) is a first priority to support vital organ autoregulated blood flow. However, stabilization of blood pressure does not guarantee adequate organ perfusion—resuscitation aimed primarily at normotension risks leaving the patient in persistent compensated shock.[17] Unfortunately, there is no single best resuscitation end point for all clinical circumstances. An approach seeking to normalize a combination of both global and regional perfusion markers is most prudent (**Box 159.3**).

### *Empiric Fluid Challenge*

Empiric volume challenges remain the standard means of early fluid resuscitation. Volume expansion is achieved by infusing serial aliquots of isotonic fluid under direct observation. This strategy is appropriate for acute undifferentiated shock or for obvious or suspected hypovolemia. Crystalloid (10 to 20 mL/kg) or colloid (4 to 7 mL/kg) should be infused rapidly over a period of 15 minutes with serial boluses titrated to the clinical end point objective while monitoring for adverse effects. A positive clinical response to volume loading confirms volume responsiveness but does not predict further response to therapy. Failure to recognize patients not responding to fluid may contribute to overly aggressive volume therapy and delay alternative care measures.

Total volume requirements are difficult to predict at the onset of resuscitation and are often underestimated. Classic hypovolemia, as occurs with acute hemorrhage or fluid loss, may stabilize rapidly with appropriate volume expansion. The 3 : 1 rule of hemorrhage resuscitation suggests that 3 volumetric units of crystalloid are required to replete an extracellular fluid deficit of 1 unit of blood loss. However, experimental models have confirmed that with severe hemorrhage, volume requirements exceed the 3 : 1 suggestion. Pathologic vasodilation and capillary leak contribute to the need for ongoing volume replacement. Exaggerated transcapillary fluid shifts are common with early burns, peritonitis, and pancreatitis. Crystalloid requirements average greater than 60 mL/kg in the first hours of septic shock but may be as high as 200 mL/kg to normalize perfusion.[18,19]

### *Predicting Volume Responsiveness*

The utility of fluid administration to improve stroke volume depends on a number of variables, including venous tone and ventricular function. Critically ill patients may manifest continued hypoperfusion despite initial empiric volume resuscitation. As an example, only half of hypotensive patients with sepsis are stabilized with volume resuscitation alone.[19] In the absence of overt clinical hypovolemia or ongoing fluid loss, volume responsiveness should not be assumed. Continued fluid therapy does not have any impact on macrocirculatory flow in up to 50% of critically ill patients.[20]

Volume or preload responsiveness refers to the ability to augment stroke volume with fluid administration. In contrast to an empiric volume challenge, volume responsiveness is gauged before fluid administration, and the resulting information is used to guide whether fluid administration is a solution to reverse clinical hypoperfusion. Fluid loading in volume-unresponsive patients is optimally avoided because it delays appropriate therapy and contributes to fluid excess that contributes to organ dysfunction, including hypoxemic respiratory failure and abdominal compartment syndrome.[4] A more rational approach for patients who remain hypoperfused after initial empiric management incorporates selection and titration of subsequent therapy under the guidance of objective cardiovascular monitoring.

A target central venous pressure (CVP) of 8 to 12 mm Hg is recommended to maximize preload before instituting pressor and inotropic support.[21] Unfortunately, there is no consistent threshold CVP to reliably estimate response to fluid administration.[22] Values that are considered low, normal, or high can be found in patients who respond positively to fluid.[20]

Dynamic hemodynamic indices are more dependable signs of volume responsiveness. Respirophasic variation in stroke volume during positive pressure mechanical ventilation is among the most useful signs of fluid responsiveness.[20] Respiratory collapse of the inferior vena cava (IVC) is another helpful indicator. Minimal IVC variation is associated with supranormal CVP and a low probability of fluid responsiveness. Inspiratory IVC collapse greater than 50% indicates a high probability of augmenting stroke volume with fluid therapy.

## FLUID SELECTION

Early resuscitation and ongoing replacement of fluid deficits may be performed with a variety of fluids. Because each possesses specific benefits and potential disadvantages in given clinical scenarios, an understanding of fluid composition is important. Isotonic solutions are effective volume expanders (**Table 159.2**). Electrolyte disorders (including hypernatremia and hyponatremia) take secondary priority to isotonic volume loading in hypoperfused patients. Hypotonic solutions are ineffective and inappropriate volume expanders.

### *Crystalloids*

Isotonic sodium-based crystalloids are distributed to the extracellular compartment, which includes the vascular space. Partitioning within the extracellular fluid leaves 25% of the infused volume within the circulation. Normal saline and lactated Ringer (LR) solution are two isotonic resuscitation solutions in common use. LR solution, also known as Hartmann solution, was developed as a more physiologic alkalinizing replacement solution; bicarbonate is generated by lactate metabolism via the Cori cycle.

The clinical superiority of any single crystalloid remains unproved, and selection of fluid should be based on the source of the hypovolemia, associated electrolyte derangements, and volume requirements. Normal saline provides a supraphysiologic chloride load that induces metabolic acidosis when administered in large volumes. This is advantageous in correcting the volume and electrolyte disturbances (hypochloremic metabolic alkalosis) associated with loss of gastric secretions (e.g., profuse vomiting, gastric outlet obstruction, nasogastric suctioning). LR solution provides a more physiologic electrolyte balance and is often preferred for large-volume resuscitation. LR is recommended for trauma resuscitation but is incompatible with blood. Isotonic bicarbonate (i.e., three ampules of sodium bicarbonate in 1 L of sterile water) is an alternative resuscitation fluid for patients with coexisting metabolic acidosis.

### *Colloids*

Colloid solutions are composed of electrolyte preparations reinforced with macromolecules designed to preserve colloid oncotic pressure. Vascular retention of colloid makes these formulations more efficient volume expanders with a longer duration of action than is the case with crystalloids. Crystalloid solutions require two to four times more volume for equivalent resuscitation. Dilutional hypoalbuminemia, transcapillary fluid shift, and interstitial and pulmonary edema may therefore be limited with colloid use. When dosed to the same end points, colloids and crystalloids are equally effective. Randomized clinical trials have failed to prove clinical superiority of one fluid class, with comparable rates of mortality and lung dysfunction.[23,24] Traumatic brain injury remains one important exception in which isotonic albumin is associated with a higher risk for adverse outcomes when compared with equivalent crystalloid.[23,25] Crystalloid solutions remain the standard ED choice for resuscitation and confer a significant cost advantage over colloid solutions.

Human albumin and hydroxyethyl starch (HES) are the colloids primarily used in clinical practice in the United States. Human albumin solutions are heat-sterilized

**Table 159.2 Intravenous Fluid Composition and Distribution**

| | *Electrolytes (mEq/L)* | | | | | | | | | *Distribution* | |
|---|---|---|---|---|---|---|---|---|---|---|---|
| **SOLUTION** | **Na** | **K** | **Ca** | **Mg** | **Cl** | **$HCO_2$** | **LACTATE** | **mOsm/L** | **pH** | **ECF (%)** | **ICF (%)** |
| **Crystalloid** | | | | | | | | | | | |
| NS (0.9%) | 154 | | | | 154 | | | 308 | 5 | 100 | |
| LR | 130 | 4 | 2.7 | | 109 | | 28 | 273 | 6.5 | | |
| 1 L water with 3 ampules $HCO_3$ (150 mEq) | 130 | | | | | 130 | | | | | |
| 3% NaCl | 513 | | | | 513 | | | 1027 | 5 | | |
| 7.5% NaCl | | | | | | | | 2400 | | | |
| 0.45% NaCl | 77 | | | | 77 | | | 154 | 5 | 67 | 33 |
| 0.20% NaCl | 34 | | | | 34 | | | 77 | 5 | | |
| $D_5W$ | | | | | | | | 278 | 4 | 33 | 67 |
| **Colloid** | | | | | | | | | | | |
| Hextend | 143 | 3 | 5 | 1 | 124 | | 28 | 307 | 5.9 | | |
| Hespan | 154 | | | | 154 | | | 310 | 5.5 | | |
| Human albumin 5% | 145 | | | | 95 | | | 300 | | | |

*$D_5W$*, 5% Dextrose in water; *LR*, lactated Ringer solution; *NS*, normal saline.

derivatives of donor plasma. Isotonic 5% albumin is recommended for resuscitation of patients with severe hypoalbuminemia and end-stage liver disease, but there is little outcome evidence to support this position.[21,26,27] HES, a semisynthetic polymerized amylopectin compound, has supplanted dextran and gelatin-based colloids. A 6% solution provides volume expansion equivalent to that of 5% albumin. The renal dysfunction and coagulopathy that complicated early-generation synthetic colloids do not appear to be clinically significant with new-generation HES solutions.

### *Hypertonic Solutions*

HYPERONCOTIC ALBUMIN Infusions of hyperoncotic albumin (20% to 25%) result in vascular expansion greater than two times the volume administered. Besides the obvious benefits of small-volume resuscitation, improved portability, and more rapid hemodynamic stabilization, hyperoncotic albumin has additional advantages. Synergistic interaction with administered drugs and primary antioxidant effects are explanations hypothesized for the improved morbidity linked to hyperoncotic albumin administrated to patients with complicated hypoalbuminemic states.[27] End-stage liver disease is one important example in which hyperoncotic albumin attenuates renal dysfunction and death in patients with spontaneous bacterial peritonitis or those undergoing large-volume paracentesis.[28-30]

HYPERTONIC SALINE Hypertonic sodium solutions rapidly expand intravascular volume by mobilizing water from the interstitial and intracellular spaces. A small infusion expands plasma several times the volume infused. Used alone, the hemodynamic impact of hypertonic crystalloid is transient. Hypertonic crystalloid is often used in combination with hyperoncotic colloid (6% dextran or 10% HES) to sustain vascular expansion. Animal resuscitation models have demonstrated additional benefits, including enhanced cardiac output, improved microcirculatory flow, and attenuated inflammatory response. Hypertonic saline is safe, but data are insufficient to conclude that it is better than isotonic crystalloid for the resuscitation of patient with burns, trauma, or sepsis.[31] Severely traumatized patients with associated traumatic brain injury remain an exceptional use for hypertonic saline, but outcome evidence is mixed.[32,33]

## SPECIAL TREATMENT CONSIDERATIONS

### *Minimal-Volume Resuscitation of Hemorrhagic Shock*

Traditional resuscitation of hemorrhagic shock prioritized rapid restoration of circulating blood volume with crystalloid and blood products. Strategic limited-volume resuscitation for uncontrolled hemorrhage dates back to the early 1900s and reemerged in the 1980s.

The rationale is that the increased intravascular pressure and hemodilution resulting from aggressive fluid resuscitation compounds the blood loss by precipitating rebleeding from hemostatic sites. Animal models of uncontrolled hemorrhage reveal that aggressive fluid administration reduces oxygen delivery and results in higher mortality. The widely recognized Houston experience showed a mortality benefit in penetrating trauma victims, but the results have yet to be matched by other investigators.[34,35] In this strategy, hypotensive patients with a source of uncontrolled life-threatening hemorrhage receive IV fluids titrated to sustain critical organ flow until definitive surgical control is achieved (see Box 159.3). Conventional resuscitation ensues once surgical hemostasis is achieved.

The degree and duration of permissive hypotension remain to be clarified, although current recommendations target a systolic blood pressure of 70 mm Hg. Patients with concomitant traumatic brain injury are not candidates for this strategy.

## BURN RESUSCITATION

Patients with partial-thickness and full-thickness burns exhibit marked fluid shifts related to denuded skin, injured tissue, and the systemic inflammatory response. Early anticipation of these large fluid requirements prevents underresuscitation. The Parkland formula remains the most commonly used guide for acute burn resuscitation. Formula calculations are based on the time of injury rather than the time until medical attention and incorporate prehospital fluid administration. All burn formulas provide only estimates of fluid requirements. The requirements must be modified and individualized based on patient response because volume needs may substantially exceed formula approximation.[36] LR solution is the resuscitation crystalloid preparation of choice for acute burn management. In addition to burn formula replacement, maintenance fluid requirements should be allocated. Urine output greater than 1 mL/kg/hr is a traditional end point of acute burn resuscitation and may be augmented by the perfusion end points discussed earlier.

### *Oral Rehydration Therapy*

Oral rehydration therapy is a valuable tool for maintenance and correction of mild to moderate dehydration secondary to gastroenteritis in children and adults. It remains underused in the United States despite worldwide success, guideline support, and evidence from controlled trials.[37] When used as per published guidelines, oral rehydration therapy is comparable with IV therapy, but with reduced hospitalization and improved safety and expense. Small aliquots of fluid (as low as 5 mL, depending on patient size and tolerance) are administered by bottle, spoon, syringe, or nasogastric tube at regular 2- to 5-minute intervals to meet deficit and maintenance goals. After patient and family education, appropriate fluid selection is the most important factor in successful oral rehydration therapy.

Many common household fluids, including fruit juice, sport drinks, carbonated beverages, and soups, contain poorly tolerated concentrations of sugar and salt. Commercial (e.g., Rehydralyte, Pedialyte) and reconstituted liquids (oral rehydration salts or home recipe) are balanced, low-carbohydrate enteral solutions. One recipe for an oral rehydration solution containing home ingredients consists of 1 L of water, 8 teaspoons of sugar, and 1 teaspoon of salt.

### *Maintenance Fluid Therapy*

The goal of maintenance fluid therapy is normal body fluid composition and volume. Fluid orders anticipate daily fluid requirements, ongoing losses, and coexisting electrolyte abnormalities. Though often ordered concurrently, the estimated physiologic fluid (true maintenance) should be consciously distinguished from therapy aimed to replace an existing fluid deficit.

**Table 159.3** Pediatric Maintenance Fluid Estimate Formulas*

| BODY WEIGHT | DAILY MAINTENANCE (mL/DAY) | HOURLY MAINTENANCE (mL/HR) |
|---|---|---|
| 1-10 kg | 100 mL/kg | 5 mL/kg |
| 10-20 kg | 1000 mL plus 50 mL/kg | 40mL plus 2 mL/kg |
| 20-80 kg | 1500 mL plus 20 mL/kg† | 60mL plus 1 mL/kg† |

*Note that the following two formulas calculate disparate rates. The difference between these calculated rates is clinically insignificant. Sodium and chloride—2 to 3 mEq per 100 mL water; potassium—1 to 2 mEq per 100 mL water. $D_5$NS with 20 mEq KCl is a common maintenance solution for most euvolemic pediatric patients and provides 20% of the daily calories at a routine maintenance rate. Comorbid conditions or electrolyte abnormalities may require modification.

†To a maximum of 2400 mL/day or 100 mL/hr.

Routine water and electrolyte maintenance is based on normal energy expenditure, sensible loss from urine and stool, and insensible loss from the respiratory tract and skin. Calculations assume euvolemia and are adjusted for body mass. The greater per-kilogram fluid requirements in children are proportionate to their TBW and metabolism (**Table 159.3**).

All maintenance prescriptions should be individualized—energy expenditure, fluid losses, and electrolyte status vary with disease and dictate the rate and electrolyte modifications. For example, exfoliative skin disease, increased work of breathing, and fever enhance insensible loss. Measurable nasogastric, fistula, ostomy, and urinary drainage can be estimated and replaced per drained volume. Limitation of fluid and potassium is an important disease-specific modification for patients with renal insufficiency.

Hypotonic solutions (e.g., 0.45% and 0.2% sodium chloride) with or without dextrose and potassium are popular fixed-combination maintenance solutions. Hospitalized patients often suffer impaired free water excretion because of nonosmotic release of antidiuretic hormone, which makes them vulnerable to hyponatremia. The serum sodium concentration provides a simple and accurate marker of hydration status. Isotonic maintenance solutions should be considered in all patients (including children), especially those with a serum sodium concentration of less than 138 mEq/L.[38-40] Glucose infusions are best formulated by adding dextrose to an electrolyte solution (e.g., LR solution, 0.45% or 0.9% normal saline) rather than using 5% dextrose in water, which behaves as electrolyte-free water on sugar metabolism.

## REFERENCES

*References can be found on Expert Consult @ www.expertconsult.com.*

# Acid-Base Disorders 160

*Matthew T. Robinson and Alan C. Heffner*

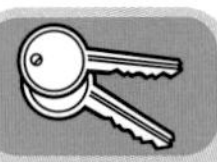

**KEY POINTS**

- Normal pH or serum bicarbonate values can mask an important, underlying acidosis in the setting of a mixed disorder.
- An elevated anion gap is a sign of metabolic acidosis and should be calculated on each chemistry sample.
- Arterial and venous blood gas sampling is a useful emergency department test because of the strong association between arterial and venous $HCO_3^-$ and pH.
- Correlation between venous $PCO_2$ and arterial $PCO_2$ is lacking, although venous $PCO_2$ levels may be used as a screening tool for hypercapnia.
- Admission lactate level and standard base excess are markers of illness severity that correlate with patient morbidity and mortality in the hospital.
- The urine ketone dipstick test is highly sensitive for serum ketosis.
- Venous and arterial lactate samples are equivalent.
- Indiscriminate use of sodium bicarbonate for the treatment of undifferentiated metabolic acidosis should be avoided.

## PATHOPHYSIOLOGY

### REGULATION OF ACID-BASE BALANCE

The normal hydrogen ion ($H^+$) concentration in serum is approximately 40 nanoequivalents per liter. This is approximately 1/1,000,000 the concentration of the other major serum ions, but the small size and high charge density of protons make them highly reactive and capable of inducing conformational and functional changes in body proteins. Rigid control of the free $H^+$ concentration is therefore essential to life.

Daily metabolism produces an acid load of 150 mmol of nonvolatile (fixed) acid and 12,000 mmol of volatile acid ($CO_2$). Physiologic, pathologic, and dysregulated endogenous production, as well as externally administered product, can all increase the systemic acid load.

Maintenance of systemic homeostasis in the setting of acid-base changes occurs via three main mechanisms:

1. Chemical buffering
2. Alterations in alveolar ventilation
3. Alterations in renal $H^+$ excretion

#### *Chemical Buffering*

Extracellular buffers, including plasma proteins, phosphates, and bicarbonate, are the earliest defense against acidosis. The most prominent extracellular buffer is bicarbonate, which is highly abundant and acts as a dynamic buffer by independently regulating $PCO_2$ through changes in alveolar ventilation. This feature increases buffering capacity by more than 10-fold. Buffering also occurs within the intracellular compartment but is delayed as $H^+$ equilibrates over a period of hours. Intracellular buffers, including bone, inorganic phosphates, proteins, and hemoglobin, are eventually responsible for more than 50% of the overall chemical buffering capacity.

#### *Alterations in Alveolar Ventilation*

Alterations in alveolar ventilation provide compensation for acute acid-base disturbances. According to the Henderson-Hasselbalch equation, serum pH can be determined as follows:

$$pH = 6.1 + pK_a + \log[HCO_3^-]/0.03\,(PCO_2)$$

Stimulation of peripheral chemoreceptors triggers changes in ventilation within minutes. By altering $PCO_2$ through variations in minute ventilation, the $HCO_3^-/PCO_2$ ratio remains relatively constant, and alterations in pH are thereby mitigated. The effectiveness of the ventilatory response is acutely limited by differences in the solubility of $CO_2$ and $H^+$ within the central nervous system (CNS). The hyperventilation induced by systemic acidosis is incomplete as a result of local alkalosis sensed by the central chemoreceptors as $CO_2$ diffuses more rapidly across the blood-brain barrier.

#### *Alterations in Renal Hydrogen Ion Excretion*

Because of the inability of $HCO_3^-$ to effectively buffer $H_2CO_3$ produced through acute $CO_2$ retention as described, renal compensation is centrally important in the response to primary respiratory disorders. Renal compensatory mechanisms include enhanced proton excretion and increased $HCO_3^-$ resorption. Renal compensation for acute acid-base disorders begins immediately; however, the full effect is not appreciated for 5 or 6 days.

#### *Nomenclature*

The normal range of serum pH is 7.38 to 7.42. Acidemia is defined by serum pH below 7.38. Likewise, alkalemia is defined by serum pH above 7.42. These terms describe the absolute directional change of measured pH but say nothing about the processes that alter pH from normal. The processes that alter pH are termed *acidosis* and *alkalosis*.

Acid-base disorders are often complex—pH may be normal in the setting of an obvious acid-base disorder because of the presence of a second or even a third coexisting acid-base process. For example, patients with a mixed disorder may have a normal or alkalemic pH during ketoacidosis if a concomitant alkalosis (metabolic or respiratory) is also present. It is therefore important to note that a normal pH does not exclude an important acid-base disorder.

## DIAGNOSTIC INTERPRETATION

Primary acid-base processes are divided into respiratory or metabolic disorders by examining $PCO_2$ and serum bicarbonate. Primary elevations in $PCO_2$ signify respiratory acidosis, whereas decreased serum bicarbonate identifies metabolic acidosis. Diagnostic assessment of acid-base disorders requires accurate measurement of these plasma variables, in addition to calculated values, to unmask mixed disorders. Coupling the clinical history and physical assessment with these values reveals important clues about the causative illness.

Serum testing includes direct evaluation of pH, $PCO_2$, and $HCO_3^-$ through arterial and venous blood sampling; calculation of the anion gap from serum chemistries; and additional measures (e.g., the standard base excess) in an attempt to quantify the metabolic component of acid-base disorders (see the "Facts and Formulas" box for basic formulas used in this chapter).

$SI = \frac{SV}{BSA}$ **FACTS AND FORMULAS**

pH = 6.1 + Log[$HCO_3^-$]/0.03 × $PCO_2$

Anion gap = Unmeasured anions − Unmeasured cations = $Na^+$ − [$Cl^-$ + $HCO_3^-$]

Delta gap = Δ Anion gap − Δ $HCO_3$ = [Calculated anion gap − 10] − [24 − Measured serum $HCO_3$]

Calculated Sosm (mOsm/kg) = 2 ($Na^+$) + BUN/2.8 + Glucose/18 + Ethanol/4.8

Osmolal gap = Measured Sosm − Calculated Sosm

**Correction Formulas**

Corrected anion gap = Anion gap + 2.5 (Normal albumin − Measured albumin)

**Compensation Formulas**

Metabolic acidosis: $PCO_2$ = 1.5 ($HCO_3^-$) + 8

Metabolic alkalosis: Increase in $PCO_2$ = 0.6 × Increase in $HCO_3^-$

Respiratory acidosis

- Acute: [$HCO_3^-$] increases by 1 mEq/L for each 10–mm Hg increase in $PCO_2$
- Chronic: [$HCO_3^-$] increases by 4 mEq/L for each 10–mm Hg increase in $PCO_2$

Respiratory alkalosis

- Acute: [$HCO_3^-$] decreases by 2 mEq/L for each 10–mm Hg decrease in $PCO_2$
- Chronic: [$HCO_3^-$] decreases by 5 mEq/L for each 10–mm Hg decrease in $PCO_2$

*BUN*, Blood urea nitrogen; *Sosm*, serum osmolarity.

## ARTERIAL AND VENOUS BLOOD GASES

The ability to substitute venous blood gas samples for arterial samples is appealing because of the pain, difficulty, and complications associated with arterial sampling. Arterial pH and venous pH vary by less 0.04 in most situations.[1-3] Patients in clinical shock are an important exception, however, because arteriovenous $PCO_2$ (and therefore pH) can vary significantly.

Despite incomplete correlation between venous and arterial $PCO_2$, venous $PCO_2$ may be used to screen for arterial hypercapnia. In hemodynamically normal patients, $PCO_2$ higher than 45 mm Hg is sensitive (but less than 50% specific) for the detection of arterial hypercapnia, which is defined as $PCO_2$ higher than 50 mm Hg. Venous blood gas screening led to a 29% reduction in arterial sampling in one study.[4] Finally, arterial blood gas analysis enables precise interpretation of respiratory compensation when needed.

### *Standard Base Excess*

Although the serum bicarbonate level may describe an acid-base disorder, the amount of acid or base added to the system cannot be calculated unless $PCO_2$ is held constant. The concept of the standard base excess (SBE) was introduced to address this problem and is defined as the quantity of strong acid or base required to restore plasma pH to 7.40 when $PCO_2$ is held constant at 40 mm Hg. A negative value indicates excess acid, whereas a positive value indicates excess base.

SBE has been studied extensively as a resuscitation end point in trauma and as a marker of tissue acidosis. Preresuscitation base excess values are reliably linked to the degree of tissue acidosis and serve as independent predictors of mortality in critically ill patients. Base excess has been shown to correlate with hypovolemia, length of hospital stay, and transfusion requirements, whereas the rate of normalization correlates with patient survival.[5,6]

### *Lactate*

Lactic acid is generated through the reduction of pyruvate with the reduced form of nicotinamide adenine dinucleotide (NADH) as follows:

$$\text{Pyruvate} + \text{NADH} \rightleftharpoons \text{Lactate} + \text{NAD}^+$$

Lactate is produced by skeletal muscle, brain, intestines, and kidneys, with normal blood lactate levels maintained below 2 mmol/L and the threshold for lactic acidosis defined by a serum level higher than 4 mmol/L.

Arterial lactate sampling is considered the most reliable measure for detecting hyperlactatemia; however, venous and capillary sampling is also used. Central venous sampling is highly correlated with arterial lactate measurements. Peripheral venous samples are sufficient to screen for hyperlactatemia but retain poor specificity (57%) when compared with arterial samples.[7] Elevations in venous lactate should be confirmed with arterial sampling.

## ANION GAP

Within serum, the requirement for electroneutrality dictates that the net serum cation charge equal the net total anion charge. The calculated difference in commonly measured serum ions is termed the anion gap (AG). It is important to note that the AG represents anions that are present but unmeasured (at least historically) and that an AG is present during health. Fortunately, the difference between unmeasured anions and unmeasured cations may change (increased or decreased AG) and therefore provide a clue to disease states (**Box 160.1**).

The greatest utility of the AG is identification and discrimination of metabolic acidosis. The potential for a mixed acid-base disturbance to mask acidosis by normalizing pH and serum bicarbonate highlights the importance of calculating the AG on every chemistry sample. An increased AG almost always signifies a process causing a "wide-gap" metabolic acidosis. Furthermore, calculation of the AG assists in discriminating the cause of undifferentiated metabolic acidosis (e.g., AG versus non-AG processes carry different differential diagnoses).

When acids are added to the system, bicarbonate is replaced by the acid anion (X) as follows:

$$HX + NaHCO_3 \rightarrow NaX + H_2O + CO_2$$

Titration and replacement of bicarbonate by unmeasured organic acid produce a relative equimolar elevation in the AG.

In contrast, bicarbonate loss (or addition of protons) can occur in the absence of an endogenous or exogenous anion contribution.

$$HCl + NaHCO_3 \rightarrow NaCl + H_2CO_3 \rightarrow CO_2 + H_2O$$

Hyperchloremia maintains electroneutrality without altering the AG. Gastrointestinal and renal losses are the most common causes of non-AG metabolic acidosis (**Box 160.2**).

**BOX 160.1 Causes of Measured Changes in the Anion Gap**

**Increased Anion Gap**

Increased unmeasured anions
- Organic acids: lactate, ketones, phosphate, sulfate
- Toxins and metabolites: formate (methanol), oxalate (ethylene glycol), salicylates
- Severe volume depletion (hyperalbuminemia)
- IgA paraproteinemia

Decreased unmeasured cations
- Calcium, magnesium, potassium
- Laboratory error
- Metabolic alkalosis
- Respiratory alkalosis

**Decreased Anion Gap**

Laboratory error
- Overestimation of chloride or bicarbonate
- Underestimation of sodium
- Bromide intoxication (overestimation of chloride)
- Iodine intoxication (overestimation of chloride)

Decreased unmeasured anions
- Hypoalbuminemia

Increased unmeasured cations
- Lithium
- Paraproteins (myeloma)
- Bromide intoxication
- Hypermagnesemia
- Hypercalcemia
- Hyperlipidemia
- IgG gammopathy
- Polymyxin B

The historical range for the AG was $12 \pm 4$ (8 to 16 mEq/L). With the adoption of ion-specific electrodes, chloride is measured at a higher concentration such that the currently accepted range of AG is $7 \pm 3$ (4 to 10 mEq/L). More importantly, the AG must be corrected for individual patients. Albumin accounts for 80% of the AG in health. Consequently, large and important deviations may occur if serum albumin is assumed to be normal. AG is thus commonly corrected for serum albumin to improve sensitivity of the AG as a screening tool.[8] The correction factor is calculated as follows:

$$\text{Corrected AG} = \text{Calculated AG} + 2.5\,[\text{Normal} - \text{Measured albumin (g/dL)}]$$

### *Delta-Delta Calculation*

The AG is also useful for investigating the presence of mixed metabolic disturbances. In simple AG acidosis, bicarbonate is presumably titrated in a one-to-one fashion by organic acid such that the following relationship is noted:

$$\text{Increase in AG} = \text{Decrease in } HCO_3^-$$

The difference between the change in the AG and the change in serum bicarbonate is called the delta gap, or delta-delta calculation. Deviations from this stoichiometric relationship indicate a mixed metabolic disturbance. When the change (delta) in the AG is greater than the change in bicarbonate, a preexisting or concomitant metabolic alkalosis is present. Alternatively, a change in AG less than the change in bicarbonate identifies a coexisting non-AG acidosis. A delta gap higher than 6 is generally considered significant.[9]

### *Serum Osmolar Gap*

Osmolarity is defined as the number of particles within a volume of fluid (mmol/L), and osmolality is defined as the number of particles in a mass of fluid (mmol/kg). The terms are used interchangeably because the density of water is 1 kg/L. The size of the particle contributing to serum osmolality (Sosm) is unimportant; that is, small ions contribute equally with large proteins.

Sosm is elevated in the presence of osmotically active particles such as alcohols, glycols, and sugars. The difference in measured and calculated Sosm is termed the osmolar gap. An elevated osmolar gap confirms the presence of unmeasured osmotically active particles, which may be helpful

**BOX 160.2 Causes of Non–Anion Gap Metabolic Acidosis**

**Gastrointestinal $HCO_3^-$ Loss**

Diarrhea

**Renal $HCO_3^-$ Loss**

Renal tubular acidosis (types 1, 2, and 4)
Hyperaldosteronism
Renal failure

**Ingestions**

Ammonium chloride
Hyperalimentation

**Other**

Treatment phases of ketoacidosis

when investigating the cause of unexplained AG acidosis. Osmolar gaps greater than 10 mOsm/kg are considered abnormal and may reflect the presence of a toxic alcohol as the source of the acidosis. However, delayed evaluation after the ingestion of toxic alcohol will show little to no elevation in the osmolar gap as a result of metabolism of the offending alcohol. Likewise, normal osmolar gap values are imprecisely defined, with ranges of −13 to +14.0 mOsm/kg noted in healthy patients.[10,11] This wide variation in the normal range may lead to a normal osmolar gap in the presence of a significant ingestion.

### *Evaluation of Mixed Acid-Base Disorders*

By applying the formulas for AG, delta gap, and expected physiologic compensation, a stepwise approach to the evaluation of simple and mixed acid-base problems can be developed.[12] This process is summarized in **Box 160.3**.

Additionally the clinical history is centrally important for proper interpretation of acid-base disorders (**Box 160.4**).

**BOX 160.3 Five-Step Approach to Acid-Base Disorders**

**Rule 1: Determine the pH status (alkalemia or acidemia: >7.44 or <7.40)**

**Rule 2: Determine whether the primary process is respiratory, metabolic, or both**

- Alkalemia
- Respiratory alkalosis: if $P_{CO_2}$ substantially <40 mm Hg
- Metabolic alkalosis: if $HCO_3^-$ >25 mEq/L
- Acidemia
- Respiratory acidosis: if $P_{CO_2}$ >44 mm Hg
- Metabolic acidosis: if $HCO_3^-$ <25 mEq/L

**Rule 3: Calculate the anion gap***

- Anion gap = $Na^+ + (Cl^- + HCO_3^-)$
- Increased anion gap (>10 mEq/L) may indicate metabolic acidosis
- Increased anion gap (>20 mEq/L) always indicates metabolic acidosis

**Rule 4: Check the degree of compensation**

- Metabolic acidosis: $P_{CO_2} = 1.5\,[HCO_3^-] + 8$
- Metabolic alkalosis: increase in $P_{CO_2}$ = 0.6 increase in bicarbonate
- Respiratory acidosis
  - Acute: $[HCO_3^-]$ increases by 1 mEq/L for each 10–mm Hg increase in $P_{CO_2}$
  - Chronic: $[HCO_3^-]$ increases by 4 mEq/L for each 10–mm Hg increase in $P_{CO_2}$
- Respiratory alkalosis
  - Acute: $[HCO_3^-]$ decreases by 2 mEq/L for each 10–mm Hg decrease in $P_{CO_2}$
  - Chronic: $[HCO_3^-]$ decreases by 5 mEq/L for each 10–mm Hg decrease in $P_{CO_2}$

**Rule 5: Determine whether there is a 1:1 relationship between the change in the anion gap and the change in serum bicarbonate**

- Each 1-point increase in the anion gap should be accompanied by a 1-mEq/L decrease in bicarbonate
- If bicarbonate is higher than predicted, a metabolic alkalosis is also present
- If bicarbonate is lower than predicted, a non–anion gap metabolic acidosis is present

Modified from Whittier WL, Rutecki GW. Primer on clinical acid-base problem solving. Dis Mon 2004;50:122-62.

*For every 1 g/dL that albumin is less than normal (4.2 g/dL), add 2.5 to the calculated anion gap.

## SPECIFIC ACID-BASE DISORDERS

### RESPIRATORY ACIDOSIS

Normal ventilatory control is regulated through central receptors that respond to elevated $P_{CO_2}$ and through peripheral chemoreceptors in the carotid bodies that respond to hypoxia. Because the ventilatory response to hypercapnia is much stronger than that to hypoxemia, only minor elevations in $P_{CO_2}$ are required to increase minute ventilation. As a result of this vigorous response and the ability to significantly increase minute ventilation, respiratory acidosis almost always develops as a consequence of impaired alveolar ventilation and not from increased production of $CO_2$.

Elevated $P_{CO_2}$ causes a decrease in arterial pH and a variable, acute increase in plasma $HCO_3^-$ as a result of shifts in equilibrium reactions and a similar, but chronic increase as a result of renal compensation through enhanced $H^+$ excretion and $HCO_3^-$ retention. $CO_2$ functions as a volatile acid:

$$H^+ + HCO_3^- \rightarrow H_2CO_3 + H_2O + CO_2$$

Under normal conditions, this acid load is immediately buffered by intracellular and extracellular nonbicarbonate buffers. The acute rise in $P_{CO_2}$ elicits a similar elevation in $HCO_3^-$ through a highly predictable relationship:

$[HCO_3^-]$ increases by 1 mEq/L for each 10–mm Hg increase in $P_{CO_2}$

In chronic respiratory acidosis, elevations in $P_{CO_2}$ are partially protective, with larger amounts of $CO_2$ able to be excreted at lower minute ventilation. The system also adapts to chronically elevated $CO_2$ by enhancing renal $H^+$ excretion and $HCO_3^-$ retention, thereby attenuating the ventilatory response to hypercapnia. The result of chronic respiratory acidosis is that the ventilatory drive becomes dependent on a hypoxic stimulus.

The renal compensatory response in patients with chronic respiratory acidosis requires 3 to 5 days to develop and may be predicted by the following equation:

$[HCO_3^-]$ increases by 4 mEq/L for each 10–mm Hg increase in $P_{CO_2}$

### RESPIRATORY ALKALOSIS

Respiratory alkalosis is produced through alveolar hyperventilation and results in a decrease in arterial $P_{CO_2}$ and an increase in arterial pH. Plasma $HCO_3^-$ is variably decreased, acutely because of shifts in equilibrium and later because of renal $HCO_3^-$ wasting. The decreased $P_{CO_2}$ causes a decreased volatile acid load with secondary release of $H^+$ from nonbicarbonate buffers (Buf) as follows:

**BOX 160.4 Acid-Base Interpretation Based on Clinical History**

**Case 1**

A 65-year-old man with a history of chronic obstructive pulmonary disease has a fever, increased shortness of breath, cough, and sputum production. The following arterial blood gas and serum $HCO_3^-$ values are obtained:

- pH = 7.27
- $P_{CO_2}$ = 65 mm Hg
- $HCO_3^-$ = 29 mEq/L
- $P_{O_2}$ = 70 mm Hg

Review shows decreased pH and elevated $P_{CO_2}$, indicative of respiratory acidosis. The chronicity of the acidosis can be evaluated by calculating the expected metabolic compensation:

- Acute: $[HCO_3^-]$ increases by 1 mEq/L for each 10–mm Hg in $P_{CO_2}$
- Expected $HCO_3^-$ = 24 + 2.5 = 26.5
- Chronic: $[HCO_3^-]$ increases by 4 mEq/L for each 10–mm Hg in $P_{CO_2}$
- Expected $HCO_3^-$ = 24 + 10 = 34

Comparing these values with the measured $HCO_3^-$ reveals that $HCO_3^-$ falls between the two calculated levels. Based on the history, the clinical diagnosis is acute on chronic respiratory acidosis.

**Case 2**

A 65-year-old man with a history of chronic obstructive pulmonary disease has had diarrhea for 1 week and his baseline $P_{CO_2}$ is 65 mm Hg.

Based on his history, the patient's $HCO_3^-$ is lower than predicted, which represents acute metabolic acidosis in the presence of chronic respiratory acidosis.

**Case 3**

A 65-year-old man being treated long-term with diuretic therapy has an acute exacerbation of asthma.

His history indicates acute respiratory acidosis with an expected $P_{CO_2}$ of 26.5 mm Hg. The elevated serum $HCO_3^-$ indicates acute respiratory acidosis with concomitant metabolic alkalosis.

The renal compensatory response in chronic respiratory acidosis requires 3 to 5 days to develop and may be predicted by the following equation:

- $[HCO_3^-]$ increases by 4 mEq/L for each 10–mm Hg increase in $P_{CO_2}$

$$HCO_3^- + HBuf \rightarrow H_2CO_3 + Buf \rightarrow CO_2 + H_2O$$

The expected $[HCO_3^-]$ can be calculated from the following equation:

$[HCO_3^-]$ decreases by 2 mEq/L for each 10–mm Hg decrease in $P_{CO_2}$

In chronic respiratory alkalosis, renal adaptive mechanisms result in diminished $H^+$ secretion and enhanced $HCO_3^-$ excretion. This combined response begins within hours and is completed within 2 to 3 days. The expected response may be calculated as follows:

**BOX 160.5 Diabetic Patient with Mixed Acid-Base Disorder**

A 26-year-old woman with a history of diabetes mellitus is vomiting and has had generalized malaise for the past 3 days.

Laboratory evaluation shows the following:

- $Na^+$ = 134; $K^+$ = 4.6; $Cl^-$ = 94; $HCO_3^-$ = 20 mEq/L; pH = 7.38; $P_{CO_2}$ = 35 mm Hg

Step 1: Arterial blood gas analysis shows that the patient is minimally acidemic

Step 2: Serum bicarbonate is less than 25 mEq/L, indicative of metabolic acidosis

Step 3: The anion gap is elevated: 134 – 94 – 20 = 20

Step 4: Respiratory compensation is appropriate: 1.5 $[HCO_3^-]$ + 8 = [1.5 × 20] + 8 = 38 mm Hg

Step 5: Calculation of the delta gap reveals that the change in $HCO_3^-$ (24 – 20 = 4 units) is significantly less than the change in anion gap (20 – 10 = 10 units). This indicates the presence of a concomitant metabolic alkalosis that is masking the significant anion gap acidosis. These findings are explained by vomiting-induced alkalosis in a patient with diabetic ketoacidosis

$[HCO_3^-]$ decreases by 5 mEq/L for each 10–mm Hg decrease in $P_{CO_2}$

Ventilation is primarily controlled through peripheral, central, and pulmonary mechanical receptors. Peripheral chemoreceptors respond to changes in $P_{CO_2}$ and $O_2$, so it is not surprising that many cases of hyperventilation stem from hypoxemia.

## METABOLIC ACIDOSIS

Metabolic acidosis is induced by the addition of $H^+$ ions or by the loss of $HCO_3^-$. Addition of $H^+$ may occur as a result of exogenous administration or endogenous production of acids associated with pathologic states. Loss of bicarbonate occurs primarily through gastrointestinal or renal wasting, with acidosis being produced by driving the equilibrium reaction to the left:

$$H^+ + HCO_3^- \rightleftharpoons H_2CO_3 \rightleftharpoons CO_2 + H_2O$$

As discussed previously, the initial response to acidosis is extracellular and intracellular buffering, combined with respiratory compensation via increased alveolar ventilation. These protective mechanisms attempt to minimize free $H^+$ within the system until a full renal response excretes the excess acid load.

It is important to remember that compensatory responses do not fully normalize pH. If a normal pH is seen in a patient with metabolic acidosis, a second acid-base disorder must be present. The typical laboratory pattern of metabolic acidosis is decreased pH and bicarbonate with a compensatory decrease in $P_{CO_2}$ (**Box 160.5**).

Enhanced alveolar ventilation is triggered through pH-mediated stimulation of peripheral chemoreceptors. Minute

**BOX 160.6 Metabolic Acidosis with Inadequate Respiratory Compensation**

A 68-year-old woman exhibits dyspnea and coughing.

**Vital Signs:**

Blood pressure, 100/50; heart rate, 120 beats/min; temperature, 101.3° F

**Laboratory Data:**

$Na^+$ = 142; $Cl^-$ = 106; $HCO_3^-$ = 6 mEq/L; lactate = 8.8 mEq/L; pH = 7.08; $P_{CO_2}$ = 24 mm Hg; $P_{O_2}$ = 70 mm Hg

Review of the laboratory test results reveals an anion gap acidosis. Calculation of the expected respiratory compensation is as follows:

$$\text{Expected } HCO_3^- = 1.5\,[HCO_3^-] + 8 = 1.5(6) + 8 = 17$$

The expected $P_{CO_2}$ is lower than the actual $P_{CO_2}$, which is producing a relative respiratory acidosis and indicating a need for ventilatory assistance

**BOX 160.7 Four-Year-Old Boy with Diarrhea for 5 Days**

Physical examination reveals dry mucous membranes.

**Vital Signs:**

Blood pressure, 80/50; heart rate, 170 beats/min; temperature, 99.1° F; respiratory rate, 44 breaths/min

**Laboratory Data:**

$Na^+$ = 134; $K^+$ = 4.8; $Cl^-$ = 114; $HCO_3^-$ = 3; pH = 6.98; $P_{CO_2}$ = 13 mm Hg; $P_{O_2}$ = 110 mm Hg

Step 1: The patient is found to be acidemic on examination of arterial blood gases

Step 2: Serum bicarbonate is less than 25 mEq, indicative of the presence of metabolic acidosis

Step 3: The anion gap is elevated: 134 – 116 – 3 = 15

Step 4: Respiratory compensation is appropriate: 1.5 × $[HCO_3^-]$ + 8 = [1.5 × 3] + 8 = 12.5

Step 5: Calculation of the delta gap reveals that the change in $HCO_3^-$ (24 – 3 = 21 units) is significantly greater than that the change in anion gap (15 – 10 = 5 units). This indicates the presence of a concomitant non–anion gap acidosis that is overshadowing the anion gap acidosis. The mixed acidosis can be clinically explained by the presence of diarrhea (non–anion gap acidosis) with dehydration (anion gap acidosis)

ventilation is augmented via increased tidal volume (hyperpnea) and later followed by an increased respiratory rate (tachypnea), depending on the degree of acidosis. The expected $P_{CO_2}$ is calculated by the following equation:

$$P_{CO_2} = 1.5 \times (HCO_3^-) + 8 \pm 2$$

This equation assesses the adequacy of respiratory compensation. A $P_{CO_2}$ that is significantly higher or lower than this calculated value signals the presence of a secondary respiratory acidosis or alkalosis, which may have a profound impact on treatment decisions (**Box 160.6**).

This protective effect lasts only a few days, however, because the chronically diminished $P_{CO_2}$ paradoxically signals renal bicarbonate wasting. The final effect is that arterial pH in chronic metabolic acidosis is the same, with or without respiratory compensation.

Causes of metabolic acidosis are classified according to the presence or absence of an elevated AG. However, even in the absence of an AG, there may be accumulation of unmeasured anions.

Non-AG acidoses are those that add HCl to the system. The acid anion in these cases is chloride; because of its inclusion in the AG equation, no change in the gap is noted. The most common causes of non-AG acidosis include renal and gastrointestinal bicarbonate wasting (**Box 160.7**).

## METABOLIC ALKALOSIS

Metabolic alkalosis is characterized by the net gain of base equivalent, as reflected by elevated plasma bicarbonate. Direct proton loss from extracellular fluid produces an elevation in serum bicarbonate by shifting the following equilibrium reaction to the right:

$$H_2CO_3 \rightarrow H^+ + HCO_3^-$$

The elevated plasma pH produces compensatory hypoventilation to increase $P_{CO_2}$. Because serum pH is determined by the ratio of $HCO_3^-$ to $P_{CO_2}$ and not by the absolute $HCO_3^-$ level, this compensatory response acts to minimize the change in serum pH.

Metabolic alkalosis is the second most common acid-base disorder and is found in approximately one third of hospitalized patients. It can be caused by several processes: increased $H^+$ loss, typically through renal or gastrointestinal wasting; increased bicarbonate resorption; infusion or ingestion of bicarbonate; intracellular shifts in $H^+$; or contraction of extracellular fluid around a stable $HCO_3^-$ pool (**Box 160.8**).

Because of the kidneys' ability to excrete excess $HCO_3^-$, maintenance of metabolic alkalosis requires impairment of this process. The majority of the filtered bicarbonate is reclaimed in the proximal tubule, with approximately 10% of $HCO_3^-$ being reabsorbed in the distal segments. Type B cells in the cortical collecting tubule may also actively secrete excess bicarbonate. Maintenance of metabolic alkalosis requires failure of these mechanisms. This generally results from contraction of extracellular volume, which stimulates $Na^+$ retention and enhanced activity of the $Na^+$-$H^+$ antiporter in the proximal tubule.

Hyperaldosteronism induced by extracellular fluid depletion also plays a role in maintaining alkalosis by increasing $H^+$ secretion in the distal nephron through activation of $H^+$-transporting adenosine triphosphatase ($H^+$-ATPase). Hypokalemia and hyperaldosteronism maintain the alkalosis through stimulation of proximal and distal bicarbonate resorption, transcellular exchange of $K^+$ and $H^+$, and increased ammoniagenesis.

The most frequent causes of metabolic alkalosis are loss of gastric secretion and use of diuretics. Loss of gastric secretion generates an equimolar gain in $HCO_3^-$ for the lost $H^+$. Likewise, loss of gastric secretion is associated with a contracted

**BOX 160.8 Causes of Metabolic Alkalosis**

**Loss of Hydrogen**
Gastrointestinal
- Vomiting, nasogastric suction
- Antacid therapy
- Bulimia
- Chloride-losing diarrhea (villous adenoma)

Renal
- Loop and thiazide diuretics
- Mineralocorticoid excess (hyperaldosteronism, drug or medication)
- Cushing disease
- Bartter syndrome
- Gitelman syndrome
- Chronic hypercapnia
- Low chloride intake
- High-dose carbenicillin
- Hypercalcemia, milk-alkali syndrome

**Intracellular $H^+$ Shift**
Massive blood transfusion
$NaHCO_3$ administration
Milk-alkali syndrome

**Contraction Alkalosis**
Loop or thiazide diuretics
Gastric loss
Sweat loss (cystic fibrosis)

volume of extracellular fluid, which maintains alkalosis through volume depletion and hyperaldosteronism. Diuretics also induce an alkalosis through secondary hyperaldosteronism associated with hypovolemia, hypokalemia, and enhanced distal $H^+$ secretion.

The respiratory compensation for metabolic alkalosis is variable. On average, $P{CO_2}$ can be predicted as follows:

$$\text{Increase in } P{CO_2} = 0.6 \text{ increase in } HCO_3^-$$

Compensation rarely results in a $P{CO_2}$ greater than 55 mm Hg. Significant deviations from this compensatory response indicate a superimposed respiratory acidosis or alkalosis.

The signs and symptoms of alkalosis are commonly related to the associated volume contraction. Weakness, fatigue, coma, seizure, carpopedal spasm, respiratory depression, and neuromuscular irritability are observed, probably related to decreased ionized calcium as a result of alkalemia. Neuromuscular signs and symptoms are uncommon in patients with metabolic alkalosis because of the slow movement of charged $HCO_3^-$ into the CNS.

Urine chloride helps determine the cause and treatment of the metabolic alkalosis. Urine chloride levels less than 20 mEq/L indicate appropriate renal chloride avidity and imply that the source of the metabolic alkalosis is extrarenal. Accordingly, fluid and chloride repletion is the mainstay of therapy in these saline- or chloride-responsive conditions. In contrast, urine chloride levels higher than 40 mEq/L indicate renal chloride wasting and implicate altered renal function at a source of the metabolic alkalosis.

## TREATMENT

### METABOLIC ACIDOSIS

Initial treatment of metabolic acidosis includes reversing the source of the metabolic acidosis and treating with exogenous bicarbonate when indicated. A second priority is assessing the adequacy of respiratory compensation and providing ventilatory support as needed. Respiratory exhaustion with concomitant respiratory acidosis compounds the patient's dilemma.

Alkali therapy is aimed at reversing the acid-induced organ dysfunction. However, the effects of bicarbonate therapy are complex. Indiscriminate use may be more deleterious than helpful. Sodium bicarbonate infusions introduce an additional volatile acid load because bicarbonate produces $CO_2$ on reaction with water (serum):

$$\text{HBuf} + HCO_3^- \rightarrow \text{Buf}^- + H_2CO_3 \rightarrow CO_2 + H_2O$$

This additional $CO_2$ load must be excreted by the lungs to have an impact on pH. Additionally, $CO_2$ diffuses freely across cell membranes and paradoxically exacerbates intracellular and CNS acidemia. Sodium bicarbonate is associated with complications that include hypertonicity, hypernatremia, hypervolemia, increased organic acid (lactate) production, and impaired oxygen unloading.

Use of bicarbonate infusions is appropriate for bicarbonate-wasting acidoses or toxic acidosis because systemic alkalinization facilitates removal of toxin through ion trapping. However, supplemental bicarbonate in patients with organic acidoses (lactic acidosis and ketoacidosis) has not been shown to affect outcome. In these states, therapy should be aimed at addressing the underlying cause of the acidosis and promoting regeneration of bicarbonate through metabolism of the accumulated anions. In hyperchloremic acidosis, no anions exist for the regeneration of bicarbonate, and therefore infusions can promptly reverse the acidemia and restore serum bicarbonate.

When used, the goal of bicarbonate infusion is to increase pH to 7.1 to 7.2 and restore buffering capacity (>12 mEq/L $HCO_3^-$). Overzealous administration risks paradoxic alkalemia on metabolism of organ acids. The bicarbonate deficit may be calculated with the Henderson-Hasselbalch equation or by estimating the deficit at 1 mEq/kg and infusing one half the amount over a period of 20 to 30 minutes, with the remainder being infused over the next 2 to 4 hours. Bicarbonate also makes an excellent resuscitation or maintenance fluid. Isotonic bicarbonate is prepared by combining three ampules of sodium bicarbonate (50 mEq) with 1 L of sterile water, which creates an isotonic solution of 130 to 150 mEq/L $NaHCO_3$ (depending on removal of water before instillation). During this time, acid-base and volume status must be carefully monitored to avoid overshooting the pH correction.

### METABOLIC ALKALOSIS

Metabolic alkalosis is best treated by correcting the underlying cause of the alkalosis. Examination of urine chloride allows causes to be classified as saline responsive or saline resistant.

The majority of cases of metabolic alkalosis are saline responsive. Volume depletion is reversed with 0.9% normal saline. Concomitant hypokalemia is an important maintenance factor that should be reversed with potassium chloride. The total body potassium deficit may be profound and is often underappreciated.

Saline-resistant alkaloses display excessive mineralocorticoid activity, such as hyperaldosteronism, Cushing syndrome, and renal artery stenosis. Treatment of saline-resistant causes (urine chloride >20 mEq/L) is directed at the other causes of the metabolic alkalosis. Potassium deficits should be corrected by supplementation or direct antagonism of aldosterone with agents such as spironolactone. In patients with metabolic alkalosis and concomitant edematous states (e.g., congestive heart failure, cirrhosis, nephrotic syndrome), acetazolamide enables bicarbonate and volume excretion.

## REFERENCES

***References can be found on Expert Consult @ www.expertconsult.com.***

# Alcoholic Ketoacidosis 161

Christopher R. Carpenter

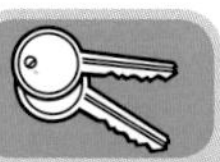

**KEY POINTS**

- Alcoholic ketoacidosis accounts for up to 20% of cases of ketoacidosis.
- The characteristic example is an alcoholic person who abruptly abstains and has signs and symptoms such as vomiting, abdominal pain, malnutrition, and an anion gap metabolic acidosis, but no measurable alcohol levels.
- Initial glucose levels may be low, normal, or high.
- A ratio of β-hydroxybutyrate to acetoacetate in excess of 10:1 is pathognomonic for alcoholic ketoacidosis, whereas a 3:1 ratio is more common in diabetic ketoacidosis.
- Treatment emphasizes hydration with dextrose-containing solutions and thiamine; resolution of the acidosis usually occurs within 6 to 12 hours.
- Mortality from uncomplicated alcoholic ketoacidosis is less than 1%.

## DEFINITION AND EPIDEMIOLOGY

The diagnosis of alcoholic ketoacidosis (AKA) is established when an alcoholic patient is found to have an anion gap metabolic acidosis without historical or laboratory evidence suggesting an alternative cause. AKA may develop after protracted vomiting in malnourished, chronic alcoholics who consume a daily average of 200 g of ethanol. AKA generally occurs with equal frequency in adult men and women between 20 and 60 years of age. Its incidence and prevalence remain undefined. Up to one half of patients are likely to suffer recurrence. It is unclear whether these individuals have a genetic predisposition to AKA or whether they repeatedly reproduce the hormonal milieu that precipitates ketoacidosis. Almost one fifth of cases of ketoacidosis are alcoholic ketoacidosis.[1-3]

## PATHOPHYSIOLOGY

The term *alcoholic acidosis* describes a syndrome of four types of metabolic acidosis that occur in alcoholics and vary in severity: ketoacidosis, lactic acidosis, acetic acidosis, and loss of bicarbonate in urine. AKA arises from a complicated interplay of the metabolic effects of alcohol in fasted, dehydrated alcoholics who abruptly stop their intake of ethanol.[4]

β-Hydroxybutyrate is the predominant ketoacid.[5] Metabolism of ethanol to acetaldehyde is catalyzed by alcohol dehydrogenase in the liver and results in accumulation of the reduced form of nicotinamide adenine dinucleotide (NADH) relative to the oxidized form of nicotinamide adenine dinucleotide ($NAD^+$). The altered ratio of NADH/$NAD^+$ is the rate-limiting step in alcohol metabolism and favors the conversion of acetoacetate to β-hydroxybutyrate, as illustrated in **Figure 161.1**.

Impaired insulin effects, dehydration, and hormonal responses propagate the accumulation of ketoacid. Ethanol consumption, acute starvation, and catecholamine release cause a relative insulin insufficiency that acts to favor lipolysis and limit glycogen storage. The formation of ketone bodies is further promoted by a dehydration-induced stress response–related release of cortisol, growth hormone, glucagons, and catecholamines. It is unclear whether the elevated levels of cortisol and growth hormone observed in patients with AKA initiate or sustain this process. Ketone bodies in the form of β-hydroxybutyrate are produced as a result of the NADH/$NAD^+$ ratio induced by ethanol metabolism, as well as the lipolytic effect of counterregulatory hormones. Renal excretion of ketone bodies becomes impaired because of dehydration, volume contraction, and diminished renal clearance. Accumulation of ketoacid ensues.

Lactic acidosis is a common, concurrent acid-base disorder, in addition to ketoacidosis. Although lactic acidosis may result from another cause such as sepsis or seizures, alcohol consumption can cause mild accumulation of lactic acid by two distinct mechanisms. First, the elevated NADH/$NAD^+$ ratio can shift the pyruvate–lactic acid equilibrium in favor of lactic acidosis. Second, the thiamine deficiency common in chronic alcoholics prohibits the alternative oxidation of pyruvate to acetyl coenzyme A because thiamine is a coenzyme in this reaction.[6,7]

## PRESENTING SIGNS AND SYMPTOMS

AKA typically develops in severe alcoholics whose recent binge drinking has abruptly and recently stopped. The sudden alcohol cessation is often due to an alcohol-related disease

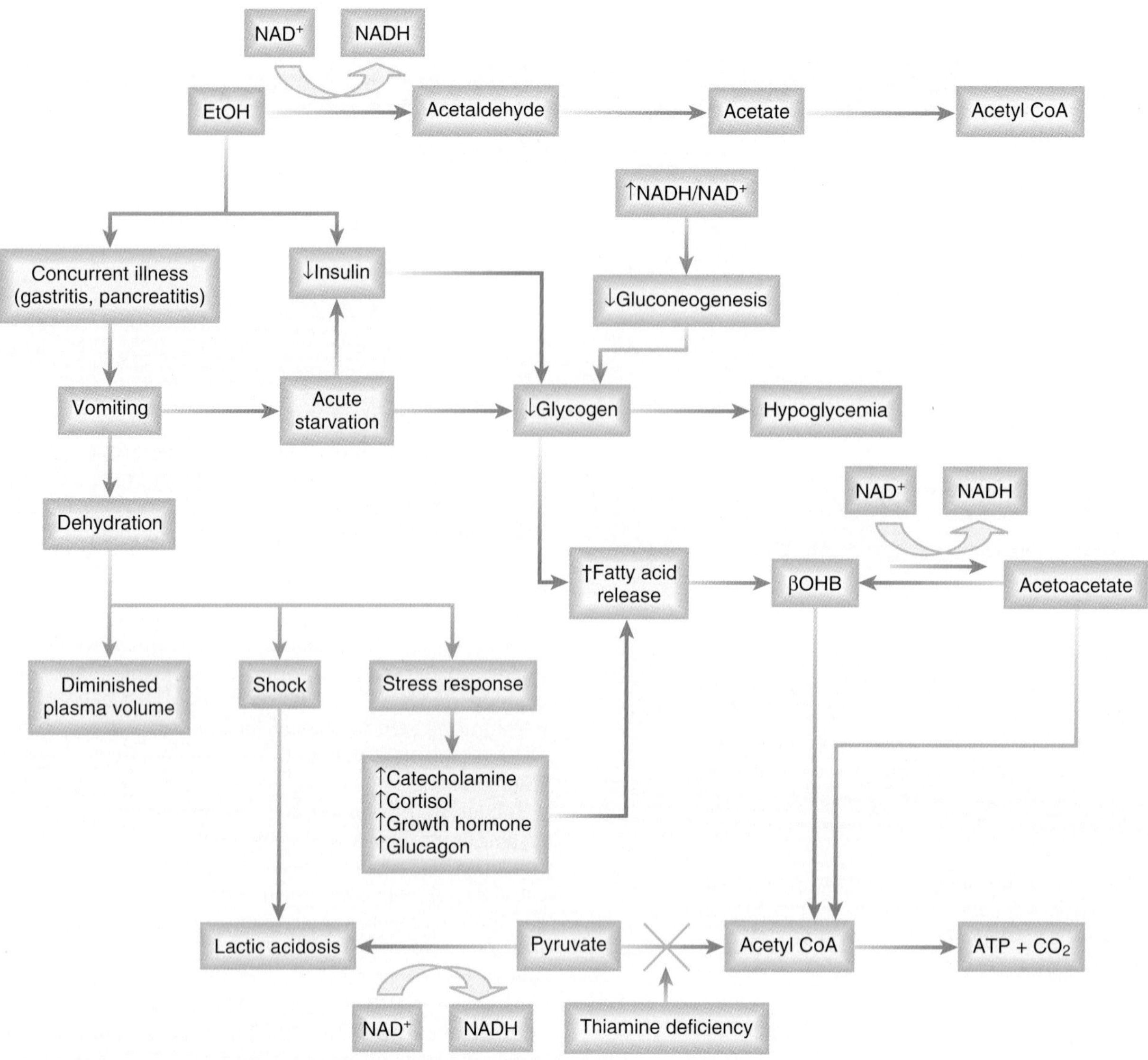


**Fig. 161.1 Pathophysiology of alcoholic ketoacidosis.** Alcohol dehydrogenase in hepatocyte cytosol metabolizes ethanol to acetaldehyde, which is then transported into the mitochondria for metabolism to acetate. Acetate is activated by adenosine triphosphate (ATP), coenzyme A (CoA), and acetate thiokinase to form acetyl CoA, which can (1) be oxidized to carbon dioxide ($CO_2$) by the citric acid cycle, (2) form ketone bodies, or (3) be converted to fat. Insulin depletion results from a number of influences, including endogenous suppression from malnutrition, the direct suppressive effects of ethanol, and α-adrenergic suppression from catecholamines. Volume depletion stimulates the counterregulatory release of catecholamines, cortisol, growth hormone, and glucagon. Glycogen depletion from malnutrition and alcoholic liver disease stimulates enhanced fatty acid release, which is further promoted by catecholamines. The relative increase in NADH over $NAD^+$ resulting from the metabolism of ethanol drives several reactions to produce βOHB and lactate. Thiamine deficiency favors the conversion of pyruvate to lactate rather than acetyl CoA. *ATP*, Adenosine triphosphate; *EtOH*, ethyl alcohol; *$NAD^+$*, oxidized form of nicotinamide adenine dinucleotide; *NADH*, reduced form of nicotinamide adenine dinucleotide; *βOHB*, β-hydroxybutyrate.

such as gastritis, pancreatitis, hepatitis, or pneumonia. Concurrent starvation, abdominal pain, and protracted vomiting are common features.

Patients typically have a clear sensorium, are not confused, and are able to provide a complete history, although there are case reports of encephalopathic manifestations. **Box 161.1** summarizes the sensitivity of signs and symptoms for AKA.

Tachycardia and tachypnea are typically the most remarkable findings on examination. Tachycardia results from volume depletion and early alcohol withdrawal, whereas tachypnea is generally a physiologic response to the ongoing metabolic acidosis. Hypotension and hypothermia are rare. Fever usually indicates a separate, concurrent infectious process. Abdominal examination may reveal hepatomegaly, hepatic tenderness, epigastric discomfort, or severe and diffuse tenderness. The presence of hypotension, fever, peritoneal signs, bloody stools, trauma, or altered mental status mandates a search for alternative causes of these physical findings.

**BOX 161.1 Prevalence of Signs and Symptoms of Alcoholic Ketoacidosis**

Nausea (76%)
Vomiting (73%)
Abdominal pain (62%)
Dyspnea (20%)
Heart rate higher than 100 beats/min (58%)
Respiratory rate higher than 20 breaths/min (49%)
Abdominal tenderness (43%)
Altered mental status (18%)

$SI = \frac{SV}{BSA}$ **FACTS AND FORMULAS**

Osmolar gap = [2 (Na) + (glucose/18) + (BUN/2.8) + (EtOH/4.6)].

An osmolar gap greater than 25 mOsm/kg is specific for methanol or ethylene glycol.

A β-hydroxybutyrate level greater than 386 μmol/L has been proposed as a forensic pathology cutoff to identify "keto-alcoholic death." Levels higher than 2500 μmol/L can be fatal.

*BUN*, Blood urea nitrogen; *EtOH*, ethanol.

## DIFFERENTIAL DIAGNOSIS

Alcoholic patients are predisposed to a variety of complications that may precipitate AKA, including gastritis, peptic ulcer disease, Boerhaave syndrome, pancreatitis, and hepatitis. In addition, intoxicated patients are at increased risk for infectious complications such as aspiration pneumonia. Evaluation for alcohol-related conditions should occur in parallel with evaluation and management of presumed AKA.

## DIAGNOSTIC TESTING

AKA is one of the many conditions that cause an anion gap metabolic acidosis, which is partly summarized by the mnemonic CAT-MUDPILES, as shown in the Tips and Tricks box. When an anion gap is present, an osmolar gap can help distinguish between these various entities. Additional rare causes of an anion gap metabolic acidosis include sulfuric acidosis, short bowel syndrome, formaldehyde, nalidixic acid, methenamine mandelate, rhubarb ingestion, and inborn errors of metabolism such as the methylmalonic acidemias.

**TIPS AND TRICKS**

"CAT-MUDPILES" Mnemonic
**C** = Carbon monoxide, Cyanide
**A** = Alcoholic ketoacidosis
**T** = Toluene
**M** = Methanol*
**U** = Uremia
**D** = Diabetic ketoacidosis
**P** = Paraldehyde, Phenformin
**I** = Iron, Isoniazid
**L** = Lactic acidosis
**E** = Ethylene glycol*
**S** = Salicylates, Strychnine, Starvation

*Osmolar gap, greater than 25 mOsm/kg.

The acid-base disorder in AKA is usually a mixed anion gap metabolic acidosis and respiratory alkalosis. pH ranges from 6.7 to 7.6, and the anion gap ranges from 20 to 40. Hypoalbuminemia is common in alcoholics and may lower the observed anion gap.

Glucose levels may be low, normal, or elevated. Diabetic alcoholics with modest elevations in glucose (>250 mg/dL) pose a particular diagnostic challenge because they may have diabetic ketoacidosis (DKA) or concurrent DKA and AKA. A useful distinguishing feature in these cases is the β-hydroxybutyrate–acetoacetate ratio, which is 1 : 1 normally, 3 : 1 with DKA, and 10 : 1 with AKA.

Because the nitroprusside reaction used in a urine dipstick tests for DKA, a negative urine dipstick test for "ketones" does not exclude AKA. In such instances, the dipstick may show paradoxic worsening of urine ketones as AKA resolves with treatment and β-hydroxybutyrate is converted to acetoacetate.[8,9]

Hypokalemia and hypophosphatemia are common with AKA, particularly as treatment progresses. Alcohol levels are generally zero, although case reports have noted the presence of AKA even when ethanol is detectable.[10-12]

## TREATMENT

Treatment of AKA is directed at correcting three deficits: volume depletion, glycogen depletion, and the elevated $NADH/NAD^+$ ratio. Intravenous fluid and glucose are highly effective treatments. Administration of dextrose-containing solutions to hypoglycemic or euglycemic patients stimulates NADH oxidation and replaces glycogen stores, which results in more rapid correction of acidosis than with saline alone. Antiemetics should be provided.

Initially normal levels of magnesium, potassium, and phosphorus decrease during treatment and require repletion. Intravenous thiamine supplementation (100 mg) provides theoretic prophylaxis against Wernicke encephalopathy and may help reverse the lactic acidosis. Exogenous insulin and bicarbonate therapy is rarely indicated.[12-14]

## DISPOSITION

Mortality in patients with AKA is less than 1%. Adverse outcomes are typically associated with concurrent alcohol-related complications rather than with the ketoacidosis itself. Admission for uncomplicated AKA is indicated for patients with intractable vomiting or abdominal pain of unclear cause.

If a thorough evaluation fails to reveal additional acute health issues, the acidosis can be treated and resolved within 6 to 12 hours. Discharged patients should have appropriate follow-up to address issues of chronic alcohol abuse. Patients may also benefit from an alcohol rehabilitation program (see Chapter 199). Discharge instructions should advise patients of their predisposition for recurrent episodes of AKA, as well as the potentially detrimental effect of alcohol abuse on other aspects of their health. Return precautions should include intractable vomiting, caloric starvation, and increasing abdominal pain.

## REFERENCES

***References can be found on Expert Consult @ www.expertconsult.com.***

# Diabetes and Hyperglycemia 162

*Matthew N. Graber*

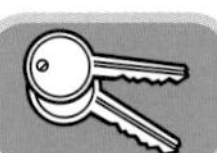

**KEY POINTS**

- Type 1 diabetes mellitus is defined as an absolute deficiency of insulin and type 2 as a relative insulin deficiency. These terms replace older definitions.
- The primary treatment modality for hyperglycemic emergencies is hydration with normal saline. In patients with diabetes, insulin therapy must follow evaluation of electrolyte levels.
- The majority of ketones in patients with diabetic ketoacidosis consist of β-hydroxybutyrate, but standard laboratory tests evaluate for acetoacetate. Hence, the standard "ketone" studies may not reflect this disease process.
- Intravenous bolus insulin has no role in any hyperglycemic condition or emergency, including diabetic ketoacidosis.
- Subcutaneous insulin is the preferred route for the treatment of hyperglycemia. A continuous intravenous insulin infusion may be warranted in patients with severe emergency conditions such as diabetic ketoacidosis; however, subcutaneous insulin has been suggested to be as efficacious for mild to moderate disease.
- Patients with diabetic ketoacidosis have a significant potassium deficit and require supplementation.
- Intravenous administration of dextrose-containing fluid should be initiated in patients with diabetic ketoacidosis when their glucose level is at or below 250 mg/dL to minimize the risk for hypoglycemia.

## DIABETES MELLITIS

### SCOPE

Glucose is critical to function of the central nervous system because it is the primary fuel for these tissues. Plasma levels of glucose are strictly regulated—even after a large oral glucose load or exercise the serum level should not deviate from a range of 70 to 150 mg/dL.

### EPIDEMIOLOGY

More than 23 million individuals in the United States have diabetes mellitus, and this number continues to increase at an accelerated rate, partially because of the worsening obesity epidemic in this country. In almost 6 million of these individuals, however, the diabetes is undiagnosed. In addition to the cost of life and morbidity associated with this disease, the financial expense is enormous. In 2007 the estimated direct and indirect cost of treating diabetes mellitus in the United States was $116 billion and $58 billion, respectively.[1]

### STRUCTURE AND FUNCTION

Insulin is a 51–amino acid protein produced by the beta cells of the islet of Langerhans in the endocrine pancreas. After the initial protein, preproinsulin, is translated on the rough endoplasmic reticulum, it is cleaved serially first to proinsulin and then to insulin and C peptide. Insulin and its C peptide are stored in a 1 : 1 ratio in secretory granules and released primarily in response to glucose and, to a lesser extent, amino acids. Release can be further potentiated or inhibited by a number of gastrointestinal and systemic hormones.

On release, insulin binds to its membrane-spanning receptor. Binding induces a conformational change in the structure of the receptor so that it becomes enzymatically active; it is now a functional tyrosine kinase that can initiate anabolic pathways.

A newer classification system of diabetes mellitus reflects the pathophysiology of the disease and long-term treatment options. The new system identifies four types of diabetes mellitus: type 1, type 2, gestational diabetes, and "other" (**Table 162.1**).

Type 1 diabetes mellitus (note the Arabic numbering) has replaced older terms such as type I, insulin-dependent, and juvenile-onset diabetes mellitus. These older terms became confusing for a multitude of reasons. For example, a small subset of "type II" diabetics fail oral hypoglycemic treatment and must be treated with an insulin regimen; are these patients "insulin dependent"? With increasing worldwide childhood obesity, more and more childhood diabetics are being seen who are not "insulin dependent," and yet their disease cannot be classified as "adult onset."

Type 1 diabetes mellitus can best be defined as an absolute deficiency of insulin. The mechanism is complex and occurs in approximately 5% of all patients with diabetes mellitus. The process usually begins years before symptoms appear when the patient is exposed to an antigen (e.g., viral infection) that is similar in structure to a protein found in islet beta cells. The immune system begins to produce a humoral and cell-mediated assault on these antigens that leads to progressive destruction of the cells. Destruction of beta cells results in a decrease in insulin levels, and eventually a critical point is

**Table 162.1 Comparison of the Four Types of Diabetes Mellitus**

| | TYPE 1 | TYPE 2 | GESTATIONAL | OTHER |
|---|---|---|---|---|
| Insulin production | No | Yes | Yes | Dependent on the degree of damage to the pancreas |
| Previous names | Type I, juvenile, insulin dependent | Type II, adult onset, non–insulin dependent | | |
| Usual onset | Sudden | Insidious | Insidious | Dependent on the mechanism |
| Genetic predisposition | Moderate | Strong | Moderate | Dependent on the mechanism |

reached at which insulin requirements are no longer met and hyperglycemia ensues.

The other categories include patients with relative insulin deficiency; it is important to note that the majority of hyperglycemic patients in the remaining groups do produce insulin, and thus it is easier to conceptualize their insulin deficiency as a balance between insulin and other counterregulatory hormones (e.g., epinephrine, glucagon, cortisol, growth hormone).

Type 2 diabetes mellitus has replaced older terms such as *type II, non–insulin-dependent,* and *adult-onset diabetes mellitus.* The process leading to this type of diabetes also begins years before the onset of overt clinical symptoms. For a multitude of reasons, most commonly obesity, peripheral tissues become increasingly resistant to the effects of insulin. Such resistance leads to increased production of insulin by beta cells, which allows years of relative glucose control. Eventually, the relative insulin resistance can no longer be met by increasing beta cell production, and the patient begins to experience hyperglycemia. Additionally, the beta cells may begin to "burn out" and ultimately produce progressively less and less insulin. The onset of clinical symptoms may be insidious in an otherwise healthy patient or abrupt when significant illness produces a spike in the counterregulatory hormones (e.g., epinephrine, glucagons, cortisol, growth hormone) that tends to increase plasma glucose levels. This abrupt onset occurs because a type 2 diabetic is not able to increase insulin production to counteract this rise, as would a nondiabetic.

The third category is gestational diabetes mellitus, which occurs in about 2% to 5% of all pregnancies, most often in the second or third trimester. It is believed to occur in a manner similar to that of type 2 diabetes. Pregnancy induces increased levels of human placental lactogen, estrogen, and cortisol—all hormones that tend to increase plasma glucose levels. Pregnant women are usually able to produce insulin in sufficient quantities to combat this increase in glucose-elevating hormones; however, susceptible women cannot. This condition most often resolves after delivery, but as one would expect, these women are susceptible to the development of type 2 diabetes later in life. Gestational diabetes mellitus can cause fetal complications, mostly as a result of increased fetal plasma glucose levels. In response to this elevated glucose derived via placental blood, the fetal pancreas increases plasma insulin production, which results in increased fetal birth weight.

The fourth category—"other"—is a catchall that contains all other causes of diabetes mellitus, including genetic anomalies causing malfunctioning insulin protein, insulin receptors, and beta cells in general, as well as other immune-mediated causes. Any significant insult to the exocrine pancreas—be it trauma, chronic pancreatitis, or cystic fibrosis—may result in this type of diabetes. Many common drug-induced causes of diabetes mellitus fall into this category (**Box 162.1**), as well as endocrinopathies such as hyperthyroidism, Cushing syndrome, and pheochromocytoma. Infectious causes include congenital rubella and cytomegalovirus. Less common causes include genetic disorders that may be associated with diabetes mellitus, including Down syndrome, Klinefelter syndrome, Turner syndrome, Prader-Willi syndrome, Huntington chorea, and porphyria.

**BOX 162.1 Drugs That May Cause Diabetes Mellitus***

| | |
|---|---|
| Pentamidine | Octreotide |
| Nicotinic acid | β-Adrenergic agonists |
| Glucocorticoids | Thiazides |
| Thyroid hormone | Phenytoin |
| Diazoxide | Interferon alfa |

*"Other" category.

## CLINICAL PRESENTATION

The signs and symptoms of diabetes mellitus can be quite varied. The classic manifestations are discussed here, but it is important to note that many patients do not have these symptoms. Typically, patients with type 1 diabetes have had years of progressively decreasing insulin secretion as a result of beta cell destruction. However, most often an infection or other stressor acutely increases levels of the counterregulatory hormones and the patient is unable to counter this spike with an insulin surge. Hyperglycemia (generally defined as a fasting glucose level > 126 mg/dL) then ensues, and the patient suddenly seeks care in the emergency department (ED).

As the plasma glucose level increases and eventually surpasses the threshold of the kidneys to reabsorb glucose, the patient begins to spill glucose into urine. This leads to osmotic diuresis and ensuing polyuria and polydipsia.

## DIAGNOSTIC TESTING

All patients with a history of diabetes mellitus should have an early point-of-care glucose assay performed when seen in the ED.[2] At a minimum, diabetic patients with systemic complaints or complaints common to hyperglycemia require glucose testing at the time of first assessment. It is important to note that if serial tests are to be performed, there is a small but significant difference between capillary and venous blood glucose levels.[3] Additionally, any patient with altered mental status or new neurologic concerns should also have glucose levels tested because patients with hypoglycemia or hyperglycemia may exhibit these changes.

The purpose of laboratory testing in a hyperglycemic patient is to differentiate simple hyperglycemia from DKA and less commonly from HHS. It is important to note that no reliable historical or physical examination findings are sensitive or specific enough to confirm or exclude these acute and serious complications of diabetes in hyperglycemic patients.[4] A bicarbonate level below 15 mmol/L with an elevated anion gap (varies depending on the laboratory, but the upper limit is generally approximately 16 mEq/L) strongly suggests DKA. A more complete laboratory evaluation for hyperglycemia includes venous pH, β-hydroxybutyrate (BHB), and possibly serum osmolality. Additional laboratory tests may be necessary as dictated by the clinical picture. It has recently been suggested that acetoacetate (ACA), the standard ketone assayed for by serum and urine "ketone" assays, is neither sensitive nor specific for the diagnosis of DKA.[5,6]

## TREATMENT

Patients with significant hyperglycemia, diabetic ketoacidosis (DKA), or hyperglycemic hyperosmolar state (HHS) are almost universally dehydrated and intravascularly depleted. Even though this is certainly more so in the latter two conditions, all conditions require hydration. The initial treatment is intravenous (IV) hydration with normal saline (NS). Insulin is *not* the initial treatment of these diabetic complications.

# HYPERGLYCEMIA

## PATHOPHYSIOLOGY

Hyperglycemia ensues when the endocrine pancreas cannot produce enough insulin to decrease plasma levels of glucose appropriately (>126 mg/dL in a fasting patient). In type 1 diabetes, this is due to an absolute deficiency; in the other types of diabetes, it is due to a relative deficiency of insulin in comparison with the levels of counterregulatory hormones. In this way, glucose levels increase in plasma and eventually overwhelm the renal glucose threshold, thereby resulting in spillage of glucose into urine. By osmosis, water is pulled into urine, which leads to increased urination and dehydration. This in turn leads to increased thirst and polydipsia. The degree of hyperglycemia and dehydration varies greatly from patient to patient and even in the same patient on different occasions.

## DIAGNOSIS AND DIAGNOSTIC TESTING

The purpose of laboratory testing in a hyperglycemic patient is to differentiate simple hyperglycemia from DKA and less commonly from HHS.

It is important to ascertain the probable cause of the hyperglycemia. Although dietary indiscretion and medication noncompliance do play a role, these diagnoses should be considered only after excluding more serious causes. The most concerning causes can be grouped into two classes: infection and infarction.

Complete a thorough evaluation for possible sources of infection in all diabetic patients.[7] Chest radiography is indicated to search for pneumonia in patients with historical and physical examination findings suggesting pneumonia, patients in whom a thorough history and physical examination cannot be obtained, clinically ill patients, and patients at the extremes of age.

Infarction-related causes of hyperglycemia include acute coronary syndrome (acute myocardial infarction and unstable angina), pulmonary embolism, and cerebrovascular accident. It is important to note that acute coronary syndrome is very likely to be manifested in an atypical manner in diabetic patients (e.g., new-onset congestive heart failure without any history of chest pain or dyspnea without chest pain).[8] Any hyperglycemic patient with these findings should undergo a complete ED evaluation for acute coronary syndrome. A computed tomography scan of the brain or chest may be required if cerebrovascular accident or pulmonary embolism is a concern.

## TREATMENT

Because hyperglycemia is most often associated with some degree of dehydration, the primary modality of treatment should be rehydration with NS. Early insulin therapy is contraindicated before determining electrolyte levels. After the patient is significantly rehydrated, laboratory studies have excluded additional complications such as DKA, and electrolyte status has been stabilized, subcutaneous insulin can be administered.

IV bolus administration of insulin has no role in the treatment of hyperglycemia. Administration of insulin via a continuous drip is not indicated, except in very special circumstances in which exceedingly tight glucose control is required (e.g., during a progressing cerebral vascular accident) for the treatment of simple hyperglycemia. In fact, very tight glucose control in an ill patient has been suggested to have no effect on patient outcome other than significantly increased rates of hypoglycemia.[9] The dose of insulin depends on the degree of hyperglycemia after hydration and the patient's previous exposure to insulin therapy. Patients with known diabetes treated with insulin therapy may be given their usual dose after hydration. Patients new to insulin may be given low-dose subcutaneous insulin with the goal of decreasing glucose to acceptable levels at a rate of 100 mg/dL/hr.

A guideline for subcutaneous regular insulin dosing is presented in **Table 162.2**. This guideline is appropriate for hyperglycemic patients who have little to no previous experience with subcutaneous insulin. Those managed with insulin

**Table 162.2 Regular Subcutaneous Insulin Dosing Guideline***

| GLUCOSE LEVEL | DOSAGE |
|---|---|
| >250 mg/dL | 2 units |
| >300 mg/dL | 4 units |
| >350 mg/dL | 6 units |
| >400 mg/dL | 8 units |
| >450 mg/dL | 10 units |
| >500 mg/dL | 12 units |

*See text for a discussion of modifications of this guideline. Patients treated with regular insulin regimens should be given their usual dosage if appropriate for their condition.

regimens may do better with one approximating their typical dosage. In addition, this guideline assumes that the patient has first been rehydrated and remains hyperglycemic.

It is important to note that euglycemia may not be a realistic or even appropriate goal in these patients while they are in the ED; longer-term (over a period of days to weeks) personalization of an insulin or oral hypoglycemic regimen by the patient's primary care provider or inpatient physician is preferred. The ED goal may be simply to rehydrate the patient and then use subcutaneous insulin to further decrease the patient's glucose level. Targeting a "normal glucose" level in patients new to insulin therapy is fraught with risks, mostly notably hypoglycemia. Moreover, no target "maximum allowable glucose level" before discharge of the patient has been established.

## NEW-ONSET TYPE 2 DIABETES

**Box 162.2** summarizes the clinical and diagnostic findings in patients with new-onset diabetes. In the past these patients were admitted to the hospital without question and a new drug or insulin regimen started. This practice has changed in the last decade because it is now recognized that medications can be started in the outpatient setting without exposing these patients to the inherent risks associated with hospitalization.

### TREATMENT AND DISPOSITION

The initial medication for patients with new-onset diabetes is most often a low-dose sulfonylurea. A good choice of sulfonylurea is glyburide (1.25 to 2.5 mg orally once a day) or glipizide (2.5 to 5 mg orally once a day). These doses may not allow strict glucose control but are appropriate early therapy and pose little risk for hypoglycemia. When starting these medications, patients should be instructed to take them with an early meal or breakfast and to eat regular meals throughout the day. Metformin (850 mg orally once a day) is an appropriate choice for initiating diabetes therapy when a nonsulfonylurea drug is preferred. This drug, when used alone in initial therapy, poses a very low risk for hypoglycemia and may be a good choice for obese patients.[10]

**BOX 162.2 Diagnosis of New-Onset Diabetes Mellitus**

Diabetes mellitus is diagnosed in patients with symptoms of uncontrolled diabetes, including polyuria, polydipsia, and weight loss, and a random glucose level higher than 200 mg/dL.

Diabetes mellitus is also diagnosed in patients with a fasting plasma glucose level higher than 125 mg/dL.

Fasting glucose levels higher than 110 mg/dL suggest impaired glucose metabolism; these patients should be discharged and scheduled for follow-up with a primary care provider.

Fasting glucose levels higher than 95 mg/dL in pregnant patients are consistent with the diagnosis of gestational diabetes mellitus.

Data from American Diabetes Association. Diagnosis and classification of diabetes mellitus. Diabetes Care 2004;27:S5-10; and Metzger BE, Coustan DR. Summary and recommendations of the Fourth International Workshop-Conference on Gestational Diabetes Mellitus. The Organizing Committee. Diabetes Care 1998;21(Suppl 2):B161-7.

All patients with new-onset diabetes should have follow-up arranged in an expedited manner. Patients with comorbid conditions or acute disease should be admitted for inpatient evaluation and treatment.

## DIABETIC KETOACIDOSIS

The signs and symptoms of patients with DKA seen in the ED can be incredibly variable. For this reason it is important to remember that although there is a classic manifestation of DKA, there are no typical findings. The emergency physician should not be lulled into a false sense of security by a hyperglycemic patient who "looks good." DKA should be considered a spectrum of disease, and patients can progress from "looking good" to "being ill" very quickly. Thus any patient in the ED with hyperglycemia requires a laboratory evaluation.[4]

### EPIDEMIOLOGY

The approximate incidence of DKA is 5 to 8 cases per 1000 diabetics per year. Mortality has remained approximately 4% to 5% for the last decade in patients in whom DKA is diagnosed and treatment begun early in the disease course. Some estimates of mortality in patients in whom diagnosis and treatment are delayed run as high as 14%.[11] Other estimates suggest that in as many as 20% of patients DKA is misdiagnosed; these patients therefore have a significantly increased risk for death.

### PATHOPHYSIOLOGY

A hyperglycemic patient has a deficiency in insulin; type 1 diabetics have an absolute deficiency and type 2 diabetics have a relative deficiency. When this deficiency is significant,

**BOX 162.3 Primary Causes of Diabetic Ketoacidosis Seen in Emergency Department Patients***

Infection (35%)
Inadequate insulin (30%)
Initial manifestation (20%)
Other illness (e.g., infarction) (10%)
Unknown (5%)

*The approximate percent distribution is shown in parentheses.

patients are unable to uptake glucose from blood into cells and must rely on the metabolism of fat for energy. Fatty acids from blood are metabolized in the liver to three ketone bodies: ACA, BHB, and acetone. Acetone is a minor component and may be removed from the body via the lungs; this is often manifested as a fruity odor on the breath. The other ketone bodies are in equilibrium with their ratio determined by the redox state and relative levels of nicotinamide adenine dinucleotide (NAD) to NADH (the reduced form of NAD); consequently, the majority of ketones generated during DKA are in the form of BHB. The increasing level of BHB causes an acidosis and leads to significant electrolyte shifts, including shift of potassium out of cells into blood. Because of the continued hyperglycemia, the patient experiences hyperglycemic osmotic diuresis, which leads to significant renal potassium loss and total body potassium depletion. The acidosis also causes a decrease in serum bicarbonate levels and eventually overwhelms this buffering system and results in decreased serum pH.

These changes lead to the classic findings of DKA, including dehydration, Kussmaul breathing (deep, sighing type of respiration caused by acidosis-induced stimulation of the central respiratory center, which may be seen in other forms of acidosis), abdominal discomfort, vomiting, and often altered mental status.

## CLINICAL PRESENTATION

The causes of DKA are many, and they are similar to those of hyperglycemia (**Box 162.3**). The onset may be due to any significant stressor (classically an infection or infarction) or may be due to a deficiency of insulin, usually because the insulin dosage is insufficient, oral therapy is ineffective, or the patient is not compliant with therapy. It is important to note that diabetic patients may have acute conditions—for example, patients with diabetes and pneumonia—and may therefore need increased insulin administration temporarily or DKA will develop; in these cases the cause of the ketoacidosis is both infection and inadequate insulin administration.

## DIFFERENTIAL DIAGNOSIS, DIAGNOSTIC TESTING, AND TESTING PITFALLS

The differential diagnosis of DKA is summarized in **Box 162.4**. In any patient who may have DKA, the laboratory evaluation shown in **Box 162.5** should be performed. No single standard laboratory diagnosis has been established for DKA; however, any diagnosis should include the factors noted in **Box 162.6**. It should be stressed that the diagnosis of DKA is based mainly on clinical findings; although laboratory evaluation is important, common complicating factors often make

**BOX 162.4 Differential Diagnosis of Diabetic Ketoacidosis**

Hyperglycemic hyperosmolar state
Simple hyperglycemia
Toxic alcohol ingestion
- Methanol
- Ethylene glycol

Uremia
Toxin overdose
- Isoniazid
- Iron
- Salicylates

Lactic acidosis
Alcoholic ketoacidosis
Rhabdomyolysis

**BOX 162.5 Recommended Laboratory Evaluation for Hyperglycemia**

Basic chemistry panel ($Na^+$, $K^+$, $Cl^-$, serum bicarbonate, blood urea nitrogen, creatinine, glucose)
Venous pH
Urinalysis
Ketones (serum β-hydroxybutyrate preferred)
If diabetic ketoacidosis is suspected or confirmed, add magnesium, phosphate, ECG
If the initial glucose level is higher than 600 mg/dL or a hyperglycemic hyperosmolar state is suspected, add plasma osmolality
As clinically indicated, cardiac enzymes, serial ECG, lipase, ventilation-perfusion scan, CTPA, CT of the head

*CT*, Computed tomography; *CTPA*, computed tomographic pulmonary angiography; *ECG*, electrocardiography.

**BOX 162.6 Classic Diagnostic Test Findings in Patients with Diabetic Ketoacidosis***

Glucose level of 250 mg/dL or higher
Elevated β-hydroxybutyrate†
At least two of the following three:
- pH lower than 7.30
- Serum bicarbonate lower than 18 mmol/L‡
- Anion gap greater than 15 mEq/L‡

*The diagnosis of diabetic ketoacidosis will ideally be made with the above findings; however, it is important to note that the clinical scenario dictates the relative importance of each finding, as discussed in the text.
†β-Hydroxybutyrate is the preferred ketone, but most laboratories substitute blood acetoacetate.
‡These values may vary depending on the laboratory.

laboratory diagnosis difficult. Each of the components of the laboratory diagnosis is fraught with limitations and qualifications.

Hyperglycemia is commonly considered the cornerstone of the work-up; however, DKA in the presence of "euglycemia" is not an uncommon finding. In fact, approximately 30% of patients with DKA have a glucose level lower than 300 mg/dL,[12] and some studies suggest that the longer patients are in a state of DKA, the more likely they are to be euglycemic.[13] The reasons for this are manyfold. Patients with DKA often have gastrointestinal disturbances that cause vomiting and therefore limited oral intake, with the result that liver glycogen stores will be depleted and gluconeogenesis, which may be inhibited during acidosis,[14] will be the sole source of glucose production. It has also been suggested that patients with poorly controlled diabetes do not store glucose as liver glycogen as readily or efficiently as do nondiabetic individuals or patients whose disease is well controlled. Liver disease of any cause will also limit or prevent glycogen storage and gluconeogenesis.

Acidosis, or decreased serum bicarbonate, and an elevated anion gap are the basic components of the diagnosis. Patients with DKA often vomit considerably and lose acid through this mechanism. They can also become exceptionally dehydrated, which leads to stimulation of the renin-angiotensin system and promotes the loss of both potassium and hydrogen ion in the distal tubule of the kidneys. Medications such as diuretics and antacids may also cause a metabolic alkalosis.

Although the majority of patients have a low serum bicarbonate level and pH, as well as an elevated anion gap, approximately 10% will have at least one of these factors reported as normal.[5] It should be noted that venous pH is perfectly acceptable and there is no reason to obtain an arterial sample.[15]

The final component of the diagnosis is the presence of ketones. As discussed previously, the majority of ketones are in the form of BHB, but the standard laboratory urine and serum examinations assay for ACA. Recent work has suggested that ACA is neither sensitive nor specific for DKA, whereas BHB appears to be very sensitive and specific for this disease.[5,6,16] Additionally, ACA levels may not be high enough to be detected, especially in the dilute urine of a patient experiencing hyperglycemic osmotic diuresis. However, as the patient is rehydrated and treatment begins, serum BHB is converted to ACA. Thus, in a not-uncommon scenario, a hyperglycemic patient is initially negative for urine ketones but after rehydration and treatment begins to "suddenly spill" them and is falsely labeled as worsening and beginning to be in DKA when in fact the patient already was in DKA but the diagnosis was missed because the urine examination tested for the "wrong" ketone.

## TREATMENT

A treatment plan for DKA is outlined in **Box 162.7**. Early treatment is similar to that for hyperglycemia. Patients usually exhibit moderate to severe dehydration and should receive NS. The average patient without a history of congestive heart failure or renal failure often requires 5 to 8 L of fluid over the

**BOX 162.7 Treatment Plan for Patients with Diabetic Ketoacidosis**

This regimen is recommended for the average adult patient and must be tailored to the individual patient. Patients in whom volume overload is a concern (e.g., with a history of congestive heart failure or renal impairment) may need more gentle hydration. Those with a greater degree of dehydration may require greater amounts of normal saline (NS).

**Intravenous Fluids**

Administer 2 L NS over first 1 to 2 hours; a third liter may be administered over an additional hour.

Change from NS to ½ NS after the patient's clinical hydration status begins to improve (usually after 2 to 3 L).

Change from ½ NS to $D_5$ ½ NS when the patient's glucose level reaches 250 mg/dL.

**Electrolytes**

No insulin should be given until the patient's potassium level is known.

Potassium replacement (oral administration is preferred, but the intravenous route can be used if the patient cannot tolerate oral replacement) should be started as follows:

- $K^+$ higher than 5.0 mEq/L—no acute replacement needed.
- $K^+$ 3.5 to 5.0 mEq/L—give a single oral dose of 40 mEq/L of KCl.
- $K^+$ lower than 3.5 mEq/L—give two oral doses of 40 mEq/L of KCl. Ensure that $K^+$ is 3.5 mEq/L or higher before starting insulin.

**Insulin**

Intravenous bolus insulin has no role in the treatment of diabetic ketoacidosis.

After the patient is hemodynamically stable, start a regular insulin drip at 0.05 to 0.1 U/kg/hr. Early evidence suggests that mild to moderate diabetic ketoacidosis may be treated with insulin subcutaneously.[17]

When the patient's anion gap has resolved to less than 15 mEq/L, administer a long-acting insulin (e.g., glargine) subcutaneously at the patient's usual dose or as below:

- Calculate the total insulin units given by the intravenous route over the last 4 hours. Multiply this total by 6, which equals the total 24-hour dose (T24D) of insulin needed.
  - T24D × 0.5 = units of insulin glargine to give subcutaneously now.
  - Turn insulin infusion off 2 hours after glargine insulin has been given subcutaneously.
  - The remaining total daily dose of insulin is given as a prandial short-acting insulin (aspart or lispro) divided into three doses.
  - Example: A patient received 12 units of regular insulin intravenously over the last 4 hours. Multiply 12 × 6 = 72 units T24D. Give half the total daily dose as glargine; therefore, 36 units of glargine insulin is given subcutaneously. The remaining units (36) are divided by three and given as 12 units aspart subcutaneously with three meals.

course of the hospitalization. Potassium levels must be checked and hypokalemia corrected concurrent with the administration of insulin because patients may have significant (often hundreds of milliequivalents) total body potassium depletion. Insulin will drive extracellular potassium into cells and, because of the total body depletion, may cause an exaggerated serum hypokalemia that may lead to cardiac arrhythmia.

Other electrolytes such as magnesium and phosphorus are less crucial and may be administered as usual. Correction of even moderate hypophosphatemia has not been shown to be beneficial in these patients. It is therefore recommended that only severe hypophosphatemia (<1 mmol/L) or moderate hypophosphatemia with clinical findings such as respiratory muscle weakness or cardiomyopathy be corrected.[18] If necessary, potassium chloride may be replaced with potassium phosphate for this purpose. Hypomagnesemia may be corrected with IV magnesium sulfate.

Bicarbonate therapy rarely has a place in the treatment of patients with DKA. Although administration of bicarbonate to a patient with metabolic acidosis may seem logical, it is rarely helpful and may cause multiple, significant complications.[19,20] Because bicarbonate cannot cross the blood-brain barrier but carbon dioxide can, administration of bicarbonate may allow increased carbon dioxide to enter cerebrospinal fluid and cause a paradoxic cerebrospinal fluid acidosis. Additionally, bicarbonate administration may worsen the hypokalemia by driving potassium into cells. Studies have clearly shown administration of bicarbonate to a patient with DKA and a pH of at least 6.8 to be of no benefit.[19] No studies specifically support the administration of bicarbonate for any pH in patients with DKA. If bicarbonate administration has any role, it may be only in a patient with shock and impending or present cardiovascular collapse secondary to marked acidosis and dehydration.

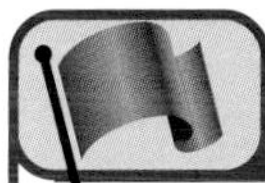

**RED FLAGS**

**Pitfalls in the Treatment of Diabetic Ketoacidosis**

Administration of insulin before correcting potassium deficiencies. This can lead to clinically significant hypokalemia and cardiac arrhythmias.

Not repeating serum chemistry panels every 2 hours and beside glucose testing every hour to adjust the administration of fluids, insulin, and electrolytes. This should be continued for at least 2 hours after discontinuing the insulin drip.

Administration of insulin should begin only after the initial hydration and electrolyte correction. IV bolus insulin has no role in treatment. Administration of IV bolus insulin leads to a supraphysiologic serum insulin level that can cause a significant drop in plasma potassium levels and cardiac arrhythmias.[21] It may also cause hypoglycemia and cerebral and pulmonary edema, and it has been theorized to lead to changes in gene-regulated protein synthesis that may exert its effects for weeks.[22,23] Additionally, because IV regular insulin has a plasma half-life of less than 5 minutes, a continuous, low-dose infusion reaches a steady-state level quickly.[24]

The standard insulin protocol has been to start a drip of regular insulin at 0.1 U/kg. More recently it has been suggested that lower doses may work as well with less risk for hypokalemia, and some authors have even suggested the use of subcutaneous insulin.[25]

Patients treated by insulin drip are at risk for hypoglycemia and hypokalemia, as mentioned previously, and therefore require regular electrolyte and glucose assays. The author recommends alternating a bedside glucose assay with a basic chemistry panel every hour and charting a flow sheet as shown in **Table 162.3**. Potassium can then be supplemented as necessary. The patient's fluid should be changed to $D_5$ ½ NS (5% dextrose solution in ½ NS) when the glucose level reaches 250 mg/dL. When the anion gap has resolved to 15 mEq/L or less, the patient should be given subcutaneous insulin at the usual dose or at a dose similar to those detailed in Box 162.7. Two hours later, the insulin drip can be discontinued; this approach allows subcutaneous insulin administration and the insulin drip to overlap by 2 hours.

It is not necessary nor should it be expected for the pH to return to normal before discontinuing the insulin drip. Because the treatment regimen by itself will often cause hyperchloremic acidosis, monitoring the anion gap is more helpful than monitoring the pH. In a patient with normally functioning kidneys, the chloride level and pH will then be slowly corrected over a period of hours to days. In a patient who has otherwise recovered, mild acidosis at this point should not prevent discharge.

Cerebral edema has long been the most feared complication of pediatric DKA. It occurs in approximately 1% of all cases but carries a mortality rate quoted to be as high as 50%. It has long been held that the treatment regimen, especially rapid rehydration, has been responsible for this complication.

**Table 162.3** Typical Flow Sheet for Diabetic Ketoacidosis

| TIME | TEST | Na | K | Cl | $HCO_3$ | AG | pH | GLUCOSE | CURRENT IVF | CURRENT Tx |
|---|---|---|---|---|---|---|---|---|---|---|
| 6:55 | FS Glu | | | | | | | 388 | | |
| 7:00 | Chem | 130 | 3.0 | 100 | 8 | 22 | | 410 | NS | KCl |
| 7:00 | VBG | | | | 7 | | 7.0 | | NS | KCl |
| 8:00 | Chem | 132 | 3.8 | 106 | 8 | 18 | | 302 | NS | Insulin |
| 9:00 | FS Glu | | | | | | | 250 | ½ NS | Insulin |

*Chem*, Chemistry; *FS Glu*, point-of-care glucose; *IVF*, intravenous fluids; *KCl*, potassium chloride; *NS*, normal saline; *Tx*, treatment; *VBG*, venous blood gas.

However, no data support this belief, and the current literature strongly suggests that there is no casual relationship between cerebral edema in pediatric patients with DKA and their treatment regimen[17]; instead, it is more likely that the degree of illness better correlates with the likelihood of this deadly complication. Treatment is similar to that for other causes of cerebral edema while the standard management of DKA continues.

## DISPOSITION

All discharged patients should begin an insulin regimen. Oral hypoglycemic medications are insufficient after treatment of DKA.

Patients being treated with an insulin drip need to be monitored closely for all the reasons discussed previously; they are usually admitted to an intensive care unit or other specialized unit that can closely monitor their glucose, electrolytes, and clinical status.

If patients with DKA are hungry and have no other contraindication, they should be allowed to eat. Eating a normal meal will decrease the likelihood of hypoglycemia and hypokalemia.

## HYPERGLYCEMIC HYPEROSMOLAR STATE

HHS is a comparatively uncommon but nonetheless serious complication of diabetes mellitus, with a mortality rate as high as 50%.[11] It has had many other names in the past, including hyperosmolar nonketotic coma, hyperglycemic hyperosmolar coma, and hyperosmolar nonacidotic diabetes mellitus. The term *hyperglycemic hyperosmolar state* is more appropriate because not all patients with HHS are nonketotic and certainly not all are in coma or have altered mental status.[26]

## PATHOPHYSIOLOGY

Like DKA, HHS is initiated by a relative lack of insulin; however, the insulin deficiency is usually significantly less profound than that of DKA. Very low levels of insulin (or a low ratio of insulin to counterregulatory hormones) are necessary to prevent ketoacidosis; as insulin levels increase, further gluconeogenesis and glycogen metabolism are sequentially switched off. Because just small amounts of insulin are needed to prevent ketosis, only limited amounts of ketones are produced during HHS. The patient becomes successively more dehydrated secondary to the glucose-driven osmotic diuresis. The dehydration may eventually lead to impaired renal function and an inability to excrete the continually produced glucose, thereby resulting in severe hyperglycemia.[27]

## CLINICAL PRESENTATION

Typically, these patients may state that they cannot or do not wish to drink liquids; patients with HHS may thus have an impaired thirst sensation or may be unable to obtain water (e.g., elderly or bedridden, psychiatric, or jailed patients).

Despite many similarities between DKA and HHS, they differ in some very important ways (**Table 162.4**). As discussed earlier in regard to DKA, patients with HHS may often have atypical findings. The diagnosis of HHS is associated with glucose levels higher than 600 mg/dL, but the average glucose level is approximately 900 mg/dL, and it is not uncommon for the glucose level to be well in excess of 1000 mg/dL.

## DIAGNOSTIC TESTING AND TESTING PITFALLS

Diagnostic criteria for HHS are summarized in **Box 162.8**. As with DKA, it needs to be stressed that the diagnosis is based mainly on clinical findings; although laboratory evaluation is important, common complicating factors often make laboratory diagnosis difficult.

When considering the diagnosis, any treatment before collection of samples for laboratory tests must be noted. These patients are severely dehydrated and hyperglycemic; any fluid administration—for example, by the emergency medical service—will significantly decrease their glucose level. In this context it is not uncommon for HHS to be diagnosed in

**Table 162.4 Comparison of Classic Laboratory Findings in Patients with Diabetic Ketoacidosis and Hyperglycemic Hyperosmolar State**

| FINDING | DKA | HHS |
|---|---|---|
| Osmolarity (mOsm/L) | Normal (280-300) | >320 with AMS<br>>350 with normal MS |
| Glucose (mg/dL) | Usually 250-600 | >600 |
| Insulin | Absent to low | Low to normal |
| Ketones (BHB) | Present | Absent |
| pH | <7.35 | Mildly low to normal |
| $HCO_3$ | <15 | Mildly low to normal |
| Onset | Variable | Usually slow onset over days to weeks |

*AMS*, Altered mental status; *BHB*, β-hydroxybutyrate; *DKA*, diabetic ketoacidosis; *HHS*, hyperglycemic hyperosmolar state; *MS*, mental status.

**BOX 162.8 Diagnostic Testing Criteria for Patients with Hyperglycemic Hyperosmolar State**

Glucose higher than 600 mg/dL
Normal pH (classically, however, patients are often mildly acidotic)
No significant ketosis*
Serum osmolarity
- >320 mOsm/L with any mental status changes, *or*
- >350 mOsm/L

*Acetoacetate is often present, typically with no to low β-hydroxybutyrate.

patients with an initial glucose level of just 500 mg/dL. Serum osmolarity may also decrease to a lesser degree with initial fluid resuscitation.

Absence of ketosis is required to differentiate pure HHS from pure DKA. However, many patients lie in a spectrum between these two entities and may form a small amount of BHB. Additionally, because most laboratories actually assay for ACA, as discussed earlier, mild ketoacidosis is common secondary to anorexia and vomiting. Another classic finding of HHS is a "normal pH." However, it is not uncommon to have a mild acidotic hyperosmolar state secondary to lactic acidosis caused by lack of perfusion to peripheral tissues from the severe dehydration. In fact, approximately one half of patients with HHS are believed to have a mild anion gap metabolic acidosis.[28] In addition, the pH may temporarily decrease further during the initial fluid resuscitation as the peripherally produced lactic acid is returned to the liver for processing.

## TREATMENT

A treatment plan for HHS is summarized in **Box 162.9**. As with simple hyperglycemia and DKA, the primary treatment is fluid resuscitation with NS. The average fluid deficit is 9 L.[29] Resuscitation includes administration of boluses of 1 to 2 L of NS initially, followed by administration of NS until there is improvement in vital signs that suggests improved hemodynamics, as indicated by the onset of urine output and an improved clinical hydration state. Fluids then can be changed to ½ NS.

Failure to change the fluid at this point is apt to lead to significant and clinically detrimental hypernatremia. Fluid administration can be guided further by the following:

1. Patients should have approximately 50% of their fluid deficit met in the first 12 hours of treatment.
2. Glucose levels should fall no faster than 100 mg/dL/hr after the initial resuscitation is completed.

Electrolytes also require aggressive monitoring and replacement. Total body deficits of potassium, magnesium, and phosphate cannot be gauged accurately from the initial laboratory assays and should be supplemented aggressively once urine output has been established. Note that although the initial measured potassium may be normal or even high, the patient is still severely potassium depleted. Therefore, potassium supplementation must be started early in the course of

**BOX 162.9 Treatment Plan for Patients with Hyperglycemic Hyperosmolar State**

This regimen is recommended for the average adult patient and must be tailored to the individual patient. Patients in whom volume overload is a concern (e.g., with a history of congenital heart failure or renal impairment) may need more gentle hydration. Those with a greater degree of dehydration may require greater amounts of normal saline (NS).

**Insulin**

Intravenous bolus insulin has no role in the treatment of patients with hyperglycemic hyperosmolar state (HHS), nor does insulin of any kind have a role during the early resuscitation phase of treatment.

After early fluid and electrolyte administration and when the patient is hemodynamically stable, start a regular insulin drip at 0.05 to 0.1 U/kg/hr. Note that some authorities suggest significantly lower doses, starting around 2 U/hr, in an average-sized adult and adjusting the rate based on the decrease in glucose levels.

Do not allow glucose levels to decrease at a rate greater than 100 mg/dL/hr.

**Intravenous Fluids**

Administer 2 L of NS over the first 1 to 2 hours and continue until the patient is hemodynamically stable

Change from NS to ½ NS when approximately half the fluid deficit is replaced during the first 12 hours of treatment

**Electrolytes**

Patients with HSS have significant total body depletion of potassium, phosphate, and magnesium; repletion should be started in the emergency department with the goal of reaching approximately normal blood levels during treatment, but total body repletion of these electrolytes may take days.

- Potassium replacement (oral administration is preferred, but the intravenous route can be used if the patient cannot tolerate oral replacement) should be started as follows:
  - $K^+$ higher than 5.0 mEq/L—no acute replacement is needed.
  - $K^+$ 3.5 to 5.0 mEq/L—give a single oral dose of KCl, 40 mEq/L.
  - $K^+$ lower than 3.5 mEq/L—give two oral doses of KCl, 40 mEq/L. Ensure that the $K^+$ level is 3.5 mEq/L or higher before starting insulin.
- Magnesium replacement—unless the patient is in renal failure and not able to produce urine, early administration of magnesium is mandatory:
  - Begin intravenous piggyback (IVPB) administration of 2 g of $MgSO_4$ over a 2-hour period and continue administration over the course of treatment.
  - Magnesium must be supplemented along with phosphate to prevent the development of clinically significant hypocalcemia.
- Phosphate replacement
  - Potassium phosphate can be substituted for a portion of the potassium chloride.
- Patients being treated for HHS are at risk for refeeding syndrome and should receive thiamine supplementation.
  - An initial IVPB dose of 100 mg of thiamine in the emergency department is an appropriate early intervention.
- When the patient has clinically improved with a glucose level lower than 300 mg/dL, intravenous insulin may be switched to subcutaneous insulin in a manner similar to that for diabetic ketoacidosis (see Box 162.7).

treatment and certainly before the initiation of any insulin therapy.

Phosphate and magnesium supplementation may be more essential in the management of HHS than in the treatment of DKA. Because HHS characteristically develops over a period of days to weeks, total body stores of these electrolytes are more likely to have been significantly affected by the osmotic diuresis. Although compelling studies are lacking, it is probably of greater urgency to supplement these electrolytes early in the course of treatment.[30,31]

Insulin administration should begin only after the patient has been fluid-resuscitated to the point of hemodynamic stability and potassium replacement has been started. Insulin has no role in the initial treatment of HHS—early administration can lead to cardiovascular collapse.

The effective osmolarity of the vasculature in patients with HHS is dependent on the high level of glucose present. This level may decrease slowly with the administration of NS as sodium begins to replace glucose in maintaining proper tonicity. However, if insulin is administered early before appropriate NS resuscitation is attained, this cannot happen. Insulin will drive glucose intracellularly, thereby effectively and quickly decreasing intravascular tonicity, which may lead to acute and catastrophic cardiovascular collapse. Additionally, early insulin administration will drive potassium intracellularly and risk the same hypokalemia-induced arrhythmias discussed earlier in the treatment of DKA.

After early fluid and electrolyte administration and when the patient is hemodynamically stable, insulin therapy can begin. Typically, a drip of regular insulin is started at 0.05 to 1 U/kg/hr; many authorities suggest low doses of 2 to 4 U/hr. This is then titrated to control the rate of decrease in glucose to approximately 50 to 100 mg/dL/hr. As with DKA and hyperglycemia, IV bolus administration of insulin has no role in the treatment of HHS.

## DISPOSITION

Patients should be admitted to the intensive care unit because frequent neurologic examinations and regular laboratory studies are required during the first 24 hours of treatment. Electrolyte supplementation will need to be adjusted regularly based on the results of these laboratory tests. As with patients with DKA, if patients being treated for HHS are hungry, their mental status has returned to baseline, and no other contraindications are present, there is no reason that they should not eat. They are often ravenously hungry, and eating will act naturally to decrease the likelihood of hypoglycemia and acute electrolyte deficiencies.

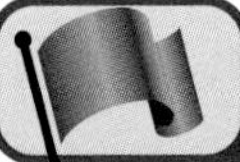

**RED FLAGS**

**Pitfalls in the Treatment of Hyperglycemic Hyperosmolar State**

Hypernatremia may be caused by failure to change normal saline to ½ normal saline after the resuscitation phase of treatment has concluded.

Early administration of insulin may lead to:
- Total cardiovascular collapse
- Clinically significant hypokalemia, which may result in cardiac instability

Failure to replete electrolytes during fluid administration may lead to cellular and cerebral edema and cardiovascular instability.

Seizures occurring in a patient in a hyperglycemic hyperosmolar state should not be treated with phenytoin (Dilantin) because this drug is known to decrease endogenous insulin secretion.

## REFERENCES

*References can be found on Expert Consult @ www.expertconsult.com.*

# Hypoglycemia 163

*Wesley H. Self and Candace D. McNaughton*

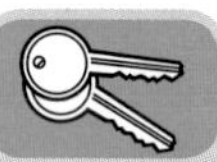

**KEY POINTS**

- Every patient with an acute neurologic abnormality must be evaluated for hypoglycemia by rapid bedside measurement of the blood glucose concentration.
- The most common cause of hypoglycemia is exogenous insulin or sulfonylurea use as a treatment of diabetes, although hypoglycemia can be the initial feature of a large array of serious illnesses, including sepsis, liver disease, renal disease, and cancer.
- A blood glucose concentration lower than 60 mg/dL in a symptomatic patient should be corrected immediately with the administration of glucose, either orally or intravenously, or with intramuscular glucagon.
- Patients treated for hypoglycemia in the emergency department should be discharged only if a readily identifiable cause of the hypoglycemia was identified and if the risk for recurrence is minimal.

## SCOPE

Hypoglycemia is common, life-threatening, and readily treatable. It often occurs in diabetic patients as a side effect of glucose-lowering therapy and can easily be identified and treated in this setting.

## DEFINITION

Hypoglycemia is an abnormally low blood glucose concentration that causes symptoms of autonomic hyperactivity (anxiety, irritability, palpitations, trembling) or neurologic dysfunction (inattention, lethargy, altered consciousness, seizure, coma), or any combination of these symptoms. Definitive diagnosis requires fulfillment of the Whipple triad: symptoms consistent with hypoglycemia are present, the blood glucose concentration is low, and the symptoms resolve when blood glucose recovers to the normal range. An exact threshold for defining "low blood glucose" has not been firmly established because of variations in the concentration at which different people begin to experience symptoms, but a blood glucose concentration lower than 60 mg/dL is generally considered abnormally low.

This work was supported by the Office of Academic Affiliations, Department of Veterans Affairs, VA National Quality Scholars Program with resources and use of the facilities at VA Tennessee Valley Healthcare System, Nashville, TN.

## EPIDEMIOLOGY

Patients who use insulin or oral hypoglycemic medications are at the greatest risk for hypoglycemia. These patients experience mild, self-treated hypoglycemic episodes about twice per week.[1] Severe hypoglycemia, which requires the assistance of another person to regain euglycemia, is experienced at least once per year by 27% of patients treated with intensive insulin regimens.[2] Hypoglycemia is the cause of death in approximately 3% of people with insulin-dependent diabetes.[3] Patients taking oral hypoglycemic agents also commonly experience hypoglycemia. Although these episodes are generally associated with milder symptoms, they occur in more than 30% of patients each year.[4] Sulfonylureas are the most widely used oral hypoglycemic agents. In 2004, 4148 sulfonylurea overdoses were reported to American poison control centers; of these, 36% occurred in children younger than 6 years, 21% required treatment of hypoglycemia, 2.5% were life-threatening, and 0.22% were fatal.[5] The incidence of hypoglycemia is expected to rise as tight glycemic control continues to be emphasized for the 17 million Americans with diabetes.

Hypoglycemia in nondiabetic patients is quite rare and should raise concern about the possibility of a severe underlying illness, alcohol ingestion, or inappropriate exposure to insulin or an oral hypoglycemic agent.

## NORMAL GLYCEMIC CONTROL

### INSULIN

Unlike other organs, the brain cannot synthesize glucose or store a significant glycogen supply and therefore requires an uninterrupted flow of glucose from the bloodstream for normal function and survival. Under normal physiologic conditions, the blood glucose concentration is maintained within a narrow range (70 to 110 mg/dL) through a balance of catabolic processes that increase blood glucose and anabolic processes that decrease blood glucose. Insulin, a protein released from pancreatic beta cells in response to rising blood glucose levels, is the hormone responsible for initiating anabolic glucose metabolism. It promotes glycolysis, inhibits glycogenolysis and gluconeogenesis in the liver, inhibits proteolysis in skeletal muscle, and inhibits lipolysis and promotes lipogenesis in adipose tissue. Insulin secretion is inhibited during fasting to maintain euglycemia and essentially ceases when the blood glucose concentration falls below 80 mg/dL.

### COUNTERREGULATORY HORMONES

The hormones glucagon, epinephrine, cortisol, and growth hormone promote catabolic glucose metabolism as part of the counterregulatory response and oppose the actions of insulin. When the blood glucose concentration drops below 65 to 70 mg/dL, glucagon is secreted from pancreatic alpha cells, and epinephrine is released from the adrenal medulla and sympathetic neurons. These hormones inhibit the entry of glucose into cells, stimulate glycogenolysis and gluconeogenesis, mobilize amino acids to act as gluconeogenic precursors, activate lipolysis, and inhibit insulin secretion.

Glycogenolysis increases blood glucose within minutes and can maintain euglycemia in a well-nourished person for 24 hours. Gluconeogenesis requires several hours to raise blood glucose levels and is the principal mechanism responsible for maintaining euglycemia if fasting is extended beyond 24 hours. Secretion of cortisol from the adrenal cortex and growth hormone from the anterior pituitary gland is a delayed response to blood glucose falling below 60 to 65 mg/dL; these hormones are not involved in the correction of acute hypoglycemia but act to maintain euglycemia over a period of days to weeks.[6,7]

A clinically important consequence of the counterregulatory response is the Somogyi phenomenon. A nighttime insulin dose that is too large causes hypoglycemia during sleep, and the counterregulatory response causes rebound hyperglycemia at the morning glucose check. Increasing the nighttime insulin dose in response to morning hyperglycemia will cause dangerous overnight hypoglycemia and exacerbate the morning hyperglycemia. Paradoxically, decreasing the nighttime insulin dose in this case would lower the morning blood glucose concentration and is the appropriate treatment.

Many of the symptoms of hypoglycemia are caused by an acute increase in glucagon (which causes nausea, vomiting, and abdominal pain) and epinephrine (which causes anxiety, trembling, palpitations, tachycardia, and sweating). The hypoglycemic symptoms caused by epinephrine, called autonomic or hyperepinephrinemic symptoms, function as a warning that mild hypoglycemia has developed; the patient can then correct the hypoglycemia by eating before neurologic impairment ensues. Hypoglycemia unawareness, or the development of hypoglycemia without the normal autonomic symptoms to warn the patient, increases the risk for severe hypoglycemia.

Patients with type 1 and advanced (insulin-dependent) type 2 diabetes may have an impaired counterregulatory reaction. In these patients, the glucagon response is often nonexistent and the epinephrine response is greatly attenuated.[8] This impaired counterregulatory response predisposes patients to severe hypoglycemia by blunting the glycemic response to falling blood glucose levels and thereby leaving the patient with no early warning symptoms of hypoglycemia. Furthermore, even one episode of hypoglycemia blunts the epinephrine response to future hypoglycemia and can result in hypoglycemia-associated autonomic failure.[9] In this manner a vicious cycle of recurrent hypoglycemia can develop. Avoidance of hypoglycemia for several weeks improves hypoglycemia awareness and restores the epinephrine component of the counterregulatory response.[8]

## CAUSES OF HYPOGLYCEMIA

Hypoglycemia occurs in patients with a relative excess of insulin in comparison with the hormones of the counterregulatory response. Such excess can occur through the administration of exogenous insulin, an increase in endogenous insulin, or inhibition of the counterregulatory response. This section highlights the most important causes of hypoglycemia, the mechanisms by which they act, and the context in which they are likely to be observed in the emergency department (ED) (**Table 163.1**).

### EXOGENOUS INSULIN AND ORAL HYPOGLYCEMIC AGENTS

Administration of insulin or an oral hypoglycemic medication is the most common cause of hypoglycemia. In a patient with diabetes who is being treated with an established regimen of insulin or an oral hypoglycemic medication, hypoglycemia can develop for a number of reasons (**Table 163.2**).

Oral hypoglycemic medications include the sulfonylurea and meglitinide drug classes, both of which increase endogenous pancreatic secretion of insulin. Other classes of antihyperglycemic oral medications, including biguanides, α-glucosidase inhibitors, and thiazolidinediones, do not increase insulin levels and do not induce hypoglycemia when used in isolation. However, when used in addition to insulin or an oral hypoglycemic medication, these medicines can precipitate hypoglycemia that is more refractory to treatment.

The time to peak effect and duration of action of insulin preparations and oral hypoglycemic medications dictate management and disposition (**Table 163.3**). Patients often cannot reliably recall which type of insulin they use; a helpful characteristic is that glargine and all rapid- and short-acting insulins are clear liquids whereas neutral protamine Hagedorn (NPH) and Ultralente appear cloudy.

Diabetes caused by chronic pancreatitis is associated with a concomitant deficiency of glucagon because of the loss of pancreatic alpha cells, thus making these patients very susceptible to the hypoglycemic effects of insulin and oral hypoglycemic medications. These medications can also cause hypoglycemia in a nondiabetic patient when taken accidentally, in a suicide attempt, or as part of a factitious disorder or Munchausen by proxy syndrome. Factitious disorder and Munchausen by proxy syndrome should be considered in cases of unexplained hypoglycemia in healthy patients, especially in female health care workers and family members of a person with diabetes.

### ADDITIONAL CAUSES OF HYPOGLYCEMIA

Alcohol ingestion (ethanol), the second most common cause of hypoglycemia in the ED, inhibits the counterregulatory response by suppressing hepatic gluconeogenesis. It has minimal effects on glycogenolysis. Therefore, alcohol

**Table 163.1** Causes of Hypoglycemia

| CAUSE (EXAMPLES) | COMMENT |
|---|---|
| Exogenous insulin (treatment of diabetes or hyperkalemia, factitious disorder, Munchausen by proxy) | Hypoglycemia caused by excessive insulin administration. Most common cause of hypoglycemia |
| Oral hypoglycemic agents (sulfonylureas, meglitinides) | Induce secretion of insulin from pancreatic beta cells |
| Alcohol (ethanol) | Inhibition of hepatic gluconeogenesis. Hypoglycemia usually requires concomitant fasting |
| Sepsis | Inhibition of hepatic gluconeogenesis and increased peripheral glucose utilization |
| Liver disease (hepatitis from infections or toxins, cirrhosis, Reye syndrome, HELLP syndrome, hepatoma, metastatic tumors) | Inhibition of hepatic gluconeogenesis and glycogenolysis |
| Renal disease | Decreased clearance of insulin and reduced mobilization of gluconeogenic precursors |
| Congestive heart failure | Hepatic congestion causes inhibition of gluconeogenesis and glycogenolysis |
| Starvation (prolonged fasting, anorexia nervosa, pyloric stenosis, pediatric gastroenteritis) | Depletion of glycogen stores and gluconeogenic precursors |
| Hormone deficiency (cortisol, growth hormone, epinephrine, glucagon, hypopituitarism) | Failure of the counterregulatory mechanism of glucose metabolism. The hormone deficiency may be either congenital or acquired |
| Medications not used for the treatment of diabetes mellitus (ACE inhibitors, acetaminophen, acetazolamide, aluminum hydroxide, beta-blockers, benzodiazepines, *Bordetella*-pertussis vaccine, chloroquine, chlorpromazine, cimetidine, ciprofloxacin, colchicine, diphenhydramine, disopyramide, doxepin, ecstasy, EDTA, etomidate, ethionamide, fluoxetine, furosemide, haloperidol, imipramine, indomethacin, isoniazid, lidocaine, lithium, maprotiline, mefloquine, monoamine oxidase inhibitors, nefazodone, orphenadrine, pentamidine, phenytoin, propoxyphene, quinine, quinidine, ranitidine, ritodrine, selegiline, terbutaline, tetracyclines, trimethoprim-sulfamethoxazole, warfarin) | Induce hypoglycemia rarely and unpredictably, usually in otherwise healthy individuals |
| Insulinoma | Excessive, unregulated endogenous insulin secretion from a tumor of pancreatic beta-cell origin |
| Nesidioblastosis | Excessive insulin secretion by hypertrophic pancreatic beta cells |
| Non–islet cell tumors (sarcoma, carcinoid, melanoma, leukemia, hepatoma, teratoma, colon, breast, prostate, stomach, mesothelioma) | Various mechanisms, including secretion of insulin-like growth factors, increased metabolic demand, production of insulin autoantibodies |
| Post–gastric surgery status (gastric bypass, gastrectomy, pyloroplasty) | Rapid dumping of glucose into the small intestine causes an exaggerated insulin response; nesidioblastosis may have a role |
| Inborn errors of metabolism (errors in glycogen synthesis, glycogenolysis, gluconeogenesis, mitochondrial beta oxidation, amino acid metabolism) | Congenital defect prevents normal metabolism from maintaining euglycemia |
| Idiopathic ketotic hypoglycemia | Fasting intolerance, possibly caused by deficiency in alanine as a gluconeogenic precursor |
| Autoimmune | Antibodies against insulin or the insulin receptor augment the effects of insulin |
| Akee fruit | Unripe akee, a fruit found in Jamaica, contains toxins that inhibit hepatic gluconeogenesis |
| Vacor rat poison | Damages pancreatic beta cells, which initially causes release of insulin and hypoglycemia but eventually results in impaired insulin secretion and diabetes mellitus. Banned in the United States |
| Transient neonatal hypoglycemia (prematurity, intrauterine growth retardation, severe infant distress syndrome, perinatal asphyxia, maternal hyperglycemia, erythroblastosis fetalis, beta-agonist tocolytic agents) | Occurs in the immediate newborn period. Rarely seen in the ED |
| Persistent neonatal hypoglycemia (mutation in the sulfonylurea receptor gene, glutamate dehydrogenase gene, glucokinase gene) | Occurs in the immediate newborn period. Rarely seen in the ED |

*ACE*, Angiotensin-converting enzyme; *ED*, emergency department; *EDTA*, ethylenediaminetetraacetic acid; *HELLP*, hemolysis elevated liver enzymes, and low platelet count.

**Table 163.2 Potential Causes of Hypoglycemia in a Diabetic Patient with an Established Regimen of Insulin or an Oral Hypoglycemic Agent**

| MECHANISM | EXAMPLES |
|---|---|
| Decreased glucose availability | Missed or unusually light meal<br>Impaired gluconeogenesis:<br>Alcohol ingestion |
| Increased glucose use | Unusually heavy exercise<br>Illness, especially infection, with increased metabolic demands |
| Increased dose of drug | Patient or provider mistake in delivering too much drug:<br>Patient with memory problem causing repeated doses<br>Patient with visual impairment causing inaccurate dosing<br>Inaccurate glucometer leading to excessive insulin dose<br>Provider change in shift and poor documentation<br>Insulin pump malfunction or programming error<br>Intentional overdose:<br>Suicide attempt<br>Factitious disorder<br>Munchausen by proxy<br>Pharmacy medication filling error<br>Physician prescribing error |
| Increased availability of drug | Renal insufficiency (insulin and sulfonylureas are excreted renally)<br>Liver failure (many sulfonylureas are metabolized hepatically)<br>Drug interactions:<br>Warfarin inhibits metabolism of chlorpropamide and tolbutamide<br>$H_2$ blockers inhibit metabolism of glipizide and glyburide<br>Ciprofloxacin inhibits metabolism of glyburide[10]<br>Clarithromycin displaces glyburide from serum proteins[11] |

typically requires concomitant fasting to deplete glycogen stores before hypoglycemia ensues. The classic example of alcohol-induced hypoglycemia is a malnourished alcoholic who undertakes a prolonged binge. However, fasting for only 6 hours before significant alcohol consumption in an otherwise healthy person can cause hypoglycemia. Although hypoglycemia is rare (less than 1%) in intoxicated patients in the ED,[12,13] the hypoglycemic episodes seen in EDs in lower socioeconomic urban areas involve alcohol 50% of the time.[14]

Critical illness can cause hypoglycemia in patients with and without diabetes. Sepsis is the third most common cause of hypoglycemia. The mechanism involves increased peripheral utilization of glucose and hepatic hypoperfusion impairing gluconeogenesis. Meanwhile, severe liver disease induces hypoglycemia via failure of hepatic gluconeogenesis and glycogenolysis. Renal failure can also cause hypoglycemia; the mechanism is not completely understood but probably involves delayed clearance of insulin and reduced mobilization of gluconeogenic precursors. The kidney is just a minor contributor to gluconeogenesis, and this loss is not thought to play a significant role in hypoglycemia caused by renal failure. Congestive heart failure can also lead to hypoglycemia, probably via hepatic vascular congestion impairing gluconeogenesis and glycogenolysis.

Starvation, as in the case of anorexia nervosa, depletes glycogen stores and gluconeogenic precursors and can eventually lead to hypoglycemia. Hypoglycemia as a complication of anorexia nervosa is a late finding and implies a very grave prognosis.[15]

Insulinomas are tumors of pancreatic beta-cell origin that secrete insulin without the normal feedback mechanisms, thus producing unexplained hyperinsulinemia and hypoglycemia in otherwise healthy people. Insulinomas are rare, with an incidence of 4 per 1 million per year.[16] Early diagnosis is important because these tumors are curable with surgery before they lead to potentially fatal hypoglycemia. Nesidioblastosis is characterized by hypertrophied (nonneoplastic) beta-cell tissue that oversecretes insulin and can also be manifested as unexplained hypoglycemia.

Non–islet cell tumors, including hepatomas, carcinoids, sarcomas, and melanomas, can cause hypoglycemia by several mechanisms: a paraneoplastic syndrome caused by secretion of insulin-like growth factors, multiple metastases to the liver with impaired hepatic function, massive tumor burden with increase metabolic demand for glucose, and production of autoantibodies to insulin or the insulin receptor. Autoantibodies that augment the effects of insulin can also occur in conjunction with autoimmune diseases such as systemic lupus erythematosus and Graves disease.

Vague autonomic symptoms after eating were once labeled postprandial hypoglycemia, alimentary hypoglycemia, or functional hypoglycemia. This poorly understood mimic of hypoglycemic symptoms has never been linked to depressed blood glucose concentrations.[17] However, after gastric surgery, including gastric bypass, gastrectomy, and pyloroplasty, patients can experience a true postprandial or alimentary hypoglycemia. Traditionally, the mechanism was thought to be rapid emptying of carbohydrates into the small intestine causing an exaggerated insulin response, or dumping syndrome. Recent evidence suggests that nesidioblastosis (beta-cell hyperplasia causing hyperinsulinism) plays a role in postprandial hypoglycemia following gastric surgery.[18]

Medications other than those used for the treatment of diabetes have been associated with hypoglycemia (see Table 163.1).[19] Quinine, quinidine, pentamidine, and disopyramide stimulate release of insulin from pancreatic beta cells and have the potential to cause severe hypoglycemia. Commonly used drugs that may cause hypoglycemia include salicylates (mechanism unknown), acetaminophen (hypoglycemia occurs only in overdose with liver damage), angiotensin-converting enzyme (ACE) inhibitors (the mechanism may involve increased insulin sensitivity), and beta-blockers (inhibit the counterregulatory response of epinephrine). ACE inhibitors and beta-blockers typically cause hypoglycemia only when used concomitantly with insulin or oral hypoglycemic agents. Nonselective beta-blockers (e.g., propranolol) have more hypoglycemic potential than do selective $beta_1$-blockers (e.g., metoprolol) and can occasionally cause hypoglycemia in the absence of antidiabetic medications, especially in children.

**Table 163.3 Features of Insulin Preparations and Oral Antidiabetic Agents Relevant to the Emergency Department Management of Hypoglycemia**

| | | USUAL TIMING OF HYPOGLYCEMIC EFFECT IN ADULTS (HR) | | |
|---|---|---|---|---|
| **DIABETIC MEDICINE** | **RISK FOR HYPOGLYCEMIA?** | **ONSET** | **PEAK** | **DURATION** |
| Rapid-acting insulins | Yes | | | |
| Aspart (NovoLog) | | ¼-½ | 1-2 | 3-5 |
| Glulisine (Apidra) | | ¼-½ | 1 | 4-5 |
| Lispro (Humalog) | | ¼-½ | 1-2 | 3-5 |
| Short-acting insulins | Yes | | | |
| Regular | | ½-1 | 2-4 | 6-10 |
| Semilente | | 1-2 | 3-8 | 10-16 |
| Intermediate-acting insulins | Yes | | | |
| Lente | | 3-4 | 6-14 | 16-24 |
| NPH | | 1-3 | 4-12 | 18-24 |
| Long-acting insulins | Yes | | | |
| Glargine (Lantus) | | 2-4 | None | ≈24 |
| Ultralente | | 4-8 | 8-12 | 18-36 |
| Sulfonylureas, first generation | Yes | | | |
| Acetohexamide (Dymelor) | | — | 3 | 12-18 |
| Chlorpropamide (Diabinese) | | — | 2-7 | 60 |
| Tolazamide (Tolinase) | | — | 4-6 | 12-24 |
| Tolbutamide (Orinase) | | — | 3-4 | 6-12 |
| Sulfonylureas, second and third generation | Yes | | | |
| Glimepiride (Amaryl) | | — | 2-3 | 16-24 |
| Glipizide (Glucotrol) | | — | 1-3 | 12-24 |
| Glipizide extended release (Glucotrol XL) | | — | 6-12 | 24 |
| Glyburide (DiaBeta, Glycron, Glynase PresTab, Micronase) | | — | 2-6 | 12-24 |
| Meglitinides | Yes | | | |
| Nateglinide (Starlix) | | — | ½-1 | 4-6 |
| Repaglinide (Prandin) | | — | ½-1 | 4-6 |
| Biguanides | No | | | |
| Metformin (Glucophage) | | | — | |
| α-Glucosidase inhibitors | No | | | |
| Acarbose (Precose) | | | — | |
| Miglitol (Glyset) | | | | |
| Thiazolidinediones | No | | | |
| Rosiglitazone (Avandia) | | | — | |
| Pioglitazone (Actos) | | | | |

## CAUSES OF HYPOGLYCEMIA IN PEDIATRIC POPULATIONS

Children are predisposed to hypoglycemia because they have small glycogen stores and a large brain-to-body mass ratio. Neonates are at significant risk for hypoglycemia as a result of developmental immaturity of gluconeogenesis and ketogenesis combined with temporary impairment of glycogenolysis because of the stress of delivery. Neonates of mothers with poorly controlled diabetes are further predisposed to hypoglycemia as a result of the hyperinsulinemia induced by maternal hyperglycemia. Additionally, inborn errors of metabolism, such as glucose-6-phosphatase deficiency, galactosemia, and carnitine deficiency, can be manifested as hypoglycemia in neonates.

Gastroenteritis increases the risk for hypoglycemia by decreasing intestinal absorption of carbohydrates and by increasing metabolic demands of the illness. Reid and Losek[20] found that 9% (18 of 196) of children aged 1 month to 5 years seen in an ED with gastroenteritis and dehydration had hypoglycemia, although none of the children exhibited altered mental status.

Idiopathic ketotic hypoglycemia is the most common cause of clinically significant hypoglycemia in nondiabetic children aged 7 months to 5 years. This syndrome is characterized by fasting intolerance and may be caused by a deficiency of alanine, an amino acid substrate for gluconeogenesis.[21] During a 10- to 16-hour fast, the counterregulatory response converts triglycerides to ketone bodies and causes a mild metabolic acidosis and ketonuria, but it fails to maintain euglycemia. Affected children tend to be slender but not malnourished, with weight percentile below height percentile. These children often have a concurrent illness and are seen in the ED in the morning with a blood glucose concentration of 35 to 60 mg/dL, bicarbonate value of 14 to 19 mmol/L, and ketonuria. The syndrome typically remits by 6 years of age as lean body mass and alanine levels increase.

## CLINICAL PRESENTATION

The signs and symptoms in patients with hypoglycemia are divided into two categories: those caused by elevated levels of glucagon and epinephrine as part of the counterregulatory response (autonomic or hyperepinephrinemic symptoms) and those cause by insufficient supply of glucose to the brain (neuroglycopenic symptoms). Autonomic symptoms typically appear when the blood glucose concentration drops below 60 mg/dL and include anxiety, irritability, nausea, vomiting, palpitations, trembling, flushing, hunger, and sweating. Neuroglycopenic symptoms emerge below a blood glucose concentration of 50 mg/dL and include inability to concentrate, inattention, headache, lethargy, dizziness, blurry vision, agitation, confusion, and focal neurologic deficits.[5] When the blood glucose concentration drops below 30 mg/dL, seizures and coma may ensue.[1] Permanent brain damage and death are rare but occur when the hypoglycemia is severe and left untreated. Predicting who will have permanent neurologic impairment is difficult in the ED, but elderly patients, those with concurrent hypoglycemia, and in particular those with previous strokes are vulnerable to incomplete recovery.

The signs and symptoms of hypoglycemia are not uniformly present with each episode. Recurrent episodes in the same person tend to be symptomatically similar, but hypoglycemia can be manifested differently among individuals. Variations include the blood glucose threshold at which symptoms develop, the severity of symptoms at a given glucose concentration, the predominance of certain symptoms, and their order of appearance. The severity of neuroglycopenic symptoms depends on many factors other than the nadir of blood glucose, including the patient's general state of health and age; integrity of the counterregulatory response; and the severity, duration, timing, and number of previous hypoglycemic episodes. For example, Osoria et al. showed that nondiabetic, neurologically normal people who were administered exogenous insulin to decrease their blood glucose concentration to 30 mg/dL experienced only subtle neuroglycopenic symptoms and no alteration in consciousness.[22] Hypoglycemic episodes blunt the symptoms of future hypoglycemia. Therefore, lower blood glucose concentrations with recurrent episodes will be symptomatically silent and predispose the patient to repeated severe hypoglycemia, which can cause cumulative cognitive decline.[23]

Other than previous hypoglycemic episodes, additional features that increase the risk for hypoglycemia in diabetic patients include the use of insulin, longer duration of insulin use, higher doses of insulin, glycosylated hemoglobin values that are initially high and fall rapidly with therapy, adolescent age, and male gender.[2] Use of an insulin pump does not alter the risk for hypoglycemia when compared with multiple daily insulin injections.

## DIFFERENTIAL DIAGNOSIS

The signs and symptoms of hypoglycemia are associated with a long list of diagnoses. The causes of hypoglycemia create an equally long list (see Tables 163.1 and 163.2).

Hypoglycemia should be considered in any patient with an acute neurologic abnormality, however obvious or subtle, especially if it involves an alteration in mental status. Classic examples include a diabetic patient who collapses during exercise, an alcoholic patient with seizures, and patients in coma after an overdose of oral medications. More challenging findings include strokelike focal neurologic deficits, psychotic-like bizarre and combative behavior, and septiclike hypotonia and lethargy in an infant. Hypoglycemia should be included in the differential diagnosis of each of the following diseases: stroke, transient ischemic attack, seizure, traumatic brain injury, narcolepsy, multiple sclerosis, psychosis, and drug intoxication.

Furthermore, the blood glucose concentration should be checked in all patients requiring ED resuscitation because critical illness can cause hypoglycemia. Losek[24] found that 18% (9 of 49) of pediatric patients undergoing nontraumatic ED resuscitation were hypoglycemic. Additionally, hypoglycemia should be considered in all accidental and intentional drug ingestions, in children with prolonged vomiting and diarrhea, and in all diabetics encountered in the ED.

## DIAGNOSTIC TESTING

### GLUCOMETRY

The optimal method for diagnosing hypoglycemia is rapid determination of the blood glucose concentration through point-of-care testing with a bedside glucometer. Bedside glucometers measure the concentration of glucose in whole blood, whereas laboratory tests measure the glucose concentration in plasma or serum. Because of the relative paucity of glucose in blood cells, whole blood concentrations of glucose are approximately 15% lower than plasma concentrations. Newer models of bedside glucometers calculate an estimated plasma glucose concentration based on the measured whole blood concentration. Although bedside glucometers that undergo routine quality control have adequate accuracy to direct immediate therapy, laboratory tests of glucose concentration are more accurate than bedside glucometers, especially in the extreme high and low ranges of blood glucose concentration.

The accuracy of bedside glucometry and laboratory tests of serum glucose concentration can be compromised by several mechanisms.[25] Bedside glucometers are less accurate with hematocrit levels above 55 or below 30 because of variations in the relative amount of blood cells and plasma. Artificially low serum glucose measurements are seen with hemolytic anemia (nucleated red blood cells consume glucose in the collection tube[26]), with leukemia (leukocytes consume glucose[27]), and when blood is collected in a tube lacking a glycolysis-suppressing agent such as fluoride. An artificially high glucose concentration may be reported by bedside glucometry during an acetaminophen overdose because of interference with the measuring technique.[28]

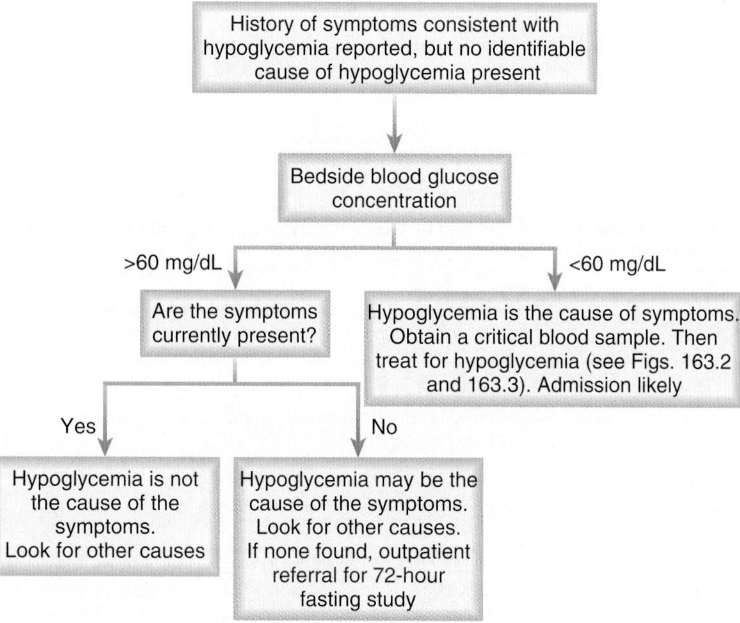


**Fig. 163.1 Approach to determine whether a patient's symptoms are the result of hypoglycemia when no cause of the hypoglycemia is readily apparent.**

## URINALYSIS

Urine ketones are expected in hypoglycemia when the counterregulatory hormones are in relative abundance in comparison with insulin because the counterregulatory response induces the production of ketone bodies from lipolysis. Therefore, urine ketones are typically present in hypoglycemia not caused by hyperinsulinemia and absent in hypoglycemia caused by hyperinsulinemia. An exception to this rule is hypoglycemia caused by an enzymatic defect in fatty acid oxidation, which prevents the synthesis of ketone bodies.

## EXTENDED LABORATORY TESTING

Other diagnostic tests that are useful in selected cases, especially for critically ill hypoglycemic patients, include liver function tests, blood alcohol concentration, salicylate level, acetaminophen level, random cortisol level, chest radiograph, urine cultures, blood cultures, electrocardiogram, and cardiac markers. Recent evidence suggests that hypoglycemia may be associated with cardiac ischemia. Desouza et al. found that ischemic electrocardiographic changes were more common during hypoglycemia than during euglycemia or hyperglycemia in diabetic patients with coronary artery disease.[29] Thus an evaluation for ischemic heart disease is indicated for patients with hypoglycemia and risk for coronary artery disease.

## CRITICAL BLOOD SAMPLE

In nondiabetic patients without an immediately identifiable cause of hypoglycemia who have symptoms consistent with hypoglycemia, a normal glucose reading on a bedside glucometer excludes hypoglycemia irrespective of symptoms (**Fig. 163.1**). No further testing for hypoglycemia is indicated—other possible causes of the symptoms should be suspected.

If a symptomatic patient does have a low glucose concentration by bedside glucometer, a blood sample should be drawn as early as possible for the following laboratory tests: glucose, insulin, C peptide, proinsulin, glucagon, growth hormone, cortisol, β-hydroxybutyrate, insulin antibodies, and sulfonylurea drug levels. This so-called critical blood sample will be essential later, after the patient's ED course, for determining the cause of the hypoglycemia. The critical blood sample is most important for the evaluation of first-time occurrences of hypoglycemia; recurrent cases of medication-induced hypoglycemia do not require such extensive testing. Treating the hypoglycemia before obtaining the critical blood sample will limit its usefulness, but in a life-threatening situation, the first duty of the emergency physician (EP) is to reverse the hypoglycemia and only secondarily to facilitate a diagnostic evaluation.

# TREATMENT

Stabilization of a patient with hypoglycemia begins with the primary assessment. A bedside glucose measurement should be obtained, intravenous (IV) access secured, supplemental oxygen initiated, and a cardiac monitor applied. Intubation should not proceed until hypoglycemia has been treated because treatment of hypoglycemia may completely restore baseline mentation.

Treatment of hypoglycemia involves repletion of blood glucose via oral or IV administration of exogenous glucose or glucagon administration to stimulate endogenous glucose production. The specific treatment modality depends on the patient's age, whether the patient's mental status allows safe oral ingestion, and whether IV access can be established (**Fig. 163.2**).

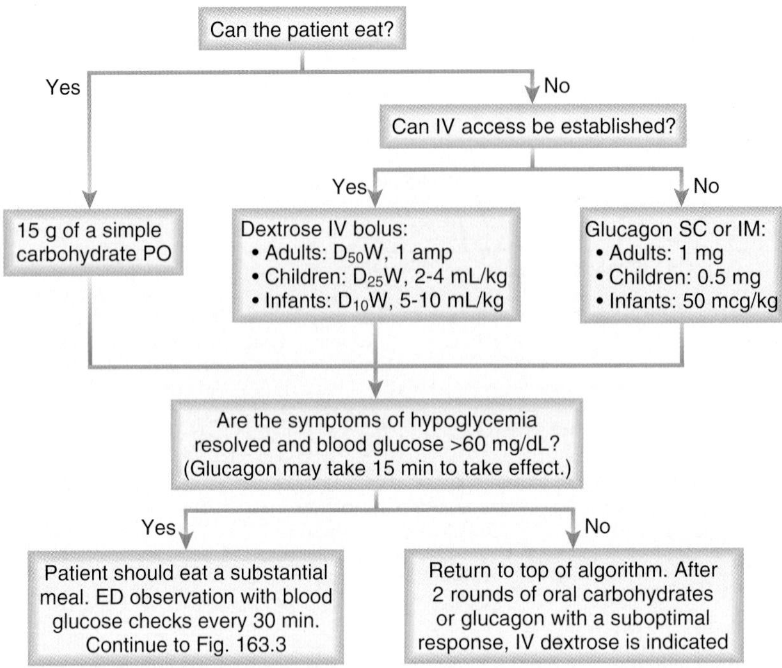


**Fig. 163.2 Initial treatment of hypoglycemia.** *$D_{50}W$*, 50% Dextrose in water; *ED*, emergency department; *IM*, intramuscularly; *IV*, intravenous; *PO*, orally; *SC*, subcutaneously.

## METHODS OF ADMINISTRATION

### Oral Administration

Oral repletion of glucose is appropriate if the patient can eat without risk for aspiration. An initial oral dose is 15 g of a simple carbohydrate such as glucose, fructose (fruit juice), or sucrose (table sugar). Dextrose is the *d*-isomer of glucose and for practical purpose can be considered synonymous with glucose. Commercially available oral glucose products include tablets (4 to 5 g per tablet), gels (15 to 45 g per tube), and nutritional bars (15 to 24 g per bar). Alternatively, an equivalent carbohydrate dose can be given as 6 oz of regular soda or juice or 1 tablespoon of honey, jelly, or table sugar.

α-Glucosidase inhibitors (acarbose, miglitol) interrupt the intestinal absorption of oral sucrose; therefore, if oral repletion is planned for a patient taking one of these medications, sucrose products, including soda, candy, and table sugar, should be avoided in favor of glucose products. Oral repletion with simple carbohydrates increases the blood glucose concentration within minutes and lasts about 20 minutes.

### Intravenous Administration

If a patient's mental status prohibits oral repletion and IV access can be obtained, an IV dextrose bolus is the treatment of choice. The IV dose in adults is 1 ampule of 50% dextrose in water ($D_{50}W$), which contains 25 g of glucose it may be repeated up to three times. The increase in blood glucose concentration in response to 1 ampule of $D_{50}W$ is unpredictable; it ranges from about 40 to 350 mg/dL and averages about 160 mg/dL. The glycemic response to a bolus of dextrose peaks within 5 minutes and lasts about 30 minutes.[30,31]

Because hypertonic solutions such as $D_{50}W$ sclerose small veins, children younger than 8 years should be given IV $D_{25}W$ as a bolus of 2 to 4 mL/kg. Infants should be given IV $D_{10}W$ 5 to 10 mL/kg. These doses deliver 0.5 to 1 g of glucose per kilogram of body weight. As in adults, repeated boluses of dextrose are appropriate if an incomplete response is seen.

The rare complications of dextrose administration include hypokalemia, hypophosphatemia, dilutional hyponatremia, and fluid overload. Electrolyte levels should be monitored if repeated boluses or continuous infusions are given.

### Intramuscular Administration

If oral glucose repletion is not possible and IV access cannot be established, intramuscular (IM) or subcutaneous (SC) glucagon becomes the treatment of choice. IM or SC dosing is 1 mg of glucagon for adults, 0.5 mg for children younger than 8 years, and 50 mcg/kg for infants. Glucagon stimulates glycogenolysis and reverses the symptoms of hypoglycemia after about 10 minutes; the peak glycemic response occurs in 30 minutes and the duration of action is 1 to 2 hours. Glucagon can be repeated after 10 minutes if neurologic recovery is incomplete, but dextrose is preferred if IV access can be established in the interim.

Glucagon is ineffective in patients with depleted glycogen stores, including alcoholic, malnourished, and elderly patients. Adverse effects include significant nausea and vomiting about 60 minutes after administration, so protection of the airway from vomiting and potential aspiration is a priority if mental status does not improve.

## MONITORING AND REPEATED GLUCOSE ADMINISTRATION

The glycemic response to oral carbohydrates, IV dextrose, and glucagon is transient. It is essential to monitor for signs of recurrent hypoglycemia and recheck glucose levels every 30 minutes for 4 hours after euglycemia is achieved. The patient should also eat a substantial meal with protein, fat, and complex carbohydrates to rebuild glycogen stores and maintain euglycemia. If the glucose concentration falls toward hypoglycemic levels again, a continuous dextrose infusion ($D_5W$ or $D_{10}W$) should be started. Patients with intact pancreatic insulin secretion, including nondiabetic and some patients with type 2 diabetes, are at risk for rebound hypoglycemia 1 to 2 hours after receiving dextrose boluses or glucagon because of an endogenous insulin response induced by these therapies.

Hypoglycemia caused by short-acting insulin, alcohol, and idiopathic ketotic hypoglycemia usually responds rapidly to initial replacement and does not recur. Recurrent hypoglycemia is expected when the cause of the hypoglycemia is ongoing, as with sulfonylureas, long-acting insulin, and critical illness. In these cases, continuous IV infusion of dextrose is often necessary.

## ADJUNCTIVE TREATMENTS

### *Octreotide*

Octreotide is used as a supplemental treatment of sulfonylurea- and insulinoma-induced hypoglycemia. It is a synthetic analogue of the hormone somatostatin and a potent inhibitor of pancreatic insulin secretion. Although octreotide does not treat existing hypoglycemia, it can prevent recurrent hypoglycemia and reduce the amount of dextrose supplementation needed.[32,33] In sulfonylurea-induced hypoglycemia, octreotide should be used instead of continuous dextrose infusions and glucagon whenever possible because dextrose and glucagon stimulate further insulin secretion from the sulfonylurea-primed pancreatic beta cells.

The most effective octreotide dose has not been established. One recommended adult dose is 50 to 100 mcg of SC octreotide every 6 hours; continuous IV infusions of octreotide (100 to 125 mcg/hr) have also been used successfully. A recommended pediatric dose is SC octreotide, 4 to 5 mcg/kg/day divided every 6 hours. No significant side effects of octreotide have been demonstrated when used for hypoglycemia.

### *Diazoxide*

Diazoxide, a rarely used antihypertensive medication, also inhibits pancreatic insulin secretion and can be used for sulfonylurea-induced hypoglycemia. It is considered a second-line therapy in comparison with octreotide because of lower efficacy and greater risk for toxicity.[34] Side effects include hypotension and sodium retention. The IV adult dose is 300 mg of diazoxide given over a 1-hour period; the IV pediatric dose is 1 to 3 mg/kg given over a 1-hour period. Doses can be repeated every 4 hours as needed.

### *Other Adjunctive Treatments*

When hypoglycemia is caused by a massive overdose of SC insulin, one case report suggests that needle aspiration or surgical excision of the SC reservoir may reduce the systemic absorption of insulin.[35]

Early administration of activated charcoal is indicated for sulfonylurea overdose and accidental pediatric sulfonylurea ingestion. Maximum efficacy is achieved if the charcoal is given within 1 hour of the ingestion. Glipizide undergoes enterohepatic circulation; peak plasma concentrations may be decreased by multiple doses of activated charcoal. Because of the delayed peak effects of extended-release glipizide, whole-bowel irrigation can be considered for overdoses of this preparation.

Urine alkalization can reduce the half-life of chlorpropamide from 49 hours to 13 hours through increased renal excretion. However, urine alkalization does not appear to be useful in reducing the duration of effect of other hypoglycemic agents.[36]

## RISKS ASSOCIATED WITH PRESUMPTIVE TREATMENT

It has been suggested previously that dextrose be given to all patients with undifferentiated altered mental status as part of the "coma cocktail," which consists of oxygen plus IV administration of 1 ampule of $D_{50}W$, 100 mg of thiamine, and 0.4 mg of naloxone. This practice was challenged in the 1980s when animal and retrospective human studies suggested that hyperglycemia may be detrimental to the injured brain, particularly in the setting of acute stroke, cardiac arrest, hypotension, and head trauma.[37] The true risk of administering a small glucose load to a euglycemic or hyperglycemic patient with a brain injury has not been established but is thought to be small. Hypoglycemia, in contrast, is known to be detrimental, especially to the injured brain. Therefore, the current recommendation is to obtain a bedside glucose measurement in patients with altered mental status and administer dextrose only when the blood glucose level is lower than 60 mg/dL. Treatment should be initiated empirically only when a glucometer is not immediately available.

Traditional teachings also warn that dextrose should never be given to patients with altered mentation without a preceding dose of thiamine because of the risk of precipitating Wernicke encephalopathy. Thiamine is a cofactor for two essential reactions in the glycolysis–tricarboxylic acid cycle (conversion of pyruvate to acetyl coenzyme A and α-ketoglutarate to succinate). Theoretically, without adequate supplies of thiamine, the energy contained in glucose cannot be converted to adenosine triphosphate, so substrates for the thiamine-dependent reactions accumulate in the brain and cause Wernicke encephalopathy. Administering dextrose to a thiamine-deficient patient increases the production of these substrates, but no clinical evidence has shown that a dextrose load dosed to reverse hypoglycemia precipitates Wernicke encephalopathy if thiamine is not given first.[38] When treating a patient with altered mental status and confirmed hypoglycemia or with possible hypoglycemia without access to a bedside glucometer, EPs should administer thiamine and dextrose simultaneously if possible. Dextrose administration should not be delayed if thiamine is not immediately available, even in alcoholic patients. Hypoglycemia should be corrected immediately, and thiamine should be administered as soon as possible.

## PERSISTENT ALTERED MENTAL STATUS

If hypoglycemia is the sole cause of the altered mental status, restoration of euglycemia should lead to reversal of the neurologic symptoms within minutes. In the case of a seizure caused by hypoglycemia, the altered mentation may persist for a short period while the patient recovers from the postictal state. If a patient's mental status remains altered for more than 15 minutes after return to euglycemia and there is no history of seizure, a secondary cause must be considered. The EP should return to the primary assessment and consider a broad differential diagnosis, including traumatic brain injury, anoxic brain injury, stroke, alcohol intoxication, opioid intoxication, central nervous system infection, liver failure, and renal failure. The coma cocktail should be given in full, if not administered earlier. Rapid-sequence intubation, computed tomography of the brain, and lumbar puncture may be indicated. If a lumbar puncture is performed, a low cerebrospinal fluid glucose value is not necessarily a sign of central nervous system infection because this value remains depressed for several hours after a low blood glucose concentration has been corrected.[39]

## DISPOSITION

### DISCHARGE

Patients with hypoglycemia caused by a short-acting, easily reversed mechanism that is unlikely to recur may be considered for discharge (**Box 163.1**). A history of recurrent episodes of hypoglycemia may be an indication for hospital admission to adjust medications. When taken in massive doses, even short-acting insulin preparations can cause delayed, recurrent hypoglycemia because of altered pharmacokinetics. Renal failure also increases the half-lives of insulin preparations and can cause unexpected recurrent hypoglycemia.

For patients who are discharged from the ED, insulin doses should be reduced by 25% for the next 24 hours to reduce the risk for recurrent hypoglycemia. Patients should be educated about how to prevent hypoglycemia (see the "Patient Teaching Tips" box), and short-term follow-up with a primary care physician should be arranged.

Children with known idiopathic ketotic hypoglycemia can also be discharged home after the hypoglycemia has been reversed and an uneventful ED observation completed. Parents should be educated to avoid prolonged fasts in these children and to provide a bedtime snack. An initial diagnosis of idiopathic ketotic hypoglycemia should not be made in the ED; patients with symptoms consistent with this diagnosis require admission to exclude other potential causes of hypoglycemia.

**BOX 163.1 Minimum Requirements for Discharge from the Emergency Department (ED) After a Hypoglycemic Episode**

Hypoglycemia fully and rapidly reversed without continuous infusion of dextrose
Uneventful 4-hour ED observation with serial blood glucose measurements in the normal range and not trending downward
Full meal eaten in the ED
Cause of the hypoglycemia known and recurrence unlikely (i.e., short-acting insulin)
Accidental hypoglycemia
Isolated hypoglycemic episode (no other recent severe hypoglycemic events or frequent mild hypoglycemic events)
No major concurrent illnesses
Patient understands how to prevent future episodes
Patient can accurately monitor blood glucose at home
Responsible adult will monitor the patient for the next several hours
Follow-up with a primary care physician arranged

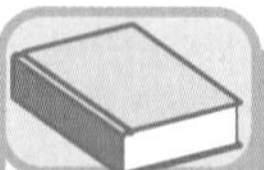

**PATIENT TEACHING TIPS**

Know the symptoms of hypoglycemia. Train yourself to estimate your blood glucose concentration through your symptoms.
Carry fast-acting carbohydrates with you at all times. Immediately take 15 to 30 g when you experience symptoms of hypoglycemia. Do not delay to check your blood glucose level. After the symptoms resolve, eat a small snack of complex carbohydrates and protein (cheese or peanut butter and crackers).
Stop driving immediately if you experience symptoms of hypoglycemia.
Even moderate alcohol consumption increases the risk for hypoglycemia.
Train friends and family when and how to administer glucagon. These people should know where the glucagon kit is and should practice mixing the glucagon mixture. Know the expiration date on your glucagon kit.
The risk for hypoglycemia is increased in the hours to days after an initial hypoglycemic episode. You should increase your vigilance and check your blood glucose more frequently in the 24 hours following a hypoglycemic episode.
Call your doctor for a hypoglycemic episode requiring fast-acting carbohydrates that you cannot readily explain and the use of glucagon.
Call 911 for an incomplete response to glucagon or oral fast-acting carbohydrates or a seizure.
More information is available through the American Diabetes Society (www.diabetes.org).

### OBSERVATION AND ADMISSION

Patients who do not meet the criteria outlined in Box 163.1 require admission or monitoring in an observation unit for at least 24 hours (**Fig. 163.3**). Because of the risk for recurrence, hospitalization is recommended for those with hypoglycemia caused by an oral hypoglycemic medication or an intermediate- or long-acting insulin. Hypoglycemia caused by sulfonylureas tends to be prolonged and severe, and intensive care unit admission may be necessary, especially if a continuous dextrose infusion is needed in addition to octreotide to maintain euglycemia. Experience with hypoglycemia caused by the meglitinides is limited, so these patients should be managed similar to those with sulfonylurea-induced hypoglycemia.

Patients with hypoglycemia that cannot be completely reversed in the ED, as well as patients with hypoglycemia caused by massive insulin overdoses, starvation, sepsis, liver failure, and adrenal insufficiency, should be admitted to the intensive care unit.

Psychiatry consultation is appropriate for cases of hypoglycemia involving suicide attempts, factitious disorder, and Münchausen by proxy.

### PATIENTS TREATED IN PREHOSPITAL SETTING

Emergency medical service (EMS) personnel frequently treat hypoglycemia in the prehospital setting. After treatment and resolution of the symptoms, patients often refuse transport to the ED. Recent studies suggest that the risk for recurrent hypoglycemia is not different in patients transported to the ED and those released on the scene.[40,41] Mechem et al.[42] reported that 9% (9 of 103) of patients who initially refused transport to the ED contacted EMS again within 3 days because of recurrent hypoglycemia. Similarly, Lerner et al.[43] found that 8% (3 of 38) of patients released by EMS experienced recurrent hypoglycemia in 24 to 48 hours. However, caution is advised because fatal cases of hypoglycemia have occurred following release by EMS.[42] EMS personnel should encourage all patients with symptomatic hypoglycemia, especially those who do not meet the criteria listed in Box 163.1, to be transported to the ED.

## SPECIAL CONSIDERATION: ACCIDENTAL PEDIATRIC SULFONYLUREA INGESTION

Children are particularly susceptible to the effects of sulfonylureas, and significant hypoglycemia can develop after the ingestion of a single tablet.[44,45] Therefore, all pediatric patients with possible sulfonylurea ingestion should be evaluated in the ED. If hypoglycemia is present on arrival at the ED, treatment as outlined previously with dextrose, octreotide, oral feedings, and hospital admission is indicated. The optimal management of a child who ingested a sulfonylurea or is thought to have done so and who has a normal blood glucose concentration is debated in the literature, with recommendations varying from mandatory admission to 8-hour ED observation.[45-48]

Two studies provide the best available data for directing the management of asymptomatic pediatric sulfonylurea ingestions. In a retrospective study of pediatric patients after sulfonylurea ingestion, Quadrani et al.[49] found that 27% (25 of 93) had a blood glucose concentration lower than 60 mg/dL 30 minutes to 16 hours after ingestion, with the mean time to development of hypoglycemia being 4.3 hours. All four patients in whom hypoglycemia developed after 8 hours had received a continuous dextrose infusion while euglycemic during the observation period. It is thought that the dextrose infusions delayed the onset of hypoglycemia in these patients.

In a prospective study of pediatric sulfonylurea ingestions, Spiller et al.[50] found that hypoglycemia developed in 29% (54 of 185). In all but one of the hypoglycemic patients, low blood glucose developed within 8 hours of ingestion. The lone patient in whom hypoglycemia developed after 8 hours had been given a continuous dextrose infusion after a blood glucose measurement of 62 mg/dL at 3 hours.

In both studies, hypoglycemia developed more than 8 hours after ingestion only in patients who received prophylactic

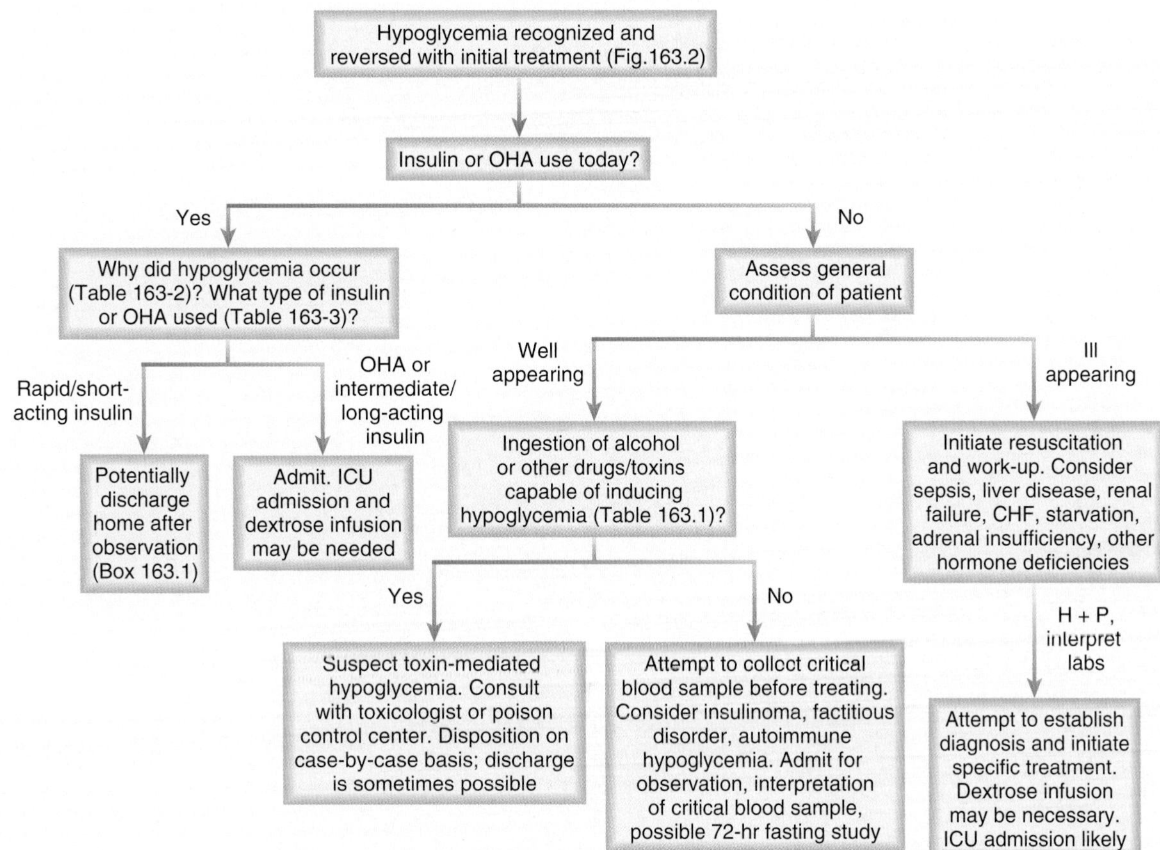


**Fig. 163.3 Approach to a hypoglycemic adult in the emergency department.** *CHF*, Congestive heart failure; *H + P*, history and physical examination; *ICU*, intensive care unit; *OHA*, oral hypoglycemic agent.

dextrose infusions. These infusions probably masked early hypoglycemia and potentially stimulated further pancreatic insulin secretion.

An 8-hour ED observation period for pediatric patients with asymptomatic sulfonylurea ingestion appears to be safe when the following protocol is used. An blood glucose measurement should be obtained immediately. Activated charcoal should be administered if the child is initially seen within 1 hour of ingestion and there is little risk for vomiting and aspiration. For an asymptomatic patient with a blood glucose concentration higher than 60 mg/dL, oral carbohydrates should be encouraged but no IV dextrose given. The blood glucose concentration should be checked every 30 to 60 minutes; a decrease in concentration to below 60 mg/dL is an indication for an IV dextrose bolus and hospital admission.

If the patient remains asymptomatic and blood glucose remains higher than 60 mg/dL for 8 hours after ingestion, the patient may be discharged with appropriate return precautions. However, hospitalization is advised if IV dextrose is administered at any time, if the ingestion involved extended-release glipizide (Glucotrol XL—a sulfonylurea with peak effects possibly delayed longer than 8 hours), or if the ingestion may have been intentional.

## REFERENCES

***References can be found on Expert Consult @ www.expertconsult.com.***

# Sodium and Water Balance 164

*Michael C. Wadman and Lance H. Hoffman*

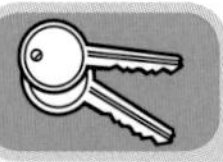

**KEY POINTS**

- Most signs and symptoms of clinically significant hyponatremia are related to an increase in cellular volume in the central nervous system and subsequent cerebral edema.
- Hyposmolar hypovolemic hyponatremia, the most common type of hyponatremia encountered in the emergency department, is seen in patients with severe total body water depletion in excess of sodium loss.
- Diagnostic criteria for the syndrome of inappropriate secretion of antidiuretic hormone (ADH) include hyposmolar hyponatremia, inappropriately concentrated urine, and exclusion of other causes of hyposmolar euvolemic hyponatremia such as hypothyroidism and adrenal insufficiency.
- Hypovolemic hypernatremia, the most common cause seen in the emergency department, results from severe total body water depletion.
- Patients with central diabetes insipidus produce dilute urine because of a decrease in ADH secretion from the hypothalamus; those with nephrogenic DI exhibit a decreased response to ADH at the renal tubule.
- Osmotic demyelination syndrome, the most serious complication of the treatment of hyponatremia, occurs when the administration of relatively hyperosmolar intravenous fluid causes intracellular water to rapidly diffuse out of central nervous system cells.
- The most serious complication of therapy for hypernatremia is the development of cerebral edema secondary to excessively rapid rehydration.

## SCOPE

Water accounts for 60% of total body weight and is divided between two spaces or compartments: intracellular and extracellular. Osmotic equilibrium between the extracellular and intracellular spaces depends on free flow of water through a solute-impermeable/water-permeable membrane barrier. Water balance describes the normal state of equilibrium, with osmolality, the ratio of solute to free water, being constant between the two spaces when water diffuses freely across the membrane. The predominant solute of the extracellular space is sodium.

Various disease states may alter water balance and lead to abnormally high or low sodium levels that may result in significant disability or death from either the causative disease, the direct effects of the sodium concentration, or the ill effects of inappropriate treatment. The signs and symptoms range from subtle constitutional symptoms to seizure and coma. Suspicion for disorders of water balance depends on assessment of existing risk factors and the clinical information available at the time of arrival at the emergency department (ED).

Hyponatremia is diagnosed when the serum sodium level is lower than 135 mEq/L, but clinical signs and symptoms most often occur when sodium falls below 130. Hyponatremia most commonly occurs in the very young and the very old, with prevalence increasing with advancing age. Hyponatremia is observed in infants given tap water as a home remedy for gastroenteritis and in elderly patients with a poorly regulated thirst mechanism or an inability to procure fluids because of immobility (or both).[1,2]

Hypernatremia, a plasma sodium level higher than 145 mEq/L, most commonly results from inadequate water intake. In the very young, this situation usually occurs secondary to water loss exceeding intake, such as with diarrheal illness; in the geriatric population, hypernatremia may result from a poor sense of thirst or an inability to obtain adequate fluids because of physical or mental impairment. Hypernatremia is less common than hyponatremia, but it is associated with a far greater mortality rate of approximately 50%, primarily from the causative disease states in elderly patients and from the direct neurologic effects of the high sodium concentration in the very young.[3]

## PATHOPHYSIOLOGY

Water balance is regulated through the homeostatic mechanisms of thirst and renal excretion. High serum osmolality is detected by hypothalamic osmoreceptors and leads to secretion of antidiuretic hormone (ADH) and stimulation of thirst. ADH regulates plasma osmolality by increasing free water absorption in the kidney. Low plasma osmolality results in suppression of ADH and the production of dilute urine.

Hypovolemia stimulates thirst, as well as the secretion of ADH and aldosterone. Aldosterone is synthesized in the adrenal cortex and is secreted in response to hypovolemia via the renin-angiotensin-aldosterone axis. Aldosterone acts by increasing sodium absorption at the distal tubule, which leads to expansion of intravascular volume.

### HYPONATREMIA

The low osmolality of the intravascular space and the relatively high osmolality of the intracellular space results in an osmotic gradient and diffusion of water into the cell. The resulting cellular edema is generally well tolerated by most tissues, except when it occurs in a confined space such as the central nervous system (CNS). The initial, rapid response to the increase in CNS cellular volume is diffusion of electrolytes and water out of the cell, which leads to a partial reduction in glial cell volume. Continuing hyponatremia over the next 48 to 72 hours generates slow diffusion of organic osmolytes, primarily large amino acids, out of the cell, thereby further reducing cell volume.[4] Treatment of hyponatremia with intravenous fluid (IVF) may then lead to a state of relative hyperosmolality in the extracellular space with resultant diffusion of water out of the cell and continued reduction in cellular volume. This cycle creates the most serious treatment complication of hyponatremia: osmotic demyelination syndrome (otherwise known as central pontine myelinolysis).[5]

### HYPERNATREMIA

In hypernatremia, water diffuses out of the cell along the osmotic gradient, which results in loss of cellular volume. In the acute phase, electrolytes and water rapidly diffuse into the cell to partially restore cellular volume. With ongoing hypernatremia, slow redistribution of osmolytes occurs and water diffuses into the cell. With treatment, the relatively hyposmolar IVF leads to an osmotic gradient that promotes further diffusion of water into the cell. The size of the larger organic osmolytes prevents rapid diffusion out of the cell and results in the most serious treatment complication of hypernatremia: cerebral edema.[6,7]

## CLINICAL PRESENTATION

### HYPONATREMIA

Most signs and symptoms of significant hyponatremia are related to an increase in CNS cellular volume and subsequent cerebral edema. The rapid compensatory mechanisms of the acute phase produce more obvious signs and symptoms, whereas the slow, adaptive phase of the chronic state results in minimal symptomatology.

The signs and symptoms of hyponatremia depend on both the rate of change and the absolute plasma sodium concentration. An acute fall in the serum sodium level below 120 almost always results in symptoms, whereas a more gradual decline to this level may go undetected.

Symptoms of hyponatremia include nausea, headache, and general malaise with sodium levels of 125 to 130 and lethargy, confusion, agitation, psychosis, and seizures as the sodium level falls to the range of 115 to 120; severe symptoms develop at 110 regardless of the rate of change. Severe CNS signs observed with hyponatremia include a decreased level of alertness, focal or generalized seizure activity, and signs of brainstem herniation such as unilateral dilated pupil, posturing, and respiratory arrest.[8]

### HYPERNATREMIA

The signs and symptoms of hypernatremia depend on age. Infants exhibit restlessness, tachypnea, characteristic high-pitched crying, alternating irritability and lethargy, and hypotonia. Elderly patients have nausea, weakness, altered mental status, agitation, irritability, lethargy, stupor, coma, and seizures. The severity of the CNS symptoms correlates with serum sodium levels.[9]

## DIFFERENTIAL DIAGNOSIS AND CLASSIFICATIONS

### HYPONATREMIA

The differential diagnosis of hyponatremia begins with determination of serum osmolality (**Fig. 164.1**).[4] Osmolality is measured by osmometry in the laboratory or is calculated according to the following formula:

$$\begin{aligned}\text{Plasma osmolality} = {} & [2 \times \text{Na}^{+}\ (\text{mEq/L})] \\ & + [\text{glucose}\ (\text{mg/dL})/18] \\ & + [\text{BUN}\ (\text{mg/dL})/2.8]\end{aligned}$$

(BUN = blood urea nitrogen).

Depending on serum osmolality, the patient is classified as being either hyposmolar (plasma Osm < 275), isosmolar (275 to 290), or hyperosmolar (>290). In hyposmolar patients, clinical assessment of the patient's volume status further differentiates hyponatremic patients as hypovolemic, euvolemic, or hypervolemic.

Hyposmolar hypovolemic hyponatremia, the most common type of hyponatremia encountered in the ED, is seen in patients with severe depletion of total body water (TBW) in excess of sodium loss.[10] Urine osmolality and sodium determinations allow further narrowing of the differential diagnosis. Dilute urine (urine osmolality > 100 mOsm/kg) suggests polydipsia or beer potomania. In patients with urine osmolality greater than 100 mOsm/kg, urinary sodium levels lower than 20 mEq/L indicate an extrarenal source of the sodium and water loss. Extrarenal causes of hyponatremia include gastrointestinal problems such as vomiting or diarrhea and skin loss from severe burns. Urinary sodium levels higher than 20 mEq/L suggest a renal source of the sodium and water loss, such as sodium-losing nephropathy, hypoaldosteronism, diuretic excess, or osmotic diuresis.

Hyposmolar euvolemic hyponatremia is most commonly associated with the syndrome of inappropriate secretion of antidiuretic hormone (SIADH) (**Box 164.1**). ADH, or vasopressin, decreases free water excretion and results in inappropriately concentrated urine (urine osmolality >100 mOsm/kg) and a urine sodium concentration higher than 20 mEq/L. SIADH may result from various malignancies, pulmonary disorders, CNS diseases, and several drugs.[11-13] Diagnostic criteria for SIADH include hyposmolar hyponatremia, inappropriately concentrated urine, and exclusion other causes of hyposmolar euvolemic hyponatremia such as hypothyroidism and adrenal insufficiency.

Hyposmolar hypervolemic hyponatremia occurs in patients retaining water in excess of sodium, which leads to an edematous state. Such patients with congestive heart failure, cirrhosis, or nephrotic syndrome retain sodium in response to a decreased effective intravascular volume, which results in a

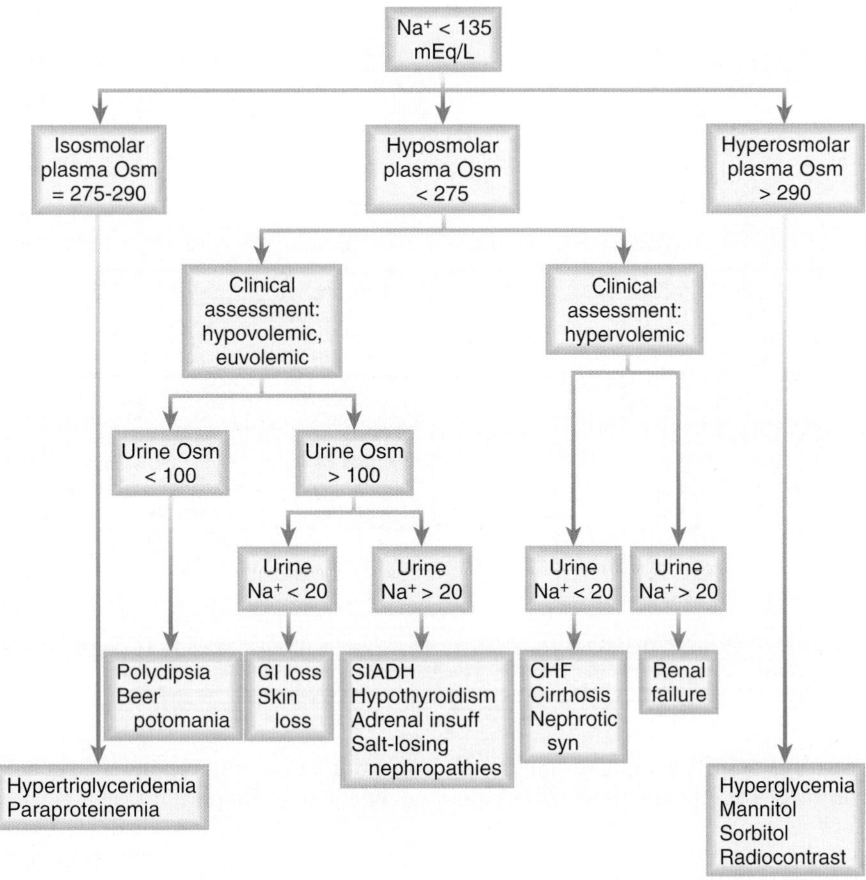


**Fig. 164.1 Diagnostic algorithm for hyponatremia.** *CHF*, Congestive heart failure; *GI*, gastrointestinal; *Osm*, osmolality; *SIADH*, syndrome of inappropriate antidiuretic hormone secretion. (Adapted from Kumar S, Berl T. Sodium. Lancet 1998;352:220-8.)

**BOX 164.1 Causes of Inappropriate Antidiuretic Hormone Secretion**

**Central Nervous System Disease**
Encephalitis, meningitis, abscess, cerebrovascular accident, subdural hematoma, subarachnoid hemorrhage, tumors

**Drugs**
Amiodarone, carbamazepine, clofibrate, chlorpropamide, theophylline, cyclophosphamide, vincristine, tricyclic antidepressants, selective serotonin reuptake inhibitors, ecstasy (3,4-methylenedioxymethamphetamine), nonsteroidal antiinflammatory drugs, exogenous vasopressin, antipsychotic drugs

**Pulmonary Disease**
Abscess, pneumonia, empyema, tuberculosis, aspergillosis, cystic fibrosis

**Malignancy**
Carcinoma (lung, oropharyngeal, gastrointestinal, genitourinary), lymphoma, sarcoma

urine sodium level lower than 20 mEq/L, whereas patients with renal failure produce a urine sodium level higher than 20 mEq/L.

Isosmolar hyponatremia, or "pseudohyponatremia," is observed when laboratory determination of the sodium concentration is affected by large molecules that increase the nonaqueous, sodium-free plasma fraction, which leads to a corresponding decrease in the concentration of sodium per unit volume of serum. The large molecules responsible for pseudohyponatremia are usually derived from a paraproteinemia (as with multiple myeloma) or from hyperlipidemia. Many newer laboratory methods for determination of sodium measure only the aqueous serum component, thereby eliminating the possibility of pseudohyponatremia.

Hyperosmolar hyponatremia commonly results from hyperglycemia. The high osmolality of the extracellular compartment secondary to high serum glucose drives water out of cells and dilutes the concentration of sodium. In the evaluation of a patient with hyperosmolar hyponatremia, a decrease in plasma sodium of 1.6 mEq/L for every 100-mg/dL increase in serum glucose provides an estimate of the degree of hyponatremia. A similar situation may also occur in patients receiving mannitol, sorbitol, or radiocontrast media.

## HYPERNATREMIA

**Figure 164.2** is an algorithm for the diagnosis of hypernatremia.[4] Hypernatremia may also be classified as hypovolemic, euvolemic, or hypervolemic.

Hypovolemic hypernatremia, the most common cause seen in the ED, results from severe depletion of TBW. Urine sodium measurement allows determination of an extrarenal or renal source of the water loss. Levels lower than 10 mEq/L suggest an extrarenal source of the water loss, such as the skin

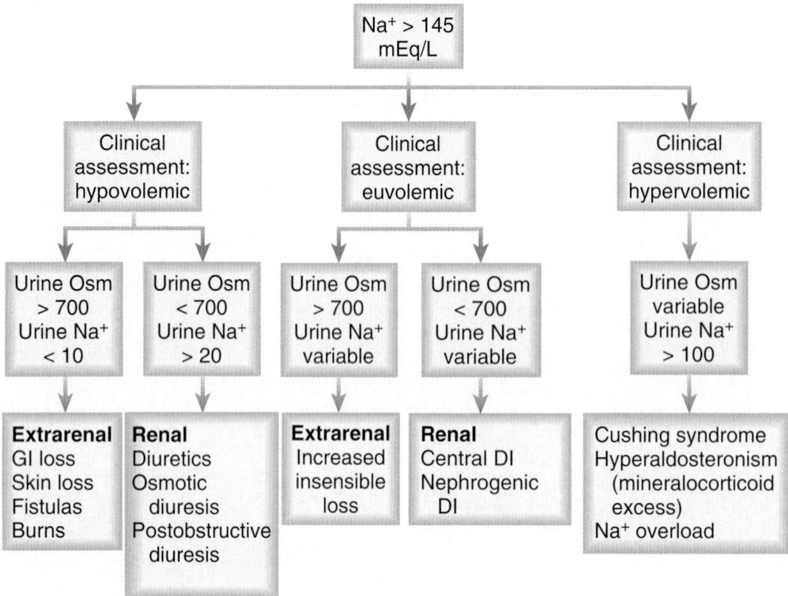


**Fig. 164.2 Diagnostic algorithm for hypernatremia.** *DI*, Diabetes insipidus; *GI*, gastrointestinal; *Osm*, osmolality. (Adapted from Kumar S, Berl T. Sodium. Lancet 1998;352:220-8.)

(excessive sweating or severe burns) or the gastrointestinal system (vomiting or diarrhea). Levels higher than 20 mEq/L suggest renal causes such as excessive diuretic use, osmotic diuresis, postobstructive diuresis, or intrinsic renal disease.[6]

Euvolemic hypernatremia results from water loss without solute loss, with the majority of water loss most notably being from the intracellular space. Water loss occurs from both extrarenal and renal sources. Extrarenal sources include insensible skin and respiratory loss, coupled with lack of water intake because of impaired thirst mechanisms or inability to procure fluids. Urine osmolality is typically high (>700 mOsm/kg) as a result of secretion of ADH. Urine sodium levels vary. Renal water loss occurs secondary to diabetes insipidus (DI) of central or nephrogenic origin and results in dilute urine (urine osmolality < 700 mOsm/kg). Patients with central DI produce dilute urine because of a decrease in ADH secretion from the hypothalamus; those with nephrogenic DI exhibit a decreased response to ADH at the renal tubule.[6]

Hypervolemic hypernatremia is the least common cause seen in the ED patient population. Usually iatrogenic in hospitalized patients, it is observed in the ED as a result of sodium overload from improperly prepared infant formula or home remedies, excessive use of salt tablets, and hyperaldosteronism.

## DIAGNOSTIC TESTING

Accurate laboratory determination of the serum sodium level is critical for accurate diagnosis and proper treatment of hyponatremia and hypernatremia. Clinical information confirms the laboratory results. The possibility of errors in laboratory analysis or blood sampling should be considered when the sodium level and clinical information conflict. A common sampling error occurs when blood samples are obtained proximal to an intravenous (IV) line. When the results are in doubt, a new sample should be obtained to ensure accuracy.

Blood tests for the evaluation of sodium imbalance include plasma osmolality, sodium, potassium, BUN, glucose, and thyroid-stimulating hormone. Although most laboratories will report a plasma osmolality measured by osmometry, determination of sodium, glucose, and BUN allows calculation of osmolality. Plasma osmolality guides the initial classification of hyponatremia as true hyposmolar, hyperosmolar, or isosmolar. The diagnosis of true hyposmolar hyponatremia excludes paraproteinemia, hyperlipidemia, and hyperglycemia as causes of the low laboratory sodium levels. Normal thyroid-stimulating hormone and potassium levels exclude possible thyroid or adrenal causes of euvolemic hyposmolar hyponatremia.

Relevant urine studies include urine osmolality and urine sodium. High urine osmolality indicates the possibility of SIADH, whereas a low value suggests DI, excessive fluid intake, or hyperaldosteronism. Urine sodium levels obtained before the initiation of therapy provide diagnostic information regarding the source of the free water loss.

## TREATMENT

### HYPONATREMIA

Osmotic demyelination syndrome (ODS), the most serious complication of the treatment of hyponatremia, occurs when the administration of relatively hyperosmolar IVF causes intracellular water to rapidly diffuse out of CNS cells. Patients typically improve transiently after IVF administration, only to deteriorate a week after treatment. Signs and symptoms include altered mental status, dysarthria, vertigo, parkinsonism, pseudobulbar palsy, diffuse spastic hypertonia, quadriparesis, and coma. To minimize the risk for ODS, the absolute change in serum sodium over a 48 hour period must not exceed 15 to 20 mEq/L. Additional risk factors for the development of ODS include alcoholism, malnutrition, and liver transplantation.[5]

In patients with severe neurologic symptoms (seizures, coma, or respiratory arrest) and laboratory-confirmed hyposmolar hypovolemic hyponatremia, the likelihood of cerebral edema outweighs the potential risk for treatment-related ODS secondary to rapid correction of the hyponatremic state. In this clinical situation, administration of hypertonic saline (HTS, 3%) is suggested for the first 2 to 4 hours or less if the patient's condition improves with a maximum rate of sodium correction of 1.0 to 2.0 mEq/L/hr. Seizure risk usually declines with a serum sodium correction of approximately 5 mEq/L. Patients with acute hyponatremia for less than 48 hours may tolerate more rapid correction of the sodium concentration. Hyponatremic patients with less severe symptoms usually have a more chronic condition. The risk for ODS outweighs the benefits of rapid correction in this group, and the recommended rate of sodium correction is less than 0.5 mEq/L/hr.[8,14]

The following formula calculates the required volume of IVF needed to correct serum sodium to the desired level:

$$\text{Required fluid volume (L)} = \frac{(\text{Na}_{\text{desired}} - \text{Na}_{\text{measured}})(\text{TBW})}{\text{Na}_{\text{IVF}} - \text{Na}_{\text{measured}}}$$

TBW in liters equals the patient's mass in kilograms multiplied by a constant that depends on the patient's gender and age (young men, 0.6; young women and elderly men, 0.5; elderly women, 0.4).[15] See the "Facts and Formulas" box to determine the sodium content of 1 L of commonly used IVF.

$SI = \frac{SV}{BSA}$ **FACTS AND FORMULAS**

Sodium Content of Commonly Used Intravenous Fluids

| Intravenous Fluid | $Na^+$ (mEq/L) |
|---|---|
| $D_5W$ | 0 |
| 0.45% Saline | 77 |
| 0.9% Saline | 154 |
| 3% Saline | 513 |

*$D_5W$, 5% Dextrose in water.*

For an 80-kg elderly man with seizures and a serum sodium level of 110 mEq/L, the goal of the emergency physician is to increase serum sodium to 115 mEq/L, with the probable effect being cessation of seizure activity. Using 3% saline, the required volume of IVF to attain a serum sodium level of 115 mEq/L is (115 – 110)(80)(0.5)/(513 – 110), which equals 0.496 L (496 mL) of 3% saline to be infused over approximately a 2- or 3-hour period.

Some authors do not endorse the use of formulas to guide the treatment of hyposmolar hyponatremic patients with seizures. Instead, they recommend an empiric IV bolus of 100 mL of 3% HTS, followed by up to two repeated doses if the seizures have not resolved, with the goal of increasing serum sodium 5 to 6 mEq/L in the first 1 to 2 hours of treatment. Monitoring of serum sodium after the second IV bolus and every 2 hours during HTS therapy is required to guide further therapy. HTS is discontinued once serum sodium levels have increased by 10 mEq/L in the first 5 hours or if the symptoms resolve. Further recommendations include avoidance of both overcorrection and an absolute increase exceeding 15 to 20 mEq/L in the first 48 hours of treatment.[16]

Most patients with euvolemic and hypervolemic hyponatremia require restriction of free water intake to 800 to 1000 mL/day. Patients with severe hyponatremia may need IVF to replace the total body sodium deficit.

## HYPERNATREMIA

ED management of hypernatremia requires restoration of plasma volume. The choice of IVF depends on the clinical situation, but 0.9% normal saline (NS) is appropriate in the initial resuscitative treatment phase, with subsequent conversion to a hypotonic IVF such as 0.45% NS when euvolemia is attained.

Once the serum sodium level is known, the goal rate of correction of the sodium concentration is 0.5 to 1.0 mEq/hr, not to exceed 10 mEq/L over a 24-hour period. One approach to correcting the water imbalance resulting in hypernatremia is to calculate the free water deficit and then replace the deficit over a 48-hour period under the assumption that plasma sodium increases approximately 5 mEq/L for each liter of water replaced. The free water deficit is calculated as follows:

$$\text{Free water deficit (L)} = \frac{(\text{Na}_{\text{measured}} - \text{Na}_{\text{desired}})(\text{TBW})}{\text{Na}_{\text{measured}}}$$

In this formula, TBW equals patient mass (kg) multiplied by a constant that depends on the patient's gender and age (young men, 0.6; young women and elderly men, 0.5; elderly women, 0.4). It is important to distinguish acute hypernatremia (<48 hours' duration) from chronic hypernatremia (>48 hours' duration) during ED management because this information has implications for the safe rate of correction of the patient's free water deficit. Five percent dextrose in water ($D_5W$) and 0.45% NS are the fluids most commonly used to replace a free water deficit. Refer to the "Facts and Formulas" box for the sodium content of 1 L of commonly used IVF. The free water deficit in patients with acute hypernatremia is usually replaced over a period of 2 days, whereas the free water deficit in patients with chronic hypernatremia is usually replaced over a period of 3 days to minimize risk for the development of cerebral edema.

For a 55-kg elderly woman with somnolence and dehydration of gradual onset, normal vital signs, a serum sodium level of 158 mEq/L, and a target sodium level of 140 mEq/L, her free water deficit in liters is (158 – 140)(55)(0.4)/158, or 2.506 L (2506 mL). Therefore, she will require approximately 2.5 L of $D_5W$ infused over a 3-day period to slowly correct her serum sodium to normal to minimize her risk for the development of cerebral edema.

Another correction method is to calculate the effect of 1 L of a given IVF on the patient's sodium level by using the following formula and values described by Androgué and Madias (**Box 164.2**)[7]:

$$1\text{ L IVF} = \frac{\text{Na}_{\text{IVF}} - \text{Na}_{\text{measured}}}{\text{TBW} + 1}$$

**BOX 164.2 High-Risk Neurologic Complications Occurring in Hyponatremic Patients**

**Acute Cerebral Edema**
Postoperative menstruating patients
Elderly women taking thiazide diuretics
Pediatric patients
Patients with psychiatric polydipsia
Patients with hypoxemia

**Osmotic Demyelination Syndrome**
Alcoholic patients
Malnourished patients
Patients with hypokalemia
Patients with burns
Elderly women taking thiazide diuretics

Adapted from Lauriat SM, Berl T. The hyponatremic patient: practical focus on therapy. J Am Soc Nephrol 1997;8:1599-607.

Calculation of the decrease in serum sodium for each liter of IVF administered permits close monitoring of the response to therapy. This method may facilitate changes during the course of therapy based on measured sodium levels.

The most serious complication of therapy for hypernatremia is the development of cerebral edema secondary to excessively rapid rehydration (see Box 164.2). In the chronic hypernatremic state, large organic osmolytes that slowly accumulated in CNS cells during the adaptive phase are unable to rapidly diffuse into the extracellular space when a relatively hypotonic fluid is administered.

## REFERENCES

***References can be found on Expert Consult @ www.expertconsult.com.***

# Potassium 165

*Megan Boysen Osborn*

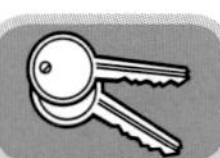

**KEY POINTS**

- Insulin enhances the activity of the sodium-potassium adenosine triphosphate pump, with a resultant decrease in extracellular potassium. Patients with diabetes mellitus are predisposed to hyperkalemia because of impaired insulin feedback and subsequently poor intracellular transfer of potassium.
- Asthmatic patients treated with bronchodilator therapy or epinephrine are predisposed to hypokalemia.
- Renal failure is responsible for the majority of cases of critical hyperkalemia seen in the emergency department.
- Calcium normalizes electrocardiographic manifestations of hyperkalemia within minutes of administration; however, the clinical effects are generally short-lived. Doses may need to be repeated within 30 minutes.
- Regular (short-acting) insulin administered as a 10-unit intravenous bolus will begin to lower serum potassium concentrations within 10 to 20 minutes, and the clinical effect lasts several hours. An ampule of 50% dextrose in water should be given concurrently to prevent hypoglycemia.
- Nebulized albuterol in 10- to 20-mg continuous treatments will transiently decrease serum potassium by 1 mEq/L over a 1- to 2-hour period.
- Definitive treatment of hyperkalemia is elimination of potassium. Hemodialysis is indicated for severe cases of hyperkalemia; when potassium-free dialysate is used, hemodialysis can reduce serum potassium by 1.5 mEq/hr.

## PERSPECTIVE

Potassium is the major intracellular cation and is closely regulated by the sodium-potassium adenosine triphosphatase ($Na^+$,$K^+$-ATPase) pump. Hypokalemia and hyperkalemia are electrolyte abnormalities common to both hospitalized and emergency department (ED) patients.[1]

Hypokalemia is observed more frequently than hyperkalemia and affects a broader range of patients; diuretic therapy accounts for as much as 80% of clinically significant cases seen in the ED.[2] Hypokalemia is defined as a serum potassium level lower than 3.5 mEq/L. It is further classified as mild (3 to 3.5 mEq/L), moderate (2.5 to 2.9 mEq/L), and severe (<2.5 mEq/L).

Hyperkalemia, a disorder that affects patients with underlying renal insufficiency almost exclusively,[1] is defined as a potassium level higher than 5.0 mEq/L. Hyperkalemia is further classified as mild (5 to 6 mEq/L), moderate (6.1 to 7 mEq/L), and severe (>7 mEq/L).

Both disorders can result in cardiac dysfunction, arrhythmia, and death.

## PATHOPHYSIOLOGY

Total body potassium ($K^+$) is approximately 50 mEq/kg, or 3500 to 4000 mEq, in a normal-sized adult. For conversion purposes, 1 mEq of potassium is equivalent to 39.09 mg. Potassium is the major intracellular cation, and more than 98% of total body potassium is stored in the intracellular space. Intracellular fluid concentrations of potassium range from 150 to 160 mEq/L, with the highest amounts sequestered either in muscle (75%) or in bones and cartilage (8% to 10%).[2]

Extracellular potassium makes up less than 2% of total body stores, only two thirds of which is measurable in serum sampling. The normal range of plasma concentrations reported by most laboratory testing is 3.5 to 5 mEq/L; this small fraction is not reflective of total body potassium. Strict regulation of the ratio of intracellular to extracellular potassium (150 to 4 mEq/L) maintains a critical voltage gradient across cell membranes and plays a crucial role in establishing membrane potentials in cardiac and neuromuscular cells.[1] The $Na^+$,$K^+$-ATPase transmembrane pump continuously maintains this gradient by actively transporting potassium into and sodium ($Na^+$) out of cells[1] (**Fig. 165.1**). Large changes in the intracellular potassium concentration have little effect on the ratio of intracellular to extracellular potassium. Conversely, even small changes in the extracellular concentration significantly affect this ratio, the transmembrane potential gradient, and the function of cardiac and neuromuscular tissue.[1]

All potassium disorders result from one of three disturbances[3]: impaired potassium intake, impaired distribution of potassium between the intracellular and extracellular spaces, and impaired renal excretion of potassium (**Fig. 165.2**).

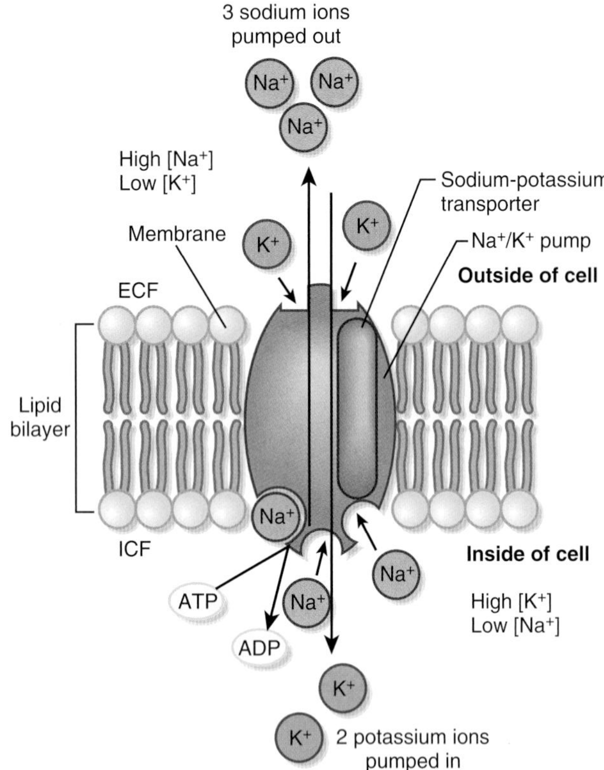


**Fig. 165.1 The Na⁺,K⁺-ATPase pump.** *ADP*, Adenosine diphosphate; *ATP*, adenosine triphosphate; *ECF*, extracellular fluid; *ICF*, intracellular fluid.

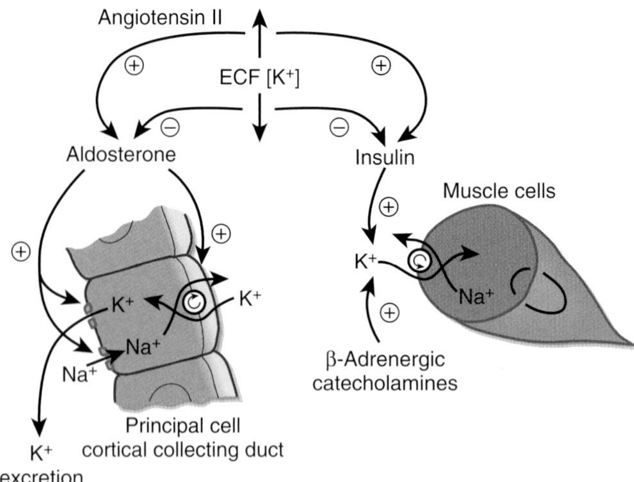


**Fig. 165.2 Regulators of potassium homeostasis.** *ECF*, Extracellular fluid.

## CLINICAL PRESENTATION

### HYPOKALEMIA

Approximately 20% of hospitalized patients are found to have subtherapeutic serum potassium levels.[1] Despite this disease prevalence, most patients are asymptomatic, and only 5% of these patients have clinically significant hypokalemia.

In the outpatient setting, roughly 18% of patients have mild hypokalemia, which is generally asymptomatic. The vast majority of these cases (80%) are caused by potassium-wasting diuretic medications.[2] Men and women are affected equally.

Symptoms of hypokalemia are determined by the degree of hypokalemia, the cell or organ type affected, and the general health of the patient. Healthy patients with gradual-onset hypokalemia are usually asymptomatic and have mild to moderate potassium depletion.

The effects of low serum potassium levels can range from vague myalgias to life-threatening paralysis or dysrhythmias. Because potassium is the major intracellular ion that maintains the charge gradient across cell membranes, any alteration in its concentration will have broad effects on muscle, cardiac, and gastrointestinal tissue. Skeletal muscle cells are the first to be affected, with patients experiencing cramping, fasciculations, and tetany. In patients with underlying ischemic heart disease or congestive heart failure, hypokalemia-induced dysrhythmia with mild to moderate potassium depletion is more likely to develop.

**Box 165.1** summarizes the clinical findings of hypokalemia.

#### *Mild Hypokalemia (3 to 3.5 mEq/L)*

Patients without significant comorbid conditions tolerate mild hypokalemia very well. Muscular symptoms are generally absent, although occasionally patients experience mild cramping or early muscle fatigue. Hypokalemia may affect smooth muscle function in the gastrointestinal tract with resultant constipation or abdominal cramping, or both. Cardiac and neurologic symptoms are absent.

#### *Moderate Hypokalemia (2.5 to 2.9 mEq/L)*

Muscular symptoms become more pronounced as the degree of hypokalemia worsens; the weakness is generalized, but proximal and lower extremity muscle groups are typically affected to a greater degree.[2] Cardiac manifestations may include palpitations, non–life-threatening dysrhythmias (premature atrial contractions, premature ventricular contractions), and atrial fibrillation. Electrocardiographic (ECG) changes occur but do not correlate with the degree of hypokalemia (**Box 165.2; Fig. 165.3**).

Hypokalemia may precipitate or worsen encephalopathy in patients with severe liver disease. Potassium depletion increases renal production of ammonia, which readily crosses the blood-brain barrier in the setting of alkalosis.[2] Hypokalemia also inhibits the release of insulin and may cause hyperglycemia in patients with preexisting glucose intolerance or non–insulin-dependent diabetes mellitus. The renal complications of moderate hypokalemia reflect vasopressin resistance to the tubular reabsorption of water; symptoms include nocturia, polydipsia, and polyuria.[2]

#### *Severe Hypokalemia (<2.5 mEq/L)*

Alcoholics have the greatest risk for severe hypokalemia. Musculoskeletal symptoms include pronounced fasciculations, tetany, and rhabdomyolysis. Myolysis may cause a transient release of intracellular potassium that can mask the inciting hypokalemic state. In rare cases, life-threatening ascending paralysis and loss of deep tendon reflexes can result in quadriplegia.[2]

Cardiac manifestations of severe hypokalemia worsen the previously mentioned ECG abnormalities. Of great

**BOX 165.1 Clinical Findings in Hypokalemia**

**Gastrointestinal**
Ileus (nausea, vomiting, distention)

**Vascular**
Postural hypotension (decreased peripheral resistance and autonomic dysfunction)

**Cardiac**
Ventricular arrhythmias
Cardiac arrest
Bradycardia, tachycardia
Premature ventricular contractions, premature atrial complexes
Electrocardiographic abnormalities (see Box 165.2)
Enhanced digitalis toxicity

**Respiratory**
Hypoventilation, respiratory distress
Respiratory failure

**Neurologic**
Lethargy
Changes in mental status
Paralysis

**Muscular**
Cramping, restless legs syndrome
Decreased muscle strength, paralysis
Fasciculations, tetany
Decreased deep tendon reflexes
Rhabdomyolysis

**Renal**
Nephrogenic diabetes insipidus
Metabolic alkalosis
Impaired urinary concentrating ability (polyuria)
Increased ammonia production and hydrogen ion excretion
Hypokalemic nephropathy (interstitial renal disease)

**Other**
Cushingoid appearance (edema)
Inhibition of insulin release
Aldosterone inhibition
Negative nitrogen balance

Modified from Zull DN. Disorders of potassium metabolism. Emerg Med Clin North Am 1989;7:771-94.

**BOX 165.2 Electrocardiographic Abnormalities in Mild to Moderate Hypokalemia**

Low, flattened, or inverted T waves
Potassium concentration usually less than 3.5 mEq/L
Decreased or depressed ST segment
Increased PR interval
Increased QRS duration
U waves
- Taller than T waves
- Seen in septal leads ($V_2$, $V_3$)

Prominent R wave
Atrial or ventricular arrhythmias

Adapted from Cohn JN, Kowey PR, Whelton PK, et al. New guidelines for potassium replacement in clinical practice. Arch Intern Med 2000;160: 2429-46; and Zull DN. Disorders of potassium metabolism. Emerg Med Clin North Am 1989;7:771–94.

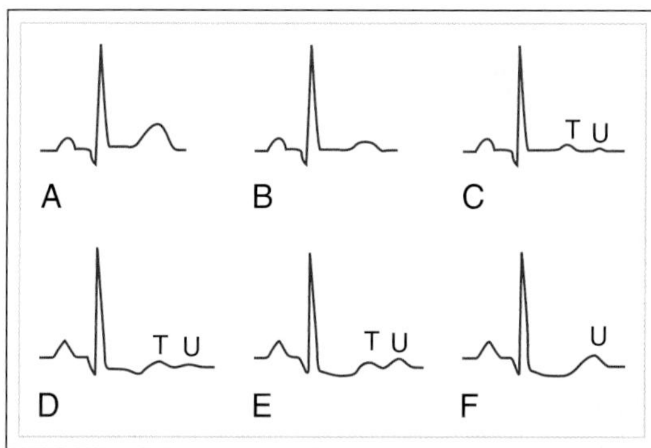


**Fig. 165.3 Electrocardiographic findings in hypokalemia.** **A,** Normal. **B,** Mild T-wave flattening (the earliest change). **C,** U wave associated with T-wave flattening. **D,** Slight ST depression and a "pseudo–P pulmonale" pattern. **E,** ST depression is more noticeable, and the U wave increases in amplitude. **F,** The U wave overtakes the T wave—"QU" prolongation.

concern is the development of potentially life-threatening ventricular arrhythmias in patients with preexisting cardiac disease. Ventricular ectopy ranges from premature ventricular contractions to couplets, bigeminy, trigeminy, and episodes of ventricular tachycardia, torsades de pointes, and ventricular fibrillation. In the setting of myocardial infarction or digitalis toxicity, hypokalemia-induced ventricular dysrhythmias are directly proportional to the degree of potassium depletion.[2]

## HYPERKALEMIA

Hyperkalemia is often asymptomatic and discovered only on routine laboratory screening. When symptoms do occur, conduction abnormalities at the cellular level promote cardiac and neuromuscular findings. ECG abnormalities may not be present even with severe hyperkalemia; ventricular fibrillation may be the first cardiac manifestation.

### *Mild Hyperkalemia (5 to 6 mEq/L)*

Mild hyperkalemia is generally asymptomatic. Patients with underlying cardiac disease occasionally report palpitations or other well-tolerated disturbances in rhythm.

### *Moderate Hyperkalemia (6.1 to 7 mEq/L)*

Patients with moderate hyperkalemia may exhibit ECG abnormalities, including peaked T waves and prolongation of the PR interval and QRS complex[4] (**Figs. 165.4 to 165.7; Box 165.3**).

Neuromuscular symptoms similar to those seen with hypokalemia can occur. Muscle cramps and weakness are the most commonly reported complaints.

### *Severe Hyperkalemia (>7 mEq/L)*

Progressively worsening hyperkalemia can result in significant conduction abnormalities, heart block, potentially life-threatening arrhythmias, and asystole. Symptoms such as palpitations, syncope, chest pain, and dyspnea (from left-sided heart failure) may be present. Ascending paralysis and tetany may result.

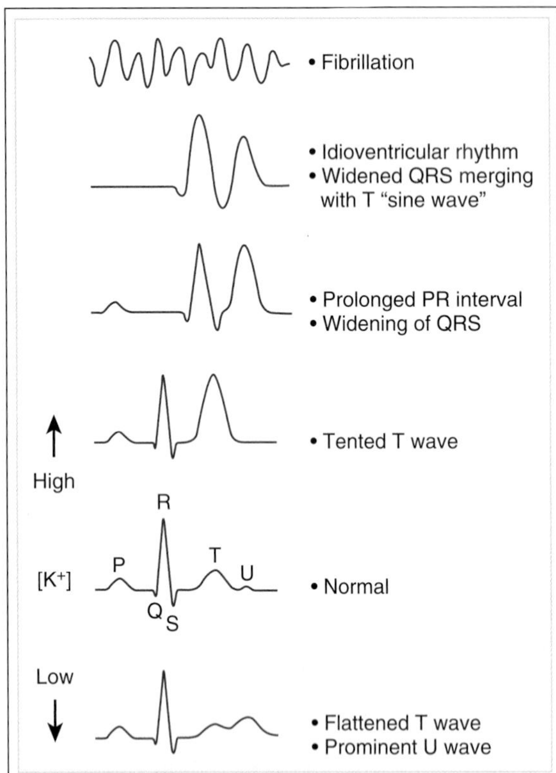


**Fig. 165.4 Electrocardiographic findings in hyperkalemia.** (Adapted from Gennari FJ. Disorders of potassium homeostasis: hypokalemia and hyperkalemia. Crit Care Clin 2002;18:273-88.)

## DIAGNOSTIC TESTING

### HYPOKALEMIA

Historical elements that may mandate measurement of serum potassium include potential causes of inadequate intake (malnutrition, alcoholism) and excessive wasting (diarrhea, vomiting, polyuria). Long-standing use of diuretics, $\beta_2$-agonists, or laxatives should also prompt potassium screening.

In the ED, evaluation should focus on identification of hypokalemia by laboratory testing, classification of disease severity, correlation with findings on physical examination,

**BOX 165.3 Electrocardiographic Manifestations of Hyperkalemia**

**Mild Hyperkalemia**
Peaked T waves
Shortened QT interval (early repolarization)

**Moderate Hyperkalemia**
Prolonged PR interval
Diminished P-wave amplitude
Widened QRS
Bundle branch blocks
Second- and third-degree heart block

**Severe Hyperkalemia**
Absence of P wave
Atrioventricular nodal block
Widened QRS
Sine wave
Ventricular fibrillation
Asystole

Adapted from Mattu A, Brady WJ, Robinson DA. Electrocardiographic manifestations of hyperkalemia. Am J Emerg Med 2000;18:721-9.

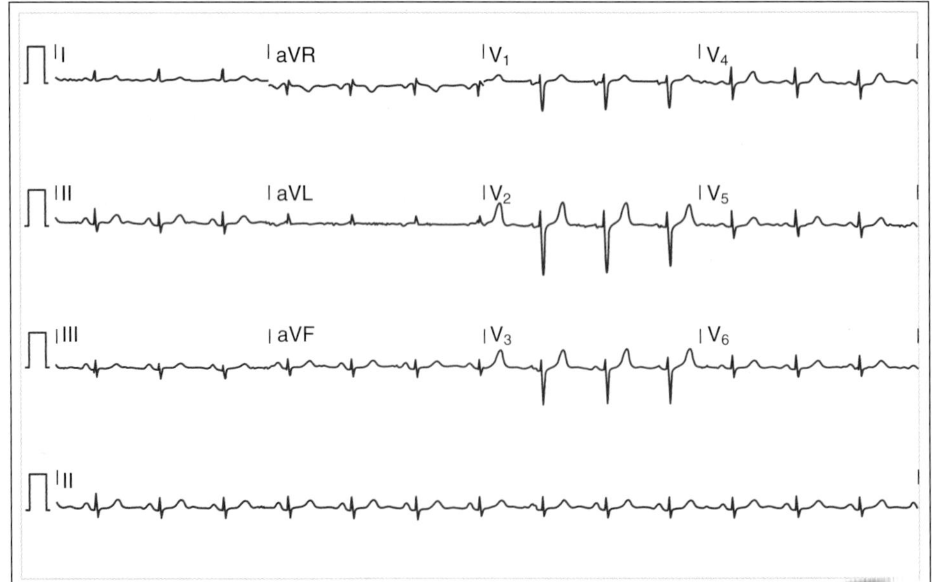


**Fig. 165.5 Baseline electrocardiogram in a patient 1 month before emergency department evaluation ($K^+$ = 4.3 mmol/L).**

and correction or stabilization of potentially life-threatening conditions.

If hypokalemia is identified, screening for hypomagnesemia and hypophosphatemia is necessary; these coexistent entities are difficult to distinguish from hypokalemia by physical examination alone. Urine pH higher than 6 suggests type I renal tubular acidosis; urine electrolytes and venous blood gas analysis should be obtained to search for a corresponding normal–anion gap metabolic acidosis.

If the patient is taking digoxin, a serum digoxin level is indicated; hypokalemia potentiates digitalis toxicity and increases the likelihood of cardiac dysrhythmias. Additional laboratory testing and imaging can be performed later in the inpatient or outpatient setting.

## HYPERKALEMIA

Patients with hyperkalemia be asymptomatic or have life-threatening cardiovascular disturbances. Historical features that should raise suspicion for hyperkalemia include known acute or chronic renal insufficiency, potassium supplementation, and ECG changes following an incomplete hemodialysis session. End-stage renal dialysis patients who have missed a scheduled dialysis session should be placed on a cardiac monitor and immediately be screened for ECG abnormalities and electrolyte disturbances.

The first sign of hyperkalemia may be abnormal ECG findings on arrival at the ED. If hyperkalemia is suspected in an asymptomatic renal patient with abnormal ECG findings, a complete serum chemistry panel should be obtained, as well

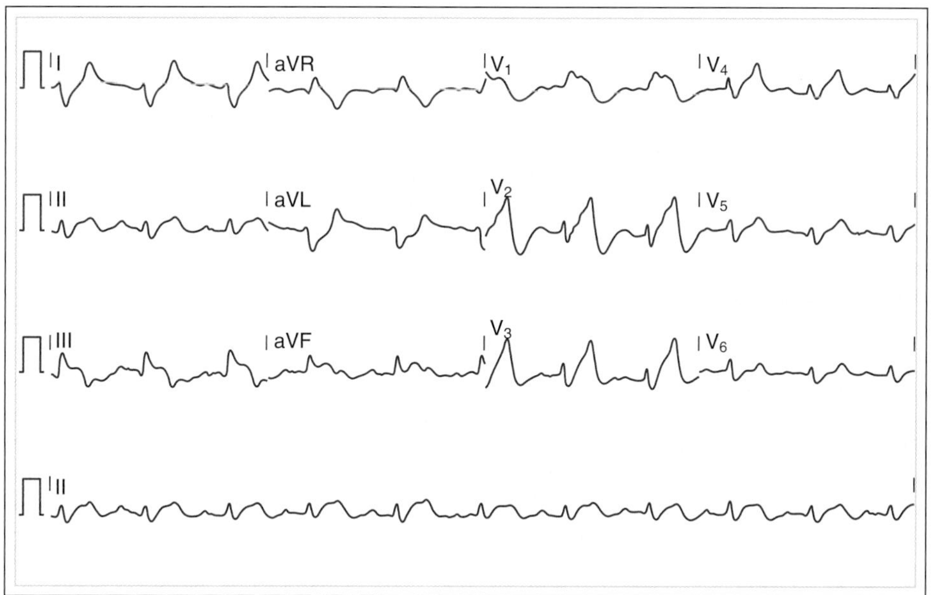


**Fig. 165.6** Patient with severe hyperkalemia on arrival at the emergency department ($K^+$ = 8.3 mmol/L).

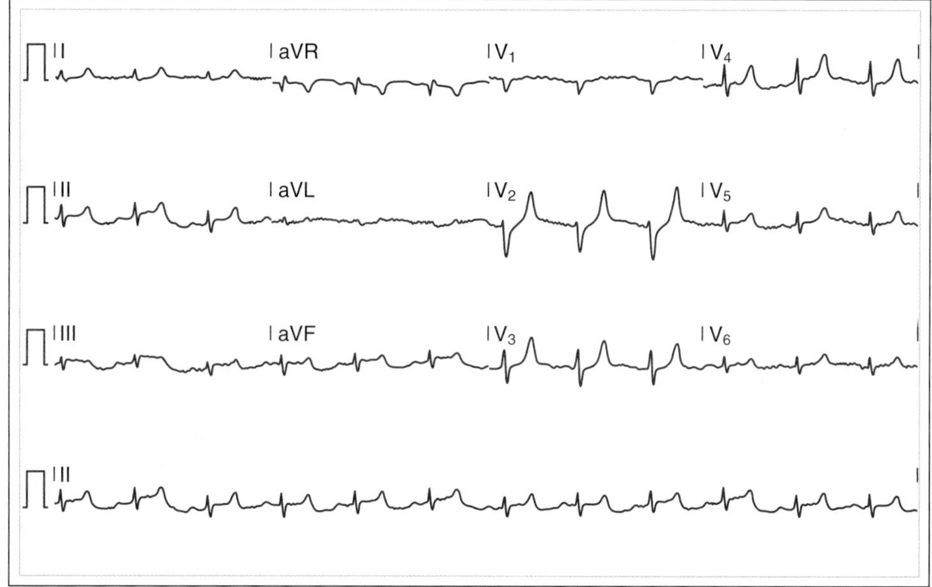


**Fig. 165.7** Patient during treatment of severe hyperkalemia, now with mild to moderate hyperkalemia ($K^+$ = 6.3 mmol/L).

**Table 165.1 Treatment of Hypokalemia**

| FORMULATION | DOSAGE REGIMEN | INDICATION |
|---|---|---|
| Oral KCl | 20-80 mEq/day divided 2-3 times per day | Non-urgent correction and/or maintenance therapy with diuretic use |
| Oral KCl liquid (recheck serum $K^+$ in 24-72 hr) | 40-60 mEq per dose | Rapid elevation in patients requiring urgent, but not emergency correction |
| Intravenous KCl | 10-20 mEq/hr (recheck serum $K^+$ after giving 60 mEq) | For patients with severe symptoms or inability to tolerate oral therapy |

Adapted from Zull DN. Disorders of potassium metabolism. Emerg Med Clin North Am 1989;7:771-94; and Schaefer TJ, Wolford RW. Disorders of potassium. Emerg Med Clin North Am 2005;23:723-47.

as a whole blood potassium level measured by venous blood gas analysis. Arterial or venous blood gas sampling is generally the most efficient method of obtaining an accurate measurement of the potassium concentration.

Additional laboratory tests useful in the ED evaluation of hyperkalemia include serum calcium, creatinine, digoxin, and blood pH. Other testing can be deferred to the inpatient setting.

## TREATMENT (Table 165.1)

### HYPOKALEMIA

#### *Patients with Cardiovascular Disease*

Optimal goals for serum potassium repletion are predicated on the underlying pathology. Patients with a history of congestive heart failure, coronary artery disease, or dysrhythmias and hypertensive patients being treated with diuretic medications should have a serum potassium level of at least 4 mEq/L. These patients require oral supplementation for even mild, asymptomatic hypokalemia with potassium chloride tablets (20 to 40 mEq daily).[5] If the patient is taking a potassium-sparing diuretic, the dose should be decreased.

#### *Asymptomatic Mild Hypokalemia*

Healthy patients with asymptomatic, mild hypokalemia (3 to 3.5 mEq/L) do not require pharmacologic potassium supplementation. Treatment should be focused on minimizing further potassium loss and increasing oral intake. Patients should be encouraged to eat a diet rich in potassium (**Box 165.4**). Potassium-wasting diuretics should be decreased or eliminated, as blood pressure allows. Use of substances that contain glycyrrhizic acid (e.g., licorice, chewing tobacco, laxatives) should be avoided.[1,6]

#### *Symptomatic Mild and Moderate Hypokalemia*

Potassium supplementation is required for patients with symptomatic mild or moderate (<3 mEq/L) hypokalemia. Potassium supplements are available in several forms: potassium chloride, potassium phosphate, potassium citrate, potassium acetate, potassium gluconate, and potassium bicarbonate. Potassium chloride is the preferred formulation for most ED cases of hypokalemia. Potassium phosphate may be beneficial in certain cases of diabetic ketoacidosis.[6] Oral potassium supplements are available as tablets, powder, or elixir.

**BOX 165.4 Foods Rich in Potassium**

**Highest Content (>1000 mg/100 g)**
Figs
Molasses

**Very High Content (>500 mg/100 g)**
Dates, prunes
Nuts
Avocados
Bran
Wheat germ
Lima beans

**High Content (>250 mg/100 g)**
Vegetables—spinach, tomatoes, broccoli, beets, potatoes
Fruits—bananas, cantaloupe, oranges, mangos, kiwi
Meat—beef, pork, veal, lamb

Adapted from Cohn JN, Kowey PR, Whelton PK, et al. New guidelines for potassium replacement in clinical practice. Arch Intern Med 2000;160:2429-36.

Dosing ranges from 20 to 80 mEq/day; doses greater than 40 mEq should be divided and given either two or three times per day. Oral therapy should be monitored daily because serum potassium levels will rise within 48 to 72 hours.[6] Healthy patients who require daily oral supplementation can be discharged from the ED safely if repeated serum potassium measurements can be monitored by the primary care physician for 1 to 2 days. Patients who are elderly, have significant comorbid conditions, or have poor access to follow-up should be admitted to the hospital for a 24-hour observation period.

Magnesium deficiency should be suspected in patients who fail to respond to oral potassium therapy within 96 hours. Magnesium promotes activity of the $Na^+,K^+$-ATPase pump, which will replenish intracellular fluid concentrations in the first days of potassium supplementation.[6]

#### *Severe Hypokalemia*

Intravenous (IV) potassium replacement is indicated for patients with severe hypokalemia (<2.5 mEq/L) or moderate hypokalemia accompanied by cardiac arrhythmias, familial periodic paralysis, or severe myopathy.[6]

Replacement consists of 100 mEq of potassium chloride in 1 L of normal saline (or 5% dextrose in water [$D_5W$]) infused

**Table 165.2 Treatment of Hyperkalemia**

| MEDICATION | DOSAGE REGIMEN | ONSET | DURATION |
|---|---|---|---|
| **Cardiac Stabilization** | | | |
| Calcium chloride | 1 ampule (10 mL) over 2-5 min | 1-3 min | 30-40 min |
| Calcium gluconate | 10 mL of a 10% solution | 1-3 min | 20-60 min |
| **Transcellular Shift** | | | |
| Insulin | 10 units IV with 50 mL of 50% dextrose (one ampule of $D_{50}W$) *or* 10 units in 500 mL $D_{10}W$ over a 1-hr infusion | 10-20 min | 2-4 hr |
| Albuterol nebulized over 20-60 min | 10-20 mg in 4 mL NS | 20-30 min | 2-4 hr |
| **Elimination** | | | |
| Kayexalate | 30 g PO | 2 hr PO | 4-6 hr |
| | 50 g PR | 1 hr PO | 4-6 hr |
| Lasix (furosemide) | 20-40 mg IVP | Variable | Variable |
| Hemodialysis | | Minutes | Variable |

Adapted from Zull DN. Disorders of potassium metabolism. Emerg Med Clin North Am 1989;7:771-94; and Schaefer TJ, Wolford RW. Disorders of potassium. Emerg Med Clin North Am 2005;23:723-47.

*$D_{10}W$*, 10% Dextrose in water; *IV*, intravenously; *IVP*, intravenous push; *NS*, normal saline; *PO*, orally; *PR*, rectally.

at a rate of 100 to 200 mL/hr (10 to 20 mEq/hr). If the patient has any form of heart block or renal insufficiency, the initial infusion rate should be reduced to 50 mL/hr (5 mEq/hr).

In rare instances of extreme hypokalemia or life-threatening clinical findings, potassium may be infused at a rate of 40 to 60 mEq/hr (400 to 600 mEq/L of normal saline at 100 mL/hr) for a short period (10 to 20 minutes). Therapy should be monitored with great caution. Serum potassium levels should be rechecked after every 40 to 60 mEq infused.

IV potassium supplementation can cause excruciating phlebitis and cardiac arrest if directly injected into a vessel—potassium should never be administered as an IV push. Peripheral IV lines can be used for rates of 10 to 20 mEq/hr or less. In cases of moderate hypokalemia, potassium infusions should remain at 10 mEq/hr. To minimize the risk for phlebitis, a central line is necessary for infusion rates greater than 20 mEq/hr (see earlier indications). There is a theoretic concern for cardiac arrest when potassium is administered via central venous access—splitting the potassium infusion rate over two peripheral lines may be preferable.[2]

In general, patients receiving IV potassium supplementation require telemetry monitoring and frequent repeated potassium measurements (up to every 1 to 3 hours after the initial infusion begins). Significant potassium depletion may take days to correct. As serum potassium levels approach 3.5 mEq/L, patients should be converted to oral therapy if possible. IV potassium supplementation should be discontinued if any ECG signs of hyperkalemia are noted or if a single potassium measurement is higher than 3.5 mEq/L.

Unstable ventricular arrhythmias resulting from severe hypokalemia should be managed according to standard practice guidelines. Severe neuromuscular manifestations may endanger adequate respiratory effort and therefore mandate aggressive airway stabilization. Any volume depletion should be corrected, and coexisting medical conditions that may exacerbate the effects of hypokalemia should be addressed.[1]

## HYPERKALEMIA

Management of hyperkalemia focuses on three goals of care: cardiac stabilization, transcellular shift of potassium from extracellular fluid to intracellular fluid, and elimination of excess potassium (**Table 165.2**). Only potassium excretion is a definitive treatment step—other actions serve to temporarily stabilize the cell membrane in an effort to prevent hemodynamic collapse.

## CARDIAC STABILIZATION: CALCIUM

IV calcium rapidly antagonizes the adverse effects of moderate to severe hyperkalemia on cell membrane potential in cardiac myocytes. Calcium can be administered as IV calcium chloride or calcium gluconate, even in patients who are normocalcemic. IV preparations of calcium chloride contain three times more calcium per ampule than do calcium gluconate formulations. Calcium chloride is more likely than calcium gluconate to cause tissue necrosis if it extravasates.[7] Calcium normalizes ECG manifestations of hyperkalemia

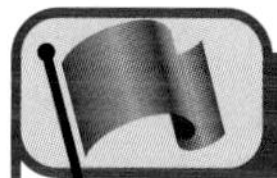

**RED FLAGS**

**Calcium Supplementation**

Calcium chloride may cause significant skin necrosis if extravasated.

Calcium should not be administered with solutions that contain sodium bicarbonate because calcium carbonate ($CaCO_3$) will precipitate.

Intravenous calcium boluses should be avoided in hyperkalemic patients with suspected digoxin toxicity because of the risk for cardiac tetany or fatal arrhythmia. Slow calcium infusions (over a 30-minute period) require close monitoring of these patients.

within minutes of administration; however, the clinical effects are generally short-lived. Doses may need to be repeated within 30 minutes or if no effects are observed within 5 to 10 minutes of the initial dose. Calcium should be administered to patients with hyperkalemia-induced ECG changes, and caution should be exercised in patients taking digoxin.

### Transcellular Shift: Insulin and Albuterol

Potassium can be temporarily shifted from the extracellular to the intracellular compartment through stimulation of the $Na^+,K^+$-ATPase pump by insulin or a $\beta_2$-agonist such as albuterol. Although either of these agents can temporize moderate hyperkalemia when given alone, studies suggest that combination therapy with both agents may be more efficacious.

Insulin forces a transcellular shift of potassium into liver and muscle cells. Regular (short-acting) insulin administered as a 10-unit IV bolus will begin to lower serum potassium concentrations within 10 to 20 minutes, and the clinical effect lasts several hours. An ampule of $D_{50}W$ should be given concurrently to prevent hypoglycemia; patients who are already hyperglycemic (>250 mg/dL) do not require supplemental dextrose. Blood glucose should be rechecked 1 hour after insulin administration because hypoglycemia may develop despite initial supplementation with dextrose.

Albuterol is the most readily available $\beta_2$-agonist used to treat hyperkalemia in the ED. Nebulized albuterol in 10- to 20-mg continuous treatments will decrease serum potassium by 1 mEq/L over a 1- to 2-hour period.[8] Though not approved for use in the United States, IV administration of albuterol shifts potassium into the intracellular fluid compartment even more rapidly. Once routinely used for treatment of hyperkalemia, the use of sodium bicarbonate has been challenged. Recent studies have demonstrated that sodium bicarbonate may only enhance urinary elimination of potassium and does not function at a cellular level. It may especially have a deleterious effect on anuric patients and worsen the degree of intracellular acidosis.[9]

### Elimination: Resin Exchange (Kayexalate) and Dialysis

Definitive treatment of hyperkalemia is elimination of potassium. For patients with renal insufficiency, resin exchange (Kayexalate) and dialysis are the mainstays of therapy. Potassium-wasting diuretics (thiazides, loop diuretics) may be taken by patients with normal renal function and mild asymptomatic hyperkalemia. Sodium bicarbonate infusion may also promote renal secretion of potassium but is no longer considered a first-line agent in the treatment of hyperkalemia.

Sodium polystyrene sulfonate (Kayexalate) is an inert resin that exchanges sodium for potassium in the intestinal tract. One gram of Kayexalate removes approximately 0.5 to 1 mEq of potassium in exchange for 2 to 3 mEq of sodium.[8] The usual dose of Kayexalate is 30 to 60 g given orally or rectally. Oral Kayexalate begins to reduce total body potassium within several hours of administration, and the clinical effect lasts 4 to 6 hours. Rectal Kayexalate has a shorter time to onset than the oral formulation but is less efficacious.

Emerging literature questions the efficacy and safety of Kayexalate. Although Kayexalate reliably decreases serum potassium when administered over a period of several days, recent literature reviews suggest that the acute effects of the resin may not be as significant as once thought.[10] Colonic necrosis, ischemic colitis, colonic bleeding, and perforation have been reported when Kayexalate is combined with 70% sorbitol.[9] Kayexalate is often premixed with 33% sorbitol to prevent resin-induced constipation, and there is little evidence to suggest that Kayexalate with 33% sorbitol causes significant colonic pathology at standard doses.[11] Very rare instances of colonic injury have been observed when 33% sorbitol is coadministered with Kayexalate as an enema to patients after recent colon surgery.[10,11] High-dose Kayexalate precipitates pulmonary edema by increasing extracellular sodium in fluid-overloaded patients.

Hemodialysis is the most rapid method of potassium elimination in patients with persistent, symptomatic, or severe hyperkalemia. If a potassium-free dialysate is used, serum potassium may decrease as much as 1.5 mEq/L/hr. Stable patients may be transferred to an inpatient hemodialysis unit for therapy under strict cardiac monitoring. Patients with ECG abnormalities, hypotension, significant volume overload, or respiratory distress should undergo dialysis in the ED or intensive care unit. Cell membrane stabilization with IV calcium, IV insulin or glucose, and inhalational albuterol is necessary to prevent arrhythmia while awaiting emergency hemodialysis.

## REFERENCES

*References can be found on Expert Consult @ www.expertconsult.com.*

# Calcium, Magnesium, and Phosphorus 166

*Katrina A. Leone*

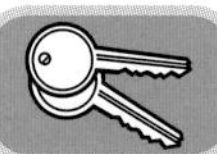

**KEY POINTS**

- Regulation of calcium, magnesium, and phosphorus is interrelated, and abnormalities in one are highly correlated with other electrolyte abnormalities.
- Severely depressed mental status and precipitation of arrhythmias are the most dangerous consequences of severe abnormalities in calcium, magnesium, or phosphorus.
- Proper correction of electrolyte deficiencies requires knowledge of the various oral and intravenous electrolyte preparations available.

$SI = \frac{SV}{BSA}$ **FACTS AND FORMULAS**

| | |
|---|---|
| Normal serum calcium level | 8.5-10.5 mg/dL (2.1-2.6 mmol/dL) |
| Normal ionized calcium level | 4.5-5.6 mg/dL (1.1-1.4 mmol/L) |
| Normal serum magnesium level | 1.8-2.5 mg/dL (0.74-0.94 mmol/L) |
| Normal serum phosphorus level | 2.5-4.5 mg/dL (0.81-1.45 mmol/L) |
| Total serum calcium level corrected for albumin: | For every 1 g/dL in albumin, serum calcium drops 0.8 mg/dL |
| Corrected calcium (mg/dL) | Measured calcium (mg/dL) + 0.8[4.4 − albumin (g/dL)] |

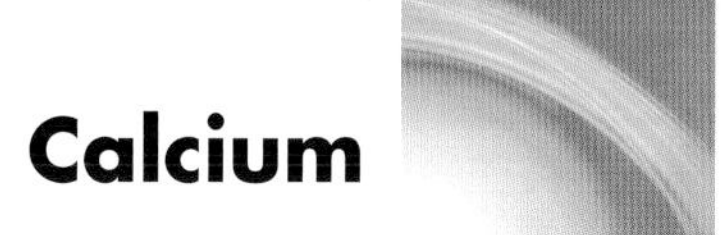

## Calcium

Approximately 99% of total body calcium is located in bone as the calcium phosphate salt hydroxyapatite. Of the remaining total body calcium, 45% is bound to albumin; 10% is complexed with circulating ions such as bicarbonate, phosphate, citrate, or sulfate[1]; and the remaining 45% is found in the free, ionized form. The normal range for serum calcium is 8.5 to 10.5 mg/dL, with some variability among different laboratories. The normal range of ionized (unbound) calcium is 4.5 to 5.6 mg/dL, but this is often reported in the international units (SI units) of mmol/L, with the normal range being 1.1 to 1.4 mmol/L. This ionized fraction is responsible for the physiologic actions of calcium and is not dependent on albumin levels. The total serum calcium level can be corrected for the amount of serum albumin (see the "Facts and Formulas" box), but such correction can be unreliable, so an ionized calcium level should be obtained whenever true hypercalcemia or hypocalcemia is a concern.

The plasma concentration of calcium is tightly maintained within the normal range by a feedback-regulated endocrine system that balances interactions among the small intestines, kidneys, bones, parathyroid glands, thyroid gland, and bloodstream. The key regulatory molecules in this system include calcium, phosphorus, parathyroid hormone (PTH), and 1,25-dihydroxyvitamin D (calcitriol)[1,2] (**Fig. 166.1**).

## HYPERCALCEMIA

### EPIDEMIOLOGY

Hypercalcemia is defined as a total serum calcium level greater than 10.5 mg/dL and is often divided into categories to describe the severity of symptoms as mild (10.5 to 11.9 mg/dL), moderate (12 to 13.9 mg/dL), and severe (>14 mg/dL).

The prevalence of hypercalcemia is approximately 0.5% to 3% in hospitalized adults.[3] Hyperparathyroidism is the most common cause of hypercalcemia, and the incidence of primary hyperparathyroidism is approximately 21 cases per 100,000 person-years.[4]

The paraneoplastic syndrome hypercalcemia of malignancy is the second most common cause of hypercalcemia and occurs in approximately 10% to 30% of patients with cancer. Multiple myeloma and lung, breast, and prostate malignancies are most often associated with this disorder. It is typically seen in the end stages of disease and indicates a poor prognosis.[5]

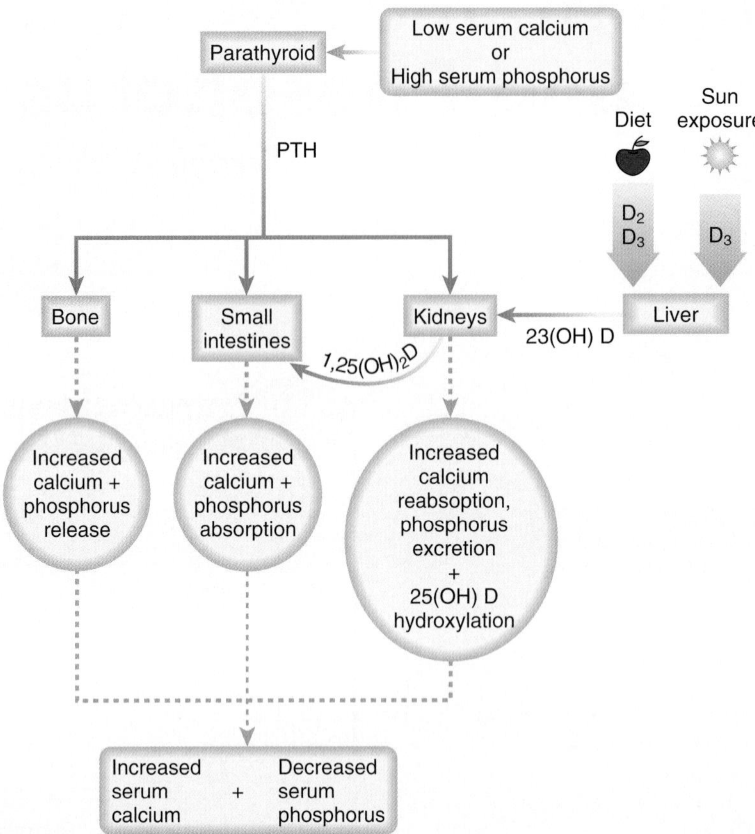


**Fig. 166.1 Calcium homeostasis.** Parathyroid hormone (PTH) is released from the parathyroid glands in response to hypocalcemia and hyperphosphatemia. PTH acts on bone, the small intestines, and the kidneys to effect a rise in serum calcium and a net decrease in serum phosphorus. Hydroxylation of inactive forms of vitamin D occurs in the liver and kidneys. 1,25(OH)$_2$D facilitates intestinal absorption of calcium and phosphorus. *1,25(OH)$_2$D*, 1,25-Dihydroxyvitamin D; *25(OH) D*, 25-hydroxyvitamin D; *$D_2$*, vitamin $D_2$; *$D_3$*, vitamin $D_3$.

## PATHOPHYSIOLOGY

Under normal conditions, excess calcium is excreted together with sodium in the proximal tubules of the kidneys. With hypercalcemia, dehydration caused by vomiting, poor oral intake, and osmotic diuresis results in reabsorption of sodium instead of excretion. This concurrent calcium reabsorption exacerbates the underlying hypercalcemia. PTH regulates the renal excretion of calcium. The excess production of PTH in primary hyperparathyroidism results in inappropriate calcium reabsorption. Causes of primary hyperparathyroidism include solitary adenomas (most common), ectopic adenomas in the mediastinum, diffuse hyperplasia of one or more parathyroid glands, and parathyroid carcinoma.[6] These parathyroid abnormalities may be independent or a component of the multiple endocrine neoplasia syndromes (MEN 1 or 2a).

Bone acts as a pool of calcium that is regulated by the balance between osteoblast and osteoclast activity. Calcium is released from bone by relative overactivation of osteoclasts and is enhanced by PTH. Prolonged hyperparathyroidism results in osteopenia.

The small intestines are the location of calcium absorption from the diet. Absorption is facilitated by vitamin D. Inactive forms of vitamin $D_3$ are synthesized in the skin in response to exposure to sunlight; vitamin $D_2$ is ingested from a normal diet. Vitamins $D_2$ and $D_3$ are subsequently converted into the active form 1,25-dihydroxyvitamin D (calcitriol) by enzymatic hydroxylation first in the liver and then in the kidney. Calcitriol acts on villi of the small intestines to augment absorption of calcium and phosphorus. Calcitriol also acts on bone to increase osteoclast activity. Excessive ingestion of vitamin D supplements is a rare cause of hypercalcemia. A serum 25-hydroxyvitamin D concentration greater than 125 nmol/L (50 ng/mL) is considered to be excessive, and greater than 500 nmol/L (200 ng/mL) is potentially toxic.

In the paraneoplastic syndrome hypercalcemia of malignancy, the majority of cases of hypercalcemia arise from tumor secretion of parathyroid hormone–related protein (PTHrP), a PTH homologue that acts on tissues like PTH does. Osteolytic bone metastases and ectopic tumor production of calcitriol and PTH cause the remaining cases of hypercalcemia of malignancy.[5]

Milk-alkali syndrome is the third most common cause of hypercalcemia severe enough to result in hospitalization.[7] The clinical definition of milk-alkali syndrome is hypercalcemia, alkalosis, and renal failure in a patient ingesting excessive amounts of calcium and an alkali. Diagnosis is based on the patient history when other causes of hypercalcemia are excluded. Over-the-counter calcium carbonate supplements are commonly used for dyspepsia and prevention of

**BOX 166.1 Signs and Symptoms of Hypercalcemia**

**Neurologic**
Fatigue
Weakness
Delirium
Coma

**Gastrointestinal**
Anorexia
Nausea and vomiting
Constipation or ileus
Peptic ulcers
Pancreatitis

**Renal**
Osmotic diuresis
Nephrolithiasis
Nephrocalcinosis

**Cardiac**
QT-interval shortening
ST-segment elevation
Bradydysrhythmias

**Musculoskeletal**
Muscle weakness
Bone pain
Osteopenia

osteoporosis and are currently the most frequent cause of milk-alkali syndrome. Historically, ingestion of milk and sodium bicarbonate for the treatment of peptic ulcer disease was the most common cause of milk-alkali syndrome, but this medication regimen went out of favor with the availability of $H_2$ receptor antagonists and proton pump inhibitors. Serum PTH is low in these patients, indicative of no concurrent hyperparathyroidism.

Several medications rarely cause hypercalcemia. Thiazide diuretics, lithium, and the vitamin A derivatives all-*trans*-retinoic acid and *cis*-retinoic acid have been implicated. Some systemic illnesses also have the potential to cause hypercalcemia, including the granulomatous diseases sarcoidosis, leprosy, coccidiomycosis, histoplasmosis, and tuberculosis. The mechanism of hypercalcemia in these conditions is thought to be production of calcitriol by macrophages within granulomas.[8] Additionally, rare inherited disorders such as familial hypocalciuric hypercalcemia cause hypercalcemia.[9]

## PRESENTING SIGNS AND SYMPTOMS

Patients often become symptomatic from hypercalcemia at levels near 12 mg/dL, and nearly all patients with levels higher than 14 mg/dL will be symptomatic. Hypercalcemia affects a broad array of organ systems (**Box 166.1**).

Neurologic symptoms progress with increasing serum levels of calcium and range from mild cognitive impairment and depression to drowsiness, altered mental status, delirium, and obtundation.

Gastrointestinal symptoms include anorexia, constipation, nausea, vomiting, and paralytic ileus. Pancreatitis secondary to hypercalcemia is a well-described clinical phenomenon, but the exact mechanism of the development of this condition is still unclear. There is also an association between hypercalcemia and the development of peptic ulcer disease, in addition to a link between milk-alkali syndrome and antacid use in the treatment of this condition.

A common renal manifestation of hypercalcemia is osmotic diuresis manifested as polyuria and excessive thirst. Nephrolithiasis and nephrocalcinosis are hallmarks of hypercalcemia. In patients with primary hyperparathyroidism, up to 20% have a history of symptomatic nephrolithiasis. Case series of patients with kidney stones have demonstrated a 2% to 8% incidence of primary hyperparathyroidism.[10] It is thought that excessive calciuria combined with dehydration and decreased urine output leads to stone formation.

Cardiac manifestations of hypercalcemia are generally manifested as asymptomatic electrocardiographic (ECG) changes. Shortening of the QT interval (QTc <0.4 msec) is common, and ST elevations that may mimic acute myocardial infarction have been reported[11,12] (**Fig. 166.2**). Symptomatic cardiac manifestations are rare and generally limited to bradydysrhythmias.

Musculoskeletal symptoms of hypercalcemia include muscle weakness, bone pain, and osteopenia.

## DIFFERENTIAL DIAGNOSIS AND MEDICAL DECISION MAKING

The serum calcium level is generally reported when a basic or comprehensive metabolic panel is ordered. Special consideration of hypercalcemia should be included in the evaluation of vague chief complaints such as fatigue, weakness, nausea and vomiting, abdominal pain, and altered mental status.

Discovery of significant hypercalcemia on laboratory testing should prompt a directed history for idiopathic causes of hypercalcemia, including ingestion of calcium or vitamin D supplements and use of thiazide diuretics or lithium. Evaluation for hyperparathyroidism, granulomatous diseases, and neoplasms should follow if a cause is not discovered on the history.

## TREATMENT

Initial therapy for hypercalcemia includes correction of dehydration and facilitation of renal excretion of calcium through volume reexpansion with normal saline at a rate of 200 to 500 mL/hr. Patients with severe hypercalcemia may require several liters of fluid resuscitation. For example, in a case series of patients with severe hyperparathyroid crisis requiring parathyroidectomy, a mean of 16 ± 6 L of isotonic fluid was administered over a period of several days before surgery.[6]

Loop diuretics may be used to facilitate forced calcium excretion in urine. Evidence for the effectiveness of loop diuretics is poor, and they should be used only after normovolemia has been achieved.

An additional therapy that has been studied most extensively in patients with hypercalcemia of malignancy is the use of bisphosphonates. These medications act on osteoclasts and limit release of calcium from bone. Their maximum calcium-lowering effects do not occur until several days after administration and can last for several weeks to months.[13-15] Side effects of the bisphosphonates include hypophosphatemia, hypomagnesemia, osteonecrosis of the jaw, and postadministration acute phase reactions (fever, arthralgias, fatigue, malaise, myalgias). **Table 166.1** summarizes the dosing regimens for available bisphosphonates.

A treatment of hypercalcemia that is immediately effective in lowering serum calcium is calcitonin. Calcitonin inhibits urinary reabsorption of calcium and osteoclast maturation. The most commonly available form of this medication is

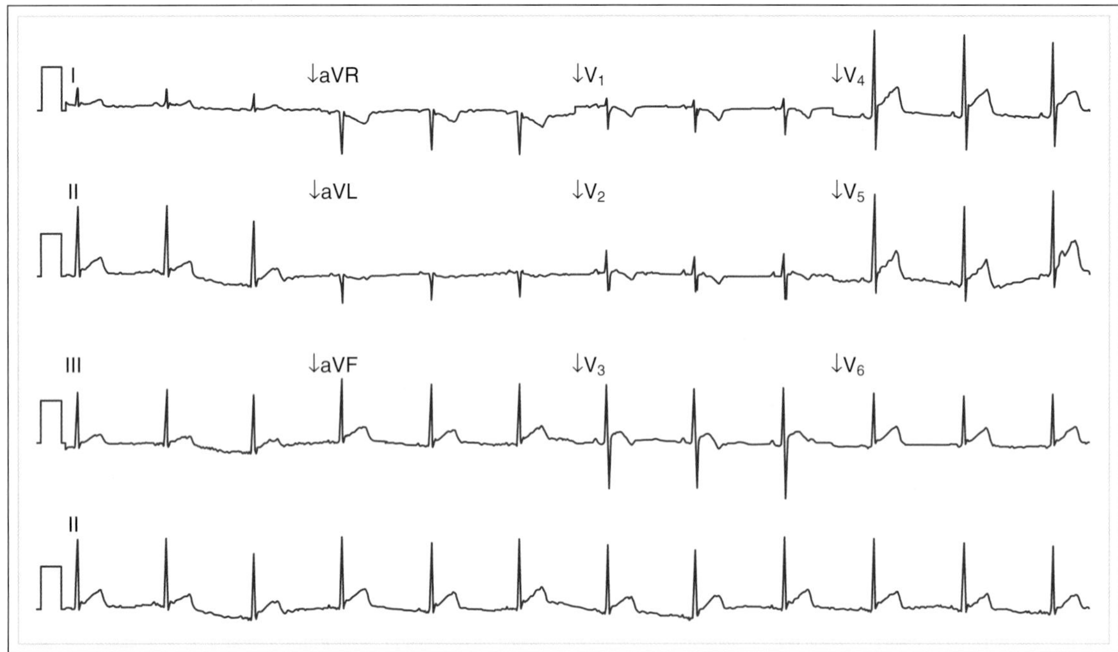


**Fig. 166.2 Electrocardiographic manifestations of hypercalcemia.** Note the shortened QT interval, T-wave inversions, and ST-segment elevation. (Courtesy Loren K. Rood, MD, Indiana University School of Medicine, Indianapolis.)

**Table 166.1 Bisphosphonates Available in the United States for the Treatment of Hypercalcemia of Malignancy**

| | DOSE* | INFUSION TIME | MEDIAN TIME TO RELAPSE OF HYPERCALCEMIA |
|---|---|---|---|
| Pamidronate | 60 or 90 mg | 2-4 hr | 17 days |
| Zoledronic acid | 4 or 8 mg | 15 min | 30-40 days |

Adapted from Major P, Lortholary A, Hon J, et al. Zoledronic acid is superior to pamidronate in the treatment of hypercalcemia of malignancy: a pooled analysis of two randomized, controlled clinical trials. J Clin Oncol 2001;19:558-67.

*Higher doses are reserved for patients with severely elevated calcium levels.

salmon calcitonin administered at 4 to 8 U/kg subcutaneously every 8 to 12 hours. Lowering of the serum calcium level can occur as quickly as 2 hours after administration, but the effects are generally modest (lowering calcium by up to 3.8 mg/dL)[16] and short-lived. Tachyphylaxis to this treatment occurs within 2 days. Side effects of salmon calcitonin include flushing, nausea, vomiting, and abdominal cramps.

Glucocorticoids inhibit conversion of 25-hydroxyvitamin D to calcitriol, which causes a decrease in intestinal absorption of calcium and an increase in renal calcium excretion. Efficacy in lowering serum calcium has been demonstrated only in the treatment of certain types of lymphoma that secrete calcitriol, vitamin D intoxication, and the granulomatous diseases.[8] Additionally, administration of glucocorticoids may delay tachyphylaxis to calcitonin, so they are often used in conjunction with salmon calcitonin. A common regimen for the treatment of hypercalcemia is hydrocortisone, 200 to 300 mg/day intravenously for 3 to 5 days.

An older medication for the treatment of hypercalcemia that has primarily been supplanted by use of the bisphosphonates is gallium nitrate. Gallium nitrate acts to lower serum calcium by inhibition of osteoclast activity. It is also thought to inhibit PTHrP. The typical dose is 200 $mg/m^2$/day of gallium nitrate for 5 days by continuous infusion. The need for several days of continuous infusion is a significant drawback to the use of this medication. Because of risk for nephrotoxicity, gallium nitrate is generally indicated only when bisphosphonates are contraindicated or in refractory cases of hypercalcemia of malignancy when tumors exhibit a high level of PTHrP secretion.

An important step in the treatment of all causes of hypercalcemia is discontinuation of vitamin D and calcium-containing products. In the setting of milk-alkali syndrome, discontinuation of supplements and fluid resuscitation are often the only treatments required. Hemodialysis may be indicated for patients with severe hypercalcemia complicated by renal failure or for cases refractory to other therapies.

## FOLLOW-UP, NEXT STEPS IN CARE, AND PATIENT EDUCATION

Hospital admission is indicated for patients with symptomatic hypercalcemia, especially in the setting of altered mental status, dehydration, or acute renal failure. Definitive treatment of any underlying diseases causing hypercalcemia should be

**Table 166.2 Recommended Daily Dietary Intake of Vitamins and Minerals by Age and Sex**

| | | 4-8 | | 9-13 | | 14-18 | | 19-30 | | 31-50 | | 51+ | |
|---|---|---|---|---|---|---|---|---|---|---|---|---|---|
| | 1-3 | F | M | F | M | F | M | F | M | F | M | F | M |
| Vitamin D (mcg) | 5 | 5 | 5 | 5 | 5 | 5 | 5 | 5 | 5 | 5 | 5 | 10 | 10 |
| Calcium (mg) | 500 | 800 | 800 | 1300 | 1300 | 1300 | 1300 | 1000 | 1000 | 1000 | 1000 | 1200 | 1200 |
| Magnesium (mg) | 80 | 130 | 130 | 240 | 240 | 360 | 410 | 310 | 400 | 320 | 420 | 320 | 420 |
| Phosphorus (mg) | 460 | 500 | 500 | 1250 | 1250 | 1250 | 1250 | 700 | 700 | 700 | 700 | 700 | 700 |

From U.S. Department of Agriculture Center for Nutrition Policy and Promotion. Report of the Dietary Guidelines Advisory Committee on the Dietary Guidelines for Americans, 2010. Available at http://www.dietaryguidelines.gov. Accessed 1/14/2011.
*F*, Female; *M*, male.

undertaken, as clinically appropriate. This may include parathyroidectomy for primary hyperparathyroidism or initiation of therapy for malignancy. Patients should be educated about the proper use of dietary supplements or antacids containing calcium and vitamin D (**Table 166.2**).

# HYPOCALCEMIA

## EPIDEMIOLOGY

Hypocalcemia is defined as a serum calcium level lower than 8.5 mg/dL, although symptoms of hypocalcemia typically do not occur until serum calcium is below 7.0 to 7.5 mg/dL or ionized calcium is below 2.8 mg/dL (0.7 mmol/L).[17] The incidence of hypocalcemia has not been well quantified.

## PATHOPHYSIOLOGY

The most common cause of hypocalcemia is hypoparathyroidism, which is defined as inadequate release of PTH from the parathyroid glands. Inappropriate release of PTH results in poor calcium absorption from the gastrointestinal tract, excessive excretion of calcium in urine, and sequestration in bone.

The most common cause of hypoparathyroidism is neck surgery, specifically parathyroidectomy, followed by thyroidectomy and then other neck surgeries. Autoimmune destruction of the parathyroid glands also causes hypoparathyroidism. Antiparathyroid antibodies are found in more than 30% of patients with isolated hypoparathyroidism and in more than 40% of patients with hypoparathyroidism accompanied by other autoimmune diseases. Infiltration of the parathyroids as a result of sarcoidosis, Wilson disease, hemochromatosis, or amyloidosis is a rare cause of hypoparathyroidism.

Pseudohypoparathyroidism is defined as a blunted renal response to PTH and is manifested similar to hypoparathyroidism as low serum calcium and elevated phosphorus levels; PTH in this setting is normal or elevated. Several genetic pseudohypoparathyroid syndromes are associated with hypocalcemia, as well as abnormal skeletal development, dysmorphic features, and abnormal development.

Vitamin D deficiency (rickets) is rarely symptomatic in adults unless hypocalcemia develops. The majority of patients with vitamin D deficiency have osteopenia with potential for the development of osteoporosis and pathologic fractures. It is most common in elderly, hospitalized, or institutionalized persons. These patients have impaired skin production of vitamin D in response to sun exposure because of aging, a low amount of sun exposure, or dietary deficiency. Individuals with darker skin that is highly pigmented by melanin are at higher risk than lighter-skinned individuals for vitamin D deficiency secondary to relative underproduction of vitamin D in response to sun exposure. Measurement of 25-hydroxyvitamin D is considered the best measure of body vitamin D stores. Serum levels of 25-hydroxyvitamin D below 30 to 50 nmol/L (<12 to 20 ng/mL) are considered deficient.

Pancreatitis causes hypocalcemia when peripancreatic fat combines with extracellular calcium to form insoluble salts. This processes is called saponification. Other causes of hypocalcemia include sepsis, critical illness, chronic renal failure, and massive transfusion of blood anticoagulated with citrate.

DiGeorge syndrome is a rare genetic disorder caused by deletion of a portion of chromosome 22 at the location 22q11.2. Hypocalcemia is a common component of this syndrome because of parathyroid agenesis or dysgenesis. Children with this disorder may exhibit hypocalcemia shortly after birth, and many require lifelong treatment for prevention of hypocalcemia.

The electrolyte abnormalities hyperphosphatemia and hypomagnesemia also cause hypocalcemia. Drugs and toxins implicated as causes of hypocalcemia include bisphosphonates, cisplatin, ketoconazole, phenytoin, phenobarbital, proton pump inhibitors, $H_2$ receptor antagonists, aminoglycosides, phosphate-based enemas or laxatives, and exposure to hydrofluoric acid.

## PRESENTING SIGNS AND SYMPTOMS

The primary symptoms of hypocalcemia are manifestations of calcium's critical role in the contraction and relaxation of skeletal and smooth muscle, as well as neurotransmission (**Box 166.2**). Neurologic symptoms often include both sensory and motor complaints. Sensory findings include perioral and extremity paresthesias. The most common motor abnormalities are neuromuscular irritability, including muscle cramps, hyperreflexia, carpal-pedal spasms, tetany, and seizures. Smooth muscle manifestations of hypocalcemia include

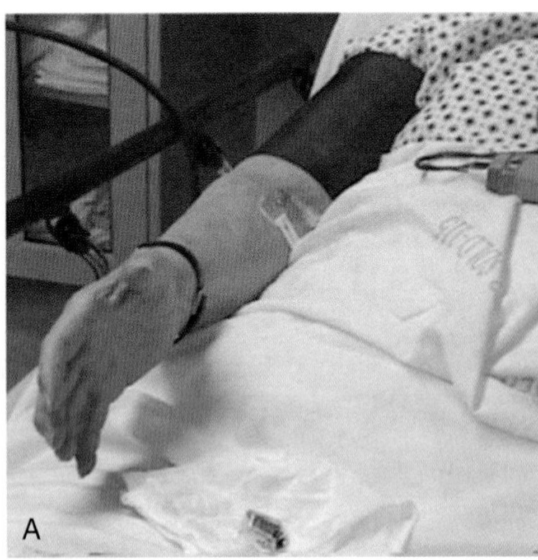


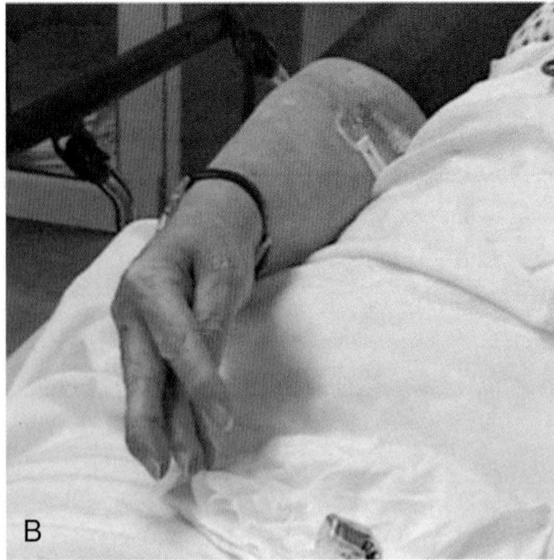


**Fig. 166.3 Trousseau sign in a patient with hypocalcemia and hypomagnesemia.** A 51-year-old woman had a serum calcium level of 5.4 mg/dL. **A,** Patient's hand at rest. **B,** Patient's hand demonstrating carpal spasm 90 seconds after inflation of the blood pressure cuff to 10 mm Hg above systolic pressure. (From Meininger ME, Kendler JS. Images in clinical medicine. Trousseau's sign. N Engl J Med 2000;343:1855.)

**BOX 166.2 Symptoms of Hypocalcemia, Hypomagnesemia, and Hyperphosphatemia**

**Neuromuscular**
Paresthesias
Cramps
Carpal-pedal spasms
Tetany
Seizures

**Cardiovascular**
QT-interval prolongation
Bradycardia
Congestive heart failure
Hypotension
Dysrhythmias (torsades de pointes)

**Pulmonary**
Laryngospasm
Bronchospasm

**Psychiatric**
Irritability
Depression
Altered mental status

bronchospasm, laryngospasm, biliary and small bowel cramping, dysphagia, bladder dysfunction, and painful menses or preterm labor from uterine contractions. Laryngospasm can be life-threatening.

Two well-recognized findings on physical examination that are pathognomonic for hypocalcemia are the Chvostek and Trousseau signs. The Chvostek sign is defined as facial muscle spasm elicited by tapping the facial nerve 1 to 2 cm anterior to the tragus of the ear. This sign is neither sensitive nor specific for hypocalcemia, with 25% of healthy people having a positive sign and only 71% of hypocalcemic patients having a positive sign.[17] The Trousseau sign is more reliable, with only 1% to 4% of healthy people having a positive sign and 94% of hypocalcemic patients having a positive sign. The Trousseau sign is defined as carpal and digit spasm elicited by occluding the brachial artery with a sphygmomanometer inflated to 20 to 30 mm Hg above systolic blood pressure for 3 minutes (**Fig. 166.3**).

Neuropsychiatric manifestations of hypocalcemia include irritability, depression, anxiety, confusion, hallucinations, psychosis, and extrapyramidal symptoms (tremor, akathisia, slurred speech, dystonia, muscle rigidity, bradyphonia, and bradykinesia).

In addition to neuromuscular and neuropsychiatric abnormalities, cardiac conduction abnormalities and dysrhythmias may occur. The most common cardiac manifestation is QT prolongation, but bradycardia, congestive heart failure, hypotension, and triggered ventricular dysrhythmias, including torsades de pointes, may occur (**Fig. 166.4**).

In patients with chronic hypocalcemia, skin and ophthalmologic abnormalities may become notable. Cataracts in the lenses of the eyes, brittle nails, and coarse or dry hair and skin are typical.

## DIFFERENTIAL DIAGNOSIS AND MEDICAL DECISION MAKING

Hypocalcemia found on routine laboratory evaluation should prompt evaluation for hypoparathyroidism, vitamin D deficiency, renal or liver failure, hypomagnesemia, and hyperphosphatemia.

The emergency physician should consider ordering a total serum calcium or ionized calcium level in patients with a new seizure, psychosis or altered mental status, extrapyramidal symptoms, paresthesias, muscle spasms, congestive heart failure, prolonged QTc interval, or torsades de pointes.

In patients requiring massive blood transfusion, hypocalcemia should be prevented by regular assessment of calcium levels and early administration of intravenous calcium.

Calcium administration should be performed with caution in hypocalcemic patients being treated with digoxin because of the risk for precipitation of digoxin toxicity.

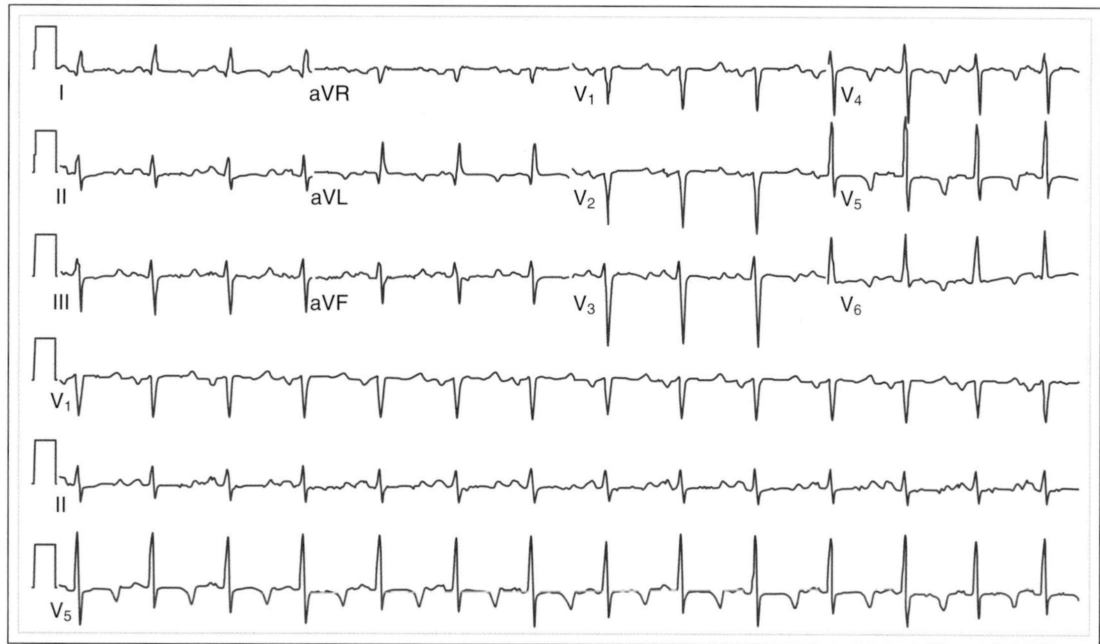


**Fig. 166.4 Prolongation of the QT interval on an electrocardiogram in a patient with hypocalcemia.** (Courtesy Richard Parks, MD, Indiana University School of Medicine, Indianapolis.)

## TREATMENT

The goals of therapy for hypocalcemia are to stop the uncomfortable symptoms of tetany and muscle spasm and prevent seizures, dangerous dysrhythmias, and laryngospasm. Severe, symptomatic hypocalcemia should be treated with a 10% intravenous solution of calcium gluconate or calcium chloride. The 10% solution of calcium chloride contains nearly three times the elemental calcium per milliliter as the 10% solution of calcium gluconate (**Table 166.3**). The dose of 10% calcium gluconate is 10 to 30 mL infused intravenously over a 10-minute period (provides 93 to 279 mg of elemental calcium). The dose of 10% calcium chloride is 10 mL infused intravenously over a 10-minute period (provides 270 mg of elemental calcium). The effects of a single bolus administration of intravenous calcium are temporary, so repeated boluses or a continuous infusion may be required in the setting of severe hypocalcemia or an ongoing process of calcium loss (pancreatitis or after parathyroidectomy). The rate of continuous infusion of calcium gluconate is 0.5 to 1.5 mg/kg/hr of elemental calcium, and it is generally supplied as 100 mL of 10% calcium gluconate in 900 mL of 5% dextrose in water (0.5 to 1.5 mL/kg/hr). Calcium chloride should be administered through a central vein. It is highly irritating to smaller peripheral veins and can cause phlebitis, and extravasation into subcutaneous tissues can result in significant local tissue necrosis.

Supplementation of calcium and vitamin D is the mainstay of therapy for chronic hypocalcemia. Virtually all forms of chronic hypocalcemia are associated with some degree of vitamin D deficiency. Vitamin D is available in a variety of forms. Selection of the appropriate form is based on the underlying cause of the vitamin D deficiency and the patient's ability to appropriately hydroxylate the supplement in the liver and kidney (**Table 166.4**).

**Table 166.3 Comparison of Intravenous Solutions of Calcium for the Treatment of Hypocalcemia**

| SOLUTION | ELEMENTAL CALCIUM (IN 10 mL) | DOSE |
|---|---|---|
| 10% Calcium chloride (1 g/10 mL) | 270 mg | 10 mL IV over 10-min period |
| 10% Calcium gluconate (1 g/10 mL) | 93 mg | 10-30 mL IV over 10-min period |

Adapted from Maeda SS, Fortes EM, Oliveira UM, et al. Hypoparathyroidism and pseudohypoparathyroidism. Arq Bars Endocrinol Metab 2006;50:664-73.

Oral calcium is available as a variety of salts, each with a different concentration of elemental calcium (**Table 166.5**). Calcium carbonate is generally preferred because it has the highest concentration of elemental calcium per tablet and thus fewer tablets are required to reach the appropriate dose of 1 to 1.5 g of elemental calcium daily.[17] In the elderly, calcium citrate is preferred because it is more easily absorbed in the setting of low gastric acid.[18]

## FOLLOW-UP, NEXT STEPS IN CARE, AND PATIENT EDUCATION

Patients with mild, chronic, and asymptomatic hypocalcemia can follow up with their primary physician as an outpatient. Initiation of calcium and vitamin D supplementation should be considered for symptomatic individuals in discussion with the patient's primary physician.

**Table 166.4 Comparison of Vitamin D Supplement Preparations**

| SUPPLEMENT | HEPATIC HYDROXYLATION REQUIRED | RENAL HYDROXYLATION REQUIRED | DOSAGE FORMS | NOTES |
|---|---|---|---|---|
| Ergocalciferol (vitamin $D_2$) | + | + | 50,000 IU | Considered equivalent |
| Cholecalciferol (vitamin $D_3$) | + | + | 400, 1000, 2000, 5000 IU | |
| Calcidiol (25-hydroxyvitamin D) | – | + | Not available | |
| Calcitriol (1,25-dihydroxyvitamin D) | – | – | 0.25, 0.5 mcg | Available PO and IV, expensive |

The biologic activity of 40 IU is equivalent to 1 mcg.

Adapted from Maeda SS, Fortes EM, Oliveira UM, et al. Hypoparathyroidism and pseudohypoparathyroidism. Arq Bars Endocrinol Metab 2006;50:664-73; and Tohme JF, Bilezikian JP. Hypocalcemic emergencies. Endocrinol Metab Clin North Am 1993;22:363-75.

**Table 166.5 Comparison of Calcium Salt Preparations**

| SUPPLEMENT | ELEMENTAL CALCIUM CONTENT | AMOUNT OF SALT REQUIRED TO OBTAIN THE RECOMMENDED DAILY DOSE FOR ADULTS (1 g ELEMENTAL CALCIUM/DAY) |
|---|---|---|
| Calcium carbonate | 40% | 2.5 g |
| Calcium phosphate | 38% | 2.6 g |
| Calcium chloride | 27% | 3.7 g |
| Calcium citrate | 21% | 4.8 g |
| Calcium lactate | 13% | 7.7 g |
| Calcium gluconate | 9% | 11.1 g |

Adapted from Maeda SS, Fortes EM, Oliveira UM, et al. Hypoparathyroidism and pseudohypoparathyroidism. Arq Bars Endocrinol Metab 2006;50:664-73.

Patients with profound or life-threatening symptoms or any patients requiring intravenous calcium supplementation should be admitted to a monitored setting and may require intensive care unit admission. Goals of inpatient admission include serial monitoring of calcium levels, further calcium replacement, and evaluation for critical illnesses and other causes of hypocalcemia. Telemetry monitoring should be used because of the risk for precipitation of ventricular arrhythmia.

## Magnesium

Approximately 50% of total body magnesium is found in bone as a component of hydroxyapatite, similar to calcium. The remaining magnesium is located primarily intracellularly. Only 1% of total body magnesium is found in the extracellular space, with this amount further divided into protein-bound (30%) and ionized fractions.[19]

The balance between gastrointestinal absorption and renal excretion determines the serum magnesium level, with bone acting as a buffer to increase serum magnesium when levels are low. Neither gastrointestinal absorption nor renal excretion of magnesium is hormonally regulated. Circulating PTH regulates bone metabolism. Because serum magnesium levels influence release of PTH from the parathyroid glands, magnesium has an effect on serum calcium and phosphorus levels. The kidneys have the ability to reabsorb all but 0.5% of the filtered magnesium in the setting of hypomagnesemia and excrete up to 80% in the setting of hypermagnesemia.[20] The normal serum range of magnesium is 1.8 to 2.5 mg/dL (0.74 to 0.94 mmol/L). No ionized magnesium laboratory test is available.

The recommended daily intake of elemental magnesium for adults is 320 mg for women and 420 mg for men. Dietary sources of magnesium include fish, nuts, cereals, and green vegetables. A variety of magnesium salt formulations are used therapeutically as laxatives and magnesium supplements (**Table 166.6**).

Magnesium acts as a cofactor for an extensive number of intracellular enzymatic reactions and is necessary for protein and DNA synthesis, as well as for adenosine triphosphate (ATP) function and glucose metabolism.[21] It is also critical for neuromuscular conduction and muscle contraction.

**Table 166.6 Common Magnesium-Containing Preparations**

| SUPPLEMENT | ELEMENTAL MAGNESIUM CONTENT (%) | AMOUNT OF ELEMENTAL MAGNESIUM IN COMMON PREPARATIONS |
|---|---|---|
| Magnesium oxide | 61 | 242 mg in 400-mg tablet |
| Magnesium hydroxide (milk of magnesia) | 42 | 167 mg in 400 mg/5 mL oral suspension |
| Magnesium citrate | 16 | 48 mg in 290 mg/5 mL oral solution |
| Magnesium gluconate | 5 | 27 mg in 500-mg tablet |
| Magnesium chloride | 12 | 64 mg in 535-mg tablet |
| Magnesium sulfate solution | 10 | 500 mg in 10 mL of a 50% solution (5 mg $MgSO_4$/10 mL) |
| Magnesium sulfate Epson salts | 10 | 98 mg in 1 g of salts |
| Magnesium lactate | 12 | 10 mg in 84-mg tablet |
| Magnesium aspartate | 10 | 122 mg in 1230-mg tablet |

Adapted from Guerrera MP, Volpe SL, Mao JJ. Therapeutic uses of magnesium. Am Fam Physician 2009;80:157-62.

# HYPOMAGNESEMIA

## EPIDEMIOLOGY

Hypomagnesemia is defined as a serum magnesium level lower than 1.8 mg/dL, but most patients are not symptomatic until lower levels are reached. Two older studies demonstrated an incidence of hypomagnesemia of approximately 10% in the general hospitalized population and up to 65% in the intensive care unit patient population.[22,23] It is unclear whether this incidence has changed over time. The incidence of hypomagnesemia in patients seen in the emergency department has not been determined.

## PATHOPHYSIOLOGY

Magnesium is absorbed over the entire length of the gastrointestinal tract. Absorption is passive in the small bowel. Active transcellular absorption occurs in the colon. The direction of passive flow of magnesium can change to favor magnesium excretion into the bowel lumen in patients with conditions such as excessive diarrhea, vomiting, persistent nasogastric suction, or bulimia.[19,24] Failure to properly absorb dietary magnesium because of malabsorption syndromes such as short gut syndrome, gastric bypass, steatorrhea, celiac disease, and radiation-induced enteritis can result in chronic hypomagnesemia.

Failure of renal magnesium absorption occurs in settings of osmotic diuresis as a result of hypercalcemia, hyperglycemia, and mannitol administration. Renal tubular, glomerular, and interstitial diseases may also result in an inability to properly reabsorb magnesium.

Hypomagnesemia may be triggered by acute pancreatitis secondary to saponification of fatty acids. A baseline poor dietary intake of magnesium from chronic alcohol abuse that precipitates pancreatitis may also contribute to hypomagnesemia in these patients.

Other causes of hypomagnesemia include acidosis, chronic alcoholism, non–magnesium-containing laxative abuse, and several drugs, including diuretics, aminoglycosides, amphotericin B, cisplatin, and cyclosporine.

## PRESENTING SIGNS AND SYMPTOMS

Hypomagnesemia is highly correlated with abnormalities in other electrolytes. Hypokalemia is common because magnesium is necessary for proper function of the sodium-potassium adenosine triphosphatase ($Na^+$,$K^+$-ATPase) pump, which maintains an appropriate transcellular potassium gradient. Hypomagnesemia impairs secretion of PTH, causes renal and bone resistance to PTH, and causes intestinal resistance to vitamin D, thereby resulting in hypocalcemia.[19]

Similar to hypocalcemia, hypomagnesemia results in significant neuromuscular hyperexcitability. The Chvostek and Trousseau signs may be present.

Magnesium has been demonstrated to be helpful in the treatment of dangerous arrhythmias, especially torsades de pointes and atrial fibrillation, thus suggesting that hypomagnesemia plays a role in the development of these arrhythmias. ECG changes associated with hypomagnesemia include prolongation of the PR and QTc intervals and the development of U waves (**Fig. 166.5**).

## DIFFERENTIAL DIAGNOSIS AND MEDICAL DECISION MAKING

Magnesium levels should be checked and normalized in patients with known or suspected hypocalcemia or hypokalemia and in patients with weakness or sensory-motor complaints. Assessment of the underlying cause of hypomagnesemia, especially in the setting of gastrointestinal losses, is necessary.

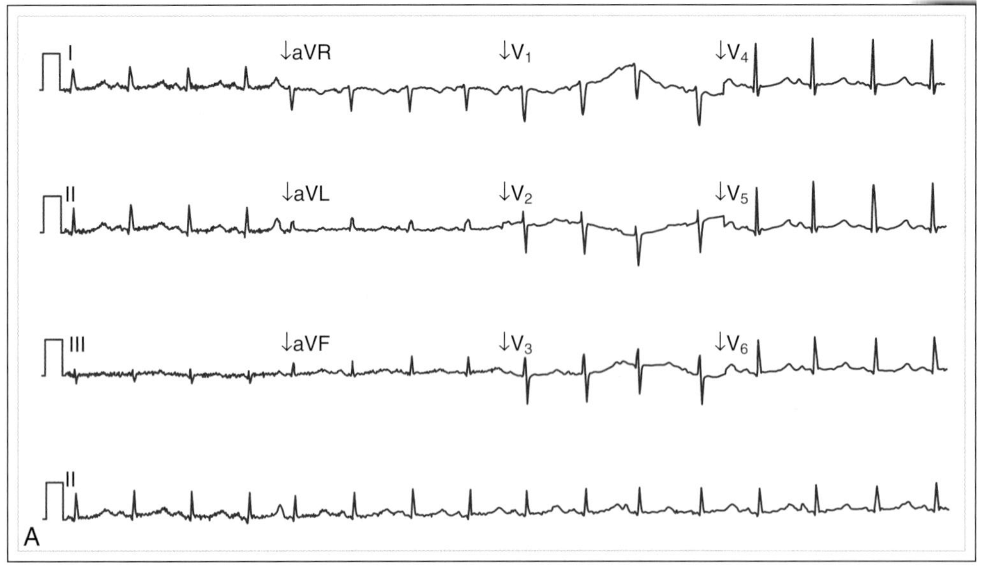


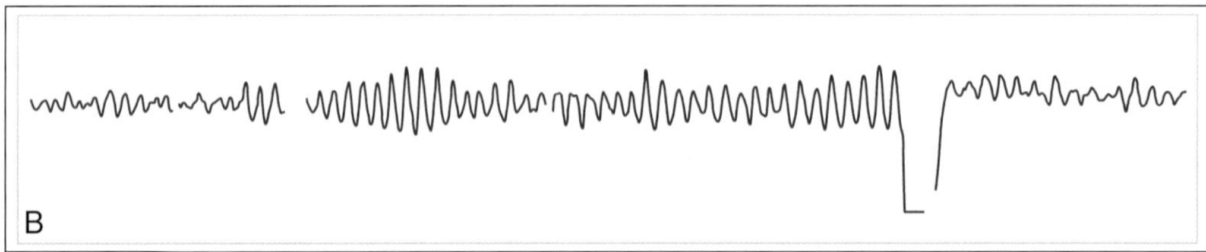


**Fig. 166.5** **A,** Prolongation of the QT interval on an electrocardiogram in a patient with hypomagnesemia. **B,** Deterioration of the same patient's rhythm to torsades de pointes, which was corrected with intravenous magnesium. (Courtesy Loren K. Rood, MD, Indiana University School of Medicine, Indianapolis.)

## TREATMENT

Treatment of hypomagnesemia is slow intravenous infusion of 2 to 4 g of a 50% magnesium sulfate solution. It may be repeated as necessary, to a maximum dose of 8 g/day. This maximum dose is often exceeded in patients being treated with continuous infusions of magnesium sulfate for preeclampsia or tocolysis, so continuous monitoring for signs of hypermagnesemia are indicated in these patients.

## FOLLOW-UP, NEXT STEPS IN CARE, AND PATIENT EDUCATION

Hospital admission is indicated for patients with life-threatening complications of hypomagnesemia, including seizures and cardiac arrhythmias. Mild, chronic hypomagnesemia can be treated on an outpatient basis with supplementation of magnesium salts. Dietary or lifestyle changes, including cessation of alcohol abuse, may be necessary to completely rectify the hypomagnesemia.

# HYPERMAGNESEMIA

## EPIDEMIOLOGY

Hypermagnesemia is defined as a serum magnesium level higher than 2.5 mg/dL. Hypermagnesemia is rare because of efficient renal excretion of excessive magnesium. In 1990 a published series of more than 1000 hospitalized adult patients demonstrated a 5.7% prevalence of hypermagnesemia in this population.[25] There are multiple case reports in the emergency medicine literature of hypermagnesemia caused by iatrogenic and accidental overdoses.[26]

## PATHOPHYSIOLOGY

In the setting of iatrogenic or accidental overdose of magnesium, renal excretion of magnesium can be overwhelmed. The imbalance of absorption over excretion is worsened in the setting of acquired or chronic renal insufficiency, especially in patients with a glomerular filtration rate lower than 30 mL/min. Symptomatic hypermagnesemia is seen most often in the setting of iatrogenic administration of intravenous magnesium or after an overdose of magnesium-containing supplements or enemas. Concomitant use of anticholinergic or opiate medications that slow gastrointestinal motility can increase the risk for toxicity from magnesium-containing medications.[27]

Magnesium acts as a nonspecific calcium channel blocker. This property results in cardiac conduction abnormalities and hypotension in patients with acute elevations in magnesium.

## PRESENTING SIGNS AND SYMPTOMS

The symptoms of hypermagnesemia progress in a dose-related fashion (**Table 166.7**). Early signs of hypermagnesemia

**Table 166.7 Symptoms of Hypermagnesemia**

| MAGNESIUM LEVEL | SYMPTOMS |
|---|---|
| 5-8 mg/dL | Nausea, vomiting, flushing, hyporeflexia |
| 9-12 mg/dL | Somnolence, areflexia, hypotension, bradycardia, prolongation of the QRS, PR, and QT intervals |
| >15 mg/dL | Respiratory depression, complete heart block, paralysis, coma |
| >20 mg/dL | Asystole, death |

Adapted from Birrer RB, Shallash AH, Totten V. Hypermagnesemia-induced fatality following Epson salt gargles. J Emerg Med 2002;22:185-8.

include headache, nausea, vomiting, flushing, and hypotension as a result of peripheral vasodilation. Reflexes diminish and are eventually lost. Mental status worsens from somnolence to coma. Muscle weakness can progress to include the muscles of respiration and result in ventilatory failure and the need for endotracheal intubation and mechanical ventilation. At higher magnesium levels, cardiac complications begin to develop, with progression from bradycardia to atrioventricular block, intraventricular conduction block, complete heart block, or asystole.

## DIFFERENTIAL DIAGNOSIS AND MEDICAL DECISION MAKING

Hypermagnesemia should be included in the differential diagnosis of patients with altered mental status, cardiac arrhythmias, hypotension, and shock. A directed history of use of over-the-counter antacids, laxatives, and enemas should be elicited when hypermagnesemia is suspected or found on laboratory analysis.

## TREATMENT

The mainstay of treatment of hypermagnesemia is cessation of the use of any magnesium-containing medications. Fluid resuscitation with isotonic saline followed by diuretic therapy to encourage renal clearance of excessive magnesium is indicated. In patients with significant cardiac complications of hypermagnesemia, 10 to 20 mL of 10% calcium gluconate should be administered and repeated every 5 to 10 minutes as needed. Intravenous calcium administration antagonizes the natural calcium channel–blocking properties of magnesium. Hemodialysis may be required in the setting of hypermagnesemia and renal failure.

## FOLLOW-UP, NEXT STEPS IN CARE, AND PATIENT EDUCATION

Hospital admission to a monitored setting or intensive care unit is indicated in the setting of severely elevated magnesium levels, especially with levels that place the patient at risk for hypotension, cardiac conduction abnormalities, or ventilatory failure.

Patients should be educated about the appropriate use of magnesium-containing antacids and laxatives and be made aware of the possibility of overdose when these medications are not used appropriately.

# Phosphorus

Eighty percent to 85% of total body phosphorus is contained in bone, complexed with calcium and magnesium as hydroxyapatite. Less than 1% of total body phosphorus is found extracellularly in plasma; the remaining phosphorus is located intracellularly. Phosphorus is the most abundant intracellular anion.

Phosphorus exists as organic and inorganic forms—it is the inorganic forms that are measured in the laboratory determination of serum phosphorus. Within the range of typical body pH, inorganic phosphorus exists as a balance between the phosphate anions $H_2PO_4^-$ and $HPO_4^{-2}$. At neutral pH the ratio of $H_2PO_4^-$ to $HPO_4^{-2}$ is 1 : 4. The normal serum range of phosphorus is 2.5 to 4.5 mg/dL (0.81 to 1.45 mmol/L).[28]

Adequate phosphorus levels are important for multiple life-sustaining processes. Phosphorus is a key component of ATP, which is required for the generation of energy to carry out cellular processes. It is a part of the phospholipids that make up cell membranes, as well as DNA and RNA. Phosphorus is also necessary for 2,3-diphosphoglycerate in red blood cells, which facilitates release of oxygen from hemoglobin.

The balance between gastrointestinal absorption, bone anabolism and catabolism, and renal excretion determines serum phosphorus levels. Passive absorption of phosphorus from the diet occurs in the small intestines. Vitamin D–dependent active absorption also occurs and is responsible for approximately 30% of phosphorus absorption.[29] Foods rich in phosphorus include animal proteins, milk, eggs and multiple food preservatives.[30]

Excretion of phosphorus occurs in the kidneys. Serum phosphorus is freely filtered by the glomeruli, with 80% to 90% being reabsorbed though an $Na/PO_4$ cotransporter in the proximal tubules. PTH enhances the excretion of phosphorus by inhibiting this transporter. When PTH is released from the parathyroid gland, it acts on bone to release calcium and phosphorus. It also stimulates the kidney to increase production of 1,25-dihydroxyvitamin D, which results in increased gastrointestinal absorption of calcium and phosphorus. Both these mechanisms result in efficient increases in serum calcium, but the increase in serum phosphorus is modest. When combined with the increased excretion of phosphorus by the kidneys in response to PTH, the net effect of a rise in PTH is a decrease in serum phosphorus and an increase in serum calcium (see Fig. 166.1).

# HYPOPHOSPHATEMIA

## EPIDEMIOLOGY

Hypophosphatemia is rare in the general population, occurs in only 2% to 3% of hospitalized patients,[31,32] but is much more common in the setting of critical illness, in which the incidence of phosphorus levels lower than 2.5 mg/dL ranges from 24% to 100%, depending on the intensive care unit population studied.[33]

## PATHOPHYSIOLOGY

There are three predominant mechanisms of hypophosphatemia.[33] Acute hypophosphatemia occurs in the setting of forces that drive phosphate excessively from the extracellular space into the intracellular space. Respiratory alkalosis and treatment of diabetic ketoacidosis with insulin are two common examples of this form of hypophosphatemia. Refeeding syndrome, in which severely malnourished patients are fed a diet high in carbohydrate, is a rare cause of hypophosphatemia but may be encountered in the treatment of patients with severe anorexia nervosa.

Increased urinary excretion of phosphorus (as seen in primary and secondary hyperparathyroidism) and decreased intestinal absorption of phosphorus are the two other mechanisms of hypophosphatemia. Decreased dietary intake of phosphorus, excessive use of phosphate-binding antacids, vomiting, nasogastric suctioning, diarrhea, vitamin D deficiency, and malabsorption are all causes of decreased intestinal absorption of phosphorus. Chronic alcoholism can result in both dietary deficiency and excessive renal excretion of phosphorus.

## PRESENTING SIGNS AND SYMPTOMS

The symptoms of hypophosphatemia worsen with falling serum levels. Patients with mild hypophosphatemia, or serum levels in the range of 2.0 to 2.5 mg/dL, are often asymptomatic. With moderate hypophosphatemia in the range of 1.0 to 2.0 mg/dL, patients may experience myalgias, muscle weakness, and anorexia. Severe hypophosphatemia, defined as a serum phosphorus level lower than 1.0 mg/dL, results in paresthesias, tremor, confusion, decreased deep tendon reflexes, cardiac arrhythmias and impaired cardiac contractility, impaired respiratory muscle function, seizures, and coma.

Rhabdomyolysis can occur in the setting of severe hypophosphatemia secondary to an inability to maintain muscle membrane integrity as a result of ATP deficiency.

## DIFFERENTIAL DIAGNOSIS AND MEDICAL DECISION MAKING

When hypophosphatemia is discovered, causes of respiratory alkalosis should be considered, including hyperventilation from salicylate toxicity, anxiety, pain, alcohol withdrawal, and chronic obstructive pulmonary disease.

Hypophosphatemia should be excluded in patients with myalgias, weakness, and rhabdomyolysis. Phosphorus levels should be monitored in patients being treated for diabetic ketoacidosis.

## TREATMENT

Patients with severe phosphorus deficiency (serum phosphorus <1 mg/dL) should receive intravenous replacement in the form of either sodium phosphate or potassium phosphate. Potassium phosphate is preferred in patients with concomitant hypokalemia. Multiple studies have examined the safety of various doses and rates of administration of intravenous phosphorus supplementation. Doses up to 45 mmol and rates of 20 mmol/hr have been demonstrated to be safe when administered through a central venous catheter.[31,33] The typical dose recommended for adults is 0.08 to 0.16 mmol/kg (2.5 to 5 mg/kg) administered over a period of 2 to 6 hours.[34] Intravenous administration of phosphate-containing supplements can precipitate hypocalcemia, as well as hyperkalemia when potassium phosphate is used.

Mild hypophosphatemia (serum phosphorus level of 1 to 2 mg/dL) may be treated with oral phosphate-containing supplements at a dose of up to 1000 to 2000 mg daily, divided three or four times per day. A combination sodium phosphate and potassium phosphate tablet is available (K-Phos Neutral) that contains 250 mg of phosphorus, 298 mg (13 mEq) of sodium, and 45 mg of potassium (1.1 mEq). Cow's milk is a rich dietary source of phosphorus that contains approximately 1 mg of phosphorus per 1 mL of milk.[35]

## FOLLOW-UP, NEXT STEPS IN CARE, AND PATIENT EDUCATION

Patients with severe hypophosphatemia are often critically ill and require admission for management of their underlying illnesses. Patients with severe, symptomatic hypophosphatemia should be admitted for replacement therapy and monitoring of electrolytes.

# HYPERPHOSPHATEMIA

## EPIDEMIOLOGY

Hyperphosphatemia is defined as a serum phosphorus level higher than 4.5 mg/dL, with severe hyperphosphatemia being defined as serum levels higher than 14 mg/dL. The most common cause of hyperphosphatemia is chronic renal failure requiring hemodialysis. Nearly 90% of these patients are managed with phosphorus-binding therapy and diets low in phosphorus to limit hyperphosphatemia.[36]

## PATHOPHYSIOLOGY

In patients with chronic renal failure, gastrointestinal absorption of phosphorus continues, but renal excretion ceases. Hemodialysis removes approximately 800 to 1000 mg of phosphorus per session,[30] which is less than the typical dietary intake of phosphorus—a mainstay of treatment of hyperphosphatemia is limiting dietary intake and absorption of phosphorus. Excessive phosphorus combines with calcium to form salts that are deposited in the soft tissues of the body. Deposition in the soft tissues of the heart, kidneys, and vasculature has the potential to cause abnormalities in cardiac electrical conduction and cardiac muscle relaxation and contraction, as well as renal disease, coronary artery disease, and peripheral vascular disease. Some evidence indicates that calcium phosphate salt deposition increases mortality in patients undergoing hemodialysis.[36]

Causes of acute elevations in phosphorus include hemolysis, tumor lysis syndrome, and rhabdomyolysis. All three conditions result in rapid breakdown of cellular membranes, which allows stores of intracellular phosphate to quickly be released into the extracellular space. Unless concomitant renal insufficiency is present or ongoing cellular destruction is occurring, the hyperphosphatemia in these conditions is self-limited because renal excretion soon exceeds extracellular phosphate shifting when supportive care is given.

Vitamin D toxicity and overuse of phosphate-containing antacids or enemas have been reported as causes of acute hyperphosphatemia resulting from excessive gastrointestinal absorption. An additional cause of chronic hyperphosphatemia is hypoparathyroidism. In the setting of impaired PTH secretion, renal excretion of phosphorus is decreased.

## PRESENTING SIGNS AND SYMPTOMS

The symptoms of hyperphosphatemia are generally the consequence of associated renal failure and hypocalcemia and include altered mental status, seizures, dysrhythmias, prolongation of the QTc interval, muscle weakness, and neuromuscular excitability (see Box 166.2).

## DIFFERENTIAL DIAGNOSIS AND MEDICAL DECISION MAKING

Acute hyperphosphatemia should prompt evaluation for acute renal failure, rhabdomyolysis, tumor lysis syndrome, and hemolysis. Calcium, magnesium, and potassium levels should be assessed in patients with hyperphosphatemia because many of these electrolyte abnormalities occur simultaneously.

## TREATMENT

In the setting of acute hyperphosphatemia it is necessary to treat the underlying cause. This includes limiting further cell breakdown as much as possible in patients with hemolysis, tumor lysis syndrome, and rhabdomyolysis. Increasing renal excretion of phosphorus with fluid resuscitation, alkalinization of urine with sodium bicarbonate, and diuretic therapy are also indicated.

In the setting of chronic hyperphosphatemia secondary to hypoparathyroidism or chronic renal failure, the mainstays of therapy are to reduce the dietary intake and gastrointestinal absorption of phosphorus.

Phosphate-binding salts are frequently used in the treatment of hyperphosphatemia in patients with renal failure.[36] The cheapest and best-tolerated phosphate binders are calcium carbonate and calcium acetate. These medications may increase deposition of calcium phosphate salt in soft tissues, but considerable debate exists about the cost-effectiveness and side effect profile of alternative phosphate binders. Gastrointestinal side effects of nausea and diarrhea are common. Magnesium hydroxide, magnesium carbonate, sevelamer hydrochloride, sevelamer carbonate, and lanthanum are alternative phosphate-binding salts used for the treatment of hyperphosphatemia in patients with renal failure.

## FOLLOW-UP, NEXT STEPS IN CARE, AND PATIENT EDUCATION

Patients with severe, acute hyperphosphatemia, especially in the setting of acute renal failure or symptomatic hypocalcemia, require admission for supportive care. Many patients with chronic hyperphosphatemia are asymptomatic and require only outpatient follow-up for dietary modifications or adjustment of phosphate-binding salt regimens.

## SUGGESTED READINGS


Amanzadeh J, Reily Jr RF. Hypophosphatemia: an evidence-based approach to its clinical consequences and management. Nat Clin Pract Nephrol 2006;2:136-48.

Moe SM. Disorders involving calcium, phosphorus, and magnesium. Prim Care 2008;35:215-37, v-vi.

Pellitteri PK. Evaluation of hypercalcemia in relation to hyperparathyroidism. Otolaryngol Clin North Am 2010;43:389-97.

Phitayakorn R, McHenry CR. Hyperparathyroid crisis: use of bisphosphonates as a bridge to parathyroidectomy. J Am Coll Surg 2008;206:1106-15.

Tonelli M, Pannu N, Manns B. Oral phosphate binders in patients with kidney failure. N Engl J Med 2010;362:1312-24.


## REFERENCES

*References can be found on Expert Consult @ www.expertconsult.com.*

# 167 Thyroid Disorders

*Sarah Stewart de Ramirez and Frederick Korley*

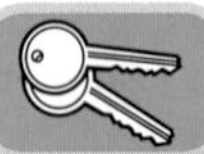

**KEY POINTS**

- Hypothyroidism secondary to iodine deficiency is the most common endocrine disorder worldwide.
- Primary hypothyroidism results from dysfunction of thyroid tissue. Secondary hypothyroidism is a component of panhypopituitarism that results from pituitary disease.
- Severe hypothyroidism is a rare condition characterized by altered mental status, hypothermia, and primary thyroid dysfunction. Myxedema is seen in most cases; true coma is not.
- Patients with suspected severe hypothyroidism should receive empiric, low-dose intravenous levothyroxine.
- Thyroid storm, the most extreme form of thyrotoxicosis, is a rapidly fatal condition.
- Antithyroid medication should be given at least 1 hour before the administration of iodine for the treatment of thyroid storm.
- Emergency department testing for thyroid disease includes serum thyrotropin, or thyroid-stimulating hormone, and free thyroxine measurements.

## PERSPECTIVE

Hypothyroidism is a deficiency of thyroid hormones resulting in a hypometabolic state. Iodine deficiency accounts for most cases of hypothyroidism and goiter in underdeveloped countries; Hashimoto thyroiditis is a more commonly recognized cause in westernized societies.

Thyrotoxicosis describes any condition characterized by an excess of free thyroid hormones in the circulation. The term is frequently used interchangeably with hyperthyroidism; however, hyperthyroidism refers only to disease states in which the thyroid gland produces an excess of thyroid hormones.

## EPIDEMIOLOGY

Abnormal thyroid function is by far the most common endocrine disorder worldwide and is second only to diabetes mellitus in the United States. Thyrotoxicosis is a rare condition that is 10 times more prevalent in women than in men (2% versus 0.2%).[1] It is uncommon before the age of 15 years.[2] Although most manifestations of thyrotoxicosis do not represent a true emergency, the extreme case of so-called thyroid storm does. Early detection and treatment of this condition may prevent progression to shock and death.

## ANATOMY

The thyroid gland derives its name from the shape of the nearby thyroid cartilage (from the Greek, meaning "shield"). Although it varies, the isthmus is usually centered over the third tracheal ring. Normal adult thyroid dimensions are a height of 5 cm, thickness of 1.5 cm, isthmus thickness of 0.5 cm, volume of 10 cm, and weight of 12 to 20 g. Thyroid thickness greater than 2 cm is considered abnormal.

The thyroid gland is palpable on physical examination in nonobese patients; thyroid nodules and some cancers are sometimes noted on palpation. Rarely, ectopic thyroid gland tissue is found at the base of the tongue.

## PHYSIOLOGY

Thyrotropin-releasing hormone (TRH) is synthesized in the hypothalamus and regulates the production of thyroid-stimulating hormone (TSH), or thyrotropin, in the anterior pituitary gland. Principal cells in the thyroid bind TSH, which activates the production and release of thyroid hormones.

The thyroid is highly efficient in its absorption and extraction of iodine. Iodine is added to tyrosine to make up diiodotyrosine (DIT); two molecules of DIT combine to form thyroxine ($T_4$), much of which is stored in the thyroid gland. $T_4$ is released into the circulation largely bound by thyroid-binding globulin (TBG). Even though levels of TBG vary widely, this protein is seldom involved in a disease process.

Triiodothyronine ($T_3$) is formed by peripheral conversion of $T_4$ in tissues. When compared with $T_4$, $T_3$ is four to six times more active, exhibits less affinity for TBG, and has a much shorter half-life (12 hours versus 6 days). $T_3$ and $T_4$ exert feedback on the hypothalamus and TRH levels, thereby completing a regulatory loop.

$T_3$ and $T_4$ stimulate metabolic activity in tissues throughout the body. Both hormones are associated with growth and development early in life.

## GOITER

Goiter refers to a visible enlargement of the thyroid gland that may result from euthyroid, hyperthyroid, or hypothyroid states. The presence of a goiter mandates a detailed review of systems and appropriate thyroid testing to determine the functional status of the tissue. The most common cause of goiter is iodine deficiency. Other causes include Hashimoto thyroiditis, Graves disease, nodules, cancer, and lithium therapy.

Goiters are usually benign, but thyroid malignancy must be considered in each case. Three rare but potentially life-threatening emergencies can result from continued enlargement of a malignant goiter. First, partial or complete obstruction of the jugular veins may occur, especially in hypercoagulable patients. Clot extension from a partially obstructed jugular vein can impede venous drainage from the brain. Second, invasive or extremely large goiters have been reported to cause airway compromise. Third, malignant involvement of the carotid sheath structures can result in devastating morbidity.

## HYPOTHYROIDISM

## PATHOPHYSIOLOGY

Primary hypothyroidism implies a condition of thyroid tissue dysfunction. Causes include Hashimoto thyroiditis, surgical ablation, iodine I 131 ablation, and iodine deficiency. Idiopathic cases are frequently observed as well. The most common cause of hypothyroidism in industrialized countries is Hashimoto thyroiditis, an autoimmune disease of unclear cause.

Secondary hypothyroidism refers to pituitary dysfunction that results in a low TSH level and subsequent poor stimulation of otherwise normal thyroid tissue. Pituitary dysfunction generally affects more than one endocrine axis (panhypopituitarism); hypothyroidism is never the only resultant condition. Secondary hypothyroidism is seen with Sheehan syndrome and space-occupying lesions (adenomas) of the pituitary gland.

Hypothyroidism is 3 to 10 times more common in women than in men. Its incidence increases with age and obesity; 1% of young girls are affected as compared with 6% of older women. Smoking has been identified as an independent risk factor for hypothyroidism, but the reason for the observed association is unknown. Hypothyroidism has no racial or ethnic predilection. Symptoms of hypothyroidism are more apparent during the winter months in moderate and cold climates.

Iodine deficiency is the major worldwide cause of both hypothyroidism and cretinism; the latter is characterized by growth and mental retardation. Selenium deficiency appears to worsen the cretinism. Iodine deficiency is rare in the United States but affects approximately one in three persons worldwide, particularly in mountainous regions. Iodine deficiency has been decreasing because of supplementation programs sponsored by the World Health Organization. Excessive supplementation and diets high in seafood may contribute to thyroiditis.

## CLINICAL PRESENTATION

Hypothyroidism is a deficiency of thyroid hormones that results in decreased metabolic activity. It mimics many conditions commonly encountered in the emergency department (ED) and is accompanied by a myriad of indolent symptoms (**Boxes 167.1 and 167.2**).

In a recent study of the incidence of newly diagnosed primary overt hypothyroidism in adults seen in a Taiwanese ED, the most common symptoms were fatigue (50%), dyspnea (45%), chest tightness (20%), constipation (14%), and cold intolerance (9%). The majority of these patients were seen during winter months. In only 21% was hypothyroidism diagnosed by the emergency physician.[3]

Clinicians should maintain a high index of suspicion for hypothyroidism in patients with new-onset depression.

### SEVERE HYPOTHYROIDISM (MYXEDEMA COMA)

Patients with severe hypothyroidism may have mild to moderate hypothermia, depression, lack of energy, and altered mental status. Myxedema coma is a misnomer often used for severe hypothyroidism; not all patients with severe hypothyroidism are truly comatose, whereas most (but not all) patients with hypothyroid coma have myxedema. Myxedema coma best describes a patient in extremis secondary to a severe hypothyroid state (**Box 167.3**).

**BOX 167.1 Symptoms of Hypothyroidism**

| | |
|---|---|
| Fatigue | Irritability |
| Cold intolerance | Coarse hair |
| Weakness | Dry skin |
| Weight gain | Myalgias |
| Depression | Arthralgias |
| Decreased mental function | Brittle fingernails |
| | Myxedema |
| Constipation | Menstrual irregularity |
| Decreased libido | Peripheral neuropathy |

**BOX 167.2 Signs of Hypothyroidism**

| | |
|---|---|
| Prolonged reflexes | Bradycardia |
| Hypothermia | Facial edema |
| Narrow eyebrows | Periorbital edema |
| Peripheral neuropathy | Pale, dry skin |
| Hoarse voice | Sparse axillary and pubic hair |

**BOX 167.3 Findings in Patients with Severe Hypothyroidism (Myxedema Coma)**

| | |
|---|---|
| Decreased mentation | Nonpitting edema |
| Hypothermia | Delayed or absent deep tendon reflexes |
| Bradycardia | |
| Hypotension | Hypoglycemia |
| Periorbital edema | Hyponatremia |

## DIAGNOSIS

Historical symptoms and physical signs suggestive of hypothyroidism justify testing. The incidence of this disease is so high in elderly women that screening of these patients, even though they are asymptomatic, is performed by many primary care physicians.

Markers of primary hypothyroidism include a high serum TSH level and a low unbound free $T_4$ ($FT_4$) level in the presence of classic signs and symptoms. Symptomatic patients with even minimally elevated TSH may benefit from low-dose thyroxine supplementation.

There is disagreement about the level of TSH and $FT_4$ required to begin treatment in asymptomatic individuals. Several sources recommend thyroxine supplementation for asymptomatic patients with a serum TSH level that is three times the upper limit of normal, regardless of a low or low-normal $FT_4$ level.

Secondary hypothyroidism, generally a component of panhypopituitarism, is marked by low TSH, low $FT_4$, and low serum cortisol levels. Both thyroid and steroid replacement is required, and further diagnostic evaluation (e.g., pituitary imaging, endocrine testing) is indicated.

Hypothyroid patients may also have low serum sodium levels and elevated total cholesterol, both of which may resolve with thyroxine therapy.

## TREATMENT

### MILD HYPOTHYROIDISM

Treatment is initiated with levothyroxine, 1.6 mcg/day. In patients with primary thyroid disease, TSH should be monitored every 30 days. Those being treated with levothyroxine do not require monitoring of $FT_4$. Although mild hypothyroidism is not an emergency per se, initiating treatment for symptomatic patients (in consultation with an endocrinologist) is appropriate if the diagnosis is established in the ED. Routine follow-up is necessary.

### SEVERE HYPOTHYROIDISM (MYXEDEMA COMA)

Management of severe hypothyroidism consists of standard ED resuscitation measures, including consideration and empiric treatment of potential sepsis. The only treatment step specific for severe hypothyroidism is intravenous (IV) administration of levothyroxine. Empiric administration of low-dose levothyroxine is appropriate in patients in whom a serum TSH level cannot be obtained in timely fashion. ED treatment of myxedema coma is summarized in **Box 167.4**.

Note that previous studies have deemed $T_3$ supplementation to be unsafe; however, because of the low incidence of myxedema coma, large clinical trials of $T_3$ have not been performed.

**BOX 167.4 Emergency Department Treatment of Myxedema Coma**

Provide airway support and supplemental oxygen as needed. Check bedsid e glucose.
Obtain serum laboratory tests: complete blood count, comprehensive metabolic panel, thyroid-stimulating hormone, free thyroxin, cortisol.
Evaluate for other causes of altered mental status; for example, infection, medication or recreational drug effect, intracranial pathology.
Consider broad-spectrum antibiotics.
Support temperature with passive rewarming.
Administer 0.3 to 0.5 mg of levothyroxine intravenously; decrease to 0.1 mg in patients with suspected heart disease.
Give stress-dose steroid therapy as appropriate.

## DISPOSITION

Patients with mild hypothyroidism may be managed as outpatients with referral to a primary care physician and an endocrinologist. Patients with severe hypothyroidism should be admitted to the hospital for further management.

## THYROTOXICOSIS

Thyrotoxicosis is caused by at least one of four potential mechanisms:

1. Overproduction of thyroid hormones by the thyroid gland
2. Unregulated release of thyroid hormones secondary to destruction of thyroid cells (thyroiditis)
3. Ingestion of thyroid hormones
4. Production of thyroid hormones from ectopic foci (**Fig. 167.1**)

## CAUSES

### GRAVES DISEASE

Graves disease, the most common cause of hyperthyroidism, accounts for approximately 60% to 80% of cases of hyperthyroidism in the United States. It is the most common autoimmune disorder in North America. In this disease, thyroid-stimulating immunoglobulins (an IgG antibody) bind to and activate thyrotropin receptors on thyroid cells, thereby mimicking the action of TSH. Continued binding of the antibody to the TSH receptor leads to excessive production of $T_3$ and thyroid enlargement.[4]

### THYROIDITIS

Thyroiditis describes conditions in which inflammatory changes lead to the destruction of thyroid cells, which results in the excess release of thyroid hormones. This is followed by depletion of circulating thyroid hormones and subsequent euthyroid and, eventually, hypothyroid states.

Autoimmune destruction of thyroid cells is seen in patients with Hashimoto thyroiditis, painless sporadic thyroiditis, and painless postpartum thyroiditis. Hashimoto thyroiditis is characterized by high levels of serum antithyroid antibodies. This

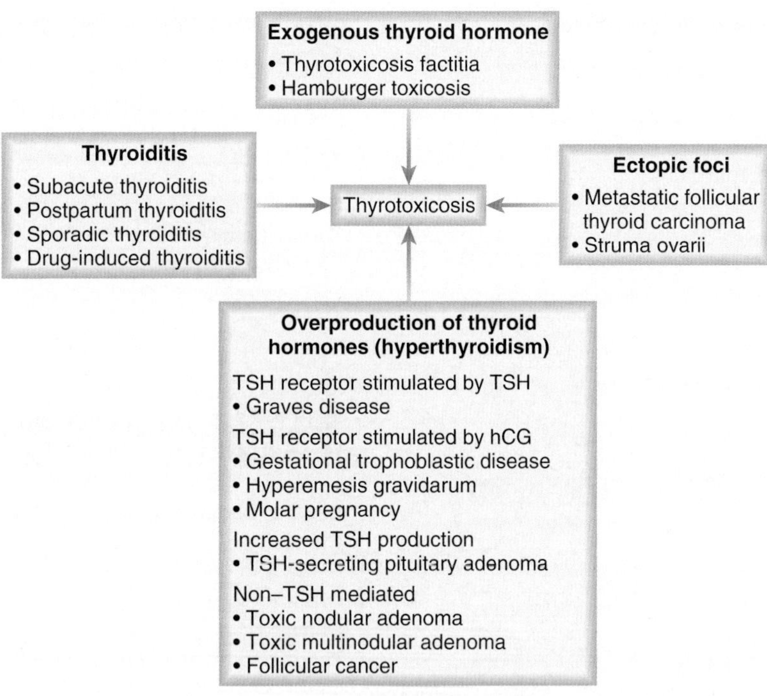


**Fig. 167.1 Causes of thyrotoxicosis.** *hCG*, Human chorionic gonadotropin; *TSH*, thyroid-stimulating hormone.

condition is the most common cause of hypothyroidism in the United States.[5] Painless postpartum thyroiditis occurs in up to 10% of American women. Its onset is usually 1 to 6 months after delivery. Approximately 80% of women recover normal thyroid function within a year. The chance of recurrence with subsequent pregnancies is 70%.[6]

Painful subacute (de Quervain) thyroiditis is the most common cause of thyroid pain. It is a self-limited disorder that is frequently preceded by an upper respiratory infection. Suppurative thyroiditis is a very rare condition that is caused by bacterial, fungal, or mycobacterial infection of the thyroid gland. It may be seen in severely immunocompromised patients. Additionally, amiodarone and lithium can cause drug-induced thyroiditis.[7]

### NON–THYROID-STIMULATING HORMONE–MEDIATED HYPERTHYROIDISM

Hyperthyroidism is sometimes caused by a benign, monoclonal, autonomously secreting thyroid nodule known as toxic adenoma (Plummer disease). When more than one nodule is present, it is referred to as toxic multinodular goiter. This condition is the second most common cause of thyrotoxicosis and accounts for 5% to 15% of all cases of thyrotoxicosis. In the United States, toxic multinodular goiter is primarily seen in persons older than 50 years and accounts for more than 40% of all cases of thyrotoxicosis in this age group.[8] Similarly, thyroid follicular cell cancer can likewise lead to excessive production of thyroid hormones.

### OTHER CAUSES

Increased secretion of thyrotropin by a pituitary adenoma can also cause thyrotoxicosis. Alternatively, thyroid hormones may be produced from sites outside the thyroid gland. This occurs in cases of metastatic follicular thyroid carcinoma and struma ovarii (an ovarian teratoma that contains thyroid tissue).

Human chorionic gonadotropin can also stimulate TSH receptors to produce excess thyroid hormones in patients with gestational trophoblastic disease and hyperemesis gravidarum.

## CLINICAL PRESENTATION

Thyrotoxicosis can be asymptomatic (subclinical hyperthyroidism) or feature mild, moderate, or severe symptoms that result from a surge in catecholamines. Patients with classic thyrotoxicosis may appear nervous, irritable, and tremulous. They may complain of unintentional weight loss, palpitations, exertional dyspnea, heat intolerance, thinning of their hair, irregular menses, increased frequency of bowel movements, and sleep disturbance. On physical examination, patients may have a palpable goiter, warm moist skin, sinus tachycardia out of proportion to fever, or atrial fibrillation on electrocardiography.[9]

Patients with Graves disease may have the following physical findings: goiter, periorbital ecchymosis, chemosis, proptosis, lid retraction, and lower extremity edema.[4,10] Patients with painful subacute thyroiditis may have fever, malaise, myalgias, fatigue, and neck pain in addition to the symptoms of thyrotoxicosis mentioned previously.

### VARIATIONS

#### *Pregnancy*

Women of childbearing age represent the peak incidence of thyroid disease; however, this presents a clinical dilemma

**BOX 167.5 Precipitants of Thyroid Storm**

Sepsis
Surgery
Iodinated contrast medium
Withdrawal of antithyroid medications
Myocardial infarction
Cerebrovascular accident
Trauma (e.g., strangulation)
Ingestion of thyroid hormone

**BOX 167.6 Differential Diagnosis of Thyroid Storm**

Sepsis
Serotonin syndrome
Malignant hyperthermia
Neuroleptic malignant syndrome
Sympathomimetic toxidrome
Pheochromocytoma
Panic attacks

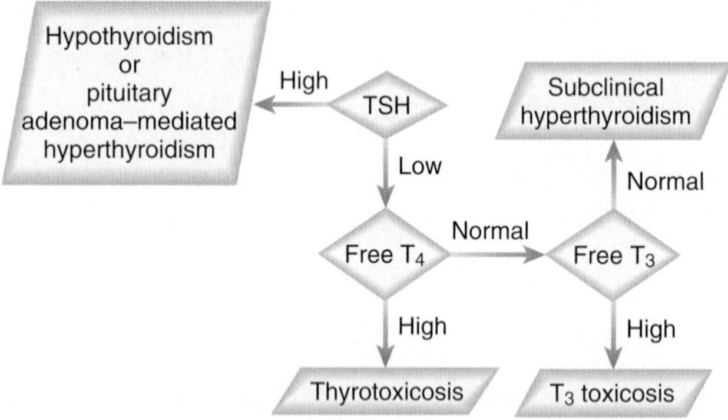


**Fig. 167.2 Interpretation of thyroid-stimulating hormone (TSH), free $T_4$ ($FT_4$), and free $T_3$ ($FT_3$) levels.**

because thyrotoxicosis can mimic the normal physiologic changes of pregnancy. In addition to the symptoms mentioned previously, pregnant patients may have inappropriate weight gain for gestational age, fetal intrauterine growth retardation, and tachycardia that does not slow with a Valsalva maneuver or with fluids.[11]

### *Elderly Patients*

Patients older than 60 years may not exhibit signs of increased catecholamine levels[12]; instead, older adults may have a small goiter, slow atrial fibrillation, weight loss, and severe depression. This manifestation is termed *apathetic thyrotoxicosis.*[13] Other findings in the elderly include atrial fibrillation and congestive heart failure.

### THYROID STORM

Thyroid storm represents the extreme manifestation of thyrotoxicosis. Approximately 1% to 2% of patients with thyrotoxicosis progress to thyroid storm. Common precipitants of this condition are listed in **Box 167.5**. Patients in thyroid storm may exhibit fever, signs of congestive heart failure, agitation, psychosis, and coma. It is a rapidly fatal condition with a mortality rate of 20% to 30% in hospitalized patients.[14]

## DIAGNOSIS

The most useful ED tests for diagnosing thyrotoxicosis are TSH and $FT_4$ measurements. The algorithm in **Figure 167.2** provides an interpretation of variable TSH, $FT_4$, and free triiodothyronine ($FT_3$) levels. **Box 167.6** lists conditions that should be considered in the differential diagnosis.

**BOX 167.7 Emergency Department Testing for Patients in Thyroid Storm**

Bedside serum glucose
Complete blood count, chemistry panel
Blood and urine cultures
Chest radiograph
Urinalysis
Thyroid-stimulating hormone, free thyroxine

Patients with painful subacute thyroiditis will have an elevated serum erythrocyte sedimentation rate and C-reactive protein levels. **Box 167.7** lists the tests that should be obtained in the ED for patients in thyroid storm. If thyrotoxicosis is suspected, an endocrinologist may schedule further testing to confirm the diagnosis and determine the cause. Such tests may include measurement of total $T_3$, thyroid autoantibodies, and radioactive iodine uptake; ultrasonography; and fine-needle biopsy.

## TREATMENT

A beta-blocker should be started in patients with mild symptoms to provide symptomatic relief from tremors, palpitations, tachycardia, sweating, and anxiety (**Fig. 167.3**). It is important to withhold other treatment until the cause of the thyrotoxicosis is confirmed.[15] Treatment options include antithyroid medications, radioactive iodine ablation, and surgery. The risks and benefits of these treatments must be weighed by the patient and the endocrinologist.

Treatment of most forms of thyroiditis is supportive. Patients with persistent tachycardia should be given beta-blockers. Patients with painful subacute thyroiditis should be treated with nonsteroidal antiinflammatory drugs, IV fluids, and beta-blockers.

### THYROID STORM

Medications are administered to stop the synthesis, release, and peripheral effects of thyroid hormones. The order in which antithyroid medications and iodide are given is very important.

First, the synthesis of new thyroid hormone is blocked by the oral administration of 200 mg of propylthiouracil (PTU) every 4 hours or 25 mg of methimazole every 6 hours. (PTU and methimazole should not be given together.) In addition to

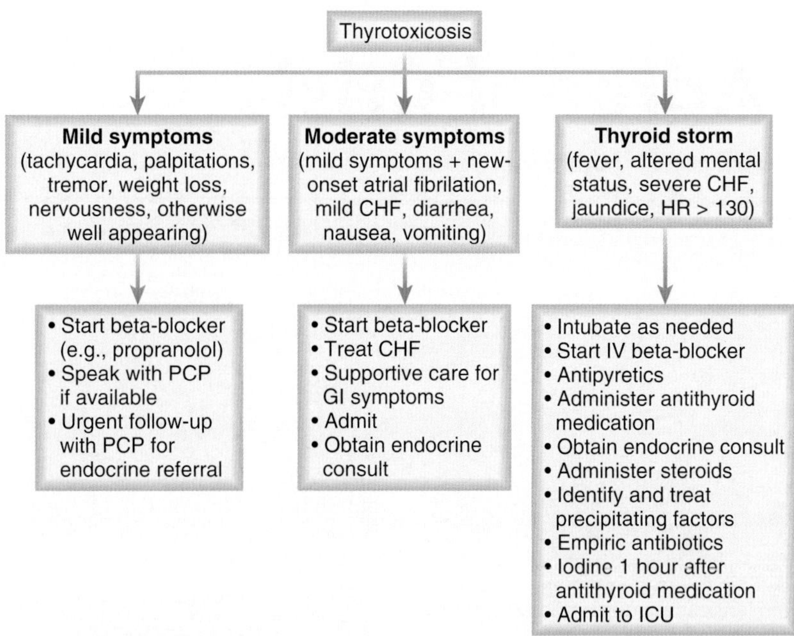


**Fig. 167.3 Emergency department treatment of thyrotoxicosis.** *CHF*, Congestive heart failure; *GI*, gastrointestinal; *HR*, heart rate; *ICU*, intensive care unit; *IV*, intravenous; *PCP*, primary care physician.

blocking the synthesis of new thyroid hormones, PTU also blocks the peripheral conversion of $T_4$ to $T_3$. Methimazole has a longer half-life than PTU does and can therefore be administered less frequently to stable patients. No U.S. Food and Drug Administration–approved IV formulation of these medications is currently available. For patients who cannot tolerate oral medications, PTU tablets should be dissolved in 60 mL of Fleet enema and administered rectally.

Next, release of thyroid hormones is inhibited with iodine. This should be done no sooner than 1 hour after administering the antithyroid medications. Formulations of potassium iodide include Lugol 10% solution (8 drops given orally every 6 hours) and saturated solution of potassium iodide (5 drops given orally every 5 hours), which is highly concentrated and more palatable.

Other supportive therapy that should be initiated includes beta-blockers (e.g., esmolol, metoprolol, propranolol) to counteract the catecholamine surge and acetaminophen for fever; aspirin and other salicylates should be avoided because they decrease thyroid protein binding and increase the amount of free thyroid hormones in circulation.

Patients in thyroid storm may have concomitant adrenal insufficiency that may or may not lead to refractory hypotension. Treatment consists of hydrocortisone, 100 mg intravenously every 8 hours, or dexamethasone (Decadron), 8 mg given intravenously.[8,16,17]

## DISPOSITION

Patients with mild symptoms of thyroid disease may be discharged with beta-blocker therapy and primary care follow-up instructions. Those with moderate symptoms should be admitted to the hospital for supportive care and endocrinology consultation. Patients with severe symptoms or thyroid storm should be admitted to the intensive care unit.

## SUGGESTED READINGS

Brent GA. Clinical practice. Graves' disease. N Engl J Med 2008;358:2594-605.
Chen YJ, Hou SK, How CK, et al. Diagnosis of unrecognized primary overt hypothyroidism in the ED. Am J Emerg Med 2010;28:866-70.
Cooper DS. Hyperthyroidism. Lancet 2003;362:459-68.
Pearce EN, Farwell AP, Braverman LE. Thyroiditis. N Engl J Med 2003;348:2646-55.
Ringel MD. Management of hypothyroidism and hyperthyroidism in the intensive care unit. Crit Care Clin 2001;17:59-74.

## REFERENCES

*References can be found on Expert Consult @ www.expertconsult.com.*

# 168 Adrenal Crisis

*Brian K. Nelson*

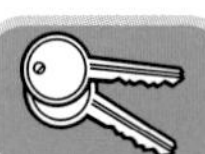

**KEY POINTS**

- Adrenal crisis is an uncommon cause of shock.
- An inappropriate adrenal response may contribute to shock in patients with sepsis, trauma, myocardial infarction, and other conditions associated with extreme physiologic stress.
- The diagnosis of acute adrenal crisis may be challenging because the symptoms are often nonspecific (e.g., weakness, fatigue, gastrointestinal symptoms, abdominal, flank, or back pain).
- Laboratory findings include hyponatremia, hyperkalemia, hypoglycemia, lymphocytosis, and eosinophilia.
- Adrenal crisis may result from either primary adrenal insufficiency or secondary adrenal suppression as a result of exogenous steroids or from failure of the hypothalamic-pituitary-adrenal axis. In the latter, mineralocorticoid replacement is not necessary, but thyroid supplementation may be lifesaving.
- Emergency department management includes aggressive fluid resuscitation, correction of electrolyte abnormalities, maintenance of euglycemia, and administration of glucocorticoids and mineralocorticoids.
- Treatment should begin with initial suspicion of adrenal crisis, not at the time of laboratory confirmation. Interventions are indicated when the cause of the shock is obscure, the patient fails to respond to volume and pressors within 1 hour, or the diagnosis of adrenal insufficiency is confirmed.

## EPIDEMIOLOGY

Most cases of primary adrenal insufficiency are autoimmune mediated, but other common causes include infection and hemorrhage. Onset is generally indolent, although acute adrenal crisis accounts for approximately 25% of all cases. Primary adrenal insufficiency has an estimated incidence of 50 per 1 million persons. Secondary insufficiency as a result of chronic glucocorticoid administration is more common than primary insufficiency in the United States; 2% of the population is estimated to have relative insufficiency that becomes manifested only at times of physiologic stress.[1]

## PATHOPHYSIOLOGY

Adrenal insufficiency is an uncommon disease with nonspecific manifestations, including fatigue, nausea, vomiting, hyperpigmentation, hypotension, and weight loss. Failure to recognize and treat the often subtle signs and symptoms of adrenal crisis can result in significant morbidity and mortality.

Acute adrenal crisis may complicate a variety of conditions that are related to an inadequate neuroendocrine response to stress. Crisis may result from primary adrenal failure or may occur secondary to failure of the hypothalamic-pituitary-adrenal axis. Failure may result from a primary process or may be secondary to suppression by exogenous steroid administration.

## ANATOMY

The adrenal glands are retroperitoneal structures that lie within the fascia of Gerota, superior and medial to the kidneys. Their blood supply arises from the aorta and the renal and inferior phrenic arteries. Blood flows from the arteries through a sinusoidal system and collects in single veins draining into either the inferior vena cava or the left renal vein for the right and left adrenals, respectively. The adrenal glands are encapsulated and divided into a cortex and a catecholamine-producing medullary zone. The cortex is further subdivided into the zona glomerulosa, which produces mineralocorticoids, and the zona fasciculata and zona reticularis, which secrete glucocorticoids and androgens.

## ADRENAL PRODUCTS

Cholesterol is converted to pregnenolone, an adrenal precursor of more than 50 separate chemical pathways and by-products. Of these, the most clinically important glucocorticoid is cortisol, the most important androgen is dehydroepiandrosterone acetate, and the most important mineralocorticoid is aldosterone.

## FEEDBACK LOOPS

Adrenocorticotropic hormone (ACTH) is the major regulator of cortisol and adrenal androgen production. ACTH is regulated by corticotropin-releasing hormone and antidiuretic hormone. Cortisol levels feed back on corticotropin-releasing hormone production. The renin-angiotensin system regulates aldosterone production.

### CORTISOL PHYSIOLOGY

ACTH and cortisol levels vary by circadian rhythm. They both reach their nadir at about 4 AM and peak at approximately 8 AM. Serum levels also peak within minutes of stress-induced release of corticotropin-releasing hormone in the central nervous system. Most circulating cortisol is bound to protein (75% to corticosteroid-binding globulin and 15% to albumin); only 10% is "free cortisol" (unbound).

### TARGETS OF ACTION

Mineralocorticoids act at the renal tubules to maintain $Na^+$, $K^+$, and water balance. Glucocorticoid subunits enter various cell nuclei and modify the expression of a wide range of genes in different organ systems (**Table 168.1**). Cortisol is capable of targeting the mineralocorticoid receptors at pharmacologic doses, although at physiologic levels it is converted to inactive cortisone on entering the kidney.

### CLINICAL APPLICATION

Adrenal insufficiency is classified as primary, secondary, or relative. Causes of primary insufficiency are numerous (**Table 168.2**). Secondary insufficiency is most commonly due to exogenous steroid withdrawal. Relative adrenal insufficiency occurs in individuals who may have normal glucocorticoid levels but exhibit an inadequate response of the hypothalamic-pituitary-adrenal axis to major stress.

Relative adrenal insufficiency is one of the most important subtypes of adrenal insufficiency encountered in emergency medicine. It should be considered in any seriously ill patient who fails to respond to the usual interventions. This condition is most commonly observed in patients with severe sepsis, but it may develop in any patient with uncompensated shock that is resistant to adequate fluid resuscitation and vasopressors.

**Table 168.1** Actions of Glucocorticoids

| FUNCTION/ TARGET SYSTEM | ACTION |
|---|---|
| Metabolism | Stimulate gluconeogenesis<br>Promote lipolysis<br>Induce muscle protein catabolism<br>Increase plasma glucose during stress |
| Endocrine | Inhibit insulin secretion, promote peripheral insulin resistance<br>Increase epinephrine synthesis |
| Inflammatory | Cause demargination of granulocytes, suppress adhesion<br>Reduce circulating eosinophils and lymphocytes<br>Decrease production of inflammatory cytokines |
| Cardiovascular | Increase contractility and the vascular response to vasoconstrictors |
| Renal | Increase the glomerular filtration rate; pharmacologic doses act at mineralocorticoid receptors |

## PRESENTING SIGNS AND SYMPTOMS

Patients with primary and secondary adrenal insufficiency typically have chronic complaints. Those with primary disease may exhibit weakness, fatigue, anorexia, nausea, vomiting, weight loss, hypotension, hyperpigmentation, hyponatremia, and hyperkalemia. The hyperpigmentation is initially generalized and later becomes evident in the mucous membranes, palmar creases, nail beds, and nipples. Gastrointestinal disturbances are present in about half of patients with postural symptoms. Salt craving is a less common complaint. Associated endocrinopathies may complicate the initial findings (see Table 168.2).

Patients with secondary adrenal insufficiency typically have normal mineralocorticoid levels and therefore less serious volume or electrolyte abnormalities. The chronic findings of secondary adrenal insufficiency are classically nonspecific in nature and consist of weakness, lethargy, anorexia, and myalgias. Hyperpigmentation is not a feature of secondary adrenal insufficiency.

## TYPES OF ADRENAL INSUFFICIENCY

### ACUTE ADRENAL INSUFFICIENCY

Although most patients with subacute or chronic adrenal insufficiency are identified during outpatient evaluation, some patients in whom it has not yet been diagnosed will be encountered in the emergency department (ED) with acute insufficiency. Such patients may have either primary or secondary insufficiency and seek care because of physiologic stress that cannot be met with appropriate rises in adrenal hormones. The majority of these patients will exhibit shock, nausea, vomiting, confusion, fever, and abdominal pain.

### ACUTE ADRENAL HEMORRHAGE

Acute adrenal hemorrhage is a rare condition that should be suspected in seriously ill postoperative patients and in those with antiphospholipid syndrome, severe sepsis, or shock. Such patients have the general features of acute adrenal crisis and focal findings of abdominal, flank, or back tenderness. Abdominal examination may reveal a surgical abdomen.

Treatment should begin on suspicion of this diagnosis. Early intervention has been shown to reduce mortality in postoperative patients and those with antiphospholipid syndrome; the timing of therapy does not appear to affect the usually high mortality associated with this condition in patients with sepsis or severe shock. Only a minority of patients will be found to have hyponatremia or hyperkalemia. The diagnosis is confirmed through imaging studies[2,3] (**Fig. 168.1**).

**Table 168.2 Causes of Primary Adrenal Insufficiency**

| CAUSE | ASSOCIATED FACTORS |
|---|---|
| Autoimmune adrenal atrophy (80% of cases) | |
| Associated endocrinopathies | Hypoparathyroidism, hepatitis, type 1 diabetes mellitus, hypogonadism, hypothyroidism |
| Infections | Disseminated tuberculosis, cytomegalovirus, histoplasmosis, human immunodeficiency virus, candidiasis |
| Genetic diseases | Congenital adrenal hyperplasia, adrenoleukodystrophy, familial glucocorticoid deficiency |
| Metastatic malignancy or lymphoma | |
| Adrenal hemorrhage | |
| Infiltrative disorders | Amyloidosis, hemochromatosis |
| Drugs | Ketoconazole, suramin |

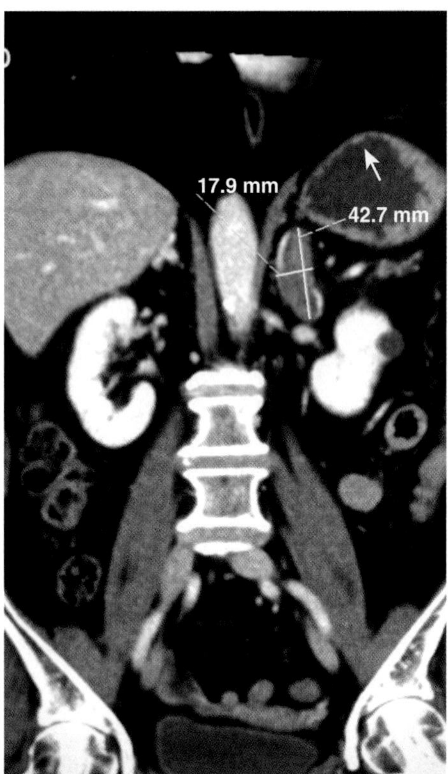


**Fig. 168.1 Coronal section showing left adrenal hemorrhage.** The right adrenal demonstrates a usual inverted "Y" appearance.

## RELATIVE ADRENAL INSUFFICIENCY IN CRITICALLY ILL PATIENTS*

It is estimated that approximately 2% of the U.S. population has an inadequate adrenal response to stress. The incidence of relative adrenal insufficiency in critically ill patients has been reported to be as low as 0% and as high as 77%.[12,15]

Diagnosis and treatment of relative adrenal insufficiency are controversial. Disagreement exists about the incidence of disease, the normal range of serum cortisol levels in response to stress or corticotropin testing in the seriously ill, the dose of corticotropin to be administered for testing, and the indications for, optimal dosing of, and desired efficacy of steroids in the critically ill.[4-13,15]

The use of steroids for sepsis has been explored. Well-designed trials of supraphysiologic doses of steroids have demonstrated no beneficial effect. Two recent randomized clinical trials of corticosteroids in septic shock populations with new criteria for relative adrenal insufficiency and lower dosages of steroids have been completed with conflicting results. Entry criteria differed somewhat between the studies. At present, the following conclusions can be drawn:

1. There is evidence that the use of "low-dose" hydrocortisone may be beneficial for severe septic shock refractory to fluid resuscitation and vasopressors if given early in the course of the shock (within 8 hours).[15]
2. Delayed administration of steroids in resuscitated patients is not beneficial and may be harmful.[6]

## DRUG-INDUCED ADRENAL INSUFFICIENCY

A number of medications may cause reversible adrenal insufficiency. Examples include ketoconazole, rifampin, phenytoin, and etomidate. Use of etomidate as an induction agent for rapid-sequence intubation (RSI) of critically ill patients is controversial. A single dose can cause relative adrenal insufficiency for up to 48 hours, but the clinical significance of this degree of suppression is unclear.[14,16,17] In two retrospective and one prospective observational studies of single-dose etomidate RSI in the ED, no significant difference was found in in-hospital mortality.[18-20] In a randomized study of trauma patients requiring RSI, those receiving etomidate had longer intensive care unit and hospital length of stay and more ventilator days and required more red blood cell transfusions and fresh frozen plasma.[21] In an a priori substudy of the CORTICUS trial, use of etomidate in the 72 hours before study inclusion was associated with higher mortality.[22] However, the

* See references 4 to 14.

**BOX 168.1 Differential Diagnosis**

**Vomiting and Hypotension**
Gastroenteritis with dehydration, sepsis, myocardial infarction, peptic ulcer disease, pancreatitis, cholecystitis, surgical disease

**Weakness and Fatigue**
Anemia, hypopituitarism, depression, neuromuscular disorders

**Hyponatremia**
See Chapter 164, Sodium and Water Balance

survival curves did not separate until 10 to 18 days after the administration of etomidate, thus leading to questions about how the drug could have caused the deaths because relative adrenal suppression usually resolves within 72 hours of a single dose.

The benefits of etomidate for RSI should be weighed against the need for an adrenal stress response. Alternative induction agents can be considered for patients being treated chronically with steroid therapy, for trauma victims, and for those at risk for severe sepsis. Supplemental corticosteroids may be administered empirically for 24 hours if etomidate is used.

## DIFFERENTIAL DIAGNOSIS

The differential diagnosis of adrenal crisis includes most other conditions known to cause shock (**Box 168.1**). These same conditions may induce relative adrenal insufficiency, and therefore their diagnosis does not exclude a concurrent adrenal crisis.

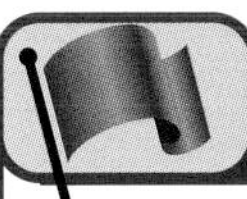

**RED FLAGS**

Conditions that promote shock may induce concurrent relative adrenal insufficiency; diagnosis of one condition does not exclude a second occult disease.

Induction doses of etomidate may cause relative adrenal insufficiency for up to 72 hours after rapid-sequence intubation in critically ill patients.

## DIAGNOSTIC TESTING

Empiric treatment of patients with suspected acute adrenal crisis should not be delayed for confirmatory laboratory testing. The initiation of glucocorticoid therapy should be accompanied by a concurrent, single measurement of serum cortisol. Levels below 15 mcg/dL in a patient with severe sepsis or shock suggest adrenal crisis. Laboratory standards for adrenal function were established in normal subjects and are thus not applicable to populations under physiologic stress.

Adrenal function testing begins with the administration of 250 mcg of synthetic ACTH. A rise in serum cortisol to greater than 8 mcg/dL within 30 minutes is considered a normal response. Such a finding excludes primary insufficiency but does not evaluate hypothalamic-pituitary-adrenal axis–related causes of secondary insufficiency. The hypothalamic-pituitary-adrenal axis is usually tested afterward with a metapyrone or insulin-hypoglycemia challenge. Critically ill patients in whom serum cortisol fails to rise by more than 9 mcg in serial measurements should be considered nonresponders who require glucocorticoid therapy.

The classic finding of concurrent hyponatremia and hyperkalemia may indicate subacute or chronic adrenal insufficiency in the appropriate clinical setting.

Imaging studies may identify adrenal tumors or hemorrhage that may be responsible for the insufficiency. Incidental adrenal pathology is observed in approximately 2% of abdominal scans. Tumors may be benign or malignant, primary or metastatic.[19,20]

## TREATMENT

For the purposes of immediate resuscitation before testing, a functional parameter is used: a patient in shock who fails to respond to fluids and vasopressors within 1 hour should be treated empirically for adrenal insufficiency.

### HYDROCORTISONE

Patients with adrenal crisis should receive intravenous (IV) hydrocortisone replacement. The initial adult dose of hydrocortisone is 100 mg every 6 hours. In children the dose can be given as 50 to 75 mg/m$^2$/day divided into four IV doses. The dose can be tapered as the patient's condition stabilizes. Severely ill patients, particularly those exhibiting septic shock, may require longer durations of treatment.

### DEXAMETHASONE

Stable patients may be given IV dexamethasone, 4 mg every 6 hours. Dexamethasone allows a corticotropin stimulation test to be conducted because it does not immediately suppress hypothalamic activity. Dexamethasone has little mineralocorticoid activity, however, and should therefore be avoided in patients with adrenal crisis.

### FLUDOCORTISONE

Mineralocorticoid therapy is available only in oral form in the United States. Parenteral hydrocortisone, 100 mg given every 6 hours, has sufficient mineralocorticoid activity to adequately treat critically ill patients who cannot tolerate oral medications. As their condition stabilizes and patients are able to take medications by mouth, hydrocortisone is tapered and oral fludrocortisone, 0.05 to 0.1 mg, is added each morning. Patients with secondary adrenal insufficiency do not require mineralocorticoids.

### OTHER TREATMENT CONSIDERATIONS

Patients with primary failure of the hypothalamic-pituitary-adrenal axis may have concurrent clinical hypothyroidism and require thyroxine supplementation. All patients with adrenal insufficiency should undergo prompt correction of volume status, electrolyte imbalance, and hypoglycemia.

Patients with incidental laboratory findings may be referred for outpatient management if they have no clinical evidence of acute adrenal insufficiency or excess, aldosterone excess, or pheochromocytoma. Adrenal masses larger than 6 cm will probably be removed, as well as those that demonstrate endocrine activity.

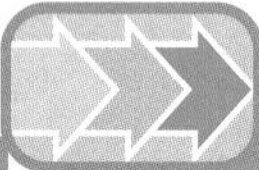

**PRIORITY ACTIONS**

**Do:**

Use a bedside glucometer and administer 50% dextrose in water as needed.
Administer a 20-mL/kg bolus of normal saline.
Begin vasopressors when shock persists despite volume resuscitation.
Check serum electrolytes, thyroid-stimulating hormone, and free thyroxine levels.
Check a random serum cortisol level.
Administer 100 mg of hydrocortisone intravenously every 6 hours.
Search for comorbid conditions, particularly causes of sepsis.

**Do Not:**

Withhold glucocorticoids while awaiting laboratory results.
Attempt endocrine stimulation testing in acutely ill patients.

**Disposition**

Patients with shock or obtundation should be admitted to a critical care unit. Those who quickly respond to treatment may be considered for admission to an unmonitored floor. Patients with mild symptoms, known disease, and reliable follow-up can be treated in the emergency department and be discharged to the care of their personal physician (see Tables 168.1 and 168.2).

**DOCUMENTATION**

History of steroid administration and withdrawal
Risk factors for adrenal crisis: malignancy, tuberculosis, cytomegalovirus infection, human immunodeficiency virus infection, infiltrative disorders
Record of initial serum glucose, sodium, potassium, and volume status

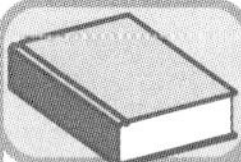

**PATIENT TEACHING TIPS**

Absolute lifelong compliance with outpatient medication regimens is mandatory.
Double the steroid doses during times of physiologic stress and minor illness.
Seek medical attention if nausea and vomiting occur; they may be symptoms of adrenal crisis and might prevent tolerance of needed oral medications.

## SUGGESTED READINGS

Annane D, Sebille V, Charpentier C, et al. Effect of treatment with low doses of hydrocortisone and fludrocortisone on mortality in patients with septic shock. JAMA 2002;288:862-71.
Cuthbertson BH, Sprung CL, Annane D, et al. The effects of etomidate on adrenal responsiveness and mortality in patients with septic shock. Intensive Care Med 2009;35:1868-76.
Hildreth AN, Mejia VA, Maxwell RA, et al. Adrenal suppression following a single dose of etomidate for rapid sequence induction: a prospective randomized study. J Trauma 2008;65:573-9.
Sprung CL, Annane D, Keh D, et al. Hydrocortisone therapy for patients with septic shock. N Engl J Med 2008;358:111-24.
Tekwani KL, Watts HF, Rzechula KH, et al. A prospective observational study of the effect of etomidate on septic patient mortality and length of stay. Acad Emerg Med 2009;16:11-4.

## REFERENCES

*References can be found on Expert Consult @ www.expertconsult.com.*

# Rhabdomyolysis 169

*Bruce D. Adams and Charles B. Arbogast*

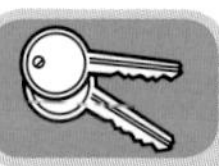

**KEY POINTS**

- The most common causes of rhabdomyolysis include substance abuse, direct muscle injury, infection, strenuous physical activity, medications, and toxic ingestions.
- Only 50% of patients with rhabdomyolysis complain of specific muscle symptoms, and less than 10% have muscle tenderness on examination.
- Acute kidney injury is a potential major complication of rhabdomyolysis.
- Aggressive fluid resuscitation decreases the likelihood of kidney injury.
- Rhabdomyolysis and crush syndrome often emerge as the leading causes of delayed mortality in mass casualty incidents involving building collapse.
- Early hemodialysis is indicated when severe hyperkalemia, refractory metabolic acidosis, or crush injury is present.
- Use of supplemental calcium or loop diuretics should be avoided if possible in the setting of rhabdomyolysis.

## DEFINITION AND EPIDEMIOLOGY

Rhabdomyolysis is a condition characterized by injury to skeletal muscle that results in release of the intracellular contents into the extracellular fluid and circulation. Authoritative thresholds for creatine kinase (CK) range between 1000 and 10,000 U/L, but some definitions additionally mandate the presence of myoglobinuria (**Box 169.1**).

Rhabdomyolysis can occur secondary to trauma, exertion, muscle hypoxia, genetic defects, infections, changes in body temperature, metabolic and electrolyte disorders, drugs and toxins, and idiopathic causes. Various categorizations of rhabdomyolysis have been proposed: traumatic versus atraumatic, reversible versus irreversible, endogenous versus exogenous, and hereditary versus acquired. More than half of all cases of rhabdomyolysis are multifactorial (**Box 169.2**).

Rhabdomyolysis afflicts more than 25,000 individuals in the United States each year. Morbidity and mortality vary tremendously depending on etiology, available treatment, time course, and comorbid factors. Acute kidney injury is a potential major complication of rhabdomyolysis and worldwide occurs in 15% to 45% of cases. In contrast, 7% to 10% of cases of acute kidney injury in the United States are caused by rhabdomyolysis.[1] Mortality generally ranges from 3% to 10% but can be as high as 25% in mass casualty incidents that involve crush injuries.

Certain populations appear to be at increased risk for the development of rhabdomyolysis. Alcohol and recreational drug abusers, patients taking numerous medications, military recruits, and athletes training well above their level of conditioning are of particular concern. Athletes with a predominance of type II fast twitch fibers (typically sprinters and weight lifters) are at higher risk for rhabdomyolysis than are those with a majority of type I slow twitch fibers (e.g., marathon runners). A large number of genetic disorders are linked to rhabdomyolysis as well.

## PATHOPHYSIOLOGY

Rhabdomyolysis is a condition characterized by injury to skeletal muscle that alters the integrity of the cell membrane. Despite the large number of causes of rhabdomyolysis, the underlying pathology involves direct damage to the sarcolemma or depletion of adenosine triphosphate (ATP) within the myocyte resulting in an unregulated increase in intracellular calcium. This leads to constant contraction, energy depletion, and eventual necrosis and death of the muscle cell with release of its intracellular contents into the circulation.[2] The most important products released include potassium, phosphorus, myoglobin, CK, aspartate transaminase, alanine transaminase, lactate dehydrogenase, urate, cytokines, and purines.

## CAUSES OF RHABDOMYOLYSIS

### DIRECT MUSCLE INJURY

Traumatic rhabdomyolysis is primarily the result of motor vehicle crashes, occupational injuries, or environmental tragedy (i.e., mine collapse, earthquakes, war). Muscle compression may also occur during torture and abuse, long-term confinement in the same position (as with orthopedic injuries or during restraint of psychiatric patients), prolonged surgical interventions with improper positioning (high lithotomy or

**BOX 169.1 Suggested Definition of Clinical Rhabdomyolysis**

Absolute creatine kinase > 15,000 U/L

*or*

Creatine kinase > 5000 U/L *and* any of the following:

- Crush injury
- Acute kidney injury or overt failure
- Myoglobinuria
- Acidosis, disseminated intravascular coagulation, hypocalcemia, or hyperkalemia
- Massive muscle injury
- Prolonged extrication or initial evaluation delayed longer than 4 hours

lateral decubitus position), and coma. Compression causes muscle ischemia as tissue pressure exceeds capillary perfusion pressure. Additionally, direct mechanical injury to the sarcolemma causes an incipient rise in intracellular calcium. Calcium activates destructive enzymes within the cell that facilitate necrosis and death of the myocyte.

## INFECTION

Bacterial, viral, parasitic, and rickettsial infections have been associated with rhabdomyolysis. The most common viral cause is influenza. Viruses cause rhabdomyolysis both by direct muscle invasion and by endotoxins and exotoxins that are responsible for skeletal muscle injury and subsequent release of myoglobin. *Legionella* is the most common bacterial cause, with its myotoxic effects mediated through an

**BOX 169.2 Causes of Rhabdomyolysis**

**Direct Muscle Injury**
Burns
Electrical injury
Lightning injury
Sickle cell disease
Trauma, crush, compression

**Ischemic Injury**
Compartment syndrome
Compression
Sickle cell disease
Vascular occlusion (embolism, thrombosis)
Vasculitis

**Excessive Muscular Activity**
Acute dystonia
Contact sports
Delirium tremens
Isometric exercise
Lethal catatonia
Overexertion in untrained athletes
Psychosis
Seizures
Sports, basic training, marathon running
Status asthmaticus

**Drugs of Abuse**
Amphetamines
Caffeine
Cocaine
Methylenedioxymethamphetamine (MDMA; "ecstasy")
Ethanol
Gasoline
Heroin
Lysergic acid diethylamide (LSD)
Marijuana
Mescaline
Methamphetamines
Opiates
Phencyclidine (PCP; "angel dust")
Toluene

**Medications**
Amphotericin B
Antihistamines
Azathioprine
Barbiturates
Benzodiazepines
Butyrophenones
Chlorpromazine
Cimetidine
Codeine
Clofibrate
Colchicine
Corticosteroids
Cotrimoxazole
Cyclosporine
Erythromycin
3-Hydroxy-3-methylglutaryl–coenzyme A (HMG-CoA) reductase inhibitors
Inhalational anesthetics
Isoniazid
Itraconazole
Lindane
Lithium
Lovastatin
Methadone
Monoamine oxidase inhibitors
Narcotics
Neuroleptic agents
Organic solvent
Pentamidine
Phenothiazine
Phenylpropanolamine
Phenytoin
Procainamide
Quinine
Salicylates
Serotonergic agents
Succinylcholine
Theophylline
Total parenteral nutrition

endotoxin. *Salmonella* and *Streptococcus* also induce rhabdomyolysis through direct myocyte invasion and inhibition of glycolytic enzymes.

## EXCESSIVE MUSCLE CONTRACTION

Strenuous exercise by both trained and untrained athletes can cause rhabdomyolysis. The degree of muscle injury is related to the duration and intensity of the exercise, and damage is frequently confined to the lower extremities. Muscle injury is exacerbated by hot, humid conditions; lack of heat acclimatization; prolonged, profuse sweating; and insufficient intake of salt. Patients at increased risk include athletes, marathon runners, new military recruits ("march myoglobinuria"), outdoor workers, and persons unaccustomed to strenuous exercise ("white collar rhabdomyolysis").

Pathologic causes of excessive muscle activity such as status epilepticus, myoclonus, dystonia, tetanus, chorea, and mania also lead to rhabdomyolysis. Additionally, patients suffering from a multitude of intoxications, including isoniazid, strychnine, amoxapine, loxapine, theophylline, water hemlock, and lithium, may experience excessive motor activity and seizures producing rhabdomyolysis.

Excessive muscle activity causes rhabdomyolysis through dehydration, increased activity of heat-sensitive degradative

**BOX 169.2 Causes of Rhabdomyolysis—cont'd**

**Medications—cont'd**
Tricyclic antidepressants
Trimethoprim-sulfamethoxazole
Vasopressin
Zidovudine

**Metabolic Disorders**
Diabetic ketoacidosis
Hyperaldosteronism
Hypernatremia
Hypokalemia
Hyponatremia
Hypophosphatemia
Hypothyroidism
Nonketotic hyperosmolar coma
Renal tubular acidosis
Thyrotoxicosis

**Genetic Disorders**
***Affecting Carbohydrate Metabolism***
Adenine deaminase deficiency
Amylo-1,6-glucosidase deficiency
Cytochrome disturbances
α-Glucosidase deficiency
Lactate dehydrogenase deficiency
Myophosphorylase deficiency (McArdle disease)
Phosphofructokinase deficiency
Phosphoglycerate kinase deficiency
Phosphoglycerate mutase deficiency

***Affecting Lipid Metabolism***
Carnitine deficiency
Carnitine palmitoyltransferase deficiency
Short- and long-chain acyl-coenzyme A dehydrogenase deficiency

***Affecting Purine Metabolism***
Duchenne muscular dystrophy
Myoadenylate deaminase deficiency

**Immunologic Diseases**
Dermatomyositis
Polymyositis

**Infection**
***Bacterial***
Gas gangrene
Group A β-hemolytic streptococci
Legionnaires disease
*Salmonella*
Septic shock
*Shigella*
*Staphylococcus aureus*
*Streptococcus pneumonia*
Tetanus

***Viral***
Adenovirus
Coxsackievirus
Cytomegalovirus
Echovirus
Epstein-Barr virus
Hepatitis
Herpes simplex virus
Human immunodeficiency virus
Influenza A and B
Parainfluenza
Rotavirus

***Other***
Parasites—trichinosis
Rickettsial—Rocky Mountain spotted fever

**Temperature Related**
Heat stroke
Hyperthermia
Hypothermia
Malignant hyperthermia
Neuroleptic malignant syndrome

**Toxins**
Brown recluse spider bite
Carbon monoxide
Centipede bite
Cyanide
Ethylene glycol
Haff disease
Hymenoptera sting
Isopropyl alcohol
Mercuric chloride
Methanol
Quail ingestion
Snake venom
Tetanus toxin
Toluene
Typhoid toxin
Water hemlock

enzymes, and depletion of cellular energy (ATP) with prolonged exercise. These insults lead to failure of the sarcolemmal sodium-potassium adenosine triphosphatase ($Na^+,K^+$-ATPase) and $Ca^{2+}$ pumps, which results in increased intracellular calcium and cell necrosis.

### MEDICATIONS

Drugs in almost every category have been implicated as a cause of rhabdomyolysis. The medications of most concern are the lipid-lowering agents, including 3-hydroxy-3-methylglutaryl–coenzyme A (HMG-CoA) reductase inhibitors (lovastatin, simvastatin) and fibric acid derivates that decrease triglyceride synthesis (gemfibrozil and clofibrate). HMG-CoA reductase inhibitors block the production of coenzyme Q, which plays an important role in the production of ATP in mitochondria. The resultant decrease in ATP production leads to cell death and subsequent rhabdomyolysis. Patients with preexisting renal dysfunction are at increased risk.

Immediate withdrawal of these drugs is mandatory if patients complain of muscle dysfunction or if their CK level rises to more than three times normal. The risk for drug-induced muscle disease is aggravated by the simultaneous administration of danazol, nicotinic acid, cyclosporine, itraconazole, or erythromycin. The combination of HMG-CoA reductase inhibitors with gemfibrozil also carries a high rate of myotoxicity.

### DRUGS OF ABUSE

Substance abuse is one of the most common causes of rhabdomyolysis, largely because of the high incidence of ethanol abuse and its direct toxicity to the myocyte membrane. Other drugs of abuse implicated in cases of rhabdomyolysis include cocaine, heroin, methamphetamine, phencyclidine hydrochloride (PCP), lysergic acid diethylamide (LSD), 3,4-met hylenedioxymethamphetamine (MDMA; "ecstasy"), benzodiazepines, and barbiturates. Most abused drugs cause muscle damage through direct toxic effects or immunologic reactions to the contaminants found mixed with the drug. Cocaine is also toxic to the sarcolemma and induces vasospasm resulting in ischemia. Cocaine increases energy demands of the cell that outstrip energy production.

Besides its direct toxicity, ethanol has multiple additional mechanisms by which it causes muscle damage. Its sedative and hypnotic properties may cause prolonged immobilization of a body part, with external compression of its blood supply leading to ischemia. Rhabdomyolysis can be induced by excessive motor activity when associated with alcohol-related seizures and delirium tremens. Poor nutrition inhibits the rate of ethanol metabolism, and the resultant higher blood ethanol concentration at the cell membrane for prolonged periods leads to increased sarcolemmal damage.

### TOXINS

Toxins that cause direct myocyte damage include venom from the European adder, the Australian tiger snake, the Australian king brown snake, the death adder, and North and South American rattlesnakes. These snakes deploy a single venom with multiple myocyte toxins that cause direct muscle injury and rhabdomyolysis. Stings from Africanized bees (killer bees) and honeybees mediate rhabdomyolysis through myotoxins. Quail fed hellebores or hemlock have also been associated with outbreaks of rhabdomyolysis (coturnism). Outbreaks of Haff disease occur intermittently in the United States as a result of contaminated fish.

Toxins that act at the molecular level by interfering with the production of ATP are capable of producing damage to skeletal muscle. Carbon monoxide, cyanide, hydrogen sulfide, and phosphine inhibit electron transport in mitochondria; salicylates and chlorphenoxy herbicides uncouple oxidative phosphorylation; and iodoacetate and sodium fluoroacetate inhibit glycolysis in the Krebs cycle.

### GENETIC DISORDERS

Rhabdomyolysis can result from genetic defects in glycolysis, glycogenolysis, fatty acid oxidation, and mitochondrial function. These disorders cause inappropriate use of carbohydrate and lipids, which leads to an imbalance between energy supply and demand in myocytes.

Genetic defects should be suspected in patients in whom the cause of rhabdomyolysis is obscure. Symptoms often begin before the age of 20 years, and attacks occur intermittently. Examples include recurrent rhabdomyolysis after minimum to moderate exercise, after viral infections starting in childhood, or in patients with a family history of rhabdomyolysis. In glycogenolytic disorders, the mode of inheritance is usually autosomal dominant; phosphoglycerate kinase deficiency is X-linked.

Diagnosis of an inherited muscle enzyme defect is based on muscle biopsy findings demonstrating abnormally increased glycogen or lipid deposits, as well as histochemical staining demonstrating a decrease or absence of specific enzymes.

## PRESENTING SIGNS AND SYMPTOMS

Common symptoms include myalgias, fatigue, and red or brown urine; however, atypical findings are customary for rhabdomyolysis. Only 50% of patients complain of specific muscle symptoms, and less than 10% have muscle tenderness. Liberal testing for rhabdomyolysis is therefore warranted in high-risk populations. Rhabdomyolysis should be considered in patients with hyperkalemia, disseminated intravascular coagulation (DIC), sepsis, cardiovascular collapse, compartment syndrome, heat stroke, altered mental status, and acute kidney injury. These patients may have occult primary rhabdomyolysis or suffer from rhabdomyolysis as a complication of their primary disease process.

## MEDICAL DECISION MAKING AND DIAGNOSTIC TESTING

### CREATINE KINASE

CK is the enzyme responsible for reversible transfer of the terminal phosphate group of ATP to creatine to form phosphocreatine. Serum CK begins to rise 2 to 12 hours after the destruction of more than 200 g of muscle, with the peak level occurring between 1 and 3 days. Levels decline within 3 to 5 days after the muscle injury ceases. Serum CK levels remain elevated longer than those of myoglobin because of relatively slow plasma clearance (serum $t_{1/2}$ = 1.5 days). CK decreases at a steady rate of 39% per day. Rhabdomyolysis is suspected at minimum thresholds for CK of between 1000 and 10,000 U/L.

A rise in serum CK follows the rise in serum myoglobin. Three isoenzymes of CK exist in human tissues: MM, MB, and BB. The predominant source of the CK-MM isoenzyme is skeletal and cardiac muscle; CK-BB is found in brain tissue and CK-MB mainly in cardiac muscle. In rhabdomyolysis, the primary CK isoenzyme elevated is CK-MM. Creatine phosphokinase is a serum marker of CK-MM reported by many clinical laboratories.

### MYOGLOBIN

Myoglobin is a small protein with a free circulating concentration that is very low under normal physiologic conditions. Myoglobin functions as an oxygen reservoir in muscles; serum myoglobin levels rise within 1 hour of skeletal muscle damage. Myoglobin levels become normal within 1 to 6 hours after the cessation of muscle injury because of rapid clearing both by renal excretion and by metabolism to bilirubin.

When myoglobin levels reach 15 mg/L, it can be detected by urine dipstick, and at 1 g/L it may cause the color of urine to appear dark, like cola. Myoglobinuria does not always result in dark urine, however; discoloration depends on (1) the amount of myoglobin released from muscle into plasma, (2) the glomerular filtration rate, and (3) the urine concentration.

### URINALYSIS

The urine dipstick is a commonly used screening test for rhabdomyolysis. The orthotoluidine test on the urine dipstick will react in the presence of either myoglobin or hemoglobin. A report of "large blood" on the urine dipstick and absence of red blood cells on microscopy classically suggests the presence of free myoglobin in urine. **Figure 169.1** shows the typical urine appearance in the setting of myoglobinuria. Unfortunately, clinical data do not fully support this screening practice, with microscopic hematuria occurring in about 30% of patients with rhabdomyolysis. In addition, myoglobinuria may be transient and not identified at the time of urinalysis despite the presence of significant clinical rhabdomyolysis. Dipstick testing will detect a urine myoglobin level higher than 1.0 mg/dL, which correlates with a serum value of approximately 100 mg/dL.

Other common findings on urinalysis include the presence of tubular casts, proteinuria, and evidence of acute tubular necrosis.

### RENAL FUNCTION TESTS

Though not consistently observed in all analyses, creatinine has at times been shown to rise faster with rhabdomyolysis than with other causes of acute renal failure. Markedly high creatinine levels or a relatively low ratio of blood urea nitrogen to creatinine should raise suspicion for rhabdomyolysis (**Box 169.3**).

## COMPLICATIONS

Following sufficient muscle damage, extrusion of cellular contents into the general circulation causes several complications, including acute renal failure, metabolic derangements, DIC, compartment syndrome, and peripheral neuropathy.

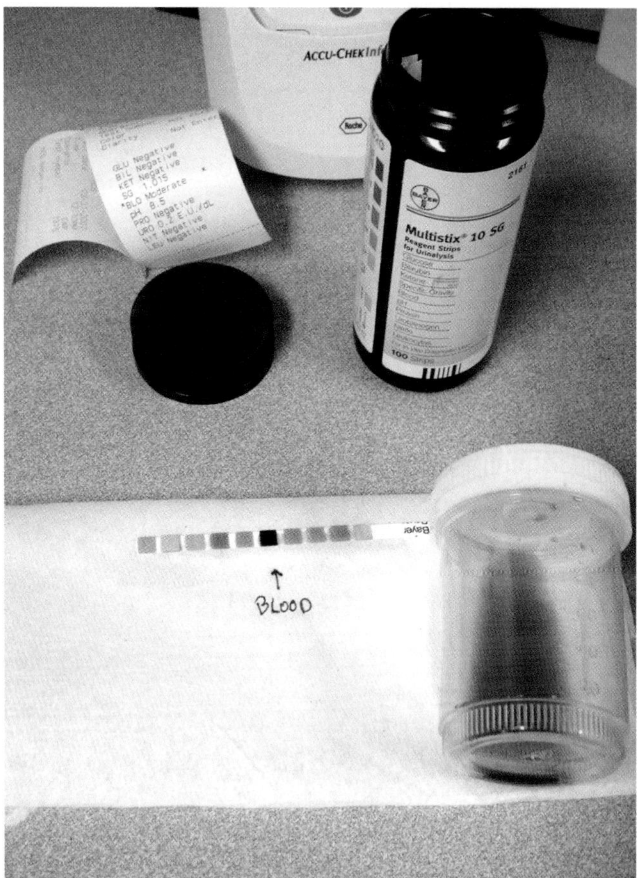


**Fig. 169.1 Myoglobinuria.** The dipstick is strongly positive for blood, with no red blood cells seen on microscopy. (From Roberts JR, Hedges JR. Clinical procedures in emergency medicine. 5th ed. Copyright 2009 Saunders, an imprint of Elsevier.)

### ACUTE KIDNEY INJURY

Acute kidney injury is the most important cause of morbidity in patients with rhabdomyolysis. Rhabdomyolysis induces acute kidney injury by three main pathophysiologic mechanisms. First, the heme protein in myoglobin exerts direct toxicity on renal tubular cells by initiating lipid peroxidation. This toxicity is potentiated by an acidic urine. Second, myoglobin precipitates in the renal tubules and causes intraluminal cast formation and tubular obstruction. Degradation of intratubular myoglobin results in the release of unbound iron, which catalyzes free radical production and further enhances the ischemic damage. Third, renal vasoconstriction is promoted by platelet-activating factor and endothelin.

Acute kidney injury caused by rhabdomyolysis may be oliguric (most common), nonoliguric, or occasionally anuric. It typically results in a higher anion gap acidosis and higher uric acid levels and often leads to a more rapid increase in serum creatinine than do other forms of acute kidney injury. Fractional excretion of sodium is often less than 1%, in contrast to other forms of acute tubular necrosis. It is difficult to predict the patients in whom acute kidney injury will develop based on laboratory values at initial evaluation.[3]

### METABOLIC AND ELECTROLYTE DERANGEMENTS

Hyperkalemia occurs in 10% to 40% of patients with rhabdomyolysis. It is the most serious electrolyte derangement

**BOX 169.3 Laboratory Abnormalities Observed with Rhabdomyolysis**

**Potassium**
Elevated
Risk for acute kidney injury

**Bicarbonate**
Decreased (20 mEq/L)
Metabolic acidosis

**Uric Acid**
Elevated (>7 mg/dL)
Marker of acute renal failure

**Sodium**
Usually normal
Can decrease with mannitol therapy
Use serum osmolarity values as a guide

**Phosphate**
Elevated
Risk for precipitation of calcium phosphate
May need phosphate binders if phosphate >7 mg/dL

**Creatine Kinase**
Elevated
Associated with creatine kinase level of 15 to 75,000

**Blood Urea Nitrogen**
Elevated (>20 mg/dL)

**Creatinine**
Elevated

**Calcium**
Initially low, sometimes markedly so
Rebound phase may demonstrate hypercalcemia

**Liver Function Tests**
Sometimes elevated
Serum aspartate transaminase, lactate dehydrogenase, aldolase, muscle enzyme levels elevated

**Troponin**
Normal
Suspect myocardial damage as a cause (or effect) if elevated
Seven percent false-positive rate for troponin I

**Anion Gap**
Sometimes elevated
May be predictive of acute renal failure

**Prothrombin Time, Partial Thromboplastin Time, D-Dimer**
Disseminated intravascular coagulation in up to 30% of severe cases
Associated with higher mortality

observed with rhabdomyolysis because of its potential lethal effect on cardiac rhythm and function. More than 15 mmol of potassium is released with necrosis of only 150 g of muscle and results in an acute 1.0-mmol/L increase in extracellular potassium. The degree of increase is further dependent on renal function, which is often concurrently impaired.

Hypocalcemia is the most common metabolic complication of rhabdomyolysis; low calcium levels are present early and are usually asymptomatic. Hypocalcemia results from deposition of calcium salts in necrotic muscle secondary to hypophosphatemia and decreased 1,25-dihydroxycholecalciferol. Soft tissue calcifications can be seen on radiographs of the involved limbs. Hypocalcemia should be treated only if severe symptoms or hyperkalemia develops and leads to cardiac arrhythmias, muscular contraction, and seizures. Later, as calcium is mobilized from tissues, serum calcium levels rise and symptomatic hypercalcemia may develop. Hypercalcemia usually occurs in patients with acute renal failure during the diuretic phase, typically when urinary output is greater than 1500 mL/24 hr. Hypercalcemia also occurs more frequently if $Ca^{2+}$ is supplemented in the hypocalcemic stage. Volume expansion alone is usually adequate treatment, but diuretics may be needed.

Hyperphosphatemia is caused by leakage of phosphate from injured myocytes and is higher in azotemic patients. Phosphate binders should be used when phosphate levels exceed 7 mg/dL. Hypophosphatemia may be seen later in the disease course but rarely requires treatment. Hypermagnesemia may occur in patients with renal insufficiency. Standard management is appropriate. Hyperuricemia is especially common in crush injury as a result of the release of muscle adenosine nucleotides, which are subsequently converted to uric acid in the liver. Uric acid levels typically correlate with serum CK levels.

Organic acids, especially lactic acid, are released from hypoxic, necrotic muscle cells and produce a pronounced anion gap acidosis.

## COMPARTMENT SYNDROME

Most striated muscles are contained within rigid compartments formed by fascia and bones. When the muscle is traumatized, marked swelling and edema occur within a closed osteofascial compartment, and muscle perfusion is reduced to a level below that required for cellular viability. As intracompartmental pressure rises above 30 to 35 mm Hg, compartment syndrome develops and significant muscle ischemia ensues and requires decompressive fasciotomy. **Figure 169.2** shows an example of compartment syndrome.

Classic signs and symptoms of compartment syndrome include pain, pallor, paresthesias, poikilothermia, paralysis, and pulselessness. Paresthesias are the most reliable sign—muscle edema exerts pressure on peripheral nerves, which results in neuronal ischemia, paresthesias, and paralysis. Decompressive fasciotomy reverses the peripheral neuropathies within a few days to weeks, although symptoms may be permanent in a minority of patients.

## DISSEMINATED INTRAVASCULAR COAGULATION

DIC occurs in patients with severe rhabdomyolysis when extensive injury results in multisystem organ failure. Although this disorder is more common with severe trauma and crush injury, rhabdomyolysis from medical causes may lead to DIC. Severe bleeding is most pronounced on days 3 to 5 of illness. If severe bleeding does not occur, spontaneous improvement can be expected by days 10 to 14. When severe bleeding does occur, infusion of fresh frozen plasma (to replace coagulation factors) and transfusion of platelets may be indicated.

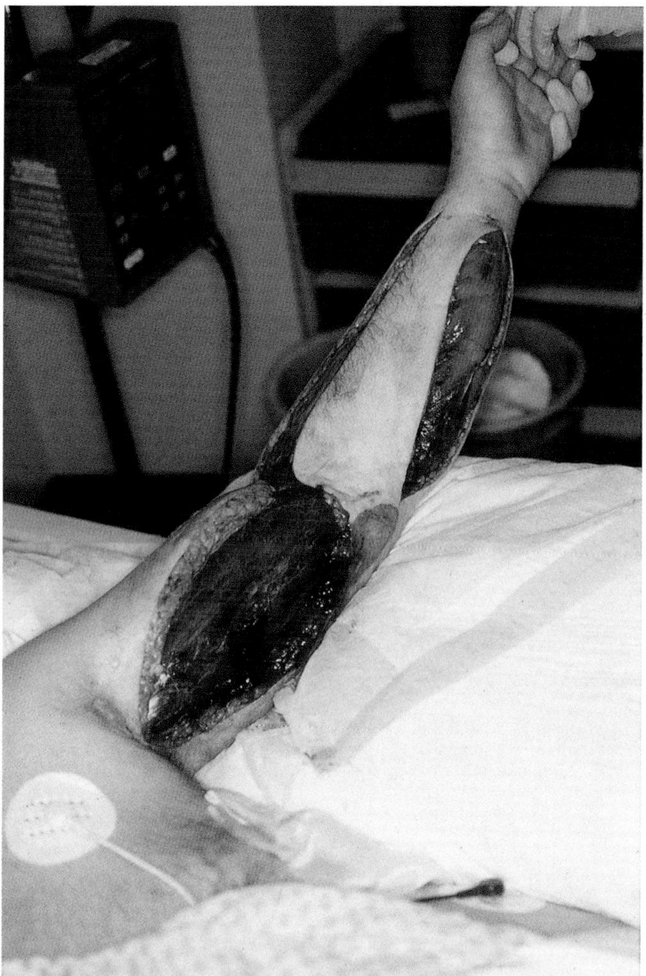

**Fig. 169.2 Compartment syndrome.** This man was in coma from a heroin overdose and had been lying on his arm for a number of hours. He was hypotensive, in renal failure, comatose, and on a ventilator. The entire arm was swollen and rhabdomyolysis was suspected correctly. Because of the coma, he was unable to voice any complaint of pain. When he awakened 20 hours later, the pain was severe, and measurement of compartment pressure demonstrated the need for fasciotomy. Heroin can cause rhabdomyolysis and hypotension on reperfusion, and certainly prolonged pressure on the muscles may have exacerbated the condition. (From Roberts JR, Hedges JR. Clinical procedures in emergency medicine. 5th ed. Copyright 2009 Saunders, an imprint of Elsevier.)

## HEPATIC DYSFUNCTION

Hepatic dysfunction occurs in approximately 25% of patients with rhabdomyolysis. The proteases released from injured muscle may be implicated in hepatic inflammation.

# TREATMENT

## GENERAL MEASURES

Rhabdomyolysis is physiologically and clinically similar to cell degradation states such as tumor lysis syndrome and sepsis. An organized, aggressive treatment strategy should focus on clinical end points similar to those for other cell lysis conditions. The emergency treatment of rhabdomyolysis, in an early goal-directed fashion, is summarized in **Figure 169.3**.

The main goal of therapy is prevention of acute renal failure through high-volume resuscitation.[4] The two most common reasons for the development of acute kidney injury are slow fluid resuscitation and inadequate fluid resuscitation. Normal saline is superior to lactated Ringer solution for the treatment of rhabdomyolysis because normal saline is not associated with risk for phosphate toxicity. More than 10 L of normal saline is typically administered in the first 24 hours of therapy to maintain high-volume dilute urine output.

Initial fluid administration with normal saline is titrated to achieve a goal urine output of 200 to 300 mL/hr. It is important that intravenous (IV) fluid resuscitation be started as soon as possible; fluid resuscitation before the extrication of crushed and trapped patients is preferred. After diuresis is established and urine pH is less than 6.5, fluids are changed to a more alkaline solution (i.e., 75 mmol of sodium bicarbonate added to 1 L of one-half isotonic saline), with the rate titrated to achieve the goal of 200 to 300 mL/hr of urine output. Alternating normal saline with sodium bicarbonate is also an option. If urine pH is higher than 6.5, normal saline is continued. Mannitol, an osmotic diuretic, can be considered in this situation, but only after adequate fluid repletion has been attained.

With moderate to severe alkalemia (serum pH higher than 7.5), acetazolamide can be considered. The goal urine output remains 200 to 300 mL/hr. Fluid repletion is continued until the CK level falls below 5000 to 10,000 U/L and the myoglobinuria clears.

If initial diuresis is not achieved with fluid replacement alone or the patient has contraindications to further fluid replacement, additional diuretics should be considered and a nephrologist consulted for possible renal replacement therapy.

Vital signs, cardiac rhythm, and urine output should be monitored continuously. Medication dosages should be adjusted according to renal function, and drugs that are potentially nephrotoxic should be avoided.

## PHARMACOLOGIC THERAPY

### *Mannitol*

Mannitol theoretically exhibits several protective mechanisms. It is a potent diuretic that may increase myoglobin solubility and excretion in the renal tubules, thereby reducing cast formation. It decreases sodium reabsorption in the kidney, which may promote renal conservation by decreasing the energy requirement of the renal medulla. Additionally, mannitol is probably a potent oxygen free radical scavenger. Mannitol also improves compartment pressures in compartment syndromes that result from crush injuries.

The available literature regarding the effectiveness of mannitol in preventing kidney injury from heme pigment is conflicting. No randomized, controlled trial has supported the general use of mannitol for rhabdomyolysis. However, limited evidence suggests that mannitol along with sodium bicarbonate may be beneficial when CK levels are higher than 20,000 to 30,000 U/L.

Mannitol therapy can be given in both an intermittent and continuous fashion. Intermittent therapy is preferred, with a dose of 0.5 to 1 g/kg (averaged as 400 g over a 60-hour

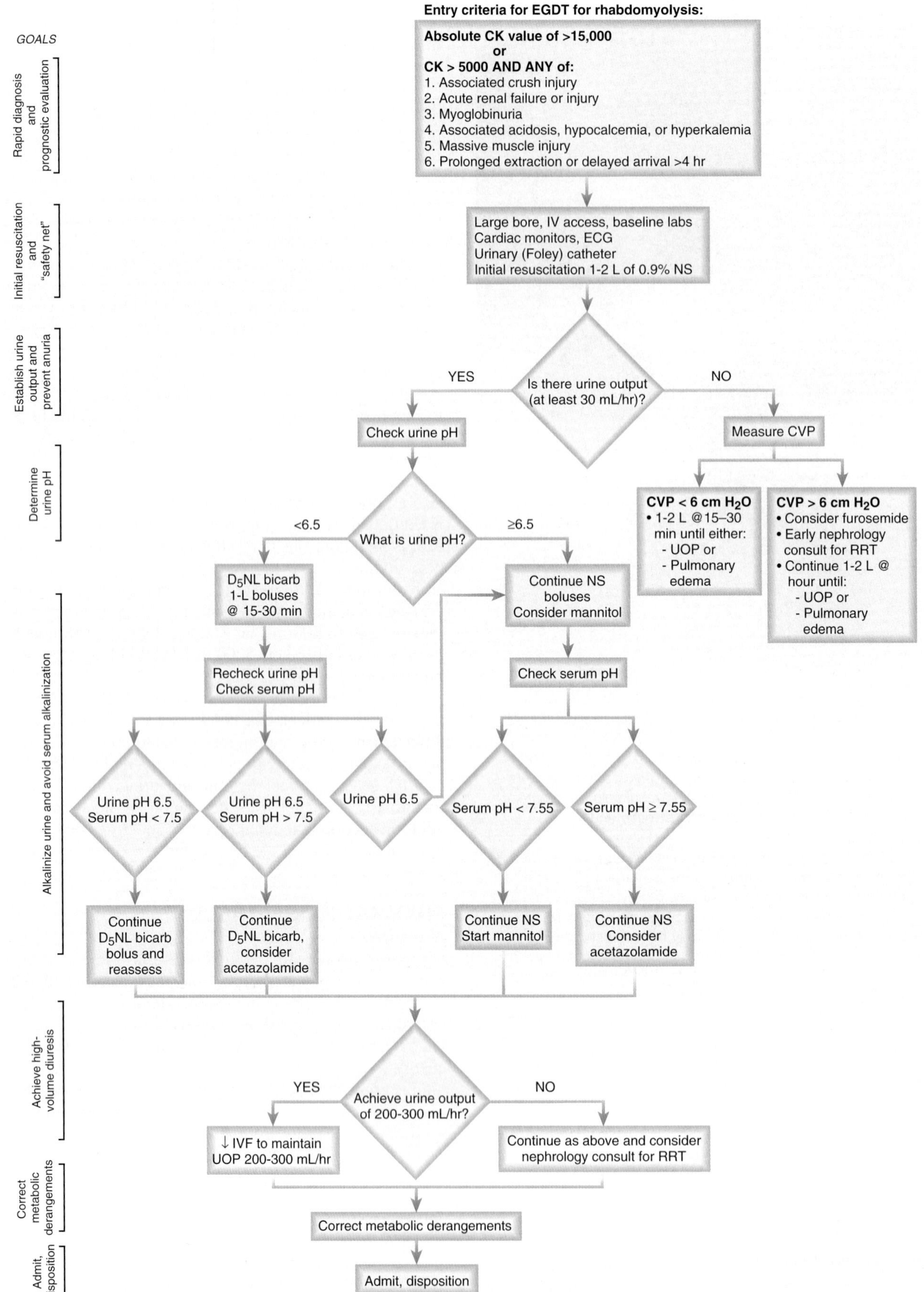


**Fig. 169.3 Early goal-directed therapy for rhabdomyolysis.** *CK*, Creatine kinase; *CVP*, central venous pressure; *$D_5$NL bicarb*, 5% dextrose in normal sodium bicarbonate solution; *EGDT*, early goal-directed therapy; *IV*, intravenous; *IVF*, intravenous fluid; *NS*, normal saline; *RRT*, renal replacement therapy; *UOP*, urinary output.

period) to achieve a urine output of 300 mL/hr. Serum sodium and osmolarity should be checked frequently to avoid a hyperosmolar state. Acute kidney injury is more likely to occur with doses higher than 200 g/day and a cumulative dose higher than 800 g.

### *Sodium Bicarbonate*

Patients with idiopathic rhabdomyolysis may not need bicarbonate therapy, but severely injured or hypotensive patients generate a tremendous organic acid load that often requires treatment with supplemental sodium bicarbonate. Bicarbonate infusion of more than 500 mEq in 24 hours may be indicated. Urine alkalinization with sodium bicarbonate potentially reduces heme protein precipitation and cast formation. As with mannitol, no randomized, controlled trials have demonstrated that sodium bicarbonate therapy is more effective than normal saline alone. Caution should be exercised when administering large doses of bicarbonate because treatment may exacerbate hypocalcemia, alkalemia, and related arrhythmias.

### *Acetazolamide*

Acetazolamide prevents the complications of serum alkalemia caused by bicarbonate therapy. It promotes the excretion of sodium bicarbonate in the renal tubules, thereby inhibiting cast formation. When serum pH exceeds 7.50, a standard dose of acetazolamide (250 mg) may be administered.

## RENAL REPLACEMENT THERAPY AND HEMODIALYSIS

Early hemodialysis is not necessary unless crush injuries or certain complications have occurred (e.g., severe hyperkalemia, refractory metabolic acidosis, oliguria or anuria, volume overload). Early consultation with a nephrologist is warranted. Myoglobin molecules can be removed by hemofiltration, but not by hemodialysis or peritoneal dialysis.

Reductions in morbidity and mortality have been observed in victims of mass casualty incidents who underwent dialysis within 4 to 6 hours of injury.

## EXPERIMENTAL THERAPY

Several promising experimental therapies for rhabdomyolysis have been studied in animal models but have not been well tested in humans. Nitric oxide may prevent acute renal failure by promoting renal vasodilation, and lazaroids (21-aminosteroids) inhibit oxidant-induced lipid peroxidation in animals. Other experimental treatment modalities include deferoxamine (an iron chelator), glutathione, vitamin E, carvedilol, and dantrolene.

## AVOID CALCIUM SUPPLEMENTATION AND LOOP DIURETICS

Patients with rhabdomyolysis often have acute hypocalcemia. The hypocalcemia results from deposition of calcium salts in necrotic muscle. Supplemental calcium administration should be avoided if possible because it can exacerbate the cytoplasmic injury. During the rebound and recovery phases of rhabdomyolysis, calcium is remobilized and hypercalcemia becomes a true risk. Only if the patient is symptomatic or if severe hyperkalemia is present should calcium be considered, and even then other measures to ameliorate the hyperkalemia should be undertaken first.

Loop diuretics (e.g., furosemide) should generally be avoided because they contribute to urine acidification and tubular cast formation. Forced diuresis is best facilitated with mannitol. Under alkalemic conditions, acetazolamide can be considered.

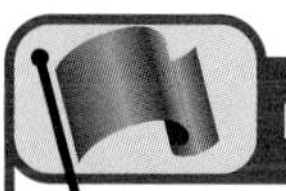

**RED FLAGS**

**Cautions for a Physician**

Hypercalcemia can develop after recovery of acute renal failure secondary to rhabdomyolysis. Calcium administration should be avoided during renal failure unless the patient has symptomatic hypocalcemia or severe hyperkalemia.

With the large volume of fluid administration typically needed in patients with rhabdomyolysis, it is important to monitor the patient closely for any evidence of fluid overload.

If mannitol is used, serum sodium and osmolarity should be checked frequently to avoid a hyperosmolar state. Acute kidney injury may occur with doses higher than 200 g/day and cumulative doses higher than 800 g.

If alkalinization of urine is initiated, there is a potential for worsening of hypocalcemia. It can also lead to hypokalemia. Urine pH, serum bicarbonate, serum calcium, and serum potassium should be monitored, and if urine pH does not rise after 4 to 6 hours or symptomatic hypocalcemia develops, alkalinization should be stopped.

## CRUSH SYNDROME: DISASTER AND MASS CASUALTY CONSIDERATIONS

Delayed extrication from debris causes delayed resuscitation—rhabdomyolysis and crush syndrome often emerge as the leading causes of delayed mortality. Crush syndrome, perhaps the most dramatic manifestation of rhabdomyolysis, results from both the initial blunt force trauma and the marked reperfusion injury that occurs after release of the crushing pressure. Commonly, crush syndrome will occur epidemically because of structural failure from earthquakes or warfare with resultant entrapment of victims beneath debris. Although acute renal failure is the most life-threatening manifestation, crush syndrome can occur with failure of any organ system, much like rhabdomyolysis. Frequently, management of the obvious concomitant traumatic injuries can overshadow the emergency of crush syndrome.

Crush syndrome and compartment syndrome act synergistically on the degradation of muscle. Acute musculoskeletal compartment syndrome can damage myocytes and induce rhabdomyolysis. Rhabdomyolysis in turn exacerbates the inflammatory cascade associated with crushing of the muscle compartment, thereby worsening compartment pressures. Crush syndrome may worsen acute renal failure.

During mass casualty situations in which crush injuries would be expected (earthquakes, building collapse, bombings), it is important to start IV volume restoration in all survivors as quickly as possible (see the Tips and Tricks box "Management of Crush Syndrome"). Emergency medical service and ED personnel should be instructed to begin IV resuscitation even before the victims have actually been extricated from the scene. This may involve placing an IV line in a confined space on any free limb.

The International Society of Nephrology can be contacted to respond to a mass casualty incident with emergency renal therapy equipment through its Disaster Relief Task Force (http://www.isn-online.org/isn/society/about/isn_20011.html).

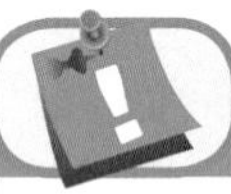

**TIPS AND TRICKS**

**Management of Crush Syndrome**

**Prehospital Phase**

Begin high-volume intravenous fluid resuscitation before extrication from collapsed buildings.

Remove constrictive jewelry and clothing.

Flaccid paralysis may mimic spinal cord injury (but rectal tone will be normal).

Prehospital amputation may be necessary to allow extrication of the victim.

"Physiologic amputation" (application of a tourniquet above the point of injury) may minimize the release of toxic substances into the circulation, thereby reducing rates of rhabdomyolysis; ice or dry ice should be applied distal to the tourniquet.

**Hospital Phase**

Anticipate the need for renal replacement therapy and hemodialysis resources.

The decision for amputation can be aided by use of the mangled extremity severity score (MESS). A MESS score of 7 or higher is a 100% positive predictor of amputation.

Avoid early aggressive surgical débridement unless vascular compromise is obvious.

## SURGICAL THERAPY

Surgical therapy is a consideration for patients with rhabdomyolysis caused by crush syndrome. Amputation removes damaged muscle that serves as the source of cellular toxins.

Physiologic amputation can act as temporizing measure when immediate surgical care is not available, particularly in the setting of disasters or military combat. To perform physiologic amputation, one or two tourniquets are applied firmly to the extremity above the level of injury or entrapment, and dry ice is applied distal to the tourniquet. Combat surgery hospitals beginning in World War II through current conflicts have performed this procedure with success. Physiologic amputation rapidly reduces myoglobin and other intracellular toxins associated with crushed, ischemic, or septic extremities. This can dramatically reduce myoglobinuria and reperfusion injury. Physiologic tourniquets have allowed definitive surgery to be delayed for up to 32 days. Emergency physicians must be aware, however, that physiologic amputation will inevitably result in loss of the affected limb.

Early prophylactic fasciotomy increases the need for transfusions and the risk for both sepsis and death. Fasciotomy is not indicated unless signs of compartment syndrome are observed.[5]

## FOLLOW-UP, NEXT STEPS IN CARE, AND PATIENT EDUCATION

Most patients with rhabdomyolysis should be admitted to a telemetry floor staffed by a physician or to an intensive care unit. If there is uncertainty regarding the diagnosis or severity, patients should be admitted for observation, testing, and treatment.

Rhabdomyolysis can be associated with acute kidney injury. Patients with renal failure should be admitted to the hospital and a nephrologist consulted early in the treatment course.

Patients with minimal elevations in CK and no identifiable complications may be managed as an outpatient if urgent follow-up with a primary care provider can be ensured.

## SUGGESTED READINGS

Bosch X, Poch E, Grau J. Rhabdomyolysis and acute kidney injury. N Engl J Med 2009;361:62-72.

Bywaters E, Beall D. Crush injuries with impairment of renal function. Br Med J 1941;1:427-32.

Fernandez WG, Hung O, Bruno GR, et al. Factors predictive of acute renal failure and need for hemodialysis among ED patients with rhabdomyolysis. Am J Emerg Med 2005;23:1-7.

Giannoglou GD, Chatzizisis YS, Misirli G. The syndrome of rhabdomyolysis: complications and treatment. Eur J Intern Med 2008;19:568-74.

Lippi G, Cervellin G, Comelli I. Rhabdomyolysis: historical background, clinical, diagnostic and therapeutic features. Clin Chem Lab Med 2010;48:749-56.

## REFERENCES

***References can be found on Expert Consult @ www.expertconsult.com.***

# Pituitary Apoplexy 170

*Brian K. Nelson*

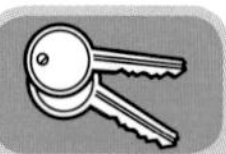

**KEY POINTS**

- Pituitary apoplexy is a rare but serious condition caused by hemorrhage or infarction of the pituitary gland.
- Patients are seen acutely with severe headache, meningismus, visual field deficits, cranial nerve palsies, loss of visual acuity, and altered mental status.
- Acute hypopituitarism may develop following pituitary apoplexy. Treatment of impending adrenal crisis is mandatory.
- Emergency consultation with a neurosurgeon who has expertise in pituitary surgery and management is required.

## EPIDEMIOLOGY

Pituitary adenomas are common, with a prevalence of 3% to 27% in various autopsy series. They are rarely diagnosed in life, with a reported incidence of 4 per 100,000 in a Finnish population and a prevalence of 77 per 100,000 in a British one.[1,2] Apoplexy occurs in a minority of such lesions and can occasionally be seen with normal glands. Because of the relative rarity of this condition, pituitary apoplexy may be confused with more common entities such as subarachnoid hemorrhage. Delay in diagnosis and treatment may lead to blindness, permanent cranial nerve palsies, or death.[3,4]

## PATHOPHYSIOLOGY

The two lobes of the pituitary gland sit within an enclosed space known as the sella turcica. Blood supply to this gland is one of the richest of all mammalian tissues.

The anterior lobe receives the portal hypophyseal vessel from the hypothalamus. Differentiated cells in the anterior lobe secrete specific hormones, including growth hormone (GH), adrenocorticotropic hormone (ACTH), prolactin (PRL), thyroid-stimulating hormone (TSH), and gonadotropins: luteinizing hormone (LH) and follicle-stimulating hormone (FSH).

The posterior lobe is an extension of the hypothalamus and secretes two hormones: antidiuretic hormone (or arginine vasopressin) and oxytocin. The pituitary stalk and the portal vessel pass through a small diaphragm that separates the sella turcica from the middle fossa. This anatomic arrangement places the pituitary at risk for infarction or hemorrhage when a mass increases pressure in the sella or compresses the stalk and vessels. Higher intrasellar pressures are associated with poor outcomes.

Pituitary tumors are common and many are asymptomatic. They are classified by size (microadenoma, <10 mm; macroadenoma, >10 mm) and by the hormone produced. Of tumors that cause clinical symptoms, the most commonly secreted hormones are PRL, which leads to hypogonadism; GH, which promotes acromegaly; and ACTH, a cause of Cushing disease.

Tumors involved in apoplexy are typically nonfunctional and unsuspected macroadenomas. In patients undergoing an endocrine stimulation test for hypogonadism, hypothyroidism, or adrenal insufficiency, apoplexy may occasionally develop secondary to stimulation of a macroadenoma. Treatment of a pituitary tumor can also precipitate apoplexy, particularly in cases of surgery, irradiation, or bromocriptine administration. Other reported risk factors include pregnancy (Sheehan syndrome), head trauma, recent cardiac surgery, anticoagulation, hypertension, diabetic ketoacidosis, and ovarian stimulation medications.[5]

Most patients with pituitary apoplexy have no identifiable risk factor. Apoplexy may occur in normal glands.

## PRESENTING SIGNS AND SYMPTOMS

### CLASSIC

The findings in patients with pituitary apoplexy vary from mild headache to sudden collapse and coma. Most patients exhibit severe frontal or retroorbital headache, vomiting, impaired visual acuity, visual field defects, hypopituitarism, and subsequent adrenal crisis. A minority have ocular palsies, obtundation, meningismus, blindness, or long-tract signs. The visual field deficit is classically bitemporal upper quadrantopia or hemianopia. Associated cerebral infarction occasionally occurs secondary to vasospasm from subarachnoid hemorrhage or direct compression of the internal carotid artery by tumor. **Table 170.1** lists the frequency of signs and symptoms reported in four case series.[3,5-7]

**Table 170.1 Signs and Symptoms of Pituitary Apoplexy**

| SIGN OR SYMPTOM | FREQUENCY (% INCIDENCE) |
|---|---|
| Headache | 63-97 |
| Visual field deficit | 43-82 |
| Hypopituitarism | 81 |
| Adrenal crisis | 65 |
| Vomiting | 50 |
| Visual impairment | 60 |
| Complete blindness | 10 |
| Ocular palsies | 40-46 |
| Meningismus | 25 |
| Altered mental status | 13 |
| Hyponatremia | 12 |
| Long-tract signs | 5 |

Data from references 1, 3, 4, 5.

## VARIATIONS

### *Hypopituitarism*

Most cases of hypopituitarism are diagnosed in the outpatient setting because of their subacute or indolent manifestation. Patients with hypopituitarism exhibit sequential signs and symptoms of GH deficiency, hypogonadism, hypothyroidism, and adrenal insufficiency. They are typically weak, hypopigmented, and overweight and appear chronically ill. Body hair and genitalia are diminished. Severe cases may be complicated by bradycardia and hypotension.

### *Asymptomatic Pituitary Tumors*

Silent tumors are incidental microadenomas found during imaging studies ordered for an unrelated condition. Patients with silent tumors have no symptoms attributable to cell type.

## DIFFERENTIAL DIAGNOSIS AND MEDICAL DECISION MAKING

Common neurologic emergencies can be confused with pituitary apoplexy (**Box 170.1**). The sudden onset of severe headache suggests subarachnoid hemorrhage. Obtundation and meningeal signs suggest meningitis, cerebral hemorrhage, or cerebral venous thrombosis. Cranial nerve findings in the setting of altered mental status may indicate cavernous sinus thrombosis or midbrain infarction. Rare hypothalamic and pituitary compressive or destructive processes may closely mimic apoplexy because of accompanying headaches and visual field deficits. Two such mimics are lymphocytic hypophysitis and Rathke cleft cysts. Pediatric craniopharyngiomas and several primary and metastatic lesions in adults may also compress the pituitary gland and mimic apoplexy. Generally, deficits in visual acuity and visual fields raise suspicion for apoplexy in the appropriate clinical setting.

**BOX 170.1 Differential Diagnosis**

Sudden severe headache with or without changes in mental status or long-tract signs
- Subarachnoid hemorrhage, meningitis, cerebral hemorrhage, mass, infarction, intracranial venous thrombosis

Severe headache with decreased visual acuity, ocular palsies, or visual field changes
- Complicated migraine, cavernous sinus thrombosis, cerebellar hemorrhage, midbrain infarction

Signs of hypogonadism, hypoadrenalism, or hypothyroidism
- Causes of hypopituitarism, including remote head injury, lymphocytic hypophysitis, iatrogenic surgical or radiation injury, and infections (particularly tuberculosis and mycotic infections); consider primary hypoadrenalism and hypothyroidism

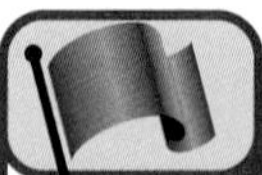

**RED FLAGS**

The following signal the need for immediate surgical decompression:
- Changes in mental status
- Rapidly progressive course
- Severe vision loss

## DIAGNOSTIC TESTING

Visual acuity and confrontational visual field testing should be performed when the diagnosis of pituitary apoplexy is considered. Samples should be obtained for electrolytes, renal function, liver function, clotting screen, blood counts, random cortisol, thyroxine, TSH, PRL, insulin-like growth factor, GH, LH, FSH, and testosterone in men and estradiol in women.[8] A non–contrast-enhanced computed tomography scan of the head will exclude the diagnosis of acute subarachnoid hemorrhage. Endocrine simulation testing could worsen the condition and should be deferred. Computed tomography is not sufficiently sensitive to exclude a pituitary process. Contrast-enhanced, diffusion-weighted magnetic resonance imaging allows the best visualization of pituitary tumors and details of the hemorrhage and infarction within them (**Fig. 170.1, *A* and *B***).[9]

## MANAGEMENT

Parenteral hydrocortisone (100 mg every 6 hours) or dexamethasone (4 mg every 12 hours) is given to decrease tumor edema and treat impending adrenal crisis. Obtunded or comatose patients should be intubated.

There is controversy regarding conservative treatment with steroids versus surgical intervention.[8,10,11] Patients with minimal or improving visual symptoms are sometimes managed medically. Definitive treatment is pituitary decompression, most often through a transsphenoidal approach. The outcome depends on the severity of symptoms at initial

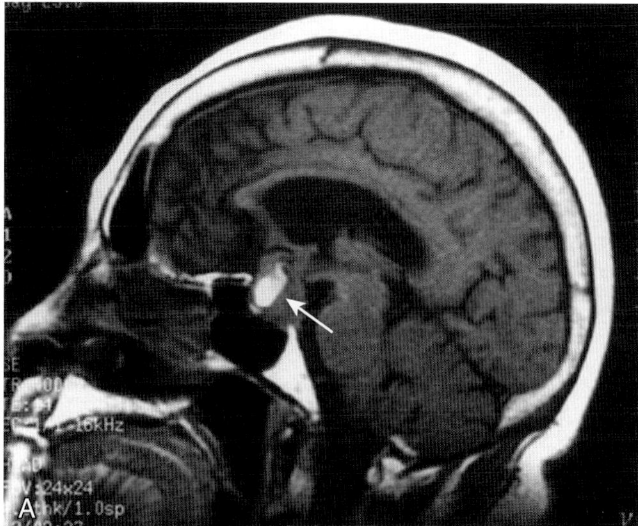

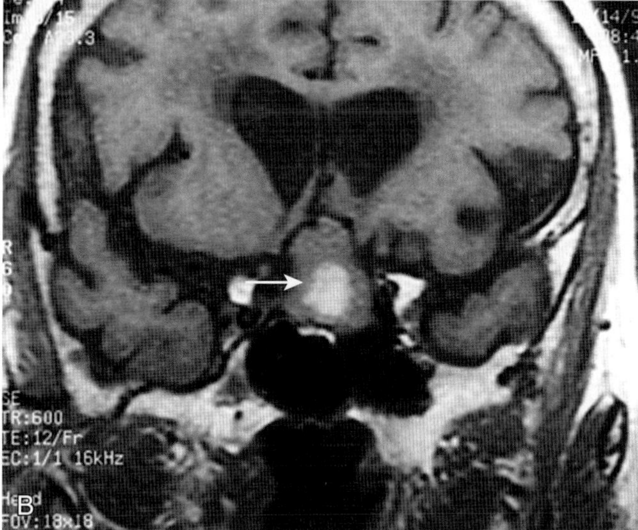

**Fig. 170.1** **A,** Magnetic resonance imaging of the brain showed a 3 × 2 × 2-cm pituitary macroadenoma with bleeding in the center *(arrow).* **B,** The tumor shown in coronal section *(arrow).* (From Basaria S, Turchin A, Krasner A. Apoplexy in recurrent pituitary adenoma. Postgrad Med J 2001;77:23.)

evaluation and prompt decompression of the sella turcica. Early diagnosis and treatment improve outcome and visual acuity; any residual hypopituitarism generally persists.[6,7]

## DISPOSITION

Patients with pituitary apoplexy require emergency consultation with a neurosurgeon experienced in pituitary surgery. Admission to a neurologic intensive care unit should be accompanied by consultation with a medical intensivist and endocrinologist.

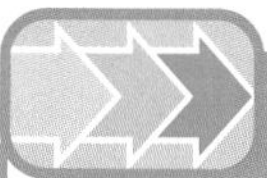

**PRIORITY ACTIONS**

**Do:**

Fingerstick glucose test; treat if hypoglycemic.

Draw blood for serum cortisol, thyroid-stimulating hormone, and free $T_4$ (thyroxine).

Administer parenteral hydrocortisone, 100 mg four times daily, or dexamethasone, 4 mg twice daily.

Provide fluid and electrolyte support.

Perform computed tomography to exclude subarachnoid hemorrhage, followed by magnetic resonance imaging.

Initiate early consultation with an endocrinologist and neurosurgeon with pituitary expertise.

Admit the patient to a neurologic critical care unit.

**Do Not:**

Withhold glucocorticoids while awaiting laboratory results.

Attempt endocrine simulation testing in the emergency department.

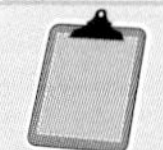

**DOCUMENTATION**

Onset, location, and severity of the headache

Mental status

Complete neurologic examination, including visual acuity and confrontational visual fields

Initial glucose, electrolytes, volume status

Results of initial imaging studies

Patients with subacute or chronic panhypopituitarism should be evaluated by an endocrinologist for initiation of therapy and further management. Asymptomatic pituitary tumors can be safely followed in the outpatient setting because such cases rarely progress to apoplexy.

## SUGGESTED READINGS


Biousse V, Newman NJ, Oyesiku NM, et al. Precipitating factors in pituitary apoplexy. J Neurol Neurosurg Psychiatry 2001;71:542-5.

Maccagnan P, Macedo CL, Kayath MJ, et al. Conservative management of pituitary apoplexy: a prospective study. J Clin Endocrinol Metab 1995;80:2190-7.

Rajasekarn S, Vanderpump M, Baldeweg S, et al. UK guidelines for the management of pituitary apoplexy. Clin Endocrinol (Oxf) 2011;74:9-20.

Semple PL, Webb MK, de Villiers JC, et al. Pituitary apoplexy. Neurosurgery 2005;56:65-72.


## REFERENCES

*References can be found on Expert Consult @ www.expertconsult.com.*

# Meningitis, Encephalitis, and Brain Abscess 171

*Amandeep Singh and Susan B. Promes*

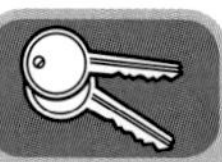

**KEY POINTS**

- There is significant overlap among the initial clinical presentations of meningitis, encephalitis, and brain abscess.
- The four most common bacteria responsible for adult bacterial meningitis are *Streptococcus pneumoniae, Neisseria meningitides, Haemophilus influenzae* type B, and *Listeria monocytogenes.* Group B *Streptococcus* remains the predominate cause of meningitis in infants less than 2 months of age.
- The classic constellation of fever, neck stiffness, headache, and change in mental status are seen in less than 50% of cases of acute bacterial meningitis.
- Cranial computed tomography (CT) scan, prior to lumbar puncture, is recommended in patients with a history of immunocompromised state, history of central nervous system (CNS) disease, new-onset seizure, abnormal neurologic examination, papilledema, altered mental status, or altered level of consciousness.
- Empiric therapy in patients with high clinical suspicion for CNS infection should not be delayed for neuroimaging or lumbar puncture.
- Although epidemiologic clues and assessment of risk factors should be sought in all patients with encephalitis, herpes simplex virus and arboviruses remain the most common causes of nonepidemic and epidemic outbreaks of encephalitis, respectively, in the United States.
- Acyclovir should be initiated in all patients with suspected encephalitis, pending the results of diagnostic studies.
- Risk factors for the development of intracranial abscess include inadequately treated subacute or chronic ear, nose, mastoid, and dental infection; endocarditis; congenital heart disease; and having undergone neurosurgical procedures.
- Patients with intracranial abscess often present with mild headache symptoms in the weeks to months prior the emergency department visit. The classic triad of fever, headache, and focal neurologic deficit is seen in less than 20% of patients with brain abscess.

## MENINGITIS

### EPIDEMIOLOGY

The combination of routine vaccination against *Streptococcus pneumoniae*, *Haemophilus influenzae type B*, and *Neisseria meningitides*, maternal screening for and intrapartum treatment of group B *Streptococcus (Streptococcus agalactiae)*, and enhanced efforts to reduce the contamination of processed foods by *Listeria monocytogenes* have all led to a significant decrease in the incidence of acute bacterial meningitis (ABM). Data from the Emerging Infections Programs Network, established by the Centers for Disease Control and Prevention (CDC), have noted a decrease in the incidence of meningitis from 2.0 cases per 100,000 population in 1998 to 1999 to 1.38 cases per 100,000 population in 2006 to 2007.[1] During this same time the case fatality rate decreased to 14.3%. Projecting these data on a national level reveals an estimated 4100 cases and 500 deaths from bacterial meningitis annually in the United States.[1]

### ETIOLOGY

A 10-year review (1998 to 2007) of 3188 cases of bacterial meningitis noted that *S. pneumoniae* accounted for the greatest proportion of cases (58%), followed by group *B. streptococcus* (18.1%), *N. meningitides* (13.9%), *H. influenzae* (6.7%), and *L. monocytogenes* (3.4%).[1] Among infants less than 3 months of age, group B *Streptococcus* and gram-negative rods account for most cases of ABM. After 3 months of age, *S. pneumoniae* and *N. meningitidis* become the predominant pathogens. *L. monocytogenes* is primarily seen in infants less than 1 month of age, in adults more than 50 years old, and in immunocompromised patients. *Staphylococcus aureus* is acquired mainly nosocomially and occurs predominantly after neurosurgical procedures or following penetrating head trauma. *S. aureus* may be acquired in the community setting, linked to predisposing conditions such as endocarditis, injection drug use, and compromised immune systems.

## PATHOPHYSIOLOGY

ABM develops after encapsulated bacteria, which have colonized the nasopharynx and/or oropharynx, penetrate the intravascular space and enter the subarachnoid space through vulnerable sites within the blood-brain barrier.[2] Once the pathogens enter the central nervous system (CNS), they replicate rapidly, thus consuming glucose and liberating protein within the cerebrospinal fluid (CSF). The ensuing inflammatory reaction occurs in response to the liberation of bacterial cell wall and cell membrane components (e.g., lipopolysaccharide, peptidoglycan, lipoteichoic acid) and the induction of proinflammatory mediators. These events culminate in injury to the vascular endothelium that results in increased vascular permeability to the blood-brain barrier, meningeal inflammation, and cerebral vasculitis. The accompanying cerebral edema and increase in intracranial pressure (ICP) contribute to CNS hypoperfusion and cell death.

Other routes of pathogen entry include direct inoculation of the CNS, seen in trauma or surgery, through direct infection and seeding of parameningeal structures (e.g., from endocarditis or concurrent infection), contact and aspiration of maternal intestinal and genital tract secretions during birth.

## PRESENTING SIGNS AND SYMPTOMS

Patients with ABM typically appear ill and often present within 24 to 72 hours of symptom onset. **Table 171.1** reviews the presenting signs and symptoms of adults with ABM.[3] The cardinal symptoms of ABM (i.e., fever, neck stiffness, change in mental status, and headache) are seen in combination in less than half of all patients. Nearly 95% of patients will present with at least two of these cardinal symptoms, which provides the rationale for performing a lumbar puncture in patients who are lethargic or confused and develop a fever. The absence of these four findings typically excludes the diagnosis of ABM.

The headache described by patients with ABM can be moderate to severe in intensity, generalized, often with an occipital or nuchal component, and unlike "normal" headaches. Photophobia is commonly present, as is nausea. Worsening of the headache while the examiner rapidly turns the patient's head from side to side (at a rate of two to three times per second), the so-called *jolt accentuation test,* has been reported to be helpful in identifying patients with ABM,[4] but a recent study questioned the utility of this finding.[5]

Although neck pain may be infrequently reported, the objective finding of neck stiffness is seen in more than 80% of patients. Examining the neck for rigidity, during gentle forward flexion, with the patient in the supine position best assesses neck stiffness, whereas difficulty in lateral motion of the neck is a less reliable finding. Patients with severe meningeal irritation may spontaneously assume the tripod position (also called the *Amoss sign* or the *Hoyne sign*) with the knees and hips flexed, the back arched lordotically, the neck extended, and the arms brought back to support the thorax.[6] The *Kernig sign* is performed with the patient lying supine and the hip and knee flexed to 90 degrees. A positive sign is present when extension of the knee from this position elicits resistance or pain in the lower back or posterior thigh. The classic *Brudzinski sign* refers to spontaneous flexion of the knees and hips during attempted passive flexion of the neck. A separate sign described by Brudzinski, the *contralateral reflex,* is present if passive flexion of one hip and knee causes flexion of the contralateral leg. The presence or absence of *Kernig* or *Brudzinski signs* has been shown to have little positive or negative predictive value in the diagnosis of ABM, unless severe meningeal inflammation is present.[7]

**Table 171.1** **Findings in 696 Episodes of Bacterial Meningitis**

| SIGN OR SYMPTOM | FREQUENCY (%) |
|---|---|
| Duration of symptoms ≤ 24 hr | 48 |
| Fever (temperature ≥ 38° C) | 77 |
| Headache | 87 |
| Nausea or vomiting | 74 |
| Neck stiffness | 83 |
| GCS ≤ 14 (AMS) | 69 |
| GCS ≤ 8 (coma) | 14 |
| Rash | 26 |
| Focal neurologic deficit | 33 |
| Seizures | 5 |
| Arthritis | 7 |

From Van de Beek D, de Gans J, Spanjaard L, et al. Clinical features and prognostic factors in adults with bacterial meningitis. N Engl J Med 2004;351:1849-59.

*AMS,* altered mental status; *GCS,* Glasgow Coma Scale.

Atypical presentations of ABM occur in infants, older adults, and immunocompromised patients. Infants with bacterial meningitis may present with fever or hypothermia, hypoglycemia, poor feeding, seizures, or irritability (excessive or abnormal crying). On examination, the findings of jaundice, ill appearance, a bulging fontanelle, meningeal irritation (including neck stiffness, the Kernig sign, and the Brudzinski sign), fever higher than 40° C, and increased general body tone predict bacterial meningitis.[8]

Older and immunocompromised patients may also present atypically. These populations are associated with a higher rate of misdiagnosis that contributes to an increase in the morbidity and mortality following an episode of acute meningitis. A lower proportion of fever, headache, and nausea or vomiting is present in these subgroups.[9] Neck stiffness has a lower sensitivity and specificity for meningitis in older patients. Finally, these populations may present to the emergency department (ED) with altered mental status and/or altered level of consciousness but without a fever.

## DIFFERENTIAL DIAGNOSIS

The differential diagnosis of patients presenting with fever, headache, and altered mental status includes other forms of meningitis (e.g., nosocomial meningitis, aseptic meningitis), encephalitis, and cerebral abscess. The diagnosis of meningitis is challenging in patients who present atypically. In a review of 156 cases of meningitis in patients who presented to a single tertiary care hospital, 66 cases were initially misdiagnosed in the ED as an alternative infection (i.e., sepsis of unclear origin, pneumonia, urinary tract infection), metabolic encephalopathy, or nonspecific conditions (e.g., weakness, malaise, degenerative state). Higher percentages of these patients were more than 65 years of age, and these patients were also noted to have lower proportions of fever, headache, nausea or vomiting, and neck stiffness.[10]

Nosocomial meningitis may result from invasive CNS procedures (e.g., craniotomy, placement of ventricular catheters, lumbar puncture [LP], intrathecal infusions of medication, or spinal anesthesia), head trauma, and metastatic infection in patients with hospital-acquired bacteremia. Meningitis that develops after neurosurgical procedures or following penetrating cranial trauma is often caused by infection from *S. aureus*, coagulase-negative staphylococci (especially *Staphylococcus epidermidis*), or facultative and aerobic gram-negative bacilli (including *Pseudomonas aeruginosa*). Most cases of meningitis associated with basilar skull fractures are caused by *S. pneumoniae*, *H. influenza*e, and group A β-hemolytic streptococci.

*Aseptic meningitis* refers to a disorder in which patients have clinical and laboratory evidence of meningeal irritation with negative results of routine bacterial cultures. Precise epidemiologic data on the incidence of aseptic meningitis are lacking, but aseptic meningitis is associated with an estimated 26,000 to 42,000 hospitalizations per year in the United States. The origin of aseptic meningitis is varied (**Box 171.1**). Enteroviruses, the leading causes of viral meningitis in adults and children, account for 50% to 75% of all cases of aseptic meningitis. Additional causes include other infections (mycobacteria, fungi, spirochetes), parameningeal infections, medications (especially nonsteroidal antiinflammatory drugs), and malignant disease. The signs and symptoms of bacterial meningitis significantly overlap with those of aseptic meningitis. This overlap led to the development of several decision rules to distinguish the two conditions. The most useful pediatric score appears to be the Bacterial Meningitis Score. This score classifies patients 1 month to 18 years old as being at very low risk of bacterial meningitis if they lack all the following criteria: positive CSF Gram stain, CSF absolute neutrophil count (ANC) of at least 1000 cells/mcL, CSF protein of at least 80 mg/dL, peripheral blood ANC of at least 10,000 cells/mcL, and a history of seizure before or at the time of presentation.[11]

**BOX 171.1 Etiology of Aseptic Meningitis**

**Viral Meningitis**
- Enteroviruses (e.g., coxsackievirus, echovirus, poliovirus)
- Herpes simplex viruses (HSV)
- Human immunodeficiency virus (HIV)
- West Nile virus (WNV)
- Varicella-zoster virus (VZV)
- Lymphocytic choriomeningitis virus (LCM)

**Other Pathogens**
- *Mycobacterium tuberculosis*
- *Treponema pallidum* (syphilis)
- *Borrelia burgdorferi* (Lyme disease)
- *Rickettsia rickettsiae* (Rocky Mountain spotted fever)
- Agents of ehrlichiosis
- *Cryptococcus neoformans*
- *Coccidioides immitis*

**Carcinomatous Meningitis**
- Large cell lymphomas
- Acute leukemia
- Certain solid tumors (e.g., breast cancer, lung cancer, melanoma, gastrointestinal tumors)

**Drug-Induced Meningitis**
- Nonsteroidal antiinflammatory drugs (NSAIDs)
- Trimethoprim-sulfamethoxazole
- Intravenous immune globulin

## MEDICAL DECISION MAKING

### ROUTINE LABORATORY TESTS

Routine testing of patients with suspected meningitis should include complete blood cell count (CBC), serum electrolytes, bicarbonate, serum urea nitrogen (BUN), creatinine, and glucose (**Table 171.2**). Serum lactate determinations and blood cultures are also indicated in patients with suspected meningitis.

Several newer tests have shown potential in distinguishing bacterial meningitis from nonbacterial meningitis. These tests include serum procalcitonin,[12] serum C-reactive protein,[13] CSF cortisol,[14] and CSF lactate.[15] Additional tests employing common biochemical laboratory techniques (e.g., latex agglutination, enzyme-linked immunosorbent assay, polymerase chain reaction [PCR] assay, microarrays) have shown significant promise in identifying the specific pathogen responsible for infection.

### NEUROIMAGING BEFORE LUMBAR PUNCTURE

Selected patients with meningitis may warrant a computed tomography (CT) scan of the head, to identify patients with lesions that place them at risk for herniation from LP and to diagnose conditions that would make LP unnecessary if the patient's work-up was limited to the LP (e.g., tumor, cerebral abscess). Unfortunately, cranial CT has inadequate sensitivity for identifying patients at risk for brain herniation. A systematic review on this subject found only a handful of cases of brain herniation that occurred following a normal cranial CT scan.[16] Despite this limitation, generally accepted criteria for obtaining a cranial CT scan before LP are listed in **Box 171.2**. For maximal sensitivity in those patients with suspected or confirmed human immunodeficiency virus infection, contrast-enhanced cranial CT should be performed at the same time as the nonenhanced cranial CT.

**Table 171.2** Suggested Laboratory Testing in Suspected Meningitis

| BLOOD TEST | COMMENT |
|---|---|
| Complete blood count | WBC typically elevated with left shift, although normal or low values in infants and immunosuppressed patients |
| Electrolytes | Hyponatremia (Na < 135 mmol/L) seen in 30% of cases of ABM |
| Bicarbonate | Alkalosis seen with excessive vomiting, acidosis seen with poor tissue perfusion |
| BUN, creatinine | Renal function tests essential for antibiotic dosing and timing |
| Glucose | Useful in calculating the CSF/serum glucose ratio and in the initial evaluation of altered mental status or altered level of consciousness |
| Lactate | Has prognostic information (i.e., correlates with mortality) and used to identify candidates for early goal-directed therapy |
| Blood cultures | Positive results in 50% to 75% of patients with ABM when obtained before antibiotic administration |

*ABM,* Acute bacterial meningitis; *BUN,* blood urea nitrogen; *CSF,* cerebrospinal fluid; *Na,* sodium; *WBC,* white blood cell count.

**BOX 171.2 General Recommendations for Computed Tomography Before Lumbar Puncture**[17]

History of immunocompromised state
History of central nervous system disease (e.g., mass lesion, stroke, focal infection)
New-onset seizure (or new-onset seizure within 1 week of presentation)
Papilledema on funduscopic examination (or elevated optic nerve sheath diameter on ultrasound)
Abnormal neurologic examination
Altered mental status
Altered level of consciousness

Hasbun R, Abrahams J, Jekel J, et al. Computed tomography of the head before lumbar puncture in adults with suspected meningitis. N Engl J Med 2001;345:1727-33.

## LUMBAR PUNCTURE AND CEREBROSPINAL FLUID ANALYSIS

Although the diagnosis of bacterial meningitis rests on CSF examination, CSF analysis alone cannot reliably distinguish bacterial and aseptic meningitis.[13] In addition to measuring the opening pressure, the examiner should obtain four tubes of CSF, each containing 1 to 2 mL of fluid, and send them for analysis. Typically tube 1 (and/or tube 4) is sent for cell count and differential, tube 2 for protein and glucose, tube 3 for Gram stain and culture, and tube 4 for special testing or additional cultures.

In ABM, the opening pressure is usually elevated to 20 to 50 cm $H_2O$, although values may be lower in pediatric patients. Between 15% and 20% of adults with bacterial meningitis have a CSF opening pressure lower than 20 cm $H_2O$.

The appearance of the CSF can range from clear to cloudy, depending on the presence of significant concentrations of cells, bacteria, and protein. The CSF white blood cell (WBC) count can be significantly elevated, usually in the range of 1000 to 5000 cells/mm$^3$, although this range can be quite broad (<100 to >10,000 cells/mm$^3$). Up to 20% of adults with bacterial meningitis have a CSF WBC count lower than 1000 cells/mm$^3$, and one third of these adults have a CSF WBC count of less than 100 cells/mm$^3$.[18] Classically, a CSF neutrophil predominance is present (seen in 80% to 95% of cases). In 10% of cases, such as in neonatal meningitis or patients infected with *L. monocytogenes*, a CSF lymphocyte predominance can be seen.[18] In resource-depleted environments, a urinary reagent strip to determine the presence of leukocyte esterase can be used as a marker for the presence of WBCs in the CSF and a point of care glucose device can be used to rapidly obtain a CSF glucose concentration.

Despite the classic teachings on CSF findings (**Table 171.3**), the absence of one or more typical findings is commonly seen in patients with confirmed ABM. For example, in a review of 296 episodes of ABM, 50% of patients had a CSF glucose concentration of approximately 40 mg/dL, 44% had a CSF protein level lower than 200 mg/dL, and 13% had a CSF WBC count lower than 100 cells/mm$^3$.[19] In another series of 696 episodes of ABM, 12% had none of the characteristic CSF findings of ABM.[3]

Overall, the sensitivity of CSF Gram stain in bacterial meningitis ranges from 60% to 90%, depending on the concentration of the bacteria in the CSF.[20] Sterilization of bacteria can begin to occur as soon as 15 minutes after the initiation of antibiotic therapy. A positive CSF Gram stain result is highly specific for bacterial meningitis. The following patterns are important to recognize: gram-positive diplococci suggest pneumococci; gram-negative diplococci suggest meningococci; small pleomorphic gram-negative coccobacilli suggest *H. influenzae;* gram-positive rods and coccobacilli suggest *L. monocytogenes.*

## TREATMENT

Recommendations for empiric antimicrobial therapy for ABM are based on the patient's age and predisposing conditions.

A reasonable approach to immunocompetent patients with highly suspected meningitis or meningoencephalitis consists of empiric treatment with ceftriaxone (or cefotaxime), vancomycin, and acyclovir, along with dexamethasone (**Table 171.4**). Acyclovir is given to cover herpes simplex virus (HSV) encephalitis, the most common cause of nonepidemic encephalitis in the United States, whose presentation can significantly overlap with that of suspected meningitis. A more conservative approach to pharmacotherapy is reasonable for stable, immunocompetent patients with normal mentation and alertness in whom CNS infection is less strongly suspected.

Treatment with high-dose dexamethasone (0.15 mg/kg intravenously, maximum dose, 10 mg, every 6 hours) before

**Table 171.3** Cerebrospinal Fluid Findings in Meningitis

| PARAMETER (NORMAL) | BACTERIAL MENINGITIS | VIRAL MENINGITIS | FUNGAL MENINGITIS | TUBERCULOSIS MENINGITIS | NEOPLASTIC MENINGITIS |
|---|---|---|---|---|---|
| Opening pressure (6-20 cm $H_2O$) | >20 cm $H_2O$ | Normal to mildly elevated | >20 cm $H_2O$ | >20 cm $H_2O$ | >20 cm $H_2O$ |
| CSF WBC (<5 cells/mL) | >1,000 cells/mL | <1,000 cells/mL | <500 cells/mL | <500 cells/mL | <500 cells/mL |
| PMNs (<80%)<br>Lymphocytes (<10%) | >80% | <50%<br>>50% | <50%<br>>80% | <50% | <50% |
| CSF glucose (>40 mg/dL) | <40 mg/dL | >40 mg/dL | <40 mg/dL | <40 mg/dL | <40 mg/dL |
| CSF protein (<50 mg/dL) | >150 mg/dL | <100 mg/dL | >100 mg/dL | >100 mg/dL | >100 mg/dL |

*PMN,* Polymorphonuclear leukocytes; *WBC,* white blood cell count.

**Table 171.4** Empiric Antimicrobial Therapy for Suspected Meningitis

| PREDISPOSING FACTOR | ANTIMICROBIAL REGIMEN |
|---|---|
| Age < 1 mo | Cefotaxime 50 mg/kg IV q6h or |
| | *and* |
| | Ampicillin 50 mg/kg IV q8h |
| Age 1 mo-50 yr | Ceftriaxone 50 mg/kg (maximum dose, 2 g) IV q12h or Cefotaxime 50 mg/kg (maximum dose, 2 g) IV q6h |
| | *and* |
| | Vancomycin 15 mg/kg IV q12h |
| | *and* |
| | Acyclovir 10 mg/kg IV q8h |
| | *and* |
| | Dexamethasone 0.15 mg/kg (maximum dose, 10 mg) IV q6h |
| Age > 50 yr | Ceftriaxone 50 mg/kg (maximum dose, 2 g) IV q12h or Cefotaxime 50 mg/kg (maximum dose, 2 g) IV q6h |
| | *and* |
| | Vancomycin 15 mg/kg IV q12h |
| | *and* |
| | Ampicillin 50 mg/kg (maximum dose, 2 g) IV q4h |
| | *and* |
| | Acyclovir 10 mg/kg IV q8h |
| | *and* |
| | Dexamethasone 0.15 mg/kg (maximum dose, 10 mg) IV q6h |
| Postoperative neurosurgical patients | Ceftazidime 50 mg/kg (maximum dose, 2 g) IV q8h or Cefepime 50 mg/kg (maximum dose, 2 g) IV q8h |
| | *and* |
| | Vancomycin 15 mg/kg IV q12h |
| Patients with penetrating skull trauma | Ceftriaxone 50 mg/kg IV (maximum dose, 2 g) IV q12h or Cefotaxime 50 mg/kg IV (maximum dose, 2 g) IV q6h |
| | *and* |
| | Vancomycin 15 mg/kg IV q12h |

*IV,* Intravenously; *q4h, q6h, q8h, q12h,* every 4, 6, 8, and 12 hours, respectively.

or concurrent with the first dose of antibiotics is thought to attenuate the inflammatory response and to lead to better outcome in children (excluding neonates) and adults with meningitis.[20] The rationale for this approach is provided by animal studies showing that hearing loss is temporally associated with the severe inflammatory changes induced by bacterial meningitis and that dexamethasone reduces CSF synthesis of cytokines, CSF inflammation, and cerebral edema.

Antibiotics should not be delayed for CT or LP when the clinical suspicion of ABM is high. Although no prospective clinical data are available on the relationship of the timing of antibiotics with clinical outcome in patients with bacterial meningitis, several retrospective reviews examined this issue and concluded that an association may exist between delayed administration of antibiotics and worse overall outcome.[18]

Chemoprophylaxis is indicated for high-risk contacts (e.g., household, school, or work contacts) of patients with documented *N. meningitidis* or *H. influenza* type B infection, including health care providers who intubated the patient without first donning a face mask. Other health care providers do not require prophylaxis. First-line treatment is with rifampin, 10 mg/kg intravenously (to a maximum of 600 mg per dose) every 12 hours for four doses. Alternatives are ceftriaxone, ciprofloxacin, and sulfisoxazole.

## FOLLOW-UP, NEXT STEPS OF CARE, AND PATIENT EDUCATION

There is substantial overlap between the clinical presentation of bacterial meningitis, which is a life-threatening illness requiring rapid diagnosis, treatment, and hospital admission, and aseptic meningitis, which can often be monitored in an outpatient setting without antibiotic therapy. When a patient's presentation is ambiguous, the emergency clinician should take into account the underlying risk factors for bacterial meningitis, the results of the physical examination, and the findings on CSF analysis. Patients with CSF profiles consistent with bacterial meningitis require hospital admission for administration of parenteral antibiotics and further monitoring. The disposition of well-appearing patients with CSF leukocytosis and findings consistent with viral meningitis is more variable. Management options include hospital admission and treatment with parenteral antibiotics or discharge with 24- to 48-hour follow-up if the patient is reliable.

The overall prognosis of ABM is poor. Mortality rates range from less than 5% for infection with *H. influenzae* to 10% with *N. meningitidis* to 20% with *S. pneumoniae.*

During hospitalization, focal neurologic deficits are seen in 50% of patients, and seizures occur in 15% of patients.[3] Cardiopulmonary failure occurs in nearly 30% of patients, and mechanical ventilation is required in almost 25% of patients. Two thirds of patients with ABM have mild or no disability using a Glasgow outcome scale. Approximately 15% of patients have moderate to severe disability following infection. The most common neurologic findings on discharge are as follows: eighth nerve cranial palsy, which occurs in nearly 15% of survivors; hemiparesis, occurring in 4% of survivors; and sixth nerve cranial palsy, occurring in 3% of survivors.[3] Aphasia, quadriparesis, third nerve cranial palsy, and seventh nerve cranial palsy are all rare.

**Table 171.5** Causes of Encephalitis Among Hospitalized Patients

| DIAGNOSIS | FREQUENCY (%) |
|---|---|
| Encephalitis, unspecified cause | 72 |
| Herpetic encephalitis | 14 |
| Immune-mediated encephalitis | 8 |
| Other viral encephalitis with identified cause | 4 |
| Bacterial encephalitis | 1 |
| Fungal, parasitic, or protozoal encephalitis | <1 |

# ACUTE ENCEPHALITIS

## EPIDEMIOLOGY

*Encephalitis* refers to inflammation of brain parenchyma that may coexist with inflammation of the meninges *(meningoencephalitis)* or spinal cord *(encephalomyelitis).* The overall incidence of encephalitis is reported to be 3 to 4 cases per 100,000 population. Most cases of encephalitis are often not recognized or misdiagnosed because routine care and time are sufficient for many cases to improve. Children less than 1 year of age, patients more than 65 years of age, and immunocompromised patients are at greatest risk for acute encephalitis.[21] Viral infection is the most common identifiable cause of encephalitis, although infections with other pathogens and noninfectious causes (i.e., immune-mediated encephalitis) have been described (**Table 171.5**).

## ETIOLOGY

Many of the viruses that cause meningitis can also cause encephalitis, but certain viruses are more likely to cause encephalitis and are responsible for most cases. These include the herpes family viruses (e.g., HSV, human herpesvirus-6 [HHV-6], varicella-zoster virus [VZV], cytomegalovirus [CMV]), arboviruses (e.g., La Crosse virus, St. Louis virus, West Nile virus [WNV], Western Equine virus, Eastern Equine virus), and enteroviruses.[22] Although HSV is the most common cause of nonepidemic, acute focal encephalitis in the United States, the arboviruses can account for as many as 50% of cases during epidemics.

Few pyogenic bacteria cause encephalitis without overt meningitis. Syphilis, leptospirosis, brucellosis, tuberculosis, and listeriosis can be associated with encephalitis. Occasionally, encephalitis is a presenting manifestation of cryptococcosis, histoplasmosis, blastomycosis, or coccidiomycosis.

**Table 171.6** Clinical Features of Common Viral Encephalitis

| VIRUS | PRIMARY SITE OF CNS INFECTION | CLINICAL MANIFESTATIONS |
|---|---|---|
| Herpes simplex | Frontal and temporal lobe | Fever, hemicranial headache, taste and smell hallucinations, language and behavior abnormalities, memory impairment, seizures; SIADH |
| West Nile | Anterior horn cells | Abrupt onset of fever, headache, stiff neck, and vomiting; other clinical features including tremors, myoclonus, parkinsonism, and poliomyelitis-like flaccid paralysis |
| La Crosse | Cortical areas | Seizures, disorientation, focal neurologic signs; seen in late spring to early fall; primarily in school-age children |
| St. Louis | Substantia nigra, pons, thalamus, cerebellum | Tremor, myoclonus, opsoclonus, nystagmus, ataxia, stupor, disorientation; SIADH and urinary symptoms (dysuria, urgency, incontinence) |
| Eastern Equine | Basal ganglia, thalamus, brainstem | Headache, altered mental status, seizures; primary seen in summer |

*CNS,* Central nervous system; *SIADH,* syndrome of inappropriate antidiuretic hormone.

## PATHOPHYSIOLOGY

Access of viruses to the CNS can occur by either hematogenous or neuronal routes.[23] For example, after an insect bite with local arboviral replication in the skin, transient viremia ensues, followed by penetration of the blood-brain barrier and the development of encephalitis. Other agents can enter through the respiratory or gastrointestinal tract or through blood transfusion or organ transplantation. Several herpes family viruses (e.g., HSV, VZV) and the rabies virus reach the CNS through retrograde travel along neuronal axons where they have gained access to nerve endings.

## PRESENTING SIGNS AND SYMPTOMS

The syndrome of acute encephalitis shares many clinical features with acute meningitis. Patients with either syndrome may present with fever, headache, and altered level of consciousness. Although mental status changes early in the disease course are more common in patients with encephalitis, this finding does not reliably differentiate patients with encephalitis from those with bacterial meningitis. Acute encephalitis should be considered in febrile patients presenting with the following clinical features, singly or in combination: new psychiatric symptoms, cognitive defects, and diffuse or focal neurologic signs such as hemiparesis or seizure. Patients with encephalitis typically have prominent cognitive and mental changes such as lethargy, aphasia, amnestic syndrome, confusion, stupor, or even coma. In most cases, some concomitant meningeal irritation complicates the encephalitic component, and this condition is referred to as meningoencephalitis.

Clinically distinguishing among the various infectious encephalitides is difficult because of the large degree of overlap in symptoms. Epidemiologic clues that may help in directing the investigation into a cause include the following: the season of the year; the geographic locale; the prevalence of the disease in the local community; and the patient's travel history, recreational activities, occupational exposure, insect contact, animal contact, vaccination history, and immune status. Viral affinity for certain CNS locations can provide clues to the diagnosis (**Table 171.6**).[22]

## DIFFERENTIAL DIAGNOSIS

Several conditions mimic the clinical presentation of acute encephalitis, notably meningitis (both bacterial and aseptic) and intracranial abscess. These conditions commonly manifest with fever, headache, altered mental status, altered level of consciousness, and focal neurologic deficits. Encephalitis should be distinguished from conditions causing encephalopathy (e.g., secondary to metabolic disturbances, hypoxia, ischemia, drugs, intoxications, organ dysfunction, or systemic infection). Encephalopathy is defined by a disruption of brain function in the absence of a direct inflammatory process in the brain parenchyma.

The physician should try to distinguish between infectious encephalitis and postinfectious or postimmunization encephalitis or encephalomyelitis. These conditions are presumed to result from an immunologic response to an antecedent antigenic stimulus provided by the infecting microorganism, immunization, or other antigens as part of the initial infection or vaccination. One example of immune-mediated encephalitis is acute disseminated encephalomyelitis (ADEM), a condition seen more commonly in children. ADEM is characterized by the abrupt onset of neurologic symptoms several days after viral illness or vaccination, generally in the absence of fever. Patients can have multifocal neurologic signs, including optic neuritis with brain and spinal cord demyelinating lesions. Disturbances in consciousness can range from stupor and confusion to coma. Treatment includes corticosteroids, plasma exchange, and intravenous immune globulin.

## MEDICAL DECISION MAKING

Routine testing of patients with suspected encephalitis should include CBC, serum electrolytes, bicarbonate, BUN, creatinine, and glucose. Serum lactate determinations and blood cultures may also be indicated in patients with suspected encephalitis.

A CT scan of the brain should be performed before LP in patients suspected of having a CNS infection who also present with altered mental status, altered level of consciousness, seizures, or focal neurologic deficit. Additionally, patients with

**BOX 171.3 Findings Suggestive of Herpes Simplex Virus Encephalitis**

Red blood cells in atraumatic lumbar puncture
Computed tomography or magnetic resonance imaging findings of edema or hemorrhage in the frontal and/or temporal lobes
Electroencephalographic pattern of periodic, asymmetrically sharp waves

a compromised immune status or with a history of CNS disease (e.g., mass lesion, stroke, focal infection) should have a CT scan prior to LP. Most patients with encephalitis have a normal CT scan; however, patients with encephalitis may show diffuse cerebral edema or, in HSV encephalitis specifically, focal edema, with or without parenchymal hemorrhages in the frontal and/or temporal lobes. Magnetic resonance imaging (MRI) is considered more sensitive and is the preferred imaging method in patients with suspected encephalitis.

Electroencephalography (EEG) is a sensitive indicator of cerebral dysfunction and may demonstrate cerebral involvement during the early stages of encephalitis. Although EEG is rarely useful in identifying a pathogen, it has a characteristic pattern of discharge in patients with HSV encephalitis (i.e., temporal focus that produces asymmetric sharp and slow waves, occurring at intervals of 2 to 3 seconds). Furthermore, EEG has a role in identifying patients with nonconvulsive seizure activity who are confused, obtunded, or comatose.

The findings on CSF analysis of patients with encephalitis may be close to normal or similar to those seen in viral infections causing aseptic meningitis (i.e., increased CSF WBC count, usually < 250 cells/mm$^3$, normal or mildly elevated CSF protein, and normal or mildly reduced CSF glucose).[21] Red blood cells in an atraumatic LP suggest HSV encephalitis, but they can be present in other conditions (e.g., other viral encephalitides, amebic encephalitis, acute necrotizing hemorrhagic leukoencephalitis) (**Box 171.3**). CSF analysis is essential in patients with suspected acute encephalitis, and a CSF sample should be sent for routine analysis to exclude ABM. An additional CSF sample should be sent for nucleic acid amplification tests (e.g., PCR). A positive CSF PCR result is very helpful for documenting infection caused by a specific pathogen, but a negative PCR result cannot exclude this diagnosis. Viral cultures of CSF specimens are of limited value in patients with encephalitis and are not routinely recommended.

## TREATMENT

The treatment of acute encephalitis is mainly supportive.[22] This includes optimization of fluid balance and electrolytes, symptomatic treatment of fever, headache, and nausea, airway protection, management of ICP, and management of seizures. Effective therapy exists for HSV and VZV infection (i.e., acyclovir, 10 mg/kg intravenously every 8 hours). Anecdotal reports of improvement have also been described with the combination of ganciclovir (5 mg/kg intravenously every 12 hours) and foscarnet (90 mg/kg intravenously every 12 hours) for CMV or HHV-6 infection and with pleconaril (5 mg/kg orally every 8 hours) for severe enteroviral disease.[22]

**BOX 171.4 Recommended Empiric Treatment for Suspected Acute Encephalitis**

Acyclovir 10 mg/kg IV every 8 hours
PLUS
Ceftriaxone 50 mg/kg IV (maximum dose, 2 g) every 12 hours
PLUS
Vancomycin 15 mg/kg IV (maximum dose, 500 mg) every 6 hours
PLUS
Dexamethasone 0.15 mg/kg IV (maximum dose, 10 mg) every 6 hours
Note: Ampicillin, 2 g IV every 4 hours, added for patients more than 50 years old and in patients with compromised immunity

IV, Intravenously.

A reasonable approach to immunocompetent patients with a high suspicion of meningitis, encephalitis, or meningoencephalitis consists of empiric treatment with ceftriaxone, vancomycin, and acyclovir, along with dexamethasone (**Box 171.4**). These therapies should be initiated as soon as possible after blood cultures are obtained, but before CT or LP are performed. A more conservative approach to pharmacotherapy is reasonable for immunocompetent patients with normal mentation and alertness who are less likely to have CNS infection.

A key decision point in the continuation of therapy rests with the results of the Gram stain. Whereas acyclovir can be discontinued or omitted in patients with a positive Gram stain result, acyclovir should be continued or initiated in patients with a negative Gram stain result. Currently, acyclovir is given to less than one in three patients in the ED who ultimately have the diagnosis of encephalitis.[24] Corticosteroids should be continued regardless of the results of the Gram stain. The use of corticosteroids in patients with HSV encephalitis is associated with improved outcome.

## FOLLOW-UP, NEXT STEPS IN CARE, AND PATIENT CARE

Patients with all but the mildest cases of encephalitis should be admitted to the hospital. The overall risks of death and morbidity from encephalitis are 3% to 4% and 7% to 10%, respectively. These rates are greatly influenced by the infectious pathogen and by the immune response elicited by the host. Infections with HSV, rabies virus, and Eastern Equine virus and infections in immunocompromised, pediatric, and geriatric patients are all associated with a worse outcome. Before the advent of routine treatment with antiviral therapy, the mortality rate of untreated HSV encephalitis was greater than 70%, with less than 5% of the survivors returning to a normal lifestyle. The current mortality rate of HSV encephalitis in patients treated with acyclovir is less than 30%.[25,26] Mortality rates of Eastern Equine, St. Louis, and La Crosse, and WNV encephalitis are greater than 30%, 20%, 10% to 15%, and 7.5%, respectively.

As with overall mortality from encephalitis, the prognosis depends on the specific etiologic agent and host factors. Significant lifelong morbidity may result from acute encephalitis. In one series that examined outcome after acyclovir-treated HSV encephalitis, 40% of surviving patients at 1 month had moderate to severe disability. Nearly 75% of the long-term survivors reported memory impairment, and approximately 50% had personality or behavioral abnormalities.[22]

# INTRACRANIAL ABSCESS

## EPIDEMIOLOGY

A *brain abscess* is a focal, intracerebral infection that begins as a localized area of cerebral inflammation and develops into a collection of pus surrounded by a well-vascularized capsule. With an incidence of 0.9 cases per 100,000 population, approximately 2500 cases of brain abscess are diagnosed each year in the United States.[26] In the general population, brain abscess is a disease of young male patients. Case series have reported male-to-female ratios of 2 : 1 to 3 : 1.[27] Although brain abscess can occur in any stage of life, most cases occur during the third and fourth decades. Additional risk factors for development of brain abscess are listed in **Box 171.5**.

**BOX 171.5 Identified Risk Factors for the Development of Brain Abscess**

- Immunocompromised patients (acquired immunodeficiency syndrome, transplantation, neutropenia)
- Contiguous source of subacute or chronic infection (e.g., sinusitis, otitis media, mastoiditis, odontogenic infection, meningitis)
- Endocarditis
- Chronic pulmonary infection (e.g., lung abscess, empyema)
- Other infection (e.g., intraabdominal, pelvic, skin, bone)
- Penetrating head injury
- Earlier neurosurgical procedure
- Congenital heart disease
- Intrapulmonary right-to-left shunt in patients with pulmonary arteriovenous malformation

## ETIOLOGY

The bacterial pathogens responsible for the development of brain abscess depend on the age and immune status of t he patients and the site of the primary infection. Streptococci (especially *Streptococcus milleri* and viridans streptococci) are the most common cause of pyogenic brain abscess resulting from extension from the nasopharynx and oropharynx. Anaerobic bacteria (e.g., *Bacteroides, Prevotella melaninogenica, Peptostreptococcus, Fusobacterium,* and *Actinomyces*) are additional major causes of brain abscesses, often as part of a polymicrobial infection. *S. aureus* and *Propionibacterium acnes* are seen in patients with endocarditis, in patients who have undergone neurosurgical procedures, and in patients with penetrating head trauma. Opportunistic bacterial pathogens, such as *Nocardia asteroides, M. tuberculosis, and L. monocytogenes*, as well as infection from fungal and parasitic sources, can be seen in immunocompromised patients.

## PATHOPHYSIOLOGY

Bacteria can invade the brain by contiguous spread from nearby structures, by hematogenous invasion, or from direct implantation during surgery or penetrating head trauma. The most common contiguous infections include sinusitis, otitis media, and mastoiditis.[28] Odontogenic infections (particularly involving those involving the molar teeth) account for up to 10% of cases. Hematogenous spread from distant sites of infection has been implicated in approximately 25% of brain abscesses. Endocarditis and pulmonary infections are among the most commonly reported distant foci of infection, but other sites of infection (e.g., intraabdominal, pelvic, skin, bone) can lead to the development of brain abscess. Direct implantation from invasive neurosurgical procedures or from penetrating head trauma, especially injury associated with a gunshot wound or retained foreign bone fragments, can also lead to the development of a brain abscess.[29] No primary site or underlying condition can be identified in approximately one third of patients with brain abscess.

In pediatric patients, congenital heart disease is a significant risk factor for the development of a brain abscess. It accounts for 25% to 50% of the cases of brain abscesses in some pediatric series.[30] Patients with cyanotic congenital heart disease have low-perfusion regions in their brain as a result of chronic severe hypoxemia and metabolic acidosis, as well as increased viscosity of the blood from secondary polycythemia, which may serve as a focus of infection. Furthermore, right-to-left shunting of the venous blood in the heart bypasses the pulmonary circulation, where phagocytes normally filter bacteria in the bloodstream.

## PRESENTING SIGNS AND SYMPTOMS

The presenting symptoms of a brain abscess are often nonspecific and vary according to several factors, including the location and size of the abscess, the underlying immune status of the host, and the virulence of the infecting organism. Common presenting signs and symptoms in brain abscess are shown in **Table 171.7**. Patients with intracranial abscess often have a subacute onset of illness and rarely appear toxic. Because the initial presentation is often nonspecific, the diagnosis may be initially missed in the ED, and the patient may return for subsequent visits when symptoms persist. On average, the diagnosis is made 13 to 14 days after the onset of symptoms, although symptoms can last from a few hours to several months. The most common signs and symptoms of brain abscess are headache, mental status change, focal neurologic deficit, and fever.[31] The clinical triad of headache, fever, and focal neurologic deficit is present in less than 20% of cases.

**Table 171.7 Common Presenting Signs and Symptoms in Brain Abscess**

| SIGN OR SYMPTOM | FREQUENCY (%) |
|---|---|
| Fever | 37-75 |
| Headache | 56-94 |
| Nausea or vomiting | 31-77 |
| Neck stiffness | 11 |
| Altered level of consciousness | 10-100 |
| Focal neurologic deficit | 49-75 |
| Seizure | 12-47 |
| Papilledema | 6-50 |

## DIFFERENTIAL DIAGNOSIS

The differential diagnosis in patients presenting with fever, headache, and focal neurologic deficits includes other intracranial abscesses (e.g., intracranial epidural abscess, subdural empyema), as well as meningoencephalitis. Selected patients with severe alcohol withdrawal, anticholinergic poisoning, diabetic ketoacidosis, seizures, stroke, acute psychosis, CNS tumor or mass, or other infections can present with signs and symptoms mimicking a CNS infection.

Intracranial epidural abscess is an extraaxial infection occurring in the virtual space between the dura mater and the skull. It most often occurs as a complication of neurosurgery, but it can result from spread of infection to the epidural space from the paranasal sinuses, middle ear, or mastoid process. An intracranial epidural abscess often has an insidious onset, with symptoms developing over several weeks to months. Patients present with headache, fever, and signs of increased ICP. Nuchal irritation and neurologic symptoms are unusual because the infection is typically frontal or temporal in location, and tight adherence of dura to the overlying skull limits its spread and protects the underlying brain parenchyma. The Pott puffy tumor is a rare clinical entity characterized by a frontal brain epidural abscess with overlying osteomyelitis, typically occurring as a complication of frontal sinusitis.

Subdural empyema is an infection that occurs in the potential space between the dura mater and the arachnoid, typically as a result of direct spread from paranasal sinusitis, otitis media, or mastoiditis. Unlike the epidural space, the subdural space is less restrictive, resulting in wider spread of the empyema. This spread of infection can cause inflammation of the brain parenchyma, in addition to a mass effect (and increased ICP) from the diffuse abscess. Common causative organisms are anaerobes, aerobic streptococci, staphylococci, *H. influenzae*, *S. pneumoniae*, and other gram-negative bacilli. Patients present with signs and symptoms consistent with a CNS infection, such as headache, fever, signs of increased ICP, altered level of consciousness, focal neurologic deficits, and seizures. High-resolution contrast-enhanced CT scanning is the standard technique for quick and noninvasive diagnosis of subdural empyema, although the diagnostic neuroimaging modality of choice is MRI with gadolinium enhancement.

## MEDICAL DECISION MAKING

Routine testing of patients with suspected brain abscess should include CBC, serum electrolytes, bicarbonate, BUN, creatinine, and glucose. Serum lactate determinations and blood cultures are also indicated in patients with suspected brain abscess. LP is inadvisable because of the likely presence of increased ICP and the subsequent risk of herniation.

The diagnosis of brain abscess is made by contrast-enhanced cranial CT or MRI. Nonenhanced cranial CT can identify approximately 90% of mature brain abscesses,[32] but it is considered inadequate to exclude the diagnosis. The classic contrast-enhanced cranial CT appearance of a mature brain abscess is that of a ring-enhancing mass lesion with a hypodense center that is frequently surrounded by a substantial amount of edema. Contrast-enhanced cranial CT is highly sensitive (>95%) for identifying this type of lesion.[29] Unfortunately, ring-enhancing lesions seen on CT images are not specific for brain abscess; cystic and necrotic neoplastic lesions, hematomas, demyelinating diseases, thrombosed giant aneurysm, and infarcted brain tissue may have the same CT characteristics. Both nonenhanced and enhanced cranial CT may miss lesions that are early in their maturity (i.e., during the "cerebritis" stage of brain abscess formation), small lesions, and lesions of the posterior circulation. Gadolinium-enhanced MRI is considered the gold standard for diagnostic imaging for this disease.

## TREATMENT

Successful management of confirmed intracranial abscess involves a combination of broad-spectrum antibiotics and radiologically guided surgical drainage. Once the diagnosis is established, a neurosurgeon and an infectious disease specialist should be consulted. A sample of the infected tissue or fluid (pus) must be obtained quickly, to guide the initial therapy. The initial antibiotic regimen is based on the presumptive source of the abscess and on the Gram stain results, if available. Additional consultation with an oral-maxillofacial or ear, nose, and throat specialist may be required, depending on the extent of the primary infection. The principles of effective treatment of brain abscess are outlined in **Box 171.6**. Effective empiric antibiotic regimens for brain abscess are listed in **Table 171.8**.

Although the benefit of corticosteroids in treatment of brain abscess remains unclear, dexamethasone (10 mg intravenous loading dose, followed by 4 mg intravenously every 6 hours) is recommended when a substantial mass effect can be demonstrated on imaging. Unnecessary or prolonged use of corticosteroids should be avoided because of numerous side effects, including decreased penetration of antibiotics across the blood-brain barrier and into the abscess cavity.

## FOLLOW-UP, NEXT STEPS IN CARE, AND PATIENT CARE

Patients with brain abscess should be admitted to a monitored setting where serial neurologic examinations can take place. The sudden worsening of headache accompanied by neck

**BOX 171.6 Principles of Effective Treatment for Brain Abscess**

- Combined medicine and surgical team approach
- If possible, sample of infected material obtained before initiation of antibiotics in the emergency department
- Empiric coverage based on site of primary infection and initial Gram stain results
- Surgery reserved for the following:
  - Abscess larger than 2.5 cm
  - Traumatic brain abscess
  - Cerebellar or brainstem abscess
  - Periventricular brain abscess
  - Encapsulated fungal abscess
  - Multiloculated abscesses
  - Placement of ventriculostomy in patients with increased intracranial pressure
- Corticosteroid and anticonvulsant therapy as indicated

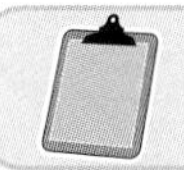

**DOCUMENTATION**

- The most important procedure to document in a patient presenting with suspected brain abscess is a good neurologic examination.
- Consider intracranial abscess in patients who have had recent, subacute, or chronic sinus, ear, mastoid, dental, or cardiac infection and new headache or focal neurologic deficit.
- Although this disease has nonspecific symptoms early in its course, litigation often focuses on the failure to diagnose brain abscess. Consistent documentation of return precautions in patients with headache and fever may limit time to diagnosis and your exposure if the case becomes litigated.

**Table 171.8** Antibiotic Regimen for Brain Abscess

| LIKELY SOURCE OF INFECTION | ANTIBIOTIC REGIMEN |
|---|---|
| Contiguous site: odontogenic source | Penicillin G 3 to 4 million units IV q4h<br>*and*<br>Metronidazole 15 mg/kg IV loading dose, followed by 7.5 mg/kg IV q8h |
| Contiguous site: nonodontogenic source (e.g., sinusitis, otitis media, mastoiditis) | Ceftriaxone 50 mg/kg IV (maximum dose, 2 g) IV q12h *or*<br>Cefotaxime 50 mg/kg IV (maximum dose, 2 g) IV q6h<br>*and*<br>Metronidazole 15 mg/kg IV loading dose, followed by 7.5 mg/kg IV q8h |
| Hematogenous spread of infection (e.g., bacteremia, endocarditis) | Ceftriaxone 50 mg/kg IV (maximum dose, 2 g) IV q12h *or*<br>Cefotaxime 50 mg/kg IV (maximum dose, 2 g) IV q6h<br>*and*<br>Metronidazole 15 mg/kg IV loading dose, followed by 7.5 mg/kg IV q8h<br>*and*<br>Vancomycin 15 mg/kg IV q12h |
| Postoperative neurosurgical patients | Ceftazidime 50 mg/kg IV (maximum dose, 2 g) IV q8h *or*<br>Cefepime 50 mg/kg IV (maximum dose, 2 g) IV q8h<br>*and*<br>Vancomycin 15 mg/kg IV q12h |
| Patients with penetrating skull trauma | Ceftriaxone 50 mg/kg IV (maximum dose, 2 g) IV q12h *or*<br>Cefotaxime 50 mg/kg IV (maximum dose, 2 g) IV q6h<br>*and*<br>Vancomycin 15 mg/kg IV q12h |

*IV,* Intravenous(ly); *q4h, q6h, q8h, q12h,* every 4, 6, 8, and 12 hours, respectively.

stiffness is an ominous sign in the patient with a periventricular brain abscess and may indicate rupture of the abscess into the ventricles.

Intracranial abscesses are associated with significant mortality and permanent neurologic morbidity. With the development of rapid diagnostic imaging, effective antibiotics, and improved surgical technique, reports from contemporary case series place the overall mortality from brain abscess at less than 10%. However up to 20% of the survivors will have severe neurologic disability or end up in a vegetative state. Neurologic morbidity and overall mortality are related to the initial level of consciousness at the time of diagnosis, host immune status, and response to initial therapy. Seizures occur in approximately 25% of patients with brain abscess.[33] A frontoparietal location of the brain abscess or underlying valvular heart disease predicts seizure development in the presence of brain abscess.

## REFERENCES

*References can be found on Expert Consult @ www.expertconsult.com.*

# 172 Sepsis

*Michael J. Schmidt*

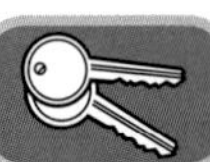

**KEY POINTS**

- Sepsis encompasses a spectrum of diseases: infection with signs of a systemic inflammatory response, severe sepsis, and septic shock.
- Treatment in the emergency department includes early, presumptive administration of antibiotics and early, aggressive fluid resuscitation, with the use of central venous pressure monitoring and vasopressors when appropriate to optimize resuscitation.
- Patients with severe sepsis and septic shock must be monitored closely and should be admitted to an intensive care unit.

## EPIDEMIOLOGY

In the United States alone, more than 750,000 cases of sepsis occur, and approximately 215,000 deaths result from this disease annually.[1] Over the 25-year period between 1972 and 1997, little change occurred in the mortality rate (ranging from 40% to >60%) for patients with septic shock.[2] More recent advances in the early treatment of severe sepsis and septic shock have shown improvements in mortality and thus promise for patients and their treating physicians.[3-5]

## PATHOPHYSIOLOGY

*Sepsis* is defined as a condition in which an identified or suspected source of infection leads to a systemic inflammatory process, known as the systemic inflammatory response syndrome (SIRS) (**Box 172.1**). *Severe sepsis* refers to sepsis that has progressed to cellular dysfunction and organ damage or evidence of hypoperfusion, whereas *septic shock* refers to sepsis with persistent hypotension despite adequate fluid resuscitation. SIRS can develop when an exaggerated response of the body's immune system to infection results in the release of inflammatory cytokines (tumor necrosis factor-α, interleukin-1, and interleukin-6) as the immune cells encounter the organisms' endotoxins.[6] These cytokines can lead to activation of the coagulation cascade with subsequent thrombosis and disseminated intravascular coagulation, as well as the release and activation of nitric oxide, thought to be the key mediator in vasodilation and shock.[4,7] Progression of shock can lead to poor oxygen delivery and use at the tissue level, thereby creating an environment in which lactic acid is generated and mixed venous oxygenation is impaired.

## PRESENTING SIGNS AND SYMPTOMS

The patient with classic severe sepsis or septic shock appears ill, with fever (less commonly hypothermia) and chills, an increased respiratory rate, and tachycardia. Patients may have cold skin showing outward signs of decreased perfusion (**Fig. 172.1**), and they may have mental status changes.

The presentation may or may not direct the clinician to the potential source of infection. For example, dyspnea and crackles on a lung examination may point to a pneumonia source, or left lower quadrant tenderness on an abdominal examination may point to diverticulitis as the source. Determining the site of infection in the emergency department (ED) may be difficult, and even retrospectively, an initial source is not determined in up to 15% of patients (**Box 172.2**).[8]

More objective measures (SIRS criteria, lactate level, mixed venous oxygenation) are used to determine whether a patient has sepsis because patients can sometimes appear surprisingly well even when they have severe sepsis or septic shock. Their only complaint may be fever, even though other SIRS criteria and hypotension may be present, especially in relatively younger, healthier, immunocompetent patients (see Fig. 172.1).

## DIFFERENTIAL DIAGNOSIS AND MEDICAL DECISION MAKING

The differential diagnosis of sepsis includes many other life-threatening emergencies, including toxidromes (sympathomimetic, anticholinergic), thyrotoxicosis or myxedema coma, neuroleptic malignant syndrome, heat stroke, withdrawal (ethanol, sedative-hypnotics), pulmonary embolism, and other causes of shock (anaphylactic, cardiogenic, hypovolemic).

The diagnostic work-up may vary among patients, but most patients require standard testing to start. Serum lactate has

**BOX 172.1 Definition of Systemic Inflammatory Response Syndrome**

The presence of two or more of the following four items constitutes sepsis:

- Temperature lower than 36° C or higher than 38° C
- Heart rate greater than 90 beats per minute
- Respiratory rate greater than 20 breaths per minute or partial pressure of arterial carbon dioxide lower than 32 mm Hg
- White blood cell count lower than 4000 or higher than 12,000 cells/$mm^3$ or more than 10% bands

**BOX 172.2 Most Common Sites of Infection (in order of frequency)**

- Lung (pneumonia)
- Abdominopelvic region
- Urinary tract
- Soft tissue (cellulitis)
- Other: blood, central nervous system (meningitis), bone (osteomyelitis), joint, heart (endocarditis)

become an important risk stratification tool because both the initial serum lactate level and lactate clearance have been shown to be important predictors of mortality.[9,10] Further work-up should be guided by the suspected source of infection. For example, concern about a possible abdominopelvic infection (e.g., diverticulitis, acute cholecystitis) may warrant a computed tomography scan of the abdomen or pelvis or a right upper quadrant ultrasound scan, whereas concern about a possible central nervous system infection (e.g., meningitis) may warrant lumbar puncture. A procalcitonin level determination may be helpful in guiding therapy and predicting outcomes, whereas future molecular assays may help in more rapid identification of pathogens.[11,12] The diagnostic evaluation is important, but aggressive treatment in advance of test results is essential.

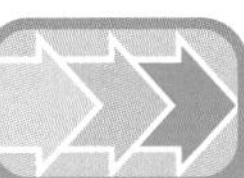

**PRIORITY ACTIONS**

**Diagnostic Testing**

- Blood cultures before antibiotic administration
- Complete blood count
- Chemistry panel
- Lactic acid level
- Urinalysis
- Urine culture
- Chest radiograph
- Prothrombin time and partial thromboplastin time if concern exists about disseminated intravascular coagulation
- Further imaging or invasive diagnostic testing (e.g., lumbar puncture, paracentesis) as indicated

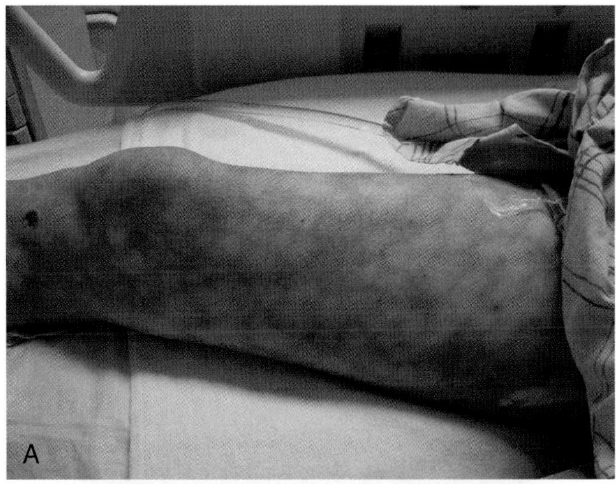


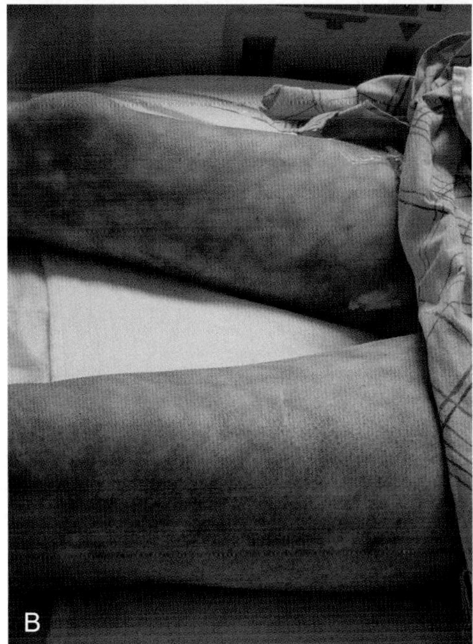


**Fig. 172.1 A and B, Skin mottling.** This patient presented to the emergency department with septic shock and showed extreme signs of hypoperfusion. He underwent early goal-directed therapy and actually survived to discharge from the hospital.

## TREATMENT

Intubation may be necessary to provide airway protection (i.e., for decreased mental status) or to decrease the work of breathing and improve oxygenation. Etomidate causes measurable, albeit transient, adrenal suppression (see Chapter 168), but the use of a single dose of etomidate as an induction agent in the ED to facilitate rapid-sequence intubation remains clinically indicated.[13] Corticosteroids can be considered in patients with persistent hypotension unresponsive to fluids.

High-volume fluid resuscitation is required for patients with sepsis, even frail older patients, so two large-bore intravenous lines are required. Aggressive resuscitation with intravenous crystalloid (or colloid) fluids should be initiated immediately. The administration of 2 L of normal saline, or a 20 to 30 mL/kg bolus of fluids, is a good starting point.

Antibiotics should be administered early in the patient's course. Central venous access can be established to monitor central venous pressures, to administer intravenous fluids and medications such as vasopressors, and to obtain mixed venous oxygen saturation measurements. Foley catheterization should be performed to monitor urine output. All patients should have continuous cardiac monitoring and pulse oximetry.

## SEPSIS BUNDLES

The Institute for Healthcare Improvement developed recommendations for early, initial treatment of the patient with severe sepsis or septic shock (**Box 172.3**).[14] These recommendations are based on the best current available evidence from the Surviving Sepsis Campaign's management guidelines.[15]

**BOX 172.3 Institute for Healthcare Improvement Sepsis Resuscitation Bundle**

- **A.** Serum lactate measured
- **B.** Blood cultures obtained before antibiotic administration
- **C.** Antibiotics administered within 3 hours of emergency department presentation
- **D.** In the event of hypotension or lactate greater than 4 mmol/L (36 mg/dL):
  1. Deliver an initial minimum of 20 mL/kg of crystalloid (or colloid equivalent).
  2. Apply vasopressors for hypotension not responding to initial fluid resuscitation to maintain mean arterial pressure higher than 65 mm Hg.
- **E.** In the event of persistent hypotension despite fluid resuscitation or lactate greater than 4 mmol/L (36 mg/dL):
  1. Achieve central venous pressure higher than 8 mm Hg.
  2. Achieve central venous oxygen saturation greater than 70%.

From Institute for Healthcare Improvement: Sepsis. 2011. http://www.ihi.org/IHI/Topics/CriticalCare/Sepsis.

## ANTIMICROBIAL THERAPY

Patients should receive antibiotic coverage, early and presumptively. Coverage should be directed at the source, if known, but broad-spectrum antibiotics are generally advisable. Early administration of adequate antibiotics favors improved outcomes, whereas delays in administration result in increased mortality for this patient population.[16,17]

## EARLY GOAL-DIRECTED THERAPY

Early goal-directed therapy has generated great interest and is influencing treatment for patients with severe sepsis or septic shock.[3] Mortality is reduced by early identification of patients with severe sepsis (identified as patients with lactic acid >4 mmol/L) or septic shock (identified as patients with systolic blood pressure <90 mm Hg after 20 to 30 mL/kg of fluid) and by early aggressive hemodynamic monitoring and optimization using specific resuscitation end points (central venous pressure, mean arterial pressure, mixed venous oxygen saturation). Early goal-directed therapy is summarized in **Figure 172.2**.

## VASOPRESSORS

In patients with persistent hypotension (mean arterial pressure < 65 mm Hg or systolic blood pressure < 90 mm Hg) despite initial fluid resuscitation (20 to 30 mL/kg), vasopressors should be used to maintain organ perfusion. First-line agents include norepinephrine, at 2 to 20 mcg/minute, or dopamine, at 5 to 20 mcg/kg/minute.[15] Norepinephrine (Levophed) may improve survival in patients with septic shock who require vasopressor therapy, and this agent may be better at correcting hypotension while avoiding potential arrhythmias more commonly seen with dopamine.[18,19] Vasopressin, at 0.01 to 0.04 units/minute, can be considered as an additional agent in patients with hypotension refractory to initial vasoactive

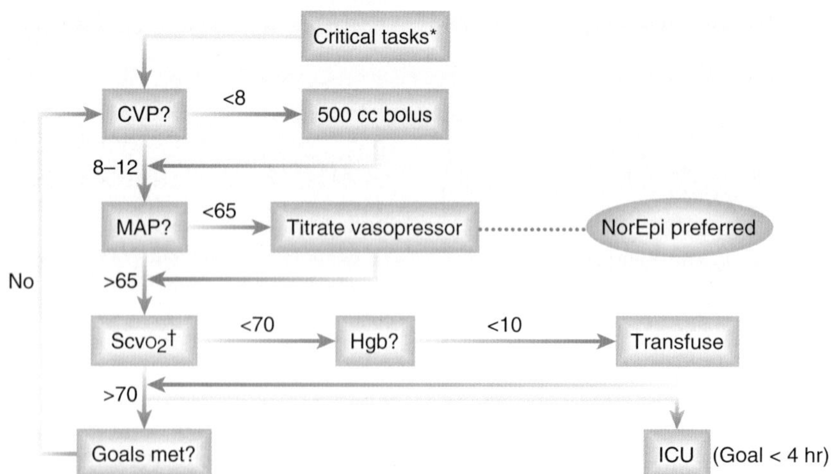


**Fig. 172.2 Early goal-directed therapy.** *CVP,* Central venous pressure; *Hgb,* hemoglobin; *ICU,* intensive care unit; *MAP,* mean arterial pressure; *NorEpi,* norepinephrine; *Scvo2,* central venous oxygen saturation.

medications because it appears to have synergistic effects.[20] Other second-line agents include phenylephrine and epinephrine.

### LOW-DOSE CORTICOSTEROIDS AND ACTIVATED PROTEIN C

In addition to being less conducive to administration in the ED, low-dose corticosteroids and activated protein C have limited scope, and their use continues to be debated.[4,5,21,22] In a large, multicenter trial, corticosteroids were not shown to improve survival and were also associated with an increased risk of superinfection.[21] Shock was reversed more rapidly with corticosteroids when reversal was achieved, and previous studies showed improved survival.[5] Corticosteroids can still be considered in patients poorly responsive to fluids and vasopressors.[15] If given, corticosteroids can be administered in the form of intravenous hydrocortisone (200 to 300 mg/day as a continuous infusion or as 50-mg boluses). Adrenocorticotropic hormone stimulation testing is not necessary.

Activated protein C promotes fibrinolysis and inhibits thrombosis and inflammation. Recombinant human activated protein C, or drotrecogin alfa (activated), can be considered in high-risk patients with severe sepsis or septic shock. Identification of appropriate patients (those with an Acute Physiology and Chronic Health Evaluation II [APACHE II] score ≥25), contraindications (risk of bleeding), and cost currently limit the utility of this agent in the ED.

## FOLLOW-UP, NEXT STEPS OF CARE, AND PATIENT EDUCATION

Patients with severe sepsis or septic shock warrant admission to an intensive care unit. An elevated lactate level is evidence of hypoperfusion. Patients without evidence of hypoperfusion, end-organ damage, or hypotension may be admitted to a medical ward. Reliance on improved vital signs alone can be misleading, and additional objective measures (serum lactate concentration, mixed venous oxygenation) are required to exclude shock states. Close monitoring of all patients is warranted because signs and symptoms can progress.

## SUGGESTED READINGS

De Backer D, Biston P, Devriendt J, et al. Comparison of dopamine and norepinephrine in the treatment of shock. N Engl J Med 2010;362:779-89.

Dellinger RP, Carlet JM, Masur H, et al. Surviving Sepsis Campaign: international guidelines for management of severe sepsis and septic shock: 2008. Crit Care Med 2008;36:296-327.

Rivers E, Nguyen B, Havstad S, et al. Early goal-directed therapy in the treatment of severe sepsis and septic shock. N Engl J Med 2001;345:1368-77.

Shapiro NI, Howell MD, Talmor D, et al. Serum lactate as a predictor of mortality in emergency department patients with infection. Ann Emerg Med 2005;45:524-8.

Sprung CL, Annane D, Keh D, et al. Hydrocortisone therapy for patients with septic shock. N Engl J Med 2008;358:111-24.

## REFERENCES

***References can be found on Expert Consult @ www.expertconsult.com.***

# 173 Infections in the Immunocompromised Host

*Fredrick M. Abrahamian*

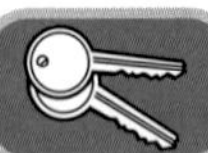

**KEY POINTS**

- Neutropenia is a significant risk factor for infections in patients with malignant diseases. Empiric antibiotic therapy should be administered to all neutropenic febrile patients and to afebrile neutropenic patients who have new signs and symptoms consistent with infection.
- Neutropenia is defined as an absolute neutrophil count of less than 500 cells/$mm^3$ or an absolute neutrophil count expected to decrease to less than 500 cells/$mm^3$ during the next 48 hours.
- Splenectomized patients are at higher risk of fulminant infection by *Streptococcus pneumoniae, Haemophilus influenzae,* or *Neisseria meningitidis.*
- Prolonged corticosteroid therapy (>3 to 4 weeks) at doses of more than 20 mg per day places the patient at risk of hypothalamic-pituitary-adrenal suppression and infectious complications.
- Malignant otitis externa, rhinocerebral mucormycosis, emphysematous pyelonephritis, emphysematous cholecystitis, and Fournier gangrene occur predominantly in diabetic patients.

## PERSPECTIVE

Immunocompromised patients frequently visit emergency departments (EDs) for evaluation and treatment of various conditions. Infectious complications are common, and they are a diagnostic priority because clinical presentations are often subtle and atypical. This chapter covers infections in patients with malignant disease, in patients receiving immunosuppressive and corticosteroid therapy, in patients who have undergone solid organ or bone marrow transplantation, and in diabetic patients. Human immunodeficiency virus infection is discussed in Chapter 175.

## MALIGNANCY, NEUTROPENIA, AND FEVER

### EPIDEMIOLOGY

Fever associated with neutropenia is often a presenting sign of infection in patients receiving chemotherapy for cancer. Patients with severe neutropenia (absolute neutrophil count < 100 cells/$mm^3$) or prolonged neutropenia (>7 days' duration) are at higher risk of bacteremia.[1]

### PATHOPHYSIOLOGY

Patients with malignant diseases are predisposed to infections from various organisms, including bacterial, fungal, and viral pathogens. Patients with malignant disease are more prone to infections because of impairment of normal host defenses (e.g., neutropenia associated with acute leukemia), complications associated with tumor growth and spread (e.g., bronchial obstruction from bronchogenic carcinoma that results in pneumonia), the use of chemotherapeutic agents and corticosteroids, a history of splenectomy, and infections associated with intravascular catheters or other implanted devices.[2]

Neutropenia is a significant risk factor for infections in patients with malignant disease, and it can be a result of the condition itself (e.g., acute leukemia) or a consequence of the myelosuppressive effects of agents used in disease management. The 2010 guidelines of the Infectious Disease Society of America (IDSA) for the use of antimicrobial agents in neutropenic patients with cancer defined neutropenia as an absolute neutrophil count of less than 500 cells/$mm^3$ or an absolute neutrophil count expected to decrease to less than 500 cells/$mm^3$ during the next 48 hours.[1] The frequency and severity of infection are inversely proportional to the neutrophil count, and susceptibility to infection increases when the neutrophil count falls to less than 1000 cells/$mm^3$.[3] In addition, vulnerability to infection increases with longer periods of neutropenia. The same guidelines also defined fever, in the absence of obvious environmental causes, as a single oral temperature measurement of 38.3° C (101° F) or higher or a temperature of 38.0° C (100.4° F) or higher for at least 1 hour.[1]

In addition to the neutrophils, other components of cell-mediated immunity, such as lymphocytes, monocytes, or macrophages, may also become deficient or defective in certain types of cancers (e.g., lymphoma, leukemia, Hodgkin disease). Many organisms may be responsible for infections in patients with these types of cancers that impair cell-mediated immunity[2] (**Box 173.1**). These patients most often undergo an extensive work-up to establish the etiologic agent of infection. Special attention also needs to be paid to patients who have undergone splenectomy. These patients are at a higher risk of developing fulminant infection by *Streptococcus pneumoniae, Haemophilus influenzae,* or *Neisseria meningitidis.*

Approximately 60% of bacterial infections are the result of gram-positive cocci, and 35% are caused by gram-negative bacilli.[2] Bacteremia complicates approximately 20% of the

**BOX 173.1 Organisms Often Associated with Infections in Patients with Impaired Cell-Mediated Immunity**

**Bacteria**
*Nocardia, Salmonella, Listeria, Legionella, Pseudomonas, Mycobacterium* species

**Fungi**
*Cryptococcus neoformans, Aspergillus, Candida* species

**Viruses**
Cytomegalovirus, herpes simplex virus, varicella-zoster virus

**Parasites**
*Toxoplasma gondii, Giardia lamblia*

**BOX 173.2 Most Common Causes of Bacteremia in Febrile Neutropenic Patients**

*Staphylococcus aureus*
*Staphylococcus epidermidis*
*Streptococcus pneumoniae*
*Streptococcus pyogenes*
Viridans streptococci
*Enterococcus faecalis*
*Enterococcus faecium*
*Corynebacterium* species
*Escherichia coli*
*Klebsiella* species
*Pseudomonas aeruginosa*

infections. The most common causes of bacteremia in febrile neutropenic patients are listed in **Box 173.2**.[1,4] Anaerobes are uncommon culprits of infection in neutropenic patients, except in the presence of clinical features of oral mucositis or perirectal or intraabdominal infections.[2,5]

Fungal infections most commonly involve *Candida* and *Aspergillus* species and are typically encountered in patients with prolonged neutropenia, or they manifest as secondary infections in patients who have received broad-spectrum antibiotics. Fungal infections can cause fever following recovery from chemotherapy-induced neutropenia. Candidal infections commonly manifest with thrush and esophagitis, and less frequently as acute disseminated candidiasis. Aspergillus infections usually manifest with sinus and pulmonary infections. This organism infects catheter sites and the gastrointestinal tract, and it causes thrombosis and infarction of blood vessels. Both *Candida* and *Aspergillus* are difficult to grow on blood cultures. Identification of these fungi requires multiple blood cultures, as well as other diagnostic tests (e.g., nasal endoscopy, biopsy of lesions).

## PRESENTING SIGNS AND SYMPTOMS

Neutropenic patients may have fever as their only presenting feature of infection, without other specific clinical manifestations of infection. Cellulitis, pustulation, or lymphadenopathy may be diminished. A pulmonary infiltrate may be absent on initial radiographs. Meningitis and urinary tract infection may cause minimal pleocytosis and pyuria, respectively. Pain at any site should heighten the suspicion of occult infection despite the absence of typical physical signs of infection.

## MEDICAL DECISION MAKING

The initial evaluation often includes broad diagnostic testing, including serum chemistry studies, complete blood cell count, liver and renal function tests, urinalysis, blood and urine cultures, and radiographic evaluations (e.g., plain chest radiographs). Blood cultures should be drawn before the initiation of antimicrobial therapy. When a catheter-related infection is suspected, blood cultures should be simultaneously drawn through the central venous catheter and the peripheral vein.[6] Urine cultures are especially indicated if the patient has signs and symptoms of urinary tract infection, if a urinary catheter is present, or if the urinalysis results are abnormal. A chest radiograph is indicated if the patient has any respiratory abnormalities or chest discomfort. A negative chest radiograph does not rule out the presence of a pulmonary infection in a neutropenic patient. In this population of patients, multiple studies have shown that high-resolution computed tomography (CT) scanning of the chest is a better diagnostic test than plain chest radiographs for the early detection of pneumonia.[7-9] Unless clinically indicated, routine lumbar puncture and cerebrospinal fluid examination are not recommended.[4]

## TREATMENT

Empiric antibiotic therapy should be administered promptly to all neutropenic febrile patients and to afebrile neutropenic patients who have signs and symptoms consistent with infection. **Box 173.3** depicts recommended initial antimicrobial therapy for the management of febrile neutropenic patients.[1,4,5] The 2010 IDSA guidelines[1] advocated that high-risk patients should receive intravenous antimicrobial monotherapy with any one of these agents: piperacillin-tazobactam, cefepime, ceftazidime, meropenem, or imipenem. Other antimicrobials such as vancomycin or metronidazole can be added in the presence of specific clinical situations (see Box 173.3).

When a catheter-related infection is suspected, empiric intravenous antibiotic therapy with vancomycin should be initiated[6] (see Box 173.3). Peripheral venous catheters should be removed if the patient shows signs of infection at the site (e.g., drainage of pus, erythema) or evidence of septic shock with no other source of infection. Prompt removal of the catheter is warranted when intravascular catheterization is complicated by septic thrombophlebitis.[6] The diagnosis can be made by ultrasonography with color Doppler imaging. Emergency physicians (EPs) should involve the oncologist and the infectious disease specialists in the decision-making process when considering removal of a central line.

Antiviral agents should not be initiated empirically as initial therapy in the ED for all patients with neutropenic fever. However, the presence of lesions resulting from herpes simplex virus or varicella-zoster virus warrants the initiation of antiviral agents (e.g., acyclovir, valacyclovir), even if these

**BOX 173.3 Recommended Initial Antimicrobial Therapy for the Management of Febrile Neutropenic Patients***

**Oral Therapy†**

Ciprofloxacin plus amoxicillin-clavulanate

**Intravenous Therapy**

Piperacillin-tazobactam or cefepime or ceftazidime or antipseudomonal carbapenem (e.g., imipenem, meropenem)

Vancomycin if any one of the following clinical situations exists: suspected catheter-related infection, skin and soft tissue infection, pneumonia, hemodynamic instability

Metronidazole if either of the following clinical situations exists: abdominal or *Clostridium difficile* infections

*Selection of the empiric regimen should be based on knowledge of the local antibiotic susceptibility pattern, prevalence of methicillin-resistant *Staphylococcus aureus* (MRSA) and other resistant organisms within the community, and potential drug interactions and toxicities within each patient.

†Indicated only for low-risk patients (see text and Box 173.4).

**BOX 173.4 Factors Associated with a Lower Risk of Complications and a Favorable Prognosis in Adult Patients Presenting with Neutropenic Fever**

Absolute neutrophil and monocyte counts 100 cells/mm$^3$ or higher
Age less than 60 and more than 16 years
Cancer in partial or complete remission
No symptoms or only mild to moderate symptoms of illness
Outpatient status at the time of fever onset
Temperature lower than 39.0° C
Normal findings on chest radiographs
Absence of hypotension
Respiratory rate of up to 24 breaths per minute
Absence of chronic pulmonary diseases and diabetes mellitus
Absence of confusion or other signs of mental status alteration
Absence of blood loss and dehydration
No history of fungal infection or receipt of antifungal therapy during the 6 months before presentation with fever

pathogens are not suspected as the cause of fever.[1] Cytomegalovirus (CMV) is an uncommon cause of fever in neutropenic patients, unless these patients undergone bone marrow transplantation. Empiric use of granulocyte or granulocyte colony-stimulating factor transfusions is not recommended for the treatment of established fever and neutropenia.[1]

Antifungal agents (e.g., amphotericin B) should not be initiated empirically in the ED as initial therapy for all patients with neutropenic fever. When antifungal agents are considered, administration is best done in consultation with specialists. In patients with persistent fever (≥4 days) despite adequate antimicrobial therapy and in whom no specific cause of infection has been found, empiric antifungal therapy is often initiated by the specialists.[1]

## ADMISSION

In general, almost all febrile neutropenic patients should be admitted to the hospital (in isolation) for intravenous antibiotic therapy and continued diagnostic work-up. Numerous studies, mostly in adult patients, have examined the identification of variables and scoring indexes that predict a low risk of severe infection among febrile neutropenic patients[10-12] (**Box 173.4**). The most current IDSA guidelines recommended consideration of oral therapy only in low-risk adults who can be vigilantly observed and who have timely access to continued medical care.[1] If outpatient therapy is considered, EPs should always involve the oncologist and the infectious disease specialists in the decision-making process.

### IMMUNOSUPPRESSIVE AND CORTICOSTEROID THERAPY

Chemotherapeutic agents induce variable degrees of myelosuppression. These agents can affect both the number and function of various cell lines such as neutrophils, lymphocytes, monocytes, and macrophages. The effect depends on the type of agent and the duration of exposure. Immunosuppression can be prolonged even after completion of therapy. The potential organisms and treatment of neutropenic fever associated with treatment-induced immunosuppression mirror the condition itself (see Boxes 173.1 to 173.3).

Like antitumor agents, corticosteroids can induce myelosuppression of various cell lines (e.g., lymphocytes, macrophages, immunoglobulins) and can increase the patient's susceptibility to infections by various types of organisms. The risk of infection is directly related to the underlying condition, the dose of corticosteroid, and the duration of therapy.[13] Prolonged treatment (>3 to 4 weeks) at doses of more than 20 mg per day places the patient at risk for hypothalamic-pituitary-adrenal suppression and infectious complications.[13] In addition to pyogenic bacteria, infections can also involve *Mycobacterium, Aspergillus,* and *Listeria* species.[14] Because steroids can suppress fever, the absence of fever does not exclude the possibility of infection. Fever in patients who are receiving long-term corticosteroid therapy is infectious in origin until proven otherwise.

### SOLID ORGAN TRANSPLANTATION

The two major complications of solid organ transplantation are infections and organ rejection. These two entities have similar clinical presentations and are very difficult to differentiate with certainty based only on the initial signs and symptoms. When these complications are suspected, the patient should be isolated and admitted to the hospital. Initial evaluation in the ED includes the liberal use of blood tests (e.g., serum electrolytes, complete blood cell count, liver enzymes), urinalysis, cultures, arterial blood gas measurements (especially for patients who have undergone lung transplantation), radiographic evaluations (e.g., plain chest radiographs), and drug levels (e.g., cyclosporine). The transplant team should be notified of the patient's clinical presentation and situation

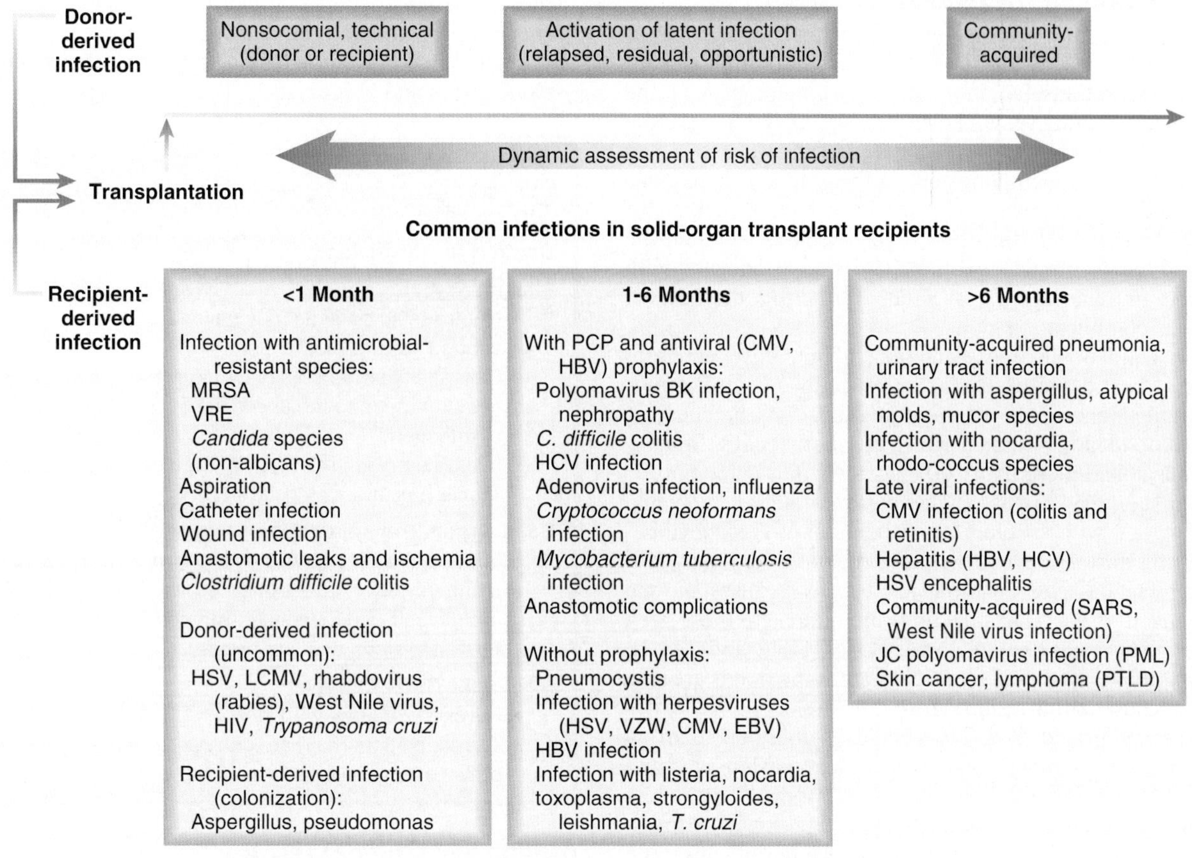


**Fig. 173.1 Timeline of common infections in solid organ transplant recipients.** *CMV,* Cytomegalovirus; *EBV,* Epstein-Barr virus; *HBV,* hepatitis B virus; *HCV,* hepatitis C virus; *HIV,* human immunodeficiency virus; *HSV,* herpes simplex virus; *LCMV,* lymphocytic choriomeningitis virus; *MRSA,* methicillin-resistant *Staphylococcus aureus; PCP, Pneumocystis carinii* pneumonia; *PML,* progressive multifocal leukoencephalopathy; *PTLD,* post-transplantation lymphoproliferative disorder; *SARS,* severe acute respiratory syndrome; *VRE,* vancomycin-resistant *Enterococcus faecalis; VZV,* varicella-zoster virus. (From Fishman JA. Infection in solid-organ transplant recipients. N Engl J Med 2007;357:2601-14.)

The choice of antimicrobial therapy depends on the presenting clinical situation. After stabilization, the patient may require transfer to a transplant center for further evaluation.

All recipients of solid organ transplants undergo similar immunosuppressive therapies after transplantation, and as a result of these standardized regimens, a predictive temporal pattern of infections (i.e., timetable of infections) is recognized (**Fig. 173.1**).[15,16] This posttransplantation timetable is best divided into three periods: the first month, 1 to 6 months, and more than 6 months after transplantation. Opportunistic pathogens (e.g., *Pneumocystis jiroveci* [formerly *Pneumocystis carinii*], *Aspergillus fumigatus, Listeria monocytogenes, Nocardia asteroides*) are more likely to cause infections during the period from 1 to 6 months after transplantation. Prophylaxis against *Pneumocystis jiroveci* and CMV has reduced the incidence of infection by these organisms in transplant recipients.

Of all the pathogens, CMV is the single most important infectious agent affecting the recipients of solid organ transplants.[15,17] The onset of infection is usually after the first month of transplantation. The clinical presentation is variable and can range from flulike illness (e.g., fever, myalgia) to pneumonitis and encephalitis. Laboratory abnormalities can include leukopenia, thrombocytopenia, mild atypical lymphocytosis, and mild hepatitis. The transplanted organ is more susceptible to infection by CMV than are native organs. CMV also has immunosuppressive properties that can render patients more susceptible to opportunistic infections.[15,17] The diagnosis is made by either tissue biopsy or demonstration of viremia. For a symptomatic patient with a confirmed diagnosis, the treatment of choice is intravenous ganciclovir.

In transplant recipients, unexplained fever or headache mandates exclusion of central nervous system (CNS) infection. Evaluation should include a CT scan of the head and lumbar puncture. Because of immunosuppression, these patients may not have a high fever or signs of meningeal inflammation. Common organisms that cause CNS infections include *A. fumigatus, L. monocytogenes, Cryptococcus neoformans,* herpes viruses (e.g., CMV, Epstein-Barr virus), and *Toxoplasma gondii.*

*Aspergillus* infections, most often caused by *A. fumigatus,* are associated with a high rate of mortality in solid organ transplantation. This pathogen can be associated with various infections such as fungemia, wound infections, and sinus, pulmonary, and CNS infections. CNS infections caused by *Aspergillus* may be complicated by abscess or aneurysm formation. *Aspergillus* infection, especially in the disseminated form, is more often seen in liver transplant recipients.

## BONE MARROW TRANSPLANTATION

The risk of infection in recipients of bone marrow transplants depends on various factors, such as the extent of immunosuppression before transplantation, the type of the transplant, the occurrence of graft-versus-host disease (GVHD), and the degree of immunosuppressive therapy. GVHD occurs when immunologically functioning cells in the graft attack antigens on the cells in the recipient. The clinical manifestation of GVHD is variable and involves organs such as the skin, the liver, and the gastrointestinal tract. GVHD is associated with profound immunosuppression, thus furthering the risk of infectious complications.

As in solid organ transplantation, a predictive temporal pattern of host defense defects and infectious complications occurs after bone marrow transplantation. This timetable is also best divided into three periods: the first 30 days, from 31 to 100 days, and more than 100 days after transplantation.[18]

The first 30 days are associated with profound leukopenia, often coupled with absolute neutropenia and lymphocytopenia. During this period, bacteremia is the most common identifiable infectious complication. The bacterial causes and the management of bacterial infections are similar to those seen in other neutropenic patients (see Boxes 173.2 and 173.3). *Candida, Aspergillus,* and recurrent herpes infections are also common causes of infection during this period.[18]

The second period, from 31 to 100 days after bone marrow transplantation, is more notable for defects in humoral and cell-mediated immunity. Leukopenia during this stage is less profound when compared with the earlier period after transplantation. Acute GVHD typically occurs during this time frame, thus prolonging the state of immunosuppression. Many organisms can cause infections in this period (see Boxes 173.1 and 173.2). The most common cause of severe viral illness during this period is CMV, which can lead to interstitial pneumonitis characterized by fever, diffuse pulmonary infiltrates, hypoxia, and the acute respiratory distress syndrome. Treatment of CMV pneumonia includes intravenous ganciclovir and CMV immunoglobulin.

The development of chronic GVHD and a delay in the development of humoral and cell-mediated immunity contribute to infectious complications during the third period (i.e., >100 days) after transplantation. Common bacterial organisms causing infections in this period include encapsulated organisms such as *S. pneumoniae* and *H. influenzae. Candida, Aspergillus,* and varicella-zoster virus are also common causes of infection during this time frame.[18]

## DIABETES MELLITUS

Diabetes mellitus affects several aspects of the immune system. Functional properties of polymorphonuclear leukocytes, monocytes, and lymphocytes such as adherence, chemotaxis, and phagocytosis are depressed in patients with diabetes. These effects are exaggerated in patients with concomitant acidosis. Other alterations in the immune system can include reduced cell-mediated immune responses, impaired pulmonary macrophage function, and abnormal delayed-type hypersensitivity responses. No significant alternations are shown to occur with humoral immunity.[19,20]

Certain community-acquired infections are more common in patients with diabetes (e.g., lower respiratory tract infections, urinary tract infections, skin and mucous membrane infections). The risk of recurrence of such infections is also higher in diabetic patients. Some specific types of infections also occur predominantly in diabetic patients (e.g., malignant otitis externa, rhinocerebral mucormycosis, emphysematous pyelonephritis and cholecystitis, Fournier gangrene).[19,20]

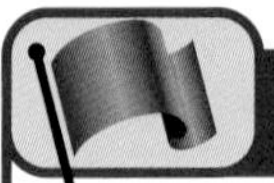

**RED FLAGS**

**Caution for Physicians**

**Malignancy, Neutropenia, and Fever**

- Neutropenic patients may have fever as their only presenting feature of infection.
- Pain at any site should heighten the suspicion of occult infection despite the absence of typical physical signs of infection.
- Initiate empiric antimicrobial therapy in all neutropenic febrile patients.

**Solid Organ Transplantation**

- Infections and organ rejection in a solid organ transplant recipient have similar clinical presentations and are difficult to differentiate with certainty based only on the initial signs and symptoms.

**Malignant Otitis Externa**

- Fever is commonly absent.
- The condition may be confused with nonmalignant otitis externa and perichondritis.

### *Malignant Otitis Externa*

Malignant otitis externa is primarily a disease of older diabetic patients. The infection involves the external auditory canal and the adjacent temporal bone. It can also involve the cranial nerves (e.g., facial nerve) and vascular structures. The primary causative organism is *Pseudomonas aeruginosa.* Signs and symptoms of malignant otitis externa include severe otalgia, otorrhea, edema, and cellulitis of the external auditory canal, diminished hearing, and trismus. Fever is commonly absent. Initially, the condition may be confused with nonmalignant otitis externa and perichondritis. The diagnostic work-up should include an evaluation of the extent of soft tissue involvement with radiographic studies such as contrast CT scan (preferred as the initial radiographic modality) or magnetic resonance imaging. Patients should be admitted for intravenous antimicrobial therapy (e.g., ciprofloxacin, ceftazidime, imipenem). Simultaneously, topical antipseudomonal eardrops should also be initiated. The otolaryngologist should be consulted promptly for initiating further diagnostic tests (e.g., obtaining deep tissue samples for culture and exclusion of epidermal carcinoma), as well as surgical intervention (e.g., débridement of necrotic tissue).

### *Mucormycosis*

Mucormycosis results from infection by fungi of the order Mucorales. Most infections in humans are caused by the species *Mucor* and *Rhizopus.* The spores produced by these fungal species are ubiquitous in the environment. The disease caused by Mucoraceae almost exclusively occurs in immunocompromised individuals. A frequent predisposing condition associated with Mucorales infection is diabetes mellitus. The most common clinical manifestations are rhinocerebral and pulmonary mucormycosis.

Rhinocerebral mucormycosis involves infection of the sinuses with extension into surrounding structures (e.g., bones, orbits, brain, cavernous sinus, carotid artery, and jugular veins). Clinical manifestations depend on the extent of disease and can include fever, headache, lethargy, facial and periorbital pain and swelling, and nasal congestion (with or without discharge). On examination, the patient may have proptosis, chemosis, ulceration, and necrotic lesions on the palate or nasal mucosa, cranial nerve palsies, and hemiparesis. A vital clue to the diagnosis is the characteristic black necrotic eschars on the nasal turbinates. The definitive diagnosis is confirmed by performing biopsy and cultures of the necrotic tissue. Radiographic evaluation in the ED should include contrast CT scan or magnetic resonance imaging (preferred) of the head and neck. Management of rhinocerebral mucormycosis includes aggressive resuscitation and glycemic control, initiation of amphotericin B, and emergency surgical consultation for drainage of sinuses and débridement of infected tissues. Because the definitive diagnosis is often difficult to make in the ED, empiric broad-spectrum antimicrobial therapy for presumed bacterial infection or coinfection should be initiated.

Pulmonary mucormycosis is a rare, rapidly progressing type of pneumonia with a high mortality rate. Risk factors for acquiring the disease include diabetes, neutropenia, and other immunosuppressive conditions. Diabetic patients have impaired pulmonary macrophage function, an important mechanism in host defense against Mucoraceae. Patients may present with mild to massive hemoptysis; otherwise, pulmonary mucormycosis has no specific differentiating clinical manifestation. Chest radiography may demonstrate patchy or diffuse infiltrates, solitary nodules, or cavitary lesions. A predilection exists for involvement of the upper lobes. The definitive diagnosis requires bronchoscopy or lung biopsy. The management of pulmonary mucormycosis includes aggressive resuscitation and glycemic control, initiation of amphotericin B, and surgical consultation for potential resection of isolated pulmonary disease.

### Emphysematous Pyelonephritis

Emphysematous pyelonephritis is a life-threatening, fulminant, suppurative, and necrotizing infection involving the renal parenchyma and perirenal tissues. The disease occurs primarily in diabetic patients and in women more frequently than in men, and it more often involves the left kidney.[21] Patients frequently present in severe sepsis or septic shock. Emphysematous pyelonephritis can be complicated by obstruction of the renoureteral system and by the presence of renal or ureteral stones.

The diagnosis is confirmed radiographically by demonstration of gas in the renal parenchyma or perinephric space. The imaging modality of choice is noncontrast CT scan of the abdomen and pelvis. Intravenous contrast studies can be obtained for better delineation of abscess or vascular structures. Although plain film radiography may show the presence of renal calculi or gas, radiography is of limited value because of its inability to reveal detail. Renal ultrasound scanning is inferior to CT scanning for the localization of gas. Precise localization of gas is important in the differentiation of emphysematous pyelonephritis from emphysematous pyelitis (gas confined to the collecting system).[21] Therapeutically, the distinction between the two disorders is crucial. Emphysematous pyelonephritis usually requires nephrectomy, whereas emphysematous pyelitis often requires medical management, with a drainage procedure only if it is associated with obstruction.[21]

Common organisms isolated from cultures of urine, blood, or aspirate material in patients with emphysematous pyelonephritis include *Escherichia coli* (most common), *Klebsiella pneumoniae, Proteus mirabilis, Enterococcus* species, and *P. aeruginosa*. Management includes intensive resuscitation, initiation of broad-spectrum antibiotics, and immediate surgical consultation and intervention. Antimicrobial therapy can include a combination of a β-lactam–β-lactamase inhibitor antibiotic with antipseudomonal activity (e.g., piperacillin-tazobactam) and an aminoglycoside (e.g., gentamicin). Surgical measures depend on the condition of the patient and the extent of disease and can include percutaneous catheter drainage, incision and drainage, or nephrectomy. Early surgical intervention (e.g., drainage, nephrectomy) in combination with broad-spectrum antibiotics has decreased mortality from emphysematous pyelonephritis.[22,23]

### Emphysematous Cholecystitis

Emphysematous cholecystitis is a rare condition primarily of older diabetic men. The clinical presentation can resemble that of typical acute cholecystitis (i.e., fever, nausea, vomiting, right upper quadrant abdominal pain). Gangrene and perforation of the gallbladder are frequent complications. Contrast CT scan of the abdomen is the imaging modality of choice for the diagnosis of emphysematous cholecystitis. The infection is often polymicrobial, with gram-negative bacilli (e.g., *E. coli*) and anaerobes (e.g., *Clostridium perfringens*). Management includes initiation of broad-spectrum antibiotics (e.g., piperacillin-tazobactam or a combination of ceftriaxone with metronidazole) and emergency cholecystectomy.

### Skin and Soft Tissue Infections

Soft tissue infections in diabetic patients frequently involve the feet. The most common factor predisposing patients to diabetic foot infection is foot ulceration, and it is often related to peripheral neuropathy.[24] Complications can include fulminant and life-threatening septicemia, osteomyelitis, fasciitis, and amputation.

Acute infections in patients with diabetic foot infections who have not recently received antibiotics are often monomicrobial infections with aerobic gram-positive cocci (e.g., *Staphylococcus aureus,* ß-hemolytic streptococci). Chronic wounds or those that have been treated previously with antibiotics are polymicrobial infections commonly resulting from *S. aureus,* β-hemolytic streptococci, *E. coli, P. aeruginosa,* and *Bacteroides fragilis*.[19,24] Depending on the prevalence in the community, community-associated methicillin-resistant *S. aureus* (CA-MRSA) should also be considered a culprit in these infections.[25]

The initial assessment should include plain radiography for the exclusion of foreign bodies and for evaluation of osteomyelitis.[26] This study also serves as a baseline for future comparisons. The ability to see or touch bone with a sterile surgical probe suggests underlying osteomyelitis. Wound specimens for aerobic and anaerobic cultures, although not usually necessary for mild infections, are best obtained by biopsy, ulcer curettage, or aspiration and are preferred to swab specimen.[24]

Management of diabetic foot infection should include initiation of antimicrobial therapy, glycemic control, débridement of devitalized and necrotic tissue, application of sterile dressing, and off-loading pressure at the ulcer.[19,24] The choice of antimicrobial therapy depends on the duration and the severity of the infection, the history of recent antibiotic therapy, the local antibiotic susceptibility pattern, and the prevalence of CA-MRSA and other resistant organisms within the community. Patients discharged home should have early follow-up to ensure proper wound healing.

Fournier gangrene, a form of necrotizing fasciitis involving the male genitalia, is typically seen in older diabetic patients. Clinical features can include crepitus, bullous skin lesions, pain out of proportion to physical findings, and marked systemic toxicity. The infection is most often polymicrobial, involving aerobic and anaerobic streptococci, *S. aureus, E. coli, Pseudomonas, Clostridium,* and *Bacteroides* species.[20] Early recognition, hemodynamic stabilization, the use of broad-spectrum antibiotics (e.g., vancomycin plus piperacillin-tazobactam plus clindamycin), and emergency surgical débridement are the mainstays of therapy. Other potential adjunctive therapeutic modalities such as hyperbaric oxygen therapy should not take precedence over early surgical intervention.

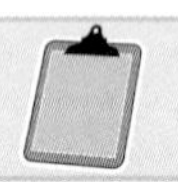

### DOCUMENTATION

**Malignancy, Neutropenia, and Fever**

- Document the duration of fever and signs and symptoms of infection.
- Document well the conversations with the oncologist or infectious disease specialist (time contacted, name of the person, recommendations, treatment plans).

**Solid Organ Transplantation**

- Document well the conversations with the transplant team (time contacted, name of the person, recommendations, treatment plans).

**Diabetic Foot Infection**

- Document when bone is visible or palpable with a probe.

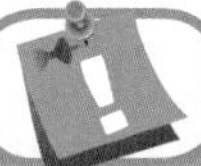

### TIPS AND TRICKS

**Malignancy, Neutropenia, and Fever**

- Suspect occult infection when a patient complains of pain in any bodily area despite the absence of signs of infection.
- Pay special attention to the oral cavity, perineum, toes, bone marrow aspiration sites or sites, and vascular catheters for signs of infection.
- Look for a splenectomy scar. Splenectomized patients are at a higher risk of infection with *Streptococcus pneumoniae, Haemophilus influenzae,* and *Neisseria meningitidis.*

**Rhinocerebral Mucormycosis**

- A vital clue to the diagnosis is the presence of characteristic black necrotic eschars on the nasal turbinates.

## SUGGESTED READINGS

Fishman JA. Infection in solid-organ transplant recipients. N Engl J Med 2007;357:2601-14.

Freifeld AG, Bow EJ, Sepkowitz KA, et al. Clinical practice guideline for the use of antimicrobial agents in neutropenic patients with cancer: 2010 update by the Infectious Diseases Society of America. Clin Infect Dis 2011;52:e56-e93.

Grayson ML, Gibbons GW, Balogh K, et al. Probing to bone in infected pedal ulcers: a clinical sign of underlying osteomyelitis in diabetic patients. JAMA 1995;273:721-3.

Mermel LA, Allon M, Bouza E, et al. Clinical practice guidelines for the diagnosis and management of intravascular catheter-related infection: 2009 update by the Infectious Diseases Society of America. Clin Infect Dis 2009;49:1-45.

## REFERENCES

***References can be found on Expert Consult @ www.expertconsult.com.***

# Viral Infections 174

*Deepi G. Goyal, Kristine M. Thompson, and Annie T. Sadosty*

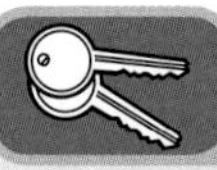

**KEY POINTS**

- If herpes infection of the skin, central nervous system, or other location is suspected, initiate treatment with valacyclovir or acyclovir.
- When patients have respiratory symptoms, the use of face masks, proper hand hygiene, and prudent patient isolation may help minimize the spread of infectious agents.
- Oral acyclovir should be offered to patients with chickenpox who are more than 13 years old, but treatment must be initiated within 24 hours of the onset of the rash.
- When a patient presents with a viral syndrome in the late summer or early fall and has significant muscle weakness, consider West Nile virus.
- Patients with cutaneous pain may be in the early stage of herpes zoster infection because the skin sensation may precede the rash by several days.

## PATHOPHYSIOLOGY

A virus can be viewed as genomic machinery surrounded by a structure that allows it to bind and deliver the contents to a host cell.[1] The structural envelope also determines the mode of transmission of the virus and provides the immunologic basis for host immunity and vaccines. Viral genomes may be composed of either RNA or DNA, and they may be single or double stranded and either circular or linear.

Viruses gain entry into a host organism when the host is exposed to the virus through respiratory droplets, contaminated food or water, or body fluids or tissues. Once the host is inoculated, the virus may cause infection by reproducing locally (e.g., influenza virus causing respiratory infections), or it may be disseminated to distant sites (e.g., varicella zoster virus [VZV]). Many viruses, such as Epstein-Barr virus (EBV), cytomegalovirus, and hepatitis B and C viruses, can cause persistent infections. Although latent, these infections can be reactivated, with resulting acceleration of viral replication and subsequent acute infection.

Virulence is often mediated by the surface proteins involved in cellular attachment and entry. By producing a protein that attaches to the structural cell coat, some viruses can enhance their infectivity.

## HERPES

The word *herpes* derives from a Greek word meaning "to creep." This designation refers to the tendency of herpes viruses to creep along nerve pathways. Currently, at least eight identified herpesviruses cause human disease. Each has distinguishing clinical characteristics. Herpes simplex viruses (HSV-1 and HSV-2) are the agents of herpes genitalis, herpes labialis, and herpes encephalitis. VZV causes chickenpox and herpes zoster (shingles). EBV most commonly causes mononucleosis, but it has also been implicated in several lymphoproliferative syndromes. Cytomegalovirus may also manifest as mononucleosis, although it is more commonly associated with invasive disease in immunocompromised patients. Human herpesvirus 6 is the causative agent of roseola infantum. Human herpesvirus 8 has been linked to Kaposi sarcoma and Castleman disease. More recently, herpes B virus has been linked to fatal human encephalitis. Human herpesvirus 7 has been described, but it is not completely understood. As research advances, more herpes strains will likely be identified.

## HERPES SIMPLEX VIRUS

### EPIDEMIOLOGY

According to the U.S. Centers for Disease Control and Prevention, one out of five of the total adolescent and adult population in the United States is infected with HSV-2. The incidence is even higher for HSV-1, which infects approximately 80% of the U.S. population. HSV-1 most commonly infects the lips and leads to lesions referred to as "cold sores," but it can also produce genital lesions. HSV-2 is most often associated with genital herpes, but this virus can infect the mouth during oral sex. The most common locations for herpes simplex lesions are the mouth and the genitals, but infections of the eyes, brain, fingers, face, and esophagus are also seen (**Table 174.1**).

**Table 174.1 Herpes Simplex Infections**

| TYPE AND CAUSE | SIGNS AND SYMPTOMS | TREATMENTS |
|---|---|---|
| Oral herpes (herpes labialis)<br>Commonly HSV-1, but can also be HSV-2 | Blisters on the lips or tongue, painful swallowing, often called cold sores or fever blisters | Valacyclovir for 1-2 days for severe primary infection<br>Topical agents (penciclovir, docosanol cream, acyclovir cream) may shorten duration of symptoms if started early |
| Genital herpes<br>Equally split between HSV-1 and HSV-2 | Women: flulike illness; nerve pain; itching; abdominal pain; dysuria; blisters around the vagina, buttocks, urethra, in the vagina, or on the cervix<br>Men: lesions on the shaft or head of the penis, buttocks, or thigh | **Primary**<br>Acyclovir or valacyclovir<br>Penciclovir cream, steroid ointments, or topical lidocaine jelly for pain<br>**Secondary**<br>Acyclovir, valacyclovir, or famciclovir for severe outbreaks<br>Preventive and suppressive dosing schedules available |
| Ocular herpes<br>Usually HSV-1 | Keratitis, usually in one eye<br>May progress to stromal keratitis, which is a major cause of corneal blindness | Trifluridine drops; acyclovir or vidarabine ointments are equally effective<br>Artificial tears<br>Consult ophthalmology |
| HSV encephalitis<br>Usually HSV-1 in adults, HSV-2 in newborns | Fever, headache, stiff neck, seizures, focal weakness, altered mental status, psychosis | Acyclovir IV started immediately in suspected cases |
| Herpetic whitlow<br>HSV-1 or HSV-2 | Itching, pain, or swelling of infected finger followed by blisters lasting 2-3 wk<br>Often associated with thumb sucking in children and occupational exposure in adults (health care workers) | Topical acyclovir<br>Commonly acquired from oral or genital lesions, which should be identified and treated appropriately |
| Bell palsy | Focal weakness following distribution of peripheral cranial nerve VII | Acyclovir, valacyclovir, or famciclovir in combination with a steroid taper (data regarding efficacy conflicting)*<br>Eye protection (topical lubricants, eye patch at night) |
| HSV esophagitis<br>Usually HSV-1 in immunocompromised patients | Dysphagia | Acyclovir IV |

*HSV,* Herpes simplex virus; *IV,* intravenously.

*Allen D, Dunn L. Acyclovir or valacyclovir for Bell's palsy (idiopathic facial paralysis). Cochrane Database Syst Rev 2004;4:CD001869 [update of Cochrane Database Syst Rev 2001;4:CD001869]; and Salinas R. Bell's palsy. Clin Evid 2003;10:1504-7 [update in Clin Evid 2006;15:1745-50].

## PRESENTING SIGNS AND SYMPTOMS

The first time a patient experiences a herpes simplex outbreak (primary infection), he or she often notes a prodrome of symptoms such as fever, muscle aches, headache, malaise, and swollen lymph nodes up to a week before the skin eruptions appear. The first sign of infection of the skin appears 2 to 12 days after initial exposure and begins as cutaneous edema. This edema is quickly followed by the development of small, grouped vesicles on an erythematous base. The lesions typically dry out and heal within 7 to 10 days, although they can last up to 3 weeks. The symptoms almost always recur and are often heralded by a prodrome of skin itching, pain, or paresthesias at the site of infection. Recurrent outbreaks often occur at the same site as the primary infection, but they tend to be milder and have a shorter duration. These recurrences can erupt in intervals of days, weeks, or years, and the triggers vary by patient.

## DIAGNOSTIC TESTING

Herpes simplex is typically identified clinically by the characteristic skin lesion of a thin-walled blister on an inflamed base. Definitive testing is available, and the Tzanck smear uses scrapings from lesions to identify the giant cells with inclusion bodies indicative of HSV infection. Although this test is the most readily available, it is not very sensitive. Viral cultures can be accurate if material is collected early in the illness when intact vesicles are sampled, but the sensitivity wanes with the duration of symptoms. Polymerase chain reaction testing is available and is considered the "gold standard." It is the fastest and most accurate for testing cerebrospinal fluid (CSF). Serum immunologic studies can be used to identify specific strains of the virus, but most of these tests are time consuming and expensive. Although one point-of-care test is available for HSV-2, it is not widely used, and treatment in the emergency department is most often based on clinical suspicion.

## TREATMENT AND DISPOSITION

As yet, no cure for herpes simplex exists. Some of the most exciting research is in the area of vaccination. Several vaccines in clinical trials have the potential to eliminate infection.[2] Until then, herpes symptoms are managed using several different antiviral medications that help to reduce outbreaks and shorten the course of illness (see the "Facts and Formulas" box). The most commonly used agents are nucleosides and nucleotide analogues that block viral reproduction. They include acyclovir, valacyclovir, famciclovir, and penciclovir. Patients with a first episode of genital herpes, even with mild symptoms, should receive antiviral therapy to decrease progression to severe or prolonged symptoms.[3] For acute outbreaks, valacyclovir and famciclovir are the most commonly prescribed medications, but they must be started within 1 day of lesion onset or during the prodrome that precedes some outbreaks.[3] Once-daily valacyclovir can reduce the transmission rate of genital herpes by 50% to 75%.[4] Low-dose suppressive therapy is also available for patients with frequent outbreaks. Foscarnet is a pyrophosphate analogue that can be used for treatment of HSV strains that have become resistant to the nucleosides and nucleotide analogues.

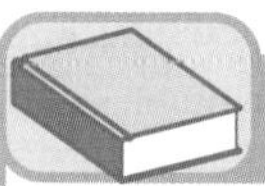

**PATIENT TEACHING TIPS**

**Herpes Simplex Symptom Relief**

Keep blisters and sores clean and dry. Avoid talcum powder, synthetic materials in underwear, and tight-fitting clothing.

Ice packs and over-the-counter analgesics may alleviate pain.

Urinating in the shower or bath may alleviate dysuria.

Avoid sexual contact during both outbreaks and prodromes.

$SI = \frac{SV}{BSA}$ **FACTS AND FORMULAS**

**Antiviral Medications**

Acyclovir is available in oral, injectable, and topical forms. The method of administration is determined by the site and severity of infections. It has good penetration into most tissues including cerebrospinal fluid. Compliance is difficult to achieve with acyclovir because of the need for frequent doses.

Valacyclovir is an oral antiviral that is converted to acyclovir in the intestine and liver. It delivers a higher concentration of drug in the bloodstream and requires less frequent dosing.

Famciclovir is converted to penciclovir within the infected cells. It has a much longer half-life than acyclovir and therefore requires less frequent dosing.

Penciclovir is currently available only in a topical preparation.

Foscarnet is a pyrophosphate analogue and is used for treatment of strains of herpes simplex virus that have become resistant to the nucleosides and nucleotide analogues. It is available in an intravenous form, but it is more toxic than acyclovir.

Cidofovir is used in acquired immunodeficiency syndrome and in bone marrow transplant recipients with severe infections.

# VARICELLA-ZOSTER VIRUS

## EPIDEMIOLOGY

VZV is the organism that causes varicella (chickenpox) and herpes zoster (shingles). Before the initiation of the varicella vaccination program, chickenpox was a very common illness, and 90% of cases occurred in children less than 10 years of age. Although most cases were uncomplicated, chickenpox led to 11,000 hospitalizations and 100 deaths every year before the introduction of the varicella vaccine. Adolescents and adults who contracted the illness tended to have a more prolonged and severe course. Since the introduction of widespread vaccination, the incidence of chickenpox has declined by 81%, thus leading to an 88% decline in varicella-related hospitalizations.[5]

Herpes zoster (shingles) occurs when the latent varicella virus is reactivated in the sensory ganglia. The lifetime incidence of herpes zoster is approximately 10% to 20% of the

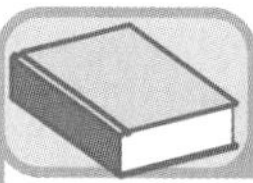

**PATIENT TEACHING TIPS**

**Preventing Transmission of Herpes Simplex**

Avoid touching the sores. Wash your hands frequently.

Keep personal items (e.g., towels, razors) separate during an outbreak because the virus can live for 2 hours on cloth and for 4 hours on plastic.

Viral shedding occurs without any symptoms in one third to one half of cases, and the virus can be transmitted through fluids to other people.

Use condoms (male or female) during any sexual activity, even when lesions are not present.

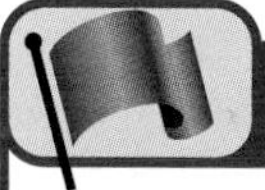

**RED FLAGS**

**Varicella and Herpes Zoster**

- Instruct patients about measures to prevent transmission to others.
- Admit all patients with primary varicella who are immunocompromised.
- Consult an ophthalmologist if the infection is periorbital.
- Use caution when recommending nonsteroidal antiinflammatory drugs in children with chickenpox.
- Look for evidence of complications (pulmonary, central nervous system, bacterial superinfection) in both primary and secondary varicella-zoster virus infections.
- Be sure to arrange follow-up for patients with shingles because long-term pain management may be required.

population, and most symptomatic infections occur in older or immunocompromised patients. In 2005, a safe, effective live attenuated vaccine was approved by the U.S. Food and Drug Administration and was recommended by the Advisory Committee on Immunization Practices after clinical trials demonstrated a significant reduction in morbidity secondary to herpes zoster and postherpetic neuralgia.[6] An observational study reported a significant reduction in incidence of herpes zoster in patients 60 years old or older who received the vaccine regardless of age, race, or the presence of chronic diseases.[7]

## PRESENTING SIGNS AND SYMPTOMS

A primary infection (chickenpox) is characterized by a diffuse, pruritic, vesicular rash 10 to 21 days after exposure. Patients with the illness typically experience a prodrome of 1 to 2 days of fever and malaise, followed by the eruption of macular lesions that progress to papules and then to vesicles that rupture and crust. Most often, the first lesions appear on the face or trunk and then spread to the extremities. Lesions may also involve the mucous membranes of the oropharynx, respiratory tract, vagina, cornea, and conjunctiva. The distinguishing feature of this rash is the presence of lesions in various stages in a single affected area. Patients less than 1 year old or more than 15 years old have the highest risk of complications, including skin infections, central nervous system involvement, and pneumonia. Chickenpox in pregnant women or neonates can lead to life-threatening pneumonitis, and primary infection during pregnancy may result in the congenital varicella syndrome.

As the patient recovers from a primary infection, the virus establishes a latent infection in the sensory dorsal root ganglia. Reactivation of this latent infection leads to the clinical symptoms of shingles. Patients frequently report a prodrome of fever, malaise, headache, and skin sensitivity before the eruption of the characteristic rash of grouped vesicles. The lesions typically crust by 7 to 10 days and resolve in 3 to 4 weeks. Pain is the most common symptom of shingles and is typically described as a burning sensation. The infection typically covers one dermatome, but it can occasionally affect neighboring dermatomes. Postherpetic neuralgia occurs in 10% to 15% of cases and is the most frequent complication of VZV. People who are more than 60 years old account for half of these cases. *Postherpetic neuralgia* is defined as the persistence of sensory symptoms more than 30 days after the onset of zoster. Herpes zoster ophthalmicus is a vision-threatening condition that requires ophthalmologic consultation. It is caused by involvement of the ophthalmic branch of cranial nerve V. The Hutchinson sign (a lesion on the tip of the nose) suggests the diagnosis, but it is not always present. Other complications include herpes zoster oticus (Ramsay Hunt syndrome) and disseminated herpes zoster, which can be identified by the rash crossing the midline or involving several dermatomes.

## CHICKENPOX

Most cases of chickenpox follow a benign, uncomplicated course, and full recovery without chronic sequelae is expected. Treatment of varicella is aimed primarily at symptomatic relief. Acetaminophen is recommended for discomfort and fever. A small study from 1999 suggested a link between ibuprofen and necrotizing fasciitis in children with varicella.[8] Although subsequent investigations have not been able to provide causal evidence, antiinflammatory medications continue to be associated with higher risk of invasive group A streptococcal infections, and these agents are not recommended in children with chickenpox.[9] Another prominent symptom is severe pruritus, leading to excoriations and scarring. Oral antihistamines, calamine lotion, and oatmeal baths may be helpful.

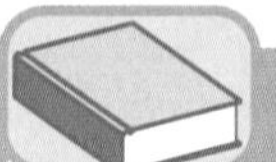

### PATIENT TEACHING TIPS

**Varicella**

Eighty percent of susceptible household contacts will contract chickenpox when they are exposed to chickenpox or shingles.

Patients are infectious for approximately 48 hours before the onset of rash until the vesicles are crusted over (usually approximately 4 to 5 days after the appearance of the lesions).

Illness tends to occur 10 to 21 days after exposure.

Patients who have been vaccinated may still develop chickenpox or shingles, but the illness is generally less severe.

People with shingles are contagious to those who have never had chickenpox or the vaccine, but you cannot "catch" shingles from someone else.

Avoid contact with pregnant women while you are infectious.

Do not give children with chickenpox aspirin because of its association with Reye syndrome.

Oatmeal baths, calamine lotion, and oral antihistamines may help to alleviate pruritus.

Consider mittens for small children to prevent excoriation and scarring.

Acetaminophen should be given for discomfort and fever.

A return visit to the emergency department is needed if signs of skin infection or pneumonia or changes in behavior or level of consciousness occur or if oral hydration cannot be maintained.

Several antiviral medications are active against VZV. Clinical studies have shown that these drugs may shorten the duration of illness and severity of cutaneous symptoms, but they have not been shown to reduce transmission or complications. To maximize clinical benefit, these agents should be given within 24 hours of rash onset. The decision to start antiviral therapy is based on the characteristics of the host and the extent of infection. Antiviral therapy is not recommended for cases of chickenpox in healthy children with uncomplicated infections or for use as postexposure prophylaxis. The physician should offer oral antiviral therapy to patients who are more than 13 years of age, who have chronic cutaneous or pulmonary disorders, and who are receiving long-term salicylate or steroid therapy. The most common treatment for

**Table 174.2 Varicella Complications**

| COMPLICATION | CLINICAL FEATURES |
|---|---|
| Bacterial infection of skin lesions | Impetigo, cellulitis, or local abscesses<br>Most common complication in young children |
| Invasive group A streptococcal infection | Necrotizing fasciitis<br>Streptococcal toxic shock syndrome<br>Suspect in localized swelling, erythema, pain out of proportion to examination, or fever >4 days |
| Pneumonitis | Cough, tachypnea, dyspnea 4 days after onset of illness<br>Most common life-threatening complication in adults<br>Rare in young children<br>Diffuse infiltrate on chest radiograph |
| Encephalitis | Altered level of consciousness, confusion, fever, vomiting, headache, seizure<br>Most common life-threatening complication in children |
| Cerebellar ataxia | Benign, typically full recovery in 30 days<br>Ataxia, vomiting, tremor, change in speech |
| Reye syndrome | Associated with use of aspirin in children with chickenpox; nausea and vomiting early symptoms<br>Markedly elevated liver function tests with normal bilirubin and hypoglycemia<br>Progressive cerebral edema nearly always fatal |
| Congenital varicella syndrome | Various abnormalities including limb atrophy<br>Risk ≈2% if illness contracted before 20 weeks of gestation<br>No reported cases from vaccination during pregnancy to date |

children is oral acyclovir, at 20 mg/kg (maximum, 800 mg/dose) four times daily for 5 days. Adults should receive 800 mg four times daily for 5 days. An obstetrician should be consulted before therapy is initiated in pregnant or peripartum women because treatment recommendations range from no treatment to admission for intravenous acyclovir. All immunocompromised patients and those who develop complications should be given intravenous acyclovir and admitted (**Table 174.2**).

## SHINGLES

Pharmacologic treatment of shingles is controversial. Most patients recover within 1 to 2 weeks without therapy. Up to 15% will develop postherpetic neuralgia, a potentially chronic, debilitating pain syndrome. Therapeutic trials support the use of antiviral medications to shorten the course of the acute illness and accelerate resolution of the painful neuritis,[10] but conflict exists regarding the ability of these drugs to prevent postherpetic neuralgia. No clear difference in efficacy among the currently available antiviral medications (acyclovir, famciclovir, and valacyclovir) has been reported. Acyclovir has been studied more extensively, but the dosing regimen of five times daily limits compliance. Valacyclovir is rapidly metabolized to acyclovir, and its dosing schedule makes compliance much more likely. Steroid therapy may heal the rash more quickly, but it has not been shown to prevent postherpetic neuralgia and is not routinely recommended.[11] Pain control is difficult in patients with acute shingles and postherpetic neuralgia. Opioids, lidocaine patches, and topical capsaicin have all been shown to provide pain relief, yet no single therapy has emerged as superior to the others. Gabapentin and amitriptyline are considered second-line agents and should be initiated in the primary care setting because patients taking these medications require close follow-up. A summary of treatment recommendations is provided in the "Priority Actions" box. Most patients with herpes zoster may be discharged to home. The exceptions include patients who are immunosuppressed or who have disseminated disease.

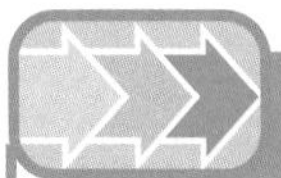

**PRIORITY ACTIONS**

**Treatment of Herpes Zoster (Shingles)**

- Consider treatment with antiretroviral therapy for all eligible patients with zoster regardless of age.
- Antiretroviral therapy is strongly recommend for persons more than 50 years who have moderate or severe pain, moderate or severe rash, or involvement of nontruncal dermatomes.
- Initiate therapy as soon as possible, ideally within 72 hours of the onset of the rash.
- Prescribe valacyclovir, 1000 mg three times daily for 7 days, or famciclovir, 500 mg three times daily for 7 days (use acyclovir if cost is an issue).
- Analgesia including opioids must be provided. Consider lidocaine patches or topical capsaicin.
- Referral to primary care is needed because postherpetic neuralgia can become a chronic, debilitating disorder best managed in the outpatient setting.

# INFLUENZA

## EPIDEMIOLOGY

Influenza viruses cause epidemic respiratory illnesses that can range from mild to severe to deadly. The virulence of influenza has tremendous year-to-year variability. In the 30-year period between 1976 and 2006, annual flu deaths ranged from a low of 3000 to a high of 49,000.[12] Influenza causes disease in all age groups. During peak influenza season, the percentage of primary care office visits for influenza-like illness ranges from 3.3% to 7.1%.[13] Each year, approximately 20% of children and 5% of adults develop symptomatic influenza infection.[14] Although children have the highest infection rates, the rates of serious infection and death are highest in patients more than 65 years old or less than 2 years old and in patients with coexisting comorbidities.

The virus is classified as type A, B, or C, based on differences in the composition of its matrix and nucleus protein. Human disease is caused only by influenza A and B. Influenza A is further subtyped based on the antigenicity of the hemagglutinin and neuraminidase surface glycoproteins. Currently, 16 hemagglutinin and 9 neuraminidase subtypes have been identified.[15] Influenza B viruses are not further subtyped. Hemagglutinin facilitates the entry of the virus into host cells, and neuraminidase assists in the release of the progeny virions from the infected cells. These antigenic determinants are the primary basis for human immunity, thus reducing the likelihood and severity of infection in persons with prior exposure to a particular subtype. Immunity to one subtype, however, confers little to no immunity to another subtype. Antigenic variation in the surface glycoproteins causes the influenza virus to change constantly and enables it to evade immune recognition and produce repeated outbreaks of disease.

Influenza is spread through respiratory droplets that may lodge on fomites. The typical incubation period is 1 to 4 days. Adults can be infectious the day before and 5 days after symptom onset, but children can have a longer period of asymptomatic infectivity both before and after symptoms. The average number of secondary cases caused by an index case ranges from 5 to 25. In comparison, the average number of secondary cases of severe acute respiratory syndrome (SARS) caused by a single case ranges from 2.2 to 3.7.[16]

## SIGNS AND SYMPTOMS

Uncomplicated cases of influenza are characterized by the abrupt onset of constitutional and respiratory symptoms such as fever, myalgias, headache, malaise, sore throat, and rhinitis. Accompanying gastrointestinal symptoms such as vomiting and diarrhea are more common in children than in adults. A meta-analysis attempting to identify specific symptoms or combinations that could predict influenza infection found that the combination of fever and cough during influenza season was the only clinical criterion that reliably increased the likelihood of influenza.[13] Fortunately, weekly influenza surveillance data are readily available in the United States at the Centers for Disease Control and Prevention website (www.cdc.org). Surveillance data can be used not only to determine the incidence of influenza in the community, but also to ascertain the predominant circulating type of influenza.

## TESTING, TREATMENT, AND DISPOSITION

Influenza testing can be performed by culture, immunofluorescence, reverse transcriptase polymerase chain reaction, or rapid tests. Because testing time is typically less than 30 minutes for the rapid diagnostic tests, these are commonly available in emergency departments. Whereas the specificity of these tests is high, the sensitivity is low. One must take care when interpreting test results because a negative result does not rule out influenza infection.[17] Current guidelines encourage testing only when results will change the clinical care of the patient or influence the clinical care of other patients. Given the poor sensitivity of these tests and the recommendation that treatment not be delayed pending results, most patients do not benefit from testing.

Options for controlling influenza include immunoprophylaxis with vaccines, treatment with antiviral agents, and chemoprophylaxis. Available vaccines include inactivated influenza vaccine injection and intranasal live attenuated influenza vaccine.

Although antiviral agents are not a substitute for influenza vaccination, they can offer marginal benefit in controlling symptoms. Two classes of available agents are as follows: the adamantines (amantadine and rimantadine), which display activity against influenza A; and the neuraminidase inhibitors (zanamivir and oseltamivir), which have activity against both influenza A and B. To be effective, all these agents must be started within 48 hours of symptom onset, a feature that limits the use of these agents to patients seeking care promptly.

## PANDEMIC INFLUENZA

Influenza pandemics occur when a new virus emerges that is spread easily from person to person and to which humans have little to no immunity.[18] Three major pandemics occurred in the twentieth century. Pandemic influenza differs from seasonal influenza in that young, healthy individuals are at increased risk of serious complications.

Aquatic birds likely serve as the largest reservoir for influenza viruses. Nearly all strains of influenza A circulate among wild birds, which can infect domestic fowl. Although these avian influenza viruses are not readily transmissible among humans, individuals in close contact with infected fowl may become infected. Concern exists that an avian influenza virus may mutate and trigger a pandemic. The virus that caused the catastrophic pandemic from 1918 to 1919 originated from an avian source and appears to have subsequently infected humans and adapted to allow spread among persons.[19] The viruses causing the pandemics of 1957 and 1968, conversely, seem to have infected an animal (either human or pig) and reassorted with another influenza virus, resulting in the emergence of a new virus that was readily capable of human transmission.

In 2009, a novel influenza A virus (H1N1) caused a worldwide pandemic and resulted in an estimated 59 million illnesses and 12,000 deaths in the United States.[20] Although the overall case fatality rate was less than 0.5%, most serious illnesses occurred in children and young adults, with a relative sparing of adults more than 60 years old. In addition to the usual array of chronic medical conditions associated with increased morbidity, pregnancy and obesity were associated with a 4 to 15 times higher risk of hospitalization or death.

Although the overall case fatality rate for the 2009 pandemic was lower than that of seasonal influenza, several lessons were learned. Physical interventions such as hand hygiene, masks, gowns, and gloves were all found to reduce transmission.[21] Similarly, resources were effectively mobilized to develop and distribute a novel vaccine that was effective at limiting disease spread. Despite effective methods to limit spread, several challenges were identified as well. Shortages of supplies during the pandemic were a significant problem. Surgical masks, N95 respirators, disinfectant wipes, and antiviral medications were all in short supply, particularly in the early stages of the pandemic.

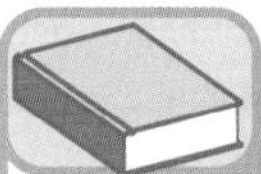

**PATIENT TEACHING TIPS**

**Suspected Influenza**

Symptoms of influenza (flu) include fever, headache, tiredness, cough, sore throat, muscle aches, and occasionally nausea, vomiting, and diarrhea.

Rest, drink plenty of fluids, and take medications to control fever as directed by your physician.

Flu is spread very easily from person to person through coughs and sneezes and respiratory droplets and secretions.

Wash your hands frequently with soap and water whenever you are in contact with others.

Cover your nose and mouth when sneezing or coughing.

Frequently clean the surfaces of objects that may have come in contact with respiratory secretions, and use a household disinfectant labeled by the Environmental Protection Agency as having activity against bacterial and viruses.

Monitor for symptoms of increased difficulty breathing, and seek care with a medical provider should this occur.

If you have other medical conditions including asthma or heart disease, see a medical provider immediately if you notice worsening symptoms.

Never give aspirin to children or teenagers with the flu without first consulting your doctor.

Receiving the influenza vaccine in the fall can prevent flu infection.

# MONONUCLEOSIS

## EPIDEMIOLOGY

In the United States, the annual incidence of infectious mononucleosis ranges between 345 and 671 cases per 100,000.[22] EBV is the principal cause, and by adulthood nearly all persons have been infected. Other viruses such as cytomegalovirus and human immunodeficiency virus can cause syndromes that resemble acute mononucleosis.

## PRESENTING SIGNS AND SYMPTOMS

In developing nations, EBV is generally a disease of the very young and is often asymptomatic or minimally symptomatic. In industrialized nations, people contract primary EBV infections at slightly later ages. In the United States, approximately one third of cases manifest during adolescence and early adulthood.[23] Nearly half these patients develop clinically evident mononucleosis that can manifest classically or with typical or atypical variations of the classic presentation.

### CLASSIC PRESENTATION

The incubation period for primary EBV infection is approximately 1 to 2 months. The disease is communicable, and saliva exchange is the most common mode of transmission. Classically, acute mononucleosis manifests in adolescence with fever, malaise, myalgias, and sore throat. The examination reveals impressive exudative tonsillitis and diffuse lymphadenopathy. The physician should palpate carefully for an enlarged spleen because splenomegaly occurs in approximately half of these patients. Symptoms usually abate within a few weeks, but prostration can occur for up to a few months.

### TYPICAL VARIATIONS

#### *Hepatitis*

Intrahepatic cholestasis occurs with mononucleosis. Hepatic transaminases commonly rise to levels approximately three times normal, but jaundice is present in fewer than 10% of patients.[24] Most patients recover fully.

#### *Rash*

A nonspecific maculopapular rash frequently develops after ampicillin or amoxicillin administration.

#### *Splenic Rupture*

Fifty percent of patients with acute mononucleosis develop splenic enlargement.[24] The feared complication of mononucleosis is splenic rupture. Spontaneous splenic rupture occurs in 0.1% of patients with mononucleosis.[25] Splenic rupture, traumatic or spontaneous, usually occurs within 3 weeks of the onset of symptoms.[24]

#### *Fulminant Infection*

In healthy hosts, fatal or fulminant EBV infection is rare. Fatal infectious mononucleosis usually results from a rare virus-associated hemophagocytic syndrome. In these patients, the classic presentation is further coupled with fulminant hepatic dysfunction, pulmonary infiltrates, cytopenias, and rash.[23]

## DIAGNOSTIC TESTING

If performed, laboratory studies may point toward mononucleosis as the cause of the patient's viral syndrome (**Table 174.3**). Ultrasonography may reveal hepatosplenomegaly.

**Table 174.3 Laboratory Findings in Acute Mononucleosis**

| TEST | ABNORMALITIES | COMMENT |
|---|---|---|
| Complete blood count | ↑White blood cell count, ↓ platelets, atypical lymphocytosis | Neutropenia and thrombocytopenia usually mild |
| Liver function tests | ↑Aspartate aminotransferase, ↑alanine aminotransferase, ↑bilirubin | Transaminases elevated in most patients; <10% clinically jaundiced, however |
| Monospot | Positive monospot | Heterophile antibodies detectable in second week of illness and transiently present; heterophile antibodies possibly absent in young children |
| EBV-specific antibody testing | EBV viral capsid antigen immunoglobulin M assay | Utility for short-term decision making limited by slow turnaround time |

↑, Increased; ↓, decreased; *EBV,* Epstein-Barr virus.

## TREATMENT AND DISPOSITION

No specific therapies for EBV mononucleosis exist. Patients are supported through the illness by management of their symptoms. Many patients with mononucleosis can be managed as outpatients. Severely ill patients, those with refractory symptoms (pain, dehydration), and those at risk for severe complications should be admitted.[26]

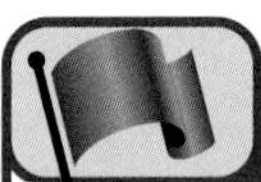

**RED FLAGS**

**Mononucleosis**

To allow the inflamed spleen to recover, restrict the patient's athletic activity until symptoms resolve and until the spleen returns to normal size. Most authorities recommend refraining from vigorous exercise for at least 3 weeks.[26] A longer period may be necessary in cases of persistent splenomegaly.

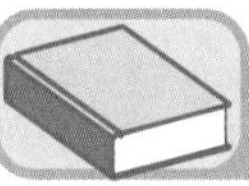

**PATIENT TEACHING TIPS**

**Mononucleosis**

Mononucleosis is a communicable disease. Avoid sharing saliva while you are ill.

Keep well hydrated, and control your fever with acetaminophen or ibuprofen, if the fever is bothersome.

Mononucleosis causes inflammation and enlargement of the spleen, an organ in your upper abdomen. Avoid abdominal impact.

Return if you worsen, if you have concerns, or if you develop abdominal pain.

Follow your physician's instructions about symptom management.

Be aware of the risk of splenic rupture, and follow your physician's instructions about returning for symptoms consistent with splenic injury.

# SEVERE ACUTE RESPIRATORY SYNDROME

## EPIDEMIOLOGY

In February of 2003, reports of an outbreak of unexplained pneumonia that killed 5 of 305 afflicted individuals emerged in southern China.[27] The disease was characterized by flulike symptoms with high fever, myalgias, nonproductive cough with dyspnea, lymphopenia, and infiltrates on chest radiography. The disease often progressed to cause respiratory failure and carried a mortality rate of 11%. The SARS epidemic serves to remind us how global travel contributes to the epidemic spread of disease. A Chinese physician who was treating patients in the afflicted region then traveled to Hong Kong, where 10 guests at his hotel were secondarily infected. These guests then traveled to Singapore, Vietnam, Canada, and the United States, thus creating the first global epidemic spread by air travel. Over the next 100 days, more than 8422 individuals were infected and 916 died in 30 countries.[28] Over the next several months, SARS spread to more than 20 countries on 4 continents. The World Health Organization launched a global initiative to characterize and contain this new infection and demonstrated how concerted efforts can successfully contain epidemics. By March of 2003, the offending virus was identified as a coronavirus, termed *SARS coronavirus* (SARS-CoV), and the genome was mapped by April of that year. Through a remarkable globally concerted effort involving international surveillance and quarantines, SARS was effectively contained by the summer of 2003.[29] The last new case was reported in April of 2004, in a scientist studying the virus in a laboratory in China (**Table 174.4**).

Relative to other pandemic infectious agents, the infectivity of SARS-CoV is generally low, but in some cases, a single person can infect a large number of people.[27] The greatest population at risk during an epidemic seems to be health care workers because they are often in close contact with infected patients. During the 2003 epidemic, 20% of those infected were health care workers.[28]

**Table 174.4 Features of Severe Acute Respiratory Syndrome That May Help with the Clinical Diagnosis**

| | EXAMPLE | CAUTION |
|---|---|---|
| Clinical history | Sudden onset of flulike prodrome, fever, dry cough, nonrespiratory symptoms (e.g., diarrhea, myalgia, headache, chills or rigors) | Take a travel history, occupational history, history of hospitalization, and history of contact with health care facility or person with SARS; the absence of any of these factors in the history should not automatically exclude the diagnosis of SARS |
| Clinical examination | No correlation with chest radiology changes | Lack of respiratory signs, particularly in groups such as older patients |
| Bedside monitoring | Hypoxia | Temperature may not be elevated on admission; the respiratory rate should be documented |
| Hematology investigations | Low lymphocyte count, raised C-reactive protein, prolonged activated partial thromboplastin time | These changes are nonspecific and are not always seen in SARS |
| Biochemistry investigations | Raised lactate dehydrogenase, hepatic transaminases, creatine phosphokinase | These changes are nonspecific and are not always seen in SARS |
| Radiology investigations | Chest radiography changes poorly defined, patchy progressive changes | May present as a lobar pneumonia; pneumothorax and pneumomediastinum may also occur |
| Microbiology investigations | Investigation for community-acquired and hospital-acquired pneumonias including atypical pneumonias | Concurrent infections possible |
| Virology investigations | Investigation for other causes of atypical pneumonia | SARS-coronavirus test results interpreted with caution, based on assessment of population risk of SARS at local level and individual risk of SARS |
| Treatment | Lack of response to antibiotic treatment for community-acquired pneumonia, including atypical pneumonia | No response to standard antibiotic treatments in all viral pneumonias and some bacterial pneumonias; as yet, no proven treatment for SARS; supportive measures recommended |

Adapted from World Health Organization: WHO guidelines for the global surveillance of SARS: Updated recommendations, October 2004. www.who.int/csr/resources/publications/WHO_CDS_CSR_ARO_2004_1.pdf.

*SARS*, Severe acute respiratory syndrome.

**Table 174.5 Manifestations of West Nile Virus Infection**

| | SYMPTOMS | PROGNOSIS |
|---|---|---|
| West Nile fever | Acute onset of the following:<br>Fever<br>Headache<br>Fatigue<br>Malaise<br>Myalgia<br>Weakness | Symptoms possibly lasting a few days to several weeks<br>Median time for full symptomatic recovery: 60 days<br>Fatigue and muscle weakness possible for 1 mo after acute disease |
| Neuroinvasive West Nile virus | Meningitis<br>Fever<br>Headache<br>Stiff neck<br>Encephalitis<br>Fever<br>Headache<br>Altered level of consciousness<br>Focal neurologic deficits<br>Tremors and movement disorders<br>Poliomyelitis<br>Acute onset of limb weakness without sensory symptoms | Symptoms possibly lasting several weeks<br>Possibly permanent neurologic deficits |

# WEST NILE VIRUS

## EPIDEMIOLOGY

West Nile virus had not been reported in the Western Hemisphere until the first case was discovered in New York City in 1999.[30] Since then, more than 12,000 cases of neuroinvasive disease and more than 1200 deaths have been reported in the United States.[31] West Nile virus is a member of the Japanese encephalitis complex that includes Japanese encephalitis and St. Louis encephalitis. Birds serve as the primary reservoir for the virus. Mosquitoes become infected when they feed on afflicted birds. No known animal-to-human or human-to-human cases of transmission have occurred other than those in recipients of blood or organ transplants.[32]

## PRESENTING SIGNS AND SYMPTOMS

Approximately 80% of persons infected with West Nile virus are asymptomatic.[33] Of those in whom symptoms develop, most will have West Nile fever, but less than 1% will have neuroinvasive disease. Characteristics of each of these illnesses are presented in **Table 174.5**. The incubation period for West Nile Virus infection ranges from 2 to 14 days.

## DIAGNOSTIC TESTING

In most cases of infection with West Nile virus, no diagnostic testing is necessary because symptoms are usually mild and self-limited. In patients with neuroinvasive disease, testing may be necessary to differentiate the disease from other central nervous system infections requiring specific therapy. The CSF in patients with neuroinvasive disease may have lymphocyte-predominant pleocytosis. West Nile virus–specific immunoglobulin M in serum or CSF provides evidence of recent infection, but it may persist for up to 16 months.[34] West Nile virus can also be diagnosed by using acute and convalescent serum antibody titers, as well as by nucleic acid amplification, to detect virus in CSF, serum, or tissues.

## TREATMENT AND DISPOSITION

Most cases of infection with West Nile virus are asymptomatic. Almost all patients who do have symptoms have West Nile fever. Although West Nile fever is self-limited, it can last from days to months and can produce long-term sequelae. One study found that in patients hospitalized for West Nile virus infection, only 37% had total recovery at 12 months after symptom onset.[35] Persons more than 65 years old and patients with other comorbidities have a higher incidence of long-term sequelae. Although this statement is skewed to the most serious infections, West Nile virus infection can have sequelae that outlast the acute phase of the disease.

## REFERENCES

***References can be found on Expert Consult @ www.expertconsult.com.***

# 175 Human Immunodeficiency Virus Infection

Ellen M. Slaven

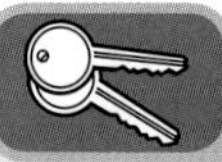

**KEY POINTS**

- In the United States, more than 1.1 million people are estimated to be living with human immunodeficiency virus/acquired immunodeficiency syndrome (HIV/AIDS), and approximately 50,000 new infections occur each year.
- When the CD4 cell count falls to less than 200 /μL (from a normal level of approximately 1000 cells/μL), opportunistic infections are more likely to develop.
- The Centers for Disease Control and Prevention continue to emphasize "opt out" routine HIV screening during any health care encounter, including in the emergency department, for patients between the ages of 13 and 64 years, to allow for earlier detection and treatment and to prevent transmission.
- Current treatment recommendations include early initiation of antiretroviral therapy in asymptomatic patients with CD4 cell counts of up to 500/μL.

In 1981, the first report of *Pneumocystis (carinii) jiroveci* pneumonia (PCP), in 5 healthy young men, heralded the arrival of a previously unknown pathogen and the disease it caused, later identified as human immunodeficiency virus (HIV) and acquired immunodeficiency syndrome (AIDS). Since then, the infection has spread globally and has led to the untimely deaths of more than 25 million people. In the United States alone, more than 1.1 million people are estimated to be currently living with HIV/AIDS, and more than 50,000 new infections occur each year. Many of those infected, estimated to be more than 20%, may be unaware of their own HIV infection.

Despite some early advances in decreasing the yearly incidence of new infections, progress appears to have stalled. In certain subpopulations, the prevalence of HIV infection rivals that of some sub-Saharan African countries, such as men who have sex with men in New York City and black men in Washington, D.C. Injection drug users remain a high-risk group.

The mainstay of transmission of HIV infection is sexual exposure. The sharing of needles for illicit drug use also leads to transmission of HIV. An HIV-infected mother has approximately a 30% chance of passing the virus to her newborn, but with treatment, the risk plummets to less than 1%. Health care workers have a less than 0.3% chance of becoming infected with HIV following an accidental stick with a contaminated needle. Only in rare cases is HIV now transmitted through infected blood products (estimated to be less than 1 transmission per 500,000 blood transfusions) (**Table 175.1**).

The HIV virions enter the host and primarily target the lymphocytes, particularly a subset of T lymphocytes known as CD4 cells. The virus establishes itself within the cells, where it prepares strands of DNA from its own viral RNA and the cells' own enzyme reverse transcriptase. The new viral DNA becomes integrated within the lymphocytes' DNA, and new virions are produced. The new virions are released from the host cell by budding and are free to invade other uninfected cells.

Initially, viral replication goes unchecked, and the high level of viremia may lead to symptoms such as fever, rash, pharyngitis, and enlarged lymph nodes. This stage is a transient illness, lasting days to several weeks, and has been termed acute HIV infection, or acute retroviral syndrome.

The immune system eventually responds to the viremia and suppresses viral replication. The viral load diminishes, and the symptoms of the acute infection resolve. Low-grade viral production continues at a steady state, and the host and virus reach a balance of viral suppression and continued viral production. This chronic steady state may be maintained for years until the immune system eventually is overwhelmed.

Infection with HIV is a progressive disease. Following years of viral replication, and eventual destruction of CD4 cells, the immune system begins to fail. During the chronic phase of infection, patients have a predictable decline of approximately 70 CD4 cells/μL/year. When the CD4 count approaches 200 cells/μL (from a normal level of approximately 1000 cells/μL), opportunistic infections (e.g., PCP, Kaposi sarcoma, pulmonary tuberculosis) begin to appear. When the CD4 cell count falls to less than 50 cells/μL, immunosuppression is profound.

## TESTING

The detection of HIV-specific antibodies in serum or plasma establishes the diagnosis of HIV infection. Tests of HIV antibodies are highly sensitive and specific. The enzyme-linked immunosorbent assay (ELISA) is the most commonly used screening test for HIV because of its high sensitivity and rapid results. All positive test results should be confirmed by

**Table 175.1** Risk of Human Immunodeficiency Virus Infection

| ROUTE OF TRANSMISSION | PER 10,000 EXPOSURES | PERCENTAGE OR INCIDENCE |
|---|---|---|
| Transfusion of contaminated blood | 9000 | Almost 100% |
| Transfusion of blood after screening | — | 1/500,000 |
| Mother-to-child without treatment | 3000 | 30% |
| Mother-to-child with treatment | — | <0.01% |
| Needle stick in health care worker | 30 | 0.3% |
| Unprotected receptive penile-vaginal intercourse | 10 | — |
| Unprotected insertive anal intercourse | 6 | 0.01-1.0% |
| Unprotected insertive vaginal intercourse | 5 | 0.01-1.0% |
| Unprotected receptive penile-vaginal intercourse with genital ulcers | 100 | 0.1-10% |
| Unprotected receptive oral intercourse | 1 | — |
| Unprotected insertive oral intercourse | 0.5 | — |

Western blot. The Western blot test uses electrophoresis to separate HIV proteins, which produce a colored band after reacting with specific antibodies found in a sample of blood. It is the most commonly used confirmatory test and is considered the "gold standard."

Following the initial HIV infection, antibody production occurs at such low levels that antibodies are undetected by most assays. This window period, in which HIV antibody testing leads to false-negative results, lasts approximately 4 weeks. In this setting, testing directly for the viral antigen p24 or polymerase chain reaction (PCR) testing for viral RNA may be performed. The U.S. Food and Drug Administration (FDA) has approved a newer test that detects both p24 antigen and antibodies to HIV. This highly sensitive assay, the ARCHITECHT HIV Antigen/Antibody (Ag/Ab) Combo, will be instrumental in detecting early stages of infection.

## RAPID ASSAYS

Rapid assays for detecting HIV-specific antibodies in serum can yield results in less than 30 minutes. These tests have high sensitivity and specificity and have proven effective for screening. HIV-specific antibodies may be detected in oral fluids, whole blood, serum, and plasma. Many people find oral fluid testing more acceptable than blood testing. Unfortunately, the rapid tests suffer from the same limitation as ELISA. They produce false-negative results during the window period. Positive results on rapid assays require confirmation with the Western blot.[1]

## OPT-OUT TESTING

In 2006, the U.S. Centers for Disease Control and Prevention (CDC) revised the recommendations for HIV screening to include routine (i.e., nontargeted) testing in all health care settings, including emergency departments (EDs). Understanding that an estimated 20% of patients infected with HIV are unaware of their status and that ongoing HIV transmission continues at a steady rate, the new recommendations highlight the need to expand screening. Additionally, the number of persons who are newly diagnosed with HIV and who already have advanced disease is unacceptably high. Routine testing will also decrease the number of "late testers" and provide earlier entry to care. Testing now should be done on all patients 13 to 64 years old, regardless of risk factors, at all health care facilities where the prevalence of undiagnosed HIV infection is greater than 0.1%. Patients are to be informed of the testing and have the opportunity to decline or opt out of it. General consent for medical care is sufficient for testing, and special written consent for HIV testing is not required, except in the few states that continue to require written consent. Pretest and post-test counseling is no longer required.[2]

# MONITORING INFECTION AND TREATMENT

Monitoring the progression of infection with HIV has been likened to a runaway train on railroad tracks that lead to the edge of a cliff. The CD4 cell count is analogous to the distance between the train and the cliff, and the viral load is analogous to the speed of the train.

Close monitoring of the level of viremia and of the CD4 cell counts is crucial in the management of the HIV-infected patient. PCR testing quantitatively measures the viral RNA in copies per milliliter of plasma, the viral load. Untreated patients typically have viral loads of up to 1,000,000 copies/mL of HIV RNA. One goal of antiretroviral therapy is to decrease the viral load sufficiently to be undetectable, as occurs when fewer than 5 to 50 copies/mL of HIV RNA are present. The CD4 cell counts provide prognostic information. Patients with CD4 cell counts higher than 200 cells/μL rarely develop opportunistic infections, and those with counts higher than 50 cells/μL rarely die of HIV/AIDS.

**BOX 175.1 Signs and Symptoms of Acute Human Immunodeficiency Virus Infection**

| | |
|---|---|
| Fever | Myalgias |
| Rash | Arthralgias |
| Headache | Nausea |
| Lymphadenopathy | Vomiting |
| Pharyngitis | Diarrhea |

Viral resistance to antiretroviral medications is an emerging phenomenon that may require alteration of a particular antiretroviral regimen. Two types of tests measure HIV resistance. The first is genotype testing, in which the sequences of the relevant viral genes are determined. The sequences reveal the presence or absence of mutations associated with antiretroviral resistance. Second, phenotypic tests excise relevant viral genes and insert them into a standard test virus. The test virus is then exposed to various antiretroviral medications to determine resistance.

## ACUTE INFECTION

Acute HIV infection, also termed acute retroviral syndrome or primary HIV infection, is a self-limited stage that develops in the first few weeks following initial infection. During this period, viral replication is rapid and ongoing, leading to high viral loads. The CD4 cell count may decrease transiently during the acute phase. The signs and symptoms are nonspecific and most commonly include fever and rash (**Box 175.1**). Approximately one third of patients are asymptomatic. The average duration of illness is 14 days, but this stage may last from a few days to more than 10 weeks.[3]

In time, the immune system recovers. CD8 cells proliferate, and the humoral immune system produces antibodies that lead to diminishing viremia. With the falling viral load, symptoms also subside. Testing for HIV-specific antibodies (e.g., ELISA) during the early phase often produces false-negative results because of the low levels of antibodies. Testing for viral p24 antigen and PCR testing of HIV RNA are other options.

As many as one half of all new HIV transmissions are estimated to occur from persons newly infected with HIV themselves. These people are likely to have extremely high viral loads, and many are unaware of their own HIV infection and therefore continue risky behaviors. The importance of establishing the diagnosis of acute HIV infection lies in early therapy for the individual and the decrease in transmission to others.

Current guidelines recommend antiretroviral therapy (ART) for symptomatic acute HIV infection. Early treatment decreases the viral load set-point, preserves immune function, suppresses the development of viral mutations, reduces transmission, and may slow the progression to AIDS.

Acute HIV infection is often not recognized in the primary care setting because the nonspecific symptoms resemble an influenza-like illness. When patients with febrile influenza-like illnesses are evaluated, clinicians need to consider inquiring about recent (past 2 to 6 weeks) high-risk behaviors. If suspicion of acute HIV infection arises, testing should include a plasma HIV RNA assay (viral load), or p24 antigen, in addition to HIV-specific antibody testing (ELISA). Consultation with an infectious disease specialist is warranted to arrange for further testing, to assist with initial ART, and to arrange a link to future care of the patient.

## OPPORTUNISTIC INFECTIONS

Opportunistic infections continue to be responsible for considerable morbidity and mortality in people infected with HIV. The introduction of ART has been profoundly beneficial in decreasing the number and severity of opportunistic infections. Unfortunately, not all HIV-infected people worldwide have access to ART, and resistance to ART continues to advance. The following sections discuss examples of opportunistic infections likely encountered in the ED.

### CENTRAL NERVOUS SYSTEM INFECTIONS

#### *Toxoplasmosis*

The protozoan *Toxoplasmosis gondii* is capable of causing focal encephalitis in HIV-infected patients with severe immune suppression. This condition is rarely identified in patients with CD4 cell counts higher than 200 cells/μL, and it is most commonly found in those with CD4 cell counts lower than 50 cells/μL. Symptoms include headache, fever, and confusion. More advanced encephalitis may cause seizures and coma. Physical examination findings may include focal weakness or stupor.

The diagnosis is suggested by a contrast-enhanced computed tomography scan of the brain showing classic, multiple ring-enhancing lesions. Serologic testing for antitoxoplasmosis immunoglobulin G antibodies is helpful if the result is positive, but a negative test result cannot exclude the disease. The definitive diagnosis requires detection of the organism in a clinical sample (e.g., brain biopsy). Most patients are given empiric therapy based on a compatible clinical syndrome, typical radiographic appearance, and serologic results. Favorable response to therapy, both clinically and radiographically, supports the diagnosis. Brain biopsy is reserved for patients who fail to respond to treatment. A combination of pyrimethamine, sulfadiazine, and leucovorin (to prevent the hematologic toxicity of pyrimethamine) is the treatment of choice. Treatment is given for at least 6 weeks. Prophylactic anticonvulsants are not indicated in patients without seizures.

### PULMONARY INFECTIONS

#### *Pneumocystis pneumonia*

*Pneumocystis (carinii) jiroveci* is the organism causing PCP. Despite a decline in the incidence of PCP as a result of ART and prophylaxis, many patients who are diagnosed with PCP are unaware of their underlying HIV infection. PCP is most likely to occur in patients with CD4 cell counts lower than 100 cells/μL.

Patients with PCP tend to experience a subacute illness with a dry cough, fever, and progressive dyspnea that worsens over the course of days to weeks. On physical examination, one may note tachycardia, tachypnea, and fine crackles on auscultation of the lungs. The patient may also have oropharyngeal candidiasis. Radiographs of the chest may be normal in the early stage of infection, but the common findings are bilateral and diffuse interstitial infiltrates.

The definitive diagnosis is by recovery of the organism from the lung. Expectorated sputum samples have a very low diagnostic yield and are not recommended. Bronchoalveolar lavage is the preferred method of obtaining clinical specimens. Many patients are treated empirically based on the clinical presentation, presence of hypoxia, and elevation of lactate dehydrogenase level to more than 500 mg/dL (a common but nonspecific finding in PCP). The drug of choice is trimethoprim/sulfamethoxazole, orally for mild to moderate disease and intravenously for more severe infection. Those patients with severe disease, as defined by a room air oxygen pressure of less than 70 mm Hg, should receive additional treatment with corticosteroids in the ED. The current recommendations are for a regimen of prednisone, 40 mg orally twice daily for 5 days, then 40 mg orally once daily day for 5 days, then 20 mg orally once daily for an additional 11 days.

### GASTROINTESTINAL INFECTIONS

#### *Mucocutaneous Candidiasis*

*Candida* species are frequent pathogens of the oral, pharyngeal, and esophageal mucosa. *Candida albicans* is the most common culprit. Infection is most often found in patients with CD4 cell counts lower than 200 cells/μL. Infection limited to the oropharynx may be mild, without symptoms, and patients may be unaware of the disease. Esophageal candidiasis more likely produces symptoms of odynophagia, burning chest discomfort, and fever.

Clinically, candidiasis appears as patches of whitish lesions on the oropharyngeal mucosa. These lesions are painless and are easily scraped off. Scrapings from these lesions may be examined microscopically with the use of potassium hydroxide to search for yeast. Scrapings may also be cultured. The diagnosis is generally made based on clinical findings. The presence of oral candidiasis, in combination with symptoms of odynophagia, suggests esophageal involvement. The definitive diagnosis of esophageal disease requires endoscopic visualization and sampling of the lesions.

Topical antifungal therapy, such as nystatin oral suspension or clotrimazole troches for 5 to 7 days, may be adequate for mild cases of oropharyngeal candidiasis. Systemic therapy with oral fluconazole is indicated for patients with recurrent disease and esophageal involvement. The safety and convenience of fluconazole (200 mg orally on the first day and then 100 mg orally once daily for a total of 7 to 14 days) make it preferable to topical therapy.

### DISSEMINATED INFECTION

#### Mycobacterium Avium *Complex*

Organisms that comprise the *Mycobacterium avium* complex (MAC) are ubiquitous in the environment and are capable of causing disseminated and multiorgan disease in patients with profound immunosuppression. Patients at highest risk are those whose CD4 cell counts have fallen to less than 50 cells/μL. Early symptoms of disseminated MAC infection may be mild and intermittent. As the illness progresses, nonspecific symptoms of fever, diarrhea, weight loss, and fatigue develop. Some clinicians refer to these symptoms as "the dwindles." Physical examination reveals few clues. Patients may be cachectic. Lymphadenopathy may be present, and anemia may result in pallor. The diagnosis of disseminated MAC is confirmed by isolating the organism from cultures of blood or bone marrow. Treatment of disseminated MAC infection is with a combination of antimycobacterial agents. The agents of choice are clarithromycin, ethambutol, and rifabutin.

### OPHTHALMOLOGIC INFECTIONS

#### *Cytomegalovirus Retinitis*

Investigators once estimated that approximately one third of patients with AIDS would develop cytomegalovirus (CMV) retinitis, but with the introduction of potent ART regimens, new cases of CMV retinitis have greatly declined. Retinitis is the most common form of CMV disease, although gastrointestinal and neurologic manifestations of CMV infection are not unusual. CMV disease is found primarily in patients with profound immunosuppression (i.e., CD4 cell counts < 50 cells/μL). Patients with CMV retinitis may be asymptomatic, but typical symptoms include "floaters" (dark spots within the visual field that move), scotomata, or visual field defects. Symptoms primarily occur unilaterally. The diagnosis is suggested by findings on funduscopic examination, including the classic fluffy yellow-white retinal lesions. Hemorrhage into these retinal lesions leads to the appearance of "ketchup and mustard" lesions. Oral valganciclovir (900 mg orally once daily for 21 days) is the initial treatment of choice for CMV retinitis. Treatment of sight-threatening infections includes the addition of ganciclovir intraocular implants.

## IMMUNE RECONSTITUTION INFLAMMATORY SYNDROME

Immune reconstitution syndrome is an inflammatory condition that occurs in approximately 25% of patients following the initiation of ART for HIV infection. As immune function improves, worsening symptoms of preexisting infections, either previously treated or subclinical, develop within weeks to months after beginning ART. This paradoxical clinical deterioration in spite of immune recovery is commonly associated with mycobacterial (*Mycobacterium tuberculosis* and MAC) and herpesvirus infections (herpes zoster and cytomegalovirus). This syndrome tends to be self-limited, and ART is rarely interrupted. Therapy is supportive. Specific treatment of the responsible opportunistic infection may be warranted, and nonsteroidal antiinflammatory medication and steroids may be used for symptomatic relief.

## ANTIRETROVIRAL THERAPY

The life expectancy of persons newly infected with HIV continues to increase because of advances in ART. Incredibly, most HIV-infected patients who are receiving ART will die of something other than AIDS. The goal of treatment is complete viral suppression to lower than detectable levels, to prevent viral replication and mutation that may lead to resistance. Additionally, viral suppression protects the immune system from eventual destruction. With the development of new ART, physicians increasingly design regimens that are long lasting and well tolerated, and they are more able to construct subsequent lines of therapy that can continue viral suppression. Advances in newer classes of drugs (e.g., integrase inhibitors, fusion inhibitors) offer the promise of more potency and fewer adverse effects. The development of fixed-dose combinations

**BOX 175.2 Antiretrovirals**

**Nucleoside Reverse Transcriptase Inhibitors**
- Abacavir (Ziagen)
- Didanosine (ddI, Videx)
- Emtricitabine (Emtriva)
- Lamivudine (Epivir, 3TC)
- Stavudine (Zerit, d4T)
- Zidovudine (Retrovir, AZT)

**Non-nucleotide Analogue Reverse Transcriptase Inhibitor**
- Tenofovir (Viread)

**Non-nucleoside Reverse Transcriptase Inhibitors**
- Delavirdine (Rescriptor)
- Efavirenz (Sustiva)
- Etravirine (Intelence)
- Nevirapine (Viramune)

**Protease Inhibitors**
- Atazanavir (Reyataz)
- Darunavir (Prezista)
- Fosamprenavir (Lexiva)
- Indinavir (Crixivan)
- Nelfinavir (Viracept)
- Ritonavir (Norvir)
- Saquinavir (Invirase)
- Tipranavir (Aptivus)
- Lopinavir/ritonavir (Kaletra)

**Fusion Inhibitors**
- Enfuvirtide (Fuzeon) (subcutaneous injections)
- Maraviroc (Selzentry)

**Integrase Inhibitor**
- Raltegravir (Isentress)

**Fixed Dose Combinations**
- Zidovudine/lamivudine (Combivir)
- Zidovudine/lamivudine/abacavir (Trizivir)
- Lamivudine/abacavir (Epzicom)
- Emtricitabine/tenofovir (Truvada)
- Efavirenz/emtricitabine/tenofovir (Atripla)
- Lopinavir/ritonavir (Kaletra)

revolutionized the treatment of HIV by allowing fewer pills and less frequent dosing, thereby enhancing the tolerability of therapy. The combination pill containing efavirenz, emtricitabine, and tenofovir is dosed by one pill once a day.

Currently, 23 antiretrovirals are available (**Box 175.2**). The early initiation of ART can prevent the progressive destruction of the immune system that occurs even when a patient is asymptomatic and has been shown to reduce mortality markedly. Safety and tolerability of new ART regimens and increasing evidence of the detrimental effects of uncontrolled viremia led to changes in the latest management guidelines. The 2010 International AIDS Society-USA Panel revised recommendations for adults with HIV infection to include initiating ART for all asymptomatic patients with a CD4 cell count of up to 500/μL.[4] Additionally, ART is recommended, regardless of CD4 cell count, for all symptomatic patients, as well as those who are pregnant, those with hepatitis B or C coinfection, patients with HIV-associated nephropathy, persons with active or high-risk coronary artery disease, persons more than 60 years old, patients with acute HIV infection, or persons with a high risk of HIV transmission.

Antiretroviral medications are primarily prescribed by specialists in the field and are given in various combinations to prevent the development of drug resistance. The recommendations include the combination of nucleoside and nucleotide analogue reverse transcriptase inhibitors (emtricitabine and tenofovir) with a non-nucleoside reverse-transcriptase inhibitor (efavirenz), a ritonavir-boosted protease inhibitor (atazanavir/ritonavir), or the integrase inhibitor (raltegravir). The precise combination selected depends on the patient's individual condition. The FDA approved six fixed-dose combination pills that greatly simplified therapy and enhanced adherence.

### ADVERSE EFFECTS

Investigators have estimated that approximately 25% of all patients will discontinue ART because of side effects. Adverse reactions may be mild to potentially life-threatening (**Table 175.2**). Distinguishing between these adverse effects and possible symptoms of infection with HIV or opportunistic pathogens is often difficult for clinicians. Emergency physicians must be familiar with the frequently encountered, and possibly deadly, adverse effects of ART.

Common adverse effects are primarily gastrointestinal (e.g., nausea, vomiting, diarrhea). More severe reactions include lactic acidosis. Patients often present with nonspecific symptoms such as fatigue, shortness of breath, nausea, and weight loss, and laboratory testing confirms the diagnosis by demonstrating an elevated anion gap metabolic acidosis and a serum lactate level higher than 3 mmol/L. Treatment is supportive, with immediate discontinuation of ART. Hepatotoxicity with transaminitis is primarily associated with protease inhibitors and the non-nucleoside reverse transcriptase inhibitors and warrants discontinuation of ART. Abacavir may cause a hypersensitivity reaction, usually seen within the first 6 weeks of initiating therapy, characterized by fever, myalgia, malaise, nausea, vomiting, anorexia, and rash. Symptoms progressively worsen with continued administration. Treatment is again supportive, and abacavir must be permanently discontinued. Consultation with an infectious disease expert is prudent in the management of adverse effects of ART.

## PROPHYLAXIS AGAINST COMMON OPPORTUNISTIC INFECTION

Patients infected with HIV infection and who are severely immunosuppressed are at risk for many opportunistic infections. Long-term antimicrobial prophylaxis has been demonstrated to be beneficial in preventing several common opportunistic infections (**Table 175.3**).

## POSTEXPOSURE PROPHYLAXIS

### OCCUPATIONAL EXPOSURE

Although the risk of occupational transmission of HIV to health care workers is quite small, it is not zero. Percutaneous exposure to blood from an HIV-infected patient carries an

**Table 175.2** Adverse Effects of Antiretroviral Agents

| AGENTS | ADVERSE EFFECTS* |
|---|---|
| **Nucleoside Reverse Transcriptase Inhibitors** | |
| Abacavir | Rash<br>Hypersensitivity* |
| Didanosine | Pancreatitis*<br>Peripheral neuropathy<br>Transaminitis |
| Emtricitabine | Headache<br>Rash<br>Hyperpigmentation |
| Lamivudine | Headache |
| Stavudine | Peripheral neuropathy |
| Zidovudine | Headache<br>Myalgias<br>Anemia (elevated mean corpuscular volume) |
| **Non-nucleotide Analogue Reverse Transcriptase Inhibitors** | |
| Tenofovir | Lactic acidosis*<br>Hepatitis<br>Renal insufficiency |
| **Non-nucleoside reverse transcriptase inhibitors** | Rash |
| Delavirdine | Severe rash*<br>Hepatitis<br>Fatigue |
| Efavirenz | Hepatitis*<br>Severe rash<br>Central nervous system effects or abnormal dreams |
| Etravirine | Elevation of liver function tests |
| Nevirapine | Stevens-Johnson syndrome*<br>Severe rash*<br>Hepatitis*<br>Fever<br>Headache |
| **Protease Inhibitors** | Dyslipidemia<br>Lipodystrophy<br>Hyperglycemia<br>Elevations of liver function tests |
| Atazanavir | Jaundice |
| Darunavir | Rash |
| Fosamprenavir | Rash |
| Indinavir | Nephrolithiasis |
| Lopinavir/ritonavir | Taste perversion |
| Nelfinavir | Enteritis |
| Ritonavir | Taste perversion |
| Saquinavir | Oral ulcers |
| Tipranavir | Rash |
| **Fusion Inhibitors** | |
| Enfuvirtide | Injection site reactions<br>Neutropenia |
| Maraviroc | Hepatitis<br>Myalgias or arthralgias |
| **Integrase Inhibitor** | |
| Raltegravir | Elevation of liver function tests<br>Rash |

*Severe adverse effect warrants discontinuation of all antiretrovirals.

**Table 175.3** Prophylaxis Against Opportunistic Infections

| OPPORTUNISTIC INFECTION | INDICATION | RECOMMENDED ANTIMICROBIAL |
|---|---|---|
| *Pneumocystis* pneumonia | CD4 cell count < 200 cells/μL ***or*** history of oropharyngeal candidiasis | TMP/SMX 1 DS/ day PO |
| Toxoplasmosis | CD4 cell count < 100 cells/μL | TMP/SMX 1 DS/ day PO |
| Disseminated *Mycobacterium avium* complex | CD4 cell count < 50 cells/μL | Azithromycin 1200 mg/wk PO |

*DS,* Double strength; *PO,* orally; *TMP/SMX,* trimethoprim-sulfamethoxazole.

estimated risk of transmission of approximately 0.3%. Similar exposures to mucous membranes are associated with a 0.09% risk of transmission, and the risk of transmission following exposure to nonintact skin is even lower. The CDC provides recommendations for the management of health care workers exposed to HIV and for postexposure prophylaxis (PEP). These recommendations are based on the severity of the exposure and the viral load of the source patient (**Box 175.3**).[5] Health care workers with low-risk exposures are recommended to take the basic two-drug regimens. A small-volume blood exposure to mucous membranes or nonintact skin from a source patient who is asymptomatic or who has a low viral load (<1500 RNA copies/mL) represents a low risk of infection (**Box 175.4**). Those with high-risk exposures are recommended to take the expanded three-drug regimen of PEP. Percutaneous exposure to a source patient with a high viral load is considered to carry a higher risk.

No PEP is recommended for any type of exposure if the source patient is HIV negative. Saliva, tears, nasal secretions,

**BOX 175.3 Occupational Transmission of Human Immunodeficiency Virus to Health Care Workers**

**High-Risk Exposure**
Percutaneous exposure
- Large, hollow-bore needle
- Deep puncture
- Visibly bloody device
- Needle from source patient's artery or vein

Source patient
- Symptomatic HIV infection
- Acquired immunodeficiency syndrome
- Acute HIV infection
- High viral load

Large volume of blood/prolonged contact with mucous membranes or nonintact skin

**Low-Risk Exposure**
Percutaneous exposure
- Solid needle
- Superficial injury

Source patient
- Asymptomatic HIV infection
- Viral load known to be <1500 RNA copies/mL

Small volume of blood (a few drops) in contact with mucous membranes or nonintact skin

**BOX 175.4 Recommended Regimens for Postexposure Prophylaxis**

**Basic Regimen**
Zidovudine plus lamivudine (Combivir) twice daily
*or*
Tenofovir plus emtricitabine (Truvada) once daily

**Expanded Regimen**
Basic regimen plus:
Lopinavir and ritonavir (Kaletra) once or twice daily
*or*
Darunavir/ritonavir once daily

sputum, gastric fluids, urine, and feces are not infectious unless they are visibly bloody. All medications should be initiated as soon as possible, and all regimens should be continued for 28 days. Initiating PEP 72 hours after exposure is not effective, and it is generally not recommended. Available resources include a 24-hour telephone help line (PEPline: 888-448-4911) and online information from the National HIV/AIDS Clinicians' Consultation Center at www.nccc.ucsf.edu.

## NONOCCUPATIONAL EXPOSURE

In 2005, the CDC published recommendations for antiretroviral PEP following sexual exposure, injection drug use, or other nonoccupational exposure to HIV.[6] A 28-day course of ART is now recommended for persons seeking care less than 72 hours after nonoccupational exposure to blood, genital secretions, or other potentially infectious bodily fluid from a source known to be HIV positive.

**BOX 175.5 Recommendations for Nonoccupational Postexposure Prophylaxis**

**Negligible Risk**
nPEP not recommended regardless of source's HIV status

**Substantial Risk**
Source HIV positive: nPEP recommended

**Indeterminate Risk**
Source HIV status unknown: nPEP recommended if source patient at high risk for HIV

*nPEP,* Nonoccupational postexposure prophylaxis.

Nonoccupational PEP (nPEP) is not always effective, and antiretroviral medications may produce harmful adverse effects, so all persons should be evaluated on a case-by-case basis. For example, persons who engage in high-risk behaviors, resulting in frequent exposures to HIV and the use of multiple and repeated courses of antiretrovirals, should not take nPEP. They should instead be counseled on risk-reduction strategies. All persons should be tested for baseline HIV infection. Additionally, they should be evaluated for other sexually transmitted diseases because the presence of these diseases may increase the risk of transmission of HIV.

Substantial exposure risk is defined as exposure of vagina, eyes, rectum, mouth, or other mucous membranes, or nonintact skin, or percutaneous contact, with blood, semen, vaginal secretions, rectal secretions, breast milk, or any bodily fluid that is visibly contaminated with blood from a source that is HIV positive. Negligible exposure risk is defined as exposure of vagina, eyes, rectum, mouth, or other mucous membranes, or nonintact skin, or percutaneous contact, with urine, nasal secretions, saliva, sweat, or tears if not visibly contaminated with blood, regardless of the known or suspected HIV status of the source. If the source's HIV status is unknown, the source should be tested, if possible. The first dose of nPEP may be given initially, and no further doses are given if the source is determined to be HIV negative. If the source's HIV status cannot be determined and the person seeking care had a substantial risk exposure, consideration of the source patient's risk of having HIV is warranted. High-risk populations include men who have sex with men, commercial sex workers, those who inject drugs, those with history of incarceration, persons from countries where the HIV seroprevalence is at least 1%, or sexual partners of persons at high risk. Perpetrators of sexual assault are considered to have a high risk for HIV. Substantial exposure to high-risk populations warrants nPEP (**Box 175.5**).

Once the decision has been made to initiate nPEP, ART should be administered promptly. The basic regimens recommended for occupational PEP are also recommended for nPEP (see Box 175.4).[7] The expanded regimens are reserved for patients exposed to a source population in which background resistance of HIV to ART is high.

Persons who are given nPEP must be counseled on the potential adverse effects, in particular nausea, vomiting, and diarrhea, and must be offered symptomatic therapy such as antiemetics or antimotility drugs. All persons receiving nPEP should have prompt follow-up care provided by their primary care practitioners or an infectious disease specialist.

## PREVENTION OF HIV INFECTION

Exciting data have revealed fundamentally new, effective approaches to prevent HIV transmission. The Center for the AIDS Program of Research in South Africa (CAPRISA) study demonstrated the effectiveness and safety of a 1% vaginal gel formulation of tenofovir for the prevention of HIV acquisition in women.[8] A double-blind, randomized controlled trial comparing tenofovir gel with placebo demonstrated a reduction in risk of HIV transmission by more than one half. This microbicide gel allows women around the world to play a greater role in HIV prevention when compared with relying on their partners to use condoms.

The second landmark report was the Preexposure Prophylaxis Initiative (iPreEx) trial.[9] This study, conducted in six countries, included 2499 HIV-negative men who had sex with men to evaluate whether antiretroviral medications could prevent the transmission of HIV. A once-daily antiretroviral combination pill of emtricitabine and tenofovir was compared with placebo. The participants were followed for an average of 14 months. The antiretroviral group demonstrated a 44% reduction in the incidence of HIV compared with the placebo group, and a subset of participants with enhanced compliance had an even greater risk reduction of 73%. This trial clearly showed that preexposure prophylaxis is generally safe, well tolerated, and effective. Together, these two reports demonstrate significant advances in the prevention of HIV transmission.

## REFERENCES

***References can be found on Expert Consult @ www.expertconsult.com.***

# Fungal Infections 176

*Richard Paula*

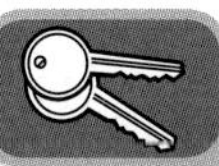

**KEY POINTS**

- Fungi can cause significant human disease.
- Human fungal infection is overwhelmingly caused by the following organisms: *Aspergillus, Blastomyces, Candida, Coccidioides, Cryptococcus, Histoplasma, Paracoccidioides, Sporothrix,* and *Zygomycetes.*
- Fungal infection rates have dramatically increased after the arrival of improved diagnostic capabilities and a growing population of immunosuppressed patients.
- Invasive fungal infections carry an extremely high mortality rate, and recognition with rapid treatment by an observant emergency physician prevents morbidity.

## GENERAL EPIDEMIOLOGY

The risk of fungal infections is tied to both geography and immune status. Immunocompromised individuals are exponentially more likely to suffer from fungal infection. Immunocompetent patients do acquire significant, often invasive fungal disease, especially in endemic areas. In 3 counties in the southwestern United States, coccidioidomycosis in immunocompetent patients who were more 65 years old occurred with an incidence of 40 in 100,000. In addition to the best-known endemic areas, smaller areas in Africa and Asia are known to harbor pockets with high rates of infection. Fungal infections are a scourge in hospitals, and they account for significant numbers of nosocomial infections. Previously published data showed that 10% of all nosocomial infections were fungal,[1] and *Candida* was responsible for 83% of those infections.[2]

### RISK FACTORS

Outside the endemic areas of concern, the significant risk factor for fungal infection is immune dysfunction. One of the reasons for the extended life expectancy of immunocompromised patients is the ability to recognize the increased susceptibility of these patients to fungal disease. Patients with selective specific immune deficiency often contract specific fungal infections. Different weaknesses in immune-mediated host defenses allow varying types of infection. Candidal infections offer a clear example of this point. Granulocytes primarily prevent bloodborne candidiasis, and this becomes apparent in neutropenic patients, who are at greater risk to develop *Candida*-induced fungemia and sepsis. Contrast this situation with the T-cell–mediated defense that prevents mucosal *Candida* proliferation. This property explains why almost 90% of patients with human immunodeficiency virus (HIV) infection have oropharyngeal colonization, and more than half develop clinical thrush. Some fungal organisms, such as *Histoplasma capsulatum* and *Coccidioides immitis,* change form during active infection of the host, and others remain exclusively in the yeast form. This adaptation allows *Histoplasma* and *Coccidioides* to infect healthy individuals.

### ANATOMY

Fungal disease may occur in any organ system (central nervous system [CNS], cardiovascular system, respiratory system, skin, eyes); no system is spared. The type of infection is often associated with a specific risk factor or endemic exposure. The anatomic location of infection may be noted by the presenting symptoms. A particular area of infection may help to identify a specific deficiency in a patient's immune system. Certain immune deficiencies are associated with specific fungal disease manifestations.

## PRESENTING SIGNS AND SYMPTOMS

No specific presenting signs or symptoms are pathognomonic of fungal infection. Certain patient populations are more likely to contract fungal infections (**Table 176.1**).

Depending on the site of infection, presenting symptoms vary. The important signs of fungal infection are indicated by indirect evidence found in the patient's history. Patients who have a history suggestive of greater risk for fungal infection should be evaluated and treated more extensively. For example, when a patient with acquired immunodeficiency syndrome (AIDS) presents to the emergency department (ED) after a recent admission for pneumonia with recurrent symptoms of pneumonia, the incidence of fungal infection, specifically *Candida,* is much higher. The patient needs cultures specifically for *Candida* and requires prompt antifungal therapy in the ED, in addition to broad-spectrum antibiotics covering health care–associated pneumonia.

**Table 176.1 Predisposing Factors in Fungal Infections**

| PATIENT RISK FACTOR | COMMON FUNGAL INFECTION |
|---|---|
| Human immunodeficiency virus infection (acquired immunodeficiency syndrome) | Candidiasis, cryptococcosis, aspergillosis |
| Recent organ transplantation | Candidiasis, aspergillosis |
| Neutropenia | Candidiasis, aspergillosis |
| High-dose steroids | Zygomycosis, candidiasis |
| Recent antibiotic treatment | Candidiasis |
| Diabetes | Candidiasis, zygomycosis |
| Recent or ongoing hospitalization | Candidiasis, aspergillosis |
| Recent abdominal surgery or burns (especially with intensive care unit stay) | Candidiasis |
| Travel to endemic area | Histoplasmosis, blastomycosis, coccidioidomycosis |

## ORGAN-SPECIFIC CLINICAL FINDINGS

### Pulmonary Disorders

Patients with fungal pneumonia present similarly to patients with other types of pneumonia. They have fever, dry or productive cough, fatigue, shortness of breath, or hemoptysis. The chest radiographic appearance also resembles that of other pneumonias. No specific finding is associated with particular fungal infections; lobar and interstitial infiltrates are both common. Certain fungal infections occasionally manifest with visible masslike lesions (e.g., blastomycosis, aspergillosis), and other infections form cavitary lesions (e.g., sporotrichosis), but these are the exception and not the rule. Fungal pneumonia causes varying symptoms and radiologic appearances. In one review,[3] aspergillosis was the most common fungal cause of pneumonia in patients with cancer. Other reviews reported aspergillosis as the most common cause of pneumonia in immunocompromised patients. Healthy, immunocompetent individuals are overwhelmingly more likely to have one of the endemic fungal infections.

### Central Nervous System Disorders

Almost all the common fungal pathogens can cause CNS infection. The best known is *Cryptococcus* because of its propensity to cause meningitis in 50% to 60% of infected, immunocompromised patients. CNS infections may also be seen in much lower proportions in healthy individuals. Histoplasmosis leads to meningitis in approximately 1% of symptomatic individuals. Almost all patients with fungal meningitis present after known fungal infections and are hospitalized patients with severe immunodeficiency. This is not the case in many HIV-infected patients with cryptococcal meningitis. Patients with cryptococcal meningitis have varying presentations, often including a headache for weeks, fever, nausea, or frank mental status decline. Such patients require lumbar puncture and prompt antifungal therapy.

### Sepsis

Fungal sepsis is rare, but it is highly fatal. The Recombinant Human Activated Protein C Worldwide Evaluation in Severe Sepsis (PROWESS) trial[4] demonstrated a fungal sepsis mortality rate of nearly 56% that was more than double the nonfungal sepsis mortality rate of 28% to 30%. Suspicion is necessary to identify these patients early. A patient with a history of recent hospitalization, immunosuppression from organ transplants, or abdominal surgery has a dramatically increased risk of disseminated fungal infection causing sepsis. Cultures with specific fungal organism media should be sent, followed by initiation of antifungal therapy.

### Ear, Nose, and Throat Disorders

Fungal infections in the craniofacial area may be progressive and often fatal (e.g., zygomycosis), or they may be chronic and need referral for eventual diagnosis and treatment (e.g., allergic fungal sinusitis). Zygomycosis is rare, but it is also extremely invasive and may manifest as facial pain and swelling. Patients with diabetes, especially those with diabetic ketoacidosis, require a thorough craniofacial examination to look for the characteristic black exudate. Craniofacial computed tomography (CT) scanning hastens the diagnosis when zygomycosis is suspected. Most patients with fungal sinusitis present with common sinusitis symptoms: facial pressure, congestion or drainage, swelling, and allergic "shiners." Although most of these patients may be treated conservatively, patients with ongoing symptoms, nasal polyps, or evidence of facial deformity or bone erosion on CT will need rapid ear, nose, and throat follow-up and evaluation for débridement and antifungal therapy.

### Rheumatic Disorders

Patients with disseminated fungal infections often complain of polyarthritis. Specifically, sporotrichosis spreads to the elbow or knee, and blastomycosis spreads to the weight-bearing joints or spine. Patients with cutaneous evidence of sporotrichosis or blastomycosis who have joint pain and swelling need aspiration and specific fungal analysis of the synovial fluid.

### Cutaneous Disorders

The most common fungal infections in humans are the superficial cutaneous fungal infections (e.g., tinea), which are detailed in Chapter 184. Certain fungal species may start as cutaneous lesions and disseminate to invasive disease, or they may begin as pulmonary disease and disseminate to form cutaneous lesions. The latter type is a form of blastomycosis characterized by a primary pulmonary infection that spreads, leading to cutaneous lesions in 75% of patients with disseminated disease. Sporotrichosis behaves similarly, but in an opposite fashion, because most patients with disseminated disease initially have cutaneous lesions. Both infections manifest as raised verrucous lesions with irregular borders that are painless and are often seen on the face or neck. Either infection can develop into the verrucous form or can become an extremity ulcer. Potassium hydroxide (KOH) scraping identifies these lesions as fungal.

### *Vulvovaginal Disorders*

*Candida* is well known to cause a vulvovaginal infection that is common among sexually active women. This infection is often seen after a course of antibiotics, or it may appear spontaneously. Patients describe itching, burning of the labia, and a thick, white discharge. The incidence is increased in women taking oral contraceptives and in patients with diabetes. Adequate treatment is usually provided by over-the-counter antifungal creams, but patients may require oral medication if the infection is recurrent or severe.

## DIAGNOSTIC TESTING

Fungi are usually visible in a tissue or fluid sample with the aid of KOH solution, which destroys nonfungal cell structures. This approach identifies only fungi that are easy to sample. In cases of pneumonia or fungemia, this type of testing is not usually possible. Most fungi can be cultured, and species such as *Coccidioides* and *Candida* grow readily on most agars. Other species, such as *Histoplasma* and *Aspergillus,* are much more difficult to grow and require antigen testing such as enzyme-linked immunosorbent assay to confirm infection. *Zygomycetes* requires special stains and is often a laboratory contaminant. It may be erroneously discarded if the laboratory is not told that it is a possible pathogen. Emergency physicians should call their particular hospital or outpatient microbiology laboratory to determine the best method of identification.

## SPECIFIC FUNGAL INFECTIONS

### BLASTOMYCOSIS

Blastomycosis is caused by the fungus *Blastomyces dermatitidis.* This infection occurs primarily in healthy individuals who are exposed in one of the endemic areas (**Table 176.2**). Pulmonary infections are typical, especially in the acute phase, and are contracted though inhalation of the dormant form. After attaining body temperature, the organism transforms into the yeast form and develops a greater ability to infect. Many patients acquire the infection and have chronic pneumonia for years, often diagnosed as reactive airway disease, before the infection is discovered. Patients with chronic pulmonary infections often develop extrapulmonary manifestations of the disease. These patients frequently have cutaneous lesions, and frank meningitis occurs in 10% of disseminated cases. If CNS involvement is suspected, a simple lumbar puncture is inadequate because results are routinely negative; ventricular fluid collection is required to confirm the diagnosis.

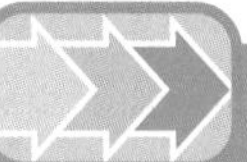

**PRIORITY ACTIONS**

**Differential Diagnosis**

**Shortness of Breath or Productive Cough?**

Does the patient have evidence of pneumonia that did not respond to antibiotics?

Does the patient have a noninfectious cause of the infiltrate such as pulmonary embolism or congestive heart failure?

If not, fungal pneumonia should be suspected and treated. Although some controversy exists regarding treatment of mild fungal pneumonia with antifungal therapy, initiating therapy in the emergency department is prudent and recommended.

**Headache or Mental Status Changes?**

Does a patient with poorly controlled HIV infection have a significant or prolonged headache? Are mental status changes associated with this headache?

Does the patient have a normal brain computed tomography scan?

If so, a lumbar puncture with the patient in the lateral decubitus position should be performed. The opening pressure should be recorded and the cerebrospinal fluid examined for evidence of fungal infection along with bacterial and viral causes.

**Organ or Bone Graft Transplant Patient with a Fever?**

Does the fever have another cause? Is the patient hemodynamically stable?

If a transplant recipient has a fever while taking antibiotics or appears to have sepsis, initiating antifungal therapy after obtaining appropriate cultures is appropriate and important.

**Difficult or Painful Swallowing?**

Does the patient have evidence of an esophageal foreign body or a bacterial infection such as with streptococci?

If not, *Candida* esophagitis should be suspected in patients with HIV infection or other immunocompromised states and in healthy individuals after recent antibiotic exposure.

Patients who are not tolerating oral fluids need to be admitted for hydration and evaluation for esophagogastroduodenoscopy.

**Verrucous Lesion or Extremity Ulcer?**

Does the patient work with plant material such as roses or moss?

If so, scrape the lesions and send sample for a potassium hydroxide preparation. If the patient has no sign of systemic disease, discharge with oral fluconazole and follow-up instructions.

*HIV,* Human immunodeficiency virus.

**Table 176.2** Endemic Areas of Common Fungi

| FUNGUS | ENDEMIC AREA |
|---|---|
| *Coccidioides* | Southwestern United States |
| *Blastomyces* | Mississippi, St. Lawrence, and Ohio River valleys |
| *Histoplasma* | Mississippi and Ohio River valleys |

Patients with pulmonary blastomycosis present with pneumonia: cough, fever, chills, malaise, and classic pneumonia symptoms. The chest radiographic findings can be an infiltrate or a masslike structure. This masslike appearance explains why blastomycosis is regularly diagnosed at bronchoscopy. Patients from endemic areas with symptoms resembling pneumonia and who present with mass lesions on radiography should be treated for blastomycosis, in addition to being given appropriate antibiotics. The organism can be identified by sputum smear or culture. Identification of the organism is considered to be diagnostic of infection because colonization does not occur, as it may with other fungi such as *Candida.* Blastomycosis does not generally clear without treatment, and untreated patients have mortality rates higher than 50%. Treating pulmonary blastomycosis is best done with the azoles, either itraconazole or ketoconazole for immunocompetent hosts. If the patient has life-threatening, disseminated disease or is immunocompromised, amphotericin B remains the most commonly recommended therapy.

## HISTOPLASMOSIS

Histoplasmosis is caused by the fungus *H. capsulatum.* Infections regularly occur in healthy, immunocompetent individuals. The disease is prevalent in endemic areas, but it has a much greater geographic spread than blastomycosis. *Histoplasma* is found in caves, chicken coops, and ships hulls all over the world. Pulmonary infections are typical, and infection is often contracted through inhalation of the dormant mold form. This mold form is then activated by increased body temperatures, thus causing proliferation. Histoplasmosis has a much greater affinity for extrapulmonary symptoms than blastomycosis; spreading infection causes pericarditis, rheumatologic symptoms, and CNS involvement. Active infection depends on the load of inoculation. Lighter exposures do not produce disease, and published rates of infections higher than 50% occur in endemic areas without evidence of symptoms.

The common presentation of symptomatic histoplasmosis-induced pneumonia is indolent, with flulike symptoms, malaise, fever, and headache in almost 100% of patients. Chest radiography is highly variable, and findings may be normal, but patchy alveolar infiltrates and hilar adenopathy are common. Disease disseminates in approximately 10% of patients, mostly immunocompromised persons, and it leads to pericarditis in 10%, arthritis and arthralgias in 10%, and meningitis in 10%. Symptoms in disseminated infection are associated with pancytopenia, with significant elevations in lactate dehydrogenase, and this condition must be differentiated from thrombotic thrombocytopenic purpura.

Identification of histoplasmosis is complicated. Culture is difficult because the organism is dangerous to laboratory personnel and must be held more than a month before results can be reported as negative. Antigen testing is helpful, but many individuals have been exposed, and complement fixation rates as high as 5% may suggest the diagnosis when it is not present. The polysaccharide antigen test is preferred, although it has problems because it cross-reacts with blastomycosis and coccidioidomycosis.

When treatment is discussed, to the physician should remember that most healthy patients without chronic or disseminated infections recover without any treatment. The current literature suggests a period of observation for otherwise healthy patients with symptomatic histoplasmosis. In making the decision to treat, the side effects of therapy must be weighed against the high likelihood of spontaneous recovery. Admittedly, this was much more of an issue before azole therapy because the side effects of treatment with amphotericin B ("amphoterrible") were sometimes worse than the infection itself.

Recommendations are to initiate treatment with oral itraconazole for a minimum of 6 weeks in patients who are hypoxic or who have not improved after 3 weeks of observation. Infected immunocompromised patients or patients with disseminated or life-threatening infections are treated best with lipid formulations of amphotericin B, with the addition of a steroid taper if pulmonary involvement is severe. Itraconazole has been used successfully in patients with HIV infection who have not developed AIDS.

## COCCIDIOIDOMYCOSIS

Coccidioidomycosis is caused by the soil fungus *C. immitis,* which is endemic to the southwestern North American continent. Famously responsible for San Joaquin Valley fever, this organism regularly infects healthy persons. A dramatic increase in infections has been observed, with more than 100,000 infections annually in the United States alone. The increase mirrors population growth within the endemic geographic area. Infection occurs through inhalation of the mold form and subsequent transformation at body temperature into a more virulent spherule. Many infections are not symptomatic, and estimates in the literature reflect that 40% to 70% of exposed individuals never show evidence of disease. Coccidioidomycosis becomes disseminated in only 10% of cases, and much of the time only to the skin, where it frequently forms abscesses. Meningitis occurs in fewer than 5% of cases. Most complications are local, with pulmonary cavitation and chronic pneumonia responsible for the 20% of cases judged as severe.

Although primary infection usually remains in the lungs, extrapulmonary symptoms are common. Fever, chills, cough, pleuritic chest pain, and malaise are hallmarks of disease. Arthralgias and rash are also common, hence the designation "desert rheumatism." Because only 50% of symptomatic patients have abnormal chest radiographs, the diagnosis is easy to overlook. When apparent, abnormal findings include hilar adenopathy, diffuse infiltrates, and pleural effusions. Cavitation occurs in 5% of untreated patients, and it often appears as a solitary, peripheral lesion.

Identification of *Coccidioides* is significantly easier than detection of other fungi because of the rapid growth of this organism. Most growth media produce identifiable organisms in 2 to 3 days. Mature spherules may also been seen in tissue biopsies with special stains, and antibody detection is helpful. Unlike in histoplasmosis, colonization is rare. Complement immunoglobulin M identification is considered a sign of active infection, and it disappears over time. Results of immunoglobulin G testing continue to remain positive in patients with chronic infection, but they also resolve when the infection clears.

Treatment of coccidioidomycosis is not always necessary because the infection often resolves without intervention. The Infectious Diseases Society of America (IDSA) reported[5] that no evidence indicated that treating the mild form of pneumonia reduces morbidity or prevents chronic infection. Therefore, the recommendations are to treat only the following groups: immunocompromised patients, patients with severe pneumonia, and patients with suspected high inoculum loads such as after laboratory accidents. Certain ethnic groups, individuals with African or Filipino ancestry, are at greater risk of disseminated infection and should be considered more thoroughly for treatment. The precise definition of severe pneumonia is left to the physician's judgment. Therapeutic options are similar to those in other fungal diseases, with azole therapy as first-line treatment. Some literature suggests a benefit of itraconazole over fluconazole.[3] Both drugs are associated with considerable relapse rates in chronic disease, and this is why a 3-month course of therapy is recommended. Disseminated disease may still be treated with the azoles if the patient is not immunocompromised. Patients with life-threatening cases require amphotericin. Patients with CNS involvement were traditionally treated with intrathecal amphotericin B. More recently, this approach was challenged by using high-dose azole therapy, and response rates were high, at 60% to 90%. However, cure was not observed, only suppression, and current thought is that a combination of intrathecal amphotericin B and intravenous azole therapy will work best.

## ASPERGILLOSIS

The *Aspergillus* species that infects humans is most commonly *Aspergillus fumigatus,* and it is responsible for 90% of infections. *Aspergillus flavus* is less common, but it is much more likely to cause sinus disease. *Aspergillus* is a saprophyte, a soil-loving species found worldwide. Aspergillosis casts a wide spectrum of disease. It can benignly colonize immunocompetent hosts, it can cause chronic allergic symptoms, or it can devastatingly lead to overwhelming fungal sepsis in immunocompromised patients. Infection is usually contracted through inhalation of the conidia form, which progresses to the hyphae form at increased body temperature. The hyphae form is much more aggressive and difficult for the human immune system to combat. Because of the pathogenicity of the hyphae form, infection occurs in normal and immunocompromised hosts.

Immunocompetent hosts who acquire aspergillosis frequently manifest disease in the form of sinusitis. The theory of the continuum of sinus disease termed allergic fungal sinusitis is controversial. *Aspergillus* has been recovered from 13% of adults with allergic fungal sinusitis. The origin is obscured by the finding that the evidence points in both directions, toward either inflammatory or infectious disease. What are not debated are the secondary effects. The accumulation of mucinous debris leads to nasal polyps and possibly more invasive disease, causing bone erosion and facial deformity. Patients with nasal polyps should be promptly referred to an ear, nose, and throat specialist because surgical débridement is currently thought necessary for cure. Because of the complex nature of the disease, therapy should not be initiated until ear, nose, and throat consultation has been obtained, unless evidence of concomitant bacterial sinusitis is present. If clinical evidence of anatomic distortion is present, facial CT scanning is helpful in determining the extent of disease. Sinusitis is the most common form of aspergillosis in immunocompetent hosts, and pulmonary disease, particularly aspergilloma, often occurs in patients who are chronically diseased but not immunocompromised.

The long-recognized fungal ball or aspergilloma infects individuals with preexisting cavitary disease, such as tuberculosis, sarcoidosis, or bullous chronic obstructive pulmonary disease. These patients continue to have an infection rate of 10% to 15%. Symptoms, most commonly cough and hemoptysis, are difficult to discern from those of the chronic disease state in these patients. Aspergillomas are usually easily identified on plain chest radiography or on CT scans. Classic therapy involves surgical resection, and admission with surgical consultation is recommended.

Aspergilloma is the contained form of pulmonary aspergillosis. Invasive pulmonary aspergillosis is far more dangerous and must be addressed quickly. The immunocompromised patient, in particular the transplant recipient, is at great risk of contracting pulmonary aspergillosis. The incidence of *Aspergillus* in the bronchial tree of transplant recipients has been reported at 20% to 40%. Patients with AIDS have experienced an increase in invasive aspergillosis, and the current incidence has been reported at 1% to 2%. Symptoms of invasive pulmonary aspergillosis are variable, but they usually involve a combination of fever, cough, malaise, hemoptysis, and pleuritic chest pain. Heavily immunosuppressed patients present late and may have only fatigue as their first symptom, followed by massive hemoptysis or sepsis. Diagnosis in these patients is challenging, and no "gold standard" for diagnosis exists. Findings on plain radiography may be normal. Chest CT is more helpful in identifying disease, but it is not specific for aspergillosis. Serum culture for *Aspergillus* is highly specific, but it has a very low yield. Enzyme-linked immunosorbent assay may be better, although sensitivity has been reported to be as low as 60% and as high as 100%. Clinical suspicion is important, and even though no randomized study has proven the value of empiric therapy, initiating therapy before an official diagnosis has been confirmed is prudent and may be lifesaving. Even treated patients have a 20% to 100% mortality rate.

Therapy for invasive aspergillosis traditionally consisted of amphotericin B, but reported cure rates were as low as 40%. In 2002, a randomized study comparing voriconazole with amphotericin B demonstrated a significantly higher survival rate of 71% versus 58%, respectively.[6] The study also reported an unfortunately high rate of adverse events that occurred with amphotericin B therapy in 24% of the trial participants, almost double the 13% rate in the voriconazole-treated group. The IDSA recommended voriconazole as first-line treatment for invasive disease in their most recent guidelines.[7]

## CRYPTOCOCCOSIS

*Cryptococcus neoformans* is an arboreal fungus found worldwide, with a predilection for the excrement of certain bird species, particularly pigeons. This disease was described in the 1950s to be similar to tuberculosis in terms of progression of disease in healthy individuals. Currently, *Cryptococcus* rarely infects immunocompetent individuals and is mainly linked to morbidity in HIV-infected individuals. Before the AIDS epidemic, infection rates were 0.8 per million in persons who were not infected with HIV. These rates spiked to 66 per 100,000 in patients with advanced HIV infection and then dropped again in that population with the advent of highly active antiretroviral therapy. Although *Cryptococcus* is not responsible for significant disease in otherwise healthy individuals, it is known to cause widespread asymptomatic colonization. Most adults have serum antibodies to *Cryptococcus*. A study of children in New York City demonstrated seroconversion before the age of 10 years.[8]

Infection is thought to occur through inhalation of contaminated propagules (microscopic plant material), although aerosolized pigeon dander has yielded a potentially infectious yeast form of the fungus. Patients who manifest pulmonary cryptococcosis have common pneumonia symptoms: cough, fever or chills, and pleuritic chest pain. *Cryptococcus* has a well-known predilection for CNS involvement, and even though infection may be through inhalation, 50% to 60% of patients with cryptococcosis have CNS involvement. Patients with cryptococcal meningitis have varying presentations: often headache for weeks, fever, nausea, or frank mental status decline. Any HIV-infected patient with significant headache or mental status changes should be evaluated by lumbar puncture for cryptococcal meningitis.

The diagnosis is made with India ink examination of infected cerebrospinal fluid. Of HIV-infected patients with infected cerebrospinal fluid, 80% have organisms visible with India ink staining. Systemic involvement is often present in these patients and may be confirmed with either serum culture or latex agglutination, although latex agglutination is more accurate, with a sensitivity and specificity of more than 90%. Latex agglutination should be added to the cerebrospinal fluid studies to increase the likelihood of diagnosis.

Treatment should begin immediately in ill-appearing patients, even before lumbar puncture. The current literature points to combination therapy for CNS cryptococcosis in immunocompromised patients. Randomized trials showed that flucytosine, in combination with either amphotericin B or fluconazole, is superior to any single agent. In less severe infection such as symptomatic pneumonia in healthy individuals, oral fluconazole as monotherapy is sufficient. Revised IDSA recommendations include newer liposomal amphotericin formulations found to be effective in severe disease. Details regarding amphotericin B lipid complex (ABLC), L-amphotericin B, and amphotericin B colloidal dispersion (ABCD) are beyond the scope of this text.[9]

## CANDIDIASIS

*Candida* is the most common fungal pathogen seen by physicians. It is common in healthy individuals and in immunocompromised patients, and it is a frequent cause of nosocomial infection. More than 100 species of *Candida* have been identified. *Candida albicans* remains the most common species, but a rise of other species has been reported. The increase in non-*albicans* species is thought to be related to improved identification methods, the longer life span of immunocompromised patients, and a significant increase in the number of patients living with implantable devices.

*Candida* is a ubiquitous organism, existing as a yeast form and reproducing with buds and hyphae. It lives for long periods on surfaces, especially in hospital environments, but it does not commonly cause laboratory contamination. *Candida* can infect any organ and is sometimes seen as having a commensal relationship with healthy humans. *Candida* infection is fought by multiple components of the immune system. T-cell–mediated attacks prevent mucosal overcolonization, and granulocytes help to prevent candidemia. Evidence of these mechanisms is seen in the common occurrence of thrush in patients with AIDS and of *Candida* sepsis in neutropenic patients. The most common infection with *Candida* is vulvovaginal candidiasis. Although identification of vulvovaginal and oral candidiasis is almost always made clinically, identifying candidiasis in other disease states is a challenge.

Candidiasis may be diagnosed on sight, as is often the case with thrush or vulvovaginal infections. The diagnosis may be aided by a simple scraping and KOH preparation that will show the yeast or hyphae forms of the fungus. Culture is still the most common method of identification. *Candida* grows on most agars and is an unlikely contaminant. Unfortunately, the specificity of the culture is not matched by the sensitivity, and although the blood culture remains important, results can be misleading. In patients with autopsy-proven systemic candidiasis, the rate of recovery from blood cultures was only 40% to 60%. Because of the low sensitivity and increased incidence of invasive candidiasis, enzyme-linked immunosorbent assay and polymerase chain reaction testing are becoming more popular. Antigen testing should be pursued when invasive disease is suspected or identification of a particular species of *Candida* is important, such as in organ transplantation or in recent bone graft recipients. When patients develop invasive disease, treatment should be instituted when it is suspected, not when it is confirmed.

Treatment of invasive disease is much different from treatment of mucocutaneous infection. *Candida* can infect any organ system and has become a deadly cause of sepsis. It is now one of the top five causative organisms in sepsis. *Candida* sepsis has a mortality rate of 50%. Many of these cases are nosocomial, and *Candida* is responsible for approximately 9% of all nosocomial infections. Along with immunocompromised patients, patients with burns, patients with recent abdominal surgery, newborns, and patients receiving total parental nutrition are at risk for invasive candidiasis. Traditional treatment of disseminated candidiasis has been with amphotericin B, but intravenous fluconazole was equally effective in randomized trials in neutropenic patients. The IDSA guidelines stated that either drug may be used. Patients with recent azole exposure may have developed resistant organisms, and caspofungin should be added to the initial therapy.[10] No convincing studies exist to prove the value of initial treatment of septic immunocompromised patients with antifungal agents, although multiple guidelines have suggested that septic patients who are at high risk for candidemia may benefit from empiric antifungal therapy. Less invasive forms of candidiasis are much more prevalent and are commonly seen in EDs.

Oral candidiasis may occur in healthy individuals after antibiotic use or in HIV-infected patients. Initial episodes should be treated with clotrimazole troches or nystatin. If this approach is not curative or if the condition recurs, oral azole therapy should be started. Oral fluconazole and itraconazole solutions are equivalent, and both are superior to other oral therapies. HIV-infected patients with oral thrush who complain of odynophagia or retrosternal chest pain likely have esophageal involvement and should be admitted for systemic azole therapy and culture of *Candida* to check for resistance.

Vulvovaginal candidiasis is a common diagnosis, and 50% of women have received the diagnosis by the age of 25 years. This disorder is common after antibiotic use and is more frequent in women taking oral contraceptives. Infrequently, it can be the first sign of diabetes, and anyone who is diagnosed with vulvovaginal candidiasis for the first time should have a spot blood glucose check as a screening examination. Vulvovaginal candidiasis can be diagnosed by the combination of symptoms, visual inspection of the genitals, and KOH preparation of the scraping. Although coinfection may exist, if symptoms do not resolve, further evaluation is necessary. Patients often treat vulvovaginal candidiasis with over-the-counter agents before they see the physician. If treatment has not been attempted by patients, an over-the-counter cream should be suggested as first-line therapy. When over-the-counter treatment fails, a higher-concentration prescription azole cream is second-line therapy. An alternative is single-dose oral therapy with fluconazole or itraconazole.

## SPOROTRICHOSIS

Sporotrichosis, or rose cutter's disease, is caused by the fungal saprophyte *Sporothrix schenckii.* The fungus is found in the soil of tropical and subtropical environments, but it can be present in more austere areas, especially in greenhouses. Sporotrichosis is almost always identified as the cutaneous form in healthy individuals, although it can become disseminated through the pulmonary or cutaneous forms in immunocompromised patients. Outbreaks do occur occasionally, especially when heavy colonization is found in packed sphagnum moss that is used to protect plants (e.g., saplings, rose bushes) during transportation. More common is the sporadic case seen in plant workers, such as rose cutters.

The noninvasive form of the disease is caused by inoculation from a thorn or a skin tear during plant handling. Symptoms usually occur 3 to 4 weeks after exposure, and they begin with a small, erythematous area, usually on the forearm or hand. The lesion becomes indurated and often verrucous, and then it spreads locally to cause lymph node swelling. The lesions are not painful, but they may become superinfected with skin flora. In healthy individuals, the lesions grow very slowly and may appear the same for months. The reason for physician visits is often the cosmetic appearance. In immunocompromised patients, these skin lesions may spread. Disseminated sporotrichosis causes arthritis, often of the elbow or knee, and immunocompromised patients with suggestive skin lesions and joint effusions should be evaluated for fungal joint disease. Smaller numbers of patients with disseminated disease have pulmonary involvement. Symptoms in these patients are similar to those in patients with other types of fungal pneumonia, with presenting productive cough and pleuritic chest pain. The chest radiograph is nonspecific; interstitial infiltrates, nodules, and cavitary lesions can be seen. Systemic illness causes constitutional symptoms such as fatigue, weight loss, and, uncommonly, fever.

The diagnosis is made with KOH examination of the cutaneous lesion scrapings. If a more specific diagnosis is required, or if extracutaneous disease is suspected, *S. schenckii* is easily cultured on various media, and it is identified by latex agglutination. *Sporothrix* is not considered a contaminant, and its presence signifies disease.

Treatment of the cutaneous form of the disease has traditionally been with saturated solution of potassium iodide (SSKI). Although theories exist, exactly how this solution works to combat sporotrichosis is unknown. The main problem with SSKI is the side effect profile. When used for more than a month, SSKI has a disabling effect on thyroid hormone production, especially in children. Itraconazole is more efficacious and has fewer side effects. Other azoles may also be used. Therapy is long, often lasting 3 to 4 months, and it should continue for a month after resolution of lesions. Patients with disseminated disease can also be treated with intravenous azoles.

## ZYGOMYCOSIS

*Zygomycosis* is now the preferred term for the former mucormycosis. The preference stems from the use of zygomycosis to refer to an invasive form of disease produced by any of several *Zygomycetes* organisms: *Absidia corymbifera, Rhizomucor pusillus,* and *Rhizopus arrhizus.* Zygomycosis is rare, and it is almost always diagnosed in immunocompromised patients. In these patients, zygomycosis is invasive, rapidly progressive, and usually fatal. The rhinocerebral form has a mortality rate of 80% to 90%. The severity of disease is likely related to the particular affinity this group of fungi has for blood vessels. These fungi have been termed angiotrophic because of the widespread invasive blood vessel disease. This predilection for blood vessel invasion leads to ischemia, necrosis, and emboli.

Zygomycosis exists predominantly in the rhinocerebral, pulmonary, gastrointestinal, and cutaneous systems, and it may disseminate. The different forms are witnessed in particular subgroups of immunocompromised patients. The rhinocerebral form is seen in diabetic patients, especially during diabetic ketoacidosis, and in patients receiving high-dose or long-term steroids. Patients with leukemia or neutropenia often have the pulmonary form. Organ transplant recipients represent the group with the fastest-growing incidence of disease; zygomycosis represented less than 1% of fungal disease in transplant recipients in 2001, and it now represents 20%.

Symptoms of the rhinocerebral form are insidious and consist of local pain or swelling, nasal congestion, headache, fever, or epistaxis. *Rhizomucor* leaves a distinctive black exudate, "black pus," that is a foreboding sign of disease. Pulmonary involvement causes cough, fever, and occasional hemoptysis, and it is usually diagnosed in extremely ill-appearing patients. Gastrointestinal involvement is also seen in significantly ill patients, and it causes hematochezia, nausea, and emesis, eventually leading to intestinal ischemia.

The diagnosis is made by tissue biopsy with microscopic examination and culture. Special stains are often needed to identify the organism accurately, and the laboratory must be made aware that the physician is looking for *Zygomycetes.* Culture is available, but these organisms are common laboratory contaminants and are not considered diagnostic unless serial cultures are combined with direct tissue examination. Treatment should not wait for confirmation. The high mortality rate demands that treatment be initiated when the diagnosis is considered.

Rapid treatment may still not prevent death. The mortality rate of general zygomycosis is 50%, with a mortality of 80% to 90% in the rhinocerebral form. Amphotericin B is the recommended first-line therapy because the traditional azoles are not effective for zygomycosis. Members of a newer class of extended-spectrum azoles, voriconazole and posaconazole, have achieved success in patients in whom amphotericin therapy has failed.

## MEDICATION

Antifungal therapy is the primary treatment for known or suspected fungal infections. Current therapy is transitioning from amphotericin B toward more potent forms of azole medications. Amphotericin B has been used for decades for nearly every type of fungal infection and is still recommended primarily in certain situations. Because of the many situations that call for antifungal therapy, recommending one particular drug over another is impossible. A newer generation of azole medications, the triazoles, is supplanting amphotericin. These medications, including voriconazole and fluconazole, have shown superior rates of improvement and cure compared with amphotericin B. In the most serious infections such as systemic aspergillosis and zygomycosis, voriconazole and posaconazole have been directly compared with amphotericin B and have had higher cure rates and lower side effects.[11] In less serious, but symptomatic infections, fluconazole is superior or equal to amphotericin B, with a dramatically lower side effect profile.

## REFERENCES

***References can be found on Expert Consult @ www.expertconsult.com.***

# Helminths, Bedbugs, Scabies, and Lice Infections 177

Sara Lary and Kathleen J. Clem

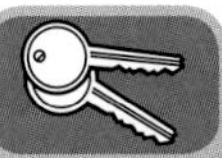

**KEY POINTS**

- Immigration and travel continue to increase the parasitic diseases seen in emergency departments.
- Consider parasitic infections in patients presenting with abdominal pain, diarrhea, unexplained fever, rash, or eosinophilia.
- History of illness, travel, occupation, recreation, and behavior is paramount in diagnosing parasitic disease.

## HELMINTHS

### EPIDEMIOLOGY

Helminth infections are estimated to affect 1 billion people in developing countries, namely, sub-Saharan Africa, Latin America, and Asia. Most commonly seen in resource-poor areas with poor sanitation, helminthiases are increasingly recognized in refugees, immigrants, rural populations, and international travelers.

### PERSPECTIVE

Parasite morbidity includes anemia, growth stunting, undernutrition, disfigurement, reduced work capacity, and increased susceptibility to other infections. Complications can include elephantiasis, blindness, gastroenterologic and urinary obstruction, and bladder cancer. Despite the widespread distribution of helminthic disease, research funding comprises less than 1% of global dollars spent.[1]

### CLASSIFICATION

Two major phyla are responsible for human disease: Nemathelminthes (roundworms) and Platyhelminthes (flatworms). Nematodes are categorized by their migration route. *Enterobius* and *Trichuris* are found intraintestinally, whereas filarial worms live in tissue and lymphatics. Platyhelminthes is further divided into two classes: cestodes, or tapeworms; and trematodes, or flukes.

## Nemathelminthes (Roundworms)

Nematodes range in length from 1 mm to up to 50 cm. Intestinal nematodes include *Ascaris, Necator,* and *Ancylostoma,* which develop in soil, whereas *Strongyloides* and *Enterobius* can be directly transmitted from person to person. With the exception of *Strongyloides,* most helminthes do not undergo replication within the host. Nematodes causing human disease include *Dracunculus* and filarial worms such as *Wucheria, Brugia,* and *Onchocerca*.

## INTESTINAL ROUNDWORMS: *ASCARIS*

### EPIDEMIOLOGY

Ascariasis infects approximately 25% of the world's population.[1,2] It is prevalent in warm countries and areas of poor sanitation and is endemic to the southern United States. Ova can remain infective for several years. They are sensitive to temperatures higher than 65° C or lower than 20° C, direct sunlight, and organic solvents. *Ascaris lumbricoides* reaches up to 40 cm and is characterized by a constricted area at the junction of the first and middle thirds. The golden brown ovoid eggs measure 60 by 40 mcm.

### TRANSMISSION AND LIFE CYCLE

Ascariasis is transmitted by ingesting mature eggs from contaminated soil or in conjunction with human feces used as fertilizer. Infection may cross into nonendemic areas through vegetable transport and tainted water. Children frequently contract the disease by playing in dirt.

Fertilized eggs become infective in soil 3 to 4 weeks after excretion. When the eggs are swallowed, the larvae hatch in the duodenum, penetrate the intestinal wall, and migrate through the portal venous system to the liver. The larvae migrate through the right side of the heart, the lungs, and into the tracheobronchial tree. Over 2 weeks, the larvae are carried up the trachea to the larynx, where they move into the esophagus and are swallowed a second time, to reach the small intestine, where they mature. Female *Ascaris* worms lay eggs 2 to 3 months after ingestion and produce up to 240,000 eggs per day. The life span of *Ascaris* is 6 months to 1 year. *Ascaris* coexists with *Trichuris trichiura* in the United States, predominantly in the Appalachian Mountains.

## PRESENTING SIGNS AND SYMPTOMS

Many patients are asymptomatic or have mild symptoms, and the infection ends after expulsion of the adult worms. Ectopic migration is possible,, and it causes severe clinical manifestations. The pulmonary larval migration occurs 9 to 12 days after egg ingestion and may manifest with cough, bloody or mucoid sputum, pleurisy, and fever.

Eosinophilia develops during this pulmonary migration and may manifest as eosinophilic pneumonitis, known as Loeffler syndrome. Chest radiographs may demonstrate small, rounded infiltrates that are transient and usually resolve after several weeks. Loeffler syndrome is seen mainly in ascariasis, but it also may occur in other parasitic infections such as hookworm infestation and strongyloidiasis. Allergic reaction can occur with reinfection. Two to 3 months after ingestion, the parasite matures in the small intestine and can cause abdominal pain, nausea, vomiting, anorexia, diarrhea, constipation, volvulus, or intussusception. Biliary obstruction and intestinal inflammation can manifest as an acute surgical abdomen, mimicking acute appendicitis or cholecystitis. Liver abscesses and pancreatitis are possible when the female worm migrates up the common bile duct. Protein malnutrition and intestinal obstruction are more likely to occur in heavily infected children rather than in adults.

## DIAGNOSIS AND MEDICAL DECISION MAKING

The diagnosis can be made from the passage of worms in the stool or by finding eggs in the feces. A single stool specimen sent for ova and parasite examination is usually sufficient. As the worm transverses the esophagus, it may be coughed out. In eosinophilic pneumonitis, larvae may be isolated from sputum or gastric aspirate.

Gastrointestinal radiographic examination may visualize adult worms on contrast studies, ultrasound scans of the pancreatic-biliary system, plain abdominal films, and endoscopic retrograde cholangiopancreatography (ERCP). ERCP can be therapeutic in extracting worms. Serologic antibody tests include complement fixation, precipitin, agar gel diffusion, immunoelectrophoresis, and the radioallergosorbent test.

# INTESTINAL ROUNDWORMS: *NECATOR* AND *ANCYLOSTOMA* (HOOKWORMS)

## EPIDEMIOLOGY

Hookworm infestations of *Ancylostoma duodenale* prevail in southern Europe, northern Asia, and North Africa, whereas *Necator americanus* is the main species affecting the Western Hemisphere and equatorial Africa. Worldwide, 1 billion persons are believed to be infected with hookworms.[3] The frequency of infection is a general indication of the local level of hygiene and sanitation. Disease burden from hookworms results in iron-deficiency anemia and hypoproteinemia.

## TRANSMISSION AND LIFE CYCLE

Hookworm infection is contracted by penetration of the skin or oral mucosa by filariform larvae. Persons who walk barefoot on contaminated soil or who eat contaminated vegetables become infected. Transplacental infection and transmammary infection are also possible. Eggs are passed in the stools to the soil, where they hatch into rhabditiform larvae that develop into filariform larvae. The larvae penetrate the skin or mucosa directly and reach the alveoli through the circulation. The larvae then ascend the airway, enter the esophagus, are swallowed, and reach the small intestine, where they mature.

Adult worms use hooks to attach to the intestinal mucosa, and they suck blood directly from the host. The time frame from skin invasion to egg appearance is 6 to 8 weeks. *Ancylostoma* adults live on average for 6 to 8 years, and the life span of *Necator* ranges from 2 to 5 years, but both species of worms can survive for more than a decade.

## PRESENTING SIGNS AND SYMPTOMS

Presentation includes rash, cough, low-grade fever, abdominal pain, diarrhea, generalized weakness, weight loss, heme-positive stools, and eosinophilia. Early larval invasion of the skin causes pruritus and erythematous maculopapular or vesicular dermatitis, known as "ground itch." Sensitized hosts may have serpiginous tracts as larvae migrate through the subcutaneous tissue, similar to cutaneous larva migrans.

Transient pneumonitis can occur as larvae travel through the lungs. Epigastric pain, inflammatory diarrhea, and eosinophilia may develop with early intestinal invasion. Loss of plasma protein results from malabsorption and increased intestinal permeability and may cause anasarca.

Chronic hookworm infection leads to iron deficiency. In malnourished patients, infection can cause severe anemia and growth delay. Infection in pregnancy may lead to low fetal birth weights and birth defects. Pica and geophagy are observed in infected children.

## DIAGNOSIS AND MEDICAL DECISION MAKING

Multiple stool specimens for ova and parasite studies or concentration techniques may be necessary to confirm the diagnosis. The parasite burden may be estimated using the Beaver stool or Kato 50 adult slide smear method. The polymerase chain reaction (PCR) technique can identify a hookworm from a single egg.

Hookworm infection may be confused with pneumonia, anemia, and malnutrition from other causes. Hypochromic microcytic anemia, coupled with eosinophilia or hypoproteinemia, indicates a heavy infection.

## TREATMENT

Oral iron supplementation is usually sufficient to correct mild anemia, although blood transfusion may be needed to correct more severe anemia. Vaccine development is currently under way, based on canine and sheep models.[3]

# INTESTINAL ROUNDWORMS: *STRONGYLOIDES*

## EPIDEMIOLOGY

*Strongyloides stercoralis* is found in the tropics, subtropics, and in temperate areas, and it affects an estimated 55 million to 100 million persons.[4] *Strongyloides* is endemic to Southeast Asia, Latin America, the West Indies, Bangladesh, Pakistan, Africa, Spain, and the Appalachian region of the United States. *S. stercoralis* is an unusual helminth in its ability to replicate within the human host, thus resulting in continuous autoinfection. The infection is often difficult to eradicate, especially in immunocompromised hosts (**Box 177.1**). The larvae can disseminate and can cause systematic disease and mortality.

## TRANSMISSION AND LIFE CYCLE

In addition to replication within the human host, *Strongyloides* can survive in a free-living cycle in soil. The rhabditiform larvae can directly transform into infective filariform larvae or a free-living soil form. The filariform larvae penetrate skin or mucosa, travel to the alveoli, and ascend the airway. The larvae are then swallowed and reach the small intestine. The host has no adult male worms, and the 2-mm female worms reproduce by parthenogenesis, hatching eggs within the intestinal mucosa. Rhabditiform larvae migrate to the intestinal lumen and either pass into the feces or directly transform into filariform larvae and cause autologous reinfection.

**BOX 177.1 Strongyloidiasis in the Immunocompromised Patient**

Immunocompromised hosts are at risk for hyperinfection syndromes, in which filariform larvae cause colitis, malabsorption, ulcerative enteritis, ileus, systemic dissemination, gram-negative sepsis, meningitis, pneumonia, intraabdominal abscess, or acute respiratory distress syndrome. Immunosuppressive therapy, especially glucocorticoids, should be avoided in patients suspected to have *Strongyloides* infection because hyperinfection and iatrogenically caused fatal outcomes may result. Additional risk factors for hyperinfection and disseminated strongyloidiasis include infection with human T-cell lymphotropic virus-1, solid organ transplantation, hematologic malignant disease, hypogammaglobulinemia, uremia, malnutrition, diabetes mellitus, and chronic alcohol consumption.[4] *Strongyloides* does not appear to be a common opportunistic pathogen in human immunodeficiency virus (HIV)–positive patients, and the risk of hyperinfection is not increased with HIV coinfection.[4]

## PRESENTING SIGNS AND SYMPTOMS

Patients may be asymptomatic or have mild abdominal discomfort, cough, dyspnea, wheezing, and peripheral eosinophilia. Ten percent of patients present with wheezing as their primary complaint.[5] If adult worms invade the duodenojejunal mucosa, the symptoms can mimic those of peptic ulcer disease, and small bowel obstruction may occur.

Fluctuating eosinophilia is a common finding. Strongyloidiasis may also manifest with urticaria, usually recurrent along the buttocks and wrists. These urticarial serpiginous eruptions are called larva currens, and they are pathognomonic findings.

## DIAGNOSIS AND MEDICAL DECISION MAKING

Stool examinations need to be repeated 3 to 5 times. An immunosorbent assay for aspiration or biopsy of duodenojejunal contents is also available. Serum immunoglobulin G (IgG) antibodies can be detected with enzyme-linked immunosorbent assay (ELISA). In disseminated strongyloidiasis, sputum, bronchoalveolar lavage samples, and surgical drainage fluids should be examined for larvae. Eosinophilia greater than 5% or a finding of more than 400 eosinophils/microliter is consistent with *Strongyloides* infection.[5]

Strongyloidiasis can mimic gastroenteritis, gastritis, colitis, irritable bowel syndrome, asthma, and pneumonia. It may also cause meningitis or sepsis.

## TREATMENT

Strongyloidiasis must be treated to avoid hyperinfection. In patients coinfected with human T-cell lymphotropic virus-1 (HTLV-1), treatment failures are common. A regimen of ivermectin plus thiabendazole or ivermectin plus albendazole is recommended for patients with disseminated disease.

# INTESTINAL ROUNDWORMS: *ENTEROBIUS* (PINWORMS)

## EPIDEMIOLOGY

Enterobiasis is worldwide in distribution and is commonly found in young children. Pinworms are most common in developed countries with temperate or colder climates. The adult worms are 6 to 12 mm in length and 0.3 to 0.5 mm in diameter. The eggs are 50 by 25 mcm and are asymmetrically flattened on one side.

## TRANSMISSION AND LIFE CYCLE

Eggs are ingested orally, hatch in the stomach, and pass through to the intestine, where they invade the glandular crypts. The adult worms live in the cecum and appendix and survive for approximately 2 months. Whether pinworms cause appendicitis is not known. The female pinworm migrates out through the rectum and onto the perianal skin to deposit her eggs. Rarely, the worms invade the abdominal cavity and cause threadworm granulomas of the liver, ovary, kidney, spleen, and lung. Transmission of pinworms occurs by direct anus-to-mouth spread from contact with an infected person. It can also be caused by airborne eggs that are shaken free from contaminated clothing or bed linens. Autoinfection is common because patients scratch the pruritic anal area and then bite their nails or put their fingers in their mouth. The whole cycle takes 2 to 4 weeks.

## PRESENTING SIGNS AND SYMPTOMS

Pruritus ani is the main symptom and varies from mild itching to acute pain, generally worse at night. Pinworm disease is essentially an allergic reaction to the release of eggs and other secreted materials from the gravid female. Associated scratching and excoriation can cause secondary bacterial infection. Vulvitis can occur when pinworms enter the vulva and cause a mucoid discharge with pruritus vulvae. Insomnia, restlessness, loss of appetite, weight loss, irritability, and enuresis may be associated with pinworm infection.

## DIAGNOSIS AND MEDICAL DECISION MAKING

The eggs are rarely seen in the feces, but they are observed when the adult worms migrate to the anus or vulvar area, particularly at night. The "Scotch tape test" is done by pressing a piece of clear sticky tape against the perianal region and then mounting the tape on a slide. The eggs are identified with light microscopy. Patients usually have no eosinophilia or associated anemia.

## TREATMENT

The entire family is treated simultaneously, to avoid reinfection. All bedding and contaminated clothing should be washed. Fingernails should be kept short. Frequent hand washing and bathing may reduce reinfection. Eradication of the parasite may necessitate repeated courses of treatment.

# TISSUE NEMATODES: *TRICHINELLA*

## EPIDEMIOLOGY

Trichinosis has a worldwide distribution. Eight species of *Trichinella* infect humans. *Trichinella spiralis* and *Trichinella pseudospiralis* are found worldwide. *Trichinella nativa* is found in the Arctic; *Trichinella nelsoni* occurs in eastern Africa; *Trichinella britovi* is found in Europe, Asia, and western Africa; and *Trichinella murrelli* occurs in North America. *Trichinella papuae* and *Trichinella zimbabwensis* have also been identified. Human infection results from ingestion of poorly cooked infected meat, particularly pork. Cattle, horse, dog, and wild game meat are also potential sources.

## TRANSMISSION AND LIFE CYCLE

The encysted larvae are released from their capsule by digestive enzymes in the intestine. The larvae then penetrate the intestinal mucosa and mature into adults. After mating, the male worms die, and the female worms discharge larvae to the tissues. After travelling through the circulation, the larvae encyst in muscle and may calcify. Cysts can be seen in the diaphragm, masseter and intercostal muscles, musculature of the larynx, tongue, eye, and heart, and the brain.

The main methods of infection prevention are thorough cooking and regular meat inspection. *Trichinella* larvae in meat may be killed by heating to a temperature of 77° C or freezing to 15° C for 3 weeks. Both encysted and free *Trichinella* larvae remain viable for years.

## PRESENTING SIGNS AND SYMPTOMS

The presenting symptoms depend on the level of infection and the location of the larvae. Two phases are recognized: intestinal and muscular. Enteric invasion may cause diarrhea, fever, nausea, vomiting, and abdominal pain during the first week of infection and is often confused with food poisoning. During the second week, the larvae migrate into the muscles and cause hypersensitivity reactions with fever, eosinophilia, rash, headache, cough, and myalgias.

Cardinal clinical findings of trichinellosis include cachexia, edema, splinter hemorrhages, dehydration, ongoing fever, and pruritus. Myocarditis, encephalitis, nephritis, congestive heart failure, pneumonitis, hemiplegia, severe pain, psychiatric disturbances, and epilepsy may develop and lead to death.

## DIAGNOSIS AND MEDICAL DECISION MAKING

Eosinophilia is a hallmark of trichinellosis. No relationship exists between the level of eosinophilia and the clinical course of disease. Other laboratory manifestations of trichinosis include leukocytosis and elevated creatine phosphokinase, lactate dehydrogenase, and myokinase levels. The diagnosis is made by identification of larvae in blood or tissue. Serologic assays are available, including ELISA, indirect immunofluorescence, and latex agglutination. The circulating antibody can be detected by serologic tests between 2 and 4 weeks after infection. Immunofluorescence is positive 2 to 3 weeks after infection. If serologic test results are equivocal, larvae may be found in muscle by trichinoscopy. This procedure is performed during the muscular phase approximately 7 days from onset of symptoms with samples taken from the deltoid, biceps, gastrocnemius, or pectoralis major muscle.

Trichinosis resembles many conditions: typhoid, encephalitis, myositis, and tetanus. Trichinosis may also be confused with collagen disorders such as periarteritis nodosa and rheumatoid arthritis.

### TREATMENT

For light infections, supportive therapy with analgesics, rest, and antipyretics usually suffices. Patients with severe hypersensitivity reactions such as myositis, myocarditis, and central nervous system (CNS) disease may benefit from corticosteroids tapered over 2 to 3 weeks. Corticosteroids are not indicated for mild disease because the use of these agents can increase the number of circulating larvae.

## TISSUE NEMATODES: FILARIA

### EPIDEMIOLOGY

Filarial nematodes are estimated to infect 170 million persons.[1] Four main species cause most serious infections: *Wucheria bancrofti, Brugia malayi, Onchocerca volvulus,* and *Loa loa. W. bancrofti* is found in Africa, South America, Asia, the Pacific islands, and the Caribbean. *Brugia* species are found mainly in Southeast Asia, Asia, and Indonesia.

### TRANSMISSION AND LIFE CYCLE

Mosquitoes transmit infective *Wucheria* and *Brugia* larvae during a blood meal. *Onochocerca* and *Loa loa* larvae are carried by the black and tabanid flies, respectively. The larvae mature into adults that remain alive in the lymphatics or subcutaneous tissues for years. Microfilariae are produced by the adult worms, which are ingested by mosquitoes and develop into infective larvae over a period of weeks.

### PRESENTING SIGNS AND SYMPTOMS

Most infected persons remain asymptomatic, and few progress to acute or chronic disease. Common presentations include hydrocele, adenolymphangitis, microscopic hematuria and proteinuria, and lymphangiectasia. Acute adenolymphangitis is a form of retrograde lymphangitis accompanied with high fevers, lymphadenitis, and often thrombophlebitis.

*W. bancrofti* infection involves the genital lymphatics, and it often manifests with epididymitis and scrotal pain. Travelers to endemic regions may develop acute edema, urticaria, and local lymphadenitis, especially of the femoral, axillary, inguinal, or epitrochlear lymph nodes.

### DIAGNOSIS AND MEDICAL DECISION MAKING

Parasite detection is key for definitive diagnosis. Blood and hydrocele fluid may demonstrate microfilariae, although blood draws should be timed based on the periodicity of the endemic species suspected. ELISA and rapid-format immunochromatographic card tests are available for *W. bancrofti* antigens. In addition, PCR assays for *W. bancrofti* and *Brugia* DNA are available.

High-frequency ultrasound with Doppler imaging of the breast and scrotum may reveal dilated lymphatics containing moving adult worms, known as the filarial dance sign. The broad cross-reactivity of filarial antigens with other helminths often confounds the serologic test results. In addition, endemic populations may become sensitized through mosquito exposure without actual infection.

### TREATMENT

*Wolbachia* bacterial endosymbionts are present in most filarial worms, with the exception of *L. loa.* When patients are treated with diethylcarbamazine, a hypersensitivity reaction to the intracellular *Wolbachia* may occur and may progress to encephalopathy. Diehtylcarbamazine should not be used as treatment, except for *Loa loa*, because the hypersensitivity reaction can lead to hypotension or angioedema. Chemotherapy and vaccine development directed against *Wolbachia* are under investigation.[6]

## TISSUE NEMATODES: *ONCHOCERCA*

### EPIDEMIOLOGY

*O. volvulus* is responsible for river blindness, a leading cause of infectious blindness in Africa, South America, and the Middle East.

### TRANSMISSION AND LIFE CYCLE

Blackfly vectors bite humans and transmit larvae into the skin. Nodules form in a few months to years, and the developed adults release microfilariae into the dermis. Adult worms can live for a decade or two.

### PRESENTING SIGNS AND SYMPTOMS

Onchocerciasis results from inflammatory reactions to the microfilaria that can affect skin, eyes, and lymph nodes. An intensely pruritic papular rash is common. Atrophy and pigmentation changes can occur in long-term infection. Subcutaneous nodules, or onchocercomas, contain adult worms and are common over bony prominences. Conjunctivitis, uveitis, chorioretinitis, and optic atrophy result from ongoing optic inflammation; neovascularization and scarring of the cornea lead to corneal opacity and eventual blindness. Lymphadenopathy is also common.

### DIAGNOSIS AND MEDICAL DECISION MAKING

The removal of an adult worm from onchocercomas or of microfilariae from skin snips leads to the definitive diagnosis. The Mazzotti test, involving a small dose of diethylcarbamazine (50 mg/kg) and subsequent observation for worsening rash or pruritus, can aid in diagnosis. Topical diethylcarbamazine (10% in lotion) can be applied to the skin as a localized Mazotti test; it is considered safer than an oral test. If there are *Onchocerca microfilariae* present in the ocular chamber, diethylcarbamazine treatment can lead to ocular damage.

# Platyhelminthes (Flatworms)

The cestodes, or tapeworms, are segmented. Humans serve as intermediate hosts for *Taenia solium, Echinococcus, Hymenolepis, Sparganosis, Coenurosis,* and *Dipylidiasis* species. *Taenia saginata* and *Diphyllobothrium* also can infect humans, although these species cannot complete their life cycle within human hosts. Tapeworm eggs are transmitted by the fecal-oral route and are endemic in areas with poor sanitation and livestock.

## CESTODE: *TAENIA SOLIUM* (PORK TAPEWORM)

### EPIDEMIOLOGY

*Taenia* has a worldwide distribution and is highly endemic in Latin America, Africa, Eastern Europe, Central and South Asia, and the Middle East.[7] Approximately 45 *Taenia* species and subspecies are currently recognized.[8] *T. solium* infection of the CNS, or neurocysticercosis, is a leading cause of acquired epilepsy and may result in more than 50,000 deaths annually.[9]

The most distinctive feature of *Taenia* infection is that humans can serve as both the definitive host and the intermediary host. When humans are infected by the larval stage, the infection is known as cysticercosis. Infection with the adult tapeworm is associated with taeniasis. For *T. saginata* and *T. solium,* humans serve as the final obligatory host. Infection is uncommon in infants and vegetarians.

### TRANSMISSION AND LIFE CYCLE

Humans acquire the infection by ingestion of undercooked pork containing cysticerci (larval cysts). The cysts contain protoscolices. After ingestion, the protoscolices are released and attach to the intestinal wall. Each protoscolex can become an adult tapeworm. The head of the worm generally resides in the jejunum. Adult worms contain 800 to 900 proglottids. Maturation occurs over 2 to 4 months. The mature proglottids are hermaphroditic, become gravid, and contain 1000 to 2000 eggs. These eggs are passed in the stool. Pigs acquire the infection from soil contaminated with human feces, and then larvae are activated, penetrate tissues, and encyst within 2 to 3 months.

### PRESENTING SIGNS AND SYMPTOMS

Most patients are infected by a single worm. The symptoms are usually mild, or the patient may be asymptomatic. Because tapeworms can survive for years in an otherwise healthy host, symptomatic patients may have a protracted clinical course. Complaints are nonspecific and include indigestion, anorexia, diarrhea, constipation, and vague abdominal pain.

Severe signs and symptoms may include intestinal obstruction, appendicitis, and perforation. The worms occasionally migrate to the biliary system, respiratory tract, uterine cavity, or nasopharynx. If cysts are in the CNS, the patient may present with seizures, meningitis, stroke, or signs of increased intracranial pressure. Approximately 30% of patients with neurocysticercosis have residual calcification, and less than 20% have seizures.[7] Parasite invasion of the ventricles can result in obstructive hydrocephalus. Extraparenchymal disease leads to a worse prognosis, secondary to invasive cyst growth and increased cerebrospinal fluid (CSF) debris and inflammation.[7] Classic calcified lesions from prior infections are often seen on computed tomography (CT) or magnetic resonance imaging (MRI).

### DIAGNOSIS AND MEDICAL DECISION MAKING

Infection is confirmed by finding the eggs or proglottids in the feces. The mobile proglottids often move with discharge, and some patients may feel their passage. Because the eggs are often eliminated intermittently, several stool specimens may need to be obtained. ELISA, DNA probes, and co-proantigen assays are available. The enzyme-linked immunoelectrotransfer blot (EITB) assay is quite specific and sensitive.

Neurocysticercosis is usually diagnosed by the characteristic CNS cystic lesions, which are nodular calcifications 5 to 20 mm in diameter, with or without ring enhancement on CT or MRI. Although calcified lesions are identified more easily on CT, MRI is more sensitive for ring enhancement and cystic lesions. The CSF may show pleocytosis, elevated protein, and occasionally low glucose concentrations.

### TREATMENT

Calcified cysts do not warrant antiparasitic therapy.[10] Patients with seizures may be treated with antiepileptics, and occasionally endoscopic surgery or ventriculoperitoneal shunting is necessary to relieve obstructive hydrocephalus. Corticosteroids may help mitigate cerebrovascular complications and may be used in the treatment of cysticercotic encephalitis.

## CESTODE: *ECHINOCOCCUS*

### EPIDEMIOLOGY

Echinococcosis is caused by the larval invasion of *Echinococcus granulosus, Echinococcus multilocularis,* and *Echinococcus vogeli.* These cestodes are ubiquitous, with particularly heavy endemicity in Central Asia, the Mediterranean, the Middle East, South America, and eastern Africa. *E. multilocularis* is confined to the Northern Hemisphere. *E. granulosus* causes cystic echinococcosis, with 3 million cases, and *E. multilocularis* is responsible for the alveolar variant, with half a million cases.[11] Canines are the definitive hosts and pass echinococcal eggs in feces. Intermediate mammalian hosts then ingest the eggs, and eventually cysts develop. The cycle is continued as canines eat infected meat.

## TRANSMISSION AND LIFE CYCLE

*E. granulosus* has three proglottids, one of which is gravid and releases eggs. After ingestion of the parasite, embryos penetrate the intestinal mucosa and enter the portal circulation. Fluid-filled hydatid cysts are formed in organs, commonly the lungs and liver. Within these hydatid cysts, brood capsules that house new larvae develop.

## PRESENTING SIGNS AND SYMPTOMS

The cysts grow over several years, and patients are usually asymptomatic until large cyst size or encroachment causes abdominal pain, palpable masses, biliary colic, or, if in the lungs, dyspnea, cough, pleurisy, or hemoptysis. Cyst rupture may provoke an anaphylactic or allergic reaction with eosinophilia, fever, pruritus, and rash. Less commonly, the cysts can invade bone, CNS, cardiac tissue, and other intraabdominal structures.

## DIAGNOSIS AND MEDICAL DECISION MAKING

Radiographs, CT, ultrasound, and MRI can all reveal cysts. Additional testing of aspirated fluids may reveal protoscolices. In addition, immunoblotting techniques are available for serologic antigen testing.

## TREATMENT

Treatment depends on cyst size, location, and symptoms. Ultrasound staging is recommended. Percutaneous aspiration, infusion of scolicidal agents, and reaspiration (PAIR) is less invasive and is preferred over surgical removal. If cysts are superficial, honeycombed, connected to the biliary systems, or intrapulmonary, PAIR is not recommended. For complicated cysts, surgical intervention is warranted.

# CESTODE: *DIPHYLLOBOTHRIUM* (FISH TAPEWORM)

## EPIDEMIOLOGY

*Diphyllobothrium* species are estimated to infect more than 20 million people. Although an overall decline in North America, Europe, and Asia has been reported, outbreaks have occurred in Russia, Japan, South Korea, Italy, France, Switzerland, and South America.[12] *Diphyllobothrium* also enjoys a range of hosts, from humans to foxes, bears, sea birds, and other fish-eating mammals.

## TRANSMISSION AND LIFE CYCLE

The fish tapeworm, or *Diphyllobothrium latum,* holds the dubious honor for longest tapeworm known to humankind, with adult worms measuring up to 10 to 25 m. The adult tapeworms consist of 3000 to 4000 proglottids and produce up to 1 million eggs a day; they may survive for decades in the human host. Egg-laden feces enter lakes, rivers, and deltas, and the eggs hatch into embryos.

Crustaceans, usually *Cyclops* or *Diaptomus* species, ingest the free-swimming embryos, known as coracidia. The coracidia penetrate the crustacean intestinal wall and develop into a procercoid. The crustacean host is eaten by a freshwater or marine fish, and additional development takes place. The procercoid larva migrates into fish tissue and organs and sometimes encysts. Multiple predatory fish, such as perch, pike, burbot, walleye, snook, Alaska blackfish, salmon, whitefish, trout, and Japanese anchovy have been implicated as hosts.[12] After the host ingests a meal of undercooked or raw fish, *Diphyllobothrium* matures in the human gastrointestinal tract within a few weeks.

## PRESENTING SIGNS AND SYMPTOMS

Most *Diphyllobothrium* infections are asymptomatic or are characterized by mild gastrointestinal upset. Acute abdominal pain, cholecystitis, cholangitis, and intestinal obstruction are rare. Approximately 2% of infected persons demonstrate megaloblastic anemia secondary to tapeworm absorption of vitamin $B_{12}$. In older patients and in patients with chronic infections, neurologic manifestations of vitamin $B_{12}$ deficiency may arise.

## DIAGNOSIS AND MEDICAL DECISION MAKING

Stool examination reveals eggs and segment chains. After ingestion by the human host, adult worms usually begin producing eggs within 15 to 45 days, so results of early stool studies may be negative.

## TREATMENT

Intraduodenal Gastrografin has been used to remove large cestodes. Heating fish to 54° C for 5 minutes or freezing to −18° C for 24 hours kills *Diphyllobothrium.* Placing fish in a 12% brine solution kills the eggs.[12]

# TREMATODA (FLUKES)

## EPIDEMIOLOGY

Trematodes represent a diverse group of flatworms, or flukes, that cause human infection through invasion of blood, intestines, biliary system, and lungs. *Schistosoma* is perhaps the best known of the flukes. *Clonorchis* and *Opisthorchis* species cause biliary inflammation and obstruction and predispose patients to cholangiocarcinoma. *Paragonimus* and *Fasciolopsis* species cause granulomatous disease in the pulmonary and intestinal systems, respectively.

## TRANSMISSION AND LIFE CYCLE

The life cycle of most trematodes involves a mammalian definitive host and intermediate snail hosts. Sexual reproduction occurs in the mammalian host, with subsequent asexual reproduction in snail hosts. Ova are excreted in feces or sputum, and they become miracidia that then undergo asexual reproduction in often multiple intermediate hosts. Free-living cercariae larvae and encysted metacercariae infect the definitive host. Transmission to humans is through ingestion or direct dermal penetration.

# TREMATODA: *SCHISTOSOMA*

## EPIDEMIOLOGY

Human schistosomiasis, also known as bilharziasis, remains a serious health threat in Africa, Southeast Asia, South America, and the Middle East.[1] Schistosomiasis is a complex of acute and chronic parasitic infections caused by digenetic blood nematodes. Infections with *Schistosoma haematobium* (bladder fluke), *Schistosoma mansoni, Schistosoma japonicum, Schistosoma mekongi,* and *Schistosoma intercalatum* (intestinal flukes) cause illness in humans. Schistosomes have been documented to infect humans for thousands of years and are associated with agricultural civilizations of the great river valleys. Hematuria, most likely caused by *S. haematobium,* occurred in ancient Egypt and Mesopotamia.[13]

## TRANSMISSION AND LIFE CYCLE

The adult fluke lays eggs that leave the definitive host through the feces or urine, depending on the species and the host location. A freshwater species of snail is required as an intermediate host for each species of fluke. In general, the miracidium (larval stage) emerges from the egg in freshwater, enters the snail host, and then undergoes multiplication. The cercaria (final larval state) leaves the snail.

These larvae penetrate the tissues of humans through contact in infested freshwater. The cercaria then loses its tail, becomes a schistosomulum, and migrates to blood vessels to become an adult. Adults migrate into intestinal veins and vesical veins *(S. haematobium)* and lay eggs in the vasculature. The ova transmigrate through the lumen and are voided in feces or urine. Ova that reach freshwater complete the life cycle in intermediate hosts.

## SIGNS AND SYMPTOMS

Patients may be asymptomatic initially, or they may show mild pruritic maculopapular skin lesions within hours to days after exposure to cercariae. Four to 8 weeks after invasion, some patients may present with fever, eosinophilia, lymphadenopathy, and hepatosplenomegaly. Acute schistosomiasis or Katayama fever resembles serum sickness, and it appears to be related to antigen excess during sexual maturation of the parasite. It is associated with a mortality rate of up to 25%.[13]

Chronic schistosomiasis persisting for months to years after primary exposure is more common. A granulomatous reaction to *Schistosoma* eggs, coupled with host cell–mediated inflammatory response lead to organomegaly and obstruction. Patients may present with abdominal pain, hematemesis, ascites, hematuria, dysuria, vulvar or perianal lesions, dyspnea on exertion, fatigue, cough, chest pain, or seizures, depending on the site of infection and the involvement of the body system.

Eggs induce an immune response as they travel to the liver, intestine, bladder, and rarely, to the brain or spinal cord. Granuloma formation in the bowel wall with *S. mansoni* or *S. japonicum* may cause bloody diarrhea, cramping, and colonic polyposis. *Schistosoma* can also cause pulmonary and CNS disease, with sequelae including pulmonary hypertension, cor pulmonale, epilepsy, and transverse myelitis.[13]

Egg retention and granuloma formation in the urinary tract with *S. haematobium* can lead to hematuria, urinary tract infections, glomerulonephritis, obstructive uropathy, dysuria, and bladder polyps and ulcerations. *S. haematobium* is considered a carcinogen in squamous cell bladder cancer.[13]

## DIAGNOSIS AND MEDICAL DECISION MAKING

Geographic history and clinical presentation are key considerations in diagnosing schistosomiasis. The diagnosis can also be aided by recovery of eggs in feces or urine, but Kato thick smear microscopy must be ordered specifically. Hatching assays on fresh stool specimens help to distinguish active from treated infection. Dead eggs may be shed for up to a year. Peripheral eosinophilia supports the diagnosis. Gross and microscopic hematuria is common in patients infected by *S. haematobium.*

Imaging techniques such as ultrasonography, echocardiography, and radiography can help pinpoint organ system involvement. ELISA testing is available and confirms past exposure, although it cannot discriminate between acute and chronic infection. The EITB test also yields good results. In some cases, colonic biopsy is necessary to visualize parasite eggs in the bowel wall.

Acute schistosomiasis should be suspected in patients recently returning from endemic areas who present with fever, headache, malaise, arthralgias or myalgias, bloody diarrhea, and right upper quadrant abdominal pain, especially if they have a history of freshwater swimming or bathing.

**BOX 177.2 Helminth Immunomodulation**

"The hygiene hypothesis suggests that microbes and worms are important for shaping and tuning the development and function of our immune system."[18]

As developed countries experience better sanitation and reduced exposure to infectious disease agents, the immune system may be left "uneducated" and may develops "incorrect" or uncontrolled inflammation responses: rhinitis, atopic dermatitis, asthma, inflammatory bowel disease, multiple sclerosis, and type 1 diabetes mellitus.[17] Helminth infections as therapies have been observed to decrease colitis in both murine and human models. A few studies have shown benefit from *Trichuris* infection in patients with inflammatory bowel disease; similar results have been reported in patients with multiple sclerosis.[14,16-18] Much more research is needed to characterize human-helminth immunomodulatory dynamics. Genetics and environment play important roles.

## TREATMENT

Early treatment with cidal drugs may exacerbate Katayama fever, and concomitant steroid therapy is recommended. Patients with long-term infection may require procedures such as bladder stents, endoscopic treatment, or surgery.

Helminths cause a large burden of disease, yet their coevolution with humans and adaptation to our immune defenses may be beneficial (**Box 177.2**). Numerous epidemiologic and experimental studies have noted the low prevalence of allergy and autoimmune disease among populations with chronic helminth infections. Helminth infections generally cause a skewed type 1 helper T-cell (Th2) response. The Th1 arm of the immune system is often suppressed or downregulated. Populations with chronic helminthiases may not clear microbial infections adequately or respond optimally to vaccination.[14,15] *Schistosoma* and *Onchocerca* infections appear to decrease tetanus and tuberculosis vaccine efficacy, and *Ascaris* infection similarly dampens the immune response to *Mycoplasma* pneumonia vaccination.[16]

# Bedbugs

## EPIDEMIOLOGY

Bedbugs, or cimicids, are insects that have plagued humankind since ancient Egypt.[19] These ectoparasites are found in temperate and tropical regions worldwide, and global infestations are increasing. Much media attention has been paid to bedbugs, and millions of dollars have been spent in the hospitality and private sectors. Travelers, backpackers, immigrants, guest workers, the homeless, and persons sharing close quarters, such as military barracks and dormitories, are potential hosts and vectors.

## TRANSMISSION AND LIFE CYCLE

Cimicids are wingless, obligate hematophages. Both sexes require blood meals. *Cimex lectularius* and *Cimex hemipterus* are the two species that prefer human hosts. Adults are oval, flat, approximately 5 mm in length, and reddish brown. Adults can survive for up to 12 months, perhaps even 2 years, without feeding.[20] Nymphs tend to be lighter in color. Bedbugs usually conceal themselves during the day, often in bedding, carpet, wallpaper, or any crevice, usually within 1 to 2 m of a host.

## PRESENTING SIGNS AND SYMPTOMS

Most persons bitten by bedbugs are asymptomatic, perhaps bearing miniscule puncture wounds to exposed extremities, face, and neck. Those who seek medical attention commonly present with 2- to 5-mm pruritic maculopapular, erythematous lesions at bite sites. If not excoriated or superinfected, these lesions resolve spontaneously within a week. Occasionally, some patients experience local popular rashes or diffuse urticaria. Bullous rashes, folliculitis, cellulitis, and eczematoid dermatitis may develop after a few days.

Anaphylaxis and asthma have also been reported, and they may be related to increased exposure with subsequent feedings.[21] Saliva of bedbugs contains a protein, nitrophorin, that may be responsible for cutaneous reactions.[21] Beyond the physical irritation, bedbugs are responsible for anxiety, stigma, and insomnia.

## TREATMENT

Topical antipruritics such as paroxime, doxepin, or corticosteroids may alleviate dermal irritation. Oral antibiotics may be necessary if lesions become secondarily infected by skin flora. For anaphylactic and urticarial reactions, supportive therapy including epinephrine, antihistamines, and corticosteroids is warranted. Much speculation remains about bedbugs as vectors for multiple diseases. Although human immunodeficiency virus (HIV) can be detected in bedbugs after a concentrated blood meal days later, no viral replication has been found, nor has virus been detected in the feces. Similarly, hepatitis B virus antigen has also been detected weeks after a feeding, but no internal replication has been observed.[21] Concern about insecticide resistance is widespread.[21,22]

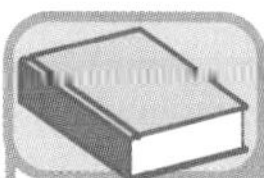

**PATIENT TEACHING TIPS**

Inspect bedding carefully. Signs of bedbugs can be seen on infested mattresses and in bed frames.

Affected areas should be thoroughly cleaned. Bedding, infested furniture, and carpets should be placed in airtight plastic bags, steam cleaned, or thrown away.

Plastic mattress covers can be placed to prevent nocturnal emergence of the insects.

# Scabies

## EPIDEMIOLOGY

Scabies is a common parasitic infection caused by the mite *Sarcoptes scabiei* var. *hominis,* an arthropod of the order Acarina. Worldwide prevalence is estimated at 300 million.[23] Scabies is endemic in sub-Saharan Africa, South and Central America, India, the South Pacific, and among Aboriginal communities in Australia. Additionally, infestations are sporadic in industrial countries. Overcrowding, poor hygiene and poor nutrition, poverty, war, and dementia are predisposing factors. Despite the stigma of scabies as an infection of the poor, scabies affects all ethnic and socioeconomic groups.

## TRANSMISSION AND LIFE CYCLE

These obligate parasites complete their entire life cycle on humans. Scabies mites measure 0.2 to 0.5 mm in length, naked to the human eye. Only the female mite burrows into the skin, where the mite tunnels at a rate of 2 mm/day. The parasite can survive approximately 36 hours away from the human host. Each mite lays approximately 10 to 25 eggs and then dies in the stratum granulosum. Larvae hatch in 3 to 4 days, molt, then leave the burrow for the surface, copulate, and continue the cycle. Maturation is complete in 15 days.

The number of mites infesting a person usually ranges from 5 to 15, although thousands may be present in patients with crusted scabies. Symptoms of infestation usually manifest 3 to 6 weeks after the mite is acquired, but they may appear as soon as 1 day after the mite is acquired in cases of reinfestation, as a result of a hypersensitivity reaction. The primary mode of transmission is direct skin-to-skin contact. Investigators estimate that a 15- to 20-minute encounter is sufficient to transmit the mite. Transmission through shared clothing or other objects is rare, but it may occur with crusted scabies. Mites crawl at a rate of 2.5 cm/minute on human skin. The greater the parasite load, the greater is the chance of transmission. Sexual transmission also occurs. Immunocompromised hosts, including those who are HIV positive, HTLV-1 positive, undergoing immunosuppressant therapies, and malnourished, are at higher risk for developing crusted (Norwegian) scabies.

## SIGNS AND SYMPTOMS

Intense, intractable, pruritic dermatitis with erythematous papulovesicular lesions characterize scabies infections. The itch is usually worse at night or after a hot shower. Skin burrows, gray serpiginous lines 1 to 10 mm in length, are pathognomonic findings. In adults, burrows and nodules are usually found in interdigital web spaces, axillary folds, extremities, buttocks, nipples, and genitals. Very young children and immunocompromised persons may have facial and neck lesions. Lesions to palms and soles, pinkish brown nodules, and acral pustules are unique to infested infants.

Crusted, or Norwegian, scabies is usually confined to immunocompromised, older, cognitively impaired, and institutionalized patients. Presumably, the lack of scratching may allow superinfection to occur.[24] Crusted scabies represents a hyperinfection with thousands to millions of mites present. The lesions appear hyperkeratotic, similar to psoriatic papules, and can cover large areas of the scalp, face, neck, and extremities. Skin crusts may be loose or adherent, flaky or thick. Nail involvement is common with crusted scabies, as are eczematization and impetigo. Large flakes of epidermis slough off, carrying mites and furthering transmission. In crusted scabies, high levels of IgE and IgG and peripheral eosinophilia are present.[24]

Nodular scabies manifests with pruritic, violaceous nodules localized to the groin, axilla, and male genitalia. These nodules may represent a variant hypersensitivity reaction because mites are not found within them. Rarely, bullous lesions may occur with scabies, perhaps because of superinfection with *Staphylococcus.* Pyodermas, or bacterial skin infections, may be secondary to scabies infections, especially in the tropics.[25]

## DIAGNOSIS AND MEDICAL DECISION MAKING

The diagnosis is primarily clinical. Patients complain of generalized and intense pruritus, usually sparing the face and head. Symptoms are often out of proportion to examination findings. The definitive diagnosis is made by identification of mites, eggs, or mite fecaliths on microscopic evaluation of burrow scrapings. Obtaining multiple superficial skin samples from characteristic lesions is helpful. This is done by gently scraping laterally across the skin with a scalpel. If the number of mites is low, as is commonly the case in classic scabies, mites may not be identified. Skin biopsy may also be performed.

Enhanced microscopy techniques, such as epiluminescence microscopy and noncomputed dermoscopy, may also identify scabies products in burrows. ELISA and PCR assays can also aid in detection of scabies antibodies and help in determining the efficacy of treatment.

Scabies may mimic several diseases, including bullous pemphigoid, urticaria, chronic lymphocytic leukemia, B-cell lymphoma, necrotizing vasculitis, lupus erythematous, secondary syphilis, atopic dermatitis, and urticaria pigmentosa.

## TREATMENT

Empiric treatment is not recommended in the absence of a history of prolonged skin-to-skin exposure, typical eruption, or both. The infested patient and close physical contacts should be treated simultaneously, regardless of whether symptoms are present. Crusted scabies is very easily transmitted, and patients who have been even minimally exposed should be treated. Crusted scabies requires hospital admission, and keratolytics improve penetrance of topical therapy penetration. Usually, at least three consecutive topical treatments are required. Pruritus normally persists after treatment and may worsen as release of mite antigens exacerbates the hypersensitivity reaction. Most recurrent cases can be traced to untreated contacts.

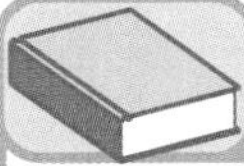

**PATIENT TEACHING TIPS**

Scabies is a benign, easily treated disease commonly called "the itch."

It causes a pruritic rash and spreads rapidly among people in close proximity.

Transmission among family members and within institutional settings is common.

Itching can persist for up to 4 to 6 weeks after the completion of treatment.

Schools do not ordinarily provide the level of contact necessary for transmission.

Keep fingernails well trimmed!

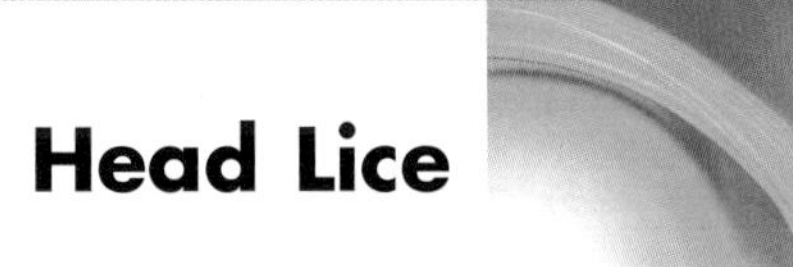

# Head Lice

## EPIDEMIOLOGY

Lice are epidemic throughout the world. *Pediculus humanus* species are permanent ectoparasites that require multiple blood meals a day. Infections are becoming more difficult to treat because of increasing resistance to common pediculicides. Lice prevalence is estimated at 6 to 12 million cases annually in the United States alone and more than 1 million globally.[26-28]

Head lice *(P. humanus capitis)* most commonly afflict children 3 to 12 years old. Body lice *(P. humanus corporis)* can transmit *Rickettsia* species, the causative agents of endemic typhus and trench fever. Louse-borne relapsing fever caused by *Borrelia recurrentis* is also transmitted by *Pediculus humanus corporis*. Unlike body lice, head lice are not vectors for any known diseases.

## TRANSMISSION AND PATHOPHYSIOLOGY

*Pediculus* species carry out their entire life cycle on the human host and survive only briefly in the environment. One female head louse can lay up to 150 eggs during her 1-month life span. Eggs (nits) are cemented onto hair shafts of the host and hatch in 1 week; full maturation to adult stages is completed in another week. If nits are found less than 1 cm from the scalp, an active infestation is considered highly likely. Because human hair grows at a rate of 1 cm/month, and nits can remain attached to hair for up to 6 months, the presence of nits a few centimeters from the scalp may not represent an active infestation.[26] Lice are transferred directly from host to host. Eggs are transferred from louse-infested clothing or personal articles such as shared combs, headphones, beds, and hats. Head lice can live up to 55 hours without a host.

## PRESENTING SIGNS AND SYMPTOMS

Signs and symptoms may include pruritus and pruritic papules at the site of infestation, especially in occipital and retroauricular regions. Saliva and fecal excretions of the louse may cause a local hypersensitivity reaction including fever, conjunctivitis, malaise, cervical lymphadenopathy, and a rash, mimicking a viral exanthem. If a secondary bacterial infection occurs, the lesion may resemble mange. Patients often identify the presence of a parasite before they present for treatment.

## DIAGNOSIS AND MEDICAL DECISION MAKING

The diagnosis is made by identifying lice or nits on the patient. Using a fine-toothed comb and placing any removed lice or nits on a light-colored surface and viewing them with a magnifying device may assist in the identification. The head louse is a gray-white, 3- to 4-mm insect. Currently, no antibody or serologic tests exist. The diagnosis is based on clinical suspicion, with confirmation on finding *Pediculus* adults, nymphs, or nits.

## TREATMENT

Three main avenues exist for treatment: mechanical removal, topical agents, and oral therapy (**Table 177.1**). Children can return to school immediately after completion of the first application of a topical insecticide. Wet hair combing to remove *P. humanus capitis* nits and adults is not as effective as the use of topical agents. Infested clothing and bed linen should be washed in hot water, dry cleaned, or discarded.

**Table 177.1** Treatment of Helminth Infections

| ORGANISM | TREATMENT | PRECAUTIONS AND COMMENTS |
|---|---|---|
| **Roundworms: Intestinal** | | |
| *Ascaris* | Albendazole 400 mg PO × 1<br>Mebendazole 500 mg PO × 1<br>Mebendazole 100 mg PO bid × 3 days<br>Pyrantel pamoate 11 mg/kg × 1 | Maximum dose, 1 g |
| | Ivermectin 150-200 mcg/kg PO × 1 | Lactating/pregnant women<br>Weight > 15 kg |
| *Necator, Ancylostoma* | Albendazole 400 mg PO × 1<br>Mebendazole 500 mg PO × 1 or 100 mg PO bid × 3 days<br>Pyrantel pamoate 11 mg/kg PO × 3 days<br>Supplemental iron PO | Maximum dose, 1 g |
| *Strongyloides:* simple | Ivermectin 200 mcg/kg PO × 2 days; ± repeat in 1-2 wk | Lactating/pregnant women<br>Weight > 15 kg |
| | Albendazole 400 mg PO bid × 3-7 days; ± repeat in 1-2 wk | |
| *Strongyloides:* disseminated | Ivermectin 200 mcg/kg PO once daily; continue +2 wk after symptom resolution<br>+ Albendazole or thiabendazole | Lactating/pregnant women<br>Weight > 15 kg |
| | Albendazole 400 mg PO bid; continue +2 wk after symptom resolution<br>Thiabendazole 25 mg/kg PO bid; continue +2 wk after symptom resolution | |
| *Enterobius* | Albendazole 400 mg PO × 1<br>Mebendazole 100 mg PO × 1<br>Pyrantel pamoate 11 mg/kg PO × 1 | Maximum dose, 1 g<br>TOC for pregnant women |
| *Trichuris* | Albendazole 400 mg PO × 3 days<br>Mebendazole 200 mg PO × 3 days<br>Ivermectin 200 mcg/kg PO × 3 days | Lactating/pregnant women<br>Weight > 15 kg |
| **Roundworms: Tissue** | | |
| *Trichinella:* mild | Supportive therapy | |
| *Trichinella:* hypersensitivity | Corticosteroid taper | |
| *Trichinella:* enteric only | Albendazole 15 mg/kg/day PO × 10-15 days, may repeat in 5 days<br>Mebendazole 5 mg/kg/day PO × 10-15 days, may repeat in 5 days<br>Corticosteroids if severe disease | |
| Cutaneous larva migrans | Albendazole 400-800 mg/day PO × 3-5 days<br>Ivermectin 200 mcg/kg PO × 2 days | |
| Lymphatic filariasis<br>*Wucheria bancrofti*<br>*Brugia malayi* | Diethylcarbamazine 6 mg/kg/day PO × 12 days<br>Albendazole 400 mg PO bid × 21-30 days<br>Doxycycline 200 mg PO once daily × 8 wk | Hypersensitivity reaction |
| | Albendazole 400 mg PO × 1 + diethylcarbamazine 6 mg/kg PO × 1<br>*or*<br>Ivermectin 200-400 mcg/kg PO × 1 | Microfilariacidal only<br>Lactating/pregnant women<br>Weight > 15 kg |
| *Loa loa* | Diethylcarbamazine 8-10 mg/kg/day PO × 21 days<br>Diethylcarbamazine 300 mg/week for prophylaxsis | Microfilariacidal only |
| *Mansonella ozzardi* | Ivermectin 200 mcg/kg PO × 1 | Lactating/pregnant women<br>Weight > 15 kg |
| *Mansonella perstans* | Mebendazole 100 mg PO bid × 30 days<br>Albendazole 400 mg PO bid × 10 days | Often not effective |
| *Mansonella streptocerca* | Diethylcarbamazine 6 mg/kg/day PO × 14-21 days<br>Ivermectin 150 mcg/kg PO × 1 | Lactating/pregnant women<br>Weight > 15 kg |

**Table 177.1 Treatment of Helminth Infections—cont'd**

| ORGANISM | TREATMENT | PRECAUTIONS AND COMMENTS |
|---|---|---|
| *Onchocerca* | Ivermectin 150-200 mcg/kg PO × 1; can repeat in 3-6 mo | Microfilariacidal only<br>Mazzotti reaction |
| | Doxycycline 100-200 mg PO once daily × 6 wk<br>Mebendazole 1 g PO bid × 28 days | Pulmonary eosinophilia |
| **Flatworms: Cestoidea** | | |
| *Taenia solium:* intestinal | Praziquantel 10-20 mg/kg PO × 1<br>+ Cimetidine | Hepatic impairment, does not inactivate eggs released from dead adult worms |
| | Niclosamide 2 g PO | |
| *Taenia solium:* neurocysticercosis | Praziquantel 50-60 mg/kg/day PO × 15-30 days + steroids<br>albendazole 15 mg/kg/day PO × 8-30 days<br>If > 60 kg, then 400 mg PO bid × 8-30 days<br>+ Anticonvulsants and corticosteroids:<br>Dexamethasone 16-24 mg/day PO<br>Followed by prednisone 1 mg/kg/day PO<br>Taper over 2-3 wk<br>± Endoscopic surgery/ventriculoperitoneal shunt | Hepatic impairment<br>Maximum, 800 mg/day |
| *Echinococcus* | Nonsurgical cysts: albendazole 10-15 mg/kg/day or mebendazole 40-50 mg/kg/day for 3-6 months<br>Surgical adjuncts: albendazole 15 mg/kg/day PO, start minimum of 4 days before procedure and continue for 8 weeks after procedure<br>Intraoperative: praziquantel 40 mg/kg/day PO<br>PAIR 90% ethanol or 20% hypertonic saline | Neutropenia and liver toxicity with prolonged albendazole and mebendazole use |
| | Praziquantel 50 mg/kg/day PO × 2 wk | Hepatic impairment |
| *Diphyllobothrium latum* | Praziquantel 25 mg/kg PO × 1 | |
| *Diphyllobothrium* other spp. | Praziquantel 10 mg/kg PO × 1<br>Niclosamide 2 g PO × 1 adults<br>1 g PO × 1 pediatrics >6 yr old | |
| **Flukes: Trematoda** | | |
| *Schistosoma* | Praziquantel 40-60 mg/kg/day PO × 1 day | Age > 4 yr<br>Hepatic impairment |
| **Other Flukes** | | |
| *Clonorchis*<br>*Fasciola*<br>*Opisthorchis*<br>*Paragonimus* | Praziquantel 75 mg/kg/day PO × 1-2 days<br>Albendzole 10 mg/kg/day PO × 7 days | Hepatic impairment |
| **Bedbugs: *Cimex* spp.** | Antipuritics ± corticosteroids | |
| **Scabies: *Sarcoptes* spp.** | Permethrin 5% topical, 8-14 hr; wash off ± repeat 1 wk | Age > 2 mo<br>First-line treatment in United States<br>Resistance reported |
| | Lindane 1% topical, 6 hr then wash; can repeat in 1 wk | Lactating/pregnant women<br>Increased seizure risk<br>Aplastic anemia risk<br>Weight > 50 kg<br>Age > 6 mo<br>Resistance reported |
| | Crotamiton 10% topical bid × 5 days<br>***or*** × 1 for 48 hr total | Lactating/pregnant women |
| | Benzyl benzoate 10-25% 2-3 × in 1 day | Lactating/pregnant women<br>Age > 2 yr<br>Not available in United States<br>Effective in permethrin-resistant scabies |

*Continued*

**Table 177.1 Treatment of Helminth Infections—cont'd**

| ORGANISM | TREATMENT | PRECAUTIONS AND COMMENTS |
|---|---|---|
| | Sulfur 2-10% petroleum, 2-3 days | Dermatitis<br>Stains clothing<br>Not available in United States |
| | Sulfur 10% may be more effective than permethrin for crusted scabies[23] | |
| | Malathion 0.5% 8-12 hr | Lactating/pregnant women<br>Age > 6 mo<br>Not available in United States |
| | Ivermectin 0.8% topical | Lactating/pregnant women<br>Weight > 15 kg |
| | Ivermectin 200 mcg/kg PO × 1; repeat in 2 wk<br>***or*** Ivermectin 250-350 mcg/kg PO × 1 | |
| **Lice: *Pediculus humanus capitis*** | Permethrin 1% topical 8-14 hr; wash off ± repeat 1 wk<br>May use 5% topical if >2 mo old | Resistance reported |
| | Lindane 1% topical, 6 hr then wash; can repeat in 1 wk | Lactating/pregnant women<br>Increased seizure risk<br>Aplastic anemia risk<br>Weight > 50 kg<br>Age > 6 mo<br>Resistance reported |
| | Malathion 0.5% topical 12 hr | Age > 6 mo<br>Flammable<br>Ovicidal<br>Resistance reported[29] |
| | Carbaryl 0.5% topical | Carcinogenic[26]<br>Available in United Kingdom |
| | Benzyl alcohol 5%, topical 10 min; repeat in 10 days | Age > 6 mo<br>Approved in United States[30,31] |
| | Ivermectin 200 400 mcg/kg PO × 1; repeat in 7-10 days | Lactating/pregnant women<br>Weight > 15 kg |
| | Ivermectin 200 mcg/kg PO days 1, 2, 10 | Good option in resource-poor area[36,37] |
| | Spinosad 0.9% cream 10 min; wash | Under development[32] |
| | Dimethicone 4% lotion | Used in United Kingdom, Europe, Brazil[33,34] |
| | Essential oils: lavender, coconut, citronella, anise, ylang-ylang | No investigative trials[35] |
| | Occlusive dressings: petroleum jelly<br>Mayonnaise, olive oil | Anecdotal home remedies |
| | LouseBuster 30 min | Expensive<br>Special training required<br>No case-control trials[27] |

*bid,* Twice daily; *PAIR,* percutaneous aspiration, infusion of scolicidal agents, and reaspiration; *PO,* orally; *tid,* three times daily.

## SUGGESTED READINGS

Frankowski BL, Bocchini JA Jr, Committee on School Health the Committee on Infectious Diseases. Head lice. Pediatrics 2010;126:392-403.

Goddard J, DeShazo R. Bed bugs (Cimex lectularius) and clinical consequences of their bites. JAMA 2009;301:1358-66.

Hicks M, Elston DM. Scabies. Dermatol Ther 2009;22:279-92.

Hotez PF, Brindley PJ, Bethony JM, et al. Helminth infections: the great neglected tropical diseases. J Clin Invest 2008;118:1311-21.

Jackson JA, Friberg IM, Little S, Bradley JE. Review series on helminths, immune modulation and the hygiene hypothesis: immunity against helminths and immunological phenomena in modern human populations: coevolutionary legacies? Immunology 2008;126:18-27.

## REFERENCES

*References can be found on Expert Consult @ www.expertconsult.com.*

# Tetanus 178

*Lisa D. Mills*

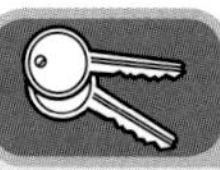

**KEY POINTS**

- Puncture wounds pose the highest risk for tetanus. Tetanus also occurs following clean, minor wounds, abscesses, and cellulitis.
- Keep current the tetanus immunization status of patients with any injury, even minor, clean wounds.
- Give tetanus immune globulin to patients with wounds, other than clean, simple wounds, who have never completed a primary tetanus immunization series.
- Tetanus is a clinical diagnosis. Begin treatment when the diagnosis is suspected in any patient with unexplained rigidity.
- Tetanus treatment consists of tetanus immune globulin, antibiotics, and local wound care.

## EPIDEMIOLOGY

Tetanus is a rare disease in the United States, with only 20 cases reported in 2003. In 1990 to 2000, the average number of cases in the United States was 50 per year. The average annual incidence from 1995 to 2000 was approximately 0.16 cases per million population.[1,2] Tetanus is more common among people 60 years old or older (0.35 cases per million population), patients 60 years old or older who have diabetes (0.70 cases per million population), and Hispanic persons (0.37 cases per million population). Injecting drug users are at unique risk for tetanus and accounted for 15% of cases of tetanus from 1998 to 2000.[1] Most (74%) injecting drug users who developed tetanus reported injecting heroin, and 100% reported "skin popping" rather than intravenous injection.[3]

Tetanus morbidity and mortality remain high, even with appropriate treatment. Current vaccination status decreases the severity of the disease and the likelihood of death from tetanus. In 1998 to 2000, 18% of patients with tetanus died. Of fatal cases, 75% occurred in patients who were 60 years old or older. No patients with an up-to-date vaccination status died of tetanus.[1]

## PERSPECTIVE

Although clinical cases are rare, emergency physicians (EPs) often are the first, and sometimes only, point of contact for patients. As a result, physicians must maintain an awareness of the clinical presentation of the disease. The diagnosis can be suspected but not confirmed in the emergency department (ED).

In addition to recognizing the clinical presentation of tetanus, EPs play a vital role in the prevention of the disease. Primary pediatric vaccination and regular decennial booster vaccination are the mainstays of disease prevention and severity modulation.[4] Herd immunity does not occur with tetanus. Therefore, only people who receive the vaccination benefit from immunization. In the United States, the prevalence of tetanus immunity decreases by age, after 40 years of age. At 40 years of age, 80% of the population is immune to tetanus. By the age of 80 years, only 30% of the population remains immune. This decrease is most striking in women and Mexican Americans.[5] Only 36% of persons age 65 years old or older report receiving tetanus vaccination in the past 10 years.[6,7] Most cases of tetanus and fatalities resulting from tetanus are in patients who either have never been vaccinated or have not had a booster in the past 10 years.[8] EPs have the opportunity to provide booster vaccination at times of minor to severe injury and skin infection. In light of pertussis epidemics,

$SI = \frac{SV}{BSA}$ **FACTS AND FORMULAS**

**Tetanus Booster Based on Age**

| | |
|---|---|
| Infant to 7 years | DTap (diphtheria, tetanus, acellular pertussis) |
| | DT (pediatric diphtheria, tetanus preparation), if pertussis is contraindicated |
| Age 7 to 10 years | dT |
| | Tdap, if not previously given once in primary series |
| Age 11 to 18 years | Tdap (tetanus, diphtheria, acellular pertussis) preferred |
| | Td (tetanus, diphtheria) acceptable |
| Adult | Td |
| | In people aged 11 to 64 years, if primary series not completed, can substitute Tdap for one Td; substitution should be done in people aged 11 to 18 years who have not completed a primary series |

From Centers for Disease Control, September 2005. Available at http://www.cdc.gov/mmwr/preview/mmwrhtml/00041645.htm

**Table 178.1 Tetanus Wound Characteristics and Risks**

| | MOST THREATENING | MOST COMMON |
|---|---|---|
| Location of injury | Face | Lower extremity<br>Upper extremity<br>Head and trunk |
| Type of injury | Puncture wound<br>Crush injury<br>Burn<br>Chronic ulcer | Puncture wound<br>Laceration<br>Chronic wound<br>Abrasion |
| Patients | Diabetic patients<br>Age > 60 yr<br>Neonates<br>No prior tetanus immunization | Intravenous drug users<br>Age > 60 yr<br>Hispanic ethnicity<br>Diabetic patients<br>No prior tetanus immunization<br>Last immunization >10 yr ago |

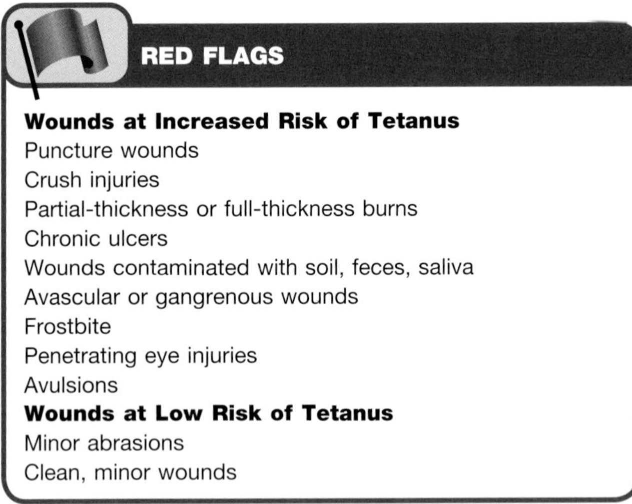

**RED FLAGS**

**Wounds at Increased Risk of Tetanus**
Puncture wounds
Crush injuries
Partial-thickness or full-thickness burns
Chronic ulcers
Wounds contaminated with soil, feces, saliva
Avascular or gangrenous wounds
Frostbite
Penetrating eye injuries
Avulsions
**Wounds at Low Risk of Tetanus**
Minor abrasions
Clean, minor wounds

providers should also consider a patient's pertussis immunization status when choosing the tetanus vaccine.

## ANATOMY

Most cases of tetanus are associated with acute trauma (**Table 178.1**), but many cases are associated with abscesses, cellulitis, chronic ulcers, dental infections, frostbite, and gangrene. In one study of injecting drug users with tetanus, 69% had an abscess at the injection site.[3] Tetanus affects postpartum women, with an increased risk after unsanitary birth or abortion practices.[1]

Puncture wounds are the most frequent type of acute trauma associated with tetanus. Puncture wounds include nail injuries to the foot, splinters, barbed wire injuries, tattoos, drug injection, penetrating eye injuries, and spider bites. Crush injuries, burns, and eye injuries are also portals of tetanus infection. In patients with tetanus, approximately 50% of injuries are located on the lower extremity, 36% on the upper extremity, 10% on the head or trunk, and 5% on other areas.[1]

The occurrence of tetanus following minor or trivial wounds is well documented in the literature. Tetanus results from minor wounds and abrasions when proper wound care is not administered.[2,9-12] Nearly half of the wounds that resulted in tetanus in 1998 to 2000 occurred indoors.[1]

## PATHOPHYSIOLOGY

Clinical tetanus is caused by two exotoxins produced by *Clostridium tetani,* a gram-positive, anaerobic rod. The bacterium produces spores that are heat resistant, surviving autoclaving at 250° F for 10 to 15 minutes, and resistant to treatment with phenols and common chemical agents. The bacterium dies with heat or oxygen exposure. The bacterium and spores are widely disseminated in soil, intestines of farm animals and pets, and feces. Spores exist on human skin and contaminated heroin. In anaerobic conditions, such as puncture wounds and crush injuries, spores germinate.

*C. tetani* enters the body through a wound and produces two exotoxins: tetanolysin and tetanospasmin. Tetanolysin causes local cell death and creates an anaerobic environment in the wound site.[13] Tetanospasmin interferes with the transmission of inhibitory impulses in the central nervous system. It creates a presynaptic blockage of the inhibitory Renshaw cells and Ia fibers of alpha motoneurons that transmit gamma-aminobutyric acid (GABA) and glycine. Renshaw cells that transmit acetylcholine are not affected as strongly. Tetanospasmin binding prevents inhibitory signals in the central nervous system.

Tetanus becomes a systemic disease as the toxin spreads through the body. Tetanospasmin binds to nerve terminals, is internalized, and travels in retrograde fashion to the cell synapse. The toxin travels at 75 to 250 mm/day, and it affects synapses of shorter nerves before synapses of longer nerves.[14] The toxin also travels by lymphatic and blood flow to remote nerves. The toxin exhibits local effects first and then spinal motor effects. The autonomic system is the last to be affected because of the length of the nerves. Tetanospasmin also inhibits acetylcholine release, a process that leads to flaccid paralysis between episodes of spasticity.[15]

The result of the general loss of inhibitory signals is rigidity with periods of spasticity. The reflex inhibition of antagonizing muscles is lost, thus allowing agonist and antagonist muscle groups to contract simultaneously. Autonomic disinhibition occurs late in the disease. Toxin binding appears to be irreversible; the growth of new nerve terminals is required to overcome the effects.[16]

## CLINICAL PRESENTATION

The average incubation period from time of injury to the onset of symptoms is 7 to 10 days, with a range of 1 to 60 days. Shorter incubation times are associated with more severe clinical presentation and a poor prognosis.[8,16] Tetanus is usually an afebrile disease until autonomic instability occurs late in the disease. Fever suggests coinfection of the wound or other infectious causes. Generalized tetanus, or tetanus affecting the whole body, is the most common form of tetanus.

In the first week of illness, the patient presents with rigidity and muscle spasms. Tetanus most commonly affects the cranial nerves first. The most common first symptoms and signs are trismus, neck stiffness, and dysphagia. Muscle spasm progresses diffusely to involve the facial muscles, thus causing the classic facial grimace risus sardonicus. Disinhibition of the neck muscles causes neck extension. Truncal rigidity follows head and neck involvement.

The general increased tone is interrupted by acute spastic events that can involve any muscle groups. These spastic events can be spontaneous or caused by tactile, visual, or auditory stimuli. Agonist and antagonist muscle groups can simultaneously contract. The contractions are painful and can be strong enough to break long bones and avulse tendons. Opisthotonos is a classic spastic event in tetanus. Abdominal rigidity can mimic an acute abdomen. Spasticity of the trunk and diaphragm can interfere with respiration. Laryngeal spasm interferes with the gag reflex or can occlude the airway.

Before modern mechanical ventilation, death resulted from respiratory failure or aspiration.[17] With modern mechanical ventilation, death is more commonly caused by autonomic events.[18,19]

The second week of illness involves autonomic instability in addition to the muscle spasms. The sympathetic nervous system is more strongly affected. Sudden increased autonomic tone, with elevated circulating catecholamine levels, increased vascular tone, hypertension, and tachycardia alternate with profound hypotension, bradycardia, and even cardiac arrest. Cardiac dysrhythmias occur, and the patient may develop hyperpyrexia at this point.[20-23]

Recovery begins in the third or fourth week. Muscle spasms decrease, but rigidity may persist. The duration of recovery, in those who survive, ranges from 2 to 4 months, as new axon terminals grow. Most patients return to their baseline with no residual deficit.[8]

### VARIATIONS

Local tetanus is an uncommon presentation of the disease in which only focal symptoms occur. Muscle spasticity is limited to the area adjacent to the wound. Local tetanus can progress to generalized tetanus, and the disease is generally milder. The exception is in cases of cephalic tetanus.

Cephalic tetanus is another rare form of disease. Cephalic tetanus follows a head or facial wound or, rarely, otitis media. The cranial nerves are initially affected. Spasticity or flaccid paralysis may be the presentation. Cephalic tetanus generally progresses rapidly to generalized tetanus and is associated with a severe course.[24]

Neonatal tetanus is generalized tetanus of the neonate. It occurs in infants born to mothers who are inadequately immunized. The port of entry is usually the umbilicus, with increased risk if the umbilicus is cut with a nonsterile instrument or is packed with contaminated material, such as soil, dung, or clay. Symptoms manifest on day 3 to 9 of life.[25]

The initial presentation is failure to feed in a child who previously fed normally. Neonatal tetanus progresses to generalized tetanus as described previously. The mortality rate of neonatal tetanus, when treated, is 25% to 90%.[26] Thirteen cases of neonatal tetanus were diagnosed in the United States from 1992 to 2000. In these cases, 85% of the neonates had not been vaccinated because of parental religious or philosophic objections.[27]

**BOX 178.1 Differential Diagnosis of Tetanus**

- Dystonic reaction
- Seizure
- Hysteria
- Craniofacial infection
- Meningitis
- Encephalitis
- Strychnine poisoning
- Hypocalcemia
- Black widow spider envenomation
- Intracranial hemorrhage
- Rabies
- Bell palsy
- Ischemic stroke

Because tetanus is a rare disease in the United States, it is difficult to suspect and diagnose (**Box 178.1**). Tetanus should be considered in the differential diagnosis of patients with rigidity or spasticity. The disease can be found in the setting of a minor or trivial injury that may not be remembered by the patient or family.[2,9-11] Tetanus is more common in patients without vaccination or without booster in the last 10 years. Unusually, from 1998 to 2000, 6% of tetanus cases occurred in patients who reported being up to date on tetanus vaccination.[1]

Older patients and patients with chronic illness may have a decreased immune response to vaccination and therefore may lack protective antibody levels to tetanus in spite of appropriate vaccination. This situation is increasingly true in patients aged 65 years or older.[28,29]

## DIAGNOSTIC TESTING

The diagnosis of tetanus is clinical. The *Vaccine-Preventable Diseases Surveillance Manual* defines tetanus as "the acute onset of hypertonia or by painful muscular contraction (usually, initially of the jaw and neck) and generalized muscle spasms without other apparent medical cause."[27] No laboratory tests confirm or refute the diagnosis of tetanus. The organism is rarely recovered from wounds and can be cultured from patients without clinical tetanus. Serologic testing to detect anti-etanus antibody levels plays a small role in the diagnosis of the disease. Patients can develop tetanus with "protective" levels of antibody.[27] The aim of testing is to rule out other causes of rigidity and spasticity. If tetanus is suspected, begin treatment immediately. Do not delay treatment, because no confirmatory test exists.

Check the patient's electrolytes, primarily to evaluate for hypocalcemia. Order a strychnine level determination if concern exists about exposure to strychnine, with the understanding that illegally imported pesticides contain strychnine.[30-32] Ask patients about pesticide exposure, and consider accidental ingestion in children.[33,34]

Obtain a computed tomography scan of the head if an acute intracranial event is considered. A lumbar puncture is necessary only if meningitis or encephalitis is included in the differential diagnosis. Examination of cerebrospinal fluid is

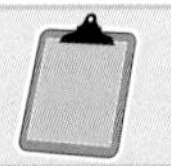

**DOCUMENTATION**

**History**
Document the history of onset of symptoms and symptom progression and the history of trauma, even minor, healed wounds, including the location of the wound. Involve witnesses, especially if the patient is having difficulty with speech or breathing. Obtain an immunization history in as much detail as possible. Ascertain allergies or reactions to medications and immunizations.

**Physical Examination**
Conduct a detailed neurologic examination. Evaluate the cranial nerves with motor function. Test for inducible spasticity (spatula test or other stimuli). Assess for compromise of respiration, ventilation, or airway protective reflexes.

**Studies**
Document review of any studies, even if results are normal. Exclusion of other disease is an important aspect of the diagnosis of tetanus.

**Medical Decision Making**
Document reasoning for excluding other, more common diagnoses or the reason for continued consideration of multiple diagnoses while concurrently treating the patient. Note findings in favor of tetanus.

Document the choice of medications for spasticity, including those for deep sedation or muscle relaxation.

Document the indications for intubation or assessment of adequate airway reflexes, ventilation, and respiration.

**Procedures**
Document wound care, including copious irrigation, incision and drainage, and débridement. Document rapid-sequence induction and intubation, the timing of consultation with the surgeon for extensive wounds, and the timing of the order for tetanus immune globulin.

**Hospital Course**
Document the patient's response to treatment.

Document the timing of interventions, including antibiotics, tetanus immune globulin, and intensive care consultation.

Document the indications for change in care, including intubation, deeper sedation, and additional medications.

noncontributory in tetanus, except to rule out other disorders. Because of unpredictable muscle spasms, performance of lumbar puncture on a patient with generalized tetanus may require intubation and deep sedation or muscle relaxation.

The spatula test has been used to distinguish tetanus from other forms of spasticity. In this test, a blunt instrument such as a tongue blade is used to touch the oropharynx. A patient without tetanus gags and attempts to expel the instrument. In a patient with tetanus, the stimulus triggers masseter spasm, resulting in a reflex bite of the blade.[35] Although this test is reported to have a sensitivity of 94% and a specificity of 100%, the results may not be applicable to the United States, where tetanus is rare.

## MANAGEMENT

Management of tetanus has two aspects: prevention and treatment. Each time an EP sees a patient with a wound, the opportunity for prevention exists. Treatment of tetanus is multifaceted and includes systemic treatment of the toxin, supportive treatment of the muscle spasms, and wound care.

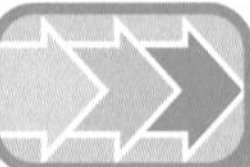

**PRIORITY ACTIONS**

Suspect tetanus in patients with rigidity.

- Control airway and ventilation.
- Administer tetanus immune globulin.
- Administer antibiotics.
- Aggressively treat spasticity.
- Débride wounds and incise abscesses.

### PREVENTION

Prevention through vaccination and proper wound care remains the mainstay of therapy for tetanus. Update the patient's tetanus immunization, and administer tetanus immune globulin according to Centers for Disease Control and Prevention guidelines (**Fig. 178.1**). Maintain the patient's current tetanus immunization status in cases of cellulitis, abscesses, eye injuries, chronic ulcers, burns, injecting drugs, minor abrasions, acute lacerations, punctures, and crush injuries (**Figs. 178.2 to 178.4**). Clean wounds to remove any contaminants.

Some patients have decrease in tetanus titers earlier than 10 years. For this reason, patients with wounds that are not clean or are more than minor should receive a tetanus booster at 5 years after the last booster.[27] Clinical tetanus does not confer immunity. Therefore, survivors of tetanus require immunization when they are clinically stable. Pregnant women can receive tetanus prophylaxis, if indicated.[36-38] No confirmed risk to the fetus has been determined from tetanus-diphtheria or tetanus immune globulin.[36]

### TREATMENT

#### *Antitoxin Therapy*

Administer tetanus immune globulin at a dose of 3000 to 5000 units intramuscularly to the pediatric or adult patient. Some sources recommend infiltration of some immune globulin around the wound site, if identified.[27] Intravenous immune globulin has tetanus antitoxin and may be administered if tetanus immune globulin is not available in a reasonable amount of time.

#### *Antibiotic Therapy*

Metronidazole is the drug of choice for tetanus. Administer intravenously, 1 g every 12 hours or 500 mg every 6 hours, to adult patients. Administer intravenous metronidazole at 30 mg/kg/day, divided every 8 or 12 hours, to pediatric patients. Penicillin G is the second choice of antibiotics. Penicillin antagonizes GABA with unknown clinical significance. The dose of penicillin is 24 million units intravenously,

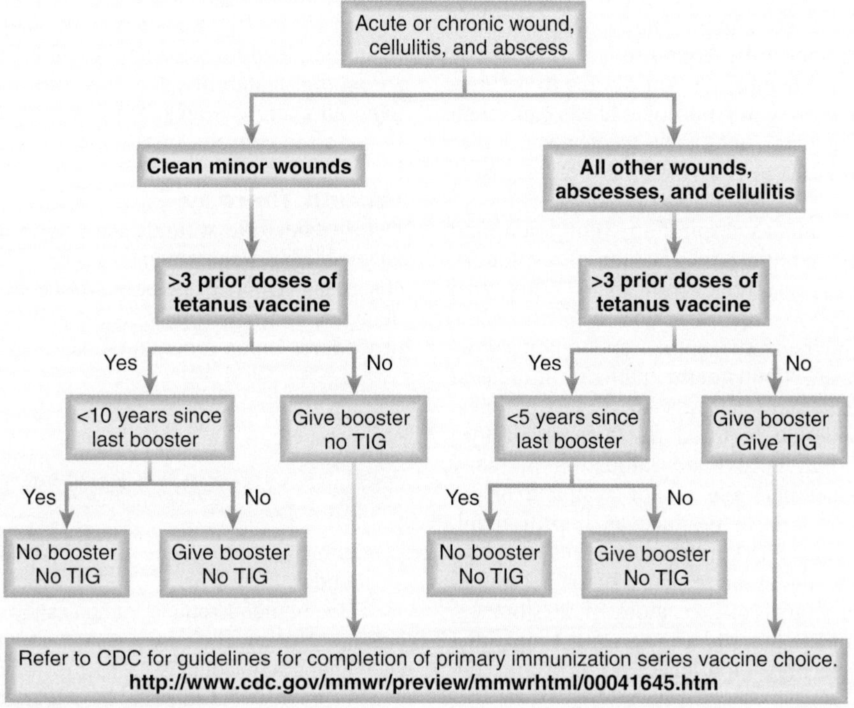


**Fig. 178.1 Approach to tetanus prevention.** *CDC,* Centers for Disease Control and Prevention; *TIG,* tetanus immune globulin.

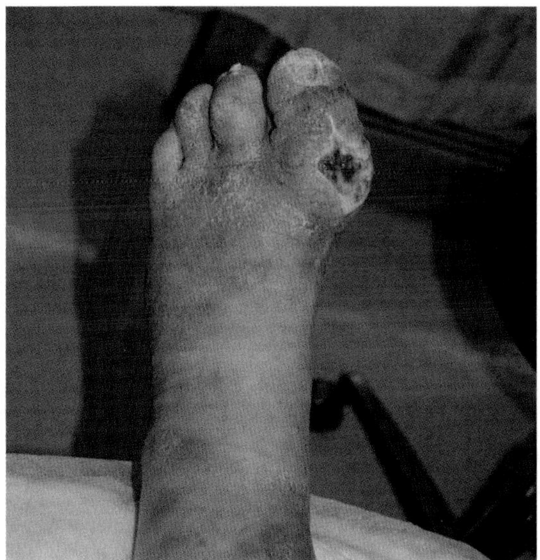

**Fig. 178.2** Chronic ulcers, especially in diabetic patients, pose an increased risk for tetanus.

divided every 4 to 6 hours, for adults. The pediatric dose of penicillin G is 100,000 to 250,000 units/kg/day, divided every 6 hours.[39-43] Erythromycin, doxycycline, tetracycline, chloramphenicol, and clindamycin are alternatives if metronidazole and penicillin are contraindicated.[43,44]

### Supportive Therapy

Muscle spasms are controlled with large doses of benzodiazepines to augment GABA activity. Continuous infusions improve effectiveness. Control pain with generous doses of morphine or another opiate, but avoid meperidine. If

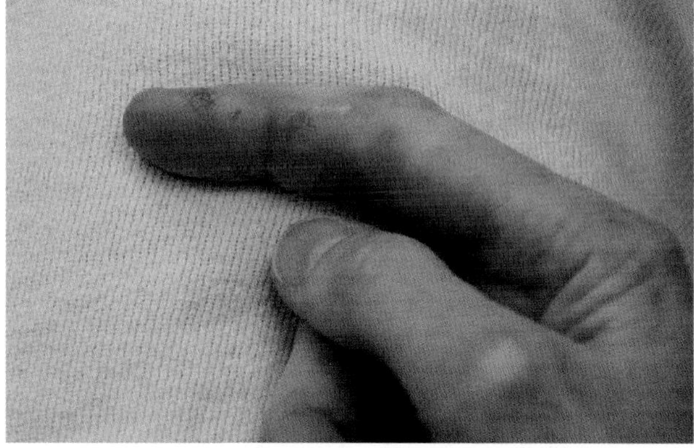

**Fig. 178.3** Even subtle abrasions and puncture wounds present an increased risk for tetanus.

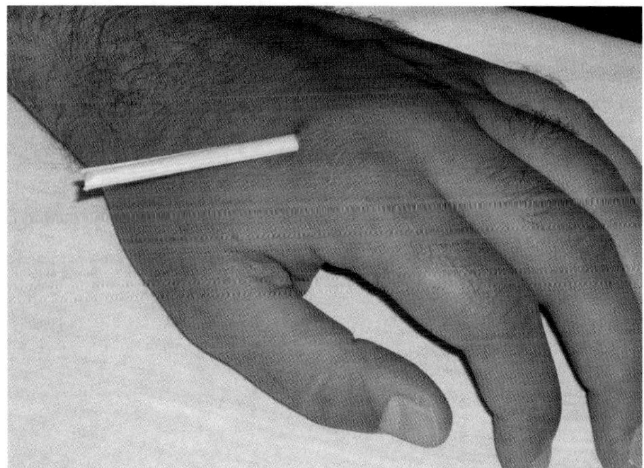

**Fig. 178.4** A puncture wound to the hand from this organic material introduces a significant tetanus inoculum.

respiratory depression results from sedation, intubate the patient. Magnesium in a continuous intravenous infusion has been used as an adjunct to benzodiazepines in the treatment of muscle spasms. Magnesium contributes to respiratory depression.[45-48] Sedation with propofol at levels equivalent to those used during general anesthesia decreases muscle rigidity and spasm. Intubate the patient before using propofol.[49,50]

Closely monitor the patient's respiration, ventilation, and airway reflexes. Intubate patients with any sign of respiratory or ventilatory compromise resulting from truncal or laryngeal spasm.

If deep sedation with benzodiazepines and opioids fails to control muscle spasm, intubate the patient. Intrathecal baclofen has been used with success in a few patients. The large doses of baclofen required result in respiratory depression and coma that necessitate intubation in many patients.[49,50] If intrathecal baclofen is not available on an emergency basis or if it fails to produce an improvement, administer a neuromuscular blocking muscle agent.

Patients with tetanus are at increased risk of aspiration because of the loss of laryngeal reflexes, atony of the stomach, and forceful contraction of the abdominal wall. Empty the patient's stomach to decrease the chances of aspiration.

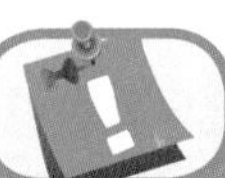

**TIPS AND TRICKS**

| Type of Wounds | Wound Care Tips |
|---|---|
| Puncture | Copiously irrigate. Remove foreign bodies as indicated. |
| Simple laceration | Copiously irrigate. |
| Complex laceration | Copiously irrigate. Débride nonviable tissue. |
| Abscess | Incise and drain. Débride avascular tissue. |
| Cellulitis | Débride any necrotic tissue. |
| Crush | Copiously irrigate. Débride avascular tissue. |
| Abrasion | Copiously irrigate. |
| Avulsion | Copiously irrigate. Débride nonviable tissue. |

Autonomic instability is a late finding and is not likely to be treated in the ED. Sedation with morphine and maintenance of a quiet, low-stimulus environment are critical in decreasing autonomic instability.[48,51,52] Esmolol has been used to control hyperadrenergic states. Propranolol and labetalol are both linked to increased mortality.[52,53]

### *Wound Therapy*

Débride necrotic wounds with wide margins, to remove the anaerobic environment and to arrest *C. tetani.* Incise and drain abscesses. Débride necrotic tissue at abscess sites. Do not delay débridement or incision and drainage. Perform these procedures on an emergency basis.

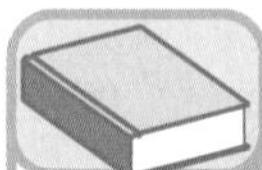

**PATIENT TEACHING TIPS**

Inform all patients of the risk of tetanus for even minor, clean wounds.

Recommend routine immunization every 10 years, even without injury.

Encourage patients to record tetanus boosters in their own records and to notify their primary care doctor of vaccination boosters.

Update tetanus immunization before pregnancy and childbirth.

The tetanus-diphtheria booster is believed to be safe in pregnancy and is given if an acute indication exists.

## DISPOSITION

Admit patients with tetanus to the intensive care unit. Consult a surgical service on an emergency basis if wound or abscess management requires surgical intervention.

## REFERENCES

***References can be found on Expert Consult @ www.expertconsult.com.***

# Rabies 179

*Lisa D. Mills*

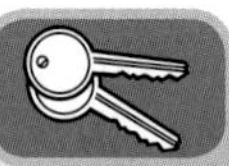

**KEY POINTS**

- Prevention of rabies through postexposure prophylaxis is the main treatment and the only one proven to be beneficial.
- Once signs or symptoms of rabies manifest, the disease is nearly 100% fatal.
- The postexposure prophylaxis regimen recommended by the World Health Organization should not be modified in any way.
- Initiate prophylaxis for any high-risk exposure, even if the wound is healed and the event is remote.
- Treatment of symptomatic rabies is experimental and requires consultation with the health department, the Centers for Disease Control and Prevention, or an infectious disease specialist. It should not begin in the emergency department.

## PERSPECTIVE

Rabies in humans remains rare in the United States. Only 36 cases were reported in the United States in the 20 years from 1980 to 2000,[1,2] but rabies exposures in the United States require that approximately 40,000 people receive postexposure prophylaxis annually.[3] Human rabies cases in the United States continue to occur, with 2 cases detected in 2008, 4 in 2009, and 1 in 2010.[4] International travelers are at increased risk of exposure to rabies and may return to the United States to receive postexposure prophylaxis or rabies treatment. Rabies is a fatal disease.[1,2,5,6] Only 6 people are known to have survived the disease.[7-13] The low rate of occurrence of the disease challenges physicians to consider this in the differential diagnosis of encephalitides.

Postexposure prophylaxis, if started before clinical signs of rabies develop, is highly effective. With strict adherence to protocol, including wound care, passive immunization, and vaccination with a cell culture vaccine, postexposure prophylaxis prevents rabies.[2,14-16] Emergency physicians (EPs) should know when to begin rabies postexposure prophylaxis, when to delay it, and when postexposure prophylaxis is not indicated, and they should also know state and local resources for rabies information.

## ANATOMY

Rabies is transmitted when saliva or neural tissue from an infected host contacts open wounds or mucous membranes of a recipient. This transmission can occur through bites, aerosolized tissue, or tissue transplantation. Rabies virus is not transmitted by blood, feces, or urine. Rabies is not transmitted across intact skin.[2]

Once the virus is in a new host, it performs one of two actions. Some virus replicates at the site of the bite in nonnerve tissue. The virus then enters peripheral nerves and travels to the central nervous system (CNS). Some virus does not replicate at the site, but rather immediately enters the peripheral motor and sensory nerves for transport to the CNS. During this time, the virus is in an eclipse phase, and it is difficult to detect with diagnostic tests.[17] The virus travels at speeds of 15 to 100 mm/day by retrograde axoplasmic flow.[6] When the virus enters the CNS, the incubation time ends. Incubation times range from 2 weeks to several years, and the average is 2 to 3 months.[6,17] Once in the CNS, the virus replicates and spreads by cell-to-cell transfer. The virus then travels by anterograde axoplasmic flow to nervous and nonnervous tissue. At the onset of clinical symptoms, the virus is disseminated throughout the body.

## PATHOPHYSIOLOGY

Rabies is caused by a negative-stranded RNA virus that belongs to the Lyssavirus family. The virus envelope fuses to the host cell membrane, and the virion penetrates the cell, where it replicates and buds new virus.

The virus causes inflammation in the CNS, both encephalitis and myelitis. Perivascular lymphocytic infiltration occurs with lymphocytes, polymorphonuclear leukocytes, and plasma cells. Cytoplasmic eosinophilic inclusion regions (Negri bodies) in neuronal cells are associated with rabies, but they are not sensitive or specific for the diagnosis of rabies.[17] Viral replication in dorsal root ganglia causes ganglionitis, and it is responsible for the first clinical symptoms of the disease.[5]

## CLINICAL PRESENTATION

The first clinical symptoms of rabies are neuropathic pain, paresthesias, or pruritus at the inoculation site. These symptoms were present in 61% of cases in the United States.[5,18] A prodromal, flulike illness may mark the onset of clinical rabies. Brain involvement causes encephalitis, manifesting as delirium with periods of lucidity. Two major clinical forms of the disease exist: furious and paralytic.

*Furious rabies* is a manifestation of brainstem encephalitis. Hyperexcitability, autonomic dysfunction, and hydrophobia mark furious rabies. Spasms are induced with olfactory, visual, auditory, and tactile stimuli, causing aerophobia and hydrophobia. These spasms are painful, and the patient remains aware of the pain. Spasms are more prominent in the furious form of the disease. Focal neurologic signs are usually absent in furious rabies. The spasms are differentiated from tetanus by a lack of rigidity or trismus between spastic episodes. Involvement of the autonomic nervous system causes hypersalivation, profuse sweating, tachycardia, and hypertension.

*Paralytic rabies* results in quadriplegia.[19] It is more common after the bite of a vampire bat in South America. Peripheral neuropathy is responsible for the paralysis in paralytic rabies. Because peripheral nerves are involved, patients lose deep tendon reflexes. The paralysis occurs in an ascending pattern and is associated with pain and fasciculations. The anal sphincter is involved in the quadriplegia.[6] Death results from paralysis of bulbar and respiratory muscles.

At some point in the course of the disease, spontaneous inspiratory spasms occur in all patients with rabies. These painful inspiratory spasms can escalate to opisthotonos, generalized clonus, and respiratory arrest. Inspiratory spasms persist until death. Without treatment, clinical rabies is uniformly fatal in 2 to 10 days.

### VARIATIONS

Consider rabies in patients with a clinical presentation of encephalitis.[20] Atypical presentation of disease is increasingly acknowledged, but it remains poorly described in the literature. Atypical presentations make the suspicion of rabies very difficult, especially if a clear history of rabies exposure is not presented.

## DIFFERENTIAL DIAGNOSIS

The furious form of rabies is rapidly progressive and is fatal in 1 to 5 days (**Table 179.1**). The paralytic form of rabies is more slowly progressive, and patients live for up to a month. However, clinical rabies is considered a fatal disease regardless of the clinical manifestation.

**Table 179.1** Differential Diagnosis of Rabies

| MOST THREATENING FURIOUS RABIES | MOST COMMON PARALYTIC RABIES |
|---|---|
| Delirium tremens | Poliomyelitis |
| Intoxication with stimulants or hallucinogens | Guillain-Barré syndrome |
| Strychnine poisoning | Botulism |
| Tetanus | Tick paralysis |
| Encephalitis of other origin | Paralytic shellfish poisoning |
| Meningitis | Ciguatera toxin poisoning |
| African sleeping sickness | African sleeping sickness |
| | Herpes B virus encephalitis |

## DIAGNOSTIC TESTING

In the early stage of the disease, tests may show negative results.[6] The "gold standard" for the diagnosis of rabies is direct fluorescent antibody testing of the brain. Brain biopsy exclusively for the diagnosis of rabies is discouraged.[21,22]

Multiple testing techniques exist for the diagnosis of rabies during life. Discuss with the pathologist the preferred sample at your institution. Serum, saliva, and skin samples are commonly used, whereas cerebrospinal fluid, urine, and lacrimal fluid are occasionally tested.[6,23] Do not withhold empiric antirabies therapy to obtain diagnostic studies.

Perform a lumbar puncture for analysis of cerebrospinal fluid for meningitis and encephalitis. Sedate the patient, if necessary, to control spasms. Send cerebrospinal fluid for diagnostic studies according to the patient's geographic exposure. Perform a toxicologic screen to evaluate for intoxication, but remember that intoxicants may be incidental findings.

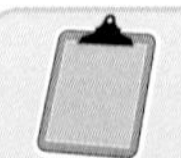

**DOCUMENTATION**

**Rabies Exposure**

**History**

Exposure type: bite, nonbite

Details of animal involved: species, vaccination history, domestic feral or wild, healthy or ill, provoked or unprovoked in domestic animal, animal detained or escaped

Animal control contacted or not

Patient's rabies vaccination history

**Physical Examination**

Neurovascular, tendons, wound size and depth, tenderness, visible contaminants, tattooing, discoloration, infection, masses, range of motion

**Studies**

Radiograph for tooth, if bite

Urine pregnancy test in women of childbearing capacity

**Medical Decision Making**

Indication for rabies PEP or not, including type of exposure, likelihood of infection of animal, ability to observe animal; discussion with health department or CDC

**Procedures**

Wound care

Wound infiltration with rabies immune globulin, if given

Wound closure, if performed

**Patient Instructions**

Documentation of discussion with patient regarding need for multiple vaccinations, if PEP initiated

Documentation of discussion with patient regarding need to stay in contact with animal control for animal undergoing observation or for euthanized animal

Wound care instructions

*CDC*, Centers for Disease Control and Prevention; *PEP*, postexposure prophylaxis.

## RABIES TRANSMISSION

Rabies is transmitted only by mammals, both domestic and wild. Common wild animals known to contract and transmit rabies include foxes, skunks, raccoons, coyotes, and bats. Dogs, cats, cattle, and other domestic animals can also contract and transmit rabies.

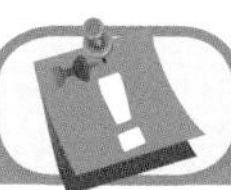

### TIPS AND TRICKS

**Zoonotic Rabies Reservoirs**

| Continent or Geographic Region | Primary Animal Reservoir |
|---|---|
| Africa | Dog, mongoose, antelope |
| Asia | Dog |
| Europe | Fox, bat |
| Middle East | Wolf, dog |
| North America | Fox, skunk, raccoon, bat (insectivorous) |
| South America | Dog, vampire bat |

Patients commonly present after bites and scratches from small rodents, both wild and domestic. In these circumstances, wound care and reassurance are all that is required. Rats, mice, squirrels, chipmunks, hamsters, and guinea pigs do not transmit rabies. Rabbits and other lagomorphs have not been found to have rabies and have never been known to cause rabies.

Postexposure prophylaxis is virtually never indicated after a bite from or exposure to any rodent, so the health department should be consulted before initiating postexposure prophylaxis if the animal's behavior was suspicious and prophylaxis appears clinically indicated.

To assess the likelihood of rabies exposure, it is helpful to know the distribution of rabid animals in the area. The local or state health department can provide information about rabies prevalence and animal vectors. A list of state health department contact numbers is available through the Centers for Disease Control and Prevention (CDC) at http://www.cdc.gov/ncidod/dvrd/rabies/Links/Links.htm. Moreover, the CDC can be contacted at 877-554-4625 after hours or if the local or state health department is unavailable (http://www.cdc.gov/ncidod/dvrd/rabies/professional/professi.htm).

If the animal involved can carry rabies, determine whether the patient had an exposure (see the "Facts and Formulas" box). Consider any breach in the skin that was caused by teeth to be a bite exposure.[2,23] Exposure to aerosolized virus in a laboratory or cave setting constitutes a nonbite exposure. Saliva, neural tissue, or other infectious material contacting open wounds or mucous membranes constitutes an exposure. Contact of infectious material with intact skin does not constitute an exposure, nor does contact with noninfectious material, such as feces, blood, or urine, or petting a rabid animal. Do not provide postexposure prophylaxis to patients who have not had an exposure.[2]

If an exposure has occurred, the decision to begin postexposure prophylaxis is multifactorial. The type of animal, the epidemiology of rabies in the region of the exposure, and the

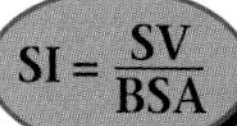

### FACTS AND FORMULAS

**Exposure**
Bite
Contamination of wound with saliva or infectious material
Mucous membrane contact with saliva or infectious material
Exposure to aerosolized virus
Transplant of infected organ
Bite, scratch, or mucous membrane contact with bat

**Unlikely Exposure**
Contact with dry secretions

**Nonexposure**
Contact with intact skin
Petting of rabid animal
Contact with feces, blood, or urine

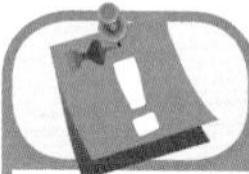

### TIPS AND TRICKS

**Postexposure Prophylaxis**

| Status | Postexposure Prophylaxis Regimen |
|---|---|
| Unvaccinated | Wash the wound thoroughly with soap and water. |
| | Treat the wound with a virucidal agent (povidone-iodine). |
| | Administer RIG, 20 units/kg. Infiltrate as much as possible into wound and tissue immediately adjacent to the wound. Administer the remaining dose intramuscularly, remote from the tetanus vaccination site. |
| | Administer 1 mL tetanus vaccine intramuscularly. Use the deltoid muscle in adults. Use the deltoid or anterior thigh in small children. Avoid the site of RIG administration. |
| | Instruct the patient to receive four more vaccinations, on days 3, 7, 14, and 28. |
| Previously vaccinated | Wash the wound thoroughly with soap and water. |
| | Treat the wound with a virucidal agent (povidone-iodine). |
| | Do *not* administer RIG. |
| | Administer 1 mL tetanus vaccine intramuscularly. Use the deltoid muscle in adults. Use the deltoid or anterior thigh in small children. |
| | Instruct the patient to receive one more vaccination, on day 3. |

*RIG*, Rabies immune globulin.

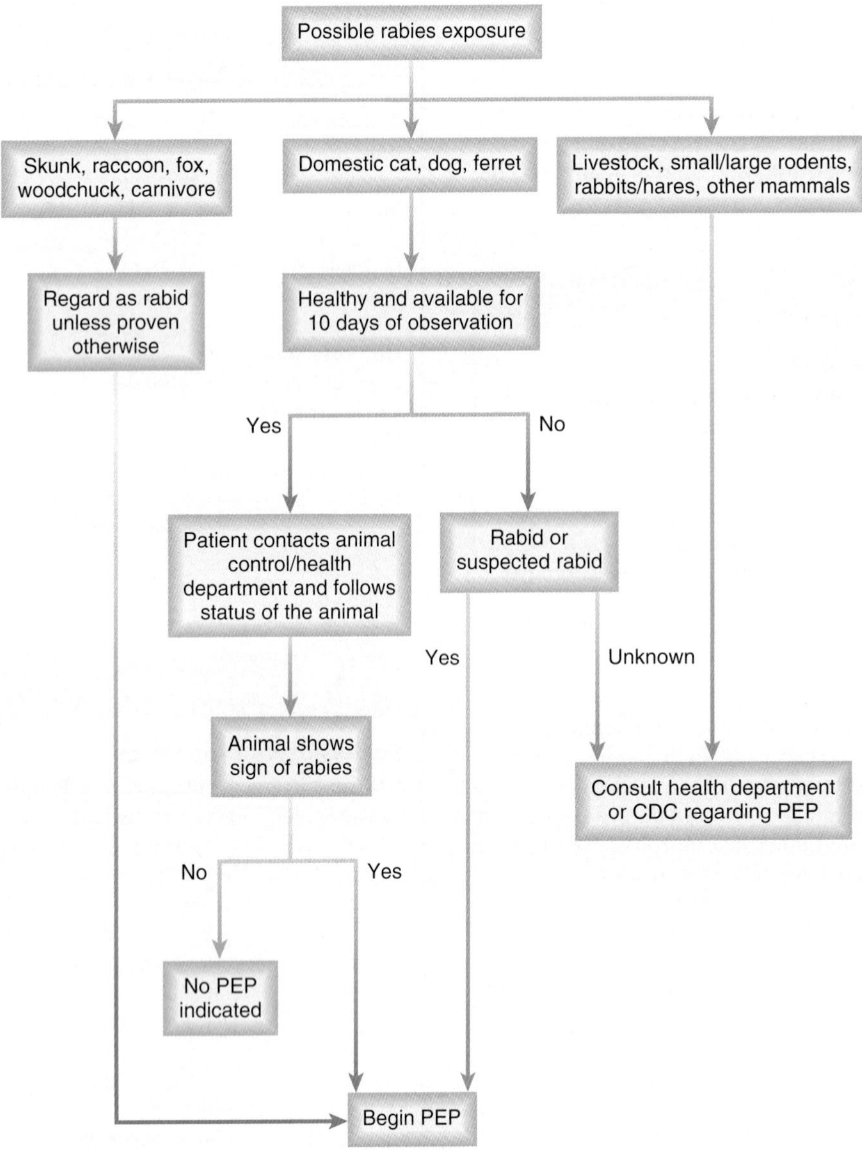


**Fig. 179.1 Approach to assessing rabies exposure and initiating postexposure prophylaxis (PEP) in the United States.** *CDC,* Centers for Disease Control and Prevention.

health of the animal all contribute to the decision. **Figure 179.1** provides an algorithm for the decision to start postexposure prophylaxis in humans. If an exposure involved a wild animal of a species that is a rabies vector, in a rabies-endemic area, begin postexposure prophylaxis immediately (see the "Tips and Tricks: Postexposure Prophylaxis" box). Do not await laboratory results. If the animal involved is an unlikely vector, postexposure prophylaxis can be withheld in consultation with the health department or CDC, as long as the animal can be tested for rabies, with results available within 48 hours.[6]

If a wild animal that is a potential vector for rabies is responsible for an exposure but is unable to be captured, begin postexposure prophylaxis immediately (see the "Tips and Tricks: Postexposure Prophylaxis" box).[6] If a wild animal responsible for an exposure is caught, it should be immediately and humanely euthanized and tested. Wild animals should never be observed for signs of rabies because the time course of rabies in mammals other than dogs, ferrets, cats, and humans is not understood.[6]

Bats are common wildlife reservoirs of rabies in the United States, and prophylaxis is indicated even after seemingly trivial exposure. Rabies has been transmitted from unimportant or unrecognized exposures to bats.[2] Consider direct human-to-bat contact to be a likely exposure, even in the absence of a known bite. Begin rabies postexposure prophylaxis on all bites, scratches, and mucous membrane exposures to bats. Strongly consider postexposure prophylaxis in anyone who has had contact with a bat, even people who may be unaware of injury.[2] Strongly consider postexposure prophylaxis in a person who is near a bat and is uncertain whether contact has occurred, such as a person who awakens in a room with a bat.[24]

If the animal responsible for an exposure is a pet cat, dog, or ferret that is not currently showing signs of rabies, the animal can be observed for 10 days under the care of a veterinarian.[25,26] A currently vaccinated dog or cat is unlikely to have rabies, but vaccination failures have been reported. Therefore, even vaccinated animals should be reported to the health department for observation.[6]

If the animal remains healthy, postexposure prophylaxis need not be started. If any suspicion exists that the animal is rabid, begin postexposure prophylaxis (see the "Tips and Tricks: Postexposure Prophylaxis" box). Postexposure prophylaxis can be terminated if laboratory results show that the animal does not have rabies. If the domestic animal is not identifiable, contact the local health department to determine whether postexposure prophylaxis is indicated in your area.

In the case of a healthy, known pet that is not suspected of having rabies, provide the patient with information regarding the local health department and the need for animal quarantine by local animal control. The patient bears the responsibility of maintaining contact with the health department and animal control regarding the status of the animal. EPs are not expected to perform these functions for the patient. The CDC considers postexposure prophylaxis a medical urgency, not an emergency. Therefore, it is reasonable, in the low-risk exposures outlined in Figure 179.1, to delay postexposure prophylaxis. In this case, the patient will follow up with the health department or animal control and will return to a physician for postexposure prophylaxis, based on the finding in the animal.[2]

### TRAVEL OUTSIDE THE UNITED STATES

Tens of thousands of people die of rabies worldwide, most commonly after being bitten by an infected dog. In developing countries of Africa, Asia, and Latin America, rabies is common. Preexposure vaccination is indicated only if the patient will have a high likelihood of contact with animals, will remain for an extended period of time, and will have difficulty obtaining postexposure treatment. Even if preexposure prophylaxis is administered, postexposure treatment is still needed.

The World Health Organization (http://www.who.int/rabies/epidemiology) reports that rabies is present on every continent except Antarctica. Of 145 countries reporting, 45 note no cases of rabies. These rabies-free countries include selected islands such as New Zealand, Japan, Fiji, and Barbados, as well as certain developed European countries such as Greece, Portugal, and Scandinavian countries. In Latin America, Chile and Uruguay are noted to be free of rabies.

If a patient has had an exposure outside the United States, contact the CDC regarding the risk and the need for postexposure prophylaxis. Presume that prophylaxis should be initiated unless convincing evidence is present to the contrary. Initiate prophylaxis even if the wound is healed and the exposure was remote.

If a patient has begun postexposure prophylaxis outside the United States, obtain as much information as possible regarding the treatment before the patient's return to the United States. Contact the CDC or state or local health department regarding how to continue postexposure prophylaxis in this patient.

Human-to-human transmission of rabies is possible. Documented cases have involved inoculation through saliva by biting or kissing.[27] Human-to-human transmission has also occurred from the transplantation of infected organs.[28,29] When providing routine health care to a person with rabies, the use of appropriate contact isolation practices prevents rabies exposure in the health care provider.[2,30] No known case of transmission of rabies to a health care worker from a patient exists.[5] Treat persons who have been stuck with a contaminated needle from a patient with rabies as a rabies exposure. The concern is that the needle may contain neural tissue.

Incubation periods of up to 6 years have been reported for rabies.[17] For this reason, if exposure to rabies may have occurred, start postexposure prophylaxis regardless of the time from the exposure.[6] Adhere to the postexposure prophylaxis protocol as with any other exposure (see the "Tips and Tricks: Postexposure Prophylaxis" box).

## WOUND TREATMENT AND RABIES PREVENTION

Postexposure prophylaxis consists of three steps: wound care, conferring of passive immunity, and active immunization. When World Health Organization guidelines for postexposure prophylaxis are followed, postexposure prophylaxis is effective. Postexposure prophylaxis failures have all involved deviation from the guidelines.[2]

The first step in rabies postexposure prophylaxis is local wound care. Copiously irrigate the wound with soap and water. Follow with treatment with a virucidal agent, such as povidone-iodine. Wound care alone decreases the chance of contracting rabies.[31] Failures of postexposure prophylaxis have been attributed to inadequate local wound care.[2]

The second step in postexposure prophylaxis is passive immunization. It takes approximately 7 days to develop an antibody response to rabies vaccine. Rabies immune globulin (RIG) provides passive immunization until the antibody response begins. Administer 20 units/kg of RIG. This dose is the same for pediatric and adult patients. Infiltrate as much RIG as possible into the wound and tissue immediately surrounding the wound. Administer the remaining dose of RIG intramuscularly at a site remote from the vaccination site.

If the patient presents with a bite or wound that is already infected, clean the wound appropriately. Débride and incise the wound as needed. RIG can be infiltrated safely into an infected wound following proper local wound care.[6]

The third step in postexposure prophylaxis is vaccination (see the "Tips and Tricks: Postexposure Prophylaxis" box). Three cell culture vaccines are available in the United States: human diploid cell vaccine (HDCV), rabies vaccine adsorbed (RVA), and purified chick embryo cell vaccine (PCEC). These vaccines are all equally efficacious, and the dose and administration are the same for all three types.

Administer 1 mL of vaccine intramuscularly. The vaccine is administered intramuscularly into the deltoid muscle of adults. The vaccine can be administered intramuscularly into the deltoid or anterior thigh of a child. Vaccine failures have been recorded for administration of vaccine into sites other than the deltoid of adults.[32] Do not administer vaccine into the same intramuscular region as RIG was administered. Do not use the same syringe to administer vaccine and RIG.

The first day of vaccination is day 0. Inform the patient that four additional vaccinations are required, on days 3, 7, 14, and 28. The subsequent doses are the same, 1 mL intramuscularly. Postexposure prophylaxis should not be modified or discontinued unless the animal is found by laboratory testing to be free of rabies. If interruption of the postexposure prophylaxis schedule occurs, contact the local health department or the CDC to determine the new schedule.

Some people have been previously vaccinated against rabies. If they are exposed to rabies, previously vaccinated people undergo a modified vaccination regimen with two doses of vaccine, one dose on day 0 and one dose on day 3 (see the "Tips and Tricks: Postexposure Prophylaxis Vaccination" box). Administer a 1-mL intramuscular dose of vaccine in the deltoid muscle. Instruct the patient to receive another dose of vaccine on day 3. Do *not* administer RIG to anyone who has been previously immunized. Provide local wound care, as with any exposure.

Because rabies is considered a fatal disease, postexposure prophylaxis is not withheld during pregnancy. Inform pregnant patients that no known fetal anomalies have been linked to rabies postexposure prophylaxis,[33-35] but extensive testing in humans has not been performed. When possible, discuss the case with the patient's obstetrician.

Patients who are immunocompromised as a result of chronic illness or immune-modulating drugs require monitoring for immune response. Administer the same dose of vaccine and RIG, and provide appropriate wound care. If possible, discuss the case with the patient's primary physician or infectious disease specialist. Refer the patient to the patient's primary physician or infectious disease specialist for the remainder of the vaccination course and the appropriate antibody titers. Monitoring for immune response is outside the scope of emergency medicine.

## TREATMENT

Rabies is considered a fatal disease.[5] Only six known cases of survivors of clinical rabies have been reported, and in five of these cases, patients had some form of rabies immunization before the onset of clinical disease. Four of the six survivors had neurologic devastation.[8-11]

### SYMPTOMATIC RABIES

Once clinical signs or symptoms of rabies have begun, no reliably successful rabies treatment is known. Treatments are all considered experimental and have included antiviral therapy with ribavirin, vidarabine, and interferon alfa.[5,36,37] Rabies vaccine has not been demonstrated to have a beneficial effect in animal models when it is administered after the onset of clinical disease. RIG is of unknown benefit in clinical disease, but it is administered.[5] Ketamine has been used to induce coma and has been shown to decrease viral replication in rat models. This drug is of unknown clinical benefit in humans.[38] Corticosteroids are associated with increased mortality in laboratory studies. Avoid corticosteroids in patients suspected of having rabies encephalitis.[5] Because of the lack of an effective therapeutic regimen, the treatment of rabies involves consultation with local or state health departments and the CDC, in conjunction with an infectious disease specialist and intensive care specialist, when available. The responsibility of the EP is to maintain a level of suspicion for rabies in a patient with signs of encephalitis, to consult for definitive diagnosis and management of rabies, and to provide supportive care while the patient is in the emergency department (ED). The determination of an effective antiviral regimen for a patient with suspected or confirmed rabies is outside the scope of practice of emergency medicine.

When rabies is suspected, consult the local or state health department, the CDC, or an infectious disease specialist for emergency treatment guidance. Give RIG, 20 units/kg intramuscularly, if significant delay in consultation is encountered. Provide supportive care to the patient. Spasms are painful, and the patient remains aware through much of the clinical course of the disease. When it is not contraindicated because of other comorbidities, administer ketamine by continuous intravenous infusion to sedate the patient and to alleviate the pain of rabies.[5] Intubate the patient if the patient has lost protective

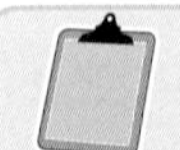

**DOCUMENTATION**

**Clinical Rabies**

**History**

- History of potential rabies exposure, including any bat or laboratory exposure
- Symptoms: onset, duration, progression
- Risk factors for other forms of encephalitis

**Physical Examination**

- Neurovascular features, tendons, wound size and depth, tenderness, visible contaminants, tattooing, discoloration, infection, masses, range of motion

**Studies**

- Lumbar puncture: send routine studies and request that laboratory retain extra cerebrospinal fluid for encephalitis studies to be ordered by consultant
- If pathologist available, discuss preferred diagnostic tissues (if after hours, diagnostic studies can be sent during admission)
- Screening for drugs of abuse

**Medical Decision Making**

- Recommendations of infectious disease consultant, CDC, health department regarding treatment
- Indications for sedation
- Response to sedation
- Indication for intubation

**Procedures**

- Lumbar puncture
- Rapid-sequence induction
- Intubation

**Patient Instructions**

- Documentation discussion with patient or family regarding suspicion of rabies and poor prognosis

*CDC,* Centers for Disease Control and Prevention.

airway responses as a result of progression of the disease or because of sedation from medications. Unlike in bacterial infectious emergencies, delay in beginning antiviral agents is acceptable. Because of the lack of a standard of care in the treatment of rabies, the decision to begin antiviral therapy is best made in conjunction with consultants.

## DISPOSITION

Patients who have had an exposure to a healthy pet that is undergoing 10 days of observation should be referred to animal control or to the health department. It is the patient's responsibility to stay in contact with animal control for information regarding the health of the animal.

Patients who have received the first treatment of postexposure prophylaxis are treated as outpatients. When possible, patients should continue the postexposure prophylaxis with a primary care physician or the health department, to ensure continuity of care. If not possible, the patient can return to the ED for the remainder of the postexposure prophylaxis. Patients with suspected clinical rabies require admission to the intensive care unit.

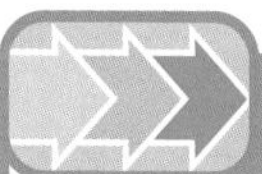

**PRIORITY ACTIONS**

**Clinical Rabies**

Assess the patient for rabies exposure.
If exposure is likely or possible, contact the health department or the CDC for treatment recommendations.
Consult an infectious disease specialist, when available.
Consult an intensive care specialist.
Administer rabies immune globulin, 20 units/kg intramuscularly, if obtaining consultant recommendations is delayed.
Administer ketamine by intravenous infusion if the patient is in pain or is experiencing agitation.
Have the patient admitted by an intensive care specialist.
Defer vaccine administration and antiviral therapy to the health department or CDC or an infectious disease specialist.

*CDC*, Centers for Disease Control and Prevention.

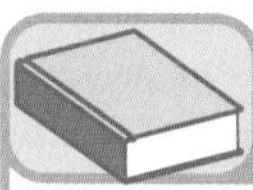

**PATIENT TEACHING TIPS**

Avoid contact with bats, including prevention of bat colonies.
Seek medical care after exposure to bats.
Avoid direct contact with wildlife.
Avoid contact with any ill-appearing animal and with animals exhibiting bizarre behavior.
Do not approach unknown cats or dogs.
Seek medical attention for domestic animal bites.
Any person bitten by a wild animal should seek medical attention.

## REFERENCES

*References can be found on Expert Consult @ www.expertconsult.com.*

# 180 Tick-Borne Diseases

*Jonathan A. Edlow*

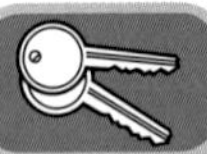

**KEY POINTS**

- Many patients with tick-borne diseases (TBDs) do not recall a tick bite; the history should focus on activities that predispose to tick exposure.
- Because some of the TBDs are fatal if untreated, consider these diseases in patients with fever of unknown source, especially in "tick season."
- TBDs most often can be strongly suspected or diagnosed clinically, and treatment should be initiated before definitive laboratory confirmation.

## EPIDEMIOLOGY

Untreated, tick-borne diseases (TBDs) can be associated with significant morbidity or mortality. Definitive treatments exist for the more serious diseases. TBDs usually can be confidently diagnosed clinically, based on pathognomonic or suggestive physical or laboratory findings that are available in the emergency department. Confirmatory laboratory testing is rarely available in real time and is often unnecessary for initial medical decision making. Therefore, physicians must understand both classic and atypical presentations and must be prepared to treat these illnesses based on clinical suspicion.

Because these illnesses frequently occur in the absence of a known tick bite, physicians must consider TBDs when patients present in the correct epidemiologic context and with a recognizable syndrome. This chapter considers these diseases in syndromic groups (patterns of presentation), rather than individually. Individual TBDs are listed in **Table 180.1** (North America) and **Table 180.2** (worldwide). Travelers may import the TBDs from one location to another.

Epidemiologic context is a key principle in diagnosing TBDs. As in a criminal investigation, the practitioner must assess the tick's means, motive, and opportunity to transmit a TBD. The means has to do with tick anatomy—the ability to bite a mammal, usually without the mammal's knowledge. This factor is crucial because most TBDs require many hours of tick attachment to transmit the infectious agent. The motive has to do with tick physiology; ticks require a blood meal from a host to live and transform to their next life stage. Opportunity relates to patient and geographic factors, that is, epidemiologic context. Taking a history that focuses on this epidemiologic context is essential to the diagnosis of all TBDs. Ask whether the patient has been bitten by a tick, but remember that most patients with TBDs do *not* recall a tick bite. For example, only approximately 25% of patients with Lyme disease (smaller ticks) and only two thirds of patients with Rocky Mountain spotted fever (RMSF) (larger ticks) recall the bite. Questions directed at whether a tick *could have* bitten the patient should be asked:

- How do you spend your time?
- What is your job?
- What hobbies and recreational activities do you enjoy?
- Where have you traveled recently?

As for the season, most TBDs are acquired from April through September, but "tick season" depends on the stage of a disease, geography, and local weather patterns for that geographic area. For example, Lyme arthritis could manifest in January from a bite in July, and a warm spell in late fall in North Carolina could result in a case of RMSF that develops in November.

## PATHOPHYSIOLOGY AND TICK ANATOMY

Two families of ticks are important in human TBDs. Hard (Ixodidae) ticks tend to attach and feed for days, whereas soft ticks (Argasidae) feed in minutes to hours. **Table 180.3** lists some characteristics of these different types of ticks. Because the hard ticks, which transmit most of the human TBDs, feed for so long, tick removal during the first 24 hours of attachment provides one strategy for disease prevention, a concept best studied in the context of Lyme disease. **Figures 180.1 to 180.3** show various stages of *Ixodes scapularis, Dermacentor variabilis,* and *Amblyomma americanum* ticks.

Because multiple TBDs are covered in this chapter, specific pathophysiology for each of the TBDs is covered in the next section.

**Table 180.1** Tick-Borne Diseases of North America

| DISEASE | PATHOGEN OR AGENT | MAJOR TICK VECTOR |
|---|---|---|
| Lyme disease | *Borrelia burgdorferi* | *Ixodes scapularis,* others |
| Babesiosis | *Babesia microti* | *Ixodes scapularis* |
| Anaplasmosis, granulocytic | *Anaplasma phagocytophilum* | *Ixodes scapularis* |
| Anaplasmosis, monocytic | *Ehrlichia chaffeensis* | *Amblyomma americanum* |
| Rocky Mountain spotted fever | *Rickettsia rickettsiae* | *Dermacentor variabilis* |
| Tularemia | *Francisella tularensis* | *Dermacentor variabilis, Dermacentor andersoni,* and *Amblyomma americanum* |
| Relapsing fever | *Borrelia* species (various) | *Ornithodoros* species |
| Colorado tick fever | Coltivirus | *Dermacentor andersoni* |
| Tick paralysis | Neurotoxin | *Dermacentor variabilis,* others |
| Q fever | *Coxiella burnetii* | *Dermacentor variabilis* |

**Table 180.2** Other Important Tick-Borne Diseases Worldwide

| DISEASE | PATHOGEN OR AGENT | MAJOR TICK VECTOR |
|---|---|---|
| Mediterranean spotted fever | *Rickettsia conorii* | *Rhipicephalus sanguineus* |
| Other spotted fevers | Other rickettsial species | Varies |
| Tick-borne encephalitis | Flavivirus | *Ixodes ricinus,* others |
| Relapsing fever | Various *Borrelia* species | Various *Ornithodoros* species |

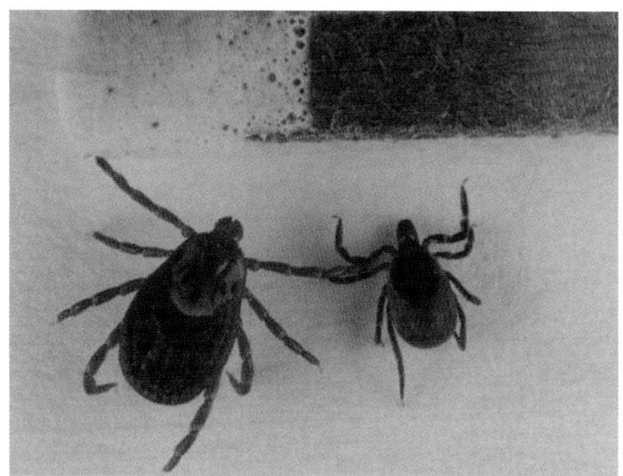

**Fig. 180.2 A *Dermacentor variabilis* tick next to an *Ixodes scapularis* tick.** This photograph shows an adult *D. variabilis (left)* tick next to an adult *I. scapularis (right)* tick, both next to a common match for scale. In cases of Rocky Mountain spotted fever, even with this larger tick vector, 30% to 40% of patients are not aware of a tick bite. (Photograph by Darlyne Murawski.)

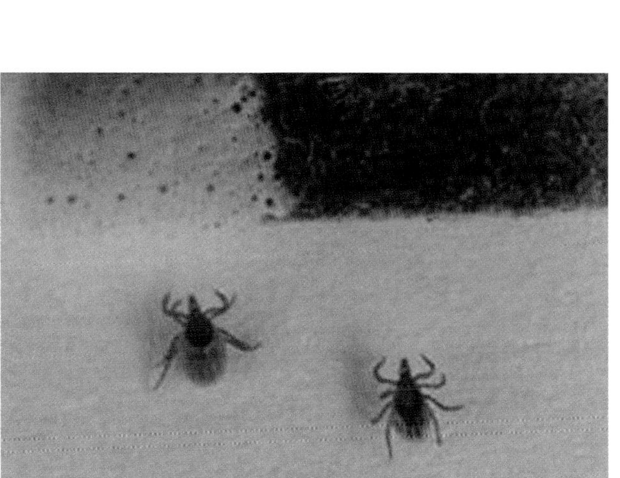

**Fig. 180.1 *Ixodes scapularis* ticks, nymphal stage.** Two nymphal *I. scapularis* ticks are shown next to a common household match. The tick on the *left* has been feeding on a mouse for 48 hours and is larger than the unfed tick on the *right*. Seen in three dimensions, the fed tick is more spherical, whereas the unfed tick is flatter. (Photograph by Darlyne Murawski.)

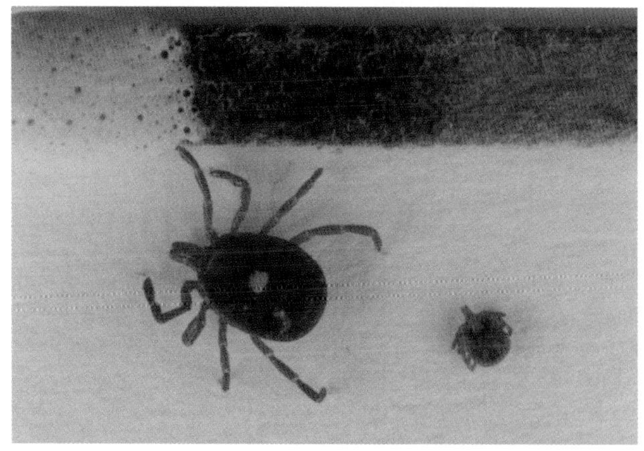

**Fig. 180.3 *Amblyomma americanum* tick.** An adult female Lone Star tick next to a nymph of the same species. This tick is responsible for transmission of human monocytic anaplasmosis and Master disease. (Photograph by Darlyne Murawski.)

**Table 180.3** Common Ticks Related to Human Disease

| TICK GENUS | HARD OR SOFT | FEEDING DURATION | DISEASES CAUSED |
|---|---|---|---|
| *Ixodes* | Hard | Days | Lyme disease, babesiosis, human granulocytic anaplasmosis |
| *Amblyomma* | Hard | Days | Human monocytic anaplasmosis, Master disease, tick paralysis |
| *Dermacentor* | Hard | Days | Rocky Mountain spotted fever, tularemia, tick paralysis, Colorado tick fever |
| *Rhipicephalus* | Hard | Days | Mediterranean spotted fever |
| *Ornithodoros* | Soft | Minutes to hours | Relapsing fever |

**Table 180.4** Tick-Borne Disease Syndromes

| SYNDROME | DISEASE | CHARACTERISTICS OF TYPICAL CASES |
|---|---|---|
| Localized rash (without or without fever) | Erythema migrans (Lyme disease) | Large, flat, red rash, sometimes with central clearing at the site of the tick bite |
| | Tularemia (ulceroglandular) | Shallow ulcer, usually acral at the site of the tick bite, associated with regional lymphadenopathy |
| Febrile illness without rash | Anaplasmosis | High fever, chills, headache, myalgias |
| | Babesiosis | High fever, chills, headache, fatigue, myalgias |
| | Lyme disease | Flulike illness without respiratory or gastrointestinal manifestations |
| | Rocky Mountain spotted fever | Severe headache, fever, myalgias |
| | Tularemia | High fever without localizing findings except respiratory symptoms in tularemic pneumonia |
| | Q fever | Nonspecific febrile illness |
| | Colorado tick fever | Fever (saddle-back curve), headache, myalgias |
| Febrile illness with generalized rash | Rocky Mountain spotted fever | As above with rash; rash beginning as maculopapular, then possibly evolving into petechial and skin necrosis |
| | Lyme disease | Multiple erythema migrans lesions (smaller, no punctum, less complexity than primary erythema migrans lesions) |
| | Anaplasmosis | Nonspecific maculopapular rash |
| Acute neurologic illness | Tick paralysis | More commonly in children, especially in young girls with the tick embedded in the scalp |

## PRESENTING SIGNS AND SYMPTOMS

TBDs most commonly manifest as one of four syndromes (**Table 180.4**):

- Localized rash (with or without fever)
- Febrile illness without prominent rash
- Febrile illness with diffuse rash
- Acute neurologic symptoms

Other possible presentations are possible, especially with respect to atypical presentations of any of these diseases and, most notably, Lyme disease. The other signs and symptoms of Lyme disease are discussed separately.

Before discussing the individual syndromes and diseases, the physician should know that as often as 20% of the time, a single tick bite results in multiple infections. Therefore, a patient may develop the rash of Lyme disease along with babesiosis or anaplasmosis. This possibility has implications with respect to the manifestations of the diseases and also the choice of antimicrobials.

### LOCALIZED RASH (WITH OR WITHOUT FEVER)

A localized rash from TBD occurs in early Lyme disease and ulceroglandular tularemia. Tularemia has multiple presentations, but the ulceroglandular form, which accounts for 80% of cases, usually starts with a papule that evolves into an ulcer on an extremity at the site of a tick bite (or animal exposure). The lesion evolves into a necrotic eschar and is often associated with regional lymphadenopathy, fever, and other systemic signs.

Mediterranean spotted fever and some of the African spotted fevers also manifest with a local eschar at the site of a tick bite, sometimes called a "tache noire."

Erythema migrans (EM), the rash of early localized Lyme disease, is an important condition that emergency physicians should be familiar with because antibiotic treatment at this stage almost always leads to excellent outcomes. Lyme disease is by far the most common vector-borne illness in North

America. EM develops at the site of the tick bite roughly 7 to 10 days later (range, 3 to 33 days), usually as flat erythema that is neither pruritic nor painful, although it can be either. The classic description of a target or bull's-eye lesion with central clearing is not the most common. Most EM rashes are uniformly red. EM can be darker in the center, vesicular, or necrotic. Know the spectrum of morphology of EM to avoid misdiagnosis of this infection (**Figs. 180.4 to 180.6**).

The location of EM tends to be at the sites where ticks feed or experience an impediment to further movement (groin, popliteal fossa, axilla, an elastic underwear strap, or the hairline in children). Although the rash can be anywhere, it tends not to occur acrally, and the torso is another common location. Size is another important feature; EM becomes large, 16 cm on average. Cellulitis, a common diagnostic competitor, rarely attains this size without fever, significant tenderness, and other systemic findings.

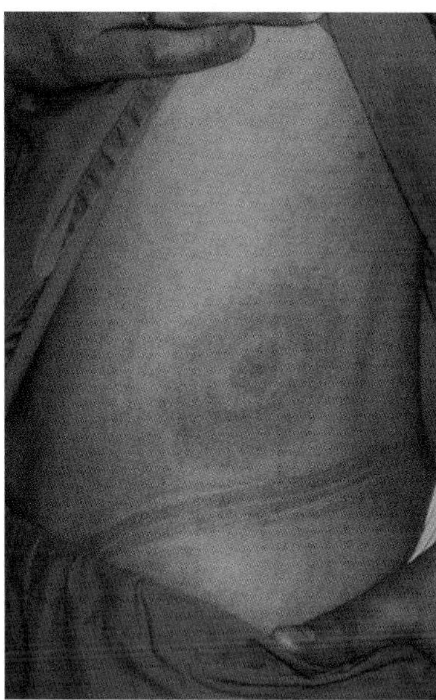

**Fig. 180.4 Classic erythema migrans.** Note the location (torso) and the bull's-eye appearance in this patient with fever and localized rash, which was flat and neither painful nor pruritic. A suggestion of a central punctum, the location of the tick bite, is evident.

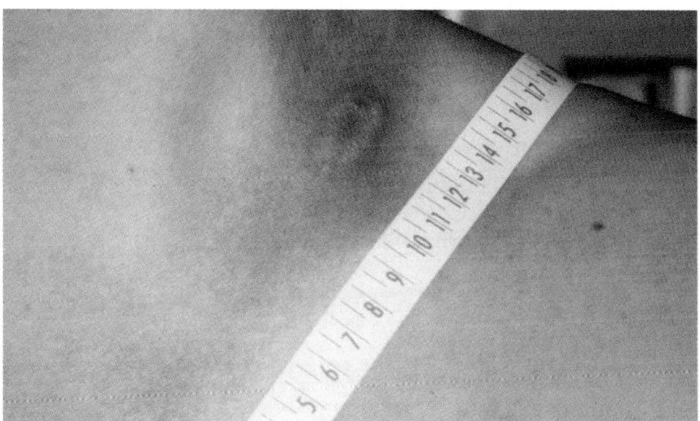

**Fig. 180.5 Erythema migrans with a raised, vesicular center.** This patient presented in early July after having pulled a tick off himself 7 days earlier. Approximately 18 hours after starting doxycycline, the patient had a Jarisch-Herxheimer reaction (abrupt onset of chills, tachycardia, intensification of rash), which occurs with treatment of spirochetal diseases.

Some patients with EM have fever, headache, myalgias, neck pain or stiffness, and other systemic symptoms. The fever is usually low grade, and high fevers suggest coinfecting babesiosis or anaplasmosis. Roughly 10% to 20% of patients with early Lyme disease have multiple cutaneous lesions (see later).

Although EM has always been thought to be pathognomonic of Lyme disease, EM-like lesions have been reported in the southeastern and central states; this has been called Master disease or southern tick-associated rash illness (STARI).[1] Although these patients' rashes have some differences from classic EM in patients from Lyme-endemic states, significant overlap can occur in individual patients. Other novel *Borrelia* species may cause this lesion, and these patients should also be treated with antibiotics, similar to patients with Lyme disease.

## FEBRILE ILLNESS WITHOUT PROMINENT RASH

Most TBDs can manifest as a nonspecific febrile illness. These diseases are babesiosis, anaplasmosis, tularemia, Colorado tick fever, relapsing fever, and Q fever. Lyme disease can also manifest this way, although the frequency of this presentation is unclear. Typical patients with RMSF do not have a rash until the third to the sixth day of illness, and in as many as 15% of patients, a rash never appears. If RMSF is a real diagnostic possibility on epidemiologic grounds, treat with empiric antibiotics even in the absence of a rash. Finally, all these diseases that typically present without rash are sometimes associated with nonspecific, usually maculopapular rashes.

Anaplasmosis (formerly called ehrlichiosis), a relatively newly described illness, has a presentation similar to that of

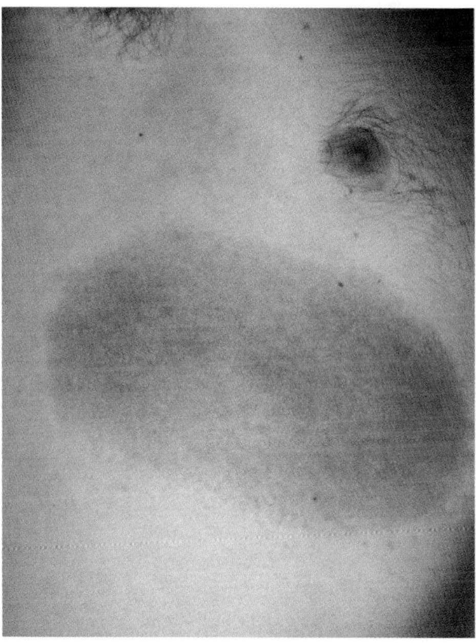

**Fig. 180.6 Erythema migrans with a homogeneous color.** This young man had a rash that had been ascribed to a spider bite but was growing larger. The rash was painless, thus making a spider bite much less likely. The patient also had a tender, palpable lymph node in the right axilla.

RMSF but without the rash. The two most common forms in humans are granulocytic and monocytic (terms based on the tropism of the organisms toward white blood cells). These patients complain of high fever, headache, and myalgias. The spectrum of disease is wide, and published series likely emphasize sicker patients. As in RMSF, some patients have prominent encephalitis, noncardiogenic pulmonary edema, and shock.

Babesiosis, a malaria-like parasitic infection transmitted by *I. scapularis,* is diagnosed with increasing frequency in areas of the United States where this tick is active. The usual agent in North America is *Babesia microti.* Infection results in a wide spectrum of illness ranging from asymptomatic seroconversion to mild flulike illness, to malaria-like illness, or even overwhelming sepsis and death. Fever, fatigue, headache, sweats, and chills are the most common symptoms. Hepatosplenomegaly may be present. Complications include hemolysis and renal failure, noncardiogenic pulmonary edema, and coma. Patients with babesiosis can be ill for weeks to months and may have subacute or chronic illness. Splenectomized patients have an unusually fulminant course.

Colorado tick fever is a viral illness that occurs in the Rocky Mountain states and southwestern Canada and is transmitted by *Dermacentor andersoni* at elevations of 1200 to 3300 m. Only a few hundred cases are diagnosed annually in the United States. The presentation is nonspecific (fever, headache, and myalgias), but the fever often follows a characteristic "saddle-back" pattern (two periods of 2 to 3 days of fever, punctuated by an afebrile interval). Occasionally, a small, red, painless papule is seen, and less commonly, patients have a nonspecific generalized rash. Pharyngitis, lower gastrointestinal symptoms, and central nervous system (CNS) symptoms may also occur in some cases.

Q fever manifests as a nonspecific febrile illness sometimes associated with hepatitis or pneumonia. Hepatitis is particularly common. Other organ systems, especially the heart and CNS, may be affected, and a few patients also exhibit a nonspecific maculopapular rash. Q fever may become chronic, and in these patients, it often affects the heart (endocarditis), blood vessels, and liver. The diagnosis is established by serologic methods and by polymerase chain reaction because the organism is very rarely cultured.

Typhoidal tularemia manifests as a nonspecific febrile illness and headache and is uncommon. Tularemic pneumonia may develop. One outbreak of this form of the disease that occurred on Martha's Vineyard (an island off the coast of Massachusetts) likely resulted from inhalation of ticks aerosolized by power lawn mowers.

Relapsing fever is caused by various *Borrelia* species transmitted by *Ornithodoros* species, soft ticks that feed for very short times. This illness is characterized by intervals of fever interspersed with afebrile periods. The explanation of these episodes is that the *Borrelia* organisms undergo antigenic shifting, thus presenting a new antigen to the patient's immune system. After an incubation period of approximately 1 week, patients develop fever, headache, myalgias, and chills. Abdominal pain and altered mental status are common. Untreated, most patients improve and then suffer a relapse from the new antigenic variety 1 week later. Complications include focal neurologic findings (including seventh nerve palsy), myocarditis, and ruptured spleen.

## FEBRILE ILLNESS WITH GENERALIZED RASH

Many TBDs can manifest with fevers in which a generalized rash is a prominent manifestation of the illness. RMSF is the most dramatic of these illnesses; patients present with fever, headache, myalgias, and rash. The classic triad of fever, headache, and rash in a patient with a recent tick bite is seen in a few patients. Even with the larger tick vector, only approximately two thirds of patients recall the tick bite. In addition, the rash of RMSF does not develop until the third to the sixth day of the illness. The rash begins as a maculopapular rash that becomes petechial and finally may evolve into frank ecchymosis. The classic description of a rash that begins acrally and spreads centrally does not always apply. Thus, the rash can vary from nonexistent to frank skin necrosis. Because the organisms cause small vessel vasculitis, the manifestations are based on the particular organs affected. Patients can present with a surgical abdomen, an illness resembling meningitis, myocarditis, renal failure, or circulatory collapse. Untreated, RMSF has a mortality rate of 25% to 40%. Therefore, considering this diagnosis in any febrile patient with the correct epidemiologic context is important, because early antibiotic treatment reduces the mortality rate to less than 5%.[2]

Early disseminated Lyme disease with secondary EM is the other TBD that manifests as fever and generalized rash. Secondary lesions occur approximately 20% of the time and imply hematogenous spread of the organism. The secondary lesions differ from the primary EM lesion in that they tend to be smaller, lack the central punctum, and exhibit less central clearing.

## ACUTE WEAKNESS

The one TBD that is not caused by an infectious agent is tick paralysis. This illness can be caused by several tick species that produce neurotoxins. Patients present with gait instability, acute ascending weakness, and sometimes cranial nerve findings that suggest Guillain-Barré syndrome.[3] Children, often girls with long hair, are more frequently affected, and the scalp of these patients must be very carefully inspected. The diagnosis is established by finding an engorged tick, the removal of which is also the treatment of this rare disease.

Despite (or perhaps because of) the rarity of this disorder, consider this entity in all patients with acute onset of weakness. Cases have been reported in the Philadelphia area (acquired locally) and in Los Angeles (likely contracted in Montana). The neurologic findings resolve over 6 to 24 hours. Finding the tick precludes the need for more expensive and invasive evaluation and prevents deaths. Patients have no fever and no alteration of consciousness.

Lyme disease can also manifest with different kinds of focal weakness resulting from meningoradiculitis; the deficit depends on which nerve roots are involved. Of course, any febrile illness can lead to overall nonlocalizing malaise.

## OTHER MANIFESTATIONS OF LYME DISEASE

Lyme disease has been traditionally divided into three phases (**Table 180.5**). Early localized disease is characterized by EM, although some authors include flulike illness in this stage. Early disseminated disease typically involves the skin, heart, joints, and nervous system. Late disseminated disease generally affects the joints, nervous system, and (in Europe) the skin. Although early disseminated Lyme disease has many

**Table 180.5 Common Manifestations and Treatment of Lyme Disease**

| STAGE | MANIFESTATION | TREATMENT |
|---|---|---|
| Early localized | Localized erythema migrans | Oral amoxicillin, doxycycline, or cefuroxime axetil for 10-30 days |
| Mild early disseminated | Disseminated erythema migrans<br>Conjunctivitis<br>Early arthritis<br>Seventh nerve palsy with normal cerebrospinal fluid<br>Carditis with PR interval <0.30 | Ceftriaxone, cefotaxime, or penicillin G for 21-30 days |
| Severe early disseminated | Early neurologic manifestations with abnormal cerebrospinal fluid*<br>Carditis with PR interval >0.30 or higher degrees of heart block | Ceftriaxone, cefotaxime, or penicillin G for 2-3 wk |
| Late disseminated | Late neurologic manifestations (encephalopathy, peripheral neuropathy)<br>Lyme arthritis | Intravenous antibiotics for 2-4 wk<br>Oral antibiotics for 30-60 days |

*Manifestations include cranial neuropathy, lymphocytic meningitis (with or without radiculitis or plexitis), transverse myelitis, and cerebellitis. Controversy exists regarding parenteral antibiotics if seventh nerve palsy is the only manifestation (and cerebrospinal fluid pleocytosis).

potential manifestations, the common and important manifestations for emergency physicians are cranial nerve palsy, meningitis, carditis, and arthritis.

Any cranial nerve can be affected, but seventh nerve palsy is by far the most common. Bilateral facial involvement is not uncommon in patients with Lyme-induced facial palsy. Controversy exists regarding the appropriateness of lumbar puncture in these patients. The major question is this: Should the presence of pleocytosis mandate parenteral therapy or not? Although this question has no definitive answer, many physicians favor lumbar puncture and treat the patient parenterally if the cerebrospinal fluid shows abnormalities. A European study suggested that this approach is not necessary.[4] Lyme meningitis, which can occur with or without other neurologic abnormalities, can be surprisingly "quiet" with respect to symptoms. Headache may be mild and intermittent, and meningeal signs are often absent.

Carditis occurs in 5% to 10% of untreated patients, usually in young male patients. It has a predilection for the conduction system and often leads to complete heart block. Although temporary cardiac pacing is indicated, permanent pacemakers are rarely necessary. Arthritis is usually a late finding, but it can also occur in the early disseminated phase.

## DIFFERENTIAL DIAGNOSIS AND MEDICAL DECISION MAKING

The differential diagnosis in these patients depends on the specific presenting syndrome and is largely covered in the previous section. A complete differential diagnosis of EM includes various other acute rashes.[1] Physicians should diagnose early localized Lyme disease and tick paralysis by history and physical examination. Fifty percent of patients with EM have a negative Lyme serologic test result; therefore, no testing is necessary because a negative result should not dissuade the physician from diagnosing EM and treating it. Serologic testing is not indicated in most patients with EM.

The differential diagnosis of undifferentiated fever is enormous and includes just about every cause of fever. In patients with fever and generalized rash, one must consider bacteremia and viremia, especially meningococcemia and streptococcal and staphylococcal sepsis. Physicians should also treat suspected RMSF empirically without waiting for diagnostic test confirmation. **Table 180.6** gives clues to the diagnosis of TBDs.

**Table 180.6 Clinical Clues (History, Physical Examination, or Laboratory) Suggesting the Diagnosis of a Tick-Borne Illness Manifesting as a Nonspecific Febrile Illness***

| DISEASE | CLUES |
|---|---|
| Anaplasmosis | Faint rash possible<br>Low white blood cell or platelet count<br>Elevated hepatic transaminases |
| Babesiosis | Findings of hemolysis<br>History of splenectomy<br>Presence of faint rash, hepatomegaly, or splenomegaly |
| Lyme disease | Careful skin examination for any rash consistent with erythema migrans<br>Bradycardia from heart block<br>Associated seventh nerve palsy or lymphocytic meningitis |
| Colorado tick fever | Saddle-back fever curve |
| Rocky Mountain spotted fever | Maculopapular or petechial rash<br>Normal white blood cell count or low platelet count<br>Hyponatremia<br>Peripheral edema |
| Relapsing fever | Recurring episodes of fever with afebrile intervals |
| Tularemia | Acrally located ulcer<br>Regional lymphadenopathy<br>Possible associated pneumonia |

*Apart from an epidemiologic context suggesting a tick-borne disease.

Physicians can often confidently diagnose babesiosis (**Fig. 180.7**), anaplasmosis (**Fig. 180.8**), and relapsing fever (**Fig. 180.9**) on the basis of a blood smear. Although numerous antigen and antibody tests are available for all these diseases, the results of these tests are hardly ever available in real time.

For later manifestation of Lyme disease, the Centers for Disease Control and Prevention currently recommend a two-step testing procedure (screening enzyme-linked immunosorbent assay followed by a confirmatory Western blot). Newer tests, especially the C-6 peptide, hold promise for a single-tier test. In these patients, the physician must carefully interpret the serologic results in the context of the patient's symptoms, clinical course, and epidemiologic features.

In patients with acute weakness, tick paralysis can be confused with Guillain-Barré syndrome, myasthenia gravis, botulism, hypokalemic paralysis, organophosphate poisoning, transverse myelitis, and spinal cord compression.

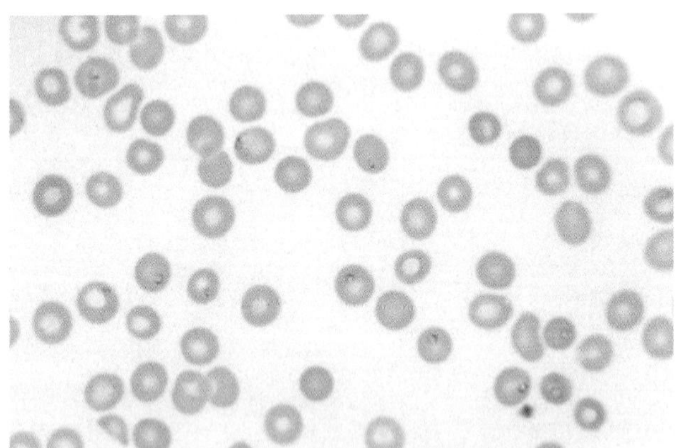

**Fig. 180.7 Blood smear showing babesiosis.** This figure shows intraerythrocytic ring forms in multiple red blood cells from a patient with a high parasite count.

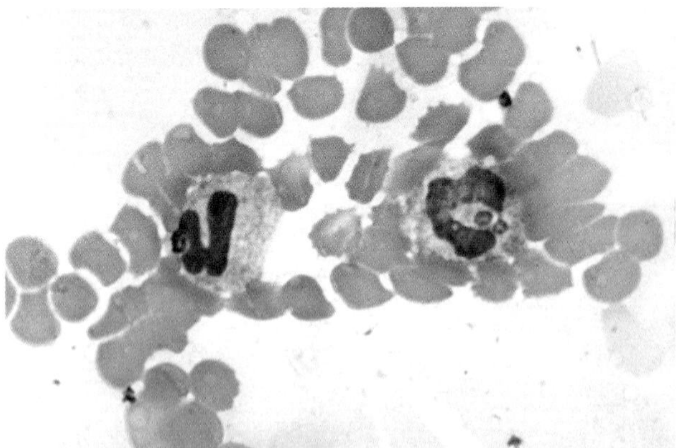

**Fig. 180.8 Blood smear showing a morula in a patient with anaplasmosis.** This blood smear shows two morulae (intracellular clumps of anaplasma organisms in the white blood cell to the *right*) that can be diagnostic in a patient with anaplasmosis. (Courtesy of Dr. J. S. Dumler.)

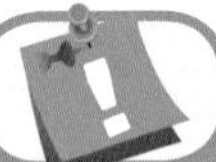

### TIPS AND TRICKS

- Most patients with Lyme disease and approximately one third of patients with Rocky Mountain spotted fever (for which the tick vector is much larger) do not have a history of a known tick bite.
- Treat patients with presumed Rocky Mountain spotted fever with a tetracycline even if a rash is not yet present.
- Remember that up to 20% of patients with tick-borne disease have more than one infection transmitted by the same tick bite.
- Examine the whole body, and particularly the scalp, in all patients presenting with acute significant weakness or a clinical picture resembling Guillain-Barré syndrome. This is especially important in young children and occurs most often in young girls.
- In early localized Lyme disease with erythema migrans, serologic testing is not indicated or helpful, unless the clinical findings and situation are very atypical or ambiguous. Serologic test results are normal approximately 50% of the time.
- In children, even those younger than 9 years of age, with life-threatening cases of Rocky Mountain spotted fever or anaplasmosis, use intravenous doxycycline initially.

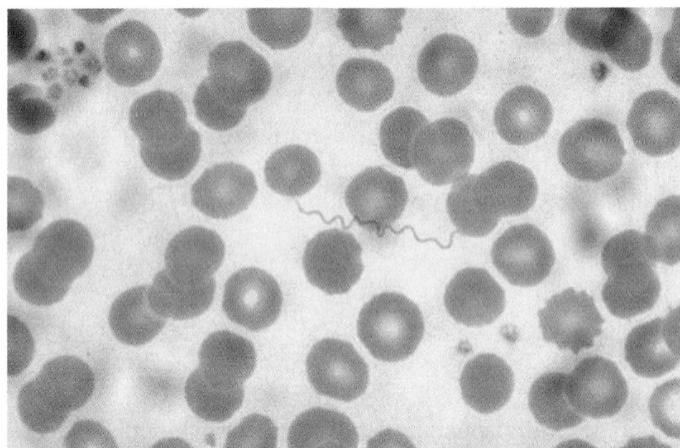

**Fig. 180.9 Blood smear showing relapsing fever *Borrelia*.** This blood smear shows a spirochete in the blood from a patient with relapsing fever.

## TREATMENT

Tick removal is best accomplished by using fine forceps applied close to the skin and gradually pulling the tick upward and outward. Because ticks use a cement-like substance to embed, this removal procedure may take steady gentle pressure over a minute or two. Try to remove the entire tick. Retained mouth parts may cause a foreign body reaction or a staphylococcal or streptococcal skin infection, but they have no implications in terms of TBD transmission.

No specific antimicrobial therapy exists for Colorado tick fever or tick-borne encephalitis. The definitive treatment for tick paralysis is tick removal; improvement often begins within hours.

**Table 180.7 Treatment of the Tick-Borne Diseases***

| DISEASE | ANTIMICROBIAL TREATMENT | OTHER ISSUES |
|---|---|---|
| Anaplasmosis (formerly called ehrlichiosis) | Doxycycline | Even in children, IV doxycycline indicated |
| Babesiosis | Clindamycin and quinine<br>Atovaquone and azithromycin | In severely affected patients, consider exchange transfusion |
| Rocky Mountain spotted fever (and other rickettsial spotted fevers) | Doxycycline or chloramphenicol. | Even in children, IV doxycycline indicated |
| Relapsing fever | Doxycycline | Some patients with carditis require a temporary pacemaker |
| Tularemia | Streptomycin, gentamicin, or doxycycline | |
| Q fever | Doxycycline | |
| Tick paralysis | None | Tick removal constitutes treatment; ICU observation often necessary |
| Colorado tick fever, tick-borne encephalitis | None | Supportive care |

*ICU,* Intensive care unit; *IV,* intravenous.

*The choices of antibiotics, route, dose, and duration should be made on a case-by-case basis, depending on the severity of illness, allergies, age of patient, pregnancy, and other individual factors.

Table 180.5 shows the treatments for specific manifestations of Lyme disease. Treat patients with the remaining bacterial TBDs with specific antimicrobial therapy (**Table 180.7**). Data suggest a trend toward shorter courses of antibiotics in patients with early Lyme disease.[5,6]

The threshold to treat should be low, and frequently the decision to treat is based purely on presentation and epidemiologic context. Although tetracyclines are generally contraindicated in children less than 9 years of age, short courses of intravenous doxycycline are indicated in children with life-threatening manifestations of RMSF or anaplasmosis.

## FOLLOW-UP, NEXT STEPS, AND PATIENT EDUCATION

Most patients with TBDs can be treated as outpatients with primary care follow-up. Patients with syndromes requiring intravenous antibiotics, cardiac pacing, or intensive care for CNS, respiratory, renal, or circulatory failure should be admitted to an appropriate inpatient setting. Consultation with specialists is on a case-by-case basis.

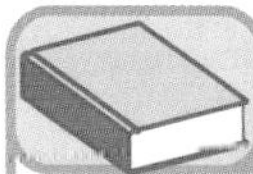

**PATIENT TEACHING TIPS**

If you cannot avoid tick exposure, do daily tick checks, and carefully remove any ticks found.

If you become ill and have either been bitten by a tick or been exposed to ticks, be sure to mention this to your doctor, even if you develop new symptoms weeks or months later. The tick bite could possibly cause delayed problems.

## SUGGESTED READINGS


Anderson JF. The natural history of ticks. Med Clin North Am 2002;86:205-18.

Borg R, Dotevall L, Hagberg L, et al. Intravenous ceftriaxone compared with oral doxycycline for the treatment of Lyme neuroborreliosis. Scand J Infect Dis 2005;37:449-54.

Dattwyler RJ, Luft BJ, Kunkel MJ, et al. Ceftriaxone compared with doxycycline for the treatment of acute disseminated Lyme disease. N Engl J Med 1997;337:289-94.

Demma LJ, Traeger MS, Nicholson WL, et al. Rocky Mountain spotted fever from an unexpected tick vector in Arizona. N Engl J Med 2005;353:587-94.

Edlow JA. Erythema migrans. Med Clin North Am 2002;86:239-60.

Edlow JA. Lyme disease and related tick-borne illnesses. Ann Emerg Med 1999;33:680-93.

Klempner MS, Hu LT, Evans J, et al. Two controlled trials of antibiotic treatment in patients with persistent symptoms and a history of Lyme disease. N Engl J Med 2001;345:85-92.

Krause PJ, Telford 3rd SR, Spielman A, et al. Concurrent Lyme disease and babesiosis: evidence for increased severity and duration of illness. JAMA 1996;275:1657-60.

Masters EJ, Olson GS, Weiner SJ, Paddock CD. Rocky Mountain spotted fever: a clinician's dilemma. Arch Intern Med 2003;163:769-74.

Nadelman RB, Nowakowski J, Fish D, et al. Prophylaxis with single-dose doxycycline for the prevention of Lyme disease after an *Ixodes scapularis* tick bite. N Engl J Med 2001;345:79-84.

Philipp MT, Wormser GP, Marques AR, et al. A decline in C6 antibody titer occurs in successfully treated patients with culture-confirmed early localized or early disseminated Lyme borreliosis. Clin Diagn Lab Immunol 2005;12:1069-74.

Tick-borne diseases, part I: Lyme disease. Infect Dis Clin North Am 2008;22(2)[entire issue].

Tick-borne diseases, part II. Infect Dis Clin North Am 2008;22(3)[entire issue].


## REFERENCES

***References can be found on Expert Consult @ www.expertconsult.com.***

# 181 Tuberculosis

D. Matthew Sullivan

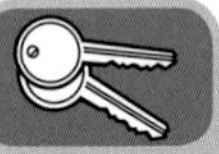

**KEY POINTS**

- Despite advances in diagnosis and therapy, tuberculosis (TB) remains a leading cause of death worldwide.
- TB begins as a primary infection (usually in the lung, but other organ systems may be involved) that enters a latent period.
- Immunocompromised patients are at increased risk of reactivation of the disease and the development of active TB.
- The presentation of TB can be very broad and should remain in the differential diagnosis in all patients who present with systemic signs of infection.
- Therapy for TB should include multiple drugs to which the mycobacterium is susceptible and should continue for at least 6 to 12 months.
- Because of the risk of multidrug-resistant TB, an initial four-drug regimen with isoniazid, rifampin, ethambutol, and pyrazinamide is recommended.

## PATHOPHYSIOLOGY

*Mycobacterium tuberculosis* is a small, slow-growing bacterium that is transmitted by inhalation of droplet nuclei. As infected persons talk, cough, or sneeze, numerous nuclei are expelled into the surrounding air. Only a few inhaled droplets are needed to infect, so an increased length of exposure to the pathogen and the number of bacilli present correlate with infectivity.[1]

Inhaled bacilli travel down the bronchi and lodge within an alveolus. Activated macrophages then ingest the bacilli, which replicate and ultimately cause lysis. Monocytes are attracted and differentiate into macrophages, which again consume the mycobacteria and form a tubercle. The tubercle travels through the lymphatic and hematogenous systems and lodges in the lung apices, lymph nodes, meninges, vertebra, long bones, or kidney.

Two to 3 weeks after infection, cell-mediated immunity converts the tubercle to a granuloma by means of CD4 helper T cells. This process arrests the local infection for most immunocompetent hosts. At that time, the only sign of the disease may be a positive reaction to the purified protein derivative (PPD) skin test.

A delayed hypersensitivity response uses cytotoxic killer CD8 suppressor T cells to kill the other nonactivated macrophages with bacilli. This process creates local tissue destruction and the formation of a caseating granuloma. In immunocompromised patients, this caseous center may expand and then calcify to form a Ghon complex in the lung. If the infection is uncontrolled, primary tuberculous pneumonia may ensue, or infection may spread through blood and lymph, with resulting disseminated TB.[2]

Active TB develops months to years later in those patients with decreased capacity for cell-mediated immunity, such as patients with malnutrition, comorbidities, and immunosuppression. Patients with acquired immunodeficiency syndrome are especially prone to develop active disease. As the caseating granuloma liquefies and releases numerous bacilli, a delayed hypersensitivity response is initiated, and local tissue destruction follows. Ultimately, erosion through a bronchial wall creates a cavitary lesion and the development of pneumonia. The high oxygen tension of the cavity lends itself to replication of bacilli and persistent disease.

## CLASSIC PRESENTATION

The symptom constellation of cough, night sweats, and hemoptysis, commonly associated with TB, is of little benefit in the early identification of disease because TB often has no early symptoms. Late symptoms are wide ranging and do not always involve the respiratory tract. Extrapulmonary manifestations of TB are seen in 20% of patients when the host is immunocompetent and are even more common when the host is immunocompromised.[3] In patients with one or more risk factors for TB (**Table 181.1** and **Box 181.1**),[4] a detailed history helps to refine the pretest probability for the diagnosis of TB.

Early stages of infection are most often asymptomatic in the normal host. Unless cell-mediated immunity is impaired, symptoms may manifest only after reactivation of the infection. Patients may present with a combination of systemic symptoms including cough, fatigue, fever, anorexia, malaise, and weight loss. An indolent cough that has progressed over more than 2 weeks should raise the clinical suspicion of pulmonary TB.[5] Hemoptysis signifies erosion into the bronchial

**Table 181.1 Tuberculosis Rates (per 100,000 Population) Among Five Racial and Ethnic Populations: United States, 2003**

| RACE OR ETHNICITY | RATE* |
|---|---|
| White, non-Hispanic | 1.4 |
| American Indian/Alaska Native | 8.0 (5.7) |
| Hispanic | 10.5 (7.5) |
| Black, non-Hispanic | 11.5 (8.2) |
| Asian/Pacific Islander | 29.4 (21.0) |

From American Thoracic Society, Centers for Disease Control and Prevention, Infectious Diseases Society of America. Treatment of tuberculosis. MMWR Recomm Rep 2003:52:1-77 [erratum appears in MMWR Recomm Rep 2005;53:1203; dosage error in text].

*Numbers in parentheses represent risk for tuberculosis compared with white non-Hispanics.

**BOX 181.1 Populations at Risk for Contracting Tuberculosis**

Persons with human immunodeficiency infection
Persons with exposure to a known case
Persons of Asian, African, or Latin American descent
Migrant farmers
Homeless persons
Persons of low income
Older persons
Nursing home residents
Correctional facility residents
Intravenous drug users
Persons with occupational exposure

Adapted from American Thoracic Society, Centers for Disease Control and Prevention, Infectious Diseases Society of America. Controlling tuberculosis in the United States. Am J Respir Crit Care Med 2005;172:1169-1227.

**Table 181.2 Differential Diagnosis of Tuberculosis**

| Pulmonary Tuberculosis |
|---|
| Severe systemic symptoms? |
| Bacterial pneumonia |
| Geographic distribution for fungal infection? |
| Histoplasmosis |
| Coccidioidomycosis |
| Blastomycosis |
| HIV infection? |
| *Mycobacterium avium* infection |
| *Mycobacterium kansasii* infection |
| *Pneumocystis jiroveci* (formerly *carinii)* infection |
| Cavitary lesion? |
| *Klebsiella pneumoniae* infection |
| *Staphylococcus pyogenes* infection |
| Aspiration pneumonia |
| Carcinoma |
| Pulmonary infarction |
| Wegener granulomatosis |
| Bullous disease |
| Mediastinal lymphadenopathy? |
| Lymphoma |
| Sarcoidosis |
| **Extrapulmonary Tuberculosis** |
| Lymphadenitis? |
| Scrofula |
| Lymphoma |
| Metastatic cancer |
| Fungal disease |
| Cat-scratch disease |
| Sarcoidosis |
| Toxoplasmosis |
| Reactive or bacterial adenitis |
| Bone or joint infection? |
| Pott disease |
| Bacterial abscess |
| Synovitis |
| Sterile pyuria? |
| Appendicitis |
| Pelvic inflammatory disease |
| Diverticulosis or diverticulitis |
| Mesenteric adenitis |
| Headache and altered mental status? |
| Bacterial meningitis |
| Viral meningitis |
| Encephalitis |

*HIV,* Human immunodeficiency virus.

tree and is unlikely to be an early symptom of pulmonary TB. When the clinical suspicion is raised, the physical findings in pulmonary TB may include fever, pleural effusion, focal pneumonic ausculatory findings, and adenopathy.

## VARIATIONS

Extrapulmonary manifestations clinically conform to the site of infection, and care should be taken to include TB in the differential diagnosis in patients who present with the following conditions:

- Diffuse adenopathy of the neck (scrofula)
- Recurrent urinary tract infections, scrotal mass, prostatitis, epididymitis, or orchitis (genitourinary TB)
- Headache, fever, meningeal signs, or altered mental status (TB meningitis)
- Focal neurologic deficits, cranial nerve abnormalities, cerebellar dysfunction, or seizure (central nervous system tuberculomas)
- Joint or spinal pain (Pott disease)
- Chest pain or dullness to percussion (pleural TB)
- Multiple organ system disease (disseminated TB)

## DIFFERENTIAL DIAGNOSIS

Depending on the clinical symptoms at presentation, TB may mimic numerous systemic diseases. Radiographic findings, sputum smears, and skin tests help in the diagnosis of TB. The "gold standard" diagnostic test is culture, and results may not be available for several weeks (**Table 181.2**).

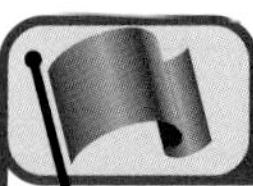

**RED FLAGS**

- Failure to consider extrapulmonary tuberculosis in the differential diagnosis
- Tuberculosis in immunocompromised patients or those at the extremes of age
- Tuberculosis in patients with risk factors for multidrug-resistant tuberculosis
- Patients with social concerns who may not be able to fulfill directly observed therapy

## DIAGNOSTIC TESTING

Latent TB in asymptomatic patients is clinically difficult to identify. Targeted population screening has been advocated as a means to identify early disease while it is still in the more easily treated latent period. Current recommendations are to perform a PPD skin test on patients who would benefit from therapy for latent TB and who are at high risk of developing active TB (**Box 181.2**).[6] Currently, the foundation of screening is skin testing with PPD in patients at risk for TB. Patients who harbor latent TB and who have intact cellular immunity demonstrate a hypersensitivity reaction at the site of PPD placement that can be graded and evaluated with a well-established scale reflecting positivity or negativity (**Table 181.3**).[6] This type of screening is not particularly sensitive in immunocompromised patients, older patients, newly infected patients, or very young children. Additionally, the PPD test lacks the specificity to distinguish among other *Mycobacterium* infections.[7] Newer whole-blood antigen-stimulated interferon-γ release assays are available that have high sensitivity and specificity, are not affected by prior bacille Calmette-Guérin vaccination, and do not have a waning response over time.[4,7] As genomic testing becomes more widely available, the ability to predict disease progression based on the genetic expression of an individual patient may play an important role in diagnosis.[8]

The advent of auscultation and radiography greatly advanced the diagnosis of TB in the eighteenth and nineteenth centuries.[9] Despite technical advances in diagnostic tests, history, physical examination, and conventional radiography remain cornerstones in the diagnosis of TB in the emergency department (ED). Frequently, patients who present to the ED with symptoms of pulmonary or extrapulmonary TB have limited prior access to care, and heightened suspicion is required. Once a history is obtained that suggests active pulmonary disease, patients should be isolated (in a negative-pressure room, if possible), and a chest radiograph should be obtained. The identification of an upper lobe infiltrate suggests the presence of active disease (**Figs. 181.1 and 181.2**). Chest radiography is not highly sensitive, particularly in the immunocompromised patient, in whom reticulonodular and miliary patterns of disease may be present.[10] The clinical syndrome of normal chest radiographs with sputum culture-positive TB is well described in patients with human immunodeficiency virus (HIV) infection and low CD4 counts.[11] In these patient populations, a high clinical suspicion for disease mandates that sputum studies be ordered.

**BOX 181.2 Indications for a Purified Protein Derivative Skin Test**

Increased risk of exposure to infectious cases
- Close contacts of persons with known active TB
- Health care workers where TB is treated

Increased risk of TB infection
- Foreign-born persons from a country with a high prevalence of TB
- Homeless persons
- Persons living or working in long-term care facilities

Increased risk of active TB once infection has occurred
- Persons infected with human immunodeficiency virus
- Intravenous drug users
- Persons receiving immunosuppressive therapy
- Patients with end-stage renal disease
- Patients with silicosis
- Diabetic patients
- Patients with hematologic malignant diseases
- Patients with prior gastrectomies
- Patients with prior jejunoileal bypass
- Persons with severe malnutrition
- Persons with recent TB infection

From Myers JP. New recommendations for the treatment of tuberculosis. Curr Opin Infect Dis 2005;18:133-40.
*TB*, Tuberculosis.

Unfortunately, sputum Gram stain with carbolfuchsin and phenol or auramine O staining for the identification of acid-fast bacilli (AFB) is unreliable in the ED evaluation of patients suspected to have TB. In addition to the variability in performance inherently linked to the skill of the laboratory technical staff, and the availability of rapid test results at all times of day, the sensitivity of a single AFB smear remains low (<50%), far too low for the safe discharge of the high-risk patient.[12] This situation necessitates further management by the inpatient team or close follow-up with the local health department for further sputum smears in those patients who are deemed safe for discharge. The additive value of three morning sputum smears is helpful for excluding the diagnosis of active pulmonary TB. When AFB smears are identified, distinguishing among *Mycobacterium* species is not possible, and the definitive diagnosis should be confirmed with sputum culture.

Sputum culture is not part of the ED evaluation of a patient with suspected TB. Cultures traditionally take 4 to 8 weeks to grow. Cultures are sensitive in more than 80% of cases of infiltrative pulmonary TB and in more than 90% of cases of cavitary TB.[13] Newer methods of radiometric culture systems with radiolabeled carbon-14 yield faster results (1 to 3 weeks).

The advent of nucleic acid amplification tests and of polymerase chain reaction identification greatly increased the sensitivity (97% to 99%) for the diagnosis of TB from a single sample, and accurate results can be obtained in hours. Additional strain typing for *M. tuberculosis* with restriction fragment length polymorphism is available to identify the organism's DNA.[14] Even for large centers, these tests are time and resource consuming to perform on an as-needed basis, and they are impractical for use in the ED work-up of patients

**Table 181.3 Evaluation of Purified Protein Derivative Skin Testing Results**

| INDURATION SIZE | CONSIDERED POSITIVE IN |
|---|---|
| ≥5 mm | Recent contact with TB-positive patient<br>Chest radiographic findings consistent with prior TB<br>HIV-infected patients<br>Immunosuppressed patients<br>Organ transplant recipients |
| ≥10 mm | Recent immigrants from countries with a high prevalence of TB<br>Intravenous drug users<br>Homeless and low-income populations<br>Residents or employees of nursing homes, hospitals, homeless shelters, correctional facilities<br>Risk factors for reactivation TB (diabetes, renal failure, malignant disease)<br>Medically underserved populations<br>Children < 4 years old<br>Children and adolescents exposed to TB-positive adult |
| ≥15 mm | People with no risk factors |

From Myers JP. New recommendations for the treatment of tuberculosis. Curr Opin Infect Dis 2005;18:133-40.
*HIV,* Human immunodeficiency virus; *TB,* tuberculosis.

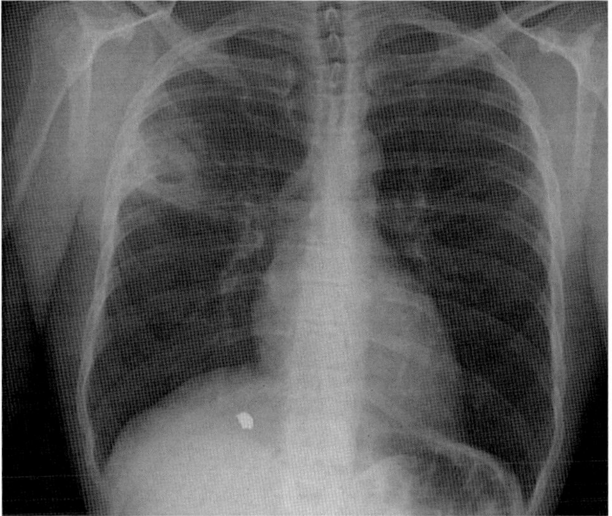

**Fig. 181.1 Right upper lobe cavitary lesion.**

with suspected TB. The utility of these newer tests in smear-negative individuals has been called into question with reports of lower sensitivities (70%) in this population.[15]

Extrapulmonary TB is often confirmed by biopsy of affected tissues and lymph nodes. Blood culture, urine culture, and culture of other body fluids are used to aid in the diagnosis of extrapulmonary TB, with varying sensitivities, depending on the host and the site of culture. The diagnosis of pleural TB is facilitated with pleural biopsy and culture; yields are 86% in immunocompetent patients and 47% in immunocompromised patients.[16]

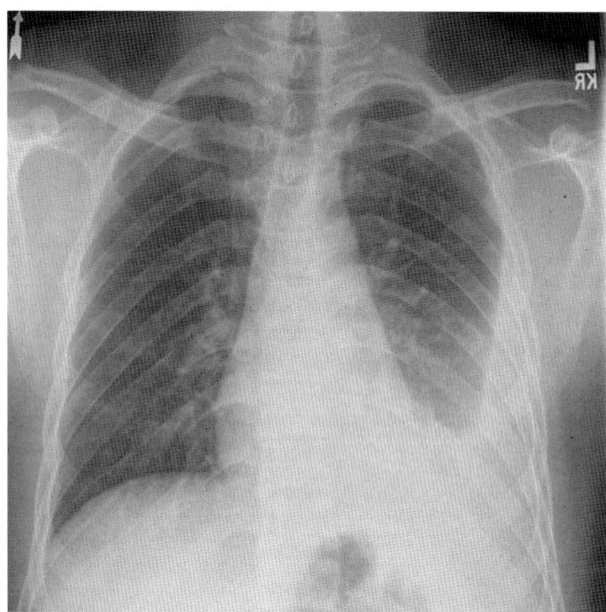

**Fig. 181.2 Left lower lobe infiltrate with effusion.**

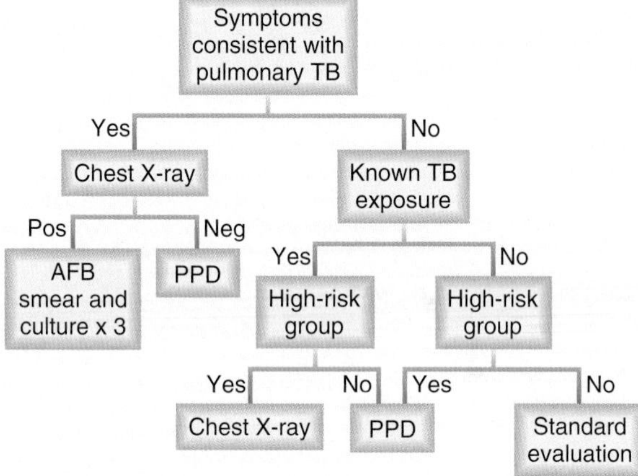


**Fig. 181.3 Algorithm for patients suspected to have tuberculosis (TB).** *AFB,* Acid-fast bacillus; *Neg,* negative; *Pos,* positive; *PPD,* purified protein derivative.

Ultimately, the diagnosis of TB remains firmly grounded in the clinician's analysis. A high suspicion of disease, coupled with appropriate testing for the given presentation, will translate into clinical success (**Fig. 181.3**).[17]

## PROCEDURES

Historically, bleeding, leeches, cupping, application of animal excrement, "touching" by kings, pleurocentesis, and the isolation of patients in sanatoriums were used to treat TB. More modern medical times have seen the use of surgical pneumonectomy, thoracoplasty, pneumothorax, and phrenic nerve interruption as potential therapeutic procedures.[9] The only procedure infrequently used today is surgical resection.

## TREATMENT AND DISPOSITION

### PULMONARY TUBERCULOSIS

Prevention of the spread of TB is paramount in the treatment regimen, and involvement of the local health department ensures a higher success rate. Empirically in the ED, start patients with suspected TB on a drug regimen after obtaining sputum for AFB smears and cultures.

Treatment consists of two phases: the initiation (bactericidal) phase, lasting 2 months; and the continuation (sterilizing) phase, usually lasting 4 to 7 months. Because of the risk of multidrug-resistant organisms, at least two drugs should be used. The American Thoracic Society, the Centers for Disease Control and Prevention, and the Infectious Diseases Society of America recommend an initial four-drug cocktail of isoniazid (INH), rifampin (RIF), pyrazinamide (PZA), and ethambutol (ETH) for 2 months (**Table 181.4**).[4] Directly observed therapy increases completion rates for pulmonary TB and prevents the spread of disease.[18-20]

Immunocompetent patients become noninfectious 2 to 4 weeks after initiating therapy if the organism is susceptible. If the initial treatment regimen fails, then at least two additional drugs should be added.[20] Usually, PZA or another

**Table 181.4 Antituberculosis Medications**

*FDA-Approved First-Line Agents*

| DRUG | MECHANISM | DAILY DOSE | SIDE EFFECTS | MONITORING NEEDED |
|---|---|---|---|---|
| Isoniazid | Inhibition of cell wall synthesis | Adults: 5 mg/kg<br>Peds: 10-15 mg/kg (max, 300 mg) | Hepatic; peripheral neuropathy | Prior liver disease; elevation in liver enzymes |
| Pyrazinamide | Sterilizing effect | Adults: 20-25 mg/kg<br>Peds: 20-30 mg/kg (max, 2.0 g) | Hepatic; exacerbates gout | Prior liver disease; if used in combination with rifampin for latent tuberculosis |
| Rifampin | RNA synthesis interference | Adults: 10 mg/kg<br>Peds: 10-20 mg/kg (max, 600 mg) | Orange body fluids; influenza-like syndrome | None needed; watch for drug interactions |
| Ethambutol | Inhibition of cell wall synthesis; possible increased permeability of cell wall | Adults: 15-20 mg/kg<br>Peds: 15-25 mg/kg (max, 1.0 g) | Peripheral neuritis; optic neuritis | Baseline and monthly visual acuity and color discrimination test needed |

*FDA-Approved Second-Line Agents*

| DRUG | DAILY DOSE |
|---|---|
| Cycloserine | Adults: 10-15 mg/kg; peds: 10-15 mg/kg (max, 1.0 g) |
| Ethionamide | Adults: 15-20 mg/kg; peds: 15-20 mg/kg (max, 1.0 g) |
| Rifapentine | Adults: 10 mg/kg/wk dose; peds: not applicable (max, 600 mg) |
| Capreomycin | Adults: 15 mg/kg; peds: 15-30 mg/kg intramuscularly/intravenously (max, 1 g) |
| *p*-Aminosalicylic acid (PAS) | Adults: 8-12 g; peds: 200-300 mg/kg (peds max, 10 g) |
| Streptomycin | Adults: 15 mg/kg; peds: 20-40 mg/kg (max, 1 g) |

*Non–FDA-Approved Drugs*

Rifabutin
Aminoglycosides
Fluoroquinolones

*Drugs Used in Drug-Resistant Tuberculosis Treatment*

Clarithromycin
Amoxicillin/clavulanate
Linezolid

Data from Sahbazian B, Weis SE. Treatment of active tuberculosis: challenges and prospects. Clin Chest Med 2005;26:273-82; American Thoracic Society, Centers for Disease Control and Prevention, Infectious Diseases Society of America. Controlling tuberculosis in the United States. Am J Respir Crit Care Med 2005;172:1169-227; and American Thoracic Society, Centers for Disease Control and Prevention, Infectious Diseases Society of America. Treatment of tuberculosis. MMWR Recomm Rep 2003:52:1-77 [erratum appears in MMWR Recomm Rep 2005;53:1203; dosage error in text]; and Centers for Disease Control and Prevention. Treatment of tuberculosis. MMWR Morb Mortal Wkly Rep 2003;52:4.
*FDA*, Food and Drug Administration; *max*, maximum; *peds*, pediatric patients.

first-line agent is coupled with a second-line agent such as ethionamide or a fluoroquinolone.[5]

## Special Populations

PATIENTS INFECTED WITH HUMAN IMMUNODEFICIENCY VIRUS Because of specific drug interactions and resistance, HIV-infected patients present a challenge to standard treatment protocols. Many of the anti-TB drugs have overlapping toxicities with the antiretroviral agents, and some anti-TB drugs may decrease the concentration of certain antiretroviral agents as a result of cytochrome system interactions.[21] HIV-infected patients should not receive once-weekly INH-RIF combinations because of high relapse rates. Patients with CD4 counts lower than 100 cells/mL should receive the anti-TB regimen at least three times a week because of the potential for RIF resistance. If sputum cultures are still positive at 2 months, the continuation phase of treatment may need to be extended to 7 months.[20] Coordination with the infectious disease specialist during treatment of these patients is important.

MULTIDRUG-RESISTANT ORGANISMS By definition, *multidrug-resistant TB* is disease that is resistant to two or more first-line agents, usually INH and RIF. Multidrug-resistant TB results from improper treatment regimens, noncompliance with therapy, and spontaneous mutations of the mycobacterium (**Box 181.3**).[4] These patients should be treated with alternative drug regimens that include at least three drugs to which the organism is susceptible and that have not been previously administered. Ideally, one of these drugs should be injectable.[4]

PREGNANCY Pregnant patients may be treated with INH, RIF, and ETH. These drugs do cross the placenta, but they are not known to have any teratogenic effects.[4] Adjuvant pyridoxine should be given to decrease the potential for the development of peripheral neuropathy.[4]

CHILDREN Disseminated TB occurs more frequently in children, so treatment of initial infection should be aggressive. Children may be treated with the same drug regimen as adults, with the exclusion of ETH. A regimen of 2 months of RIF, INH, and PZA, followed by 4 months of RIF and INH, has a treatment success of 95%. Children must have directly observed therapy. Children with disseminated TB, TB meningitis, and HIV infection may need an extended treatment period of 9 to 12 months.

**BOX 181.3 Risk Factors for Multidrug-Resistant Tuberculosis**

- Human immunodeficiency virus infection
- Intravenous drug use
- Recent immigration from a country with a prevalence of multidrug-resistant TB
- Cavitary lung lesion
- Homelessness
- Incarceration
- History of gastrectomy or ileal bypass
- Prior failed TB treatment
- Noncompliance with treatment regimen

From American Thoracic Society, Centers for Disease Control and Prevention, Infectious Diseases Society of America. Controlling tuberculosis in the United States. Am J Respir Crit Care Med 2005;172:1169–227.
*TB,* Tuberculosis.

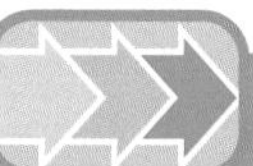

**PRIORITY ACTIONS**

- Isolate patients who have risk factors for pulmonary tuberculosis.
- Recognize that immunocompromise may distort the classic presentation.
- Maintain a high level of suspicion for tuberculosis across multiple organ systems.
- Ensure that patients with suspected tuberculosis are managed in conjunction with your local health department.

### EXTRAPULMONARY TUBERCULOSIS

Most patients with extrapulmonary TB infections may be treated with the same drug regimen as patients with pulmonary TB. In patients with TB pericarditis or meningitis, corticosteroids are added to prevent pericardial constriction and neurologic sequelae, respectively.[12] A regimen of 6 to 9 months of treatment is adequate for most infections, but patients with meningeal infection require 9 to 12 months of therapy.[4]

### LATENT TUBERCULOSIS

Patients with latent TB who are at high risk of developing active TB need empiric therapy. Before INH is initiated, patients require a chest radiograph and clinical evaluation to exclude active TB. The preferred treatment regimen for latent TB is daily INH for 9 months.[4]

### *MYCOBACTERIUM BOVIS* BACILLE CALMETTE-GUÉRIN VACCINE

Bacille Calmette-Guérin is an attenuated strain of *Mycobacterium bovis* that is the only current vaccine for TB. It was developed by Albert Calmette and Camille Guérin in the early twentieth century and remains the most commonly used vaccine in the world. Unfortunately, its efficacy may be waning as a result of mutations and deletions in the bacterium. Interest in creating alternative improved vaccines has been renewed.[22,23]

## DISPOSITION

Most patients with TB may be treated as outpatients as long as directly observed therapy can be ensured, usually by the health department. Admit patients with significant comorbidities, severe disease, a need for parenteral therapy, HIV infection, multidrug-resistant TB, and social situations that would render outpatient therapy unsuccessful.

## SUGGESTED READINGS

American Thoracic Society, Centers for Disease Control and Prevention, Infectious Diseases Society of America. Controlling tuberculosis in the United States. Am J Respir Crit Care Med 2005;172:1169-227.

Blumberg HM, Leonard Jr MK, Jasmer RM. Update on the treatment of tuberculosis and latent tuberculosis infection. JAMA 2005;293:2776-84 [erratum appears in JAMA 2005;294:182; dosage error in text].

National Tuberculosis Controllers Association, Centers for Disease Control and Prevention. Guidelines for the investigation of contacts of persons with infectious tuberculosis: recommendations from the National Tuberculosis Controllers Association and CDC. MMWR Morb Mortal Recomm Rep 2005;54:1-37.

## REFERENCES

***References can be found on Expert Consult @ www.expertconsult.com.***

# Epidemic Infections in Bioterrorism 182

*Amer Z. Aldeen*

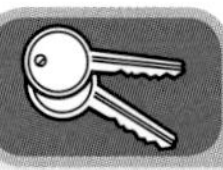

**KEY POINTS**

- Anthrax is the agent considered most likely to be used in a bioterrorist attack.
- Suspect a bioterrorism attack when large groups of patients present in a short time period with respiratory or neurologic symptoms, or when an index patient has characteristic findings.
- Use isolation precautions, and give antibiotics based on clinical suspicion, before diagnostic confirmation.
- Always draw blood cultures and send Gram stains in suspicious cases.
- Refer to the Centers for Disease Control and Prevention (CDC) website (www.bt.cdc.gov) for more detailed information on bioterrorism threats, and report any confirmed cases to the CDC.

## PERSPECTIVE*

Biologic agents have the potential to cause as many casualties in a densely populated area as a nuclear weapon. If used in a terrorist attack on civilian populations, biologic weapons could also result in widespread social disruption and complete exhaustion of health care resources.[1,5-7]

The Centers for Disease Control and Prevention (CDC) classified the major bioterrorist threats into three categories, based on the overall danger to the American public.[8] Category A agents are the most easily weaponized and disseminated, cause the highest mortality, produce extensive social disruption, and require special public health preparedness systems. Category B agents do not cause as high mortality as category A agents, but they still result in considerable morbidity and require enhancement of current surveillance systems. Category C agents are the third-highest priority and comprise new and emerging agents that are concerning because of their potential to cause significant morbidity. The list of category A, B, and C agents is given in **Table 182.1**.

Bioterrorism agents are most dangerous to humans when these agents are in aerosolized form.[6] Particles smaller than 10 mcg effectively reach the alveoli. Certain agents (e.g., anthrax, botulinum) are more resistant to environmental degradation than others (e.g., plague). Some agents (e.g., plague, smallpox) may be transmitted from person to person, thus causing high rates of dissemination and requiring strict isolation measures. Until biologic contaminants are excluded, pulmonary isolation measures should be instituted in all these patients. At present, only anthrax and smallpox have vaccines licensed by the U.S. Food and Drug Administration, and both vaccines require complex administration schedules.[9]

Surveillance and management protocols should be instituted at the hospital level for dealing with large numbers of patients who present with respiratory complaints over a short period of time. If surveillance methods do indicate a bioterrorist attack, the community must work to prevent widespread contamination, to help curb the strain on health care resources. A joint report by the CDC and the U.S. Department of Health and Human Services in February 2007 established guidelines to limit the spread of a pandemic infection.[10] Measures such as the recommendation that ill individuals stay home from work or school, cancellation of large public gatherings, and the use of strict hygiene techniques in the workplace could help avert a health care crisis.

## ANTHRAX†

Anthrax is caused by *Bacillus anthracis,* a gram-positive, aerobic, spore-forming bacillus. It is considered to be the biologic agent most likely to be used in a terrorist attack. A bioterrorist attack with powder containing anthrax spores in the United States in 2001 resulted in 22 confirmed cases. The bacteria are simple to obtain and grow. The resulting spores can be aerosolized, are extremely resistant to environmental degradation, and can cause untreated mortality rates up to 50% in exposed individuals. A 1970 World Health Organization study estimated that 50 kg of anthrax spores released in a city with half a million people could cause almost 100,000 deaths.

Anthrax causes cutaneous, gastrointestinal, and pulmonary disease. Human infection, usually cutaneous, typically occurs naturally from exposure to domesticated farm animals, such as sheep and cattle. Cutaneous anthrax is responsible for more than 90% of naturally occurring infections. It initially manifests as an erythematous patch, followed by degeneration into necrotic cellulitis with black eschar similar to a brown recluse spider bite. Gastrointestinal anthrax is extremely rare and causes hemorrhagic gastroenteritis and systemic toxicity.

Inhaled anthrax, the bioterrorist threat, causes the highest mortality of all the forms of anthrax. The clinical syndrome is divided into three phases, none exhibiting findings that would allow a clinician to identify the disease definitively. The first phase mimics a nonspecific viral syndrome and is followed by the second phase, which is a 2-day recovery period. The third phase resembles severe bacterial pneumonia, with sudden onset of fever, chills, cough, dyspnea, and respiratory failure. Hematogenous spread can cause meningitis and

*See References 1 to 4.

†See References 5, 6, 11, 12.

**Table 182.1 Centers for Disease Control and Prevention Categories of Bioterrorism Agents**[13]

| BIOLOGIC AGENT | DISEASE |
|---|---|
| **Category A** | |
| Variola major virus | Smallpox |
| *Bacillus anthracis* | Anthrax |
| *Yersinia pestis* | Plague |
| *Clostridium botulinum* | Botulism |
| *Francisella tularensis* | Tularemia |
| Filoviruses and arenaviruses | Viral hemorrhagic fevers |
| **Category B** | |
| *Coxiella burnetii* | Q fever |
| *Brucella* spp. | Brucellosis |
| *Burkholderia mallei* | Glanders |
| *Burkholderia pseudomallei* | Melioidosis |
| Alphaviruses (equine viruses) | Encephalomyelitis |
| *Rickettsia prowazekii* | Typhus fever |
| Toxins (e.g. ricin) | Toxic syndromes |
| *Chlamydia psittaci* | Psittacosis |
| Food threats *(Salmonella, Escherichia coli)* | Gastroenteritis |
| Water threats *(Vibrio, Cryptosporidium)* | Gastroenteritis |
| **Category C** | |
| Nipah virus | Encephalitis |
| Hantaviruses | Hantavirus pulmonary syndrome |
| Tick-borne hemorrhagic fever viruses | Crimean-Congo hemorrhagic fever |
| Flaviviruses | Yellow fever |
| Multidrug-resistant *Mycobacterium tuberculosis* | Tuberculosis |

***Category A Agents: General Information***[5,6,14]

| Disease | Pathogen | Incubation (Days) | Diagnosis | Characteristics Feature |
|---|---|---|---|---|
| Anthrax | *Bacillus anthracis* | 4-6 | Gram stain, culture, ELISA | Hemorrhagic mediastinitis |
| Smallpox | Variola major virus | 12-14 | Clinical, culture | Same-stage vesicles |
| Plague | *Yersinia pestis* | 2-8 | Gram stain, culture, Wright stain | Rapid respiratory failure |
| Tularemia | *Francisella tularensis* | 1-14 | Culture, DFA | Extremely infectious, HEENT and pulmonary signs |
| Botulism | *Clostridium botulinum* | 2 hr-8 days | Clinical, bioassays | Descending flaccid paralysis, cranial neuropathies |
| Viral hemorrhagic fevers | Lassa, Ebola, Marburg, dengue, Crimean-Congo hemorrhagic fever viruses | 2-21 | ELISA, PCR | Nonspecific viral symptoms, rash, MODS |

**Table 182.1 Centers for Disease Control and Prevention Categories of Bioterrorism Agents—cont'd**

*CATEGORY A AGENTS: TREATMENT, PROPHYLAXIS, AND MORTALITY*[5-7,14,15]

| Disease | Vaccine | Postexposure Prophylaxis | Treatment | Untreated Mortality |
|---|---|---|---|---|
| Anthrax | Yes | Ciprofloxacin 500 mg PO bid × 60 days *or* Amoxicillin 500 mg PO tid × 60 days *or* Doxycycline 100 mg PO bid × 60 days | Ciprofloxacin 400 mg IV/ 500 mg PO × 14 days *or* Doxycycline 100 mg IV bid × 60 days *or* Penicillin 4 million units IV q4h × 14 days | 45-90% |
| Smallpox | Yes | Vaccinia IG 0.6 mL/kg IM within 3 days | Supportive care only | 30-95% |
| Plague | No | Doxycycline 100 mg PO bid × 7 days *or* Ciprofloxacin 500 mg PO bid × 7 days | Streptomycin 15 mg/kg IM bid × 14 days *or* Gentamicin 1.5 mg/kg IM/IV tid × 14 days *or* Ciprofloxacin 400 mg IV bid until improved, then 750 mg PO bid × 14 days *or* Doxycycline 100 mg IV bid until improved, then 100 mg PO bid × 14 days | 100% |
| Tularemia | Yes | Doxycycline 100 mg PO bid × 14 days *or* Ciprofloxacin 500 mg PO bid × 14 days | Streptomycin 10 mg/kg IM bid × 14 days *or* Gentamicin 1.5 mg/kg IV tid × 14 days *or* Ciprofloxacin 400 mg IV until improved, then 500 mg PO bid × 14 days | 5-30% |
| Botulism | Yes | None | Botulism antitoxin from CDC | 60% |
| Viral hemorrhagic fevers | No | None | Ribavirin 30 mg/kg IV × 1, then 16 mg/kg IV q6h × 4 days, then 8 mg/kg IV q8h × 6 days | 10-90% |

Adapted from Centers for Disease Control and Prevention: Bioterrorism agents/diseases. http://emergency.cdc.gov/agent/agentlist-category.asp.
*bid,* Twice daily; *CDC,* Centers for Disease Control and Prevention; *DFA,* direct fluorescent antigen; *ELISA,* enzyme-linked immunosorbent assay; *HEENT,* head, eyes, ears, nose, throat; *IM,* intramuscularly; *IV,* intravenously; *MODS,* multiple organ dysfunction syndrome; *PCR,* polymerase chain reaction; *PO,* orally; *q,* every; *tid,* three times daily.

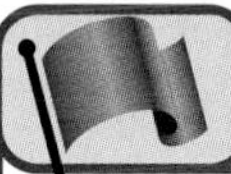

**RED FLAGS**

- Most cases caused by bioterrorism agents manifest initially as nonspecific viral syndromes.
- Inhalational anthrax and pneumonic plague are extremely difficult to distinguish clinically and radiographically, and Gram stain may be necessary.
- Cutaneous anthrax is often mistaken for a brown recluse spider bite.
- Consider smallpox if large numbers of patients who have already had chickenpox present with a diffuse vesicular rash.
- Botulism may resemble organophosphate toxicity or a variant of Guillain-Barré syndrome.

Data from References 5-7, 13, 14.

necrotizing enteritis. Results of common laboratory tests may be abnormal, but all these tests lack sufficient sensitivity and specificity. Chest radiographs characteristically show mediastinal widening consistent with hemorrhagic mediastinitis. Computed tomography has better sensitivity for mediastinal lymphadenopathy and should be performed in suspected cases when radiographs are normal.

The findings are not sufficiently distinctive from those of other bacterial illnesses to ensure early clinical identification. An astute clinician, noting mediastinal widening on radiographs, should send blood cultures, initiate presumptive antibiotics, and maintain vigilance. Blood cultures and enzyme-linked immunosorbent assay for antibodies to *B. anthracis* are extremely sensitive. Ciprofloxacin is the first-line agent for treatment and postexposure prophylaxis, but doxycycline or amoxicillin may also be used. Decontamination of spores must be accomplished with bleach solution because alcohol does not adequately kill anthrax. Novel immunotherapies involving antibodies to anthrax toxin components are currently under development.

## SMALLPOX[‡]

Variola major virus, a double-stranded DNA virus in the Poxviridae family, causes smallpox. The last confirmed, naturally occurring case of smallpox occurred in 1977. Since then, the

[‡]See References 6, 7, 14.

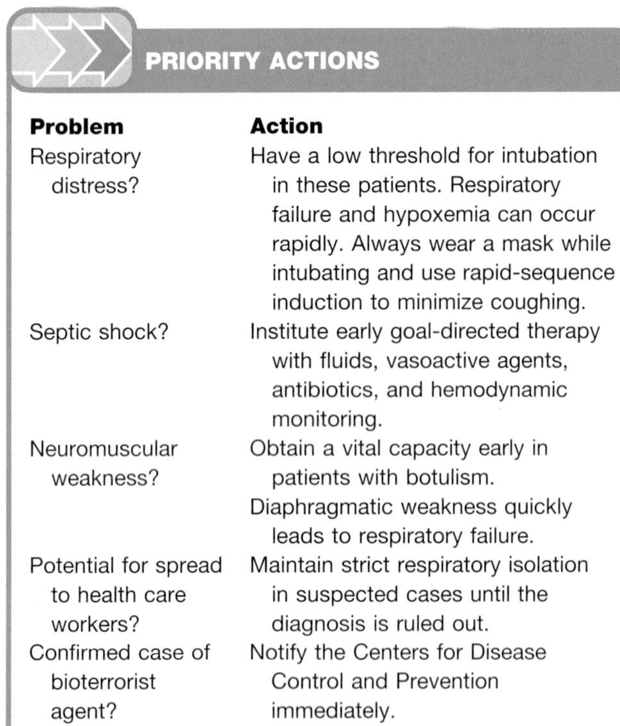

**PRIORITY ACTIONS**

| Problem | Action |
|---|---|
| Respiratory distress? | Have a low threshold for intubation in these patients. Respiratory failure and hypoxemia can occur rapidly. Always wear a mask while intubating and use rapid-sequence induction to minimize coughing. |
| Septic shock? | Institute early goal-directed therapy with fluids, vasoactive agents, antibiotics, and hemodynamic monitoring. |
| Neuromuscular weakness? | Obtain a vital capacity early in patients with botulism. Diaphragmatic weakness quickly leads to respiratory failure. |
| Potential for spread to health care workers? | Maintain strict respiratory isolation in suspected cases until the diagnosis is ruled out. |
| Confirmed case of bioterrorist agent? | Notify the Centers for Disease Control and Prevention immediately. |

Data from References 5-7, 13, 14.

existence of variola major virus has been restricted to laboratories in the United States and the former Soviet Union. Because of the extreme contagiousness of the virus, lack of adequate antiviral therapy, and dissolution of the vaccination program, smallpox has extremely high potential to cause considerable morbidity and mortality as a bioterrorism agent. Mortality rates approach 30% in nonimmunized victims.

Classic smallpox infection initially manifests as a nonspecific viral syndrome 2 weeks after exposure, followed by ulcerated lesions in the oropharynx and face. The characteristic vesicular lesions then develop diffusely over the next few days, which when patients are the most contagious. The vesicles eventually transform into pustules and then crust over in the course of 2 weeks. Chickenpox lesions from varicella-zoster virus may be confused with smallpox lesions. Smallpox lesions are characteristically concentrated on the face and extremities (more than the trunk), are in the same stage of development, and usually follow a viral prodrome lasting several days.

Two uncommon variants of smallpox are important to consider because of their high mortality rates. Flat-type smallpox causes soft, macular skin lesions and multiorgan dysfunction, and it has a mortality rate of 95%. Hemorrhagic-type smallpox results in a hyperacute, diffuse bleeding diathesis and is always fatal.

The treatment of smallpox is purely supportive. Postexposure prophylaxis consists of vaccination, which is effective only if it is administered within 4 days of exposure. Vaccinia immunoglobulin may provide some benefit after smallpox exposure and may reduce dermatologic complications after smallpox vaccination. Strict isolation precautions are indicated, including respiratory isolation for confirmed cases and quarantine of exposed individuals.

## PLAGUE[§]

Plague, the infamous "Black Death" of the Middle Ages, is caused by *Yersinia pestis,* a gram-negative, facultative anaerobic coccobacillus. Fleas are the main vector, and rodents are the main reservoir. Bubonic plague, an acute febrile form of lymphadenitis, and septicemic plague still occur naturally in parts of Africa, Asia, and the southwestern United States.

A bioterrorist attack from aerosolized droplets would likely cause pneumonic plague, which is highly contagious and impossible to distinguish clinically from severe community-acquired pneumonia. Hemoptysis is more commonly seen in pneumonic plague than in inhalational anthrax. Buboes, the necrotic lymph nodes characteristic of bubonic plague, are notably absent in pneumonic plague.

No findings on complete blood count, chemistry studies, or imaging tests are sufficiently specific for the diagnosis. Chest radiographs are usually abnormal, exhibiting either alveolar infiltrates or pleural effusions. Blood cultures are positive in 90% of cases, and gram-negative coccobacilli with bipolar stain uptake are seen in more than 70% of cases. First-line treatment of pneumonic plague is with streptomycin or gentamicin. Mortality approaches 100% without administration of antibiotics within 24 hours of overt signs of infection.

## BOTULISM[||]

Botulinum toxin is the most potent poison known. It is produced by the gram-positive, anaerobic, spore-forming bacillus, *Clostridium botulinum.* Food contamination and aerosolization are the likely mechanisms of a bioterrorist attack with botulinum toxin. Once absorbed, the agent causes irreversible inhibition of presynaptic acetylcholine release. The classic clinical picture starts with cranial neuropathies, followed by descending flaccid paralysis resulting in diaphragmatic weakness and requirement for mechanical ventilation. Mental status, sensation, and body temperature are usually normal. Botulism is not transmitted from human to human.

A specific bioassay exists to confirm the diagnosis, and clinicians should suspect botulism in any patient with descending flaccid paralysis. Treatment is with supportive care, mechanical ventilation, and antitoxin (available from the CDC). Antitoxin therapy binds to circulating toxin and is most effective when it is given within 24 hours of the onset of neurologic signs. Antibiotic therapy does not improve outcomes in patients with aerosolized or food-borne botulism and does not play a role in this toxin-mediated bioterrorist threat. A pentavalent botulinum toxoid vaccine is currently under development.

## TULAREMIA[¶]

Like anthrax and plague, tularemia occurs naturally as a zoonotic infection, transmitted by arthropods in rabbit, deer, and

[§]See References 5 to 7.
[||]See References 6 and 7.
[¶]See References 5 to 7.

**DOCUMENTATION**

| | | |
|---|---|---|
| History | General | Timing of symptoms, presence of viral prodrome, known exposure, travel to endemic area, close contacts, allergies to antibiotics, history of inflammatory skin disease |
| | Constitutional | Fever, chills, headache, myalgias, malaise |
| | Respiratory | Dyspnea, cough, hemoptysis, sputum color |
| | Gastrointestinal | Diarrhea, abdominal pain, hematochezia |
| | Neurologic | Weakness, paralysis, stiff neck |
| | Dermatologic | Rash, lesions, jaundice |
| Physical examination | General | Respiratory distress, handling of secretions, toxic appearance, coughing |
| | Head, ears, eyes, nose, and throat | Oropharyngeal lesions, drooling |
| | Lungs | Crackles, wheezes, decreased sounds, dullness to percussion |
| | Abdomen | Tenderness, distention, bowel sounds, hepatosplenomegaly, rectal examination |
| | Neurologic | Mental status, cranial nerves, meningismus, motor weakness |
| | Skin | Rash, lymphadenopathy, jaundice, necrosis |
| Studies | Chest radiograph | |
| | Chest computed tomography | |
| | Gram stain | |
| | Vital capacity (if neurologic weakness is present) | |
| Medical decision making | CDC notification if diagnosis is confirmed | |
| | Time of antibiotic order and administration | |
| Procedures | Intubation and mechanical ventilation: risks, benefits, rapid-sequence induction method, confirmation chest radiograph results, intensive care unit notification | |
| | Lumbar puncture: risks, benefits, methods, cerebrospinal fluid results | |
| Patient instructions | Return instructions, warning signs, follow-up | |
| | Recommend close contacts to seek evaluation | |
| | Mandatory completion of postexposure prophylaxis | |
| | CDC website for further information | |

Data from References 6, 7, 13.
*CDC,* Centers for Disease Control and Prevention.

squirrel reservoirs. Tularemia is caused by *Francisella tularensis,* a gram-negative coccobacillus that is a potential bioterrorism agent because of its extremely high infectivity, ease of spread, and significant morbidity. Only 10 organisms are required to cause pulmonary illness. Six forms of tularemia exist: glandular, ulceroglandular, oculoglandular, oropharyngeal, typhoidal, and pneumonic.

Aerosolized bacteria causing pneumonic tularemia would be the primary threat in a bioterrorist attack. The clinical syndrome of pneumonic disease can resemble a nonspecific viral illness, meningitis, or pneumonia. Respiratory failure and shock are far less common with tularemia than with inhalational anthrax or pneumonic plague. Although mortality of tularemia is lower than that of other diseases caused by category A agents, and even though human-to-human transmission does not occur, the ability of *F. tularensis* to cause illness after seemingly insignificant exposures is prodigious. Treatment is with aminoglycosides or fluoroquinolones, and postexposure prophylaxis is with fluoroquinolones or doxycycline.

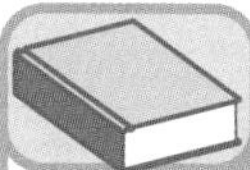

**PATIENT TEACHING TIPS**

Use the Centers for Disease Control and Prevention website (www.bt.cdc.gov) for further information about bioterrorism agents.

Finish postexposure prophylaxis completely.

Return immediately if you have worsening:

- Fever, chills, lightheadedness, fatigue
- Shortness of breath, cough
- Rash
- Headache, stiff neck

Tell your close contacts to be evaluated if they are symptomatic.

Stay home from work or school until you are beyond the incubation period of the suspected agent or no longer symptomatic.

Adapted from Reference 13.

**Table 182.2** Characteristics of Viral Hemorrhagic Fevers

| ILLNESS | VECTOR/RESERVOIR | CONTAGIOUS? | MORTALITY(%) | VACCINE |
|---|---|---|---|---|
| Dengue | Mosquito/monkey | No | 1-50 | No |
| Ebola/Marburg | Unknown/monkey | Yes | 25-90 | Experimental |
| Crimean-Congo | Tick/domestic animals | Yes | 15-30 | No |
| Rift Valley | Mosquito/sheep | No | <50 | Experimental |
| Lassa | Mice | Yes | 15-25 | Experimental |
| South American | Mice | Yes | 15-30 | No |

Data from References 6 and 14.

**Table 182.3** Differentiation of Aerosolized Bioterrorist Threats Causing Respiratory Illness

| FINDING | ANTHRAX (INHALATIONAL) | PLAGUE (PNEUMONIC) | TULAREMIA (PNEUMONIC) | VIRAL HEMORRHAGIC FEVERS |
|---|---|---|---|---|
| Dyspnea | + | + | + | ± |
| Odynophagia | – | – | + | ± |
| Hemoptysis | ± | + | – | ± |
| Headache | ± | – | ± | + |
| Stiff neck | ± | ± | – | + |
| Rash | – | – | ± | + |
| Fever | + | + | + | + |
| Leukopenia | – | – | – | + |
| DIC | ± | + | ± | + |
| Blood cultures | + (always) | + | – | + (viral culture) |
| Gram stain | Gram-positive bacilli | Gram-negative coccobacilli | Gram-negative coccobacilli | N/A |
| Chest radiograph | Widened mediastinum, pleural effusions | Patchy alveolar infiltrates, pleural effusions | Hilar adenopathy, pleural effusions | Patchy alveolar infiltrates (only when ARDS occurs) |
| Renal failure | ± | ± | – | ± |
| Hepatic failure | – | – | – | ± |

Data from References 5-7, 14.
*ARDS,* Acute respiratory distress syndrome; *DIC,* disseminated intravascular coagulation; *N/A,* not applicable.

## VIRAL HEMORRHAGIC FEVERS[#]

Viral hemorrhagic fevers (VHFs) represent a group of zoonotic diseases caused by RNA viruses that are currently geographically isolated to specific world regions. The dearth of vaccines, postexposure prophylaxis, and treatment options combined with high mortality rates would make these agents especially dangerous if they were weaponized in a bioterrorist attack. The characteristics of the individual viruses are listed in **Table 182.2**. Clinical features common to all VHFs include fever, myalgias, headache, and rash. Most patients exhibit thrombocytopenia, leukopenia, and either renal or hepatic failure (**Table 182.3**). The diagnosis is made by serologic testing or viral culture. Treatment is purely supportive, although ribavirin may provide some benefit. Mortality ranges from 1% for dengue to almost 90% for Ebola hemorrhagic fever.

## REFERENCES

***References can be found on Expert Consult @ www.expertconsult.com.***

[#]See References 6 and 14.

# Food- and Water-Borne Infections 183

David K. Zich

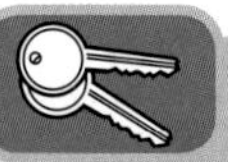

**KEY POINTS**

- In patients who develop clinical illness from food-borne and water-borne pathogens, most symptoms resolve spontaneously without intervention.
- Significant mortality does occur. Each year, thousands of people in the United States and millions of people in developing countries die of acute gastroenteritis.[1]
- Proper treatment can lead to significant relief for the patient, but inappropriate medications may complicate the clinical picture, lengthen the carrier state, or trigger potentially life-threatening conditions.
- Developing a systematic approach to gastrointestinal disease is essential to eliminate unnecessary testing and to restore health as quickly as possible while minimizing adverse and dangerous effects of intervention.

## PATHOPHYSIOLOGY

The portion of the gastrointestinal tract affected by food- and water-borne illnesses depends on the pathogen. Staphylococcal food poisoning is caused by a toxin that has no effect on the intestinal mucosa. Instead, once absorbed, the toxin acts directly on nausea centers in the brain and thus causes severe nausea and vomiting.

Infections of the small intestine may disrupt ionic exchange and result in increased chloride secretion and sodium retention within the bowel lumen. Water follows, thereby overwhelming absorption capacity, and diarrhea ensues. Viruses create diarrhea by distorting the epithelium and interfering with absorptive capabilities. This process results in loss of fluid, electrolytes, and, in some cases, fats and sugars. Because of the high secretory capabilities of the small intestine, infection of this region can lead to large-volume, watery diarrhea. In patients with large fluid losses, significant electrolyte disturbances and acidosis may occur, more commonly with infections of the small intestine.[2] Given the predominant location of the small intestine, cramping and discomfort are localized more often to the upper abdomen.

Invasive organisms primarily affect the distal ileum and large intestine. Common invasive organisms include *Campylobacter, Salmonella, Shigella, Yersinia,* and *Entamoeba histolytica.* These pathogens penetrate the intestinal lining and create an intense inflammatory response. This process results in losses of fluid and, in some cases, varying amounts of blood. The large intestine has less secretory function. Therefore, infections of this region are more likely to cause smaller, frequent episodes of diarrhea that is more apt to contain mucus or blood when compared with small intestine infections. Severe alterations in electrolytes and acid-base balance are less common. Symptoms of large intestine infections tend to be felt in the lower quadrants, and in some cases they may mimic appendicitis, with focal right lower quadrant pain.

Small bowel and large bowel are both susceptible to toxin-producing organisms that induce diarrhea through direct damage to the epithelium, thereby disrupting the regulation of fluid balance. Because the lactase enzyme responsible for breakdown of lactose is present primarily in the epithelial surface, any infection that causes significant epithelial damage may lead to temporary lactose intolerance. Whereas bacterial toxin-induced diarrhea tends to be isotonic, virally induced diarrhea causes losses primarily of sodium, potassium, and bicarbonate.

## PRESENTING SIGNS AND SYMPTOMS

Presenting signs and symptoms vary widely, depending on the pathogen causing the disease. Many parasites that infect the intestines cause no discernible symptoms. Asymptomatic chronic bacterial carrier states can occur in otherwise healthy individuals. When symptoms do occur, they are limited in most patients to vomiting and diarrhea of varying degrees. Rarely, patients have more systemic symptoms. *Listeria monocytogenes* infections, more common in pregnant women, cause fever, myalgias, headache, and neck stiffness. Scombroid poisoning from fish can cause symptoms of a severe allergic reaction, and ciguatera poisoning, also from fish, can cause neurologic symptoms including severe paresthesias and dysesthesias.

Although food containing preformed toxins can cause illness within 1 to 6 hours, most acute gastroenteritis has at least a 12- to 48-hour incubation period (**Table 183.1**). Typically, the onset is gradual and is often noticed as mild dyspepsia after eating a meal. This is the meal often suspected by the patient to be the cause of the illness. However, the

**Table 183.1** Symptom Onset Time

| ORGANISM OR PATHOGEN | SYMPTOM ONSET |
|---|---|
| Scombroid fish (poisoning) | 5-60 min; average, 20-30 min |
| *Staphylococcus* | 1-6 hr |
| *Bacillus cereus* | 2-14 hr; average, 2-4 hr |
| Ciguatera fish (poisoning) | 2-6 hr, ≥24 hr |
| *Clostridium perfringens* enterotoxin | 6-24 hr |
| *Vibrio parahaemolyticus* | 4-48 hr; average, 8-12 hr |
| *Salmonella* | 8-48 hr |
| *Shigella* | 24-48 hr |
| *Plesiomonas shigelloides* | 24-48 hr |
| Cholera and noncholera *Vibrio* species | 24-48 hr |
| Enterotoxigenic *Escherichia coli* | 24-72 hr |
| Norovirus or rotavirus | 24-72 hr |
| *Campylobacter* | 2-5 days |
| *Yersinia* | 1-14 days; average, 2-4 days |
| *Aeromonas hydrophila* | 1-5 days |
| Hemorrhagic *Escherichia coli* O157:H7 | 3-8 days |
| *Cryptosporidium* and *Isospora* | 5-10 days |
| *Clostridium difficile* | Days to month;, average, 5-14 days |
| *Giardia* | 1-3 wk |
| *Entamoeba histolytica* | 1 wk-1 yr |

pathogen has usually been incubating for the last 1 to 2 days and is just starting to cause symptoms.

Within 1 to 2 hours after the initial dyspepsia, nonbloody vomiting often begins. If bleeding does occur, the most common cause is a Mallory-Weiss tear. This results when forceful ejection of gastric contents creates a tear in the mucosa at the junction of the esophagus and the stomach. It rarely occurs during the first episode of vomiting, and treatment is almost always supportive. An initial presence of blood, or a persistent predominance of gross blood, should prompt a search for noninfectious causes of vomiting such as a bleeding peptic ulcer or esophageal varices.

Diarrhea can occur simultaneously with vomiting, or it may be delayed for up to 48 hours after vomiting begins. In some cases, diarrhea may be the only component of clinical illness. Gross diarrheal blood is more common than hematemesis and varies by pathogen (**Box 183.1**). Dysentery, defined as a diarrheal stool containing gross blood, can be accompanied by fever, abdominal pain, and tenesmus.

**BOX 183.1 Infectious Causes of Bloody Diarrhea**

**Frequently**
*Campylobacter*
*Plesiomonas shigelloides*
Hemorrhagic *Escherichia coli*
*Entamoeba histolytica*

**Occasionally**
*Salmonella*
*Yersinia*
*Vibrio parahaemolyticus*

**Rarely**
*Shigella*
*Aeromonas hydrophila*
*Clostridium difficile*

## DIFFERENTIAL DIAGNOSIS

Vomiting and diarrhea can result from other pathologic states, or they may be iatrogenic, such as from a medication side effect. Vomiting and diarrhea can herald an endocrine emergency such as in adrenal crisis, or they may represent a completely benign event, such as diarrhea after long-distance running. Maintaining a level of suspicion for other causes is essential, to minimize the chance of missing a more dangerous disorder or to reassure a patient when the cause is benign. The following subsections describe additional diagnoses to consider.

### VOMITING AND DIARRHEA

#### *Toxic Ingestions and Overdoses*

Accidental or intentional ingestion of toxic chemicals or medication overdoses frequently manifest with abdominal pain, nausea, vomiting, and sometimes diarrhea. Depending on the situation, patients may not be forthcoming with an accurate history unless they are specifically questioned.

#### *Prescription Drugs*

Nausea, vomiting, and diarrhea are some of the most common side effects of many different prescriptions drugs, from antibiotics to chemotherapy agents. Patients with acquired immunodeficiency syndrome (AIDS) often take antiviral medications that cause such a high incidence of vomiting that antinausea medications are prescribed prophylactically. A careful history of new medications or changes in dose will help rule out medications as a cause.

#### *Opiate Withdrawal*

Nausea and vomiting are quite common in acute opiate withdrawal. In addition, a patient usually experiences agitation,

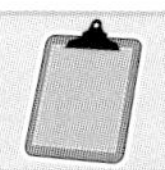

**DOCUMENTATION**

**History**
- Onset and duration
- Amount of vomiting
- Amount of diarrhea
  - Presence of blood in either
- Associated symptoms
  - Fever
  - Headache
  - Neurologic symptoms
  - Pain
- Ingestion of suspicious foods in last 7 days
  - Raw or undercooked (sushi)
  - Well or wilderness water
  - Picnics
- Exposure to people with similar symptoms
- Recent travel
  - Camping or hiking (consider *Giardia*)
  - International travel (consider simple traveler's diarrhea or a more serious cause such as cholera, depending on location)
- Recent antibiotics or hospitalizations (consider *Clostridium difficile*)
- Pregnancy (increased risk of *Listeria monocytogenes*)
- Past medical history
  - Abdominal surgical procedures (consider partial obstruction)
  - Irritable bowel syndrome/inflammatory bowel disease
  - Immunocompromised state
  - Diabetes (look for ketoacidosis)
- Medications
  - Antibiotics (consider *Clostridium difficile*)
  - Warfarin (case reports of extreme international normalized ratio elevation in severe diarrhea have been published)
- Social history
  - Alcohol or illicit drugs (consider symptoms of withdrawal)
  - Sexual activity (consider pregnancy, gynecologic cause, and multiple causes in men who have sex with men)
- Animal exposure
  - New pets in house (10% of dogs and cats excrete *Salmonella*)
  - Slaughterhouse workers, farm workers, veterinarians (e.g., *Bacillus anthracis, Coxiella burnetii*)
- Family history
  - Irritable bowel syndrome or inflammatory bowel disease

**Physical Examination**
- Vital signs
  - Tachycardia
  - Hypotension or orthostasis
  - Fever
- Oropharynx examination (ulcerations seen in anthrax or Crohn disease)
- Abdominal examination
  - Focal tenderness
  - Rebound or guarding
  - Distention
  - Bowel sounds
- Extremities: edema
- Neurologic: hot or cold sensation, paresthesias, and dental pain (ciguatera)

diffuse aches, and diaphoresis. Patients experiencing opiate withdrawal often have hypertension along with tachycardia and tachypnea. Patients may not always admit their illicit drug use, thus making the diagnosis more challenging.

### *Malignant Disease*

Brain tumors cause vomiting through neurogenic activation of the vomiting centers of the brain, usually in conjunction with increases in intracranial pressure. Gastric cancers lead to nausea and vomiting in advanced stages as gastric plasticity decreases. Infiltrative malignant diseases such as Kaposi sarcoma and lymphomas, especially in immunocompromised patients, can invade the intestinal wall and cause diarrhea. Colon cancers usually do not manifest with diarrhea until very late in the course when they obstruct solid matter, and liquid flows around the obstruction. Patients usually report gradual difficulty moving their bowels long before diarrhea begins.

### *Irritable Bowel Syndrome*

Irritable bowel syndrome manifests predominantly as either constipation or diarrhea, sometimes accompanied by diffuse, crampy abdominal pain, although it rarely involves vomiting. Fever is absent, and no blood should be seen in the stool unless hemorrhoids are present. Patients may have a history of a stressful trigger, and they can often tell what is typical for a flare of this syndrome.

### *Inflammatory Bowel Disease*

Inflammatory bowel disease flares usually manifest with gradually worsening abdominal pain and diarrhea, often bloody. Vomiting is less likely unless significant bowel stricture occurs in patients with Crohn disease.

## VOMITING WITHOUT DIARRHEA

Vomiting is a symptom and not a diagnosis. Gastroenteritis can be diagnosed only if signs of gastritis enteritis are clearly present, based on clinical evaluation. Vomiting can also be caused by many toxic and metabolic disorders and organ dysfunction. Ingestions, carbon monoxide, and other poisonings often incite vomiting without other signs. Early hepatitis, biliary disease, and early appendicitis may cause vomiting, with few other signs. Other important causes of isolated vomiting include those discussed in the following paragraphs.

### Obstruction

A history of abdominal surgery should raise suspicions of a possible intestinal obstruction. On physical examination, abdominal distention is common, and hypoactive, high-pitched bowel sounds are in contrast to the hyperactive bowel sounds usually found in gastroenteritis.

### Cyclic Vomiting

The challenge in patients with cyclic vomiting is in determining the rare episode when the symptoms may be caused by gastroenteritis, instead of being an exacerbation of the underlying disorder. Diarrhea is rare, fever should not be present, and a history of stressful triggers is often identifiable when the episode results from an exacerbation of cyclic vomiting.

### Intracranial Disease

Headache is a common complaint that often accompanies acute gastroenteritis. However, vomiting also frequently occurs simultaneously with headaches caused by migraines, intracranial hemorrhage, or tumor. When the history of a headache is elicited, the physician must consider the following factors so that more dangerous disease is not overlooked. Headache that started before the onset of vomiting, or headache as the primary focus of the patient, is concerning. Similarly, a sudden, severe headache occurring while vomiting may indicate an aneurysmal rupture resulting from increased intracranial pressure during the Valsalva maneuver.

### Myocardial Infarction

Atypical presentations of myocardial infarction are important to recognize. Vomiting without diarrhea in a patient with significant risk factors should prompt consideration of a cardiac cause. The concomitant presence of shortness of breath and diaphoresis, with or without chest pain, further increases the probability of myocardial infarction.

### Early Pregnancy

"Morning sickness" is most common within the first 13 weeks of gestation. However, pregnancy-associated nausea and vomiting may be more severe at other times of day and may continue well past the first trimester. Not unusually, vomiting is the first symptom a woman experiences before she is aware of the pregnancy. Vomiting without diarrhea, symptoms spanning several days, and hunger between episodes should arouse suspicion of pregnancy as the cause. Inquiring about breast tenderness and missed or irregular menstrual periods can help to elicit the diagnosis. A pregnancy test should be standard in the evaluation of any woman of childbearing age who presents with symptoms of acute gastroenteritis.

## FOCAL PAIN

Patients with acute gastroenteritis often complain of abdominal pain, but the quality of this pain tends to be crampy and migratory secondary to increased intestinal motility and spasm. Mild, constant midepigastric pain is also common after vomiting because of gastritis and abdominal wall muscle exertion. In rare cases, *Campylobacter* and *Yersinia* may cause isolated cecitis, characterized by focal right lower quadrant pain in the absence of vomiting or diarrhea that mimics acute appendicitis. Severe, focal, unrelenting pain should prompt a search for other causes, however.

### Focal Inflammation

Causes of focal inflammation including gastritis, pancreatitis, cholecystitis, diverticulitis, and appendicitis are suspected when pain is isolated to these respective areas.

### Gynecologic Emergencies

These conditions include tubo-ovarian abscess, ovarian torsion, ruptured ectopic pregnancy, and pelvic inflammatory disease. A pelvic examination and pregnancy test are essential in the evaluation of women who complain of concomitant pelvic or lower abdominal pain.

## DIFFUSE PAIN

### Perforated Viscus

A history of peptic ulcer disease, recent gynecologic or gastrointestinal instrumentation, or fever with peritoneal signs should raise the suspicion of perforated viscus.

### Ischemic Bowel

In patients with risk factors for peripheral vascular disease, diffuse abdominal pain along with nausea and diarrhea after eating may indicate compromised blood flow to the intestines. The onset may be more gradual in patients with slowly progressive atherosclerosis, or it may be abrupt from an embolic event to the intestinal vasculature. The physical examination is often unimpressive, given the severity of the stated discomfort (hence the finding of "pain out of proportion to examination"). A high index of suspicion should be maintained, especially in the older population, because missing the diagnosis can lead to significant morbidity and even death.

# DIAGNOSTIC TESTING

Diagnostic testing is often overused in infectious gastroenteritis. With symptoms lasting less than 24 hours in otherwise healthy individuals who are not at the extremes of age, no diagnostic testing is indicated, other than a pregnancy test in women of reproductive age. Exceptions include patients with severe symptoms, multiple grossly bloody stools, or hemodynamic instability, as well as testing for epidemiologic purposes if food poisoning or a bioterrorism event is suspected.[3,4]

Laboratory or radiologic evaluation may be helpful in several situations. A bedside urine evaluation for ketones may be useful to document dehydration and to guide intravenous fluid management. In patients whose symptoms have persisted for more than 24 hours, electrolyte determinations and tests of kidney function may be indicated. If a chemistry panel is obtained, calculation of the anion gap should be done to prevent missing clues to diabetic or alcoholic ketoacidosis, toxic ingestions, or other serious conditions. Mild elevations in liver function tests are very nonspecific in acute gastroenteritis, but marked elevations could be an indication of hepatitis A infection.

Although the diagnostic yield is generally low, stool culture in patients who have unrelenting diarrhea may detect a treatable cause that can significantly shorten the course of illness.[5] Typically, positive results take at least 2 to 3 days, and symptoms have often resolved by the time results return. For patients who develop diarrhea 3 days or more after being hospitalized, bacterial stool cultures have not been found to be helpful.[6] Testing for ova and parasites has not shown to be cost effective unless the patient is at identifiable risk. This group includes patients with diarrhea persisting for several days after international travel to endemic regions, persons who ingest untreated water while camping or hiking, those with exposure to daycare centers, men who have sexual contact with other men, and persons who have sexual contact with patients with AIDS.[7] If parasitic infection is suspected, three separate specimens from different time periods must be sent for ova and parasites before the test can be considered negative. *Clostridium difficile* testing should be performed for anyone with persistent diarrhea and a history of antibiotic use in the previous 3 months. In patients with severe diarrhea, *C. difficile* testing should be considered even in the absence of recent antibiotic exposure or recent hospitalization. The reason is the emergence of a hypervirulent strain, designated NAP1/BI/O27, that has caused illness in otherwise healthy individuals without the traditional risk factors for *C. difficile* colitis.[8]

The recommended diagnostic work-up in patients with AIDS and in others who are severely immunocompromised is more aggressive. Studies in these patients tend to yield more positive results, and symptoms are less apt to resolve without intervention. Stool should be sent for culture just as in immunocompetent patients. *C. difficile* testing should be performed because this remains the most common pathogen detected in patients with human immunodeficiency virus infection and diarrhea. Three separate specimens should be sent to be examined for ova and parasites, given the intermittent shedding of organisms. In addition, stool should be sent for acid-fast smear to detect *Cryptosporidium, Isospora,* and *Cyclospora.* Finally, in severely immunocompromised patients with a CD4 count lower than 100 cells/microliter, a trichrome stain should be ordered to test for microsporidium.[9] Unlike in immunocompetent patients, in whom blood cultures are of extremely limited use, blood culture results in immunocompromised patients may be positive in up to 40% of cases and may yield a diagnosis even in the absence of positive stool culture results.[10] Fungal blood cultures should also be considered, to detect *Mycobacterium avium* complex. In this population, if severe diarrhea persists despite negative evaluations, the patient will need endoscopic evaluation for mucosal biopsy and additional cultures.

For patients with severe abdominal pain or distention, an obstructive plain radiographic series or abdominal computed tomography scan with oral and intravenous contrast can help to differentiate other more serious causes of their symptoms. Abdominal computed tomography scans without contrast, or with oral contrast alone, may be sufficient, depending on the experience of the radiologist conducting the examination.

A complete blood count is usually of little value, with rare exceptions. The stress of vomiting often causes transient leukocytosis that does not correlate with the severity or cause of illness. Hemoglobin and hematocrit determinations may be helpful in patients with hemorrhagic diarrhea for assessment of anemia. Eosinophilia may indicate an allergic or parasitic origin. Macrocytic anemia can occur with infection involving *Diphyllobothrium latum*, and low platelet counts can be seen in infections such as Q fever *(Coxiella burnetii).*

In patients with an acute onset of vomiting and diarrhea, documentation of gross blood in the stool is helpful. Checking for occult blood has not been proven to be sensitive or specific. When gross blood is absent, hemoccult testing provides little to no insight into the causative pathogen and should not be used to guide treatment. Similarly, fecal leukocyte testing has low sensitivity and specificity and should not be used to justify empiric antibiotic treatment.[11,12]

To reiterate, most cases occur in young, otherwise healthy individuals who have had symptoms for less than 24 hours. In this population, minimal to no testing should be the rule.

## TREATMENT AND DISPOSITION

Emergency treatment of gastroenteritis begins with airway, breathing, and circulation. Airway and breathing are rarely an issue unless large-volume hematemesis is present. Boerhaave syndrome, disruption of esophageal varices while vomiting, and severe cases of anthrax are some of the few causes of massive hematemesis.

If the patient is hemodynamically unstable, immediate intervention is required. The patient should receive fluid resuscitation with two large-bore intravenous catheters or a central line, and the physician should consider causes of illness other than simple gastroenteritis. If the patient has a recent history of international travel, review of the previous location's endemic pathogens is essential. Countries such as Haiti have had outbreaks of cholera *(Vibrio cholerae)* that can lead to circulatory collapse in as little as 24 hours.

For patients who have severe allergic symptoms after ingesting fish and scombroid is suspected, treatment should be initiated with antihistamines.

For patients experiencing neurologic symptoms such as paresthesias, dysesthesias, reversal of hot and cold sensation, or even altered mental status after eating fish, ciguatera poisoning should be suspected. Although not universally accepted, mannitol, 1 g/kg of a 20% solution over 30 minutes, has dramatic effects on improving symptoms.[13-15]

Most patients are stable, however, and are suffering from nausea, vomiting, crampy abdominal pain, and possibly diarrhea without other significant symptoms. For this group, the mainstays of treatment consist of rehydration and alleviation of symptoms through antiemetics (**Fig. 183.1**). The use of empiric antibiotics is not indicated in most cases.

For those patients who are hemodynamically stable and whose vomiting can be controlled, oral rehydration is adequate and is often greatly underused. Ketonemia has been implicated in gastroenteritis. In patients with significant dehydration, nausea and vomiting may continue because of circulating ketones long after the initial infectious cause has been eradicated by the body. In this circumstance, proper administration of intravenous fluids may be all that is required to resolve the patient's symptoms. If a patient is unable to tolerate oral intake, intravenous normal saline solution is adequate for initial hydration. For patients with significant ketosis, switching to dextrose-containing compounds after initial rehydration may help to restore normal metabolic function more quickly.

Many choices of antiemetics and routes of administration are available. When choosing a medication, one should consider pregnancy class, cost, and side effects, particularly the extrapyramidal side effects of the phenothiazines and

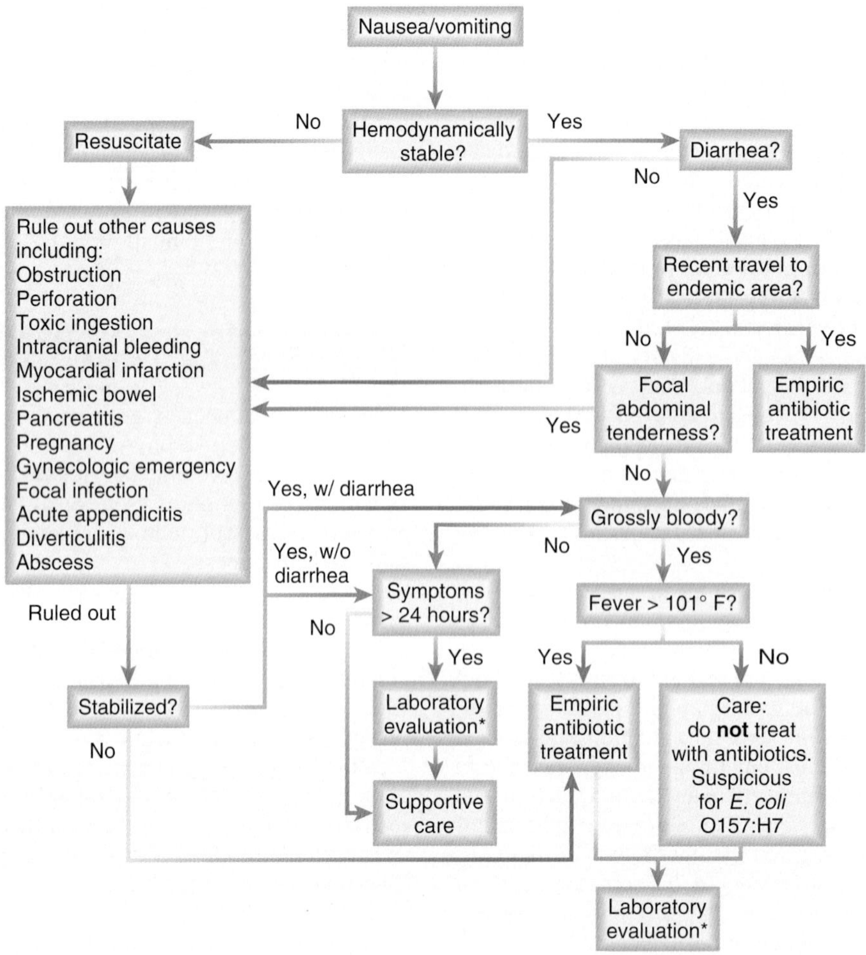


*Laboratory evaluation should include BUN/Cr level (with calculation of the anion gap), general chemistries, and diarrheal stool (if available) for culture, ova and parasites, and *C. difficile*.

**Fig. 183.1 Treatment algorithm for adults without significant comorbid illness.** *BUN*, Blood urea nitrogen; *Cr*, creatinine.

metoclopramide. **Table 183.2** gives the characteristics of common antiemetic agents. If one agent fails, a switch to a different class of agent is recommended, rather than repeat administration of an agent of the same class.

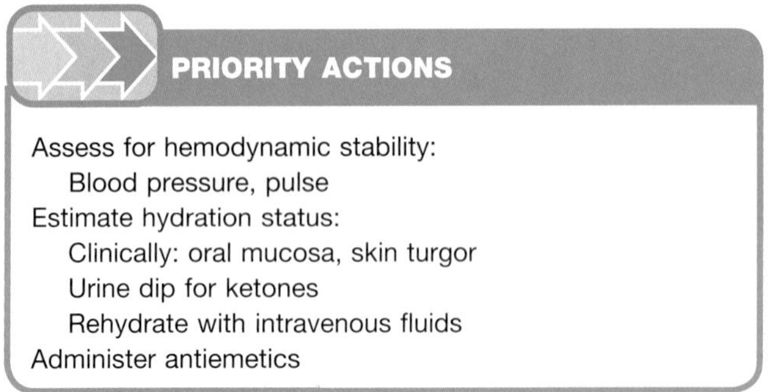
**PRIORITY ACTIONS**

Assess for hemodynamic stability:
- Blood pressure, pulse

Estimate hydration status:
- Clinically: oral mucosa, skin turgor
- Urine dip for ketones
- Rehydrate with intravenous fluids

Administer antiemetics

The hazards of using antidiarrheal agents in acute gastroenteritis appear to have been overstated. For afebrile patients without grossly bloody diarrhea or a high suspicion of *C. difficile* colitis from recent antibiotic use, antimotility agents such as loperamide or atropine-diphenoxylate can be safely administered. Use of these drugs is recommended for large-volume diarrhea that compromises hydration status or is otherwise hindering a patient's ability for self-care.

Antibiotics are rarely indicated in the empiric treatment of acute gastroenteritis, for many reasons. Viruses remain the most common causes of acute gastroenteritis in the general population, and these infections resolve without intervention. Most bacterial causes are self-limited and are eradicated by the host defenses in a short time. Common adverse reactions of most antibiotics are nausea or diarrhea, occurring in up to 10% of patients. Although certain antibiotics are more prone to causing *C. difficile* colitis, any antibiotic can predispose patients to this complication. Administering antibiotics to patients with non-*typhi Salmonella* infections is ineffective and may lead to a prolonged carrier state. If the patient has contracted illness from *Escherichia coli* serotype O157:H7, antibiotics will have no effect on the symptoms but may lead to an increased incidence of hemolytic-uremic syndrome. Finally, empiric treatment with antibiotics contributes to the alarming development of resistant pathogens in the general patient population. Empiric antibiotics are usually ineffective, may complicate the picture, may even harm the patient, and contribute to the formation of resistant organisms.

**Table 183.2** Commonly Used Drugs

| GENERIC NAME | BRAND NAME | PREGNANCY CLASS | DRUG CLASS | ROUTE | COST | COMMON SIDE EFFECTS |
|---|---|---|---|---|---|---|
| Prochlorperazine | Compazine | C | Phenothiazine | PO/PR/IM/IV | Inexpensive | Akathisia, drowsiness, extrapyramidal effects, risk of death in patients with dementia-related psychosis who are taking antipsychotic drugs |
| Droperidol | Inapsine | C | Butyrophenone | IM/IV | Inexpensive | Akathisia, drowsiness, extrapyramidal effects, QT prolongation, risk of death in patients with dementia-related psychosis who are taking antipsychotic drugs |
| Promethazine | Phenergan | C | Nonselective antihistamine | PO/PR/IM/IV | Inexpensive | Extreme sedation, anticholinergic effects, severe tissue injury if extravasation occurs during IV administration; subcutaneous route contraindicated |
| Trimethobenzamide | Tigan | C | Nonselective antihistamine | PO/PR/IM (adults only) | Inexpensive | Extreme sedation, hypotension, anticholinergic effects |
| Metoclopramide | Reglan | B | Dopaminergic blocker | PO/IM/IV | Inexpensive | Restlessness, extrapyramidal effects |
| Ondansetron | Zofran | B | Selective 5-$HT_3$ antagonist | PO/ODT/IM/IV | Expensive | Less frequent: headache, dizziness, agitation; beware of serotonin syndrome in patients also taking SSRIs |
| Granisetron | Kytril | B | Selective 5-$HT_3$ antagonist | PO/IV | Expensive | Less frequent: headache, drowsiness, taste changes, prolonged QT interval; beware of serotonin syndrome in patients also taking SSRIs |
| Dolasetron | Anzemet | B | Selective 5-$HT_3$ antagonist | PO/IV | Expensive | Less frequent: headache, dizziness, fatigue, prolonged QT interval; beware of serotonin syndrome in patients also taking SSRIs |
| Palonosetron | Aloxi | B | Selective 5-$HT_3$ antagonist | IV | Expensive | Less frequent: headache, prolonged QT interval; beware of serotonin syndrome in patients also taking SSRIs |

*5-$HT_3$*, 5-Hydroxytryptamine 3; *IM*, intramuscular; *IV*, intravenous; *ODT*, orally disintegrating tablet; *PO*, oral; *PR*, rectal; *SSRIs*, selective serotonin reuptake inhibitors.

The indications for empiric antibiotics are very narrow. If a patient appears toxic, has a fever higher than 101° F and bloody diarrhea, or is hemodynamically unstable, antibiotics may be helpful. Grossly bloody diarrhea alone is not an indication for empiric antibiotic use, and again, bloody diarrhea may be caused by *E. coli* O157:H7. This serotype does not usually cause a fever, and therefore empiric antibiotics prescribed for grossly bloody diarrhea in conjunction with a temperature greater than 101° F should not raise concerns of inducing hemolytic-uremic syndrome.

Another indication for empiric antibiotics involves acute gastroenteritis in the setting of travel to areas endemic for traveler's diarrhea. The most common pathogens include enterotoxigenic *E. coli, Shigella, Salmonella,* and *Campylobacter*. In many cases, prompt use of a fluoroquinolone can lead to relief of symptoms within hours. Unfortunately, resistance to this class of drugs and to many other antibiotics is rising throughout the world, and treatment failures are becoming more common. Of the foregoing pathogens, *Campylobacter* has a high enough resistance to fluoroquinolones that erythromycin is now the drug of choice in these infections. For continued empiric treatment of traveler's diarrhea in patients who do not respond to fluoroquinolones, azithromycin may be used. Sending stool cultures before the initiation of antibiotics can be helpful, given the high rates of resistance, in anticipation of potential treatment failures. **Table 183.3** gives specific antibiotic regimens for symptomatic patients in whom the pathogen is identified.

In general, patients who are hemodynamically unstable at any point in their stay, who have persistent pain, or who continue to vomit frequently should be admitted until oral intake can be tolerated and pain improves. If a noninfectious origin has not been ruled out and symptoms continue, admission should also be considered. Patients with severe comorbid illness, and those who take multiple medications that would be affected by poor oral intake or malabsorption, may also need to be admitted.

Diabetic patients may be particularly challenged by acute gastroenteritis. Infection combined with an inability to take hypoglycemic medications may increase their blood glucose concentrations and may exacerbate their dehydration. Diabetic patients may become hypoglycemic, given their decreased intake in the setting of long-acting hypoglycemic medications, and physicians should have a low threshold for

**Table 183.3 Antibiotic Regimens for Identified Pathogens**

| ORGANISM OR PATHOGEN | ANTIBIOTIC TREATMENT | COMMENT |
|---|---|---|
| Unknown (if empiric therapy deemed necessary) | Ciprofloxacin 500 mg bid × 3 days<br>*or*<br>TMP-SMX DS bid × 3 days | Resistance high in tropics |
| Unknown with recent antibiotic exposure; treat empirically for *Clostridium difficile* colitis | Metronidazole 500 mg PO tid × 10 days<br>*or*<br>Vancomycin 125 mg PO qid × 10 days | Also effective IV<br><br>Not effective IV |
| *Campylobacter* | Erythromycin 500 mg bid × 5 days<br>*or*<br>Azithromycin 500 once daily × 3 days | Not fluoroquinolones because of resistance |
| *Salmonella* | Ciprofloxacin 500 mg bid × 7-10 days<br>*or*<br>Azithromycin 1 g, then 500 mg once daily × 7 days<br>*or*<br>Ceftriaxone IV | <br><br>Total 7 days<br>For inpatient treatment |
| *Coxiella burnetii* | Doxycycline 100 mg PO bid × 15-21 days | |
| *Listeria monocytogenes* | Usually self-limited, efficacy of oral antibiotics unknown; susceptible to ampicillin and TMP-SMX<br>For suspected or known bacteremia, parenteral antibiotics required:<br>Ampicillin 2 g IV q4h with or without gentamicin (first week only) × 14 days<br>*or*<br>TMP-SMX 20 mg/kg/day of trimethoprim IV divided q6h × 14 days | |
| *Shigella* | Ciprofloxacin 750 mg PO once daily × 3 days<br>*or*<br>Azithromycin 500 mg once daily × 3 days | |
| *Yersinia* | For severe symptoms:<br>Doxycycline 100 mg IV bid + tobramycin or gentamycin 5 mg/kg/day once daily × 7-10 days | Supportive care if mild symptoms |
| *Vibrio parahaemolyticus* | Does not shorten the course | In vitro susceptibilities to ciprofloxacin |
| Hemorrhagic *Escherichia coli* O157:H7 | Antibiotics not effective; may be detrimental | |
| *Aeromonas* or *Plesiomonas* | Azithromycin 500 mg PO once daily × 3 days<br>*or*<br>Ciprofloxacin 750 mg once daily × 3 days | |
| *Staphylococcus* | Antibiotics not effective | |

**Table 183.3 Antibiotic Regimens for Identified Pathogens—cont'd**

| ORGANISM OR PATHOGEN | ANTIBIOTIC TREATMENT | COMMENT |
|---|---|---|
| *Clostridium perfringens* enterotoxin | Antibiotics not effective | |
| *Bacillus cereus* | Antibiotics not effective | |
| Cholera and noncholera *Vibrio* species | Ciprofloxacin 1 g × 1 ***or*** Doxycycline 300 mg × 1 dose ***or*** Azithromycin 500 mg PO once daily × 3 days | |
| Scombroid fish (poisoning) | Antihistamines; antibiotics not effective | |
| Ciguatera fish (poisoning) | Antibiotics not effective<br>Mannitol 1 g/kg 20% solution over 30 min for symptom relief | |
| Enterotoxigenic *Escherichia coli* | Ciprofloxacin 750 mg once daily × 1-3 days ***or*** Azithromycin 1 g PO x 1 | |
| *Clostridium difficile* | Metronidazole 500 mg PO tid × 10 days ***or*** Vancomycin 125 mg PO qid × 10 days | Also effective IV<br>Not effective IV |
| Norovirus or rotavirus | Antibiotics not effective | |
| *Cryptosporidium* | Antibiotics poorly effective | |
| *Isospora* or coccidia | TMP-SMX DS bid for 10 days ***or*** Ciprofloxacin 500 mg bid × 7 days | 87% effective |
| *Giardia* | Tinidazole 2 g PO × 1 ***or*** Nitazoxanide 500 mg PO bid × 3 days ***or*** Metronidazole 250 mg tid × 5 days ***or*** Paromomycin 25-35 mg/kg/day divided tid × 7 days | In pregnancy |
| *Entamoeba histolytica* | Metronidazole 500 mg tid × 10 days followed by Paromomycin 25-35 mg/kg/day divided tid × 7 days | |
| Enterobius vermicularis | Albendazole 400 mg × 1 ***or*** Mebendazole 100 mg chewed × 1 ***or*** Pyrantel pamoate 11 mg/kg (maximum, 1 g) × 1 | Repeat dose × 1 in 2 wk<br>Repeat dose × 1 in 2 wk<br>Repeat dose × 1 in 2 wk |
| *Taenia saginata* or *Taenia solium* | Praziquantel 5-10 mg/kg PO × 1 ***or*** Niclosamide 2 g PO × 1 | |
| *Diphyllobothrium latum* | Praziquantel 5-10 mg/kg PO × 1 ***or*** Niclosamide 2 g PO × 1 | |

From DuPont HL. Bacterial diarrhea. N Engl J Med 2009;361:1560-1569.
*bid,* Twice daily; *DS,* double strength; *IV,* intravenously; *PO,* orally; *qid,* four times daily; *tid,* three times daily; *TMP-SMX,* trimethoprim-sulfamethoxazole.

admitting these individuals. If an insulin-dependent patient is discharged, a basal rate of insulin must be continued. Cutting the usual dose of insulin in half, or instructing the patient to take the long-acting insulin only and checking blood glucose levels regularly, may be sufficient. Discussion with the primary care physician before discharge facilitates outpatient management.

Patients with persistent nausea but no vomiting can usually be discharged with an antiemetic and careful instructions for maintaining hydration. Persistent diarrhea alone is not an indication for admission, unless the patient is immunocompromised and has significant dehydration on presentation.

$SI = \frac{SV}{BSA}$ **FACTS AND FORMULAS**

**Homemade Oral Rehydration Solution**

½ teaspoon salt
½ teaspoon baking soda
4 tablespoons sugar
All in 1 L of water

The most common cause of acute gastroenteritis is viral.

Of bacterial causes, the three most common are *Campylobacter, Salmonella,* and *Shigella.*

*Escherichia coli* O157:H7 is more common in patients with grossly blood stools.

Nonbloody bacterial stool cultures are positive 1% to 5% of the time in immunocompetent adults.

Grossly bloody bacterial stool cultures are positive up to 20% of the time in immunocompetent adults.[16]

A pathogen can be identified in 80% to 85% of patients with acquired immunodeficiency syndrome and diarrhea.[17]

Dietary recommendations are always of great concern to patients on discharge. Many complex regimens involve significant dietary restrictions, based on limited scientific data. Patients should be advised that the number-one priority is to stay hydrated. If solid foods do not sound appealing, then they should not be encouraged. For patients with mild diarrhea or persistent nausea, water or commercially available sports drinks should be adequate. These drinks are not properly balanced for more severe dehydration. If the patient is having large volumes of diarrhea or fluid losses, a balanced glucose and electrolyte solution with or without starches is recommended. Oral rehydration solutions are available in many pharmacies. An effective solution can be made at home by adding one-half teaspoon of salt, one-half teaspoon of baking soda, and four tablespoons of sugar to 1 L of water.[18]

Once a patient becomes interested in solid foods, a bland diet of bananas, rice, apples, and toast (the BRAT diet) traditionally has been recommended. No data support the BRAT diet, and patients should be encouraged to eat small amounts of whatever appeals to them, with a few exceptions. Both caffeine and alcohol have direct stimulatory effects on the bowel and therefore may worsen symptoms. In addition, a few patients encounter temporary lactose intolerance after gastroenteritis. If dairy products exacerbate symptoms, then refraining from these products for 1 to 2 weeks should allow the intestines to restore their normal function.

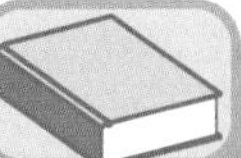

**PATIENT TEACHING TIPS**

**Prevention of Transmission**

- Wash hands well.
- Separate drinking glasses, towels, and preferably bathrooms.

**Diet**

- Start drinking sips of liquids.
- If tolerated, advance to full liquids.
- Once hungry, eat small amounts of whatever sounds good, with the exception of alcohol and caffeine-containing foods and drinks because these may exacerbate the symptoms.
- If dairy products exacerbate symptoms, avoid for 1 to 2 weeks as a temporary measure because lactose intolerance is not uncommon.

**Further Action**

- Return to the emergency department if vomiting persists, if pain in the abdomen increases, if fever increases, or if signs of dehydration develop.

## COMPLICATIONS

Significant complications are fortunately quite rare following gastroenteritis. The following are important to keep in mind when treating a patient with current symptoms or a recent history of acute gastroenteritis.

### LACTOSE INTOLERANCE

The most common minor complication is temporary lactose intolerance, which usually resolves spontaneously. As symptoms of the primary infection improve, patients may ingest milk products. However, if dairy products result in worsening bloating and cramping symptoms, then patients are advised to avoid these products for 1 to 2 weeks. Rarely does the intolerance become more chronic. Similarly, steatorrhea, or fat malabsorption, may occur transiently, particularly after a rotavirus infection, but it also resolves spontaneously.

### PROFOUND INTERNATIONAL NORMALIZED RATIO ELEVATIONS IN PATIENTS TAKING WARFARIN

Case reports in patients taking warfarin have noted significant coagulopathies occurring in acute gastroenteritis. Although these disorders are usually associated with episodes lasting several days, one case occurred after a single day of diarrhea. The mechanism is presumed to be a decreased vitamin K level in the body, from both decreased oral intake and malabsorption within the intestine.[19,20] Prothrombin time and international normalized ratio should be checked in patients taking warfarin, and close follow-up with repeat blood tests can prevent potential bleeding complications.

## ESOPHAGEAL INJURY

Any patient who is forcefully retching may suffer a tear in the mucosal surface of the esophagus, called a Mallory-Weiss tear, and this can lead to blood in the vomitus. Patients usually have little to no associated pain, and bleeding almost always resolves spontaneously, but occasionally, endoscopic intervention is required to acquire hemostasis. A more serious complication results when complete transmural disruption occurs in the esophagus. Known as Boerhaave's syndrome, it is usually accompanied by significant pain and is associated with a high mortality. A chest radiograph is almost always positive for mediastinal or intra-abdominal free air. Emergent surgical consultation and aggressive resuscitative management are essential.

## BOWEL NECROSIS

*Clostridium perfringens* normally causes self-limited gastroenteritis. However, in rare cases, it can lead to enteritis necroticans, which rapidly progresses to shock and death.

## DIABETIC KETOACIDOSIS

Diabetic patients may become significantly dehydrated in combination with high blood glucose levels, especially if these patients are unable to take their usual oral hypoglycemic agents. In severe circumstances, acute gastroenteritis may lead to diabetic ketoacidosis, coma, and death. A low threshold for electrolyte testing and measurement of the anion gap can help to detect the patient in danger of this complication.

## THROMBOTIC THROMBOCYTOPENIC PURPURA AND HEMOLYTIC-UREMIC SYNDROME

*E. coli* 0157:H7 hemorrhagic colitis has been associated with the hemolytic-uremic syndrome and with thrombotic thrombocytopenic purpura. Using antibiotics to treat gastroenteritis caused by this pathogen does nothing to eradicate the disease, but it may increase the incidence of these complications.

## NEUROLOGIC COMPLICATIONS

*Campylobacter* has been associated with a more severe form of Guillain-Barré syndrome that occurs even in patients with asymptomatic infections who have no signs of gastroenteritis.[21] Most neurologic symptoms from ciguatera poisoning resolve in days to weeks, but some long-term dysesthesias have been documented up to 2 years later.[13] *Shigella* can cause seizures and other neurologic symptoms, especially in children.

## OTHER ORGAN SYSTEM INVOLVEMENT

Although rare, invasive bacterial pathogens have been associated with systemic complications such as cholecystitis, pancreatitis, meningitis, endocarditis, and osteomyelitis.[22] Patients suffering from amebic colitis resulting from *E. histolytica* can develop a hepatic abscess. *Bacillus anthracis* may cause a spectrum of illness from minimal symptoms to shallow oral ulcers, massive lymphadenopathy with tissue edema, and fulminant upper and lower gastrointestinal bleeding. Severe cases of *C. difficile* colitis have led to protein-losing enteropathy with ascites and peripheral edema.[23]

## SUGGESTED READINGS

Cohen SH, Gerding DN, Johnson S, et al. Clinical practice guidelines for *Clostridium difficile* infection in adults: 2010 update by the Society for Healthcare Epidemiology of America (SHEA) and the Infectious Disease Society of America (IDSA). Infect Control Hosp Epidemiol 2010;21:1-25.

DuPont HL. Bacterial diarrhea. N Engl J Med 2009;361:1560-9.

Fleckenstein JM, Bartels SR, Drevets PD, et al. Infectious agents of food- and water-borne illnesses. Am J Med Sci 2010;340:238-46.

## REFERENCES

***References can be found on Expert Consult @ www.expertconsult.com.***

# 184 Skin and Soft Tissue Infections

Ellen M. Slaven

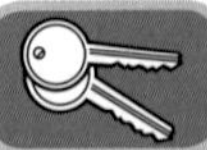

**KEY POINTS**

- Uncomplicated subcutaneous abscesses in otherwise healthy patients require incision and drainage alone, without antibiotic therapy.
- Cellulitis with induration may harbor a deep purulent collection despite the lack of fluctuance on physical examination. Ultrasound or needle aspiration may be used to assist in the search for areas of pus that require incision and drainage.
- Cellulitis with purulence should be treated with antibiotics that are active against community-acquired methicillin-resistant *Staphylococcus aureus* (CA-MRSA), and cellulitis without purulence should be treated with antibiotics active against *Streptococcus* species.
- Patients with mild diabetic foot infections may be treated with oral agents that target gram-positive organisms, including CA-MRSA.
- Emergency physicians must always search for signs of necrotizing infection to exclude the deadly diagnosis early in the management of skin and soft tissue infections.
- Emergency consultation with a surgeon is mandated when a suspicion of necrotizing skin and soft tissue infection arises.

## COMMUNITY-ACQUIRED METHICILLIN-RESISTANT *STAPHYLOCOCCUS AUREUS*

Since the late 1990s, an epidemic of skin and soft tissue infections has been caused by community-acquired methicillin-resistant *Staphylococcus aureus* (CA-MRSA). Currently in the United States, CA-MRSA is the most common cause of skin and soft tissue infection in patients presenting to emergency departments. Patients who develop these infections have been previously healthy, and most have not been exposed to health care settings or prior antibiotic therapy.[1]

CA-MRSA is distinguished from hospital-acquired MRSA (HA-MRSA) not only by the location of acquisition, but also by the type of infection produced. HA-MRSA causes wound infections, sepsis, endocarditis, and metastatic infections, but CA-MRSA causes predominantly purulent skin infections. HA-MRSA rarely carries the Panton-Valentine leukocidin that is believed to be a potent virulence factor found in most CA-MRSA strains. In addition, HA-MRSA is generally resistant to many antibiotics, whereas CA-MRSA tends to be resistant predominantly to β-lactam agents but remains susceptible to many other antibiotics, such as trimethoprim-sulfamethoxazole and the tetracyclines. Unfortunately, the designation of these staphylococcal strains based on the site of acquisition has led to confusion now that newly developed CA-MRSA infections have been increasingly identified within hospitals.

In 2011, the Infectious Disease Society of America released its long-anticipated first clinical guidelines for the treatment of MRSA infections, including CA-MRSA, in adults and children.[1] The panel of experts provided an evidence-based framework for the clinical evaluation and treatment of skin and soft tissue infections and more invasive infections such as bacteremia and pneumonia.

## SUPERFICIAL SKIN INFECTIONS

### IMPETIGO

*Impetigo* is most commonly encountered in preschool-age children. It is a superficial infection involving the epidermis and is highly contagious. Impetigo is readily spread from one site to another on one child and just as easily from one child to another. Two types of impetigo are recognized. The classic *nonbullous impetigo* begins with a vesicular lesion that becomes purulent. The vesicle then ruptures and reveals the typical, honey-colored crusted lesion. The face and extremities are commonly involved. *Streptococcus pyogenes* (group A *Streptococcus*) is the pathogen. The infection is self-limited and generally heals without scarring. Treatment is aimed at rapid resolution and prevention of transmission. The second type of impetigo, *bullous impetigo,* is caused by a toxin-producing strain of *S. aureus.* The appearance of bullous impetigo is of a flaccid, bullous lesion that may become filled with purulent fluid. Approximately 10% to 20% of all cases of impetigo are the bullous type.

Treatment with topical mupirocin is effective in patients with mild impetigo. Patients with more severe infections require systemic therapy with cephalexin for 7 days. Azithromycin (500 mg orally on day 1, then 250 mg orally on days 2 to 5) is an alternative for patients who are allergic to penicillin. Empiric therapy for CA-MRSA bullous impetigo should be reserved for patients in whom this standard treatment fails.

### ERYSIPELAS

*S. pyogenes* is the primary pathogen responsible for the intradermal infection known as *erysipelas,* or Saint Anthony's fire. This infection also involves the lymphatic drainage of the skin and produces a bright, erythematous raised area of skin. It is very well demarcated. The diagnosis is based on clinical appearance. The rash is common in older persons and in young children. Seventy percent of infections occur on the lower leg, and approximately 20% of infections occur on the face. The onset is quite sudden, fever may be present, and the rash is frequently very painful.

The drug of choice is penicillin. Admission to the hospital for intravenous antibiotics and supportive care may be indicated for patients who suffer from serious comorbidities or for patients who appear toxic. Azithromycin is an alternative agent. Always examine the feet carefully for signs of fissuring and include topical antifungals for treatment of tenia pedis because fissures may be a portal of entry for streptococci.

## CELLULITIS

*Cellulitis* results from bacterial infection of the dermis and the subcutaneous fat. Infection may arise following the entry of bacteria into the dermis through small breaks in the skin, larger wounds, or preexisting dermatitis. The infection may be limited to a small patch, or it may spread to include extensive areas of skin. Cellulitis is manifested by erythematous, warm, tender regions of skin that frequently spread. Lymphangitis and lymphadenitis may be present. Fever, chills, and malaise are common associated symptoms.

The pathogens of cellulitis are rarely identified in any particular patient, but they are thought to be primarily *S. pyogenes* (less commonly, other β-hemolytic streptococci such as groups B, C and G) and *S. aureus.* Culture of material aspirated from the involved skin is not routinely performed because of the invasive nature of the procedure and the low diagnostic yield. Blood cultures are of little value; only approximately 2% to 5% of these cultures yield results. A newer distinction has been proposed between nonpurulent cellulitis, which is believed to be more likely caused by *Streptococcus* species, and cellulitis that is associated with purulence and is probably caused by *S. aureus*. (See the later discussion of purulent skin infections.)

Patients with mild cases of nonpurulent cellulitis may be treated on an outpatient basis with an antibiotic effective against *Streptococcus* species such as cephalexin or dicloxacillin. The precise length of therapy is determined by the patient's response to therapy. A 5- to 10-day course of antibiotics is recommended. Empiric coverage for CA-MRSA should be reserved for patients who do not respond to β-lactam agents.

In patients with cellulitis who require hospital admission (e.g., those with extensive disease or underlying immunocompromises those who appear toxic), blood cultures are often obtained. Although the diagnostic yield of blood cultures is quite low, these cultures may provide useful information for patients who are significantly ill. Radiography may provide valuable information about patients with significant cellulitis, in particular to establish the presence of gas or foreign bodies. Patients with nonpurulent cellulitis who require admission may be treated with intravenous antibiotics, such as oxacillin, nafcillin, or cefazolin. For patients allergic to penicillin, azithromycin or levofloxacin may be substituted. Empiric coverage for CA-MRSA may be reserved for patients who do not improve during β-lactam therapy.

## PURULENT SKIN INFECTIONS

Small, superficial pustular infections arising from the hair follicle are usually caused by *S. aureus* and are referred to as *folliculitis.* The lesions of folliculitis tend to be approximately 2 to 5 mm in diameter, they are isolated to the epidermis, and they generally produce pruritus rather than pain. Treatment consists of warm, moist compresses and topical antibiotic ointment, such as mupirocin. If systemic therapy is desired (because of a lack of response to topical therapy, extensive infection, or the presence of underlying immunocompromising medical condition), an agent active against CA-MRSA is recommended (**Table 184.1**).

*Furuncles* begin as simple folliculitis and extend deeper into the subcutaneous tissue and surrounding dermis. Furuncles are also called boils or subcutaneous nodules. These painful lesions tend to erupt in areas with hairy skin, in particular the face, axilla, and buttock.

When multiple adjacent furuncles coalesce, a large, purulent mass develops in the subcutaneous tissues. This is a *carbuncle.* These lesions tend to occur in areas of overlying thick skin, such as the nape of the neck, back, and posterior thighs. Carbuncles appear as erythematous soft tissue masses, and they may contain several orifices capable of draining purulent material. Diabetes is a risk factor for the development of carbuncles. These lesions are quite painful and are frequently associated with fever.

Incision and drainage are required for both furuncles and carbuncles. Carbuncles generally require drainage in the

**Table 184.1** Antibiotics for Community-Acquired Methicillin-Resistant *Staphylococcus aureus* Skin Infections

| DEGREE OF INFECTION | ANTIBIOTIC REGIMEN |
|---|---|
| Mild | Trimethoprim-sulfamethoxazole (double strength) 1 PO bid<br>Clindamycin 300 mg PO qid<br>Doxycycline 100 mg PO bid<br>Linezolid 600 mg PO bid |
| Moderate to severe | Vancomycin 15-20 mg/kg/dose IV q8-12h (not to exceed 2 g/dose)<br>Clindamycin 600 mg IV q8h<br>Linezolid 600 mg IV q12h<br>Daptomycin 4 mg/kg IV q24h<br>Telavancin 10 mg/kg IV over 60 min q24h* |

*bid,* Twice daily; *IV,* intravenously; *PO,* orally; *q,* every; *qid,* four times daily.

*Women of childbearing potential must have a serum pregnancy test before administration of telavancin because of the possibility of fetal malformations.

operating room to provide sufficient analgesia and complete drainage. Antibiotics are indicated in patients with furuncles that are complicated by surrounding cellulitis and in all patients with carbuncles, and the selected antibiotic should be active against CA-MRSA (see Table 184.1).

*Subcutaneous abscesses* are collections of purulent material in the subcutaneous tissues, and they may occur anywhere on the body. The overlying skin may be uninvolved and may appear intact, or it may be erythematous and indurated. A pustule may be noted, or the overlying skin may be thin and in various stages of breakdown as the purulence drains spontaneously. Cellulitis of the surrounding dermis may also be noted. Purulent material must be sought out in patients who have cellulitis with moderate induration because pus may lie deep beneath the surface, without any signs of pustules or fluctuance. Ultrasound scanning or aspiration with a large-gauge needle (following local anesthesia) may reveal occult purulent collections. Incision and drainage are required for all subcutaneous abscesses. Antibiotics are not indicated for uncomplicated subcutaneous abscesses in healthy patients. The indications for antibiotic use are listed in **Table 184.2**.

Recurrent subcutaneous abscesses are common in this era of CA-MRSA. All patients should be educated regarding proper wound care, including keeping the incision site covered with a clean and dry bandage, regular hand washing, cleaning of surfaces that may become contaminated in the home, and avoiding shared personal items, such as razors. Attempts at decolonization may be beneficial for patients with recurrent abscesses or when intrapersonal transmission occurs with a household. These efforts, however, may be more successful after the patient has recovered and no longer has an open moist wound that may likely continue to harbor staphylococci. Regimens for decolonizing are not clearly defined. Some experts recommend intranasal mupirocin, twice daily for 5 to 10 days, in conjunction with daily chlorhexidine body washes for 5 to 10 days. Oral antibiotic therapy is not recommended for decolonization.

For outpatient management in patients with *purulent cellulitis,* empiric therapy with an agent active against CA-MRSA is recommended (see Table 184.1). The high cost of linezolid makes it a less desirable choice.

Intravenous vancomycin (15 to 20 mg/kg/dose actual body weight every 8 to 12 hours, not to exceed 2 g per dose) is the drug of choice for patients admitted with purulent cellulitis. Alternatives include clindamycin (600 mg orally or intravenously [IV] three times a day), linezolid (600 mg orally or IV twice daily), daptomycin (4 mg/kg/dose IV once daily), or telavancin (10 mg/kg/dose IV once daily).

No scientific data exist to support the routine culturing of purulent skin infections. Most patients improve with antibiotic therapy and incision and drainage, and microbiologic data are unnecessary. Most experts agree that cultures should be obtained when patients present with serious infections, when a course of outpatient antibiotics has failed, or when infections are complicated by underlying immune compromise, thus requiring hospitalization.

**Table 184.2 Indications for Antibiotic Therapy for Subcutaneous Abscesses**

| Abscesses in Patients with Compromised Immune Systems |
|---|
| Diabetes |
| Acquired immunodeficiency syndrome |
| Liver disease |
| Organ transplantation |
| Medications, such as long-term corticosteroid therapy |
| Chemotherapy |
| Extremes of age |
| **Abscesses Complicated by Other Conditions** |
| Cellulitis |
| Lymphangitis |
| Fever |
| Sepsis |
| Abscesses located on the central face |
| Extensive or severe disease (e.g., multiple abscesses) |
| Lack of response to incision and drainage alone |

## DIABETIC FOOT INFECTIONS

With more than 16 million diabetic patients in the United States and a 3-year incidence of foot ulceration of 6% among them, emergency physicians are likely to treat many patients with diabetic foot infections. The ulcers may begin as small lesions, but these sites are prone to infection and are associated with great morbidity and mortality. Fifteen percent of diabetic patients with foot ulcerations require amputation, and the 3-year mortality is almost 30%.[2]

Diabetic foot infections are diagnosed by their clinical appearance. Laboratory testing and radiography may be helpful to support the presence of infection or to define complications. The white blood cell count and erythrocyte sedimentation rate may be elevated in the presence of infection, but these tests are neither sufficiently sensitive nor definitively specific. Blood glucose testing is important because infections often lead to hyperglycemia. Uremia is known to impair healing. Radiographs may reveal the bony changes of osteomyelitis or subcutaneous gas produced by a necrotizing infection.

Obtaining a sample for microbiologic testing is worthwhile, particularly in the setting of severe infection. Swabbing the surface of an infected ulcer, or capturing purulent material as it makes its way to the surface, is likely to result in culture of contaminating bacteria, not necessarily the offending pathogen. Aspiration of deep-lying purulent material and sampling of tissue obtained during débridement are superior methods of acquiring material for microbiologic testing. The management of diabetic foot infections is directed by the severity of infection. Emergency physicians must assess the extent and depth of infection and the presence of foreign bodies or necrosis.

Aerobic gram-positive cocci, in particular *S. aureus,* including CA-MRSA, are the most predominant pathogens in diabetic foot infections. Patients with *mild infections,* defined as superficial when the lesions have less than 2 cm of surrounding cellulitis and are lacking abscess or necrosis, may be treated with antibiotics targeting *S. aureus*, including CA-MRSA (see Table 184.1). Moderate to severe infections tend to be caused by gram-positive cocci in addition to gram-negative bacilli and anaerobes. *Moderate infections* are defined as those with cellulitis extending more than 2 cm, lymphangitis, spread to deep tissues, or the presence of abscess or necrosis. *Severe infections* cause systemic toxicity, including features such as fever, hypotension, confusion, acidosis, or azotemia. Empiric therapy for these polymicrobial infections requires a broad-spectrum regimen until the results of microbiologic culture are available. When a limb- or life-threatening infection is present, imipenem and vancomycin or linezolid are recommended (**Table 184.3**). Surgical consultation should be considered for all diabetic patients with foot infections that may be complicated by abscess or necrosis.

## NECROTIZING INFECTIONS

Necrotizing skin and soft tissue infections comprise a group of potentially limb- and life-threatening diseases caused by various virulent pathogens. The common theme is infection leading to ischemia and necrosis of skin, subcutaneous tissue, fat, fascia, and even muscle. These infections are also characterized by their capacity to progress rapidly. During the initial presentation of patients with necrotizing skin and soft tissue infections, emergency physicians are not able to discern the depth of the infection precisely, nor can they identify the particular pathogen or pathogens. The most important component of the emergency physician's initial evaluation is to detect, or at least suspect, the presence of necrosis based on clinical findings alone. Be cautious when intense, localized pain is otherwise unexplainable, and consider the presence of an infection. Early use of antibiotics and consultation with surgeons may allow for lifesaving surgical débridement.[3]

**Table 184.3 Empiric Antimicrobial Therapy for Infections of the Diabetic Foot**

| DEGREE OF INFECTION | ANTIBIOTIC REGIMEN |
|---|---|
| Mild | Clindamycin 300 mg PO qid |
| Moderate to severe | Ampicillin-sulbactam 3 g IV q6h<br>*or*<br>Piperacillin-tazobactam 4.5 g IV q6h<br>*and*<br>Vancomycin 15-20 mg/kg/dose IV q8-12h (not to exceed 2 g/dose)<br>*or*<br>Linezolid 600 mg IV or PO q12h<br>*Levofloxacin 500 mg IV q24h<br>*and*<br>Clindamycin 900 mg IV q8h |
| Limb- or life-threatening infections | Imipenem 500 mg IV q6h<br>*and*<br>Vancomycin 15-20 mg/kg/dose IV q8-12h (not to exceed 2 g/dose)<br>*or*<br>Linezolid 600 mg IV or PO q12h<br>*Aztreonam 2 g IV q8h<br>*and*<br>Metronidazole 7.5 mg/kg IV q8h<br>*and*<br>Vancomycin 15-20 mg/kg/dose q8-12h (not to exceed 2 g/dose) |

*IV,* Intravenously; *PO,* orally; *q,* every; *qid,* four times daily.
*Alternative regimens for patients with severe β-lactam allergy.

*Gas gangrene,* or clostridial myonecrosis, is the classic necrotizing skin and soft tissue infection. It often develops after a wound is contaminated with soil containing *Clostridium perfringens.* Another virulent bacterium, *Vibrio vulnificus,* can also cause necrotizing soft tissue infections. Particularly during warm months, *V. vulnificus* may cause infections in patients with wounds that are exposed to salt or brackish waters. Additionally, *S. pyogenes* can produce necrotizing soft tissue infections in previously healthy patients.

Many patients with necrotizing skin and soft tissue infections are found to be infected with multiple pathogens. An example is *Fournier gangrene.* This highly lethal infection of the perineum is commonly diagnosed in men with diabetes. This infection tends to be "mixed" because several pathogens, such as *Streptococcus* species, Enterobacteriaceae, and anaerobes (e.g., *Bacteroides* species), are recovered from culture.

When a necrotizing skin and soft tissue infection is suspected, no diagnostic testing, in particular imaging studies, should delay consultation with a surgeon. Although many diagnostic imaging studies have been employed in attempts to confirm and exclude necrotizing skin and soft tissue infections, none is superior to surgical exploration. A plain radiograph may demonstrate the presence of gas within the tissues, but it does not exclude a diagnosis of necrosis. Ultrasound scanning and computed tomography may identify gas within the tissues, in addition to deep-seated abscesses. Computed tomography and magnetic resonance imaging may show edema in the subcutaneous tissues or muscle and enhancement of inflamed fascia. None of these studies are adequately sensitive to exclude the presence of necrosis.

The definitive diagnosis of necrotizing skin and soft tissue infection is made by surgical exploration with direct visualization of the affected tissues and histologic examination of a frozen section biopsy specimen. Early surgical débridement is the definitive therapy.

Microbiologic studies, including blood cultures and culture of purulent material aspirated from a deep source, are indicated. Simply obtaining a swab from an open wound is likely to yield only contaminating bacteria. Infected tissue and fluids obtained during surgical débridement should also be cultured.

Antimicrobial therapy is vitally important early in the management of necrotizing skin and soft tissue infections. Antimicrobial therapy alone without surgical débridement leads to a mortality rate approaching 100%.

Surgical consultation must be obtained as soon as the presence of a necrotizing soft tissue infection is suspected. **Box 184.1** lists common clinical indicators that mandate surgical consultation.

Early empiric antimicrobial regimens require broad-spectrum antimicrobial activity, including coverage for gram-positive, gram-negative, and anaerobic bacteria and for pathogens with multidrug resistance, such as MRSA. No excellent options for monotherapy are available in this setting. Tigecycline is a broad-spectrum intravenous agent that is active against gram-positive, gram-negative, and anaerobic bacteria, including MRSA, but it is not as effective against *Pseudomonas* species, and safety concerns have limited its utility in this setting. Combination regimens include the

**Table 184.4** Antimicrobial Regimens for the Empiric Treatment of Necrotizing Skin and Soft Tissue Infections

| CONVENTIONAL REGIMEN | ALTERNATE REGIMEN FOR PATIENTS WITH SEVERE β-LACTAM ALLERGY |
|---|---|
| Imipenem 500 mg IV q6h<br>***or***<br>Piperacillin/tazobactam 4.5 g IV q6h<br>***and***<br>Vancomycin 15-20 mg/kg/dose q8-12h (not to exceed 2 g/dose)<br>***or***<br>Linezolid 600 mg IV or PO q12h | *Clindamycin 900 mg IV q8h<br>***and***<br>Gentamicin 5 mg/kg IV q24h<br>***and***<br>Vancomycin 15-20 mg/kg/dose q8-12h (not to exceed 2 g/dose)<br>***or***<br>Linezolid 600 mg IV or PO q12h |

*IV*, Intravenously; *q*, every.

**BOX 184.1 Clinical Indicators of the Potential for Necrotizing Soft Tissue Infections**

Cellulitis that is rapidly advancing
Cellulitis with the following features:
- "Pain out of proportion" to physical examination
- Pain-restricted limb movement
- Crepitus
- Hemorrhagic bullae
- Ecchymosis
- Necrotic or black tissue

carbapenems (imipenem or meropenem) or piperacillin-tazobactam combined with either vancomycin or linezolid (**Table 184.4**). Clindamycin and linezolid inhibit bacterial protein synthesis and may be beneficial by blocking toxin production in several organisms responsible for necrotizing skin and soft tissue infections, in particular streptococcal and clostridial infections. All patients with necrotizing skin and soft tissue infections, even those with suspected yet unproven infections, should be admitted to the hospital for intravenous antibiotic therapy and surgical evaluation.

## REFERENCES

***References can be found on Expert Consult @ www.expertconsult.com.***

# Antibiotic Recommendations 185

Ellen M. Slaven

The proper selection of antibiotic therapy in the setting of the emergency department (ED) is often complicated. The offending pathogen is rarely known with certainty, and emergency physicians must contend with diseases caused by emerging microbes, such as human immunodeficiency virus and the coronavirus that causes sudden acute respiratory syndrome. Many common bacterial pathogens have developed novel antimicrobial resistance patterns, such as drug-resistant *Streptococcus pneumoniae* and *Escherichia coli*, and some well-known bacteria have developed new strains, such as community-acquired methicillin-resistant *Staphylococcus aureus* (CA-MRSA). Complicating this challenge is a perpetually growing list of new antimicrobial agents, and emergency physicians clearly must remain diligent to keep current with the ever-changing arena of infectious diseases that are frequently encountered in the ED.

Fortunately, many helpful resources are available, such as local hospital antibiograms and hospital-specific protocols. National guidelines such as the Surviving Sepsis Campaign and the Centers for Disease Control and Prevention (CDC) guidelines for sexually transmitted diseases provide helpful references. The annually updated *Sanford Guide to Antimicrobial Therapy* remains an invaluable up-to-date tool literally found within one's pocket.

In general, antibiotic therapy is empiric, based on epidemiologic data of the most likely encountered pathogen. Critically ill patients benefit from early and appropriate antibiotic therapy and therefore initially require broad-spectrum therapy, unless a specific pathogen has been identified. Whenever possible, the safest, least expensive, and easiest to administer antibiotic should be prescribed. Oral therapy is preferable over parenteral, and single-dose regimens eliminate concerns regarding compliance when compared with multidose regimens.

Recommendations for antibiotic therapy in the ED for selected infectious diseases are outlined in the sections that follow.

## ODONTOGENIC INFECTIONS

Penicillin (Pen Vee K, 500 mg orally [PO] four times daily for 5 to 7 days) is indicated for dentoalveolar abscesses, such as periapical abscesses. Clindamycin (300 mg PO four times daily for 5 to 7 days) is an alternative for penicillin-allergic patients. Significant abscesses (i.e., those causing facial swelling) require emergency drainage in addition to antibiotics. For patients admitted to the hospital with severe infection, ampicillin-sulbactam (1.5 g intravenously [IV] every 6 hours) is preferred. Clindamycin (900 mg IV every 6 hours) is again a suitable alternative.

## PHARYNGITIS

Penicillin (Pen Vee K, 500 mg PO four times daily for 10 days) remains the drug of choice for group A streptococcal pharyngitis. A single intramuscular injection of benzathine penicillin (600,000 units if the patient's weight is < 27 kg and 1.2 million units if it is >27 kg) may be administered to enhance compliance.

Patients with allergy to penicillin may be treated with azithromycin (500 mg PO on day 1, then 250 mg PO every day for 4 days). Group A *Streptococcus* has not developed resistance to penicillin, but approximately one third of isolates are resistant to macrolides or clindamycin. Linezolid (400 mg PO twice daily for 10 days) may be used for resistant strains.

## ACUTE SINUSITIS

Mild symptoms of acute sinusitis may initially be treated with decongestants and analgesics. Reserve antibiotics for those in whom such conservative therapy fails and in patients with more severe symptoms, such as severe maxillary or facial pain and fever. High-dose amoxicillin is the preferred agent (adults: 1 g PO three times daily for 10 days; children: 90 mg/kg/day PO divided three times daily for 10 days).

## OTITIS EXTERNA

Hydrocortisone, polymyxin B, and neomycin combined (Cortisporin otic, 4 drops in affected ear four times daily for 7 days) remain the standard therapy for otitis externa. If the tympanic membrane is perforated, a preferred combination of ciprofloxacin with hydrocortisone (3 drops in affected ear twice daily for 7 days) is indicated because of the ototoxicity of neomycin. Removal of debris from the ear canal promotes enhanced entry of the medication deep into the canal. When the canal is sufficiently swollen, a wick may need to be carefully placed to allow medication penetration.

## OTITIS MEDIA

A prudent approach is to withhold antibiotics for 48 hours in afebrile children with otitis media who are more than 2 years old and are without pain. Treat with high-dose amoxicillin for 7 days (adults: 1 g PO three times daily; children: 90 mg/kg/day PO divided three times daily). Alternative therapy is with azithromycin (adults: 500 mg PO on day 1, then 250 mg PO every day for 4 days; children: 10 mg/kg [maximum, 500 mg] PO on day 1, then 5 mg/kg [maximum, 250 mg] PO every day for 4 days).

## ACUTE BACTERIAL MENINGITIS

The treatment of acute bacterial meningitis is guided by epidemiologic risk factors; likely pathogens are determined primarily by the age of the patient and by exposure following trauma or surgical intervention. The goal of treatment is to administer antibiotics within 30 minutes of the patient's arrival to the ED.

A Cochrane Review of more than 4000 patients with acute bacterial meningitis concluded that the use of adjunctive steroids decreases neurologic sequelae including hearing loss. Dexamethasone should be given intravenously 15 minutes before or concomitantly with the first dose of antibiotics and continued for 4 days (adults: 10 mg every 6 hours; children: 0.15 mg/kg every 6 hours).

Neonates (<1 month old): Combination treatment with ampicillin (200 mg/kg/day IV divided every 6 hours) and cefotaxime (300 mg/kg/day IV divided every 6 hours) targets the most common pathogens, which are group B *Streptococcus, E. coli,* and *Listeria* species.

Age 1 month to 50 years: Ceftriaxone (adults: 2 g IV every 12 hours; children: 100 mg/kg/day [maximum, 2 g] IV divided every 12 hours) with vancomycin (adults: 15-20 mg/kg [maximum, 2 g] IV every 12 hours; children: 15 mg/kg [maximum, 2 g] IV every 6 hours) provides coverage against *S. pneumoniae* (including penicillin-resistant strains), *Neisseria meningitidis*, and *Haemophilus influenzae* (although now rare because of the Hib vaccine).

Age greater than 50 years: Ampicillin (2 g IV every 4 hours), ceftriaxone (2 g IV every 12 hours), and vancomycin (15 to 20 mg/kg [maximum, 2 g] IV every 12 hours) are combined to cover *S. pneumoniae, Listeria* species, and gram-negative bacilli.

Postoperative/trauma: *S. pneumoniae, S. aureus* (including MRSA), and gram-negative bacilli (including *Pseudomonas aeruginosa*) are common pathogens in this setting; thus, ceftazidime (2 g IV every 8 hours) combined with vancomycin (15 to 20 mg/kg [maximum, 2 g] IV every 12 hours) is recommended.

## COMMUNITY-ACQUIRED PNEUMONIA

Both the Infectious Diseases Society of American and the American Thoracic Society provide guidelines for the management of community-acquired pneumonia. For outpatient management of otherwise healthy patients, azithromycin (500 mg PO on day 1, then 250 mg PO every day for 4 days) or doxycycline for 7 to 10 days (age > 8 years: 100 mg PO twice daily for 7 days) remains an excellent option.

If the patient has comorbid illness, then a respiratory fluoroquinolone (with enhanced activity against *S. pneumoniae*) is indicated, such as levofloxacin (750 mg PO every day), moxifloxacin (400 mg PO every day), or gemifloxacin (320 mg PO every day). Telithromycin is not recommended here out of concern for hepatotoxicity.

For inpatients, combination therapy is recommended for with ceftriaxone (2 g IV every 24 hours) and azithromycin (500 mg IV every 24 hours). Alternatives include intravenous respiratory fluoroquinolones levofloxacin (750 mg IV every day) or moxifloxacin (400 mg IV every day).

Patients admitted to the intensive care unit should be treated with either levofloxacin (750 mg IV every day) or moxifloxacin (400 mg IV every day), with the addition of either vancomycin (15 to 20 mg/kg [maximum, 2 g] IV every 12 hours) or linezolid (600 mg IV every 12 hours) if MRSA is suspected (i.e., after influenza, severe disease with hemoptysis, and necrotizing features). If the patient has a life-threatening illness or suspicion of *P. aeruginosa* (i.e., an alcoholic patient, or one with underlying bronchiectasis or malignant disease), also add piperacillin-tazobactam (4.5 g IV every 6 hours) or aztreonam (2 g IV every 6 hours).

### PEDIATRIC PATIENTS

Neonates with pneumonia require treatment for group B *Streptococcus, Listeria* species, and gram-negative bacilli. The combination of ampicillin (50 mg/kg IV every 12 hours) and gentamicin (2.5 mg/kg IV first dose) is recommended.

Children treated as outpatients require coverage for *S. pneumoniae,* and high-dose amoxicillin (100 mg/kg divided every 8 hours) is commonly used. An alternative is azithromycin (10 mg/kg [maximum, 500 mg] PO on day 1, then 5 mg/kg [maximum, 250 mg] PO every day for 4 days). If the patient is hospitalized, then use ceftriaxone (50 mg/kg IV every day) for children younger than 5 years. Add azithromycin (10 mg/kg [maximum, 500 mg] divided IV every 12 hours) if children are older than 5 years. For severe infection, add vancomycin (15 mg/kg IV every 6 hours).

## CHOLECYSTITIS

Enterobacteriaceae such as *E. coli* and *Proteus* species are the most common pathogens in cholecystitis, as well as other biliary tract infections, and antibiotic selection must take into consideration adequate activity against these gram-negative bacilli. Other pathogens include anaerobes and enterococci. A regimen of piperacillin-tazobactam (3.375 g IV every 6 hours) alone or ciprofloxacin (500 mg IV every 12 hours) with metronidazole (1 g IV first dose) is recommended, in addition to surgical intervention.

## DIARRHEA (DYSENTERY)

Mild to moderate diarrhea is best managed with antimotility agents and fluids. Severe diarrhea (i.e., more than six unformed stools/day, the presence of fever, or bloody stools) is an indication for antimicrobial therapy. Fluoroquinolones, either ciprofloxacin (500 mg PO twice daily) or levofloxacin (500 mg PO every day), remain the drugs of choice. Trimethoprim-sulfamethoxazole ([TMP-SMX] 1 double-strength [DS] tablet PO twice daily) is an alternative. All regimens are recommended for 3 to 5 days. If the patient has recently received antibiotic therapy and *Clostridium difficile* colitis is considered, then add metronidazole (500 mg PO three times daily) for 10 to 14 days.

## URINARY TRACT INFECTION

Growing concern exists about widespread and increasing resistance of *E. coli* to TMP-SMX and ciprofloxacin. In 2009, the rate of resistance to each of these two agents was greater than 25% in many regions of the United States. Knowledge of local antibiotic resistance patterns in urinary pathogens may assist in the empiric treatment of urinary tract infections. TMP-SMX (1 DS tablet PO twice daily for 3 days) is the drug of choice if the local rate of resistance to TMP-SMX is less than 20%. Ciprofloxacin (250 mg PO twice daily for 3 days) or levofloxacin (250 mg PO every day for 3 days) is an alternative if the local rate of resistance to fluoroquinolones is less than 20%. (Moxifloxacin and gemifloxacin have low urinary concentrations and are not recommended.) An alternative for uncomplicated urinary tract infections is nitrofurantoin (100 mg PO four times daily for 7 days) or fosfomycin (3 mg PO once).

Pyelonephritis is initially treated with ciprofloxacin (500 mg PO twice daily for 7 days) or levofloxacin (250 mg PO every day for 7 days). Hospitalized patients may receive ciprofloxacin IV (400 mg twice daily) or levofloxacin (750 mg every day) for 14 days. Urinary cultures must be obtained to assess for possible resistance to fluoroquinolones. An alternative regimen is ampicillin (2 g IV every 6 hours) plus gentamicin (5 mg/kg IV every 24 hours), or piperacillin-tazobactam alone (3 g IV every 6 hours) for 14 days.

## SEPSIS

Patients with sepsis who do not have a clear source of infections require early broad-spectrum antibiotics; the goal is intravenous antibiotic administration within the first hour of their presentation to the ED. Imipenem (500 mg IV every 6 hours) plus vancomycin (15 to 20 mg/kg [maximum, 2 g] IV every 12 hours) or piperacillin-tazobactam (4.5 mg IV every 6 hours) with vancomycin (15 to 20 mg/kg [maximum, 2 g] IV every 12 hours) is recommended. In penicillin-allergic patients, a combination of ciprofloxacin (400 mg IV every 12 hours), metronidazole (1 g IV every 12 hours), and vancomycin (15 to 20 mg/kg [maximum, 2 g] IV every 12 hours) may be prescribed.

Neonatal sepsis (<1 month of age) may be empirically treated with ampicillin (25 mg/kg IV every 8 hours) and cefotaxime (50 mg/kg IV every 12 hours). Vancomycin (15 mg/kg IV every 12 hours) should be added if MRSA is a potential concern.

Empiric therapy of childhood sepsis is with ceftriaxone (100 mg/kg in every 24 hours) plus vancomycin (15 mg/kg [maximum dose, 2 g] IV every 12 hours).

## CELLULITIS

A newer paradigm has been proposed by the Infectious Diseases Society of America for the treatment of cellulitis in the era of CA-MRSA. This protocol is based on the detection of purulent material associated with cellulitis and the likely presence of CA-MRSA.

Dry cellulitis, or cellulitis not associated with exudates, purulence, or abscess formation, is likely caused by β-hemolytic streptococci, such as *Streptococcus pyogenes*, and should be treated with an antibiotic targeting these organisms; that is, cephalexin (500 mg PO four times daily) or dicloxacillin (500 mg PO four times daily) for 5 to 10 days. The precise duration of therapy should be dictated by the clinical response.

Cellulitis associated with an underlying abscess or with purulent exudates must be treated with an agent that is active against CA-MRSA, such as TMP-SMX (1 DS tablet PO twice daily), clindamycin (300 mg PO four times daily) or doxycycline (100 mg PO twice daily) for 5 to 10 days. Vancomycin (15 to 20 mg/kg [maximum, 2 g] IV every 12 hours) remains the drug of choice for patients requiring hospitalization. Clindamycin (900 mg IV every 8 hours) is an alternative. Linezolid (600 mg IV every 12 hours) is not recommended as first-line therapy, primarily because of its higher cost.

Skin and soft tissue infections that are limb- or life-threatening should be treated empirically with imipenem (500 mg IV every 6 hours) and vancomycin (15 to 20 mg/kg [maximum, 2 g] IV every 12 hours).

## MAMMALIAN BITES

Prophylaxis against infection following the bite of an animal must provide coverage against *Pasteurella* species, *S. aureus*, and anaerobes. Amoxicillin-clavulanate (875/125 mg PO twice daily) is the primary oral agent and should be prescribed for 3 days. Dual therapy with clindamycin (300 mg PO four times daily) plus ciprofloxacin (500 mg PO twice daily), also for 3 days, is an alternative regimen for patients with penicillin allergy.

Outpatient treatment of an established soft tissue infection resulting from an animal bite may be implemented with the same antibiotics used for prophylaxis, only for a longer duration (i.e., 7 to 10 days). Patients hospitalized with severe infection may be treated with one of the β-lactam–β-lactamase inhibitors (ampicillin-sulbactam, 1.5 g IV every 6 hours, or piperacillin-tazobactam, 3.375 g IV every 6 hours). Alternatively, clindamycin (900 mg IV every 8 hours) with a fluoroquinolone (ciprofloxacin, 400 mg IV every 12 hours, or levofloxacin, 500 mg IV every 24 hours) may be given.

## SEXUALLY TRANSMITTED DISEASES

### URETHRITIS AND CERVICITIS

Dual therapy with ceftriaxone (250 mg intramuscularly [IM] once) for coverage of penicillin and fluoroquinolone-resistant *Neisseria gonorrhoeae* and azithromycin (1 g PO) for *Chlamydia trachomatis* is recommended. The more recently recognized *Mycoplasma genitalium* is also covered by azithromycin. For patients with severe penicillin allergy, 2 g of azithromycin PO may be given.

## SYPHILIS

The treatment of syphilis has remained essentially unchanged since the 1940s, when penicillin was introduced. Today, penicillin remains the drug of choice for syphilis.

For primary, secondary, and early latent (<1 year) syphilis, a single injection of benzathine penicillin G (2.4 million units IM) is recommended. Patients with severe penicillin allergy may be treated with doxycycline (100 mg PO twice daily) for 14 days.

Late latent syphilis, syphilis of unknown duration, and tertiary syphilis are treated with three injections, 1 week apart, of benzathine penicillin G (2.4 million units IM). Doxycycline (100 mg PO twice daily) for 4 weeks is an alternative.

Neurosyphilis requires intravenous administration of aqueous crystalline penicillin G (4 million units every 4 hours for 10 to 14 days).

## CHANCHROID

Fortunately, the painful genital ulcers of chancroid, caused by the difficult to detect *Haemophilus ducreyi*, have declined in prevalence in the United States. Single-dose therapy is recommended with azithromycin (1 g PO) or ceftriaxone (250 mg IM).

## EPIDIDYMITIS AND PROSTATITIS

Men 35 years of age and younger who have either epididymitis or prostatitis must be treated with antimicrobial agents that target the sexually transmitted pathogens *N. gonorrhoeae* and *C. trachomatis* with ceftriaxone (250 mg IM once) and doxycycline (100 mg PO twice daily for 10 days). In contrast, men older than 35 years are more likely to be infected with Enterobacteriaceae, and fluoroquinolones are recommended; that is, ciprofloxacin (500 mg PO twice daily) or levofloxacin (750 mg PO every day) for 10 to 14 days.

# SUGGESTED READINGS

Brouwer MC, McIntyre P, de Gans J, et al. Corticosteroids for bacterial meningitis. Cochrane Database Syst Rev 2010;(9):CD004405.

Centers for Disease Control and Prevention. Sexually transmitted diseases: treatment guidelines, 2010. MMWR Morb Mortal Wkly Rep 2010;59:1-109.

Gilbert DN, Moellering RC, Eliopoulous GM, et al. The Sanford guide to antimicrobial therapy. 40th ed. Sperryville, Va: Antimicrobial Therapy; 2010.

Liu C, Bayer A, Cosgrove S, et al. Clinical practice guidelines by the Infectious Diseases Society of America for the treatment of methicillin-resistant *Staphylococcus aureus* infections in adults and children: executive summary. Clin Infect Dis 2011;52:285-92.

Mandell LA, Bartlett JG, Dowell SF, et al. Update of practice guidelines for the management of community-acquired pneumonia in immunocompetent adults. Clin Infect Dis 2003;37:1405-33.

Niederman MS, Mandell LA, Anzueto A, et al. Guidelines for the management of adults with community-acquired pneumonia: diagnosis, assessment of severity, antimicrobial therapy, and prevention. Am J Respir Crit Care Med 2001;163:1730-54.

# Wound Repair 186

*Robert Lockwood*

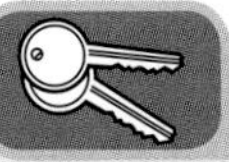

**KEY POINTS**

- Thoughtful consideration of the patient, characteristics of the wound, and selection of an appropriate technique for closure is the most important aspect of wound care.
- Antibiotics are not a substitute for adequate wound preparation, irrigation, and exploration.
- Following gross decontamination, the pressure of an irrigating stream must be sufficient to overcome the adhesive force of bacteria (5 to 12 psi).
- Proper skin eversion and suture placement make a difference and take no significantly greater amount of time than does hastily managing a wound.
- Address tetanus status and allergies in all patients.
- Immobilization, a clean moist environment, elevation, and avoidance of sun are the key elements of aftercare.
- Diligent documentation needs to include information regarding the patient's characteristics, the wound's appearance, previous care, assessment of the functionality of surrounding structures before and after intervention, and steps taken to reduce infection, as well as the actual closure technique.

Within the broad scope of emergency medical treatment, wound repair plays a prominent role. Wounds occur in all types of people—from the youngest toddlers to frail elderly grandparents. In contrast to many other conditions requiring treatment in the emergency department (ED), wounds (typically) occur independently of patients' other medical issues. However, each patient's unique substrate for healing is one of the two most significant factors affecting satisfactory wound healing. The second significant consideration is the characteristics of the wound itself.

## EPIDEMIOLOGY

Approximately 12 million wounds are treated in EDs in the United States each year.[1] Data on the true incidence of wounds are limited because many are thought to be treated away from the ED or urgent care setting. Of individuals with wounds seen in the ED, the majority are men.[2] Wounds can clearly occur anywhere on the body, but lacerations on the upper extremities, head, and neck constitute the majority of cases encountered in EDs.

## PATHOPHYSIOLOGY

Skin, the largest organ in the body, has numerous functions, most prominently heat exchange, prevention of infection, and provision of a tactile interface with the environment. The layers of skin—epidermis, dermis, and connective tissue—all play different roles in wounds and healing. The thickest and most important layer, the dermis, serves as structural integument, supports conveyance of nutritional and waste products, and contains cutaneous nerves (**Fig. 186.1**).

Disruption of the skin may be caused by an infinite number of means, from simple cutlery accidents to industrial mishaps or intentional violence. Wounds that disrupt the full depth of skin are fundamentally different from those that affect only the superficial layers. Wounds that affect merely the epidermis may typically be cleansed and dressed appropriately with less concern for complications. However, it is imperative to assess seemingly superficial wounds in a diligent manner to ensure that more significant injuries are absent.

After injury, a continuum of coagulation, hemostasis, inflammation, tissue formation, and tissue remodeling quickly ensue. Each of these steps is influenced by the patient's condition and the clinician's wound repair skills. Clearly achieving hemostasis is a primary concern for wound repair, both to prevent exsanguination and to allow adequate visualization of the wound, as well as closure of it. Any delay in wound closure allows the later three steps of inflammation, tissue formation, and remodeling to proceed naturally, which will probably result in skin that is functional but scarred.

The aesthetic qualities of a scar are influenced by its thickness, color, and height or degree of depression. Thickness is most dependent on the width of the healing wound and on whether additional granulation tissue is necessary to fill gaps (as in secondary intention). The height of a scar is altered by the alignment and apposition of the healing skin edges, as well as by tensile and shear forces across the wound and the amount of inflammation preceding the formation of scar tissue. The increased height of a hypertrophic scar is the result of

Acknowledgment and thanks to Dr. E. Parker Hays, Jr., for his work on the first edition.

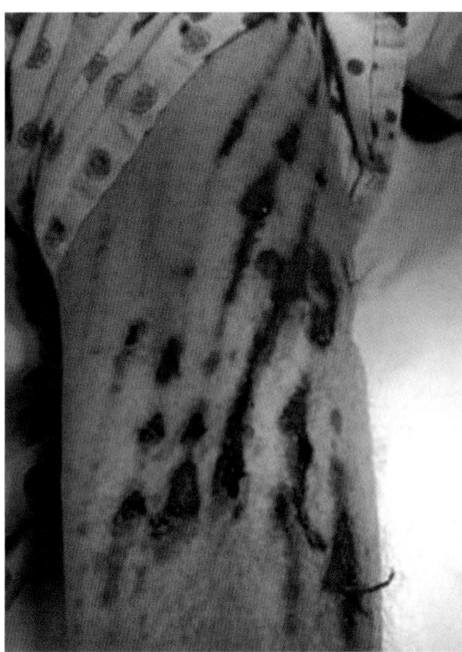

**Fig. 186.1 Skin anatomy.** The layers of skin—epidermis, dermis, and connective tissue—all play important roles in wound healing. The dermis is the most important and thickest, but it thins with age or steroid use. Note the tearing appearance of the skin of this elderly patient, who fell on an escalator.

redundant tissue. If it extends beyond the original margins of the wound, it is called a keloid. Depressed scars create shadowing (consider the visibility of age-associated wrinkles), which makes them appear darker than the neighboring reflective surfaces. The color of a scar results from its vascularity and pigmentation with respect to surrounding healthy tissue. Melanocytes do not produce pigment at the same rate in injured and healing tissue or in scars as they do in normal tissue.

All these factors in scar formation vary among individuals. Some patients heal very well, whereas hypertrophic keloids invariably develop in others. However, steps to improve outcomes generally remain the same in emergency management.

## PRESENTING SIGNS AND SYMPTOMS

Wound repair may be sought intentionally or be required following evaluation of other complaints, such as a syncopal event. It is not uncommon for patients to be entirely unaware of their wounds (as in trauma) or to be unimpressed with the severity of their lesion because of more painful conditions, such as a fracture. For all these reasons, a thorough physical examination plus evaluation of all wounds is required. Through this evaluation and assessment of the patient's unique situation, an appropriate approach may be undertaken to address a wound. The overall risk for infection and the likelihood of complications can be predicted by considering wound and host factors. A major pitfall of wound management is fixation on the wound without sufficient attention to the host. For example, a 4-cm linear laceration on the arm of a healthy 18-year-old patient has a different prognosis than the same wound on the shin of a 73-year-old diabetic patient with peripheral vascular disease (**Box 186.1**).

**BOX 186.1 Wound and Patient Factors**

**Wound Factors**
Location
Mechanism
Degree and type of contamination
Proximity to adjacent structures
Timing of closure
Antibiotics

**Patient Factors**
Extremes of age
Vasculopathies
Diabetes
Immunosuppression (iatrogenic or intrinsic)
Renal dysfunction
Extremes of size: obesity or cachexia

## DIFFERENTIAL DIAGNOSIS AND MEDICAL DECISION MAKING

### PATIENT EVALUATION

With an infinite variety of medical conditions and circumstances requiring ED management, each patient has a unique environment for wound healing. Hosts also change over time: thinning of the dermis, varying degrees of vascular compromise, increased likelihood of fractures, and medication use. Assessment of patient status before the injury, as well as prediction of the patient's capacity for healing, is important before initiating wound repair.

A wound is the physical manifestation of an injurious force exerted on the body. Accordingly, careful evaluation of the patient as a whole is critical. A common pitfall is focusing on the most visible injury and not recognizing other lesions that were caused by one event, such as trauma. Understanding the injurious mechanism also enables better prediction of the wound's severity. As an example, blunt force injuries have significantly greater potential for diffuse tissue nonviability and are consequently more prone to infection.[3] Once all injuries have been catalogued, each may be addressed. Important considerations include knowing how the patient was injured (shear, abrasion, compression), whether the location of the wound is in a cosmetically or functionally vital area, and whether potentially confounding influences on the potential for healing are present.

### INJURY TO UNDERLYING STRUCTURES

When sufficiently breached, skin fails in its protective role and may allow underlying structures to be injured (**Fig. 186.2**). Diligent assessment of the functionality of surrounding anatomic structures is of utmost importance.

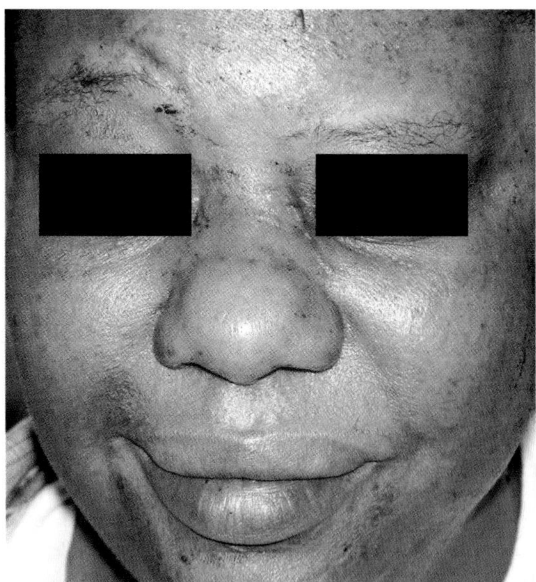

**Fig. 186.2 Injury to underlying structures.** Missing an associated nerve, tendon, vascular, or bony injury is a significant pitfall in wound care. This patient had partial facial nerve palsy from her injury that was slightly exacerbated by anesthesia, but it resolved almost completely over time.

Tendon function should be assessed throughout its range of motion. It may help to ask the patient to estimate the position of a body part at the time of the injury, especially with hand injuries. Tendons may be partially lacerated but their range of motion may remain intact, thereby misleading the practitioner. Patients' complaints of pain or subjectively decreased range of motion, despite objectively normal findings on examination, should raise suspicion for partial disruption.

Nerves can be injured by the wounding mechanism itself or by iatrogenic maneuvers, especially indiscriminate ones. Clamping, blind probing, and injudicious débridement may all disrupt adjacent nerves. The hands and face are at greatest risk because nerves run in close proximity to the vasculature; zealous attempts to control bleeding vessels can result in damage to adjacent nerves. Injected anesthetics may also injure nerves as a result of pressure necrosis in finite spaces. Examples include injections into the olecranon grooves or foramina in the hard palate of the mouth.

Muscles are highly vascular tissue and are often disrupted with deep wounds. Because muscles are dynamic units, subsequent hematomas, scars, or infection can result in dysfunction. Unnecessary débridement should be avoided and bleeding controlled with direct pressure. Muscle can usually be repaired by securing the surrounding structures, thereby placing the cut surfaces of the muscle in direct apposition. Muscle tissue should be repaired directly only when the foregoing maneuver is insufficient.

Occasionally, a wound is the first sign of an underlying fracture, either because the skin was injured with the force carried onto the bone or because the broken bone edges penetrated the skin from inside.

## FOREIGN BODIES

Foreign bodies can be driven into wounds through innumerable routes of entry. Common situations include shattered glass in motor vehicle accidents, vegetative material in wounds during outdoor pursuits, and puncture wounds through footwear. Foreign bodies increase the risk for infection and may prevent healing. The following section on puncture wounds specifically addresses foreign bodies in these situations. For additional discussion of foreign body evaluation and management, see Chapter 187.

**BOX 186.2 Wounds Requiring Specialty Consultation**

- Open fractures of long bones
- Disruption of joint capsules
- Extensive débridement
- Nerve disruption
- Vascular disruption
- Injury to special facial structures, such as the eyelids or lacrimal ducts
- Significant injuries to genitourinary structures
- Disruption of skin that was previously repaired surgically, as in grafts

# TREATMENT

The emergency physician (EP) can close most wounds; some situations requiring specialist consultation are listed in **Box 186.2**.

## WOUND PREPARATION

To meet the goals of reducing risk for infection, minimizing damage to underlying structures, and forming a functional and cosmetically acceptable scar, preparation of the wound can be tantamount to or may surpass closure in importance. An appropriately prepared wound has been anesthetized, has been decontaminated of large particles or foreign bodies, has minimized bacterial counts, and has edges amenable to optimal repair.

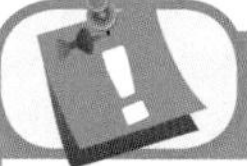

**TIPS AND TRICKS**

**Wound Preparation**

- Always place the patient in a comfortable position, preferably supine.
- Remove as much gross contamination as possible before pressure irrigation.
- Lidocaine with epinephrine may be used in most areas of the body.
- Water is an acceptable initial irrigating fluid for many wounds.
- Hair does not need to be removed.

### *Sterile Technique*

Use of sterile fields, gloves, caps, masks, and gowns is de rigueur in operating room surgery but not as well established in routine wound closure. Studies have shown that the use of sterile versus nonsterile boxed gloves in routine wound management may not have a significant effect on the rate of infection.[4] Powdered gloves should be avoided because of their association with granuloma formation, and EPs must be aware of possible latex allergy.

### Anesthesia

In general, anesthesia should precede significant efforts at cleansing, irrigation, exploration, and closure. Despite long-held dogma, lidocaine with epinephrine can be used in most areas of the body, including the majority of hand wounds and digital blocks.[5] For a complete discussion of local and regional anesthesia, please see Chapter 188.

### Wound Cleansing and Irrigation

The goals of wound cleansing and irrigation are to remove gross contaminants and particulate matter, reduce bacterial counts in the wound, and avoid impeding the host's responses and natural defenses. In general, ideal wound irrigation requires sufficient pressure and volume while providing drainage and preventing operator exposure. If large particles are present, gross decontamination should be performed before pressure irrigation. A sink, an intravenous infusion set, or holes made in the plastic top of a saline solution bottle can be used to make a spray of water for removing leaves, dirt, and other large contaminants. Following gross decontamination, the pressure of the irrigating stream must be sufficient to overcome the adhesive force of bacteria (5 to 12 psi). Such pressure can be produced with a 35- or 50-mL syringe and a 19-gauge catheter or a commercial device with an integrated splash cup.[6] Excessive pressure during irrigation may actually cause additional harm and should be avoided.

The volume of irrigant sufficient to decontaminate wounds is unresolved. However, because bacteria may be present in all sections of a wound, all surfaces of a wound should be exposed to the irrigating stream.

The composition of irrigating fluid has been debated and studied inconclusively, but no significant inferiority has been demonstrated for normal saline. Antiseptics such as povidone-iodine kill bacteria in wounds, but they can also kill fibroblasts and harm normal tissue in the process, particularly if the antiseptics are not diluted to less than the typical 10% preparations. Anecdotally, some clinicians reserve diluted povidone-iodine irrigation for grossly contaminated or high-risk wounds and use saline solution for other wounds, but no conclusive evidence supports this approach.[7] At the other end of the spectrum, some studies demonstrate favorable results when irrigation with tap water is used rather than sterile water or saline solution.[8] The benefits of using water for irrigation include ease of use and drainage and some modest cost savings. Tap water may be used for irrigation of wounds on body parts well suited to it (e.g., the hand), either alone or as an adjunct to subsequent pressure irrigation, depending on the risks associated with the individual wound and host. In summary, the composition of the fluid is much less important than its mechanical action in decontaminating a wound.

### Wound Edge Preparation

Hair does not generally need to be removed. Shaving has been shown to increase the rate of infection. Hair that directly and substantially interferes with proper suture placement can be clipped near the wound edges with scissors.

In general, one should not débride any more than is absolutely necessary to remove clearly devitalized tissue. An irregular, undulating wound may be superior to a straight, linearly excised wound because the longer surface area results in better tensile strength across the healing wound and it maintains the natural contours and marks of the original skin. If débridement is necessary, high-quality forceps and a No. 15 scalpel blade should be used.

### Planning the Repair

The first decision to be made is whether to close a wound primarily. The time elapsed since the injury, the degree of contamination, host factors, and wound factors all play a role in deciding the best option. Primary closure refers to mechanical apposition of the wound edges with subsequent wound healing. Delayed primary closure is the same technique carried out 4 to 5 days after the injury.[9] At this point the host's defenses against infection have been mustered locally, and the risk for subsequent infection with primary closure declines significantly. In secondary closure (secondary intention), gaps between the wound edges become filled with granulation tissue by the body and reepithelialization subsequently occurs.

No well-accepted studies have established firm guidelines for the timing of closure on different portions of the body. Nonetheless, many clinicians agree that certain wounds on the face and head, especially in pediatric patients, have such a low risk for infection that they may be closed after protracted times from injury, including up to 1 to 2 days later. However, wounds of the same size on the hand or forearm of adults probably do have a higher risk for infection after passage of a similar amount of time from injury.[10]

If the decision is made to close a wound primarily, various options are available. As with almost all decisions in wound management, more than one alternative may be correct, but one option is often best. Methods available for closure include sutures, staples, tissue adhesives, and wound tape or strips.

### Wound Closure Techniques

SUTURE REPAIR Sutures offer the most detailed and meticulous closure option, arguably the greatest tensile strength across the wound, and the best choice for certain considerations such as the amount of time that they must remain in the body. However, sutures can be time-consuming to place, require the discomfort of anesthesia, and typically require removal later. Additionally, a suture is a foreign body with attendant risk for infection and inflammation. In particular, EPs should avoid placing deep sutures in a high-risk wound. Monofilament, braided, absorbable, and nonabsorbable sutures also have varying risk for infection, as well as raise other concerns.

Selection of sutures for a wound should be based on size, absorbability, tissue reactivity, risk for infection, and ease of use. In general, nonabsorbable and monofilament sutures are the easiest to use and have the least tissue reactivity and risk for infection. They are best for percutaneous closure. Traditionally, absorbable suture is used for subcutaneous closure. However, some cutaneous closures can be done with absorbable suture, thus obviating the need for removal.[11,12]

At a minimum, four basic suture patterns should be at the command of EPs: the simple interrupted suture, the corner

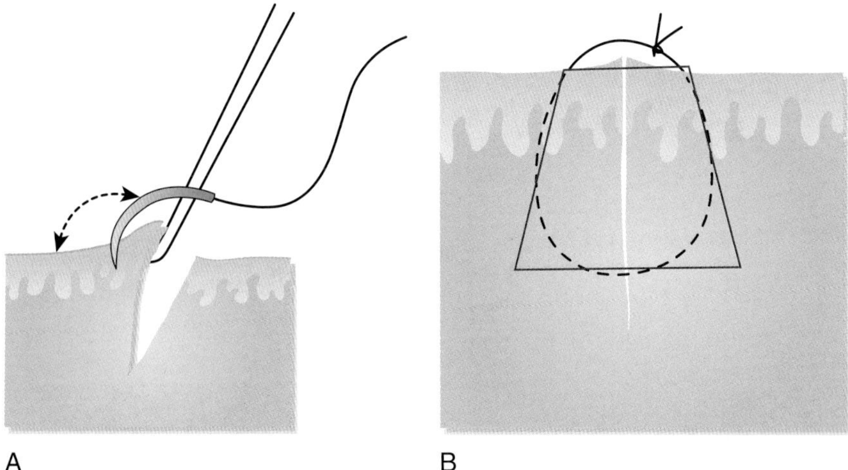


**Fig. 186.3** **A** and **B,** Simple interrupted suture. This is easy to do, harder to master. Enter the skin pointing away from the wound edge and exit the skin pointing toward it to achieve a trapezoidal cross section and slightly everted skin edges.

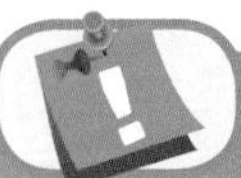

**TIPS AND TRICKS**

**Suture Placement**

Use longitudinal traction to assess how the wound edges correspond and affix the wound (even temporarily) to maintain appropriate alignment.

If you place a suture that seems poor, use the spot to place another knot and remove the original one.

Muscle can typically be repaired by aligning adjacent tissue.

Do not place sutures in high-risk wounds.

The goal of suturing is to have a trapezoidal stitch to disperse tensile force.

Sutures should be removed at the earliest appropriate time.

stitch, and two mattress suture techniques. One should master the simple interrupted pattern first and then move to the others and subsequently to more advanced subcuticular and plastic techniques as required (**Fig. 186.3**, *A* and *B*).

*Simple Interrupted Suture* Though simple in name, proper placement of an interrupted suture requires fastidious practice. Effecting proper wound apposition with regard to the height of each plane of skin and eversion of the closed product will result in more exact healing and a flatter scar. The angle of entry is often suggested to be 90 degrees; however, because the goal is to achieve a trapezoidal cross-sectional stitch with a wider base than top, the angle of entry can exceed 90 degrees. Simply stated, the needle should enter the skin pointing away from the wound edge and should exit the skin on the opposite side of the wound pointing toward the wound edge.

*Running Suture* The tenets of eversion and alignment of skin planes are the same if the suture is continued in running fashion. After starting at one end with a simple interrupted pattern, the needle end of the suture is run along the length of the wound. Tying the needle end of the suture to the last-placed loop finishes the suture.

*Running Subcuticular Sutures* Subcuticular sutures are more difficult to master. They are useful in that the entire suture remains under the surface of the skin and typically does not need to be removed because absorbable sutures are used. However, many wounds that were previously closed with subcuticular running suture and were of low tension and of some cosmetic importance are now amenable to closure with tissue adhesive.

*Deep Sutures* Subcutaneous or deep sutures are useful to eradicate a large dead space that could accumulate hematoma and to give structural support to the wound and skin. By drawing the skin edges closer together, these sutures also reduce the tension needed to close the wound percutaneously or may allow closure of the skin with tissue adhesive (**Fig. 186.4**, *A* and *B*).

*Corner Stitch* A corner suture should be considered when a Y- or V-shaped incision is encountered. The shape of the wound should be assessed for the most advantageous flap to secure into an apex. A corner suture encompasses both percutaneous and subcutaneous portions, but as a single first stitch it can achieve excellent overall wound alignment and thus facilitate placement of subsequent interrupted sutures to finish closing the wound (**Fig. 186.5**, *A* and *B*).

*Mattress Sutures* Both horizontal and vertical mattress sutures provide, as a single benefit, better eversion of the wound edges than other sutures do. The horizontal mattress pattern has the additional benefit of some added speed by covering more linear wound length with each knot tie. However, it does result in more pressure on the epidermis by the suture material, which can have cosmetic effects. Horizontal mattress sutures may be useful to evert a problematic section of wound that has a tendency to roll inward. It may then either be replaced with interrupted sutures to hold it in place or be left as is with timely suture removal. Similarly, an isolated vertical mattress suture may be useful to effect better skin eversion (**Fig. 186.6**).

## Staples

Staples can be used in many places where sutures would also be appropriate. Staples also have the benefits of speed and ease of placement and removal. However, staples may offer somewhat less meticulous closure and have a tendency to leave punctate marks alongside the linear scar. For this reason they should not be used for facial lacerations, on fine skin, or

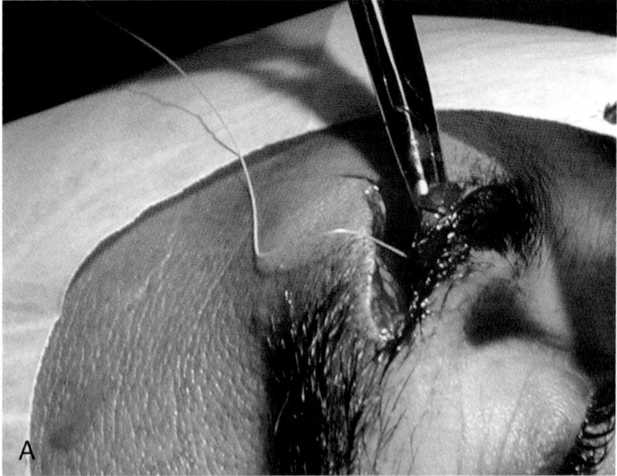


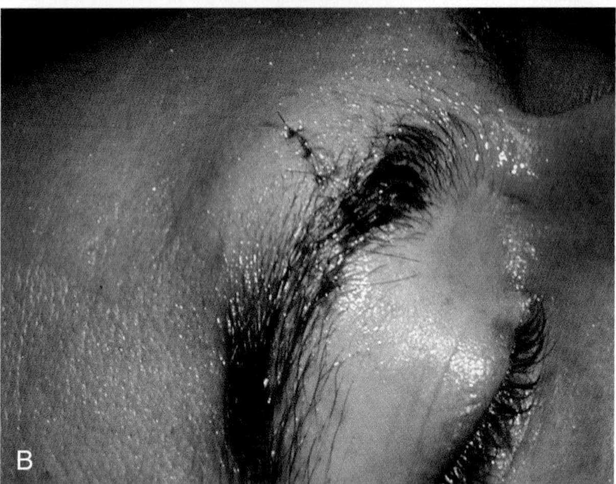


**Fig. 186.4** A and **B,** Deep suture. Use deep sutures with a buried knot to bring wounds closer together and to decrease tension on the edges of the skin.

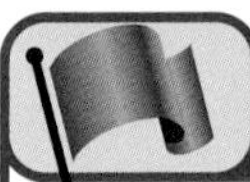

**RED FLAGS**

**Wound Repair**

Insufficient preparation will also create issues with wound treatment and resolution.

Tendons may be partially torn or lacerated while range of motion remains intact. Thorough evaluation of any suspected lesion is thus warranted.

Excessively tight sutures—or those without appropriate angles—place an undue amount of pressure on the epidermis that increases the risk for tissue dehiscence and decreases the probability of a good cosmetic outcome.

Negligence in providing appropriate aftercare and home care instructions increases the likelihood that the patient will return to the emergency department and decreases the prospects for good recovery from the injury.

in other areas where cosmesis is of particular importance. Although staples are frequently used to close scalp wounds, it is wise to ask patients about their preferred sleeping position and whether they wear headgear in sports or work because staples can be uncomfortable if direct pressure is applied

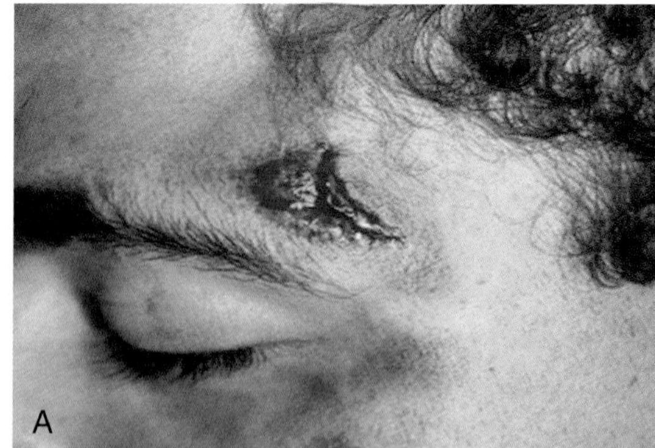


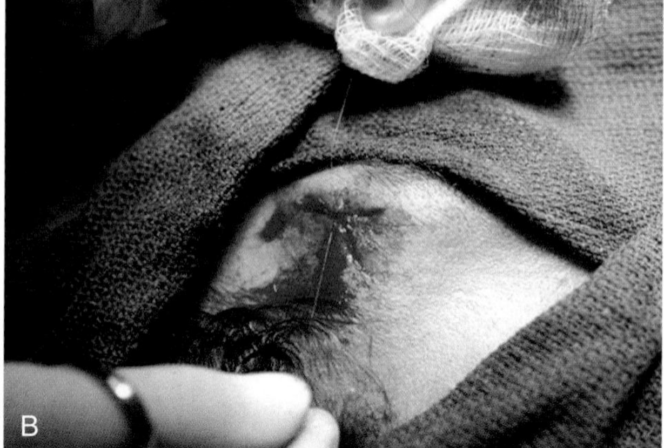


**Fig. 186.5** A and **B,** Corner suture. Use this stitch to secure a triangular flap into an apex for rapid reapproximation of the wound architecture.

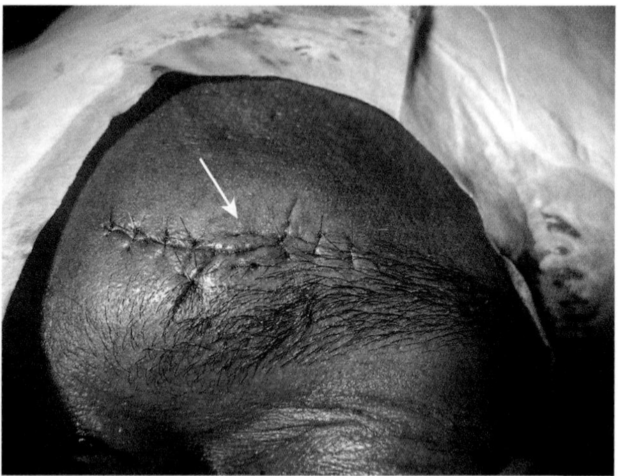

**Fig. 186.6** **Mattress sutures.** When wound sections are difficult to properly evert, consider a mattress suture. A single horizontal mattress suture *(arrow)* corrected a depressed area of the laceration.

against them during wound healing. Staples are most often used to close wounds on the proximal ends of extremities.

### *Tissue Adhesives*

Tissue adhesives have been approved for use in the United States since 1998. The majority of products today consist of 2-octylcyanoacrylates. These compounds are similar to cyanoacrylate, commonly known as superglue. Additional modifications to the chemical composition have been made in

**Table 186.1** Special Wound Locations

| LOCATION | ANATOMIC CONSIDERATIONS | PITFALLS | REPAIR TIPS | AFTERCARE |
|---|---|---|---|---|
| Scalp | Thick connective tissue layer | Bleeding, hematoma formation; low risk for infection but serious if it occurs | Gain hemostasis first. Remove only hair interfering with placement or tying of sutures. Close horizontal galea defects. Close skin with 3-0 or 4-0 horizontal mattress suture or with staples | Pressure dressing if chance for hematoma |
| Lip | Vermilion border, wet-dry line, muscle | Cosmetic deformity, infection | Ensure meticulous alignment. Use traction with the first landmark suture | Antibiotics considered for through-and-through or significant devitalized tissue |
| Cheek | Branches of the facial nerve, parotid duct | Damage to infrastructure, cosmetic deformity | Assess function before and after anesthesia and repair. Do not clamp anything | Sun protection or avoidance |
| Intraoral areas | Mucosa over muscular layers and specialized structures | Infection, missed associated damage | Sew inside first. Reirrigate and close the skin | Peroxide and water rinses |
| Tongue | Highly vascular and muscular | Bleeding, hematoma with deformity, dysfunction | Close if >1 cm, apt to trap food, or cosmetically or functionally impairing. Stabilize the tongue and close the wound with chromic gut | Peroxide and water rinses |
| Eyebrow | Hairs exit the skin obliquely | Cosmetic deformity | Ensure meticulous alignment. Do not shave it. Avoid pressure on tender bone. Evacuate hematomas. Débride parallel to hairs | Ointment dressing |
| Eyelid | Levator palpebrae, medial and lateral canthus ligaments, lacrimal canaliculi | Damage to these structures or to the globe, cosmetic deformity | Assess damage carefully. Repair only extramarginal lacerations with 6-0 polypropylene or nylon | Referral for any wound with other damage or involving the margin |
| Ear | Cartilage between two skin layers | Infection, cosmetic deformity, hematoma | Débride judiciously, but leave no cartilage exposed. Close the skin with 5-0 or 6-0 polypropylene or nylon | Use of dressing to obliterate dead space |

an effort to reduce tissue reactivity, increase pliability of the finished bond, and make the substance more suitable for use on human skin. Studies have demonstrated antibacterial properties of these products as well.[13]

These substances were originally thought to replace suture closure in 25% to 32% of wounds, but it is unclear how often they are actually used in lieu of traditional repair. The most common use of tissue adhesives is for low-tension, nongaping wounds on the face, particularly in pediatric patients. Wounds that would otherwise be closed with 5-0 or 6-0 suture may be considered for adhesive repair. Adhesives are also useful for small avulsion injuries with flaps and occlusion over abrasion injuries as a protective barrier. The material is not suitable for use within the wound itself. Tissue adhesives should not be used in areas of high tension (e.g., across joint surfaces) or to close significantly gaping wounds. Aftercare is similar to that for other repair mechanisms, but the tissue adhesive will gradually slough off without assistance.

### *Wound Tape and Strips*

Wound tapes or strips may be an option for wounds in which placement of a foreign body (i.e., suture) may be disadvantageous, in initial management of wounds that may undergo delayed primary closure, or in wounds with a protracted time until treatment. Many wounds that were previously closed with wound tapes or strips are now amenable to closure with tissue adhesive. Examples of wounds and their preferred and alternative closure methods are presented in **Table 186.1**.

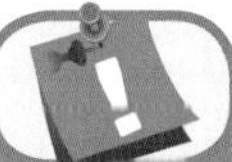

**TIPS AND TRICKS**

**Placement of Adhesive**

Place the patient so that any excess adhesive runs away from important structures such as the eyes.

Have both hands free to place the adhesive; an aide may be useful.

Because each brand of adhesive is different, ensure that the number of coats recommended for the product is applied.

Maintain the wound in the desired position for a sufficient amount of time.

### Puncture Wounds

By their nature, puncture wounds are different from other lacerations in mechanism, risk, and prognosis. No definitive studies exist to guide evaluation, acute management, or risk stratification of puncture wounds. Despite years of publications, the data available are largely retrospective and observational. What is clear is that plantar puncture wounds, in particular, are commonplace and that many patients do not go to the ED for evaluation. One self-reported survey indicated that 44% of persons had experienced a plantar puncture wound at some time during their life. However, perhaps only half of those wounded underwent medical evaluation.[14] It has been assumed that puncture wounds may have a higher complication or infection rate than other wounds, but the true incidence is unknown. Wounds on the plantar surface of the foot that become infected may have very serious complications, including osteomyelitis, osteochondritis, and septic arthritis. The bones of the foot are in close proximity to the skin, and the mechanism of injury typically includes significant force of the weight of the body on the penetrating object.

Evaluation of plantar wounds includes the same delineation of host and wound factors as mentioned previously. Additional considerations with puncture wounds include possible penetration of a sock and shoe by a nail or by objects with various degrees of contamination.

Many authors believe that the timing of arrival at the ED also guides initial evaluation and treatment. Patients seen within 24 hours of injury tend to have lower rates of cellulitis at the time of evaluation, but they may also have a greater possibility of useful manipulative intervention. Patients seen after 24 hours may have concerns about infection and may be more likely to require invasive exploration for foreign material in the wound.[15] One study indicated that 3% of plantar puncture wounds had a foreign body after initial cleansing without exploration.[16]

Reasonable recommendations for the management of plantar puncture wounds include consideration of enlargement of the wound and tissue exploration or excision when the puncture wound mechanism is significant. Concerning mechanisms include puncture of protective footwear while wearing socks, wounds in immunocompromised patients, and wounds caused by organic or contaminated objects. In the last instance, thorns, sharp pieces of wood, and other vegetative matter may be more difficult to identify, and these materials carry a higher risk for bacterial infection. It is also reasonable to consider excision of tissue if particulate foreign material is found in the wound. In the instance of thin needles, either hypodermic or sewing, radiography may be useful for identification, but exploration is not typically needed in these patients if no foreign body is identified.

Anesthesia of the sole of the foot is mandatory to allow a good degree of wound care and possible exploration or excision. Ankle blocks are relatively easy to perform, they can provide adequate anesthesia for the plantar surface, and they obviate the need for painful injections into the thick connective tissue of the sole (see Chapter 188).

Patients with overt signs of infection should be assumed to have a foreign body in the wound. A thorough radiographic, ultrasonographic, and local search for foreign bodies should be conducted. In the presence of infection or when the clinician decides to use prophylactic antibiotics, a fluoroquinolone may be the best choice because of improved *Pseudomonas* coverage.[17]

## FOLLOW-UP, NEXT STEPS IN CARE, AND PATIENT EDUCATION

Too often, aftercare equals afterthought with underemphasis, lack of instruction and documentation, and inadequate knowledge of evidence-based principles. As in other aspects of laceration and wound care, the aims of aftercare are to optimize the chance of a wound healing without infection and with a functional, aesthetically pleasing scar. Generally accepted principles that promote wound healing include maintenance of a clean environment, immobilization, and elevation to reduce edema.

Application of an antibiotic ointment is commonly recommended. Whether the petroleum vehicle promotes a moist environment for reepithelialization or the antibiotics have an actual effect is unclear, but at least one study supports the use of these ointments.[18] Immobilization should be considered at least until epithelialization occurs (usually 2 days) or considerably longer in wounds subjected to high tension (e.g., laceration over the kneecap or shin). Optimal times for removal of sutures (for a wound that is not under tension) from various body parts are listed in **Table 186.2**.

The patient's scar represents a permanent reminder of the wound, but the medical record is also an enduring account of the events. As a simple guideline with regard to wound documentation, "if you did it or said it, write it" (see the "Documentation" box). Critical elements of record keeping include a description of the mechanism, the patient's history, and previous home care of the wound; documentation of the function of surrounding structures before and after any medical maneuvers; and description of the steps taken to reduce infection, search for foreign bodies, and close the wound. Furthermore, the instructions given to patients need to include precautions for return, signs of infection, and step-by-step short- and longer-term instructions for aftercare of the wound. Pitfalls in documentation are inadequately addressing the search for a foreign body, irrigation, and assessment of surrounding function, as well as failure to describe the wound's length and complexity.[19]

**Table 186.2** Optimal Time for Removal of Sutures

| LOCATION | OPTIMAL TIME FOR REMOVAL |
|---|---|
| Hands or fingers | 7-9 days |
| Forearms | 10-12 days |
| Feet | 10-12 days |
| Lower extremity | 10-12 days |
| Torso (chest or back) | 10-12 days |
| Scalp | 5-7 days |
| Face | 3-5 days |

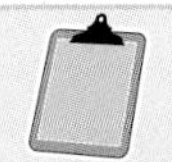

**DOCUMENTATION**

**Wound Repair**

**History**

Detailed mechanism, hand dominance, timing, type of material, whether the object broke on impact or was already broken, whether the wound was soiled, whether anything was pulled out of the wound, FB sensation, paresthesia, weakness, tetanus immunization status, medical conditions that may impair healing or compromise immune function, intravenous drug use, and persistent pain, infection, or drainage

**Physical Examination**

Position of the hand at rest (if the hand is involved), detailed neurovascular examination distal to the injury including two-point discrimination, ability to perform active range of motion and the presence of pain with passive motion, wound size and depth, tenderness, visible contaminants, infection, tattooing, discoloration, signs of infection, and masses

**Studies**

Documentation of radiographic results before and after FB removal (if done) or any other injuries

**Medical Decision Making**

Reasons to pursue or not pursue FB work-up, factors involved in attempting FB removal or leaving in place, and referral or consultation

Documentation of reasons to refer to a surgeon on an outpatient basis and discussion of the case with the referral physician

**Procedures**

Documentation of whether the entire extent of the wound base was visualized in a bloodless field with adequate anesthesia and whether the tendons were visualized through full range of motion (when appropriate)

**Patient Instructions**

Documentation of discussion with the patient regarding the possibility of a retained FB, tendon or nerve injury, warning signs, what to do to care for the wound and what not to do, when to return, and when follow-up should occur

*FB*, Foreign body.

## PATIENT TEACHING

Patients frequently ask, "Will there be a scar?" The inevitable and appropriate answer is yes. However, scars can be minimized by recognition of the aforementioned factors. Patients can serve as their own case controls; earlier scars give clues to how an acute wound may heal. Beyond the initial wound aftercare outlined previously, patients who have a tendency to form hypertrophic or keloid scars should be identified by the EP and informed of treatment options available to decrease the size of the scar. Although many methods have been studied, the only treatments with sufficient prospective data to support their use are silicone gel sheets and intralesional corticosteroid injections.[20,21] Additionally, pressure or paper taping and massage over developing scars are simple measures that may be initiated soon after initial wound healing. Sunscreen use is important during the first 6 months to 1 year. Certain topical preparations have been promoted to improve scars aesthetically. Vitamin E cream is popular and available over the counter, but no well-conducted study exists to show its effectiveness for acute lacerations, and at least one study has shown a detrimental effect.[22] An onion extract (Mederma) is promoted as a way to make scars "appear" softer and smoother. One prospective study is cited in the company's literature, but no large studies have yet been published to support its use.[23]

Aftercare of wounds is largely directed and conducted by patients themselves. Consequently, patients need a thorough list of return precautions, including signs of infection: increased redness, pus from the wound, more swelling than they think is appropriate, and excessive pain. Any of these situations should be reason to return to the ED.

In addition, a persistent foreign body sensation may represent just that, and the patient should return for further evaluation. Some EDs perform a routine wound check at 48 hours, although for uncomplicated wounds in an informed patient, this approach is not necessary. The timing of suture removal and sun avoidance or the use of sunscreen should be discussed in relation to aftercare. A preprinted sheet detailing "if-then" scenarios and expected occurrences is useful. Because many wounds are treated at home, information on what types of wounds require evaluation in the ED in the future may result in better prehospital home care and more effective use of ED resources.

## SUGGESTED READINGS


Capellan O, Hollander J. Management of lacerations in the emergency department. Emerg Med Clin North Am 2003;21:205-31.

Dire DJ, Coppola M, Dwyer DA, et al. Prospective evaluation of topical antibiotics for preventing infections in uncomplicated soft-tissue wounds repaired in the ED. Acad Emerg Med 1995;2:4-10.

Holger JS, Wandersee SC, Hale DB. Cosmetic outcomes of facial lacerations repaired with tissue adhesive, absorbable, and nonabsorbable sutures. Am J Emerg Med 2004;22:254-7.

Mustoe TA, Cooter RD, Gold MH, et al. International Advisory Panel on Scar Management, 2002: international clinical recommendations on scar management. Plast Reconstr Surg 2002;110:560-71.

Singer AJ, Hollander JE, Quinn JV. Evaluation and management of traumatic lacerations. N Engl J Med 1997;337:1142-8.


## REFERENCES

***References can be found on Expert Consult @ www.expertconsult.com.***

# 187 Soft Tissue Injury

*Matthew R. Levine and Navneet Cheema*

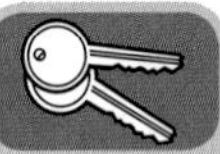

**KEY POINTS**

- Retained foreign bodies (FBs) can cause pain, infection, delayed healing, nerve and tendon injury, masses, and functional impairment.
- Specific injuries, such as those caused by broken glass or surfaces with gravel and stepping on objects, are particularly prone to retained FBs.
- Wounds should be explored for FBs with adequate anesthesia and lighting in a bloodless field.
- Plain radiographs are useful in evaluating for radiopaque FBs and should be ordered commonly.
- Plain films may miss nonradiopaque FBs such as wood, plastic, and vegetative matter. They may also miss radiopaque FBs that are tiny, obscured by bone, or in areas that are difficult to obtain quality images, such as the face or sole of the foot.
- Ultrasound scans and portable fluoroscopic studies may aid in localization and removal of FBs. Computed tomography and magnetic resonance imaging are rarely indicated.
- Neither exploration nor imaging alone can rule out an FB. The two should be used in combination in most instances. No wound is too small or superficial to harbor an FB.
- Careful discharge instructions are crucial and can minimize the morbidity and medicolegal risk associated with retained FBs. Patients should be informed that it is impossible to detect all FBs, be told what to expect in the event of a missed FB, and be given appropriate referral should these circumstances arise.
- Direct exploration of wounds plus visualization of tendons placed through a full range of motion is necessary for proper evaluation of tendon injuries.
- A detailed neurovascular examination is required to identify possible nerve lacerations.
- Most tendon and nerve lacerations can be repaired on an outpatient basis. Ensuring appropriate and timely follow-up is important.

## RETAINED FOREIGN BODIES

### EPIDEMIOLOGY

Open wounds are frequent reasons for emergency department (ED) visits. The true incidence of foreign bodies (FBs) in wounds is unknown, but with more than 5 million estimated lacerations repaired in EDs in 2007,[1] wound FBs surely occur in such a significant number that all emergency physicians (EPs) will encounter them. Wound FBs are frequently missed on initial evaluation. Seventy-five of 200 FBs encountered in a hand clinic were missed by the initial physician.[2] Furthermore, missed FBs pose high medicolegal risk for EPs, with one report listing it to be among the top three causes of litigation after wound care.[3]

Most wound FBs are wood, glass, or metal. The upper extremity is the most common location (58%), followed by the lower extremity (36%). The head and neck (4%) and the trunk (1%) are far less common. Most cases will be seen on the day of injury (75%), but some (8.7%) will initially be evaluated weeks, months, or years later.[4]

### PATHOPHYSIOLOGY

A retained FB can lay harmlessly dormant for a long period and then can react with surrounding tissue. When a tissue reaction occurs, several sequelae are possible. An infection may occur. The patient's body may dissolve, extrude, or encapsulate the FB and form a granuloma, and subsequent rupture of the granuloma from minor trauma can cause delayed infection. The extent of tissue reaction depends primarily on the chemical composition of the material. Inert material causes less tissue inflammation, whereas reactive material can cause intense tissue reactions (**Box 187.1**) and rarely even allergic reactions. Even when an FB does not cause a tissue reaction, it can have other effects. The FB may cause local compression on neighboring structures such as nerves, tendons, joints, or vessels, thereby causing pain or structural damage. Local migration or, more rarely, distant embolization can also occur.

The most threatening FBs are reactive. Wood is especially toxic to soft tissue and virtually always requires removal. FBs causing infection and pain and FBs that are near vital structures such as nerves, tendons, vessels, and joints are also potentially dangerous. Hand FBs tend to migrate locally but rarely embolize, whereas proximal forearm FBs are more likely to embolize.

### PRESENTING SIGNS AND SYMPTOMS

The classic example of a wound FB is a patient who sees or knows that foreign material is present in a wound, such as a splinter, glass in the sole of the foot that the patient cannot remove, or an obviously soiled wound. Alternatively, it is also common for a patient to have a wound and not to know that foreign material is present. The chief complaint of such patients is simply that they have a wound. Certain mechanisms are highly suggestive of wound FBs (**Box 187.2**).[5-8] Some unique wound FBs include shrapnel, fishhooks, bullets and BBs, cactus spines, and marine material (**Table 187.1**). Some patients may exhibit sequelae of a retained FB from the near or distant past, such as a mass, persistent pain, infection, functional impairment as a result of nerve or tendon injury, arthritis, vascular injury, or embolization.

Neither the presence nor the absence of FB sensation on the part of the patient can confidently rule in or exclude an FB. In a series of 164 wounds caused by glass, 41% that contained glass caused an FB sensation, with a positive predictive value of 31% and a negative predictive value of 89%.[5]

The most important aspect of the physical examination is wound exploration. The wound should be explored in a bloodless field, which may require tourniquets or lidocaine with epinephrine infiltration if direct pressure is insufficient. Adequate anesthesia is crucial. The wound should be visualized completely and with range of motion of the involved digit. The wound can be probed with an instrument. Sometimes an FB is detected only by the grating sound of a metal probe against it. Probing the wound with the examiner's finger exposes the examiner to puncture wounds and should not be done. The wound can be palpated through the skin with two hands, one stationary as a "stabilizer" and the other mobile as a "mover." Puncture wounds should be palpated for the exquisite tenderness that may be elicited in the presence of an FB. The function of nearby nerves and tendons should also be evaluated.

**BOX 187.1 Inert and Reactive Foreign Bodies**

| Inert Foreign Bodies | Reactive Foreign Bodies |
|---|---|
| Glass | Wood |
| Most metals | Thorns |
| Plastic | Other vegetative matter |
| | Clothing |
| | Skin fragments |

## DIFFERENTIAL DIAGNOSIS AND MEDICAL DECISION MAKING

No wound is too small or superficial to harbor an FB, and thus the possibility of an FB must be considered for all wounds. Most wound FBs are initially diagnosed by physical

**BOX 187.2 Scenarios Suggestive of Foreign Bodies in Wounds**

History of stepping on glass
History of punching through a window
Motor vehicle collision wounds from glass
Wounds on the sole of the foot
Puncture wounds
Head wounds from glass
Objects that fragment while in one's hand
Fall onto gravel or soil
Pain at a site of intravenous drug use
Foot laceration while walking in a stream
Wound infection, especially if persistent
Perioral wounds in the presence of broken teeth
Persistent wound pain
Failure to heal, persistently draining wound

**Table 187.1 Treatment—Special Circumstances**

| TYPE OF FOREIGN BODY | TIPS AND COMMENTS |
|---|---|
| Fishhooks | Anesthetize the area, advance the tip of the fishhook through the skin, cut the barb, and withdraw the hook. |
| Splinters | Do not pull long splinters out because they tend to fragment. Instead, excise along the long axis or elliptically. |
| Needle tips | Removal may require excision of a block of tissue. |
| Shrapnel | When extensive, emergency department removal of all shrapnel may not be feasible or indicated. Remove as much as reasonably possible, with a focus on dangerous locations, and refer the patient for further treatment. |
| Bullets, BBs | These items are often left in situ, but objects larger than 4.5 mm in diameter tend to track skin and clothing into wounds, so visualize, irrigate, and leave open when possible. Remove these objects only if they are easily accessible or in the pleura (risk for lead poisoning). |
| Cactus spines | Use fine-tipped forceps or glue to remove them. |
| Marine envenomations | Treatment (hot water immersion, vinegar, shaving) depends on the type of spine or nematocyst. |
| Traumatic tattooing | Sources include pencils and blacktop. Débride with a scrub brush. Management is difficult. Consider referral to dermatology or plastic surgery for dermabrasion or laser treatment. |

examination (78%), but many are diagnosed primarily by imaging studies (22%).[4] Exploration alone is insufficient to rule out an FB,[5,9,10] even when the entire wound is thought to be visualized. Therefore, imaging should be used liberally. Selection of the proper imaging modalities requires knowledge of the radiographic properties of the material (**Box 187.3** and **Figs. 187.1 through 187.3**). Even when a suspected FB is not radiopaque, plain film radiographs with an underpenetrated soft tissue technique could be considered because other useful soft tissue or bony findings and reactions may be present. Furthermore, failure to order radiographs has been associated with unsuccessful legal defense in cases of retained FBs.[11] Ultrasound scanning is particularly useful for nonradiopaque FBs (**Fig. 187.4**).[7] Low-power portable fluoroscopy, when available, is useful to aid in removal of radiopaque FBs. Computed tomography and magnetic resonance imaging are rarely indicated. However, computed tomography may be useful for ocular or periorbital FBs (**Table 187.2**).[12,13]

After an FB is diagnosed, the next step is to decide whether to attempt removal or to leave the FB in place. Not all FBs require removal. If an FB is deep, small, inert, away from vital structures, and asymptomatic, attempts at removal may be more destructive than helpful (**Box 187.4**). Irrigation is an important intervention that not only cleans the wound but also often removes tiny FBs and particulate matter that would otherwise be difficult to localize.

**BOX 187.3 Radiopaque and Nonradiopaque Foreign Bodies**

**Radiopaque Foreign Bodies**
Glass
Metal
Bone
Teeth
Pencil tips, graphite
Gravel

**Nonradiopaque Foreign Bodies**
Wood (only 15% seen on radiographs)
Most plastic
Thorns
Cactus spines
Vegetative matter

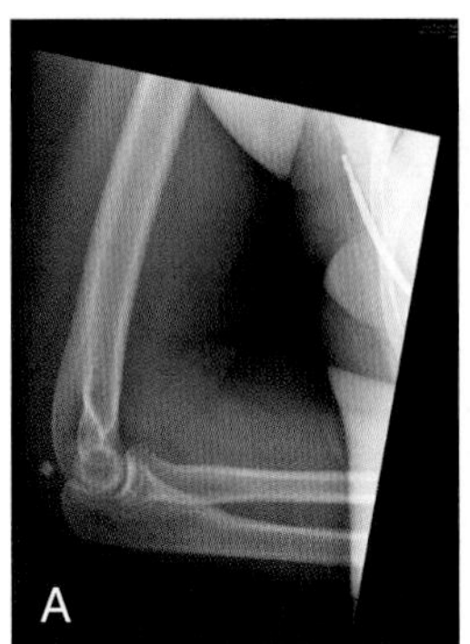


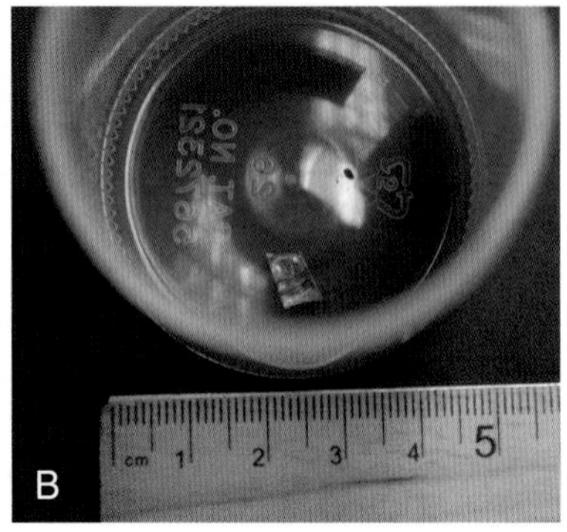


**Fig. 187.1** This patient had a laceration over the olecranon after a motor vehicle collision. A radiograph reveals a foreign body (**A**). A piece of glass was removed (**B**).

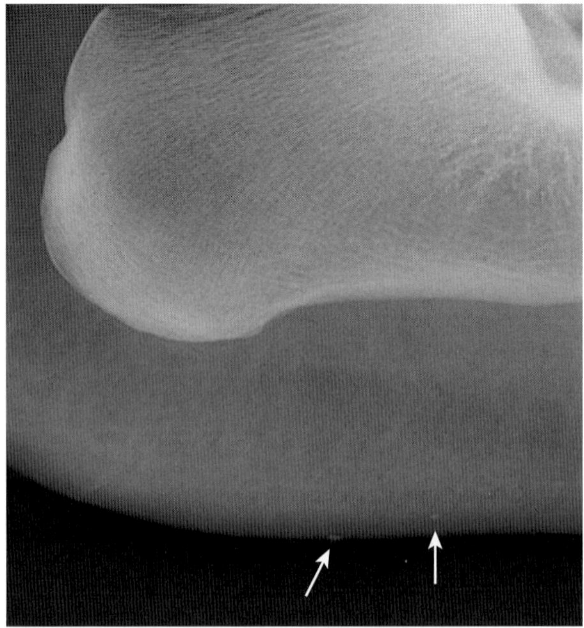

**Fig. 187.2** This patient sustained multiple superficial wounds to the sole of the foot while running barefoot through gravel. A radiograph performed after all gross material was removed revealed two residual foreign bodies *(arrows)*. The bits of gravel were removed.

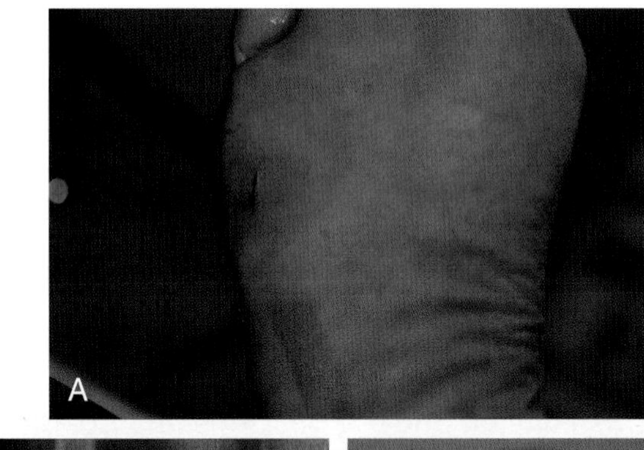


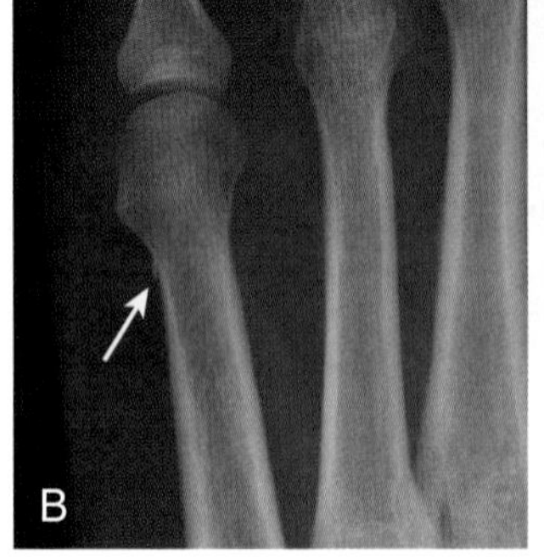


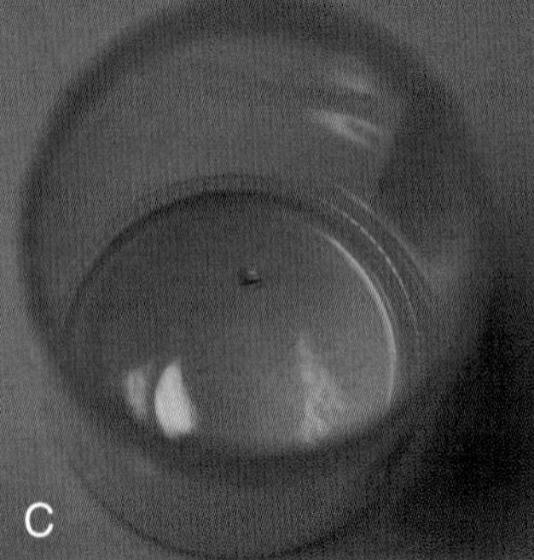


**Fig. 187.3** This patient stepped on broken glass (**A**). The radiograph, when magnified and scrutinized, showed a possible foreign body *(arrow)* in the proximity of the wound (**B**). The wound was explored and a glass foreign body was removed (**C**). This is an example of the limitations of radiographs for detection of foreign bodies, even those that are radiopaque, in certain locations such as the sole of the foot because of the thickened tissue and multiple bony structures that may obscure the foreign body. This is why wound exploration is also important.

## TREATMENT (see the "Tips and Tricks" box)

Exploration is best done while the EP is seated comfortably with optimal anesthesia, hemostasis, lighting (even headlamps), and equipment. Fine-tipped forceps, retractors, special pickups, and magnifying loupes are particularly helpful. Many explorations require extending the incision for better exposure. The EP should listen during probing for a grating sound of the FB against the instrument. Blind grasping is destructive to tissue and should be avoided. The use of portable fluoroscopy or ultrasound scanning, if readily available, should be considered to facilitate removal. A time limit for the procedure should be set in advance because it is easy to become involved and determined to recover an FB that may be too difficult to remove in the ED setting. The patient should be aware of this time limit.

Wounds that are contaminated or may still contain FBs should be left open or packed. Antibiotics should probably be prescribed for these patients. EPs should be sure to pad or splint areas with retained FBs before patients are discharged. If all FBs have been removed and the wound has been thoroughly cleansed, closure may be appropriate. An algorithm for an approach to FBs is presented in **Figure 187.5**.

If all FBs have been removed and the wound has been cleaned adequately, the patient is unlikely to require further referral. If concern still exists about a retained FB, the area should be padded or splinted, antibiotics should be prescribed,

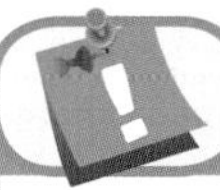

### TIPS AND TRICKS

**Foreign Body**

**Hemostasis**
Direct pressure
Tourniquets
Lidocaine with epinephrine when safe

**Anesthesia**
Nerve blocks for difficult locations (sole of the foot)

**Irrigation**
High pressure: a 30-mL syringe with an 18-gauge angiocatheter generates 6 to 8 psi

**Exploration**
Good lighting
Equipment: loupes, fine-tipped forceps helpful
Possible need to extend the incision
Incision perpendicular to the long axis of long, thin foreign bodies (splinters, needles) for localization
Bloodless field and adequate anesthesia required
Listening for grating sounds of the foreign body against the probe
Ultrasound or fluoroscopic guidance helpful
Time limit needed

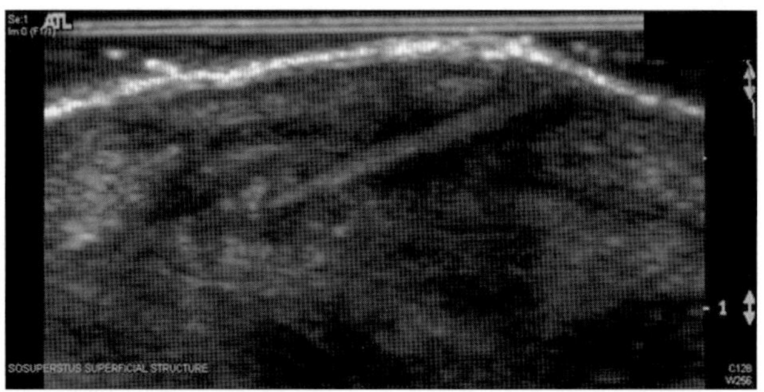

**Fig. 187.4 Ultrasound scan showing a wood foreign body with characteristic acoustic shadowing deep to the foreign body.**

**Table 187.2 Features of Available Imaging Techniques**

| IMAGING MODALITY | POSITIVE FEATURES | NEGATIVE FEATURES |
|---|---|---|
| Radiography | Inexpensive<br>Easy to obtain and read<br>99% sensitive for radiopaque objects >2 mm* | Misses nonradiopaque foreign bodies<br>Sensitivity falls for objects <2 mm<br>Two-dimensional still picture may not aid in removal |
| Ultrasound | Detects all materials†<br>Live bedside images may aid removal<br>Consider for wood, plastic<br>No radiation exposure | Operator dependent<br>Gel complicates use during removal of foreign bodies<br>Difficult in large open wounds, web spaces<br>False-positive results: sesamoids, calcification<br>False-negative results: gas, hematoma, near bone or scar |
| Portable fluoroscopy | Low radiation exposure<br>Can aid in real-time removal<br>For difficult removal of radiopaque foreign bodies | Misses nonradiopaque foreign bodies<br>Often limited availability |
| Computed tomography | Good for periorbital, intraocular, intracranial foreign bodies<br>May help in bony areas<br>High resolution may enhance detection | Costly<br>Impractical<br>More radiation exposure |
| Magnetic resonance imaging | May help for some difficult plastic foreign bodies<br>High resolution may enhance detection<br>No radiation exposure | Costly<br>Impractical<br>Potential harm if metal foreign body present |

*Courter BJ. Radiographic screening for glass foreign bodies: what does a "negative" foreign body series really mean? Ann Emerg Med 1990;19:997-1000.
†Horton LK, Jacobson JA, Powell A, et al. Sonography and radiography of soft-tissue foreign bodies. AJR Am J Roentgenol 2001;176:1155-9.

**BOX 187.4 Indications for Removal of Foreign Bodies**

Significant pain
Functional impairment, restriction of motion
Reactive material: wood, thorn, other vegetative material, clothing
Cause of infection
Cause of psychologic distress
Contamination: tooth, soil
Toxicity: venomous spines, lead poisoning from bullets
Allergic reaction
Impingement of nerve, tendon, vessel
Intraarticular or periarticular location
Intravascular location
Location near fractured bone
High potential to migrate toward anatomic structures or to embolize
Cosmetic concerns: tattooing, masses

From Lammers RL, Magill T. Detection and management of foreign bodies in soft tissue. Emerg Med Clin North Am 1992;10:767-81.

and the patient will require consultation or referral to a surgical specialty such as hand, orthopedic, plastic, or general surgery. Such referral can almost always take place on an outpatient basis unless severe infection or important structural damage is present.

## FOLLOW-UP, NEXT STEPS IN CARE, AND PATIENT EDUCATION

Admission is seldom indicated. Admission scenarios may include severe infections and FBs that are going to be removed in the operating room. Documentation and patient education are important aspects of all wound cases. (See the "Documentation", "Patient Teaching Tips", "Red Flags", and "Priority Actions" boxes.)

# TENDON AND NERVE LACERATIONS

## EPIDEMIOLOGY

Lacerations are one of the most common chief complaints of patients seen in the ED. It is estimated that a total of

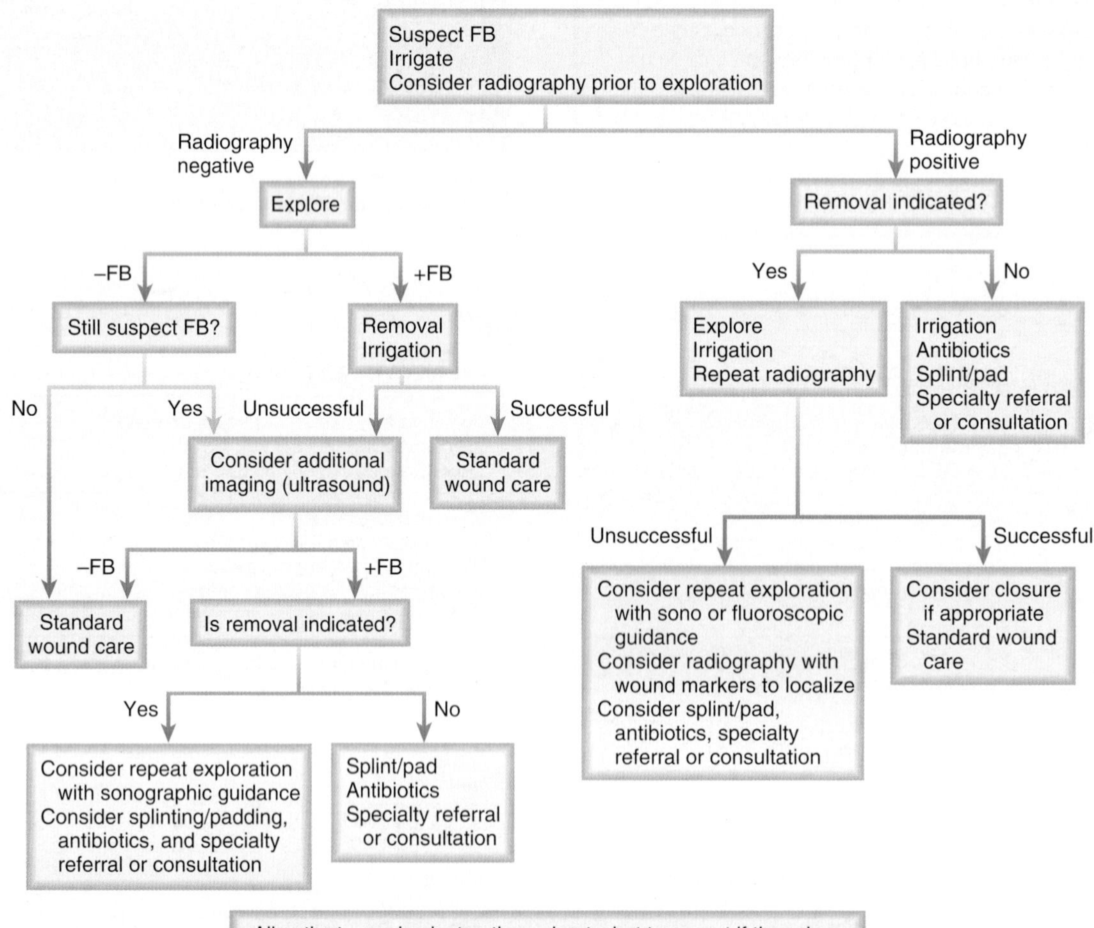


**Fig. 187.5** Approach to managing a wound foreign body (FB).

6,400,000 open wounds were treated in EDs in the United States in 2004, thereby making open wounds anywhere on the body the third leading primary diagnosis group. Approximately one third of all open wounds are located on the upper extremity (specifically the fingers, hand, or wrist).[14] An improperly functioning or insensate digit as a result of tendon or nerve injury can lead to markedly impaired function and significant subsequent morbidity. Wound claims, particularly of the hand, are a leading cause of litigation.[3] Although lacerations about the foot and ankle are also relatively common, given the importance and prevalence of hand injuries, this part of the chapter focuses primarily on tendon and nerve lacerations of the hand.

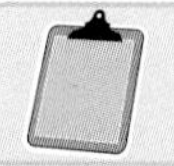

**DOCUMENTATION**

**Soft Tissue Injury**

**History**

Detailed mechanism, hand dominance, timing, type of material, whether the object broke on impact or was already broken, whether the wound was soiled, whether anything was pulled out of the wound, FB sensation, paresthesia, weakness, tetanus immunization status, medical conditions that may impair healing or compromise immune function, intravenous drug use, and persistent pain, infection, or drainage

**Physical Examination**

Position of the hand at rest, detailed neurovascular examination including two-point discrimination, ability to achieve active range of motion and the presence of pain with passive motion, wound size and depth, tenderness, visible contaminants, infection, tattooing, discoloration, signs of infection, and masses

**Studies**

Documentation of radiographic results before and after removal of FBs or any other injuries

**Medical Decision Making**

Reasons to pursue or not pursue FB work-up, factors involved in attempting FB removal or leaving in place, and referral or consultation

Documentation of reasons to refer to a surgeon on an outpatient basis and discussion of the case with the referral physician

**Procedures**

Documentation of whether the entire extent of the wound base was visualized in a bloodless field with adequate anesthesia and the tendon was visualized through full range of motion (when appropriate)

**Patient Instructions**

Documentation of discussion with the patient regarding the possibility of a retained FB, tendon or nerve injury, warning signs, what to do, when to return, and when follow-up should occur

*FB*, Foreign body.

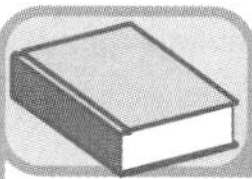

**PATIENT TEACHING TIPS**

Inform patients with wounds of the remote possibility of a missed foreign body because there is no way to truly guarantee that all foreign material has been identified and removed.

After the first couple days, a normal wound should show consistently gradual improvement in pain, swelling, and discoloration.

Inform patients that a retained foreign body may result in persistent pain, loss or impairment of function, a mass, infection, or injury to a nerve, tendon, vessel, or joint. These complications may develop even months or years later.

If any of the foregoing situations develop, the patient should know to return to the emergency department or should have received specialty referral.

Warn the patient to return for signs of infection, including redness, discharge, pain, and swelling.

Warn patients who have documented partial tendon lacerations, depending on the degree of laceration and findings on subsequent examination, that the referring physician may or may not repair the injury.

Inform all patients of the possibility of tendon or nerve lacerations not visualized on examination.

If a nerve or tendon laceration has been documented, ensure that the patient understands the importance of timely follow-up.

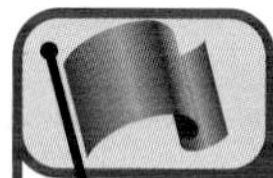

**RED FLAGS**

**Complications of Retained Foreign Bodies**

Infection, possibly recurrent
Persistent pain
Functional impairment
Granuloma formation
Psychologic distress
Migration, embolization
Delayed healing
Nerve, tendon, joint, vascular injury

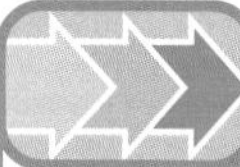

**PRIORITY ACTIONS**

**Maintaining a High Index of Suspicion for Foreign Bodies in All Wounds**

Appropriate use of imaging
Wound exploration
Decision whether to attempt removal of the foreign body in the emergency department
High-pressure irrigation, wound cleansing
Appropriate use of antibiotics
Specialty referral, consultation for retained foreign bodies
Proper discharge instructions

## PATHOPHYSIOLOGY

The hand is one of the most multifaceted and complex musculoskeletal systems in the body. The precision and fine motor functions of the hand are a direct result of its intricate structure. The frequency and importance of hand injuries necessitate that EPs have a thorough understanding of the anatomic and functional complexity of the hand.

The nerve supply to the hand is provided by the radial, ulnar, and median nerves. The radial nerve is purely sensory in the hand (motor function of the radial nerve includes wrist extension). The median and ulnar nerves provide the entire motor function of the hand and some sensory function as well (**Fig. 187.6**). Each digit has two neurovascular bundles located near the palmar aspect of the finger, one on the radial side and the other on the ulnar side.

The extensor tendons are located on the dorsal surface of the forearm, wrist, and hand. Nine extensor tendons pass under the extensor retinaculum. The extensor tendons join to become the extensor expansion and then separate into six fibroosseous compartments. In each digit, the extensor expansion then divides into a central slip attaching to the middle phalanx and two lateral bands joining with the tendons of the lumbricals and then continuing on to attach to the base of each distal phalanx. See **Figure 187.7** for extensor tendon zone classification.

The flexor tendons are located on the volar side of the forearm, wrist, and hand. A single tendon (the flexor pollicis longus) inserts on the distal phalanx of the thumb, and two flexor tendons go to each of the remainder digits. Each digit has a superficial flexor tendon that inserts at the base of the middle phalanx and a deep flexor tendon that inserts at the base of the distal phalanx.

The superficial location of the tendons and nerves of the hand combined with the lack of overlying subcutaneous tissue predisposes these structures to injury. Injuries to the tendons have been grouped into anatomic zones for easy understanding and classification. The most widely accepted classification system is that of Verdan. This system uses eight zones, from zone I at the distal interphalangeal joint level to zone VIII at the distal forearm level. This system has been modified to five zones for the flexor tendons (**Fig. 187.8**).[15] Although the Verdan system is no longer used to determine treatment options, knowledge of the zones is useful for prognosis.

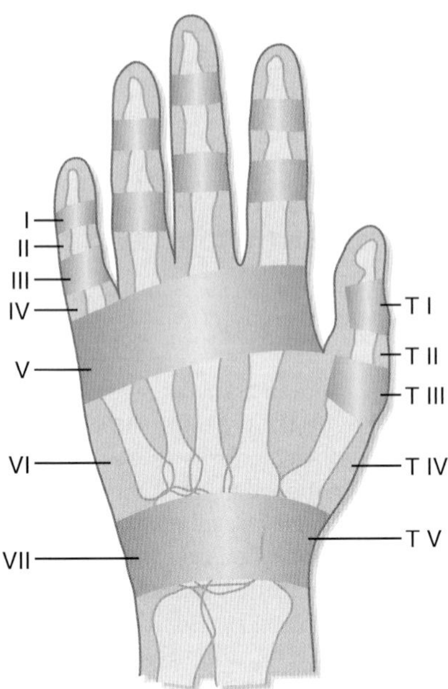


**Fig. 187.7 Zone classification of extensor tendon injuries.** (Redrawn from Lyn E, Antosia RE. Hand. In: Marx JA, Hockberger RS, Walls RM, eds. Rosen's emergency medicine. 6th ed. Philadelphia: Mosby; 2006. p. 576-621.)

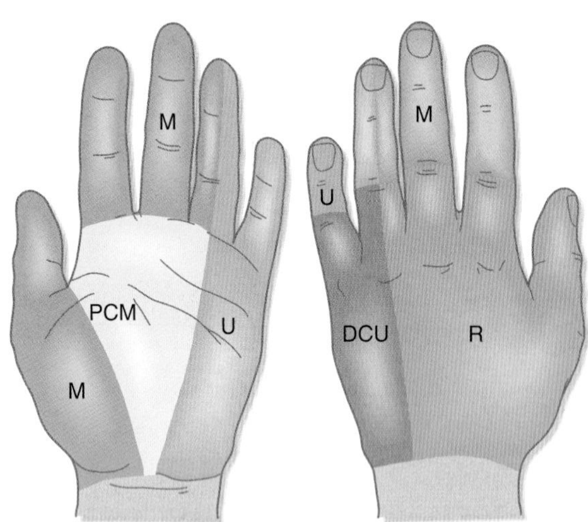


**Fig. 187.6 Cutaneous nerve supply in the hand.** *Left*, Palmar aspect; right, dorsal aspect; *DCU*, dorsal cutaneous branch of the ulnar nerve; *M*, median; *PCM*, palmar cutaneous branch of the median nerve; *R*, radial; *U*, ulnar. (Redrawn from Lyn E, Antosia RE. Hand. In: Marx JA, Hockberger RS, Walls RM, eds. Rosen's emergency medicine. 6th ed. Philadelphia: Mosby; 2006. p. 576-621.)

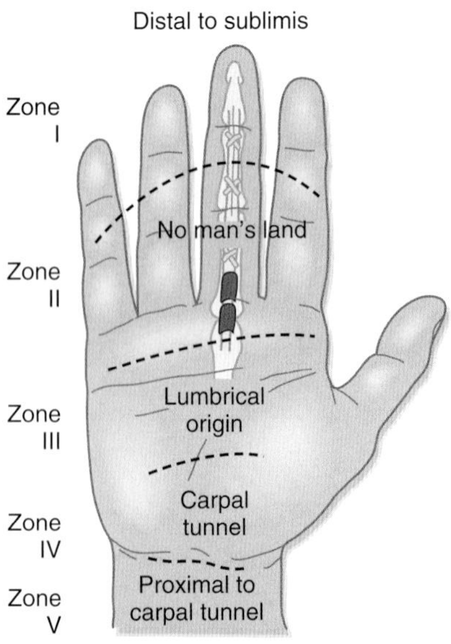


**Fig. 187.8 Zone classification of flexor tendon injuries.** (From Canale ST, editor. Campbell's operative orthopaedics. 10th ed. Philadelphia: Mosby; 2003.)

## PRESENTING SIGNS AND SYMPTOMS

Any patient with a laceration about the hand or wrist may have sustained a tendon or nerve laceration regardless of how superficial the wound may appear. In a study of 226 patients with upper extremity lacerations that were less than 2 cm in length, 59% were found to have at least one injury to a deep structure.[16] Depending on the degree of injury, the patient may have no obvious injury other than a laceration through the skin.

Patients with nerve lacerations typically have a complaint of numbness or tingling distal to the laceration. In cases of injury to the radial, ulnar, or median nerves, the corresponding motor distribution is affected. Unless a motor deficit is noted, the clinical finding of a nerve injury may easily be missed.

The normal resting position of the hand—flexed fingers, with the little finger having the greatest degree of flexion and the index finger the least—may be altered in patients with a complete tendon laceration (**Fig. 187.9**). Flexor tendon disruption is indicated when the injured finger lies in complete extension while the others are in slight flexion. When the patient has an extensor tendon injury, the affected digit is held in full flexion while the others are held in slight extension or the normal position of function. Partial lacerations may not be evident based on the position of the finger. Limited or painful movement, especially if more severe than would be expected with the laceration, suggests partial tendon involvement.

## DIFFERENTIAL DIAGNOSIS AND MEDICAL DECISION MAKING

The most important aspects of the diagnosis of tendon or nerve laceration are a thorough history and physical examination. Basic historical details should include the time and mechanism of injury, position of the hand when injured, hand dominance, tetanus status, previous hand injuries, and occupation and hobbies (musician or anyone requiring fine motor control). Patients should be specifically asked about loss of motion, weakness, pain, and any numbness or tingling.

Examination of the hand begins with an overall assessment of the position of the hand and fingers. Pallor, gross deformity, or digits lying in abnormal positions should be noted and compared with the other fingers and hand. Next, the sensation and motor strength of the hand should be assessed to detect nerve injury. As stated previously, the radial, ulnar, and median nerves provide sensation to the hand. Because of the overlap in sensory innervation, it is best to test nerves in the area least likely to have dual innervation. The median nerve is tested at the palmar surface of the index finger, the ulnar nerve at the palmar surface of the little finger, and the radial nerve at the dorsal surface of the web space between the thumb and index finger.

Various stimuli can be used to test sensory function of the hand. Gross touch with a blunt object is the least specific. It can be useful for rapid screening to test for nerve injury, especially when compared with the other hand. A more accurate method for assessing nerve function is two-point discrimination. A paper clip can be used. A patient with a normally innervated fingertip should be able to distinguish two simultaneously delivered stimuli 6 mm or more apart from each other. Most patients can detect a difference down to 3 mm. When identification of stimuli separated by 8 mm or more is not reported by the patient, the examination is clearly abnormal.

Accurate evaluation of two-point discrimination to assess for nerve injury is not always possible at the time of injury. The patient's pain and anxiety, as well as factors such as the presence of hand calluses, can interfere with this test. Any subjective "numbness" reported by the patient must be taken seriously, and consultation with a hand specialist should be considered. Under these circumstances, it is common to close the skin wound and refer the patient for evaluation within a few days of the initial injury.

A systematic examination of the hand and wrist includes assessment of active and passive range of motion of the wrist and digits. To check specifically for extensor tendon injuries, the patient should actively extend each finger and then extend each finger against resistance. In evaluating the flexor tendons, the superficialis and profundus tendons should be tested independently, with the patient actively flexing individual proximal and distal interphalangeal joints (**Fig. 187.10**). Examiners

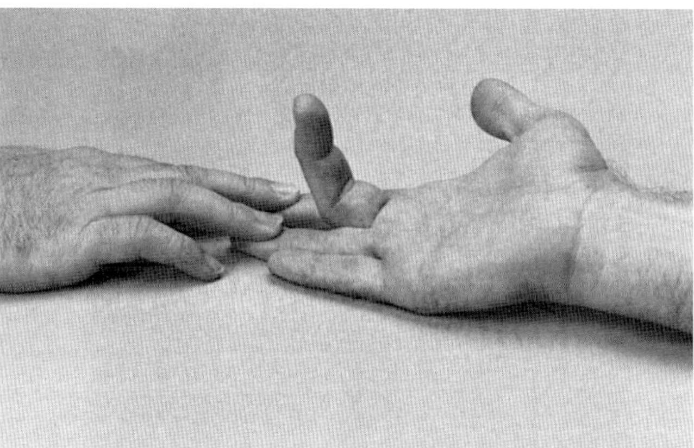

**Fig. 187.9 Examination to assess the function of the flexor digitorum superficialis.** (From Lyn E, Antosia RE. Hand. In: Rosen's emergency medicine. 6th ed. Philadelphia: Mosby; 2006. p. 576-621.)

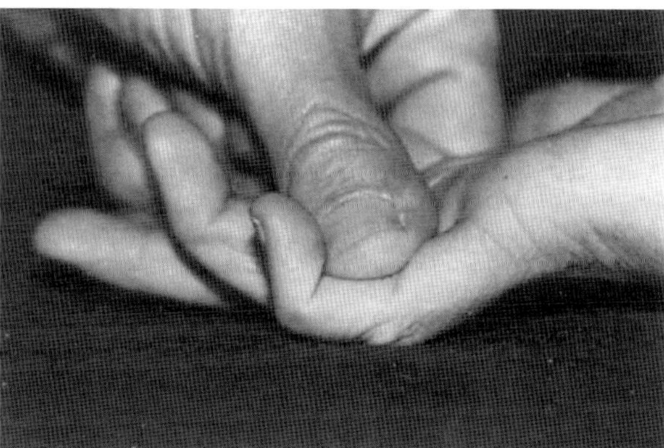

**Fig. 187.10** To test for an intact profundus tendon, the examiner maintains the digit in extension while the patient attempts to flex the terminal phalanx. (From Lyn E, Antosia RE. Hand. In: Rosen's emergency medicine. 6th ed. Philadelphia: Mosby; 2006. p. 576-621.)

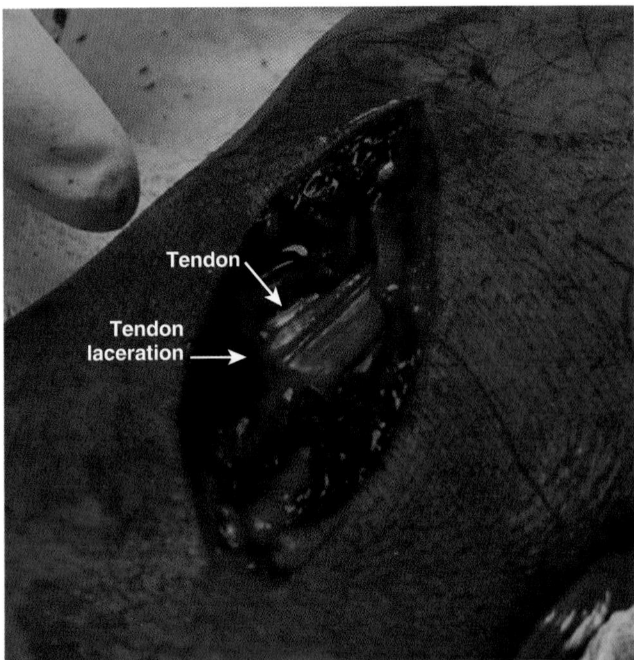


**Fig. 187.11 A gaping wound explored in a bloodless field.** The shiny tendon is visible, as is the tendon laceration.

should be sure to check tendon motion against resistance because patients with partial tendon lacerations may have normal range of motion.

The next step is exploration of the wound (**Fig. 187.11**), which is best done with the EP seated comfortably with optimal anesthesia, hemostasis, lighting, and equipment. Adequate anesthesia is crucial. Failure to provide adequate exposure of deeper wound structures because of the patient's discomfort often leads to missed injuries. The wound should be explored in a bloodless field. A tourniquet may be required if direct pressure is insufficient to achieve such a field. The wound should be visualized completely and with full range of motion of the involved digit.

Additional studies or imaging techniques are indicated to evaluate for FBs, fractures, and avulsions. They are not useful in evaluating tendon or nerve lacerations. Ultrasonography may be a viable diagnostic tool in evaluating tendon injuries, although at this time it has not been studied in the ED.[17]

## TREATMENT

All motor branches of the ulnar and median nerve should be repaired. Both consultation in the ED and referral the following day after discussion with the referring physician are appropriate (**Box 187.5**). Digital nerve injuries proximal to the distal interphalangeal crease on the radial aspect of the index and middle fingers, the ulnar side of the little finger, and both sides of the thumb should be repaired. The timing of repair for simple, clean nerve injuries is somewhat controversial; some data show better results with repair in 6 to 12 hours, whereas other data show acceptable results with delayed repair.[18] Satisfactory return of function can occur after nerve repair or a graft performed within 3 months of injury.[19] Any patient with a suspected nerve injury should be referred to a specialist for evaluation and possible repair.

**BOX 187.5 Indications for Immediate Consultation in the Emergency Department for Nerve or Tendon Laceration**

Multiple or extensive lacerations
Inability to close the wound
Contamination: tooth, soil
Joint involvement

Patients with tendon lacerations (partial or complete) require early referral to a surgeon. Most surgeons recommend repairing complete lacerations primarily within 12 to 24 hours after the injury. However, data on delayed primary (<10 days) or early secondary (2 to 4 weeks) repair show little difference in outcomes when compared with the traditional immediate repair.[20] Repair of partial tendon lacerations is still controversial, and most hand surgeons now repair only lacerations that involve more than 50% of the tendon surface. Regardless of whether the laceration is full or partial, primary coverage of the injured tendon by skin suturing after wound irrigation protects the tendon and retards infection, but it should be undertaken only after consultation with the specialist who will perform the definitive repair.

Extensor tendon injuries are underestimated by EPs. Because of the superficial location and thin overlying subcutaneous tissue, these tendons are often injured. Their superficial location makes repair easier; in the past these injuries have been repaired by EPs, although it is generally best to coordinate with a surgeon willing to provide repair and follow-up. Zones VII and VIII are associated with significant retraction of tendons, and given the proximity of many tendons, multiple tendons may be injured. Therefore, injuries to tendons in these zones are more difficult to repair and may have worse outcomes.

Flexor tendon injuries are more difficult to repair. These injuries are more complicated because both superficial and deep tendons are present and both may be injured. Injuries in zones II and IV have a much worse prognosis as a result of the propensity to form adhesions within a confined space. Overall, ED consultation with a specialist or early referral after discussion with the specialist who will perform the definitive repair should be ensured for any confirmed nerve or tendon injury (extensor and flexor), overlying lacerations should generally be sutured after discussion with the definitive treating physician, a splint should be applied, and the EP should consider antibiotic coverage if appropriate.

## FOLLOW-UP, NEXT STEPS IN CARE, AND PATIENT EDUCATION

Most patients with tendon and nerve lacerations can be discharged home safely from the ED. Educating the patient regarding expectations and the importance of follow-up is of utmost importance. All patients with documented or suspected lacerations of a tendon or nerve require evaluation by the appropriate surgeon. ED consultation and early referral following discussion with a specialist are both appropriate courses of action. If severe infection or important structural damage is present, ED consultation may be more prudent than outpatient follow-up. The area should be splinted appropriately and antibiotics prescribed if indicated. Flexor injuries should be splinted with the wrist in 30 degrees of flexion, the metacarpophalangeal joints flexed 70 degrees, and the interphalangeal joints flexed 10 to 15 degrees. A metal protective splint is recommended for patients who are going to return to work. All but very minor hand wounds are best followed up within 48 hours for removal of the dressing and inspection of the wound for signs of infection. (See **Box 187.6** for complications.)

**BOX 187.6 Complications of Tendon Injury**

Triggering
Synovial adhesions
Entrapment
Delayed tendon rupture

## SUGGESTED READINGS

Anderson MA, Newmeyer WL, Kilgore ES. Diagnosis and treatment of retained foreign bodies in the hand. Am J Surg 1982;144:63-7.

Avner JR, Baker MD. Lacerations involving glass: the role of routine roentgenograms. Am J Dis Child 1992;146:600-2.

Courter BJ. Radiographic screening for glass foreign bodies: what does a "negative" foreign body series really mean? Ann Emerg Med 1990;19:997-1000.

Lee DH, Robbin ML, Galliott R, et al. Ultrasound evaluation of flexor tendon lacerations. J Hand Surg [Am] 2000;25:236-41.

Levine MR, Gorman SM, Young CF, et al. Clinical characteristics and management of wound foreign bodies in the ED. Am J Emerg Med 2008;26:918-22.

Steele MT, Tran LV, Watson WA. Retained glass foreign bodies in wounds: predictive value of wound characteristics, patient perception, and wound exploration. Am J Emerg Med 1998;16:627-30.

Tuncali D, Yavuz N, Terzioglu A, et al. The rate of upper-extremity deep-structure injuries through small penetrating lacerations. Ann Plast Surg 2005;55:146-8.

## REFERENCES

***References can be found on Expert Consult @ www.expertconsult.com.***

# 188 Local and Regional Anesthesia

*Heather Murphy-Lavoie and Tracy Leigh LeGros*

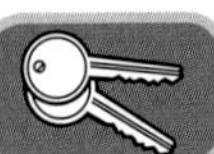

**KEY POINTS**

- Alternatives to local infiltration for anesthesia include topical anesthesia and regional nerve blocks.
- Comfortable wound repair requires adequate anesthesia.
- Local infiltration may be inadequate or suboptimal in certain situations.
- For the safety and efficacy of regional anesthesia, the clinician must have a detailed understanding of the local anatomy.
- Ultrasound is a very useful adjunct to regional anesthesia.

## PERSPECTIVE

Adequate anesthesia is essential for many situations in the emergency department (ED), such as acute wound repair, removal of foreign bodies, drainage of abscesses, removal of ingrown toenails, joint reductions, and management of fractures. To achieve anesthesia safely and accurately, the clinician must have a thorough understanding of the various agents that can be used, the methods of administration, and the techniques for achieving regional anesthesia.

## SELECTION OF ANESTHETIC AGENTS

### MECHANISM OF ACTION

Local anesthetics usually have an aromatic ring structure connected to a tertiary amine by either an ester or an amide link. This link determines the class of the agent, ester or amide. Local anesthetics work by reversibly binding to and blocking neuronal sodium channels, thereby blocking conduction of the nerve impulse. Their potency, onset, and duration of action are determined by their ability to access and bind these sodium channels. The higher the lipid solubility, the higher the potency of the anesthetic. The higher their protein binding, the longer the duration of action. Onset of action is determined by the $pK_a$, or the pH at which the agent exists in equal amounts of its ionized and un-ionized forms. The closer the $pK_a$ is to physiologic pH, the faster the onset of action.[1] Most local anesthetic agents are associated with a burning sensation that lasts several seconds before the onset of anesthesia. Patients should be warned of this sensation before administration (**Table 188.1**).

### TOXICITY

Local anesthetic agents exert toxic effects primarily on the cardiovascular system and central nervous system (CNS). The severity of toxicity is directly related to lipid solubility and therefore the potency of an agent. Accordingly, bupivacaine is much more likely than lidocaine to cause toxicity. The likelihood of toxicity also rises with increased vascularity and systemic absorption. Absorption rates by anatomic location, from highest to lowest, are as follows:

Intercostal > Intratracheal > Epidural > Brachial plexus > Mucosal > Distal peripheral nerve > Subcutaneous

An intercostal block has the highest potential for toxicity; therefore, the maximum amount of anesthetic agent recommended for this location is only one tenth of the maximum for peripheral nerve blocks.[1] All sites are associated with a certain degree of risk, especially when accidental intravascular injection is likely.

Signs of CNS toxicity with local anesthetics are presented in **Box 188.1**.

If exposure is not halted, toxicity can progress to seizures, coma, respiratory depression, and cardiorespiratory arrest. Higher doses result in cardiovascular toxicity and lead to tachycardias, sinus arrest, atrioventricular dissociation, hypotension, and full arrest. Premedication with benzodiazepines may blunt the CNS toxicity, and in these cases the first sign of toxicity to develop may be cardiovascular collapse.[2,3] Amides are metabolized by the liver, and patients with hepatic dysfunction may be predisposed to systemic toxicity. Esters are metabolized by plasma pseudocholinesterase, and therefore patients with pseudocholinesterase deficiency, such as those with myasthenia gravis, are at higher risk for systemic toxicity. In addition, metabolites of prilocaine (a component of EMLA cream) and benzocaine have been associated with methemoglobinemia.

**Table 188.1** Local Anesthetic Agents

| AGENT | POTENCY* | COST PER 10 mL† | PKA‡ | ONSET | DURATION (HR) | MAXIMUM DOSE (MG/KG) |
|---|---|---|---|---|---|---|
| Lidocaine | 2 | $0.76 | 7.8 | Fast | 2-3 | 4.5 (7 when given with epinephrine) |
| Mepivacaine | 2 | $4.60 | 7.6 | Fast | 2-4 | 7 (not to exceed 400 mg) |
| Tetracaine | 4 | $7.31 | 8.2 | Moderate | 3 | 3 |
| Ropivacaine | 4 | $4.43 | 8.1 | Moderate | 3-8 | 3 |
| Bupivacaine | 5 | $1.68 | 8.1 | Moderate | 4-10 | 2 (3 when given with epinephrine) |

Data from Crystal C, Blankenship R. Local anesthetics and peripheral nerve blocks in the emergency department. Emerg Med Clin North Am 2005;23:477-502; and Salam G. Regional anesthesia for office procedures. Part 1: head and neck surgeries. Am Fam Physician 2004;69:585-90.

*This table assumes equal concentrations of agents compared (e.g., 1%).

†Available at www.medscape.com.

‡$pK_a$ = the pH at which the agent exists in equal amounts of its ionized and un-ionized forms.

**BOX 188.1 Signs of Central Nervous System Toxicity**

- Tingling
- Numbness
- Dysarthria
- Lightheadedness
- Vertigo
- Tinnitus
- Metallic taste in mouth
- Difficulty focusing
- Agitation
- Apprehension
- Twitching in the face, extremities
- Seizures
- Change in mental status, coma

## SYSTEMIC AGENTS

### *Lidocaine*

Lidocaine is the most commonly used local anesthetic agent. Its low cost, rapid onset, duration, and toxicity profile make it ideal for most routine applications. The maximum dose of lidocaine is 4 to 4.5 mg/kg (e.g., a 70-kg patient should receive no more than 300 mg, or 30 mL of a 1% solution). The maximum dose may be increased to 7 mg/kg when lidocaine is given with epinephrine but will also cause an increase in sympathomimetic side effects (tachycardia and hypertension) and a theoretically higher risk for infection because of diminished blood supply to the affected area. The pain of injection can be reduced either by warming lidocaine to body temperature before administration[4] or by buffering it with sodium bicarbonate (1 mL sodium bicarbonate to 9 mL of 1% lidocaine).[2,5]

### *Mepivacaine*

Mepivacaine is structurally similar to lidocaine and has a similar onset of action and a slightly longer duration. As with bupivacaine, this longer duration of action is associated with a slightly higher risk for toxicity. The toxicity of mepivacaine is between that of lidocaine and bupivacaine, which corresponds to its intermediate duration of action.

### *Tetracaine*

Tetracaine is an ester agent. It is most commonly used in the ED for corneal anesthesia and as a component of LET (lidocaine 4%, epinephrine 0.1%, tetracaine 0.5%).

### *Ropivacaine*

Ropivacaine is a relatively new amide local anesthetic that was approved by the U.S. Food and Drug Administration (FDA) in 1996. Being the *S*-isomer of bupivacaine, ropivacaine is very similar in terms of onset of action, is slightly less potent, has a slightly shorter duration of action, and is associated with a 70% lower likelihood of cardiac toxicity. It also costs almost twice as much as bupivacaine.

### *Bupivacaine*

Bupivacaine is slightly more potent than lidocaine and lasts longer, but its onset of action is delayed. The maximum dose of bupivacaine is 2.5 mg/kg (e.g., a 70-kg patient should receive no more than 175 mg, or 35 mL of a 0.5% solution), which can be increased to 3 mg/kg if this agent is given with epinephrine. The high potency and protein binding of bupivacaine increase its risk for systemic toxicity when compared with lidocaine.

## ALLERGIC REACTIONS

True allergic reactions to local anesthetics are relatively rare. They are usually secondary to the preservative rather than to the agent itself. If an allergy is reported but not verified, the emergency physician should consider using a preservative-free agent, such as cardiac lidocaine from the "code" cart. Other options include switching classes (allergy to esters is more common than allergy to amides, and cross-reactivity is common within the class) or using benzyl alcohol,[6] diphenhydramine,[7] ice, or normal saline injection. An easy way to determine the class of an agent is to remember that all amides have two i's in their names and the esters only have one. If a patient is truly allergic to lidocaine, none of the anesthetic agents with two i's should be used (diphenhydramine is an exception to this rule of thumb because it is not classically considered an anesthetic agent).

## TOPICAL AGENTS

### *Lidocaine, Epinephrine, and Tetracaine*

LET (lidocaine 4%, epinephrine 0.1%, tetracaine 0.5%) is an excellent and safe topical anesthetic agent. It can be premixed by the hospital pharmacy and stored in the refrigerator for use in the ED. It is applied to wounds by soaking a cotton ball in LET and then securing the cotton ball to the wound for 15 to 30 minutes. Blanching of the skin around the wound indicates adequate anesthesia. Additional injected anesthetic may be required, but its application should be much more comfortable for the patient after LET pretreatment. LET (or any mixture containing epinephrine) should, by convention, not be used on the ear, nose, penis, or digits because of its vasoconstrictor effects.[8,9]

### *EMLA*

EMLA (eutectic mixture of local anesthetics: 2.5% lidocaine and 2.5% prilocaine) is approved by the FDA only for use on intact skin, although successful use in open wounds has been reported in the medical literature. Approximately 1 hour of topical application of EMLA is required to achieve local anesthesia, a characteristic that limits its usefulness in emergency cases. Infants younger than 3 months are at theoretically higher risk for the development of methemoglobinemia from EMLA because of inadequate levels of methemoglobin reductase.[1,8,9]

### *Liposomal Lidocaine*

ELA-Max is a relatively new proprietary mixture of 4% liposomal lidocaine that has been approved by the FDA for the temporary relief of pain from minor cuts and abrasions. Its onset of action is much shorter than that of EMLA (only 30 minutes), and it carries a much lower risk for methemoglobinemia because it does not contain prilocaine. This formulation may replace EMLA for most topical indications.[8,9]

# REGIONAL NERVE BLOCKS

## INDICATIONS

Regional nerve blocks are used for areas that are not amenable to local infiltration, such as the palms, the soles, and the fat pads of fingers and toes. Other advantages are avoidance of local tissue distortion and the ability to anesthetize large areas with fewer injections and less anesthetic agent. This reduces both the likelihood of toxicity and overall discomfort to the patient. Specific examples of common indications for regional nerve blocks are drainage of paronychia or felons; treatment of hand, foot, ear, and digit lacerations; débridement of road rash; treatment of nail bed injuries and ingrown toenails; and dental extraction. Regional nerve blocks also alleviate the pain associated with long-bone fractures and joint dislocations. Ultrasound guidance is recommended for injections into deep structures, such as femoral and scalene nerve blocks.

## GENERAL TECHNIQUE

The physician should explain the procedure to the patient and obtain consent (after carefully documenting any known allergies). The procedure is performed as follows:

1. Prepare the skin with povidone-iodine or other antiseptic skin solution.
2. Identify the area's landmarks.
3. Induce a superficial skin wheal at the injection site to reduce the discomfort of further manipulation.
4. Advance the needle to the target area while asking the patient to report any paresthesias.
5. If the patient does report paresthesias, thus indicating that the needle is within the nerve sheath, withdraw the needle 1 to 2 mm, aspirate to ensure that the needle is not in a vessel, and inject the agent slowly.

The agent of choice is usually lidocaine. Bupivacaine may be preferable when longer duration of action is desired.

## UPPER EXTREMITY BLOCKS

### *Median Nerve*

The median nerve provides sensation to the palmar surface of the radial half of the hand and the first through fourth fingers (**Fig. 188.1**). The median nerve is accessed between the palmaris longus tendon and the flexor carpi radialis tendon at the proximal wrist crease (**Fig. 188.2**). The patient should be instructed to oppose the thumb and fifth digit with the wrist flexed to allow visualization of these landmarks. The needle is inserted perpendicularly between the palmaris longus and flexor carpi radialis tendons and is then advanced until a "pop" is felt as the flexor retinaculum is penetrated. The needle is then advanced 0.5 cm past the retinaculum,

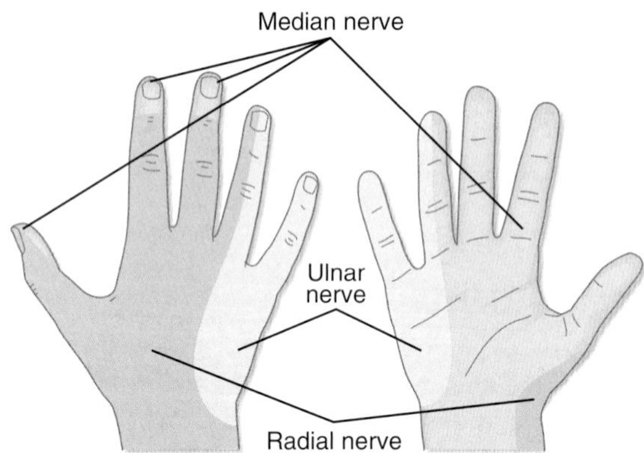


**Fig. 188.1** Sensory nerve distribution of the hand.

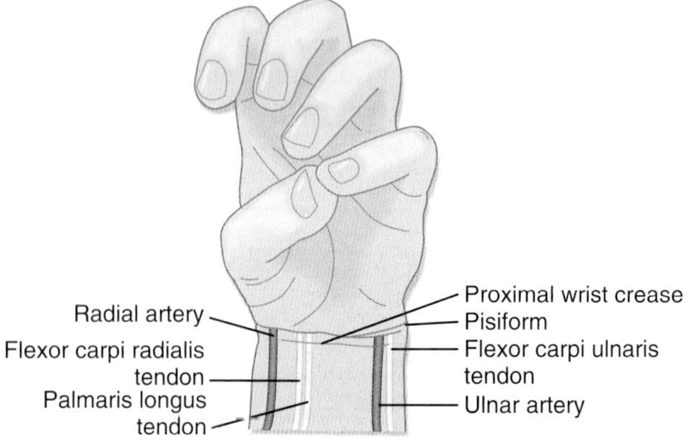


**Fig. 188.2** Landmarks for wrist nerve blocks.

aspiration is performed to verify that the needle is not in a vessel, and 5 mL of anesthetic agent is injected slowly as the needle is withdrawn.

### Ulnar Nerve

The ulnar nerve provides sensation to the palmar surface of the ulnar half of the hand and the fourth and fifth fingers (see Fig. 188.1). The ulnar nerve travels very close to the ulnar artery, deep to the flexor carpi ulnaris, so extra care must be taken to avoid intraarterial injection. The landmarks for this block are the flexor carpi ulnaris and the proximal wrist crease (see Fig. 188.2). The patient should be instructed to flex the wrist, and the operator should palpate the tendon proximal to the pisiform. With the lateral approach, the needle is advanced 1 to 1.5 cm horizontally under the flexor carpi ulnaris tendon, aspiration is performed to ensure that the needle is not located intraarterially, and 5 mL of anesthetic agent is slowly injected while the needle is withdrawn.

The ulnar nerve also gives off several subcutaneous branches that travel from the lateral border of the flexor carpi ulnaris to the dorsal midline. These branches are blocked by subcutaneous injection of an additional 5 to 10 mL in a superficial ringlike wheal from the lateral aspect of the proximal wrist crease to the dorsal midline (see Fig. 188.2).

### Radial Nerve

The radial nerve provides sensation to the dorsal radial aspect of the hand and the first through third digits (see Fig. 188.1). The radial nerve travels lateral to the radial artery at the wrist and gives off superficial cutaneous branches that travel laterally to the dorsal midline. The landmarks for this block are the proximal wrist crease and the radial pulse (see Fig. 188.2). The needle is inserted perpendicularly, just lateral to the radial pulse and 1 to 2 mm below the depth of the artery. Aspiration is performed and 3 to 5 mL of anesthetic agent is injected as the needle is slowly withdrawn. The subcutaneous branches are blocked with a superficial ringlike wheal, starting at the initial injection site and tracking to the dorsal midline (see Fig. 188.2).

### Digital Nerves

Each finger has two sets of nerves, called the dorsal and palmar digital nerves, that travel in the 2-, 4-, 8-, and 10-o'clock positions around the digit (**Fig. 188.3**). These four branch form two root nerves at the metacarpal-metatarsal heads. The most common approach for a digital nerve block is the proximal-most aspect of the finger or toe, where the nerves travel in the most consistent path. A skin wheal is formed on the dorsal surface of the finger or toe. The needle is then directed to the 2-, 4-, 8-, and 10-o'clock positions, respectively. After aspiration is performed, 0.5 to 1 mL of agent is injected at each site. Epinephrine and other vasoconstricting agents should not be used in this location because of the risk for critical ischemia.

### Interscalene Nerve

An ultrasound-guided interscalene nerve block is a useful method of inducing anesthesia for shoulder dislocations and is especially useful in patients who have a contraindication to procedural sedation or high opiate tolerance.[10] Deep to the sternocleidomastoid muscle on the lateral anterior aspect of the neck is where the anterior and middle scalene muscles lie. The interscalene nerve bundle appears between the anterior and middle scalene muscles and has the appearance of three small round pealike structures (**Fig. 188.4**). Under direct visualization with ultrasound, 30 mL of 1% lidocaine should be

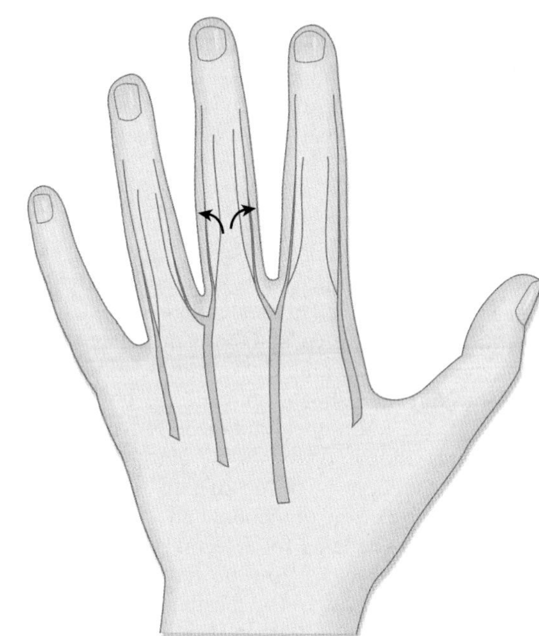

**Fig. 188.3 Landmarks for a digital nerve block.**

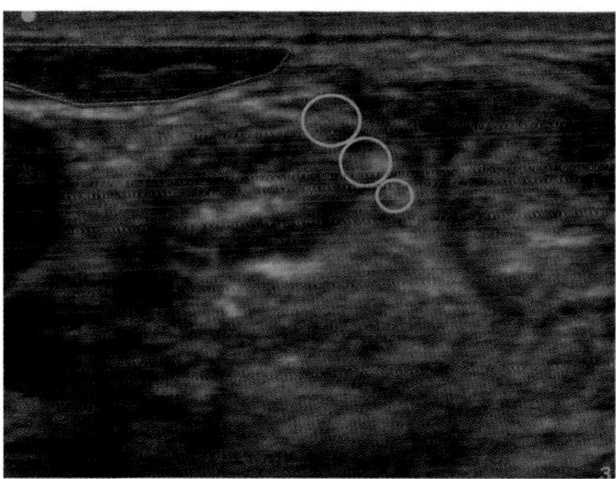

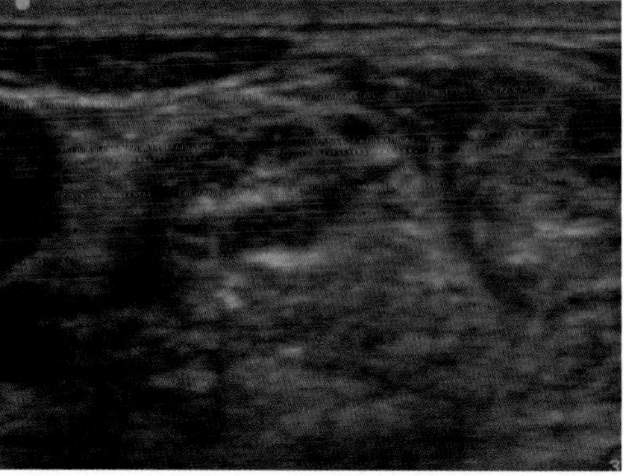

**Fig. 188.4 Ultrasound-guided interscalene nerve block.** (Courtesy Christine Butts, MD, and Shawn D'Andrea, MD.)

injected adjacent to the nerve bundle. Use of a 20-gauge spinal needle is recommended because its noncutting nature may be less likely to result in nerve laceration. Of note, it is important to visualize the needle tip throughout the entire procedure to ensure proper positioning and avoid damage to surrounding structures. After approximately 10 to 30 minutes, shoulder anesthesia should allow painless reduction. Temporary paralysis of the hemidiaphragm will occur and is usually asymptomatic; however, this procedure would be contraindicated in anyone who cannot tolerate a 30% reduction in pulmonary function. Occasionally, the cervical sympathetic chain may be affected and result in hoarseness and Horner syndrome. Patients should be advised of these possibilities when consent is obtained for the procedure.

### Bier Block

A Bier block involves the intravenous injection of a regional anesthetic into an extremity on which a tourniquet has been placed. Its use is relatively uncommon in the ED, but its advantage is the concomitant creation of a bloodless field. Peripheral intravenous access should be established in the target extremity at least 10 cm distal to the tourniquet. In addition, access should be established in a backup extremity in the event that access for resuscitation is needed. Because of its safely profile, 0.5% lidocaine without epinephrine is the agent of choice. This can be mixed by dilution of 1% lidocaine with an equal part of normal saline. The usual dose is 1.5 to 3 mg/kg.

A pneumatic tourniquet is applied over cotton padding proximal to the injury on the arm. The arm is elevated for at least 3 minutes to exsanguinate it before inflation of the tourniquet. With the arm elevated, the cuff is inflated to 250 mm Hg (or in a child, to 50 mm Hg greater than systolic pressure). The extremity is then lowered, and the agent is injected slowly. Onset of action is 3 to 5 minutes. Tourniquet time should be monitored carefully and should not exceed 1 hour. If the procedure is brief, the tourniquet should be left in place for at least 30 minutes after injection of the anesthetic to avoid a systemic bolus and higher risk for toxicity.

At the completion of the procedure and waiting period, the tourniquet should be deflated for 5 seconds and reinflated for 1 to 2 minutes; this cycle should be repeated three or four times to ensure slow release of the anesthetic into the systemic circulation. The patient should then be monitored for at least 30 minutes for signs of toxicity.[1]

## LOWER EXTREMITY BLOCKS

### Femoral Nerve and Three-in-One Block

The femoral nerve block and the three-in-one block (femoral, obturator, and lateral femoral cutaneous nerves) are useful for patients with fractures of the femur or hip. In view of the proximity of the femoral artery and vein to the target nerve, careful palpation of the pulse and aspiration are crucial to the safety of this procedure. Ultrasound can greatly improve the safety and accuracy of this procedure and has been shown to reduce the need for opiate analgesia and the amount of anesthetic required[11] (**Fig. 188.5**). The landmarks for this procedure are the inguinal ligament and the femoral artery (**Fig. 188.6**). The femoral artery is palpated 1 to 2 cm distal to the inguinal ligament. The operator's nondominant hand is kept on the femoral pulse throughout the procedure to reduce the likelihood of intraarterial injection, especially if ultrasound is not being used to visualize the injection. With a perpendicular and slightly cephalad approach, the needle is inserted 0.5 to 1 cm lateral to the pulse until paresthesias are elicited, the patella moves involuntarily, or the needle begins to pulsate laterally. To anesthetize only the femoral nerve, 10 to 20 mL of agent should be injected. To anesthetize all three nerves, 30 mL of agent should be injected in a cephalad direction into the femoral sheath while distal pressure is maintained to ensure proximal tracking of the anesthetic agent.[1,3,11,12]

### Sural Nerve

The sural nerve supplies sensation to the heel and lateral aspect of the foot (**Fig. 188.7**). Landmarks for this block are the lateral malleolus and the Achilles tendon (see Fig. 188.7). The needle is inserted just lateral to the Achilles tendon, 1 cm above the lateral malleolus, and directed toward the fibula. When contact with the fibula is made, the needle is withdrawn 1 mm, aspiration is performed, and 5 mL of agent is injected as the needle is withdrawn slowly.

### Peroneal Nerves (Superficial and Deep)

The superficial peroneal nerve supplies sensation to the dorsum of the foot and toes, whereas the deep peroneal nerve supplies the first web space (see Fig. 188.7). The landmarks for these blocks are the extensor hallucis longus tendon, the anterior tibialis tendon, and the anterior lip of the tibia (see **Fig. 188.8**). The superficial peroneal nerve travels anteriorly between the extensor hallucis longus tendon and the lateral malleolus. The deep peroneal nerve travels under the extensor hallucis longus tendon. For a superficial peroneal nerve block, the needle is inserted just lateral to the hallucis longus tendon and is directed toward the lateral malleolus. The agent is injected in a ringlike fashion from the extensor hallucis longus to the lateral malleolus. For a deep peroneal nerve block, the needle is inserted between the anterior tibialis tendon and the extensor hallucis longus tendon, 1 cm above the base of the medial malleolus, and directed 30 degrees laterally under the tendon. The needle is advanced until it touches the tibia (less than 1 cm) and then withdrawn 1 mm, and 5 mL of agent is injected while the needle is slowly withdrawn.

### Saphenous Nerve

The saphenous nerve provides sensation to the medial aspect of the foot and the arch (see Fig. 188.7). The landmarks for this block are the medial malleolus and the anterior tibialis tendon (see Fig. 188.8). The patient is instructed to dorsiflex the foot to enable the anterior tibialis tendon to be located at the anterior lip of the tibia. The saphenous nerve travels superficially between the anterior tibialis tendon and the medial malleolus. The needle is inserted at the anterior lip of the distal end of the tibia, just lateral to the tibialis tendon, and directed toward the medial malleolus. Five milliliters of agent is injected subcutaneously, in a ringlike fashion, from the anterior tibialis tendon to the medial malleolus.

### Posterior Tibial Nerve

The posterior tibial nerve supplies sensation to the distal two thirds of the plantar surface of the foot (see Fig. 188.7). The landmarks for this block are the medial malleolus, the posterior tibial artery, and the Achilles tendon (see Fig. 188.8). The

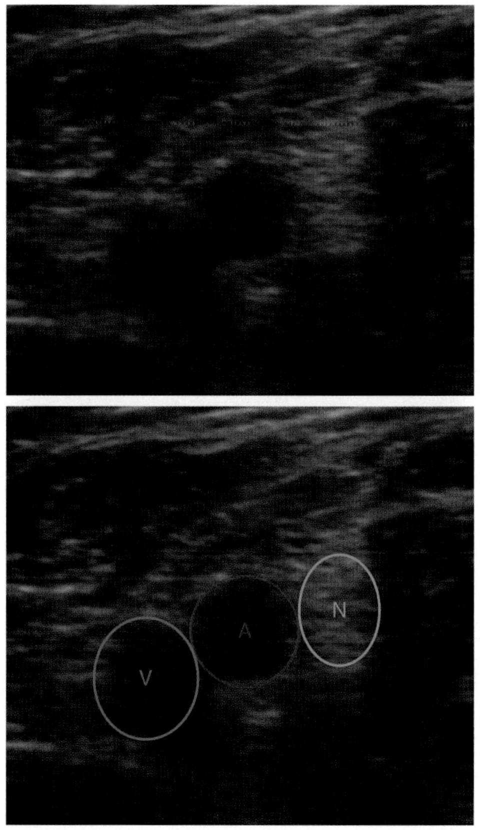


**Fig. 188.5 Ultrasound-guided femoral nerve block.** *A*, Artery; *N*, nerve; *V*, vein. (Courtesy Christine Butts, MD, and Shawn D'Andrea, MD.)

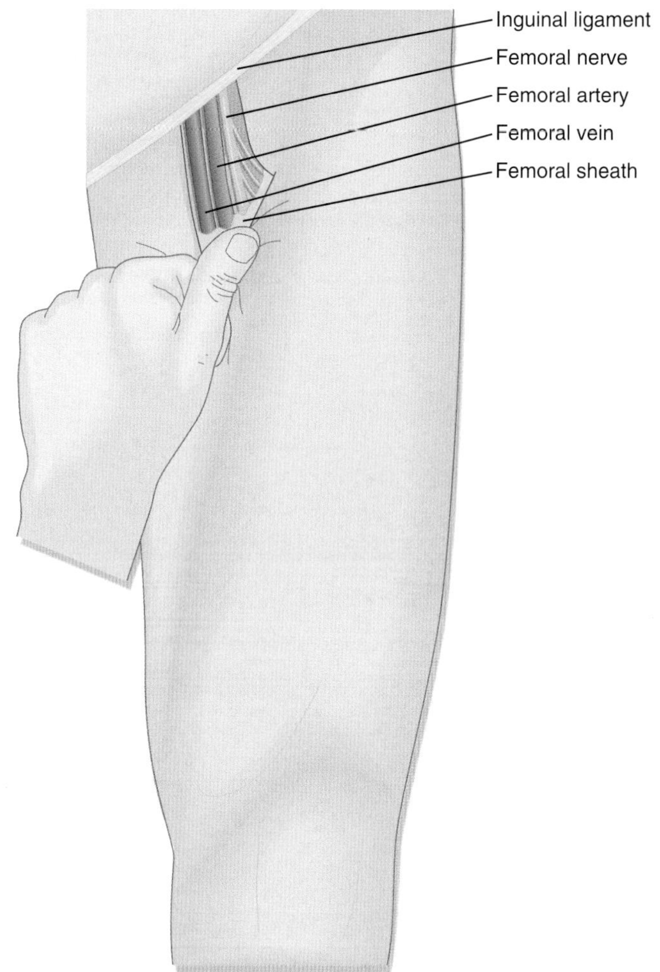


**Fig. 188.6 Landmarks for a femoral nerve or three-in-one nerve block.**

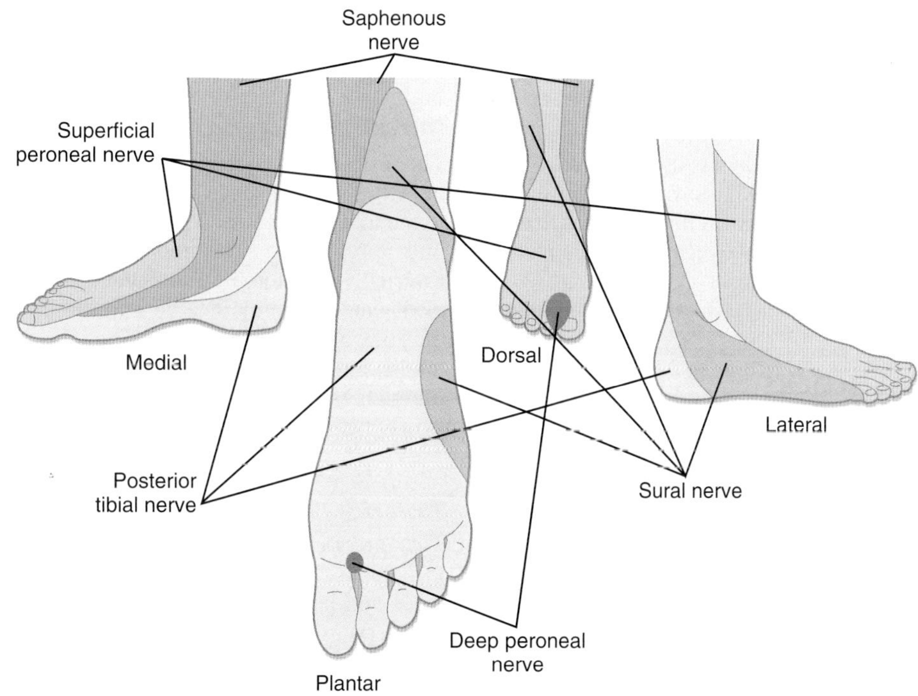


**Fig. 188.7 Sensory nerve distribution of the ankle.**

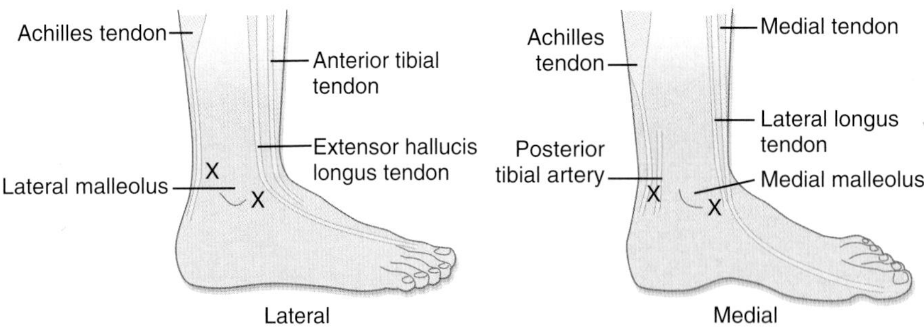


**Fig. 188.8 Landmarks for ankle nerve blocks.**

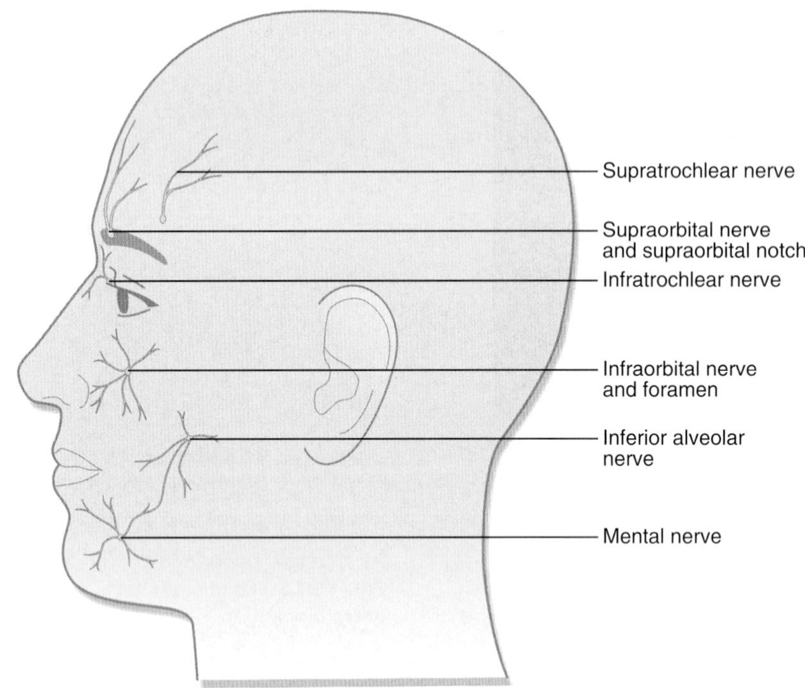


**Fig. 188.9 Distribution of the facial nerves.**

needle is inserted just anterior to the Achilles tendon at a level 1 cm above the medial malleolus. The needle is directed just posterior to the posterior tibial artery toward the posterior aspect of the tibia. It is advanced until it hits the tibia and is then withdrawn 1 mm. Five milliliters of agent is then injected while the needle is slowly withdrawn.

## FACIAL AND ORAL BLOCKS

### *Supraorbital Nerve*

The supraorbital nerve exits the supraorbital notch along the supraorbital rim. Along with the supratrochlear and infratrochlear nerves, it supplies sensation to the forehead (**Figs. 188.9 and 188.10**). For a nerve block, the supraorbital notch is palpated, and 1 to 3 mL of agent is injected at this location. If inadequate anesthesia is obtained, a subcutaneous wheal is made down the supraorbital rim with 5 mL of agent to anesthetize branches of the supratrochlear and infratrochlear nerves. Placing a finger just below the eyebrow decreases the incidence of eyelid swelling.[2]

### *Infraorbital Nerve*

The infraorbital nerve exits the infraorbital foramen and branches into the superior alveolar nerves supplying sensation to the midface region (see Figs. 188.9 and 188.10). The intraoral approach is recommended. While holding one finger externally over the inferior border of the infraorbital rim, the physician inserts the needle into the labial mucosa, opposite the apex of the first premolar. The needle is advanced parallel to the long axis of the tooth until it is palpated near the foramen. After aspiration, 2 to 3 mL of agent is injected slowly near but not into the foramen.

### *Anterior Superior Alveolar Nerve*

The anterior superior alveolar nerve supplies sensation to the ipsilateral central and lateral incisors, as well as the canine tooth and half the upper lip (see Fig. 188.10). For block of this nerve, the needle is inserted with the bevel facing bone, superior to the apex of the canine, and directed to the canine fossa. After aspiration, 2 mL of agent is injected (see Fig. 188.10).

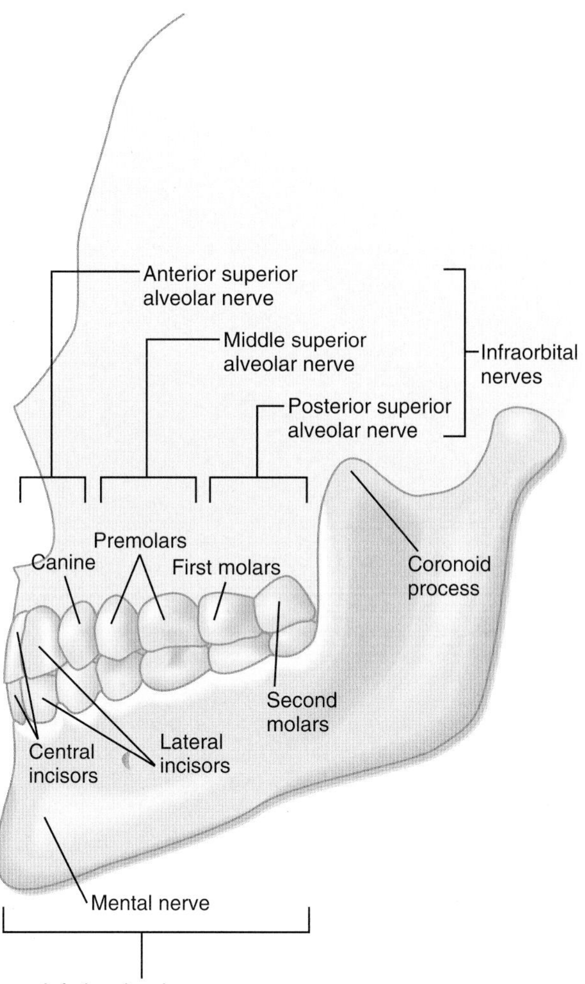


**Fig. 188.10 Landmarks for facial nerve blocks.**

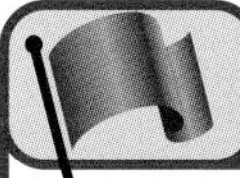

**RED FLAGS**

- Be wary of allergy to anesthetic agents; consider applying a preservative-free agent, crossing an anesthetic class, or using benzoyl alcohol.
- Always aspirate before injecting to avoid accidental intravascular injection.
- Perform a thorough neurologic evaluation before initiating local anesthesia.
- Ask the patient to tell you whether paresthesias develop.
- If paresthesias develop, withdraw the needle 1 to 2 mm before making the injection.
- Monitor the patient closely for any signs of toxicity.
- To reduce the incidence of toxicity, use the smallest effective dose of an anesthetic agent.

### *Posterior Superior Alveolar Nerve*

The posterior superior alveolar nerve provides sensation to the ipsilateral maxillary molars (see Fig. 188.10). After the cheek is retracted laterally, the needle is inserted into the mucosal reflection, just distal to the distal buccal root of the upper second molar. The needle is advanced 2 to 2.5 cm along the curvature of the maxillary tuberosity, at which point 2 to 3 mL of agent is injected to effect a nerve block. The operator should beware of the pterygoid plexus and must be sure to perform aspiration before making an injection.

**TIPS AND TRICKS**

- Inject anesthetic agents slowly, in increments of no more than 3 mL, and aspirate before injecting.
- Maintain verbal contact with the patient to help screen for dysarthria and changes in mental status.
- Use a small needle (27- to 30-gauge for local infiltration, 25- or 27-gauge for nerve blocks).
- Use warmed or buffered lidocaine.
- Use a small-caliber syringe to reduce the pressure and pain associated with injection.
- Administer 1 to 2 mL of anesthetic for digital blocks, 5 mL for most other blocks.

### *Middle Superior Alveolar Nerve*

The middle superior alveolar nerve provides sensation to the ipsilateral premolars and sometimes the first maxillary molars (see Fig. 188.10). For a block of this nerve, the needle is inserted with the bevel facing bone, superior to the apex of the upper second premolar tooth, and 2 mL of agent is injected.

### *Inferior Alveolar Nerve*

The inferior alveolar nerve supplies sensation to the ipsilateral mandibular teeth, lower lip, and chin (see Figs. 188.9 and 188.10). The coronoid process of the mandible is palpated, and the cheek is retracted laterally. A triangle is visualized in the mucosa posterior to the molars. The needle is inserted into this triangle, 1 cm above the occlusal surface of the molars, and advanced until it contacts the mandible. The needle is retracted slightly, aspiration is performed, and 2 mL of agent is injected slowly. If the needle does not contact the mandible and is directed posteriorly toward the parotid gland, temporary Bell palsy may be elicited if the facial nerve is unintentionally anesthetized. Injection of more agent while the needle is withdrawn will anesthetize the lingual nerve as well.

## MENTAL NERVE

The mental nerve branches off the inferior alveolar nerve to supply sensation to the ipsilateral part of the chin (see Figs. 188.9 and 188.10). This nerve emerges from the mental foramen inferior to the second premolar (see Fig. 188.10). For a mental nerve block the foramen is palpated, and then through an intraoral approach, the needle is inserted in the

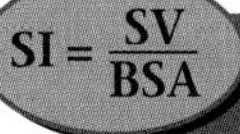


**FACTS AND FORMULAS**

- The names of all amide anesthetic agents contain two i's.
- The maximum dose of lidocaine is 4.5 mg/kg without epinephrine and 7 mg/kg with epinephrine.
- One milliliter of a 1% solution of lidocaine contains 10 mg of lidocaine.

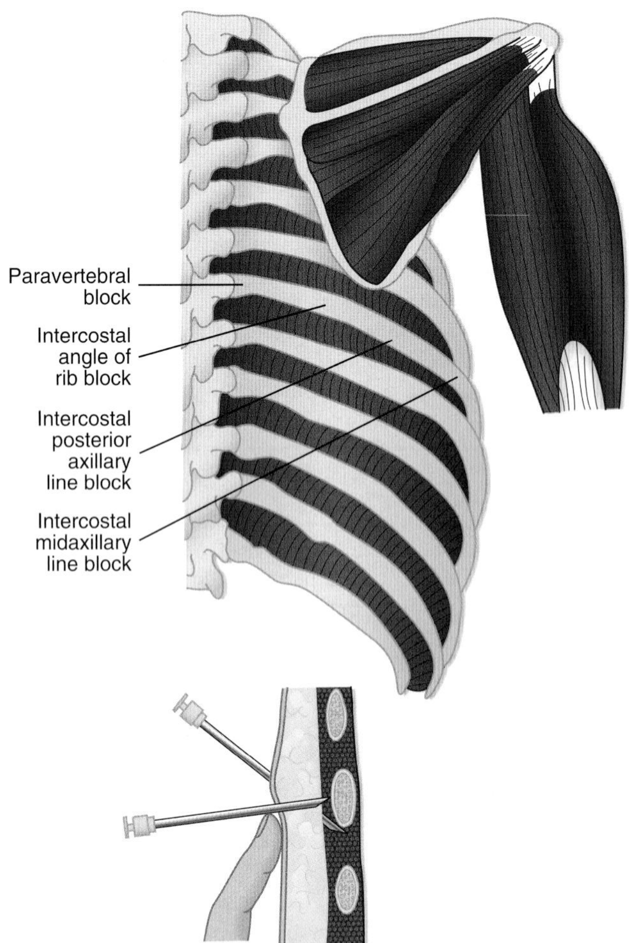


**Fig. 188.11** Landmarks for an intercostal nerve block.

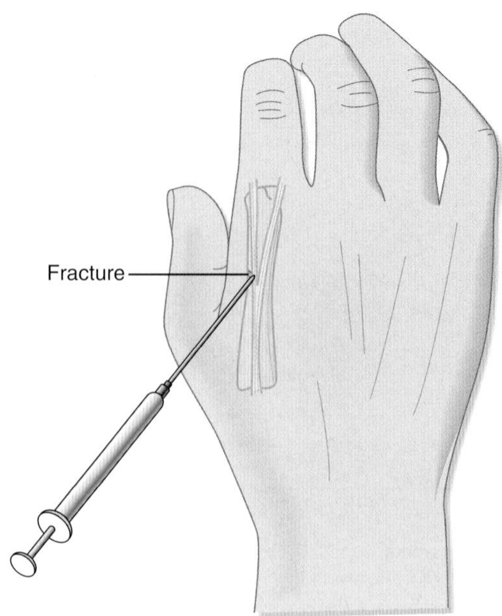


**Fig. 188.12** Landmarks for a hematoma block.

mucobuccal fold and advanced until it can be palpated over the foramen. After aspiration is performed, 1 to 3 mL of agent is slowly injected.

### Nerve Block of an Individual Tooth (Supraperiosteal Block)

The operator can block the nerve of a single tooth by having the needle enter the mucobuccal fold with the bevel facing bone and injecting 1 to 2 mL of agent at the apex of the tooth, close to the periosteum. It may take longer than most blocks to achieve complete anesthesia because the agent has to penetrate the cortex of the bone to reach the nerve root (5 to 10 minutes).

### Ear Block

Because several different nerves supply sensation to the ear, an ear block requires a superficial skin wheal around the entire anterior and posterior auricular aspect of the face and scalp (see Fig. 188.10).

## MISCELLANEOUS NERVE BLOCKS

### Intercostal Nerve Block

An intercostal nerve block is perhaps one of the most dangerous nerve blocks because of greater systemic absorption of agent injected in this area and a 1.4% incidence of pneumothorax.[13] However, significant pain relief from rib fractures can be obtained with this method. In most cases, opiate analgesia is probably a safer method of pain control. The injured rib is palpated posterior to the posterior axillary line, and the skin is retracted superiorly over the rib. The needle is inserted 5 mm over the rib, the retracted skin released, and the needle walked gently down the inferior edge of the rib. The needle is then advanced 2 to 3 mm, aspiration is performed, and 2 to 5 mL of agent is injected. If pain control is inadequate, this procedure can be repeated for two ribs above and two below the injured area (**Fig. 188.11**).

### Hematoma Block

The hematoma of a fracture can be locally anesthetized to relieve the pain associated with relocation of a displaced fracture. This block is most commonly used for metacarpal fractures. Two milliliters of agent is usually sufficient. In this case, if aspiration of blood confirms placement of the needle within the hematoma, care should be taken to avoid anatomic locations of known vessels (**Fig. 188.12**).[3]

## SUGGESTED READINGS

Christos S, Chiampas G, Offman R, et al. Ultrasound-guided three-in-one nerve block for femur fractures. West J Emerg Med 2010;11:310-3.
Crystal C, Blankenship R. Local anesthetics and peripheral nerve blocks in the emergency department. Emerg Med Clin North Am 2005;23:477-502.
Eidelman A, Weiss J, Lau J, et al. Topical anesthetics for dermal instrumentation: a systematic review of randomized, controlled trials. Ann Emerg Med 2005;46:343-51.
Fletcher A, Rigby A, Heyes F. Three-in-one femoral nerve block as analgesia for fractured neck of femur in the emergency department: a randomized controlled trial. Ann Emerg Med 2003;41:227-33.
Wedmore I, Johnson T, Czarnik J, et al. Pain management in the wilderness and operational setting. Emerg Med Clin North Am 2005;23:585-601.

## REFERENCES

*References can be found on Expert Consult @ www.expertconsult.com.*

# Thermal Burns 189

*Jeffrey Druck*

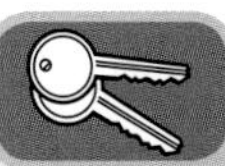

**KEY POINTS**

- Many patients who initially appear to have a mild airway burn injury still require early intubation because critical edema will develop. Intubate; do not observe.
- Extremely high doses of narcotics (three to five times normal) are usually required to control pain in patients with severe burns.
- Patients with severe burns have large fluid requirements, which are best determined initially by standard calculations.
- The best measure of adequate fluid replacement is urine output.
- Cold water can help relieve the pain of first- and second-degree burns, but patients with significant burns involving more than 9% of their total body surface area should not have cold applied.
- Burn centers have improved mortality rates, so transfer to a burn center should be considered early in the patient's management.
- Empiric oral or intravenous antibiotic administration is not indicated, but topical antibiotics are.

## EPIDEMIOLOGY

Approximately 500,000 patients sustain nonfatal burn injuries in the United States each year.[1] Only 6% of these patients require hospitalization, so most are treated as outpatients.

Serious burns are some of the most challenging critical care cases. Approximately 8% of all burns result in death. Furthermore, care must be optimized because long-term disability can be moderated if initial resuscitation is adequate, infections are minimized, and specialty care by burn experts is promoted.

## PATHOPHYSIOLOGY

Knowing the anatomy of the skin is essential to understanding burn pathophysiology (**Fig. 189.1**). Burns are classified according to the depth of injury (**Table 189.1** and **Fig. 189.2**). First- and second-degree burns are partial-thickness burns and have a better prognosis. Full-thickness burns (third and fourth degree) are insensate and require skin grafts (unless <1 cm) or reconstruction because of destruction of the epidermis and dermis. Based on the depth of the burn, the ability to heal can be predicted. Because the dermis itself is the living tissue, the depth of burn into the dermis determines how likely wounds are to heal and what degree of scarring can be expected.

The severity of the burn depends on the duration of contact with the burn agent, the heat and conductivity of tissues, the heat of the burn agent, heat transfer (conduction, convection, or radiation), and the heat capacity of the burn agent.

Burns damage by two methods: first, by direct injury to the cellular structure of the tissue and, second, by the release of local mediators. Three zones are discussed with burn injuries: the zone of coagulation, the zone of stasis, and the zone of hyperemia. The zone of coagulation is the necrotic area of cell death as a result of direct thermal injury. Surrounding this area is the zone of stasis, which has decreased blood flow and is at risk for cell death within 24 hours but may initially appear as living tissue. Cell mediators such as thromboxane $A_2$ are predominantly responsible for transforming this area into the zone of coagulation. Outside this zone is the zone of hyperemia. The zone of hyperemia is defined as the outside area of tissue affected by the burn, usually blanching on touch, but with intact blood flow and high potential to recover from the initial insult.

The secondary effects of burns, such as histamine release and edema, are thought to result from cellular mediators. Aggregated platelets from the burn release serotonin, whereas histamine is derived from mast cells within the burned skin.

## PRESENTING SIGNS AND SYMPTOMS

Frequently, occupational exposure causes burns. Direct contact with flame, scalds, injuries caused by heated equipment or arc welding, gasoline fires, and cooking accidents are all common. In children or elderly patients with burn injuries, the concern for abuse is always present (see the "Red Flags" box).

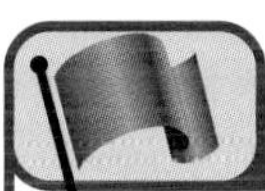

**RED FLAGS**

Burns inconsistent with the mechanism: concerning for nonaccidental trauma or abuse

Circular burns consistent with cigarette butt burns

Burns on the lower extremities without burns on the soles: consistent with forced immersion scald burns

Any perineal burn (area not exposed during normal activities)

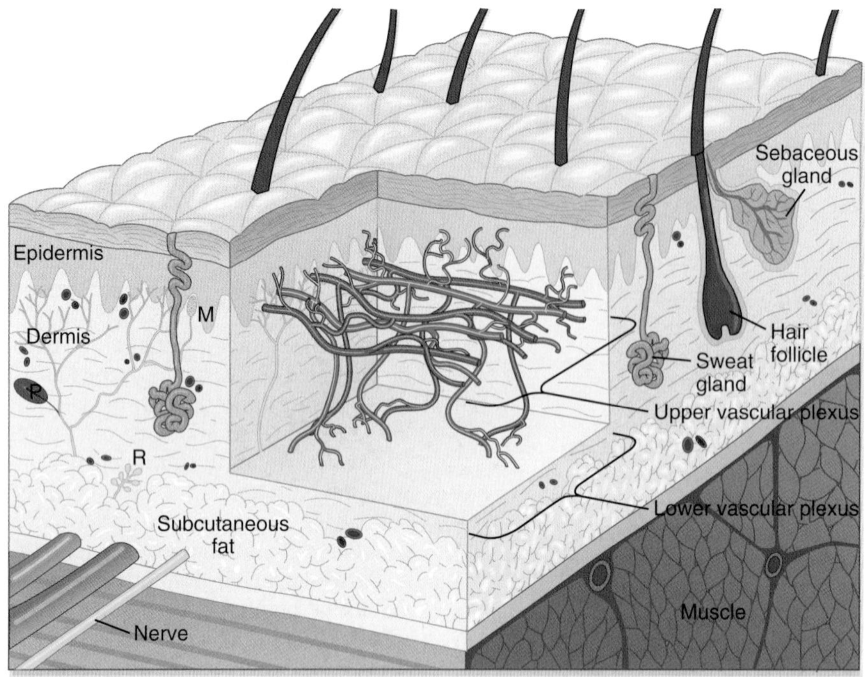


**Fig. 189.1 Schematic representation of a cross section of human skin.** The two major layers of human skin, the epidermis and the dermis, overlie subcutaneous fat and muscle. Arterioles *(red)*, venules *(blue)*, and lymph vessels *(yellow)* of the dermis form a lower and an upper vascular plexus. Capillary loops extend toward the epidermis from the upper plexus of blood vessels into the dermal papillae, approximately one loop per dermal papilla. Sensory and autonomic nerves *(yellow* fibers*)* are also arranged in a lower and an upper plexus at the junction of the dermis and subcutaneous fat and in the upper dermis. Sweat glands and hair follicles with their associated sebaceous glands are also integral components of skin. (From Adkinson NF, Yunginger JW, Busse WW, et al, editors. Middleton's allergy: principles and practice. 6th ed. St. Louis: Mosby; 2003.)

**Table 189.1** Types of Burns

| DEGREE OF BURN | DEPTH | PAIN LEVEL | BLANCHING | COLOR | EXAMPLE |
|---|---|---|---|---|---|
| First degree | Epidermal | Painful | Blanches | Erythematous | Sunburn |
| Superficial second degree | Superficial dermal | Painful | May blanch, usually blisters | Erythematous | Scald injury |
| Deep second degree | Deep dermal | Painful to pinprick | Does not blanch | Pale and mottled | Hot grease burn |
| Third degree | Full thickness | Insensate | Does not blanch | Hard, leathery eschar, often black | House fire (sustained burn) |
| Fourth degree | Deep organ involvement | Insensate | Does not blanch | Burn involving bone, fat, or muscle apparent | Extensively sustained burn |

One issue that is often of concern is the depth of burns. Determining between deep partial-thickness and superficial partial-thickness burns is difficult because it may take time for a definitive area of demarcation to develop. The usual method of distinction, blistering (which occurs with deep partial-thickness burns, or second-degree burns), can be delayed; however, it is the only distinction that is available early. Third-degree burns are insensate.

With all burn patients, assessment of the airway is critical. Signs of deep injury are stridor, soot in the mouth, and singed nasal hairs; any of these signs should indicate the need for close monitoring and more aggressive airway management. Swelling can occur rapidly in burned tissues, so signs of airway involvement should suggest earlier intubation because decompensation may occur rapidly.

## DIFFERENTIAL DIAGNOSIS AND MEDICAL DECISION MAKING

In each patient with a burn, the airway is still the most important component. Burn victims are often also subject to smoke inhalation or thermal injury to respiratory tissue from superheated air, and these injuries take priority over any others. Carbon monoxide, cyanide, and other inhaled toxins should be considered. The most threatening injuries are deep burns,

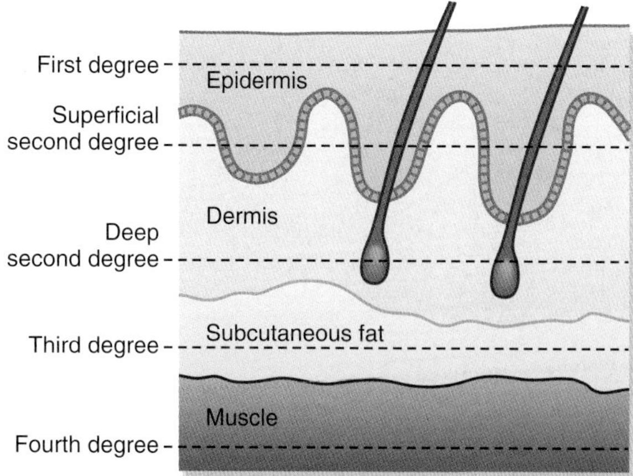


**Fig. 189.2 Depth of burns.** First-degree burns are confined to the epidermis. Second-degree burns extend into the dermis (dermal burns). Third-degree burns are full-thickness burns through the epidermis and dermis. Fourth-degree burns involve injury to underlying tissue structures such as muscle, tendon, and bone. (From Townsend CM, Beauchamp RD, Evers BM, et al, editors. Sabiston textbook of surgery. 17th ed. Philadelphia: Saunders; 2004.)

**BOX 189.1 Criteria of the American Burn Association for Referral to a Burn Unit**

- Partial-thickness burns involving greater than 10% total body surface area
- Burns that involve the hands, face, feet, genitalia, perineum, or major joints
- Third-degree (full-thickness) burns in any age group
- Electrical burns, including lightning injury
- Chemical burns
- Inhalation injury
- Burn injury in patients with preexisting medical disorders that could complicate management or recovery or could affect mortality
- Patients with concomitant burn injury and trauma in which the burn injury poses the greatest risk for morbidity or mortality
- Burned children in hospitals without qualified personnel or equipment for the care of children
- Burn injury in patients who require special social, emotional, or long-term rehabilitative intervention

Adapted from American Burn Association. Burn unit criteria. Available at http://www.ameriburn.org.

burns covering a significant proportion of body surface area, and respiratory burns (**Box 189.1**).

Aside from the ABCs (airway, breathing, circulation), the most important aspect of burn assessment is estimation of burn depth and burn surface area. Burn depth can be assessed by evaluating the degree of blanching, noting the presence of blistering of the skin, and checking for the presence of pain. Total burn surface area is best assessed by using a Lund and Browder chart (**Fig. 189.3**). Alternatively, a patient's palmar surface (not including the fingers) can be used as a crude measure of 1% of the patient's body surface area.

Children's body surface area is significantly different from that of adults. A child's head and torso account for a much larger percentage of body surface area than in an adult. Patients with serious burns need specific burn unit care and require transfer if such care is unavailable at the institution.

In patients with severe burn injuries, burn shock can occur. Hypovolemic shock develops from alterations in capillary permeability. Cell death can result in severe hyperkalemia, although this condition is usually a delayed finding.

## TREATMENT

The first intervention for burn victims is assessment of the airway. Smoke inhalation is a common issue, so all patients who do not need immediate intubation should be given 100% humidified oxygen via a nonrebreather mask. Because edema can progress in minutes to hours and the full extent of respiratory damage may not become evident until 12 hours after the initial injury, patients with evidence of airway damage should be intubated prophylactically, before the airway becomes edematous (see the "Priority Actions" box).

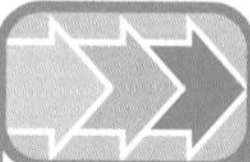

**PRIORITY ACTIONS**

- Address the patient's respiratory status, with high suspicion for airway injury that will worsen; intubate if necessary, and supply supplemental oxygen otherwise.
- Assess the size and depth of the burn injury.
- Provide anesthesia and pain management. Patients may require extremely high doses of narcotics (three to five times normal).
- Start appropriate fluid management and consider placement of a Foley catheter for assessment of fluid status.
- Dress wounds appropriately.
- Evaluate for the need for escharotomies.
- Consider the need for burn unit referral.

Because of the expected hypovolemic state of these patients, two large-bore intravenous lines should be placed. Although placement of intravenous lines through burned skin is not optimal given that they allow another portal for infection into an open wound, it is preferable to having no intravenous access at all.

Fluid requirements are a key facet in the management of a burn patient. Two specific formulas are most commonly used. The Parkland formula is used to estimate fluid replacement in adults. This formula gives suggested fluid replacement in addition to maintenance fluid amounts over a 24-hour period; half of this fluid should be given over the first 8 hours, with the remaining half administered over the following 16 hours. The original Parkland formula used lactated Ringer solution as the fluid of choice.[2]

For children, the Galveston formula is recommended for calculation of fluid repletion. The Galveston formula suggests that lactated Ringer solution with 5% dextrose should be used as the fluid of choice because of the lack of glycogen stores in the pediatric population. Again, half of the total amount should be given in the first 8 hours, with the remainder administered within the next 16 hours. Maintenance fluid should be

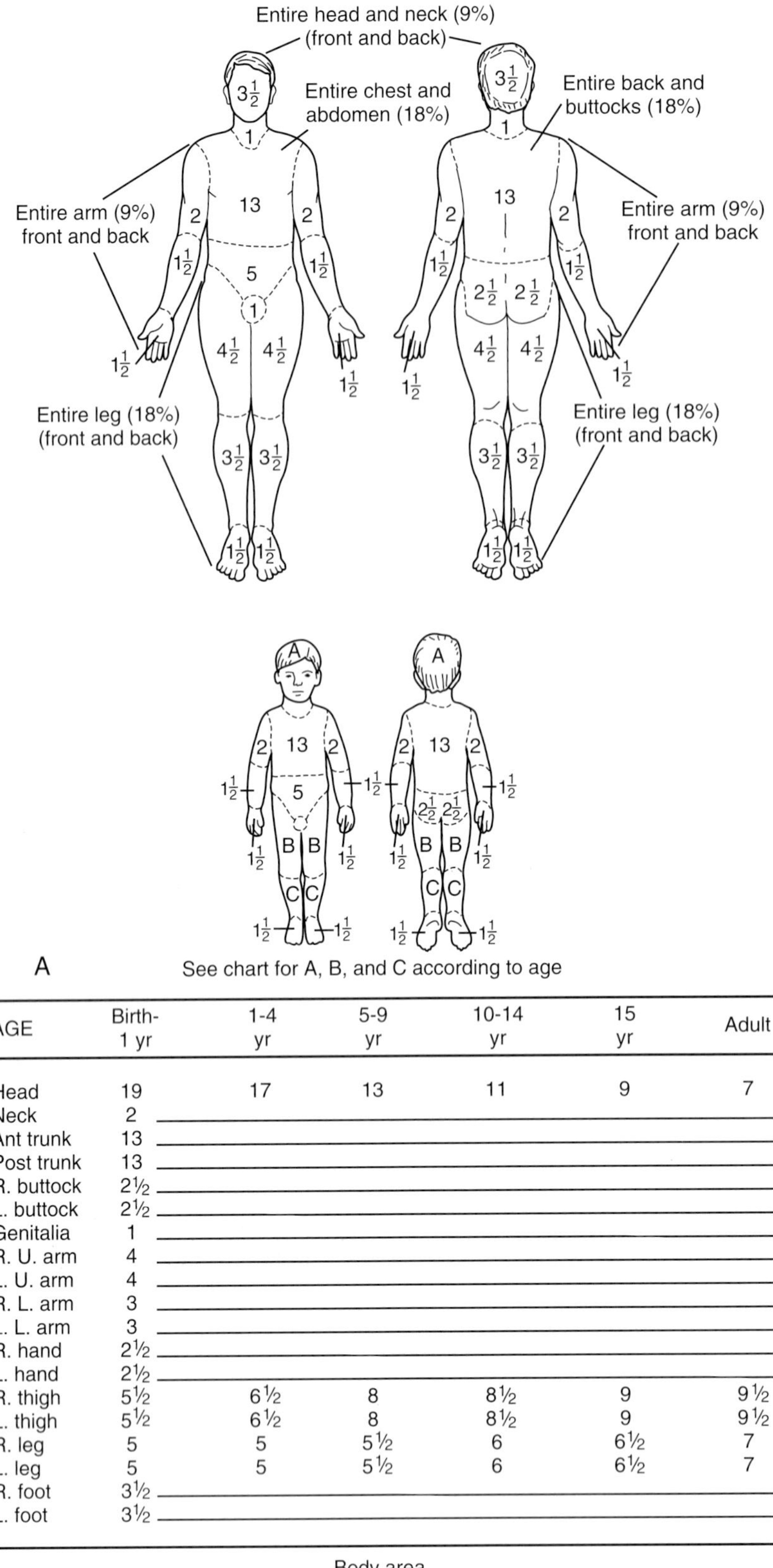


| AGE | Birth-1 yr | 1-4 yr | 5-9 yr | 10-14 yr | 15 yr | Adult |
|---|---|---|---|---|---|---|
| Head | 19 | 17 | 13 | 11 | 9 | 7 |
| Neck | 2 | | | | | |
| Ant trunk | 13 | | | | | |
| Post trunk | 13 | | | | | |
| R. buttock | 2½ | | | | | |
| L. buttock | 2½ | | | | | |
| Genitalia | 1 | | | | | |
| R. U. arm | 4 | | | | | |
| L. U. arm | 4 | | | | | |
| R. L. arm | 3 | | | | | |
| L. L. arm | 3 | | | | | |
| R. hand | 2½ | | | | | |
| L. hand | 2½ | | | | | |
| R. thigh | 5½ | 6½ | 8 | 8½ | 9 | 9½ |
| L. thigh | 5½ | 6½ | 8 | 8½ | 9 | 9½ |
| R. leg | 5 | 5 | 5½ | 6 | 6½ | 7 |
| L. leg | 5 | 5 | 5½ | 6 | 6½ | 7 |
| R. foot | 3½ | | | | | |
| L. foot | 3½ | | | | | |

Body area

B

**Fig. 189.3** **A,** The Lund and Browder charts are somewhat more accurate than the rule of nines in estimating the total body surface area burned. **B,** The proportion of total body surface area of individual areas, according to age. When compared with adults, children have larger heads and smaller legs. Other areas are relatively equivalent throughout life. The rule of nines is not accurate in determining the percentage of total body surface area burned in children. *Ant*, Anterior; *L*, left or lower; *Post*, posterior; *R*, right; *U*, upper. (From Roberts JR, Hedges J, editors. Clinical procedures in emergency medicine. 4th ed. Philadelphia: Saunders; 2004.)

$SI = \frac{SV}{BSA}$ **FACTS AND FORMULAS**

| | | | |
|---|---|---|---|
| Parkland formula | Adults | Lactated Ringer solution, 4 mL × patient's weight (in kg) × percent TBSA | 50% in first 8 hours; 50% divided over next 16 hours (goal mean arterial pressure > 60 mm Hg and urine output >0.5 mL/kg/hr for adults) |
| Galveston formula | Pediatric patients | 5% dextrose in lactated Ringer solution 5000 mL/TBSA burned (in m²) + 2000 mL/TBSA (in m²)/24 hr | 50% in first 8 hours; 50% divided over next 16 hours (goal urine output 1 mL/kg/hr) |

*TBSA*, Total body surface area.

also added, and particular attention should be paid to maintaining body temperature (see the "Facts and Formulas" box).

Despite these formulas, fluid resuscitation is more accurately based on appropriate urine output, which is 0.5 mL/kg/hr in adults and up to 1 mL/kg/hr in children. When one is uncertain about the patient's fluid status, as may occur with congestive heart failure or pulmonary edema, a Swan-Ganz catheter may be necessary to provide guidance. Some controversy exists about the optimal fluid to use in burn patients. Although current guidelines specify crystalloid only initially, more recent studies suggest a probable role for colloid solutions.[3,4]

All burns should be gently cleansed of debris with normal saline solution. Superficial burns (superficial second- and first-degree burns) should be dressed with topical antimicrobial dressings, with frequent dressing changes planned (every 6 hours). A degree of controversy exists about the best antimicrobial dressing. No clearly superior agent has been reported in the literature.[5] One commonly used agent, silver sulfadiazine, should not be applied to the face because of concerns about staining. A good option, particularly for the face, is a simple, over-the-counter antibiotic ointment. For mild burns, aloe vera cream is also acceptable. Biosynthetic dressings are another option, but because of cost and availability, these dressings are usually limited to inpatient burn management. A recent study showed a combination of hyaluronic acid plus silver sulfadiazine to be superior to just silver sulfadiazine alone.[5]

Deeper burns may require débridement and grafting. Specific recommendations should be discussed with the local burn center. If burns are in areas that can be elevated, they should be; this approach decreases the amount of subsequent edema that develops in the burn areas. Controversy also exists about whether burn blisters should be sterilely incised or left alone. No definitive data on the subject are available, but the general consensus appears to be that unless a blister prevents the application of a dressing, it should be left intact.

Pain management is beneficial to the patient and is important to address early. Third-degree (full-thickness) burns are insensate, but more superficial burns are exquisitely painful. Most burns vary in depth and are painful, so early intravenous administration of morphine or hydromorphone (Dilaudid) is indicated for patients with extensive or deep burns. First-degree burns can be managed with oral nonsteroidal antiinflammatory medications as a first-line therapy, although narcotics may be required. Superficial partial-thickness burns require oral narcotics for pain control.

Occasionally, a burn covers such a large area that it poses a risk for respiratory or vascular compromise. For example, a circumferential burn on an extremity can compromise the vascular supply to that extremity, whereas a nearly circumferential full-thickness burn on the chest can prevent chest movement and result in an inability to ventilate. Through escharotomies these constricting bands of tissue can be released (**Table 189.2**). The basic method of performing an escharotomy is to incise the constricting band of tissue down to subcutaneous fat. Fasciotomies for compartment syndrome may also be required with thermal burns that cause edema and subsequent increased compartmental pressure.

Much discussion has centered around empiric antibiotic administration. No data support the empiric use of antibiotics for acute burn wounds, except in topical form, as recommended for superficial burn wounds.[6]

Application of cold inhibits the production of lactate, release of histamine and thromboxane, and sequelae such as edema, microvascular congestion, and progressive ischemia. Cold should be used for small burns but not for large burns because hypothermia could result. Ice should not be applied directly because frostbite can increase tissue injury. Cold water can help relieve the pain of first- and second-degree burns, but patients with significant burns involving more than 9% of their total body surface area should not have cold applied.

**TIPS AND TRICKS**

**Escharotomy**

Consider local anesthesia (lidocaine).

Pack the wound with gauze impregnated with topical antibiotic.

Treat the escharotomy wound as part of the burn.

**Anesthesia**

Large doses of intravenous narcotics may be necessary.

Intubated patients still have pain—address it.

**Dressings**

First, ensure adequate anesthesia.

Gently clean the wound with normal saline solution.

Assess the depth of each wound individually.

For superficial wounds, dress with a topical antibiotic and cover with gauze.

For deep wounds, consider burn unit referral, surgical débridement, or application of a dry dressing.

**Table 189.2 Eschar Treatment**

| TYPE OF ESCHAR | RECOGNITION | APPROACH |
|---|---|---|
| Chest eschar | Burn across the chest with difficulty expanding the chest, possible increased peak pressures if on a ventilator | Anesthetize and cut to subcutaneous fat on the chest in the anterior axillary lines from the clavicles to the inferior costal margins; connect these incisions superiorly and inferiorly, with possible other transverse incisions needed if ventilation is still not possible. |
| Extremity eschar | Burn of the extremity with vascular compromise in the extremity | Anesthetize and cut to subcutaneous fat on the medial and lateral sides of the extremity from 1 cm proximal to the eschar to 1 cm distal to the eschar, with care taken at sites where vascular or neurologic injury may occur. |
| Neck eschar | Circumferential burn of the neck | Anesthetize and cut to subcutaneous fat on the lateral and posterior aspects of the neck; avoid the carotid or jugular venous structures. |
| Penile eschar | Circumferential burn of the penis | Anesthetize and cut to subcutaneous fat on the midlateral portions of the penis; avoid the dorsal penile vein. |
| Hand eschar | Circumferential burn of the hand with evidence of vascular compromise | Anesthetize and cut to subcutaneous fat on the lateral side of each finger, the palmar crease, and between the metacarpals on the dorsum of the palm. |
| Abdominal wall eschar | Burn of the abdominal wall with evidence of increasing intraabdominal pressure (elevated bladder pressure) | Anesthetize and cut to subcutaneous fat on the lateral sides of the abdominal wall. |

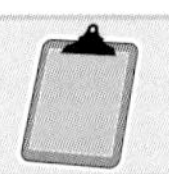

## DOCUMENTATION

**History**

Circumstances of the burn, timing, type of material burning, presence of associated trauma, presence of other victims, presence of voice change, presence of pain or paresthesias, weakness, tetanus status, medical conditions that may impair healing or compromise immune function, family situation

**Physical Examination**

Respiratory examination including signs of airway injury (soot in mouth, singed nasal hairs), neurovascular examination of all extremities, skin examination including wound size and depth, tenderness, neurologic examination, signs of concomitant trauma

**Studies**

None necessary unless associated with trauma; consideration of a chest radiograph for assessing pulmonary baseline status

**Medical Decision Making**

Reasons for intubation, reasons for transfer, initial cause of the thermal injury, follow-up plan

**Procedures**

Documentation regarding the need for escharotomy; if necessary, documentation of reversal of signs for escharotomy after the procedure

**Patient Instructions**

Documentation of discussion with the patient regarding the possibility of worsening injury and the warning signs of infection and vascular compromise; instructions on what to do and when to return

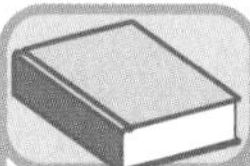

## PATIENT TEACHING TIPS

Inform all burn patients about the remote possibility that the burn may worsen over the next 24 hours, with tissue death possibly requiring grafts.

After the first couple of days, a normal wound should exhibit consistently gradual improvement in pain, swelling, size, and tissue color.

Inform patients that a burn may result in a scar and probably will; the size and shape of the scar can be addressed by a plastic surgeon, who may need to perform a scar revision to obtain the desired cosmetic result.

If any of the foregoing situations develop, the patient should know to return to the emergency department or to follow up with specialty referral.

Assure patients that if they follow these instructions, additional steps can then be taken to optimize recovery.

Care of a partial-thickness burn: Check the burn every day for signs of infection, such as increased pain, redness, swelling, or pus. If you see any of these signs, go to your doctor right away. To prevent infection, avoid breaking blisters. Change the dressing every day. First, wash your hands with soap and water. Then gently wash the burn and put antibiotic ointment on it. If the burn area is small, a dressing may not be needed during the day.

Burned skin itches as it heals. Keep your fingernails cut short and do not scratch the burned skin. The burned area will be sensitive to sunlight for up to 1 year. Sunscreen has been shown to decrease how severe scars appear and should be used regularly.

## FOLLOW-UP, NEXT STEPS IN CARE, AND PATIENT EDUCATION

Patients with major burns should receive care in a specialized burn center (see Box 189.1). Minor burns can be cared for on an outpatient basis with close follow-up and instructions for assessing for infection. Patients should be informed of what to expect over the days and weeks following their burn (see the "Patient Teaching Tips" box). All patients with concern for possible nonaccidental burns should be evaluated by both social services and law enforcement, and patients with self-inflicted injuries should be referred for psychiatric care. Any pediatric patient suspected of suffering abuse should be admitted to the hospital, even if the burn itself does not meet admission criteria, so that social services can ensure the child's safety (see the "Red Flags" box).

## REFERENCES

***References can be found on Expert Consult @ www.expertconsult.com.***

# 190 Chemical Burns

*Jeffrey Druck*

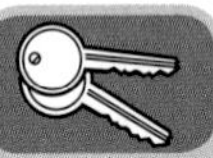

**KEY POINTS**

- Copious, immediate irrigation is the most important treatment of chemical burns.
- Elemental metal burns are the only chemical burns that should not be irrigated with water. Instead, wipe the material off with dry gauze and protect yourself from contamination.
- Identifying the cause of a chemical burn may be difficult, but the use of external resources (material safety data sheet, paramedics, employers, poison center) will help characterize the agents.
- Patients who exhibit no further signs of systemic toxicity may require only a chemistry panel and an electrocardiogram to complete an assessment.
- Patients with hydrofluoric acid burns require topical treatment with calcium gluconate gel, local infiltration of calcium gluconate, or for the most severe cases, intraarterial administration of calcium gluconate.

## EPIDEMIOLOGY

Chemical burns are an unusual type of burn because the tissue injury is caused by the chemical reaction rather than by thermal damage. Chemical burns are common at work, at home, or in association with hobbies. One study found 22% of all pediatric burns to be a result of chemical burns,[1] whereas other studies have estimated the percentage of admitted burned patients with chemical burns to be between 10% and 14%.[2,3] With the recent concerns over terrorism, chemical agents have been emphasized as a possible method of attack, so knowledge of chemical burns is critical in the education of today's emergency physicians. In addition, failure to recognize chemical burns or to treat them appropriately can have a detrimental impact not only on patients but also on care providers.

## PATHOPHYSIOLOGY

Different chemical burns affect tissue by different mechanisms. **Table 190.1** provides different categories of chemical agents and their mechanism of tissue damage. Most chemical burns involve skin; accordingly, knowledge of skin anatomy is key to understanding the pathophysiology of various chemical burns because of the link to treatment. A direct injury results when the epidermis is penetrated. Systemic absorption is possible once the injury extends through the dermis.

## PRESENTING SIGNS AND SYMPTOMS

A classic example of a chemical burn is an industrial worker who "got something" on his or her arm and pain and sloughing of the skin developed over the next few minutes. The burning may have continued despite irrigation. An alternative example may be someone who got something on his or her clothes and noticed burning and a "rash" after touching the clothing.

In our modern times, chemical agents may be used in a terrorist attack, so multiple victims with similar burns and systemic toxicity should trigger concern for a mass casualty event. In addition, burns that appear to worsen over short periods may not be thermal burns, as initially thought, but instead may be chemical.

## DIFFERENTIAL DIAGNOSIS AND MEDICAL DECISION MAKING

With chemical agents, the initial complaint may be a red, burning rash; because some agents cause a delayed onset of symptoms, chemical burns should be considered in the differential diagnosis of all rashes. However, there is usually a direct cause-and-effect relationship that makes the diagnosis easy. Treatment, however, varies with the agent, identification of which may be more difficult. The most important task is to identify the offending agent. Various resources can be used, but the best source of information is usually patients themselves. The job site may provide clues, but the employer should also have the material safety data sheet available. Paramedics or others can bring in bottles of the agent, which may have a list of ingredients. The presence of systemic symptoms may also suggest specific agents.

Although the specific agent may be difficult to identify without other information, further testing can assist in the diagnosis. pH paper can be used on the wound to determine the presence of acid or base. A chemistry panel may suggest acidosis, whereas hypocalcemia may suggest exposure to hydrofluoric acid.

The gowns and gloves readily available in the hospital are not sufficient for many substances. Most chemicals penetrate these materials immediately. Relatively inexpensive, chemical-resistant, multilayer suits are available. Furthermore, respiratory precautions may be indicated for some agents. For these reasons, both hospital and community resources may be required for safe and expedient decontamination.

## HAZARDOUS MATERIALS

The U.S. Department of Transportation requires color-coded identification of the type of material transported. These identifying codes are widely used. Additionally, a standard four-number code should be present to identify or characterize the agent more specifically. **Figure 190.1** indicates the general categories and identifying colors, which include the following:

- Explosives (solid orange)
- Nonflammable gases (solid green)
- Flammable liquids (solid red)
- Flammable solids (white and red stripes)
- Oxidizers and peroxides (solid yellow)
- Poisons and biohazards (solid white)
- Radioactive materials (half white, half yellow, with a black radiation symbol)
- Corrosives (half white, half black)
- Other (usually white)

**Table 190.1 Chemical Agents and Their Mechanisms of Tissue Damage**

| TYPE OF CHEMICAL AGENT | MECHANISM OF TISSUE DAMAGE | EXAMPLE OF AGENT |
|---|---|---|
| Acids | Coagulative necrosis | Sulfuric acid |
| Alkali agents | Saponification and liquefactive necrosis | Calcium hydroxide |
| Desiccants and vesicants | Dehydration of cells through exothermic reactions, release of amines within cells | Nitrogen mustards |
| Oxidizing and reducing agents | Denaturing of proteins and direct cytotoxic effects | Bleach |
| Protoplasmic poisons | Formation of salts with cellular proteins | Picric acid |

## TREATMENT

The first step in caring for patients with chemical burns is removal of the offending agent. This involves copious irrigation with several liters of either water or normal saline solution. All contaminated clothing should be removed, with care taken to ensure that health care providers are not exposed.

### ELEMENTAL METALS: DO NOT IRRIGATE

Regardless of the type of offending agent, copious irrigation is the first step, with one exception: elemental metals. Elemental sodium and potassium cause exothermic reactions when exposed to water, in addition to forming toxic alkali agents. Patients with these injuries should undergo specific decontamination and removal of the offending metal by brushing it off with gauze. The poison center may provide advice about proper disposal of the metal.

**Figure 190.2** is an algorithm for the management of patients with possible chemical burns.

### OCULAR EXPOSURE

Ocular chemical burns are highly morbid injuries. The initial therapy of copious irrigation cannot be emphasized enough. Lid retraction with eversion is a key procedure to remove all chemical particles. Testing for the continued presence of chemicals can be accomplished with pH paper, but it is important to wait a minimum of 5 minutes after irrigation to make sure that the pH of the irrigation fluid is not being checked. Patients with burns caused by certain chemicals may require admission for continuous irrigation. Any patient with ocular exposure that results in corneal burns (identified by fluorescein examination) should have an ophthalmology consultation. Other elements of the examination are similar to any eye examination and include visual acuity, slit-lamp examination, and visual field evaluation. Tap water is recommended as the initial irrigating agent (because it is the most easily obtained and time until irrigation is a key element), but normal saline, lactated Ringer solution, and buffered solutions all work effectively.[4]

### INGESTIONS

Although discussion of the management of caustic chemical ingestion is beyond the scope of this chapter, two key concepts should be emphasized. First, the primary issue is maintenance of the airway. Second, the extent of burn is usually limited to the initial exposure, and decontamination of the gastrointestinal tract is difficult and not recommended; the only substance that has been suggested is water, but because of possible exothermic reactions resulting from attempted water

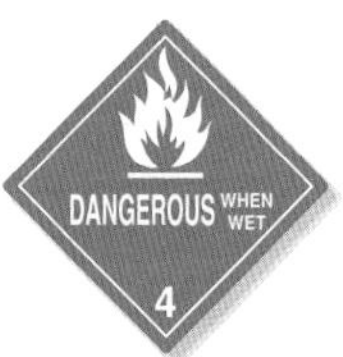

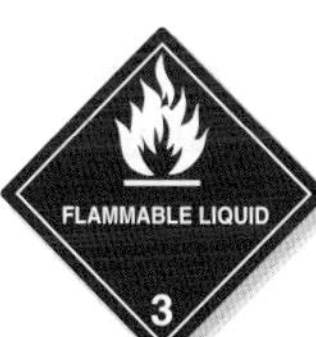

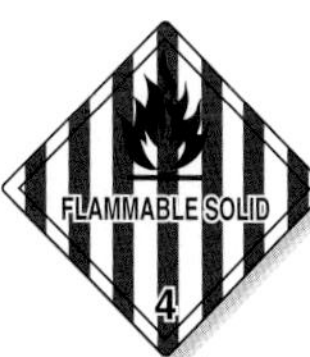

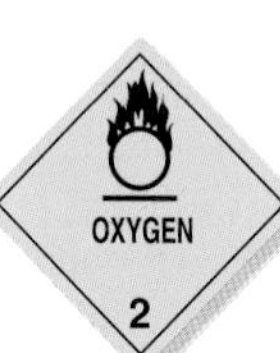

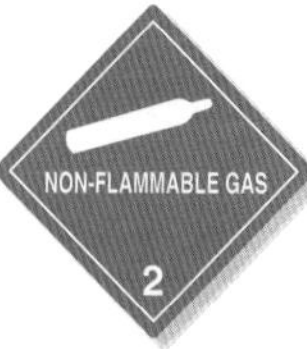


**Fig. 190.1 General categories and identifying colors for hazardous materials signs.**

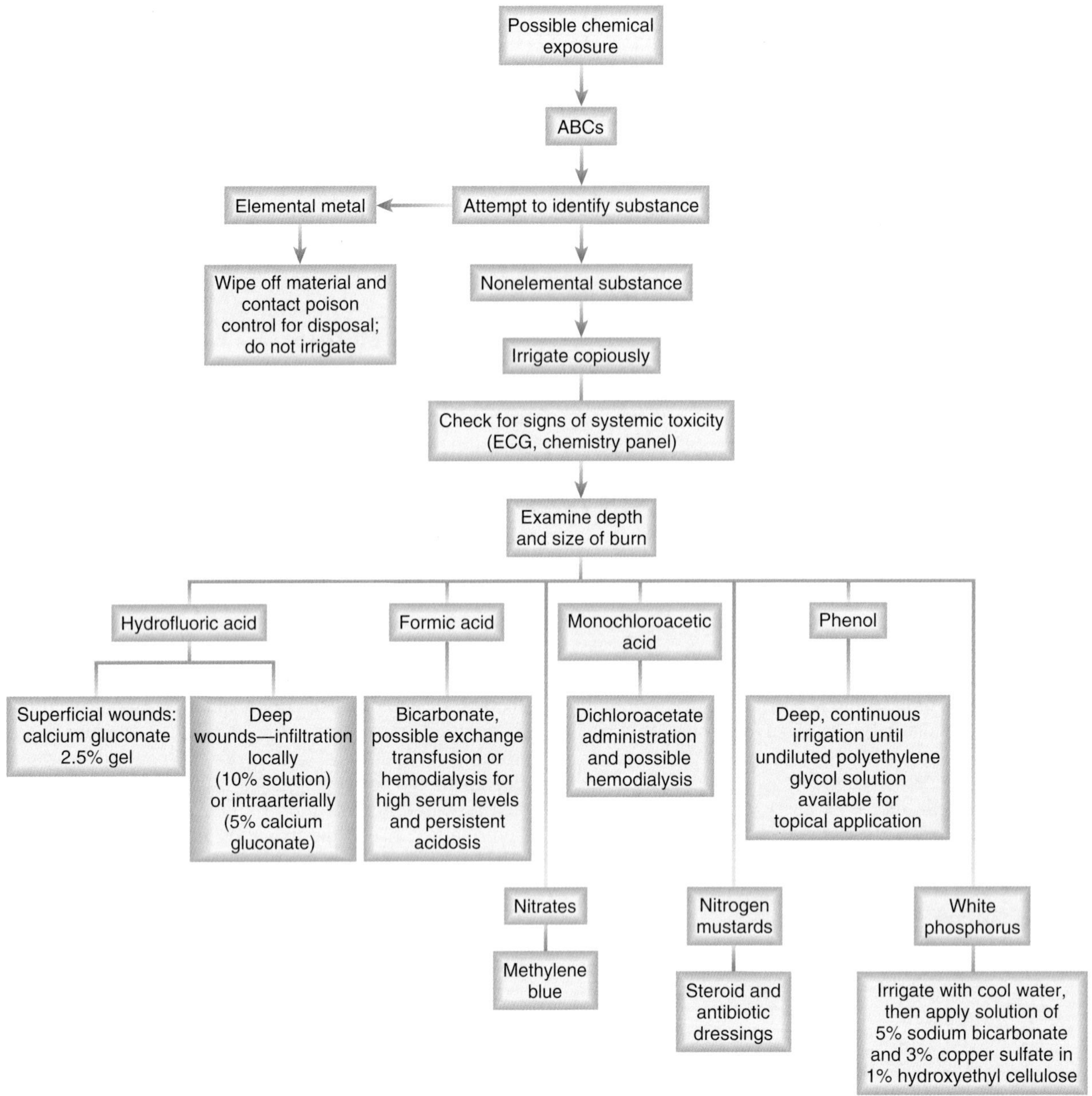


**Fig. 190.2 Algorithm for the treatment of chemical burns.**

irrigation, water decontamination of the gastrointestinal tract is controversial. Endoscopy is the only method for definitive assessment of the degree of injury, but the common complications of perforation and mediastinitis should also be assessed.[5] Some recent studies suggest that not every patient with a chemical burn involving the esophagus requires endoscopy, but consultation with gastroenterology and toxicology is recommended.[6]

## INHALATIONAL INJURY

Again, the primary issue in patients with inhalational injury is maintenance of the airway. For a variety of chemicals, the initial chest radiograph and the absence of respiratory symptoms belie the serious pulmonary edema or tracheobronchitis that may develop even days later. Consultation with the local poison control center while supportive measures are being instituted is the recommended pathway of care.

## DIRECTED THERAPIES

Specific agents are known to cause specific toxicities. If the substance is known, therapy should be directed against that toxicity (**Table 190.2**).

### *Hydrofluoric Acid*

Hydrofluoric acid is used in glass etching, automotive and industrial wheel cleaning, brick cleaning, semiconductor manufacturing, metal purification, and other industries. Immediate irrigation is indicated, as with other chemical injuries, but hydrofluoric acid can cause progressive tissue damage. Extensive exposure of an uncovered arm or leg can

**Table 190.2 Specific Therapies for Chemical Burns**

| AGENT | SPECIFIC TOXICITY | ADDITIONAL TREATMENT |
|---|---|---|
| Hydrofluoric acid | Severe hypocalcemia and continued liquefactive necrosis | Superficial wounds: calcium gluconate 2.5% gel<br>Deep wounds: local infiltration (10% solution) or intraarterial injection (5% solution) of calcium gluconate |
| Formic acid | Severe acidosis | Bicarbonate administration, possible exchange transfusions or hemodialysis for high serum levels and persistent acidosis |
| Cement (alkali burn) | Persistent burns when exposed to water if not irrigated away completely | Thorough irrigation |
| Phenol | Systemic absorption causing central nervous system depression, coma, and death | Because a more dilute solution is absorbed more rapidly, deep, continuous irrigation is performed until undiluted polyethylene glycol solution is available for topical application; all other treatment is supportive for systemic symptoms |
| White phosphorus | Continued thermal burning resulting from burns on exposure to oxygen; systemic absorption causing acidosis and electrocardiographic abnormalities, possibly sudden death | Removal of as much phosphorus as possible through irrigation with cool water, then placement of a solution of 5% sodium bicarbonate and 3% copper sulfate in 1% hydroxyethyl cellulose |
| Elemental metals (sodium, potassium) | Exothermic reaction when exposed to water | Wiping away of material and contacting a poison control center for disposal instructions |
| Nitrates | Methemoglobinemia | Administration of methylene blue |
| Monochloroacetic acid | Systemic lactic acidosis | Administration of dichloroacetate and possible hemodialysis |
| Nitrogen mustards | Vesicle formation | Steroid and antibiotic dressings after copious irrigation |

be fatal. Pain may be delayed but can subsequently continue for hours or days. The hydrofluoric acid ion does not dissociate but rather penetrates tissues deeply and reacts with calcium and magnesium. Hypocalcemia can result.

Patients with mild, limited superficial exposure can be treated with topical calcium gluconate, which must usually be mixed in the emergency department by combining calcium gluconate powder with commonly available lubricant jelly. Affected fingers and hands can be placed in a medical glove that contains the solution.[7]

Subcutaneous infiltration of 10% calcium gluconate may help relieve the pain, but it also irritates the tissue. Slow infiltration with the smallest available needle, preferably 30 gauge, or dilution of the solution may minimize tissue damage. Intraarterial administration of 10 mL of calcium gluconate mixed in 50 mL of 5% dextrose in water through the radial or ulnar artery via an arterial line over a 4-hour period may be beneficial for severe exposures to the hand.

Cardiac dysrhythmias may result from systemic hypocalcemia and hypomagnesemia. The electrocardiogram should be monitored for QT prolongation. Calcium and magnesium should be administered as needed.

## FOLLOW-UP, NEXT STEPS IN CARE, AND PATIENT EDUCATION

After determination of the offending agent and copious irrigation until no further chemical remains (for acids and bases, this can be determined with pH paper), disposition of the patient should be based on the presence of systemic symptoms, the size and depth of the burn, the nature of the agent, and access to appropriate follow-up. All patients should be warned about scarring and the potential for infection. The circumstances of the exposure should be verified, and appropriate state and local authorities should be notified about exposures in industrial incidents.

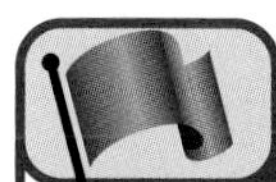

**RED FLAGS**

**Scenarios Suggestive of Specific Types of Chemical Burns**

| Scenario | Suspicious Agent |
|---|---|
| Circumferential lower extremity burns above the sock line | Cement |
| Burn in a glass etcher | Hydrofluoric acid |
| Burn from fireworks | White phosphorus |
| Mass exposure (terrorist attack) | Nitrogen mustard |

## REFERENCES

*References can be found on Expert Consult @ www.expertconsult.com.*

# 191 Approach to the Adult Rash

*Heather Murphy-Lavoie and Tracy Leigh LeGros*

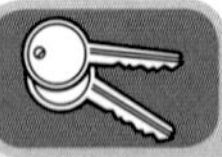

**KEY POINTS**

- Rashes are a common reason for a visit to the emergency department. Some rashes are simple and straightforward. However, others represent the initial complaint of a patient with a life-threatening disease.
- Fever with a rash is key to recognizing some of the more dangerous conditions.
- The key for differentiating a diffusely erythematous rash includes the presence or absence of the Nikolsky sign.
- Key factors for differentiating a maculopapular rash include its distribution and target lesions.
- A vesiculobullous rash is also differentiated by distribution; a localized or diffuse distribution helps narrow the differential diagnosis.
- Petechial/purpuric rashes are differentiated by the presence or absence of palpable lesions.
- Petechiae do not blanch with pressure.
- Palpable purpura occurs in vasculitic diseases secondary to inflammation or infection.
- Nonpalpable purpura is characteristic of thrombocytopenic conditions.
- Bullous rash with mucosal involvement is worrisome, and steroid therapy may be warranted.
- A careful history and physical examination are crucial for narrowing the differential diagnosis of an unknown rash.

## EPIDEMIOLOGY

Evaluation of rashes ranks highly among the top 20 reasons for visits to the emergency department.

A well-reasoned algorithmic approach to the evaluation of rashes might aid the emergency medicine specialist in identifying the most common and potentially lethal rash syndromes. Although an exhaustive review of all potential fungal, parasitic, and viral causes of rash is beyond the scope of this chapter, the algorithms presented will equip physicians to quickly recognize the most common and critical rashes. Pediatric rashes are discussed in detail in Chapter 18. Additionally, the most life-threatening rashes are discussed in more detail in Chapter 192.

## PATHOPHYSIOLOGY

A rash is a skin eruption that has a defined morphology and location. The morphology of the rash is usually distinct and related to the pathophysiologic dysfunction of the skin. Most severe rashes begin as exanthems (from the Greek *exanthema*, which means "breaking out," and *anthos*, which means "flowering"). These rashes subsequently take on a particular morphology, characteristic lesions, or distribution. **Table 191.1** delineates the most common terms used for skin lesions. Understanding these terms helps one better document progression of disease and facilitates communication with consulting physicians.

## PRESENTING SIGNS AND SYMPTOMS

Eliciting the initial distribution and progression of a rash is essential. Additionally, the involvement of palms, soles, and mucous membrane is of key importance. It should be kept in mind that dysphasia, as well as eye or genital irritation, may be a manifestation of as mucosal involvement and is often the initial symptom of several life-threatening conditions. The rash's rapidity of progression is also an essential in diagnosis. **Box 191.1** categorizes these important findings.

### PHYSICAL EXAMINATION TIPS

Evaluation of vital signs is essential. Fever and hypotension, in particular, are ominous findings that mandate expedited and intensive care. Additional findings of concern on physical examination include a new-onset heart murmur or nuchal rigidity. Generalized lymphadenopathy is present with many illnesses, including mononucleosis, human immunodeficiency virus (HIV) infection, other infections, serum sickness, and drug reactions.

To ensure that lesions on the back, buttocks, and perineum are identified, patients should be completely undressed. Patients are often unaware of lesions present in these locations. Shoes and socks should also be removed, especially in diabetic patients. Toenails should be inspected closely for signs of systemic disease or fungal infection. Some fungal foot infections can cause an id (autoeczematization) reaction and exacerbate eczema in the upper extremities. Treatment of the fungal infection will be necessary to control the dermatitis. Additionally, the fingers, toes, palms, and soles should be examined closely for the distribution of the rash and stigmata of endocarditis.

**Table 191.1 Common Terms for Skin Lesions**

| TERM | DESCRIPTION |
|---|---|
| Lesion | Single small diseased area |
| Macule | Circumscribed area of change without elevation |
| Rash | Skin eruption that is more extensive than a single lesion |
| Papule | Solid raised lesion < 1 cm |
| Nodule | Solid raised lesion > 1 cm |
| Plaque | Raised confluence of papules > 1 cm |
| Pustule | Fluid-filled area containing purulence |
| Vesicle | Fluid-filled area < 1 cm containing clear fluid |
| Bullae | Fluid-filled area > 1 cm |
| Petechiae | Pinpoint flat round spots < 3 mm caused by intradermal bleeding that do not blanch |
| Purpura | Hemorrhagic area > 3 mm that does not blanch |
| Exanthem | Rash outside the body (skin) |
| Enanthem | Rash inside the body (mucous membranes) |

**BOX 191.1 Distribution and Progression of a Rash**

**Distribution and Spread**

Begin peripherally, then spread centrally
- Rocky Mountain spotted fever
- Erythema multiforme
- Vasculitides

Begin centrally, then spread peripherally
- Viral exanthems
- Smallpox

**Involvement of Palms and Soles**

Diffuse involvement (more serious and lethal)
- Rocky Mountain spotted fever
- Erythema multiforme
- Stevens-Johnson syndrome
- Toxic epidermal necrolysis
- Syphilis
- Bacteremic endocarditis

Localized involvement
- Contact dermatitis
- Infectious process

**Involvement of Mucous Membranes**

Toxic epidermal necrolysis
Stevens-Johnson syndrome
Pemphigus vulgaris
Kawasaki disease
Viral syndromes

**Rapidity of Rash Progression**

Spread in minutes
- Urticarial anaphylaxis

Spread in hours
- Meningococcemia

Spread in days
- Drug reactions

## SPECIFIC SIGNS

Two signs are important in the evaluation of these rashes: the Nikolsky sign and the Asboe-Hansen sign. A positive Nikolsky sign (**Fig. 191.1**) is noted when slight rubbing of the skin results in exfoliation of the outermost layer with lateral extension of the erosion into the intact skin. The area of denuded skin is pink and tender. The Asboe-Hansen sign (indirect Nikolsky sign or Nikolsky II sign) is extension of a blister into normal skin with the application of light pressure on the top of the blister. All patients with tender, blistering, or sloughing skin should be evaluated serially for these important signs.

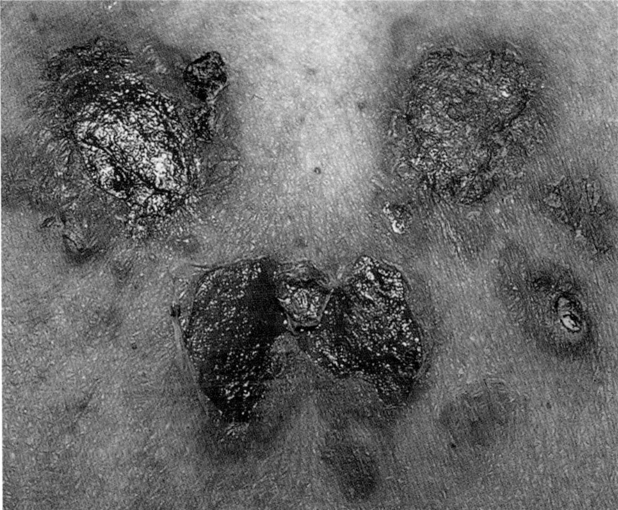

**Fig. 191.1** Fragile blisters rupture easily to form painful erosions. Finger pressure separates normal-appearing epidermis and produces an erosion (Nikolsky sign). Pressure on the edge of a blister spreads the blister into unaffected skin (Asboe-Itansen sign). (From Habif TP, editor. Clinical dermatology, 5th ed. Philadelphia: Mosby; 2009. Figure 16-14.)

# DIFFERENTIAL DIAGNOSES AND MEDICAL DECISION MAKING

History taking is an essential component in formulating appropriate differential diagnoses and guiding medical decision making. Inquiry regarding the patient's travel, medical, occupational, recreational, and medicinal history is required. Once the history and physical examination are complete, in-depth evaluation of the rash is in order. The differential diagnoses can be narrowed by categorizing the rash as erythematous, maculopapular, petechial/purpuric, or vesiculobullous.

## TRAVEL HISTORY

Lyme disease is common in the mid-Atlantic, central, western, and northeastern parts of the United States. Patients who have recently traveled to the Caribbean may have dengue fever. In addition, patients reporting recent camping and travel through

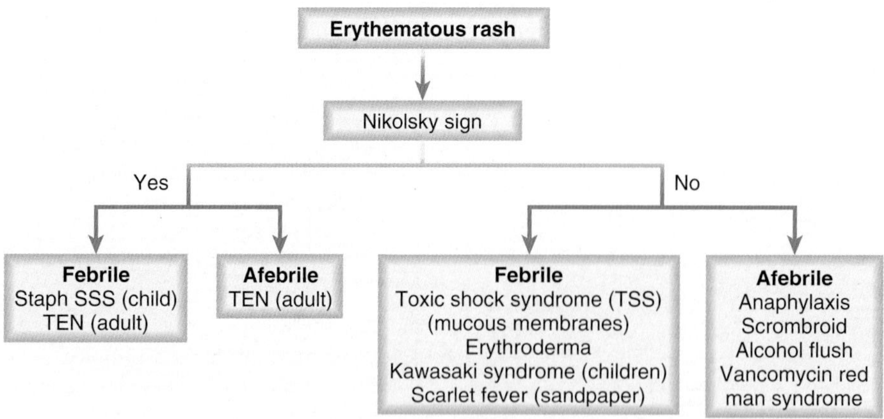


**Fig. 191.2 Algorithm for erythematous rashes.** *SSS*, Scalded skin syndrome; *TEN*, toxic epidermal necrolysis (From Murphy-Lavoie H, LeGros TL. Emergent diagnosis of the unknown rash: an algorithmic approach. Emerg Med 2010;42[3]:6-17.)

wooded areas are candidates for Rocky Mountain spotted fever (RMSF) and other tick-borne illnesses.

## MEDICAL, OCCUPATIONAL, AND RECREATIONAL HISTORY

Patients with diabetes, HIV infection, or a history of intravenous drug abuse and patients undergoing chemotherapy are at risk for diseases associated with high morbidity and mortality (meningococcemia, thrombotic thrombocytopenic purpura [TTP], necrotizing fasciitis, disseminated zoster, Stevens-Johnson syndrome [SJS], toxic epidermal necrolysis [TEN], and sepsis). Persons with valvular heart disease are at increased risk for endocarditis. College students, military personnel, and employees of daycare facilities are more likely to contract meningococcemia. Hunters and campers are at risk for tick-borne illnesses.

## MEDICINAL HISTORY

Potentially lethal drug reactions such as SJS, TEN, anaphylaxis, and angioedema mandate specific and emergency interventions, but discontinuing the offending agent is the initial step. This will reduce the risk for death by 30% daily! Additionally, many patients self-treat rashes before seeking medical care. Steroid creams, in particular, may significantly alter the morphology of the rash. It is important to note any treatments before initial evaluation.

## THE ALGORITHMIC APPROACH

### *Erythematous Rashes*

These rashes are characterized by diffuse redness of the skin as a result of capillary congestion. Erythematous rashes are differentiated by the presence or absence of fever and the Nikolsky sign (**Fig. 191.2**).[1] If a Nikolsky sign is present, the diagnosis is narrowed substantially, usually to TEN in adults and to staphylococcal scalded skin syndrome (SSSS), generally in infants and young children. If fever is present without a Nikolsky sign, the differential diagnosis includes Kawasaki disease, scarlet fever, erythroderma, and toxic shock syndrome (TSS). Patients with an erythematous rash but without a fever or Nikolsky sign may be having an anaphylactic reaction or a reaction to vancomycin, scombroid, or alcohol exposure. Please refer to Chapter 18 for review of SSSS, Kawasaki disease, and scarlet fever. Refer to Chapter 192 for review of TEN, TSS, and erythroderma.

### *Maculopapular Rashes*

The term *maculopapule* is a portmanteau of macule and papule. Maculopapular rashes are differentiated by the distribution of the rash and systemic toxicity (**Fig. 191.3**). Patients with centrally distributed rashes who appear toxic and febrile have a wide differential diagnosis; however, it is paramount that patients living in endemic areas be assessed for Lyme disease. Those with centrally distributed rashes but no signs of toxicity usually have either a drug reaction or pityriasis rosea. Patients with peripherally distributed rashes have a broader differential diagnosis that is dependent on systemic toxicity, the presence or absence of target lesions, and whether the rash is located on the flexor or extensor surfaces. Target lesions (**Fig. 191.4**) are pathognomonic for SJS or erythema multiforme (EM). The target lesion of Lyme disease is usually a single large bull's eye that measures at least 5 cm in diameter (erythema migrans). Patients with peripheral lesions and systemic toxicity but without target lesions require emergency evaluation for meningococcemia, RMSF, and syphilis. Nontoxic patients with a peripherally distributed rash and no target lesions require further assessment for flexor involvement (scabies or eczema) or extensor involvement (psoriasis). Please refer to **Table 191.2** for review of EM minor and major. See Chapter 18 for review of viral exanthems. Please refer to Chapter 192 for review of Lyme disease, meningococcemia, RMSF, SJS, and syphilis.

### *Petechial/Purpuric Rashes*

These rashes can be especially challenging and are associated with devastating differential diagnoses; however, an algorithmic approach can help the physician narrow the diagnosis with confidence (**Fig. 191.5**). By definition, petechiae do not blanche with pressure; additionally, remembering the cause of palpable versus nonpalpable lesions is paramount. Palpable (raised) purpura occurs in vasculitic diseases secondary to inflammation or infection. Nonpalpable purpura (flat, subcutaneous hemorrhages) are seen with thrombocytopenic conditions. Patients with petechial/purpuric rashes and fever or toxicity require emergency evaluation. If the lesions are

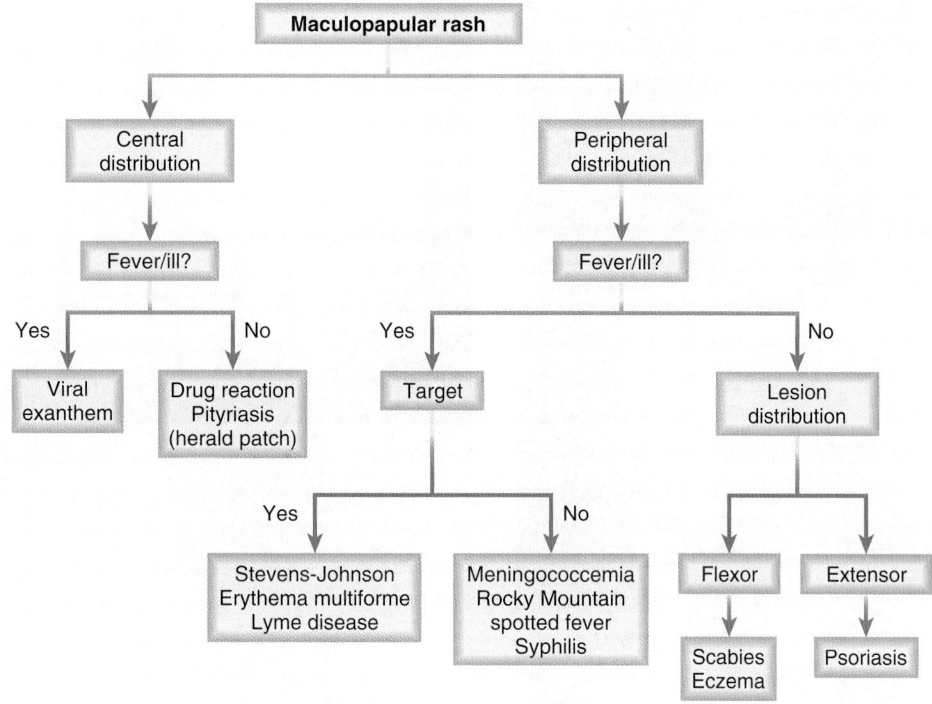


**Fig. 191.3 Algorithm for maculopapular rashes.** (From Murphy-Lavoie H, LeGros TL. Emergent diagnosis of the unknown rash: an algorithmic approach. Emerg Med 2010;42[3]:6-17.)

palpable, the differential diagnosis includes meningococcemia, disseminated gonococcal disease, endocarditis, RMSF, and Henoch-Schönlein purpura (HSP). Those with petechial/purpuric rashes and fever or toxicity but without palpable lesions may have purpura fulminans, disseminated intravascular coagulopathy (DIC), or TTP. If the patient is afebrile and has a petechial or purpuric rash, the diagnosis may be far simpler and less ominous. Nontoxic patients with palpable lesions may have a vasculitis; those with nonpalpable lesions may have idiopathic thrombocytopenic purpura (ITP). A detailed history may elucidate the cause of a vasculitis by identifying a key drug use history, recent illness, or an underlying symptom characteristic of the triggering disease.[5] In patients with ITP, it is important to exclude other causes of thrombocytopenia, including HIV infection, hepatitis, autoimmune disease, liver or renal disease, cancer, infection, pregnancy, alcohol use, and exposure to heparin or other inciting drugs or agents. Patient with ITP also require a full assessment of their risk for complications because of their thrombocytopenic condition, including age older than 60 years, engagement in athletic sport activities, peptic ulcer disease, menorrhagia, and intracranial hemorrhage.[4] Please refer to **Table 191.3** for review of disseminated gonococcemia, secondary vasculitis, and ITP. **Box 191.2** lists a vasculitis classification scheme, and these conditions are discussed in more detail in Chapter 110. Please refer to Chapter 18 for review of HSP and Chapter 192 for review of meningococcemia, endocarditis, RMSF, TTP, and purpura fulminans/DIC.

**BOX 191.2 Vasculitis Classifications**

**Large Vessel Vasculitis**
Temporal arteritis
Takayasu arteritis

**Medium Vessel Vasculitis**
Polyarteritis nodosa
Kawasaki disease

**Small Vessel Vasculitis**
Wegener granulomatosis
Churg-Strauss syndrome
Microscopic polyangiitis
Henoch-Schönlein purpura
Essential cryoglobulinemic vasculitis
Cutaneous leukocytoclastic vasculitis

## *Vesiculobullous Rashes*

Vesiculobullous rashes provoke significant angst in many physicians (**Fig. 191.6**). However, the differential diagnosis can be greatly simplified by categorizing patients with these rashes as febrile or afebrile and noting whether the distribution of the rash is diffuse or localized. Patients with a diffuse vesiculobullous rash and a fever may have varicella or a more devastating illness such as smallpox, disseminated gonococcal disease, or purpura fulminans/DIC. Necrotizing fasciitis and hand-foot-and-mouth disease are characterized by localized lesions and fever. In afebrile patients with a diffuse vesiculobullous rash, the differential diagnosis includes bullous pemphigus (BP) and pemphigus vulgaris (PV). One of the distinguishing features is based on the Nikolsky sign. A positive Nikolsky sign is seen with PV but is absent in BP. These

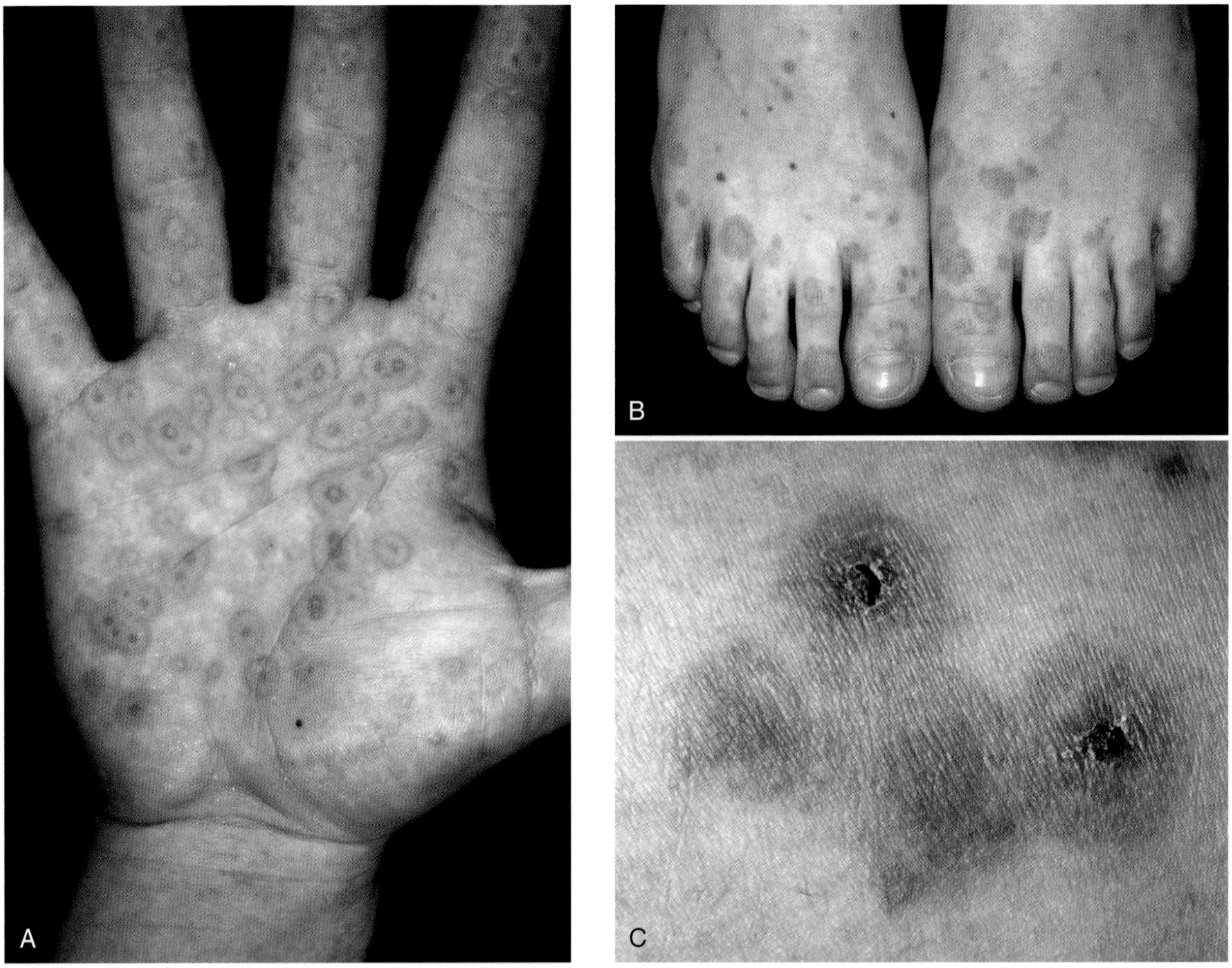

**Fig. 191.4** Target lesions on the palms and soles are highly characteristic of erythema multiforme. Lesions begin as dull red macules with a vesicle developing in the center. The periphery becomes cyanotic. (From Habif TP, editor. Clinical dermatology, 5th ed. Philadelphia: Mosby; 2009. Figure 18-4.)

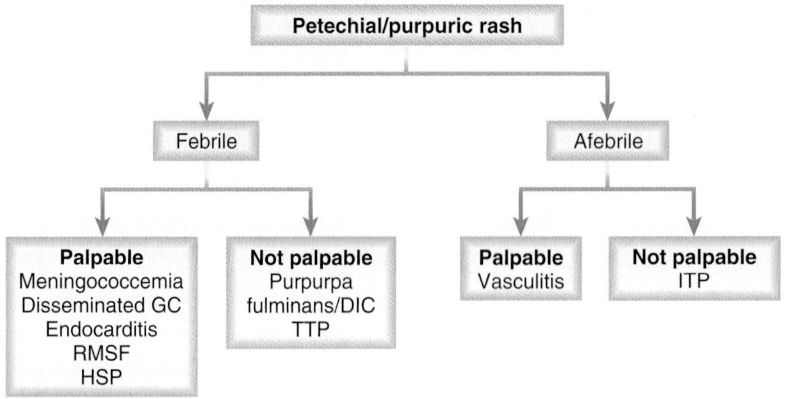


**Fig. 191.5 Algorithm for petechial/purpuric rashes.** *GC*, Gonococcal disease; *HSP*, Henoch-Schönlein purpura; *ITP*, idiopathic thrombocytopenic purpura; *RMSF*, Rocky Mountain spotted fever; *TTP*, thrombotic thrombocytopenic purpura. (From Murphy-Lavoie H, LeGros TL. Emergent diagnosis of the unknown rash: an algorithmic approach. Emerg Med 2010;42[3]:6-17.)

**Table 191.2 Erythema Multiforme**

| | | |
|---|---|---|
| Causes | Possibly autoimmune<br>Unknown in 50% | |
| Exposures | Infections: herpes simplex, *Mycoplasma*, fungi<br>Drug exposures: sulfa and other antibiotics, anticonvulsants | |
| Classification | Erythema multiforme minor | Erythema multiforme major |
| Description | Mild, self-limited rash | Severe, life-threatening disease with significant mucous membrane involvement[2] |
| Prodromal symptoms | No prodromal symptoms | Mild upper respiratory infection with moderate fever<br>Cough, sore throat, chest pain<br>Vomiting and diarrhea<br>Rash appears in 1-2 wk |
| Rash characteristics | Symmetric extremity lesions that develop into target lesions | Begins as a maculopapular rash that evolves into target lesions; rapidly progressive with centripetal spread |
| Distribution | Lower extremities | Palms, soles, dorsa of hands, face, and extensor surfaces |
| Mucous membrane involvement | None | Significant mucous membrane involvement<br>Eye involvement (10%); often bilateral, purulent conjunctivitis |
| Pruritic | Yes | No |
| Diagnosis | Confirmed with biopsy | Confirmed with biopsy |
| Treatment | Usually outpatient management<br>Symptomatic support<br>Analgesics<br>Cold compresses<br>Topical steroids<br>Treatment of the cause<br>Discontinue use of the offending agent<br>Dermatology follow-up | Usually inpatient management<br>Treatment of the cause<br>Discontinue use of the offending agent<br>Fluid and electrolyte balance<br>Analgesics<br>Wound care (avoid silver sulfadiazine)<br>Soothing oral solutions[3]<br>Dermatology consultation[3]<br>Ophthalmologic consultation[3]<br>Intravenous steroids may increase complications |
| Physical examination pearl | In contrast to Stevens-Johnson syndrome or toxic epidermal necrolysis, the target lesions of erythema multiforme are discrete rather than confluent, and the skin is not usually tender. The skin is very tender with toxic epidermal necrolysis | |

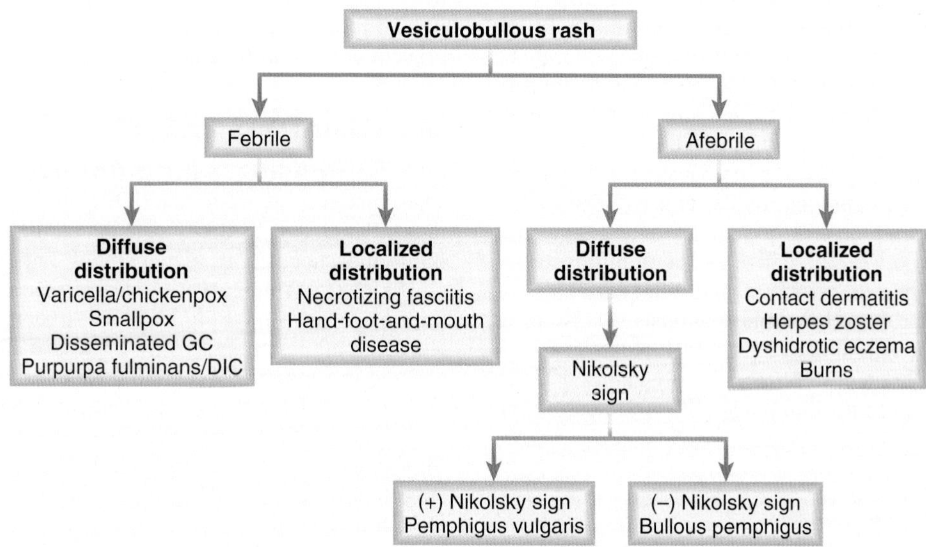


**Fig. 191.6 Algorithm for vesiculobullous rashes.** *DIC*, Disseminated intravascular coagulopathy; *GC*, gonococcal disease. (From Murphy-Lavoie H, LeGros TL. Emergent diagnosis of the unknown rash: an algorithmic approach. Emerg Med 2010;42[3]:6-17.)

**Table 191.3 Selected Petechial/Purpuric Rashes**

| | DISSEMINATED GONOCOCCEMIA | SECONDARY VASCULITIS | IDIOPATHIC THROMBOCYTOPENIC PURPURA |
|---|---|---|---|
| Causes | *Neisseria gonorrhoeae*<br>More frequent in women<br>Associated with menses | Infection or inflammation<br>Malignancy<br>Collagen vascular disease<br>Sarcoid<br>Drug reactions[5,6]<br>Antibiotics, analgesics<br>Urticaria<br>Cryoglobulinemia<br>Transplantation | Isolated thrombocytopenia (peripheral destruction) as a result of IgG antibodies against platelet membrane proteins[4]<br>Preceding infection common |
| Signs and symptoms | Petechial rash<br>Fever<br>Constitutional symptoms[7]<br>Arthralgias<br>May be migratory<br>Two thirds are polyarthralgias<br>Tenosynovitis | Rash (usually asymptomatic)<br>Nonthrombogenic palpable purpuric crops on lower extremities and buttocks (88%)[5]<br>Necrotic or crusted ulcers[5]<br>Nonspecific symptoms[5]<br>Fever, joint pain<br>Diarrhea, abdominal pain<br>Pruritus | Bleeding diathesis<br>Bruising<br>Hemorrhagic bullae on mucous membranes<br>Epistaxis<br>Menorrhagia<br>More acute manifestation in children<br>More chronic manifestation in adults |
| Work-up | Cultures<br>Blood<br>Cervical, penile<br>Throat<br>Gram stain<br>Sexually transmitted disease screens | Detailed history<br>Skin biopsy<br>Direct immunofluorescence | Exclude other thrombocytopenias<br>Assess increase in bleeding risk[7] |
| Treatment | Ceftriaxone intravenously<br>Ciprofloxacin for cephalosporin-allergic patients | Nontoxic patients<br>Discharge<br>Close follow-up<br>Admission for ill patients<br>Hypertension<br>Pulmonary hemorrhage<br>End-organ damage<br>Changes in mental status<br>Ill appearance | Hospital admission<br>High-dose intravenous glucocorticoids<br>Intravenous immunoglobulin<br>Platelets for severe hemorrhage (immediately after intravenous immunoglobulin)<br>Emergency hematology consultation<br>Bone marrow evaluation<br>Patient > 60 yr<br>Consideration of splenectomy for persistent thrombocytopenia[8] |

entities are regularly confused, and it is essential to differentiate them urgently. It is important to remember that both BP and PV have strong associations and known triggers. For those with BP, the list of drug triggers includes furosemide, ibuprofen, captopril (or other thiol-containing compounds), penicillamine, and antibiotics. Patients with PV have similar drug triggers (with the addition of rifampin). Please refer to **Table 191.4** for additional associations for PV and BP. The differential diagnosis is simpler and less of an emergency in a patient who is afebrile with a localized vesiculobullous rash; contact dermatitis, herpes zoster, dyshidrotic eczema, and burns are included in the differential diagnosis. Please refer to Table 191.4 for a discussion of PV and BP. Refer to Chapters 18 and 192 for review of varicella and Chapter 192 for review of smallpox, purpura fulminans/DIC, and necrotizing fasciitis.

## TREATMENT

The type of rash, the overall health and physical reserves of the patient, and the rapidity of diagnosis determine treatment. Many of these diseases are associated with significant morbidity and mortality, and a high index of suspicion is required to prevent a delay in diagnosis.

## ERYTHEMATOUS RASHES

### *Febrile Patients with a Positive Nikolsky Sign*

These patients are systemically ill and require intensive treatment. Patients with SSSS usually require hospitalization for fluid and electrolyte management and supportive wound and skin care. Young, well-appearing patients with SSSS and minimal skin sloughing may be managed as outpatients. However, adult patients with SSSS have a 60% mortality rate and require much closer monitoring. Antibiotics are usually recommended, but is it unclear whether they measurably alter the course of the disease. Please refer to Chapters 18 and 192 for further review. Patients with TEN require immediate discontinuation of the offending agent, wound care, eye care, fluid and electrolyte resuscitation, and admission to either an intensive care unit (ICU) or burn unit. Intravenous immune globulin (IVIG) may be helpful, but it has yet to be approved by the Food and Drug Administration for this use. Most

**Table 191.4 Pemphigus Vulgaris and Bullous Pemphigus**

| | PEMPHIGUS VULGARIS | BULLOUS PEMPHIGUS |
|---|---|---|
| Causes | Generalized mucocutaneous autoimmune blistering | Chronic, cutaneous, autoimmune blistering |
| Characteristics | Patients 50-60 yr old<br>Initial mucosal involvement (60%)<br>Progression to nonpruritic skin blisters[9]<br>Possible skin sloughing<br>Nikolsky and Asboe-Hansen signs | Older patients (average age, 65 yr)<br>Infant incidence rising<br>Initial mucosal involvement (10-25%)[9]<br>Rash is generalized and bullous |
| Associations | Autoimmune disease<br>Myasthenia gravis<br>Thymoma<br>Triggers (drugs, emotional stress) | Triggers<br>Lichen planus/psoriasis<br>Ultraviolet radiation, x-ray therapy<br>Childhood vaccines<br>Drugs |
| Clinical sign | Positive Nikolsky sign | Negative Nikolsky sign |
| Diagnosis | Clinical findings<br>Skin biopsy | Clinical findings<br>Histopathologic evaluation of blister edges |
| Treatment | Hospital admission<br>Fluid and electrolyte balance<br>Pain control<br>Infection monitoring<br>Immunosuppressant drugs[9,10] | Supportive care<br>Oral or topical steroids<br>Tetracycline<br>Immunosuppressive agents<br>Dapsone<br>Dermatology consultation<br>Otolaryngologic consultation (mucosal involvement)<br>Ophthalmologic consultation (ocular involvement)[10] |
| Prognosis | Generally poor<br>50% mortality (before steroids)<br>10-20% with steroids[3] | Better prognosis<br>Less oral involvement<br>May persist for years (waxing and waning)<br>May be fatal in frail patients |

physicians recommend against steroid use. It is important to avoid sulfadiazine on these wounds because sulfa is a common offending agent.

### Febrile Patients Without a Positive Nikolsky Sign

These patients are systemically ill and require intensive treatment. Patients with TSS require immediate removal of the infective material, intravenous antibiotics, fluid resuscitation, ICU admission, and consideration of the use of IVIG. Erythroderma is a devastating and overwhelming disease. All patients require admission, fluid and electrolyte monitoring, skin care, antihistamines, prevention of secondary infection, treatment of the underlying cause, and topical steroids. Systemic steroids are controversial. Recovery is long and recurrences are common. Patients with Kawasaki syndrome require high-dose aspirin immediately, hospitalization, and IVIG. Those with scarlet fever require penicillin to prevent local suppurative complications and acute rheumatic fever. Please refer to Chapter 18 for review of scarlet fever. Refer to Chapter 192 for review of erythroderma. Refer to Chapters 18 and 192 for review of Kawasaki disease and TSS.

### Afebrile Patients Without a Nikolsky Sign

These patients have exposure reactions. Anaphylaxis is a medical emergency that calls for immediate intervention. These patients require intravenous access, cardiac monitoring, high-flow oxygen, fluid resuscitation, airway management as indicated (laryngeal edema), inhaled β-agonists (wheezing or stridor), corticosteroids or aminophylline (for refractory bronchospasm), and epinephrine. The use of epinephrine is not contraindicated in this emergency. However, there is a death correlation associated with delay in administration. Scombroid toxicity is treated with antihistamines and supportive care. Complications are rare, and usually no further treatment is needed. Patients who experience an alcohol flush reaction require supportive care and should limit their alcohol consumption because their symptoms are due to an accumulation of acetaldehyde, a known carcinogen. Vancomycin red man syndrome is a drug-induced infusion reaction characterized by flushing and an erythematous rash secondary to mast cell degranulation. Hypotension and angioedema may occur and require close monitoring. Treatment consists of antihistamines. An extreme vancomycin-induced drug reaction results in an overwhelming exfoliative dermatitis that requires hospital admission, fluid and electrolyte management, skin and wound care, topical steroids, and treatment of complications.

## MACULOPAPULAR RASHES

### Central Maculopapular Rashes in Febrile or Ill-Appearing Patients

These patients usually have viral exanthems. They are typically ill appearing with fever but are not moribund. Most patients respond to supportive care. Please refer to Chapter 18 for a discussion of pediatric exanthems.

### Central Maculopapular Rashes in Well-Appearing Patients

These patients may be having a drug reaction. Many drugs have been implicated: antibiotics, nonsteroidal antiinflammatory drugs (NSAIDs), chemotherapeutic agents, anticonvulsants, and psychotropics, among others. Treatment includes discontinuation of the offending agent, and most care is supportive. Severe reactions, such as SJS, TEN, and hypersensitivity reactions, require hospital admission, meticulous wound care, and intensive support. Pityriasis is also in the differential diagnosis of well-appearing patients with central maculopapular rashes, and usually no treatment is required because it is generally a self-limited disease. For symptomatic pruritus, zinc oxide and calamine lotion are useful.

### Peripheral Maculopapular Rashes in Febrile or Ill-Appearing Patients with Target Lesions

These patients may have EM major (refer to Table 191.2 for review). SJS and Lyme disease are also in the differential diagnosis. Treatment of SJS involves discontinuation of the offending agent, optimization of fluid and electrolyte balance, meticulous wound care, and ICU admission. For patients with Lyme disease, doxycycline is first-line treatment in nonpregnant adults. Children are treated with amoxicillin. Refer to Chapter 192 for further review of SJS and Lyme disease.

### Peripheral Maculopapular Rashes in Febrile or Ill-Appearing Patients Without Target Lesions

These patients may have meningococcemia, RMSF, or syphilis. Patients with meningococcemia require intravenous ceftriaxone, with vancomycin added in cases of diagnostic uncertainty or to cover resistant streptococcal meningitis. Dexamethasone reduces neurologic sequelae if administered early and before antibiotics if possible. These patients also require admission and continuous surveillance for end-organ damage and complications. RMSF is always in the differential diagnosis in patients with these rashes or in those in whom meningococcemia is suspected. With any diagnostic uncertainty, one should treat for both illnesses. Doxycycline is the drug of choice in all nonpregnant patients with RMSF, even children. Pregnant patients may be treated with chloramphenicol, although doxycycline should also be considered because it is simply more effective. Secondary syphilis is also a diagnostic possibility in these patients and should be treated with intramuscular penicillin G in all patients. Benzathine penicillin should not be used because it does not penetrate cerebrospinal fluid. Pregnant patients allergic to penicillin should undergo desensitization. Nonpregnant, penicillin-allergic patients may be treated with doxycycline.

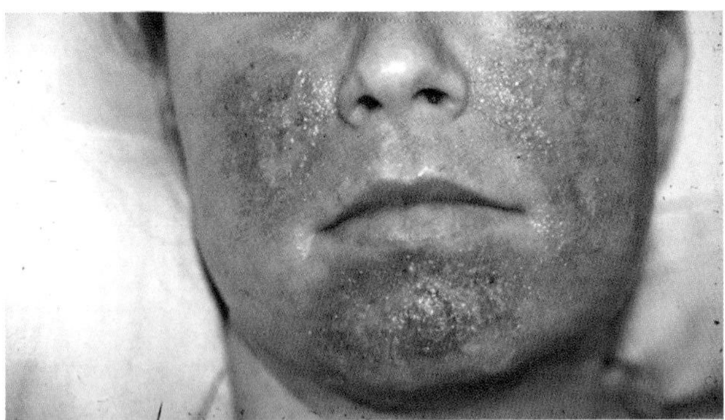

Fig. 191.7 Eczema.

Refer to Chapter 192 for further information on meningococcemia, RMSF, and syphilis.

### Peripheral, Flexural, Maculopapular Rashes in Well-Appearing Patients

These patients may have scabies or eczema. Scabies usually responds to household hygiene, a scabicide, and antihistamines. Eczema (**Fig. 191.7**) is treated with topical steroids, cold compresses, and ultraviolet light.

### Peripheral, Extensural, Maculopapular Rashes in Well-Appearing Patients

These patients may have psoriasis and usually respond well to the use of moisturizers, salicylic acid, light therapy, sun exposure, topical steroids, oatmeal baths, stress reduction, and dermatologic follow-up.

## PETECHIAL/PURPURIC RASHES

### Palpable Petechial/Purpuric Rashes in Febrile Patients

These patients have wide differential diagnoses with high morbidity and mortality. Meningococcemia and RMSF were discussed in the section related to the treatment of maculopapular rashes. Treatment of disseminated gonococcemia is reviewed in Table 191.3. Patients with endocarditis require early recognition, intensive therapy, broad-spectrum antibiotics to cover methicillin-resistant *Staphylococcus* (with subsequent guidance by blood cultures), and cardiology consultation. See Chapter 192 for further information on endocarditis. HSP is a small vessel vasculitis that is usually self-limited, and treatment is supportive. NSAIDs are used to reduce joint and soft tissue pain. Patients with significant bleeding, intussusception, and renal failure require admission for HSP. Please refer to Chapter 192 for review of endocarditis and Chapter 18 for review of HSP.

### Nonpalpable Petechial/Purpuric Rashes in Febrile Patients

Purpura fulminans and DIC are acutely life-threatening disorders that require emergency hematology consultation and ICU admission. First-line therapy is treatment of the underlying cause. Folate, vitamin K, fresh frozen plasma, cryoprecipitate, platelets, and red blood cell transfusions are given as needed. Heparin is also used for associated thrombi. These patients are very ill, and use of these therapies is best done in consultation with the ICU team and a hematologist. TTP is a devastating disease with greater than 90% mortality if not treated properly. Treatment includes emergency hematology consultation, treatment of the underlying cause, fresh frozen plasma (as a temporizing measure), plasmapheresis, and ICU admission. It is important to avoid platelet administration because it will precipitate more thrombus formation. Exchange transfusions can reduce mortality to 10%, and facilities without these capabilities should consider early transfer. Please refer to Chapter 192 for further review of purpura fulminans/DIC and TTP.

#### *Petechial/Purpuric Rashes in Afebrile Patients*

These patients may have a vasculitis (palpable rash) or ITP (nonpalpable rash). Please refer to Table 191.3 and Box 191.2 for reviews of these petechial/purpuric rashes.

### VESICULOBULLOUS RASHES

#### *Febrile Patients with a Diffuse Rash*

These patients may have varicella, smallpox, disseminated gonococcemia, or purpura fulminans/DIC. Varicella is a childhood viral exanthem (chickenpox) that is intensely pruritic. Treatment is supportive and consists of wet dressings, soothing baths, calamine lotion, surveillance for secondary infection, and antihistamines. The role of acyclovir in healthy children is unclear. Immunocompromised patients are at risk for significant complications. Maternal infection in the first trimester may result in devastating congenital varicella syndrome, whereas perinatal maternal infection predisposes to disseminated neonatal herpes. Smallpox is a dreaded variola infection against which 50% of the U.S. population has not been vaccinated. Care is supportive, and all personnel with smallpox exposure require quarantine and vaccination. The mortality rate is 30% in those who are unvaccinated. Treatment of disseminated gonococcemia is reviewed in Table 191.3. Treatment of purpura fulminans/DIC was reviewed with petechial/purpuric rashes. Please refer to Chapter 18 for review of varicella and Chapter 192 for review of smallpox and purpura fulminans/DIC.

#### *Febrile Patients with a Localized Rash*

Necrotizing fasciitis is in the differential diagnosis for these patients. It is an acutely toxic bacterial infection with very high mortality. Treatment consists of prompt surgical débridement, broad-spectrum antibiotics, and adjunctive hyperbaric oxygen therapy. Hand-foot-and-mouth disease is a highly contagious viral illness that requires symptomatic care for the painful oral ulcers. Complications are rare; however, infection during the first trimester of pregnancy may result in spontaneous abortion. Please refer to Chapter 192 for review of necrotizing fasciitis and Chapter 18 for review of hand-foot-and-mouth disease.

#### *Afebrile Patients with a Diffuse Rash*

These patients have either BP or PV. Both these diseases and their treatments are reviewed in Table 191.4.

#### *Afebrile Patients with a Localized Rash*

These patients may have herpes zoster, dyshidrotic eczema, or a local burn. Herpes zoster or shingles (caused by varicella virus) is a self-limited illness that will resolve without intervention. However, treatment is required for immunocompromised patients and those with ocular involvement or disseminated disease and is recommended for individuals older than 50 years, especially those with significant pain. High-risk patients require intravenous acyclovir, judicious administration of corticosteroids, ophthalmologic consultation (eye involvement), fluid and electrolyte monitoring, pain management, and supportive care. Treatment of dyshidrotic eczema was reviewed in the section on maculopapular rashes. Treatment of burns depends on the type, whether induced by trauma, chemicals, radiation, or heat. Treatment is also guided by the depth, severity, and surface area involved. Severe burn injuries are treated with intravenous fluid administration, early intubation (for airway involvement), removal or neutralization of the source of the injury, meticulous wound care, pain management, surgical intervention (early skin grafts or flaps, débridement, or escharotomy), and adjunctive hyperbaric oxygen therapy.

## FOLLOW-UP AND PATIENT EDUCATION

### PATIENTS WITH ERYTHEMATOUS RASHES

Follow-up is dependent on the cause of the rash, the patient's baseline immunologic health, disease complications, treatment side effects, and patient resources. Toxic patients with an erythematous rash require admission, intensive treatment, and close follow-up because all these diseases are associated with either very high morbidity and mortality or the potential for devastating complications. Patients with TSS require education regarding infective bacterial material. Those with SSSS, erythroderma, TSS, and TEN require close surveillance for secondary infections and wound care therapy. Patients with Kawasaki syndrome and scarlet fever require pediatric or primary care follow-up for monitoring of complications. Patients with severe exposure reactions (anaphylaxis and vancomycin) require intensive treatment, critical care monitoring, and close follow-up for complications related to end-organ damage or the exfoliative dermatitis associated with vancomycin-induced erythroderma. Less serious exposure reactions (scombroid and alcohol flush) require primary care follow-up and patient education regarding exposure toxicities.

### PATIENTS WITH MACULOPAPULAR RASHES

Patients with viral exanthems, drug reactions, and scabies have self-limited illnesses and benefit by close follow-up and patient education with their primary care provider regarding exposures and potential complications. Those with eczema, psoriasis, or pityriasis should be referred to a dermatologist for initial consultation and primary care follow-up. Patients with SJS or EM require close outpatient management for complications and wound care follow-up. Those with meningococcemia, RMSF, Lyme disease, or syphilis require primary care follow-up in conjunction with infectious disease consultation and monitoring.

### PATIENTS WITH PETECHIAL/PURPURIC RASHES

Patients with meningococcemia, disseminated gonococcemia, RMSF, and endocarditis require close primary care follow-up, as well as infectious disease consultation and monitoring. Additionally, follow-up of endocarditis should include cardiologist involvement. Patients with HSP should be monitored by their primary care physician for resolution of symptoms and for complications. Patients with purpura fulminans/DIC, ITP, and TTP must be monitored by a primary care provider, a hematologist, and a wound care specialist as needed. Those with vasculitis benefit from continued monitoring by their primary care provider, with dermatology consultation and wound care as appropriate.

## PATIENTS WITH VESICULOBULLOUS RASHES

Patients with varicella, hand-foot-and-mouth disease, herpes zoster, dyshidrotic eczema, and contact dermatitis benefit from close primary care follow-up for pain control and monitoring for complications. Patients with smallpox, disseminated gonococcemia, and necrotizing fasciitis should follow up with their primary care physician, an infectious disease specialist, and a wound care specialist as needed. Patients with necrotizing fasciitis should also receive follow-up from their attending surgeon. Patients with purpura fulminans/DIC require close monitoring for continued improvement by a primary care physician and a hematologist. Wound care may be needed. Those with BP and PV benefit from close primary care follow-up, as well as dermatologic consultation and wound care.

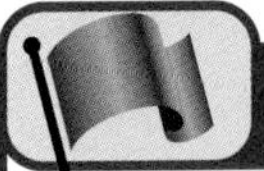

**RED FLAGS**

- Fever and petechiae/purpura
- Mucous membrane involvement
- Hemorrhagic bullae
- Nikolsky sign
- Nonpalpable petechiae with neurologic symptoms

## SUGGESTED READINGS

Carr DR, Houshmand E, Heffernan MP. Approach to the acute, generalized, blistering patient. Semin Cutan Med Surg 2007;26:139-46.

Mukasa Y, Craven N. Management of toxic epidermal necrolysis and related syndromes. Postgrad Med J 2008;84:60-5.

Murphy-Lavoie H, LeGros T. Emergent diagnosis of the unknown rash, the algorithmic approach. Emerg Med 2010;42(3):6-17.

Nguyen T, Freedman J. Dermatologic emergencies: diagnosing and managing life-threatening rashes. Emerg Med Pract 2002;4:1-28.

Rothe MJ, Bernstein ML, Grant-Kels JM. Life-threatening erythroderma: diagnosing and treating the "red man." Clin Dermatol 2005;23:206-17.

## REFERENCES

*References can be found on Expert Consult @ www.expertconsult.com.*

# Rash in the Severely Ill Patient 192

*Heather Murphy-Lavoie and Tracy Leigh LeGros*

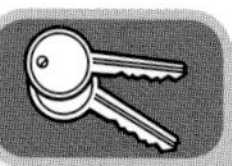

**KEY POINTS**

- Identification of rash morphology is paramount for elucidating the differential diagnoses of potentially lethal rashes.
- History taking must include occupation, travel, medications, comorbid conditions, and immune status.
- Complete and serial physical examinations are needed for proper evaluation of any patient with a potentially lethal rash.
- Blood cultures and early antibiotic administration are crucial because most potentially lethal rashes have an infectious cause.
- The clinical manifestations of Rocky Mountain spotted fever and meningococcemia are very similar. With any diagnostic uncertainty, treat for both.
- Petechial and purpuric rashes are marked by high morbidity and mortality.
- Petechiae and fever are very concerning. These patients may decompensate rapidly and require aggressive care.
- Palpable petechiae are due to vasculitides and may have an infectious cause.
- Nonpalpable petechiae are most often associated with thrombocytopenia.
- Hemorrhagic bullae are ominous.
- Patients with toxic epidermal necrolysis and other skin-sloughing diseases desquamate extensively and may require admission to a burn unit.

## INTRODUCTION

Early in the disease process, life-threatening rashes may occur in relatively well-appearing patients. However, these patients may deteriorate rapidly, and early resuscitative measures, including pressure support with central venous access, aggressive respiratory care, and broad-spectrum antibiotic therapy, are crucial. Early recognition of these potentially lethal rashes is facilitated by morphologic classification and refined by serial physical examination.

## PATHOPHYSIOLOGY

The pathophysiology of rashes in severely ill patients is broad and depends on the cause. Most of these rashes result from devastating bacterial infections, viral infections, tick bites, drug reactions, vasculitides, or environmental triggers. Many of these diseases also have a high predisposition in those with comorbid conditions.

## PRESENTING SIGNS AND SYMPTOMS

### HISTORY TAKING

The history is of paramount importance in the diagnosis of a patient with a rash. Of particular concern is an accounting of any recent travel, the patient's own geographic location, medical and occupational history, animal exposure, and medication regimens. **Table 192.1** classifies rashes in severely ill patients by exposure to geographic regions and animals.

### PHYSICAL EXAMINATION

At the start it is very important to evaluate the vital signs of toxic-appearing patients with rashes. Fever and hypotension are of particular concern and mandate expedited and intensive care. A complete examination should include evaluation for any new-onset heart murmur, changes in mental status, and nuchal rigidity. Of particular importance are the onset and progression of the rash; involvement of the palms, soles, and mucous membranes; and the age of the patient. An algorithmic approach can aid greatly in the identification of systemically ill patients with a rash. **Table 192.2** categorizes rash characteristics in severely ill patients.

### PHYSICAL SIGNS

Two signs are important in the evaluation of these rashes, the Nikolsky sign and the Asboe-Hansen sign. A positive Nikolsky sign (Fig. 191.1) is noted when slight rubbing of the skin results in exfoliation of the outermost layer with lateral extension of the erosion into intact skin. The area of denuded skin is pink and tender. The Asboe-Hansen sign (indirect Nikolsky sign or Nikolsky II sign) is extension of a blister into normal skin with the application of light pressure on top of the blister. All patients with tender, blistering, or sloughing skin should be evaluated serially for these important signs.

**Table 192.1 Rashes in Severely Ill Patients by Geographic and Animal Exposure**

| | DISEASE | DISEASE HIGHLIGHTS |
|---|---|---|
| **By Geographic Exposure** | | |
| Northeastern ⅔ of United States | Lyme disease | Erythema migrans<br>Bull's-eye formation |
| Caribbean | Dengue fever | Breakbone fever<br>Flushed skin and petechiae |
| Continental U.S. except Vermont and Maine | Rocky Mountain spotted fever | *Rickettsia rickettsii*<br>Maculopapular and centripetally spreading rash |
| Colombia | "Tobia fever" | |
| Brazil | "Sao Paulo fever" | |
| Mexico | "Fiebre Manchada" | |
| **By Animal Exposure** | | |
| | **DISEASE** | **DISEASE HIGHLIGHTS** |
| Farm animals, especially pregnant ones: cattle, goats, sheep | Q fever | Maculopapular truncal rash (20%); usually present with culture-negative endocarditis |
| Rats | Rat-bite fever | Constitutional symptoms, endocarditis, hepatitis, enteritis, and a rash around an open sore that may spread and appear red or purple; ulcerations of the hands and feet; wounds are slow to heal and may recur |
| Herbivores (plant eaters): buffalo, cattle, horse, deer, goat, rabbit, sheep, birds | Anthrax | Boil-like lesion that forms an ulcer with a painless black eschar<br>Exposure to infected or dead animals or their products |
| Bioterrorism | | |

**Table 192.2 Rash Characteristics in Severely Ill Patients**

| | |
|---|---|
| Centripetal progression | RMSF, EM major |
| Centrifugal progression | Viral exanthems, smallpox |
| Rash with palm and sole involvement | EM, RMSF, bacteremic endocarditis, syphilis, erythroderma |
| Rash with mucous membrane involvement | EM major, TEN, SJS, pemphigus vulgaris, syphilis |
| Rash with rapid spread | Urticaria, anaphylaxis, meningococcemia, erythroderma |
| Rash with hypotension | Meningococcemia, TSS, RMSF, TEN, SJS |
| 0-5 yr | Meningococcemia, Kawasaki disease, viral exanthems |
| >65 yr | Bullous pemphigus, sepsis, meningococcemia, TEN, SJS, TSS |

*EM*, Erythema multiforme; *RMFS*, Rocky Mountain spotted fever; *SJS*, Stevens-Johnson syndrome; *TEN*, toxic epidermal necrolysis; *TSS*, toxic shock syndrome

## DIFFERENTIAL DIAGNOIS AND MEDICAL DECISION MAKING

### ALGORITHMIC APPROACH TO CLASSIFICATION

It is helpful to first define the rash into one of four types: erythematous, maculopapular, vesiculobullous, or petechial/purpuric (see Chapter 191 for more detailed review). Erythematous rashes can then be further classified into those with or without a positive Nikolsky sign. Maculopapular rashes may be subdivided into those with or without target lesions. Vesiculobullous rashes should be differentiated into those with a localized or a diffuse distribution. Petechial/purpuric rashes should be classified into those with palpable or nonpalpable rash morphology (**Table 192.3**).

### ERYTHEMATOUS RASHES

Erythematous rashes are characterized by diffuse redness of the skin as a result of capillary congestion.

Toxic patients with an erythematous rash may have specific signs that narrow the differential diagnosis. The combination of an erythematous rash in a toxic patient with a positive Nikolsky sign reduces the differential diagnosis substantially, usually to toxic epidermal necrolysis (TEN) in adults and staphylococcal scalded skin syndrome (SSSS)

**Table 192.3** Differential Diagnoses of Severely Ill, Febrile/Toxic Patients with a Rash

| ERYTHEMATOUS | | MACULOPAPULAR | | VESSICULOBULLOUS | | PETECHIAL/PURPURIC RASH | |
|---|---|---|---|---|---|---|---|
| **Positive Nikolsky Sign** | **Negative Nikolsky Sign** | **Positive Target Lesions** | **Negative Target Lesions** | **Localized Distribution** | **Diffuse Distribution** | **Palpable Rash** | **Nonpalpable Rash** |
| TEN (adults)<br>SSSS (children) | TSS<br>Kawasaki disease (children)<br>Erythroderma | SJS<br>Lyme disease (erythema migrans) | RMSF<br>Syphilis<br>Meningococcemia | Necrotizing fasciitis | Varicella<br>Smallpox<br>Purpura fulminans/ DIC | RMSF<br>Endocarditis<br>Meningococcemia | TTP<br>Purpura fulminans/ DIC |

*DIC*, Disseminated intravascular coagulopathy; *RMSF*, Rocky Mountain spotted fever; *SJS*, Stevens-Johnson syndrome; *SSSS*, staphylococcal scalded skin syndrome; *TEN*, toxic epidermal necrolysis; *TSS*, toxic shock syndrome; *TTP*, thrombotic thrombocytopenic purpura

**Table 192.4** Selected Erythematous Rashes

| | TOXIC EPIDERMAL NECROLYSIS | STAPHYLOCOCCAL SCALDED SKIN SYNDROME | TOXIC SHOCK SYNDROME | ERYTHRODERMA (RED MAN SYNDROME) |
|---|---|---|---|---|
| Associations and triggers | Sulfa drugs<br>Anticonvulsants<br>Antivirals<br>NSAIDs<br>Allopurinol | Common illness:<br>Children<br>Neonates<br>Rare in adults:<br>Chronic illness<br>Renal failure<br>Immunodeficiency | Tampon use<br>Nasal packing[1]<br>Surgical wounds[1]<br>Postpartum[1] | Lymphoma<br>Leukemia<br>Medications<br>Cancer<br>Skin disorders<br>Many drugs<br>Heavy metals |
| Predispositions or increased risk[2] | Women<br>HIV infection<br>Head injury patients<br>Brain tumor patients<br>Lupus patients | Children < 5 yr<br>Males 2:1 | Recent varicella infection<br>Soft tissue infections<br>Major surgery | Generalized erythema<br>Scaling, sloughing<br>Nail, hair loss |
| Symptoms | Sudden diffuse erythema<br>Toxic appearing<br>Tender skin, blistering<br>Skin sloughing<br>Significant mucous membrane involvement | Scarlatiniform<br>Abrupt fever<br>Very tender skin<br>Blisters, sloughing<br>No mucous membrane involvement | Shock<br>Fever<br>Diffuse erythematous rash<br>Desquamation of extremities | >90% skin exfoliation<br>Large tissue loss<br>Fever, chills[3]<br>Fatigue[3]<br>Intense pruritis[3] |
| Clinical signs | Positive Asboe-Hansen sign<br>Positive Nikolsky sign | Positive Nikolsky sign | Negative Nikolsky sign | Negative Nikolsky sign |
| Mortality | 30-35% with optimal care | Children (<5%)<br>Adults (50-60%)[4,5] | 30-70%<br>Secondary to end-organ and multisystem organ damage | 20-40% |
| Treatment | Stop offending agent<br>Wound care<br>Eye care<br>Fluid, electrolyte balance<br>ICU or burn unit | Antibiotics<br>Fluid, electrolyte balance<br>Wound care | Remove infective material<br>IV antibiotics<br>Fluid resuscitation<br>ICU admission<br>Consider IVIG | Cancer work-up<br>Admission<br>Fluid, electrolyte balance<br>Wound care<br>Topical steroids[6]<br>Antihistamines |

*HIV*, Human immunodeficiency virus; *ICU*, intensive care unit; *IV*, intravenous; *IVIG*, intravenous immune globulin; *NSAIDs*, nonsteroidal antiinflammatory drugs.

in infants and young children. Alternatively, the differential diagnosis for toxic and febrile patients with an erythematous rash as well as a negative Nikolsky sign includes toxic shock syndrome (TSS), Kawasaki disease, and erythroderma (see Table 192.3). **Table 192.4** details the symptoms, signs, mortality, and treatment of the aforementioned erythematous rashes. SSSS, TSS, and Kawasaki disease are also covered in Chapter 18.

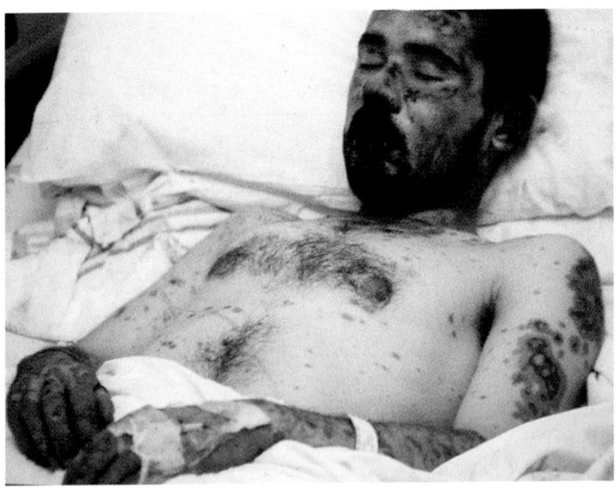

**Fig. 192.1** Toxic epidermal necrolysis.

### *Toxic Epidermal Necrolysis*

TEN (Lyell disease) is the most serious cutaneous drug reaction. It is most commonly associated with sulfa drugs; however, it has other important triggers as well. TEN is manifested as the sudden onset of diffuse erythema with tender skin and blistering. The skin cleavage is full thickness with positive Nikolsky and Asboe-Hansen signs and significant skin sloughing (**Fig. 192.1**). These patients are toxic and exhibit significant mucous membrane involvement. Symptoms occur first around the eyes, spread caudally (shoulders and upper extremities), and then progress to involve the entire body. Several populations are predisposed to TEN and others are at high risk (see Table 192.4). However, one group deserves expanded mention. It is important to consider that patients infected with human immunodeficiency virus (HIV) who are on a chronic regimen of trimethoprim-sulfamethoxazole prophylaxis and other polypharmacy have a 1000 times greater risk for TEN than do those without HIV.[2,7]

### *Staphylococcal Scalded Skin Syndrome*

Also known as Ritter disease or dermatitis exfoliativa neonatorum,[4] SSSS is manifested as a scarlatiniform, erythematous rash caused by a staphylococcal infection that blisters and sloughs (positive Nikolsky sign). Children younger than 5 years are at highest risk.

### *Toxic Shock Syndrome*

This toxin-mediated staphylococcal or streptococcal infection is historically associated with tampon use, although any staphylococcal or streptococcal source can precipitate TSS. Up to 45% of cases are unrelated to menses. Patients are overtly toxic, febrile, and in shock with a diffuse erythematous rash that eventually leads to desquamation of the hands and feet. The mortality associated with TSS is 30% to 70% and is usually due to multisystem organ failure and end-organ damage. Complications include azotemia, rhabdomyolysis, encephalopathy, thrombocytopenia, and liver dysfunction.

### *Kawasaki Disease*

This childhood illness is also known as mucocutaneous lymph node syndrome or infantile polyarteritis. It is a vasculitis of unknown cause, although infective and autoimmune theories abound. It affects many organ systems, including the skin, mucous membranes, lymph nodes, and blood vessels. Diagnostic criteria include high fever for at least 5 days, diffuse erythroderma of the skin, strawberry tongue, significant cervical lymphadenopathy, conjunctival injection, peeling of the fingers and toes, and edema of the extremities.[8] Thrombocytosis may also be present. By far the most serious complication is vasculitis of the coronary arteries, which leads to coronary vessel aneurysms, myocarditis, and myocardial infarction (even in the very young). Treatment consists of high-dose aspirin (given immediately), hospitalization with supportive care, and very importantly, intravenous immune globulin (IVIG) because Kawasaki disease does not respond to antibiotics.[8,9]

### *Erythroderma*

Erythroderma, also known as exfoliative dermatitis, is an erythematous, scaling rash that involves more than 90% of the skin.[10] Erythroderma is also termed red man syndrome when a primary cause cannot be identified.[10] The rash begins as a very generalized erythema. The skin begins to scale and slough, along with nails and hair.[11] The skin is inflamed and may lose pigmentation in dark-skinned individuals. This is an overwhelming disease process in which large tissue burdens of exfoliated scales are lost en masse daily; these patients are, in essence, "burn victims." They have marked increases in skin perfusion and profound temperature dysregulation that result in significant heat loss, increased basal metabolic rate, fluid loss, edema, and hypoalbuminemia.[10] Although this disease primarily affects adults, it does occur in younger populations who have other skin or connective tissue disorders (lupus, sarcoid, psoriasis, SSSS, atopic dermatitis, or seborrheic dermatitis). Patients with rapid disease progression usually have a history of cancer or SSSS or an inciting medication reaction. Those with gradual symptomatology generally have a skin disorder history. The work-up for these patients should be conducted in close consultation with a dermatologist, who can aid in identification of the primary lesions, which can be a difficult task. All patients warrant cancer evaluation and treatment of the underlying cause. Laboratory studies include a sedimentation rate, complete blood count, comprehensive metabolic panel, HIV testing, skin scrapings, skin biopsies, and wound cultures.[6] All patients warrant admission. In pediatric patients, erythroderma and fever are predictors of hypotension and may reflect TSS.[12] Systemic steroids are controversial and may worsen psoriasis and SSSS. Recovery is long and recurrences common in the case of red man syndrome. Mortality ranges from 20% to 40% and in many instances is due to factors unrelated to the disease process itself.[3,13]

## MACULOPAPULAR RASHES

The term *maculopapule* is a portmanteau of macule and papule. Maculopapular rashes are differentiated according to the distribution of the rash and systemic toxicity (**Table 192.5**). Patients who appear toxic and febrile have a wide differential diagnosis; however, it is paramount that patients living in endemic areas be assessed for Lyme disease. Target lesions (see Fig. 191.4) are pathognomonic for Stevens-Johnson Syndrome (SJS) and erythema multiforme (EM). Refer to Chapter 191 for review of EM. A full discussion of

**Table 192.5** Maculopapular Rashes

| | ROCKY MOUNTAIN SPOTTED FEVER | MENINGOCOCCEMIA | SECONDARY SYPHILIS | LYME DISEASE | STEVENS-JOHNSON SYNDROME |
|---|---|---|---|---|---|
| Characteristics | Febrile and toxic<br>Rash begins on ankles and wrists<br>Spotless fever in 20% | Fever, shock<br>Rash begins on ankles and wrists<br>Changes in mental status | Constitutional symptoms<br>Meningeal signs<br>Pruritic<br>Optic neuritis<br>Nephropathy<br>GI distress | Fever<br>Meningeal signs<br>AV nodal block<br>Arthralgias<br>Myalgias<br>Neuritis<br>Bell palsy | Toxic<br>Constitutional symptoms |
| Clinical signs | No target lesions<br>Involves the palms and soles | No target lesions<br>No palm and sole involvement | No target lesions<br>Involves the palms and soles<br>Condylomata lata | Single target lesion<br>Erythema migrans | Diffuse target lesions<br>Involves the palms and soles<br>Involves mucous membranes |
| Mortality | 30% if untreated<br>5% with prompt therapy | 100% if untreated<br>10-20% with prompt therapy | Death from:<br>Gumma<br>CV syphilis<br>Neurologic syphilis | Rarely lethal<br>Significant morbidity | 10-30% |
| Treatment | Admission<br>Serologic testing<br>Early antibiotics | Cultures<br>Admission<br>Early antibiotics | HIV testing<br>Serologic testing<br>Early antibiotics | Tick bite biopsy<br>Serologic testing<br>Early antibiotics | Stop offending agent<br>ICU admission<br>Fluid and electrolyte balance<br>Wound care |

*AV*, Atrioventricular; *CV*, cerebrovascular; *GI*, gastrointestinal; *HIV*, human immunodeficiency virus.

TEN was presented in the previous section (erythematous rashes); however, TEN and Lyme disease may also be associated with target lesions. Toxic patients with a maculopapular rash but no target lesions require emergency evaluation for Rocky Mountain spotted fever (RMSF), syphilis, and meningococcemia (see Table 192.3).

### Stevens-Johnson Syndrome

SJS is often a drug reaction, although infections and malignancies have been implicated. Previously, SJS was thought to be linked with EM, but it has recently been reclassified on the spectrum with TEN.[2] These patients have diffusely distributed target lesions that include the palms and soles. Significant mucous membrane involvement is present as well (**Fig. 192.2**). Patients with SJS are toxic with many constitutional symptoms. Treatment involves discontinuation of the offending agent and optimization of fluid and electrolyte status. Steroid treatment is controversial. Both SJS and TEN have greater mortality (10% and 30%, respectively) than do EM major (mortality less than 5%) and minor (negligible morbidity and mortality). Patients with SJS require intensive care unit (ICU) admission.[2,5,8,14-16]

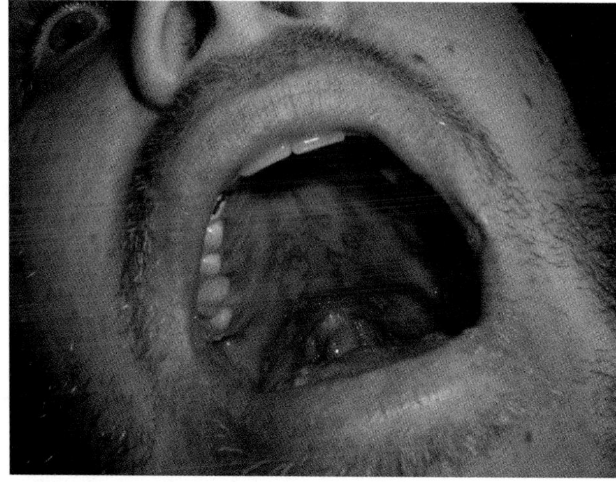

**Fig. 192.2 Erosion of the palate in Stevens-Johnson syndrome.**

### Lyme Disease

This tick-borne illness is caused by *Borrelia burgdorferi*. The patient generally has erythema migrans (a large annular target lesion with a dark red border and central clearing) at the site of the tick bite (**Fig. 192.3**). The rash begins with tick inoculation and may therefore be central or peripheral in location.[6] As the infection spreads hematogenously over a period of days to weeks, the patient may experience a variety of systemic symptoms, including a secondary rash (annular lesions), fever, meningitis, atrioventricular nodal block, migratory arthralgias, and myalgias. Neuritis occurs as well and is often manifested as Bell palsy (which may be bilateral); however, any nerve can be affected. The diagnosis is made clinically, although biopsy of the site of the tick bite is often diagnostic. Serologic tests are positive after several weeks but do not differentiate active from inactive infection. Though rarely lethal, Lyme disease can be accompanied by significant morbidity, usually related to neurologic and rheumatic complications. Doxycycline is first-line the treatment in nonpregnant adult patients. Children may be treated with amoxicillin. Ceftriaxone is indicated for those with significant neurologic or cardiac involvement.

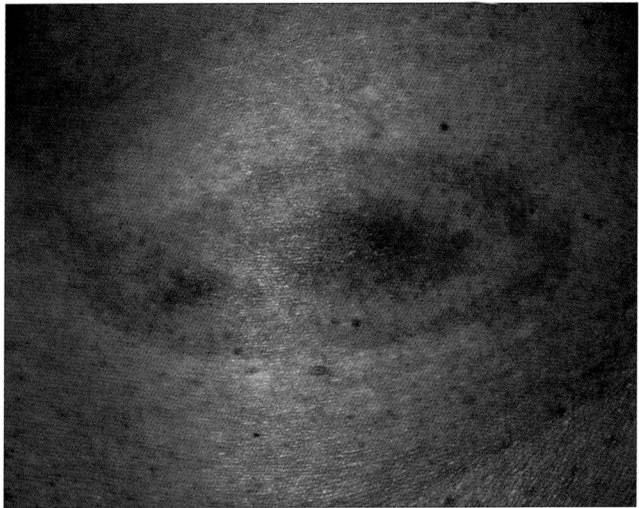

**Fig. 192.3 Annular erythema migrans spreading centrifugally.** The peripheral erythematous border may or may not be sharply demarcated and is usually 1 to 2 cm in width. (From Bolognia JL, Jorizzo JL, Rapini RP, eds. Dermatology. 2nd ed. Philadelphia: Mosby; 2008.)

### *Rocky Mountain Spotted Fever*

This tick-borne illness *(Rickettsia rickettsii)* has been recorded from Canada to Mexico and in every mainland state in the union except Vermont and Maine. Although history taking is essential, only 50% can recall a tick bite.[1] The RMSF-associated erythematous, maculopapular rash begins on the wrists and ankles and spreads over the entire body (including the palms and soles). In its early stage the rash consists of reddish macules that blanch, only to become petechial and purpuric later. In up to 20% of patients, the rash is absent (spotless fever).[1] Regardless of whether the rash is present, these patients are highly febrile and toxic. The diagnosis is clinical! Do not await confirmatory antibody tests to begin treatment (they will be negative in the acute period). These patients may appear to have meningococcemia. If the clinician is unsure of the diagnosis, it is essential to treat for both diseases. Lumbar puncture in a patient with RMSF will show leukocytosis with 25% neutrophils, elevated protein, and low to normal glucose. If not recognized and treated early, the mortality associated with RMFS is higher than 30%. However, mortality decreases to 5% with prompt appropriate antibiotic therapy. The neurologic deficits are permanent in 15% of cases.[15,17-20] Doxycycline is the drug of choice in all nonpregnant patients, even children. Pregnant patients may be treated with chloramphenicol, although doxycycline may also be considered in especially sick pregnant patients because chloramphenicol simply does not work as well.[1,15,17-20]

### *Secondary Syphilis*

Syphilis is an infection caused by the spirochete *Treponema pallidum*. Primary syphilis is characterized by a painless chancre (punched-out base with rolled edges).[21] It resolves completely and without scar formation in about 3 to 6 weeks. Secondary syphilis develops about 4 to 10 weeks after emergence of the chancre.[22] The patient will have many constitutional symptoms: malaise, headache, sore throat, fever, joint and muscle aches, decreased oral intake, meningeal symptoms, generalized lymphadenopathy, and a rash.[21,23] The rash of secondary syphilis is maculopapular, symmetric, nonpruritic, and diffuse. It may also involve the palms and soles, as well as the oral mucosa.[22,23] Patients may also have other skin findings, including condylomata lata (painless, gray to white verrucous lesions in the groin and other moist regions) and patchy alopecia. These patients can become very ill, with gastrointestinal distress, hepatitis, arthritis, optic neuritis, proctitis, and nephropathy. The diagnosis is made clinically, and a high index of suspicion is required. Testing for HIV is also recommended. The sensitivity of the Venereal Disease Research Laboratory (VDRL) and rapid plasma reagin (RPR) tests approaches 100% for secondary syphilis.[24] Because false-positive testing does occur, confirmatory fluorescent treponemal antibody absorption testing (FTA-ABS) is also performed.[24] The sensitivity of FTA-ABS for secondary syphilis also approaches 100%.[24] Treatment consists of intramuscular administration of penicillin G for all patients.[23] Bicillin LA is preferred over Bicillin CR due to increased concentrations of benzathine penicillin G. Penicillin G is also the only treatment for pregnant women. Pregnant patients with allergies should undergo desensitization and then treatment with penicillin.[23] Nonpregnant patients allergic to penicillin may be treated with doxycycline.[22]

### *Meningococcemia*

Meningococcemia is caused by infection with *Neisseria meningitidis*, a gram-negative intracellular diplococci that causes fulminant septicemia and has a predilection for adolescents and children younger than 4 years. Without proper treatment, meningococcemia is invariably fatal; mortality remains at 10% to 20% even with immediate therapy.[1] Patients are ill appearing, febrile, and in shock and have changes in mental status and a rash that develops within 24 hours of toxicity. The rash is initially erythematous and maculopapular (beginning on the wrists and ankles) and then spreads (sparing the palms and soles) and becomes a petechial vasculitis that is palpable. Early in the illness, meningococcemia can be mistaken for RMSF. Treatment of both is mandatory when there is any diagnostic uncertainty. The diagnosis is confirmed by Gram stain and blood or CSF culture. Gram staining of a specimen from a meningococcal skin lesion is more sensitive than a CSF Gram stain (72% versus 22%, respectively).[1] Lumbar puncture in patients with meningitis will show leukocytosis with a predominance of neutrophils, low glucose, and high protein. Complications include disseminated intravascular coagulopathy (DIC), acute respiratory distress syndrome, renal failure, multisystem organ failure, and adrenal hemorrhage (Waterhouse-Friderichsen syndrome). Ceftriaxone is first-line therapy. Vancomycin should be added in cases of diagnostic uncertainty to cover resistant streptococcal meningitis. Dexamethasone has been shown to reduce neurologic sequelae if administered early (before antibiotics, if possible). Rifampin prophylaxis for close contacts is recommended; alternatives include single-dose ciprofloxacin and intramuscular ceftriaxone.[1] A vaccine is available and is now recommended routinely for children 11 to 18 years of age.

## VESICULOBULLOUS RASHES

Vesiculobullous rashes provoke significant angst in many physicians; however, the differential diagnosis for febrile and toxic patients can be greatly simplified by discerning whether the rash is localized or diffuse. Ill patients with a diffuse vesiculobullous rash and a fever may have varicella or a more devastating illness such as smallpox or purpura fulminans/DIC. Toxic patients with localizing lesions require evaluation for necrotizing fasciitis (see Table 192.3).

### *Necrotizing Fasciitis*

This acutely toxic disease is caused by group A β-hemolytic streptococci and may also be synergistic with *Staphylococcus aureus, Vibrio vulnificus*, anaerobes, or polymicrobial infections.[25] Predisposing factors include intravenous drug use, diabetes, malignancy, acquired immunodeficiency syndrome, alcoholism, and other immunosuppressive states.[25,26] Importantly, these patients have pain out of proportion to the findings on examination and more toxicity than typical for cellulitic disease. Hemorrhagic bullae are often evident superficially, and the disease spreads rapidly along fascial planes. Crepitation may be present and can be seen as subcutaneous gas on radiographs. Treatment is prompt surgical débridement and broad-spectrum antibiotics. Adjunctive hyperbaric oxygen therapy has also been shown to significantly reduce mortality and amputation rates in these patients.[27] Mortality in patients with necrotizing fasciitis ranges from 0% to 75% (average mortality, 35%) and is dependent on the infective organisms, patient population, treatment protocols, and resources (including the availability of hyperbaric oxygen therapy).

### *Varicella*

Chickenpox (varicella-zoster virus or herpesvirus 3) is usually a benign, self-limited infection with an incubation period of 10 to 21 days. Infectivity is present 48 hours before the onset of fever and continues until all lesions have crusted.[28] Symptoms include conjunctival and catarrhal manifestations followed by a rash.[28,29] The rash appears in various stages at same time (papules, vesicles, crusted) and is described historically as "dew drops on a rose petal."[28] Children should not be given aspirin for fever because of concerns related to Reye syndrome. All patients should avoid those who are pregnant, elderly, or immunocompromised. Complications from varicella include staphylococcal or streptococcal secondary infections, visceral complications (15% mortality rate in the immunocompromised), neurologic complications (most common in children), pneumonia (most common in adults), and perinatal varicella (30% mortality rate).[28-32] Prevention involves immunization, which decreases the rate of occurrence and severity. Please refer to Chapter 18 for further review of varicella.

### *Smallpox*

Few differential considerations invoke more fear or dread than smallpox. Although smallpox was eradicated in 1980, isolates still exist in the United States and Russia.[33] Moreover, nearly 50% of the U.S. population has never been vaccinated against smallpox. Infection by the variola virus is manifested in two forms (major and minor), and only humans are infected (no carrier state). It is spread by inhalation or direct contact. Infection results in a silent viremia for 2 weeks, followed by the sudden onset of fever, severe headache, nausea, malaise, and a sore throat.[33,34] During this time an enanthem that is fine, erythematous, and macular may be found on the posterior pharynx, soft palate, and tongue.[35] It is followed by the exanthem, which begins on the face and spreads centrifugally to encompass the entire body (including the palms and soles in 50%) within 24 hours. These lesions start as macules, then papules, and finally pustules that crust over in several weeks. The lesions are always in the same stage of development. Any suspected cases should be reported to the Centers for Disease Control and Prevention at once. Vaccinated personnel should obtain viral swabs of the patient's throat or pustular skin lesions. Strict respiratory and contact isolation is mandatory. Supportive care with attention to eye care (keratitis) is indicated. The mortality rate positively correlates with the extent of the rash (10% to 80%; mean, 30%).[33] Death usually occurs as a result of overwhelming toxemia. Complications include blindness and diffuse scarring.

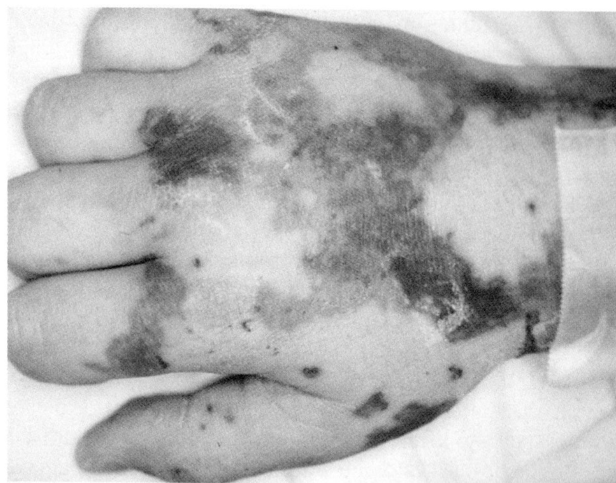

**Fig. 192.4 Meningococcal purpura fulminans in overwhelming meningococcal meningitis.**

### *Purpura Fulminans/Disseminated Intravascular Coagulopathy*

This acutely life-threatening disorder is associated with previous infection (often meningococcus or gram-negative organisms), sepsis, pregnancy, massive trauma, end-stage malignant disease, hepatic failure, snake bites, transfusion reactions, or anything that can precipitate DIC. It is characterized by fever, shock, rapid subcutaneous hemorrhage (ecchymotic purpura, hemorrhagic bullae), tissue necrosis, widespread petechiae, bleeding from multiple sites, widespread organ failure, and DIC (**Fig. 192.4**). The pathophysiology of this disease spectrum involves activation of the coagulation cascade with thrombin and fibrin formation. This leads to occlusion of vessels and end-organ damage with the consumption of platelets and clotting factors. Overactivation of the fibrinolytic system then occurs with resultant endogenous fibrinopeptide A production and bleeding. Laboratory findings include thrombocytopenia, schistocytes, prolongation of the prothrombin time (PT) and partial thromboplastin time (PTT), increases in fibrin degradation products and D-dimer levels, and a decrease in fibrinogen levels. The lower the fibrinogen levels, the higher the mortality. Emergency hematology/

oncology consultation and ICU admission are mandatory. First-line therapy is treatment of the underlying cause. Folate, vitamin K, fresh frozen plasma (FFP), cryoprecipitate, platelets, and red blood cell transfusions are given as needed; heparin is also used for associated thrombi. Antithrombin III is a promising investigational drug but has not been approved by the Food and Drug Administration (FDA). A metaanalysis of trials showed a reduction in mortality from 47% to 32% with the administration of antithrombin. Knowing when to use each of these agents is a tricky balancing act and is best done in consultation with a hematologist.[36,37]

### PETECHIAL/PURPURIC RASHES

These rashes can be especially challenging and are associated with devastating differential diagnoses. However, an algorithmic approach can help the physician narrow the diagnosis with confidence (see Table 192.3). It is helpful to determine early whether the rash is palpable or nonpalpable. Palpable (raised) purpura occurs in vasculitic diseases secondary to inflammation or infection. In toxic and febrile patients with palpable petechial/purpuric lesions, the differential diagnoses includes RMSF, endocarditis, and meningococcemia. Nonpalpable purpura (flat, subcutaneous hemorrhages) occurs in thrombocytopenic conditions. Toxic and febrile patients with petechiae or purpura but without palpable lesions may have purpura fulminans/DIC or thrombotic thrombocytopenic purpura (TTP).

#### *Bacteremic Endocarditis*

Endocarditis is a systemic infectious process caused most commonly by *Streptococcus viridans*, coagulase-negative staphylococci, and *S. aureus*.[38] Patients with endocarditis have various constitutional symptoms that mimic other diseases (tuberculosis, heart failure, and malignancy). Early in its course, patients may not appear to be toxic. However, the symptoms progress to fever, new cardiac murmur, weakness, anemia, fatigue, malaise, weight loss, and rash. Risk factors include valvular disorders, intravenous drug use, immunodeficiency, dialysis, poor dental hygiene, and chronic in-dwelling vascular access.[39] Associated skin findings are pathognomonic and include petechiae (most common finding and may involve the eyelids and conjunctiva), Roth spots (exudative, edematous hemorrhagic retinal septic emboli), splinter hemorrhages, Janeway lesions (macular erythematous or hemorrhagic spots on the palms and soles), and Osler nodes (painful, violaceous nodules in the pulp pads of finger and toes).[40] The diagnosis is confirmed with transesophageal echocardiography and by identification of valvular vegetations. Treatment consists of broad-spectrum antibiotics to cover methicillin-resistant *S. aureus* (MRSA) and, thereafter, guidance by culture of blood (three sets) obtained before antibiotic therapy. Endocarditis is associated with significant morbidity; mortality is 25% to 40% for *S. aureus* endocarditis and 19% for *S. viridans* endocarditis.

#### *Thrombotic Thrombocytopenic Purpura*

Patients with TTP have fever, jaundice, and a diffuse, nonpalpable petechial/purpuric rash in a distinct manifestation. The classic pentad of symptoms includes fever, thrombocytopenia, hemolytic anemia, neurologic deficits, and renal failure. It is more common, however, to observe the clinical triad of thrombocytopenia, hemolytic anemia, and elevated lactate dehydrogenase. This triad of findings alone is sufficient for the diagnosis and initiation of treatment. Numerous conditions are associated with TTP, including HIV infection, lupus, pregnancy, malignancy, and transplantation. Drugs associated with TTP include clopidogrel, cyclosporine, and quinine. Laboratory studies reveal that unlike DIC, the PT, PTT, and fibrin level are often normal. Schistocytes and helmets cells are seen on blood smears and indicate hemolysis. The pathophysiology of TTP involves platelet aggregation and thrombus formation with diffuse organ and tissue damage. Treatment includes emergency hematology/oncology consultation, plasmapheresis, FFP, ICU admission, and treatment of the underlying cause. Importantly, FFP can be used as a temporizing measure, but patients with TTP should be transferred to a facility with the capability of performing plasmapheresis. Platelet administration is to be avoided because it will precipitate more thrombus formation.[41] The mortality associated with TTP is higher than 90% if not properly treated. Exchange transfusion can decrease the mortality to 10%.[41,42] Facilities without the ability to perform exchange transfusions must consider emergency transfer to an appropriate facility.

## TREATMENT

### ERYTHEMATOUS RASHES

Treatment of these rashes can be found in Table 192.4. These highly lethal rashes require intensive treatment and continuous monitoring for complications. Patients with TEN may benefit from IVIG, although this indication is not yet approved by the FDA. Most physicians recommend against steroid use. Sulfadiazine should not be used on the wounds because sulfa is the most common offending agent.[43] Treatment of SSSS in young, well-appearing patients with minimal skin sloughing may be conducted on an outpatient basis (mortality < 5%). By contrast, adult SSSS has a mortality that can be as high as 60%.[4,5] Treatment of Kawasaki disease involves hospitalization, supportive care, and immediate high-dose aspirin to prevent coronary artery vasculitis, coronary vessel aneurysms, myocarditis, and myocardial infarction. Importantly, IVIG must be administered because Kawasaki disease does not respond to antibiotics.[9,10] Treatment of erythroderma involves recognition that recovery is long and recurrences common.

### MACULOPAPULAR RASHES

Treatment of these rashes can be found in Table 192.5. Though rarely lethal, Lyme disease can be associated with significant morbidity, usually related to neurologic and rheumatic complications. Doxycycline is the first-line treatment of Lyme disease in nonpregnant adult patients. Children may be treated with amoxicillin. Ceftriaxone is indicated for those with significant neurologic or cardiac involvement. Treatment of RMSF consists of doxycycline. It is the drug of choice in all nonpregnant patients, even children. Pregnant patients may be treated with chloramphenicol, although doxycycline may also be considered in especially sick pregnant patients because chloramphenicol simply does not work as well.[1,15,17-20] Patients with SJS are toxic and have many constitutional symptoms, but the use of steroids is controversial at this time. Meningococcemia is a dreaded disease with many complications. Ceftriaxone is first-line therapy. Vancomycin should be added in cases of diagnostic uncertainty to cover resistant streptococcal meningitis. Dexamethasone reduces neurologic sequelae if administered early.

### VESSICULOBULLOUS RASHES

Treatment of necrotizing fasciitis involves prompt surgical débridement, broad-spectrum antibiotics, and fluid resuscitation. Adjunctive hyperbaric oxygen therapy significantly reduces mortality and amputation rates.[27] Varicella is a self-limited illness in most patients, although complications can be devastating. Treatment of varicella is reviewed in Chapter 18. Smallpox is a devastating illness whose care is primarily supportive, with attention to eye care for keratitis. Death usually occurs as a result of overwhelming toxemia. In a similar manner, purpura fulminans is a disease with high morbidity and mortality. First-line therapy involves treatment of the underlying cause and administration of blood products (FFP, cryoprecipitate, platelets, and red blood cells). Folate, vitamin K, and heparin are also given. Antithrombin III is a promising investigational drug that has not yet been approved by the FDA. A metaanalysis of trials showed a reduction in mortality from 47% to 32% with the administration of antithrombin. Hematologist consultation is essential.[36,37]

### PETECHIAL/PURPURIC RASHES

Treatment of RMSF, meningococcemia, and purpura fulminans was discussed in a previous section. Bacterial endocarditis is a disease that requires consultation with cardiology and infectious disease specialists. Treatment consists of broad-spectrum antibiotics to cover MRSA and, thereafter, guidance by culture of blood (three sets) obtained before antibiotic therapy. Treatment of TTP includes ICU admission, emergency hematology consultation, plasmapheresis, FFP, and treatment of the underlying cause. Importantly, FFP is only a temporizing measure. Patients must be treated definitively with plasmapheresis (exchange transfusion) or be transferred. Platelet administration will precipitate more thrombus formation.[41,42]

## FOLLOW-UP AND PATIENT EDUCATION

Most of these illnesses are devastating with significant morbidity and mortality. Invariably, most patients will require close follow-up not only with their primary care provider (PCP) but also with infectious disease specialists, dermatologists, and cardiologists, and some will require surgical interventions.

### ERYTHEMATOUS RASHES

Patients with TEN require primary care follow-up, wound care, and dermatologic referral. Ophthalmologic consultation is needed for eye involvement. Those infected with HIV also require infectious disease follow-up. Patients with SSSS require PCP follow-up, as well as wound care and referral for any evidence of end-organ damage. Patients recovering from TSS require wound care and PCP monitoring during recovery and surveillance for end-organ damage. Recovery from Kawasaki disease requires PCP follow-up and cardiology referral. Patients with erythroderma require PCP follow-up, dermatologic referral, and wound care. Recovery is long for these patients, and recurrences are common.

### MACULOPAPULAR RASHES

Patients recovering from SJS require PCP and dermatologic follow-up. Significant mortality and morbidity are associated with SJS, and monitoring for end-organ damage is required. Patients discharged with a diagnosis of either Lyme disease, RMSF, syphilis, or meningococcemia require close PCP follow-up, as well as continued monitoring by an infectious disease specialist.

### VESSICULOBULLOUS RASHES

Patients with necrotizing fasciitis require continued surgical monitoring, wound care, and possibly adjunctive hyperbaric oxygen therapy. Those in whom varicella is diagnosed require PCP follow-up and wound care as needed. Those with smallpox will require management by an infectious disease physician. Patients with purpura fulminans need continuous, close monitoring with a PCP and a hematologist.

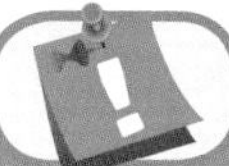

**TIPS AND TRICKS**

Drug reactions: Stop the offending agent and all related compounds at once. This will reduce the risk for death by 30% daily!

Toxic epidermal necrolysis and Stevens-Johnson syndrome: Usually caused by drugs.

Endocarditis, meningococcemia, and Rocky Mountain spotted fever: May be manifested as either a maculopapular (early) or petechial/purpuric rash (late) morphology. Serial examinations are mandatory!

Meningitis: The gold standard for diagnosis is cerebrospinal fluid analysis.

Meningitis prophylaxis: Should be given to close contacts, including classmates, household members, and medical personnel who had contact with respiratory droplets.

Rocky Mountain spotted fever: Doxycycline is the drug of choice, even in children. Pregnant patients may be treated with chloramphenicol, but doxycycline should be considered if the patient is especially ill.

Meningitis versus Rocky Mountain spotted fever: If the diagnosis is not clear, treat both!

Streptococcal toxic shock syndrome: 80% have an associated skin or soft tissue infection. Look for it early because drainage is a critical component of treatment.

Necrotizing fasciitis: Pain out of proportion to findings on examination. Always complete a full genitourinary examination on all ill-appearing patients because many are too toxic to adequately relate symptoms.

Fingers and toes: Must be evaluated for signs of endocarditis (Janeway lesions, Osler nodes, splinter hemorrhages).

Tissue samples: Can be of immense value in certain instances. Tzanck smears are sensitive for herpes infections. Potassium hydroxide preparations can identify yeast infections. Gram stains will identify gonococcals and anthrax organisms. Punch biopsies with a Gram stain will aid in the identification of meningococcemia and Rocky Mountain spotted fever.

### PETECHIAL/PURPURIC RASHES

Patients with RMSF or meningococcemia will require PCP follow-up in conjunction with an infectious disease specialist. Those with TTP or purpura fulminans/DIC need close PCP follow-up, as well as close monitoring by a hematologist. Patients treated for endocarditis will require PCP and cardiology follow-up.

## SUGGESTED READINGS

Carr DR, Houshmand E, Heffernan MP. Approach to the acute, generalized, blistering patient. Semin Cutan Med Surg 2007;26:139-46.

Mukasa Y, Craven N. Management of toxic epidermal necrolysis and related syndromes. Postgrad Med J 2008;84:60-5.

Murphy-Lavoie H, LeGros T. Emergent diagnosis of the unknown rash, the algorithmic approach. Emerg Med 2010;42(3):6-17.

Nguyen T, Freedman J. Dermatologic emergencies: diagnosing and managing life-threatening rashes. Emerg Med Pract 2002;4(9):1-28.

Rothe MJ, Bernstein ML, Grant-Kels JM. Life-threatening erythroderma: diagnosing and treating the "red man." Clin Dermatol 2005;23:206-17.

## REFERENCES

***References can be found on Expert Consult @ www.expertconsult.com.***

# The Emergency Psychiatric Assessment 193

*Douglas M. Char*

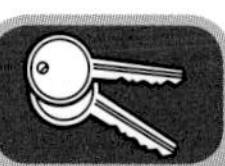

**KEY POINTS**

- The emergency psychiatric evaluation is a focused medical assessment with the primary goal of distinguishing between acute medical and psychiatric conditions.
- Primary mental disorders include disturbances in thought, mood, or personality. The onset of such disorders generally occurs at younger ages.
- Delirium and dementia are causes of global cognitive impairment that may be mistaken for psychiatric disease in emergency department patients, especially the elderly.
- Approximately 50% of patients seeking emergency psychiatric services have a poorly treated or undiagnosed medical illness contributing to their symptoms.
- Provisional diagnoses should drive the need for and extent of diagnostic testing.
- Acute interventions should improve the patient's cooperation, reduce agitation, prevent secondary harm, and initiate treatment of the primary mental disorder.

## PERSPECTIVE

The primary purpose of the emergency psychiatric evaluation is to distinguish between medical and psychiatric causes of disturbed behavior and thoughts. Comorbid medical conditions must be addressed to ensure appropriate and safe admission of patients to a psychiatric facility.

## EPIDEMIOLOGY

Cases of psychiatric illness in emergency department (ED) patients have increased 15% in the past decade and now account for 6% of ED visits. Declining inpatient psychiatric beds and limited community mental health resources complicate the care for this population of patients.[1]

Pediatric ED visits for psychiatric illness are less well studied, although the predominance of cases occur in the adolescent age group. Suicide prevention is the overriding concern. Teen suicide has tripled since 1950 and is the third leading cause of death in adolescents.[2]

## PATHOPHYSIOLOGY

Controversy surrounds the "medical clearance" process, more appropriately referred to as the "focused medical assessment." The evidence available to guide emergency practice remains limited and conflicting. Much of the debate revolves around the differing expectations and priorities of emergency physicians (EPs) and psychiatric consultants. The responsibilities of the EP are to obtain an appropriate history, identify the degree of stress, rule out medical cause, recognize the need for developing specific interventions, arrange psychiatric consultation, and plan disposition.[3]

## DEFINITIONS

The fourth edition of the *Diagnostic and Statistical Manual of Mental Disorders* (DSM-IV) distinguishes "mental disorders that are due to a general medical condition" from "primary mental disorders."[4] The terms *organic* and *functional* are no longer used to differentiate between illnesses of medical and psychiatric origin (**Box 193.1**). Clinical practice teaches us that the separation between mental and medical causes is often blurred.

Primary mental disorders include disturbances in thought, mood, or personality. Memory impairment, disorientation, and inattention are rarely features of primary mental disorders.

Delirium and dementia are medical conditions characterized by global impairment in cognitive function. A primary mental disorder may be mistakenly diagnosed in patients with delirium or dementia. It is important to differentiate between these conditions and other psychiatric disorders.

### DELIRIUM

The diagnosis of delirium consists of four key elements. (1) Delirious patients have impaired attention and concentration. (2) They demonstrate alterations in consciousness that fluctuate over time. (3) A delirious patient may become acutely agitated or lethargic because of disturbances in the sleep-wake cycle. (4) Abnormal cognition and speech may be apparent.

**BOX 193.1 Medical Causes of Disturbed Behavior versus Primary Mental Disorders**

**Medical Causes of Disturbed Behavior**
Delirium
Dementia
Intoxication and withdrawal
Infections
Metabolic or endocrine disorders
Medications

**Primary Mental Disorders and Psychiatric Illness**
Cognitive disorders (thought)
Affective disorders (mood)
Somatoform disorders
Hysteria
Dissociative states
Disruptive behavioral, conduct disorders
Eating disorders

Sensory perceptions, delusions, and hallucinations are prominent.

The onset of delirium is usually acute, with development over a period of hours to days. Determination of a patient's baseline cognitive function and onset of symptoms is essential in distinguishing delirium from dementia.

## DEMENTIA

Pervasive disturbance of cognitive function is the hallmark of dementia. Deficits commonly involve memory, judgment, personality, and language. Patients have no clouding of consciousness. The earliest sign of dementia is subtle memory loss, which may promote anxiety, depression, and psychosis. Patients with dementia may experience an acute worsening of symptoms when stressors overwhelm their intellectual and physiologic reserves. As the disease progresses, patients become less capable of recognizing concomitant medical illnesses (**Table 193.1**).

**Table 193.1 Clinical Factors That Help Differentiate Delirium and Dementia from Psychiatric Disease**

| CHARACTERISTIC | DELIRIUM | DEMENTIA | PSYCHIATRIC ILLNESS |
|---|---|---|---|
| **Symptoms** | | | |
| Age at onset | <12 or >40 yr | Usually elderly, >50 yr | 13-40 yr |
| Onset | Acute | Gradual or insidious | Gradual |
| Symptom course | Rapid, fluctuating | Stable and progressive | Stable |
| Duration | Days to weeks | Months to years | Months to years |
| Reversibility | Usually | Rarely | Rarely |
| **History** | | | |
| Past medical history | Substance abuse, medical illness | Comorbid conditions of aging | Previous psychiatric history |
| Family history | Unusual | History of dementia | History of psychiatric illness |
| **Physical Examination** | | | |
| Vital signs | Usually abnormal | Usually normal | Usually normal |
| Involuntary activity | May have tremors, asterixis, etc. | None unless coexistent disease | None |
| **Mental Status** | | | |
| Affect | Emotional liability | Flat affect with advanced disease | Flat affect |
| Orientation | Usually impaired | Impaired with advanced disease | Rarely impaired |
| Attention | Impaired | Slow to focus | Disorganized |
| Hallucinations | Primarily visual | Rare | Primarily auditory |
| Speech | Slow, incoherent, dysarthric | Usually coherent | Usually coherent |
| Consciousness | Decreased to impaired | Normal (clear) | Alert |
| Intellectual function | Usually impaired | Impaired | Intact |

## PRESENTING SIGNS AND SYMPTOMS

Most patients requiring emergency psychiatric assessment exhibit some form of altered mental status, psychosis, or self-harm. Common psychiatric problems seen in the ED include substance abuse and addiction, affective disorders, anxiety disorders, antisocial personality disorders, and severe cognitive impairment. ED visits for mental health disorders occur when events cannot be managed at home or when caretakers cannot control behavior or provide adequate support.

In addition to cognitive (thought) and affective (mood) disorders, pediatric providers must also be aware of disruptive behavioral or conduct disorders, such as attention-deficit/hyperactivity disorder and eating disorders. These disorders may be the primary reason for the pediatric or adolescent ED visit. Primary mental disorders are usually manifested in patients between 12 and 40 years of age. In older patients, various causes of delirium and dementia are more common than primary mental disorders.

The prevalence of coexisting medical illness in psychiatric patients has been reported to be as high as 50%.[1] Untreated medical illness often causes deterioration of baseline cognitive function in patients with a known psychiatric disorder. The prevalence of medical disease in patients seen in the ED with an acute exacerbation of an existing mental illness may be as high as 80%.[3] Up to 50% of patients demonstrate a causal relationship between acute medical and psychiatric complaints.[5] Five groups are regarded to be at high risk for medical illness: older patients, patients with history of substance abuse, patients without a psychiatric diagnosis, patients with preexisting medical disorders, and patients from a lower socioeconomic level.[6]

The EP must answer six key questions during the focused medical assessment:

1. Is the patient stable or unstable?
2. Is the behavior the result of an underlying medical illness?
3. What is the severity of the primary mental disorder?
4. Is psychiatric consultation necessary?
5. Does the patient need to be detained to facilitate emergency treatment?
6. What capability does the psychiatric facility have to treat medical conditions?

### HISTORY

A focused history of the present illness that reviews current symptoms, elicits precipitating circumstances, assesses risk severity, and establishes a time course should be obtained. Critical historical elements include past medical and psychiatric illnesses, medication use (**Table 193.2**), substance abuse or addiction, and a family history of psychiatric illnesses.

Patients with cognitive or affective disorders are often unable to provide a coherent clinical history. Friends, family members, and prehospital providers are useful sources of additional information. The patient's baseline cognitive function may be obtained from the medical record or solicited through discussion with primary care providers.

For children and teens, the history should concentrate on the precipitant of the mental health crisis. Particular areas to review include school performance, relationship with family and peers, living situation, family composition, sexuality, and neighborhood environment. When developmentally appropriate, the history should be obtained from both the child and the caretaker. Up to 20% of adolescents have a serious behavioral or medical problem.[2]

### PHYSICAL EXAMINATION

An organized and thorough physical examination should be performed. Cursory examination of psychiatric patients is unacceptable. Uncooperative or fully dressed patients may hide weapons, illicit drugs, evidence of physical abuse, or signs of medical illness. Younger patients are more likely to receive a cursory examination.[7]

The patient's vital signs should be scrutinized for evidence of shock, metabolic derangement, or infection. Search for signs of impaired organ and tissue perfusion. Check for hypoxia and abnormal respiratory effort. Look for abrasions or contusions that may represent recent trauma or unsuspected head injury. Identify subtle, focal weakness or neglect suggestive of possible neurologic impairment. Evaluate for other signs of neurologic disease, including dysesthesia (distortion of sense), apraxia (loss of the ability to carry out purposeful movements), agnosia (inability to recognize sensory stimuli), left-right disorientation, aphasia, or an inability to follow commands. Sensory illusions can be associated with neurologic conditions or intoxications. Visual, tactile, and olfactory hallucinations are generally attributable to medical disease (**Table 193.3**).

The mental status examination is critical and should assess the patient's level of consciousness, appearance, behavior, mood, affect, language, thought form and content, perceptions, and cognition. Much of this information can be obtained indirectly by observing the patient during the interview. Standardized assessment tools such as the Folstein Mini-Mental Status Examination (MMS) or the Quick Confusion Scale (QCS) allow detection of subtle deficits (**Tables 193.4 and 193.5**). Given the demands of a busy ED, many EPs find administering a formal MMS impractical—abbreviated tools are often preferred. Scores of less than 12 on the shorter QCS six-question battery have been shown to correlate with impaired cognition.[8]

## DIFFERENTIAL DIAGNOSIS AND MEDICAL DECISION MAKING

Patients with disturbed behavior or thought processes should be presumed to have a medical origin of their condition. Patients with chronic illnesses such as thyroid disease, diabetes mellitus, reactive airway disease, heart failure, stroke, and dementia may have a sudden and dramatic impairment in cognition or affect. Life-threatening causes of delirium should be considered in all patients with psychiatric disturbances. Primary mental disorders should be diagnosed only after serious medical conditions have been convincingly excluded (**Box 193.2**).

Diagnostic criteria such as those provided in the DSM-IV aid in establishing a provisional psychiatric diagnosis in the ED. Although standardized criteria are useful, interrater agreement among emergency psychiatrists is variable.[9]

Multiaxial diagnoses serve to organize complex clinical information and acknowledge the interplay of medical and psychiatric disease. Axis I diagnoses reflect mental disorders,

**Table 193.2 Medications That Cause Psychiatric Symptoms**

| DRUG CLASS | REACTIONS |
|---|---|
| Amphetamines | Bizarre behavior, hallucinations, paranoia, agitation, anxiety, mania, nightmares |
| Antibiotics | Cephalosporins: Euphoria, delusions, depersonalization, illusions<br>Fluoroquinolones: Psychosis, confusion, agitation, depression, hallucinations, paranoia, tics, mania<br>Sulfonamides: Confusion, disorientation, depression, euphoria, hallucinations |
| Anticholinergics | Confusion, memory loss, disorientation, depersonalization, delirium, auditory and visual hallucinations, fear, paranoia, incoherent speech, agitation, bizarre behavior, flushing, dry skin, retrograde amnesia |
| Antidepressants | Monoamine oxidase inhibitors: Mania or hypomania<br>Selective serotonin reuptake inhibitors: Mania, hypomania, hallucinations<br>Tricyclics: Mania or hypomania, delirium, hallucinations, paranoia, irritability, dysphoria |
| Antiepileptics | Agitation, confusion, delirium, depression, psychosis, aggression, mania, toxic encephalopathy, nightmares |
| Antihypertensives | Angiotensin-converting enzyme inhibitors: Mania, anxiety, hallucinations, depression, psychosis<br>Beta-blockers: Depression, psychosis, delirium, anxiety, nightmares, hallucinations<br>Calcium channel blockers: Depression, delirium, confusion, psychosis, mania<br>Thiazide diuretics: Depression, suicidal ideation |
| Barbiturates | Hyperactivity, visual hallucinations, depression, confusion, dyskinesia |
| Benzodiazepines | Rage, hostility, paranoia, hallucinations, delirium, depression, nightmares, antegrade amnesia, mania, disinhibition |
| Dopamine receptor agonists | Hallucinations, paranoia, delusions, confusion, mania, hypersexuality, anxiety, depression, nightmares |
| Histamine receptor antagonists | Histamine-1: Hallucinations<br>Histamine-2: Delirium, confusion, psychosis, mania, aggression, depression, nightmares |
| Nonsteroidal antiinflammatory agents | Depression, paranoia, psychosis, confusion, anxiety |
| Opioids | Nightmares, anxiety, agitation, euphoria, dysphoria, depression, paranoia, psychosis, hallucinations, dementia |
| Procaine derivatives | Fear of imminent death, anxiety, hallucinations, illusions, delusions, agitation, mania, depersonalization, psychosis |
| Salicylates | Agitation, confusion, hallucinations, paranoia |
| Statins (HMG-CoA reductase inhibitors) | Anxiety, depression, obsessions, delusions |
| Steroids | Anabolic: Psychosis, mania, depression, anxiety, aggressiveness, paranoia<br>Corticosteroids: Psychosis, delirium, mania, depression, hyperactivity, disinhibition |

Modified from Drugs that may cause psychiatric symptoms. Med Lett Drugs Ther 2002;44:59-62.
*HMG-CoA*, 3-Hydroxy-3-methylglutaryl coenzyme A.

axis II diagnoses identify personality disorders, axis III diagnoses include general medical conditions, and axis IV and V diagnoses include psychosocial stressors and adaptive functioning (**Fig. 193.1**). When evaluating children and teens, complaints should be considered within the context of their physical and social developmental stage.

## DIAGNOSTIC TESTING

A commonly held belief is the presumed inability of psychiatric patients to relate an accurate history or report signs and symptoms to guide testing. No literature supports this view. Directed testing based on patient complaints is often appropriate.

No standardized or widely accepted ED protocol exists for performing a focused medical assessment of psychiatric patients.[10] Differentiation between medical and psychiatric disease is best accomplished by a detailed history and physical examination. However, it should be noted that many psychiatric facilities have limited medical diagnostic capabilities and that the ED assessment may be the only medical evaluation and source of laboratory testing or imaging that the patient receives.[11]

**Table 193.3 Physical Examination Findings and Medical Causes of Abnormal Behavior**

| ORGAN SYSTEM | FINDING | POTENTIAL MEDICAL CONDITION |
|---|---|---|
| General | Hyperthermia | Thyrotoxicosis, vasculitis, alcohol withdrawal, sedative-hypnotic withdrawal, meningitis, inflammatory processes |
| | Hypothermia | Sepsis, dermal disease, endocrine disorders, CNS dysfunction, intoxication |
| | Hypotension | Shock, Addison disease, hypothyroidism, adverse drug reactions, dehydration |
| | Hypertension | Hypertensive encephalopathy, stimulant abuse, anticholinergic excess |
| Abdomen | Distention | Constipation, hepatic encephalopathy with ascites, obstruction, perforation of a viscus with sepsis |
| | Masses | Liver disease, cancer, obstruction |
| Cardiovascular | Bradycardia | Hypothyroidism, Stokes-Adams syndrome, elevated intracranial pressure |
| | Tachycardia | Hyperthyroidism, infection, heart failure, pulmonary embolism, alcohol intoxication or withdrawal |
| | Arrhythmias | Toxins, embolic strokes, electrolyte abnormalities |
| Neurologic | Confusion | Hypoxia, infection, toxins, electrolyte abnormalities, trauma, meningitis, encephalitis |
| | Seizures | Infections, head trauma, intoxication, poisonings, primary seizure disorder, meningitis |
| | Motor deficits | Stroke, encephalopathy, neuropathy, spinal trauma, movement disorders |
| | Aphasia | Stroke, head trauma, CNS disease |
| | Headache | Head trauma, meningitis, vasculitis, stroke, toxins, hypertensive emergencies |
| | Visual deficits | Head trauma, increased intracranial pressure, meningitis, cerebritis, ocular trauma, poisoning |
| Pulmonary | Tachypnea | Metabolic acidosis, pulmonary embolism, pneumonia, cardiac failure, fever |
| | Wheezing, stridor | Reactive airway disease, airway foreign body, hypoxia |
| | Rales | Pneumonia, pulmonary effusions, heart failure |
| Skin | Abrasions and contusion | Closed head injury, intracranial hemorrhage |

*CNS*, Central nervous system.

**Table 193.4 Mini-Mental Status Examination**

| CATEGORY | TEST BEHAVIOR | SCORE |
|---|---|---|
| Orientation | What is the (year) (season) (date) (day) (month)?<br>Where are we (state) (country) (town) (hospital) (floor)? | 5<br>5 |
| Registration | Name 3 objects (1 second to say each). Ask the patient to name all 3 after you have said them. Give 1 point for each correct answer. Repeat until all 3 have been learned. Count and record trials ________. | 3 |
| Attention and calculation | Serial 7s, backward from 100. 1 point for each correct answer. Stop after 5 answers. Alternatively, spell "world" backward. | 5 |
| Recall | Ask for the 3 objects named above. Give 1 point for each correct answer. | 3 |
| Language | Name a pencil and watch.<br>Repeat the following "No ifs, ands, or buts."<br>Follow a 3-stage command (e.g., "Take this paper in your hand, fold it in half, and put it on the floor.")<br>Read and obey the following: CLOSE YOUR EYES.<br>Write a sentence.<br>Copy the design shown (two intersecting pentagrams). | 2<br>1<br>3<br>1<br>1<br>1 |

From Folstein M. "Mini-Mental State" a practical method for grading the cognitive state of patients for the clinician. J Psychiatr Res 1975;12:189-98.

Maximum score = 30. A score of less than 23 indicates cognitive impairment.

**Table 193.5 Quick Confusion Scale***

| QUESTION | RESPONSE | WEIGHT | SCORE |
|---|---|---|---|
| What year is it? | 0 or 1 | × 2 | ______ |
| What month is it? | 0 or 1 | × 2 | ______ |
| Give a memory phrase | *John Brown, 42 Market Street, New York* | | |
| What time is it? | 0 or 1 (if within an hour) | × 2 | ______ |
| Count backward from 20 to 1 | 0, 1, or 2 (2 if no errors, 1 if 1 error, 0 if 2 or more errors) | × 1 | ______ |
| Say the months in reverse | 0, 1, or 2 (2 if no errors, 1 if 1 error, 0 if 2 or more errors) | × 1 | ______ |
| Repeat the memory phrase | 0, 1, 2, 3, 4, or 5 (score for each portion correct) | × 1 | ______ |

From Stair TO, Morrissey J, Jaradeh I, et al. Validation of the quick confusion scale for mental status screening in the emergency department. Int Emerg Med 207;2:130-2.

*A score lower than 12 suggests an alteration in cognition.

**BOX 193.2 Life-Threatening Causes of Delirium**

Hypoxia
Hypoglycemia
Hypertensive encephalopathy
Intracranial hemorrhage
Thyrotoxicosis
Sepsis
Arrhythmia
Wernicke encephalopathy
Intoxication or withdrawal
Meningitis or encephalitis
Status epilepticus
Poisonings
Hepatic failure
Renal failure

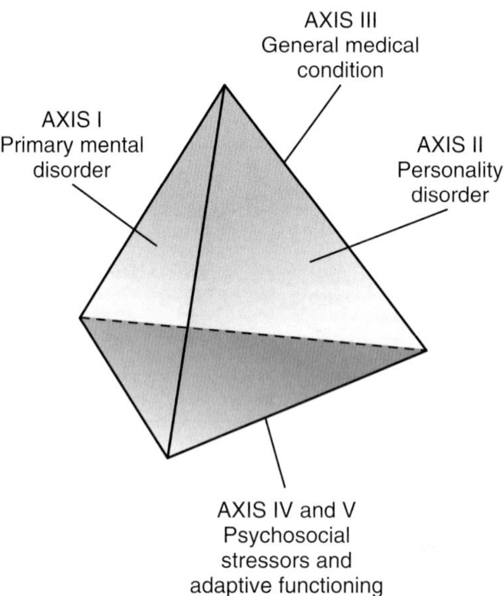


**Fig. 193.1 Multiaxial diagnosis data from the fourth edition of the *Diagnostic and Statistical Manual of Mental Disorders* (DSM).** (From First MB, Frances A, Pincus HA, editors. DSM-IV-TR handbook of differential diagnosis. Arlington, Va: American Psychiatric Association; 2002.

Screening tests commonly ordered as part of the emergency psychiatric evaluation include pulse oximetry, complete blood count, chemistry panel with glucose, electrocardiogram, urine toxicology screen, urine pregnancy testing, and serum alcohol level. Testing of liver and thyroid function, as well as computed tomography imaging of the brain, should be based on the history (or previous diagnosis) and findings on physical examination. Chest radiography, lumbar puncture, arterial blood sampling, and electroencephalography are rarely indicated as screening tests in the evaluation of patients with suspected psychiatric illness.[12,13]

The 2006 American College of Emergency Physicians (ACEP) clinical policy "Critical issues in the diagnosis and management of the adult psychiatric patient in the emergency department" posed three questions related to diagnostic testing[14]:

1. What testing is necessary to determine medical stability in alert, cooperative patients with normal vital signs, a noncontributory history and physical examination, and psychiatric symptoms?
2. Do the results of a urine drug screen for drugs of abuse affect management in alert, cooperative patients with normal vital signs, a noncontributory history and physical examination, and a psychiatric complaint?
3. Does an elevated alcohol level preclude the initiation of a psychiatric evaluation in alert, cooperative patients with normal vital signs and a noncontributory history and physical examination?

EPs are frequently asked to perform detailed screening laboratory and radiographic testing to exclude any medical illness that may be causing or contributing to the patient's psychiatric symptoms. Early studies of the coexistence of medical illness in patients with psychiatric symptoms argued for the routine use of laboratory testing, although they did not specify which components of the history and physical examination were included or performed on all patients.[14] These studies involved patients admitted directly to mental health facilities without a medical screening examination. When routine testing is performed, abnormal results are often clinically insignificant.[13,15-17] Patients who are delirious, have abnormal vital signs, or display altered cognitive states mandate more extensive evaluations. The 2006 ACEP consensus panel noted that routine laboratory testing is of limited utility in teens and younger adults. The value of routine laboratory testing in younger children with psychiatric symptoms has not been studied in ED populations.[2]

EPs and emergency psychiatrists often disagree on the necessity for a urine toxicology screen as part of emergency focused medical assessment. Although many surveyed EPs find a urine drug screen to be unnecessary, psychiatrists may use the test to determine a cause of the patient's symptoms or aid in disposition and long-term care of a patient.[13,18] Retrospective studies suggest that the sensitivity of routine toxicologic testing for the diagnosis of a medical cause of isolated psychiatric complaints is just 20%.[19] Schiller et al. prospectively tested approximately 400 patients and found no difference in terms of inpatient or outpatient disposition or hospital length of stay.[17] The ACEP recommends against routine testing for drugs of abuse in alert, awake, cooperative patients. They acknowledged that receiving psychiatric facilities often require such testing but urged that testing not delay psychiatric assessment or admission or transfer.

Acute intoxication may impair the ability to conduct a comprehensive psychiatric examination. It can also mimic or alter psychiatric symptoms and delay proper patient disposition. Psychiatric facilities will often refuse the transfer of intoxicated patients. No data have been found to support a specific blood alcohol concentration at which psychiatric evaluation can be accurately initiated. Adequate decision-making capacity is often unrelated to the patient's serum ethanol level. Cognitive function should be assessed on an individual basis. The consensus panel recommended that the patient's cognitive abilities, rather than a specific blood alcohol level, be the basis on which clinicians initiate psychiatric assessment.

Diagnostic testing of psychiatric patients in the ED should accomplish one of the following goals: (1) detect or exclude the presence of a condition that has treatment consequences, (2) determine the relative safety or appropriate dose of potential alternative treatments, or (3) provide baseline information useful for monitoring response to treatment. ED protocols should be based on local disease prevalence, common clinical findings, the potential for needed treatment, and the likelihood of admission or extended monitoring. In some states, emergency medicine and psychiatry organizations have created consensus guidelines regarding ED medical assessment of psychiatric patients in an effort to reduce unnecessary resource utilization.[3]

A few studies have suggested that it may be possible to identify patients with psychiatric complaints who can safely bypass the traditional ED focused medical assessment and be directed for primary psychiatric evaluation.[20,21] These studies suggest that patients must be alert with normal vital signs, not be under the influence of drugs or alcohol, and have a history of psychiatric illness that is consistent with their current symptoms. The availability of immediate online medical control is critical.

## TREATMENT

Acute behavioral disturbances mandate emergency care that is time and resource intensive. Treatment should be directed at the underlying cause of the disordered thought process or behavior, if known. Emergency psychiatric interventions are guided by three principles: (1) improve patient cooperation, (2) reduce agitation, and (3) reduce the risk for secondary harm.

Patient and staff safety is of paramount importance. Suicidal patients need to be monitored closely and protected from self-harm. Agitated patients constitute a threat to themselves and to others. Rapid administration of psychotropic or anxiolytic medications (or both) is a safe and effective method for controlling potentially dangerous patients. Seclusion, sitters, and the use of physical restraints may be required temporarily. Chapters 194 to 197 provide specific treatment recommendations for psychotic, violent, and suicidal patients. Disease-appropriate treatments of the various causes of delirium and dementia are reviewed elsewhere in this text.

## FOLLOW-UP AND NEXT STEPS IN CARE

The emergency psychiatric focused medical assessment should result in one of four outcomes: (1) a medical cause of the chief complaint is identified, (2) a primary mental disorder is suspected, (3) the symptom or condition is self-limited and resolves, or (4) the cause of the abnormal behavior or disordered thought process remains unclear and mandates further evaluation (medical admission) (**Box 193.3**).

Patients without an apparent medical cause of their confusion, disordered thought, or bizarre behavior require psychiatric evaluation. Most of these patients will probably need to be admitted to a psychiatric service for extended observation and therapy. Some individuals may need to be held involuntarily according to individual state laws.

Discharge may be considered for patients whose symptoms resolve rapidly after minimal treatment or after a short period of observation. Three discharge criteria must be

**BOX 193.3 Potential Outcomes of the Emergency Psychiatric Evaluation**

A medical cause of the abnormal behavior or thought process is identified and treatment is initiated.

A primary mental disorder is suspected and psychiatric consultation is obtained.

The patient's condition is self-limited and has resolved. Discharge criteria are met.

The cause of the abnormal behavior or disordered thought process remains unclear. Further evaluation mandates admission to a medical service with psychiatric consultation.

**Table 193.6 Common Pitfalls in the Emergency Psychiatric Evaluation**

| PITFALL | INCORRECT RATIONALE | RESULTANT ERROR |
|---|---|---|
| Inappropriate or premature referral to psychiatry | Bizarre, disruptive behavior is less urgent or serious than the medical complaints of other ED patients. Initial decisions are often based on a single symptom or historical feature. | Provider bias and faulty assumptions lead to incorrect diagnoses. |
| Bizarre behavior or thoughts are "diagnostic" of primary mental disorders | Delusions, hallucinations, and disorganized thoughts are usually signs of primary psychosis. | These symptoms are nonspecific and may reflect delirium. |
| Premature referral of violent patients to psychiatry | Violent patients place staff and others at risk and disrupt the flow of care in the emergency department. | Violent behavior may be the result of an underlying medical illness. |
| Allowing biased staff to hinder evaluation and guide care | Certain patients (alcoholics, drug abusers, suicidal individuals) create their own disease and do not deserve urgent intervention. | Blaming patients for their illness does not correct the behavior or address the underlying psychiatric disease. |
| Provider convinced that the patient is insincere | The provider does not believe the threats or complaints of seemingly unreliable patients. | The potential for serious or lethal outcomes may be underestimated. |
| Discharging elderly patients with "dementia" | Dementia cannot be treated. | The provider presumes that all elderly patients are permanently impaired (60% of dementias are treatable). |

met: (1) patients should be able to care for themselves or should have an appropriate caregiver at home, (2) patients cannot be actively suicidal or homicidal, and (3) patients should not have any unresolved symptoms of an acute medical illness.

If subacute medical conditions are identified in patients requiring psychiatric admission, the accepting psychiatric service must be capable of providing appropriate care and follow-up. Untreated medical illnesses may complicate psychiatric interventions and result in repeated visits to the ED (**Table 193.6**).

## SUGGESTED READINGS

Baren JM, Mace SE, Hendry PL, et al. Children's mental health emergencies—part 2. Pediatr Emerg Care 2008;24:485-98.

Lukens TW, Wolf SJ, Edlow JA, et al. Clinical policy: critical issues in the diagnosis and management of the adult psychiatric patient in the emergency department. Ann Emerg Med 2006;47:79-99.

Szpakowicz M, Herd A. "Medically cleared": how well are patients with psychiatric presentations examined by emergency physicians? J Emerg Med 2008:35:369-72.

Zun LS. Evidence-based evaluation of psychiatric patients. J Emerg Med 2005;28:35-9.

## REFERENCES

*References can be found on Expert Consult @ www.expertconsult.com.*

Derby Teaching Hospitals
N... Foundation Trust
Lib... ...nd Knowledge ...

# Psychosis and Psychotropic Medication 194

*Tae Eung Kim and Lynda Daniel-Underwood*

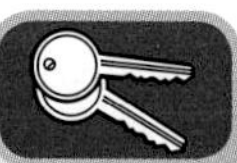

**KEY POINTS**

- Psychosis refers to symptoms that demonstrate impairment in thought content and process.
- Patients with schizophrenia, bipolar disease, substance abuse, or depression may have psychotic features over time.
- Most psychotic disorders are initially manifested during adolescence and young adulthood.
- Typical antipsychotic medications have high affinity for dopamine receptors and are more effective in treating hallucinations and delusions, the "positive" symptoms of schizophrenia.
- Atypical antipsychotic medications have high affinity for serotonin receptors. These agents are more effective in treating the "negative" behavioral symptoms associated with psychosis.

## DEFINITIONS AND EPIDEMIOLOGY

Psychosis describes syndromes that impair both thought content and thought process. Disturbances in thought content include perceptions that are not based in reality, whereas disturbances in thought process reflect thoughts that are disorganized and illogical in form. Psychotic symptoms include visual, tactile, or olfactory hallucinations; delusions; impairment of concentration and attention; and disorientation. Schizophrenia is the disorder that is most often associated with psychosis. Bipolar disorder, major depression, and substance abuse are examples of psychiatric diagnoses that can also cause symptoms of acute psychosis.

The 1-year prevalence of the schizophrenic disorders is 1.1%. One in every 100 persons in the United States suffers from psychotic symptoms.[1] Episodes of psychosis are generally precipitated or exacerbated by psychosocial stressors. Psychosis may be acute or chronic. As is often the case with the first manifestation of schizophrenia, acute psychotic episodes prompt patients to seek emergency care for their bizarre behavior or troubling perceptions.

## PATHOPHYSIOLOGY

The dominant theory used to explain the pathophysiology of psychotic thought is the dopamine hypothesis. This theory suggests that psychosis is probably the result of excessive dopamine transmission in the mesolimbic pathway of the brain. Evidence offered for the behavioral influence of this neurotransmitter is based on the observed effects of antipsychotic medications on dopamine pathways of the brain. Dopamine receptor antagonists ($D_2$ receptor antagonists) improve disturbed thoughts in psychotic patients. The efficacy of the typical (first-generation) antipsychotic agents depends on the degree to which these drugs block $D_2$ receptor activity.

Competing theories that describe the pathophysiology of psychosis are also based on neurotransmitter activity. These theories generally cite the effects and interplay of serotonin and glutamate with dopamine.

## PRESENTING SIGNS AND SYMPTOMS

Most psychotic disorders are initially manifested in adolescence and young adulthood. The median age at the onset of symptoms of a psychiatric disorder is 16 years. By the age of 38 years, symptoms will have developed in more than 90% of patients with a mental disorder.[1] The typical example of a newly psychotic patient is a young person brought to the emergency department (ED) by family or friends who are concerned about the patient's bizarre behavior or unusual beliefs. The "positive" symptoms of psychosis, including hallucinations and delusions, are often more obvious and distressing than the "negative" symptoms, which are affective and generally develop more insidiously.

The key features of psychotic symptoms are perceptions and beliefs that are not based in reality. Such disturbances include hallucinations, illusions, and delusions.

*Hallucinations* are sensory perceptions that are apparent only to the patient experiencing them. Auditory hallucinations are the most common and are typically described as hearing voices of people who are not present. Hallucinations that involve other senses (visual, olfactory, or tactile) are less frequently reported and may be the result of medical illness. Patients who are hallucinating appear to be preoccupied or distracted as they respond to internal stimuli.

*Illusions* refer to misperceptions about a patient's surroundings, whereas hallucinations are wholly internal and are not prompted by an environmental stimulus.

*Delusions* are misinterpretations of events or perceptions that lead psychotic patients to erroneously attribute experiences to unlikely or bizarre beliefs. Unlike cultural beliefs, delusions are explanations that are not shared by others. Most delusions involve a sense of control. For example, patients with delusions of persecution may believe that they are under hostile surveillance or that people are plotting against them. Grandiose delusions cause patients to believe that they are endowed with supernatural powers or are able to affect events outside their sphere of influence.

Psychosis may also be manifested as disorganization in thought process, with patients expressing ideas and words that are not coherently linked. Thoughts are described as tangential when the patient switches from one topic to another without logical association. When thoughts become more disorganized, the patient may start using neologisms, or self-created nonsense words. Speech may later regress into an incomprehensible jumble of unassociated phrases that may be described as a word salad.

The negative symptoms of psychosis reflect a loss of function, such as the ability to express affect, generate speech, or become motivated. These symptoms may be overlooked because they are often perceived as less obviously disturbing than "positive" symptoms, but they can also significantly impair the lives of psychotic patients.

## DIFFERENTIAL DIAGNOSIS

First manifestations of psychosis are uncommon in young children and older adults; delirium or dementia should not be confused with true psychotic behavior. Causes of delirium may become evident through abnormal vital signs or subtle findings on physical examination, either of which should prompt a search for medical conditions that may mimic psychiatric disease. Examples of medical causes of delirium that may be mistaken for psychosis include ingestion of toxins, substance abuse, and brain tumors. Additionally, certain medical conditions may precipitate psychosis or exacerbate chronic underlying mental disorders.

## DIAGNOSTIC TESTING

A detailed discussion of the emergency psychiatric evaluation can be found in Chapter 193.

## PSYCHOTROPIC MEDICATIONS

### TYPICAL (FIRST-GENERATION) ANTIPSYCHOTIC AGENTS

Typical antipsychotic medications have high affinity for $D_2$ receptors, thus blocking dopamine overactivity in the mesocortical pathway. $D_2$ antagonism accounts for the clinical profile of these agents, which are useful in treating the positive symptoms of schizophrenia, namely, hallucinations and delusions.[2] Haloperidol (Haldol) is the prototypic agent of this drug class (**Table 194.1**).

Typical antipsychotic agents also decrease dopaminergic activity in the nigrostriatal pathway at therapeutic doses. This adverse effect leads to increased cholinergic activity, which promotes extrapyramidal symptoms (EPSs) such as dystonia, akathisia, and other movement disorders. Tardive dyskinesia is thought to arise from upregulation (supersensitivity) of postsynaptic dopamine receptors in the nigrostriatal pathway after prolonged receptor blockade. Concomitant administration of benztropine (Cogentin) may slow the development of EPSs.

### ATYPICAL (SECOND-GENERATION) ANTIPSYCHOTIC AGENTS

Atypical antipsychotic medications have higher affinity for serotonin ($5\text{-}HT_{2A}$) receptors than for $D_2$ receptors. Serotonergic neurons in the dorsal raphe nuclei interact with dopaminergic neurons in the nigrostriatal pathway and modulate the clinical effects. Atypical antipsychotic agents are characterized by a lower incidence of EPSs and show a diverse range of binding activities at other receptor sites as well. Serotonin and other neurotransmitter blockade may account for the beneficial effects of atypical antipsychotic agents against negative behavioral symptoms by increasing dopamine activity in the prefrontal cortex (**Table 194.2**).

**Table 194.1** Typical Antipsychotic Medications (Dopaine$_2$ Receptor Antagonists)

| DRUG | USUAL DOSE | COMMENTS |
|---|---|---|
| Haloperidol (Haldol) | 5-10 mg IM or IV*<br>1-2.5 mg PO in elderly patients<br>≤20 mg PO per dose | Onset: 30-60 min<br>Risk for adverse effects (extrapyramidal symptoms, akathisia)<br>Pregnancy class C |
| Chlorpromazine (Thorazine) | 25 mg IM | Faster time to onset<br>Prolonged sedation<br>Pregnancy class C |
| Droperidol† (Inapsine) | 5-10 mg IM<br>2.5-5 mg IV | Onset: 3-5 min<br>Arousal time: 2 hr<br>Prolongation of QT interval reported at low doses†<br>Pregnancy class C |

$D_2$, Dopamine 2; *IM*, intramuscularly; *IV*, intravenously; *PO*, orally.

*Administration of haloperidol intravenously is off label because of the risk for QT prolongation and arrhythmia.

†A "black box" warning was mandated by the Food and Drug Administration in 2001 given the risk for fatal tachyarrhythmias.

**Table 194.2** Atypical Antipsychotic Medications (Serotonin and $D_2$ Receptor Antagonists)

| DRUG | USUAL DOSE | COMMENTS |
|---|---|---|
| Clozapine (Clozaril) | 12.5 mg PO bid | Used for refractory schizophrenia<br>May cause agranulocytosis, diabetes, weight gain<br>Pregnancy class B |
| Risperidone (Risperdal) | 2 mg PO liquid or ODT | May cause weight gain, elevation of prolactin levels, extrapyramidal symptoms<br>Pregnancy class C |
| Olanzapine (Zyprexa) | 10 mg IM, may repeat in 2 hr to a maximum of 30 mg/day<br>10-15 mg SL (ODT), maximum of 20 mg/day | Strong antihistamine effect, sedating<br>Controls positive, negative, and affective symptoms<br>May promote weight gain, diabetes<br>Causes the least change in QT intervals<br>Pregnancy class C |
| Ziprasidone (Geodon) | 10 mg IM q2h or 20 mg IM q4h | Promotes the greatest QT prolongation of the class<br>Pregnancy class C |

*bid*, Twice daily; $D_2$, dopamine 2; *IM*, intramuscularly; *ODT*, orally disintegrating tablet; *PO*, orally; *q2h*, every 2 hours; *SL*, sublingually.

## PARTIAL RECEPTOR AGONISTS

Partial receptor agonists demonstrate variable clinical effects, as influenced by the receptor-binding affinity of the agent and the patient's endogenous levels of neurotransmitter. One available partial agonist, aripiprazole (Abilify), appears to be an effective and possibly a superior treatment option for patients with schizophrenia. It does not completely block the mesolimbic system (associated with "negative" symptoms and cognitive impairment), nor does it completely stimulate the nigrostriatal or tuberoinfundibular pathways responsible for EPSs and elevated prolactin levels.[2] Aripiprazole thus has a low side effect profile and is taken orally at a dose of 10 to 30 mg/day.

## BENZODIAZEPINES

Benzodiazepines are commonly used to treat psychotic agitation because of their efficacy and tolerability. These agents increase the effects of γ-aminobutyric acid (GABA) on the chloride ionophore of the GABA-benzodiazepine receptor complex, thereby causing sedation and sleepiness. Benzodiazepines are generally administered in combination with typical antipsychotic medications to sedate agitated or violent patients. An added benefit of the administration of benzodiazepines is the treatment of alcohol withdrawal if that is the cause of the agitation.[3] Adverse effects, including oversedation and diminished respiratory drive, are minimal at low doses. Rare reports have noted "frontal disinhibition" leading to increased impulsive behavior with benzodiazepine use in patients with previous head injury or mental retardation[4] (**Table 194.3**).

**Table 194.3** Benzodiazepines

| DRUG | USUAL DOSE | COMMENT |
|---|---|---|
| Lorazepam (Ativan) | 2-4 mg PO or 1-2 mg IM | Half-life: 6-20 hr<br>Treats aggressive behavior<br>Pregnancy class D |
| Clonazepam (Klonopin) | 1-2 mg IM | Rapid onset, long half-life<br>Pregnancy class D |
| Diazepam (Valium) | 5-10 mg PO or 2-5 mg IM | Half-life: 20 hr IM<br>Pregnancy class D |

*IM*, Intramuscularly; *PO*, orally.

# TREATMENT

Pharmacologic management in the ED can be difficult because of the constellation of nonspecific behavior observed in psychotic patients with an undifferentiated psychiatric or medical condition. Haloperidol remains the most accepted pharmacologic treatment of psychosis of uncertain origin. More recently, combination therapy using benzodiazepines with typical antipsychotic agents has been shown to provide superior results. Combination therapy allows rapid, safe sedation, in addition to control of the psychotic features.

Any agitation or violent behavior associated with psychosis should be managed as soon as a patient arrives in the ED. Verbal warnings should precede the use of chemical or physical restraint. The least restrictive method of restraint is preferable to facilitate a safe and complete diagnostic evaluation.[5,6]

# DISPOSITION

In many jurisdictions, patients may be held against their will by police officers or attending medical staff if they are determined to be gravely disabled, a danger to themselves, or a danger to others because of a mental disturbance. The goal of involuntary restraint is to provide treatment that may improve the patient's decision-making capacity and allow time for evaluation of any undiagnosed illnesses. Patients may be discharged from the ED if their psychotic behavior is well controlled, if medical and surgical concerns are addressed, if they have accompanying family or friends, and if aftercare is readily available.

# REFERENCES

*References can be found on Expert Consult @ www.expertconsult.com.*

# 195 The Violent Patient

Eric Isaacs

**KEY POINTS**

- Patient risk factors for violent behavior include evidence of agitation (e.g., pacing), substance abuse, a previous history of violence, arrival at the emergency department in police custody, and male gender.
- Disarming protocols and deescalation techniques are critical methods for prevention of violence.
- Agitated or violent behavior is frequently caused by medical conditions, such as hypoglycemia or intoxication.
- Violent patients should be given a verbal warning before they are restrained. Physical restraint should be supplanted by chemical restraint when safety allows.
- Medical complications of incorrect or prolonged physical restraint include hyperthermia, acidosis, rhabdomyolysis, and death.
- Sedation should be tailored to the suspected cause of the agitation, as well as the desired depth and length of sedation.
- A combination of an intramuscular benzodiazepine (lorazepam) and a butyrophenone (haloperidol) provides consistent sedation for many causes.

## EPIDEMIOLOGY

The goal of caring for a violent patient is first to protect everyone involved and also to diagnose and treat important medical and psychiatric conditions (see the "Priority Actions" box). These goals are best achieved if warning signs of violence are recognized and the safest and most effective means of behavioral control are used.

The epidemiology of violence in the emergency department (ED) is inexact; past surveys suggest that as many as 80% of events are unreported.[1] Still, clear evidence indicates that most EDs experience violent patients routinely. Of greater concern, ED caregivers are often victims. More than 70% of ED nurses have reported being the victim of physical violence during their career.[2] The rate of assault on health care workers is 8 per 10,000, as compared with 2 per 10,000 for all private-sector industries, with the ED being one of the highest-risk areas.[3]

Violence may range from verbal threats to physical assault. Of reported events in one survey, 90% of cases involved the patient and 10% involved family or visitors. A few staff members may be confronted by former patients outside the ED or may become victims of stalking.

Nearly 60% of EDs in the United States have reported an armed threat on a staff member within 5 years.[4] Weapons may be carried by patients, family members, visitors, or even staff members. Patients most likely to carry weapons include those with schizophrenia or paranoid ideation and individuals who have been the victims of gunshot wounds. Many violent patients are intoxicated with alcohol or drugs.

Violence threatens the career longevity of ED staff. Violent events should be regularly reported to police and hospital administration to raise awareness of this societal problem and to encourage safer practice environments.

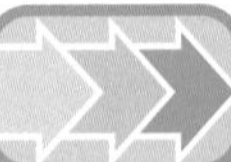

**PRIORITY ACTIONS**

**Goals for the Care of Violent Patients in the Emergency Department**

Recognize risk factors and warning signs before violence occurs.

Use deescalation (communication) techniques to prevent violent behavior.

Control the patient and situation to minimize further violence.

Diagnose and treat reversible causes of agitation.

Protect the patient and others through appropriate restraint methods.

## HOW TO PREDICT VIOLENCE

Violent behavior rarely erupts without warning. Risk factors for violence include an escalating psychiatric illness (e.g., schizophrenia, personality disorders, mania), alcohol and drug abuse, a previous history of violence, arrival at the ED in police custody, and male gender (**Box 195.1**). The use of risk factors to predict violent behavior has not been tested in cohorts of emergency physicians; psychiatrists have been only 60% accurate in predicting violence when using risk factors alone.[5]

**BOX 195.1 Risk Factors for the Use of Concealed Weapons and Violent Behavior in the Emergency Department**

**Concealed Weapons**
Schizophrenia
Paranoid ideation
Victims of gunshot wounds

**Violent Behavior**
Schizophrenia
Personality disorders
Mania
Substance abuse or intoxication
Previous history of violent behavior
Arrival in police custody
Male gender

Verbal and nonverbal clues provide evidence of impending violence. As patients become more agitated, the level of their voice may rise and their hand gestures may be more pronounced and expressive. Patients may exhibit restlessness on their gurney or may pace. Providers should trust their instincts when they become uncomfortable with an agitated patient. Emotional stress, prolonged waiting times, and gaps in communication create a provocative and unsupportive environment.

## INTERVENTIONS

Standardized methods should be used to confiscate concealed weapons. Metal detectors are used in some EDs and are recommended when possession of weapons by patients or visitors is frequent. For patients, a policy of routine undressing and gowning will minimize the likelihood of using hidden weapon when performed in an unbiased manner, regardless of the chief complaint.

Preparation of the examination room can facilitate safety. As many objects as possible should be removed from examination rooms that routinely hold violent or agitated patients. Panic buttons should be available for use by staff in any room where agitated patients are interviewed. Ideally, examination rooms should have two exits so that neither the clinician nor the patient feels trapped. Restless patients may become more agitated when physical outlets are constrained, so both the patient and caregiver must have unobstructed, rapid egress. Staff members should remove personal objects that could be used to cause injury by an assaultive patient. Such objects include neckties, large dangling earrings, and stethoscopes kept around the neck.

## DEESCALATION TECHNIQUES

Early attention and preferential treatment may defuse anger born of impatience. If at triage, an agitated patient should be taken directly to a treatment room. Volatile patients should be removed from contact with other persons to decrease stimuli and avoid tension.

Essential violence prevention techniques include interpersonal skills that convey respect and unconditional positive regard. Improper behavior does not have to be accepted by ED staff, but no disrespect to the person should be conveyed. Start by stating explicitly that "this emergency department is a safe place" and the patient will be cared for well. Make the patient physically comfortable. Offer food or drink both as an expression of caring and also to minimize irritability. Do not surprise the patient; announce your arrival with a knock on the door or a verbal greeting. Ask permission to touch the patient before doing so. When speaking to the patient, use a calm and soothing voice. Listen attentively and intuitively to overt words and actions while attempting to assess underlying motivations and driving impulses. Additionally, listening will reassure the patient, and it is a caring act. Use straightforward speech and always be honest.

Even as the person receives genuine, unconditional care, boundaries of acceptable behavior should be set and consequences must be consistent. Inappropriate behavior is unacceptable and patients should be told the ramifications. Some patients do not have the ability to cope with the stressful environment and become verbally or physically uncontrolled. Other patients respond to limit setting and rules. Most require anxiolytics. Early use of a low-dose benzodiazepine often helps patients cope and prevents later escalation. No action or treatment should ever be punitive. Chemical restraint, physical restraint, seclusion, and arrest are predictable consequences of inappropriate behavior, but early medical therapy is compassionate and usually prevents escalation.

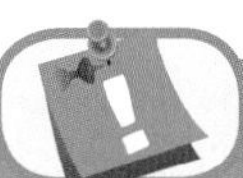

**TIPS AND TRICKS**

**Deescalation Techniques Useful for Prevention of Violence in the Emergency Department**

**Do**
Disrobe and gown all patients regardless of the chief complaint.
Disarm all patients at triage through the use of metal detectors.
Remove dangerous objects from the examination room.
Remove personal objects that can be used as weapons (tie, stethoscope).
Provide preferential, timely, and attentive care.
Make the patient comfortable (offer food, blankets).
Ask permission to enter the room and to examine or touch the patient.
Use a calm voice.
Explain anticipated waits, delays, and testing.
Set limits and ramifications for inappropriate behavior.

**Do Not**
Block exits from the examination room.
Shout or yell at patients.
Argue or challenge patients.
Allow your emotions to overcome your judgment and behavior.

Health care providers can escalate a patient's behavior through their own instinctive, impulsive, natural human conduct.[6] Anger or frustration should never inspire unprofessional behavior or decisions. Physical and emotional distance may minimize the emotional reactions. A buffer zone of at least four body widths between the provider and the patient is recommended.

When a caregiver feels the urge to shout, argue, or engage in a staring match with a patient, the caregiver is inadvertently reciprocating the violence of the patient. Controlling these natural instincts is an important professional skill that for many requires cultivation and practice. Other caregivers must cultivate a willingness to engage sufficiently because their instinct is to disengage. Too much distance can be equally detrimental. Finding the optimal emotional and physical distance to be effective and caring is a practiced art. If caregivers are too distant, they will be aloof, condescending, or disengaged. If caregivers are too close, they may become stimulated by the patient's disorder. The right distance enables control and effectiveness.

## MEDICAL CLEARANCE

Agitated or violent behavior is frequently caused by treatable medical conditions. Reversible causes of altered mental status and violent behavior should be considered during the initial evaluation of the patient. Such causes include substance abuse, intoxication, glucose abnormalities, hypoxia, trauma, abnormal temperature (hypothermia and hyperthermia), infection, stroke, hypertension, and seizures. Older adults with new agitated behavior, delirium, or psychosis should undergo an extensive inpatient medical evaluation before a first-time psychiatric unit admission.

## TREATMENT

### PHYSICAL RESTRAINT

#### *Rationale*

The use of restraint is indicated when verbal attempts have failed and action must be taken to prevent injury to the patient or staff. Restraint should be used only to facilitate diagnosis and treatment. It is inappropriate to use restraint as punishment or simply to quiet a disruptive patient.[7]

The Supreme Court case *Youngberg v. Romero 1982* provided exception from assault statutes for physicians who restrained patients to protect the patient or others. This physician decision must be made carefully, as rarely as possible, and only under compelling circumstances to ensure safety.

The Joint Commission has published clear guidelines regarding monitoring, documentation, and the application of physical restraint (**Box 195.2**). Protection of the patients' rights, dignity, and well-being is of utmost importance. The decision to apply physical restraint should be assessment driven; the provider must evaluate the individual patient in some way before a restraint is applied. It is inappropriate to maintain standing protocols. The selection of restraint should be individualized, and the least restrictive method is preferred; for instance, it is not necessary to restrain an agitated elderly patient with dementia in the same manner as an aggressive, muscular patient with cocaine intoxication. Hospitals must provide adequate training such that competent staff members are available for the safe application of physical restraint at all times.

**BOX 195.2 Guidelines for the Application of Physical Restraint**

Protect the patient's rights, dignity, and well-being.
Use of restraint is assessment driven.
Use the least restrictive method.
Trained, competent staff should provide safe application of restraint.
A time-limited order must be noted on the chart.
Document why restraint is necessary—be specific.
Protect yourself and others.
Act in the best interests of the patient.
Use restraints to facilitate medical evaluation or treatment.
Nursing documentation should be very thorough.
Monitoring and reassessment of the patient's clinical condition and needs are essential.

Adapted from The Joint Commission: 2006-2007. Comprehensive accreditation manual for behavioral health care. Oakbrook Terrace, Ill: Joint Commission Resources; 2006.

**BOX 195.3 Systematic Process for the Application of Physical Restraint**

Minimize physician involvement if possible.
The restraint team consists of four members and an identified leader:
- The restraint team enters together.
- The restraint team is professional and nonthreatening.
- The leader is at the head of the bed.
- The leader explains the process to the patient.

Limbs are controlled by contact at the major joints.
Restraints are attached to the solid frame of the gurney.

#### *Documentation*

Documentation differs for physicians and for nursing staff. A time-limited order for restraints must be written on the chart before or shortly after restraints are applied. Providers must document why physical restraints were necessary and must cite that verbal techniques failed to calm the patient. Be specific about the patient's condition and reasons for restraint, including potential danger to the patient or others, the planned medical evaluation or treatment, and assessment of the patient's decision-making capacity. Nursing responsibilities include monitoring, frequent reassessment, and documentation of the patient's condition and personal needs. The advent of electronic medical records and computerized physician order entry presents an opportunity to direct documentation that better meets regulatory requirements.[8]

#### *Technique*

Safe application of physical restraint is best achieved through systematic, consistent, protocol-driven techniques (**Box 195.3**). Many hospitals have a restraint team of at least five members who respond to the bedside when called by any

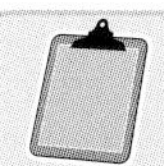

**DOCUMENTATION**

**Restraint***

**Physician**

Document why physical or chemical restraint was chosen and necessary. Cite that verbal techniques failed to calm the patient.

Record specific information about the patient's arrival, the reasons for restraint, the potential danger to self or others, the planned medical evaluation, and an assessment of the patient's decision-making capacity.

Record the initial evaluation by a licensed, independent provider within 1 hour of the patient's arrival and restraint.

A time-limited order should be charted within 1 hour of the patient's arrival.

Update restraint orders every 4 hours for adults, 2 hours for adolescents aged 9 to 17 years, and 1 hour for children younger than 9 years.[9]

**Nursing**

Frequently reassess the patient's vital signs, condition, and personal needs.

Patients should then be reassessed every 15 minutes for the following:

- Signs of injury associated with the application of restraint
- Nutrition and hydration
- Circulation and range of motion in the extremities
- Vital signs
- Hygiene and elimination
- Physical and psychologic status and comfort
- Readiness for discontinuation of restraint

*Refer to www.jointcommission.org for more information.

provider. One staff member should lead the restraint team, which usually consists of nurses, medical assistants, and security personnel. Ideally, physician involvement in restraint is minimized in an effort to preserve the physician-patient relationship as much as possible. Physicians are held responsible for the negligent application of restraint, however, so they should limit their involvement only if another experienced team member is available to lead the restraint team.

It is important for the restraint team to enter the room together in a professional but nonthreatening manner. This "show of force" frequently defuses any patient resistance. The leader should be positioned at the head of the bed, should inform the patient that he or she is to be restrained, and should explain the steps about to transpire. One member of the team is assigned to each limb and applies the restraint to that limb and to the solid frame of the bed or gurney. Limiting movement at major joints (elbow and knees) provides the most efficient and effective limb control.

Once clinically appropriate, restraints should be removed one at a time at 5-minute intervals until two restraints are left. If the patient is cooperative, the last two restraints should be removed at the same time.

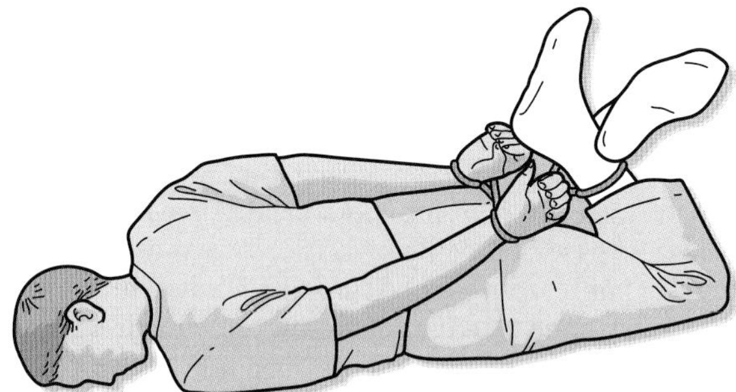

**Fig. 195.1** Incorrect method of patient restraint.

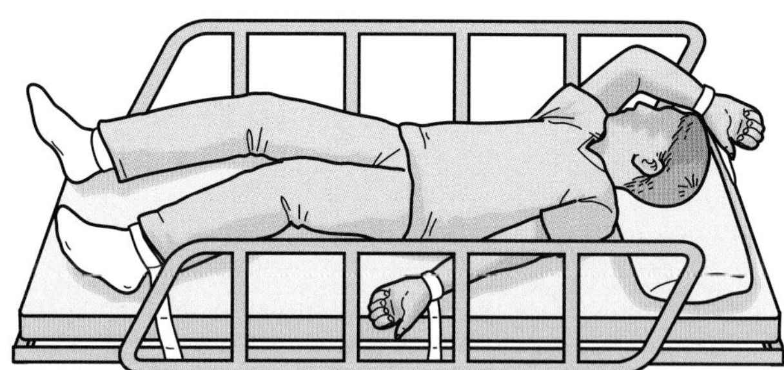

**Fig. 195.2** Proper attachment of restraints to the gurney.

## *Types of Physical Restraint*

The type of physical restraint used is frequently institution specific. Leather and soft cloth restraints are the types most commonly applied to the limbs. Leather restraints are difficult for the patient to remove and rarely compromise the distal circulation; however, they require a special key to remove and are difficult to cut off in an emergency. Soft cloth restraints may tighten as the patient struggles against them, thus causing circulatory compromise. In contrast to leather restraints, soft cloth restraints are simpler for staff to remove by untying knots or cutting with trauma shears. Vest and waist restraints ("posies") are useful for elderly patients who are at risk for wandering or falls but who not need their limbs restrained.

## *Positioning*

Restraint position may be changed depending on the patient's clinical status and the needs of the staff. Restraining a patient in the supine position is more comfortable for the patient and allows greater ease of examination. Patients with an increased risk for aspiration should be restrained on their side. Patients should not be restrained in a "hog-tied" position (**Fig. 195.1**).

Agitated patients are able to generate significant force and momentum and have been known to overturn gurneys if they are not restrained in the proper position. If all four limbs are to be restrained, the patient should have one arm up and one arm down. When only two limbs are restrained, the contralateral arm and leg should be restrained. It is more difficult to generate enough force to overturn a gurney in these positions (**Fig. 195.2**).

Special situations may arise when additional or alternative restraint is indicated. A sheet may be placed across the patient's chest and tied to the gurney as a chest restraint when movement of a patient's torso increases the risk for fall or injury despite the use of four-point limb restraint. Extra attention should be paid to the patient's respiratory status if a chest restraint is added. A firm cervical collar, such as a Philadelphia collar, may be applied to patients who bite. Some providers advocate greater patient comfort by tying the lower extremity to the contralateral bed rail. This allows more movement of the legs while preventing external rotation and extension of the knee for deriving more kicking power.

In the rare case of a patient who is loose in the ED or hospital with a knife or a needle-syringe assembly, a mattress may be used to push the patient into a wall, or two mattresses may be used to sandwich the patient and thus prevent injury to the patient, staff, or innocent bystanders.

### *Complications*

Abrasions and bruising account for the majority of complications resulting from restraint.[10] However, serious complications and death can occur if restraints are applied inappropriately or the patient is not adequately monitored.

One small subset of physically restrained patients, usually accompanied by law enforcement, suffers cardiac arrest shortly before or after arrival at the ED. For many years their demise was attributed to positional asphyxia related to the prone or hobble position.[11] Positional asphyxia results from an alteration in respiratory mechanics with ensuing decreased pulmonary function and increased cardiac output caused by the patient's position. This change in pulmonary function is not clinically relevant in normal volunteers subjected to prone restraint, however. More recent studies have found that factors related to the excited delirium are more likely to contribute to sudden death in these restrained individuals. Protracted struggle against physical restraint by patients with altered pain sensation may complicate or lead to hyperthermia, increased sympathetic tone with vasoconstriction, and release of lactic acid from prolonged isotonic muscle contractions. Profound metabolic acidosis is associated with cardiovascular collapse in many restraint-related deaths.[12] Cocaine and other sympathomimetic intoxications are frequently seen in this patient population.

Patients delivered to the ED who are restrained in a prone or hobble position should be turned onto their side. Patients who have been struggling against restraint should receive aggressive fluid resuscitation while evidence of associated metabolic acidosis or rhabdomyolysis is excluded. Aggressive chemical sedation should be administered to patients who continue to struggle against physical restraint.

## CHEMICAL RESTRAINT, ANXIOLYSIS, AND SEDATION

### *Rationale*

Chemical restraint is the administration, generally involuntarily, of medications to control a patient's dangerous behavior. Ideally, before violent behavior erupts, patients should be offered voluntary treatment with anxiolytics or sedatives to prevent the need for acute, involuntary behavioral control. Patients with the potential for violence often go to the ED voluntarily because they know that they need help and treatment. Experienced, wise caregivers offer an anxiolytic when it is evident that patients have poor self-control and a propensity for violence. Early provision of oral medication can maximize safety, patient comfort, and mutual trust. Chemical restraint is needed when verbal warnings and voluntary acceptance of low-dose anxiolytics are not prudent options. Chemical restraint is preferred over physical restraint to control a violent patient, but these methods are often properly used together for rapid control of dangerous behavior. Physical restraint should be used for as brief a period as possible. Chemical restraint should be more broadly applied because sedation and anxiolysis are preferable.

Many patients with a history of chronic psychiatric conditions know, accurately, that they have the right to refuse antipsychotic medication in nonemergency settings. However, this right does not extend to patients who are acutely combative and in whom violent behavior threatens life or limb by failure to become calm through verbal or physical means.[13] Although it is difficult to accurately predict the cause of agitated behavior, the choice of chemical restraint agent should be tailored to the suspected cause of agitation, the optimal duration of sedation, and the depth of sedation needed.

### *Butyrophenones*

Butyrophenones (haloperidol and droperidol) constitute the main class of typical antipsychotic medications recommended for an undifferentiated patient with acute agitation in the ED.[14] The butyrophenones are considered high-potency antipsychotic agents because of their strong affinity for the dopamine 2 ($D_2$) receptor in comparison with other typical antipsychotic agents. As a result of this affinity, the butyrophenones are more effective, cause less hypotension, and have fewer anticholinergic effects than older agents do.

Absolute contraindications to the use of butyrophenones include allergy to this class of drugs, anticholinergic drug intoxication, and a history of Parkinson disease. Relative contraindications include pregnancy, lactation, and hypovolemia. Butyrophenones are widely reported to decrease the seizure threshold, yet no conclusive evidence supports this observation, particularly in patients with sympathomimetic use.[15]

The most common complications of the use of butyrophenones are related to extrapyramidal symptoms, which occur in less than 10% of patients within the first 24 hours of ED care. Dystonic reactions and akathisia are the most common manifestations of extrapyramidal symptoms requiring treatment in the ED. Akathisia is frequently misdiagnosed as psychiatric decompensation when it is manifested as restlessness, pacing, tension, and irritability.[16] Extrapyramidal symptoms are treated with either benztropine (Cogentin), 2 mg, or diphenhydramine (Benadryl), 50 mg, intramuscularly or intravenously. Doses may be repeated every 5 minutes up to three times. Relief is rapid and dramatic in most cases. Benzodiazepines may be added for patients who do not respond initially. Many international providers use haloperidol in combination with promethazine because of its antihistamine and sedating properties. Studies show that this combination provides deeper sedation and requires less additional medication at 4 hours than an atypical antipsychotic does alone.[17]

As with other neuroleptic agents, neuroleptic malignant syndrome has been reported with the use of butyrophenones (**Table 195.1**). This potentially fatal complex of autonomic instability is marked by high fever, muscle rigidity, and altered mental status. Aggressive symptomatic treatment includes cooling, benzodiazepines, dantrolene, and discontinuation of the offending agent.[18]

HALOPERIDOL (HALDOL) Haloperidol may be given in 2.5- to 10-mg increments at 30- to 60-minute intervals for adults. Its onset of action is between 15 and 30 minutes and

**Table 195.1 Managing Acute Complications of Sedation with Antipsychotic Agents**

| PROBLEM | TREATMENT |
|---|---|
| Acute dystonic reaction | Discontinue antipsychotic medication<br>Benztropine (Cogentin), 2 mg IM<br>Discharge with benztropine (Cogentin), 2 mg PO qd for 3 days<br>***or***<br>Diphenhydramine (Benadryl), 50 mg IM<br>Discharge with diphenhydramine (Benadryl), 25-50 mg PO qid for 3 days |
| Akathisia | Benztropine (Cogentin), 1-2 mg IM/IV/PO qd to bid<br>***or***<br>Diphenhydramine (Benadryl), 50 mg IM/IV/PO tid to qid<br>Lorazepam (Ativan), 1-2 mg PO |
| Hypotension | Lie the patient flat |
| Profound hypotension or cardiac arrest | Normal saline bolus, 250-500 mL (repeat as tolerated and clinically necessary)<br>Phenylephrine (Neo-Synephrine), 0.005-0.02 mg/kg (0.35-1.4 mg for 70-kg adult) as a bolus IV every 10-15 min as needed |
| Increased temperature without other signs of NMS | Discontinue antipsychotic medication |
| Increased temperature with signs of NMS (lead pipe rigidity, diaphoresis, labile blood pressure, tachycardia, urinary incontinence, altered mental status) | Monitor closely for signs of NMS<br>Cool the patient<br>Add a benzodiazepine for sedation<br>Discontinue antipsychotic medication<br>Use active cooling measures<br>Add a benzodiazepine for sedation<br>Consider neuromuscular blockade (paralysis) if temperature >40° C<br>Institute aggressive hydration and alkalinization of urine to prevent renal failure from rhabdomyolysis<br>Dantrolene indicated for malignant hyperthermia but of unproven clinical benefit for NMS |

*bid*, Twice daily; *IM*, intramuscularly; *IV*, intravenously; *NMS*, neuroleptic malignant syndrome; *PO*, orally; *qd*, once daily; *qid*, four times daily; *tid*, three times daily.

its duration is 4 hours. Although a dosage ceiling has not been established, it is unusual to require more than three doses to achieve adequate sedation for an acute episode. It is rare to administer more than 60 mg in a 24-hour period.[19]

Though uncommon, the use of haloperidol in violent pediatric patients is well described. The pediatric dose of haloperidol is 0.075 mg/kg/day, repeated up to every hour (orally) or every 30 minutes (intramuscularly) at a dose of up to 2 mg/day in patients younger than 12 years. Of note, younger children are at greater risk for extrapyramidal symptoms than adolescents are because of increased $D_2$ receptor activity at younger ages.[20,21]

Although haloperidol is frequently given intravenously, this is an off-label use of the medication. Food and Drug Administration (FDA) approval is only for intramuscular or oral use. Prolongation of the QT interval has been observed with high-dose (e.g., 50 mg) intravenous haloperidol.

Haloperidol remains an effective and inexpensive option for the treatment of acute aggression. It is well tolerated if coadministered with an anticholinergic agent.[20]

DROPERIDOL (INAPSINE) Droperidol has a long history of use for the treatment of acute agitation in the ED. Studies have shown the superiority of droperidol over haloperidol within the first 30 minutes of intramuscular administration. The FDA issued a "black box" warning for droperidol in 2001, however, because of the risk for QT prolongation and ventricular dysrhythmias causing sudden cardiac death. Some authors analyzed the case records cited by the FDA and presented cogent arguments supporting continued use of this drug; these investigators questioned the reasoning behind the "black box" warning.[22-24] Administration of droperidol for the treatment of violent patients and migraine headaches is now considered an off-label use of the drug. Droperidol is still approved for intravenous administration to prevent and treat postoperative nausea and vomiting.

Droperidol may be given in 2.5- to 5-mg increments intravenously at 15-minute intervals for adults. The intramuscular dose is 5 to 10 mg. Its onset of action is between 3 and 10 minutes. More than two doses are rarely required to achieve adequate sedation for an acute episode. The time to arousal is approximately 2 hours.[19] Droperidol was found to produce more consistent moderate sedation than occurs with midazolam and the combination of droperidol and midazolam together.

Conduction abnormalities can develop with the administration of butyrophenones in high doses. The FDA "black box" warning for droperidol also referred to some cases of conduction abnormalities at low doses. Experts recommend obtaining an electrocardiogram before administering droperidol to patients in the ED, a recommendation that is impractical with an acutely agitated or violent patient. Although many authors disagree with the conclusions of the FDA, it is prudent to avoid the use of butyrophenones in elderly patients, critically ill patients, or patients with known preexisting heart disease.[18]

### *Benzodiazepines*

Benzodiazepines are preferred first-line agents for the acute management of agitation.[12] Benzodiazepines are particularly useful for agitation caused by the ingestion of sympathomimetic agents and alcohol withdrawal. Sedation and mild respiratory depression are the most prominent side effects of benzodiazepines. Therefore, these drugs are quite safe in patients with most medical comorbid conditions. Lorazepam and midazolam are the two prototypic benzodiazepines used for the treatment of violent patients in the ED.

LORAZEPAM (ATIVAN) Observational studies have reported that lorazepam is at least as effective as haloperidol in treating patients with acute agitation. Lorazepam is given in 0.5- to 2-mg increments as frequently as every 15 minutes, depending on the patient's level of sedation and respiratory status. Intramuscular injection is the most common route of administration and is quite reliable. Lorazepam has a shorter half-life than some parenteral benzodiazepines and lacks active metabolites. Lorazepam may also be given intravenously, orally, and sublingually. The time of onset after intravenous or intramuscular injection is between 15 and 30 minutes, and the drug's effect lasts more than 3 hours. Sublingual or oral administration of lorazepam is a viable alternative route for patients who are cooperative and would benefit from rapid relief of anxiety (**Table 195.2**). Lorazepam is classified as a class D agent in pregnancy and thus should be avoided in pregnant and lactating women. Pediatric dosing of lorazepam is 0.05 mg/kg with doses of 0.5 to 2 mg orally or intramuscularly. Onset is 30 minutes orally and 15 minutes intramuscularly. The duration of effect is 6 hours orally or intramuscularly.[20]

MIDAZOLAM (VERSED) Midazolam is particularly beneficial if rapid sedation is required and prolonged sedation is less important. The first ED study describing midazolam for this indication used an intramuscular dose of 5 mg, which provided rapid sedation with a mean time to onset of 18 minutes and arousal at a mean time of 82 minutes.[25] Another study reported the effective sedation time to be 45 minutes for midazolam and more than 2 hours for other agents.[26] Fewer cardiorespiratory effects are seen with the intramuscular administration of midazolam; most authors have reported no difference in vital signs or oxygen saturation in comparison with other agents used to sedate agitated or violent patients when the 5-mg dose was administered.[20,25] However, other authors have reported increased respiratory depression in patients suffering from alcohol intoxication.[27] The intramuscular dose should be decreased by half in elderly patients or when midazolam is used in combination with opioid agents. Larger doses of midazolam (e.g., 10 to 15 mg intramuscularly) result in greater need for airway adjuncts.[28]

Treatment of oversedation and respiratory depression from the use of benzodiazepines in agitated or violent patients is supportive care (**Fig. 195.3**). Supplemental oxygen, repositioning, and airway adjuncts such as nasal trumpets suffice in most cases. Active airway management, including jaw thrusts, use of bag-valve-mask ventilation, or endotracheal intubation, is rarely necessary. It is prudent to avoid the use of flumazenil (Romazicon) because of the frequency of epileptogenic coingestion and the use of combination therapy with butyrophenones.

**Table 195.2 Medication Recommendations for Patients Willing to Take Oral Medications**

| CLINICAL SCENARIO | RECOMMENDED ORAL MEDICATION |
|---|---|
| No information on past history | Lorazepam |
| Psychosis in the past; delirium or dementia | Risperidone |
| Cardiac arrhythmias or conduction defects | Lorazepam |
| Diabetes or hyperglycemia | Lorazepam and haloperidol, ziprasidone |
| Obesity | Lorazepam |
| Pediatric ages | Haloperidol, lorazepam, atypical antipsychotic agents, antihistamines |

COMBINATION THERAPY The combination of lorazepam, 2 mg, and haloperidol, 5 mg, for sedation of agitated psychotic patients was found to be superior to either agent alone when investigators considered the speed of sedation and frequency of side effects. The duration of sedation was longer in patients receiving combination therapy.[29] Lorazepam, haloperidol, and benztropine (Cogentin, 1 mg) can be administered in the same intramuscular syringe.

### *Atypical Antipsychotic Medications*

Second-generation (atypical) antipsychotic drugs became feasible options for the treatment of agitated and violent patients in the ED with approval of the first intramuscular formulation in 2001. Several such medications are now available in intramuscular or rapidly absorbable formulations and are indicated for the treatment of acute agitation in selected patient populations. This class of antipsychotics acts by blocking both $D_2$ and serotonin (5-HT) receptors and provides more tranquilization than sedation. The increased serotonin receptor activity results in fewer extrapyramidal effects. Second-generation antipsychotic agents are available in oral preparations, which allows easier conversion to long-term therapy when compared with the benzodiazepines and butyrophenones.

Atypical antipsychotic agents have been used in off-label fashion for the treatment of behavioral disorders in elderly patients for several years. In 2005, the FDA distributed an advisory describing a higher death rate in demented patients receiving atypical antipsychotic medications versus placebo. It is unclear how this advisory applies to the limited use of these drugs in the ED for acutely agitated elderly patients.

ZIPRASIDONE (GEODON) Ziprasidone is approved for the treatment of acute agitation in schizophrenic and bipolar/manic patients. Ziprasidone has not been extensively studied

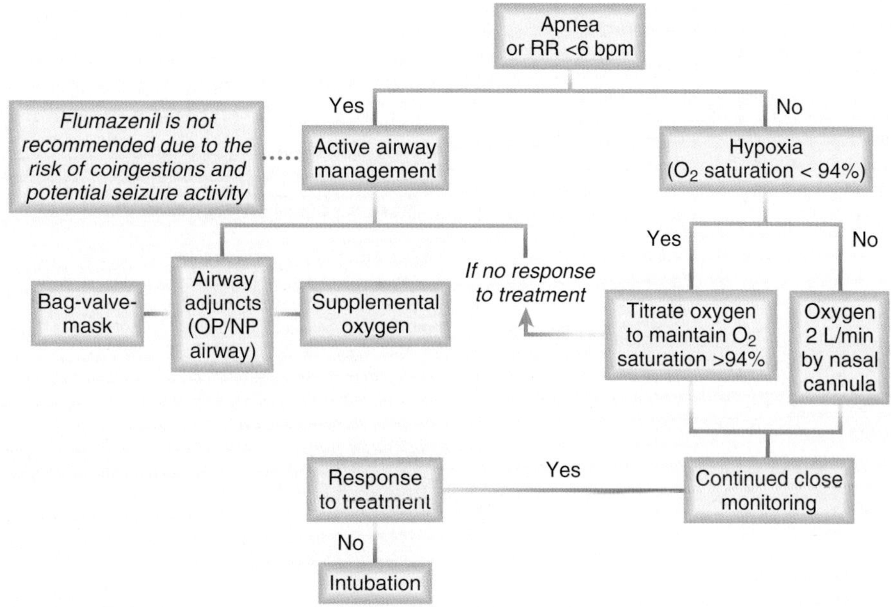


**Fig. 195.3 Respiratory depression after the administration of sedative medication (respiratory rate [RR] < 10 breaths per minute [bpm]).** $O_2$, Oxygen; *OP/NP*, oropharyngeal/nasopharyngeal.

in patients with undifferentiated causes of agitation in the ED. The typical dose is 10 mg intramuscularly every 2 hours or 20 mg intramuscularly every 4 hours. Ziprasidone is associated with the greatest change in the QT interval of the atypical antipsychotics, comparable with the QT prolongation seen with haloperidol. In addition, ziprasidone needs to be diluted and is not as readily available for use as other agents.[16] No dosing information is available for the use of ziprasidone in children with agitation, but the drug is used for the treatment of Tourette syndrome at a dose of 5 to 40 mg/day.[26]

OLANZAPINE (ZYPREXA) Olanzapine is also approved for the treatment of acute agitation in schizophrenic and bipolar/manic patients in the ED. Olanzapine is available in either an intramuscular or oral disintegrating tablet formulation at 5 to 10 mg. Olanzapine is strongly sedating and demonstrates 160 times the antihistamine potency of diphenhydramine. Olanzapine causes the smallest change in QT interval of the atypical antipsychotics. Long-term use of the drug is associated with weight gain and hyperglycemia.[26] The manufacturer does not recommend the combination of intramuscular olanzapine with a parenteral benzodiazepine. Olanzapine has been approved for use in children at a dose of 0.1 mg/kg. Children younger than 12 years may receive 2.5 mg orally or intramuscularly. Children older than 12 years may be administered the adult dose. Its onset of action is 30 minutes orally and 10 to 20 minutes intramuscularly, with a duration of action of up to 24 hours.[20]

RISPERIDONE (RISPERDAL) Risperidone is equivalent to haloperidol for the treatment of psychosis, and it is possibly more effective in treating aggressive behavior. Risperidone may be administered orally in the ED as a liquid formulation or as a rapidly disintegrating tablet at a dose of 1 to 3 mg. Although both methods of oral administration are easier with a cooperative patient, the liquid formulation can be mixed in a beverage or administered orally by syringe to resistant patients. The mean time until sleep was 43 minutes in one study. Risperidone has fewer anticholinergic properties, thus resulting in less confusion and sedation than with other atypical antipsychotic agents. Pediatric dosing of risperidone is 0.025 to 0.05 mg/kg. Children younger than 12 years may receive a dose of 0.25 to 0.5 mg orally. Pubertal pediatric patients may be administered a dose of 0.5 to 1 mg orally. Doses may be repeated two to four times until sedated. Its onset of action is 30 minutes with a peak concentration in 1 to 2 hours.[20]

ARIPIPRAZOLE (ABILIFY) Aripiprazole is approved for the treatment of acute agitation in patients with schizophrenia and bipolar mania. It is available as a 9.75-mg intramuscular injection and may be repeated every 2 hours. Doses should not exceed more than 30 mg/day. Aripiprazole is equivalent to haloperidol with regard to control of agitation without oversedation.[16] An oral dose of 2 mg is recommended for pediatric patients because of autism-related irritability or bipolar mania.

## NEXT STEPS

Patients may demonstrate resolution of their agitation in the ED as a result of sleep or the metabolism of offending drugs and alcohol. Patients may be considered for discharge if they have normal mental status without agitation on waking, as long as other acute medical and psychiatric conditions have been addressed. Patients who continue to exhibit violent or threatening behavior, abnormal vital signs, or evidence of psychiatric decompensation require further medical or psychiatric care.

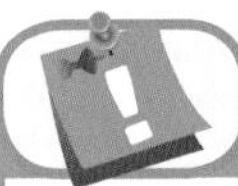

**TIPS AND TRICKS**

Violence rarely erupts without warning.
- Primary prevention: Control factors leading to violence.
- Secondary prevention: Respond to previolent behavior.
- Tertiary prevention: Limit injury once violence is present.

Avoid the "us versus them" mentality: Unprofessional staff behavior can elicit violent eruptions by patients.

R-E-S-P-E-C-T goes a long way toward helping patients regain their composure.

Be aware of your own reactions: You can make the situation worse.

"GOT IVS": The seven do-not-forget reversible causes of altered metal status and violent behavior:
- Glucose
- Oxygen
- Trauma/temperature
- Infection
- Vascular (stroke, hypertension)
- Seizure/status epilepticus

Document, document, document: If restraint is the right thing to do, be sure to say why.

Different situations require different medications and treatment; one drug is not good for all circumstances, so tailor your treatment to the situation.

Agitated or violent patients who elope from the ED before full evaluation or resolution of their symptoms represent a significant legal risk to providers, as well as a risk to the safety of themselves and other individuals. Legal authorities should be notified of the elopement of such patients.

## SUGGESTED READINGS

Allen MH, Currier GW, Carpenter D, et al. The expert consensus guideline series: treatment of behavior emergencies 2005. J Psychiatr Pract 2005;11(Suppl 1):6-108.

Hill S, Petit J. The violent patient. Emerg Med Clin North Am 2000;18:301-15.

Marco CA, Vaughan J. Emergency management of agitation in schizophrenia. Am J Emerg Med 2005;23:767-76.

Sorrentino A. Chemical restraints for the agitated, violent, or psychotic pediatric patient in the emergency department: controversies and recommendations. Curr Opin Pediatr 2004;16:201-5.

Zun LS. A prospective study of the complication rate of use of patient restraint in the emergency department. J Emerg Med 2003;24:119-24.

## REFERENCES

***References can be found on Expert Consult @ www.expertconsult.com.***

# Self-Harm and Danger to Others 196

*Nicole Malouf, Benjamin F. Jackson, and Keith Borg*

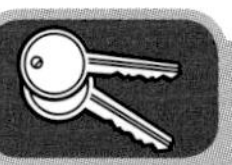

**KEY POINTS**

- Risk factors that increase the likelihood of self-harm include depression and other mental disorders, alcohol or substance abuse, separation or divorce, physical or sexual abuse, and significant medical conditions such as human immunodeficiency virus infection, cancer, and dialysis-dependent renal failure.
- Psychiatric illness and substance abuse increase the likelihood of homicidal ideation.
- Although adolescent and young adult female patients are more likely to be treated in the emergency department after a suicidal gesture, older men are more likely to commit suicide.
- In the United States, all 50 states provide physicians the legal right to commit any patient who is a threat to either self or others.
- Health professionals are required to inform individuals directly if they are at risk for harm from a homicidal patient. Police should also be notified of such risk.
- Any patient discharged from the emergency department after appropriate psychiatric evaluation should agree to immediately seek medical care if thoughts of violence or self-harm return.

## EPIDEMIOLOGY

Patients with suicidal or homicidal ideation are encountered frequently in the emergency department (ED). Approximately 0.4% of all ED visits in the United States involve suicidal patients, and suicide accounted for 34,598 deaths in 2007 (almost twice the number of deaths by homicide, 18,361), which makes it the 10th leading cause of death overall.[1] For Americans aged 15 to 24 years, suicide ranks as the third leading cause of death.[2] This age group also accounts for more ED visits for attempted suicide and self-injury than any other age group does. More than 1200 children and adolescents complete suicide annually in the United States,[3] and it is estimated that 11 attempted suicides occur per suicide death.[1] More than 40% of individuals 16 years or older who completed suicide were evaluated in an ED in the year before their terminal act.[3]

Although the rate of attempted suicide was highest in female patients 15 to 19 years old, nearly five times as many males died by suicide in this age group. About six times as many males as females died by suicide in the 20- to 24-year age group, and older, non-Hispanic white men have a suicide rate than is staggeringly higher than the national average for the general population. Of patients with evidence of self-harm, poisoning was the cause of death in 13% of males and 40% of females, suffocation in 24% of males and 21% of females, and firearms in 56% of males and 30% of females.[1] Self-mutilation (by cutting or piercing) was observed in 20% of patients evaluated in the ED for a suicidal gesture. One third of suicidal patients were admitted for inpatient management, one third were transferred to an off-site facility, and one fifth were referred to outpatient psychiatric services.[4]

Intentionally harmful behavior also constitutes a growing problem in children, adolescents, and young adults. It has been estimated that the prevalence of mental illness among youth in Canada and the United States approaches 15% to 20%, with an anticipated 50% increase by 2020. Pediatric mental health complaints account for 1.6% of all annual ED visits in the United States and 1% of all annual ED visits in Canada.[2,5]

Homicide ranks as the most common cause of death in black males 15 to 24 years of age and is the second leading cause of deaths for all youths in this age group. In 2005 alone, more than 5000 deaths by homicide occurred in this age group, and in 2006 this age group received medical care for more than 750,000 cases of nonfatal violent injury.[6]

A focused risk assessment is the primary objective for the emergency provider caring for a patient who is threatening harm to self or others. Risk assessments vary widely, depending on the circumstances of the patient, comorbid disease, mental status, and other social issues. The main challenge to effective risk assessment is the lack of a specific diagnostic test to stratify threat in suicidal or homicidal patients. No interventional test is currently available to determine who is at greatest risk for injury—data for risk stratification come from psychologic autopsy, which is the study of patient characteristics in completed suicides. Predictive data for outcomes of these patients after ED evaluation are lacking. This chapter focuses on the directed examination and evaluation of patients who pose threats of harm to self or others.

## PATHOPHYSIOLOGY

Numerous factors influence the likelihood of self-harm, including depression and other mental disorders, alcohol or substance abuse, separation or divorce, physical or sexual abuse, and significant medical conditions such as human immunodeficiency virus infection, cancer, and dialysis-dependent renal failure (see the "Red Flags" box). Previous suicide attempters also have more concurrent general medical conditions, alcohol or substance abuse, work hours missed, and current suicidal ideation than do nonattempters.[7] More than 90% of people who die by suicide have a mental health disorder, a substance abuse disorder, or both.[1] Depression is a significant and common risk factor to address because one in three patients encountered in the ED have moderate to severe depression. In adult male ED patients, depression is more strongly associated with the likelihood of perpetrating violent behavior than excessive alcohol consumption is.[8]

Besides the presence of risk factors, poorly understood biologic factors probably influence self-harm. Serotonin levels have been studied in suicidal patients, and data suggest that lower levels of cerebral 5-hydroxyindoleacetic acid (a serotonin metabolite) are found in patients who attempt suicide.[9-11] Increasing serotonin levels through pharmacotherapy with drug classes such as tricyclic antidepressants or selective serotonin reuptake inhibitors is a common treatment of depression and suicidal ideation.

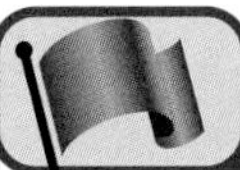

**RED FLAGS**

Potentially lethal attempt
Patient found accidentally
Trauma incongruent with an accident (single-car motor vehicle crash, pedestrians struck by a vehicle)
Intoxicated or altered patients
Previous suicide attempts
History of mental illness, especially depression or schizophrenia
History of alcohol or substance abuse
Male gender
Widowed or divorced status
Elderly status
Family history of suicide, mental disorders, or substance abuse
Family history of child maltreatment, including physical or sexual abuse
Access to firearms
Incarceration
Feelings of hopelessness
Impulsive or aggressive tendencies
Barriers to accessing mental health treatment
Loss (relationship, work, financial)
Physical illness (especially human immunodeficiency virus infection, cancer, end-stage renal disease)
Easy access to lethal methods (stored pills, firearms)
Unwillingness to seek help because of stigma attached to mental illness, substance abuse, and suicidal ideation
Conflicting cultural or religious beliefs
Local epidemics of suicide
Isolation
Presence of breast implants

Data from American Psychiatric Association. Practice guideline for the assessment and treatment of patients with suicidal behaviors. November 2003. Available at http://www.psych.org/psych_pract/treatg/pg/prac_guide.cfm; and Villeneuve P, Holowaty E, Brisson J, et al. Mortality among Canadian women with cosmetic breast implants. Am J Epidemiol 2006;164:334-41.

## PRESENTING SIGNS AND SYMPTOMS

Patients may seek treatment in the ED after considering or attempting to harm themselves or others. These actions range from unsuccessful, yet serious gestures to the use of suicidal ideation for secondary gain. Clinical suspicion should always be high, and patients' complaints must be taken seriously. Careful, open-ended, nonjudgmental questioning can help discern the level of risk by understanding the patient's intent.

In addition, emergency physicians should be cognizant of interactions with adolescent patients and consider screening either formally or informally for suicidal ideation. A recent study evaluated the feasibility of screening nonpsychiatric patients for suicide risk and targeted patients between the ages of 10 and 21 years. In this study interval, 37 of 50 patients with psychiatric complaints screened positive for suicide risk. However, 27 of 106 patients evaluated for nonpsychiatric complaints also screened positive for suicide risk. Each of the patients underwent formal psychiatric consultation, and none of the patients with nonpsychiatric complaints warranted hospitalization but were provided with available outpatient psychiatric services. Interestingly, screening of nonpsychiatric patients did not increase the overall length of stay.[3]

Injured patients with a concerning mechanism (ingestion, single-person car accident, fall) should be screened for suicidal ideation and intent. If an attempt is uncovered, the provider should solicit the patient's feelings about survival. It is important to understand why patients survived as a predictor of immediate or ongoing risk for harm. The following questions should be considered:

Was the patient found accidentally?
Did a low-risk gesture precede a phone call for help?
Is the patient sad to have survived?
Is the patient having increasing thoughts of suicide?
Does the patient have a plan? Has the patient gathered the means to act on that plan?
Is the patient feeling depressed or hopeless, or does the patient appear withdrawn?
What are the patient's risk factors for future suicidal ideation or attempts?

A practice guideline of the American Psychiatric Association summarized large amounts of retrospective data regarding risk factors in patients who committed suicide.[12] The relative importance and clinical utility of such risk factors can be challenging, however. Seemingly innocuous patient data may represent significant risk, as evidenced by studies demonstrating a higher suicide rate in women who received breast implants.[13] Such epidemiologic studies are difficult to translate into clinical practice, but they do provide an understanding of the complexity of risk stratification in suicidal and homicidal patients.

## DIFFERENTIAL DIAGNOSIS AND MEDICAL DECISION MAKING

The differential diagnosis of self-harm includes minor depression, major depression, suicidal ideation, suicidal gestures, and suicidal attempts of varying lethality and intent. Other alternative diagnoses can be difficult to establish in the ED. One such alternative is the threat of suicide for secondary gain; very little is written or researched about patients with such intents. The goal of secondary gain is often hospitalization to avoid incarceration, legal prosecution, homelessness, or other social problems. A second alternative diagnosis is intentional self-mutilation, such as cutting or hair pulling. This is differentiated from suicidal ideation by its nonlethal intent and frequency of the behavior. Self-mutilation is believed to be a maladaptive response to stress.

### MOST COMMON AND MOST THREATENING PRESENTATIONS

Common manifestations of suicidality include minor threats or ideation of suicide by nonlethal means (**Box 196.1**). The most frequent ED scenarios involve young female patients who report a recent ingestion. Depressive symptoms are also common.

Men are far more likely to complete suicide.[4] Threatening scenarios include attempts with potentially lethal consequences, a history of previous attempts, traumatic attempts that are difficult to recognize (e.g., single-car motor vehicle crashes), and elderly men with suicidal ideation.

## DIAGNOSTIC TESTING

Diagnostic testing in patients with threats of harm to self should focus on the mechanism of the suicidal attempt and any significant comorbid disease (including alcohol and drug abuse). Specific testing may help in evaluating certain treatable ingestions, such as acetaminophen or salicylates; in many cases, however, no specific testing is required. Imaging should be ordered appropriately for patients whose harmful actions involve jumping, hanging, or other traumatic injuries. Screening laboratory tests may be required to arrange for transfer or admission to a psychiatric facility, although such testing has little diagnostic value in the ED evaluation and treatment of suicidal or homicidal patients.[14]

**BOX 196.1 Most Threatening and Most Common Scenarios**

**Most Threatening**

- Suicide attempt with potentially lethal means
- Accidental discovery of a suicide attempt
- Elderly men with suicidal ideation
- Suicidal ideation with a clear plan or history of previous attempts
- Homicidal ideation with a plan or means

**Most Common**

- Depressive thoughts or expressions ("Life is not worth living")
- Suicidal gestures such as nonlethal ingestions
- Cutting
- Threatening suicide for secondary gain

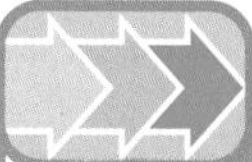

**PRIORITY ACTIONS**

- Evaluate for any immediate life threats from a suicide attempt or current ideation.
- Place the patient in a setting in which constant monitoring is possible.
- Minimize the patient's risk to self, staff, and others.

## TREATMENT

Patients who have attempted suicide must be evaluated immediately to determine the lethality of the reported or suspected method of harm. Once the threat assessment is complete, the patient should be placed in a closely monitored setting. Physical or chemical restraint and suicide precautions may be required in certain circumstances. Suicide precautions include undressing and gowning the patient, removal of potential weapons or harmful items, one-on-one or video supervision, and security escort for travel and transfer. Careful questioning and examination of the patient should establish the level of risk and cooperation.

All 50 states provide the physician the ability to commit any individual who is a threat either to self or to others or who is unable to care for himself or herself. This psychiatric hold is time limited (usually 72 hours) to permit emergency evaluation and treatment of the patient. The specific actions and documentation required to commit a patient vary by state jurisdiction. Adherence to the process is very important, and the decision to act should be made with appropriate gravity. Documentation of the reason for committal should be provided in clear detail, and supplementary historical information from family, police, or others should also be included in the chart.

*Tarasoff v. Regents of the University of California* was a landmark legal decision in 1976 that established an obligation by the health care professional to warn a specific individual at identifiable risk for harm, thus overriding the patient's confidentiality. To fulfil this obligation, both the threatened individual and the police must be informed of the intentions of the homicidal patient. Patients who have an intention to hurt or kill an identifiable individual should be committed and evaluated by a psychiatrist. Discussions with legal and psychiatric colleagues should clarify who will perform any required notification.

Contracts for safety are pacts that include a patient's promise to seek immediate evaluation should thoughts of violence or self-harm increase. Current American Psychiatric Association guidelines do not recommend contracts for safety in emergency situations,[12] although such understandings should be reinforced with any patient who is discharged after psychiatric evaluation in the ED.

## DISPOSITION

Once the initial challenges of medical assessment have been met, the practitioner should determine the safest and most appropriate disposition for the individual patient's social condition (**Fig. 196.1**). Psychiatric consultants often aid in the necessary evaluation, admission, or follow-up of at-risk patients. If the clinician has significant concerns, the patient should be admitted or transferred to an appropriately safe inpatient setting. Patients may need to be committed for involuntary psychiatric admission if they are not willing to sign in voluntarily.

One prospectively validated tool that is valuable for use in the ED is the Modified SAD PERSONS Scale developed by Hockberger and Rothstein in 1988 (**Table 196.1**). The scale uses a series of criteria that allow easy review of risk factors and assist in the identification of conditions that should

**TIPS AND TRICKS**

Establish referral patterns with consultants and mental health services in advance.

Know your local resources for inpatient and outpatient psychiatric care.

Do not be judgmental or condescending. Despite being in crisis, patients perceive your degree of concern or lack of compassion.

Do not allow staff to make pejorative comments in which they "instruct" patients how to complete a future suicide attempt.

Deescalate the situation by using calming mannerisms, voice, and tone.

Be safe—stay between the door and the patient.

Do not approach violent patients alone.

Ask permission to sit down beside the patient and have a conversation. Be willing to listen.

Involuntary commitment is frequently reportable on job applications and physician licensure. Voluntary commitment is seen as asking for help. This distinction can be used to persuade patients to agree to admission and to seek future help without long-term repercussions.

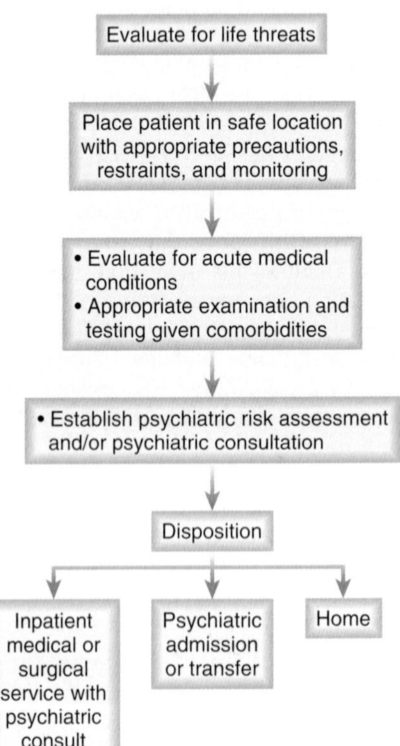


**Fig. 196.1** Algorithm for the evaluation and treatment of suicidal or homicidal patients.

**Table 196.1 Modified SAD PERSONS Scale of Hockberger and Rothstein: Based on the SAD PERSONS Mnemonic**

| PARAMETER | FINDING | POINTS |
|---|---|---|
| **S**ex | Male<br>Female | 1<br>0 |
| **A**ge | <19 yr<br>19-45 yr<br>>45 yr | 1<br>0<br>1 |
| **D**epression or hopelessness | Present<br>Absent | 2<br>0 |
| **P**revious attempts or psychiatric care | Previous suicide attempts or psychiatric care<br>Neither | 1<br>0 |
| **E**xcessive alcohol or drug use | Excessive<br>Not excessive or none | 1<br>0 |
| **R**ational thinking loss | Lost as a result of an organic brain syndrome or psychosis<br>Intact | 2<br>0 |
| **S**eparated, divorced, or widowed | Separated, divorced, or widowed<br>Married or always single | 1<br>0 |
| **O**rganized or serious attempt | Organized, well thought out, or serious<br>Neither | 2<br>0 |
| **N**o social support | None (no close family, friends, job, or active religious affiliation)<br>Present | 1<br>0 |
| **S**tated future intent | Determined to repeat or ambivalent about the prospect<br>No intent | 2<br>0 |
| **SCORE*** | **MANAGEMENT** | |
| 0-5 | May be safe to discharge, depending on circumstances | |
| 6-8 | Requires emergency psychiatric consultation | |
| 9-14 | Probably requires hospitalization | |

Adapted from Hockberger RS, Rothstein RJ. Assessment of suicide potential by non-psychiatrists using the SAD PERSONS score. J Emerg Med 1988;6:99-107.

*The score equals the points for all 10 parameters: minimum score, 0; maximum score, 14. The higher the score, the greater the risk for suicide. A patient with a score of 5 or less rarely requires hospitalization.

prompt admission. Patients with a low score are less likely to have adverse events.[15] However, patients testing positive for anxiety and hopelessness with concurrent depression are at increased risk to commit suicide.[7]

As evidence suggests from multiple studies, the following four items have also demonstrated high sensitivity and specificity for predicting suicidality in adolescents:

Are you here because you tried to hurt yourself?
In the past week, have you been having thoughts about hurting yourself?
Have you tried to hurt yourself in the past other than this time?
Has something very stressful happened to you in the past few weeks?[3,16,17]

For homicidal patients or victims of violent injury, it is incumbent on the provider to assess the risk for retaliatory violence. Because retaliation often occurs in the weeks immediately following an incident and commonly involves firearms, the following screening questions (known as the "FiGHTS" mnemonic) may aid the ED clinician in determining an adolescent's risk for carrying handguns:

**F**ights: During the last 12 months, have you been in a physical fight?
**G**ender: Male
**H**urt: During the last 12 months, have you been in a fight in which you were injured and had to be treated by a physician or nurse?
**T**hreatened: During the last 12 months, have you been threatened with a weapon (knife or gun) on school property?
**S**moker: Have you ever smoked cigarettes regularly (1 cigarette per day for 30 days)?[6]

A positive screen for suicidal or homicidal ideation or intent should prompt further evaluation and management, but patients may be discharged home if they are deemed safe after medical evaluation and psychiatric consultation (**Box 196.2**). Among patients discharged from the ED, significant predictors of return visits within 30 days include lack of a caregiver at the time of discharge and a history of a previous suicide attempt.[18] A treatment plan, return precautions, and conditions for safety should be clear, well documented, and understood by all parties involved (including friends, family, and caregivers of the patient, especially when children or adolescents are involved).

**BOX 196.2 Reassuring Factors for Safe Discharge**

Care established for mental, physical, and substance abuse disorders
Follow-up in 1 to 2 days
Family and community support
Problem-solving and conflict resolution skills
Cultural and religious beliefs that discourage suicide and support the patient

From American Psychiatric Association. Practice guideline for the assessment and treatment of patients with suicidal behaviors. November 2003. Available at http://www.psych.org/psych_pract/treatg/pg/prac_guide.cfm.

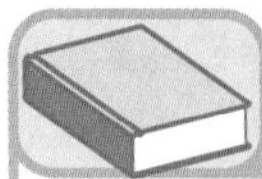

**PATIENT TEACHING TIPS**

Patients who are going to be discharged must be sober.
Contract for safety: patients must state that they will not harm themselves and that they will return to the emergency department if thoughts of violence or self-harm return.
Patients must be discharged to a safe environment, such as home with supportive friends or family who are able to offer needed assistance.
It should be made clear that if patients' conditions change, they should return to the emergency department for reevaluation. Patients should be made welcome to do so at any time.
Resources for outpatient follow-up should be appropriate to the social situation.
If possible, confirm that patients have a designated time and place for follow-up.

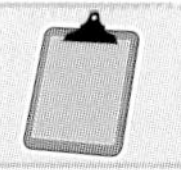

**DOCUMENTATION**

Document the patient's risk factors, psychiatric history, medical history, and discussions with supplemental historians (friends, family, police).
Record the process of admission or discharge and make note of risk stratification and medical decision making.
- Example: "This patient is deemed stable for discharge because he has contracted for safety, has mental health follow-up tomorrow morning (which has been confirmed by telephone), is going home with family who are supportive, has no firearms or stockpile of pills at home, and has no concurrent medical or other high-risk social issues."

Carefully document the reasons for psychiatric committal, and give specific examples.
Document discussions and decision making with psychiatric consultants.

## SUGGESTED READINGS

American Psychiatric Association. Practice guideline for the assessment and treatment of patients with suicidal behaviors. November 2003. Available at http://www.psych.org/psych_pract/treatg/pg/prac_guide.cfm.
Cunningham R, Knox L, Fein J, et al. Before and after the trauma bay; the prevention of violent injury among youth. Ann Emerg Med 2009;53:490-500.
Newton AS, Hamm MP, Bethell J, et al. Pediatric suicide-related presentations: a systematic review of mental health care in the emergency department. Ann Emerg Med 2010;56:649-59.

## REFERENCES

*References can be found on Expert Consult @ www.expertconsult.com.*

# 197 Anxiety and Panic Disorders

*Christopher S. Kang and Benjamin P. Harrison*

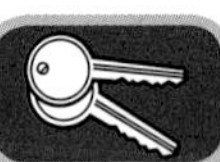

**KEY POINTS**

- Anxiety disorders are the most common psychiatric illnesses diagnosed in adolescents and older adults, are increasingly being seen in urban emergency departments, and occur more frequently in women than in men.
- Potentially life-threatening medical disorders may feature somatic and cognitive signs and symptoms that often mimic anxiety on initial evaluation.
- Most anxiety disorders have significant familial aggregation, with the inheritability of panic disorder approaching a rate of 40%.
- Panic attack is a discrete episode of sudden, intense apprehension, fearfulness, or terror that is often associated with feelings of impending doom.
- Benzodiazepines are the recommended first-line agents for the pharmacologic management of anxiety.

## DEFINITION AND EPIDEMIOLOGY

Anxiety is defined as an unpleasant emotional state consisting of psychologic and physiologic responses to the anticipation of real or imagined danger.[1] Regardless of whether the observed disease prevalence is related to the escalating complexity and stress of traumatic events and modern life, evolving access to medical and behavioral health care, the inherent nature of the emergency department (ED), or an increased awareness of psychiatric disorders, anxiety is common in patients who seek emergency care.[2,3]

In the United States, anxiety disorders have a 12-month prevalence of 18% and a lifetime prevalence that approaches 25%. Anxiety-related conditions cost more than $42 billion in medical expenses and lost worker productivity in 1990 alone.[4-6] Patients with anxiety disorders use outpatient and emergency care more often and generate higher medical costs than do patients without anxiety disorders.[7]

Anxiety disorders are increasingly being seen in urban EDs and, particularly panic disorder, occur more frequently in women than in men.[3,8] These conditions are the most common psychiatric illnesses diagnosed in children, adolescents, and older adults.[9,10] Anxiety disorders may significantly affect a patient's quality of life and overall health. Anxiety is commonly associated with depression, other mood disorders, and substance abuse.

Numerous potentially life-threatening medical disorders feature symptoms that often mimic anxiety on initial evaluation. Emergency physicians must be able to discern such serious medical conditions from a principally anxious patient.

## PATHOPHYSIOLOGY

Anxiety disorders are caused by a combination of biologic factors and environmental influences.[11] Despite increased basic science and clinical research, a specific explanatory mechanism or model to describe the exact causes of anxiety has yet to be identified.

The genetic epidemiology of anxiety disorders has been confirmed by numerous studies and metaanalysis. Most anxiety disorders have significant familial aggregation, and the inheritability of panic disorder approaches a rate of 40%.[12]

Several neurotransmitters play integral roles in the pathophysiology of stress and mood and anxiety disorders. Decreased γ-aminobutyric acid and serotonin receptor sensitivity are common in most anxiety disorders. Overactivity of the central norepinephrine system and elevated sensitivity to lactate and carbon dioxide are prominent findings in panic disorder. Cholecystokinin and increased excitatory neurotransmission by glutamate may contribute to the evolution of conditioned fear.[13,14] Evolving research suggests that dopamine and corticotropin-releasing factor play a role in both mood and anxiety disorders.[14,15]

An environmental factor is integral to the development of anxiety. Stressful childhood experiences, such as abuse and divorce, contribute to generalized anxiety and panic disorders.[11] Caffeine and other socially accepted stimulants (e.g., taurine, ginseng), as well as recreational substances (e.g., cocaine, methamphetamine, γ-hydroxybutyrate, jimson weed, salvia), often promote symptoms of anxiety.[16,17] Finally, increasing exposure to violence, natural disasters, terrorism, and other traumatic events has caused greater numbers of people to suffer from acute stress reactions, anxiety, depression, and posttraumatic stress disorder.[18,19]

## CLINICAL PRESENTATION

Anxiety may be accompanied by many somatic and cognitive signs and symptoms, as listed in **Box 197.1**.[9,10,20] The physical symptoms of acute anxiety are similar to those of excitation, such as chest pain, dry mouth, dyspnea, lightheadedness, and palpitations. Symptoms of subacute or chronic anxiety include fatigue, insomnia, and menstrual abnormalities. An anxious patient may have normal findings on physical examination or may exhibit tachycardia, tachypnea, and diaphoresis.

Psychologic symptoms of anxiety include distractibility, emotional lability, noncompliance, and recurrent or obsessive thoughts. An anxious patient may be easily startled, demonstrate pressured speech, or suffer repetitive behavior.

Children may not be able to articulate their fear or anxiety. As a result, an anxious pediatric patient may have seemingly disparate chief complaints, such as nonspecific abdominal pain and headache. During examination, anxious pediatric patients may have a temper tantrum or may appear more clingy or needy than expected.[9]

A panic attack may be the feature of most anxiety disorders.[21] A panic attack is a discrete episode of intense fear or discomfort in the absence of real danger that meets specific symptomatic criteria. The intensity of a panic attack usually peaks within 10 minutes and resolves within 30 minutes. Panic attacks are often accompanied by at least 4 of 13 discreet somatic and cognitive symptoms.[22]

### BOX 197.1 Symptoms and Signs of Anxiety

**Somatic Symptoms**
Abdominal pain
Amenorrhea or dysmenorrhea
Chest tightness or pain
Choking sensation
Dry mouth
Dyspnea
Erectile dysfunction
Fatigue
Frequent or loose stools
Frequent urination
Headache
Increased flatulence
Lightheadedness
Muscle tightness
Nausea
Palpitations
Paresthesias

**Cognitive Symptoms**
Amnesia
Apprehension
Depersonalization
Derealization
Distractibility
Emotional lability
Fear
Flashbacks or recurrent images
Intrusive thoughts
Irritability
Racing thoughts

**Physical Signs**
Atypical affect
Avoidance
Diaphoresis
Hyperkinesis
Hypervigilance
Pressured speech
Repetitive behavior
Restlessness
Startle response
Stiffness
Tachycardia
Tachypnea
Temper tantrum
Tremor

## DIFFERENTIAL DIAGNOSIS, DIAGNOSTIC CRITERIA, AND TESTING

As evidenced by the broad range of associated signs and symptoms, anxiety disorders are part of an extensive differential diagnosis. Anxiety may represent a primary psychiatric condition or may be secondary to a medical illness. More than a dozen different anxiety disorders have similar physical symptoms and signs (**Box 197.2**).[22]

The first and most important step in evaluating an anxious patient is to search for potential medical causes of the patient's symptoms. As noted in **Table 197.1**, many different medical conditions and medications mimic, manifest, produce, or exacerbate anxiety.[17,23-25] Thorough evaluation of all of the patient's recent and past medical problems, current medications and supplements (including those available over the counter), family history, and social history (especially substance use and social stressors) may preclude an exhaustive and unnecessary medical work-up.[26] The onset of a new behavioral symptom at a late age or the report of any feature that is not typically associated with anxiety increases the likelihood of a medical cause.

An appropriate physical examination helps identify or eliminate potential causes of anxiety. Abnormal vital signs and characteristic toxidromes often signal the presence of a medical illness or drug-associated condition. A focused neurologic examination, including mental status, is critical to the diagnosis of intracranial disease.[27]

Myocardial infarction, angina pectoris, and dysrhythmias may have clinical findings similar to those of a panic attack. Several studies have indicated that up to 30% of patients with chest pain who are evaluated in the ED meet the diagnostic criteria for panic disorder. Alternatively, more than 40% of patients with panic disorder had documented coronary artery disease in a related study.[28]

Nearly 25% of medical conditions that cause symptoms of anxiety are endocrine disorders such as hypoglycemia, hyperthyroidism, and hypoparathyroidism.[29] Approximately 30% to 50% of female hyperthyroid patients suffer from panic and generalized anxiety disorders.[30]

Transient ischemic attacks, temporal lobe seizures, and brain tumors may promote anxiety. Up to 50% of patients with intracranial tumors, such as pituitary adenomas and metastatic disease, may have psychiatric manifestations.[31]

Exacerbations of asthma and chronic obstructive pulmonary disease may mimic the hyperventilation and respiratory distress observed during a panic attack. A patient with acute pulmonary embolism may exhibit chest tightness, dyspnea, diaphoresis, and apprehension.

An appropriate screening evaluation with laboratory and ancillary tests should be considered for anxious patients whose findings are not consistent with a past episode. At minimum, a chemistry panel, complete blood count, pregnancy test, prescription drug levels, and toxicology screen are often necessary. If indicated, additional tests such as an electrocardiogram, computed tomography of the brain, thyroid levels, or lumbar puncture may also be obtained.

## TREATMENT

Treatment of an anxious patient should begin with the creation of a calm, quiet clinical environment. An empathetic tone and willingness to listen will relieve some of the patient's anxiety,

## BOX 197.2 Definitions of Anxiety Disorders

**Panic attack** is a discrete period characterized by the sudden onset of intense apprehension, fearfulness, or terror; it is often associated with feelings of impending doom.

**Agoraphobia** is anxiety about or avoidance of places or situations from which escape may be difficult (or embarrassing) or in which help may not be available in the event of a panic attack or panic-like symptoms.

**Panic disorder without agoraphobia** is characterized by recurrent, unexpected panic attacks about which persistent concern exists.

**Panic disorder with agoraphobia** is characterized by both recurrent, unexpected panic attacks and agoraphobia.

**Agoraphobia without history of panic disorder** is characterized by the presence of agoraphobia and panic-like symptoms without a history of unexpected panic attacks.

**Specific phobia** is characterized by clinically significant anxiety provoked by exposure to a specific fear, object, or situation; it often leads to avoidance behavior.

**Social phobia** is characterized by clinically significant anxiety produced by exposure to certain types of social or performance situations; it often leads to avoidance behavior.

**Obsessive-compulsive disorder** is characterized by obsessions (which cause marked anxiety or distress) or compulsions (which serve to neutralize anxiety).

**Posttraumatic stress disorder** is characterized by the recurrent mental experience of an extremely traumatic event accompanied by symptoms of increased arousal and avoidance of stimuli associated with the trauma.

**Acute stress disorder** is characterized by symptoms similar to those of posttraumatic stress disorder that occur immediately after an extremely traumatic event.

**Generalized anxiety disorder** is characterized by at least 6 months of persistent and excessive anxiety and worry.

**Anxiety disorder due to a general medical condition** is characterized by prominent symptoms of anxiety that are judged to be a direct physiologic consequence of a general medical condition.

**Substance-induced anxiety disorder** is characterized by prominent symptoms of anxiety that are judged to be a direct physiologic consequence of drug abuse, medication use, or toxin exposure.

**Anxiety disorder not otherwise specified** is included for coding disorders with prominent anxiety or phobic avoidance that do not meet the criteria for any of the specific anxiety disorders.

Data from American Psychiatric Association. Diagnostic and statistical manual of mental disorders. 4th ed, text rev. Washington, DC: American Psychiatric Association; 2000. pp. 429-30.

**Table 197.1** Medical Conditions Associated with Anxiety

| SYSTEM OR CAUSE | CONDITION |
|---|---|
| Cardiac | Angina, arrhythmias, hypertensive urgency or emergency, mitral valve prolapse, myocardial ischemia, Takotsubo syndrome |
| Endocrine | Addison disease, carcinoid syndrome, Cushing syndrome, diabetes, parathyroid disease, pheochromocytoma, postpartum depression, thyroid disease |
| Exogenous | Caffeine or stimulant use, dietary supplement use, herbal remedies, acute intoxication (alcohol, amyl nitrate, cocaine, γ-hydroxybutyrate, khat, lysergic acid diethylamide [LSD], methamphetamine, salvia, yohimbine), monosodium glutamate, tyramine-containing foods in combination with monoamine oxidase inhibitors, withdrawal (alcohol, benzodiazepine, heroin, sedative) |
| Gastrointestinal | Dyspepsia, gastroesophageal reflux disease, irritable bowel syndrome, liver failure |
| Immunologic | Allergic reaction and mastocytosis |
| Infectious | Acute or evolving infection, human immunodeficiency virus infection, neurosyphilis |
| Medication | Amphetamine/dextroamphetamine (Adderall), albuterol, anticholinergics, digitalis, dystonic reaction, agents for erectile dysfunction, estrogen, histamine 1 and 2 blockers, selective serotonin reuptake inhibitors, serotonin syndrome, theophylline |
| Metabolic | Electrolyte abnormalities (calcium, glucose, magnesium, phosphorus, potassium, sodium, urea), nutritional deficiencies (vitamin deficiency such as $B_{12}$ and folate), porphyrias, Wilson disease |
| Neurologic | Brain tumors, cerebrovascular accidents (including transient ischemia attack), degenerative disorders (Huntington chorea, multiple sclerosis, myasthenia gravis), delirium, dementia (Alzheimer type), encephalitis, meningitis, seizure disorder (nonconvulsive and temporal lobe) |
| Psychiatric | Conversion disorder, depression, insomnia or sleep disorders, mania, psychosis, schizophrenia, stress disorder or stressors (e.g., abuse, finances, marital or relationship, trauma) |
| Pulmonary | Asthma, chronic obstructive pulmonary disease, pulmonary embolism, upper respiratory infection |

as well as facilitate an appropriate medical evaluation. The presence of a trusted, supportive friend or family member may also be helpful.

Benzodiazepines are the recommended first-line agents for pharmacologic management and may be given orally to patients in the ED for minimal to moderate symptoms. In those with severe symptoms, intravenous lorazepam, diazepam, and midazolam should be administered. Lorazepam may be given in 0.5-mg doses, whereas diazepam and midazolam may be given in 1- to 2-mg increments. For milder, less urgent symptoms and limited outpatient use, the recommended dose of clonazepam and alprazolam is 0.25 to 0.50 mg.[21,32] Buspirone, monoamine oxidase inhibitors, selective serotonin reuptake inhibitors, and recently, cognitive behavioral therapy are used by psychiatrists for the outpatient treatment of anxiety disorders.[33-36]

## DISPOSITION

Most anxious patients may be discharged home after appropriate ED evaluation and stabilization. Immediate psychiatric consultation is recommended for anxious patients who report suicidal or homicidal ideation, who are severely depressed or unable to care for themselves, or who may not have reliable follow-up. Coordination with a behavioral health resource or case management–based intervention may also improve follow-up care.[37] Anxious patients discharged from the ED should be instructed to seek care from their primary physician or mental health provider as soon as possible.

## REFERENCES

***References can be found on Expert Consult @ www.expertconsult.com.***

# 198 Conversion Disorder, Psychosomatic Illness, and Malingering

*Glen E. Michael and J. Stephen Huff*

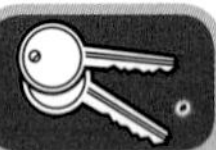

**KEY POINTS**

- Somatization disorder, conversion disorder, and hypochondriasis are psychologic reactions to stressful circumstances that are neither intentional nor planned.
- Malingering and factitious disorders involve deliberate actions of deceit of which the patient is aware.
- Somatoform conditions feature complaints and symptoms that cannot be attributed to medical illness.
- Emergency department evaluation of patients with suspected somatoform disorders should focus on the search for a medical cause of the reported symptoms and exclusion of life-threatening illness.
- Identification and appropriate referral of patients with somatoform illness are secondary objectives of the emergency department encounter.
- As with other psychiatric and medical diagnoses, thorough documentation is required when somatization is suspected.

## EPIDEMIOLOGY

Somatoform conditions include the following diagnoses: somatization disorder, conversion disorder, somatoform pain disorder, hypochondriasis, body dysmorphic disorder, and undifferentiated somatoform illness. The boundaries between these disorders can be subtle, and it has recently been proposed that four of these conditions—somatization disorder, somatoform pain disorder, hypochondriasis, and undifferentiated somatoform illness—should be reclassified under a single common rubric called complex somatic symptom disorder (CSSD).[1] Further classification of somatoform disorders is continually evolving as research better defines their distinctive characteristics.[1-3]

The reported prevalence of somatoform conditions ranges from 50% to 65% in ambulatory settings.[4,5] When definitions are narrowed to include only patients meeting strict diagnostic criteria for somatization disorder, the lifetime prevalence drops to less than 3%.[6] Accurate classification is difficult because some patients exhibit somatoform symptoms in the presence of demonstrable medical illness.

True somatization disorder (or Briquet syndrome, after Paul Briquet, who first described the illness in 1859) is typically manifested before 30 years of age and is far more common in women than in men. Although many patients somatize, somatization disorder is ultimately diagnosed in few.

Acknowledgment and thanks to Dr. Marshall for his work on the first edition.

## DEFINITIONS

*Somatization disorder* is characterized by the presence of multiple chronic distressing somatic symptoms that are not medically explained. Patients with this condition tend to be highly anxious about their symptoms, even in the face of evidence that their condition is not medically serious. In the draft of the upcoming *Diagnostic and Statistical Manual of Mental Disorders* (DSM-V), this condition has been renamed CSSD.[1]

*Hypochondriasis* is preoccupation with or excessive fear of illness despite negative testing and reassurance from a health care professional. Hypochondriasis is more common than somatization disorder and has a prevalence of 4% to 9% in general medical practice.[7] It peaks in men in the fourth decade and in women in the fifth, with no significant predilection by gender. Hypochondriasis is increasingly being described in geriatric populations.[8] It has been renamed the "predominant health anxiety" subtype of CSSD in the proposed draft of DSM-V.[1]

*Somatoform pain disorder*, an important and particularly challenging somatoform illness, is characterized by somatoform symptoms that are manifested predominantly as pain. In the proposed draft of DSM-V, this condition is reclassified as the "predominant pain" subtype of CSSD.[1]

*Conversion disorder* is a condition in which patients complain of sensory or motor symptoms as a manifestation of stress or unconscious conflict that cannot be attributed to a pathophysiologic process. Conversion disorder is more common in women and members of lower socioeconomic groups. Its onset typically begins in adolescence, and it follows a discontinuous course. Conversion disorder has also been observed in military, mass casualty, and industrial accident settings without a female preponderance of the disorder.[9] Estimates of prevalence vary considerably as a result of inconsistent classifications and definitions of the disorder.

*Body dysmorphic disorder* is characterized by a preoccupation with an imagined defect in physical appearance. Although it is currently classified under somatoform disorders, body dysmorphic disorder more closely resembles obsessive-compulsive disorder and as a result may be moved to the anxiety disorders section of the DSM-V.[1] This disorder is commonly encountered by primary care providers, plastic surgeons, and the body enhancement industry.

*Factitious disorders*, including malingering, feature deliberate manufacturing of symptoms or illness. The combined prevalence of all factitious disorders ranges from 1% to 5%, again with a female preponderance. The term *Munchausen syndrome* (after the famous 18th-century raconteur Baron von Munchausen) is reserved for chronic or "career" medical imposters, and it represents the extreme form of the disorder. However, cases of Munchausen syndrome tend to involve male patients.[10]

*Malingering and symptom exaggeration* are probably underreported. In one study, "39% of mild head injury, 35% of fibromyalgia/chronic fatigue, 31% of chronic pain, 27% of neurotoxic, and 22% of electrical injury claims resulted in diagnostic impressions of probable malingering."[11] Malingering is most often exhibited by patients who are either trying to avoid an unpleasant circumstance, such as military duty or a prison term, or attempting to secure some form of compensation, such as occupational health or personal injury plaintiff claims. Malingering can result in criminal charges.[12]

*Factitious disorder by proxy* or *Munchausen syndrome by proxy* deserves special mention because it may represent a form of child abuse. It is typically defined as the intentional production or feigning of physical or psychiatric illness in a child by the child's guardian, although it has also been reported in caregivers of geriatric patients. Factitious disorder by proxy can be active (symptom producing) or passive (neglect). Munchausen syndrome by proxy is rare and occurs in roughly 2.8 per 100,000 children younger than 1 year and 0.5 per 100,000 children younger than 16 years.[13] As with the other factitious illnesses, the deceptive nature of the disorder makes it extremely difficult to detect and study.

## PATHOPHYSIOLOGY

Somatoform illnesses represent emotional stress experienced as physical symptoms. Both somatization and hypochondriasis are commonly associated with depression and anxiety, and somatization is classified as a potential initial symptom of depression.[14] This strong association with depressive disorders has led to the practice of treating somatization with antidepressant medications. Hypochondriasis and depression coexist in roughly 40% of cases. Twenty percent of patients with hypochondriasis have a diagnosis of panic disorder, and 10% have an obsessive-compulsive disorder.[15] As the number of reported physical symptoms rises in patients with somatoform illness, the likelihood of an underlying psychiatric disorder increases proportionately.[16]

A significant correlation does not appear to exist between psychiatric illness and factitious disorder, unlike somatization and hypochondriasis. Malingering is observed in individuals with antisocial and psychopathic personalities, but the nature of this association remains unclear.

## PRESENTING SIGNS AND SYMPTOMS

### CLASSIC FEATURES

*Somatization* is exhibited by patients who are chronically and persistently "sick" with numerous vague complaints and symptoms involving many organ systems; review of systems is often globally "positive." Patients' symptoms are distressing to them, and their suffering is authentic even if medically inexplicable. Patients maintain a very strong conviction of illness despite multiple negative diagnostic work-ups, hospital admissions, specialist referrals, and surgical procedures. An example of the breadth of symptoms associated with somatoform disorders can be seen in the diagnostic criteria listed in **Box 198.1**.

Patients with *hypochondriasis*, like somatizers, are convinced that they are gravely ill. Although a somatizer focuses on symptoms, a patient with hypochondriasis focuses on disease states and invests great personal energy in seeking multiple extensive reassurances from the health care system. Patients with hypochondriasis are typified by health anxiety leading to strong convictions of illness and fixation with the body and its functions. Ominous implications are often attributed to mundane or insignificant findings, and symptoms are exaggerated out of proportion to any actual organic illness.

*Conversion disorder*, in contrast to somatization disorder, is the acute, often episodic onset of one symptom or sign involving limited body parts or organ systems. Complaints are generally sensory or motor in nature and often occur in response to an identified stressor. Unlike malingering or factitious disorders, the malady is not consciously feigned or deliberate. Examples of conversion disorder typically seen in the ED include pseudoseizures, altered mental status, paralysis, and movement disorders.[17] Other common conversion symptoms are presented in **Box 198.2**.

**BOX 198.1 *Diagnostic and Statistical Manual of Mental Disorders* (Fourth Edition, Text Revision) Criteria for Somatization Disorder**

1. Pain in at least four distinct locations or circumstances (e.g., headache, backache, chest pain, dysuria, dyspareunia)
2. Two or more gastrointestinal symptoms (e.g., nausea, vomiting, diarrhea, constipation, but not pain)
3. One or more sexual dysfunction symptoms (e.g., impotence, lack of libido, menorrhagia, but not pain)
4. One or more neurologic conversion symptoms (also see Box 198.2) (e.g., paresthesia, paralysis, ataxia, blindness, pseudoseizure)

Symptoms are not medically explainable or may represent an exaggeration of symptoms attributable to an organic illness.

Symptoms must not be deliberately produced.

Adapted from American Psychiatric Association. Diagnostic and statistical manual of mental disorders. 4th ed, text rev. Washington, DC: American Psychiatric Association; 2000.

One of the more unusual conversion disorders is *pseudocyesis*, or "hysterical pregnancy," which includes the physical symptoms of pregnancy (even amenorrhea) in the absence of a true gestation.

*La belle indifférence*, a seemingly incongruous disinterest in one's illness, is classically associated with conversion reactions. However, la belle indifférence may be seen with organic disease states such as stroke. La belle indifférence should not be used alone to differentiate between conversion and organic disorders.[18]

Patients who *malinger* and those who have *factitious disorder* tend to limit themselves to exaggerations of symptoms of a previously diagnosed illness or to symptoms that are difficult to investigate and disprove; examples include pain of any variety, psychiatric conditions such as suicidality, and the pseudoneurologic symptoms of tingling, amnesia, and seizures. Less commonly, patients with factitious disorder inflict injury or disease on themselves. Deliberate misuse of medications such as hypoglycemic agents has been described in health care workers.[10]

Unlike the somatoform disorders, malingering and factitious behavior involve feigned illness. Even though they are aware of their deception, patients with factitious disorder (unlike malingerers) are helpless to control the behavior.[19] To illustrate the differences among somatoform disorder, factitious disorder, and malingering, one can use the example of nonepileptic or pseudoseizures, which can be seen in each condition. A patient with a somatoform disorder suffers a nonvolitional convulsion in response to a psychologic stressor, a patient with factitious disorder has an uncontrollable compulsion to feign a nonepileptic convulsion to gain attention and the sick role, and a patient who malingers feigns a convulsion as part of a ruse to achieve a specific end. What sets malingering apart from factitious disorder is the patient's intentional pursuit of an identifiable, tangible goal or gain.[20]

**BOX 198.2 Common Conversion Symptoms**

| | |
|---|---|
| Anesthesia | Vertigo, dizziness |
| Paresthesia | Diplopia |
| Paralysis | Blindness |
| Ataxia | Deafness |
| Syncope | Tremor |
| Seizure | Globus hystericus |
| Coma | Dysphagia |

### VICTIMS OF INTIMATE PARTNER VIOLENCE

Among patients who tend to use emergency care frequently, an important subgroup consists of victims of intimate partner violence (see Chapter 93). Intimate partner violence results in high levels of psychologic stress for the victim. Many of these patients repeatedly seek care in the ED with somatoform behavior.[21] Physicians must screen for ongoing abuse when new or recurrent physical symptoms cannot be attributed to a medical condition. Just as with current abuse, patients with a past history of physical, sexual, or psychologic abuse also tend to use medical services more frequently.

## DIFFERENTIAL DIAGNOSIS AND TESTING

In the emergency department (ED), the brevity of the clinical encounter and a diagnostic focus on life threats make accurate identification of patients with somatoform disorders difficult. Even when demonstrable medical disease is present, symptoms and severity are modulated by the psychologic well-being of the patient. Even though it stands to reason that many patients somatize to some degree, clearly a subset exists in whom such behavior represents a disorder.

The goals when evaluating somatoform illness are identification of the condition and appropriate referral. In the ED, life-threatening conditions on the differential diagnosis are excluded first, other potentially serious medical illnesses are excluded second, and somatoform causes are excluded last, if at all.

Classic findings can make one suspect a somatoform illness; however, such behavior is insufficient for psychiatric diagnostic criteria. Synopses of the characteristics of somatoform disorders can be found in **Table 198.1**. It is useful to categorize these illnesses as nondeliberate (somatization,

**Table 198.1 Characteristics of Somatoform Disorders**

| DISORDER | HALLMARKS |
|---|---|
| Somatization disorder | Multiple, chronic vague symptoms occurring in different organ systems<br>Many past medical evaluations<br>Associated psychiatric disorder |
| Conversion disorder | Acute, episodic<br>Limited symptoms and body parts<br>Motor or sensory complaints predominant |
| Hypochondriasis | Health anxiety<br>Fixation on diagnoses and body functions |
| Factitious disorder | Compulsive urge to feign illness by report or deed |
| Malingering | Feigned illness for the purpose of avoiding something unpleasant or to gain some reward |

conversion disorder, and hypochondriasis) and deliberate (factitious disorders and malingering).

The symptoms experienced by a patient with a nondeliberate somatoform illness are perceived as very real. Diligent history taking often uncovers telling patterns. Useful questions to consider include the following: Are these complaints chronic? Do they correlate with identifiable stressors? Does the patient hold a conviction of a particular illness or imminent death? Does the patient have a lifelong history of "illness"? What has been done for this patient in previous visits, by previous providers? What is new today? Obtaining answers to these questions, along with a careful physical examination, can help direct the emergency evaluation while at the same time reassuring patients that they are being taken seriously. Respect ultimately aids in disposition because these patients are far more likely to comply with a plan when they believe that a provider has their best interests at heart.

Concerns about making the diagnosis of a somatoform illness should not preclude a thorough ED evaluation because many medical conditions can be mistaken for somatization, particularly when the findings are atypical. **Box 198.3** provides examples of medical conditions that can mimic somatoform behavior.

As a general rule, patients with nondeliberate somatoform illness acquiesce to invasive diagnostic testing, whereas those with factitious disorders and malingerers are more reluctant. The presence of two or more of the following features is suggestive of malingering behavior: mention of a medicolegal context of the visit, discrepancy between subjective and objective assessment of the degree of stress and disability, poor compliance with evaluation and treatment, and antisocial personality disorder.[19] Malingering is very difficult to prove, even in the presence of high clinical suspicion and deliberate investigation, and surveillance of the patient is often required.[22] Determination of malingering is usually the purview of specialists such as neuropsychologists.

Various maneuvers are purported to assist in identifying factitious symptoms, as shown in **Table 198.2**. Waddell's "behavioral responses to examination," as applied to a chief complaint of back pain, are one example. Although the Waddell signs provide a compelling method of detecting feigned illness, the predictive value of such maneuvers is generally poor and correlates with an unfavorable treatment outcome.[23]

Tests for factitious paralysis have also been proposed but are similarly nonspecific.[24] The abductor test is one such test: with true paresis, the unaffected leg abducts when the patient attempts to abduct the affected leg against resistance. The Hoover test involves placing the examiner's hand under the "weakened" lower extremity and asking the supine patient to raise the unaffected leg; downward pressure with the affected leg is considered positive for feigned paralysis. Prudent caution is warranted in the interpretation of any diagnostic maneuver that is infrequently performed.

**BOX 198.3 Medical Conditions That May Be Mistaken for Somatization**

| | |
|---|---|
| Multiple sclerosis | Uremia |
| Thyroid disorders | Periodic paralysis |
| Guillain-Barré syndrome | Lupus |
| Porphyria | Pituitary disorders |
| Botulism | Addison disease |
| Myasthenia gravis | Wilson disease |
| Parathyroid disorders | Carbon monoxide exposure |
| Insulin derangements | Medication side effects |

## TREATMENT

No specific treatment of nondeliberate somatoform illness exists. Psychiatric comorbid conditions such as depression, anxiety, and substance abuse should be addressed. Cognitive behavioral therapy has shown promise in the minority of patients willing to be referred.[25,26]

Whether to use medication to treat symptoms believed to be somatoform in origin is as much an ethical question as a medical one. This quandary often develops when considering analgesics for chronic pain syndromes. In accordance with the principles of beneficence and nonmaleficence, one may want to spare a patient potential side effects and addiction; this is

**Table 198.2 Physical Examination Maneuvers Purported to Differentiate Factitious from Organic Conditions**

| TEST | SYMPTOM | DESCRIPTION | RELIABILITY OF TEST |
|---|---|---|---|
| Hoover | Leg paresis | Cup the heel of the weakened leg with the examiner's hand, and have the patient raise the unaffected leg. The paresis is nonorganic if downward pressure is exerted on the hand. | Poor |
| Abductor | Leg paresis | Instruct the patient to abduct the weakened leg against resistance. In true paresis, the opposite leg should consensually abduct. | Poor |
| Arm drop | Arm paresis | Raise the paretic arm above the patient's face and then release. If the dropped arm misses the face, a nonorganic cause is suggested. | Poor |
| Midline split | Sensory loss | Test facial sensation. Sharp demarcation of sensory loss at the midline suggests a nonorganic cause. | Poor |

Adapted from Greer S, Chambliss L, Mackler L, et al. Clinical inquiries: what physical exam techniques are useful to detect malingering? J Fam Pract 2005;54:719-22.

countered by the harm of leaving a patient in pain or consigning the patient to withdrawal if he or she is a chronic user of analgesics.

The final common pathway of pain is the perception of pain, and even imagined pain can be very real. Given that emergency providers do not primarily manage somatoform illness, it is not unreasonable to provide short-term "bridging" prescriptions on a case-by-case basis to patients with appropriate follow-up arrangements. Patients who seek care only to acquire narcotics are not considered to be suffering from somatoform illness; rather, they may have substance abuse, addiction, or illegal market motivations.

## FOLLOW-UP AND NEXT STEPS IN CARE

It is not generally recommended that a patient with a somatoform illness be confronted. Instead, the patient should be reassured that the symptoms do not represent an imminent threat. Even in cases of malingering, neuropsychologists rarely confront patients; most use descriptive terminology rather than the diagnosis "malingering."[27]

Good charting practices are critical when somatization is suspected. The history of the present illness and review of systems should include liberal use of patient quotes to convey the character of the visit to subsequent providers. Findings on physical examination also need to be documented carefully because they may be the reason to pursue or defer diagnostic intervention. Discharge instructions should ideally include times, dates, and names of follow-up visits; doses of medications; and specific return criteria.

The final discharge diagnosis should reflect the chief complaint (e.g., "leg pain") rather than the suspected somatoform behavior. This is particularly true of feigned illness because these diagnoses may have criminal implications. Exceptions to this rule are suspected intimate partner violence or Munchausen syndrome by proxy, which deserve special consideration. In both these instances, a high index of suspicion for the condition is appropriate, and interventions such as reporting or activating protective services may be required.

## SUGGESTED READINGS

Dula D, DeNaples L. Emergency department presentation of patients with conversion disorder. Acad Emerg Med 1995;2:120-3.

Greer S, Chambliss L, Mackler L, et al. Clinical inquiries: what physical exam techniques are useful to detect malingering? J Fam Pract 2005;54:719-22.

Mendelson G, Mendelson D. Malingering pain in the medicolegal context. Clin J Pain 2004;20:423-32.

Stone J, Smyth R, Carson A, et al. La belle indifférence in conversion symptoms and hysteria: systematic review. Br J Psychiatry 2006;188:204-9.

## REFERENCES

***References can be found on Expert Consult @ www.expertconsult.com.***

# Addiction 199

*Randall S. Jotte*

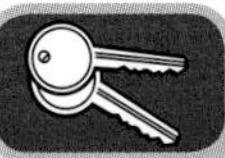

**KEY POINTS**

- Drug abuse and alcohol abuse irrevocably change brain physiology; addiction represents a brain disorder.
- The acute manifestations of substance abuse and dependency arise from drug-specific patterns of intoxication and withdrawal.
- Acute pharmacologic detoxification is accomplished through the administration of a long-acting medication in the same category as the drug of dependence, thereby blocking withdrawal symptoms.
- Anticraving medications are psychotropic agents that reduce the desire for drugs or alcohol in detoxified patients and prevent relapse into compulsive substance abuse.

## SCOPE, EPIDEMIOLOGY, AND DEFINITIONS

Addiction is a personal state of inner tyranny. Addicts hold traditional concerns of family, work, health, and the law as secondary to one primal urge—getting the drug or drink. Many are familiar with the destructive effects of drugs or alcohol for the addict on the street, but most are unaware of the cumulative consequences of addiction on society.

From several viewpoints the problem is vast. Regarding alcohol, the Centers for Disease Control and Prevention reports that approximately 79,000 deaths are attributable to excessive alcohol use annually in the United States, which makes it the third leading lifestyle-related cause of death for the nation. In addition, excessive alcohol use accounts for 2.3 million years of potential life lost annually—an average of about 30 years of potential life lost for each death.[1] Concerning drugs, the Substance Abuse and Mental Services Administration of the U.S. Department of Health and Human Services reported that in 2009, 21.8 million Americans used an illegal drug during the month before the survey, which represents 8.7% of the population aged 12 years or older. Illegal drugs include marijuana or hashish, cocaine (including crack cocaine), heroin, hallucinogens, inhalants, and nonmedical use of prescription-type psychotherapeutics.[2]

Many of those abusing or dependent on alcohol or drugs, or both, disproportionately consume public health care resources, particularly emergency services. Between 1992 and 2000, alcohol-related visits to U.S. emergency departments (EDs) averaged 76 million per year, which accounted for 7.9% of the total ED visits.[3] The Drug Abuse and Warning Network reported that in 2007, 1.9 million ED visits were associated with drug misuse or abuse. Although the overall number of ED visits attributable to drug misuse and abuse was stable from 2004 to 2007, ED visits involving nonmedical use of pharmaceuticals with no other drug involvement rose significantly (73%), as did the nonmedical use of pharmaceuticals with alcohol (36%).[4]

The societal burdens of substance abuse extend well beyond EDs. The U.S. Office of National Drug Control Policy reported that incarcerated offenders were often under the influence of drugs when they committed their offenses and that offenders often commit crimes to support their drug habit. In addition, trafficking in illicit drugs tends to be associated with the commission of particularly violent crimes.[5]

The cumulative economic cost of substance abuse is astounding. In 1998, alcohol abuse in the United States cost approximately $185 billion, with 47% of this cost simply being due to lost productivity at work.[6] The same year, drug abuse in the United States cost $143 billion.[7] When adjusted for 2010 dollars, abuse of both drugs and alcohol costs the nation $440 billion—the equivalent of 80% of all revenue raised to fund public education for grades prekindergarten through 12.[8] Substance abuse is as much a public crisis for our nation as it is a personal crisis for the addict.

To address the problem of substance-related disorders, we must understand the clinical condition. To understand, we must speak the same language by sharing a common terminology. In general, these disorders are classified not by the quantity of the cause but rather by the effect.

With *substance abuse*, adverse consequences occur but the pattern has not yet deteriorated into a state of dependence. More specifically, the American Psychiatric Association defines substance abuse as "a maladaptive pattern of substance use" revealed by the recurrent and significant consequences arising from repeated use of the substance: failure to fulfill major role obligations, recurrent use in situations in which it is physically hazardous, multiple substance-related legal problems, and recurrent social and interpersonal problems[9] (**Box 199.1**). Although the consequences of use are significant, some degree of control is present.

In contrast, *substance dependence* is defined as severe impairment or absence of control. Use is compulsive and occurs under the ever-present threats of tolerance and withdrawal. As stated earlier, the American Psychiatric

**BOX 199.1 Criteria for Substance Abuse**

**A.** A maladaptive pattern of substance use leading to clinically significant impairment or distress, as manifested by one (or more) of the following occurring within a 12-month period:
  1. Recurrent substance use resulting in failure to fulfill major role obligations at work, school, or home (e.g., repeated absences or poor work performance related to substance use; substance-related absences, suspensions, or expulsions from school; neglect of children or household)
  2. Recurrent substance use in situations in which it is physically hazardous (e.g., driving an automobile or operating a machine when impaired by substance use)
  3. Recurrent substance-related legal problems (e.g., arrests for substance-related disorderly conduct)
  4. Continued substance use despite having persistent or recurrent social or interpersonal problems caused or exacerbated by the effects of the substance (e.g., arguments with spouse about the consequences of intoxication, physical fights)

**B.** The symptoms have never met the criteria for substance dependence for this class of substance.

From First MB, Frances A, Pincus HA. Substance-related disorders. In: DSM-IV-TR guidebook. Washington, DC: American Psychiatric Publishing; 2004.

**BOX 199.2 Criteria for Substance Dependence**

A maladaptive pattern of substance use leading to clinically significant impairment or distress, as manifested by three (or more) of the following occurring at any time in the same 12-month period:

1. Tolerance, as defined by either of the following:
   - **a.** Need for markedly increased amounts of the substance to achieve intoxication or the desired effect
   - **b.** Markedly diminished effect with continued use of the same amount of the substance
2. Withdrawal, as manifested by either of the following:
   - **a.** The characteristic withdrawal syndrome for the substance (refer to criteria A and B of the criteria sets for withdrawal from the specific substances)
   - **b.** The same (or a closely related) substance is taken to relieve or avoid withdrawal symptoms
3. The substance is often taken in larger amounts or over a longer period than was intended.
4. There is a persistent desire or unsuccessful efforts to cut down or control substance use.
5. A great deal of time is spent in activities necessary to obtain the substance (e.g., visiting multiple doctors, driving long distances), use the substance (e.g., chain smoking), or recover from its effects.
6. Important social, occupational, or recreational activities are given up or reduced because of substance use.
7. The substance use is continued despite knowledge of having a persistent or recurrent physical or psychologic problem that is likely to have been caused or exacerbated by the substance (e.g., current cocaine use despite recognition of cocaine-induced depression, continued drinking despite recognition that an ulcer was made worse by alcohol consumption).

From First MB, Frances A, Pincus HA. Substance-related disorders. In: DSM-IV-TR guidebook. Washington, DC: American Psychiatric Publishing; 2004.

Association more specifically defines substance dependence as a cluster of cognitive, behavioral, and physiologic symptoms indicating continued use of the substance despite significant substance-related problems[9] (**Box 199.2**).

*Tolerance* is reflected by the "need for increasing amounts of the substance to achieve intoxication or desired effect … or diminished effect with continued use of the same amount of the substance."[9]

*Withdrawal* is a physiologic response manifested by the characteristic "withdrawal" syndrome for the particular substance or use of the same or a closely related substance to relieve or avoid such symptoms.[9]

*Addiction* is a term of more general public reference that includes drug and alcohol dependence but also includes other inherent self-destructive behavioral patterns, such as eating disorders, compulsive gambling, and excessive sexual behavior.

This chapter focuses on drug- and alcohol-related disorders. Although multiple agents of abuse exist, most substances commonly encountered in the ED can be classified as either central nervous system depressants (alcohol, sedatives, hypnotics, and anxiolytics) or stimulants (cocaine, amphetamines, and sympathomimetics).

## PATHOPHYSIOLOGY AND ANATOMY

Insight into the pathophysiology of substance-related disorders has progressed substantially in recent years. Neuropharmacologic animal studies and human imaging modalities, in particular, positron emission tomography and functional magnetic resonance imaging brain scans, have identified the neurochemical processes and anatomic structures most affected in states of substance abuse and dependence.

Addiction changes brain physiology, thus prompting designation of this condition as a brain disorder.[10] Addictive substances alter multiple neurotransmitter pathways within the brain, including *N*-methyl-D-aspartate (NMDA) and γ-aminobutyric acid (GABA) receptors, as well as the endogenous opioid, serotonin, and dopamine systems.[11] Changes particularly occur within the mesolimbic system of the brain. Projecting from the ventral tegmental area to the nucleus accumbens, olfactory tubercle, frontal cortex, and amygdala, the mesolimbic system is regarded as the "reward center" of the brain[12] (**Fig. 199.1**). These neurocircuits presumably evolved to reward survival-enhancing behavior, including productive familial and social interactions, reproduction, and other such behavior. Some suggest that mesolimbic dopamine is a direct mediator of reward, whereas others emphasize that dopamine signals an interest in reward or the expectation that reward is forthcoming. Either way, evidence suggests that the common reinforcing and incentive effects of addictive substances are substantially mediated by increasing extracellular dopamine within the mesolimbic system. On an elementary level, this drug-induced efflux of dopamine is pleasurable.[10]

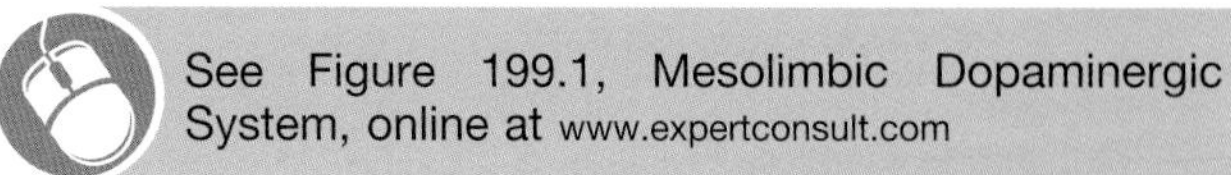

See Figure 199.1, Mesolimbic Dopaminergic System, online at www.expertconsult.com

As addicts and clinicians mutually recognize, artificially inducing the mesolimbic system with drugs and alcohol for these pleasant effects is accompanied by grave shortcomings. Neurochemical pleasure circuits, overwhelmed by excessive stimulation, adapt by desensitizing.[13] Evaluation by multiple disciplines, including anatomic, behavioral, biochemical, and electrophysiologic studies, commonly shows that dopamine neurons function insufficiently in addicts. A hypodopaminergic state develops.[10] The dopamine deficiency associated with acute withdrawal is manifested clinically as acute dysphoria, depression, irritability, and anxiety. Neurochemically, baseline levels of the "reward" neurotransmitters are depressed.[12] The traditional social and behavioral stimulants of the mesolimbic system that function effectively in the nonaddictive state, such as family and positive affirmation from work or friends, become inadequate to generate a significant perception of pleasure. Drugs and alcohol are the sole stimuli sufficient to activate the impaired mesolimbic neurocircuits and generate pleasure.[13] Yet even though the baseline mesolimbic system remains hypodopaminergic in addicts, the system remains hyperresponsive to abused drugs and alcohol, thereby conferring long-lasting vulnerability even after extensive periods of abstinence.[10] The most promising avenues of treatment for addicts are pharmacologic agents aimed at restoring these dopaminergic neurocircuits.[10]

Not all individuals are equally susceptible. Those with risk-taking and novelty-seeking traits favor the use of addictive drugs. Psychiatric conditions, in particular, schizophrenia, bipolar disorder, and attention-deficit/hyperactivity disorder, are associated with increased risk for substance abuse and dependency. A dual diagnosis of substance abuse and mental disorder has especially unfavorable implications for both management and outcome.[14]

Genetic factors clearly increase the risk for addiction. First-degree relatives of alcoholics (e.g., parents, siblings, children) have a threefold to fourfold greater prevalence of alcohol abuse than the general population does.[15] Men whose parents were alcoholics have an increased likelihood for alcoholism even when adopted at birth and raised by nonalcoholic parents.[14] Genetic factors, as revealed by studies in identical twins, account for approximately half of the risk for alcohol abuse.[15]

Some of this genetic predilection for addiction is expressed through enzymatic variants. For instance, highly active forms of aldehyde dehydrogenase increase alcohol metabolism and decrease the negative side effects of alcohol intake, thereby enhancing consumption and addiction (**Fig. 199.2**). In contrast, less active variants of aldehyde dehydrogenase (i.e., the ALDH2*2 allele initially detected in eastern Asian populations) allow accumulation of acetaldehyde, the toxic intermediary by-product of alcohol metabolism. Sensitivity to alcohol increases with a subsequent reduction in the rates of alcoholism.[16] Genetic influence is also expressed through neurotransmitter variants. Neuropeptide Y, a 36–amino acid peptide neurotransmitter, regulates appetite, anxiety, and reward. A functional Lue7Pro polymorphism in the neuropeptide Y gene increases the risk for alcohol dependence by 7.3%, primarily in European Americans.[17] Although the initial use of a drug or alcohol is a willful act, for those predisposed to abuse or dependency, some if not most of what follows is progressively beyond their control.

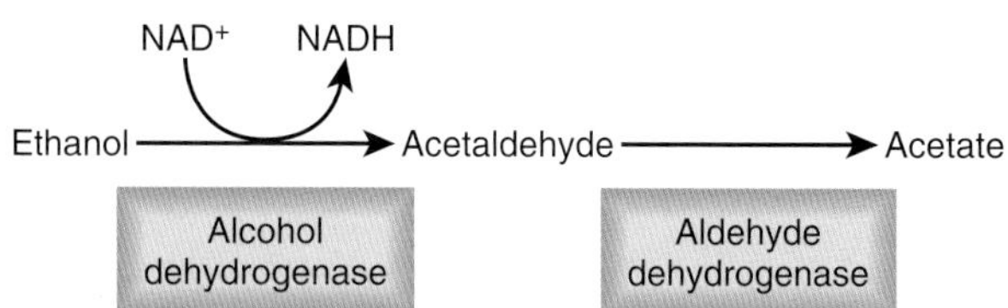


**Fig. 199.2 Metabolism of alcohol.** *NAD$^+$*, Oxidized form of nicotinamide adenine dinucleotide; *NADH*, reduced form of nicotinamide adenine dinucleotide.

## PRESENTING SIGNS AND SYMPTOMS

The signs and symptoms of substance abuse and dependency result from acute states of intoxication and withdrawal. Although some manifestations are specific to the substance, common patterns exist.

Acute intoxication with central nervous system depressants—alcohol, sedatives, hypnotics, and anxiolytics—is characterized by dysfunctional behavioral and neurologic changes. Individuals suffer mood swings and impaired social or occupational functioning. Poor judgment prevails, often reflected by inappropriate sexual or aggressive behavior. Neurologic dysfunction occurs along a clinical spectrum determined by the degree of intoxication and ranges from slurred speech, incoordination, and unsteady gait to impairment of memory and attention, stupor, and coma (**Box 199.3**). In contrast, acute withdrawal from central nervous system depressants is manifested as physiologic and behavioral agitation. Psychomotor distress can be significant, with transient visual, tactile, or auditory hallucinations. Patients experience autonomic hyperactivity, evident as tachycardia and diaphoresis. Nausea and vomiting may be prevalent, as well as hand tremors. Generalized seizures can occur. Mentally, emotionally, and physically miserable, such patients cannot function.[9]

Though also central nervous system depressants, opiates confer somewhat unique states of intoxication and withdrawal. Because of the rapid but variable degrees of tolerance that develops to opiates, incremental doses are required to achieve euphoria. However, the unreliable concentration of opiates in street drugs complicates attempts by addicts to self-administer a specific dose. Overdosage frequently results in extreme drowsiness and potentially coma and death from respiratory depression (**Box 199.4**). In contrast, opiate withdrawal is an extremely unpleasant, conscious experience. Patients experience severe dysphoria, diaphoresis, vomiting, and diarrhea.[9]

**BOX 199.3 Diagnostic Criteria for Intoxication with Alcohol, Sedatives, Hypnotics, or Anxiolytics**

**A.** Recent use of a sedative, hypnotic, or anxiolytic
**B.** Clinically significant maladaptive behavioral or psychologic changes (e.g., inappropriate sexual or aggressive behavior, mood lability, impaired judgment, impaired social or occupational functioning) that developed during or shortly after sedative, hypnotic, or anxiolytic use
**C.** One (or more) of the following signs developing during or shortly after sedative, hypnotic, or anxiolytic use:
1. Slurred speech
2. Incoordination
3. Unsteady gait
4. Nystagmus
5. Impairment in attention or memory
6. Stupor or coma

**D.** The symptoms are not due to a general medical condition and are not better accounted for by another mental disorder

From First MB, Frances A, Pincus HA. Substance-related disorders. In: DSM-IV-TR guidebook. Washington, DC: American Psychiatric Publishing; 2004.

**BOX 199.4 Diagnostic Criteria for Opioid Intoxication**

**A.** Recent use of an opioid
**B.** Clinically significant maladaptive behavioral or psychologic changes (e.g., initial euphoria followed by apathy, dysphoria, psychomotor agitation or retardation, impaired judgment, or impaired social or occupational functioning) that developed during or shortly after opioid use
**C.** Pupillary constriction (or pupillary dilation as a result of anoxia from a severe overdose) and one (or more) of the following signs developing during or shortly after opioid use:
1. Drowsiness or coma
2. Slurred speech
3. Impairment in attention or memory

**D.** The symptoms are not due to a general medical condition and are not better accounted for by another mental disorder

From First MB, Frances A, Pincus HA. Substance-related disorders. In: DSM-IV-TR guidebook. Washington, DC: American Psychiatric Publishing; 2004.

The signs and symptoms of acute intoxication with central nervous system stimulants—cocaine, amphetamines, and sympathomimetics—are determined by the pattern, route, and amount of drug used, as well as the specific agent. Intermittent "binge" use is often accompanied by euphoria and heightened psychomotor and autonomic activity (e.g., tachycardia, hypertension, seizures, cardiac arrhythmias, chest pain). Chronic daily users have a contrasting scenario. Psychomotor depression and affective blunting may be present, often in the setting of hypotension, bradycardia, and respiratory insufficiency (**Box 199.5**). Withdrawal from central nervous system stimulants occurs after a period of heavy and prolonged use. The withdrawal symptoms of dysphoria, suicidal ideation, extreme fatigue, and hypersomnia are the antithesis of those of acute intoxication.[9]

Emergency physicians often encounter a particularly challenging if not frustrating clinical scenario arising from addiction—drug-seeking activity. Those seeking drugs may engage in "doctor shopping" by visiting multiple outpatient clinics, EDs, and pain management clinics to obtain prescriptions for controlled substances. At times, "scam" situations are presented, such as chronic toothaches, lost or stolen prescriptions, or multiple drug allergies. While recognizing the need to evaluate each situation separately, the physician must be particularly vigilant when patients insist on specific controlled substances, self-assert a high tolerance to medications, or issue veiled threats. Additional clues to drug-seeking behavior are listed in **Box 199.6**. When in doubt, the signs and symptoms can often be validated through contact with the patient's personal physician, review of recently issued prescription drugs with the patient's pharmacist, or perusal of previous medical records.[18]

**BOX 199.5 Diagnostic Criteria for Cocaine and Amphetamine Intoxication**

**A.** Recent use of cocaine or amphetamine
**B.** Clinically significant maladaptive behavioral or psychologic changes (e.g., euphoria or affective blunting; changes in sociability; hypervigilance; interpersonal sensitivity; anxiety, tension, or anger; stereotyped behavior; impaired judgment; impaired social or occupational functioning) that developed during or shortly after the use of cocaine or amphetamine
**C.** Two (or more) of the following developing during or shortly after cocaine or amphetamine use:
1. Tachycardia or bradycardia
2. Pupillary dilation
3. Elevated or lowered blood pressure
4. Perspiration or chills
5. Nausea or vomiting
6. Evidence of weight loss
7. Psychomotor agitation or retardation
8. Muscular weakness, respiratory depression, chest pain, or cardiac arrhythmias
9. Confusion, seizures, dyskinesias, dystonias, or coma

**D.** The symptoms are not due to a general medical condition and are not better accounted for by another mental disorder

From First MB, Frances A, Pincus HA. Substance-related disorders. In: DSM-IV-TR guidebook. Washington, DC: American Psychiatric Publishing; 2004.

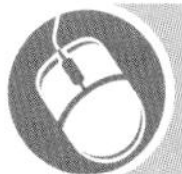

See Box 199.6, Drug-Seeking Behavior, online at www.expertconsult.com

## DIFFERENTIAL DIAGNOSIS

The differential diagnosis of substance abuse–related disorders is limited (**Box 199.7**). Hypochondriasis and somatization disorders are generally difficult to distinguish from true addiction in a single ED encounter. Pseudoaddiction describes behavior similar to that of addiction but arising from mismanaged pain. Pseudoaddiction patients are highly focused on obtaining medications, though usually through appropriate routes. They may be "clock watchers" and be focused on the scheduled delivery of approved analgesics. When suspecting a disruption in their expected regimen, a pseudoaddict may become deceptive or overly dramatic in attempts to ensure treatment. As noted, distinguishing between addicts and pseudoaddicts is challenging in an isolated encounter. In a broader perspective, however, pseudoaddicts generally function well once their pain is treated effectively, usually with long-acting opioids.[19]

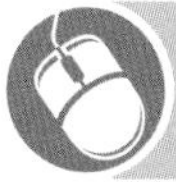

See Box 199.7, Differential Diagnosis of Substance-Related Disorders, online at www.expertconsult.com

## DIAGNOSTIC TESTING

In contrast to the increasing reliance on technology in diagnosing other medical disorders, the clinical interview remains the best tool for the diagnosis of substance-related disorders. Patients should be questioned about the quantity and frequency of use in an empathetic, nonjudgmental manner. Problems and symptoms current and past should be addressed, including any other family members with substance-related disorders. A number of screening tools are available: CAGE, the Michigan Alcoholism Screening Test (MAST), the Alcohol Use Disorders Identification Test (AUDIT), and the Drug Abuse Screening Test (DAST). These interview tools consist of anywhere from 4 to 28 "yes or no" or multiple choice questions and require from 30 seconds to 7 minutes to complete.[20]

When substance use is suspected, toxicologic analysis is recommended to establish or confirm a diagnosis. Qualitative analysis is generally sufficient to substantiate drug use, although quantitative levels are indicated for ethanol.

## TREATMENT AND DISPOSITION

The treatment goals of substance abuse, in particular, substance dependency, are twofold: detoxification and prevention of relapse (**Table 199.1**). These objectives are approached through two strategies: pharmacotherapy and behavioral therapy.

Detoxification is a pharmacologic process. The principle of pharmacologic detoxification is straightforward. Patients receive a long-acting medication in the same category as the drug of dependence, thereby blocking withdrawal symptoms.

**Table 199.1 Treatment**

| AGENT | DETOXIFICATION | ANTICRAVING |
|---|---|---|
| Ethanol | Benzodiazepines | Naltrexone<br>Acamprosate<br>Disulfiram<br>Topiramate* |
| Opiates | Opioid agonists<br>Methadone<br>Buprenorphine<br>$\alpha_2$-Agonists<br>Clonidine<br>Lofexidine† | Methadone<br>Buprenorphine<br>Naltrexone |
| Cocaine | Benzodiazepines | Topiramate‡<br>Modafinil‡<br>Vigabatrin‡<br>Disulfiram‡<br>Propranolol‡ |
| Methamphetamine | Benzodiazepines | None |

*Food and Drug Administration (FDA) approved as an anticonvulsant but potentially effective in preventing alcohol relapse.

†Use in Britain; not currently FDA approved for use in the United States.

‡FDA approved for another indication.

The dosage of this medication is gradually reduced under medical supervision.[21]

Alcoholics are detoxified with benzodiazepines: lorazepam, diazepam, and chlordiazepoxide. These drugs act by decreasing the hyperautonomic state of alcohol withdrawal by facilitating inhibitory GABA transmission.[22] Simultaneous therapy is directed not at alcohol withdrawal per se but rather at frequently associated comorbid conditions, such as malnutrition, and includes thiamine, multivitamins, folate, and magnesium.

Opiate detoxification is managed with two classes of medications: opioid agonists and $\alpha_2$-agonists. The time-tested opioid agonist of broadest use is methadone. The 36-hour half-life of methadone far exceeds the 3- to 4-hour half-life of heroin. Methadone may be prescribed only by maintenance programs approved by the Food and Drug Administration (FDA) and designated state authorities. However, methadone may be used by physicians for temporary maintenance or detoxification if an addicted patient is admitted to the hospital for an illness other than opioid addiction. Methadone may also be used in an outpatient setting when administered daily for a maximum of 3 days while a patient awaits admission to a licensed methadone treatment program.[23] Buprenorphine, a partial $\mu$-receptor opioid agonist, has a half-life of 20 to 25 hours and may be prescribed by physicians who have received a waiver by the Drug Enforcement Agency (DEA). $\alpha_2$-Agonists are a commonly used detoxification therapy for mild to moderate opiate withdrawal symptoms in the ED. Activation of presynaptic $\alpha_2$ receptors inhibits sympathetic outflow.[24] Currently, only clonidine is available in the United States. However, lofexidine, another $\alpha_2$-agonist similar to clonidine but with a lower incidence of associated hypotension, has been used effectively in Britain for opioid detoxification for more than a decade. Lofexidine will probably be submitted to the FDA for approval based on recent clinical trials.[25]

Withdrawal from central nervous system stimulants, in particular, cocaine and methamphetamine, is acutely managed with benzodiazepines. As noted earlier, these drugs diminish the hyperautonomic withdrawal state by increasing inhibitory GABA transmission.

## PREVENTION OF RELAPSE

Prevention of relapse is the second, yet most critical component of treatment because it primarily determines overall morbidity and mortality. Pharmacologic and behavioral therapies, though considered separately, appear to be most effective if combined.

In the past 25 years, a new class of psychoactive medications has emerged that show substantial promise in the treatment of addiction disorders. These "anticraving" medications reduce desire for the drug or alcohol in detoxified patients and deter relapse into compulsive substance abuse.[21]

Three medications have been approved by the FDA for the prevention of alcohol relapse: naltrexone, acamprosate, and disulfiram. As noted earlier in the section "Pathophysiology and Anatomy," alcohol increases extracellular dopamine in the nucleus accumbens.[21] In mice pretreated with naltrexone, an opioid μ-receptor antagonist, the alcohol-induced increase in dopamine is blocked. These mice do not self-administer alcohol.[26] Similarly, in a study of 99 alcoholic men, naltrexone-treated subjects reported reduced alcohol craving and drinking and decreased alcohol-related euphoria. Relapse rates in naltrexone-treated men were also significantly lower.

Naltrexone can be administered in two formats: an oral daily dosage of 50 mg and depot intramuscular injections of 380 mg every 4 weeks. A metaanalysis of 18 trials of naltrexone for alcohol dependence demonstrated a decrease in the risk for relapse with naltrexone when compared with placebo (relative risk, 0.64; 95% confidence interval, 0.51 to 0.82), as well as a reduction in craving and return to drinking and an increase in time to the first drink. The effect size for reducing relapse was modest (number needed to treat, 7).[27]

Not unexpectedly, daily dosing regimens with naltrexone limit compliance. Depot injections of naltrexone every 4 weeks both enhance compliance and establish more stable therapeutic levels. Three extended-release injectable formulations of naltrexone are available: Vivitrol, Naltrel, and Depotrex.[27]

Acamprosate was approved by the FDA in 2004 for the maintenance of abstinence in detoxified alcohol-dependent patients. The neurochemical effect of acamprosate is attributed to modification of glutamate neurotransmission.[27] Administered orally three times daily, acamprosate is less convenient than either oral or depot naltrexone. In addition, the impact of acamprosate on abstinence is unclear. Several largely positive clinical trials in Europe were contradicted by three negative clinical trials in the United States and Australia. Thus the clinical benefits of acamprosate are equivocal.[27]

Disulfiram blocks aldehyde dehydrogenase, an enzyme fundamental to alcohol metabolism. When someone consumes alcohol while taking disulfiram, acetaldehyde, an intermediate and relatively toxic by-product, accumulates 5- to 10-fold relative to normal circumstances. A most disagreeable clinical consequence, the "disulfiram reaction," develops. Diaphoresis, headache, dyspnea, hypotension, flushing, palpitations, nausea, and vomiting can all occur. Individuals taking disulfiram have poor compliance because of the unpleasantness of this effect.[21] Disulfiram is administered at 500 mg/day for 1 to 2 weeks, followed by an average maintenance dose of 250 mg/day. Reviews of efficacy show mixed results.[27]

Topiramate, though approved by the FDA as an anticonvulsant, has shown promise in preventing alcohol relapse. A multisite U.S. trial showed that topiramate reduced the percentage of heavy drinking days when compared with placebo (43.8% versus 51.8%) in 371 men and women with alcohol dependence over a period of 14 weeks. Topiramate was also more effective than placebo in improving the secondary outcomes of percent days abstinent and number of drinks per day.[28]

Additional agents under investigation for the prevention of relapse include baclofen, nalmefene, selective serotonin reuptake inhibitors, and ondansetron, among others.[29]

Three medications have been approved by the FDA for the prevention of relapse from opiates: methadone, buprenorphine, and naltrexone. Methadone and buprenorphine act as complete (methadone) or partial (buprenorphine) μ-receptor agonists. Conceptually, methadone and buprenorphine provide long-term replacement therapy for the brain disorder of addiction, comparable with the use of prednisone in patients with adrenal insufficiency or levothyroxine in those with hypothyroidism. Naltrexone, a μ-receptor antagonist, blocks the euphoric effects of opioids. Compliance is relatively poor with naltrexone.[21]

Unfortunately, no medications have been approved by the FDA for the prevention of relapse from cocaine addiction. However, five agents that are FDA-approved for other indications have been found in randomized, controlled trials to be effective for cocaine addiction. Topiramate, modafinil, and vigabatrin affect glutamate and GABA neurotransmission. The mechanism of two others, disulfiram and propranolol, is unknown.[21]

Clinical trials have yet to demonstrate any clear therapeutic options for prevention of relapse from methamphetamine.[30]

## DISPOSITION

ED patients with substance-related disorders should be referred to behavioral change programs. Success is determined by the pharmacologic anticraving therapy available to prevent relapse and the patient's intrinsic motivation for change.

Multiple behavioral therapies are available to diminish the likelihood of relapse. Contingency management is based on the operant conditioning principle that behavior resulting in positive consequences is more likely to recur. Patients meeting specific drug-free goals receive incentives or rewards. Cognitive behavioral and skills training emphasizes a functional analysis of drug use by taking into account the antecedents and consequences of drug use. Addicts then learn to identify situations at high risk for drug use and relapse. Through rehearsal and role-playing, addicts develop strategies to either avoid such situations or cope effectively. Motivational enhancement therapy (MET) seeks to develop the individual's inner drive for change. Couples and family treatment takes into account the familial and social systems in which substance use commonly occurs. Alcoholics Anonymous (AA) provides a facilitative form of behavioral therapy that consists of a 12-step program based on self-assessment and fellowship activities.[31]

As noted earlier, pharmacologic and behavioral therapies appear to be most effective when used together. To assess this assumption, from 2001 through 2004 the National Institute on Alcohol Abuse and Alcoholism (NIAAA) compared the efficacy of acamprosate, naltrexone, and placebo in combination with behavioral treatments among 1383 recently alcohol-abstinent volunteers (median age, 44 years) from 11 U.S. academic sites in the nationwide clinical study COMBINE (Combining Medications and Behavioral Intervention). Patients receiving medical management with naltrexone, combined behavioral intervention (CBI), or both fared better on drinking outcomes. Acamprosate showed no evidence of efficacy, with or without CBI. No combination produced better efficacy than did naltrexone or CBI alone in the presence of medical management. Placebo pills and meeting with a health care professional had a positive effect above that of CBI during treatment. Naltrexone with medical management could be delivered in health care settings, thus serving alcohol-dependent patients who might otherwise not receive treatment.[32,33]

## TREATMENT EFFICACY

### Alcohol

The diversity of pharmacologic and behavioral therapies complicates analysis of treatment efficacy. Furthermore, individuals with substance-related disorders differ. No single treatment has been shown to be effective for all.

To better understand the value of particular therapies for alcoholism, the NIAAA initiated Project MATCH (Matching Alcoholism Treatment to Client Heterogeneity) in late 1989. A total of 1726 patients were recruited at treatment facilities throughout the United States. Two parallel cohorts represented the primary formats of treatment: outpatients recruited directly from the community and "aftercare" patients consisting of those who had just completed an inpatient or intensive day hospital treatment program. The three treatment arms included MET, cognitive behavioral therapy (CBT), and a Twelve-Step Facilitation (TSF) program grounded on the 12-step principles of AA but based on professionally delivered individualized therapy rather than therapy in peer groups.[34]

Project MATCH revealed several notable findings. Most significantly, linking patients to specific behavioral therapies added little to treatment outcome. This disputed the notion that specific patient–behavioral treatment matching is essential for effective treatment of alcoholism. In addition, when compared with their status before treatment, drinking and negative consequences declined regardless of which of the three treatments the participants received. In the outpatient group, 10% more patients receiving TSF achieved continuous abstinence than did those receiving the other two treatments (24% for TSF as opposed to 15% for CBT and 14% for MET).[34]

Overall, more "aftercare" patients (35%) than "outpatients" (19%) were able to sustain complete abstinence during the year after treatment despite the fact that aftercare patients entered the study with more alcohol dependence symptoms. Although this finding may suggest that an initial period of closely supervised abstinence from alcohol is important to outcome, patients were not randomly assigned to the two cohorts, and other factors may have contributed.

### Opiates

Since 1964, methadone has been the mainstay of opiate pharmacotherapy. Studies have shown that moderate- to high-dose treatment with methadone (80 to 120 mg) reduces or eliminates opiate use in outpatient settings. A placebo-controlled study of methadone involving 100 male narcotic-addicted subjects evaluated both long-term retention in treatment and criminal activity. After initial stabilization of acute withdrawal symptoms with methadone, subjects were randomized to treatment with either methadone or placebo. At 32 weeks, the placebo group had a 10% retention rate as compared with a 76% retention rate in the methadone group. At 156 weeks, 2% of the control group and 56% of the methadone group were still in treatment. Approximately one third of subjects in the methadone group continued to use illicit opiates. Felonious behavior was also positively affected by methadone. Criminal activity in the placebo group, measured by conviction per man-month, was double that of the methadone group.[35]

## REFERENCES

*References can be found on Expert Consult @ www.expertconsult.com.*

# 200 Anorexia Nervosa and Bulimia Nervosa

*Jason E. Liebzeit*

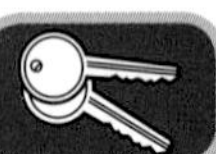

**KEY POINTS**

- Patients with anorexia or bulimia are at increased risk for life-threatening metabolic derangements and cardiac dysrhythmias that mandate hospital admission.
- The most common cause of death from anorexia is cardiac arrest secondary to conduction delays or ventricular dysrhythmias.
- Urgent outpatient psychiatric referral is appropriate for well-appearing patients who are able to adequately care for themselves.

## DEFINITIONS AND EPIDEMIOLOGY

*Anorexia nervosa* ("anorexia") is a disturbance in body perception that results in fear of gaining weight and refusal to maintain a minimally normal body weight. *Bulimia nervosa* ("bulimia") is an obsessive self-evaluation of body shape and weight that leads to a characteristic cycle of binge eating and subsequent actions that prevent weight gain.

Though similar in their relationship with food, these diseases represent two separate psychiatric entities with distinct clinical sequelae. Distinguishing features include the body mass index or height-matched weight and, in women, the presence of regular menstruation. Amenorrhea is a key finding of anorexia in postmenarchal women. Diagnosis requires fulfillment of all criteria listed in the text revision of the fourth edition of the *Diagnostic and Statistical Manual of Mental Disorders* (DSM-IV-TR) (**Box 200.1**). These diseases do not coexist in the same patient; a patient has either anorexia or bulimia, but never both simultaneously.[1]

Anorexia can be divided into the restricting or binge eating–purging subtypes. Restricting patients commonly eat only 300 to 700 calories each day, or they engage in excessive exercise to ward off weight gain. Binge-purging behavior involves intentional vomiting or the inappropriate use of laxatives, enemas, or diuretics in response to even small amounts of consumed food. Bulimia is similarly divided into purging and nonpurging. The subtypes are based on the behavior occurring at the time of diagnosis.[2]

Anorexia and bulimia are diseases nearly exclusively encountered in North America, western Europe, and Japan. Childhood anxiety disorders may increase the likelihood of these disorders, although no clear cause has been identified for either illness. Women suffer from anorexia and bulimia more frequently than men do. The lifetime prevalence of anorexia varies from 0.3% to 1% for women; men are estimated to have one tenth of that prevalence. Bulimia is more common than anorexia, with a lifetime prevalence of 1% to 3% in women. Similarly, only 10% of bulimic patients are male; these men are more likely to suffer from premorbid obesity. The incidence is further increased in male wrestlers.[3]

## PRESENTING SIGNS AND SYMPTOMS

Emergency department (ED) patients with anorexia or bulimia generally complain of symptoms related to associated disease states or complications; they rarely seek primary treatment of their psychiatric illness. ED visits provide an opportunity for both intervention and education. Recognition of these underdiagnosed diseases creates an opportunity for early consultation and referral. Medical care alone is often of transient utility. Successful cure of both anorexia and bulimia requires intensive individual or family psychotherapy.

### CLASSIC PRESENTATION

The typical patient with anorexia is an otherwise successful mid- to late-adolescent girl exhibiting marked cachexia. The patient may demonstrate a remarkable lack of insight regarding her appearance. Common complaints include fatigue, cold intolerance, abdominal pain, and amenorrhea. Weakness, especially symptomatic orthostasis, features prominently in the patient's review of systems. Emaciation is the most notable clinical feature. Bradycardia and hypotension are common findings. Lanugo, or the fine body hair commonly seen on the extremities and trunk, may be present. Signs of nutritional deficiency may be present in patients with the food-restricting subtypes.

Patients with the purging subtypes of both bulimia and anorexia share physical findings, although bulimic patients may have a more normal-appearing body habitus. Purging through vomiting often results in erosion of dental enamel, particularly on the lingual ("back") side of the teeth. Manual induction of vomiting leads to calluses on the dorsal aspect of the fingers as a result of recurrent contact with the teeth, a finding known as the Russell sign. Benign parotid salivary enlargement is common.

**BOX 200.1 *DSM-IV-TR* Diagnostic Criteria Differentiating Anorexia and Bulimia**

| ANOREXIA NERVOSA | BULIMIA NERVOSA |
|---|---|
| 1. Refusal to maintain weight greater than or equal to 85% of expected<br>2. Fear of gaining weight despite being underweight<br>3. Disturbance in body perception, excessive influence of body shape or weight on self-evaluation, or denial of seriousness of current weight<br>4. In women of appropriate age, amenorrhea (defined as at least three consecutive missed menses) while not on hormones<br>Subtype as either restrictive or binge-purge | 1. Recurrent episodes of binge eating:<br>a. More food in a discreet period than most people would eat in similar circumstances<br>b. Sense of lack of control over eating episodes<br>2. Recurrent inappropriate compensatory behavior to prevent weight gain (vomiting, exercise, laxatives, diuretics)<br>3. Bingeing and compensatory behavior occurring at least twice per week for 3 months<br>4. Undue influence of body shape or weight on self-evaluation<br>5. This disturbance does not occur during an episode of anorexia |

From American Psychiatric Association. Diagnostic and statistical manual of mental disorders. 4th ed, text rev (DSM-IV-TR). Washington, DC: American Psychiatric Association; 2000.

### ATYPICAL PRESENTATION

Advances in the management of severe anorexia and bulimia have extended life expectancy for those afflicted. Long-standing anorexia or bulimia affects normal physiology, as with any chronic disease. Notably, gastrointestinal motility may slow and lead to chronic nausea, gastroparesis, impaction, or obstruction. Rare complications of these eating disorders that may be encountered in the ED are discussed in the following section.

"Late-onset" eating disorders are increasingly being recognized in elderly patients; the clinical features and diagnostic criteria are the same, with the exception of amenorrhea in postmenopausal women.[4]

## COMPLICATIONS

- Arrhythmia: Disruption of normal cardiac conduction is the most life-threatening medical complication of anorexia. Prolongation of the QTc interval is ominous. Cardiac arrest resulting from conduction delays or ventricular dysrhythmias is the most common cause of death from anorexia.[5]
- Elevated abdominal pressure: Patients engaging in binge eating may experience severe gastric dilation that significantly increases intraabdominal pressure, either with or without intestinal obstruction. This increased pressure may ultimately result in cardiac arrest from direct mechanical force or decreased venous return.[6,7]
- Dehydration and renal insufficiency: Insufficient fluid intake may occur with anorexia. With bulimia, prerenal hypovolemia arises from fluid losses as a result of excessive vomiting or laxative abuse.
- Starvation and vitamin deficiency: These conditions result from inadequate caloric intake.
- Osteopenia: Pubescent anorexia or severe bulimia may cause hypoestrogenemia and resultant undermineralized bone. Bone pain or pathologic fractures may ensue.
- Electrolyte abnormality: This condition results from either insufficient intake or excessive gastrointestinal losses.
- Esophageal and gastric trauma: Repetitive, forceful vomiting may lead to Mallory-Weiss tears or Boerhaave syndrome. Gastric distention occurs with binging.
- Nausea and constipation: Gastrointestinal motility decreases with starvation. Native colonic contraction decreases with laxative abuse, thereby leading to colonic distention and constipation.
- Rectal prolapse: This condition results from muscle weakening secondary to laxative abuse.
- Congestive heart failure: Cardiomyopathy may be caused by starvation states or by ipecac abuse.
- Refeeding syndromes: Peripheral edema, hypophosphatemia, and dysrhythmias are common features associated with resumption of appropriate caloric intake.
- Inattention and changes in mental status: Chronic disease may lead to decreases in both gray matter and white matter along with concurrent ventricular enlargement. Starvation-associated hypoglycemia or other electrolyte abnormalities may affect mental status.

## ASSOCIATED COMORBID CONDITIONS

- Anxiety disorders: The lifetime prevalence is 64% in eating-disordered patients versus 13% in the general population. Obsessive-compulsive disorder and social phobia are common.[8]
- Depression.
- Substance abuse: This is often seen in patients with binge-type bulimia.[9]
- Personality disorders: Obsessive-compulsive personality disorder is associated with anorexia; cluster B disorders are more frequently identified in patients with bulimia.[9]

## DIFFERENTIAL DIAGNOSIS

Evaluation of a patient with cachexia must be thorough. A notable lack of subjective complaints in an emaciated patient may be cause to suspect anorexia. The differential diagnosis of anorexia and bulimia is narrow because the patient's behavior is an essential component of the disease. Catabolic states associated with increased caloric consumption, such as infection or hypermetabolism, should be differentiated from inadequate caloric intake (**Box 200.2**).

## DIAGNOSTIC TESTING

No ancillary tests are available to confirm the diagnosis of anorexia or bulimia. The diagnosis is made by following the

**BOX 200.2 Limited Differential Diagnosis of Cachexia**

**Excessive Caloric Consumption**
Hyperthyroidism
Infection
Malignant disease
Advanced acquired immunodeficiency syndrome

**Inadequate Caloric Intake**
Superior mesenteric artery syndrome
Depression
Psychotic disorders
Malabsorption syndromes

**Table 200.1 Diagnostic Laboratory Findings**

| LABORATORY ABNORMALITY DIAGNOSIS | FINDING |
|---|---|
| Hypokalemia, hypochloremia, alkalosis (elevated $HCO_3^-$ or pH); elevated amylase | Excessive vomiting |
| Hypokalemia, acidosis (decreased $HCO_3^-$ or pH) | Diarrhea |

*HCO3⁻*, Bicarbonate.

guidelines set forth in the DSM-IV-TR. Screening tools have been developed to aid in the diagnosis of both these eating disorders; the SCOFF questionnaire proposed by Morgan et al. is one such tool. Answering "yes" to two or more of the SCOFF questions is 100% sensitive for both anorexia and bulimia.[10] The SCOFF screen includes the following questions: Do you induce vomiting because you feel uncomfortably full? Do you worry that you have lost control over how much you eat? Have you recently lost more than 14 lb in the last 3 months? Do you think you are fat even when other people say you are too thin? Does food dominate your life?

Laboratory tests aid in identification of the potentially life-threatening physiologic abnormalities commonly seen in an eating-disordered patient. Serum electrolytes, including phosphorus, are critical in the evaluation of patients with suspected anorexia or bulimia. Hypokalemic, hypochloremic metabolic alkalosis is the most common finding in patients with induced vomiting. Laxative abuse results in metabolic acidosis from intestinal loss of bicarbonate. Endocrine abnormalities may be encountered in patients with chronic disease; insufficient thyroid hormone may cause hypotension, hypothermia, and bradycardia. An elevated serum amylase level may serve as useful evidence of surreptitious vomiting, although the degree of increase in the serum value itself has little clinical significance (**Table 200.1**).

An electrocardiogram should be obtained for all patients with suspected anorexia or bulimia. Although bradycardia is a common benign finding in anorexia, other arrhythmias are likely to result in morbidity and mortality. Prolongation of the QTc interval is the most concerning electrocardiographic abnormality and may be present despite normal electrolytes.

Intracranial imaging reveals loss of gray matter.[8] Such imaging studies are indicated only for patients with altered mental status or trauma (see the "Priority Actions" box).

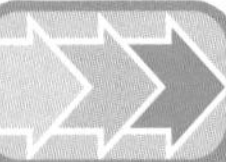

**PRIORITY ACTIONS**

Primary survey
- Fluid resuscitation
- Cardiovascular stabilization

Obtain an electrocardiogram
Laboratory evaluation: complete blood count, electrolytes, glucose, phosphorus
Chest radiography in cases of excessive vomiting or ipecac abuse
Do *not* initiate nutritional support in the emergency department

## TREATMENT

ED management should focus on correcting any abnormalities detected during the medical evaluation. Cardiovascular compromise requires immediate intervention. Arrhythmias are managed according to standard advanced cardiac life support guidelines. Electrolytes and glucose should be normalized, and body temperature should be regulated. Aggressive fluid resuscitation should be avoided because it may result in sudden congestive heart failure. The mechanical sequelae of purging (esophageal rupture, Mallory-Weiss tears, or rectal prolapse) respond to conventional treatment discussed elsewhere in this text.

Nutritional support is not a priority in the ED. For outpatients, the intake goal should be 1200 to 1500 kcal/day with weekly increases; weight gain should be limited to 0.5 to 0.9 kg (1 to 2 lb) each week. Inpatient feeding has been associated with life-threatening arrhythmias and transient edematous states; such refeeding is best managed in a monitored medical unit.

Sophisticated and concurrent psychologic, social, dietary, and medical support is crucial for both inpatients and outpatients. Selective serotonin reuptake inhibitors, in particular fluoxetine, have been associated with increased compliance in the outpatient treatment of bulimia and may also address the anxiety states commonly encountered with eating disorders. Antidepressants should not be initiated in the ED without the collaboration of the treating psychiatrist or primary physician.[11,12]

## DISPOSITION

Patients generally consent to hospital admission for the treatment of symptomatic somatic complaints. Voluntary admission for psychiatric treatment is often more difficult to arrange. Lack of insight into the disordered eating clouds a patient's appreciation of the severity of the disease. Adult patients whose weight is at least 25% less than that expected for their height are candidates for admission.

Telemetry monitoring is indicated when arrhythmias or QTc abnormalities are present. Additionally, refeeding may promote cardiovascular complications, for which continuous monitoring is required. Critical care admission should be reserved for patients with unstable vital signs or dangerous metabolic abnormalities.

Current guidelines suggest psychiatric or medical admission for any child or adolescent with rapid weight loss. Parents or guardians may request inpatient admission when outpatient management has failed. Psychiatric admission for minors is typically easier to accomplish than for adults. Early inpatient treatment is associated with a decreased risk for both arrhythmias and loss of cortical volume. Admission should be advocated for all patients who lack home support or who are otherwise at risk for failure of outpatient treatment (**Box 200.3**).[13,14]

Barring clear impairment of decision-making capacity, involuntary admission of adults is rare. The judicial system in the United States generally recognizes that a patient's actions supersede stated intent, thus supporting hospitalization of patients who are at significant risk for self-harm. For example, an anorexic patient may deny suicidality despite behavior that clearly resulted in a life-threatening dysrhythmia. Involuntary admission should be considered for patients with such profound lack of insight, as well as for those who lack decision-making capacity.[5,15]

**BOX 200.3 Admission Guidelines**

**Medicine**
Weight less than 25% of expected
Need for intravenous electrolyte replacement
Gastrointestinal dysmotility
Heart failure

**Telemetry**
QT abnormality
Stable arrhythmia (i.e., premature ventricular contractions)

**Intensive Care**
Unstable vital signs
Life-threatening metabolic derangements

## SUGGESTED READINGS

American Psychiatric Association Work Group on Eating Disorders. Practice guideline for the treatment of patients with eating disorders (revision). Am J Psychiatry 2000;157(Suppl):1-39.

Morgan JF, Reid F, Lacey JH. The SCOFF questionnaire: a new screening tool for eating disorders. West J Med 2000;172:164-5.

Yager J, Andersen AL. Anorexia nervosa. N Engl J Med 2005;353:1481-8.

## REFERENCES

***References can be found on Expert Consult @ www.expertconsult.com.***

# Introduction to Oncologic Emergencies 201

*Jeremy D. Sperling*

**KEY POINTS**

- Fever in a neutropenic patient with cancer is assumed to be a life-threatening infection; antibiotic therapy must be started immediately.
- Hypercalcemia is common in malignant disease and is often missed. Presenting symptoms may include weakness, vomiting, and mental status changes.
- Tumor lysis syndrome causes acute renal failure, hyperkalemia, hyperphosphatemia, and hypocalcemia; it is a rare but life-threatening complication of chemotherapy.
- Adrenal insufficiency and pericardial tamponade are causes of hypotension.
- Pleural effusions commonly cause dyspnea in the oncology patient. However, always exclude life-threatening causes of dyspnea (e.g., pulmonary embolism, pneumonia, pericardial tamponade) in this patient population.

## EPIDEMIOLOGY

As the population ages, cancer prevalence is expected to increase.[1] In 2010, the United States population had more than 1.5 million new cancer diagnoses and more than 569,000 cancer deaths.[2] The American Cancer Society estimated that the number of new cancer cases will double from 2000 to 2050.[1] At the same time, aggressive treatment strategies, whether involving surgery, chemotherapy, or radiation, are helping oncology patients to live longer and at times overcome their cancer. In fact, U.S. cancer death rates decreased by 1% per year from 2001 through 2006.[2] Since the 1970s, the 5-year survival rate for all cancers has increased from 50% to 68% in the United States.[2] Declines in cancer deaths are the result of many factors, including better screening, early detection strategies, public health risk reduction programs, and improved medical and surgical treatment. Emergency physicians (EPs) are routinely called on to recognize and treat emergency complications of cancer and cancer therapies. Interventions that the EP makes to keep a patient alive acutely may allow the patient's chemotherapy or radiation therapy to work for an overall cure. Today, oncology patients treated in the emergency department (ED) are increasingly more likely to survive to hospital discharge, even if they are admitted to an intensive care unit.[3]

## TRIAGE

Some oncologic emergencies require timely action. One example is the patient with fever and potential neutropenia; this patient requires rapid assessment and early antibiotic administration. Other oncologic emergencies requiring immediate intervention include airway or respiratory complications, spinal cord compression, and possible cerebral herniation.

## ISOLATION AND INFECTIOUS CONTROL ISSUES

Each year, approximately 1.9 million nosocomial infections occur in U.S. hospitals, and approximately 88,000 patients die.[4] Immunocompromised patients with cancer, especially neutropenic patients and bone marrow transplant recipients, are at increased risk for these infections. At-risk patients should be identified on ED arrival and should not be allowed to spend a significant amount of time in waiting rooms or busy ED hallways, where they can be exposed to infections from other patients. Ideally, bone marrow transplant recipients and potentially neutropenic patients should be placed in single rooms with positive air pressure at 12 or more air exchanges per hour. Positive air pressure decreases the number of infectious particles that enter a patient's room. If such a room is unavailable, the next best option is to place the patient in an individual room with the door closed. Patients with a potential airborne illness (e.g., tuberculosis) are the exception; they should be placed in a negative pressure room to protect other patients and the ED staff.

As with all patients, careful hand washing is essential when dealing with the neutropenic patient. However, when providing noninvasive care, the use of sterile gowns, masks, and gloves does not provide any extra protection. To avoid bacterial contamination, neutropenic patients should generally be offered only cooked (or pasteurized) food and bottled water. However, data supporting this type of "neutropenic diet" is quite limited and may unnecessarily restrict the patient's nutritional options.

## ONCOLOGIC HISTORY

Although obtaining a complete past medical history from a patient with cancer is not always possible or necessary for the EP, certain questions may prove crucial and are unique to the oncology patient. Pertinent information includes the type of cancer, the stage of the cancer (the extent of its spread), previous cancer-related complications, and previous cancer treatments including surgery, chemotherapy, and radiation therapy. The timing of recent treatments and the names of specific chemotherapeutic agents that have been used are important because these treatments may be the direct cause of the patient's current illness. Oncology patients may have complicated past medical histories. Reliable sources such as hospital records (if the patient has recently been admitted) or the patient's oncologist should be used to obtain pertinent data quickly.

Early in the ED encounter with an oncology patient, the patient should be asked whether he or she has any specific wishes or advanced directives. Specifically, patients should be asked whether they have a "do not resuscitate" or "do not intubate" order or a health care proxy. Many patients with cancer, especially those with late-stage disease, may have very defined treatment objectives in mind (e.g., intravenous hydration but no invasive procedures or tests). These objectives and wishes should be documented in the chart and respected. Early inquiry about the patient's wishes and expectations will help to guide treatment appropriately.

## FEVER

Fever is a very common chief complaint for oncology patients who present to the ED, especially for those undergoing chemotherapy. Fever can be the first sign of a life-threatening infectious process. In particular, neutropenic patients are highly susceptible to almost any type of bacterial or fungal infection. Fever in the setting of neutropenia must be assumed to be a life-threatening bacterial infection, and antibiotic therapy should be started immediately (see the "Facts and Formulas" box for the definition of neutropenic fever). Besides the immediate infectious risks, a neutropenic fever episode may delay or end future chemotherapy treatment and therefore may compromise the overall chances for a cancer cure.

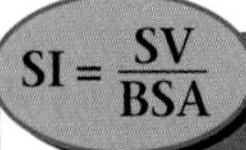


**FACTS AND FORMULAS**

**Neutropenic Fever Defined**

Fever: Temperature ≥ 38.3° C once or ≥38.0° C for >1 hour

Neutropenia: Absolute neutrophil count < 500/mm$^3$ or <1000/mm$^3$ with a predicted decline to <500/mm$^3$

## EPIDEMIOLOGY

Neutropenic fever is the most common emergency indication for hospital admission among oncology patients. The in-hospital mortality rate in patients with neutropenic fever is approximately 9.5%, and it increases if the patient has any associated comorbidities.[5] Patients with neutropenic fever have a mean (median) length of stay of 11.5 (6) days, at a mean cost of more than $19,000 per case.[5]

## PATHOPHYSIOLOGY

Chemotherapy can severely damage a patient's normal defense mechanisms, including both humoral and cellular immunity, thus leaving the patient defenseless to combat infection. Chemotherapy can weaken or destroy neutrophils, T lymphocytes, macrophages, monocytes, and immunoglobulin production. Radiation and chemotherapy also affect the patient's mechanical barriers against infection. In particular, they damage the integrity of the mucous membranes and skin. All this injury to the patient's immune system takes place in an individual who already has cancer and therefore may already have either a weakened immune system or compromised physiologic factors.

## DIFFERENTIAL DIAGNOSIS AND MEDICAL DECISION MAKING

Although the prudent approach is to assume that fever in an oncology patient is from an infectious source, infection is not the only reason that oncology patients may have a fever. Fever can sometimes be a manifestation of the underlying malignant process itself or a side effect of a chemotherapeutic agent. Chemotherapeutic agents such as bleomycin and cytosine arabinoside have been noted to cause fevers. Lymphomas, leukemias, and renal cell carcinoma have been recognized as sources of fever without any concurrent infection, and at times, fever can be their initial presenting symptom. Thrombophlebitis, medications, and transfusion reactions can also be rare causes of fever.

## DIAGNOSTIC TESTING

The EP should search for an infectious source of the fever. A minimum evaluation should include at least two blood cultures, a urinalysis and urine culture, a chest radiograph, a complete blood count with differential (to confirm neutropenia), and baseline chemistry studies including kidney and liver function. Blood cultures should be obtained from all indwelling vascular catheters that are present. At least one blood culture should be drawn from a peripheral vein. Further diagnostic testing should be driven by the patient's symptoms or physical examination findings. For example, an abdominal and pelvic computed tomography (CT) scan should be ordered if an intraabdominal source of the fever is possible. Other sources to consider culturing in the appropriate clinical setting are the oropharynx, cerebrospinal fluid, peritoneal fluid, pleural fluid, stool, and any purulent skin lesions.

## TREATMENT

Empiric, broad-spectrum antibiotics should be started as early as possible for patients in the ED who have neutropenic fever. Antibiotics should not be delayed while awaiting confirmation of the neutropenia but rather should be started on all febrile patients at high risk (e.g., recent chemotherapy).[6] Additionally, antibiotics should not be delayed while the EP looks for an infectious source. An obvious source is very often not identifiable in the ED. Rapid antibiotic administration is the likely reason for substantial mortality reductions among bacteremic patients with cancer. With the incorporation of this early antibiotic strategy, a large European research group found an overall mortality decrease from 21% to 7% over a 16-year period.[7]

Patients should be started empirically on antibiotics that reflect the resistance patterns and bacterial profiles of the treating institution. Most institutions have antibiotic protocols based on these bacterial patterns. Gram-positive organisms such as *Staphylococcus aureus, Staphylococcus epidermidis,* and viridans streptococci are currently more predominant than gram-negative organisms as the source of neutropenic fever. However, gram-negative organisms can be more virulent (e.g., *Pseudomonas*), and therefore the patient must always be empirically treated for these pathogens.

Single-agent intravenous antibiotics regimens are currently recommended for hemodynamically stable patients whose medical condition is uncomplicated.[6,8] Potential monotherapy regimens include cefepime, piperacillin-tazobactam, or a carbapenem (e.g., imipenem-cilastatin, meropenem).[6,8] Double coverage with an aminoglycoside (e.g., gentamicin, tobramycin) or a fluoroquinolone (e.g., levofloxacin) should be considered if antibiotic resistance is strongly suspected, if the patient is in shock, or if this approach is needed to manage other complications. Vancomycin should not be started empirically for neutropenic fever.[6,8] No significant difference in morbidity or mortality was found in a meta-analysis of 13 randomized control trials when a standard neutropenic antibiotic regimen was compared with the same regimen plus a glycopeptide (e.g., vancomycin).[9] However, one should consider starting vancomycin if the infection is suspected to originate from an indwelling central venous catheter, a soft tissue infection, or hospital-associated pneumonia or if the patient is in septic shock.[6,8] A lower threshold for adding vancomycin should be used if the institution has a high rate of methicillin-resistant *S. aureus* (MRSA) or resistant viridans streptococcal strains.

Long indwelling catheters should generally be left in place and not removed in the ED. Many catheters in this patient population are buried subcutaneously and are not easily removed. Removal of the catheter in the ED should be considered if the tunnel is grossly infected or if the infected catheter has produced septic emboli or endocarditis.

Granulocyte colony-stimulating factors (G-CSFs) are used by oncologists with certain chemotherapy regimens to decrease the incidence of neutropenic episodes. Current guidelines recommend the prophylactic administration of a G-CSF with chemotherapy to patients who, based on age, past medical history, chemotherapy toxicity, and tumor characteristics, have a greater than 20% chance of developing febrile neutropenia.[8,10] This G-CSF prophylaxis regimen with chemotherapy has been shown to be effective; for example, in patients with small cell lung cancer, it decreases the incidence, duration, and severity of neutropenic fever.[11] Commonly used G-CSFs for prophylaxis are daily injections of filgrastim or lenograstim or a once per chemotherapy cycle injection of pegfilgrastim. Adverse side effects of G-CSF use include bone, joint and musculoskeletal pain and flulike symptoms.[12]

The use of a G-CSF in the acute setting of neutropenic fever is controversial. A meta-analysis of 13 studies with 1518 patients found that patients with neutropenic fever who were treated with G-CSFs had shorter hospitalizations and neutrophil recovery times but only a marginally significant benefit in infection-related mortality and no significant benefit in overall mortality.[12] Because the effects of G-CSFs on mortality are not clear and because these agents are very expensive, a G-CSF should not be given routinely in the ED for neutropenic fever. Rather, until more convincing evidence exists, G-CSFs should be given only after discussion with the patient's oncologist and considered only for patients who are at high risk for infectious complications or who have prognostic factors predictive of a poor outcome.[10,13]

## FOLLOW-UP AND NEXT STEPS

Nearly all patients with neutropenic fever require admission. Outpatient management could be considered for carefully selected low-risk patients within a well-designed institutional protocol and in concert with the patient's oncologist. Certain decision rules have attempted to determine which neutropenic patients are at low risk for complications and therefore could be eligible for outpatient treatment with oral antibiotics. The most commonly cited decision rule for assessing low-risk patients is the Multinational Association for Supportive Care in Cancer (MASCC) index score[6,8] (**Table 201.1**). In its initial

**Table 201.1 Multinational Association for Supportive Care in Cancer Index Score for Identifying Low-Risk Patients at Neutropenic Fever**

| BURDEN OF ILLNESS* | SCORE |
|---|---|
| No or mild symptoms/moderate symptoms* | 5/3 |
| No hypotension | 5 |
| No chronic obstructive pulmonary disease | 4 |
| Solid tumor or no previous fungal infection | 4 |
| No dehydration | 3 |
| Outpatient status† | 3 |
| Age < 60 yr | 2 |
| Add together points to obtain score (maximum score, 26) | |
| Risk of complication: high risk < 21; low risk ≥ 21 | |

From Klastersky J, Paesmans M, Rubenstein EB, Boyer M. The Multinational Association for Supportive Care in Cancer Risk Index: a multinational scoring system for identifying low-risk febrile neutropenic cancer patients. J Clin Oncol 2000;18:3038-51.

*Burden of illness: 5 for no or mild, 3 for moderate, 0 for severe.

†Outpatient status means onset of fever as an outpatient.

validation study, the MASCC index score was found to have a positive predictive value of 91%, a specificity of 68%, and a sensitivity of 71%.[14] The MASCC decision rule is likely best applied to select patients who can quickly undergo conversion to oral antibiotics as inpatients and, in the absence of early complications, be targeted for early hospital discharge. If the patient is discharged, an oral antibiotic regimen is prescribed; ideally, the patient is observed taking the first dose in the ED. The two most common regimens used are a quinolone alone (e.g., ciprofloxacin) or a quinolone plus amoxicillin-clavulanate.[15]

## INFECTIOUS CAUSES OF FEVER UNIQUE TO THE PATIENT WITH CANCER

### NEUTROPENIC ENTEROCOLITIS (TYPHLITIS)

Typhlitis (neutropenic enterocolitis) is an inflammatory process of the ileum and colon that affects neutropenic patients. Typhlitis is most commonly associated with acute leukemia, but it can be seen with other malignant conditions. Typhlitis usually occurs in patients undergoing chemotherapy, although it occasionally occurs in patients who are not. Presenting clinical symptoms may include fever, lower abdominal pain, and diarrhea, which can be bloody or watery. Other potential symptoms include abdominal distention and nausea or vomiting. On physical examination, the patient's abdomen may be generally tender, or the tenderness may be localized to the right lower quadrant. CT scan can make the diagnosis and rule out other potentially dangerous abdominal processes (e.g., appendicitis, diverticulitis). Typical CT scan findings of typhlitis are diffuse submucosal thickening of the affected bowel wall, generally the terminal ileum or ascending colon. Other CT scan findings may include paracolonic fluid and gas in the bowel wall. Uncomplicated cases should be treated with broad-spectrum antibiotics (covering aerobic and anaerobic pathogens, including *Pseudomonas aeruginosa*), bowel rest, and supportive care. Patients who present with perforation, obstruction, bleeding, or gangrenous bowel require prompt surgical consultation. The mortality rate of typhlitis is quite high; in one case series, six of nine patients died of sepsis.[16]

### FUNGAL INFECTIONS

Fungal infections increasingly are the likely source of the infection when neutropenic patients with cancer have persistent fevers despite ongoing broad-spectrum antibiotics. *Candida albicans* is the most common fungal pathogen in these cases, but aspergillosis, cryptococcus, and other fungal infections can occur. In oncology patients with neutropenic fever, invasive candidiasis and aspergillosis are associated with high mortality rates (36.7% and 39.2%, respectively).[5] Patients with leukemia, in particular, have increasing incidences of fungal infections, especially with *Candida* species. Empiric antifungal therapy should be considered in neutropenic patients with persistent fever despite 4 to 7 days of antibiotic therapy.[8]

### INVASIVE FUNGAL SINUSITIS

Invasive fungal sinusitis affects immunocompromised patients and has a high mortality rate. *Aspergillus* and species of the Mucoraceae family (usually *Rhizopus*) are the most common fungi involved; they can destroy both tissue and bone. Fungal infection of the paranasal sinuses becomes acute invasive fungal sinusitis as it spreads through tissues to the orbit or the central nervous system. Patients with acute invasive fungal sinusitis may appear severely ill. Symptoms include fever, nasal congestion, headache, maxillary tenderness, periorbital swelling, and even mental status changes. Conversely, in an immunocompromised patient with cancer, symptoms may be subtle because the patient may not mount enough of an inflammatory response to produce clinical symptoms. Therefore, the clinician must maintain a high index of suspicion in this patient population. If the disease is suspected, immediate consultation with an otorhinolaryngologist for surgical débridement is imperative. A CT scan of the sinuses may be helpful to define the extent of the disease, but imaging should not delay surgical consultation. Intravenous antifungal therapy should be initiated with amphotericin B; however, antifungal therapy may not be effective without wide surgical débridement.

# Electrolyte Disturbances in the Oncology Patient

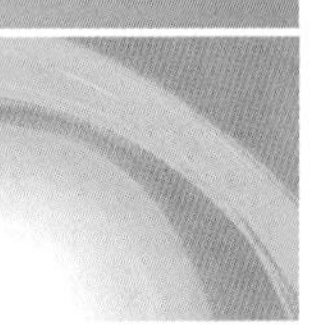

## TUMOR LYSIS SYNDROME

### PERSPECTIVE

Tumor lysis syndrome (TLS) is the constellation of metabolic abnormalities that occur in response to the rapid destruction of malignant cells, generally from the initiation of chemotherapy (**Table 201.2**). The sudden death of many malignant cells results in the release into the bloodstream of their intracellular contents, and this causes sudden increases in potassium, phosphorus, and uric acid levels. TLS is generally

**Table 201.2 Tumor Lysis Syndrome: Electrolyte Disturbances and Treatment**

| DISTURBANCE | TREATMENT |
|---|---|
| Hyperkalemia | Sodium polystyrene sulfonate, regular insulin and glucose, calcium gluconate; if severe: dialysis |
| Hyperphosphatemia | Aluminum hydroxide; if severe: dialysis |
| Hypocalcemia | Calcium gluconate (only if symptomatic) |
| Uremia | IV hydration; IV rasburicase (recombinant urate oxidase) |
| Renal failure | Dialysis |

*IV*, Intravenous.

predictable. It usually occurs with the initiation of chemotherapy in a patient with newly diagnosed cancer. Acute lymphoblastic leukemia, acute myeloid leukemia, and non-Hodgkin lymphoma (especially Burkitt lymphoma) are the most common cancers associated with TLS.[17] Less commonly, TLS occurs in other leukemias, in multiple myeloma, or after the treatment of some solid tumors such as breast and lung cancer. When initiating chemotherapy, oncologists generally take measures to prevent TLS in at-risk patients by pretreatment with aggressive hydration, diuresis, and allopurinol (in an attempt to decrease uric acid formation). Rarely, TLS develops spontaneously. When it does, it is usually in the setting of relapsing or newly diagnosed (but untreated) cancer.

## PATHOPHYSIOLOGY

TLS most frequently occurs when the patient has a high tumor burden that is very sensitive to chemotherapy. Chemotherapy rapidly destroys malignant cells; intracellular nucleic acids are released and are broken down into uric acid. Uric acid, which is renally excreted, precipitates in the renal tubules. The precipitation may obstruct flow and can result in renal failure. Clearly, patients with baseline renal dysfunction are at even greater risk. Potassium, found in high concentrations intracellularly, is released with the destruction of the malignant cells. Because of worsening renal function secondary to uric acid precipitation, the kidneys are unable to clear this excess potassium, and the result can be dangerously high potassium levels. Phosphorus is similar to potassium; it is concentrated intracellularly and is generally excreted by the kidney. Therefore, phosphorus levels also rise. The excess phosphorus congregates with available calcium to form calcium phosphate crystals that cause the calcium level to drop. These crystals may precipitate in the renal tubules and worsen renal function.

## PRESENTING SIGNS AND SYMPTOMS

TLS manifests with symptoms reflective of the metabolic abnormalities that are present (e.g., hyperkalemia, renal failure). Therefore, symptoms may be nonspecific. Symptoms of hyperkalemia tend to be vague and may include palpitations, paresthesias, fatigue, muscle cramps, nausea, and weakness; examination findings may include nonfocal reduced muscle strength or decreases in deep tendon reflexes. Mild hypocalcemia causes muscle cramps, paresthesias, and minor mental status changes. With severe hypocalcemia, the patient may have significant mental status changes, tetanic contractions, seizures, hypotension, or dysrhythmias. Classic physical examination findings include the Chvostek sign (facial twitching or spasms with tapping over the facial nerve anterior to the ear) and the Trousseau sign (carpal spasm with inflation of a blood pressure cuff above the systolic blood pressure). Very high levels of phosphorus can cause vomiting, diarrhea, lethargy, and even seizures.

## DIAGNOSTIC TESTING

Laboratory evaluation should include, at minimum, blood urea nitrogen, creatinine, potassium, calcium, magnesium, phosphorus, uric acid, albumin, and urinalysis. The measurement of ionized calcium may be helpful. An electrocardiogram (ECG) should be obtained because it can quickly help diagnose significant hyperkalemia or hypocalcemia. A chest radiograph may be useful if the EP is concerned about fluid overload secondary to renal failure.

## TREATMENT

Despite the widespread oncologic practice of prophylactic measures to prevent TLS, the EP occasionally must manage this potentially life-threatening syndrome. A high index of suspicion must be kept for this clinical entity, especially in high-risk patients who recently started chemotherapy or who may have baseline renal insufficiency. Patients with suspected TLS should be placed on continuous cardiac monitoring because they are at risk for cardiac dysrhythmias. Treatment should be focused on closely monitoring electrolytes and renal function, correcting electrolyte abnormalities, and ensuring appropriate hydration. Patients who do not have acute renal dysfunction should be aggressively hydrated with normal saline solution. Aggressive hydration helps renal blood flow and the excretion of potassium, uric acid, and phosphorus. After adequate hydration, furosemide or mannitol may be added to increase urine output.

Hyperkalemia and hyperphosphatemia should be promptly treated. Only symptomatic hypocalcemia should be treated because infusing calcium into a hyperphosphatemic patient increases the risk of calcium phosphate formation and deposition throughout the body, including in the renal tubules. In clinically significant TLS (e.g., renal dysfunction, hyperuricemia), rasburicase, a recombinant form of urate oxidase, can be used. Urate oxidase is an enzyme (not found in humans) that converts uric acid to allantoin, which is 5 to 10 times more water soluble than uric acid. The recommended rasburicase dose is 0.1 to 0.2 mg/kg/day intravenously in 50 mL of normal saline solution over 30 minutes.[17] Rasburicase is contraindicated in patients with glucose-6-phosphate dehydrogenase deficiency. Allopurinol, which has been traditionally used in the prevention and treatment of TLS, works by decreasing uric acid production through competitive inhibition of the enzyme xanthine oxidase, which turns xanthine into uric acid. Once uric acid is present, allopurinol's effect is limited; therefore, allopurinol is not very useful in the acute treatment of TLS. [17] Finally, when renal failure develops and becomes severe (e.g., uncontrolled hyperkalemia, uncontrolled hypertension, fluid overload), emergency hemodialysis is indicated.

Controversy exists regarding the practice of urine alkalinization, which consists of adding sodium bicarbonate to intravenous fluids in an effort to help excrete uric acid. The theory is that alkalinization (with a goal of achieving a urine pH of 7 to 7.5) decreases uric acid precipitation in the renal tubules and increases uric acid excretion in the form of urate. Although a sodium bicarbonate infusion may help to eliminate uric acid, it may also worsen hypocalcemia and increase phosphate and calcium precipitation, potentially in the heart and kidneys, and therefore worsen renal function. Because hydration alone may achieve adequate uric acid excretion, routine urine alkalinization is not currently recommended.[17]

# HYPERCALCEMIA

## EPIDEMIOLOGY

Hypercalcemia is the most common metabolic abnormality found in patients with cancer. At some point in their illness, at least 10% to 30% of patients with cancer develop hypercalcemia.[18] Unfortunately, the diagnosis is frequently missed and left untreated because the symptoms are nonspecific and are often attributed to other causes (e.g., chemotherapy, infection). Hypercalcemia is most commonly found in breast and lung cancer, but it also occurs in multiple myeloma, leukemias, lymphomas, and cancers of the head, neck, kidney, and gastrointestinal tract.[18]

## PATHOPHYSIOLOGY

Primary hyperparathyroidism is the most common cause of an elevated calcium level in patients who do not have cancer. In malignant disease, hypercalcemia is related not to parathyroid hormone activity, but rather to increased osteoclastic activity in bone. A few mechanisms are responsible for this increased osteoclastic activity. First, metastasis of solid tumors can cause extensive direct bone destruction. Some cancer cells release osteoclast-activating factors. Some cancers produce a parathyroid-like hormone that acts on bone by increasing calcium uptake and also acts on the kidneys by decreasing calcium excretion.

## PRESENTING SIGNS AND SYMPTOMS

Symptoms of hypercalcemia are generally nonspecific. Symptom severity depends more on how rapidly the calcium level has escalated, rather than on the actual calcium level. Symptoms include general weakness, constipation, nausea and vomiting, dehydration, polyuria and polydipsia, personality changes, and bone and muscle pains. Severe symptoms include confusion, drowsiness, and even coma. No physical examination findings are specific only to hypercalcemia. However, the diagnosis must be considered when evaluating an oncology patient with any degree of mental status alteration (from mild confusion to obtundation), hyporeflexia, or dehydration.

## DIAGNOSTIC TESTING

If hypercalcemia is suspected, an ECG should be performed and laboratory tests sent for, at minimum, creatinine, potassium, calcium, phosphate, alkaline phosphatase, and albumin. QT shortening on the ECG may provide the quickest method of diagnosing hypercalcemia. In patients with higher calcium levels, the ECG may have a variety of finding, including T-wave changes, bradycardia, or heart block. The calcium level reported in a basic metabolic profile reports the calcium concentration in serum, the normal value of which is 9 to 11 mg/dL. Calcium levels greater than 12 mg/dL should generate concern, and levels higher than 14 mg/dL require immediate intervention. However, calcium levels correlate poorly with actual symptoms. Because calcium is present both in an ionized form and a protein-bound form, the concentration of calcium depends on plasma protein concentrations. A corrected calcium level should be calculated to assess whether hypercalcemia is truly present (see the "Facts and Formulas" box). The corrected calcium concentration is based on the albumin level. After this calculation, if any uncertainty remains, an ionized calcium level should be obtained.

$SI = \frac{SV}{BSA}$ **FACTS AND FORMULAS**

**Corrected Calcium Formula**

Corrected calcium (mg/dL) =
Measured serum calcium (mg/dL) + 0.8 ×
(4.0 g/dL − Measured albumin g/dL)

Notes:
Corrected calcium (normal range) = 9 to 10.6 mg/d
4.0 g/dL = Average albumin level

## TREATMENT

Correcting hypercalcemia not only improves symptoms, but it also may decrease the risk of death during hospitalization.[19] For initial treatment of significant hypercalcemia, aggressive intravenous hydration with normal saline solution should be started. Hypercalcemic patients may be significantly volume depleted and require intravenous fluids. Saline hydration dilutes the calcium concentration, promotes urinary excretion of calcium, and treats dehydration. Patients with severe hypercalcemia should be placed on continuous cardiac monitoring, and their urine output should be closely monitored (with a Foley catheter if necessary).

Electrolyte studies should be obtained every few hours to monitor the calcium level and to ensure that the saline hydration does not cause significant hypokalemia or hypomagnesemia. If the patient is in renal failure and will not tolerate aggressive saline hydration, dialysis may be needed to correct the calcium level.

In addition to saline hydration, a bisphosphonate should be considered (e.g., pamidronate, zoledronic). Bisphosphonates work by inhibiting osteoclastic activity through prevention of osteoclast attachment to bone and interference with osteoclast recruitment; this process decreases bone reabsorption. Pamidronate, the most commonly used bisphosphonate, can be administered at 60 mg intravenously over 2 to 24 hours for moderate hypercalcemia and at 90 mg over 2 to 24 hours for severe hypercalcemia. Another bisphosphonate, zoledronic acid, 4 mg intravenously, may be more effective.[20]

Calcitonin should be considered next. Calcitonin inhibits bone reabsorption and increases renal excretion of calcium. The effects of calcitonin are short-lived, but they can be seen within 4 hours. Calcitonin is administered at 4 to 8 units/kg either intramuscularly or subcutaneously.

Even though loop diuretics (e.g., furosemide) are unlikely to lower the calcium level significantly, they may be useful if the patient becomes volume overloaded and needs diuresis. Before a diuretic is administered, the patient should have demonstrated adequate urine output; this will ensure that the diuretic will not worsen a volume-depleted state.

Other possible treatments for hypercalcemia include gallium nitrate, mithramycin, and corticosteroids (e.g., hydrocortisone). These agents can be administered in consultation with the patient's oncologist. Finally, patients with mild calcium elevations or minimal symptoms can be treated with oral hydration.

## FOLLOW-UP, NEXT STEPS, AND ADMISSION AND DISCHARGE

Patients with mild calcium elevations can be discharged after hydration in the ED. Discharge can be considered if patients have no other active issues and if close follow-up can be arranged with their oncologist. Patients with significant symptoms (e.g., dehydration, altered mental status) should be admitted, as should patients with baseline renal insufficiency, because they are more difficult to treat.

# HYPOTENSION

## DIFFERENTIAL DIAGNOSIS AND MEDICAL DECISION MAKING

The causes of hypotension or shock in an oncology patient in the ED vary to some degree from those seen in the general ED population (**Box 201.1**). Common causes of hypotension and shock, such as sepsis and hypovolemia (e.g., secondary to gastrointestinal losses or bleeding), are also common in the oncology patient. Severe dehydration is a particular problem because many cancers or cancer treatments make oral intake very difficult and may cause vomiting or diarrhea. Certain clinical entities such as pericardial tamponade and adrenal insufficiency appear with increased frequency in this patient population. Cardiac tamponade is discussed in Chapter 202, but the EP must always consider this disorder in any patient with cancer who presents with hypotension, shock, or dyspnea. Some causes of hypotension are unique to the patient with cancer, such as myocardial dysfunction from a chemotherapeutic agent (e.g., doxorubicin). Because oncology patients are immunocompromised at baseline, they may require more intensive management and may suffer a worse outcome if hypotension is not addressed promptly.

**BOX 201.1 Differential Diagnosis of Hypotension in the Patient with Cancer**

Sepsis
Acute adrenal insufficiency
Pericardial tamponade
Severe dehydration
- Secondary to hypercalcemia, anorexia, mucositis, or chemotherapy-induced vomiting or diarrhea
- Secondary to an inability to tolerate oral intake as a result of obstruction or cancer

Hemorrhage secondary to tumor or thrombocytopenia
Pulmonary embolism (massive)

# ADRENAL INSUFFICIENCY

## PATHOPHYSIOLOGY

In the oncology patient, adrenal insufficiency is most commonly a result of previous treatment with high-dose steroids used in chemotherapy protocols. Many patients with cancer may have subclinical or mild adrenal insufficiency that is not asymptomatic until a significant stress (e.g., infection, dehydration) develops. Adrenal insufficiency can be primary if the adrenal glands are destroyed in some way (e.g., hemorrhage, infarction) or secondary if dysfunction of the hypothalamic-pituitary-adrenal axis causes a deficiency of adrenocorticotropic hormone. Previous exogenous steroid use is a secondary cause. Metastatic infiltration of the adrenal glands is not uncommon because of the adrenal's rich blood supply; however, metastatic infiltration rarely causes adrenal insufficiency. In one study, only 4.3% (20 of 464) of patients with metastasis to the adrenal glands on CT scan had or developed symptomatic adrenal insufficiency before they died.[21] Metastasis to the adrenal glands is most common in lung cancer, gastrointestinal malignant disease (stomach, esophagus, liver, pancreas, and bile duct), lymphoma, kidney cancer, and breast cancer.[21]

## PRESENTING SIGNS AND SYMPTOMS

Adrenal insufficiency manifests with vague symptoms such as fatigue, weakness, nausea, vomiting, nonspecific abdominal pain, dehydration, and altered mental status. Laboratory analysis may show any combination of hyponatremia, hyperkalemia, or hypoglycemia. When severe, acute adrenal insufficiency ("adrenal crisis") produces significant hypotension secondary to distributive shock that may not respond to aggressive fluid resuscitation. The EP must have a high index of suspicion for this entity because the symptoms are often vague and can be incorrectly attributed to other causes.

## DIAGNOSTIC TESTING

According to consensus guidelines, adrenal insufficiency (in the setting of critical illness) can be diagnosed with either a random total cortisol level of less than 10 mcg/dL or by cortisol level nonresponse (less than 9 mcg/dL) to the 250-mcg short corticotropin-stimulation test.[22] The short corticotropin-stimulation test can be performed by administering 250 mcg of cosyntropin intravenously after a baseline cortisol level is obtained. The cortisol level is repeated 30 and 60 minutes later. If the patient has adrenal insufficiency, the cortisol level response will be less than 9 mcg/dL (the difference between the baseline level and the highest response).[23] In an effort to increase the sensitivity of detecting adrenal insufficiency, the corticotropin-stimulation test with 1 mcg was studied, but further outcome data are needed.[24] If etomidate, which selectively inhibits 11-β-hydroxylase, is used in the ED course (specifically in the previous 4 hours), it may interfere with the cortisol response to corticotrophin. This may give a false-positive result to the corticotropin-stimulation test and the clinician may falsely conclude that the patient is adrenally suppressed.[25]

## TREATMENT

The treatment of adrenal insufficiency consists of glucocorticoid replacement. The most commonly recommended glucocorticoid is hydrocortisone (initial dose, 100 mg intravenously). Dexamethasone may be preferred over hydrocortisone because dexamethasone is less likely to interfere with the corticotropin-stimulation test, which can be performed later by the inpatient team or in the ED to confirm the diagnosis. A serum cortisol level can be obtained before steroid therapy is initiated. Hypotension, or dehydration is likely to be present and should be treated with fluid resuscitation (either with normal saline solution or 5% dextrose in normal saline). Any electrolyte abnormalities, especially hypoglycemia, should be promptly corrected.

# Myocardial Dysfunction Secondary to Chemotherapy

As in the general population, the most common cause of cardiac dysfunction or cardiogenic shock in the oncology population is coronary artery disease. Oncology patients, like any other patient who presents in congestive heart failure or cardiogenic shock, must be evaluated for myocardial infarction. However, a few chemotherapeutic agents, most notably the anthracyclines, can cause cardiomyopathies and congestive heart failure (**Table 201.3**). A newer drug, trastuzumab (Herceptin), which is a recombinant monoclonal antibody used in the treatment of breast cancer, has been associated with reductions in left ventricular ejection fraction and episodes of congestive heart failure.[26]

# Dyspnea and Airway Issues in the Oncology Patient

## AIRWAY MANAGEMENT

### PATHOPHYSIOLOGY

When managing the airway of the oncology patient, the EP must keep some unique issues in mind. Challenging airway situations may develop in patients with certain head, neck, and laryngeal cancers or with cancers of the esophagus, thyroid, or lung whose tumor has impinged on or distorted the airway. Metastatic lesions to the bronchial tree, mediastinal structures, or lymph nodes of the neck may also cause difficulties. The major concern in these patients is that typical rapid-sequence intubation with a paralytic agent may turn a nonobstructing airway lesion into a lesion that, in a patient without any muscular tone, completely obstructs the airway and makes endotracheal intubation and bag-valve mask ventilation difficult or impossible.

### TREATMENT

Clues to a potentially hazardous airway may include complaints of dyspnea (especially if it is worse in the supine position), stridor, hemoptysis, difficulty with handling secretions, hoarseness, or a recent change in voice. If the EP is concerned about paralyzing the patient, a few options exist.

**Table 201.3 Chemotherapy Agents That Cause Cardiac Toxicity**

| AGENT OR DRUG CLASS | TOXICITY |
|---|---|
| Anthracyclines (e.g., doxorubicin, daunorubicin, epirubicin, idarubicin) | Myocardial cell death, fibrosis, left ventricular dysfunction, CHF |
| Mitoxantrone (drug class: anthracenedione) | Cardiomyopathy similar to that caused by anthracyclines |
| 5-Fluorouracil | Coronary vasospasm or ischemia |
| Cyclophosphamide | Acute hemorrhagic myopericarditis |
| Trastuzumab (Herceptin) | Decrease in left ventricular ejection fraction, CHF |
| Taxanes (paclitaxel, docetaxel)* | Dysrhythmias (atrial or ventricular), bradycardia |
| Radiation therapy (to lung, breast, or mediastinum) | Coronary artery disease, chronic pericarditis, valvular disease, dysrhythmias |

*CHF,* Congestive heart failure.
*These effects may be acute.

One option is to give the patient topical and nebulized lidocaine and a small dose of a sedative (e.g., midazolam, etomidate) and then perform direct laryngoscopy. If the vocal cords can be visualized with this approach and no obvious concerns for airway obstruction are noted, the patient should be either directly endotracheally intubated or intubated with typical rapid-sequence intubation using a paralytic agent. If airway control is not an emergency, awake fiberoptic intubation may be a prudent approach. Whatever method is taken, a cricothyroidotomy kit should be at the bedside, in the event that endotracheal intubation proves impossible. Even cricothyroidotomy may be difficult if the patient has significant alterations in neck anatomy secondary to neck cancer or previous neck radiation.

Specialist consultation (e.g., pulmonology, oncology, thoracic surgery) may be helpful if concern exists that a malignant tumor may be impinging on the airway, but the airway does not need to be secured on an emergency basis. In this nonemergency setting, a specialist may use one of several treatment options, including self-expanding stents (placed by rigid bronchoscopy), airway dilatation (by flexible bronchoscopy), laser therapy, radiation, or chemotherapy.

Difficult airways may arise in oncology patients who have severe mucositis or bleeding disorders. Mucositis, especially, may make the tissues of the airway and oropharynx extremely friable, and the tissues may bleed easily with any manipulation; this problem makes standard endotracheal intubation more challenging. Many patients with cancer have significant thrombocytopenia. Special care must be taken with these patients because multiple or traumatic airway attempts may cause significant bleeding into the airway that may be difficult to control. Rarely performed, nasotracheal intubation, which may cause trauma to the nasal passages, should be avoided in patients with mucositis or bleeding disorders.

## MALIGNANT PLEURAL EFFUSIONS

### PRESENTING SIGNS AND SYMPTOMS

Pleural effusion is a common cause of dyspnea in the patient with cancer who presents to the ED. Malignant pleural effusions are most commonly seen in patients with lung and breast cancers but are also seen with lymphoma and ovarian and gastric cancers. The diagnosis of a malignant pleural effusion is associated with increased 6-month mortality. The dyspnea of pleural effusions is generally progressive and may occasionally be associated with cough or chest pain. A chest radiograph usually enables the EP to make this diagnosis. Ultrasound can be useful to diagnose pleural effusion quickly and can simultaneously exclude pericardial effusion or cardiac tamponade. A chest CT scan can confirm the diagnosis and may be especially helpful because it can simultaneously rule out other life-threatening causes of dyspnea (e.g., pulmonary embolism, pneumonia).

### TREATMENT

Thoracentesis should be performed for highly symptomatic patients. Removing pleural fluid may provide instant relief; however, some patients may not respond. Unfortunately, the reaccumulation rate after thoracentesis alone is nearly 100% at 1 month.[27] Traditionally, a blind approach was incorporated. Bedside ultrasound scanning makes this procedure much simpler and safer. If thoracentesis is performed for the first presentation of pleural effusion, the fluid should be sent for cytologic study because it may prove useful diagnostically. In general, unless a pleural effusion must be tapped for diagnostic purposes or to provide symptomatic relief, no need exists to tap the effusion in the ED. A chest radiograph should be performed at the completion of the procedure, to ensure that pneumothorax has not developed. More definitive treatment of the pleural effusion should be coordinated by the patient's oncologist and will be tailored based on the patient's prognosis, severity of symptoms, and type of malignant disease. Multiple treatment options exist, including supplemental oxygen, radiation therapy, chemotherapy, chemical pleurodesis, and long-term indwelling pleural catheter placement.

# Emergency Side Effects of Oncology Treatment

Although some chemotherapeutic agents have unique side effects (**Table 201.4**), a few side effects are more universal. Bone marrow depression is a very common side effect of most agents. Nausea, vomiting, diarrhea, and mucositis are also quite common. The severity of these symptoms varies, depending on the particular chemotherapy agent.

# Global Issues

## PAIN

Pain in the oncology patient may represent an acute process, the progression of disease, or inadequate outpatient treatment. In a survey of physicians directly involved in cancer care (oncologists, hematologists, surgeons, and radiation therapists), 86% believed that most of their patients with cancer-related pain were being undermedicated, and 76% reported performing poor pain assessments for their patients.[28] After potentially dangerous or reversible causes of pain have been ruled out and the patient's pain is under control, usually in response to high doses of intravenous narcotics, a plan for outpatient pain control should be created with the patient and

**Table 201.4 Chemotherapeutic Agents and Their Toxicities***

| CHEMOTHERAPY AGENT (TRADE NAME) | DRUG CLASS | COMMON OR NOTEWORTHY TOXICITIES | INDICATIONS FOR USE (TYPES OF CANCER) |
|---|---|---|---|
| Alemtuzumab (Campath) | Monoclonal antibody | BMD, infusion-related/anaphylactoid reactions, cardiomyopathy, CHF, arrhythmias | B-cell CLL, T-cell leukemia |
| Altretamine (Hexalen) | Alkylating agent | BMD, neurologic toxicity | Ovarian |
| Anastrozole (Arimidex) | Aromatase inhibitor | Bone and joint pain, headache, hot flashes, thrombophlebitis | Breast |
| Asparaginase (Elspar) | Enzyme | Anaphylaxis, coagulopathy, pancreatitis, acute renal failure, hyperglycemia, fever, seizure, altered mental status | ALL, AML, CML, CLL |
| Bevacizumab (Avastin) | Monoclonal antibody | BMD, GI perforation, hemorrhage (GI, hemoptysis, epistaxis) | Colon, lung, breast |
| Bicalutamide (Casodex) | Antiandrogen | Hepatotoxicity, CHF, MI | Metastatic prostate |
| Bleomycin (Blenoxane) | Antibiotic (antitumor) | Pulmonary fibrosis, pneumonitis, fever, pericarditis, anaphylaxis, mucocutaneous reactions | Multiple |
| Busulfan (Myleran, Busulfex) | Alkylating agent | BMD, addisonian symptoms, pulmonary fibrosis, CHF, AV block, cardiac tamponade | CML, AML |
| Capecitabine (Xeloda) | Pyrimidine analogue | BMD, ulcerations, diarrhea, mucositis, palmar-plantar erythrodysesthesia | Breast, GI |
| Carboplatin (Paraplatin) | Alkylating agent (platinum) | BMD, anaphylactic-like reactions, peripheral neuropathy | Multiple |
| Carmustine (BCNU) | Nitrosourea alkylating agent | BMD, hepatotoxicity, pulmonary fibrosis nephrotoxicity | Multiple |
| Cetuximab (Erbitux) | Monoclonal antibody | Infusion reactions (dyspnea, angioedema, fever, hypotension), rash, pulmonary toxicity | Colon, head and neck |
| Chlorambucil (Leukeran) | Alkylating agent | BMD, erythema multiforme, hepatotoxicity, peripheral neuropathy | Leukemia, lymphoma |
| Cisplatin (Platinol) | Alkylating agent (platinum) | BMD, nephrotoxic, tinnitus, hearing loss, peripheral neuropathy, hypersensitivity reactions | Multiple |
| Cladribine (Litak) | Purine analogue | BMD, neurotoxicity, fever, nephrotoxicity | Leukemia, lymphoma |
| Cyclophosphamide | Alkylating agents | BMD, hemorrhagic cystitis, SIADH, fever, acute hemorrhagic myopericarditis, pulmonary fibrosis | Multiple |
| Cytarabine | Pyrimidine analogue | BMD, fever, hepatotoxicity, mucositis, peripheral neuropathy, ataxia, skin exfoliation, pulmonary infiltrates | Leukemia, lymphoma |
| Dacarbazine (DTIC) | Alkylating agent | BMD, hepatotoxicity, nephrotoxicity, fever | Melanoma, Hodgkin lymphoma |
| Dactinomycin (Cosmegen) | Anthracycline | BMD, fever, rash, hepatitis | Sarcomas |
| Daunorubicin (Cerubidine) | Anthracycline | Cardiac damage, CHF, BMD | Kaposi sarcoma |
| Doxorubicin | Anthracycline | Cardiac damage, CHF, BMD | Multiple |
| Epirubicin (Ellence) | Anthracycline | Cardiac damage, CHF, BMD | Multiple |
| Etoposide (Eposin, Vepesid) | Podophyllotoxin (topoisomerase II inhibitor) | BMD, peripheral neuropathy, fever, hypersensitivity reactions, CHF, TEN | Multiple |

**Table 201.4 Chemotherapeutic Agents and Their Toxicities—cont'd**

| CHEMOTHERAPY AGENT (TRADE NAME) | DRUG CLASS | COMMON OR NOTEWORTHY TOXICITIES | INDICATIONS FOR USE (TYPES OF CANCER) |
|---|---|---|---|
| Exemestane (Aromasin) | Aromatase inhibitor, (hormone agent) | Hot flashes, sweats, arthralgias, fractures, CHF, MI, CVA | Breast |
| Fludarabine (Fludara) | Purine nucleotide analogue | BMD, autoimmune hemolytic anemia, neurotoxicity, blindness, fever | CLL, AML |
| 5-Fluorouracil | Pyrimidine analogue | BMD, cerebellar problems, coronary vasospasm, ischemia, conjunctivitis, mucositis | Multiple |
| Flutamide (Eulexin) | Antiandrogen | Hot sweats, hepatotoxicity, hepatic failure | Prostate |
| Gemcitabine (Gemzar) | Nucleoside analogue | BMD, neuropathy, hemolytic-uremic syndrome, hepatotoxicity | Multiple |
| Gemtuzumab ozogamicin (Mylotarg) | Monoclonal antibody | BMD, hypersensitivity reactions (anaphylaxis), infusion-related reactions, hepatotoxicity | AML |
| Ibritumomab tiuxetan (Zevalin) | Monoclonal antibody | Infusion reactions, cutaneous/ mucocutaneous reactions, BMD | Non-Hodgkin lymphoma |
| Idarubicin (Idamycin) | Anthracycline | Cardiomyopathy, CHF, BMD | AML |
| Ifosfamide (Ifex, Mitoxana) | Alkylating agent | BMD, nephrotoxicity, neurotoxicity, hemorrhagic cystitis, metabolic acidosis | Multiple |
| Letrozole (Femara) | Aromatase inhibitor | Arthralgias, sweats, fractures, PE, MI | Breast |
| Leuprolide (Lupron) | Gonadotropin-releasing hormone agonist | Flushing, CHF | Prostate, breast |
| Lomustine (CeeNU) | Nitrosourea alkylating agent | BMD, hepatotoxicity, pulmonary fibrosis, nephrotoxicity | Multiple |
| Mechlorethamine (Mustargen) | Alkylating agent, nitrogen mustard | BMD, dermatitis, erythema multiforme | CLL, CML |
| Megestrol (Megace, Ovaban) | Progesterone derivative | Hot sweats, PE, DVT, adrenal insufficiency | Breast, endometrial, renal call |
| Melphalan (Alkeran) | Alkylating agent | BMD, pulmonary fibrosis, hypersensitivity reaction | Multiple |
| Mercaptopurine (Purinethol) | Purine analogue | BMD, pancreatitis, hepatotoxicity | ALL |
| Methotrexate | Folate antagonist | BMD, hepatotoxicity, nephrotoxicity | Multiple |
| Mitomycin (Mutamycin) | Antitumor antibiotic | BMD, nephrotoxicity, hemolytic-uremic syndrome | Multiple |
| Mitoxantrone (Novantrone) | Antitumor antibiotic | Cardiotoxicity, CHF, BMD, hepatoxicity | Multiple including AML and prostate |
| Nilutamide (Nilandron) | Antiandrogen | Hot flashes, impairs ability to adjust eyes from light to dark, pneumonitis, pulmonary fibrosis | Metastatic prostate |
| Oxaliplatin (Eloxatin) | Alkylating agent (platinum) | BMD, hypersensitivity reactions, peripheral neuropathy, neuropathic throat pain, abdominal pain, colitis, fever | Colorectal |
| Paclitaxel (Taxol) | Taxane (mitotic inhibitor) | BMD, fever, cardiac arrhythmias, peripheral neuropathies, neuromyopathy, hypersensitivity reactions (with dyspnea, hypotension, anaphylaxis) | Multiple, including breast |
| Panitumumab (Vectibix) | Monoclonal antibody | Rash, infusion reactions, dyspnea, PE, pulmonary fibrosis | Colorectal |

*Continued*

**Table 201.4** Chemotherapeutic Agents and Their Toxicities—cont'd

| CHEMOTHERAPY AGENT (TRADE NAME) | DRUG CLASS | COMMON OR NOTEWORTHY TOXICITIES | INDICATIONS FOR USE (TYPES OF CANCER) |
|---|---|---|---|
| Pemetrexed (Alimta) | Antimetabolite | BMD, skin peeling, lung injury | Lung (non–small cell), mesothelioma |
| Pentostatin (Nipent) | Purine analogue (antimetabolite) | BMD, fever, rash, hypersensitivity reactions, neurotoxicity | Leukemias |
| Procarbazine (Matulane) | Alkylating agent | BMD, neurotoxicity, peripheral neuropathy, rash | Multiple, including Hodgkin lymphoma |
| Rituximab (Rituxan, MabThera) | Monoclonal antibody | Fevers, BMD, fatal infusion reactions, severe mucocutaneous reactions, cardiac arrhythmias, MI, hypersensitivity reactions, nephrotoxicity | Lymphomas and leukemias |
| Sorafenib (Nexavar) | Multikinase inhibitor | Rash, hand-foot-mouth skin reaction, cardiac ischemia, MI, bleeding | Renal cell, liver |
| Streptozocin (Zanosar) | Alkylating agent | Nephrotoxicity, fever, altered mental status | Islets of Langerhans, carcinoid, pancreas |
| Sunitinib malate (Sutent) | Receptor tyrosine kinase inhibitor | Cardiotoxicity (arrhythmias, cardiac dysfunction, MI), QT prolongation (torsades de pointes), bleeding, BMD, rash, hepatotoxicity | Renal cell, GI stromal |
| Tamoxifen (Nolvadex) | Nonsteroidal antiestrogen | Hot flashes, sweating, CVA or PE (both very rare) | Breast, multiple myeloma, pancreatic |
| Temozolomide (Temodar) | Alkylating agent | BMD, headache, seizures, constipation | Brain, multiple myeloma |
| Teniposide (Vumon) | Podophyllotoxin (topoisomerase II inhibitor) | BMD, hypersensitivity reactions | Acute lymphoid leukemia, non-Hodgkin lymphoma, lung (small cell) |
| Thalidomide (Thalomid) | Immunomodulatory agent | Rash, neuropathy, thromboembolic disease, altered mental status, teratogenicity | Multiple, including multiple myeloma |
| Thioguanine (Tabloid) | Purine analogue | BMD, hepatotoxicity | Acute myeloid leukemia |
| Thiotepa | Alkylating agent | BMD, rash, hypersensitivity reaction | Multiple, including breast, bladder, ovarian |
| Topotecan (Hycamtin) | Topoisomerase I inhibitor | BMD, abdominal pain, fever, dyspnea | Multiple, including lung, ovarian |
| Toremifene (Fareston) | Nonsteroidal antiestrogen | Hot flashes, sweating, dizziness, thromboembolic disease (rare) | Breast (metastatic) |
| Tositumomab (Bexxar) | Monoclonal antibody | BMD, fever | Non-Hodgkin lymphoma |
| Trastuzumab (Herceptin) | Monoclonal antibody | Acute cardiomyopathy, CHF, infusion reactions (fever, anaphylaxis, angioedema), rash, fever, abdominal pain, BMD | Breast, gastric |
| Tretinoin (Vesanoid) | Retinoid | "Retinoic acid syndrome" consisting of fever, dyspnea, effusions, hepatic, renal and multiorgan failure; fever, headache, chest pain, dyspnea | Acute promyelocytic leukemia |
| Vinblastine (Velbar, Velsar) | Vinca alkaloid | BMD, peripheral neuropathy, hypertension, acute dyspnea or chest pain | Multiple |
| Vincristine (Oncovin) | Vinca alkaloid | SIADH, neuromuscular effects, peripheral neuropathy | Multiple |

**Table 201.4 Chemotherapeutic Agents and Their Toxicities—cont'd**

| CHEMOTHERAPY AGENT (TRADE NAME) | DRUG CLASS | COMMON OR NOTEWORTHY TOXICITIES | INDICATIONS FOR USE (TYPES OF CANCER) |
|---|---|---|---|
| Vindesine (Eldisine) | Vinca alkaloid | BMD, neurotoxicity, peripheral neuropathy, fever, acute respiratory distress | Esophageal, lung (non–small cell) |
| Vinorelbine (Navelbine) | Vinca alkaloid | Acute dyspnea, acute bronchospasm, acute respiratory distress syndrome, neuropathy, SBO, BMD | Breast, lung (non–small cell), ovarian |

Data from MICROMEDEX Healthcare Series. www.thomsonhc.com/hcs/librarian; and Merck Manual Online Medical Library for Healthcare Professionals. www.merck.com/media/mmpe/pdf/Table_149_3.pdf.

*ALL,* Acute lymphoid leukemia; *AML,* acute myeloid leukemia; *AV,* atrioventricular; *BMD,* bone marrow destruction or myelosuppression; *CHF,* congestive heart failure; *CLL,* chronic lymphocytic leukemia; *CVA,* cerebrovascular accident; *DVT,* deep venous thrombosis; *GI,* gastrointestinal; *MI,* myocardial infarction; *PE,* pulmonary embolism; *SBO,* small bowel obstruction; *SIADH,* syndrome of inappropriate antidiuretic hormone; *TEN,* toxic epidermal necrolysis.

*This chart is not meant to be all inclusive. When dealing with a patient who is receiving a chemotherapeutic agent in the clinical setting, use an up-to-date online resource. Nausea and vomiting are common side effects of most chemotherapeutic agents and are not included in this table. See Box 201.2 for a list of most highly emetogenic chemotherapeutic agents. Bone marrow myelosuppression, mucositis, and diarrhea can also be caused to some degree by most chemotherapy agents.

in consultation with the patient's oncologist. Oncologists tend to use an escalating approach to outpatient pain management, starting with nonsteroidal antiinflammatory drugs, then weaker opioids (e.g., codeine), and finally stronger opioids (e.g., morphine, fentanyl). Some physicians question this escalating approach, especially in advanced cancer, and instead start with small doses of stronger opioids and titrate upward as needed. Because the pain in patients with cancer is ongoing, pain medication with longer half-lives or continuous action, such as very-long-acting oral opioids or a transdermal opiate patch, is preferred. Additional short-acting medications should be provided for breakthrough pain; breakthrough dosing often needs to be 10% to 20% of the patient's 24-hour total opiate dose. A new or escalating-dose opioid prescription should be accompanied by a prescription for a laxative because constipation is the most common side effect of opioid therapy.

**BOX 201.2 Chemotherapeutic Agents with the Highest Emetogenic Potential***

| | |
|---|---|
| Altretamine | Doxorubicin |
| Carmustine | Epirubicin |
| Cisplatin | Mechlorethamine |
| Cyclophosphamide | Procarbazine |
| Dacarbazine | Streptozocin |

From Schwartzberg L, Szabo S, Gilmore J, et al. Likelihood of a subsequent chemotherapy-induced nausea and vomiting (CINV) event in patients receiving low, moderately or highly emetogenic chemotherapy (LEC/MEC/HEC). Curr Med Res Opin 2011;27:837-45.

*These agents have greater than 90% incidence of emesis without coadministration of an antiemetic. Emetogenic potential is generally dose dependent.

## NAUSEA AND VOMITING

Nausea and vomiting, of all the side effects of chemotherapy, are often considered the worst adverse effects. Occasionally, nausea and vomiting can be severe enough to cause patients to discontinue their treatment. Poor antiemetic control with previous chemotherapy, female sex, low alcohol intake, and younger age are all associated with a higher risk of emesis after chemotherapy.[29] In an effort to reduce the risk of emesis and to increase the tolerability of the treatment, chemotherapy regimens usually include an antiemetic drug. Chemotherapeutic agents with the highest emetogenic potential are listed in **Box 201.2**.[30]

Conversely, nausea and vomiting can be the initial symptoms of a potentially life-threatening issue. Nausea or vomiting can be the first sign of a neurologic condition (e.g., increase in central nervous system pressure, brain metastasis, intracranial bleeding), a gastroenterologic disorder (e.g., bowel obstruction), or even a metabolic problem (e.g., hypercalcemia).

Patients who complain of nausea or vomiting in the ED should be treated promptly with a strong antiemetic and appropriate hydration. Serotonin receptor antagonists (e.g., ondansetron, granisetron) are among the most commonly used antiemetics for patients with cancer. Other commonly used antiemetics in this patient population include phenothiazines (e.g., prochlorperazine), benzamides (e.g., metoclopramide), corticosteroids (e.g., dexamethasone), and benzodiazepines (e.g., lorazepam).

## MUCOSITIS

### PATHOPHYSIOLOGY

Mucositis is inflammation and ulceration of the mucous membranes, and it occurs in up to 58% of patients with cancer, depending on their diagnosis.[31] Mucositis most commonly manifests in the mouth, but it can occur anywhere in the gastrointestinal, genitourinary, or respiratory tracts. Because mucositis is a breakdown of the normal integrity of mucous membranes, it is associated with an increased risk of infection. Oral mucositis is a side effect of chemotherapy or radiation, or it can result from certain cancers, such as oral cancers

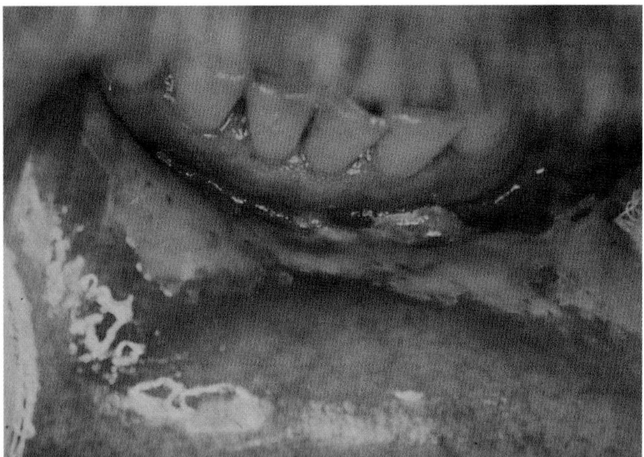

**Fig. 201.1. Oral mucositis caused by radiation therapy.** (From Keefe ZDM, Logan RM. Oral complications of cancer and its treatment. In: Walsh TD, Caraceni AT, Fainsinger R, et al, editors. Palliative medicine. Philadelphia: Saunders; 2008.)

and leukemia. Patients obtaining either radiation for head and neck cancers or chemotherapy with 5-fluorouracil, anthracyclines, or irinotecan and patients who are bone marrow transplant recipients have high rates of mucositis (**Fig. 201.1**).

## PRESENTING SIGNS AND SYMPTOMS

Oral mucositis is quite painful and causes significant difficulties with swallowing. Oral mucositis can cause altered taste, halitosis, and dry mouth. Painful swallowing and altered taste may adversely affect the patient's oral intake and may result in dehydration. Oral mucositis can result in difficulty with speaking. In severe cases, mucositis can be secondarily infected with bacteria or fungi and can bleed.

## TREATMENT

Patients who present to the ED with oral mucositis should be given proper pain control, which may include the use of opiates. Any secondary infections, such as oral candidiasis or herpes simplex, should be treated. A bland, soft diet is recommended, as well as ice chips or other cold products to keep the oral mucosa moist. Special attention to oral hygiene is essential for at-risk patients with cancer, including the use of a soft toothbrush, frequent saline or baking soda rinses, prophylactic anticandidal rinses (e.g., nystatin), and adequate general nutrition. Optimal mucositis treatment is still in question and requires further research. Protocols vary at different institutions. A 2010 Cochrane systematic review did not find any high-level evidence-based treatment options.[32] Although not an ED option, low-level laser therapy was the only potentially useful intervention found in two or more clinical trials.[32]

## SUGGESTED READINGS


Coiffier B, Altman A, Pui CH, et al. Guidelines for the management of pediatric and adult tumor lysis syndrome: an evidence-based review. J Clin Oncol 2008;26:2767-78.

Freifeld AG, Bow EJ, Sepkowitz KA, et al. Executive summary: clinical practice guideline for the use of antimicrobial agents in neutropenic patients with cancer. 2010 update by the Infectious Diseases Society of America. Clin Infect Dis 2011;52:427-31.

Santarpia L, Koch CA, Sarlis NJ. Hypercalcemia in cancer patients: pathobiology and management. Horm Metab Res 2010;42:153-64.

Tam CS, O'Reilly M, Andresen D, et al. Use of empiric antimicrobial therapy in neutropenic fever. Intern Med J 2011;41:90-101.


## REFERENCES

***References can be found on Expert Consult @ www.expertconsult.com.***

# Cardiovascular and Neurologic Oncologic Emergencies 202

*Manish Garg and Jacob Ufberg*

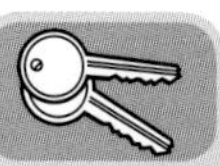

**KEY POINTS**

- Early symptoms of cardiac tamponade are tachypnea and dyspnea with exertion.
- The superior vena cava (SVC) syndrome is caused by obstruction of blood flow through the SVC by compression or vascular thrombosis.
- Headaches from brain tumors are often described as tension-type headaches, but more frequently they have associated nausea and are sometimes worse with body positioning that increases intracranial pressure (i.e., leaning forward).
- In patients with spinal cord compression from malignant disease, pain may precede neurologic changes by several weeks. At the time of presentation to the emergency department, some motor weakness is usually evident.
- Corticosteroids and radiation therapy are typical initial treatments for spinal cord compression from malignant disease.

## Cardiovascular Oncologic Emergencies

### PERSPECTIVE

Two primary cardiovascular oncologic emergencies encountered in the emergency department (ED) are cardiac tamponade and superior vena cava syndrome. Generally, both have subacute presentations and result from mechanical obstruction of normal cardiovascular function. Patient morbidity and mortality can be improved by early recognition and management directed at relieving the cardiovascular obstruction or preventing secondary injury.

## CARDIAC TAMPONADE

### EPIDEMIOLOGY

Malignant cardiac involvement is common, occurring in 11% to 12% of patients with cancer. Of these patients, three fourths have epicardial involvement, and one third of these patients have a pericardial effusion.[1] The most common malignant primary tumor that progresses to involve the pericardium is lung cancer. Breast cancer, gastrointestinal cancers, melanoma, sarcoma, lymphoma, and leukemia account for most other cases. These tumors invade the pericardium through direct or metastatic spread. Less commonly, malignant primary pericardial tumors such as mesothelioma and sarcoma or benign tumors such as angioma, fibroma, or teratoma may occur. In a study conducted from 1996 to 2005, malignant disease was the primary cause of medical cardiac tamponade (65%), followed by unknown causes (10%), viral disease (10%), and anticoagulant medication–related intrapericardial bleeding (3%).[2]

### PATHOPHYSIOLOGY

The pericardium is a fibroelastic sac surrounding the heart that normally contains a thin layer of fluid. When a larger amount of fluid accumulates and exceeds the elastic limit of the pericardium, the heart begins to compete for the now fixed amount of intrapericardial space. As more fluid accumulates, the cardiac chambers become compressed, and diastolic compliance lessens.

Throughout this process, the decline in intrathoracic pressure associated with inspiration continues to be transmitted through the pericardium to the heart. Thus, venous return to the heart is still increased with inspiration. However, the free wall of the right ventricle cannot expand to accommodate this increased volume, thus leading the intraventricular septum to bow to the left. The result is decreased left ventricular filling during inspiration. When the size of the effusion progresses further, total venous return diminishes, and cardiac output and blood pressure deteriorate.

*Cardiac tamponade* is generally classified as acute or subacute. In *acute* cardiac tamponade, the relatively stiff pericardium can become rapidly filled with blood that causes tamponade with only a small effusion. This generally occurs in the setting of trauma, myocardial or aortic rupture, or invasive medical interventions. In *subacute* cardiac tamponade, a much larger effusion accumulates slowly and allows the pericardium to stretch over time. This type of tamponade occurs most commonly in the setting of malignant disease or renal failure, and it may not occur until the amount of pericardial fluid reaches 2 L or more. In either setting, very little additional fluid may cause cardiac tamponade once the limits of pericardial elasticity have been reached.

## PRESENTING SIGNS AND SYMPTOMS

### CLASSIC

Cardiac tamponade is a physiologic continuum, from mild to severe. Classically, patients present with tachypnea and dyspnea on exertion. As the disease progresses, patients may have shortness of breath at rest, peripheral edema, or orthopnea. Patients with severe disease may be obtunded on presentation, thus obscuring the diagnosis of cardiac tamponade. A history of malignant disease or symptoms and signs of malignant disease such as weight loss, fatigue, or anorexia may help to guide the clinician toward a diagnosis of malignant pericardial effusion.

### PHYSICAL FINDINGS

Patients with pericardial tamponade most commonly present with shortness of breath, hypotension, and often with clear lungs. Unfortunately, physical examination holds little value for diagnosing the presence of a pericardial effusion. However, as a malignant effusion becomes large enough to cause cardiac tamponade, some distinct physical findings may become evident. The Beck triad, first described in 1935, consists of increased jugular venous pressure, hypotension, and muffled heart sounds. However, this triad is most useful in acute cardiac tamponade, and it may be uncommon or difficult to assess in patients with atraumatic cardiac tamponade.[3]

Sinus tachycardia is seen in most patients with cardiac tamponade. This physiologic response allows for maintenance of cardiac output despite decreased cardiac filling volumes. Patients may present with slightly lower heart rates if they are taking beta-blocking medications or if they suffer from hypothyroidism. Significant tamponade also manifests with absolute or relative hypotension. Patients with early tamponade may present with normotension or even hypertension, especially if they have preexisting hypertension.

*Pulsus paradoxus* is defined as a drop of more than 10 mm Hg in systolic blood pressure during normal inspiration. Most patients with moderate to severe cardiac tamponade have pulsus paradoxus, which is often palpable in the peripheral arteries. As cardiac output drops, however, pulsus paradoxus may be difficult to measure without invasive monitoring. Pulsus paradoxus results when the effusion limits expansion of the free wall of the right ventricle as venous return increases during inspiration. The right ventricle is then forced to expand by bulging the intraventricular septum into the left ventricle, thus leading to greatly reduced filling and stroke volume during inspiration.

To quantify pulsus paradoxus noninvasively, a sphygmomanometer is used in the standard fashion. The cuff is inflated to more than the systolic blood pressure and then is slowly deflated until the first Korotkoff sounds are audible only during exhalation. This condition is typified by hearing Korotkoff sounds for several beats during exhalation, followed by silence during inspiration, and then followed by Korotkoff sounds for several beats during exhalation. The pressure is noted on the sphygmomanometer at this point, and slow deflation is continued until all beats are audible. The amount of pulsus paradoxus is determined by subtracting the pressure at which all beats are heard from the pressure at which beats were heard only during exhalation.

Multiple conditions may alter the physiology of cardiac tamponade and may cause pulsus paradoxus to be absent. The most common conditions are elevated left ventricular diastolic pressures and increased heart rate. Other conditions include severe hypotension, irregular rhythm, atrial septal defect, regional cardiac tamponade, and severe aortic regurgitation.

## MEDICAL DECISION MAKING AND DIAGNOSTIC TESTING

### ELECTROCARDIOGRAPHY

The electrocardiogram is abnormal in most, but not all, patients with pericardial effusion. The most common findings are nonspecific ST-segment and T-wave abnormalities and sinus tachycardia. The electrocardiogram may mimic that seen in acute pericarditis.

Low QRS voltage may be a sign of a large pericardial effusion, but it is more likely to be associated with tamponade physiology. In one small study, Bruch et al.[4] studied 43 patients with a pericardial effusion. Of those patients, 14 of 23 with tamponade demonstrated low-voltage QRS complexes, as opposed to none of the 23 patients with effusion but without tamponade[4] (**Fig. 202.1**). Electrical alternans (**Fig. 202.2**), demonstrated as beat-to-beat alterations in the amplitude of the QRS complex, is relatively specific but not very sensitive for cardiac tamponade. Electrical alternans may also rarely occur in patients with very large effusions without tamponade. Electrical alternans is caused by swinging of the heart in the pericardial effusion, and it generally disappears after removal of even modest amounts of pericardial fluid.

### CHEST RADIOGRAPHY

The typical finding on chest radiograph is an enlarged cardiac silhouette (the "water bottle"–shaped heart), as seen in **Figure 202.3**. In most cases, the lung fields are clear unless preexisting lung disease (e.g., malignant disease) is present. Cardiac tamponade may manifest without an enlarged cardiac silhouette if a small, rapidly accumulating effusion is the cause.

### ECHOCARDIOGRAPHY AND EMERGENCY MEDICINE BEDSIDE ULTRASOUND

Echocardiography and emergency medicine bedside ultrasound play crucial roles in the diagnosis of cardiac tamponade. The first steps are to suspect a problem and to perform a screening cardiac ultrasound examination[5] (**Fig. 202.4**).

Echocardiographic findings indicative of cardiac tamponade include the presence of pericardial fluid with accompanying diastolic collapse of the right atrium and right ventricle. During atrial relaxation at the end of diastole, pericardial pressure is maximal, whereas right atrial volume is minimal. This situation results in right atrial collapse that, if lasting more than one third of the cardiac cycle, is sensitive and

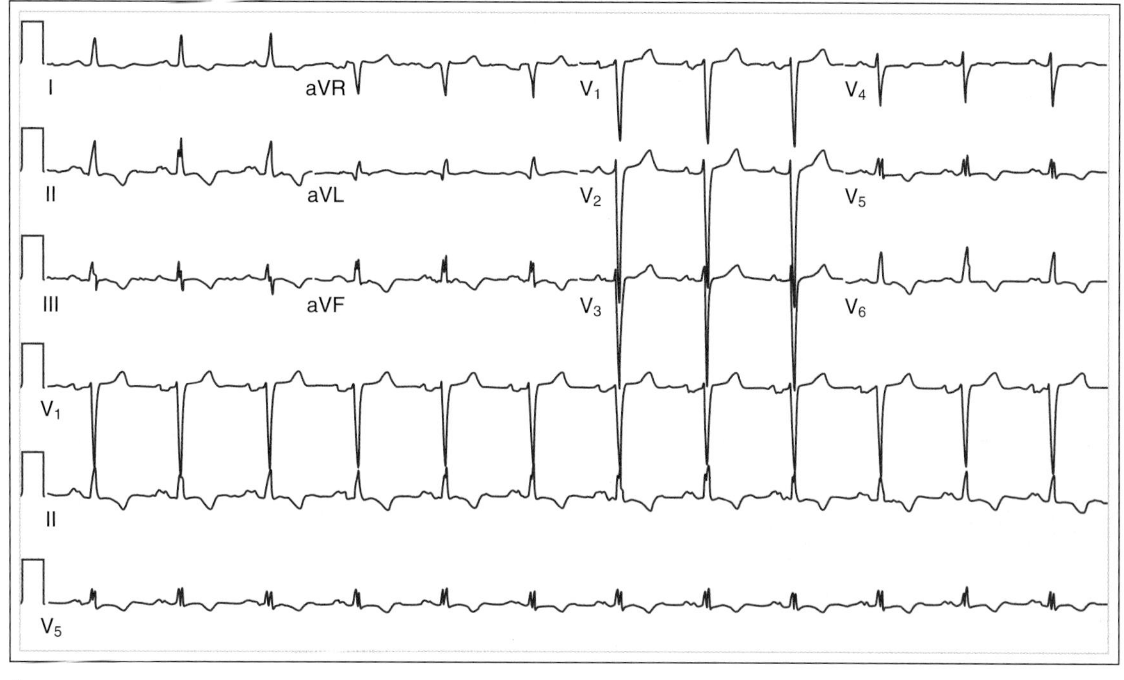


A

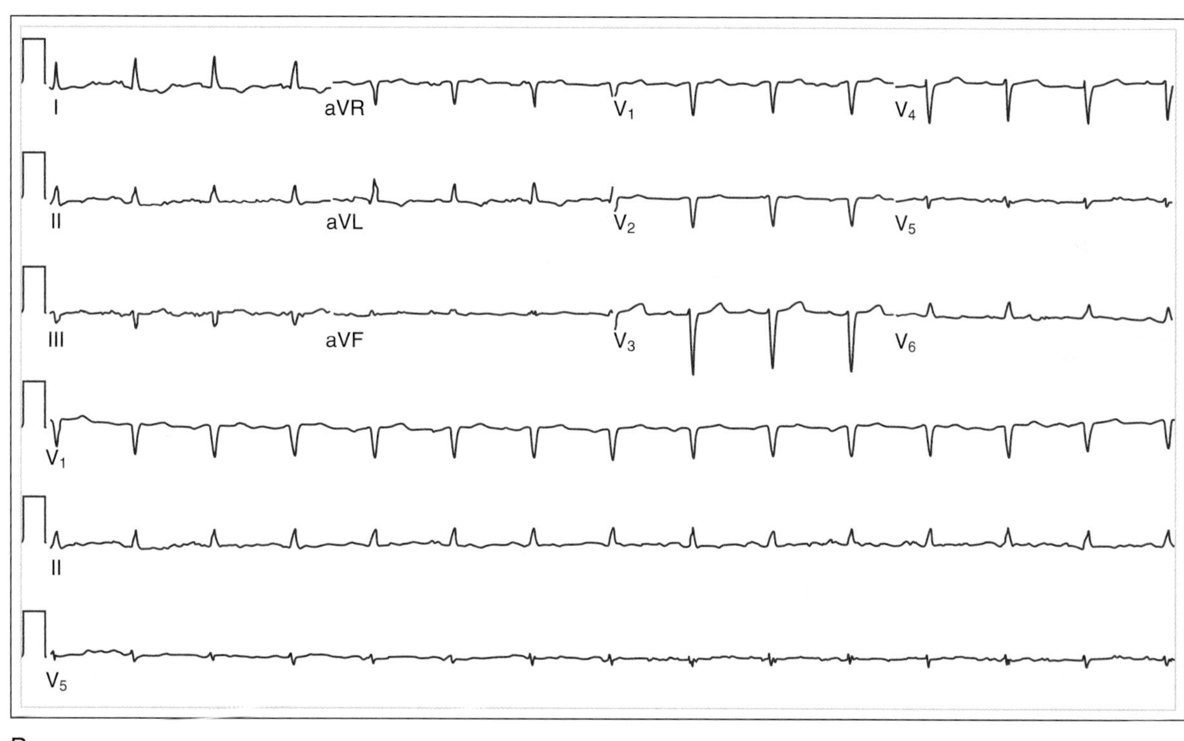


B

**Fig. 202.1** **A,** Patient's electrocardiogram on a prior visit to the emergency department (ED). **B,** Patient's electrocardiogram on presentation to the ED with cardiac tamponade.

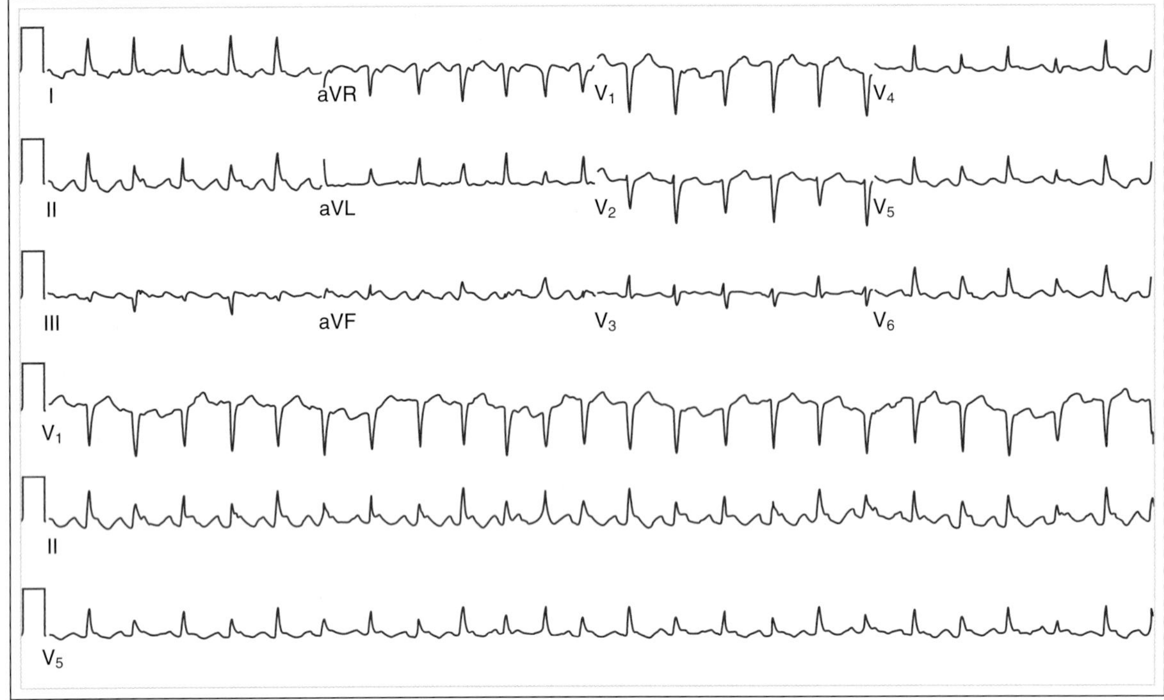

A

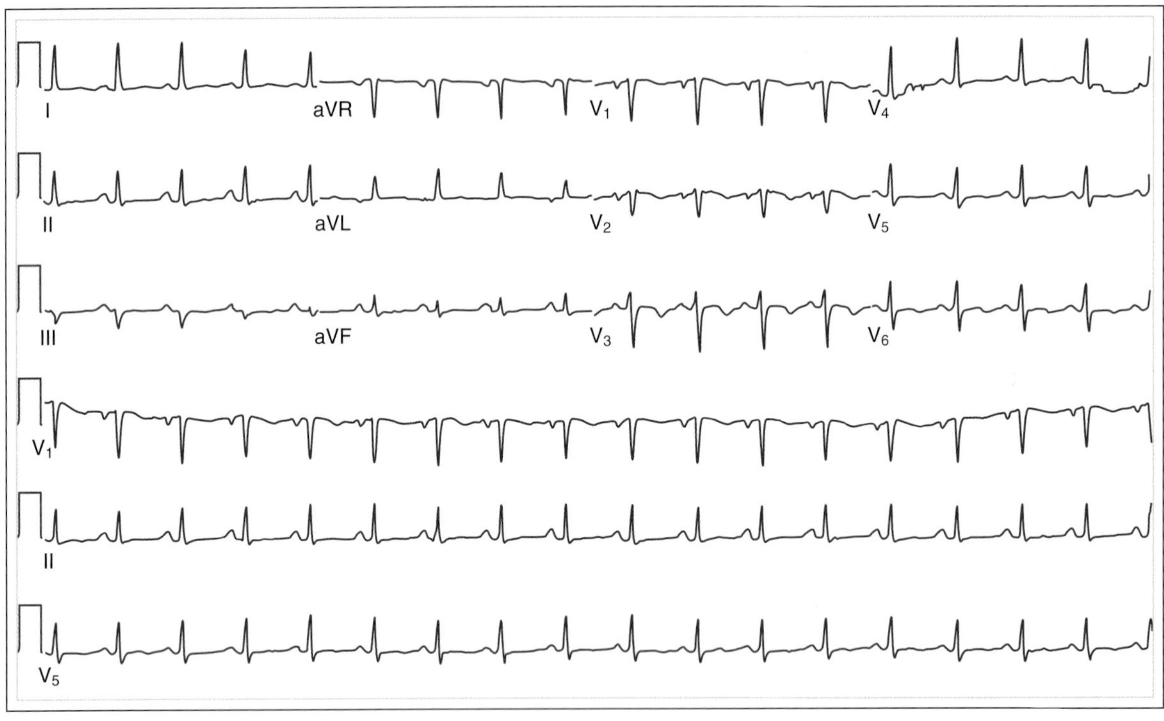


B

**Fig. 202.2** **A,** Electrocardiogram demonstrating electrical alternans most notable in the lead II rhythm strip. This patient's electrocardiogram also has atrial flutter with 2:1 conduction. **B,** Electrocardiogram performed on the same patient several days after drainage of his pericardial effusion.

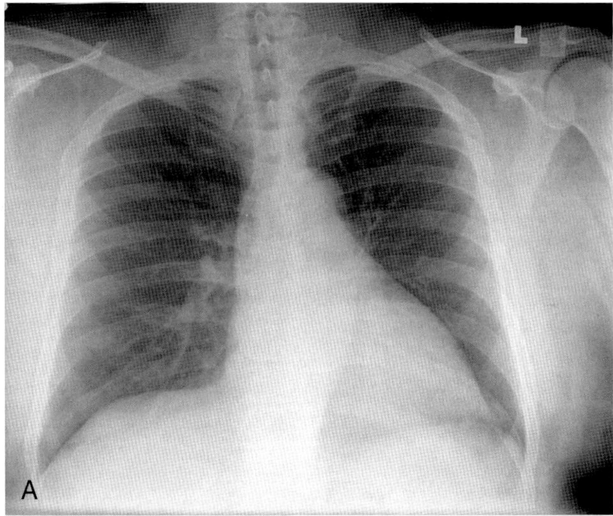


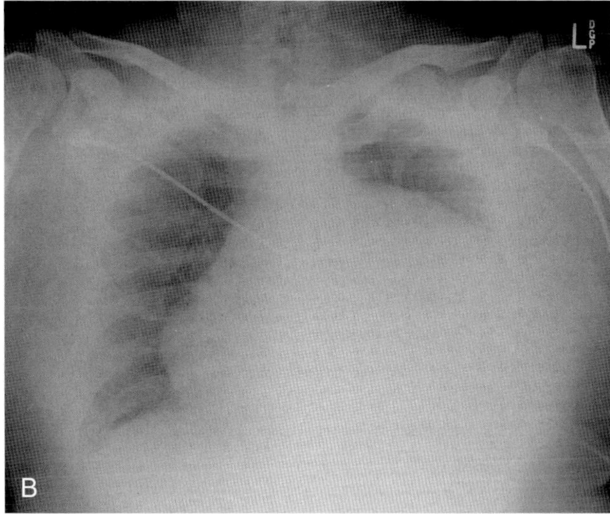


**Fig. 202.3 A,** Patient's chest radiograph 1 year before presentation with cardiac tamponade. **B,** Same patient's chest radiograph on presentation to the emergency department with cardiac tamponade.

specific for cardiac tamponade. Right ventricular diastolic collapse occurs early in diastole when ventricular volume is minimal. Left atrial collapse is less common, but it is also very specific for cardiac tamponade. Collapse of the left ventricle is uncommon because of its greater muscular thickness.

As discussed earlier, left- and right-sided volumes vary with the respiratory cycle. During inspiration, the atrial and ventricular septa bulge to the left. During expiration, the atrial and ventricular septa bulge rightward.

## TREATMENT

Patients with mild hemodynamic compromise require urgent drainage of pericardial fluid. If the patient is sufficiently stable, cardiology and cardiothoracic surgery consultation may be appropriate to decide whether emergency catheter drainage or surgical creation of a pericardial window is the most appropriate therapy. In such cases, the emergency physician (EP) should be prepared to perform emergency pericardial drainage if the patient's clinical condition should deteriorate.

Patients with severe hemodynamic compromise require immediate removal of pericardial fluid. Pericardiocentesis should be performed to remove as much of the pericardial effusion as possible. Percutaneous aspiration of even 50 to 100 mL has been demonstrated to reverse cardiac tamponade physiology temporarily.

Pericardiocentesis may be performed under electrocardiographic or echocardiographic guidance. Echocardiographic guidance is preferred when available, because it allows greater precision of procedure direction and needle angle. Placement of an indwelling catheter is advisable, to prevent reaccumulation of fluid. The technique used for pericardiocentesis can be found in the "Tips and Tricks" box. Fluid obtained from pericardiocentesis should be sent for Gram stain, culture, acid-fast stain and culture, cytologic study, carcinoembryonic antigen determination, and polymerase chain reaction evaluation. Complications of pericardiocentesis are listed in **Box 202.1**.

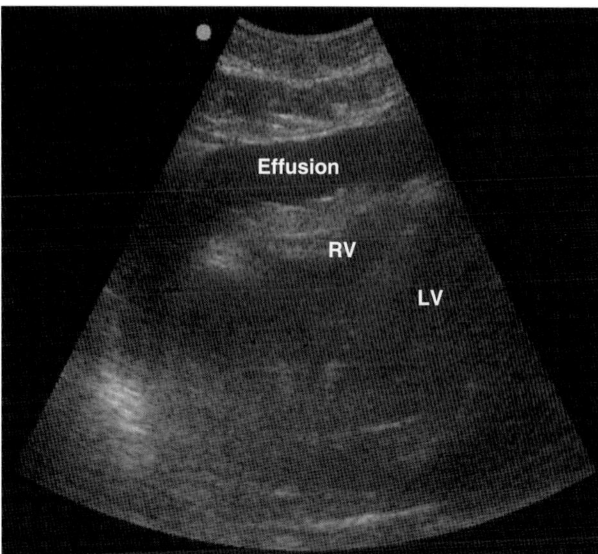


**Fig. 202.4 Bedside ultrasound image showing large pericardial effusion.** The patient subsequently had 2 L drained from this effusion. *LV,* Left ventricle; *RV,* right ventricle.

**BOX 202.1 Complications of Pericardiocentesis**

| | |
|---|---|
| Cardiac arrest (rare) | Postprocedure pulmonary edema |
| Cardiac chamber laceration | "Dry tap" |
| Coronary vessel laceration | Pericardial-pleural shunt |
| Cardiac tamponade | Air embolism or pneumopericardium |
| Lung laceration with pneumothorax | Liver laceration |
| Dysrhythmia | |

## DISPOSITION AND PROGNOSIS

Patients with cardiac tamponade are admitted to the hospital, typically in a cardiac care or intensive care unit (see the "Priority Actions" box). Emergency referral to cardiology for a

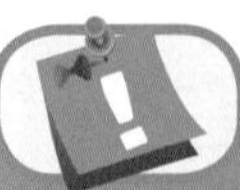

**TIPS AND TRICKS**

**Technique for Pericardiocentesis Using Ultrasound Guidance**

- Using bedside ultrasound, locate the ideal site of skin puncture where the largest fluid collection lies closest to the skin surface. This site is usually located on the left anterior chest wall. The clinician can choose either to mark the skin or to use the ultrasound device with a sterile sheath for dynamic guidance at this point.
- Prepare the skin in sterile fashion, and anesthetize the skin if time permits.
- Attach a 20-mL syringe to an 18-gauge spinal needle.
- Insert the needle at the site and trajectory determined by bedside ultrasonography. Take care to avoid the neurovascular bundle at the lower rib border and the internal mammary artery, which lies 3 to 5 cm lateral to the sternal border.
- Gently aspirate as the needle is advanced until fluid is obtained.
- Aspirate as much fluid as possible using the three-way stopcock.
- Alternately, use an over-the-needle catheter or the Seldinger technique if prolonged drainage is necessary. The Seldinger technique is performed using the same methods as outlined, but the clinician may use a thin-walled 18-gauge needle to pass a guidewire, followed by a catheter (e.g., a pigtail catheter) that may be left in place.

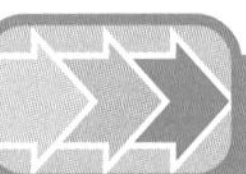

**PRIORITY ACTIONS**

- Consider malignant pericardial effusion in patients with a history of cancer who have tachypnea and dyspnea on exertion.
- Determine whether the patient has cardiac tamponade physiology by physical examination (i.e., Beck triad, pulsus paradoxus) or diagnostic evaluation (i.e., emergency bedside ultrasound).
- Perform an emergency pericardiocentesis or refer to cardiology for a pericardial window, based on hemodynamic instability.
- Assess for postprocedure reversal of tamponade physiology and for complications.
- Admit to a cardiac care or intensive care unit so that vital sign monitoring and follow-up diagnostics can be performed.

pericardial window procedure is determined if the patient is hemodynamically stable for the procedure. Documenting the hemodynamic instability and emergency intervention is important (see the "Documentation" box). Initial in-hospital mortality is high for patients with malignant effusion and pericardial tamponade; the median survival is 150 days, and the 1-year mortality rate is 76.5%. This mortality results jointly from the underlying cancer and the cardiovascular compromise.[2]

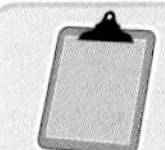

**DOCUMENTATION**

- Vital signs, examination findings, and diagnostics supporting hemodynamic instability and cardiac tamponade physiology
- Informed consent for the emergency pericardiocentesis
- Postintervention assessment of vital signs, examination findings, or diagnostics to support therapeutic reversal of tamponade and improved patient clinical condition
- Code status to support the patient's wishes given the underlying cancer history and invasiveness of the procedure

# SUPERIOR VENA CAVA SYNDROME

## EPIDEMIOLOGY

The superior vena cava (SVC) may become obstructed either acutely or subacutely, thus causing SVC syndrome. This condition may be caused by extrinsic mass, infiltration of the SVC by contiguous pathologic processes, or thrombosis. In the preantibiotic era, syphilitic aortic aneurysms, fibrosing mediastinitis, and complications of untreated infections were the most common causes of SVC syndrome.

Currently, malignant disease is the cause of SVC syndrome in 85% of cases. Bronchogenic carcinomas account for most cases, and small cell and squamous cell carcinomas are far the most common causes. Although lung cancer is the leading cause of SVC syndrome, the overall incidence of SVC syndrome in patients with lung cancer is low, at 2% to 4%. The next most common malignant cause of the SVC syndrome is non-Hodgkin lymphoma because of its frequent presentation as a mediastinal mass. Metastatic cancers account for a small proportion of cases of SVC syndrome. Patients with SVC syndrome rarely experience immediately life-threatening complications in the absence of concurrent central airway obstruction.[6,7]

Benign causes of SVC syndrome account for 10% to 15% of cases. In the patient with cancer, the most common benign cause is the presence of indwelling vascular devices such as hyperalimentation lines and chemotherapy ports or lines, which induce thrombosis of the SVC. Other causes include fibrosing mediastinitis resulting from histoplasmosis, as well as other infections.

## PATHOPHYSIOLOGY

SVC syndrome is caused by one of several mechanisms. The first is direct compression by tumor or by enlarging lymph nodes (from inflammation or metastatic disease). The second is direct invasion of the SVC by tumor or other pathologic processes. The third is obstruction of the SVC by thrombus. Thrombus may additionally occur in up to 50% of patients with one of the other causes of SVC syndrome, and it may account for some treatment failures when therapy is directed at the underlying malignant disease.[8] With compression of the

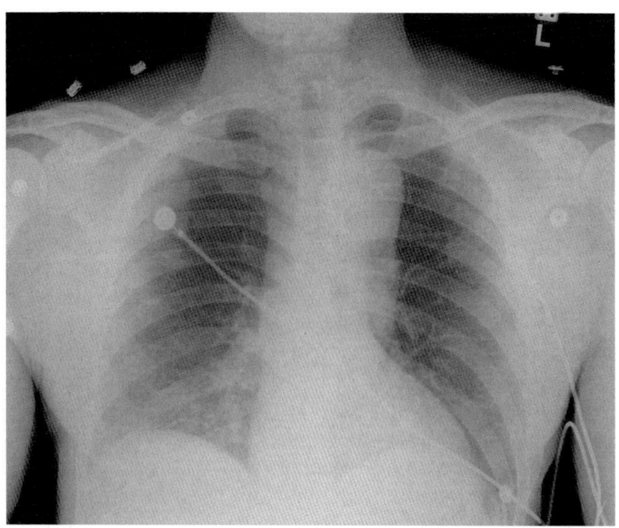


**Fig. 202.5 Chest radiograph showing widened mediastinum.**

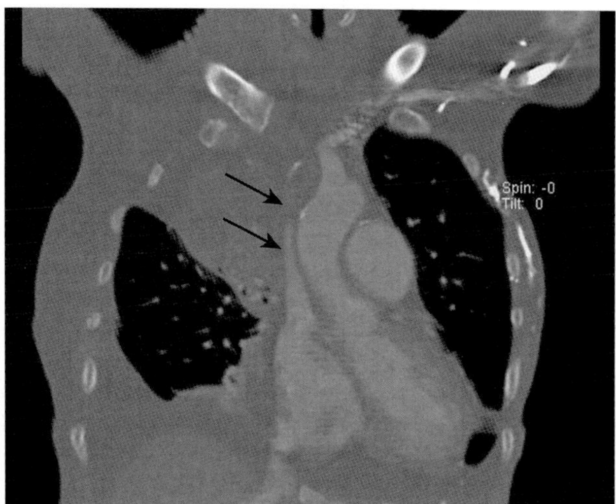


**Fig. 202.6 Computed tomography scan showing blockage of the superior vena cava** *(arrows).*

SVC, the patient has increased resistance to venous blood flow, which is diverted through collateral venous networks.

## PRESENTING SIGNS AND SYMPTOMS

The physical examination of the patient with SVC syndrome is often diagnostic. Most patients have facial edema or dilation of chest wall or neck veins. Some patients have cyanosis, arm edema, or plethora. A patient with the SVC syndrome who does not have visible upper body venous dilation is rare.[9] An indwelling central venous device may be a clue to the diagnosis in thrombotic causes of SVC syndrome.

Dyspnea, one of the most common symptoms of SVC syndrome, occurs in more than half of patients. Patients may complain of fullness or swelling of the face, trunk, or upper extremities that may be exacerbated by positional changes such as bending over or lying down. Contrary to previous beliefs, catastrophic neurologic events appear to be quite rare.[6,7] Findings of cerebral edema, laryngeal edema or upper airway stridor, or hemodynamic compromise represent the greatest emergencies.

## MEDICAL DECISION MAKING AND DIAGNOSTIC TESTING

The initial test of choice when SVC syndrome is suspected is chest plain film radiography. Most of these radiographs are abnormal; one series found 84% of films to be abnormal. The most common abnormal findings were mediastinal widening in 64% (**Fig. 202.5**) and pleural effusion in 26%.[9] A mass may also be seen in the superior mediastinum, right hilum or perihilum, or right upper lobe. Less commonly, right upper lobe collapse or rib notching may be apparent. However, a normal chest radiograph does not rule out the possibility of SVC syndrome.[9]

The next test is a contrast-enhanced computed tomography (CT) scan (**Fig. 202.6**). CT defines the level and extent of blockage, provides detail on the amount of collateral flow, and is often able to identify the cause of obstruction. The presence of collateral vessels with compression of the SVC on CT is a reliable indicator of SVC syndrome, with a sensitivity of 96% and a specificity of 92%.[10,11]

## TREATMENT

Rarely, SVC syndrome requires emergency care, as in the case of cerebral edema, airway obstruction, or hemodynamic compromise. In these situations, airway and vascular support and a specialist to assist in managing the obstruction are required. More commonly, symptomatic therapy should be instituted, including elevation of the head of the bed, oxygen, and bed rest. Diuretics and steroids have been used without clear evidence of efficacy. Anticoagulation may be of benefit in patients with thrombotic causes, after the origin is determined. Endovascular stenting has been successful in symptomatic improvement, and it has been steadily gaining favor as a treatment modality.

## DISPOSITION AND PROGNOSIS

All patients diagnosed with the SVC syndrome should be admitted to the hospital (see the "Priority Actions" box). The

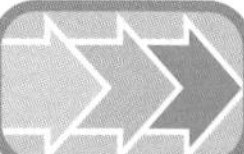

**PRIORITY ACTIONS**

- Diagnose the SVC syndrome in a patient with lung cancer or lymphoma with head or neck swelling, engorged upper extremity veins, plethora, or dyspnea.
- Determine whether the patient has any emergency obstructive SVC syndrome findings of cerebral edema, airway obstruction, or hemodynamic compromise, and provide supportive measures and specialist consultation on an emergency basis.

*SVC,* Superior vena cava.

level of care should be chosen based on the clinical stability of the patient. Oncology specialists should be consulted to help begin the work-up necessary to establish a histologic diagnosis, if one is not already known.

Survival of patients with the SVC syndrome depends on the underlying diagnosis and the treatments chosen. The median survival is 6 months, but it may differ considerably based on the type of malignant disease.

# Neurologic Oncologic Emergencies

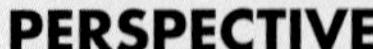

## PERSPECTIVE

The primary neurologic oncologic emergencies encountered in the ED can be divided into those that affect the central nervous system (CNS), including altered mental status, increased intracranial pressure (ICP), and seizures from brain tumors or metastatic lesions, and those that affect the peripheral nervous system, such as epidural spinal cord compression (ESCC). Generally, these emergencies involve acute to subacute presentations and result from mechanical obstruction of normal neurologic function. Patient morbidity and mortality can be improved by early recognition and management directed at relieving the neurologic obstruction or preventing secondary injury.

## CENTRAL NERVOUS SYSTEM EMERGENCIES

### EPIDEMIOLOGY

The most important CNS manifestations include altered mental status, elevated ICP, and seizures. Brain tumors represent a diverse group of neoplasms that can originate primarily from the CNS or metastatically through hematogenous spread from distant organs.

Although brain tumors account for only 2% of all tumors, they have significant sequelae. The 5-year survival rate of patients of all ages and all races who have malignant brain tumors is 33%; for children less than 14 years old, it is 62%; and for adults 65 years or older, it is 4.9%.[12] In children, brain tumors are the most common solid malignant tumors and the second leading cause of cancer death after leukemia. **Box 202.2** illustrates the differences in primary tumor types between adults and pediatric patients.

Brain metastases are more common than primary tumors in adults and account for more than half of all intracranial brain tumors. In adults with systemic malignant diseases, brain metastases occur in 10% to 30% of patients. The most common primary tumors responsible for brain metastases in adults are carcinomas, and they include lung cancer, renal cell cancer, melanoma, breast cancer, and colorectal cancer. In children with systemic malignant diseases, brain metastases occur in 6% to 10% of patients. The most common primary tumors responsible for brain metastases in children are sarcomas, neuroblastomas, and germ cell tumors.

In general, a slight male predominance is seen in the incidence of malignant brain tumor. Whites have the highest incidence, with a descending incidence in Latinos and African Americans, and the lowest incidence in Native Americans and Asian Americans.[12] The rising incidence of brain tumors in industrialized countries is thought to be mostly a result of environmental exposures and improved detection using diagnostic imaging.

Although cancers typically are indolent in their evolution, the neurologic manifestations may be acute or chronic, and they may be local or distant from the primary source. Rapid diagnosis and treatment are imperative to prevent irreversible damage, primarily from cerebral hypoxia, inflammation, or swelling, which can have catastrophic consequences. The long-term prognosis of patients with cancer and significant neurologic complications is poor, and recurrence of illness is common despite optimal management.

### PATHOPHYSIOLOGY

The pathogenesis of tumor-related neurologic dysfunction involves disruption of the blood-brain barrier leading to vasogenic edema. This condition is caused primarily by factors that increase the permeability of the tumor vessels (vascular endothelial growth factor, glutamate, and leukotrienes) and by the absence of tight endothelial cell junctions in tumor blood vessels. This process culminates in leakage of protein-rich

**BOX 202.2 Approximate Differences in Primary Tumor Types Between Adults and Children**

**Adults**

| 50% | 20% | 15% | 10% | 4% | 2% |
|---|---|---|---|---|---|
| Glioma > | Meningioma > | Pituitary tumor > | Astrocytoma > | CNS lymphoma > | Craniopharyngioma |

**Children**

| 50% | 25% | 10% | 10% | 5% |
|---|---|---|---|---|
| Astrocytoma > | Medulloblastoma > | Ependymoma > | Glioma > | Craniopharyngioma |

*CNS*, Central nervous system.

fluid into the extracellular space, predominantly in the white matter of the brain. When this peritumoral edema begins to accumulate, the synaptic transmission can be disrupted and thus can lead to altered neuronal excitability and neurologic sequelae (**Fig. 202.7**). Vasogenic edema is what causes patients to suffer from headaches, nausea or vomiting, seizures, cognitive dysfunction, focal neurologic deficits, encephalopathy, or increased ICP leading to syncope or fatal herniation. Intratumoral hemorrhage, obstructive hydrocephalus, and tumor embolization can also have tumor-related consequences, but these entities are much less common than vasogenic edema.

Brain metastases arrive through hematogenous spread. They are usually located in two places. The first is directly at the junction of the gray and white matter, where smaller vessels begin to trap tumor cells. The second is at terminal "watershed areas" of arterial circulation. Metastases distribute according to weight and blood flow and are seen in the cerebral hemispheres (80%), in the cerebellum (15%), and in the brainstem (5%). Pelvic (prostate and uterine) and gastrointestinal tumors commonly metastasize to the posterior fossa, whereas small cell lung carcinoma distributes equally through all regions of the brain.

## PRESENTING SIGNS AND SYMPTOMS

A classic presentation to the ED for brain metastasis is a patient with known cancer who has a sudden onset of a neurologic deficit or change in mental status, syncope, or seizure. Patients with primary or metastatic disease can present with either generalized or focal signs or symptoms. Generalized symptoms include headaches, nausea or vomiting, generalized seizures, cognitive dysfunction, and loss of consciousness. Focal symptoms include weakness, sensory loss, aphasia, focal seizures, and visual spatial dysfunction.

Headache is the most common symptom of brain tumor, and headaches occur in approximately 40% to 50% of patients with primary or metastatic brain tumors. In one retrospective review, headaches were described variably, but most were described as tension-type headaches. The patients described the headaches as bifrontal and worsening ipsilateral to the lesion.[13] Tumor-related headaches were differentiated from tension headaches by complaints of nausea and vomiting or especially by worsening of the headache with changes in body positioning that increased ICP (i.e., leaning forward). Worsening of the headache typically occurred following maneuvers that increase intrathoracic pressure, such as coughing, sneezing, or the Valsalva maneuver.

Tumor-related headaches tend to be worse at night because of small increases in the partial pressure of carbon dioxide, recumbency, and decreased cerebral venous return. Headaches related to increased ICP are thought to be mediated by the pain fibers of cranial nerve V in the dura and blood vessels. Headaches associated with increased ICP can be the result of large mass lesions or of restriction of cerebrospinal fluid outflow causing hydrocephalus. Classically, increased ICP is manifested by the classic triad of headache, nausea and vomiting, and papilledema. Thus, a careful ophthalmologic examination is requisite for all patients with complaints of headache.

Seizure represents the most common presenting symptom of gliomas and cerebral metastases. In these tumor types, one study showed that seizure was the initial complaint in

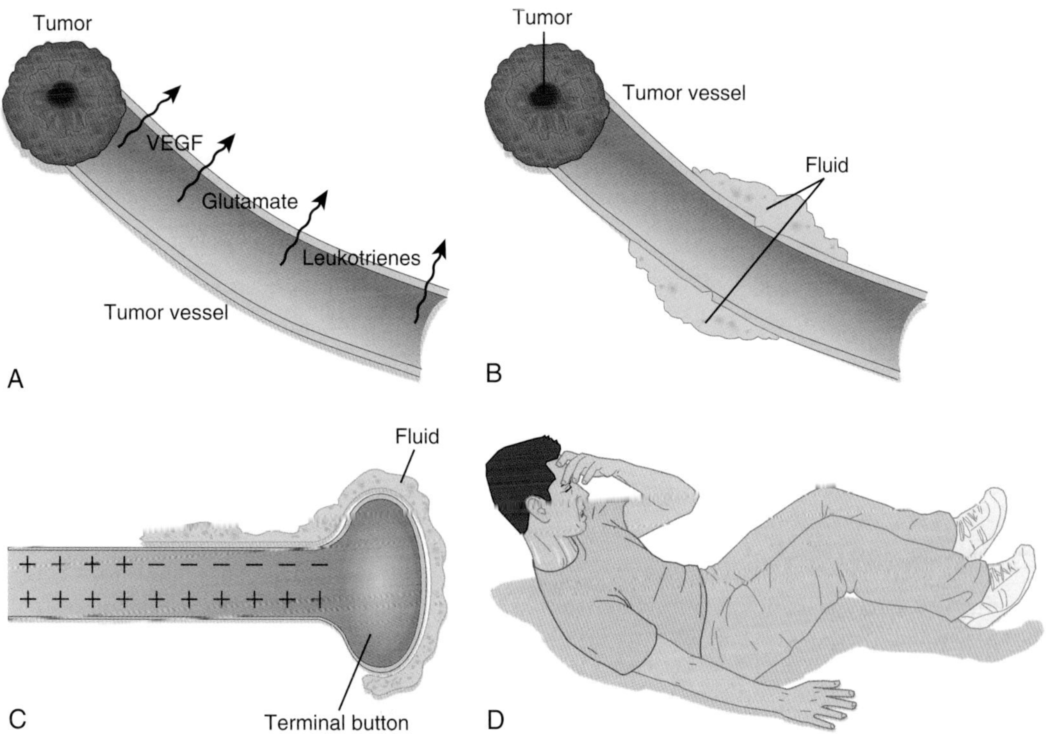


**Fig. 202.7 Pathophysiology of vasogenic edema. A,** Tumor vessel with factors that increase vascular permeability. *VEGF,* Vascular endothelial growth factor. **B,** Protein-rich fluid leaking into extracellular spaces. **C,** Disruption of synaptic transmission. **D,** Neurologic sequelae.

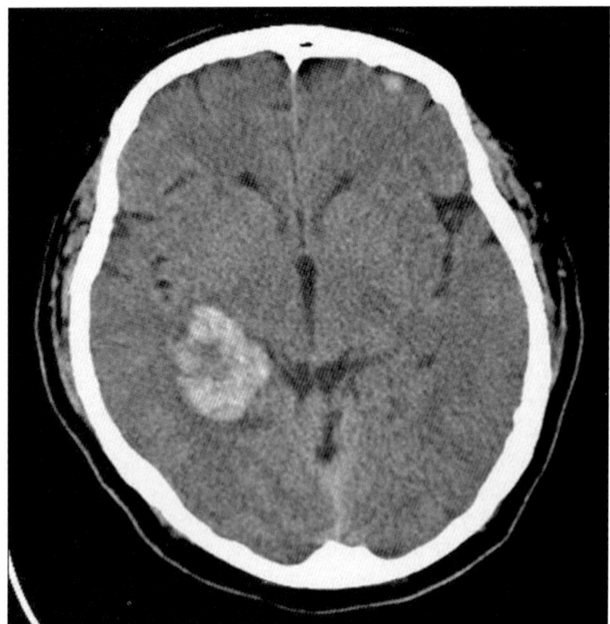

**Fig. 202.8 Noncontrast computed tomography scan of the head showing an intratumoral hemorrhage.**

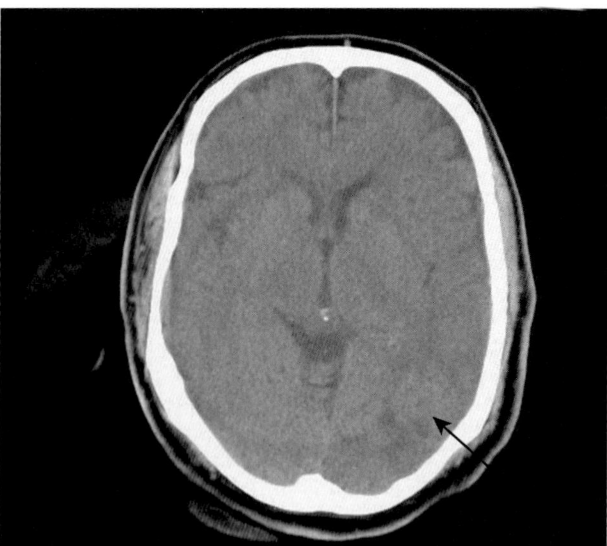

**Fig. 202.9 Noncontrast computed tomography scan of the head showing a brain tumor** *(arrow).*

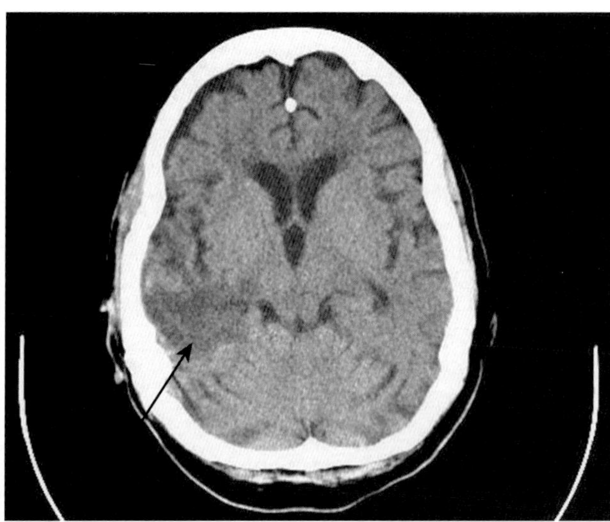

**Fig. 202.10 Noncontrast computed tomography scan of the head showing peritumoral edema** *(arrow).*

approximately 20% to 25% of patients.[14] Patients who present with seizure activity usually have smaller primary tumors or fewer metastatic lesions in the brain compared with other presenting symptoms, because the seizure leads to earlier diagnostic imaging and diagnosis. Seizures can be generalized or focal, depending on the location in the brain of the tumor. Frontal lobe tumors may cause tonic-clonic movements in an extremity, and occipital lobe tumors may cause visual disturbances. Temporal lobe seizures may cause abrupt personality changes. Patients with a history of tumor-related seizures commonly present in a similar fashion on each visit, with or without a prodromal phase followed by a postictal period. If the seizures are generalized, the patient will be fatigued and sleepy; if the seizures are focal, however, the patient may have Todd paralysis.

Acute mental status change describes a deficit in cognitive function and is a presenting complaint in approximately 30% to 35% of patients with brain metastases.[15] Cognitive dysfunction includes memory problems and mood or personality changes. Patients commonly present with fatigue, low energy, increased urge to sleep, and apathy toward daily activities.

## MEDICAL DECISION MAKING AND DIAGNOSTIC TESTING

Diagnostic neuroimaging is the standard for confirming brain tumors and subsequent neurologic manifestations of oncologic emergencies. For the EP, CT scanning is the initial test of choice because of its speed and availability. Contrast-enhanced magnetic resonance imaging (MRI) is the preferred study for primary and metastatic brain tumors, but it does not need to be performed on an emergency basis (**Figs. 202.8 through 202.12**).

## TREATMENT

The main goals of treatment for neurologic manifestations of oncologic emergencies are to preserve and maintain cerebral oxygenation and perfusion, to decrease inflammation and swelling, and to identify and correct the underlying condition. In the severely neurologically depressed patient with a declining Glasgow coma scale and an inability to protect the airway, rapid-sequence endotracheal intubation should be performed, with supplemental oxygen administered to prevent cerebral hypoxia. Before intubation, care should be taken to prevent a rise in ICP, and appropriate choices for sedation and paralytic agents should be used.

Pretreatment with 1 to 1.5 mg/kg of lidocaine to blunt the rise in ICP from intubation has limited supporting evidence, but it can be used as an adjunct. Etomidate is the best choice for sedation, at a dose of 0.3 mg/kg, and it induces general anesthesia without raising ICP or dropping blood pressure.

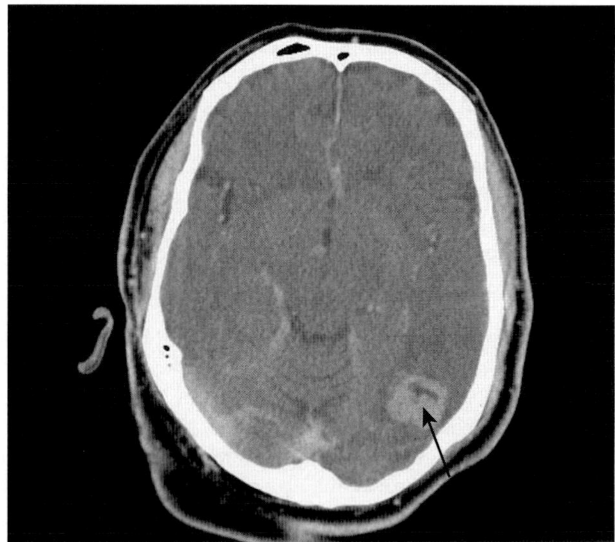

**Fig. 202.11 Contrast computed tomography scan of the head showing a brain tumor** *(arrow).*

Another agent for sedation, propofol, at a dose of 2 mg/kg, induces general anesthesia without raising ICP with the advantage of rapid onset of action and a short half-life. A defasciculating dose of a nondepolarizing agent (e.g., 0.01 mg/kg of vecuronium) may help to blunt the fasciculations caused by succinylcholine (1.5 mg/kg).

Diagnostic neuroimaging must be performed immediately following stabilization to ascertain the underlying cause of neurologic dysfunction. Once the patient is stabilized and the brain is adequately oxygenated, secondary treatments must be performed to protect the brain from further injury such as increasing edema or herniation.

Corticosteroids, specifically dexamethasone, help to reduce the inflammatory response by decreasing the permeability of tumor capillaries and by clearing edema through transport of fluid into the ventricular system. Dexamethasone is the standard agent of choice because of its antiinflammatory effects and its relative lack of mineralocorticoid activity, which may cause fluid retention. The initial dose is typically a 10-mg loading dose. If the drug is given orally, absorption is completed within 30 minutes. Tumor-related weakness is very responsive to dexamethasone treatment.

Reduction of ICP and improvement of neurologic symptoms usually begin within hours. The permeability of the blood-brain barrier has been found to improve within 6 hours, and changes in MRI demonstrating decreased edema have been shown within 2 to 3 days. The long-term side effects of corticosteroid use include gastrointestinal complications, steroid myopathy, and opportunistic infection.

If steroids alone cannot effect adequate reduction of ICP, increasing ICP can evolve into a medical emergency leading to herniation. The neurologic intensive care specialist will consider placement of a ventriculostomy to monitor the ICP and to drain cerebrospinal fluid to reduce ICP. The goal of ICP monitoring and treatment should be to keep ICP to less than 20 mm Hg and cerebral perfusion pressure (CPP) between 60 and 75 mm Hg. In the patient who has required intubation, the head of the bed should be elevated 30 degrees to decrease ICP.

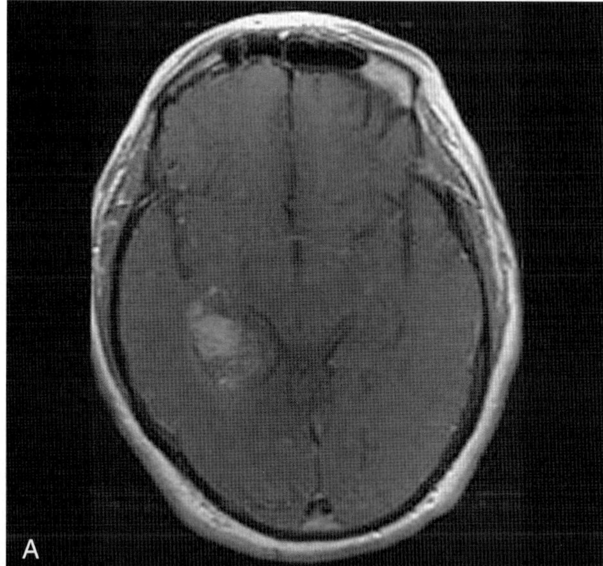



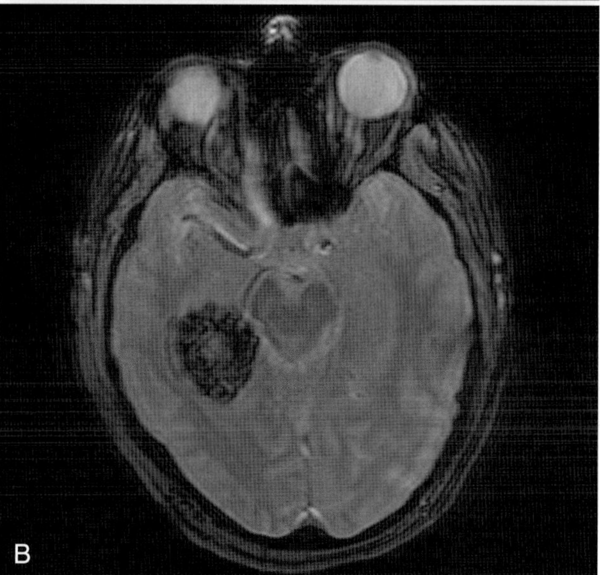



**Fig. 202.12 A and B,** Magnetic resonance images showing brain tumor with hemorrhage and edema.

Osmotic agents (e.g., mannitol, at a dose of 1 g/kg) reduce ICP by 50% in 30 minutes, peak after 90 minutes, and last 4 hours. Loop diuretics (e.g., furosemide, 1 mg/kg) also decrease ICP without increasing serum osmolality. The use of mannitol or diuretics can be discussed with the neurologic intensive care specialist. Hyperventilation to reduce ICP is controversial; if it is performed after discussion with the neurologic intensive care specialist, however, all efforts should be made to keep the partial pressure of carbon dioxide between 30 and 35 mm Hg. Sedation should also be continued to reduce metabolic demand.

Blood pressure control should attempt to maintain CPP higher than 60 mm Hg, because systemic hypotension and resultant low CPP actually increase ICP. Pressors can be used safely without further increasing ICP if the blood pressure becomes too low. Hypertension should generally be treated only when CPP is higher than 120 mm Hg and ICP is higher than 20 mm Hg, to prevent further damage. The patient should be kept euvolemic with 0.9% normal saline to ensure that no hypotension from hypovolemia or hydrocephalus from hypervolemia occurs. The patient should also be kept in the normal osmolarity range (295 to 305 mOsm); hyponatremia may be managed with hypertonic saline after discussion with the intensive care specialist because its use is controversial. Euglycemia (80 to 120 mg/dL) should be maintained for metabolic needs.

Antiemetic medications should be used so that vomiting does not increase ICP. Barbiturate therapy can be considered to reduce ICP based on the ability of these drugs to reduce brain metabolism and cerebral blood flow. Pentobarbital is often used, with a loading dose of 5 to 20 mg/kg as a bolus, followed by 1 to 4 mg/kg/hour. Treatment should be assessed based on ICP, CPP, and the presence of unacceptable side effects such as hypotension. Continuous electroencephalographic monitoring is generally used. Therapeutic hypothermia has not been reliably studied in increased ICP secondary to oncologic emergencies and is not currently standard management. Treatment alternatives to assist in the care of acute vasogenic edema are listed in the "Tips and Tricks" box.

**TIPS AND TRICKS**

**Treatment Alternatives for Patients with Acute Vasogenic Edema**

- Corticosteroids
  - Dexamethasone (10-mg loading dose)
- Osmotic agents or diuretics
  - Consider mannitol (1 g/kg).
  - Consider furosemide (1 mg/kg).
- Antiemetics (*phenothiazine of choice* or ondansetron for refractory vomiting)
- Euvolemia (0.9% normal saline solution)
- Euglycemia (80 to 120 mg/dL)
- Normal osmolarity (295 to 305 mOsm)
  - Consider hypertonic saline after discussion with specialist.
- Blood pressure control (CPP > 60 mm Hg and CPP < 120 mm Hg when ICP > 20 mm Hg)
  - Consider pressors for hypotension.
  - Consider calcium channel blockers or beta-blocking agents for hypertension.
- Ensure airway protection with intubation if necessary.
- Consider pretreatment with an agent to blunt increased ICP (e.g., 1.5 mg/kg lidocaine).
- Choose a sedative agent that does not increase ICP (e.g., etomidate 0.3 mg/kg or propofol 2 mg/kg).
- Consider a defasciculating dose of a nondepolarizing agent before a depolarizing agent (e.g., 0.01 mg/kg vecuronium before 1.5 mg/kg succinylcholine).
- Elevate the head of the bed to 30 degrees.
- Consider hyperventilation after discussion with a specialist (ensure Pco2 30 to 35 mm Hg).
- Consider antiseizure medication or barbiturate therapy (i.e., lorazepam, 2- to 5-mg bolus, or pentobarbital, 5-to 20-mg/kg bolus, then 1 to 4 mg/kg/hour).

*CPP*, Cerebral perfusion pressure; *ICP*, intracranial pressure; *P*$CO_2$, partial pressure of carbon dioxide.

The main goals of treatment in tumor-related seizures are to ensure adequate oxygenation and perfusion and to stop prolonged seizures or evolving status epilepticus. In addition to supplemental oxygenation and steps to ensure that the patient is not injured, the initial choice of medication is a benzodiazepine such as lorazepam (2 to 4 mg intravenous loading dose). If the seizure is refractory, and monotherapy with escalating doses of benzodiazepines is not working, consider the addition of phenobarbital (20 mg/kg intravenous loading dose) or phenytoin (18 mg/kg intravenous loading dose).

Prophylactic anticonvulsants are commonly considered in patients with diagnosed brain tumors but who have not had a seizure. Prophylactic anticonvulsants were reviewed by the Quality Standards Subcommittee of the American Academy of Neurology, and the summary recommendation stated that prophylaxis did not affect the frequency of subsequent seizures and should not be used in patients with either primary or metastatic brain tumors. Thus, the subcommittee believed the 5% to 25% subsequent seizure risk in brain tumors was outweighed by the deleterious interactions of anticonvulsants with cytotoxic drugs and corticosteroids. In postoperative seizure, the subcommittee recommended that anticonvulsants should be tapered and discontinued after the first postoperative week in patients who have not had a seizure, particularly in patients who are medically stable and are experiencing anticonvulsant-related side effects.

## DISPOSITION AND PROGNOSIS

Once stabilized, patients presenting with neurologic complications of cancer require admission to the hospital (priority actions for the management of cerebral oncologic emergencies are listed in the "Priority Actions" box). Patients with significantly depressed neurologic function require intubation, neuroprotective interventions, and intensive monitored care by a neurologic intensive care specialist. Patients who are awake, hemodynamically stable, and protecting their airway

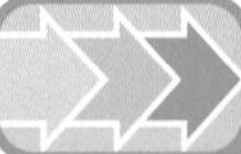

**PRIORITY ACTIONS**

- Consider a central nervous system emergency in patients with a history of cancer who have mental status change, headache, cognitive dysfunction, seizure, syncope, or focal findings.
- Address life-threatening emergencies with prompt interventions (i.e., intubation to prevent anoxic brain injury; antiepileptic medications for status epilepticus).
- Prevent secondary brain injury by directing therapies to maintain oxygenation and perfusion of the brain and to reduce inflammation and neurologic sequelae of the tumor.
- Obtain prompt neurologic specialist input with the assistance of medical oncology for brain monitoring and admission management.

require admission to a general unit with neurology and medical oncology evaluation. Careful documentation of change in neurologic status is important (see the "Documentation" box). The prognosis of patients with CNS oncologic emergencies is generally poor.

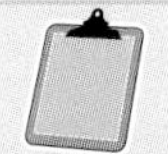

**DOCUMENTATION**

- Fundus examination for evidence of papilledema
- Serial neurologic examinations to assess for a change in condition
- Seizure precautions
- Continuous electroencephalographic monitoring for seizure activity (especially in intubated or paralyzed patient)
- Serial blood pressure and cerebral perfusion pressure measurements
- Time of neurologic consultant evaluation and recommendations and interventions
- Management to prevent secondary brain injury
- Code status to support the patient's wishes given the underlying cancer history and neurologic outcome

# EPIDURAL SPINAL CORD COMPRESSION

## EPIDEMIOLOGY

Neoplastic ESCC is a common complication of metastatic cancer that has been documented to occur in 5% of patients with cancer.[16] The most widely accepted definition of ESCC includes any radiographic indentation of the thecal sac. Although the cauda equina is not technically considered part of the spinal cord, the pathophysiology of compression of the cauda equina is the same as that of the spinal cord. Thus, compression of the thecal sac by malignant disease at this level is also referred to as ESCC.

The most common tumors are prostate, breast, and lung cancers (each accounting for 15% to 20% of all cases), which tend to metastasize to the vertebral column. Other important tumors are renal cell carcinoma, multiple myeloma, non-Hodgkin lymphoma, and plasmacytoma, which make up most of the remaining cases. In children, the most common causes are sarcomas, neuroblastomas, Hodgkin lymphoma, Wilms tumor, and germ cell tumors. The most common vertebral levels of involvement for ESCC for all age groups are the thoracic spine (60% to 78%), followed by the lumbar spine (16% to 33%), followed by the cervical spine (4% to 15%); multiple levels are involved in up to 50% of patients.[17] Delays in diagnosis and treatment remain common, and reports from multiple countries describe poor neurologic outcome in half or more of patients diagnosed with ESCC, including motor weakness, bladder dysfunction, and inability to ambulate.[18-20]

## PATHOPHYSIOLOGY

The most common method for hematogenous spread to the spinal column is by direct arterial embolization of tumor cells. The seeding of these cells creates a destructive and expansive mass in the vertebral body. As the vertebral body weakens, both the tumor and collapsed bony fragments place pressure on the epidural space and subsequently on the thecal sac that results in ESCC.

## PRESENTING SIGNS AND SYMPTOMS

The most common presenting symptom of ESCC is back pain, which occurs in more than 80% of patients.[16] In general, pain precedes the onset of neurologic symptoms by several weeks. The pain is generally slowly progressive, although abrupt worsening of pain may signal a pathologic compression fracture. The pain may worsen with recumbency, movement, or the Valsalva maneuver, or it may develop a radicular quality. The radicular pain may be bilateral, especially in thoracic lesions.

Motor weakness is present in most patients with ESCC at the time of diagnosis. When the cauda equina is compressed, the deep tendon reflexes may also be depressed. Laterally situated tumors may cause isolated motor radiculopathy or radiculopathy superimposed on bilateral lower extremity weakness. Weakness tends to be most pronounced in patients with thoracic lesions.

Sensory findings are present in more than half the patients with ESCC. Patients often report ascending numbness or paresthesias. When a sensory level is present, it is generally several levels below the actual level of spinal cord compression. Cauda equina lesions result in saddle anesthesia, whereas higher lesions often spare these sacral dermatomes. Like motor symptoms, sensory symptoms can occur in a radicular pattern.

Bowel dysfunction and bladder dysfunction are often late findings, but these disorders are frequently present by the time

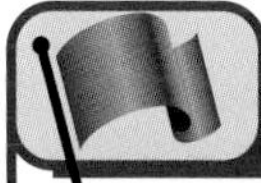

**RED FLAGS**

**Malignant Epidural Spinal Cord Compression Cautions for the Physician**

- Back pain in a patient with prostate, lung, or breast cancer
- Repeat patient visits for accelerating back pain with risk factors for cancer without a plan for diagnostic imaging
- Not including ESCC in the differential diagnosis of a patient with urinary retention with risk factors for cancer
- Assuming that the ESCC is limited to the lumbar spine
- Not documenting a thorough neurologic examination, including strength, sensation, rectal tone, or reflex testing, in a patient suspected of malignant ESCC

*ESCC*, Epidural spinal cord compression.

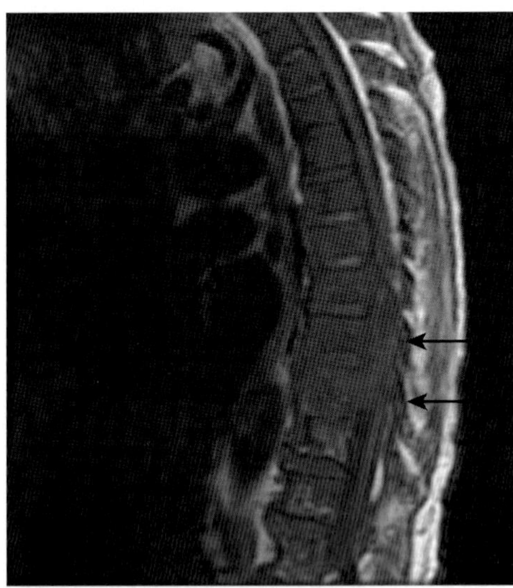

**Fig. 202.13 Magnetic resonance image demonstrating compression of the thecal sac** *(arrows).*

of diagnosis of ESCC. The most common presenting symptom is urinary retention, which may be potentiated by the use of narcotic analgesics for the back pain. Other signs and symptoms of myelopathy that may indicate ESCC include diminished proprioception, ataxia, spasticity, reflex hyperactivity, and autonomic dysfunction. The presenting signs and symptoms of ESCC are difficult to diagnose, and cautions for the physician are listed in the "Red Flags" box.

## MEDICAL DECISION MAKING AND DIAGNOSTIC TESTING

Although plain radiography is easily accessible in the ED and is able to predict ESCC in most patients with an evident lesion, it is still generally inadequate. Between 10% and 17% of patients have ESCC without findings on plain radiography.[16]

MRI and myelography (or CT myelography) remain the cornerstones of diagnosis of ESCC. MRI holds several advantages in that it is accurate, reliable, noninvasive, and able to image the entire thecal sac regardless of whether myelographic block is present (**Fig. 202.13**).

In general, definitive imaging is necessary when ESCC is suspected. Imaging should be performed on an emergency basis in any patient with evidence of neurologic dysfunction suspected to be caused by ESCC. In patients with cancer who have new or worsening back pain without any evidence of neurologic dysfunction and a normal plain radiograph, it is probably reasonable to allow urgent outpatient definitive imaging.

## TREATMENT

When epidural metastatic lesions are found in the investigation for ESCC, therapy is indicated for any patients who have not had prolonged paraplegia (more than several days). The cornerstones of therapy are corticosteroids, radiation therapy, and, in some cases, surgery.

The value of corticosteroids to relieve edema contributing to spinal cord compression is well documented. What remains controversial is the dosage of dexamethasone. Initial bolus doses of anywhere from 10 to 100 mg have been used, with no clear answer on the most appropriate dosage. Subsequent lower doses may be given orally as directed by the consultant specialist. Steroids should be given immediately, even before MRI scanning, if ESCC is strongly suspected or if ESCC is suspected and appropriate imaging will be delayed for any reason.

Neurosurgery should be consulted immediately for cases of ESCC. The consultant will weigh the neurologic status of the patient and clinical variables such as life expectancy to tailor a treatment plan for the patient including radiation therapy or surgery.

## DISPOSITION AND PROGNOSIS

Patients with ESCC are admitted to the hospital, and they should have early ED consultation by a neurosurgeon (see the "Priority Actions" box). In general, the outcomes of patients following ESCC heavily depend on the neurologic status of the patient at the time of diagnosis, and documentation is very important (see the "Documentation" box). Although the median survival of patients diagnosed with ESCC is 6 months, the outcome is better in patients who are ambulatory at the time of diagnosis. Patients with lung cancer as the source of metastatic disease have poorer prognosis than those with breast or prostate cancer.

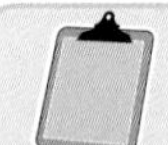

### DOCUMENTATION

- Thorough neurologic examination, including motor, sensory, genitourinary (including rectal tone), and reflex testing
- Serial neurologic examinations to assess for a change in condition
- Time of neurologic consultant evaluation and recommendations and interventions
- Code status to support the patient's wishes given the underlying cancer history and neurologic outcome

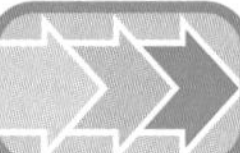

### PRIORITY ACTIONS

- Consider ESCC in patients with a history of cancer with back pain and focal neurologic dysfunction.
- Treat with dexamethasone.
- Obtain prompt neurologic specialist input because preintervention neurologic function predicts the postintervention neurologic outcome.

*ESCC,* Epidural spinal cord compression.

## SUGGESTED READINGS

Cornily J, Pennec P, Castellant P, et al. Cardiac tamponade in medical patients: a 10-year follow up survey. Cardiology 2008;111:197-201.

Forsyth PA, Posner JB. Headaches in patients with brain tumors: a study of 111 patients. Neurology 1993;43:1678-83.

Mandavia DP, Hoffner RJ, Mahaney K, Henderson SO. Bedside echocardiography by emergency physicians. Ann Emerg Med 2001;38:377-82.

Sun H, Nemecek AN. Optimal management of malignant epidural spinal cord compression. Hematol Oncol Clin North Am 2010;24:537-51.

Wan JF, Bezjak A. Superior vena cava syndrome. Hematol Oncol Clin North Am 2010;24:501-13.

## REFERENCES

***References can be found on Expert Consult @ www.expertconsult.com.***

# 203 White Blood Cell Disorders

*Eric Goralnick*

**KEY POINTS**

- White blood cell disorders are the result of cell overproduction, underproduction, or dysfunction.
- Hematologic malignant diseases have variable initial presentations and significant associated complications.
- Rapid evaluation and intervention are essential to minimize morbidity and mortality in the immunocompromised patient.

## EPIDEMIOLOGY

The National Cancer Institute estimated that approximately 137,260 new cases and 54,020 deaths from hematologic malignant diseases (leukemias, lymphomas, and plasma cell disorders) occurred in 2010. On January 1, 2007, approximately 908,512 men and women living in the United States had a history of hematologic malignant disease. In adults, non-Hodgkin lymphomas and chronic lymphocytic leukemia are the most common of these diseases.[1] Of a total of 26,446 childhood cancers (age 1 to 19 years) diagnosed in the United States from 2001 to 2003, leukemias were the most common (26.3%). The lymphoid leukemias were the type with the highest incidence. Lymphomas, comprising 14.6% of new childhood malignant diseases, were the third most common cancers.[1,2] A history of malignant disease is a common feature in the emergency department (ED) patient population. In a retrospective review of 5640 patients in a community teaching hospital with an annual ED census of 31,000, cancer history was identified in 5% of patients. Ten percent of patients with oncology-related visits died during the admission, and 48% died within 1 year of the ED visit.[3]

## PATHOPHYSIOLOGY

White blood cells (WBCs), or leukocytes, are the primary cells responsible for the inflammatory and immune response. WBCs include granulocytes (neutrophils, eosinophils, basophils) and mononuclear cells (T and B lymphocytes, monocytes). These cells are all produced from a common stem cell in the bone marrow, and they differentiate through various cytokines including colony-stimulating factors and interleukins. Normal blood leukocyte counts are 4.34 to 10.8 $\times 10^9$/L, with neutrophils representing 45% to 74% of cells, bands representing 0% to 4%, lymphocytes representing 16% to 45%, monocytes representing 4% to 10%, eosinophils representing 0% to 7%, and basophils representing 0% to 2%.[4] WBC disorders are the result of cell overproduction, underproduction, or dysfunction (**Box 203.1**). The WBC count with differential lacks specificity and sensitivity but is the most frequent laboratory test ordered by emergency physicians.[5]

### LEUKOPENIA

Leukopenia, or a WBC count less than $1.5 \times 10^9$/L, is most clinically relevant with significant neutropenia and its complications (primarily increased risk of infection, further outlined in Chapter 201). Although neutropenia is most common in patients with bone marrow suppression secondary to chemotherapy, **Box 203.2** outlines a differential diagnosis of certain infections that characteristically manifest with neutropenia. Lymphocytopenia is a nonspecific finding that is present in many bacterial, fungal, viral, and protozoan infections.[6]

### LEUKOCYTOSIS

Leukocytosis, or an increased number of WBCs, is defined as an elevation in the total number of circulating WBCs greater than 2 standard deviations above the age-based mean circulating WBC count. This disorder is most commonly secondary to infections or systemic stressors; however, an increase in a subset of WBCs (neutrophilia, monocytosis, lymphocytosis, eosinophilia, or basophilia) may guide the differential diagnosis. Bacteria are the culprit in two thirds of infection-related cases of neutrophilia.[7] **Box 203.3** outlines infectious causes of lymphocytosis, with *Bordetella pertussis* being the rare bacterial exception. Eosinophilia is classically caused by multicellular parasites that invade tissue, most commonly seen in invasive parasitic disease, but it may also be seen in protozoan and fungal infections.[8]

### MORPHOLOGIC CHANGES

In addition to altered numbers, changes in cellular morphology found in a peripheral blood smear may aid in the diagnosis. A left shift (or greater percentage of immature cells, such as metamyelocytes) may be present in severe infection. Intracellular abnormalities including toxic granulations,

**BOX 203.1 Differential Diagnosis of White Blood Cell Disorders by Pathogenesis**

### Overproduction

***Stress (Infections, Inflammation)***

***Drugs***

- Corticosteroids
- Granulocyte colony-stimulating factor
- Acetylcholine
- Adrenergic agents
- Heparin
- Lithium
- Histamine
- Lead
- Iron

***Neoplastic Disease***

**Primary Hematologic**

- Myelodysplastic syndromes
- Acute leukemias
  - Acute myelogenous leukemia
  - Acute lymphocytic leukemia
- Chronic leukemias
  - Chronic lymphocytic leukemia
  - Chronic myelogenous leukemia
  - Hairy cell leukemia
  - Large granular lymphocytic leukemia
- Non-Hodgkin lymphoma

**Cancers Metastatic to Bone**

- Most commonly breast, lung, prostate, and lymphomas

### Underproduction

***Drug or Toxin Suppression***

- Cancer chemotherapy
- Phenytoin
- Penicillins
- Sulfa

***Aplastic Anemia***

***Malignant Disease (Leukemia, Myelodysplastic Syndrome)***

***Vitamin $B_{12}$ or Folate Deficiency***

### Dysfunction

***Increased Splenic Sequestration***

- Cirrhosis
- Gaucher disease

***Diabetes Mellitus***

- Impaired polymorphonuclear neutrophil function

***Chronic Renal Failure***

- Impaired polymorphonuclear neutrophil and lymphocyte function

***Drugs***

- Corticosteroids

Adapted from Lepin HD, Powell BL. White cell disorders. In: Halter JB, Ouslander J, Tinetti M, et al, editors. Hazzard's geriatric medicine and gerontology. 6th ed. New York: McGraw-Hill; 2009.

**BOX 203.2 Infections That May Cause Neutropenia in the Normal Host**

**Bacterial**

- Salmonellosis
- Tularemia
- Brucellosis
- Rickettsial disease (Rocky Mountain spotted fever)
- Miliary tuberculosis

**Viral**

- Measles
- Varicella (chickenpox)
- Rubella
- Influenza
- Infectious hepatitis
- Yellow fever
- Sandfly fever
- Human immunodeficiency virus infection
- Colorado tick fever
- Dengue fever

**Protozoan and Parasitic**

- Malaria
- Kala-azar
- Relapsing fever

Adapted from Hoffman R, Benz Jr EJ, Shattil SJ, et al, editors. Hematology: basic principles and practice. 5th ed. Philadelphia: Churchill Livingstone; 2009.

**BOX 203.3 Infections That May Cause Lymphocytosis**

**Acute Infection**

- Pertussis
- Infectious mononucleosis
- Infectious hepatitis
- Acute infectious lymphocytosis
- Toxoplasmosis
- Cytomegalovirus

**Chronic Infection**

- Tuberculosis
- Brucellosis
- Syphilis
- Rickettsial disease

Adapted from Hoffman R, Benz Jr EJ, Shattil SJ, et al, editors. Hematology: basic principles and practice. 5th ed. Philadelphia: Churchill Livingstone; 2009.

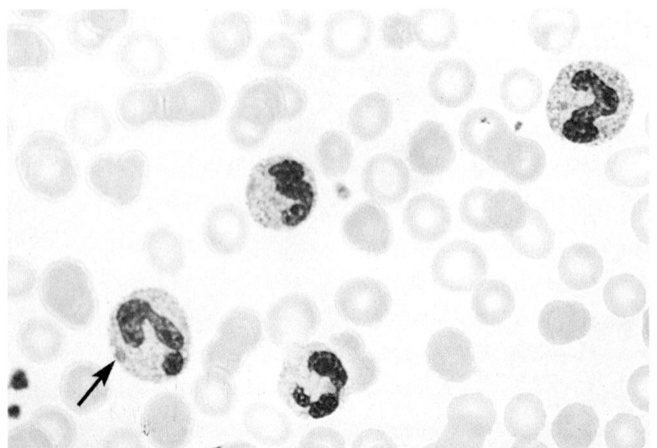

**Fig. 203.1 Reactive changes in neutrophils.** Neutrophils containing coarse purple cytoplasmic granules (toxic granulations) and blue cytoplasmic patches of dilated endoplasmic reticulum (Dohle bodies; *arrow*) are observed in this peripheral blood smear prepared from a patient with bacterial sepsis. (From Kumar V, Abbas, AK, Fausto N, Aster J, editors. Robbins and Cotran pathologic basis of disease. 8th ed. Philadelphia: Saunders; 2009.)

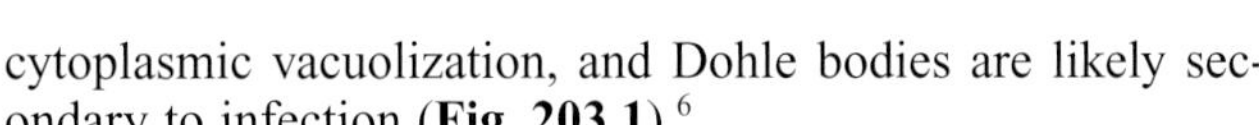

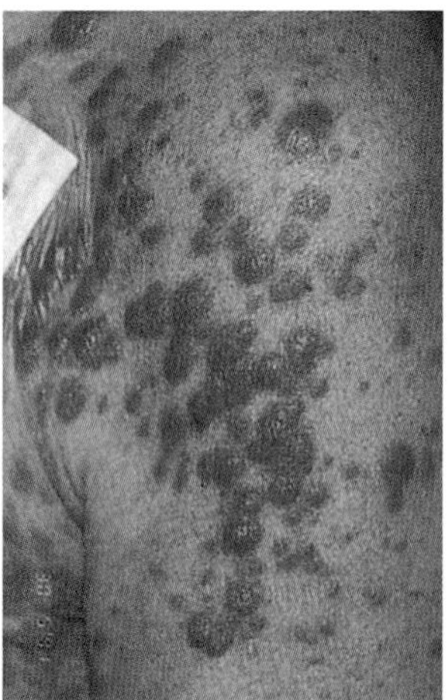

**Fig. 203.2 Leukemia cutis in a patient with monoblastic leukemia.** (From Miller KB, Pihan G. Acute myeloid leukemia. In: Hoffman R, Benz Jr EJ, Shattil SJ, et al, editors. Hematology: basic principles and practice. 5th ed. Philadelphia: Churchill Livingstone; 2009.)

cytoplasmic vacuolization, and Dohle bodies are likely secondary to infection (**Fig. 203.1**).[6]

### WHITE BLOOD CELL MALIGNANCY

Although WBC disorders have a vast differential diagnosis, the remainder of this chapter focuses on hematologic malignant diseases. Leukemias, lymphomas, and plasma cell disorders are the main general categories of these malignant diseases.

Leukemias are a result of failure of differentiation of hematopoietic precursor cells that leads to unchecked proliferation of blasts, either immature myeloid or lymphoid cells, which impede the normal manufacturing of red blood cells, WBCs, and platelets in the bone marrow. Anemia, bleeding, and infection are a result of decreased normal cell production. Eventually, blasts multiply and migrate throughout other hematopoietic organs including the spleen and lymph nodes. In acute leukemias, WBC counts vary greatly (25% of patients have counts <5000/microliters, 25% have counts >50,000/microliters, and 50% have counts between 5000 and 50,000/microliters), but anemia, thrombocytopenia, and blasts are common. Bone marrow aspiration and biopsy are used to diagnose leukemias definitively.

Lymphomas are a vast group of malignant diseases defined by clonal proliferation of malignant lymphocytes. The World Health Organization lymphoma classification defined 27 types of lymphomas categorized primarily by the primary clonal cells: B cells, T cells, or natural killer cells. Lymphocytosis and varied characteristic cells are present on a peripheral blood smear. Lymph node and bone marrow biopsy also aid in the diagnosis.

Monoclonal proliferation of immunoglobin-secreting plasma cells characterizes plasma cell disorders. These conditions include multiple myeloma, monoclonal gammopathies, Waldenström macroglobulinemia, heavy-chain diseases, cryoglobulinemia, and primary amyloidosis. These diseases are diagnosed by using serum or protein electrophoresis and bone marrow analysis.

## PRESENTING SIGNS AND SYMPTOMS

Nonspecific presentations of liquid malignant diseases are common, but prompt recognition of these signs and symptoms is essential for rapid treatment of immunocompromised patients. Initial presentations of malignancy vary greatly from subtle historical features or physical findings to in extremis shock states typically resulting from complications and grave immunodeficiency. Patients with known malignant disease also have variable presenting complaints based on the type of malignant disease, the burden of disease, and current oncologic therapeutic regimens.

### ACUTE MYELOGENOUS AND LYMPHOID LEUKEMIAS

#### *Acute Myelogenous Leukemia*

Patients with leukemia present with signs and symptoms secondary to the invasion of other organs by leukemic cells and decreased production of normal hematopoietic cells. Fever, malaise, and a viral-like syndrome are common presenting symptoms. Diffuse bony tenderness, as a result of expansion of the intramedullary space or periosteal infiltration by leukemic cells, is the initial symptom in 25% of patients.[9]

Acute myelogenous leukemia (AML) typically affects all three cells lines and results in anemia, thrombocytopenia, and neutropenia. Pallor, dyspnea, and chest pain reflect anemia, whereas petechiae, ecchymosis, and excessive bleeding are a result of thrombocytopenia. One third of patients will have significant infections on diagnosis.[10] Splenomegaly occurs in up to 50% of patients, and lymphadenopathy is rare.[9]

AML has several skin manifestations. Raised, nontender plaques or nodules (leukemia cutis) are manifest in many forms of leukemia, but they are most commonly seen in AML (**Fig. 203.2**).[11] Tender, pseudovesicular, erythematous plaques are a characteristic feature of Sweet syndrome, which may precede the diagnosis of AML by months (**Fig. 203.3**). Gingival hyperplasia may also be present (**Fig. 203.4**).

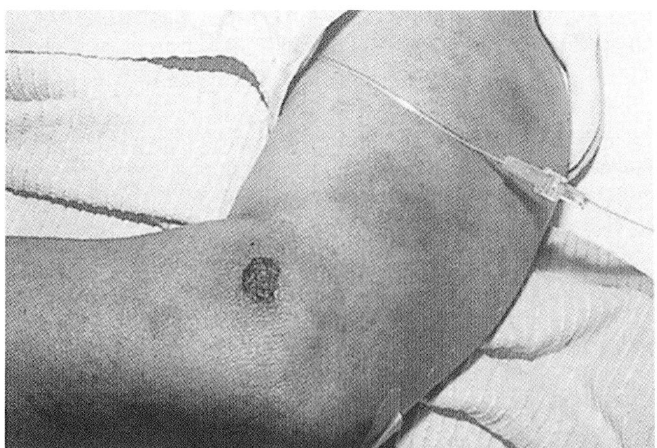

**Fig. 203.3 Sweet syndrome in a patient with acute myeloid leukemia.** Tender, pseudovesicular, erythematous plaques are a characteristic feature of this syndrome. (From Cohen PR. Acral erythema: a clinical review. Cutis 1993;51:175, with permission.)

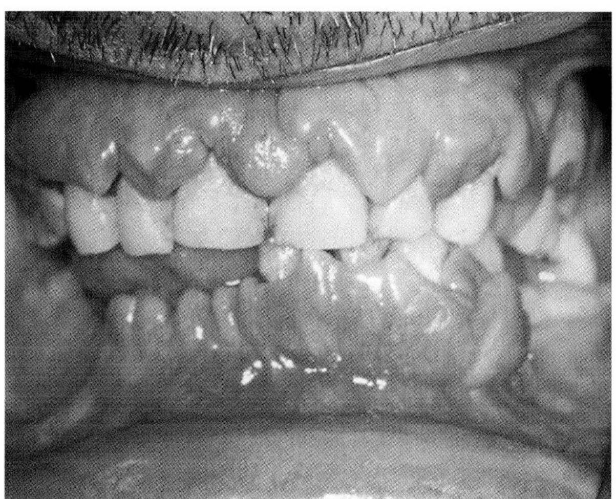

**Fig. 203.4 Generalized gingival hyperplasia in a patient with leukemia.** (Courtesy of Dr. Edward V. Zegarelli. In: Ibsen OAC, Phelan JA, editors. Oral pathology for the dental hygienist. 4th ed. St. Louis: Mosby; 2004.)

Central or peripheral nervous system signs and symptoms on initial presentation are rare, although cranial nerve palsies (most commonly fifth and seventh) or meningeal signs have been documented.[10]

## CHRONIC LYMPHOCYTIC LEUKEMIA

Chronic lymphocytic leukemia has a wide spectrum of presentations, but most commonly patients are diagnosed after an incidental finding such as enlarged lymph nodes (present in two thirds of patients at diagnosis), a palpable spleen (found in 40% of presenting patients), hepatomegaly (present in 10% of patients with a new diagnosis), or abnormal blood test results. Fatigue, lethargy, decreased appetite, weight loss, and decreased exercise tolerance are nonspecific, but they are again indicative of the effects of compromised hematopoiesis of all three cell lines. Central nervous system infiltration is rare; symptoms are more likely secondary to opportunistic infections.[12]

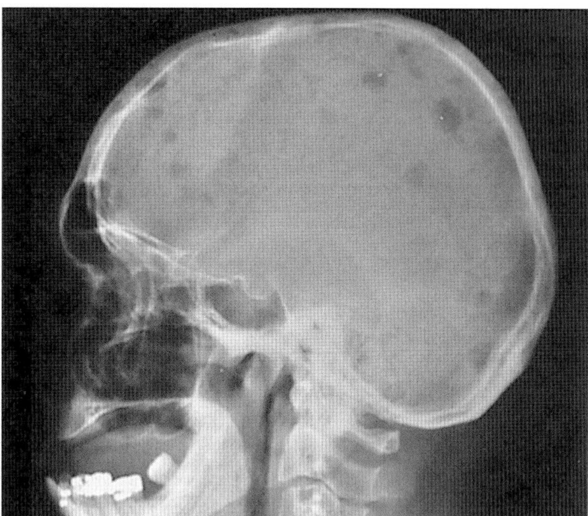

**Fig. 203.5 Lytic lesions.** (From Kyle RA, Rajkumar SV. Plasma cell disorders. In: Goldman L, Ausiello DA, editors. Cecil textbook of medicine. 22nd ed. Philadelphia: Saunders; 2004. pp. 1184–1195.)

## CHRONIC MYELOGENOUS LEUKEMIA

Thirty percent to 50% of patients diagnosed with chronic myelogenous leukemia are asymptomatic. Splenomegaly is present in 50% to 60%, and hepatomegaly occurs in 10% to 20% of new cases. Lymphadenopathy is rare.[13]

## NON-HODGKIN LYMPHOMA

Presentation of non-Hodgkin lymphoma is extremely variable, but patients most commonly seek medical evaluation for incidental painless, firm cervical, axillary, or inguinal adenopathy. Chest pain, cough, superior vena cava syndrome, abdominal pain, back pain, spinal cord compression, and symptoms of renal insufficiency may be present. Fevers, night sweats, and weight loss are also common symptoms.

## HODGKIN LYMPHOMA

Fever, night sweats, and weight loss are the classic "B" symptoms associated with Hodgkin lymphoma. Other classic signs are systemic pruritus and painful lymphadenopathy after drinking alcohol. Painless, rubbery, supradiaphragmatic lymphadenopathy, particularly of the neck and supraclavicular nodes, is common. Less than 10% of patients will have a subdiaphragmatic presentation.[14]

## PLASMA CELL DISORDERS

Fatigue and bone pain are the most common presenting symptoms of multiple myeloma.[15] Pain may be secondary to characteristic lytic lesions or pathologic fractures (**Fig. 203.5**). Focal weakness or paresthesias may be secondary to nerve root or spinal cord compression from extramedullary expansion of bony lesions.

## DIFFERENTIAL DIAGNOSIS, MEDICAL DECISION MAKING, AND TREATMENT

Once the diagnosis of a hematologic malignant disease is suspected, laboratory evaluation should be performed, including a complete blood cell count with manual differential, peripheral blood smear, chemistry studies (including uric acid,

**BOX 203.4 Differential Diagnosis of White Blood Cell Disorders by Signs and Symptoms**

**Fever (Nonlocalizing)**
- Granulocytopenia
  - Bacterial → fungal → breakthrough fungemia
  - Since the late 1990s, great increase of gram-positive organisms, often MRSA
- Cell-mediated immunodeficiency
  - Viral
  - Mycobacterial, fungal, nocardial, listerial
- Humoral immune deficiency
  - B-cell, splenectomy related

**Abdominal Pain**
- Chemotherapy-related nausea and dehydration
- Splenomegaly
- Obstructive adenopathy: jaundice, uropathy, or small bowel obstruction
- Organ-specific pain
  - Ascites or spontaneous bacterial peritonitis
  - Portal vein thrombosis
- Mesenteric ischemia
- Typhlitis (neutropenic enterocolitis)
- Zoster
- Constipation (opioid)
- Hypercalcemia
- Psychogenic (e.g., depression)

**Dyspnea**
- Pneumonia
- Pulmonary embolism
- Pleural effusion
- Pericardial effusion
- *Pneumocystis* pneumonia
- Acute respiratory distress syndrome
- Chemotherapeutic and radiographic toxicity
- Hyperviscosity leukostasis
- Paraneoplastic syndromes
- Heart failure
  - Chemotherapy related
- Adrenal insufficiency
- Thymus: pain and dyspnea with T-cell ALL infiltration
- Bronchiolitis obliterans organizing pneumonia
- Mass effect and obstruction
- Anemia
- Chronic obstructive pulmonary disease
- Anxiety disorder
- Superior vena cava syndrome

**Malaise and Body Pains**
- Elevated uric acid levels or gouty arthritis
- Osteolytic lesions
- Osteopenic fractures (corticosteroid induced)
- Hypercalcemia
- Oral mucositis
- Skin lesions
  - Systemic (hairy cell) vasculitis
  - Leukemia cutis
- Hyperviscosity leukostasis
- Tumor lysis syndrome
- Renal failure
- Anorexia of malignancy[17]
- Amyloidosis pains (accumulation of monoclonal plasma cells in tissues and organs, frequently the heart)[12]

*ALL,* Acute lymphocytic leukemia; *MRSA,* methicillin-resistant *Staphylococcus aureus.*

creatinine, potassium, phosphorus, and calcium), coagulation factors, and blood type and screen. If the patient is febrile, blood cultures (aerobic, anaerobic, and fungal) should also be obtained, and empiric antibiotics should be initiated early because many of these patients have functional neutropenia, even in the setting of normal neutrophil count, and are at high risk of bacteremia or sepsis.[16] Diagnostic imaging should be ordered based on the focality of patients' symptoms, but a chest radiograph is a general starting point to evaluate any of the intrathoracic complications associated with these malignant diseases. An electrocardiogram should be performed to evaluate for evidence of electrolyte abnormalities.

Patients presenting with hyperleukocytosis (an extreme elevation of the blast count or WBC count $>100,000/mm^3$) and many different symptoms affecting multiple organ systems are at an increased risk of hyperviscosity syndrome (see Box 203.5), a medical emergency with mortality rates as high as 40%.[17] Metabolic and electrolyte abnormalities are common. The most serious complication is tumor lysis syndrome, a result of the massive cell lysis, which releases intracellular urate, phosphate, and potassium (please refer to Chapter 201 for details on tumor lysis syndrome).

## CARDINAL PRESENTATIONS AND COMPLICATIONS OF PATIENTS WITH KNOWN WHITE BLOOD CELL CANCER

Abdominal pain, dyspnea, fever, and malaise are all key chief complaints that require a comprehensive ED evaluation in patients with WBC disorders. **Box 203.4** lists the differential diagnosis of these complaints.

### ABDOMINAL PAIN

Gastrointestinal symptoms are the most common chief complaints of patients with cancer who present to the ED.[3] Immunosuppressed patients represent a diagnostic challenge, because classic examination findings of an acute abdomen may be replaced by nonspecific signs or systems such as tachycardia, hypotension, and altered mental status.[18]

In addition to disorders present in the immunocompetent host, disorders secondary either to the malignant disease or to the therapy used to combat it should be considered. Opportunistic infections, intestinal obstruction, perforation, typhlitis, and venoocclusive disease of the liver (Budd-Chiari syndrome) should be considered in the differential diagnosis of

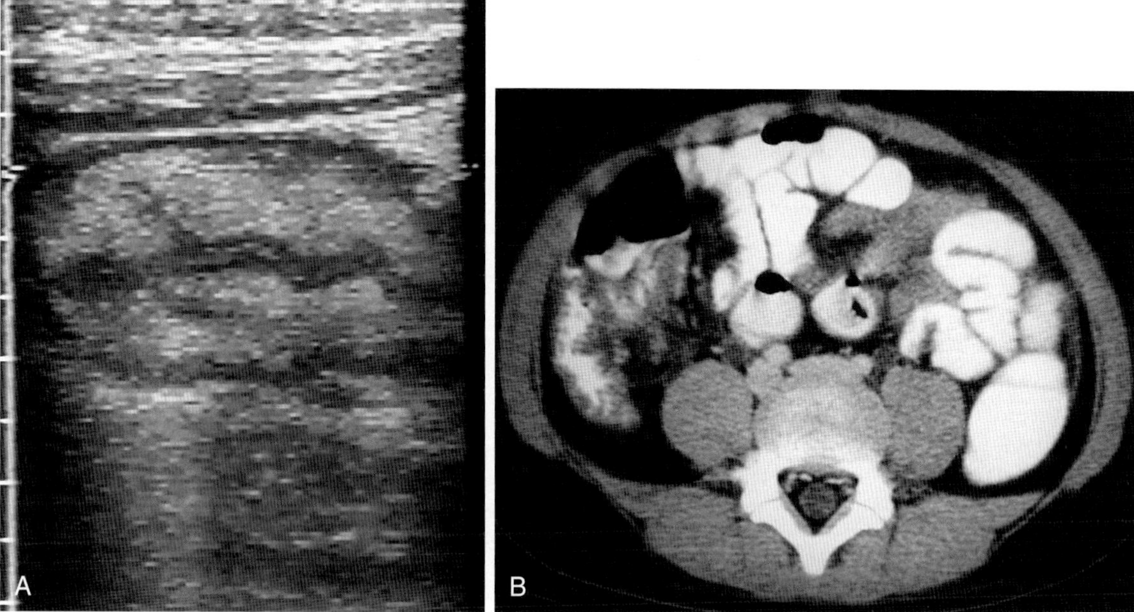


**Fig. 203.6 Typhlitis. A,** Ultrasound scan showing thickened bowel wall. **B,** Axial computed tomography showing thickening of the wall of the ascending colon. (From Adam A, Dixon AK, editors. Grainger and Allison's diagnostic radiology. 5th ed. Philadelphia: Churchill Livingstone; 2007.)

a patient with cancer who has an acute abdomen. In a retrospective series of patients with acute leukemia who developed severe abdominal infections during chemotherapy-induced neutropenia, 68% presented with enterocolitis (primarily bacteremia, but also fungal and viral infections).[19] A broad diagnostic strategy, including abdominal diagnostic imaging (computed tomography [CT] or ultrasound, or both), is usually necessary in the thorough evaluation of these patients.

Typhlitis, or neutropenic enterocolitis, is a necrotizing inflammation of the ascending colon or cecum that is a common cause of the acute abdomen in a neutropenic patient (**Fig. 203.6**).[18] Although the incidence varies (from 0.8% to 26%), typhilitis has a mortality rate of 50% and higher.[20] The pathogenesis is unclear, but theories have implicated failed mucosal integrity secondary to chemotherapy or the migration of bacteria causing bowel necrosis and hemorrhage secondary to the effects of neutropenia.[21] Several case reports have described typhlitis as a presentation of acute leukemia.[22,23] Signs and symptoms vary. In a retrospective case review of 10 patients, all presented with fever, and some had abdominal pain (most commonly right lower quadrant), nausea, diarrhea, and hypotension.[24] CT imaging shows bowel wall thickening and cecal distention. Ultrasound imaging may show bowel wall thickening but is not specific. Therefore, CT is recommended in addition to ultrasound, to assess potential complications, including colonic wall hemorrhage, pneumatosis intestinalis, pneumoperitoneum, and abscesses, more thoroughly.[25] Broad-spectrum antibiotics (covering enteric gram-negative organisms, *Pseudomonas,* and anaerobes including *Clostridium difficile*), bowel rest, surgical evaluation, and supportive care are recommended.

Hepatic venous outflow obstruction caused by thromboses, or Budd-Chiari syndrome, results from a hypercoagulable state or direct tumor invasion of the hepatic venous system. Venous stasis and hepatic congestion lead to cell death and eventual liver failure.[26] Symptoms include ascites, hepatomegaly, abdominal pain, jaundice, and, in severe cases, variceal bleeding and portal hypertension. Ultrasound scanning with Doppler is the initial imaging modality of choice; it has a sensitivity of more than 85%, but CT and magnetic resonance imaging are alternatives.[27] The initial management strategy consists of sodium restriction, diuretics, anticoagulation, and periodic paracentesis. Portosystemic shunting or liver transplantation is indicated for severe forms of Budd-Chiari syndrome.[26]

## DYSPNEA

Patients presenting to the ED with dyspnea should be approached with a rapid assessment of respiratory status and should be given immediate resuscitative care in the form of supplemental oxygen, assisted ventilation, or intubation with mechanical ventilation. Despite this initial universal approach to the dyspneic patient, investigation of the broad differential diagnosis is essential to formulating an emergency management plan.

Acute respiratory failure is the most common cause of admission to the intensive care unit (ICU) in patients with cancer, and it has an incidence of 10% to 50% and an overall mortality rate of 50%.[28] Patients with leukemia and lymphoma have a higher incidence of respiratory insufficiency as the cause of ICU admission than do patients with solid tumors.[28]

Common causes of acute respiratory failure in these patients include pulmonary infections (pneumonia), cardiogenic or noncardiogenic pulmonary edema, antineoplastic (chemotherapy or radiation) therapy-induced lung injury, venous thromboembolism, diffuse alveolar hemorrhage (DAH), airway obstruction, and underlying disease progression.[29]

Pneumonia is the most common cause of respiratory failure in patients with hematologic malignant diseases. *Streptococcus pneumoniae* and *Haemophilus influenzae* are the most common organisms in patients with leukemia and myeloma (impaired B-cell immunity). Patients with Hodgkin lymphoma (impaired T-cell immunity) are more likely to be infected with *Pneumocystis jiroveci,* mycobacteria and fungi, and viruses (including cytomegalovirus and herpes simplex virus). Presentation may be atypical. Although fever is common, cough and sputum are not, and findings on chest radiography may be normal. Chemotherapy-induced neutropenia can give rise to infection with *Staphylococcus aureus*, gram-negative bacilli (*Pseudomonas* and *Klebsiella*), and opportunistic fungi (*Aspergillus*).[30] Debilitation, malnourishment, prolonged bed rest, and central nervous system metastasis predispose oncologic patients to increased aspiration risk.[31]

Pulmonary edema may be cardiogenic, noncardiogenic, or a combination thereof because of several inciting events, including the use of cardiotoxic chemotherapeutic agents, infection, radiation, or transfusions. These patients are at a high risk of developing acute respiratory distress syndrome (ARDS).

Chemotherapy- and radiation-induced lung injury comprises another syndrome that may manifest with exertional dyspnea, low-grade fevers, and a nonproductive cough during or up to several months after treatment. The various diagnoses include interstitial pneumonitis, acute lung injury, ARDS, capillary leak syndrome, organizing pneumonia, hypersensitivity reaction, bronchospasm, and DAH.[30] On examination, bilateral inspiratory crackles may be auscultated, and diffuse or patch ground-glass opacities are seen on chest radiography and CT. Each syndrome requires a multipronged approach, but cessation of the culprit chemotherapeutic agent and treatment with systemic corticosteroids are general management principles.

Venous thromboembolism (deep venous thrombosis or pulmonary embolism) is an important cause of morbidity and mortality in patients with cancer and may be a predictor of worse overall prognosis.[32] Chemotherapeutic agents, intrinsic procoagulant tumor activity, indwelling catheters, immobilization, and surgery are risk factors for venous thromboembolism in oncologic patients. Ten percent of patients with lymphoma develop venous thromboembolism.[33] Presenting symptoms of dyspnea, pleurisy, and palpitations and signs of tachypnea, hypoxia, and dysrhythmias should prompt a thorough evaluation for venous thromboembolism.

DAH is common in patients with leukemia or multiple myeloma, after bone marrow transplantation, and in patients with thrombocytopenia (platelets < 50,000/mm$^3$). Total body irradiation, thoracic irradiation, and increased age are all risk factors for DAH.[30] Patients present with progressive dyspnea, cough, and fever but rarely hemoptysis. Chest radiography may show diffuse interstitial and alveolar infiltrates, and the diagnosis is confirmed by bronchoscopy. Supportive therapy includes corticosteroids, platelet transfusions, and mechanical ventilator support.

Transfusion-related acute lung injury may develop in those patients receiving red blood cells, platelets, or fresh frozen plasma. Patients develop fever, hypotension, hypoxemia, pulmonary hypertension, and noncardiogenic pulmonary edema within 6 hours of transfusion.[34] Treatment is supportive and often requires ventilatory support.

Airway obstruction may be secondary to locally advanced tumors in the airway or metastatic lesions to the mediastinum or tracheobronchial tree. Lymphoma may develop mediastinal masses that may cause stridor, dyspnea, hemoptysis, or cough.

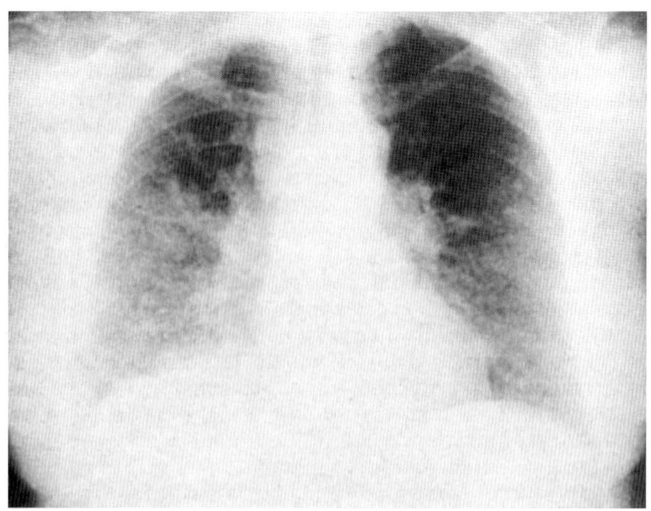

**Fig. 203.7 Chest radiograph showing pulmonary leukostasis in a patient with monoblastic leukemia and a white blood cell count of 150,000/mm$^3$.** (From Miller KB, Pihan G. Acute myeloid leukemia. In: Hoffman R, Benz Jr EJ, Shattil SJ, et al, editors. Hematology: basic principles and practice. 5th ed. Philadelphia: Churchill Livingstone; 2009.)

Chest radiography, CT, and bronchoscopy are used in combination to establish a diagnosis and guide therapy. Definitive airway management is difficult but may be essential in these patients. Eventual treatment may consist of stents, lasers, radiation therapy, or chemotherapy.

## PAIN

The most common complaint of patients with cancer who present to the ED is pain, with nausea or vomiting and weakness a close second and third most frequent chief complaints.[3] Although pain is nonspecific, the ED physician needs to be aware of critical, life-threatening diagnoses that may manifest with pain.

Hypercalcemia may occur in up to 30% of patients with cancer, and they may present with vague symptoms of nausea, vomiting, abdominal pain, or myalgias.[35] Hypercalcemia may lead to progressive neurologic symptoms, coma, renal failure, and arrhythmias. In multiple myeloma, hypercalcemia results from bone osteoclastic bone resorption. Lymphomas and myelomas hydroxylate vitamin D into 1,25-dihydroxyvitamin D (1.25(OH)2D), the active form of vitamin D, thus enhancing intestinal absorption of vitamin D and resulting in hypercalcemia.[35] This diagnosis is critical in this patient population because approximately 50% of these patients will die within 30 days.[36] The diagnosis is best made by using ionized calcium, and an electrocardiogram may show a shortened QT interval. The cornerstone of management is aggressive intravenous and oral hydration. Once volume repletion is achieved, loop diuretics are used for calcium excretion. Bisphosphonates, calcitonin, and steroids are other adjuncts, depending on the response to treatment and the primary cause of the elevated calcium concentration. Please refer to Chapter 201 for further details on hypercalcemia.

Acute blood hyperviscosity results from elevations of serum proteins (hyperviscosity syndrome) or WBCs (hyperleukocytosis) in the blood circulation. Leukocytosis and leukostasis (**Fig. 203.7**) have mortality rates that range from 20%

**BOX 203.5 Hyperviscosity Syndrome Presentation and Management**

**History**
- Waldenström macroglobulinemia
- Multiple myeloma
- Sjögren syndrome
- Rheumatoid arthritis
- Systemic lupus erythematosus
- Cryoglobulinemia
- Diabetes
- Human immunodeficiency virus infection

**Physical: Triad of Symptoms**
- Bleeding
- Visual disturbances
- Focal neurologic signs
  - Vertigo
  - Paresthesias
  - Headaches
  - Ataxia

**Diagnosis**
- Clinical
- Increased viscosity
  - More than 4 cp (normal, 1.4 to 1.8 cp)

**Management**
- Supportive
  - Judicious fluid resuscitation
  - Correction of electrolyte derangements
  - Antibiotics if underlying infection
- Plasma exchange
  - Indication: seizure or coma
  - Phlebotomize 1 to 2 units
  - Replace volume with normal saline solution
- Plasmapheresis
  - Establish central venous access
  - Contact plasmapheresis team
- Chemotherapy for underlying malignant disease

Adapted from Adams BD, Baker R, Lopez JA, Spencer S. Myeloproliferative disorders and hyperviscosity syndrome. Emerg Med Clin North Am 2009;27:459-76.

**BOX 203.6 Hyperleukocytosis Syndrome Presentation and Management**

**History**
- Leukemia
  - More common in AML and ALL
- Dyspnea
- Chest pain
- Neurologic symptoms
- Malaise

**Physical**
- Respiratory distress
- Altered mental status
- Focal neurologic deficits
- Limb ischemia

**Diagnosis**
- Laboratory values
  - Leukostasis: WBC > $100 \times 10^9$/L (AML), WBC > $400 \times 10^9$/L (ALL)
- Chest radiography
  - Normal, interstitial or alveolar infiltrates, pleural effusions

**Management**
- Leukapheresis
  - Central venous access
- Hydroxyurea
- Intravenous hydration

Adapted from Adams BD, Baker R, Lopez JA, Spencer S. Myeloproliferative disorders and hyperviscosity syndrome. Emerg Med Clin North Am 2009;27:459-76.

*ALL,* Acute lymphocytic leukemia; *AML,* acute myelogenous leukemia; *WBC,* white blood cell.

to 40%, and these conditions therefore represent an emergency diagnosis.[17] **Boxes 203.5 and 203.6** outline the presentations and management of both conditions.

## NEXT STEPS OF CARE: ADMISSIONS (INPATIENT AND OUTPATIENT)

Overall patient disposition is based on clinical assessment, the ability to follow-up with a primary care physician or oncologist, and the patient's home environment.

A patient with a new diagnosis of malignant disease may require an in-depth work-up that may be more rapidly facilitated by admission and coordination between oncology staff and primary care physicians.

For patients with a known cancer diagnosis, positive pressure isolation rooms should be considered in patients with significant neutropenia, in bone marrow transplant recipients, or in patients with other high-risk immunocompromised states (after intensive chemotherapy or solid organ transplantation). Intensive care monitoring should be reserved for patients who are critically ill, usually from complications of immunocompromise or chemotherapy.

## SUGGESTED READINGS

Matasar MJ, Zelenetz AD. Overview of lymphoma diagnosis and management. Radiol Clin North Am 2008;46:175-98.

Mattu A, editor. Cancer emergencies. Emerg Med Clin North Am 2009;27:174-354.

Menon, KV, Shah V, Kamath PS. The Budd Chiari syndrome. N Engl J Med 2004;350:578-85.

Nau KM, Lewis WD. Multiple myeloma: diagnosis and treatment. Am Fam Physician 2008;78:853-9.

Swenson KK, Rose MA, Ritz L, et al. Recognition and evaluation of oncology-related symptoms in the emergency department. Ann Emerg Med 1995;26:12-7.

## REFERENCES

***References can be found on Expert Consult @ www.expertconsult.com.***

# 204 Emergency Management of Red Blood Cell Disorders

*Ugo A. Ezenkwele*

**KEY POINTS**

- Anemia is the absolute reduction in the amount of oxygen-carrying pigment hemoglobin (Hgb) that represents a relative decrease in the capacity of blood to carry oxygen to the tissues.
- Anemia is not a diagnosis. It is an indication of an underlying disease, disorder, or deficiency.
- Transfusion of red blood cells provides immediate correction of low Hgb levels helpful in the context of either severe anemia (in which the Hgb is <8.0 g/dL) or life-threatening anemia (in which the Hgb is <6.5 g/dL).
- Most cases of anemia (chronic) do not require acute interventions and drug therapy in the emergency department (ED). Patients can be referred for follow-up to their primary care physician or gastroenterologist.
- The cardinal features of acute chest syndrome are fever, pleuritic chest pain, referred abdominal pain, cough, lung infiltrates, and hypoxia.
- Pneumococcal sepsis is a leading cause of death among infants with sickle cell anemia because a damaged spleen cannot clear pneumococci from the blood.
- Transfusions are not needed for the usual anemia or episodes of pain associated with sickle cell disease.
- Splenic sequestration is life-threatening and requires intensive care admission with transfusion and possible splenectomy.
- ED-based pain management protocols have been shown to decrease ED visits and hospitalizations and to increase use of primary care clinics by patients with sickle cell disease.
- Patients with severe pain should be given an opiate parenterally at frequent, fixed intervals until the pain has diminished, at which time the dose of the opiate can be tapered and then stopped, and oral analgesic therapy can be instituted.
- For polycythemia vera, phlebotomy is the only therapy indicated for isolated erythrocytosis when its mechanism cannot be established.

## PERSPECTIVE

The red blood cell (RBC) disorders include a distinct group of disease entities that are diverse in presentation yet similar in their emergency diagnosis and management. These disorders include anemia (acute, chronic), sickle cell anemia, and polycythemia vera (PV). Patients with both malignant and nonmalignant hematologic disease may present with dramatic and often life-threatening complications. Emergency management of these disorders requires a thorough understanding of the underlying pathologic processes, as well as a concise and systematic approach to diagnosis, stabilization, and treatment.

# ANEMIA

## EPIDEMIOLOGY

Anemia is more common than is generally realized. The World Health Organization defines *anemia* as a condition characterized by hemoglobin (Hgb) levels lower than 13 g/dL in men or lower than 12 g/dL in women.[1] Data from the National Center for Health Statistics that likely underestimate the frequency of anemia indicated that approximately 3.4 million U.S residents have anemia, and that the groups with the highest prevalence are women, African Americans,[2] older persons, and those with the lowest incomes. Using laboratory data from the general U.S. population, the second National Health and Nutrition Survey reported anemia to be the most prevalent in infants, teenage girls, young women, and older men.[3] In another survey, the prevalence of anemia declined significantly among U.S women and children from 1988 to 2002, but the cause of this decline was unknown.[4] In persons 65 years and older, anemia was present in 11.0% of men and 10.2% of women, and the prevalence rose to more than 20% in people 85 years and older. One third of the cases of anemia were the result of nutritional deficiencies, and one third of cases were secondary to chronic illness, including but not limited to chronic renal disease.

## PATHOPHYSIOLOGY

Anemia is classified into three broad categories: (1) disorders of decreased RBC production, (2) disorders of increased RBC destruction, and (3) disorders resulting from RBC loss. Disorders in each of these categories may manifest differently and ultimately have their own management approaches (**Table 204.1**).

RBCs, or erythrocytes, contain fluid Hgb encased in a lipid membrane and are the predominant cellular component of blood. RBCs make up 45% of the blood volume and are responsible for carrying oxygen from the lungs to the peripheral tissues. A 70-kg person has approximately 30 trillion RBCs, resulting in approximately 300 million RBCs in each drop of blood. The normal RBC is composed of three types of Hgb: Hgb A (97%), Hgb F (1%) or fetal Hgb, and Hgb $A_2$ (2%).[5] Hgb A is composed of two β-globin chains and two α-globin chains bonded to four iron-containing heme groups. Hgb production requires iron, the synthesis of the protoporphyrin ring, and the production of the globin chains. Reductions in any of these processes result in anemia.

RBC precursors develop in bone marrow at rates usually determined by the body's demand for sufficient circulating Hgb to oxygenate tissues adequately. Once produced, the mature RBC remains in circulation for approximately 120 days before it is engulfed and destroyed. Given the life span, chronic anemias that are caused by RBC underproduction generally develop and progress slowly over weeks to months. In contrast, acute anemias that are caused by bleeding or hemolysis generally occur rapidly over days to weeks. The tempo of anemia development depends on the pace of bleeding or hemolysis in relation to RBC production. The aggressiveness of intervention and management depends on the acuteness of onset and the severity of the clinical presentation.

## PRESENTING SIGNS AND SYMPTOMS

Because anemia either can be a primary disorder or can occur secondary to other systemic processes, a careful history and physical examination provide valuable insight into the potential cause. All patients require a focused yet thorough history. For critically ill and noncommunicative patients, the history

**Table 204.1 Classification of Anemia**

| CATEGORY | CLASSIFICATION | DISEASE PROCESS |
|---|---|---|
| Decreased RBC production (hypoproliferative) | Microcytic | Iron deficiency<br>Thalassemia<br>Sideroblastic<br>Chronic disease (neoplasm, infection, diabetes, uremia, thyroid disease, cirrhosis) |
| | Normocytic | Primary bone marrow problem (aplastic, myeloid metaplasia, myelofibrosis, myelophthisic anemia, Diamond-Blackfan anemia)<br>Secondary bone marrow problem (uremia, liver disease, endocrinopathy, chronic inflammation) |
| | Macrocytic | Folic acid deficiency<br>Liver disease<br>Vitamin $B_{12}$ deficiency<br>Scurvy<br>Hypothyroidism<br>Chemotherapy, immunosuppressive therapy |
| Increased RBC destruction (hemolytic) | Intrinsic | Membrane disorder (spherocytosis, sickle cell, stem cell disorder, elliptocytosis, spur cell) |
| | Extrinsic | Hemoglobin disorder (thalassemia, autoimmune, hemoglobinopathies)<br>Infections (hepatitis and cytomegalovirus, Epstein-Barr virus, typhoid fever, *Escherichia coli*)<br>Medications (penicillin, antimalarials, sulfa drugs, or acetaminophen)<br>Leukemia or lymphoma<br>Autoimmune disorders (systemic lupus erythematosus, rheumatoid arthritis, Wiskott-Aldrich syndrome, ulcerative colitis)<br>Enzyme defect (G6PD) |
| RBC loss (hemorrhagic) | Acute or chronic | Gastrointestinal tract<br>Traumatic<br>Intraperitoneal<br>Extraperitoneal<br>Gynecologic<br>Urinary<br>Pelvic<br>Drug related<br>Epistaxis, hemoptysis |

*G6PD*, Glucose-6-phosphate dehydrogenase; *RBC*, red blood cell.

should be obtained from caretakers, paramedics, or primary care physicians.

The extent of the symptoms, whether mild or life-threatening, depends on several contributing factors. If anemia develops acutely, compensatory adjustments may not have enough time to take hold, and consequently, the patient may have more pronounced symptoms than if the anemia developed over weeks to months. Furthermore, underlying chronic comorbidities such as myocardial ischemia and transient cerebral ischemia may be unmasked in the presence of anemia.

## ACUTE ANEMIA

Patients with anemia resulting from acute bleeding present with hypovolemia. The combined effects of hypovolemia and anemia may cause tissue hypoxia or anoxia through diminished cardiac output, resulting in decreased oxygen-carrying capacity (anemic hypoxia). When the Hgb concentration falls to less than 7.5 g/dL as a result of losses ranging from 5% to 15% in blood volume, the resting cardiac output rises significantly, with an increase in both heart rate and stroke volume. These patients are symptomatic at rest and may be aware of this hyperdynamic state; they often complain of palpitations, lightheadedness, dizziness, or a pounding pulse. Larger losses cause progressive increases in heart rate, decreases in arterial blood pressure, and evidence of organ hypoperfusion. Hypovolemic shock is seen when vital organ systems such as the kidneys, the central nervous system, and the heart are affected. In the emergency department (ED), a source of blood loss may be readily apparent on evaluation (e.g., trauma with hemorrhage from the extremities, gastrointestinal bleeding, menstrual blood loss); however, this may not be the case in, for example, aortic dissection or retroperitoneal hemorrhage.

Mild to moderate hypovolemia may be tolerated in the young patient. In older patients, however, these responses are modified by the rapidity of blood loss and by characteristics such as comorbid illnesses, preexisting volume status, Hgb values, and the use of medications that have cardiac or peripheral vascular effects (e.g., beta-blockers, antihypertensive agents). Therefore, the emergency physician (EP) should elicit a thorough and focused history, including medications, while assessing the airway, stabilizing breathing, and initiating resuscitation as needed.

## CHRONIC ANEMIA

Because anemia can be a primary disorder or can occur secondary to hypoproliferation or chronic blood loss, a careful history and physical examination provide valuable insight into the potential cause. Individuals with mild anemia are often asymptomatic and are able to sustain a relatively normal level of function at Hgb levels that are significantly lower than normal. Other patients may present with myriad nonspecific symptoms (**Box 204.1**). Because fatigue is nonspecific, determining the concomitant presence of a systemic inflammatory disorder, infection, or malignant disease may be critical in determining the underlying causes of anemia.

Past medical history is quite informative. For instance, a history of diabetes mellitus is associated with significantly impaired renal production of erythropoietin.[6] Certain medications are associated with bone marrow depression. Therefore, all pharmacologic agents, both prescribed drugs and over-the-counter agents, including alternative medications, should be reviewed. Occupational history is relevant, as in the case of welders, who may have been exposed to lead or other agents potentially toxic to the bone marrow. Social history is important because a history of intravenous drug use may suggest the possibility of human immunodeficiency virus infection, which can be associated with anemia.[7] Dietary history is relevant. For example, the finding of pica in adults (most commonly from the ingestion of nonfood items) is well known to be associated with iron deficiency anemia. A family history of anemia is important; for example, adults with congenital hereditary spherocytosis often develop symptoms later in life.

Physical findings in either acute or chronic anemia are myriad and often nonspecific, and they may relate to the underlying disease process and the duration (**Table 204.2**). Pathognomonic findings are not the norm. Furthermore, patients with chronic anemia usually do not have the typical physical findings associated with acute anemia.

**BOX 204.1 Chronic Anemia**

Fatigue
Weakness
Irritability
Headache
Dizziness (vertigo, especially postural)

**Table 204.2 Physical Findings in Anemia**

| ORGAN | FINDING |
|---|---|
| Skin | Pallor<br>Usefulness limited by color of skin, Hgb concentration, and fluctuation of blood flow to skin<br>Palmar crease color a better indicator, if as pale as surrounding skin, Hgb usually <7 g/dL |
| Hematologic | Purpura, petechiae, and jaundice |
| Cardiovascular | Tachycardia<br>Wide pulse pressure<br>Orthostatic hypotension<br>Hyperdynamic precordium<br>Systolic eject murmur over pulmonic area |
| Respiratory | Tachypnea<br>Rales |
| Gastrointestinal | Hepatomegaly and/or splenomegaly<br>Ascites<br>Masses<br>Positive result on Hemoccult test |
| Ophthalmologic | Pale conjunctiva<br>Scleral icterus<br>Retinal hemorrhages |
| Neurologic | Peripheral neuritis or neuropathy<br>Mental status changes |

*Hgb,* Hemoglobin.

**Table 204.3 Differential Diagnosis of Anemia**

| CATEGORY | DIFFERENTIAL DIAGNOSIS | CBC CLUES |
|---|---|---|
| Microcytic | Iron deficiency anemia | Elevated RDW<br>Thrombocytosis |
| | Thalassemia | Normal or elevated RBC count<br>Normal or elevated RDW |
| | Anemia of chronic disease | Normal RDW |
| Normocytic | Hemolysis | Normal or elevated RDW<br>Thrombocytosis |
| | Bleeding | Unchanged |
| | Nutritional anemia | Elevated RDW |
| | Anemia of chronic disease | Normal RDW |
| | Primary bone marrow disease | Elevated RDW<br>Leukocytosis<br>Thrombocytosis<br>Monocytosis |
| Macrocytic | Alcohol use, liver disease | Normal RDW<br>Thrombocytopenia |
| | Drug induced | Elevated RDW |
| | Bone marrow disorder | Elevated RDW |
| | Hypothyroidism | Normal RDW |
| | Hemolysis | Normal or elevated RDW |
| | Nutritional | Elevated RDW |

*CBC,* Complete blood cell count; *RBC,* red blood cell; *RDW,* red blood cell distribution width.

## DIFFERENTIAL DIAGNOSIS AND DIAGNOSTIC TESTING

The differential diagnosis of anemia is myriad, as documented in **Table 204.3**. Once anemia is suspected, the initial diagnosis involves the complete blood count (CBC). The variables to focus on when examining the CBC are hematocrit (as a general indicator of anemia or polycythemia), mean corpuscular volume ([MCV] a key parameter for the classification of anemias), RBC distribution width (a relatively useful parameter in the differential diagnosis of anemia), RBC count (an increased RBC count associated with anemia is characteristic in the thalassemia trait), platelet count (to detect either thrombocytopenia or thrombocytosis), and white blood cell (WBC) count with differential (usually gives important clues to the diagnosis of acute leukemia and chronic lymphoid or myeloid disorders, as well as clues to the presence of leukopenia and neutropenia).[8]

The first step in approaching anemia is to classify the process as microcytic (MCV < 80 fL), normocytic (MCV, 80 to 100 fL), or macrocytic (MCV > 100 fL). Clues to the diagnostic possibilities for the three major classes are listed in Table 204.3.

Along with anemia, another characteristic laboratory feature of hemolysis is reticulocytosis, the normal response of the bone marrow to the peripheral loss of RBCs. Patients with aplastic anemia or some other insult to the bone marrow from drugs or toxins have a reduced reticulocyte count. Some patients require special correction of their reticulocyte count (see the "Facts and Formulas" box).

$SI = \frac{SV}{BSA}$ **FACTS AND FORMULAS**

Corrected reticulocyte count (%) = Observed count × Measured count (%) / 45%

Finch reticulation production index = Corrected reticulocyte count (%) / Expected maturation time (days)

- Patients with hemolytic anemias may require a *Finch reticulocyte count,* which corrects for the anemia and the expected maturation time.
- For example, a 2-day life span (versus a 1-day life span, typically) is used for immature reticulocytes. The Finch count is the measured reticulocyte count, multiplied by the measured hematocrit level, divided by 45, and then divided by 2.
- Patients with sickle cell disease may use a simple corrected reticulocyte count.
- This is the *measured reticulocyte count,* multiplied by the measured hematocrit level, divided by 45.
- Normal reticulocyte counts are 0.5% to 1%.

Finch CA, Marshall PN, Brecher G, et al. Method for reticulocyte counting. NCCLS proposed standard H16-P. Villanova, Penn: National Committee for Clinical Laboratory Standards; 1985.

Blood type and cross should be sent to the blood bank so that type-specific or type-matched and crossmatched blood can be readied. Other tests to obtain are unconjugated bilirubin and lactate dehydrogenase. These values are increased when RBCs are destroyed. In patients with severe intravascular hemolysis, the binding capacity of haptoglobin is exceeded rapidly, and free Hgb is filtered by the glomeruli, thus leading to decreased haptoglobin and increased hemoglobinuria or urobilinogen levels.

Imaging studies are disease specific and depend on the patient's symptoms. Chest radiographs are indicated in all patients with significant anemia. Cardiomyopathy may be present in patients with chronic anemia. An electrocardiogram is required for older patients, those with chest pain, patients with profound anemia, or those who have an underlying disease or increased risk factors for cardiac ischemia.

Patients with blood loss may benefit from an ultrasound examination, which is a quick, noninvasive, and relatively simple bedside test useful for diagnosing intraperitoneal bleeding. The focused abdominal sonography for trauma (FAST) examination detects blood in the hepatorenal fossa, paracolic gutters, splenorenal area, and pelvis. Ultrasound is also useful for detecting pregnancy-related bleeding, especially that emanating from a ruptured ectopic pregnancy. Stable patients with intraabdominal blood loss benefit from computed tomography (CT) scanning. CT scanning has sensitivities similar to those of ultrasound, yet it identifies causes, including retroperitoneal, pelvic, and subcapsular sites, more clearly.

A nasogastric tube may be indicated in the acute setting to diagnose and manage an ongoing upper gastrointestinal hemorrhage. Bile must be aspirated to rule out bleeding proximal to the ligament of Treitz. Once upper gastrointestinal bleeding is established, esophagogastroduodenoscopy is the study of choice for determining the source of bleeding and for treatment. Emergency esophagogastroduodenoscopy can be performed in the ED, and its use is indicated in the hemodynamically unstable patient. Consultation with a gastroenterologist is required. Sigmoidoscopy or colonoscopy may be useful in diagnosing and treating lower gastrointestinal bleeding, but it is rarely helpful in the acute setting.

## TREATMENT

After anemia is identified by a CBC determination in the ED, management is aided by an approach that categorizes anemia as a symptom caused by the decrease in Hgb, rather than as an isolated diagnosis (see the "Priority Actions" box). Like fever, anemia is a symptom of disease that requires investigation to determine the underlying origin.

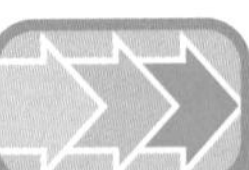

### PRIORITY ACTIONS

1. Determine the patient's hemodynamic status. The need for transfusion is often limited to those in hypovolemic shock.
2. If the patient is unstable, initiate resuscitation with crystalloids.
3. Once the patient is stabilized, blood transfusions are widely used as a rapid and effective therapeutic intervention in the context of either severe anemia (Hgb $< 8.0$ g/dL) or life-threatening anemia (Hgb $< 6.5$ g/dL).[9]
4. Look for the underlying cause and attempt to correct it.

*Hgb,* Hemoglobin.

Patients with long-standing or chronic anemias are able to compensate and do not require transfusion, especially if the Hgb is greater than 9.0 g/dL. Patients who are expected to respond to the administration of a specific agent such as folic acid, iron, or vitamin $B_{12}$ can usually be spared transfusions. If the anemia has precipitated an episode of congestive heart failure or myocardial ischemia, prompt administration of packed RBCs is indicated. For some patients in the ED, treatment can be begun without waiting for a definitive outpatient evaluation. For example, prenatal vitamins and iron replacement can be begun in the pregnant patient with anemia. In symptomatic pregnant patients, parenteral iron is preferred.[10] Megaloblastic anemia resulting from folic acid or vitamin $B_{12}$ deficiency can be treated with parenteral cobalamin (1000 g/day) or oral folic acid (1 mg/day). Erythropoietin therapy remains an option for patients undergoing elective surgical procedures or receiving chemotherapy and in patients with chronic heart failure or acquired immunodeficiency syndrome. In the acute setting, however, specifically in symptomatic heart failure, the role of erythropoietin therapy remains to be defined.[11,12]

## DISPOSITION

Fortunately, most patients have chronic anemia without blood loss and can be managed conservatively. In many cases, acute interventions and drug therapy are not indicated in the ED, and patients can be referred for follow-up to their primary care physicians.

Emergency consultation and hospital admission are required for patients presenting with hypovolemia or active bleeding who demonstrate a considerable drop in Hgb and hematocrit values when compared with previous values. A Hgb value of less than 8.0 g/dL in a symptomatic patient is enough to warrant admission for replacement of blood products. Patients who have underlying disease such as cardiac ischemia or congestive heart failure and who are now symptomatic and complaining of chest pain, tachypnea, or shortness of breath because of their anemia also require admission. Patients with new-onset or worsening pancytopenia require urgent consultation. Finally, admission is indicated for those patients who may not comply with follow-up or those in whom the clinician anticipates the need for an extensive work-up. Admission is to a medical ward bed, intermediate unit, or intensive care bed, depending on the patient's presenting symptoms.

# SICKLE CELL ANEMIA

## EPIDEMIOLOGY

Sickle cell disease (SCD), characterized by lifelong hemolytic anemia and many different painful and debilitating vasoocclusive events, occurs in 70,000 to 80,000 U.S. residents of African, Mediterranean, or Middle Eastern descent. In the United States, the life expectancy for patients with SCD is shortened by approximately 30 years, whereas in Africa, where comprehensive medical care is less readily available, death in early childhood is usual.[13] Eight percent of African Americans are heterozygous carriers of the sickle cell trait; approximately 40% of their Hgb is Hgb S. They do not have anemia and need neither treatment nor occupational restrictions.

## PATHOPHYSIOLOGY

SCD is an inherited condition caused by a point mutation in the β-globin gene (Hgb B) that causes the substitution of valine for glutamic acid at position 6 of the β-globin chain (Glu6Val). This mutation results in the abnormal Hgb S[14] (**Fig. 204.1**). When deoxygenated, Hgb S polymerizes, thus damaging the sickle RBC. These sickle cells are short-lived

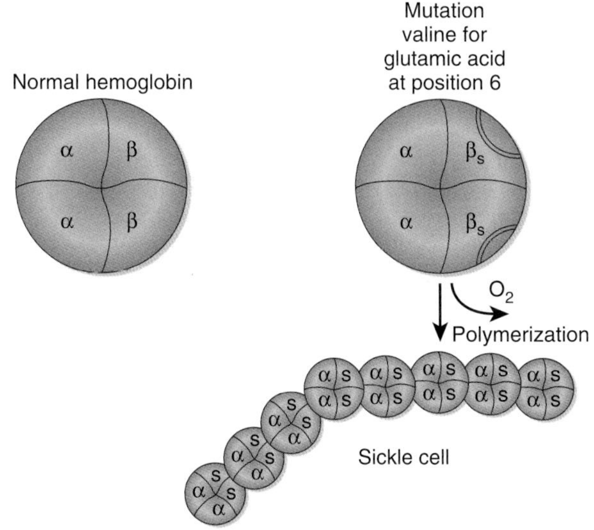


**Fig. 204.1 Sickle cell disease.**

and interact with endothelial cells, WBCs, platelets, and other plasma components to initiate the vasoocclusive manifestations associated with SCD.[15] Among hemolytic anemias, the vasoocclusive features of SCD are unique. By occluding small blood vessels and sometimes large vessels, sickle cells cause vascular injury (**Fig. 204.2**).

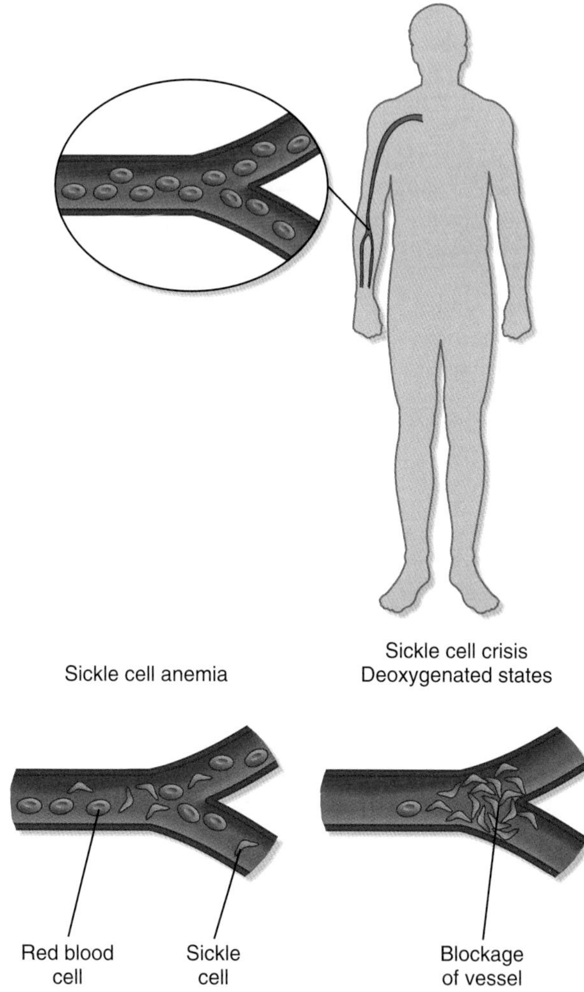


**Fig. 204.2 By occluding small blood vessels and sometimes large ones, sickle cells cause vascular injury.**

## PRESENTING SIGNS AND SYMPTOMS

Vasoocclusion, which is responsible for most of the severe complications of SCD, can occur wherever blood flows. The clinical features of SCD are outlined in **Table 204.4**.

### PAINFUL EPISODES

Acute painful crisis in SCD is a frequent complication and considerably diminishes the quality of life of patients with this disease. Approximately 60% of patients have an episode of severe pain. A few patients have severe pain almost constantly. Episodes of pain are sometimes triggered by infection, extreme temperatures, or physical or emotional stress, but more often they are unprovoked and begin with little warning.

### ACUTE CHEST SYNDROME

The *acute chest syndrome* is the leading cause of death and hospitalization among patients with SCD. Affecting approximately 40% of all patients with sickle cell anemia, it is the second most common reason for hospitalization and the leading cause of intensive care unit admission and premature death in patients with SCD.[16] Its cardinal features are fever, pleuritic chest pain, referred abdominal pain, cough, lung infiltrates, and hypoxia.[17] It is most common but least severe in children, can occur postoperatively, and when recurrent, can lead to pulmonary hypertension, restrictive lung disease, and eventually right-sided heart failure and death.[16]

**Table 204.4 Clinical Complications of Sickle Cell Disease**

| TYPE | CLINICAL FEATURES |
|---|---|
| Vasoocclusive complications | Pain crises<br>Acute chest syndrome<br>Splenic sequestration<br>Cerebrovascular crisis<br>Priapism<br>Liver disease<br>Leg ulcers<br>Spontaneous abortion<br>Osteonecrosis<br>Renal crisis<br>Retinopathy |
| Infectious complications | Osteomyelitis<br>*Escherichia coli* sepsis<br>*Streptococcus pneumoniae* sepsis |
| Hemolytic complications | Cholelithiasis<br>Anemia<br>Aplastic anemia |

Asthma has been associated with multiple complications of SCD, including acute chest syndrome. Asthma is an independent risk factor for mortality in children with SCD, and it confers a twofold higher risk of death.[18]

## CEREBROVASCULAR CRISIS

Cerebrovascular disease is the second leading cause of mortality and a common cause of morbidity in sickle cell anemia: approximately 10% of patients have a clinical stroke by age 20 years, and another 22% have evidence of silent infarction on magnetic resonance imaging. Manifestations of neurologic complications may include overt clinical stroke or subtler neuropsychological abnormalities often associated with subclinical stroke. Risk factors for ischemic stroke presentation in SCD include prior transient ischemic attacks, a decrease in steady-state Hgb, a history of acute chest syndrome, and an increase in systolic blood pressure. Risk factors for hemorrhagic stroke include a decrease in steady-state Hgb and an increase in steady-state WBC.

## RIGHT UPPER QUADRANT SYNDROME

*Right upper quadrant syndrome* is manifested by any or all of the following features: hyperbilirubinemia, abdominal pain, fever, right upper quadrant abdominal tenderness, hepatomegaly, abnormalities on liver function testing, and hepatic failure. Possible causes include cholelithiasis, viral hepatitis, biliary cholestasis, and hepatic ischemia. Cholelithiasis occurs in children as young as 3 to 4 years of age and is eventually found in approximately 70% of patients; this condition often necessitates cholecystectomy once right upper quadrant pain is identified.

The three acute hepatic syndromes seen in SCD are acute hepatic cell crisis, acute hepatic sequestration crisis, and sickle cell intrahepatic cholestasis. Intrahepatic cholestasis is benign and may be associated with severe hyperbilirubinemia that resolves in 7 to 10 days, especially in children.[19] A syndrome more common in adults is associated with fever, leukocytosis, abdominal pain, and deteriorating liver function, as indicated by measurement of liver enzymes. This hepatic crisis usually progresses to hepatic failure, coagulopathy, encephalopathy, and death.

## PRIAPISM

Priapism is a sustained, painful, and unwanted erection of the penis that pathophysiologically is the result of an accumulation of sickled RBCs in the corpora cavernosa that cause ischemia or low flow. Approximately 30% of male patients with SCD who are less than 20 years old report at least one episode of priapism, whereas frequencies of 30% to 45% are estimated for adult men. This condition is most common in patients with the greatest amount of hemolysis. Postpubertal male patients tend to have more prolonged episodes of priapism and have a less favorable prognosis for future potency.[20] One sequela is impotence; therefore, for the EP, the utmost priority in these patients is detumescence, especially within the first 12 hours.

## SPLENIC SEQUESTRATION

Splenic sequestration, caused by sickled cells trapped in the splenic circulation, results in precipitous decreases in Hgb concentration and rapid enlargement of the spleen. This condition may be life-threatening. It is common in infants and young children and is less common in older children and adults because the spleen is significantly fibrotic in these patients by the age of 5 years. *Acute splenic sequestration crisis* generally is defined as an acute drop in Hgb levels (>2 g/dL) associated with splenomegaly, reticulocytosis, and signs of intravascular volume depletion. Drops in Hgb levels greater than 4 g/dL are associated with 35% mortality. Splenic sequestration carries a 15% mortality rate and is the second leading cause of death among children. It may manifest as hypotension (caused by shock from worsening anemia) associated with an enlarged, tender spleen. Fatigue, listlessness, and pallor have also been described. An association between this crisis and acute viral infections exist, especially parvovirus B19 infection.

## TRANSIENT APLASTIC CRISIS

Aplastic crisis occurs in children with sickle cell anemia in response to transient suppression of erythropoiesis, most often because of infection with parvovirus B19, the same etiologic agent that causes erythema infectiosum ("fifth disease"). This crisis is usually a unique event in the life of a patient and suggests the induction of long-lasting, protective immunity. Although self-limited, aplastic crisis can cause severe, occasionally fatal, anemia that precipitates congestive heart failure, cerebrovascular accidents, and acute splenic sequestration. WBC and platelet counts may fall somewhat during transient aplastic crisis, especially in patients with functioning spleens. Aplastic crisis may be also be precipitated by other infections, including infections with *Streptococcus pneumoniae,* other streptococci, *Salmonella,* and Epstein-Barr virus. Children present with signs of severe anemia, such as tachycardia and pallor.

## STREPTOCOCCUS PNEUMONIAE SEPSIS

The incidence of invasive *S. pneumoniae* infection is 20- to 100-fold higher in children with SCD than in the general population. Penicillin prophylaxis for children with sickle cell anemia reduces the incidence of invasive pneumococcal infection by 84%, independent of pneumococcal immunization status.

# DIFFERENTIAL DIAGNOSIS AND DIAGNOSTIC TESTING

Patients with SCD frequently require immediate medical attention because of the severity of their disease and its potential complications. Understanding the various presenting symptoms and staying alert for severe manifestations of the disease are important for EPs (see the "Priority Actions" box). Diagnostic testing is often focused, depending on the presenting symptoms. In most patients, however, a basic set of laboratory tests should be obtained. Baseline laboratory values are helpful, as well as knowledge of the patient's medication history, the severity and frequency of previous crisis, and any surgical complications.

Emergency management depends on clinical presentation and can be symptom specific. Patients with known SCD should have a CBC and a reticulocyte count. These tests are necessary to help screen for severe anemia, aplastic crisis, sequestration crisis, and infection. A major drop in Hgb (e.g., >2 g/dL) from baseline values indicates a hematologic crisis.

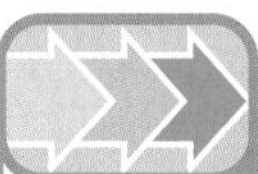

**PRIORITY ACTIONS**

**Bony Pain?**
Does the patient have evidence of trauma or infection?
If not, consider osteomyelitis. Although *Salmonella* is commonly described, *Staphylococcus aureus* is the predominant organism. Admit for intravenous antibiotics.

**Diffuse or Isolated Pain?**
Does the patient have any identifiable triggers (i.e., infection, dehydration, hypoxia, pregnancy, cold exposure, acidosis, recent flight in unpressurized aircraft)?
If yes, assess and treat underlying cause. If not, consider whether this is a usual vasoocclusive crisis; inquire about onset, duration, location, and a history of previous episodes. Treat with analgesics, preferably opiates.

**Abdominal Pain, Nausea, and Vomiting?**
Does the patient have pancreatitis, appendicitis, peptic ulcer disease, diverticulitis, colitis, or renal colic?
If not, consider symptomatic cholelithiasis, acute hepatic crisis, or splenic sequestration. Obtain right upper quadrant ultrasound imaging, check transaminases, and consider surgical consultation. Consider transfusion for severe anemia.

**Focal Neurologic Deficits (Hemiplegia, Aphasia, Paresthesias) or Seizures?**
Does the patient have hypertension, coronary artery disease, or atrial fibrillation with a possible thromboembolic phenomenon?
If not, consider vasoocclusion in the cerebral circulation. Obtain an emergency computed tomography scan and neurologic consultation, and consider red blood cell apheresis.

**Productive Cough with Fever?**
Does the patient have high fever, leukocytosis, positive Gram stain, or evidence of pneumonia on radiographs?
If not, consider acute chest syndrome, especially with low-grade temperature and vasoocclusive symptoms elsewhere. Obtain a chest radiograph and blood cultures. Admit for observation and possible exchange transfusion.

**Child with Fever Greater Than 101.3° F?**
Does the patient have pneumonia, pyelonephritis, cholangitis, cholecystitis, osteomyelitis, or meningitis?
If not, consider sepsis. Obtain a complete blood count, urinalysis, urine and blood cultures, chest radiograph, and lumbar puncture. Pneumococcal sepsis is a leading cause of childhood mortality, with a 14% mortality rate.

**Pallor, Fatigue, Listlessness, or Recent Viral Illness?**
Consider aplastic anemia. Obtain a reticulocyte count. Treatment is supportive and depends on the degree of anemia and hemodynamic instability.

**Abdominal Pain with Enlarged Spleen?**
Splenic sequestration is life-threatening and requires intensive care admission with transfusion and possible splenectomy.

**Painful, Erect Penis?**
Does the patient have paraphimosis, phimosis, or recent trauma?
If not, consider priapism. Obtain urology consultation, and initiate oral terbutaline or pseudoephedrine. Intracavernosal injection with α-adrenergic agonist is warranted. Also, treat with hydration, analgesia, ice packs, and exchange transfusions.

If the reticulocyte count is normal, splenic sequestration is the probable cause. If the reticulocyte count is low, bone marrow failure is the probable cause. An infection is indicated by major elevations in the WBC count (e.g., >15,000/mm$^3$) accompanied by a left shift and significant bandemia. In interpreting these values, the EP should know that most patients with SCD have chronic anemia (hematocrit of 20% to 30%), mild leukocytosis, elevated reticulocyte counts, and thrombocytosis.

Serum electrolytes, blood urea nitrogen, and creatinine levels are essential to determine when hydration status and metabolic function are concerns. However, these values are not always needed, especially in mild disease. Any toxic-appearing patient in respiratory distress requires arterial blood gas analysis, to establish a baseline and to diagnose acid-base abnormalities. Continuous pulse oximetry monitoring is warranted and reliable.

A type and crossmatch are sent to the blood bank, in case transfusion is required. Measurement of prothrombin and partial thromboplastin times are indicated to evaluate for hypercoagulable states, especially in patients demonstrating evidence of thrombotic disease, including stroke, and myocardial ischemia.

Patients with abdominal pain require liver function tests and serum lipase evaluations. An elevated baseline indirect bilirubin level may be normal because of chronic hemolysis. Extreme elevation may indicate cholelithiasis and cholecystitis. Patients with chest pain require an electrocardiogram to screen for myocardial ischemia.

The urine must be examined for evidence of infection if the patient has fever or signs of urinary tract infection. Hematuria and isosthenuria are often present in patients with SCD. If signs of urinary tract infection are present, a urine Gram stain and culture should be obtained. Patients with fever without clear evidence of pneumonia, cholecystitis, pyelonephritis, or apparent source require blood cultures, preferably two sets.

Imaging studies are also symptom specific. A chest radiograph is indicated in all patients with respiratory symptoms, including productive cough and tachypnea. Radiographic findings in acute chest syndrome may be normal in the early stages of presentation. Bone radiographs are necessary in patients with localized bony pain if osteomyelitis is suspected. Although not readily available in the ED, bone scans may be used to confirm the diagnosis. Ultrasonography is necessary in patients with abdominal pain to rule out cholecystitis, cholelithiasis, hepatomegaly, and splenomegaly. Patients with new neurologic signs and symptoms require CT scanning or magnetic resonance imaging of the head.

## TREATMENT

Treatment of SCD is evolving. The description of barriers to effective pain management is interesting and has been well documented.[21] EPs tend to undertreat their patients because they fear patients' dependence on pain medication, which in reality is present in only 1% to 3% of patients.[22] Patients with SCD who are in pain are also misunderstood because they display a different attitude to their severe pain than do trauma or oncology patients. Although patients with SCD complain of severe pain, they may engage in activities that are inconsistent with the traditional image of the patient in severe pain, such as watching television or talking on the telephone. These patients are therefore often perceived as exaggerating their pain to receive additional narcotics, whereas these activities may actually be learned distractions or coping mechanisms. Another example is the sleeping patient who, when awakened, reports unrelenting pain. This situation may stem from an imbalance between the sedative and analgesic effects of opiates or a need for sleep despite the pain. The result is a lack of trust between patients and health care providers. In centers specializing in sickle cell crises, the attitudes toward pain tend to be better understood, and treatment outcomes are superior, compared with EDs.

Oral analgesics suffice for treating mild to moderate pain. Patients with mild to moderate pain seem to find no difference between intravenous and oral morphine. Most opiates have comparable efficacy and safety profiles, but morphine (0.1 mg/kg) is considered the drug of choice for treatment of acute sickle cell pain. Hydromorphone (1.5 mg) may be used if morphine is unable to achieve effective analgesia. In children, studies emphasize oral dosing of potent opioids (weight-based dosing) and nonsteroidal antiinflammatory drugs, home treatment, and reduced reliance on EDs departments or inpatient admission.[23] A pain protocol, if available, should be used (**Box 204.2**). ED-based pain management protocols have been shown to decrease ED visits and hospitalizations and to increase use of primary care clinics by patients with SCD.[24]

Patients in severe pain should be given an opiate parenterally and preferably initiated within 15 to 20 minutes. The opiate should be dosed at frequent (15 to 30 minutes), fixed intervals, not as needed, until the pain has diminished, at which time the dose of the opiate can be tapered and then stopped, and oral analgesic therapy can be instituted.[25]

When available and appropriate for the treatment of acute pain, patients prefer patient-controlled analgesia (PCA) to scheduled dose or continuous infusion of morphine.[26] When used to treat acute pain episodes, PCA results in similar pain relief with lower morphine consumption when compared with continuous infusion of morphine. Furthermore, when introduced in the ED for the treatment of acute pain, PCA use was associated with a shorter elapsed time between onset of pain and treatment.[27] These data, along with clinical experience, suggest that PCA has emerged as a standard for the treatment of acute pain, and, if possible, it should be started in the ED.

The use of meperidine is discouraged because of the risk of seizures. Many opioid side effects can be ameliorated by drug therapy directed at the side effect (e.g., antiemetics to treat nausea and vomiting, antihistamines to treat itching, laxatives to treat constipation).[28] Antiinflammatory drugs and intravenous methylprednisolone may provide an opiate-sparing effect, but concern exists about their negative effects on bone healing. In addition, painful crises seem to recur frequently after treatment with methylprednisolone.

Urgent replacement of blood is often required for sudden severe anemia occurring in children when blood is sequestered in an enlarged spleen or when parvovirus B19 infection causes transient aplastic crisis. For aplastic crisis, clinical management is supportive and depends on the degree of anemia and cardiovascular compromise. Simple transfusions are administered to raise the Hgb to approximately 10 g/dL and the hematocrit to approximately 30% if the reticulocyte count is less than 1% to 2% with no signs of spontaneous recovery. Increasing the Hgb level to more than 11 g/dL is not recommended because of increased viscosity and risk of vaso-occlusion. For shock caused by splenic sequestration, emergency management is aimed at restoring circulating blood volume and hemodynamic stability through the infusion of crystalloids and volume expanders and by repeated simple or exchange blood transfusions. Ultimately, splenectomy may be performed because sequestration has been shown to recur in 50% of patients and represents a life-threatening event. Admission is required for patients with aplastic crisis and

**BOX 204.2 Emergency Department–Based Pain Protocol**

- Determine patients' previous known requirement for analgesia.
- Determine drug allergies and document the type of reaction.
- All patients should receive ibuprofen, 600 mg PO × one dose, unless a contraindication exists.
- Morphine is the drug of choice; hydromorphone is preferred in morphine-allergic patients.
- Evaluate pain: patients with severe pain requiring IV opioids or moderate pain able to take PO opioids.

**Severe Pain**

- Administer morphine, 5 to 10 mg IV initial dose, then 4 to 6 mg every 5 to 10 minutes, or hydromorphone, 1.5 mg IV initial dose, then 0.5 to 1 mg IV every 5 to 10 minutes.
- Titrate to comfort.
- Start IV PCA.
- If PCA demands fewer than 3, wean off IV PCA, and discharge with a standing dose of ibuprofen, Percocet (acetaminophen and oxycodone), morphine SR, or hydromorphone.
- If PCA demands more than 3, admit the patient.

**Moderate Pain**

- Administer morphine liquid, 10 mg PO × one dose or hydromorphone tablet, 2 mg PO × one dose.
- Reassess at 10 minutes.
- If no relief occurs, treat with IV opioids.
- If relief occurs, discharge the patient with a standing dose of ibuprofen, Percocet (acetaminophen and oxycodone), morphine SR, or hydromorphone.

*IV,* Intravenous(ly); *PCA,* patient-controlled analgesia; *PO,* oral(ly); *SR,* sustained release.

splenic sequestration. Transfusions are not needed for the usual anemia or episodes of pain associated with SCD.[28]

Treatment of acute chest syndrome is supportive and may include supplemental oxygen to maintain arterial oxygen saturation at more than 92%. Analgesia and incentive spirometry can minimize chest wall splinting and thus prevent atelectasis and hypoxemia.[28] Pulse oximetry in patients with SCD has been shown to correlate with arterial oxygen content. Antibiotics should be given to treat infections with *S. pneumoniae, Haemophilus influenzae,* and atypical organisms such as *Mycoplasma, Legionella,* and *Chlamydia.* Frequently, a macrolide with a third-generation cephalosporin is chosen. In acute chest syndrome, simple transfusion has been demonstrated to be more effective than exchange transfusion.[29] Given the increased proclivity of patients with SCD to develop alloantibodies, the potential negative effects of a higher Hgb level after exchange, and the time and the expense of both the pheresis procedure and the vascular access insertion, EPs should initiate simple transfusions first in the event that the Hgb is less than 30%.

Acute hepatic cell crisis manifests with tender hepatomegaly, worsening jaundice, and fever. This syndrome usually resolves within 3 to 14 days with supportive care alone, but it can progress to liver failure, which carries a dismal prognosis. Exchange transfusion should be considered for patients with signs of progressive liver dysfunction.

Sepsis is a leading cause of death, especially in younger children. Management incorporates the following: (1) treatment of the infection with source control and antimicrobial agents; (2) rapid and targeted resuscitation from shock with administration of fluid (and, if appropriate, blood products), vasopressors, or inotropic agents; (3) adjuvant therapy with recombinant human activated protein C or corticosteroids in carefully selected patients; and (4) supportive measures such as lung-protective ventilation for acute respiratory distress syndrome. Appropriate cultures of blood and material from other sites should be quickly obtained, and broad-spectrum intravenous antibiotics should be started within the first hour after severe sepsis or septic shock is recognized. All patients who have high fevers and who are not receiving prophylactic penicillin should receive intravenous ceftriaxone as a precaution against meningitis from *S. pneumoniae* and *Neisseria meningitidis.* Patients with osteomyelitis should be treated for infection with *Salmonella* and *Staphylococcus aureus.* Patients with presumed urinary tract infections, especially pyelonephritis, should receive treatment for *Escherichia coli* infection.

Hydroxyurea increases the production of Hgb F in patients with sickle cell anemia and thus ameliorates the disease clinically. The only successful therapeutic strategy so far for SCD is based on the use of hydroxyurea to increase the RBC content of Hgb F. Substantial reductions in pain rate, acute chest crises, and transfusion requirements have been achieved with hydroxyurea therapy. Long-term follow-up (9 years) of hydroxyurea-treated patients showed a 40% reduction in mortality with this therapy. The use of this agent in the ED is limited. Other interventions as described previously should be initiated earlier.

Novel therapies may include dipyridamole (Persantine), which has been shown to be a powerful inhibitor of the deoxygenation-induced fluxes of sickled cell polymerization, especially in dehydrated cells in vitro. However, more clinical trials are needed to demonstrate this benefit in vivo. Low-dose, longer-acting glucocorticoids, especially dexamethasone, have shown a benefit in the management of acute chest syndrome. However, more research is also needed. More recent studies and ongoing clinical trials have hypothesized that inhaled nitric oxide may be beneficial in managing various clinical conditions, including sickle cell anemia.[30] However, because the delivery of inhaled nitric oxide may have more limited applicability in the clinical setting as a result of inherent administration problems, the oral administration of L-arginine (precursor of nitric oxide) shows promise as a potential treatment for vasoocclusive crises and acute chest syndrome.[31]

## DISPOSITION

Patients with SCD who have uncomplicated painful crises and who receive hydration and adequate pain relief in the ED can be discharged. Adequate pain relief can be achieved on a variable basis for different patients, and no set rule exists about when this occurs. Some practitioners advocate for either temporal observation in the ED (6 hours) or a set amount of parenteral analgesics, most commonly opioids (two or three trials). Failure to achieve adequate pain relief requires inpatient admission (see the "Red Flags" box).

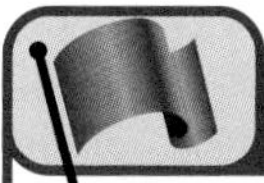

**RED FLAGS**

**Indications for Hospital Admission**

- Inability to control pain
- Inability to maintain adequate hydration
- Acute chest syndrome
- Bacterial infection with unexplained fever, leukocytosis
- Cerebrovascular crisis (new neurologic sign or symptom)
- Priapism
- Splenic sequestration
- Aplastic or hemolytic crisis
- Acute abdomen, especially right upper quadrant syndrome
- Noncompliance with follow-up schedules
- Uncertain diagnosis

In the absence of contraindications (temperature > 38° C, respiratory signs or symptoms, low arterial oxygen saturation, tachycardia, or hypotension) and if adequate pain relief is attained, patients can be discharged home on a regimen of oral analgesics for 1 week, with continuity of care arranged. Patients who have minor infections can be discharged with oral antibiotics, more commonly amoxicillin-clavulanate, azithromycin, or levofloxacin. Primary care physicians should be contacted, and specialist care (hematology) referral should be arranged. Finally, counseling is indicated to prevent future crises, given the chronic nature of SCD. Preventive measures include advising the patient to adhere to an immunization schedule (especially pneumococcal, influenza, and hepatitis vaccines), to maintain biannual health care visits, and to take advantage of oral penicillin prophylaxis for patients with frequent infections.

# POLYCYTHEMIA VERA

## EPIDEMIOLOGY

PV is traditionally classified as a myeloproliferative disorder, which is a broad category of clonal stem cell diseases that include myelofibrosis with myeloid metaplasia and chronic myeloid leukemia.[30] The true incidence and prevalence of PV are unknown. PV is relatively rare, occurring in 0.6 to 1.6 persons per million population. The disease has been recognized since the early twentieth century, and the initial description as presented by Osler has not changed. Fortunately, PV has the survival characteristics of a benign disease, and much still needs to be learned. For the EP, understanding the complications of the disease ultimately aids in its management.

## PATHOPHYSIOLOGY

The Greek term *polycythemia* is synonymous with the word *erythrocytosis,* and it literally translates as "many cells in the blood." *Absolute polycythemia* is a condition with increased RBC mass. Numerous primary and secondary polycythemic disorders lead to absolute polycythemia.[32]

Primary and secondary polycythemias can be either acquired or congenital. Congenital polycythemias may result from inherited appropriate responses to tissue hypoxia, acquired conditions characterized by autonomous erythropoietin production (secondary polycythemias), defects in hypoxia sensing (either primary or secondary polycythemia), or inherited intrinsic defects in RBC precursors that render erythroid progenitors hypersensitive to erythropoietin (primary familial and congenital polycythemia).[32]

PV, the most common primary polycythemia, is caused by the somatic change of a single hematopoietic stem cell, thus leading to clonal hematopoiesis. The molecular defects responsible for PV are unknown.

## PRESENTING SIGNS AND SYMPTOMS

Symptoms of PV are related to hyperviscosity, sludging of blood flow, and thromboses, which lead to poor oxygen delivery and symptoms that include headache, dizziness (vertigo), tinnitus, visual disturbances, angina pectoris, and intermittent claudication. Hypertension is common in patients with PV.

Bleeding manifestations in PV involve primarily the skin and mucous membranes, findings suggesting defective primary hemostasis, and include ecchymosis, epistaxis, menorrhagia, and gingival hemorrhage. Gastrointestinal hemorrhage occurs less frequently but can be severe, necessitating hospitalization and blood transfusion, and it is often associated with the use of aspirin.[33] This type of bleeding pattern is consistent with platelet defects (quantitative or qualitative) or von Willebrand disease.

Thrombosis, hemorrhage, and systolic hypertension result from the hyperviscosity associated with RBC mass expansion. Historically, thrombosis, both venous and arterial, occurred in up to 40% of patients during the course of the illness.

Dyspepsia and gastric or peptic ulceration appear to be more common in patients with PV than in the general population. The most serious complication other than thrombosis is pruritus.

Physical findings in PV are the result of manifestations of the myeloproliferative process and include splenomegaly (present in 75% of patients) and hepatomegaly (present in ~30% of patients). Plethora or a ruddy color results from the marked increase in total RBC mass. This manifests in the face, palms, nail beds, mucosa, and conjunctiva.

## DIFFERENTIAL DIAGNOSIS AND DIAGNOSTIC TESTING

PV is a clinical diagnosis. Diagnostic tests are nonspecific, sometimes uninformative, and none of them establish clonality. The diagnosis is currently facilitated through the laboratory measurement of RBC mass, plasma volume, and arterial oxygen saturation and determination of oxygen pressure at 50% Hgb saturation. In the ED, elevated RBC counts and hematocrit values (including Hgb levels) are used to make this diagnosis. Generally, Hgb concentrations of at least 20 g/dL or hematocrit values of at least 60% in male patients and 56% in female patients can be presumed to indicate a myeloproliferative disorder. Direct measurement of the RBC mass should show an increase, with a normal or slightly decreased plasma volume. However, this nuclear medicine test uses radiochromium-labeled RBCs to measure actual RBC and plasma volume and is not readily available. If RBC mass results are available, the Polycythemia Vera Study Group diagnostic criteria can be used (**Table 204.5**).

The arterial oxygen saturation and carboxyhemoglobin levels are important to rule out hypoxia as a secondary cause of erythrocytosis.

**Table 204.5 Polycythemia Vera Study Group Criteria for the Diagnosis of Polycythemia Vera**

| DIAGNOSTIC GROUP | CRITERIA |
|---|---|
| Category A | Total red blood cell mass<br>In male patients, ≥36 mL/kg; in female patients, ≥32 mL/kg<br>Arterial oxygen saturation ≥ 92%<br>Splenomegaly |
| Category B | Thrombocytosis with a platelet count >400,000/mL<br>Leukocytosis with a white blood cell count >12,000/mL<br>Leukocyte alkaline phosphatase > 100 units/L<br>Serum vitamin $B_{12}$ concentration > 900 pg/mL or binding capacity > 2200 pg/mL |
| Diagnosis | A1 plus A2 plus A3<br>A1 plus A2 plus any two criteria from category B |

## TREATMENT

In the absence of other manifestations of disease, phlebotomy is the only therapy indicated for isolated erythrocytosis when the mechanism cannot be established. Phlebotomy can be initiated in the ED; however, a hematology consultation is required. Other agents such as aspirin, various antihistamines, synthetic androgens, and phototherapy have been described, and initiation of these therapeutic adjuncts can be carried out on an inpatient basis.

Finally, splenectomy is an option for patients with painful splenomegaly or repeated episodes of thrombosis that cause splenic infarction. At this juncture, inpatient evaluation is warranted, and surgical consultation should be obtained.

## DISPOSITION

Patients requiring phlebotomy should be admitted. Bleeding and hemodynamically unstable patients require inpatient evaluation. In many patients with newly identified PV, drug administration and other interventions are not indicated in the ED setting. Asymptomatic patients can be referred to the hematologist for accurate determination of the underlying disease process, including measurements of RBC mass and karyotyping of bone marrow cells.

## SUGGESTED READINGS

Field JJ, Knight-Perry JE, Debaun MR. Acute pain in children and adults with sickle cell disease: management in the absence of evidence-based guidelines. Curr Opin Hematol 2009;16:173-8.

Givens M, Rutherford C, Joshi G, Delaney K. Impact of an emergency department pain management protocol on the pattern of visits by patients with sickle cell disease. J Emerg Med 2007;32:239-43.

Goodnough LT, Bach RG. Anemia, transfusion, and mortality. N Engl J Med 2001;345:1272-4.

Prchal JT. Polycythemia vera and other primary polycythemias. Curr Opin Hematol 2005;12:112-6.

Tefferi A, Hanson CA, Inwards DJ. How to interpret and pursue an abnormal complete blood cell count in adults. Mayo Clin Proc 2005;80:923-36.

## REFERENCES

***References can be found on Expert Consult @ www.expertconsult.com.***

# 205 Platelet Disorders

*Taku Taira*

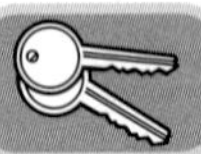

**KEY POINTS**

- Immune thrombocytopenic purpura (ITP) is a diagnosis of exclusion.
- Immunomodulation, in patients with suspected ITP, should be done in consultation with a hematologist.
- Thrombocytopenia with microangiopathic hemolytic anemia is sufficient to make the diagnosis of thrombotic thrombocytopenic purpura (TTP) and to initiate plasma exchange.
- TTP should be considered in patients with severe preeclampsia or HELLP (hemolysis, elevated liver enzymes, low platelets) syndrome.
- TTP and hemolytic uremic syndrome (HUS) are distinguished by the primary organ dysfunction: brain in TTP and kidney in HUS.
- TTP-HUS is distinguished from disseminated intravascular coagulation by the lack of coagulation abnormalities.
- Drug-induced thrombocytopenia should be considered in patients with acute or chronic exposure to implicated medications.
- Heparin-induced thrombocytopenia leads to thromboses in both arterial and venous beds.
- Patients with primary or essential thrombocythemia are at risk for both thrombotic and bleeding complications.
- Patients with essential thrombocythemia and thrombotic complications should be treated with cytoreductive treatments and considered for platelet pheresis.
- Pulses are maintained in patients with essential thrombocythemia who have thromboses.

## PERSPECTIVE

Patients presenting with primary platelet disorders are rare in the emergency department (ED). Although emergency physicians commonly encounter patients with thrombocytosis, thrombocytopenia, and dysfunctional platelets, these disorders are usually observed in the context of another illness. When abnormalities of the platelet count are discovered, the challenge is to identify the primary process and determine whether the patient has an associated life-threatening condition (**Box 205.1**).

## IDIOPATHIC OR IMMUNE THROMBOCYTOPENIC PURPURA

### EPIDEMIOLOGY

Immune thrombocytopenic purpura (ITP) is an autoimmune disorder characterized by isolated thrombocytopenia. The estimated incidence is 100 cases per 1,000,000 patients, and half of the cases are seen in children. In children, the gender distribution is equal, whereas in adults, women are three times more likely to be affected than are men.[1] ITP is defined as chronic if it lasts for longer than 6 months. Eighty percent of children with ITP have the acute form, whereas 80% of adults with ITP develop the chronic illness.[2]

### PATHOPHYSIOLOGY

Thrombocytopenia in ITP is primarily the result of accelerated platelet destruction. Autoantibodies bind to platelet antigens and thus lead to accelerated clearance by macrophages found primarily in the spleen and the liver. This increased clearance is magnified by decreased production caused by intramedullary destruction of platelets and megakaryocyte inhibition.[3] Thrombocytopenia, in turn, leads to bleeding through loss of the integrity of the vascular wall and deficits in thrombus formation.

### PRESENTING SIGNS AND SYMPTOMS

ITP is classically described as occurring after a prodromal infection. This presentation accounts for 60% of cases in patients 1 to 10 years of age. Outside this age range, thrombocytopenia occurs without any preceding symptoms and is often found incidentally.

Patient's symptoms of bleeding depend on the severity of the thrombocytopenia. Patients with platelet counts higher than 50,000/mm$^3$ are asymptomatic. Patients with platelet counts lower than 50,000/mm$^3$ may report easy bruising with

**BOX 205.1 Differential Diagnosis of the Patient with Thrombocytopenia**

**Possible Disorders**

- ITP
- TTP-HUS
- HELLP syndrome or preeclampsia
- Acute infections or sepsis
- Drug-induced thrombocytopenia
- DIC
- Malignant hypertension
- Hematopoietic malignant diseases
- Myelodysplastic syndromes

**Physical Examination Findings**

- Petechiae
- Subconjunctival hemorrhage
- Guaiac-positive stools
- Bruising

**Laboratory Findings**

- ITP
  - Isolated thrombocytopenia
  - No other cytopenias
  - Normal chemistries and normal coagulation studies
- TTP-HUS
  - Thrombocytopenia
  - Anemia
  - Schistocytes
  - Negative Coombs test
  - Elevated lactate dehydrogenase
  - Normal coagulation studies
  - Signs of organ dysfunction (i.e., creatinine, troponin, LFT elevations)
  - Increased reticulocyte and decreased haptoglobin
- DIC
  - Thrombocytopenia
  - Anemia
  - Elevation of coagulation studies
  - Elevated D-dimer
  - Elevated fibrin split products
- Heparin-induced thrombocytopenia
  - Thrombocytopenia (relative or absolute)
  - Normal coagulation studies
  - Elevated platelet factor 4 antibodies

*DIC*, Disseminated intravascular coagulation; *HELLP*, hemolysis, elevated liver enzymes, low platelets; *ITP*, immune thrombocytopenic purpura; *LFT*, liver function test; *TTP-HUS*, thrombotic thrombocytopenic purpura–hemolytic uremic syndrome.

minor trauma, whereas patients with platelet counts between 10,000 and 30,000/mm$^3$ can have spontaneous petechiae and bruising. Patients with platelet counts lower than 10,000/mm$^3$ are at risk for internal bleeding, including intracranial hemorrhage (ICH).[4]

ICH is the major cause of mortality in patients with ITP.[1] The mortality rate of patients with ITP and ICH is greater than 50%.[5] Atraumatic ICH secondary to ITP is rare, estimated to occur in 0.1% to 1% of patients with ITP. In one report of patients with ICH, 70% had platelet counts lower than 10,000/mm$^3$.[5] Despite the rarity of this complication, patients with ITP and any cranial or neurologic complaint should be evaluated for ICH.

## DIFFERENTIAL DIAGNOSIS AND MEDICAL DECISION MAKING

Primary and secondary forms of immune-mediated destruction of platelets are recognized. ITP generally refers solely to the primary form of this disease. The secondary form is associated with rheumatic disease, connective tissue disorders, malignant disease, drug exposure, immune deficiencies, and infections, including human immunodeficiency virus infection and hepatitis C. Because no specific diagnostic criteria exist for ITP, it is a diagnosis of exclusion.

The importance of pursuing alternative diagnoses is highlighted by the associated morbidity and mortality of the other diagnoses. The patient's history can point toward an alternate cause of the thrombocytopenia. Constitutional symptoms such as fever or weight loss suggest malignant disease or infection. Recent initiation of medications such as heparin, clopidogrel, or vancomycin may indicate drug-induced thrombocytopenia.

In ITP the remainder of the laboratory evaluation should be within normal limits. Thrombocytopenia with other abnormalities suggests alternative diagnoses. For example, thrombocytopenia with anemia is found in patients with thrombotic thrombocytopenic purpura (TTP) or hemolytic uremic syndrome (HUS). Thrombocytopenia and additional cytopenias are found in leukemia and myelodysplastic disorders. Thrombocytopenia and coagulation abnormalities are found in disseminated intravascular coagulation (DIC).

The peripheral blood smear should be examined. The smear can differentiate true thrombocytopenia from spurious causes of thrombocytopenia such as platelet clumping, platelet satellitism, and abnormally large platelets. Furthermore, the peripheral blood smear can identify manifestations of the primary cause of thrombocytopenia, such as schistocytes in TTP-HUS, evidence of parasitic infections, or findings suggestive of leukemia.

In the patient with suspected ITP, the physician must identify the degree of any bleeding complications. A careful skin examination can quantify the degree of petechiae or bruising. Rectal examination can identify gastrointestinal bleeding. Additionally, any intracranial symptoms, especially in the context of trauma, should be evaluated by computed tomography for possible ICH.

Patients with a history of ITP often have relapses. Most adults with ITP have one or more relapses, commonly during a steroid taper. Relapses are also seen in patients treated with intravenous immune globulin (IVIG) after steroids have failed. Patients with an ITP relapse are treated in the same manner as patients with an initial presentation of ITP. Patients with ITP relapse should also have a nonemergency surgical consultation for possible splenectomy.

## TREATMENT

ITP is treated by immunomodulation. The first-line treatment is with parenteral steroids. Most patients presenting with ITP are well and do not need treatment in the ED and can be managed with an early referral to a hematologist. Treatment should be started in patients who are ill, have bleeding complications, need emergency surgery, or have severe thrombocytopenia.

Initiation of treatment should be coordinated with a hematologist, for several reasons. Early leukemia can manifest with isolated thrombocytopenia, especially in pediatric patients. Leukemia should also be considered in adults who have prominent and persistent constitutional symptoms. In a patient who is presenting with leukemia, empiric steroids can lead to alteration of the bone marrow aspirate that causes difficulty and delay in diagnosis.

Steroids are usually started at a dose 1 to 1.5 mg/kg of prednisone per day. IVIG (usual dose of 1 g/kg) is reserved for infants and patients with severe disease or internal bleeding. Anti-D immune globulin is used as an adjunct in Rh-positive patients (usual dose of 75 mcg/kg). Patients with a recurrence of ITP are treated in the same manner as patients with an initial presentation of ITP and should be considered for escalation of therapy. Patients who have chronic or refractory ITP should be considered for splenectomy. The rate of remission of ITP after splenectomy in children is 70% to 80%. The remission rate in adults is unpredictable, ranging from 60% to 70%.[1] Platelet transfusion leads to a rapid but transient increase in platelet count and is therefore indicated only in certain settings, such as in patients with bleeding complications, patients undergoing emergency surgery, and those with severe thrombocytopenia.

## FOLLOW-UP, NEXT STEPS OF CARE, AND PATIENT EDUCATION

Most patients with suspected ITP are treated and managed as outpatients. However, patients with severe thrombocytopenia —defined as a platelet count lower than 10,000/mm$^3$, patients with head trauma, and those with bleeding complications—should be admitted. Patients should be considered for admission if their platelet count is lower than 30,000/mm$^3$, if they work in a profession (e.g., construction) in which trauma is inevitable, or if the diagnosis is in question. Ultimately, disposition should be based on the patient's appearance, the severity of thrombocytopenia, concomitant use of antiplatelet agents, and the patient's access to expeditious follow-up.

Patients who are managed as outpatients should be advised to avoid any antiplatelet agents. Patients, especially children, should limit their activities in situations associated with possible trauma (e.g., construction work, contact sports, gym class). Discharge instructions should instruct patients to return if they have any signs of bleeding, abdominal pain, trauma, or neurologic symptoms.

# THROMBOTIC MICROANGIOPATHIES

## PERSPECTIVE

The thrombotic microangiopathies are a group of disorders characterized by intravascular aggregation of platelets that leads to organ ischemia. These disorders include TTP and HUS. Although the two diseases have different names, they share a common mechanism, as well as overlapping clinical features. TTP and HUS are generally believed to lie on a spectrum of disease, as opposed to being distinct clinical entities. Therefore, they are discussed together.

## EPIDEMIOLOGY

TTP and HUS are rare diseases. TTP has an estimated prevalence of 4 to 11 cases per million people,[6] and HUS has an incidence of 1 to 10 cases per 100,000.[7] TTP is associated with black race, female sex, and obesity.[8] Pregnant and peripartum patients account for 12% to 25% of patients with TTP.[9]

Despite the rarity, TTP and HUS are associated with significant morbidity and mortality. Untreated TTP has a mortality rate of 90%,[10] and adults with typical HUS have a 45% mortality rate.[11] Children less than 10 years of age have a 15% chance of developing HUS in the setting of diagnosed *Escherichia coli* O157:H7 infection.[12] Although 90% of children with typical Shiga toxin–associated HUS recover with supportive care,[13,14] they have a 12% rate of death or permanent end-stage renal disease and a 25% incidence of hypertension and proteinuria.[13] Shiga toxin–associated HUS is the most common cause of acute renal failure in childhood, and it accounts for 4.5% of pediatric patients who undergo long-term renal replacement therapy.[7] Commonly cited risk factors for developing HUS include antibiotic administration, use of antimotility agents, and age younger than 10 years.[15]

## PATHOPHYSIOLOGY

The underlying process of the thrombotic microangiopathies is organ dysfunction resulting from intravascular aggregation of platelets that leads to consumptive thrombocytopenia and organ ischemia from thrombosis. The platelet aggregation, in turn, causes mechanical destruction of red blood cells and microangiopathic, nonimmunologic anemia.

In classic HUS, the inciting event is typically an infection with Shiga toxin–releasing bacteria, most commonly *E. coli* O157:H7 and non-O157:H7 subtypes.[12] The toxin produced by the bacteria is systemically absorbed, thus leading to widespread microvascular injury and consequent thrombosis. For unknown reasons, most cases of thrombosis in HUS occur in the renal vasculature. Ten percent of cases of HUS are atypical and are not triggered by Shiga toxin.[16] The triggers in atypical HUS include pregnancy, autoimmune disorders, drug toxicity, malignant disease, drug reactions, and preceding infections.[17]

Most patients with TTP have an acquired deficit in the protease ADAMTS-13 that is typically caused by autoantibody destruction. This deficit in ADAMTS-13 leads to the inability to cleave von Willebrand factor multimers and causes intravascular platelet aggregation and thrombosis.[14] Genetic susceptibility to the development of TTP has been described but is not well characterized.[16] Although most patients with TTP are characterized as having idiopathic TTP, ADAMTS-13 antibodies have also been associated with medications (e.g., quinine, ticlopidine, clopidogrel[8,18]), pregnancy, autoimmune disorders, direct drug toxicity, and hematopoietic stem cell transplantation.[8] TTP is treated with plasma exchange, which is thought to work by both removing the autoantibodies against ADAMTS-13 and replacing ADAMTS-13 activity.

## PRESENTING SIGNS AND SYMPTOMS

The presenting symptoms of both TTP and HUS depend on the severity of the organ dysfunction, the anemia, and the thrombocytopenia. TTP is classically defined by the pentad of thrombocytopenia, anemia, neurologic abnormalities, renal failure, and fever. Fever is typically low grade and is not usually a prominent feature of the syndrome. The neurologic abnormalities in TTP can range from seizures and fluctuating focal deficits to transient confusion. Patients with HUS typically present with signs and symptoms of renal failure including oliguria or anuria, edema, and hypertension. Ninety percent of patients with HUS have typical HUS, with a prodrome of watery diarrhea, which becomes bloody on the third day of illness, that is caused by a Shiga toxin–producing bacterial infection. Despite the distinctions made between TTP and HUS, 25% of patients with HUS can have neurologic abnormalities, and patients with TTP often have renal failure. When both renal impairment and neurologic dysfunction are present, the patient is considered to have TTP if the neurologic abnormalities are prominent and HUS if renal failure is prominent. In both diseases, patients can have symptoms caused by thrombosis and ischemia in any organ, including the heart, bowel, lungs, and pancreas, as well as having symptoms caused by anemia or thrombocytopenia.

Despite the classic descriptions of both TTP and HUS, the most common symptoms are nonspecific. Patient typically present with complaints of abdominal pain, nausea, vomiting, and weakness and are frequently misdiagnosed as having gastroenteritis, sepsis, or transient ischemic attack.[8] Even when the diagnosis is made, 10% of patients with an initial diagnosis of TTP in one report were eventually found to have sepsis or systemic cancer.[19]

## DIFFERENTIAL DIAGNOSIS AND MEDICAL DECISION MAKING

Making the diagnosis of TTP-HUS is challenging. Clinical suspicion is essential. The diagnosis is clinical, with no "gold standard" findings, and the signs and symptoms can be subtle, especially early in the disorder. These are also rare conditions that have clinical overlap with sepsis and DIC. The importance of making the diagnosis is emphasized by the 90% mortality rate of TTP and the knowledge that plasma exchange is a curative treatment.

Several elements of the patient's history should alert the clinician to the possibility of TTP-HUS. HUS should be considered in children with symptoms of renal failure after a diarrheal illness. TTP should be considered in patients presenting after initiating antiplatelet agents, especially in the first 3 to 14 days. Although TTP is considered an acute illness, one fourth of patients report symptoms for several weeks before diagnosis.[8]

TTP has been described in patients of all ages, but it is seen primarily in adults. The diagnosis of TTP should be considered in any patient with thrombocytopenia and anemia without a readily apparent cause. The anemia of TTP is microangiopathic hemolytic anemia, which is associated with schistocytes and elevated lactate dehydrogenase levels. The hemolysis is nonimmunologic and therefore should elicit a negative Coombs test result. The dyad of thrombocytopenia and microangiopathic hemolytic anemia, with or without renal or neurologic abnormalities, is sufficient to establish the diagnosis of TTP and to start plasma exchange. Additional signs of hemolysis include elevated serum lactate dehydrogenase levels secondary to red blood cell fragmentation and organ ischemia, an elevated reticulocyte count, and low haptoglobin levels. These patients should have no coagulation abnormalities.

Because of the clinical overlap and the divergent treatment of sepsis, DIC, and TTP-HUS, the physician should focus on the distinguishing features. Fever is part of the pentad of TTP but tends to be low grade. High fevers, associated with rigors, or the identification of an infectious source, point toward sepsis. A new coagulation abnormality suggests DIC as the cause of thrombocytopenia and anemia.

Pregnant and peripartum patients with suspected TTP are a diagnostic and clinical challenge. Pregnant patients account for a large percentage of cases of TTP,[9] and clinical overlap exists between TTP and preeclampsia-HELLP (hemolysis, elevated liver enzymes, low platelets) syndrome. Clinically, the two diseases have vastly divergent treatment. Patients with TTP and preeclampsia-HELLP have thrombocytopenia, microangiopathic anemia, renal disease, and neurologic abnormalities. Both diseases are seen primarily in the second and third trimesters. Distinguishing features include more severe hypertension in preeclampsia. The renal dysfunction in patients with preeclampsia is typically proteinuria, compared with the frank renal failure and oliguria seen in TTP-HUS. The thrombocytopenia in preeclampsia tends to be milder and corrects rapidly after delivery. The neurologic abnormalities in preeclampsia are typically headache, scotoma, and seizure, unlike the cerebrovascular accident or mental status change seen in TTP. Pregnant patients with possible TTP should have care coordinated among obstetrics, hematology, and nephrology.

Examination of the peripheral blood smear can be useful in patients with suspected TTP-HUS. In addition to identifying schistocytes, it can differentiate true thrombocytopenia from spurious causes of thrombocytopenia, as well as identifying alternative diagnoses such as leukemia. Hematology and nephrology should be involved in these cases to coordinate plasma exchange and dialysis.

## TREATMENT

The treatment for TTP is plasma exchange.[10] Plasma exchange halts the thrombosis by removing the autoantibodies against ADAMTS-13 and replacing the ADAMTS-13. Plasma exchange should start within 24 hours of presentation. If plasma exchange is not available or will be severely delayed, plasma infusion at 30 mL/kg/day may be attempted. Immunosuppression with glucocorticoids is used as an adjunct in patients with idiopathic ITP and in patients who have exacerbations after plasma exchange is stopped or in patients who have a relapse after remission.[20] The dose of prednisone is 1 to 2 mg/kg/day. Some weak evidence indicates that additional immunosuppression with cyclophosphamide or vincristine may be beneficial, but it is not routinely recommended.[8] When clopidogrel or ticlodipine is the suspected cause, the medication must be discontinued.

The treatment of HUS varies among patient populations. The treatment of children with typical Shiga toxin–associated HUS centers around aggressive supportive care, including fluid and electrolyte management, blood pressure management, red blood cell transfusion, and dialysis when indicated. Plasma exchange or plasma infusion is not routinely indicated for the treatment of typical HUS. Plasma exchange should be considered in patients with HUS that is not associated with Shiga toxin–associated diarrhea,[16] in adults, in patients with neurologic abnormalities, and in those who are very ill.[7]

## FOLLOW-UP, NEXT STEPS OF CARE, AND PATIENT EDUCATION

All patients with TTP-HUS should be admitted to the hospital for further management. Even if patients appear well, TTP has no outpatient management. Patients with HUS need electrolyte and fluid management. Patients should be admitted to telemetry beds because of the possibility of myocardial ischemia.

Patients should be educated about the possibility of long-term sequelae, including renal failure, permanent neurologic disability, and myocardial dysfunction, as well as the possibility of relapse. The long-term prognosis depends on various factors, including age, degree of organ dysfunction, prompt treatment with plasma exchange, and length of time undergoing dialysis. Children universally do better than adults. Young children with typical (Shiga toxin diarrhea–associated) HUS have the best prognosis of all patients with TTP-HUS. Patients with typical HUS are unlikely to have a recurrence, whereas patients with idiopathic TTP have a 50% relapse rate.[8]

# DRUG-INDUCED THROMBOCYTOPENIA

## EPIDEMIOLOGY

The diagnosis of drug-induced thrombocytopenia is challenging. More than 150 drugs have been implicated (**Box 205.2**),[21] but the epidemiology is not well characterized because of the dual lack of consistent, high-quality reporting and diagnostic criteria. This rare disease has an estimated incidence of 10 cases per 1,000,000 patients, but it occurs more frequently in hospitalized patients and in older persons.[22] Reported incidences of thrombocytopenia induced by specific medications have ranged from 0.0003% with quinine to 1% with gold salts and abciximab. This diagnosis is important to consider because the only effective treatment is discontinuation of the medication. Drug-induced thrombocytopenia does not respond to immunomodulation, as do conditions such as ITP.

Heparin-induced thrombocytopenia (HIT) must be considered separately from all other forms of drug-induced thrombocytopenia. HIT is more common than other drug-induced thrombocytopenias, with an incidence as high as 5% in high-risk populations.[23] Additionally, it has a much higher rate of both morbidity and mortality from thrombotic complications, which can persist after the heparin is discontinued and platelet levels return to normal. The risk of developing thrombocytopenia is 10 times higher in patients who are exposed to unfractionated heparin, when compared with those receiving low-molecular-weight heparin.[24]

**BOX 205.2 Drugs Commonly Implicated in Drug-Induced Thrombocytopenia**

Heparin (unfractionated and low-molecular-weight heparin)
Quinine or quinidine
Rifampin
Trimethoprim-sulfamethoxazole
Methyldopa
Acetaminophen
Digoxin
Vancomycin
Amiodarone
Cimetidine
Haloperidol

Date from George J, Raskob G, Shah S, et al. Drug-induced thrombocytopenia: a systematic review of published case reports. Ann Intern Med 1998;129:886-90.

## PATHOPHYSIOLOGY

In drug-induced thrombocytopenia, the drop in platelets is an immunologic process. The drugs themselves are not immunogenic. When the drug is bound to the platelet, however, the drug-platelet complex induces antibody production. The key feature of most of these antibodies is that they are not true autoantibodies because they do not bind to the platelet if the drug is not bound. Very rarely, drugs can induce true autoantibodies that can bind to the platelet in the absence of the drug. This phenomenon is most commonly seen during treatment with gold salts, but it also occurs with procainamide, sulfonamides, and interferon-$\alpha$ and -$\beta$.[22]

Binding of the antibodies to the platelet or the platelet-drug complex leads to immune destruction of the platelet and thrombocytopenia through the reticuloendothelial system, primarily in the spleen. In addition to the immune destruction of the platelets, the antibodies in HIT lead to platelet activation, which causes thrombosis.

## PRESENTING SIGNS AND SYMPTOMS

Most patients with drug-induced thrombocytopenia, including HIT, are asymptomatic. Patients presenting with bleeding complications are common in platelet dysfunction. These complications include findings such as petechiae, easy bruising, epistaxis, and other mucocutaneous bleeding. The typical time course is 5 to 7 days after exposure to a new medication. Patients previously sensitized to a medication can have a dramatic and rapid drop in platelets. The development of HIT can, in rare circumstances, be remote from the drug exposure.

In contrast to the other type of drug-induced thrombocytopenia, 20% to 50% of patients with HIT present with thrombotic complications. Of these thromboses, 70% are venous, and 30% are arterial.[25] The clinical presentation of patients with thrombotic complications from HIT depends on the vascular bed that is involved. The venous thromboses are most commonly deep vein thromboses and pulmonary emboli, but they also include cerebral and adrenal venous thromboses. The arterial thromboses are reported in the limbs, aorta, cerebral, and coronary vasculatures.

## DIFFERENTIAL DIAGNOSIS AND MEDICAL DECISION MAKING

The thrombocytopenia of HIT can either be absolute (<150,000/mm$^3$) or relative (decrease of >50% from baseline.) Patients almost universally have detectable levels of antibodies against platelet factor 4. Other drugs with drug-induced thrombocytopenia do not have readily available testing for drug-platelet antibodies.

Because immunologic testing is not often available or available in a timely fashion, the diagnosis and initial management must often be empiric. Drug-induced thrombocytopenia should resolve within several days of discontinuation of the medication.

## TREATMENT

The most important therapeutic intervention is discontinuation of the offending medication. Most of these antibodies have activity against the platelets only when the drug is bound, thus stressing the importance of identification and discontinuation of the drug. In most patients, the thrombocytopenia resolves without further intervention.

Patients with severe thrombocytopenia or bleeding should be treated with platelet transfusion. Immunomodulating medications such as corticosteroids, IVIG, and plasma transfusion have been tried, without any conclusive evidence supporting their efficacy.[22]

Patients with thromboses from HIT must be treated with direct thrombin inhibitors (e.g., lepirudin, argatroban, bivalirudin). When choosing among these medications, the physician must consider that lepirudin and bivalirudin are renally excreted, whereas argatroban is hepatically metabolized. This distinction is especially important because of the high rate of iatrogenic bleeding complications. Furthermore, because lepirudin is highly immunogenic, patients with recurrent HIT should not be treated with lepirudin more than once. Warfarin monotherapy in active HIT is contraindicated, but warfarin may be started in patients with platelet counts higher than 150,000/mm$^3$ and therapeutic levels of anticoagulation. Care should be taken to remove all sources of heparin, including catheter ports and dialysis tubing.

## FOLLOW-UP, NEXT STEPS OF CARE, AND PATIENT EDUCATION

The determination of disposition of a patient with suspected drug-induced thrombocytopenia should start with a search for other conditions that cause thrombocytopenia, most importantly sepsis. Next, the implications of discontinuing the medication and the question whether an acceptable alternative exists must be considered. Patients treated as outpatients should have urgent follow-up to evaluate for signs of bleeding and serial blood counts to ensure the resolution of the thrombocytopenia.

# THROMBOCYTOSIS

## EPIDEMIOLOGY

Thrombocytosis is usually an incidental finding in a patient in the ED. Most patient have secondary thrombocytosis, from an acute or chronic condition such as infection or malignant disease. Even in the extremes of thrombocytosis with platelet counts greater than 1,000,000/mm$^3$, 88% of patients have reactive thrombocytosis.[26]

The other main cause of thrombocytosis is essential thrombocythemia (ET), which is one of the myeloproliferative disorders. ET is a relatively rare disease with an estimated incidence of 2.5 cases per 100,000 patients.[27] In contrast to reactive thrombocytosis, patients with ET are prone to both bleeding and thrombotic complications.

## PATHOPHYSIOLOGY

Platelet production and homeostasis are primarily controlled by the effects of thrombopoietin on the megakaryocytes. Thrombocytosis can either be primary or secondary. In primary thrombocytopenia (ET), the thrombocytosis results from the clonal proliferation of megakaryocytes. Secondary thrombocytosis is caused by the effects of various catechols and cytokines,[28] as well as increased production of thrombopoietin in the liver in response to inflammatory stimuli.[29]

## PRESENTING SIGNS AND SYMPTOMS

Thrombocytosis is typically an incidental finding. Because most patients with thrombocytosis have secondary thrombocytosis, the presenting symptoms relate to the underlying condition and not to the thrombocytosis itself. The underlying conditions can be transient or sustained. Secondary thrombocytosis can be caused by a clinically occult process such as malignant disease or a chronic inflammatory condition. Patients with secondary thrombocytosis do not have any thrombotic or bleeding sequelae even in the extremes of thrombocytopenia unless it is a sequela of the underlying disorder.

Patients with ET can present with both bleeding and thrombotic complications. Thrombotic complications are more common that bleeding complications, with a ratio of 11 : 1, and arterial thrombosis is more common than venous thrombosis, with a ratio of 3 : 1.[30]

The bleeding complications are similar to those seen with thrombocytopenia and qualitative platelet disorders. Findings may include petechiae, hematuria, and gastrointestinal bleeding. Counterintuitively, these bleeding complications are more likely to occur in the extremes of thrombocytosis.[28]

The thrombotic complications of ET are common. Fifty percent of patients with ET have at least one thrombotic complication in the first 9 years from diagnosis.[30] The thrombotic complications have an unusual distribution. In addition to deep vein thromboses, patient are at risk for developing venous thromboses of the cerebral, hepatic, and portal veins. Most arterial complications are cerebrovascular, accounting for symptoms ranging from migraine-like symptoms to transient ischemic attack and stroke.[30,31] Despite its relative rarity, ET is classically associated with digital ischemia and erythromelalgia, which is characterized by patchy burning or throbbing pain in the extremities. Associated skin findings range from mottling, to erythema, to absent. Erythromelalgia can progress to gangrene and necrosis if it is not treated. In addition, patients with ET are at extreme risk for pregnancy-related complications, including fetal growth retardation and recurrent spontaneous abortions, because of placental thromboses.

## DIFFERENTIAL DIAGNOSIS AND MEDICAL DECISION MAKING

No known signs, symptoms, or laboratory findings distinguish ET from secondary thrombocytosis. Because of the lack of diagnostic criteria, ET is a diagnosis of exclusion, and the initial diagnosis and treatment should be focused on excluding an underlying cause of secondary thrombocytosis. ET can be secondary to acute and chronic conditions, medication reactions, stress, and clinically occult conditions. Tests such as C-reactive protein and erythrocyte sedimentation rate, as well as fecal occult blood testing, can point toward an underlying inflammatory or malignant condition.

The main differentiating feature between secondary and ET is that secondary thrombocytosis does not have associated thrombotic or bleeding complications attributable to the thrombocytosis. Even so, that primary disease process can put the patient at increased risk for both thrombotic and bleeding sequelae. Patients with ET are at risk for spontaneous transformation of the disorder into acute leukemia. The main clue to leukemic transformation is involvement of multiple cell lines.

## TREATMENT

Treatment of ET depends on the presentation. Patients with ET are commonly receiving a combination of aspirin and cytoreductive therapy. Typical agents include hydroxyurea, anagrelide, or interferon-α. Hydroxyurea is teratogenic, and the safety of interferon-α in pregnancy is not known, so patients with ET and newly diagnosed pregnancy should be counseled appropriately.

Patients with symptomatic ET must be treated aggressively. Patients with arterial thrombotic complications should have a combination of aspirin and cytoreductive therapy with hydroxyurea, anagrelide, or interferon-α. In addition, patients should be considered for platelet pheresis especially if they have cerebral and digital ischemia.[28] ED initiation of treatment for asymptomatic patients with suspected ET is not indicated. Patients should be referred to hematology and to their primary care physician for further evaluation.

Patients with secondary thrombocytosis do not need any specific treatment for the thrombocytosis. Diagnostic work-up and treatment should all be directed toward the underlying condition.

## FOLLOW-UP, NEXT STEPS OF CARE, AND PATIENT EDUCATION

Patients with known ET with either thrombotic or hemorrhagic complications should be admitted. Patients with asymptomatic thrombocytosis that has no clear underlying cause can be treated as outpatients, with coordination with their physicians and a hematologist. Patients with suspected ET should be instructed to return to the ED for any neurologic complaints or unexplained burning or throbbing pain in the extremities or bleeding.

## SUGGESTED READINGS

Cines D, Blanchette V. Immune thrombocytopenic purpura. N Engl J Med 2002;346;995-1008.

George JN. Clinical practice: thrombotic thrombocytopenic purpura. N Engl J Med 2006;354:1927-35.

McMinn J, George J. Evaluation of women with clinically suspected thrombotic thrombocytopenic purpura-hemolytic uremic syndrome during pregnancy. J Clin Apher 2001;16:202-9.

Moake JL. Thrombotic microangiopathies. N Engl J Med 2002;347:589-600.

Schafer AI. Thrombocytosis. N Engl J Med 2004;350:1211-9.

## REFERENCES

***References can be found on Expert Consult @ www.expertconsult.com.***

# Bleeding Disorders 206

*Michael Levine and Joshua N. Goldstein*

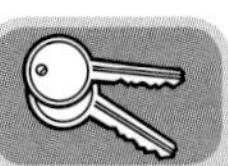

**KEY POINTS**

- Bleeding disorders are common and can be classified as congenital or acquired.
- A thorough history, including medication history, can help screen for many potential bleeding disorders.
- The prothrombin time is a measurement of abnormalities in the tissue factor pathway, whereas the activated partial thromboplastic time is a measurement of abnormalities in the contact activation pathway.
- Hemophilia A and B are both X-linked conditions, and factor replacement may be needed as prophylaxis or treatment for bleeding. Recombinant factor VIIa can be used to treat patients with inhibitors.
- von Willebrand disease is the most common congenital bleeding disorder. Treatment options vary, depending on the severity of the condition and bleeding, but they include desmopressin, aminocaproic acid, tranexamic acid, and factor replacement.
- Common causes of acquired coagulopathies include trauma, massive transfusion, disseminated intravascular coagulation, drugs, and toxins.
- The definitive treatment of disseminated intravascular coagulation is reversal or treatment of the underlying cause.

## EPIDEMIOLOGY

Under normal physiologic conditions, a constant balance exists between clot formation and clot breakdown, with a preference favoring anticoagulation.[1] Hemostasis results from a complex interaction among the vascular endothelium, platelets, the coagulation cascade, and the fibrinolytic system. Any disorder that affects this interplay can alter the equilibrium, thereby producing either excessive thrombosis or excessive hemorrhage.

Broadly speaking, bleeding disorders can be either inherited or acquired. Of the inherited disorders, the von Willebrand syndromes and hemophilia A are the most common, with a prevalence between 1 per 100 individuals and 1 per 100,000 individuals. Less common inherited disorders include deficiencies of factors II, V, VII, X, XIII, and fibrinogen, with a prevalence between 1 and 2 per 100,000 individuals.[2] The most common acquired bleeding disorders are drug induced, from therapeutic administration of agents expressly intended to decrease the risk of thrombosis. Oral anticoagulants are taken by up to 2% of the population and up to 8% of persons more than 65 years old, and the use of antiplatelet agents is vastly more common than that.[3] Patients with inherited bleeding disorders will likely present to the emergency department (ED) for treatment of abnormal bleeding at some point during their lifetime,[4] and ED visits for bleeding in patients who are taking antithrombotic agents are not uncommon.[5] The clinician must be familiar with these disease states to provide prompt care because treatment delays can increase morbidity and mortality.[4,6]

## PHYSIOLOGY AND BIOLOGY OF HEMOSTASIS

### COAGULATION CASCADE

The coagulation cascade (**Fig. 206.1**) is typically thought of as two pathways working separately. In reality, however, the tissue factor pathway (formerly called the extrinsic system) and the contact activation pathway (formerly called the intrinsic system) function intimately with each other to produce thrombin, a critical enzyme in the coagulation system.[1,7]

Tissue factor typically resides on smooth muscle cells, fibroblasts, and pericytes.[8-10] Binding of tissue factor to factor VII results in an activated factor VII (factor VIIa). Factor VIIa subsequently catalyzes the conversion of factors IX and X to their active forms (factors IXa and Xa, respectively).

The contact activation pathway begins with the activation of factor XII by the high-molecular-weight enzymes kininogen and prekallikrein.[1] This activation subsequently triggers a series of reactions leading to the conversion of X to Xa, the first step of the common pathway. The exact relevance of the contact activation pathway is debatable, however, because its activation is not needed in trauma-initiated coagulopathy.[1] Furthermore, with the exception of a deficiency of factor XI, deficiencies in enzymes involved in the contact activation pathway generally do not produce substantial coagulopathies.[1]

The common pathway starts with the conversion of factor X to Xa, which, in turn, converts prothrombin to thrombin. Ultimately, thrombin catalyzes the conversion of fibrinogen to fibrin.

### PLATELET FUNCTION

Following injury to the vascular endothelium, endothelin is released, resulting in vasoconstriction. In addition, injury to the vascular endothelium results in tissue factor exposure, with subsequent binding of platelets to the endothelium.[8,10] Platelet adhesion primarily involves the binding of platelets to damaged endothelium by von Willebrand factor (vWF).[11,12] Additional platelet activation occurs through the release of numerous mediators including adenosine diphosphate (ADP), epinephrine, thromboxane $A_2$, and thrombin.[11] Ultimately,

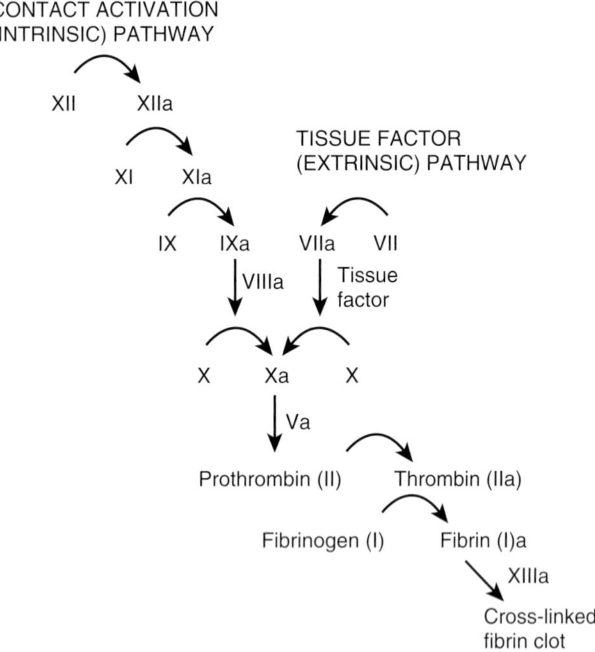


**Fig. 206.1 Coagulation cascade.**

platelet activation and aggregation require glycoprotein IIb/IIIa.[11] Thrombus stability, however, requires fibrin, which is formed from the coagulation cascade on the surface of platelets.[11]

## PRESENTING SIGNS AND SYMPTOMS

The optimal management of the patient with a bleeding disorder involves, as always, aggressive resuscitative measures (e.g., focus on ensuring adequate airway, breathing, and circulation). However, those patients with bleeding disorders also require specific therapies targeted toward the underlying disease state. Diagnostic laboratory tests and factor or product replacement should be administered on an individualized basis.

A careful history must be obtained from the patient, including the exact nature of the bleeding disorder, if known. A history regarding xenobiotic usage and past bleeding episodes should be obtained, including a history of previous bleeding with mild procedures (e.g., prolonged bleeding following tooth extractions), menstrual history (e.g., particular heavy or prolonged bleeding), and prior transfusion history. In addition, the clinician should question the patient regarding current bleeding, including the presence of dermal (petechiae, purpura, or ecchymosis), gastrointestinal (melena, hematochezia, or hematemesis), genitourinary (hematuria), mucosal membrane (gingival or epistaxis), and musculoskeletal (hemarthrosis) hemorrhage.

## DIFFERENTIAL DIAGNOSIS AND MEDICAL DECISION MAKING

The initial assessment of a patient with a known or suspected bleeding disorder begins with a thorough history and physical examination. Laboratory studies can be used to assess the severity of the disorder and to support a diagnosis. The initial laboratory studies that should be obtained when evaluating such patients include a complete blood count, prothrombin time (PT; a measure of the tissue factor pathway), and an activated partial thromboplastin time (aPTT; a measure of the contact activation pathway). A fibrinogen count can also assist in the initial management. These laboratory tests can help screen for clinically significant factor deficiencies, such as hemophilia A or B, as well as hypofibrinogenemic states. Additional tests may be indicated, depending on the condition of interest. For example, the concentration of D-dimers may be helpful in establishing the diagnosis of disseminated coagulation (DIC), whereas factor concentrations may be useful in assessing the severity of hemophilia. Patients with acute fulminant hepatic failure may demonstrate abnormalities similar to those seen in DIC. In such cases, factor V, VII, and VIII levels can be obtained. Although factor V levels are likely to be decreased in both DIC and liver failure, factor VIII levels are normal or elevated in liver failure–induced coagulopathy, yet markedly decreased in DIC-induced coagulopathy. Factor VII levels are also reduced in coagulopathy resulting from hepatic failure. Mixing studies can be performed to determine whether a factor deficiency or inhibitor is present in patients with prolonged aPTT.[13] Examination of the peripheral blood film can be very helpful in patients with unexplained bleeding disorders.

## COAGULATION CASCADE DEFECTS

Platelet-related defects are discussed in Chapter 205.

### HEREDITARY DEFECTS

#### *Hemophilia A and B*

Hemophilia A and hemophilia B are X-linked recessive disorders involving factors VIII and IX, respectively. Clinically, hemophilia B is indistinguishable from hemophilia A. However, nearly half of all cases of hemophilia A, the most common form of hemophilia, represent de novo mutations, in which boys are born to parents without the disease.[1] These disorders can be classified as mild, moderate, or severe, corresponding to a plasma coagulation factor concentration of 6% to 30%, 2% to 5%, or 1% or lower, respectively.[14] Those patients with a mild form of the disease generally have bleeding only after trauma or surgery. In contrast, patients with the severe form of the disease have an average of 20 to 30 bleeding episodes annually, and bleeding occurs spontaneously or after minor trauma.[14] Hemarthrosis is one of the most common forms of bleeding in severe forms of hemophilia.[1] Historically, treatment involved transfusions of plasma concentrates of coagulation factors.[14] However, such an approach was associated with the acquisition of numerous infectious diseases, including human immunodeficiency virus infection or hepatitis, as well as the development of inhibitors to the clotting factors.[14,15] Now, both plasma and recombinant-derived factor VIII and IX exist. Treatment can be administered as an on-demand regimen, in which therapy is given based on bleeding, or in a prophylactic regimen. Because the plasma half-life of factor IX is longer than of factor VIII (18 to 24 hours versus 8 to 12 hours), dosing of factor replacement is less frequent for hemophilia B than for hemophilia A.[16]

**Table 206.1** Common Treatment Strategics for coagulopathies*

| | TREATMENT OPTIONS | NOTES |
|---|---|---|
| **Disease-Induced Coagulopathy** | | |
| Factor V deficiency | FFP | |
| Factor VIII deficiency | Recombinant factor VIIIa | 1 U/kg IV increases plasma factor VIII concentrations by 2%. A typical dose will be 40 U/kg for severe bleeding. |
| | Recombinant factor VIIa can be used for those with inhibitors to factor VIII | 90 mcg/kg IV |
| Factor IX deficiency | Recombinant factor IXa | 1 U/kg IV increases plasma factor IX concentrations by 1%. A typical dose will be 80 U/kg for severe bleeding. |
| Factor X deficiency | FFP or PCC | |
| Factor XI deficiency | FFP | |
| von Willebrand disease | DDAVP<br>Aminocaproic acid<br>Tranexamic acid | 0.3 mcg/kg IV<br>50-60 mg/kg IV q4-6h<br>10-15 mg/kg IV q8-12h |
| Congenital fibrinogen disorders | FFP<br>Cryoprecipitate<br>Fibrinogen concentrates† | |
| Coagulopathy of trauma | FFP<br>Platelets | |
| Disseminated intravascular coagulation | Cryoprecipitate<br>Platelets | Primary treatment is to treat the underlying cause |
| Transfusion-related coagulopathy | FFP<br>Platelets | |
| **Drug/toxin–Induced Coagulopathy** | | |
| Heparin | Protamine | 1 Unit reverses 100 U UFH |
| Factor Xa inhibitors | rFVIIa<br>FFP | 90 mcg/kg IV |
| Warfarin | Vitamin K, FFP, PCC | |
| Crotalid envenomation | Crotalidae polyvalent immune Fav (ovine); CroFab | |

* Many etiologies of coagulopathy do not require factor replacement or transfusion. If these products are to be administered, the specific agent is listed in the table. However, for many conditions, no blood product should be transfused. The text can help guide when specific therapies should be administered.

†Where licensed.

*DDAVP*, Desmopressin; *FFP*, fresh frozen plasma; *PCC*, pool complex concentrates.

**Table 206.1** shows a common treatment regimen. Minor bleeding requires factor replacement to achieve factor concentrations of 30% of normal (typically 30 units/kg). In contrast, major hemorrhagic events, including hemarthrosis and large muscle bleeding, requires factor replacement to achieve factor concentrations of at least 50% (typically 50 units/kg). Life-threatening hemorrhage requires factor replacement to achieve factor concentrations of at least 80% (typically 80 units/kg).[16] In general, each unit per kilogram of body weight of factor VIII increases plasma factor VIII concentrations by 2%, whereas each unit per kilogram of body weight of factor IX increases plasma factor IX concentrations by 1%.[16] In patients with life-threatening bleeding, however, in vivo factor concentrations should be followed to ensure adequate replacement. When patients with hemophilia A have developed inhibitors to factor VIII, recombinant factor VIIa (rFVIIa) (90 mcg/kg) has been used.[4]

### von Willebrand Disease

von Willebrand disease (VWD) is the most common hereditary bleeding disorder. Although laboratory evidence of this disorder is present in up to 2% of the population, clinically relevant bleeding occurs much less commonly.[17] vWF has two roles in maintaining hemostasis. First, vWF forms a link between platelets and the vascular endothelium of injured blood vessels. Second, vWF serves as a plasma carrier for factor VIII.[18] The primary defect in VWD is a quantitative deficiency (types I, III) or a qualitative defect (type II) in vWF.[1,17] However, because vWF serves as a plasma carrier and stabilizer for factor VIII, VWD is also associated with a secondary decrease in factor VIII.[17]

Mucocutaneous bleeding is the most common clinical manifestation of VWD. Epistaxis, hematomas, and menorrhagia are relatively common. Patients with type III disease, the most severe form, develop spontaneous hemarthrosis resembling that seen in hemophilia.[18] The diagnosis can be confirmed by obtaining a vWF antigen, vWF ristocetin cofactor assay, and factor VIII activity. Minor bleeding, including mucosal bleeding, usually does not warrant specific treatment. For more severe bleeding, however, antifibrinolytic agents and desmopressin should be administered (see Table 206.1) Desmopressin produces a transient increase in factor VIII and vWF three to five times higher than baseline within 1 hour of intravenous administration, and it should be administered at a dose of 0.3 mcg/kg intravenously. Antifibrinolytic agents include aminocaproic acid (50 to 60 mg/kg every 4 to 6 hours) and tranexamic acid (10 to 15 mg/kg every 8 to 12 hours).[17] For those patients with life-threatening bleeding, factor VIII and vWF concentrates may be needed.[4]

### *Miscellaneous Factor Deficiencies*

Numerous other congenital coagulation factor deficiencies are recognized. Defects in factor V can result in either hemorrhagic or thrombotic complications.[19] Factor V deficiencies can be classified as either type I (low or unmeasurable antigen level) or type II (normal or mildly low antigen level). Parahemophilia, a severe form of the type I variety, is generally associated with mild bleeding.[19,20] No factor V–specific concentrate is available, so bleeding, if it occurs, should be treated with fresh frozen plasma (FFP) (see Table 206.1).[20]

Factor X, a vitamin K–dependent clotting factor, is the first enzyme in the common pathway in the coagulation cascade. Factor X deficiency is one of the rarest inherited coagulation disorders.[21] Patients with severe deficiency usually develop hemorrhage early in life, including umbilical stump bleeding. Patients with less severe deficiency, in contrast, typically develop bleeding only following trauma or menorrhagia, for example.[21,22] In addition to congenital deficiencies, several states are associated with acquired factor X deficiency, including liver disease, vitamin K deficiency, myeloma, and various malignant diseases.[21] In addition, the AL, but not the AA, form of amyloidosis has been associated with acquired factor X deficiency.[21] Sodium valproate use is associated with a transient form of factor X deficiency.[23] If bleeding occurs, the patient should receive FFP or prothrombin complex concentrates (PCC) (see Table 206.1).

A deficiency of either factor XI or factor XII (Hageman trait) is rarely associated with clinically relevant bleeding.[24-26] Severe forms of factor XI deficiency can be clinically relevant, however, and bleeding is best treated with the administration of FFP (see Table 206.1). Factor XI is more common among individuals of Ashkenazi heritage.

### *Congenital Fibrinogen Disorders*

Congenital fibrinogen disorders include hypofibrinogenemia and afibrinogenemia. Patients frequently present at birth with umbilical stump bleeding.[27] In older individuals, life-threatening bleeding is rare, but it can include gastrointestinal hemorrhages and central nervous system bleeding.[27] In contrast to patients with various factor deficiencies, patients with fibrinogen defects typically do not have significant spontaneous bleeding, and when bleeding does occur, it is typically less severe and primarily associated with trauma or surgery.[2] Fibrinogen deficiency can be treated with FFP, cryoprecipitate, or (where licensed) fibrinogen concentrates (see Table 206.1).

## ACQUIRED DEFECTS

### *Drugs*

Numerous pharmaceutical agents can produce coagulopathy by interfering with the coagulation cascade at various levels. Furthermore, salicylates, ADP antagonists (e.g., ticlopidine, clopidogrel, prasugrel, and ticagrelor), and glycoprotein IIb/IIIa inhibitors (abciximab, eptifibatide, and tirofiban) can result in hemorrhage, but they induce platelet dysfunction, rather than disorders in fibrin formation. In addition, innumerable drugs can cause thrombocytopenia with prolonged use. Drugs that alter platelet function are discussed elsewhere (see Chapter 205).

Warfarin is a vitamin K antagonist, which inhibits the cyclic conversion of vitamin K 2,3-epoxide to vitamin K quinone, as well as the conversion of vitamin K quinone to the active form of vitamin K, vitamin K quinol. The inhibition of these enzymes prevents the $\gamma$-carboxylation of the vitamin K–dependent clotting factors, namely, factors II, VII, IX, and X, along with protein C and protein S.[28] Patients taking warfarin frequently present to the ED either because of a supratherapeutic international normalized ratio (INR), which was checked during an outpatient visit, or because of hemorrhage. The treatment of an elevated INR depends on the clinical circumstances.[29,30] For example, if a patient is asymptomatic but has an incidental INR of 4, simply withholding a dose of warfarin may be appropriate, whereas a patient with an intracranial hemorrhage with an INR of 2 requires aggressive reversal. **Table 206.2** outlines the recommended guidelines for warfarin reversal. In general, if vitamin K is to be administered, oral and intravenous routes are preferred because subcutaneous and intramuscular administration leads to poor and erratic absorption.[31]

Heparin products can be classified as either unfractionated heparin (UFH) or low-molecular-weight heparin (LMWH). Commonly used LMWHs include dalteparin, enoxaparin, tinzaparin, and ardeparin. Traditionally, UFH was the primary xenobiotic used for both prophylaxis and treatment of venothromboembolic disease.[32] However, because of increased ease of administration, a lack of need for laboratory monitoring, and a more predictable dose-response curve, the use of LMWH has substantially increased.[32] UFH produces anticoagulation by binding to antithrombin III, thereby producing a conformational change. The modified antithrombin III–heparin complex is a potent inhibitor of factors IIa and Xa. UFH also has some activity against factors IXa, XIIa, and kallikrein.[33,34] The LMWHs, in contrast, also bind to antithrombin III, but they have greater effect on factor Xa. Comparing the LMWHs with UFH, the LMWHs have a higher ratio of antifactor Xa to IIa than does UFH.[32,34]

The anticoagulant effects of heparin are measured by following the aPTT. Monitoring is typically not needed for the LMWHs. However, if monitoring is desired, an antifactor Xa level should be obtained 4 hours after subcutaneous

**Table 206.2 Guidelines for Warfarin Reversal**

| INR | CHEST GUIDELINES | AUSTRALASIAN SOCIETY OF THROMBOSIS AND HAEMOSTASIS |
|---|---|---|
| 2-5; no bleeding | Lower or omit dose | Lower or omit dose |
| 5-9; no bleeding | Hold 1-2 doses *or* 1-2.5 mg PO vitamin K* | Hold warfarin; if bleeding risk high, 1-2 mg PO or 0.5-1 mg IV vitamin K |
| ≥9; no bleeding | Hold warfarin; give 5 mg PO vitamin K | Hold warfarin; if bleeding risk low, give 2.5-5 mg PO vitamin K or 1 mg IV vitamin K If high risk, give 1 mg IV vitamin K, consider PCC, FFP |
| Serious bleeding | Hold warfarin; give 10 mg IV vitamin K, supplemented by FFP, PCC, or rVIIa | Hold warfarin; give 5-10 mg IV vitamin K, PCC, and FFP |
| Life-threatening bleeding | Hold warfarin; give FFP, PCC, or rVIIa, supplemented by 10 mg IV vitamin K | |

Date from Ansell J, Hirsh J, Hylek E, et al. Pharmacology and management of the vitamin K antagonists: American College of Chest Physicians evidence-based clinical practice guidelines. Chest 2008;133:160S-98S; and Baker RL, Coughlin PB, Gallus AS, et al. Warfarin-reversal: consensus guidelines, on behalf of the Australasian Society of Thrombosis and Haemostasis. Med J Aust 2004;181:492-7.)

*FFP,* Fresh frozen plasma; *INR,* international normalized ratio; *IV,* intravenous; *PCC,* prothrombin complex concentrates; *PO,* oral; *rVIIa,* recombinant factor VIIa.

injection.[35] Heparin reversal is accomplished by the intravenous administration of protamine sulfate (see Table 206.1). Each unit of protamine sulfate reverses 100 units of UFH. Because protamine sulfate primarily reverses factor IIa, and not Xa, its use in patients with LMWH produces only a partial reversal.[36]

Factor Xa inhibitors can inhibit factor Xa either indirectly (idraparinux or fondaparinux) or directly (rivaroxaban). Unlike the LMWH agents, which inhibit both factors IIa and Xa, the factor Xa inhibitors produce no inhibition of factor IIa. Rivaroxaban, which is available orally, is considered a direct factor Xa inhibitor because it binds directly to factor X, unlike idraparinux and fondaparinux, which bind to antithrombin III.[32] In the event of life-threatening hemorrhage in patients taking a factor Xa inhibitor, no consensus on therapy exists, although some investigators have recommended rFVIIa for this purpose.[37] Outcome data are insufficient to recommend the routine administration of rFVIIa for the reversal of factor Xa inhibitors; the use of rFVIIa for this purpose must be weighed against the potential for thromboembolic events.

## *Coagulopathy of Trauma*

Coagulopathy is common among trauma patients. Nearly 25% of critically ill trauma patients are found to have some laboratory or clinical evidence of coagulopathy on admission. This coagulopathy is related to injury severity but not to fluid resuscitation.[38] Coagulopathy, along with hypothermia and acidosis, is part of the "triad of death" because its development produces synergistic effects that can ultimately culminate in mortality.[39]

The mechanism by which this process occurs is unclear. First, local tissue damage after trauma is thought to result in exposure to tissue factor from the damaged endothelium, thereby activating the coagulation cascade. In addition, traumatic brain injury results in the release of brain-specific thromboplastins, leading to consumption of clotting factors.[40] Finally, severely injured trauma patients can present in shock. This leads to diffuse endothelial disruption and early production of factors II, V, VIII, and X. Furthermore, shock results in decreased clearance of thrombin, thereby leading to activation of protein C with resultant inactivation of factors Va, VIIIa, and plasminogen activator inhibitor-1.[40,41] Acidemia alters coagulation protease function, increases fibrinogen degradation, and further contributing to coagulopathy. Hypothermia, which is common in trauma patients, results in coagulopathy secondary to decreased activity of factor VIIa, inhibition of coagulation protease activity, and impaired platelet function.[39,40]

Treatment of patients with trauma-induced coagulopathy begins with basic resuscitation, including the removal of wet clothes, as well as the application of warmed blankets, warmed fluids, and maintenance of high ambient heat. Coagulopathy can be treated with FFP (see Table 206.1). In the setting of acute blood loss, platelet transfusions can be given to maintain a platelet count of at least $50 \times 10^9/L$.[42] rFVIIa has been used on an off-label basis in numerous studies as a treatment of trauma-induced coagulopathy. Although the use of rFVIIa may be associated with reduced transfusion of blood products, no effect on outcome has yet been demonstrated.[41] Its use must be weighed against its associated cost, lack of clear proven benefit, and potential for thromboembolic complications.

## *Transfusion-Related Coagulopathy*

The administration of large volumes of fluids to actively bleeding patients can lead to a dilution of clotting factors and platelets that contributes to coagulopathy.[43] Furthermore, the aggressive use of colloids (e.g., hydroxyethyl starch) is associated with migration of plasma proteins to the interstitial space, with a resulting reduction of plasma concentrations of factors VII and vWF, as well as impaired platelet function.[43] The liberal use of crystalloid fluids, especially lactated Ringer solution with racemic lactate, is associated with a significant increase in immune mediators.[44]

The term *massive transfusion* commonly refers to the replacement of one's blood volume within 24 hours, or the replacement of 50% of the total blood volume within 3 hours.[45] The transfusion of large volumes of packed red blood cells (PRBCs), as occurs during a massive transfusion, is associated with numerous complications, including coagulopathy.[46] In the military setting, the use of massive transfusion protocols has been associated with improved survival. In the civilian trauma setting, however, mortality benefit from such protocols is conflicting. An example of such a protocol includes a set transfusion ratio of FFP to PRBCs of 1 : 2 or 1 : 1.[41,47,48] Many protocols also include platelets, which are transfused at a ratio of FFP to PRBCs to platelets of 1 : 1 : 1.

### Toxin

Pit vipers include rattlesnakes, copperheads, and cottonmouths. Pit viper envenomations, especially those from rattlesnakes, can lead to local pain and edema, myotoxicity, and hematotoxicity. Initial evaluation of these patients should include a complete blood count, fibrinogen, and prothrombin time. Thrombocytopenia, hypofibrinogenemia, and coagulopathy can develop quickly after an envenomation. Because the venom does not result in thrombin production, fibrin is not cross-linked. This lack of thrombin production and fibrin cross-linkage separates crotalid-induced coagulopathy from true DIC.[49] Afibrinogenemia, which can occur following envenomation, is not a result of a consumptive coagulopathy, but rather of primary fibrinogenolysis.[50] Furthermore, despite profoundly abnormal laboratory findings, because the patient is able to produce endogenous thrombin, hemostasis remains intact, and gross hemorrhage remains rare.[49]

Treatment of pit viper–induced coagulopathy and thrombocytopenia is with antivenom. Crotalidae polyvalent immune Fab (ovine) (CroFab) is the only available antivenom currently approved for the management of pit viper envenomation in the United States. A full review of pit viper envenomations is beyond the scope of this chapter, but in general, stable patients should receive an initial dose of four to six vials intravenously over 1 hour.[51] In the absence of life-threatening hemorrhage, blood products are not indicated, despite the presence of critically abnormal platelets, PT, or fibrinogen.[52]

Following therapy with CroFab for rattlesnake envenomation, late hematotoxicity can occur. Patients can develop recurrence, in which severe thrombocytopenia or coagulopathy can occur days after therapy, even if these laboratory abnormalities were not initially present. Thus, these patients should have a fibrinogen, PT, and complete blood count assessed 2 to 4 days and again 5 to 7 days after envenomation.[51,53]

### Disseminated Intravascular Coagulation

In the setting of severe systemic illness or injury, the body's coagulation processes can become activated, thereby resulting in widespread, excessive microvascular thrombosis. This thrombosis can result in impaired end-organ perfusion that contributes to multisystem organ failure. Because of this extreme, disproportionate activation of the coagulation system, consumptive coagulopathy can occur, in which platelets, clotting factors, and protease inhibitors are consumed. Intravascular fibrin strand formation results in the shearing of red blood cells, with subsequent development of microangiopathic hemolytic anemia.[54] Thus, this condition, DIC, results in excessive clot formation, bleeding, or both simultaneously.[55] DIC does not occur as a primary process but is always secondary to some underlying disorder, including sepsis, trauma, malignant disease (particularly metastatic adenocarcinoma, acute promyelocytic leukemia), tumor lysis syndrome, and obstetric conditions (e.g., abruptio placentae, placenta previa, amniotic fluid embolism, HELLP [hemolysis, elevated liver enzymes, low platelets] syndrome, uterine atony), among others.[54,56]

DIC can be considered either acute or chronic.[54] The diagnosis of DIC can be confirmed by the finding of several laboratory abnormalities, including the presence of thrombocytopenia, prolongation of the PT and aPTT, hypofibrinogenemia, elevated D-dimer, and the presence of schistocytes on peripheral smear. Not all these laboratory abnormalities need to be present to make the diagnosis of DIC, and no single laboratory test can confirm or exclude the diagnosis.[54,56] The primary treatment of DIC is to treat the underlying inciting cause.[54,55] Platelet transfusion is indicated only in those patients with active bleeding or in those who are at risk for significant bleeding. Such patients include those with platelet counts lower than $50 \times 10^9$/L who need an invasive procedure or those with platelet counts lower than 10 to $20 \times 10^9$/L.[55] Cryoprecipitate can be used to correct severe hypofibrinogenemia (<50 mg/dL) in patients with active bleeding.[54] No role exists for routine transfusion of cryoprecipitate in the absence of bleeding.

The use of low-dose heparin in patients with DIC has been suggested in an effort to reduce thrombin generation. This practice is controversial, however, because convincing data supporting its use are lacking.[54,55]

## SUMMARY OF AGENTS USED TO TREAT BLEEDING DISORDERS

Table 206.1 shows many of the agents used to correct various coagulopathies. FFP contains most coagulation factors in varying concentrations; some factor shave mildly to moderately decreased concentrations following thawing. Blood type (ABO) compatibility is required, but Rh factor is not. Each unit of plasma is approximately 200 to 250 mL of fluid. In contrast to FFP, which contains all clotting factors, cryoprecipitate contains fibrinogen, fibronectin, VWF, and factors VIII and XIII. It is the only widely form of concentrated fibrinogen currently available. Six bags of cryoprecipitate will raise the fibrinogen approximately 45 mg/dL. Finally, prothrombin complex concentrate (PCC) is a generic term for several different plasma-derived coagulation products that were designed as concentrates of factor IX and that contain varying amounts of factors II, VII, IX, X, and proteins C and S. Different formulations are available in different countries.

## REFERENCES

***References can be found on Expert Consult @ www.expertconsult.com.***

# Leadership and Emergency Medicine 207

J. Stephen Bohan

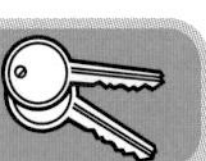

**KEY POINTS**

- The value of leadership lies in its ability to form individuals into a group directed to a goal.
- Even small groups benefit from a leader.
- People seek leadership.
- The soul of leadership is integrity.
- The substrate of leadership is change.
- Leadership and management are different.

## PERSPECTIVE

The library of books on leadership is large and heterogeneous, although most of these books focus on large organizations, predominantly business. Most describe general principles, whereas some are specific to gender or career stage or are targeted to CEOs or school principals. None are specific to emergency medicine, and few are written for physicians. This chapter isolates the characteristics possessed by recognized leaders and then applies these characteristics to the context of emergency medicine.

## SCOPE

The nature of the practice of emergency medicine means that leadership is a constant requirement. Few patients can be managed by one person, and many patients require the simultaneous attention of multiple people. A universal acknowledgment is that better care is delivered when such a group works under effective leadership. This same phenomenon is present at the department level. Thus, leadership is an everyday requirement that is vital to the agreed mission of the emergency medicine: respectful and good care for anyone, any time, irrespective of any restriction. The leader is an enabler of the goal of "always getting better" at this mission at every level: direct patient care, department operations and development, and national policy matters.

## LEADERSHIP QUALITIES

Plato pointed out that it is difficult to say what quality is but that one recognizes it when one sees it. The same can be said, to a large extent, about leadership. Everyone recognizes an outstanding leader, but, despite listing various characteristics, it remains difficult to say what exactly makes that individual a leader worthy of note.

What is a leader? What do leaders do? Are leaders really managers, or is it the other way around? Can one learn leadership? Are leaders necessary? How big must a group be before it needs a leader?

### GROUP SIZE AND LEADERSHIP

Certainly, 2 people walking down a street do not need a leader, but observation tells us that 15 people walking down a street, as a group, do need leadership even for this simple task. The action as a group makes leadership necessary. Whenever one person acts in concert with another and is recognized to do so by others, then that group, as small as 2 individuals, needs a leader if for no other purpose than to communicate the needs and wants of the pair to the outside world. Obviously, leading a pair is easier than leading a group of 3, and so the complexity grows with each individual.

In large organizations (e.g., a university, a firm such as General Electric or Wal-Mart, the U.S. Navy), the leadership responsibility is divided at different levels. The chief executive officer (CEO) is expected to lead on matters of policy and general direction of the institution or corporation. As one travels down the chain of responsibility, the ratio of leadership to managerial skill changes.

### MANAGER VERSUS LEADER

Managers direct processes, whereas leaders create change. Managers are given goals and are responsible for the tasks required to achieve that goal. The responsibility of a leader is to make the organization better by creating goals. The leader generates or adopts and then adapts the "better idea" to the needs of the organization.

> *"The reasonable man adapts himself to the world; the unreasonable one persists in trying to adapt the world to himself. Therefore, all progress depends on the unreasonable man."*
>
> George Bernard Shaw

This process requires the leader to have a skill set for each of several roles:

**Visionary:** The ability to see that options exist.

**Decision maker:** The ability to choose among options. These options may be self-generated or given to the leader by others, but decisions need to be explicit and timely, neither too early (insufficient data, inadequately prepared staff) or late (problem requiring change is now too large, with a different set of options prevailing). Making decisions is hazardous, but leaders cannot be adverse to risk. Recognized leaders rarely revisit decisions and always look forward.

**Informant:** The ability to inform the members of the organization effectively of the nature of the change and the direction it will take them and also inform related individuals outside the organization of how they will be affected.

**Tone setter:** Setting the tone (creating the atmosphere) that will allow the change to develop is actually more important than any policy that directs the change.

All these roles (visionary, decision maker, informant, tone setter) require unfailing attention to interpersonal skills for the simple reason that someone else, and various others at various levels, will, of necessity, be executing the change.

## CHARACTER

The *primum non nocere* of interpersonal skills is character. Recognition by others that the leader is a person of character is the bedrock of the respect needed to take people to a goal.

*"He listens, he is honest and he always takes the high road."*

Cheryl Kane, street nurse, Boston Health Care for the Homeless, about her boss, Robert Taube

Character and selfishness are mutually exclusive. The leader must see and be seen to understand that the needs of the organization override individual interests and that "doing the right thing" is always in the interests of the organization. This includes recognizing that the needs of the organization are best served when the appropriate needs of the individual are properly served in the context of the community that is the organization. Character requires commitment, focus, and a willingness to undertake and exercise responsibility, including accepting responsibility for failures. Failures will always occur as change proceeds. The absence of failures means that change is not happening.

*"Most things you try will fail."*

Richard Pearle, MD, CEO Kaiser Permanente Northern California

*"If you are not succeeding, you need to double your failure rate."*

Thomas Watson, founder IBM

Individuals of character rarely if ever complain, never gossip, and always follow through on what they said they would do. They are, and are seen to be, committed to making the organization and the individuals in it better. They hold themselves and others accountable while being loyal. Loyalty is a two-way street. The leader must be loyal to relevant external agents (the larger organization, the community, and its needs) while simultaneously acknowledging subordinates though recognition and by supporting them in time of personal need. Leaders are readily distinguishable from sycophants.

*"Never complain, never explain."*

Anonymous

## STRATEGIC POSITIONING: OUT IN FRONT

If the prime role of the leader is to take the organization to a different place, then he or she needs to be "out in front." With a combination of knowledge of the organization as it currently exists and a clear vision of the goal of what it should look like in the future, both near and long term, the leader needs to pull the organization forward by using the respect that he or she enjoys as the rope.

The position out in front is not to place the leader on a pedestal, nor is it to isolate the leader in any way. In fact, the distance between the leader and the group is actually crucial. When it is too close, the leader is just another member of the group participating in the group think, whereas when it is too far, the leader is not seen to have any relationship with the group at all. Walking and talking too fast put more and more distance between the leader and the group and erode the necessary organic relationship between leader and followers.

For example, if the drum major is 10 yards ahead of the band, he is leading it; if he is 50 yards ahead, he has no useful relationship with it. His signals are difficult to see and difficult to interpret if they can be seen, and the musical cues are dropped, with results that one would expect. This principle is true irrespective of the nature of the organization.

*"Take no credit; share no blame."*

Anonymous

## COMMUNICATION

The person of character readily gains respect. This respect makes people willing to listen to what the individual has to say but, more important, makes them willing to talk to the leader because when integrity is recognized, trust exists. The individual telling his or her story is seeking, even demanding, attention and should receive it. That attention should be undivided because listening is the overarching virtue of a leader. The decision that follows is often viewed by the narrator as less important than the fact that the story was heard.

*"Many a man would rather you heard his story than granted his request."*

Lord Chesterfield

There is much to be learned in listening. Buried beneath the words are essential truths about the individual and the job that he or she does, as well as the barriers that faced while doing it.

Discerning the nature and number of barriers to success at each level is a hallmark of a leader. It also implies the intention and action to remove those barriers and to allow individuals to succeed in their tasks.

Over and over, when individuals in large organizations are asked what could be improved in both their workplace and the organization as a whole, they reply "better communication." By this, they imply the need to be listened to but also to be told "what is going on." People left on the outside of the information stream feel powerless and neglected. Because a major purpose of any communication is to inform, the leader must be a successful informant. The message must be clear, so it must be simple and declarative. Avoidance of the passive voice enhances clarity. Jargon of any sort, whether medical, administrative, or managerial, should be avoided. The message must have a human touch to communicate not only the information but also sympathy with the recipient. To do this successfully in both written and oral forms takes practice and perhaps some coaching.

In the end, the whole purpose is to communicate the goal of the group and how any change promotes that goal. The goal itself must be a "good" something that makes both the group and the community better, and it must be easily recognized as such. Effective communication aids in this recognition. The "good" is a reflection of the leader's beliefs, the underpinning of the leader's character. The beliefs are then known and are seen to be the moral context in which goals and directives are enunciated. This sense of morality implies a sense of fairness and justice.

## FAIRNESS AND JUSTICE

Fairness and justice imply the absence of a special relationship between a leader and other individuals. Experience tells us that these relationships prevent us from viewing the object of our friendship or affection objectively, thus suggesting unequal regard among all individuals of the organization. The wise and successful leader develops successful acquaintanceship with members of his group but rarely friendship and never affection. This dispassionate approach is absolutely necessary to treating members of the group fairly and justly. Should affection develop, one of the individuals should leave the organization forthwith.

*"Get your luvin' at home."*

Peter Rosen

Also necessary for developing a sense of equity and fairness is the willingness to abide by the rules, whatever those rules may be. If the conclusion is that the rules are silly, counterproductive, or antiquated, then the successful leader will revise or remove them, but never ignore them.

## MANAGING LEADERSHIP

Were one to possess and be able to exercise all the foregoing necessary virtues, one would be "the" natural leader, but such is only occasionally the case. Thus, one must have the ability to recognize one's own weaknesses and "staff them." This can be done by delegation. One may be excellent at decisional activities but a less than magnetic communicator. In that case, communication can, for some large part, be delegated, all the while taking precautions to ensure that the message is recognized as coming from the leader. The same holds for most activities, including fiscal, personnel management, and community affairs.

It is an unequivocal fact that some people possess leadership talent, whereas others do not. These other individuals may possess other talents that are useful for the organization, such as insight, salesmanship, or the ability to absorb and relate financial information. The successful organization places the individual with a particular talent needed in the position in which that talent is useful, and the individual, once placed, does the same all the way down through the organization. Having individuals in positions for which they have no talent is impairing both for the organization and for the individual, and if this position happens to be a leadership role, then the impairment reverberates widely. Having individuals succeed is a fundamental necessity to the success of the organization. Removing unsuccessful people from positions for which they have no talent is never a bad thing. Keeping them in the position in which they are not succeeding does a substantive disservice both to the organization and to themselves as it perpetuates dysfunction and delays their placement into positions in which they can succeed.

## LEARNING AND KNOWLEDGE

Leaders must be knowledgeable. This requires being informed and trusting the informant. Thus, hiring trustworthy people is a key to success. This team of reliable informants helps the leader to "prepare relentlessly, to get the facts straight, to never assume anything." Each episode of "doing the right thing and doing it correctly" sets an example of the standard expected of others. Just as a single adverse headline in a newspaper, truthful or not, can undo decades of reputation building, being mistaken even once on factual matters can serve to diminish credibility, a virtue on which leadership rests. This fact supports the notion that, as in everything else, successful leadership comes from talent supplemented by hard work. One can learn important elements of leadership, or at least improve on them.

Preeminent musicians practice several hours per day, as do star athletes. The skills of leadership are as amenable to improvement as any other skill. Presentation skills can be improved through education and practice. Focusing on individuals, for example, by learning and remembering names and personal facts of members of the team or work force, can alter the regard in which the leader is held, as can attendance at team social events. All these behaviors take initiative, time, and effort to learn and perform. Leadership is never a leisurely stroll in the park; attention can never lapse.

# EFFECTIVE LEADERSHIP

Leadership is about promoting and managing change. Changing people is more challenging than changing material. The effective leader is one who regularly succeeds in driving change. The methods for this entail all the previously mentioned characteristics and character traits. Communication must be regular but not frequent, simple, consistent and persistent. It should antedate the effective date of the change by a period measured in months and should become more frequent as date nears. The communication should be seen to be personal, should explain the value of the change to the group, and should continue well into the implementation period, until the change is stabilized in the culture of the institution or group. The use of e-mail is not an effective means of staff behavior change.

## LEADERSHIP IN EMERGENCY MEDICINE

The scale of leadership in emergency medicine is usually small: the physician group, the department, the organization. The principles remain identical, however, irrespective of the size of the requirement. Leaders must be respected because without respect no willingness exists on the part of the group to listen to and adopt the goals enunciated. The fundamental requisite for respect is character and then, not far behind, is being good at the job. Technical skill (and "interpersonal skills" are actually a technique of the job) is necessary but not sufficient because it does not replace or make up for character deficiencies. Thus, anyone interested in being a leader in emergency medicine must devote a substantive amount of attention to becoming a respected clinician. This includes being completely knowledgeable about the core scientific knowledge, as well as having sufficient interpersonal skills to be respected by both patients and other staff members. With character and clinical skill in place, a leader in emergency medicine usually requires a record of academic accomplishment in addition to the record of administrative accomplishment (e.g., quality programs, emergency medical service activities, community outreach, fiscal management) that is needed in all emergency departments irrespective of size or mission.

An alternative to this traditional view exists. This alternative view holds that leadership skill is the most important attribute, as opposed to being the best physician. In other words, the person who is the best leader, be it a nurse, a physician, or an administrator, should be the leader.

> *"Asking who the boss should be is like asking who should sing tenor in a quartet, it is the person who can sing tenor."*
>
> Henry Ford

The record of accomplishment is the interface between the bedrock of character and clinical skill and the leadership position. Once a position is achieved, what successful leaders do in emergency medicine differs little from what successful leaders do in any other organization. The exception is that leaders in emergency medicine are more often expected to continue clinical activities, whereas in other organizations, especially large ones, no such expectation of "working on the shop floor" exists. On a local level, leaders seek to move the organization forward, including the physician group and hospital activities, both internal and external to the department, that affect the department. On a regional and national level, the principles remain the same; only the scale changes. Regional and national leaders in emergency medicine seek to initiate and manage change, be it through education, legislation, or offering new structures in national and state policy or new ways of thinking about processes. They set and move toward goals by seeking to align talent and job requirements, to make the workplace hospitable and just, thereby reducing costly employee turnover, and to inform peers, other members of the organization, the public, and politicians. They listen, act, take responsibility, and pause and reflect often.

## SUGGESTED READINGS

Campbell MJ. Five gifts of insightful leaders. Newton, MA: Charlesbank Press; 2006.
Gikley RW. The 21st century health care leader. San Francisco: Jossey-Bass; 1999.
Harvard Business Review. Harvard Business Review on leadership. Boston: Harvard Business School Press; 1998.
Maxwell J. The 21 indispensable qualities of a leader. Nashville, TN: Nelson Business; 1999.
Morrell M, Capparell S. Shackletons's way. New York: Penguin; 2001.

# 208 Quality and Patient Safety in Emergency Medicine

Azita G. Hamedani, Jeremiah D. Schuur, Cherri D. Hobgood, and Elizabeth A. Mort

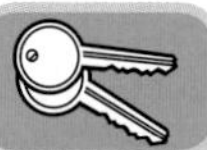

**KEY POINTS**

- The great variability in local and regional clinical practice patterns indicates that the U.S. population does not consistently receive high-quality health care. Problems with overuse, underuse, and misuse of health care resources have been documented.
- Two watershed Institute of Medicine reports brought the quality problems in health care to center stage. These reports championed that health care should be safe, effective, patient-centered, timely, efficient, and equitable.
- The greatest sources of quality problems in health care are not "bad apples" (i.e., incompetent providers), but rather "bad systems," specifically systems that promote, or at least do not mitigate, predictable human errors.
- Medical errors and adverse events are caused by both active and latent failures, as well as factors (e.g., error-producing conditions or reliance on heuristics) that lead to cognitive errors (e.g., slips, lapses, premature closure). Diagnostic errors are a leading cause of patient safety issues in emergency medicine. High-reliability organizations are preoccupied with failures and serve as models for health care.
- Both public and private sectors have a strong movement away from purchasing health care services by volume and toward purchasing value (defined as health care value per dollar spent). Future reimbursement models will inevitably center on performance measurement and accountability, with a likely shift in level of financial risk borne from payer to provider.

## HISTORY OF HEALTH CARE QUALITY

Efforts to assess quality in health care extend back to Dr. Ernest A. Codman, an early twentieth-century surgeon at Massachusetts General Hospital in Boston. Codman was the first to advocate for the tracking and public reporting of "end results" of surgical procedures and initiated the first morbidity and mortality conferences.[1] Such public information would allow patients to choose among surgeons and surgeons to learn from better performers. Codman was clearly ahead of his time. The medical establishment resisted having their "results" measured and publicized, and Codman was accordingly ostracized by his peers. In 1913, however, the American College of Surgeons adopted Codman's proposal of an "end result system of hospital standardization" and went on to develop the Minimum Standard for Hospitals. These efforts led to the formation of the forerunner of today's Joint Commission (JC) in the 1950s. The JC's accreditation process, local hospital quality reviews, professional boards, and other systems that developed allowed the medical profession and hospitals to judge the quality of their work and be held accountable only to themselves for most of the twentieth century.

The academic science of quality management in health care is credited to Dr. Avedis Donabedian's efforts in the 1980s. Donabedian advocated for evaluating health care quality through assessment of *structure* (e.g., physical plant, personnel, policies and procedures), *process* (how things are done), and *outcome* (final results).[2] His ideas were first adopted in public health and later spread to administration and management. Shortly thereafter, Dr. Donald Berwick, a Harvard Medical School (Boston) pediatrician, building on a systems approach to quality management, introduced the theory of continuous quality improvement into the medical literature. In his landmark *New England Journal of Medicine* article,[3] Berwick remarked the that the "Theory of Bad Apples" relies on inspection to improve quality (i.e., find and remove the bad apples from the lot). In health care, those who subscribe to this theory seek outliers (deficient health care workers who need to be punished) and advocate a blame and shame culture through reprimand in settings such as morbidity and mortality conferences. The "Theory of Continuous Improvement," however, focuses on the average worker, not the outlier, and on systems problems, rather than an individual's failure.

Examples of bad systems abound in medicine. One example provided by Berwick involves the reported deaths resulting from an inadvertent mix-up of racemic epinephrine and vitamin E.[4] Newborns in a nursery received the epinephrine instead of the vitamin in their nasogastric tubes. If presented as the mix-up of a benign medication for a potentially toxic one, it is viewed as appalling, and blaming individual negligent behavior is easy. Yet when one notes that the two bottles were nearly identical, one can understand why the system "is perfectly designed to kill babies by ensuring a specific—low but inevitable—rate of mixups." The Theory of Continuous Improvement suggests that quality can be improved by improving the knowledge, practices, and engagement of the average worker and by improving the systems environment in which they work. The "immense, irresistible quantitative power derived from shifting the entire curve of production upward even slightly, as compared with a focus on trimming the tails" is what makes a systems focus so attractive (**Fig. 208.1**).

Although Berwick and others were publishing new studies critiquing health care's approach to quality and safety throughout the 1980s and 1990s, not until the publication of two reports by the Institute of Medicine (IOM) did quality and safety capture the public's attention: *To Err is Human: Building a Safer Health System,*[5] in 1999, and *Crossing the Quality Chasm: A New Health System for the 21st Century,*[6] in 2001.

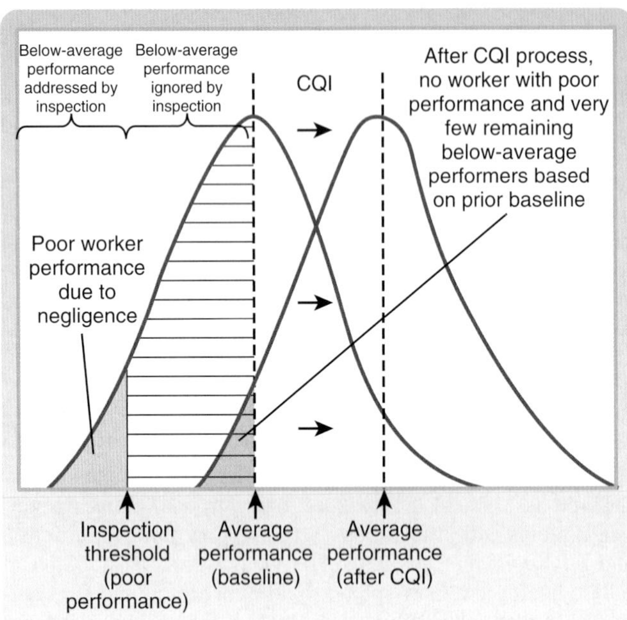


**Fig. 208.1 Inspection versus continuous quality improvement (CQI).**

*To Err is Human* focused the attention of the U.S. public on patient safety and medical errors in health care. The report's most famous sound bite, that medical errors result in the deaths of two jumbo jetliners full of patients in U.S. hospitals each day, gained traction with lawmakers, employers, and patient advocacy groups. This estimate, that 44,000 to 98,000 deaths occur per year in the United States as a result of medical error, would make hospital-based errors the eighth leading cause of death in the United States, ahead of breast cancer, acquired immunodeficiency syndrome, and motor vehicle crashes. These statistics were derived from two large retrospective studies. In the Harvard Medical Practice Study,[7] nurses and physicians reviewed more than 30,000 hospital records and found that adverse events occurred in 3.7% of hospitalizations. Of these adverse events, 13.6% were fatal, and 27.6% were caused by negligence. The Colorado-Utah study[8] reviewed 15,000 hospital records and found that adverse events occurred in 2.9% of hospitalizations. Negligent adverse events accounted for 27.4% of total adverse events in Utah and for 32.6% of those in Colorado. Of these negligent adverse events, 8.8% were fatal. Extrapolation of results from these two studies provided the upper and lower limits for deaths associated with medical errors for the IOM report. In both studies, compared with other areas of the hospital, the emergency department (ED) had the highest proportion of adverse events resulting from negligence.

*Crossing the Quality Chasm* focused more broadly on redesign of the health care delivery system to improve the quality of care. The report begins by stating: "The American health care delivery system is in need of fundamental change. … Between the health care we have and the care we could have lies not just a gap, but a chasm." The report goes on to detail that this chasm exists for preventive, acute, and chronic care and reflects *overuse* (provision of services when potential for harm exceeds potential for benefit), *underuse* (failure to provide services when potential for harm exceeds potential for benefit), and *misuse* (provision of appropriate services, complicated by a preventable error, such that the patient does not receive full benefit). The report first defined six domains for classifying quality improvement for the health care system (**Table 208.1**). Together, the IOM reports solidified a key

**Table 208.1 Institute of Medicine's Six Aims for Quality Improvement**

| AIM | DEFINITION |
|---|---|
| **Health Care Should Be:** | |
| Safe | "Avoiding injuries to patients from care that is intended to help" |
| Effective | "Providing services based on scientific knowledge (avoiding underuse and overuse)" |
| Patient centered | "Providing care that is respectful of and responsive to individual patient preferences, needs, and values and ensuring that patient values guide all clinical decisions" |
| Timely | "Reducing waits and sometimes harmful delays for both those who receive and those who give care" |
| Efficient | "Avoiding waste, in particular waste of equipment, supplies, ideas, and energy" |
| Equitable | "Providing care that does not vary in quality because of personal characteristics such as gender, ethnicity, geographic location, and socioeconomic status" |

Adapted from Committee on Quality Health Care in America. Crossing the quality chasm: a new health system for the 21st century. Washington, DC: National Academies Press; 2001.

concept—quality problems are generally not the result of bad apples but of bad systems. In fact, well-intentioned, hard-working people are routinely defeated by bad systems, regardless of training, competence, and vigilance.

## COSTS IN HEALTH CARE

In 2009, the United States spent $2.5 trillion, or $8000 per person, on health care.[9] Although we spend well over twice as much per capita on health care than any other industrialized country, we repeatedly fare poorly when compared with other systems on quality and outcomes.[10] Half of the U.S. population admits to being very worried about paying for health care or health care insurance.[11] One in four persons in the United States reports that his or her family has had problems paying for medical care during the past year.[12] Close to half of all bankruptcy filings are partly the result of medical expenses.[13] U.S. businesses similarly feel shackled by health care costs, with reports of companies spending more on health care than on supplies for their main products. In Massachusetts, annual health care costs in school budgets outpaced state aid for schools and forced schools to make spending cuts in books and teacher training.[14] The increased cost of U.S. health care threatens the ability of our society to pay for other needed and wanted services.

## VARIABILITY IN HEALTH CARE

Although the number of errors coupled with increasing health care costs paints a negative picture, the variability of care is both more concerning and a source for optimism. Dr. John (Jack) E. Wennberg's work in regional variability has illustrated the differences in cost, quality, and outcomes of U.S. health care since the 1970s. In 1973, Wennberg and Gittelsohn[15] first identified the extreme degree of variability that exists in clinical practice by documenting that 70% of women in one Maine county had hysterectomies by the age of 70 years, as compared with 20% in a nearby county with similar demographics. Not surprisingly, the rate of hysterectomy was directly proportional to the physical proximity of a gynecologist. Similarly, residents of New Haven, Connecticut are twice as likely to undergo coronary artery bypass grafting (CABG), whereas patients in Boston are twice as likely to undergo carotid endarterectomy, even though both cities are the home of top-rated academic medical centers.[16]

Dr. Wennberg's work in regional variability led to the creation in the 1990s of the Dartmouth Atlas Project, which maps health care use and outcomes for every geographic region in the United States, and details care down to the referral region of each hospital. Atlas researchers, notably Dr. Elliott Fisher et al.,[17,18] have looked at the pattern of health care delivery and have found no clear association between the volume, intensity, or cost of care and patient outcomes. According to the Dartmouth Atlas Project, patients in areas of higher spending receive 60% more care, but the quality of care in those regions is no better, and at times worse, when key quality measures are compared.[17,18] More widely reported in the lay press was the finding that Medicare spends twice the national average per enrollee in McAllen, Texas than it does any other part of the country, including other cities in Texas, without better-quality outcomes.[19] The increased expense comes from more testing, more hospitalizations, more surgical procedures, and more home care. Variability in practice pattern, however, is not limited to overuse, but also includes underuse. McGlynn et al.[20] found that, in aggregate, the U.S. population receives only 55% of recommended treatments, regardless of whether preventive, acute, or chronic care is examined.

The findings of the Dartmouth Atlas Project have frequently been cited as a rationale for health care reform law. The Project's underlying methodology, however, has been scrutinized. Some investigators have questioned whether it appropriately adjusts for the costs of medical practice in different regions. Others have pointed out the limitations of focusing analysis on health care costs incurred by patients over the 2 years before their deaths and attributing these costs to the hospital most frequently visited.[21] A study by Romley et al.[22] reported an inverse relationship between hospital spending and inpatient mortality. Although great variability clearly exists in clinical practice, what is not clear is how to translate maps of geographic variation into health care policies that improve quality and contain costs.

One attempt at decreasing practice variability has been the rapid proliferation of clinical practice guidelines. Guidelines have been developed by physician specialty societies, hospitals, employers' consortia, and government agencies (e.g., the Agency for Healthcare Research and Quality). The physician community, however, has been slow to adopt guidelines for several reasons. Some physicians disparage guidelines as "cookbook medicine," whereas others point to the limited evidence on which these guidelines are built. Fear that deviation from guidelines may lead to more malpractice claims has also dampened enthusiasm for their use. Although clinical practice guidelines, order sets, and electronic decision support may not individually be the magic bullet for decreasing unwarranted clinical practice variability, all health care efforts should aim to be safe, effective, patient centered, timely, efficient, and equitable.

## INSTITUTE OF MEDICINE AIM: PATIENT SAFETY

Echoing the ancient axiom of medicine, *Primum non nocere*, or "First, do no harm," patients expect not to be harmed by the very care that is intended to help them. As such, patient safety is the most fundamental of the IOM's six domains. **Tables 208.2** and **208.3** provide the IOM's Patient Safety and Adverse Event Nomenclature.

### ACTIVE AND LATENT FAILURE TYPES

Failures in the ED fall into two main failure types: active and latent. *Active failures* are unsafe acts or omissions at the level of the front-line operator, such as the emergency physician (EP), nurse, or care provider, and the effects are felt almost immediately. This is sometimes called the *sharp end* of care. *Latent failures* are failures of the system that can lie dormant, or latent, for years. Despite, or perhaps because of, their obscurity, latent failures can cause multiple types of operator, or active, failures, yet go unnoticed to the casual observer; thus, they pose the greatest threat to safety in the complex ED system. Masked as the cause of incidents, these failures are powerful in joining with other factors to breach the system's

**Table 208.2 Institute of Medicine's Patient Safety and Adverse Event Nomenclature**

| TERM | DEFINITION |
|---|---|
| Safety | Freedom from accidental injury |
| Patient safety | Freedom from accidental injury; involves the establishment of operational systems and processes that minimize the possibility of error and maximize the probability of intercepting errors when they occur |
| Accident | An event that damages a system and disrupts the ongoing or future output of the system |
| Error | The failure of a planned action to be completed as intended or the use of a wrong plan to achieve an aim |
| Adverse event | An injury caused by medical management rather than by the underlying disease or condition of the patient |
| Preventable adverse event | Adverse event attributable to error |
| Negligent adverse event | A subset of adverse event meeting the legal criteria for negligence |
| Adverse medication event | Adverse event resulting from a medication or pharmacotherapy |
| Active error | Error that occurs at the front line and whose effects are felt immediately |
| Latent error | Error in design, organization, training, or maintenance that is often caused by management or senior-level decisions; when expressed, these errors result in operator errors but may have been hidden, dormant in the system for lengthy periods before their appearance |

Adapted from Kohn LT, Corrigan J, Donaldson MS, McKenzie D. To err is human: building a safer health system. Washington, DC: National Academies Press; 2000.

**Table 208.3 Active and Latent Failure Types**

| FAILURE TYPE | CHARACTERISTICS |
|---|---|
| Active | Committed by those whose actions have immediate adverse consequences (e.g., direct patient care providers [sharp end])<br>Cognitive errors<br>Slips<br>Lapses<br>Mistakes<br>Rule based<br>Knowledge based<br>Violations<br>Low morale<br>Poor examples from senior staff<br>Maladaptive decision styles<br>Authority gradient<br>Overconfidence or underconfidence |
| Latent | Resulting from the actions or decisions of those not directly involved in the workplace (e.g., management or senior clinicians [blunt end])<br>Excessive workloads or inadequate staff<br>Inadequate knowledge, experience, or training<br>Lack of supervision<br>High-stress environment<br>Poor communication systems<br>Poor maintenance of work environment<br>Rapid organizational change<br>Conflict between institutional mission and values<br>Production pressure<br>Overcrowding<br>Poor feedback<br>Poor design characteristics |

From Aghababian R, editor. Essentials of emergency care. 2nd ed. Sudbury, Mass: Jones and Bartlett; 2006.

defences and coalesce in errors. In large part, latent failures are the result of decisions affecting daily ED operations, decisions often made by persons not directly involved in care delivery; for example, managers, designers, procedure writers, and drug manufacturers.

Active and latent failures are plentiful in the ED. An active failure occurs when a triage nurse accidentally measures a pediatric patient's weight in pounds but writes down the weight in a chart box labeled kilograms instead. A similar error occurs when an EP orders antibiotics for a pediatric patient based on milligrams per kilograms (mg/kg) but uses weight in pounds instead. A latent failure exists when a patient with a pending pregnancy test undergoes computed tomography imaging before the positive result returns, or a patient with a pending creatinine test is given intravenous contrast before the abnormal results are acknowledged by the ordering provider.

## REASON'S "SWISS CHEESE" MODEL

Described by James Reason in 1990,[23] the "Swiss cheese" model of human error has four levels of human failure useful to evaluating a medical error (**Fig. 208.2**). The first level depicts active failures, which are the *unsafe acts* of the operator that ultimately led to the error. The next three levels depict latent failures *(preconditions for unsafe acts, unsafe supervision, and organizational influence),* which are underlying holes (or *hazards*) that allow errors to pass through to the sharp end. As with slices of Swiss cheese, when the levels of error are not aligned, an active failure can be caught before it causes harm—a near miss. With the right alignment, however, patients can be harmed by predictable human errors when systems are not appropriately designed to protect them.

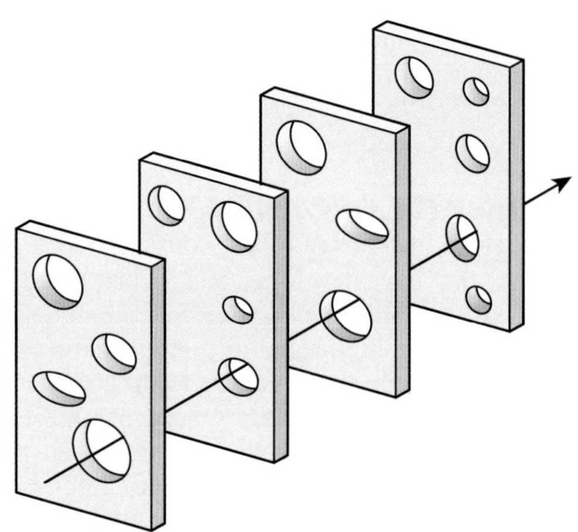

**Fig. 208.2 Reason's "Swiss cheese" model.** (Adapted from Reason J. Human error. Cambridge: Cambridge University Press; 1990.)

## COGNITIVE ERRORS

Cognitive errors fall into three distinct types: skill based, rule based, and knowledge based. Consider the act of driving a car or putting on your shoes. At some point, most of us acquired the requisite skills to accomplish these tasks quickly and efficiently without having to think about them. *Skill-based cognitive performance* refers to such acts. In the clinical setting, experienced clinicians approach the tasks of preparing a wound, tying a suture, or starting a central line in like fashion. Such clinical actions require little cognitive decision making. Skill-based errors are known as slips and lapses. *Slips* arise when actions fail to proceed as planned; for example, when a physician chooses an appropriate medication and writes 10 mg when the intention was to write 1 mg. Slips are errors in execution resulting from a failure of attention or perception often caused by interruptions or altered routines. In lay terms, slips are often equated with minor incidents. In the ED, patients can die as a result of slips. *Lapses* also result in failure to execute a plan, but whereas slips are observable, memory-based lapses are not. Pressing the wrong button on a defibrillator because you are interrupted and lose your train of activity is a slip; not being able to *recall* the correct energy to defibrillate ventricular stimulation is a lapse.

Any task departure from skills-based processing requires either a rules-based or a knowledge-based approach. *Rules-based processing* occurs when the clinician applies a known rule to make a decision. Rules, typically applied in the form "if X, then Y," come from past experience, explicit instructions, or clinical guidelines. Traditional medical education is full of experienced-based rules, often termed clinical pearls. For example, the advice not to discharge a patient with abnormal vital signs is based on clinicians' cumulative experience of reviewing adverse events after ED discharges. In contrast, the use of formalized clinical decision rules or guidelines (e.g., the Ottawa ankle rules to determine need for radiographs in ankle injuries) is another form of rule-based processing. *Knowledge-based processing* is when medical knowledge is applied and analytic processes are used to execute a plan of care. Errors of rule-based and knowledge-based cognition are known as mistakes. In rules-based errors, the wrong rule is selected, applied, or linked to the situation. Knowledge-based errors result when incomplete or incorrect knowledge is applied or flawed analytic processes are used, resulting in a poor plan of care. A mistake in medicine may involve selecting the wrong drug or treatment because of an incorrect diagnosis.

As clinicians gain experience, they engage to greater extent in skill-based and rule-based processing and to a lesser degree in knowledge-based processing. This shift in cognitive processing creates an interesting paradox with respect to the types of errors clinicians are most likely to commit. Although the rate of their knowledge-based errors is substantially reduced, highly trained individuals are more likely to experience skill-based errors, which are errors that arise from processes requiring the least amount of cognitive function.

EP are at particular risk for cognitive errors related to the core tasks of the specialty of emergency medicine—the rapid evaluation of patients with undifferentiated complaints and the high-risk decisions that must be made with incomplete information.

## HEURISTICS

Medical decision making in the ED is also characterized by a reliance on heuristics. *Heuristics* are shortcuts, rules of thumb, or any kind of abbreviated thinking that accomplishes quick and efficient decision making. Although they often serve EPs well, heuristics sometimes fail, thus leading to poor outcomes.

The four most commonly applied heuristics in emergency medicine are representativeness, availability, anchoring, and premature closure. The *representativeness heuristic* is applied when a clinician makes a subjective judgment of the similarity of a particular patient's presentation to that of most patients who present with a particular condition. The more *un*representative the patient's presentation is, the greater is the chance that the diagnosis will be delayed or missed. Representativeness errors appear most often in settings of high diagnostic uncertainty, such as that typifying the ED, and they are more likely to be committed by clinicians with lower levels of experience. An example is the evaluation of a patient for thoracic aortic dissection, a relatively rare diagnosis. Although the classic symptom of a sudden onset of tearing thoracic chest pain that radiates to the back is not present in most cases, most physicians are less likely to consider this diagnosis without a representative presentation.

Another heuristic that can lead to errors in decision making is *availability*. Certain encounters are more prevalent in our memories, perhaps because they have occurred more recently, but more often because they are emotionally salient. When making diagnoses, human nature leads to an overreliance on encounters that are vivid and to place less importance on those least salient. For example, if a physician has a particularly vivid experience of missing an acute myocardial infarction (AMI) in a young person, the physician may become overcautious in managing similar patients with chest pain. Availability may similarly be increased by indirect experience: a recent discussion with a colleague, a case presentation at rounds, or an article reviewing a particular case. In contrast, availability is decreased by long intervals since encountering a particular disease, or never having previously seen it.

*Anchoring* results when physicians commit early to a diagnosis and give it undue weight when considering the available data. One way of avoiding anchoring is to ask "What else could this be?" and always to be disciplined in thinking about the differential diagnosis. The tendency to look for evidence that bolsters an original hypothesis is referred to as *confirmation bias.* Instead of ignoring conflicting data, EPs must look for disconfirming evidence that rejects the initial contention. If anchoring occurs early in a presentation and EPs operate under a strong confirmation bias, they are sure to miss diagnoses. For example, an older patient who presents with epigastric pain and a bulge in the abdomen could have either an incarcerated hernia or an AMI. A clinician who anchors on the diagnosis of incarcerated hernia can easily explain away tachycardia as the result of pain, and subtle electrocardiographic changes as nonspecific, rather than identifying them as the pattern of an early AMI.

Finally, *premature closure* occurs when a physician makes a quick diagnosis (often based on pattern recognition and not confirmed by appropriate testing), then stops collecting data, and fails to consider other possible diagnoses. Premature closure can occur in any case, but it is especially common when EPs take care of patients who seem to have an exacerbation of a known disorder. For example, a patient with a history of migraine is assumed to have another migraine, rather than an acute presentation of subarachnoid hemorrhage. Another example is a patient with chest pain and ST-segment elevation on the electrocardiogram who is assumed to be suffering from an acute coronary syndrome, rather than thoracic aortic dissection leading to coronary artery dissection.

Awareness of such cognitive biases is crucial, and simply knowing what they look like can help in overcoming them. Avoiding reflexive thinking and taking the time to think about how we think can help to minimize or avoid errors. Decision support tools, such as templated charts with potential diagnoses, or more sophisticated electronic tools that are queued by patient complaints and history, can help physicians overcome some of these biases.

## ERROR-PRODUCING CONDITIONS IN THE EMERGENCY DEPARTMENT

The ED ranks among the top three hospital locations with the highest risk of error, along with the intensive care units and operating rooms. This finding is not surprising when one considers the combinations of error-producing conditions that exist in the typical ED. Many different providers (e.g., physicians, nurses, technicians) work closely together to care simultaneously for multiple patients of varying medical acuity who present with any imaginable chief complaint, from the most life-threatening to the most poorly defined, with whom these providers typically have no prior relationship. Providers are bombarded with multiple interruptions, and they struggle at times with understaffing and overcrowding while working through disruptive sleep cycles. As such, error-producing conditions in the ED include *diagnostic uncertainty, low signal-to-noise ratio* (i.e., the incidence of a serious condition or diagnosis [e.g., cauda equine syndrome] is low compared with more common and more benign diagnoses [e.g., musculoskeletal back pain]), *high cognitive load*, and *poor feedback.* Lack of continuity of care and unreliable and untimely feedback of patient diagnoses and outcomes make it difficult for EPs to refine their clinical skills continuously. A national survey of U.S. EDs documented commonly reported problems in four major areas: physical environment, staffing, inpatient coordination, and information coordination and consultation. The surveys suggest that the U.S. EDs have substantial room to reduce the latent conditions for errors.

## HIGH-RELIABILITY ORGANIZATIONS

In the ED, we can learn from other industries (e.g., aviation, nuclear power) that have developed and incorporated systems allowing for early error corrections or prevention and leading them to function as high-reliability organizations.[24] Such industries tightly couple the process of doing work with the process of learning to do it better. Operations are expressly designed to reveal problems as they occur. When problems arise, no matter how trivial, they are addressed quickly. High-reliability organizations share the following six traits:

*Preoccupation with failure*. These organizations are willing to examine any systems failure to identify causes. Even very small events are evaluated as opportunities to remove systems errors before they coalesce to create large, catastrophic system failures. The organizations have a strong culture of safety.

*Reluctance to simplify interpretations*. Such organizations seek materials and accurate appraisals of any failure. They do not simply blame individual workers and then consider the case closed.

*Sensitivity to operations*. These organizations methodologically approach each task with an eye toward improvement, by probing the systems factors that contributed to the failure.

*Commitment to resilience*. These organizations continually address a deficit until resolution occurs.

*Understanding of expertise*. These organizations defer decisions to the person who has the requisite knowledge, rather than the requisite rank.

*Clarity in mission and vision*. A common view of the world allows team members to communicate accurately.

Understanding the importance of a culture of safety in the strive for high quality, Johns Hopkins Hospital (Baltimore) researchers implemented a comprehensive, unit-based safety program (CUSPS) at almost 150 individual units in the hospital.[25] This program ultimately led to the establishment of an organization-wide culture of safety at the hospital. Although in the past, organizations focused many resources on building a *culture of safety*, patient safety leaders have shifted to advocating for a *just culture,* one that balances *safety* with *accountability*.[26] Whereas a culture of safety allows evaluation of suboptimal medical outcomes without fear of punitive action toward individuals, a culture of accountability also encourages providers to do the right thing, especially when doing the right thing is easy. A notable example is facilitating hand hygiene through provision of soap dispensers in key locations while holding providers accountable for their individual behavior through direct observation and feedback.

# INSTITUTE OF MEDICINE AIM: TIMELINESS

Timeliness is a core mission of the specialty of emergency medicine. In a little more than one decade, ED visits have grown by nearly 25%, whereas at least 10% of EDs have closed nationally. This situation has caused many EDs to experience increased waiting room times, length of stay, and boarding of inpatients in the ED.[27] In fact, up to 25% of patients are not seen by an EP within acuity-based recommended times,[28] and patients with AMI have experienced a 150% increase in wait times over this period.[29] Deaths in the waiting room reported in the lay press serve as a stark reminder of the consequences of systems failures on individual patients.[30]

Although one goal of health care reform is to decrease ED visits, to date, large-scale health systems reforms have not been able to do this. In fact, given aging demographics (older patients have a higher ED use rate) and patient preferences (for rapid acute care at the time of their choosing), current crowding trends are likely to continue. Furthermore, if efforts at health care reform lead to an increased number of insured patients, Massachusetts' experience of requiring individual to obtain health insurance (the individual mandate) suggests that more, rather than fewer, ED visits can be expected in the near term.[31]

A growing body of evidence links prolonged ED length of stay, ED crowding, and boarding of inpatients in the ED to lower quality care and worse patient outcomes. ED crowding has been associated with worse-quality care for patients with AMI, acute coronary syndromes, and hip fractures.[32-34] For example, cardiac patients boarded in the ED for longer than 8 hours are less likely to receive guideline-recommended therapies and are more likely to have recurrent MIs. Given prolonged wait times to evaluation in the ED, one study evaluated the safety of managing potential cardiac patients in the ED waiting room.[35] Although approaches such as this, to improve safety in the crowded ED, are reasonable short-term solutions, they do not address the primary latent failure of ED crowding, which is the inability to evaluate and treat patients in the appropriate location in a timely fashion.

Given the challenge of addressing quality and safety issues in a crowded ED, many departments are redesigning their operations and patient flow models to improve the timelines of care. Most notably, newer models of care have been developed to replace the traditional model of ED care that was serial (e.g., patient triage, then nursing evaluation, then physician evaluation, then laboratory or diagnostic testing, then decision on final disposition) and uniform (regardless of patient's clinical needs). Newer models of care have several common features: optimizing front-end operations, developing multiple pathways through the ED that attempt to match a patient's acuity and resource needs, eliminating duplicate evaluations, maximizing the use of limited ED beds, and facilitating rapid discharge of patients.[36] One example is vertical patient flow, a model in which a cohort of patients, rapidly identified on arrival to the ED, is evaluated, managed, and either admitted or discharged in advance (or in lieu) of occupying a traditional ED bed.[37] These patients (often a subset of Emergency Severity Index [ESI] 3 patients) require greater medical decision making and more resources than do fast-track patients, but they do not require a room and a stretcher for evaluation. Because these patients do not need to be disrobed in a private room for most of their ED visit, they can sit in recliners in an internal waiting room for most of their ED visit.

## INSTITUTE OF MEDICINE AIM: PATIENT-CENTERED CARE

The IOM report identified patient-centered care as a core element of quality. Although many physicians equate patient-centeredness with patient satisfaction, satisfaction is only one component of patient-centeredness. Patient-centered care respects individual patients by addressing the values, ethnicity, social situation, and information needs of each patient.[38] Although patient satisfaction surveys have been used for a long time in emergency medicine, only more recently have EPs begun to implement changes that strive to make emergency care more inclusive and responsive to patients' values, needs, and wishes. Two notable examples are the move to include families in resuscitations[39] and the use of structured decision aids to guide joint medical decision making.[40-41] Historically, family members were kept out of ED resuscitation rooms when their loved one was undergoing advanced resuscitation (e.g., cardiopulmonary resuscitation). Studies show that family members benefit from their involvement at the end of the patient's life because the resuscitation, instead of being traumatic, often helps bring closure to a tragic event. A second example is using structured decision aids to engage patients in complex diagnostic decisions, such as whether to conduct cardiac risk stratification in the ED, in the hospital, or in the outpatient environment. When presented with well-designed decision aids, patients are both less likely to request more resource-intensive testing and more likely to be satisfied with their care.

## INSTITUTE OF MEDICINE AIMS: EFFECTIVE, EFFICIENT, AND EQUITABLE CARE

According to the IOM, *effective* care should be based on best evidence, thus avoiding inappropriate underuse or overuse. The literature supports the care of some common patient presentations (e.g., syncope, sepsis). Much room for improvement remains, however, because much of emergency practice is without a strong basis in the literature. In this relatively new specialty that deals with a diverse patient population under challenging clinical conditions, conducting methodologically rigorous clinical research has been difficult. Much of the evidence that has been cited to justify emergency practice is from other populations, clinical venues, and focus on nonemergency outcomes. This situation is illustrated by the paucity of level I recommendations in the American College of Emergency Physicians Clinical Policies. As in other areas in which clinical practice has been studied, tremendous provider-to-provider variability exists in emergency medicine. The hope is that minimizing this variability by developing evidence-based guidelines will allow EPs to provide effective care more reliably.

According to the IOM, *efficient* care avoids waste. Although most ED administrators may define efficiency by the rapidity with which patients are processed through the ED, most health policy analysts view efficiency as a measure of the quality of care delivered for the amount of resources consumed. Efficiency is akin to value and can be improved by reducing waste or improving quality, while holding all else constant.

Unfortunately, ED care is widely viewed by the medical community as inefficient. This view is often based on comparisons of charges and costs for ED visits and primary care physician visits for simple presentations, such as sore throat or ear infections. The true marginal cost of such patient visits in the ED is open to debate, however, given the high fixed expenses associated with operating a clinical environment 24 hours a day, 365 days a year. More problematic is the view that all emergency visits are avoidable and examples of failures of the health care delivery system. Clearly appropriate ED visits for patients range from heart attacks and strokes to stab wounds and motor vehicle accidents.

EPs can respond to the push for increased efficiency in the health care system by looking for ways to deliver their care with less waste. For example, efficiency measures focused on appropriateness of imaging studies are likely to be defined. By reducing inappropriate and unnecessary testing, EPs can improve the efficiency of emergency care without reducing quality or access.

The IOM defined *equitable* care as care that does not vary in quality based on personal characteristics (e.g., race, gender, geographic location, socioeconomic status). Although most EPs pride themselves on providing equal care to all, regardless of ability to pay and personal background, studies have documented racial disparities in emergency care.[42-45] Significant room exists for future research on equality of emergency care because it has received little research attention.

## SPECIAL FOCUS: CARE COORDINATION

Appropriate care coordination around transitions of care is a topic that cuts across multiple domains of quality. The totality of care cannot be timely, efficient, and patient centered if it is poorly coordinated during the many hand-offs that occur in health care. For example, almost 20% of Medicare beneficiaries are rehospitalized within 30 days of hospital discharge, and half of these patients did not have an intervening primary care visit.[46]

Care coordination is especially important for "hot spotters," patients who are extreme outliers in health care use and cost.[47] Although 10% of patients account for two thirds of all U.S. health care costs (**Fig. 208.3**), these extreme outliers (top 1%) can account for a significant fraction of costs by themselves. Intensive outpatient care for complex high-needs patients can significantly reduce health care costs. So far, these efforts have viewed ED visits as systems failures and have not engaged emergency caregivers, but such programs will likely be more successful if they integrate coordination of care plans between the outpatient providers and the local ED providers.

More directly affecting ED care are the hand-offs between physicians at change of shift or on patient admission. Communication errors are the root cause of most safety events that occur in the ED. Many quality lapses occur when critical information is lost in such transitions. Many barriers to effective communication exist, including the need to balance conciseness with completeness, the lack of a standardized approach, and ambiguous time stamp for when transition of care occurs. Nonetheless, Cheung et al.[48] provided with strategies to improve hand-offs, including reducing the number of unnecessary hand-offs, limiting interruptions and distractions, communicating outstanding tasks and anticipated changes along with a clear care plan, encouraging questioning of assessment, and signaling a clear moment in transition of care.

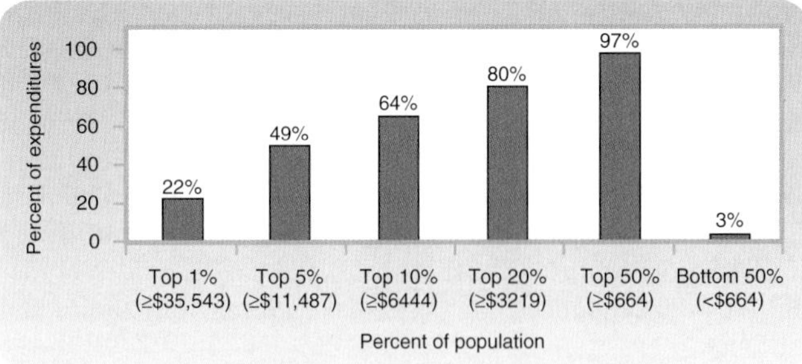


**Fig. 208.3 The high concentration of U.S. health care expenditures.** (Modified from Conwell LJ, Cohen JW. Characteristics of people with high medical expenses in the U.S. civilian noninstitutionalized population, 2002. Statistical brief no. 73. Rockville, Md: Agency for Healthcare Research and Quality; 2005. [http://www.meps.ahrq.gov/mepsweb/data_files/publications/st73/stat73.pdf].)

## SPECIAL FOCUS: FROM "NEVER EVENTS" TO "SERIOUS REPORTABLE EVENTS"

The most high-profile patient safety errors have been those that were serious and preventable. This is not surprising because explaining to a patient or patient's family how a system allows such events to occur again and again is difficult. For example, at one hospital in Rhode Island, neurosurgeons operated on the wrong side of a patient's brain three times over the course of 3 years, and an additional two other wrong-site surgical procedures occurred in this time.[49,50] Such errors were initially labeled "never events"—events that should never occur. However, as the number of preventable events (e.g., hospital-acquired infections) grew, maintaining the paradigm of never events became difficult. Instead, the focus was changed from events that should never occur to ones that should not occur.

As such, in 2002, in an effort to develop a single standard list of serious medical errors requiring reporting, the National Quality Forum convened a multidisciplinary group that developed a consensus list of Serious Reportable Events in Healthcare (SREs). The goal of defining SREs was to guarantee that serious patient safety events would undergo systematic review to determine causes and contributing factors and that the findings would be used to improve care and avoid future events. Given public reporting requirements and potential nonpayment, SREs represent an important hospital patient safety priority.

## FINANCIAL STRATEGIES TO IMPROVE HEALTH CARE QUALITY AND VALUE

### CENTER FOR MEDICARE AND MEDICAID SERVICES

As the country's largest insurer and purchaser of health care services, the Centers for Medicare and Medicaid Services (CMS) is very interested in making sure its health care dollars are being well spent. Toward the aim of increased transparency and accountability, CMS launched a public reporting effort in 2004. Initially, participation in Hospital Compare (www.hospitalcompare.hhs.gov) was voluntary, and only quality measures related to pneumonia, AMI, and congestive heart failure were reported. Since then, the number of measures reported on this website has dramatically increased, and it includes risk-adjusted death and readmission rates, as well as patient satisfaction.

In 2007, the CMS rolled out a Physician Quality Reporting Initiative (PQRI), which has since been renamed the Physician Quality Reporting System (PQRS). Initially, physician groups received a 2% bonus for participating in the program. By 2014, that amount will decrease to 0.5%. Starting in 2016, physicians who do not participate in PQRS will see a 2% reduction in their Medicare payments. EPs have notably had one of the highest participation rates among all the specialties.

In January 2011, the CMS launched a Physician Compare website. Although it started with simple provider-specific information (e.g., whether a physician accepts Medicare and uses electronic prescribing), by 2015 it is expected to have public reports of physician-specific quality measures, including patient satisfaction. Developing physician profiles is replete with challenges.[51] One of the most important unintended consequences of physician profiling is risk aversion (physician's avoiding complex or high-risk patients), which inevitably leads to decreased health care access for minorities and economically disadvantaged populations.[52-54] Most problematic has been physician cost profiling because current methods misclassify physician ranking one fourth of the time.[55] The reliability of these profiling schemes therefore is paramount.

The Affordable Care Act established an Innovation Center within the CMS to test innovative payment and health care delivery models, aimed at reducing health care expenditures and improving quality. For example, the Innovation Center will likely link payment to hospitals to their ability to reduce hospital-acquired infections and readmissions. The effectiveness of such financial incentive programs has been drawn into question. Looking at data from the United Kingdom's Quality and Outcomes Framework, researchers did not find any improvement in outcome measures for patients treated before or after the introduction of the incentive program.[56]

## FUTURE REIMBURSEMENT MODELS

In both public and private sectors, a strong movement is leading away from purchasing health care services by volume and toward purchasing value (defined as health care value per dollar spent).[57,58] Reimbursement models are evolving to motivate providers to be more cost and quality conscious. Since 2000, several schemes have emerged that have been called pay-for performance (P4P) programs. Many of these programs were simply fee-for-service models, with either a bonus or withhold based on achieving certain performance thresholds.

A newer, emerging reimbursement model is bundled payment, in which hospitals and providers share in the accountability for delivering value. Geisinger Health System's ProvenCare program[59] defined and implemented best practices for patients undergoing CABG and then offered risk-based pricing to insurers. Specifically, preoperative, inpatient, and postoperative care within 90 days was packaged into a fixed price and touted in the lay press as a "CABG warranty." The success of this program in improving care and reducing costs brought the concept of bundled payments to the center stage of health care reform.

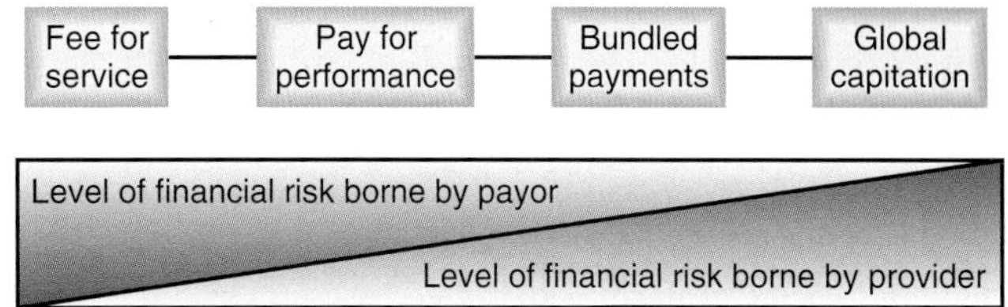


**Fig. 208.4 Health care reimbursement models.**

Global or capitated payment is also reemerging as a viable way to reimburse for care. Blue Cross/Blue Shield of Massachusetts reported that its global payment system improved patient care during its first year, including decreasing avoidable ED visits by 25% through one of its contracts.[60] Under an alternative quality contract, physicians are provided a monthly per-patient budget, as well as bonuses for improving care. Future reimbursement models will inevitably center on performance measurement and accountability, with a likely shift in level of financial risk borne from payer to provider (**Fig. 208.4**).

To be fiscally viable within potential future reimbursement models, health care providers are being encouraged to organize themselves into accountable care organizations (ACOs).[61-63] ACOs are meant to encompass various provider arrangements (e.g., integrated delivery systems, multispecialty group practices, physician-hospital organizations, independent practice associations) that lead involved parties (e.g., physician group and hospital) to be jointly accountable for improving patient care and reducing spending. Unlike an HMO, this needs to be accomplished within the context of patients' choice to visit providers internal or external to the ACO for which their care is attributed. Ideally, ACOs will be able to bend the cost curve of increasing health care expenditures. Many different prototypes have been reported in the lay and medical literature. Certification of ACOs for participation in the Affordable Care Act's Shared Savings Program for Medicare still must occur. A fine balance will need to be reached because a liberal policy may lead to provider mergers and market dominance that have driven up costs in the past.

## MEASURE DEVELOPMENT

Future reimbursement models will depend on development of methodologically sound quality measures, and particularly on measures of outcomes of care. The most easily accessible outcome measures (e.g., mortality rate, readmission rates) are important but nonspecific measures of quality.

To date, numerous organizations have developed quality of care measures ranging from academic researchers, to individual hospitals and health systems, to federal agencies and their contractors. Although virtually anyone can develop a potential measure, several organizations have taken the lead in reviewing and endorsing measures of quality of care.

The American Medical Association's Physician Consortium for Performance Improvement is composed of all the medical specialty societies and leads projects to develop measures for individual specialties and for conditions that cross specialties (e.g., stroke). Similarly, the National Center for Quality Assurance has taken the lead in developing measures of care for insurance plans and health care systems. The National Quality Forum (NQF) is a public-private venture whose mission is to improve health care by endorsing consensus-based national standards for measurement and public reporting of health care quality data. Payers and government agencies, such as CMS rely on the NQF to endorse valid performance measures.

Emergency medicine faces a unique challenge in developing and commenting on potential quality measures. Because EPs care for patients with all types of conditions, many specialties and condition-specific quality measure sets could measure and judge emergency care. As such, the American College of Emergency Physicians and the Society for Academic Emergency Medicine have lobbied to have EPs included in quality measure development panels that affect emergency medicine.

Without representation, poorly framed, yet nationally endorsed, quality measures may negatively affect emergency care. For example, the initial measure set for community-acquired pneumonia was developed using low-quality evidence from cross-sectional Medicare studies. EPs contended that these measures had many unintended consequences, including the administration of inappropriate antibiotics and excessive use of blood cultures.[64] As more research was published showing that these measures were not linked to improved patient outcomes, the CMS revised the measures (**Box 208.1**).

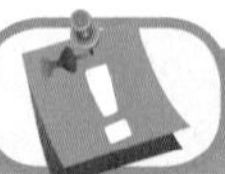

**TIPS AND TRICKS**

**Quality in the Emergency Department**

- Do what is right for the patient regardless of timing (e.g., off hours) or circumstances (e.g., overcrowding).
- At change of shift, briefly evaluate patients turned over to your care so that you have a baseline in mind should an acute deterioration in a patient's condition occur.
- Before discharge, make sure to review all laboratory results and radiographs even if you expect the results to be normal.
- Explain diagnostic uncertainties at discharge so that the patient will seek care if his or her condition deteriorates.
- In general, think twice before:
  - Discharging a patient against the preference or comfort of the patient or family.
  - Discharging a patient against the advice of another physician.
  - Discharging a patient who was seen in the past 48 hours for the same condition.
  - Discharging a patient with narcotic pain medications without a clear diagnosis.
  - Ruling out a critical diagnosis based on a negative result of a suboptimal test.
  - Discharging a patient with abnormal vital signs.

## HEALTH CARE QUALITY LAPSES AND INDIVIDUAL PROVIDERS

Despite an increased focus on transparency and systems improvement (**Box 208.2**), physicians and hospitals continue to underreport their errors and quality lapses. Too often, providers react to medical errors with shame, fear, and secrecy. To most physicians, the admission of wrongdoing has the dual effect of causing humiliation in front of patients and peers and introducing fear of lawsuits into everyday life. Ofri[65] reported, "No doctor will easily confess to error when a core sense of self is at risk. … Unless we can defuse the shame and loss of self that accompany admitting medical errors, there will always be that taut inner core of resistance."

**BOX 208.1 Blood Cultures for Community-Acquired Pneumonia**

This measure serves as an example of a measure with a poor scientific basis and little regard for implementation feasibility. These guidelines were developed and approved without adequate input from the emergency medicine community. Despite feedback and modification, the current measures are not evidence based, they require laborious chart review, and performance is more easily improved by modifying documentation than by improving processes of care.

- **1998 and 2000**: Clinical guidelines for CAP published by specialty societies recommend routine blood cultures for patients admitted with CAP (e.g., the Infectious Disease Society of America).
- **2000**: A technical panel charged to develop CAP quality measures from the Oklahoma Foundation for Medical Quality reviews the guidelines and recommends blood cultures in pneumonia as a CAP measure to CMS and the Joint Commission.
- **2000**: Once approved by CMS and the Joint Commission, the measures are then submitted and endorsed by the National Quality Forum.
- **2002**: The measures are adopted as National Hospital Quality Measures, and results are reported on the Hospital Compare website.
- **2004 and 2006**: Because of feedback from emergency physicians, the measures were revised several times to limit the eligible population. The first revision limited the applicable patient population to those admitted to an ICU within the first 24 hours of their stay. The second revision further refined the eligible population as the subset of patients with CAP who have cultures drawn in the ED.
- **2011**: Current CAP measures are as follows:
  - The proportion of patients admitted to the ICU within 24 hours of hospital arrival because of pneumonia who have blood cultures obtained within 24 hours of arrival
  - The proportion of patients who have blood culture drawn in the ED who have the culture drawn before antibiotic administration

*CAP*, Community-acquired pneumonia; *CMS*, Centers for Medicare and Medicaid Services; *ED*, emergency department; *ICU*, intensive care unit.

In most emergency medicine residency programs, the morbidity and mortality conference is the most widely used error-based teaching conference. The culture of this conference helps shape physicians' view of medical errors. One step in the right direction is for senior EPs to share their own mistakes with the next generation of physicians in an open and safe manner and to encourage reporting of errors, especially when appropriate peer-review protected systems are in place. Another cultural change is for EDs and hospitals to adopt policies encouraging rapid and open admissions of error to patients. Although individual physicians can adopt this strategy, it may be most effective if adopted by an institution and supported with changes in the way patients are compensated for medical errors. In 2001, the University of Michigan adopted a program of full disclosure of medical errors with offers of compensation. This approach both decreased the number of lawsuits and the time to resolution, without increasing the overall amount spent on medical malpractice.[66]

**BOX 208.2 Quality Improvement Toolkit**

**Investigate**

- *RCA* (root-cause analysis): This is an attempt to learn the underlying systems cause of problems (e.g., equipment, staffing, policies and procedures, information systems), frequently by asking "why" five times until the root cause is identified; it is facilitated by use of a fishbone diagram.
- *FMEA* (failure modes and effects analysis): This is a systematic, proactive method for evaluating a process to identify where and how it may fail and to assess the relative impact of different failures to identify the parts of the process that are most in need of change.

**Mitigate**

- *Standardization*: Consistency minimizes errors caused by varied processes (e.g., using the same tube thoracostomy set throughout the hospital).
- *Simplification*: The more steps a process has, the more likely it will be that a given process will go wrong (e.g., different admitting procedures for different services within the same hospital).
- *Checklist*: This was made famous by Provonost's Keystone Initiative, which showed that a simple checklist for central venous catheter placement in the ICU could substantially decrease the infection rate.
- *Forcing function*: Systems designs make it difficult to do the wrong thing (e.g., gas connectors on anesthesia machines are designed so that oxygen and nitrous oxide tanks can be attached only to proper ports, thus eliminating the potential of a fatal mix-up) or make it easy to do the right thing (e.g., opt-out provisions for deep venous thrombosis prophylaxis as part of inpatient order sets decrease the rate of subsequent pulmonary embolus).

**Improve**

- *PDCA* (plan, do, check, act): Identify a problem, plan a solution, execute the plan on a small scale, measure performance, check to see whether the plan resulted in the desired outcome, make changes to improve the plan, and/or execute the plan on a larger scale. In terms of improving the daily practice of medicine, PDCA cycles are more useful than formal studies (e.g., randomized trials) and erratic trial and error approaches.
- *LEAN*: with the use of value stream maps, lean thinking identifies value-added and non–value-added steps in every process, with the goal of driving out waste so that all work adds value and serves the patient's needs.

## REMAINING CHALLENGES

Although more than a decade has passed since the IOM reports were published, studies still show that nearly 20% of patients continue to be harmed by their care.[67] In addition, one in seven Medicare beneficiaries will experience adverse events while hospitalized, and SREs (e.g., wrong site surgery) continue to occur.[68] Furthermore, physician involvement in quality improvement activities varies considerably and will become mandatory only as each specialty board incorporates quality improvement into its maintenance of certification programs.[69] The American Board of Emergency Medicine requires a "patient care practice improvement activity" for those diplomates recertifying in 2013 and beyond.

No one can predict today what our health care system will look like in 3, 5, or 10 years. Current visions of bundled payment systems and ACOs are based more on theory than on experience. What one can be certain of is that pressure to address the rising costs of health care and the variable and often inadequate quality and safety of health care will continue. These pressures will lead to dramatic changes in the way physicians and hospitals are organized. The ED of 2020 may contain many more or many fewer patients, depending on how the system evolves. Yet EPs are uniquely qualified to understand quality and safety throughout health care systems and to mobilize multidisciplinary teams to address these challenges. EP engagement in improving care from the ED to the greater health care delivery system is needed now more than ever.

**TIPS AND TRICKS**

**Tell the Truth: Disclosure of Medical Errors**

Physicians may not be providing the information patients want about errors. Although physicians disclose the adverse event, they often avoid stating that an error occurred, why the error happened, or how recurrences could be prevented. Physicians should disclose the following minimal information about harmful errors, even if not requested by the patient:

- An explicit statement that an error occurred
- A basic description of the error, why the error happened, and how recurrences will be prevented
- Emotional support, including an apology

Adapted from Gallagher TH, Waterman AD, Ebers AG, et al. Patients' and physicians' attitudes regarding the disclosure of medical errors. JAMA 2003;289:1001-7.

## SUGGESTED READINGS

Berwick DM. Continuous improvement as an ideal in health care. N Engl J Med 1989;320:53-6.

Committee on Quality Health Care in America. Crossing the quality chasm: a new health system for the 21st century. Washington, DC: National Academies Press; 2001.

Croskerry P, Cosby KS, Schenkel S, Wears RL. Patient safety in emergency medicine. Philadelphia: Lippincott Williams & Wilkins; 2009.

Fisher ES, Wennberg DE, Stukel TA, et al. The implications of regional variations in Medicare spending. Part I: the content, quality, and accessibility of care; Part II: health outcomes and satisfaction with care. Ann Intern Med 2003;138:273-87, 288-298.

Kohn LT, Corrigan JM, Donaldson MS, editors. To err is human: building a safer health system. Washington, DC: National Academies Press; 1999.

## REFERENCES

***References can be found on Expert Consult @ www.expertconsult.com.***

# Conflict Resolution in Emergency Medicine 209

*Gus M. Garmel*

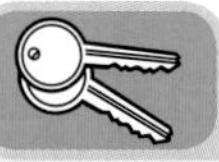

**KEY POINTS**

- Conflict is the result of discordant expectations, goals, needs, agendas, communication styles, and backgrounds between or among individuals. *At least* two perspectives contribute to conflict.
- Conflict in emergency medicine (EM) may occur with patients, family members, nurses, consultants, residents, students, hospital administrative staff, or agents inside and outside the emergency department.
- The goals of effective conflict resolution are to optimize immediate outcomes and to establish a solid foundation for subsequent interactions. Success depends on one's communication style, awareness of other's needs and psyche, and understanding of relationship dynamics.
- Successful conflict resolution requires a systematic and structured approach. Recognizing each participant's principal interests and underlying positions is important. Having a strong BATNA (best alternative to a negotiated agreement) is beneficial. Possessing a "win-lose" attitude interferes with successful conflict resolution.
- Not all conflict in EM can be resolved immediately, if at all; some resolutions require the assistance of a third party.
- Efforts to prevent conflict before it happens are recommended whenever possible.

*The problem with conflict is not its existence, but rather its management.*[1]

Conflict is inevitable. Opportunities for conflict in emergency medicine (EM) are numerous because individuals with different backgrounds and divergent agendas interact over important concerns (e.g., patient care or resource use). By nature, these interactions take place under time constraints, which often exacerbate conflict. Many interactions between emergency physicians (EPs) and patients, family members, staff members, or consultants occur with limited or no previous working relationship or when prior interactions have been problematic. As such, involved parties may be unable to reflect on prior successful interactions, an approach that often decreases the likelihood of intense exchange.[2]

Controversy exists about the *value* of conflict. Many believe that, at its best, conflict is disruptive. Most agree that, at its worst, conflict is destructive to team harmony and patient outcomes. However, conflict also serves as a creative force, providing both initiative and incentive to solve problems.

This chapter describes conflict in general, identifies contributing factors, and offers several examples specific to EM. The importance of effective communication in conflict resolution is presented, as well as its role in de-escalating, limiting, and preventing conflict. This chapter offers strategies to facilitate successful conflict resolution. Conflict resolution ultimately benefits patients, staff, and EPs by optimizing patient care, decreasing patient morbidity, improving patient safety, and maximizing an individual's or health care team's overall satisfaction.

*Communication,* in the form of language and interaction, and *power,* in terms of how conflict is managed (or mismanaged), are tremendously important in the dynamics of groups. EM is very much about group dynamics because physicians, nurses, and other staff members must consistently demonstrate successful teamwork to offer patients the best possible outcomes. Louise B. Andrew, MD, JD, stated "… conflict is often the result of miscommunication, and may be 'fueled' by ineffective communication."[3]

Three important sources of conflict have been identified: resources, psychological needs of individuals or groups, and values. *Resource-based* conflicts relate to limited resources, common in EM. *Psychological needs* include power, control, self-esteem, and acceptance. These needs often exist under the conflict's surface and can be difficult to identify or address. *Values* (beliefs) are fundamental to conflict. Core values, such as religious, ethical, financial, or those involving patient care are difficult to change and therefore generally assume a large role in conflict. Value differences among people or groups (e.g., health care professionals and physicians with different training) may result in repeated conflicts. The expectations that EPs have of hospital and emergency department (ED) staff regarding work ethic or efficiency, for example, often result in conflict (perceived or real). Under these circumstances, people feel as if their integrity is being questioned, and this is one reason that value-based conflicts are extremely difficult to resolve.

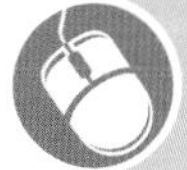

For additional information about sources and types of conflict, see the online version of this chapter at www.expertconsult.com

Conflict in medicine is relatively easy to understand if one considers physician attributes, such as a tendency toward perfectionism and delayed social development. These characteristics are highly adaptive to doctoring, reinforced by training, and rewarded by society. These traits may be maladaptive when it comes to communicating and interacting with nonphysicians, however, with resulting conflict and poor conflict management.

The ED environment is particularly predisposed to conflict for many reasons. Differences in professional opinion and value systems among staff members and patients are contributing factors. EPs must interact with individuals in all areas of health care, at any time of day or night, and during periods of great stress. EPs are unlikely to know everyone on every service with whom they must interact. This challenges EPs because they are not familiar with each medical staff members' idiosyncrasies, preferred practice pattern, or communication style. These interactions create even greater difficulties for new EPs, who lack histories of favorable reputations or successful relations with hospital staff, thus significantly increasing the likelihood of conflict.

## EXAMPLES OF CONFLICT

Conflict in EM results from a mismatch of expectations among patients, family members, providers, or consultants, as well as among nurses, ED staff, or ancillary staff outside the ED. Patients and family members may have unrealistic expectations about their ED experience, not to mention the pain or fear that brought them to the ED. Nurses may have unrealistic expectations of physicians and generally have widely differing backgrounds. Although gender representation of EPs has become more equal, older EPs tend to be male, whereas nurses are predominantly female. Misunderstandings and communication problems exist in the workplace between genders and age groups. Additionally, each time a consultant is contacted, his or her practice, social life, or sleep is disrupted. This added workload alone may ignite conflict.

Numerous additional factors further explain the high likelihood of conflict in EM. Diversity in training, experience, and perspective often result in differences of opinion between EPs and colleagues from other areas of medicine, including nursing. For example, conflict arises simply because EPs do not want to send someone home who should not go home, whereas hospital-based physicians or specialists may prefer not to admit (or may be pressured not to) patients who do not require admission. These two opposing "forces" create conflict.

The responsibility of patient advocacy assumed by EPs and ED staff often creates conflict because it may not coincide with the interests of the patient or family members. If a patient's decision-making capacity is impaired or their legal advocate is not present, EPs have the duty to act in the best interest of the patient, state, or society, regardless of the patient's wishes. One common challenge occurs when a patient with a history of substance abuse and chemical dependency demands narcotics for "pain." An EP's refusal to prescribe narcotics is certain to create conflict. Conflict also occurs when a patient or family member desires admission to the hospital without medical justification, a test that is not indicated or available (or may be harmful), or consultation with a specialist that is medically unnecessary or inappropriate at that time. Other times, an EP may believe that it is in the patient's best interest to be admitted to an inpatient medical service even if hospitalization may not influence the ultimate outcome, and this creates conflict with the admitting service. Conflict may also develop between two services over which service will admit a patient. The EP must mediate this dispute while keeping the patient's needs and interests at the discussion's forefront.

Perhaps the area most likely to create conflict is ineffective or incomplete communication between or among two or more parties. Given cultural and language differences among patients, families, nurses, staff, and consultants, communication challenges prime the ED for conflict. Frustration, unmet expectations, time constraints, and limitations on staffing, equipment, space, and privacy may be overwhelming if communication is suboptimal or barriers to effective communication exist.

Because the specialty of EM is so complex and has tremendous liability associated with its practice environment, many areas of potential conflict have been addressed at federal, state, and local levels. Hospital policies and bylaws have established guidelines addressing these issues, in an attempt to prevent conflict before it occurs. Despite these policies, conflict still occurs. EM organizations are addressing these and other areas of potential conflict, based on the needs of emergency patients and professionals. As health policy and the specialty of EM evolve, new challenges will be identified, with more issues requiring resolution (**Box 209.1**).

**BOX 209.1 Areas of Conflict Related to Emergency Medicine**

1. Differences in education, background, values, belief systems, and interpersonal styles of communication between EPs and others
2. Commitment to patient satisfaction
3. Final patient disposition (and who determines this)
4. Timing of follow-up care and outpatient tests for released patients
5. Telephone conversations required for patient care issues
6. Lack of professional respect from primary physicians or consultants
7. Dual advocacy expected by others for the EP
8. Teaching hospitals with house staff who may lack communication and conflict resolution skills, have less commitment to the hospital, patients, or ED staff because of temporary scheduling at that hospital or ED, and sense a lack of input, ownership, and control over patients' (or their own) lives
9. Patient transfers to or from the ED
10. Time limitations and urgency
11. Practice variability, including patient hand-offs
12. High patient acuity and volume
13. Space issues and patient privacy
14. Federal or hospital reporting mandates
15. EM practice, such as caring for multiple patients with limited information, with risk of great morbidity and mortality
16. Threat of litigation related to high stakes, clinical challenges, and patient's lack of previous personal relationship with EPs

*ED*, Emergency department; *EM*, emergency medicine; *EP*, emergency physician.

Many challenging situations that result from the nature of EM practice are less likely to create conflict than in previous decades because hospital administrators seem more willing to collaborate with ED leadership to prevent conflict before it occurs. Many EM leaders are sharpening administrative skills to allow them greater success when exchanging ideas with hospital leaders. Opportunities for communication, education, and problem solving in areas prone to conflict, especially during "business hours," are in the best interest of patients and the entire medical staff.

## IMPORTANCE OF COMMUNICATION

Effective communication is extremely important to the process of conflict resolution. For effective communication to occur, mutual respect and concern must exist between parties. This includes respect for an individual's professional and personal choices. Many physicians have difficulty interacting with individuals who do not share similar values, such as work ethic, practice style, or lifestyle.

Communication is difficult for various reasons, especially because many physicians are poor listeners. Physicians interrupt patients early and often; these patterns are likely present during communication with colleagues and team members, especially during stressful situations. In the ED, time constraints make communication challenging, as does the fact that most communication occurs in a public area. Communication often is done by telephone or electronically, which eliminates visual cues. Furthermore, individuals may have unique or differing agendas that make it even more difficult to communicate efficiently, let alone effectively. Past interactions affect future communications. Previous negative interactions are far more likely to be remembered than are positive interactions. The personalities of different specialists often clash, thus contributing to the likelihood of conflict.

The role of stress on physician communication must not be overlooked. Besides patient care stressors, contacting physicians about patient care issues, particularly at night, is stressful for EPs. It is especially difficult for EPs to contact physicians with hospital leadership roles, with reputations of demeaning behavior, or in senior positions that may affect partnership opportunities or future employment. These situations may directly or indirectly result in less than optimal patient care when an EP's desire to avoid conflict takes priority. Fortunately, instruction in communication and conflict resolution is required not only in EM training programs but also by medical schools and other residency training programs.

## COSTS OF CONFLICT

What are the costs associated with conflict in EM? Staff morale is likely to be low in EDs with high levels of conflict. Staff turnover and dissatisfaction with the work environment are likely to be high. Management will probably need to address an increasing number of complaints about the ED from it and other areas of the hospital, and that takes up valuable administrative time. Conflict interferes with patient satisfaction, throughput, quality of care, and patient safety. Pride in the ED may decline, thus further reducing morale and creating a potentially debilitating negative spiral.

Conflict (and poor conflict resolution) increases the likelihood that the ED is an unpleasant place to work; this increases stress and decreases everyone's job security. Reductions in physician reimbursement, staff salaries, and positions may result, causing even greater professional dissatisfaction. Medical errors are likely to occur more frequently, errors that further compromise patient care and reduce patient outcomes. The emotional and financial costs to patients, staff members (especially nurses), consultants, managers, and administrators are immeasurable if an EP frequently creates conflict and does not possess the skills to identify his or her contribution, to minimize it, or to resolve it promptly.

## CONFLICT RESOLUTION IN EMERGENCY MEDICINE

If conflict is a disruptive yet inevitable force in EM, conflict resolution and the skills necessary to achieve it are key factors for favorable patient care. Conflict management starts with effective communication among parties. Successful conflict resolution therefore requires parties to demonstrate a willingness to listen fully to the concerns of each other, without interrupting or planning a reply. Expressing a willingness to find common ground may help resolve conflict or at least de-escalate it. A healthy approach to conflict resolution includes treating the other person with respect, active listening (e.g., paraphrasing, demonstrating understanding), and clarifying one's own needs and perspective.

Conflict resolution for today's interactions is crucial to tomorrow's triumphs because future conflict is inevitable. Individuals likely adapted their approach to conflict management based on what "worked" for them in childhood, or from observing mentors. Conflict itself is not necessarily problematic, but how individuals (or organizations) deal with it may be. Five distinct responses to conflict can be plotted using the axes of *assertiveness* (the extent that individuals attempt to satisfy their own concerns) and *cooperativeness* (the extent that individuals attempt to satisfy the concerns of others) (**Fig. 209.1**). Each of these responses to conflict or approaches to resolving it has advantages and disadvantages and circumstances when it may prove effective or ineffective. For example, an EP preferring the *accommodating* style (low assertiveness and high cooperativeness) may have poor patient outcomes over time. The *competing* style employed by many EPs may create quick results necessary for patient care, but it is unpopular.

Although most complex, the *collaborating* style is the method to adopt whenever possible. Its outcome generally causes both sides to win. Collaboration is one of the main tenets of *principled negotiation*. Characterized by high assertiveness and high cooperativeness, this style is best used for learning, integrating solutions, and merging perspectives. Exploring issues in depth and confronting differences often result in increased commitments and improved relationships among involved parties. Despite the time constraints of EM, the collaborating style can be integrated into patient care activities by an EP and used successfully in conflict resolution

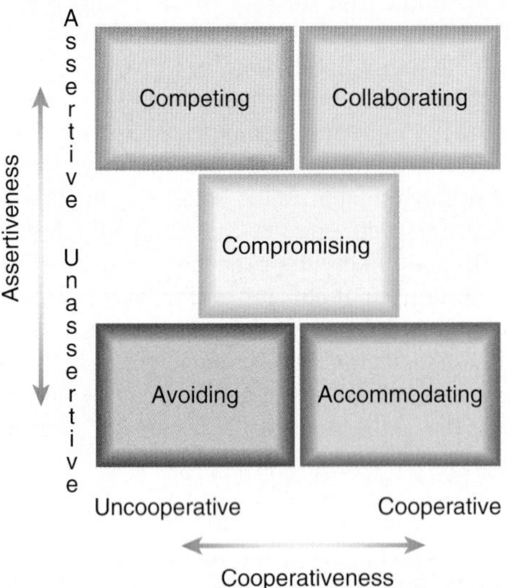


**Fig. 209.1** Matrix illustrating five distinct responses to conflict plotting axes of *assertiveness* (extent to which an individual attempts to satisfy his or her own concerns) and *cooperativeness* (extent to which an individual attempts to satisfy the other person's concerns). (Adapted with permission from Thomas-Kilmann Conflict Mode Instrument.)

**BOX 209.2 Principles of Conflict Resolution in Emergency Medicine**

1. Establish common goals (e.g., to deliver the best or most appropriate patient care possible in a patient-centered fashion).
2. Communicate effectively.
3. Do not take conflict personally.
4. Avoid accusations and public confrontations.
5. Compromise.
6. Establish specific commitments and expectations (e.g., Who will see the patient? At what time? Who will assume responsibility for care, including admission or discharge orders and/or instructions?).
7. Accept differences of opinion.
8. Use ongoing communications (invest in future interactions).
9. Consider a neutral mediator for situations that are not working and become disruptive or emotionally problematic.
10. Be pleasant.

Data from Marco CA, Smith CA. Conflict resolution in emergency medicine. Ann Emerg Med 2002;40:347-9.

if understood and practiced. This approach generally preserves relationships for future interactions while achieving appropriate outcomes.

Conflict resolution in EM has a critical role with respect to patient care, as well as positive interpersonal and group relations. Successful communication is integral to promoting positive interactions among individuals, in an effort to prevent (or minimize) conflict before it becomes detrimental. Poor communication among individuals may potentiate ongoing conflict and misunderstanding. Building alliances with colleagues may reduce the likelihood and amount of conflict. Team building within the ED and hospital, to promote constructive, creative, and cooperative approaches to conflict management, is vital to success.

## CHALLENGES TO CONFLICT RESOLUTION

EPs take for granted that difficult interactions occur as part of their daily experience. Some EPs may not find conflict particularly challenging or stressful. Successful EPs must be leaders within the ED, even if outside staff members are uncomfortable with their leadership style. This may be particularly true during stressful situations, when EPs gravitate toward the competing style of conflict resolution. Individuals who seldom use the ED (e.g., patients, families, consultants, hospital administrators) may not be comfortable with the environment or its interactions because its structure and culture are "foreign" to them. Unfortunately, the ED does not always provide the kind of service that health care professionals have come to expect. For example, a surgeon in the operating room has instruments handed to him or her in exactly the way he or she prefers by a designated individual. This is done in both the patient's and the surgeon's best interests. In the ED, however, staffing shortages or more pressing cases may cause a consultant to be "ignored." This situation often results in problems for everyone because consultants may take their frustration out on EPs or ED staff. Conflict within the ED is the likely outcome.

## STRATEGIES FOR SUCCESSFUL CONFLICT RESOLUTION

With all this conflict occurring in the ED, successful EPs apply strategies to reduce or resolve it, to preserve the best possible patient and provider satisfaction without compromising patient care. Drs. Marco and Smith described 10 reasonable principles for conflict resolution in EM (**Box 209.2**).[4] EPs should make it their "standard of care" to refrain from hostile communication and instead persuade others using kindness and intellect, focusing on patient advocacy and safety.

O'Mara focused on the interrelationship between communication and conflict resolution. She wrote that "each relationship presents its own potential for ongoing communication dynamics, which may include conflict and misunderstanding" and added that "appreciating alternative viewpoints and a willingness to adapt are prerequisites for managing interpersonal conflict."[5]

## RELATIONSHIPS IN THE EMERGENCY DEPARTMENT

Certain unique aspects of the EP-patient interaction may lead to conflict. First, the nature of this interaction is new, intense, unexpected, brief, and unselected. Neither the patient nor the EP chose the other. Furthermore, the balance of power in any doctor-patient relationship is unequal. Each participant has a different perspective on the nature of the emergency condition. Anxiety, pain, cost of care, lost wages, disability, morbidity, and mortality are of great concern to patients. Furthermore, the timing of care—how long is appropriate to wait for pain relief, test results, consultants, an admission bed, or discharge instructions—creates conflict (and at times open hostility). In these situations, mismatched expectations and perspectives between a patient and an EP result in conflict that can be intensified by stress, pain, and social, cultural, and language differences.

EPs have numerous interactions with nursing that must be successful as often as possible even though they occur under stress. Positive or negative exchanges between physicians and nurses are likely remembered during subsequent interactions; nurses typically interpret an EP's words, communication style, and body language in the context of prior interactions. Research clearly demonstrates that the doctor-nurse relationship has a significant impact on patient care.

Conflict resolution between EPs and staff members may be difficult to achieve, especially if interactions occur infrequently. In almost all situations, the earlier and more directly problem interactions are addressed, the more likely it is that future interactions and outcomes will be positive. These difficulties should be addressed in a nonthreatening, collegial, and supportive environment, in addition to removing personal issues from the problem. If this approach is neither possible nor successful, a skilled, unbiased outsider may be needed (particularly if differences in age, gender, cultures, ethnicity, rank, or position exist).

Additional strategies to foster successful conflict resolution in EM include social or educational meetings with colleagues and staff outside the ED. EPs who participate in medical staff affairs or who serve on hospital committees share time with colleagues when stress is not maximal. Positive interactions and sharing of common interests during these activities are likely to build alliances that may reduce the amount and intensity of conflict. This strategy will almost certainly improve conflict resolution in the future.

The book *Getting to Yes* describes using *principled negotiation,* which decides issues on their merit to resolve conflict, rather than through a haggling process focused on what each side says it will and will not do.[6] This method suggests looking for mutual gains whenever possible. When interests conflict, individuals should insist that the result of negotiation be based on fair standards, independent of the will of the other side.

Preparation is an important element before negotiations begin, although this is sometimes difficult in EM. Several opportunities exist to increase preparation before consultation (which is a negotiation). Making efforts to have the patient's identifying information available at the start of the conversation, reviewing the laboratory and radiographic results before the call if possible, and clearly stating specific goals of the contact help reduce conflict before it occurs. Communicating in the consultant's language and refraining from making suggestions (even obvious ones) unless asked are excellent strategies.

*Getting to Yes* recommends that negotiators develop their best alternative to a negotiated agreement (BATNA), which serves as the basis for exploring and evaluating options.[6] This approach involves thinking carefully about what would happen if a negotiated agreement cannot be reached, while simultaneously serving as an impetus to engage in a process with agreement as the outcome. Communication that begins with careful, empathic listening helps resolve conflict and allows the other party to feel heard. Avoiding negative comments or ridicule (especially public) and depersonalizing the conflict are healthy approaches to its management. This allows the other party to maintain self-esteem and self-respect. Remaining objective and maintaining composure while focusing on the issues are important. One must be careful when responding to emotions; silence can be powerful and may de-escalate conflict.[7]

**BOX 209.3 Positive Outcomes of Conflict Resolution**

1. Improved communication with patients and colleagues
2. Reduced stress levels and improved staff morale
3. Increased workplace productivity (and possibly reimbursement), with reduced expenditures related to conflict
4. Promotion of healthy relationships with colleagues and staff
5. Improved patient, staff, and physician satisfaction
6. Decreased staff turnover (increased staff retention)
7. Improved recruitment
8. Prevention of future conflict, or at least resolution of future conflict more effectively and expeditiously
9. Decreased medical error with improved patient safety
10. Improved overall patient care

## BENEFITS OF CONFLICT RESOLUTION

Dr. Andrew recommended "paraphrasing the communication back to the complainer" and "expressing a willingness to find a common ground."[3] These recommendations are critical because conflict is often generated (and many times escalated) by the fear that a concern was not heard or validated. Dr. Andrew described four A's that assist with conflict resolution:

1. *Acknowledge* the conflict ("I understand your concern. I can tell you are not pleased with what has taken place.").
2. *Apologize* (blamelessly) for the situation ("I'm sorry this situation occurred.").
3. *Actively* listen to the concern ("Please go on. I want to hear more about this.").
4. *Act* to amend ("I promise I will act to fix this situation and [try] to make certain it doesn't happen again to someone else.").[3]

Skillful negotiating techniques embody an empowering, active, constructive, and positive approach to resolving difficulties and often yield successful outcomes or incremental change over time. Numerous benefits result from successful conflict resolution, with short- and long-term impact (**Box 209.3**).

**BOX 209.4 Comprehensive Approach to Successful Conflict Resolution**

1. Accept the existence of the conflict.
2. Focus on the big picture.
3. Separate the person from the problem.
4. Clarify and identify the nature of the problem creating conflict.
5. Deal with one problem at a time, beginning with the easiest.
6. Engage the respective parties in an environment of impartiality.
7. Listen with understanding and interest, rather than evaluation.
8. Validate issues and concerns.
9. Identify areas of agreement; focus on common interests, not on positions.
10. Attack data, facts, assumptions, and conclusions, but not individuals.
11. Brainstorm realistic solutions in which both parties benefit.
12. Use and establish objective criteria, when possible.
13. Do not prolong or delay the process.
14. Implement the plan.
15. Evaluate and assess the problem-solving process after implementing the plan (follow up periodically).

## SUMMARY

Conflict has been described as a natural consequence of incompatible behaviors and unmet expectations.[7] The preferred strategy to manage conflict is to prevent its occurrence, which is not easy in EM. Effective communication among individuals and within groups in which parties are respected and heard produces an environment of trust. This results in the likelihood that conflict will be resolved more effectively. EPs should be aware of their behaviors and styles of interaction that increase conflict in an environment predisposed to conflict. Furthermore, EPs must strive to understand principles of conflict and conflict resolution, including effective communication, strong interpersonal and listening skills, and the tenets of professionalism because they may help achieve successful EM practices (**Box 209.4**).

## REFERENCES

***References can be found on Expert Consult @ www.expertconsult.com.***

# Informed Consent and Assessing Decision-Making Capacity in the Emergency Department

# 210

*Diane B. Heller*

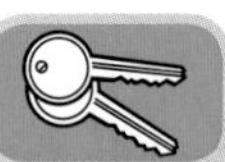

**KEY POINTS**

- To respect patient autonomy and abide by the law, the physician must obtain informed consent from a patient before examination and treatment.
- To satisfy the requirement for informed consent, three elements must be present: (1) disclosure of information by the physician must be adequate, (2) the patient's decision must be voluntary, and (3) the patient must possess decision-making capacity.
- Decision-making capacity is a medical determination made by the treating physician and is specific to the clinical decision at issue.
- The emergency department environment poses unique challenges to determination of decision-making capacity.
- To possess decision-making capacity, a patient must have the ability to (1) communicate a choice, (2) understand relevant information, (3) appreciate the significance of information to the patient's own individual circumstances, and (4) use reasoning to arrive at a decision.

## INFORMED CONSENT

### BACKGROUND

The concept of informed consent is based on both ethical and legal obligations that have evolved over the past century. The ethical foundations of informed consent are that the physician must strive to balance the goals of acting in the best interest of the patient while respecting the patient's autonomy to decide what is best for his or her own body. Currently informed consent requires an active role on the part of the patient, as well as respect for the patient's wishes by the emergency physician (EP).[1]

The legal foundation of informed consent centered initially on protection of the patient from battery or unwanted touching. In 1914, Justice Cardozo succinctly stated that "Every human being of adult years and sound mind has a right to determine what shall be done with his own body."[2] The presumption is that every adult has the right to accept or decline recommended treatment from a physician.

When the patient is a minor, the general rule is that informed consent must be obtained from a parent before a physician may proceed with nonemergency treatment. However, EMTALA[3] (Emergency Medical Treatment and Active Labor Act) permits a physician to evaluate every patient, including minors, to assess whether an emergency medical condition exists and to stabilize any such condition.[4] Many exceptions exist to the general rule of parents consenting for their minor children. For example, a minor may have the ability to consent to treatment of sexually transmitted diseases or drug addiction. These exceptions vary from state to state, however, so it is important to be familiar with the local laws where you practice.

Today, in the absence of a recognized exception to the requirement for informed consent, failure to obtain consent properly may also result in liability under the legal theories of privacy or negligence. In the emergency department (ED), we often find ourselves in circumstances in which the so-called emergency exception applies. The emergency exception states that consent is implied in cases in which an immediate threat to the life or health of the patient exists, when the proposed treatment is necessary to address the emergency condition, and when one is unable to obtain express consent of the patient or someone authorized to consent on the patient's behalf. In these instances the EP may presume that the patient would consent to the emergency treatment, and the EP does not need to obtain express consent before proceeding with treatment.[5]

### ELEMENTS

To satisfy the requirements of informed consent, three elements must be met. First, the physician must provide the patient with adequate disclosure of information to enable the patient to make an informed decision. Second, the patient must make the decision voluntarily. Finally, the patient must have the capacity to make the decision.

The scope of information to be disclosed is well established in theory but challenging in practice. The physician must disclose (1) the nature of the disease or problem and the nature and purpose of the proposed treatment or procedure; (2) the potential benefits and risks associated with the proposed treatment or procedure, as well as the likelihood that they will occur; and (3) alternative approaches, as well as the benefits and risks of such alternatives.[6]

Fulfillment of the disclosure element in the ED poses several challenges. For example, the time for patient-physician interaction is often limited in the ED. In addition, a quiet and private setting for discussion is often unavailable. Furthermore, the EP is typically working with limited knowledge about the full scope of the patient's medical history, intellectual capabilities, and emotional state.[7] It is the EP's responsibility, however, to minimize the impact of these challenges and to provide information that will maximize the likelihood that the patient will participate effectively in the decision-making process.

The second element, that consent must be given voluntarily, is not as well delineated in the medical literature or by the courts. Although it is obvious that outright threats or forced treatments violate this tenet, there are subtle ways in which a physician may coerce a patient into making a decision that are also unacceptable. For example, if a physician tells a patient that pain medicine will be withheld until the patient agrees to undergo a computed tomography (CT) scan, the voluntary nature of the patient's decision will be compromised. Additionally, the physician cannot withhold or distort information to alter a patient's decision. The physician must present information in a way that aids the patient in making the decision and leaves the patient feeling that he or she has an actual choice in the matter.

The final element—and the focus of the remainder of this chapter—is that the patient must possess decision-making capacity. Decision-making capacity refers to a patient's ability to participate in and make a meaningful decision regarding diagnosis and treatment. The treating physician must determine whether the patient is able to make a specific decision regarding his or her medical care. However, the physician must start with the presumption that an adult patient has the capacity to give informed consent and, absent evidence to the contrary, health care decisions should be deferred to the patient. If the physician determines that the patient lacks the capacity to make medical decisions, the physician must then determine how to proceed. If the patient has specifically expressed health care wishes through an advanced directive, these wishes should be honored. Similarly, if the patient has designated an individual to make health care decisions for him or her, that person should be contacted to make decisions on behalf of the patient. In other instances, family members should be contacted to help make health care decisions.

Although psychiatric consultation may be helpful in assessing decisional capacity in patients, it is not required. Formal legal procedures also exist to assist in the determination, but evaluations of capacity are routinely made without recourse to the court system. The process is usually performed solely by the treating EP in the ED. Indeed, the EP assesses decision-making capacity as part of routine interactions with every patient treated.

## DECISION-MAKING CAPACITY

*Decision-making capacity* is a clinical term that is specific to the particular medical decision at issue. If the physician determines that the patient lacks decision-making capacity, the patient can be denied the right to make meaningful decisions regarding his or her medical care.

To possess decision-making capacity, the patient must exhibit the following four abilities: (1) to communicate a choice, (2) to understand relevant information as it is communicated, (3) to appreciate the significance of the information to his or her own individual circumstances, and (4) to use reasoning to arrive at a specific choice.[7,8] When patients cannot demonstrate these abilities, they lack the capacity to give informed consent for their medical care.

In all instances the physician must balance the interests of protecting the patient from harm while respecting patient autonomy. The level of scrutiny that a physician applies to evaluating capacity therefore varies depending on the decision to be made and the risks and benefits of the proposed medical care. For example, if a patient with a superficial abrasion refuses the application of a bandage, the EP should exercise a very low level of scrutiny when assessing the patient's capacity to make decisions. If the same patient, however, refuses a CT scan after head trauma with prolonged loss of consciousness, the EP should scrutinize the patient's capacity at a much higher level. This general approach to evaluating decision-making capacity is often referred to as the sliding scale model. Determination of capacity can be made only with reference to the particular facts surrounding an individual decision by the patient; as the risks associated with a decision increase, the level of capacity needed to consent to or refuse the intervention also increases.[9]

### WHEN TO EXERCISE ADDITIONAL CARE IN ASSESSING CAPACITY

Assessing a patient's decision-making capacity is an implicit part of every medical encounter in the ED. The process is generally spontaneous and straightforward and takes place as the EP examines and talks with the patient. The EP's starting point is always the presumption that an adult patient has the requisite capacity to consent to or refuse medical treatment. Under certain circumstances, however, a more detailed and direct inquiry into a patient's decision-making capacity must be performed (see the "Red Flags" box). Although no accepted rules exist regarding when the EP must delve more deeply into this issue, certain situations should alert an EP to the need to assess a patient's decision-making capacity more carefully.[10]

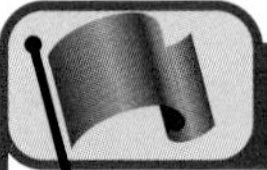

**RED FLAGS**

**Signs That a More Careful Evaluation of Capacity Might Be Warranted**

Patients who refuse recommended treatment (especially if they refuse to discuss their decision)

Patients with a change in mental status

Patients who frequently change their mind or make inconsistent decisions

Patients with known risk factors for impaired decision making, such as the following:

- Chronic psychiatric or neurologic conditions
- Cultural or language barriers
- Educational-level concern or developmental delay issues
- Significant stress, anxiety, or untreated pain
- Extremes of age: older than 80 years because of an increased risk for dementia; younger than 18 years because of a potential need for parental involvement

The most common situation that triggers a more detailed inquiry into a coherent patient's decision-making capacity occurs when the patient chooses a course of treatment contrary to the one recommended by the EP or refuses treatment entirely. Simple disagreement with an EP's recommendation, however, is not grounds for declaration of a lack of capacity. If the EP believes that the patient's choice is not reasonable, it may trigger the start of an inquiry, but it is not the end of the inquiry. As discussed earlier, refusal of treatment is more worrisome if the consequences of the patient's decision are great. Furthermore, if the patient is unwilling to discuss the reasons behind his or her refusal, the EP should be even more concerned about performing a careful evaluation of the patient's decision-making capacity before simply accepting the patient's choice.

A second general area that should raise the EP's concern regarding decision-making capacity is when a patient has an abrupt change in mental status. Although the reasons for the change in mental status may be as varied as infection, stroke, head trauma, or ingestion of mind-altering substances, the result is the same. The EP is under an obligation to conduct a more careful evaluation of the patient's capacity to participate in decisions on medical care. The simple existence of a change in mental status, however, does not automatically preclude a patient from possessing the requisite capacity. It is simply a situation that should trigger the EP to make a more detailed inquiry.

A third broad area that should prompt the EP to evaluate the patient's capacity more carefully is the presence of a known risk factor for impaired decision making. Risk factors may include known psychiatric conditions such as severe depression or schizophrenia.[8] Although the presence of mental illness does not automatically preclude a patient from having the right to participate in his or her medical care, in such an instance it may be helpful to seek the opinion of a psychiatrist. If cultural or language barriers are present or if concerns exist about a patient's level of education, the EP should also exercise heightened scrutiny of the patient's decision-making capacity. In these instances the EP must take steps to compensate for these factors to ensure that the patient has the greatest opportunity to participate in his or her medical care. The EP should arrange for a translator when necessary and should take additional time to explain the issues in terms that the patient can more readily understand. Extremes of age are also known risk factors for impaired decision making. Although not every patient over a certain age exhibits dementia, the EP must be aware of the increased prevalence of this condition in elderly patients. Other common risk factors in the ED are extreme pain, stress, and anxiety, each of which can impair a patient's ability to receive or process information.[11]

Although the foregoing situations are by no means all-inclusive, they represent instances that should put an EP on notice that a more careful and detailed evaluation of capacity may be needed. Again, none of these circumstances will alter the presumption that an adult possesses the requisite capacity to participate in his or her medical care. They simply mark the need for a more detailed inquiry. In each of these instances the EP should take additional care when documenting the care of the patient, as well as his or her interactions with the patient. Specifically, the physician should document any evaluation that is conducted of the patient's capacity (see the "Documentation" box).

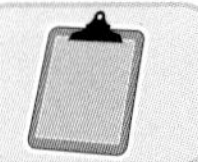

**DOCUMENTATION**

**When Capacity Is at Issue**

If any of the "red flag" situations exist or if there are other reasons to have heightened concern regarding a patient's decision-making capacity, the emergency physician (EP) should take care to document the following elements carefully:

- Whether the patient exhibits each of the elements of decision-making capacity
- The patient's medical condition
- The proposed treatment or procedure and its necessity
- The urgent or emergency nature of the proposed treatment or procedure
- Actions by the EP to maximize patient capacity
- Actions by the EP to minimize impediments to patient capacity
- Availability and involvement of family members or surrogate decision makers
- Psychiatric consultation when obtained

## SUGGESTED QUESTIONS TO AID IN THE DETERMINATION OF CAPACITY

The final determination of a patient's decision-making capacity depends on whether the EP believes that the patient exhibits the four abilities required for capacity: (1) to communicate a choice, (2) to understand relevant information as it is communicated, (3) to appreciate the significance of the information to his or her own individual circumstances, and (4) to use reasoning to arrive at a specific choice. Thus the EP's inquiry should consist of focused questions to evaluate each of these areas[11,12] (see the "Tips and Tricks" box).

The first requirement, communicating a choice, can be evaluated simply by asking the patient what he or she wants to do. Stability of the choice is also important. Although this may not be a factor given the urgency of many procedures in the ED, if the proposed treatment or procedure will not occur immediately, the EP should confirm that the patient's choice remains the same after a certain period. If, for example, patient A agrees to a lumbar puncture for his headache, the EP can simply confirm the patient's decision after preparations for the procedure have been made.

To test the patient's ability to understand relevant information, the EP may start out by simply asking the patient to paraphrase what he or she has been told. Patients should use their own words and not simply parrot back the information recited by the physician. The EP can also ask pointed questions such as "What is your understanding of your condition and the options that we have discussed?" Patient should be able to explain, in their own words, the nature of the condition, the available options, and the risks and benefits of these options. This includes their understanding of what will happen if they do nothing. In the foregoing example of a lumbar puncture, patient A needs to understand the risks of the procedure, as well as the possibility that a negative CT scan without a negative lumbar puncture may mean that he still has a life-threatening condition.

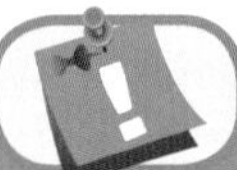

**TIPS AND TRICKS**

**Questions to Ask Patients to Facilitate the Determination of Decision-Making Capacity**

The ability to communicate a choice:
- Have you decided what you want to do?
- We have discussed many things; have you made a decision?

The ability to understand relevant information as it is communicated:
- What is your understanding of your medical condition?
- What are the possible diagnostic tests or treatments of your condition?
- What are some of the risks of the options that we have discussed?
- How likely is it that you will have a bad outcome?
- What could happen if you choose to do nothing at this time?

The ability to appreciate the significance of the information to one's own individual circumstances:
- Why do you think your doctor has recommended this specific test or treatment for you?
- Do you think that the recommended test or treatment is the best option for you?
- Why do you think that this is the best option for you at this time?
- What do you think will happen if you accept (or refuse) this option?

The ability to use reasoning to arrive at a specific choice:
- Why have you chosen the option that you did?
- What factors influenced your decision?
- What weight did you give to these different factors?
- How do you balance the positives and negatives (or risks and benefits)?

To satisfy the third element of decision-making capacity, the EP must be sure that patients understand how the information discussed relates to them as an individual. The EP can ask patients whether they think that the proposed option is the best option and why. The EP should also explore what patients think will happen in the future if they choose the proposed option. Using the foregoing example, this may be as simple as the fact that patient A will need to spend several hours in the ED waiting for the results of the lumbar puncture or that he may experience a postprocedural headache that will interfere with work the following day.

To evaluate the patient's ability to reason, the EP should ask the patient why he or she has chosen a specific option. The EP can inquire what factors influenced the patient's decision and what weight was given to these factors. In the foregoing example, patient A may tell the EP that he cannot wait for a lumbar puncture after the CT scan because he has to pick up his daughter after school or that he has had similar headaches in the past and therefore thinks that this headache is not serious. Alternatively, patient A could tell the EP that he believes that when the procedure is performed, the EP will inject radioactive material into his body because the EP is trying to kill him. Sometimes simple questions yield very complex and interesting answers that can aid the EP's determination of capacity.

In addition to asking focused questions relevant to capacity, the EP has the option of obtaining a consultation from a psychiatrist if time allows. Although no requirement mandates that a psychiatrist be involved, it may be helpful in certain circumstances. First, it can never hurt to obtain a second opinion when making a determination of capacity. Second, psychiatrists are skilled at interviewing patients. Third, they are experts in diagnosing mental illnesses that may impair a patient's decision-making ability. Involvement of a psychiatrist does not relieve EPs of their responsibility to take part in determination of capacity. Decision-making capacity relies on the communication of adequate medical information that is unique to the patient's condition and proposed treatment. Only the treating EP can ensure adequate disclosure of this information, and the EP cannot delegate this task to a psychiatrist.

## CONCLUSION

In every encounter in the ED, it is the treating EP's responsibility to ensure that the patient gives informed consent for medical care. This consent must be given voluntarily by a patient with the requisite decision-making capacity, and the patient must receive adequate information to make the decision. Although some evaluation of decision-making capacity is an inherent part of every patient-physician encounter, certain situations should alert the EP to the need for a more detailed inquiry. To this end, the EP should ask questions in the clinical interview that specifically address the requisite elements of capacity.

## REFERENCES

***References can be found on Expert Consult @ www.expertconsult.com.***

# Regulatory and Legal Issues in the Emergency Department 211

*Paul D. Biddinger*

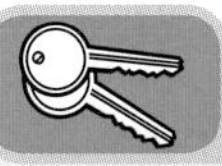

**KEY POINTS**

- Individual states have the authority to regulate the practice of emergency medicine within their borders. The state public health department generally administers this authority.
- The Joint Commission is a private organization with a mission to improve the safety and quality of medical care. Although participation in the accreditation program is voluntary, most hospitals in the United States seek Joint Commission accreditation, and therefore most emergency departments are subject to its standards.
- Certain federal laws, such as the Emergency Medical Treatment and Active Labor Act (EMTALA) and the Health Insurance Portability and Accountability Act (HIPAA), create additional obligations for emergency departments and physicians. Emergency physicians can place themselves at significant legal and financial risk if they are not aware of these obligations.
- EMTALA requires emergency physicians to provide appropriate screening and stabilization for all patients seen in their institutions with an emergency complaint. EMTALA further regulates access to "on-call" specialists, as well as transfer of patients between health care facilities.
- HIPAA has changed the way in which physicians and hospitals collect, store, and share health information. Although the regulations are complex, physicians can best adhere to the regulations when they access or share health information only on a "need-to-know" basis and attempt to obtain the patient's permission for sharing such information whenever possible.
- Most states have special reporting requirements for victims of child abuse and certain infectious diseases. Some states have additional requirements, such as to report victims of other violent crimes, patients who seize and have a driver's license, or animal bites. Emergency physicians should be familiar with the reporting requirements in the jurisdiction in which they practice.

## BACKGROUND

The medical care delivered in the emergency department (ED) is subject to a significant number of local, state, and federal regulations, as well as nongovernmental standards, that are designed to ensure quality care for each individual, ensure equity in care among all patients undergoing emergency evaluation, and protect vulnerable patients who may not be able to adequately advocate for themselves. Emergency physicians should be aware of the regulatory environment in which they practice because ignorance of these regulations (especially with respect to regulations of the Emergency Medical Treatment and Active Labor Act [EMTALA] and the Health Insurance Portability and Accountability Act [HIPAA]) may place both an individual physician and the institution at significant financial and legal risk.

## PUBLIC HEALTH AUTHORITY

Each state has the right to license and regulate both the health care facilities and providers within its jurisdiction. Generally, the state public health authority (state health department) administers this right. Even though all emergency physicians are, of course, aware that they, nurses, and other medical professionals obtain their medical licenses from the state department of public health, relatively few know of the extent to which their hospitals and associated departments (e.g., hospital EDs, operating rooms, computed tomography scanners, cardiac catheterization laboratories) must obtain similar permissions to deliver health care or the extent to which hospitals may be subject to review in the event of a perceived or reported problem. In addition to state regulation, hospitals are also generally subject to "Conditions for Coverage (CFC)" and "Conditions of Participation (CoP)" from the Center for Medicare and Medicaid Services (CMS) of the federal government. According to the CMS, the CFC and CoP are the "minimum health and safety requirements that hospitals must meet to participate in the Medicare and Medicaid program." Although the CFC and CoP are not generally required of hospitals for licensure, hospitals are mandated by federal law to meet the standards if they wish to receive Medicare and Medicaid reimbursement for their services. Because Medicare and Medicaid funding is a substantial part of most hospitals' revenue, most hospitals adhere to the CMS CFC and CoP regulations, as well as those of the state health department.

Because the responsibility to regulate and monitor health care institutions is so great, most states and the CMS share, delegate, or "deem" some portions of this regulatory authority to national expert organizations to help them oversee the quality of health care delivered in their state.[1] The most visible of these expert organizations is the Joint Commission, formerly known as the Joint Commission on Accreditation of

Healthcare Organizations (JCAHO). Other organizations to which states frequently delegate regulatory authority include the American College of Surgeons, which sets standards for trauma centers, and the American Burn Association, which sets standards for burn centers. In addition to delegating portions of their authority to national organizations, state departments of public health may also delegate portions of their authority over health care institutions to local public health officials. One example is the receipt of reports of suspected or confirmed cases of reportable communicable disease.

In no case does any sharing of authority supersede the state's ability to regulate and oversee health care quality. Indeed, although some states and the CMS recognize Joint Commission accreditation as evidence of meeting acceptable standards, both states and the CMS can always perform their own inspections of facilities, in addition to the Joint Commission surveys. Furthermore, whenever there is a question or concern regarding specific care delivered, the state public health authority generally carries out the site inspection and investigation on its own.

## THE JOINT COMMISSION

The Joint Commission is a private, not-for-profit organization. Its mission is to "continually improve the safety and quality of care provided to the public through the provision of health care accreditation and related services that support performance improvement in health care organizations."[2] Broadly, the Joint Commission sets standards that hospitals must meet to receive accreditation (and generally, by extension, licensure from the state) and receive funding from the CMS. These standards cover a broad range of subjects from patient rights, to patient care, to infection control. The Joint Commission also integrates outcomes and other performance measures into its standards. To maintain their accreditation, health care organizations must undergo a site survey by Joint Commission staff every 3 years. Laboratories must undergo a site survey every 2 years for the same accreditation.

Over the years the Joint Commission has created a number of special programs and work groups with particular relevance to the ED, including groups specifically examining ED overcrowding and hospital emergency preparedness. The most overarching of the Joint Commission programs related to the ED is the set of National Patient Safety Goals (**Table 211.1**). These goals have been revised and expanded over the years to appropriately reflect the changes in clinical care that have evolved, as well as to address systemic sources of error in medications as they are identified.

Although many departments and practitioners frequently see the Joint Commission requirements as a burden, especially at the time of their site visit, it is important to remember that the purpose of the requirements is to enhance patient safety and reduce opportunities for error. By developing programs that satisfy the Joint Commission requirements, EDs and individual physicians will decrease their risk for adverse events and better mange their medical liability.

Two specific programs that institutions are required to use to help them achieve the national patient safety goals are the "do-not-use list" and the "universal protocol." The universal protocol was developed by The Joint Commission to prevent "wrong site, wrong person, wrong procedure" surgery and is required of accredited institutions. Although the universal protocol has clear safety benefits for some of the patients cared for in the ED, many emergency physicians remain uncertain of which specific procedures require use of the universal protocol. Even though it is difficult to conceive that repair of a laceration or emergency intubation could be

**Table 211.1 2011 Joint Commission National Patient Safety Goals**

| | |
|---|---|
| Identify patients correctly | Use at least two ways to identify patients. For example, use the patient's name and date of birth. This is done to make sure that each patient gets the medication and treatment meant for them.<br>Make sure that the correct patient gets the correct blood type when they receive a blood transfusion. |
| Improve staff communication | Quickly get important test results to the correct staff person. |
| Use medications safely | Label all medications that are not already labeled; for example, those in syringes, cups, and basins.<br>Take extra care with patients who take medications to thin their blood. |
| Prevent infection | Use the hand-cleaning guidelines from the Centers for Disease Control and Prevention or the World Health Organization.<br>Use proven guidelines to prevent infections that are difficult to treat.<br>Use proven guidelines to prevent infection of the blood from central lines.<br>Use safe practices to treat the part if the body on which surgery was performed. |
| Check patient medications | Find out what medications each patient is taking. Make sure that it is OK for the patient to take any new medications with the current ones.<br>Give a list of the patient's medications to the next caregiver or patient's regular doctor before the patient goes home.<br>Give a list of the patient's medications to the patient and the patient's family before the patient goes home. Explain the list.<br>Some patients may get medications in small amounts or for a short time. Make sure that it is OK for these patients to take these medications with their current ones. |
| Identify patient safety risks | Find out which patients are most likely to try to commit suicide. |

performed on the wrong limb or wrong patient, it is possible that tube thoracostomy, lumbar puncture, or central venous cannulation (among other procedures) could be performed in the ED on the wrong patient, especially when a patient's visit spans different shifts or when consultation services are requested to perform procedures. Thus, for the appropriate circumstances and procedures, EDs must develop and use a universal protocol that includes provisions for a hard-stop "timeout" in which the physician and nursing staff stop to ensure that informed consent has been given, that the procedure is warranted, and that it is performed on the correct patient at the correct site before selected procedures are performed.

The do-not-use list is a compilation of medical abbreviations that have been identified as the most likely sources of error found when orders are either miswritten or misinterpreted (or both) (**Table 211.2**). The growing use of computerized order entry systems and computerized prescription writing programs is likely to decrease the number of these types of errors; however, physicians who write handwritten orders must be familiar with the prohibited abbreviations, and departments should bar them from use in clinical practice.

## EMERGENCY MEDICAL TREATMENT AND ACTIVE LABOR ACT

One of the most confusing, misinterpreted, and misquoted set of regulations in emergency medicine is EMTALA. Even the name itself can be confusing because the regulations are sometimes inexactly referred to as "COBRA," which refers to the broader Consolidated Omnibus Reconciliation Act in which the original EMTALA statutes were enacted. First enacted in 1986 and significantly revised in 2003, EMTALA originated as a response to several well-publicized allegations of patient "dumping" in which patients were alleged to have been turned away or transferred from EDs without appropriate care. Broadly, EMTALA creates two major requirements for hospitals that have a dedicated ED and participate in CMS programs. First, patients who "come to" the emergency department and request care must receive an appropriate medical screening examination. Second, for patients with an identified "emergency medical condition," the emergency physician must either provide appropriate stabilization or arrange transfer to another facility and meet several additional specific requirements pertaining to the transfer.[3] Although

**Table 211.2** 2010 Joint Commission Do-Not-Use List

| DO NOT USE | POTENTIAL PROBLEM | USE INSTEAD |
|---|---|---|
| **Official Do-Not-Use List*** | | |
| U (unit) | Mistaken for "0" (zero), the number "4" (four), or "cc" | Write "unit" |
| IU (international unit) | Mistaken for IV (intravenous) or the number 10 (ten) | Write "international unit" |
| Q.D., QD, q.d., qd (daily)<br>Q.O.D., QOD, q.o.d., qod (every other day) | Mistaken for each other<br>Period after the Q mistaken for "I" and the "O" mistaken for "I" | Write "daily"<br>Write "every other day" |
| Trailing zero (X.0 mg)†<br>Lack of leading zero (.X mg) | Decimal point is missing | Write X mg<br>Write 0.X mg |
| MS<br>$MSO_4$ and $MgSO_4$ | Can mean morphine sulfate or magnesium sulfate<br>Confused for one another | Write "morphine sulfate"<br>Write "magnesium sulfate" |
| **Additional Abbreviations, Acronyms, and Symbols‡** | | |
| > (greater than)<br>< (less than) | Misinterpreted as the number "7" (seven) or the letter "L"<br>Confused for one another | Write "greater than"<br>Write "less than" |
| Abbreviations for drug names | Misinterpreted because of similar abbreviations for multiple drugs | Use metric units |
| @ | Mistaken for the number "2" (two) | Write "at" |
| cc | Mistaken for U (units) when poorly written | Write "mL" or "ml" or "milliliters" ("mL" is preferred) |
| µg | Mistaken for mg (milligrams), thereby resulting in a 1000-fold overdose | Write "mcg" or "micrograms" |

*Applies to all orders and all medication-related documentation that is handwritten (including free-text computer entry) or on preprinted forms.

†Exception: A "trailing zero" may be used only when required to demonstrate the level of precision of the value being reported, such as for laboratory results, imaging studies that report size of lesions, or catheter or tube sizes. It may not be used in medication orders or other medication-related documentation.

‡For *possible* future inclusion in the official do-not-use list.

EMTALA applies to hospitals that receive CMS funding, it applies to all patients, not simply those with Medicare or Medicaid insurance.

The first requirement under EMTALA, the "medical screening examination," must be provided to all individuals who go to the ED requesting an evaluation for a medical condition. Although the specific components of this examination remain ill defined, it is generally agreed that an examination should be performed so that the clinician can say with "reasonable clinical confidence" that an emergency condition is not present that may place an individual's health (or the health of an unborn child) in serious jeopardy, seriously impair body functions, or represent serious dysfunction of body organs. Furthermore, this medical screening examination must be provided without regard to the ability to pay, insurance status, race, citizenship, or gender.

The second requirement under EMTALA is to provide appropriate stabilization for an emergency medical condition, once identified. In general, this means that an appropriate level of medical care must be provided in the ED or in the hospital (or in both) for the acute medical problem of the patient, again without regard to the ability to pay, insurance status, race, citizenship, or gender. This provision of EMTALA also has implications for on-call physicians. As part of Medicare, hospitals must maintain on-call physicians who are able to provide the medical services needed to treat an emergency medical condition after the medical screening examination. Although the list of on-call physicians is not required by Medicare to be comprehensive, the specialties represented in the on-call list must be appropriate to best meet the needs of its patients within the hospital's capability. If a hospital does not maintain an appropriate on-call roster or if an on-call physician does not show up to care for a patient with an unidentified emergency medical condition within a reasonable amount of time, that hospital and the on-call physician may be liable under EMTALA statutes.

In the event that the ED or the hospital (or both) are unable to provide appropriate stabilization, EMTALA allows transfer of patients from one facility to another under certain, very specific conditions. First, the patient must request the transfer and a physician must state in writing that the medical benefits of the transfer outweigh its risks. Second, the hospital that receives the transferred patient must be "appropriate" and have both the space and qualified personnel to treat the emergency medical condition (**Box 211.1**).[4]

Penalties for violations of EMTALA statutes can be significant for both the physician and the institution. Both the physician and the hospital can be liable for fines of up to $50,000 per violation, and both can be excluded from future participation in CMS programs. Generally, malpractice insurance specifically excludes EMTALA violations. Furthermore, hospitals that receive patients transferred in violation of EMTALA statutes may bring a civil suit against the transferring institution to recover the financial loss created by the inappropriate transfer.

**BOX 211.1 Key Provisions of the Emergency Medical Treatment and Active Labor Act**

Anyone who goes to the main hospital property with an emergency medical complaint must receive a medical screening examination and appropriate stabilization.

Hospitals must maintain appropriate on-call lists of specialists to care for identified emergency medical conditions.

Patients may not be transferred from a higher level of care to a lower level of care.

All patients transferred from one facility to another must be accepted by a physician at the receiving facility before transfer.

When transferring a patient to another hospital, the responsibility to choose the appropriate means of transport (i.e., private vehicle, basic life support, advanced life support, critical care transport) lies with the sending physician.

Institutions with specialty care services must accept transfers from hospitals without such services, provided that they have the space and capability at that time to deal with the patient's needs.

Patients with an emergency condition must be stabilized before transport to another facility except if (1) the receiving facility has specialty services that the sending facility lacks and the benefits outweigh the risks of transfer and (2) the patient requests the transfer and understands the risks.

Patients may refuse transfer from one facility to another.

**TIPS AND TRICKS**

**Medical Screening Examination**

Must be performed on all patients without regard to their ability to pay

Must be performed before financial interview

Not the same as triage

Must be performed by a medical professional granted authority by hospital bylaws

Must be sufficient to rule in or rule out an emergency medical condition

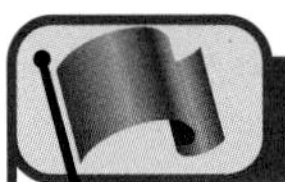

**RED FLAGS**

**Emergency Medical Condition**

Acute symptoms

May result in serious injury or impairment of function to an organ or body part if not treated immediately

Could jeopardize the health of the patient or unborn child

Includes severe pain, psychiatric disturbance, active labor, and substance abuse, among others

## HEALTH INSURANCE PORTABILITY AND ACCOUNTABILITY ACT

HIPAA was initially enacted in 1996 in an attempt to make it easier for individuals to transfer their medical records and health care coverage and also to provide greater accountability among providers to limit fraud.[5] Subsequent federal rules defining privacy standards under HIPAA have substantially

**BOX 211.2 Health Insurance Portability and Accountability Act**

Requires institutions and providers to develop policies and procedures to protect patients' unique health information
Allows institutions and health care providers to use protected health information for treatment, payment, and normal health care operations with minimal restrictions as long as patients consent to its use
Requires written permission for any use of protected health information outside normal health care operations
Gives patients the right to access, copy, and amend their health record
Allows certain health information to be disclosed without the patient's consent only under very narrowly defined conditions (e.g., for public health reporting)
Provides significant penalties for violations

changed the way in which health care providers and health plans collect, store, and share health information.

Health care providers, institutions, health plans, and health care clearinghouses are all required to conform to HIPAA standards (**Box 211.2**). Accordingly, they are all known as "covered entities." Broadly, HIPAA standards require that all covered entities have appropriate policies and procedures in place to ensure the privacy of all personally identifiable health information that they store and also that personally identifiable health information be shared only with the patient's permission and only in appropriate circumstances.[6] Being covered entities under HIPAA means that health care providers, institutions, and health plans may share health information with one another, when appropriate, without needing to verify the privacy protection of one another. Each covered entity is assumed to have appropriate electronic and physical access controls to patients' medical records and electronic data and to conduct routine audits of its data security procedures.

From the perspective of the emergency physician, HIPAA means that personal health information should be obtained or accessed only when it is relevant to immediate care of the patient. Furthermore, personal health information should be disclosed only to other covered entities and only with the patient's permission. Sanctions for violating HIPAA standards include civil and criminal penalties with fines of up to $250,000 or imprisonment for up to 10 years (or both) for knowingly misusing a patient's identifiable health information.[7]

## SPECIAL CIRCUMSTANCES

### MANDATORY REPORTING

Most state public health authorities have mandatory reporting requirements designed to protect vulnerable members of society. Some types of mandatory reporting have to do with the characteristics of the victim. The most common mandatory report of this type is a suspected case of child abuse or neglect. In addition, some states also mandate reporting of suspected elder abuse or abuse of the mentally handicapped.[8] Other types of mandatory reporting have to do with the characteristics of the event. The most common type of this mandatory report is the requirement that health care providers contact police when treating victims of gun violence. Other examples of mandatory reporting may include knife injuries, unusual infections, animal bites, or major burns. Sexual assault represents a unique circumstance in which frequently health care providers are required to report that they treated the victim of such a crime but are not required to report the identity of the patient. This is because it is generally believed that mandatory reporting of individual identities would discourage some victims of sexual assault from seeking medical care.

### SEXUAL ASSAULT

In addition to reporting certain types of injuries and certain forms of mistreatment, emergency physicians should also be aware of the regulations and procedures in their environment with respect to collection of possible evidence of crimes. Use of an evidence "kit" for a sexual assault victim is commonplace in EDs across the country, but procedures for maintaining the chain of custody of the kit and its ownership can vary substantially. Moreover, the manner in which clothes, valuables, and other items removed from a victim of violence are collected, stored, and transferred to law enforcement personnel can have a significant impact on the legal outcome of a case. Emergency physicians should generally be familiar with the basic principles of how to properly handle and store such potential evidence.

**TIPS AND TRICKS**

Know the relevant public health regulations and reporting requirements in your area.
Understand that patient safety initiatives and Joint Commission requirements generally improve care for patients, decrease the chance of error, and therefore decrease emergency physicians' overall medical-legal risk.
Develop mechanisms to perform medical screening examinations on all patients encountered in the emergency department in a timely manner.
Ensure that patients transferred between health care institutions (1) have an accepting physician at the receiving institution, (2) have a signed consent form for transfer when possible, (3) are sent with complete copies of their medical record and any relevant radiographic images, and (4) are transferred by staff with the appropriate level of training and monitoring capability.
Access protected health information only when it is directly relevant to the medical care that you provide.
Be sure to obtain written permission whenever possible when sharing protected health information.
Use caution when restraining patients or preventing them from leaving the emergency department. Make sure that such decisions are supported by the appropriate regulations, careful clinical documentation, and written medical orders.

## RESTRAINTS

Finally, the manner in which patients with acute psychiatric complaints such as suicidality, homicidality, or psychosis are monitored and restrained in EDs is generally regulated by the state health authority. Use of physical or chemical restraint in a manner inconsistent with state laws or regulations can expose providers to significant liability.[9] Emergency physicians should always carefully document the reasons for such restraint and the reasons why less restrictive measures could not be used or were insufficient. In some states, in addition to writing the appropriate medical orders to support their decisions, emergency physicians may need to complete specific forms when either physically or chemically restraining a patient or when preventing a patient from leaving the ED for safety concerns.

## REFERENCES

***References can be found on Expert Consult @ www.expertconsult.com.***

# Medical-Legal Issues in Emergency Medicine 212

*Gregory L. Henry and Geetika Gupta*

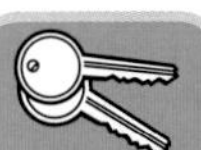

**KEY POINTS**

- Establish a trusting and positive doctor-patient relationship
- Understand the medical-legal system
- Manage concerns specific to the current-day emergency department
- Manage specific high-risk medical complaints

Medical-legal considerations are an integral part of every doctor-patient interaction. This chapter provides an overview of the important balance between the practice of medicine and legal implications.

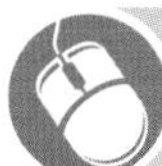

For a more in-depth version of this chapter, see www.expertconsult.com

## ESTABLISHING A TRUSTING AND POSITIVE PHYSICIAN-PATIENT RELATIONSHIP

### BE SERVICE ORIENTED

The key is to understand that as an emergency physician (EP), when you arrive at work, you check all your prejudices at the door. Remember that you may never be able to solve a patient's chronic medical problem, but showing genuine concern and providing a positive patient experience will go a long way toward relieving the patient's fears. **Box 212.1** is a list of simple rules that should help facilitate the doctor-patient interaction.

### CHARTING AND THE MEDICAL RECORD

The only things that really go to court with a physician are the patient's medical record and the physician's credibility. The chart is the only document that the plaintiff attorney has to understand what happened and to be able to decide whether bringing legal action is worthwhile.

Multiple issues with regard to a chart accompany every lawsuit. **Box 212.2** is a list of simple rules that should help facilitate the key points for a sound medical chart.

**BOX 212.1 Rules for Physician-Patient Interactions**

It does not matter how long they waited; it was too long. Never argue with patients over the amount of time that they waited.

Never use excuses, such as you are working short staffed or "I've been here all day."

Apologize for the wait. As soon as you have apologized for the wait, you have at least acknowledged that the patient's time is as valuable as yours and you understand that waiting is not a comfortable situation.

Thank the patient the family for coming in.

Trivialization of minor complaints can lead to a dissatisfied patient. Most patients believe that they have a legitimate reason to be in the emergency department. To be informed that it is the doctor's perception that theirs is not an *emergency* never helps the doctor-patient interaction and does not prevent further emergency department visits.

### DISCHARGE INSTRUCTIONS

Approximately half the lawsuits in emergency medicine revolve around discharge instructions and the discharge program given to patients. **Box 212.3** gives a few paramount rules for discharge instructions.

## UNDERSTANDING THE MEDICAL-LEGAL SYSTEM

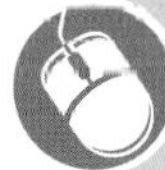

Information on this topic can be found online at www.expertconsult.com

## CONCERNS SPECIFIC TO THE CURRENT-DAY EMERGENCY DEPARTMENT

The function of this section is to delineate areas where emergency medicine and the law come into direct contact on a regular basis. The emergency department (ED) is under increasing stress to serve and aid the growing number of

**BOX 212.2 Legibility and Decipherability**

Handwritten entries on a chart must be legible to the average person. Action can now be brought by hospitals against physicians for poor handwriting.

**Electronic Medical Records**

The electronic medical record (EMR) is legible but often very sparse in the medical decision-making section. An advantage of the EMR is that all entries are time-stamped, thereby giving a better account of the emergency department (ED) visit. Its biggest disadvantage is automated and templated charting. This can be a downfall and cause to question the chart's accuracy, particularly if obvious mistakes are present.

**Timeliness of Making a Record**

All events and entries made on the chart should be timed. This is critical to fully understand what transpired during the ED visit.

**Address Nursing Charting**

Emergency physicians (EPs) should also routinely read nursing notes during the shift. If there are discrepancies between the EP and nursing assessments, they can be addressed while the patient is in the ED.

**Altering the Medical Record**

Corrections should be made in an obvious and straightforward manner. All additions and corrections to the chart need to be dated and timed. Nefarious correction of the medical chart is now a federal crime.

**Comments on the Chart**

The chart is a legal document protected by both state and federal law. The chart should reflect the objective observations of concerned health care personnel.

uninsured patients. No other specialty in medicine is subjected to laws by the national government to screen and stabilize all individuals entering the ED regardless of their ability to pay for the services.

## OWNERSHIP OF PATIENTS

The legal relationship of parties is that the physician is "the retained agent and servant of the patient." When a patient is in your department, he or she is your patient from a legal standpoint, and thus the physician cannot abrogate responsibility by saying that the patient belongs to another physician.

## COMBATIVE PATIENTS

The ED has the duty to restrain patients when they constitute a danger to self or others by virtue of a physical or mental condition (**Box 212.4**). Determination of mental and physical capacity is the key issue. Patients who lack capacity will depend on the substitute judgment of the EP. Belligerent patients who have capacity require law enforcement to handle the situation.

## CIVIL COMMITMENT

Again, the role of the ED is to secure the patient so that the patient does not cause harm to self or others and to fill out a first certification detailing the behavior and physical findings that justify civil commitment.

**BOX 212.3 Rules for Discharge Instructions**

All instructions should be time specific.
- Time-specific instructions such as "Return in 6 hours for reexamination of your abdomen or sooner if worse" are clear and to the point. The patient knows what to do and when to do it.

Instructions should be action specific.
- Although discharge instructions need to be brief and to the point, they need to provide knowledge to the patient about the disease process. It is important to discharge an informed customer.

Abbreviations in discharge instructions should be avoided.

Instructions should be doctor specific.
- It is preferable that the patient be given names and phone numbers for all the physicians with whom the patient is to follow up.

**BOX 212.4 Rules for Restraining Combative Patients**

Restraint methods should be appropriate.
- Both chemical and physical restraints are still commonly used to control patients who constitute a threat.

The need for restraints must be documented.
- The specific mode of restraint needs to be written as an order, and the patient's basic personal needs require proper nursing care.

All restrained patients require reevaluation.
- This is done at specific intervals to determine the continued need for restraints.

Emergency physicians rarely become involved legally in restraint cases.
- The exception is battery/assault cases in which they (1) fail to document the reason for restraint and (2) fail to follow their own hospital emergency department's restraint policy.

- Most states require a second certification process to be done in a specified time frame by a mental health professional.
- Ruling out organic causes of disease is necessary.
- The primary goal of the initial evaluation is to arrange for the patient to be reevaluated by mental health professionals.

# Transfers

The Emergency Medical Treatment and Active Labor Act (EMTALA) is the rule by which a patient can legally be transferred or discharged out of the ED to another facility. **Box 212.5** contains a set of guidelines for complying with the EMTALA.

## REPORTABLE ILLNESSES

The legal system and the ED function together as essentially an officer of the court. In all 50 states, child abuse, elder abuse, and assaults are reportable conditions. The EP also maintains a duty to third parties who may not be present in the ED. Therefore, when a patient has a gunshot or stab

**BOX 212.5 Key Points of the Emergency Medical Treatment and Active Labor Act**

Informed refusal can allow a patient to exempt himself or herself from EMTALA regulations. The emergency physician and the nurse involved in the case should carefully note this on the patient's chart.

The patient should be stabilized such that the acts of transfer and moving the patient to a higher level of care have a reasonable probability of providing a better outcome for the patient.

A hospital that usually and customarily receives patients should accept these patients unless their capabilities, at that time, are overwhelmed and they are unable to find room. This fact should be noted on the records when trying to procure transfer of a patient.

Failure to comply can lead to hefty fines to the institution and physician.

**BOX 212.6 Against Medical Advice**

Patients who leave against medical advice are using a form of informed refusal. The legal process contains the following:

- Document the mental capacity of the patient.
- Provide the patient a diagnosis or potential diagnosis in a form that the patient can understand.
- Explain the risk and benefits of what can happen if the patient does not take the advice of health care workers.
- While being compliant with the Health Insurance Portability and Accountability Act, communicate with family or friends who are with the patient so that they may also be involved in persuading the patient to receive medical care.
- Have a witness, such as a nurse or family member, sign the document.
- Document all of the above.

wound, other people may be at risk, and failure to report such injuries could place the patient and institution in danger.

## LEGAL BLOOD DRAW FOR ALCOHOL TESTING

This varies from state to state because some states have given the police warrant authority to obtain blood whereas in others a court order is required. It is the ED's responsibility to comply with the law. The police have the right to discarded body contents (e.g., vomitus, urine, feces) once such material passes into the public domain. An EP is also obligated under the EMTALA to offer a medical screening examination to all individuals arriving for a blood draw.

## INCIDENT REPORTS

Incident reports are a part of the quality assurance system. In most states, incident reports are protected from both discovery and judicial admissibility. The function of such reporting is to improve care. Incident reports should not be filed in a patient's chart.

## RESPONSE TO IN-HOUSE EMERGENCIES

All contracts should be written such that the EP will respond if not required to remain in the ED because of the acuity level of other patients. The hospital always has the alternative of putting a patient on a cot and bringing the patient to the ED. In many states, response to in-house emergencies is considered part of an in-house Good Samaritan statute. This again varies from state to state and should be confirmed by EPs at each site where they are required to perform this duty.

## WRITING ORDERS FOR ADMITTED PATIENTS

The EP's medical liability carrier may have questions regarding orders written on already hospitalized patients. The best ways to limit exposure on the writing of inpatient orders are as follows:

- Limit all orders.
- Write only true admitting orders and not continuing care orders.
- Make it clear when Dr. X, the attending physician, assumes care of the patient.

## PRESCRIPTIONS FROM THE EMERGENCY DEPARTMENT

Any prescription requiring a Drug Enforcement Agency prescription number should have proper warnings documented, usually on the ED general discharge instructions. In addition, one should avoid writing prescriptions for nonregistered patients (i.e., the nurse or technician you are working with). There is no medical liability coverage for this practice.

## MIDLEVEL PROVIDERS, RESIDENTS, AND EMERGENCY PHYSICIAN SUPERVISION

Midlevel providers (MLPs) practice under the EP's license. EPs should sign off on charts only after they have been reviewed by them. The EP is ultimately responsible for the actions of the MLP.

All resident work must be supervised if it is to be billed for under any federal program. All violations of this mandate are considered criminal violations of the federal law, and the current act has no exemptions.

## PATIENTS WHO LEAVE BEFORE EXAMINATION OR AGAINST MEDICAL ADVICE OR WHO ELOPE

The last health care professional to see the patient should write a note about why the patient left and attest that the patient had the mental capacity to make such a decision at that time (**Box 212.6**).

Elopement is a similar process in which the patient disappears in the middle of a work-up. Document what actions were taken to find the patient. For example:

- Search the ED.
- Have security check the parking and smoking areas.
- Call the patient's contact phone number.

## RETURN VISITS

In emergency medicine, "bounce-back patients" should often be reevaluated as new-visit patients. Disease processes may often become evident only after the second or third visit.

## CHANGE OF SHIFT

A note should be made in the chart that the patient's care was transferred to another physician at a particular time and that discussion was held with this other physician so that he or she is properly engaged in continuing care of the patient. The discharging doctor—the second physician to see the patient—generally assumes the duty to make certain that the patient's care is complete. Repeating the examination and evaluation of vital signs is recommended before discharge.

## LABORATORY STUDIES, RADIOGRAPHS, AND ELECTROCARDIOGRAMS

The ED should have a process to detect what has been ordered and to account for the results received. A system is needed in which each variance in laboratory or radiographic test should be handled within the ED.

## HEALTH INSURANCE PORTABILITY AND ACCOUNTABILITY ACT

The doctor-patient relationship and patient records are protected by federal law under the Health Insurance Portability and Accountability Act (HIPAA). Protection and release of this information are mandated by the HIPAA. Please refer to Chapter 211 for a more in-depth discussion.

## DUTY TO A THIRD PARTY

Various therapies may render a patient incapacitated in some way and thereby place the patient and a third party in danger. Issuing a prescription requiring a Drug Enforcement Agency number means that the EP is accepting some responsibility to inform the patient about use of the drug. Other devices that make the patient incapable of normal functioning (e.g., the use of crutches, eye patches, various splints) may also place the patient and others at risk. Discussion of this situation on the chart is useful should the need to provide defense arise.

## MINORS

Emancipated minors are those who live outside the home, provide their own financial support, have borne a child, or make their own life decisions. Such emancipation is given through the act of a probate court. In most states, children who arrive for treatment and who are older than 12 years may have questions of child abuse, substance abuse, sexually transmitted disease, and pregnancy treated without parental consent.

## TELEPHONE ORDERS AND TELEPHONE ADVICE

In general, the ED should not give telephone advice. Answering machine devices that advise the patient to come into the ED or to call 911 are often the most useful.

# SPECIFIC HIGH-RISK MEDICAL COMPLAINTS

The following is a system-based collection of high-risk situations commonly found in the ED that have caused considerable medical-legal consternation.

**BOX 212.7 Orthopedic Conditions**

If you think enough of an injury to have it radiographed, you should think enough of it to splint it.

One radiograph does not rule out a fracture. The emergency physician should never guarantee that something is not broken.

*Calcaneal fracture*: Examination of the lumbar spine is indicated.

*Spinal fractures in children*: The thought process must include the possibility of child abuse.

*Traumatic femoral fracture*: Other chest, abdominal, and cervical spine injuries must be considered.

**BOX 212.8 Eye, Ear, Nose, and Throat Rules**

Proper use of a laryngeal mask airway or bag-valve-mask apparatus can frequently control and provide adequate ventilation for patients.

*Eye foreign body sensation*: Make sure that there is no organic cause of the injury, no retained foreign body, and no contact lens use. Prescribe tetanus toxoid, antibiotics, and close ophthalmology follow-up.

*Nasal septal hematoma*: Document the presence or absence of a septal hematoma.

*Ear cartilage injury*: Prescribe antibiotics and timely referral to otolaryngology.

## ORTHOPEDICS

It is always wise for the EP to let patients know that this is the beginning of a process. Orthopedic management includes recognition, reduction, retention, and rehabilitation (**Box 212.7**). The ED is only the first part of what may be a long and complex process.

## EYE, EAR, NOSE, AND THROAT OR AIRWAY

Airway, in emergency medicine, is everything. Cases involving the airway are major problems because of the serious neurologic injuries that can result (**Box 212.8**).

## WOUNDS

All wounds seen in the ED are potentially contaminated and have foreign material almost by definition (**Box 212.9**). Lawsuits in emergency medicine wound management are based on three critical issues: foreign body, nerve injury, and tendon injury.

## POISONING

"Accidental poisoning" must be clearly reviewed and the potential for abuse or neglect considered. A patient with an intentional overdose should be placed under suicide precautions while actively treating the patient for the effects of the overdose. An EP may consult with poison control.

## PSYCHIATRY

In emergency medicine, the major issue with psychiatry is that the physician must be able to delineate organic disease manifested as abnormal behavior (**Box 212.10**).

**BOX 212.9 Rules for Wound Care**

Never guarantee that no foreign bodies are left in a wound.
Glass does show on radiographs. Liberal use of radiography in shattered glass–type wounds is advisable.
A laceration chart that does not comment on foreign body, nerve, and tendon assessment is probably inadequate.
Splint wounds in the hand.
*Tendon injuries*: Deep wounds should be observed through a range of motion to make certain that the tendon injury is not hidden by soft tissue. Repair of tendons is rarely an emergency procedure. These wounds can be properly irrigated and closed loosely, and tendon repair can be performed later, within a reasonable period.
*Nerve injuries*: Proper documentation of nerve function and follow-up in a timely manner are needed, but immediate intervention is rarely, if ever required.
*Wound infections*: Higher-pressure irrigation through a syringe is preferable.
*Bite wounds*: Immobilization, intravenous antibiotics, elevation, and follow-up in a timely manner is recommended.
*Follow-up and suture removal*. Arranging for follow-up and suture removal is important. Having the wound rechecked in 48 hours and arranging for proper interventions will essentially go a long way in preventing any legal actions concerning wound infections or retained foreign bodies.

**BOX 212.10 General Considerations for Psychiatric Patients**

The emergency physician (EP) is ultimately responsible for the patient regardless of the opinions of the consulting psychiatric worker.
The EP should adhere to guidelines of the Joint Commission on restraining and reevaluating patients.
The EP cannot say that a patient is free of organic disease, only that the patient is capable of being evaluated by a psychiatric service.
Abnormal vital signs should not be ascribed to psychiatric disease. Clues to organic disease include unexplained abnormal vital signs, tremors, and abnormal speech patterns.

## CHEST PAIN

This condition is still the largest risk issue in emergency medicine. Between 20% and 25% of malpractice funds expended in emergency medicine are related to the complaint of chest pain. The groups of diseases that constitute most of these cases are acute coronary syndromes, aortic dissection, and pulmonary embolism (**Box 212.11**).

## ABDOMINAL PAIN

Lawsuits related to abdominal pain in emergency medicine are highly age and sex dependent because of difficulties in diagnosis. Excellent evidence suggests that up to 50% of the time a patient with a complaint of abdominal pain leaves the ED without a specific diagnosis proved by testing. Short-term follow-up is the key because examination is merely a snapshot of a moving picture. If a patient's examination shows peritonitis, remember that computed tomography has a 5% to 8% error rate for appendicitis. Clinical judgment should rule (**Box 212.12**).

**BOX 212.11 Rules for Chest Pain**

There is no single description of the pain that rules out a cardiopulmonary source of the complaint.
One electrocardiogram and one cardiac marker are not adequate to rule out acute coronary syndrome.
D-dimer is helpful only if negative in a low-risk patient.
Do not rationalize abnormal vital signs.
The emergency physician should not write prescriptions for nitroglycerin. Unstable chest pain is unstable angina until proved otherwise.
Response to a gastrointestinal cocktail proves nothing. It is in no way related to being able to separate myocardial from esophageal disease.

**BOX 212.12 Rules for Abdominal Pain**

If the patient still has an appendix, it could be appendicitis. The emergency physician should not avoid this discussion with the patient.
Repeated evaluations may be the safest and single best test for abdominal pain.
A few white blood cells or red cells in urine do not equal a urinary tract infection; there may be some other cause of the problem, such as an inflammatory process or aortic pathology.
In elderly patients with new-onset abdominal or flank pain, think aortic disease as an important rule-out diagnosis.

## BACK PAIN

Evaluation of back pain is a daily occurrence in the ED. More than 6 million annual visits have been reported. The evaluation should be systematic and consider the red flags to warrant imaging for ruling out diagnoses with high morbidity and mortality, including ectopic pregnancy, abdominal aortic aneurysm, aortic dissection, spinal cord compression syndrome, and inflammatory conditions (**Box 212.13**).

## UROLOGIC ISSUES

In emergency medicine, urologic emergencies are few. Diagnoses that require emergency intervention are testicular torsion and sexually transmitted diseases. A patient who is being treated for possible sexually transmitted diseases should be asked about partners and should be informed that these partners will also require evaluation and treatment. It is also fair to warn the patient that the public health department will be involved if cultures are positive. The health department has a duty to third parties who have been involved with the patient

**BOX 212.13 Rules for Back Pain Evaluation**

If the patient is a childbearing female, pregnancy should be ruled out.
If the patient is older than 50 years, the differential diagnosis should include aneurysm and dissection.
If the patient is immunocompromised or an intravenous drug abuser or has a history of cancer, squamous cell cervical carcinoma and inflammatory pathology should be considered.
A directed neurologic examination should be performed and bowel and bladder dysfunction should be assessed.

**BOX 212.14 Rules for Headache Emergencies**

If a computed tomography scan is obtained for subarachnoid hemorrhage, a spinal tap should be performed to confirm the negativity.
If this is a sudden onset of the worst headache in the patient's life, it is prudent to rule out subarachnoid hemorrhage.
A sudden onset of neck pain can indicate a subarachnoid hemorrhage. One third of subarachnoid hemorrhages occur in the posterior fossa.
Patients with fever, photophobia, meningismus, and suspicion of meningitis should have antibiotics started promptly and then undergo a lumbar puncture when feasible.

to seek them out and provide therapy. It may be best for the patient to understand the need to inform contacts and to advise such contacts that they may be at some risk.

## ELEVATED BLOOD PRESSURE

Elevated blood pressure is often found in the ED. Most commonly it is related to the stress or pain of the situation involving the chief complaint. It is not the standard to lower all elevated blood pressure. It is recommended that the absence of end-organ dysfunction be documented and that the patient understand the sequelae of elevated blood pressure. Timely follow-up is recommended to address this issue with the patient's primary care physician.

## HEADACHE EMERGENCIES

Headache is one of the most common chief complaints in emergency medicine (**Box 212.14**). The EP must consider the possibility of subarachnoid hemorrhage, meningitis, or carbon monoxide poisoning in every patient with headache.

## SPINAL CORD INJURY

Spinal cord injuries are relatively rare, but they carry a devastating societal and financial cost. During the patient's evaluation, the EP should properly document immobilization, and there should be no hurry to remove such immobilization. Document an appropriate neurologic examination on arrival of the patient. Obtain a magnetic resonance image for patients with evidence of motor, bowel, or bladder dysfunction.

**BOX 212.15 Rules for Trauma Patients**

A systematic approach involving the use of advanced trauma life support should be carried out.
The goal is to stabilize and transfer the patient to higher tertiary centers if definitive resources are not available.
Keep the patient immobilized until injury has been ruled out.
Head-injured patients should not be admitted merely for observation but should be sent to a center where intervention can take place if it is actually required.

## SEIZURES AND SYNCOPE

Seizures and syncope can be lethal from multiple perspectives. Injury to the patient and reoccurrence are real potential problems. Precautions for safety should be initiated in the ED as soon as possible. If the patient is discharged, warnings about driving and the operation of machinery are important for protection of the public in general. Such warnings should be indicated in some way on the patient's chart.

## TRANSIENT ISCHEMIC ATTACKS AND STROKE

Transient ischemic attacks and stroke are becoming larger issues. The American College of Emergency Physicians has gone on record as specifically stating that tissue-type plasminogen activator is not the standard of care for stroke. Lack of rapid evaluation of patients with a transient ischemic attack and the initial use of aspirin therapy have been the source of many ED lawsuits. Patients with transient ischemic attacks represent a high-risk group and require timely intervention.

## TRAUMA

All EPs should know what they can and cannot do and should move quickly to ensure that the patient receives the actual help needed (**Box 212.15**). Administration of blood and treatment of shock are critical.

## OBSTETRIC AND GYNECOLOGIC ISSUES

With regard to obstetric and gynecologic issues, it is important for the EP to realize that there may be two patients and not one (**Box 212.16**).

## PEDIATRICS

The number of pediatric medical-legal cases in emergency medicine has actually decreased as rates of immunization and the various diseases that can be immunized against have increased. The keys to pediatrics are examination and early reexamination. Child abuse is a serious social problem in EDs. In general, you should never accuse anyone of abusing his or her child. You merely state that an investigative process is required because of the findings. It is important to emphasize that "they" make us do this type of investigation in these situations. Abuse and neglect are often difficult to separate in the ED, and such distinction needs to be made through social services. When in doubt, however, the child's safety is paramount, and admitting a child for observation can certainly be a reasonable use of the hospital facility. Certain specific disease entities, such as sudden infant death syndrome, unusual burns, vaginal infections, certain types of fracture,

**BOX 212.16 Rules for Obstetric and Gynecologic Issues**

Missed ectopic pregnancies have decreased dramatically in the United States as a medical-legal problem since the widespread use of β-human chorionic gonadotropin testing and ultrasound scanning.
A negative ultrasound does not rule out an ectopic pregnancy.
Sudden loss of consciousness or shock in a young female patient should raise the possibility of a ruptured ectopic pregnancy until proved otherwise.
Eclampsia is the second most common obstetric and gynecologic emergency. It can be present up to 2 weeks postpartum.
In postpartum febrile female patients, ultrasound scans to check for retained products of conception and infection within the uterus are as important as checking the urine.
Women who are 5 months into gestation and have sustained trauma to the abdomen should undergo a period of fetal monitoring in the labor and delivery department.

**BOX 212.17 Rules for Pediatrics**

Fever in children younger than 36 months needs a probable source.
Close follow-up is necessary.
Splint musculoskeletal injuries for reevaluation in a week.
Consider child abuse in children who visit the emergency department frequently.

and repeated toxic ingestions, should always be considered suggestive of child abuse until further information is obtained (**Box 212.17**).

## SUGGESTED READINGS

Fisher R, Ury W. Getting to YES. Negotiating agreement without giving in. New York: Penguin; 1991.
Henry G, Sullivan D. Emergency medicine risk management: a comprehensive review. 2nd ed. Dallas: American College of Emergency Physicians; 1997.
Mayer T, Cates R. Leadership for great customer service: satisfied patients, satisfied employees. Chicago: Health Administration Press; 2004.
Salluzzo R, Mayer T, et al, editors. Emergency department management: principles and applications. St. Louis: Mosby; 1997.

# 213 Documentation

*James K. Takayesu*

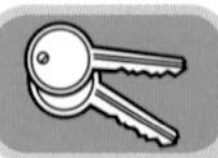

**KEY POINTS**

- The emergency department (ED) chart must be adequate to support billing and accurate to prevent claims of fraud against the emergency physician.
- Most reimbursement comes from the five levels of the evaluation and management codes and is dependent on a combination of historical and physical examination data, medical decision making, and diagnostic assignments.
- Billing for critical care requires more than 30 minutes of physician attention to a patient and obviates the level-specific evaluation and management charting requirements.
- Billing for observation requires separate documentation in the ED chart.
- The emergency physician is legally accountable for claims based on the ED chart, including the potential for audits of electronic medical records by the Centers for Medicare and Medicaid Services and criminal penalties in cases of upcoding, such as assumption coding.

## INTRODUCTION

Documentation in the emergency department (ED) medical record serves three basic functions:

1. To provide a detailed record of a patient's medical conditions and treatments
2. To minimize the medical liability risk of emergency physicians (EPs) by documenting the thought process behind treatment plans
3. To support the charges billed to the patient by clearly substantiating the services rendered

Documentation in the ED chart must be both adequate to support reimbursement claims and accurate to prevent claims of billing fraud. What is not documented does not get reimbursed—in effect, it did not happen. Understanding the fundamentals of coding and billing from the ED chart is essential to ensure a revenue stream that supports the financial viability of the ED. This revenue is critical in enabling professional autonomy, continuing medical education, and improvements in ED patient care and technology. Revenue from patient care is obtained through two parallel billing structures: hospital billing and professional billing. This chapter focuses on professional billing.

## CURRENT PROCEDURAL TERMINOLOGY CODES

Before publication of the Current Procedural Terminology (CPT) codes, third-party payers had their own idiosyncratic list of physician services and their respective codes, thus making consistent and reliable procedural billing extremely difficult. CPT coding was published by the American Medical Association (AMA) in 1966 in an attempt to standardize reimbursement for medical procedures. These codes are used to report physician services for claims processing and for local, regional, and national service utilization comparisons by the Centers for Medicare and Medicaid Services (CMS). CPT codes are reviewed annually by the AMA CPT Editorial Committee with input from various specialty physician organizations to account for new procedures and changes in reimbursement patterns.

A CPT code is a unique five-digit code that represents a service in contemporary medical practice that is being performed by physicians.[1] Some common examples of emergency procedures and physician fees are listed in **Table 213.1**. The AMA Relative Value Update Committee assigns a relative value unit (RVU) to the code to reflect the complexity of the service relative to other physician services. The Resource-Based Relative Value Scale ranks services according to three factors: (1) the relative work of the physician, (2) the cost of performing the service, and (3) the risk involved in the service to both the patient and the provider. Each of these factors is assigned a numerical value, which when added together gives a total RVU for the service. This RVU is then multiplied by a geographically adjusted monetary conversion factor to arrive at an actual fee for the services provided (see Table 213.1).

## EVALUATION AND MANAGEMENT

The evaluation and management (E&M) codes are five CPT codes (see Table 213.1) that account for approximately 85% of all EP reimbursement. These five codes categorize the complexity of the encounter. Coders (and hence payers) rely on the documentation of historical information, physical

**Table 213.1 Sample Fee Schedule for Blue Cross/Blue Shield of Massachusetts Emergency Medicine Procedure and Physician Fees, Effective September 1, 2004**

| PROCEDURE CODE | PROCEDURE | FEE |
|---|---|---|
| 10060 | Drainage of skin abscess | $102.98 |
| 10120 | Removal of foreign body | $78.37 |
| 12001 | Repair of superficial wound(s) | $104.75 |
| 12032 | Layer closure of wound(s) | $208.87 |
| 16020 | Treatment of burn(s) | $68.77 |
| 23650 | Shoulder dislocation | $308.73 |
| 29125 | Application of forearm splint | $48.75 |
| 29130 | Application of finger splint | $32.58 |
| 30901 | Control of nosebleed | $73.45 |
| 31500 | Insertion of emergency airway | $135.95 |
| 62270 | Spinal fluid tap, diagnostic | $76.92 |
| 69210 | Removal of impacted earwax | $40.66 |
| 99235 | Observation/hospital same date | $220.62 |
| 99236 | Observation/hospital same date | $274.84 |
| 99281 | ED visit (level 1) | $24.61 |
| 99282 | ED visit (level 2) | $41.29 |
| 99283 | ED visit (level 3) | $91.68 |
| 99284 | ED visit (level 4) | $142.32 |
| 99285 | ED visit (level 5) | $222.63 |
| 99291 | Critical care, first hour | $245.68 |
| 99292 | Critical care, additional 30 min | $122.89 |

*ED*, Emergency department.

examination, and medical decision making (MDM) to determine the complexity of the visit. The last digit of each CPT code is used to denote the "level" of service (**Table 213.2**). Services provided between the hours of 10 PM and 8 AM may be coded with an additional code, 99053.[2] Each progressive level of service requires incrementally more documentation to support the level of coding. The EP must be sure to document an adequate history of the present illness (HPI), review of systems (ROS), and past medical, family, and social history (PMFSHx) to support each level of the chart. This requirement increases substantially for level 4 and 5 charts (**Tables 213.2A and 213.2B**). The HPI should include a variety of descriptors of the chief complaint, including the relevant location, quality, severity, timing, context, and associated symptoms. The ROS and PMFSHx can be recorded by ancillary staff (resident, nurse practitioner, and others) or on a form completed by the patient but must have a notation supplementing or confirming that this information has been reviewed by the attending physician.

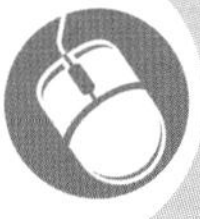

See Table 213.3A, Charting Requirements for Charts by Level, and Table 213.3B, Emergency Department Observation Codes and Descriptions, online at www.expertconsult.com

Certain statements commonly used in medical documentation deserve specific mention. The PMFSHx should contain specific historical information obtained from the interview. Truncating the ROS with "all other systems negative" is adequate to meet documentation requirements for a level 5 visit; however, it should be used cautiously. When used indiscriminately in low-acuity patients, it may raise concern for upcoding and subject the EP to an audit.[3] The designation "unable to obtain secondary to acuity or mental status" is appropriate for patients from whom no history can be obtained. EPs should document the specific clinical condition that prevents them from obtaining the history, as well as the specific source of the historical information obtained, such as nursing home records, family members, or electronic records.

MDM is the most complex and least clinically intuitive. MDM should capture in text the complexity of the decision-making process and reflect the intellectual workload of the EP. It should include at minimum two of the following three elements: the number of possible diagnoses or treatments, the tests or records reviewed, and the potential risk to the patient, including complications of treatment or possible morbidity or mortality (**Table 213.4**). When applicable, EPs should also list all major comorbid conditions affecting their decision making, consultations, and discussions with primary care providers.

In assigning diagnoses, EPs should list all diagnoses applicable to the patient's current situation, including abnormal vital signs.[4] For example, a hypotensive patient with diverticulitis and fever should have the diagnotic assignments of "hypotension," "diverticulitis," and "pyrexia." Language that does not connote a specific diagnosis, such as "rule out," "probable," "motor vehicle accident," "possible," "chronic," or "mild," should be avoided. Including a breadth of diagnoses to paint a more thorough and accurate clinical picture of the clinical workload involved will maximize billing.[5]

## CRITICAL CARE

Critical care (E&M code 99291) is the E&M of an unstable, critically ill, or injured patient for which the EP's constant cognitive attendance is required.[1] Many intensive care unit admissions qualify for critical care billing because they involve "a critical illness or injury that acutely impairs one or more vital organ systems such that there is a high probability of imminent or life threatening deterioration in the patient's condition."[6] Common clinical conditions that should prompt consideration of critical care include sepsis, abdominal aortic aneurysm, ruptured ectopic pregnancy, trauma, stroke, subarachnoid hemorrhage, atrial fibrillation with a rapid ventricular response, acute coronary syndrome, severe asthma, chronic obstructive pulmonary disease requiring bilevel positive airway pressure, diabetic ketoacidosis, and hyperkalemia. The first 30 minutes, up until 74 minutes of care, is billed with this code, after which additional increments of 30 minutes (code 99292) may be billed. The physician must be engaged

**Table 213.2** Evaluation and Management Code Examples

| VISIT LEVEL | CPT CODE | DESCRIPTION | EXAMPLES |
|---|---|---|---|
| Level 1 | 99281 | Problem focused | Suture removal<br>Tetanus-diphtheria immunization<br>Insect bite |
| Level 2 | 99282 | Expanded problem focused, low complexity | Sunburn<br>Conjunctivitis<br>Minor extremity trauma without radiograph indicated |
| Level 3 | 99283 | Expanded problem focused, moderate complexity | Corneal foreign body<br>Vaginal discharge without abdominal pain<br>Extremity trauma with radiograph indicated<br>Minor head injury |
| Level 4 | 99284 | Detailed | Renal colic<br>Hip fracture<br>Abdominal pain<br>Head injury with loss of consciousness<br>Motor vehicle accident victim arriving by ambulance |
| Level 5 | 99285 | Comprehensive | Acute myocardial infarction<br>Chest pain requiring admission<br>Gastrointestinal bleeding, active<br>Transient ischemic attack<br>Dyspnea<br>Altered mental status<br>Headache with stiff neck |

*CPT*, Current Procedural Terminology.

**Table 213.4** Medical Decision Making Correlated with Chart Billing Level

| | MEDICAL DECISION-MAKING COMPLEXITY | | | |
|---|---|---|---|---|
| | **MINIMAL** | **LOW** | **MODERATE** | **HIGH** |
| Diagnoses considered (number) | Minimum | Limited | Multiple | Extensive |
| Data or testing required or reviewed (number) | None or minimum | Limited | Moderate | Extensive |
| Clinical impression or potential risk to the patient | Minimum | Low | Moderate | High |
| Chart billing level | 99281 or level 1 | 99282 or level 2 | 99283 or level 3; 99284 or level 4 | 99285 or level 5 |

in work directly related to the individual patient's care. Because of the implied severity of the patient's condition, none of the history or physical examination requirements apply to qualify for critical care billing. Certain procedures associated with critically ill patients may be "bundled" with the critical care payment and thus are not billable separately. Such procedures include arterial blood gas, electrocardiogram (ECG), chest radiograph, and pulse oximetry interpretation; gastric intubation; temporary transvenous pacing; ventilator management; vascular access; cardiopulmonary resuscitation (CPR); and defibrillation.

## BILLING COMPLIANCE

Accuracy is essential to avoid issues of fraud and abuse. All EPs are individually responsible and accountable for correct processing of the claims associated with their charts. It is incumbent on EPs to document the visit accurately without underrepresenting or overrepresenting the encounter's complexity.[4,5] Using electronic macros with identical documentation of HPI and MDM across different patient encounters can be a red flag to billing auditors.[7] Cutting and pasting text verbatim is strongly discouraged by the CMS. Ancillary providers and scribes may be used to document information on the chart but must have their own electronic signature.

Recovery Audit Contractors (RACs) are auditing groups hired by the CMS to review the documentation supporting claims to detect and correct payments that are not supported by adequate documentation of a clinical encounter.[8] RACs review claims on a postpayment basis by using two types of review, automated (no medical record needed) or complex (complete medical record required). A RAC employs a staff consisting of nurses, therapists, certified coders, and a physician to review reimbursements with the goals of lowering inappropriate reimbursement rates by the CMS, providing public accountability of health care expenditures, and providing feedback to EPs submitting claims that do not comply with Medicare reimbursement rules.

Documentation is perhaps most important when it comes to protecting EPs from claims of fraud in providing care. Procedures or services that are billed for and not documented, regardless of whether they occurred, are considered fraudulent and are subject to criminal penalties. Assumption coding is defined as billing at a higher level than what the chart supports. For example, a patient with chest pain and changes on the ECG who is admitted on intravenous heparin qualifies for a level 5 encounter. However, if the EP seeing this patient documents only a four-element HPI, 5 physical examination points, moderate-complexity MDM, and "rule out myocardial infarction" as the diagnosis, the evidence provided by this chart is inadequate to support billing above level 4. If this chart were reviewed, the EP would be liable for filing a fraudulent claim. To protect physicians from such pitfalls, physician groups or hospitals should have compliance review committees in place to review charts in a systematic fashion to ensure that EP documentation and chart coding are appropriate and consistent for the patient services rendered.[6]

## PROCEDURAL BILLING

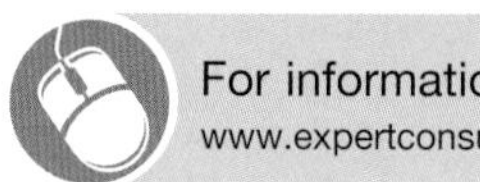

For information on this topic, see www.expertconsult.com

## OBSERVATION CARE

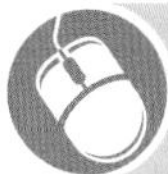

For information on this topic, see www.expertconsult.com

## HOSPITAL BILLING AND CAPTURABLE REVENUE

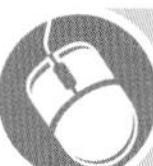

For information on this topic, see www.expertconsult.com

## SUGGESTED READING

Centers for Medicare & Medicaid Services. Recovery audit program. Available at www.cms.hhs.gov/RAC. Accessed June 7, 2012.

## REFERENCES

***References can be found on Expert Consult @ www.expertconsult.com.***

# 214 Ethics of Resuscitation

*Tammie E. Quest and Dave W. Lu*

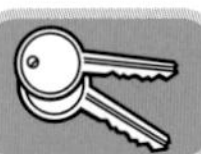

**KEY POINTS**

- Resuscitation colloquially comprises a spectrum of care that includes intravenous fluids, oxygen, cardiac pressors, and antibiotics.
- Cardiac arrest is the moment of death, when cardiac or respiratory effort ceases. Noninitiation of cardiopulmonary resuscitation (CPR) in the event of death is called "natural death."
- In the event of cardiac arrest, CPR is universally presumed unless patients have previously expressed a desire to be treated otherwise.
- The ethical principles of autonomy, beneficence, nonmaleficence, and justice must be considered in discussions regarding resuscitation.
- Emergency physicians (EPs) should be prepared to guide patients and families in the recommendation regarding initiation of CPR in the event of cardiac arrest based on goals of care. EPs should also be able to discuss the usual outcomes of cardiac arrest in terms of survival and disability and be comfortable describing nonresuscitation as "natural death."
- When discussing prognoses in patients with a chronic progressive medical illness, it may be helpful to explain that the best medical outcome that can be hoped for is that the patient returns to his or her "baseline status" or condition before admission.
- EPs should be able to recognize and treat the syndrome of imminent death and provide comfort measures regardless of the initiation of CPR.

## PERSPECTIVE

In the United States, universal presumed consent for cardiopulmonary resuscitation (CPR) after cardiac arrest is standard medical practice unless patients have previously expressed an explicit desire to be treated otherwise. Once a patient is in the hospital setting, however, the ethical choice to initiate or continue CPR and other life-prolonging measures should be based on the clinician's best prediction of expected medical outcomes, as well as the wishes and goals of the patient and his or her designated medical decision maker.

CPR holds a unique position in medicine and society. It is the only medical intervention that the patient must take steps to refuse in advance because of presumed consent, even if the clinician does not believe that it is beneficial or medically warranted. Ethical dilemmas surrounding the initiation, continuation, and cessation of resuscitation are common.

Patient autonomy, nonmaleficence (doing no harm), beneficence (promoting good or well-being), and justice (being fair) are the guiding principles of medical ethics.[1] For a patient to make autonomous decisions about resuscitation preferences, the patient (or designated medical decision maker) should be given the best information available to weigh his or her medical care options. The Jonsen model for ethical decision making suggests that the following four "ethical quadrants" be weighed: medical indications, patient preferences, quality of life, and contextual features.[2]

Despite much debate and discussion, medicine and society have not been able to agree on a common and accepted definition of the term *medical futility*.[3] One suggested paradigm of medical futility characterizes a medical intervention as futile when its goal will not probably be achieved.[3] Although one common medical goal of clinicians who perform CPR after cardiac arrest is return of spontaneous circulation, the patient, surrogate, and clinician may have other equally important goals, including neurologic outcome and quality of life after resuscitation. Timely discussion between the clinician and the patient or his or her designated decision maker regarding the goals of care is paramount to ensure quality end-of-life care.

Noninitiation of CPR is increasingly being described as "allow natural death." It is of utmost importance for clinicians to understand that before CPR, a host of interventions may be used to extend life but, in the event of death, the option may be to not attempt CPR. For example, research suggests that in cancer patients for whom all aggressive interventions (antibiotics, fluids, pressors, airway support) have been tried, in the event of death the success of CPR in achieving survival to discharge is zero.[4]

On the road to eventual death, patients may have a constellation of physical, psychologic, and emotional symptoms that can be treated. The majority of patients who are critically ill are not in active cardiac arrest at initial encounter but are at high risk for it. Emergency physicians (EPs) most often care for these patients at high risk for cardiac arrest and may find themselves ethically driven to discuss with patients and families the appropriateness of resuscitative efforts to reverse death in the event of cardiopulmonary arrest.

## EPIDEMIOLOGY

Out-of-hospital cardiac arrest (OHCA) has an incidence of 52.1 per 100,000 population, which makes it the third leading cause of death in North America.[5] The survival rate of patients experiencing OHCA after treatment by emergency medical services is approximately 8%, but it varies widely among regions.[5] For patients who suffer in-hospital pulseless cardiac arrest, survival to hospital discharge depends widely on the characteristics of the arrest and patient comorbid conditions (**Table 214.1**). Research suggests that when talking with patients, physicians can describe the overall likelihood of survival to discharge as 1 in 8 for patients who undergo CPR and 1 in 3 for patients who survive CPR.[6] Many of the patients who survive to discharge will be discharged to institutionalized settings. Poor prognostic indicators of survival after cardiac arrest include cancer, dementia, sepsis, cardiac disease, elevated serum creatinine, and African American race.[6] Despite these well-publicized numbers in the medical literature, EPs should be aware that patients and their families may have very different expectations of resuscitative efforts after cardiac arrest. Popular U.S. television programs, for example, incorrectly suggest that the immediate survival rate after cardiac arrest approaches 75%, with 67% of patients being portrayed as surviving to hospital discharge.[7]

**Table 214.1 Survival After In-Hospital Cardiopulmonary Resuscitation***

| | |
|---|---|
| Incidence of in-hospital cardiopulmonary resuscitation | 2.73 events per 1000 admissions |
| Incidence higher for nonwhite patients | 2.53/1000 in white patients<br>4.35/1000 in black patients<br>3.85/1000 for other races |
| Survival to discharge | 18.3% |
| Lower survival rates for patients who were: | Men<br>Older<br>Not white<br>Categorized as having a higher chronic illness burden<br>Admitted from a skilled nursing facility<br>Received care in a metropolitan or teaching hospital |

Data from Ehlenbach WJ, Barnato AE, Curtis JR, et al. Epidemiologic study of in-hospital cardiopulmonary resuscitation in the elderly. N Engl J Med 2009;361:22-31.

*Medicare data from 1992 to 2005 involving 433,895 cases of in-hospital cardiopulmonary resuscitation in patients 65 years or older.

## PATHOPHYSIOLOGY

Cardiac arrest is the sudden, abrupt loss of heart function.[8] The most common underlying reason for patients to die suddenly after cardiac arrest is coronary heart disease. Most cardiac arrests that lead to sudden death occur as a result of arrhythmias such as ventricular tachycardia or ventricular fibrillation. A patient's chances of survival after cardiac arrest are reduced by 7% to 10% with every minute that passes without CPR and defibrillation. Few attempts at resuscitation succeed after 10 minutes.[8]

## PRESENTING SIGNS AND SYMPTOMS

One classic scenario illustrating many of the ethical dilemmas surrounding resuscitation is a patient who arrives at the ED critically ill with possible impending cardiac arrest or with signs of active dying (**Table 214.2**). Decisions must be made quickly regarding which life-extending measures will be used while also simultaneously ensuring relief of patient distress. If a patient is likely to deteriorate rapidly or shows signs of imminent death, a discussion regarding resuscitation should be initiated with the patient or the appropriate surrogate. The EP should make a clinical assessment that includes evaluation of the goals of care, determination of the presence or absence of an advance directive, and a recommendation regarding the utility of CPR to meet the patient's goals of care. Table 214.2 lists the signs of active dying in the setting of a chronic progressive incurable illness, such as late-stage cancer, dementia, or failure to thrive.

## DIFFERENTIAL DIAGNOSIS AND MEDICAL DECISION MAKING

Before discussions with patients and families about critical illness, the EP may be able to initiate several easy medical

**Table 214.2 Signs of Active Dying in Patients with Chronic Illness**

| | EARLY | MID | LATE |
|---|---|---|---|
| Recognition | Confinement to bed<br>Loss of both interest in and ability to consume nutrition<br>Cognitive changes: either hypoactive or hyperactive, with delirium or increasing sleepiness | Further decline in mental status—obtunded<br>"Death rattle"—from pooled oral secretions that are not cleared because of loss of the swallowing reflex<br>Fever is common | Coma<br>Cool extremities<br>Altered respiratory pattern—either fast or slow<br>Fever is common<br>Death |
| Time course | The time to traverse the three stages can be less than 24 hours or up to 10 to 14 days. Once a patient enters the process, it is difficult to accurately predict the time course, which may cause considerable family distress if the dying patient seems to "linger." | | |

interventions to provide important and valued information for patients and their families to inform the medical recommendation. Bedside glucose testing and pulse oxygen saturation measurements, for example, may be sought. Rapid measurement of serum electrolytes (potassium in particular) may yield a quick overview of the patient's renal or acid-base status. Bedside ultrasonography is a minimally invasive way to diagnose potentially lethal catastrophes such as pericardial tamponade and rupture of an abdominal aortic aneurysm. Bedside electrocardiography may detect myocardial infarction. Good clinical information can help guide decision making.

### TIPS AND TRICKS

**Prognostication**

The safest prognostication that the emergency physician can make about a patient's outcome is that at best the patient may return to his or her baseline or the condition in which he or she was right before the precipitating event that brought the patient to the emergency department. For example, if the patient has end-stage dementia at baseline and is unable to care for himself, the best outcome from cardiac arrest would be survival to return to his previous baseline end-stage dementia, with the same level of assistance still being needed.

**Goals of Care Assessment**

The emergency physician should be prepared to assess the goals of care to make a recommendation regarding resuscitation: (1) establish what the patient or surrogate understands; (2) determine what the patient or surrogate expects; (3) discuss resuscitation in plain language, void of medical jargon; (4) respond to emotion; and (5) make a clinical recommendation or plan.

**Do-Not-Resuscitate Orders**

Such orders should not imply limits on any other interventions besides cardiopulmonary resuscitation in the event of cardiac arrest. The emergency physician should clearly distinguish other therapies that will be used, aside from cardiopulmonary resuscitation, in the event of death. It is a common mistake to "overinterpret" the meaning of "do not resuscitate" to exclude a host of life-sustaining treatments before cardiac arrest.

## TREATMENT

Temporizing measures that might "buy time" for discussion of the medical and ethical grounds for resuscitation, for examination of the medical record, or for contact of a provider more familiar with the patient should be considered on a case-by-case basis.

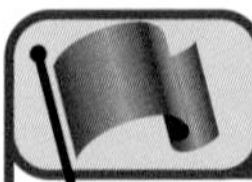

### RED FLAGS

Emergency physicians should advise patients and surrogates on the utility of resuscitation based on best available evidence to achieve a patient-centered meaningful outcome.

Patients who have do-not-resuscitate orders may desire life-sustaining treatments up to and until cardiac arrest.

## FOLLOW-UP, NEXT STEPS IN CARE, AND PATIENT EDUCATION

The medical condition and comorbid conditions of individual patients make each person's survival rate highly variable. Discharge survival rates and function in patients with chronic, progressive terminal illnesses such as end-stage cancer, heart failure, and pulmonary and neurologic diseases, for example, tend to be extremely poor. Increasingly, language such as "allow natural death" and "do not resuscitate" suggests that no attempt be made to initiate CPR in the event of physiologic death. However, other measures—oxygen, fluids, nutrition, pain control—may still be initiated to support patient comfort.

Patients or their medical decision makers who choose to forgo measures such as CPR may also, but not necessarily, choose a more global comfort approach to their end-of-life care. The EP should be able to provide palliative measures and support this comfort care (**Table 214.3**). It is important to recognize, however, that these patients may still need

**Table 214.3 Support of a Comfort Approach**

| | |
|---|---|
| Clearly define the goals of treatment | Once imminent death is recognized, discuss with family and confirm the treatment goals. When assuming a comfort approach, make a supportive statement, such as "You are doing the right thing."<br>Discuss with family stopping interventions that do not contribute to comfort. |
| Provide good palliative care | To contral oral/respiratory secrections ("death cattle"), use antimuscarinic blockers such as glycopyrrolate, 0.2 mg intravenously (onset, 1 min); atropine, 0.1 mg intravenously (onset, 1 min); atropine eyedrop 1%, 2 drops sublingually (onset, 30 min); or hyoscyamine hydrobromide, 1.5 mg transdermally (onset, 12 hr).<br>Use morphine (1-2 mg IV/SC every 5 min or 5 mg orally every 1 hr as starting dose) to control dyspnea or tachypnea. It can be very disturbing for family members to see loved ones in a coma breathing at 40 breaths/min. The goal should be to keep the respiratory rate in the range of 10 to 15 breaths/min.<br>Provide excellent mouth and skin care. |
| Determine disposition | According to symptom burden, patients may require assignment to the intensive care unit to ensure that the treatment goals remain on target and that the medical aspects of palliative care are met (control of pain and dyspnea, for example) despite a "do-not-resuscitate" status. |

intensive in-hospital care. In some cases, transfer of a patient from the emergency department to a hospice may be possible. More often, patients are admitted to the hospital and may require temporary intensive care to assess the goals of care and adequately achieve comfort. For a patient who is undergoing advanced life support measures, such as invasive ventilation and cardioactive drugs, a time-limited trial may help the patient and his or her family feel more comfortable delineating the goals of care.

## SUGGESTED READINGS

Beauchamp TL, Childress JF. Principles of biomedical ethics. 6th ed. New York: Oxford University Press; 2008.

Ehlenbach WJ, Barnato AE, Curtis JR, et al. Epidemiologic study of in-hospital cardiopulmonary resuscitation in the elderly. N Engl J Med 2009;361:22-31.

Ewer MS, Kish SK, Martin CG, et al. Characteristics of cardiac arrest in cancer patients as a predictor of survival after cardiopulmonary resuscitation. Cancer 2001;92:1905-12.

Jonsen AR, Siegler M, Winslade WJ. Clinical ethics: a practical approach to ethical decisions in clinical medicine. 7th ed. New York: McGraw-Hill Medical; 2010.

Nichol G, Thomas E, Callaway CW, et al. Regional variation in out-of-hospital cardiac arrest incidence and outcome. JAMA 2008;300:1423-31.

## REFERENCES

***References can be found on Expert Consult @ www.expertconsult.com.***

# 215 Emergency Medical Services and Disaster Medicine

*Jennifer Avegno and Jeffrey M. Elder*

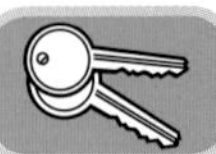

**KEY POINTS**

- Emergency medical services (EMS) consist of a heterogeneous group of entities that vary according to urbanization, training procedures, skill level of practitioners, resources, and scope.
- Although EMS research is developing rapidly, controversy exists over the role of EMS interventions and protocols in commonly encountered conditions such as trauma and cardiovascular emergencies.
- Disaster medicine encompasses planning, resource allocation, and health care response to any event—natural or man-made—that overwhelms the resources of a particular locality.
- Weapons of mass destruction have the potential to cause severe physical damage and health concerns that require specific, targeted planning and coordination for emergency care personnel.

## INTRODUCTION AND HISTORY

An emergency medical services (EMS) system can be defined as "a coordinated arrangement of resources (including personnel, equipment, and facilities) organized to respond to medical emergencies, regardless of the cause."[1] Modern EMS systems in the United States have their origins largely in battlefield medicine.[2-6] Indeed, it was a surgeon in the Napoleonic military campaign who pioneered the concept of rapid response to injured soldiers in the field of combat.[3] Baron Larrey, the "father of modern prehospital care," developed a systematic approach to combat trauma in which ambulances transported wounded soldiers from the battlefield to organized medical stations. In the American Civil War, ambulances were placed under structured medical direction. Successive advances in technology and EMS organization in later wars resulted in significantly decreased mortality rates for battle combatants who were transported to field hospitals.[5]

Although civilian "rescue societies" and ambulance services existed from the mid-1800s, the most significant nonmilitary advancement in EMS occurred in the 1950s with the establishment of life support training programs through the Chicago Fire Department. From this effort the basis for the now widely accepted emergency medical technician (EMT) and paramedic training programs were formed.[2] By the 1960s, some regions had nascent ambulance systems with paramedics trained in advanced life support (ALS) techniques, although others developed a separate system of "heartmobiles" with physicians on board to provide care only for cardiac emergencies.[7]

The need for sophisticated, coordinated EMS systems was brought to the national spotlight in 1966 with publication of the National Academy of Sciences paper titled "Accidental Death and Disability: The Neglected Disease of Modern Society." This paper noted that few people were trained in advanced resuscitation, no widely accepted standards had been established for training ambulance personnel, and communication systems and supplies were lacking. This report spurred a national, organized effort to increase awareness of traumatic disease and the need for development of a comprehensive EMS system.[5] Congress responded with the National Highway Safety Act of 1966 and the EMS Systems Act of 1973, which authorized federal grants to state, local, and regional governments for the development of EMS systems within a specified "systems approach" framework.[8] In 1981, however, guaranteed federal funding for EMS was replaced with state block grants and increased financial insecurity.[4] Currently, nearly 1 million people are certified in some form as emergency response personnel, and nearly 20 million patients are treated in the EMS system annually, but heterogeneity in system design, scope, and certification requirements persists.[9]

## EMS SYSTEM DESIGN

EMS systems are, arguably, some of the most complex organizational entities in modern society. They include representatives from municipalities of every size, law enforcement, fire and safety, health care, transportation services, and community groups. Federal governing bodies define the necessary components of EMS systems but do not directly oversee organization or management. Coordination between agencies is essential but often difficult to achieve.[1] Ideally, EMS system design is centered around the particular needs of the community that it serves, with one standard characteristic: emergency medical personnel act as on-scene "physician surrogates" to provide appropriate life support techniques.[7] Common models categorize different systems in terms of control by the public or private agencies, rural or urban communities, and single-tiered or multitiered systems.

### PUBLIC AND PRIVATE AGENCIES

Public EMS systems are often part of the local fire department organization and are more common in large urban counties or cities. This structure developed in the early days of EMS systems as a result of logistic concerns: fire stations were located at tactical points throughout communities and had experience in emergency response. Firefighters could be trained in basic life support (BLS) techniques and thus could function as both fire/safety and emergency medical personnel. Alternatively, public EMS systems may be municipal "third-service" entities that do not fall directly under fire or police organization but may be interconnected with these agencies under a larger public safety institutional structure. Public EMS systems are generally funded through a combination of local taxes, user fees, and patient insurance.

Private EMS systems may be hospital based, locally owned, or subsidiaries of a large national corporation. Depending on the community, these organizations may provide interfacility transfers, as well as respond to local 911 calls. In some areas, private firms constitute the designated first or second responder for all calls and also provide routine transport of nonemergency patients (e.g., scheduled patient trips to dialysis or rehabilitation facilities). Financing generally depends on individual patient insurance and user fees, with occasional government subsidies. Hospital-based systems may be based out of one hospital or a larger hospital organization. If they are under the control of a state or county-run hospital, they may operate under public authority in concert with other safety agencies.

Public-private hybrids are quite common. A local government may contract with one or both types of EMS systems for fulfillment of specified emergency services in a particular region. For example, fire department personnel may be the designated first responders for all 911 calls, but a private or public ambulance may transport all patients from the scene to the hospital. Financing may involve direct patient billing, reimbursement from local government, or a designated fee for services.

### RURAL AND URBAN EMS SYSTEMS

The design of and challenges faced by EMS systems are often significantly different between rural and urban areas. In general, rural systems developed later than urban ones and are more likely to be staffed with unpaid volunteers.[3] These volunteer-based organizations may be public or private and are generally nonprofit entities. Volunteers are usually citizens with outside employment who offer their services on an unpaid basis for emergency response, training, and community education. Funding is largely through taxes and municipal support, although private donations and fund-raising are often necessary. Volunteer EMS systems face many challenges that are representative of rural systems as a whole, namely, high cost to cover large geographic areas with few citizens, high response times, lower levels of training, and relatively low patient volumes.[10,11] Urban EMS systems have their own distinct set of difficulties, among them high patient volumes, traffic congestion, and limited resources.

Evidence suggests that rural emergency morbidity and mortality is significantly greater than that for comparable urban patients. Reasons for this difference include longer response and scene times, lower patient volumes, and less overall training for first responders.[12-15] Technologic advances such as "E911" (enhanced 911) show some promise in significantly reducing emergency responders' transport time to the scene.[16] Adapting specific on-scene protocols and increasing access to high-quality medical care (prehospital and in-hospital) in rural areas have also been suggested as possibilities to decrease the gap in rural-urban adverse outcomes.[15]

### SINGLE-TIERED AND MULTITIERED SYSTEMS

EMS systems are further divided by hierarchic types. In single-tiered systems, all dispatched calls are serviced by a single level of first responder and vehicle. In contrast, multitiered systems have variable types and levels of personnel, equipment, and vehicles available for response. A typical multitiered model includes both "first responders"—police or fire department personnel who are strategically geographically located throughout the area—and a second-tier response of more skilled paramedics and EMS personnel. First responders generally have limited training in BLS techniques such as lifesaving airway maneuvers, hemorrhage control efforts, and cardiopulmonary resuscitation (CPR). The second-tier response can usually provide advanced emergency techniques and transport to the hospital.

In addition to the basic first-response, advanced transport system just described, other multitiered EMS designs may be used. Examples include police or fire first response with private ambulance transport, ground first response with air transport, BLS transport with an ALS intercept vehicle as needed, and separate ALS response and transport vehicles. All systems are designed, in theory, to minimize EMS response, scene, and transport time while providing the highest possible quality of patient care.

## EMS SYSTEM ORGANIZATION, TRAINING, AND TRANSPORT TYPES

### DISPATCH AND MEDICAL CONTROL

In the United States, 99% of the population has access to 911 for emergency calls.[7] Most dispatch centers use E911, a system whereby the caller's location is shown on the dispatch operator's screen. Formal training for 911 dispatch personnel exists, and national guidelines that advocate for certification standards have been established.[17] There is a trend toward consolidation of all emergency calls into one 911 center, where dispatchers take calls and then directly relay information to the appropriate EMS or public safety agency. Dispatch actions and instructions may be shaped by established guidelines that allow adaptation to the situation at hand or by more rigid protocols that detail a specific plan of action. Some agencies may rely on computerized algorithms to assist dispatch; a controlled trial of British nonurgent emergency calls found that using a computerized decision tool plus either nurse or paramedic input resulted in more than half the calls triaged as not needing an emergency ambulance. However, only 20% of these callers chose to cancel the ambulance, and this group had similar hospital admission rates as those triaged as needing emergency transport.[18]

EMS systems rely heavily on both online (direct) and off-line (indirect) medical control. Physician involvement in EMS medical control developed as physicians spent less time directly in the field and paramedics increased their training and ability to act as physician surrogates. Every EMS system is headed by a medical director, a physician with or without specialty training who has direct authority over operation of the system, performance of emergency personnel, and patient care. Standardized guidelines and requirements for EMS medical direction have been published by the American College of Emergency Physicians (ACEP).[19,20]

Online medical direction involves direct communication about patient care between on-scene emergency responders and the EMS medical director or a designated representative. Depending on the region, online medical control may be provided by a single centralized facility (base station) such that all calls requiring medical control—regardless of their destination—are handled by one institution. In other areas, each receiving hospital may have its own medical control and handle calls specifically directed toward that facility. The personnel responsible for direct medical control must be knowledgeable about specific protocols or regional system capabilities to provide accurate information about patient care in the field and appropriate transport.

The evidence basis for improved patient outcomes with online medical control is mixed. It has been shown to significantly increase on-scene time, and orders given rarely deviate from existing protocols.[21-23] However, there is some evidence that online medical direction may decrease the use of inappropriate resources while preserving outcomes in some patients.[24] The greatest benefits of online direction may be in resolving difficult ethical or medicolegal situations on scene and in notifying receiving hospitals of incoming critical patients so that resources can be assembled and are ready before arrival of the patient.

Off-line medical direction refers to written protocols that guide common patient interactions, as well as continuing education and quality assurance initiatives. EMS systems have specific protocols for commonly encountered situations that, ideally, should improve patient outcomes and reduce time at the scene. Protocols should be developed on the basis of patient history, mechanism of injury, physiologic characteristics, local hospital capability, and transport times. Medical directors should be active in developing and implementing protocols, as well as in training responders in their application and quality evaluation of patient records.[25] Research indicates that use of well-developed standing protocols significantly reduces on-scene time and decreases inappropriate treatment in the field.[26] Furthermore, diagnostic accuracy plus agreement with physician assessment of patients is generally high.[27]

### EMS RESPONDER PERSONNEL

Before the National Academy of Sciences paper on trauma in the 1960s, few standardized training programs existed for EMS personnel. Subsequent creation of the Department of Transportation resulted in a formalized 70-hour curriculum for basic EMT certification. Passage of the EMS Systems Act of 1973 provided millions of dollars for EMS training, equipment, and research and identified basic elements that must be included in all EMS systems (**Fig. 215.1**).[28] However, until recently, heterogeneity of regional systems persisted such that a 1996 survey identified more than 40 different types of EMS personnel certification across the country.[29]

In general, EMS personnel are categorized into four skill levels: first responders, EMT-basic (EMT-B), EMT-intermediate (EMT-I), and EMT-paramedic (EMT-P). First responders undergo roughly 50 hours of training in basic first aid, CPR, uncomplicated obstetric delivery, simple wound and fracture care, and use of automated external defibrillators (AEDs). EMT-B personnel receive first-responder training plus an additional 50 to 60 hours of education in triage, extrication, transfer, oxygen and self-medication assistance, and possibly advanced airway techniques. Most U.S. ambulances are staffed with at least one EMT-B. EMT-I requirements often vary by state but generally include intravenous access and monitoring and possibly advanced airway and life support measures. EMT-Ps undergo EMT-B training plus at least 250 to 500 additional hours of education, including in-hospital experience. They are skilled in advanced airway and life support techniques, vascular access, monitoring, and administration of medication per local protocols.

Recognition of the wide regional variation in training standards and skill levels led to development of the National Highway Traffic Safety Administration National EMS Scope of Practice Model in 2005. This consensus document promotes national standardization in training and education to improve consistency within and among agencies, increase public understanding of EMS roles, and move toward a coordinated national EMS system.[9] The model advocates four separate and sequential levels of certification—emergency medical responder, EMT, advanced EMT, and paramedic—and clearly defines minimum educational levels and skill sets for each. Most states have already implemented or are in the process of testing these national guidelines for local use.

There is some evidence basis for the current multilevel EMS personnel system. Early EMS research found a significant reduction in mortality from cardiac arrest with the use of paramedic responder crews versus EMT-Bs.[30,31] Outcomes in trauma have also been shown to improve significantly when ALS-capable ambulances are on scene as compared with BLS personnel.[32,33] However, other studies evaluating paramedic- and non–paramedic-containing crews found mixed results. In general, on-scene time is significantly longer for crews in which one or all of the responders are paramedics.[34,35] Paramedic crews had higher skill levels and provided more on-scene interventions, but some authors suggest that their presence on every ambulance may not be warranted.[36]

## EMS VEHICLES, EQUIPMENT, AND TYPES OF TRANSPORT

Equipment available on emergency transport vehicles varies by both type of vehicle and the skill level of responder personnel on board. Joint guidelines developed by the ACEP and the American College of Surgeons detail the minimum necessary supplies for appropriate patient care.[36] Items needed for basic-level interventions include ventilation and airway equipment, monitors and defibrillators, immobilization devices and bandages, mobile communication devices, obstetric and pediatric specialty equipment, and infection control and injury prevention measures. Ambulances with advanced life support

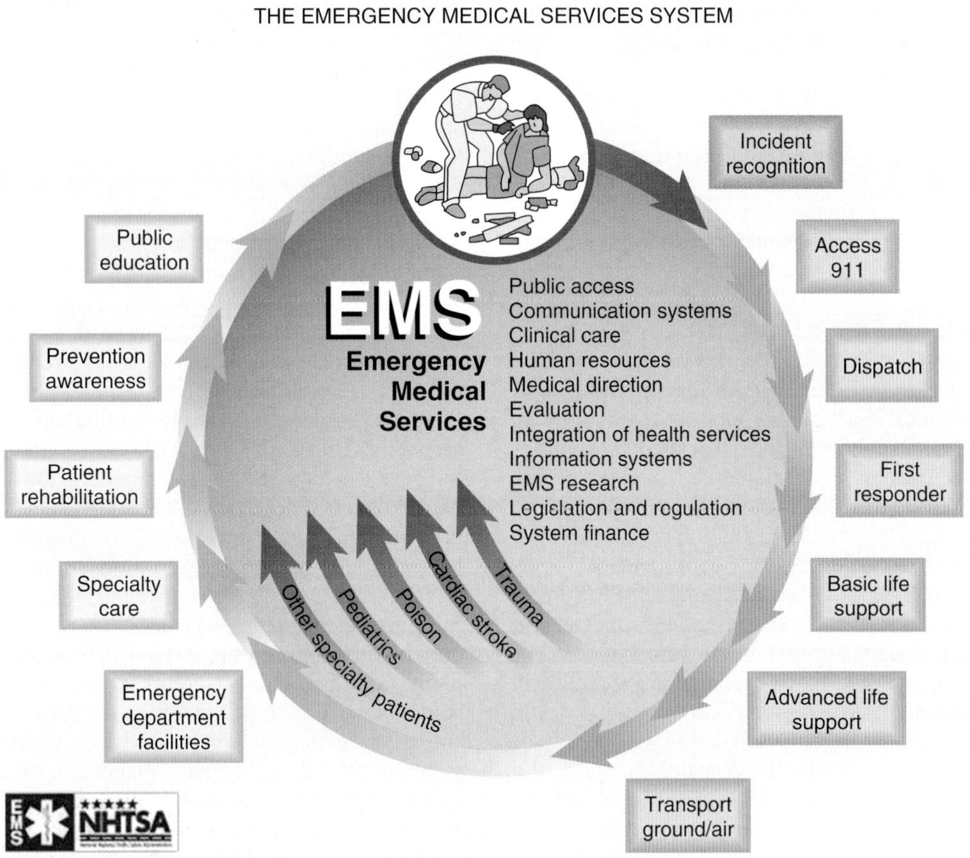

THE EMERGENCY MEDICAL SERVICES SYSTEM

Incident recognition
Access 911
Dispatch
First responder
Basic life support
Advanced life support
Transport ground/air
Emergency department facilities
Specialty care
Patient rehabilitation
Prevention awareness
Public education

EMS
Emergency Medical Services

Public access
Communication systems
Clinical care
Human resources
Medical direction
Evaluation
Integration of health services
Information systems
EMS research
Legislation and regulation
System finance

Trauma
Cardiac stroke
Poison
Pediatrics
Other specialty patients

NHTSA

**Fig. 215.1 Functions and personnel of emergency medical services.**

capability (EMT-I or EMT-P) should contain all the aforementioned basic equipment plus vascular access material, advanced airway and ventilation tools, advanced cardiac life support and other protocol-driven medications, more sophisticated monitoring, and advanced diagnostic equipment (e.g., glucometer, pulse oximeter). In addition, all vehicles should have some measure of extrication equipment for use in patient rescue.

## AIR MEDICINE TRANSPORT

Although a full description of air ambulance systems is beyond the scope of this chapter, this method of transportation plays a crucial role in the transport and transfer of critically ill patients. Ground emergency transport remains the mainstay of prehospital transport and transfer; however, air medical services can have a significant impact on patient care in selected conditions.[37,38] The benefits of air ambulance transport are largely attributed to increased speed and higher crew skill levels; however, safety, cost, and limited evidence to support improved outcomes are major concerns.

The literature on selected prehospital air transport focuses largely on trauma patients and presents mixed evidence for its use. Retrospective evaluations of trauma patients have shown a significant decrease in mortality with helicopter transport[39,40]; however, several studies have found no difference in patient outcomes for both trauma and nontrauma conditions[36-38] and that air transport is overused and costly.[40-44] Criteria for air transport can vary widely by EMS system, and overtriaging is common.[45]

The National Association of EMS Physicians has published guidelines regarding the use of various methods of air transport, as well as which patients are most likely to benefit from its use. In general, helicopters are best used for transport involving a shorter distance (less than 100 miles) but are subject to weather concerns. Fixed-wing aircraft are preferable for distances greater than 100 miles and are less dependent on inclement weather, but they must land at airports (thereby prolonging transport time). Severely injured trauma patients at some distance from a regional trauma center are most likely to benefit from air transport or transfer; critically ill nontrauma, cardiac, pediatric, and possibly obstetric patients may also have improved outcomes in selected situations.[46]

The safety of both patients and medical staff is a prominent issue in air medical transport. As the number of flights has increased in recent years, so has the number of aircraft accidents. Between 2002 and 2005, 55 crashes occurred and resulted in 54 fatalities; the incidence of aircraft accidents per number of flights increased as well.[47] Patient safety in flight is also of concern; an estimated 5% of patients suffer a "critical event" (decompensation or deterioration) during transport.[45] Factors such as weather, time of the day, terrain, communication difficulties, and medical crew training have been found to be associated with adverse events, but more study is needed to improve air transport safety.

## CURRENT CONTROVERSIES IN EMS

Research on the influence of EMS systems on patient outcome is a growing field. Ideally, well-designed studies should investigate the impact of EMS system design, training, personnel, and operation on community needs and patient outcomes. Most studies to date have focused on several broad topics: cardiovascular emergencies, prehospital interventions, trauma, and response times.

### CARDIOVASCULAR EMERGENCIES

Some of the earliest organized EMS research focused on cardiac arrest and early CPR and defibrillation. A 20-year review of EMS systems in 29 cities found that systems with a single emergency responder were associated with lower rates of survival of patients in cardiac arrest than were two-responder (EMT and paramedic) systems, largely because of early CPR in the latter.[48] Time to defibrillation has consistently been found to improve outcomes after cardiac arrest.[49,50] A 25-year retrospective review of cardiac arrest with EMS intervention found that survival rates remained unchanged; however, the authors suggested that improvements in EMS delivery, such as dispatcher-assisted bystander CPR and early defibrillation, balanced the adverse temporal trends that would otherwise have increased mortality rates.[51] New life support guidelines emphasize the role of EMS dispatch in instructing hands-only CPR to bystanders and widespread use of AEDs, both of which are considered to be an important adjunct to trained EMS response.[52,53]

### PREHOSPITAL RESUSCITATIVE INTERVENTIONS

Advanced resuscitative techniques, such as endotracheal intubation and intravenous fluid administration, are frequently performed by skilled paramedics on critically ill patients. Common thinking has been that earlier intervention should improve outcomes; however, solid evidence supporting prehospital intubation is lacking. Although studies are most frequently observational, the literature available suggests that EMS intubation does not improve morbidity and mortality and may in some cases worsen patient outcomes.[47,54] Similarly, a recent large multicenter study found that prehospital intravenous fluid administration was associated with increased mortality in nearly all subsets of trauma patients, particularly those with penetrating trauma, hypotension, and severe head injury.[55] This evidence indicates that a "less is more" or "scoop and run" approach to EMS transport may be safer for patients.

### TRAUMA

Much research on EMS response to trauma focuses on response times and the perceived benefit of "regionalization" of trauma care—that is, linking prehospital systems with participating hospitals, public health agencies, and other care providers within a certain region to achieve optimal system efficiency and outcomes.[56] Regional systems generally have specific protocols governing EMS responder actions and transport to specialized trauma centers when appropriate. Even though patients transported directly to designated trauma centers in lieu of the closest facility have more critical injuries, mortality generally remains low, largely because of decreased prehospital time until direct transfer to the specialty hospital.[57]

Despite the advantages of regionalization, the effect of EMS transport to a trauma center may not always be significant. Some evidence suggests that critically ill patients transported to a trauma center by EMS arrive at the hospital significantly faster than did patients in private vehicles but have no significant improvement in mortality rates, complications, or length of stay.[58]

### RESPONSE TIME

EMS response time is often used as a benchmark of overall system performance, with accepted standards of 4 minutes for BLS and 8 minutes for ALS arrival.[59] Specifically, national guidelines recommend medical intervention within 4 to 6 minutes of EMS activation for patients in cardiac or respiratory arrest, although such intervention may include dispatcher-assisted bystander CPR or AED use.[60] Studies of set response time criteria have shown mixed results. Retrospective and post hoc analyses of urban EMS transport show a possible survival benefit for patients transported to hospitals in 4 minutes or less, although the advantage was not significant for those not in cardiac arrest.[59,61] E911 systems—in which caller location is available instantly—can decrease response times because they help plan more direct routes to the scene and reduce the likelihood of ambulance crews becoming lost.[16] Furthermore, response times should be targeted to specific regional needs and may be maximized by a strong community-wide first-responder presence, strategic placement of ambulances based on historical call data, mobile mapping or global positioning systems, and adequate fleet maintenance.[5,61]

From their earliest beginnings as purely military organizations to the complex heterogeneous models in place today, EMS systems have evolved into critical providers of health care and a critical component of modern emergency medicine. In 2010, EMS was approved by the American Board of Medical Specialties as the sixth subspecialty of emergency medicine, with development of standard examination and certification procedures underway. This further solidifies EMS as a distinct clinical subspecialty involving the prehospital care of sick and injured patients, regardless of specific local or regional system design.

## DISASTER MEDICINE

### INTRODUCTION AND HISTORY

Disaster medicine can be defined as "a sudden and extraordinary misfortune that overwhelms the immediate ability to manage or compensate."[2] Increasing attention has been focused on this nascent medical specialty in recent years with such high-profile disasters as the September 11, 2001, terrorist attacks and severe natural disasters such as hurricanes, earthquakes, and tsunamis. With each successive disaster and its medical and public health response, more is learned and planning can be refined for the next event.

Although the existence of apathy toward disaster planning (and resource allocation toward this end) is well documented,[62,63] major and minor disasters occur with regular and increasing frequency. In the past hundred years, millions of lives have been lost internationally from natural disasters. In 2005, Hurricane Katrina–related flooding was responsible for more than 1500 fatalities along the U.S. Gulf Coast. Worldwide, flooding of the Yangtze River in China caused 3 million casualties in 1931, deaths from the Indian Ocean tsunami in 2004 approached 300,000, and the devastating 2010 Haiti earthquake killed more than 230,000 and displaced up to an additional 2 million. Over the years, earthquakes, landslides, volcano eruptions, and massive fires have resulted in staggering economic losses, population displacement, disease, and death. Research suggests that losses from natural disasters are probably only going to rise because of growing population density (particularly in high-risk areas) and increased hazards as a result of rapidly expanding technology (i.e., transportation of more dangerous materials, fire threats in high-rise buildings, vulnerable financial and economic infrastructure).[62]

Despite the clear threats from natural disasters, much of the focus of disaster medicine in recent years has been placed on intentional, man-made events—namely, terrorism and mass casualty incidents. Even before the devastating terrorist attacks on New York City in 2001, researchers predicted that the probability of exactly such an event was extremely high.[64] Despite performing a mass casualty drill just 3 days before September 11, none of the existing protocols or triage systems proved adequate for the resulting event.[65] Subsequent creation of the Department of Homeland Security (DHS) has provided federal agency support for and focus on expanded research into and development of all aspects of disaster planning for man-made incidents.

## DEFINITIONS AND CLASSIFICATIONS

In general, disasters are classified by their relationship to the hospital setting, inciting event (natural or man-made), and the anticipated necessary response. Internal events occur solely within a particular hospital or medical center (e.g., power outage, building collapse), whereas external events involve some part of the larger community. This system is most useful in preparing the facility to either receive patients from outside or deal with internal problems; however, many disasters have both internal and external effects, and such a narrow classification scheme is not easily applicable to a variety of situations. In terms of anticipated response, most disasters are classified into one of three categories. Level I disasters are those in which local emergency response teams and organizations are adequate to manage the event alone. Level II incidents require a regional approach and mutual aid from surrounding areas. Level III events overwhelm local and regional efforts and require state or federal support.[63]

## DISASTER PLANNING

Although The Joint Commission (TJC) requires all health care facilities to conduct two disaster drills per year, disaster planning is rarely emphasized or sufficient. Many factors contribute to the inadequacy of most hospital or regional disaster plans, namely, the unexpected and sudden nature of most events (thus making prospective evaluation impossible), poor record keeping, faulty assumptions on which significant parts of the plan are based, and failure of communication and command structures.[66] For disaster plans to be effective, they must be based on valid assumptions of what may occur in a variety of event settings. Furthermore, the planning process must include all systems and organizations that will be affected by the disaster and have a role in its aftermath, and all parties must have a working knowledge of the plan, the chain of command, and their role in it.[62]

Critical to the development of an appropriate plan is a hazards analysis of particular events to which a hospital or region is most susceptible. In this manner, organizations can plan effectively for the types of disasters that they are most likely to experience. A standard tool for evaluating hospitals' disaster plans is available through the Agency for Healthcare Research and Quality.[67] Frequent rehearsals of disaster plans are of utmost importance. A written plan is useless unless it is thoroughly understood and practiced by all parties involved.[62] Rehearsals should be varied and include single-agency drills, tabletop exercises with participating community organizations, functional experiences with state and local emergency operations centers, and a full-scale interagency real-time drill. The latter should be as realistic as possible, with mock patients, evolving scenarios, and full community-wide participation. Equally important to any disaster plan is the "afteraction"—discussion of the drill or real-life event with a focus on identification and rectification of problems and appropriate refinement of the plan.[68]

A good disaster plan should cover both internal agency and external community needs and focus on all phases of the inciting event: prodrome/mitigation, impact, rescue, and recovery.[2,63] Interhospital plans should involve all departments responsible for patient care and infrastructure and detail clear policies related to the chain of command and physical control centers, communication and public relations, record keeping, personnel needs, and equipment and resource supply. External planning should involve all local agencies responsible for protection and care of citizens. The Incident Command Structure (ICS) provides a means to delineate a clear chain of command and management structure during critical events. Developed after a series of devastating California wildfires in the 1970s, this model provides for an overall incident commander of any disaster event who oversees predesignated public relations, logistics, finance, supply, and organizational section chiefs. Each section has a variety of personnel with specific duties and areas of focus who report to the chiefs at regular intervals. The ICS is frequently revised and is designed to be flexible, predictable, and accountable, with improved documentation, common language, and cost efficiency.[69]

## DISASTER RESPONSE

Response to a catastrophic event requires rapid mobilization and efficient use of available resources. Clear and defined roles should be established for prehospital providers, health care facilities, and all levels of governmental agencies involved in public safety and welfare. The usual standard of medical care may not be possible or desirable in the acute postdisaster period, and alterations in practice will probably be necessary, within accepted boundaries.[70]

### *Prehospital Disaster Response and Triage*

Though fully capable of responding to individual emergency calls, most local EMS systems are often not able to respond adequately to a widespread or overwhelming event.[71] The concept of prehospital triage, used routinely by EMS, is of utmost importance in managing disasters. Unlike routine triage—where the aim is to identify those few critically ill patients who require immediate, aggressive resource utilization—disaster triage attempts to "do the most good for the most people" and often requires that seriously injured

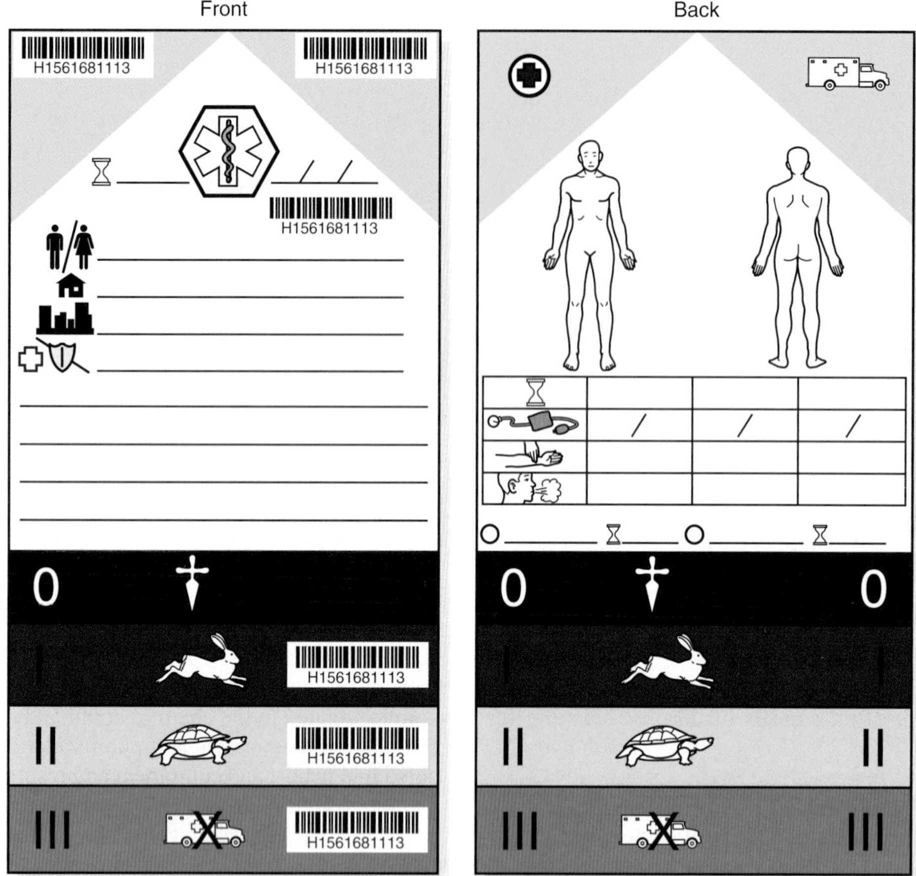


**Fig. 215.2** Example of a simple disaster triage tag.

victims receive little to no immediate care. Disaster triage models attempt to rapidly identify individuals who will benefit most from immediate stabilization with the least amount of available resources.

The simplest method of triage assigns each patient a color-coded tag with frequent opportunities for reassessment (**Fig. 215.2**). Green tags are given to patients who require minor, nonimmediate medical intervention. Yellow tags indicate potentially serious injuries, but ones that are relatively stable and can wait a short period. Red tags designate patients who have life-threatening, but potentially treatable injuries that require immediate medical care. Black tags signify dead or critically ill patients who will not survive without significant use of resources and time unavailable under disaster conditions. For example, an apneic victim of a large-scale blast injury with significant head and abdominal injuries may be tagged "black" because the immediate resuscitative and stabilization needs of the victim would require an inordinate use of personnel and equipment given the number of victims and likelihood of a meaningful outcome.

Tag systems are combined with triage models to provide specific algorithms for classification of patients. Widely used in the United States, the START (Simple Triage and Rapid Assessment) system triages mass casualty patients by several simple variables: breathing, ambulation, radial pulse, and ability to follow commands (**Fig. 215.3**). Patients are categorized as "green" if they are initially ambulatory with minor injuries. "Yellow" victims are those who may be unable to walk but are breathing with respiratory rates lower than 30 breaths/min, are well perfused (capillary refill longer than 2 seconds), and can follow simple commands. Patients with respiratory rates higher than 30 (with or without airway positioning), delayed capillary refill, or inability to follow simple commands are tagged as "red," and the need for immediate lifesaving attention is assessed. Apneic patients are tagged as "black," and no further interventions are performed. Refinement of this model has led to specific, but still simple modifications for pediatric patients.[72]

The SAVE (Secondary Assessment of Victim Endpoint) model was developed as an adjunct to the START system. After primary assessment with START, secondary triage is performed with SAVE to assess the following: prognosis if only minimal treatment is performed and prognosis with just the available resources on site or at the disaster medical aid center. Patients are sent to a treatment area only if treatment will reduce morbidity or mortality within the delayed time to definitive care without consuming a disproportionate amount of resources.[73] The SAVE protocol provides specific guidelines based on age, injury location (head, extremity, spine, chest, and abdomen), and type of injury (burns, crush injuries, blunt or penetrating trauma) and suggests treatment priorities in order of likelihood of success (**Box 215.1**).

The START system has been shown to have high sensitivity, be quick to administer, and easily be taught to first

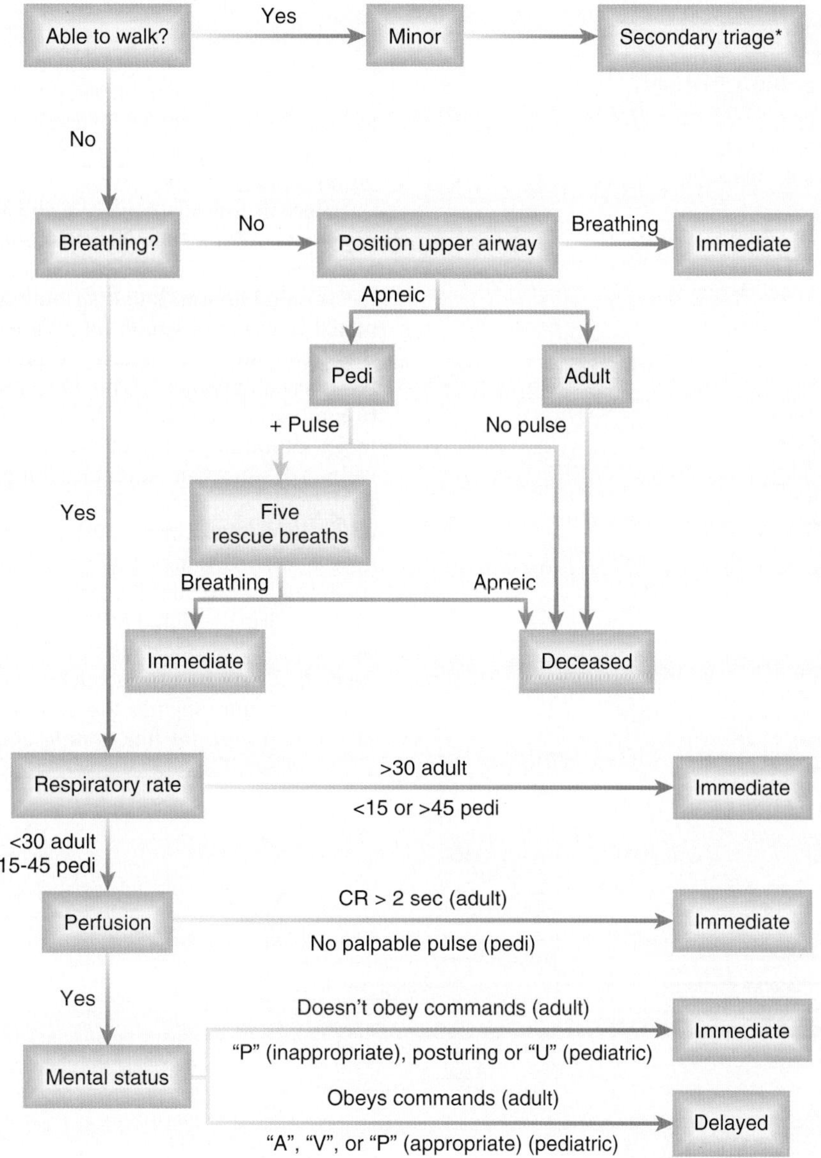


**Fig. 215.3 Combined START (Simple Triage and Rapid Treatment)/JumpSTART triage algorithm.** *When using the JumpSTART algorithm, first evaluate all children who did not walk under their own power. *A*, Alert; *CR*, capillary refill time (seconds); *Delayed*, treatment may be delayed for hours to days; *Immediate*, requires immediate lifesaving treatment; *JS*, JumpSTART; *P*, pain; *Pedi*, pediatric (patient); *U*, unresponsive; *V*, voice.

responders.[74,75] However, real-time use of the START system during the terrorist attacks in New York City in 2001 proved ineffective. Because of the dynamic nature of the event, the loss of communications, and the fact that rescue personnel were in personal danger, the START system was abandoned.[65] International triage systems (Careflight, Triage Save, and Sort) are comparable with START in prediction of critical injury,[76] but currently no national triage guideline exists. The SALT (**s**ort, **a**ssess, **l**ifesaving intervention, **t**reatment/**t**ransport) model was developed by a multidisciplinary panel of disaster experts to provide such a national standard.[74] This model includes anatomic and physiologic considerations, as well as assessment of available resources (**Fig. 215.4**).

## Hospital and Agency Disaster Response

With proper triage and communication, the prehospital disaster response can successfully reduce the burden of any mass incident on receiving health care facilities.[66,77] TJC requirements necessitate that hospitals prepare for both internal and external events; these plans should easily be integrated in the event of a combined internal and external disaster. Internal and external events may involve different roles for emergency department (ED) staff. In an internal disaster, the ED's main focus is generally to treat individuals within the institution who may be injured, with actual management and control of the situation being left to other in-hospital departments

**BOX 215.1 Secondary Assessment of Victim Endpoint Protocol Treatment Priorities (in Descending Order)**

Temporary airway management
Pressure dressings to stop bleeding
Simple pneumothorax
Treatment of shock after control of bleeding
Advanced airway techniques
Limb manipulation for vascular supply
Burns—25% mortality
Chest trauma
Spinal injury
Fasciotomies, amputations
Open wound care, closure
Head injury; GCS score ≥ 8
Abdominal trauma
Head injury; GCS score < 8
Burns—50% mortality
Burns—75% mortality
Head injury; GCS score 3

From Benson M, Koenig KL, Schultz CH. Disaster triage: START, then SAVE—a new method of dynamic triage for victims of a catastrophic earthquake. Prehosp Disaster Med 1996;11:117-24.
GCS, Glasgow Coma Scale.

according to the institution's incident command protocol. The possibility of ED evacuation should be part of any hospital plan and be well thought out and rehearsed for maximum speed and safety. In an internal disaster, resources and outside aid should be sufficient for patient care and evacuation such that critically ill patients can be treated or evacuated (or both) with highest priority.

External disasters usually result in sudden and often overwhelming volumes of patients at one or more local health care facilities. Ideally, controlled prehospital triage should result in even and appropriate distribution of patients to local hospitals; however, research on a variety of disasters has shown that frequently, the majority of patients do not arrive at hospitals via ambulance.[66] This fact can cause significant disruption of carefully planned dispersion of resources and lead to rapid saturation of the closest or most familiar facilities, as well as difficulty in patient tracking and timely hospital notification. Hospitals should be prepared for significant communication breakdown, restricted access, limited outside help, mass influx of victims with a variety of injuries, and personnel limitations. For example, hospitals in the flood zone of Hurricane Katrina suffered prolonged austere conditions because of protracted physical inaccessibility, primitive communications, and lack of timely outside aid. Other prolonged mass casualty events, such as the 2009 H1N1 influenza pandemic, affect both hospital functioning and the community at large

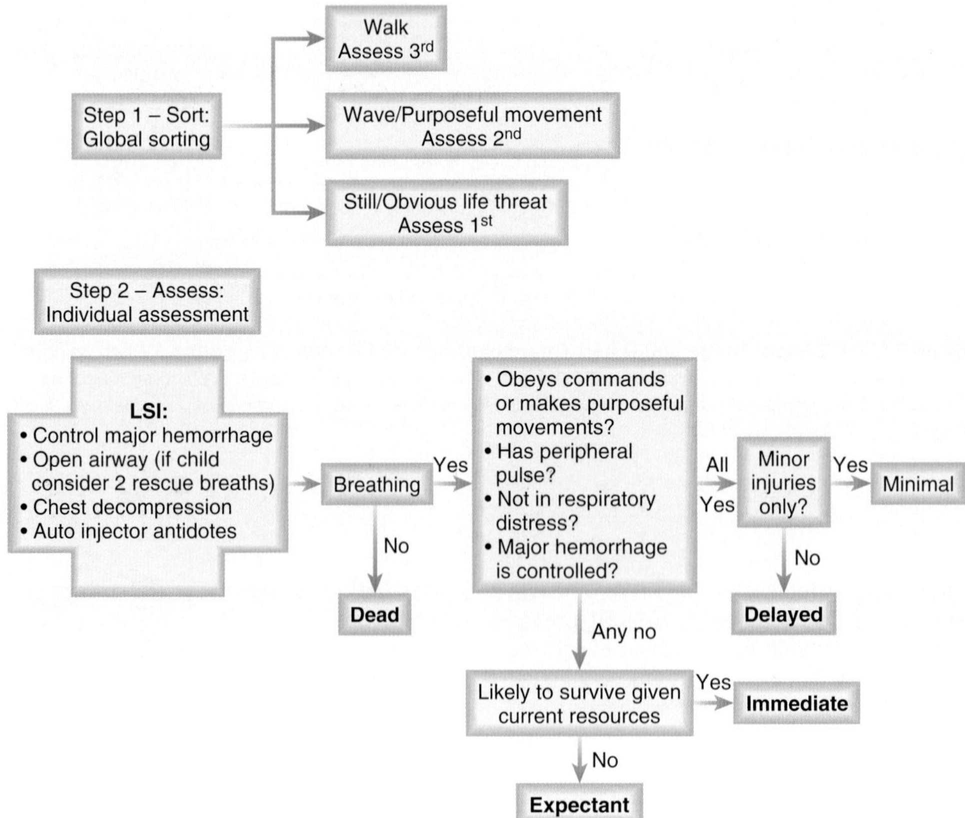


**Fig. 215.4 Proposed SALT (*s*ort, *a*ssess, *l*ifesaving *i*ntervention, *t*reatment/*t*ransport) mass casualty incident national triage guidelines.** (Adapted from Lerner EB, Schwartz RB, Coule PL, et al. Mass casualty triage: an evaluation of the data and development of a proposed national guideline. Disast Med Public Health Prep 2008;2(Suppl 1):S25-34. Available at http://www.dmphp.org/content/vol2/Supplement_1/images/medium/7FF1.gif).

and create chronic resource shortages both internally and externally.

When local and regional resources are overwhelmed in a disaster, national governmental and private agencies may be needed for assistance. The largest and most important source of aid comes from the federal government through the DHS. This department was founded after the 2001 terrorist attacks on New York City and combined many different government agencies that were responsible in some way for public health or safety. The Emergency Preparedness and Response subdirectorate of the DHS combined the Federal Emergency Management Agency (FEMA) and the National Disaster Medical Service (NDMS), as well as the Federal Bureau of Investigation, Energy, and Justice Department agencies, to oversee federal disaster response and training. FEMA has several thousand full-time and reserve employees who are responsible for planning and coordinating a federal response to disaster, as well as on-scene deployment of resources. NDMS provides medical assistance to disaster areas in the form of volunteer health care personnel, resources and infrastructure for delivery of care, veterinary and mortuary teams, and preevent training of first responders. Nongovernmental organizations such as the Red Cross (and, internationally, the United Nations) often partner with federal agencies to coordinate response and allocation of resources after catastrophes.

Although FEMA search-and-rescue teams are ideally deployed within 6 hours after declaration of a disaster and can provide basic scene and patient stabilization, federal resources are often delayed for several days. Evidence suggests that local response to disasters has the most lifesaving potential because outside aid generally arrives too late for meaningful immediate medical care.[78]

## WEAPONS OF MASS DESTRUCTION AND HAZARDOUS MATERIALS

Traditional disaster medicine developed mainly in response to natural events such as floods, earthquakes, tornadoes, and other disasters. However, increasing sophistication and spread of man-made disasters in recent years have brought these types of catastrophic incidents to the forefront of focus and research. Potential agents available to terrorists include chemical, biologic, nuclear, radiologic, and explosive devices (generally referred to as weapons of mass destruction [WMD]); although the overall likelihood of an attack is low, the consequences may be cataclysmic. One gram of botulin toxin has the potential to kill 1 million people,[79] and the effects of nuclear and radioactive agents can reach across continents. The response to WMD events may differ significantly from the traditional disaster models described earlier, with shifting priority on decontamination, agent-specific triage, and special resources and personnel.

Preparing for biologic and chemical attacks is difficult and must be adaptive. Disease surveillance programs that link a community are essential for detection and prompt response because biologic agents may not be detected for days to weeks.[80,81] Predisaster emphasis should be on hazard analysis, as well as training and stockpiling of antidotes for the most likely agents to be used. The Strategic National Stockpile is a national reserve of medical supplies, antidotes, and medications managed by the Centers for Disease Control and Prevention and strategically placed in states for rapid availability following a mass casualty event.

In both biologic and chemical attacks, early evacuation and containment of the "hot zone" (the area of maximum contamination) is critical to mitigate injuries and spread. The hot zone should have a clear and strict entry and exit, separate "clean" and "dirty" areas, and continuous monitoring. Primary emphasis should be given to decontamination and safety of first-responder personnel, not only to ensure a strong medical response but also to limit unintentional dissemination of the contaminant. Accurate risk assessments should be communicated to the public and updated frequently.

Traditionally, preparation for WMD has used the more common hazardous materials (HAZMAT) exposure training methods. These models may not, however, be appropriate.[64,82] HAZMAT events assume an exposure away from health care facilities, where response teams with maximum personal protection and extensive decontamination equipment work to rescue and decontaminate small numbers of victims. Large-scale exposure to WMD may encompass public areas and health care facilities, thereby compromising response efforts and calling into question the traditional decontamination methods.[83] For example, in the 1995 Japanese subway nerve gas attacks, several thousand people were potentially exposed, yet fewer than 100 were killed or seriously injured. However, thousands arrived at hospitals by private vehicle without on-scene decontamination, which quickly overwhelmed the facilities and potentially exposed scores of essential medical personnel.[80]

## THE ROLE OF EMERGENCY PHYSICIANS IN DISASTER MEDICINE

Published ACEP policy advocates a leadership role for emergency physicians in all aspects of disaster research, planning, and implementation.[84] The traditional focus of disaster medicine—to do the most good for the greatest number of people—may seem to be at odds with the traditional emergency medical principles of aggressive resource utilization for selected critically ill patients. However, the emergency physician is generally the best-trained individual to coordinate medical control, supervise triage, connect with other municipal and public health agencies, and oversee direct patient care during a catastrophic event. Several formal disaster medicine fellowships exist for emergency medical physicians, and disaster training is included in the emergency medical residency curriculum. Advances in research and increased global attention to natural and man-made disasters create exciting potential for emergency physicians to lead the development of disaster medicine as a discipline.

## REFERENCES

***References can be found on Expert Consult @ www.expertconsult.com.***

# 216 Patient-Centered Care

*Kevin Klauer and Kirsten G. Engel*

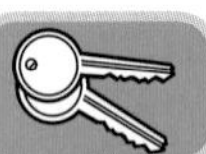

**KEY POINTS**

- Patient-centered care is an approach to patient-provider interactions in which providers work together with patients and their families in an effort to ensure that the patient's personal experience and preferences are an integral part of the care process.
- A patient-centered approach to care confers many benefits in the acute care setting and can be critical in overcoming barriers to the communication process in the emergency department.
- The practice of patient-centered care involves both personal elements that individual providers can integrate into their daily interactions, as well as system-level elements that can be implemented and supported on the departmental and institutional level.

## INTRODUCTION

Patient-centered care (PCC) is an approach to patient-provider interactions that promotes a collaborative partnership among health care providers, patients, and their families. In clinical practice, emphasis is placed on understanding patients and their clinical presentation within the larger context that includes their family, personal views, preferences, values, past experiences, and cultural factors. By embracing each patient as an individual, a patient-centered approach seeks to ensure high-quality care that consistently meets the needs and preferences of patients and their families.

## GOALS

The goals of this chapter are as follows:

1. To review the evolution and core features of PCC and its importance to clinical practice in emergency medicine
2. To discuss practical, realistic approaches and strategies in the following three domains of daily clinical practice, which can facilitate the delivery of PCC:
   a. Personal issues—practice considerations for the individual provider that can promote PCC
   b. Systems issues—practice considerations on a departmental level and from a systems perspective that can promote PCC
   c. Critical issues—practice considerations for special circumstances when PCC can be particularly important

## BACKGROUND

The concept of PCC gained attention with the influential Institute of Medicine reports in 1999 ("To Err Is Human") and 2001 ("Crossing the Quality Chasm"). The first report outlined mechanisms to improve patient safety, including efforts to engage patients in their care and enhance their understanding of their treatment.[1] Two years later, "Crossing the Quality Chasm" identified PCC as one of the six aims intended to improve the quality of health care in our country.[2]

In 2006, the American College of Emergency Physicians (ACEP) and the American Academy of Pediatrics issued a joint policy statement supporting patient and family-centered care as an important means of improving satisfaction, safety, and quality of care for patients and their families.[3]

The emergency department (ED) environment is inherently challenging to the communication process between patients and providers, and a patient-centered approach to care can be particularly valuable in this setting. ED providers routinely confront significant time constraints, unpredicted interruptions, and overcrowding while caring for patients with life-threatening illness and injury.[4-7] Given these circumstances, it is essential that ED providers possess skill in rapidly establishing rapport and engaging patients in critical decision making. A patient-centered approach to care is vital in overcoming barriers to the communication process through an understanding of the many situational and personal factors that characterize a patient's visit to the ED. In many cases, fear, anxiety, and uncertainty, as well as preconceived and often unrealistic expectations, play an important role, and these factors must be recognized and appropriately managed to effectively communicate with patients.[3]

A patient-centered approach to care provides clear benefits to the immediate patient-provider interaction, but it also appears to have a positive impact on important outcomes for the patient and provider. Although research in this area is challenging, early work indicates that PCC improves patient satisfaction and may also enhance adherence and health outcomes.[8-12]

## PERSONAL ISSUES

As individual providers, there are many simple things that we can do every day in the ED during our patient interactions that facilitate the provision of PCC. The following sections highlight practical approaches and strategies that can be realistically incorporated into clinical practice on a daily basis. Our discussion will consider three areas: communication, operational considerations, and humanistic considerations.

## COMMUNICATION

Communication is the process of information exchange and is a central and critical aspect of our care of patients in the ED. As providers, we must solicit and receive information, establish the diagnosis, understand the social situation, and make an appropriate plan for care. In addition, we must provide our patients with information to facilitate understanding of their treatment and diagnosis, improve adherence to instructions, and ensure good outcomes.

Communication has two major components: verbal and nonverbal. These components work together and complement one another, with both having an impact on information exchange.

Verbal communication in our interactions with patients includes several key elements:

1. Introduce yourself, including your name and role.
2. Allow patients to speak and complete their thoughts while avoiding interruptions whenever possible. Be sure that you address all the patient's medical concerns.
3. Use clear, nontechnical language.
4. Give patients the opportunity to ask questions.
5. Review information to confirm patient understanding (i.e., treatment, diagnostics, follow-up, discharge instructions).

Nonverbal communication is just as powerful as verbal communication with respect to its impact on patient-provider interactions. Facial expressions, body language, and physical space or touch are several aspects of nonverbal communication. Although nonverbal communication is more subtle and may seem less vital than verbal communication, it is essential to recognize the importance of nonverbal elements and their role in supporting or undermining the words that we use. This component is particularly critical in our efforts to convey courtesy, compassion, and respect.

Nonverbal communication in our interactions with patients has several key elements:

1. Greet patients and family members with a handshake when appropriate.
2. Make consistent eye contact and commit your complete attention to the interaction.
3. Use calm, compassionate body language.
4. Consider appropriate use of physical touch to provide comfort while being sensitive to cultural issues.
5. Avoid nonverbal cues of discontent.

## OPERATIONAL CONSIDERATIONS

Interactions between providers and patients progress through several important stages of the ED visit. Provision of PCC relies on effective engagement of patients during each of these critical junctures. Although a systems approach to PCC is discussed later in this chapter, some practical considerations for incorporating patient-centered care into daily practice are reviewed here and include examples of appropriate phrases and statements for each stage of the ED visit.

### *Intake*

When a patient first enters the ED, it is critical to engage the patient quickly with effort to minimize time between arrival and the first interaction. Patients often feel anxious or frightened by the ED environment and typically experience distress and frustration because of the event or abrupt change that has prompted the need for their visit. Providers should be sensitive to these feelings by immediately delivering expressions of caring and concern, acknowledging the patient's discomfort and circumstances, and providing reassurance.

"I am sorry to hear about your injury (or that you are not feeling well). We are happy that you are here and will work as quickly as possible to help you feel better."

### *Assessment*

During the initial assessment phase, it is important that patients be given the opportunity to express their concerns and symptoms and to feel that they have been heard. Repeating a brief summary and highlighting patients' key issues can help assure them that their concerns are being given appropriate consideration.

"So, let me make sure that I've heard everything you said about your symptoms. As I understand it, you have had ..."

As the diagnostic and treatment plan is developed, it is also important that this plan be shared with the patient and that there be clarity and agreement about the intended testing strategy, its anticipated duration, and overall expectations for the visit and ultimate disposition. This approach facilitates a collaborative relationship between the provider and patient, which is a key element of patient-centered care.

"In order to better understand what might be causing your symptoms, we are going do a series of tests, including ... This is expected to take ... I will come back and talk to you about the results when I receive them."

### *Waiting and Delays*

In any situation, when a patient needs to wait or experiences a delay in care, it is vital that providers reconnect with the patient and provide explanations and reassurance. Previous research has demonstrated that patients have greater tolerance for these circumstances if they are well informed about the causes and the anticipated duration.[13]

"I know you are waiting, and I want to make sure you know that we have not forgotten about you. We expect that ..."

### *Disposition*

When the evaluation has been completed, and patients are ready for discharge or admission, it is critical that the treatment and management plan be reviewed with them in detail and that they be given the opportunity to ask questions. Using an open-ended statement to elicit questions may help set an expectation that questions are welcome and anticipated.

"What questions do you have?" may be preferable to a more closed approach such as "Do you have any questions?"

## HUMANISTIC CONSIDERATIONS

An additional core element of PCC is the consideration of a patient's illness and signs and symptoms in the larger context of the patient's personal experiences and background. As providers, we are well aware that similar illnesses or conditions can yield diverse reactions and responses in different patients or populations. These differences reflect variation in patients' personal views, cultural beliefs, preferences, values, past experiences, and fears. Provision of PCC means simply that we do not disregard these differences but, instead, actively seek to understand them, embrace them, and incorporate them into our clinical practice and plan of care. We should view each patient as an individual (not a disease process or diagnosis) and recognize that each brings a unique story and circumstance to the ED.

In the real world, these humanistic elements of PCC are often met by important challenges. We discuss these issues here and consider how one can begin to recognize and minimize such barriers to the practice of PCC in a busy ED.

### *Time: Making the Most of What We Have*

All too often, ED providers face time constraints and significant clinical demands that are perceived as obstacles to providing care with a humanistic approach. It seems impossible for us to have the time to explore individual patients' personal experiences, values, or beliefs.

Although it is not easy to create more time during a busy shift, we can make sure to take advantage of the opportunities that we do have and optimize our available resources. During assessment and evaluation in the ED, patients often share thoughts and give small clues that are important to understanding their social situation, motivation, and values. We need to be sure to explore these avenues because this additional information can help us connect with our patients and create a plan that better incorporates their perspectives and needs. This extra effort may prevent the conflict or frustration that will lead to larger, more time-consuming obstacles and challenges. Each of us can surely think of a situation in which we disregarded a patient's expression of anxiety or uncertainty about a plan (e.g., admission to the hospital) that later resulted in a difficult and prolonged interaction (e.g., trying to convince the patient to go upstairs when the bed was ready).

In addition, ED providers need to enlist the support of all available resources, including social workers, nursing staff, and consulting services, to evaluate and support each patient's needs. These interactions can help us better understand our patients and their personal circumstances, even when we are unable to pursue this level of detailed information independently.

Overall, it is important to keep in mind that "technically excellent" patient care (including the "right" diagnosis, correct management plan, and appropriate disposition) is not "the best" patient care unless it reflects some understanding of the patient's personal story.

### *Provider Emotions: Leaving Our Personal Reactions and Feelings at the Door*

As is true for our patients, providers have a history and past personal and professional experiences that can lead to intense emotional responses. When we care for patients, our personal feelings, reactions, and judgments can significantly influence how we interact with patients and families. To provide PCC, it is critical that we learn to acknowledge our feelings, recognize how they are affecting us, and minimize any negative impact that they may have on our patient-provider encounters.

## SYSTEMS ISSUES

Historically, the care provided in most health care settings has been provider centric and focused on flow and outcomes from the provider's perspective. The ED is no exception. Until recently—the last decade and especially in the past few years a patient-centered approach to care was seldom considered in ED operations, and when it was, its weight and priority were often too far down the list to be given serious consideration. However, the tide has turned. Patient satisfaction has been recognized as a driver for hospital market share. Not surprisingly, the topic in patient satisfaction surveys most important to hospital administrations is the likelihood to return or refer others. This focus on patient satisfaction has helped prompt a change in the culture of medicine that has resulted in PCC. Although satisfying our patients to improve hospital market share is important, it is not the only factor influencing this shift in paradigm. The current state of our medical-legal system, compliance with governmental regulations (including pay-for-performance initiatives), and the demand for operational efficiency are all critical stimuli for turning to an approach that is patient centered. Although patient-centered care can be provided on a case-by-case basis, a systems approach is necessary to develop a patient-centered culture.

### PATIENT SATISFACTION

Satisfying patients is at the core of developing a culture that is patient centered. Although many providers will summarily dismiss the value of the patient's perception of the care rendered, this viewpoint is only partially valid and is misguided. Certainly, patients are not qualified to judge the technical adequacy of the medical care provided. However, they are more than qualified to judge whether the system and providers cared about their comfort, communicated their treatment plans, addressed their pain, and informed them about wait times and delays. It should not be a surprise to anyone that these same concepts are represented in almost every commercial and noncommercial patient satisfaction survey tool currently in use.

So, EDs need to be in the business of making patients happy. Those that are not will quickly learn that their competitors are more than happy to do so. The ED is the operational "front door" of most hospitals. In 2008, the National Ambulatory Medical Care Survey, 2006, reported that the ED was the source of 50.2% of all nonobstetric admissions to U.S. hospitals. Furthermore, if an ED is not interested in making a good impression on the community and embracing patient satisfaction as a core competency, many chief executive officers will look for ED staffing solutions that will provide the appropriate emphasis on this important goal. Although individual interactions can be standardized and scripted to improve patients' experience, as discussed previously, operational efficiency goes a long way toward pleasing patients.

Common themes in the literature are that provider interpersonal communication skills, delivery of information and explanations, and perceived wait times most strongly correlate with patient satisfaction. Although actual wait times are less likely to predict satisfaction or a lack thereof, patients with a length of stay of 8 hours are generally less satisfied than their counterparts waiting only 4 hours.[14] Operational efficiency is not only critical to ensuring patient satisfaction but is also a key factor associated with a patient-centered approach to care.

### OPERATIONAL EFFICIENCY

Operational metrics such as overall length of stay, door-to-provider time, provider-to–decision making time, and decision making–to-disposition time are nationally recognized measures of operational efficiency. These metrics should be measured and performance improvement initiatives tailored toward a more efficient experience for the patient.

Operational efficiency not only provides a positive impact on patient satisfaction but also promotes patient safety; both are critical to PCC. In other words, patients are happier when they are seen more quickly and have a shorter length of stay. In addition, when throughput is more efficient, an ED's bed capacity can be used more effectively, more patients can be seen, patients who leave without being seen can be avoided, and the likelihood of deterioration of patients in the waiting room can be reduced. For instance, if the average length of stay for admitted patients is 6 hours in one ED versus 3 hours in another, with both seeing 50,000 patients a year and having 40 ED beds and an admission rate of 50%, 205 patient care hours would be saved in the more efficient ED on a daily basis. Thus, the more efficient ED can see 68 more admitted patients than the less efficient ED. Of course, the operational efficiency of admitted patients is dependent on many factors inside and outside the ED.

A truly patient-centered culture will address ED crowding and ED boarding of admitted patients as a hospital system issue, not an isolated ED issue. We know that boarding often results in inefficient bed management in the hospital and leads to delays in the time that it takes to execute a decision for admission. A policy statement released by the ACEP in January 2011 clarified the definition of boarded patients:

"In order for emergency departments to continue to provide quality patient care and access to that care, ACEP believes a 'boarded patient' is defined as a patient who remains in the emergency department after the patient has been admitted to the facility, but has not been transferred to an inpatient unit."

Furthermore, it has been proved that the heavy demand on ED resources during times of crowding is an impediment to providing high-quality care and compromises patient safety. Although a thorough discussion of throughput metrics is beyond the scope of this chapter, it is important to note the critical nature of these metrics when considering the patient as the primary stakeholder in these processes.

The time from decision making to actual disposition (departure from the ED) may be viewed by many as being beyond the control of the ED, as well as by many institutions that do not view boarding as an institutional issue. However, intake is a process that is solely owned by the ED. Yes, intake processes are adversely affected by boarding and lack of availability of hospital resources, but nimble EDs can create the necessary "work-arounds" to stay patient centric in their approach. Bedside registration is an excellent tool to improve door-to-bed times. Registration is often a non–value-added step, from the patient's perspective, that is frequently placed ahead of patient care. Not only does this have potential Emergency Medical Treatment and Active Labor Act (EMTALA) implications, it also delays the care provided. Because there is often considerable downtime during an ED visit, it is ideal for the registration process to be conducted during these times, not at the critical front-end portion of the visit. Some would argue that care cannot begin until a chart can be generated and ordering in the hospital's information system can begin. This argument holds no water because very little information is actually needed to generate a patient identification capable of initiating care, and this information can be obtained during the triage process.

The shortfall is that bedside registration does not ensure that a provider will get to patients any quicker than if they were in the waiting room. Thus this may not affect the more important metric of door-to-provider (doctor) time. However, placing a provider in triage does. Whether a physician or midlevel provider, placement of a provider at triage with the nurse can initiate the visit without the need for formalized ED bed placement. Furthermore, many low-acuity patients may be discharged directly from triage, after completion of their care, and never need an ED bed. Standing orders may be a bridge to initiate care. However, standing orders are often overly broad in application and result in unnecessary tests being ordered, and they do not take the place of the provider in evaluating and initiating management of the patient.

## MEDICAL-LEGAL FACTORS

The two primary factors associated with filing medical malpractice claims or lawsuits are bad patient outcomes and unhappy patients. Although the relatively frequency of medical malpractice claims is fairly low, with a range of approximately 1 in 25,000 to 40,000 ED encounters, it is difficult to find definitive correlations between patient satisfaction and lawsuits. However, the preponderance of the literature more than strongly suggests that poor patient satisfaction results in more patient complaints. Additional data suggest a strong correlation with patient complaints and risk management events and medical malpractice lawsuits. In one study, a 1-point decrease in patient satisfaction survey results correlated with a 6% increase in the incidence of risk management events (claims, lawsuits, and incident reports). In this same study, 75% of 483 claims were associated with communication errors, thus emphasizing the need for improved communication between patients and providers.[15] Patients who are well informed about their care are less likely to be taken by surprise by changes in their condition, medication side effects, and failure of treatment. To that end, treatment and diagnostic plans should be discussed with patients and their significant others, results should also be discussed with them, therapeutic response to treatments needs to be assessed, and final disposition plans need to be discussed and agreed and comprehension acknowledged and confirmed. Although many busy EDs defer some of these tasks to nursing, it is of vital importance that the physician at least reinforce these communications. However, it is ideal for the physician to be the primary provider to conduct communications with the patient.

Patient handoffs are another aspect of a patient-centered culture that is both an operational and a risk management concern. Up to 24% of medical malpractice claims result from faulty handoffs. Handoffs are transitions in care from one provider to another and often from one care setting to another. To ensure that errors are avoided, the quality of care is not compromised, and patient safety is preserved, a standardized approach should be taken to handoffs in the ED. Recommended steps include a face-to-face encounter by the incoming and outgoing providers, an explanation of the active problem list and any outstanding diagnostics, and the expectations for disposition. In addition, it is useful to advise the patient that the handoff is occurring and even introduce the patient to the incoming provider.[16]

Yet another new focus on PCC that is intertwined with risk management is error disclosure. Disclosing errors is now a patient safety requirement from the Joint Commission. Concealing medical errors is unethical, immoral, and unwise. Furthermore, every hospital must have a policy outlining the requirements for disclosure of medical errors. The decision to disclose should not be based on the severity of the error or the provider's perception of patient impact. If the error occurred, the patient has the right to know that it occurred, regardless of how others value the importance of this information. Such a policy should include notification of the hospital risk manager and ED leadership (i.e., medical director, nurse manager). It is also important to note that disclosure is an excellent risk management tool. Appropriate settlements can be reached, litigation avoided, and indemnity and defense expenses reduced. Moreover, if a medical error is concealed and a lawsuit is filed, the error will invariably be identified through the discovery process. Once it appears that the providers intended to "cover up" the error, there is no viable defense, and no jury in the United States will be sympathetic with defendants who were flagrantly dishonest.

## COMPLIANCE

The federal government has long been interested in PCC. Consider the patient implications with the Civil Rights Act of 1964, the Health Insurance Portability and Accountability Act (HIPAA), and EMTALA. Clearly, the federal government has embarked on many initiatives that are patient centered. The Civil Rights Act requires that any institution accepting federal compensation for rendered care must provide medical interpretive services for limited English-proficient patients. Not doing so is in violation of this statute and may constitute civil rights violations on behalf of the patient. Medical interpreters are not only required to be fluent in the language that they are interpreting but must also have experience in medical interpretation. In other words, finding someone in the hospital who speaks a language (i.e., a Spanish-speaking housekeeper) is not sufficient. It is also important to recognize that the use of family members is not a viable substitute unless the patient refuses formal medical interpretation. If there is a problem, complaint, or bad outcome, the only witness to the interaction between providers and the patient will be the interpreter. It is unwise for that sole witness to be a nonimpartial family member.

HIPAA focuses on the patient's right to due care being given to their protected health information. This information, sensitive to the patient, must be handled in accordance with this statute to protect the patient's privacy. EMTALA requires that all patients who go to the hospital, its "campus," and related buildings with an emergency medical condition have a medical screening examination (MSE) performed, regardless of their ability to pay. The MSE also includes stabilization of any identified emergency medical condition. Thus, through the course of compliance and performing the MSE, the care of most ED patients is completed. Though not a financially viable program for hospitals and emergency medicine, it is certainly a patient-centered initiative that allows access to care for all emergency patients (**Box 216.1**).

Compliance with federally mandated programs is essential for a hospital to maintain an individual provider's Medicare provider number. Without these numbers, participation in federally funded programs such as Medicare and Medicaid is prohibited.

**BOX 216.1 Operational Strategies for Patient-Centered Emergency Care**

Minimize door-to-doctor time.
Initiate diagnostics as soon as possible after arrival (by physician evaluation, provider in triage, or standing orders).
Assess and address pain promptly.
Build processes to notify the physician of returned results and prompt delivery of the results.
Promote diagnostic efficiency (only appropriate testing, obtaining laboratory tests at the time of insertion of an intravenous line).
Make decisions promptly once sufficient data have returned.
Use computerized discharge instructions at the second-grade educational level (language appropriate).
Provide medical interpretive services (also avoids violation of the Civil Rights Act of 1964).
Formalize processes for disclosure of medical errors.
Draft policies for EMTALA compliance.
Draft policies for HIPAA compliance.
Formalize the patient handoff process.
Formalize the approach to and emphasis on patient satisfaction.
Foster a culture of excellent communication.

*EMTALA*, Emergency Medical Treatment and Active Labor Act; *HIPAA*, Health Insurance Portability and Accountability Act.

# CRITICAL ISSUES

## ADVANCED DIRECTIVES

In the ED setting we frequently care for patients with life-threatening illnesses who are faced with important choices regarding their management. As emergency providers we need to develop skill in helping patients and their families understand their disease and prognosis, consider the acute issues that they are confronting, and make choices that reflect their personal priorities and goals. The process of discussing and establishing goals of care is a large and important topic that incorporates many of the core principles of PCC. Advanced directives represent a critical subset of this area that we encounter frequently and often cannot be deferred to a later time.

As we approach a patient and family for a discussion of advanced directives, we should be guided by the fundamental elements of PCC. We must embrace our patients (and their families) as unique entities and consider their personal story and circumstances as we provide clinical information and guidance in their decision making. With this approach we are able to support the patient and family in choosing the best path for them while recognizing that there is no absolute "right" choice or plan.

## FAMILY-WITNESSED RESUSCITATION

Interest in the practice of family-witnessed resuscitation (FWR) began in the 1980s after studies surveying families of survivors of sudden death found that their most frequent criticisms centered on frustrations with inadequate information and updates during resuscitation.[17] Additionally, it was noted that families of critically ill or dying patients often complained about feeling helpless, uninformed, and uninvolved.[18] As a result of these findings and some requests by family members to be present during resuscitation procedures, standard practices excluding families began to come into question.[19,20]

Within the field of emergency medicine there has been significant debate regarding whether families should be allowed to accompany their relatives who are undergoing critical resuscitation. Proponents of this practice advocate that family members should have the choice to be present during these desperate efforts, which are often the final moments of patients' lives. However, many medical professionals are strongly opposed to the idea and cite a wide range of concerns: that relatives will interfere with or misunderstand medical efforts, that the events will be too upsetting for relatives to bear, and that family presence will create additional stress and anxiety for the medical team.[21-25]

Research to date demonstrates that families who are allowed to be present during resuscitation procedures recognize the practice as beneficial to both themselves and their ill relatives. Family members perceive their presence as important not only to provide support and reassurance to the patient but also to relieve their own anxiety by reducing feelings of helplessness and the "agony of waiting."[26] Relatives also report that being present with a dying loved one eased their subsequent bereavement process.[20,26,27]

Research findings also indicate that the anticipated problems or expected complications of FWR fail to occur in clinical practice.[27-29]

In recent years FWR has been recognized as being fundamentally consistent with a patient- and family-centered approach to care.[30] FWR provides the opportunity to engage and empower a patient's loved ones during the most critical moments of serious injury or illness. The open door facilitates a connection and partnership between the provider and family that can have significant downstream effects on this relationship and, ultimately, the grief and bereavement process.

In the future, more research is needed to fully assess the consequences of FWR for all participants in the resuscitation process and for different clinical situations and patient populations. However, it is clear that research alone will not resolve this debate because our emotional responses as providers may defy research results. As emergency providers we must focus our energy on helping ourselves and others remain open-minded to the possibility of benefit from these practices and consider their role in our efforts to provide patient- and family-centered care.

### INFORMED REFUSAL

In emergency medicine we often encounter patients who refuse our recommended care, and our interactions with these individuals can be frustrating and challenging. Many factors can lead to refusal, and ultimately we must accept a patient's choice to refuse our recommendations. However, when we encounter these situations in our daily practice, a few important concepts should be considered.

First, we must work hard to ensure that we use the basic principles of PCC in our efforts to discuss this issue with our patients. We must explore the situation from their perspective—their past experience, social circumstances, fears, and anxiety—to help us understand the factors that are leading to their refusal. Second, we must set aside our personal reactions and feelings as we engage in these interactions. In particular, we cannot allow our own emotions and responses to patients prevent us from making a genuine effort to connect with them and to help them understand how our recommendations may be compatible with their personal views and preferences.

In the end, we must accept that sometimes our efforts will not be successful and we have to understand how to approach these situations. Informed refusal stems from the doctrine of informed consent, and the same basic tenets apply. Patients need to possess the medical decision-making capacity to consent or refuse care (e.g., conscious, alert, and oriented to person, place, time, and situation), and they need to be informed of the risks and benefits of the proposed treatment and the risks and benefits of alternatives, including no treatment at all. Patients need to demonstrate their understanding of this discussion. The standard for informed consent or refusal is what a reasonable patient would want to know. This is vastly different from the former physician standard regarding what a reasonable physician would inform the patient about. Informed refusals should be well documented in the medical record, and it is important to recognize that signing a refusal or against-medical-advice form does not necessarily meet the required elements for informed refusal. Merely signing a form does not document which risks associated with refusal were discussed with the patient.

## CONCLUSION

PCC is emerging as a primary initiative in many care settings. The ED is no exception. Whether the goal is patient satisfaction, improved patient safety, reduced risk, improvement in hospital market share, operational efficiency, or compliance with governmental mandates, patient-centeredness is the correct focus and emphasis for the future. Any initiatives considered should first be vetted in the context of the patient's perspective and the impact that such endeavors may have on the patient. What is wrong for our patients is wrong for us.

## REFERENCES

***References can be found on Expert Consult @ www.expertconsult.com.***

# 217 Health Care Disparities and Diversity in Emergency Medicine

*Lisa Moreno-Walton and Christian Arbelaez*

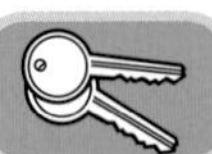

**KEY POINTS**

- The U.S. population is changing rapidly and becoming more diverse.
- Improvement in access to care for racial and ethnic minorities has not proved effective in ameliorating health care disparities.
- A diverse workforce that mirrors the patient population is a key and important step toward reducing health care disparities.
- Cultural competency helps health care providers understand how to approach patients from different backgrounds by improving communication and building trust in the doctor-patient relationship.
- Cultural competency is integral to clinical competency.

## INTRODUCTION

As the globalization of trade, technology, investment, and migration create a more diverse U.S. population, we are increasingly becoming aware of disparities in economics, health care, and human rights. Our nation was founded on the concept that "all men are created equal,"[1] and equal treatment and equal access are the goals toward which we strive. Nowhere else in medicine is the commitment to equality as obvious as it is in emergency departments (EDs), where the sole criteria for moving to the front of the line is severity of illness. Other specialties now restrict the days and hours during which they are available to patients and tell their patients at discharge from the hospital to go the ED if they have any problems or concerns. Changes in the economy have resulted in a significant increase in the percentage of uninsured.[2] Only the ED provides medical care 24 hours a day, 365 days a year for every patient with any complaint. As advocates for our patients, emergency physicians (EP) are at the forefront of the promotion of diversity and the elimination of disparities in health care, not just at home but throughout the world.

The definitions of some important terms, broadly and more specifically as they relate to emergency medicine (EM), will help provide a common understanding and language for the reader[3] (**Box 217.1**). Awareness of the history of disparities in access to quality health care (**Box 217.2**),[4-17] the benefits of clinical research (**Table 217.1**),[18-23] and medical education and EM practice (**Box 217.3**) will create a contextual framework within which the reader can appreciate all that has been accomplished, as well as the tasks that remain, as we work toward the ideals of diversity and cultural competency.

## IDENTIFYING ISSUES OF DISPARITY

In 2003 the Institute of Medicine (IOM) was charged by Congress to examine racial and ethnic disparities in health care. Their landmark report, "Unequal Treatment: Confronting Racial and Ethnic Disparities in Healthcare,"[24] brought the issue of health care disparities to national attention. The report concluded that "Racial and ethnic minorities tend to receive a lower quality of healthcare than non-minorities, even when access-related factors, such as patients' insurance status and income, were controlled." The report defined disparities as "racial or ethnic differences in the quality of healthcare that are not due to access-related factors or clinical needs, preferences, and appropriateness of intervention."[24]

According to the U.S. Census Bureau, there are currently more than 300 million Americans: 65% white, 16% Hispanic, 13% black, 5% Asian, and 1% American Indian.[25] Yet according to a report by the American Medical Association, only 6.4% of practicing physicians are Hispanic and 4.5% are black.[26] Recognizing the changing patient demographics and the unchanging demographics of the physician workforce, the Association of American Medical Colleges (AAMC) Executive Council adopted a definition of *underrepresented in medicine* (URM) as "those racial and ethnic populations that are under-represented in the medical profession relative to their numbers in the general population." Before this, the AAMC used the term "under-represented minority," which specifically targeted African Americans, Mexican Americans, Native Americans, and mainland Puerto Ricans. A much broader definition of diversity includes race, ethnicity, socioeconomic status, sexual orientation, religion, disability, age, language, and geographic diversity.[27]

## UNDERSTANDING CULTURAL COMPETENCY

Diversity and cultural competency have emerged as the two main forces for eliminating disparity in medicine. When patients have contact with the health care system, they bring their culture and all that it encompasses, including their beliefs, values, identity, and links to the community. When people of different cultures and backgrounds come together, diversity is achieved. The Office of Minority Health (OMH) defines cultural and linguistic competence as "a set of congruent behaviors, attitudes and policies that come together in a system, agency or among professionals that enables effective work in cross-cultural situations."[28] The educational concepts for cultural competency are centered on the provider's ability to acquire the knowledge, attitude, and skills necessary to elicit an explanatory model of illness from the patient and to incorporate it into the medical decision-making process. Ultimately, this concept empowers the physician to navigate the cross-cultural experience with any patient from any cultural background by enabling greater understanding of the patient's perspective and social context. The OMH published their standards for culturally and linguistically appropriate services in health care in 2002.[29] Another conceptual model by the Agency for Healthcare Research and Quality describes how integrating nine major cultural competency techniques can potentially improve the ability of physicians and health care systems to deliver appropriate services to diverse populations.[30]

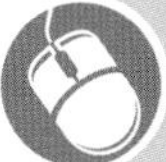

See bonus section, Diversity and Cultural Competency, in online version of chapter at www.expertconsult.com

**BOX 217.1 Definitions**

*Culture*: Customary beliefs, social forms, and material traits of a racial, religious, or social group; also, the characteristic features of everyday existence shared by people in a place

*Disparity*: Lack of parity, the state of being dissimilar or unequal

*Diversity*: Inclusion of different types of people in a group or organization

**BOX 217.2 History of Health Care Disparities**

1619-1865: Contaminated drinking water led to frequent outbreaks of disease among slaves.[4] Slaves develop a system of care involving indigenous herb root doctors and midwives.[5]

1824: The Bureau of Indian Affairs is established and provides limited health care to Native Americans on reservations.[6]

1852: The first hospital for the care of blacks is opened: Jackson Street Hospital, Augusta, Georgia.[7]

1862: The only government-funded hospital for blacks, Freedmen's Hospital in Washington, DC, is established.[8]

1948: Executive Order 9981 mandates the integration of Veterans Administration hospitals.[9]

1955: The Indian Health Service is commissioned.[10]

1965: The Johnson administration announces that federal Medicaid and Medicare payments will be denied to segregated hospitals.[11]

1990: A metaanalysis of 485 articles confirms that migrant health care is confined almost exclusively to charity migrant clinics and virtually nothing is known about the health status of the workers.[12]

2004: At every age, blacks have higher blood pressure than nonblacks.[13]

2005: A total of 16.5% of American Indians, 10.4% of Hispanics, and 6.6% of whites are diabetic.[14]

2006: African Americans are more likely than whites to die of coronary artery disease. They and Hispanics are less likely to be offered bypass or angioplasty. Blacks have worse cancer survival rates, are more likely to undergo amputation for complications of diabetes, and are less likely than whites to be referred for transplant evaluation. Hispanics and Native Americans are least likely to be offered cholesterol management services.[15]

2009: Of all patients in whom human immunodeficiency virus infection was diagnosed this year, 52% were black.[16]

2010: Twenty percent of the population lives in rural areas, where only 9% of physicians practice.[17]

**Table 217.1 History of Disparities in Research**

| | |
|---|---|
| Nazi human experimentation: 1938-1945 | Josef Mengele, MD, was one of the notorious physicians who performed burning, boiling, freezing, beating, hanging, and poisoning experiments on human prisoners of war who were predominantly racial and ethnic minorities in Europe.[18] |
| Tuskegee Study of Untreated Syphilis in the Negro Male: 1932-1972, Taliaferro Clark, MD | The U.S. Public Health Service conducted a study on the natural course of syphilis in black males; they were often not informed of their diagnosis and were deliberately prevented from seeking and obtaining treatment, even after penicillin became widely available.[19] |
| Willowbrook: 1963-1966 | Saul Krugman, PhD, deliberately infected mentally handicapped children with hepatitis B virus to study the effects of gamma globulin on the disease.[20] |
| Nuremberg Code: 1948 | It arose from the trials of Nazis for crimes against humanity and addressed consent by and protection of subjects of human research.[21] |
| Declaration of practice, Helsinki: 1964 | The World Medical Association establishes good clinical practices in human research (standards revised in 1975, 1983, 1989, 1996, 2000, 2002, 2004, and 2008).[22] |
| Belmont Report: 1979 | Boundaries were established between practice and research and basic ethical principles of human research.[23] |

**BOX 217.3 History of Disparities in Medical Education**

1783: Dr. James Durham, a former slave, becomes the first African American physician. He sets up practice in New Orleans after apprenticeship training.
1837: Dr. James McCune Smith is the first African American to obtain an MD degree. He has to go to the University of Glasgow to do so. He sets up practice in New York City.
1847: Dr. David J. Peck is the first African American to graduate from a U.S. Medical School (Rush Medical College).
1849: Two African American men receive MD degrees from Bowdoin College, Maine.
1850: There are 13 African American doctors: 9 in New York City and 4 in New Orleans.
1857: Dr. Elizabeth Blackwell becomes the first woman to graduate from a U.S. medical school and founds the New York Infirmary for Women and Children.
1867: Dr. Blackwell founds the Women's Medical College of Pennsylvania
1868 and 1876: Eight Negro medical schools were established, but only two are still open: Meharry, Tennessee (1876), and Howard, Washington, DC (1868).
1889: Dr. Susan La Flesche Picotte is the first American Indian woman to earn an MD degree; she receives it from the Women's Medical College of Pennsylvania.
1890: There are 909 African American doctors, as compared with 1734 in 1900 and 4500 in 1960.
1891: Dr. Daniel Hale Williams opens the first black-owned hospital (Provident Hospital in Chicago).
1905: Being denied membership in "mainstream" medical associations, Dr. Williams establishes the National Medical Association.

Over the course of time there has been an evolution in the education and assessment of cultural competency in undergraduate and graduate medical education. The Liaison Committee on Medical Education has codified the following criteria: "Students must demonstrate an understanding of the manner in which people of diverse cultures and belief systems perceive health and illness and respond to various symptoms, diseases, and treatments."[31] Similarly, the Accreditation Council for Graduate Medical Education (ACGME) has defined its competency standards within two of the six core competencies: patient care and interpersonal communication skills.[32]

## EXPLORING SOLUTIONS

The Sullivan Alliance, composed of former members of the IOM and the Sullivan Commission, a group commissioned by Duke University and the Kellogg Foundation to study diversity in the health care workforce, aimed to transform the health professions by providing a comprehensive framework of 62 recommendations from both reports.[33,34] The AAMC has led several efforts targeted at the critical steps referenced by the Sullivan Alliance. Recognizing the challenges that medical schools and academic medical centers face when implementing the recommendations, the AAMC published several road maps that highlight some of the legal, practical, and subtle barriers and describe the different levels of commitment required throughout the organization.[35]

## MOVING TOWARD PARITY IN HEALTH CARE

Even though access to care has improved remarkably for racial minorities over the past 2 centuries, it is important to realize that they "are disproportionately affected by multiple barriers to care: financial, linguistic, cultural, logistical, organizational, institutional and systemic. Disturbingly, providing disadvantaged populations with adequate access to care may not be sufficient to eliminate racial/ethnic disparities in health."[36] In the Health Disparities and Inequities Report of 2011 by the Centers for Disease Control and Prevention, minority groups were overrepresented in every diagnostic category monitored except suicide and drug-induced death, where whites prevailed.[37] To highlight the importance of patient-centered, culturally competent care, the AAMC developed the Tool for Assessing Cultural Competence Training (TACCT), which provides a framework for designing, implementing, and integrating an effective cultural competency educational program.[38] The TACCT is a self-administered assessment tool that can be used to identify the strengths and weaknesses of a program's educational curriculum. ACGME's Toolbox of Assessment Methods is an excellent resource that includes assessment methods and references to articles where more in-depth information can be found. The design, implementation, and assessment of effective cultural competency curricula must be flexible, be tailored to the institution, maximize existing resources, and be linked to a data collection component to measure and monitor for success.

The 2003 Academic Emergency Medicine national consensus conference "Disparities in Emergency Health Care" went further by addressing issues of unconscious personal bias, disparities profiling, and the need for epidemiologic and clinical research directed at making an impact on outcomes and improving physician-patient communication.[37]

## MOVING TOWARD JUSTICE IN RESEARCH

Several particularly shocking acts of injustice and abuse in clinical research (see Table 217.1) culminated in governmental intervention to protect the human rights of research subjects. In the United States, the Belmont Report remains the standard by which institutional review boards (IRBs) ensure that subjects of human research are treated with respect for persons, beneficence, and justice. The report states that "injustice arises from social, racial, sexual, and cultural biases institutionalized in society. Thus, even if individual researchers are treating their research subjects fairly, and even if IRBs are taking care to assure that subjects are selected fairly within a particular institution, unjust patterns may nevertheless appear in the overall distribution of the burdens and benefits of research."[39] Theoretically, diseases that predominantly affect racial and ethnic minorities and low socioeconomic groups should have the same opportunity to be studied as diseases predominantly affecting males, whites, and the middle class. In recent decades there has been concern regarding the lack of inclusion of women as subjects of research[40] and inadequate inclusion of blacks and Hispanics in research on human immunodeficiency virus.[41] Because trauma is predominantly a disease of racial and ethnic minorities, the poor, and the undereducated and because these populations are regarded as vulnerable by IRBs, there are significant barriers to conducting trauma research. Several EM researchers have questioned whether there exist vulnerable populations in conditions in which acute loss of decisional capacity makes all patients equally vulnerable.[42] Others question whether the standard informed consent process, refused more often by black than by white patients, may not introduce bias into research studies by underrepresenting disease among minority patients.[43] Because EM research is predominantly conducted by EP scientists, our specialty must continue to take the lead in ensuring that all patients have equal access to the benefits of research while being equally respected and protected from potential abuse.

## MOVING TOWARD DIVERSITY IN MEDICAL EDUCATION AND PRACTICE OF EMERGENCY MEDICINE

Increasing the diversity of the medical student population and ensuring that physicians are trained to be culturally competent have been cited as key strategies in addressing health care disparities and preparing health care systems for the challenges of the 21st century. The concept of concordance,[44] another factor in favor of increasing diversity of the physician workforce, has been well documented in the literature. Yet despite increasing evidence of the benefits of physician diversity, we have been slow to change. In 2004, 6.6% of U.S. medical students were Latino and 7.3% were African American. Today, although 16% of the U.S. population is Latino and 13% is African American, only 7.9% of medical students are Latino and 7.1% are African American.[45] In 2008 there were 25,516 practicing EPs: 78% white and 12% URM (1474 African American, 1365 Hispanic/Latino, and 156 American Indian).[46] In 1963, Dr. W. Montegue Cobb, in discussing the reasons for the dearth of black physicians in the country, cited "failure to become oriented toward medicine and its exacting requirements early enough."[7] The National Medical Association and the National Hispanic Medical Association continue to take the lead in nurturing URM high school and college students to consider medicine as a career. The Diversity Interest Group[47] of the Society for Academic Emergency Medicine (SAEM) provides virtual and real-time advisement and support to minority students interested in EM. "Mentoring in Medicine,"[48] an organization started by EPs, provides a pipeline program beginning at the elementary school level to encourage URM children in their desire to become health care professionals and to facilitate this desire through mentoring, tutoring, and linkage to resources.

## LEADERSHIP STRATEGIES IN EMERGENCY MEDICINE

Our specialty has been a leader in both clinical care and education by raising awareness, promoting discussion, and developing strategies around diversity and cultural competency. Professional organizations, consensus conferences, and work groups have convened leaders from the broad membership of EM to develop and publish policy statements, recommendations, and tools for implementation in residency programs and clinical and academic departments.

## ORGANIZATIONAL LEADERSHIP

The SAEM's Diversity Statement asserts that "attaining diversity in emergency medicine residencies and faculty that reflect our multicultural society is a desirable and achievable goal. SAEM encourages all academic medical centers to recruit, retain, and advance a faculty reflective of the community served. SAEM encourages its members to respect, support, and embrace the existing cultural differences of its membership. SAEM encourages the development of didactic, educational, research, and other programs to assist academic emergency medicine departments to improve the diversity of their faculties and residencies."[49]

The American College of Emergency Physicians Policy Statement on Workforce Diversity in Health Care Settings states that "hospitals and emergency physicians should work together to promote staffing of hospitals and their emergency departments with qualified individuals who reflect the ethnic and racial diversity in our nation.... Attaining diversity with well-qualified physicians in emergency medicine residencies and faculties that reflects our multicultural society is a desirable goal."[50]

The American Academy of Emergency Medicine (AAEM) makes a statement on diversity within the AAEM and Emergency Nurses Association Joint Position on a Code of Professional Conduct by stating that "the ideal for emergency nurses and physicians is to practice in an optimal working environment where there is respect for diversity."[51]

In 2008, the Council of Residency Directors in EM convened the Promoting Diversity in Emergency Medicine Workgroup and, in 2009, published a set of primary recommendations, secondary considerations, and tools to help EM residency training programs and academic departments promote diversity.[52]

## BARRIERS AND CHALLENGES

EPs provide continuous care to patients from varying ethnic, cultural, and social backgrounds, frequently the most disadvantaged and vulnerable populations. The fast-paced and unpredictable clinical setting of the ED presents challenges that include time constraints, limited information, and inadequate resources. The health care team must establish rapport quickly and gain the trust of both patient and family. Patients who are acutely ill, sometimes with a language barrier, represent significant challenges for EPs and are at the highest risk of suffering from unconscious bias, disparities in care, and worse outcomes.

The major challenge to diversifying the physician workforce rests with the establishment of an educational pipeline, beginning in elementary school and continuing mentorship through residency training and on into faculty leadership roles. Barriers at the academic faculty level include inadequate recruitment efforts for qualified URM physicians and inadequate efforts toward retention and promotion.[53] Clinical and academic departments are often remiss by spending limited educational time devoted to cultural competency, which they may believe is not as important as clinical competency. Individual physicians may be resistant to acknowledging that disparities exist in their health care delivery or may be reluctant to admit to the possibility of subconscious bias.

## FUTURE DIRECTIONS

Elimination of disparities and the development of a diverse, culturally competent workforce will require the collective effort of individual providers, EM residency programs, faculty practices, hospital administration, and medical school leadership in embracing the goals of delivering equal care to all. In closing the health care disparities gap, EM leaders and educators will play a critical role by recognizing disparity as an important issue in medicine and by developing methods of addressing the knowledge and attitudinal barriers that propagate the problem. As the population continues to become more diverse, we will need to quickly expand the professional pipeline from high school to faculty leadership positions to meet the public's need. Development and implementation of cultural training that is compliant with the ACGME core competencies should provide our residency graduates with the skills that they need to be effective, culturally competent practitioners. Increasing workforce diversity and ensuring cultural competency are the most important strategies for eliminating racial and ethnic disparities in health care.

## REFERENCES

***References can be found on Expert Consult @ www.expertconsult.com.***

# Introduction to Cost-Effectiveness Analysis 218

*Emilie S. Powell and Brian W. Patterson*

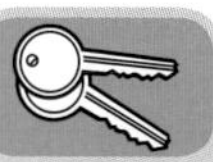

**KEY POINTS**

- Cost-effectiveness analysis (CEA) is a method for evaluating and comparing the outcomes and costs of interventions designed to improve health.
- CEA is an increasingly important component of the medical literature because it drives both clinical and policy decisions that affect the practice of emergency medicine.
- The output of any CEA model is contingent on appropriate and accurate input data.
- The primary outcome of importance in a CEA is the incremental cost-effectiveness ratio, or ICER, which represents the incremental change in cost and effectiveness when choosing one strategy over another.
- CEA model outcomes incorporate a degree of uncertainty based on input data, which is quantified in the process of sensitivity analysis.

## WHAT IS COST-EFFECTIVENESS ANALYSIS?

A key skill for emergency physicians is effective integration of new interventions into existing clinical practice. Physicians have classically been trained and have become comfortable with more traditional methodologies of evaluating new interventions and treatment modalities, such as randomized controlled trials, but are often less comfortable in applying techniques such as cost-effectiveness analysis (CEA). As health care resources become more limited, costs rise, and treatment options expand, interventions and treatments are increasingly being compared and evaluated on the basis of cost.[1]

CEA falls under the broad umbrella of comparative effectiveness research, which refers to any study that compares the effectiveness of two or more strategies with or without regard to cost. CEA is a method for evaluating and comparing the outcomes and costs of interventions designed to improve health.[2] Although many methodologies fall under the umbrella of CEA, they all share the common goal of reporting outcomes as a cost per achieving a unit of health effect (i.e., lives saved, year of life gained, quality-adjusted year of life gained). CEA tracks costs and effectiveness for a number of strategies by using both real and modeled data, compares the cost-effectiveness of the strategies, and then accounts for uncertainty in the data through sensitivity analyses.[3]

## HOW DOES COST-EFFECTIVENESS ANALYSIS AFFECT THE EMERGENCY PHYSICIAN?

CEA is becoming an increasingly important input into health policy decisions; however, the methodology does have limitations. CEA cannot incorporate all aspects of a decision, and the results are only as good as the data available to input into the analyses. Economic analyses such as CEA cannot capture every input necessary to make health care decisions and should not be reported as scientific fact, but models and their results may be reported as aids in decision making.[4] An additional criticism of CEA is that although the economic models have become increasingly complex to better represent reality, they have also become increasingly opaque to the lay reader, thus making it difficult for those without a background in economics to personally interpret the results.[1] Despite these limitations, CEA offers the benefit of adding perspective to difficult questions regarding treatment choices in the setting of limited resources.[2,5,6] If emergency physicians are to act as decision makers in our changing practice environment, it is essential to have an understanding of the basic principles of CEA.

## METHODOLOGY IN COST-EFFECTIVENESS ANALYSIS

### COMPONENTS OF A COST-EFFECTIVENESS ANALYSIS

CEA has four main components: inputs (costs and effectiveness and the perspective from which these variables are determined), the model, primary outcomes, and sensitivity analyses. Inputs are known values gathered from primary research, previously published literature, or estimation and are incorporated into a model. The model is the computational framework created to combine these known values along with clinical probabilities to output the overall cost-effectiveness of an intervention or set of interventions. Uncertainty in the model is evaluated and reported through sensitivity analyses.

All CEAs starts with a focused clinical question that drives collection of data for analysis and allows appropriate interpretation of results. As an example for the proceeding sections, we will consider a hypothetic CEA created to answer a clinical question. Suppose an emergency department (ED) is attempting to create a cost-effective strategy for stratification of cardiac risk in low-risk patients with chest pain. After a normal electrocardiogram and two negative cardiac enzyme tests, these low-risk patients could either be sent home or be admitted to the hospital for an exercise stress test. A CEA could be created to answer the following question: "Among low-risk patients seen in the ED with chest pain, is adding admission for an exercise stress test more cost-effective than discharging the patient directly home?"

## INPUTS

### *Perspective*

An important characteristic of any CEA is the perspective from which the analysis is conducted. The cost and effectiveness of an intervention may vary depending on the perspective. Common perspectives include those of the patient, the insurer, the employer, the hospital, or society, to name a few. For instance, from the perspective of an insurer, the cost of an intervention for a patient whom it insures is simply the amount of money paid to physicians and hospitals. However, from the perspective of an employer who provides health care insurance, the cost of an intervention additionally includes loss of productivity while the employee is ill and undergoing the intervention. The choice of perspective is of critical importance in performing and interpreting a CEA because it determines the relevance of the study for decision making.

Although one can perform a CEA from a vast number of perspectives, the most common is the societal perspective, which will be used for our example. In a CEA conducted from the societal perspective, the analyst considers all parties affected by the intervention and all costs related to the intervention, regardless of who experiences these costs and effects. Because the societal perspective includes all costs and health effects, it does not necessarily give an individual group the information necessary to make decisions on which interventions to implement. However, the societal perspective is used most commonly because it has several benefits.[3] It is standardized and therefore allows comparison of various interventions across a broad spectrum of disciplines in medicine and society when making policy decisions. It is fair: if all decisions in health care were made from a societal standpoint, resources would be allocated to provide the most benefit to the most people. Moreover, although other perspectives may be more useful for individual groups, these perspectives do not necessarily take into account the cost or harm seen by those outside the sphere of the analyst's perspective that the societal perspective takes into account.

### *Costs*

Costs may be gathered from several different sources: institutional data, Medicare or other payment records, or elsewhere in the published literature. In our example study, the costs associated with the hospital stay, such as the cost of an exercise stress test and hospital admission, could be taken from institutional data. Because the study is conducted from a societal perspective, the true cost of these interventions to the hospital (as opposed to hospital charges) would need to be calculated. Other costs included in the study, such as the cost of a day of missed work and the cost of outpatient medical treatment of coronary artery disease (CAD), could be taken from the economic or medical literature. When evaluating a CEA, it is important to verify that the authors included all relevant costs for the stated perspective of the study and that these costs are plausible.

### *Effectiveness*

In CEA, each strategy has an associated effectiveness. The effectiveness (sometimes referred to in the economic literature as utility) can be expressed with a number of different metrics. The most common measure is "life-years gained" or "lives saved." Traditionally, most medical and public health studies use "life-years," whereas CEAs in transportation and environmental policy use "lives saved."[7]

Even though life-years may be used alone as an effectiveness measure, they are generally adjusted to account for quality of life or disability. Without adjustment, two interventions would have the same effectiveness based on life-years even if one substantially increased quality of life without any extension in life expectancy. The most common adjustment unit is the quality-adjusted life-year (QALY), although other units such as disability-adjusted life-year are sometimes used.[8]

Several methods can be used for quality-adjusting life-years to arrive at QALYs. All methods seek to find the value placed on various disease states among a group representing the interests of either a patient population or society. One commonly used method is known as the time trade-off. In a time trade-off, subjects are asked to choose between remaining in a particular health state for a fixed length of time or "trading off" that time for some shorter amount of time in perfect health. The ratio of time traded gives the QALY equivalent for the health state. For instance, if respondents would choose to equate 6 months of perfect health with 1 year in a health state, each year in that state would be worth 0.5 QALYs. Another commonly used method for quality adjustment is the standard gamble. Respondents choose between remaining in a health state or taking a gamble on a treatment that will either kill them or restore them to perfect health. If a patient in a particular health state is willing to take a 50-50 chance of dying or being restored to perfect health, that state is valued at 0.5 QALYs.

These methodologies for quality adjustment have limitations. Not all patients will value quality of life and disease states the same. The life-year–to-QALY conversion is not standard or universal, and when evaluating a CEA, one should verify that the adjustments seem appropriate. Controversy exists regarding the most appropriate derivation method, and the different approaches to derive QALYs may deliver different results even with the same respondent.

In our example model we could track the effectiveness of several outcomes. Our first outcome could be a disease-free outcome; this would represent the average quality-adjusted life span of CAD-free patients following discharge from the ED after a negative work-up. Another outcome would be a true diagnosis of CAD. Patients found to have CAD in the hospital would probably have a lower quality-adjusted life expectancy than those without CAD but would benefit from treatment of the disease. A third outcome would be patients discharged from the ED after a false-negative work-up; that is, those who have CAD but are sent home thinking that they are well. These patients would probably have the shortest life expectancy.

### *Clinical Probabilities*

To build a model, in addition to the cost and effectiveness of the strategies, a set of clinical probabilities must be created to govern how patients flow through the model. Similar to cost and effectiveness measures, these probabilities can be derived from a number of sources, from primary institutional data to educated estimation. Our model would include population characteristics such as the prevalence of CAD, as well as test characteristics such as the sensitivity and specificity of an exercise stress test in detecting clinically relevant CAD. Anywhere a chance node lies on a decision tree, a model must contain a corresponding set of probabilities that dictate the outcomes from that node.

### *Discounting*

An important aspect of economic analyses is the practice of discounting. Many CEAs take into account costs and health states that occur years in the future from the time of an intervention. To compare future costs and utilities with those occurring in the present, future costs and utilities are devalued at a constant yearly rate to reflect their lower opportunity cost. For example, if one needs to pay for a health intervention, clearly it is preferable to pay the same sum of money 10 years from now rather than paying today because the sum of money used for payment in the future could be invested in the meantime to generate further revenue. Therefore, a discount rate is applied to compare present and future events. The discount rate for all costs and utilities is generally approximately 3% to 5% per year in health economic analyses. Even though this value is commonly used, there is little agreement among economists regarding what represents an appropriate discount rate and exactly how this rate should be calculated.[9,10]

## THE MODEL

Mathematic models are used in CEA to simulate the chain of events surrounding alternative interventions so that the costs and outcomes related to the choice of one medical intervention over another can be tracked. Although it is theoretically possible to complete a CEA by measuring every variable prospectively, the broad scope of most CEAs necessitates at least some component of mathematic modeling.[11,12] A successful model is transparent, internally consistent, reproducible, and interpretable.[13] Multiple modeling methodologies are used in modern CEAs; here we will cover the two most common: decision tress and Markov models. Decision trees depict decisions and chance events as branches of a tree. Computerized decision trees can track the costs and outcomes associated with various health interventions. Graphic branches in the tree represent a chain of related events, and nodes in the branches represent decisions, such as a choice between competing strategies, or chances, such as the chance of a complication developing after an intervention. **Figure 218.1** depicts a simple decision tree.

Certain situations are difficult to model with decision trees alone; especially problematic are episodic or recursive disease states (i.e., a chronic disease with frequent exacerbations). For these situations more complex models, such as Markov models, are used. A Markov model consists of a set of health states, as well as allowable transitions between these states. The model moves forward with discrete steps in time; at each time step the model allows patients to transition between states along allowable transitions according to predefined transition probabilities. Markov models can be constructed independently or be inserted into decision trees. If in our example CEA we wish to model CAD in more detail and specifically include ischemic congestive heart failure states, we could use a Markov model as depicted in **Figure 218.2**.

## PRIMARY OUTCOMES

The most basic outcome from any CEA is a cost-effectiveness ratio (CE ratio), in which the cost of an intervention is placed in the numerator and the measure of effectiveness in the

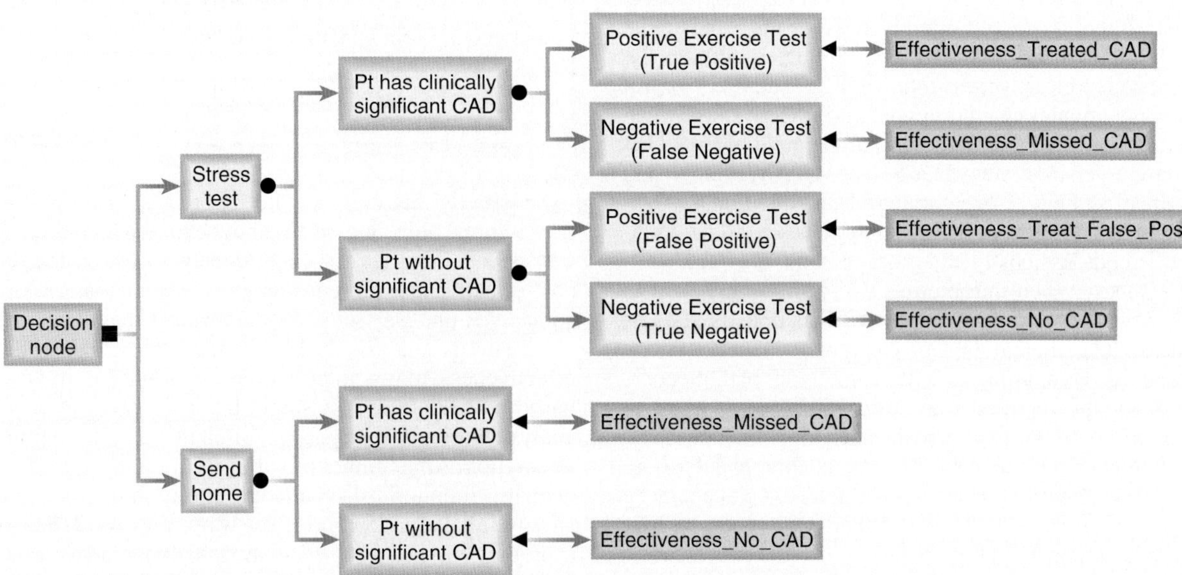


**Fig. 218.1 Sample decision tree.** The *square* represents a decision node, *circles* represent chance nodes, and *triangles* represent terminal nodes. Costs are tracked at each branch along the chain, and each terminal node is associated with an effectiveness. Clinical probabilities are documented below the nodes. *CAD*, Coronary artery disease; *Pt*, patient.

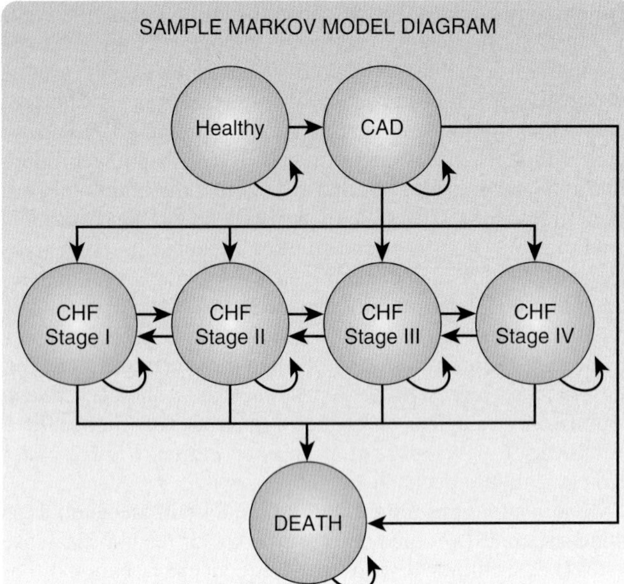


**Fig. 218.2 Sample Markov model.** *Circles* represent health states, and *arrows* represent allowable transitions between states. Each *arrow* is associated with a transition probability that governs the percentage of patients who make that transition at each time step. *Arrows* that point back at the same *circle* indicate the associated chance of remaining in the same state. The model can track cost and effectiveness associated with staying in a particular health state, as well as with making the transition between states. *CAD*, Coronary artery disease; *CHF*, congestive heart failure.

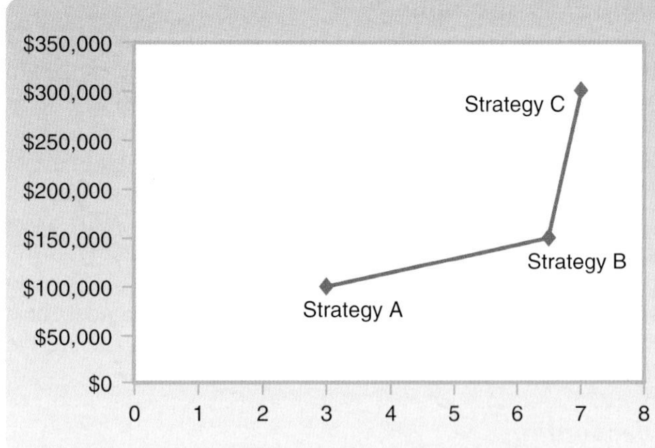


**Fig. 218.3 Cost-effectiveness frontier.** The total cost of a strategy is plotted against each strategy's effectiveness. This graph gives a representation of the additional life years gained for the additional cost of a strategy. The slope of the line connecting two points is mathematically equivalent to the incremental cost-effectiveness ratio.

denominator; for instance, "dollars per QALY." The CE ratio can then be compared with a predetermined "willingness to pay" to determine whether the intervention is cost-effective. Frequently, from a societal perspective a CE ratio is not particularly useful by itself because it involves a large number of societal costs and outcomes. It is often more useful to view the cost-effectiveness of one intervention versus another. The cost-effectiveness frontier graphically shows this difference, with cost on the y-axis and effectiveness on the x-axis (**Fig. 218.3**). To numerically compare two strategies, we use the incremental cost-effectiveness ratio (ICER). The ICER represents the incremental change in cost and effectiveness when choosing one strategy over another. For example, if the ICER for strategy A versus strategy B is $10 per QALY, by choosing to implement strategy A over strategy B, an additional $10 is spent for one additional QALY. A strategy is said to be dominant if it is both less costly and more effective than the comparator strategy. When interpreting ICERs it is important to remember two key points. First, the ICER is only as good as the value of the comparators. One can always make a strategy look good by comparing it with something bad. Second, ICERs should be reported only when positive. A negative ICER can mean one of two opposite scenarios: the new strategy is dominant, or the new strategy is dominated (more costly and less effective). The cost-effectiveness plane may be used as an intuitive way to understand and report ICERs between two strategies[14] (**Fig. 218.4**).

## SENSITIVITY ANALYSES

The point estimate of cost-effectiveness provided from a model is known as the "base case."[15] There is likely to be some uncertainty associated with the inputs of any model, and expressing this uncertainty in the outcome is a critical component of any CEA.[9,12] The degree to which a model's outcome changes with changes in particular inputs is referred to as its sensitivity. Examination of uncertainty in a CEA consists of varying input parameters and measuring the effects on results through sensitivity analyses. Sensitivity can be calculated on a number of levels.

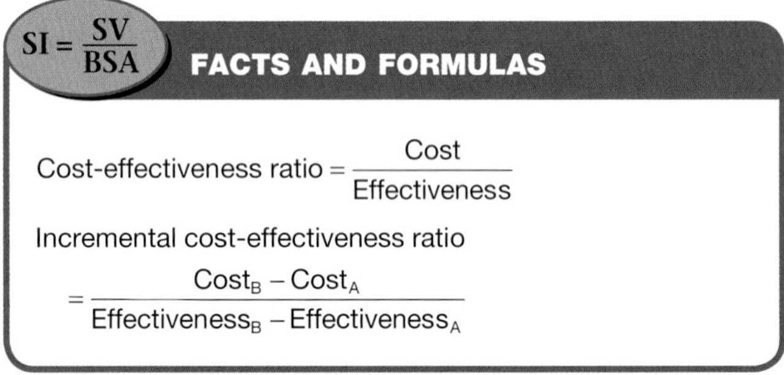

$SI = \frac{SV}{BSA}$ **FACTS AND FORMULAS**

$$\text{Cost-effectiveness ratio} = \frac{\text{Cost}}{\text{Effectiveness}}$$

Incremental cost-effectiveness ratio

$$= \frac{\text{Cost}_B - \text{Cost}_A}{\text{Effectiveness}_B - \text{Effectiveness}_A}$$

Sensitivity analyses may be reported as a threshold value (i.e., a threshold value on an input beyond which the intervention is cost-effective) or continuously, in which the resultant cost-effectiveness is considered across a range of input values.[16] A one-way sensitivity analysis is the most basic form of sensitivity analysis. It demonstrates the variability in cost-effectiveness of an intervention or group of interventions based on variation of a single input. A two-way sensitivity analysis varies two variables simultaneously to capture their interaction. Any number of parameters can be varied simultaneously, although it is challenging to graphically depict sensitivity analyses beyond two way. **Figure 218.5** depicts examples of one- and two-way sensitivity analyses for our example model, as well as an example of a tornado diagram, another commonly used methodology for reporting sensitivity. Tornado diagrams give a graphic representation of the magnitude of a number of one-way sensitivity analyses simul-

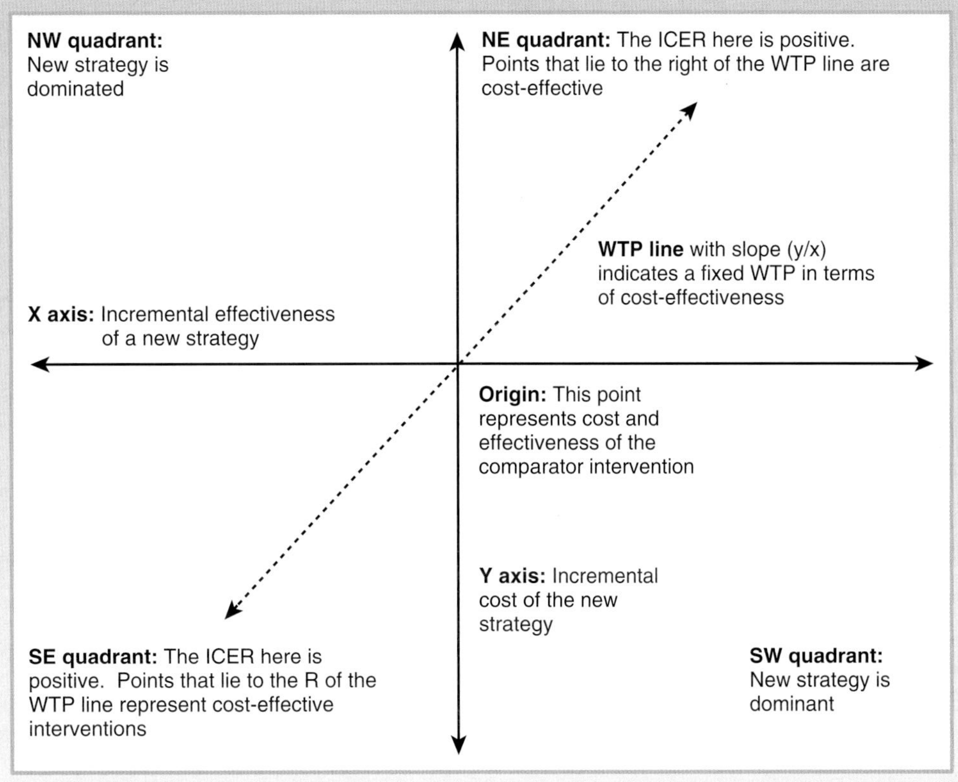


**Fig. 218.4 Incremental cost-effectiveness plane.** *ICER*, Incremental cost-effectiveness ratio; *WTP*, willingness to pay.

taneously but do not incorporate interaction between these variables.

The goal of multivariate sensitivity analysis is to gain a sense of model uncertainty by varying all variables simultaneously. It allows the generation of true confidence intervals of the inputs. The confidence interval for an ICER is dependent on the confidence intervals of all model inputs, as well as the structure of the model. Several methods have been described for empiric calculation of confidence intervals, but there is no consensus method. Most commonly, "bootstrap methods" are used, in which iterative methods are used to create confidence intervals from the data after the model has been run.[17]

The most common bootstrap method for calculating multivariate sensitivity is the Monte Carlo method. In a Monte Carlo analysis, each input in a model is replaced by a distribution representing the uncertainty surrounding the input variable. For instance, in our sample decision tree we may know that the incidence of CAD in the patient population in question is 0.1, with a 95% confidence interval of 0.05 to 0.15, normally distributed. To perform a Monte Carlo sensitivity analysis, we would replace our incidence point probability with a normal distribution of probabilities with a mean of 0.1 and standard deviation of 0.025. We would perform a similar replacement for all model inputs with uncertainty. The model would then be run many times (generally at least 1000).[17] For each iteration of the model, the computer picks a value for each input based on the probability distribution. In the case of our CAD incidence distribution, most iterations would have values near the mean of 0.1, but some iterations would pick outlier values such that over the course of 1000 runs, the values picked would form the distribution specified. Each model run creates an individual ICER. These ICERs then form a distribution, the characteristics of which (standard deviation and confidence intervals) reflect the uncertainty of the model as whole.

Several methods can be used for reporting confidence intervals generated from multivariate sensitivity analyses. In an ICE scatterplot (**Fig. 218.6**), individual runs of a multivariate Monte Carlo analysis are plotted as individual points on a cost-effectiveness plane.[18] **Figure 218.7** shows a sample cost-effectiveness acceptability curve in which individual model runs are compiled to form a probability distribution that reflects the likelihood that a given intervention is cost-effective at a given willingness to pay.[17]

## EVALUATING A COST-EFFECTIVENESS ANALYSIS

See **Box 218.1** for a sample approach to critically evaluating a CEA. Though not the only approach or an all-inclusive list, it provides a framework for assessing the impact of a particular study on a clinical question. See "Suggested Readings" for more in-depth analysis.[12,19-22]

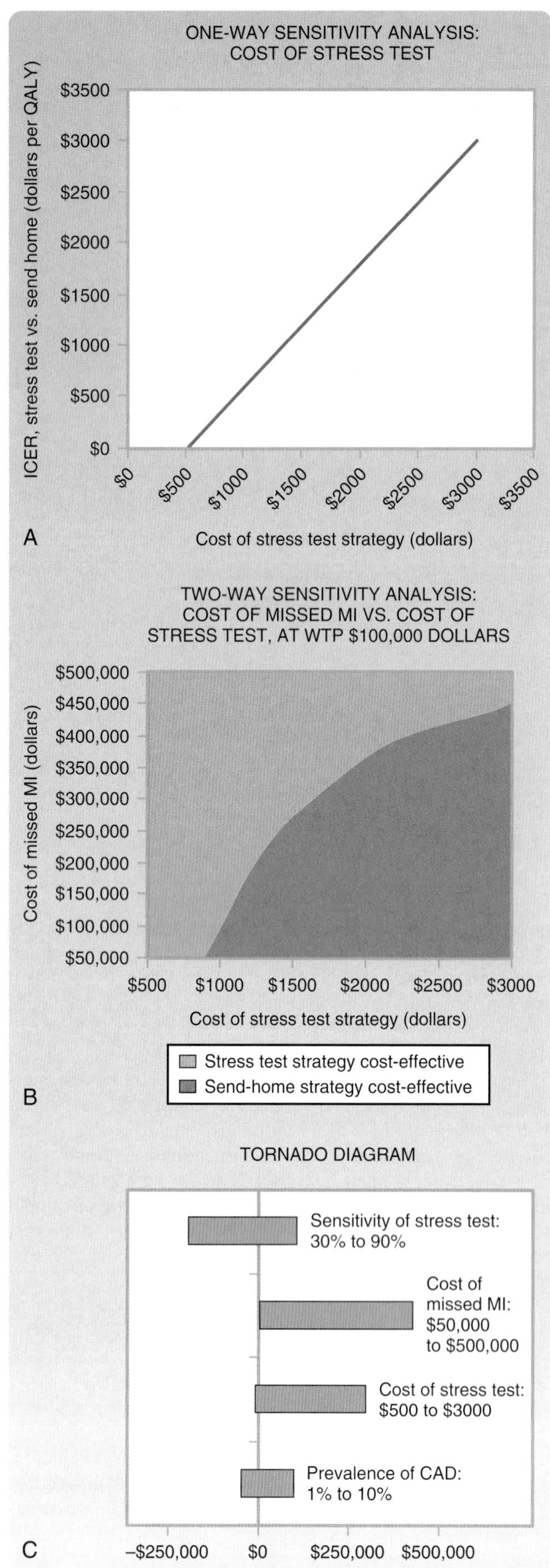


**BOX 218.1 Template for Critiquing a Cost-Effectiveness Analysis**

1. What is the research question being asked?
   a. From what perspective is the analysis conducted, and is this appropriate?
   b. What population is specifically modeled or studied?
   c. Are all appropriate interventions or strategies included in the comparison?
   d. Was the choice of units describing the costs and effectiveness of the evaluated strategies appropriate?
2. What is the quality of the evidence?
   a. Are the sources of model parameter values stated clearly?
   b. Is uncertainty of the source data described (ranges given for all parameters)?
   c. Is the search strategy used to identify model data described and adequate?
   d. Were future costs and consequences discounted appropriately?
3. Is the model's design valid?
   a. Is the structure of the model consistent with the stated research question?
   b. Are the disease states in the model driven by a sound biologic model of the underlying disease (as opposed to data available during construction of the model)?
   c. Were all important and relevant costs and consequences for each alternative identified and valued credibly?
   d. Are model assumptions clearly stated and reasonable?
   e. Is the model as transparent and reproducible as possible while adequately representing the disease and interventions studied?
4. Are the base case results presented?
   a. Are all strategies present in the base case results?
   b. Are appropriate incremental cost-effectiveness ratios calculated for all relevant comparisons?
5. Was an appropriate sensitivity analysis performed?
   a. Do the ranges of possible variable values accurately reflect the uncertainty of the data?
   b. Was a multivariate sensitivity analysis performed?
   c. Are outputs of the sensitivity analysis reported appropriately?
6. Is the model externally consistent?
   a. Are any relevant studies or models identified for comparison?
   b. Does the discussion include and address all points of concern?

**Fig. 218.5 A-C,** Sensitivity analyses. *CAD*, Coronary artery disease; *ICER*, incremental cost-effectiveness ratio; *MI*, myocardial infarction; *QALY*, quality-adjusted life year; *WTP*, willingness to pay.

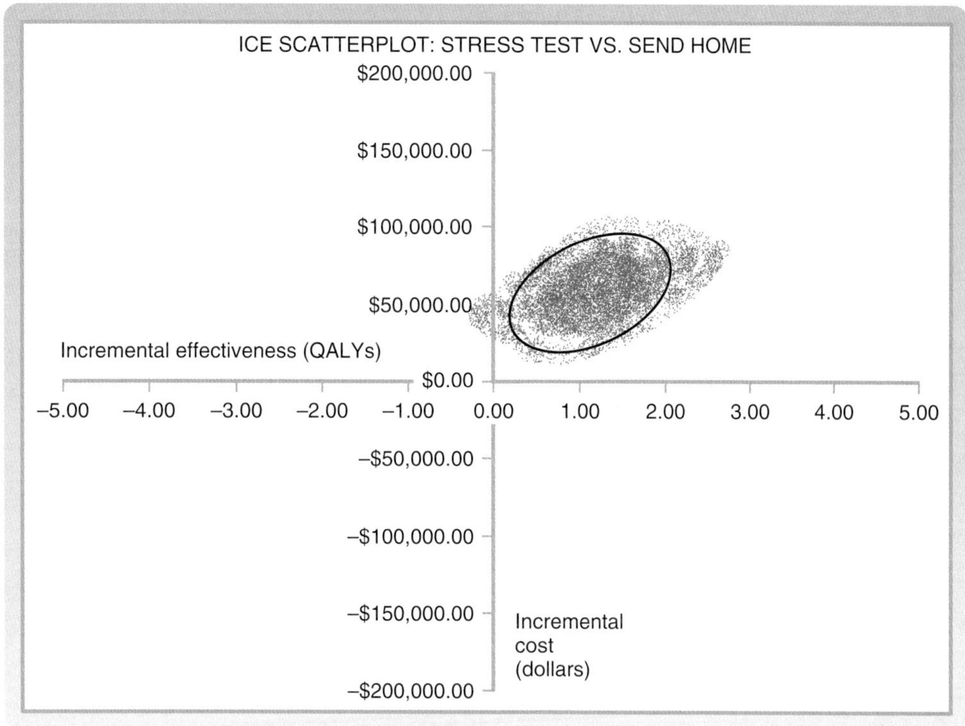


**Fig. 218.6 Monte-Carlo sensitivity analysis: ICE scatterplot.** *ICE*, Incremental cost-effectiveness; *QALYs*, quality-adjusted life years.

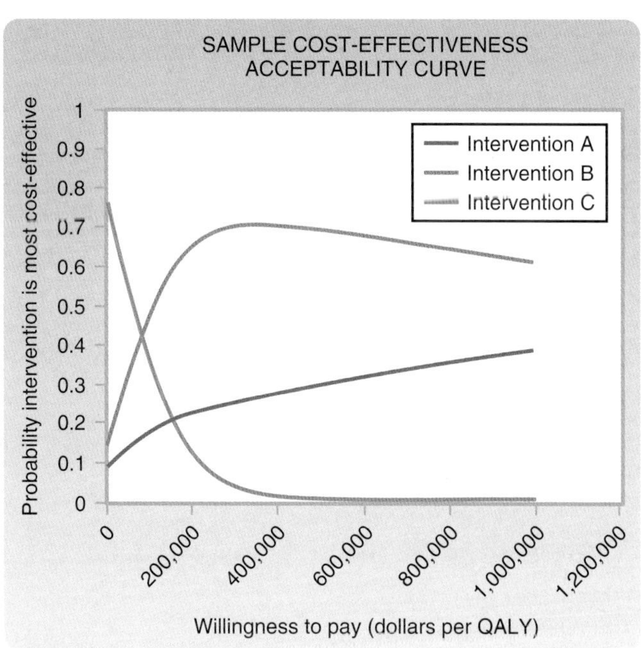


**Fig. 218.7 Cost-effectiveness acceptability curve.** This curve displays the output of a multivariate sensitivity analysis as a function of willingness to pay. At each dollar value, the y-value of the line corresponds with the probability that the intervention is the most effective without exceeding that dollar value per effectiveness unit. *QALY*, Quality-adjusted life year.

## SUGGESTED READINGS

Black WC. The CE plane: a graphic representation of cost-effectiveness. Med Decis Making 1990;10:212-4.

Cost-effectiveness analysis. In: Jamison DT, Breman JG, Measham AR, et al, editors. Priorities in health. Washington, DC: International Bank for Reconstruction and Development/The World Bank Group; 2006. p. 39-57. Full text available online at http://files.dcp2.org/pdf/PIH/PIH.pdf.

O'Brien BJ, Briggs AH. Analysis of uncertainty in health care cost-effectiveness studies: an introduction to statistical issues and methods. Stat Methods Med Res 2002;11:455-68.

Russell LB, Gold MR, Siegel JE, et al. The role of cost-effectiveness analysis in health and medicine. Panel on Cost-Effectiveness in Health and Medicine. JAMA 1996;276:1172-7.

Sox HC, Blatt MA, Higgins MC, et al. Medical decision making. Woburn, Mass: Butterworth-Heinemann; 1988.

## REFERENCES

*References can be found on Expert Consult @ www.expertconsult.com.*

# Index

Note: Page numbers followed by *f* refer to figures, by *t* to tables, by *b* to boxes, and by *e* to online-only content.

**F**

**W**

Derby Teaching Hospitals
NHS Foundation Trust
Library and Knowledge Centre

WITHDRAWN